MW01527363

Spine Surgery

Techniques, Complication Avoidance, and Management

THIRD EDITION

VOLUME TWO

EDITOR

Edward C. Benzel, MD
Chair
Department of Neurosurgery
Neurological Institute
Cleveland Clinic
Cleveland, OH

VIDEO EDITOR

Todd B. Francis, MD, PhD
Clinical Spine Fellow
Center for Spine Health
Neurological Institute
Cleveland Clinic
Cleveland, OH

ELSEVIER
SAUNDERS

CONTRIBUTORS

Khalid M. Abbed, MD
Chief
Yale Spine Institute;
Director
Minimally Invasive Spine Surgery
Department of Neurosurgery
Yale University School of Medicine
New Haven, CT

Kalil G. Abdullah, BS
Cleveland Clinic Lerner College of Medicine
Cleveland, OH

Steven S. Agabegi, MD
Michigan Orthopaedic Institute
Southfield, MI

Basheal M. Agrawal, MD
Associate Professor and Vice Chair
Department of Neurosurgery
University of Wisconsin
Madison, WI

Manzoor Ahmed, MBBS
Staff Radiologist
Imaging Institute
Neuroradiology Section
Cleveland Clinic
Cleveland, OH

Michael Ahrens, MD
Consultant (Oberarzt)
Spinecenter
Roland Klinik
Bremen, Germany

Yunus Alapan, BS
Research Assistant
Yildiz Technical University
Istanbul, Turkey

Rodolfo E. Alcedo-Guardia, MD
Neurosurgery Resident
University of Puerto Rico Medical Sciences Campus
San Juan, Puerto Rico

Joseph T. Alexander, MD
Assistant Professor
Department of Neurosurgery
Wake Forest University School of Medicine
Winston-Salem, NC

Neel Anand, MD
Professor and Chair
Department of Neurosurgery
Louisiana State University Health Science Center
Shreveport, LA

D. Greg Anderson, MD
Professor
Departments of Orthopaedic Surgery and Neurological Surgery
Thomas Jefferson University
Philadelphia, PA

Lilyana Angelov, MD, FRCS(C)
Staff
Brain Tumor and Neuro-Oncology
Gamma Knife Center;
Center for Spine Health;
Taussig Cancer Institute;
Section Head
Spinal Radiosurgery and Neurological Surgery
Neurological Institute
Cleveland Clinic
Cleveland, OH

John A. Anson, MD
Las Vegas, NV

Ronald I. Apfelbaum, MD
Professor Emeritus
Department of Neurosurgery
University of Utah
Salt Lake City, UT

Paul M. Arnold, MD, FACS
Professor of Neurosurgery
University of Kansas Medical Center;
Attending Neurosurgeon
University of Kansas Hospital
Kansas City, KS

Harel Arzi, MD
Spine Fellow
Department of Neurosurgery
University of Kansas Medical Center
Kansas City, KS;
Chaim Sheba Medical Center
Ramat Gan, Israel

Ferhan A. Asghar, MD
Assistant Professor
Department of Orthopaedic Surgery
University of Cincinnati
Cincinnati, OH

Michelle Aubin, MD
Resident
University of Massachusetts School of Medicine
Worcester, MA

Basem I. Awad, MD
Department of Neurosurgery
Mansoura University Hospital
Mansoura, Egypt

Christopher Baggot, MD
Resident
Department of Neurological Surgery
School of Medicine and Public Health
University of Wisconsin–Madison
Madison, WI

Lissa C. Baird, MD
Chief Resident
Division of Neurosurgery
University of California–San Diego Medical Center
San Diego, CA

Jamie Baisden, MD
Associate Professor
Department of Neurosurgery
Medical College of Wisconsin
Milwaukee, WI

Nevan G. Baldwin, MD, FACS
Clinical Associate Professor
Texas Tech University
Lubbock, TX

Perry A. Ball, MD
Associate Professor
Departments of Surgery and Anesthesiology
Dartmouth Medical School
Hanover, NH;
Staff Neurosurgeon
Dartmouth-Hitchcock Medical Center
Lebanon, NH

Eli M. Baron, MD
Neurosurgeon and Spine Surgeon
Cedars-Sinai Medical Center
Los Angeles, CA

H. Hunt Batjer, MD
Professor and Chair
Northwestern University Feinberg School of Medicine;
Chair
Department of Neurological Surgery
Northwestern Memorial Hospital
Chicago, IL

Andrew M. Bauer, MD
Resident Physician
University of Wisconsin
Madison, WI

Thomas W. Bauer, MD, PhD
Departments of Orthopaedic Surgery and Pathology
Cleveland Clinic
Cleveland, OH

James R. Bean, MD
Neurosurgical Associates at Central Baptist
Lexington, KY

Gordon R. Bell, MD
Director
Center for Spine Health
Neurological Institute
Cleveland Clinic
Cleveland, OH

J. Brad Bellotte, MD
Chief
Department of Neurosurgery
Hamot Medical Center
Erie, PA

David M. Benglis, Jr., MD
Complex Spine Fellow
Department of Neurosurgery
University of Miami
Miami, FL

Gregory Bennett, MD
Clinical Director
Neurosurgery
Erie County Medical Center
Buffalo, NY

Edward C. Benzel, MD
Chair
Department of Neurosurgery
Neurological Institute
Cleveland Clinic
Cleveland, OH

Darren L. Bergey, MD
Loma Linda University Medical Center
Loma Linda, CA

Marc L. Bertrand, MD
Associate Professor
Department of Anesthesiology
Dartmouth Medical School
Hanover, NH;
Director
Graduate Medical Education
Dartmouth-Hitchcock Medical Center
Lebanon, NH

Sigurd Berven, MD
Associate Professor in Residence;
Co-Director
Spine Fellowship;
Director
Resident Education Program
University of California–San Francisco
San Francisco, CA

Tarun Bhalla, MD
Resident
Department of Neurosurgery
Neurological Institute
Cleveland Clinic
Cleveland, OH

Aaron J. Bianco, MD
Spine Fellow
Warren Alpert Medical School
Brown University
Providence, RI

Dani S. Bidros, MD
Resident
Department of Neurosurgery
Neurological Institute
Cleveland Clinic
Cleveland, OH

Mark H. Bilsky, MD
Professor
Weill Medical College of Cornell University;
Memorial Sloan-Kettering Cancer Center;
Attending Surgeon;
Chief
Multi-Disciplinary Spine Tumor Center
Memorial Hospital for Cancer and Allied Diseases
New York, NY

Barry D. Birch, MD
Department of Neurosurgery
Mayo Clinic Scottsdale
Scottsdale, AZ

Frank S. Bishop, MD
Director
Comprehensive Spine Center
Neuroscience & Spine Institute
Kalispell Regional Medical Center
Kalispell, MT

Kevin Blaylock, CPA
Oklahoma Spine Hospital
Oklahoma City, OK

Maxwell Boakye, MD, FACS
Assistant Professor
Department of Neurosurgery
Stanford School of Medicine
Stanford, CA

Scott D. Boden, MD
Professor of Orthopaedics and Director
Emory Orthopaedics & Spine Center
Emory University;
Staff Physician
Department of Orthopaedic Surgery
Atlanta VA Medical Center
Atlanta, GA

Christopher Bono, MD
Assistant Professor
Orthopaedic Surgery
Harvard Medical School;
Chief
Orthopaedic Spine Service
Brigham and Women's Hospital
Boston, MA

Charles L. Branch, Jr., MD
Professor
Wake Forest School of Medicine;
Chair
Neuroscience Service Line
Wake Forest Baptist Medical Center
Winston-Salem, NC

Darrel S. Brodke, MD
Professor and Vice Chair
Department of Orthopaedics
University of Utah
Salt Lake City, UT

Nathaniel Brooks, MD
Fellow
Center for Spine Health
Neurological Institute
Cleveland Clinic
Cleveland, OH

Cristian Brotea, MD
Clinical Instructor
New York Medical College;
Associate Director
Spine Service
Westchester Medical Center
Valhalla, NY;
Sound Shore Medical Center
New Rochelle, NY;
White Plains Hospital
White Plains, NY

Samuel R. Browd, MD, PhD
Assistant Professor of Neurological Surgery
University of Washington;
Attending Neurological Surgeon
Seattle Children's Hospital
Seattle, WA

Harlan Bruner, MD
Assistant Professor
Department of Neurosurgery
University of Minnesota
Minneapolis, MN

John Butler, MD
Coastal Neurosurgical Associates
Wilmington, NC

David W. Cadotte, MD
Department of Surgery
Division of Neurosurgery
University of Toronto;
Resident
Division of Neurosurgery
Toronto Western Hospital
Toronto, Ontario, Canada

David W. Cahill, MD*
Department of Neurosurgery
College of Medicine
University of South Florida
Tampa, FL

John R. Caruso, MD
Neurological Specialists, LLC
Hagerstown, MD

Jeroen Ceuppens, MD
Department of Neurosurgery
University Hospital Gasthuisberg
Leuven, Belgium

Saad B. Chaudhary, MD
Assistant Professor
Department of Orthopaedic Surgery
New Jersey Medical School–University of Medicine and Dentistry of New Jersey
Newark, NJ

Morgan N. Chen, MD
Assistant Clinical Professor of Orthopaedics
Mount Sinai School of Medicine
New York, NY;
Attending Surgeon
Saint Charles Hospital
Port Jefferson, NY

Thomas C. Chen, MD PhD
Associate Professor
Departments of Neurosurgery and Pathology
Keck School of Medicine;
Director
Surgical Neuro-oncology;
Co-Director
University of Southern California Neuro Spine Program
Los Angeles, CA

Tanvir Choudhri, MD
Assistant Professor and Director
Neurosurgery Spine Program
Department of Neurosurgery
Mount Sinai Medical Center
New York, NY

Adam Conley, MD
Resident
Department of Neurosurgery
Virginia Commonwealth University Medical Center
Richmond, VA

Camille Connelly, MD
Resident
Department of Orthopaedic Surgery
University of Cincinnati College of Medicine
Cincinnati, OH

Edward S. Connolly, MD
Professor
Department of Neurosurgery
Ochsner Clinic Foundation
Louisiana State University School of Medicine
New Orleans, LA

Kevin Cooper, MD
Spine Medical Center of Pascagoula
Pascagoula, MS

Paul R. Cooper, MD
Professor of Neurosurgery
New York University School of Medicine
New York, NY

Domagoj Coric, MD
Chief of Neurosurgery
Carolinas Medical Center
Charlotte, NC;
President
North Carolina Spine Society
Raleigh, NC

Jean-Valery C.E. Coumans, MD
Assistant Professor
Department of Neurosurgery
Massachusetts General Hospital
Boston, MA

Sorin Craciunas, MD
Staff Neurosurgeon
Bagdasar-Arseni Hospital
Bucharest, Romania

Albert E. Cram, MD, FACS
Professor Emeritus
Department of Surgery
University of Iowa
Iowa City, IA

*Deceased.

Charles H. Crawford III, MD
Assitant Professor
Department of Orthopaedic Surgery
University of Louisville;
Adult and Pediatric Spine Surgeon
Norton Leatherman Spine Center
Louisville, KY

H. Alan Crockard, MD
The National Hospital for Neurology and Neurosurgery
London, United Kingdom

William T. Curry, Jr., MD
Assistant Professor
Department of Surgery
Harvard Medical School;
Attending Neurosurgeon
Massachusetts General Hospital
Boston, MA

Joseph F. Cusick, MD
Professor
Medical College of Wisconsin
Madison, WI

Scott D. Daffner, MD
Assistant Professor
Department of Orthopaedics
Robert C. Byrd Health Sciences Center
University of West Virginia School of Medicine
Morgantown, WV

Nader S. Dahdaleh, MD
Fellow Associate
Department of Neurosurgery
University of Iowa
Iowa City, IA

Sedat Dalbayrak, MD
Chair
Department of Neurosurgery
Trabzon Numune Teaching and Research Hospital
Trabzon, Turkey

Mark D. D'Alise, MD, FACS
Neurosurgical Associates
Complex Reconstructive Spinal Surgery
Lubbock, TX

Russell C. DeMicco, DO
Staff Physician
Center for Spine Health
Neurological Institute
Cleveland Clinic
Cleveland, OH

Michael DePalma, MD
President and Director of Research
Virginia Spine Research Institute, Inc.;
Medical Director
Interventional Spine Care Fellowship
Virginia Spine Physicians, PC
Richmond, VA

Harel Deutsch, MD
Assistant Professor
Department of Neurosurgery
Rush University Medical Center
Chicago, IL

Denis DiAngelo, MD
Associate Professor
School of Biomechanical Engineering
University of Tennessee Health Science Center
Memphis, TN

Curtis A. Dickman, MD
Associate Chief
Spine Section;
Director
Spinal Research
Division of Neurological Surgery
Barrow Neurological Associates
Phoenix, AZ

Christian P. DiPaola, MD
Assistant Professor
Memorial Medical Center
University of Massachusetts
Worcester, MA

Gary A. Dix, MD, FRSC(C)
Clinical Professor of Neurosurgery
George Washington University Hospital
Washington, DC;
Attending Neurosurgeon
Anne Arundel Medical Center
Annapolis, MD

John Doyle, MD
Associate Professor
Department of Neurology;
Chief
General Neurology Division
University of Pittsburgh
Pittsburgh, PA

Thomas B. Ducker, MD
Professor of Neurosurgery (retired)
Johns Hopkins Hospital;
University of Maryland Medical Center
Baltimore, MD;
Anne Arundel Medical Center
Annapolis, MD

Michael Ebersold, MD
Professor of Neurosurgery
Mayo Clinic College of Medicine;
Department of Neurological Surgery
Luther Middlefort Clinic–Mayo Health System
Eau Claire, WI

Bruce L. Ehni, MD
Associate Professor
Department of Neurosurgery
Baylor College of Medicine;
Neurosurgery Section Chief
Operative Care Line
DeBakey VA Medical Center
Houston, TX

Kurt Eichholz, MD
Resident
Department of Neurosurgery
University of Iowa
Iowa City, IA

Marc Eichler, MD, FACS
Chief of Neurological Surgery
Trinity Medical Center
Newton Centre, MA

John P. Eickman, MD
Wake Forest School of Medicine;
Resident
Wake Forest Baptist Medical Center
Winston-Salem, NC

Samer K. Elbabaa, MD, FAANS
Director
Division of Pediatric Neurosurgery;
Assistant Professor
Department of Neurosurgery
St. Louis University School of Medicine
St. Louis, MO

J. Bradley Elder, MD
Assistant Professor
Department of Neurological Surgery
The Ohio State University Medical Center
Columbus, OH

Richard Ellenbogen, MD, FACS
Professor and Chair
Department of Neurological Surgery
University of Washington School of Medicine
Seattle, WA

Sanford E. Emery, MD
Professor and Chair
Department of Orthopaedics
West Virginia University
Morgantown, WV

Nancy E. Epstein, MD
Clinical Professor
Department of Neurological Surgery
Albert Einstein College of Medicine
Bronx, NY;
Chief
Neurological Spine and Education
Winthrop University Hospital
Mineola, NY;
President
Long Island Neurological Associates, PC
Long Island, NY

Thomas J. Errico, MD
Professor
Department of Orthopaedic Surgery and Neurosurgery;
Director
Spine Surgery Fellowship Program;
Director
International Spine Surgery Fellowship Program
NYU Medical Center Hospital for Joint Diseases
New York, NY

Malik Fakhar, BS
Cleveland Clinic
Cleveland, OH

Steven M. Falowski, MD
Fellow
Department of Neurosurgery
Rush University Medical Center
Chicago, IL

Ehab Farag, MD, FRCA
Staff Anesthesiologist;
Assistant Professor of Anesthesiology
Cleveland Clinic
Cleveland, OH

Chad W. Farley, MD
Deparment of Neurosurgery
University of Cinncinnati
Cincinnati, OH

Michael G. Fehlings, MD, PhD
Department of Surgery
Division of Neurosurgery
University of Toronto;
Krembil Chair in Neural Repair and Regeneration
Division of Neurosurgery
Toronto Western Hospital
Toronto, Ontario, Canada

Frank Feigenbaum, MD, FAANS
Midwest Neurosurgery Associates
Kansas City, MO

Lisa A. Ferrara, PhD
President and CEO
OrthoKinetic Technologies, LLC
Southport, NC;
President and CEO
OrthoKinetic Testing Technologies, LLC
Shallotte, NC

Richard G. Fessler, MD, PhD
Professor
Department of Neurosurgery
Northwestern University Feinberg School of Medicine
Chicago, IL

David Fiorella, MD, PhD
Professor
Clinical Radiology and Neurosurgery
Cerebrovascular Center
Stony Book University Medical Center
Stony Brook, NY

Jeffrey S. Fischgrund, MD
Professor
Department of Orthopaedics
Oakland University School of Medicine
Rochester, MI;
Director
Spine Surgery Fellowship
William Beaumont Hospital
Royal Oak, MI

Kevin T. Foley, MD
Professor
Neurological Surgery
Semmes-Murphey Neurologic and Spine Institute
Memphis, TN

Ricardo Fontes, MD
Department of Neurosurgery
Rush University Medical Center
Chicago, IL

Todd B. Francis, MD, PhD
Clinical Spine Fellow
Center for Spine Health
Neurological Institute
Cleveland Clinic
Cleveland, OH

Kai-Ming G. Fu, MD, PhD
Department of Neurosurgery
University of Virginia
Charlottesville, VA

Brian R. Gantwerker, MD
The Craniospinal Center of Los Angeles
Los Angeles, CA

Mark Garrett, MD
Chief Resident
Department of Neurosurgery
Barrow Neurological Institute
St. Joseph's Hospital and Medical Center
Phoenix, AZ

Rasha Germain, MD
Chief Resident
Department of Neurosurgery
Barrow Neurological Institute
St. Joseph's Hospital and Medical Center
Phoenix, AZ

John W. German, MD
Associate Professor
Division of Neurosurgery
Albany Medical College
Albany, NY

Alexander J. Ghanayem, MD
Associate Professor and Chief
Department of Orthopaedic Surgery
Division of Spine Surgery
Loyola University Medical Center
Maywood, IL

George M. Ghobrial, MD
Resident
Neurological Surgery
Thomas Jefferson University Hospital
Philadelphia, PA

Zoher Ghogawala, MD
Clinical Assistant Professor
Department of Neurosurgery
Yale University;
Attending Physician
Department of Neurosurgery
Yale–New Haven Hospital
New Haven, CT;
Lecturer in Neurosurgery
Tufts University
Boston, MA;
Attending Physician
Department Neurosurgery;
Director
Wallace Clinical Trials Center
Greenwich Hospital
Greenwich, CT;
Attending Physician and Chair of Neurosurgery
Lahey Clinic
Burlington, MA

Paul A. Glazer, MD
Assistant Clinical Professor
Department of Orthopedic Surgery
Harvard University;
Spine Surgeon
Beth Israel Deaconess Medical Center
Boston, MA

Vijay K. Goel, PhD
Distinguished University Professor
Departments of Bioengineering and Orthopaedic Surgery;
Endowed Chair and McMaster-Gardner Professor of Orthopaedic Bioengineering;
Co-Director
Engineering Center for Orthopaedic Research Excellence
Univeristy of Toledo
Toledo, OH

Jan Goffin, MD, PhD
Professor
Catholic University of Leuven;
Chair
Department of Neurosurgery
University Hospital Gasthuisberg
Leuven, Belgium

Ziya Gokaslan, MD
Donlin M. Long Professor of Neurosurgery, Oncology, and Orthopedic Surgery;
Vice Chair
Department of Neurosurgery;
Director
Spine Division
Johns Hopkins University Hospital
Baltimore, MD

Harry S. Goldsmith, MD, FACS
Clincal Professor
Department of Neurosurgery
University of California–Davis School of Medicine
Sacramento, CA

Sohrab Gollogly
University of Utah
Salt Lake City, UT

L. Fernando Gonzalez, MD
Assistant Professor
Department of Neurological Surgery
Division of Neurovascular Surgery and Endovascular Neurosurgery
Jefferson Medical College
Thomas Jefferson University
Philadelphia, PA

Jorge A. Gonzalez-Martinez, MD
Associate Staff
Epilepsy Center;
Department of Neurosurgery
Neurological Institute
Cleveland Clinic
Cleveland, OH

Jeffrey D. Gross, MD
Medical Director
O.A.S.I.S. Wellness Center
Laguna Niguel, CA

Yabo Guan, PhD
Department of Neurosurgery
Medical College of Wisconsin
Milwaukee, WI

İlker Gulec, MD
Vice Chief
Department of Neurosurgery
Antalya Teaching and Research Hospital
Antalya, Turkey

David Gwinn, MD
Staff Orthopaedic Spine Surgeon
Department of Orthopaedics and Rehabilitation
Walter Reed Army Medical Center
Washington, DC

Elad Hadar, MD
Associate Professor
Department of Neurosurgery
University of North Carolina School of Medicine
Chapel Hill, NC

Alexander Hadjipavlou, MD, MSc, FACS, FRCS(C)
Professor
Orthopaedic Surgery and Rehabilitaton
University of Crete
Heraklion, Crete, Greece

Mark N. Hadley, MD, FACS
Charles A. and Patsy W. Collat Professor of Neurological Surgery;
Program Director
Neurosurgery Residency Training Program
University of Alabama
Birmingham, AL

Regis W. Haid, Jr., MD
Atlanta Brain and Spine Care
Atlanta, GA

Fadi Hanbali, MD, FACS
Clinical Associate Professor
Department of Neurosurgery
Texas Tech University HSC;
Faculty Neurosurgeon
Sierra Medical Center;
Providence Memorial Hospital;
University Medical Center of El Paso
El Paso, TX

Ran Harel, MD
Faculty
Spine Surgery Unit
Sheba Medical Center
Ramat-Gan, Israel

Jurgen Harms, MD
Center for Spine Surgery;
Department of Orthopedics and Traumatology
Klinikum Karlsbad-Langensteinbach
Karlsbad-Langensteinbach, Germany

Colin B. Harris, MD
Spine Fellow
Department of Orthopedics
Rush University
Chicago, IL

James S. Harrop, MD
Associate Professor of Neurologic and Orthopedic Surgery
Jefferson Medical College
Philadelphia, PA

Blaine L. Hart, MD
Professor
Department of Radiology
University of New Mexico School of Medicine
Albuquerque, NM

Robert A. Hart, MD
Professor and Spine Fellowship Director
Oregon Health & Science University
Portland, OR

Reyaad A. Hayek, MD
Associate Professor
Department of Radiology
University of New Mexico School of Medicine
Albuquerque, NM

Robert F. Heary, MD
Professor
Department of Neurological Surgery
New Jersey Medical School–University of Medicine and Dentistry of New Jersey
Newark, NJ

Joshua E. Heller, MD
Assistant Professor
Neurological Surgery
Thomas Jefferson University
Philadelphia, PA

Fraser C. Henderson, MD
Chief
Division of Neurosurgery
Doctors Community Hospital
Lanham, MD

Ann M. Henwood, MSN, CNS, RN
Department of Neurosurgery;
Advanced Practice Nurse
Center for Spine Health
Neurological Institute
Cleveland Clinic
Cleveland, OH

Yoshitaka Hirano, MD
Center for Spine and Spinal Cord Disorders
Southern Tohoku General Hospital
Iwanuma, Miyagi, Japan

Girish K. Hiremath, MD
Staff Neurosurgeon
Riverside Methodist Hospital
Columbus, OH

Patrick W. Hitchon, MD
Professor
Departments of Neurosurgery and Bioengineering;
Director of Spine Surgery
University of Iowa College of Medicine;
Department of Neurosurgery
University of Iowa Hospitals and Clinics
Iowa City, IA

Daniel J. Hoh, MD
Assistant Professor
Department of Neurological Surgery;
Joint Assistant Professor
Department of Neuroscience
University of Florida
Gainesville, FL

Paul J. Holman, MD
Assistant Professor
Department of Neurosurgery
Weill-Cornell Medical College
New York, NY;
Staff Neurosurgeon
Methodist Neurological Institute;
Department of Neurosurgery
Methodist Hospital
Houston, TX

Noboru Hosono, MD, PhD
Chief
Spine Surgery
Osaka Kosei-nenkin Hospital
Osaka, Japan

John K. Houton, MD
Associate Professor
Department of Neurological Surgery
Montefiore Hospital;
Albert Einstein/Jaboni Hospital
Bronx, NY

Augusto T. Hsia, Jr., MD
Staff
Center for Spine Health
Neurological Institute
Cleveland Clinic
Cleveland, OH

Thomas A. Kopitnik, MD
University of Texas Southwestern Medical Center
Dallas, TX

Panagiotis Korovessis, MD
Department of Pathology
General Hospital "Agios Andreas"
Achaia, Greece

Tyler Koski, MD
Assistant Professor
Department of Neurological Surgery
Northwestern University
Chicago, IL

Robert J. Kowalski, MD
Clearwater, FL

Chandan Krishna, MD
Resident Neurosurgeon
Department of Neurosurgery
Methodist Neurological Institute;
Methodist Hospital
Houston, TX

Ajit A. Krishnaney, MD
Staff
Center for Spine Health
Cerebrovascular Center
Department of Neurosurgery
Neurological Institute
Cleveland Clinic
Cleveland, OH

Varun R. Kshettry, MD
Resident
Department of Neurosurgery
Neurological Institute
Cleveland Clinic
Cleveland, OH

Charles Kuntz IV, MD
Associate Professor and Vice Chair
University of Cincinnati College of Medicine;
Mayfield Clinic and Spine Institute
Cincinnati, OH

Steven M. Kurtz, PhD
Research Professor
Biomedical Engineering
Drexel University;
Corporate Vice President
Exponent
Philadelphia, PA

John A. Lancon, MD, FAAP, FACS, FAANS
Affiliate Faculty
University of Mississippi Medical Center;
Chief of Neurosurgery
St. Dominic Jackson Memorial Hospital;
Consultant
Regency Hospital of Jackson;
Mississippi Methodist Rehabilitation Hospital
Jackson, MS

Jorge Lastra-Power, MD
Assistant Professor
Neurosurgery Section
University of Puerto Rico
San Juan, Puerto Rico

Elizabeth Demers Lavelle, MD
Assistant Professor of Anesthesiology
SUNY Upstate Medical University
Syracuse, NY

William F. Lavelle, MD
Assistant Professor;
Orthopaedic Spine Surgeon
SUNY Upstate Medical University
Syracuse, NY

Nathan H. Lebwohl, MD
Chief of Spinal Deformity Surgery
Department of Orthopaedics
University of Miami Miller School of Medicine
Miami, FL

Joon Y. Lee, MD
Associate Professor
Department of Orthopaedic Surgery
University of Pittsburgh Medical Center
Pittsburgh, PA

Lawrence G. Lenke, MD
Jerome J. Gilden Professor of Orthopaedic Surgery;
Professor of Neurological Surgery;
Co-Chief Adult/Pediatric Scoliosis and Reconstructive Spinal Surgery
Washington University School of Medicine;
Chief
Spinal Service
Orthopaedic Surgery
Shriners Hospital for Children
St. Louis, MO

Steven P. Leon, MD, FACS
Clinical Assistant Professor
Weill–Cornell Medical College
New York, NY;
Brookhaven Memorial Hospital Medical Center
Patchogue, NY;
St. Charles Hospital and Rehabilitation Center
Port Jefferson, NY

Allan D. Levi, MD, PhD, FACS
Professor of Neurosurgery
University of Miami;
Chief of Neurosurgery
University of Miami Hospital;
Chief of Neurospine
Jackson Memorial Hospital
Miami, FL

Isador H. Lieberman, MD, FRCSC
Director
Scoliosis and Spine Tumor Program
Texas Back Institute;
Texas Health Hospital
Plano, TX

Timothy Lindley, MD, PhD
Fellow Associate
Department of Neurosurgery
University of Iowa Hospitals and Clinics
Iowa City, IA

James K.C. Liu, MD
Resident
Department of Neurosurgery
Neurological Institute
Cleveland Clinic
Cleveland, OH

Andrew D. Livingston, MD
Resident Neurosurgeon
Department of Neurosurgery
Methodist Neurological Institute;
Methodist Hospital
Houston, TX

Bjorn Lobo, MD
Resident
Department of Neurosurgery
Neurological Institute
Cleveland Clinic
Cleveland, OH

S. Scott Lollis, MD
Assistant Professor of Surgery
Department of Neurosurgery
Dartmouth Medical School
Hanover, NH;
Attending Neurosurgeon
Dartmouth-Hitchcock Medical Center
Lebanon, NH

Donlin M. Long, MD
John Hopkins University Medical School
Baltimore, MD

Miguel Lopez-Gonzalez, MD
Chief Resident
Department of Neurosurgery
Neurological Institute
Cleveland Clinic
Cleveland, OH

Robert G. Louis, MD
Department of Neurosurgery
University of Virginia
Charlottesville, VA

Daniel C. Lu, MD, PhD
Assistant Professor
Department of Neurosurgery
University of California–Los Angeles
Los Angeles, CA

Mark G. Luciano, MD
Staff
Pediatric Surgery and Neurosciences
Department of Neurosurgery
Neurological Institute
Cleveland Clinic
Cleveland, OH

Andre Machado, MD, PhD
Director
Center for Neurological Restoration;
Staff
Center for Spine Health and Pain Management
Department of Neurosurgery
Neurological Institute
Cleveland Clinic
Cleveland, OH

Dennis J. Maiman, MD, PhD
Professor and Chair
Department of Neurosurgery
Medical College of Wisconsin;
Attending Neurosurgeon
Children's Hospital of Wisconsin;
Froedtert Memorial Lutheran Hospital
Milwaukee, WI

David G. Malone, MD
Oklahoma Spine and Brain Institute
Tulsa, OK

Lisabeth L. Maloney, MD
Associate Professor of Anesthesiology
Dartmouth Medical School
Hanover, NH;
Director
Anesthesiology Residency Program
Dartmouth-Hitchcock Medical Center
Lebanon, NH

Antonios Mammis, MD
Resident
Department of Neurological Surgery
New Jersey Medical School–University of Medicine and Dentistry of New Jersey
Newark, NJ

Satyajit Marawar, MD

Edward Marchan, MD
Resident Physician
Department of Radiation Oncology
Emory University
Atlanta, GA

Nicolas Marcotte, MD
Staff Neurosurgeon
New England Baptist Hospital
Boston, MA

Joseph Maroon, MD
Clinical Professor and Vice Chair
Department of Neurosurgery
University of Pittsburgh Medical Center
Pittsburgh, PA

Michael Martin, MD
Assistant Professor
Department of Neurosurgery
University of Oklahoma
Oklahoma City, OK

Mitchell Martineau, MSN
Oklahoma Spine and Brain Institute
Tulsa, OK

Eric M. Massicotte, MD
Associate Professor
University of Toronto;
Coordinator of Spine Fellowship;
Director
Undergraduate Studies for Neurosurgery
University Health Network
Toronto, Ontario, Canada

Virgilio Matheus, MD
Resident
Department of Neurosurgery
Neurological Institute
Cleveland Clinic
Cleveland, OH

Hidenori Matsuoka, MD
Southern Tohoku General Hospital
Koriyama, Japan

Paul K. Maurer, MD
Professor
Department of Neurosurgery
University of Rochester;
Chief
Department of Neurosurgery
Unity Health System
Rochester, NY

Eric A.K. Mayer, MD
Staff
Center for Spine Health;
Center for Neurological Restoration
Neurological Institute
Cleveland Clinic
Cleveland, OH

Daniel J. Mazanec, MD
Associate Professor
Cleveland Clinic Lerner College of Medicine of Case Western Reserve University;
Associate Director
Center for Spine Health
Neurological Institute
Cleveland Clinic
Cleveland, OH

Paul C. McAfee, MD
Part-time Associate Professor
Departments of Orthopedic Surgery and Neurosurgery
Johns Hopkins Hospital;
Chief of Spinal Surgery
St. Joseph Hospital
Baltimore, MD

Bruce M. McCormack, MD
Clinical Faculty
University of California–San Francisco Medical Center
San Francisco, CA

Paul C. McCormick, MD, MPH
Herbert and Linda Gallen Professor of Neurological Surgery
Columbia University College of Physicians and Surgeons
New York, NY

William McCormick, MD
Schwartzapfel Novick
West Islip, NY

Robert A. McGuire, Jr., MD
Professor and Chair
Department of Orthopaedic Surgery and Rehabilitation
University of Mississippi Medical Center
Jackson, MS

Michael D. McKibben, JD
Bradley Arant Boult Cummings, LLP
Birmingham, AL

Robert F. McLain, MD
Professor of Surgery
Cleveland Clinic Lerner College of Medicine at Case Western Reserve University;
CCF Adjunct Professor
Department of Chemical and Biomedical Engineering
Cleveland State University;
Staff Spine Surgeon
Center for Spine Health
Neurological Institute
Cleveland Clinic
Cleveland, OH

D. Mark Melton, MD
Resident
Department of Neurosurgery
University of South Florida College of Medicine
Tampa, FL

Muhammad Zeeshan Memon, MD
Department of Neurosurgery
Neurological Institute
Cleveland Clinic
Cleveland, OH

Umesh S. Metkar, MD
Spine Surgeon
Department of Orthopedics
Carolina Pines Regional Medical Center
Hartsville, SC

Vincent Miele, MD
Assistant Professor of Neurological Surgery and Orthopaedic Surgery
Department of Neurosurgery;
Chief
Neurosurgery Spine Section;
Director
WVU Neurosurgery Southern Division
West Virginia University
Morgantown, WV;
Faculty
Cleveland Clinic Spine Research Lab
Cleveland, OH

Amrendra S. Miranpuri, MD
Resident
University of Wisconsin School of Medicine and Public Health;
Resident
University of Wisconsin Hospital and Clinics
Madison, WI

Junichi Mizuno, MD
Associate Professor
Department of Neurological Surgery
Aichi Medical University School of Medicine
Aichi, Japan

Sergey Mlyavykh, MD
Institute of Traumatology and Orthopaedics
Nizhni Novgorod, Russia

Michael T. Modic, MD
Chair
Neurological Institute;
Staff
Diagnostic Radiology
Cleveland Clinic
Cleveland, OH

Hikaru Morisue, MD, PhD
Instructor
Department of Orthopaedic Surgery
Kawasaki Municipal Hospital
Kawasaki-shi, Kanagawa-ken, Japan

Michael A. Morone, MD
Deaconess Billings Clinic
Billings, MT

Thomas E. Mroz, MD
Assistant Professor
Cleveland Clinic Lerner College of Medicine;
Director
Spine Surgery Fellowship;
Neurological Instititute
Center for Spine Health
Cleveland Clinic
Cleveland, OH

Jeffrey P. Mullin, MD
Resident
Department of Neurosurgery
Neurological Institute
Cleveland Clinic
Cleveland, OH

Praveen V. Mummaneni, MD
Associate Professor and Vice Chair
Department of Neurosurgery
University of California–San Francisco
San Francisco, CA

F. Reed Murtagh, MD
Professor
Department of Radiology
University of South Florida;
Department of Diagnostic Imaging
Moffitt Cancer Center
Tampa, FL

Ryan D. Murtagh, MD
Assistant Professor
Department of Radiology
University of South Florida;
Department of Diagnostic Imaging
Moffitt Cancer Center
Tampa, FL

John S. Myseros, MD
Associate Professor
Departments of Pediatrics and Neurosurgery
George Washington University School of Medicine;
Attending Neurosurgeon
Children's National Medical Center
Washington, DC;
Attending Neurosurgeon
Inova Fairfax Hospital for Children
Fall Church, VA

Sait Naderi, MD
Professor and Chair
Department of Neurosurgery
Umraniye Teaching and Research Hospital
Istanbul, Turkey

Dileep Nair, MD
Director
Intraoperative Monitoring;
Section Head
Adult Epilepsy
Department of Neurology
Cleveland Clinic
Cleveland, OH

Hiroshi Nakagawa, MD, DMSc
Professor Emeritus
Aichi Medical University Nagakute
Aichi-gun, Aichi, Japan;
Director
Spine Center
Kushiro Kojinkai Memorial Hospital
Kushiro City, Japan

Anil Nanda, MD, FACS
Professor and Chair
Department of Neurosurgery
Louisiana State University Health Science Center
Shreveport, LA

Chris J. Neal, MD
Department of Neurosurgery
National Naval Medical Center
Bethesda, MD

Russ P. Nockels, MD
Professor
Departments of Neurosurgery and Orthopedics;
Vice Chair
Department of Neurosurgery;
Director
Complex Spinal Surgery
Loyola University Medical Center
Maywood, IL

Chima Ohaegbulam, MD
Resident
Department of Neurosurgery
Brigham and Women's Hospital
Boston, MA

Eijiro Okada, MD, PhD
Assistant Professor
Department of Orthopaedic Surgery
Keio University School of Medicine
Tokyo, Japan

Bernardo Jose Ordonez, MD
Neurosurgical Associates
Norfolk, VA

Jennifer Orning, MD
Resident Physician
University of North Carolina Hospitals
Chapel Hill, NC

R. Douglas Orr, MD
Attending Staff
Center for Spine Health
Neurological Institute
Cleveland Clinic;
Chair of Surgery
Lutheran Hospital
Cleveland, OH

John O'Toole, MD
Assistant Professor
Department of Neurosurgery
Rush University Medical Center
Chicago, IL

A. Fahir Ozer, MD
Professor
Department of Neurosurgery
Koe University;
American Hospital
Istanbul, Turkey

Richard J. Parkinson, MD
Visiting Neurosurgeon
Department of Neurosurgery
St. Vincent's Clinic
Darlinghurst, New South Wales, Australia

Robert S. Pashman, MD
Director of Scoliosis and Spinal Deformities
Cedars-Sinai Institute for Spinal Disorders
Los Angeles, CA

Nirav J. Patel, MD
Cerebrovascular and Skull Base Fellow
Macquarie University
Sydney, New South Wales, Australia

Vishal C. Patel, MD

Stanley Pelofsky, MD
Oklahoma Spine Hospital
Oklahoma City, OK

Noel I. Perin, MD, FRCS
Professor
Department of Neurosurgery;
Director
Minimally Invasive Spine Section
NYU Medical Center
New York, NY

Olga Perlmutter, MD
Leading Scientific Fellow
Neurosurgery Department
Research Institute of Trauma and Orthopaedics
Novgorod, Russia

Frank M. Phillips, MD
Professor
Department of Orthopaedic Surgery;
Co-Director
Spine Fellowship
Rush University Medical Center
Chicago, IL

Rick Placide, MD, PT
Assistant Clinical Professor
Department of Physical Medicine and Rehabilitation
Virginia Commonwealth University;
Spine and Orthopaedic Surgeon
OrthoVirginia;
Chief
Orthopaedic Surgery
Chippenham Medical Center
Richmond, VA

Paul Porensky, MD
Neurosurgical Resident
Department of Neurological Surgery
The Ohio State University Medical Center
Columbus, OH

Srinivas Prasad, MD
Assistant Professor
Departments of Orthopaedic Surgery and Neurosurgery
Thomas Jefferson University
Philadelphia, PA

Mark L. Prasarn, MD
Assistant Professor
Division of Orthopaedic Surgery
University of Texas;
Memorial Hermann Hospital
Houston, TX

Gregory J. Przybylski, MD
Professor of Neuroscience
Seton Hall University
South Orange, NJ;
Director of Neurosurgery
New Jersey Neuroscience Institute at JFK Medical Center
Edison, NJ

Doron Rabin, MD
St. Luke's University Health Network
Fountain Hill, PA

Ashraf A. Ragab, MD
University of Mississippi Medical Center
Jackson, MS

Sharad Rajpal, MD
Staff Neurosurgeon
Boulder Neurological and Spine Associates
Boulder, CO

Y. Raja Rampersaud, MD, FRCSC
Assistant Professor
Division of Orthopedic Surgery
University of Toronto;
Spinal Program
Krambil Neuroscience Center
Toronto Western Hospital
University Health Network
Toronto, Ontario, Canada

Peter A. Rasmussen, MD
Director
Cerebrovascular Center
Neurological Institute
Cleveland Clinic
Cleveland, OH

Wolfgang Rausching, MD
Research Professor
Clinical and Applied Anatomy and Pathology
Uppsala University Hospital
Uppsala, Sweden

Gary L. Rea, MD, PhD
Assistant Professor
Department of Neurosurgery
The Ohio State University
Columbus, OH

Davis L. Reames, MD
Chief Resident
Department of Neurosurgery
University of Virginia
Charlottesville, VA

Glenn R. Rechtine II, MD
Professor
Department of Orthopaedic Surgery
University of South Florida
Tampa, FL;
Professor
Department of Orthopaedic Surgery
Univerity of Rochester
Rochester, NY;
Associate Chief of Staff
Bay Pines Veterans Administration Health Care System
Bay Pines, FL

PREFACE

I stated in the front matter of the second edition of this book that "[it] was bigger and better than the first." The same is true for this third edition: It is without question much bigger and better than its predecessors.

The purpose of this book (to assist the spine surgeon with the avoidance, identification, and management of complications) has not changed. Its presentation, however, has: It is more colorful; the contributors are more seasoned—and, hence, they have refined the information transmission process, as well as the dialogue employed. This edition is easier to read, more organized, and much more user friendly. In this third edition good contributions from the prior editions were made better. Some have been eliminated; others have been added; new topics are addressed; and antiquated topics have been dropped.

This edition remains a *techniques* book but provides much, much more. In addition to the "*how* tos," it provides significant discussion regarding the "*when* tos," the "when *not* tos," and the "*whys*" associated with the decision-making process.

Decision making is, indeed, the central focus of this text. Decision making is facilited by understanding both the triumphs and the mistakes made by our predecessors. This book liberally provides such understanding. In addition to technique, it focuses on ethics, logic, nonoperative management, and controversies. Perhaps more important than any other factor, it focuses on the fundamentals. The fundamental disciplines of anatomy, biomechanics, and physiology provide the foundation for all we do as spine surgeons. I am perpetually compelled to focus on this foundation and have striven to do so in the pages that follow.

Risk Taking

Surgeons are risk takers and surgery is a risk-taking process. The patient places himself or herself in the hands of the surgeon, and the ensuing decision-making process involves the resolution (or the attempts at such) of many technical and quality-of-life–related issues and dilemmas. A surgical procedure may be warranted if the sum of the costs (both financial and personal) and risks is less than the sum of the benefits. This risk/benefit analysis should be of paramount concern and should be emphasized by the surgeon and realized by the patient. This book is designed to help surgeons achieve these goals, by minimizing the *risk-taking* component and by maximizing the *benefit* component of this "equation."

Repetition

We learn most effectively by having data presented in a repetitive manner, often from different perspectives, using differing techniques (e.g., written, mathematical, or visual).

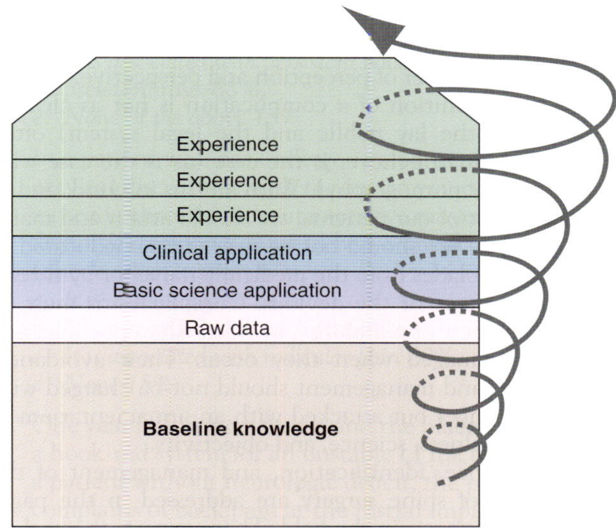

FIGURE 1. The spiral of learning.

The true understanding of a concept or body of knowledge involves the *spiral of learning*, which often involves multiple exposures to information so that a solid database (foundation of knowledge) is acquired. New (raw) data are then added and assimilated. This "expanded" knowledge base can then be applied to, and enhanced by, additional basic science, clinical input, and applications. This entire process is perpetually refined and reshaped by new experiences, such as clinical encounters or through reading and other sources of learning (Fig. 1). Repetition is the mother of learning. Repetition is, indeed, good—very good.

What Is a Complication?

The definition of what constitutes a complication is usually unclear and often argued. In a way, it's like pornography: "I cannot define it, but I know it when I see it."

> *I shall not today attempt further to define the kinds of material I understand to be embraced within that shorthand description ["hard-core pornography"]; and perhaps I could never succeed in intelligibly doing so. But* I know it when I see it, *and the motion picture involved in this case is not that.* [Emphasis added.]
>
> —Justice Potter Stewart, concurring opinion in *Jacobellis v. Ohio 378 U.S. 184 (1964)*, regarding possible obscenity in *The Lovers.*

Perhaps complications and pornography alike do not require strict definition, which may be too confining and, in the case of complications, detract from the purpose of focusing on its mitigation—i.e., *doing what's right!*

CONTENTS

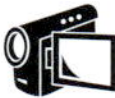

To view corresponding videos, please visit the Spine Surgery video collection online at expertconsult.com.

VOLUME ONE

SECTION 1 History

SECTION 2 The Fundamentals

VOLUME TWO

4.7 Tumors, Vascular Malformations, and Related Lesions

4.8 Pediatric Spinal Surgery and Related Conditions

4.9 Adjunctive Surgical Considerations

SECTION 5 Spinal Instrumentation

SECTION 6 Motion Preservation Strategies

CONFLICT OF INTEREST

In order to minimize bias, the disclosure of potential conflicts of interest is imperative. The following contributors to this book have disclosed financial relationships with industrial partners. These relationships could bias the author's opinion and, therefore, should be considered accordingly.

Author	Industrial Partner
Lilyana Angelov	BrainLab
Edward C. Benzel	AxioMed, Cervical Spine Research Society, Computational Biodynamics, DePuy, Elsevier Publishing, OrthoMEMS, Rawlings, Stryker, Thieme Publishing, Turning Point
Christopher Bono	Deputy Editor of Journal of the American Academy of Orthopedic Surgeons
Darrel S. Brodke	Amedica, DePuy, Medtronic, Pioneer, Vertiflek
Charles H. Crawford III	Alphatec, Medtronic, Synthes
Gary A. Dix	Alphatec, Biomet, DePuy Spine, Globus, ISTO, Pioneer, Spine Wave
Ehab Farag	Hospira
David Fiorella	Codman & Shurtleff, Cordis, Covidien EV3, Microvention, Micrus Endovascular, Nfocus Medical, Siemens
Jeffrey S. Fischgrund	Baxter, Cervical Spine Research Society, Lumbar Spine Research Society, Relievant, Salient, Smith & Nephew, Stryker, Trans1
Jan Goffin	Medtronic
Regis W. Haid, Jr.	Globus Medical, Medtronic, Nuvasive
Fraser C. Henderson	Computational BioDynamics
Patrick W. Hitchon	DePuy Spine
Brian J. Kistler	Synthes
Joon Y. Lee	Stryker
Isador H. Lieberman	Alphatec Spine, Axiomed Spine Corporation, Collplant, CrossTrees Medical, Mazor Surgical Technologies, Merlot OrthopediX, NOC2 Healthcare, Orthofix, Pearl Diver, Stryker Spine, Synthes Spine, Trans1, Zyga
Eric M. Massicotte	DePuy Canada, Medtronic
Junichi Mizuno	Ammtec
Thomas E. Mroz	Globus Medical, PearlDiver
Praveen V. Mummaneni	DePuy Spine, Quality Medical Publishers
Hiroshi Nakagawa	Stryker
R. Douglas Orr	Medtronic
Frank M. Phillips	Nuvasive
K. Daniel Riew	Amedica, Benvenue Medical, Biomet, Cervical Spine Research Society, Expanding Orthopedics, Korean American Spine Society, Medtronic Sofamor Danek, Nexgen Spine, Osprey, Paradigm Spine, PSD, Spinal Kinetics, Spineology, Vertiflex

Meic H. Schmidt	Aesculap, NREF
Christopher I. Shaffrey	AO, Biomet, Department of Defense, DePuy, Medtronic, National Institutes of Health, North American Clinical Trials Network
Daniel Shedid	Baxano, DePuy Spine
Justin S. Smith	Biomet, DePuy Spine, Globus, Medtronic
Volker K.H. Sonntag	Medtronic
Robert F. Spetzler	Boston Scientific, Dicom Grid, EmergeMD, iCO Therpeutics, Katalyst/Kogent, Neurovasc, RSB Spine, Stereotaxis, Synergetics, Zeiss
Michael P. Steinmetz	Biomet Spine, Medtronic Power Division
Brian J. Sullivan	Globus Medical
Daisuke Togawa	Medtronic Sofamore Danek
Michael Y. Wang	Aesculap Spine, Biomet, DePuy
William A. Wilson IV	Computational BioDynamics
Hansen A. Yuan	BreakAway Imaging, DePuy Spine, Medtronics, Pioneer Surgical

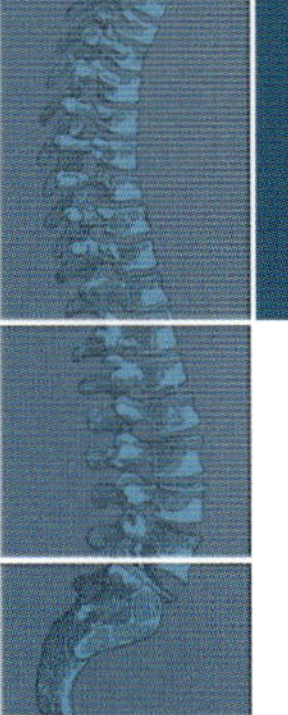

4.7 Tumors, Vascular Malformations, and Related Lesions

CHAPTER 101

Intramedullary Spinal Cord Lesions

Paul C. McCormick | John A. Anson

Surgery, once used for the diagnosis of intramedullary spinal cord tumors alone, now represents the most effective treatment of benign well-circumscribed tumors (which constitute the majority of intramedullary neoplasms).[1-9] Long-term tumor control or cure, with preservation of neurologic function, can be achieved in most patients with microsurgical removal alone.[2,5,10] The benign nature of most intramedullary neoplasms, advances in microsurgical techniques, early clinical diagnosis with MRI, and the ineffectual or inconsistent treatment response of most intramedullary tumors to radiation therapy largely account for the expanded role of surgery in the management of these lesions.[4,11,12] Therefore, optimization of surgical treatment is the key to successful management of patients with intramedullary masses. This includes early diagnosis and aggressive primary treatment, the avoidance of technical and judgmental errors and their associated complications, and a strict adherence to contemporary microsurgical technique.

Patient Evaluation

The predominant benefit of surgery for an intramedullary tumor is prophylactic. Preservation, rather than restoration, of neurologic function is the most likely outcome after successful surgical treatment. In fact, significant improvement of a severe or long-standing preoperative neurologic deficit rarely occurs after a technically successful surgical excision. Surgical morbidity is also greater in patients with more significant preoperative deficits. This creates a therapeutic irony in which the risk of surgery is actually less in patients with minimal or no objective neurologic deficit. Thus, early clinical diagnosis and, if possible, definitive initial treatment are critical to successful clinical management of most intramedullary tumors. A therapeutic dilemma arises, however, in the asymptomatic patient in whom an incidental intramedullary spinal cord lesion has been discovered. A posterior column deficit is a common consequence of a dorsal median myelotomy; thus, some degree of morbidity often accompanies even the most successful surgical removal.[13] In completely asymptomatic patients, therefore, observation with serial clinical and radiologic follow-up may be an appropriate management strategy. This is also true for patients with conditions such as neurofibromatosis or von Hippel-Lindau disease.

Because of the slow growth rate of benign tumors and the availability of MRI, most patients with intramedullary tumors are diagnosed before the onset of significant neurologic deficit. Gadolinium-enhanced MRI is the procedure of choice for imaging and preoperative evaluation of an intramedullary tumor. Spinal cord enlargement and tumor enhancement are the characteristic findings (Fig. 101-1). Polar cysts are often present. Ependymomas are usually symmetrically located and exhibit uniform tumor enhancement, whereas astrocytomas are associated with a more variable appearance with respect to tumor margins and enhancement patterns (Fig. 101-2). Prediction of these tumor types on MRI appearance is often inaccurate, predominantly because of the variability of presentation on MRI scans, and is therefore avoided because it may unfairly influence the surgical objective. Hemangioblastomas usually appear as intensely enhancing eccentric masses or nodules. There is often diffuse spinal cord enlargement that may extend a considerable distance from the tumor (Fig. 101-3). The cause of this tumor enlargement is most likely vasogenic edema.[14]

Patient Selection

Whereas early diagnosis is routinely achieved with gadolinium-enhanced MRI, the sensitivity of MRI has far exceeded its specificity. Acute inflammatory conditions or demyelinating conditions such as multiple sclerosis or transverse myelitis are exquisitely imaged with MRI. These are not surgical lesions, and biopsy for diagnosis usually reveals only a nonspecific inflammatory response. This rarely provides a specific diagnosis, a prognosis, or treatment options. In most cases, patients with these conditions can be distinguished on the basis of clinical presentation and MRI appearance. These patients usually have symptoms of either acute or subacute onset of significant neurologic deficit. MRI typically shows patchy or focal gadolinium enhancement that may be confined to the white matter (Fig. 101-4). Spinal cord enlargement is subtle or, more likely, absent. In contrast, patients with benign intramedullary tumors usually experience a significant spinal cord enlargement with minimal, if any, objective neurologic deficit. Thus, a patient who shows symptoms of an acute or subacute onset of a significant neurologic deficit in the absence of obvious spinal cord enlargement usually harbors a nonsurgical inflammatory lesion.

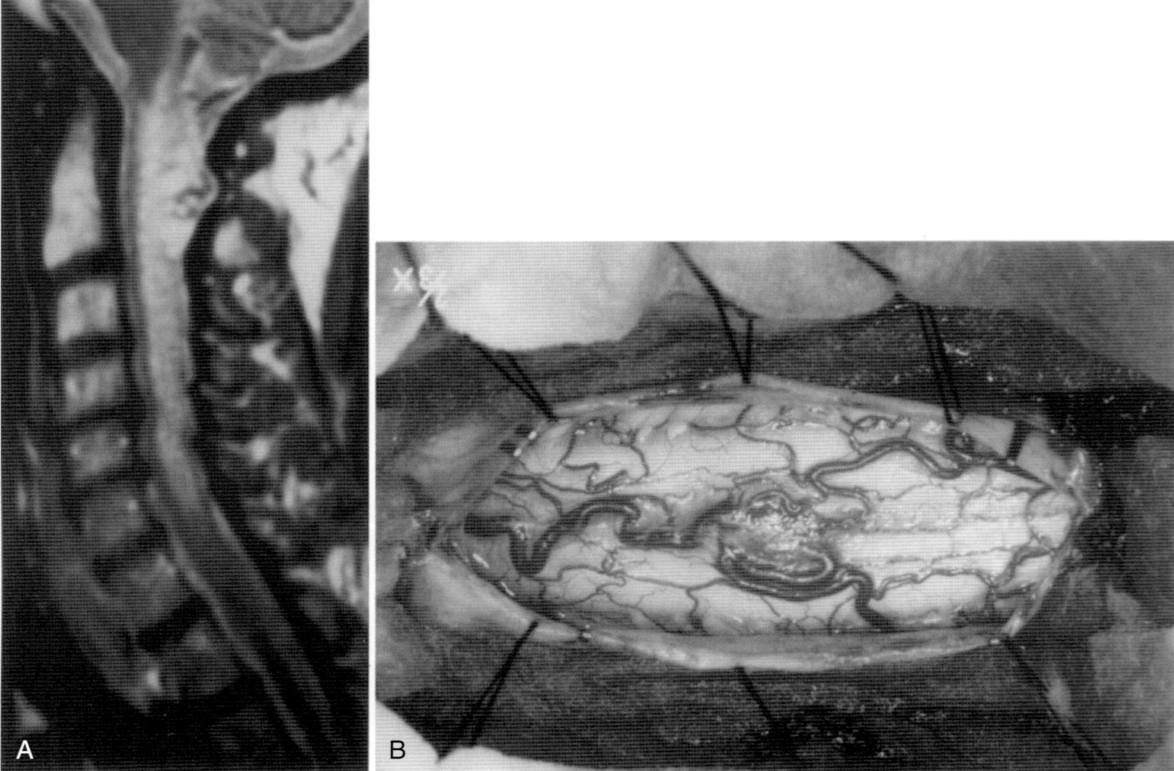

FIGURE 101-3. **A,** A sagittal MRI demonstrates a focal dorsal mass at the C2 level. Note diffuse spinal cord enlargement. **B,** An intraoperative photograph demonstrates orange pia-based hemangioblastoma with associated epipial draining veins.

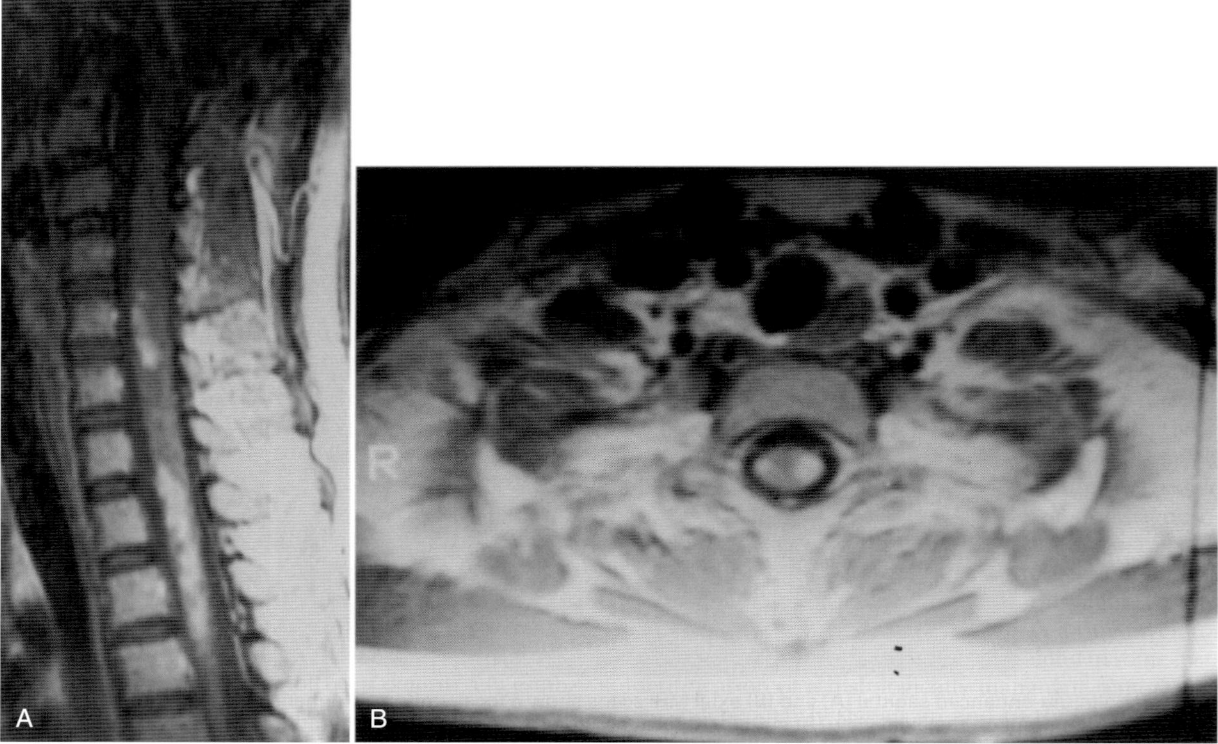

FIGURE 101-4. Gadolinium-enhanced sagittal (**A**) and (**B**) axial MRI scans in a patient with acute onset of significant neurologic deficit demonstrate patchy white matter enhancement without spinal cord enlargement. The clinical presentation and radiographic appearance are consistent with transverse myelitis. Surgery is not indicated in this patient.

identification of an ependymoma reassures the surgeon that a plane must exist and that surgical removal should continue.

Surgical Technique

After intubation and administration of perioperative steroids and antibiotics, the patient is turned to the prone position. A Mayfield skull clamp is used for cervical and upper thoracic lesions above the T6 level. Neck flexion and head elevation (i.e., military prone position) reduce the spinal curvature at these levels. Sensory and motor evoked potential monitoring may be used throughout the procedure. The acquired data, however, rarely influence the surgical technique or the surgical objective.[19]

A midline incision and subperiosteal bony dissection are made, and a standard laminectomy is performed. This should extend to at least one segment above and one segment below the solid tumor component. The facet joints are preserved, if possible. Delayed instability rarely occurs after laminectomy for intramedullary tumor removal in adults. Although laminoplasty may be a reasonable option, it is not required.

Strict hemostasis must be secured before the dura is opened to prevent ongoing contamination into the dependent microsurgical field. Wide, moist, cottonoid "wall-offs" cover the exposed muscles. Oxidized cellulose (Surgicel) is generously spread over the lateral gutters to prevent contamination of the operative field with blood. The dura mater is opened in the midline and tented laterally to the muscles with sutures (Fig. 101-5A).

The arachnoid is opened separately, and the spinal cord is inspected for any surface abnormality. Most glial tumors appear with only localized spinal cord enlargement. The spinal cord may be rotated. Occasionally, the overlying spinal cord may be thinned or even transparent secondary to a large or eccentrically located tumor or polar cyst. Ultrasonography is useful for tumor localization and assurance of adequate bony exposure.

Rarely, an exophytic component of a benign glial tumor may extend into the subarachnoid space through a nerve root entry zone. Malignant neoplasms may replace surface spinal cord tissue or fungate through the pia into the subarachnoid space. Most hemangioblastomas arise from the dorsal half of the spinal cord with a visible pial attachment (see Fig. 101-3B).[3,7] The size of the pial attachment may bear no relationship to the underlying embedded portion of the tumor.

Exposure of most intramedullary glial neoplasms is through a dorsal midline myelotomy. Eccentrically located tumors that abut the pia may be exposed via an off-midline myelotomy that extends longitudinally from both ends of the visible tumor.

The dorsal midline septum is identified as the midpoint between corresponding dorsal root entry zones. Bipolar cautery marks the dorsal midline over the extent of the intended myelotomy. The myelotomy is begun with a microknife in an avascular pial segment at the point of maximum spinal cord enlargement. The pia is a white, glistening fibrocartilaginous membrane that is tightly applied to the outer glial limiting membrane of the spinal cord. The pia is sharply incised over the entire extent of the tumor. Midline crossing epipial vessels are sequentially cauterized and divided. The myelotomy is deepened by gentle spreading with blunt microforceps and dissectors. Fibrous gliosis at the polar margins of the tumor may require sharp dissection with a microknife. The myelotomy continues until the entire rostrocaudal extent of the dorsal tumor surface has been identified (see Fig. 101-5B). Although the myelotomy must extend a few millimeters beyond the solid portion of the tumor, it is not necessary to completely expose polar cysts. Sizes #6-0 pial sutures are placed and clipped laterally to the dura to maintain gentle traction (see Fig. 101-5C). Evaluation of the tumor–spinal cord interface and frozen-section biopsy examination (to a lesser extent) determine the appropriate treatment objective. Ependymomas are usually characterized by a glistening reddish or brownish-red surface that may be slightly lobulated (see Fig. 101-5C) Blood vessels often course over the tumor surface. These tumors are clearly distinguishable from the surrounding spinal cord on the basis of color and texture. Although unencapsulated, these tumors do not infiltrate and can be easily distinguished and separated from the surrounding spinal cord. Astrocytomas are more heterogeneous with respect to physical characteristics and abut the spinal cord. Intratumoral cysts are quite common, but tumor color and consistency are variable. In adults, most astrocytomas appear as a definable intramedullary mass with a gradual and indistinct transition between the tumor mass and surrounding spinal cord (see Fig. 101-2C). This reflects the infiltrative nature of these neoplasms.

The technique of tumor removal depends on its juncture with the spinal cord and its size. Development of the tumor–spinal cord juncture is preferred for circumscribed tumors with a well-defined plane. The dorsal tumor surface is exposed with pial sutures and gentle, blunt lateral displacement of the overlying dorsal hemicords with dissectors. Fibrous and vascular attachments that tether the spinal cord to the tumor surface are systematically cauterized and divided. The development of the lateral and polar tumor margins is facilitated by forceps traction on the tumor and gentle pial suture and manual dissector countertraction on the spinal cord (see Fig. 101-5D). Larger tumors require internal decompression with an ultrasonic aspirator or laser to allow better visualization and mobilization of the lateral and ventral tumor margins. Infiltrating tumors are removed using an "inside-out" technique. Internal decompression is continued peripherally until the clear distinction of the tumor and spinal cord is no longer obvious (see Fig. 101-2C).

The technique of hemangioblastoma removal differs because of its vascularity and pial attachment. Internal decompression is not an option (because of the vascularity). Instead, the pial attachment should be circumferentially incised (Fig. 101-6A). Systematic cautery on the tumor surface shrinks the tumor bulk to allow adequate mobilization and dissection from the surrounding spinal cord. Small polar longitudinal myelotomies may improve visualization of large tumors embedded in the spinal cord, with only a small exposed pial surface attachment (Fig. 101-6B). After completion of tumor resection, the pial sutures are removed. No attempt is made to suture the dorsal hemicords. The subarachnoid space is copiously irrigated with warm saline. Meticulous multilayer closure is then performed to prevent cerebrospinal fluid (CSF) leakage. This is particularly important in patients who have undergone previous surgery and radiation therapy. There is a high risk of CSF fistula in these patients. An autologous thoracodorsal fascia dural patch graft may be used after biopsy of infiltrative or malignant tumors.

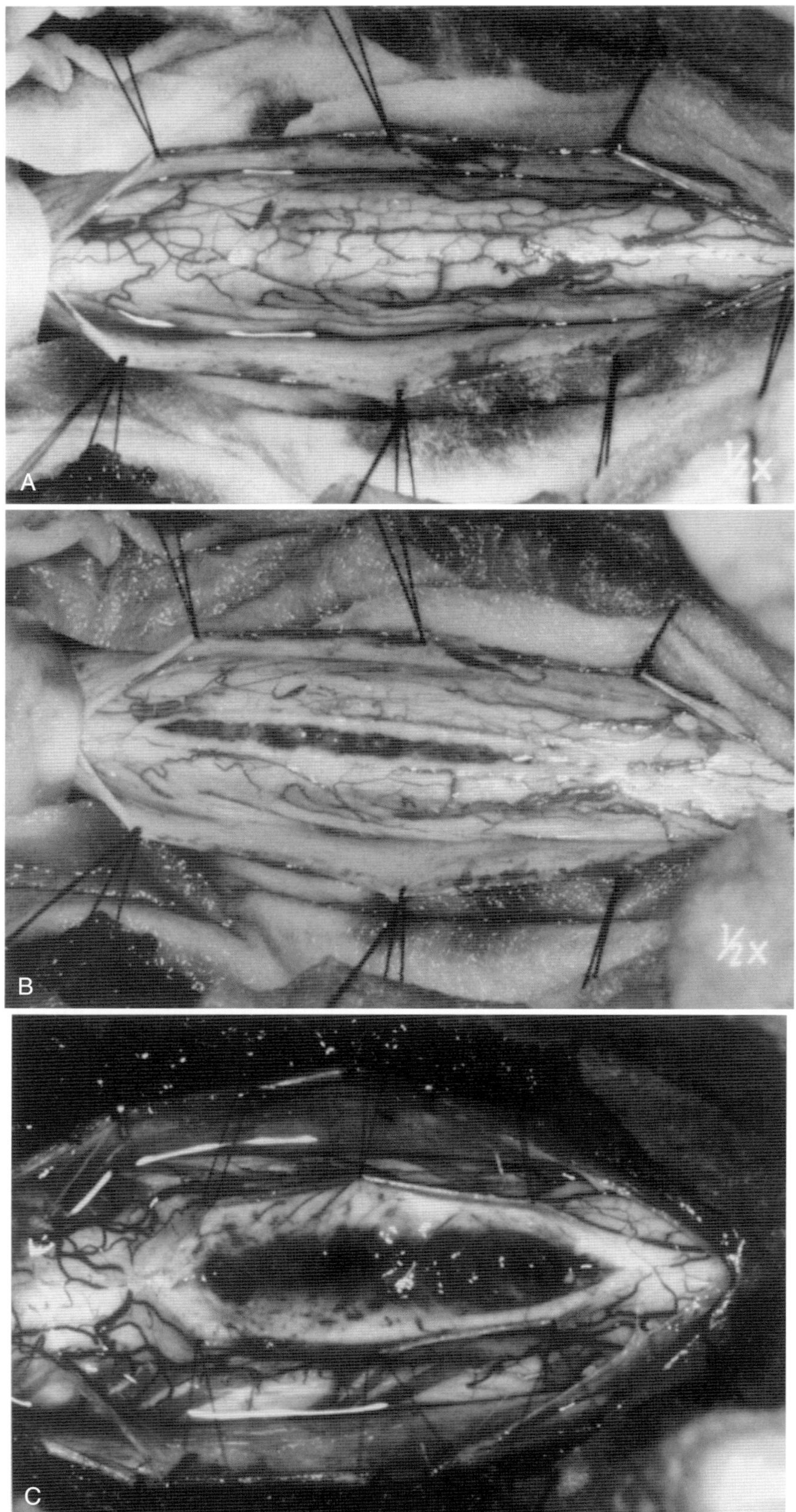

FIGURE 101-5. **A,** Initial exposure of the spinal cord. The dura mater is tented to the muscles with suture. Surgicel and cottonoid wall-offs are placed in the lateral gutters to prevent blood drainage into the dependent operative field. The spinal cord is swollen without visible surface abnormality. **B,** A midline myelotomy has been performed. The tumor is encountered at a depth of about 2 mm. The myelotomy extends over the entire rostrocaudal extent of the tumor mass. **C,** A photograph after exposure of the dorsal tumor surface demonstrates glistening appearance of an intramedullary ependymoma that is clearly separate from the surrounding spinal cord. Exposure is maintained with pial traction. Sutures are hung over the edge of the wound by mosquito clamps.

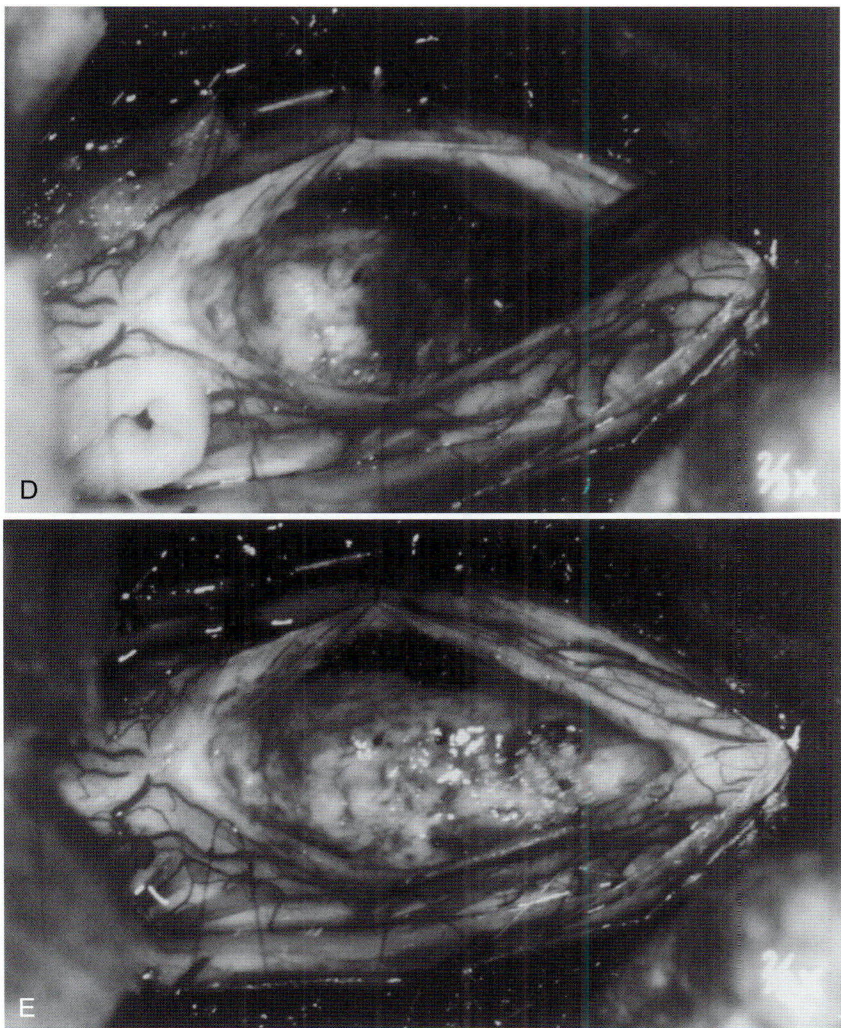

FIGURE 101-5, cont. D, Development of the lateral and ventral tumor margins is performed with forceps traction on the tumor against gentle countertraction on the surrounding cord tissue. **E,** An intraoperative photograph after gross total resection of an intramedullary ependymoma shows clean tumor margins without evidence of residual tumor.

Postoperative Management

Postoperative management is standard. Early mobilization is encouraged to prevent complications of recumbency such as deep venous thrombosis and pneumonia. Paretic patients are particularly vulnerable to thromboembolic complications. Sequential compression devices, initially placed immediately prior to surgery, are continued postoperatively until the patient is adequately mobilized. Subcutaneous heparin (5000 units twice a day) or low-molecular-weight heparin (enoxaparin 40 mg every day) may also be considered on or about postoperative day 2 but may increase the risk of wound hematomas. Orthostatic hypotension may occasionally occur after removal of upper thoracic and cervical intramedullary neoplasms. This is usually a self-limiting problem that can be managed with liberal use of fluids and more gradual mobilization. A posterior fossa syndrome occasionally occurs after removal of a high cervical intramedullary neoplasm. This is effectively managed with steroids, although a spinal tap may be required to rule out meningitis. Open CSF fistulae are aggressively managed. An early return to the operating room for wound revision is recommended to prevent this complication in selected cases. Closed CSF pseudomeningoceles can be managed more expectantly because they frequently spontaneously resolve.

Despite confident gross total resection, benign intramedullary tumors present a continued risk of recurrence. Long-term clinical and radiographic follow-up is warranted in these patients. An early postoperative MRI (6–8 weeks after surgery) establishes the completeness of resection and serves as a baseline against which further studies can be compared. Serial gadolinium-enhanced MRI scans are obtained yearly because radiographic evidence of tumor recurrence usually precedes clinical symptoms. Surgical reexploration, if clinically appropriate, can then be performed with minimal surgical morbidity. Exposure of the spinal cord at reoperation can be technically difficult. There is often tethering of the spinal cord to the dural suture line at the previous myelotomy site. If the dura was not closed at the previous surgery, then the spinal cord may be densely adherent to the thick epidural scar. In either case, normal dura should be exposed above and below the tethered segment, even if additional bone removal is required. The dura mater or scar is opened as an ellipse

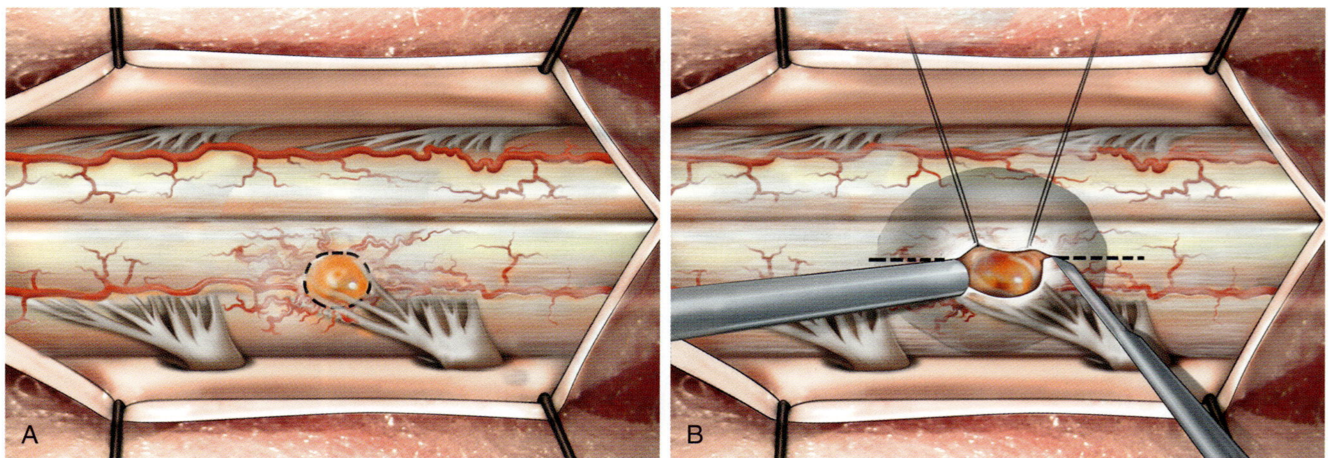

FIGURE 101-6. Illustration of superficial hemangioblastoma (**A**) showing circumferential incision (*dotted line*) at the margin of hemangioblastoma and normal pia. For tumors with a large intramedullary extension with only a small surface component, longitudinal myelotomies (*dotted lines*) are performed (**B**).

around the tether. Meticulous sharp dissection is carried centrally to free the dorsal surface of the spinal cord.

Nearly all patients experience dorsal column dysfunction postoperatively. This probably results from the dorsal midline myelotomy. Patients often complain of numbness or paresthesias with minimal objective discriminative or proprioceptive deficits. These subjective complaints usually improve with time but do not resolve totally. Postoperative neurologic function usually correlates with the preoperative neurologic deficit. The new onset of significant objective neurologic deficits uncommonly occurs in patients with minimal or no preoperative deficits. Conversely, worsening of an existing preoperative deficit often occurs postoperatively.

Summary

Surgery represents the only established effective treatment modality for benign intramedullary neoplasms. Optimization of surgical outcome, therefore, is the most important treatment consideration. Aggressive initial management, appropriate judgment and technique, and adherence to strict microsurgical techniques are the most effective methods of avoiding complications and ensuring an optimal treatment outcome.

KEY REFERENCES

Aghakhani N, David P, Parker F: Intramedullary spinal ependymomas: analysis of a consecutive series of 82 adult cases with particular attention to patients with no preoperative neurological deficit. *Neurosurgery* 62:1279–1285, 2008.

Gomez DR, Missett BT, Wara WM, et al: High failure rate in spinal ependymomas with long-term follow-up. *Neuro-oncology* 7:254–259, 2005.

Lee J, Parsa AT, Ames CP, et al: Clinical management of intramedullary spinal ependymomas in adults. *Neurosurg Clin North Am* 17(1):21–28, 2006.

Raco A, Esposito V, Lenzi J, et al: Long-term follow-up of intramedullary spinal cord tumors: a series of 202 cases. *Neurosurgery* 56:972–981, 2005.

Woodworth GF, Chaichana KL, McGirt MJ, et al: Predictors of ambulatory function after surgical resection of intramedullary spinal cord tumors. *Neurosurgery* 61:99–105, 2007.

REFERENCES

The complete reference list is available online at expertconsult.com.

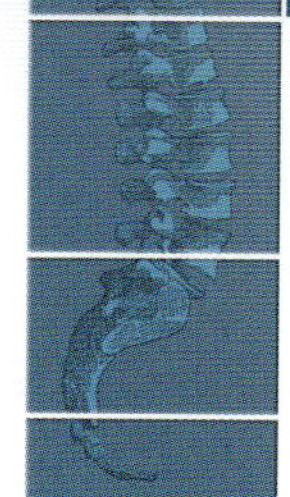

CHAPTER 102

Intradural Extramedullary Spinal Lesions

Basheal M. Agrawal | Barry D. Birch | Paul C. McCormick | Daniel K. Resnick

Before the advent of microsurgical techniques, surgery of many spinal cord neoplasms consisted primarily of open biopsy and radiation therapy.[1-3] Recent technologic advances in neurosurgery and diagnostic imaging have expanded the role for operative treatment of spinal tumors. Although Horsely performed the first successful excision of a spinal tumor in 1887, and Elsberg and Frazier advocated resection of spinal tumors in the early part of the 20th century, consistently acceptable morbidity and mortality were not realized until recently.[4-7] MRI has facilitated preoperative localization and surgical planning. The use of intraoperative neurologic monitoring and ultrasound has led to reduced operative morbidity. Advances in microsurgical techniques as well as the development of ultrasonic aspiration and laser technology have established microsurgical removal as the most effective treatment for benign intradural extramedullary tumors.

Incidence and Pathology

Tumors of the spine are anatomically classified by their relationship to the dura mater and spinal cord parenchyma. Intradural tumors can be intramedullary or extramedullary, and extramedullary tumors account for approximately three fourths of all intradural spinal tumors.[1,5,8,9] Intradural spinal neoplasms make up approximately 10% of primary central nervous system tumors in adults,[1,10] and about two thirds are extramedullary, histologically benign, and well circumscribed. Meningioma, schwannoma, and filum terminale ependymoma are the most common histopathologic lesions in the intradural extramedullary space. Meningiomas and nerve sheath neoplasms account for 80% of extramedullary spinal cord tumors, and filum terminale ependymomas make up 15% of these lesions. The remaining 5% includes paragangliomas, drop metastases, and granulomas, all of which are rare.

Meningiomas

Meningiomas arise from arachnoid cap cells embedded in the dura mater near the nerve root sleeve, reflecting their predominant lateral location and meningeal attachment. Other possible cells of origin include fibroblasts associated with the dura or pia mater, which may account for the occasional ventral or dorsal location of these tumors. Meningiomas occur in all age-groups, but most arise in people between the fifth and seventh decades of life. Women account for 75% to 85% of cases, and about 80% of tumors are thoracic.[11-13] The upper cervical spine and foramen magnum are also common sites[14] (Fig. 102-1). Here, meningiomas often occupy a ventral or ventrolateral position and may adhere to the vertebral artery near its intradural entry and initial intracranial course. Low cervical and lumbar meningiomas are infrequent. Most spinal meningiomas are

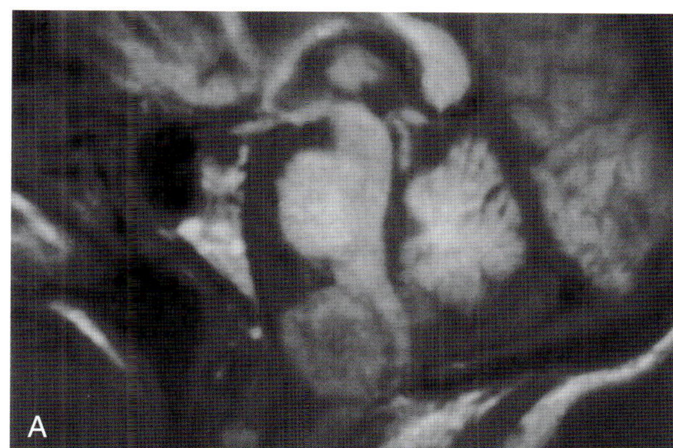

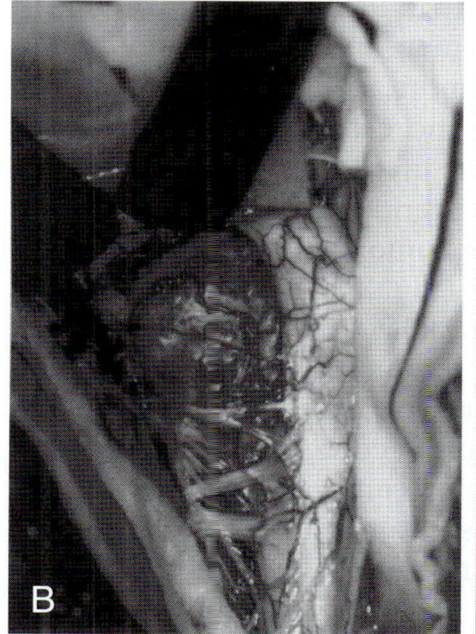

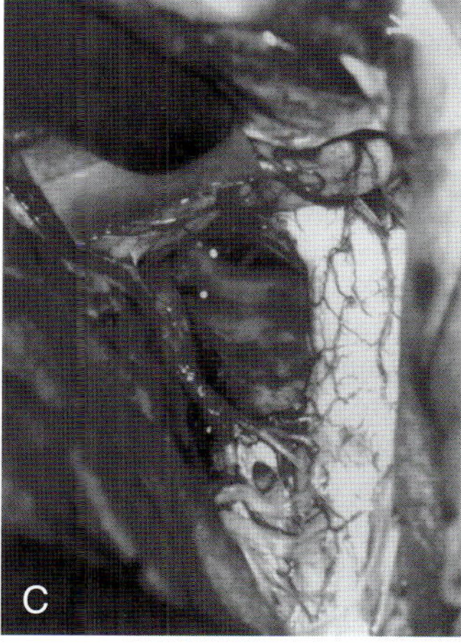

FIGURE 102-1. Foramen magnum meningioma. **A,** T1-weighted MRI demonstrating ventral location with dorsal displacement of the spinal cord. **B,** Dorsolateral approach prior to resection. **C,** Appearance after gross total resection.

dorsal midline tumors. Bowel and bladder functions are not significantly impaired until late in the clinical course. Filum ependymomas are characterized most frequently by back pain and subsequent asymmetrical radiation to both legs. Increased pain on recumbency, an important clinical feature of extramedullary tumors, is most often associated with large cauda equina lesions. Subarachnoid hemorrhage has also been reported as a presenting feature of an extramedullary tumor.[39]

Imaging Evaluation

The mainstay of imaging diagnosis for all spinal cord tumors is MRI. It provides spatial and contrast resolution of neural structures that is unattainable by any other imaging modality. Plain radiographs are of little use in the modern diagnosis of spinal cord tumors because they do not image soft tissue adequately. However, the effects of intraspinal tumors on the vertebral elements are sometimes evident. Nerve sheath tumors can cause enlargement of the intervertebral foramina. This finding may be important in patients imaged for other reasons. Myelography alone has a very limited role in the workup of spinal cord tumors and is seldom performed without subsequent CT. Intradural extramedullary tumors typically produce rounded filling defects of the dye column on a plain myelogram. CT and CT myelography (myelo-CT) greatly enhance anatomic details compared to plain radiographs and myelography. CT provides excellent visualization of osseous structures, but soft tissue detail is inferior to that provided by MRI. For extramedullary tumors, myelo-CT allows excellent visualization of tumors arising in the region of the neural foramen, and accompanying bony changes are well demonstrated. MRI with and without intravenous contrast is the optimal initial radiographic examination for patients suspected of having an intradural extramedullary spinal lesion.

Lesion signal abnormalities, CSF capping, and spinal cord or cauda equina displacement identify most extramedullary masses in a technically adequate MRI study.[40] The diagnosis of lipoma, neurenteric cysts (dermoid or epidermoid), arachnoid cysts, or vascular pathology can often be established on the basis of imaging characteristics alone. Gadolinium-enhanced images markedly increase the sensitivity of MRI, particularly for small tumors.

Most extramedullary tumors are isointense or slightly hypointense with respect to the spinal cord on T1-weighted images. Nerve sheath tumors are more likely to be hyperintense to the spinal cord than meningiomas on T2-weighted images. Cauda equina tumors usually demonstrate increased signal intensity with respect to CSF on both T1 and T2 pulse sequences. However, small cauda equina tumors are easily overlooked on noncontrast scans.[40,41]

Virtually all extramedullary spinal tumors demonstrate some degree of contrast enhancement. Meningiomas typically exhibit intense uniform enhancement, although nonenhancing calcifications or intratumoral cysts may be seen. Enhancement of the adjacent dura, a "dural tail," strongly supports the diagnosis of meningioma (Fig. 102-4). Although most nerve sheath tumors and filum ependymomas also demonstrate uniform contrast uptake, heterogeneous enhancement from intratumoral cysts, hemorrhage, or necrosis is frequent (Fig. 102-5).

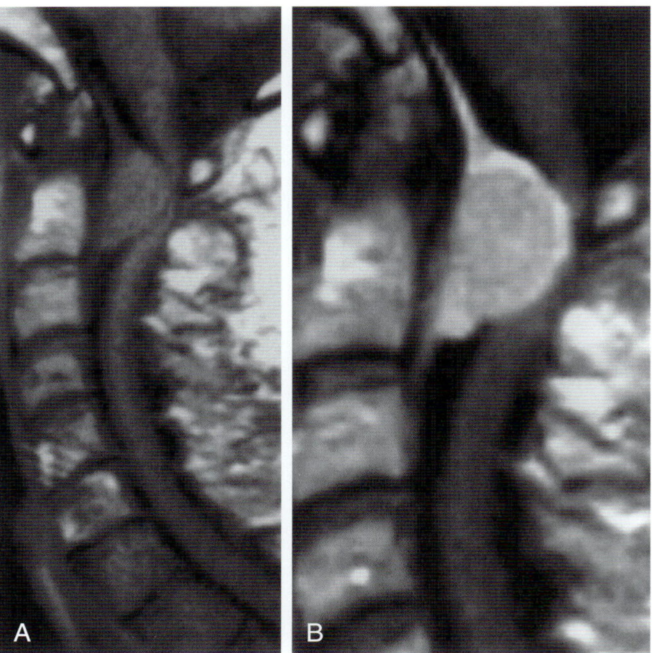

FIGURE 102-4. High cervical meningioma. Sagittal T1-weighted MRIs before (**A**) and after (**B**) intravenous gadolinium. Enhancing dural tails are evident.

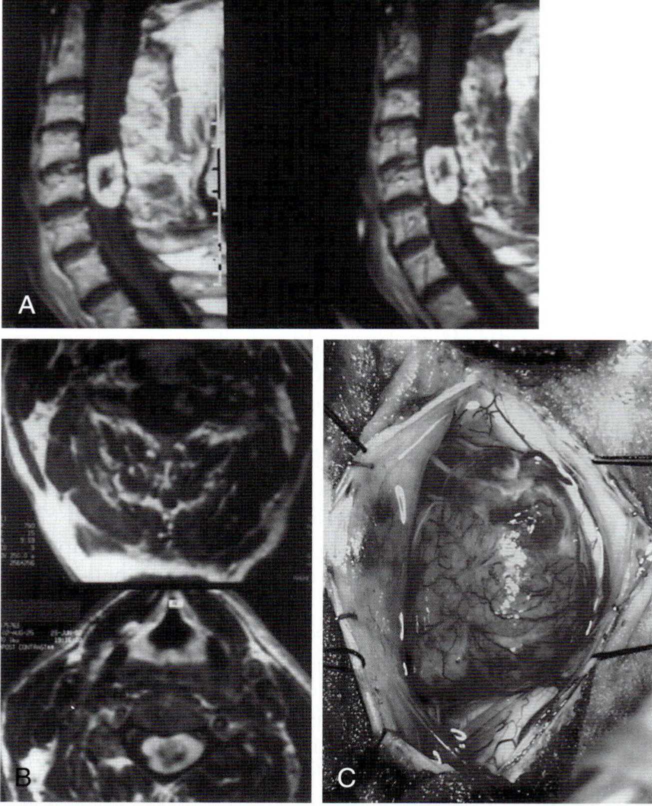

FIGURE 102-5. Cystic schwannoma. Sagittal (**A**) and axial (**B**) T1-weighted MRIs after intravenous gadolinium, denonstrating a small apical syrinx and heterogeneous enhancement. **C,** Intraoperative photograph showing encapsulated tumor with a densely adherent arachnoid layer.

Currently, myelography and myelo-CT are not often used for the evaluation of intradural pathology. Nevertheless, the spatial resolution of myelo-CT remains superior to that of MRI. For tumors that are closely applied to the surface of the spinal cord and when the MRI is equivocal with respect to an intramedullary or extramedullary location, myelo-CT can sometimes provide better resolution. The intradural or extradural distribution of a paraspinal or dumb-bell–shaped tumor is also better visualized with myelo-CT than with MRI (see Fig. 102-2C).

Management

After clinical and imaging evaluation reveal a lesion that is believed to be a spinal cord tumor, tissue diagnosis is necessary. The surgical objective for most intradural extramedullary spinal cord lesions is gross total removal, and surgical planning must proceed accordingly. Immediately preoperatively, patients are given high-dose glucocorticoids, if spinal cord manipulation is anticipated, and intravenous antibiotics. Mechanical venous thromboembolism prophylaxis and a Foley catheter are used. Most tumors are accessible with the patient in the prone position. For cervical lesions, stabilization of the head and neck in pins is necessary as and aid to microscopic dissection. Adequate exposure is crucial and is dictated by the location and extent of the lesion. Intraoperative monitoring with somatosensory-evoked potentials and motor-evoked potentials should be considered; this monitoring is especially useful with intramedullary extension of tumor. Spontaneous and triggered electromyography can be used to identify nerve roots in filum pathology.[42] Such monitoring does not uniformly protect against neural injury, and false-positive alarms are frequent. Surgical decision making must incorporate the patient's preoperative neurologic status, the likely pathology of the tumor, and technical challenges presented by a particular lesion. Intraoperative ultrasound is often useful in localizing and delineating the extent of the pathology if it is not obvious on inspection. Competent dural closure is essential. Steroids are tapered postoperatively, and early mobilization and rehabilitation are encouraged.

Surgical Considerations

The optimal treatment of intradural extramedullary tumors is surgical excision. For nerve sheath lesions, this can be accomplished in nearly all cases through standard laminectomy.[7] Recurrences are rare when gross total removal has been achieved. Most nerve sheath tumors are dorsal or dorsolateral to the spinal cord and are easily seen after opening the dura mater (Fig. 102-6). Ventral tumors may require dentate ligament section to achieve adequate visualization, and lumbar tumors may be covered by the cauda equina or conus medullaris. The nerve roots must be separated to provide adequate visualization.

Laminectomy provides adequate exposure for spinal meningiomas in most cases. Unilateral laminectomy and facetectomy can be used for eccentrically located or ventral tumors. Large ventral tumors can also be approached satisfactorily through standard dorsal exposures because they have already provided the necessary spinal cord retraction. Suture retraction on a divided dentate ligament or on noncritical dorsal

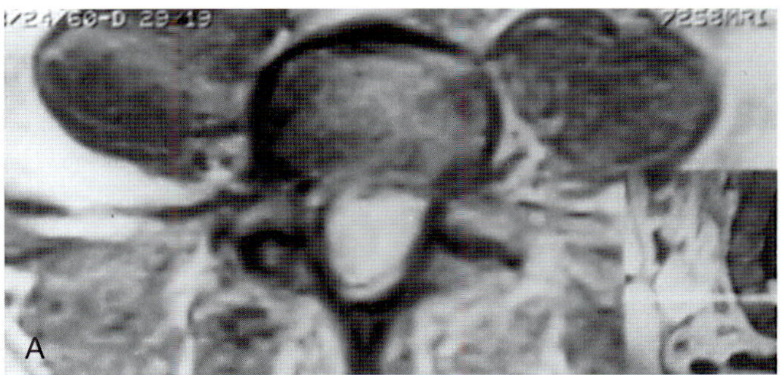

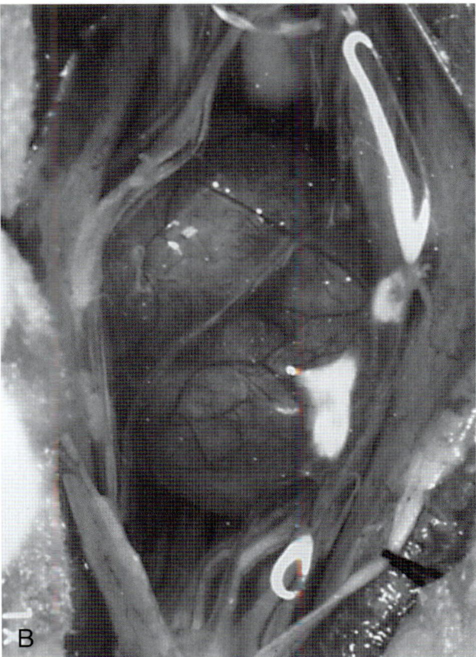

FIGURE 102-6. Cauda equina schwannoma. **A,** Axial T1-weighted MRI after intravenous gadolinium; a homogeneously enhancing lesion is apparent. **B,** Dorsolateral location is evident with displacement of the cauda equina ventrolaterally.

nerve roots provides additional ventral exposure. Depression of the paraspinal muscle mass with table-mounted retractors further facilitates ventral access. Alternatively, a costotransversectomy or lateral extracavitary approach can be used for ventral thoracic tumors. The extreme lateral approach is used when there is a significant ventral tumor component above the foramen magnum.[43] Resection of ventrally located cervical nerve sheath tumors through a ventral corpectomy approach has also recently been reported.[44] Similarly, a thoracoscopic approach to ventral thoracic tumors has also been decribed.[45] Both of these techniques have been described via case reports, however, and the reader is cautioned that intradural tumor resection from a ventral approach is technically challenging.

The role of surgery in treating filum terminale ependymomas depends on the size of the tumor and its relationship to the surrounding roots of the cauda equina. Gross total en bloc resection should be attempted whenever possible. This can usually be accomplished for small and moderate-sized tumors that remain well circumscribed within the fibrous coverings of the filum terminale and are easily separated from the cauda equina nerve roots. A portion of uninvolved filum terminale is generally present between the tumor and spinal cord. Amputation of the afferent and efferent filum segments is required for tumor removal. Internal decompression is not used for small and moderate-sized tumors because it can increase the risk of CSF dissemination. Recurrences after successful en bloc resection are rare.

Adjuvant Therapy

The effects of postoperative radiation therapy on spinal meningiomas and nerve sheath tumors have not been extensively studied. Radiation treatment can be considered for subtotally resected lesions that are recurrent and histologically and clinically aggressive. It is probably best to wait until reoperation is complete before instituting therapy. In one series, 3.5% of patients receiving radiation therapy experienced neurologic worsening attributable to the therapy.[46]

Biologically aggressive filum ependymomas, which are more common in the younger population, demonstrate early tumor recurrence and can be treated with radiation therapy. If significant tumor burden is present after initial surgery, however, as in the case of known CSF dissemination, postoperative radiation therapy is given as a primary adjunct. Postoperative radiation therapy is delayed in situations where piecemeal total or near total removal has been accomplished. In these cases, tumor recurrences can be treated with repeat surgery and followed by radiation therapy. Although the response of spinal cord ependymomas to radiation therapy is unpredictable, there is some evidence that long-term control can be achieved with radiation therapy in some patients.[47] This response cannot be predicted individually. Because prior radiation therapy markedly increases the morbidity of future surgical prospects, it is generally delayed in situations where further surgery may be contemplated. The role of stereotactic radiosurgery in the management of inoperable or recurrent tumors is currently being evaluated as well and may be useful in reducing surgical morbidity of tumors adherent to the spinal cord.[48,49]

Recently, a phase III study was conducted looking at the use of etoposide as salvage chemotherapy in patients with recurrent spinal cord ependymomas. Ten patients were treated, and five achieved stable disease status. However, most of these patients had intramedullary tumors, so these results may not be relevant to the more benign tumors of the cauda equina.[50]

Operative Technique

Meningiomas

A variety of strategies can be used for removal of spinal meningiomas. Dorsal and dorsolateral lesions are delivered away from the spinal cord with traction on the open dural margins, and circumscribing excision of the dural origin completes the removal. For lateral and ventral tumors, the arachnoid over the exposed portion of the tumor is incised and reflected so that the dissection can proceed directly on the tumor surface (Fig. 102-7). The rostral and caudal tumor poles should be identified. Small cotton pledgets can be placed in the spinal lateral canal gutters on either side of the tumor to minimize blood spillage into the subarachnoid space. The exposed tumor surface is then cauterized to diminish tumor vascularity and to shrink tumor mass. Large tumors are bisected and debulked through a central trough. The tumor segment apposing the spinal cord is then delivered into the resection cavity with gentle traction and surface dissection. The remaining dura-based tumor is amputated from the dural attachment, and the attachment is then extensively coagulated. Alternatively, the dural base can be excised and replaced with a thoracodorsal fascia patch graft. All blood and debris are irrigated from the subarachnoid space with warm saline, and arachnoid adhesions holding the cord in a deformed position are divided. These maneuvers can diminish the risk of postoperative complications such as spinal cord tethering, arachnoiditis, delayed syrinx formation, and hydrocephalus, which occasionally complicate extramedullary tumor removal. Rarely, a spinal meningioma extends through a dural nerve root sleeve and appears as a dumbbell–shaped tumor. The techniques for removal are similar to those described here for nerve sheath tumors.

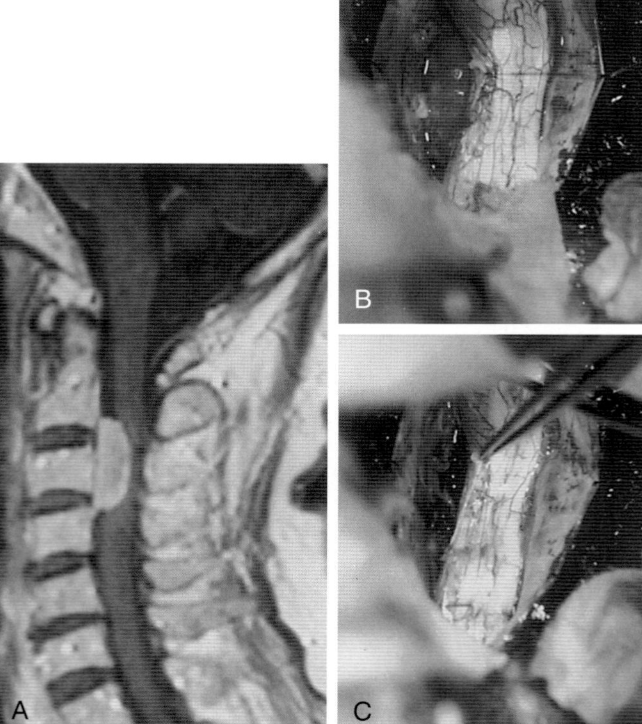

FIGURE 102-7. Ventral cervical meningioma. **A,** Sagittal T1-weighted MRI after intravenous gadolinium. **B,** Exposure after arachnoid dissection and section of the dentate ligaments. **C,** Appearance after gross total resection.

Nerve Sheath Tumors

Surgical exposure of nerve sheath tumors depends on the specific anatomy of the lesion. Tumors that are small and strictly intradural can be approached via dorsal laminectomy. Ventrally located tumors may require facetectomy, transthoracic, or far lateral approaches. Once exposure is achieved, a plane of dissection directly on the tumor surface must be identified.

There is usually an arachnoid membrane tightly applied to the tumor surface (see Fig 102-5C). This is the fenestrated arachnoid layer that separately ensheaths each dorsal and ventral nerve root within the subarachnoid space.[51] This layer is sharply incised and reflected off the tumor surface. The tumor capsule is cauterized to diminish vascularity and shrink tumor volume. Tumor removal requires identification and division of the proximal and distal nerve root tumor attachments, which may not be immediately apparent with large tumors. Internal decompression with a laser or ultrasonic aspirator is used in such cases. Sacrifice of the nerve rootlets of origin is usually required for tumor removal. Occasionally, some fascicles of the nerve rootlet can be preserved, especially for smaller tumors. It is usually possible, however, to preserve the corresponding intradural nerve root because the fenestrated arachnoid sheaths allow anatomic separation of the dorsal and ventral nerve roots to a point just distal to the dorsal root ganglion. In a typical case involving dorsal root tumor origin, for example, it is possible to preserve the ventral root, which is tightly applied to the ventral tumor surface. Extension of a dumb-bell–shaped tumor through the root sleeve, however, usually necessitates resection of the entire spinal nerve.[51] This rarely causes significant nerve deficit, even at the cervical and lumbar enlargements. The function of the involved root has probably already been compensated for by adjacent roots. A very proximal tumor origin may be partially embedded in the epipial tissue or may elevate the pia to occupy a subpial location. The tumor-cord junction may be difficult to develop in these cases and requires resection of a segment of pia to effect complete removal.

Filum Ependymomas

The exposure for resection of filum ependymomas is standard dorsal laminectomy over the involved levels. Removal consists of developing a clean arachnoid plane around the lesion and separating it from the involved nerve roots. Large filum terminale ependymomas, however, can present significant problems for surgical resection. These tumors have been present for many years and involve a risk of CSF tumor dissemination. Unencapsulated, pliable neoplasms can insinuate among the roots and within the arachnoid sheaths of the cauda equina, compartmentalized by innumerable arachnoid septae. Filum ependymomas can also spread as contiguous tumor sheaths along the arachnoid septae that act as scaffolding for surface growth. CSF dissemination may occur because of the subarachnoid location. Tumor removal in these cases is necessarily piecemeal and is almost always subtotal. Dense tumor attachments to the roots of the cauda equina present significant risks of postoperative deficits because of the manipulation required for removal.

Outcome

The results of surgery for intradural extramedullary spinal cord tumors are usually excellent. Neurologic morbidity is typically less than 15%, and mortality is extremely uncommon.[7,52] Complications are generally related to wound healing and CSF leakage. Most patients have not received radiation therapy; therefore, conservative treatment with lumbar drainage is sufficient management for CSF leakage in most cases. Neurologic complications, such as new deficits or exacerbation of existing ones, are uncommon but are most often associated with manipulation of the cauda equina. Motor and sensory deficits typically improve after surgery, but return of bladder function is variable. Improvement in preoperative deficits is typical and may be dramatic early in the postoperative period. Recovery is related to the duration and severity of the existing deficit and the age of the patient.

Meningiomas

Recurrence of spinal meningiomas after total resection is about 1% at 5 years and 6% at 14 years. Subtotally resected lesions have average recurrence rates of approximately 15%.[11,13] Dural resection versus coagulation apparently does not significantly affect recurrence.[13] Meningiomas with extradural spread or en plaque lesions are more difficult to remove and tend to recur more frequently. These lesions are also associated with greater degrees of postoperative morbidity. These factors must be balanced when planning the extent of resection.

Nerve Sheath Tumors

Total removal of neurofibromas and schwannomas not associated with neurofibromatosis is generally curative.[7,53] However, tumors with extensive paraspinal involvement that are subtotally resected have a definite propensity to recur. Deficits resulting from sacrifice of the involved nerve roots are usually minor and well tolerated. Patients with multiple lesions from neurofibromatosis should usually be observed. Resection is reserved for progressive and symptomatic focal lesions.

Filum Ependymomas

Neurologic deterioration after removal of filum ependymomas is more frequent than that associated with nerve sheath tumors and meningiomas.[23,40,54] Lesions involving the conus medullaris or intimately adherent to many roots of the cauda equina carry the highest risk of postoperative morbidity. Recurrence after gross total resection is rare, and subtotally removed lesions recur in approximately 20% of cases. Survival after total removal is almost 100%.[7,23] Incompletely resected lesions treated with postoperative radiation therapy are associated with 5- and 10-year survival rates of 69% and 62%, respectively.[47,55] Subtotally removed lesions should be frequently followed by MRI.

Summary

Treatment of intradural extramedullary spinal cord lesions remains a gratifying area of neurosurgery. Advances in imaging sensitivity and refinement of microsurgical skills have allowed removal alone to be viewed as definitive treatment in most cases. Early diagnosis and aggressive definitive treatment, when possible, optimize the management of most of these neoplasms.

KEY REFERENCES

Kernohan JW, Sayre GP: *Tumors of the central nervous system*, fascicle 35, Washington, DC, 1952, Armed Forces Institute of Pathology.

McCormick PC: Anatomic principles of intradural surgery. *Clin Neurosurg* 41:204–223, 1994.

McCormick PC, Post KD, Stein BM: Intradural extramedullary tumors in adults. *Neurosurg Clin North Am* 1:591–608, 1990.

Nittner K: Spinal meningiomas, neurinomas and neurofibromas, and hourglass tumours. In Vinken PH, Bruyn GW, editors: *Handbook of clinical neurology*, New York, 1976, Elsevier, pp 177–322.

Sloof JL, Kernohan JW, MacCarthy CS: *Primary intramedullary tumors of the spinal cord and filum terminale*, Philadelphia, 1964, WB Saunders.

Solero CL, Fornari M, Giombini S: Spinal meningiomas: review of 174 operated cases. *Neurosurgery* 25:153–160, 1989.

Sonneland PRW, Scheithauer BW, Onofrio BM: Myxopapillary ependymoma: a clinicopathologic and immunocytochemical study of 77 cases. *Cancer* 56:883–893, 1985.

St Amour TE, Hodges SC, Ross JS, et al: *MRI of the spine*, New York, 1994, Raven Press. pp 299–434.

REFERENCES

The complete reference list is available online at expertconsult.com.

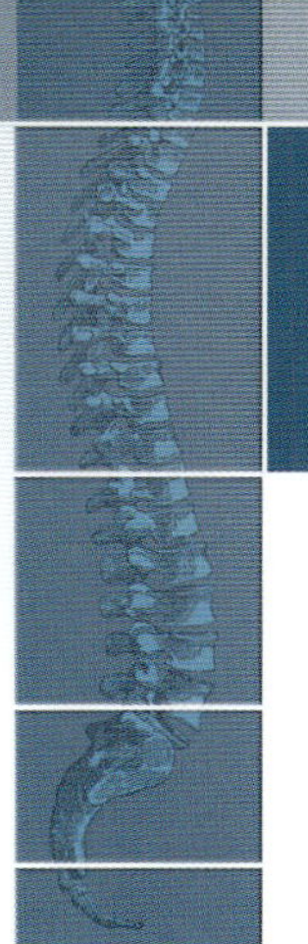

CHAPTER 103

Spinal Intradural Vascular Malformations

Jonathan A. White | Thomas A. Kopitnik | H. Hunt Batjer

Spinal vascular malformations are a family of lesions involving abnormalities of the arteries or veins surrounding the spinal column, spinal cord, and nerve roots. They are relatively rare[1-3] and may manifest as a hemorrhage, myelopathy, radiculopathy, or back pain.[4-7] These lesions can be divided into two broad categories: those that are intradural and those whose abnormal arterial connections are extradural. Extradural lesions are the most common and account for approximately 80% of spinal vascular malformations and are considered in another chapter. This chapter discusses the intradural lesions and includes glomus arteriovenous malformations (AVMs), juvenile AVMs, and intradural direct arteriovenous fistulas (AVFs). Cavernous malformations of the spinal cord and intradural spinal aneurysms are also discussed. In addition to detailing the symptoms, diagnosis, treatment, natural history, and outcomes of these lesions, the demographics and symptoms of these lesions are contrasted with those of the extradural lesions.

History and Nomenclature

The early classification of spinal AVMs occurred prior to the advent of spinal angiography. Patients with signs and symptoms of myelopathy underwent surgery, and the lesions were characterized based on their pathologic appearance.[8-17]

With the advent of spinal angiography in the 1960s, a more refined nomenclature developed based on the pattern of arterial input and venous drainage.[18-20] This resulted in the creation of the terms *type I*, *type II*, and *type III AVMs* still in common use today.[2,21,22]

A type I lesion is a dural AVF whose single or, occasionally, multiple arteriovenous connections lie within the dura of the nerve root sheath and result in a dilated, arterialized coronal venous plexus.[23,24] Prior to angiography, this dilated vein was erroneously felt to be the site of pathology rather than the arteriovenous connection that is the true source of pathology. Surgical treatment consisted of stripping the veins, often with poor results.[25] With the recognition of the fistulous component of this lesion, surgical therapy has been directed at ligation of the abnormal arteriovenous connection and has led to significantly better outcomes.

Type II lesions, or glomus AVMs, are analogous to intracranial AVMs and consist of a tightly packed nidus of vessels over a short segment of the spinal cord. These lesions tend to manifest at an earlier age than the type I lesions and tend to occur at the cervicothoracic junction rather than at the thoracolumbar junction.[1,26] Like type I lesions they may be amenable to surgical excision. Type III lesions, or juvenile AVMs, arise in single or multiple adjacent somites and therefore are frequently both extradural and intradural and may involve soft tissue and bone in addition to the spinal cord and dura.[27,28] In the cord they form a diffuse nidus with normal spinal cord existing between loops of abnormal vessels. The embryologic term *metameric* was historically used in connection with these lesions because it connotes involvement of tissue derived from the entire somite.[15] Surgical cure of these metameric or type III lesions (juvenile AVMs) is difficult and often requires a multidisciplinary approach.

Shortly after the introduction of the type I to III classification an additional type IV lesion was proposed by Heros et al.[13] This lesion is a direct connection between an intradural artery and a vein in the subarachnoid space without a definable nidus. The lesions are frequently ventral and involve the anterior spinal artery. Surgical cure is possible when the lesions are small. Embolization may be a helpful adjuvant and may be palliative for the larger lesions.

The understanding and classification of spinal vascular malformations continue to evolve. Recently, a type V spinal AVM was proposed based on the observation that some type III AVMs are outside the spinal cord and dura and are therefore not truly metameric.[29] Their epidural location drastically changes the potential for treatment. Spetzler et al.,[30] in addition to their other nomenclature contributions, have proposed that juvenile AVMs of the conus medullaris be considered a separate category of spinal AVM because complex juvenile lesions at the level of the conus may have a more favorable prognosis with surgical resection.

With the advent of MRI, cavernous malformations of the spinal cord have been identified with increasing frequency.[1,7-9,16,31-53] Like their intracranial counterparts, they are sinusoidal venous channels that appear with stair-step neurologic decline from repeated hemorrhage. Some controversy exists over the indication for surgical resection of these lesions. Intradural spinal aneurysms are also being diagnosed with increasing frequency and may be traumatic, flow related from AVM feeding vessels, or rarely congenital such as an aneurysm of a posterior inferior cerebellar artery that has a spinal origin. These lesions appear with subarachnoid hemorrhage and may require direct surgical repair or endovascular vessel sacrifice.

Embryology and Vascular Anatomy

The fetal spinal vascular network develops in four stages.[54] The first, or *primitive segmental,* stage, occurs between weeks 2 and 3 of gestation. During this stage, 31 pairs of segmental vessels originate from paired dorsal aortas and grow toward the neural tube along the developing nerve roots. The segmental vessels divide into ventral and dorsal branches and form capillary networks on the ventrolateral surface of the neural tube. These networks ultimately develop into paired primitive ventral arterial tracts, the precursors of the anterior spinal artery. The anterior spinal artery develops when these paired ventral arterial tracts fuse during the third stage of development.

The second, or *initial,* stage occurs between weeks 3 and 6 of development and is significant for development of dorsal arterial anastomoses, separate and distinct from the ventral spinal vascular system. At this stage, longitudinal venous channels also develop on both the ventral and dorsal spinal cord surfaces. These venous channels eventually expand and give rise to an interconnected capillary network. It is within this second stage that maldevelopment theoretically leads to the genesis of vascular malformations that persist after birth and into adulthood.

The *transitional* stage is the third embryologic stage of spinal vascular development and occurs between the sixth week and fourth month of fetal growth. The major development in this stage is the formation of the adult pattern of vascular supply. The primitive ventral longitudinal arterial tracts fuse, and the number of segmental arteries supplying the spinal cord is reduced.[55] By 10 weeks' gestational age, adult patterns of superficial spinal cord vessels are present. The last stage, called the *terminal* stage, occurs after 4 months of development and is the phase of maturation and increased tortuosity of the major spinal cord vessels.

The most likely stage of embryologic development at which spinal vascular malformations can arise is the second stage (3–6 weeks). Maldevelopment in this stage leads to persistence of thin-walled tortuous vessels that exhibit primitive capillary interconnections, arteriovenous shunts, and poorly developed elastic and medial layers that closely resemble intracranial angiomas.[11] The concept that intradural vascular malformations are congenital and are the result of fetal vascular maldevelopment is supported by the fact that 20% of patients with intradural AVMs have other associated congenital vascular anomalies (Table 103-1). Furthermore, these malformations are present in younger patients and are distributed throughout the entire spinal axis. This favors a common dysembryogenic basis of intradural spinal and other vascular malformations.

In the adult, the anterior spinal artery arises from the fusion of a contribution from each of the vertebral arteries. It supplies the ventral two thirds of the spinal cord, including the lateral corticospinal tracts. It narrows as it descends but is reinforced by blood vessels at some segmental levels of the spinal column. At each segmental level a dorsal ramus of the intercostal artery enters the intervertebral foramen and gives rise to three branches: a dural branch, a radicular branch, and a medullary branch. The radicular and dural branches go to the nerve root and dura, respectively, and the medullary branch augments the flow to the anterior spinal artery. As mentioned, in fetal life during the third stage of vascular development most of the medullary branches involute, leaving the distal portion of the cord relatively ischemic. In the upper lumbar region at one segmental level the medullary artery does not involute and augments the supply of blood to the cord. This retained medullary vessel arises somewhere between T8 and L4, most often on the left, and is known as the *arteria radicularis magna,* or *artery of Adamkiewicz*. This still leaves a zone relatively vulnerable to ischemia in the upper thoracic region. The paired posterior spinal arteries run the length of the spine and supply the dorsal third of the spinal cord.

Venous drainage of the cord follows the arterial supply. Radial veins coalesce from the cord and anastomose to become the coronal venous plexus, a plexus of veins on the cord surface. At segmental levels, medullary veins leave the coronal plexus and exit the intervertebral foramen to join the epidural venous plexus. This epidural plexus communicates with the venous sinuses of the cranial dura and drains into ascending lumbar veins and the azygous venous system.

TABLE 103-1

Congenital Vascular Anomalies Associated with Intradural Spinal Arteriovenous Malformations

Congenital Anomaly	Reference
Brain arteriovenous malformation	Brion et al.[10]; Bruni et al.[33]; Di Chiro and Wener[18]; Hebold[17]; Jellinger et al.[91]
Cerebral aneurysm	Aminoff and Logue[4]; Djindjian[6]; Djindjian et al.[71]; Hebold[17]
Vascular agenesis	Hebold[17]
Rendu-Osler-Weber syndrome	Doppman et al.[21]; Hebold[17]
Klippel-Trénaunay-Weber syndrome	Cogen and Stein[68]; Hebold[17]; Heros et al.[78]
Soft tissue hemangiomas	Djindjian et al.[58]
Hemangioblastomas	Hall et al.[14]

Glomus Arteriovenous Malformations

Glomus, or type II, spinal AVMs are high-flow malformations in which a tightly packed malformation nidus is located within a short segment of the pia or the spinal cord parenchyma. They may occur anywhere along the longitudinal axis of the spinal cord, although some reports indicate a higher incidence of glomus AVMs in the cervicothoracic junction.[1,26] The feeding arteries of glomus AVMs usually arise from distinct medullary arteries and also supply the spinal cord.[56] The malformations are frequently found in the ventral aspect of the spinal cord and derive their blood supply from medullary branches of the anterior spinal artery. Venous drainage is through the coronal venous plexus, and, unlike dural (type I) AVMs, the venous drainage usually occurs in both a rostral and a caudal direction[57] (Fig. 103-1). With dural lesions, caudal venous drainage is extremely rare.

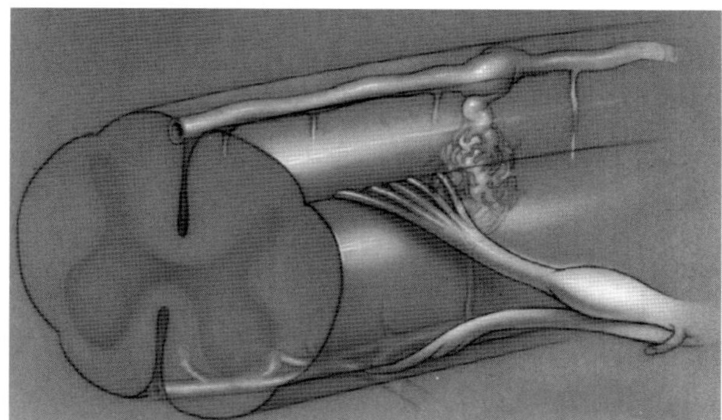

FIGURE 103-1. Spinal cord glomus arteriovenous malformation with arterial feeding from the anterior spinal artery and bidirectional venous drainage.

The clinical symptoms of glomus-type intramedullary AVMs is usually apoplectic in nature because of sudden hemorrhage from the malformation. These AVMs usually become symptomatic before adulthood and frequently appear with subarachnoid hemorrhage (SAH). Neurologic symptoms often involve the upper extremities, if the nidus is in or near the cervical portion of the spinal cord. By comparison, upper extremity involvement is exceedingly rare in the more commonly observed dural (type I) AVMs. There is no gender predilection for intradural AVMs, whereas at least 85% of spinal dural AVMs occur in males. SAH or intramedullary hemorrhage occurs in 50% of patients with intradural vascular malformations and is attributed to the frequently associated presence of arterial or venous aneurysms.[1,58,59] Of 54 patients with confirmed intradural spinal AVMs who were studied at the National Institute of Health, 30 patients (52%) had experienced SAH and 24 patients (44%) had aneurysms associated with either the draining or feeding vasculature.[59] SAH occurs as the initial symptom most commonly in glomus-type malformations, whereas weakness is most common in any other spinal vascular malformation.

At the time of diagnosis, most patients with intradural AVMs have some motor and sensory deficit. Spastic paraparesis and pain and temperature sensory deficits are the most frequent neurologic findings during onset.[59] A bruit heard over the affected dermatome may also be present. With intradural AVMs, specific neurologic symptoms reflect the location of the nidus along the longitudinal axis of the spinal cord. Strenuous activity or postural changes rarely exacerbate the symptoms of intradural glomus-type AVMs, although this is a common finding with dural type I lesions or juvenile (type III) spinal malformations.

The differential diagnosis encompasses numerous conditions that may mimic the symptoms of an intradural AVM. Because of the relatively rare incidence of intradural spinal vascular malformations, other diagnoses are more tenable. They include degenerative diseases, neoplasms, infections, trauma, demyelinating or neurodegenerative diseases, and developmental and acquired conditions. The apoplectic nature of spinal SAH, which occurs in at least one half of patients with intradural glomus AVMs, is the single distinguishing event that strongly implicates an intradural vascular malformation as the etiology.

Adequate and appropriate radiologic investigation is paramount for confirming the diagnosis of an intradural vascular malformation. Plain spine radiographs may be useful to rule out other pathology and have been found by some to be abnormal in patients with high-flow intradural AVMs. Rosenblum et al.[59] found that 15% of patients with intradural AVMs had widened interpeduncular distances on plain spine radiographs. No increase in spinal canal dimension was observed with type I dural lesions.

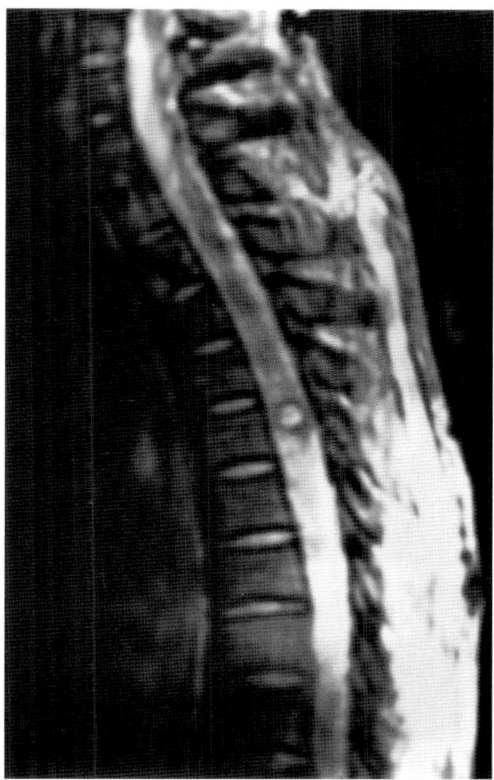

FIGURE 103-2. Sagittal MRI of glomus arteriovenous malformation.

Although total spine myelography was the radiologic test of choice for many years, most patients now undergo MRI as a screening test instead of myelography (Fig. 103-2). Although the sensitivity of myelography and CT for detecting a spinal AVM is high, the anatomic information is nonspecific.[60] Selective spinal angiography with high-resolution digital imaging remains the diagnostic test of choice to provide the most precise anatomic information (Fig. 103-3).

The indications for surgical resection of glomus, or type II, spinal AVMs are difficult to generalize because of the rarity of these lesions, the variability of symptoms, and their poorly understood natural history. Several authors have reported excellent results with surgical resection of glomus AVMs, although extrapolation of these results, obtained by highly specialized microvascular surgeons, to a general neurosurgical practice would be grossly misleading.[61] Rosenblum[59] reported a series of 43 patients who underwent surgery to resect intradural spinal malformations. In 22 patients (51%) the neurologic status was unchanged, 14 patients (33%) improved, and 6 patients (14%) were neurologically worse after surgery. In this series, residual malformation was detected in one third of the patients who underwent postoperative angiography.[59] This finding is extremely important if the natural history of intramedullary spinal AVMs parallels that of cranial AVMs, because partial resection

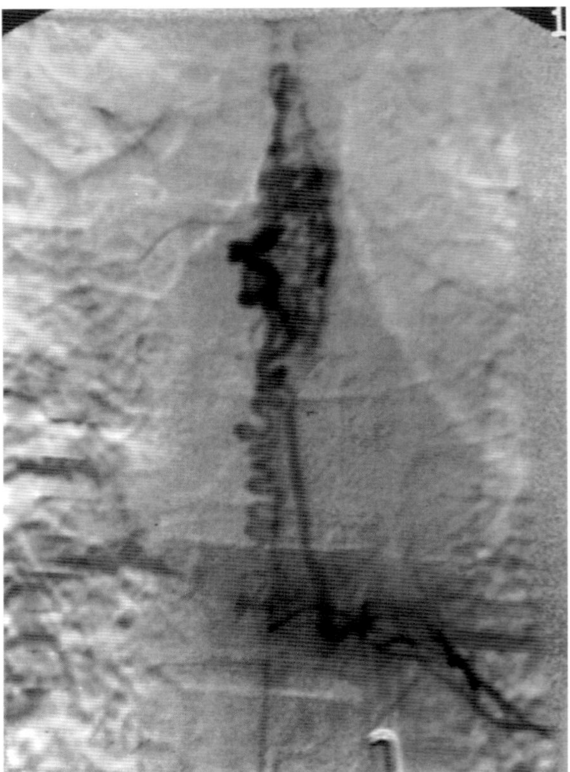

FIGURE 103-3. Anteroposterior spinal arteriogram of juvenile spinal arteriovenous malformation.

offers no benefit but poses a tremendous risk. A more recent series reported that 6 of 15 (40%) patients improved, 8 of 15 (53%) patients were stable, and 1 (7%) patient became worse after resection of a type II lesion.[62]

Favorable features for surgical resection of a glomus AVM include the radiographic appearance of a compact nidus located in an accessible portion of the spinal cord and an informed patient who understands the risks and the potential benefits of the procedure.[63] The operative procedure requires precise localization of the nidus and adequate exposure to minimize spinal cord manipulation. Use of the operative microscope and microsurgical technique is mandatory to minimize trauma to the spinal cord. Dissection is initially directed at the feeding vessels entering at the periphery of the lesion. The plane of dissection is deepened until the arterial supply has been eliminated and only venous drainage remains. The venous drainage is divided, and the nidus delivered out of the spinal cord. The presence of an intramedullary clot is helpful for defining the periphery of the nidus, although SAH hampers visualization. It is best not to attempt surgery in the period immediately after an acute spinal SAH; it should be delayed.

The embolization of type II spinal AVMs through endovascular techniques can be a useful adjunct to surgical resection. Preoperative embolization may reduce the blood flow and the number of vessels supplying the malformation and thus decreases the technical difficulty of surgical resection. The risk of embolization of glomus AVMs is the inadvertent occlusion of radiculomedullary afferent vessels supplying vital regions of the adjacent spinal cord parenchyma and potential worsening of the patient's neurologic status.[64] Embolization has been advocated as a sole treatment for these lesions in some cases[65] and has been shown to favorably alter the hemodynamics of the lesions.[66] The high tendency toward revascularization and the need for frequent repeat procedures are significant limitations of this strategy. Newer embolic agents such as the nonadhesive liquid agent Onyx may reduce the revascularization rate.[67]

Juvenile Arteriovenous Malformations

Juvenile, or type III, spinal AVMs are extremely rare, formidable lesions that constitute approximately 7% of all spinal AVMs.[68,69] These AVMs can be distinguished from glomus, or type II, malformations by several characteristics. Juvenile spinal AVMs are exceedingly rare, large, high-flow intramedullary AVMs. They usually have multiple feeding vessels over several spinal segments and often extend into and involve the epidural space, vertebrae, paravertebral musculature, and soft tissues[27,28] (see Fig. 103-3). Juvenile malformations may have integumentary representation with cutaneous extension of the AVM within the somites corresponding to the spinal level of involvement.[70] They are frequently located in the cervical or upper thoracic region and involve several spinal segments. The entire transverse area of the spinal cord is usually involved with malformation, and functional neural tissue is present within the interstices of the lesion (Fig. 103-4).

Subarachnoid, or intramedullary, hemorrhage is an uncommon occurrence in juvenile type III spinal AVMs.[59] The typical symptom is one of progressive neurologic deterioration that occurs during early adulthood or adolescence. Postural changes, Valsalva maneuver, and pregnancy have been reported to exacerbate the clinical symptoms.[4,46,71-73] There may be an overlying bruit if significant soft tissue involvement is present.[68]

Due to the extensive involvement of the spinal cord, type III spinal AVMs can only rarely be removed with acceptable morbidity.[18,19,69,74] Touho et al.[75] and Spetzler et al.[73] have reported cases of successful removal of juvenile spinal AVMs in patients who had a definable nidus within the spinal cord. Malis[69,74] described his experience in the treatment of spinal AVMs. He reported a series of 43 patients in which 3 underwent attempted surgical resection of type III malformations. In this series one patient died, one had no improvement of severe neurologic deficits, and one patient was left paraplegic after attempted surgical resection.[69,74] Ommaya et al.[22]

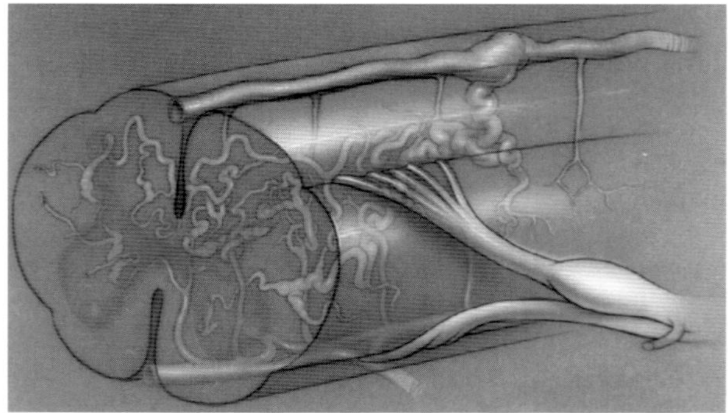

FIGURE 103-4. Spinal cord juvenile arteriovenous malformation with multiple arterial feeders and functional neutral tissue within the interstices of the lesion.

and Djindjian[6] have reported some success with arterial embolization as the sole treatment regimen. Hall et al.[14] reported delayed recanalization of spinal AVMs that had previously undergone complete angiographic embolization as the only treatment. Similarly, Bao and Ling[76] reported that 17 of 22 (75%) patients with a type III lesion, treated with embolization, required repeat embolization because of recanalization or clinical recurrence. Cyanoacrylate, a more permanent liquid embolic agent, may provide higher cure rates but is difficult to control.[76]

Intradural Arteriovenous Fistulas

True intradural or perimedullary AVFs are very rare, with only a few cases reported over the past decade.[77-80] Heros et al.[78] suggested classifying true intradural fistulas separately from previously described spinal AVMs and proposed referring to them as type IV spinal AVMs. Others have subsequently reported similar cases that could be classified as type IV spinal AVMs.[4,80] These lesions are direct AVFs that involve the normal arterial supply of the spinal cord and drain into the coronal venous plexus that often becomes dilated and aneurysmal. Of those cases reported in the United States, 10 of 14 patients had AVFs involving the anterior spinal artery, whereas 4 of the patients reported on by Tomlinson et al.[78,80] had posterior spinal artery supply of the fistula.

Three types of intradural extramedullary fistulas have been described based on radiographic appearance and intraoperative observations. The first type may be a simple connection between an elongated but normal-caliber, anterior spinal artery and the coronal venous plexus as described by Aminoff et al.[77] The second type consists of a dilated anterior spinal artery with a fistulous connection to a dilated aneurysmal venous system, similar to the case reported by Heros et al.[78] The third type consists of a large fistula from multiple arterial pedicles with rapid blood flow and a massively dilated system of draining veins.[13,81,82]

The etiology of intradural direct AVFs remains unclear, although a congenital etiology is a likely possibility. In the patients reported by Aminoff et al.[77] and Heros et al.,[78] the symptoms and history were inconsistent with fistulas of an acquired nature. Wakai et al.[82] have also reported a similar case in a 9-year-old child in whom an unusual intradural AVF was treated. This patient suffered two distinct SAHs separated by approximately 1 year. The patient underwent three negative cerebral arteriograms before an MRI was obtained that demonstrated a spinal intradural AVF. The typical symptoms are usually related to progressive neurologic deterioration rather than hemorrhage, although SAH can occur and may be a repetitive occurrence if the fistula remains undiagnosed and untreated. In patients with these rare lesions, symptoms of progressive myelopathy may be due to compressive mass effect from venous aneurysms, arterial vascular steal phenomenon, venous hypertension, or subacute intraparenchymal hemorrhage.

The diagnosis is usually confirmed with selective spinal angiography. Treatment is contingent on the precise localization and anatomic delineation of the fistula. Surgical interruption of the AVF is the definitive treatment when feasible. Because of the frequent involvement of the anterior spinal artery and the commonly ventral location of the fistulas, complex ventral spinal approaches are often necessary to adequately expose the fistula for resection.[78,83] When the arterial feeders are separated from the venous outflow, complete removal of the dilated venous structures is hazardous and usually unnecessary.

If the fistula is of giant proportions and the risks of surgical intervention are deemed too great, endovascular occlusion techniques may be considered. Hall et al.[14] reported six patients who were followed after complete embolization of spinal AVMs. Three patients underwent endovascular treatment of type I spinal AVFs, whereas three others underwent embolization of glomus malformations as the sole treatment modality. All but one patient developed recanalization of the malformation, and four of the six patients had symptomatic recurrence.[14] Definitive treatment of spinal intradural direct AVFs by endovascular techniques is feasible, but the long-term efficacy remains to be demonstrated. Furthermore, endovascular occlusion of feeding arteries in too proximal a location may result in delayed recruitment of collateral arterial channels, whereas extremely distal occlusion may compromise an already tenuous venous outflow and precipitate neurologic deterioration.[13,79] Endovascular treatment as the sole modality is perhaps most useful with giant AVFs and least appropriate for small fistulas of the first type.

Cavernous Angiomas

Spinal cavernous malformations are rare and represent 5% to 12% of all spinal vascular malformations.[40] Most spinal cavernous malformations arise within the vertebral bodies, although many reports of intradural and intramedullary cavernous malformations exist.[1,7-9,16,51-53] Cavernous angiomas occur throughout the nervous system. They are vascular malformations, pathologically composed of closely opposed, blood-filled spaces lined by a single layer of epithelium. The vessel walls of the malformation vary from thin capillary-sized vessels to thick, hyalinized vessels densely packed with collagen. Typically, there are no elastic fibers and no smooth muscle within the walls,[46] and the vessels of the cavernous malformations are arranged in a sinusoidal network without intervening neural tissue. The neural parenchyma surrounding these malformations is often gliotic and hemosiderin laden.[45,49] According to McCormick and Nofzinger,[45] spinal cavernous malformations are pathologically indistinguishable from cerebral cavernous malformations.

The clinical symptoms of patients with intradural spinal cavernous malformations usually include progressive paraparesis and sensory loss, along with pain. Symptoms may exist or progress over many years. In the pre-MRI era, diagnosis was difficult, and cavernous angioma was often confused with multiple sclerosis.[44,84] Symptoms appear most commonly during the fourth decade, although as many as 10% may occur in children.[85] Females account for 70% of patients diagnosed with spinal cavernous malformations.[34,46] These lesions may occur anywhere along the neuroaxis and occur with equal frequency in the cervical and thoracic cord. The average size at diagnosis is 17 mm and is similar to cranial cavernous malformations; no correlation between size and the incidence of hemorrhage has been shown.[86] Familial cavernous malformations account for 50% of all cases of CNS cavernous angiomas, and in these cases, genetic transmission is believed to be autosomal dominant.[16,87] Spontaneous development of new cavernomas has been documented in rare patients followed for existing lesions,[50] and patients with cavernous malformations of the spine have an increased risk of multiple neuroaxis cavernous malformations.[88]

Cavernous malformations produce symptoms through repetitive hemorrhages. Typically, hemorrhage is associated with small amounts of bleeding into the surrounding neural parenchyma. In rare cases of intradural extramedullary cavernomas, SAH has been reported.[31,33,38,48,51] In a literature review by Canavero et al.,[34] the risk of hemorrhage was estimated to be 1.6% per person-year of exposure. This is roughly two times the estimated annual risk of hemorrhage with cranial cavernous malformations. Pregnancy appears to statistically increase the risk of hemorrhage, as does a cervical location of the cavernoma.[34,52]

Before the availability of MRI, cavernous malformations of the spinal cord were difficult to visualize radiographically. Myelography is uniformly unreliable and may only reveal subtle widening of the spinal cord. CT may also demonstrate pathologic spinal cord widening or the presence of acute hemorrhage, calcifications, or a syrinx cavity. Angiography is uniformly negative and carries unnecessary risk because the diagnosis can be confirmed with MRI. MRI is the diagnostic procedure of choice for intradural cavernous malformations and is virtually 100% reliable. The appearance of spinal cavernous malformations on MRI is similar to that of cerebral lesions. There is typically mixed signal intensity on both T1- and T2-weighted images that variably enhance with gadolinium (Fig. 103-5). Regions of acute hemorrhage, edema, or hemosiderin deposition may be observed immediately surrounding these lesions. Hemosiderin deposition produces a ringlike region of decreased signal intensity on both T1- and T2-weighted images.[37]

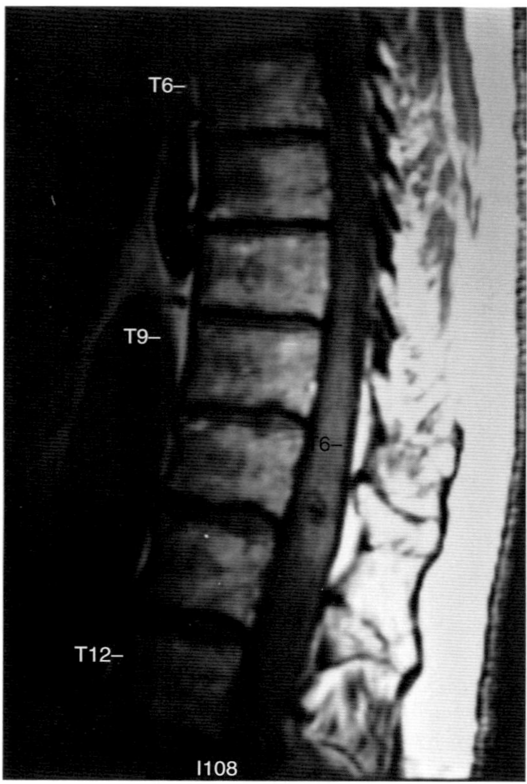

FIGURE 103-5. T1-weighted sagittal MRI of thoracic cavernous malformation.

Optimal treatment of a spinal cavernous malformation remains unclear. In the review of 57 patients by Canavero et al.,[34] the single most important factor relating to outcome was neurologic status at onset of symptoms. When neurologic status was poor, patients typically did poorly with surgical treatment. In their review, the age of the patient, site of the lesion, duration of the condition, and extent of removal had no significant effect on outcome. Because neurologic improvement is common after a bleeding episode, the reported improvement with surgical resection may be coincidental.

The goal of microsurgical removal of cavernous malformations is to prevent further hemorrhage and subsequent neurologic deterioration. Intraoperative ultrasonography is useful for precise intraoperative localization and for limiting the length of the myelotomy.[42] After exposure of the involved spinal cord, slight staining of the dorsal surface is often observed. A myelotomy is made over the region of staining, and microsurgical technique under high magnification is used to dissect the gliotic plane surrounding the lesion. Bleeding on the periphery of the malformation is usually due to low-flow, low-pressure vessels that are easily controlled with bipolar electrocoagulation. The resected lesions resemble small "berries" of vascular tissue similar to cerebral cavernous malformations. Preoperative treatment of patients with high-dose steroids and the use of intraoperative somatosensory evoked potentials may be useful to minimize the inherent morbidity of intramedullary spinal cord surgery.

Although some surgeons have reported good results with radiosurgery for occult vascular malformations of the brain, others have reported poor results and have pathologically confirmed posttreatment radiation necrosis when brainstem lesions have been treated with stereotactic radiosurgery.[89,90] Because of the lack of evidence of therapeutic benefit and the risk of radionecrosis, microsurgical resection, if clinically warranted, appears to be the only therapeutic treatment option. There is no apparent indication for radiosurgery in the treatment of spinal cavernous malformations.

KEY REFERENCES

Cogen P, Stein BM: Spinal cord arteriovenous malformations with significant intramedullary components. *J Neurosurg* 59:471, 1983.

Heros RC, Debrun GM, Ojemann RG, et al: Direct spinal arteriovenous fistula: a new type of spinal AVM. *J Neurosurg* 64:134, 1986.

Krayenbuhl H, Yasargil MG, McClintock HG: Treatment of spinal cord vascular malformations by surgical excision. *J Neurosurg* 30:427, 1969.

Oldfield EH, Doppman JL: Spinal arteriovenous malformations. *Clin Neurosurg* 34:161, 1986.

Spetzler RF, Detwiler PW, Riina HA, et al: Modified classification of spinal cord vascular lesions. *J Neurosurg* 96(Suppl 2):145, 2002.

REFERENCES

The complete reference list is available online at expertconsult.com.

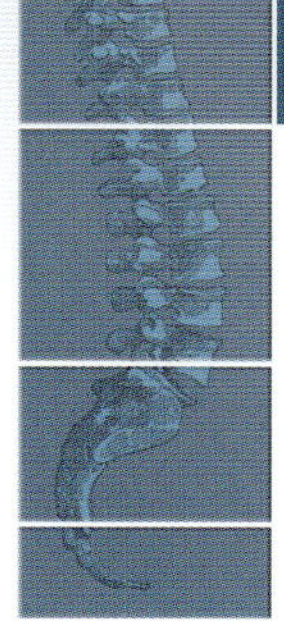

CHAPTER 104

Spinal Dural Vascular Malformations

H. Hunt Batjer | Tarun Bhalla | Alejandro Spiotta | Peter A. Rasmussen | Robert F. Spetzler

The most common type of spinal cord arteriovenous malformation (AVM) is the spinal-dural arteriovenous fistula (SDAVF), also known as a type I spinal AVM. First described by Gaupp[1] in 1888 as "hemorrhoids of the pia mater," spinal-dural AVMs have recently become better recognized and understood with the advent of modern superselective neuroangiography. As a distinct subtype of spinal AVMs, these lesions require specific treatments that differ from those for intradural or intraparenchymal vascular malformations. At present, these AVMs are best treated surgically, although endovascular techniques may play an increasing role in the future.

Spinal Vascular Anatomy

A comprehensive knowledge of the vascular anatomy of the spinal cord is necessary to understand the pathologic and clinical aspects of SDAVFs and their differentiation from other spinal AVMs. The spinal cord receives its blood supply from three separate longitudinal vessels: one anterior spinal artery and two posterior spinal arteries (Fig. 104-1).

The anterior spinal artery is formed by the convergence of branches from each of the distal intradural vertebral arteries and descends in the anterior median sulcus. Additional contributions are received from radiculomedullary arteries branching from the vertebral, ascending cervical, intercostal, and lumbar arteries. These arteries make a characteristic hairpin turn as they join with the anterior spinal artery. The largest of these is the artery of Adamkiewicz, or arteria radicularis magna. Usually arising from a lower intercostal artery on the left side, this vessel supplies the ventral two thirds of the thoracic spinal cord and conus medullaris. Another large radicular artery from the C5 or C6 level often predominates in the cervical region and is known as the artery of cervical enlargement. As they enter the dura mater at the level of the nerve root sleeve, the radiculomedullary arteries give off small branches that supply the dura. These are the vessels that form the enlarged arterial feeders to SDAVFs.

The posterior spinal arteries course along the dorsolateral aspect of the spinal cord behind the dorsal nerve roots. They also receive supply from radiculomedullary arteries. The two posterior spinal arteries supply the dorsal one third of the spinal cord, including the posterior columns and portions of the lateral columns of the spinal cord. They join with the distal anterior spinal artery at the end of the conus medullaris to form the cruciate anastomosis.

The venous drainage of the spinal cord is via small radial veins that run from the center to the periphery of the cord and into the coronal venous plexus that ascends and descends along its dorsal surface. These surface veins converge to form medullary veins that exit at the root sleeve. The coronal veins along the dorsal spinal cord surface become dilated and tortuous in patients with SDAVFs, often

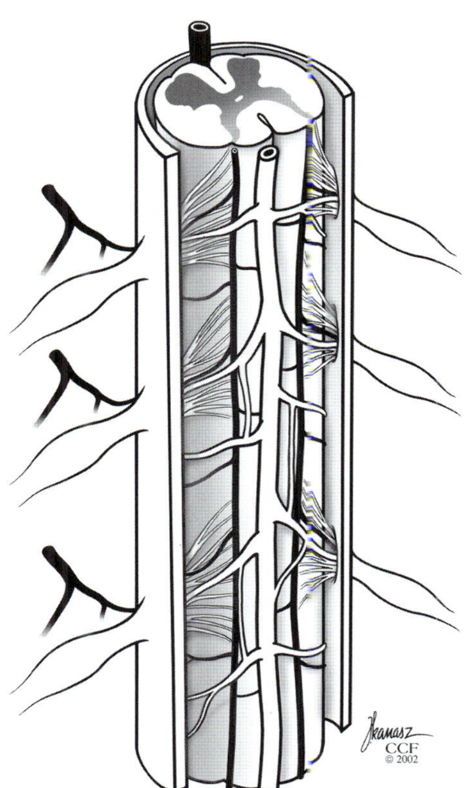

FIGURE 104-1. Normal vascular anatomy of the spinal cord. The radiculomedullary artery enters the dura at the root sleeve, supplying the anterior and posterior spinal arteries. (Copyright Cleveland Clinic Foundation.)

forming a convoluted vascular mass along the dorsal aspect of the spinal cord.

Classification

Although this chapter addresses only SDAVFs, the classification system for spinal AVMs should be understood to appreciate the differences between these lesions and other types of AVMs. Recognizing and properly categorizing spinal AVFs, particularly distinguishing between dural and intramedullary lesions, is important for treatment decisions. Historically, spinal-dural AVMs were first referred to as *angioma racemosum venosum* by Wyburn-Mason[2] in his 1943 monograph. This was later shortened to just angioma racemosum by Bergstrand et al.[3] and Krayenbuhl et al.[4] Malis[5] later referred to them as *long dorsal AVMs*. Currently, *dural AVF* or *type I spinal AVM* is the most appropriate term.[6,7]

Type II spinal AVMs, also known as *glomus AVMs*, represent intramedullary AVMs with a true compact nidus.[2,5] Type III spinal AVMs are also known as *juvenile AVMs* and are much less common. They are larger, more extensive lesions that often involve intramedullary, extramedullary, and extradural spaces over more than one spinal level.[5,8] Last, type IV AVMs are intradural extramedullary AVFs that were first described by Djindjian et al.[9] and later classified as type IV lesions by Heros et al.[10] Unlike type I dural AVFs that arise from dural branches, these lesions are fed from the anterior spinal artery or, less commonly, from the posterior spinal artery. They flow directly into an enlarged venous outflow tract, lie outside the spinal cord and its pia mater, and vary in size and flow.[11]

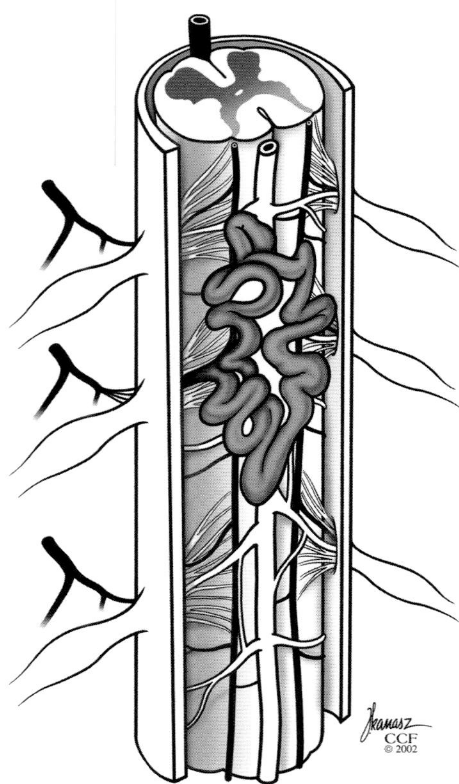

FIGURE 104-2. Spinal dural arteriovenous fistula. The nidus is located in the dura mater at the root sleeve, at which it is usually supplied by a single arterial feeder and at which it drains into an enlarged intradural (medullary) vein running to the dorsal venous plexus. (Copyright Cleveland Clinic Foundation.)

Pathophysiology

It is important to understand that the clinical signs and symptoms develop because of venous hypertension of the spinal cord. The fact that the patient has a small AVM of the dura is inconsequential. What is of utmost importance, however, is that the venous outflow of this AVM is into the coronal venous plexus of the spinal cord. This leads to venous congestion of the plexus, stagnation of arterial flow through the spinal cord, decreased perfusion pressure, ischemia, and edema formation.

It is easiest to think of SDAVFs as consisting of two relevant compartments: a vascular malformation (AVM) nidus located in the spinal dura and the medullary vein and coronal venous plexus draining the AVM. Usually, a single radiculomedullary artery enters the dural root dorsolaterally at the dural root sleeve. This artery supplies an AVM that is typically embedded within the dura mater around the proximal nerve root sleeve and/or adjacent spinal dura (Fig. 104-2). The venous outflow of the AVM is then via retrograde flow through a medullary vein that has anastomosis with the coronal venous plexus. This medullary vein and coronal venous plexus is obvious on the superselective spinal angiogram. This medullary vein and coronal venous plexus are normal but dilated from the flow through the AVM lying in the dural wall.

The radiculomedullary arterial feeder tends to be separate from the branch that normally penetrates the dura to supply the anterior or posterior spinal arteries. Occasionally, however, a single vessel supplies both the malformation and the anterior spinal artery.

Although most SDAVFs have a single arterial feeder, some may have two arterial feeders that enter at separate levels.[5,12] The additional feeders appear to travel within the dura mater to the fistula nidus located in the wall of the dura, where they converge and communicate with the intradural efferent medullary vein. No valves are present within the radial veins or coronal plexus and, therefore, the increased pressure is transmitted to the spinal cord parenchyma. It is critical to recognize the additional feeding branches when these are present, because failure to obliterate all inflow channels can lead to recurrence of the AVF.[13]

On angiography, the nidus appears as a small area of fine vessels near the neuroforamen. From there, outflow of the fistula passes intradurally through the medullary vein and then into the dorsal venous plexus along the spinal cord surface. This plexus becomes dilated and tortuous because of the arterialized venous pressure and may extend over the full length of the cervical, thoracic, and lumbar spine.

Clinical Characteristics

Most patients with type I dural AVFs are between the ages of 40 and 70, with few showing symptoms before age 30. Over 80% of patients are male, and no familial tendency has been identified.[14,15] This differs from types II and III spinal AVMs, which typically appear in patients younger than age 40 and have less male predominance. This age discrepancy suggests that type I lesions may be acquired rather than congenital.

The typical pattern of symptoms and clinical course was first described by Aminoff and Logue,[16,17] and this description has been supported by other more recent reports.[13-15,18] The most common symptom associated with dural AVFs is pain, which may be local, radicular, or nonspecific. Most patients also experience leg weakness and sensory changes by the time of diagnosis.[14,15] Spastic paraparesis, along with loss of pain and temperature sensation, is the most common neurologic pattern. Most patients have a distinct sensory level corresponding to the level of the vascular nidus. Disturbances of bladder, bowel, and sexual function are less common initially but become more frequent over time.

Most patients experience a gradual onset of symptoms and a slowly progressive clinical deterioration.[16,17] Only 10% to 15% of patients experience an acute onset of symptoms, in contrast to patients with types II and III AVMs that lead to an acute onset of symptoms in more than 50% of patients. The progressive neurologic deterioration occurring with these lesions was first documented by Aminoff and Logue.[17] At 6 months after onset of symptoms, only 56% of patients had unrestricted activity, and 19% were severely disabled. At 3 years after onset, only 9% had no restrictions, and 50% were severely disabled.

Because of the infrequency and gradual course of SDAVFs, symptoms are often present long before the diagnosis of SDAVF is made. In the series of 55 patients studied by Symon et al., only 33% were diagnosed within 1 year of symptom onset, and 66% were not diagnosed for more than 3 years.[15] In fact, given the large amount of edema found on T2-weighted MRI, many patients will have undergone spinal cord biopsy in search of a tumor prior to proper diagnosis. On rare occasions, onset of symptoms can be acute, caused by thrombosis within the draining medullary veins. This produces a catastrophic, acute necrotizing myelitis that is often referred to as Foix-Alajouanine syndrome.[19] Subarachnoid hemorrhage (SAH) is extremely uncommon with SDAVMs.[14,15] In contrast, other types of spinal AVMs, particularly type II lesions, have a significant incidence of SAH.

Exercise and certain postures can exacerbate symptoms in patients with dural AVMs.[14-16] Because almost all dural AVMs have rostrally directed venous outflow, the greater venous hydrostatic pressure in the upright position may explain why symptoms worsen with standing.[20] Types II and III AVMs, which have both rostral and caudal venous drainage, do not produce symptoms that change with position. Worsening symptoms have also been associated with physical activity, probably because of increased draining venous pressure during systemic hypertension.[21]

The key to making a timely diagnosis of an SDAVF lies with a physician being aware of this condition and having a high clinical suspicion for the presence of this lesion.

Radiologic Evaluation

Since the first diagnosis of spinal AVM was made by myelography in 1927,[20] most patients have undergone myelography as part of their radiologic evaluation. Although the typical findings of tortuous channels outlined by intrathecal contrast are almost pathognomonic for spinal AVM, in recent years myelography has largely been replaced by MRI as the initial imaging study.[22] Irregular, serpentine flow void signals suggest vessels can often be seen along the dorsal surface of the spinal cord (Fig. 104-3). MRI can also differentiate type I from type II and type III lesions, and it is the test of choice for visualizing spinal cord cavernous malformations. Moreover, T2-weighted MRI images often suggest extensive edema of the cord.[23,24]

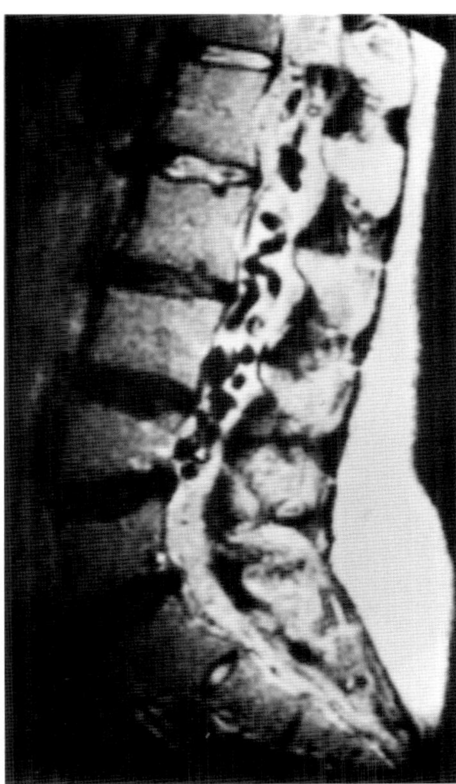

FIGURE 104-3. MR showing the typical serpiginous flow void within the canal, suggesting the presence of a type I dural arteriovenous fistula.

The definitive radiologic study for SDAVFs is selective spinal angiography. Aortography may demonstrate the general location of the AVM; however, this large-volume contrast injection may limit the extent of the superselective injections available because of contrast load reasons. Generally, bilateral selective injections of radiculomedullary branches are performed in both anteroposterior and lateral views to demonstrate the precise location, extension, hemodynamic characteristics, and venous drainage of the lesion. Multiple levels above and below the nidus must be studied to identify any additional feeding vessels. It is also essential to visualize the anterior spinal artery above and below the AVM to determine whether it has a supply in common with the AVM. Although this is a rare configuration with dural AVFs, it is a critical factor in planning treatment. Most dural AVFs are located along the dorsal aspect of the spinal cord, although 15% of patients may have dilated veins ventral to the spinal cord, and almost all of these lesions are found in the midthoracic to lower thoracic or thoracolumbar region.[5,14,15] This distribution differs from that of other types of spinal AVMs, which occur throughout the length of the spinal cord. If there is high clinical and radiographic suspicion of the presence of an SDAVF, selective angiography is not complete until all

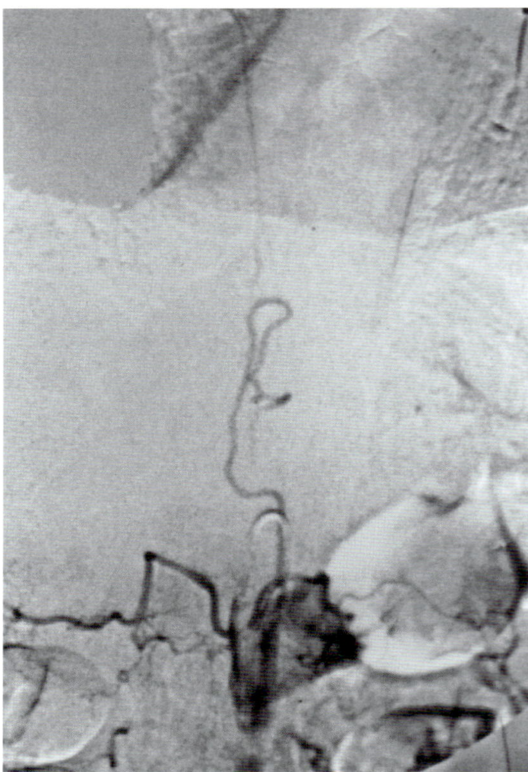

FIGURE 104-4. Spinal angiogram showing the characteristic appearance of a spinal dural arteriovenous malformation. The feeding vessel goes into the cluster of small vessels at the nidus in the root sleeve dura, which then drains into the dilated dorsal coronal venous plexus.

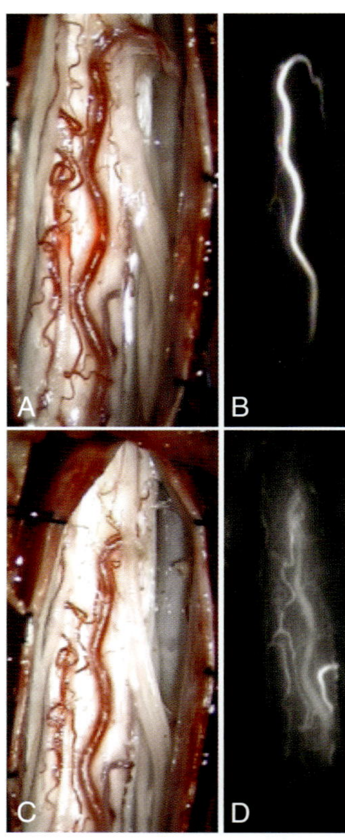

FIGURE 104-5. A, Intraoperative photograph of a spinal dural arteriovenous fistula. The intradural vein is seen entering from the dura and communicating with the enlarged dorsal venous plexus. The fistulous connection is identified by direct visualization and by indocyanine green (ICG) angiography (**B**). **C,** Following surgical obliteration, the arterialized vein shrinks in size and no longer displays early arterial phase on ICG angiography (**D**).

possible vessels that may contribute to the spinal vasculature have been imaged. This includes vertebral, external carotid, and sacral arteries. Occasionally, before this can be accomplished, the maximum volume of contrast that the patient's kidneys can safely tolerate is reached. Therefore, scheduling the spinal angiogram over 2 days' time enables completion of the examination.

Characteristically, the radiculomedullary feeding vessel is observed to disperse into a cluster of small abnormal vessels within or adjacent to the dura inside the neural foramen (Figs. 104-4 and 104-5). The transition from artery to vein, representing the AVF itself, is usually observed at the medial margin of this cluster. When additional feeders are present, they usually run within the dura to the level of the fistula. Flow is then seen progressively throughout the dilated dorsal venous plexus that typically extends for three to five spinal segments, but occasionally, dilated veins are seen extending over the full length of the cervical, thoracic, and lumbar regions. The blood flow is slow through the intradural veins, and 16 to 20 seconds is often required for contrast to clear.[13] Associated arterial or venous aneurysms are extremely uncommon with dural AVFs, in contrast to intramedullary lesions.

Venous drainage from dural AVFs is typically in a rostral direction,[14] unlike that from intramedullary AVFs, which drain both rostrally and caudally. It has been suggested that this rostral drainage of dural AVFs, along with their occurrence in the lower spine, is additional evidence for an acquired etiology of dural AVFs.[14] The pattern of venous drainage through anatomically normal, but dilated, venous channels, despite increased hydrostatic pressure, supports theories that a diminished, rather than an increased, venous outflow may be associated with the formation of dural AVFs. Congenital malformations would be expected to occur along the entire spinal axis, as seen with intramedullary AVMs.

Complete neuroradiologic evaluation of these lesions allows for planning accurate surgical and possible endovascular treatment.

Endovascular Treatment

Embolization of SDAVFs has been reported, most commonly with cyanoacrylate "glue" or with polyvinyl alcohol (PVA) particles.[18,22,25-27] Because the spinal arteries do not participate in the dural fistula, these lesions are potentially well suited for endovascular treatment, with minimal risk to the normal spinal cord.

The goal of endovascular treatment is the same as that for surgery, namely, to interrupt the fistula itself, including the distal feeding vessel and, most importantly, the proximal efferent intradural arterialized vein.[28] Because most patients improve after obliteration of the fistula, thus making excision of the venous plexus unnecessary, several authors[27,29,30] have recommended embolization as the initial treatment of choice.

The most important factor that determines the feasibility of embolizing a dural AVF is the normal supply to the spinal cord. An anterior spinal artery supplied by the same arterial feeder as the AVF is a relative contraindication to embolization.[26,31] Inability to selectively catheterize the radiculomedullary artery because of its size or configuration is another contraindication. The second most important factor that determines the feasibility of embolization is the durability of the embolic agents. Previous reports concerning the use of PVA suggest a high rate of recurrence within only a few months of treatment.[1,26] Experience with the use of PVA would indicate that this material is not a permanent embolic agent. Cyanoacrylate glues such as *n*-butyl cyanoacrylate (NBCA) are likely to be more permanent.

In addition to treatment failure, the complications of endovascular treatment include direct clinical or neurologic deterioration. Neurologic deterioration after embolization is usually due to inadvertent occlusion of feeding arteries to the normal spinal cord because of an unrecognized connection, improper placement or dislodgement of the catheter, improper particle size, or failure to discontinue embolization when the fistula is occluded.[26,31,32] With dural AVFs, the greatest risk of deterioration is from occlusion of the venous drainage at a site considerably distal from the fistula.[33] This would occlude normal venous drainage of the spinal cord. Distal occlusion can aggravate venous hypertension, impede normal blood flow through the spinal cord, and potentially cause enlargement or rupture of the AVF.

Several large series of patients, in which surgical and endovascular treatments were compared, showed comparable clinical results with the two approaches.[22,26,27] Failures included a number of patients in whom the dural AVF could not be successfully obliterated initially, patients in whom interruption of the fistula had failed at a later stage, and one patient who became paraplegic after the cyanoacrylate embolus migrated into the distal veins.[22,26,27,34]

Late recanalization after initial obliteration with PVA particles is a well-recognized phenomenon.[18,22,25,35] Of 17 patients with these lesions reported from the Mayo clinic, 14 underwent embolization with PVA particles or microfibrillary collagen.[18] Although initial obliteration of the AVM was accomplished in all but one patient, delayed follow-up angiography demonstrated recanalization in 13 of the 15 patients studied, with the average time for recanalization being only 5 months. Similar results have been reported from the National Institutes of Health in two of three patients[25] and by Djindjian et al.,[35] who found recanalization in 10 of 12 patients. PVA is not an adequate embolization material for the sole treatment of these lesions and should be used only for preoperative embolization of lesions that will then be treated surgically. Recanalization is less common after embolization with cyanoacrylate glue.[34] However, the distal extent of embolization with glue is more difficult to regulate because of its polymerization characteristics, making complications from normal venous obstruction more likely. In addition, microcatheters have been glued in place with the use of cyanoacrylates. Because of the greater risk of complications with glue and the high rate of recanalization with particulate embolization, direct surgical treatment is generally considered preferable in suitable patients.

As newer liquid embolic agents, such as Onyx, with better material properties become available, the role of endovascular treatment of these lesions holds significant promise[36,37] for future therapy.

Surgical Treatment

Although Krause[38] performed the first surgical exposure of a spinal AVM in 1910, the first successful surgical treatment of an SDAVF, at the T9 sensory level, was reported by Elsberg[39] in 1916 in a patient with paraparesis. He ligated and excised a large "vein" that traversed the dura adjacent to the T8 nerve root and the patient made a complete neurologic recovery. A number of subsequent reports, however, described poor results,[3,40,41] and it was not until the advent of modern neuroangiography, which allowed preoperative evaluation of these lesions, that therapy improved.[4,42]

For many years the standard surgical treatment for dural AVFs included stripping the enlarged venous plexus from the dorsal spinal cord.[5,42,43] It subsequently become clear, however, that this extensive resection is unnecessary and, also, potentially dangerous. Obliteration of the AVF alone is sufficient to eliminate the AVM in the dural sleeve. Surgery is much safer without resection of the dorsal veins, because manipulation of the spinal cord is minimized, risk to normal vessels is diminished, and the operation is shortened. In addition to complicating the surgery, resection of the dorsal vessels may injure the spinal cord by interrupting its normal venous drainage because the radial veins have no anastomotic system within the spinal cord parenchyma.[13]

The authors' approach to type I spinal AVFs is to obliterate the dural fistula surgically by interrupting the arterialized medullary vein without resection of the enlarged dorsal veins. The surgical technique is as follows: Patients are positioned on a Wilson frame, a Jackson table, or chest rolls, and the appropriate level is verified by radiology. A standard approach to the dorsal spinal elements is performed. A laminectomy is performed using a high-speed air drill. Alternatively, a one-piece laminectomy may be performed as in a laminoplasty.

Once the laminectomy is completed, the operating microscope is used. The dural surface is carefully examined for evidence of the nidus, although it is often located too far laterally to be seen easily. After meticulous hemostasis is achieved, the dura is opened longitudinally, with care being taken to leave the underlying arachnoid intact. The dura mater is retracted laterally using #4-0 sutures. The arachnoid is then opened separately under the microscope. After dividing the small arachnoid adhesions to the spinal cord, it is held up to the dural edges with small hemoclips. The intradural arterialized vein is located, the preoperative angiogram serving as a guide.

An emerging adjunctive method for delineating intraoperative vascular anatomy is indocyanine green (ICG) angiography. Employing this method, the operating field is illuminated by near-infrared excitation light and ICG is injected intravenously. The intravenous fluorescence is imaged instantly with a video camera integrated into the microscope, allowing differentiation between arterial, capillary, and venous phases (see Figs. 104-5A and B). Recently, its use has been reported in the surgical treatment of cerebral arteriovenous malformations,[44] the resection of tumors encasing the extracranial vertebral artery,[45] and during surgical obliteration of SDAVF.[46-48]

After identification, the offending vessel is carefully dissected free from surrounding tissues and the arachnoid. This should be done with sharp dissection with microscissors.

It is best to avoid blunt dissection, which can tear small vessels from the radial spinal cord veins and cause bleeding and impaired venous drainage. After the intradural arterialized vein is freed, it is coagulated with bipolar cautery and divided. Alternatively, a temporary aneurysm clip can be applied to the vessel, and observation of the coronal venous plexus for a color change to a more purplish hue may provide the surgeon with reassurance prior to definitive occlusion. At this point, the inner dural surface should be carefully inspected and coagulated. Care should be taken to identify and interrupt any other feeding vessels running in or under the dura from adjacent levels. When the nidus and efferent vein have been obliterated, the large dorsal veins should have decreased turgor and flow. The surgeon should allow several minutes for direct inspection because the venous plexus can remain arterialized for 5 to 10 minutes as a result of the sluggish venous outflow. Microvascular Doppler imaging can be of assistance if insonation is performed before and after venous interruption. ICG angiography can be obtained a second time to verify the eradication of AV shunting at this time (see Figs. 104-5C and D). If the veins do not become blue and soft after 5 to 10 minutes, additional feeders should be sought and interrupted. There is no need to resect or strip the dorsal venous plexus from the dorsal surface of the spinal cord. Attempting this only causes bleeding and interferes with normal venous drainage of the spinal cord and may lead to venous infarction.

Once the dural fistula has been completely obliterated, the arachnoid is let down from its dural clips but not sutured. The dura is closed with a running suture (#4-0 to #6-0) in a watertight fashion. The lamina segment may be replaced, usually being reattached with #2-0 sutures or craniotomy plates. It is brought laterally to abut the bone on one side to improve refusion. Instrumentation and fusion are rarely indicated. The wound is then closed in the usual fashion. A drain is not routinely placed.

All patients undergo postoperative spinal angiography, usually the day after surgery, which includes selective bilateral angiography of the spinal level involved and of two levels above and below the lesion. If residual flow through the AVF is present, reoperation is performed. With this basic approach, good surgical results were achieved in 24 patients with SDAVFs.[12] Of the 24 patients, 17 improved, 6 remained unchanged, and 1 worsened slightly.

Similarly, good results after obliteration of the dural AVF alone have been reported by others (Table 104-1). One of the largest series was reported by Symon et al.,[15] who operated on 50 of 55 patients with dural AVFs. Through a limited laminectomy, this group identified the communication between the AVM and the dorsal venous plexus. If the nidus was accessible on the dura, it was coagulated or excised. If the nidus was separated from the coronal plexus by several levels, it was left undisturbed, and the intradural arterialized vein was interrupted. Improvement after surgery was related mainly to preoperative disability, with 65% of patients with severe preoperative disabilities and 80% of moderately disabled patients showing improvement. The authors[15] stressed that attempts to resect the coronal venous plexus are unnecessary and potentially damaging. Although previously considered a factor, spinal cord compression by these enlarged veins is improbable. Furthermore, because obliteration of the fistula causes collapse of the veins, resection to "decompress" the spinal cord is not a reasonable indication.

Rosenblum et al.[14] reported surgical results in 27 patients with spinal-dural AVMs and 54 patients with intradural AVMs. After surgical obliteration of the AVF, 72% of patients improved and 28% stabilized, in comparison with surgical results in 43 patients treated for intramedullary AVMs, in which 33% improved, 51% remained unchanged, and 14% worsened. Outcome after surgery did not correlate with the presence or degree of preoperative sensory loss or with the rate of neurologic deterioration. There was a direct correlation, however, between preoperative and postoperative motor function.

Similarly, good results were described by Oldfield et al.[13] in five patients treated by coagulating and excising the cluster of abnormal vessels at the nidus and by dividing the intradural arterialized vein. In all patients, neurologic function improved progressively within days of surgery.

Summary

Although SDAVFs are rare lesions, it is important to recognize and treat them appropriately. If left untreated, they almost invariably cause progressive neurologic deterioration, with paraparesis, sensory symptoms, and urinary disturbances, as well as pain. Unlike intradural spinal AVMs, these lesions usually appear in men older than age 40, have a gradual onset of symptoms that is often affected by activity, and usually localize to the lower half of the spinal column. Spinal cord dysfunction is produced by venous hypertension and not by compression or vascular steal as once thought.

TABLE 104-1

Reported Results of Surgical Series of Fistula Obliteration for Spinal Dural Arteriovenous Fistulas

Reference	Year	No. of Patients with Surgery	No. of Patients Improved	No. of Patients Stabilized	No. of Patients Worsened
Ommaya et al.[49]	1969	9	5	4	0
Oldfield et al.[13]	1983	5	4	1	0
Symon et al.[15]	1984	46	32	?	?
Rosenblum et al.[14]	1987	27	19	7	0
Mourier et al.[22]	1989	20	10	9	1
Anson and Spetzler[28]	1994	24	17	6	1
Totals		131	87	27	2

After initial diagnosis by MRI or myelography, selective spinal angiography is critical for precise characterization of the number and nature of the arterial feeders, as well as of the intradural draining vein. Although endovascular treatment can be of short-term effectiveness, at present it carries greater risk and has a poorer outcome than does surgery. Surgical treatment should be aimed at complete obliteration of the dural nidus and intradural efferent draining vein, without resection of the enlarged dorsal venous plexus. With appropriate surgical treatment, the outcome in patients who are not already severely disabled is excellent, and risk is minimal.

KEY REFERENCES

Aminoff MJ, Logue V: Clinical features of spinal vascular malformation. *Brain* 97:197–210, 1974.

Aminoff MJ, Logue V: The prognosis of patients with spinal vascular malformations. *Brain* 97:211–218, 1974.

Djindjian M, Djindjian R, Rey A, et al: Intradural extramedullary spinal arteriovenous malformations fed by the anterior spinal artery. *Surg Neurol* 8:85–93, 1977.

Djindjian R, Merland JJ, Djindjian M, et al: Embolization in the treatment of medullary arteriovenous malformations in 38 cases (In French). *Neuroradiology* 16:428–429, 1978.

Heros RC, Debrun GM, Ojemann RG, et al: Direct spinal arteriovenous fistula: a new type of spinal AVM. Case report. *J Neurosurg* 64:134–139, 1986.

Hettige S, Walsh D: Indocyanine green video-angiography as an aid to surgical treatment of spinal dural arteriovenous fistulae. *Acta Neurochir (Wien)* 152:533–536, 2010.

Masaryk TJ, Ross JS, Modic MT, et al: Radiculomeningeal vascular malformations of the spine: MR imaging. *Radiology* 164:845–849, 1987.

Oldfield EH, Di Chiro G, Quindlen EA, et al: Successful treatment of a group of spinal cord arteriovenous malformations by interruption of dural fistula. *J Neurosurg* 59:1019–1030, 1983.

Warakaulle DR, Aviv RI, Niemann D, et al: Embolisation of spinal dural arteriovenous fistulae with Onyx. *Neuroradiology* 45(2):110–112, 2003.

REFERENCES

The complete reference list is available online at expertconsult.com.

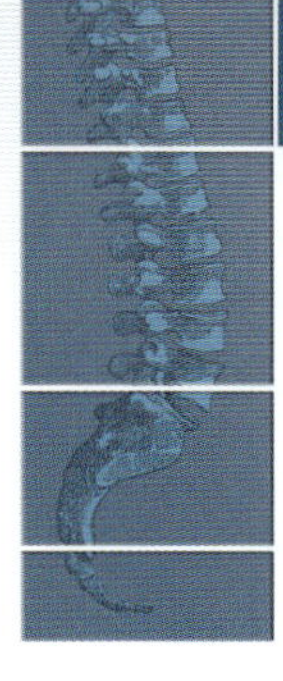

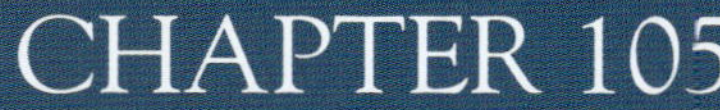

CHAPTER 105

Cauda Equina Syndrome

Michael G. Fehlings | Seth M. Zeidman | Neilank Jha | Y. Raja Rampersaud

Cauda equina syndrome (CES) is a complex of symptoms and signs, including low back pain, unilateral or bilateral radiculopathy, lower extremity motor weakness, sensory disturbance including saddle anesthesia, and loss of visceral function (i.e., bladder and bowel incompetence ranging from frequency to bladder and anal sphincter paralysis, and erectile dysfunction), that results from either acute or chronic cauda equina compression (Box 105-1). This syndrome is characterized by a variable clinical presentation that depends on the anatomic location (lumbar, sacral, or coccygeal/focal central or complete compression), rapidity, and duration of compression of the cauda equina. Motor weakness involving the lumbar, sacral, and coccygeal roots in isolation or in combination is often present. Hypesthesia or anesthesia is often present in the dermatomal distribution of L3 to Coc1, inclusive. Radicular signs and symptoms may be either unilateral or bilateral. Bowel or bladder dysfunction is common and is the source of the hallmark signs and symptoms of CES. The knee and ankle jerk may be absent. There are typically no upper motor neuron findings, and the Babinski sign is absent. CES, particularly if unrecognized and untreated, often results in paraplegia, severe paraparesis, permanent bladder and bowel incontinence, or sexual dysfunction.

Pathophysiology

Spinal nerve root compression commonly occurs in conditions such as acute herniated disc, spinal stenosis, trauma (e.g., burst fractures), metastatic or primary tumors of the spine, or spinal infections (e.g., epidural abscess) (Box 105-2). Acute CES most commonly presents secondary to lumbosacral intervertebral disc prolapse (Fig. 105-1). However, the pathophysiology of the symptoms and signs related to spinal nerve root compression remains poorly defined.

Several experimental studies have assessed the pathophysiologic mechanism of CES. Delamarter et al.[1,2] developed an animal model of CES, subjecting 30 beagle dogs to L6-7 laminectomy and cauda equina compression. Neurologic recovery was assessed in animals undergoing 75% constriction of the cauda equina followed by immediate, early, or delayed decompression. The first group was constricted and immediately decompressed. The remaining groups were constricted for 1 hour, 6 hours, 24 hours, and 1 week, respectively, before being decompressed. Evoked potentials were measured before and after surgery, before and after decompression, and 6 weeks after decompression. Six weeks after decompression, all dogs were killed, and the neural elements were analyzed histologically. After compression, all 30 dogs had significant lower extremity weakness, tail paralysis, and urinary incontinence. All dogs recovered significant motor function by 6 weeks after decompression. The dogs with immediate decompression typically recovered neurologic function within 2 to 5 days. The dogs receiving 1- and 6-hour compression recovered within 5 to 7 days. Dogs receiving 24 hours of compression remained paraparetic for 5 to 7 days, with bladder dysfunction persisting for 7 to 10 days and tail dysfunction for up to 4 weeks. The dogs with compression for 1 week were paraparetic and incontinent during the duration of cauda equina compression. They recovered the ability to walk by 1 week and regained bladder and tail control by the time of euthanasia. Immediately after

BOX 105-1. Clinical Features of Cauda Equina Syndrome

- Low back pain
- Unilateral or bilateral radiculopathy
- Motor weakness of the lower extremities
- Sensory disturbance including saddle anesthesia
- Loss of visceral function (i.e., bladder and bowel incontinence)

BOX 105-2. Causes of Cauda Equina Syndrome

- Disc herniation
- Trauma
- Spinal stenosis
- Tumors: primary and secondary
- Infection
- Arteriovenous malformation
- Hemorrhage (subarachnoid, subdural, epidural)
- Ankylosing spondylitis
- Iatrogenic causes
- Continuous spinal anesthesia
- Postsurgery
- Postintradiscal therapy
- Postchiropractic manipulation

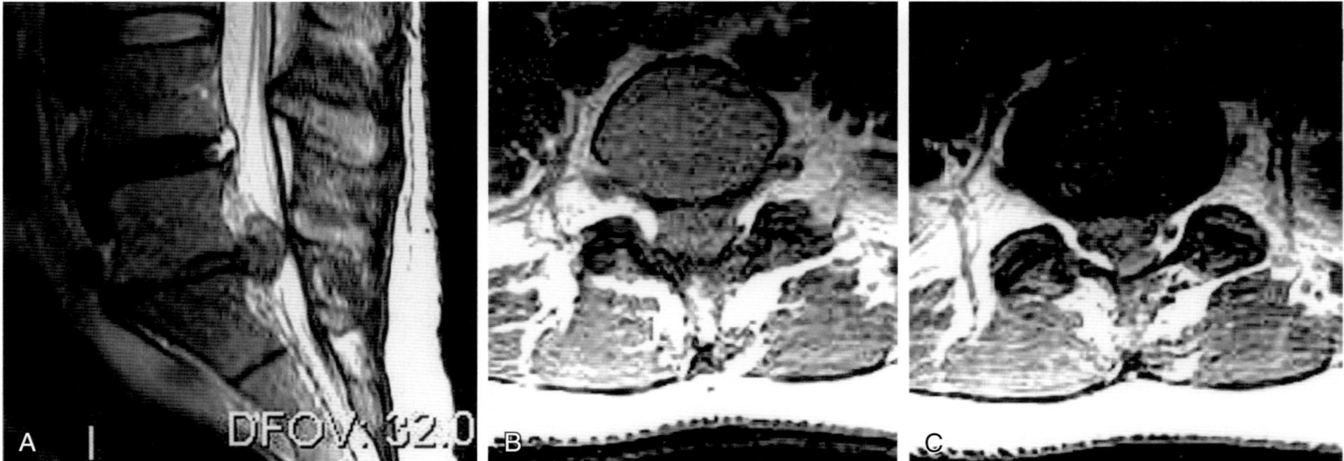

FIGURE 105-1. Thirty-year-old woman with acute cauda equina syndrome secondary to a large herniated disc at the L5-S1 level. The patient's initial symptoms included urinary retention (postvoid residual = 200 mL), saddle anesthesia, and S1 motor-sensory radiculopathy. **A,** T2-weighted midsagittal MRI. **B,** Axial MRI demonstrating complete occlusion of the spinal canal at L5-S1. **C,** Axial MRI caudal to area of maximal compression (**B**) demonstrating displacement of the S1 roots and compression of the central sacral roots. Patient underwent urgent surgical (<24 hours of bladder symptoms) decompression with complete recovery of bladder function, sensation, and radiculopathy.

compression, all five groups demonstrated at least 50% deterioration of the posterior tibial evoked potential amplitudes.[2] Delamarter et al.[2] demonstrated axoplasmic flow blockade and wallerian degeneration of the motor nerve roots distal to the constriction and of the sensory roots proximal to the site of constriction, as well as dorsal column degeneration. Severe arterial narrowing occurred at the level of the constriction with venous congestion of the roots and dorsal root ganglia of the seventh lumbar and first sacral nerves.[1] Evoked potentials were the most sensitive predictor of neural compression, revealing neurologic abnormalities before the appearance of neurologic signs and symptoms.[1] Cystometrograms were not sensitive until severe compression was achieved. Bladder dysfunction was correlated with axoplasmic flow blockade and early sensory changes during neurovenous congestion.

Olmarker et al.[3-7] developed an experimental model of acute, graded compression of the cauda equina in pigs that accurately mimics the neural and vascular anatomy of the human cauda equina. There were structural and vascular differences between spinal nerve roots and peripheral nerves that could contribute to differences in compression susceptibility between these two parts of the nervous system. Pressure transmission from the balloon to the nerve roots permitted determination of occlusion pressures for the arterioles, capillaries, and venules of the cauda equina.[7] Arteriolar blood flow ceased when the applied pressure approached the mean arterial blood pressure. Capillary blood flow was dependent on flow in connected venules, and the blood flow in some venules ceased at 5 to 10 mm Hg despite venous occlusion pressures ranging from 5 to 60 mm Hg. Compression up to 200 mm Hg for 2 hours did not induce a no-reflow phenomenon upon compression release. However, transient hyperemia was noted at all pressure-time relations studied, indicating nutritional deficit in the compressed segment during compression. Signs of edema were observed in nerve roots exposed to compression for 2 hours at either 50 or 200 mm Hg. The nutritional supply to the cauda equina was impaired at low pressure levels (<10 mm Hg).[4,5] Thus diffusion from adjacent tissues with a better nutritional supply, including the cerebrospinal fluid, could not compensate completely for compression-induced effects on the transport of nutrients. However, a certain nutritional supply to the compressed segment was present even at 200 mm Hg compression. A rapid compression rate resulted in more pronounced effects on the nutritional supply than did a slow compression rate. Nutritional impairment was observed both within and outside the compressed nerve segment. An increase in vascular permeability was induced by compression at 50 mm Hg for 2 minutes.[6] The magnitude of this permeability increase was dependent on both the magnitude and the duration of compression. The permeability increase was more pronounced for the rapid compression onset rate than for the slow compression onset rate at all pressure-time relations studied. Reduction of muscle action-potential amplitude in tail muscles, after stimulation cranial to the compression zone, was induced by compression at 100 and 200 mm Hg for 2 hours.[4,6]

Pedowitz et al.[8] and Rydevik et al.[9,10] presented an experimental model of compression-induced functional changes of the porcine cauda equina that permits electrophysiologic investigation of the neurophysiologic changes induced by nerve root deformation. In several studies, they compared the effects of various pressures and durations of acute compression on spinal nerve root conduction in the pig cauda equina. Changes in both afferent (compound nerve action potentials) and efferent (compound motor action potentials) conduction were induced at an acute pressure threshold of 50 to 75 mm Hg. Higher compression pressures produced a differential recovery in afferent and efferent conduction.[9,10] Efferent conduction and afferent conduction were monitored during compression for 2 or 4 hours with compression pressures of 0 (sham treatment), 50, 100, or 200 mm Hg. Recovery was monitored for 1.5 hours. No significant deficits in spinal nerve root conduction were observed with 0 or 50 mm Hg compression, whereas significant deficits were induced by 100 and 200 mm Hg compression. Variance analysis demonstrated significant effects of compression pressure and duration on conduction, with a significant difference between efferent and afferent conduction at the end of the recovery period, suggesting a synergistic interaction between biomechanical and microvascular mechanisms in the production of nerve root conduction deficits.[8]

Compression of the spinal nerve roots often occurs at multiple levels simultaneously; however, the basic pathophysiology of multilevel compression is poorly defined. Using a thermal diffusion technique, Takahashi et al.[11] quantitated intraneural blood flow in the uncompressed segment between two compressive balloons in the porcine cauda equina. At 10 mm Hg compression, there was a 64% reduction of total blood flow in the uncompressed segment compared with precompression values. Total ischemia occurred at pressures 10 to 20 mm Hg less than the mean arterial blood pressure. After two-level compression at 200 mm Hg for 10 minutes, there was a gradual recovery of the intraneural blood flow toward the baseline. Recovery was less rapid and less complete after 2 hours of compression. Double-level compression of the cauda equina induced blood flow impairment, not only at the sites of compression but also in the intermediate nerve segments located between two compression sites, even at very low pressures.

Cauda Equina Syndrome Secondary to Disc Herniation

Epidemiology

CES secondary to a large central disc herniation is a relatively uncommon entity, but its clinical importance far exceeds its rarity (see Fig. 105-1). CES secondary to lumbar disc herniation is an absolute indication for surgical intervention.[12]

The incidence of CES has been estimated to range from 1.2% to 6%. In 1970, Raaf[13] reported an incidence of 2% in 624 patients with protruded discs. In 1972, Spangfort[14] reported a 1.2% incidence in 2504 cases, and his review of the literature found a total incidence of approximately 2.4%. In 1986, Kostuik et al.[15] reported a 2.2% incidence of CES in patients admitted for lumbar laminectomy. In 1990, Gleave and MacFarlane[16] reported cauda equina paralysis secondary to lumbar disc prolapse in 3.2% of cases; this probably overestimated the true incidence because they did not consider nonoperatively treated patients.

Clinical Syndrome

CES can mimic the typical presentation of a lumbar intervertebral disc herniation with low back pain and unilateral radiculopathy. However, back and perianal pain often predominates, and radicular symptoms may be minimal. Severe back pain, often out of proportion with the radicular pain, should alert the physician to a possible CES lesion and mandates periodic evaluation to exclude a progressive neurologic deficit. Accurate diagnosis may be delayed if the lesion is incomplete or evolving. CES often presents with abnormal radicular signs and normal or upper motor neuron lesion activity, but it can present as a lower motor neuron lesion.

Clinical presentation varies depending on the level and location of the disc herniation. For example, a large central disc herniation can compress several or all of the traversing cauda equina roots. A disc at L2-3 with complete compression may present with motor-sensory disturbance from L3 (+L2) to S5. An L5-S1 disc may cause CES without motor or sensory loss in the lower extremities. This scenario happens when the herniation is focally central and compresses the lower centrally located sacral nerve roots, serving bowel and bladder function, but leaves the S1 roots unaffected. If slowly progressive, large central disc herniations can also mimic the presentation of an intraspinal tumor.

When compromised, the centrally placed sacral fibers to the lower abdominal/pelvic viscera produce the symptoms characterizing cauda equina compression. Initial leg pain may be followed by foot numbness and difficulty with ambulation. Sensory deficits are common and often involve the lower sacral roots. Perianal numbness, saddle dysesthesia or anesthesia, and a loss of the anal reflex or diminished rectal tone characterize the syndrome. Difficulty with urination, including either frequency or retention with overflow incontinence, can develop relatively early in the clinical course. The onset of bladder and rectal paralysis with saddle anesthesia should be viewed with a high index of suspicion in any patient with backache and sciatica. In men, a recent history of impotence can often be elicited. This should be clarified as to whether the impotence is pain mediated or neurologically (unable to obtain an erection) mediated.

Some reports contend that bilateral sciatica is a necessary component of CES, but a number of large series refute this notion. In a review of 31 patients by Kostuik et al.[15] in 1986, sciatica was bilateral in 14 patients and unilateral in 17. Severe saddle anesthesia was indicative of a poor prognosis, particularly for return of bladder and bowel function.[15] However, any correlation of factors such as severity of somatic signs and symptoms, symptom duration before surgical decompression, and the size and location of disc protrusion with recovery of bowel and bladder function was unclear. In a review of 58 patients by Doman et al. in 2009, urinary retention of more than 500 mL alone or in combination with two or more of the following symptoms—bilateral sciatica, urinary retention, or rectal incontinence—were the most important predictors of MRI-confirmed cauda compressions.[17]

Clinical Course

Tay and Chacha[18] reported eight cases observed over a 5-year period that fell into three clinical groups. The first group of patients noted sudden onset of symptoms without previous back problems. The second group noted recurrent episodes of backache and sciatica, with the most recent episode resulting in cauda equina involvement. The final group of patients had slowly evolving backache and sciatica that progressed to cauda equina paralysis. Disc prolapse occurred between the L5 and S1 vertebrae in 50% of the patients, most of whom had no limitation in straight-leg raising. Urgent myelography and disc removal within 2 weeks of symptom onset resulted in substantial recovery of motor and bladder function within 5 months after surgery. Sensory and sexual function recovery was incomplete for as long as 4 years postoperatively.[18] Patients at the preclinical and early stages have better functional recovery than patients in later stages after surgical decompression.[19]

Choudhury and Taylor[20] reported on 42 patients with lumbar disc disease and herniation who presented with CES. Simple disc herniation accounted for the syndrome in only five cases. Associated structural lesions were noted in the remaining 37 cases, and operative manipulation and trauma during disc removal through an interlaminar approach was reported in two patients.[20]

Lafuente et al.[21] noted sacral sparing and preservation of sphincter control in 8 of 14 cases of cauda equina compression from central lumbar disc herniation and postulated that the triangular shape of the lumbar spinal canal may be one factor for this constellation of findings, because the increase in linear strain on the stretched roots of the cauda equina is least in the more centrally placed lower sacral roots. Kostuik et al.[15] identified two distinct modes of presentation. The first was an acute mode (in 10 patients) in which there was an abrupt onset of severe symptoms and signs and a slightly poorer prognosis after decompression, especially for the return of bladder function. The second mode of presentation (in 21 patients) had a more protracted onset, characterized by prior symptoms for varying time intervals before the gradual onset of CES. All patients reported preoperative urinary retention. Bladder function was the most seriously affected function preoperatively and remained so postoperatively. The prognosis for return of motor function was good. Of 30 patients receiving surgery, 27 regained normal motor function.[15]

Diagnostic Imaging

Diagnosis and treatment are often delayed because of lack of recognition of the condition and failure to appreciate the surgical imperative for its treatment. Once cauda equina compression is recognized or suspected, MRI is the investigation method of choice. If an MRI is contraindicated, of poor quality because of motion artifact (patients with CES are often in severe pain), or unavailable, CT-myelography is recommended. CT alone can be misleading in cases of complete canal occlusion (Fig. 105-2).

Surgical Therapy

Urgent surgical intervention should commence after diagnosis. Choudhury and Taylor[20] advocated wide laminectomy with excision of the overhanging facet joints and adequate visualization of the lumbar nerve roots. This yielded good or excellent results in 95% of patients and fair results in the remainder. No postoperative spinal instability or significant morbidity was reported.[20]

A routine microdiscectomy interlaminar approach necessitates retraction on already severely compromised nerve roots. Furthermore, because of the extent of compression, these roots often have no available canal space; thus, retraction not only increases traction but also may cause direct compression (against the disc or the overlying lamina). For the same reason, the use of large punches with a thick foot plate is also not recommended (compresses underlying roots against the herniated disc) (Fig. 105-3). Consequently, the authors advocate a wide bilateral decompression (laminectomy and medial third facetectomy). To avoid iatrogenic compression of the cauda equina, the surgeon can perform the laminectomy using a high-speed bur to thin out the lamina and then curettes and small punches lateral to the area of maximal compression to release the medial portion of the lamina (see Fig. 105-3). Once the lamina is released, it can be safely lifted away from the cauda equina. The decompression should be adequate enough to allow access lateral to the thecal sac and traversing roots at the level of the affected disc space and/or the sequestered fragment. The surgeon should carefully perform retrieval of the herniated fragment to avoid creating a further mass effect and therefore increased traction on the less mobile central sacral roots. This can be accomplished by performing a lateral anulotomy and discectomy and then pushing the central fragment back into the disc space with a reverse-angle curette. If the fragment is sequestered, it should be manipulated in a lateral direction using a nerve hook or angled curette and then retrieved. Before closure, the surgeon should confirm adequate decompression.

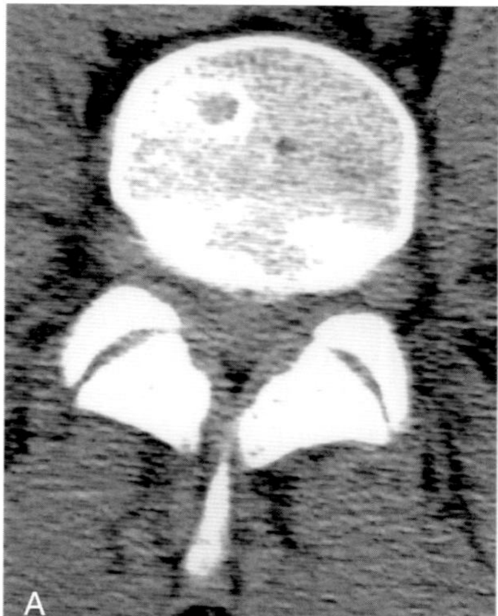

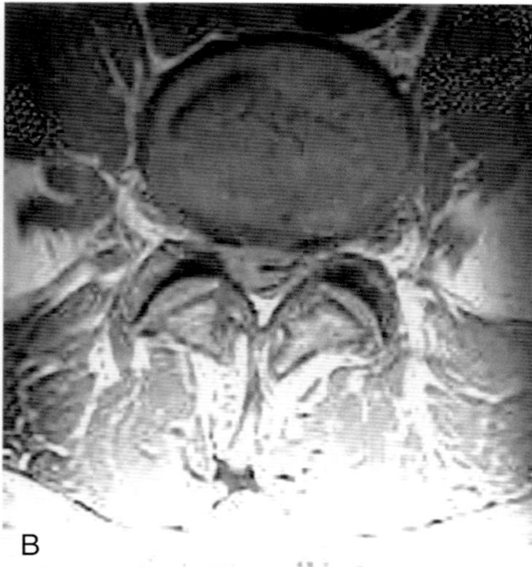

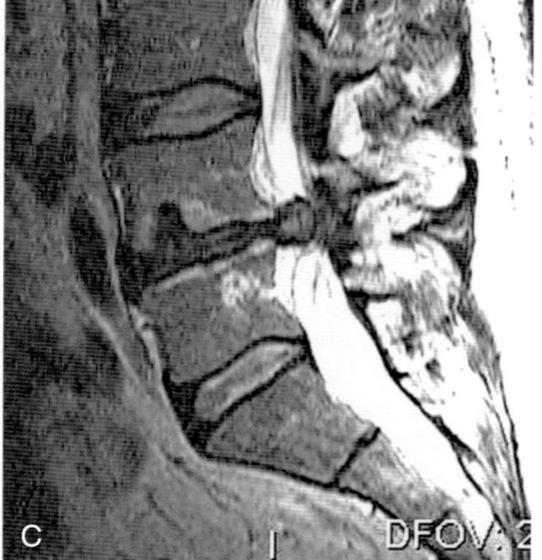

FIGURE 105-2. A, Axial CT at L4-5 of a 43-year-old male patient with right L5 radiculopathy and abnormal perineal sensation. Axial (**B**) and sagittal (**C**) MRIs of the same patient. As can be seen, the contrasting effect of epidural fat or cerebrospinal fluid in CT can be lost because of massive disc herniations causing near or complete occlusion of the spinal canal. This patient's CT was interpreted as equivocal for an L4-5 disc herniation. Consequently, MRI and CT-myelography are the imaging modalities of choice for the evaluation of cauda equina syndrome.

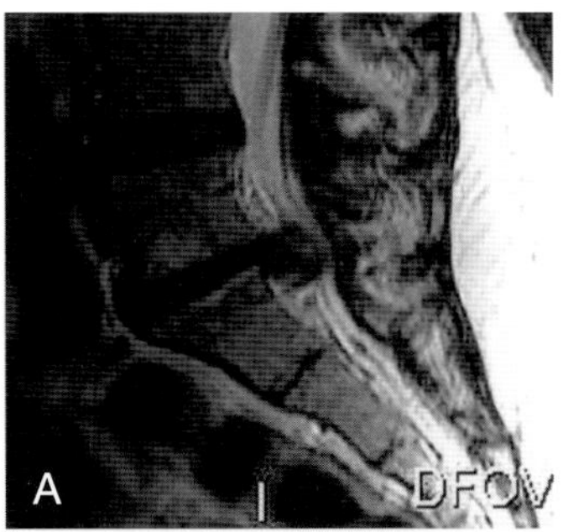

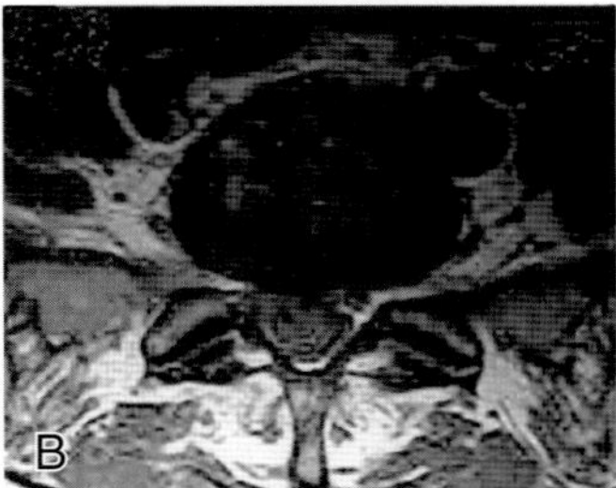

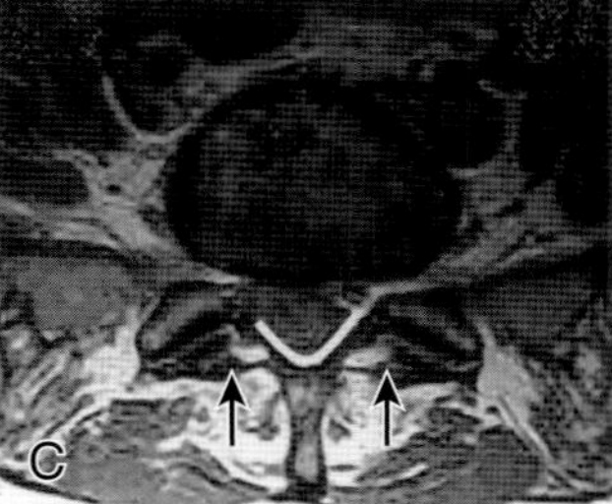

FIGURE 105-3. Sagittal (**A**) and L5-S1 axial (**B**) MRIs of a 45-year-old woman with cauda equina syndrome demonstrating severe compression of the cauda equina. **C,** The cauda equina (*outlined in white*) is draped over the disc and compressed between the disc and lamina. Removal of the lamina (medial to the *black arrows*) by sublaminar placement of standard spinal punches (see text) would obviously cause further compression of the roots. Wide bilateral laminectomy is required to gain safe access to the disc. Following appropriate decompression of the cauda equina, care must be taken when retrieving large disc fragments to avoid excessive traction or mass effect on the tented traversing nerve roots.

Timing of Surgical Intervention

Controversy persists regarding the definition, cause, diagnosis, and timing of surgical intervention for CES resulting from lumbar disc herniation. Conventional wisdom has been that early detection of CES is essential to maximize the probability of neurologic recovery after decompressive laminectomy and discectomy.[22] Some investigators have gone so far as to advocate the necessity for decompression within 6 hours of presentation.[23] However, data supporting immediate intervention are far from clear.

Kostuik et al.[15] reported 31 patients with CES secondary to a central disc lesion. The average time to surgical decompression after initial presentation ranged from 1.1 days for the group with more acute lesions to 3.3 days for the second group. There was no correlation between these times and return of function. The authors recommended early surgery but noted that decompression did not have to be immediate.[15]

Shapiro[24] studied 14 patients with acute CES from herniated lumbar discs who all presented with bilateral sciatica and leg weakness; 93% had bladder or bowel dysfunction. All patients were emergently studied with CT, myelography, or MRI. Nine patients had large or massive herniations, and five had smaller herniations superimposed on preexisting stenoses. The time to surgery ranged from less than 24 hours to more than 30 days. Postoperatively, six patients (43%) were normal, four patients (28.5%) had chronic pain and numbness, and four patients (28.5%) had persistent incontinence and weakness. Of the 10 patients without postoperative incontinence, 7 underwent surgery within 48 hours of onset. Of the four patients with persistent incontinence, all underwent surgery 48 hours or more after presentation.[24]

The onset of bladder paralysis is an important indicator for urgent surgery. Dinning and Schaeffer[25] reported a significant difference in the outcome of patients operated on within 24 hours of bladder paralysis compared with those operated on after this period. Thus it would appear that urgent decompression is superior to delayed surgery with regard to the recovery of neurologic function, but the necessity to perform immediate surgery (within 6 hours of presentation) is less clear. Hussain et al.[26] recently reported on 20 patients with CES from herniated lumbar disc. Nine patients underwent emergent decompression (<5 hours from time of presentation to the surgical unit), and the remainder had their surgery the next day but within 24 hours. At a mean of 16 months follow-up, there was no difference in urologic or quality of life outcome between the emergent and delayed groups.[26] Qureshi and Sell conducted a prospective longitudinal inception cohort study of 33 patients undergoing surgery for CES. They reported a significantly better outcome in patients who were continent of urine at presentation compared with those who were incontinent.[27]

Cauda Equina Syndrome Resulting from Intradural Disc Rupture

There is a strong association between the presence of intradural disc rupture and the development of CES. Dinning and Schaeffer[25] reported that intradural sequestration of disc fragments occurs in 7.5% of cases, although in most other series the rate is less than 1%. Spangfort[14] detected no differences in age or sex distribution. Lower lumbar discs were the most commonly affected levels; however, there was a significantly larger number of high lumbar herniations leading to this problem than to other disc syndromes. Myelography typically demonstrates complete block, and at surgery, intradural fragments of sequestrated disc material can be found (Fig. 105-4). Intradural exploration or transdural sequestrectomy avoids traction on already compromised nerve roots and is often safer than extradural sequestrectomy.

Cauda Equina Syndrome Secondary to Trauma

Patients with sacral fracture or dislocation and CES have been reported. Schnaid et al.[28] reported CES complicating acute lumbosacral fracture or dislocation 3 weeks postinjury. Isolated transverse sacral fractures are rare, but extensive neurologic deficits may accompany these injuries. Extradural hemorrhage can accompany these fractures and produce a serious neurologic deficit requiring urgent sacral laminectomy.[29]

Hilibrand et al.[30] reported CES associated with acute spondylolytic spondylolisthesis after major trauma. The deformity progressed from grade III to grade V (spondyloptosis), and the patient developed CES. The patient was treated with dorsal reduction and arthrodesis followed by an anterior arthrodesis, and the neurologic deficits resolved. Although

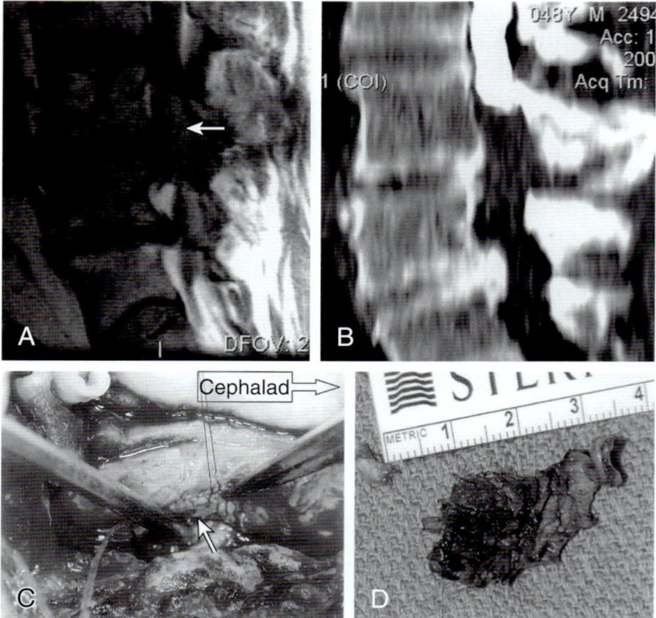

FIGURE 105-4. Patient is a 48-year-old man who presented with a 2-week history of severe low back pain and 24-hour history of progressive frank cauda equina syndrome with complete loss of erectile, bladder, and bowel function, as well as right bilateral L4-S1 leg weakness. He had undergone a right L3-4 microdiscectomy 2 years previously. **A,** T1-weighted sagittal MRI demonstrating intradural disc herniation (*arrow*). Because of uncontrollable pain, the patient was unable to lie flat for the rest of the MRI and underwent a CT-myelogram in the lateral decubitus position. **B,** Sagittal reformatted CT demonstrating complete myelographic block at the rostral aspect of the L3 vertebral body. Patient underwent urgent (<12 hours from presentation to emergency) surgical decompression. **C,** Intraoperative picture demonstrating wide decompression, release of previous epidural scar, and small defect (5 mm) in the dura. The defect was enlarged, and a massive intradural sequestered disc fragment (*white arrow*) was removed (**D**). At 2 years follow-up, the patient has some residual right L5 weakness; a functional bladder with normal postvoid residuals; good, but not normal, bowel function; and incomplete erectile dysfunction that has responded to medical management.

minor or repetitive trauma is often associated with spondylolysis, high-energy trauma may produce a more severe form of spondylolysis with spondylolisthesis. These deformities are more unstable, with instability similar to that of a fracture-dislocation, and they have a greater propensity to progress than does the usual form of spondylolytic spondylolisthesis.[30]

Dorsal dural lacerations associated with lumbar burst fractures can occur and are produced by dural impaction within a fractured lamina. Neural elements can be extruded outside the dura mater and be trapped in a lamina fracture. Preoperative appreciation of this diagnosis is imperative and is based on clinical presentation, fracture pattern, and radiographic findings. Denis and Burkus[31] recommended extraction of entrapped neural elements from the fractured lamina by laminoplasty of the dorsal neural arch. Neurologically impaired patients with lumbar burst fractures and radiographic evidence of dorsal displacement of the neural elements in the lamina fracture should undergo dorsal exploration of the spinal canal, extraction of cauda equina neural elements, and repair of the dural laceration before any spinal reduction maneuver is attempted.[31]

Intradural lumbar arachnoid diverticulas are rare but can cause mild compression of the cauda equina and produce debilitating symptoms. A chronic posttraumatic lumbar intradural arachnoid cyst causing CES has been reported.[32]

Cauda Equina Syndrome Secondary to Primary or Secondary Neoplasms

Primary extradural or intradural tumors may rarely present with acute CES.[23] For example, myxopapillary ependymomas of the conus or filum may present acutely with subarachnoid hemorrhage and cauda equina dysfunction.[33,34] There are reported cases of paraganglioma of the cauda equina causing compression requiring urgent treatment.[35]

Metastatic tumors to the lumbosacral spine can create CES by one of two means: (1) cauda equina compression by epidural tumor or (2) vertebral instability resulting in canal compromise and subsequent cauda equina compression (Fig. 105-5). The most common clinical manifestation is pain with or without concomitant nerve root signs. Regardless of the cause, the major goal of treatment is prompt decompression of the neural elements with stabilization or, at a minimum, avoidance of destabilization of the spine.

Indications for surgical intervention in patients with CES secondary to metastatic tumors include unknown tumor with rapid compression, previous irradiation precluding further radiotherapy, radioresistant tumor, neurologic deterioration during radiotherapy, and pathologic fracture/instability producing neural compression.

Spiegelmann et al.[36] reported a patient with acute myelogenous leukemia with CES as the presenting symptom. Staff et al. reported two patients with metastatic lobular breast adenocarcinoma presenting as CES.[37] There have been eight reported cases in the literature of intradural spinal metastasis from renal cell carcinoma causing CES.[38] Woo et al.[39] reported 97 Chinese patients with multiple myeloma, of whom 23.7% had cauda equina or spinal cord compression. Predictive features for spinal cord compression include paraprotein type, hemoglobin level, and extent of bone lesion at

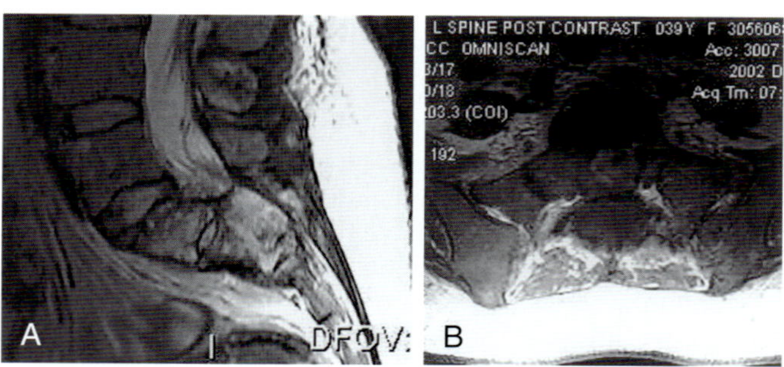

FIGURE 105-5. Sagittal (**A**) and L5-S1 axial (**B**) MRIs of a 39-year-old woman with low back pain and urinary incontinence. She had no leg symptoms. MRI demonstrated multiple spinal metastases of unknown origin with complete compression of the sacral cauda equina by tumor extending posterior from the body of S2. Patient underwent urgent surgical decompression and postoperative palliative radiation. She had rapid resolution of her pain, but at 6-month follow-up, she still required in-and-out catheterization. Her tumor is an adenocarcinoma, but extensive investigations have not identified the origin.

initial hematologic diagnosis. They concluded that vertebral cortex involvement predisposes the patient to spinal cord compression.[39] Rarely, patients with gynecologic tumors may present with acute CES.[23]There have been two reported cases of CES due to leptomeningeal carcinomatosis of the ovary.[40]

Cauda Equina Syndrome Secondary to Ankylosing Spondylitis

CES may occur as a neurologic complication of long-standing ankylosing spondylitis. The syndrome is uncommon, and its pathophysiology is poorly defined. There are several case reports of slowly progressive CES in patients with long-standing ankylosing spondylitis, with loss of lower spinal motor and sensory root function. The pathogenesis of CES in ankylosing spondylitis may be demyelination, postirradiation ischemia, or compression from spinal arachnoiditis, or it may arise in association with massive dural ectasia.[41-43]

Symmetrical neurologic deficits typically progress slowly and occur late in the evolution of spondylitis, long after the onset of the condition and well after the rheumatologic symptoms have abated. The initial symptom is typically disturbance of sphincter control with subsequent changes in ankle reflexes and cutaneous sensation, particularly in the sacral dermatomes. Variable lower nerve root involvement has been reported. Typical findings include cutaneous sensory impairment of the lower limbs and perineum with sphincter disturbances. Motor impairment occurs less commonly, and associated pain is inconsistent. Eventually, patients experience cutaneous sensory loss in the fifth lumbar and sacral dermatomes and develop a lower motor neuron urinary sphincter disturbance with loss of rectal sphincter tone and with incontinence or severe constipation. Some patients have mild to moderate weakness in the lumbosacral myotomes or pain in the rectum or lower limbs.[44]

A cauda equina–like syndrome with neuropathic bladder is a rare but well-described complication of long-standing ankylosing spondylitis. Diverticulas from the subarachnoid space may erode into the lumbosacral vertebrae. These spinal diverticulas can be demonstrated by CT.[45] Electromyographic (EMG) abnormalities are typically consistent with multiple lumbosacral radiculopathies.[44] In the setting of ankylosing spondylitis, MRI is valuable in excluding other spinal lesions because it excludes the presence of extrinsic compression of the cauda equina.[46]

The clinical diagnosis of CES can be adequately confirmed with plain radiology, EMG, and CT. CT and MRI represent noninvasive means of establishing the diagnosis of CES in patients with ankylosing spondylitis.[43] MRI of the CES in patients with ankylosing spondylitis aids in the diagnosis and may provide valuable insight into the pathophysiology of this condition.[47] The features observed on MRI are pathognomonic, allowing accurate noninvasive diagnosis of the disorder.[48]

CT-myelography of the lumbosacral spine typically shows dilation of the spinal canal and lumbar sac with multiple dorsal arachnoid diverticulas eroding the laminae and spinous processes. Young et al.[49] found no compressive lesions with myelography, and foraminal encroachment was not seen. The pathogenesis of these erosions may be related to arachnoiditis in the early phase of the spondylitis.[50] Recognition of this syndrome, coupled with CT of the lower spinal canal, allows the clinician to avoid myelography, a procedure that is often difficult to perform in these patients because of associated spine abnormalities.

Early investigators concluded that surgery for CES secondary to ankylosing spondylitis was neither beneficial nor indicated and that it should be avoided.[43,44] However, surgery may be indicated in some patients, particularly when there is nerve root compression by the arachnoid cysts and when the patient is treated before irreversible damage to the cauda equina has occurred.[51]

Cauda Equina Syndrome Secondary to Arteriovenous Malformation or Hemorrhage

Spinal subdural hematoma is a rare cause of cauda equina compression that can occur in patients with a bleeding diathesis. Johnson et al.[52] reported a case of subacute lumbar subdural hematoma that was demonstrated by MRI. Laus et al.[53] reported three cases of CES resulting from epidural hematoma secondary to warfarin (Coumadin)-induced coagulopathy. They recommended anticoagulant correction with appropriate medications and hemoderivatives, with surgical treatment for the severe cases. Schmidt et al.[54] presented a patient with acute CES from a ruptured aneurysm in the sacral canal. The lesion was associated with pathologic enlargement of the lateral sacral arteries bilaterally, which occurred to provide cross-pelvic collateral flow in response to the diversion of the right internal iliac artery for renal transplantation. The patient showed signs and symptoms of spontaneous spinal epidural hemorrhage. In addition to angiography and partial embolization of the vascular supply, contrast-enhanced, high-resolution CT was essential in the diagnosis and treatment of this aneurysm.[54] Brown and Stambough reported a case of CES caused by an epidural hematoma secondary to a rupture of a synovial cyst.[55] In the literature it is reported that patients who have undergone exploration and evacuation of spinal epidural hematoma experienced the most extensive neurologic recovery within 6 hours of diagnosis. Patients who were surgically treated within 8 hours of diagnosis demonstrated less recovery.[56,57]

CES caused by massive spontaneous subarachnoid hemorrhage from an intradural angioblastic meningioma of the filum terminale has been reported.[58] Kulali et al.[58] reviewed six cases of spontaneous spinal subarachnoid hematoma caused by subarachnoid hemorrhage from a spinal tumor with acute compression of the adjoining nervous structures. Likewise, Malbrain et al.[34] reported a patient with acute CES resulting from intratumoral and spinal subarachnoid hemorrhage from a filum terminale ependymoma after therapy with oral anticoagulants. Only 13 cases of spinal subarachnoid hemorrhage caused by cauda equina ependymoma have been reported.

Cauda Equina Syndrome Secondary to Pregnancy

CES is rarely associated with pregnancy, with few cases reported in literature. Curtin and Rice reported a case of CES in a 37-year-old woman in the first trimester of pregnancy, due to a prolapsed lumbar disc.[59] Chow et al. reported a case of CES immediately following caesarean section.[60] We recommend that vigilance be maintained in the neurologic surveillance of pregnant women with known disc disease.

Iatrogenic Cauda Equina Syndrome

Postsurgical Cauda Equina Syndrome

Postoperative CES may develop as a result of intraoperative injury or after a normal baseline postoperative neurologic examination. CES developing postoperatively is often reversible if recognized and corrected expeditiously. Delay in diagnosis or treatment can result in a permanent neurologic deficit. Postoperative CES may develop because of hematoma formation, malpositioned or excessively large autologous fat graft, epidural abscess, or failure to relieve spinal stenosis.

Laus et al.[61] analyzed the complications resulting from the surgical treatment of lumbar stenosis and reported 4 cases of CES in 96 patients undergoing multiple bilateral laminectomies. Maurice-Williams and Marsh[62] reported four cases of cauda equina lesions after dorsal surgery for severe dysplastic spondylolisthesis: three cases after in situ fusion and one case after decompressive laminectomy. The mechanism of nerve root injury was postulated to be mechanical, occurring during decortication before bone grafting.[62]

Schoenecker et al.[63] identified 12 patients who developed CES after in situ bilateral dorsolateral arthrodesis for grades III or IV lumbosacral spondylolisthesis. No mention of direct cauda equina injury was noted in the operative reports. Five of the 12 patients eventually recovered completely. The remaining seven patients had a permanent residual neurologic deficit, manifested by complete or partial inability to control the bowel and bladder. Schoenecker et al.[63] postulated that preoperative sacral nerve root dysfunction in a patient with lumbosacral spondylolisthesis is an indication for cauda equina decompression concomitant with the arthrodesis. They recommended immediate decompression, including resection of the dorsal rostral rim of the dome of the sacrum and the adjacent intervertebral disc for acute CES after in situ arthrodesis for spondylolisthesis.

McLaren and Bailey[64] reported six cases of acute CES after lumbar discectomy in a series of 2842 lumbar discectomies. Five patients had coexisting bony spinal stenosis at the level of the disc protrusion that was not decompressed at the time of surgery. Inadequate decompression played a role in the postoperative neurologic deterioration. Bowel and bladder recovery was good when the cauda equina was decompressed early, sensory recovery was universally good, and motor recovery was poor if a severe deficit developed before decompression. McLaren and Bailey[64] advised urgent decompression of postoperative CES if cauda equina compression is radiographically confirmed. Bowen and Ferrer[65] reported a case of CES that resulted from displacement of a hook plate into the canal at L5, eroding the dura and pressing on the nerve roots. Removal of the hook and fusion of L5 and S1 relieved the symptoms. Mulder et al. reported a case of cauda equina compression by hydrogel dural sealant after a laminotomy and discectomy. The dural sealant was used to stop an iatrogenic cerebrospinal fluid leak at L4-5. Postoperative imaging and operative findings confirmed swelling and migration of the material.[66] Iatrogenic CES following lumbar puncture is rare, but can cause significant morbidity.[67]

The overall incidence of neurologic deficit after lumbar spine surgery is approximately 0.2%. The development of postoperative CES in patients undergoing lumbar discectomy is a well-documented complication. Dimopoulos et al. presented two cases of postoperative CES in patients undergoing single-level lumbar microdiscectomy. They found that intraoperative somatosensory evoked potential monitoring may be useful in predicting the development of CES in patients undergoing this operation.[68] We use electrophysiologic monitoring, including somatosensory evoked potentials, as an intraoperative adjunct when decompressing lesions involving the cauda equina. During resection of large tumors involving nerve roots or during surgery for congenital malformations such as tethered cord, intraoperative stimulation of nerve roots and recording of EMG activity from selected muscles including the tibialis anterior, gastrocnemius, and perianal sphincter are performed.[69,70]

Cauda Equina Syndrome after Intradiscal Therapy

Automated percutaneous lumbar discectomy to manage contained herniated lumbar discs has a low associated morbidity. Epstein[71] reported cauda equina injury after a left-sided L5-S1 automated percutaneous discectomy. Despite delayed surgery, which included excision of a sequestrated L5-S1 disc and intradural exploration, S1 radiculopathy, sacral numbness, and overflow incontinence persisted. Onik et al.[72] reported CES secondary to a Nucleotome probe (Clarus Medical, Minneapolis, MN) placed in the thecal sac, reviewed the landmarks for the thecal sac, and emphasized the preventable nature of this complication.

Hedtmann et al.[73] reported two patients who developed CES after intradiscal collagenase therapy to treat large extruded disc fragments. Smith et al.[74] similarly reported three cases of acute disc herniation causing cauda equina compression syndrome after chemonucleolysis. All three patients had myelographic blocks and, despite emergency decompression procedures, were left with residual neurologic deficits.

Postchiropractic Cauda Equina Syndrome

CES has been implicated as a potential complication of spinal manipulation. Multiple cases of CES have been reported to result from chiropractic lumbar spinal manipulation.[75-77] Haldeman and Rubinstein[78] identified 10 reported cases of CES in patients who underwent manipulation between 1911 and 1989 and presented 3 new cases in which cauda equina symptoms occurred after lumbar manipulation. Kostuik et al.[15] reported three patients who developed CES after chiropractic manipulation of the spine. Solheim et al. reported a case of a72-year-old man receiving anticoagulation therapy for chronic atrial fibrillation who developed CES due to a spinal epidural hematoma immediately following a chiropractic manipulation. Caution should be shown in patients seeking chiropractic treatment while receiving antithrombotic therapy.[79]

Cauda Equina Syndrome Secondary to Continuous Spinal Anesthesia

CES may occur after continuous spinal anesthesia.[80] In the described cases, there was evidence of a focal sensory block and, to obtain adequate analgesia, the patients were given a dose of local anesthetic that was greater than the dose usually administered with a single-injection technique. The combination of maldistribution and a relatively high dose of local anesthetic was postulated to result in neurotoxic injury. The increased incidence of CES associated with the use of microcatheters and continuous spinal anesthesia prompted the U.S. Food and Drug Administration to issue a safety alert.[80]

Cauda Equina Syndrome Caused by Infection

CES can manifest in association with lumbar spinal infections that result in an epidural abscess or pathologic fracture (Fig. 105-6). CES typically results from direct compression of the cauda equina, but may also occur secondary to subarachnoid vascular injury or thrombosis.[81] Management consists of early detection, antibiotic and surgical decompression, and debridement with or without spinal stabilization.[82]

Arend et al.[83] described a patient who developed toxic shock syndrome, meningitis, and CES several days after lumbar laminectomy. Enterotoxin-producing *Staphylococcus aureus* was cultured from the surgical wound and the cerebrospinal fluid. The patient recovered from toxic shock syndrome but remained partially paralyzed. CES was postulated to result from the neurotoxic effects of the intrathecally produced *S. aureus* exotoxins.[83]

Crawfurd et al.[84] presented five patients who were HIV positive who had symptoms initially thought to be indicative of lumbar disc lesions. Signs of nerve root or cauda equina compression were noted in all five patients, but lumbar imaging studies demonstrated no evidence of compressive lesions. Therefore, physicians must exercise caution in diagnosing nerve root compression in HIV-positive patients. Likewise, Zeman and Donaghy[85] reported a case of CES in the context of acute infection with HIV and emphasized the importance of considering the possibility of primary HIV infection in a wide range of self-limiting neurologic disorders.

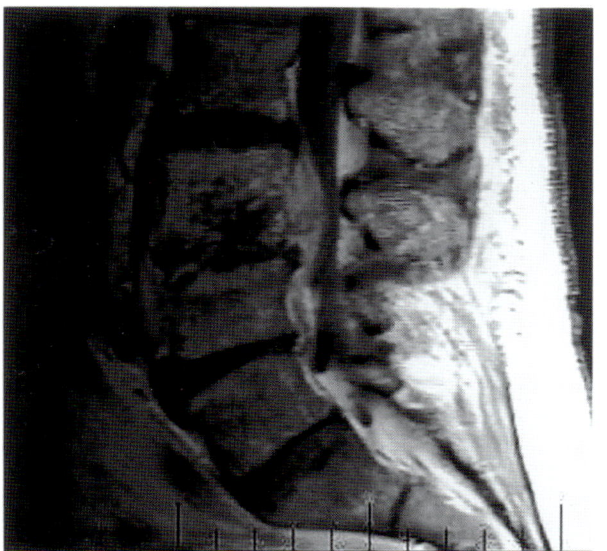

FIGURE 105-6. Gadolinium-enhanced T1-weighted MRI of a 70-year-old diabetic woman with cauda equina compression from an epidural abscess.

Diagnostic Pitfalls

Tullberg and Isacson[86] reported on 19 patients with normal lumbar myelograms and symptoms consistent with CES. Two patients had thoracic lesions—one with a tumor and the other with a herniated disc—who were discovered on a second myelogram. One patient was considered to have hysterical paresis. In three other patients, the symptoms were attributed to diseases not related to the spine. Thirteen patients recovered spontaneously. The authors concluded that the prognosis for patients with signs of compression of the cauda equina is favorable, provided the myelography results are normal and surgical exploration is not indicated. However, if severe unexplained symptoms persist and the CT-myelogram is normal, the authors recommend myelography of the thoracic spine.[86]

A large number of patients present to neurosurgical units with symptoms suggestive of CES without radiologic evidence of pathology. In these cases, a high level of suspicion should be maintained. If lumbosacral compression is not demonstrated, then imaging studies should be pursued to rule out a proximal lesion.[87]

Prognosis for Recovery of Bladder Dysfunction

CES must be considered for prompt surgical intervention because spontaneous neurologic recovery is uncommon. If incontinence is present, prompt surgery can possibly lessen the likelihood of future urinary dysfunction and maintain whatever function still remains. Similarly, severe paresis or paraplegia merits the consideration for prompt and generous decompression. Patients with CES should undergo emergent radiologic evaluation and urgent surgical intervention if indicated.

Gleave and MacFarlane[16] reviewed 932 patients who underwent surgery for prolapsed lumbar intervertebral disc and identified a group of 33 with acute urinary retention. No identifiable factor predisposed this group of patients to CES. The mean duration of bladder paralysis before operation was 3.6 days. Ultimately, 79% of patients claimed full recovery of bladder function, but only 22% were left without sensory deficits in the limbs or perineum. There was no correlation between recovery and the duration of bladder paralysis before surgery, except in three patients in whom there was no sciatica and in whom the correct diagnosis was delayed for many days. Retention developing less than 48 hours after acute prolapse was associated with a worse prognosis.

Hellstrom et al.[88] urodynamically evaluated bladder function after surgery in 17 patients with CES caused by lumbar intervertebral disc herniation. At the 3-year follow-up, 10 patients (59%) reported normal bladder function, whereas 7 patients (41%) noted obstruction or incontinence. Urodynamic function was normal in four patients (24%), three patients (18%) had no detrusor contraction, two patients (12%) used the detrusor but strained during voiding, and three patients (18%) had an unstable detrusor; the remaining five patients (29%) had either an increased bladder capacity or a decreased maximal flow rate. Neurologic findings were normal in two patients (12%). Bladder function is often substantially disturbed in patients with asymptomatic CES, and therefore urodynamic testing is warranted in all patients with CES. Urgent surgical intervention may improve long-term bladder function. Regeneration of the autonomic nervous supply to the bladder and genitals often requires several months or even years.

Nielsen et al.[89] reported that among 1972 patients undergoing surgery for lumbar disc herniation in a 7-year period (from 1971 to 1978), CES was diagnosed in 26 patients. Twenty-two patients had follow-up visits 4 to 72 months postoperatively (average, 37 months). At follow-up, half of the patients had a history of normal micturition, and only six patients had a serious complaint of micturition. One third of the patients were free from lumbar or sciatic pain, whereas two thirds complained of distressing pain and neurologic symptoms. The urodynamic investigation revealed complete bladder emptying in all but one patient. In half of the patients, normal detrusor contraction was demonstrated, whereas one third of the patients voided by straining only. Preoperative micturition symptoms exceeded 2 days in almost all patients voiding by straining. This finding indicates a connection of early diagnosis and treatment with the degree of detrusor damage.

Summary

CES is a complex of low back pain, saddle anesthesia, bowel and bladder dysfunction or incontinence that is often associated with radiculopathy, and lower-extremity motor weakness that occasionally progresses to paraplegia.

Patients with CES should undergo rapid radiologic evaluation and surgical intervention. It is prudent to adhere to a few simple principles during evaluation of patients with acute back pain or lumbosacral trauma (Box 105-3). It is important to maintain a high index of suspicion for the diagnosis of CES and its implications both diagnostically and prognostically. It is essential that these patients are specifically asked about urinary incontinence and retention and that their bladder and bowel functions are monitored vigilantly. If the clinician is suspicious, he or she should obtain a postvoid residual urine volume. In addition, trauma patients often receive an indwelling catheter at the time of admission to the emergency department. This catheter should be removed and checked for postvoid residual urine volume as quickly as possible. A rectal examination and evaluation of perianal sensation is mandatory when assessing any patient with acute onset of severe back pain or significant lumbosacral trauma. Imaging studies to determine the nature of the lesion (e.g., disc herniation, fracture, hematoma, tumor) must be performed expeditiously. If one imaging study (e.g., MRI) is inadequate, a complementary study (e.g., CT-myelography) should be obtained. If surgical management is indicated, meticulous surgical technique is critical so as to avoid additional nerve root traction or compression.

BOX 105-3. Recommendations for Evaluating Patients with Acute Back Pain or Lumbosacral Trauma

Maintain a high index of suspicion
Perform a rectal examination
Perform appropriate imaging studies
Perform early operation

KEY REFERENCES

Domen PM, Hofman PA, van Santbrink H, et al: Predictive value of clinical characteristics in patients with suspected cauda equina syndrome. *Eur J Neurol* 16(3):416–419, 2009.

Gleave JR, MacFarlane R: Prognosis for recovery of bladder function following lumbar central disc prolapse. *Br J Neurosurg* 4:205–209, 1990.

Pedowitz RA, Garfin SR, Massie JB, et al: Effects of magnitude and duration of compression on spinal nerve root conduction. *Spine (Phila Pa 1976)* 17:194–199, 1992.

Rooney A, Statham PF, Stone J: Cauda equina syndrome with normal MR imaging. *J Neurol* 256(5):721–725, 2009.

Shi J, Jia L, Yuan W, et al: Clinical classification of cauda equina syndrome for proper treatment. *Acta Orthop* 81(3):391–395, 2010.

Tullberg T, Isacson J: Cauda equina syndrome with normal lumbar myelography. *Acta Orthop Scand* 60:265–267, 1989.

REFERENCES

The complete reference list is available online at expertconsult.com.

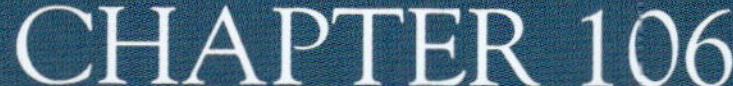
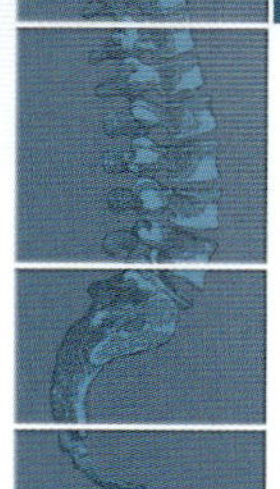

CHAPTER 106

Primary Bony Spinal Lesions

Patrick W. Hitchon | Timothy Lindley | Michael Ebersold

General Discussion

Primary tumors of the spine are extraordinarily uncommon. The incidence of primary spinal neoplasms has been estimated to be between 2.5 and 8.5 per 100,000 per year,[1] the equivalent of an estimated 7500 new cases per year in the United States.[2] Overall, primary spinal tumors are more common in men than women. Osteoid osteoma, osteoblastoma, osteochondroma, plasmacytoma, chordoma, and chondrosarcoma all occur more commonly in men at a nearly 2:1 ratio compared with women.[2] In a review of 6221 bone tumors at the Mayo Clinic, Dahlin and Coventry[3] found that less than 10% of all primary tumors involved the spine. In a recent, even more extensive review at the Mayo Clinic, Unni et al. (unpublished data, personal communication, 2000) reviewed 8091 skeletal bone tumors in patients who underwent surgery. Of these 8091 skeletal tumors distributed throughout the skeleton, 2334 were benign and 5757 were malignant. A further analysis of this group revealed that 510 tumors involving the spine were malignant and only 145 were benign. A more detailed grouping of the benign tumors is presented in Table 106-1. Not all patients with benign or malignant tumors undergo surgery. Therefore, these figures likely underestimate the true incidence of the disease.

The presenting symptoms of night pain, pain at rest, or progressive neurologic deficit should prompt the clinician to entertain the diagnosis of benign or malignant disease of the spine. The primary complaint of most patients with primary tumors of the spine is pain. In a recent review, more than 84% of the patients complained of pain, either localized to the back (60.2%) or radicular (24%). There was no apparent difference between the pain symptoms in patients with benign disease involving the spine and those with malignant disease involving the spine.[4] Fifty-five percent of the patients with malignant spine tumors and 35% of the patients with benign tumors demonstrated objective evidence of neurologic deficits. It is postulated that with the advent and increased availability of MRI, the number of patients presenting with neurologic deficits will decrease secondary to earlier diagnosis.

Although a rapidly progressive neurologic deficit is more suggestive of a malignant tumor or a pathologic fracture, it is not uncommon for patients with benign tumors involving the spine to experience rather rapid progressive neurologic deterioration. Nevertheless, because of the slow growth of these benign tumors of the spine, there is often a prolonged interval between the onset of symptoms and the diagnosis.

The data presented in Table 106-1, contrasted with those in Table 106-2, demonstrate the relative frequency or infrequency of these primary tumors involving the spine. In spinal tumors the distinction between tumors considered benign or malignant can be somewhat misleading. Chordoma is listed among the malignant tumors involving the spine, although tumor growth in some patients with chordoma is extremely slow. Conversely, giant-cell tumor is considered a benign tumor, although this particular lesion, in some cases, can be aggressive in nature. Early recurrence following surgery for giant-cell tumors is common, and there is even the potential for metastasis. Furthermore, progression to a high-grade sarcoma can occur in up to 10% of patients following postoperative radiation therapy.[5]

Often, plain radiographs demonstrate the site of the lesion and, in many cases, can be diagnostic. CT and MRI are often extremely valuable for defining the extent and precise location of the lesion. The need for myelography to diagnose and define benign tumors of the spine has been nearly eliminated by these two imaging advances. However, angiography can often be of significant benefit in confirming the nature of the lesion. In addition, angiography may be used for accurate definition of the vascular extent of the lesion and for preoperative embolization, when appropriate. Often, preoperative embolization can decrease the operative blood loss and therefore the postoperative morbidity. Aneurysmal bone cysts, giant-cell tumors, and hemangiomas, in particular, should be considered for preoperative embolization.

Some of the primary tumors of the spine have very characteristic imaging findings. The clinician should be aware of the classical radiographic findings associated with these tumors, because this knowledge is not only helpful for identifying the cause of the symptoms, but may also be of value by limiting additional testing and in guiding management decisions. Several of the common spinal lesions have unique features and are presented later in this chapter.

Management

Staging

Once a primary spinal tumor is suspected, thorough imaging of the lesion is required, including plain radiographs, CT, and MRI to narrow the differential diagnosis. In addition, a

TABLE 106-1

Skeletal Distribution of Benign Tumors

Tumor Type	NUMBER OF PATIENTS WITH	
	Tumors Involving the Spine	Benign Skeletal Tumors
Giant cell tumor	32	574
Osteoid osteoma	30	332
Osteoblastoma	29	87
Hemangioma	28	109
Osteochondroma	19	748
Chondroma	5	290
Chondroblastoma	1	119
Chondromyxoid fibroma	1	45
Neurilemmoma	0	14
Fibrous histiocytoma	0	9
Lipoma	0	7
Total	145	2334

Only those patients undergoing surgery and who, therefore, have tissue available for pathologic review are included in this table.
From Unni KK et al: Unpublished data, personal communication, 2000.

TABLE 106-2

Skeletal Distribution of Malignant Tumors

Tumor Type	NUMBER OF PATIENTS WITH	
	Tumors Involving the Spine	Malignant Skeletal Tumors
Myeloma	232	803
Lymphoma	82	694
Chondrosarcoma	54	892
Chordoma	51	356
Osteosarcoma	37	1649
Ewing tumor	16	514
Hemangioendothelioma	13	80
Fibrosarcoma	9	255
Secondary chondrosarcoma	7	121
Mesenchymal chondrosarcoma	4	25
Malignant giant-cell tumor	2	35
Malignant fibrous histiocytoma	2	83
Dedifferentiated chondrosarcoma	1	120
Hemangiopericytoma	1	13
Periosteal osteosarcoma	0	69
Adamantinoma	0	36
Desmoid fibroma	0	12
Total	511	5757

Only those patients undergoing surgery and who, therefore, have tissue available for pathologic review are included in this table.
From Unni KK et al: Unpublished data, personal communication, 2000.

complete systemic workup should also be performed. A CT of the chest, abdomen, and pelvis, or a positron emission tomography scan can help to identify any additional distant pathology. Ultimately, however, a tissue diagnosis is typically required to aid in preoperative planning. The decision to perform a biopsy must be a part of a comprehensive management strategy to reduce the risk of local recurrence. It has been suggested that resecting the tissue along the biopsy tract during the definitive resection could prevent recurrence caused by the contamination of surrounding tissues during the biopsy.[6]

After a histopathologic diagnosis is made, staging can be completed to aid in presurgical planning. The Enneking classification system assists in determining the goals of surgery and is a guide to adjuvent therapy. Both benign and malignant tumors can be staged and are classified as either high- or low-grade, depending on the local extent of disease and the presence of metastasis. Management strategies range from no surgical intervention to palliative surgery based on the stage.[7] The Weinstein, Boriani, Biagini (WBB) classification[8] was developed to guide a surgeon in determining the most appropriate surgical approach. In the WBB system, the vertebra is divided into 12 radiating zones (numbered 1 through 12, clockwise starting dorsally at the spinous process) and into five layers (A–E, from paravertebral to dural involvement). In addition, the longitudinal extent of the tumor is noted. Depending on the area of involvement, a surgical approach is recommended. For tumors involving only the vertebral body (zones 4–9), an anterior approach is recommended, whereas a dorsal approach is ideal for tumors involving the pedicles, facets, spinous process, and lamina (zones 3–10).

Surgery

The goal of surgical management of spine tumors is to establish a definitive diagnosis, decompress the neural elements, maintain or achieve spinal stability, and if possible, cure the patient. In the case of benign tumors involving the spinal axis, cure can often be achieved if proper consideration is given to size, extent, and location of the tumor.

Not every patient with a primary tumor of the spine is a candidate for surgery. For example, hemangioma is often an incidental finding, and surgery is not appropriate unless specific clinical symptoms or signs are present. In general, progressive neurologic loss is a rather definite indication that surgery should at least be considered in the patient with a benign lesion. The patient's age, his or her general well-being, and the expected morbidity from the surgical procedure are all factors that must be considered.

Spine tumor resection can be en bloc or intralesional.[1] En bloc resection, or spondylectomy, is the resection of the entire tumor in one piece. En bloc resections are further subdivided into marginal or wide. Marginal resection dissects through the pseudocapsule of the tumor, and wide resection provides a cuff of normal tissue (>2 mm of healthy bone, reactive periosteum, or pleura) with a margin of healthy surrounding tissue. For primary tumors, the long-term local tumor control, survival, and cure are dependent on en bloc tumor resection. For this reason, there has been resurgent interest in treating primary spinal tumors with en bloc resection. Intralesional resection is the incision into the tumor, and debulking from within. Although intralesional resection of spine tumors results in good neurologic outcomes, local recurrence rates remain high. Wide resection occurs when the excision is inclusive of the pseudocapsule. As applied to the spine, marginal en bloc resection or intralesional resection with an adjuvant (e.g., phenol, liquid nitrogen, methyl methacrylate) may be curative for aneurysmal bone cysts, giant-cell tumors, osteoid osteomas, and osteoblastomas. Evidence is mounting that wide en bloc resections for primary tumors such as chondrosarcoma, chordoma, osteogenic sarcoma, and Ewing sarcoma may effect a longer disease-free interval and a potential cure.

However, en bloc resections often require extensive procedures associated with high rates of morbidity and mortality.[9] Bandiera et al.[9] recently published the largest study to date examining the complication rates in en bloc resections of spinal tumors. They reviewed 134 consecutive attempted en bloc resections from 1990 to 2007 at a single institution. Major complications occurred in 43 cases, including three deaths. Major complications were also more common in patients who had undergone a previous failed resection at a prior institution. Of those previously treated, 72% suffered a major complication, whereas 20% with a new presentation suffered a major complication. Furthermore, with an average follow-up period of 37 months, the local recurrence rate was higher in patients treated previously elsewhere (40% vs. 16%). Thus, surgical management of primary spinal tumors is associated with high morbidity and recurrence rates, both of which can be reduced if treatment from biopsy to resection occurs at the same institution by a dedicated multidisciplinary team.

When the biopsy is performed prior to the definitive procedure, if possible, the biopsy path should be well marked and the soft tissue along the biopsy path should be resected along with the tumor at the time of surgery. Also, one must always be cautious to avoid contamination of surrounding tissues with tumor cells. In addition, resecting the dura as a margin may increase the risk of intradural seeding.[10] When a fusion is planned, bone graft should be obtained through a separate surgical setup.[5]

Radiation

Primary tumors may benefit from neoadjuvant or postoperative adjuvant radiation or chemotherapy. In general, the more benign tumors (e.g., osteoid osteoma, osteoblastoma, osteochondroma) have a poor response rate to these therapeutic modalities, and gross resection of the tumor will effect a cure. A significant concern in patients receiving radian therapy for the more benign tumors is the development of postradiation sarcomas. In a review of 59 patients who underwent operation for spinal sarcoma at Memorial Sloan-Kettering Cancer Center, 7 patients had postradiation sarcomas at a median interval of 14 years from the time of radiation.[11,12] Other tumors, such as osteogenic sarcoma and Ewing sarcoma, may benefit from neoadjuvant chemotherapy followed by resection. Chondrosarcoma and chordoma are extremely radiation therapy resistant and still chemotherapy resistant, but positive surgical margins are irradiated.

A great challenge in radiation therapy to the spine is that the dose the spinal cord can tolerate is significantly lower than the dose required to achieve local tumor control. Experience with extremity sarcomas has demonstrated good local control with 60 Gy for postoperative radiation therapy in patients with close surgical margins. For patients with gross residual disease after resection, 70 Gy is typically delivered in 200-cGy fractions. The spinal cord is thought to tolerate no more than 50 Gy when delivered in 200-cGy fractions.[11] Several strategies have evolved in an attempt to deliver tumoricidal doses of radiation while avoiding radiation-induced myelopathy. These advances include intraoperative radiation therapy, brachytherapy, proton beam therapy, high-dose conformal photon therapy, and stereotactic radiation. Each of these techniques provides a higher tumoral dose of radiation with reduced damage to surrounding tissues and potentially smaller fields than do conventional external beam techniques.

Intraoperative radiation therapy (IORT) involves the delivery of a custom-designed electron beam or high-dose brachytherapy that precisely demarcates the tumor volume. Lead shields and gold foil are used to shield the spinal cord.[13] Unfortunately, this technique is somewhat labor intensive, and dosimetry considerations are difficult to predict around the spinal cord. An alternative radiation approach is brachytherapy, or the direct application of radioisotopes within the resection cavity. Earlier attempts with the use of iodine-125 were disappointing due to difficulties with dosing near the spinal cord. However, intraoperative therapy with yttrium-90 has recently been approved by the U.S. Food and Drug Administration and has been demonstrated to be effective in the treatment of sarcoma. Yttrium-90 is a pure β-emitter with limited penetrance. DeLaney et al.[14] treated five patients with yttrium-90 plaques placed intraoperatively, including two chondrosarcomas and one osteosarcoma. With a median follow-up of 24 months, no local recurrences were observed in the chondrosarcoma or osteosarcoma patients and no treatment-related myelopathy or neuropathy was detected.[14]

Proton beam therapy[15,16] has an inherent geometric advantage over therapy with photons and electrons because of the finite range of penetration in tissues (Bragg-peak effect). Proton beams can be designed so that a uniform dose is administered to the target volume (i.e., tumor) and a minimal dose is delivered to the critical surrounding tissues (e.g., spinal cord, bowel, esophagus). Proton beam treatment plans are often supplemented with additional photon beam therapy to improve tumoral coverage. Studies have shown outstanding results for the control of chordoma and chondrosarcoma with proton beam therapy. Hug[17] reported on 33 patients with skull base chordomas and 25 patients with skull base chondrosarcomas treated to a mean dose of 70.7 cobalt gray equivalents (CGEs) with a mean follow-up period of 33 months. Local control was achieved in 76% of the chordoma patients and 82% of the chondrosarcoma patients.[17] A major drawback for proton beam therapy is the limited availability of treatment centers in the United States to accommodate the demands for treating primary tumors, particularly chordomas and chondrosarcomas. Currently, proton beam centers are located at the Loma Linda University Medical Center, Massachusetts General Hospital, Indiana University, University of Florida, M.D. Anderson Cancer Center in Houston, and INTEGRIS Cancer Campus in Oklahoma.

High-dose conformal photon therapy (3D-CRT) has made it possible to deliver cytotoxic doses to tumor volume, doses similar to proton beam radiation, without the side effect of radiation-induced myelopathy.[18-22] Similar to proton beam therapy, 3D-CRT is a method of irradiating a tumor volume with an array of photon beams that are individually shaped to conform to a 3D rendering of the target. Treatment planning considers dose inhomogeneities caused by the differing electron densities of various tissues and calculates the resulting dose distribution using sophisticated algorithms. Intensity-modulated radiation therapy (IMRT) represents an advanced form of 3D-CRT in which multileaf collimators are used to dynamically change the field shape during treatment, thus permitting the delivery of an inhomogeneous dose that conforms more tightly to the target region. Because of the precise dosimetry demands of IMRT, accurate delivery requires reproducible patient setup and positioning. Recent data suggest that IMRT may improve the clinical outcome of inoperable tumors and those tumors requiring a boost after surgical resection. Yamada et al.[23] reported on 14 patients with primary spinal malignancies and 21 with metastatic lesions treated with IMRT at Memorial Sloan-Kettering Cancer Center. Patients had unresectable disease near the spinal cord and either previously received radiation therapy or were prescribed doses beyond spinal cord tolerance. With a mean follow-up period of 11 months, local control was achieved in 81% of primary malignancies and 75% of metastatic lesions. No radiation-induced myelopathy was observed, and more than 90% reported palliation from pain, weakness, or paresthesia.[23]

Chemotherapy

Chemotherapy has not been found to be beneficial in the majority of spinal tumors. However, recent evidence has shown promise in the treatment of osteogenic sarcoma. A recent prospective randomized trial demonstrated 3-year event-free survival rates of 71% and 78% for patients with osteogenic sarcoma treated with either cisplatin, doxorubicin, and methotrexate versus muramyl tetrapeptide following resection, respectively.[24] Chordoma, also previously thought to be chemoresistant, has also been shown to be sensitive to a new class of tyrosine kinase inhibitors. Imatinib mesylate (Gleevac) is one such tyrosine kynase inhibitor that has shown promise in early clinical trials. In initial studies, imaging revealed extensive tumor necrosis in six out of six patients treated with imatinib mesylate.[2] Sunitinib (Sutent) is another tyrosine kinase inhibitor recently developed that is currently being tested on chordoma patients in clinical trials.[11] As new therapeutic strategies continue to be developed, chemotherapy holds great promise for the treatment of primary spinal tumors in the future.

Hemangioma

Hemangioma is one of the common benign lesions involving the spinal axis. It is often discovered incidentally during evaluation of patients with back or neck pain. The relatively low incidence, noted in Table 106-1, confirms that most patients with hemangioma are not treated surgically. Several studies have demonstrated that this entity may affect as much as 10% to 12% of the population.[25-33] Less than 5% of patients with hemangiomas develop symptoms.[34] Spine surgeons become involved with the treatment of hemangioma when the lesion causes spinal cord or nerve root compression. In general, decompressive surgery should be reserved for this specific group, because such surgery is usually not required for the management of pain that is not associated with neurologic involvement. In a 1993 review of spinal hemangioma from the Mayo Clinic, it was demonstrated that, in fact, it is rare for incidental hemangiomas associated with pain alone to progress to spinal cord compression.[28] Only 2 of 59 patients with previously diagnosed asymptomatic or painful lesions later developed spinal cord compression. Symptomatic hemangiomas are usually observed during adulthood and found to occur in the thoracic region.[29] Patients with asymptomatic lesions do not require further evaluation unless pain or neurologic deficits develop. Patients with painful lesions should be followed closely, with a combination of radiographic studies and periodic neurologic evaluations.

In the past, subtotal tumor removal with postoperative irradiation was often considered the treatment of choice in symptomatic tumors. The development of modern spine surgery techniques and the advancements made possible by a skilled surgical team and modern instrumentation have now made total removal of these lesions a viable option in many cases. Preoperative embolization has also significantly decreased intraoperative and postoperative morbidity.

Imaging

Plain radiography, tomography, and CT often clearly demonstrate the typical coarsened trabeculae within the involved vertebrae, with a characteristic honeycombed appearance. Gadolinium enhancement and MRI evidence of a soft tissue component are often observed (Fig. 106-1).

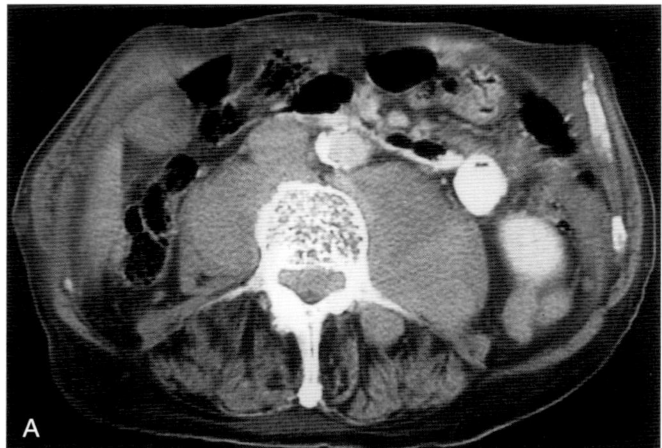

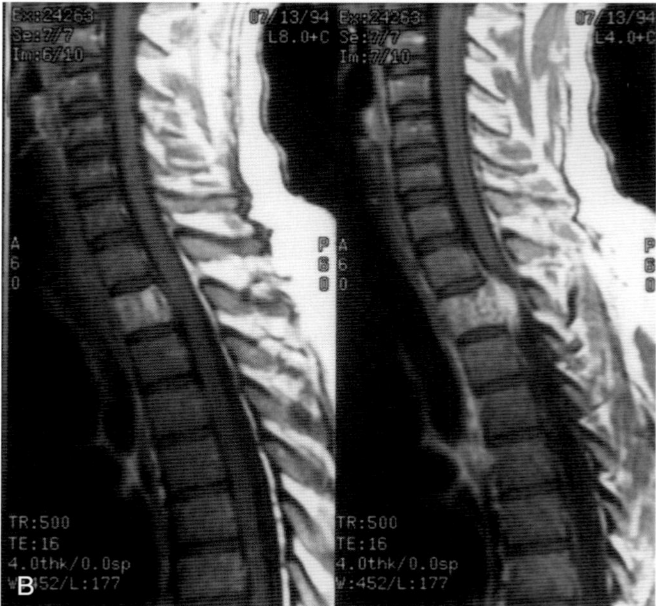

FIGURE 106-1. A, CT of vertebral body demonstrating the typical trabeculated appearance of a hemangioma of the lumbar spine. **B,** T1-weighted sagittal MRI of the thoracic spine demonstrates an indeterminate mass, later pathologically proven to be a hemangioma involving the body and right pedicle of T2. This hemangioma displaced the thecal sac and produced mild to moderate deformity of the adjacent thoracic spinal cord. In asymptomatic patients, this appearance is often an incidental finding.

Histology

Most of the trabeculae are atrophic because of the abnormal blood vessels, although some become thickened and sclerotic. Microscopically, there are two main types of trabeculae. These are characterized by cavernous or capillary vessels. In some cases, adipose tissue may be found within the lesion.[27] Spinal cord compression may arise from the expansile nature of the vertebral body, an associated soft tissue component of the tumor that rests within the spinal canal, a compression fracture of the weakened vertebral body, or, rarely, an epidural hemorrhage.

Management

The management scheme should depend on the size, extent, and location of the lesion; the patient's general age and health; and the patient's clinical course and neurologic findings. Surgical decompression is recommended if there is progressive neurologic decline. It is important for the spine surgeon to be familiar with the variety of available surgical approaches so that the most appropriate technique can be used to remove the tumor. Many patients for whom laminectomy and postoperative radiation therapy would have been recommended can now be treated using a lateral or ventral surgical approach to the lesion. Laminectomy followed by radiation therapy of lesions involving the vertebral body yielded a 93% rate of neurologic recovery, without recurrent symptoms, in a 52-month follow-up period.[31] Laminectomy without radiation therapy for subtotal tumor resections resulted in tumor control rates of 70% to 80%.[29-31] It appears that postoperative irradiation reduces the risk of tumor recurrence in patients after subtotal tumor removal. Nevertheless, because of the potential morbidity and relative lack of efficacy associated with radiation therapy, total lesion removal often should be attempted.

Vertebroplasty and kyphoplasty have also been advocated for the treatment of symptomatic hemangiomas. Studies have recently reported excellent pain relief with no evidence of posttreatment instability and preservation of vertebral body height. Such a less invasive approach may be ideal for patients who are not good surgical candidates.[35]

Eosinophilic Granuloma (Langerhans Cell Histiocytosis)

Eosinophilic granulomas are vertebral lesions found in 10% to 15% of cases of Langerhans cell histiocytosis. Most commonly, eosinophilic granulomas are identified in children younger than age 10, and spinal lesions have been reported in 6.5% to 25% of cases involving bone.[36] Eosinophilic granulomas involving the adult lumbar spine are very rare, and to date only 13 cases have been reported.[37] These self-limiting, benign lesions cause bony destruction[38] secondary to the local proliferation of histiocytes. Occasionally, multiple levels are involved and can rarely result in pain, but are more often identified incidentally.[5]

Radiographically, eosinophilic granulomas are identified as destructive bony lesions with well-demarcated borders and no evidence of a soft tissue mass. The adjacent disc spaces are well preserved (Fig. 106-2). These findings differentiate eosinophilic granulomas from other lesions in the differential diagnosis (e.g., infection, benign tumor, or malignancy).[5]

Management

Prior to any invasive treatment, a biopsy is indicated. In many cases, symptoms will resolve over time, and a conservative approach should always be considered first. The vertebral body height can be restored spontaneously if the areas of endochondral ossification were preserved and the child is young. Therefore, treatment is generally conservative with activity limitations and bracing.[36,38] A recent report described the use of percutaneous vertebroplasty to treat eosinophilic granuloma involving the cervical spine of a child, though this approach was taken only after conservative measures failed and a more aggressive approach was declined by the family.[39] In cases where vertebral body collapse results in loss of neurologic function, decompression and biopsy are warranted.[5] If the bony destruction leads to instability that persists despite a course of conservative management, arthrodesis is required.[38]

Aneurysmal Bone Cysts

Aneurysmal bone cysts (ABCs) are benign, proliferative nonneoplastic lesions that may occur in any part of the skeleton. Although this is not a tumor per se, its classical appearance and presentation should be familiar to clinicians dealing with spine lesions. ABCs make up 1% to 6% of primary spinal neoplasms, with approximately 40% to 45% involving the lumbar spine, 30% involving the thoracic spine, and 25% to 30% involving the cervical spine.[40] Lesions are often not confined to a single vertebra; instead they bridge two or more levels in approximately 40% of cases.[41,42] Although primary ABCs are of unknown cause, a secondary form of ABC has been described that arises within eosinophilic granulomas, simple bone cysts, osteosarcomas, chondroblastomas, or giant-cell tumors.[42]

ABCs of the spine typically present in young patients in their second decade, with a slight predominance in women.[43] In one series, 60% of lesions arose in the neural arch and 40% arose in the body. Pain that occurs especially at night and that is localized to the site of the mass is the most common presenting complaint.[44] The presence or absence of a neurologic deficit depends on the site of the tumor and on the degree of compression of adjacent neural elements. Symptoms and signs may vary from cord compression with myelopathic findings to radicular features of single-root involvement. The clinical course is commonly progressive over several months because of the slow growth of these lesions, although rapid growth can also occur. Imaging the anatomic delineation of ABCs is often best achieved with plain radiography and CT, which accurately define the degree of bone destruction and full extent of the lesion (Figs. 106-3A and B). MRI can be helpful for defining a spinal cord compressive component, and it readily demonstrates the full epidural extent of the mass. The rather classical appearance of the involved vertebra is that of a multiloculated, expansile, highly vascular mass with eggshell-like cortical bone and blood product fluid levels.

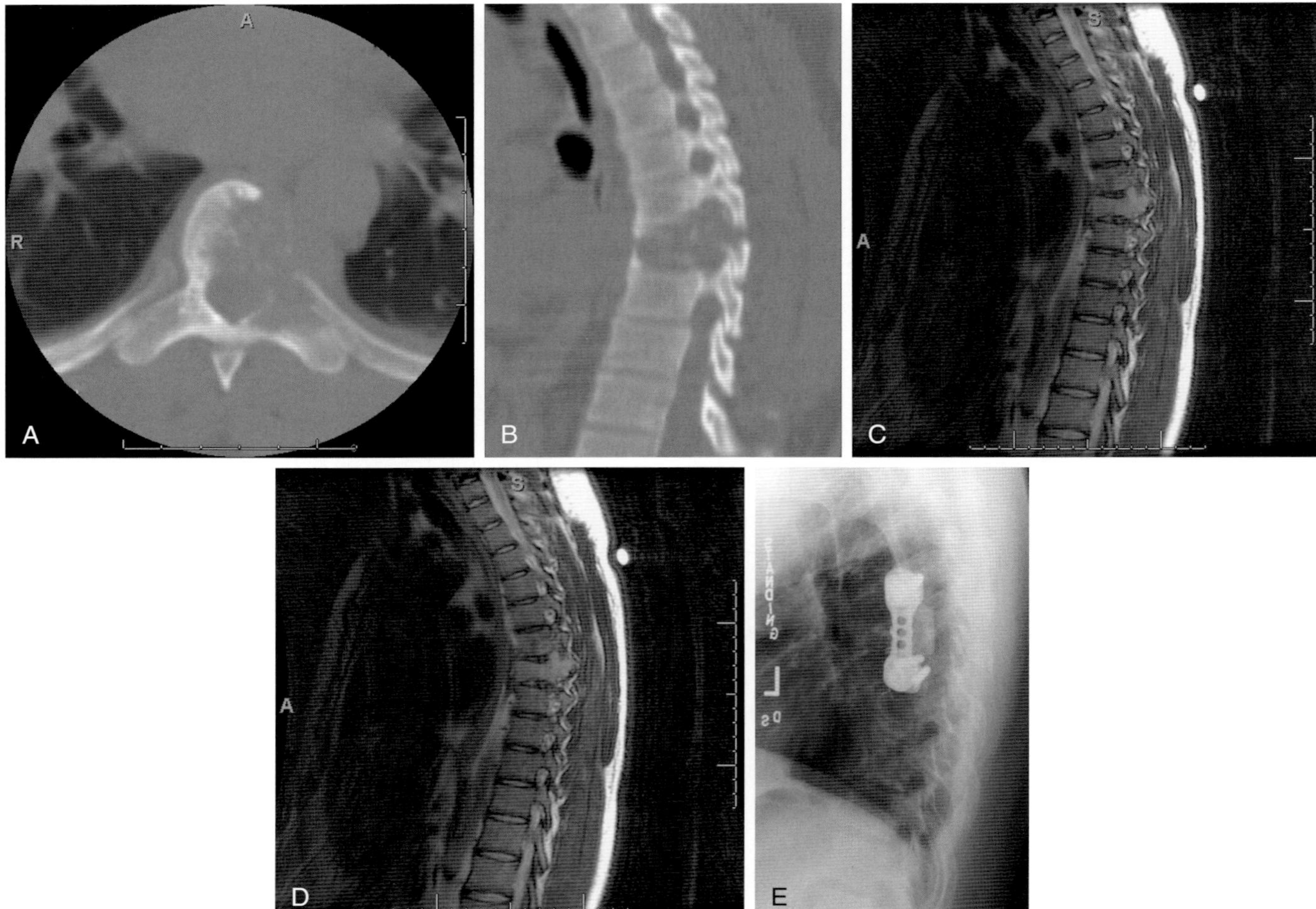

FIGURE 106-2. A 27-year-old man presents with a 2-month history of midback pain, leg weakness, and difficulty with urination. Examination showed him to be paraparetic $3/5$ bilaterally with hyperactive reflexes. Axial (**A**) and sagittal (**B**) CT scans show a lytic process involving the T7 body and left pedicle and, to a lesser extent T6. Sclerosis suggests an indolent process such as eosinophilic granuloma. **C,** MRI shows a soft tissue mass with destruction of the bone, extending into the canal and compressing the cord. There is extension of the soft tissue mass into the left paraspinal space. **D** and **E,** A left-sided transthoracic T6 partial and T7 total corpectomy was performed with humeral allograft, and screw and rod fixation. When seen 15 months later, the patient continued to have back pain and some unsteadiness, although he had no leg weakness or sphincter complaints.

Collapse of involved bodies and involvement of adjacent ribs may also be observed.

Selective spinal angiography has both diagnostic and, potentially, therapeutic value.[44] In addition to defining the relationship of the arterial supply of the lesion to the arterial supply of the cord, angiography also defines the involvement of the vertebral arteries with cervical lesions. The anatomic location of the artery of Adamkiewicz in lower thoracic or upper lumbar lesions can be defined clearly with spinal angiography. Finally, preoperative embolization is a useful adjunct that may decrease the intraoperative blood loss (Fig. 106-3C).

Histology

Microscopically, ABCs are characterized by spaces separated by septa that contain fibroblasts and giant cells. Reactive new bone is usually present. Although mitotic activity is brisk, there is no cytologic atypia. The lesions are lytic and expansile, and they extend to the cortex and occasionally violate the periosteum. Hemorrhage is common. The lesions contain sinusoidal vessels with hypervascular stroma, and multinucleated giant cells, monocytes, and macrophages are common.

Management

Rarely, spontaneous disappearance of ABCs has been reported to occur, and when discovered incidentally, conservative management could be considered. Diagnosis is generally established based on diagnostic studies (CT and MRI) without the need for a biopsy. When a biopsy is required, an open biopsy is preferred to decrease the risk of hemorrhage and improve the diagnostic value of the sample. Once a diagnosis has been established based on imaging or biopsy, several therapeutic options for ABCs have been described in the literature. The treatment options for ABCs include percutaneous injection of a fibrosing agent, arterial embolization, radiation therapy, curettage with or without bone grafting, or resection. Percutaneous injection of fibrosing agents has been shown to successfully treat ABCs. Injection of zein alcohol (Ethibloc) with histoacryl glue or of methylprednisolone with

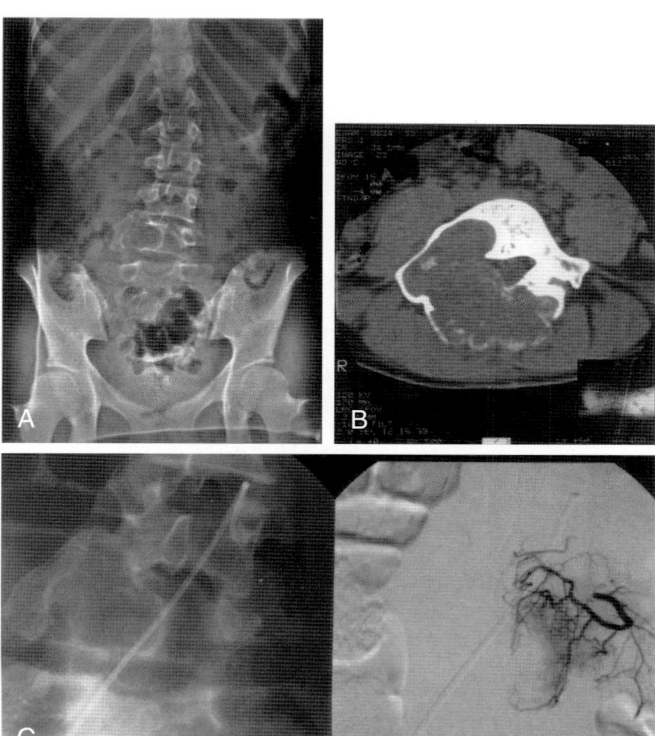

FIGURE 106-3. Aneurysmal bone cyst (ABC). **A,** Plain radiograph of lumbar spine demonstrating the typical appearance of a lytic, eccentric, expansile lesion of the vertebral body and dorsal elements of L5, as observed with an ABC. **B,** CT of lumbar spine demonstrating the lytic lesion of the dorsal elements and the vertebral body, with the tumor having an osseous shell consisting of a thin rim of cortical bone surrounding the mass. **C,** Plain and subtracted angiographic views display the typical segmental vascular supply of an ABC with vascular staining.

calcitonin has been shown to lead to successful destruction of the lesion with low recurrence rates.[40] However, injection therapies must be performed cautiously because of the presence of abnormal vascular channels and the risk of migration of the material into the vasculature. Embolic stroke resulting in death has been reported.[40]

More recently, some investigators have suggested that selective arterial embolization is the treatment of choice in cases where neither spinal instability nor neurologic deficits are identified. In such cases, it is sometimes preferable to repeat the embolization at least two times in an effort to avoid open surgery.[5] Arterial embolization preoperatively can also significantly reduce the risk of bleeding during surgery.[40]

Because of the destructive nature of ABCs and the risk of progressive instability coupled with the frequent presence of neurologic deficits secondary to compression of neural elements, complete surgical resection is often considered the treatment of choice. The approach (ventral, dorsal, or dorsolateral) depends on the exact location and extent of the lesion. An eggshell-thin cyst of subperiosteal new bone that is continuous with adjacent cortex is observed at surgery. This delineates the extent of the lesion, and its removal often results in intense bleeding. The core of the tumor consists of soft, fleshy, vascular tissue, as well as a cystic trabeculation of the interior of the mass containing unclotted blood. The mass may invade adjacent soft tissue or surround the thecal sac. Although there may be some concern about using a cell saver when removing tumors from any location in the body, there appears to be no contraindication to this procedure when removing ABCs. Despite the inherent technical difficulties of excision that are related to location and extent of the lesion, the prognosis is excellent with complete excision and recurrence rates are rare in most series.[40] Subtotal surgical excision, conversely, is followed by a high incidence of recurrence, which is usually rapid (within 1 year, and often within 4 months).[43] Likewise, curettage and bone grafting is associated with a 20% or greater recurrence rate.[40] Therefore, en bloc resection should be the goal of surgical intervention. As with all resections of spinal neoplasms, postoperative spinal instability should always be considered and instrumented fusion performed when identified.

Giant-Cell Tumor

Giant-cell tumors of the spine are locally aggressive benign primary bone tumors that constitute 4.2% of bone tumors in Dahlin and Coventry's series.[3] Approximately 6.5% of all giant-cell tumors occur in the spine,[45] with half occurring in the sacrum, followed by the thoracic and cervical spine in frequency.[46] The mean age of involvement is approximately 30 years, with a range of 13 to 62 years.[46,47] In most reviews, the incidence in women appears to outnumber that in men by a ratio of 2:1.[45] Most patients present with pain localized to the site of the lesion and, occasionally, with a neurologic deficit, depending on the location. Malignant transformation occurs in approximately 10% of cases. Some giant-cell tumors are biologically aggressive lesions. In patients with these tumors, local recurrence is common after incomplete resection.

Imaging

The diagnosis of giant-cell tumors may be made from plain radiographs and CTs (Fig. 106-4). The lesion is characterized as a destructive, expansile mass within the sacrum or other vertebrae. MRI reveals a heterogeneous, cystic, compartmentalized mass that may contain blood degradation products.

Histology

Grossly, giant-cell tumors are soft and fleshy and have a characteristic tan-brown color. Areas of necrosis and yellow discoloration may be found. Microscopically, these tumors show a combination of mononuclear cells and giant cells. The mononuclear cells are round to oval, and the nuclei are similar to those of the giant cells. Areas of necrosis and cystic change may be observed.

Management

In a review of 24 patients with giant-cell tumor of the spine, pain was the presenting symptom in all cases, and half of the patients also had a neurologic deficit.[45] All patients were treated with surgical curettage or en bloc resection, depending on the location and extent of the tumor. Ten patients had recurrences, and seven of these were treated with radiation. The most acceptable treatment approach seems to be an

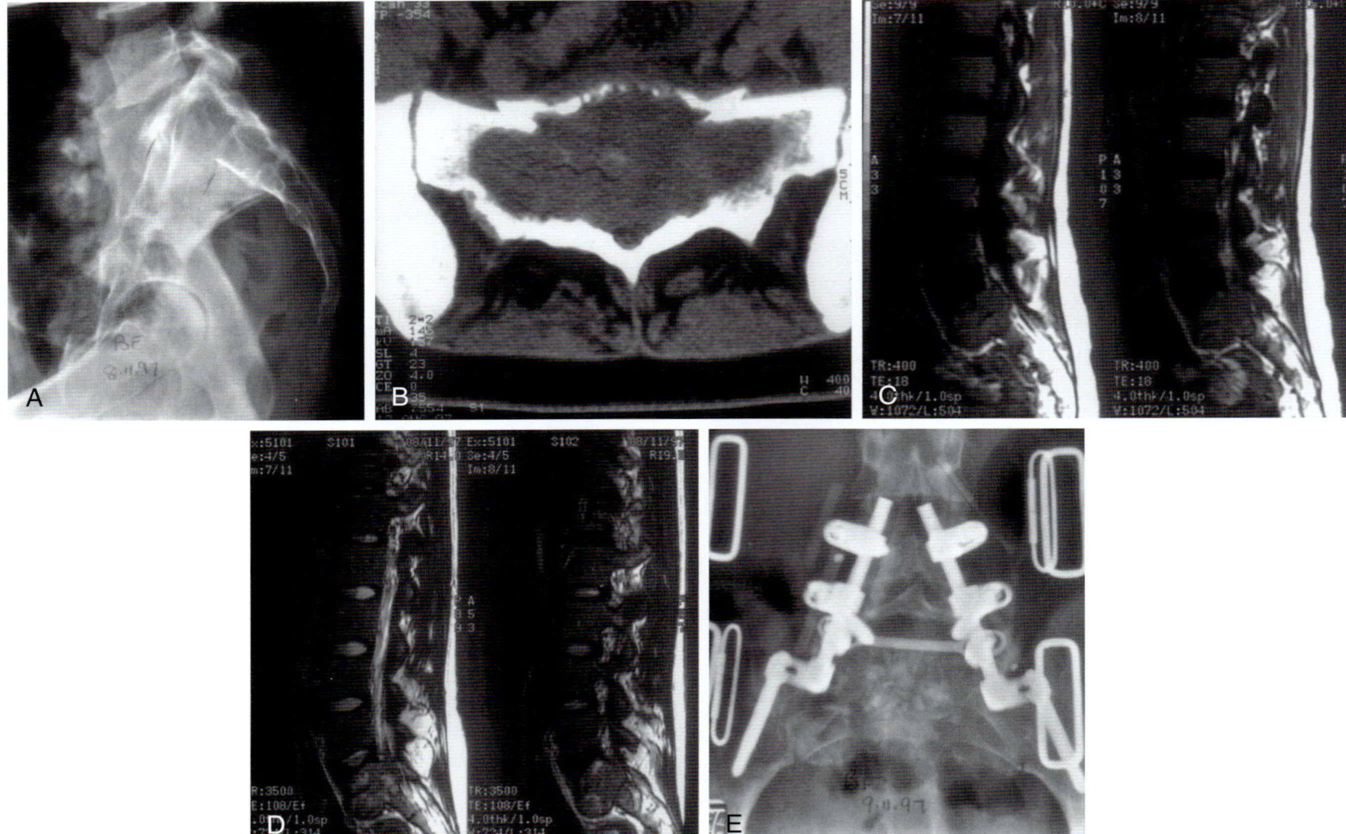

FIGURE 106-4. Giant-cell tumor in a 17-year-old girl with several years of low back pain and a 1-year history of leg weakness and urinary retention and constipation. **A,** The lateral plane film demonstrates a lytic lesion of S1, with erosion of the anterior cortex. **B,** The CT demonstrates the expansile intramedullary tumor with extension into the spinal canal. T1-weighted (**C**) and T2-weighted (**D**) MRIs reveal the bony tumor arising from S1 with extension anteriorly and posteriorly. **E,** One month following posterior decompression and stabilization, radiographs show satisfactory alignment with hardware in place. The patient later underwent anterior resections 5 and 26 months following the first operation. She is doing well, without recurrence and received no radiation.

attempted wide resection. Preoperative tumor embolization may be beneficial and advisable according to some authors.[5]

Radiation therapy may be considered with subtotal surgical excision. Giant-cell tumors can recur relatively early after even the most radical surgical excision. In such cases, it may be reasonable to consider radiation therapy if it is believed that further excisional attempts will also be unsuccessful. The 10-year success rate of radiation alone was 69% compared with 83% for postoperative radiation therapy.[5] Unfortunately, progression to a high-grade sarcoma occurs in 5% to 15% of cases following radiation treatment.[5] Therefore, radiation therapy should be reserved for patients with recurrent or residual disease after attempted resection.[48] In the spine, wide resection may cause destabilization and may necessitate instrumentation of the spine and fusion.[23] However, total excision is curative if it is achieved.[48]

Because of their location, sacral lesions pose specific problems. Complete eradication of the tumor usually necessitates sacrifice of bowel and bladder control. For this reason, some authors propose irradiation as the primary form of treatment. However, sacrectomy with attempted wide excision is warranted with acceptance of inevitable neurologic sequelae, if it is believed that such surgery can result in total tumor removal and cure.

Osteoid Osteoma

Osteoid osteoma is a relatively common benign neoplasm that occurs in the spine and accounts for 21% of surgically managed benign lesions.[49,50] Typically, it has a central nidus of interlacing osteoid and woven bone within a loose vascular stroma, surrounded by an osteosclerotic rim. These lesions are sharply demarcated from surrounding bone (Fig. 106-5). The nidus is rarely greater than 1.5 cm in diameter, and lesions larger than this are categorized as osteoblastomas. The distinction between the two lesions is often unclear, and they may represent a continuum.

Most patients are young, with half of all cases occurring in the second decade, with a marked male predominance. Typically, the neural arch elements are affected, most commonly in the lumbar spine. In a series of 33, the patients invariably presented with pain, which increased with exercise and was classically relieved with aspirin.[51] Associated features included the presence of radicular symptoms referable to the underlying root and antalgic scoliosis. A neurologic deficit was present in only two patients (both with cervical lesions). Osteoid osteoma is the most common cause of painful scoliosis in adolescents. This deformity can be corrected with resection of the osteoid osteoma alone if surgery is within 15 months

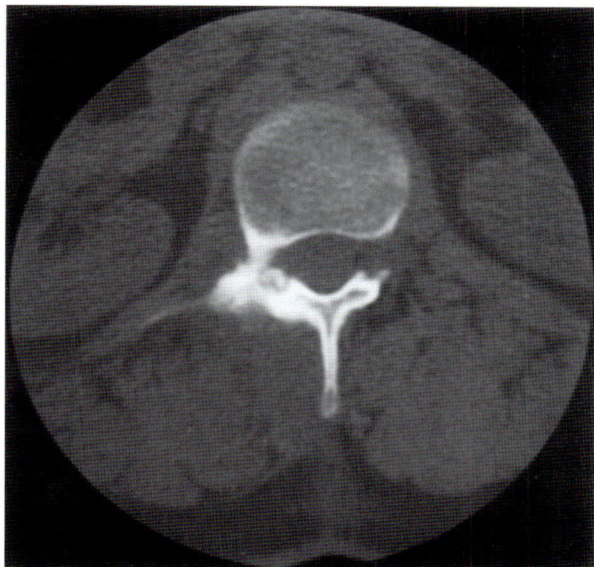

FIGURE 106-5. Osteoid osteoma. CT of the lumbar spine demonstrates the distinctive osteoblastic lesion or nidus with the associated surrounding zone of sclerosing bone in a typical osteoid osteoma. In this patient, it involves the facet joint.

of onset of symptoms or before the development of a structural curve.[51] Fifteen months appears to be the critical cut-off point after which spontaneous correction does not occur after surgery.

Imaging

Osteoid osteomas are best imaged by CT, which reveals the lucent nidus with surrounding sclerotic changes. Technetium bone scans show an intense focal increase in activity on intermediate and delayed films at the site of the lesion. However, lesions may be missed on plain radiographs and MRI scans.

Management

Because treatment with nonsteroidal anti-inflammatory drugs (NSAIDs) is so effective for pain relief, conservative therapy is an option. Long-term NSAID therapy is particularly attractive when surgical morbidity would be high due to the complexity of a given case. However, chronic NSAID treatment is associated with significant side effects, and in a small number of cases the lesion may ultimately be found to be an osteoblastoma. Therefore, the definitive treatment for osteoid osteomas is complete surgical excision.[50,52] In more than 95% of cases, resection results in almost immediate pain relief. When a complete resection is not achieved and the lesion recurs, reoperation is recommended. Radiation is not recommended, either alone or following surgery.[5] In patients who are not good surgical candidates, radiofrequency ablation has recently emerged as an additional therapeutic option. Initially avoided due to concerns of causing thermal injury to neural structures, radiofrequency ablation has since been shown to provide complete pain relief in a number of patients. The reported pain relief rates range between 77% and 100%, complication rates between 5% and 24%, and recurrence rates between 5% and 12%.[35]

Osteoblastoma

Osteoblastomas are uncommon lesions, constituting approximately 0.36% of all primary bone tumors that are treated with surgery. Thirty-three percent of these lesions occur in the spine. Osteoblastomas represent a histologic continuum of osteoid osteoma, the difference being the size of the lesions. Osteoblastomas are lesions that are greater than 1.5 cm in diameter. Patients are usually in their second or third decade at presentation,[52] and there is a male:female predominance of 2:1.7.[52] Osteoblastomas are distributed throughout the spine, and in the series by Boriani et al.,[53] 16 of 30 lesions occurred in the lumbar spine, 8 in the thoracic spine, and 6 in the cervical spine. Two thirds of these lesions are confined to the dorsal elements. As observed with other benign spinal neoplasms, pain is the most common presenting complaint, and it may be associated with scoliosis and neurologic deficit. Unlike osteoid osteomas, osteoblastomas can progressively enlarge. The radiologic workup of these lesions should include plain radiography and CT. These scans may show a well-defined, lobulated, lytic, expansile mass that usually involves the neural arch structures. Fifty percent of lesions are radiolucent with a sclerotic rim. As with osteoid osteomas, MRI is often less informative than CT for defining these lesions.[54] Unlike osteoid osteomas, bone scans often are not necessary for diagnosis but may be helpful with smaller lesions. Osteoblastomas should be treated surgically with total resection. Approximately 10% of lesions recur after surgery.

It is important to remember that both osteoid osteoma and osteoblastoma should be considered in any young patient with back or neck pain, painful scoliosis, or radicular pain. These lesions often become symptomatic before they are visible on plain radiographs.

Management

Although osteoid osteoma and osteoblastoma form a histologic continuum, and the duration of symptoms is prolonged in many cases because of diagnostic difficulties, a number of differences exist. Osteoid osteomas are small lesions that are not progressive and that have even been described to exhibit spontaneous regression. Patients with these lesions are treated most commonly because of persistent pain. Conversely, osteoblastomas demonstrate progressive enlargement, with the potential for malignant transformation. Thus, they are managed for pain, progressive enlargement, and the destructiveness of the lesion. In addition, there is a much higher recurrence rate with osteoblastomas.

Both osteoid osteomas and osteoblastomas may cause scoliosis and neurologic deficit, the latter being more common with osteoblastoma. Surgical resection is the first line of treatment, and when total is associated with cure.[55,56] With larger, aggressive lesions, radiation therapy and embolization may be considered as adjuncts to surgical resection, but the potential risks of radiation therapy must be considered, including the risk of sarcomatous transformation.

Osteochondromas

Osteochondromas constitute 9.2% of all primary bone tumors that are treated surgically, but they rarely occur in the spine (2.5% of all osteochondromas). They consist of cartilage-covered cortical bone with underlying medullary bone, both types of bone being contiguous with their counterparts in the parent bone. The cartilaginous cap undergoes ossification to form the osteochondroma.

Histologically, the cartilaginous cap and underlying bone are identical to normal bone. The tumors can be solitary or multiple, and most present in the third decade. There is a male:female predominance of 2:1. The lesions affect the transverse or spinous processes, and half of all lesions occur in the cervical spine. Lesions are best diagnosed by plain radiography and CT. Patients usually have localized pain, although neurologic deficit can also occur.[57] Rarely, osteochondromas may also be a manifestation of hereditary multiple osteochondromas. Only 1% of solitary lesions undergo malignant transformation. Surgical excision is the treatment of choice.[58-60]

Other Benign Primary Spine Tumors

The other benign tumors that affect the spine are uncommon, as evidenced from Table 106-1. However, the indications for surgical intervention for these rare lesions and the goals of treatment are similar to those for the more common spine lesions already discussed.

Plasma Cell Tumors

Plasma cell tumors of the spine (multiple myeloma and solitary plasmacytoma) are the most common type of malignant primary tumors involving the spine (see Table 106-2). Multiple myeloma is the most common plasma cell tumor, characterized by multiple bony lesions, infiltration of the bone marrow by plasma cells, and a marked reduction of normal immunoglobulins.[26,61,62] Conversely, solitary plasmacytoma constitutes only 3% of plasma cell tumors. Up to 50% of plasmacytomas occur in the spine and most commonly occur in the thoracic spine, accounting for 24 of 33 cases in a recent series, though they have been reported throughout the spine.[63] Fifty percent of patients diagnosed with plasmacytoma ultimately develop multiple myeloma, most commonly within 2 years[64] (Fig. 106-6). Patients with this condition are characterized by one or, at most, two bony lesions. A bone scan can be used to identify additional lesions.[64] The incidence of multiple myeloma is the same in both males and females, whereas with solitary plasmacytoma, a twofold to threefold higher incidence is encountered in males. A small monoclonal spike that disappears with treatment may reflect local lesions only.

Plasma cell tumors of the spine usually present with pain and, in advanced cases, with myelopathy. The duration of symptoms before diagnosis may vary; however, in general, symptoms worsen considerably in the 6 to 12 months before presentation. The diagnosis of solitary plasmacytoma is established histologically by either a needle biopsy or an open procedure. In plasmacytoma, the bone marrow is negative for plasma cell infiltrates, and serum protein electrophoresis results are normal. Multiple myeloma is usually diagnosed definitively by a bone marrow biopsy, the presence of multiple bony lesions on bone survey, and an abnormal monoclonal immunoglobulin spike on serum or urine electrophoresis.[64] Most patients with multiple myeloma present with Bence Jones proteinuria, reflecting the spillover of monoclonal immunoglobulin fragments into the urine.

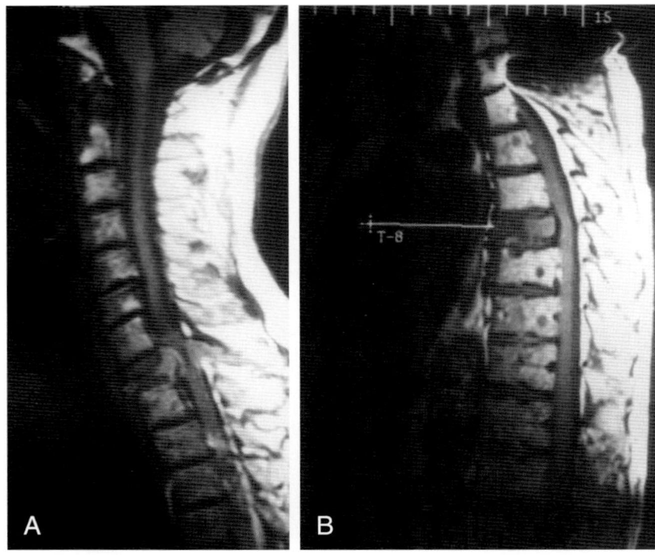

FIGURE 106-6. A 63-year-old man presenting with paraparesis and Brown-Séquard syndrome. **A,** Pathologic fracture involving T1 with retropulsion of bone and circumferential spinal cord compression by a solitary plasmacytoma (sagittal T1-weighted MRI). A bone scan and skeletal survey were negative for other lesions. **B,** A progressive increase in pain and paraparesis developed 18 months later. Sagittal T1-weighted MRI shows a pathologic fracture at T8 with spinal cord compression. Multiple other lytic lesions of bone, secondary to multiple myeloma, are also noted. Bone marrow aspirate revealed plasma cell infiltrates, and bone scan showed increased uptake in the left clavicle.

Management

The treatment of choice for solitary plasmacytoma in the absence of instability or rapid paralysis is radiation therapy. The dose of radiation to the spine for plasmacytoma varies from 35 to 50 Gy, although some oncologists favor larger doses. Local control rates of up to 96% and survival rates of up to 11 years have been reported.[64] It is recommended that patients with a diagnosis of solitary plasmacytoma be followed closely for the development of indices characteristic of multiple myeloma. Chemotherapy is generally withheld until progression to multiple myeloma is documented.[62] When the diagnosis of multiple myeloma is established, chemotherapy is indicated, although prognosis at that time is poor, with a median survival rate thereafter of 2 years and a 5-year survival rate of 18%.[47,62] Whether chemotherapy should be instituted after the diagnosis of solitary plasmacytoma of bone remains unclear.[62] Vertebroplasty can help relieve pain and improve the quality of life in patients without neurologic deficit.[65]

Because plasmacytomas are highly radiosensitive, surgical decompression and fusion are generally reserved for patients with progressive neurologic deficit and deformity. Studies have demonstrated that one can predict the risk of pathologic collapse by determining the extent of the involvement of the vertebral body.[66] It has been shown that patients with osteolytic lesions involving greater than 50% of the vertebral body are likely to require instrumentation. It has been recommended that surgical intervention be considered when the likelihood of future instability exceeds 50%, local kyphosis is greater than 20%, or there is translational deformity.[67]

Chordoma

Chordoma constitutes approximately 5% of malignant tumors involving the spine (see Table 106-2). The tumor originates from primitive remnants of the notochord. Fifty percent of all chordomas are sacrococcygeal, 40% are sphenoccipital, and the remaining 10% involve the mobile intermediate regions of the spine.[26,47,68,69] These tumors, considered to be of low-grade malignancy, are extremely difficult to resect because of their proximity to the spinal cord and cauda equina. In addition, in 5% to 10% of cases, they tend to metastasize within 1 to 10 years of the diagnosis. Fifty percent of all chordomas occur in the fifth to seventh decades of life, with a mean age of onset of approximately 50 years.[26,68,69] Men are twice as likely to be afflicted with this tumor as women.[70]

Chordomas arise from the vertebral body, with ensuing ventral and dorsal extension. Pain is the presenting symptom in 75% of cases and a radicular component in 10% of patients. More than two thirds of patients present with weakness or other neurologic deficits. Mean duration of symptoms at presentation is 14 months, with a range of 4 to 24 months.[71] In chordomas arising from the sacrum, 40% complain of rectal dysfunction, including constipation, tenesmus, or bleeding hemorrhoids. A palpable tumor on rectal examination can be identified in most patients.[1] These tumors can also affect two adjacent vertebral bodies, while sparing the intervertebral disc.

Histology

Histologically, chordomas consist of two cell types: a small, compact stellate cell that is considered to be the precursor of the more prevalent and larger physaliferous cell containing mucinous vacuoles.[1,68] These tumors have a characteristic lobular appearance on MRI. They can often be diagnosed by radiologic studies, including plain radiography. On plain radiographs, calcification can be observed in 40% of cases, and it is twice as likely to be observed by CT. Chordomas are generally avascular and are not associated with excessive intraoperative blood loss.

Grossly, chordomas appear lobulated and are often gray or partially translucent. The consistency varies from firm and focally ossified to a soft, myxoid, or semifluid material. There is generally a pseudocapsule separating the tumor from adjacent soft tissue, but the tumor is diffusely invasive within adjacent bone without clear margins.[1]

Management

Percutaneous CT-guided biopsy is generally recommended to establish a definitive working diagnosis. The optimal treatment of chordomas is wide en bloc resection.[69,70,72] The location of these lesions (close to neural structures) renders cure extremely unlikely. Some authors recommend a staged approach where first a posterior approach is performed to mobilize the posterior elements, free the dura from the tumor pseudocapsule, and place posterior instramentation, followed by an anterior approach to perform an en bloc vertebrectomy.[1] With involvement of the sacrococcygeal spine, resection can be accomplished by ventral, dorsal (Fig. 106-7), or combined approaches.[1,69,73-75] These approaches are geared for the widest possible resection of tumor, with sparing of as many nerves as possible.[69] Generally, sparing the S3 nerve root on either side may be sufficient to preserve bladder and fecal continence. Loss of sexual function also needs to be discussed with the patient preoperatively. Local recurrence in patients undergoing en bloc resection was 28%. Local recurrence in those where the tumor capsule was violated was 64%.[76]

Chordomas are not generally radiosensitive. However, because of the high risk of recurrence, postoperative radiation therapy is often recommended.[69,77,78] A retrospective study involving 21 patients with spinal chordomas favored a combination of surgery and irradiation over surgery alone.[78] There is no evidence that doses higher than 40 to 55 Gy are more likely to be associated with better results.[77] Neither is there evidence in support of treatment with more than a single fraction per day. The 40-year experience at the M.D. Anderson Cancer Center from 1954 to 1994 yielded 27 patients.[72] The median Kaplan-Meier survival estimate for the entire group was 7.4 years. The disease-free interval for patients undergoing radical resection was 2.3 years compared with 8 months for those undergoing subtotal excision ($P < .0001$). The addition of radiation to the group undergoing subtotal resection increased survival from 8 months to 2 years ($P < .02$). The often-quoted 5-year survival rate has ranged, depending on the source, from 50% to 77%, with a 10-year survival rate of 50%.[1,79] Approximately 30% of spinal chordomas develop metastases.[70]

Proton therapy has also been used as an adjuvant treatment; however; there is currently insufficient evidence to demonstrate that proton therapy is superior to conventional

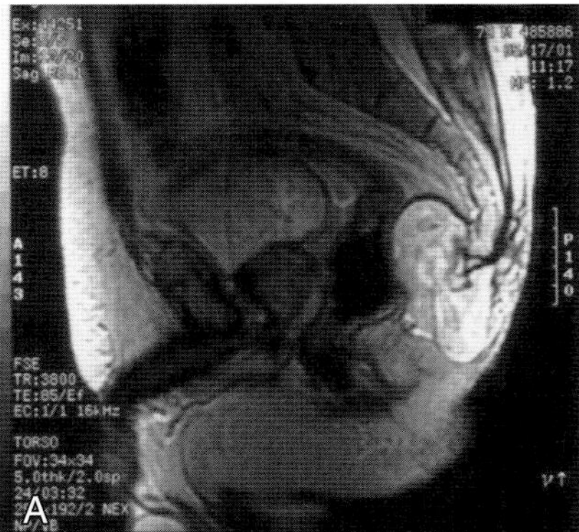

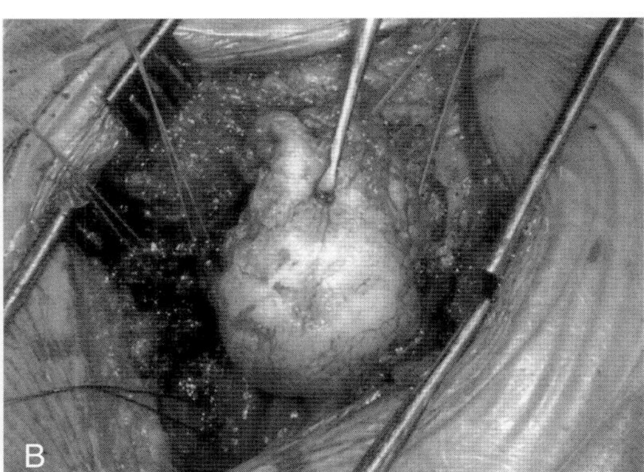

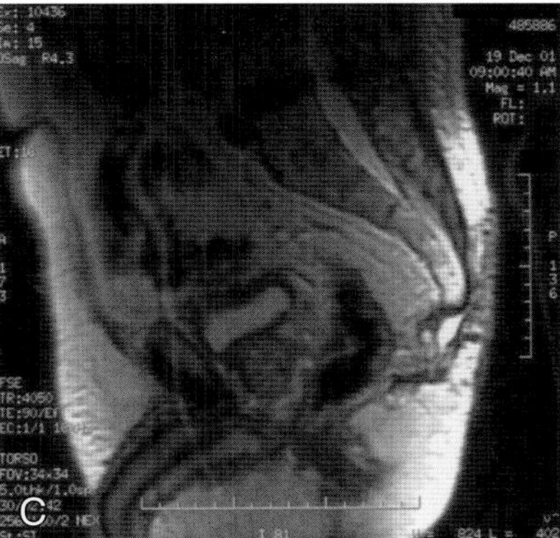

FIGURE 106-7. An 80-year-old man presenting with rectal bleeding resulting from rectal adenocarcinoma. During his workup, a presacral mass was discovered. **A,** T2-weighted MRI in the sagittal plane demonstrated a soft tissue mass arising from the lower sacrum and coccyx. **B,** Through a posterior midline approach, the chordoma was removable with distal amputation of the sacrum and coccyx. **C,** An MRI 7 months after surgery shows the resection bed devoid of tumor.

radiation therapy. In a review of the available literature, Brada et al. found the 5-year local progression-free survival rate of skull base chordomas to range from 54% to 64%.[80]

Chordomas are well known to be resistant to chemotherapy. In cases where all surgical and radiation therapy options have been exhausted, reports have been published showing responses to adriamycin-cisplatin or ifosfamide-adriamycin-platinum combinations, particularly in high-grade spindle cell sarcomas. More recently, evidence has emerged demonstrating that chordomas may be susceptible to agents targeting tyrosine kinase and angiogenesis pathways. Agents such as imatinib, erlotinib, and gefitinib have all shown promise in small series.[1]

Primary Spinal Ewing Sarcoma

Ewing sarcoma constitutes 6% of all primary malignant bone tumors[26,81]; however, primary spinal involvement occurs in only 3.5% of all patients with Ewing sarcomas.[81] This tumor afflicts males more commonly than females (2:1 ratio), and 88% of cases present in the first 2 decades of life.[26,81] In terms of the level of involvement, frequency decreases in a caudal-to-rostral progression, with more than 50% of all cases occurring in the sacrum.[26,81,82] The most common presenting feature is pain, with or without radicular involvement, depending on the level. In general, two of three patients present with a neurologic deficit (Fig. 106-8). The duration of symptoms can range from 1 to 30 months; most symptoms are 1 year or less in duration. A rectal mass may be encountered on examination, considering that there is sacral involvement in one of four patients with primary spinal Ewing sarcoma. In half of the cases, a lytic process is observed on plain radiographs, whereas other cases show blastic or mixed features.[81] A paravertebral soft tissue mass may occur independently or concurrently with bony involvement. This may be best appreciated on CT or MRI (see Figs. 106-8C and D). Confirmation of diagnosis has been accomplished more commonly by laminectomy, particularly in the presence of neurologic deficit. With the advent of CT-guided biopsies, needle aspiration has been undertaken in some patients.

Histology

Histologically, Ewing sarcoma consists of infiltrating sheets of small, round to oval cells with a scant amount of cytoplasm that tests positive for glycogen.[26] These tumors are fragile and

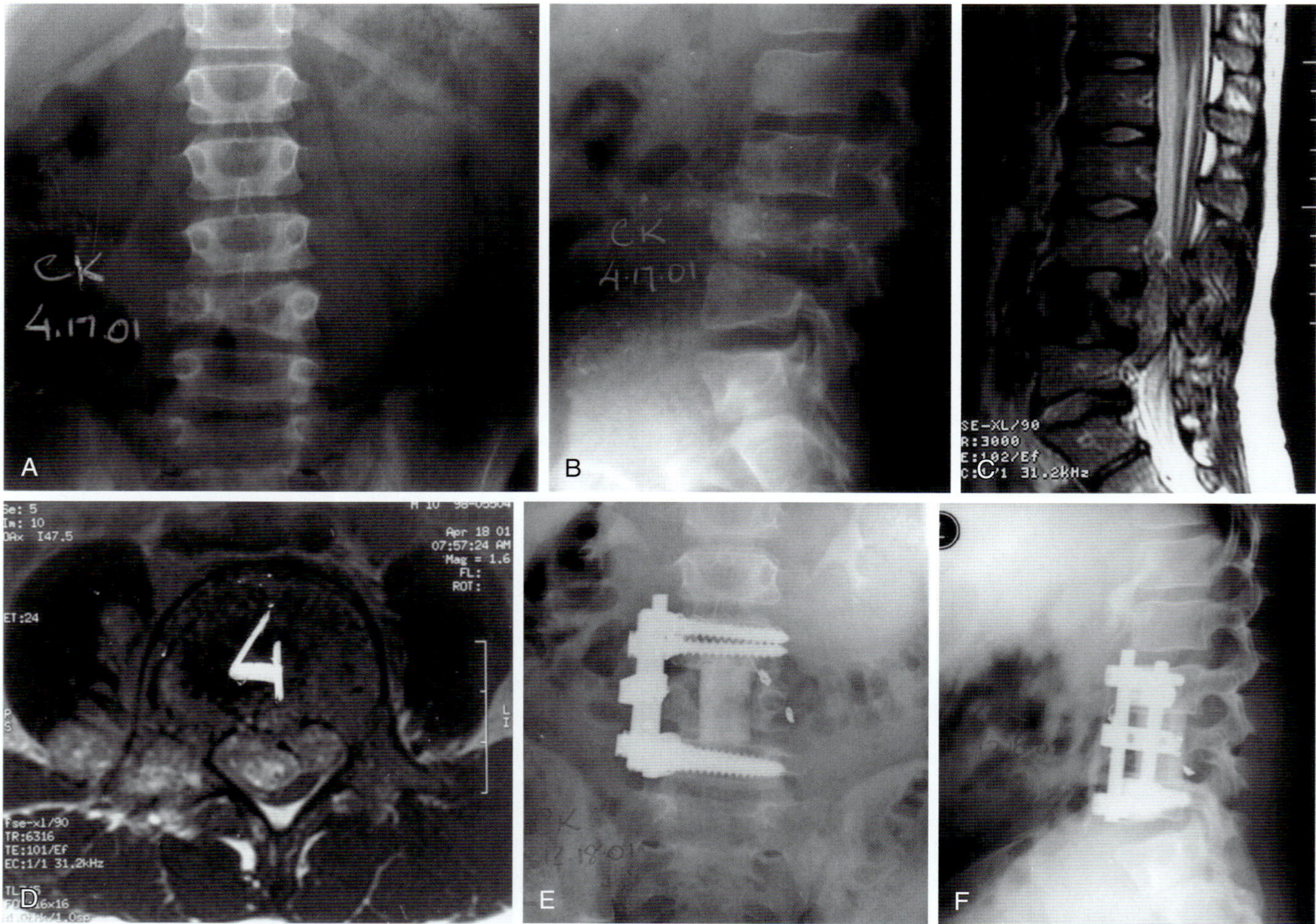

FIGURE 106-8. A 10-year-old boy presents with a 4-month history of low back pain and right leg weakness. Anteroposterior (**A**) and lateral (**B**) radiographs show a pathologic fracture of L4. T2-weighted sagittal (**C**) and axial (**D**) images show the exophytic Ewing sarcoma extending into the spinal canal and compressing the thecal sac. Because of tumor vascularity, the tumor was embolized preoperatively. Eight months postoperatively, radiographs in the anteroposterior (**E**) and lateral (**F**) projections show the alignment to be satisfactory, with the hardware and femoral allograft in place. The endovascular coils are seen in both projections.

vascular. Intraoperative bleeding can be extensive, particularly with spinal involvement. Grossly, these tumors are gelatinous in consistency and gray-white in color. The borders of these lesions are poorly outlined, with extension into the bony trabeculae as well as into the paravertebral soft tissues.

Management

Optimal treatment after diagnosis is provided by a combination of radiation therapy and chemotherapy.[82,83] Local radiation therapy to the spine is usually given at a dose of 50 to 55 Gy, with inclusion of an adequate margin as deemed appropriate by CT or MRI. Higher doses, when delivered to the spine, can be associated with postradiation myelopathy.[84] In a recent review of the data collected in the Cooperative Ewing's Sarcoma Study and the European Intergroup Cooperative Ewing's Sarcoma Study, local recurrence occurs in 22% of patients receiving radiation alone and 18.7% of those receiving surgery and radiation.[85] These recurrence rates were similar to those found in patients with Ewing sarcoma not involving the spine. Further analysis confirmed that surgical debulking prior to radiation did not improve outcomes and that surgery should be performed only if a wide resection is possible.[85]

The accepted chemotherapy protocol developed by the Intergroup Ewing's Sarcoma Study (IESS) consists of cyclophosphamide, vincristine, dactinomycin, and doxorubicin. This regimen, when administered in addition to local radiation therapy, has proven superior to a three-drug regimen with local irradiation or to a four-drug regimen with bilateral pulmonary radiation therapy.[82] The IESS protocol was tested in 342 patients and involved mostly appendicular, pelvic, and rib tumors. As expected, the most favorable results were encountered with distal appendicular disease, and the worst were encountered with pelvic involvement. Younger patients (<10 years of age) were observed to have an associated 71% 5-year survival, compared with 46% in patients older than 15 years of age. A more intense chemotherapeutic and radiation therapy protocol (the IESS-II protocol) was developed for the treatment of pelvic and sacral Ewing sarcoma.[83] With this regimen consisting of four-agent chemotherapy before and after high-dose local irradiation, a survival pattern was achieved that is comparable to that achieved for disease in nonpelvic sites. A large randomized trial was recently published that revealed that cyclophosphamide resulted in similar survival rates compared with ifosfamide when used in conjunction with vincristine, dactinomycin, and doxorubicin.[86] Furthermore, the addition of etoposide with ifosfamide improved survival in high-risk patients.[86]

The role of surgery in the treatment of spinal Ewing sarcoma remains controversial and is best performed after initial treatment with chemotherapy and radiation. Neoadjuvant therapy can reduce the size of the tumor and allow for adjacent bone to heal prior to surgical intervention. Indications for operation include high-grade epidural compression with symptomatic neurologic progression, stabilization, poor response to neoadjuvant chemotherapy or radiation therapy, and radiographic residual tumor postneoadjuvant treatment. When resection is attempted, maximal resection should be attempted. Evidence has shown that en bloc resection may improve local control but does not significantly improve survival.[87] When surgical excision is attempted, preoperative embolization is recommended[26,84] and routinely requires bony fusions with spinal implants to restore stability and prevent progressive deformity and neurologic deficit. Decompressive laminectomy alone may be associated with significant complications, including instability and progressive angulation.[81] When an adequate surgical margin is not achievable, postoperative radiation should be added to the surgical bed.

In an attempt to identify certain prognostic factors associated with Ewing sarcoma, a retrospective study was conducted with 46 patients, 43 with osseous involvement and 3 with extraosseous involvement. An attempted resection was performed in 12 patients but not in the remaining 34.[88] This analysis demonstrated that survival is improved in patients with local disease, tumors less than 500 mL in volume, peripheral involvement only, and who undergo gross total resection, compared with patients who have metastatic involvement, tumor volume greater than 500 mL, central involvement, and who do not undergo resection. This analysis suggested that aggressive surgery with radiation therapy might be an important prognostic factor. The best prognosis is provided by local irradiation and chemotherapy. A retrospective review of 36 patients who had primary involvement of the spine with Ewing sarcoma yielded a 5-year survival of 33%, with a mean survival of 2.9 years. Nine patients treated with the IESS regimen remained disease free at follow-up.[88]

In summary, all patients with Ewing sarcoma should initially be treated with chemotherapy. Surgical resection should be considered in all cases where the surgeon feels it is possible to achieve a complete resection. If the margins of the resection are less than 1 cm, as is often the case in spinal tumors, radiation therapy is added. Alternatively, chemotherapy and radiation treatment can be utilized alone when an adequate resection is not possible.[87]

Osteosarcoma

Osteosarcoma is the most common sarcoma of the spine, accounting for 3% to 15% of all primary tumors of the spine.[89] Among all sarcomas, however, spinal involvement is uncommon, present in only 37 of 1649 osteosarcomas (2.2%) (see Table 106-2). Osteosarcomas occur most commonly in the fourth decade of life,[89] have a slight predilection for males,[3] and are the most common primary malignant bone tumor in the pediatric population. In addition, osteosarcoma has one of the lowest survival rates among pediatric cancers.[87] In adults, prognosis with this tumor is especially poor. Shives et al.[90] reviewed 27 cases of spinal osteosarcoma and reported a median survival of 10 months from diagnosis.

Osteosarcomas can occur throughout the spine, though they are more common in the thoracic spine and sacrum and typically arise in the posterior elements.[89] Osteosarcomas usually arise de novo or may occur secondarily in previously irradiated bone, usually several years later (Fig. 106-9). Postirradiation osteosarcomas occurred in 16 of 600 cases in Dahlin and Coventry's series.[3] Paget disease is also a known risk factor for the development of osteosarcoma. Though as few as 1% of Paget disease patients go on to develop osteosarcoma, these patients make up as much as 50% of the patients in some registries.[89]

Diagnosis is often delayed due to the nonspecific nature of the symptoms. Pain is the most common presenting feature

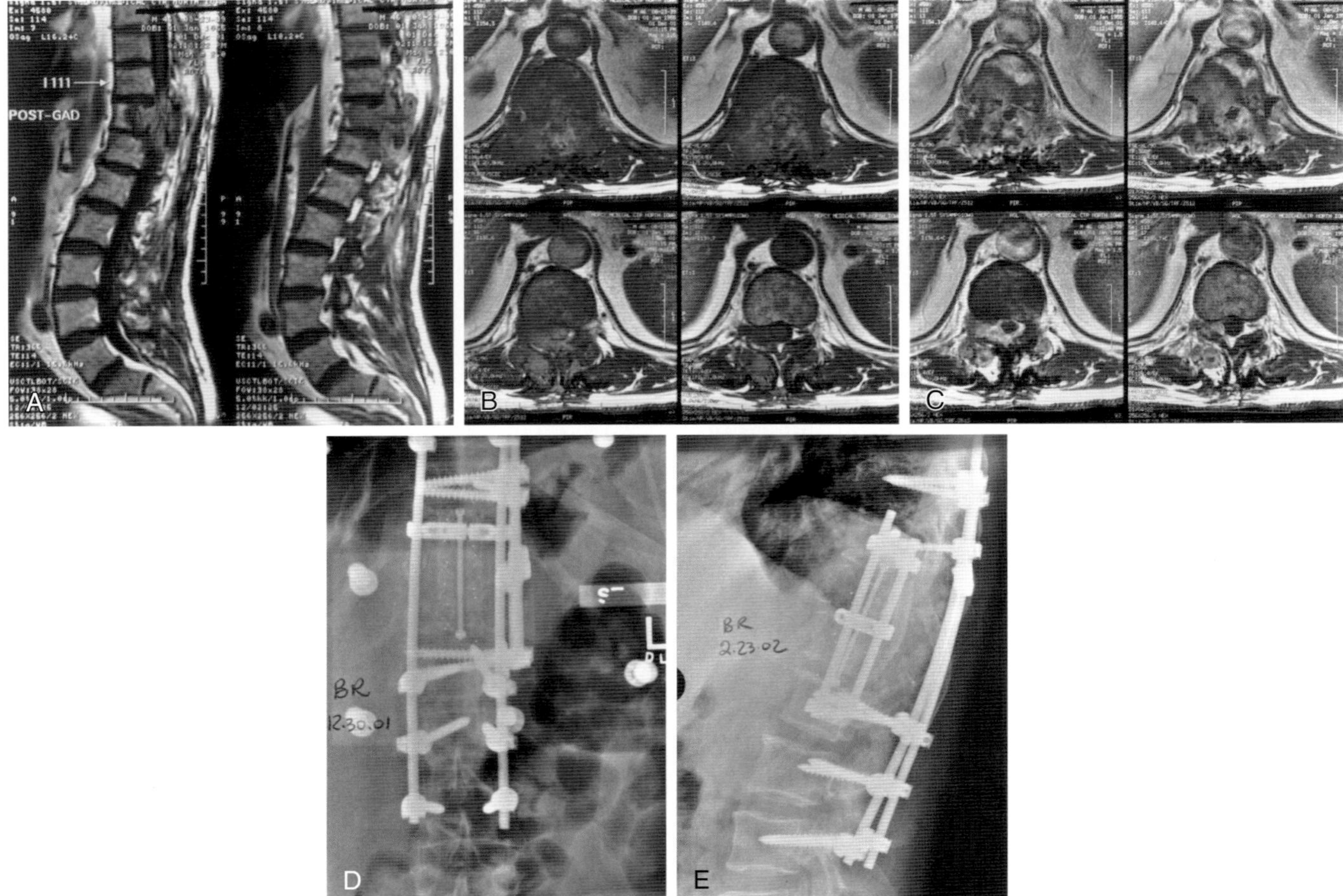

FIGURE 106-9. A 46-year-old man presented with rapidly progressive spinal pain and paraparesis of 3 months' duration. Past medical history indicated that 15 years earlier he had undergone surgery for a conus myxopapillary ependymoma. This had been followed by a full course of radiation therapy. His condition necessitated emergency decompression that revealed osteosarcoma. Sagittal T1-weighted and axial MRIs (**A**) without (**B**) and with (**C**) enhancement revealed a destructive bone tumor involving T11 and T12, with extension into the canal and neural foramina. The cord is circumferentially compressed. Three weeks following emergency decompression, the patient underwent T11-12 corpectomy, anterior stabilization, and posterior instrumentation from T8 to L3 (**D** and **E**). Motor performance improved, but pain control has remained a major problem.

and may be axial or radicular. Weakness is present in more than half of patients at the time of diagnosis, whereas loss of bowel and bladder function is generally seen only in advanced cases.

Pathologically, osteosarcomas are firm and calcified and consist mostly of sarcomatous connective tissue that forms osteoid tissue or bone. Histologically there are several different subtypes, but all osteosarcomas produce an osteoid matrix. Conventional osteosarcomas can be broken into three subtypes based on the matrix produced: osteoblastic (55%), fibroblastic (23%), and chondroblastic (22%) types.[3] Telangiectatic osteosarcomas are a separate classification of osteosarcoma that more closely resembles an ABC. In addition to the production of an osteoid matrix, there are also numerous blood-filled sinusoids.[89] Small-cell osteosarcoma is another subtype characterized by the presence of small cells with hyperchromatic nuclei and is positive for CD99. Sometimes confused for a Ewing sarcoma, small-cell osteosarcomas can be distinguished by the presence of an osteoid matrix. Similarily, epitheliod osteosarcoma is another subtype that is sometimes mistaken for a carcinoma, and again, the presence of an osteoid matrix leads to a correct diagnosis. Other reported variants include giant-cell osteosarcoma or osteoblastoma-like osteosarcoma; however, these are exceedingly rare.[89]

Radiographically, these tumors can have a fairly diverse appearance. Plain radiographs and CT scans of osteosarcomas may demonstrate osteolytic or osteoblastic changes. MRI is superior for showing tumor extent within the bone marrow and associated soft tissue and for delineating epidural tumor extension.

Management

Initial treatment with radiation as the primary treatment modality produced poor results. More recently, improvement in surgical techniques allowing more complete resections with improvement in adjuvant therapies has appeared to improve survival rates from the 10 months originally reported.[89] Multimodality therapy to treat spinal osteogenic sarcoma was originally described by Sundaresan et al.[91] in 1988. Eleven patients underwent neoadjuvant chemotherapy followed by aggressive resection and postoperative irradiation. In this limited series, there were five long-term survivors. A more recent series by Ozaki et al.[50] reported on 22 patients who received a neoadjuvant chemotherapy regimen according to the Cooperative Osteosarcoma Study Group (COSS) followed by resection. Four different chemotherapy protocols were used. All patients received preoperative high-dose methotrexate and doxorubicin in combination with a variety of other agents, including cisplatin, ifosfamide, bleomycin, actinomycin D, and alfa-interferon. COSS 96 used both preoperative and postoperative chemotherapy. Twelve patients underwent tumor resection, including two wide, three marginal, and seven intralesional excisions. Eight patients received radiation therapy. The median survival was 23 months. Patients with metastases (p = .004), large tumors (>10 cm) (p = .010), and sacral tumors (p = .048) had a worsened survival rate compared with those with no metastases, small tumors, and nonsacral tumors. There was a significant difference between the 17 patients who underwent intralesional excision or no surgery and the 5 patients who underwent marginal or wide excisions (p = .033). Postoperative irradiation extended overall survival in patients who underwent intralesional or no resection (p = .059).[50] In this series, patients received conventional external photon beam irradiation (median tumoral dose 45 Gy). No patient underwent either proton beam or IMRT irradiation.

Based on the available information, the Spine Oncology Study Group recommends that all patients with osteosarcoma of the spine are treated with neoadjuvant chemotherapy. Surgical resection should be attempted when it is felt a complete resection can be achieved and is associated with an improvement in survival and local control.[87] Postoperative radiation should also be considered to further improve survival.

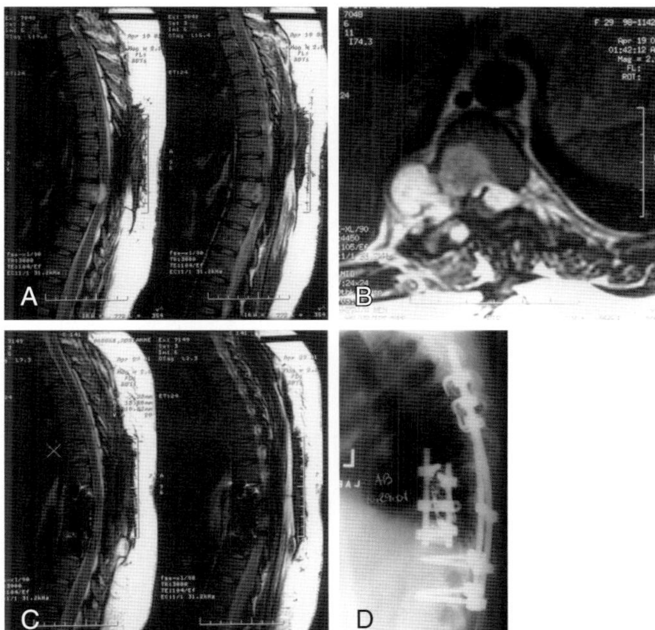

FIGURE 106-10. A 29-year-old woman presented with pain and paraparesis necessitating emergency decompression 5 months earlier. The pathologic condition was low-grade chondrosarcoma. Sagittal (**A**) and axial (**B**) MRIs show a tumor arising from the body of T10 extending into the canal compressing the cord primarily on the patient's left side. The tumor also extends into the paravertebral space on the right side. Through a right thoracotomy approach, the patient underwent a T10 corpectomy with tumor resection and anterior stabilization. Because of recurrence and paraparesis, posterior decompression with instrumentation was necessary 5 months later. **C,** Postoperative sagittal MRI shows the decompression and the hardware artifact. **D,** Plain lateral radiograph shows the anterior titanium mesh graft and the anterior and posterior screw-and-hook fixation. The patient received postoperative radiation and has subsequently required further surgery for recurrence.

Chondrosarcoma

Chondrosarcomas are primary malignant tumors arising from cartilaginous elements. They are rare tumors, constituting 892 of the 5751 malignant skeletal tumors (see Table 106-2). In this series, 54 tumors (6%) occurred in the spine. Like osteosarcomas, chondrosarcomas show a predilection for males; however, unlike osteosarcomas, they occur in middle-aged and older patients. Chondrosarcoma may arise de novo as a primary lesion or may occur as a secondary tumor from a preexisting solitary osteochondroma (1%) or from hereditary multiple exostosis (20%).[92]

Pain, the most common presenting symptom, may be indolent, leading to a delay in diagnosis. Pathologically, chondrosarcomas do not demonstrate neoplastic osteoid tissue or bone evolving from a sarcomatous matrix. Instead, they display nuclear pleomorphism, with numerous mitoses surrounded by a myxoid matrix. In addition to this conventional chondrosarcomatous appearance, variants may be subcategorized as predominantly myxoid, mesenchymal, or dedifferentiated.

Imaging

Plain radiographs and CT scans demonstrate osteolytic lesions with a calcified matrix. The amount of calcification correlates with the degree of differentiation. MRI is the study of choice for demonstrating the adjacent soft tissue and epidural extent of tumor spread. MRI also demonstrates the heterogeneity of the lesion (Fig. 106-10). Of note, lesions that are more malignant tend to have larger amounts of soft tissue components, more irregular calcification, and more extensive bone destruction.

Management

Although chondrosarcomas are slow-growing lesions, they have a relatively poor overall prognosis. Survival correlates with degree of malignancy. Because of the spinal location, total resection is usually not possible. This, combined with resistance of the tumor to chemotherapy and radiation therapy, establishes a tendency for local recurrence of tumor. However, small numbers of long-term survivors with low-grade lesions have been observed. Such patients can be treated with multiple local excisions. Complete excision is the goal of surgery, considering the propensity of the tumor for local recurrence.

In a series of predominantly low-grade chondrosarcomas, Boriani et al.[93] showed improved local control with marginal or wide resections compared with intralesional resection. In this series, 17 of 18 patients undergoing intralesional resection had a local recurrence within 36 months. Two patients who had en bloc resections but contaminated margins (i.e., intralesional resections) experienced recurrence at 12 and 32 months, respectively. At a median follow-up of 81 months, only one patient undergoing marginal or wide resection had recurrence at 48 months. The patients in this series had predominantly posterior-element tumors and no epidural extension.

Despite the relative radioresistance of chondrosarcoma, we recommend high-dose 3D-CRT, using either proton beam or IMRT, following resection in patients with high-grade tumors following either intralesional resections or en bloc excisions with positive histologic margins.

Avoidance of Complications

Advances in radiologic imaging, especially MRI and CT, have resulted in better preoperative planning. Knowing the extent and precise location of the tumor certainly can result in an optimally planned surgical approach. Improvements in preoperative angiography and embolization have significantly decreased intraoperative blood loss with some of the more vascular benign and malignant tumors. With lesions such as the ABC, the use of the cell saver has resulted in a decreased requirement for administration of blood products. This, in turn, can significantly decrease the likelihood of intraoperative or postoperative complications from transfusion. With benign lesions especially, because there is often adequate time for preoperative planning, the practice of autodonation of blood can significantly decrease the risks of transfusion reaction.

Wound healing, especially in patients who have previously undergone extensive radiation therapy, can be a significant problem. The plastic surgeon can assist significantly in planning the surgical incision to maximize options for wound closure.

Often, incomplete lesion removal results in early recurrence. When appropriate, every attempt should be made to perform the procedure definitively during the first operation. To achieve the best outcomes with the least morbidity, the surgical team dealing with these lesions must be very comfortable with a variety of ventral and dorsal approaches to the spine, so that the best method can be selected for the lesion at hand.

After the tumor has been removed and the spinal cord and nerve roots decompressed, bone grafting, with or without instrumentation, should be considered. Many of the complications that result from spine surgery involve the destabilizing effects of surgery. If spinal instability has resulted from the tumor or the surgical treatment of the tumor, it is necessary to supplement the surgical procedure with a fusion of the unstable segments.

Over time, most spinal instrumentation constructs fatigue, loosen, and fail unless bony fusion ensues. In the case of malignant disease, the limited life expectancy of the patient may, in fact, make bony fusion unnecessary. On the other hand, when clinicians are dealing with benign disease, it is important that they recognize the limitations of instrumentation without fusion. The purpose of the instrumentation is to maintain stability and proper spinal alignment while the bony fusion is occurring. A fusion is much more likely to occur if movement at the fusion site is minimized.

One of the disadvantages of using metal implants is their interference with CT and MRI. Some of the new alloys produce fewer imaging artifacts, and these alternatives, although more expensive, should be considered in some cases. Titanium implants have major advantages over stainless steel in MRI tumor recurrence. Titanium implants should be standard for spine tumor reconstruction. Other materials such as carbon fiber have been adopted to lessen artifact and improve imaging. They readily show tumor recurrence, as well as osteointegration of bone graft, on imaging.[94]

Although the goal of surgical treatment of benign tumors involving the spine is usually total removal of the pathologic process, in some situations the massive size of the lesion, its benign nature, and the overall age and status of the patient need to be considered in the decision-making process. Overaggressive surgery should be avoided. The unnecessary removal of additional bone can further compromise future stability and may necessitate more elaborate stabilization procedures than might otherwise be required.

The only legitimate method of acquiring a cure in patients with both benign and malignant tumors involving the spine is total removal of the lesion. Although total removal is often impossible to accomplish with malignant tumors, it should certainly be the goal with many benign lesions. Clearly, with a malignant, diffuse process, extremely radical resections may be unwarranted.

Management of Complications

The best way to deal with complications of spine surgery is to minimize their occurrence. Some of the more common complications include inadequate wound healing (possibly related to previous radiation therapy or infection), cerebrospinal fluid leaks, deep infections, and inadequate stabilization efforts.

Cerebrospinal fluid leaks should be treated aggressively, because a persistent leak significantly increases the likelihood of infection. Although it is occasionally possible to stop a leak by simply reinforcing the skin closure with additional sutures, methods that are more elaborate are sometimes necessary. Spinal drainage via a catheter placed somewhat remote to the wound site may decrease the pressure head and allow for proper wound healing. However, if the site of the dural injury is known, it is often more appropriate to reopen that section of the wound and repair the site of the dural leak. In other cases, unhealthy, nonviable tissue overlying the dura mater may require debridement so that more viable tissue can be approximated. For patients who have received previous radiation therapy or undergone multiple surgical procedures, the assistance of a plastic surgeon may be valuable.

A deep wound infection often complicates stabilization efforts. Clearing an infection in a previously irradiated wound may be almost impossible. Spinal instability makes it necessary to leave the instrumentation in place while the infection is brought under control. This allows time for the bony fusion to mature. In some cases, the implant can be left in place, and the construct salvaged.

The need for adequate and appropriate nutritional supplementation cannot be overstated. In addition, where the wound is open, continuous wound suction or vacuum-assisted closure, and hyperbaric oxygen can make a substantial difference.

Summary

Primary tumors that involve the spinal axis, although rare, are often best managed by surgery. It may be the only method to effect a cure in some patients. It is important for clinicians to recognize that they should be prepared to achieve a total removal of this lesion, if the potential gain justifies the morbidity. A subtotal removal may require early reoperation. Certainly, the best time to accomplish total tumor removal is at the first surgical procedure. Proper preoperative planning and, when appropriate, preoperative embolization often result in satisfactory patient outcomes.

KEY REFERENCES

Bilsky MH, Gerszten P, Laufer I, et al: Radiation for primary spine tumors. *Neurosurg Clin North Am* 19:119–123, 2008.

Boriani S, Weinstein JN, Biagini R: Primary bone tumors of the spine. Terminology and surgical staging. *Spine (Phila Pa 1976)* 22:1036–1044, 1997.

Fenoy AJ, Greenlee JD, Menezes AH, et al: Primary bone tumors of the spine in children. *J Neurosurg* 105:252–260, 2006.

McMaster ML, Goldstein AM, Bromley CM, et al: Chordoma: incidence and survival patterns in the United States, 1973–1995. *Cancer Causes Control* 12:1–11, 2001.

Ozaki T, Flege S, Liljenqvist U, et al: Osteosarcoma of the spine: experience of the Cooperative Osteosarcoma Study Group. *Cancer* 94:1069–1077, 2002.

Sundaresan N, Rosen G, Boriani S: Primary malignant tumors of the spine. *Orthop Clin North Am* 40:21–36, 2009.

Weinstein JN: Surgical approach to spine tumors. *Orthopedics* 12:897–905, 1989.

REFERENCES

The complete reference list is available online at expertconsult.com.

CHAPTER 107

Spondylectomy for Spinal Tumors

Jean-Paul Wolinsky | Daniel M. Sciubba | Jorge Lastra-Power | Ziya Gokaslan

Spondylectomy is defined as removal of an entire segment of the spine, including the vertebral body, pedicles, superior and inferior articulating processes, pars, transverse processes, lamina, and spinous process. Removal of the entire spinal segment en bloc is possible only with sacrifice of the spinal cord or the cauda equina, as the spinal cord and cauda equina lie within the spinal canal, incarcerated by the spine. Tumors within the spine can be removed either in a piecemeal fashion (intralesional) or en bloc (in one piece, without violation of the tumor margin). To achieve an en bloc resection of a tumor, the technique of a total spondylectomy can be employed (Fig. 107-1). As a point of semantics, the tumor is removed en bloc, but the spondylectomy is usually not an en bloc spondylectomy.[1]

Techniques for en bloc resection of a tumor are complex and entail significant risk to the patient; they are reserved for certain tumor pathologies that oncologically may benefit from such resection. In general, when such an operation is contemplated, the tumor should be a solitary tumor without evidence of metastasis. The usual indication for an en bloc resection is malignant primary bone tumors when resection may result in cure or long-term tumor-free survival for the patient. Such tumor pathologies include chordoma, chondrosarcoma, and osteosarcoma. Other, less aggressive primary bone tumors for which en bloc resection is contemplated include giant cell tumor, aneurysmal bone cyst, osteoid osteoma, and osteoblastoma. Exceptions to this rule occur, and in certain circumstances of solitary metastasis to the spine (such as renal cell carcinoma or breast cancer), some oncologists advocate the use of this technique for local tumor control. This is a highly contentious area of debate, and the use of en bloc resection is evolving, especially with the advent of other adjunctive therapies such as stereotactic radiosurgery for the spine.

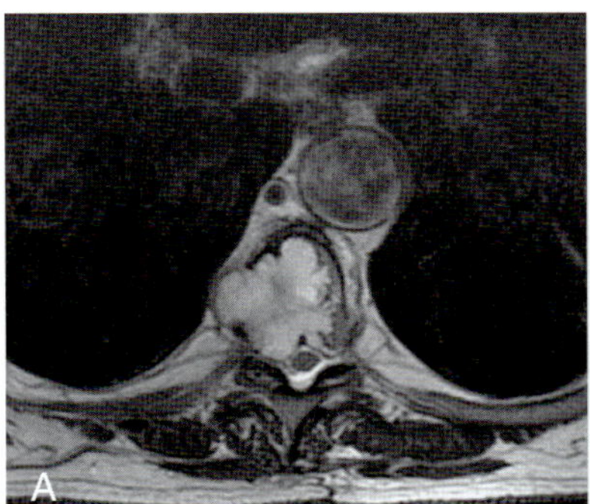

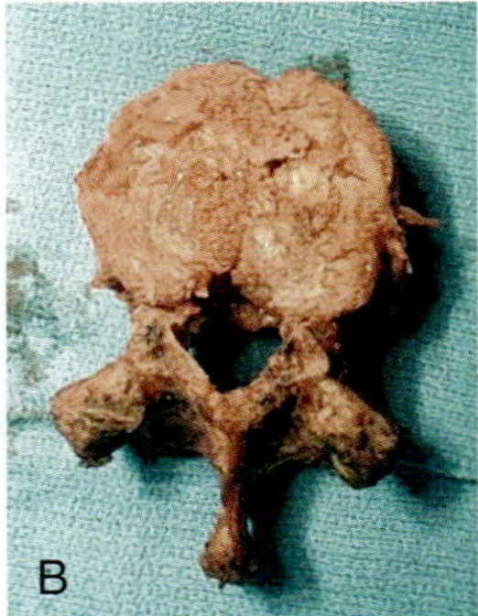

FIGURE 107-1. A, Preoperative axial T2-weighted MRI demonstrating tumor in the vertebral body without extension into the posterior elements. **B,** Pathology specimen of spondylectomy involving en bloc resection of the vertebral body and tumor; posterior elements were removed separately.

General Concepts and Surgical Planning

The anatomic location of the tumor to be removed within a particular vertebral segment or segments will dictate the steps in achieving an en bloc resection via a spondylectomy.[1] For simplicity, the planning can be divided into two stages: a preparatory stage and a stage in which the tumor is delivered. Accomplishment of the first stage, the preparatory stage, may require multiple procedures.

The goal of the preparatory stage is to free the tumor specimen from the surrounding structures so that the tumor can be delivered while the spinal cord and critical nerves are protected with minimal functional sacrifice. The goal of the delivery stage is to deliver the specimen in an en bloc fashion. As a general rule, the preparatory stage occurs on the side of the spinal cord, or thecal sac, opposite the tumor. The portion of the vertebral segment and the tumor to be removed as a single specimen are dissected as much as possible to mobilize the specimen during the preparatory stage.

In certain instances, vascular and neurologic structures may need to be sacrificed to free the en bloc specimen. The anticipated vascular complication and the deficit produced from doing so must be thoroughly understood and discussed with the patient before embarking on the treatment. Certain tumor architectures require more aggressive sacrifice that results in significant morbidity, the consequence of which must be balanced against the potential oncologic benefit and the patient's acceptance of a life with the expected permanent handicap that may result.

The vascular structures involved in the resection vary at different levels of the spine. In the cervical spine, a vertebral artery might need to be sacrificed to achieve a resection, and doing so might result in posterior fossa ischemia and stroke. In the thoracic spine, multiple segmental vessels might need to be ligated, increasing the risk of ischemia to the spinal cord. In the lumbar spine, the iliac arteries and veins might need to be manipulated or even bypassed, potentially causing ischemia to the bowel, kidneys, or lower extremities. Manipulation or sacrifice of the inferior vena cava and iliac vessels increases the chance for thrombus formation and consequent pulmonary embolus.

Neurologic sacrifice can be entertained only if the deficit that will be produced is tolerable to the patient's expectations and lifestyle acceptance. Sacrifice of a certain root alone might not produce a significant deficit, but combinations of roots sacrificed can be crippling (Table 107-1). C1-4 can usually be sacrificed without significant morbidity. Sacrifice of C3 and C4 together could result in diaphragm weakness. Cutting C5, C6, C8, or T1 usually results in profound weakness. Sacrifice in the thoracic spine (T2-12) will result in a bandlike distribution of numbness but usually has inconsequential motor loss. Sacrifice of L1 or L2 in isolation will produce weakness, but over time, patients usually are able to compensate for the loss quite well. L3 loss will result in quadriceps weakness and may require bracing of the knee to walk. L4 sacrifice can also result in quadriceps weakness, but the problem that is usually noted is proprioceptive difficulty of the knee joint. Without proper proprioception of the knee, a patient may find the knee week and can complain of the knee buckling at times during ambulation. L5 loss results in footdrop. S1 sacrifice is usually well tolerated but does results in gastocnemius weakness, which can make it difficult for a patient to stand on the toes. S4, S5, and the coccygeal nerves can usually be sacrificed without significant consequences. Loss of bilateral S2 and S3 nerve roots will result in loss of bowel, bladder, and sexual function. Unilateral S2 and S3 sacrifice usually allows a patient to have fairly normal bowel, bladder, and sexual function. Bilateral S3 sacrifice and S2 preservation will provide some function, but most patients will have difficulty with bowel, bladder, and sexual function.

TABLE 107-1

Deficits from Specific Nerve Root Sacrifice

Nerve Sacrifice	Deficit
C3 and C4	Possible diaphragm weakness
C5	Deltoid weakness
C6	Bicep weakness
C8 or T1	Hand intrinsics weakness
T2–T12	Dermatomal sensory loss
L1 or L2	Iliopsoas weakness, usually compensated over time
L3	Quadriceps weakness
L4	Quadriceps weakness, knee proprioceptive difficulty, and footdrop
L5	Footdrop
S1	Minimal deficit
Unilateral S2 and S3	Bowel/bladder/sexual function abnormal but functional
Bilateral S2 and S3	Loss of bowel/bladder/sexual function
Bilateral S3 with S2 sparing	Some bowel/bladder/sexual function
S4, S5, and coccygeal nerves	Dermatomal sensory loss

Planning for postoperative adjunct therapies is necessary in contemplating a surgical approach. If postoperative high-dose radiation therapy such as proton beam irradiation is a possibility, then this should be taken into account preoperatively. Structures that may be at risk of injury from the radiation may benefit from reposition or from protection with complex plastic surgery flaps. It may be desirable to avoid certain approaches, such as the transoral and transmandibular approaches, which have considerable risk of postoperative pharyngeal dehiscence and mandibular pseudarthrosis with adjuvant proton beam radiation therapy.

The first stage of the operation, the preparatory stage, is designed to mobilize the tumor specimen so that it can be eventually delivered and at the same time minimize the neurologic and vascular impact on the patient. This stage, as a general rule, starts on the side of the spinal cord or thecal sac opposite the tumor. The spinal segment can be thought of as a ring of bone that encases the spinal cord. In order for a portion of that ring to be delivered away from the spinal cord, a portion of it will have to be resected, creating a window that is at least as large as the diameter of the spinal canal. This will allow the spinal cord and dura to pass through this window as the remaining portion of the ring, with the specimen, is delivered away from the cord. For simplicity, this chapter describes the technique for en bloc resection starting in the thoracic spine and then the technique for the lumbar spine, and finally the technique for the cervical spine will be delineated. Nuances for each section of the spine will be discussed in more detail. This chapter does not describe the techniques of en bloc sacral resections.

Level-Specific Challenges

Thoracic Spine (T2-12)

The thoracic spine (T2-12) has a unique advantage over other spinal segments in that the nerve roots in this region can be sacrificed with minimal morbidity. In performing a multilevel spondylectomy, increasing the number of nerve roots and segmental vessels that are sacrificed increases the risk of ischemic injury to the cord. The exact tolerance of the human spinal cord for ischemia has not yet been defined, and there is probably a fair amount of variability between patients. Kato et al. have described a canine model, in which they set out to determine the number of segmental vessels that can be ligated before ischemia occurs.[2] They found that the interruption of bilateral segmental arteries of four or more consecutive levels, including the level of the Adamkiewicz artery, risks producing ischemic spinal cord dysfunction.

Tumors that are located ventrally, in the vertebral body, will need to undergo a preparatory stage from a dorsal approach. The approach is a standard midline approach with a subperiosteal exposure and exposure of the level of interest and two to three levels above and below index level(s) (Fig. 107-2A). Laterally, the exposure is carried out over the ribs for at least 6 cm on either side. Preoperatively, the MRI and CT are examined critically to understand exactly how far into the dorsal elements the tumor might extend. If the tumor extends into the pedicles and transverse process, this portion of the vertebral segment cannot be violated and must be dissected such that it can remain in continuity with the specimen[3] (Fig. 107-2B). The dorsal elements that are uninvolved with tumor at the index level(s) are removed, as are the dorsal elements above and below this level (Fig. 107-2C). Because the spinal column will be completely destabilized after the resection, instrumentation is placed at this part of the operation. The ribs at the index level(s) and the level above and below are cut 6 cm lateral to the transverse processes and, if not involved in tumor, are removed and retained as graft material. Care is taken not to injure the neurovascular bundle or pleura ventral to the rib.

The segmental vessels are traced from the rib to the foramen. A dissection plane is opened, keeping the segmental vessels ventral, opening the fatty plane between the vessel and the vertebral body. Staying in this plane with the dissection will allow the inferior vena cava and the aorta to remain ventral and away from the vertebral body and tumor. The radicular branches coming off the segmental vessels that supply the spinal roots and spinal cord are ligated and cut. Staying in this plane, keeping the segmental vessels ventral in the dissection plane, will eventually allow the dissection to be carried ventral the vertebral body and dorsal to the aorta and vena cava. As this dissection plane is developed from both the left and right sides of the patient, the aorta, vena cava, and esophagus will be kept out of the field and protected from the spine (Fig. 107-2D). A silastic sheet can be placed in this dissection plane, protecting these vascular structures and the pleura. Attention is then turned to the spinal canal. The nerve roots of the index level(s) are ligated proximal to the dorsal root ganglia and are cut. Ligating the roots proximal to

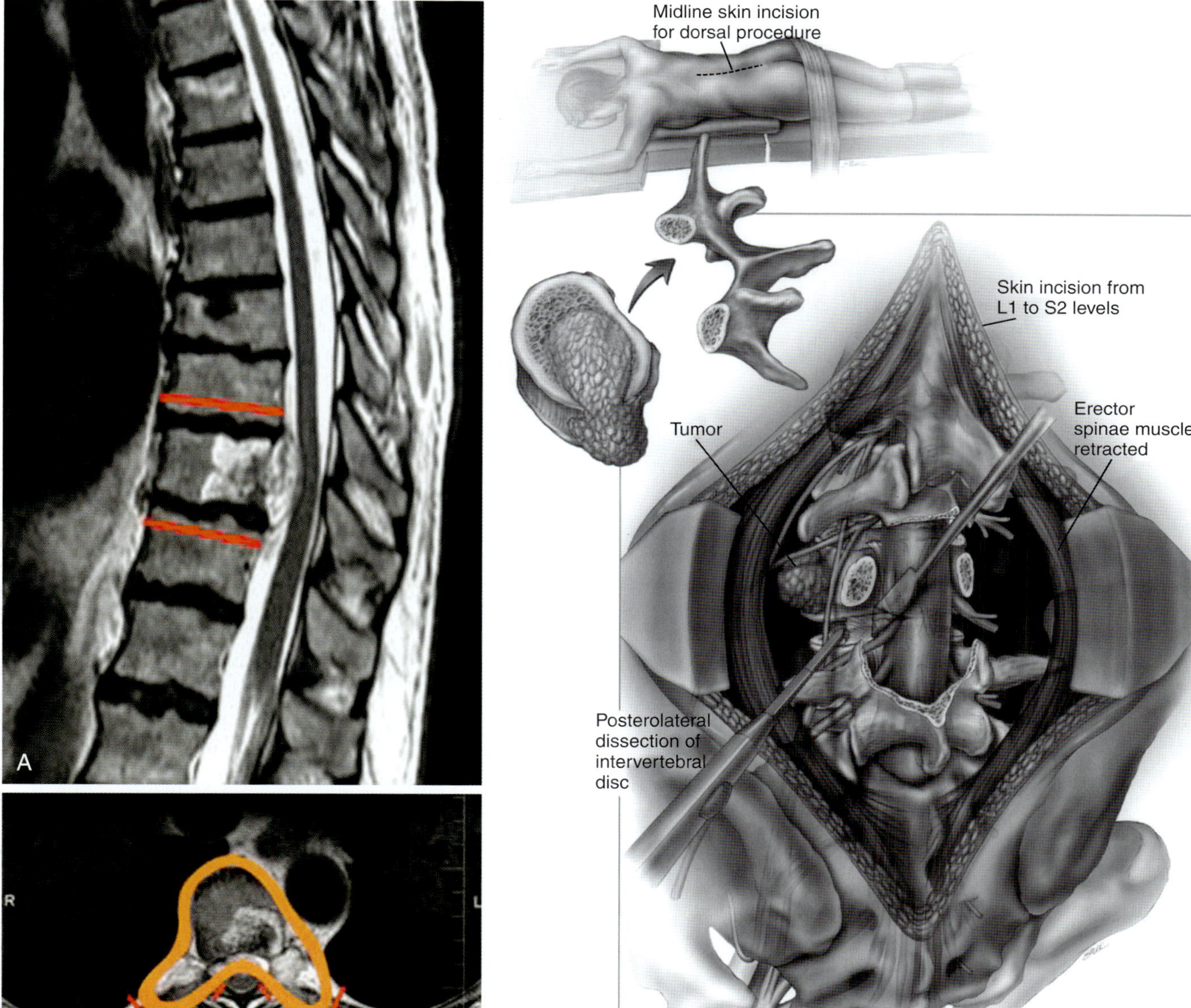

FIGURE 107-2. A, Preoperative sagittal T2-weighted MRI showing rostral and caudal planned osteotomies (*red*). **B,** Preoperative axial T2-weighted MRI showing planned laminar and rib osteotomies (*red*). The planned en bloc specimen is outlined in *orange*. **C,** Posterior exposure and removal of posterior elements.

Figure continues on following page

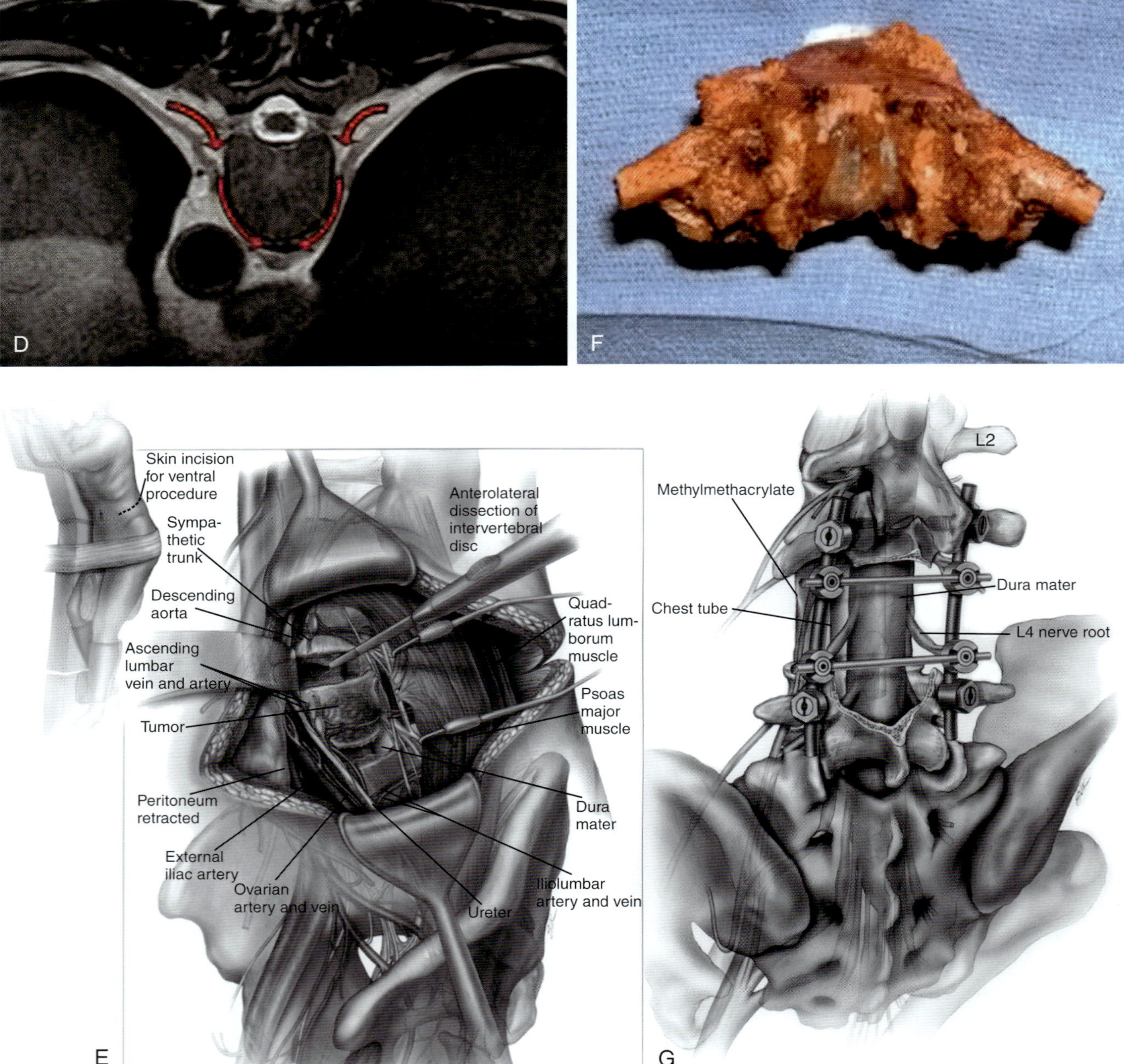

FIGURE 107-2, cont. D, Dissection plane (*red*) between vertebral body and segmental vessels. **E,** Delivery of en bloc specimen. **F,** En bloc pathology specimen. **G,** Reconstruction.

the dorsal root ganglia minimizes the chance of developing long-term chronic pain. The epidural plane is then defined, and if tumor capsule enters this plane, the epidural space is dissected, preserving the tumor capsule. Tomita saws are placed encircling the spinal column, one rostral and one caudal to the tumor. The final assembly of the instrumentation is completed, and by using the Tomita saws, the osteotomies are completed. The specimen is now free, completing the preparatory stage. The en bloc specimen is now gently rotated away from the spinal cord and delivered out through the space created by removing the ribs (Figs. 107-2E and F). The ventral vertebral defect is reconstructed, and the grafting and closure are then performed (Fig. 107-2G).

Tumors bounded by pleura, in which the pleura will need to remain with the specimen to obtain a negative margin, will need to be prepared in a slightly different fashion. Rather than approaching the tumor from an entirely dorsal approach, a ventral approach is added. The first steps of the preparatory stage are the same as those in the entirely dorsal approach. In contrast to the entirely dorsal approach, however, the ventral aspect of the spine will need to be dissected from a ventral approach to leave the pleura intact over the

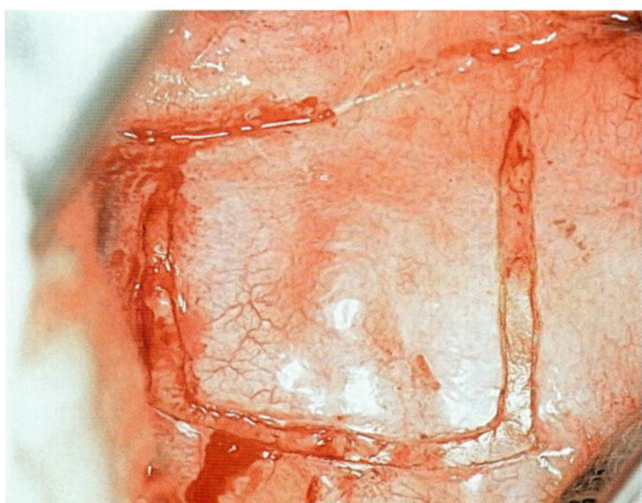

FIGURE 107-3. Pleural margin.

specimen (Fig. 107-3). The ribs need not be dissected as far laterally as is done in the entirely dorsal approach, and rather than resecting the ribs, the ribs need to be sectioned only beyond the lateral extent of the tumor. The sectioning of the pleura, osteotomies through the disc space, and then the delivery of the tumor will take place through a ventral exposure. The ventral exposure will take the form of either a thoracotomy or a thoracoscopic approach. After the exposure is completed, the segmental vessels coming off the aorta and going to the vena cava are identified, ligated, and cut. The pleura is cut in such a way as to create a margin for the tumor. The rostral and caudal osteotomies are completed, and the tumor specimen is delivered. The ventral spinal reconstruction is then completed, and the thoracotomy is closed.

The ability to sacrifice the thoracic nerve roots with little consequence allows the surgeon to approach the spine and perform the preparatory and delivery stages of an en bloc resection through an entirely dorsal approach. The need to maintain the pleura as a margin will dictate a second approach to achieve the desired resection. Because the nerve roots in the cervical and lumbar spine cannot be sacrificed without significant morbidity, in general, these segments of the spine will need at least two approaches to complete both stages of the en bloc resection.

Cervical Spine (C2-T1)

In the cervical spine, an en bloc resection of a tumor will only be realistic if the tumor is not involved in both vertebral arteries, and if the vertebral artery that remains after the tumor removal is able to provide an adequate blood supply to the posterior fossa. This will need to be determined in the preoperative period. If a cervical tumor involves one of the vertebral arteries (Fig. 107-4A) and would therefore require sacrifice of that vertebral artery, then it must be determined preoperatively whether the contralateral vertebral artery will be sufficient to provide the necessary vascular supply.[4] This determination can be made by estimating which artery is dominant. It the nondominant artery is involved in the tumor, no further investigation is usually required. If the dominant artery is involved in the tumor or dominance is not clear, then ancillary testing can be helpful. A conventional cerebral angiogram is useful in determining the patency of the circle of Willis to determine whether the anterior circulation could possibly provide the blood supply to the posterior circulation. In addition, a vertebral artery balloon occlusion test can be performed to predict functionally whether a patient will tolerate the sacrifice. Even if it is determined preoperatively that a patient may tolerate unilateral sacrifice of a vertebral artery, this must be undertaken with caution, as vasospasm, embolization, or thrombosis of the remaining vertebral artery could lead to disaster.

After it has been determined whether a vertebral artery will need to be sacrificed and that the patient will most likely tolerate the loss of the vertebral artery, the consequences of the nerve root sacrifice must be weighed by having the patient understand the postoperative disability that he or she will endure. If this is acceptable to the patient, then proceeding with the resection is a possibility. As in the thoracic spine,

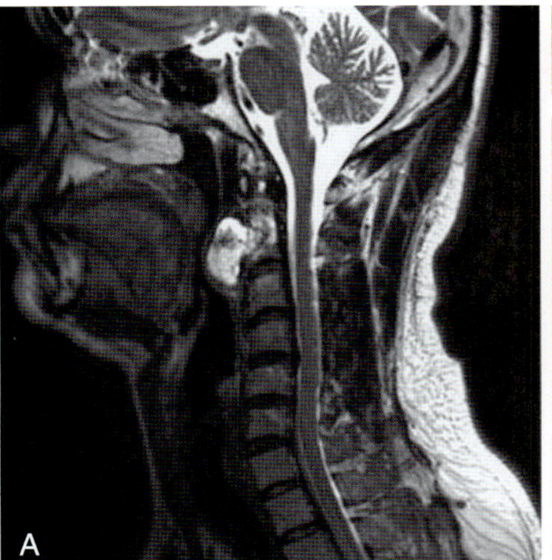

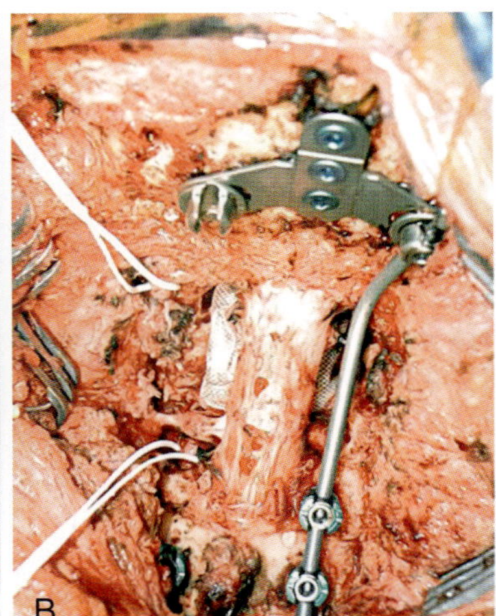

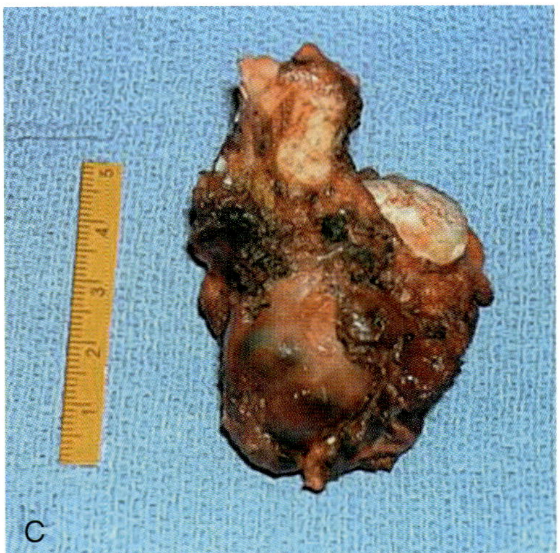

FIGURE 107-4. A, Preoperative sagittal T2-weighted MRI. **B,** Intraoperative photograph demonstrating circumferential identification (*white vessel loops*) of the left vertebral artery rostral and caudal to the tumor. **C,** En bloc pathology specimen.

the preparatory stage begins on the side of the spinal canal opposite the tumor. In general, ventrally located tumors will first be approached dorsally, and the tumor will be delivered away from the ventral aspect of the spinal cord.

During the dorsal approach, the dorsal elements of the spine are removed, exposing the normal thecal sac. A tumor that is ventrally situated and extends laterally to involve a vertebral artery and nerve roots will require that the artery and the nerve roots are sectioned during the preparatory stage. The nerve roots to be sacrificed are identified within the spinal canal and are ligated and sectioned proximal to the dorsal root ganglion. The lateral masses rostral and caudal to the tumor are carefully resected with a high-speed diamond bur. As the lateral masses are resected, the foramina for the nerve roots will be encountered. Ventral to the nerve roots lies the vertebral artery. As the vertebral artery is dissected, great care must be taken, as there is an exuberant venous plexus surrounding the vertebral artery. Bleeding from this plexus can be carefully controlled with thrombin and powdered hemostatic gelatin (Gelfoam). The vertebral artery is identified rostral and caudal to the tumor. It is circumferentially identified and then ligated and sectioned (Fig. 107-4B). Prior to ligation, a test occlusion of the vertebral artery can be made with aneurysm clips while monitoring brainstem auditory evoked potentials and the electroencephalogram. If any changes are recorded during the test occlusion, then the plan for vertebral artery sacrifice must be aborted unless a vertebral artery bypass is contemplated.

After the nerve roots and vertebral artery have been controlled, attention is turned toward the contralateral side where the vertebral artery is to be preserved. On the side where the artery is to be preserved, the artery can be skeletonized and identified to protect it during the delivery stage of the tumor. Skeletonization of this artery does carry the risk of causing vasospasm, and if this is the only remaining blood supply to the posterior fossa, this can be catastrophic. To minimize the chance of vasospasm, the vertebral artery should remain encased in the foramen transversarium if possible, and the sagittal osteotomies, lateral to the tumor, should be performed medial to the vertebral artery and foramen transversarium. At this point, the spinal instrumentation is placed, and bone graft is placed for the arthrodesis.

The ventral approach to the cervical spine will then be used to complete the preparatory stage and to deliver the tumor. A large ventral cervical exposure is performed. For high cervical tumors, a high cervical approach needs to be used, or a transoral transmandibular circumglossal approach should be considered. The temptation of a transoral transmandibular approach must be tempered by the potential consequence of the patient not being able to receive postoperative adjuvant therapy in the form of high-dose radiation therapy. Postoperative high-dose radiation therapy might not be an option, as this increases the risk of mandibular pseudarthrosis and pharyngeal dehiscence.

After the ventral cervical approach has been completed, the osteotomies rostral and caudal to the tumor need to be completed. These osteotomies need to be taken dorsally, all the way through the posterior longitudinal ligament. After these osteotomies have been completed, the specimen should be mobile, and the tumor is removed en bloc (Fig. 107-4C). The operation is then completed with a ventral reconstruction and arthrodesis.

Lumbar Spine (L1-5)

The lumbar spine is very similar to the cervical spine in regard to the challenges and limitations of nerve root sacrifice, but the lumbar spine has the advantage that it does not have the added complication of the vertebral artery. A ventrally located lumbar tumor will be approached in two stages: The preparatory stage will be a standard dorsal approach (Fig. 107-5A), and the delivery stage will be a ventral approach.[5] For L5 lesions, this will be a midline retroperitoneal or transperitoneal approach (Fig. 107-5B). For lesions above L5, this will usually be a lateral retroperitoneal approach, usually from the side that the tumor presents itself. If a tumor is located ventrally but on both sides of the vertebral body, then a midline approach for lesions rostral to L5 is considered, but this will entail significant mobilization of the aorta and inferior vena cava.

Reconstruction and Arthrodesis

Spondylectomies for en bloc tumor resection create the most unstable environment in which the spine can be placed. In addition, because such a large void is created between the remaining segments of the spine, achievement of an arthrodesis can be slow and quite challenging. Therefore, a robust reconstruction needs to be designed that can withstand the severe stress of the body on the spine and bridge the time until an arthrodesis can be achieved. In designing a specific construct after a spondylectomy procedure, an attempt to recreate all three columns should be made. Consideration should also be given to any postoperative adjuvant radiation therapy that may be given, and the implants should be designed to minimize interference with the therapy. In addition, although the goal of an en bloc resection is potential cure, postoperative monitoring with imaging for local recurrence will need to be performed, and the artifact of the implants needs to be considered. Instrumentation failure unfortunately may occur if the biomechanical stresses are not understood or if an arthrodesis is not achieved. In designing a construct, understanding how a construct might fail, what the consequences of the failure are, and how a revision operation might need to be performed should be taken into account.

Complications

Spondylectomy operations for en bloc resections of tumor are major operations. Even when the surgeon has significant experience with the spondylectomy operation, the risk of a complication is high, and the impact of the complication can be severe. During each maneuver in the course of such an operation, a complication may occur that can have a devastating impact.

The length of these operations and the blood loss during these operations increase the chance of a postoperative wound infection. Careful attention to preincision and intraoperative antibiotic dosing and aseptic technique are critical. In addition, consideration of complex plastic surgery flaps should be created to aid in wound healing, as the exposure that is necessary can result in devascularization of previously healthy tissue.

As has been mentioned, spondylectomy operations result in severe destabilization of the spine. Delayed instrumentation failures can result in cage dislodgement or dorsal

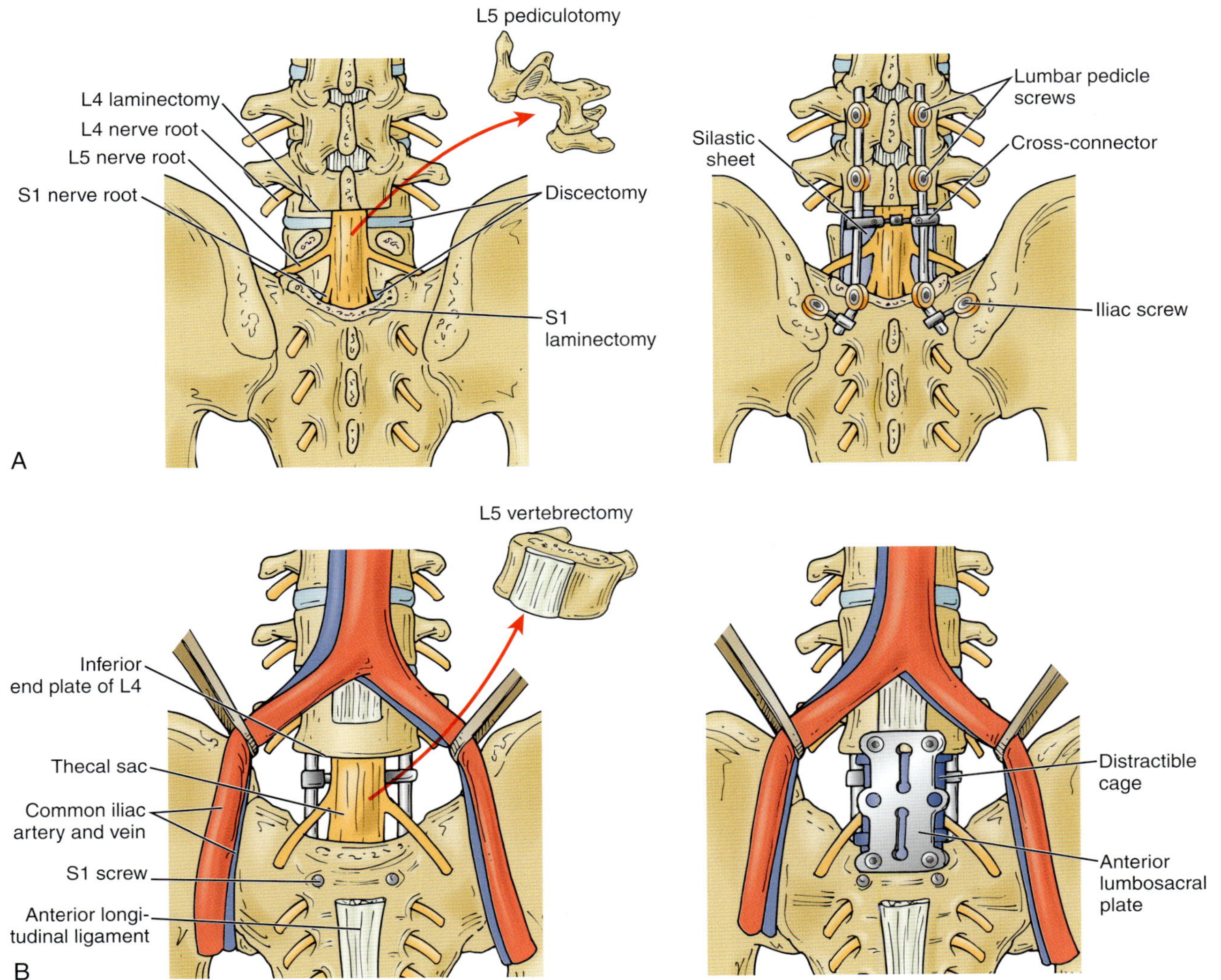

FIGURE 107-5. **A,** Illustration of the dorsal approach for en bloc resection of L5. **B,** Illustration of the ventral approach for en bloc resection of L5.

instrumentation failure, which can result in devastating vascular or neurologic injury. In addition, even if a vascular or neurologic impairment does not result from instrumentation failure, revision operations for instrumentation failure in this setting can be quite challenging, and in some circumstances impossible, dooming a potentially cured patient to a life of chronic pain.

During the dissection and mobilization of the dura mater or during ligation of a nerve root, a cerebral spinal fluid (CSF) leak can occur. Even if a CSF leak is not recognized at the time of surgery, a postoperative CSF leak may become apparent and could be the result of breakdown of a suture line or spinal fluid leaking from a ligated nerve root. If there is significant drainage of fluid from the operative drains, then a CSF leak should be suspected. Confirmation of CSF is useful by testing the fluid for the presence of B-transferrin. Although this test usually takes several days to return, it is useful for knowing whether the fluid output is CSF or serous fluid. If the fluid is CSF, then attempts at CSF diversion can be made, such as a lumbar drain to decrease the output. If the CSF is draining into the chest after a thoracotomy or dorsal pleural violation, then lumbar drainage combined with placing the thoracostomy in a water seal and putting the patient on positive pressure ventilation may help to reduce the CSF drainage. If conservative measures to control CSF drainage fail, consideration is given to reexploration and closure of the CSF leak.

Thoracic spondylectomies may result in a potential devastating complication of a chyle leak from injury to the thoracic duct. During the initial dissection, the thoracic duct may not be obvious and can be inadvertently injured. At the time of injury, this might also not be very apparent, as the chylous output may be small and the fluid can be colorless. If a chyle leak is suspected at the time of surgery, administration of cream through the nasogastric tube can stimulate the output of milky chyle and make the injury more apparent.

If a chyle leak becomes uncontrolled, the patient may have a protracted postoperative course with nutritional difficulty.

Either from a thoracotomy or during a completely dorsal approach to the thoracic spine, a pneumothorax can occur. This is best dealt with at the time of surgery by placing a thoracostomy. If the visceral pleura has not been violated, the thoracotomy can usually be removed soon in the postoperative period after serial radiographs demonstrate resolution of the pneumothorax. If the visceral pleura has been violated, then the air leak will need to be treated for a longer period of time with the thoracostomy.

Vascular injuries during spondylectomies can occur at any level of the spine. Most can be controlled and repaired. During an entirely dorsal approach for a thoracic spondylectomy, great care must be exercised in dissecting the ventral plane between the spine and the aorta and vena cava. Above T5, on the right side of the spine, the azygos vein must be identified and dissected. Maintaining the proper dissection plane is the key to avoiding a vascular injury. In addition, large veins are occasionally identified draining directly from the vertebral body. These must be carefully identified and ligated prior to any osteotomies or delivery of the specimen. During the ventral dissection of the spine, there might not be enough space for a vascular repair to be completed, and vascular control can be difficult. If this occurs, there are several options. If the specimen is ready to be delivered, the vascular injury can be temporarily tamponaded and the specimen delivered, and this should give an excellent view of the ventrally situated vascular structures. If the specimen cannot yet be delivered, continuing with the dissection without vascular control may end in exsanguination. At this point, control may be obtained by tamponade and then converting the incision to a dorsal thoracotomy or repositioning for a lateral thoracotomy.

Summary

En bloc resection via a total spondylectomy is a technically very demanding procedure. Careful preoperative planning and consideration for postoperative adjuvant therapy are needed to optimize patient outcome. Spinal reconstruction should be designed to withstand the biomechanical stresses placed on the instrumentation and lack of bony union. Plastic surgery closure should be considered to optimize wound healing and reduce postoperative wound complications.

KEY REFERENCES

Boriani S, Weinstein JN, Biagini R: Primary bone tumors of the spine. Terminology and surgical staging. *Spine (Phila Pa 1976)* 22(9):1036–1044, 1997.

Gallia GL, Suk I, Witham TF, et al: Lumbopelvic reconstruction after combined L5 spondylectomy and total sacrectomy for en bloc resection of a malignant fibrous histiocytoma. *Neurosurgery* 67(2):E498–E502, 2010.

Hsieh PC, Galia GL, Sciubba DM, et al: En-bloc excision of chordomas in the cervical spine: review of 5 consecutive cases with over 4-year follow-up. *Spine (Phila Pa 1976)* 36(24):E1581–E1587, 2011.

Hsieh PC, Li KW, Sciubba DM, et al: Posterior-only approach for total en bloc spondylectomy for malignant primary spinal neoplasms: anatomic considerations and operative nuances. *Neurosurgery* 65(Suppl 6):173–181, 2009; discussion 181.

Kato S, Kawahara N, Tomita K, et al: Effects on spinal cord blood flow and neurologic function secondary to interruption of bilateral segmental arteries which supply the artery of Adamkiewicz: an experimental study using a dog model. *Spine (Phila Pa 1976)* 33(14):1533–1541, 2008.

REFERENCES

The complete reference list is available online at expertconsult.com.

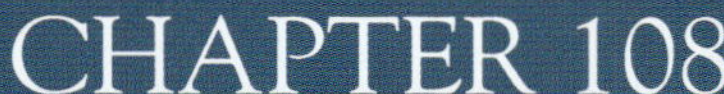
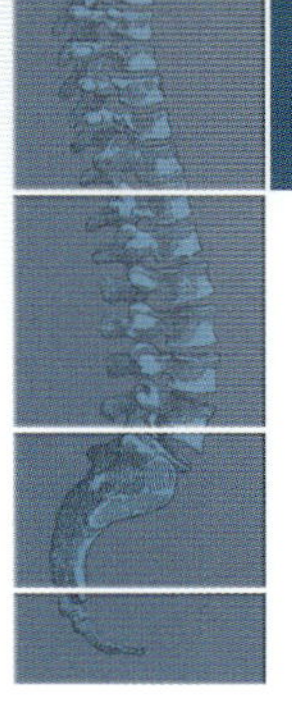

CHAPTER 108

Prognostic Factors, Surgical Outcomes, and Guidelines for Managing Metastatic Spine Cancer

Alexander Hadjipavlou | Kyriakos Kakavelakis | Panagiotis Korovessis | James W. Simmons II

Vertebral metastases constitute a major event in the course of many tumors. Quite often revealing the metastatic nature of the disease, they also constitute a new crossroads in treatment orientation and provoke a marked emotional modification in the caregiver-patient relationship.

The spine is the most common site for skeletal metastasis.[1] Approximately 5% to 10% of all cancer patients develop spine metastasis.[2,3] Although Jaffee[1] reported in 1958 a 70% incidence of vertebral metastasis, others asserted that spinal involvement ranges from 33.4% to 56%.[4-6] Spinal cord compression occurs in 10% to 25% of treated patients with preexisting spinal metastasis.[2,6-12] It is well established that if metastatic vertebral disease is left untreated, it may lead to paraplegia,[13-16] which is the most dreadful complication of metastatic vertebral disease. In this situation, surgery plays an important role. Several surgical options exist; however, their indications and outcomes must be scrutinized for better medical care. The discovery of vertebral metastases intensifies an already complex situation requiring highly technical management, sustained coherence of the entire care-provider team, and their awareness of the patient's increased need to be heard, informed, and supported.

Constructing reasonable guidelines for monitoring patients with vertebral metastases, it is important to understand the patient's expectations after surgery and what constitutes prognostic factors.

Surgical Outcomes

The following are essential when evaluating surgical outcomes for vertebral metastases:

- Overall neurologic status
- Ambulation
- Sphincter control
- Pain and suffering
- Survival rates
- Local recurrences
- Complications (including immediate postoperative mortality)
- Reoperation rate
- Overall patient satisfaction

According to published reports, the anticipated improvement after surgery is expected to range from 55% to 87% of cases as a result of overall upgrade of neurologic deficit (Table 108-1); 36% to 89% because of restoration of sphincter control (Table 108-2); 47% to 100% due to pain relief (Table 108-3); and 40% to 100% as a result of restoration of ambulation (Table 108-4). Apparently restoration of ambulation after dorsal decompression alone fares worse. The anticipated survival rates are depicted in Table 108-5. The complication rates range from 12% to 32% (Table 108-6). In our series of 70 patients, the complication rate was 25%, including two deaths. In one case, surgery was aborted, while in progress, because of massive intraoperative bleeding, despite preoperative transarterial embolization of the region.[17] Other complications were profuse bleeding in nine patients, infections in three, wound dehiscence in three, and incomplete surgery in three patients. The 4- to 6-week

TABLE 108-1

Reported Overall Neurologic Improvement after Surgery

Study	Improvement
Kostuik J et al.[68]	55%
Ernstberger T et al.[80]	57%
Weigel B et al.[18]	58%
King GJ et al.[19]	60%
Villavicencio AT et al.[81]	60%
Rompe JD et al.[82]	63%
Atanasiu JP et al.[30]	64%
O'Neil J et al.[32]	68%
Harrington KD[37]	68%
Hatrick N et al.[83]	69%
Tomita T et al.[72]	73%
Hammerberg KW[66]	74%
Bauer HCF[84]	76%
Gokalsan ZL et al.[46]	76%
Onimus M et al.[85]	79%
Hosono N et al.[86]	81%
King et al.[19]	88%
Hertlein H et al.[87]	88%
Shimizu K et al.[34]	87%

TABLE 108-2

Restoration of Sphincter Control after Surgery

Study	Successful Restoration
King GJ et al.[19]	36%
Kocialkowski A, Webb JK[88]	43%
Kostuik J et al.[68]	47%
Sinardet D et al.[89]	51%
Tomita T et al.[72]	77%
Klekamp J, Samii H[31]	89%

TABLE 108-3

Pain Relief

Study	Success Rate
Sinardet D et al.[89]	47%
Touboul E et al.[90]	71%
Hirabayashi H et al.[25]	77%
Kocialkowski A, Webb JK[88]	79%
Kostuik J et al.[68]	81%
Sundaresan N et al.[91]	85%
Ernstberger T et al.[80]	85%
Villavicencio AT et al.[81]	85%
King GJ et al.[19]	88%
Weigel B et al.[18]	89%
Hatrick N et al.[83]	90%
Hammerberg KW[66]	91%
Gokalsan ZL et al.[46]	92%
Hertlein H et al.[87]	92%
Harrington KD[37]	94%
O'Neil J et al.[32]	94%
Hosono N et al.[86]	94%
Atanasiu JP et al.[30]	95%
Tomita T et al.[72]	95%
Shimizu K et al.[34]	100%
Bilsky MH et al.[92]	100%

mortality rates after surgery, reoperation rates for complications, and local recurrences after surgery are listed in Tables 108-7, 108-8, and 108-9, respectively. Local tumor recurrence is more likely to occur in patients with certain tumors and particularly in those for whom chemotherapy and radiation therapy are ineffective. This is particularly the case in such cancers as renal cell carcinoma, in which the reported recurrence is expected to be as high as 40% to 50%.[18-21] The overall patient satisfaction was rated in the range of 55% to 80%.[18,22]

Therefore, it is reasonable to assume that these data can be used as the basis for what should be considered acceptable outcomes. The reported wide variation of survival rates after surgery probably reflects nonuniform representation of aggressive tumors in different series.

Prognostic Factors

It has been observed that certain factors, irrespective of treatment selection, may influence the prognosis when malignant tumors develop spinal metastases. The original claim that the histopathology of the tumor had no bearing on the ultimate prognosis[23] has not been duplicated by others.

TABLE 108-4

Restoration of Ambulation after Ventral or Dorsal Approach

Study	Successful Restoration
Livingston KE, Perrin RG[93]	40%
Kostuik J et al.[68]	44%
Gokalsan ZL et al.[46]	51%
Sinardet D et al.[89]	52%
Tomita T et al.[72]	60%
Patchel RA et al.[94]	62%
Hosono N et al.[86]	64%
King GJ et al.[19]	64%
Weigel B et al.[18]	70%
Onimus M et al.[85]	70%
Hammerberg KW[66]	76%
Hatrick NC et al.[83]	78%
Siegal T, Siegal T[95]	80%
O'Neil J et al.[32]	82%
Villavicencio AT et al.[81]	100%
Sundaresan N et al.[91,96]	100%
Restoration of Ambulation after Laminectomy Alone	
Klekamp J, Samii H[31]	23%
Kennady JC, Stern WE[97]	23%
Schoeggl A et al.[98]	33%
Wright RL[99]	35%
White WA et al.[100]	36%
Siegal T, Siegal T[95]	47%

Origin of Tumor

The origin of the primary tumors was postulated by several authors to influence the prognosis. Thus, metastatic vertebral tumors from unsuspected adenocarcinoma, stomach, esophagus, pancreas, and lungs, portend the worst possible prognosis, whereas carcinoid, thyroid, breast, prostate, and myeloma carry the best prognosis. Distinction should also be made between the different types of lung cancer.[24] In general, non–small cell lung cancer (NSCLC) patients with spinal metastases had survival rates of 37.1%, 14.6%, and 2.1% at follow-up of 6 months, 1 year, and 2 years, respectively. The median survival time was 4.5 months, and the mean, 6.2 months. However, for small-cell lung cancer (SCLC), the corresponding survival rates were 36.8%, 5.3%, and 0% at 6 months, 1 year, and 2 years follow-up, respectively. In both NSCLC and SCLC with spinal metastases, the presence of hypercalcemia or hypoalbuminemia was indicative of a gloomy prognosis, with a survival period of less than 3 months.[24]

The aggressiveness of cancer can also be classified as slow growth (breast, thyroid, prostate), moderate growth (kidney, uterus), and rapid growth (lung, stomach, liver, colon, unknown).[25-29]

Concurrent Visceral Metastases

The influence on survival with visceral metastasis was also observed by Tokuhashi et al.[28] and Tomita et al.[29] The average survival with no visceral metastases was 36.8 months (range,

TABLE 108-5

Anticipated Survival Rates after Surgery

Study	Survival Rate
3 month	
Kocialkowski A, Webb JK[88]	50.0%
Wai EK et al.[52]	76.0%
6 month	
Klekamp J, Samii H[31]	58.8%
Rompe JD et al.[82]	72.0%
Hosono N et al.[86]	78.0%
9 month	
Falicov A et al.[33]	50.0%
12 month	
Kocialkowski A, Webb JK[88]	25.0%
Klekamp J, Samii H[31]	48.8%
Rompe JD et al.[82]	50.0%
Villavicencio AT et al.[81]	65.0%
Gokalsan ZL et al.[46]	62.0%
19 month	
Rompe JD et al.[82]	4.7%
60 month	
Klekamp J, Samii H[31]	5%
Median month	
Schoeggl A et al.[98]	6.5%
Sioutos PJ et al.[35]	10%
Hirabayashi H et al.[25]	10.6%
Lewandrowski KU et al.[101]	14%
Sundaresan N et al.[102]	30%
Mean month	
Chataigner H, Onimus M[20]	8%
Hertlein H et al.[87]	8.5%
O'Neil J et al.[32]	9%
Livingston KE, Perrin RG[93]	9%
Atanasiu JP et al.[30]	11%
Ernstberger T et al.[80]	15.6%
Weigel B et al.[18]	13.1%
Wise JJ et al.[67]	15.9%
Cahill DW, Kumar R[103]	15.9%
Kocialkowski A, Webb JK[88]	12.0%

TABLE 108-6

Complication Rates

Study	Percentage Experiencing Complications
Bilsky MH et al.[7]	12%
Wai EK et al.[52]	12%
Hosono N et al.[86]	16%
Weigel B et al.[18]	19%
Jansson KA, Bauer HC[104]	20%
Wise JJ et al.[67]	25%
Klimo P Jr et al. (review of 24 surgical reports)[105]	23%
Falicov A et al.[33]	29%
Gokalsan ZL et al.[46]	32%

TABLE 108-7

Postsurgery Mortality Rates (4 to 6 weeks)

Study	Mortality Rate
Gokalsan ZL et al.[46]	3.0%
Klimo PJr et al.[105]	6.3%
Wise JJ et al.[67]	6.0%
Siegal TJ et al.[106]	6.0%
Weigel B et al.[18]	7.0%
Sundaresan N et al.[96]	8.0%
Harrington KD[37]	8.0%
Sinardet D et al.[89]	9.0%
Sioutos PJ et al.[35]	11.0%
Turner PL et al.[78]	10.0%
Hertlein H et al.[87]	10.0%
Chataigner H, Onimus M[20]	10.2%
Bilsky MH et al.[92]	12.0%
Jansson KA, Bauer HC[104]	13.0%
Kocialkowski A, Webb JK[88]	16.0%
Fidler MW[107]	18.0%

TABLE 108-8

Reoperation Rates for Complications or Local Recurrences

Study	Percentage Undergoing Reoperation
Weigel B et al.[18]	7.0%
Jansson KA, Bauer HC[104]	10.2%
Hertlein H et al.[87]	12.1%
Bauer HCF[84]	24.0%
Chataigner H, Onimus M[20]	15.8%
King GJ et al.[19]	56.2%

TABLE 108-9

Local Recurrences after Surgery

Study	Percentage Experiencing Recurrence
Falicov A et al.[33]	3.5%
Review of 9 surgical reports	8.0%
Klimo P Jr et al.[105]	
Bilsky MH et al.[92]	
Foumey DR et al.[108]	
Hammerberg KW[66]	
Hosono N et al.[86]	
King GJ et al.[19]	
Muhlbauer M et al.[109]	
Siegal T et al.[106]	
Weigel B et al.[18]	
Chataigner H, Onimus M[20]	8.4%
Nazarian S[110]	11.0%
King GJ et al.[19]	12.1%
Hirabayashi H et al.[25]	21.0%
Weigel B et al.[18]	22.0%
Bridwell KH et al.[71] (after laminectomy)	31.6%
Sundaresan N et al.[102]	32.0%
Hertlein H et al.[87]	49.0%

5–84 months), treatable visceral metastases, 16.5 months (4–31 months), and untreatable visceral metastases, 8.9 months (range, 1–24 months). The grave prognostic factor of extraskeletal metastatic lesions on the survival rate is also in agreement with Weigel et al.,[18] who demonstrated that a patient survival period without extraskeletal metastases at surgery was significantly longer than with extraskeletal metastases (23.5 months vs. 5.8 months; $P < .0001$).

Location of Spinal Lesion

The location of the metastatic lesion was also implicated as a survival factor. Atanasiu et al.[30] reported that lesions in the upper cervical spine had an adverse effect on life expectancy, with average survival of 1.8 months; however, this was challenged by Klekamp and Samii,[31] who found no differences in prognosis between the upper and lower spine.

Number of Affected Vertebrae

The number of affected vertebrae also had an influence on survival. Patients with single-level involvement had a better survival rate (average survival, 12.9 months) than did patients with multiple-level involvement (average, 7.9 months),[28,32,33] even after effective surgical treatment.[34]

Neurologic Deficit

Neurologic dysfunction was observed to be associated with survival rates. Some believe that ambulatory patients survive longer than nonambulatory patients with sphincter incontinence.[19,35] The state of sphincter incontinence as a bad prognostic sign is also emphasized by some.[36] The rate of neurologic deterioration was related to prognosis; slow progression had a good prognosis as opposed to rapid progression, which was correlated with dismal results. The latter was compounded when the onset of treatment was delayed.[36,37] However, the notion of preoperative intact neurologic status (ambulatory vs. nonambulatory) as a predictor of longer survival was challenged by others.[18,38]

Likewise, timing for adjunctive radiation treatment (preoperative radiation vs. postoperative radiation) was also questioned as a significant prognostic predictor for outcomes.[39] Weigel[18] and Hirabayashi et al.[25] emphasized that postoperative ambulation definitely has a positive prognostic influence on survival, rather than preoperative ambulation.

Timing of Surgery

The timing of treatment can also influence the results. Some authors[36,37] observed that delayed onset of treatment may compromise the effectiveness of neurologic recovery. More specifically, Fürstenberg et al.[40] addressed the timing of surgery and concluded that the effectiveness of decompression, when undertaken less than 48 hours after the development of symptoms, was significantly better for neurologic recovery (71.4%, unchanged 28.6%), compared with those with delayed surgical treatment (improvement 28.6%, unchanged 42.8%, deterioration 28.6%). Furthermore, they noted that normal bladder function may be considered a good prognostic factor for neurologic recovery after appropriate decompression.

Age

Weigel et al.[18] also reported that the patient age can be considered as a prognostic factor for survival, because patients younger than 60 years survived significantly longer than older patients (20.1 months vs. 6.2 months; $P = .028$). Age as a prognostic factor has not been incorporated into the Tokuhashi scoring system and needs to be duplicated by others.

More Than Two Prognostic Factors

A report indicates that when more than two of the "prognostic factors" are present, they have a compounding adverse effect on survival.[35] For example, lung cancer, neurologic deficit, and involvement of multiple vertebrae in the same patient would have a greater adverse effect on survival than the combined effect of the same type of lung cancer involving a single vertebra and without neurologic deficit. However, these findings have not been substantiated by others. When estimating survival, one should take into consideration that, invariably, most of the data from different reports were based on metastatic tumor of the spine that became symptomatic.

Clinical practice in surgical results and prognostic factors of metastatic spinal tumors has not undergone adequate scrutiny. The surgical information provided in this article must be available and known to everyone concerned with spinal tumors (e.g., physicians, patients, insurance) to form the basis of what should be considered acceptable surgical outcomes. Inferior results, therefore, are not acceptable, and well-designed guidelines should strive to achieve the best possible outcomes.

Instruments for Outcomes Assessment

As surgical procedures to treat vertebral metastases have increased, a greater interest has been expressed in the overall quality-of-life assessment and outcomes studies. However, few published reports exist on the assessment of these patients' health-performance status after surgery.

Patients with metastatic spinal disease often suffer from a multitude of concurrent clinical problems. Quality of life may be compromised by the effects of chemotherapy or surgery in conjunction with radiation therapy, as well as by the effects of the disease itself. Furthermore, survival may also be limited, and thus long-term follow-up is not feasible for this patient population.

Patient-based outcome studies have been recently introduced to assess the results of treatment and to provide patients, physicians, insurance providers, and government agencies with a tool with which to evaluate the different treatment methods. The objective is to measure how well the results approach the goals of treatment (i.e., restore function and control pain).

Evaluation of patient functional status should be based on (1) pain assessment, (2) profile of mood states, and (3) overall performance status. Because performance depends not only on pain and disability but also on neurologic status, a detailed neurologic assessment is an integral part of the evaluation of these patients and provides reliable and straightforward clinical documentation. However, the assessment of pain disability and bodily functional performance of the patient can be appreciated only through psychometric instruments, which should be simple and reproducible.[41]

Because treatment is seldom curative in metastatic disease,[42] the treating physician should keep in mind that patients with vertebral metastasis differ from noncancer patients. Therefore, the sensitivity of these instruments is limited to monitoring changes of the patient's feelings of well-being.[43,44]

Pain is an alarming consequence of vertebral metastatic disease. Specific efforts should be made to avoid crude assessment and try to quantify and locate the pain. The McGill Pain Questionnaire is a sensitive tool. A visual analogue scale (VAS) for pain measurement combined with a pain diagram that indicates the site of pain and its spread is a simple and reliable method for quantifying and depicting pain. The VAS, although a subjective assessment of pain, has been shown to be more reliable than other types of pain assessment.[45]

A distinction should be made between radicular pain and axial pain. Even the surgical approach may be responsible for severe pain. A report[46] detailing outcomes of pain demonstrated that in 72 patients who underwent a ventral approach through thoracotomy, 90% had postoperative pain (only 23% achieved complete resolution, 60% had significant improvement, and 8%, no change or worsening of thoracotomy pain). Quantification of pain is useful in monitoring the effectiveness of pain management, as well as in helping establish pain-control goals for the individual patient.[47]

Cancer patients often have emotional and psychological problems. Because anxiety and depression have a direct correlation with pain intensity, these two factors may need to be addressed. The Zung Self-Rating Anxiety Scale[48] and the Hamilton Depression Scale[49] are suitable instruments in this situation. The Memorial Pain Assessment Card (MPAC)[50] (Fig. 108-1) is a modified visual analogue with multidimensional characteristics, practically equivalent to a full assessment combining the McGill Pain Questionnaire, the Hamilton Depression Rating Scale (HDRS), and the Zung Self-Rating Anxiety Scale.

The Edmonton Symptom Assessment Scale (ESAS) is a validated patient-centered questionnaire designed specifically to address the overall quality of life in patients with terminal cancer.[43,44,51] ESAS measures nine domains (pain, tiredness, nausea, depression, anxiety, drowsiness, appetite, well-being, shortness of breath, and other problems). After surgery, the largest improvement is reported in the pain domain.[52]

The 36-Item Short Form Health Survey (SF-36) by Townsend et al. is a physician-determined assessment of the patient's physical disability. Patients are classified as having (1) normal, pain-free function, (2) normal function with pain, (3) significantly limited function requiring some type of assistance (e.g., a walker, cane), and (4) nonfunctional (e.g., wheelchair bound, bedridden).[53]

Other validated outcome measures in patients suffering from vertebral metastasis are the Health Utility Index Mark 3 (HUI-MARK 3; Table 108-10),[54] European Organization for Research and Treatment of Cancer Quality of Life Questionnaire (EORTC QLQ-C30),[55] Eastern Cooperative Oncology Group (ECOG; Table 108-11),[56] EuroQol 5d (EQ-5D; Fig. 108-2),[57] and Karnofsky Performance Status (PS; Table 108-12), which have been successfully applied in patients with vertebral metastases.[58]

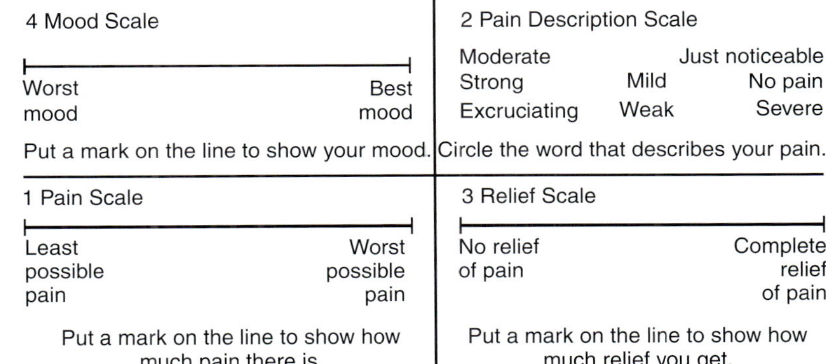

FIGURE 108-1. The Memorial Pain Assessment Card. (From Fishman B. Pasternak S, Wallenstein SL, et al: The Memorial Pain Assessment Card: a valid instrument for the evaluation of cancer pain. *Cancer* 60:1151, 1987.)

TABLE 108-10

Human Utility Index Mark 3

Scale	Description
1	FREE OF PAIN AND DISCOMFORT
2	MILD TO MODERATE PAIN Pain does not prevent activity
3	MODERATE PAIN Pain prevents few activities
4	MODERATE TO SEVERE PAIN Pain prevents some activities
5	SEVERE PAIN Pain prevents most activities

TABLE 108-11

ECOG Performance Status

Grade	ECOG
0	Fully active, able to carry on all predisease performance without restriction
1	Restricted in physically strenuous activity but ambulatory and able to carry out work of a light or sedentary nature, e.g., light housework, office work
2	Ambulatory and capable of all self-care but unable to carry out any work activities; up and about more than 50% of waking hours
3	Capable of only limited self-care; confined to bed or chair more than 50% of waking hours
4	Completely disabled. Cannot carry on any self-care. Totally confined to bed or chair.
5	Dead

ECOG, Eastern Cooperative Oncology Group.

Mobility
I have no problems in walking about ☐
I have some problems in walking about ☐
I am confined to bed ☐

Self-care
I have no problems with self-care ☐
I have some problems washing or dressing myself ☐
I am unable to wash or dress myself ☐

Usual activities (e.g., work, study, housework, family or leisure activities)
I have no problems with performing my usual activities ☐
I have some problems with performing my usual activities ☐
I am unable to perform my usual activities ☐

Pain/Discomfort
I have no pain or discomfort ☐
I have moderate pain or discomfort ☐
I have extreme pain and discomfort ☐

Anxiety/Depression
I am not anxious or depressed ☐
I am moderately anxious or depressed ☐
I am extremely anxious or depressed ☐

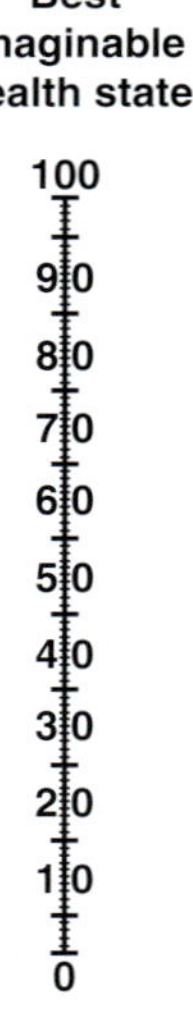

FIGURE 108-2. EQ-5D self-classifier (that consists of five dimensions) and visual analogue scale to enable the respondent to provide a health self-rating.

TABLE 108-12

Rating of Karnofsky Performance Status

Rating	Status	Description
0	Dead	Unable to care for self; requires equivalent of institutional or hospital care; disease may be progressing rapidly.
10%	Moribund Fatal processes progressing rapidly	
20%	Very sick; hospitalization necessary Active support treatment necessary	
30%	Severely disabled; hospitalization is indicated, although death not imminent	
40%	Disabled Requires special medical care and assistance	Unable to work; able to live at home and care for most personal needs; varying amount of assistance needed.
50%	Requires considerable assistance and frequent medical care	
60%	Requires occasional assistance, but is able to care for most needs	
70%	Cares for self Unable to carry on normal activity or to do active work	
80%	Normal activity with effort Some signs or symptoms of disease	Able to carry on normal activity and to work; no special care needed.
90%	Able to carry on normal activity Minor signs or symptoms of disease	
100%	Normal No complaints No evidence of disease	

From Karnofsky DA: Clinical evaluation of anticancer drugs: cancer chemotherapy. *GANN Monogr* 2:223, 1967.

The overall distribution of HUI-MARK 3 utility calculates quality-adjusted life years (QuaLY) during the 1-year postoperative period.[33]

The EORTC QLQ-C30 measures quality of life and has one global health status (QL2), five functional scales, physical functions (PF2), role functions (RF2), emotional function (EF), cognitive functions (CF), and social functioning (SF), as well as nine symptom scales.

The ECOG grading system or the Karnofsky PS is used to assess performance status. The ECOG (see Table 108-11) performance status[56] measures functional performance on a scale from 0 to 4 and is a good index of assessing the preoperative functional status.[33]

The Karnofsky PS details the condition of the patient's health status[58] (see Table 108-12). Scoring between 0 and 10% indicates poor health and total dependency on others, from 50% to 70% indicates an inability to work and requires assistance, and 80% to 100% represents the ability to carry on with normal activities. The Karnofsky PS was successfully applied by Tokuhashi et al.[59] in clinical guidance for predicting cancer patient outcomes.

Frankel et al.[60] and the American Spinal Injury Association (ASIA) impairment scores,[61] although nonspecific enough to describe nuances of the physical state of locomotion, grade the functional outcomes for neurologic assessment. Four other scales also address the state of ambulation[60,62-64] and can be used as complementary to the ASIA or Frankel scales, such as combining the Cooper and the Frankel grading systems.

Oswestry Disability Index (ODI) and SF-36 are simple tools designed to quantify disability originating from back pain. The effectiveness of these tools has not been tested in patients with metastatic spinal disease.

Surgical Guidelines

The rationale of guidelines is to achieve better treatment outcomes. Their scientific strength depends on how well evidence-based knowledge is used.[65] It is reasonable to assume that consensus-based guidelines supported by available evidence are more convincing than individual ones. Unfortunately, no such reported guidelines are available for the management of metastatic spinal tumors. Certain published guidelines are based on individual experiences without enough clinical evidence to support their effectiveness. These guidelines do not cover an integrated approach for the management of metastatic spinal tumors but are concerned with different aspects of the problem.

In 1990, Tokuhashi et al.[59] devised a guideline scoring system for the preoperative evaluation of metastatic vertebral tumor, based on the general condition of the patient, as graded by the Karnofsky PS[58] and five of the following prognostic factors: (1) number of extraspinal bone metastases, (2) number of metastases in the spine, (3) metastases to the major internal organs (lungs, liver, kidneys, and brain), (4) primary site of the cancer, and (5) severity of spinal cord impairment. Table 108-13 demonstrates the Tokuhashi prognostic scoring system for preoperative evaluation of the metastatic spinal lesions. Each parameter has a score ranging from 0 to 2 points (maximum score 12 points) that is related to the patient's prognosis: the higher the score, the better the prognosis.

Rating the preoperative health status is as follows: the score is 0 for poor condition (PS values, 10–40%); 1 for moderate (PS values, 50–70%), and 2 for good (PS values, 80–100%). For extraspinal bone metastatic foci more than three, the score is 0; between one and two metastatic foci, the score is 1; and for nonmetastatic lesions, 2. For the number of metastases in the spine, the score is 0 for more than three vertebrae; 1 for two metastases; and 2 for no more than one vertebra. For metastasis to a major internal organ, the prognosis depends on the resectability of the tumor: 0 for unremovable lesions; 1 for removable lesions, and 2 for no metastasis. For the primary site of the cancer, the score is: 0 when the expected survival is less than 3 months (lung and stomach); 1 for expected survival rate of 3 to 12 months (kidney, liver, uterus, others, unidentified), and 2 for expected survival rate of more than 12 months (thyroid, prostate, breast, rectum). Finally, the severity of spinal cord palsy was rated as 0 for Frankel grade A and B (complete paraplegia) 1 for Frankel C and D (incomplete paraplegia), and 2 for Frankel E (no paraplegia), respectively.

Excisional surgery should be performed for patients who score above 9 points, and palliative surgery for those who score less than 5 points. The patients who score between 5 and 9 points fall into a gray zone.

In 1997, Tokuhashi et al.[28] reported that the reliability for predicting the prognosis was 63.3%, tested in 128 patients with metastatic spinal tumors.

The original Tokuhashi scoring system was tested by Enkaoua et al.[26] for three types of metastatic tumors: renal cell carcinoma, thyroid cancer, and unknown primary cancer. The median survival period was 5.3 months for a score of 7 or less and 23.6 months for a score of 8 or more. For cancer of an unknown primary site, the score should be 0 because the prognosis is invariably gloomy.

Subsequently, Tokuhashi et al.[28] revised the original scoring system to improve its accuracy by providing more detailed prognostic values based on the origin of the primary tumor. The score was modified to range between 0 and 5 points. The score was designated as 0 for metastases originating in the lungs, osteosarcoma, stomach, bladder, esophagus, and pancreas; 1 for metastases from the liver, gallbladder, and unidentified sources; 2 for metastasis from other sites; 3 for renal or uterine malignancies; 4 for metastasis from the rectum; and 5 for tumors from the thyroid, breast, or prostate or a carcinoid tumor. Therefore, in the revised system, a total of 15 scores can be obtained. In the patients with a total score of less than 8 or multiple vertebral metastases, Tokuhashi et al. indicate conservative or palliative procedure (predicted survival period is less than 6 months), whereas they advocate excisional procedure when the score is 12 or more (predicted survival period, 1 year or more) and for scores between 9 and 11 (predicted survival period, 6 months or more). According to the authors, the consistency rate between the criteria for predicted prognosis and the actual survival period was high in patients within each score range (0–8, 9–11, 12–15), 86.4% in 118 patients evaluated prospectively after 1998, and 82.5% in all 246 patients evaluated retrospectively. No reports in the literature indicate that the actual value of each scoring point (0, 1, and 2) in each factor has been sufficiently scrutinized. Ogihara et al.[24] reported that the Tokuhashi preoperative scoring system for patients with lung cancer did not correlate well with the survival period. The authors found that only the performance status ECOG (PS; see Table 108-11),[56] which is similar to the Karnofsky test ,was correlated with the survival rate. However, this test was predictive only when applied postoperatively. The average survival rate for patients with a postoperative PS of 0 to 2 was 13.9 months, whereas that for patients with a postoperative PS of 3 or 4 was 2.0 months.

By using the Karnofsky PS, Weigel et al.[18] found that the postoperative general state of health was 55%, a state of health that lies halfway between total dependency (50%) and partial dependency on others (60%). No one achieved 100%. The best scores were achieved with breast tumors (80% on the index); the second best results were seen in renal cell carcinoma patients (30% of the patients scoring 80–90%); and the poorest scores were seen in patients with melanoma (mean index, 48%), tumors of other sites (43%), and lung tumors (38%).

Chantaigner et al.[20] asserted that when deciding on a surgical option in non-neurologic patients, the Karnofsky PS alone was more effective than the Tokuhashi score, which also includes the Karnofsky PS.

TABLE 108-13

Tokuhashi System for Preoperative Evaluation of Metastatic Spine Tumors

Parameters	Score
General condition (performance status)	0, 1, 2
Extraspinal bone metastatic foci	0, 1, 2
Number of metastases in the spine (vertebrae)	0, 1, 2
Metastasis to major internal organs	0, 1, 2
Primary site of the cancer (histopathology)	0, 1, 2
Spinal cord palsy	0, 1, 2
Indications for Type of Surgery	***Score***
Excisional surgery	>9
Palliative surgery	<5

Some investigators are more selective than others in applying more vigorous selection in their inclusion criteria for surgery. Therefore, the overall survival period after surgery is not accurate. In some series, surgery is not indicated when the estimated survival rate is 3 months, whereas in others, the criterion for surgery is longer than 6 months. This explains the longer survival rates with different cancer patients and particularly in lung cancer (6–12 months) in some reports.[39,66]

Harrington[37] described a classification guideline system based on both bone destruction and neurologic impairment, and distinguishes five classes of vertebral metastatic lesions (Table 108-14). He suggested surgical intervention for class IV and V lesions and conservative treatment for class I and II, while for class III, which lies in the gray zone, treatment depends on various circumstances. Harrington's[37] grading system is a practical guideline system for managing metastatic vertebral tumors, but it has some significant limitations: (1) it makes no recommendations for surgical options; (2) it does not take into account the biology of the tumor nor (3) the radiosensitivity of the metastatic lesion; and (4) it makes no provisions for the performance status of the patient. The applicability of the Harrington[37] classification system for selecting the appropriate treatment in metastatic cancer of the spine was also applied by others.[67]

Harrington[37] alluded to instability as one of the deciding factors for surgical stabilization because vertebral instability, caused by bone destruction, would provoke pain. However, he has not determined what constitutes instability in destructive metastatic lesions.

Kostuik et al.[68,69] devised a vertebral body stability model by dividing the vertebral body into six segments. More specifically, the vertebral body is divided into an anterior column consisting of the vertebral body and a posterior column consisting of the pedicles, laminae, and spinous processes. The anterior column is further subdivided into four segments: anterior right, anterior left, middle right, and middle left. The posterior column is also subdivided into right and left segments. The spine is considered stable if no more than one or two of the six segments is destroyed. The spine is considered probably unstable if three or four of the segments are destroyed, and if five or six segments are affected, the spine is considered markedly unstable. Although this has not been biomechanically tested or clinically substantiated, it may have potential applications when describing instability in the Harrington classification.

According to Taneichi et al.,[70] impending collapse is indicated (1) when more than 50% to 60% of the vertebral body is destroyed, or (2) when 25% to 30% of the vertebral structure is destroyed when there is an associated destruction of the costovertebral junction in the thoracic spine, or (3) when the destruction in the thoracolumbar spine ventrally is 35% to 40% or 20% to 25% involves the dorsal elements. Bridwell et al.[71] believe that if less than 50% of the vertebral body has been resected, vertebral body reconstruction may not be necessary.

Tomita et al.,[72] based on Enneking's grading of skeletal resection,[73] Denis's three-column classification of fracture of the spine,[74] and Weinstein's zone classification[75] (intraosseous, extraosseous, and distant spread), proposed a classification consisting of seven types of lesions (Fig. 108-3). This seems a reasonable classification for allowing the surgeon to choose the extent of surgical intervention—that is, radical excision versus stabilization alone.

TABLE 108-14

Harrington Classification Based on Structural Defect and Neurologic Deficit

Class	Neurologic Status	Structural Changes
I	Not significant	No vertebral collapse
II	Not significant	Vertebral involvement without collapse or instability (lytic or blastic lesion)
III	Major (sensory or motor)	No significant bone destruction or instability (lytic tumor)
IV	Not significant	Mechanical pain from vertebral collapse ± instability
V	Major	Retropulsion of hard discovertebral elements ± kyphotic deformity

The most recent topographic classification system reported by Boriani et al.[76] provides an excellent guideline for surgical excision of primary tumors of the spine and therefore is not specific for metastatic tumors.

A system that would encompass all these criteria would form a more comprehensive approach for the management of metastatic spinal malignancies (Fig. 108-4). For Harrington class I and II without significant neurologic involvement and without vertebral collapse, the management is nonsurgical and consists of chemotherapy, hormonal manipulation, and/or radiation therapy[37] (Fig. 108-5). However, the treatment is contingent on the origin of the metastatic tumor. For example, in renal cell carcinoma, which is resistant to radiation therapy and chemotherapy, radical excision is indicated, even in class I. For Harrington class II tumors, as in the case of multiple myeloma or small lytic metastatic lesion, considerable and immediate relief of pain can be obtained by combining chemotherapy and a cement augmentation procedure (vertebroplasty or balloon kyphoplasty). See Figure 108-6.

For Harrington category III lesions, with a neurologic deficit in the absence of major destruction of bone or spinal instability, surgery should not be entertained unless the tumor is radioresistant or unresponsive to chemotherapy.[37]

For class IV and V, surgery is the treatment of choice. For Harrington class IV, consisting of mechanical pain caused by vertebral collapse and/or instability, with a Tokuhashi score of less than 5 with the old system, or 8 with the revised system, the indications for treatment would be either conservative treatment or palliative surgery, consisting of stabilization and/or cement augmentation (Fig. 108-7).

For a Harrington class IV or V with a Tokuhashi score greater than 9 (old system) or 12 (revised system) and a Tomita B score of 6 (widespread metastases), local radical excision, if feasible combined with stabilization, would be indicated (Fig. 108-8).

When the score lies in the gray zone of 5 and 9, the use of conservative or surgical treatments depends on several factors, such as the pathology of the lesion and the status of neurologic deficit, among others—factors that may influence the final decision.

For class V, characterized by intrusion of hard discovertebral elements into the spinal canal that compromise the spinal cord, the only choice is surgery. Spinal kyphotic deformity

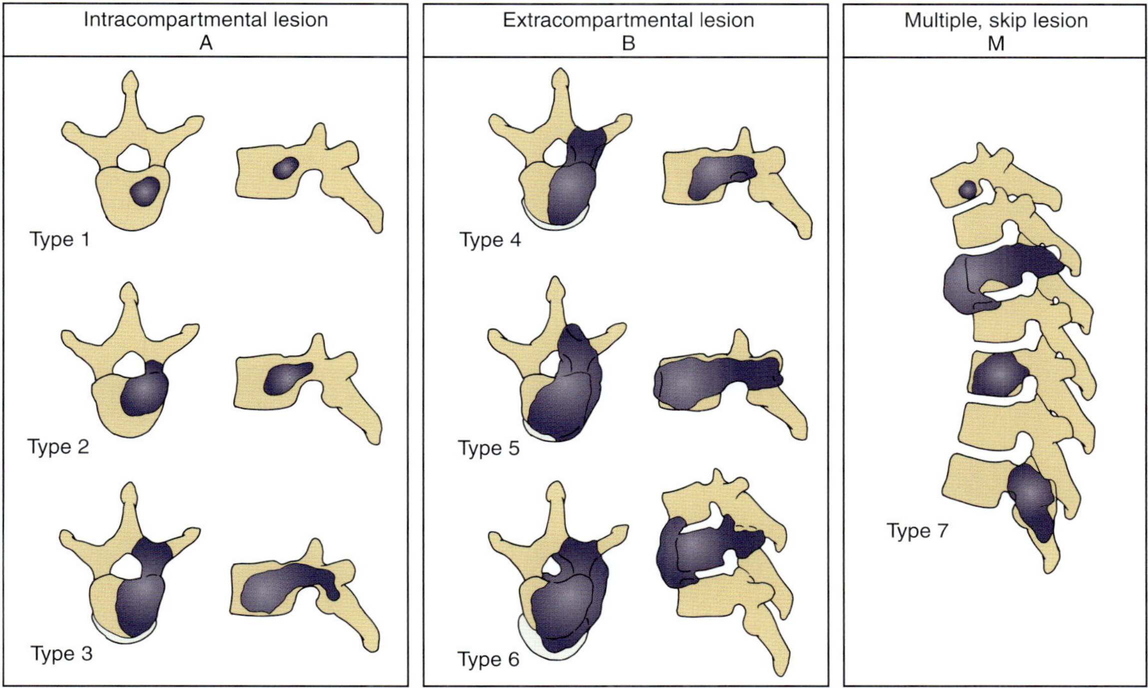

FIGURE 108-3. Tomita classification based on vertebral spread of metastasis. (From Tomita K, Kawahara N, Baba H, et al: Total en bloc spondylectomy for solitary spinal metastases. *Int Orthop* 18:291, 1994.)

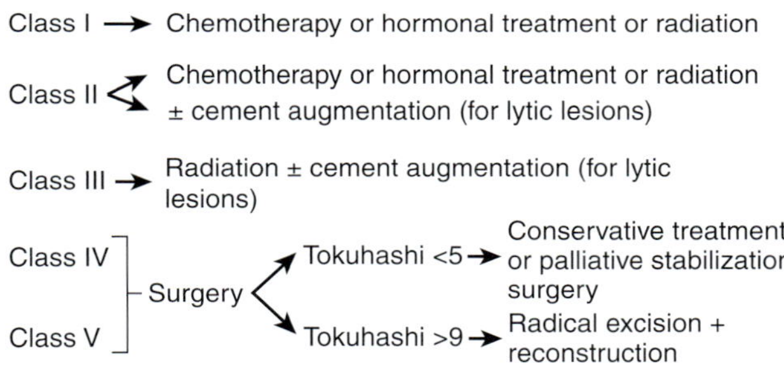

FIGURE 108-4. Treatment guidelines.

with cord compromise should be categorized as class V. In this situation, radiation has no logical place, and surgery is the treatment of choice (Fig. 108-9).

The ultimate intent of surgical management of metastatic spinal disease is to improve the patient's overall quality of life, which is definitely apparent from the cited reports. The greatest effect occurs in largely the reduction of the level of the pain. In general, a minimum life expectancy of 3 to 6 months has been accepted as a prerequisite for surgery.[67] However, even with a life expectancy shorter than 3 months, surgical intervention may be justified.[77] In this situation, palliative surgery is indicated, and the anticipated surgical intervention should be performed, with the expectation of improving the remaining global quality of life, notwithstanding the morbidity of the procedure[78] (Figs. 108-10 and 108-11). Some of the procedures for alleviating pain, such as cement augmentation (vertebroplasty, balloon kyphoplasty) and neuroaugmentation (morphine pump), are associated with minimal morbidity. Surgery is also indicated for patients who have reached spinal cord tolerance after external radiation beam treatment.

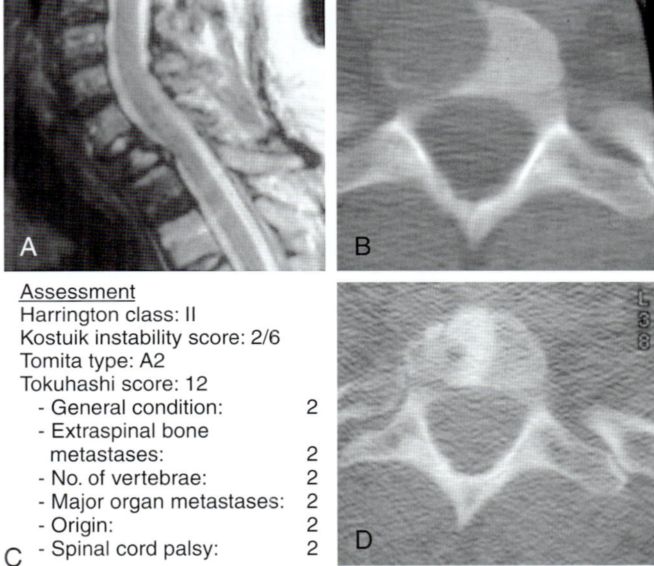

FIGURE 108-5. Metastatic lytic breast cancer as seen on midsagittal MRI (**A**) and axial CT (**B**). **C,** Assessment reveals a Harrington class II lesion with a Tokuhashi score of 12, favoring a good prognosis and nonsurgical treatment. **D,** After radiation therapy, the lesion healed and the patient was well and alive at 5 years follow-up.

It is not the purpose of this chapter to describe the available surgical techniques. In brief, the decision to use a particular approach and surgical reconstruction (ventral or dorsal) depends on the location of the tumor (e.g., vertebral body, extension into the epidural space, paraspinal region, dorsal vertebral elements) and the extent and aggressiveness of the tumor.

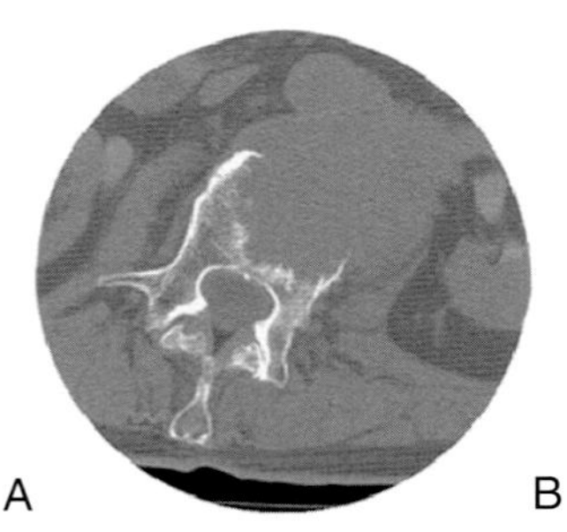

Assessment
Harrington class: II
Kostuik instability score: 3/6
Tomita type: A1
Tokuhashi score: 9

- General condition:	2
- Extraspinal bone metastases:	2
- No. of vertebrae:	1
- Major organ metastases:	0
- Origin:	2
- Spinal cord palsy:	2

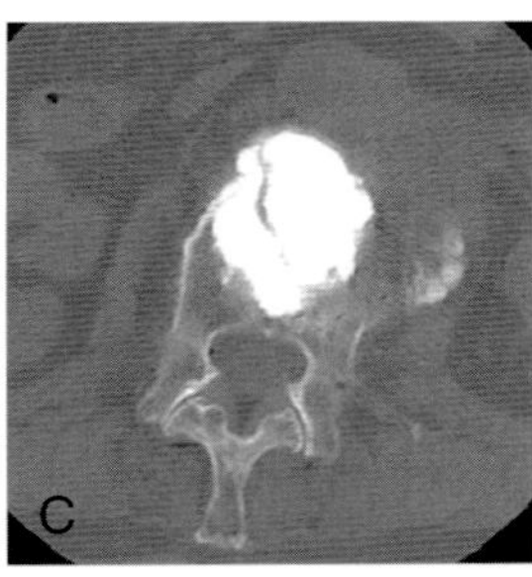

FIGURE 108-6. **A,** Lytic metastatic lesion from cancer of the breast resulting in crippling back pain as seen on axial CT. **B,** Assessment revealed a Harrington class II lesion with a Tokuhashi score of 9. **C,** The patient was treated with balloon kyphoplasty and chemotherapy. At 5-year follow-up the patient was alive and well.

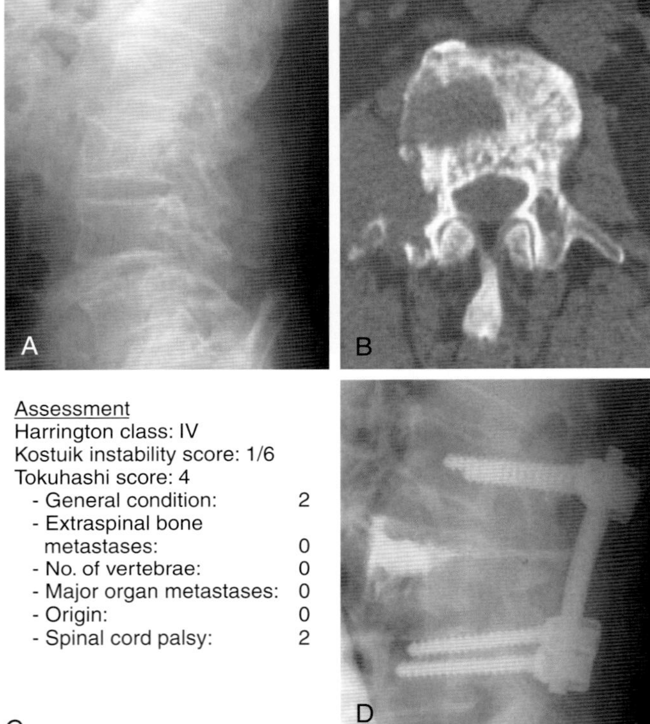

FIGURE 108-7. **A,** Lateral roentgenogram of the lumbar spine of a 67-year-old man with lung metastasis to L3 vertebra. **B,** Axial CT shows osteolytic lesion of the vertebral body. **C,** Tokuhashi score was 4, indicating a palliative surgical approach as appropriate treatment. Following minimal surgery consisting of balloon kyphoplasty and percutaneous transpedicular stabilization (**D**), the patient obtained immediate relief of pain and survived for 5 months, without neurologic complications or disability.

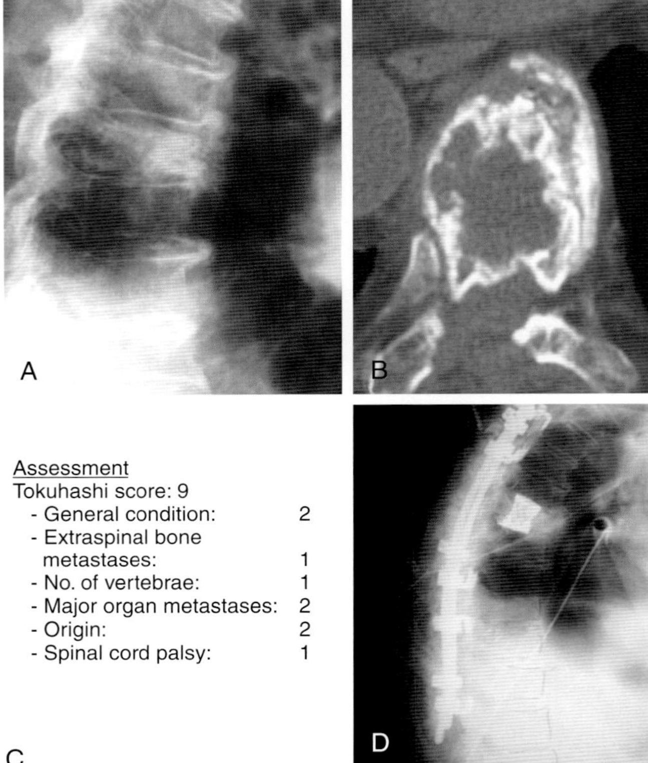

FIGURE 108-8. **A,** Lateral roentgenogram of the thoracic spine of a 72-year-old man with metastasis to the T7 vertebra from cancer of the prostate and incomplete paraplegia (ASIA C). **B,** Axial CT revealed osteolytic lesion in the vertebral body. **C,** Tokuhashi score was 9. The patient was treated with corpectomy, reconstruction with mesh cage, and posterior stabilization (**D**). This resulted in improvement of pain and neurologic rate in 15 months.

Summary

In this updated and upgraded version of a previously published chapter on this subject,[79] the conclusion remains that survival outcomes for managing metastatic spinal tumors are still gloomy. When assessing surgical outcomes, the following published parameters should form the baseline for acceptable outcomes: neurologic improvement (55–87%) restoration of ambulation (40–100%), restoration of sphincter control (36–89%), pain relief (47–100%); local recurrences (8–31%), complication (16–32%), reoperation rate for complications (7–24%), and patient satisfaction (55–80%). Furthermore, the reported mortality rate 4 to 6 weeks postoperatively ranges from 3% to 10.2%, whereas the mean survival is 8 to 15.9 months. Pain shows the greatest response. In addition, the prognostic factors that can influence the final outcomes are origin of tumor, visceral metastasis, number of affected vertebrae, state of neurologic dysfunction, and onset of surgical treatment. It is important to quantify the patient's pain, psychological distress, and performance status before establishing treatment goals. Certain outcome instruments have been validated for vertebral metastatic disease (EORTC, EQ-5D, QLOJL30, EQSD, HUI-MARK 3, ESAS, McGill Pain Questionnaire, VAS, MPAC). Appropriate surgical intervention is based on reasonable guidelines. The Harrington classification system

Assessment
Harrington class: V
Kostuik instability score: >20° kyphosis + 3/6
Tomita type: A III
Tokuhashi score: 9
- General condition: 1
- Extraspinal bone metastases: 2
- No. of vertebrae: 1
- Major organ metastases: 2
- Origin: 2
- Spinal cord palsy: 1

FIGURE 108-9. A 50-year-old woman with acute onset of leg weakness from metastatic breast cancer. Radiotherapy failed (neurologic deterioration). **A,** Sagittal CT; **B,** axial CT. **C,** Tokuhashi score was 9, indicating a good prognosis. Treatment consisted of radical corpectomy and reconstruction with titanium cage and Kaneda stabilization as seen on axial CT (**D**) and lateral radiograph (**E**). Ambulation was restored and the survival rate was over 12 months.

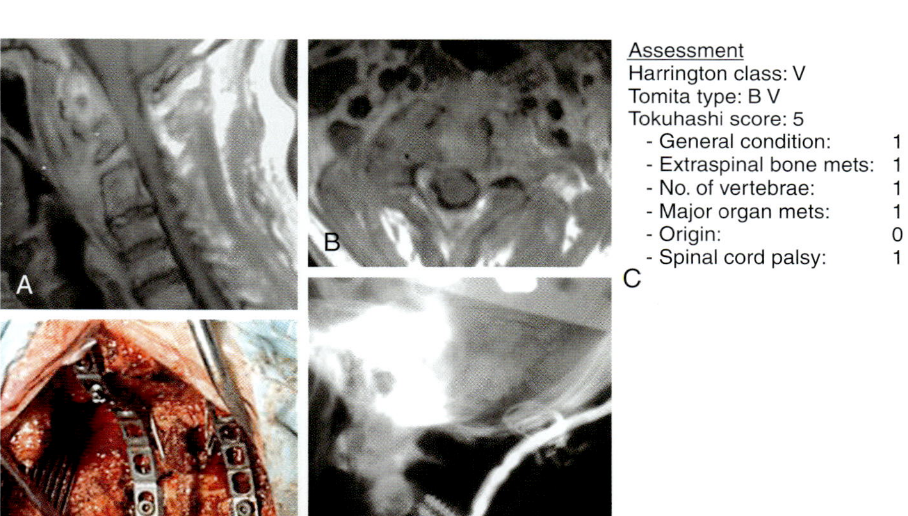

A
B
C
D
E
Assessment
Harrington class: V
Tomita type: B V
Tokuhashi score: 5
- General condition: 1
- Extraspinal bone mets: 1
- No. of vertebrae: 1
- Major organ mets: 1
- Origin: 0
- Spinal cord palsy: 1

FIGURE 108-10. A 60-year-old man with severe neck pain and leg weakness from metastatic lung cancer. Sagittal (**A**) and axial (**B**) MRIs. **C,** Tokuhashi score was 5. The patient underwent palliative treatment consisting of decompression, stabilization, and radiation (**D** and **E**). Ambulation was restored and the patient survived 11 months.

combined with the Kostuik instability model, the Tomita grading system for vertebral tumor spread, and the Tokuhashi preoperative scoring system questionnaire are excellent guides for predicting outcomes of metastatic tumors and establishing methods for selecting the most appropriate treatment. The degree of the clinical validity of these guidelines has not been vigorously tested and, therefore, is lacking strong scientific support. Although they are not consensus- or evidence-based guidelines, they are useful tools for selecting a more appropriate surgical intervention. Furthermore, they can form the basis for establishing the standards for more widely acceptable guidelines.

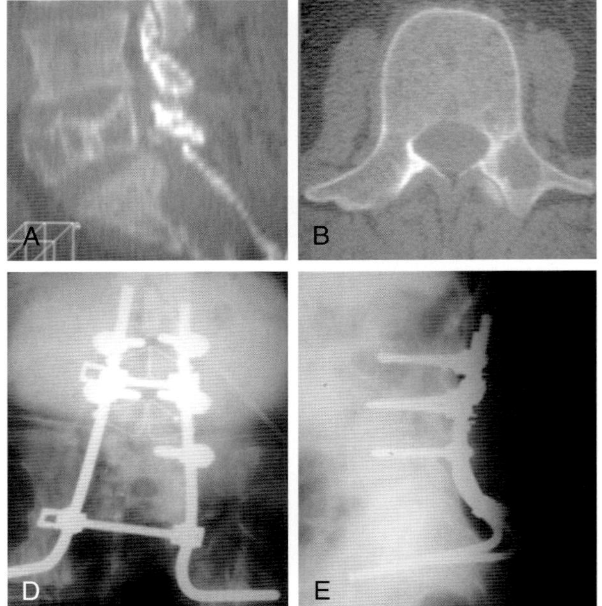

Assessment
Harrington class: V
Kostuik instability score: 3/6
Tomita type: M VII
Tokuhashi score: 8

- General condition:	1
- Extraspinal bone metastases:	2
- No. of vertebrae:	0
- Major organ metastases:	2
- Origin:	2
- Spinal cord palsy:	1

C

FIGURE 108-11. A 50-year-old man with severe back pain and increasing inability to walk from multiple myeloma. Lytic lesion as seen on sagittal (**A**) and axial CT (**B**). **C,** Assessment revealed a Tokuhashi score of 8. After a Galveston stabilization procedure (**D** and **E**), decompression, and radiation therapy, the patient's ambulation was restored completely and he survived for more than 12 months.

KEY REFERENCES

Bauer HCF: Posterior decompression and stabilization for spinal metastases: analysis of sixty-seven consecutive patients. *J Bone Joint Surg [Am]* 79:514, 1997.

Enkaoua EA, Doursounian L, Chatellier G, et al: Vertebral metastases: a critical appreciation of the preoperative prognostic Tokuhashi score in a series of 71 cases. *Spine (Phila Pa 1976)* 22:2293, 1997.

Harrington KD: Metastatic disease of the spine. *J Bone Joint Surg [Am]* 68:1110, 1986.

Karnofsky DA: Clinical evaluation of anticancer drugs: cancer chemotherapy. *GANN Monogr* 2:223, 1967.

Patchel RA, Tibbs PA, Regine WF, et al: Direct decompressive surgical resection in the treatment of spinal cord compression caused by metastatic cancer: a randomised trial. *Lancet* 366:643, 2005.

Tokuhashi Y, Matsuzaki H, Oda H, et al: A revised scoring system for preoperative evaluation of metastatic spine tumor prognosis. *Spine (Phila Pa 1976)* 30:2186, 2005.

Tokuhashi Y, Matsuzaki H, Toriyama S, et al: Scoring system for the preoperative evaluation of metastatic spine tumor prognosis. *Spine (Phila Pa 1976)* 15:1110, 1990.

REFERENCES

The complete reference list is available online at expertconsult.com.

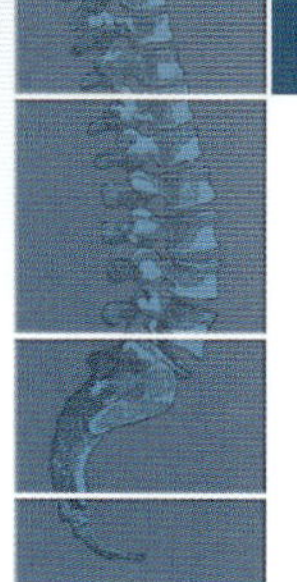

CHAPTER 109

Staging, Classification, and Oncologic Approaches for Metastatic Tumors Involving the Spine

J. Bradley Elder | Todd W. Vitaz | Mark H. Bilsky

The early diagnosis and management of metastatic spine tumors is essential to reducing pain, preserving or improving neurologic function, and improving quality of life. The three primary treatment modalities are radiation therapy (RT), surgery, and chemotherapy. Although these treatment modalities are all essential for treating metastatic spine tumors, prospective trials and prognostic guidelines have yet to definitively delineate the role of any single modality as first-line therapy. The evolution of advanced radiation techniques, such as image-guided (intensity-modulated) radiation therapy (IGRT), and noninvasive percutaneous cement augmentation procedures have added significantly to the armamentarium in the treatment of metastatic spine tumors and increased the complexity of decision making for this patient population. One recent randomized prospective study identified a subpopulation of patients who may benefit from surgery.[1] Although decision making for an individual patient remains largely based on institutional experience and the individual preferences of the treating physician,[2-3] clinical data and new decision frameworks can help guide therapy.

Decision Frameworks

Traditionally, assessment systems such as the Tomita and Tokuhashi scoring systems have been used to derive treatment for metastatic spine tumors.[2] The Tomita score takes into consideration the grade of malignancy and visceral and bone metastases. A low score indicates a good prognosis. The Tokuhashi scoring system is useful for predicting survival and evaluates performance status, tumor histology, neurologic impairment, and the numbers of bone, vertebral body, and visceral metastases.[3-5] These scoring systems were useful and validated for surgical outcomes, but the evolution of stereotactic radiosurgery has dramatically changed tumoral responses, making the surgical recommendations from these systems somewhat outdated.

At Memorial Sloan-Kettering Cancer Center (MSKCC), treatment decisions for patients with spine tumors are driven by a conceptual framework referred to as NOMS, which incorporates four fundamental considerations: neurologic (N), oncologic (O), mechanical (M), and systemic (S) disease.[6] Neurologic considerations include the presence of myelopathy or functional radiculopathy, as well as the degree of radiographic epidural spinal cord compression. Oncologic issues primarily reflect the ability to achieve local, durable tumor control, and, thus, reflect the radiosensitivity and/or chemosensitivity of the tumor. Mechanical instability is a separate assessment that evaluates the stability of the spine based on the presence of pathologic fractures, lytic bone destruction, deformity, and the presence of movement-related pain. Finally, the extent of systemic disease and medical comorbidities reflect the patient's ability to tolerate an operation, radiation, or chemotherapy and the patient's overall prognosis.

In general, the NOMS-based analysis is not intended as an algorithmic approach to patient care. Rather, this classification scheme offers a framework for discussion at multimodality treatment conferences (Fig. 109-1). Details regarding each of these four considerations are discussed later in the chapter.

Presentation

Back pain, the most common presenting symptom in patients with metastatic tumor to the bone or epidural space, often precedes the development of other neurologic symptoms by weeks or months. Back pain in a cancer patient is metastatic disease until otherwise proven. Two distinct types of back pain are encountered in patients with spine tumors: (1) biologic (i.e., tumor-related) pain and (2) mechanical pain.[7] Biologic pain is the most common presenting symptom in metastatic cancer patients. This pain syndrome is predominantly nocturnal or early morning pain that generally improves with activity during the day. A variety of causes have been proposed, including periosteal irritation, stimulation of intraosseous nerves, and increased pressure or mass effect from tumor tissue in the bone.[8] The likely genesis of biologic pain reflects the diurnal variation in endogenous steroid secretion from the adrenal gland. At night, steroid production is reduced, resulting in increased inflammatory pain caused by cytokines released by the tumor. During the day, steroid levels rise, eliminating this biologic pain. This inflammatory component of biologic pain generally responds to the administration of low-dose steroids (e.g., dexamethasone [Decadron] 4 mg three times daily). Definitive treatment of the underlying tumor with radiation or surgery often relieves this pain. Recurrence of biologic pain following treatment may be a harbinger of locally recurrent tumor.

Mechanical pain results from a structural abnormality of the spine, such as a lytic destruction of the vertebral body, resulting in instability (Fig. 109-2). Clinical symptoms and

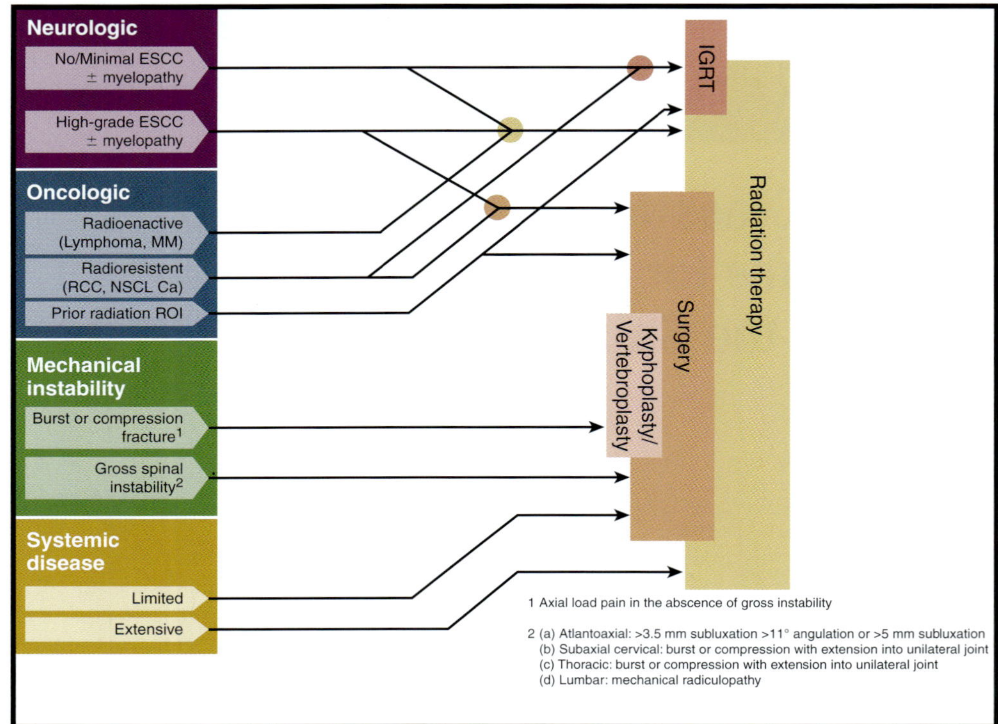

FIGURE 109-1. NOMS flowchart. Schematic diagram showing the potential treatment options based on patient-specific variables categorized into four groups. The neurologic category takes into consideration radiographic findings such as epidural spinal cord compression, as well as clinical findings such as myelopathy. The oncologic category accounts for the sensitivity of the tumor histology to radiation and whether the patient has received radiation to this area before. Mechanical instability accounts for spinal instability and fractures. Systemic disease considers the patient's overall metastatic disease burden. Treatment options based on these findings are illustrated as lines drawn from the NOMS finding to the therapeutic option. ESCC, epidural spinal cord compression; IGRT, image-guided radiation therapy; MM, multiple myeloma; NOMS, neurologic (N), oncologic (O), mechanical (M), and systemic (S) disease; NSCL Ca, Non–small-cell lung cancer; RCC, renal cell carcinoma; ROI, region of interest.

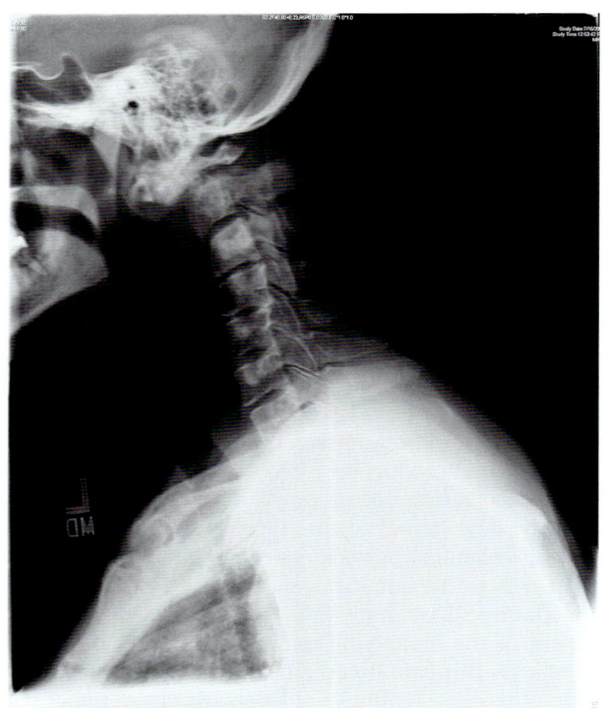

FIGURE 109-2. Mechanical instability. Lateral cervical spine plain radiograph showing fracture-subluxation of C2 due to metastatic renal cell carcinoma. (See also Figs. 109-6 and 109-15.)

radiographic correlation are important for establishing the diagnosis of instability. As opposed to biologic pain, patients with mechanical instability present with pain that is worse with movement and that is referable to the level of spinal involvement. For example, although pathologic fractures of the atlantoaxial spine may present with severe pain in flexion-extension, they virtually always have a rotational component. In the subaxial cervical spine, mechanical pain is worse with flexion and extension. Counterintuitively, patients with thoracic or thoracolumbar compression fractures often have severe pain when lying flat as opposed to sitting or standing, presumably because of extension of an unstable kyphosis (Fig. 109-3). The most common symptom of instability in the lumbar spine is mechanical radiculopathy. This lumbar pain syndrome results from an axial load narrowing the neural foramen, thus causing compression of the exiting nerve root. Mechanical pain does not typically respond to steroids but may be relieved with narcotics or an external orthosis, pending definitive therapy. Patients with intractable mechanical pain are often considered strong candidates for surgery or percutaneous cement augmentation procedures (Fig. 109-4).

Neurologic signs and symptoms often begin with radiculopathy (nerve root symptoms) and are followed by the development of myelopathy (spinal cord compression). Radiculopathy in the cervical or lumbar spine causes pain or weakness in the classic dermatomal distributions. However, thoracic radiculopathy occurs as bandlike pain at a segmental level. Myelopathy often presents with a pain level secondary to compression of the spinothalamic tracts followed by motor loss related to corticospinal tract involvement. This may be related to the pattern of tumor arising from the vertebral body compressing the anterolateral spinal cord. Loss of proprioception from involvement of the dorsal columns is often a late finding in myelopathy and results in difficulty regaining normal ambulation. Autonomic dysfunction, principally of bowel and bladder, are typically very late findings in myelopathy. The exception is compression at the level of the conus medullaris or diffuse sacral replacement where autonomic dysfunction can be a very early finding. Neurogenic bowel and bladder symptoms are almost universally associated with perineal numbness and are most often painless. In the absence of sensory changes, one should seek other causes for urinary or bowel incontinence, such as narcotics, prostatic hypertrophy, or excessive use of laxatives.

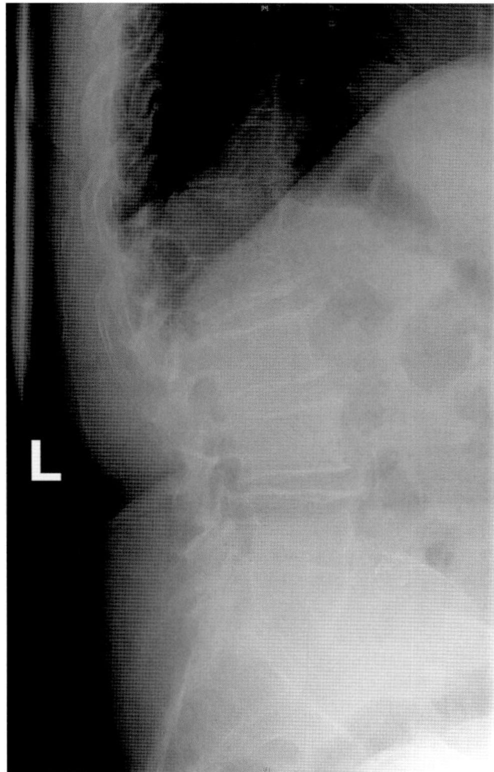

FIGURE 109-3. Pathologic compression fracture. Lateral thoracolumbar plain film showing L1 compression fracture due to multiple myeloma. Lesions at other levels, including T4 and T12, are not visualized on this film. (See also Figs. 109-4 and 109-5.)

Neurologic testing should not simply focus on sensorimotor function below the level of the lesion. This is important for several reasons. First, these patients often have multiple spine lesions and it is important to determine exactly which ones are contributing to the patient's symptoms. In addition, it is also important to adequately rule out other causes for symptoms such as brain metastasis or peripheral neuropathy. Any patient with facial weakness or other cranial neuropathies requires cranial imaging prior to surgical intervention for metastatic spine disease. In addition, focal extremity weakness with normal or decreased reflexes may be caused by plexus or peripheral nerve compression as is seen with brachial plexus metastases. Finally, adequate documentation of the patient's radiographic and neurologic status at the time of presentation is of utmost importance for judging either response or deterioration during the course of treatment.

Staging and Classification

The examination of spinal patients should include a pain assessment, quantitative neurologic score, general performance score, and quality-of-life assessment. Pain assessment can be most readily performed with a visual analogue scale. The score can be converted to reflect mild (0–4), moderate (5–6), and severe (7–10) pain.[9] The two most commonly used neurologic scales include the Frankel grading system and the American Spinal Injury Association (ASIA) score[10,11] (Table 109-1). Both assess motor function, with a score of "E" being normal and "A" being complete paralysis. Performance status reflects ambulation, medical comorbidities, and extent of disease. A patient may have normal motor strength but be unable to ambulate due to loss of proprioception, severe mechanical pain, lower extremity fracture, poor nutritional status, or poor pulmonary function. We have used the Eastern

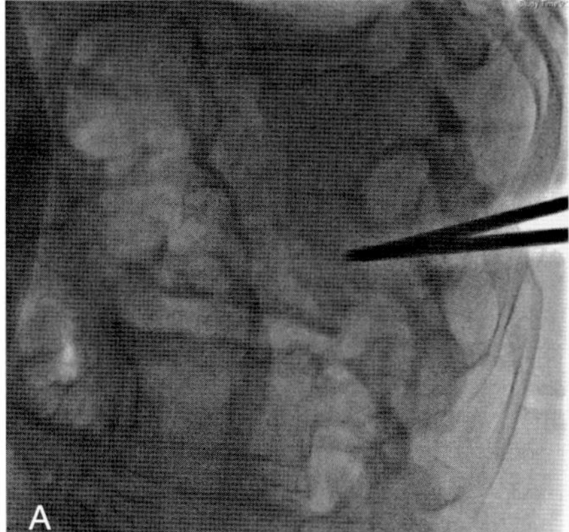

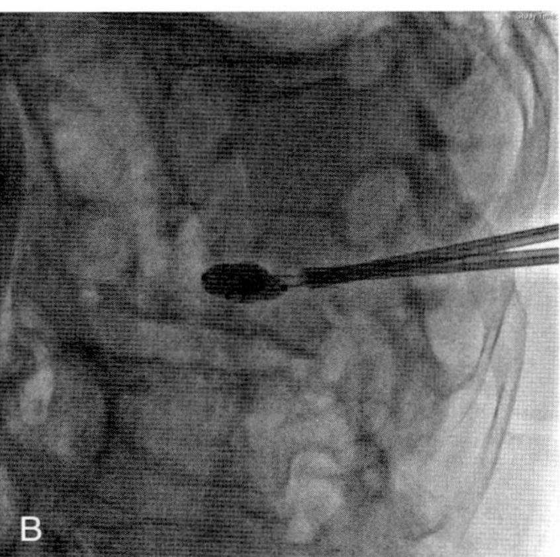

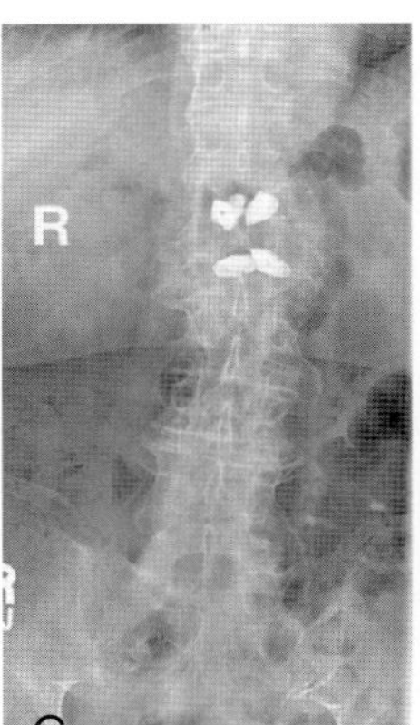

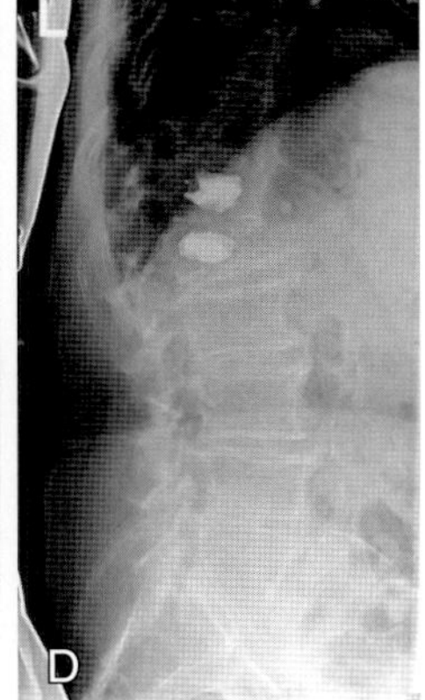

FIGURE 109-4. Kyphoplasty. Plain radiographs obtained during (**A** and **B**) and after (**C** and **D**) kyphoplasty procedure for the patient shown in Figure 109-3. **A,** Lateral plain radiograph showing percutaneous placement of bilateral Jamshidi needles into the pedicles of L1. **B,** Balloon inflation prior to instilling cement. Anteroposterior (**C**) and lateral plain radiographs (**D**) showing bilateral kyphoplasty of T12 and L1. (See also Figs. 109-3 and 109-5.)

TABLE 109-1

ASIA Impairment Scale

Grade	Description
A	Complete: No motor or sensory function below the level
B	Incomplete: Sensory but no motor function
C	Incomplete: Some motor function is preserved, but a majority of the muscle groups below the lesion have a grade <3
D	Incomplete: Some motor function preserved, but a majority of the muscle groups below the lesion have a grade >3
E	Normal sensory and motor function

ASIA, American Spinal Injury Association.

TABLE 109-2

ECOG Performance Status

Grade	Description
0	Fully active, able to carry on all predisease performance without restriction
1	Restricted in physically strenuous activity but ambulatory and able to perform light work
2	Ambulatory and capable of all self-care but unable to perform work activities (bedridden <50% of the time)
3	Capable of only limited self-care (bedridden >50% of the time)
4	Completely disabled, not capable of any self-care (bedridden 100% of the time)

ECOG, Eastern Cooperative Oncology Group.

TABLE 109-3

Review of Primary Cancers with Spinal Metastases seen at M.D. Anderson Cancer Center, 1984–1994

Primary Site	Percentage of All Spine Metastases (n = 11,884)
Breast	30.2
Lung	20.3
Blood	10.2
Prostate	9.6
Urinary tract	4.0
Skin	3.1
Unknown primary	2.9
Colon	1.6
Other	18.1

Adapted from Gokaslan ZL, York JE, Walsh GL, et al: Transthoracic vertebrectomy for metastatic spinal tumors. *J Neurosurg* 89(4): 599–609, 1998.

TABLE 109-4

Radiosensitivity of Various Metastatic Spine Tumors

Sensitivity	Tumor Histology
High	Lymphoma
	Myeloma
Intermediate	Breast
	Prostate
Low	Sarcoma
	Renal Cell
	Lung
	Colon

Cooperative Oncology Group (ECOG) performance status as a functional assessment[12] (Table 109-2). It is important to include both neurologic and performance status when reviewing outcomes in cancer patients.

Metastatic tumors to the spine are classified based on numerous features, including histology, location, and pattern of tumor. The most common spine metastases are listed in Table 109-3. These tumors are further classified into relatively radioresistant and radiosensitive groups (Table 109-4), which influences the decision to use radiation as first-line therapy. Tumors may further be divided by the level and extent of spinal element involvement (e.g., vertebral body, dorsal element, or circumferential) and degree of epidural compression (see later discussion). Thorough radiographic imaging is essential for treatment decisions.

Imaging

Advances in imaging techniques have improved the sensitivity of detecting spinal metastases and the specificity of differentiating other processes that involve the spine. MRI has revolutionized assessment of metastatic spine tumors, but many imaging modalities, including plain radiographs, bone scan, CT scan, myelogram, and positron emission tomography (PET), play a role in evaluating metastatic spinal tumors. The goal of imaging is to be 100% sensitive and specific in identifying tumor, giving precise anatomic detail, identifying distant metastases, and showing recurrent tumor following the placement of instrumentation. No single imaging modality accomplishes all of these goals, of course, but understanding the advantages and disadvantages of different imaging modalities allows the clinician to better decide patient screening and treatment planning.

Plain radiographs are often ordered as the first test to evaluate the cancer in a patient with new-onset back pain; however, plain films are relatively poor screening tests for metastases (Fig. 109-5). Visualization of a radiolucent defect on plain radiographs typically requires at least 50% destruction of the vertebral body. Additionally, metastatic tumor often infiltrates the bone marrow of the vertebral body without destroying the cortical bone. Compression and burst fractures are readily identified. Plain radiographs can identify sagittal (kyphosis) and coronal (scoliosis) plane deformities in a weight-bearing state, whereas spinal deformities imaged in a supine position by MRI or CT may be reduced and, thus, remain undetected. Dynamic flexion and extension films may be used to detect instability, although in our experience they are rarely necessary and may put the patient at risk for progressive spinal cord injury. Following surgery, plain films are the best imaging modality for assessing spinal alignment and structural integrity of the instrumentation.

Bone scans (using technetium-99m methylene diphosphonate [99mTc-MDP]) are more sensitive than plain radiographs for detecting spinal metastases[13] (Fig. 109-6). The advantage of a bone scan is its ability to screen the entire skeleton with a single image. Patients with spinal tumors often have other bone involvement that may be causing symptoms or require intervention. For example, a patient with L2 vertebral body

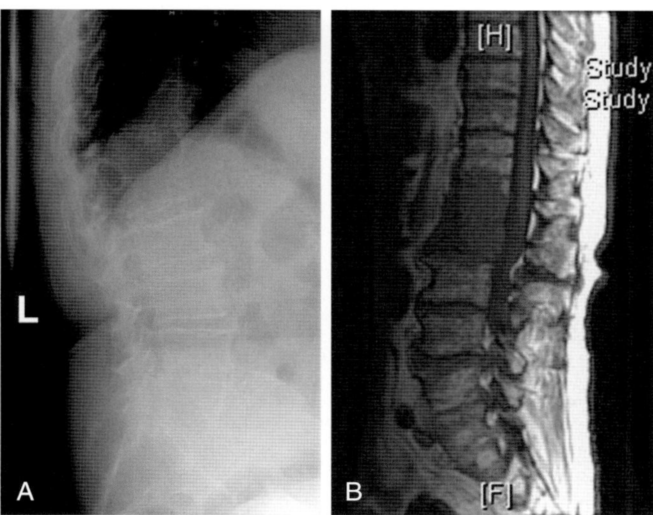

FIGURE 109-5. Comparison of plain film to MRI. **A,** Lateral plain radiograph of thoracolumbar spine showing a compression fracture at L1. This is the same film as Figure 109-3. **B,** MRI showing disease at T12 and L1. The T12 disease could not be appreciated on the plain film. (See also Figs. 109-3 and 109-4.)

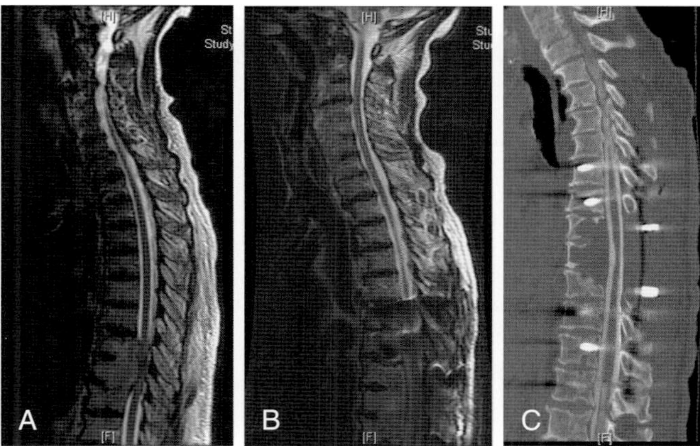

FIGURE 109-7. Comparison of MRI and CT myelogram after spine instrumentation. **A,** Preoperative T2-weighted MRI demonstrating severe spinal cord compression due to metastatic disease at T8-10. **B,** Postoperative T2-weighted MRI showing postsurgical changes and instrumentation. Note the artifacts caused by the pedicle screws that prevent complete visualization of the spinal canal. **C,** Postoperative CT myelogram allows better appreciation of the decompression of the thecal sac and spinal canal.

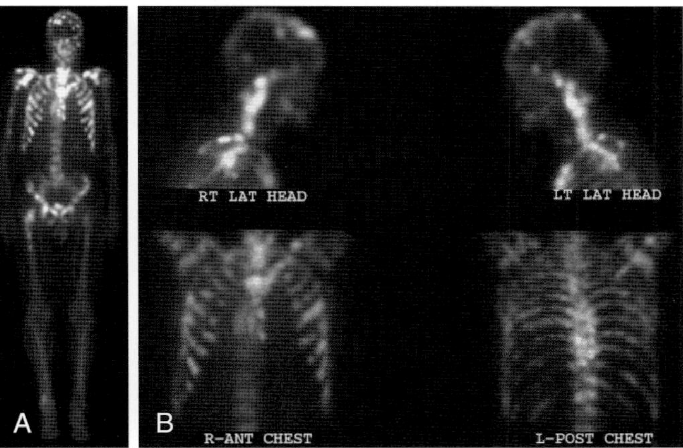

FIGURE 109-6. The bone scan is more sensitive than plain films for detecting metastatic disease. The images are total body (**A**) and head and chest views (**B**) showing numerous osseous metastases involving the skull, spine, ribs, pelvis, and long bones. Comparison of the lateral head and neck bone scan views to the plain radiograph of the same patient shown in Figure 109-2 demonstrates the increased sensitivity of bone scans for detecting osseous metastases. (See also Figs. 109-2 and 109-15.)

disease causing nerve root compression may have a concomitant, symptomatic tumor in the pelvis, hip, or femur. However, bone scans rely on an osteoblastic reaction or bone deposition to detect spinal metastases so that rapidly progressive, destructive tumors may not be detected.[13,14] Bone scans are relatively insensitive for multiple myeloma and tumors confined to the bone marrow and have a low specificity for tumor.[14] Fractures, degenerative disease, and benign disorders of the spine (Schmorl nodes, hemangioma) all may be positive. Additionally, paraspinal tumors that enter the epidural space through the neuroforamen can result in back pain and progressive neurologic symptoms that often are not detected on bone scan. In a review by Avrahami et al., 21 out of 40 patients (52%), with previously diagnosed tumor and symptoms referable to the spine had a negative CT and bone scan, but tumor was seen on MRI.[15] Frank et al. reviewed a series of 95 patients, 28% of whom had a negative bone scan with MRI scan showing tumor and a discordance rate between the two imaging modalities of 31%.[16]

Until MRI became widely available, myelogram and CT were the best diagnostic modalities for assessing acute spinal cord compression. Risks associated with myelography, including acute neurologic decompensation in patients with high-grade blocks, have diminished its role.[17,18] CT continues to be useful both for assessing the degree of bone destruction and for determining when bone rather than tumor is causing spinal cord compression. For patients who have had spinal reconstruction with placement of metallic instrumentation, including titanium, it may be difficult to obtain accurate images of the spinal canal with MRI, and CT myelogram may be helpful for ruling out recurrent epidural disease and spinal cord compression[19-21] (Fig. 109-7). Myelography and postmyelogram CT images continue to be used for imaging for these patients. Also, CT myelograms are currently used for radiosurgery treatment planning to specifically identify the location of the spinal cord or cauda equina.[22]

MRI is the most sensitive and specific modality for imaging spinal metastases. Sagittal screening images of the entire spine reveal bone, epidural, and paraspinal tumor.[23] The extent and degree of spinal cord compression can be readily appreciated, especially on T2-weighted images (Table 109-5). Hybrid scans of the brachial or lumbosacral plexus may reveal tumor in patients with extremity weakness that is not entirely related to spinal cord or root involvement. Leptomeningeal metastases and intradural metastases are often well visualized but require the use of contrast agents (gadolinium diethylene triamine pentaacetic acid [Gd-DPTA])[24] (Fig. 109-8).

Common imaging sequences used to evaluate spinal metastases are T1- and T2-weighted MRI.[25] Tumor on a T1-weighted image is hypointense relative to the normal marrow signal (Fig. 109-9A) and typically enhances after administration of gadolinium (Fig. 109-9B). The ports from prior

TABLE 109-5

Memorial Sloan-Kettering Cancer Center Epidural Spinal Cord Compression Grading Scale

Grade*	Description
0	No subarachnoid space compression
1	Subarachnoid space partially obliterated without spinal cord compression
2	Subarachnoid space partially obliterated with spinal cord compression
3	Subarachnoid space completely obliterated with cord compression

*Determined at level of worst compression.

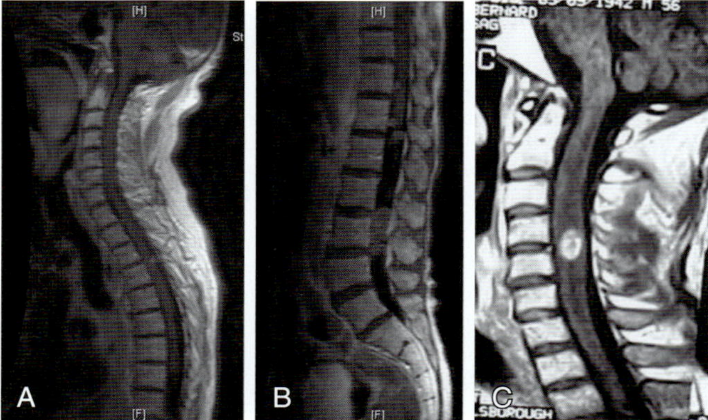

FIGURE 109-8. T1-weighted MRI after administration of gadolinium may reveal leptomeningeal disease or intramedullary metastases. Leptomeningeal disease is demonstrated at the T3-4 level (**A**) and the T11-12 and L2-4 levels (**B**) in a patient with gastric cancer. **C,** An intramedullary metastasis at the C4-5 level in a patient with prostate cancer.

spinal radiation can be discerned on T1-weighted images as hyperintense signal change and may assist in making acute therapeutic decisions when radiation port films are not available. Tumor is hyperintense relative to marrow on standard T2-weighted imaging and produces a myelogram effect with cerebrospinal fluid appearing hyperintense (Fig. 109-9C). Unfortunately, using the recently developed timesaving fast-spin echo, T2 techniques may decrease tumor conspicuity. This decreased conspicuity can be compensated for using short-tau inversion recovery (STIR) techniques. STIR images show enhanced contrast between the lipid marrow (hypointense) and tumor (hyperintense)[26-28] (Fig. 109-9D). They may be the most sensitive screening modality for tumor but give less anatomic detail than standard T1 or fast spin echo T2 images.[29] Because of the high rate of multiple noncontiguous lesions, we suggest screening the entire spine with sagittal sequences followed by axial cuts through any areas of abnormality. At our institution, a screening assessment of the entire spine is obtained specifically to evaluate the T1- and T2-weighted STIR images. The degree of compression is based on the axial T2- and/or axial T1-weighted postcontrast images.

The conversion of spine tumor assessment from CT-myelogram to MRIs left a void in describing the degree of spinal cord compression. For instance, no correlate existed on MRI for a complete myelographic block. NOMS decision making is often made based on the neurologic assessment of

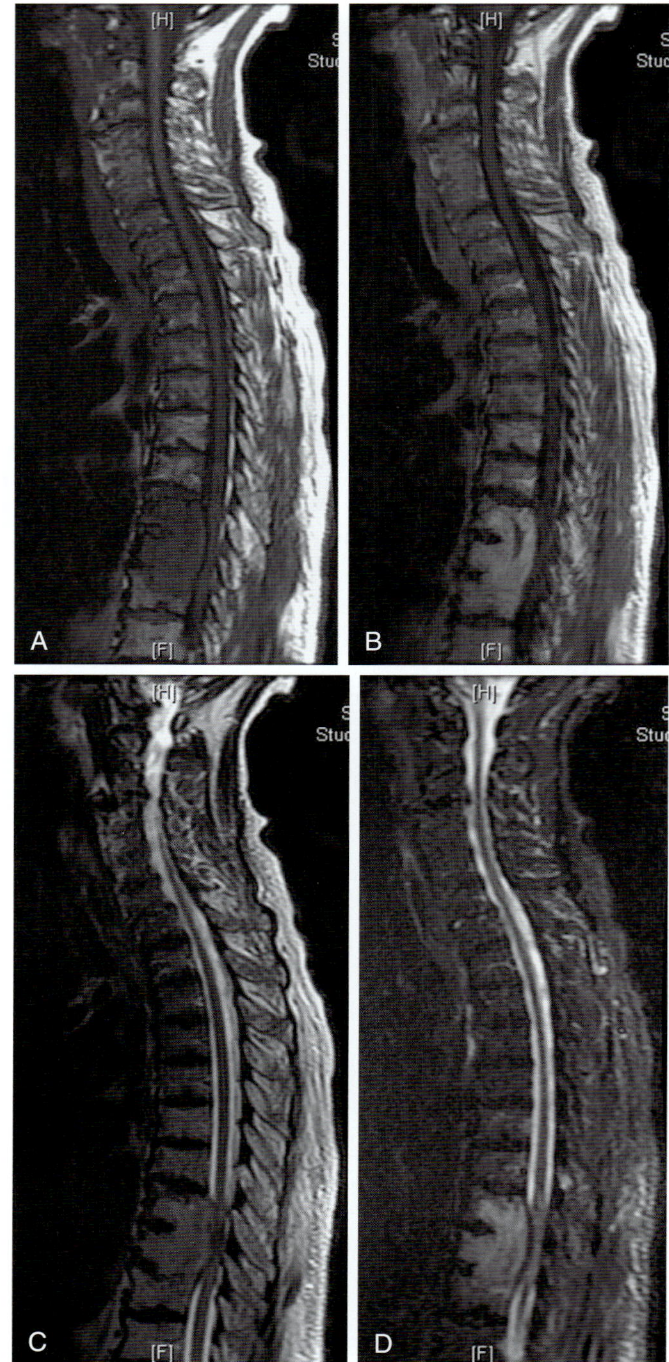

FIGURE 109-9. Different MRI sequences showing the cervicothoracic spine in a patient with thyroid cancer and multiple spine metastases. **A,** T1-weighted MRI, the tumor at T8-10 is dark compared with the bone marrow of unaffected vertebrae. **B,** T1-weighted MRI after administration of gadolinium shows an enhancing tumor that is now brighter than unaffected vertebrae. **C,** The tumor is also brighter than other vertebrae on T2-weighted MRI. **D,** Distinction between tumor and marrow is made easier using the short-tau inversion recovery (STIR) sequence because fat in the marrow is assigned an intensity of 0, although the resolution of a STIR sequence is lower than that of a T2-weighted image.

the degree of spinal cord compression in combination with relative radioresistance of the tumor.[6] A recent review by the Spine Oncology Study Group showed greater interrelater and intrarelater reliability using T2-weighted images than with T1-weighted pre- or postcontrast images in the assessment of spinal cord compression.[29A] The newly revised epidural spinal cord compression (ESCC) grading system assesses tumors on T2-weighted axial images and assigns a score from 0 to 3. Grade 0 indicates tumor within bone only without any involvement of the epidural space. Grade 1 is subarachnoid space impingement by tumor extending from the bone, but no compression or deformation of the spinal cord. For radiosurgery planning purposes, ESCC grade 1 was subdivided into 1a (epidural abutment), 1b (epidural impingement), or 1c (epidural impingement with spinal cord abutment). Grade 2 indicates spinal cord compression and deformation, but spinal fluid is still visualized at the level of compression. Grade 3 is spinal cord compression with obliteration of all cerebrospinal fluid space at the level of cord compression. Grade 3 is the magnetic resonance (MR) radiographic equivalent of a complete block on myelogram (Fig. 109-10; see also Table 109-5).

Although MRI is an excellent screening tool for metastatic tumor spread to bone, differentiating tumor from osteomyelitis, osteoporotic compression fractures, and previously treated tumor may be difficult. The T1- and T2-signal characteristics are similar in all of these conditions. Osteomyelitis is more likely to cause changes in the end plate and disc space, whereas tumor rarely, if ever, involves the disc space. Based on these imaging characteristics, osteomyelitis can be differentiated from tumor with 97% accuracy.[30] Unfortunately, patients with tumor may secondarily become infected, rendering the imaging patterns unreliable in these situations.[31]

Osteoporotic compression fractures are extremely common in the cancer population and have been differentiated from pathologic fractures with 94% accuracy based on T1-weighted imaging characteristics.[32] Osteoporotic fractures are more commonly thoracic, lack signal change, have bandlike abnormality and do not involve the pedicle, or have contour abnormality. Pathologic fractures show homogeneously decreased signal and have convex vertebral contours. Pathologic fractures may involve the pedicles and are more commonly located in the lumbar spine.

Oncologists often rely on imaging changes to determine the efficacy of treatment; however, response to RT or chemotherapy is difficult to assess in bone tumors because of the lack of signal change on MRI. On T1-weighted images, both treated and viable tumors appear hypointense relative to normal marrow signal. In a study of breast cancer patients, only 3% had a reduction in the volume or number of vertebral

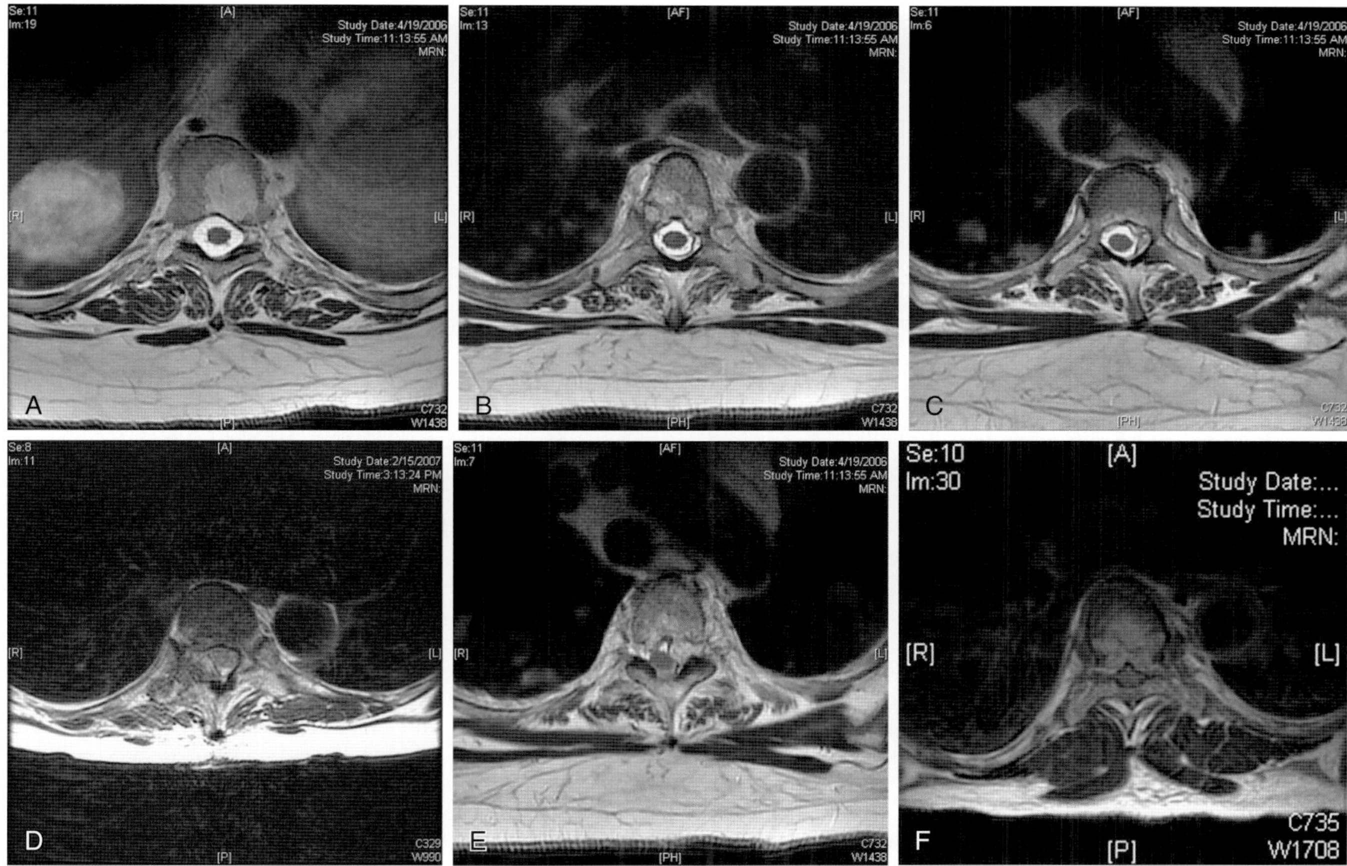

FIGURE 109-10. The epidural spinal cord compression grading scheme described in Table 109-5 is illustrated here with representative axial T2-weighted MRI. Grade 1 is epidural disease without spinal cord compression and is divided into three grades. **A,** Grade 0—bone involvement only. **B,** Grade 1a—abutment of the thecal sac. **C,** Grade 1b—indentation of the thecal sac. **D,** Grade 1c—abutment of the spinal cord. **E,** Spinal cord compression or deformation, but cerebrospinal fluid (CSF) is still found at this level. **F,** Spinal cord compression with obliteration of all CSF space at this level.

bodies involved on imaging, and there was no correlation between changes in signal intensity and clinical response to therapy.[33] In a palliative care situation, clinical response to therapy (resolution of tumor-related pain) may suffice despite the absence of radiographic change. Therapeutic decisions for some metastatic tumors (e.g., Ewing sarcoma, neuroblastoma, and seminoma) rely on differentiating viable from necrotic tumor. Traditional MRI sequences do not change significantly after treatment. Current investigations are examining the use of MR perfusion to differentiate viable from necrotic tumor.

Recent work has explored the use of 2-[^{18}F] fluoro-2-deoxy-D-glucose (FDG-PET) for differentiating osteoporotic or traumatic fractures from pathologic compression fractures and to determine viability of previously treated bone tumors.[34-36] Additionally, on T1-weighted images, bone edema may appear hypointense similar to tumor signal and FDG-PET may be useful in directing the biopsy to a specific hypermetabolic site in the vertebral body, thereby increasing the chance of successfully making a diagnosis. Laufer et al. reviewed 82 patients with hematologic and solid tumor malignancies. All patients underwent biopsy within 6 weeks of their PET scan. The mean standard uptake values (SUVs) were 7.1 for malignant tumors compared with 2.1 for benign lesions ($P < .02$). A 100% concordance was identified with an SUV cutoff of 2 in solid tumor malignancies with lytic or mixed lytic sclerotic bone involvement. Sclerotic bone lesions often have low SUVs secondary to the paucity of tumor cell, and PET is less predictive in differentiating osteoblastic tumors from benign pathology.[37] Similar work relating SUVs to the presence of tumor found a threshold cutoff of 2.5 that predicted tumor.[38] Improved diagnostic accuracy can be achieved by combining PET with CT since ^{18}(F)-FDG PET/CT has a greater specificity for detecting spine metastases than either ^{18}(F)-FDG PET or CT alone[39] (Fig. 109-11). Other radionuclide scans may be helpful for screening specific tumor types, including iodine-109 scans for papillary thyroid cancer, *meta*-iodobenzylguanidine (MIBG) scans for neuroblastoma, and somatostatin scans for neuroendocrine tumors.

Metabolic and Physiologic Issues

Cancer patients are prone to numerous metabolic and physiologic abnormalities either as the result of their disease process or due to side effects of previous treatments. Therefore, assessment for many of these abnormalities must be performed prior to considering treatment. Hypercalcemia occurs in approximately 10% to 20% of all cancer patients, with lung and breast tumors being the most common primaries.[40] The pathophysiologic abnormalities that lead to this condition are believed to be secondary to the multifactorial effects of increased bone turnover and increased calcium reabsorption in the proximal renal tubules. However, immobilization and dehydration have also been shown to be contributing factors, especially in patients with end-stage disease.[40] These homeostatic abnormalities are now thought to be the result of secretion of a parathyroid-related protein as well as secretion of cytokines such as transforming growth factor-beta (TGF-β), interleukin-1 (IL-1), and tumor necrosis factor (TNF).[41] Hypercalcemia is commonly treated with IV fluid rehydration and bisphosphonate administration; left untreated, it can result in cardiac or kidney dysfunction, and even death in extreme cases.[42]

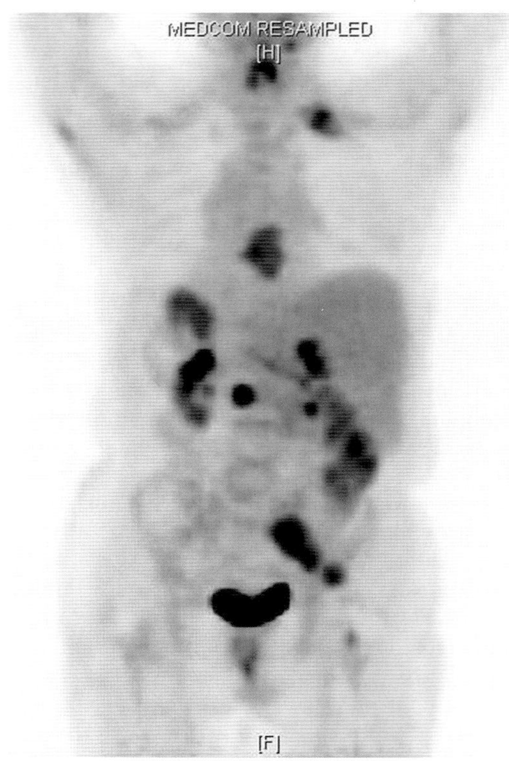

FIGURE 109-11. Whole-body representation generated from a positron emission tomography (PET)/CT showing multiple areas of osseous metastatic disease (*dark*) in a patient with thyroid cancer.

Coagulation abnormalities also occur commonly in this patient population. This can be attributed both to their cancer diagnosis as well as to an association with neurosurgical procedures.[43] Coagulopathies can result from metastatic tumor spread to the liver or more commonly from the toxic side effects of chemotherapeutic agents. In addition, frequent blood transfusions that some of these patients receive may result in antiplatelet antibodies, which may be resistant to replacement transfusions. Thrombocytopenia may result from diffuse bone marrow replacement or wide field irradiation, but commonly results from chemotherapy or common medications, such as heparin. A blood panel for heparin-induced thrombocytopenia (HIT) is obtained for patients taking heparin or heparin analogues who are thrombocytopenic, and the medication should be stopped. Treatment for coagulopathies depends primarily on the underlying cause.[44]

Diminished pulmonary reserve is another abnormality that is encountered quite commonly in patients with metastatic tumors. For example, patients undergoing thoracotomy for the treatment of lung cancer may be left with marginal reserve capacity. This is also seen as a result of multiple lung metastases, interstitial pulmonary fibrosis secondary to chemotherapy, pleural effusion, and the consequences of smoking. At our institution, all patients obtain a chest radiograph, and any patients with prior thoracotomy, any previously mentioned risk factor, or a history of dyspnea have their cases evaluated with preoperative pulmonary function tests.

Cancer patients are also at an increased risk for developing deep venous thrombosis (DVT).[45] The etiology is thought to be multifactorial and not simply a result of immobility. Many solid tumors release cytokines and other tissue factors that have procoagulant effects. We have found perioperative prophylaxis with pneumatic compression boots and subcutaneous dalteparin (Fragmin, 5000 units SQ bid) to be helpful in decreasing the rate of postoperative DVT, but not foolproof. Patients immobilized with paresis or pain, routinely undergo Doppler ultrasounds prior to surgery. Any DVT identified preoperatively is managed with inferior vena cava filter placement. Leon et al. showed a benefit to prophylactic filter placement for patients undergoing major spine surgery.[46] Risk factors for pulmonary embolism included malignancy, prior history of thromboembolism, bedridden more than 2 weeks prior to surgery, staged or multilevel procedures, and prolonged surgery (>8 hours). Consideration for placement of removable vena cava filters should be given to any tumor patient with a significant paresis or plegia who will need to intermittently discontinue full-dose anticoagulation. Postoperatively, DVTs are treated with either inferior vena cava filters or anticoagulation.

Many patients treated for spinal cord compression are also undergoing active chemotherapeutic treatment for either their primary disease or to control metastatic disease. A major concern is that many of these agents affect blood counts for several days after their administration. This may place patients at risk for neutropenia, anemia, or thrombocytopenia, all of which can have devastating consequences if not considered preoperatively.

Estimating Tumor Burden in Other Regions

The presence of distant metastases to extraspinal sites and active disease at the primary site are not contraindications to spine surgery, but recognizing the extent of disease is important for decision making. In patients with diffusely metastatic or rapidly progressive tumor, options such as irradiation may be more appropriate. However, we often determine the appropriateness of surgical interventions based more on the patient's overall medical condition than the tumor load. Even in cases with limited life expectancy (3–6 months), decompression and stabilization may help preserve neurologic function, and thus quality of life, as well as palliate pain symptoms with an acceptable level of morbidity.

At MSKCC, tumor staging is usually performed in conjunction with the primary oncologists, who have a better appreciation of the patient's disease in terms of overall aggressiveness and pace of progression.[6] This workup is typically performed with radiographic studies, including CT with and without contrast of the chest, abdomen, and pelvis. PET-CT is more commonly used as a screening method. Serum markers can also be used to screen for the presence or progression of tumors, such as prostate-specific antigen (PSA, prostate carcinoma), CA-125 (breast carcinoma), and carcinoembryonic antigen (CEA, colon carcinoma). These markers are remarkably sensitive and may be an early indicator of tumor recurrence. In hormone-refractory prostate carcinoma with spine involvement, the PSA often serves as a marker for tumor recurrence well in advance of scheduled surveillance MRI.

Pain Control

The adequate control of cancer-related and postoperative pain can be very challenging in this population. A significant number of these patients may have chronic pain syndromes and require large doses of narcotics, typically in the form of delayed-release oral or transdermal preparations.[47,48] This makes postoperative pain control difficult because of tolerance to these agents. At our institution, all patients receive narcotics via patient-controlled analgesia (PCA: morphine, fentanyl, or hydromorphone [Dilaudid]) postoperatively for several days with frequent dosing modifications until pain is adequately controlled. Following this, they are switched to equianalgesic doses of oral or transdermal medications. It is often helpful to obtain the input from pain management specialists for those patients with significant preoperative symptoms or high dose requirements.

Treatment

Three modalities are currently used to treat spinal metastases: (1) systemic chemotherapy or hormonal therapy, (2) RT, and (3) surgery. The first modality—chemotherapy or hormonal therapy—can be divided into antitumor drugs and drugs that prevent or ameliorate the effects of tumor, such as steroids or bisphosphonates.

Antitumor Chemotherapy

Antitumoral chemotherapy currently plays a relatively limited role in the treatment of spinal metastases. However, antitumor chemotherapy has an important role in the treatment of chemosensitive tumors, such as neuroblastoma, Ewing sarcoma (primitive neuroectodermal tumor [PNET]), osteogenic sarcoma, germ cell tumors, and lymphoma.[49] At MSKCC, chemotherapy is often considered the primary treatment for patients with these tumors even in the presence of epidural compression (Fig. 109-12). Chemotherapy and hormones may be useful in the treatment of prostate and breast carcinoma, but local therapy with radiation and/or surgery is commonly used for symptomatic metastases.

Steroids. Steroids are typically used for two indications in patients with metastatic spine tumors. The first is for the control of biologic pain. Typically, the administration of low doses will have profound effects on the level of pain in patients with this type of symptoms. The second indication is for the control of vasogenic edema to help reduce or stabilize neurologic symptoms in preparation for definitive radiation or surgical treatment. The optimal dose used to treat patients with acute spinal cord compression is controversial.[50-54] Doses range from moderate (16 mg/day in divided doses) to high (96 mg/day in divided doses) with or without a 10- to 100-mg load. It is unclear whether higher-dose steroids improve neurologic outcomes compared with moderate-dose steroids, but significantly more complications result from the higher doses.[55] In a case-control series from a single institution, total side effects seen in the moderate- and high-dose steroids were 8% and 29%, respectively.[55] Complications from steroids include hyperglycemia, gastrointestinal hemorrhage, intestinal perforation, and avascular necrosis of the hip. The use of steroids during radiation is also controversial, but these drugs are commonly used in symptomatic patients with high-grade spinal cord compression to prevent spinal cord swelling and neurologic decompensation. In patients fully ambulatory without spinal cord compression, steroids may not be needed. In a case series of 20 patients treated with conventional radiation, all maintained ambulation without toxicity.[56]

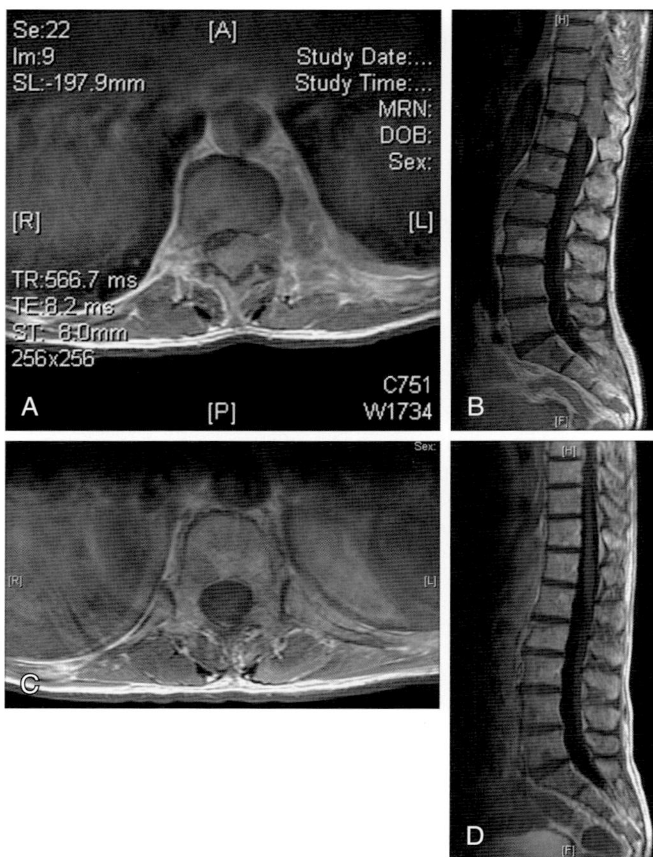

FIGURE 109-12. Multiple myeloma (MM) often responds rapidly to radiation. A patient with MM and spine disease at multiple sites presented with worsening back pain. T1-weighted MRI after gadolinium administration showed severe cord compression (grade 3) from T10-12: axial (**A**) and sagittal (**B**) views. Ten days later, after receiving 24 Gy in eight fractions, T1-weighted MRI after gadolinium administration: axial (**C**) and sagittal (**D**) views showed the tumor was no longer present in the spinal canal (grade 0).

In a patient with an undiagnosed spinal mass, steroids should be withheld prior to biopsy because of the oncolytic effect of these drugs on certain tumors such as lymphoma and thymoma.[57] The exception may be patients with high-grade spinal cord compression and myelopathy in whom a delay in steroid administration may affect neurologic outcome.

Bisphosphonates. Bone destruction that occurs secondary to bone metastases results from a combination of osteoclast activation and osteoblast inhibition. Tumor cells secrete substances such as parathyroid hormone-related protein, TGF-β, cytokines, and interleukins that affect the balance between osteoblastic bone formation and osteoclastic bone turnover.[58-60] These substances lead to osteoclast activation and thus increased bone turnover. Therefore, these cells are thought to play a central role in the development of bone metastasis, and inhibition of these cells may limit the progression of such metastases.[61-64] In multiple myeloma, the molecular mechanisms of osteoclast activation have been extensively studied. Multiple myeloma cells induce stromal cells to secrete cytokines, such as IL-6, TNF-β, and insulin-like growth factor. These cytokines up-regulate the receptor activator for nuclear factor κ B ligand (RANKL) expression, inducing the creation and activation of osteoclasts.[65-68] Osteoprotegerin normally inhibits RANK-RANKL signaling, but the level of osteoprotegerin is markedly decreased in multiple myeloma patients. This inhibition leads to increased osteoclast activation and lytic bone destruction.[69] In addition to osteoclast activation, multiple myeloma results in osteoblast inhibition. This inhibition prevents osteogenesis, adding significantly to the resultant lytic destruction of bone. Recent evidence suggests that gene expression of the secreted glycoprotein *dickkopf 1 (DKK)* inhibits the Wnt signaling pathway, which is essential for the growth and differentiation of osteoblasts.[70,71] Increased expression of DKK1 has been associated with lytic bone destruction in multiple myeloma patients.[72]

Other work has further characterized the extracellular cues, intracellular signaling cascade, and gene expression profiles that mediate osteolytic metastasis in various types of cancer, primarily breast cancer.[73,74] This work helps to explain the tendency of certain cancers to metastasize to bone, particularly the spine.

Bisphosphonates are a class of drugs recently studied as a potential treatment for cancer patients. Bisphosphonates are synthetic derivatives of pyrophosphates that reduce skeletal complications in cancer patients.[75-77] These agents inhibit osteoclast activity and, thus, reduce or inhibit further bone resorption; however, bisphosphonates do not promote the deposition of new bone.[78] This occurs as a result of down-regulation and apoptosis of osteoclasts, which decreases bone turnover.[58]

Oral bisphosphonates are not generally effective. The IV preparations used to prevent skeletal events in cancer patients include zoledronic acid (4 mg) and pamidronate (90 mg) administered every 3 to 4 weeks. Although zoledronic acid is more expensive, the injection can be given in 15 minutes compared with the 2 hours required for pamidronate. Clodronate and ibandronate are two additional bisphosphonates that have been explored in European studies for multiple myeloma patients, but are not currently approved in the United States. Multiple randomized clinical studies have shown that the use of these medications can significantly decrease the rate of skeletal-related events, such as pathologic fractures, compression fractures, hypercalcemia, and need for radiation to bone metastases in patients with breast cancer and multiple myeloma.[77,79-93] In addition, some studies in patients with breast cancer have shown that use of these compounds prior to development of bony metastasis may decrease the rate of future bone metastasis and skeletal-related complications when compared to the group receiving the placebo.[94-97] Other work does not show benefit in breast cancer patients in terms of bone metastases or fractures.[98] Berenson et al. reported the results of the Myeloma Aredia Study Group, in which 392 patients were randomized to receive placebo or pamidronate every 4 weeks for 21 cycles.[81] Skeletal-related events (SREs) were defined as pathologic fractures, the need for radiation therapy or surgery, or progression to spinal cord compression. At 21 months' follow-up, the mean number of annual SREs was 2.1 in the placebo group compared with 1.1 in the pamidronate group (P = .008). The median time to first SRE was 10 months in the placebo group and 21 months in the pamidronate group (P < .001).

These findings have been confirmed by laboratory experiments, which have shown that these agents decrease the adherence of tumor cells to bone structures.[99-101] However, studies evaluating the efficacy of these compounds for prostate cancer have shown mixed results.[102-108] In addition to protecting against skeletal complications, these medications have also been found to be useful in controlling bone pain.[109-115] Despite their ability to minimize bone metastasis and control tumor-related pain, none of these compounds have ever been shown to improve survival.[77,90,92,96]

The American Society of Clinical Oncology has published practice guidelines for the administration of bisphosphonates in patients with multiple myeloma.[116] Zoledronic acid or pamidronate is recommended for patients with lytic bone destruction or compression fracture from osteopenia. Additionally, for patients with diffuse osteopenia based on plain radiographs or a bone mineral density test in the absence of lytic disease or compression fractures, the recommendation is to start therapy. Patients on bisphosphonates are monitored for renal failure with monthly serum creatinine levels prior to administration of therapy. Patients are also monitored every 3 to 6 months for proteinuria. Other routine blood tests include measuring calcium, magnesium, and hemoglobin. Adverse side effects from bisphosphonates include transient myalgias, arthralgias, and flulike symptoms.[77-91] Side effects from bisphosphonates are uncommon, but may be debilitating. Gastrointestinal side effects predominate, especially esophagitis and diarrhea; however, administration with a full glass of water may limit many of these complaints. Other problems such as fever, fatigue, or headache have also been described.[91,92] Recently, osteonecrosis of the jaw (ONJ) has been described in conjunction with bisphosphonates. Zervas et al.[117] reported a 9.5-fold increase in this complication using zoledronic acid compared with pamidronate. To date, the role of bisphosphonates remains unclear in the genesis of ONJ as most patients are additionally receiving chemotherapy, radiation, and steroids. A number of patients with ONJ have poor dentition or recent dental work. Patients may benefit from pretreatment comprehensive dental care.

Treatment Decisions

Although chemotherapies and hormonal therapies play a role in the treatment of metastatic spine tumors, radiation therapy or surgery is considered the principle initial treatment. Technologic advances in both radiation and surgery have dramatically changed decision making over the past 10 years. From a surgical perspective, ventral transcavitary and dorsolateral approaches as well as segmental ventral and dorsal instrumentation improved outcomes for tumor patients.[118-140] Percutaneous cement augmentation provides significant pain relief in the presence of pathologic fracture. Additionally, the evolution of spine stereotactic radiosurgery (SSRS) provided unprecedented local tumor control for radioresistant tumors. The NOMS framework integrates these technologic advances into the decision making for metastatic spine tumors.

The neurologic and oncologic decisions regarding surgery versus radiation are typically made in combination. The essential considerations from a neurologic perspective are the degree of spinal cord compression with or without myelopathy and, from an oncologic perspective, the radiosensitivity of the tumor. Historically, variable radiosensitivity based on tumor histology was recognized but was not part of the decision-making process, because the results from surgery were so poor. In the 1970s, RT replaced laminectomy without instrumentation as first-line therapy for patients with spinal metastasis with epidural compression. This was based on several comparative studies that showed no difference in outcome between patients undergoing external photon beam RT versus those receiving laminectomy without dorsal segmental fixation (often in combination with RT).[17,141-157] In these older series, approximately 75% of patients were nonambulatory at the time of presentation.[158] Patients undergoing RT alone showed a 79% rate of maintaining ambulation, and paraparetic patients showed a 42% rate of return to ambulation. Both ambulatory and nonambulatory patients had a 21% risk of neurologic decompensation during RT. Patients undergoing laminectomy alone, or those receiving postoperative RT, had a 48% to 67% rate of maintaining ambulation, and paraparetic patients had a 33% rate of recovering ambulatory status. A range of 17% to 52% of patients showed neurologic decompensation following surgery with or without the addition of postoperative RT. The posttreatment morbidity was significantly less from RT than from surgery.

Radiosensitive Tumors

As advanced surgical approaches provided the ability to decompress and stabilize the spine with acceptable morbidity, the differential in radiation responsiveness became essential for decision making. Patients with radiosensitive tumors can be treated successfully with conventional external beam radiation (cEBRT), often delivered as 30-Gy doses in 10 fractions, regardless of the degree of epidural spinal cord compression. These tumors often respond dramatically, so that even with high-grade ESCC and myelopathy, radiation will decompress the spinal cord. Maranzano and Latini have the best functional results after radiation therapy, with 76% of patients ambulating after radiation and 51% of nonambulatory patients regaining ambulation.[159] The study included 209 evaluable cases that underwent 30-Gy RT using two different fractionated dosing schedules. Patients with favorable tumor histology (lymphoma, myeloma, and seminoma) received 10 fractions in 2 weeks. Patients with less favorable histology received 5 Gy daily for 3 days followed by five daily doses of 3 Gy after a 4-day rest. The results depended greatly on tumor histology, with liver, bladder, and RCC showing significantly less recovery than did breast and hematologic malignancies (i.e., lymphoma and myeloma). For example, breast carcinoma demonstrated an 80% response rate compared with hepatocellular carcinoma with a 20% response rate.

Radioresistant Tumors

As noted, traditionally radioresistant tumors respond poorly to cEBRT, but SSRS has changed the concept of radioresponsiveness even for tumors such as RCC, lung adenocarcinoma, colon carcinoma, and melanoma. As initial therapy, high-dose single-fraction radiation can be effectively delivered to tumors in the absence of high-grade ESCC (ESCC 0 to 1b). Yamada et al. reported outcomes in 103 solid-tumor metastases treated in a dose escalation from 18 to 24 Gy in a single fraction. All tumors were resistant to cEBRT with the exception of six breast carcinomas. The local control was 90%, with failures occurring at a median of 9 months. Minimal toxicity was noted with grade 1 and 2 skin or esophageal tumors. No evidence of myelopathy or functional radiculopathy was encountered. Dose constraints were maintained at less than 14 Gy to a single voxel (single point in a three-dimentional image set) on the spinal cord and less than 16 Gy to the cauda equina.[160] In a recent update of 248 treated lesions in 229 patients with a median follow-up of 17 months (range, 6–58 months), patients who received 24 Gy had a radiographic tumor control of 95%, whereas those who received 18 to 23 Gy demonstrated a local control of only 80% (P = .048) (see Fig. 109-1). Tumor local control was not affected by traditional factors that influence outcome for cEBRT, such as tumor histology or size. Other investigators have found that even traditionally radioresistant tumors, such as melanoma and RCC, respond as well as radiosensitive histologies such as breast cancer when SSRS was given.[161-163] However, others have found that histology does make a difference in tumor control when SSRS is utilized, with RCC and melanoma doing significantly worse.[164]

Surgery

Surgery is currently indicated as initial therapy in patients with high-grade spinal cord compression from radioresistant tumors with myelopathy and spinal instability (Box 109-1). From a practical standpoint, symptomatic spinal cord compression requires expeditious decompression of the epidural space. As noted, most solid tumors are relatively radioresistant to cEBRT, with response rates of 20%, thus making cEBRT unreliable in terms of spinal cord and neurologic salvage. SSRS can treat radioresistant tumors but requires a margin on the spinal cord to deliver a cytotoxic dose. In all of the surgical spine literature, only 12 publications described the outcome of surgical decompression and stabilization of spinal cord or root compression secondary to metastatic tumors.[1,130-131,165-174] Patchell et al. provide the only prospective randomized trial with evidence of the efficacy of surgical decompression for high-grade spinal cord compression.[1] The remaining four prospective cohort studies and seven retrospective chart reviews fall under very low quality evidence. Generally, the results of surgical decompression in patients with spinal cord compression are superior to those for a radiation series, and this is particularly applicable to radioresistant tumors.[175] In the surgical series, 74% to 100% of patients were ambulatory after decompression, with 57% to 82% of nonambulatory patients recovering the ability to ambulate.[118,120,126-129,131-139]

Patchell et al. conducted a randomized, multi-institutional trial comparing external beam radiation (30 Gy in 10 fractions) to decompressive surgery and instrumentation followed by external beam radiation therapy in symptomatic patients with spinal cord compression.[1] Spinal cord compression was defined as displacement of the spinal cord, and neurologic symptoms ranged from pain only to myelopathy resulting in loss of ambulation. Hematologic malignancies and markedly radiosensitive tumors, such as germ cell tumors, were excluded, as were patients with other neurologic comorbidities (e.g., brain metastases). Other exclusion criteria included discontiguous epidural disease, an expected survival time of less than 3 months, and the inability to tolerate the proposed treatment. The protocol defined instability according to the Cybulski[176] criteria or bone in the spinal canal, but instability was not an indication for exclusion.

In this study, 101 patients were randomized, and the primary tumor histology was lung carcinoma in 26 patients with 13 in each group. Patients undergoing surgery and RT had statistically significant improvement compared with those who received radiation alone in terms of the following: overall ambulation, 84% versus 57% (P = .001); maintenance of ambulation, 94% versus 74% (P = .024); recovery of ambulation, 62% versus 19% (P = .012); bowel and bladder continence, 155 versus 17 days (P = .016); narcotic requirement, 0.4 mg versus 4 to 8 mg (P = .002); and survival, 122 days versus 100 days (P = .033). Notably, 57% of patients in the radiation group maintained ambulation, but the duration was only 13 days compared with ambulation until death (122 days) in the surgical group. As the study followed an intent-to-treat analysis, all three patients who recovered ambulation in the radiation cohort crossed over to the surgical group. No patient in the radiation group recovered ambulation without surgery.

Improved surgical outcomes have been seen using techniques that provide exposure for more radical tumor resection than laminectomy. Reconstruction following these aggressive approaches is now possible using rigid dorsal segmental fixation and ventral instrumentation.[177] These include ventral transcavitary and dorsolateral transpedicular approaches. The decision to use a particular surgical approach depends on the location of the bone, epidural, and paraspinal tumor, the type of reconstruction required, patient comorbidities, the extent of disease, and the surgeon's experience. Regardless of the approach, the goal is decompression of the spinal canal with the maximal possible cytoreduction of the tumor.

As with RT, factors that affect outcome include preoperative neurologic and functional status and favorable tumor histology. Kelkamp and Samii reviewed 101 patients operated on for metastatic spinal tumor prior to receiving adjuvant therapy (RT or chemotherapy) for their spinal tumor.[126] The operations included dorsolateral (79%), ventral transcavitary (12%), and ventral and dorsal approaches (9%). Ninety-six percent of patients who were ambulating preoperatively maintained ambulation for at least 3 months. Only 22% of nonambulatory patients regained ambulation over the same duration. This maintenance or recovery of function is similar to the RT data presented by Maranzano and Latini.[159] Additionally, 89% of patients maintained continence for 3 months, but only 31% regained autonomic function. Patients with favorable tumor histology (e.g., breast, kidney, thyroid, and prostate) had significantly better neurologic outcome and survival than those with unfavorable histologies (lung, gastrointestinal tract, and unknown primary). As has been seen in other studies, local recurrence rates are significant.[131] In this

BOX 109-1. Surgical Indications

Primary Surgery
Radioresistant tumor
Spinal instability
Incapacitating radicular pain
Pathologic fracture with bone in the canal
Circumferential epidural tumor (unless highly radiosensitive)
Occult primary tumor

Surgery Following Radiation/Chemotherapy
Progressive neurologic symptoms
Tumor progression with high-grade compression
Spinal instability

study, 58% recurred after 6 months, 69% at 1 year, and 96% after 4 years. Factors predictive of low recurrence rates included preoperative ambulatory status, favorable tumor histology, cervical level, low number of affected vertebral bodies, complete resection, and elective surgery.

A review of multiple series shows complication rates from surgery ranging from 10% to 52%.[118,120-137,178] Complications include DVT, myocardial infarction, and pneumonia. Surgical complications include failed fixation requiring revision and postoperative hematoma. Wound dehiscence and infection are complications predominantly seen with dorsolateral approaches in up to 15% of cases. We have found that trapezius or latissimus dorsi rotation flaps provide excellent soft tissue coverage and markedly reduce the morbidity from this complication.[179] Mortality rates are as high as 13%[178] and are frequently related to the patient's medical or oncologic condition.

The second indication for surgery is mechanical instability because radiation treatment has no ability to stabilize an unstable spine. Definitions of instability are still being developed for pathologic fractures. In general, patients with unstable fractures demonstrate severe movement-related pain that is characteristic of specific spinal levels in correlation with radiographic findings. Burst or compression fractures of the thoracic and lumbar spine often present with axial load pain but do not require instrumented fixation. The pain from these fractures frequently improves after a few days of bedrest and limited activity. Alternatively, the fractures may respond to percutaneous cement augmentation, using vertebroplasty or kyphoplasty.[180-182] Definitive therapy with radiation provides local tumor control without the need for surgery.

Patients requiring instrumented fusion of the atlantoaxial region have pain with flexion, extension, and rotation. However, patients presenting with C1-2 pain and normal spinal alignment or minimal subluxation respond well to external beam RT. These patients can be placed in a hard collar during treatment and for 6 weeks following the completion of RT. Patients with fracture subluxations greater than 5 mm or greater than 3.5 mm subluxation and 11 degrees of angulation between C1 and C2 with movement-related neck pain require instrumented spine fixation.[183,184]

In the subaxial cervical and thoracic spine levels, simple burst and compression fractures may create kyphosis but often do not manifest instability pain. A burst or compression fracture with extension into a unilateral joint, on the other hand, is often unstable. Instability pain in the subaxial cervical and thoracic spine is often produced with extension, which causes unremitting pain as the patient straightens an unstable kyphosis. Patients with thoracic or thoracolumbar instability often give a history of sleeping upright in a chair because they cannot lie flat due to pain.

As in the subaxial cervical and thoracic spine, lumbar pathologic burst fractures are frequently stable. Lumbar spine fractures may present with mechanical radiculopathy, in which the patient develops severe radicular symptoms when the spine is axially loaded on sitting or standing. This condition results from narrowing of the neural foramen and, in our experience, does not commonly respond to radiation therapy. Mechanical radiculopathy is often seen in the presence of a burst fracture with extension of tumor into the neural foramen.

Systemic Disease Assessment

The systemic disease assessment reflects what the patient can tolerate physiologically from the standpoint of the systemic disease and medical comorbidities. The systemic disease assessment is typically aimed at survival prediction and whether the patient is likely to withstand surgery with an acceptable risk of medical complications. Several authors have developed scoring systems that attempt to predict survival and potential benefit in patients with metastatic disease to the spine.[185-187] However, these scores are based on historical data without the benefit of current adjuvant therapies, and there remains a high variability in the outcome of individual patients. As such, a poor "score" on these instruments should be interpreted with caution and should not preclude surgical intervention in otherwise satisfactory candidates.

Treatment Decision Making

At MSKCC, radiation therapy is the first-line treatment for most patients who present with metastatic spine tumors. Surgery is reserved for a variety of indications based on the four categories described earlier as NOMS: neurologic, oncologic, biomechanical, and systemic disease (see Fig. 109-1).[6] Patients with radioresistant tumors (e.g., sarcoma, RCC), spinal instability, and/or a pathologic fracture with bone in the spinal canal are considered for surgery prior to radiation therapy.[7] Patients with significant mechanical or radicular pain complaints may only marginally improve with radiation therapy alone and may benefit from surgical decompression and stabilization. Another frequently reported indication for surgery is lack of a diagnosis, but this can often be accomplished with CT-guided needle biopsy or thoracoscopic biopsy.

After RT that has reached spinal cord tolerance, patients are considered for surgery based on progression of neurologic symptoms, radiographic progression of tumor, and spinal instability. Patients with residual radiographic tumor following radiation or chemotherapy may be considered for curative surgery (e.g., osteogenic sarcoma, Ewing sarcoma, germ cell tumor). Contraindications to surgery include a limited life expectancy, significant medical comorbidities, and extensive disease.[3] Additionally, paraplegic patients are rarely operated on because of the significantly low rate of recovery, particularly after 24 hours.

Case Presentations

The following three case presentations illustrate some of the ways patients with a specific cancer, RCC, can present, as well as some of the different treatment methodologies used for spine metastases.

Mechanical Back Pain Requiring Dorsolateral Decompression

Case 1

A 62-year-old male is newly diagnosed with RCC. He presented with progressive neck and low back pain. By the time he was admitted to the hospital, he had severe mechanical

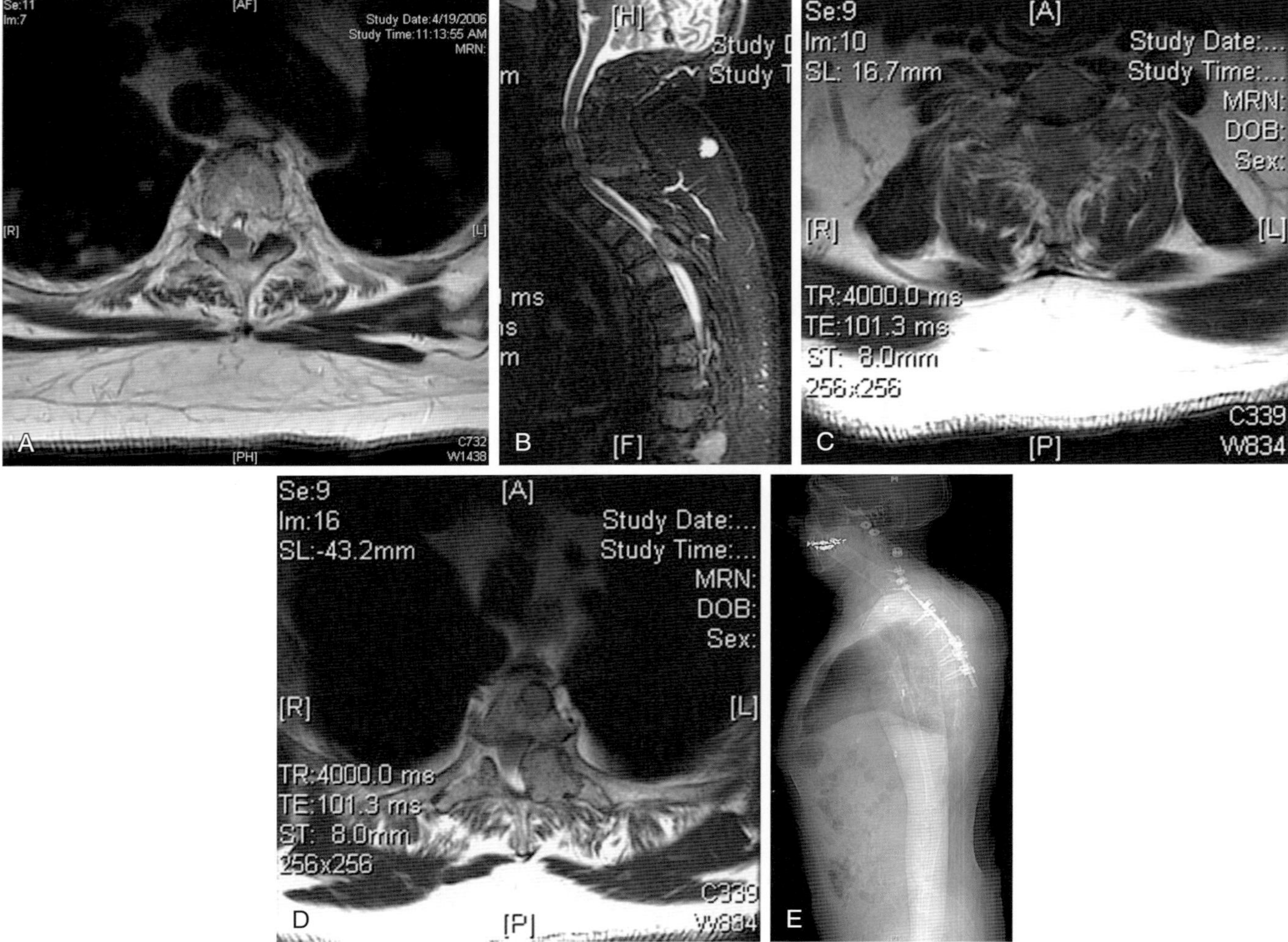

FIGURE 109-13. Case 1. MRI sequences of a patient with widely metastatic renal cell carcinoma. **A,** Sagittal T1-weighted MRI after gadolinium. **B,** Sagittal MRI STIR sequence. Axial T1-weighted MRI after gadolinium at C7 (**C**) and T3 (**D**). Lateral sequence (**E**) obtained prior to a CT myelogram after surgery shows the hardware in good position.

back pain centered at his upper thoracic spine that was worse with movement and when he was supine but better when he was sitting up. MRI showed numerous osseous metastases to his spine (Fig. 109-13). These lesions were associated with minimal spinal canal involvement except for the C7 and T3-4 lesions. The patient underwent embolization of these lesions followed by a dorsolateral decompression and instrumentation. His pain was significantly reduced (mechanical), and he underwent radiation to treat the remaining lesions.

Biologic Pain Treated with Image-Guided Radiation Therapy

Case 2

A 63-year-old male presented with low back pain that was worse at night and improved during the day. He had been treated previously with surgery for a thoracic spine lesion and had recently been removed from a clinical trial due to worsening symptoms and generalized poor health. He underwent IGRT to adjacent lesions in the lower thoracic and upper lumbar spine and ultimately achieved significant reduction in pain (oncologic) and improvement in his quality of life (Fig. 109-14).

Mechanical Instability

Case 3

A 72-year-old male presented with a 4-week history of worsening neck pain. He had a known history of widely metastatic RCC. The pain worsened with any head movement. Workup revealed metastatic disease causing a fracture-subluxation at C2. The patient underwent occipitocervical fusion followed by IGRT. Two months after treatment, his tumor showed no radiographic evidence of progression, and his pain was significantly reduced (Fig. 109-15; see also Figs. 109-2 and 109-6).

Surgical Decision Making

Once the decision to operate has been made, several other issues must be still considered. The first is whether preoperative embolization is indicated. At MSKCC, embolization is

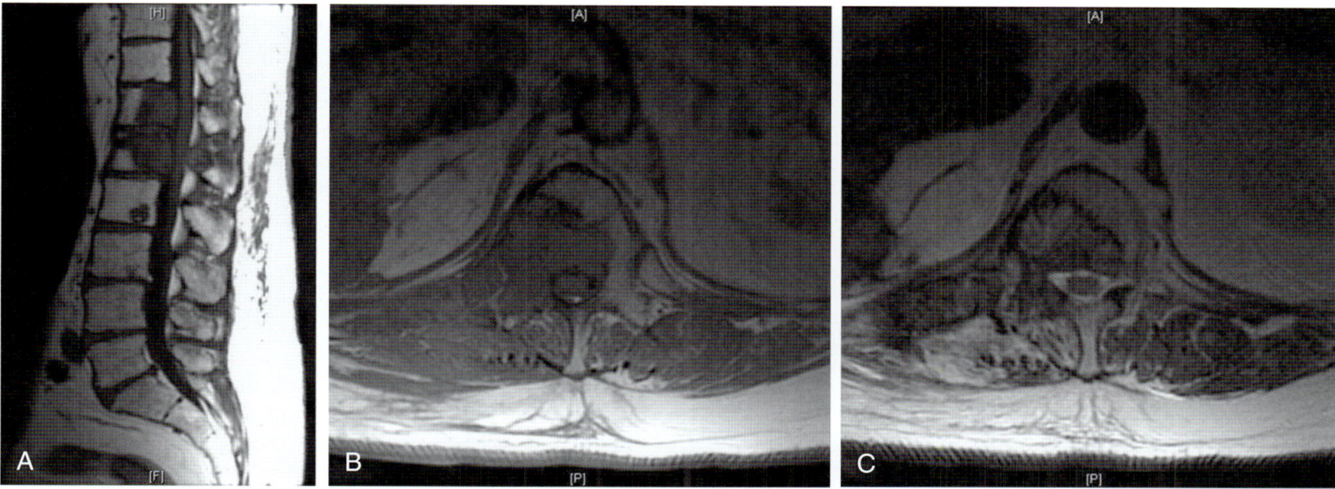

FIGURE 109-14. Case 2. MRI sequence of a patient with newly diagnosed renal cell carcinoma showed spine metastases at T12, L1, and L2 that were amenable to image-guide radiation therapy. **A,** Sagittal T1-weighted MRI showing the tumor to be darker than normal bone marrow. Larger lesions involve the dorsal aspects of T12 and L1, while a smaller lesion is found in L2. **B,** Axial T1-weighted MRI shows the lesion within the vertebral body and extending dorsally within the right pedicle and rib at T12. **C,** Axial T2-weighted MRI demonstrates grade 1b epidural spinal cord compression.

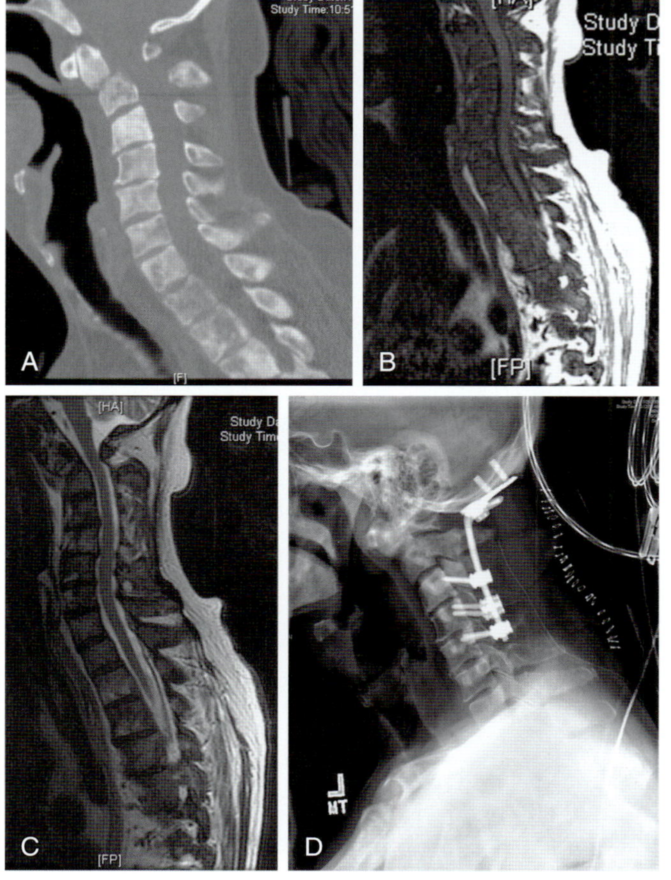

FIGURE 109-15. Case 3. A patient with renal cell carcinoma (same patient as Figs. 109-2 and 109-6) presented with neck pain. **A,** Sagittal reconstruction of a cervical spine CT shows the fracture-dislocation at C2, which can also be visualized on T1-weighted MRI (**B**) and T2-weighted MRI (**C**). **D,** Dorsal instrumentation from the occiput to C5 shown in this lateral plain radiograph of the cervical spine provided stabilization and improved his pain.

performed for vascular tumors (e.g., RCC, papillary thyroid carcinoma, leiomyosarcoma) 1 or 2 days prior to surgery as this has been shown to dramatically reduce intraoperative blood loss (Fig. 109-16).[188-190] In our series of 140 patients operated on via a dorsolateral approach with circumferential instrumentation, embolization successfully reduced operative blood loss for vascular tumors (i.e., renal, thyroid, angiosarcoma) to the same level as those not requiring embolization (1900 mL and 1620 mL, respectively).[191]

The next issue is whether instrumentation and bone grafting are necessary. Instrumentation following surgical decompression is indicated for a majority of patients undergoing surgical intervention for metastatic spine disease.[192] This is based on the fact that many of these patients have preexisting mechanical instability as a result of tumor-related bone destruction, iatrogenic instability as a result of intraoperative bone removal, or are at risk for delayed instability secondary to tumor progression. The addition of instrumentation prevents the delayed development of mechanical back pain and often only adds 30 to 60 minutes to the case. Many of these patients require longer fusion segments as opposed to patients with degenerative disease because of tumor involvement in surrounding bone, the risk of adjacent segment progression, and the high probability of osteoporosis. Autogenic bone grafting is routinely performed in cases of dorsal decompression and instrumentation, but the expectation of arthrodesis is limited due to the limited life expectancy, as well as the effects of radiation and chemotherapy.[193] The routine use of external orthoses is not supported because these can compromise pulmonary function and wound healing in patients with minimal reserves.

Another issue concerns whether the type of tumor resection should be either en bloc or intralesional. En bloc spondylectomy as described by Tomita et al. is a technique based on sound oncologic principles.[194] The intent of this surgery is en bloc resection of a tumor with negative histologic margins. This surgery is feasible as a one- or two-stage procedure, but is technically quite demanding and has higher morbidity

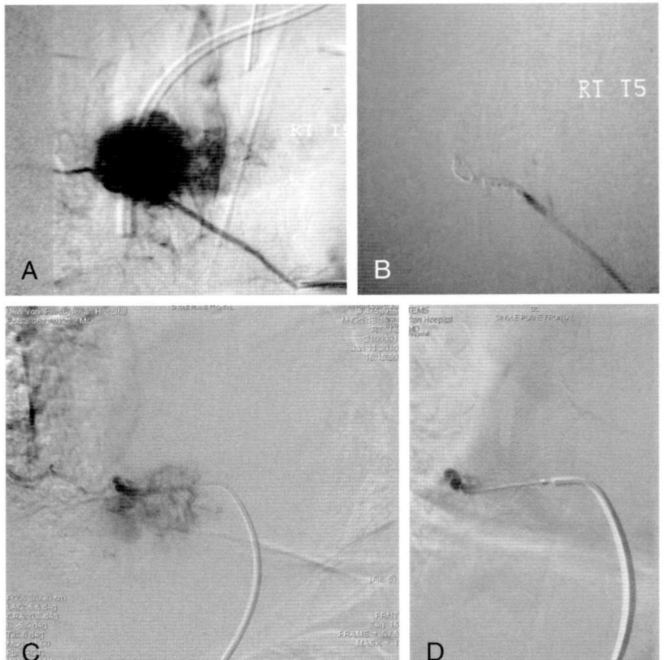

FIGURE 109-16. Embolization may decrease intraoperative bleeding. **A,** Metastatic disease at T5 is visualized as a tumor "blush" due to high vascularity of the tumor after injecting contrast through a catheter located in a segmental vessel. **B,** After selective embolization, the tumor blush is no longer seen. **C,** A less pronounced blush is demonstrated in this lesion at T8. **D,** At T8, selective embolization obliterated the vascular supply.

rates.[195-198] However, results are encouraging, both in terms of functional outcome and local control.

In most cases, though, surgery for spinal metastases is palliative, and in few cases will attempts at negative histologic margins influence clinical outcome.[199] Based on anatomic considerations, the majority of patients with metastatic tumors are not candidates for this type of surgery because of extensive epidural disease, multilevel vertebral body involvement, and large paraspinal masses. The evolution of SSRS has largely obviated the need to consider en bloc resection even in patients with solitary metastases and a long life expectancy. SSRS provides superb durable control that is independent of histology.

Thoracoscopic vertebral body resection for tumor has been reported in small series.[200,201] This relatively noninvasive approach has proven useful for removing ventral thoracic discs and ventral releases for scoliosis corrections. The potential use for most tumors requiring resection is probably limited. We currently reserve this technique for when CT-guided biopsies fail.

Summary

The diagnosis and treatment of spinal metastases requires a multidisciplinary approach. Careful examination of the patients, their symptoms, and radiographic and laboratory studies will help avoid treatment-related complications. Regardless of the treatment, diagnosis before the development of significant neurologic and functional deficits improves outcomes.

KEY REFERENCES

Bilsky M, Smith M: Surgical approach to epidural spinal cord compression. *Hematol Oncol Clin North Am* 20(6):1307–1317, 2006.

Gerszten PC, Burton SA, Ozhasoglu C, et al: Stereotactic radiosurgery for spinal metastases from renal cell carcinoma. *J Neurosurg Spine* 3(4): 288–295, 2005.

Maranzano E, Latini P: Effectiveness of radiation therapy without surgery in metastatic spinal cord compression: final results from a prospective trial. *Int J Radiat Oncol Biol Phys* 32(4):959–967, 1995.

Patchell RA, Tibbs PA, Regine WF, et al: Direct decompressive surgical resection in the treatment of spinal cord compression caused by metastatic cancer: a randomised trial. *Lancet* 366(9486):643–648, 2005.

Wang JC, Boland P, Mitra N, et al: Single-stage posterolateral transpedicular approach for resection of epidural metastatic spine tumors involving the vertebral body with circumferential reconstruction: results in 140 patients. Invited submission from the Joint Section Meeting on Disorders of the Spine and Peripheral Nerves, March 2004. *J Neurosurg Spine* 1(3): 287–298, 2004.

Yamada Y, Bilsky MH, Lovelock DM, et al: High-dose, single-fraction image-guided intensity-modulated radiotherapy for metastatic spinal lesions. *Int J Radiat Oncol Biol Phys* 71(2):484–490, 2008.

REFERENCES

The complete reference list is available online at expertconsult.com.

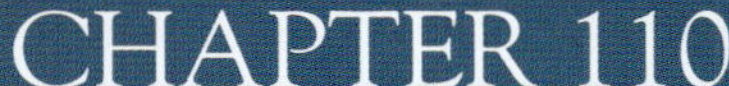

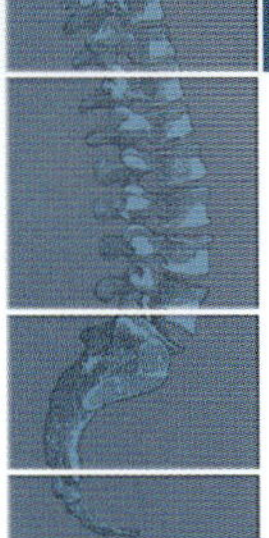

CHAPTER 110

Metabolic Bone Disease

Daniel J. Mazanec | Tagreed Khalaf | R. Douglas Orr

Metabolic bone diseases include a diverse group of skeletal disorders characterized by reduced bone mass (osteoporosis), defective bone mineralization (osteomalacia), or an accelerated rate of bone turnover (Paget disease). Clinical consequences of these conditions that are of interest to the spine specialist include vertebral fragility fracture and resultant deformity, bone pain, spinal stenosis, and, rarely, cauda equina syndrome. Surgical treatment may be compromised by metabolic bone disease. Pagetic bone is highly vascular, increasing the risk of excess bleeding. Pedicle screw loosening is more likely in osteoporotic bone.

Beyond immediate surgical concerns, medical evaluation and treatment of the underlying metabolic bone disease is crucial to a successful long-term outcome. For many patients, the presenting symptom of previously unrecognized and untreated osteoporosis is a painful vertebral fragility fracture. Unfortunately, the majority of patients who have experienced a fracture do not receive appropriate treatment for osteoporosis. Approximately 50% of female patients who have sustained a compression fracture do not receive osteoporosis treatment.[1] The rate of treatment after fracture is even lower for men. A recent retrospective study of 1171 men aged 65 or older demonstrated that only 7.1% of osteoporotic subjects and 16.1% of those with a hip or vertebral fracture received medication for osteoporosis.[2] This represents a significant missed opportunity to reduce the risk of future fractures, particularly since the likelihood of refracture approaches 10% to 20% within 1 year of the initial fracture.

Osteoporosis

Definition

Osteoporosis is defined as "systemic skeletal disease characterized by low bone mass and microarchitectural deterioration of bone tissue with a consequent increase in bone fragility and susceptibility to fracture."[3] Although the diagnosis of osteoporosis in asymptomatic individuals is typically based on bone density measurement alone, this definition emphasizes the important role of unmeasured ultrastructural abnormalities that contribute to the clinical end point of fracture. In fact, the incidence of hip fracture increases between the ages of 50 to 90 years seven times more than predicted on the basis of decline in bone density alone.[4]

Prevalence and Costs

The prevalence of osteoporosis increases with age in both men and women. It is estimated that currently about 10 million Americans older than 50 years of age have osteoporosis.[5] This number is expected to increase to more than 14 million people in 2020.[6] Though osteoporosis is commonly conceived of as a disease of women, more than 30% of people with osteoporosis are men. The clinical consequence of osteoporosis is fracture. The 2004 U.S. Surgeon General's report on Bone Health and Osteoporosis concluded that osteoporosis results in approximately 1.5 million fragility fractures annually. Vertebral compression fractures are the most common, accounting for about 700,000 fractures per year. More than 50% of women and 30% of men will experience a vertebral compression in their lifetime. As many as 20% of people who suffer from a vertebral fragility fracture will experience another within 1 year.[5]

Beyond the personal suffering and functional impact, the economic burden to society of osteoporosis is considerable. The estimated cost of caring for the greater than 2 million osteoporotic fractures in 2005 was estimated to be $17 billion.[6,7] These figures are expect to increase by 50% by 2025, when the annual fracture incidence will surpass 3 million and costs will exceed $25 billion. A significant portion of this anticipated increase is a result of the growing problem of osteoporosis in the Hispanic population.[6]

Pathophysiology

Peak bone mass is achieved by about age 30 years in both sexes. Differences in peak bone mass account for some of the variation in osteoporosis risk between men and women as well as between racial and ethnic groups. For example, African American women have higher bone densities than non-Hispanic women at all ages and are at lower risk for fractures of the spine and hip.[8] Since achievement of genetically determined peak bone mass occurs primarily before the age of 20 years, osteoporosis in later life may, in part, be regarded as a pediatric disease with geriatric consequences.[9] Juvenile calcium intake is positively associated with bone mass in the fourth decade of life.[10]

Age-related bone loss begins in the fourth decade and continues throughout life in men and women. By the eighth or ninth decade of life, women have lost approximately 35% of their cortical bone mass and 50% of their trabecular bone mass.[11] Men lose about 60% as much during their lifetimes. Menopause in women is associated with a period of accelerated loss of trabecular bone that persists for about 10 years. Thereafter, bone loss from trabecular and cortical sites continues at a slower rate, similar to that of men. Skeletal sites that are predominantly trabecular in composition, including vertebral bodies and distal forearm bones, are therefore at greatest risk for earlier osteoporosis. Rates of Colles and vertebral fractures in women rise sharply after menopause.[12]

The major cause of primary age-related osteoporosis in both men and women is loss of gonadal function. In young adults, skeletal remodeling is an ongoing process with closely coupled bone resorption and formation. In estrogen-deficient women, bone resorption as assessed by biochemical markers increases by 90%, while bone formation markers increase only 45%, reflecting an imbalance between bone formation and resorption with net bone loss.[12] Estrogen has multiple effects on both osteoclast and osteoblast function. Estrogen suppresses osteoclast development by suppressing RANKL production as well as regulating production of osteolytic cytokines including interleukin-1, interleukin-6, tumor necrosis factor alpha, and prostaglandins.[12,13] Estrogen plays a role in bone formation by stimulating production of growth factors by osteoblasts.[14] The principal risk factors for primary osteoporosis in women are related to estrogen deficiency: postmenopausal status; nulliparity; late menarche; early menopause (before age 45), either natural or surgical; and secondary amenorrhea related to exercise or eating disorders. As in women, estrogen plays a critical and dominant role in maintaining bone density in men. While androgens are important determinants of muscle mass in males, serum estradiol levels are more predictive of bone density. Peripheral aromatization of androgens to estrogen is important in maintaining estradiol levels above the threshold required to maintain skeletal homeostasis.[2]

In older men and women, other factors contribute to age-related bone loss, including physiologic hyperparathyroidism, vitamin D deficiency, and secretion of various bone-resorbing cytokines.[7,12] Recent studies suggest a remarkably high level of vitamin D deficiency among older adults. In a recent study, more than 50% of older North American women currently treated for osteoporosis were found to have suboptimal vitamin D levels.[15] In the patients with fractures or falls, the prevalence of vitamin D deficiency exceeds 90%.[16] In most studies of older adults, the prevalence of low serum vitamin D levels is unrelated to gender, race, latitude, or global location.[17]

Risk Assessment

In addition to the changes in bone density related to decline in gonadal function in both men and women, multiple lifestyle factors, medical disorders, and drugs may exacerbate or accelerate "age-related" bone loss (Box 110-1).[18] Approximately 50% of men with osteoporosis have underlying "secondary" causes, and as many as one third of women with osteoporosis are found to have other conditions beyond estrogen deficiency.[2,19,20] In men with osteoporosis, the most common secondary causes are hypogonadism, glucocorticoid use, and alcoholism. In women, secondary causes are more common in perimenopausal women and include glucocorticoid use, thyroid hormone excess, hypoestrogenemia, and anticonvulsant treatment.[18]

BOX 110-1. Risk Factors for Osteoporosis

Diet
Malabsorption syndrome
Dietary calcium deficiency
Excess alcohol

Disease
Osteogenesis imperfecta
Renal tubular acidosis
Rheumatoid arthritis
Liver disease
Multiple myeloma
Leukemia

Drugs
Glucocorticoids
Heparin
Anticonvulsants
Methotrexate

Endocrine Disorders
Hypogonadism
Cushing disease
Hyperparathyroidism
Hypothyroidism
Premature menopause
Anorexia nervosa
Athletic amenorrhea

Lifestyle
Sedentary
Smoking
High-protein diet

Measurements of bone mineral density alone are insensitive as predictors of risk of clinical fragility fractures. More than 90% of these fractures occur in individuals who do not have osteoporosis as defined by bone density measurement criteria.[21] Incorporating assessment of clinical risk factors for bone loss and fracture risk into predictive models for fragility fracture, with or without bone mineral density measurement, greatly enhances the assessment of fracture risk in both men and women.[22] The World Health Organization (WHO) has developed such a fracture risk assessment tool (FRAX), which incorporates multiple risk factors including body mass index, personal history of previous fracture, history of parental hip fracture, current smoking, history of long-term glucocorticoid use, rheumatoid arthritis, and daily alcohol consumption of three or more units.[23] The tool also includes the presence or absence of other secondary causes of osteoporosis, including hypogonadism, inflammatory bowel disease, prolonged immobility, organ transplantation, type 1 diabetes, and thyroid disorders. FRAX is available to clinicians online (www.shef.ac.uk/FRAX) and provides estimates of the 10-year probability of hip fracture and major osteoporotic fracture.

Morbidity and Mortality

Osteoporosis is similar to hypertension as a disorder with a long asymptomatic interval before resulting in clinical manifestation. If unrecognized and untreated in its preclinical phase, osteoporosis may result in significant morbidity and mortality. Fragility fractures are the single most morbid and clinically significant consequence of osteoporosis, occurring most frequently in the vertebral body, proximal femur, and distal radius.[5]

The presence of a vertebral fracture, even if asymptomatic, increases the risk of future vertebral fracture fivefold and doubles the risk of hip fracture.[1] In addition, these patients may experience chronic low back pain, loss of height, and kyphosis, leading to symptomatic biomechanical changes in the spine.[7] Pulmonary compromise may become evident as a result of the kyphosis and compression fractures manifested by restrictive lung disease with decreased vital capacity.[24] On average, each thoracic vertebral fracture reduces pulmonary vital capacity by 9%.[24,25] In addition, shortening of the thoracic spine may result in compression of the abdominal contents, resulting in symptoms of early satiety and bloating. This may result in anorexia and weight loss, which is a great concern in a population of individuals who are already frail.

Patients with compression fractures also experience lower levels of functional performance compared with controls, including difficulty with performance of activities of daily living. These patients may become more sedentary as a result, with progressive deconditioning and further bone loss. The constellation of the preceding symptoms, as well as low self-esteem due to body image changes, may result in depression in up to 40% of individuals with osteoporosis. Patients who are at greater likelihood of developing depression are those with more than one compression fracture, those who are older, and those who are more socially isolated.[24]

Patients with a compression fracture were found to have a 23% higher age-adjusted mortality rate in a recent prospective cohort study of almost 10,000 women age 65 years or older.[26] The mortality rate is even greater in patients with hip fractures, reaching 20% more than age-matched controls in the first year after hip fracture.[7] Increased mortality after hip fracture is usually due to coexisting illness or deep venous thrombosis with pulmonary embolism from the relative immobilization associated with the fracture.[27] Patients who survive the hip fracture often have limited ability to perform activities of daily living and require prolonged institutional care. In individuals over 75 years of age, hip fracture mortality is greater in men than in women: 20.7% and 7.5%, respectively.[2,6]

Diagnosis of Osteoporosis

A painful fracture is the most obvious clinical consequence of osteoporosis, but as many as 70% of osteoporotic spine fractures are asymptomatic.[28] While a clinical diagnosis of osteoporosis may be made in the presence of a fragility fracture in the absence of bone mineral density measurement, low bone mass is recognized as a more sensitive diagnostic parameter in the absence of symptoms.[29] Low bone mass is also a strong predictor of future fracture risk. The WHO has defined osteoporosis and osteopenia on the basis of bone mineral density (BMD) (Table 110-1). A T score is defined as the number of standard deviations above or below the average BMD for healthy young white females. The Z score is defined as the number of standard deviations above or below the average BMD for age- and sex-matched controls. Osteoporosis is present when the T score is at least −2.5. Severe osteoporosis is defined as a T score of at least −2.5 in the presence of one or more fragility fractures. Z scores are used preferentially to assess bone loss in premenopausal women and males younger than 50 years of age. A low Z score (<−2.0) represents bone loss in excess of age-expected loss and suggests that secondary causes of bone loss may be present.[18,30] The WHO thresholds were chosen on the basis of fracture risk in postmenopausal Caucasian women. Similar diagnostic threshold values for men are less well defined. However, several studies have demonstrated that the age-adjusted fracture risk for any given BMD is similar in men and women.[31] The International Society for Clinical Densitometry (ISCD) advises that the WHO criteria be used in postmenopausal women and in men age 50 and older but not in premenopausal women or men less than 50 years old, as the fracture risk is not the same in younger men and women.

TABLE 110-1

Osteoporosis and Osteopenia: World Health Organization Criteria

Classification	Criteria
Normal	BMD up to ±1 SD of the main of the young adult reference range
Osteopenia	BMD between 1 and 2.5 SD below the main of the young adult reference range
Osteoporosis	BMD greater than 2.5 SD below the mean of the young adult reference range
Severe osteoporosis	BMD greater than 2.5 SD below the mean of the young adult reference range in the presence of one or more insufficiency fractures

BMD, bone mineral density; SD, standard deviation.

Several technologies are available to measure bone mass, including forearm single-photon absorptiometry, spine and hip dual-photon absorptiometry, and quantitative ultrasound of the calacaneus. While multiple studies have shown that these various measurement techniques may predict osteoporotic risk,[32-37] the gold standard remains dual-energy x-ray absorptiometry (DEXA) of the hip and spine for the diagnosis of osteoporosis.[8,18,30] DEXA is considered the gold standard because it has been shown to be precise (1%–2%) and to have acceptable accuracy and good reproducibility. It is also the most extensively validated test for fracture outcomes.[29,30] Other advantages of DEXA include relatively low radiation exposure, wide availability, and the capacity to measure bone density at multiple skeletal sites. The ISCD recommends obtaining BMD measurements of the spine and hip. Numerous studies have shown that BMD measured at the femur (neck or total hip) is the best for predicting hip fracture risk.[3,30,31,38] Spinal BMD is the optimum for monitoring response to treatment. The risk of hip fracture is increased 2.6 times for each standard deviation decrease at the femoral neck.[31,39] Serial BMD measurements should be performed on the same machine for the same patient, owing to variability of BMD assessment between machines of different manufacturers.

Most clinical guidelines recommend screening healthy women for osteoporosis at age 65 and testing higher-risk women earlier. The ISCD recommends screening men without risk factors for osteoporosis at age 70 and testing higher-risk men earlier. Risk factors are as noted previously. Another indication for screening is radiographic evidence of osteopenia or vertebral fracture.[30] In addition, screening is recommended for people who have diseases associated with bone loss, such as rheumatoid arthritis, as well as people initiating long-term corticosteroid therapy. Current evidence does not support routine screening of all perimenopausal women, as its value in directing preventive therapy against future fractures has not been established[8] (Box 110-2).

Bone turnover markers reflecting bone formation and resorptive activity are not recommended for routine diagnostic purposes, as they have not been found to predict bone mass or fracture risk. Indices of bone formation include alkaline phosphatase and osteocalcin. Markers for resorption include serum and urine levels of type I collagen C- and N-telopeptides. While not reliable diagnostically, they have been found helpful in clinical trials in understanding the mechanism of bone loss. Bone markers may also be helpful for monitoring response to therapy and compliance.[8]

Evaluation of patients with osteoporosis should include a thorough history and physical examination, as most of the secondary causes of osteoporosis can be excluded with a careful history and physical examination. A minimum screening laboratory profile should be considered for all patients who have been diagnosed with osteoporosis. This is particularly important in men, as 30% to 60% will have an identifiable secondary cause. Approximately 50% of perimenopausal women with osteoporosis also have a secondary cause, including hypoestrogenemia, glucocorticoid usage, thyroid hormone excess, and anticonvulsant therapy.[18] As was mentioned previously, patients with an abnormal Z score should also be studied more aggressively for secondary causes. Initial general screening should include a complete blood count, erythrocyte sedimentation rate, serum calcium, serum 25 hydroxyvitamin D, phosphorus, alkaline phosphatase, creatinine, aspartate aminotransferase, thyroid-stimulating hormone (TSH), and serum protein electrophoresis. Tannenbaum et al. looked at the yield of laboratory testing to identify secondary causes of osteoporosis in otherwise healthy women. Their findings suggest that a basic screen of serum calcium, serum parathyroid hormone (PTH), and 24-hour urinary calcium excretion in all patients, and a serum TSH in patients on thyroid replacement, provides a high diagnostic yield (86% in their study) at a low cost (mean cost of $75/patient).[40] In male patients, serum testosterone should be obtained. Additional studies such as 24-hour urinary calcium, PTH, and serum immunoelectrophoresis should be obtained selectively on the basis of risk factors and preliminary studies (Table 110-2).

BOX 110-2. Osteoporosis Screening Guidelines

- Women age 65 and older, men age 70 and older (regardless of clinical risk factors)
- Younger postmenopausal women and men ages 50 to 69 for whom there may be concern based on their clinical profile
- Women in menopausal transition who may have a risk factor for increased fracture (low body weight, high-risk medication, or prior low trauma fracture)
- Adults who sustain a fracture after age 50
- Adults taking glucocorticoids in a daily dose of ≥5 mg or equivalent for 3 months or more
- Any person being considered for pharmacologic therapy for osteoporosis
- Anyone being treated with osteoporosis to monitor effect (generally every 2 years)
- Anyone not receiving therapy in whom evidence of bone loss would lead to treatment

Prevention of Osteoporosis

Because currently available treatments for established osteoporosis reduce fracture rates by 50% to 60% at best and restore only a small portion of skeletal bone, prevention of osteoporosis remains the ideal objective in maintaining skeletal health. Optimizing peak adult bone mass is crucial, as low peak adult bone mass is a major risk factor for subsequent development of osteoporosis. Although as much as 75% of

TABLE 110-2

Screening Laboratory Tests

Test	Purpose
CBC	Evaluate for bone marrow malignancy, infiltrative process, or malabsorption
Serum calcium	Decreased in those with malabsorption or vitamin D deficiency, increased in hyperparathyroidism
Liver function	Evaluate for intrinsic liver abnormality
Alkaline phosphatase	Increased in acute fractures, prolonged immobilization, and Paget disease of the bone
TSH	Screen for hyperthyroidism
ESR	May indicate an inflammatory process or monoclonal gammopathy (associated with bone loss)
Serum 25-hydroxyvitamin D	Evaluate for vitamin D deficiency
Serum calcium	Decreased in those with malabsorption or vitamin D deficiency, increased in hyperparathyroidism
Serum phosphorus	Decreased in patients with osteomalacia
PTH	Screening for hyperparathyroidism
Creatinine	Renal failure is associated with secondary hyperparathyroidism
Serum testosterone	In all men to screen for hypogonadism
Serum estradiol	Screening for hypogonadism in premenopausal or perimenopausal women
Urinary calcium excretion	24-hour urinary excretion on a high-calcium-intake diet screens for malabsorption and hypercalciuria
SPEP/UPEP	If monoclonal gammopathy is suspected

CBC, complete blood count; ESR, erythrocyte sedimentation rate; PTH, parathyroid hormone; SPEP/UPEP, serum protein electrophoresis/urine protein electrophoresis; TSH, thyroid-stimulating hormone.

peak adult bone mass is genetically determined, nutrition and physical activity play important roles in optimizing bone mass from infancy to adulthood.[41]

Hormone Replacement Therapy

Until the Women's Health Initiative studies were reported in 2002 through 2004, perimenopausal women were typically considered for hormone replacement therapy to preserve bone and prevent the steep escalation in bone loss in the early postmenopausal years.[42-44] Although this trial demonstrated a 34% reduction in hip and vertebral fractures in postmenopausal women treated with conjugated estrogens or estrogens plus progestin, other health risks, including coronary artery disease, stroke, and venous thromboembolism, exceeded benefits. Because of the unfavorable risk-to-benefit ratio and the availability of other effective nonhormonal drugs, hormone replacement therapy is not recommended for prevention of osteoporosis in women without vasomotor or other menopausal symptoms requiring treatment.

Nutrition

Lifelong adequate intake of calcium and vitamin D is essential to achieving peak bone mass and prevention of osteoporosis. Calcium supplementation has been shown to have a positive effect on accrual of bone mass throughout childhood and adolescence.[45] Calcium supplementation has been shown to retard bone loss in postmenopausal women.[46] For children ages 3 to 8 years, 800 mg of calcium per day is recommended.[8] After age 8 and through adult life, most guidelines recommend a daily intake of 1200 to 1500 mg of calcium from both dietary and supplemental sources.[8,47] Unfortunately, more than 50% of adolescents and young adults do not ingest sufficient dairy products to achieve dietary calcium requirements.[8]

Vitamin D plays an important role in optimal calcium absorption. Vitamin D adequacy has been defined as the level of vitamin D necessary to achieve maximal suppression of PTH, while avoiding the negative skeletal effects of secondary hyperparathyroidism.[45] In adolescents, vitamin D levels correlate with bone mineral content, and the vitamin probably plays a crucial role in achieving peak bone mass.[48] In older adults, a dose-response relationship between vitamin D and fracture reduction has been demonstrated, with a 20% reduction in hip fracture risk in individuals taking higher doses.[49] As with calcium, the decrease in dairy product consumption, particularly of vitamin D enriched or fortified milk products, contributes to inadequate consumption of this vitamin. For adults, the National Osteoporosis Foundation recommends an intake of 800 to 1000 international units (IU) of vitamin D per day. The best measure of vitamin D status is the serum level of 25(OH)D. A 25(OH)D level of greater than 32 ng/mL is the target that is considered optimal to achieve full suppression of PTH for osteoporosis prevention. The requirement for other micronutrients that are important in skeletal health, including magnesium, fluoride, vitamin C, vitamin K, and potassium, are easily met by a healthy diet that includes five servings daily of fruits and vegetables.[45]

Exercise

In prepubertal and peripubertal children, active weight-bearing exercise has been demonstrated to increase bone mineral density as measured by DEXA or calcaneal ultrasound.[50,51] In premenopausal women, total weight-bearing physical activity correlates with bone density, the strongest association with physical activity being during early age periods.[52] These studies suggest that early active, weight-bearing exercise is important in achieving peak adult bone mass. There is little evidence that exercise in midlife significantly increases BMD, however.[8] In older patients, weight-bearing exercise slows bone loss but has not been shown to decrease fracture risk.[53] However, regular exercise in older patients has been shown to reduce the risk of falls by about 25%, potentially reducing the risk of osteoporotic fracture.[54] The National Osteoporosis Foundation strongly endorses lifelong physical activity at all ages, including weight-bearing exercise and muscle-strengthening exercise.

Who Should Be Treated?

Because osteoporosis, like hypertension, is a silent disease until it manifests clinically as fracture, screening for asymptomatic disease in high-risk individuals represents an initial step before treatment. BMD measurement by DEXA represents the screening tool of choice. As was noted earlier, the WHO has defined osteopenia and osteoporosis on the basis of this measurement. However, though fracture rates are highest in individuals with osteoporosis as defined by these criteria, more than 80% of postmenopausal women with fractures have T scores better than −2.5.[55] Most fractures occur in patients with BMD in the range defined as osteopenia. However, pharmacologic treatment of women with osteopenia defined by BMD in the absence of other risk factors is not cost effective.[56] Fracture risk depends not only on BMD values but also on other independent variables, including body mass index, age, history of prior fracture, parental history of hip fracture, glucocorticoid use, tendency to fall, poor mobility, and other secondary factors.[57,58] The FRAX tool described previously represents one attempt to predict fracture risk by using a model that incorporates BMD and clinical risk factors.[31] Although biochemical markers of bone remodeling have been shown to identify perimenopausal women who are at increased risk for rapid bone loss, the role of markers in predicting fracture risk and determining who should be treated is uncertain.[59]

Current guidelines recommend that pharmacologic treatment should be offered to men and women who have known osteoporosis and to those who have experienced fragility fractures.[47,60] Both the American College of Physicians and the National Osteoporosis Foundation recommend that clinicians consider pharmacologic treatment for men and women who are at increased risk for developing osteoporosis based on a analysis of risk factors. The National Osteoporosis Foundation specifically defines this population with a 10-year probability of a hip fracture greater than 3% or a 10-year risk of a major osteoporotic fracture greater than 20% based on the FRAX calculator.

Pharmacologic Therapy

Pharmacologic therapy for the treatment of osteoporosis can be classified as antiresorptive or anabolic (Table 110-3).

Antiresorptive agents work by inhibiting osteoclast activity, therefore reducing bone resorption. The current available

TABLE 110-3

Summary of Available Osteoporosis Drug Agents

Agent	Dose	Frequency of Administration	Route of Administration	Site of Fracture Prevention
Antiresorptive				
Alendronate	10 mg	Daily	Oral	Hip, vertebral, nonvertebral
	70 mg	Weekly	Oral (liquid or tablet)	
	70 mg + vitamin D	Weekly	Oral	
Risedronate	5 mg	Daily	Oral	Hip, vertebral, nonvertebral
	35 mg	Weekly	Oral	
	35 mg + 500 mg calcium	Weekly	Oral	
	75 mg	Two consecutive days per month	Oral	
	150 mg	Monthly	Oral	
Ibandronate	2.5 mg	Daily	Oral	Vertebral
	150 mg	Monthly	Oral	
	3 mg	Every 3 months	Intravenous	
Zoledronic acid	5 mg	Yearly (15 minutes duration)	Intravenous	Hip, vertebral, nonvertebral
Calcitonin	200 IU	Daily	Intranasal	Vertebral
Raloxifene	60 mg	Daily	Oral	Vertebral
Anabolic				
Teriparatide	20 μg (?)	Daily	Subcutaneous injection	Vertebral and nonvertebral

antiresorptives include bisphosphonates, selective estrogen-receptor modulators, and calcitonin.

The bisphosphonates alendronate and risedronate are approved for both the treatment and prevention of osteoporosis. Both alendronate and risedronate have been shown to reduce vertebral and nonvertebral fragility fractures by 50%.[47,61-64] Both drugs have also been shown to be effective in the treatment of glucocorticoid-induced osteoporosis.[65,66] Another bisphosphonate, ibandronate, which has been approved for the treatment of osteoporosis, has also been shown to reduce the incidence of vertebral fracture by about 50%, but reduction in hip fracture risk remains unproven. An intravenous bisphosphonate, zoledronic acid, has been demonstrated to decrease the incidence of vertebral fractures by 70%, hip fracture by 41%, and nonvertebral fractures by 25% over 3 years in a recent double-blind, placebo-controlled trial of 3889 postmenopausal women with osteoporosis.[67] Zoledronic acid is also indicated for the prevention of new clinical fractures in patients who have recently sustained a hip fracture, as it has been shown in a recent study to decrease new clinical fracture and death.[68,47]

The most common adverse event of bisphosphonates is esophagitis. A higher risk of developing atrial fibrillation with IV zoledronic acid was noted when compared to placebo (1.3% vs. 0.5%); the atrial fibrillation occurred more than 30 days after infusion in most patients.[67] The incidence of atrial fibrillation with the treatment of the other bisphosphonates is unclear, and no definitive association has been demonstrated. [47] Rarely, osteonecrosis of the jaw has been reported, mainly in cancer patients receiving high-dose intravenous bisphosphonates. In a recent review article, osteonecrosis of the jaw was rare in osteoporosis patients treated with bisphosphonates, with an estimated incidence of less than 1 case per 100,000; on the basis of the current data, there was insufficient evidence to confirm an association of osteonecrosis of the jaw and low-dose bisphosphonate usage in the treatment of osteoporosis.[69] There is currently no consensus on how long to continue bisphosphonate therapy. However, stopping therapy after 5 years for some women may be reasonable, because there appears to be residual benefit on BMD and fractures for 5 years.[70]

Calcitonin is an antiresorptive hormone for the treatment of osteoporosis in women who are at least 5 years postmenopausal. Calcitonin is administered nasally (200 IU) or subcutaneously. In a 5-year study of postmenopausal women, calcitonin reduced the vertebral fracture risk by 33% to 36% compared to placebo.[71] Calcitonin did not decrease the risk of nonvertebral fractures compared to placebo. Unlike other antiresorptives, some patient may experience an analgesic effect from calcitonin that may be of benefit in the treatment of symptomatic vertebral compression fractures.[72] This effect may be due to modulation of beta-endorphin levels.[73]

Raloxifene is an estrogen agonist/antagonist that acts as an estrogen agonist at the bone but an antagonist in uterine and breast tissue in postmenopausal women.[47,74] It is approved for both the treatment and prevention of osteoporosis and to reduce the risk of invasive breast cancer in postmenopausal women with osteoporosis.[47] Raloxifene has been shown to decrease vertebral fractures by 30% to 50% in postmenopausal women with osteoporosis. It has also been show to increase both spinal and hip BMD.[47,75,76] Reduction of hip fracture risk has not been shown. Raloxifene is associated with increased risk of venous thromboembolism and does not decrease the risk of coronary heart disease. Hot flashes are also increased (6% over placebo).[47]

Teriparatide (recombinant human parathyroid hormone 1-34) is the only currently available anabolic agent that stimulates bone formation by stimulating osteoblasts more than osteoclasts. Administered subcutaneously daily, teriparatide has been shown to increase bone mass by 10% and to decrease vertebral and nonvertebral fracture risk by more than 50%.[77] The recommended duration of treatment is a maximum of 2 years, and observational studies suggest benefit for at least 18 months after discontinuation.[78] It is common practice to follow teriparatide treatment with an antiresorptive agent, usually a bisphosphonate, to maintain or further increase BMD.[79] Several studies have also compared teriparatide with bisphosphonates, and McClung et al. found that 20 μg/day of teriparatide resulted in significantly greater increases in lumbar spine BMD (10.3%) compared to 10 mg/day of alendronate (5.5%).[80] Common side effects seen in clinical trials include hypercalcemia, leg cramps, nausea, and dizziness.[79] The most serious concern is the risk of osteogenic sarcoma, as rat studies found a dose-dependent increase in teriparatide-treated animals.[81] The risk in humans is felt to be small. Patients with an increased risk of osteosarcoma (i.e., Paget disease of the bone); a prior history of radiation therapy of the skeleton, bony metastasis, or hypercalcemia; or a history of a skeletal malignancy should not be treated with teriparatide. This agent should be reserved for patients who are at high risk for fracture or who are unresponsive to or intolerant of antiresorptive drugs.

There is no consensus on the optimal approach for monitoring therapy. The National Osteoporosis Foundation recommends that repeat BMD assessments be performed every 2 years, which is in accordance with Medicare guidelines but recognizes that testing more frequently may be warranted in certain clinical situations.[47] Poor compliance and persistence with long-term treatment are major barriers in the management of osteoporosis. Measurement of bone markers has been shown to help overcome such barriers. Suppression of biochemical markers of bone turnover after 3 to 6 months of antiresorptive therapies has been demonstrated.

Osteomalacia

Osteomalacia is a metabolic bone disorder characterized by deficient mineralization of newly formed matrix or osteoid. Overall, there may be decreased, normal, or even increased bone mass but with decreased mechanical strength. The diminished deposition of mineral is the result of disorders that lead to a low calcium-phosphate product. Because osteomalacia is commonly asymptomatic and often coexists with osteoporosis in the elderly, its prevalence is difficult to measure. Estimates range from 1% based on unselected autopsy cases to as high as 18% in elderly nursing home patients.[82] Osteomalacia in growing children before fusion of the epiphyseal growth plates is referred to as rickets.

Pathophysiology

The most common cause of osteomalacia in the United States is vitamin D deficiency. Vitamin D plays a central role in calcium and phosphate homeostasis. The two primary sources of vitamin D are dietary and endogenous skin synthesis with exposure to ultraviolet light.[83] If serum calcium falls, parathyroid hormone levels rise and stimulate renal synthesis of 1,25(OH)2D, the most active form of the vitamin. Vitamin D increases intestinal calcium and phosphate absorption, calcium and phosphate release from the skeleton, and renal calcium and phosphate reabsorption. A negative feedback loop exists as 1,25(OH)2D also stimulates osteocyte production of fibroblast growth factor 23, which acts on the kidney to increase phosphate excretion and decrease production of 1,25(OH)2D.[84] This integrated metabolic system functions to maintain serum ionized calcium and phosphate at optimal levels for bone mineralization. In contrast, when vitamin D levels are decreased, intestinal calcium absorption is reduced by as much as 45% to 65% of normal. Absorption of dietary phosphate is also impaired. This results in a reduced calcium-phosphate product at the bone mineralization front, leading to osteomalacia.

Diagnosis

When symptomatic, osteomalacia presents with diffuse bone pain and tenderness as well as proximal muscle weakness.[82] The lumbar spine, pelvis, and lower extremities are the most common sites of involvement, which is usually bilateral. Pain is typically worse with weight bearing and diminished by rest. The bone pain is due, at least in part, to insufficiency fractures in these areas. Looser's zones are thin radiolucent lines oriented at right angles to the long axis of the bone and are typically located above the lesser trochanters, pubic rami, ribs, and axillary border of the scapula and along the shaft of long bones. Looser's zones represent insufficiency fractures in inadequately mineralized bone. A technetium-99 bone scan demonstrates increased uptake in Looser's zones. The most common radiographic abnormality in patients with osteomalacia is osteopenia. Since bone mineralization is deficient in osteomalacia, bone mineral density measurements such as DEXA are reduced, risking misdiagnosis of osteomalacia as osteoporosis.[85] Laboratory findings in osteomalacia vary by etiology (Table 110-4). In vitamin D–deficient states, for example, alkaline phosphatase is elevated and serum calcium is decreased. The best serologic marker to assess a patient's vitamin D status is the 25-hydroxyvitamin D metabolite. The lower end of the normal range of this metabolite is 25 ng/dL. In osteomalacia, serum 25(OH)D levels are often less than 10 ng/dL.[82]

In rare, atypical cases, particularly when osteomalacia is suspected in patients with coexisting osteoporosis, a transiliac tetracycline-labeled bone biopsy may be indicated. Bone biopsy may also be required when a patient fails to respond as expected to appropriate treatment. In osteomalacia, the ratio of mineral to organic matrix is low. Bone histology provides the only certain method of proving the diagnosis of osteomalacia.[86]

Treatment

The objectives of treatment include relieving pain, strengthening bone by promoting mineralization, and correcting secondary hyperparathyroidism. Vitamin D–deficient patients may require initial supplementation with 50,000 IU of vitamin D_2 until levels are normal, with continued maintenance of 800 to 1000 IU daily.[82] Higher doses of vitamin D may be required in patients with osteomalacia and chronic renal failure or defective 25 hydroxylation of vitamin D due to anticonvulsant therapy.

Paget Disease of the Bone

Definition, Epidemiology, and Pathophysiology

Paget disease of the bone (PDB), also known as osteitis deformans, was first described in 1876 by Sir James Paget. It is a chronic skeletal disorder that is characterized by focal areas

TABLE 110-4

Laboratory Values of Biochemical Markers in Metabolic Bone Disease

	DISEASE			
	Osteoporosis	**Osteomalacia (abnormal vitamin D metabolism)**	**Osteomalacia (altered phosphate reabsorption)**	**Paget Disease**
Serum calcium	N	N mild ↓ severe	N	N
Serum phosphate	N	↓	↓	N
Serum alkaline phosphatase	N	↑ moderately	↑	↑↑↑
25(OH)D	N	↓	N	N
1,25(OH)2D	N	N (mild) ↑ (severe) ↓ (late)		N
Parathyroid hormone	N	↑	N	N
Urinary calcium	N	N mild ↓ severe		N
Urinary phosphate	N	↑		N
Urinary hydroxyproline	N	↑		↑↑

of excessive osteoclastic resorption along with increased and disorganized osteoblastic activity resulting in abnormal bone formation, which results in a "mosaic" pattern of lamellar bone. The osteoclasts are increased in size and number and have more nuclei than is normal.[87] The newly laid bone is associated with hypertrophy, sclerosis, and increased vascularity.[88,89] The bone is architecturally abnormal, mechanically weaker, and more susceptible to various stresses than normal bone,[89] resulting in skeletal deformity and an increased tendency for pathologic fracture.[90] PDB may involve a single bone (monostotic) or multiple bones (polyostotic). The axial skeleton is preferentially affected, and common sites of involvement include the pelvis (70%), femur (55%), lumbar spine (53%), skull (42%), and tibia (32%).[87]

The incidence of PDB has been estimated at 3% in people older than 50 years in North America and Europe.[91] The disease seldom appears before the age of 40. The prevalence increases with age and has been reported to double with each decade beyond 50, so more than 10% of people over the age of 90 have the disease.[92] The disease is slightly more prevalent in men than in women and is more common in white than nonwhite individuals.[93,94] The marked geographic variance in the prevalence of PDB of the bone suggests genetic or environmental factors in causation. Fifteen percent of patients report a family history,[95] and children or siblings of affected patients have a sevenfold higher chance of developing PDB.[87,96] Recent epidemiologic data suggest declining rates of severity and prevalence of the condition in the last 30 years, suggesting that this disorder has an environmental component.[87,92,93]

The etiology of PDB is unknown. Environmental and genetic factors may play a role. Four genetic mutations have been identified in selected patients with PDB. The most important appears to be sequestosome 1 (SQSTM1).[87] Inclusions that resemble virus particles have been detected in the osteoclasts of pagetic bone; further studies have shown that these inclusions cross-react with antibodies against the measles virus and respiratory syncytial virus. These intranuclear particles are not specific for pagetic osteoclasts and have also been found in osteoclasts of osteoporotic bone.[87,92]

History and Clinical Presentation

The majority of cases of PDB are asymptomatic. The symptomatic cases tend to present with bone pain, and about 30% of the patients will note deep, aching bone pain that is persistent throughout the day and worse at night.[92,97] Pain is often associated with bone deformities such as bending of the long bones and enlargement of the skull and a warm sensation of the affected bone due to increased blood flow. The gait abnormalities result in increases in spine and joint pain. Fractures are common and may be incomplete.[87] Most fractures heal rapidly, although malunion is quite common.[87,92] Secondary osteoarthritis is also common in PDB, and epidemiologic studies have shown hip and knee replacements to be more common in patients with PBD.[87] Spine problems are common, with spinal stenosis and radiculopathies reported. Spinal cord lesions may result in paraparesis with loss of sphincter control and spasticity of the lower extremities.[98]

Hearing loss is also common, with deafness occurring in 50% of patients owing to temporal bone distortion or fixation of the stapes.[98] Invagination of the skull may also result in vertebrobasilar insufficiency, hydrocephalus, cerebellar herniation, ataxia, or lower cranial nerve lesions. High-output cardiac failure can arise as a complication of active disease, owing to increased blood flow through the affected bone. This is proportional to the extent of the disease.[87,89] Hypercalcemia can also occur, especially in patients who are immobilized.

Sarcomatous degeneration of a pagetic area is a rare complication of the disease, occurring in 0.2% of the cases, although the overall risk of sarcoma is 30 times greater in pagetic patients than in the general population.[92] The 5-year survival rate is between 5% and 8%.[99] Malignant transformation is suspected in any long-standing disease with constant and worsening bone pain or with involvement of a new skeletal segment.[92] Sarcoma can affect any site but is most commonly found at the femur and pelvis and is rarely multifocal.[85] In a recent study that analyzed 119 patients presenting with PBD over 35 years, 18 cases degenerated into sarcoma. Malignant transformation was not found in patients who were treated with bisphosphonates, suggesting a possible preventative effect.[99]

Diagnosis

The diagnosis of PDB is made primarily by radiologic examination of the skeleton using radiographs, radionuclide bone scanning, bone biopsies (rarely), or biochemical testing of bone formation/resorption markers.

Radiographic Findings

Radiographic changes of PBD have been described in three phases. The first, or osteolytic, phase is most common in the long bones. Osteolysis can also affect any portion of the bone, but when it affects the diaphysis, it presents as a wedge-shaped radiolucent area that is clearly demarcated from the other bone. This has been described as a "blade of grass" or "flame." Osteolysis is followed by deposition of poorly mineralized osteoid with fibrosis. This finding is typical in the skull, where it is termed osteoporosis circumscripta. During the second or mixed phase, the skull develops a so-called cotton-wool appearance. In the late phase, increased bone density with trabecular and cortical thickening has been described[92,98] (Fig. 110-1). The skull may become flattened and mottled. Characteristically, the bones in PDB demonstrate local enlargement and thickening. The increase in bone size is deceptive, as pagetic bone does not have the compressive strength and deforms with weight-bearing stress.

Radionuclide bone scanning is more sensitive than radiography for the detection of metabolically active lesions, which present as "hot spots."[85] Literature regarding the usage of MRI and CT in the evaluation of PDB is scarce. There is evidence that MRI may be helpful to better distinguish pagetic bone from sarcoma compared to radiography and CT.[85]

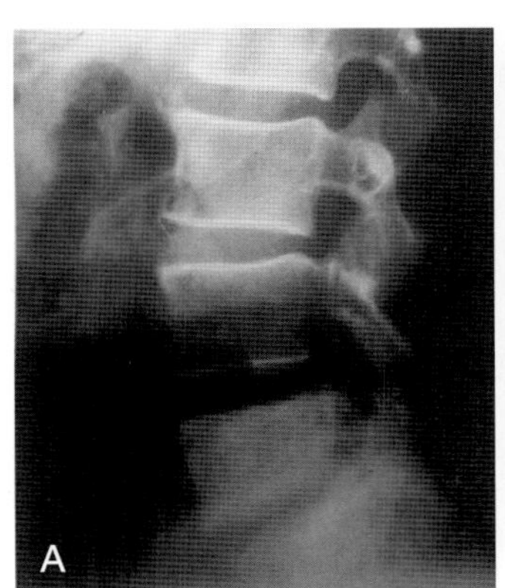

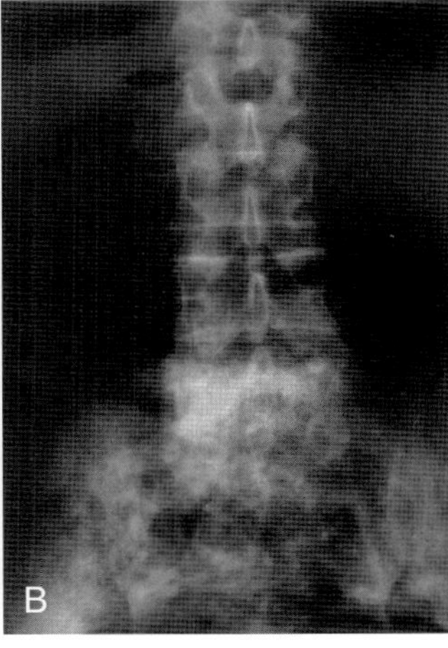

FIGURE 110-1. Lateral (**A**) and anteroposterior (**B**) radiographs of the lumbosacral spine in a patient with Paget disease of the spine. There is increased anteroposterior width of the L5 vertebral body compared to the immediately superior body. The anteroposterior view shows increased density of the bone on the right side of the L5 vertebra, the sacrum, and the ilium. There is also coarsening of the trabeculae in the same distribution, consistent with Paget disease.

Laboratory Manifestations

Serum alkaline phosphatase is elevated in 95% of untreated patients with PDB, reflecting increased bone formation. A normal level does not exclude the disease, as it may occur in monostotic disease or in patients with metabolically inactive disease. In monostotic disease, the serum bone alkaline phosphatase is the most sensitive marker. Alkaline phosphatase is also used in the monitoring of how PDB responds to treatment.

Serum osteocalcin levels may be elevated but are inconsistent and less reliable. Other indices of bone resorption, including urinary excretion of hydroxyproline and pyridinium cross-links, may correlate with disease activity.[89,92]

Treatment

The primary indication for treatment of PDB is pain. The main goals are to decrease pain and to normalize bone remodeling rates. Most patients with PDB who are asymptomatic are not treated; however, the availability of newer and safer therapeutic agents has led to changes in the indications for treatment. Patients with bone or joint pain should be treated. Asymptomatic patients who are at risk of disease complications such as hearing loss caused by skull involvement, spinal nerve entrapment due to spine disease, and fractures should be treated. Patients undergoing planned surgery at an active pagetic site should be treated with an aminobisphosphonate 3 months prior to surgery to help reduce hypervascularity and operative blood loss. Patients with anticipated prolonged immobilization should be treated to help decrease the risk of hypercalcemia. Those with early onset of the disease in areas with potential disabling deformity or when neurologic complications are anticipated should be considered for treatment.

The majority of treatment agents are directed at reducing osteoclastic activity. Calcitonin was the first therapeutic agent available for PDB, but it is no longer considered a first-line agent. The bisphosphonates are considered first in the treatment of PDB, as they strongly inhibit bone resorption and result in longer remission when compared to calcitonin.[92] Bisphosphonates are synthetic analogues of inorganic pyrophosphate that bind the surface of hydroxyapatite and are localized at the site of active bone formation. They decrease bone resorption and formation by decreasing osteoclastic activity and number.[95,96,100] Randomized placebo-controlled trials have shown that bisphosphonate therapy reduces bone turnover, improves joint pain, promotes healing of osteolytic lesions, and restores normal bone histology in Paget disease with replacement of woven bone with lamellar bone. On the basis of these findings, it is postulated that bisphosphonate therapy may help decrease bone complications; however, adequately powered studies have not been undertaken to establish this. Bisphosphonates have also anecdotally been reported to be effective in improving paraplegia in isolated patients with Paget disease of the spine and improving spinal stenosis. In addition, second-generation bisphosphonates such as pamidronate, risedronate, and zoledronic acid are preferable to the older bisphosphonates such as etidronate for treatment of PDB, as they are more effective at reducing bone turnover.[87] Alendronate (40 mg/day for 6 months) and risedronate (30 mg/day for 2 months) have shown normalization of total alkaline phosphatase in about 70% of patients with moderate to severe PDB after a course of treatment.

Pamidronate is also useful in the treatment of active PDB, leading to normalization of total alkaline phosphatase about 50% of the time.[92] In a recent randomized double-blind controlled 6-month trial, a single infusion of zoledronic acid (5 mg infused over 15 minutes) was compared to daily oral risedronate (30 mg/day for 60 days). Zoledronic acid was found to produce more rapid, more complete, and more sustained response in PDB than risedronate. Another study showed that a single intravenous dose of zoledronic acid led to favorable clinical, biochemical, and scintigraphic responses in patients with PDB starting as early as 3 months after treatment and lasting no less than 12 months.[88]

Patients receiving bisphosphonate therapy should receive 1000 to 1500 mg of calcium and 400 to 800 IU of vitamin D by diet or supplementation as new bone formation occurs throughout the process of repair in pagetic bone.[89] Focal osteomalacia has been reported in patients treated with etidronate and pamidronate despite supplementation with vitamin D and calcium.[87]

Measurements of alkaline phosphatase are used to assess the activity of PDB and monitor treatment to the bisphosphonates. Total alkaline phosphatase should be measured every 3 months for the first 6 months of therapy and every 6 months thereafter. Retreatment is indicated when there are persistent symptoms or biochemical relapse. Continuation of pain may be an indication for retreatment. In patients who are asymptomatic, retreatment should be based on biochemical markers of bone turnover.[89]

Surgical Considerations in Metabolic Bone Disease

Osteoporosis

Osteoporosis expresses itself as a surgical issue in one of two predominant ways. The first is in treatment of fractures that occurred because of the osteoporosis. The second is in the treatment of other spine pathologies such as degenerative change or deformity in the patients who have underlying osteoporosis. Osteoporosis is not in and of itself an indication for surgical intervention. The presence of osteoporosis may affect the indications for surgical intervention and may alter the operative plan.

Surgical Treatment of Osteoporotic Fractures

Most osteoporotic fractures will heal spontaneously and do not require surgical intervention.[101] A portion of osteoporotic compression fractures are persistently painful and interfere with function.[102] In recent years, many patients with such fractures have been treated with vertebral augmentation procedures such as vertebroplasty or kyphoplasty. The indications, techniques, and outcomes of these procedures are dealt with in Chapter 128.

A very small subset of osteoporotic fractures will result in a neurologic deficit, and surgery may be required to treat these fractures. The treatment goals for these fractures are to decompress the neural elements, to restore alignment, and to stabilize the fracture generally with rigid internal fixation. Ventral decompression via corpectomy and strut graft with fusion has been performed but has a relatively high failure rate of this construct.[103,104] Anterior column reconstruction followed by dorsal instrumented fusion is an option, but this procedure is extensive and has a high rate of morbidity.[105] Long-segment dorsal reconstruction with a dorsolateral corpectomy through a costotransversectomy or lateral extacavitary approaches are also options. This allows adequate decompression and reconstruction of the anterior column through a single incision. The anterior column is then reconstructed with autograft, allograft, or intervertebral body cages.[106] The addition of expandable intervertebral body cages has made the anterior column reconstruction somewhat easier.[107] These procedures are also associated with a relatively high morbidity rate. A third option is an all-dorsal procedure with the resection of the dorsal elements and a spinal column shortening through a variation of the pedicle subtraction osteotomy. This procedure corrects the kyphosis and restores anterior column weight-bearing capability, but it requires a strut graft or cage.[108-110]

Some surgeons have advocated a hybrid approach utilizing decompression and short-segment reconstruction combined with vertebral augmentation through kyphoplasty or vertebroplasty. Relatively good results have been reported with relatively low morbidity.[111-113] Long-term results of these procedures are not well known. No randomized controlled trials exist comparing these alternative options to the treatment of the neurologically compromised vertebral compression fractures.

Surgery for Degenerative Disease in the Presence of Osteoporosis

Osteoporosis does not directly cause symptoms that would lead to surgery in the absence of a fracture. However, many patients who present with typical symptoms of degenerative disease and require surgery will have associated osteoporosis.[114] The indications for surgery do not change, but the osteoporosis may affect the types of procedures that are chosen. Although osteoporosis is common in older patients with degenerative conditions, most surgeons do not routinely screen for or treat the osteoporosis prior to surgery.[115] Consideration should be given to doing so, as it may improve outcomes. Screening for osteoporosis with a DEXA scan and assessing the patient's preoperative serum calcium and vitamin D levels are likely to be warranted in older patients undergoing fusion surgery.[116]

The use of perioperative bisphosphonates in patients undergoing fusion surgery is somewhat controversial. Some studies have suggested a higher fusion failure rate; others have not.[117-120] Anabolic agents such as teriparatide may be of benefit both preoperatively and perioperatively in improving bone strength and enhancing fusion.[121-123]

Use of Instrumentation in Osteoporosis

Spine instrumentation is used in patients undergoing spine fusion. Osteoporosis weakens the holding power of the implants in bone.[124] This leads to increased rates of instrumentation failure in elective surgery in patients with osteoporosis. This in turn leads to poorer outcome and higher complication rates in osteoporotic patients undergoing spine reconstructive surgery.

Numerous strategies have been proposed for improving the outcomes of spine surgery in patients with osteoporosis. Two review articles by Ponnusamy et al.[125] and Hu[126] summarize a

BOX 110-3. Options to Improve Surgical Outcomes in Osteoporosis

Uninstrumented fusion
Increased number of fixation points
Cross-links
Neutralize forces
Triangulation
Use of osteotomies or intervertebral implants to correct deformity
Use of hooks or wires to resist pull-out
Cement augmentation of implants
Use of implants designed for osteoporotic bone
Meticulous attention to spinal balance

number of options for increasing fixation and improving outcome in osteoporotic patients. Box 110-3 summarizes some of the available options.

Uninstrumented Fusion

An obvious way of avoiding hardware failure is to avoid the use of hardware in the first place. Although hardware is commonly used in lumbar spine fusion, particularly in the presence of degenerative spondylolisthesis, studies have not shown a clear, consistent benefit of the use of instrumentation.[127-129] It is reasonable in patients with osteoporosis and stable spines to fuse without hardware. Fusion rates will be lower, but clinical results in the near term are equivalent.

Increased Number of Fixation Points

Increasing the number of fixation points decreases the loads on each individual component of the construct. Thus, the loads are distributed across more fixation points, overall construct stiffness increases, and the chance of failure decreases.[130,131]

Cross-Fixators and Triangulation

Cross-fixators have their effect by further distributing forces across the implant. They are particularly useful in rotation.[132,133] By placing the screws in a convergent fashion and adding a cross-link, further improvement in strength can be obtained through triangulation.[134] One caveat is that cross-links have been suggested to increase pseudarthrosis rates in scoliosis constructs.[135]

Use of Interbody Fusion and Osteotomies to Obtain Correction

Placement of large interbody implants across the disc space or eccentrically placed implants on the concavity can correct scoliosis. This allows the dorsal hardware to be placed as a neutralization device, and with lower loads on the screws, there should be less failure.[136-140]

In a similar vein, osteotomies can be used to obtain correction, and after closure of the osteotomies, the hardware is again placed as a neutralization device, which may lessen the risk of hardware failure.

Use of Hooks and Wires Instead of Screws

In osteoporosis, relatively more strength is lost in cancellous bone than in cortical bone. The lamina is more cortical than cancellous and loses proportionally less strength.[141] As a result, laminar hooks or wires may be an option. In addition, hooks and wires have superior holding power in pull-out and should be considered at the ends of a kyphosis construct in which pull-out is a common motor failure.[142-144]

Cement Augmentation of Pedicle Screws

Numerous studies have shown that cement augmentation improves the holding power of screws.[145-147] To date, no studies of clinical effectiveness have been published, though the technique is widely used. In our practice in long constructs, cement augmentation is used only at one or two levels at the top or bottom of a construct. If a constructs fails, the failure is usually at the end segments, and should revision be required, it is easier to do if not all segments have been cement augmented. Another interesting idea is to augment adjacent segments to lessen the risk of proximal junctional kyphosis.[148]

Use of Implants Designed for Osteoporotic Bone

A number of modifications of pedicle screws have been proposed for use in osteoporotic bone. These include hollow screws for insertion of cement,[149,150] expandable screws,[151-153] and variable pitch or thread depth screws.[153] These modifications all lead to increased pull-out strength of the implants in biomechanical testing. To date, there have been no good clinical studies showing improved outcomes with these implants.

Meticulous Attention to Spinal Balance

In studies examining outcomes of adult deformity surgery, there is a clear correlation between outcome and restoration of sagittal balance.[154] Late complications, such as implant failure or junctional kyphosis, are correlated with failure to achieve balance.[155-157] As a result, it is vitally important that surgeons performing surgery for osteoporosis pay meticulous attention to overall spinal balance, particularly the sagittal balance.

Surgical Considerations in Paget Disease of the Spine

As was mentioned previously and in this chapter, PDB can lead to spinal stenosis and neurologic compromise. Medical management will usually be successful in treating this.[158,159] In rare cases, stenosis from underlying degenerative disease may combine with PDB to create symptoms. Treatment goals and options are the same as those in degenerative disease alone. In patients with deficit due to pathologic fracture through a pagetic vertebra, surgery may be indicated.[160] Bleeding risk is higher in patients with PDB, and bisphosphonate or calcitonin treatment may lessen this risk if surgery is not urgent.[161]

A rare complication of PDB is sarcomatous degeneration. Spinal osteosarcoma in PDB is not treated differently from primary osteosarcomas.[162,163]

Surgical Considerations in Osteomalacia of the Spine

Osteomalacia has its primary effect on the spine through its effects on bone strength. Thus, its predominant effect is the same as that of osteoporosis, and the surgical considerations remain the same as those in osteoporosis. There are no specific spine pathologies related directly to osteomalacia that have a direct surgical implication.

KEY REFERENCES

Black D, Schwartz A, Ensrud K, et al: Effects of continuing or stopping alendronate after 5 years of Treatment. The Fracture Intervention Trial Long-Term Extension (FLEX): a randomized trial. *JAMA* 296:2927–2938, 2006.

Cho SK, Bridwell KH, Lenke LG, et al: Major complications in revision adult deformity surgery: Risk factors and clinical outcomes with two- to seven-year follow-up. *Spine (Phila Pa 1976)*, 2011. [Epub ahead of print].

Kanis JA, Johnell O, Oden A, et al: FRAX and the assessment of fracture probability in men and women from the UK. *Osteoporos Int* 19:385–397, 2008.

Khosla S, Riggs BL: Pathophysiology of age-related bone loss and osteoporosis. *Endocrinol Metab Clin North Am* 34:1015–1030, 2005.

Kleerekoper M, Gold DT: Osteoporosis prevention and management. An evidence-based review. *Clin Obstet Gynecol* 51:556–563, 2008.

Lyritis GP, Mayasis B, Tsakalakos N, et al: The natural history of the osteoporotic vertebral fracture. *Clin Rheumatol* 8(Suppl 2):66–69, 1989.

National Osteoporosis Foundation. *Clinician's guideline to prevention and treatment of osteoporosis*. Washington DC, 2008, National Osteoporosis Foundation.

Ponnusamy KE, Iyer S, Gupta G, Khanna AJ: Instrumentation of the osteoporotic spine: biomechanical and clinical considerations. *Spine J* 11:54–63, 2011.

REFERENCES

The complete reference list is available online at expertconsult.com.

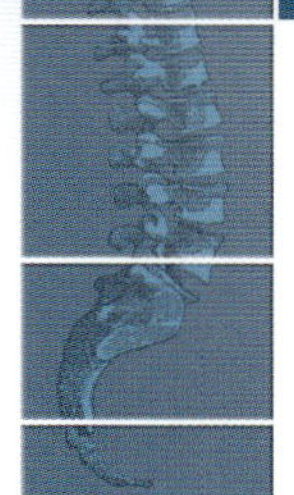

CHAPTER 111

Tumors at the Foramen Magnum: Regional Challenges

Jean-Valery C.E. Coumans | Russ P. Nockels

Tumors in the region of the foramen magnum have long challenged surgeons who confront not only the difficulties of diagnosis but also the technical obstacles of a hazardous tumor resection. Historically, determined efforts often ended in respiratory failure and death. In the 1954 series of Love et al., for example, 34 of 74 patients died postoperatively, most often as a result of respiratory failure.[1] However, with the advent of MRI and microsurgical technique, and knowledge of the regional anatomy, surgical outcome has greatly improved as reflected by the results of larger, more recent series.[2-6]

A wide array of tumors, both malignant and benign, arise in the region of the foramen magnum. Collectively they comprise about 5% of all spinal tumors and 1% of intracranial tumors.[7] It is useful to divide all foramen magnum tumors into intra-axial, intradural extramedullary, and extradural masses. Each location is associated with a specific group of tumors and special topographic relationships that present unique surgical considerations.

More than 90% of foramen magnum tumors are intradural extramedullary tumors, and most commonly occur ventrolaterally in relation to the spinal cord. The majority of these tumors are meningiomas and neurofibromas, the former being considerably more common than the latter.[2,7] Intra-axial tumors (e.g., brainstem gliomas) and extradural tumors (e.g., chordomas) comprise fewer than 10% of foramen magnum tumors.[3]

The results of surgical management of these tumors have greatly improved over the years, because, with the advent of advanced microsurgical techniques, intraoperative monitoring, and a detailed knowledge of foramen magnum anatomy, these lesions are amenable to safe surgical resection. Given the variable pathologic anatomy in the region of the foramen magnum and the availability of a variety of surgical options with varying advantages and disadvantages, the surgeon must carefully choose an appropriate surgical approach. The rational basis for this selection is outlined in this chapter, with emphasis placed on the problems presented by intradural extramedullary lesions. There has been increasing interest in the radiosurgical treatment of foramen magnum meningiomas.[8] Radiosurgery has been employed as a primary tool in patients with comorbidity or advanced age. It has also been used as adjuvant treatment in patients who have incomplete resection or aggressive tumors. In patients with inoperable tumors, conventional chemotherapy and inhibitors of epidermal growth factor receptor (EGFR), farnesyl transferase, cyclooxygenase 2 (COX-2), the protein kinase MEK-1, and the intracellar signaling pathway PI3k/Akt are being investigated.[9]

This chapter reviews the clinical features, microsurgical anatomy, and three surgical approaches to tumors in the region of the foramen magnum. It emphasizes that early diagnosis, a thorough knowledge of microsurgical anatomy, and selection of the appropriate surgical approach all contribute to an optimal patient outcome.

History

A foramen magnum tumor was first described by Hallopeau in 1874[10] in a case report of a 50-year-old woman who presented with spastic upper extremity weakness that progressed to quadriparesis with brainstem signs. The patient eventually died of respiratory failure. Autopsy revealed a foramen magnum tumor, "the size of a small chestnut," that caused compression of the lateral funiculi of the spinal cord bilaterally.

Although early attempts at surgical removal of foramen magnum tumors were met with disastrous consequences,[11,12] Elsberg and Strauss successfully removed a foramen magnum meningioma from a woman, aged 36 years, who presented with Brown-Séquard syndrome.[13] Despite several intraoperative episodes of respiratory failure, the patient enjoyed full neurologic recovery postoperatively. The report of this case in 1929 was accompanied by the first systematic evaluation of foramen magnum tumors.

In their classic 1938 treatise, Cushing and Eisenhardt divided foramen magnum tumors into craniospinal and spinocranial tumors on the basis of their predominant anatomic location and associated clinical symptomatology.[14] Since that account, several series of patients with foramen magnum tumors have been reported in the literature, with progressive improvement in outcome.[1,3-6,15-19]

Historically, most lesions have been approached dorsally. However, for ventrally and ventrolaterally located lesions, two other surgical approaches have been employed to minimize retraction of the neural structures. The transoral approach was originally described by Kanavel in 1919 in a report on the transoral removal of a bullet that was lodged between the atlas and the base of the skull.[20] Although the technique has been described most commonly as an approach to extradural lesions,[21-24] intradural lesions have also been treated this way.[25-28] Like the transoral approach, the far lateral approach was originally described to manage other lesions, and in this instance, vertebral and vertebrobasilar artery lesions were managed rather than foramen magnum tumors.[29] This approach has since been modified and adopted to deal with tumors in the region of the foramen magnum.[30,31]

Pathology and Epidemiology

Major features of the largest series of foramen magnum tumors are presented in Table 111-1. Conceptually, tumors in the region of the foramen magnum are best categorized as intra-axial, intradural extramedullary, and extradural tumors, similar to the classification used for spine tumors. Intra-axial tumors are predominantly brainstem gliomas but also include gangliogliomas, anaplastic astrocytomas, ependymomas, and cavernous hemangiomas. Caudal extension of medulloblastomas and hemangioblastomas into the foramen magnum occurs in children and adults, respectively.[32] Intradural extramedullary tumors consist mainly of meningiomas and nerve sheath tumors and a much smaller number of epidermoid tumors and paragangliogliomas.[32,33]

Extradural neoplasms are primarily osteocartilaginous tumors, of which chordoma is, by far, the most common. Chondromas and chondrosarcomas may also arise in this region.[32] Occasionally, meningiomas extend extradurally. This type of meningioma is associated with more aggressive pathologic features and clinical course.

This distribution of tumors is reflected in the series by Bruneau and George.[3] They reviewed 230 cases of extramedullary intradural and extradural tumors of the foramen magnum (intra-axial tumors were excluded). The intradural tumors that comprised almost 80% of the cases reviewed included meningiomas (60%) and neurofibromas (30%). Fifty percent of extradural tumors were chordomas. The most frequently occurring tumors (in order of decreasing frequency) were meningioma (106 cases), neurofibroma (49 cases), and chordoma (28 cases).

The topography of foramen magnum meningioma is of special interest to surgeons. Three characteristics define the lesion.[2,3] First is the compartment of origin. Tumors are divided into intradural (representing the majority of lesions), intra-extradural, and extradural (rare). The intradural lesions are further divided into three groups based on their point of attachment. Ventral tumors are attached to the ventral portion of the foramen magnum (dura, spinal root, or spinal cord) on both sides of the midline; lateral tumors originate between the midline and the dentate ligament; and dorsal tumors have a point of origin dorsal to the dentate ligament.[3] Using these strict criteria, George et al. found that among the 106 meningiomas in their series, 56% occurred laterally, 31% ventrally, and 13% dorsally.[3,33] Other authors have reported a similar distribution.[4-6,16,18] Third, the relationship to the vertebral artery is defined. Tumors arising caudal to the vertebral artery displace the lower cranial nerves upward, tumors arising above the vertebral artery displace the nerves caudally, and tumors spanning the craniocaudal extent of the vertebral artery displace the nerves unpredictably.[2,3]

The relative rarity of foramen magnum tumors belies their clinical importance. Compared with other CNS neoplasms, foramen magnum tumors occur infrequently: they account for only 5% of all spinal neoplasms and 1% of all intracranial neoplasms. Considering meningiomas alone, those occurring in the region of the foramen magnum account for only 1.2% to 3.2% of meningiomas.[6,16,18]

Among the large series, the age range of patients with foramen magnum tumors was 2 to 81 years, but the majority of these tumors occur around the fifth decade.[1,4-6,16-19,34] The average time between onset of symptoms and diagnosis was 2.5 years. The mean age was 47 years, with a female-to-male

TABLE 111-1

Series of Extramedullary Foramen Magnum Tumors

Reference	Time Span	No. of Patients	Tumor Location	Tumor Type	Age Range	Mean Duration: Symptom Onset to Diagnosis
Symonds and Meadows[19]	? yr	5	2 VL, 1 V, 1 L,1 DL	4 meningiomas, 1 neurofibroma	38–57 yr	3.5 yr
Smolik and Sachs[17]	4 yr	6	2 L, 1 DL, 1 VL	6 meningiomas	33–56 yr	2.5 yr
Stein et al.[18]	? yr	25	21 VL, 3 D, 1 L, 1 V	25 meningiomas	27–88 yr	<5 yr
Guidetti and Spallone[4]	26 yr	18	12 VL, 3 DL, 3 V	11 meningiomas, 7 neurofibromas	13–65 yr	3.5 yr
Meyer et al.[5]	58 yr	102	61 V, 21 D, 20 L	78 meningiomas, 23 neurofibromas, 1 teratoma	12–81 yr	2.25 yr
Bruneau and George[3]	10 yr	230	56% L, 31% V, 13% D	106 meningiomas, 49 neurofibromas, 28 chordomas, 32 osseous tumors,* 15 others†	47 yr (mean)	2.25 yr
Total	24.5 yr	386	38% V, 14% VL, 31% L, 14.5% D, 2% DL	NA	25.69 yr	3.2 yr

D, dorsal; DL, dorsolateral; L, lateral; NA, not applicable; V, ventral; VL, ventrolateral.

*Nineteen primary and 13 metastatic osseous tumors.

†Includes 4 melanomas, 3 hemangioblastomas, 3 dermoid or epidermoid cysts, 2 ependymomas, 1 cavernoma, 1 angiomyolipoma, and 1 cholesterin cyst.

ratio of 1.5:1.[3] These figures are consistent among authors.[4-6,18] Female predominance of meningiomas in general is also a consistent finding.

Besides neoplasms, other entities can present as foramen magnum lesions and should be considered in the differential diagnosis. Calcium pyrophosphate deposition in the transverse ligament can form a tumor-like mass that compresses the cervicomedullary junction.[35] This condition is common in the elderly and rarely becomes symptomatic. It can be diagnosed by CT, which demonstrates calcification around the odontoid. Tuberculosis can also affect the cervicomedullary junction in isolation.[36] Although uncommon, this condition should be considered in individuals with systemic tuberculosis, patients from geographic areas where it is endemic, and patients with HIV. A recent series of 29 cases of craniocervical tuberculosis describes frequent destruction of the condyles, clivus and dens, and ventral arch of the atlas. The majority of patients harbored space-occupying soft tissue masses in the epidural and paravertebral spaces, and they were large enough to cause myelopathy in 12 out of 29 cases. Cervicomedullary compression can also occur in craniometaphyseal dysplasia,[37] a sclerosing bone disorder characterized by bony encroachment of neural foramina.

Clinical Presentation

Many authors have noted that no signs or symptoms are pathognomonic for foramen magnum tumors.[16,38] As early as 1937, Symonds and Meadows observed that "the clinical picture which results from compression of the spinal cord at, or near, the level of the foramen magnum is not always easy of recognition."[19] Indeed, the clinical presentation of foramen magnum tumors usually varies and includes such ubiquitous symptoms as neck pain and limb dysesthesias, which are also associated with several more common diseases. The rarity of foramen magnum tumors may therefore cause them to be overlooked by clinicians.[39] Even a series as recent as that of Bruneau and George, which reviews 230 cases of foramen magnum tumors from 1985 to 1995, reports a misdiagnosis rate as high as 13.5%.[3]

The most common presenting symptoms of foramen magnum tumors, in order of decreasing frequency, are suboccipital or neck pain, dysesthesias of the extremities more frequent in the upper than in the lower extremities, gait disturbance, and weakness more frequent in the upper extremities than in the lower. Other common early symptoms include clumsiness of the hands, bladder disturbance, dysphagia, nausea and vomiting, headache, "drop attacks," and dizziness.[4,5,16,18] Usually a patient presents with a constellation of symptoms. Rarely, the presentation is characterized by brainstem symptoms primarily (e.g., nausea) or pure nerve dysfunction (e.g., hemifacial spasm,[40] dysphagia,[41] occipital neuralgia[42]).

Suboccipital or upper cervical pain, probably caused by irritation of the dura and C2 nerve root, is the most common presenting complaint and may precede other symptoms by months or years. C2 distribution sensory loss frequently accompanies the pain, and together, these symptoms should suggest the diagnosis of foramen magnum tumor. In the series by Stein et al.,[18] Meyer et al.,[5] and Guidetti and Spallone,[4] suboccipital or upper cervical neck pain was the initial complaint in 65% to 80% of patients. By the time of admission, 100% of Guidetti and Spallone's patients complained of neck pain.

Limb dysesthesias are frequently present and may occur in the form of a burning[4,6] or cold[13,43] sensation; proprioceptive loss is also common.[44] Weakness typically accompanies the sensory changes and tends to involve the upper extremities more than the lower, and the ipsilateral more than the contralateral side.[16] An unusual feature of the weakness is its occasional association with wasting of the intrinsic hand muscles.[45,46] Taylor and Byrnes have cogently argued, on the basis of their own experimental evidence, that foramen magnum lesions produce hand wasting by causing venous obstruction in the upper cervical cord, which leads to venous infarction in the lower cervical gray matter.[47] If the motor symptoms dominate the presentation, the combination of hyperreflexia and hand wasting can resemble the presentation of amyotrophic lateral sclerosis.

The initial neurologic examination of the patient with a foramen magnum tumor most commonly reveals weakness, sensory loss, hyperreflexia, Babinski sign, and spastic gait. Typically, the weakness first affects the ipsilateral arm and then evolves over time into a progressive spastic quadriparesis. Sensory loss may involve the modalities of pain and temperature, proprioception, or both. The burning and cold dysesthesias have been mentioned. Other less common, but still frequent, signs include nystagmus (classically, downbeat), accessory nerve palsy, and atrophy of the intrinsic muscles of the hand. Infrequent signs include atrophy of the arms and legs, papilledema, Horner syndrome, and cranial neuropathies involving cranial nerves V, VII to X, and XII.[44]

The nonspecific signs and symptoms produced by foramen magnum tumors must be distinguished from those occurring in several more common conditions. Although modern neuroimaging has lessened this problem, the neurosurgical literature is replete with examples of tumors in the region of the foramen magnum that were misdiagnosed on initial presentation. Even a recent series of foramen magnum tumors found a 13.5% incidence of misdiagnosis.[3] The failure to establish the correct diagnosis most commonly occurs because a foramen magnum tumor has not been included in the differential diagnosis.[48] The clinical entities most commonly confused with foramen magnum tumors include cervical spondylosis, multiple sclerosis, syringomyelia, intramedullary tumors, carpal tunnel syndrome, normal pressure hydrocephalus, Chiari malformation, and amyotrophic lateral sclerosis.

Surgical Anatomy

A thorough knowledge of foramen magnum anatomy is critical to safe surgical exposure in this region. For a more detailed review of the microsurgical anatomy, the reader is referred to the elegant anatomic studies of Oliveira et al.,[49] Rhoton et al.,[50] and Wen et al.[51]

Osseous Structures

The foramen magnum is formed by the occipital bone, which consists of three parts: basilar, lateral, and squamosal. The basilar part is formed by a fusion between the occipital bone and the clivus. The lateral parts consist of the occipital condyles, which articulate with the atlas. Behind and above the foramen is the occipital squama, whose internal surface is marked by a prominent midline ridge—the internal occipital crest, which serves as the attachment for the falx cerebelli. The ventral margin of the foramen magnum is termed the basion and the opposite margin, the opisthion. The shape of the foramen magnum varies. It is generally oval in shape, and the wider portion is located dorsally.[49] It measures on average 35 mm in length and 29 mm in width. The foramen magnum transmits the medulla oblongata; the meninges; the ascending portion of the spinal accessory nerve; and the vertebral, anterior, and posterior spinal arteries.

The occipital condyles are located lateral to the ventral half of the foramen magnum. The occipital condyles are oval, and their inferior surface is convex. They are oriented in a dorsolateral-to-ventromedial direction. They articulate with the superior facet of the atlas, which overlies its lateral mass. The anatomy of the occipital condyles, as it pertains to the transcondylar approach, has been reviewed.[52]

The hypoglossal canal is located within the occipital bone, ventral to the junction between the ventral and middle third of the occipital condyles.[51] The hypoglossal nerve is the only structure that travels through the hypoglossal canal. The jugular foramen is located lateral to the ventral half of the occipital condyles, at the junction of the petrous part of the temporal bone and the occipital bone. It is irregular in shape and has a smaller anterior division and a larger posterior division. The anterior division transmits the inferior petrosal sinus and the glossopharyngeal nerve. The posterior division transmits the vagus and spinal accessory nerves, the internal jugular vein, and the meningeal branches of the ascending pharyngeal and occipital arteries.[49]

Muscles

The muscles of the foramen magnum region can be divided into superficial and deep layers. The muscles of the superficial layer consist of the trapezius, the sternocleidomastoid, the splenius capitis, and the longissimus capitis. The trapezius arises from the medial third of the superior nuchal line, and extends medially to the ligamentum nuchae and laterally to the spine of the scapula and the lateral third of the clavicle. The sternocleidomastoid attaches to the lateral half of the superior nuchal line and the adjacent portion of the mastoid process, as well as to the sternum and medial clavicle. The splenius capitis attaches to the lateral part of the superior nuchal line and to the spinous processes of C7 to T4. Lateral to this muscle lies the longissimus capitis. This muscle arises from the articular processes of the last four cervical vertebrae and the transverse processes of the first five thoracic vertebrae. It inserts in the dorsal part of the mastoid process.

Deep to the splenius capitis is the semispinalis capitis. This muscle arises from the tip of the transverse processes of the first six thoracic vertebrae and inserts between the superior and inferior nuchal lines. The deepest layer comprises a group of four small suboccipital muscles: the rectus capitis posterior major and minor and the obliquus capitis inferior and superior. The rectus capitis posterior major is attached to the spinous process of C2 and inserts into the lateral part of the inferior nuchal line. The rectus capitis posterior minor arises from the tubercle of C1 and insets into the medial part of the inferior nuchal line. The superior obliquus capitis extends from the transverse process of C2 to the occipital bone, between the superior and inferior nuchal lines, laterally. The inferior obliquus capitis extends from the spinous process of C2 to the transverse process of C1.

Neural Structures

Neural structures in the region of the foramen magnum include the caudal medulla, caudal vermis, cerebellar tonsils, fourth ventricle, rostral spinal cord, lower cranial nerves, and upper cervical nerves.

The medulla blends into the spinal cord just rostral to the emergence of the dorsal and ventral rootlets that form the first cervical nerve. It is the medulla, therefore, and not the spinal cord that occupies the foramen magnum.

The dentate ligaments attach medially to the pia mater of the spinal cord and laterally to the dura mater, midway between the dorsal and ventral roots. Whereas its medial attachment is continuous, laterally the dentate ligament forms triangular processes that attach to the dura mater at intervals. Division of the upper two triangular processes may facilitate exposure of ventral tumors.

Cranial Nerves

Any of the lower four cranial nerves may be affected by lesions arising in the foramen magnum. The hypoglossal nerve is formed by a series of rootlets that arise in the ventrolateral sulcus between the pyramid and the olive, along a line that is continuous with the ventral spinal roots. The hypoglossal rootlets course ventrolaterally through the subarachnoid space on their way to the hypoglossal canal, passing dorsally in relation to the vertebral artery. If the course of the vertebral artery is short and straight, there may be no contact between the artery and the hypoglossal nerve. A tortuous vertebral artery, however, may displace the nerve dorsally and medially against the medulla, stretching and damaging its fibers.[53] Infrequently, the artery passes through the rootlets of the nerve.[49]

The glossopharyngeal, vagus, and cranial portions of the accessory nerves all arise in series along the dorsolateral sulcus, between the olive and the tuber cinereum. They exit the skull together through the jugular foramen. The cranial part of the accessory nerve is joined by a spinal part that arises as a series of rootlets between the ventral and dorsal rootlets and ascends through the foramen magnum between the dentate ligament and the dorsal roots. The hypoglossal nerve and, less commonly, the glossopharyngeal, vagus, and accessory nerves may be displaced dorsomedially by a thickened and atheromatous vertebral artery.[53]

Spinal Nerve Roots

The C1 nerve root often lacks a dorsal rootlet. The accessory nerve frequently contributes a root to the C1 nerve root when the C1 dorsal root, as is commonly the case, is absent. Before exiting the dura mater, the C1 ventral root and the dorsal root, if present, attach to the dorsal caudal surface of the intradural segment of the vertebral artery. The ventral and dorsal roots then exit the dura around the vertebral artery and unite within or just beyond the dural exit.

Vascular Structures

The arteries in the region of the foramen magnum include the vertebral and posterior inferior cerebellar arteries, the anterior and posterior spinal arteries, and the meningeal branches of the vertebral and carotid arteries.

In most individuals, the left vertebral artery is dominant. After ascending through the C1 foramina, the vertebral arteries continue medially with the C1 nerve root along a groove on the rostral surface of the dorsal arch of the atlas, behind the lateral mass. Frequently, this groove forms a complete bony canal that surrounds the vertebral artery.[49] Between C6 and C2, the vertebral arteries are thus protected dorsally by the lateral masses. However, as the arteries course dorsal to the C1 lateral mass and enter the region of the foramen magnum, they lose their dorsal bony protection.

From the rostral surface of the dorsal arch of the atlas, the arteries enter the vertebral canal by passing ventral to the lateral border of the atlanto-occipital membrane. This segment of the vertebral artery is partially covered by the atlanto-occipital membrane, the rectus capitis posterior major, and the superior and inferior oblique muscles, and, importantly, is also surrounded by a venous plexus.

Before entering the dura mater, the vertebral artery gives rise to the posterior meningeal and posterior spinal arteries, branches to the deep cervical musculature, and, infrequently, the posterior inferior cerebellar artery. Lang found only a 4% incidence of an extradural origin of the posterior inferior cerebellar artery.[54,55]

After giving off these branches, the vertebral arteries enter the dura mater just caudal to the lateral edge of the foramen magnum behind the occipital condyles, accompanied by the first cervical nerve and the posterior spinal artery.[49]

The initial intradural segment of the vertebral artery passes rostral to the dorsal and ventral roots of the first cervical nerve and ventral to the posterior spinal artery, the dentate ligament, and the spinal portion of the accessory nerve. In its ascent along the lower lateral and upper ventral aspect of the medulla, the vertebral artery remains ventral to the lower cranial nerves.[7] Variations in this relationship do exist, however, and the vertebral artery may lie dorsal to some cranial nerve rootlets.[7] Connections between the hypoglossal nerve, glossopharyngeal nerve, spinal accessory nerve, and C2 cervical root provide the anatomic substrate for various "neck and tongue" syndromes.[56]

As the vertebral arteries ascend ventromedially along the lateral and then the ventral surface of the medulla, they run adjacent to the occipital condyles, the hypoglossal canals, and the jugular tubercles and then come to rest on the clivus. At or near the pontomedullary junction, the arteries join together to form the basilar artery. The precise point at which the arteries join varies with the size and tortuosity of the vessels.[49]

The posterior inferior cerebellar artery usually originates from the intradural portion of the vertebral artery just above the foramen magnum, although it rarely arises extradurally at or below the foramen.[49] As mentioned, 4% of the posterior inferior cerebellar arteries examined by Lang arose extradurally.[54,55] In its course along the ventrolateral and then the dorsolateral medulla, this artery may pass rostrally, caudally, or between the hypoglossal rootlets or above, below, or between the rootlets of the glossopharyngeal, vagus, and accessory nerves.[56] Like the vertebral artery, the relationship between the posterior inferior cerebellar artery and the lower cranial nerves is an intimate one and frequently leads to deformation and stretching of the nerves.

After passing through or around the rootlets of the nerves, the posterior inferior cerebellar artery comes to lie dorsal to the glossopharyngeal, vagus, and accessory nerves and then takes a variable course to reach the dorsal medulla, where it bifurcates into a medial and a lateral trunk.[56] The medial trunk supplies the vermis and the adjacent cerebellar hemisphere; the lateral trunk supplies the tonsil and hemispheres.

The anterior spinal artery is usually formed by the union of the paired anterior ventral spinal arteries. These arise from the vertebral artery, supply the paramedial ventral medulla, converge, and run caudally along the ventral median fissure of the spinal cord. In a common variant, the anterior spinal artery may arise from a single vertebral artery, supplemented by supply from vertebral radicular branches at C2 or C3.[54] The posterior spinal arteries have widely variable origins. They may arise from the posterior inferior cerebellar artery or from the intradural or extradural segment of the vertebral artery.[54]

The arteries that supply the dura mater in the region of the foramen magnum include the paired anterior and posterior meningeal branches of the vertebral artery, the ascending pharyngeal artery, the meningohypophyseal trunk of the intracavernous internal carotid artery, and the occipital artery. A variable number of radiculomuscular branches also arise from the extradural vertebral artery.[54] The size and flow of any of these vessels may markedly increase when supplying a dura-based tumor of the foramen magnum.

The venous sinuses most proximal to the foramen magnum include (1) the marginal venous sinus that is formed by the dura lining the rim of the foramen magnum; (2) the occipital venous sinus that is formed by the cerebellar falx; and (3) the basilar venous plexus that is the anastomosis connecting the cavernous sinus on each side, extending along the clivus from the dorsum sellae rostrally to the ventral rim of the foramen magnum caudally.

The veins in the region of the foramen magnum are located both extradurally and intradurally. Extradural veins make up the epidural venous plexus, which is formed by veins in the epidural space, and vertebral venous plexus, which is formed by veins in the deep muscles surrounding the cervical vertebrae. Intradural veins drain the lower part of the cerebellum and brainstem and the upper part of the spinal cord. Dorsally these veins drain into the dural sinuses surrounding the foramen magnum and torcula. Ventrally and laterally they drain into the superior petrosal sinus.

Alteration of Anatomy by the Tumor

The most important consideration in the selection of a surgical approach is the topographic relationship between the tumor and the neurovascular structures. These structures include the rostral spinal nerve roots; the glossopharyngeal, vagus, accessory, and hypoglossal nerves; and the vertebral artery and its branches. Obviously, the direction of displacement of the neurovascular structures varies with the location and size of the tumor (Fig. 111-1). Although there are variations, the following guidelines generally apply:

- Dorsal midline tumors displace neurovascular structures ventrally.
- Ventral midline tumors displace neurovascular structures dorsally.
- Ventrolateral tumors displace the spinal cord and brainstem dorsomedially, the cranial and spinal nerves dorsally, and the vertebral artery and its branches ventrally.

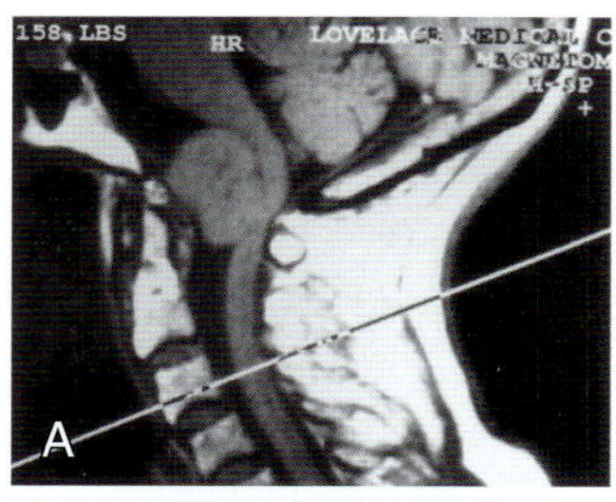

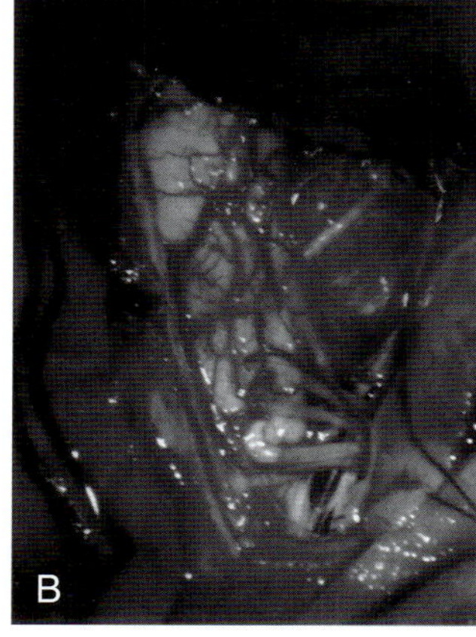

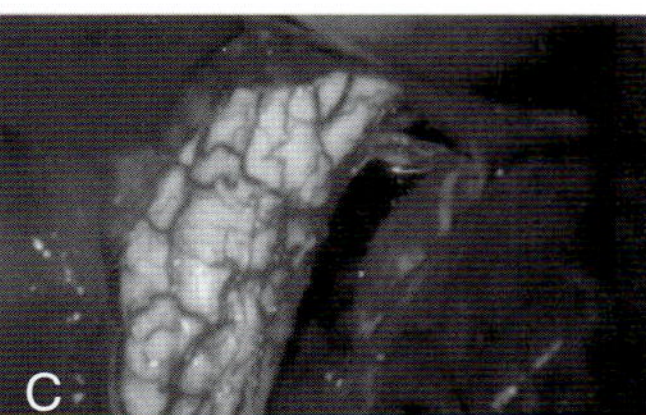

FIGURE 111-1. A 64-year-old woman presented with a progressive quadriparesis. **A,** Sagittal T1-weighted MRI of the cervicomedullary junction shows a ventrally located, well-delineated isointense mass at the foramen magnum causing dorsal displacement of the medulla and upper cervical spinal cord. **B,** Intraoperative photograph shows the tumor and its relation to the hypoglossal and accessory nerves. **C,** Intraoperative photograph after resection of the tumor. The patient experienced full neurologic recovery.

Selection of a Surgical Approach

In selecting an approach, the surgeon has to weigh the likelihood of maximally resecting the tumor with the morbidity of the approach, and his or her skill and experience with a given approach. Although many surgical approaches to the region of the foramen magnum have been described, the following three are the most common: (1) the dorsal approach, (2) the far lateral approach, and (3) the transoral approach. The advantages and disadvantages of each of these approaches are outlined in Table 111-2.[7] The approach is generally open, although the endoscopic approach has also been employed with ventral approaches.

The first step in deciding from among these approaches is to determine the topographic relationship of the tumor to the neurovascular structures.

The dorsal approach is the most familiar and least technically demanding of the three. It is best suited for dorsal midline tumors that require neither retraction of the spinal cord or brainstem nor proximal vascular control of the vertebral artery to address ventral or lateral components of the lesion. The disadvantages of this approach include its poor visualization of the spinal cord tumor junction with tumors that are more ventrolateral and its lack of provision for proximal vascular control. However, for intradural lesions located dorsal to the dentate ligament, it is the approach of choice.

In laterally located meningiomas, with an origin ventral to the dentate ligament, a far lateral approach offers advantages over a dorsal midline approach. Although it involves more dissection and greater bone removal, the far lateral approach allows the dissection of the spinal cord/tumor junction to be carried out under direct vision. It also provides excellent control of the vertebral artery.[7,57-59] It may also be used to approach ventrally located tumors because it exposes

TABLE 111-2

Advantages and Disadvantages of Surgical Approaches to the Foramen Magnum

Approach	Advantages	Disadvantages
Posterior	Most familiar Least demanding Minimal risk of infection Permits stabilization and fusion for craniocervical instability	Poor visualization of cord-tumor interface Exposure limited by neurovascular structures Limited proximal control of vertebral artery
Far lateral	Minimal risk of infection Direct visualization of cord-tumor interface Exposes anterior aspect of thecal sac Obviates need for cord retraction Excellent proximal control of vertebral artery Rarely produces craniocervical instability Permits stabilization and fusion for craniocervical instability	More complex exposure Associated with postoperative hydrocephalus Time consuming
Transoral	Obviates need for cord retraction No neurovascular obstacles in midline Exposes midline of anterior thecal sac	Deep operative field Limited lateral exposure Cord-tumor interface not seen until end of operation High risk for cerebrospinal fluid leak and meningitis Destabilizes craniocervical junction Stabilization or fusion of craniocervical junction requires separate incision No proximal control of vertebral artery

the entire ventral aspect of the thecal sac. Compared with the transoral approach, the instrumentation used in the far lateral approach is also simpler and the risk of infection is minimized. Also, in contrast to the transoral approach, destabilization of the craniocervical junction can be addressed with a fusion and instrumentation procedure. The latter is performed easily concomitantly, if required, based on the amount of removal of the occipital condyle.

The transoral approach is best suited for midline ventral tumors, especially extradural ones. Its advantages include lack of neurovascular obstacles and avoidance of any retraction of the neuraxis. The drawbacks of the transoral approach, however, are many: laterally placed or broad-based tumors are inadequately exposed; vascular control is lacking; the spinal cord/tumor junction is not observed until the end of the operation; and iatrogenic spinal destabilization, which invariably occurs, requires a separate stabilizing procedure. Furthermore, because the operative field is necessarily contaminated and because a watertight dural closure is difficult to achieve, there is a high incidence of postoperative cerebrospinal fluid (CSF) fistula and meningitis. From a technical standpoint, intradural ventral surgery is rendered difficult by the long reach through a narrow surgical corridor. Consideration has been given recently to performing these operations endoscopically or even with robot-assisted surgery, using methodologies applied previously in cardiac and prostate surgery.[60]

Preoperative Considerations

The administration of corticosteroids may improve patient symptoms during the preoperative planning stage. Patients should be informed of the possible need for a tracheotomy and gastrostomy. Prophylactic antibiotics should be administered before surgery. If the transoral approach is to be used, first obtaining nose and throat bacterial cultures may guide the choice of antibiotics.

Before induction of anesthesia, sequential compression stockings are applied as prophylaxis against deep venous thrombosis. An assessment is made of the patient's tolerance to neck flexion to avoid neurologic injury during positioning.

A lumbar drain is inserted before beginning any far lateral approach or any transoral operation in which the dura is likely to be violated. CSF can be drained at a rate of 10 to 20 mL/hour for the first 2 postoperative days. This may reduce the amount of suboccipital pain, some of which may be related to blood in the CSF. Furthermore, it reduces the need for a CSF shunting procedure after the far lateral approach. In cases of postoperative CSF leak that persists despite several days of CSF drainage, a lumboperitoneal shunt may be placed.

Electrophysiologic monitoring, including somatosensory evoked potentials, motor-evoked potentials, and brainstem auditory evoked potentials, is employed. Due to the rostral nature of the lesion, D-wave motor monitoring is not practical. The vagus nerve can be monitored using an electromyographic endotracheal tube.[61] Electromyography can also be performed on the accessory and hypoglossal nerves. Although employed uncommonly in these operations, perioperative placement of a ventriculostomy should be considered when hydrocephalus is present or seems likely to occur. Finally, the surgical approach should be selected on the basis of the location of the tumor and its relationship to the neural and osseous structures.

Dorsal Approach

The prone, three-quarter–prone (park bench), or semisitting position may be chosen. For tumors limited to the dorsal space, the prone position is the simplest and safest. For tumors that extend laterally, the three-quarter–prone position may be better. Access to the ventral foramen magnum region is further facilitated by turning the head to the side of the lesion. Three-point rigid fixation is routinely employed.

A vertical midline, vertical paramedian, or "candy-cane" incision is used. The first is adequate for true dorsal lesions; the latter two are best for more lateral lesions. Whatever incision is chosen, it must be long enough to accommodate a suboccipital craniectomy and a C1-2 laminectomy. The candy-cane incision angles rostrolaterally above the inion and can accommodate a bur hole for ventricular puncture.

After making an incision deep to the subcutaneous tissues, the underlying fascia is divided in a Y-shaped fashion. The upper limbs of the Y run along the superior nuchal line, leaving a fascial cuff attached to the bone to facilitate closure. The caudal limb of the incision extends downward in the midline to the spinous process of C2 or lower. After hemostasis is obtained, a subperiosteal dissection is carried out to expose the occipital squama and the spinous processes and laminae of C1 and C2.

Traditionally, two bur holes are next placed bilaterally in the occipital bone. After the dura mater is separated, bone cuts are made transversely and down to the foramen magnum rim with a high-speed drill. Alternatively, in younger patients without significant tension in the posterior fossa, the craniotomy can be started from the rim of the foramen magnum using the high-speed drill without bur holes. The craniotomy is carried rostrally to the caudal edge of the transverse sinus. Caudally, the dorsal rim of the foramen magnum is removed. Bilateral laminectomies are then made at the upper one or two cervical vertebrae (depending on the caudal extent of the tumor). These should be carried out widely, although disruption of the facet joints should be avoided unless absolutely necessary.

The dura mater is opened in a Y-shaped configuration. The rostral limbs of the Y are placed just below the transverse sinus, and the caudal limb is carried downward in the midline to expose the full extent of the tumor. Should the occipital sinus bleed, it may be ligated with #4-0 nylon or coagulated with bipolar cautery. Dural tack-up sutures are then placed to expose the cerebellum, the arachnoid is incised in the midline, and the cisterna magna is opened. Full exposure of tumors that attach to the roof or the floor of the fourth ventricle may require resection of a cerebellar tonsil or splitting of the inferior vermis.

Dorsally located tumors are directly accessible with this approach and usually present little risk of vascular injury or cranial neuropathy. These lesions are often amenable to en bloc resection. By contrast, ventrolateral lesions require care to avoid injury to the vertebral or posterior inferior cerebellar arteries, which may be attached to or encased by the tumor. Furthermore, ventrolateral lesions tend to displace the spinal cord dorsally, stretching one or more rootlets of the cranial nerves or rostral spinal roots over the tumor. In tumors arising ventral to the dentate ligament, tumor resection is carried out between the involved rootlets in a piecemeal fashion, with care taken to avoid injury to the radicular vessels that run along the rostral cervical nerve roots. Sectioning the dentate ligaments may improve exposure. Often, the lesion must be removed in multiple small fragments, working between rootlets of the spinal accessory nerve, to avoid excessive rootlet retraction.

The tumor capsule is best opened sharply. It is coagulated and incised. The ultrasonic aspirator can be useful for debulking the intracapsular portion of the tumor. The tumor capsule itself is dissected free from surrounding neurovascular structures and is excised along with involved dura mater. A frozen section is typically obtained intraoperatively, since other entities such as sarcoid can resemble a meningioma and may not merit a radical resection.[62]

The need for the radical resection of meningioma-involved dura mater to prevent tumor recurrence is controversial.[63,64] Curettage of the inner surface of tumor-involved dura with a Penfield dissector or a small curette, followed by bipolar coagulation, may be sufficient to prevent tumor recurrence when involved dura mater cannot be completely excised.

A watertight dural closure is necessary to prevent the development of a postoperative pseudomeningocele. In order to avoid neural compression or leakage, a dural graft may be constructed to ensure that the dura mater is not closed under tension. Autografts consisting of pericranium or fascia have excellent handling characteristics and suture well to the dura. They also avoid the risk of reaction to an implanted material that can occasionally present with a postoperative syndrome resembling aseptic meningitis.

Far Lateral Approach

The far lateral approach is best suited for tumors located ventrally or ventrolaterally.[7,57-59,61] This provides exposure of the ventral brainstem and makes excessive retraction of neural elements unnecessary. At least 15 variations exist in the far lateral approach, as described in the literature. One should therefore tailor the amount and the order of the dissection and bone removal to the pathology. It is important to weigh the added morbidity of extensive dissection against its associated gain in visualization and surgical freedom of movement.[65] Immediately after anesthesia is induced, and before surgery, a lumbar drain is inserted. The patient is then positioned in a modified "park bench" position. The lower arm is allowed to drop from the end of the table, where it is cradled in a sling. The head is flexed, rotated downward, and tilted away from the ipsilateral shoulder for maximal opening of the space between the atlas and the foramen magnum. The upper shoulder is pulled down toward the feet with tape to create a larger space for movement of the microscope. The entire body is secured with tape to allow full rotation of the table. Alternatively, this operation has been performed in the sitting position. This may provide the advantage of improved visualization due to a reduction of venous distention and bleeding, but is associated with air embolism. This is especially true when working around the vertebral artery and hypoglossal nerve, which are surrounded by a rich venous plexus.

An inverted J-shaped incision is begun at the mastoid prominence, curved to the midline, and extended caudally to the C6 level (Fig. 111-2A). The nuchal fascia is cut transversely, leaving a 1-cm cuff for reattachment. The paraspinal muscles are split and elevated from the spinous processes and lamina. The muscle flap is dissected from the suboccipital bone to the mastoid process, and the entire flap is retracted laterally and caudally with fishhooks that are attached to a table-mounted device, such as a Leyla bar (B. Braun Medical, Inc., Bethlehem, PA). The midline aspect of the wound is retracted contralaterally with fishhooks from a second Leyla bar. The lateral mass of C1 and the vertebral artery from C1 to the dura mater are exposed. Bleeding from the venous plexus surrounding the vertebral artery is controlled with bipolar cauterization and packing with oxidixed cellulose (Surgicel). Care must be taken to avoid injury to the vertebral artery or to one of its extracranial branches. Occasionally, the posterior

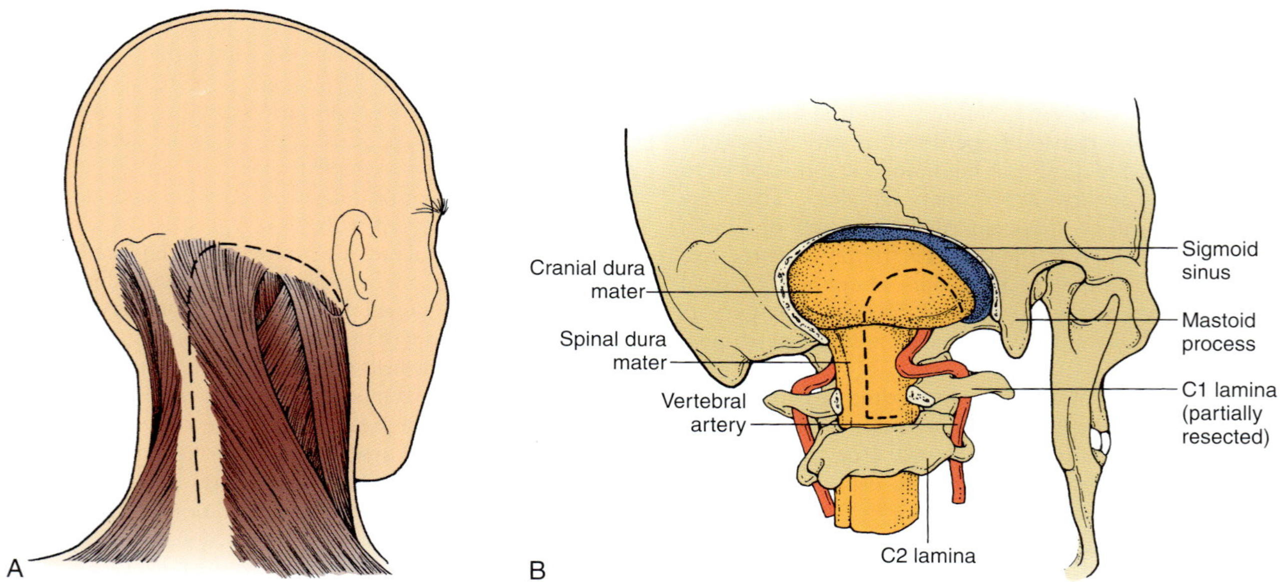

FIGURE 111-2. A, Skin incision for the far lateral approach. The inverted J-shaped incision begins at the mastoid process, curves medially to the midline, and extends caudally to the C6 level. **B,** Far lateral bone opening. A lateral suboccipital craniotomy is extended laterally to include the posterolateral one third of the occipital condyle and caudally to include the ipsilateral portion of the dorsal C1 arch.

inferior cerebellar artery arises extracranially and could be inadvertently coagulated and divided.[66] It has even been noted to originate between C1 and C2.[67] The same is true of a hypoplastic vertebral artery.[51] The dorsal arch of C1 is then removed with a high-speed drill (Midas Rex; Midas Rex Institute, Inc., Fort Worth, TX), using a B1 bit and foot plate. The ipsilateral lamina is cut at its far lateral extent, as well as on the contralateral side, slightly across the midline. The C1 arch is saved and replaced at closure.

A suboccipital craniotomy is performed with the same drill. The drilling begins at the foramen magnum and extends contralaterally across the midline and ipsilaterally as far laterally as possible. The ipsilateral rim of the foramen magnum is removed with a bone rongeur to the occipital condyle. The dorsal occipital condyle and the rostral lateral mass and facet of C1 are removed using the drill with the B1 bit. The safest technique is to drill away the inner portion of the occipital condyle, leaving a thin shell of cortical bone to protect the surrounding structures. The shell is carefully removed with small curettes and rongeurs until the dorsolateral third of the condyle has been removed (Fig. 111-2B). Bleeding from the condylar veins can be controlled easily with bone wax. The extradural vertebral artery should be protected with a small dissector while the condyle is being drilled. The hypoglossal canal is located in the ventral medial third of the condyle and is not threatened by removal of the dorsolateral third. The degree of resection of the occipital condyle varies depending on the degree of exposure needed. It is possible to perform a far lateral approach without any condylar resection.[68] Indeed, with increasing experience in the resection of these lesions, the tendency is for less resection of the condyle or for frank use of a retrocondylar approach,[69] which has the obvious advantage of eliminating the need for a fusion. At the other extreme, occasionally, a total condylectomy is necessary to remove an extradural lesion with condylar involvement.[65]

The dura mater is opened over the midline of the upper cervical spinal cord. At its caudal extent above C2, the dural incision is curved to the ipsilateral side. Rostrally, the dural opening extends in a curvilinear fashion to the rostral lateral aspect of the craniotomy. This configuration allows the dural flap to be hinged laterally, where it is tented up with #4-0 sutures. Because the occipital condyle is removed as necessary for identification of the anatomy, excellent visualization of the proximal intradural vertebral artery is achieved after the dura is opened. Minimal retraction of the cerebellar hemisphere improves the more distal exposure of the vertebral artery and the tumor (Fig. 111-3).

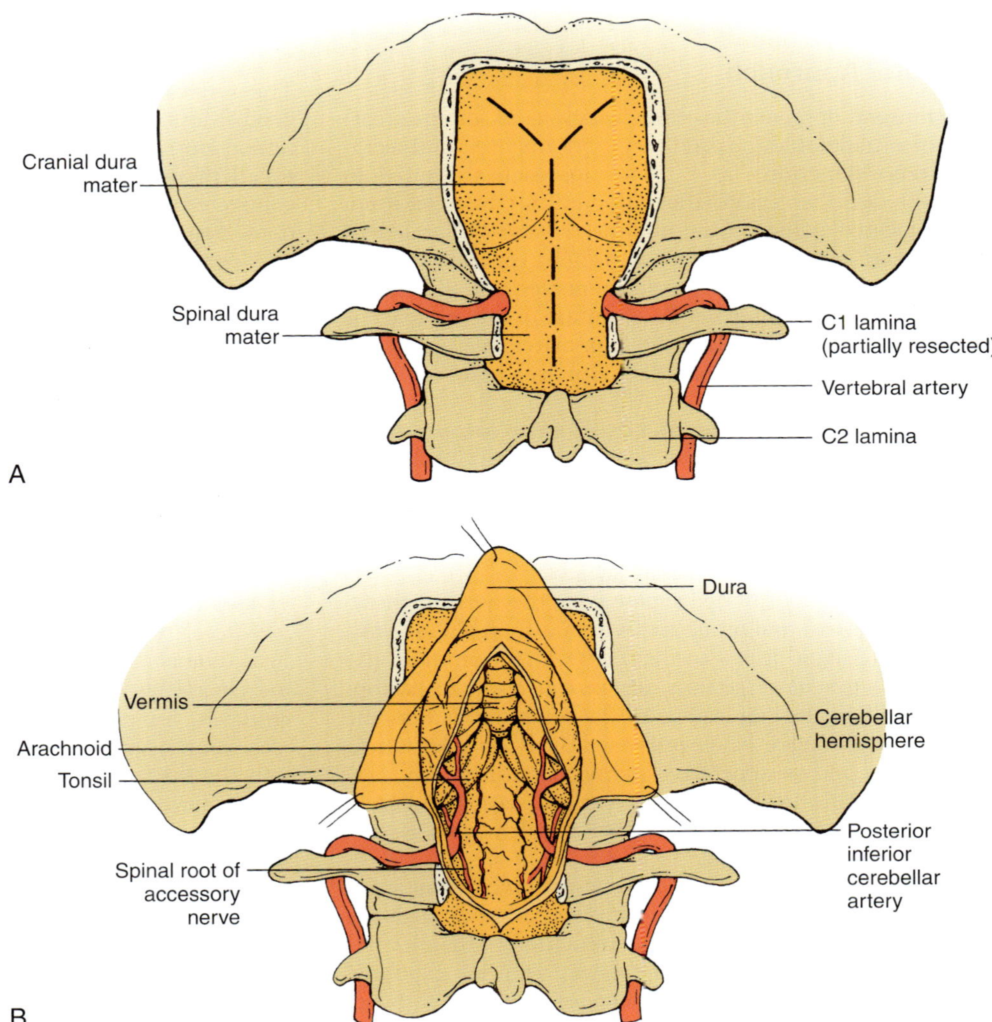

FIGURE 111-3. A, Suboccipital bone opening and dural incision. The arch of C1 has been removed. **B,** Exposure of cervicomedullary junction following suboccipital craniectomy.

After resection of the tumor, the dura mater is closed in a watertight fashion, and both the suboccipital bone flap and the C1 arch are replaced. The wound is closed in layers. If the headholder is first repositioned in a more neutral position, the nuchal fascia is easier to reapproximate.

As with any posterior fossa operation, communicating hydrocephalus can develop after the far lateral approach is performed. Postoperative CT should be performed, even in asymptomatic patients. The extensive muscle dissection involved in the far lateral approach causes considerable pain during the first 2 to 3 days after surgery. Therefore, patients should be given sufficient analgesics.

The stability of the craniocervical junction is an important issue to address following the far lateral approach.[65,70] The surgeon must carefully balance the trade-off between improving visualization and causing instability. In a series of 25 patients with a far lateral approach, Bejjani et al. performed an occipitocervical fusion in eight cases.[70] The authors delineated three indications for fusing across the occipitocervical region: (1) the presence of a painful head tilt, (2) instability on flexion-extension radiographs, or (3) complete resection of the occipital condyle. As a general rule, patients with less than 70% removal of the condyle do not require fusion. This corresponds to resection up to the hypoglossal canal. Any further resection increases the likelihood of craniocervical instability.

Transoral Approach

The transoral approach has been widely used for the treatment of extradural lesions and bony abnormalities of the craniovertebral junction.[21-24,71-76] This approach also provides the most direct access to the intradural foramen magnum lesions located at the ventral midline.[25,27,28,77-79] The lateral exposure achieved by this approach, however, is limited by the vertebral arteries, the hypoglossal nerves, and the jugular foramen structures. A further disadvantage of this approach is the inability to directly close the dura mater in a watertight fashion, leading to increased risk of CSF leak and postoperative meningitis.

Although a tracheotomy can be performed preoperatively when necessary, most surgeons use endotracheal intubation, keeping the tube depressed below the oral retractor. In all cases in which the dura mater may be penetrated or is going to be penetrated, a lumbar drain is inserted immediately after induction of anesthesia and before surgery.

The patient is positioned supine with the head in three-point fixation. An oral retraction system is then placed, with care taken to avoid injury to the teeth. Attention must also be given to tongue retraction, which can result in postoperative swelling and can lead to airway compromise. Periodic release of the tongue blade intraoperatively, in addition to preoperative and postoperative steroid administration, may help prevent this complication. Direct application of steroid ointment to the tongue and oropharyngeal mucosa is very helpful in reducing swelling.

Improved exposure of the dorsal nasopharynx is obtained by suturing the uvula to a rubber catheter passed through the nose and applying gentle upward retraction. This elevates the uvula and soft palate out of the way for C1-2 exposure. If necessary for exposure of the caudal clivus, the soft palate and uvula can be divided to expose the pharyngeal wall. The latter is incised in the midline. The soft palate incision should be brought to one side of the uvula, leaving it intact to the opposite side (Fig. 111-4A). Dissection is continued through the prevertebral musculature and prevertebral fascia, which are retracted laterally. Next, the anterior atlanto-occipital and longitudinal ligaments are detached from the clivus and the upper cervical vertebrae. The drill is then used to remove the lower third of the clivus, the ventral C1 arch, the odontoid peg, and part of the C2 body (Fig. 111-4B). Care is taken to avoid excessively lateral dissection that might injure the vertebral arteries, the hypoglossal nerves, or the jugular foramen structures. Once it is adequately exposed, the dura mater is opened in a cruciate fashion.

After excision of the tumor, the dura mater is closed. This may be accomplished by primary closure, including duroplasty, but this is difficult and is rarely watertight. The dural closure may be further sealed with fibrin glue. Where approved, a sealant (DuraSeal; Confluent Surgical, Waltham, MA) can be applied over the incision.[80] A fat graft may be used as an additional seal and to obliterate the retropharyngeal space. Finally, the longus colli is reapproximated with single interrupted polyglactin 910 (Vicryl) sutures, and the pharyngeal and soft palate mucosa are closed with running chromic gut suture.

Surgical Results

The surgical results from more recent series are generally good. Most patients with extramedullary foramen magnum tumors not only tolerate surgery well but also enjoy good to excellent neurologic recovery. The best chance to achieve complete tumor resection and to effect a cure is at the time of the first surgery.

Meyer et al. reviewed 102 patients with benign extramedullary foramen magnum tumors who underwent operation at the Mayo Clinic between 1924 and 1982.[5] They found a 5% mortality rate and an additional 5% rate of tumor-related deaths (from recurrence) within 3 years of surgery. However, the long-term survival rate was 90%, with 75% of the patients returning to productive lives and 12% being only mildly impaired.

Bruneau and George found a 77% rate of complete tumor removal, a 16% rate of subtotal removal, and only a 7% rate of partial removal. Complete tumor removal was least frequently achieved with ventrally located tumors (69%, vs. 81% for lateral tumors and 86% for dorsal tumors). Furthermore, gross total resection was more often attained among intradural tumors (83% vs. 50% for extradural tumors).[3] Bruneau and George also observed superior results with the far lateral approach, compared with the standard dorsal approach, for both ventral and lateral tumors: 86% gross total resection with the far lateral approach versus 71% with the straight dorsal approach.[3]

Samii et al. obtained a complete resection of craniocervical junction meningiomas in 25 out of 40 patients.[81] There was a marked disparity in the rate of complete removal between patients with encapsulated lesions and patients with en plaque or aggressive lesions. Incomplete tumor removal was found to be independently associated with encasement of the vertebral artery, an en plaque pattern, infiltrative growth, and an intracranial origin.

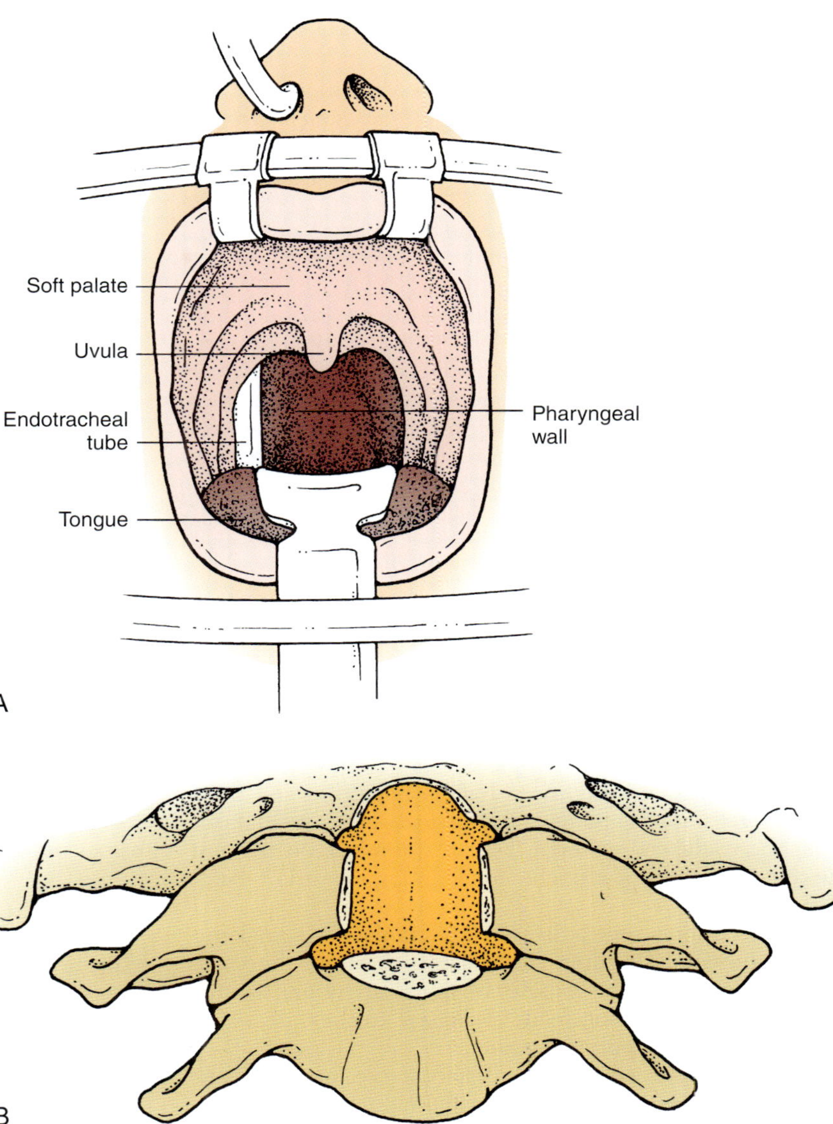

FIGURE 111-4. A, The transoral incision begins in the midline of the hard palate and is carried down to one side of the uvula. **B,** The lower third of the clivus, the ventral C1 arch, the odontoid peg, and part of the C2 body are removed using a high-speed drill with the diamond bur.

Experience with the transoral approach to intradural extramedullary tumors is limited. It is absent in the reports of both Meyer et al.[5] and Bruneau and George.[3] Among seven ventrally located intradural lesions at the craniovertebral junction, including three meningiomas, two schwannomas, a neurenteric cyst, and a basilar-anterior inferior cerebellar artery junction aneurysm, Crockard et al. achieved a total removal of both schwannomas, a subtotal removal of two of the three meningiomas, a total removal of the neurenteric cyst, and a successful clipping of the aneurysm.[22,26,27] Major postoperative complications included spinal instability (two patients), CSF leakage (three patients), and velopharyngeal insufficiency (three patients).

Chono et al. successfully removed a ventrally located foramen magnum meningioma with the transoral approach. The procedure was complicated by a CSF leak that required reoperation; a ventral occipitocervical fusion was performed.[78] Bonkowski et al. reported the successful removal of a ventrally located foramen magnum meningioma by the transoral approach that was uncomplicated by spinal instability or CSF leakage.[77] The authors' avoidance of CSF leakage may in part be related to their innovative application of a bone baffle.

The best predictors of poor outcome are the presence of a large ventrally located tumor and poor preoperative neurologic status.[1,4,5,15,18,19] Tumor-related deaths most commonly result from respiratory failure.

Complications

The intraoperative and postoperative complications of surgery in the region of the foramen magnum may be divided into categories, as formulated by Sen et al.[30] as follows: (1) neurologic, (2) CSF leakage, (3) vascular, (4) infections, and (5) systemic.

Neurologic

Neurologic complications may be caused by intradural or extradural hematoma formation, cerebellar contusion, or injury to the cranial nerves. Postoperative hematoma is best prevented by meticulous hemostasis at the time of operation. Particular attention should be paid to obtaining excellent surgical exposure to prevent undetected bleeding in areas of the wound that are not well visualized. Wide exposure also minimizes the need for excessive retraction. Routine postoperative CT may be used to detect the development of any hematoma or hydrocephalus. Cerebellar contusion is best avoided by applying only gentle retraction at the time of exposure and by providing intermittent periods of relaxation.

The glossopharyngeal, vagus, accessory, and hypoglossal nerves are vulnerable to injury during surgery in the region of the foramen magnum, particularly because of their proximity to and frequent involvement with the lesion.[82,83] Gentle and meticulous surgical technique provides the best chance of protecting these structures that may be inadvertently sectioned or stretched. In a series of ventral foramen magnum meningiomas,[61] glossopharyngeal and vagus nerve dysfunction was the most common complication postoperatively.

Injury to the glossopharyngeal or vagus nerve causes dysfunction of the pharynx and larynx. Clinically, these patients can present with hoarseness, poor cough, stridor, dysphagia, or aspiration, with the symptoms ranging from the mildly annoying to the life threatening.

Hoarseness and a poor cough may be further evaluated by indirect or fiberoptic laryngoscopy to determine the status of the vocal cord. The evaluation of dysphagia and aspiration is best made with a fluoroscopic barium swallow study that assesses the patient's ability to handle both thin and thick barium preparations and to protect the tracheobronchial tree from the swallowed material. Poor performance on this test suggests the need for a tracheotomy and nasogastric tube or a gastrostomy.

The accessory nerve is divided into cranial and spinal portions. The cranial portion carries fibers that join the vagus nerve to innervate the muscles of the pharynx and larynx. Recognition and management of damage to these fibers follows the guidelines outlined earlier.

The spinal portion of the accessory nerve innervates the sternocleidomastoid and trapezius muscles. Injury to these fibers presents clinically with inability to turn the head toward the side of the lesion (sternocleidomastoid muscle paralysis) and inability to shrug the ipsilateral shoulder (trapezius muscle paralysis). Inadvertent division of the accessory nerve should be repaired, if possible, primarily at the time of surgery. The marked decrease in range of motion of the shoulder that results from trapezius muscle paralysis may lead to adhesive capsulitis. Physiotherapy helps maintain the range of motion of the scapulohumeral joint to minimize this pathologic process.

Injury to the hypoglossal nerve results in paralysis of the ipsilateral intrinsic tongue muscles. Unilateral hypoglossal nerve injury causes the tongue to deviate toward the side of the lesion and is fairly well tolerated. Bilateral paralysis produces an immobile tongue, associated with profound difficulties in swallowing and speaking.

Concomitant lesions of the glossopharyngeal, vagus, and accessory nerves magnify the effects of a hypoglossal nerve lesion. Depending on the severity of injury, patients may require only minimal speech and swallowing therapy, or they may require a comprehensive speech and swallowing rehabilitation program with or without a tracheotomy and gastrostomy. In general, patients with preoperative cranial nerve deficits are at lower risk for postoperative aspiration pneumonia, since they have already adapted to a slowly progressive dysfunction of the lower cranial nerves.[81]

Velopharyngeal insufficiency is a unique complication of the transoral approach. Three of the seven patients of Crockard's series developed this problem postoperatively.[25] It probably results from removal of the bony support of the dorsal pharynx and should be distinguished from a cranial nerve palsy.[79] Because it appears related to bony removal, velopharyngeal insufficiency does not occur after transoral procedures for extradural lesions.[74,84] Placement of "bone baffle" has been proposed to prevent this complication.[77]

Cerebrospinal Fluid Leakage

CSF leakage is one of the more common complications of surgery in the region of the foramen magnum. Because of its association with an increased risk of CSF infection, every attempt should be made to ensure a watertight dural closure. Construction of a dural graft is often necessary to achieve this. Placement of a lumbar spinal fluid drain may also help prevent (or treat) postoperative CSF leakage. This is particularly useful during a transoral surgical approach, which is most likely to result in a postoperative CSF leak.

Once the problem is recognized, the initial management of a CSF leak is with a lumbar spinal fluid drain. If this measure fails to stop the leak, surgical reexploration and dural repair may be necessary. In addition to predisposing to meningitis, a CSF leak can produce a pseudomeningocele. This has been associated with postoperative neurologic deterioration.[85-87]

Vascular Injury

All the vessels in the region of the foramen magnum are at risk for iatrogenic injury, particularly the vertebral artery, which may be attached to, or encased by, the tumor. Good preoperative planning is the best defense against vascular injury at the time of surgery. Preoperative angiography may be useful if the MRI suggests vertebral artery involvement. This allows for preoperative embolization of vascular tumors as well. Proximal vertebral artery involvement requires extradural control. Dissection should be carried out along a plane that is parallel to the path of the artery. Blunt dissection should be avoided when separating the tumor from the artery in order to prevent irregular tears that are difficult to repair.

If sharp dissection is complicated by a major arterial laceration, the artery should be repaired primarily. Irregular tears produced by blunt dissection may require the application of a vein patch graft or the fashioning of a vein graft reconstruction. Sacrifice of a vertebral artery should be avoided and should never be done without ensuring an adequate contralateral collateral supply.

Infections

Prophylactic intraoperative antibiotics are used routinely and should be given before the skin is incised (the potential for infection starts with this step). Repeated dosing is required to maintain adequate tissue concentration of the antibiotic. Proper tissue handling helps avert tissue devitalization and desiccation that may later form the nidus for infection. Copious irrigation is performed intermittently throughout the procedure, particularly before closure. Postoperative CSF leakage, which may lead to meningitis, should be prevented or promptly recognized and addressed.

Systemic

The most common life-threatening systemic complications include lower extremity deep venous thrombosis, pulmonary embolism, and pneumonia. Intraoperative sequential compression devices should be applied before the induction of general anesthesia, which represents the period of greatest risk for formation of deep venous thrombi. Postoperatively, these devices should be continued and should be supplemented by subcutaneous injection of heparin until the patient is ambulatory.

Pulmonary care is especially important in patients with lower cranial nerve dysfunction who may suffer airway protection and swallowing difficulties and are thus at increased risk for aspiration. These patients benefit from frequent suctioning, postural drainage, and intermittent positive pressure breathing. If needed, a tracheotomy or gastrostomy is best performed early, before repeated episodes of aspiration occur.

Summary

Although early diagnosis continues to challenge clinicians, advances in the operative and perioperative management of foramen magnum tumors have greatly reduced both the morbidity and the mortality in affected patients. Intradural extramedullary tumors comprise approximately 90% of all foramen magnum tumors and include meningiomas and neurofibromas predominantly.[7]

Clinically, foramen magnum tumors are unusually variable and produce no pathognomonic signs or symptoms. Therefore, they should be considered in the differential diagnosis for any patient with neck pain and limb dysesthesias who has evidence of an upper motor neuron lesion.

There are advantages and disadvantages to each of the three surgical approaches to foramen magnum tumors discussed in this chapter. The approach used for individual patients must be tailored to the specific tumor location, tumor pathology, and relationship of the tumor to the neural and osseous structures.

KEY REFERENCES

Arnautovic KI, Al-Mefty O, Husain M: Ventral foramen magnum meningiomas. *J Neurosurg (Spine 1)* 92:71–80, 2000.

Bassiouni H, Ntoukas V, Asgari S, et al: Foramen magnum meningiomas: clinical outcome after microsurgical resection via a posterolateral suboccipital retrocondylar approach. *Neurosurgery* 59:1177–1187, 2006.

Bruneau M, Georges B: Classification system of foramen magnum meningiomas. *J Craniovertebr Junction Spine* 1(1):10–17, 2010.

de Oliveira F, Rhoton AL Jr, Peace D: Microsurgical anatomy of the region of the foramen magnum. *Surg Neurol* 24:293–352, 1985.

Wen HT, Rhoton AL, Katsuta T, et al: Microsurgical anatomy of the transcondylar, supracondylar, and paracondylar extensions of the far-lateral approach. *J Neurosurg* 87:555–585, 1997.

REFERENCES

The complete reference list is available online at expertconsult.com.

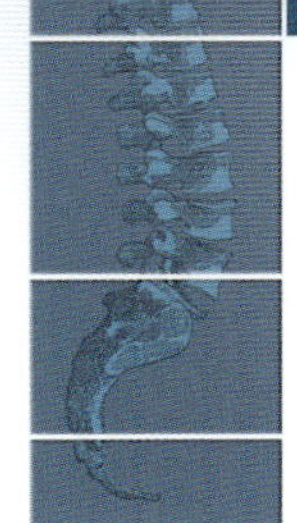

CHAPTER 112

Cervicothoracic Junction Tumors: Regional Challenges

Cristian Brotea | Michael P. Steinmetz

Incidence and Statistics

The upper thoracic vertebrae account for 15% of patients with tumors of the spine. The T1-4 region accounts for 10% of all spinal metastases.[1] Subaxial cervical spine tumors also are uncommon and constitute less than 10% of spinal metastases.[2] Due to the smaller canal size, tenuous blood supply at the cervicothoracic junction, along with unique biomechanical stresses that can lead to instability, the chance of neurologic involvement can be as high as 80%.[3]

The cervicothoracic junction is a transition zone between the more mobile cervical spine, with its lordotic alignment, and the much stiffer, kyphotic thoracic spine, stabilized ventrally by the rib cage. A variety of pathologic entities that can result in kyphotic deformity can be seen at the cervicothoracic junction, including tumor, infection, spondylosis, traumatic injury, and iatrogenic destabilization. Following surgery, the kyphotic deformity may worsen further as a result of failing to account for the unique biomechanics of the cervicothoracic junction.[4] Cervicothoracic pathology can include either primary or metastatic oncologic disease. Several studies have looked specifically at tumors in this anatomic region.[5-7] One series of 19 patients with cervicothoracic tumors had 6 patients with primary pathology, including angiosarcoma,[1] chordoma,[1] lymphoma,[2] plasmacytoma,[1] and schwannoma.[1] The other 13 patients (68%) had metastatic disease, with metastases to the lung[5] and prostate[2] being the most common. Other tumors seen were breast cancers, melanoma, and renal, ovarian, and colon cancers. Another series with 32 patients described 19 who had lung cancer and vertebral body invasion (Pancoast tumors), 11 with metastasis, 1 with chondrosarcoma, and 1 with myeloma.[6] An and Vaccaro[7] reported a group of 15 patients with cervicothoracic pathology, including 8 metastatic lesions (2 breast, 2 lung, 2 prostate, 1 thyroid, and 1 adenocarcinoma of unknown origin) and the remainder primary benign (aneurysmal bone cyst, giant cell tumor) and malignant tumors (myeloma, lymphoma, neurofibrosarcoma, and hemangioendothelioma).

Nonsurgical and Surgical Treatment

Spinal metastases, especially at the cervicothoracic junction, present unique treatment considerations. The goal of treatment is to improve or maintain neurologic function, achieve spinal stability, and attain local tumor control. The traditional methods of dealing with this pathology include radiation therapy, chemotherapy, and hormonal treatment, as well as surgery. Bilsky et al.[8] expanded on the NOMS pneumonic (neurologic, oncologic considerations, mechanical instability, and systemic disease and comorbidities), developing an algorithmic approach to decision making.

Neurologic and mechanical instability components can be detected in a patient's clinical presentation. For example, epidural spinal cord compression due to metastases can be inferred from radiographic presentation as well as the patient's signs and symptoms. A red flag for a physician is the complaint of neck and back pain mostly at night or in the early morning, resolving during the day, that is nonmechanical pain. Diurnal biologic pain is mainly due to hormonal secretion and inflammatory mediators excreted by the tumor. This is one of the earliest symptoms of bony metastasis and may correlate with tumor invasion of the vertebral body. While difficult to distinguish from tumor-related pain, pain due to mechanical instability can be a large component of the patient's complaints. It is related to movement and can correlate directly with bone and ligamentous destruction. This type of pain is described as deep and agonizing and occurs when loading the spine, as when walking or carrying objects. Flexion and extension can elicit pain in the mechanically unstable cervical and thoracic spine and occasionally can be evident on radiographic imaging. Whereas cervical instability is more evident with the patient erect, lying down can cause pain in patients with thoracic instability as the thoracic kyphotic deformity straightens. Radiculopathy may be present if instability results in foraminal compromise or if tumor has extended into the foramen.

Radiation, Chemotherapy, and Stereotactic Radiosurgery Preoperatively and Postoperatively

The ultimate goal of treatment in patients with cervicothoracic tumors is preservation or recovery of neurologic and functional status and treatment of pain. Although radiation is less invasive, has fewer complications, and traditionally has been found to be at least equivalent to surgery for the treatment of metastases, patients with epidural spinal cord compression have been shown to respond well to surgical intervention.[9] Initially, basic decompressive procedures, such as laminectomy without instrumentation, were used to resect epidural disease, although these procedures did create iatrogenic instability. Patients receiving radiation therapy as a primary treatment had 79% maintenance of ambulatory status and a 42% rate of neurologic recovery. By comparison, patients undergoing surgical intervention as mentioned above had worse odds of improving their preoperative neurologic status, with 33% chance of recovery and up to 50% of the patients worse off neurologically.[10,11]

In 1978, Gilbert and colleagues compared radiation therapy directly with laminectomy alone. They showed that patients with radiosensitive tumors, including breast cancers, myeloma, and lymphoma, had significantly better functional outcomes when compared with less radiosensitive tumors, including lung, colon, and renal cell carcinoma, regardless of the tumor treatment. Gilbert et al. helped steer primary treatment in certain metastatic diseases to radiation therapy.[12]

In the last 20 years, neurologic outcomes, specifically ambulation, have been improving with surgical treatment. Fewer than 5% of patients undergoing surgical treatment have worse neurologic outcomes after surgery, a change that can be attributed mainly to technical advances and improvement in surgical approaches and instrumentation.

In general, surgical resection of epidural metastases, if tolerated well from a medical standpoint, should be followed by radiation therapy, or possibly systemic chemotherapy or hormonal therapy. This combined approach can be used to secure local tumor control.[9] Newer techniques, including image-guided intensity-modulated radiation therapy (IGIMRT) and the cyberknife, improve the chances for tumor control in the cases of radiation therapy–resistant tumors, especially postoperatively, as opposed to conventional external-beam radiation therapy (EBRT).[13,14] At Memorial Sloan-Kettering Cancer Center, the typical tumor board protocol currently dictates that a patient with a radiosensitive tumor, regardless of the degree of spinal cord compression or myelopathy, be irradiated with standard EBRT or with single-fraction IGIMRT or chemotherapy for noncompressive masses. Patients with radioresistant tumors and a low degree of compression can undergo EBRT or IGIMRT 24-Gy single fractions, whereas the patients with higher-grade spinal compression are offered surgical decompression and fixation followed by IGIMRT.[8] Despite diligent treatment, the chance of recurrence in some of the surgical series remains high, approaching 96% at 4 years.[15]

Superior sulcus non–small-cell lung carcinomas, which are extremely difficult to treat because of their aggressiveness and invasion of adjacent spine, brachial plexus, and subclavian vessels, have been treated traditionally with radiation and surgery, yielding a 30% 5-year survival rate. More recent data suggest that induction chemoradiation (two cycles of cisplatin and etoposide with radiation) and surgical resection (thoracotomy) followed by two more cycles of chemotherapy can yield higher survival rates, of 44% at 5 years.[16]

Surgical Treatment

Surgical treatment of tumors of the cervicothoracic junction often is challenging due to the presence of major vascular and soft tissue structures requiring exquisite preoperative planning and approach. The cervicothoracic junction is unique biomechanically. This uniqueness must be accounted for when considering surgery in this region. Preoperative imaging helps define the neurovascular involvement of the tumor, guiding the direction of the surgical treatment. In the cervical spine, for example, MRI can help identify epidural spinal cord compression and vertebral artery involvement. Preoperative angiography and balloon occlusion tests may be necessary if tumor dissection or occlusion of a single vertebral artery is likely or necessary.[17] For ventral surgical approaches to the subaxial cervical spine and cervicothoracic junction, the recurrent and superior laryngeal nerve functions must be evaluated. Preoperative laryngoscopy can be used to assess bilateral vocal cord dysfunction; if present, the approach should be from the ipsilateral side. Superficial laryngeal nerve function must be evaluated by swallowing studies.

Although radiation therapy remains the treatment of choice for many patients with metastatic disease, [17] primary malignant tumors often are treated surgically for oncologic considerations, because they can be resistant to chemotherapy and radiation therapy. En bloc resection, which offers a higher probability of cure and local disease control, is preferred, but it typically is more technically demanding than an intralesional resection, especially if it extends beyond the vertebral body or dorsal elements. It may occasionally entail sacrificing the adjoining vertebral artery or an exiting nerve root.

Ideally, most hypervascular spinal tumors should undergo arterial embolization prior to surgical resection to minimize the risk of intraoperative and postoperative bleeding and enhance the surgeon's ability to safely decompress the spinal cord and maximize tumor removal.[18-20] The need for preoperative embolization is based on tumor histology, as seen in renal cell carcinoma, sarcomas (e.g., angiosarcoma and leiomyosarcoma), follicular and papillary thyroid carcinoma, hepatocellular carcinoma, germ cell tumors, and neuroendocrine tumors such as paragangliomas. The arterial blood supply must be conducive to such an attempt, because the feeder vessels must be large and accessible for microcatheterization. Some other hypervascular tumors, such as melanoma and multiple myeloma, are fed by a finer capillary network, which may not be as accessible.[18] On MRI, tumor hypervascularity may be identified as bright contrast enhancement and flow voids representing blood vessels. Hyperintensity also may be present on both T1- and T2-weighted images due to extracellular methemoglobin or hypointensity from the breakdown products of methemoglobin. Prabhu et al.[18] have recommended preoperative angiography for the following circumstances: if the tumors are of known hypervascularity, regardless of MRI findings; if the MRI suggests hypervascularity regardless of histology; or if the primary tumor origin is unknown. Cervical tumors need special consideration, because there is an increased risk of cerebral or brainstem infarction with preoperative embolization.[21] Two percent of patients experience neurologic complications, and 4% to 10% can experience local or systemic complications following embolization.[18] Therefore, only in special circumstances is embolization used for cervical malignancies.

Historical Surgical Approaches

Ventral surgical approaches to the thoracic spine initially were developed to treat Pott disease, and similar principles are used today to treat primary and metastatic tumors of the spine,

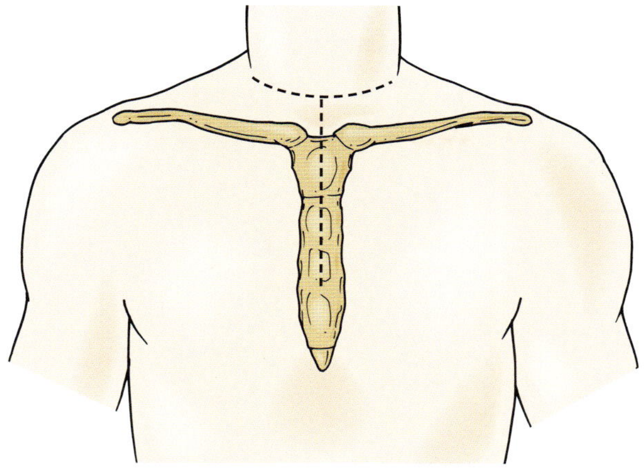

FIGURE 112-1. The T-shaped incision for the transsternal exposure of the ventral cervicothoracic junction and the upper thoracic spine. (Redrawn with permission from Benzel EC, editor: *Surgical exposure of the spine: an extensile approach,* Rolling Meadows, IL, 1995, American Association of Neurological Surgeons, p 161.)

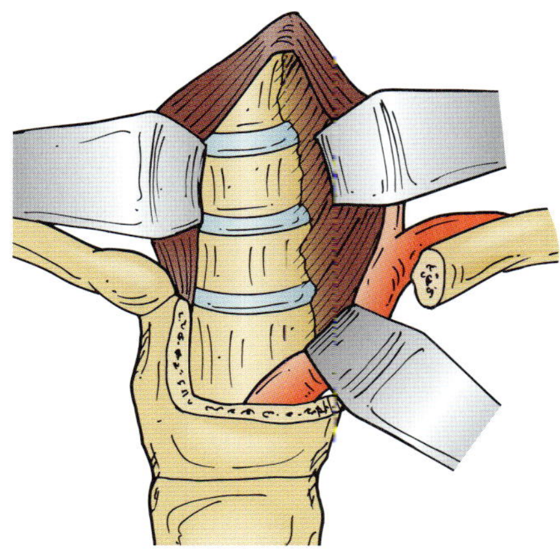

FIGURE 112-2. Resection of the manubrium and the medial part of the clavicle.

with the cervicothoracic junction being the most challenging. Menard[22] was the first to describe an approach to this pathology; he resected a portion of the rib and transverse process to gain access to a relatively small portion of the vertebral body. Capener[23] took this approach a step further by removing a longer segment of the rib, resulting in a more generous exposure and allowing ventrolateral decompression of the spinal cord.

In 1957, Nanson[24] described an oblique approach at the cervicothoracic junction that used a supraclavicular incision to gain access to the upper thoracic sympathetic ganglia. The exposure of the vertebral bodies, however, was very limited. Cauchoix and Binet[25] described a more aggressive approach to the cervicothoracic junction that involved performing a median sternotomy. This approach was essentially abandoned due to the 40% mortality rate in patients with Pott disease[26] and a 33% mortality rate in patients with cervicothoracic pathology.[3] In 1984, Sundarsan et al.[27] described a ventral approach, which involves a T-shaped incision with the transverse portion just proximal to the clavicles and a vertical component in the midline over the sternum (Fig. 112-1). Flaps are raised superiorly and inferiorly, and the external jugular vein and medial supraclavicular nerve are divided. The medial one third of the clavicle is excised, as well as a rectangular block of bone from the sternum (Fig. 112-2). Under the manubrium sterni the subclavian vein is dissected free, and the thymus may be removed for further exposure. The laryngeal nerve must be identified as the dissection continues deep between the carotid sheath laterally and the esophagus medially. The resected clavicle can be used as structural bone graft at the corpectomy site without further instrumentation.[27]

This approach was slightly modified by Birch et al.,[28] who described an osseomuscular flap containing the medial one third of the clavicle and manubrium in one piece attached to the sternocleidomastoid muscle and later reattached with wires and plate-screw fixation. There were four clavicle nonunions and one transient recurrent laryngeal nerve palsy in the 17 patients in this study. By leaving the sternocleidomastoid muscle attached, the risk of pulmonary compromise was lowered in patients with respiratory problems. Kurz and Herkowitz[29] modified this approach by only removing the medial clavicle without resecting the manubrium. Midline-crossing vascular structures limit exposure caudally to approximately T3 (Fig. 112-3). The lateral extracavitary approach to traumatic lesions of the thoracic and lumbar spine has been described for approaches as high as T3 but has limited utility with cervicothoracic junction tumors.[30]

Ventral "Trapdoor" Approach

The "trapdoor" exposure to the cervicothoracic junction has the advantage of leaving the sternoclavicular junction as well as the clavicle itself intact. Originally described by Nazzaro et al.,[31] it is a combination of the ventrolateral cervical approach, median sternotomy, and ventrolateral thoracotomy. This approach is ideal for patients with ventral pathology at the cervicothoracic junction down to the T3-4 level who need decompression and subsequent reconstruction. Patients undergoing the procedure must have their neurologic status closely monitored with motor and somatosensory-evoked potentials and intravascular volume status with the help of a central line or Swan-Ganz catheter. Lines should not be placed in the right internal jugular or subclavian vein, which will be in the field,[32] assuming a right-sided approach is utilized.

The incision is made along the ventral border of the sternocleidomastoid muscle on the right side, to the sternal notch and down to the level of the fourth intercostal space, lying over the midline of the sternum and then curving laterally over the fourth rib. Proximally, the dissection is taken deep in the usual Smith-Robinson technique[33] by incising the platysma muscle and staying in the avascular plane between the carotid sheath laterally and the tracheoesophageal viscera medially. It may be necessary to transect or ligate the omohyoid muscle and the middle thyroid vessels in order to obtain a wider exposure. Once the prevertebral fascia is reached overlying the ventral cervical spine, the longus colli muscles are visualized. Distally, a plane is identified between the manubrium and the underlying vascular structures. Once the right lung is deflated, the sternum is transected longitudinally to the level of the fourth rib, and the incision is connected to the laterally made thoracotomy dissection. A chest spreader is used to obtain deep access. The mammary artery is identified; this artery typically requires ligation.

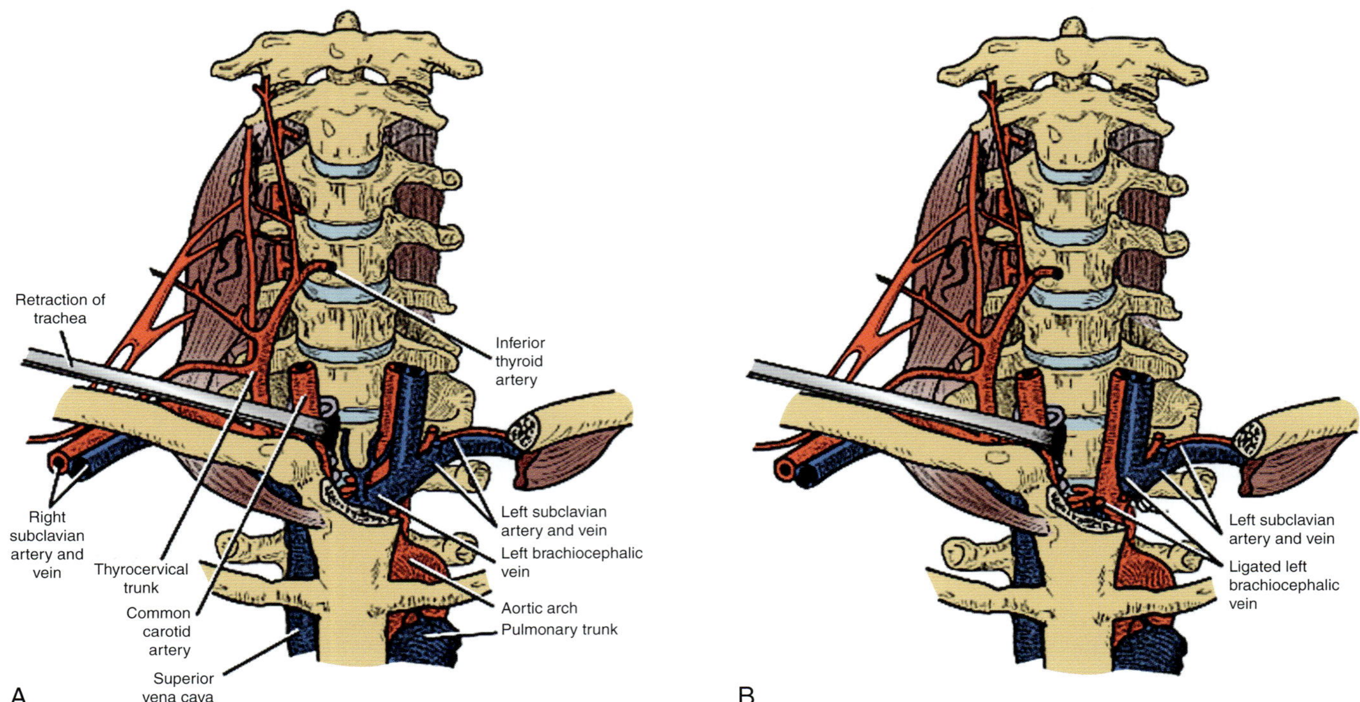

FIGURE 112-3. A, **Ventral cervicothoracic exposure is complicated by midline crossing vascular structures, as depicted. B, This limits ventral exposure to approximately T3, even if the innominate vein is ligated.** (Reprinted with permission from Benzel EC, editor: *Biomechanics of spine stabilization,* ed 2, New York, 2001, Thieme.)

Next, the vagus nerve is identified by opening the carotid sheath, and the innominate artery is dissected free to the level of the right carotid artery. The right recurrent laryngeal nerve is identified by tracing it from the right vagus nerve as it loops under the subclavian artery. The nerve is followed into the tracheoesophageal groove. This nerve, along with the aforementioned arteries, must be marked with vessel loops and protected. The cervicothoracic junction down to the level of T1 can be identified with further blunt dissection. The T3 and T4 levels are found behind the great vessels at that level, as is the junction of the mediastinal, apical, and dorsal chest wall pleurae. If the dissection is taken even further distally to T5, the azygos vein may be encountered joining the superior vena cava; it may be necessary to dissect and ligate it. Once the exposure is deemed adequate, the segmental arteries must be identified and ligated. The level should be confirmed with intraoperative fluoroscopy. In order to perform a vertebrectomy, the adjacent discs cephalad and caudad must be identified and removed. Using a high-speed diamond-tipped bur or an ultrasonic aspirator, the vertebral body may be removed to the level of the posterior longitudinal ligament (PLL). The PLL also can be removed to gain access to the ventral aspect of the thecal sac. Once the pathology is excised, the reconstruction can be performed with the help of newly developed titanium expandable cages or polymethylmethacrylate in patients with a shorter life expectancy. The column reconstruction can be augmented with a ventral plate and screws.

Risks with this approach include recurrent laryngeal nerve palsy as well as vascular damage. A dural laceration with this type of approach can be very difficult to manage. A piece of muscle can be applied over the dura with Gelfoam and fibrin glue layers. Postoperative lumbar cerebrospinal fluid (CSF) drainage may be necessary for 4 to 5 days postoperatively if CSF is visualized during surgery and a watertight closure cannot be achieved. It may be necessary to remove the chest tubes early, because intracavitary negative pressure may contribute to a continued leak. Another dreaded complication is iatrogenic injury to the esophagus, which may occur as a result of sharp deep dissection or the bur inadvertently making contact with it as it protrudes next to the retractors. Often the injury is not immediately recognized; it can present as postoperative infection, sepsis, mediastinitis, or fistula. If it is identified at the time of initial injury, the tear must be primarily repaired, the wound drained, and a nasogastric tube placed under direct visualization until it heals. Afterward, a barium swallow study should be performed to confirm that the tear is sealed. More likely, however, the injury is suggested postoperatively by the presence of crepitus in the neck or mediastinal air on chest radiograph. An esophagogram or CT scan usually can make the diagnosis definitively. At this point, reexploration has to be considered for primary repair, nasogastric drainage, and antibiotics.

Lateral Parascapular Extrapleural Approach

A straight ventral approach occasionally should be supplemented by a dorsal approach to allow for supplemental instrumentation or decompression. In 1991, Fessler et al.[34] described a lateral parascapular approach to the cervicothoracic junction that allowed access to the anterior column of the spine and simultaneous placement of dorsal instrumentation. The patient is intubated with a double-lumen endotracheal tube and placed prone on chest rolls. (We often do not use a double-lumen tube.) The incision is begun midline over the spinous processes of the subaxial cervical spine and directed distally in a curved fashion to the ipsilateral scapula. The trapezius and rhomboid muscles are identified under the deep fascia and elevated subperiosteally toward the medial border of the scapula as a musculocutaneous flap, with the interspinous ligaments and a cuff of muscles left intact for approximation later. The intact paraspinal muscles (the spinalis thoracis and longissimus thoracis) are elevated and retracted dorsally and medially. The ileocostalis group of the erector spinae musculature can be elevated and retracted either medially or laterally. These steps provide the surgeon with an excellent exposure of the upper dorsal rib cage and dorsal vertebral elements (Fig. 112-4).

At this point, the ipsilateral lung is collapsed to provide better exposure. The neurovascular bundles are stripped subperiosteally off the ribs and the costrotransverse and radiate ligaments excised sharply. The nerves and arteries are ligated and transected. Next, the thoracic cage is opened dorsally by removing ribs from their costrotransverse and costovertebral articulations laterally to the dorsal bend. Most often, only one rib is resected, but more than one may be removed if necessary. The ligated nerves are followed medially to the vertebral foramen. The sympathetic chain is identified on the lateral vertebral surface, and once the rami communicantes are transected and the segmental arteries controlled, it can be displaced ventrolaterally in a subperiosteal dissection uncovering the underlying vertebral body, pedicle, and foramina. The en bloc tumor resection/corpectomy can now be performed. If possible, the anterior and posterior longitudinal ligaments should be left intact. The resected ribs can be used as structural autograft. The nerve roots should be ligated proximal to the dorsal root ganglion to prevent formation of neuroma and postoperative neuralgia. Dorsal instrumentation also can be placed from this same approach. Complications include pneumonia, wound problems, Horner syndrome or sympathectomy, intercostal neuralgia, chest wall and medial arm hypalgesia, vascular spinal cord injury, C8 and T1 radiculopathy, CSF leak, and pneumothorax.

Dorsal Approach

Patients with cervicothoracic junction tumors that involve the dorsal elements without fixed deformity and with adequate cervical lordosis, may be approached dorsally. Surgeons must be familiar with this approach when performing multistage reconstructions that may involve the previously described ventral approach supplemented by dorsal instrumentation. Preoperative imaging including 3-foot scoliosis views is required to evaluate for any significant kyphosis or any coronal plane deformity throughout the entire spine. Flexion and extension views also may be useful to determine whether intraoperative deformity correction will be possible or if osteotomies and soft tissue releases are necessary. The choice and number of approaches are influenced by all of these factors, with some deformities necessitating combined two- or three-stage approaches. CT imaging is valuable for looking at bone quality; the specific cervicothoracic anatomy, including the size of the subaxial cervical lateral masses; C7-T3 pedicle widths; and angulations needed for instrumentation.

The patient usually is placed prone on the operating table with the head position well controlled with a three-point skull fixation device. Neck position should be checked with intraoperative fluoroscopy to prevent inadvertent fusion in an unbalanced position sagitally or coronally. Neurologic monitoring, including motor and somatosensory evoked potentials baseline values, should be obtained prior to positioning and rechecked afterward. With stenosis due to epidural pathology, cervical hyperextension can result in traumatic spinal cord injury. For these reasons, it may be necessary to perform intubation fiberoptically with the head and neck in neutral position. The arms must be carefully tucked at the sides without applying undue traction and inducing cervical plexopathy. The incision is made midline over the spinous processes at the cervicothoracic junction, exposing the lamina and lateral masses by subperiostally elevating the paraspinal muscles. In the thoracic spine, the transverse processes should be visualized to help with the placement of instrumentation and exposure of an adequate fusion bed. When only a partial vertebrectomy or hemivertebrectomy has to be achieved from a dorsal approach, the corresponding roots must be identified and ligated, following which an oblique osteotomy may be performed to isolate the pathology. Instrumentation has to be placed on the contralateral side to stabilize the segment prior to the excision.

Cervical laminectomy alone as a decompressive procedure is no longer the standard of care. In biomechanical studies, torsional stiffness decreased dramatically, a 2.5% increase in dorsal strain was noted when more than 50% of the facet had been removed at the C5-6 level, and an increase of more than 25% in dorsal strain was seen with a 75% to 100% facetectomy when compared with an intact specimen.[35] The decision to use a postoperative orthosis is complex and based on a number of factors, including patient comorbidities such as smoking, diabetes, poor nutritional preoperative status, bone density and, consequently, screw fixation, and, finally, the amount of deformity correction and the iatrogenic stresses placed on the construct.

Cervicothoracic Junction Challenges: Biomechanical Considerations

Five biomechanical studies have looked specifically at fixation at the cervicothoracic junction.[36-40] Albert et al.[36] compared a lateral mass plating system, a dorsal rod-hook system, and a ventral plate system, showing that all three systems stabilize a dorsal two-column injury similarly. The dorsal fixation systems were found to be stiffer than the others. Chapman[37] found that a lateral mass screw fixation system combined with thoracic laminar hooks can provide adequate stabilization at the cervicothoracic junction.

The degree of instability, specifically the number of columns involved, plays an important role in the surgical treatment algorithm for pathology in this region. A biomechanical cadaveric study looking specifically at dorsal stabilization at the cervicothoracic junction offered a comparison of three different fixation devices for stability with dorsal two- and three-column injuries. Kreshak et al.[38] evaluated three frequently used dorsal cervical fixation devices, including dorsal rod-screw systems and a dorsal plate-screw system. In extension, there was a significant reduction in construct stiffness with three-column injuries when compared with the fixation of the two-column injuries and the intact spine. Similar results were found with flexion testing. In lateral testing, all the fixation systems were found to be significantly stiffer than

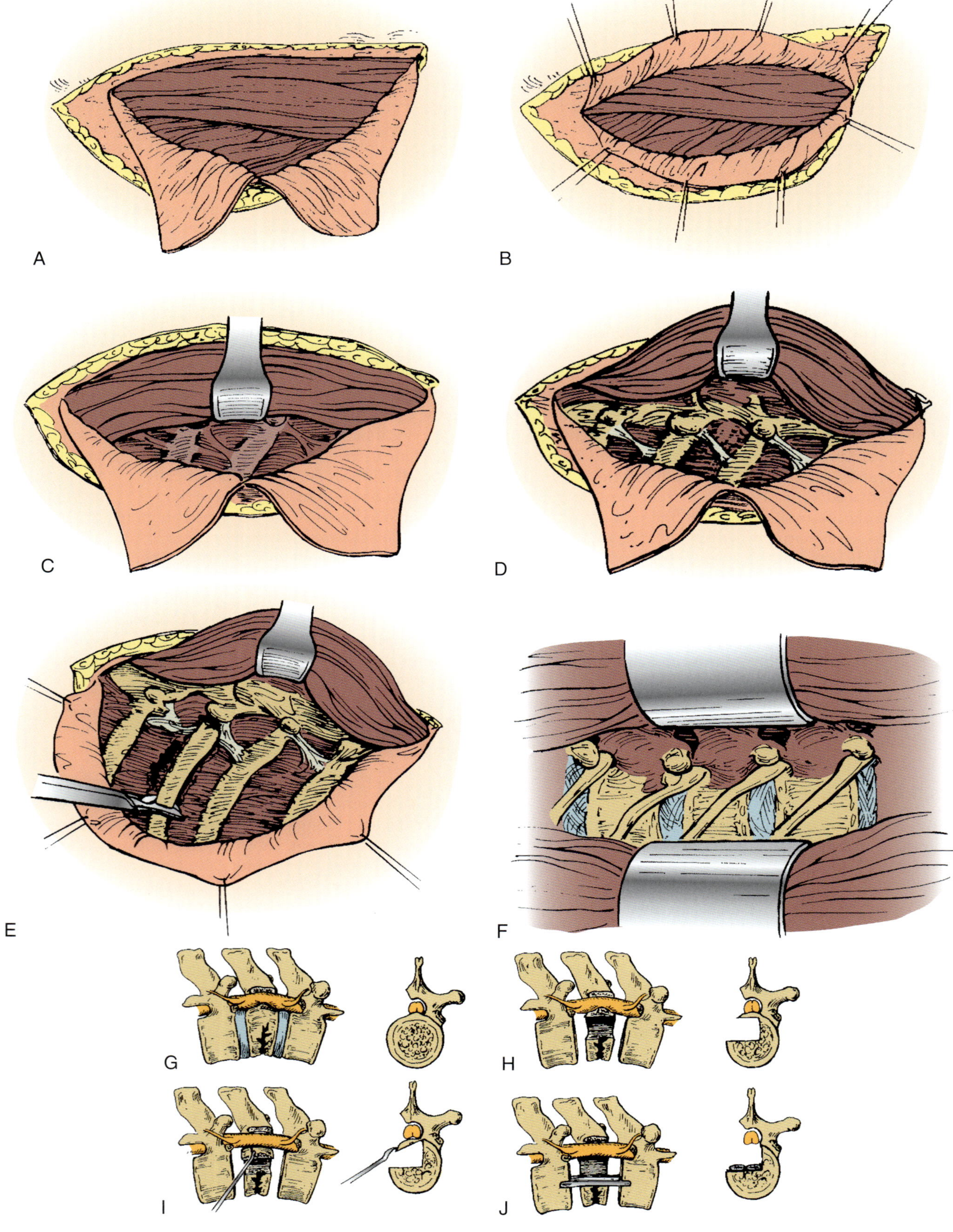
A
B
C
D
E
F
G
H
I
J

FIGURE 112-4. Fascial incisions. A T-shaped (**A**) or a paramedian straight (**B**) fascial incision may be used to transgress the thoracodorsal fascia. **C,** Incision of the thoracodorsal fascia gains access to the lateral aspect of the erector spinae muscle in the thoracic region. **D,** Retraction of the thoracic erector spinae muscles medially begins to expose the underlying ribs. **E,** In the thoracic region, the medial 6 to 10 cm of the ribs are resected. **F,** Further subperiosteal dissection along the undersurface of the ribs, pedicles, and vertebral bodies gains access to the lateral aspect of the spinal column. **G,** The appropriate pedicle is removed, and visualization of the lateral aspect of the dural sac, as well as its relationship between the ventrally situated compressive pathology, is attained. **H,** A trough is made just ventral to the dorsal aspect of the vertebral body with a high-speed bur and/or curved curet. **I,** The trough is thinned to facilitate the ventral displacement of the remaining shelf of bone away from the dural sac via a reversed-angle curet. **J,** A rib or other suitable graft is impacted into slots fashioned in the caudal aspect of the rostral vertebral body and rostral aspect of the caudal vertebral body. (Reprinted with permission from Benzel EC, editor: *Surgical exposure of the spine: an extensile approach,* Rolling Meadows, IL, 1995, American Association of Neurological Surgeons.)

the intact spine. The dorsal plate-screw system was found to be weaker in maintaining stability than the screw-rod systems. There are limitations to the plate-screw system, including the need for more surgical precision when placing the screws, difficulty in accounting for variability of the interfacet distances, and difficulty in lining up the predrilled holes in the dorsal plates with the lateral masses. It has been postulated that with a dorsal two-column injury the anterior longitudinal ligament as well as the ventral aspect of the intervertebral disc continue to provide resistance to extension, explaining the findings in this model. Dorsal fixation alone, although it provides a tension band effect in flexion, was not enough to provide stability in the three-column injury model.[38]

The data also suggest that for a two-column injury at the cervicothoracic junction, there is a trend toward increasing stiffness with prolonged dorsal thoracic fixation, with no differences recorded between the intact state and the dorsal fixation model from C5-T1, with the authors recommending fusion from C6-T2 in order to save cervical fixation points.[39] With three-column injuries, dorsal fixation alone results in excessive flexibility in flexion/extension even with instrumentation to T3. Supplementation of such fixation with anterior column instrumentation leads to increased strength of the construct, without any differences in flexion-extension and lateral bending when compared with the intact model, even if the dorsal fixation was stopped at T1. In order to reduce flexibility with axial rotation, however, the instrumentation would have to be extended to T3. For a three-column injury with corpectomy, similar recommendations were made to those for the three-column model with ventral and dorsal instrumentation.[39]

Another recent study looked at four different dorsal cervicothoracic rod-and-screw constructs, specifically at varying rod diameters and rod connector types, and tested them in flexion bending and axial rotation. There were no significant differences between a dual-diameter rod (3.5 and 5.5 mm) and a solid domino connector extending between two separate rods of the same diameters. A flexible domino connector was found to have similar stiffness but lower ultimate and yield force.[40]

The length of dorsal spinal instrumentation following decompression is a very important consideration that must be based on the patient's age, the underlying pathology, the length of the laminectomy, and the quality of the bone stock.[41] General indications for spinal fusion, as postulated by White and Panjabi, include (1) restoring clinical stability to a spine with compromised structural integrity, (2) maintaining alignment after deformity correction, (3) preventing formation of a new deformity, and (4) alleviation of pain.[42] The location of the decompression, especially at the cervicothoracic junction, must be carefully considered, because there is a higher incidence of postoperative kyphotic deformity. The normal sagittal weight-bearing axis lies dorsal to the C2-7 vertebral bodies, lowering the demand on the cervical paraspinal muscles to maintain alignment. Because laminectomy disrupts the posterior column and impairs the tension band construct dorsally, there is a tendency for the weight-bearing axis to shift ventrally. The ventral shift can lead to a kyphotic deformity, which puts the dorsal muscle groups at a significant mechanical disadvantage, requiring extra work to maintain an upright posture and leading to muscle fatigue, pain, and more kyphosis. This is even harder to achieve following dorsal cervical surgery. The use of a postoperative cervical orthosis, while it can help maintain cervical lordosis and alignment, also may lead to further paraspinal muscular atrophy. Pal and Sherk[43] have looked at each column individually at C6 and measured the axial loads. They found that 36% of the total load applied rostrally is transmitted through the two anterior columns, and most of the load is transmitted through the articular processes dorsally, again emphasizing the importance of integrity of the posterior column in load sharing.

Inoue et al.[44] had a series of 36 patients who had surgical decompression of their spinal cord tumors via laminectomy, laminoplasty, or hemilaminectomy. Those patients who underwent C7 laminectomy were found to develop kyphosis at the cervicothoracic junction with a compensatory lordosis of the cervical spine. Those who underwent laminoplasty experienced significantly less deformity.[44] Steinmetz et al.,[45] who looked at a large series of 593 total cases, found that laminectomy alone across the cervicothoracic junction led to failure in 38% of the cases. Development of postlaminectomy cervical kyphosis also has been documented in children who have undergone multilevel laminectomy.[46] De Jonge et al.[47] retrospectively looked at 76 children who had undergone noninstrumented laminectomy or laminoplasty and/or radiation therapy for malignant spine tumors. Of those, 88% developed postlaminectomy/postradiation spinal deformity. The growing spine also can be adversely affected by radiation therapy, possibly leading to asymmetrical vertebral growth and kyphosis or scoliosis. The use of instrumentation should be strongly considered in pediatric cases requiring destabilization of the dorsal elements at the cervicothoracic junction. In adults, although laminectomy is indicated in patients with cervical lordosis or straightening, it is absolutely contraindicated in the presence of preoperative kyphosis.

Cervicothoracic Junction Tumors: Instrumentation

Dorsal spinal instrumentation added to any decompressive procedure at the cervicothoracic junction should be expected to provide postoperative stability, protecting neurovascular structures from trauma and offering an optimal bed for bony fusion, allowing only micromotion at the fusion sites. These expectations are also the reason why postoperative cervical orthoses are largely unnecessary. Increased fusion rates as a result of instrumentation have been shown in single-level and multilevel discectomies with ventral plating.[48,49] There are numerous disadvantages to instrumentation, such as hardware failure, malpositioning, and stress shielding. Imaging artifact from instrumentation should be considered in oncologic cases. The latter factor can inhibit fusion and promote pseudarthrosis, which is why newer dynamically designed plates allow some settling and sharing of the load with the spacers, leading to enhanced fusion as predicted by Wolff's law, which implies that bone will remodel itself and become stronger when subjected to an external compressive load.

Certain principles must be respected when considering instrumented spinal fusion at the cervicothoracic junction. In general, focal and gradual curves as well as the apical and neutral vertebrae in two orthogonal planes, sagittal and coronal, must be identified. The neutral vertebra usually is the one least angulated and typically is located between the curves. The apical vertebra has the highest degree of segmental angulation at its rostral and caudal ends.[41] A long construct should not terminate at or near an apical vertebra[4] in either vertical plane, because loads experienced at that point would be highest due to the long moment arm of the axial load in relation to the construct. The apical vertebra is the one associated with the greatest angle (α) between adjacent vertebrae of all vertebrae, in the curve (Fig. 112-5). The second principle that must be respected is that a construct should not end at a junctional level—in this case, at the cervicothoracic junction (Fig. 112-6). It is prone to angular and translational deformation due to the difference in rigidity of the ventrally stabilized thoracic spine by the rib cage and the flexible cervical spine. Other considerations include loss of motion segments, complications related to placement of extra hardware, and cost. The quality of bone and its density also play a role and should be a consideration.[50]

Historically, dorsal hooks-rods-plate cervical compact Cotrel-Dubousset instrumentation has been described in the context of treatment of cervicothoracic junction pathologies. However, certain limitations with the instrumentation have impeded its continued use.[51] As a hook and rod system, the instrumentation required has to be longer than the levels involved with pathology because of the "claw" configuration, which requires fixation two levels above and two levels below the pathology. It obviously also must be above the levels of the laminectomy, and the hooks have to avoid levels with spinal canal stenosis. CCD hook intrusion into the spinal canal has been shown in a cadaveric study to be, on average, 27% of the diameter of the spinal canal.[52]

In the subaxial cervical spine, lateral mass screw fixation has been used often. C7 is a transitional vertebra that has characteristics common to both the cervical and the thoracic spine, with the lateral masses transitioning to the size and orientation of the thoracic transverse processes, thus offering a poorer fixation point. Panjabi et al.[53] have measured the transverse pedicle thickness and found that it increases

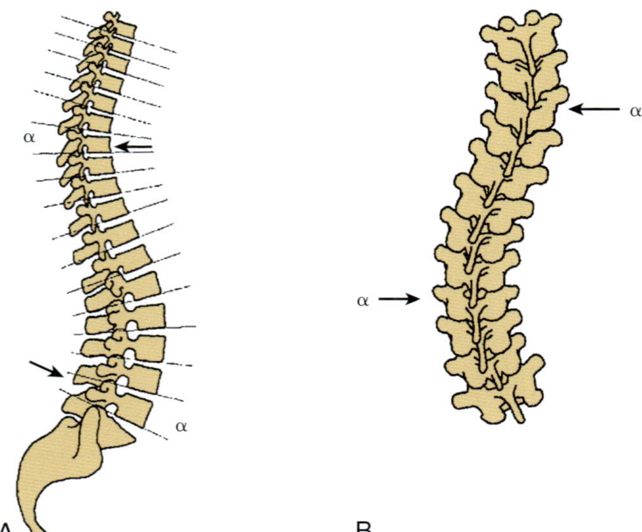

FIGURE 112-5. An apical vertebra (α) occurs at the horizon or apex of a curve, in the sagittal (**A**) or coronal (**B**) plane. It is associated with adjacent disc interspaces that have the greatest segmental angulation of all interspaces in the curve, as depicted. (Reprinted with permission from Benzel EC, editor: *Biomechanics of spine stabilization,* ed 2, New York, 2001, Thieme.)

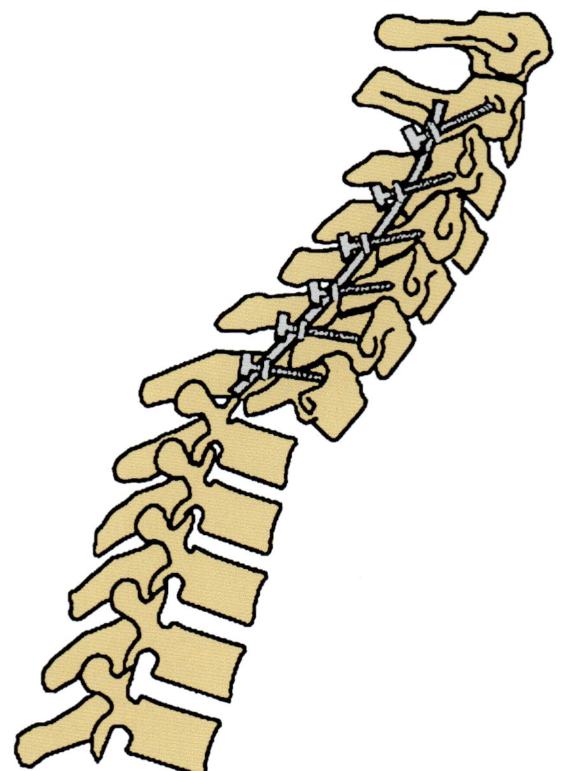

FIGURE 112-6. A long implant probably should not terminate at the cervicothoracic junction because this may result in exaggeration of deformity at the terminus of the implant. (Reprinted with permission from Benzel EC, editor: *Biomechanics of spine stabilization,* ed 2, New York, 2001, Thieme.)

from 5.1 mm at C3 to 6.6 mm at C7, which would make it amenable to transpedicular fixation. An et al.[54] measured the mediolateral and superoinferior outer pedicle diameter as 6.9 mm and 7.5 mm, respectively. The average inner diameter was 5.18 mm. The length of the pedicle was found to be 9.1 mm, with a medial angulation of 34 degrees. The recommended pedicle entry point for the C7 pedicle was 1 mm inferior to the mid-portion of the facet joint with 25 to 30 degrees of medial angulation and perpendicular to the dorsal arch.

Pedicle screw fixation, while very popular in the thoracic and lumbar spine with superior fixation characteristics, has only recently become more widely used in the cervical spine. Anatomic studies have shown the pedicle width of C3 to average 4.9 mm in men and 4.5 mm in women, with the minimum reported width of 3 mm. The C4 pedicle averages 4.7 mm in men and 4.6 mm in women, with a minimum reported width of 3.1 mm.[55] Because of this variability, measurements should be made on a case-by-case basis using CT imaging.

Several studies have specifically examined the use of distal subaxial cervical pedicle screw fixation and compared it with lateral mass fixation. The lateral mass anatomy and its particular relationship to nearby neurovascular structures have been precisely established by anatomic studies. Xu et al.[56] found that for C3-7, the average distance from the superficial, dorsal center of the lateral mass to the nerve root superiorly was 5.7 mm ± 1.5 mm. Inferiorly, the average distance was found to be 5.5 mm ± 0.8 mm. The average distance to the spinal sac from that same point was found to be 9.2 mm ± 1.4 mm. The average medial angle of the nerve root was 76.3 degrees. Closer to the cervicothoracic junction, at the C6 level, the transverse foramen was found to be located directly ventral to the dorsal midpoint of the lateral mass. These findings suggested that this point would be safe for initiation of screw insertion in the lateral masses.[56]

Pedicle screw fixation in the subaxial spine has been found to be safer with direct palpation of the medial pedicle wall. Albert et al.[57] retrospectively looked at a group of 21 patients who had pedicle screws placed at C7 with the help of a small laminoforaminotomy at C7 and by palpating the pedicle with a right-angle nerve hook. There were no neurologic complications related to screw placement and no failure of fixation related to the use of the pedicles at 1-year follow-up.[57]

In the thoracic spine, the transverse processes do not provide adequate fixation. The upper thoracic spine pedicles at T1 and T2 are larger than those found in the midthoracic spine.[37] On average, the width of the pedicles decreases caudally from 7.8 mm to 4.4 mm. The pedicle axis projects about 7 to 8 mm medial from the lateral edge of the superior facet and about 3 to 4 mm superior to the midaxis of the transverse process.[6] An et al.[54] recommended an entry point for the T1 and T2 thoracic pedicles at the midpoint 1 mm below the facet joint, whereas Mazel et al.[6] preferred 10 to 20 degrees of caudal angulation and 5 to 10 degrees of medial angulation. Mazel's entry point for screw insertion at the upper thoracic level is located at the intersection of the transverse process axis and the midline of the inferior facet. The more caudal the fixation, the less caudal and medial is the angulation of the trajectories of the pedicle screws. Some have recommended upper thoracic pedicle screw fixation with the help of laminotomy and by directly palpating the external boundaries of the pedicle to reduce pedicle wall violation.[58] However, most authors avoid using this technique due to the added time and risks; instead, they use instruments at the level of the thoracic spinal canal.[6,59] Kim et al.[59] performed a retrospective analysis of 394 patients who underwent dorsal instrumentation with a total of 3204 transpedicular screws placed using a freehand technique by two surgeons over a 10-year period. Their review showed a 6.2% violation of the pedicle cortex, with 1.7% violating the medial wall.[59] In this study, there were no neurologic, vascular, or any other soft tissue complications. The low rate of misplacement of transpedicular screws by freehand technique in the thoracic spine, however, should not give an inexperienced surgeon a false sense of security. It is still recommended to lower that risk by closely examining preoperative imaging studies and looking for any anatomic abnormalities such as unusually narrow pedicles.

Abumi et al.[60] experienced a 7% misplacement rate out of 669 cervical pedicle screws with conventional screw insertion techniques. Due to the high risks associated with transpedicular fixation at the cervicothoracic junction, including iatrogenic damage to the spinal cord, nerve roots, or vertebral artery,[55,60] computer-assisted systems were developed to minimize those risks. Richter et al.[61] dorsally instrumented 19 patients with computer assistance, placing 31 cervical pedicle screws and 10 high-thoracic pedicle screws. Postoperative CT scanning with multiplanar reconstruction for each screw did not demonstrate any misplacement greater than 2 mm or any screw-related injury to vascular, neurogenic, or bony structures. They strongly recommend computer-assisted instrumentation, especially at the C3-6 level. Certain disadvantages must be considered when using a computer-assisted instrumentation system at the cervicothoracic junction, however. Computerized systems are prone to errors and system crashes due to hardware, software, or human failure, and the surgeon must be well versed in the more traditional fixation methods. Difficulties can be encountered with registration of instrumented vertebrae where surface matching can be thrown off by small or indistinguishable bony landmarks, because most computer systems have been developed for thoracic and lumbar systems. According to Richter, "the use of a computerized assisted system for dorsal cervical spine surgery will make a good spine surgeon even better, but it can never make a bad spine surgeon a good one."[61]

Other methods of dorsal fixation at the cervicothoracic junction that have been closely examined, in addition to screws, include traditional wires and hooks. With tumors of the dorsal elements at the junction it may be difficult to use spinous process wiring or laminar hooks, which can lead to spinal canal stenosis or iatrogenic spinal cord injury.[62] Rhee et al.[62] found no significant increase in normalized stiffness in any of the lateral mass constructs with wire augmentation that were examined. The C7 pedicle screw fixation constructs demonstrated significantly higher normalized stiffness than any of the other constructs, which included lateral mass screw fixation at C7, C6 and C7 lateral mass screws, and these constructs augmented with triple wiring. There was no predictable difference in stiffness between any of the constructs while in extension. Flexion, right and left lateral bending, and axial torsion showed superior results with the C7 pedicle construct when compared with the lateral mass screws. The addition of another lateral mass screw level at C6 did show increased stiffness comparable to the C7 pedicle screws.[62] In another study, Ulrich et al.[63] showed that sublaminar wiring is inadequate, even with supplemental ventral plate fixation, in stabilizing torsional and translational loads. In an animal study, C7-T1 pedicle screw fixation was as effective as a ventral plate and dorsal wiring in stabilizing a three-column injury.[64] Dorsal wiring is adequate only in offering stability in flexion testing,[65] functioning as a supplemental tension band construct dorsally.

Outcomes and Complications Following Surgical Treatment

Ventral and dorsal approaches to the cervicothoracic junction carry specific postoperative complications, which have been discussed with the individual approaches. Recurrent laryngeal nerve injuries may be seen with low ventral cervical or cervicothoracic junction approaches, leading to unilateral vocal cord palsy with possible mild dysphagia and dysphonia. If persistent, treatment may be with medialization thyroplasty. When both recurrent largyngeal nerves are injured, vocal cord paralysis can occur, requiring permanent gastrostomy and tracheostomy.[17] Higher approaches to the ventral cervical spine carry the risks of superior laryngeal and hypoglossal nerve injury because of their approximation to the superior thyroid artery.[66]

Ventral cervicothoracic junction surgery and its complications also have been documented by Boockvar et al.[67] in a group of 14 patients, who were followed for a period of 21 months. Five patients (36%) had graft/plate failure, which needed revision, and one patient had a recurrent laryngeal nerve palsy. Surgical complications were associated with male sex, multiple levels of involvement, the use of allograft compared with autograft, and previous surgery. The authors concluded that supplemental fixation is needed when dealing with cervicothoracic junction pathology.

In An et al.'s[3] series of 15 patients with tumors, 12 presented with neurologic involvement, with 8 patients having incomplete cord syndromes and 4 having nerve root symptoms.[3] Most of the patients improved neurologically by at least 1 or 2 Frankel grades. One patient with giant cell tumor had a recurrence that required a repeat ventral procedure. Three patients died because of tumor progression: breast metastasis at T1-2, myeloma at T1, and lung tumor at T2-3.

Bilksy et al.[17] reported a series of 41 patients with subaxial cervical tumors who underwent spinal reconstruction: 12 patients from a ventral approach, 13 patients from a dorsal approach, and 16 patients from a combined approach. Thirty-three of the 41 tumors were metastatic, and 8 were primary (2 chordomas and 6 sarcomas). Twenty-five percent of the patients had surgery-related complications, including bilateral vocal cord paralysis after a right-sided trapdoor approach at the C6-7 level with the left side presumed present preoperatively, a unilateral recurrent laryngeal nerve palsy after thyroplasty, and one CSF leak. In this study, three patients experienced complications with the cervicothoracic junction instrumentation: two patients experienced pull-out of the dorsal plate screw instrumentation (with no ventral fixation performed), and the third experienced failure of the ventral graft following corpectomy of C6 and fusion with plate. No failures were noted in the patients who underwent cervicothoracic instrumentation with screws and rods. No wound issues arose following the preoperative irradiation, even though dissection sometimes was more problematic. Similar instrumentation failures were described by Lenoir et al.,[68] who looked at 30 patients who underwent surgery for destabilizing injuries at the cervicothoracic junction. One patient had mobilization of the cervical portion of a plate and another had a thoracic screw loosen. There was no direct fixation of the anterior column in these two cases.

Mazel et al.[6] retrospectively reviewed 32 patients treated for cervicothoracic junction tumors who underwent dorsal fixation with cervical lateral mass fixation and thoracic transpedicular screw fixation. Nineteen of the patients with Pancoast tumors had en bloc resections and, therefore, total and partial vertebrectomies with destabilization of the ventral two columns. Thirteen of the patients had only dorsal palliative laminectomy and cervicothoracic fixation. Two of the 32 cases failed, with both of those patients having partial or total vertebrectomies, due to the limitation of fusion length. Mazel et al. concluded that in cases of total or partial vertebrectomies, dorsal instrumentation must extend three levels above and three levels below the site of pathology. Their group had positive results with the use of autologous fibula strut graft for multilevel corpectomies and femoral head bank bone for single-level vertebrectomy.

Steinmetz et al.[45] looked at outcomes following cervicothoracic region surgical fixation by reviewing 593 patients treated over a 5-year period at the Department of Neurosurgery at the Cleveland Clinic Foundation who were followed for a mean of 20 months. Treatment failed in 14 patients, with the failures statistically associated with laminectomy and multilevel ventral corpectomies, not supplemented by dorsal fixation, as well as histories of prior cervical surgery, surgery for correction of deformity (P = .033), and tobacco use (P = .019). Three patients underwent decompression and lateral mass fixation ending at, but not crossing, the cervicothoracic junction. Two patients underwent decompression and ventral plate fixation to, but not crossing, the junction. More specifically, three out of eight patients (37.5% of patients, P = .001) who underwent laminectomy that crossed the junction without supplemental fixation and/or fusion failed. Three of 18 patients (16.7%) who underwent two- or three-level corpectomy with fixation/fusion to T1 only also failed. Finally, three of the patients experienced treatment failure after dorsal instrumentation across the cervicothoracic junction. One of those patients, who had osteoporosis, had pedicle screw fixation ending at T1. Another patient, with Ehlers-Danlos syndrome, had undergone occiput-to-T4 instrumented fixation for correction of severe swan-neck deformity, and the tapered rods fractured. Finally, a patient who underwent dorsal fusion from C4-T2 for breast metastasis also experienced failure. Interestingly, no failures occurred in association with a combined ventral-dorsal fixation ending either at C7 or below. However, with the recommendation being made to consider extension of fixation to T1 or T2, a trend toward failure was noted in cases in which the dorsal fixation was terminated at C7. Similar findings were noted by Boockvar et al.,[67] who recognized that prior cervical surgery was associated with the failure of ventral surgery at the cervicothoracic junction.

Summary

Cervicothoracic junction tumors present a unique set of challenges from a biomechanical and anatomic standpoint that need to be carefully considered prior to choosing a surgical approach. These recent techniques and considerations have significantly improved surgical outcomes in this set of patients.

KEY REFERENCES

An HS, Vaccaro A, Cotler JM, et al: Spinal disorders at the cervicothoracic junction. *Spine (Phila Pa 1976)* 19:2557–2564, 1994.
Benzel EC: *Biomechanics of spine stabilization*, ed 2, New York, 2001, Thieme.
Chapman JR, Anderson PA, Pepin C, et al: Posterior instrumentation of unstable cervicothoracic spine. *J Neurosurg* 84:552–558, 1996.
Steinmetz MP, Miller J, Warbel A, et al: Regional instability following cervicothoracic junction surgery. *J Neurosurg Spine* 4:278–284, 2006.
Tatsumi RL, Yoo JU, Liu Q, et al: Mechanical comparison of posterior instrumentation constructs for spinal fixation across the cervicothoracic junction. *Spine (Phila Pa 1976)* 32:1072–1076, 2007.
White AA, Panjabi MM: *Clinical biomechanics of the spine*, ed 2, Philadelphia, 1990, Lippincott Williams & Wilkins, p 45.

REFERENCES

The complete reference list is available online at expertconsult.com.

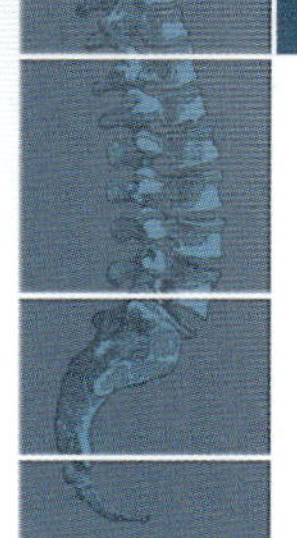

CHAPTER 113

Thoracic and Thoracolumbar Spinal Tumors: Regional Challenges

William F. Lavelle

The treatment of spinal column tumors is evolving steadily. Tumors of the thoracic and thoracolumbar regions of the spine represent a unique challenge to the spine surgeon because of the dangers posed by the surrounding neurologic and vascular structures. Each individual patient also represents a unique set of anatomic and physiologic characteristics that must be considered before the spinal tumor can be treated. Spinal tumors may be either primary or metastatic. Primary spinal tumors in the thoracic and thoracolumbar regions are uncommon, but they are tumors that may have the potential for a cure. Metastatic tumors in this region, on the other hand, represent an advanced stage of a primary cancer that may now be incurable and ultimately fatal. Any decision to perform surgery for a tumor-related condition in the thoracic or thoracolumbar spine must be carefully weighed in light of the patient's projected life-span and the morbidity associated with the surgical approach required for treating the tumor. These and related issues are discussed in this chapter.

Primary Spinal Tumors

Primary spinal tumors are an uncommon subset of the tumors affecting the thoracic and lumbar spine. A review of data from the Leeds Tumor Registry shows that 2.8% of patients had tumors of the spine.[1] In the United States, the incidence of primary tumors of the spine per 100,000 person years is estimated at 2.5 to 8.5.[2] According to the series published by Weinstein and McLain, which reviewed 82 primary neoplasms of the spine over a 50-year period, nearly two thirds of all thoracic, lumbar, and sacral tumors were malignant.[3] Rarely, these tumors present the possibility of a cure via surgical resection. A full description of primary spinal tumors is presented in Chapter 106.

Metastatic Spinal Tumors

Metastatic spinal tumors are the most common spinal tumors treated by the spine surgeon. At autopsy, 70% of patients who died of cancer have some form of vertebral metastasis.[4] Spine surgeons, therefore, must have a clear understanding of the behavior of the primary tumor. Close consultation with medical oncologists and other specialists, however, is critical. Medical and adjunctive treatments have improved the quality of life and lengthened the survival of cancer patients.

There are two primary indications for surgery in patients with metastatic disease to the spine: (1) neurologic compromise or threatened neurologic compromise, and (2) spinal instability. Surgery also may reduce pain and may aid in establishing a tissue diagnosis when other attempts at obtaining one have failed.

Tumor type has been found to correlate with outcome. More aggressive primary tumors portend a worse long-term prognosis. Wise et al. reported that the longest mean survival times after the diagnosis of spinal metastasis were for myeloma (40.3 months), breast cancer (32.3 months), and prostate cancer (26.9 months), and shortest for lung cancer (12.3 months) and adenocarcinoma.[5] The patient's neurologic status, extent of disease, nutrition, overall health, and expected length of survival are other important considerations when deciding whether the patient is a candidate for extensive spine surgery. Most surgeons agree that metastatic spinal tumor surgery should be limited to patients who have an estimated life expectancy greater than 3 months. In an effort to better determine a patent's life expectancy, Tokuhashi et al. presented a scoring system to be used in the preoperative evaluation of patients with metastatic spinal tumors.[6] Scores of 0 to 2 points are assigned for each of six parameters (Table 113-1). The patient's general health, the number of extraspinal skeletal metastases, the number of metastases to the spine, the status of metastases to internal organs, the site of the primary tumor, and the patient's neurologic status are all weighted parameters in this scoring system. In addition to using this scoring system, spine surgeons are encouraged to consult with the patient's medical and radiation oncologists, because multimodal treatment may offer the patient an even longer survival than otherwise predicted.

Surgical Margins

All discussions regarding the surgical resection of tumors, regardless of the surgical discipline, reference the type of margin that is achieved when the tumor is removed. Surgical resections may be defined as either intralesional or en bloc. An intralesional resection is, by definition, a surgical resection in which the tumor is removed in a piecemeal fashion. An en bloc resection is a tumor resection in which the capsule of the tumor itself is not violated. Intralesional resections rarely offer the possibility of complete eradication of the tumor. The reliability of an en bloc resection to relieve the patient of tumor burden depends on the margins that are obtained during the surgical resection. These margins may be described as intralesional (if the tumor capsule is violated), marginal, wide, and radical. Intralesional resections are self-explanatory. Marginal resections imply that the entirety of the tumor burden is removed, but little or no normal tissue is resected along with the tumor. Wide resection, by definition, includes a component of normal tissue that is removed along with the tumor. By taking a wide en bloc resection, the tumor tissue is not visualized at the time of the resection, as it is completely encapsulated by a margin of normal tissue. A radical resection, by definition, removes the entire organ along with the blood and lymph supply to the organ. In spine surgery, a true radical resection is rarely, if ever, possible. In the event that an en bloc resection can even be performed, a wide resection often is the only possibility.

TABLE 113-1

Tokuhashi Scoring System for Preoperative Evaluation of Patients with Metastatic Spinal Tumors

Parameter	Score
General Condition	
Poor	0
Moderate	1
Good	2
No. of Extraspinal Bone Metastases	
>3	0
1 or 2	1
0	2
No. of Metastases in the Spine	
>3	0
2	1
1	2
Metastases to Major Internal Organs	
Irremovable	0
Removable	1
None	2
Primary Site of Cancer	
Lung, stomach	0
Kidney, liver, uterus, other	1
Thyroid, prostate, breast, rectum	2
Myelopathy	
Complete	0
Incomplete	1
None	2

Data from Tokuhashi Y, Matsuzaki H, Toriyama S, et al: Scoring system for the preoperative evaluation of metastatic spine tumor prognosis. *Spine (Phila Pa 1976)* 15:1110-1113, 1990.

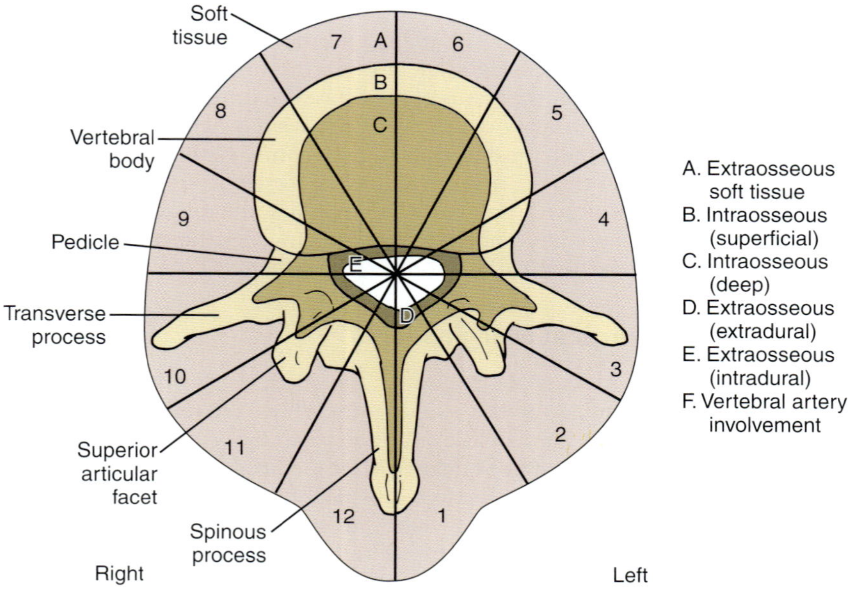

With respect to spinal tumor surgery, regional classification systems have been developed. Weinstein first popularized this type of classification system. In Weinstein's classification system, tumors were defined as intraosseous (A), extraosseous (B), and distant spread (C).[7] The zones were further subdivided with respect to the tumor's location on the vertebrae. Other groups have attempted to define spinal tumor location in a similar manner. Most recently, the Spine Oncology Study Group examined observer reliability for two of these classification systems. They found that there was moderate interobserver reliability and substantial intraobserver reliability. The Spinal Oncology Study Group thought that changing the orientation of the diagram of the zones to fit the convention of MRI and CT axial cuts made the system more user friendly (Fig. 113-1). With respect to the classification system described by Weinstein, tumors that have extraosseous extension rarely are resectable in an en bloc manner due to the risks posed to the vascular and visceral structures present in the thoracic and thoracolumbar regions.[8]

For an isolated metastatic tumor, the extent of resection has been related to patient survival. Sundaresan et al. reported that gross total resection of spinal tumors leads to a median survival of more than 2 years, compared with a historic median survival of 6 months for less aggressive resections.[9] Tomita et al. reported on 28 patients who had undergone en bloc vertebrectomy with a mean survival of

A. Extraosseous soft tissue
B. Intraosseous (superficial)
C. Intraosseous (deep)
D. Extraosseous (extradural)
E. Extraosseous (intradural)
F. Vertebral artery involvement

FIGURE 113-1. This classification system divides tumors by vertebral location. (From Chan P, Boriani S, Fourney DR, et al: An assessment of the reliability of the Enneking and Weinstein-Boriani-Biagini classifications for staging of primary spinal tumors by the Spine Oncology Study Group. *Spine [Phila Pa 1976]* 34:384–391, 2009.)

38.2 months.[10] Babat and McLain recommend that isolated metastases from less eminently lethal tumors such as breast, prostate, and kidney tumors should be managed similarly to primary tumors of the spine.[11]

Spinal Stability

One of the primary indications for surgery for tumors in the thoracic or thoracolumbar spine is the preservation of spinal stability. Kostuik et al. developed a system to evaluate the stability of spinal tumors based on the three-column classification of Denis.[12] Most spine surgeons are familiar with this model, which divides each vertebral segment into an anterior column, a middle column, and a posterior column. Unlike the Dennis classification system, these columns are further divided in half in the sagittal plane to create six zones (Fig. 113-2). Destruction of fewer than three of the six zones is considered to be stable. Further bony involvement, specifically three- and four-zone bone involvement, is considered relatively unstable. Five- to six-zone destruction is considered markedly unstable, potentially benefiting from surgical intervention (see Fig. 113-2). Other researchers have recommended that the destruction of more than 50% of the vertebral body warrants either prophylactic treatment or surgical stabilization.[13] Other modalities have been reported in the literature to be potentially helpful in this region of the spine. Specifically, minimally invasive techniques such as kyphoplasty or vertebroplasty have been found to aid both pain relief and spinal stability in this region.[14]

Dimar et al.[15] used a cadaveric model of bone destruction to examine pathologic thoracic vertebral fracture risk. This group found that the force required to cause a vertebral fracture correlated with a value they called the *vertebral strength index*, which is equivalent to the product of the remaining intact vertebral body and the bone mineral density. Despite these guidelines, there is no consensus with respect to the absolute amount of bony destruction that would compel a spine surgeon to stabilize a threatened thoracic or thoracolumbar spine. Surgeons are again reminded to consider the patient and his or her disease state as a whole.

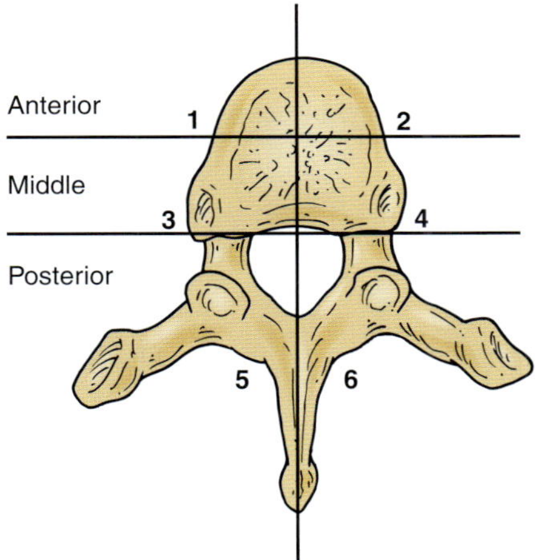

FIGURE 113-2. Regions of bony destruction described by Kostuik and Errico.[12] This classification system divides tumors by the extent of vertebral involvement. The more zones occupied by tumor, the less stable the vertebral segment.

Neurologic Stability

Few would argue that in the face of a progressive neurologic deficit, decompression surgery is necessary. Historically, surgery has involved a laminectomy despite the predominance of compressive tumors found anteriorly in the vertebral body. The results of these procedures were disappointing: only 35% of patients with an incomplete neurologic deficit experienced any appreciable improvement, and no patients with a complete neurologic deficit improved.[16]

The development of ventral surgical approaches to the thoracic and thoracolumbar spine has markedly improved patient outcomes for the surgical decompression of spinal tumors. Siegal et al. reported on 47 operative procedures performed in 40 patients with malignant epidural tumors. The indications for surgery in this group were a worsening neurologic status after previous radiation therapy in 18 procedures, the need for a tissue diagnosis in 16, a radioresistant tumor in 7, neurologic deterioration while receiving radiation therapy in 5, and a pathologic fracture-dislocation in 1 patient. Seventy percent of the procedures from this study were performed in the thoracic spine. Before surgery, all of the patients had some form of neurologic deficit. Patients were still able to walk before 12 (26%) of the procedures, were paraparetic prior to 23 procedures (49%), and were paraplegic prior to 12 procedures (26%). Bowel and bladder dysfunction was present before 25 procedures (53%). The outcome of only 44 procedures could be evaluated, because 3 patients died postoperatively. The patients were able to walk following 35 (80%) of the procedures, and were paraparetic after 8 (18%) of the procedures, and 1 patient was still paraplegic after the procedure. The patients regained normal sphincter control after 41 (93%) of the procedures. Three (6%) of the procedures were followed by the death of the patient, and complications occurred after 5 (11%) of the procedures. The authors felt that in view of the large number of patients who regained the ability to walk after ventral decompression, the role of surgical intervention as a primary treatment for epidural compression by a malignant tumor should be reconsidered.[17] Before this study, oncologists had favored the use of radiation therapy and chemotherapy alone due to the high complication rate and poor outcomes for surgical patients.[18]

Kostuik et al.[12] later compared the results of ventral and dorsal surgery for spinal tumors. They reported neurologic return in 40% of patients who underwent dorsal decompression and 71% in those with ventral decompression. Patients with ventral metastases isolated to one or two continuous segments were found to have substantially better outcomes when ventral reconstruction was performed. Weinstein and Kostuik[19] later reviewed the literature and found far better outcomes for patients undergoing ventral decompression. A satisfactory outcome was achieved in 37% of patients after a dorsal decompression and 80% of patients after a ventral decompression. As a result, interest in surgical decompressions of spinal tumors was renewed.[20]

Onimus et al.[21] reported on their series of 100 surgical decompressions of metastatic spinal tumors. Fifty-eight patients underwent a ventral approach, 33 patients underwent a dorsal decompression, and 9 patients underwent a combined approach. Mean follow-up was 13.5 months. By then, 89 patients had died in follow-up. The average survival was 10 months. The mean survival was 7 months for patients with lung metastasis, 12 months for those with breast metastasis, and 24 months for patients with prostate metastasis. Intractable pain was observed in all patients with lung cancer. All patients had been optimized on analgesic medication, with 57 patients receiving opioid-derived medications. Walking was not possible for 50 patients. Thirty-eight patients presented with at least some form of neurologic deficit. Surgical treatments included anterior surgery (58 patients), posterior surgery (33 patients), and a combined surgical approach (9 patients). The mean follow-up for this study was 13.5 months. Neurologic status was improved in 30 of 38 patients, and pain was improved in 62 patients. The authors concluded that pain depended on both the character of the bony lesion and the type of primary tumor. They also emphasized that the surgical approach should be dictated entirely by the tumor's location. Although not critically analyzed in this paper, the authors believed that even though patient survival may be limited, the surgical treatment of vertebral metastasis was beneficial in terms of functional status, such as retained ambulatory ability and retained bladder and bowel function, which were found in more than 80% of their patients.

Surgical Considerations for Patients Undergoing Radiation Therapy

The role of radiation versus surgical decompression has been well debated in the literature.[22,23] Early reports had touted the relative effectiveness of radiation in patients with spinal cancer. It is well known that radiation can interfere with wound healing, however, which is potentially disastrous in this patient population. Gilbert et al.[18] reported no significant difference in the outcome of patients who underwent laminectomy and radiation compared with patients who received radiation alone. A large number of complications were noted in the laminectomy population, including an increased incidence of spinal instability and wound complications. This study did not examine patients who had undergone ventral decompression and fusion.

In 2002, Sundaresan et al.[23] reported on the outcomes of 80 patients with solitary metastatic spinal lesions treated with a variety of surgical, medical, and radiation therapy approaches. Complete follow-up information was available on all patients. Clinical parameters, such as the neurologic grade, preoperative pain, and outcome measures, were available for analysis. Kaplan-Meier survival curves were constructed on all patients. Survival varied by tumor type, with the best prognosis noted in patients with either kidney or breast cancer. Although 48 patients (60%) had been ambulatory preoperatively, 78 (98%) were ambulatory after surgery, including 94% of those who initially had been nonambulatory. Although the patient population is heterogeneous, it was thought that a combined approach using radiation and surgery was beneficial for patients.

In 2005, a landmark article by Patchell et al. reported on the results of a randomized, multi-institutional, non-blinded trial that randomly assigned patients with spinal cord compression to either surgery followed by radiation therapy (n = 50) or to radiation therapy alone (n = 51).[24] The primary end point of the study was the ability to walk, with secondary outcomes of urinary continence, muscle strength and functional status, the need for analgesic medication, the need for corticosteroids, and, finally, survival rates examined. After an interim analysis, the study was terminated early, because significantly more patients who underwent a surgical decompression—42 of 50 patients (84%)—were able to walk, compared with the 29 of 51 patients (57%) who were able to walk after radiation alone. Surgically treated patients also were able to walk significantly longer than those who underwent radiation alone (median, 122 days vs. 13 days, $P = .003$). The need for corticosteroids, as well as analgesics, also was significantly reduced for the surgical group. Since the publication of this landmark article, most spinal oncologists believe that surgical decompression for epidural disease is the most effective means of preserving neurologic function and retaining ambulatory status.

Technical Aspects of the Surgical Approach

Dorsal Approach

As described earlier, dorsal approaches are indicated for patients who have spinal cord compression due to tumor in the dorsal elements. As also discussed earlier, one retrospective review demonstrated neurologic improvement in as few as 24% of patients undergoing a posterior decompression for a spinal tumor.[25] This study specifically examined patients who underwent a simple laminectomy (Fig. 113-3). More recently, Bauer[26] demonstrated significant neurologic improvement in patients undergoing a more aggressive dorsal approach that included pedicle resection and the removal of ventral compressive lesions, along with segmental stabilization. Seventy-six percent of patients had substantial improvement in their neurologic status, with most retaining this improvement until their deaths. Rigid segmental stabilization is thought to offer the best chance of a satisfactory outcome after an isolated dorsal decompression, because it prevents kyphosis. Familiarity with this approach is nearly universal. A midline incision is made, and the paraspinal muscles are elevated from the involved segments. A careful dorsal decompression may be completed as described in Chapter 53. In most cases, the only possible resection is an intralesional resection. However,

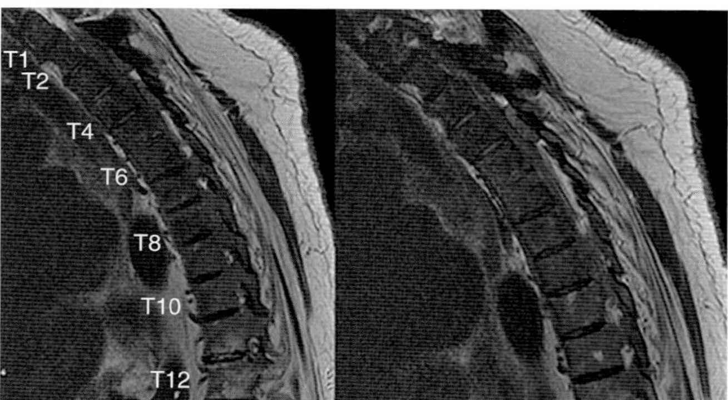

FIGURE 113-3. A 66-year-old man with known prostate cancer presented with progressive bilateral lower extremity weakness. The patient was taken for an emergent dorsal-only laminectomy, because his tumor was causing dorsal spinal cord compression.

there are occasions when a marginal resection is possible, depending on the location of the tumor in the vertebra.

Ventral Approach

In the 1980s, ventral approaches for the treatment of spinal metastasis gained popularity. Harrington believed that if the dorsal elements had minimal or no tumor involvement, their inherent tensile stability would remain intact, and a spine decompression could be accomplished entirely through the ventral approach.[27] Patients are positioned in a full lateral decubitus position with an ancillary roll placed under the dependent arm. The side (right or left) of the approach usually is dictated by the area of tumor compression. If neither side is more involved, the spine often is approached from the right side at or above T5 to avoid the arch of the aorta. Below T5, the spine is approached from the left to minimize retraction on the liver. Surgeons typically select the intercostal space one or two segments above the vertebral body for their approach. After skin incision, a rib typically is dissected in a subperiosteal fashion and resected as far dorsal as possible. The pleura usually is entered at the level of the rib bed. The segmental vessels at the levels above and below the involved vertebral body are isolated and divided. After level verification, the intervertebral discs above and below the involved level are incised and removed with a combination of curets and rongeurs. It often is necessary to remove the rib head in order to identify the pedicle of the vertebral body. The pedicle is an important landmark, because it allows the surgeon to identify the posterior aspect of the vertebral body and the location of the spinal canal. After removal of the discs above and below, as well as the rib head, the vertebral body itself can be removed. Again, in most cases the only possible resection is an intralesional resection; however, there are occasions when a marginal resection is possible, depending on the location of the tumor in the vertebra. Behind the disc space, the posterior longitudinal ligament is rather thick and offers some protection for the spinal canal. Behind the vertebral body, however, the posterior longitudinal ligament is thin and narrow, and offers little resistance to central extrusion of tumor tissue or bone fragments against the spinal cord. As the surgeon approaches the dorsal third of the vertebral body and, therefore, the spinal canal, great care must be taken to remove debris of tumor and bone without in any way increasing the already existing impingement on the spinal canal. An angled curet, usually the most effective instrument, allows material to be pulled forward out of the canal and away from the dura mater.

The upper part of the thoracic spine from the first to the third thoracic vertebrae can be exposed using a thoracoplasty approach by mobilizing the scapula ventrally and resecting the second rib. As described by Harrington, the major advantage of the ventral approach is the surgeon's ability to resect the tumor directly, decompress the neurologic structures from the side of their compromise, and "jack" open the collapsed vertebral space, thereby correcting the typical kyphotic deformity at its source.[27,28]

Access to the thoracolumbar and lumbar spine also can occur through the ventral approach. During the ventral thoracolumbar approach, both a thoracotomy and a ventral lumbar retroperitoneal approach must be completed. Again, the most common approach is through the rib just proximal to the area of interest. The rib is exposed through a subperiosteal dissection. Ventrally, the costochondral junction is incised. Retroperitoneal fat, identifiable at the thoracolumbar level, is followed into the retroperitoneal space. This is best accomplished at the T11 level (the 11th rib). Additional retroperitoneal exposure can be gained through incising the additional abdominal wall musculature. The intra-abdominal contents are bluntly dissected and reflected ventrally. Once the diaphragm is isolated, it is incised and divided one finger-breadth proximal to its insertion to avoid injury to the phrenic nerve. As the diaphragm is cut, marking sutures are inserted to facilitate reapproximation during wound closure.

An isolated retroperitoneal approach to the lumbar spine also can be completed. This approach is most useful for lesions from L1 through L4. It also may reach rostrally to T11 and T12, depending on the insertion of the diaphragm, although this exposure becomes more difficult as the crural attachments and the overlying ribs make access difficult. During this approach, the surgeon again places the patient in a lateral position and places the skin incision slightly rostral to the level of interest. The abdominal wall musculature is incised in a stepwise fashion traversing the extra oblique, the internal oblique, and finally the transversalis musculature and fascia. Just below the transversalis fascia is the peritoneum, which is bluntly reflected ventrally. Care should be taken to avoid injury to the genitofemoral nerve, which is derived from branches of the L1 and L2 nerve roots. This nerve passes through the psoas muscle and anywhere from the base of L2 through the base of L4. Additionally, the ureter, which runs between the peritoneum and the psoas muscle, should be identified and protected. The surgical results of ventral spine decompressions for metastatic disease are described in the preceding sections.

Dorsolateral Approach

A significant number of patients with spinal tumors require both ventral and dorsal decompression, as well as a ventral and dorsal stabilization. These patients often are poor candidates for a surgery that would involve two independent surgical approaches. To avoid this, a dorsolateral approach may be considered. The procedure can be performed from a single dorsolateral costotransversectomy approach, which enables a ventral and dorsal decompression, as well as segmental dorsal fixation, through a single incision. This dorsolateral approach is particularly useful for lesions in the upper thoracic spine, a difficult area to reach from a ventral thoracotomy or sternal splitting approach. The dorsolateral approach also is useful at the thoracolumbar junction, where a ventral approach necessitates taking down the diaphragm. This approach is particularly advantageous in the morbidly obese patient (see case example in Fig. 113-4).

The surgeon approaches the spine through a dorsal incision. The paraspinal muscles are elevated off of the dorsal elements. The spine itself is exposed out to the tips of the transverse process. The surgeon then identifies the rib as it passes deep to the transverse processes. The ribs at the level of interest as well as a level above and below are exposed through lateral retraction of the paraspinal musculature. Using electrocautery as well as a periosteal elevator, the rib at the level of interest is dissected free of the intercostal musculature and pleura. The rib is transected using a rongeur. The medial portion of the rib is followed in a subperiosteal fashion. Once the rib is believed to be adequately freed of

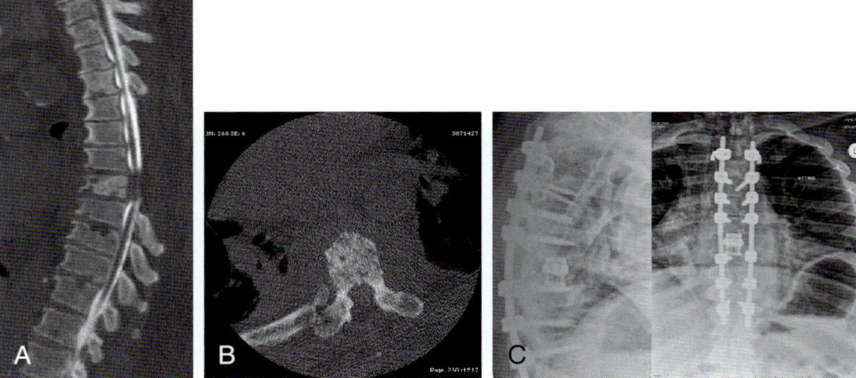

FIGURE 113-4. A 60-year-old man, who weighed 500 lbs, had undergone a previous laminectomy for a thoracic tumor. The patient presented with increasing lower extremity weakness and underwent a revision laminectomy and a dorsolateral decompression with instrumentation of the decompressed segment. The patient subsequently has had improvement in his lower extremity weakness. **A,** Sagittal reconstruction of a CT myelogram demonstrating a large compressive tumor. **B,** Axial view of a CT myelogram demonstrating a large compressive tumor. **C,** Anteroposterior and lateral radiographic views of the same patient after an extracavitary decompression and fusion.

its plural attachments, it is disarticulated from the transverse process and vertebral body. It sometimes is useful to resect the transverse process before removing the rib head. Bleeding may be encountered in this area, and should be controlled with electrocautery or an agent such as thrombin-soaked hemostatic gelatin (Gelfoam). The lateral aspect of the vertebral body may be further dissected using a periosteal elevator, such as a no. 1 Penfield dissector. A malleable retractor or a custom osteotomy retractor may be inserted to protect the underlying pleural and mediastinal structures. An exposure of this type typically allows the surgeon to approach half of the vertebral body. Bilateral exposures would facilitate the removal of the rest of the vertebral body. This approach may be combined with more extensive dorsal decompressions to perform a resection of the entire vertebra. This resection is, however, an intralesional resection and rarely is curative.

Typically, a patient will concomitantly undergo a thoracic laminectomy as well as a resection of the facet joints and pedicles. After completion of a central laminectomy, the surgeon uses a combination of Kerrisons and rongeurs to remove the facet joints and isolate the pedicle of the level of interest. The nerve root is identified exiting below the pedicle. To facilitate a more extensive ventral decompression, it may be necessary to sacrifice either one or both nerve roots at the level of interest. We recommend that, before ligating the nerve root, silk ties or clips be placed and provisionally tied to ensure that the spinal cord does not become ischemic from the occlusion of a large feeding vessel. Once the surgeon is satisfied that spinal cord ischemia is not occurring, the root may be sacrificed. We also recommend that the surgeon consider sacrificing at least one of the nerve roots if ventral spinal instrumentation is being considered. The thoracic nerve root on the side where the cage will be placed typically impedes cage placement and may cause undue traction to the spinal cord if it is manipulated to the extent that is required for cage placement.

In addition, care should be taken during this approach to avoid injury to the underlying plural structures. If the pleura is violated, a chest tube may be placed at a remote site after the completion of the surgery or, more commonly, the chest tube may be placed into the pleural rent and wound bed during closure. To protect the spinal cord from ischemia, it is recommended that the patient's mean arterial pressure be kept at greater than 65 mm. Conversely, for patients who have already failed radiation treatment, such a dorsal approach invites a high risk of wound dehiscence and infection. Because a significant amount of bone and ligament is removed, the patient is extremely unstable and would be unable to tolerate hardware removal. If an infection develops, antibiotic suppression is the most advisable form of treatment. Figures 113-4 and 113-5 show radiographic and clinical photographs of this technique.

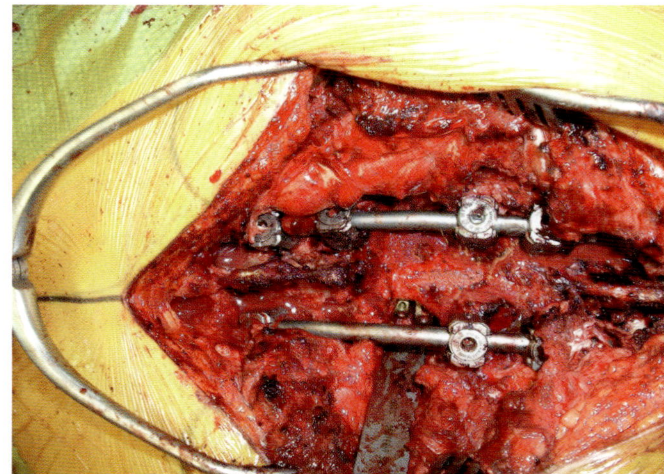

FIGURE 113-5. Clinical photograph of an extracavitary vertebral body resection.

Early results of dorsolateral approaches were reported by Dewald et al.,[13] who found that only one of five patients regained ambulatory status and that patient survival was less than 6 months. Later, Bridwell et al. found that 60% of neurologically compromised patients improved postoperatively, although they were not satisfied with their ability to thoroughly decompress the spinal cord.[29] More recently, Mülbauer et al.[30] reported that 82% of patients improved neurologically and that 70% of previously nonambulatory patients were able to walk postoperatively.

Complications

Sundaresan et al. reported that complication rates may be as high as 48% following tumor resection.[9] The complication rate was statistically higher for patients over the age of 65, those who had had prior treatment, and those with neurologic symptoms. Multiple series have found that the risk of complications is highest in previously radiated regions, because these tissues tend to be more susceptible to wound breakdown and infection.[9,26] Previously radiated tissues tend to be more friable. Significantly higher blood loss may be noted in these regions. As stated earlier, many of these tumor resections are intralesional. It may be assumed that, were patients to survive long enough, a recurrence might occur. Construct failures are another significant concern, because these patients often are malnourished and have undergone radiation therapy. Despite this, the reported failure rates have been quite low, with Bridwell reporting hardware loosening in only 1 of 25 patients[29] (4.0%) and Bauer reporting loosening in 3 of 67 patients (4.4%).[26]

Summary

The treatment of tumors located within the thoracic and thoracolumbar spine can be difficult. The kyphotic positioning of the spinal column, the tenuous vascular supply of the thoracic spinal cord, and the presence of the vital viscual structures pose unique challenges for the treating surgeon. While useful surgical techniques have been developed to aid in the treatment of these patients, the treating physician should bear in mind that each case is unique and requires sound decision making at each step from the diagnosis of the tumor through the decision to operate.

KEY REFERENCES

Kostuik JP, Errico TJ, Gleason TF, Errico CC: Spinal stabilization of vertebral column tumors. *Spine (Phila Pa 1976)* 13(3):250–256, 1988.

Nicholls PJ, Jarecky TW: The value of posterior decompression by laminectomy for malignant tumors of the spine. *Clin Orthop Relat Res* 201:210–213, 1985.

Sundaresan N, Sachdev VP, Holland JF, et al: Surgical treatment of spinal cord compression from epidural metastasis. *J Clin Oncol* 13(9):2330–2335, 1995.

Tokuhashi Y, Matsuzaki H, Toriyama S, et al: Scoring system for the preoperative evaluation of metastatic spine tumor prognosis. *Spine (Phila Pa 1976)* 15(11):1110–1113, 1990.

Weinstein JN: Surgical approach to spine tumors. *Orthopedics* 12(6):897–905, 1989.

REFERENCES

The complete reference list is available online at expertconsult.com.

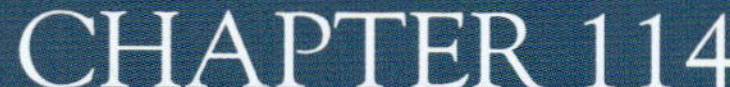
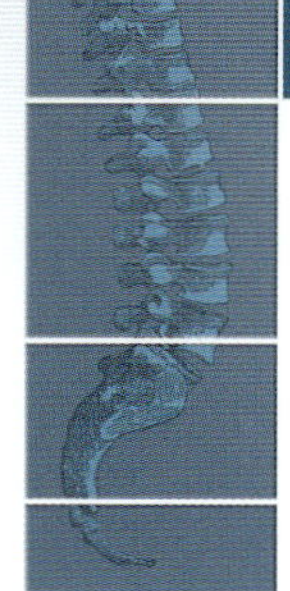

CHAPTER 114

Sacral Tumors: Regional Challenges

Sharad Rajpal | R. Douglas Orr | Michael P. Steinmetz | Donald A. Smith

Tumors of the sacrum are very rare, accounting for only 2% to 4% of all primary bone neoplasms and 1% to 7% of all primary spinal tumors.[1] Surgical resection, when possible, has the best long-term prognosis for most sacral tumors.[2] Nonetheless, the surgical treatment of tumors in this area is challenging because of the complex regional anatomy and, often, the advanced stage of cancer at the time of diagnosis. Surgeons must not only be cognizant of local anatomy from a neurologic, colorectal, urologic, and orthopaedic standpoint, but also sometimes face the difficult conflict between functional preservation of the individual and cure of the disease process. The operating strategy requires precise and rigorous preoperative planning to locate the exact levels of tissue involvement; to make an accurate assessment of the bone, muscle, nerve, and joint structures that will require resection; and to plan pelvic reconstruction.[2] This chapter focuses only on regional challenges to sacral tumors, as the anatomy and surgical approaches to the sacrum are covered more extensively elsewhere in this textbook.

Clinical Presentation

Sacral neoplasms usually grow insidiously. As a result, patients typically present with long-standing (several months to years) nonspecific symptoms, such as low-back, buttock, sacrococcygeal, or referred leg pain.[1,3,4] Conventional radiographs are not sensitive, and routine lumbar myelography, CT, and MRI studies often fail to visualize the sacrum below the S2 segment. Unfortunately, many patients are misdiagnosed with lumbar disc disease for which they undergo subsequent management.

Although aggressive tumors can present earlier, the mean time to diagnosis from onset of symptoms has been reported to be 2 years.[5] As a result of this common delay in making the appropriate diagnosis, sacral tumors may grow to advanced stages, with large dimensions and involvement of proximal organs and sacral nerves. According to Payer, an expansive space-occupying lesion of the sacrum usually leads to a specific pattern of clinical signs and symptoms throughout its natural history, depending on the anatomic location of the lesion within the sacrum, its extension, and whether there is compression or invasion of neighboring structures.[6] Some sacral tumors have characteristic syndromes of pain due to their anatomic location and pattern of growth (chordomas, for example, may produce continuous rectal pain).[7-10]

The first sign of disease may be a painless, visible sacral mass, although some patients may present with neurologic symptoms, with or without pain.[11] The most common initial manifestation is local pain from mass effect.[6] With subsequent tumor growth and impingement on and/or infiltration of local nerve roots, patients develop radicular pain, radiating into the buttocks, posterior thigh or leg, external genitalia, and perineum.[5,12] Sacral tumor pain predominates at night and can be exacerbated by Valsalva maneuvers.[5,13] Specific involvement of lumbosacral nerve roots will lead to characteristic neurologic deficits defined by the nerve or nerves involved.

Several non-neurologic clinical manifestations also can arise from sacral tumors as a result of invasion of neighboring structures. Ventral extension of a large sacral mass can present with constipation from rectal compression, as well as impede bladder emptying and uterine function.[3,14-17] Lateral extension across the sacroiliac and pelvic joints can result in local joint pain that is exacerbated by weight bearing and ambulation.[13,18] Constitutional symptoms such as weight loss, blood abnormalities, or weakness typically are more characteristic of metastatic lesions than of primary sacral tumors.[11]

By the time a sacral lesion is diagnosed, many patients may have already been mistakenly treated for lumbar spondylotic problems. Presenting factors in sacral tumors, however, may be differentiated by their insidious onset, unilaterality, and progression to involve bowel and bladder continence and/or sexual function.[6,19] A small sacral mass may even be palpable on digital rectal examination during the very early stages.[11]

Management Consideration: Biopsy

The combination of anatomic localization and imaging characteristics, when taken in the context of a specific clinical setting, often shortens the list of possible pathologic diagnoses. Preoperative biopsy is critical to establishing a surgical plan and can be reserved for those patients in whom exact knowledge of the pathologic diagnosis would influence the decision to operate or would alter the scope of surgery. If a primary rectal malignancy with local involvement of the sacrum is suspected, endoscopy with biopsy of any suspicious endoluminal lesions is appropriate. In the case of masses extrinsic to the rectal mucosa, transrectal biopsy is discouraged, because this violation of previously uninvolved tissue planes could then commit the patient to an otherwise unneeded bowel resection.

Although open biopsies and transrectal biopsies were common in the past, almost all biopsies are now performed using image guidance. The trajectory of the biopsy should be considered to allow for its easy inclusion within the boundaries of any subsequent surgical resection. Biopsy has particular relevance in hematopoietic malignancies that may be best treated with irradiation and combination chemotherapy. Lesions that are metastatic to the sacrum from remote sites are considered for operation only under special circumstances. Because this rarely occurs outside the context of a known primary tumor with widely disseminated disease, this is an uncommon indication for biopsy. In patients who are deemed unsuitable for a major operative procedure because of comorbid medical conditions, a biopsy is warranted to establish a diagnosis and direct the most appropriate therapeutic alternatives.

Most primary malignancies of the sacrum are locally aggressive tumors, metastasizing only late in the course of disease or not at all. Nonetheless, chest radiography and CT of the chest and abdomen, as well as a bone scan, are probably prudent, because evidence of remote disease may alter the decision for surgery and the method of treatment. Cancers of the rectum and pelvic organs with sacral involvement must be thoroughly staged before any consideration is given to surgery.

Tumor Classification

When considering surgical objectives in dealing with tumors of the sacrum, one must appraise the anatomic extent of the lesion and its biologic behavior. The anatomic considerations will direct the surgeon to the lesion, whereas the biologic considerations will dictate the scope of the surgery. One important variable to consider is whether the tumor is contained within its anatomic borders or has a fundamentally infiltrative or invasive nature. Approximately one half of sacral tumors are benign, encapsulated tumors and can be dealt with by lesional resection. Low-grade malignancies with infiltrative borders require more aggressive approaches with en bloc resection and a wide local excision with a circumferential margin of uninvolved tissue to effect cure. Certain higher-grade or disseminated malignancies are best treated not with surgical resection, but with radiation therapy or chemotherapy.

Sacral tumors can be classified according to four broad categories: congenital, metastatic, primary osseous, and primary neurogenic.[7] Specific tumor management considerations are described in the following sections.

Congenital Lesions

Congenital lesions include dermoid cysts, anterior and intrasacral meningoceles, perineural (Tarlov) cysts, teratomas, hamartomas, and chordomas. Chordoma is the most common primary neoplasm of the sacrum.[15,18,20-24] These tumors typically are slow-growing, locally invasive tumors that arise from remnants of the notochord. Approximately 50% of chordomas are located in the sacrum. They can reach a large size before any symptoms manifest. These tumors typically are avascular, with a large soft tissue component centered on the midline, and expand into the presacral space. Patients at diagnosis typically are 40 to 70 years of age. They may suffer from local pain, which can be sharp or dull, usually is continuous, and often is located in the rectum, or they may present with sacral radicular pain or leg weakness and/or bladder and bowel dysfunction.[3,6,17,25] Although infiltration of the gluteal muscles has been observed, the tumor does not typically involve the rectum ventrally through the presacral fascia.[14,15,17] The duration of disease-free survival depends on the degree of resection; therefore, resection should extend at least one sacral segment beyond any obvious tumor involvement.[3,14,26,27] Subtotal resection or curettage is done only when palliative treatment alone has been chosen because residual tumor is certain to progress.[28] Chemotherapy has not demonstrated convincing efficacy, and radiation is reserved for unresectable residual or recurrent disease because it has been shown to delay time to tumor progression.[29]

Metastatic Tumors

Metastatic tumors are the most common malignant neoplasm in the sacrum.[19] These tumors most often arise by hematogenous dissemination from solid organs such as the breast, lung, prostate, kidney, gastrointestinal tract, and thyroid.[30] Hematogenous malignant tumors, such as multiple myeloma, also can metastasize to the sacrum or may occur as primary lesions, as is the case with lymphoma.[19,31,32] Multiple myeloma and primary lymphoma are the second and third most common primary malignant neoplasms of the sacrum, respectively.[33] Pelvic organ tumors, such as adenocarcinoma of the rectum, can even infiltrate the sacrum directly.[11] Because of their rapid progression and locally invasive nature, metastatic tumors often are diagnosed earlier than primary sacral lesions.[31] Unfortunately, sacral involvement typically signals advanced metastatic disease: once sacral metastases are detected, 61% of cases will have distant organ involvement, and 43% of cases may have involvement of other vertebrae.[4,19]

Consequently, treatment often is limited to palliative radiation and/or chemotherapy. Palliative surgical intervention sometimes is indicated for decompression of neural or pelvic structures in the absence of active systemic disease. Sacrectomy may be indicated with an extended abdominoperineal resection or pelvic exenteration for locally invasive pelvic tumors in carefully selected patients.[7,19]

Primary Osseous Tumors

Primary osseous tumors, although histologically and biologically diverse, account for less than 10% of all primary bone tumors.[7]

Low-grade tumors, which include osteoid osteoma, osteoblastoma, osteochondroma, and aneurysmal bone cyst (ABC), often are incidental findings and can present in a variety of ways. Osteoblastoma is distinguished by a lesional diameter greater than 2 cm and can present with a poorly localized, dull ache.[34] Osteoid osteomas, on the other hand, produce localizing pain that is classically worse at night and is relieved by aspirin.[2] Osteochondromas are slow-growing, cartilage-forming lesions that favor the dorsal elements, especially the facet joints. ABCs are composed of dilated vascular channels arising within an expanded marrow cavity. They preferentially arise in the dorsal elements but may involve the entire the sacrum. ABCs typically are discovered in individuals younger than 20 years of age, and, while histologically benign, are capable of significant sacral destruction and neurologic deficit.[2,35] Most of these lesions follow an indolent course even without treatment and may even regress spontaneously. The preferred treatment is en bloc surgical resection, but curettage or subtotal resection may lead to a resolution of symptoms.

High-grade osseous tumors, which include chondrosarcoma, osteosarcoma, and Ewing sarcoma, often are very aggressive. Because these tumors respond poorly to chemotherapy and irradiation, they require a wide excision in the absence of systemic disease.[36-39] Osteosarcoma sometimes is the consequence of malignant transformation of a giant cell tumor or of Paget disease. Chondrosarcoma tends to be less aggressive. Ewing sarcoma is a small, round cell malignancy of childhood and adolescence that usually originates in bone but also may arise at extraskeletal sites. Ewing sarcoma and primitive neuroectodermal tumor are regarded as closely related members of the same family of tumors. Ewing sarcoma can occur as a primary sacral lesion but has one of the highest mortality rates of all bone tumors. Ewing sarcoma is regarded as a surgical condition only when encountered in the sacrum because of its propensity to metastasize early and because of its favorable response to both irradiation and chemotherapy.[40]

Giant cell tumors are the second most common primary tumor of the sacrum and usually peak in the third decade of life, with a predominance in women.[18,23,24,41-43] Although these tumors are histologically benign, they can degenerate into malignant sarcomatous tumors or even develop distant metastases.[18,41-44] Giant cell tumors typically are slow growing but can be locally invasive and attain a very large size by the time a diagnosis is made.[38] Because these tumors can have a high rate of recurrence, the preferred treatment is total resection, which may include a total sacrectomy if the tumor crosses the midline, involves the upper sacral segments, or involves the sacroiliac joints.[7,45] Good local control has been reported for curettage combined with bone cement and adjunctive cryosurgery.[46,47] The role of radiotherapy remains unclear, because it has been implicated in the sarcomatous transformation.[42]

Primary Neurogenic Tumors

Primary neurogenic tumors of the sacrum, which are relatively rare, include schwannomas, neurofibromas, ganglioneuromas, and ependymomas. Only about 1% to 5% of spinal schwannomas arise at this level.[48] Similar to neurogenic lesions elsewhere in the spine, they tend to originate in the spinal canal or in close relation to the nerve roots or their coverings. These tumors typically are slow growing, often are encapsulated, are intradural or extradural, and do not invade local tissue.[7] The location and slow growth of these tumors allow them to expand and fill the sacral canal and grow out of the ventral or dorsal sacral foramina to variable degrees. These tumors often remain confined to the spinal canal and may be treated with lesional excision, similar to neurogenic tumors elsewhere in the spine. In cases where the tumor is of long standing, the sacrum can become excavated from the expansion and, although the tumor maintains its bony margin, there is a "pushing" rather than an infiltrative border. Giant sacral neurofibromas, schwannomas, and ependymomas occur with equal rarity. Dorsal approaches for a curative resection are possible for schwannomas and neurofibromas, but tumors with large presacral components may require an anterior transabdominal approach.[38] Ependymomas can present both intradurally and extradurally in the sacroccygeal region and can be diagnosed in advanced stages with extensive bony destruction.[7] Ependymomas require complete en bloc resection to prevent local recurrence or neuroaxis dissemination via the cerebrospinal fluid. Ganglioneuromas are rare, slow-growing tumors that can grow in the pelvis from sacral extensions of the sympathetic chain. The preferred treatment is complete resection with a combined ventral and dorsal approach.[38]

Surgical Approaches

The complex regional anatomy, biomechanical factors, and characteristics of sacral tumors make operations in this area particularly challenging. Surgery often is performed by a multidisciplinary team that includes spine, colorectal, vascular, and plastic surgeons. Once the decision to operate has been made, the approach is dictated by several factors: the patient's preoperative status, tumor pathology, the amount of intrapelvic disease, the degree of sacral destruction (especially the sacral ala) and presence of sacroiliac joint involvement, and whether the surgical goal is palliation or cure. Patients must be carefully selected, because sacral resections can be highly morbid procedures with subsequent permanent motor or sensory deficits or loss of bowel, bladder, and/or sexual function.[7,49] In cases of planned major sacral resections, it is advisable to obtain baseline urodynamic studies to assess preoperative voiding function.

Dorsal approaches to the sacrum are the simplest and include simple laminectomy, alone or combined with sacrococcygectomy. Sacral approaches can be performed with the patient in either the prone or lateral decubitus position. The advantages of the prone position are the ease of patient positioning, its familiarity and comfort for the operator, the facilitated use of the surgical microscope, and the opportunity for participation by the assistant surgeon. The major advantages of the lateral position are good abdominal relaxation and resultant lowering of pressure within the inferior vena cava and epidural veins, gravitational drainage of blood out of the wound, and the option it affords for synchronous ventral exposure of the sacrum via the transperitoneal or retroperitoneal route. For complex resections, the sacrum may be approached ventrally and dorsally.

Sacral Laminectomy

The principles of dorsal dissection and exposure are fundamentally similar to those employed during lumbar laminectomy. The proximity of the incision to the anal orifice and the increased potential for wound contamination warrant extra care in skin preparation and surgical draping. A midline incision usually is chosen. The sacrospinalis, multifidus, and gluteus maximus muscles are reflected laterally off the sacrum, and blood vessels often are found penetrating the dorsal sacral foramina. Sacrifice of the dorsal rami is unavoidable but does not lead to serious functional consequences. Because of the physiologic lordosis at the lumbosacral junction, the S1 and S2 laminae may be perceived as sloping upward with respect to the L5 lamina. The laminectomy usually is started at the L5-S1 hiatus, because the interlaminar space provides a convenient point of entry into the rostral sacral canal. More restricted openings directly into the midsacral and distal sacral canals over a well-localized and very limited lesion are possible. The small advantage gained in preserving the integrity of the dorsal ligamentous attachments at L5-S1 usually is counteracted by the restricted exposure and the lost opportunity to orient to the thecal sac and exiting nerve roots. Because the ventral sacrum is fused, sacral laminectomy is not significantly destabilizing, as long as the sacroiliac joints remain intact. The lower sacral nerve roots and the filum terminale exit from the termination of the dural sac at the S2 level. The only other normal constituents of the sacral canal are the epidural vessels and fat.

Sacral laminectomy is an appropriate approach to pathologic conditions originating within and largely confined to the sacral canal because of the ease with which the neural elements and their coverings are exposed. Sacral laminectomy is less well suited as a definitive exposure in lesions that originate outside the sacral canal or that have developed significant extension into the pelvis via the neural foramina or through sacral replacement, or for those tumors requiring an en bloc resection.

Treatment of neurogenic tumors and cysts is the foremost indication for the sacral approach. Lesions such as schwannomas, neurofibromas, and ependymomas may burrow into the ventral and lateral sacral elements, but this is not necessarily a limitation to the use of this exposure. Rarely is the destruction so extensive as to compromise sacroiliac joint stability. The great majority of these tumors are benign and are cured by intralesional/marginal resection of the tumor and its capsule. With a dorsal approach, even large tumors can be extricated successfully from the recesses of the sacrum. Intimate involvement with functional sacral roots is the most common impediment to total surgical extirpation of such tumors. Any dural defects should be closed in a watertight fashion, using a patch graft as necessary. If a wound drain is required, low-pressure suction bulb systems are most appropriate to minimize the risk of creating a cerebrospinal fluid fistula.

Dorsal Sacrectomy

Dorsal sacrectomy, as described by MacCarty et al., is an excellent procedure for dealing with lesions of the sacrum below the level of the sacroiliac joints.[50] The ability to address the presacral extension of tumor and the potential to perform a genuine oncologic procedure including en bloc resection of tumor with a circumferential margin of uninvolved tissues distinguishes this from simple sacral laminectomy. These advantages are particularly relevant to osseous lesions of the sacrum, which more often are malignant and are more likely to present with a presacral mass. This approach usually is suitable for tumors whose superior limit can be reached on digital rectal examination; it should not be employed in cases with primary rectal involvement.

Patients are placed in a prone position over padded bolsters to allow the abdomen to hang free and minimize vena cava compression. The anus may be temporarily closed in a purse-string fashion. A midline incision is made that extends from the lumbosacral junction to the coccyx. The incision can be modified to an ellipse to incorporate any previous biopsy tract. The overlying soft tissues are reflected to expose the bony sacrum dorsally. If preoperative imaging studies indicate tumor eruption out of the sacral hiatus or dorsal foramina, the soft tissue dissection is altered to leave an island of sacrospinalis musculature and fat overlying the dorsal surface of the sacrum, and a cuff of gluteal musculature attached laterally. In these circumstances, the sacral periosteum should not be incised or dissected. The anococcygeal ligament is divided at a distance from the sphincter, and finger dissection is used to mobilize the rectum and develop the presacral space.

The sacrotuberous and sacrospinous ligaments are detached from the lateral edges of the lower sacrum to uncover the piriformis and coccygeal muscles, which are divided to reveal the lower elements of the sacral plexi. For malignant lesions, such as chordoma, the transverse sacral osteotomy should extend one whole segment rostral to the level of radiographically involved bone. This determines the level at which the sacral nerves must be divided. The procedure is facilitated through a limited sacral laminectomy immediately rostral to the level of the intended amputation. The sacral plexi and sciatic nerves are quite lateral at this point and are only rarely involved directly by tumors of the lower sacrum. The pudendal nerves exiting the greater sciatic foramen and reentering the lesser foramen also should be identified and protected, except when they are too intimately involved with the tumor to be spared. The transverse sacral osteotomy is then completed through any remaining dorsal elements and all of the ventral sacrum using an osteotome. A protected finger inserted into the presacral space at the level of the intended sacral division helps provide additional tactile guidance for the osteotomy and for the subsequent release of any soft tissue attachments. The specimen is freed circumferentially and can be removed from the field. Bleeding from the sacral stump is controlled with bone wax. Considerable care is taken to secure hemostasis in the presacral soft tissue, because a large dead-space cavity will result from the resection. The median and lateral sacral arteries and their accompanying veins usually are the major sources of this bleeding. Large-bore, closed suction wound drains are used to collapse dead space and evacuate any postoperative bleeding. The wound is reapproximated in a layered, tensionless fashion according to individual surgeon preference. This may necessitate mobilization of soft tissue flaps but generally can be achieved without resorting to more elaborate reconstructive measures.

Dorsal sacrectomy works well for smaller lesions of the midsacrum and distal sacrum that do not yet require resection through the level of the sacroiliac joint. Although MacCarty et al. described amputation as high as the first sacral segment, this method is less attractive because the ability to accurately dissect tissue planes of the upper presacrum is unpredictable from this approach and risks a major vascular injury, inadvertent entry into the rectum, or violation of the tumor capsule during attempts to osteotomize the ventral sacrum and sacroiliac joints from behind.[50] These difficulties are best addressed by combining the techniques of dorsal sacrectomy with a ventral approach for lesions requiring amputation through the level of the sacroiliac joints.

Combined Ventral and Dorsal Approach to Sacral Resection

A sequential ventral and dorsal approach to facilitate high sacral amputation was described by Bowers in 1948.[51] Transabdominal exposure was used to gain control of the hypogastric vessels and permit a safer dorsal sacrectomy. The ventral approach allows mobilization of the rectum off of the tumor under direct vision rather than by blind finger dissection. Furthermore, should the rectum be involved by tumor, either as a consequence of direct extension or because of seeding from an injudicious transrectal biopsy, it can be isolated for en bloc resection with the sacral specimen. This is impossible from the dorsal approach alone.

Localio et al. popularized a synchronous abdominosacral approach for sacral lesions.[52] They favored a lateral decubitus position to allow simultaneous ventral and dorsal exposure without requiring patient repositioning. The abdominal approach begins through an obliquely oriented flank incision centered midway between the costal margin and the iliac crest. The retroperitoneum is dissected, and the descending colon and rectum are mobilized rightward. The internal iliac arteries and veins are controlled with vessel loops, and the entire perimeter of the tumor mass is defined ventrally. Tumor vessels, which usually emanate from the lateral and median sacral arteries, are interrupted directly. The sacrum is exposed through a separate dorsal incision, and with division of the anococcygeal ligament, the two wounds become communicating. As with dorsal sacrectomy, the lateral muscular attachments onto the sacrum and sacroiliac joint are released. With the hypogastric vessels temporarily occluded, the sacrotuberous and sacrospinous ligaments are detached, and the posterior sacroiliac ligaments are divided rostrally up to the intended level of amputation. The sacrum and sacroiliac joint can then be osteotomized ventrally and dorsally under direct vision. Localio et al. suggested that this technique of synchronous abdominosacral resection resulted in less blood loss than did sequential resection.[52] Simpson et al. reported their experience with 12 patients with tumors in the cephalad part of the sacrum managed with a modified simultaneous ventral and dorsal approach via an ilioinguinal incision extended circumferentially around the body wall to the midline dorsally.[53] Although it is possible to expose the sacrum ventrally and dorsally simultaneously in the lateral position, it is more difficult to expose both of them well. The lateral position complicates efforts at soft tissue reconstruction and mechanical stabilization that are integral to the success of these procedures.

A sequential ventral and dorsal approach with pedicled rectus abdominis pull-through flap reconstruction is favored for high sacral resections (this often is performed with the aid of a plastic surgeon). The technique of surgical resection is essentially similar to that described by Stener and Gunterberg.[54] The rectus abdominis pull-through flap originally was described for reconstruction and repair of perineal wounds.[55,56] Its routine use in the closure of the large surgical voids created by high sacrectomy has virtually eliminated problems with prolonged wound drainage and breakdown.[57-59] Although the surgery is necessarily interrupted by the need for patient repositioning, the superior visibility and the working ease made possible through the sequential approach more than justify this inconvenience.

A mechanical bowel preparation is begun preoperatively, and broad-spectrum antibiotic prophylaxis is initiated. Because blood loss can be substantial (7–80 L in some series), adequate transfusion reserves and IV lines for volume resuscitation are placed in advance.[60,61] The cell saver can be used, except in cases of malignant tumor. The operation begins with abdominal exposure. Incisions for a transversely oriented myocutaneous flap based on the upper rectus abdominis muscles are outlined in the epigastrium; a midline lower abdominal entry is employed (Fig. 114-1). Although the sacrum can be exposed ventrally by bilateral extraperitoneal dissection, a transperitoneal route usually is preferred. After the bowel has been "packed off," the dorsal parietal peritoneum is opened unilaterally, the ureters are identified, and the iliac vessels are dissected bilaterally. If the rectum is to be spared, it is mobilized off of the tumor capsule ventrally after incision of the retrorectal peritoneal reflection. The tumor capsule is outlined circumferentially. Bleeding from the venous plexus in the loose areolar tissue surrounding the tumor can be profuse. Internal iliac and middle sacral arteries and veins are ligated along with any tumor vessels, and both external arteries should be preserved.[62] It may not be

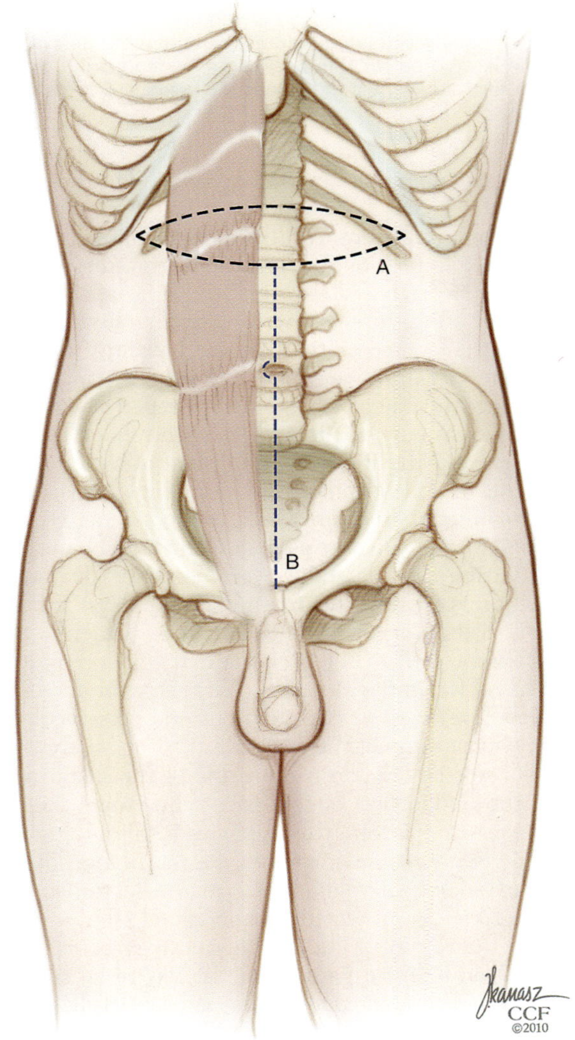

FIGURE 114-1. A sequential ventral and dorsal approach with pedicled rectus abdominis pull-through flap reconstruction is favored for high sacral resections. The ventral operation begins with abdominal exposure. Incisions for a transversely oriented myocutaneous flap (A) based on the upper rectus abdominis muscles are outlined in the epigastrium; a midline lower abdominal entry is employed (B). (Copyright Cleveland Clinic Foundation.)

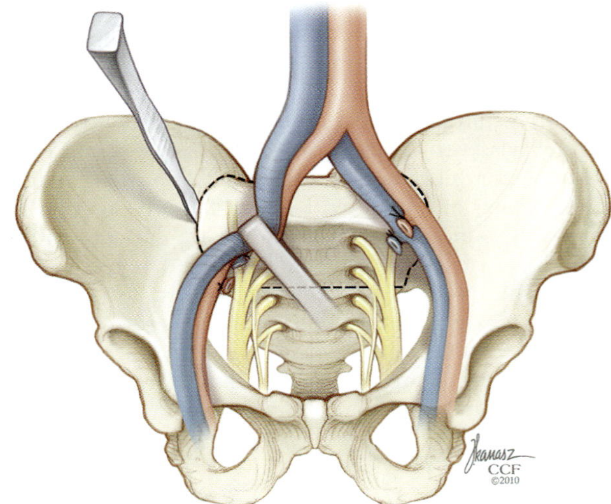

FIGURE 114-2. High sacral resections require mobilization of the iliac veins medially and laterally during the osteotomies. A chisel osteotome is favored for this because saws and drills are more apt to entrain adjacent soft tissues. (Copyright Cleveland Clinic Foundation.)

possible to attain absolute hemostasis until after the tumor is completely resected.

High sacral resections require mobilization of the iliac veins medially and laterally during the osteotomies (Fig. 114-2). The surgeon is advised to preemptively ligate the iliolumbar veins, entering through the back wall to avoid avulsion and a potential source of troublesome bleeding. The sacral foramina are visualized ventrally and serve as landmarks to guide the ventral sacral osteotomy. The peritoneal investment and periosteum are incised transversely at the sacral promontory, and the incision is reflected downward to the level of the intended amputation. Inevitably, this measure divides the sympathetic trunks and, in high sacral resections, also sacrifices the hypogastric plexus. The lumbosacral nerve trunks coursing caudolaterally over the sacral alae and the sacroiliac joints are dissected free and protected. A transverse osteotomy is then begun through the ventral sacrum at the selected level (see Fig. 114-2). Usually this incorporates the ventral sacral foramina, in which case the sacral nerves exiting at that level are first dissected out and preserved. If the osteotomy must transect the midbody of S1 above the foramina, it will not be feasible to save any of the sacral nerves. Because the midportion of the osteotomy enters the sacral canal, it is best to perform this step with a chisel to minimize the chance of premature entry into the thecal sac. The bone cuts are extended inferolaterally into the sacroiliac joints, with care taken to protect the lumbosacral trunks and any remaining sacral roots. The apically convex course of the osteotomy parallels the path of the nerves to be spared. A chisel osteotome is favored for this, as saws and drills are more apt to entrain adjacent soft tissues. The peritoneal investment and the periosteum are incised caudally as far as the greater sciatic notch, and the cortex is scored ventrally to create a stress riser that facilitates subsequent completion osteotomy from behind. Waxing the osteotomy cuts helps reduce bleeding and improves visibility. A commonly used alternative involves the passage of a Gigli saw through the sacral foramina to be picked up from the posterior approach.

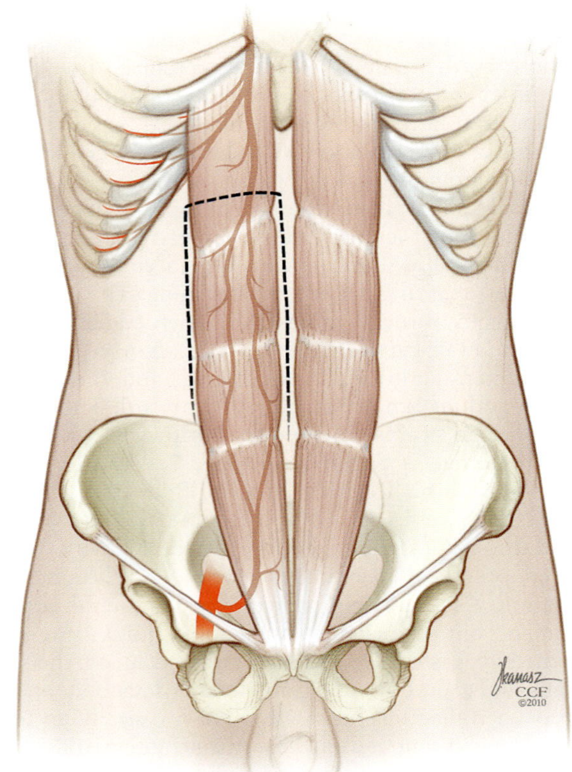

FIGURE 114-3. A rectus abdominis myocutaneous flap based on the inferior epigastric vessels is prepared. (Copyright Cleveland Clinic Foundation.)

In those cases in which the rectum is to be resected, the rectosigmoid junction is mobilized in preparation for division with a mechanical stapler. The stapled-closed stumps of bowel may then be invaginated and oversewn with serosal sutures to lessen the chances of wound soilage. The rostral and middle rectal vessels are isolated and divided, and the rectovesical or rectouterine peritoneal reflection is incised to allow access to the pelvic floor. Peritoneal adhesions between the tumor mass and the bladder or pelvic side walls should not be simply lysed, because this may indicate a need for pelvic exenteration if the surgery is to have a curative intent. Wide local excision, including bladder, prostate, vagina, cervix, or endopelvic fascia, and contained vessels, may be required in such cases.[63,64] Access for deep pelvic dissection can be enhanced through division of the symphysis pubis and introduction of a rib spreader to open the pelvic ring ventrally.

At this point, a rectus abdominis myocutaneous flap based on the inferior epigastric vessels is prepared (Fig. 114-3). The ventral abdominal wall skin island is sealed with iodine-impregnated plastic adhesive dressing and then stowed within the pelvis (Fig. 114-4). It may be helpful for the purpose of hemostasis and for anatomic demarcation during the subsequent dorsal approach to place large sheets of gelatin sponges, silicone elastomer (Silastic, Dow Corning, Midland, MI), or Gore-Tex (W. L. Gore and Associates, Inc., Elkton, MD) into the plane of dissection between the sacrectomy specimen, with any attached presacral mass and the iliac vessels, sacral plexi, and ureters remaining undisturbed. If required, a colostomy is performed, and the wound is closed layer by layer.

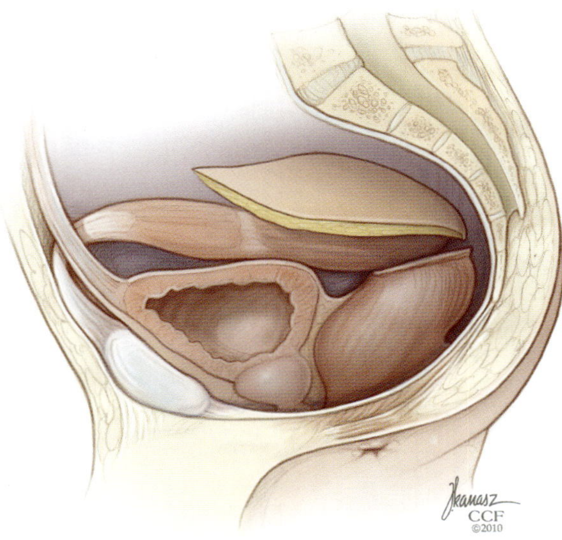

FIGURE 114-4. The rectus abdominis myocutaneous flap is then stowed within the pelvis. (Copyright Cleveland Clinic Foundation.)

The patient is then repositioned prone on a padded thoracoabdominal rest, allowing the abdomen to hang free. A dorsal midline incision extending from the L5-S1 interlaminar space to the level of the external anal sphincter is outlined (Fig. 114-5). If the rectum is to be included with the specimen, the caudal limb of the incision continues as an ellipse encircling the anus. Alternatively, the perineal dissection may be performed during the abdominal exposure if the patient is operated in the lithotomy position with the buttocks elevated on a small cushion. Any skin compromised by tumor, previous biopsy, radiation-induced change, or prior surgery should be excised with the specimen. Dissection through the soft tissues is deepened in a conical fashion: at the summit is any involved skin and at the base is the biopsy tract and any tumor erupting out of the dorsal sacrum (see Fig. 114-5). This again reemphasizes the objective of an en bloc resection with a margin of healthy, uninvolved tissues.

Rostrally, the interspinous and interlaminar ligaments at L5-S1 are dissected out to enable isolation of the thecal sac in preparation for its ligation immediately below the level of exit of the last nerve roots to be preserved. If the S2 roots are to be spared, a limited rostral sacral laminectomy is needed to allow their visualization. Dorsally, the sacrospinalis muscles are sectioned transversely, and the dorsal sacroiliac ligament is released from the ilium (Fig. 114-6). Laterally, the gluteal musculature is transected, leaving a cuff attached at its sacral origin. This uncovers the piriformis muscles, which are, in turn, divided at their musculotendinous junction. The superior gluteal vessels and nerves are found at the upper border of the piriformis, and the inferior gluteal vessels and the sciatic, pudendal, and posterior femoral cutaneous nerves are found exiting the pelvis at its lower edge. These should be identified carefully and preserved whenever possible. If rectal resection is not planned, the caudal border of the specimen is freed by division of the anococcygeal ligament just proximal to the anal sphincter. The sacrotuberous ligament is detached from the ischial tuberosity, and the coccygeal muscles are cut. The

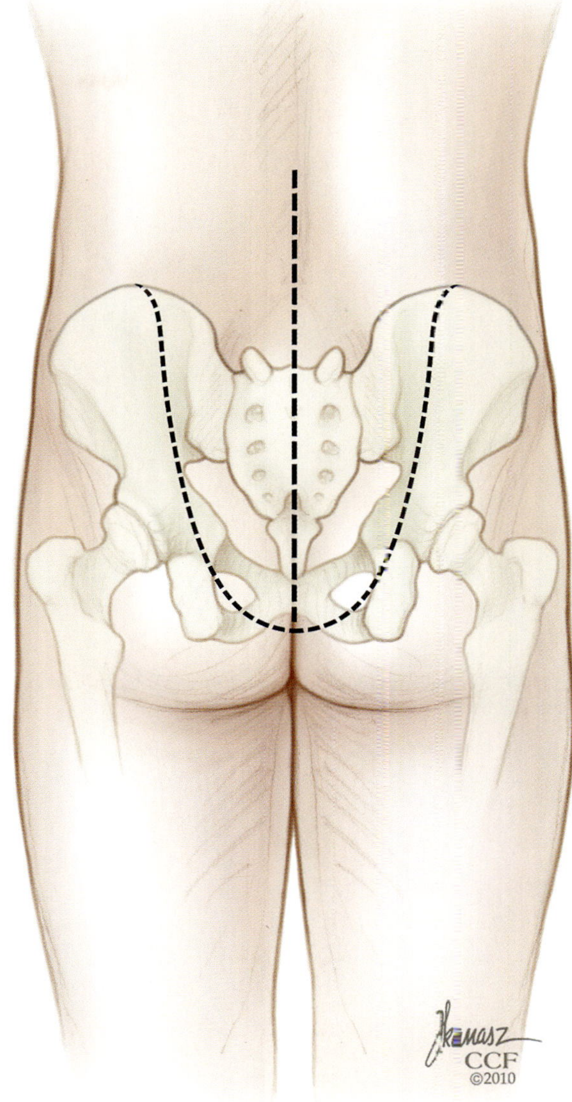

FIGURE 114-5. A dorsal midline incision extending from the L5-S1 interlaminar space to the level of the external anal sphincter is outlined. (Copyright Cleveland Clinic Foundation.)

sacrospinous ligament is conveniently detached by an osteotomy cut across the base of the ischial spine. If the rectum is to be included with the specimen, the anus is dissected circumferentially with additional division of the levator musculature.

The soft tissue dissection is now finished, and the field is prepared for completion osteotomy (Fig. 114-7). A finger is introduced through the anococcygeal interval and the greater sciatic notch on either side to redevelop the presacral space and palpate the previously outlined osteotomy cuts from within the pelvis (Fig. 114-8). This helps guide the dorsal cuts to ensure an accurate intercept with the ventral osteotomies. The osteotomy along the ilium can exit into the sciatic notch either medial or lateral to the ischial spine. The sacrum is free and can be lifted out of the wound dorsally when the

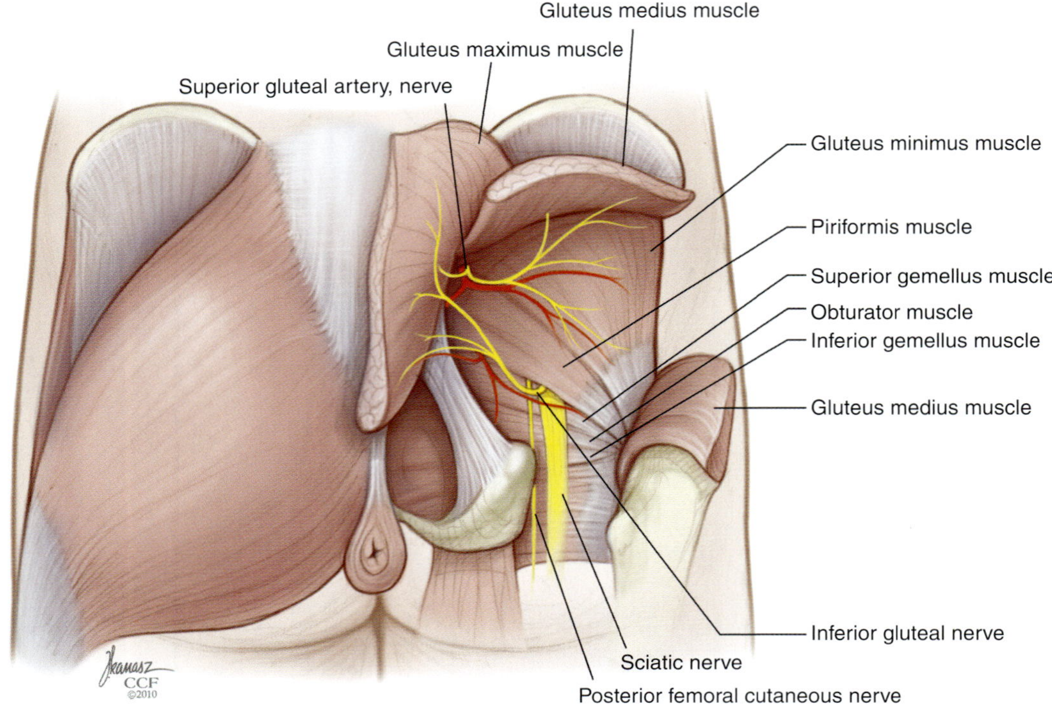

FIGURE 114-6. Dorsal muscles, nerves, and vessels should be identified carefully and preserved whenever possible. (Copyright Cleveland Clinic Foundation.)

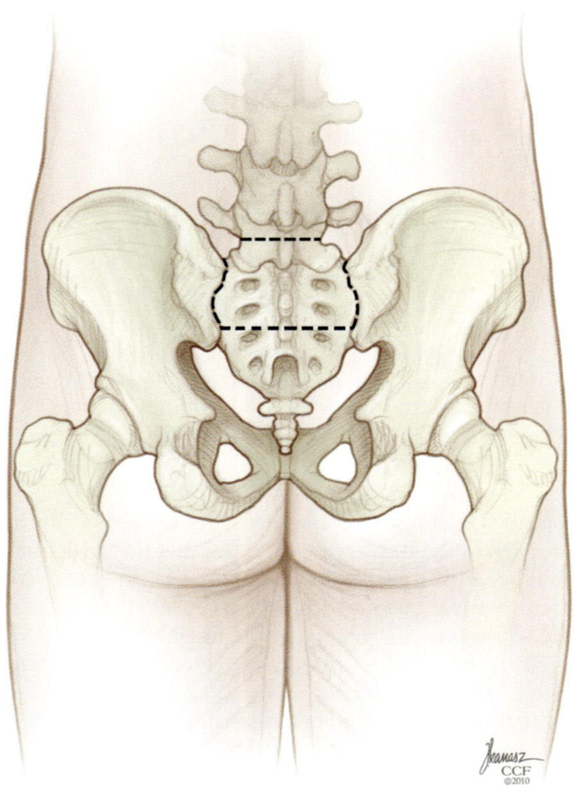

FIGURE 114-7. The soft tissue dissection is now finished and the field prepared for completion osteotomy. (Copyright Cleveland Clinic Foundation.)

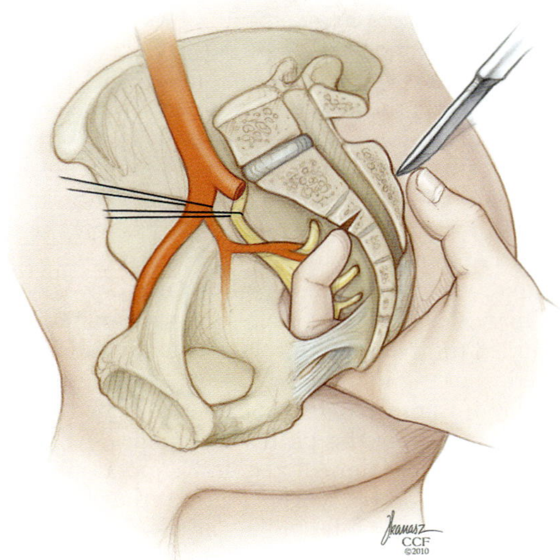

FIGURE 114-8. A finger is introduced through the anococcygeal interval and the greater sciatic notch on either side to redevelop the presacral space and palpate the previously outlined osteotomy cuts from within the pelvis. This helps guide the dorsal cuts to ensure an accurate intercept with the ventral osteotomies. (Copyright Cleveland Clinic Foundation.)

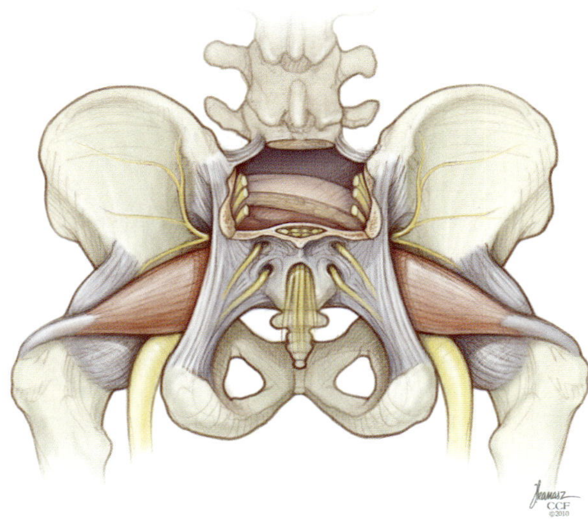

FIGURE 114-9. Following completion of the osteotomies, the sacrum is free and can be lifted out of the wound dorsally. (Copyright Cleveland Clinic Foundation.)

lower sacral roots coursing laterally toward the sacral plexi and pudendal nerves are sequentially divided (Fig. 114-9). Bleeding can be profuse at this stage—bone edges should be waxed expeditiously and bleeding from larger vessels promptly secured with ligatures or hemoclips.

Removal of the sacrum in this manner creates a large trap-door opening into the pelvis. It is desirable to obliterate as much of this dead space as possible. Toward this end, the gluteal muscles can be reapproximated to bone or to one another, a measure that also may enhance their function postoperatively by reestablishing an origin for them. Large-bore, bulb-type closed suction drains are placed into the wound after copious antibiotic irrigation. The rectus abdominis myocutaneous flap is now retrieved through the sacrectomy window, trimmed, and sewn into place in a layered fashion (Fig. 114-10). We have been far more satisfied with this reconstructive method than with the alternatives of primary closure or reconstruction with reversed latissimus dorsi flaps, gluteal flaps, or gracilis flaps. Microvascular free flap reconstruction is another option; however, it further escalates the technical requirements of an already demanding procedure. The rectus abdominis pull-through flap is recommended, especially in circumstances of previous surgery or irradiation, when the prospects for successful primary closure are remote. It largely averts problems with rectal prolapse into the wound during defecation and obviates the need for mesh closure of the dorsal peritoneal or fascial defect.

Total Sacrectomy

Tumors in which surgical extirpation requires total or near-total sacrectomy present an additional challenge because of the difficulties in reestablishing lumbopelvic stability. Integrity of the pelvic ring depends on ligamentous stabilization ventrally at the pubic symphysis and dorsally at each of the sacroiliac joints. Although the precise extent of sacroiliac joint that must be preserved to maintain clinical stability is unknown, cadaveric studies have shown that patients can bear weight as long as at least 50% of the sacroiliac joint

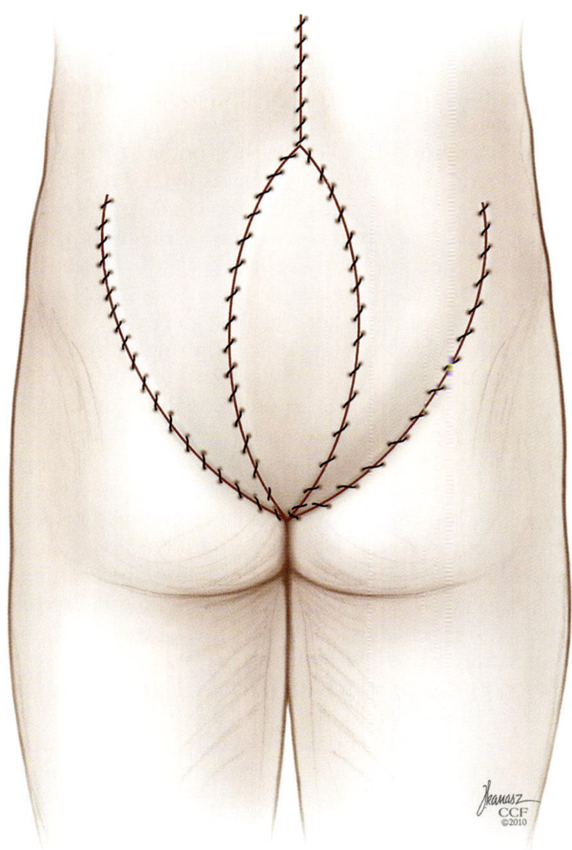

FIGURE 114-10. The rectus abdominis myocutaneous flap can be retrieved through the sacrectomy window, trimmed, and sewn into place in a layered fashion. (Copyright Cleveland Clinic Foundation.)

remains intact.[54,65] Involvement of the upper S1 segment has been regarded by some surgeons as a contraindication to surgery because of the extreme instability that would result from its resection. Certainly, if less than 50% of the sacroiliac joint remains intact, strong consideration should be given to supplemental stabilization to prevent low back pain and instability.

Only a limited number of cases of total sacrectomy have been reported in the literature. The methods of sacral resection and soft tissue reconstruction in total sacrectomy are fundamentally similar to those just discussed. Rather than a transverse osteotomy through the upper sacrum, however, the lowermost disc space is divided and the caudal end plate of L5 thoroughly denuded of soft tissue and cartilage.

With the spine functionally disconnected from the sacrum, lumbopelvic reconstruction is highly recommended but may not be mandatory.[66] Various lumbopelvic reconstruction techniques have been reported in the literature. These include sacroiliac joint screw fixation, iliac-sacral screw fixation, posterior iliosacral plating and screw fixation, custom-made prosthesis, Galveston rod fixation, iliac screws, and transiliac rods.[45,67-75] Chapter 152 provides a review of current state-of-the-art complex lumbosacropelvic reconstruction techniques.

Postoperative Considerations

Patients undergoing major sacral resections are kept in the ICU for the immediate postoperative period. Ongoing assessments are made for any blood or blood product replacements, because major fluid shifts are anticipated, and strict vigilance is required to avoid either under- or overreplacement. Clotting parameters and electrolyte status are monitored carefully in light of any fluid replacements. Keeping the patient on an air mattress is a justifiable precaution to guard against sacral decubiti and wound breakdown. Antibiotics are continued for 24 hours after removal of the last wound drain. Aggressive prophylaxis against deep vein thrombosis with sequential compression devices on the lower extremities and fractionated heparin is advised in view of recumbency, dissection of the pelvic veins, and possible neurologic deficit. Every attempt is made to mobilize the patient as soon as cardiopulmonary reserve and perceived dorsal pelvic ring stability allow. Although indwelling bladder catheters are discontinued within the first several days, one must be prepared for a high incidence of at least temporary voiding dysfunction during early convalescence. Voiding dysfunction can be dealt with appropriately by a program of scheduled intermittent catheterizations. Fecal incontinence, if persistent, generally can be accommodated with a constipating diet and prompted evacuation by digital stimulation, enema, or oral laxatives, as for spinal cord injury patients.

The level of sacral amputation correlates well with the expected neurologic deficit and postoperative function[7,76] (Table 114-1). High resection of S1 nerve roots usually results in significant motor impairment, loss of sphincter control, and sexual dysfunction. Middle resections involving S2-3 can, infrequently, lead to motor dysfunction, but saddle anesthesia and sphincter dysfunction are common. Low amputations distal to S2 typically lead to minimal deficit, with preservation of sphincter and motor function but possible sexual dysfunction. Bowel and bladder function seem to remain fairly normal when both S3 roots or the unilateral S1-5 roots are spared.[77,78] The objective of providing a patient with a true oncologic procedure, however, should not be compromised by the attempt to preserve continence. In males, the extensive dissection of the sympathetic and parasympathetic plexi will expectedly diminish erectile function and the capacity for antegrade ejaculation. Patients need to be counseled preoperatively about the potential consequences of sacral resection for anogenital and reproductive function.

Somatosensory and motor deficits that result from sacral resection usually are well compensated. If the S1 roots, lumbosacral trunks, and sciatic nerves can all be preserved, the disability in the legs is very minor. With sacrifice of the S1 roots, there is a noticeable decrease in plantar flexion power, although this is accommodated by hypertrophy of the lateral gastrocnemius muscles with time. Loss of the L5 roots or injury to the lumbosacral trunks adds to this the further difficulty of footdrop, which may be counteracted, in part, through the use of antiflexion orthoses. The glutei, which are the main physiologic extensors of the hips, often are greatly impaired after upper sacral resection as a result of detachment from their origin, denervation, or diminished blood supply. Loss of gluteal function becomes especially evident on attempts to rise from a seated posture or ascend stairs. In time, increased hamstring and adductor magnus function may help compensate for this loss. Sensory loss is rarely of a magnitude to affect protective sensibilities adversely or cause a sensory ataxia. Perineal hypesthesia is, of course, anticipated; the legs are affected to the degree that the lumbosacral trunk, the posterior femoral cutaneous nerve, and the S1 root are compromised. Generally, this is a less significant problem than are the concomitant motor deficits.

The main sources of surgical mortality in upper sacral resection are intraoperative blood loss and postoperative wound sepsis. These have generally ranged between 0 and 15% in various reports.[52,64,68,79,80] Embolization of sacral tumors is a useful adjuvant therapy that can aid in surgical management by reducing intraoperative blood loss for benign, malignant, and metastatic lesions of the sacrum.[81] Wound complications, including prolonged drainage, delayed breakdown, infections, seromas, cerebrospinal fluid leaks, and pelvic prolapse, were common in the past and probably have been underreported. Sung et al.[79] and Touran et al.[80] have acknowledged wound complication rates of 11% and 25%, respectively.

Summary

Sacral tumors pose a formidable challenge because of their rarity and the difficulty in diagnosis and treatment. Most tumors arising in the sacral canal or in the distal bony sacrum are well handled by conventional techniques. Tumors with more proximal involvement necessitating total sacrectomy, however, pose the greatest management challenges. Sacrectomy for malignant disease remains a highly morbid undertaking with a significant chance for local failure. At times, past

TABLE 114-1

Expected Dysfunction Following Sacral Tumor Resection Based on Sacral Nerve Roots Sacrificed

Sacrectomy Classification	Nerve Root Involvement	Neurologic Outcome	Comments
Hemisacrectomy	Variable	Unilateral paresis (S1), anesthesia (S2-3)	Potential preservation of sphincter and sexual function
Low	Distal to S3	Potential sexual dysfunction	Preservation of sphincter and motor function possible
Middle	S2-3 and distal	Sexual dysfunction, anesthesia, sphincter dysfunction	Functional continence possible if unilateral S2 root preserved
High	S1 and distal	Sexual dysfunction, anesthesia, continence, motor paresis (S1)	

Modified from Sciubba DM, Petteys RJ, Garces-Ambrossi GI, et al: Diagnosis and management of sacral tumors. *J Neurosurg Spine* 10:244–256, 2009, Table 2.

results have been compromised by an insufficient appreciation of the need for en bloc resection of malignant lesions with an inviolate margin of normal tissue. Otherwise, patients may be condemned to early recurrence or remote dissemination. At other times, surgical efforts have been diminished by suboptimal wound closure. The best results are achieved by drawing on the expertise of a multidisciplinary surgical team. The collaboration of oncologic, plastic, urologic, and orthopaedic surgeons may be of major assistance to the spine surgeon who undertakes a high or total sacral resection. Physical methods of tumor extirpation are relatively crude, and biologic barriers will be overcome only when these mechanical techniques can be combined with therapies directed toward the molecular genetics of the neoplastic process itself.

KEY REFERENCES

Cahill D: Surgical approaches to the lumbar spine and sacrum. In Rea G, editor: *Spine tumors*, Rolling Meadows, IL, 1994, American Association of Neurological Surgeons.

Fourney DR, Gokaslan ZL: Sacral tumors: primary and metastatic. In Fehlings M, Dickman CA, Gokaslan ZL, editors: *Spinal cord and spinal column tumors: principles and practice*, New York, 2006, Thieme, pp 404–419.

Fourney DR, Gokaslan ZL: Surgical approaches for the resection of sacral tumors. In Fehlings M, Dickman CA, Gokaslan ZL, editors: *Spinal cord and spinal column tumors: principles and practice*, New York, 2006, Thieme, pp 632–648.

Manaster BJ, Graham T: Imaging of sacral tumors. *Neurosurg Focus* 15(2):E2, 2003.

Payer M: Neurological manifestation of sacral tumors. *Neurosurg Focus* 15(2):E1, 2003.

Sciubba DM, Petteys RJ, Garces-Ambrossi GL, et al: Diagnosis and management of sacral tumors. *J Neurosurg Spine* 10(3):244–256, 2009.

Zhang HY, Thongtrangan I, Balabhadra RS, et al: Surgical techniques for total sacrectomy and spinopelvic reconstruction. *Neurosurg Focus* 15(2):E5, 2003.

REFERENCES

The complete reference list is available online at expertconsult.com.

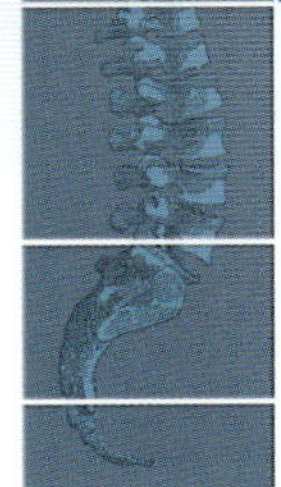

CHAPTER 115

Tarlov Cysts

Frank Feigenbaum | Jean-Marc Voyadzis |
Fraser C. Henderson

A Tarlov cyst is a bulbous enlargement of a spinal nerve root cerebrospinal fluid (CSF) space that is distinct from other meningeal cysts, such as dural ectasia or meningeal diverticula. Tarlov cysts most often are found in the sacral spinal canal, where they can produce bone erosion and compression of adjacent spinal nerve roots, resulting in a debilitating sacral radiculopathy syndrome.

Tarlov first described these cysts in 1938 during his autopsy studies of the filum terminale at the Montreal Neurological Institute.[1] Since his seminal report, numerous cases of symptomatic Tarlov cysts have been published in the literature.[2-7] With the advent of MRI, our ability to diagnose meningeal cysts, such as Tarlov cysts, has been enhanced.

The treatment of symptomatic Tarlov cysts has evolved, along with our understanding of their pathophysiology. Various therapeutic strategies have been described over the years, with more recent literature trending toward definitive surgical treatment. In this chapter the pathologic, radiographic, and clinical characteristics of Tarlov cysts are presented, and the current treatment options are discussed.

Epidemiology and Histology

Tarlov, or perineurial, cysts are one of the most common forms of meningeal cyst. Estimates of the prevalence of meningeal cysts, including Tarlov cysts, in the general population vary, but generally are in the 5% range.[8] In a study of 500 consecutive patients with back pain undergoing lumbosacral MRI, 5% were found to have one or more meningeal cysts. Among this latter group, the cyst was thought to be the source of the symptoms in 1% of the cases. Tarlov cysts, particularly those that are symptomatic, are more common among women. The reason for this is unclear, and we have postulated that there may be gender-related differences in the fundamental makeup of dura mater or spinal nerve roots that produce this epidemiologic disparity.

Tarlov distinguished perineurial cysts from other meningeal cysts based on several histologic criteria.[1,9,10] He defined them as perineurial dilations that develop between the endoneurium and perineurium, typically of the S2 or 3 nerve roots, just proximal to the junction of the dorsal root ganglion and nerve root (Fig. 115-1). Simply stated, each cyst is a dilated spinal nerve root sheath, and the individual nerve fibers of that root are found running within the cyst cavity or its inner lining. Other meningeal cyst subtypes, such as meningeal diverticula and arachnoid cysts, typically are devoid of nerve root fiber elements.

Tarlov cysts can be single or multiple, and can develop anywhere along the spine where nerve roots are present. Progressive cyst enlargement can cause significant bony erosion and impingement of adjacent spinal nerve roots, producing corresponding radiculopathies. For example, a Tarlov cyst in the sacral spinal canal arising from the S3 nerve root can cause symptomatic impingement of the ipsilateral S2 nerve root beside it, and of the S4 or S5 nerve root below (Fig. 115-2). A Tarlov cyst can also produce contralateral symptoms if it is large enough to extend across the midline and compress contralateral nerve roots. Additionally, the nerve root fibers running inside a Tarlov cyst often are attenuated and splayed out over the inner wall of the cyst. This neural fiber alteration and stretching also are suspected of causing symptoms.

Tarlov cysts occasionally can be found in combination with other meningeal cysts. For example, patients with connective tissue disorders, such as Marfan syndrome, can have Tarlov cysts and large ectatic dural cysts so extensive that the distal spinal sac extends out into the pelvis (Fig. 115-3).

The pathogenesis of Tarlov cysts remains unclear. Tarlov proposed that cyst formation could be the result of trauma, ischemic degeneration, inflammation, or hemorrhagic infiltration from the subarachnoid space.[1,9,10] Some patients with symptomatic Tarlov cysts report a history of sacral trauma, and evidence of old hemorrhage in the form of hemosiderin deposits and dystrophic calcification within Tarlov cyst walls supports prior trauma as an etiologic factor.[7,11-13] Other reports have suggested that Tarlov cysts result from arachnoidal proliferation or blockage of perineurial fluid flow.[14,15] Nabors et al. support a developmental origin, although an association between Tarlov cysts and spinal dysraphism is not as strong as that with other types of meningeal cysts.[16] Only two patients with symptomatic Tarlov cysts and spina bifida have been reported, and the relationship could have been coincidental.[7,17]

Strully et al.[18,19] and Smith[20] proposed that Tarlov cysts form as a result of increased CSF hydrostatic pressure. They point out that spinal nerve roots are in communication with the thecal sac, and that there is myelographic evidence that spinal fluid flows within the nerve roots and could produce

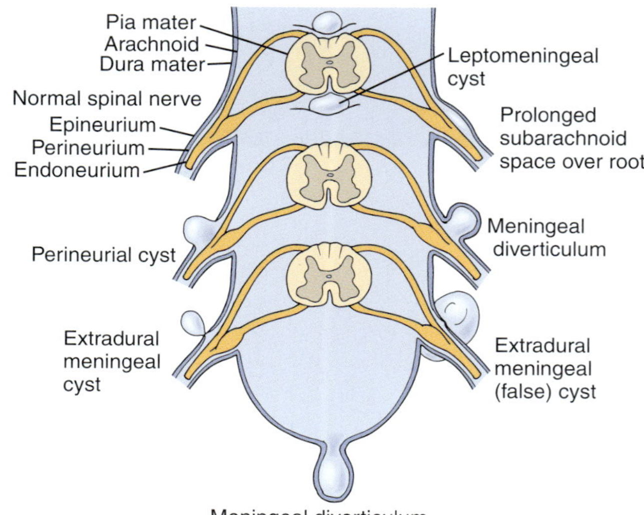

FIGURE 115-1. This diagram illustrates some of the different types of dural meningeal cysts, including the perineurial (Tarlov) cyst.

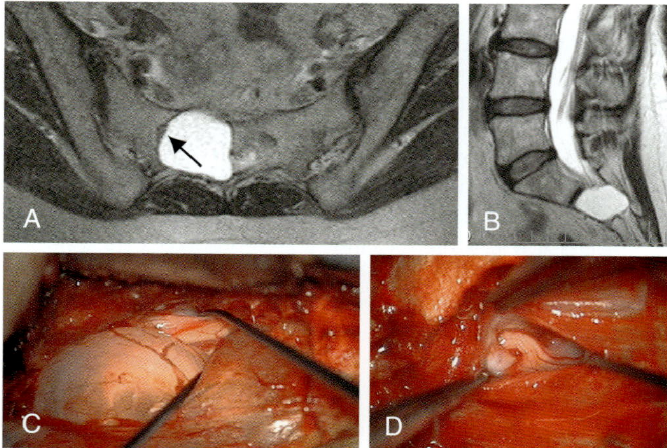

FIGURE 115-2. Axial (**A**) and sagittal (**B**) T2-weighted sacral MRIs reveal a large Tarlov cyst in the S2 region central and rightward within the spinal canal. Its contents have imaging qualities similar to those of cerebrospinal fluid (CSF), and there is widening of the spinal canal around it due to bone erosion. A compressed nerve root is seen adjacent to the cyst *(arrow)*. **C,** Intraoperatively, the compressed nerve root (upper Penfield dissector) was visualized after retracting the cyst (lower Penfield dissector). The cyst was found to arise from the S3 nerve root, and the compressed nerve root was S2. **D,** View inside a Tarlov cyst. The nerve root fibers enter the cyst through the ostium and then splay out over the cyst wall.

dilatation due to either higher hydrostatic pressure or inherent, traumatic, or iatrogenic weakness in the nerve root sheath. They also point out that the frequency and size of Tarlov cysts along the spine can be correlated with the rostral-caudal hydrostatic pressure gradient.[17,18] Several reports on patients with Tarlov cysts have documented either a history of straining or coughing or an exacerbation of symptoms by these maneuvers.[7,10,11,18] We also are aware of two cases of Tarlov cysts in patients with pseudotumor cerebri. However, no criteria have been established to determine who might benefit from CSF shunting for Tarlov cysts, and investigations are ongoing.

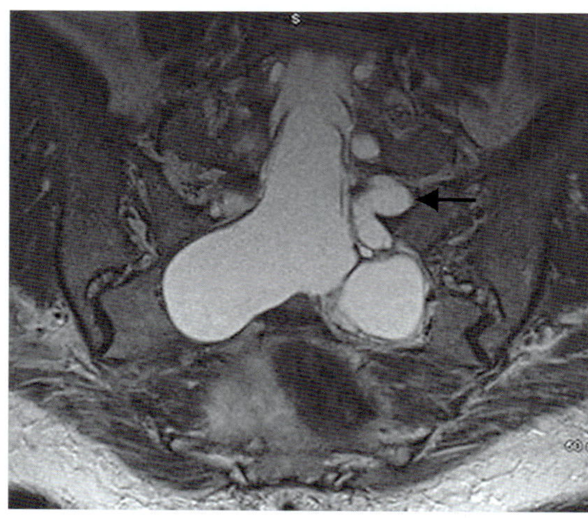

FIGURE 115-3. This coronal T2-weighted MRI of the sacrum from a patient with Marfan syndrome reveals multiple meningeal cysts. The distal spinal sac continues on as a large ectatic dural cyst eroding rightward into the sacrum. Also, multiple separate Tarlov cysts are seen adjacent to the spinal sac, particularly on the left *(arrow)*.

Diagnosis

The treatment of a symptomatic Tarlov cyst first requires a correct diagnosis. Unfortunately, many patients languish with undiagnosed or untreated symptomatic cysts due to the incorrect "rule" that Tarlov cysts always are asymptomatic, regardless of the presence of blatant compression of adjacent nerves or extensive bone erosion. Such patients often are relegated to an escalation of narcotics, injection procedures, and neuromodulatory medications as they become progressively more symptomatic. It is not uncommon to encounter patients who have developed narcotic dependency after management with extended-release morphine, transdermal fentanyl, or implanted pain pumps before they are finally referred for meningeal cyst evaluation.

Even more unfortunately, we have encountered patients with symptomatic Tarlov cysts that were misdiagnosed with a variety of other ailments and treated unsuccessfully with a variety of procedures, such as hysterectomy, laparoscopic exploration, endometriosis surgery, oophorectomy, appendectomy, surgery for piriformis syndrome, sacroiliac joint fusion with implanted cages, fusion of degenerative discs in the adjacent spine, coccygectomy, and urinary bladder procedures (Fig. 115-4).

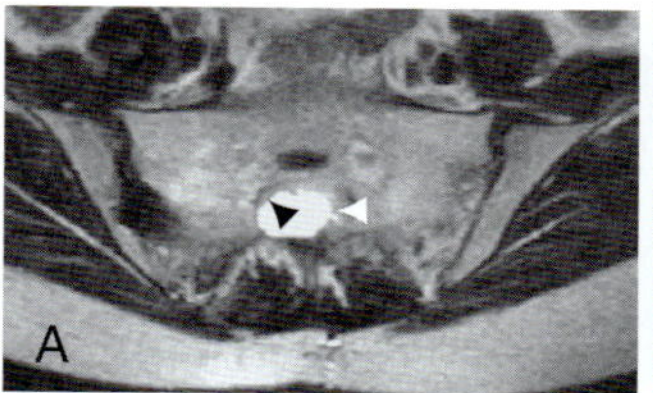

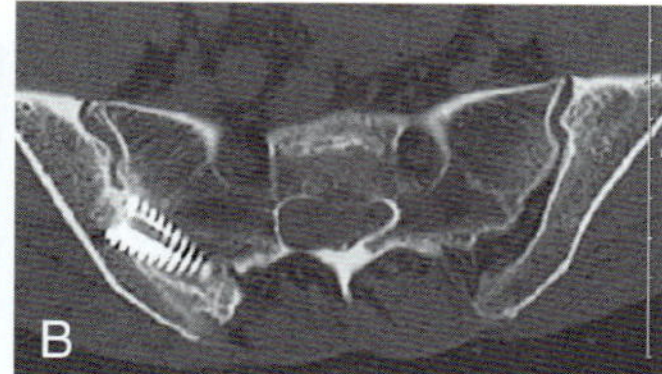

FIGURE 115-4. A, Preoperative axial T2-weighted MRI of the sacrum from a patient with a large Tarlov cyst *(white arrowhead)*. A compressed nerve root is just visible to the right of the cyst *(black arrowhead)*. **B,** This axial CT scan reveals that the patient was misdiagnosed with sacroiliac joint instability. The symptoms did not improve following insertion of a threaded titanium cage to fuse the joint. Symptoms improved only after later treatment of the Tarlov cyst, which can be seen expanding and eroding the ipsilateral spinal canal.

Symptoms

Tarlov cysts can be found anywhere spinal nerve roots are present and can produce corresponding radiculopathic symptoms. In our experience, symptomatic Tarlov cysts are most commonly encountered in the sacral region. The sacral radiculopathy pattern produced can include a multitude of symptoms, including sacral pain and numbness radiating down the backs of the legs to the bottoms of the feet in the S1 or S2 dermatomes; perineal pain; rectal pain; numbness in the S2-5 dermatomes; neurogenic bladder findings such as urgency, frequency, nocturia, and urinary retention with the need to perform a Valsalva or Credé maneuver to initiate voiding (S3-4); bowel dysfunction requiring the use of laxatives (S2-3); dyspareunia in women; and erectile/sexual dysfunction in men. Symptoms often are positional, being exacerbated by sitting or standing and improved by lying down. This finding supports the notion that symptoms are related to variations in hydrostatic cyst pressures. Cyst expansion also can produce adjacent bone erosion, resulting in painful insufficiency fractures.

Patients typically describe a crippling inability to sit, describing the feeling as being like "sitting on a rock," causing them to constantly shift from hip to hip when seated in a fruitless quest to find a comfortable position. They often are unable to participate in sitting-related activities, such as driving, working seated at a desk, dining out, or going to movies, events, and religious services. Many patients are forced to carry cushions or pillows to sit on wherever they go in an attempt to ameliorate their seated discomfort.

The severe limitation on quality of life experienced by these patients often costs them their employment, results in depression as they find themselves progressively housebound and unable to participate in social activities, and contributes to marital dysfunction and divorce. Making matters worse, some patients may be told by medical professionals that Tarlov cysts are always asymptomatic, despite obvious evidence to the contrary.

Differential Diagnosis

The surgeon should be aware of a host of disease entities that may be comorbid or confused with symptomatic Tarlov cysts.

Hydrocephalus, Benign Intracranial Hypertension, or Pseudotumor Cerebri

In addition to producing symptoms such as headaches and visual changes, increased intracranial pressure also may be a factor in the causation of Tarlov cysts. Our evaluation with spinal fluid taps revealed that 1 in 10 patients with symptomatic Tarlov cysts has consistently elevated opening pressures. To further confound the matter, patients with ongoing pressure issues can, like Tarlov patients, also experience back pain, paresthesias, and bowel and bladder changes.

Diagnosis of the subset of patients with comorbid increased spinal fluid pressure and symptomatic Tarlov cysts should rely on ruling out other causes of pain, and findings on a series of lumbar punctures that consistently reveal the CSF pressure to be elevated. An ophthalmologic examination for evidence of papilledema may be useful. However, there is no consensus on the selection criteria for shunting of patients with Tarlov cysts and its contribution to the amelioration of Tarlov cyst–related symptoms is being investigated.

Tethered Cord Syndrome

The presence of a tethered spinal cord sometimes may be overlooked in the setting of a radiographically impressive sacral Tarlov cyst. Such patients typically present with very similar symptoms, including pain and numbness in the low back or sacral region that radiates down the backs of the legs. They also can have overlapping bowel, bladder, and sexual dysfunction. As with Tarlov cysts, the onset of tethered cord symptoms may occur at any time in life, particularly following trauma, childbirth, or hyperflexion of the spine. Patients with connective tissue disorders such as Marfan or Ehlers-Danlos syndrome can have meningeal cysts, including Tarlov cysts, and occult tethered spinal cord even though the conus is at level L1-2 or above.

Unlike Tarlov cysts, however, tethered cord syndrome is associated with toe walking, flat feet or pes cavus, enuresis, and scoliosis. A spinal neurocutaneous marker sometimes may be present. The pain associated with tethered cord syndrome usually is more moderate, exacerbated by straight leg raising or other maneuvers that stretch the cauda equina, and is not affected by upright posture, as with Tarlov cysts. Muscle atrophy is prominent, and especially in the L5- and S1-related muscles. Imaging studies may reveal syringomyelia, descent of the conus to the L2 level or below, and a thickened fatty filum or a lipomeningocoele.

Spinal Stenosis and Occult Spondylolisthesis

Stenosis of the central canal or neural foramina can mimic Tarlov cyst–related symptoms and should be carefully ruled out with appropriate high-resolution imaging and dynamic radiographs. Overlapping symptoms common to both include radicular pain and numbness and urinary symptoms.

Cervical and thoracic stenosis symptoms not typical of Tarlov cysts include long-tract findings, such as spasticity and pathologic reflexes like the Babinski and Hoffman signs, and absence of the abdominal reflex. In cases of lumbar stenosis, patients usually describe pain in the lumbar area, whereas patients with symptomatic sacral Tarlov cysts complain more specifically about pain well below in the sacral region.

Other Masses

Schwannomas and neurofibromas can produce a radiculopathic pattern of symptoms similar to those of Tarlov cysts. They also can share imaging characteristics, such as a cystic appearance, lateral location in the spinal canal, and production of bone erosion and foraminal expansion (Fig. 115-5). However, Tarlov cysts do not enhance on MRI following the administration of gadolinium contrast, which is a characteristic typical of schwannomas and neurofibromas. Instead, they have signal characteristics similar to spinal fluid on all sequences, with the possible exception of differing signal when there has been hemorrhage or accumulation of stagnant, more proteinaceous, spinal fluid within a cyst.

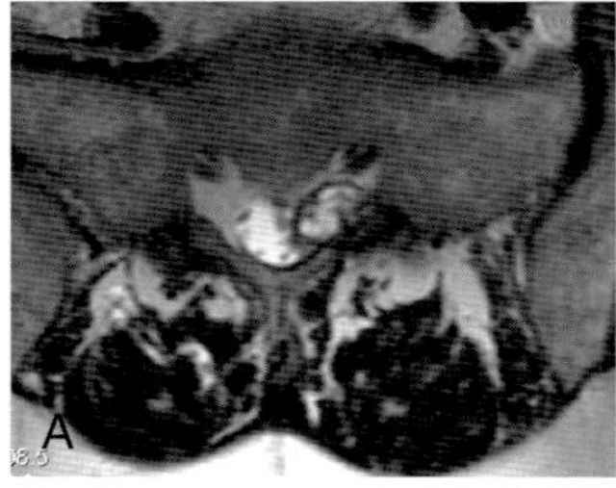
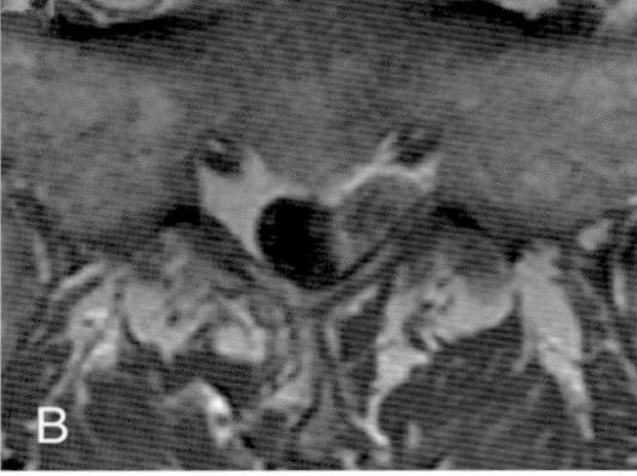

FIGURE 115-5. **A,** This left S1 foramen mass appears hyperintense on T2-weighted imaging. **B,** Unlike a Tarlov cyst, however, it enhances on T1-weighted imaging following gadolinium administration. At surgery, the lesion was found to be a schwannoma.

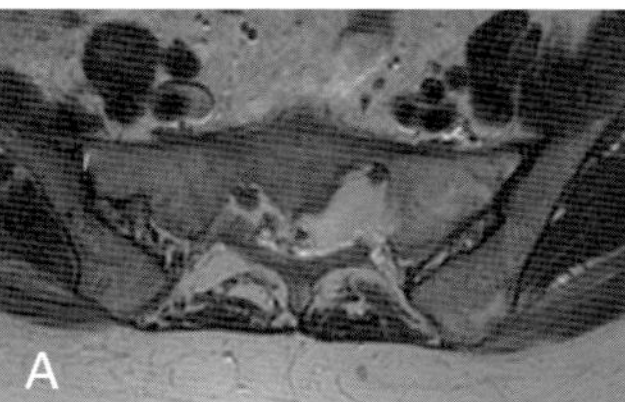
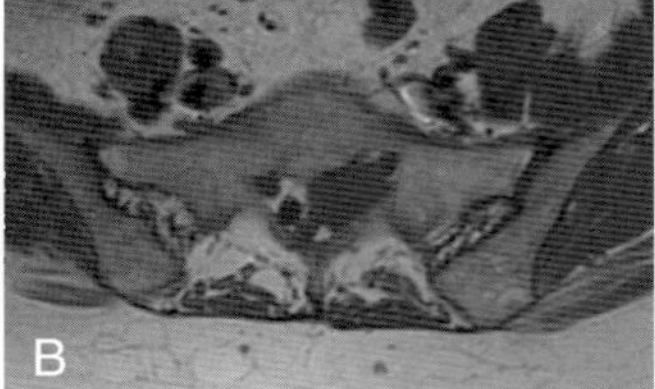

FIGURE 115-6. **A,** The cystic lesion seen centrally and to the left in the spinal canal has imaging characteristics similar to those of a Tarlov cyst on T2-weighted imaging. **B,** However, on T1-weighted imaging, the lesion is hyperintense to cerebrospinal fluid and has some areas of internal heterogeneity. Further workup with CT myelography, needle biopsy, and angiography revealed the lesion to be a large venous angioma.

We also have encountered other lesions with imaging characteristics similar to those of Tarlov cysts. For example, in one case, a large cystic lesion filling the left S1 foramen had the T2-weighted imaging appearance of a Tarlov cyst, but differed on other sequences (Fig. 115-6). Further workup revealed the lesion to be a large venous angioma within the spinal canal.

Radiography

MRI currently is the gold standard for imaging meningeal cysts.[21,22] Not only is it useful for differentiating them from other lesions, but it also can help distinguish among the different types of meningeal cysts, including Tarlov cysts. For example, Tarlov cysts typically are lateral in the spinal canal and arise from an individual spinal nerve root. Nerve root fibers often are identifiable inside the cyst on T2-weighted images (Fig. 115-7). In contrast, meningeal diverticula are found centrally in the spinal canal, and arise from the tip of the spinal sac, not from an individual nerve root. When they are large, Tarlov cysts can be seen to erode and expand the spinal canal or neural foramina and extend into the retroperitoneal pelvis (Fig. 115-8).

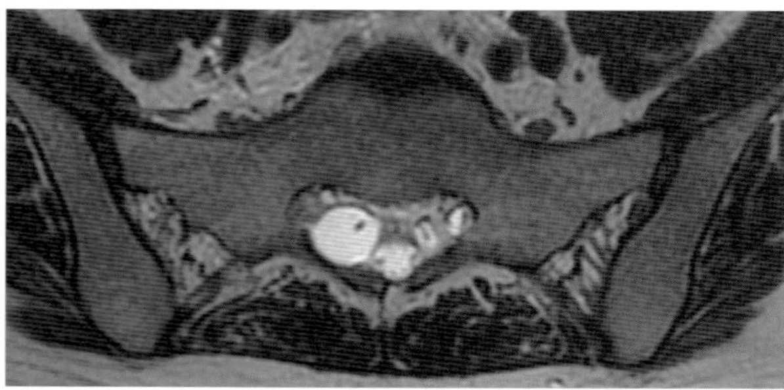

FIGURE 115-7. The nerve root fiber bundle inside this sacral Tarlov cyst is clearly seen on an axial T2-weighted MRI.

MRI also is superior for defining anatomic relationships with surrounding structures. For example, a careful review of imaging studies often reveals symptomatic cysts to be blatantly compressing adjacent nerve roots and displacing the spinal sac. Understanding these relationships preoperatively is critical for surgical planning.

CT myelography previously was used preoperatively to distinguish Tarlov cysts from other forms of meningeal cysts based on the premise that Tarlov cysts filled poorly and in a delayed fashion.[1,2,16,19] Other meningeal cysts, such as meningeal diverticula, were believed to fill more rapidly. However, these criteria are not reliable, because the extent of dye penetration into a cyst depends on the degree of its communication with the spinal sac, not on the cyst type. For example, we have encountered Tarlov cysts that communicate quite freely with the spinal sac, and filled readily on CT myelography (Fig. 115-9). Such cysts would have been erroneously categorized as non-Tarlov cysts using the more antiquated radiographic criteria.

Despite the fact that meningeal cysts, particularly Tarlov cysts, can be radiographically impressive, a careful search should be conducted to rule out other pathology that might explain the patient's symptoms. For example, a complete workup of a sacral Tarlov cyst should include not only a sacral

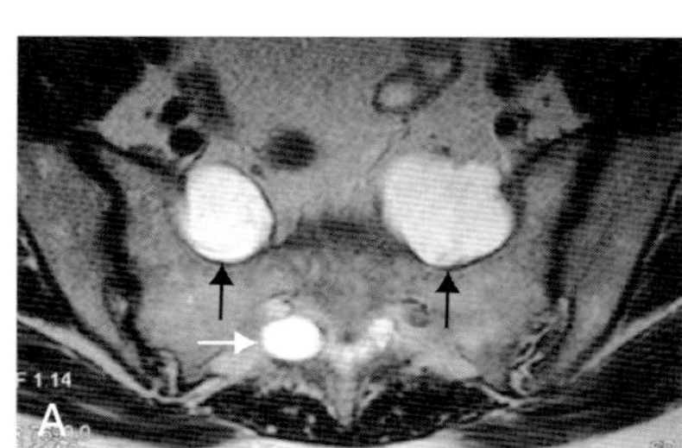
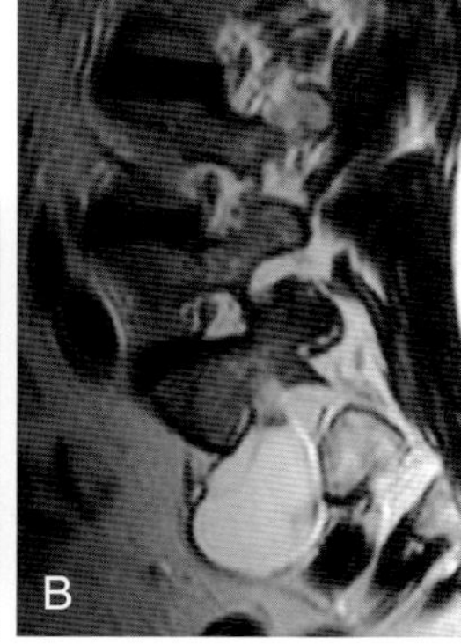

FIGURE 115-8. **A,** Two large intrapelvic Tarlov cysts are seen on this axial T2-weighted MRI (*black arrows*). Also seen is a separate Tarlov cyst within the sacral spinal canal abutting a nerve root to the right of midline (*white arrow*). **B,** On this sagittal image from the same patient, the left intrapelvic cyst can be seen extending out through the S1 neural foramen ventrally into the retroperitoneum.

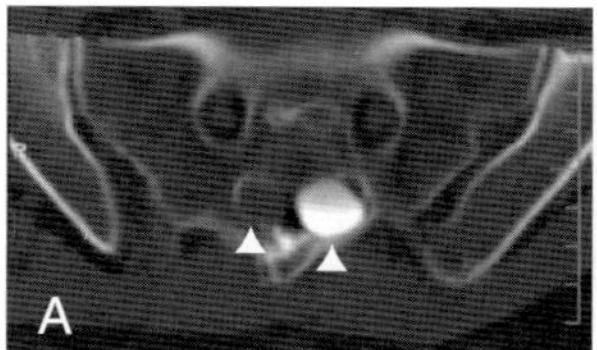
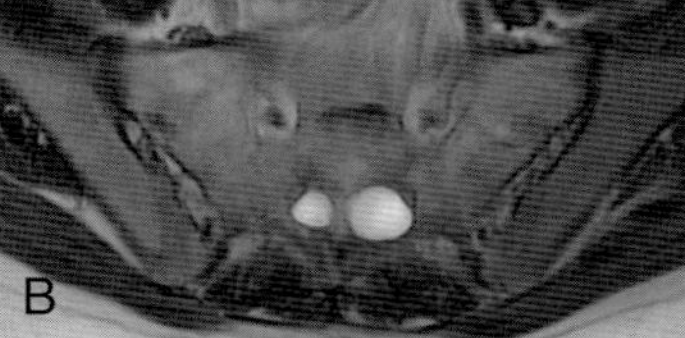

FIGURE 115-9. **A,** Side-by-side Tarlov cysts are present on this axial CT myelogram image (*arrowheads*). One fills with dye but the other does not, demonstrating that CT myelography is unreliable as a diagnostic tool for this pathology. **B,** Unlike CT, both Tarlov cysts are clearly seen on T2-weighted MRI, the preferred imaging modality.

MRI but also an MRI and flexion-extension radiographs of the lumbar spine to evaluate for disc herniations, stenosis, spondylolisthesis, metastases, hemorrhages, and other possible pathologies.

Diagnostic Cyst Aspiration

We usually avoid percutaneous procedures involving meningeal cysts due to the risks involved. However, needle aspiration occasionally is used as a diagnostic tool to determine whether a Tarlov cyst is symptomatic. When conducted with appropriate imaging to confirm correct needle placement, aspiration may temporarily decompress a cyst long enough before it refills for a patient to notice a transient improvement in symptoms. This would imply that the aspirated cyst is at least partially responsible for the patient's symptoms. Such a cyst could then be a target for treatment.

Treatment

Needle Aspiration

Unfortunately, a significant number of patients with symptomatic Tarlov cysts undergo percutaneous needle aspiration procedures as an attempt at treatment, not for diagnosis. Such procedures are ineffective, because aspirated fluid within a Tarlov cyst typically is replaced rapidly with spinal fluid through the proximal nerve root in communication with the spinal sac.[2,7,16] One study that assessed the effectiveness of percutaneous drainage of Tarlov cysts found that four of the five patients in that series suffered a recurrence of symptoms.[8] A separate report in 2001 described patients who underwent percutaneous aspiration of their cysts preoperatively.[7] None of those patients improved, and, in fact, some experienced marked worsening of their symptoms. This deterioration may have been the result of hemorrhage in the cyst wall, or nerve root injury.

In general, the use of aspiration for treatment of a Tarlov cyst is inconsistent with an understanding of the fundamental underlying pathology involved and exposes the patient to the risk of spinal fluid leakage, meningitis, hemorrhage, and nerve root injury. We therefore restrict the use of needle aspiration, using it only as a diagnostic tool in rare situations, as described in the preceding section.

Needle Aspiration and Fibrin Glue Injection

Treatment with percutaneous aspiration followed by fibrin glue injection also has been described. Authors of one report of four patients with symptomatic Tarlov cysts found that percutaneous fibrin glue therapy was effective in alleviating symptoms, although three patients developed postprocedural aseptic meningitis.[23] Blind percutaneous introduction of multiple needles into a Tarlov cyst also increases the probability of causing nerve injury.

In our experience, fibrin glue treatment fails in a large number of patients, and those patients require subsequent surgery. Unfortunately, the introduction of fibrin glue or other substrates into a Tarlov cyst makes subsequent surgical treatment more difficult because it produces scarring or coating. The neural elements within the cyst are then much harder to identify and protect during surgery. We have encountered injured nerve roots intraoperatively in several patients following prior failed fibrin glue treatment (Fig. 115-10). The fibrin glue technique is falling out of favor, both in the United States and abroad, with only a few centers with a significant experience continuing its use.

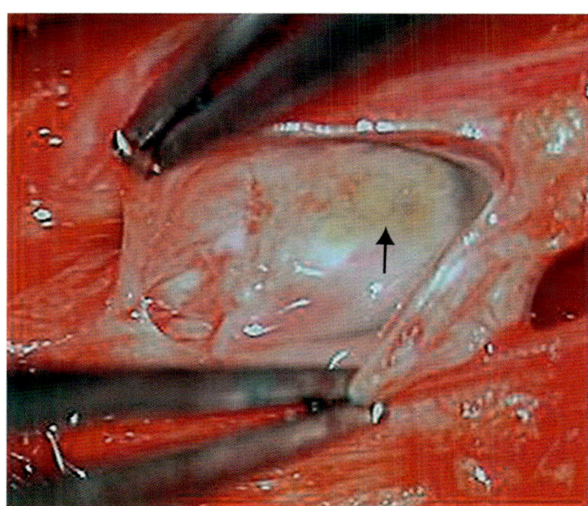

FIGURE 115-10. This intraoperative photograph reveals damage to the nerve root fibers inside the Tarlov cyst of a patient who underwent attempted treatment with percutaneous needle aspiration and fibrin glue injection. Bruising and posthemorrhagic hemosiderin deposition are seen (*arrow*). Note that the internal cyst wall has an opaque coating that makes subsequent nerve fiber identification and, therefore, surgery more difficult.

Surgical Treatment

Patient Selection

As with most spinal pathology, the selection of patients for surgical treatment is based on the correlation among symptoms, physical examination, and radiographic findings. Additionally, the size of a Tarlov cyst is an important factor in determining the probability that it is symptomatic. In general, the larger the cyst the more likely it is to produce symptoms. One study found that patients with neurologic deficits that can be radiographically correlated with Tarlov cysts greater than 1.5 cm in diameter enjoyed substantial improvement following surgery.[7] Furthermore, there was a very strong association between the presence of radicular symptoms and excellent outcome.

However, we also have encountered patients with symptomatic cysts smaller than 1.5 cm. The location of a Tarlov cyst and the extent to which it is compressing adjacent neural structures also are important factors, in addition to its size. For example, an intraforaminal Tarlov cyst in the cervical or thoracic spine arising from one spinal nerve ramus can compress the adjacent ramus of the same nerve root and produce symptoms, even though the cyst is small.

Surgery

The treatment of a symptomatic Tarlov cyst must take into account that the cyst is actually a dilated nerve root. Therefore, simple excision usually is not an option, because it can produce a critical deficit, particularly when in the lumbosacral region. This results in a treatment quandary: how does one eliminate a symptomatic Tarlov cyst without injuring the nerve root fibers inside and producing a neurologic deficit?

In the past, surgical treatments such as decompressive laminectomy, cyst fenestration, and complete cyst excision have fallen from favor due to a lack of success and unacceptable complication rates.[2,3,6,24] More recent surgical techniques have targeted the underlying pathology causing nerve root dilation, that is, the process that allows spinal fluid to accumulate within an affected nerve root.

An initial step in this direction was the description of fenestration and imbrication techniques that involve opening a Tarlov cyst.[6] The cyst is then reduced in size, either by imbrication or partial wall excision, thereby reconstituting a more normal caliber nerve root, which no longer compresses adjacent structures. However, such techniques do not prevent the continued flow of spinal fluid into the affected nerve root cyst, so they do not eliminate the risk of cyst reexpansion and spinal fluid leakage. Additionally, nerve fascicles in a Tarlov cyst often are found within the cyst wall itself, or so extensively splayed out over the internal surface of the cyst wall that they are not easily seen, even with the aid of an operating microscope. Cyst wall excision to decrease the overall size of a Tarlov cyst therefore increases the risk of producing deficits due to inadvertent nerve root fiber sectioning.

Current surgical techniques are focused on resolving the quandary of how to prevent spinal fluid flow into a symptomatic Tarlov cyst without injuring its nerve root fibers. To this end, we have focused on treatment of the ostium, where spinal fluid and nerve root fibers enter the cyst. We also have made efforts to confine cysts to prevent further compression of adjacent structures (Fig. 115-11).

Intraoperative electrophysiologic monitoring is an integral component of Tarlov cyst surgery. During the process of exposure and cyst dissection, it aids the surgeon in identifying specific nerve roots and gives feedback on the tolerance of nerves to manipulation. Thus, intraoperative monitoring can be used to assess the status of a Tarlov cyst–involved nerve root throughout the process of cyst treatment, and gives the surgeon a baseline to assess nerve function before and after cyst treatment. For example, the nerve root sleeve proximal to a treated cyst can be stimulated following cyst exploration and treatment to determine whether it is still in continuity and conducting as it was before treatment.

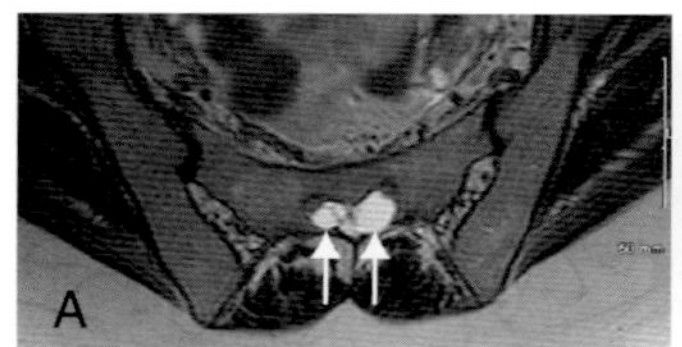

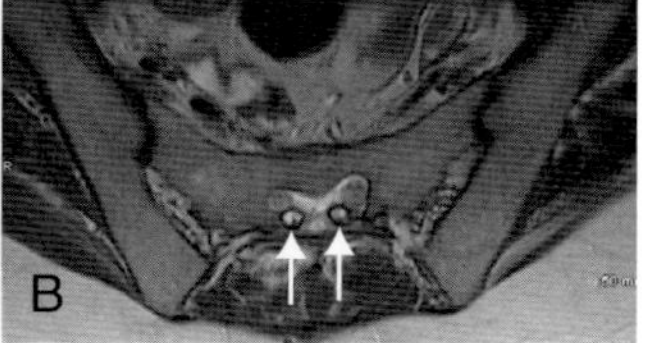

FIGURE 115-11. A, Two Tarlov cysts abutting nerve roots in the sacral spinal canal are seen on this preoperative axial T2-weighted MRI (*arrows*). **B,** Postoperatively, the treated cysts are identified (*arrows*), as are the decompressed nerve roots just ventral and lateral to each treated cyst.

Summary

Tarlov cysts are an important clinical entity in the differential diagnosis of spinal radiculopathy, sacral pain syndromes, and sacral spinal insufficiency fractures, particularly in women. The symptoms they produce can be crippling. Although the relationship remains unclear, elevated CSF pressure and trauma may play a role in their pathogenesis. MRI has enhanced our ability to diagnose symptomatic Tarlov cysts and preoperatively assess their anatomic relationships.

The management of symptomatic Tarlov cysts has progressed significantly in the last decade. Trends in the literature have favored surgical treatment in experienced hands to reduce the risk of nerve root injury and spinal fluid leakage. Treatments with percutaneous needle techniques such as aspiration or fibrin glue injection are falling out of favor due to lack of symptomatic improvement and high cyst refilling rates. In our experience, patients with large cysts and corresponding radicular symptoms are more likely to experience substantial relief from surgery. However, patients with smaller cysts also can benefit if focal nerve root compression is identified on preoperative imaging.

KEY REFERENCES

Acosta F, Quinones-Hinojosa A, Schmidt MH, et al: Diagnosis and management of sacral Tarlov cysts. *AJNR Am J Neurosurg Focus* 15:1–10, 2003.

Feigenbaum F, Henderson F: Surgical management of meningeal cysts, including perineural (Tarlov) cysts and meningeal diverticula. *Semin Spine Surg* 18:154–160, 2006.

Nabors NW, Pait TG, Byrd EB, et al: Updated assessment and current classification of spinal meningeal cysts. *J Neurosurg* 68:366–377, 1988.

North RB, Kidd DH, Wang H: Occult, bilateral anterior sacral and intrasacral meningeal and perineural cysts: case report and review of the literature. *Neurosurgery* 27:981–986, 1990.

Patel MR, Louie W, Rachlin J: Percutaneous fibrin glue therapy of meningeal cysts of the sacral spine. *AJR Am J Roentgenol* 168:367–370, 1997.

Paulsen RD, Call GA, Murtagh FR: Prevalencce and percutaneous drainage of cysts of the sacral nerve root sheath (Tarlov cysts). *AJNR Am J Neuroradiol* 15:293–297, 1994.

Strully K, Heiser S: Lumbar and sacral cysts of meningeal origin. *Radiology* 62:544–549, 1954.

Tarlov IM: Perineurial cysts of the spinal nerve roots. *Arch Neurol Psychiatry (Chic)* 40:1067–1074, 1938.

Voyadzis JM, Bhargava P, Henderson F: Tarlov cysts: a study of 10 cases with review of the literature. *J Neurosurg Spine* 95:25–32, 2001.

REFERENCES

The complete reference list is available online at expertconsult.com.

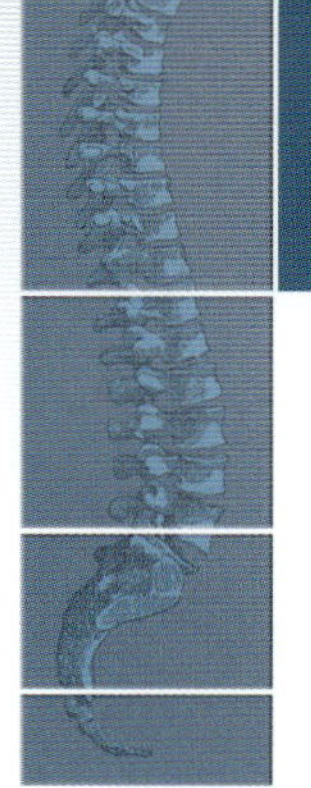

4.8 Pediatric Spinal Surgery and Related Conditions

CHAPTER 116

Occult Spinal Dysraphism and the Tethered Spinal Cord

Adam Conley | Gary W. Tye | John D. Ward | John S. Myseros

In this chapter the term *occult spinal dysraphism* describes a group of primary embryonic myelodysplastic syndromes that present with or without cutaneous manifestations and often, but not invariably, with tethering of the spinal cord. Spinal dysraphism is more common in females than in males by a ratio of at least 2:1. Although there are subtypes of occult spinal dysraphism (e.g., spina bifida associated with congenital lesions of the caudal spinal cord) that do not present with tethering of the distal cord, many do. The symptoms of spinal dysraphism with or without the presence of distal cord tethering are quite similar. Therefore, this chapter includes a discussion of the tethered cord syndrome. In addition to the tethered cord from a thickened filum terminale, the clinical entities covered in this chapter include the structural defects found in split cord syndrome, congenital dermal sinuses, and spinal lipomas.

This overlapping of structural pathology and clinical findings may present with few or minimal neurologic deficits, particularly if tension on the ascending spinal cord is not present. Symptoms such as isolated back or lower extremity pain in the young adult may be the first and only symptom referable to such a congenital lesion. Regardless, the proper surgical treatment of these anomalies is paramount to preserve and improve neurologic function, prevent potential infection, and relieve pain.

Because of the nature of these dysraphic lesions (i.e., breeching of the natural protective barriers of the distal neuraxis, such as incomplete or absent closure of the dorsal elements, enteric or subcutaneous communications with the subarachnoid space, and compromised soft tissues over the spine), repair and treatment sometimes are complicated by infection, cerebrospinal fluid (CSF) leak, and breakdown of compromised tissues. Timing of surgery, meticulous surgical technique, and close postoperative examinations, as always, may aid in avoiding potentially devastating results.

Each entity is discussed according to the following format: (1) a brief discussion of the basic embryology and pathology, (2) the clinical presentation and appropriate workup, (3) the indications for surgery, (4) a description of the technical aspects of the operative treatment (with emphasis on complication avoidance), (5) the recognition and treatment of complications, and (6) outcome.

Tethered Cord Syndrome

Pathology

The term *tethered cord syndrome*, as used in this chapter, signifies a pathologic fixation of the spinal cord in an abnormally low position so that the spinal cord, with activities and growth, undergoes mechanical stretching, distortion, and ischemia.[1] Many conditions can cause tethering of the spinal cord, including tight filum terminale, split cord malformations, lipoma, dermal sinus, and meningomyelocele. The remainder of this section addresses the care and treatment of these conditions, excluding meningomyelocele.

Presentation

The patient with a tethered cord may be either symptomatic or asymptomatic. Both groups often, but not invariably, have a midline cutaneous dorsal abnormality such as a dimple, a hairy patch or faun's patch, a hemangioma, a lipoma, or a skin tag (Figs. 116-1 and 116-2). If there is no external manifestation, the problem usually goes unrecognized until symptoms begin to develop.

Symptoms, when present, can be grouped into three general areas: sensorimotor, sphincteric, and orthopaedic. Sensorimotor symptoms can include pain, delayed walking, sensory loss (usually in the dermatomes of the lumbosacral roots), and motor weakness of the distal leg or foot (the most common symptom, presenting in 76% of cases).[2] Sphincteric symptoms usually are insidious, with frequent urinary tract infections secondary to incomplete emptying, hydronephrosis with renal involvement secondary to reflux, and fecal incontinence. In addition, these patients may develop urinary incontinence or become impotent. The orthopaedic problems are related to gait disturbance and abnormalities of the foot or scoliosis. Adult patients with tethered cords also may present with back pain that may radiate to the legs, urinary difficulties, and lower extremity weakness.[3] Patients may present either as asymptomatic in childhood and symptomatic in adulthood or as having a progression of symptoms once they reach adulthood, perhaps due to repeated microtrauma to the cord.[4] In adults, the disease may have an insidious onset or may have a predisposing factor such as exercise, lifting heavy loads, or even birth trauma.[3,5]

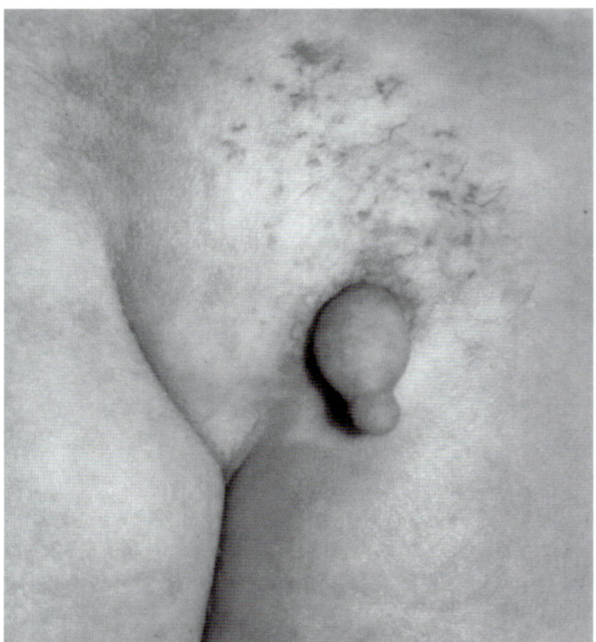

FIGURE 116-1. Skin tag and angiomatous changes in a child with a tethered cord and spinal lipoma.

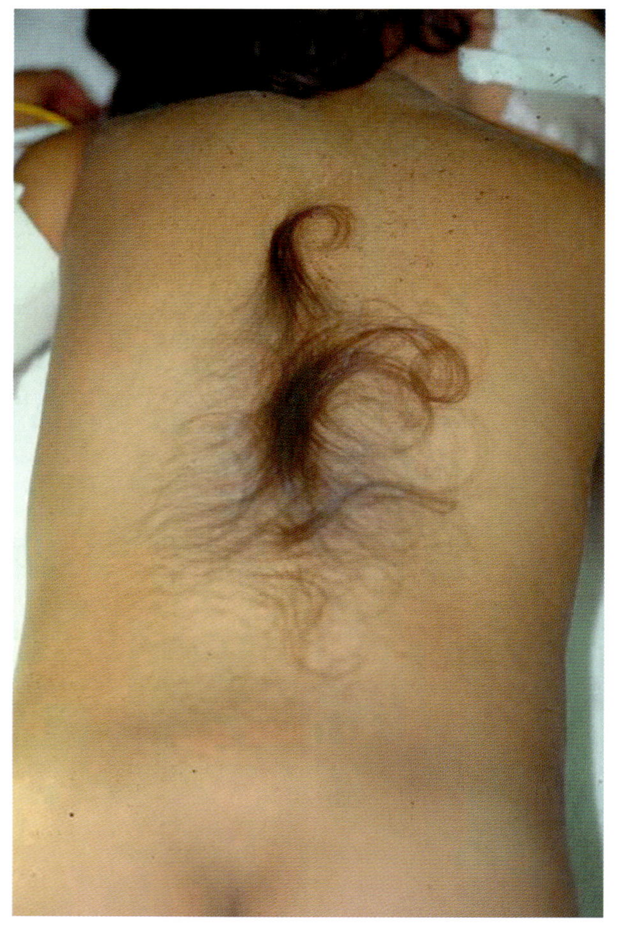

FIGURE 116-2. 5-year-old girl with faun's patch.

Diagnostic Aids

Any infant or child with a midline cutaneous lesion such as a dimple, hair patch, or hemangioma or symptoms mentioned earlier may be suspected of having a tethered cord.[6] The intention of the workup is to determine the anatomy of the anomaly.

A careful neurologic examination with attention paid to evaluation of motor and sensory function as well as sphincter tone is imperative. If the history indicates possible bladder involvement, a urologic evaluation is indicated. Plain radiographs, which may be obtained as a screening procedure, may show a widened interpedicular distance and defects at one or more levels. The procedure of choice is MRI (Fig. 116-3). Often, this is the only necessary imaging study, and treatment can be planned on the basis of MRI alone. It is prudent to image the entire spinal cord at least once to rule out other associated anomalies, such as a syrinx or a type I Chiari malformation. If there are any remaining concerns or issues, a myelogram with subsequent CT may be helpful.

Treatment

Once the problem is identified, the treatment of the tethered cord is surgical. Although controversy existed in the past (over the concept of prophylactic surgery of asymptomatic patients), most surgeons now believe that the risk of waiting for deterioration to begin is not justified, because the deficit often is not reversible. Therefore, surgery is recommended, even in the asymptomatic patient,[7] although a recent study[8] suggests that careful follow-up and monitoring for upper motor neuron signs using urodynamic assessments, in order to time surgical intervention to coincide with the appearance of upper motor neuron signs, may be possible. In adults, patients with back pain and lower extremity pain seem to benefit more than those with sphincter problems.[3]

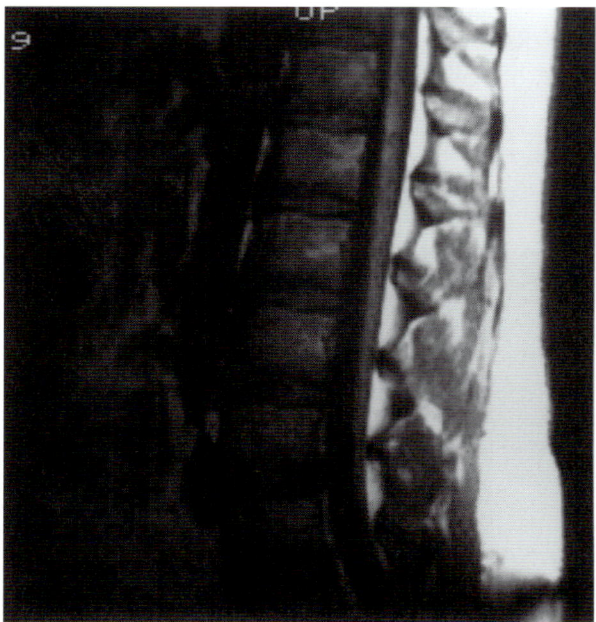

FIGURE 116-3. T1-weighted MRI demonstrating a tethered spinal cord.

The goal of surgery is to untether the spinal cord and to avoid incurring further neurologic deficit. It is crucial to expose areas of normal anatomy and then proceed to the abnormal area. The optimal surgical approach should be as low as possible in the lumbar spine so as to decrease risk of injury to the conus. Spinal deformity or instability after multilevel lumbar or thoracolumbar total laminectomy is not uncommon in children and adolescents. Limiting laminae removal and facet destruction may decrease this incidence. Fusion may be required to correct postlaminectomy deformity and to stabilize the spine. An operative approach at the L3-4 junction may be preferable to the L5-S1 level because the lumbosacral junction may present increased risk of postoperative instability.

Surgical treatment may include a single-level laminectomy with partial superior and/or inferior laminotomies. One alternative surgical approach is bilateral laminotomies at one or two lumbar levels with the use of a high-speed drill. The inferior interspinous ligament is then resected. Elevation of the lamina is done in a lobster-tail–like fashion to expose the tethered cord elements. Following surgical resection, the lamina may be replaced and sutured in place to restore the dorsal spinal column and tension band.

Care should be exercised intraoperatively because the periosteum under the lamina may appear as a separate layer and be mistaken for the dura. Once exposed, the filum often is identified in the midline and may appear fatty, fibrous, or thickened. Care should again be taken to inspect the filum to rule out the presence of attached nerve roots. Vascular supply should be identified on the ventral surface and cauterized before resection, because subarachnoid blood may potentiate nerve root adhesions. After release has been completed, and following watertight dural closure, the surgeon should assess for CSF leak by having the patient perform a Valsalva maneuver. Closure may be reinforced with fibrin glue or dural glue to further reduce the probability of CSF leak.

Electrophysiologic monitoring, especially the use of intraoperative electromyography (EMG), may be helpful. This is performed by inserting needle electrodes into the appropriate muscles and the anal sphincters under anesthesia. During surgery, the level of each root is accurately established by intradural nerve root stimulation, and before dividing any structure, it is stimulated to confirm that no neural structures are involved. The same probes that are used for a dorsal rhizotomy may be employed, although any nerve stimulator may be used. The advantage of this technique is that the response to EMG is very rapid and provides a substantial safety margin during the surgery for the tethered cord syndrome.

Complications

Several complications may occur during surgery. As with any clean neurosurgical procedure, however, the incidence of infection should be low.

CSF leak is a very uncommon complication. After careful dural closure, fibrin glue is used, and a Valsalva procedure usually is performed to check for leakage. If postoperative cutaneous leakage occurs, reoperation is mandatory. The patient should be kept flat for 3 days after surgery, with sedation if necessary.

Another potential complication is urinary retention. A Foley catheter always is inserted after induction of anesthesia and removed on the third to fifth day. If the child is unable to initiate micturition after catheter removal, intermittent catheterization is used until normal voiding is reestablished. If the child does void, a postvoid residual urine volume should be checked to verify adequate emptying. No more than 10 to 30 mL of urine should be left after the child has voided.

Outcome

The shorter the duration of symptoms, the better the prognosis.[5] A study by Archibeck et al.[9] demonstrated a 50% revision rate by 5 years after initial revision and a 57% revision rate by 2 years after the second release. In addition, 50% of patients required at least one orthopaedic procedure after tethered cord release.[9] In a study by Cornette et al.[8] of 12 patients operated on for tethered cord, none required a second operation. However, the series is small, although the follow-up period was reasonable (58 months). In terms of urologic outcome, improvement in symptoms as well as urologic dynamic parameters is expected in most patients, although few if any will return to normal.[10] Improvements may be noted in detrusor function, EMG recordings, and pressures.[11]

Split Cord Malformations

Embryology and Pathology

The term *split cord malformation* (SCM) was introduced by Pang et al.[12] in 1992 to describe diastematomyelia based on the dural tube and the nature of the septum. Two types of SCM exist: type I, diastematomyelia with septum, and type II, diastematomyelia without septum. Type II is more common.

By the end of the second week of gestation, the human embryo normally consists of a bilaminar structure: (1) an epiblast, or layer of cells next to the amnion, and (2) a hypoblast, or layer of cells next to the yolk sac. From there, the cells divide to form the primitive streak. During gastrulation, the embryo becomes trilaminar as adjacent epiblastic cells migrate medially toward the primitive streak to become mesoderm. The primitive streak begins to regress by day 16,[12] and the notochordal process begins. As the notochord elongates, it canalizes, initially forming a connection through the embryo to join the amnion and yolk sac. This connection is then lost as the open notochord separates from the endoderm and again forms a blind tube.[12]

In the split cord malformations, an adhesion forms between the ectoderm and endoderm, leading to the formation of an "accessory neurenteric canal around which condenses an endomesenchymal tract that bisects the developing notochord and causes formation of two hemineural plates."[12] Whether a type I or type II SCM is formed depends on what happens to the endomesenchymal tract. If it develops toward bone and cartilage, the result will be two dural sacs and a type I SCM. If the tract regresses or leaves a fibrous septum, a type II SCM will develop.[13]

The spinal cord above and below the split is normal. The two hemicords themselves usually are the same size, but in 10% of patients, they are grossly asymmetrical. When this occurs, the spinal cord itself, above and below the bifurcation, is asymmetrical, being smaller on the side of the smaller hemicord.

The anterior spinal artery and the central canal bifurcate to accompany each hemicord,[14] so that each has its own blood supply. The two hemicords give rise to the spinal nerve roots on their respective sides. Although splitting of the spinal cord at more than one site and cases of incomplete splitting of the spinal cord with a resultant partial cleft cord have been reported, most cases involve a single, complete cleft through the spinal cord and meninges. In cases in which there are two hemicords without an intervening septum, a single dural sac surrounds both. In such cases, symptoms may result from tethering of the cord by fibrous bands or a thickened filum terminale.

In cases in which the meninges themselves also are bifurcated, there almost always is an intervening septum. Its position is at the caudal end of the split; therefore, ascent of the neural elements is prohibited. The septum, or spur, usually is attached to both the dorsal elements and the dorsal aspect of the vertebral body. Because of the incidence of spina bifida, the spur may continue dorsally between unfused laminae. These spurs may present anywhere along the spine, but in 70% of cases they are between L1 and L5. They are less likely to occur in the thoracic spine and have only a 1% incidence in the cervical spine.[15,16] The spur initially is cartilaginous and may mature to calcified bone with time.

Other associated anomalies, such as vertebral body abnormalities, may occur. Hemivertebrae, butterfly vertebrae, blocked vertebrae, and spina bifida may contribute to a kyphoscoliosis. The scoliotic defect and segmental vertebral anomalies commonly are located near the level of the split cord malformation. In addition, many children with these anomalies have hypertrichosis over the level of the spur, clubfoot, or pes cavus. Twenty percent of cases are associated with other abnormalities of the spine, including hydromyelia, lipoma, dermal sinus, and neurenteric, epidermoid, and arachnoid cysts. Unless a preexisting myelomeningocele exists, Chiari malformations usually are not associated with split cord malformations.

Pathophysiology

The clinical symptoms most likely evolve from traction of the spinal cord against the restricting septum or bony spur.[1,17] As with other forms of tethered spinal cord, ascent of the cord within the dural sac and spinal canal is prohibited. The average age of presentation is 6½ years, with neurologic symptoms first becoming evident with the onset of walking.[16] With the onset of walking, however, increased traction of the distal spinal cord against the restricting septum results in new symptoms. To support this finding, Yamada et al.[18] have studied the oxidative metabolism of the distal spinal cord and have found a decrease when the cord is under axial tension.

Presentation

Boxes 116-1 and 116-2 include some of the presenting symptoms and physical signs of patients with split cord malformations.[19] In general, signs and symptoms fall into three categories: (1) cutaneous abnormalities, (2) pain, and (3) neurologic deficits (from spinal cord traction).

In newborns and infants in whom neurologic deficits may not yet have developed, cutaneous lesions bring the child to the attention of the neurosurgeon. Most commonly, a patch of hair or hypertrichosis is noted in the thoracic or lumbosacral midline dorsally. This hair, usually coarse and long, is sometimes referred to as *faun's tail*. The surrounding skin is associated with an intradermal angiomatous malformation, giving the skin a pinkish blue color. In addition, a dermal sinus, lipoma, abnormally protuberant spinous process, or meningocele may be associated with the spur.

BOX 116-1. Split Cord Malformation: Common Presenting Complaints

Pain
- Low backache
- Shooting pains down leg

Cutaneous abnormalities
- Hairy patch
- Prominence in lumbar midline
- Skin discoloration
- Skin defect

Symptoms arising from traction injury to spinal cord
- Limp
- Deformity or smallness of leg and foot
- Sensory disturbance
- Bladder disorder
- Impotence
- Abnormal spinal curvature

Incidental radiographic findings

Data from Mathern GW, Peacock WJ: Diastematomyelia. In Park TS, editor: *Spinal dysraphism*, Boston, 1992, Blackwell Scientific, p 91.

BOX 116-2. Split Cord Malformation: Common Physical Signs

Elicitation of pain
- Straight leg–raising test
- Flexion of spine

Cutaneous abnormalities
- Faun's tail or hypertrichosis
- Lipoma
- Prominent spinous process
- Meningocele
- Angiomatous malformation
- Dermal sinus or dimple

Neurologic abnormalities
- Short leg and hypoplasia of calf and thigh
- Varus or cavus deformity of foot
- Adducted forefoot
- Clawed toes
- Muscle weakness
- Depressed ankle and knee reflexes
- Diminished sensation in dermatomes of leg or perianal area
- Distended bladder
- Scoliosis

Data from Mathern GW, Peacock WJ: Diastematomyelia. In Park TS editor: *Spinal dysraphism*, Boston, 1992, Blackwell Scientific, p 91.

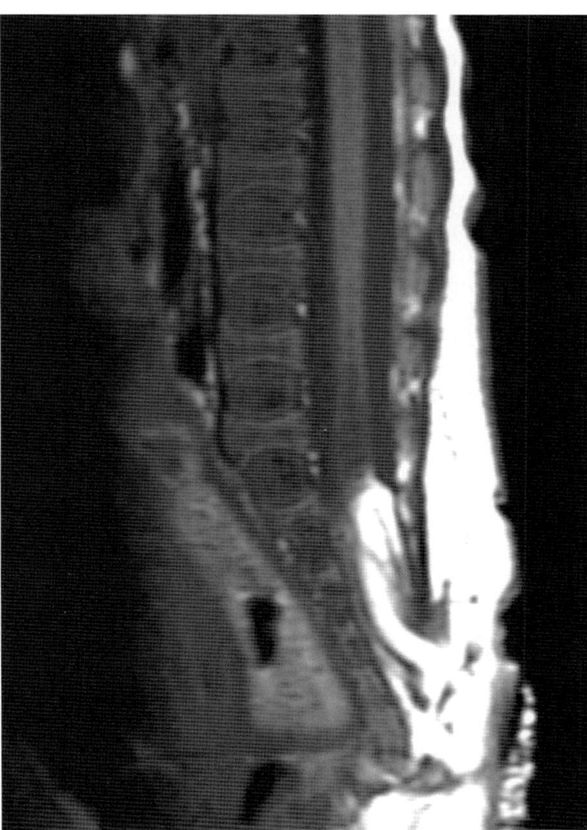

FIGURE 116-4. T1-weighted MRI demonstrating a tethered spinal cord with associated lipoma.

As the child develops, begins to walk, and acquires bowel and bladder control, the neurologic sequelae of split cord malformations usually appear. Hypoplastic lower extremity and foot deformities sometimes are present at birth. Progressive kyphoscoliosis also may become noticeable. With the onset of walking, a limp, an ulcer secondary to areas of anesthesia, and the new onset of bowel or bladder incontinence after a period of normally developed continence all indicate tethering. Although spasticity and other long-tract signs are not common, hyporeflexia and loss of sensation in the sacral dermatomes are common.

If the patient with split cord malformation has successfully progressed through development with few or none of the aforementioned symptoms, the most common complaint, particularly in older children and adults, is back or leg pain.[20] This pain may be due to subtle concomitant scoliosis or to the spinal bony deformity itself. The presence of unilateral symptoms is a key difference in the presentation of split cord malformation versus tethered cord syndrome.

Diagnostic Aids

Aids that confirm the diagnosis of split cord malformation usually are radiologic. Although plain radiographs or unenhanced CT scans of the spine may reveal the bony spur, a widened interpedicular distance, spina bifida occulta, or other segmental vertebral anomalies, MRI in all three axes can be more revealing and is the preferred procedure (Figs. 116-4 to 116-7). Associated lipomas, hydromyelia, and other intraspinal and

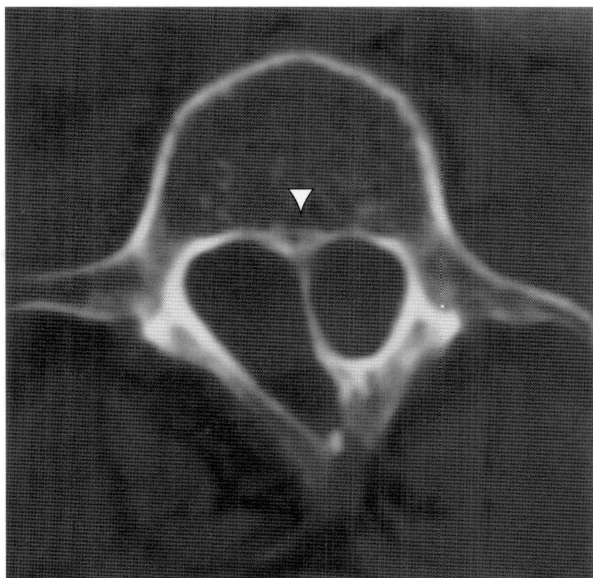

FIGURE 116-5. Plain axial CT scan revealing the bony septum *(arrowhead)* of split cord malformation.

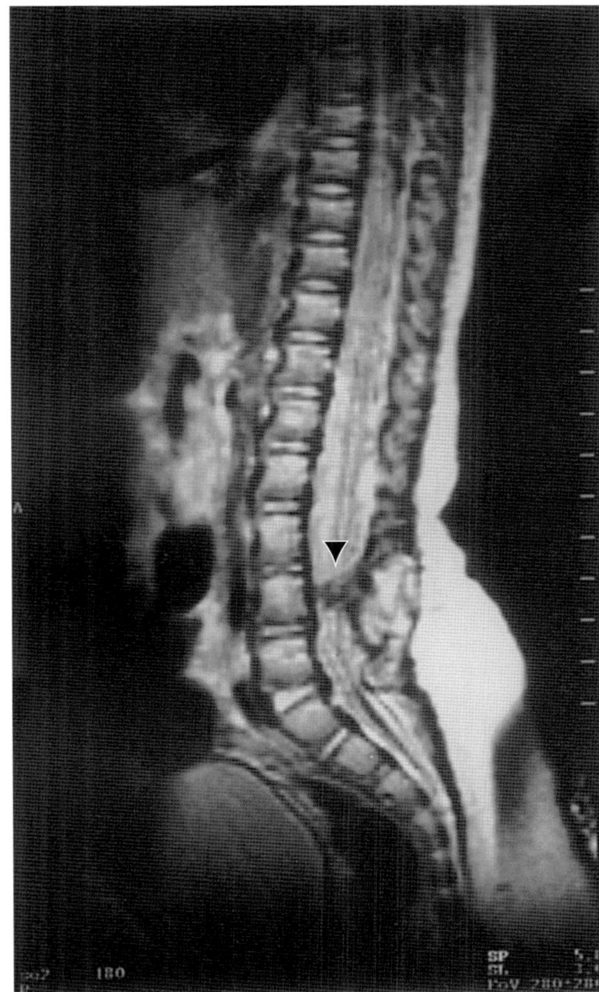

FIGURE 116-6. Sagittal T2-weighted MRI demonstrating split cord malformation, with the septum spanning from the ventral to the dorsal elements *(arrowhead)*.

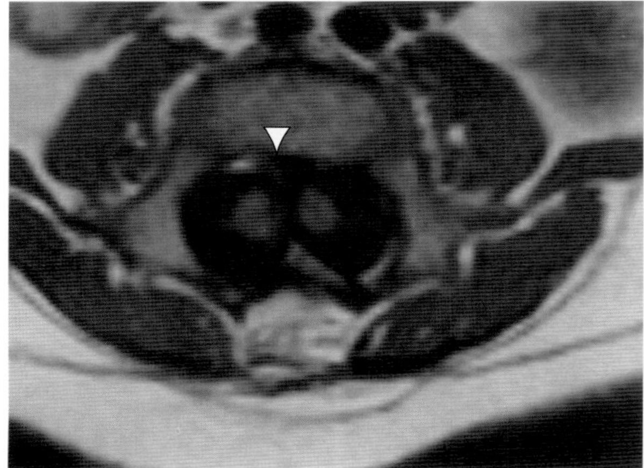

FIGURE 116-7. Axial T1-weighted MRI revealing the septum *(arrowhead)* and hemicords of split cord malformation.

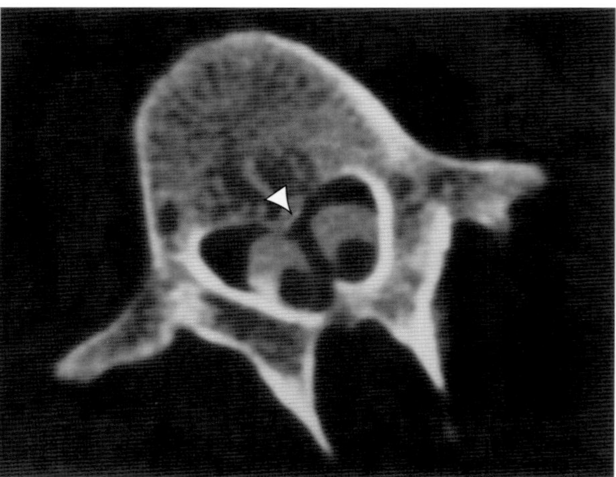

FIGURE 116-8. Axial postmyelogram CT scan demonstrating split cord malformation resulting from a nonossified fibrous septum *(arrowhead)*. Note the delineation of the hemicords.

intradural defects also may be observed incidentally, allowing for a more focused treatment approach. If there are any questions or further clarification is required, myelography and postmyelographic CT best delineate the hemicords, the dural sac, and the presence and extent of the intervening bony septum (Fig. 116-8).[21] Plain and CT myelography may reveal aberrant nerve roots, intradural bands, a thickened filum terminale, or a concomitant intradural lipoma. In addition, a recent study[22] reported an incidence of abnormal urologic dynamic studies as high as 75% in patients with SCM, despite a lack of symptoms. Therefore, obtaining preoperative and postoperative urologic dynamic studies may be of some benefit. Again, as in the tethered cord syndrome, the entire spinal cord should be imaged.

Treatment

With the exception of incidental findings of split cord malformation in newborns, any patient with signs or symptoms referable to split cord malformation should be promptly untethered to relieve symptoms, preserve function, and possibly reverse neurologic deficits. In the otherwise normal newborn, surgery should be delayed for about 3 months, because the older child will be larger, will tolerate anesthesia better, and will have developed more resilient meninges and soft tissues, allowing for more secure surgical closure.

The goal of surgery is to untether the hemicords by removing the cartilaginous, fibrous, or bony septum, as well as the dural tunnel about the septum, which itself tethers the cord. In addition, any surrounding dural adhesions restricting the motion of the spinal cord should be lysed.

Under general anesthesia, the patient should be positioned as for a laminectomy, in the prone position, either on chest rolls or on a flexed frame with adequate room for abdominal wall motion. Unless an associated tethered filum terminale that requires incision is expected, there is no need for preoperative placement of sphincter and lower extremity EMG electrodes.

Before making a standard midline incision to the lumbosacral fascia, the spine should be palpated. Occasionally, a protruding spinous process or bony spur may be felt, allowing for a more localized incision. In addition, a localizing plain radiograph with a skin marker is used and correlated with the preoperative MRI. If a cutaneous lesion, such as a patch of hair, is present, it may be beneficial to create an elliptical incision circumferentially around the defect. Because the underlying bony and soft tissue defect may not be clear, it is helpful to incise the fascia and perform a subperiosteal reflection of the paraspinous musculature at the levels above and below the level of the lesion, understanding that midline fusion defects may also exist here. The monopolar electrocautery should be used cautiously in retracting the muscles, because areas of expected protective bone may be missing. After the laminae above and below the lesion are exposed, their spinous processes are removed using a rongeur. A partial laminectomy is then performed at the caudal aspect of the lamina above the septum and the rostral aspect of the lamina below the septum. After careful curettage of the underside of both these laminae, the ligamentum flavum, if still intact, is elevated laterally with Penfield forceps and incised longitudinally through its outer layer. A blunt instrument is then gently inserted through the remaining ligament, and a small cottonoid patty is placed between the dura mater and the ligamentum flavum for protection. A small, angled Kerrison punch is then used to remove the ligamentum flavum until the dura mater is completely exposed laterally. With a no. 4 Penfield dissector, the septum is then felt over the dura from above and from below. A small-mouthed rongeur or angled Kerrison punch or high-speed drill is used to remove the lamina and overhanging bone of the involved level until only the spur is left. Because of the substantial epidural venous plexus associated in and around the bony spur and deep to the two hemicords, control of bleeding and cauterization of these vessels should be performed prior to and during the removal of the spur (Fig. 116-9). After decompression, with movement of the hemicords, it may be very difficult to maintain hemostasis. Any extruding segment of spur is removed using a rongeur, and a small dissector is used to probe and dissect the dural sheath away from the bony spicule down to the level of the dorsal vertebral body. A high-speed diamond-bit drill is then used to carefully thin down the spicule as far as possible.

At this point, the dura mater is opened along the midline above and below the spur and elliptically around the spur remnant. After the dural edges are tacked up, the two hemicords become evident. The ventral dural sac is then incised

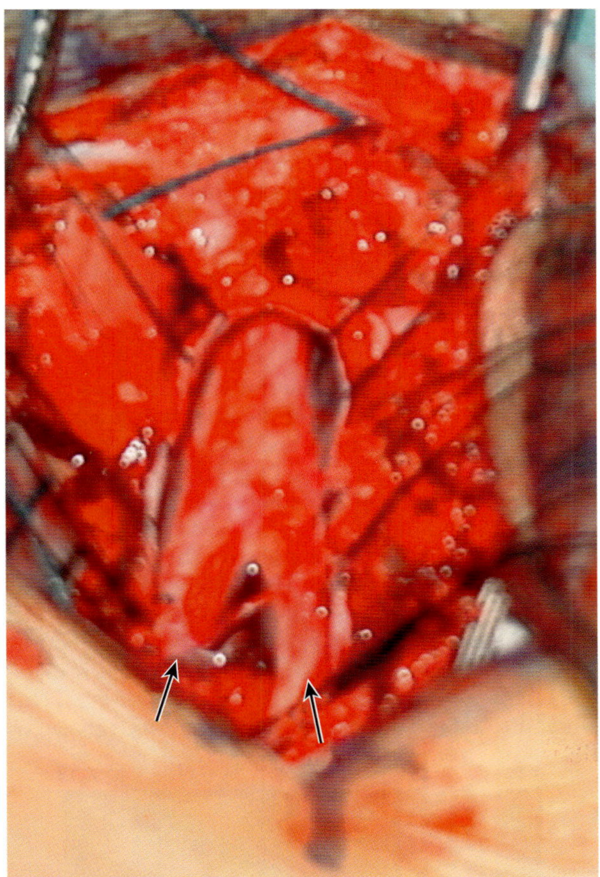

FIGURE 116-9. Intraoperative photograph showing the two hemicords *(arrows)* in a patient with split cord malformation.

along the midline above the spicule and circumferentially around it. The dural "chimney" is removed, and the resultant dural edges are teased laterally so that the remainder of the spur may be completely drilled off, with the spinal cord being protected at all times. With the removal of the spur, the entire cord may migrate rostrally. Microinstruments should be used to break or cut any additional adhesions that may be tethering the spinal cord to the dura mater. A watertight closure of the dorsal dural opening is then performed, with interrupted sutures used over the elliptical incision to avoid the unraveling of a running stitch over this area of tension; again, fibrin glue is used. The ventral dura mater does not require closure. A small drain is inserted, and the soft tissues are closed in anatomic layers. The patient should then be kept flat for 3 days postoperatively to avoid CSF leak.

Complications

If there are persistent CSF leaks from the suture line, the suture line should be oversewn or patched until the leak stops. It is not uncommon to have a small amount of CSF leakage from the suture holes of the dural closure. If it is minimal, it should not pose a problem. Although infrequent, a persistent CSF leak must be addressed to avoid incision breakdown, infection, and, possibly, meningitis. If a CSF leak from this source should occur, placing a lumbar subarachnoid drain above the incision and having the patient lie flat in bed for 3 days should allow for closure. If the leak is from the dorsal dural suture line, a drain may again avoid reoperation, but failure to stop the leak will necessitate reexploration and primary dural closure. If the meningeal tissues are found to be weak and nonresilient, a pericardium, fascia lata, or other dural graft may be required. Fibrin glue or a dura substitute (DuraGen [Integra Life Sciences, Plainsboro, NJ]) may also be of some value.

As always, postoperative epidural hemorrhage is possible. Because of the apparent increased venous drainage in the defect, hemostasis may be difficult. A delayed postoperative neurologic deficit should be worked up immediately, with either MRI or myelography. Both epidural hematomas and subdural extension secondary to ventral durotomy should be evacuated immediately. Normal coagulation studies and adequate hematologic status should be verified, and corrected if necessary. As mentioned earlier, the placement of a drain in the epidural space for 24 hours may be considered at the time of initial repair, although this should not replace meticulous surgical technique. This may prevent the accumulation of a mass lesion, and rarely does it induce leakage of CSF from the underlying suture line.

Maintaining a sterile field, administration of perioperative antibiotics, and gentle handling of tissues will aid in preventing meningitis and wound infections. If these should occur, appropriate intravenous antibiotics should be administered. The goal is to prevent a subsequent epidural or subdural empyema.

Iatrogenic traction, contusion, or direct injury with an instrument or a drill may inadvertently occur intraoperatively. Care should be exercised continuously to prevent unnecessary manipulation and traction on the spinal cord.

Outcome

In symptomatic patients, bowel and bladder dysfunction may improve up to 40% of the time; stabilization of progressive urologic symptoms also may be noted.[23] Neurologic sensorimotor deficits return to normal only 5% to 10% of the time. Patients whose main complaint is pain in general improve. Also included in improvement of pain is the dysesthetic component. A higher surgical morbidity has been reported in cases in which the bony septum is present, perhaps due to removal of the bony septum.[23] It is important to remember that preserving neurologic function is as important as improving it. Recent studies[23,24] also report that untethering the cord may have no effect on the neuro-orthopaedic syndrome (e.g., lower limb asymmetry, foot deformities), perhaps due to irreversible changes in the ligaments.

Congenital Dermal Sinus

Pathology and Embryology

Dorsal congenital dermal sinus, a subtype of spinal dysraphism not associated with spina bifida or bony abnormalities, is defined as an epithelium-lined tract from the skin of the back, usually the lumbosacral midline (although it also may occur in the thoracic and cervical spine),[13] that passes through the soft tissues toward the spine, the thecal sac, and even into the neural elements. These tracts, which usually are very thin, are thought to develop because of adhesion and failure of separation between the superficial cutaneous ectoderm and the neural tube.[25] This failure of separation usually occurs at the fourth week of fetal development, after neurulation of the tail bud. At that time, the attachment between skin and spinal cord is lengthened and thinned with the ascent of the cord and fixation of the skin. Because of its small size, the surrounding bone-forming mesoderm may produce little or no spina bifida. Also, the remainder of the vertebral body at the affected levels usually is normal. Although not usually a cause of tethering of the spinal cord, the cutaneous origin of the sinus tends to be two to three vertebral levels caudal to its adhesion to the neural elements. Congenital dermal sinus is present in 1.2% of the neonatal population.

Because of the epithelial lining and potential communication with the skin, the dermal sinus may result in an expanding dermoid or epidermoid tumor in the subdural or epidural space, in the same manner that such tumors arise from iatrogenic implantation of such elements with spinal needles.[26] These tumors may present as mass lesions or as a simple dermal sinus associated with a possible communication between the skin and subarachnoid space. Therefore, they are a nidus for infection, meningitis, and possibly abscess formation. Microscopically, they consist of dermal elements, such as sweat and apocrine glands and hair follicles.

Most dorsal dermal sinuses are lumbosacral; occipital sinuses are less common. Although about 60% of dermal sinuses end in dermoid or epidermoid tumors, only 30% of these tumors are associated with dermal sinuses.[27,28] In addition, the dermal sinus may be involved in tethering of the spinal cord, not by itself but either by a thick band of tissue attached to the spinal cord or conus medullaris or as a result of inflammatory scarring.

Pathophysiology and Presentation

Because of the low incidence of tethering with dermal sinuses, symptoms result from infectious etiologies. Bacterial causes may include *Staphylococcus aureus*, *Staphylococcus epidermidis*, *Escherichia coli*, and even *Proteus* species.[29] The tract from the bacteria-laden epidermis to the intraspinous space and even the subarachnoid space provides opportunities for intermittent, chronic, and acute infections.[30,31] Although the incidence of meningitis is higher with the presence of a concomitant dermoid or epidermoid tumor, simple tracts carry this risk as well.[32] In fact, dermal sinuses may be the cause of infection in up to one quarter of cases of intramedullary spinal abscesses, with approximately 70% of patients having neurologic deficits.[33] Because of the dimple formed in the skin over the tract, infections are noticed and addressed, often before clinical symptoms have surfaced. The dimple, or the external ostium of the sinus, usually is in the midline and may be associated with a hemangioma, a nevus, or short tufts of hair protruding from the sinus. Parents, caretakers, or physicians may notice caseous discharge from this area or perhaps some erythema or inflammation. Because of the usual lumbosacral location, fecal and skin organisms may be the cause of meningitis. Frank neurologic symptoms or neurogenic pain rarely is present unless there is compression from an associated tumor or tethering of the spinal cord or conus, as mentioned previously.

On examination, neurologic function is usually found to be preserved. The dimple should not be probed, in order to avoid lodging infection-forming organisms into the deeper sinus. Manipulation and pulling the skin around the ostium in different directions often reveal further umbilication of the tract, thus confirming that the margins of the tract are fixed to the deeper tissues. Palpation of the spine itself may reveal prominent or absent spinous processes, indicating a dorsal element malformation. It is important, however, to distinguish a low-lying dermal sinus pore from a simple pilonidal dimple, which usually is more caudal, is near the tip of the coccyx, and usually requires no further workup. However, if the dimple is over the sacrum or higher, further evaluation is indicated.

Diagnostic Aids

Although the index of suspicion for congenital dermal sinus is high solely on the basis of the examination, neuroimaging is helpful to discern its extent and the presence of associated tethering and tumors. Injection of contrast material or probing the tract is not recommended because of the risk of inducing meningitis and infection.

Ultrasound may be used to assess for the presence of spina bifida and also to evaluate for the presence of possible cyst. However, it is useful only for infants 4 to 5 months of age. The limited ability of ultrasound to detect underlying abnormalities has kept it from being used as an initial diagnostic tool.

MRI is the initial imaging modality of choice (Fig. 116-10). It is useful to follow the denser, low-signal sinus through the

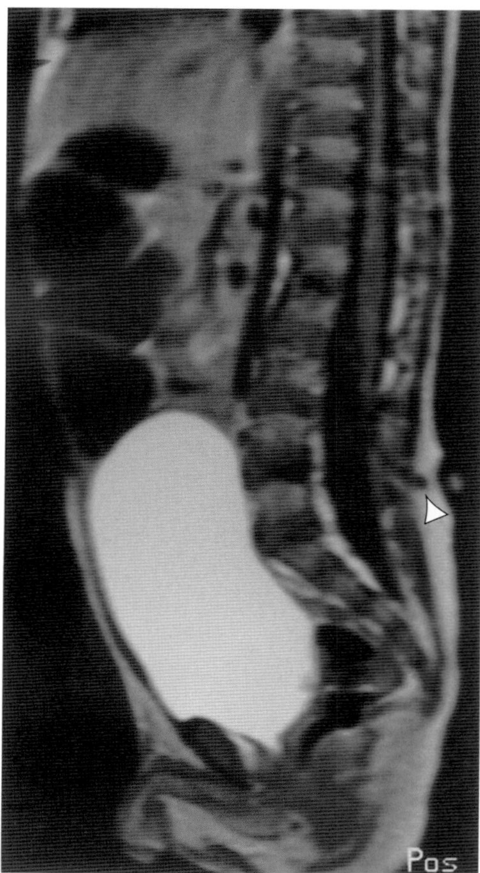

FIGURE 116-10. Sagittal T1-weighted MRI revealing a tethered spinal cord that appears to be contiguous with a dermal sinus tract *(arrowhead)*. Note the overdistended, previously undiagnosed, neurogenic bladder.

high-signal subcutaneous fat toward the dura mater. The intraspinal course of the tract, however, may not be well displayed by MRI in all cases. Dermoid and epidermoid tumors have variable signal intensity on MRI. Dermoids, with increased T1 and T2 signals compared with water (because of the cholesterol, fat, and protein content), image well. However, if chemical meningitis has been caused by leakage of the tumor, detection may be more difficult. Although epidermoid tumors contain only epithelial elements, they are equally well defined by MRI.

Axial CT imaging reveals the dense sinus tract through its course from the skin into the dura mater. Occasionally, the lumen of the tract may be visualized as a more hypodense line within the tract. CT scanning with intra-arachnoid myelographic contrast medium is the most useful method for imaging the course of the sinus in the subdural space as it ascends toward the conus medullaris.[34] Water-soluble contrast or air should be used to avoid leaving oily droplets that could act as potential foreign bodies. A lucent mass along the tubular filling defect may represent dermoid or epidermoid tumors. The use of contrast material has been reduced dramatically since the advent of MRI, however. Even in the presence of a normal MRI, if a cutaneous lesion seems to truly represent a dermal sinus in a suspicious location, surgical exploration may be warranted.

Treatment

The treatment of a true dermal sinus is surgical. Even if the MRI is normal, the sinus tract should be excised. Fewer than 25% of sacral sinuses at birth will regress to a simple dimple if left untreated. Technically, surgical excision of the dermal sinus may range from a very simple procedure (when it ends in the soft tissue) to a very difficult and complex operation (if it is adherent to the conus medullaris or is associated with one or more dermoid or epidermoid tumors). When a patient presents with soft tissue infection or meningitis, the infection first should be treated adequately with intravenous antibiotics. The surgery should not be performed until the CSF is sterile. In any case, antibiotics should be used both perioperatively and postoperatively.

Loupe or microscope magnification should be used after the dura mater is exposed. The patient is placed on chest rolls or on a frame after general anesthesia, as for a laminectomy. The skin and ostium of the sinus should be sterilized, and access should be available from the spinous process of T11 to the coccyx. A midline incision is then performed from at least two spinous processes rostral to the dimple to one spinous process below it. An elliptical incision is made around the ostium itself, including any associated nevus or other cutaneous abnormality. The skin edges around the sinus may then be secured and manipulated with a heavy silk suture or a clamp with teeth.

Use of traction on the elliptically incised skin and ostium allows for easier dissection along the tract. The tract is followed with Metzenbaum-type scissors as it dives into the soft tissues, until the lumbosacral fascia is reached. A blunter instrument, such as a small curved hemostat, is then used to follow the tract through the fascia, caudally to rostrally, while holding traction on the tract in the rostral direction. Care should be taken not to incise or avulse the tract, to prevent the remaining stump from retracting under the fascia, which makes it very difficult to locate. Care also should be exercised to avoid undue traction on the sinus tract in case it is contiguous with the neural elements. When the direction and location of the subfascial tract have been determined, the fascia above and below may be incised on either side of the spinous processes above and below the tract. Again, using subperiosteal dissection, either with a gauze and periosteum elevators or with traction and a monopolar electrocautery, the laminae are exposed. This leaves the line of spinous processes, usually with the dermal sinus tract disappearing into the interspinous ligament of the involved level. In the case of dorsal element abnormalities and spina bifida, care should be taken, particularly with the electrocautery, to protect the underlying dura mater and its contents. A no. 4 Penfield dissector is then used to probe the tract as it enters the spine, to determine the tract's position and direction. The flavum ligamentum, under upward traction with forceps, can be carefully incised. Often, the sinus tract may end in the interspinous ligament, and amputation here can be followed by thorough washing of the incision and closure. If the tract does indeed pierce the ligamentum flavum, a laminectomy above this should be performed, with rongeurs and an angled Kerrison punch. As with a standard laminectomy, if there is no access to the epidural space after bony removal, an incision through the ligamentum flavum, under traction with subsequent protection of the dura mater with a cottonoid, is warranted. The ligamentum flavum is then removed completely laterally and caudally to the tract. A small cottonoid patty should first be advanced under the ligamentum flavum and above the dura mater to avoid incision of the tract as it is neared or to avoid performing an incidental durotomy. The same is accomplished at the lamina below the tract, although only the rostral half of the spinous process, lamina, and ligamentum flavum need to be removed, because intradurally the sinus tract rarely travels caudally.

If, at this time, the tract appears to extend rostrally beyond the level of the laminectomy, the next lamina should be removed. Further exposure may be necessary until the tract is not visualized or until its termination at the conus medullaris can be visualized. The dura mater is then incised along the midline at the rostral end of the exposure, well away from the site of entry of the tract, and carefully extended in the direction of the tract. To approach the entry site, an elliptical incision is made circumferentially around the tract, and the midline incision finally is continued to the caudal end of the exposed dura mater. The dural ellipse that is incised around the tract should be kept as small as possible to preclude the need for use of graft material when closing the dura mater. Care should be taken to keep the force of suction minimal to avoid inadvertent aspiration of free-floating nerve roots. If the arachnoid has been preserved after the durotomy, it may be opened in the midline with a small hook or knife. The dural leaves may then be tacked to the musculature with #4-0 silk or woven nylon sutures.

With gentle traction on the tract, microinstruments are used to dissect away any adhesions between the tract, the dura mater, and the nerve roots. Some adhesions, particularly postmeningitic scars, may require incision. In this way the tract is followed to its attachment, usually dorsally above the tip of the conus. The sides of the tract are completely identified by using a small blunt hook, and microscissors are used to detach it. If the stump bleeds, it is lightly coagulated with bipolar forceps. After verifying the absence of other mass lesions or areas of tethering, the subarachnoid space is copiously irrigated with warm saline, and the dura mater is closed in a watertight fashion with #4-0 silk or woven nylon suture, using a graft if necessary. Fibrin glue is then applied. A drain may be placed in the epidural space and brought through the skin for 24 hours. The soft tissues are then closed in anatomic layers. Some undermining of the subcutaneous tissue occasionally is necessary to bring together the skin edges in the area of the elliptical excision. The patient should remain flat in bed for 3 days, and antibiotics should be administered postoperatively for 3 days, or longer if a previous infection was present.

If a dermoid or epidermoid tumor is encountered preoperatively or during the course of the procedure, it should be completely extirpated, with great care taken to avoid a rupture of its contents. If the tumor itself is at the end of the tract and situated within the substance of the spinal cord, it cannot be completely removed; it should be amputated with an adequate stump to avoid injuring the spinal cord.

Complications

As with other intradural procedures, CSF leakage may occur postoperatively. A Valsalva maneuver (safe to 40 mm Hg) after closing the dura mater is helpful for revealing any obvious areas of leakage. To avoid the problem of wound breakdown and postoperative meningitis, particularly with a dermal sinus and exposure to its intraluminal debris, a watertight closure (again using fibrin glue, saline irrigation before dural closure, and antibiotic irrigation after dural closure) is helpful. If meningitis should occur, the appropriate antibiotics should be administered. In the case of a superficial wound infection, the area should be opened, drained, and packed, and the patient should be treated with antibiotics. If, however, the fascia has been violated by the infection, reoperation is necessary to open the fascia, to verify a clean epidural and, if necessary, subdural space, and to close the fascia primarily. All efforts should be made to avoid leaving the dura mater exposed to the environment.

Iatrogenic injury to the conus medullaris, spinal cord, and nerve roots is minimized by gentle handling of the tissues, avoidance of traction, and protection of the neural elements. If it is thought preoperatively that the sinus may end in the conus medullaris or in a tumor adherent to the conus, somatosensory evoked potentials may be monitored during the procedure. Division of a nerve root, particularly in the absence of EMG monitoring and uncertainty as to its function, should be primarily repaired with #8-0 or #9-0 absorbable monofilament sutures. Because the incidence of postoperative neurologic deficits from dermal sinus surgery is small, no evidence supports the use of perioperative or postoperative corticosteroids for neural protection.

Emphasis should be placed on complete excision of the sinus tract. Because of its epithelial lining, the potential for dermoid or epidermoid formation remains if part of the tract remains. If a lumen is apparent in the stump of the tract after it is incised near the spinal cord or conus medullaris, it should be trimmed until no lumen is apparent, and then well cauterized.

Outcome

Most patients with simple tracts do well, and the incidence of neurologic injury is low. Even in the case of spinal cord infection, a positive outcome may be obtained. In a report by Morandi et al.,[35] 10 of 16 patients (62%) with spinal cord abscess had complete recovery.

Spinal Lipomas

Pathology and Embryology

Although associated with other forms of occult spinal dysraphism, spinal lipomas are connective tissue and fat collections that are distinct, partially or completely encapsulated, and definitely attached to the spinal cord.[36] It is thought that during the process of primary neurulation, improper disjunction of surface ectoderm and neuroepithelium may lead to inclusion of fat.[36] Distinct from lipomyelomeningoceles, isolated lipomas technically are fibrolipomas of the filum terminale or dural fibrolipomas, as defined by Emery and London.[37] In simple lipomas, the neural elements remain within the spinal canal, whereas lipomyelomeningoceles are marked by herniation of the neural elements out of the canal into the subcutaneous portion of the lipoma.[38] Strictly intradural lipomas associated with an intact dura mater are lesions of subpial fat found in the cervical and thoracic spinal cord.[39] In a large series reported by McLone and Naidich,[40] 4% of the lipomas treated surgically were intradural lipomas. More common, however, are lipomas that involve the dura mater and extend from the spinal cord to the subcutaneous tissue.[39,41,42]

Lipomas are associated with more severe bony changes than is the previously described dermal sinus, including scalloping of the dorsal vertebral body, widening of the interpedicular space, hemivertebrae, or even hypoplasia of the iliac wing.[38] These sequelae of the mass effect associated with lipomas suggest that resultant neurologic deficits occur not only by spinal cord tethering (see Pathophysiology and Presentation) but also by direct neural compression.

Pathophysiology and Presentation

Spinal lipomas, accounting for up to 35% of skin-covered lumbosacral masses, may extend to the superficial subcutaneous tissues and present in the infant as a visible and palpable mass.[43] As with other forms of the tethered cord syndrome, children with spinal lipomas may present with several complaints. At this age, before the onset of walking and the development of bladder control, a concomitant hairy patch may accompany an otherwise unnoticed lipoma. If the condition is unnoticed or disregarded, the infant without neurologic abnormalities may, with age, develop sphincter disturbance, postural and lower extremity deformities and weakness, or even verbalized discomfort.[44]

As mentioned, lipomas may cause neurologic symptoms through a combination of neural compression and spinal cord tethering. Lipomas, therefore, may present in much the same manner as do split cord malformations, a thickened filum terminale, and a congenital dermal sinus. As always, failure to attain developmental landmarks, as well as progressive loss of neurologic function, particularly lumbosacral function, should alert the health care provider to investigate the spine.

Classification

Lipomas of the conus medullaris may be classified into three categories: dorsal, caudal, and transitional. First described by Chapman, alone[45] and with Davis,[46] two distinct forms as well as a transitional form were categorized.

The dorsal variant is a lipoma that arises through a fascial defect and attaches directly to the dorsal aspect of the caudally descended conus medullaris. All nerve roots emerge from the ventral or lateral surface of the neural tissue and lie in the subarachnoid space. The lateral nerve roots are sensory, while motor roots are found more medial.

The caudal variant or terminal lipoma exits the area of the terminal filum so that the cord becomes progressively larger caudally. In this form the nerve roots may transgress the lipoma. Many of these nerve roots are thought to be nonfunctional and may be sacrificed after stimulation and monitoring. Although this caudal variant is difficult to re-form into a tubular structure, the cut end of the lipoma may retract sufficiently cephalad to reduce the probability that retethering will occur postoperatively.

The final form of lipoma described is the transitional form, which includes elements of both the dorsal and caudal variants described earlier in this chapter. Viable nerve roots pass through significant amounts of the lipoma prior to exiting. These typically are asymmetrical and are associated with a rotational component of the spinal cord. The process of distinguishing among these three types of lipoma usually is straightforward with adequate imaging, including MRI.

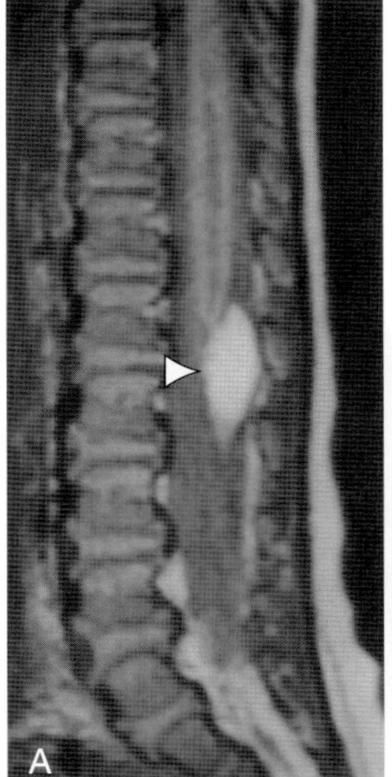

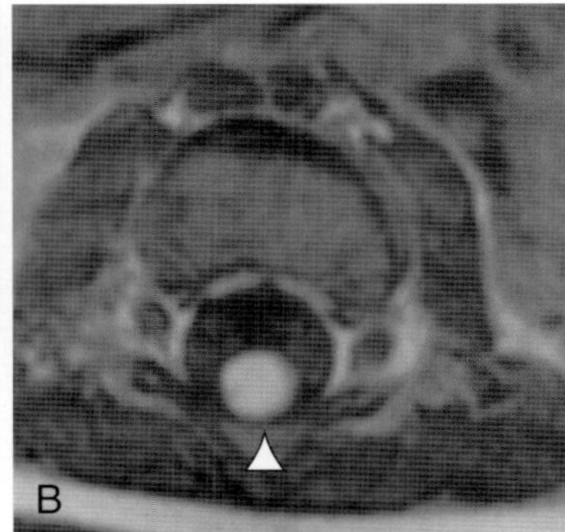

FIGURE 116-11. Sagittal (**A**) and axial (**B**) MR images of a tethered spinal cord with an intradural spinal lipoma (*arrowheads*).

Diagnostic Aids

Lipomas constitute only 1% of primary intraspinal tumors and almost always are associated with dysraphic spines.[47] Varying from intramedullary to extradural, their histologic nature and relative position to the spinal canal make them definable by both CT and MRI.[48]

Although spina bifida occulta, widening of the interpedicular distance, hemivertebrae, and vertebral body scalloping may all be observed on plain radiographic studies in the patient with a lipoma, these radiographs may be difficult to interpret. As with other spinal anomalies, lipomas usually are best worked up with MRI as the initial study (Fig. 116-11). CT usually is reserved for better definition of bony anatomy, if needed. Although not as detailed, myelograms may help define the extent of the mass (Figs. 116-12 and 116-13). Intradural lipomas are low density or even radiolucent on CT and have a high signal on T1-weighted MRI.[49] Both techniques are useful, however, in axial section. Extradural lipomas usually are more diffuse and contiguous with the nearby epidural fat. Even when epidural lipomas are not clearly visualized on CT scan and MRI, their presence should be considered.

McLone and Naidich[50] also support the use of ultrasonography in managing these lesions. The lack of calcium in immature bones allows for penetration and evaluation of structural detail, often well enough to verify the lesion, determine the extent of tethering, and proceed straight to surgery without the need for additional radiographic studies.

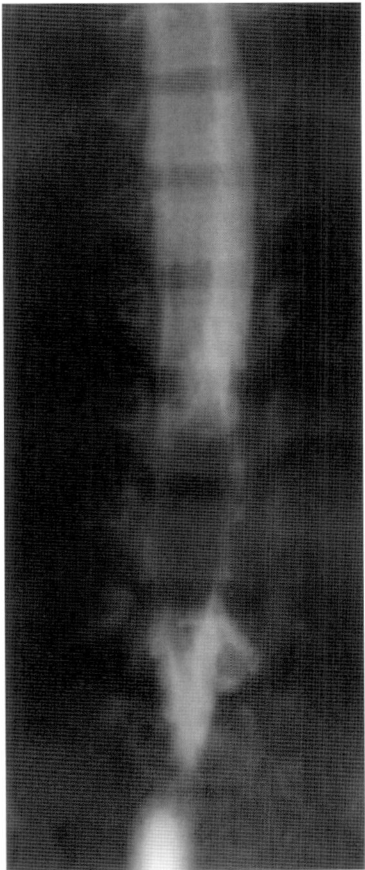

FIGURE 116-12. Anteroposterior lumbar myelogram revealing the filling defect caused by an intradural lipoma, causing a tether of the cord in the lumbosacral region.

Treatment

Whether by tethering of the filum terminale and spinal cord, direct neural compression, or both, surgery for spinal lipomas is warranted in the child with neurologic deficits. Operating on the asymptomatic patient has been controversial. However, most neurosurgeons now believe that if possible, lipomas and lipomeningoceles should be operated on before neurologic sequelae occur.[44,51,52] Unlike split cord malformations, in which involvement of the neural elements in the substance of the pathology is rare, such involvement is

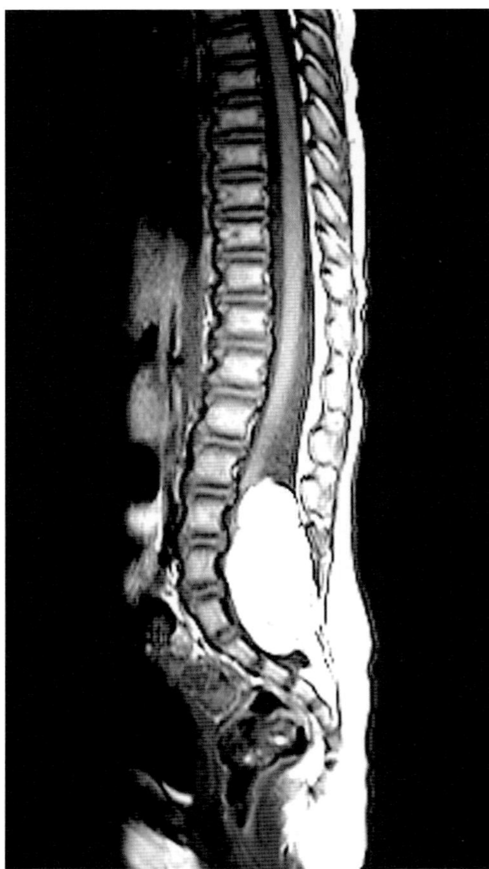

FIGURE 116-13. Sagittal T1-weighted image demonstrating large intradural spinal lipoma.

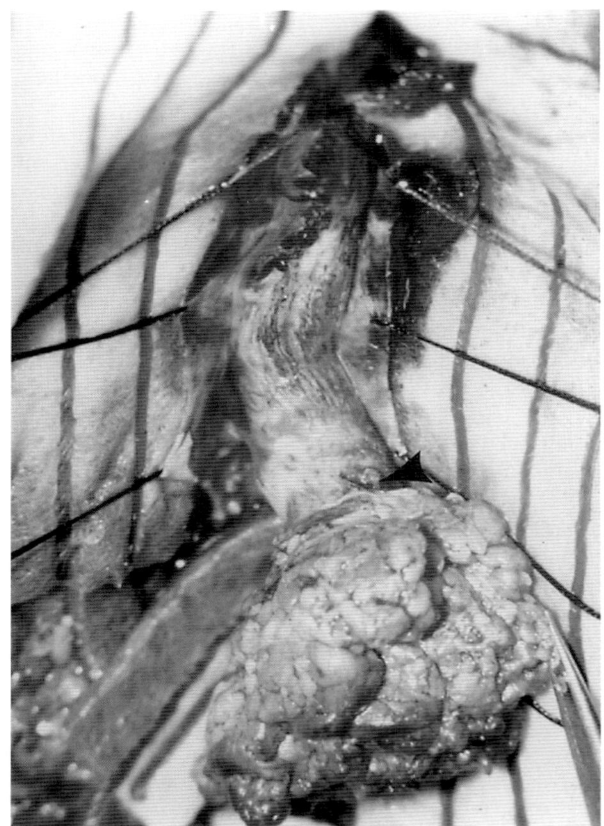

FIGURE 116-14. Intraoperative photograph showing the continuity of this large subcutaneous lipoma with the spinal cord *(arrowhead)*. Note the caudal attachment, making dissection of the nerve roots very difficult.

common in spinal lipomas. Therefore, even with detailed and defining preoperative studies, intraoperative electrophysiologic studies may be something that should be considered during resection of spinal lipomas. Not all surgeons consider this necessary. We, however, find it quite useful and do use intraoperative EMG monitoring, in which we insert needle electrodes in the muscles of the lower extremities as well as in the sphincter. Stimulation is performed with the same probes that are used for dorsal root rhizotomy. With this type of monitoring, one can ascertain whether there is undue traction on the conus medullaris and if it is safe to incise tissues that are near nerves or the spinal cord.

After sterilization of the skin, a midline incision should be performed over the palpable or visible subcutaneous portion of the lipoma. If there is no evidence of such a superficial lesion, needle localization with anteroposterior and lateral radiographs is useful. After incision of the fascia and lateral exposure of the laminae, microscopic enhancement, either with loupe magnification or the operating microscope, should be used. As with all occult dysraphic spines, care should be taken with both the scalpel and the electrocautery, because the unformed or bifid laminae may offer no protection for the thecal sac. Before the bony structures are reached, the extradural portions of the lipoma may require resection. If so, circumferential dissection of the lipoma is important so as to allow complete resection. The actual resection of the extradural portion of the lipoma usually is fairly straightforward. However, the location of the nerve roots relative to the lipoma-cord junction vary with the type of attachment that the lipoma has with the conus medullaris.[53] If the lipoma attaches to the dorsal surface of the conus, the nerve roots are ventral to the lipoma-conus interface. If, however, the lipoma is a caudal extension of the conus medullaris, the course of the nerve roots through the lipoma can be variable, and great care has to be exerted to prevent damage to neural structures (Fig. 116-14).

At the time of the durotomy, all anesthetic muscle relaxants should be avoided. Extradural lipomas that traverse the thecal sac into the intradural compartment may require resection of some dura mater. At this point, although some surgeons advocate the use of the carbon dioxide laser to vaporize the fatty lesion, we also suggest the use of the ultrasonic aspirator. Although relief of neural compression is one principle of surgery, particularly for lipomas on the dorsal surface of the spinal cord, the primary goal is to untether the spinal cord. Therefore, the surgery should be directed at accomplishing this goal. In such cases, sectioning of the filum terminale caudal to the sacral nerve roots may be required. Electrophysiologic monitoring is particularly useful at this point, not only to determine where the filum terminale may be incised and to ensure that no neural structures are coursing within the filum, but also to take care to avoid excessive manipulation of the functional nerve roots and the spinal cord. Often it is not possible or even necessary to resect the lipoma completely (Fig. 116-15). Prudence should be the rule, and one should

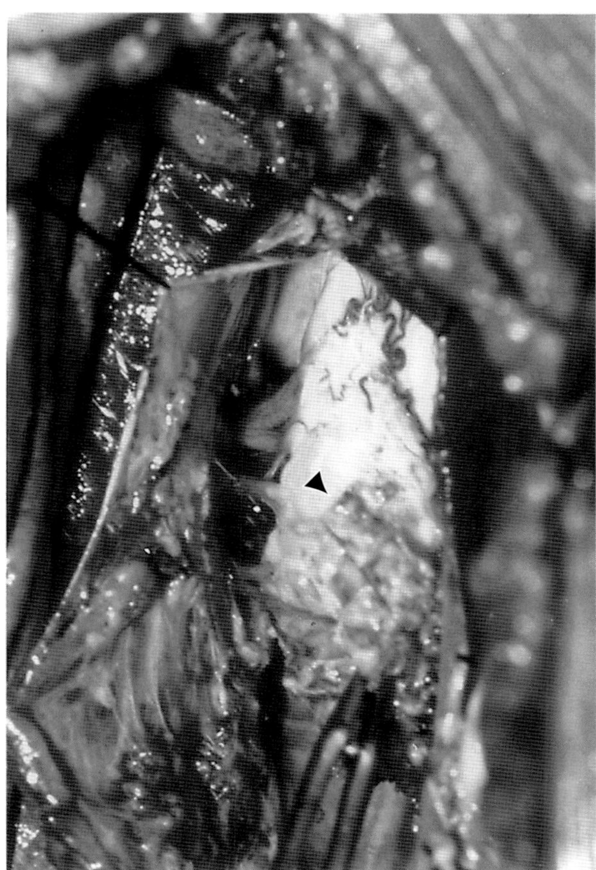

FIGURE 116-15. Intraoperative photograph demonstrating residual lipoma at the lipoma-conus interface, stimulation of which verified the presence of functional neural elements *(arrowhead)*. Note the slack nerve roots, verifying successful untethering of the cord from the dura.

not take any chance of injuring the conus medullaris or the nerve roots. It should be remembered that the primary goal of surgery is to untether the spinal cord and at the same time cause no deficits.

After removal of the lipoma, untethering of the surrounding neural structures, and possible sectioning of the filum terminale, dural closure must be watertight. Although reapproximation of two of the three meningeal layers may decrease the change of retethering, the pia and arachnoid often are incompetent after removal of the lipoma. Therefore, careful closure of the dura mater, which may include a graft, is important. As with other intrathecal operations, leaving the child flat in bed for 3 days allows for tissue healing and helps avoid collection of CSF, particularly if a large "dead space" has resulted from excision of an extradural component of the lipoma. Special techniques of closure to prevent retethering have been reported, but the patients have not been followed long enough to determine whether these techniques are better than conventional methods of closure.[54]

Complications

Infection, CSF leaks, and iatrogenic neurologic deficits are all complications that should be avoidable with meticulous surgery and disciplined technique. Preoperative administration of antibiotics is paramount, although postoperative doses depend on the surgeon's preference. Although the literature does not firmly support the use of antibiotics after elective, clean surgery, we prefer to give three postoperative doses to cover common skin flora. If postoperative infection should occur, appropriate drainage and debridement are necessary. Prolonged antibiotic treatment is indicated, and concerns about subsequent meningitis must be addressed with lumbar puncture. In the absence of obvious superficial infection, prolonged fever, or progressive worsening of neurologic function, MRI is necessary to rule out epidural abscess. In such cases, well-intentioned lumbar punctures may result in unintended meningitis.

Avoidance of CSF leaks, as previously mentioned, depends on watertight dural closure, anatomic approximation of all tissue planes, and placement of the child in the supine position postoperatively for recovery. A Valsalva maneuver at the end of the initial surgery may help expose any occult areas of leakage. Continued leaking requires decompression of the intradural pressure with a lumbar subarachnoid drain. Persistence despite these measures requires prompt reexploration, repair of obvious areas of CSF escape, and the appropriate use of dural substitutes and cryoprecipitate-based fibrin glue, with the possible addition of a lumbar subarachnoid drain. In extreme cases of dural incompetence, particularly in the face of a soft tissue defect and a potential space for CSF collection, a rotated or free-pedicle tissue flap may be required.

Immediate postoperative neurologic deficits often resolve. Manipulation of the distal spinal cord and nerve roots may result in traction injury and edema, resolution of which should imply return of neurologic function. This is not always the case, and prudence should be used while handling neural tissue during surgery. Deficits that result from definitive sectioning of the filum terminale or nerve roots are not reversible. With time, however, motor and sensory function may improve with reorganization of cortical neurons.

Outcome

Successful resection and untethering of these lipomas is now associated with little or no morbidity and mortality.[40,53,55] The best outcomes may be achieved with respect to pain, with most of the pain decreasing or disappearing within 3 months. Bladder dysfunction also may respond to resection of the lipoma in 20% to 30% of patients; of these patients, those with a spastic bladder respond best.[56] In a study by La Marca et al.,[51] 213 patients were operated on over a 20-year period, from 1975 to 1995. In patients with filum lipomas, 28 were asymptomatic and 27 were symptomatic. None of the asymptomatic patients worsened after surgery (mean follow-up, 3.4 years), and of the symptomatic group, there were no further deteriorations noted (follow-up, 6 months to 9 years). Of the group with conus lipomas, 9 of the 71 children (12.7%) operated on prophylactically later deteriorated (mean follow-up, 6.2 years) and required a second untethering operation. Symptoms of deterioration included urinary retention, pain, gait difficulty, urinary incontinence, and spasticity. In the symptomatic group (87 patients), 36 patients (41%) further deteriorated and required further surgery. At the final follow-up, however (mean, 6.6 years), 51% remained at clinical baseline and 26% improved. In a study by Xenos et al.,[57] the reoperation rate was 12% for signs of recurrent spinal cord tethering.

Emerging Technologies

Minimally Invasive Surgery

Minimally invasive or endoscopic surgical techniques have been used to treat a number of spinal pathologies in recent years. With spinal dysraphism and the tethered spinal cord presenting clinically and often repaired at a young age, minimally invasive operative techniques may be of great benefit to the patient. Recently, it has been determined that tethered spinal cords may be safely and effectively untethered using minimally invasive surgery.[58] This technique provides the advantage of reduced soft tissue injury, reduced postoperative pain, reduced postoperative scarring, and lower postoperative risk of retethering.

Minimally invasive untethering incorporates an approximately 3-cm incision with a muscle-splitting (tissue-sparing) approach, one vertebral body level below the conus. Benefits of this technique include sparing of midline structures, reduced postoperative complications, and full visualization of the filum terminale. Up to 11% of tethered cords may be found off the midline, and this approach provides visualization of the bilateral extent of the canal and full neural elements.

Carbon Dioxide Laser Detethering

Detethering of the spinal cord currently employs a number of instruments for sharp dissection during the surgical release of the tethered cord. Safely dissecting the nerve roots from the surrounding tissues requires precise microsurgical technique, although various laser technologies have been used in the past, and first were described as early as 1966.

Carbon dioxide (CO_2) lasers contain many features that make them favorable to neurosurgical procedures. CO_2 laser dissection is beneficial, in part, because CO_2 is almost completely absorbed by water and therefore does not penetrate tissue, reducing potential collateral tissue injury. Recent advancements have allowed the CO_2 laser to be passed through optical fiber; this, along with improved ergonomics, has allowed further implementation of this technology into operative practice. The unique physical properties, minimal depth of penetration, and minimal collateral nontargeted tissue damage of CO_2 laser energy make it a particularly useful tool in the release of tethered cord during the delicate operative course.

Cavitron Ultrasonic Aspiration

Cavitron ultrasonic aspiration (CUSA; Valleylab., Inc., Boulder, CO) is one alternative to the CO_2 laser. The original ultrasonic aspirator was developed in 1947 for the removal of dental plaque and was first applied to the field of eye surgery in 1967. Ultrasonic techniques became widely used in the medical and biochemical industries for sterilization, homogenization of solutions, and welding of materials. The use of the ultrasonic aspirator in neurosurgery was first reported in 1978, for the removal of intra-axial and extra-axial tumors such as meningiomas, schwannomas, and gliomas. The ultrasonic aspirator has since become a valuable tool in the neurosurgical armamentarium for the excision of intracranial and intraspinal tumors.[59] As with the CO_2 laser, the CUSA system provides efficient resection of target tissue with minimal injury to surrounding tissue or structures.

The ultrasonic aspirator has two tissue-disruptive effects at the tissue interface.[60] The first is caused by a suction effect that couples tissue to the tip and forces impacted tissue to vibrate, accelerate, and decelerate with the tip, eventually fragmenting away from unaffected tissues. The second important effect is cavitation. In cavitation, the rapidly oscillating tip produces localized pressure waves, which cause vapor pockets around cells in tissues with high water content; the collapse of these pockets then causes the tissue cells to rupture. Tissues with weak intracellular bonds, such as tumors and lipomas, are easy to fragment, whereas tissues with strong intracellular bonds, such as nerves and vessel walls, are difficult to fragment. The speed of fragmentation depends on the amplitude setting of the system.

KEY REFERENCES

Akay KM, Ershin Y, Cakir Y: Tethered cord syndrome in adults. *Acta Neurochir (Wien)* 142:1111, 2000.

Archibeck MJ, Smith JT, Carroll KL, et al: Surgical release of tethered cord: survivorship analysis and orthopedic outcome. *J Pediatr Orthop* 17:773, 1997.

Balkan E, Kilic N, Avsar I, et al: Urodynamic findings in the tethered spinal cord: the effect of tethered cord division on lower urinary tract functions. *Eur J Pediatr Surg* 11:116, 2001.

Boop FA, Russell A, Chadduck WM: Diagnosis and management of the tethered cord syndrome. *J Ark Med Soc* 89:328, 1992.

Chong C, Molet J, Oliver B, et al: The tethered cord syndrome: a review of causes. *Neurologia* 9:12, 1994.

Garzo-Mercado R: Diastematomyelia and intramedullary epidermoid spinal tumor combined with extra-dural teratoma in an adult. *J Neurosurg* 58:954, 1983.

Hilal SK, Marton D, Pollack E: Diastematomyelia in children. *Radiology* 112:609, 1974.

Yamada S, Zinke DE, Sanders DC: Pathophysiology of "tethered cord syndrome." *J Neurosurg* 54:499, 1981.

REFERENCES

The complete reference list is available online at expertconsult.com.

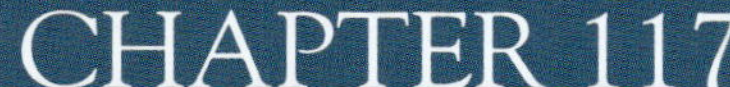
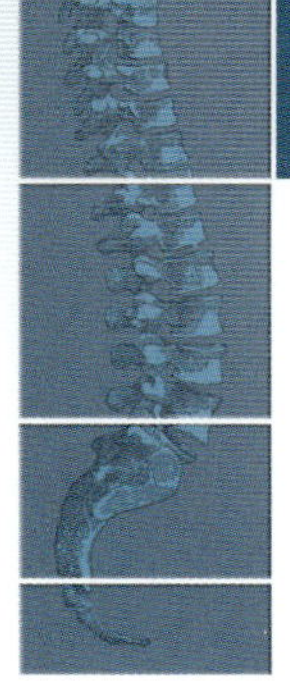

CHAPTER 117

Myelomeningocele and Associated Anomalies

Mark G. Luciano | Samer K. Elbabaa

Myelomeningocele, or spina bifida aperta, is defined as a dorsally protruding open spinal cord defect that usually is associated with spinal nerve paralysis and anomalies throughout the spinal axis. The goal of this chapter is to discuss and provide a description of the current management of myelomeningocele and its common associated anomalies in general, with special emphasis on associated spinal anomalies.

History and Epidemiology

Many epidemiologic studies have combined myelomeningocele with other defects such as anencephaly under the term *neural tube defect* (NTD). This grouping makes sense embryologically, because both myelomeningocele and anencephaly are open lesions that arise as a result of failure of primary neurulation and are separated in time by only one embryonic stage (2 days).

When describing NTD at birth, the term *incidence* is more clinically descriptive than is the term *prevalence,* because many affected fetuses abort spontaneously. NTDs exhibit wide geographic, ethnic, and gender variation. In the United States, NTD rates have declined from 1.3 per 1000 births in 1970 to 0.6 per 1000 births in 1989.[1] Worldwide, numbers range from 1 to 6 per 1000 births.[2] Superimposed on a general worldwide decrease in the incidence at birth of myelomeningocele, a number of influences cause both a reduction in prevalence at birth and an increased prevalence in the general population. Reduction of myelomeningocele at birth may result from maternal supplementation with folates and a higher rate of pregnancy termination due to availability of maternal serum α-fetoprotein testing and refined resolution of ultrasound for in utero fetal examination.

Recent improvements in neonatal and postoperative care have resulted in increased survival rates and, therefore, an increased prevalence in the general population. Zachary[3] believed that all affected infants should be operated on, even though many survivors inevitably will suffer from multiple handicaps. Worldwide, there are several variables considered and degrees of selection for candidacy for myelomeningocele treatment. The predominant factors are the level of the myelomeningocele and associated paralysis, the severity of associated hydrocephalus, and the presence of gross deformities. The overwhelming majority of untreated infants with myelomeningocele will die early in life.[4]

The evolution of myelomeningocele treatment over the last few decades also has led to a tremendous change in quality of life in affected patients. McLone[5] estimated that more than 75% of surviving infants with myelomeningocele will have normal intelligence; however, the frequency of learning disabilities is likely to be high. More than 80% will be ambulators by school age, while more than 90% will have bladder and bowel control.

Embryogenesis and Pathophysiology

During the last 100 years, various hypotheses have been proposed concerning the embryogenesis of myelomeningocele. Multiple experimental models and autopsy specimens were studied thoroughly. Myelomeningocele was produced in animal models genetically (e.g., curly tail mouse)[6] or induced by medical or environmental factors such as vitamin A,[7] valproic acid,[8] salicylates,[9] insulin,[10] and hyperglycemic[11] and hyperthermic[12] conditions.

Current theories regarding the embryogenesis of dysraphic spinal lesions in general, and of myelomeningocele in particular, invoke a primary disorder of early neural tube development. This early defect of embryogenesis occurs in the fourth week of gestation. In normal embryos, the CNS originates from the neural tube, which is the thickening of the dorsal ectoderm. By the gradual elevation of the lateral margins of the neural tube, which are termed *neural folds,* the neural groove is formed. The neural folds meet in the midline and then form the neural tube. This process begins at the mesencephalic level and proceeds rostrally and caudally, with latest tube formation in the caudal spine at the caudal level.

Four different theories have been described: simple nonclosure, overgrowth and nonclosure, reopening (overdistention), and primary mesodermal insufficiency.[7] Since its introduction, the nonclosure theory has gained almost universal acceptance because of its consistency with observations of early human embryos in which NTDs have been studied during or shortly after neural tube closure. Additional support has been provided by animal models of dysraphism, virtually all of which displayed a primary defect of neural tube closure.[13]

Myelomeningocele includes other consistent anomalies through the CNS axis, including Chiari II malformation and hydrocephalus. After studying the initial developmental defects

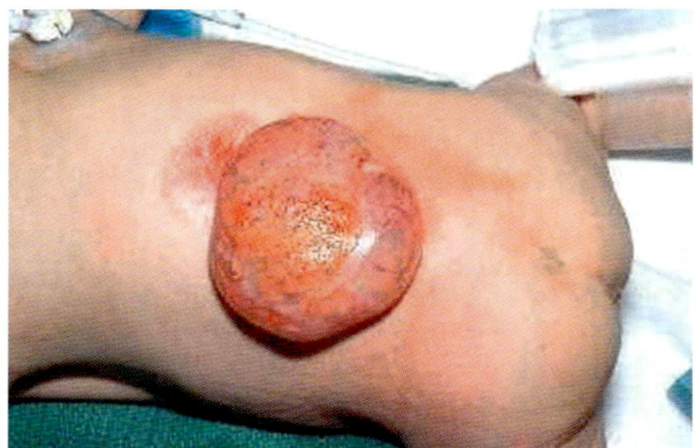

FIGURE 117-1. Preoperative photograph of a typical myelomeningocele.

of the Chiari II malformation using a genetically mutated NTD mouse model, McLone and Knepper[14] proposed a unified theory that describes and emphasizes the developmental sequence of associated anomalies. This pathophysiologic sequence starts with cerebrospinal fluid (CSF) leakage from the unclosed spinal defect. As a result, the usual distention and expansion of the developing ventricular system fails. The lack of distention of rhombencephalic vesicles alters the inductive effect of pressure on the surrounding mesenchyme and endochondral bone formation and results in small posterior fossa. Consequently, the development of the cerebellum and brainstem with a small posterior fossa leads to upward herniation and a dysplastic tentorium. Downward herniation results in a large foramen magnum and cerebellar vermis and brainstem displacement into the cervical segments (Chiari II malformation). Hydrocephalus is secondary to maldevelopment of the CSF pathways in the posterior fossa.

Most myelomeningoceles (85%) occur in the distal thoracic to lumbosacral spine. About 10% are detected in the higher thoracic area, and an additional 5% in the cervical area.[15] Typically, a neural placode (plaque), which is unfolded neural tissue, appears at the center with a pia mater on the ventral surface. The ventral and dorsal nerve roots arise from the central surface of the placode, with the dorsal roots originating more laterally. Rostrally, the placode is continuous with the normal spinal cord within the spinal canal. At the periphery of the defect, the placode is circumscribed by arachnoid membrane that fuses with the free margins of the skin, fascia, and dura mater (Fig. 117-1). At involved levels, pedicles of vertebrae are displaced laterally, creating a widened spinal canal diameter. Vertebral bodies may be normal or wedge-shaped in the anteroposterior diameter, resulting in a kyphotic deformity.[16]

Etiology

The etiology of myelomeningocele is multifactorial and heterogeneous. Experimental teratology has shown that several agents can increase occurrence rates: alcohol, carbamazepine,[17] valproic acid,[18] salicylates,[9] insulin,[10] clomiphene, influenza virus,[19] and chemotherapeutic agents have all been incriminated. Population studies, however, have provided strikingly little evidence to suggest the role of a single teratogen as the sole cause of a significant number of myelomeningoceles.[20] Maternal age and birth order also may contribute to the risk of NTDs. Most studies show an excess of first-born children in the population of NTDs.[21] In addition, most mothers of affected children are younger than 20 years of age or older than 35.[22]

Although rarely clustered in families, a mendelian pattern of inheritance is evident. The recurrence risk for siblings of an affected individual is 2% to 5%, representing a 25- to 50-fold increase in recurrence risk compared with that of the general population.[23] A multicenter NTD genetic study reviewed the identification of genes predisposing to NTD through linkage analysis and candidate gene analysis along with characteristics of a large nationally ascertained cohort of families. Results from specific assessments of *p53*, *PAX3*, and *MTHFR* failed to suggest that these genes play a major role in NTD development in these families.[24] A frequent association was found between trisomy 13 and 18 and myelomeningocele in the fetus before 24 weeks (as high as 14%) but was rare in full-term infants, suggesting fetal demise.[25]

Dietary factors related to NTDs were investigated extensively after several studies showed a progressive increase in the prevalence rate of NTDs in lower socioeconomic classes. Zinc deficiency has been considered because of a known increased risk of congenital defects in the offspring of animals fed a zinc-deficient diet,[26] but human studies have been inconclusive so far.[20]

Folic acid antagonists, such as aminopterin, were shown to cause NTDs in animal studies, and since the publication of these studies, the effect of folic acid on prevention of myelomeningocele has been studied. In one study, serum and red blood cell levels of folate were decreased in mothers of children with myelomeningocele compared with controls.[27] Folic acid and multivitamin supplementation to high-risk mothers has been demonstrated to reduce the prevalence at birth of myelomeningocele in some populations.[27,28] However, adherents to the folic acid prevention philosophy acknowledge that they cannot provide a reasonable mechanism of action.[18]

Repair of Myelomeningocele

Evaluation of the Newborn

Prenatal diagnosis and counseling have a significant effect on the preparation and decision-making process in cases of myelomeningocele.[29] Prenatal diagnosis of myelomeningocele involves the combined use of maternal serum α-fetoprotein screening and fetal ultrasonography.[30] Advances in ultrasound imaging have led to an increased rate of identification of myelomeningocele before birth. On detection, obstetricians usually refer the mother and family to a multidisciplinary team that includes a pediatric neurosurgeon, neonatologist, social worker, and spina bifida team coordinator. This referral facilitates postnatal treatment, including surgery, to be planned in a timely fashion, and informs and educates the family about the nature of myelomeningocele and its associated anomalies.[15]

Early closure of the spinal defect remains an important part of the modern management of children born with myelomeningocele. The rationale for early closure includes the prevention of ascending infection; preservation of motor, sensory, and intellectual function; establishment of a suitable environment for continued development of neural tissue; and cosmetic reconstruction.[31] Most pediatric neurosurgeons agree that closure of the open myelomeningocele within the first 24 to 48 hours after birth decreases morbidity and mortality rates. Initiating surgery after 72 hours carries a significant risk of meningitis and ventriculitis,[32] a decrease of motor function, and an increase in neurologic deficits.[15]

Postnatally, the myelomeningocele defect should be covered with a sterile dressing (wet or nonadherent dressing) before the infant is transferred to the neonatal intensive care unit. The newborn is kept in a prone or lateral recumbent position to protect the neural tissue by avoiding pressure on the placode. A thorough examination of the neonate should be conducted to assess the degree of neurologic deficit, the functional level, and associated concerns such as hydrocephalus and cardiopulmonary, genitourinary, and gastrointestinal conditions that could interfere with surgery of the myelomeningocele. Early urologic consultation is obtained with intermittent catheterization until adequate bladder function is ascertained.

A segmental motor examination should be obtained for future comparison. Observation of spontaneous hip flexion (L1-3), knee extension (L2-4), knee flexion (L5-S1), foot dorsiflexion (L4-5), and foot plantar flexion (S1-2) should be noted. If painful stimulus is required to elicit movement, it should be applied in a sensory dermatome well above those related to the lesion. Painful stimuli applied below the level of the lesion may elicit stereotypical reflex movements, which may be falsely interpreted as a functional motor segment. Gross asymmetry between the two lower extremities may indicate a more proximal lesion in the spinal cord (e.g., diastematomyelia, hemimyelocele).

More than 90% of neonates with myelomeningocele have some form of neurogenic bladder. Dribbling of urine as the neonate cries or moves is a strong indicator of future urinary incontinence, whereas periodic micturition with a good stream suggests a possibility of partial incontinence.[33] These infants also should be carefully inspected for characteristic external features that point to severe chromosomal abnormalities. Examination of the placode includes noting its shape and circumference, skin integrity, and extent of the cutaneous and epithelialized layers. The spinal column is examined for early congenital scoliosis, kyphosis, and palpable prominent laminae at the lateral margin of the lesion.

Surgical Repair

After identification of the neural placode and cerebrospinal fluid flowing from the central canal, dissection begins and is continued in a circumferential fashion, dividing the placode from the epithelial layer. This will allow the surgeon to see the pia-arachnoid attached at the periphery of the neural placode. It is essential to understand that, developmentally, the lateral edges of the ventral surface of the placode are the alar plate or the dorsal root entry zones. Dorsal nerve roots (sensory) are observed in this region. The medial portion of the ventral surface of the placode is the basal plate, which contains the ventral nerve roots (motor). Thus, the pia-arachnoid meets the neural placode at the lateral margin of the ventral surface of the placode.

The neural tissue is then gently freed from any ventral arachnoid adhesions, using microdissection techniques. When this has been completed, the flat neural placode should be free throughout its circumference and ready for dorsal reapproximation. Beginning rostrally, the pia-arachnoid neural junction of each lateral edge should be brought together in the dorsal midline. Care should be taken to engage only the pia with each pass of the suture, avoiding injury to the sensory roots.

The dura mater is located just beneath the skin edge laterally. Its lateral attachment is incised and the epidural space identified (often marked by the presence of epidural fat). The dura mater should be freed rostrally and caudally to the apices of the defect on each side so that the free edges come together in the midline dorsally. The dura mater is closed in a watertight fashion. The closure should be patulous to prevent spinal cord ischemia and tethering. Occasionally, a dural graft may be required. Intradural hemostasis should be meticulous to minimize late fibrosis and scarring. With all these surgical procedures, latex reactions should be considered.[34]

Reapproximation of the paraspinous muscles over the repair may require some lateral dissection for mobilization. In the presence of a kyphos, the paraspinous muscles can act as spine flexors because of their lateral position, which, owing to the deformity, is ventral to the neural axis of the spine. The paraspinous muscles may then be repositioned in the normal anatomic location: dorsal and paramedian. The dorsal fascia can now be reapproximated. A continuous suture with intermittent, interrupted sutures can be used for this layer to further reinforce the watertight dural closure. It is important to note that adequate mobilization of the paraspinous muscles is crucial to prevent constriction of the underlying neural elements.[15]

Closure of the skin in the midline can be facilitated by a generous blunt subcutaneous dissection for mobilization. The proper plane for this blunt dissection is just superficial to the dorsal fascia. Continuous monofilament suture is used for skin closure, which further reinforces the layer by watertight closure. Occasionally, the defect is so large that skin closure cannot be accomplished without undue tension. Consultation with a plastic surgeon may be obtained if adequate skin closure is difficult or even impossible. Several surgical techniques have been used in this situation, including local rotated skin flaps, tissue expansion,[35] relaxation of the lateral incisions with a skin graft,[36] and a Limberg-latissimus dorsi myocutaneous flap.[37]

A recent development in myelomeningocele closure involves the in utero closure of myelomeningocele defects. The rationale for fetal repair of myelomeningoceles and initial clinical outcomes have been discussed over the last few years. The development of techniques to close open neural tube malformations prior to birth has generated great interest and hope for fetal interventions and their outcomes. In most recent series of patients, intrauterine myelomeningocele repair appeared to decrease the incidence of hindbrain herniation and shunt-dependent hydrocephalus in infants with myelomeningocele, but increased the incidence of premature delivery. Long-term improvement of neurologic outcome and prevention of hindbrain herniation and hydrocephalus has yet to be proven.[38-41]

Associated Anomalies

A multitude of associated anomalies are common in infants with myelomeningocele. CNS anomalies are more common than other systemic anomalies. Microgyria, polygyria, enlargement of the massa intermedia, agenesis or dysgenesis of the corpus callosum, and cerebellar dysgenesis, along with Chiari II malformation, are common findings that can be encountered on MRI. The midbrain, especially the tectal area, can be beaked, and the aqueduct of Sylvius can be anomalous. The pons and medulla oblongata are bowed dorsally and often extend into the rostral cervical spinal canal along with the cerebellar vermis and tonsils.[15]

In a series of autopsies on infants with the myelomeningocele and Chiari malformations, cerebral and cerebellar cortical malformations were found in 92% and 72% of cases, respectively. Heterotopias (i.e., displaced, well-formed gyri and folia), heterotaxias (i.e., disordered combinations of mature neurons and germinal cells), immature germinal cell collections, microgyria, and polymicrogyria were observed. Ventricular system anomalies were present in 92% of cases in the same series, including atresia, stenosis, and forking of the cerebral aqueduct. Atresia of the third ventricle and stenosis of the fourth ventricle occurred rarely. Other uncommon findings included septum pellucidum cysts and agenesis of the olfactory tracts and bulbs.[42]

Systemic anomalies also occur and should be considered independently when assessing infants with myelomeningocele and Chiari malformations for surgical intervention. Associated systemic anomalies appear in the gastrointestinal, pulmonary, and cardiovascular systems and in the craniofacial structures.[43] The most common anomalies in the genitourinary system include hydroureter and hydronephrosis, which usually occur after long-standing neurogenic bladder. Gastrointestinal anomalies include inguinal hernia, Meckel diverticulum, malrotation, omphalocele, and imperforate anus. Cardiovascular anomalies include ventricular or atrial septal defects, patent ductus arteriosus, and coarctation of the aorta.[44]

Hydrocephalus

CSF shunting for hydrocephalus is required in approximately 80% of infants born with myelomeningocele.[45] Most clinical signs develop in the first 3 weeks of life, but clinical signs occasionally develop at an older age.[45] It is possible that the rapid onset of hydrocephalus after birth is due to the myelomeningocele acting as a compensatory reservoir that is terminated by defect closure.[16]

Both advanced gestational age and severity of posterior fossa deformity have been shown independently to correlate with the size of ventricles in infants born with myelomeningocele.[46] The sites of obstruction of CSF pathways are variable and include the aqueduct, outlet of the fourth ventricle, arachnoid space at the level of the foramen magnum, and tentorium. Wills et al.[47] showed that hydrocephalus itself has a very minor effect on intellectual development; however, prior shunt infections and ventriculitis in the neonatal period are major factors limiting intelligence.

Head circumference is below the 50th percentile in most infants born with myelomeningocele. However, serial measurements of head circumference and ultrasound examination of the head should be obtained after closure of the myelomeningocele defect to identify infants who will subsequently need shunting. A mean increase of 2 mm per day was found to have a predictive value. Infants born with overt hydrocephalus signs such as large head circumference, bulging fontanelle, split cranial sutures, and dilated scalp veins generally require early CSF diversion to relieve the intracranial hypertension and prevent myelomeningocele wound dehiscence. Signs of increased intracranial pressure in the newborn, such as bradycardia, poor sucking, apnea, and decreased spontaneous activity, indicate the need for shunting. The function of the shunt should always be considered and checked before any surgical treatment of Chiari II malformation or syringomyelia after symptoms deteriorate.[5] A common practice is to wait 5 days or more after myelomeningocele closure before shunting. Most infants will tolerate this waiting period.[16] In one series, shunt infection and malfunction rates were comparable between infants undergoing a simultaneous myelomeningocele closure and shunting procedures and those infants with the delayed-onset hydrocephalus and shunting.

Chiari Malformation and Syringomyelia

Virtually all children with myelomeningocele have a Chiari II malformation.[48] The hallmark of the Chiari II malformation is the caudal displacement of the cerebellar vermis, medulla, and lower brainstem below the level of the foramen magnum into or below the craniocervical junction. The caudal descent of the lower brainstem into the cervical canal may create a kink or spur of medulla behind the cervical spinal cord in up to 70% of patients with Chiari II malformation.[49] The cerebellum of these patients is smaller than normal; however, it resides in a proportionately smaller posterior fossa. The tentorium has a low insertion and often is hypoplastic (Fig. 117-2).

The prevalence of hydrosyringomyelia in patients with Chiari II malformation has been variably reported as 44% to 88%.[50,51] The true frequency in recent series may be underestimated secondary to collapse of the syrinx after shunting and/or Chiari decompression[52] (Fig. 117-3).

Between 20% and 33% of patients with Chiari II malformation become symptomatic from hindbrain herniation.[52] Of these symptomatic children, nearly one third do not

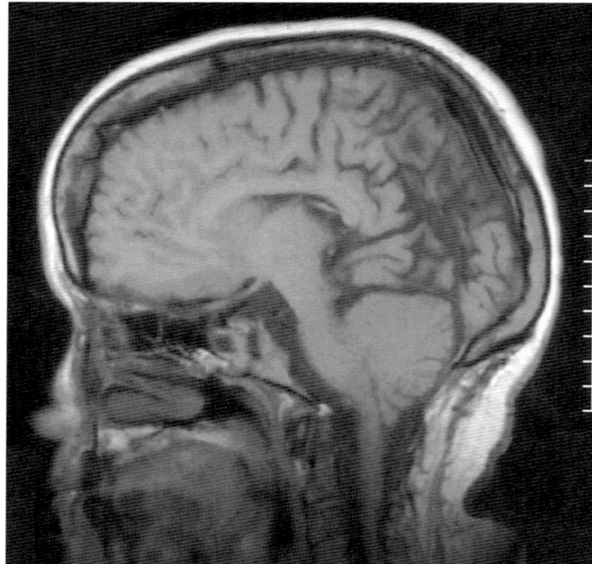

FIGURE 117-2. Sagittal T1-weighted MRI of the Chiari II malformation. Note the herniation of the cerebellar vermis through the foramen magnum, low-lying tentorium, beaked appearance of the tectal plate, and enlargement of the massa intermedia.

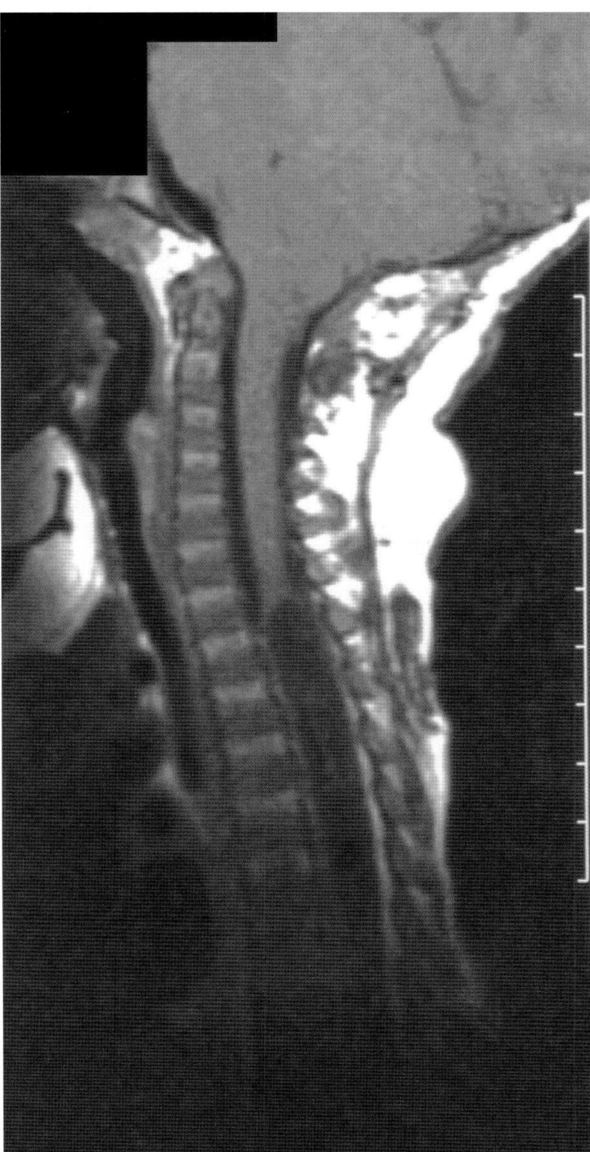

FIGURE 117-3. Sagittal T1-weighted MRI of a child with Chiari II malformation demonstrating syringomyelia of the cervical and upper thoracic spinal cord.

survive beyond infancy, making the symptomatic hindbrain herniation the leading cause of mortality in treated myelomeningocele in the first 2 years of life.[5] Between 1983 and 1992, four different retrospective studies indicated that there are basically two types of presentation that are clearly age dependent and may reflect different pathophysiologies.[48,52-54] Neonatal patients present with symptoms referable to lower cranial nerve and brainstem dysfunction, and older children present with spasticity, cerebellar signs, and weakness.[52] Infantile symptoms include swallowing difficulty, stridor, aspiration, apnea, bradycardia, arm weakness, and opisthotonic posturing.

The surgical treatment of Chiari II malformation usually consists of decompressive laminectomy at the C1 level and lower as needed, excision of the constrictive dural band at the C1 level, and a cautious suboccipital craniectomy due to the low-lying transverse sinus. Fourth ventricular exploration may be performed to ensure that a CSF outlet and dural graft may be used in closure. The timing of surgery is controversial.[53] The surgical treatment of older children can be rewarding, with almost all patients showing stabilization or return to normal function.[52] Irreversible compressive or ischemic brainstem injury has been proposed as the cause of the high mortality rate and as an argument for relatively emergent surgical intervention. Two of the retrospective studies have noted no obvious evidence of brainstem dysfunction at birth.[54] In autopsy specimens from infants with Chiari II malformation who had died, ischemic medullary hemorrhages confirmed that vascular compromise is a contributing cause.[55] It is likely that in the one third of myelomeningocele patients who become symptomatic before 3 years of age, there is a greater degree of brainstem dysmorphism, creating a brainstem at risk that would have little tolerance for compression or ischemia. In these patients, rapid deterioration would be expected, and the results of prompt surgical intervention on the initial symptoms may be favorable.[52]

The indications for surgery are clearer in patients with syringomyelia. Between 60% and 73% improved after treatment for a symptomatic syrinx, and none worsened after surgery in two series.[50,56] Typically, patients have an initial stable neurologic examination and then present with progressive spasticity and scoliosis. An expanding cervical hydrosyringomyelic cavity classically results in dissociative sensory loss of the upper extremities caused by interruption in the crossing spinothalamic tracts. Weakness, hyporeflexia, and atrophy of the upper musculature may result from involvement of the anterior horn cells. Motor and sensory findings can be asymmetrical, and a worsening scoliosis may be the sole manifestation of an expanding cavity of the thoracic spinal cord.[53,57] Also, an expanding cervical cavity can result in a worsening lower cranial nerve dysfunction.[52] Different treatment strategies have been followed. In the presence of ventriculomegaly, ventricular shunting reduces the syrinx size when there is a communication between the syrinx and the fourth ventricle (in about 10% of cases).[57,58] When a shunt is already in place, its function should be evaluated and corrected. A decompressive laminectomy and opening of the foramen of Magendie to restore normal CSF hydrodynamics is indicated when a functional shunt is confirmed.[57] Plugging of the obex, fourth ventricle-to-subarachnoid shunts, syringosubarachnoid shunts, and syringopleural shunts have all been used, but their use is controversial.[57-60] However, syrinx shunts have been used successfully when decompression alone fails to result in clinical improvement and as a primary treatment of thoracic lesions.[59]

Tethered Spinal Cord

After primary repair of myelomeningocele, late progressive neurologic deterioration commonly occurs due to a tethered spinal cord at the site of previous closure secondary to scarring and adherence of the neural placode to the dorsal dura mater[61] (Fig. 117-4). Tethered cord is the result of fixation of the spinal cord, which limits motion in the caudal-rostral direction. Yamada et al.[62] correlated the pattern of gradually developing tethered cord symptoms with impairment of oxidative metabolism and mitochondrial anoxia as a result of excessive steady traction of the spinal cord in experimental animal models.

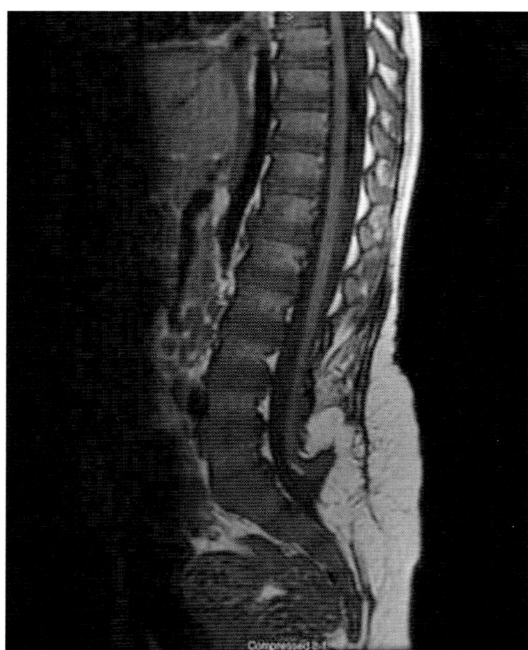

FIGURE 117-4. Sagittal T1-weighted MRI showing tethering of the spinal cord 10 years after myelomeningocele closure.

In some series, neurologic deterioration due to tethered cord occurred in 27% of children.[5] The average onset of symptoms occurs at 10 years of age and correlates with a period of accelerating growth. Presenting symptoms include gait imbalance, lower back pain, weakness in the lower extremities, bladder or bowel incontinence, scoliosis, and orthopaedic deformities. MRI of the lumbar spine is the gold standard of anatomic diagnosis. However, because all spinal cords in patients with myelomeningocele appear elongated and tethered, the decision to operate depends on the demonstration of clinical progression. The decision to treat may result from deterioration seen on a urodynamic study or ascending sensory or motor neurologic loss of function.

Surgical release involves laminectomy at the vertebral level just rostral to the defect and lysis of adhesions. Additional pathology such as hydromyelia, thickened filum terminale, dermal sinus tracts, and diastematomyelia can present in 30% of patients.[61] The stretched spinal cord tissue should appear relaxed at the completion of the procedure. Duraplasty may be considered to prevent postoperative dural adhesions in the repair of the tethered spinal cord.[63]

The timing of the surgical release of the tethered spinal cord is controversial. However, early diagnosis and early treatment are essential to provide patients with the best chance of recovery. In one report, 82% of patients who were followed closely and treated early had improvement, whereas only 54% of those not followed closely had improvement.[61] Another report showed that delayed untethering, following the onset of a neurologic deficit, may reverse some lost motor function but is unlikely to restore bladder and bowel function.[64]

Scoliosis

Deformity of the spine is common in patients with myelomeningocele. The most commonly encountered spinal deformities are scoliosis and kyphosis. Scoliotic deformities typically develop over years as a result of imbalance of the spinal musculature and abnormal posture.[65] The frequency of spinal deformities is related to the neurologic level, with nearly 100% of children with thoracic level myelomeningocele requiring corrective surgery.[66] Other important factors include age, the presence of syringomyelia,[67] and tethering of the spinal cord.[68]

Scoliosis presents in two forms in these patients: congenital and developmental.[69] Congenital scoliosis arises from vertebral anomalies, particularly hemivertebrae and segmentation defects. Developmental scoliosis, the more common type, has a delayed onset and a progressive course. It produces considerable functional decline at advanced stages and generally is believed to result from muscular imbalance, which leads to progressive deformity during growth. Scoliotic curves usually develop between 5 and 10 years of age, but most deterioration occurs between 10 and 15 years of age.[69]

The higher the level of paralysis, the greater the incidence of spinal deformity.[70] Scoliosis develops in up to 100% of patients with thoracic lesions, but in fewer than 10% of patients with sacral lesions. In a large series of 465 patients, Carstens et al.[70] showed that the patient's neurologic level of the lesion is the most important factor determining the development of scoliosis in myelomeningocele. A 3.5-degree deterioration of the angle occurred every year in patients with levels of paralysis between T3 and T12, and a 2.5-degree deterioration in patients with levels of paralysis between L1 and L3.

The natural history of untreated scoliosis in myelomeningocele is that of deformity progression, with a rate of deterioration significantly higher than in idiopathic scoliosis (Fig. 117-5). The aims of treatment are preservation of respiratory function, maintenance of sitting stability, achievement of maximal trunk length, and stabilization of the trunk.[69] Corrective bracing is used as the initial management while the child matures. Children with myelomeningocele should be examined yearly for the presence or progression of scoliosis. Once spinal curvature surpasses 30 degrees, bracing usually fails and fusion surgery is required to control progression.[65] However, spinal orthoses in children with myelomeningocele may lead to deformity of the ribs, decreased pulmonary function, ischemia of the skin, and pressure ulcerations.[71] Progressive scoliosis is often the result of other correctable neurologic pathologies such as syringomyelia, hydromyelia, tethered spinal cord, or hydrocephalus shunt malfunction.[66] Stability or improvement of the scoliosis can be anticipated following untethering of the spinal cord.[68] Tomlinson et al.[72] found that syringomyelia is associated with a high incidence of developmental scoliosis and that decompression of the syrinx either leads to improvement in, or stabilization of, the majority of scoliotic curves or postpones the need for fusion surgery. If a neurosurgical cause is discovered and treated, spontaneous improvement in the scoliosis may be seen if the curve is small in magnitude. Large curves do not resolve despite neurosurgical intervention.[73]

The definitive treatment of scoliosis in the myelomeningocele patient is spinal fusion. The entire curve must be included in the fusion. Distally, the fusion should extend to include the lumbosacral joint if there is pelvic obliquity and the patient does not walk.[66] Combined ventral and dorsal spinal fusions have been recommended because dorsal fusion alone can result in a high rate of pseudarthroses due

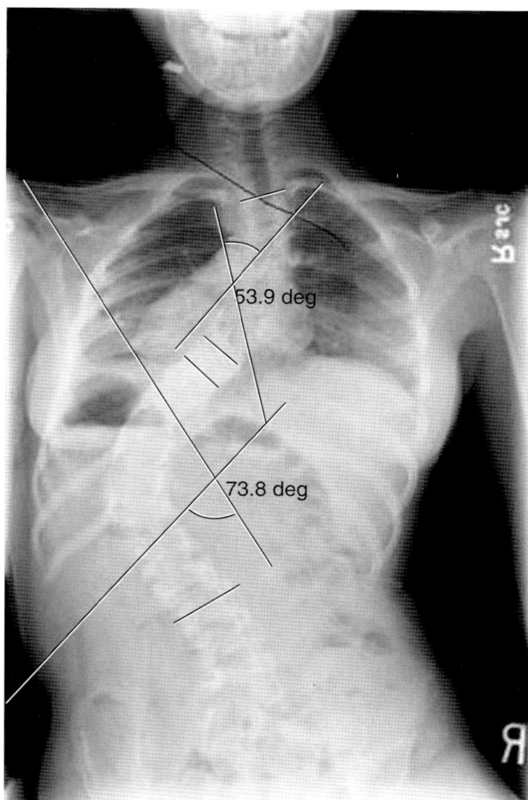

FIGURE 117-5. Sitting anteroposterior spinal radiograph shows severe scoliotic deformity in a patient with a history of lower thoracic myelomeningocele repair at birth.

to incomplete solid fusion at the defective laminar defects. Most arthroses occur at the lumbosacral junction. However, bilateral transpedicular fixation of the L5 and S1 levels can be performed as a prophylactic procedure.[74] The role of ventral fusion is controversial, and it may not be necessary for routine curves.[75] The most common complications are infection, loss of correction, and pseudarthrosis.[76]

Kyphosis

A kyphotic deformity of the spine, in association with a myelomeningocele, is present in approximately 10% of patients.[77] Progression of the kyphotic deformity can be seen in the sagittal plane of affected children.[78] Unrelenting progression of 8 degrees per year is seen in most of them.[79] Congenital kyphoses progress not only because of the deficiencies of the dorsal elements of the spine but also because of the effects of gravity during sitting and standing, as well as the subluxation of the extensor spinal muscles laterally and the unopposed psoas muscles anteriorly.[80] A kyphotic deformity can interfere with sitting and prevents supination. Common associated symptoms include skin ulceration over the gibbus and crowding of the thoracic and abdominal contents. Kyphosis usually is associated with pulmonary and digestive compromise, owing to the crowding of the lungs by the intra-abdominal contents, which are forced upward by the flexion of the trunk.[66,81] Neurologic deterioration usually is not a concern, because there is no useful neurologic function distal to the kyphosis in most children so affected.

The goal of a kyphectomy procedure is restoration of complete sagittal alignment, balance, and stability, while allowing for growth.[82] The preferred age for surgery appears to be 2 to 5 years, when the anteroposterior vertebral diameter reaches a 25-mm minimum. McLone[5] recommended that kyphectomy be performed prior to 2 years of age for children born with a thoracolumbar kyphosis and motor function at or below the L4 level. Corrective surgery also may be performed at the time of myelomeningocele closure, with resection of misaligned segments. In severe cases, this may be needed to obtain adequate closure.

Optimal surgical results require resection of the vertebral bodies at the apex of the kyphos to facilitate complete correction, without which recurrence is likely.[83] Published reports of long-term follow-up of resection of the rostral portion of the kyphotic deformity demonstrate that most patients improved, but a residual deformity persisted and that some degree of loss of correction of sagittal balance was observed over time.[82,84] A number of methods of internal fixation have been described. Aggressive deformity correction procedures that achieve satisfactory results have been described. However, this was associated with significant blood loss and a significant recurrence at 1 year of age, when limited internal fixation is used.[81]

In general, a correction of 45 degrees per vertebral level can be expected, and the lumbar lordosis can be restored, along with thoracic kyphosis and comprehensive sagittal balance. Postoperative wound breakdown, a common complication, can be managed by a postoperative full-thickness flap advancement or preoperative placement of tissue expanders.[79,81]

Other Spinal Anomalies

Other vertebral anomalies include an absence of the spinous processes and laminae, a reduction in the anteroposterior dimension of the vertebral body, an increase of the interpedicular distance, a decrease in the height of the pedicle, lateral extension of the large transverse processes, hemivertebrae, partial or complete vertebral fusion, and fusion of transverse processes.[15] Spinal cord anomalies other than open myelomeningocele include hydromyelia, diplomyelia, diastematomyelia, and defective myelinization; one or more of these were found in 88% of autopsy cases having spinal cord anomalies.[42]

Postoperative and Chronic Care

About 15% of patients with myelomeningocele are born with clinical signs of hydrocephalus, but 80% or more develop hydrocephalus in early infancy. In most instances, the clinical features and diagnosis become obvious within a week or two.[85] Performing a CSF diversion procedure (e.g., ventriculoperitoneal shunt) will relieve the ventricular pressure and tension on the myelomeningocele closure site to permit healing without CSF leakage. Third ventriculostomy may be considered for treatment of aqueductal stenosis in patients with myelomeningocele; reported success rates range between 65% and 80%. Third ventriculostomy also is a safe and effective means of treating hydrocephalus in the older myelomeningocele population even after years of shunting and offers the possibility of a long-term, shunt-independent life for selected patients.[86,87]

A thorough urologic evaluation should determine the degree of sphincter impairment, bladder dysfunction, and infection. In the United States, clean intermittent catheterization is used by 90% of children with myelomeningocele, 75% of whom perform self-catheterization.[5] Bowel management programs are easily achieved by supplementing proper nutrition, using laxatives, and taking advantage of the normal physiologic response of the gastrointestinal tract.[15]

Optimal care of a patient with myelomeningocele in the long term requires a comprehensive coordinated plan of treatment, usually in a myelomeningocele clinic that includes neurosurgery, urology, orthopaedic surgery, neurology, and rehabilitation. Neurosurgical follow-up should include periodical evaluation of the status of hydrocephalus, tethered spinal cord, Chiari II malformation, and syringomyelia. Deterioration of function must be investigated, and this investigation should begin with ensuring proper CSF diversion. Multiple surgical procedures usually include urologic and orthopaedic operations, as well as shunt revisions, Chiari decompressions, tethered cord releases, or spinal fusions.

Over the last 30 years, continual progress has been made in the outcomes of children born with myelomeningocele. Survival rates dramatically improved once it became possible to control hydrocephalus. Survival rates range between 80% and 85% at 15-year follow-up in one treated group of patients.[5] Hindbrain dysfunction caused by Chiari II malformation remains the principal cause of mortality. With an ongoing coordinated care plan, the affected patient's level of function can be expected to be maintained.[5]

KEY REFERENCES

Adinolfi M, Beck S, Embury S, et al: Levels of alpha-fetoprotein in amniotic fluids of mice (curlytail) with neural tube defects. *J Med Genet* 13:511–513, 1976.

Dias MS, Walker ML: The embryogenesis of complex dysraphic malformations: a disorder of gastrulation? *Pediatr Neurosurg* 18:229–253, 1992.

Laurence KM, James N, Miller MH, et al: Double-blind randomised controlled trial of folate treatment before conception to prevent recurrence of neural-tube defects. *Br Med J (Clin Res Ed)* 282:1509–1511, 1981.

McLone DG: Treatment of myelomeningocele: arguments against selection. *Clin Neurosurg* 33:359–370, 1986.

McLone DG: Continuing concepts in the management of spina bifida. *Pediatr Neurosurg* 18:254–256, 1992.

McLone DG, Knepper PA: The cause of Chiari II malformation: a unified theory. *Pediatr Neurosci* 15:1–12, 1989.

Park TS, Cail WS, Maggio WM, Mitchell DC: Progressive spasticity and scoliosis in children with myelomeningocele: radiological investigation and surgical treatment. *J Neurosurg* 62:367–375, 1985.

Pollack IF, Pang D, Albright AL, Krieger D: Outcome following hindbrain decompression of symptomatic Chiari malformations in children previously treated with myelomeningocele closure and shunts. *J Neurosurg* 77:881–888, 1992.

Urui S, Oi S: Experimental study of the embryogenesis of open spinal dysraphism. *Neurosurg Clin North Am* 6:195–202, 1995.

REFERENCES

The complete reference list is available online at expertconsult.com.

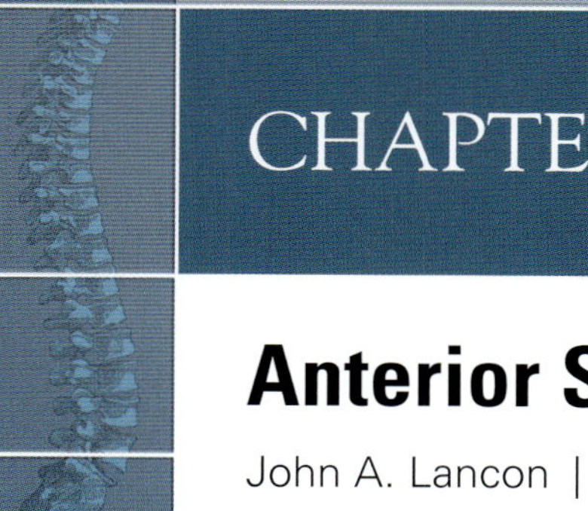

CHAPTER 118

Anterior Sacral Meningocele

John A. Lancon | Edward C. Benzel | Robert E. Tibbs, Jr.

Sacral meningocele may be congenital or acquired. Most acquired sacral meningoceles are a consequence of dural ectasia in association with the neurofibromatoses, Marfan syndrome, and Ehlers-Danlos syndrome.[1-6] These meningoceles usually are single and may expand into the intrasacral, presacral, and parasacral spaces. Traumatic avulsion of sacral nerve roots may produce sacral pseudomeningoceles in conjunction with profound neurologic deficits.[7,8] These sacs are more likely to be multiple and located in the lateral presacral space.

The congenital anterior sacral meningocele (ASM) was first described by Bryant in 1837.[9] It is rare in comparison to its dorsal counterpart. Matson noted only three examples in his analysis of 1390 cases of spina bifida cystica.[10] A congenital ASM characteristically occurs as a cystic presacral mass connected to the caudal thecal sac by a pedicle of variable size. Meningocele volumes as large as 1 to 2 L have been described.[11-13] Anorectal, genitourinary, and sacral anomalies also may be present.

In addition to the reported incidence, congenital ASM and dorsal lumbosacral meningocele differ from one another with respect to their pathogenesis, presentation, prognosis for neurologic improvement, and surgical approaches. Both anomalies may be associated with significant morbidity and mortality if not managed in a logical fashion, based on an understanding of their pathogenetic origins and surgical anatomy. This chapter reviews the pathogenesis, clinical presentation, and preoperative evaluation of congenital ASM. Needle aspiration and surgical approaches, including the transabdominal-transpelvic, presacral, parasacral, and dorsal transsacral routes, are described. In addition, guidelines for the avoidance and management of perioperative complications are reviewed.

Pathogenesis

The processes of spine and spinal cord development span the period from embryogenesis to postnatal development. Similar to more rostral vertebrae, the sacral vertebrae develop from sclerotomes. However, the sacral pattern requires additional centers of ossification. This process occurs slowly and is not completed until the third or fourth decade of life. Developmental sacral osseous anomalies (mesodermal) include sacralization of lumbar and coccygeal segments; lumbarization of the first sacral segment; stenosis or dilatation of the sacral foramina; isolated defects of the dorsal, lateral, and ventral elements; and sacral agenesis.[14]

The sacrococcygeal neural elements develop after closure of the posterior neuropore. Beneath an intact surface ectoderm, the caudal cell mass enlarges and undergoes canalization. This occurs from the 4th to 6th weeks of life, forming spinal cord segments extending from S2 to S3 to the coccygeal terminus. Extensive cellular degeneration along the distal neural tube produces a fibrous remnant at the caudal-most tip of the developing CNS. This remnant becomes the filum terminale. The ventriculus terminalis lies at the level of the S5 entry zone, marking the point of transition between the conus medullaris and filum terminale.[14] Lying at the distal end of the filum terminale, the coccygeal medullary vestige may be the origin of the intrasacral meningocele.[15-17]

Before the 9th week, spinal cord and vertebral segments are aligned level for level. With the dura mater now forming a complete covering, the spinal cord and dura mater begin to ascend in relation to the growing vertebral column, albeit at different rates. The conus medullaris rises to L3 at birth and to L1-2 by 3 months. The dural sac constricts terminally, rising only to S4 at birth and to S2-3 in the adult. Developmental sacrococcygeal neuroectodermal anomalies include meningocele, myelomeningocele, lipomyelomeningocele, myelocystocele, anomalies of the conus medullaris, tethered filum terminale, intrasacral meningocele, and caudal regression syndromes.[14]

In contrast to dorsal meningoceles that arise from failure of the posterior neuropore to close or dehiscence of a formed neural tube, a congenital ASM arises after failure of one or more sacral sclerotomes to develop. The meningeal sac expands through the sacral defect driven by cerebrospinal fluid (CSF) pulsations. The sacral defect enlarges only slightly, while the developing pelvic viscera offer less resistance to the budding meningocele. The sac enlarges tremendously in the presacral space, remaining attached to the thecal sac by a smaller pedicle. Although spontaneous regression of the meningocele does not occur after birth, progressive enlargement may occur and is associated with the development of symptoms. The large volume attained by some meningoceles causes crowding of the pelvic viscera.[11] The ventral sacral defect is usually parasagittal, less commonly midline or lateral. The typical anatomic relationships of an anterior sacral meningocele are depicted in Figure 118-1.

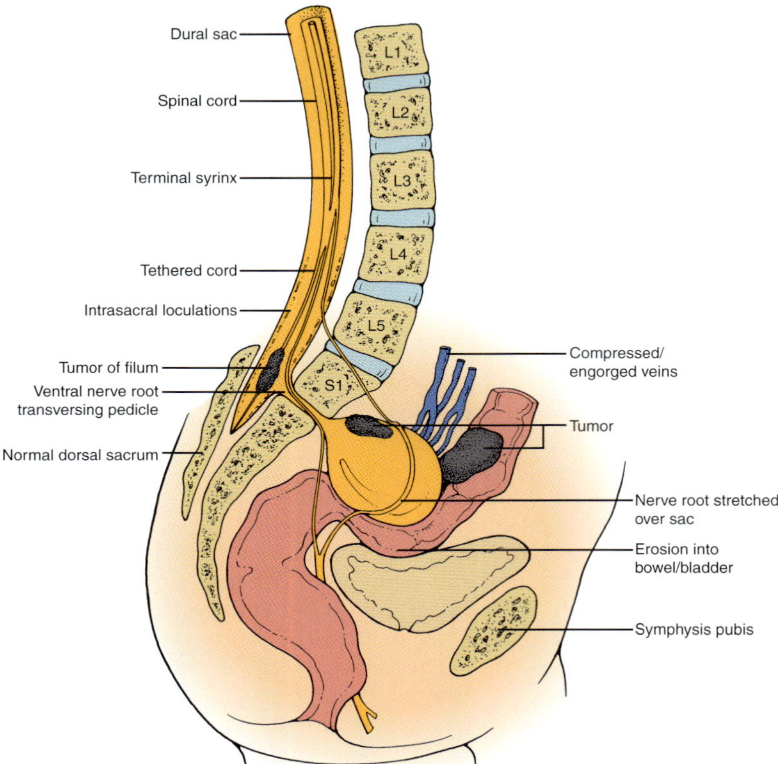

FIGURE 118-1. Illustration of a typical anatomic scenario regarding a congenital anterior sacral meningocele. Intrathecal (filum terminale), intracystic, and extracystic-intrapelvic tumors may be associated.

Complex interactions between adjacent germ cell substrata in the embryonic caudal midline give rise to varying cascades of maldevelopment, which include a spectrum of mesectodermal dystrophies. The embryologic event that initiates these patterns of maldevelopment is distinct from the insult that causes failure of the posterior neuropore to close. Although the precise event is not clearly defined, evidence for a vascular etiology exists.[14,18,19] In addition to anomalies of the conus medullaris, sacral nerve roots, and sacral dura mater, the clinical manifestations of these patterns of maldevelopment include the development of congenital tumors (e.g., dermoid, epidermoid, hamartoma, lipoma, teratoma, and teratocarcinoma) and anomalies of the colorectal, genitourinary, and reproductive systems.[2,14,20-24]

Most congenital ASMs appear to occur sporadically, although familial and X-linked dominant inheritance have been reported.[20,23,25,26] The seemingly greater incidence in females is a manifestation of the tendency toward symptomatology in the presence of sacral crowding, as well as the greater likelihood that female patients in the second and third decades of life will undergo palpation of the presacral space during routine physical examination. When cases in patients under 20 years of age are considered, the female-to-male ratio is approximately 1:1.[12,27]

Clinical Presentation

Congenital ASM has a trimodal pattern of presentation.[2,12,13,24,28-32] Some ASMs are recognized at birth, when they are discovered in association with anorectal anomalies and sacral defects (Currarino's triad).[33] Most commonly, however, ASMs present during the first and second decades of life with progressive constipation or other symptoms referable to the colorectal, genitourinary, and reproductive systems.[2,12,13,24,27,29,30-32,34,35] Less commonly, low back pain, headache, or sacral radiculopathy may be the initial manifestation.[12,13,22]

A small congenital ASM may remain occult for life, particularly in the male patient.[12,13] Occasionally, a meningocele is discovered incidentally during the initiation of routine prenatal care in a new mother. In the rare case of a pregnant woman with no prenatal care, the meningocele may present as dystocia. In this setting, the characteristically benign ASM may threaten serious morbidity and even death.

Colorectal

The most common symptom in patients with congenital ASM is chronic constipation or obstipation, usually manifesting in the first two decades of life. Fecal incontinence and soiling rarely predominate in the clinical picture. Communication between congenital ASM and the rectum may be congenital or acquired and may produce fulminant meningitis. The anal canal may be duplicated or atretic.[12,13,20]

Genitourinary

Urinary incontinence may be due to tethering of the spinal cord or direct pressure on the bladder, ureters, or S1, S2, and S3 nerve roots, or, rarely, may be the result of congenital deficits in the innervation of the lower urinary tract. Enuresis and recurrent infections affecting either the upper or the lower tract may occur. Coexisting anomalies include horseshoe-shaped kidneys and duplication of the kidneys, renal pelvis, or ureter.[12,13]

Reproductive

Dysmenorrhea, dystocia, and dyspareunia occur less commonly. Dysmenorrhea may be secondary to compression of retropelvic veins resulting in pelvic venous congestion. Duplication of the uterus and vagina and vaginal atresia may be present.[12,13,21]

Neurologic

True neurologic symptoms are rare and typically are mild when present because the distal spinal cord and nerve roots develop normally. However, progressive leg or perineal weakness, numbness, and pain may develop as a result of stretching of the sacrococcygeal nerve roots by the meningocele.[12,13,27] These patients usually will have some symptoms suggestive of involvement of the pelvic visceral innervation. Chronic pelvic pain may occur due to involvement of the pelvic autonomic plexi. Such symptoms typically are progressive and do not develop until later in life, implying the potential for reversibility after treatment if they are recognized early. Coexisting tethering of the spinal cord actually may lessen the amount of tension exerted on the nerve roots by the enlarging meningocele.[2] The presence of severe neurologic dysfunction from birth indicates a more severe myelodysraphic state and is associated with a greater tendency toward anomalous development in adjacent viscera. The patient whose clinical picture is characterized by prominent sacrococcygeal radiculopathy that worsens after a Valsalva maneuver is more likely to harbor an intrasacral meningocele or an ASM based on a large pedicle.[2,12,13,15,17] The sacrococcygeal radiculopathies are listed in Table 118-1.

Mild to moderate headache-associated symptoms may occur and are of two forms.[2,27,31,36] A high-pressure variant secondary to pressure exerted on the meningocele during pregnancy or after a Valsalva maneuver has been reported occasionally; less commonly, a low-pressure headache may occur on rising to the standing position, caused by the displacement of CSF from the thecal sac into the meningocele. Pressure-related headaches are more likely in the presence of a large communication between the thecal sac and the meningocele.[12,13]

Congenital ASM may be a cause of meningitis. Bacterial meningitis resulting from erosion of the meningocele into the bowel or bladder lumina or resulting from the presence of a congenital rectothecal or vesiculothecal fistula and aseptic meningitis resulting from leakage of an intraspinal dermoid cyst have been described.[2,23,27]

TABLE 118-1

Sacrococcygeal Radiculopathies

Level	Motor	Sensory	Autonomic
S1	Gluteus maximus	Lateral aspect and sole of foot	–
	Hamstrings	–	–
	Gastrocnemius/ soleus	–	–
	Intrinsic foot muscles	–	–
	FDL, FHL	–	–
S2	Gastrocnemius/ soleus	–	–
	FDL, FHL	Dorsal thigh	Detrusor
S3	–	Outer perineal	Detrusor
S4	–	Inner perineal	Detrusor
S5	–	Perianal	–
S0	–	Coccyx	–

FDL, flexor digitorum longus; FHL, flexor hallucis longus.

Preoperative Evaluation

The most consistent physical finding in congenital anterior sacral meningocele is a soft, cystic, retrorectal mass that appears fixed to the sacrum.[12,13] The mass is felt most commonly on rectal examination but may be felt on pelvic, abdominal, gluteal, or inguinal examination as well. A transmitted pulse wave sometimes may be appreciated with a Valsalva maneuver.[12,13] Dyck and Wilson[37] described a patient who presented with a sliding groin hernia and was found to harbor a congenital ASM. They postulated crowding of the pelvic viscera as a significant contributing factor in the development of the hernia, which contained a portion of the urinary bladder.

Although a congenital ASM usually can be felt easily on rectal or pelvic examination, the main limitation to premorbid discovery is a failure to suspect its presence. This failure is a result of both its secluded location within the deep pelvis and the great variety of typically mild, nonspecific symptoms with which it presents. The evaluation of a male or female patient presenting within the first three decades of life with progressive constipation or obstipation should include a careful history and physical examination directed toward the gastrointestinal, genitourinary, and reproductive systems. Specific examination of the sacrococcygeal innervation should be performed.

Imaging

Preoperative planning for surgery of congenital anterior sacral meningocele begins with the radiologic delineation of the surgical anatomy of the meningocele. Specific considerations are (1) confirmation of the cystic nature of the mass; (2) identification of the pedicle, associated mass lesions, and any other abnormalities of the neural, dural, or vertebral components of the sacrum; (3) determination of the relationship between the meningocele and the sacral nerve roots; and (4) determination of the relationship to the pelvic viscera. Bone window CT and MRI are the primary diagnostic studies performed.[8,38-41] Myelography and postmyelographic CT do not offer an equivalent amount of noninvasive surgically useful information.[42] Adjuvant evaluation of the pelvic viscera may provide additional useful information in selected cases.

The sacrum is difficult to evaluate with plain radiography owing to its curvilinear shape and overlying soft tissue and bowel gas patterns. The pathognomonic sickle-shaped sacral deformity, or scimitar sign, and a presacral mass may be present (Fig. 118-2). Less obvious findings include widening of isolated sacral foramina, increases in interpedicular distance or flattening of the pedicles, and abnormalities of curvature.[12,13]

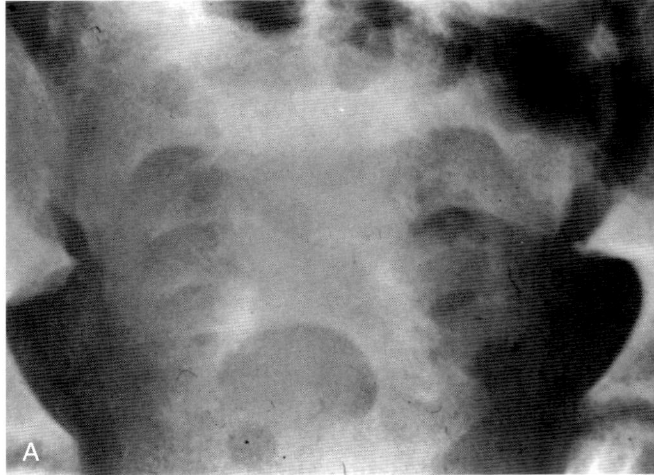

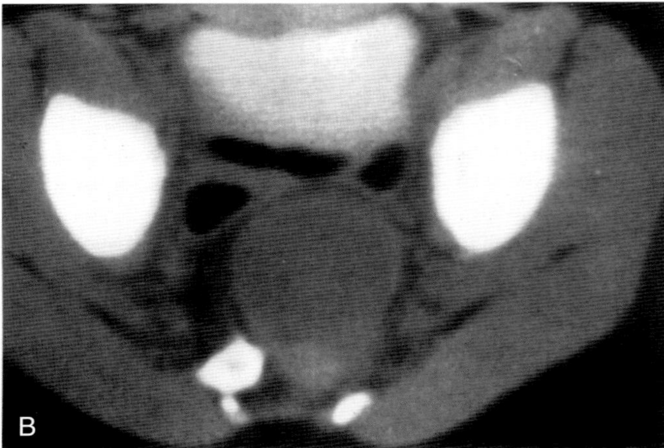

FIGURE 118-2. A, Anteroposterior radiograph of a patient with an anterior sacral meningocele. Note the classic presence of the "scimitar sign" configuration of the eroded sacrum. **B,** Pelvic CT scan demonstrating the presacral mass associated with the meningocele.

Transforaminal sacral views may better demonstrate these changes. Calcification within an associated presacral mass may be difficult to discern.

The development of myelography allowed better visualization of the meningocele and its pedicle but contributed little to the diagnosis of associated pelvic visceral anomalies. Only masses within the meningocele could be seen, and in the presence of a very small pedicle, the fistulous communication was not always demonstrated.[12,13] Delayed imaging at 24 to 48 hours and the use of large volumes of contrast material increased the chance of identifying the pedicle. Balériaux-Waha et al.[42] described the utility of CT in differentiating anterior sacral meningocele from solid masses of the presacral space. CT bone windows are particularly helpful in delineating osseous anatomy. However, as with myelography, CT (even with intrathecal contrast) may fail to demonstrate a small pedicle.

In 1988, Lee et al.[39] reported on the use of MRI to demonstrate familial anterior sacral meningoceles in a father and daughter. The authors were able to noninvasively demonstrate a horseshoe-shaped kidney, didelphic uterus, and associated pelvic teratoma, which were not shown by other imaging studies. This is a critical advantage of MRI over other diagnostic imaging studies in the evaluation of congenital ASM, considering the extensive differential diagnoses of a presacral mass (Box 118-1).[43-45]

BOX 118-1. Differential Diagnosis of a Sacral or Presacral Mass

Aneurysmal bone cyst
Anterior sacral meningocele
Chondrosarcoma
Chordoma, chondroma
Dermoid cyst
Ependymoma
Epidermoid
Fibroma
Fibrosarcoma
Gastrointestinal tract tumor
Genitourinary tract tumor
Giant cell tumor
Hamartoma
Intrasacral meningocele
Lipoma
Nephroblastoma
Neuroblastoma
Osteoblastoma
Osteomyelitis
Perineurial cyst
Pheochromocytoma
Plasmacytoma
Polycystic kidney
Reproductive tract tumors
Rhabdomyosarcoma
Seminoma
Teratoma, teratocarcinoma

In cases where ASM is present, the MRI appearance of a congenital ASM is characteristic.[39-41,46] T1-weighted images show a homogeneous low-signal cyst extending from the sacral thecal sac into the presacral space. It usually is possible to identify the communicating pedicle. The thickened filum terminale and any associated tumors may be identified. T2-weighted images show high signals, although occasionally both high and low signals may be present within the meningocele as a consequence of fluid movements during imaging (Fig. 118-3).

Management

An understanding of the pathogenesis of ASM and the anatomic confines of the sacrococcygeal region allows the surgeon to devise a systematic, logical approach to deal with each anomaly. Important surgical goals are (1) visual confirmation of the anomalous anatomy depicted by MRI, (2) aspiration of the meningocele, (3) detethering of the spinal cord, (4) ligation of the pedicle or creation of a dural sleeve around exiting nerve roots, (5) excision of associated masses, and (6) dural closure.

Five surgical approaches have been described during the evolution of the surgical treatment of congenital ASM

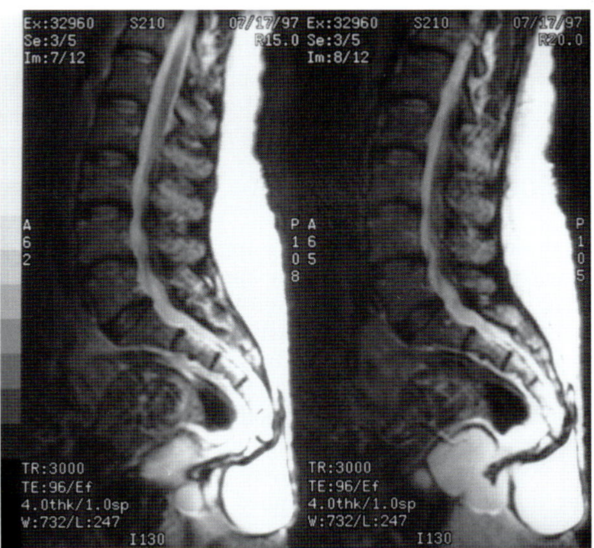

FIGURE 118-3. Axial T2-weighted MRIs of the sacral spine demonstrating a caudal anterior sacral meningocele extending into the presacral space.

(Fig. 118-4). Transrectal or transvaginal aspiration and the inferior presacral approach (e.g., Kraske approach) are associated with prohibitive risks of morbidity and mortality.[2,27,30,31,47] The oblique parasacral approach of Demel[48] and Coqui[49] was described for the rare gluteal meningocele. The ventral transabdominal-transpelvic approach was recommended by Leibowitz et al.[22] to prevent missing an occult tumor. With MRI, this approach is no longer necessary. However, it may still be useful in cases of large abdominopelvic masses or when nerve roots are known to traverse the pedicle of the meningocele. Only the dorsal transsacral approach allows the surgeon to carry out each of the aforementioned goals in a planned, logical progression, while minimizing the risks of injury to the pelvic viscera and presacral neurovascular networks.[11,50]

Aspiration

Transrectal and transvaginal aspiration were abandoned after mortality rates of 80% to 90% were reported. However, direct aspiration of the meningocele should be a deliberate goal of any surgical exposure of an anterior sacral meningocele.

Inferior Presacral Approach (Kraske-Pupovac Approach)

With the inferior presacral approach, an incision is extended from just dorsal to the rectum to the dorsal surface of the coccyx. A plane is developed in the retrorectal space, and the coccyx is excised. The pedicle is identified and ligated, after which the sac may be aspirated via direct puncture. This approach has several disadvantages. First, the pedicle and its relationship with adjacent sacral nerve roots and the filum terminale are not fully visualized. An associated mass lesion within the meningocele or ventral to it can be difficult or impossible to expose via this approach. Inadvertent entry into the bowel or bladder may occur. Finally, because any opening in the dural sac will occur in its most dependent portion, the incidence of a postoperative CSF fistula is

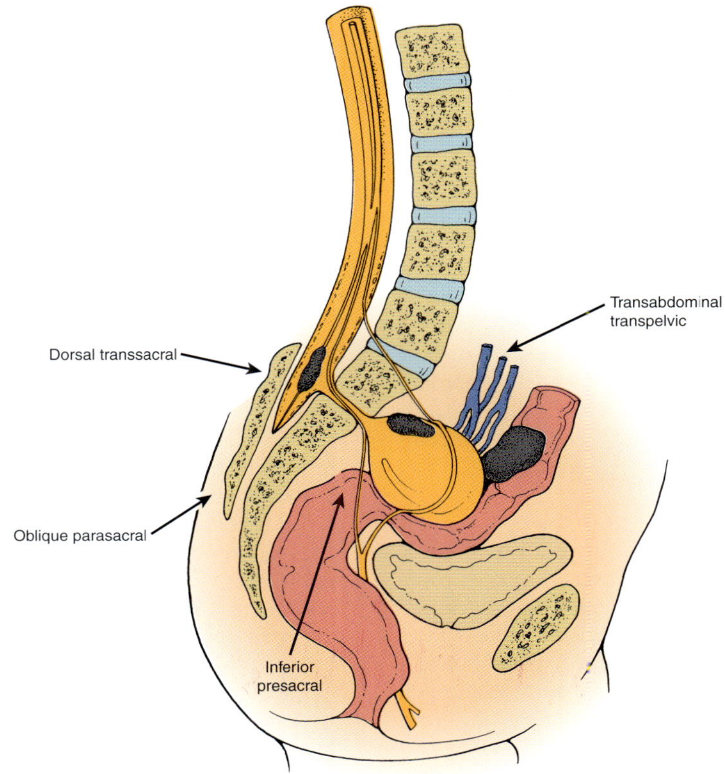

FIGURE 118-4. Depiction of the orientation of the variety of surgical approaches used for the management of anterior sacral meningoceles.

increased. Proximity of the incision to the rectum may result in postoperative wound infection, pararectal abscess formation, or meningitis. This proximity is particularly problematic in extremely young children.

Oblique Parasacral Approach (Demel and Coqui Approach)

Originally described as an approach to the rare anterior sacral meningocele presenting as a gluteal mass, the oblique parasacral approach also does not allow surgical correction of associated tethering or mass lesions. An incision on the buttocks allows identification of the gluteus maximus, which is reflected. The underlying piriformis, superior gemellus, obturator internus, inferior gemellus, and quadratus femoris muscles are identified. The superior and inferior gluteal arteries and nerves, sciatic nerve, and posterior femoral cutaneous nerves are identified in relation to the meningocele that will emerge in the space between the piriformis and quadratus femoris muscles. Although the sac may be aspirated and the protruding portion of the meningocele excised and oversewn, this approach leaves residual meningocele ventral to the sacrum and allows for further growth of the sac into the presacral or parasacral space. Unless an associated tumor has been identified in the gluteal region by preoperative imaging, this approach should not be used.

Transabdominal-Transpelvic Approach

During a transabdominal-transpelvic approach with the patient in the lithotomy Trendelenburg position, a midline incision is made from the symphysis to just above the umbilicus. The small intestine is packed off. The ureters are then identified and preserved. The peritoneum is opened on the right side of the rectum, and the meningocele is identified. The meningocele may be aspirated and the pedicle ligated, or the meningocele may be opened and the dural sac plicated around any neural elements traversing the pedicle. The primary utility of this approach is in the management of large associated abdominopelvic masses, meningoceles arising from extremely large pedicles, and cases in which multiple sacral nerve roots traverse the ostium of the meningocele. Release of an associated tethering may be difficult by this approach, and the large retropelvic veins may hinder bloodless exposure. Preoperative consultation with general or colorectal surgery colleagues is important to adequately assess the risk-to-benefit ratio of the potential exposure gained by this approach within a small pelvis.

Dorsal Transsacral Approach (Adson Approach)

The dorsal transsacral approach allows inspection of intrasacral anatomy, direct visualization of the sacral nerve roots, aspiration and collapse of the meningocele, detethering of the spinal cord, ligation of the pedicle, excision of associated tumors, and access to the sacral nerve roots for intraoperative stimulation. Rarely, a large abdominopelvic mass cannot be completely excised via this exposure. If sacral nerve roots traverse the pedicle, creation of a dural sleeve around the exiting roots may also be difficult by a dorsal exposure.[23] Because the meningocele is not excised, dissection in the presacral space is minimized. There have been no reported surgical deaths with this approach since 1965. A staged dorsal transsacral and transabdominal-transpelvic approach may be required in some cases.

Surgical Technique

Care must be taken to avoid using inappropriate surgical approaches, particularly ventral approaches, that may not provide the most direct exposure of the pathology and that, in addition, may be associated with significant morbidity. For the vast majority of cases, the dorsal transsacral approach of Adson, or a variant thereof, is recommended.[50] With this approach, the patient is positioned prone on two longitudinal chest rolls, and all pressure points are carefully padded. The bowel is prepared preoperatively. Prophylactic antibiotics are administered and continued for 48 hours postoperatively. Intraoperative monitoring, if employed, is planned in advance and is now checked. A Foley catheter, an arterial line, and two large-bore peripheral intravenous lines are placed. The skin is cleansed with 0.25% triclosan (Septisol) and alcohol and prepared with povidone-iodine (Betadine).

The skin incision is placed in the midline and extends from the level of the iliac crests to the tip of the coccyx. The dorsal sacral fascia is identified and divided, allowing reflection of the erector spinae musculature to either side. The dorsal sacral foramina and sacroiliac ligaments should not be damaged. Sacral laminectomy is then performed. In cases of a small pedicle and no associated mass, a small laminotomy of the appropriate hemisacrum may be all that is required for ligation of the pedicle and aspiration of the meningocele.

The dural sac is then opened in the midline, centered at the level of the pedicle of the meningocele. Inspection of the intrasacral anatomy is directed at identifying any intrasacral loculations, the anatomy of the sacral nerve roots, the ostium of the pedicle of the meningocele, and the relation between the sacral nerve roots and the pedicle. The filum is identified and should not be divided until the meningocele has been aspirated. All visible nerve tissue must be preserved. In the absence of a more ventral mass lesion, the pedicle is ligated. The meningocele is aspirated by way of a soft angiocatheter or ventricular catheter attached to a syringe before placement of the final stitch. Alternatively, a fascial patch may be sewn over the ostium of the meningocele. At this point, tethering may be released.

If entry into the meningocele is desired for approach to an associated mass lesion or for plication of a dural sleeve around nerve roots traversing the pedicle, an opening should be made in the ventral surface of the dural sac adjacent to the pedicle. A fibrous plane usually is found between the ventral surface of the thecal sac and the dorsal surface of the meningocele, although venous bleeding from this space occasionally may be problematic. The sac is then opened, and the associated mass lesion is excised. The thecal sac is irrigated with warm antibiotic-containing solution to remove any blood that may have run down into the exposure. A watertight closure of the dural openings with #4-0 to #6-0 monofilament or braided nylon is confirmed by a Valsalva maneuver. After closure of the dorsal thecal sac, the paraspinous tissues are reapproximated. With meticulous hemostasis, a drain is not placed. Skin closure should be cosmetic. In the infant or young child, #5-0 to #4-0

Vicryl sutures are placed in inverted fashion at the subdermal plane. The skin edges may then be held in approximation using Steri-Strips (3M Nexcare, St. Paul, MN) or #5-0 monofilament nylon in simple interrupted fashion. In the older child or adult, the subdermal closure is done with #3-0 Vicryl in a similar fashion, and the final layer is closed with #4-0 monofilament nylon in a simple interrupted manner.

Complications

Some of the operative and postoperative complications associated with the dorsal transsacral approach of Adson and the transabdominal-transpelvic approach are listed in Box 118-2. The following discussions address some of these procedures' common complications and their prevention and management.

Dural Closure

The dura mater should be handled delicately to avoid inadvertent tears that would prevent watertight closure. Cautery of dural bleeding should be minimized or avoided entirely to prevent contraction of the dural surface. Closure with #4-0 to #6-0 braided or monofilament nylon or Prolene (Ethicon 360, Somerville, NJ) sutures in watertight fashion is the most important step in preventing a postoperative CSF fistula. When a CSF leak occurs, a lumbar subarachnoid drain may be placed percutaneously into the lumbar cistern and the patient turned to the prone position. CSF drainage should be continued for 5 days, at which point the drain is clamped for 24 hours. If the leak does not recur, the drain may be removed. Failure to resolve the leak requires reoperation for primary closure. In the extremely young child, primary reexploration may be preferable to a trial of lumbar drainage to avoid having to maintain the child in a prone position for an extended period of time.

BOX 118-2. Perioperative Complications

Operative Complications
- Positioning injuries
- Prone anesthetic complications
- Wound infection
- Osteomyelitis
- Meningitis (bacterial or aseptic)
- CSF headache
- CSF fistula
- Failure to aspirate sac
- Failure to obliterate pedicle
- Failure to detether
- Premature release of tethering
- Direct injury to nerve root
- Direct injury to ureter
- Direct injury to bowel
- Direct injury to bladder

Postoperative Complications
- Ileus
- Malnutrition
- Fluid and electrolyte abnormalities
- Fecal impaction
- Urinary retention
- Urinary tract infection
- Atelectasis
- Pneumonia
- Deep venous thrombosis
- Pulmonary embolism
- Sepsis
- Decubitus
- Pain

CSF, cerebrospinal fluid.

Nerve Injury

The sacral nerve roots should be assumed to be physiologically stressed by the stretch imparted by the meningocele and may be easily injured by improper handling. They should be identified at the time of initial dural opening and handled with great care. They may be injured during drilling of the dorsal sacrum, dural opening, pedicle ligation, formation of a dural sleeve, or aspiration of the sac, and by premature release of tethering. The relation between the pedicle and the adjacent nerve roots must be clearly determined before ligation of the pedicle. Any nerve roots observed to traverse the ostium of the pedicle should be preserved, and the dural sac plicated around them. Although sacral radiculopathies may worsen transiently after surgery, they almost always improve. Conversely, damage to the presacral autonomic plexus may result in debilitating chronic pelvic pain.

Tethering

Complications related to tethering of the spinal cord result from both failure to detether and premature release of tethering. Release of a tethered spinal cord should be performed only after aspiration of the sac. This prevents sudden upward traction on the sacral nerve roots, which are already stretched tenuously by the meningocele. Failure to identify and release a tethered spinal cord may result in postoperative persistence or worsening of bowel and bladder symptoms. Because both aberrant sacral nerve roots and the filum terminale may enter the meningocele, the routine use of intraoperative electrophysiologic monitoring for identification of the filum terminale may assist with the prevention of accidental division of a sacral root.

Meningitis

Meningitis may occur secondary to bacterial contamination of the CSF by skin flora or as a result of surgical entry into the rectum or bladder. Preoperative bowel preparation and parenteral antibiotic coverage should be used. Aseptic meningitis may occur from leakage of an associated dermoid cyst or failure to remove blood that has run down into the thecal sac. Copious irrigation of the caudal thecal sac before final dural closure should always be performed and noted in the operative dictation.

Pelvic Visceral Injury

Injury to the pelvic viscera is minimized by use of the dorsal transsacral approach and by limiting dissection in the presacral space. In addition to direct injury to the ureters, rectum, and bladder and their neurovascular supply, delayed hematoma formation secondary to inadequate hemostasis of retropelvic veins and venous thrombosis with central extension are potential serious risks of transabdominal-transpelvic approaches. Retropelvic hemorrhage may be life threatening.

Postoperative Care

Urinary retention, urinary tract infection, atelectasis and pneumonia, ileus, fecal impaction, decubitus formation, sepsis, and deep venous thrombosis with pulmonary embolism may occur postoperatively. A definitive plan for bowel, bladder, pulmonary, skin, and nutritional management should be formulated for each case on an individual basis by considering preoperative and postoperative deficits. Mobilization, including physical and occupational therapy, should begin immediately after surgery.

KEY REFERENCES

Barberá J, Broseta J, Argüelles F, et al: Traumatic lumbosacral meningocele. *J Neurosurg* 46:536, 1977.

Bryant T: Case of deficiency of the anterior part of the sacrum with a thecal sac in the pelvis, similar to the tumor of spina bifida. *Lancet* 1:358, 1837.

Coller FA, Jackson RG: Anterior sacral meningocele. *Surg Gynecol Obstet* 76:703, 1943.

Currarino G, Coln D, Votteler T: Triad of anorectal, sacral, and presacral anomalies. *Am J Radiol* 137:395, 1981.

Pang D: Sacral agenesis and caudal spinal cord malformations. *Neurosurgery* 32:755, 1993.

Stern WE: Dural ectasia and the Marfan syndrome. *J Neurosurg* 69:221, 1988.

Wilkins RH, Odom GL: Anterior and lateral spinal meningocele. In Vinken PJ, Bruyn GW, editors: *Handbook of clinical neurology*, New York, 1978, Elsevier Biomedical, p 193.

REFERENCES

The complete reference list is available online at expertconsult.com.

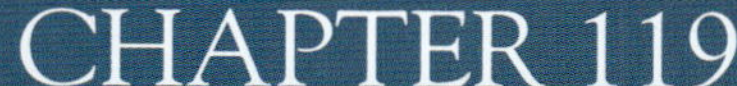

CHAPTER 119

Chiari Malformations and Syringomyelia

Samuel R. Browd | Richard Ellenbogen

Chiari malformations are commonly encountered in both pediatric and adult neurosurgical practices. Multiple variations in the anatomic development of the rhombencephalon have been described, leading to the familiar Chiari I through IV designations. Although many patients are characterized as having a Chiari malformation, and symptoms can overlap among the various Chiari types, it is unlikely that Chiari malformation represents a unified disease with a single causation. Treatment has been based on both symptomatology and imaging findings, with variations on the Chiari decompression procedure widely described in the literature. Symptom arrest or regression is the expected surgical outcome, with resolution or arrest of the spinal cord syrinx, if present. Outcomes after decompression usually are good, making Chiari decompression an effective surgical option for appropriately chosen patients.

History

John Cleland (1835–1925) was among the first to describe hindbrain herniation in a patient with myelodysplasia.[1-3] In 1883, Cleland published "Contribution to the study of spina bifida, encephalocele and anencephalus," which included an illustration and a description of patients with hindbrain herniation, in the *Journal of Anatomy and Physiology*. Julius Arnold (1835–1915) also discussed a patient with hindbrain herniation and myelodysplasia in 1894.[1,4-7] In 1891 and 1896, Hans Chiari (1851–1916) provided descriptions of hindbrain herniation in postmortem specimens in which variations I through IV were described.[5,8] Because Chiari performed the majority of the early work describing the condition, his name remains associated with the condition today.

The surgical treatment of Chiari malformations began with the technique described by Penfield and Coburn, who performed a posterior fossa decompression. In the case they described, the patient died, and subsequent early surgeries had a high rate of complications and death.[9] Gardner et al.[10-15] noted five deaths among 74 patients undergoing posterior fossa decompression. Williams[16-18] reported 5 deaths in 41 cases and also described increased neurologic deficits, increased ventricular size, and arachnoiditis in his patients. Despite these inauspicious beginnings, modern surgical techniques make Chiari surgery much safer, with the chance of a serious, irreversible injury less than 2%.

Pathophysiology

The various types of Chiari malformations are difficult to explain with a unifying theory that accounts for all the cerebral and spinal anomalies and addresses the occurrence of hindbrain herniation. Instead, the various Chiari types likely result from different causative factors but share similar radiographic and symptomatic expression. It remains unclear whether defects are a result of embryonic missteps or of other pathologic processes. While clear associations can be made with Chiari II, myelomeningocele, and folate deficiency, few other clear associations can be garnered. Few studies have demonstrated a genetic predisposition to the condition.[19]

Although causation remains unclear, mechanistic theories abound to describe Chiari I and II malformations and the common finding of syringomyelia. Gardner[11,12] posited the hydrodynamic theory, which attributes the development of hydromyelia to a "water hammer" effect caused by blockage of the foramen of Magendie whereby cerebrospinal fluid (CSF) transits the potential space of the central canal in the spinal cord, causing slow progressive dilation. Oldfield[20,21] suggested that the downward pistoning of the cerebellar tonsils seen on cine-mode MRI (cine-MRI) forces CSF via perivascular and interstitial spaces into the spinal cord, resulting in a syrinx. Regarding Chiari II, McLone et al.[22-28] posited the unified theory that CSF loss at the myelomeningocele site reduces the volume of CSF needed to distend the developing ventricular system, leading to caudal displacement of hindbrain structures. Because Chiari types I through IV represent a spectrum of conditions with various causations, research continues in an effort to understand the exact pathophysiologic processes that lead to these malformations and associated symptoms.

Signs, Symptoms, and Imaging: Pathologic Features

Chiari I

Chiari I malformation involves caudal herniation of the cerebellar tonsils more than 5 mm below the level of the foramen magnum without brainstem descent or hydrocephalus (Table 119-1) and has been associated with numerous conditions (Box 119-1). Patients typically present with nondermatomal pain in the occipital or cervical region that is exacerbated by the Valsalva maneuver.[29] Pain in younger

TABLE 119-1

Types of Chiari Malformations

Type	Description
Chiari I	>5 mm tonsillar herniation below McRae line
	No hindbrain abnormalities
	Syringomyelia possible
Chiari II	Herniation of brainstem, cerebellar vermis, fourth ventricle through foramen magnum
	Associated with myelomeningocele
	Hydrocephalus common
	Syringomyelia common
Chiari III	Foramen magnum/high cervical encephalocele
Chiari IV	Cerebellar hypoplasia or aplasia
Chiari 1.5	Low brainstem and fourth ventricle
	Caudal displacement of cerebellar tonsils
	No associated myelomeningocele
Chiari 0	Crowded posterior fossa without hindbrain herniation
	Syringomyelia

BOX 119-1. **Conditions Associated with Chiari I Malformations**

Klippel-Feil syndrome
Neurofibromatosis
Apert syndrome
Crouzon syndrome
Metopic and multisuture synostosis
Odontoid retroflexion
Pierre-Robin syndrome
Caudal regression syndrome
Costello syndrome
Paget disease
Craniometaphyseal dysplasia
Growth hormone deficiency
Cloacal exstrophy
Hemihypertrophy
Rickets
Acromegaly
Lipomyelomenigocele

BOX 119-2. **Presenting Signs and Symptoms of Chiari I and Chiari II**

Chiari I

Occipital cervical headache
Motor or sensory symptoms
Clumsiness
Ataxia
Dysphagia/dysarthria
Nystagmus
Cranial nerve dysfunction
Aspiration
Dysreflexia

Chiari II

Apnea
Stridor
Aspiration
Hypotonia
Irritability
Myelopathy
Ataxia
Nystagmus
Scoliosis
Dysarthria

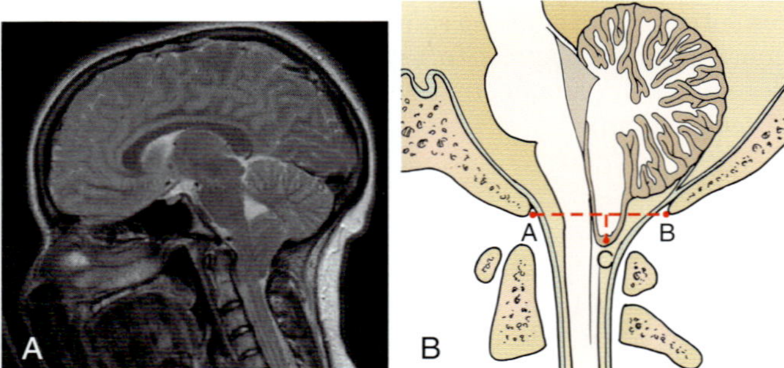

FIGURE 119-1. A, Sagittal MRI demonstrating typical Chiari I findings including 18-mm tonsillar descent. **B,** Schematic demonstrating the appropriate technique to measure the degree of tonsillar descent. The line from *A* to *B* represents the McRae line; a perpendicular line is then measured from this point to the inferior aspect of the cerebellar tonsil (*C*) .

children may manifest as irritability, crying, or failure to thrive. Sleep apnea is another common finding in younger patients. Various other symptoms are described in association with Chiari I malformation, including motor and sensory alterations, clumsiness, dysphagia, dysarthria, ataxia, and incontinence (Box 119-2). Signs on examination can include nystagmus, hyperreflexia of lower extremities, diminished upper extremity reflexes, cerebellar signs, and lower cranial nerve dysfunction, including dysarthria, palatal weakness, and decreased gag reflex. Scoliosis also can be seen in some patients, especially in the setting of an underlying spinal cord syrinx.

Multiple findings are demonstrated on imaging and at autopsy in patients with Chiari I malformation (Fig. 119-1). Abnormalities of the skull base and craniocervical junction, including a small posterior fossa, empty sella, platybasia, basilar impression, Klippel-Feil syndrome, and atlantoaxial assimilation, are seen in approximately 50% of patients. MRI is used to demonstrate cerebellar tonsils below the level of the foramen magnum, and cine-MRI routinely may show decreased flow posteriorly at the craniocervical junction.[19,30] Imaging also may demonstrate scoliosis with a leftward convexity, in contrast to the right convexity curve usually seen in idiopathic scoliosis. The fourth ventricle can be elongated, and hydrocephalus is present in 5% to 10% of cases. The cerebellar tentorium is elevated, but other brain abnormalities common in Chiari II malformation often are absent. A spinal cord syrinx is a common feature, occurring in 50% to 75% , or even more, of patients. Syrinx formation usually is seen in the lower cervical and upper thoracic cord; however, this may vary, and

BOX 119-3. Anatomic Findings in Chari II Malformation

Skeletal
Craniolacunia
Small posterior fossa
Frontal bone scalloping
Petrous bone scalloping
Clival concavity
Low-lying inion
Large occipital keel
Atlas assimilation
Klippel-Feil deformity
Basilar invagination

Intracranial
Hydrocephalus
Colpocephaly
Asymmetry of the lateral ventricles
Vertical straight sinus
Low-lying torcula
Complete or partial agenesis of corpus callosum
Polygyria
Cortical interdigitation
Enlarged massa intermedia
Tectal beaking

Spinal Cord
Split cord malformation
Syringomyelia

holochord syrinx is possible. Volumetric analysis has demonstrated reduced posterior fossa volumes and upward of 40% CSF volumes with normal brain volume.[31-33]

Chiari II

Chiari II malformation is characterized by caudal herniation of the cerebellar vermis, the brainstem, and the fourth ventricle in the setting of myelomeningocele. Hydrocephalus is common in patients with this condition, along with multiple skeletal and intracranial abnormalities (Box 119-3). After closure of the myelomeningocele and the shunting that usually is necessary, patients may display symptoms of irritability or apnea as the first sign of a Chiari II malformation. Aspiration can lead to recurrent pneumonia, and problems with dysphagia and dysarthria may be evident. Hindbrain anomalies, usually secondary to respiratory insufficiency, are the leading cause of death in myelodysplastic patients. Findings on physical examination include down-beating nystagmus, quadriparesis with hypotonia, ataxia, ocular motility defects, diminished gag reflex, and stridor (see Box 119-2). Symptom onset in older children usually indicates spinal cord tethering, shunt malfunction, or the development of spinal cord syrinx.

Among the imaging and autopsy findings in patients with Chiari II malformations, the brain may show complete or partial agenesis of the corpus callosum and septum pellucidum, prominent anterior commissure, polygyria, interdigitation of the occipital and parietal lobes, partial or complete agenesis of

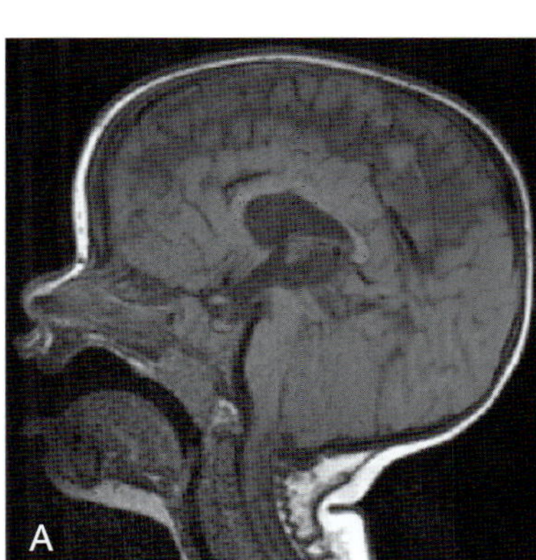

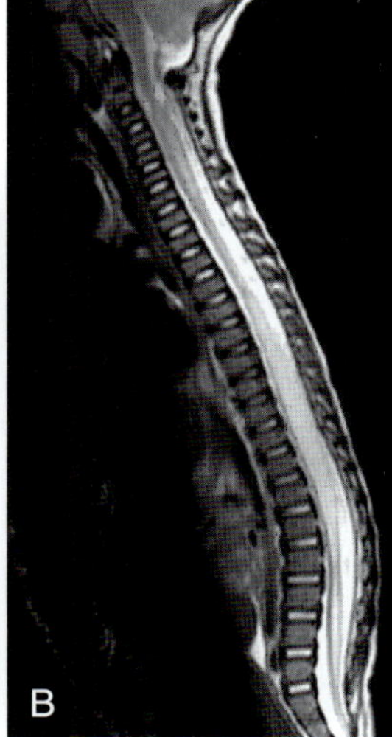

FIGURE 119-2. **A,** T1-weighted sagittal MRI of an 18-month-old boy with Chiari II malformation, recurrent aspiration, and dysphagia, demonstrating typical features of Chiari II with elongated brainstem and cerebellar tonsils in the upper cervical region. **B,** T2-weighted sagittal spine MRI of same patient demonstrating large spinal cord syrinx and low-lying cord secondary to myelomeningocele.

the olfactory bulb/tracts, enlargement of the massa intermedia, or fusion of the colliculi (i.e., tectal beaking). In addition, the cranial nerve nuclei can be malformed. The cerebellum is reduced in size, there can be dysplasia with absent folia, the medulla can be elongated and flattened with the classic medullary kink, and the cranial and upper cervical nerves can course upward. Luckenschadel, a beaten copper or fenestrated appearance on imaging, can characterize the skull. Scalloping of the petrous bone can occur. In these patients, the posterior fossa is small, and basilar impression/assimilation can be seen. Spine anomalies can include Klippel-Feil deformities and enlargement of the cervical canal. Hydrocephalus is a common feature, seen in upward of 90% of patients with Chiari II malformation, and the ventricles may demonstrate colpocephaly. The tentorium usually is low-lying, creating a more vertical straight sinus and low-lying torcula. In addition to the myelodysplasia, associated spinal cord abnormalities include split cord malformations and syrinx formation (Fig. 119-2).[34,35]

Chiari III

Occipital or cervical encephalocele—Chiari III malformation—is associated with many of the intracranial abnormalities seen with Chiari II malformations. The tissue in the encephalocele is variable in its extent and is dysplastic.

Chiari IV

Chiari IV malformation is characterized by cerebellar aplasia or hypoplasia with concomitant aplasia of the tentorium. Hindbrain herniation is absent.

Chiari 1.5

Patients with Chiari 1.5 malformation have a condition that falls somewhere between Chiari I and Chiari II. Chiari 1.5 malformation is characterized by Chiari I–type tonsillar herniation but with elongation of the brainstem and fourth ventricle.[36]

Chiari 0

Conversely, Chiari 0 malformation is characterized by syrinx formation without hindbrain herniation. It is thought that dysregulation of CSF equilibrium at the craniocervical junction contributes to the Chiari 0 malformation, and that operative findings such as arachnoid veils and adhesions account for obstruction at the foramen of Magendie or crowding at the foramen magnum.[37]

Patient Selection and Surgical Management

Diagnostic Imaging

High-resolution MR and CT imaging are critical for appropriate evaluation of the patient referred for consideration of Chiari decompression. In all patients who present for initial evaluation, it is our practice to obtain high-resolution brain MRI, including cine-MRI and constructive interference steady state (CISS) sequences, and screening sagittal MRIs of the complete spine. Cine-MRI is used to evaluate CSF pulsatility at the craniocervical junction, whereas use of a highly T2-weighted MR sequence (CISS) in the sagittal plane provides improved visualization of CSF around the cerebellum and tonsils. MRI makes it possible to measure the degree of tonsillar descent measured from the McRae line and provides some indication of CSF dynamics (on cine-MRI), reveals evidence of hydrocephalus, detects the presence or absence of a spinal cord syrinx, provides evidence of a low-lying spinal cord or tethering, and detects concurrent brain/spinal cord abnormalities (e.g., manifestations of Chiari II malformation, split cord formation, or associated scoliosis), and allows screening for associated or incidental findings. Operative candidates also undergo preoperative CT imaging to confirm that the skull thickness is sufficient for intraoperative pinning. Potential associated skull-base and cervical spine abnormalities such as atlanto-occipital assimilation, basilar invagination, and Klippel-Feil abnormalities also are evaluated with CT. Any concerns for cervical spinal stability are further evaluated with flexion-extension plain radiographs before any surgical intervention.

Surgical Indications

Chiari I

Controversy remains regarding an exact algorithm for patient selection in regard to successful and appropriate Chiari I decompression.[38,39] The initial step is to ensure that symptoms are not caused by hydrocephalus or spinal cord tethering. Evidence of hydrocephalus should lead to CSF diversion, followed by reassessment to determine whether the symptoms and imaging findings have resolved after normalization of intracranial pressure. Spinal cord tethering, while uncommon, is sought on spinal MRI. It is defined as termination of the conus below the L2-3 disc space. The filum terminale is considered abnormal if the diameter is greater than 1 mm at L5-S1.[40]

Once hydrocephalus and spinal cord tethering have been excluded or addressed, our evaluation begins with an assessment of the degree of tonsillar descent and presence or absence of a spinal cord syrinx. Like many of our colleagues, we consider a spinal cord syrinx an indicator of abnormal CSF dynamics consequent to the Chiari malformation. Patients with a spinal cord syrinx are offered surgical decompression unless they are completely asymptomatic and have only a small (<2 mm) syrinx. Patients in this small subset are monitored closely with serial imaging every 6 months and offered surgery if symptoms occur or the syrinx increases in size.[41] In several of our asymptomatic patients who were followed conservatively, the syrinx resolved over time.[42] Symptomatic patients without a syrinx pose the larger diagnostic and therapeutic challenge. Patients with more than 5 mm of tonsillar descent and clear Valsalva-induced headache or neck pain often benefit from decompression. Additional symptoms also are helpful to support the decision to offer surgery. Patients with headaches unrelated to Valsalva maneuvers who have a minimal Chiari malformation (<10 mm tonsillar descent) are the most challenging to treat and often are the least likely to benefit from operative intervention. A conservative approach often is warranted in these patients, with referral to a headache management specialist and close neurosurgical follow-up with imaging repeated yearly. Symptomatic progression or the development of a syrinx favors surgical intervention. Patients who present with more obscure neurologic findings (e.g., fussiness, head banging, nystagmus, essential hypertension, recurrent aspiration) also are a challenge, and their symptoms ideally should be correlated with radiographic findings. Surgical decompression may have a role in management of these patients, but a conservative approach often is warranted. Progressive scoliosis in the setting of a Chiari malformation is another objective finding that warrants surgical consideration.

Chiari II

In our practice, surgical decompression in the setting of Chiari II malformation is most commonly performed in children under the age of 2 years who have symptomatic brainstem dysfunction. It is critical to interrogate for shunt malfunction as a first line of evaluation in these patients. If there is any possibility of shunt malfunction, shunt exploration should be undertaken before any other procedures. After shunt malfunction has been excluded, we perform a decompression, most commonly for lower brainstem dysfunction, including respiratory failure, recurrent aspiration, progressive spinal cord syrinx, or other compelling symptoms. Outcomes for Chiari II decompression can be poor, especially if bilateral vocal cord paralysis is present preoperatively or if other signs of profound brainstem dysfunction are present. It is important to convey realistic expectations to the family when deciding on Chiari II decompression.

Surgical Technique

Anesthetic and Positioning Considerations

General endotracheal anesthesia is required for all patients. A percutaneous arterial catheter and an indwelling Foley catheter are placed, but central venous catheters usually are not used. Intubation is done either via fiberoptic guidance or with minimal neck extension. Total IV anesthesia typically is used to

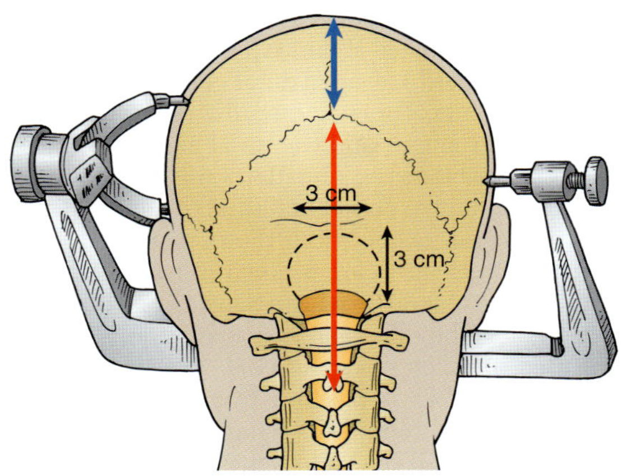

FIGURE 119-3. An incision is made from the inion to the spinous process of C2 (*red arrow*) and a separate incision is marked for the pericranial graft (*blue arrow*). The suboccipital decompression is approximately 3 × 3 cm.

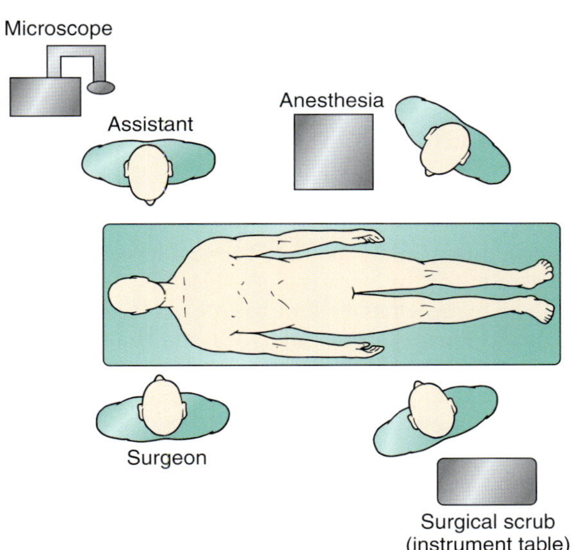

FIGURE 119-4. Patient positioning. The prone position is used with the patient in three-point Mayfield cranial fixation; the arms are positioned at the side. The head is then slightly flexed, and the table is put into a slight reverse Trendelenburg position. The head of the bed is positioned at a 90-degree angle from the anesthesiologist, with the surgeon and the assistant at the patient's head. The microscope base is brought behind the assistant, and a head-to-head configuration is used.

facilitate neurophysiologic monitoring. Once anesthesia is induced, the patient is connected to neuromonitoring devices to assess brainstem auditory evoked potentials, motor evoked potentials, and somatosensory evoked potentials. Intravenous antibiotics (usually cefazolin) are administered and redosed every 3 hours. Dexamethasone also is given every 4 hours and continued for 48 hours postoperatively. A lumbar drain is not used. Patients older than 5 years of age are put into three-point Mayfield pin fixation and positioned prone on gel rolls that run parallel to the long axis of the body. If the patient is younger than 5 years of age, we typically use a horseshoe headholder but pay considerable attention to avoiding pressure or contact of the eyes with the side of the horseshoe. We use additional foam padding to bolster the padding on the horseshoe. All contact points are meticulously padded, including the iliac crest in thin patients. We ensure that the axilla is free and the shoulders are neutrally positioned. The neck is carefully positioned in a slightly flexed position, ensuring at least two finger-breadths between the neck and chin. Airway pressures are a good indication to ensure that the amount of neck flexion is appropriate. It also is important to ensure that the chin is not touching the bed, because the patient can slide if the bed is in reverse Trendelenburg position. The arms are padded and placed at the patient's side, and a drawsheet (placed prior to positioning) is then brought over the patient's torso and secured with towel clips. Strong cloth tape and a security strap are then used to secure the patient to the operating table. After the hair is trimmed with clippers, a standard suboccipital incision is marked, starting at the inion, running along the midline, and terminating at approximately the spinous process of C2 (Fig. 119-3). The senior author (RGE) also prefers to use autologous pericranium for duraplasty, and a separate incision is marked from the inion superiorly for a length of approximately 5 cm to harvest this. Before the incision is made, the field is washed with 4% chlorhexidine soap followed by alcohol and is then dried. Chlorhexidine gluconate antiseptic (ChloraPrep, CareFusion, San Diego, CA) is used to prepare the operative field and the edge of the surrounding hair. During final preoperative positioning, the patient's head is placed at a 90-degree angle from the anesthesiologist, with surgeons situated on either side of the patient's head and the scrub technician standing across from the anesthesiologist; a Mayo stand is positioned over the patient's torso. The operative microscope is positioned for use during the intradural portion of the procedure in a head-to-head configuration with the base behind the assistant (Fig. 119-4).

Exposure

We begin by injecting the incision line with 0.25% lidocaine with epinephrine. A scalpel or Bovie cautery (Bovie Medical Corporation, Clearwater, FL) with a Colorado-tip needle is used to make the skin incision. Bovie cautery is used to continue the incision down along the avascular midline fascial sulcus. Careful hemostasis is obtained during the dissection to avoid undue blood loss and, importantly, to prevent blood from getting into the subdural space. Dissection is carried to the periosteum of the suboccipput and the posterior ring of C1. Self-retaining retractors are placed to maintain exposure. Pitfalls that must be avoided during this stage of the procedure include overaggressive dissection toward the vertebral arteries laterally and inadvertent durotomy.

The posterior ring of C1 is then removed using a combination of instruments, including rongeurs, a Kerrison punch, and/or a high-speed drill. Straight and curved curets facilitate the dissection. The lateral extent of the bone removal is the edge of the thecal sac. The suboccipital craniectomy is performed with a high-speed pneumatic or electric drill. The type of drill bit (e.g., M8, Acorn) to be used is selected based on surgeon preference. A craniectomy of approximately 3 × 3 cm is created (see Fig. 119-4). Attention is paid to careful dissection of the dura, especially along the midline keel and along the foramen magnum, because the midline keel can be quite vascular. Any bleeding can be addressed with bone wax. Epidural bleeding is controlled with bipolar cautery or liquid Gelfoam (Pfitzer, New York, NY) mixed with thrombin (Floseal, Baxter, Deerfield, IL). A large craniectomy is to be avoided because of concern over cerebellar sag and its resultant complications in the postoperative period. Pitfalls during the bony removal include low-lying torcula, excessive bone bleeding, ectatic vertebral arteries, and occipitalization of C1. During removal of the dorsal arch of C1, the lateral internal vertebral venous plexus often is encountered. This is an epidural venous plexus located between the dura and the laminae periosteum, consisting of two or more anterior and posterior longitudinal venous channels running along multiple cervical levels. Bipolar cautery is used to control venous plexus bleeding; liquid Gelfoam also can be highly effective for this type of bleeding.

The thickened ligament under C1 and the foramen magnum can be highly constrictive and should be released. The ligament is cauterized and then divided sharply; venous bleeding often is encountered during this maneuver and is controlled as previously described. The ligamentous band is resected several millimeters laterally to allow for dural expansion.

In the vast majority of infants with Chiari II malformation, the operative decompression terminates at this stage because of the concern for high blood loss from a low-lying torcula or the extensive intradural venous lakes that often are present in young patients. Other authors argue that the use of duraplasty is appropriate in these patients (WJ Oakes, personal communication), but that has not been our practice until the patients are older.

Much discussion also has revolved around the use of craniectomy without duraplasty for decompression of Chiari I malformation.[43-45] In patients without a spinal cord syrinx, we will forgo duraplasty if intraoperative ultrasound demonstrates CSF cine flow dorsal to the cerebellar tonsils and the tonsils show adequate pulsatility. We believe that syringomyelia is an indication for expansion duraplasty; however, much debate remains.

In cases in which duraplasty is to be performed, we harvest an autologous pericranial patch of approximately 3 × 3 cm from the previously marked incision superior to the inion. The patch is left to soak in bacitracin irrigation until implantation.

Dural and Arachnoid Opening

Before dural opening, we ensure that vascular clips are readily available, because the dura can be quite vascular, especially in children. The wound is irrigated copiously to remove any bone dust, and we change our gloves prior to dural opening. Once meticulous hemostasis is obtained to prevent "drip-down," we perform a standard Y-shaped dural opening starting at the level of C1. The dura is opened carefully with a no. 15 scalpel and a dental instrument, and the dural edges are coagulated to control venous bleeding. The incision is brought up to the midpoint of the dural exposure and then the edges of the Y are extended. A margin is kept from the bone edge to facilitate dural graft closure. Great care is taken to preserve the arachnoid and prevent blood from entering the subdural space. A combination of bipolar cautery, vascular clips, and cotton patties is used to accomplish this goal. The dura also can be oversewn to control brisk bleeding from the dural edge. The dural edges are then tented up using #4-0 Nurolon sutures (Ethicon, Cornelia, GA). A pledget of Gelfoam is placed in the subdural space over the cervical cord to prevent operative bleeding from escaping down the cervical subdural space (Fig. 119-5A). In cases in which the dura is tight along the cervical cord, we cut the inferior aspect of the dura laterally as described by Pirouzmand and Tucker[46] to open the dura more widely.

Once the dura is adequately opened and all bleeding is controlled, we irrigate the subdural space to flush away any blood or debris. The operative microscope is then brought in for the remainder of the intradural dissection. Under microsurgical visualization, we first open the arachnoid over the cerebellar tonsils. The cerebellar tonsils can have various configurations, and our goal is to first survey the anatomy. Once the cerebellar tonsils are identified, we begin to coagulate them carefully with bipolar cautery. As the tonsillar tissue begins to shrink, we look for the tip of the tonsil inferiorly. Due diligence must be taken to avoid injury or coagulation of lateral brainstem cranial nerves (especially accessory spinal nerves) and the posterior inferior cerebellar artery. Often, small arachnoid attachments must be sharply divided to allow the cerebellar tonsil to retract and elevate. The process is continued until the tonsil is above the level of the foramen magnum (Fig. 119-5B). The process is repeated for the contralateral cerebellar tonsil. We then inspect the outflow of CSF from the fourth ventricle/obex. Once we confirm adequate flow of CSF, the intradural portion of the procedure is concluded. Irrigation with warm saline is used before dural closure.

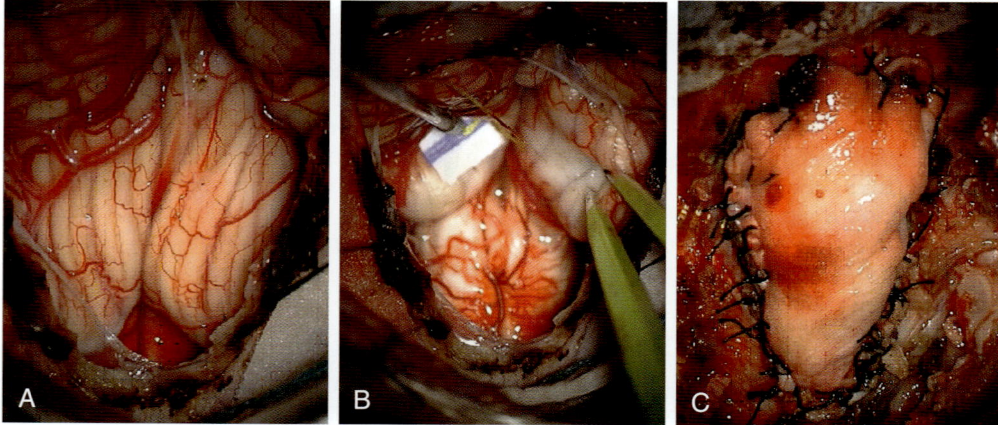

FIGURE 119-5. **A,** Intraoperative view: Note the degree of cerebellar tonsil descent. **B,** After bipolar coagulation, the cerebellar tonsils are above the level of the foramen magnum and any associated arachnoid adhesions have been lysed. **C,** Dural graft closure with autologous pericranium.

Graft Selection and Dural Closure

Many dural graft materials have been used in the long history of Chiari surgery. These include pericranium, autologous fascia lata, cadaveric dura/fascia lata, cadaveric dermis, Gore-Tex, and multiple allograft products constructed from purified bovine collagen. The senior author (RGE) prefers autologous pericranium for several reasons. Autologous tissue avoids any issues with tissue compatibility, allergies, product recalls, sterility, or remote questions of transmission of bovine illness. As previously discussed, the pericranial graft is harvested before dural opening and is soaked in bacitracin irrigation to remove any blood or debris and keep the patch hydrated. The dural closure is performed using interrupted #4-0 Nurolon sutures (Ethicon). The graft is first secured at the three corners of the opening, and then multiple interrupted sutures are placed to create a watertight closure (Fig. 119-5C). It is important not to stretch the graft, to avoid stress that can lead to suture line failure. Before the final few sutures are placed, the subdural space is flooded with saline irrigation to once again remove any debris and evacuate any air trapped under the patch. At this point, the anesthesiologist performs a Valsalva maneuver to 30 mm H_2O and then 40 mm H_2O to test the integrity of the watertight closure. Any areas that are observed to be leaking are oversewn. Once a watertight closure is obtained, we irrigate with bacitracin, then place a layer of Surgicel (Ethicon 360) over the suture line. Next we obtain 5 to 10 mL of the patient's sterile peripheral blood from anesthesia and mix it with a small amount of thrombin. As the mixture starts to coagulate, the blood is put over the suture line as a blood patch. A second layer of Surgicel is placed over the patched area. If a large defect is still present, the senior author (RGE) also will use Duraseal (Covidien, Waltham, MA) to fill the defect before closing the wound. A recent multicenter trial has found that this product is safe and effective in this setting.[47,48] The deep muscle and fascial layers are reapproximated with #0-0 and #2-0 Vicryl sutures, the dermis is reapproximated with #3-0 Vicryl sutures, and an absorbable suture such as Monocryl (Ethicon) is used in a running fashion for primary skin closure. Skin glue (Dermabond, Ethicon) is used as a sterile dressing directly over the absorbable suture line. We do not routinely place a lumbar drain either before or after the procedure.

Postoperative Care and Complications

Patients are taken for an immediate postoperative CT scan and then observed overnight in the ICU with standard monitoring. Three doses of IV antibiotics are given in this period. Dexamethasone is given every 6 hours for 48 hours and then discontinued. Pain control is generally via IV morphine. On the first postoperative day, we switch to IV ketorolac for pain control for the following 48 hours. Valium also is an excellent sedative with secondary benefits of muscle relaxation that can be started in the perioperative period. In our experience, the discomfort from the surgery generally lasts for approximately 48 hours and then improves rapidly in most patients. Analgesics and sedation are always strictly regulated to preserve an immediate neurologic examination free from the confusion that can arise with oversedation.

Possible complications are listed in Table 119-2. Immediate postoperative complications can include major complications such as posterior fossa hemorrhage requiring emergent operative clot evacuation, stroke, cranial nerve palsy, or bacterial meningitis. Fortunately, these major complications are extremely rare. Delayed complications are more common and can include aseptic meningitis, pseudomeningocele formation, hydrocephalus, and, rarely, swan neck deformities. Aseptic meningitis is treated with 7 to 10 days of high-dose steroids, including a steroid taper. Recurrent aseptic meningitis occasionally responds to serial lumbar puncture in combination with steroid administration. Pseudomeningocele formation is evaluated first by using imaging studies to ensure that hydrocephalus is not the causal factor. Once the diagnosis of hydrocephalus has been excluded, the pseudomeningocele can be treated in one of several fashions. Initially, we manage the condition conservatively as long as the incision is healing well and the pseudomeningocele is not growing. Attempts to drain the pseudomeningocele via needle puncture and use of compression dressing meet with limited success. A trial of lumbar CSF drainage for 3 to 5 days also can be successful. If the incision is in danger of breakdown or the pseudomeningocele

TABLE 119-2

Prevention and Management of Surgical Complications Associated with Treatment of Chiari Malformation

Complication	Prevention	Management
Vertebral artery injury	Avoid wide laminectomy and craniectomy; use gentle dissection; avoid lateral use of cautery; no pulling with rongeurs	Direct arterial repair; tamponade; interventional stenting or occlusion; careful watch for neurologic sequelae
Stroke	Avoid coagulation or manipulation of posterior inferior cerebellar and vertebral arteries.	Papaverine if vasospasm noted intraoperatively; postoperative stroke management
Hematoma	Meticulous hemostasis; avoid postoperative hypertension; careful graft and wound closure	Immediate postoperative CT, return to surgery if needed for clot evacuation; blood pressure control
Dural lake/bleeding	Careful preoperative identification of torcula; open dura slowly	Have hemoclips immediately available; suture dural edge to control bleeding.
Aseptic meningitis	Avoid blood in subdural/subarachnoid space	Obtain CSF for culture to rule out bacterial meningitis; high-dose steroid taper; possible serial lumbar punctures
Pseudomeningocele	Proper graft selection; meticulous graft suturing	Evaluate for hydrocephalus; tap collection; possible lumbar drain; wound exploration and revision
Cerebellar sag	Conservative posterior fossa decompression (3 × 3 cm)	Evaluate for craniovertebral instability, possible ventriculoperitoneal shunt; possible partial cranioplasty
Persistent syringomyelia	Repeat initial evaluation.	Reexploration and revision decompression; possible shunting (ventriculoperitoneal or syringosubarachnoid)

is growing despite these other interventions, we often undertake reexploration of the dural graft and repair it primarily.

Prognosis

Chiari I

The prognosis in patients with symptomatic Chiari I malformation who undergo a craniovertebral decompression is generally good, with approximately 90% experiencing improvement or stabilization of symptoms.[49] Syringomyelia improves in most patients by the third postoperative month, with an approximately 95% likelihood of the syrinx remaining small with stable or improved symptoms. Children with neurologic deficits can recover normal function if operated on in a timely fashion. Recurrent or recalcitrant syrinx is best treated with reexploration as opposed to myelotomy and syringosubarachnoid drainage. Between 5% and 10% of patients continue to experience clinically significant symptoms despite craniovertebral decompression, and alternative treatment options must be sought. These failures often demonstrate poor CSF flow at the craniocervical junction. Regarding the controversial area of duraplasty, recent meta-analysis demonstrated no significant difference between posterior fossa decompression alone and decompression and duraplasty with respect to clinical improvement or decrease in syringomyelia; however, duraplasty was associated with a lower risk of reoperation but a greater risk of CSF-related complications.[50-53] Our group still favors duraplasty in the setting of symptomatic Chiari malformation with concurrent spinal cord syrinx.

Chiari II

It is important to reiterate that definitive confirmation of a nominally functioning shunt is paramount in patients with symptomatic Chiari II malformations. Bony decompression for children under 5 years of age with symptomatic Chiari II malformation yields symptomatic improvement in about 50% of cases in our anecdotal experience. Children with profound brainstem dysfunction obviously are the least likely to benefit, but the morbid nature of the deficits makes surgical intervention a worthwhile endeavor in many cases.[54-59]

Summary

Chiari malformation is one of the most complex and challenging conditions to approach in neurosurgery. Variable signs, symptoms, and imaging findings make appropriate surgical candidate selection critical for successful outcomes. Appropriately selected patients can have dramatic, life-changing benefits from surgery that cannot be achieved with medical therapy or other interventions. The appropriate surgical treatment of Chiari malformations will remain an area of intense debate among neurosurgeons, especially in regard to the value of duraplasty. Importantly, the unprecedented access to digital media and information via the Internet gives patients a knowledge base not seen previously, and the treating surgeon should be prepared to answer a host of questions as families decide on treatment options.[60,61]

KEY REFERENCES

Armonda RA, Citrin CM, Foley KT, Ellenbogen RG: Quantitative cine-mode magnetic resonance imaging of Chiari I malformations: an analysis of cerebrospinal fluid dynamics, *Neurosurgery* 35:214–223, 1994; discussion 223–224.

Chiari H: Uber Veranderungen des Kleinhirns in Folge von Hydrocephalie des Grosshirns. *Dtsch Med Wschr* 17:1172–1175, 1891.

Milhorat TH, Chou MW, Trinidad EM, et al: Chiari I malformation redefined: clinical and radiographic findings for 364 symptomatic patients. *Neurosurgery* 44:1005–1017, 1999.

Oldfield EH, Muraszko K, Shawker TH, Patronas NJ: Pathophysiology of syringomyelia associated with Chiari I malformation of the cerebellar tonsils. Implications for diagnosis and treatment. *J Neurosurg* 80:3–15, 1994.

Tubbs RS, McGirt MJ, Oakes WJ: Surgical experience in 130 pediatric patients with Chiari I malformations. *J Neurosurg* 99:291–296, 2003.

Tubbs RS, Oakes WJ: Treatment and management of the Chiari II malformation: an evidence-based review of the literature. *Childs Nerv Syst* 20:375–381, 2004.

REFERENCES

The complete reference list is available online at expertconsult.com.

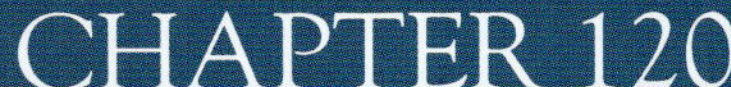

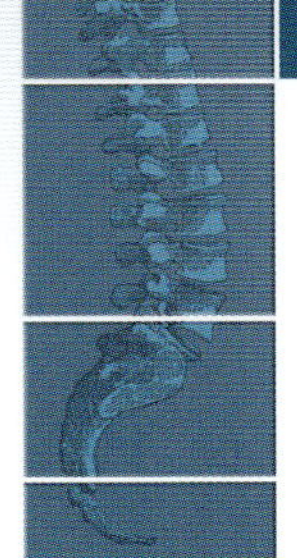

CHAPTER 120

Chiari Malformation, Chronic Fatigue Syndrome, and Fibromyalgia: A Paradigm for Care

Augusto T. Hsia, Jr. | Ajit A. Krishnaney

The Chiari malformation (CM) usually is a congenital hindbrain disorder that can be acquired in rare cases. In 1891 Hans Chiari, a pathologist, was the first to describe the deformity and group it into different categories based on the severity of tonsillar and cerebellar descent below the foramen magnum.[1]

Type I CM, occasionally called "adult" type, is the least severe form and the most common. It is described radiographically as tonsillar herniation of more than 5 mm below the foramen magnum.

Type II CM, also known as Arnold-Chiari malformation, is found almost exclusively in patients with myelomeningocele. It is characterized by herniation of the cerebellar tonsils with the adjoining vermis and part of the fourth ventricle.

Type III CM causes severe brain malformation, with caudal displacement of the cerebellum and brainstem into a high cervical meningocele. Most of these cases are not compatible with life, and infants die shortly after birth.

The incidence of Chiari malformation in a study of 22,000 brain MRIs was reported to be 1 in 1280 individuals.[2] This study probably underestimates the true incidence of Chiari malformation in asymptomatic individuals and in the general population. There is a higher preponderance of Chiari malformation I in females than in males, by a ratio of 3:2.[2]

There seems to be some evidence of genetic transmission in a subset of patients with Chiari malformation with syringomyelia.[2-4] The extent of cerebellar herniation does not necessarily correlate with subjective complaints, physical findings, and neurologic findings.[4]

Syringomyelia occurs when cerebrospinal fluid (CSF) forms a cavity within the spinal cord. Chiari malformation is the leading cause of pathologic syrinx formation. It is thought that the displaced cerebellar tonsil acts as a plug that obstructs CSF flow and may act as a miniature piston (i.e., the "piston theory") to drive CSF inside the spinal cord.[5] A syrinx cavity also can develop in other cases of CSF flow obstruction, such as spinal cord tumors, infection, or trauma. The incidence of syringomyelia in Chiari malformation I is estimated to be 50% to 75%.[6]

What Is Fibromyalgia Syndrome or Chronic Fatigue Syndrome?

Fibromyalgia syndrome is characterized by chronic widespread pain and multiple tender joints.[7,8] Most patients have coexisting fatigue, sleep disturbance, paresthesias, and morning stiffness.[8] More than 80% of patients with fibromyalgia syndrome have chronic fatigue syndrome. There are more clinical similarities than differences between the two entities. The patient is diagnosed with fibromyalgia syndrome if the predominant complaint is pain or chronic fatigue syndrome if the predominant complaint is fatigue. The prevalence of fibromyalgia is reported to be 2.1% to 5.7% in the general population and may be as high as 10% to 20% in some settings.[9-11]

In one study, fibromyalgia syndrome was found to be 13 times more common in patients following cervical spine injury as opposed to patients with lower extremity injury.[12] It also is reported that 30% to 56% of patients with fibromyalgia syndrome have coexisting mental disorders, anxiety, or depression.[13,14] Fibromyalgia can be diagnosed concomitantly in 34% of patients with chronic inflammatory arthritis (i.e., rheumatoid arthritis, systemic lupus erythematosus), and in 28% of patients with chronic spinal pain syndromes.[7]

Fibromyalgia syndrome currently is thought to be a disorder of pain regulation or "central sensitization."[15] There seems to be significant overlap in symptoms of various chronic disorders, such as irritable bowel syndrome, chronic migraines, chronic fatigue syndrome, and posttraumatic stress disorders. Patients with fibromyalgia have lower pain and heat thresholds and have higher catastrophizing and somatization behaviors in response to painful stimuli.[16] Substance P, a peptide associated with chronic pain, is elevated in the CSF of patients with fibromyalgia syndrome.[17] There seems to be a genetic predisposition as well: first-degree relatives of patients with fibromyalgia have higher rates of developing fibromyalgia syndrome. There is an increased co-aggregation of fibromyalgia syndrome with major mood disorders in families.[18]

Controversial Link between Fibromyalgia or Chronic Fatigue Syndrome and Chiari Malformation: Does It Really Exist?

In 1999, an article in *The Wall Street Journal* and an ABC *20/20* television program featuring prominent neurosurgeons suggested surgical management for patients with fibromyalgia syndrome or chronic fatigue syndrome with Chiari malformation or cervical stenosis.[8]

In 2001, in an abstract presented at the Congress of Neurological Surgeons in San Diego, Heffez reported on 64 patients with a diagnosis of fibromyalgia syndrome with signs and symptoms consistent with cervical myelopathy from either Chiari malformation or cervical stenosis who underwent surgery.[19] There was no randomization in assigning patients. At 6 months, statistically significant improvement was reported as compared with a nonsurgical control group in terms of pain, grip strength, and balance impairment. Headache also improved in 90% of patients in the surgical group compared with 45% in the nonsurgical group. Non–statistically significant improvement also was seen in the surgical group in terms of fatigue, depression, insomnia, and paresthesias.

A link between fibromyalgia syndrome and Chiari malformation has been suggested, with the recommendation that patients with fibromyalgia should be aggressively worked up for possible neurologic disorders such as Chiari malformation or cervical stenosis.[19,20] Based on the available literature, however, there is no evidence of a direct link between fibromyalgia syndrome/chronic fatigue with Chiari malformation with or without syringomyelia.[21] It is plausible to suggest that patients who have long-standing neurologic disorders (e.g., cervical myelopathy, Chiari malformation, cervical stenosis) can develop secondary fibromyalgia. This is consistent with the concept of chronic central sensitization states. Compared with the prevalence of fibromyalgia syndrome, which is 5% to 20% in the general population), the 0.77% incidence of radiographic Chiari malformation in 22,591 brain/cervical MRI scans reviewed is relatively small.[2] It could be by chance alone that they are linked. The nonstatistical improvement in fibromyalgia somatic complaints in the operated group could be explained by reduction in stress and the feeling that something "substantial" had been done. It is unclear whether these somatic symptoms referred to fibromyalgia improved permanently or if there was symptom recurrence over time, because no long-term follow-up was done.

An MRI study of consecutive patients diagnosed with fibromyalgia syndrome at two tertiary centers showed no increase in the prevalence of Chiari malformation/cervical stenosis in this group over that of the "normal" control group. In fact, 11 of 15 patients (73%) in the control group, compared with 8 of 26 patients (31%) in the fibromyalgia group, showed evidence of some degree of tonsillar herniation.[22]

How Is Fibromyalgia Diagnosed?

Diagnostic Criteria for Fibromyalgia

The diagnostic criteria described earlier in regard to palpation of tender points had limited use in general medical practice. It was cumbersome to do, and most patients ended up with more pain after their office visit. It has been a widely known secret among rheumatologists that tender points had little value except that those patients who had more trigger points probably were more distressed, and subsequent pain scores could be higher. The trigger points were of significance mainly in the research field.

In 2010, the American College of Rheumatology created simpler, clinically friendly criteria for diagnosing fibromyalgia syndrome.[23] These were designed not to replace the 1990 criteria but to provide clinically more relevant alternative criteria to diagnose fibromyalgia with similar diagnostic sensitivity and specificity. The most important change was to do away with tender point palpations and to include a widespread pain index score. The coexisting somatic symptoms that are so common in patients with fibromyalgia syndrome were highlighted.

Chiari Malformation and Syringomyelia: Clinical Diagnosis

Chiari malformation presents with symptoms related to brainstem compression, hydrocephalus, syringomyelia, or transient increase in intracranial pressure.[1]

The major presenting symptoms of Chiari malformation with syringomyelia are weakness (more pronounced in the upper extremity than in the lower extremity), pain (neck pain with extremity radiation), paresthesias or hyperesthesias, suboccipital headaches, and gait difficulties. [6,24-26]

"Hard" subjective and objective neurologic findings in Chiari malformations can be categorized based on pathophysiologic mechanisms:

Brainstem compression

- Lower cranial nerve abnormalities occur in 7.5% to 50% of cases.[6] The most commonly affected nerves are the glossopharyngeal and vagus nerves. Abnormal gag reflex, trigeminal hyperesthesia, and unilateral facial weakness can occur.[6,26]
- Direct cerebellar dysfunction with ataxia and vertigo occur in 8% to 24% of those affected.[2,6]

Intracranial pressure increase/fluctuation

- The most prominent symptom is a rather specific suboccipital headache that is worsened by the Valsalva maneuver, cough, and postural changes.[27-29] The tussive headache is the most common presenting pain complaint, seen in 54% to 80% of cases.[6,24,25]
- Pseudotumor-like syndrome with retro-orbital pain and visual changes has been reported.[24]

Progressive syrinx enlargement causing central spinal cord dysfunction

- Holocord syndrome: upper extremity weakness, hypertrophy, dissociative sensory abnormalities with intact vibration/proprioception, and hyperreflexia. These findings are present in more than 90% of patients with symptomatic syringomyelia.[6]
- Progressive scoliosis

Long tract signs

- Babinski reflex/clonus, spasticity, gait abnormality, bilateral extremity weakness, and autonomic dysregulation (i.e., bladder urgency) can occur.

In most cases of symptomatic Chiari malformation and syringomyelia, it took an average of 3 to 6 years from the start of symptoms to reach the diagnosis and begin definitive treatment.[6,24,25]

Because pain is the predominant complaint in most cases (e.g., headache, neck pain, extremity paresthesias/hyperesthesias), it is not surprising that a significant portion of patients with symptomatic Chiari malformation with syringomyelia exhibit chronic pain behavior.

Significant overlap of somatic symptoms in fibromyalgia syndrome and Chiari malformation may be seen. Muscle pain, fatigue, sleep disturbances, cognitive problems, headache, and dizziness are common in both. Chronic stress due to a significant delay in diagnosis, chronic disability, genetic susceptibility, and concomitant anxiety or depression has been suggested as a major contributing factor. Secondary gain issues in cases where trauma is involved (e.g., work injuries, motor vehicle accidents) may play a role.

The incidence of fibromyalgia in symptomatic Chiari malformation is unknown. It can be difficult to distinguish clinically between the two entities, due to overlapping symptoms. The differentiating lines are blurry at times. Usually there are more objective "hard" neurologic findings in symptomatic Chiari malformation as opposed to more subjective complaints in fibromyalgia syndrome, with a paucity of objective neurologic findings.

The pain in fibromyalgia syndrome is diffuse, as opposed to a more localized pain complaint in Chiari malformation. There also is a disproportionately higher report of somatic complaint in fibromyalgia syndrome as opposed to Chiari malformation, including fatigue, sleep disorder, cognitive abnormalities, and mood disorder.

The headache in Chiari malformation is specifically suboccipital/occipital, of variable duration, and aggravated by the Valsalva maneuver, cough, and change of body posture.[27,30] The headache pattern in fibromyalgia syndrome is more generalized and unprovoked. Most of these headaches can be classified as migraine with or without aura, tension headache, or analgesic overuse headache.[31]

Gait difficulties, poor balance, and hyperreflexia can be found in both fibromyalgia syndrome and Chiari malformation. The balance and gait difficulties in fibromyalgia syndrome can be related to deconditioning, concentration difficulties, orthostatic hypertension, and vestibular dysfunction. Except for hyperreflexia, no other objective evidence of cervical myelopathy should be elicited in primary fibromyalgia syndrome. The weakness reported in fibromyalgia syndrome generally is subjective.

It has been suggested—although not clearly proven—that the extent of pain and mood disorders in Chiari malformation/cervical stenosis is higher than in chronic pain states that have no evidence of central nervous system disorder.[32]

Most patients with Chiari malformation and syringomyelia seen in a tertiary care setting have complicated, highly variable symptomatology, with both hard and soft neurologic findings and unusually significant psychosocial distress.

Paradigm of Care in Chiari Malformation with Syringomyelia

Outside of neurosurgery, the Chiari malformation with syringomyelia disorders remain poorly understood. Most medical practitioners have very limited knowledge of these disorders, and, more importantly, only a few know how to evaluate and manage this disorder. Fibromyalgia, on the other hand, is a very common disorder and has straightforward diagnostic criteria. Despite these widely published criteria, however, some physicians still question whether fibromyalgia syndrome truly exists or is just a manifestation of significant stress, a psychiatric disorder, or some other undiagnosed illness. Delay in the diagnosis of fibromyalgia may be due to the medical practitioner's seeming lack of understanding of fibromyalgia and chronic pain states or could be due to social sensitivities in labeling patients with this syndrome. The enormous number of somatic complaints associated with fibromyalgia syndrome also may result in confusion and delay in its diagnosis.

Most patients referred to our department for evaluation of Chiari malformation have brain MRI scans showing tonsillar herniation or radiographic Chiari malformation, with or without syrinx. In most patients, we employ a multidisciplinary concept in the initial evaluation and management of symptomatic radiographic Chiari malformation. The neurosurgeon, as the lead person in the team, has the option of referring the patient to a rheumatologist if he or she has various somatic complaints consistent with fibromyalgia/chronic fatigue syndrome. The rheumatology evaluation also extends to looking for a coexisting psychosocial pathology, concurrent sleep disorders, and disability extent and distress level. A neurology referral is done if the headache complex is not clearly tussive and if there is difficulty in diagnosing and managing chronic headaches. A neurology referral also is needed if the possibility of other neurologic diseases (e.g., amyotrophic lateral sclerosis, Parkinson disease, polyneuropathy, or demyelinating neuromuscular disorders) is being entertained. The importance of good history taking and a thorough physical examination cannot be overemphasized.

Providers who routinely care for these patients must be well versed in important disease concepts, literature, and algorithmic management strategies pertaining to these disorders.

The most important imaging study for assessing the extent of anatomic tonsillar herniation and its pathophysiologic significance is a brain/spine MRI with cine CSF flow study. Obstruction of CSF flow at the craniovertebral junction and the absence of normal pulsatile flow with cine CSF MRI studies have an important physiologic significance in Chiari malformation and syringomyelia. This test is extremely sensitive in detecting abnormal tonsillar motion and the CSF flow via the foramen magnum and around the syrinx cavity.[28] Chiari-type headache correlates with tonsillar motion and subsequent reduction in the arachnoid space at the foramen magnum.[28] The results of cine phase contrast MRI are valuable in the presurgical assessment of "symptomatic" Chiari malformation. Normal studies are an independent risk factor for surgical failure, regardless of the degree of tonsillar herniation.[29] Forty percent of patients with a normal cine CSF flow study had treatment failure following surgery, compared with only 5% where there was documented CSF flow obstruction.[29]

Patients usually can be placed into one of three different categories after thorough evaluation of different specialties and review of appropriate imaging studies[4]:

1. Patients who have clinical features of a Chiari malformation, as evidenced by findings consistent with disruption of central pathways involving cerebrospinal, cerebellospinal, or sensory spinothalamic pathways (evidence of "hard" neurologic findings). Abnormalities in cine phase MRI CSF flow studies showing partial or complete CSF flow obstruction are present. These patients will likely benefit with surgery.
2. Patients who have significant somatic symptoms with features consistent with fibromyalgia and chronic fatigue syndrome. They may have radiographic Chiari malformation, but they do not have objective neurologic findings and CSF flow studies are normal. These patients will not benefit with surgery.
3. A "mixed" pattern showing possible neurologic findings attributed to brainstem compression or cord dysfunction

from a syrinx, but these are nonprogressive, mild, and "soft" findings at best. Cine CSF flow studies are normal. These patients also may present with features consistent with fibromyalgia, with significant somatic symptoms and psychosocial distress. This group is extremely challenging. These patients are managed conservatively, and very few will be considered for surgery. They are followed for evidence of neurologic deterioration. Aggressive management of coexisting fibromyalgia/chronic fatigue, chronic headaches, and depression/mood disorders is undertaken. Patients may benefit from admission to a multidisciplinary chronic pain rehabilitation program.

KEY REFERENCES

Levy WJ, Mason L, Hahn JF: Chiari malformation presenting in adults: a surgical experience in 127 cases. *Neurosurgery* 12(4):377–390, 1983.

McGirt MJ, Nimjee SM, Fuchs HE: Relationship of cine phase contrast MRI with outcome after decompression for Chiari I malformations. *Neurosurgery* 59:140–146, 2006.

Oldfield EH, Murazsko K, Shawker TH, Parronas NJ: Pathophysiology of syringomyelia associated with Chiari I malformation of the cerebellar tonsils: implication for diagnosis and treatment. *J Neurosurg* 80:3–15, 1994.

Thieme K, Turk D, Flor H: Comorbid depression and anxiety in fibromyalgia syndrome: relationship to somatic and psychological variables. *Psychosom Med* 66:837–844, 2004.

Wilke W: Can fibromyalgia and chronic fatigue syndrome be cured by surgery? *Cleve Clin J Med* 68(4):277–279, 2001.

Wolfe F, Clauw D, Goldenberg D, et al: The American College of Rheumatology preliminary diagnostic criteria for fibromyalgia and measurement of symptom severity. *Arthritis Care Res (Hoboken)* 62:600–610, 2010.

REFERENCES

The complete reference list is available online at expertconsult.com.

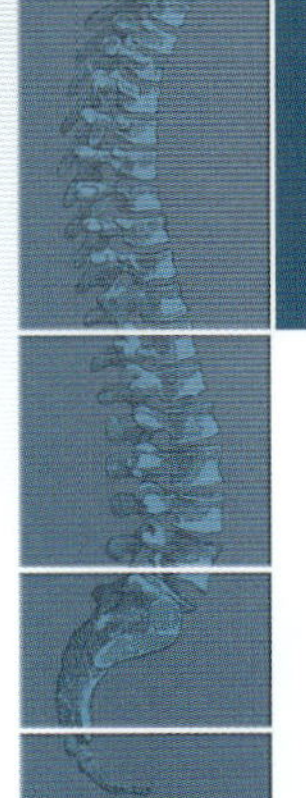

4.9 Adjunctive Surgical Considerations

CHAPTER 121

Omental Transposition and Spine Surgery: Emphasis on Revascularization and Scar Prevention

Harry S. Goldsmith

Editor's note: *In this chapter, the author has provided his unique perspective on an equally unique population of patients with impaired spinal cord function. Some, including Clifton et al. (Omental transposition in chronic spinal cord injury,* Spinal Cord *34:193–203, 1996), have discounted the author's work, while others find it intriguing. Regardless of the reader's opinion, it is included in this book in an attempt to cover all aspects of care. The reader also is referred to Chapter 72 in this book for an in-depth discussion of pharmacologic and regenerative therapeutic acute spinal cord injury strategies.*

Over the past half century there have been few therapeutic breakthroughs for the treatment of acute spinal cord injury (SCI). Recently, an attempt has been made to improve the results of these injuries by placing the omentum directly on a traumatized spinal cord (SC). Clinical evaluation of the procedure is necessary if we are to learn whether use of the omentum will be of benefit in the future treatment of acute SCI.

Pathophysiology of Spinal Cord Injury

One of the most important factors associated with an SCI is the production of vasogenic edema and extravasated blood that occurs rapidly at the site of the injury. A traumatized SC decreases the amount of localized edema that accumulates at the site of the injured SC by the dynamic movement of the fluid up and down the SC.[1] This compensatory action within the SC, however, usually is inadequate to decrease the high interstitial pressure that is caused by fluid accumulation at the site of the SCI. The swelling of the SC caused by this fluid accumulation continues within the confines of the nonyielding dura mater and the rigid spinal canal. When the interstitial pressure within the SC becomes excessive due to swelling, venous compression results. This action results in an elevated upstream venous pressure, which further enhances the capillary extrusion of blood from the porous blood vessels at the injury site. This situation causes an increase in focal osmotic pressure, which leads to a further increase in fluid accumulation. The high interstitial pressure within the SC also compresses small capillaries in the region of the SCI, which can lead to the progressive loss of capillary perfusion. This eventually can lead to complete blockage of vascular flow, causing the destruction of viable neural tissue in the area of the SC impaction.

Over the years, surgeons dealing with SCIs have appreciated the dangers of a high interstitial pressure occurring in an injured SC. This concern prompted the development of two surgical procedures—laminectomy and myelotomy—to lower the high interstitial pressure at the site of an SCI. Because the results of these attempts were unpredictable, however, they were not often used. A probable cause of these surgical failures was the inability of either operation to absorb the edema and blood accumulation that routinely develop at the site of an SCI.

The inability of edema fluid and blood to be absorbed at the site of an SCI is due to the absence of a lymphatic system in the SC. Without the absorbing mechanisms of a lymphatic system, edema fluid and blood remain at the SCI site, and the fluids eventually result in fibrosis scarring. This scarring is thought to be caused by the fibrinogen that is present in the blood that leaks from injured SC blood vessels. The fibrinogen apparently becomes activated at the SC injury site to make fibrin scar, which causes compression on blood vessels, a decrease in SC blood flow, and the blockage of axons from penetrating through the tissue (Fig. 121-1).

If healing of an acute SCI is to take place, it would appear that action should be undertaken as early as possible after injury to limit edema and blood accumulation resulting from the SCI. It has been shown that if an intact omentum pedicle is placed directly on an SC shortly after injury, absorption of edema and blood can be accomplished with little, if any, fluid accumulation or scar formation (Fig. 121-2), due to the enormous ability of the omentum to absorb fluids.[2,3] Placing the omentum directly on an injured SC apparently establishes a dynamic equilibrium between the production of blood and edema by the traumatized SC and the absorption of these fluids by the overlying omentum. Such absorption by the omentum not only decreases interstitial pressure in the area of the SCI, but, most importantly, its absorptive capability decreases the amount of blood (fibrinogen) in the injured area, thereby lessening the potential for scar formation at the injury site.

To apply the omentum directly onto an SCI location, a laminectomy is required, followed by opening of the dura

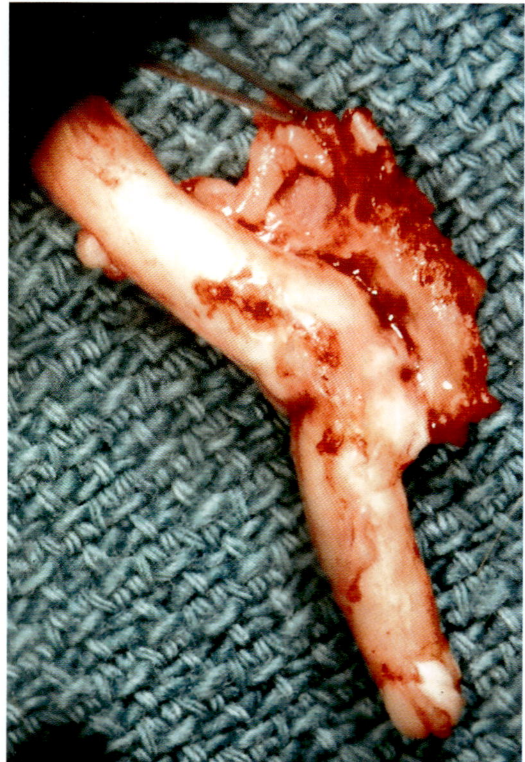

FIGURE 121-1. Spinal cord injury (450 g/cm weight injury) 1 month postoperatively. Note surface and circumferential scarring. Persistence of edema fluid also present.

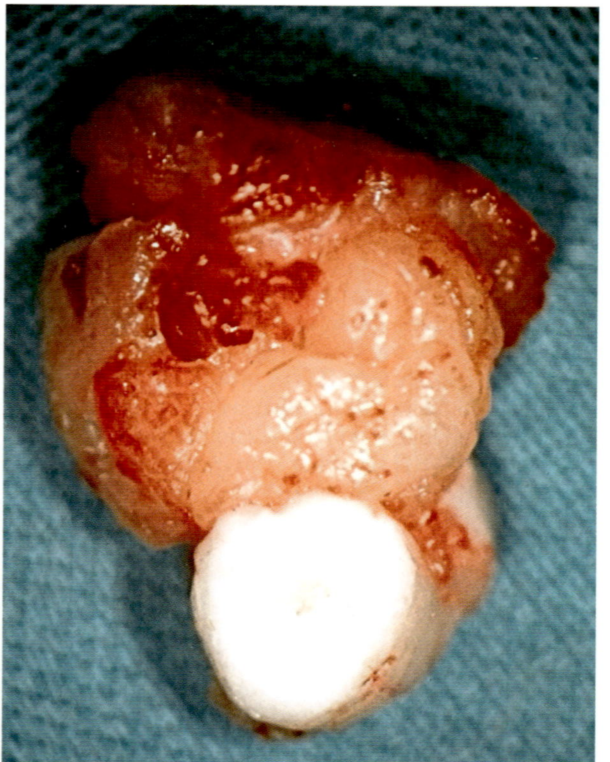

FIGURE 121-2. Omentum placed on injured spinal cord (SC; 450 g/cm weight injury) 3 weeks following injury. Note the complete adherence of the omentum to the SC with no presence of fibrosis or fluid accumulation.

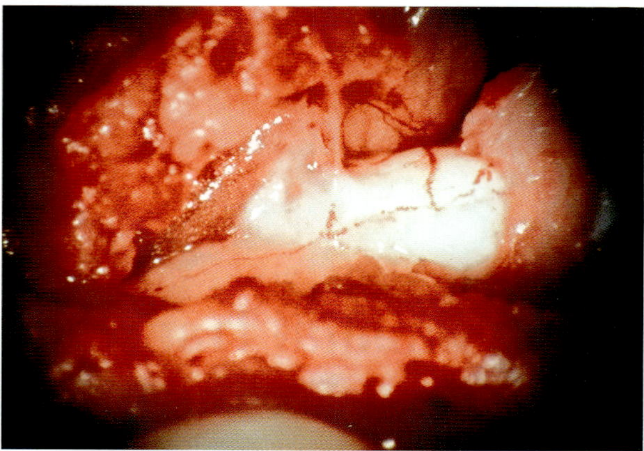

FIGURE 121-3. Early revascularization of the spinal cord (SC) is already apparent 50 hours following a 450-g/cm weight injury to the SC in a cat. Blood vessels originating from the omentum are clearly seen connecting to the SC.

mater. These maneuvers alone have a beneficial effect on an SCI, because they allow the injured SC to expand, thereby lowering the high interstitial pressure in the SC, which promotes capillary perfusion to increase in the area of the SC injury. It cannot be overemphasized that in an acute SC it is not sufficient to simply surgically stabilize the vertebral column. It appears to be necessary to open the dura mater and treat the SC directly by applying the omentum onto the injured SC, thus allowing edema absorption. This procedure must be done shortly after injury (within a few days), because a fibrotic process begins within a week of injury.

Spinal Cord Revascularization

As with any type of wound, adequate blood supply to the involved area is essential to optimize healing. Research has shown that when the omentum is laid directly on an injured SC, vascular connections penetrate from the omentum into the SC within hours.[4] This ability to revascularize the SC by the omentum was clearly proven by injecting India ink into an artery located within an intact omental pedicle that had been placed directly on a normal SC. The injected dye marker was subsequently observed on the surface of the SC, as well as in the deepest positioned capillaries that are located within the SC. It subsequently was observed in laboratory animals that omental blood vessels revascularize the SC rapidly and that a sizeable amount of blood was delivered to an uninjured SC through these omental vessels. The revascularization process was found to be even more rapid when the omentum was placed directly on an injured SC (Fig. 121-3). It is important, however, that the omentum be placed on the SCI as early following the injury as clinically possible.[5]

Spinal Cord Scarring

Clinical SCI research today is aimed primarily at determining how to improve treatment results. This is of critical importance because there has been no significant improvement in the surgical approach to such injuries over the years. It has been found, however, that absorption of blood and edema by the omentum at the site of an SCI in animals has led to functional improvement, suggesting that this approach might have a comparable beneficial effect in humans.

It is known that in animals with an acute SCI, laying an omental pedicle graft on an injured SC facilitates the absorption of blood and edema.[6] The importance of this absorptive capability is that it impedes the development of scar tissue, a step that appears to be critical in preventing the evolution of scarring in the injured SC. The idea that scar tissue markedly hinders SCI improvement is not new. Ramon y Cajal claimed over 100 years ago that functional regeneration in the SC could be accomplished if physical obstacles to central neuritic outgrowth could be removed.[7] The critical significance of scar being the physical obstacle preventing axons from penetrating through scar tissue was later brought into clearer focus by the work of Freeman at the University of Indiana in the 1950s. He clearly demonstrated that scar tissue at an SCI site prevented axons from penetrating through and making connections with neural structures in the caudal cord. Freeman wrote "that axons have a relentless compulsion to grow until they participate in return of function. If axonal regrowth is blocked by scar tissue, axons continue to grow in circles to form neuromata."[8] Cajal's and Freeman's observations strongly indicate that if scar can be eliminated from the healing process within an injured SC, functional and neuroelectrical improvement might well occur.

There appears to be no question that adequate blood supply and prevention of scar formation are crucial if SC healing is to take place. As far as revascularization is concerned, the ability of the omentum to carry out increased angiogenic activity in any area of the body is well known, especially since it has been shown that the highest concentration of vascular endothelial growth factor, the most angiogenic substance in the body, is in omental tissue.[9] Although revascularization of an injured SC obviously is important, scarring within the SC may well turn out to be the critical issue if SC healing is to occur.

The importance of eliminating SC scarring was clearly shown in a group of cats who had their SCs and dura mater totally transected at the T9 level. The transection resulted in an SC separation of 3 to 6 mm due to the elasticity of the SC. The stumps of the divided SCs were irrigated with iced saline to reduce the axoplasmic extrusion that routinely occurs following an SC transection. The gap between the divided ends of the SC was filled with collagen gel dispensed through a syringe. The collagen gel was allowed to harden for approximately 40 minutes, after which an intact pedicled omentum was placed directly on top of the collagen bridge and on the ends of the rostral and caudal SC stumps.

Blood flow measurements in the SC of animals with the omental-collagen bridge and in control animals were taken just before sacrifice, 90 days after surgery. The SC blood flow in omental-collagen animals demonstrated a 59% increase compared with the SC blood flow in normal (nontransected) control animals.[10] Also noted was a 3-to-1 increase in the blood vessel density counts in the omental-collagen–treated cats as compared with normal controls.[11]

Of particular importance in the omental-collagen bridge animals was the presence of dopaminergic and noradrenergic fibers that penetrated through the biodegrading collagen bridge with continued growth of the fibers into the distal SC stump[12] (Fig. 121-4). The axons were found to have grown at a rate of 1 mm per day for a maximum distance of 90 mm during the cats' 12-week recovery period. This penetration of axons occurred because of the absence of scar tissue.

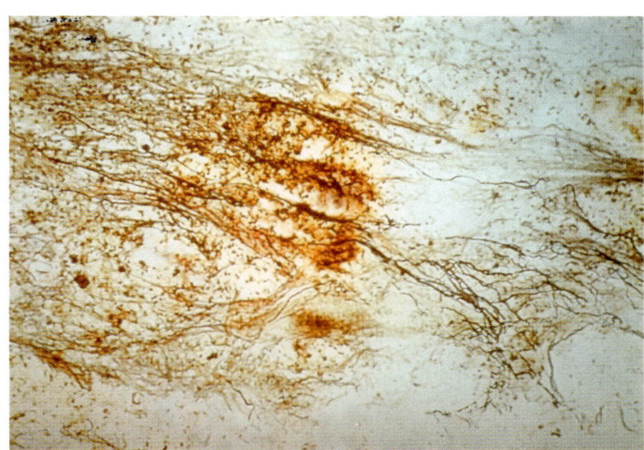

FIGURE 121-4. Axons are seen exiting from the distal end of the biodegrading omental-collagen bridge. Axons continue to grow into the distal spinal cord at the rate of 1 mm/day.

The finding that axons grew through the omental-collagen preparation was considered extremely important, but it was necessary to demonstrate whether these penetrating axons actually made synaptic connections with distal neural elements. Such penetration and connections of these axons were proven to occur by the use of the axonal marker hydroxystilbamidine (Fluoro-Gold; Fluorochrome, LLC, Denver, CO). When this dye marker was injected into the distal SC of a normal cat, the dye followed a retrograde axonal pathway up to the brain and was clearly seen in the cytoplasm and processes of neurons located in the locus coeruleus, subcoeruleus, Kolliker-Fuse nucleus, and substantia nigra. However, when cats simply had their SCs transected, the injection of Fluoro-Gold into their SCs caudal to the transection did not travel retrograde up axonal pathways toward the brain and was never observed in various locations within their brains. In contrast, when Fluoro-Gold was injected into the distal SC of cats in the presence of an omental-collagen bridge created after SC transection, Fluoro-Gold was found in the brain in the same locations as the injected Fluoro-Gold found in the brains of nontransected animals[13] (Fig. 121-5).

Histologic studies of the SCs of animals that had undergone omental-collagen reconstruction following SC transection were carefully evaluated. They showed that following the exposure of these SCs to the synaptogenic marker synaptophysin, this marker was found adjacent to preganglionic synaptic neurons located rostral and caudal to the omental-collagen bridge.[11] This finding indicated that synaptic remodeling (regeneration) by previously denervated supraspinal axons had occurred. Both the Fluoro-Gold and synaptophysin observations strongly suggested that following complete SC transection in cats, an omental-collagen bridge inserted at an SC transection site allowed disconnected supraspinal fibers to regenerate over long distances and apparently engage in synaptic remodeling with target tissue located at a distant site.

It is uncommon to encounter a patient with a transected SC. Interestingly, however, several years after successful

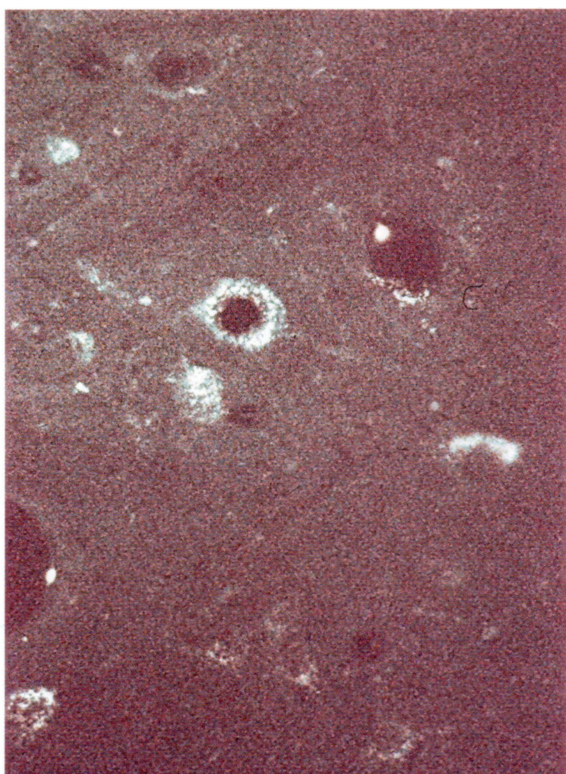

FIGURE 121-5. Retrograde axonal labeling by Fluoro-Gold shows marker in locus coeruleus neurons. Fluoro-Gold was injected in the caudal spinal cord (SC) 2 weeks before the animal's sacrifice 90 days after omental-collagen bridging of a transected SC.

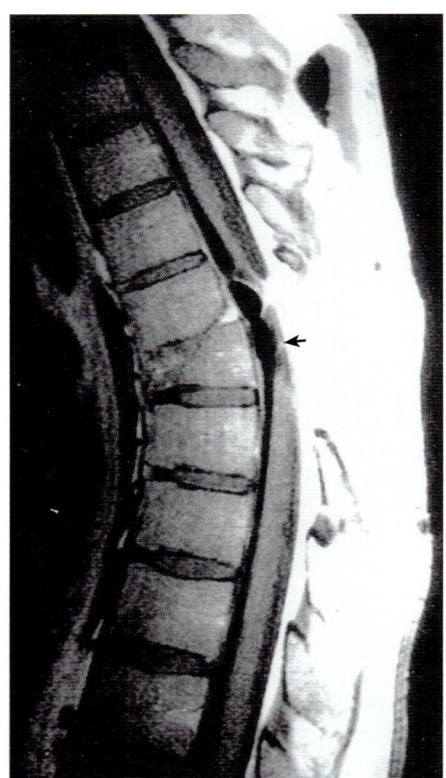

FIGURE 121-6. MRI taken shortly after injury reported as complete anatomic transection at the T6-7 level (*arrow*).

omental-collagen bridging in transected SCs in animals, a 23-year-old woman who had suffered an SCI in a high-speed skiing accident 3 years earlier was treated with this technique. An MRI taken shortly after that injury showed a complete anatomic transection of her SC at the T6-7 level (Fig. 121-6). Over the next 3 years she continued to exhibit complete motor and sensory loss below this level.

At 39 months after injury, the patient underwent reconstruction of her separated SC using the same operation that had been successfully used in cats, the omental-collagen bridge technique. At operation, a massive block of scar tissue was present between T6 and T8, resulting from the fibrotic reaction that had developed between the separated stumps of the SC. The scar tissue was surgically removed, which left an extremely large SC separation of 1.6 inches (4 cm). This defect was filled with 5 cc of collagen gel, followed by the direct application of an overlying omental pedicle onto the underlying collagen bridge.

Over the next several years, the patient regained extensive motor activity following intensive physical therapy. At the end of 4 years she could walk, but required the use of a walker (Fig. 121-7). Serial MRIs were taken of her SC on a yearly basis, and after 4 years the separated SC on MRI examination was shown to have anatomically reconstructed itself in an incontinuity longitudinal connection (Fig. 121-8). This case has been carefully documented.[14]

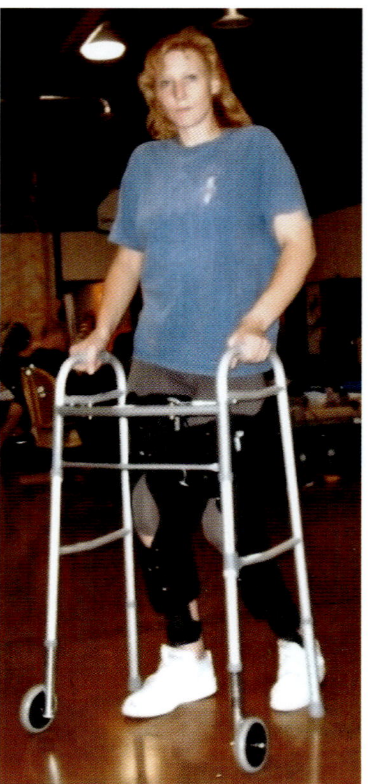

FIGURE 121-7. The patient was able to walk for long distances but required a walker because her balance did not return.

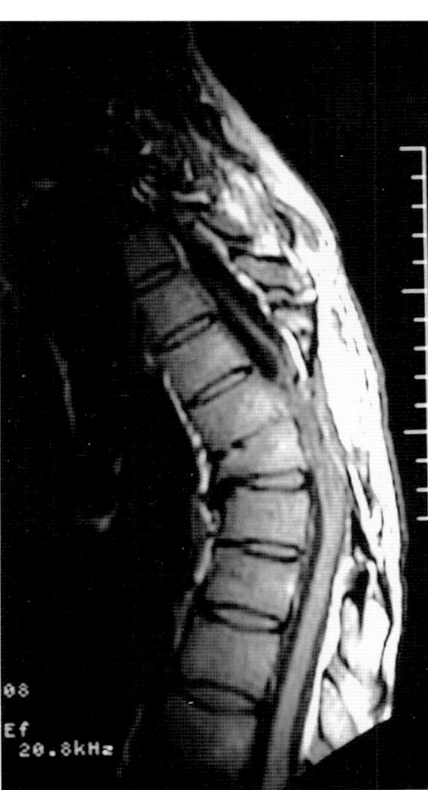

FIGURE 121-8. MRI study at 4 years after surgery showed healing of the omental-collagen bridge into a longitudinal structure connecting to the proximal and distal ends of the previously transected spinal cord.

Summary

The aim of SCI research and clinical care is to find new approaches that will improve the functional outcome of patients with an SCI.[6] An adequate blood supply is necessary for healing of an SCI to take place. Such an additional source of blood for a healing SCI can be provided by placing an omental pedicle on an acute SCI. Of even greater importance in improving the treatment of an SCI is finding a way to limit the production of scar tissue within the SC following an SCI. Such scar tissue has been known for many years to be a major physical obstacle that prevents axons from penetrating through the scar. Such action blocks connections of axons to neural tissue in the distal SC. Because the omentum can revascularize the SC and limit scarring within the SC, it seems possible that it would improve the results following surgical treatment of an acute SCI. It seems reasonable to suggest that clinical evaluation of omental transposition be undertaken, because its success could generate the clinical improvement that we continue to seek for patients who sustain an SCI.

KEY REFERENCES

de la Torre JC, Goldsmith HS: Supraspinal fiber outgrowth and apparent synaptic remodeling across transected-reconstructed feline spinal cord. *Acta Neurochir* 114:118–127, 1992.

de la Torre JC, Goldsmith HS: Coerulospinal fiber regeneration in transected feline spinal cord. *Brain Res Bull* 35:413–417, 1994.

Goldsmith HS: Treatment of acute spinal cord injury by omental transposition: a new approach. *J Am Coll Surg* 208:289–292, 2009.

Goldsmith HS, de la Torre JC: Axonal regeneration after spinal cord transection and reconstruction. *Brain Res* 589:217–224, 1992.

Goldsmith HS, Duckett S, Chen WF: Spinal cord revascularization by intact omentum. *Am J Surg* 129:262–265, 1975.

Goldsmith HS, Fonseca A Jr, Porter J: Spinal cord separation: MRI evidence of healing after omental-collagen reconstruction. *Neurol Res* 27:115–123, 2005.

Ramon y Cajal S: In May R, editor: *Degeneration and regeneration of the nervous system*, New York, 1950, Hafner Publishing, pp 749–750.

REFERENCES

The complete reference list is available online at expertconsult.com.

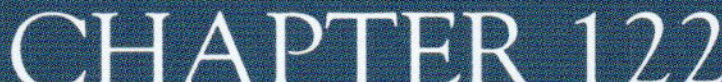
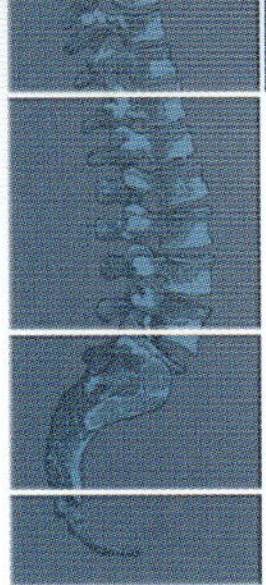

CHAPTER 122

Wound Closure

Patrick W. Hitchon | Meryl Severson | Albert E. Cram

Soft Tissue Anatomy

The first layer deep to the skin is the subcutaneous tissue. Within this layer can be found a thin membranous layer of fascia,[1] recently termed the *iliolumbar membrane*, in the back.[2] Deep to the subcutaneous tissue in the cervical spine are three layers of musculature, of which the trapezius makes up the superficial group. This muscle has descending, transverse, and ascending portions originating from the superior nuchal line of the skull, the ligamentum nuchae, the spinous processes of C7-T12, and the supraspinous ligament.[3] Immediately deep to the trapezius in the midline is the ligamentum nuchae. It is the cervical extension of the supraspinous ligament, attaches to the inion,[4] and has connections with the lesser posterior rectus, splenius, semispinalis capiti, and the lesser rhomboids.[5] The intermediate cervical muscular layer includes the splenius capitis and cervicis; semispinalis capitis and cervicis; and longissimus capitis and cervicis.[5] The splenius muscles originate from the ligamentum nuchae and the spinous processes of the lower cervical and upper thoracic vertebrae, whereas the longissimus and semispinalis muscles originate from the cervical and upper thoracic transverse processes.[5] The deep cervical musculature includes the multifidus, rotatores, spinalis, and interspinales groups.[3] Rostral to C2 the deep musculature is termed the *suboccipital musculature* and consists of the rectus and obliquus capitis groups.[3,6]

The superficial muscular group of the thoracolumbar region includes the trapezius, described in the preceding paragraph, and the latissimus dorsi, originating from the dorsal layer of the thoracolumbar fascia from the spinous processes of T7 to the sacrum and the iliac crest.[3] The thoracolumbar fascia is multilayered and arises from the aponeurosis of the transversus abdominis.[4,6] The thoracolumbar fascia attaches medially to the spinous processes of the lumbar and sacral vertebrae and caudally to the iliac crests. Laterally, it attaches to the ribs and intercostal fascia. The dorsal layer of the thoracolumbar fascia is termed the *lumbar aponeurosis* and serves as the origin of the latissimus dorsi muscle. The intermediate muscles of the trunk include the rhomboids and serratus posterior.[4] The deep muscles of the back are divided into lateral and medial tracts. The iliocostalis, longissimus, and intertransversarii muscles make up the lateral group; the rotatores, multifidus, and interspinales make up the medial group.[3] The trapezius muscle spans the entire breadth of the interscapular distance and extends from the subocciput to T12. The latissimus dorsi muscle likewise extends from T7 caudally to the sacrum. By virtue of their location and breadth, they provide a ready mechanism for the closure and repair of open spinal wounds.

Wound Closure

The basic principles and tenets of wound closure apply to surgical spinal wounds. Preoperative conditions that interfere and compromise wound healing should be corrected, where possible, to provide the best environment for closure and healing following a surgical procedure. Likewise, meticulous care should be taken throughout the operative procedure to minimize tissue damage and destruction where practicable, thereby reducing surgeon-induced impediments to wound closure/healing.

Dorsal Spinal Wounds

The technique for closure of dorsal spinal wounds is similar in the cervical and thoracolumbar regions. In procedures involving dural openings, whether intentional or inadvertent, every attempt at a watertight dural closure should be made. Nonabsorbable #6-0 polypropylene sutures generally are used, with or without a fascial autograft, or commercially available dural substitute allografts. The suture line is covered with a layer of fibrin glue, or, more recently, with the sealant DuraSeal (Covidien, Waltham, MA). Where there is concern regarding the quality of closure, a spinal drain should be placed. Failure to achieve adequate dural closure may lead to a variety of complications, including meningitis, arachnoiditis, pseudomeningocele formation, and cerebrospinal fluid (CSF) leakage from the wound. In the latter case, it is imperative to return to the operating room, readdress the CSF leak, and avoid the temptation to simply reinforce the skin closure.

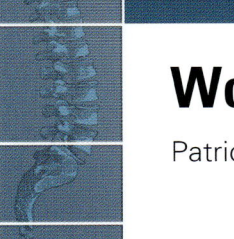

After dural closure, inspection of the deep tissues, including the resected vertebral bone edges, epidural contents, and surrounding musculature, should be performed to ensure that meticulous hemostasis has been achieved. Failure to do so may lead to postoperative hematomas, which can become symptomatic due to compression of neural structures. Epidural bleeding should be controlled with bipolar cautery or local hemostatic agents, the exposed bone edges waxed, and muscular bleeding likewise controlled with cautery. Irrigation with hydrogen peroxide often is performed in cases without dural violation, particularly in large wounds, to aid in hemostasis. Once this has been achieved, some surgeons also cover exposed dura with a local hemostatic agent.

One of the central tenets of wound approximation is the use of an orderly layered closure to optimize wound healing by eliminating dead space to reduce the risk of fluid collection and infection. After the dura has been closed and hemostasis achieved, attention should be turned to the layered closure. After extensive spinal procedures, a large potential dead space exists that is amplified in patients who have undergone laminectomy at multiple contiguous levels. The paraspinal musculature is approximated with a few large absorbable #0 sutures, with care taken not to strangulate the tissue, which can cause local muscle necrosis and severe postoperative pain. Fascial closure is performed carefully with interrupted #0 absorbable sutures. In cases of reoperation, or where radiation is anticipated, nonabsorbable braided #0 suture material is recommended. A tight closure of the fascia is recommended to reduce dead space as well as prevent possible CSF leakage. This layer also may serve as a barrier to the development of a deep infection from a superficial wound infection. Placement of a drain into the epidural and/or subfascial space should be considered in those patients with large wounds, after vascular tumor removal, after instrumented fusion procedures, and after operations for trauma. These drains diminish the occurrence of hematomas and seromas that hamper wound healing[7,8] and that also can cause neurologic deficit with neural element compression. If CSF is observed accumulating in the suction canister, the drain must be removed immediately to prevent a persistent CSF leak and complications associated with CSF overdrainage.

In larger individuals, it may be necessary to close the subcutaneous tissue in multiple layers owing to its thickness. For this, #2-0 Vicryl suture is commonly used, and the membranous superficial fascia, most easily identified in the lumbar subcutaneous tissue,[1,2] should be the target of reapproximation. The dermal tissue is reapproximated next with inverted interrupted #2-0 or #3-0 suture material, taking care to align the edges of the wound in the rostral-caudal as well as dorsal-ventral dimensions. It is important to produce wound eversion with closure of this layer to ensure the skin layer will have minimal tension after its closure, thereby improving its ability to heal. Scars from properly everted wounds tend not to widen with time, and the ridge of everted tissue always settles to normal.[9] The skin is reapproximated with either monofilament suture, staples, or, in some cases, skin adhesive application.

Ventral Spinal Wounds

Closure of wounds from ventral or lateral thoracolumbar approaches also should adhere to the basic principles of wound closure. Closure or patching of CSF leaks, meticulous hemostasis, placement of drains when appropriate, and orderly layered closure with emphasis on a watertight fascial reapproximation should be performed. These operative approaches often are performed by vascular, thoracic, or general surgeons, and the spine surgeon should participate in the subsequent closure of these wounds.

The reapproximation of anterior cervical spinal wounds, while much less tedious than posterior closures, still must be tackled in meticulous fashion. As with posterior wounds, CSF leakage should be formally addressed and the leak closed if possible. With or without closure, spinal drainage at the end of the case is recommended, and will save the surgeon several agonizing sleepless nights. The spine surgeon should be fastidious with hemostasis, because postoperative hematomas have the potential to be life threatening due to airway compromise. Placement of a drain is not a substitute for adequate hemostasis. The musculature of the neck is not reapproximated, unless it was intentionally divided, which occasionally may be the case with the omohyoid. The watertight fascial closure for the anterior neck is the platysma. It often is easily identified in young patients, but it may be quite atrophied and difficult to discern in elderly patients. In obese patients, it often is infiltrated with adipose tissue, which occasionally makes its identification difficult. The platysma often is closed with #3 Vicryl suture and is followed by reapproximation of the dermis with inverted #3 Vicryl sutures as well. Some surgeons skip deliberate closure of the dermis and instead proceed to a subcuticular closure with an absorbable monofilament suture. Skin adhesives or Steri-Strips may be placed at this point, depending on surgeon preference.

In the presence of wound dehiscence or infection before attempted closure, extensive debridement is necessary. In cases in which radiation therapy has been received preoperatively or is anticipated postoperatively, closure of the fascia should be accomplished with nonabsorbable #0 or #2 monofilament or braided nylon. Wound closure in general is uncomplicated in the cervical and lumbar region because of the thickness of the muscle layer and the lordotic curvature of the spine. An incision in the upper thoracic spine is subject to horizontal tensile forces caused by shoulder movement, and this area is notorious for dehiscence in as many as 30% of patients with cancer or spinal implants.[10] In addition to spinous process excision, a figure-8 brace may be worn postoperatively to reduce tensile forces across the vertical incision. Drains usually are left in place for 2 days, or until the drainage is less than 50 mL per 8-hour shift. Sutures are not removed until at least 2 weeks postoperatively.

When the quality of the tissue present at the wound edge or the amount of tissue damaged or missing precludes primary closure, one must consider either a skin graft or some other type of flap closure. Split-thickness skin graft can be used for closure in rare instances in which the underlying soft tissue is adequate to protect underlying structures and has adequate circulation to support survival of the skin graft. Modern electric-powered and nitrogen gas pressure–powered dermatomes make the harvest of high-quality split-thickness autograft a simple and predictable procedure. Graft may be taken from any suitable donor site, usually at a thickness between 0.012 and 0.015 inches. This is applied to the wound bed. Fixation of the graft for 4 to 5 days prevents movement between the graft and the recipient bed and usually results in graft acceptance.

Myocutaneous Flaps

Closure of large soft tissue defects currently relies heavily on the use of myocutaneous and fasciocutaneous flaps. In the back, the most commonly used musculocutaneous flap for defects of the upper third of the thoracic spine is the trapezius muscle. Variations of flap design can cover upper-third defects over a relatively wide arc of rotation, as long as the transverse cervical artery is intact. Defects in the middle third of the back are most commonly closed using the latissimus muscle, a choice based on its thoracodorsal blood supply or on the paraspinous perforators. Defects of the lower third of the back often are closed with gluteus muscle myocutaneous flaps, most often based on the inferior gluteal artery. In the lower third, the latissimus dorsi muscle also may be used. Its use must be based on a free flap using vein grafts from the thoracodorsal trunks or by anastomosis to the superior or inferior gluteal vessels, if it is to reach the caudal-most portions of the lower third of the back.

Trapezius Muscle and Myocutaneous Flaps

Because of its length, extending from the superior nuchal line to the spinous process of T12, and its width, from one acromial process to the other, the trapezius muscle is suitable for rotation, with or without overlying flaps of skin (Fig. 122-1). The blood supply to the trapezius muscle is via the type II vascular pattern characterized by one dominant vascular pedicle with other minor contributing pedicles.[11-13] The principal pedicle consists of the dorsal scapular artery, which constitutes the descending branch of the transverse cervical artery. The latter arises from the subclavian artery or thyrocervical trunk. The dorsal scapular artery courses caudally, medial to the scapula and ventral to the rhomboid muscle, supplying

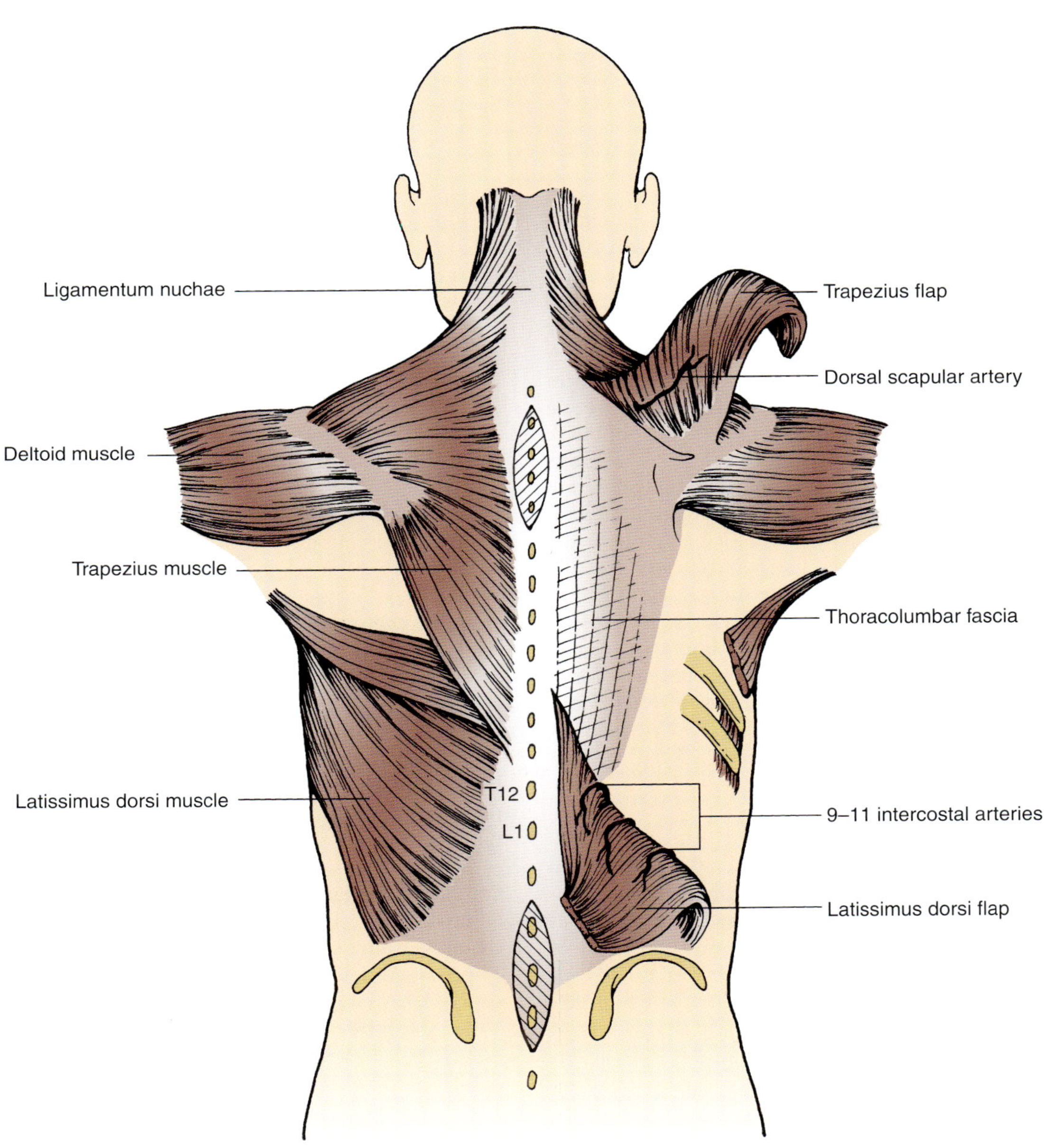

FIGURE 122-1. Normal anatomy of the trapezius and latissimus dorsi muscles (*left*). Trapezius and reverse latissimus dorsi flaps (*right*) are used for coverage of defects over the upper thoracic and lumbar spines, respectively. Mobilization of these flaps requires preservation of their blood supply.

these muscles as well as the latissimus dorsi and trapezius muscles and eventually anastomosing with the suprascapular and subscapular arteries and some of the intercostal arteries. The minor pedicle consists of branches of the occipital artery perfusing the rostral segments of the muscle.[7,14] With careful dissection, the caudal pole of the trapezius muscle can be dissected from the spinous processes and underlying latissimus and rhomboid muscles. Careful attention must be paid to preserve the integrity of its blood supply, which can be observed on the ventral aspect of the caudal and medial fibers.

Trapezius flaps, with or without attached cutaneous pedicles, can be used to repair defects overlying the kyphotic curvature of the thoracic spine. Spinal wound closure can be a challenge in patients who are being treated for thoracic spinal metastases. The apex of the thoracic kyphosis is most prone to dehiscence in patients whose wound healing capability has been compromised by chemotherapy and radiation therapy. Radiation therapy contributes to impairment of circulation by virtue of endothelial swelling and subintimal fibrosis. This results in an obstructive endarteritis with the subcutaneous tissue being replaced by dense fibrosis.[7] Shoulder movement further contributes traction on the skin edges, increasing their predilection for separation and dehiscence. This is further expedited in cases of wound infection or diabetes or in elderly patients. When such wound dehiscence fails to heal by secondary intention, alternative approaches must be sought. Failure of healing with superimposed infection can result in dural erosion and CSF leaks. Spinal drainage is insufficient to provide for dural closure in the depths of an open infected wound. Under those circumstances, extensive debridement of the wound in the operating room is necessary. Excision of all infected bone is undertaken until bleeding cancellous bone is encountered. Dural repairs are undertaken with free or pedicle fascial grafts attached to a trapezius flap. The trapezius flap can obliterate the dead space in the depths of the spinal wound, providing for an optimal watertight closure. The wound is further approximated in layers, usually over drains. The approximation usually is undertaken with heavy, nonabsorbable sutures such as #0 or #2 braided nylon, and the skin is closed with heavy #0 Prolene monofilament. It is important to maintain optimum nutritional status of the patient to enhance healing. In the presence of anemia (hemoglobin <8 g/dL), blood transfusions also will contribute to increased activity and, potentially, to wound healing. The patient is maintained in a figure-8 brace for 4 to 8 weeks.

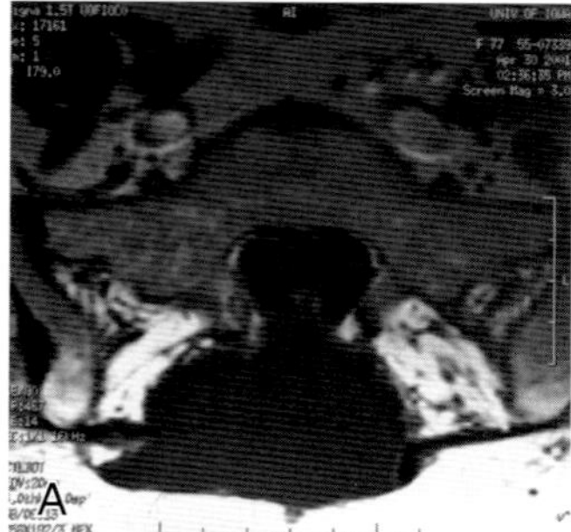

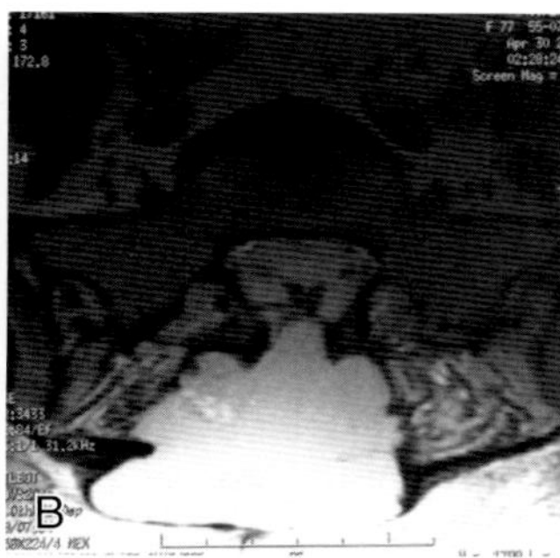

FIGURE 122-2. Postoperative axial T1-weighted (**A**) and T2-weighted (**B**) images reveal a sacral meningocele in a 77-year-old woman who underwent release of a tethered cord. Although no external cerebrospinal fluid leakage was present, the patient was symptomatic, with postural headaches and a large subcutaneous fluid collection.

Latissimus Flaps

The latissimus dorsi muscle, because of its location and blood supply, provides muscle or myocutaneous flaps for the closure of spinal defects overlying the lower thoracic and lumbar spine (see Fig. 122-1). Its blood supply is type V, consisting of one dominant vascular pedicle, which in this case is the thoracodorsal artery arising from the subclavian artery and secondary midline and paramedian pedicles. The thoracodorsal artery consists of the dorsal cutaneous branches of the intercostal and lumbar arteries.[7,11] The intercostal arteries that contribute most to the secondary pedicles are the 9th, 10th, and 11th intercostal arteries, as confirmed on cadaveric dissections.[15] These perforators usually enter the latissimus muscle approximately 5 cm from the midline. Latissimus dorsi flaps, with and without skin, are based on the thoracodorsal artery and are dissected away from the spinous process attachments. Such flaps generally are suited for repair of large thoracic wall or lateral iliac decubiti.

Reverse latissimus flaps, on the other hand, are dissected laterally or rostrally and thus maintain the blood supply of the flap from the midline paraspinal secondary vascular pedicles. The integrity of the penetrating vessels on the ventral surface of the muscle is preserved because the supply from the thoracodorsal artery is sacrificed for distal mobilization. Such latissimus dorsi flaps are referred to as *reverse flaps* and are suited for the repair of spinal defects of the lower thoracic and lumbar spines (Fig. 122-2). The muscle flap is based medially on the 9th, 10th, and 11th intercostal feeders.

The length of the pedicle is geared to the size of the spinal defect to be repaired. The portion of the latissimus dorsi muscle mobilized and its width are customized to the case at hand (Fig. 122-3). The latissimus dorsi muscle provides a large muscle mass capable of filling far larger spinal defects than is possible with trapezius muscle flaps. The reverse latissimus flap, with or without its cutaneous pedicle, when necessary, is tunneled subcutaneously to the midline incision. The site of the cutaneous pedicle is then repaired with a split-thickness skin graft. Reverse latissimus flaps are usually adequate when used unilaterally.

Bilateral large musculocutaneous latissimus flaps may be advanced medially to cover large midline spinal defects. In these circumstances, the flaps are based on the thoracodorsal artery with partial preservation of the secondary intercostal blood supply. Skin grafting may be necessary to cover the relaxing incisions made on either side of the torso to facilitate advancement.[10]

It is possible to create a large muscle or skin and muscle flap using the latissimus dorsi muscle based on a vein graft extension of the thoracodorsal artery.[12] This approach requires a microsurgical team and the harvest of saphenous or other suitable vein to interpose on both the arterial and venous circulation. The vein interposition can be performed below the subscapularis branch, and a large muscle advancement can be carried out. This overcomes the problems that occasionally occur when using the most medial portions of the flap with complete ligation of the paraspinous perforators. This medial-most portion of the flap is primarily fascial and of marginal circulation. It depends entirely on the thoracodorsal vessel for inflow. Use of the vein graft and transection of the insertion of the muscle permits safe movement of more reliable muscle and skin medially. A "V-to-Y" technique allows

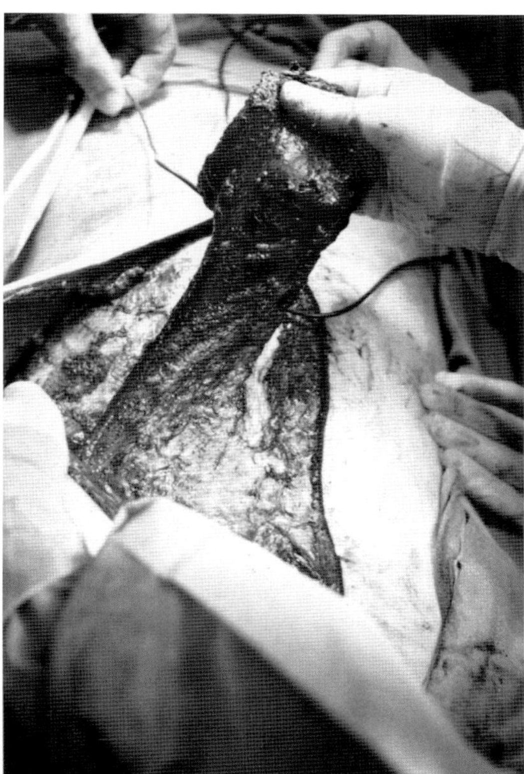

FIGURE 122-3. Surgical exploration was performed in the patient shown in Figure 122-2, and no frank cerebrospinal fluid leak was identified. This intraoperative photograph was taken while standing at the foot of the table looking toward the head. A reverse latissimus dorsi flap was harvested from the left side and used for obliteration of the dead space. The midline incision was extended rostrally, and the latissimus muscle sectioned below its insertion. The muscle head is held up and reflected into the lumbosacral incision while safeguarding its vascular supply. On follow-up, she was asymptomatic, and her lower back was flat without reaccumulation of the meningocele.

movement of relatively large skin-muscle flaps, when such flaps are needed. This technique also can be used to advance only the latissimus dorsi muscle, and the epithelial coverage is provided by application of a split-thickness graft to the exposed portion of the latissimus muscle.

Gluteus Maximus Flaps for the Sacral Region

The gluteus maximus is a large buttock muscle with a quadrilateral shape. It extends from the ilium, sacrum, coccyx, and sacrospinal aponeurosis to the greater trochanter of the femur and the iliotibial band of the fascia lata.[10] This large muscle has a type III vasculature, with two dominant arteries, the superior and inferior gluteal arteries, arising from the internal iliac artery.[11,16] Because of its location, the gluteus maximus muscle, with or without an attached skin flap, is suited for repair of sacral, ischial, trochanteric, and ilial open wounds. The muscle mass and overlying skin have sufficient size and redundancy that a unilateral myocutaneous flap often is sufficient to provide coverage for a midline defect. For the coverage of a sacral decubitus, the skin incision extends along the caudal margin of the iliac crest laterally from the edges of the wound that had been debrided. The incision is carried through the subcutaneous tissue, and a plane is created between the gluteus maximus and medius muscles. It is important to maintain the integrity of the superior gluteal artery as it enters the deep surface of the gluteus maximus muscle. However, if the superior gluteal artery interferes with the mobility of this muscle flap, it can be sacrificed for increased mobility. In instances in which this has been done, the blood supply provided by the inferior gluteal artery has proven sufficient.[16] The muscle and skin edges are then sutured to the contralateral debrided edge of the exposed wound after incision of all infected and devascularized bone. Depending on the size of the defect to be covered, the lateral caudal margin of the myocutaneous flap can extend inferiorly to the greater trochanter. The gluteus medius muscle provides adequate soft tissue padding of the iliac crest. The donor site of the skin is covered with a split-thickness skin graft. Vacuum drains usually are sufficient to avoid the accumulation of hematomas and seromas that can complicate and impede healing. The muscle flap usually is sutured in place with heavy-gauge absorbable suture such as #0 and #2 Vicryl, and the skin is sutured with monofilament nylon or Prolene. Heavy dressings are applied to prevent pressure on the flap that may impair adequate perfusion. The patient is to be kept on the side or in the prone position for at least 2 weeks subsequent to flap rotation.

The rotational advancement of gluteus-based flaps for sacral wounds has been largely replaced by V-to-Y techniques. The sacral lesion is debrided, and depending on the transverse diameter of the wound, either a single or a bilateral V incision is designed. The origins of the gluteus maximus are freed up as needed, and the muscle is dissected free at the lateral margin, dissecting medially as needed to free the flap. The superior or inferior gluteal artery must be kept intact. This myocutaneous flap is then advanced medially and sutured to the wound edge or to its mirror image flap from the opposite side, if the size of the wound dictates a bilateral approach. As the lateral portion of the flap is moved by this advancement, a linear closure of the defect results in the Y-shaped final appearance as observed in Figures 122-4 and 122-5.

Nonhealing Spinal Wounds

Impediments to wound healing are numerous and can be challenging to overcome when faced with a nonhealing spinal wound. Nonhealing wounds are costly not only in terms of dollars to the health care system but also, more importantly, in terms of the morbidity and potential for mortality for the affected patient.[17] Risk factors for poor healing include but are not limited to nutritional status, corticosteroid use, diabetes mellitus, history of radiation treatment, a variety of collagen disorders, smoking, immunosuppressant therapy, infection, neurologic deficit resulting in inability for the patient to change positions, and tissue hypoxia.[18-20] It is advantageous for the surgeon and the patient to address as many factors preoperatively as possible.

Strategies for Nonhealing Wounds

Strategies for addressing large tissue defects with flaps and grafts have been previously described. Additional strategies for nonhealing wounds include the use of vacuum-assisted closure

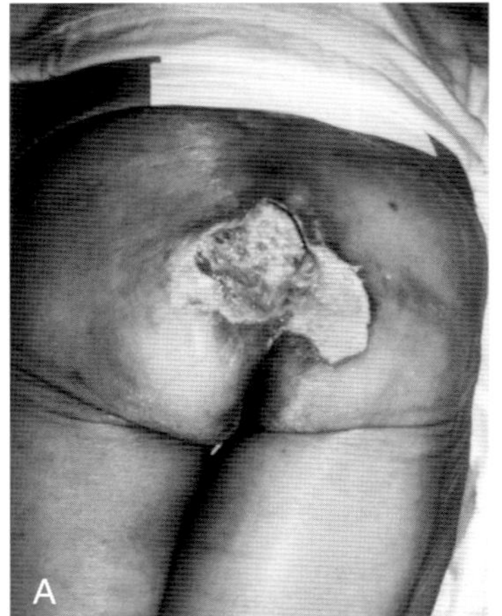

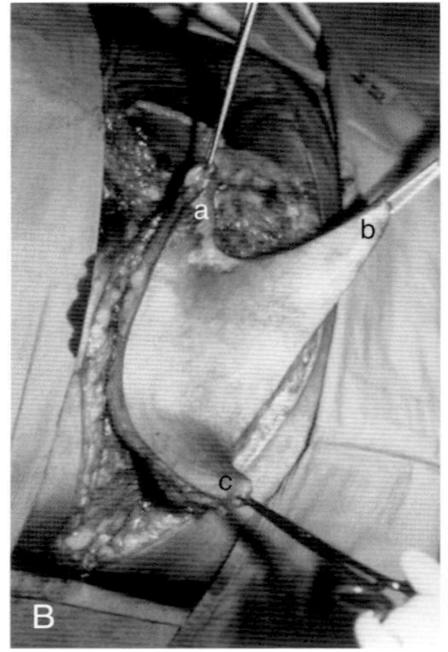

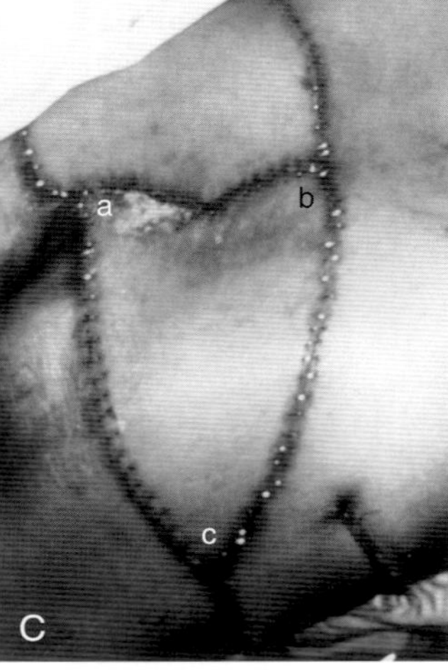

FIGURE 122-4. A, Sacral decubitus ulcer with exposure of sacrum. **B**, V-shaped myocutaneous flap. **C**, Completed bilateral gluteal myocutaneous flaps approximated in midline.

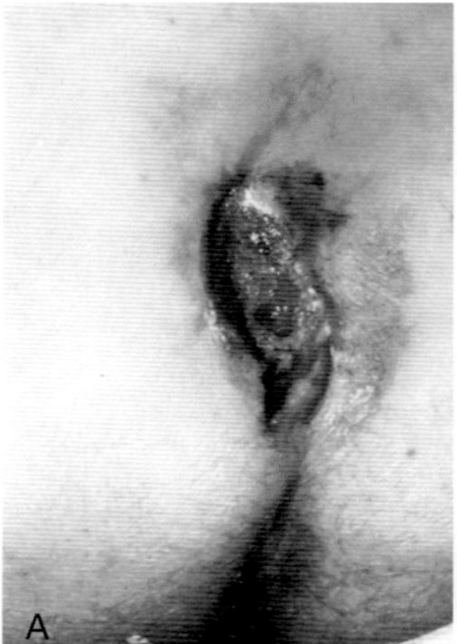

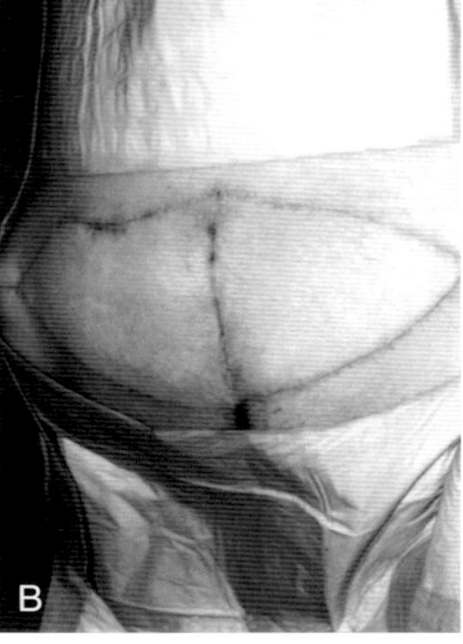

FIGURE 122-5. A, Sacral decubitus ulcer with sacral osteomyelitis. **B**, After closure.

(VAC) devices and hyperbaric oxygen therapy. Wound VAC therapy, also referred to as *negative pressure wound therapy*, involves placing a nonbioabsorbable sponge in the bed of a wound covered with an occlusive dressing connected to a suction device with a fluid collection chamber. Wound healing is enhanced by removal of wound fluid, increased angiogenesis, and up-regulation of several tissue factors.[21,22] Wound VACs have been used not only in chronic nonhealing wounds but also in cases of trauma, fasciotomy, and infection.[23-27] A variety of surgical specialties use these devices with seemingly good results,[23,27-29] and some studies have shown cost savings.[30,31] Despite their increased use, however, there are very few randomized controlled trials evaluating their efficacy. A recent *Cochrane Review* found insufficient evidence that wound VAC use improves healing of chronic wounds.[32]

Hyperbaric oxygen therapy (HBOT) is another useful adjunct in treating nonhealing wounds. HBOT involves placing a patient in a hyperbaric chamber where he or she breathes 100% oxygen for brief periods while at an increased barometric pressure. Tissue oxygen tension is more than doubled during these treatments,[33] augmenting wound healing, inducing angiogenesis, and aiding neutrophil function.[34-37] The plasma becomes supersaturated with oxygen to the point that red blood cells are not required to supply oxygen for cellular respiration.[38] HBOT is currently indicated in the treatment of the following: decompression sickness, air embolism, necrotizing fasciitis, clostridial necrosis, carbon monoxide poisoning, crush injuries, problem wounds including diabetic ulcers, refractory osteomyelitis, compromised skin grafts and flaps, thermal burns, delayed radiation injury, exceptional blood loss, and intracranial abscesses.[39] The number and length of treatments are dictated by the disease process being treated, the response of the wound to treatment, and patient tolerance. Currently, more than 600 hyperbaric chambers are in use across the United States.[39]

The usefulness of HBOT is predicated on its ability to supply oxygen to tissues at much higher concentrations than at normobaria. Before therapy is initiated, transcutaneous partial pressure of oxygen ($TcPo_2$) measurements often are made to confirm wound hypoxia and assess whether a wound may benefit from a course of HBOT.[40-43] $TcPo_2$ values near the wound are obtained with the patient inspiring air at sea level (21% oxygen), inspiring 100% oxygen at sea level, and during HBOT. If the $TcPo_2$ is in the normal range (≥40 mm Hg) while inspiring air, this confirms that the wound is not hypoxic, and alternative causes of wound nonhealing should be aggressively sought and corrected. When inspiring 100% oxygen at sea level, it has been shown that increases of less than 10 mm Hg in the $TcPo_2$ reliably predict wounds that likely will not respond to HBOT.[40] $TcPo_2$ values less than 400 mm Hg during HBOT also have been shown to predict which wounds will not respond to HBOT.[41-43]

Summary

Understanding spinal fascial and muscular anatomy is crucial when performing spinal wound closure, whether secondary to a microdiscectomy or a complicated reconstruction procedure. Following the basic tenets of wound closure, including debridement of dead tissue, elimination of dead space via an orderly layered closure, maintenance of meticulous hemostasis, and ensuring adequate vascularization of the wound bed, is crucial for optimal wound healing and closure. Large tissue defects may be treated with a variety of myocutaneous flaps, depending on the size, location, and depth of the wound. Adjunctive treatment strategies for nonhealing wounds are increasing, with current emphasis on vacuum-assisted closure devices and hyperbaric oxygen therapy in select cases.

KEY REFERENCES

Hunt TK, Hopf H, Hussain Z: Physiology of wound healing. *Adv Skin Wound Care* 13(Suppl 2):6, 2000.

Jones GA, Butler J, Lieberman I, Schlenk R: Negative-pressure wound therapy in the treatment of complex postoperative spinal wound infections: complications and lessons learned using vacuum-assisted closure. *J Neurosurg Spine* 6:407, 2007.

Mehboud AA, Ogilvie JW, Pinto MR, et al: Postoperative deep wound infections in adults after spinal fusion: management with vacuum-assisted wound closure. *J Spinal Disord Tech* 18:14, 2005.

Putz R, Pabst R, editors: *Sobotta atlas of human anatomy;* Volume 2: *Trunk, viscera, lower limb*, Philadelphia, 2001, Lippincott Williams & Wilkins.

Tibbles PM, Edelsberg JS: Hyperbaric oxygen therapy. *N Engl J Med* 334:1642, 1996.

REFERENCES

The complete reference list is available online at expertconsult.com.

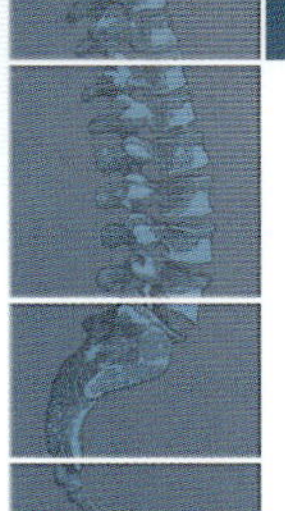

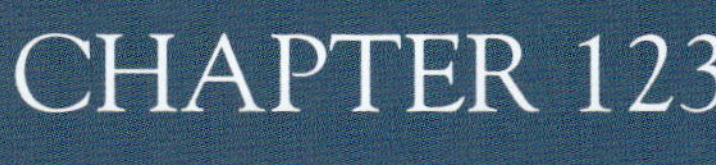

CHAPTER 123

Bone Graft Harvesting

Mehmet Zileli | Edward C. Benzel | Gordon R. Bell

Spinal surgeries typically involve neural decompression, fusion, or both. Fusion is performed to stabilize a segment, either because it is believed to be a source of pain or because of concerns regarding possible instability. Potential sources of instability include trauma, infection, tumor, or degeneration (spondylosis). Iatrogenic instability also may occur following previous spinal surgery. When instability is present, either with or without pain, fusion—using bone grafting and possibly instrumentation—often is employed. Because instrumentation provides only a temporary support, solid bony union must be achieved to provide long-term stability.

Bone Graft Specifications

Although a complete description of the myriad substances that are, or have been, used for arthrodesis is beyond the scope of this chapter, some general concepts are presented. An ideal bone graft should be incorporated rapidly, be structurally sound, have antigenic compatibility, be readily available and easily formed, have a low incidence of graft donor site complications, and be cost effective. Unfortunately, none of the grafts currently available today meet all of these requirements.

Each type of bone has its particular advantages: cortical bone graft provides good structural support, and cancellous bone graft provides more rapid incorporation. As the cellular elements in grafts die, they are slowly replaced by "creeping substitution," as the graft acts as a scaffold for new bone formation. In cortical bone this process is slower than with cancellous bone. Cancellous bone, however, is not as strong as the cortical bone and is therefore less ideally suited for structural support.

Autograft

Autografts are commonly used in spine surgery, and they remain the gold standard for fusion. An ideal autograft should include strong cortical bone for structural support and cancellous bone for more rapid incorporation and fusion.[1] Revascularization of cancellous bone is completed within several weeks, whereas the same process takes several months, or longer, for cortical bone.[2,3] Autografts commonly are used in conjunction with spinal instrumentation, but can also be used for dorsal onlay fusions without instrumentation. A significant advantage of autologous bone is that there is no risk of disease transmission.

Both cortical and cancellous grafts are commonly obtained from the iliac crest. Cortical bone can also be obtained from the fibula. In the early days of spine surgery, even the tibia was used, although the latter rarely is employed today.

Allograft

Allografts are commercially prepared and typically are obtained from cadaver bone. They are characterized by delayed vascularization and incorporation, which is believed to be due to antigenic recognition by the host. Allografts are appropriate in a variety of clinical situations.[4,5] They are most commonly used for ventral cervical interbody fusions, where single-level allografts generally lead to solid arthrodesis, similar to the fusion rate with autograft.[6] However, they incorporate relatively slowly,[7] and, if used for multilevel fusions, are associated with a pseudarthrosis rate of 63% to 70%.[7,8] Fibular allografts are preferred for cervical corpectomy, because the harvesting of a fibular autograft is associated with significant morbidity, including pedal edema, ankle pain, and the risk for peroneal nerve injury.[5]

Xenograft

Xenografts are tissues transplanted from one species to another. Xenografts give less satisfactory results than autograft or allograft, because of histocompatibility differences. Kiel (calf bone) grafts have been used in spine surgery, although their use is of historical significance only.

Additional substances also are used in conjunction with autogenous or allograft bone to augment fusion. These include autologous bone marrow and bone morphogenetic protein (BMP). The latter, when used in the cervical spine or for dorsal spine surgery, typically is used in an off-label manner. The use of BMP for ventral cervical fusions has been associated with significant complications, including airway obstruction.

Bone Graft Substitutes

Nonbiologic materials such as hydroxyapatite,[9,10] ceramic, and polymethylmethacrylate[11] also have been used, either in conjunction with, or in lieu of, of bone graft materials. They have the advantage of being able to be manufactured in a variety of sizes, shapes, and quantities. Polymethylmethacrylate is an inert substance that is rarely used, except in cases where life expectancy is severely limited, as in providing structural support in a patient with metastatic disease to the spine and a very short survival.

Bone Graft Types

The advantages and disadvantages of various autologous bone graft donor sites are discussed in this section. Preservation of the periosteum can provide a source of cells to help to form new bone to fill the defect.

Local Bone

Bone that is removed during surgical decompression commonly is used in spinal fusions. It consists of both cancellous and cortical components. It can be morselized manually with a rongeur or can be placed in a bone mill to provide a more consistent substrate for grafting.[12] The quality of local bone generally is perceived as being not as good as iliac bone grafts because of its cortical content.

Iliac Crest

The most commonly used donor site is the iliac crest. The iliac crest is a readily available source of cancellous bone, which provides rapid incorporation. Its disadvantages include donor site pain, which is a common complaint[13]; limited volume, which can be a concern for procedures requiring a copious amount of bone; and limited utility for procedures requiring a large piece of structural bone for reconstruction.

Ventral Iliac Crest Grafts

Ventral iliac crest grafts commonly are used to provide bone for various types of ventral cervical fusions (Fig. 123-1). The incision should be just caudal to the crest, to minimize discomfort that would be caused if the incision lay directly over the graft site, and should be placed approximately 3 to 4 cm lateral to the anterior superior iliac spine (ASIS) to minimize the risk of inadvertent injury to the lateral femoral cutaneous nerve. This nerve lies lateral to the ASIS in 90% of patients; in 10% it lies medial to the ASIS. When harvesting a tricortical graft for anterior cervical discectomy and fusion, an incision 6 to 8 cm long and a subperiosteal dissection of both the inner and outer wall of the ilium are performed. The iliac crest also can serve as a source of structural graft for cervical corpectomy and can provide an 8- to 10-cm length of tricortical strut graft.[14-17] Dissection of the iliacus muscle from the inner wall of the crest should be minimized to reduce the risk of hematoma formation and to reduce the risk of postoperative pain. The fascia should be closed meticulously to prevent a herniation of the pelvic contents.[18,19]

A saw or bur should be used for graft harvest rather than an osteotome to minimize the risk of graft microfracture, which may lead to graft failure. Care should be taken to keep the ventral saw cut at least 2 cm lateral to the ASIS to minimize the risk of ASIS avulsion. After obtaining the graft, the raw donor site bone surfaces should be covered with bone

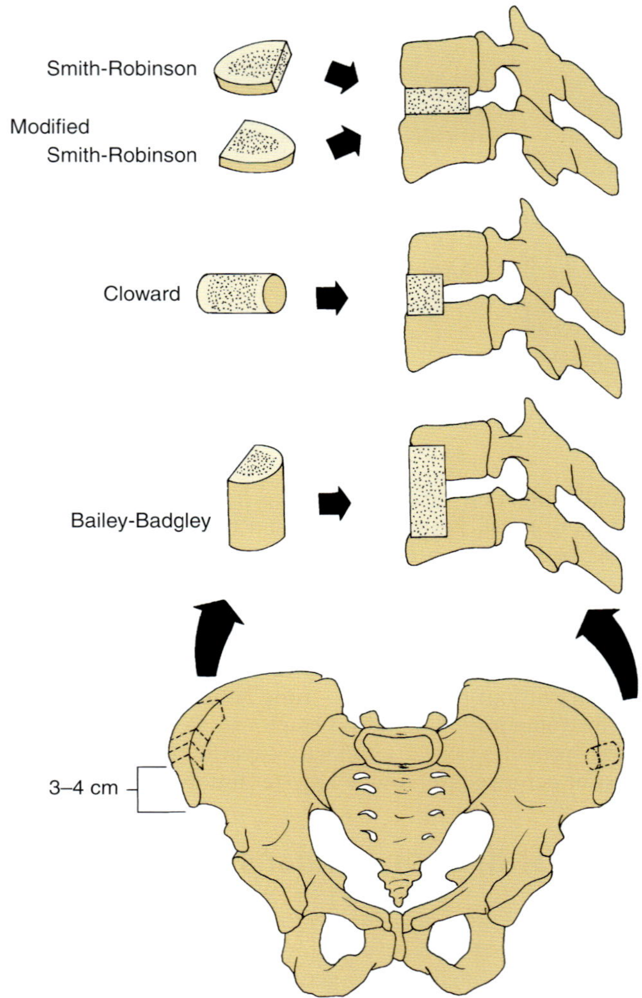

FIGURE 123-1. Ventral iliac crest graft harvesting and ventral cervical fusion techniques. The Smith-Robinson technique is shown at the top, the Cloward technique in the middle, and the Bailey-Badgley technique is illustrated at the bottom. (Redrawn with permission from White AA, Hirsch C: An experimental study of the immediate load bearing capacity of some commonly used iliac bone grafts. *Acta Orthop Scand* 42:482–490,1971.)

wax, or thrombin-soaked Gelfoam to minimize hematoma formation. A drain usually is not necessary, except for large defects.

Dorsal Iliac Crest Grafts

The dorsal iliac crest is predominantly used to obtain large quantities of dorsal onlay graft material for dorsolateral lumbar fusions. More bone is available from the dorsal iliac crest than from the ventral crest.[20] Bone graft may be obtained through the midline lumbar skin incision used to perform the concomitant decompression or through a separate lateral skin incision over the iliac crest. The midline skin incision usually is used to obtain dorsal iliac graft. The optimal site for the underlying fascial incision is 6 to 8 cm lateral to the midline. If the fascial incision is placed lateral to this point, injury to the cluneal nerves may occur, which can result in numbness or pain over the buttocks. This is more likely if a large graft is required. Laterally, the sacroiliac ligaments and

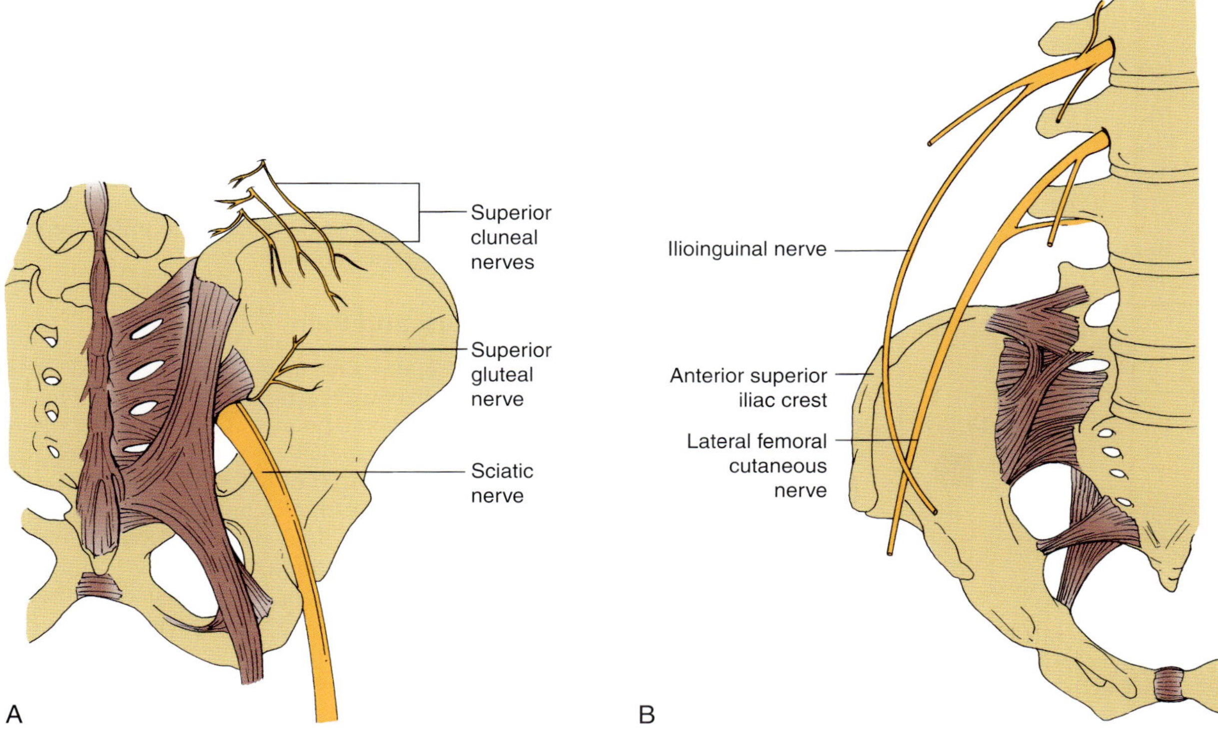

FIGURE 123-2. Possible nerve injury sites during dorsal (**A**) and ventral (**B**) iliac crest bone graft harvesting.

joints must be avoided. Care should be taken to minimize the depth of the osteotomy to avoid the sciatic notch where the superior gluteal artery and nerve could be injured. Injury to these structures is unlikely if the dissection is performed subperiosteally. Cancellous bone can be harvested with a gouge, which is helpful in removing strips of cancellous bone (Figs. 123-2 and 123-3).

When harvesting dorsal iliac crest bone for a cervical or thoracic fusion, the iliac crest graft incision can be made either obliquely just below the iliac crest, as described, or vertically.

Fibula

The fibula has the advantages of providing strength and length, and being relatively easily harvested. Its disadvantages include a slow rate of incorporation and harvest site complications. A fibular strut graft should be harvested from the middle third of the fibular shaft through a long skin incision on the lateral side of the leg, extending through the lateral intermuscular septum, preserving the periosteum (Fig. 123-4). During fibula graft harvesting, the peroneal nerve must be protected. Distally, the fibula should be harvested no more than 10 cm proximal to the ankle joint to minimize the risk of injury to the ankle syndesmosis, which is important for the stability of the ankle joint. The peroneal muscles should also be preserved. The middle third of the fibula should be osteotomized using an oscillating saw rather than an osteotome, which could cause fracture of the graft (Fig. 123-5). After fibula harvest, a few days of compressive leg wrapping with elevation of the leg will minimize swelling and discomfort.

Care must be exercised when harvesting a long segment of fibula to avoid proximal extension of the graft to the region of the neck of the fibula, where the common peroneal nerve is in jeopardy of injury. Injury to this nerve may result in pain and weakness in the foot and ankle.[21]

The advantage of a vascularized fibular graft is its more rapid incorporation. The technique of harvest and vascular anastomosis is technically demanding, and is no longer commonly employed in routine spine surgery.

Tibia

The subcutaneous ventromedial aspect of the tibia historically has been a site used occasionally for bone grafting. Currently, it is rarely used, because other, more suitable, autogenous or allograft alternatives exist. The potential morbidity associated with tibial grafts is significant, with tibial fracture being its main disadvantage. The tibia must be protected for several months to prevent fracture.[22]

Rib

Rib can be easily harvested, especially during thoracic spine operations. It is, however, a weak, poorly vascularized graft. Biomechanically it is inferior to the fibula. If taken with its artery, it is suitable for use as a vascularized strut graft.[23-25] It is used almost exclusively with thoracic or thoracolumbar fusions.

Complications of Graft Harvesting

Graft harvesting complications are common, and pain from a bone graft harvest site sometimes is more severe than the pain from the actual surgical procedure.[18,26-33] Although the

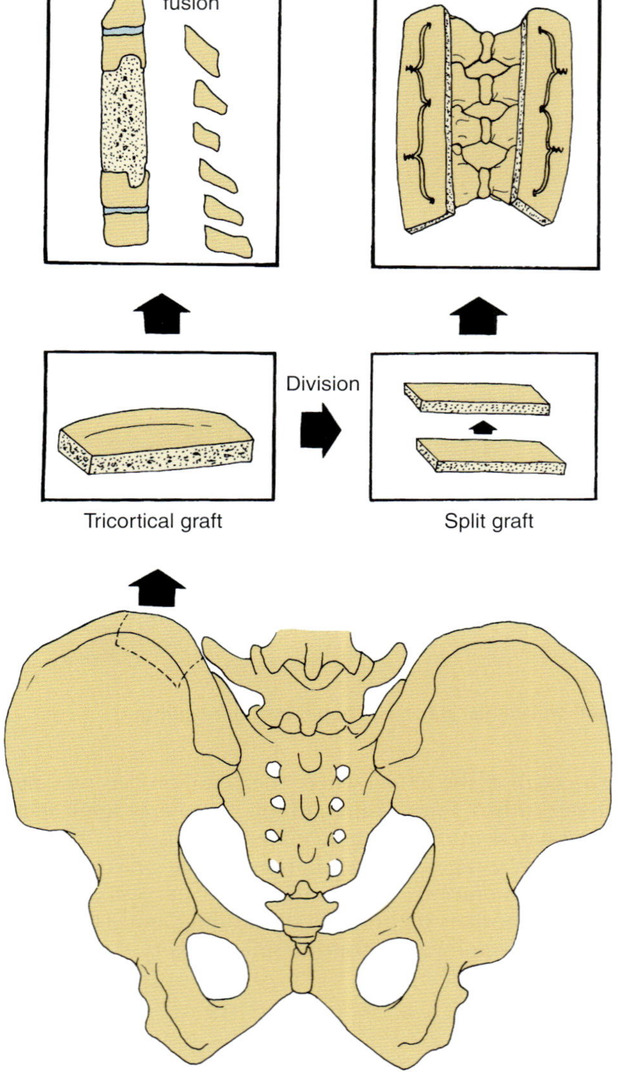

FIGURE 123-3. Dorsal iliac crest graft harvesting.

complications usually are minor, a review of 1244 cases from multiple series demonstrated that their occurrence is about 20%, whereas only a 0.2% complication rate was reported at the neck incision site.[34]

Chronic Pain

Graft donor site pain is nearly universal in the early postoperative period[13] but may be persistent in up to one third of patients[35,36] and may continue throughout the first 3 months postoperatively in up to 15% of patients.[29] One study reported that donor site pain was present for more than 10 years following surgery in more than one third of patients.[36] The reason for this chronic pain is not well understood, but it often is associated with the patient's overall pain syndrome. In addition, there are specific reasons for chronic donor site pain, including sacroiliac joint disruption, hernia through the graft site, fracture at the graft donor site (predominantly on the ventral ilium), and heterotopic bone formation.[37]

The magnitude of acute pain depends to a large extent on the size of the graft and the breadth and depth of the donor site wound. Therefore, one should consider harvesting unicortical or small tricortical grafts to minimize soft tissue injury. In addition, cancellous graft can be harvested from the dorsal iliac crest by removing the cap of the iliac crest and harvesting the cancellous bone from between the two tables of the ilium without disrupting either its inner or outer wall. In addition, the cap can be replaced to minimize the defect created to obtain the cancellous bone.

Nerve Injury and Pain

Incisions for bone grafts may injure nerves or may cause entrapment of nerves due to scar formation (see Fig. 123-2A).

The lateral femoral cutaneous nerve can be injured during ventral iliac crest harvest procedures, especially if the incision is very close to the ASIS.[38] Injury to this nerve can result in meralgia paresthetica and has been reported in 1% to 14% of cases.[32,37,38] It is characterized by numbness or dysesthesia on the ventrolateral thigh.[30,32] The nerve usually passes beneath the inguinal ligament, approximately 1 cm medial to the ASIS. However, in about 10% of cases it may pass above the inguinal ligament and just lateral to the ASIS.[39]

To avoid this complication, the incision must be kept at least 2 cm dorsal to the ASIS.[38]

The superior cluneal nerves are the most commonly injured cutaneous nerves following dorsal iliac crest bone grafting.[40] They arise from the superficial fascia, 6 to 8 cm lateral to the posterior superior iliac spine (PSIS). Injury to these nerves during dorsal iliac crest graft harvesting may cause analgesia over the buttock or painful neuromas. A hockey-stick or longitudinal incision may be helpful for avoiding this problem. Exposing the iliac crest under the deep fascia also may avoid injuring these nerves. Another technique recommended to avoid their injury is to make a separate vertical skin incision medial to the cluneal nerves.[41]

Other cutaneous nerves, such as the ilioinguinal, iliohypogastric, genitofemoral, superior gluteal, and femoral nerves may, rarely, be injured.[37]

Vascular and Other Visceral Organ Injuries

The superior gluteal artery can be injured during dorsal iliac crest graft harvesting.[42,43] This can cause severe hemorrhage. It lies between the gluteus medius and minimus muscles, and is avoided by careful subperisoteal dissection. If the artery is transected, it may retract into the pelvis, and controlling the bleeding may be difficult. Dissection of the gluteal muscles from the pelvis distally may be necessary.[43] In addition to vascular structures, the ureter and other visceral organs also may be injured.[44]

Hematoma Formation

Hematoma formation has been reported in 9% of iliac crest graft cases.[35] The bleeding typically comes from the adjacent muscles and bone surfaces and can, therefore, be minimized by the use of bone wax prior to closure. For larger bone graft defects, use of a drain may be helpful.

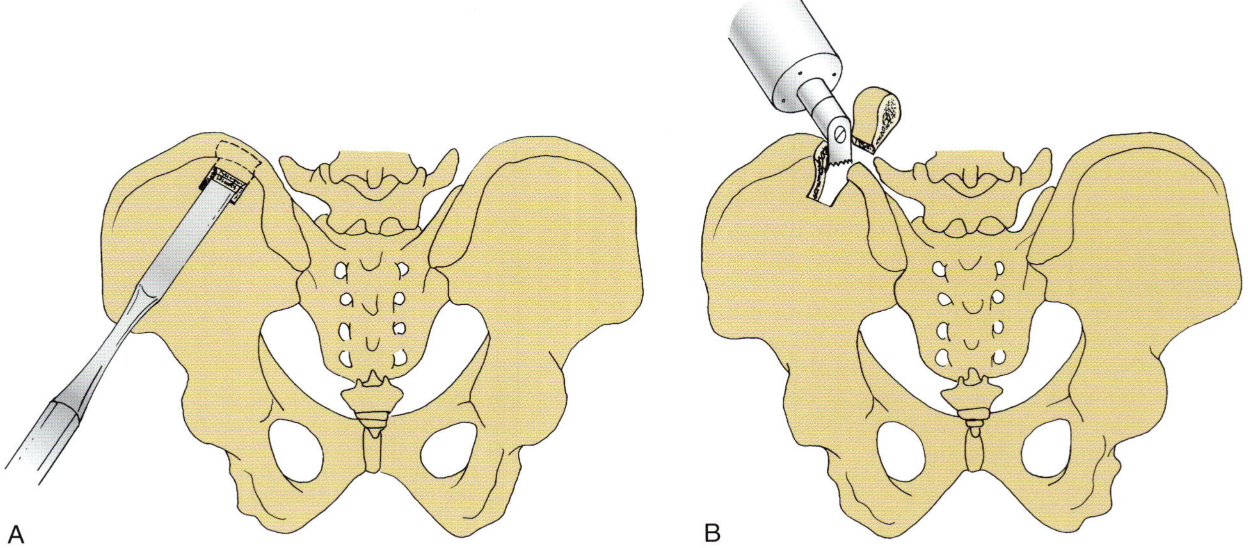

FIGURE 123-4. **A,** Unicortical graft harvesting from the dorsal iliac crest using an osteotome. **B,** Tricortical graft harvesting from the dorsal iliac crest using an oscillating saw.

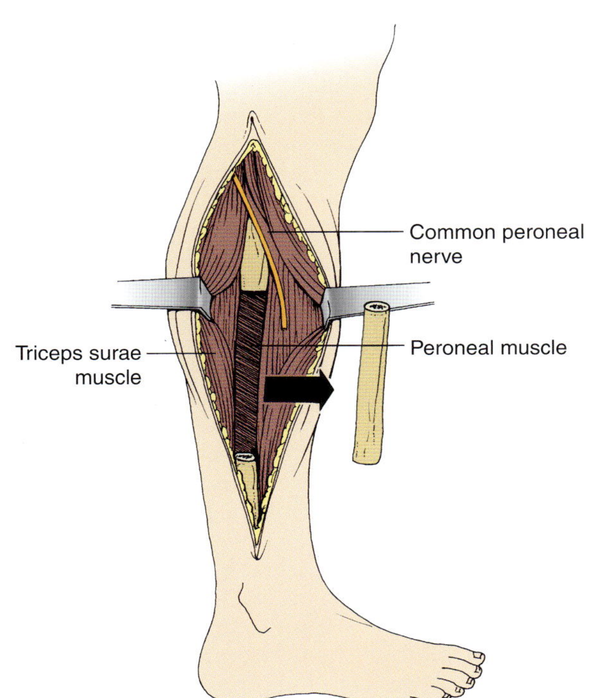

FIGURE 123-5. Fibula graft harvesting. The midportion of the fibula is removed with an oscillating saw.

Pelvic Fracture or Instability

Pelvic fracture or instability is rare, but may occur during either ventral or dorsal iliac graft harvesting procedures. Bone graft harvest performed too close to the ASIS can result in avulsion of the ASIS. Staying 2 cm behind the ASIS during bone resection will reduce the likelihood of this occurrence and also will reduce the risk of injury to the lateral femoral cutaneous nerve.[45] In addition, aggressive dorsal iliac crest grafting can result in injury to the sacroiliac joint or can produce a stress fracture to the ilium. Either of these can result in instability and can cause severe pain with ambulation.

Local Infection

Infections from the bone graft site are uncommon and have been reported in fewer than 1% of cases.[29] The risk of dorsal iliac graft site infection can be minimized by taking the bone graft through a separate facial incision, rather than from the laminectomy/fusion incision. A separate deep facial incision reduces the risk of cross-contamination between the laminectomy/fusion site and the bone graft site.

Herniation through the Graft Site

Herniation of the abdominal contents following full-thickness iliac crest grafting has been reported but is rare.[46,47]

Cosmetic Deformity

Cosmetic deformity may occur with ventral iliac crest full-thickness tricortical graft harvests. Several techniques, such as longitudinal crest splitting,[48] use of a subcrestal window technique,[29] and reconstruction with synthetic material[49] may diminish its incidence.

Where and When to Use a Bone Graft

Ventral Cervical Operations

Discectomy

Following cervical discectomy, the depth of the disc space is measured, and the graft is sized accordingly. The cartilaginous surfaces of the end plates are prepared, but the underlying cortical bone is preserved to minimize the risk of graft subsidence. A rasp or high-speed bur is used to create two parallel surfaces to optimize contact between the end plates and graft surface. A tricortical iliac crest graft of the appropriate size is harvested.

To facilitate insertion of the graft, distraction of the vertebral bodies is performed, either by cervical traction or by distracting across pins placed in the adjacent vertebral bodies (Caspar Cervical Distractor; Aesculap, Inc., Center Valley, PA).[50] Care must be exercised in gently tapping the bone into the distracted disc space to minimize risk of neural injury and to reduce the likelihood of cracking the graft. If ventral plating is not used, the graft should be recessed approximately 1 to 2 mm to lock the graft in the interspace.

After graft insertion, the cervical traction or distraction is released. The use of a plate is optional, although ventral plating currently is used in most single-level and nearly all multilevel ventral fusions. The advantage of the plate is that it facilitates fusion, reduces the likelihood of graft extrusion, and shortens the length of postoperative immobilization in a cervical orthosis.

Iliac crest grafts can be used in a three- or two-cortex construct. Three well-known graft configurations are used for ventral cervical spine surgery (see Fig. 123-1):

1. The *Smith-Robinson–type graft* is a tricortical horseshoe-type graft. Smith and Robinson have described the harvesting of the graft from the ventral iliac crest at a depth of approximately 1 cm and a width of 5 to 6 mm.[51] This graft is inserted into the intervertebral space, so that its cancellous portion is directed dorsally and the cortical surface ventrally. To prevent collapse, extrusion, or nonunion, Bloom and Raney have modified the graft position, and the cortical portion is inserted directly dorsally.[52]
2. The *Cloward-type graft* is a dowel graft. After harvesting the graft from iliac crest with a cylindrical bur, it is impacted in the intended graft site with a 1-mm, narrower bur. A special instrument set is used for graft harvesting, graft bed preparation, and graft impaction. If a Cloward type of graft is used in multilevel fusions, avascular necrosis of the vertebra may be encountered as a complication[53] if two adjacent levels are fused. The use of allograft bone rather than autograft is more common currently.[4] For multilevel fusions, a Smith-Robinson type of graft may be inserted at one disc level with a dowel graft at the adjacent space. Other alternatives for multilevel fusions include multilevel tricortical grafts (i.e., the Smith-Robinson technique) or cervical corpectomy.
3. The *Bailey-Badgley–type graft* is an iliac crest strut graft in which a trough is prepared in the ventral aspect of the vertebral body at a limited depth (0.5 cm).[19] The trough is cut to the full vertical height of the vertebra, and the discs are cleaned with a rongeur to a depth of approximately 1.2 cm.[19,34] A cortical cancellous iliac graft is then placed into the trough.

The strongest constructs are provided by the Smith-Robinson type of graft.[54] Tricortical grafts are stronger than bicortical grafts,[55] although graft breakage is a relatively uncommon complication. The optimal autologous graft has a substantial cancellous surface to facilitate bone incorporation.

Corpectomy

Reconstruction following cervical corpectomy typically involves use of either an iliac crest autograft or a fibular allograft. Iliac crest graft can be used for shorter segmental defects, but will not withstand axial stress following reconstruction for multilevel corpectomies.[5] In addition, the curved nature of the iliac crest sometimes makes it difficult to insert the graft when reconstructing a multilevel defect. The use of iliac crest autograft to reconstruct a multilevel corpectomy also leaves a significant defect in the iliac crest. A fibular allograft is used, therefore, for more than a two-level corpectomy and usually is the preferred choice for even a single-level corpectomy. We prefer to pack the medullary canal of the fibula with autogenous bone from the corpectomy to increase the healing potential of the fibular allograft.

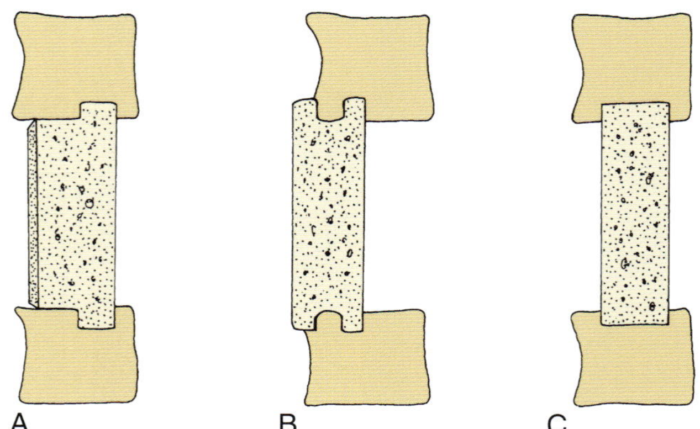

FIGURE 123-6. Cervical graft insertion after central corpectomy. **A,** T-shaped iliac crest graft. **B,** Notched fibula graft (dovetail method). **C,** Straight fibula graft ("keystone" method). The advantage of the grafts shown in **A** and **B** is that the bone graft sits on cortical bone of the end plates, thereby reducing the likelihood of graft subsidence. In **C,** the graft is countersunk through the cortical end plates into the vertebral body, thereby increasing the likelihood of graft subsidence. (Redrawn with permission from Whitecloud TS: Cervical spondylosis: the anterior approach. In Frymoyer JW, editor: *The adult spine: principles and practice,* New York, 1991, Raven, pp 1165-1185.)

Several methods are available for inserting a fibular graft into a corpectomy site (Fig. 123-6). In general, it is preferable to preserve the cortical end plates to minimize the risk of graft subsidence into the vertebral bodies. In the "keystone method" (see Fig. 123-6C) a defect is made in the midportion of both the rostral and caudal vertebral end plates.[5,56] In the "dovetail method" (see Fig. 123-6B) the bone is keyed into the ventral cortex of the vertebral body,[57] and the graft is inserted first into the rostral end, and then gently tapped into the caudal vertebra. In this instance, manual or skeletal traction may be helpful.[58] The iliac crest graft also can be tailored in a T-shaped form in which the cortical portion of the graft is faced dorsally (see Fig. 123-6A).

Ventral Thoracic or Thoracolumbar Operations

In the upper thoracic spine, a rib often is used for ventral bone grafting, since removal of a rib is commonly performed as part of the exposure. The iliac crest also can be used because the patient typically is in the lateral decubitus position and the iliac crest is readily accessible. Because the lower thoracic and lumbar vertebral bodies are relatively large, a bigger graft often is necessary. For autogenous graft, a tricortical iliac crest can be used, whereas for allograft, femur or tibia can be utilized.

Dorsal Cervical and Thoracolumbar Operations

Bone for dorsal spine surgeries usually is cancellous. Structural support is not required, because dorsal instrumentation generally is utilized and provides such support. The cancellous bone is harvested from the dorsal iliac crest, using osteotomes, gouges, and curets. Local bone from the spinous processes also can be used.

If wiring of the dorsal cervical spine is performed, a rectangular piece of iliac crest can be used following decortication of the dorsal elements. Either a unicortical, rectangular piece of bone or a bicortical piece that can then be split longitudinally can be harvested from the dorsal iliac crest and placed along the cervical spine to help maintain stability. Wires are passed through the facets or spinous processes and then through holes in the graft to help fasten the graft onto the laminar facet surfaces (see Fig. 123-3). With the introduction of cervical instrumentation, wire fixation is no longer commonly used. It has been replaced by lateral mass screws and rods, with bone grafting consisting of cancellous bone from either the dorsal iliac crest or allograft chips.

KEY REFERENCES

Hamby WB, Glaser HT: Replacement of spinal intervertebral discs with locally polymerizing methylmethacrylate. Experimental study of effects upon tissue and report of a small clinical series. *J Neurosurg* 16:311–313, 1959.

Kostuik JP, Frymoyer JW: Failures after spinal fusion: causes and surgical treatment results. In Frymoyer JW, editor: *The adult spine: principles and practice*, New York, 1991, Raven, pp 2027–2068.

Kurtz LT, Garfin SR, Booth RE Jr: Harvesting autologous iliac bone grafts—a review of complications and techniques. *Spine (Phila Pa 1976)* 14:1324–1331, 1989.

Stevenson S, Emery SE, Goldberg VM: Factors affecting bone graft incorporation—review. *Clin Orthop Relat Res* 324:66–74, 1996.

Zdeblick TA, Ducker TB: The use of freeze-dried allograft bone for anterior cervical fusions. *Spine (Phila Pa 1976)* 16:726–729, 1991.

REFERENCES

The complete reference list is available online at expertconsult.com.

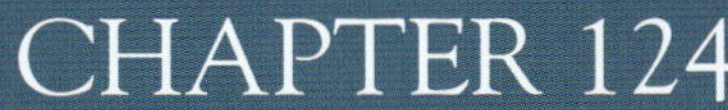

CHAPTER 124

Vascularized Bone Grafts in Spine Surgery

Alok D. Sharan | Ashwini D. Sharan

Bone grafting has had an important role in surgery since Barth first introduced bone-grafting techniques in the late 19th century.[1] Bone grafts typically have been used in the treatment of fracture nonunions, arthrodesis of joints, the filling of bone cavities, replacement of bone lost due to infection, trauma, tumor, augmentation of fracture healing, and spinal fusion. The different types of bone grafts used today include autogenous cancellous, nonvascularized autogenous cortical, vascularized autogenous cortical, allogeneic cancellous, allogeneic cortical, allogeneic demineralized bone matrix, and allogeneic inductive proteins.

Structural bone grafts commonly are used in spine surgery to provide stability in an area where a defect has been created. Currently, the gold standard for bone grafts is the autograft, which has the best biologic compatibility and leads to fewer nonunions. The most common complications associated with its use include pain at the donor site and a lack of incorporation of the graft. The advent of the use of vascularized bone grafts has provided the spine surgeon with a potentially powerful tool to use to treat difficult spine problems. This chapter presents a brief discussion of bone grafts and the basic biology of graft incorporation, along with causes of nonunion. The history of vascularized bone grafts is presented, as is a surgical technique for the donor site. The indications in spine surgery will be discussed along with a review of the results of its use in this field.

Bone Grafts in Spine Surgery

Albee first described utilizing a bone graft for spinal fusion in 1911 as a treatment for Pott disease.[2] Many advances have been made since that time, and fusion is now the standard treatment for a variety of spinal disorders. Achieving a proper fusion involves two key components: (1) preparation of the site to be fused and (2) stimulation of bone formation with the use of a bone graft. The most effective graft material currently available is autologous cancellous bone. This graft has a large surface area that allows for vascularization of the graft and incorporation with the host bone. In cases in which the fusion must span several segments, the amount of autogenous cancellous bone that is available may not be sufficient.

Autologous cortical bone is another commonly used graft in spine surgery. Unfortunately, this graft has fewer osteoblasts that survive and is associated with a slower rate of revascularization. This slower revascularization results in a slower rate of incorporation of the graft, thus limiting its use.[3] The advantage of a cortical graft, however, is that it can provide immediate structural support and that the graft is available in larger sizes. Over time, during a process called *creeping substitution*, the strength of the graft decreases. During this process, the avascular nature of the graft causes resorption by osteoclasts, while new bone is laid down by osteogenic cells originating from the recipient bed rather than the graft, a phenomenon first observed and described by Phemister in 1914.[4] This is why a cortical graft (such as a strut graft used in the treatment of kyphosis) may take up to 2 years to incorporate completely. During the process of creeping substitution, the bone graft is found to be weakest at 6 months, increasing the risk of fracture at the graft site.[5] By retaining its vascular supply and viability of the osteocytes, a vascularized bone graft provides a mechanically stronger support than a nonvascularized graft.

Vascularized Bone Grafts

The use of vascularized bone grafts parallels the developments associated with the history of vascular surgery. The beginnings of vascular surgery can be traced back to Carrel's classic paper published in 1908, "Results of the Transplantation of Blood Vessels, Organs and Limbs,"[6] in which he describes a technique whereby blood vessels can be anastomosed. Various tools for anastomosing small vessels were designed and tested in the years following that publication. Androsov designed the first vascular stapling machine,[7] Jacobsen and Suarez demonstrated the utility of the microscope in the operating room,[8] and Buncke and Schulz improved microsurgical instrumentation and performed much of the early experimental work in the field.[9] Strauch et al. used a canine model to transpose a rib to the mandible on its internal mammary pedicle in 1971,[10] and in 1973 a free vascularized rib graft was performed in a dog by McCullough and Fredrickson.[11] The first free skin flap using microvascular anastomoses was reported by Taylor in 1973,[12] and in 1975, Taylor transferred a fibula to a tibial defect as the first free vascularized bone graft in a human.[13]

The vascularized bone graft traditionally has been used in refractory nonunions or in areas where there is a large segmental defect. The need to use a more structurally supportive bone graft for kyphosis surgery resulted in the use of the first vascularized bone graft in spine surgery. Surgery for severe kyphosis secondary to infection, trauma, or deformity requires spanning multiple levels. When a nonvascular rib or fibula was used to span such a defect, the length of the graft and the slow rate of incorporation resulted in a high rate of nonunion. Bradford encountered fatigue fractures in 4 of 23 patients when a nonvascularized fibula was used for spinal kyphosis surgery.[14] These results encouraged spine surgeons to seek out alternatives to traditional bone grafts. In two separate reports, Rose et al. and Bradford described successful techniques of using a rib graft with a vascular pedicle.[15,16] Because the cross-sectional area of the rib was too small and could not provide the structural support needed for certain areas of spinal fusion, surgeons began to explore the use of the fibula as a vascularized graft.[17,18] Currently, the rib, fibula, and iliac crest are used as primary donor sites for a vascularized graft.

Indications and Principles

Based on previous studies, a vascularized bone graft is indicated for use in the following situations:

- Bone graft greater than 5 cm needed[19]
- Strut graft that will be more than 4 cm from the anterior border of the spine and thus more prone to fracture
- A pseudarthrosis after a nonvascularized bone graft
- An area of the spine that will require radiation postoperatively, as in the setting of a malignancy
- Cases of infection where placing instrumentation or avascular bone would propagate the infection
- Surgeries in which fusion is expected to be difficult to achieve, as with operations for neurofibromatosis

Surgical Technique

The three most common locations from which a vascularized bone graft can be harvested are the rib, the iliac crest, and the fibula. In spine surgery, the rib is the easiest location to harvest. Due to its thin cylindrical structure, the rib may not provide the mechanical stability necessary to fill large segmental defects. The fibula is a larger cylindrical structure that has strong mechanical properties. It can be used to span multiple levels. The disadvantage of this graft is the donor site morbidity associated with harvesting the fibula.

Preoperative Planning

Harvesting of a vascularized bone graft requires that the surgeon be well trained in microvascular techniques. Multiple types of anastomosis may be required in vessels that could be potentially scarred or traumatized. Preoperative angiography should be performed to elucidate the vasculature of the donor and recipient sites. It is important to understand that a normal arteriogram may be misleading, as scarred blood vessels may appear normal. The surgeon often will need to make an intraoperative decision regarding the viability of a blood vessel.

Fibula

The fibula is a long bone that is triangular in cross section and has a high cortical-to-cancellous bone ratio. Up to 25 cm of length can be harvested safely for long grafts. The medullary vascular supply to the fibula arises as a branch of the peroneal artery, and it enters the fibula at the junction of the proximal and middle thirds of the bone. The venous system is similar to the arterial system, with drainage occurring through the venae comitantes of the peroneal artery and the medullary sinusoidal system.

The procedure that follows is described by Vail and Urbaniak using an extraperiosteal dissection.[20] This procedure also has been described by Gore et al. in a subperiosteal plane.[21] Vail and Urbaniak report that the extraperiosteal dissection leads to decreased complaints of pain.

To obtain the fibula graft, the patient is placed supine on the operating table. The leg should be prepped from the hip to the toes and a tourniquet applied to the thigh. After the tourniquet has been inflated, the limb is exsanguinated with an elastic bandage.

A straight lateral incision is made directly over the fibula, with further dissection being performed between the posterior and lateral compartments of the calf. The peroneal muscle is separated from the anterior aspect of the fibula down to the intramuscular septum. Elevating the muscles of the anterior compartment reveals the intraosseous membrane. The muscles of the posterior compartment also are dissected extraperiosteally. The superficial peroneal nerve and a portion of the peroneal artery deep to the fibula are protected, and the fibula is divided with a Gigli saw.

The flexor hallucis longus, the posterior tibial muscle, and the remaining muscles of the anterior compartment are separated from the fibula extraperiosteally. The fibula is elevated from the wound from caudal to rostral, while the pedicle remains intact. Vascular branches entering the soleus muscle are clipped and divided. The peroneal vessels are dissected proximally to their bifurcation from the tibial vessels. The fibular diaphyseal segment, along with approximately 4 to 6 cm of the peroneal vessels, are ligated and dissected from the wound.

Aspirin often is administered postoperatively. In uncomplicated free-flap procedures, dextran and heparin play a minimal role. The donor site is closed primarily with suction drains. A splint with the foot in dorsiflexion is used for approximately 5 to 7 days, followed by active range-of-motion exercises. A radionuclide bone scan, utilizing technetium-99–labeled methylene diphosphonate, is the most useful study to assess viability of vascularized bone. It has been shown to be a reliable indicator of microvascular patency and correlates with clinical outcome if performed within the first postoperative week. Thereafter, false positives are more frequent.

Iliac Crest

Grafting of the iliac crest is based on the fact that the most reliable pedicle is the deep circumflex iliac artery. This artery has been shown to supply the majority of the bone.[22] The following technique has been described by Mezera and Weiland and is based on the original work by Taylor.[22,23]

The patient is placed supine on the operating table with a small bump under the donor hip. An incision is made from the femoral artery to a point 10 cm posterior to the anterior superior iliac spine (ASIS). The external oblique muscle is exposed and incised in line with its fibers, to a point 3 cm superior to the iliac crest. The incision is curved toward the

ASIS and parallel to the inguinal ligament so that the inguinal canal can be entered. The spermatic cord or round ligament is identified and retracted upward and medially. The fascia at this point is incised, and the deep circumflex iliac artery and vein are identified. The vessels are traced laterally, dividing the transversalis fascia, internal oblique, and transversus abdominis from the inguinal ligament. The ascending branch of the deep circumflex iliac artery will become easier to identify as the ASIS is approached. Its origin from the superficial circumflex iliac artery can be identified medially by incising the internal oblique muscle 3 cm above and behind the ASIS.

Incising the transversus muscle parallel to the iliac crest isolates the bone. The transversalis fascia is incised, the extraperitoneal fat is retracted, and a line is exposed between the transversalis and the iliacus fascia. Incising the iliacus 1 cm medial to this line exposes the periosteum of the iliac fossa. The iliacus muscle is dissected away from the rest of the bone. The attachment of the tensor fasciae latae and glutei muscles is then cut from the bone. The inguinal ligament can be divided from the origin of the sartorius muscle just medial to the ASIS.

The bone can now be osteotomized as measured to isolate it with its vascular pedicle. The flap should be allowed to sit for 20 minutes to assure its viability. Occasionally, the lateral cutaneous nerve will need to be sectioned to remove the graft, but every attempt should be made to preserve it. Using an oscillating saw, the graft can be first cut laterally and then medially to a depth of 2.5 cm. The iliac crest graft should now be ready, along with the deep circumflex iliac artery and vein. The graft can be no longer than 10 cm due to the curvature of the ilium.

During closure, careful attention must be paid to securing the layers so as to avoid abdominal herniation. The iliacus fascia and muscle should be sutured to the transversalis fascia and muscle. Next, the internal and external oblique muscles should be sutured to the glutei and the fascia lata and its muscle. Finally, the inguinal canal should be repaired and the inguinal ligament reattached laterally.

Rib

Injection studies have demonstrated that the rib receives its primary blood supply from the posterior intercostal vessels. The posterior intercostal artery is a branch off of the aorta that forms the posterior and anterior ramus. The posterior ramus provides branches to the spinal cord and the paraspinous muscles. The anterior ramus anastomoses with the anterior intercostal artery and also provides a nutrient artery to the rib. The anterior intercostal artery provides a vascular supply mainly to the periosteum and, therefore, is not as important as its posterior counterpart.

As first described by Bradford, a vascularized rib graft should be planned so that the rib removed will be long enough to span the defect. The rib to be used should be two to three segments below the rostral vertebrae.[24] The patient is placed in the lateral decubitus position. A skin incision is made over the level of the rib. The intercostal musculature is cut 0.5 to 1 cm above the rib. The rib is divided at the costochondral junction, and the intercostal musculature is then divided inferiorly to the rib, distally to proximally. A wide margin is left to avoid dividing the vascular complex. Chest retractors are placed into the wound, and the intercostal vasculature is identified. Dissection is carried out dorsally, and the rib is divided at the rib transverse process junction. At this point the rib can be mobilized along with its vascular complex. The vessels are dissected and then mobilized to the junction of the intervertebral foramen. A centimeter of rib should be dissected subperiosteally so that bone-to-bone contact can be made with the adjacent vertebra. The rib is then rotated and mobilized to span the vertebra above and below. Incising the periosteum 1 cm over the rib can test circulation to the graft. If brisk bleeding is encountered, then an intact vascular pedicle is confirmed. The chest can now be closed in the usual fashion.

Results and Complications

Results

As first reported in 1980 by Bradford, a vascularized rib graft is suitable for areas in the spine that would require strong biomechanical support.[24] This typically occurs when a large defect requires spanning. By avoiding the process of creeping substitution, the vascularized bone graft prevents microfracture and pseudarthrosis, which are commonly observed when a large nonvascularized graft is used. Most of the cases reported in the literature have used the graft in areas where mechanical support is essential, while awaiting bone graft incorporation.

Vascularized bone grafts also are useful in the setting of malignancy in cases where radiation therapy is to be employed. Often a subtherapeutic dose of radiation therapy must be applied at the site of bone fusion to minimize the occurrence of a nonunion of the bone graft.[25,26] Because of its greater number of available viable osteocytes and osteoblasts, along with its relative diminished requirement of ingrowth and neovascularization, a vascularized graft may better tolerate the deleterious effects of the radiation.[27,28]

The superior mechanical stability afforded by a vascularized graft also is useful in the setting of infection. When nonoperative therapy has failed to eradicate a spinal infection, operative intervention requires decompression of the infected bone along with fusion for stabilization. Using instrumentation or long segments of nonvascularized bone can provide a nidus for the infection. In these cases, a vascularized bone graft has been successful in aiding the speed and stability of the fusion. Table 124-1 presents a summary of different spinal uses of vascularized bone grafts.

Complications

Most complications involving vascularized bone grafts in spine surgery are related to donor site morbidities. In 1996, Vail and Urbaniak reported on complications of harvesting vascularized fibular grafts.[29] They noted that pain and motor weakness were the most prevalent complications. Sensory deficits also were noted, along with rare cases of skin breakdown secondary to loss of vascular supply. In a separate report, a functional iatrogenic valgus of the ankle joint has been reported when resection of the fibula ended too distally.[30] Other morbidities related to fibula graft harvesting include transient peroneal nerve palsy, flexor hallucis longus contracture, compartment syndrome, and fracture of the ipsilateral tibia.[31]

TABLE 124-1

Spinal Uses of Vascularized Bone Grafts

Authors	Indication	Graft Used
Bradford DS et al.[14]	Severe kyphosis	Rib
Meyers AM et al.[36]	Salvage reconstruction in severe spondylolisthesis	Fibula
Nakamura H et al.[37]	Anterior thoracic and lumbar fusion	Folded rib graft
Freidberg SR et al.[38]	Replacement of resected cervical vertebral bodies	Fibula
Govender S et al.[39]	Tuberculosis kyphosis	Rib
Wright NM et al.[40]	Anterior decompression and fusion in the setting of radiation therapy for cervical chordoma	Fibula
Asazuma T et al.[41]	Cervical kyphosis due to neurofibromatosis	Fibula
Wuisman PIJM et al.[42]	Thoracolumbar scoliotic deformity in the setting of osteogenesis imperfecta	Fibula

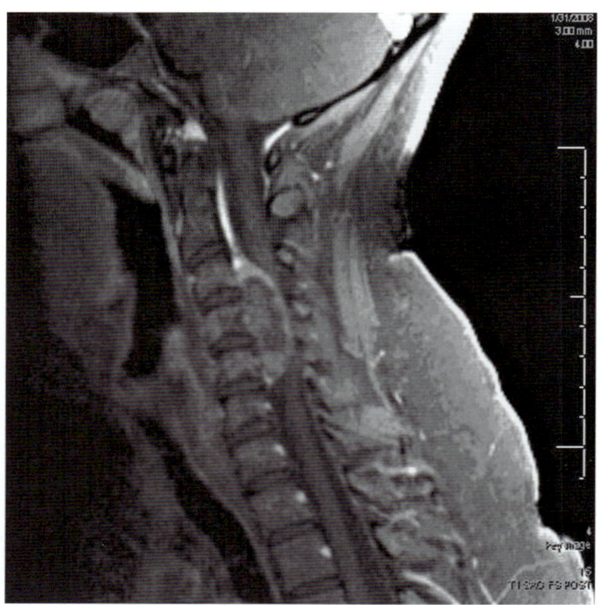

FIGURE 124-1. Sagittal MRI of the cervical spine demonstrates a mass from C3-5.

Persistent pain following removal of the iliac crest has been reported with chronic disability when a large graft is harvested.[32-34] Infection, hematoma, and fracture of the anterior superior iliac spine also have been reported.[35]

Case Presentation

A 24-year-old woman presented 3 months postpartum with right upper extremity weakness and a clumsy weak hand. Her examination was consistent with myelopathy with upper extremity strength at 2/5 motor strength. An MRI demonstrated a large epidural tumor from C3 to C6 exiting through the neural foramen, causing bony destruction of

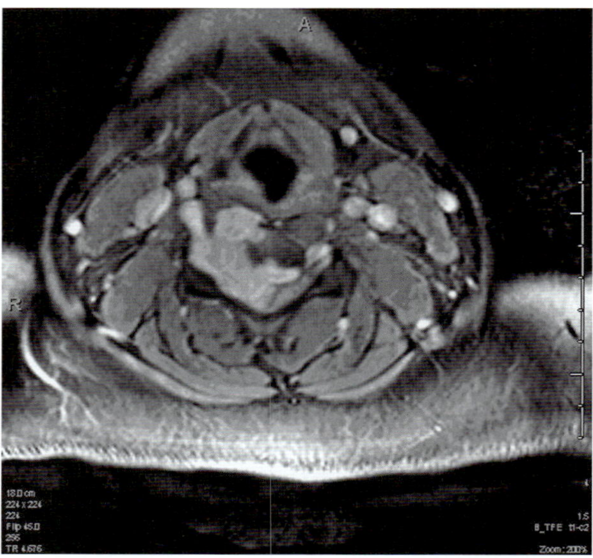

FIGURE 124-2. Axial MRI demonstrates the extent of the lesion.

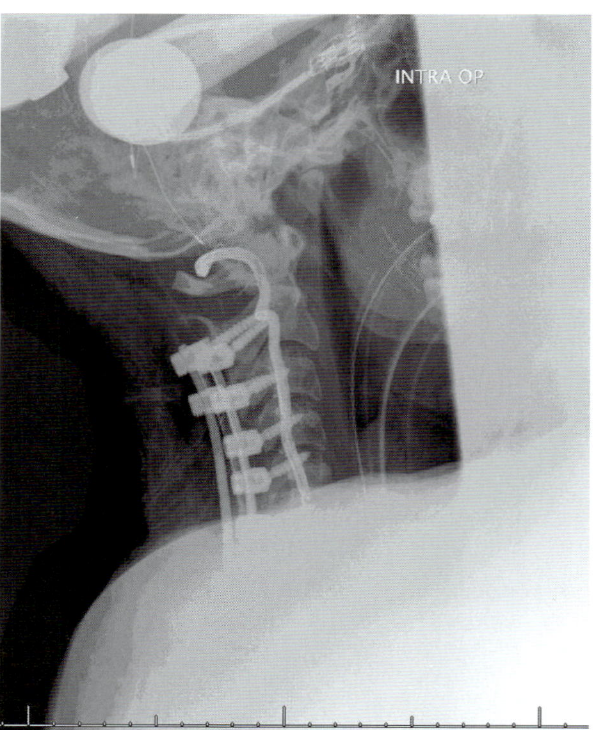

FIGURE 124-3. Lateral radiograph after completion of posterior fusion and decompression.

predominantly the C4 vertebra, as well as the C3 and C5 vertebrae (Figs. 124-1 and 124-2). A biopsy had been obtained and was suggestive of a chordoma. The patient underwent a two-staged en bloc tumor resection and reconstruction. The first stage involved a posterior C3-6 laminectomy and reconstruction from C2-T1 with disconnection of dorsal elements and tumor resection (Fig. 124-3). This was followed the next day with a C3-5 corpectomy and fusion from C2-6 with a vascularized fibula bone graft and cervical interference plate, placed ventrally, at C6 (Figs. 124-4 to 124-8).

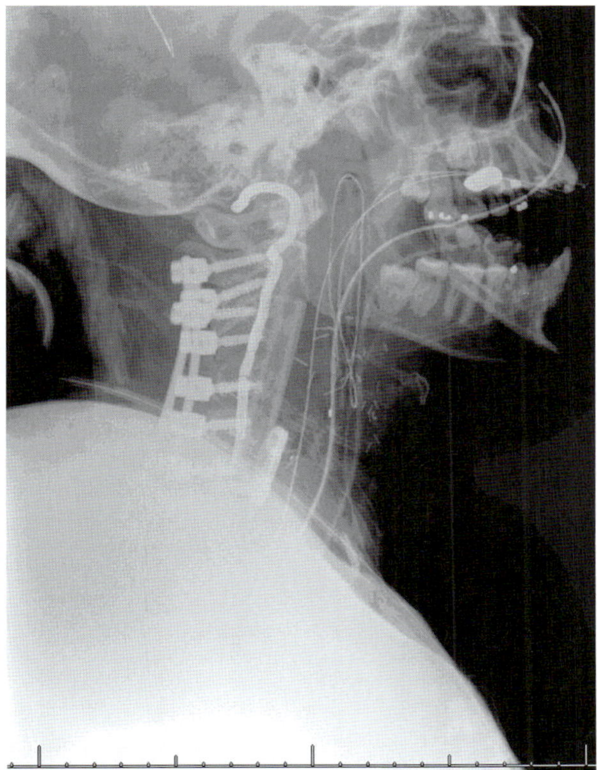

FIGURE 124-4. Lateral radiograph demonstrating placement of the anterior graft from C3-5.

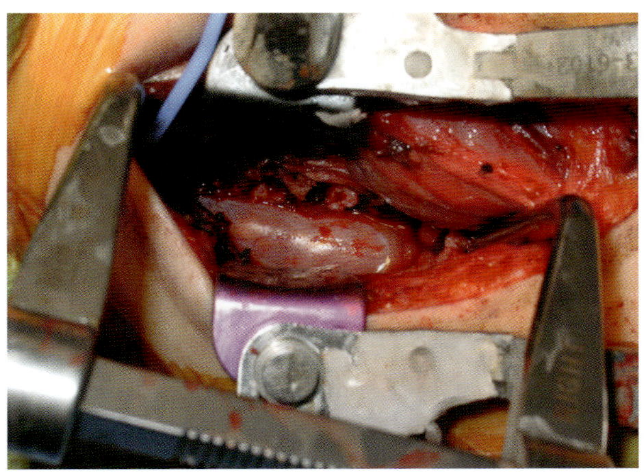

FIGURE 124-6. C3-5 corpectomy defect.

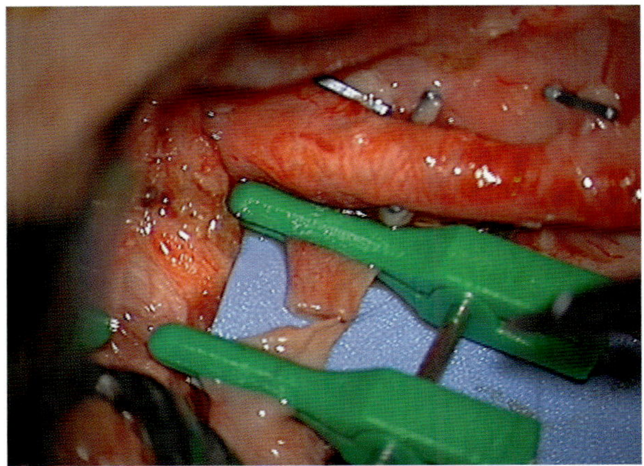

FIGURE 124-7. Anastomosis for autograft.

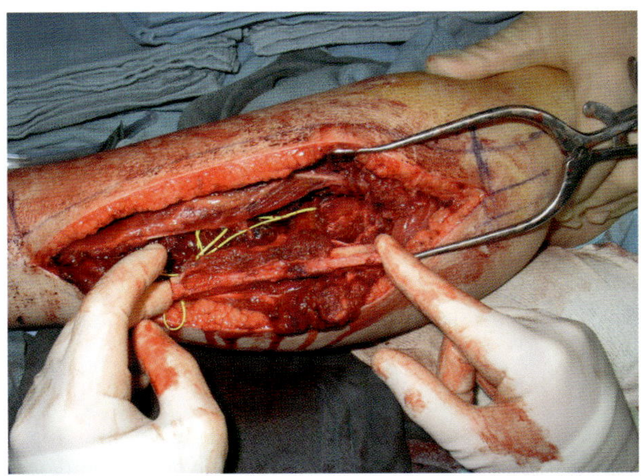

FIGURE 124-5. Harvesting the fibular graft.

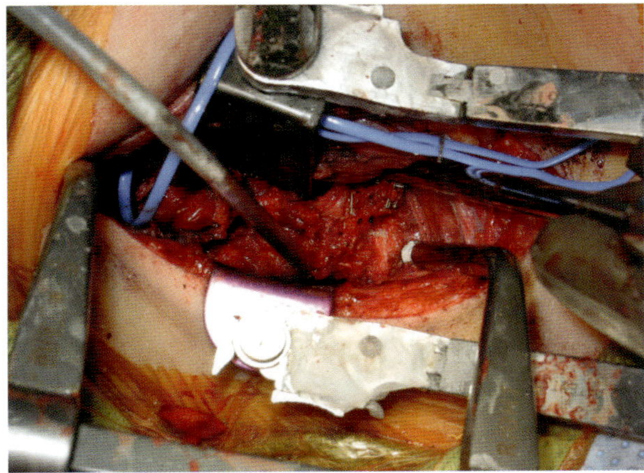

FIGURE 124-8. Placement of autograft into the corpectomy defect.

Summary

Vascularized bone grafts offer another tool for the spine surgeon to use in areas in which achieving bone union may prove difficult. It is a technically demanding procedure. As with all surgical interventions, patient selection is extremely important. Removal of the graft has known associated morbidities, and the patients should be informed of them. Overall, the vascularized bone graft provides a mechanically strong construct with a successful rate of incorporation in cases with the potential for difficulty in healing.

KEY REFERENCES

Freidberg SR, Gumley GJ, Pfeifer BA, et al: Vascularized fibular graft to replace resected cervical vertebral bodies. *J Neurosurg* 71:283, 1989.

Govender S, Suresh Kumar KP, Med PC: Long term follow-up assessment of vascularized rib pedicle graft for tuberculosis kyphosis. *J Pediatr Orthop* 21:281, 2001.

Kaneda K, Kurakami C, Minami A: Free vascularized fibular strut graft in the treatment of kyphosis. *Spine (Phila Pa 1976)* 13:1273, 1988.

Minami A, Kaneda K, Satoh S, et al: Free vascularised fibular strut graft for anterior spinal fusion. *J Bone Joint Surg [Br]* 79(1):43, 1997.

Nakamura H, Yamano Y, Seki M, et al: Use of folded vascularized rib graft in anterior fusion after treatment of thoracic and upper lumbar lesions. *J Neurosurg* 94(Suppl 2):323, 2001.

Wuisman PI, Jiya TU, Van Dijk M, et al: Free vascularized bone graft in spinal surgery: indications and outcome in eight cases. *Eur Spine J* 8:296, 1999.

REFERENCES

The complete reference list is available online at expertconsult.com.

CHAPTER 125

Pain in Spine Disease

Tatiana von Hertwig Fernandes de Oliveira | Andre Machado

Chronic axial or limb pain is common in patients with degenerative or malignant spine disease and may persist after surgical treatment. To establish a reasonable goal for the often difficult management of chronic pain, it is useful to understand the frequency of back and neck pain in the population, the frequency and severity of postlaminectomy syndrome, the pathophysiology of chronic pain, and related cognitive and behavioral concerns. Surgical issues related to compression of neural elements, biomechanics, and complication avoidance and management have been extensively covered in other chapters of this textbook.

Back pain is one of the most common complaints in the general population; more than two thirds of the population have back pain at least once during life.[1,2] Low back problems are reported to be the second leading complaint in outpatient consultations and the third complaint in hospital admissions.[1,3] Annual back pain prevalence is reported to be 15% to 45%.[4] Back pain is the most common cause of activity limitation in younger individuals,[5] and it is the third most common cause of surgical procedures in the United States, in particular, fusion surgery.[4,6] Although back pain is very common, 60% to 70% of patients with acute back pain are likely to recover in less than 3 months without functional loss. The prognosis worsens significantly when pain becomes persistent for more than 6 months, with less than 50% complete recovery.[4] The recurrence rate is also higher in patients with persistent back pain.[4] Many variables influence recovery, recurrence rates, and the probability of returning to work. Factors related to increased disability include gender (male), age, unemployment,[7] stressful work environment,[8] and compensation related to disability.[7-10] Psychological factors also influence prognosis.[11-15]

Although less common than low back pain, neck pain is also a frequent reason for seeking health care. The most common causes of neck pain include musculoskeletal disorders and degenerative disease of the cervical spine.[5,16] The lifetime prevalence of chronic neck pain ranges from 35% to 50%, and the cross-sectional prevalence is 10% to 35%.[16-18]

Most episodes of low back, neck, or related limb pain do not come to medical attention or are likely managed by primary care professionals. Specialized attention is most often required for severe, refractory, and chronic pain. However, even this smaller subsection of patients constitutes a large, imposing significant health-care challenge and burden to social security systems. The direct and indirect costs of chronic back pain have been estimated to be greater than 50 billion dollars in the United States,[8] and chronic disability secondary to chronic back pain affects more than 5 million Americans[8] (Fig. 125-1). This chapter focuses on chronic pain associated with spine disease, with emphasis on postlaminectomy syndrome and neuromodulatory treatment options.

Chronic Pain

Definition

The transition from acute to chronic pain can be defined according to time course or healing process. The first criterion is more commonly used, although different cutoff time points have been arbitrarily chosen, ranging from 1 to 6 months.[18A] Chronic pain can also be defined as pain persisting beyond the expected time of healing for the given injury.[19] This criterion avoids the need for an arbitrary cutoff but may not be as practical clinically. In this context, chronic pain is understood as pain that is not associated with

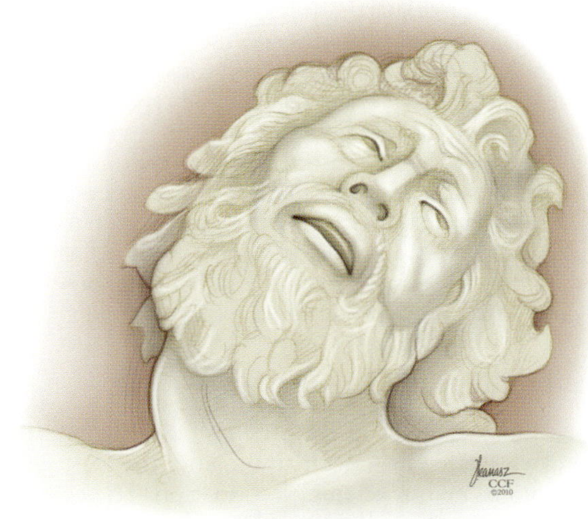

FIGURE 125-1. Pain has been a subject of interest since ancient times. (Copyright Cleveland Clinic Foundation.)

tissue injury or illness of equivalent severity. Neuropathic mechanisms may be involved in pain perpetuation as well as the influence of behavioral, social, and cognitive factors.

Nociceptive Pain versus Neuropathic Pain

Nociceptive pain is associated with tissue injury, without compromise of the nervous system itself. It is mostly described as sharp, well-defined pain, localized over the injured area. *Neuropathic pain* may develop from persistent nociceptive pain secondary to continuous sensitization of the nervous system[20] but can also occur as a result of injury directly to the peripheral or central nervous system. It usually consists of a less defined sensation, often described as burning, aching, or electrical shocks, and generally associated with altered stimulus perception, such as allodynia or hyperalgesia.

Pain-Related Pathways

Peripheral Nervous System

Noxious stimulation causes the peripheral nervous system to be activated by depolarization of receptors in the distal end of primary afferent axons, which transmit the information processed to the CNS. Only a part of the pain information processed in the periphery is transmitted to the brain because of the interference of modulatory mechanisms. Continuous or repetitive stimulation may lead to peripheral and central sensitization, contributing to the conversion of acute pain into a chronic pain syndrome. This section describes the components of the pain pathways and the mechanisms of acute pain as an introduction to the mechanisms underlying chronic pain.

Peripheral Receptors

When excited by a stimulus, the peripheral receptor acts as a transducer, transforming the initial information into chemical signals. Receptor depolarization is mediated by transmembrane potentials, triggered by external stimulation that reaches a specific threshold.[20-23] Receptors are located on the endings of sensory axons in the skin and other tissues and are composed of free, partially covered or encapsulated nerve endings. Receptors are stimulus-specific and generally do not depolarize with other types of stimuli at normal intensities. Three main modality-specific receptor subtypes are associated with spinal pain: (1) nociceptors, which respond to tissue damage; (2) mechanoreceptors; and (3) thermoreceptors.[21] These receptors include not only free nerve endings, as nociceptors, but also more specialized structures, such as partially covered receptors (Merkel discs, Ruffini endings) and encapsulated endings (Meissner, Pacini, and Golgi corpuscles; neuromuscular spindles; neurotendinous organs).[21,23,24]

Peripheral Nerve Fibers

Peripheral nerves are formed by the union of the dorsal root, which carries afferent information, and the ventral root, which contains mainly efferent information. The epineurium is formed not only by collagen and vessels but also by sympathetic fibers and polymodal receptors, forming the nervi nervorum.[24] These are possibly associated with the occurrence of chronic pain after nerve injury,[25,26] promoted by sympathetic sprouting and sensitization.

Nerve fibers are classified according to their myelinization and conduction velocity: Aα fibers are the fastest and are associated with muscle efferents. Aβ fibers are the second fastest type, carrying tactile, pressure, and proprioceptive afferents. These fibers are recruited during inflammation or other injury-related phenomena to participate in mechanisms of nociception, hypersensitivity, and sensitization.[27,28] Aδ fibers carry not only cold information but also nociception when associated with polymodal receptors. B fibers are related to autonomic activity, and C, or unmyelinated, fibers are related to nociception transmission and postganglionic autonomic function.

Pain Pathways

Painful stimuli are transmitted from the peripheral nerve to the dorsal root ganglion, dorsal root, and dorsal horn. At the level of the dorsal root entry zone, most unmyelinated and small myelinated fibers assume a more lateral position to enter the Lissauer tract (Fig. 125-2). In contradiction to the Bell-Majendie law, evidence exists that some of the nociceptive information travels not only through the dorsal root but also through the ventral root.[29-33]

The Lissauer tract comprises a bundle of longitudinal fibers and, as proposed by Ranson, is part of the pain transmission pathway.[34,35] Unmyelinated fibers make up most of the Lissauer tract,[35-37] and their central terminations are located mainly in lamina II of Rexed. Aδ fibers have a broader arborization and terminate in laminae I, II, V, and X.[35] Although some Aδ fibers terminate in the dorsal horn at the same level

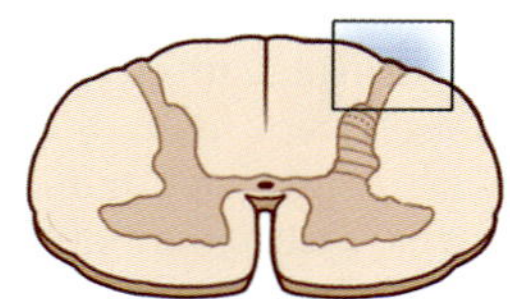

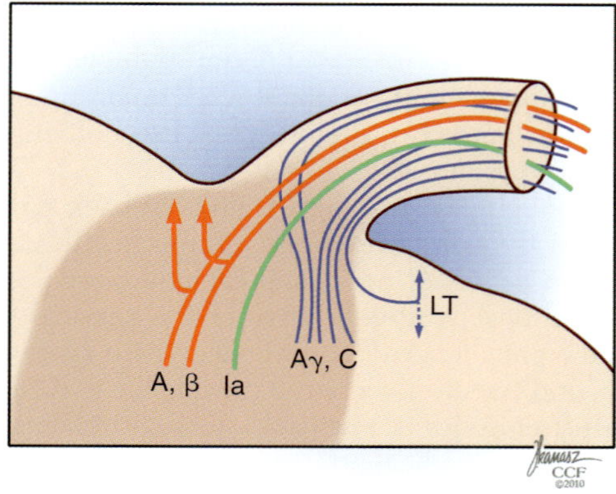

FIGURE 125-2. Diagram of dorsal root entry zone and distribution of different fibers entering the posterior aspect of the spinal cord before forming the Lissauer tract (LT), which is composed mainly of unmyelinated and small myelinated fibers. (Copyright Cleveland Clinic Foundation.)

they enter, others ascend many levels to terminate in higher segments of the cord.[35,38,39]

The dorsal horn is divided into ten laminae as defined by Rexed. Lamina I is related specifically to nociceptive and thermal information and is composed mainly of two types of cells: nociceptive-specific neurons, which respond to noxious stimuli, and wide dynamic range (WDR) cells, which respond to both noxious and non-noxious stimuli and are thought to be major contributors in the development of chronic pain.[22,40] This lamina contributes to the formation of the spinothalamic tract (STT) (Fig. 125-3) and contains primarily substance P, calcitonin gene–related peptide, and enkephalin and serotonin as neuropeptides.[22] Lamina II, also known as the substantia gelatinosa, receives nociceptive, thermoreceptive, and mechanoreceptive input.[40] Cells in this lamina project to laminae I, III, and IV[41] and contain opioid receptors,[40] corroborating the importance of lamina II in modulating nociceptive information.[22,42] Lamina III receives inputs from Aβ fibers and mechanoreceptive Aδ fibers.[22] The sprouting of the low-threshold terminals present in this layer to the more superficial laminae,[40,42] which are generally associated with nociception, suggests a role in chronic pain.[5,43] Lamina V is another important component of nociception because of its inputs from Aδ and C fibers and WDR neurons, contributing to the formation of the STT.[42,44]

The cell projections of laminae I and V, after crossing the anterior aspect of the central canal, course through the STT in the contralateral ventrolateral column to reach the ventroposterior thalamus.[40] Fibers of laminae I, VII, and IX, related to WDR neurons, project to the nonspecific intralaminar nuclei[45-47] and to the brainstem reticular formation,[48,49] periaqueductal gray matter,[50-52] and hypothalamus,[53] forming the paleospinothalamic tract[22] (see Fig. 125-3). Because the WDR neurons have larger receptive fields and respond to different kinds of stimuli when compared to the specific nociceptive neurons, they are involved in poorly localized and nondiscriminative types of pain, in addition to the transformation of acute pain into chronic pain syndrome.[22,52]

After thalamic processing, pain information is projected to the primary somatosensory cortex and secondary somatosensory cortex sequentially.[22,40,54] The thalamus also projects to the insula[20] and the anterior cingular cortex,[20] which are primarily related to the motivational and affective spheres of chronic pain[22] (see Fig. 125-3).

The role of descending pathways in pain modulation is well established,[55] starting in the periaqueductal gray matter, rostral ventromedial medulla, and dorsolateral pontine tegmentum.[20,56] The periaqueductal gray matter receives inputs from the dorsal horn, brainstem, diencephalic system, and cortex[57,58] and sends inhibitory projections to the dorsal horn.[22] It also projects back to the thalamus and orbital

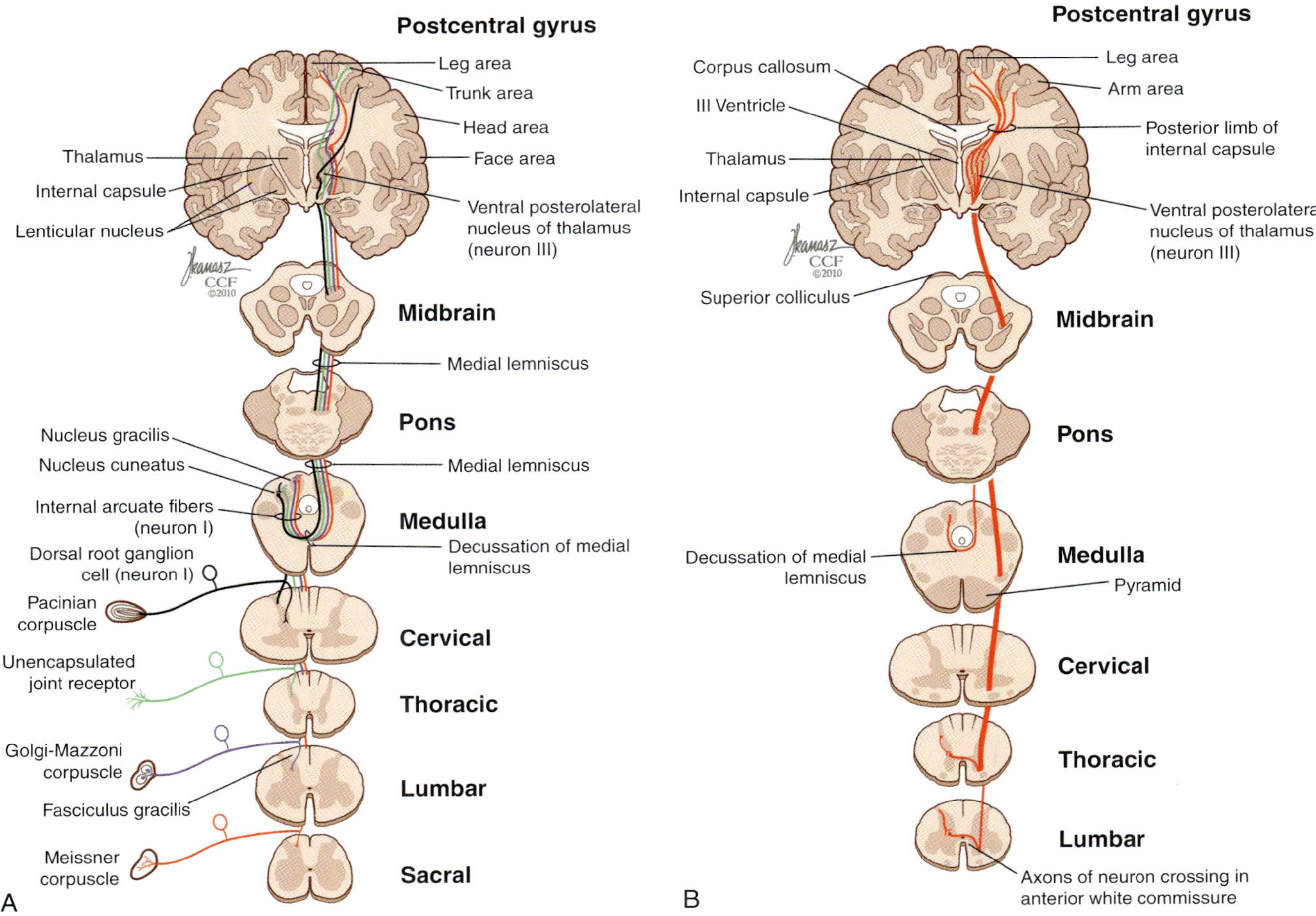

FIGURE 125-3. Diagram of the posterior columns in the spinal cord and the medial lemniscus in the brainstem (**A**) and anterior spinothalamic tract (**B**).

Figure continues on following page

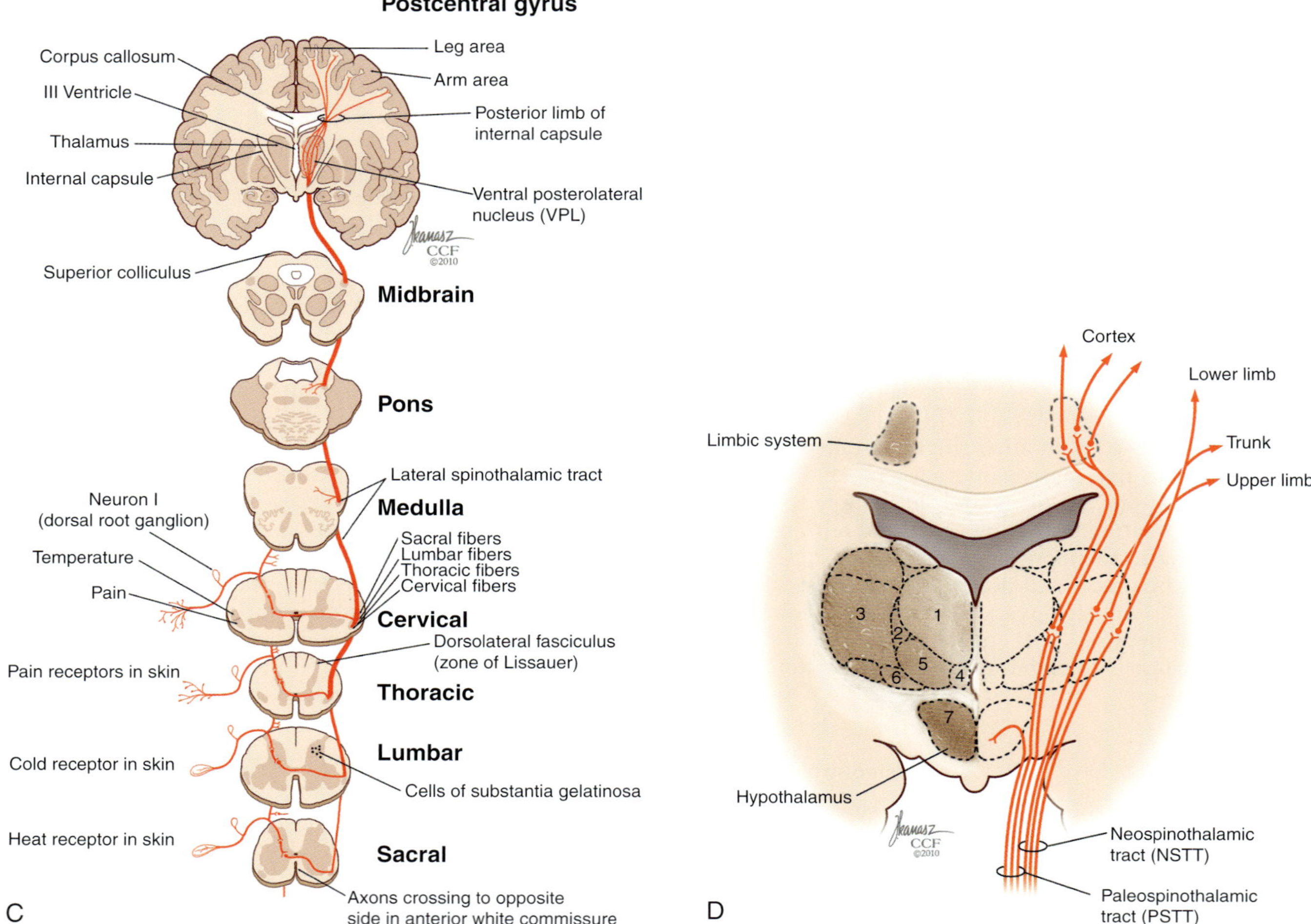

FIGURE 125-3, cont. Diagram of the lateral spinothalamic tract (**C**) and the relays of **A, B,** and **C** in the thalamus and their cortical projections (**D**). The posterior columns are responsible for the transmission of discriminative tactile and kinesthetic information, the anterior spinothalamic tract conveys light touch impulses, and the lateral spinothalamic tract conveys pain and temperature impulses. **D,** 1, dorsomedial nucleus of the thalamus; 2, intralaminar thalamic nuclei; 3, ventral posterolateral thalamic nucleus; 4, parafascicular nucleus of the thalamus; 5, centromedial nucleus of the thalamus; 6, ventral posteromedial thalamic nucleus; 7, hypothalamus. (Copyright Cleveland Clinic Foundation.)

frontal cortex,[59] possibly exerting an ascending control of nociception. Another important pathway that plays a significant role in spinal pain modulation is the noradrenergic system,[60,61] which projects extensively to the dorsal horn (Fig. 125-4). The development of chronic pain is related not only to ascending pain-facilitating mechanisms but also to reduced pain inhibition from descending and ascending modulatory mechanisms.

Physiology of Pain

During inflammation, different events occur that culminate in the generation of prolonged pain. Among these, sensitization and hyperalgesia are significant contributors. However, before continuing this discussion, it is helpful to understand some physiologic conditions involved in these mechanisms.

Each nerve fiber has different physiologic response durations, known as *adaptation*. Because C fibers are usually slowly adapting, and their responses last longer than the stimuli, the occurrence of temporal and spatial summation of painful stimuli during tissue injury may occur.[24] Properties of other fibers include a well-defined receptive field and spontaneous discharges, generated without exogenous stimuli. Summation, expansion of the receptive field, and increase in spontaneous discharges are significantly enhanced during inflammation, leading to the development of hyperalgesia and sensitization.[62] In addition to this mechanism of primary hyperalgesia, secondary hyperalgesia—increased pain sensitivity and allodynia in the surrounding uninjured area—may also occur, secondary to peripheral and central events, such as increased response to glutamate and central neuronal plasticity[63] (Fig. 125-5).

Each sensory cell has specific thresholds to respond to a given stimulus, which is lowered during inflammation. This condition is defined as *sensitization*, which is divided into peripheral and central according to the mechanisms involved.[64] Peripheral sensitization is characterized by a decreased threshold[20] and increased response to suprathreshold stimuli,[65] spontaneous nociceptive neural activity, and expansion of the receptive fields after tissue injury[66,67] (Fig. 125-6). The threshold of nociceptors is decreased as

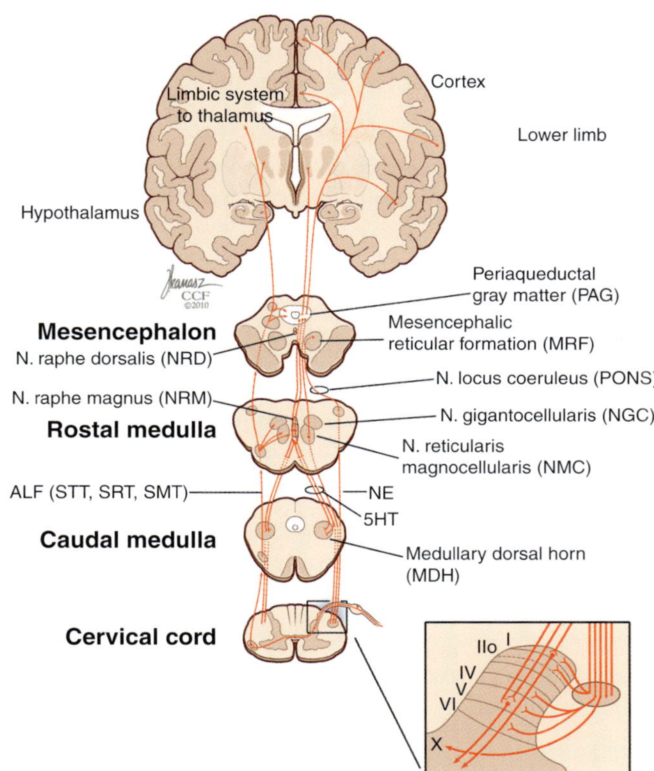

FIGURE 125-4. Diagram of descending inhibitory pain pathways and their respective projections in the dorsal horn. 5HT, serotonin; ALF, anterolateral fasciculus; NE, noradrenaline; SMT, spinomesencephalic tract; SRT, spinoreticular tract; STT, spinothalamic tract. (Copyright Cleveland Clinic Foundation.)

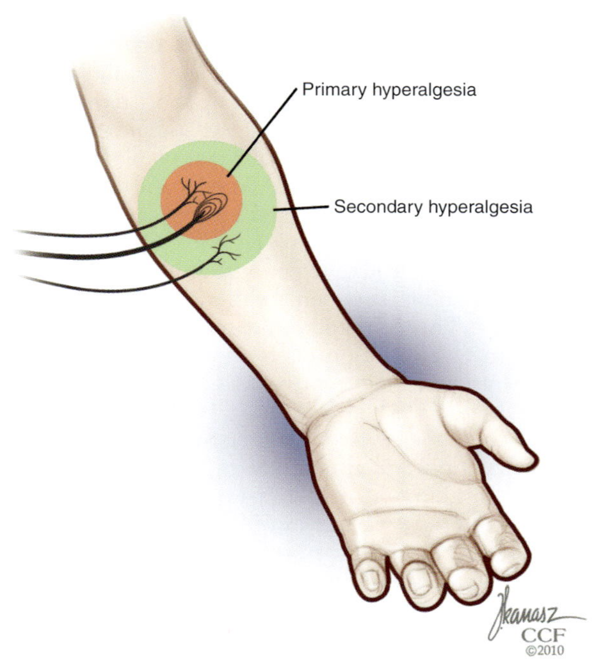

FIGURE 125-5. Primary hyperalgesia is characterized by the increase in pain sensitivity and allodynia in the area of the injured tissue. Secondary hyperalgesia involves the surrounding uninjured area. (Copyright Cleveland Clinic Foundation.)

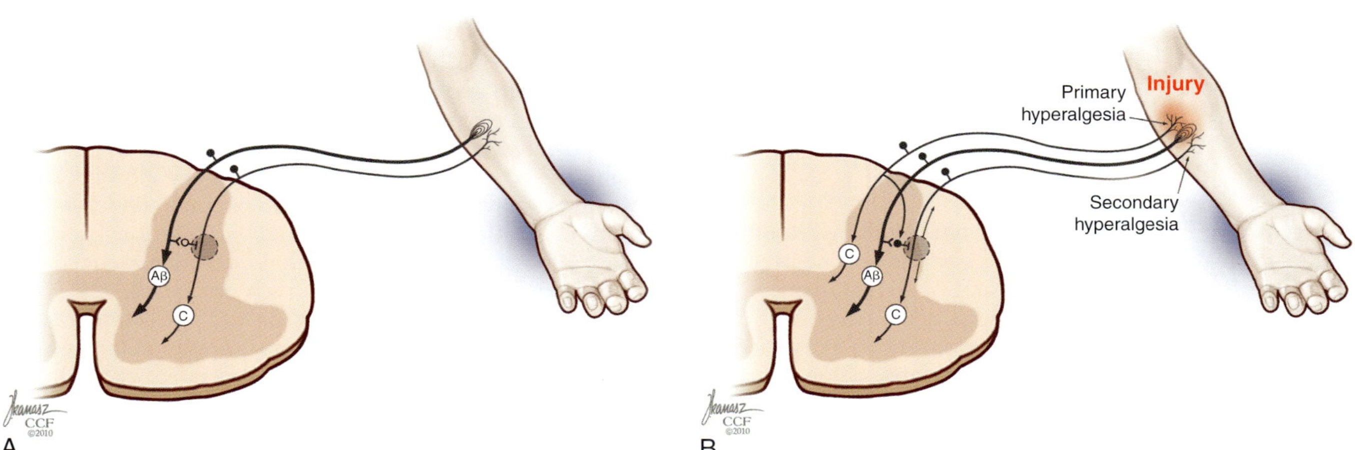

FIGURE 125-6. A, In the normal skin, stimulation of low-threshold Aβ fiber mechanoreceptors does not produce action potentials in nociceptive fibers. **B,** However, in the presence of sensitization, the decreased threshold and hyperexcitability of Aβ fibers are sufficient to generate action potentials in nociceptive afferents, leading to pain to light touch. (Copyright Cleveland Clinic Foundation.)

a result of exposed free nerve endings that fire abnormally. Sprouting of nerve terminals also generates ectopic discharges, as seen in neuromas.[22]

The increase in the number of sodium channels seen in damaged fibers[68] may lead to nociceptor hyperexcitability, which is reverted at least partially by sodium channel blockers.[69] Sympathetic sensitization is also a contributor,[20] with increased nociceptor response to catecholamines of injured[70,71] and uninjured neurons.[72,73] The sensitivity of polymodal WDR receptors is also increased in response to inflammation, causing activation that is no longer triggered preferentially by nociceptive stimuli but also by other mechanical stimuli.[20,63,64,74] Chemomediators are also involved in peripheral sensitization, with the secretion of cytokines interleukin-1β,[75] interleukin-6,[76] and tumor necrosis factor-α[77,78] by lymphocytes, macrophages, and mast cells.

Glutamate levels are increased during inflammation via macrophage and epithelial cell release, activating nociceptors via ion channels and metabotropic receptors.[79-81]

Central sensitization is mediated by short-term and long-term changes in the dorsal horn of the spinal cord.[82-85] This mediation is supported by the occurrence of allodynia in association with the recruitment of Aβ fibers and their sprouting from lamina III into lamina II and loss of regulation of nociceptive fibers.[22] Repetitive stimulation of C fibers, triggered by tissue injury, can lead to hyperexcitability and overactivity of these fibers and further perpetuation of nociceptive transmission.[22,86,87] This perpetuation of nociceptive transmission can result in magnification of the sensory input and consequent expansion of the receptive fields,[84,88-90] a phenomenon known as *wind-up*.[91-93]

A key component in the development of chronic pain is antinociception and the failure of its underlying mechanisms. The inhibitory control of pain pathways is exerted by the spinal cord via several neurotransmitters, in addition to the descending inhibitory system as discussed previously.[22] The most common inhibitory neurotransmitter in the spinal cord is gamma-aminobutyric acid, which mediates presynaptic inhibition of afferents,[94,95] decreased release of neuropeptide P, and postsynaptic inhibition of the STT.[42] Another important inhibitory pathway is the opioid system, with neurotransmitters that bind to three main receptors: mu, the most common opioid receptor in the spinal cord, which has the highest morphine affinity and mediates not only analgesia (μ1) but also respiratory depression (μ2)[22,96,97]; kappa, which binds to dynorphin; and delta, which binds to enkephalins.[42] Opioids exert their action via presynaptic and postsynaptic mechanisms,[98,99] and although they are well known for their analgesic effect, the symptoms caused by central sensitization, such as allodynia, usually do not respond well to these substances.

Cognitive and Behavioral Considerations in Chronic Pain

The gate control theory by Melzack and Wall in 1965[100] is a landmark in the understanding of chronic and neuropathic pain. The gate control theory suggested that pain is not merely transmitted by the peripheral nervous system to the CNS and proposed instead endogenous modulatory mechanisms. According to this theory, pain transmission is modulated by a gating mechanism in the dorsal horn composed of large-diameter and small-diameter fibers that close (inhibit) and open (facilitate) the pain gate.

In 1999, Melzack[101] proposed the neuromatrix theory, refining the gate control theory with additional key elements in pain processing. In the neuromatrix model, pain modulation occurs not only at the spinal level; cerebral mechanisms of pain processing and transmission are also taken into consideration, and cognitive and affective inputs are recognized to influence the final pain experience (Fig. 125-7). Several studies have corroborated further the role of cognitive and limbic systems in central pain processing.[102-105] A patient's beliefs and understanding about his or her pain syndrome, pain sensitivity, fear, anger, depression, anxiety, and catastrophic thinking influence the final pain experience.[102,106,107] Patients who are able to develop techniques to cope with pain and reduce the impact of psychological comorbidities generally have a better prognosis.[108-114]

Based on these advances in understanding of central pain processing, the evaluation of patients with chronic pain should include not only a measure of the sensory component of pain (e.g., verbal, numerical, or visual analogue scales) but also the affective and evaluative components. The McGill Questionnaire has been largely validated as a comprehensive tool for the assessment of various chronic pain conditions, including spine pain.[115] Other inventories can also be used, such as the pain disability index.[116,117] Quality-of-life measurements such as the European Quality of Life Inventory may also be useful in evaluating the impact of the pain syndrome on the patient's life and in assessing outcomes after interventions.

Work disability also plays a key role in the perpetuation of chronic pain, and its impact on long-term prognosis cannot be underestimated. Although the American Medical Association defines *disability* as "an alteration of an individual's capacity to meet personal, social, or occupational demands...because of an impairment,"[118] work disability agencies use more restricted definitions to guide benefit eligibility or ability to work.[119] Compensation for disability and unresolved litigation have a complex influence on treatment outcome. Compensation and litigation have been linked to a poor prognosis,[9,120-123] higher risk to develop chronic pain and pain behavior,[124,125] and a lower likelihood of returning to work.[126,127] Waiting for litigation and benefit disputes to resolve before discussing invasive pain interventions may improve outcomes and obviate the need for intervention.[121,128] Likewise, patients who show little interest for becoming more active or returning to work may be less likely to benefit from additional intervention.[129-131]

Postlaminectomy Syndrome

Low back pain and pain of spinal origin are among the most common chronic pain conditions in the population[132-135] and are associated with physical and psychosocial dysfunction, disability, and reduced quality of life. Although low back pain is more prevalent, neck pain is also a common reason to seek health care. Although approximately 90% of low back pain cases are nonsurgical,[136,137] the proportion of patients undergoing spine surgery has progressively increased,[6,138,139] and success rates remain variable (23–83%).[140-142] Patient selection is known to be a key factor for successful outcomes, and inappropriate indications are likely associated with a higher frequency of postlaminectomy syndrome.[139,143-145]

Postlaminectomy syndrome, also known as *failed back surgery syndrome* (FBSS), is characterized by persistent, recurrent, and chronic back pain with or without radiation to the lower extremities after surgical treatment.[20,134,146] The syndrome comprises different clinical etiologies[138] and can occur after any surgical procedure, with or without fusion or instrumentation.[138] Identification of the etiology of FBSS may assist in directing treatment, which includes medical, rehabilitative, surgical decompression or fusion, and neuromodulatory options.[147] FBSS can be associated with numerous etiologies, including ruptured discs and fragments, which are found in approximately 15% to 35% of cases[138,147,148]; degenerative changes in levels adjacent to instrumentation[149-153]; extensive fusion associated with flat back syndrome[154,155]; pseudarthrosis[156]; and instability

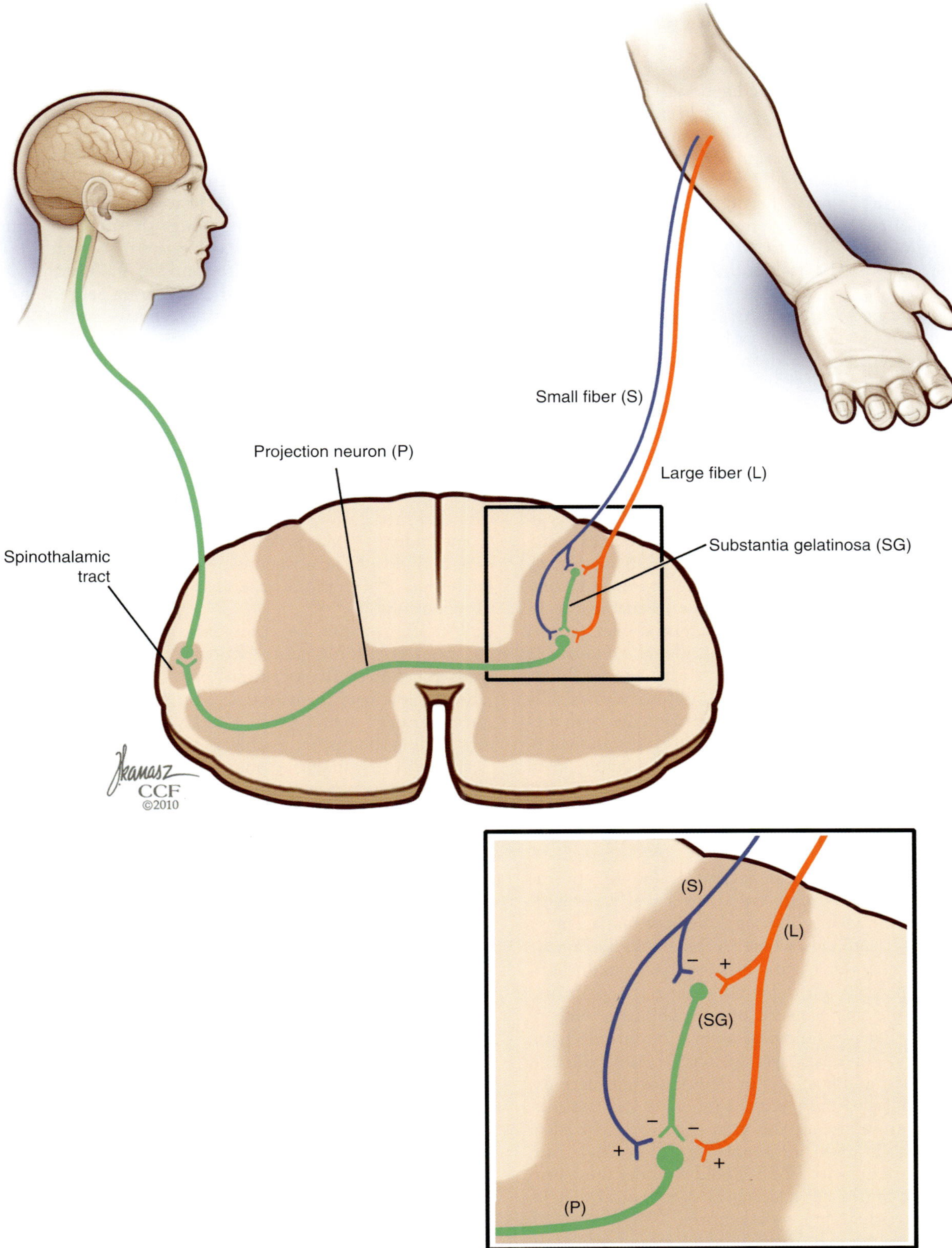

FIGURE 125-7. In the gate control theory, pain transmission is controlled by a gating mechanism in the dorsal horn that can facilitate (small fibers) or inhibit (large fibers) pain transmission. In the neuromatrix theory, cognitive and affective inputs also influence the gating mechanism. (Copyright Cleveland Clinic Foundation.)

caused by facet joint failure after decompression.[142,156] Some FBSS etiologies are associated predominantly with persistent leg pain.

Surgical treatment of spinal stenosis has failure rates of 10% to 30%.[138,147,148] Accurate diagnosis and meticulous decompression may reduce the risk of FBSS.[147] Foraminal stenosis, either residual or worsened by instability,[142,155,157] is responsible for a large proportion of FBSS cases, followed by lateral and central stenosis.[138,147,158] Recurrent or residual disc herniations causing nerve root compression are another common cause of persistent leg pain, with a highly variable incidence ranging from 10% to 50%.[138,147,148] Neuropathic pain caused by prolonged dorsal root ganglion or nerve injury is thought to be less common but may lead to severe and refractory chronic pain.[138,147,148] Arachnoiditis and epidural fibrosis, which can be caused not only by surgical manipulation but also by recurrent irritation and instability, may also lead to persistent pain.[138,142,147,148]

Although there are several alternatives for the management of FBSS, treatment is often challenging. It is common for patients and physicians to be disappointed and frustrated with outcomes. Patients may have already undergone multiple failed interventions, contributing to their psychological distress and reducing the odds that additional treatments will be successful. It is important to discuss treatment expectations beforehand with the patient and family. It is unlikely that additional treatments would be able to resolve completely chronic pain that has been refractory to medical management and surgery. In the setting of chronic back pain, a 50% improvement in pain is usually considered a reasonable outcome.[159] Good candidates for any treatment for FBSS should be motivated to return to work and have a physically active lifestyle.[159] A multidisciplinary approach has been recommended in the management of these difficult conditions, including physical therapy, rehabilitation programs, pain management, and possibly surgical intervention.[160]

Medical Management

Defining a logical algorithm is a critical step in chronic pain treatment, and conservative and reversible treatments are generally instituted first. Because medical management already has been covered elsewhere in this book, it is briefly discussed in this chapter. In this first approach, multidisciplinary assessment may allow for addressing the pain and its etiology and the management of comorbidities, such as depression and other psychological aspects of chronic pain, rehabilitation, and pharmacologic options.[161] Back pain can be associated with modifications in neuromuscular activity, altering abdominal and back muscle function and contributing to the maintenance of the pain state.[162-165] Physical therapy and rehabilitation are mainstays of low back pain treatment, and patients with FBSS should consider these programs, which are aimed at reducing biomechanical deficits and restoring strength and range of motion.[162,166-170]

The most common medications used for treatment of low back pain are nonsteroidal anti-inflammatory drugs, muscle relaxants, opioids, benzodiazepines, antidepressants, and antiepileptic drugs.[171-174] Nonsteroidal anti-inflammatory drugs can be effective for acute and chronic pain,[161,171,175,176] although long-term use of these agents is generally limited by side effects.

Muscle relaxants and benzodiazepines act predominantly on pain states perpetuated by muscle spasms and increased muscle tone and can be beneficial in the management of acute pain[171,173,177]; long-term use for chronic pain is not well established.[161,171,178] Additional care has to be taken with benzodiazepines because of the risk of aggravating depression further and exacerbating the baseline condition.[179,180]

The use of opioids in the treatment of chronic nonmalignant pain is controversial and variable.[171,181-185] Long-term use of narcotics has been linked to tolerance, addiction, and cognitive decline, which emphasizes the need for cautious use of these medications as a long-term option.[184] Their analgesic effects are dose-related and are produced in various levels of the CNS, including the substantia gelatinosa of the spinal cord, the descending antinociceptive system, and the limbic system, altering emotional response and pain behavior.[186-188] Neuropathic pain and allodynia are usually not responsive to opioids because of the activation of *N*-methyl-D-aspartate receptors (increased during central sensitization), leading to phosphorylation and inactivation of the opioid receptor.[22] In this context, the use of opioids in the treatment of nonmalignant pain is more likely beneficial for patients with mainly nociceptive pain that did not respond to other medications, without associated major psychosocial comorbidity.[189] Major long-term complications of opioid use include physical dependence,[190-192] tolerance,[184,185,190] addiction,[184,193] opioid hyperalgesia,[190,194,195] and cognitive dysfunction.[184,196-199]

Antidepressants are commonly prescribed in the management of chronic pain. Although they provide significant pain relief in various chronic pain states,[200-203] studies in chronic low back pain indicate variable efficacy.[204-207] The mechanism of action relies on activation of norepinephrine descending brainstem pathways, which is potentiated by serotonin (5-hydroxytryptamine) pathways.[208] Tricyclic antidepressants such as amitriptyline and imipramine that block the reuptake of norepinephrine and 5-hydroxytryptamine in addition to H_1, adrenergic, and cholinergic receptors tend to be the most efficacious.[208-211]

Anticonvulsants such as carbamazepine, topiramate, gabapentin, and pregabalin are also frequently tried in the medical management of neuropathic pain.[212-215] Improvements in pain scores were seen with the use of these medications,[216] mainly when radiculopathy was present,[214,217-219] although patients with axial symptoms may also have some benefit.[215] Anticonvulsants work primarily via suppression of abnormal discharge at nerve injury sites by Na^+ channel block.[220,221]

Invasive and Surgical Management

Percutaneous Procedures

Patients with FBSS and low back pain caused by ruptured discs or facet joint instability may undergo provocative discography or medial branch block, although the diagnostic usefulness of these methods remains operator-dependent and controversial.[222-225] Minimally invasive techniques can also be considered alternatives for the management of chronic pain related to FBSS. Procedures such as intradiscal electrothermal therapy and medial branch lesioning may provide functional improvement.[223,226-234] Patients with predominantly leg pain may benefit from nerve root blocks as a guide for subsequent treatments.[223,235,236] Pulsed radiofrequency lesioning of dorsal root ganglion has shown promising results in the treatment of radiculopathy associated with low back pain.[237-239] Epidural injections, performed alone or in association with spinal endoscopy, have variable long-term efficacy in this population.[223,240-245]

Reoperation

Reoperation for FBSS in the absence of a clearly defined anatomic cause is a controversial option and may not provide significant improvement of the baseline condition.[140,142,144,157,161,246] Success rates of reoperations in patients with FBSS may vary from 22% to 80% and depend on time of follow-up.[161] Usual indications to consider additional back surgery include reasonable evidence of a surgically treatable condition (instability, compression of a nerve root, or cauda equina), clinical presentation that is compatible with the anatomic lesion, failure to improve with adequate conservative treatment, and management of surgical complications that may need urgent treatment.[144,157,161] Back pain not associated with radicular symptoms, poor outcome after the first procedure, pseudarthrosis, epidural fibrosis, and psychological comorbidities all are factors associated with a worse prognosis.[140,144,145,246,247]

Intraspinal Delivery Devices

A significant proportion of patients with FBSS can fail to achieve pain relief with the previously discussed treatment options and with combined treatment. The use of long-term intrathecal infusion of pharmacologic agents can be considered an alternative in these cases.[248-252] The advantage of this route of administration is in the proximity of the drug to the receptor as it diffuses passively in the dorsal horn, allowing for lower effective doses and consequently a reduced rate of side effects.[250,252,253] Commonly used agents used include opioids, ziconotide, local anesthetics, and α_2 agonists.[250] Clinical trials are under way to evaluate the safety and efficacy of other agents for intrathecal infusion.[254-256] Although long-term intrathecal infusion of opioids is already well established for treatment of malignant pain,[249,251,257,258] the indications for nonmalignant pain are still controversial.[249,259,260] The mechanism of action may include a direct inhibition of dorsal horn cells or a modulatory effect on interneurons, blocking the central transmission of nociceptive information.[261-264] Several studies have shown promising results with short-term outcomes, even in patients with severe and refractory pain.[249,252,265-270] However, studies with long-term follow-up often describe a decrease in responsiveness over time, without success in recapturing the same extent of early benefits.[256,259,271-273]

Appropriate patient selection is an essential step for satisfactory results and includes symptoms that are refractory to less invasive therapies, response to oral doses of opioids, significant response to intrathecal opioid trial, absence of addiction history, and favorable psychosocial evaluation.[249,260,274-277] The option for intrathecal opioids may be more logical in elderly patients, for whom the goal is to achieve some degree of pain alleviation in the final years of life. Long-term management is more complicated in young patients, who are likely to increase the opioid dosage gradually over decades of use.

The intrathecal trial can be performed with sequential injections of bolus dosing with progressively increasing doses or continuous opioid infusion with an externalized catheter.[249] During the trial, the fundamental goals are to assess efficacy in alleviating the chronic pain syndrome, potential side effects, and dosage. Permanent implantation of a pump and catheter system can be considered when a significant improvement is achieved (generally ≥50% reduction in pain) with tolerable side effects.[249,250,259,274]

Different opioids may be used for intrathecal delivery; these include morphine (approved by the U.S. Food and Drug Administration [FDA]), hydromorphone, fentanyl, and sufentanil.[252,269,273,278] Their analgesic potential and side effects are strongly dependent on lipid solubility, and this should be considered when choosing the most appropriate drug for each patient.[188] Hydrophilic drugs, such as morphine, may take longer to alleviate the pain, but the concentration remains high in the cerebrospinal fluid for longer periods, allowing it to ascend to supraspinal levels, enhancing the analgesic effects.[249] Lipophilic drugs, such as fentanyl and sufentanil, have a rapid onset of action and prolonged duration but do not diffuse easily in the cerebrospinal fluid.[249,279]

The most common side effects described with intrathecal opioids include nausea, sedation, confusion, pruritus, urinary retention, myoclonus, reduced libido, and respiratory depression,[259,271,273,280] which are greater with intrathecal hydrophilic drugs.[249] Peripheral edema, usually unresponsive to diuretics, is another side effect of morphine and can be managed by changing to a lipophilic agent.[281-283] Granuloma formation is possibly the most serious long-term adverse effect of intrathecal therapy.[284] Although different agents have been related to this complication,[279,285] it seems to be more common with higher concentrations and doses.[279,286] In addition to routine imaging, screening of patients with intrathecal pump systems has been suggested to enable early detection of masses associated with the catheter tip. A panel of experts has recommended that clinicians managing these patients maintain a high index of suspicion and a low threshold for requesting imaging examination aimed at identified granulomas. Imaging should be considered not only for patients with progressive neurologic deficits but also for patients with subjective changes in neurologic status or loss of efficacy to the intrathecal infusion. Treatment options for catheter tip inflammatory masses include replacing the solution for saline and careful observation of neurologic progress. Patients with neurologic deficits or worsening neurologic examination may need surgical intervention aimed at decompression and removal of the hardware.[286-289]

Ziconotide, a blocking agent of N-calcium channels, is an intrathecal drug approved more recently by the FDA for chronic pain management. Its efficacy has been shown in the literature,[290-294] but the high incidence of serious side effects during the dose titration phase may limit its use.[279] The most common side effects include memory impairment, confusion, hallucinations, dizziness, and ataxia.[290,291,294] Second-line drugs are indicated for opioid-resistant patients and include local anesthetics and α_2 agonists, which act mainly on the neuropathic component of pain, enhancing analgesia.[256] Bupivacaine and clonidine are generally used in combination with morphine and have been shown to restore pain control and improve quality of life.[248,256,295]

The major technical complications related to intrathecal pumps include infections involving the implanted hardware, postural headaches, cerebrospinal fluid leak, pseudomeningoceles, seromas associated with the pump reservoir, and device-related complications. Although the pumps have an expected expiration time, catheter complications are more commonly the cause of premature failure of the implanted system.[296] Spinal cord injury associated with implantation of the catheter has been reported,[297] but its frequency, although thought to be low, has not been established.

Spinal Cord Stimulation

The gate control theory[100] led to the development of novel neuromodulation-based therapies for chronic pain. According to the theory, stimulation of large myelinated fibers could modulate nociceptive input.[100] Encouraging results were seen with peripheral nerve stimulation, taking advantage of the fact that large myelinated fibers can be stimulated at lower thresholds than small unmyelinated fibers.[261,298] In 1967, Shealy et al.[299] described stimulation of the dorsal columns to treat refractory lower extremity pain. Initially, the electrodes were implanted in the subdural space, but the occurrence of complications such as fibrosis and cerebrospinal fluid leak limited their use.[299,300] The technique was later modified to stimulation with epidural electrodes.[301] During the first years of use, spinal cord stimulation (SCS) was attempted in patients with various pain diagnoses, and results were variable.[302] More consistent results have been seen in subsequent series with better patient selection and technologic advances.[303-313] At the present time, it is estimated that approximately 14,000 SCS devices are implanted yearly worldwide.[302] In the United States, the most common indications for SCS are back and leg pain, whether or not associated with FBSS.[248,303,314]

SCS has been shown in well-conducted studies to be effective in alleviating leg pain associated with degenerative spine disease, improving long-term functional capacity and promoting better quality of life.[305,308,309,311,315-317] A systematic review of the literature indicated that successful outcomes after SCS (defined as ≥50% pain improvement) are seen in 59% of cases.[318] Results can vary depending on the series, technique, and patient population, ranging from efficacy rates of 12% to 88%.[315,317,319] Patients with FBSS undergoing SCS have been shown to have significantly superior pain alleviation, enhancement in quality of life, and functional status compared with patients receiving conventional medical management.[306] SCS was also found to be better than reoperation in a selected group of patients with FBSS, with greater pain relief and less crossover to the other arm of the study (reoperation).[315,320] Although SCS implants are expensive, imposing a considerably high initial cost to the health-care system, the overall treatment has been shown to be cost-effective in the long term.[315,321-328]

Patient selection is a major factor determining treatment success. The primary indication for SCS is limb neuropathic pain that is refractory to conservative management, secondary to etiologies such as peripheral nerve or nerve root damage, complex regional syndrome, FBSS, and ischemic pain.[300,320,329,330] The decision-making process for permanent implantation of an SCS system should take into account not only factors related to the pain or neurologic syndromes but also the history of previous interventions, psychological comorbidities, narcotic dependence, and outcome expectation. When a trial is performed, the short-term results of SCS can be used to exclude early nonresponders, although a positive response to the trial with greater than 50% pain relief does not guarantee good long-term results.[320,330] The trial consists of the temporary implantation of an SCS lead that is externalized for a few days.[330]

There are several technical alternatives for permanent implantation of the SCS system. Permanent implantation can be performed with cylindrical leads similar to those typically used for the externalized trials or with surgical (or paddle) leads (Fig. 125-8). Cylindrical leads can be implanted with minimally invasive percutaneous techniques but carry a higher risk of migration.[331] Surgical leads have a lower risk of migration and can be directly anchored to the spinal elements (e.g., the yellow ligament) but require a laminectomy for placement.[331,332] Modern percutaneous leads have 4 to 8 contacts, whereas paddle leads may have 16 contacts built in the lead body. Implantable pulse generators come in various sizes with different programming technologies and can be rechargeable or nonrechargeable devices.

Complications can be divided into stimulation-related, device-related, and surgical types. Stimulation-related complications include uncomfortable paresthesias or positional changes,[317] long-term loss of efficacy, and stimulation in areas not affected by the pain. Higher amplitudes may cause stimulation spread to the thoracic roots, leading to uncomfortable muscle contractions.[330,333] Because SCS is a neuromodulatory technique, adverse effects related to electrical stimulation are usually reversible and can be resolved with reprogramming of the system or turning off the stimulation. Device-related complications have been reported to affect

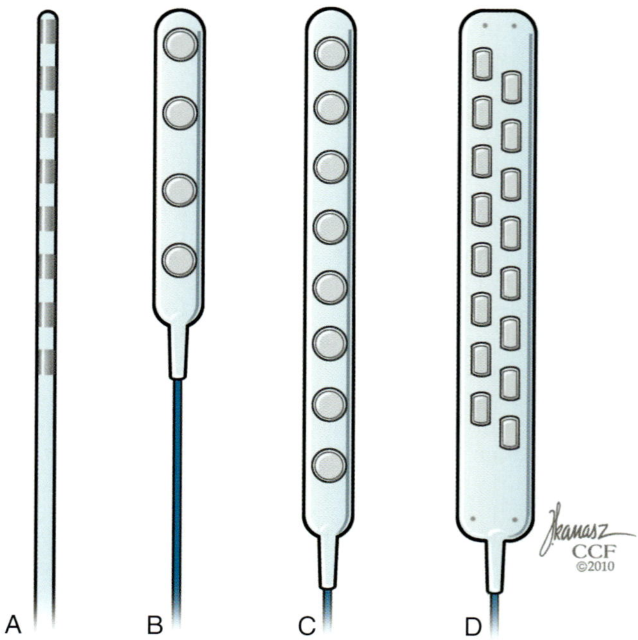

FIGURE 125-8. Different leads used for spinal cord stimulation. Cylindrical leads (**A**) are generally implanted percutaneously, whereas paddle leads (**B–D**) require a laminectomy for placement. The availability of leads with varied numbers of contacts facilitates not only the initial programming but also posterior adjustments of stimulation. (Copyright Cleveland Clinic Foundation.)

approximately 30% of patients.[330] The most common problem is migration of electrodes (more common with cylindrical leads than with paddle leads) resulting in loss of efficacy. Although reprogramming can be attempted to recapture the lost benefits, a surgical revision may be necessary.[317,333] The main complication related to the surgical procedure is infection, with a rate of approximately 4.5%.[311,331,333] Other complications include dural tear with associated spinal headaches or cerebrospinal fluid leak, postoperative hematoma, and neurologic injury, which range from 1% to 9%.[320,330]

Conclusion

Chronic back pain is a highly prevalent problem that can cause significant disability with impaired functional status and poor quality of life. Treatment of this condition is still a challenge for patients and clinicians. Patients with FBSS represent a particularly difficult group, and several treatment alternatives can be considered. Although some patients may benefit from reoperation or conservative management, SCS is a valid alternative and has been shown to be safe and effective for these patients.

KEY REFERENCES

Deer T, Krames ES, Hassenbusch S, et al: Polyanalgesic Consensus Conference 2007: recommendations for the management of pain by intrathecal (intraspinal) drug delivery: report of an interdisciplinary expert panel. *Neuromodulation* 10:300–328, 2007.

Dworkin RH, O'Connor AB, Backonja M, et al: Pharmacologic management of neuropathic pain: evidence-based recommendations. *Pain* 132:237–251, 2007.

Hassenbusch SJ, Portenoy RK, Cousins M, et al: Polyanalgesic Consensus Conference 2003: an update on the management of pain by intraspinal drug delivery—report of an expert panel. *J Pain Symptom Manage* 27: 540–563, 2004.

Kupers RC, Van den Oever R, Van Houdenhove B, et al: Spinal cord stimulation in Belgium: a nation-wide survey on the incidence, indications and therapeutic efficacy by the health insurer. *Pain* 56:211–216, 1994.

Mailis-Gagnon A, Furlan AD, Sandoval JA, et al: Spinal cord stimulation for chronic pain. *Cochrane Database Syst Rev* 3:CD003783, 2004.

Raslan AM, McCartney S, Burchiel KJ: Management of chronic severe pain: spinal neuromodulatory and neuroablative approaches. *Acta Neurochir Suppl* 97(Pt 1):33–41, 2007.

Turner JA, Sears JM, Loeser JD: Programmable intrathecal opioid delivery systems for chronic noncancer pain: a systematic review of effectiveness and complications. *Clin J Pain* 23:180–195, 2007.

REFERENCES

The complete reference list is available online at expertconsult.com.

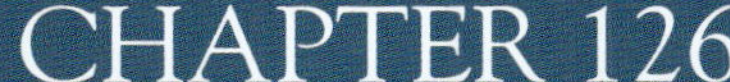
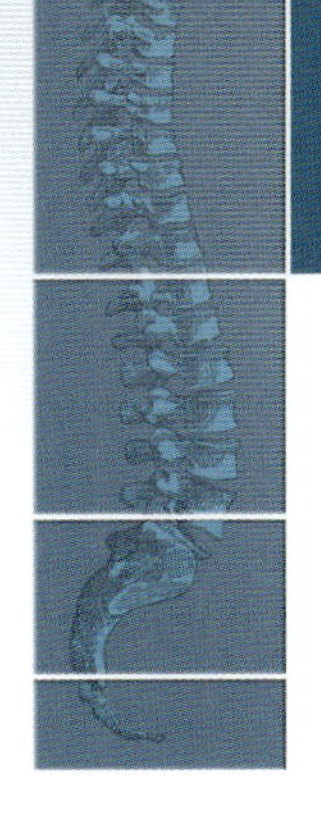

CHAPTER 126

Minimally Invasive Spinal Decompression and Stabilization Techniques I

Sait Naderi | Joseph Watson | Nevan G. Baldwin | Maurice M. Smith

Ideally, minimally invasive techniques should achieve the operative goal with minimal tissue disruption. In spinal stabilization surgery, particularly in the thoracic and lumbar regions, much of the associated morbidity is secondary to the extensive soft tissue dissection necessary to widely expose the spine for arthrodesis.

Percutaneous fixation of the thoracic and lumbar spine was used as an alternative to invasive surgery in the 1980s. At the same time, growing experience with percutaneous discectomy nurtured the development of fusion techniques to accompany decompression. The current widespread use of minimally invasive techniques in thoracic and abdominal surgery has been a catalyst for the development of less invasive ventral approaches to the spine.

The anatomic and biomechanical differences among the cervical, thoracic, and lumbar regions of the spine create completely different issues in the approach to decompression and stabilization of each region. Techniques for minimally invasive treatment are considered for each region separately; however, many of the principles of complication avoidance and management apply to all regions. There has been far more experience with techniques in the lumbar spine than in the thoracic region. Comparatively few data have yet been obtained on cervical spine approaches.

The evolution of minimally invasive spinal surgery for decompression of the neural structures began with the uniportal procedures, using the arthroscope for decompression of contained disc herniations. The first laparoscopic lumbar discectomy was reported by Obenheim in 1991.[1] The efficacy of different endoscopic surgical procedures has been documented, leading to the development of more complex and biportal arthroscopic procedures for treatment of noncontained herniations.

The use of minimally invasive surgery for fusion of motion segments of the spine was introduced at a later date. Magerl introduced this technique for percutaneous external transpedicular fixation of the thoracic and lumbar spine in the 1980s.[2] Percutaneous dorsolateral interbody fusion also was performed successfully by Leu and Schreiber, who reported on the procedure in 1991.[3] Drawbacks of these procedures included the likelihood of screw tract infection and discomfort associated with externally placed implants.

Recent advances in the evolution of minimally invasive surgery for fusion and stabilization include: (1) percutaneous interbody fusion during arthroscopic disc surgery; (2) transperitoneal and thoracoscopic placement of the interbody cage implant in the lumbar spine and thoracic spine, as well as placement of the transpedicular screw, combined with temporary subcutaneous plates in the lumbar spine; (3) placement of the plates and screws in the thoracic spine; (4) percutaneous translaminar facet screw placement; (5) percutaneous odontoid screw placement; (6) image-guided upper cervical spine instrumentation; and (7) robotic transpedicular screw placement. Other researchers simultaneously were developing techniques for fusion with new approaches, including the extreme lateral approach for lumbar interbody fusion (XLIF), transforaminal lumbar interbody fusion (TLIF), and axial interbody fusion (AxiALIF, TranS1, Wilmington, NC) techniques.

Leu[4] was one of the first to use endoscopy for spinal fusion, both ventrally and dorsolaterally. Endoscopic spinal fusion was performed first in the lumbar spine. Interest in the use of minimally invasive surgery for thoracic spine disease has increased recently. The initial results, using video-assisted thoracoscopic surgery (VATS), are encouraging, because this procedure is characterized by less pain and shorter hospital stays.[5-7]

Regan et al.[8-10] reported their results in thoracic spinal pathology using ventral and dorsal interbody grafting, with and without instrumentation. Rosenthal[11] reported the use of VATS for ventral decompression and stabilization in patients with metastatic tumors or scoliotic deformities of the thoracic spine. His technique involves endoscopic microsurgical decompression, combined with reconstructive techniques and instrumentation placed through thoracoscopic portals.

Advantages and Difficulties

The main advantages of endoscopic spine surgery are its lower morbidity, attributable to the minimally invasive approach, and cosmetic advantages. Significantly less postoperative pain is experienced by these patients because of the avoidance of extensive muscular incision and removal of ribs. There also is less impairment of pulmonary function after VATS. Dorsolateral endoscopic approaches for pedicular fixation result in less epidural bleeding, decreased incidence of perineural and intraneural fibrosis, and less venous stasis.

The most significant disadvantage of endoscopic stabilization is that it is time consuming. This aspect can be overcome, but there is a considerable learning curve. The technology and equipment costs for this approach also create a large "up front" investment requirement. All endoscopic approaches, especially thoracoscopic approaches, can be converted to open procedures, if necessary, to control bleeding or to deal with excessive adhesions.

Indications and Contraindications

Although the indications for endoscopic fusion and stabilization are similar to those for open procedures, the options are more limited. Endoscopic stabilization can be performed after decompression for burst fractures, spinal tumors, and spinal deformities (e.g., idiopathic scoliosis and Scheuermann disease), and for instability secondary to degenerative disease of one or two motion segments.

Contraindications to endoscopic dorsolateral lumbar spine fusion and stabilization include (1) considerable loss of intervertebral disc height, preventing decortication of the end plates; (2) severe spinal deformity associated with distorted neural and pedicular anatomy; (3) infection; (4) failed previous operation for interbody fusion; and (5) very large tumors requiring extensive resection.[12]

Contraindications to VATS include (1) inability to tolerate deflation of one lung, (2) significant respiratory disease, and (3) previous open thoracotomy.[13]

Contraindications to laparoscopic transperitoneal lumbar fusion and stabilization include (1) significant abdominal trauma, (2) previous transabdominal lumbar operation, and (3) previous lower abdominal laparoscopic procedure (e.g., hysterectomy).[14]

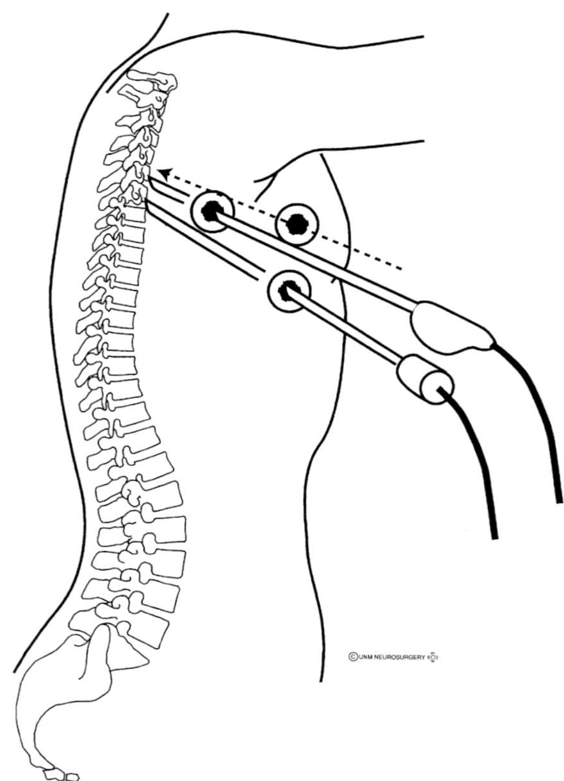

FIGURE 126-1. Thoracoscopic spinal surgery. Portal placement varies according to the level of the pathology. More portals also may be required for procedures with instrumentation to allow improved angles for hardware placement and access for retractors and other instruments.

Approaches

The anatomic features of different regions of the spine dictate a variety of endoscopic approaches for fusion and stabilization. A thoracic spine endoscopic approach necessitates VATS, whereas a lumbar spine instability requires a ventral approach, a lateral approach, a dorsolateral approach, or a combined approach. The choice of endoscopic approach in the lumbar spine is guided largely by surgeon preference.

Thoracic Spine

The most important minimally invasive technique for decompression and stabilization of the thoracic spine is VATS. This technique has been applied to a variety of thoracic spine disorders, including tumor, infection, disc disease, and deformity. VATS is performed using a double-lumen tube for deflation of the ipsilateral lung with the patient under general anesthesia and in the lateral decubitus position (Fig. 126-1).

Method

Instruments required for an open thoracotomy should be readily available for emergency use. A left- or right-sided approach may be used, depending on the pathology. Some authors prefer a right-sided approach if the pathology is not lateralized, because there is more space lateral to the azygos vein than the aorta. Consideration should be given to the position of the artery of Adamkiewicz if the intervention requires the sacrifice of one or more segmental arteries in the middle to lower thoracic region, especially T9-11 on the left.

The initial trocar should be inserted in the manner of a tube thoracostomy (over the top of the rib) in the anterior axillary line at the sixth or seventh intercostal space. Multiple working trocars may be used for instrument insertion as necessary. Soft trocars are preferred for the portals because they are less traumatic to the neurovascular bundle on the inferior rib undersurface. The size of the instrument is limited only by the intercostal distance.

The surgical levels are identified by counting ribs, preferably with fluoroscopy, and by marking in the disc space. Alternatively, ribs may be counted endoscopically from the first rib down. The rib number corresponds to the lower vertebral body at the disc space (e.g., sixth rib at T5-6). Adequate exposure of the disc space usually requires resection of the rib head, except in the lower thoracic region where the rib head may be well caudal to the disc space, permitting unobstructed access. Attention to the segmental vascular branches in the mid-bodies is advised. Stabilization across the vertebral body requires the careful division of these vascular structures. The sympathetic chain also may be identified in the surgical field through the parietal pleura. Varying anatomy of the regions of the thoracic spine dictates different exposure techniques. For the upper thoracic region, it may be necessary to elevate and support the ipsilateral arm to rotate the scapula away. In the lower thoracic region, it may be necessary to retract the diaphragm.

After exploratory thoracoscopy using a 30-degree-angle scope, a second trocar is inserted. If complete atelectasis is not achieved, a brief period of CO_2 insufflation may help to collapse the lung. As the thoracic spine is visualized through the parietal pleura, the correct level is identified by counting the ribs. Radiographic confirmation by fluoroscopy or a plain radiograph also can be obtained. The parietal pleura is then divided using monopolar cautery. After the fluoroscopic identification of the correct level, the third and fourth ports are inserted at the level of the pathology. A 0- or 30-degree-angle scope can be used. Generally, 2 to 3 cm of rib resection and partial resection of the pedicle are adequate. After using electrocautery to "clean up" the surrounding soft tissues, a discectomy with decompression is performed. Bleeding at this stage can be controlled by bipolar electrocautery, argon beam coagulation, or packing the area with hemostatic agents (e.g., Gelfoam or Surgicel).

Uncontrolled bleeding may necessitate conversion to an open procedure. Therefore, it is advisable to have an open thoracotomy setup available.

On completion of the decompression, fusion can be performed using bone chips obtained from a rib or harvested from the iliac crest. Regan et al.[10] described the placement of an interbody cage into the disc space after decompression.

Rosenthal[11] described reconstruction by homologous bone or by injection of semiliquid methylmethacrylate. He used a ventral plate and screw system (Z-plate, Sofamor-Danek, Memphis, TN) for fixation and special equipment for dilation of the skin incision during the insertion of the plate, and for insertion of instruments for handling the plates and screws in the chest cavity. These techniques allow the surgeon to address pathology resulting from degenerative disease, trauma, or metastatic disease, and then to stabilize the spine with methylmethacrylate struts, cages, or plates.[11,15-17]

After completion of the entire decompression and stabilization procedure, a tube thoracostomy is placed and the lung is reexpanded.

Complications

As with laparoscopic procedures, there is an entire complement of risks associated with the intrathoracic approach. Reported complications include prolonged atelectasis, pleural effusions, intercostal neuralgia, and diaphragmatic injury.[15-17] Time of lung collapse (i.e., length of operation) is related to the pulmonary morbidity associated with chest procedures. Therefore, until the operating surgeon has become familiar with the thoracoscopic spine procedures, he or she may expect longer operating times and some increased morbidity. In one series of thoracic endoscopic discectomies, the complication rate was 14%, which was compatible with the reported complication rate with open approaches.[18] The use of flexible portals may reduce the incidence of intercostal neuralgia, although this still occurred in 2 of 17 patients in whom the flexible portals were used.[15] Complications related to the decompression, in a series of 77 patients, were excessive epidural bleeding in one patient and transient paraparesis in another.[16] In a comparative study, Mangione et al. reported less blood loss and a shorter hospital stay, as well as a similar rate of complication after VATS, when compared with open thoracoscopic thoracic spine decompression.[19]

Operating at the wrong level is always a concern in the thoracic spine. This may be avoided by ruling out variant anatomy (e.g., accessory ribs), using preoperative radiographs, and accepting only high-quality radiographic images intraoperatively.

Lumbar Spine

A variety of laparoscopic, endoscopic, minimally invasive, and robotic techniques currently are used to stabilize and/or decompress the lumbar spine.

Fusion and Instrumentation

Laparoscopic Transperitoneal Surgery for the Lumbar Spine

The ventral endoscopic approach is limited primarily to the L4-5 and L5-S1 disc spaces because of the relation of the aorta and vena cava to the spine. The increased use of minimally invasive abdominal and retroperitoneal procedures with the laparoscope has paved the way for its use as an approach to the spine.

Despite limited enthusiasm for laparoscopic ventral discectomy for the treatment of simple disc disease,[10] interbody fusion techniques have received a warm welcome, as evidenced by the number of meeting presentations and papers on the topic.[16,20-26] The procedure has evolved from the placement of bone graft in the interspace to the use of titanium interbody distraction cages.

Technique

The ventral exposure of the lumbar spine from the peritoneal cavity is limited to L5-S1 and variably to L4-5. Laparoscopic exposure is performed in the routine manner, similar to an intra-abdominal procedure. This includes a bowel preparation, insertion of a Foley catheter and a nasogastric tube, and preincisional prophylactic antibiotics. The patient is supine in the Trendelenburg position, with the back extended using large rolls under the lumbosacral junction (Fig. 126-2). Insufflation techniques are standard, but a gasless technique also is described, which does not require specially designed instruments.[27] Assistance from a general surgeon comfortable with laparoscopy is advised.

Exposure of the L5-S1 space requires incision of the parietal peritoneum over the disc in the midline. Fluoroscopy is used to identify the disc properly. The midline sacral artery and vein must be divided. The parietal peritoneum is mobilized using blunt dissection, with bleeding controlled by bipolar electrocautery (rather than unipolar cautery), for fear of injuring the closely related autonomic plexus. At the L4-5 space the exposure can be more difficult, because the disc space often sits at the crotch of the bifurcation of the great vessels. Gentle retraction of the common iliac vein and artery is required, and it may be necessary to sacrifice segmental branches. Exposure may be facilitated by inserting Steinmann pins into the L4 vertebral body to give static retraction of the vessels.

Discectomy is performed by sharp incision of the ventral anulus fibrosus and by radical removal of disc material with curets and pituitary forceps. Fusion proceeds by distraction of the disc space and insertion of bone graft under compression.

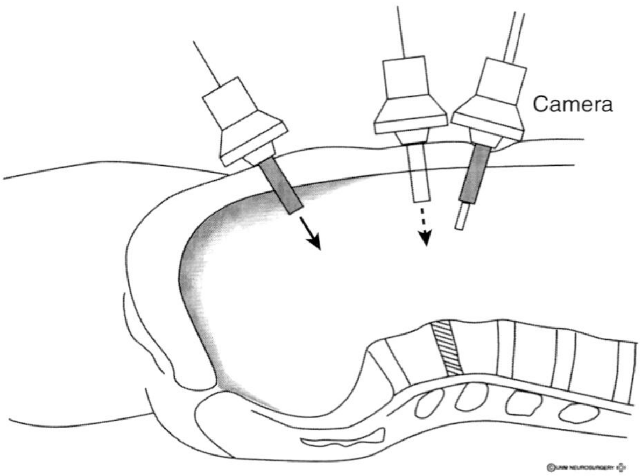

FIGURE 126-2. The transperitoneal approach to endoscopic lumbar interbody fusion. Insufflation is maintained through the caudal portal, while dissection and instrumentation are performed through the portal directly aligned with the interspace.

Currently popular is the use of a threaded titanium cage, which has been cleared by the U.S. Food and Drug Administration and is commercially available for open procedures. It also is cleared for endoscopic placement from the ventral approach. With the endoscopic placement, the procedure is outlined as follows: an estimate of graft size is made on the basis of the preoperative radiographs and specific templates provided by the manufacturer of the device. The sizes are checked in situ to confirm that adequate exposure is available. Next, a disc space distractor is placed on one side of the midline. On the other side, a circular hole is drilled (under fluoroscopic guidance to ensure a trajectory parallel to the vertebral end plates) to a depth of approximately two thirds of the diameter of the disc space. The hole is then tapped, and the titanium implant, filled with autologous bone chips, is screwed into the disc space. The distractor is then removed, and the tapping/implant procedure is repeated at the site previously occupied by the distractor. The implants should be sufficiently countersunk so that no aspect comes into contact with the overlying vascular structures. The peritoneum is then reapproximated over the site. The exposure and anatomy may dictate that only one graft be placed. However, this is not as biomechanically sound as two cages, placed side by side, especially in lateral flexion.[20] Currently, other materials such as threaded allograft dowels also are available for transperitoneal endoscopic fusion operations.

A retroperitoneal approach to the ventral aspect of the spine at levels L4-5 and L5-S1 with interbody fusion also is technically feasible. This reduces the chance of postoperative adynamic ileus and intra-abdominal adhesions. This approach also provides access to the lateral aspects of level L1-4, although the great vessels prevent midline access at these levels. Previous abdominal surgery is a relative contraindication for the transperitoneal exposure. This is not an issue with the retroperitoneal approach. An experience with 20 cases has been reported.[24]

Complications

Complications associated with transperitoneal exposure are uncommon. However, they require immediate management by experienced abdominal surgeons. An experience with 17 cases included significant ileus in four patients, which required, in two patients, an open laparotomy for bleeding. In addition, there were two graft donor site infections.[26] In another series of 22 cases, 1 iliac vein laceration was encountered, as well as 2 bone donor site infections.[16] In the small series of ventral retroperitoneal fusions, no significant complications were reported.[24] Sexual dysfunction is a dreaded complication of this approach, resulting from disruption of the sacral autonomic plexus. Several cases of transient (3 weeks) retrograde ejaculation were reported in a series using an open anterior lumbar interbody fusion technique.[20] It is recommended that, in men, reflection of the parietal peritoneum over the ventral disc space be performed with the aid of bipolar rather than monopolar electrocautery to prevent the spread of current and reduce the risk of damage to the autonomic plexus.[20,27] If Steinmann pins are used, care must be taken during removal, as well as insertion, so that the sharp tip does not lacerate a vessel, particularly the iliac vein. The hazards of the approach and drilling the disc space adjacent to the iliac vessels are ameliorated with special instruments to protect the vessels during drilling. Familiarity with these instruments is imperative.

Dorsolateral Endoscopic Transpedicular Fixation

The dorsolateral approach is performed with the patient under general anesthesia and in the prone position. After a standard arthroscopic discectomy, both end plates are decorticated. Using a pedicular jig, the guide pins are placed in the center of the pedicles under fluoroscopic control. A cannulated pedicle obturator is placed over the guidewire, and the soft tissues surrounding the pedicle are bluntly dissected. Extended-length pedicle screws are inserted under fluoroscopic control. The extensions are connected to the subcutaneous plate.

The major advantages of this form of arthrodesis are the use of local anesthesia and the lack of blood loss. When the procedure is used in conjunction with an external fixator, some of these advantages are lost, because this component of the procedure carries significant risks of infection and nerve root damage. The major disadvantage is the limited exposure, which prevents the placement of oversized bone graft into the disc space under compression and prevents placement of ventral instrumentation. The result is limited ventral column support during healing. Furthermore, the percutaneous techniques are limited with regard to their ability to decompress the spinal canal and are contraindicated in the presence of a sequestered disc rupture.

Results

Although the total experience with minimally invasive techniques in spine surgery is small in comparison with the vast experience with open procedures, the early results are encouraging (Table 126-1). Follow-up of these patients, to date, has been relatively short. Mathews et al.[21] reported successful fusion in all of their first five cases. McAfee et al.,[28] reporting the complications in the first 50 endoscopic procedures in a multicenter study, did not observe any great vessel complications. The complications reported by other authors include cage extrusion, inferior vena cava laceration, dorsal disc extrusion, prolonged ileus, and atelectasis. Zucherman and Zdeblick[29] and Novotny et al.[23] reported that 2 of 23 (9%) and 2 of 8 (25%) operated cases, respectively, were converted to open surgery.

TABLE 126-1

Recently Reported Series of Patients Undergoing Fusion and Stabilization via Endoscopic Procedures

Author	No. of Patients	Procedure
Mathews et al. (1991)[39]	4	ALIF
Novotny et al. (1994)[23]	8	TP-ALIF with cage or femoral allograft
McAfee et al. (1994)[22]	10	TP fusion
Mathews et al. (1994)[21]	5	TP with iliac crest
Kambin and Schaffer (1996)[12]	25	Lumbar posterolateral
Zuckerman et al. (1996)[14]	23	TP with cage implant
Rosenthal et al. (1996)[17]	12	Thoracoscopic with ventral plate
Regan (1996)[18]	7	Thoracoscopic with anterior instrumentation
Dickman et al. (1996)[5]	1	Thoracoscopic fusion

ALIF, anterior lumbar interbody fusion; TP, transperitoneal.
Note that cases involving decompression only are excluded from the table.

The first results of minimally invasive surgery for spine decompression and stabilization are encouraging. However, some problems persist, including long operation time, the requirement for expensive equipment, and the steep learning curve.[30] With increased experience, the rate of complications should decrease. Technologic advances should improve the safety of these operations and also may broaden the indications for the application of these techniques.

Percutaneous Translaminar Facet Screw Fixation

Percutaneous translaminar facet screw fixation using fluoroscopy was performed successfully.[31,32] Shim et al.[32] reported that this technique was a safe and useful minimally invasive dorsal augmentation method following ALIF or axiALIF.

Robotic Instrumentation

Robotic systems currently are used in a few spine centers for transpedicular and translaminar screw fixations. The results show an average accuracy level of within 1 mm relative to the surgeon's plan in both pedicle screw and translaminar facet screw applications in most of the procedures. Pechlivanis et al.[33] reported a deviation of less than 2 mm in 91.0% of cases. The major disadvantage of robotic systems is the increased cost; the major advantages include reduced radiation exposure and increased accuracy.

Extreme Lateral Approach for Lumbar Interbody Fusion

The extreme lateral approach for lumbar interbody fusion (XLIF), a modification of the retroperitoneal approach to the lumbar spine, was first presented in 2001 by Pimenta, who has performed more than 100 lateral trans-psoas surgeries since 1998. The equipment currently used in this procedure does not require additional capital expenditure. An operative microscope may be used but is not required. The XLIF technique can be safely used for interbody fusion of L3-4 and L4-5. Because of the location of the iliac bone, however, this technique cannot be applied to the L5-S1 level. Ozgur et al.[34] reported successful results using the XLIF technique.

Transforaminal Lumbar Interbody Fusion

Transforaminal lumbar interbody fusion (TLIF) also is used for interbody fusion of the lumbosacral spine. The technique requires a lumbar paramedian incision, paravertebral dissection, facet resection, discectomy, and cage placement. The upper and lower lumbar vertebrae are commonly instrumented by ipsilateral transpedicular screws.[21,35,36]

Axial Interbody Fusion

Axial interbody fusion (AxiALIF), recently developed for L5-S1 interbody fusion, uses a percutaneous paracoccygeal approach. It is indicated for minor instabilities of the L5-S1 level, for L5-S1 discogenic pains, and for pseudarthrosis of L1 screws. It can be used alone or in combination with minimally invasive L5-S1 translaminal facet screw fixation or L5-S1 transpedicular instrumentation. Early results are encouraging.[37,38]

Lumbar Discectomy

With or without laser nucleotomy, lumbar discectomy is the most commonly used minimally invasive technique.[39] Three major pathways are used to perform lumbar discectomy: dorsolateral uni- or biportal discectomy, transforaminal endoscopic discectomy, and dorsal midline endoscopic discectomy.[40-42] Dorsolateral uni- or biportal discectomy is the earliest technique, using a small incision 8 cm lateral to the midline and almost 45 degrees of working canal. A midline approach is similar to the microdiscectomy technique, whereas the transforaminal technique approaches the neural foramen first. Endoscopic discectomy provides better pain relief, shorter hospitalization stays, earlier return to work, and less paraspinal muscle atrophy.[43,44] Ruetten at al.,[40] using a transforaminal technique, reported that patients had a lower rate of low back pain after the endoscopic procedure when compared with microdiscectomy.

Complications of Endoscopic Discectomy

Complications associated with percutaneous lumbar discectomy are few, but include a 1% to 2% risk of discitis and a 1% to 2% risk of a symptomatic psoas muscle hematoma. Anecdotal evidence indicates that there is a risk of injury to the nerve roots or surrounding vascular structures.[41,45-47] As is emphasized elsewhere in this textbook, careful placement of the guidewire is crucial for the avoidance of complications with this approach. Theoretically, the risks of infection and injury to the great vessels are increased by the manipulations of bone grafting. However, this has not been demonstrated clinically.

Cervical Spine Decompression

Despite advances in available technology and interest in minimally invasive stabilization procedures in the thoracic and lumbar spine, relatively few reports on the use of these methods in the cervical spine have been published. Percutaneous discectomy and chemonucleolysis of the cervical spine reportedly have been effective in selected patients in uncontrolled trials.[48,49] Percutaneous disc access requires a ventrolateral approach. The needle entry is at the medial border of the sternocleidomastoid muscle. With the fingers of one hand acting to separate the carotid sheath and esophagus, the needle is passed under fluoroscopic control into the desired disc space. Although percutaneous decompression has been described, concomitant fusion has not been reported to date.

Microendoscopic technique has been popularized during recent years. Using a small incision for a mini-keyhole foraminotomy, nerve root can be exposed and decompression for both spondylotic changes and disc herniation can be performed.[50,51] Fessler and Khoo[50] reported less blood loss, shorter hospitalization stays, less use of narcotics, and better pain relief after cervical microendoscopic foraminotomy when compared with the open technique.

Percutaneous surgical techniques have been recently popularized in craniovertebral junction surgery. The first results after percutaneous odontoid screw fixation and C1-2 fixation are encouraging.[52,53]

Conclusion

Minimally invasive spine surgery opened new era in spine surgery. The process began with simple discectomy and was then extrapolated for complex spine procedures. These techniques were associated with shorter hospital stays, less blood loss, less muscle injury, and an earlier return to work.

KEY REFERENCES

Dickman CA, Rosenthal D, Karahalios DG, et al: Thoracic vertebrectomy and reconstruction using a microsurgical thoracoscopic approach. *Neurosurgery* 38:279–293, 1996.

Fessler RG, Khoo LT: Minimally invasive cervical microendoscopic foraminotomy: an initial clinical experience. *Neurosurgery* 51(Suppl 5):S37–S45, 2002.

Mac MJ, Regan JJ, Bobechko WP, Acuff TE: Application of thoracoscopy for disease of the spine. *Ann Thorac Surg* 56:736–738, 1993.

Ruetten S, Komp M, Merk H, Godolias G: Full-endoscopic anterior decompression versus conventional anterior decompression and fusion in cervical disc herniations. *Int Orthop* 33:1677–1682, 2009.

Sachs BL, Schwaitzberg SD: Lumbosacral (L5-S1) discectomy and interbody fusion technique. In Regan JJ, McAfee PC, Mack MJ, editors: *Atlas of endoscopic spine surgery*, St Louis, 1995, Quality Medical Publishing, p 275.

Shim CS, Lee SH, Jung B, et al: Fluoroscopically assisted percutaneous translaminar facet screw fixation following anterior lumbar interbody fusion: technical report. *Spine* 30:838–843, 2005.

REFERENCES

The complete reference list is available online at expertconsult.com.

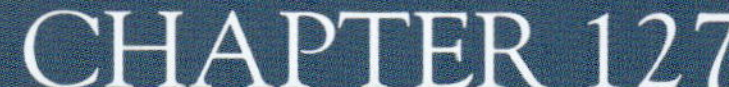
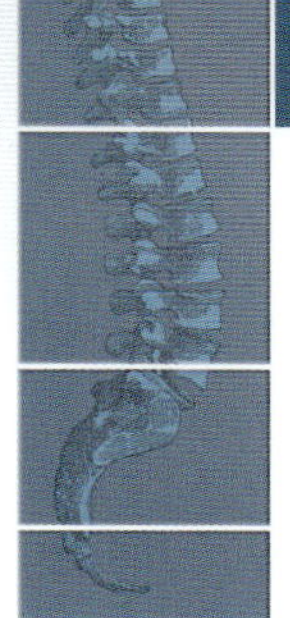

CHAPTER 127

Minimally Invasive Spinal Decompression and Stabilization Techniques II: Thoracic and Lumbar Endoscopic Approaches

Richard J. Parkinson | Isador H. Lieberman | Zachary A. Smith | Richard G. Fessler | John Regan

History

Endoscopic spine surgery refers to a rapidly evolving set of techniques potentially offering equivalent surgical outcomes with lower surgical morbidity. This includes traditional endoscopic access to a hollow cavity such as the thoracic cavity and "manufactured" cavities for spinal access. Endoscopic spine surgery does not refer to a single technique but rather to a set of tools that may be used during the approach to the spine. The philosophy behind spine endoscopy is to target the pathology and apply a therapeutic intervention while minimizing damage to surrounding nonpathologic tissues.[1-3] These endoscopic techniques are part of a trend toward less ("minimally") invasive interventions.

Endoscopy uses a fiberoptic camera and light source for visualization and magnification through a small percutaneous portal or portals.

Endoscopic inspection of the thoracic cavity was initially conceived by Bozzini in 1806.[4] Jacobaeus provided its first clinical application for diagnosing and treating tuberculosis in 1910.[5] In 1991, Lewis popularized video-assisted thoracoscopic surgery (VATS) for pulmonary diseases. Orthopaedic applications of endoscopic principles began with the advent and acceptance of knee arthroscopy. Tagaki was the first to describe and Watanabe was the first to advance diagnostic knee arthroscopy in 1918 and 1957, respectively. Cascells in 1970 and Jackson in 1972 are credited with promoting the Japanese experience with arthroscopy in North America. Over a short time, endoscopic techniques have become standard for many abdominal and knee procedures, such as cholecystectomy and meniscectomy.[6] Endoscopic spine surgery was first performed in the lumbar spine in the 1990s and, currently, experience in the lumbar spine outweighs that of thoracic endoscopic spine surgery.[7] The first description of VATS for thoracic spinal diseases was published by Mack et al. in 1993.[2] An endoscope (usually a 30- or 45-degree endoscope) may be placed during dorsal approaches to the thoracic and lumbar spine to improve visualization of the ventral spinal cord.

This chapter addresses the philosophy of endoscopic spine surgery and its specific applications in thoracic and lumbar spine surgery. These include ventral and dorsal approaches for decompression, stabilization, and lesion removal. Relevant indications and contraindications, as well as current published results and complications, are discussed. The minimally invasive philosophy has been applied to operations of increasing complexity, and recently there has been increasing interest in using these techniques for deformity or scoliosis surgery as well.

Philosophy of Spinal Endoscopy

Open surgical approaches to the spine generally involve significant soft tissue dissection that by its nature can increase surgical risk, recovery time, and long-term functional consequences. Minimally invasive approaches attempt to perform the same operation while decreasing the size of the incision and damage to otherwise normal surrounding tissues. Decreasing the collateral damage to surrounding tissue should decrease the morbidity, pain, and hospitalization while leaving an aesthetically more acceptable scar. An improvement in the functional recovery time has also been observed.

Thoracic Ventral Endoscopic Approach

Although no direct, randomized trial has compared endoscopic techniques with traditional open thoracotomy (ventral) or costotransversectomy (dorsolateral), there are many theoretical and apparent advantages to an endoscopic approach[1,3,6-24] (Box 127-1). A quality endoscopic video system affords the surgeon improved visualization through outstanding illumination and up to 15× magnification. By manipulating the endoscopic portal placement, scope angle, and camera trajectory, a parallel approach to disc space can be maintained even with significant kyphotic or coronal plane deformity, making the technique useful for thoracic scoliosis correction.

VATS requires less muscle dissection and no rib spreading, and, therefore, it probably decreases incisional pain. Decreased soft tissue/paraspinal muscle injury also allows

BOX 127-1. Advantages and Disadvantages of Thoracic Endoscopic Spine Surgery

Advantages
Improved visualization
Decreased postoperative incisional pain
Cosmetically acceptable scars
Opportunity to perform simultaneous ventral-dorsal procedures
Reduced blood loss
Reduced infection risk
Decreased compromise of respiratory mechanics and rib splinting
Decreased postoperative shoulder girdle dysfunction
Reduced intensive care and hospital stays

Disadvantages
Surgical novelty (learning curve)
Monocular visualization (triangulation, depth perception)
Loss of tactile feedback (increased working distance)
Need for second surgeon
Technical limitations in treating intraoperative complications
Anesthetic demands of double-lumen intubation and single-lung ventilation
Currently limited ability to perform endoscopic reconstruction
Currently limited ability to perform dural repair
Specialized, costly, and often single-use instruments

more cosmetically acceptable scars, lower risk of postoperative infection, and decreased compromise of respiratory and shoulder mechanics. With prone positioning, simultaneous ventral and dorsal procedures may be undertaken, obviating the need for repositioning. Simultaneous lumbar and thoracic corrections can also potentially be performed. These advantages, taken together, may reduce ICU and hospital stays, as well as operative morbidity.

On the other hand, VATS has several disadvantages over open surgery.[1,3,6-24] First, these procedures require substantially different technical skill sets than traditional, open approaches. Although the word "steep" has been associated with the learning curve for this surgical novelty, the procedure more correctly represents a "flat" learning curve in that a significant amount of time must be spent with animal, cadaveric, and proctored cases before proceeding with independent VATS spine surgery. Endoscopy changes the surgeon's binocular vision to monocular video-assisted vision. This loss of depth perception is compounded with a loss of tactile feedback associated with the long-handled instruments needed to pass through endoscopic portals. Working distance and instrument excursion increases from 4 to 30 cm. Visualization and manipulation of sensitive spinal structures also requires triangulation from widely separated starting points on the chest wall to a small thoracic disc space. Prior to embarking on endoscopic thoracic spine surgery, the surgeon must be familiar with open ventral spinal anatomy and surgical techniques. Ultimately, the surgical procedures are the same, but the methods are different enough to challenge even the most experienced spine surgeon. Other disadvantages are more technical in nature. In some centers, VATS is performed with a second, experienced thoracoscopic surgeon. In many circumstances when a spine surgeon is working with a thoracic surgeon, there is an increase in manpower during the VATS procedure. This commonly can increase operative times.

Although the insult to postoperative pulmonary mechanics may be decreased with endoscopic approaches to the thoracic spine, double-lumen intubation and single-lung ventilation are typically required. Long periods of single-lung ventilation are physiologically demanding for the patient and more technically demanding for the anesthesiologist.

VATS procedures also require additional, expensive, and often single-use equipment. Endoscopic instrumentation is constantly improving and, with these improvements, the technical limitations of thoracoscopy spine surgery are declining. Theoretical technical limitations in the ability to treat intraoperative complications endoscopically remain. In particular, it may be more difficult to obtain vascular control of major vessel hemorrhages. Similarly, options for dural repair are more limited. Finally, techniques and implants for structural grafting and spine reconstruction remain developmental. Emerging, innovative technologies are gradually addressing these limitations.

Thoracic Dorsal and Dorsolateral and Combined Open and Endoscopic Approaches

The majority of open thoracic and lumbar spine procedures continue to be performed from posterior approaches. The approaches offer relatively direct access to the bony elements and the spinal canal. However, canal exposure may result in symptomatic epidural fibrosis. The dissection and retraction of the paraspinal muscles may lead to dead space formation and extensor muscle disruption. Such disruption has been referred to as "fusion disease"[25] and may be associated with early fatigability and other long-term symptoms. Endoscopic techniques may allow for less disruption of the posterior musculature and a smaller laminotomy. Dorsal and dorsolateral approaches are also limited by the surgeon's ability to visualize the ventral dura mater. Use of an angled endoscope may also greatly improve visualization while decreasing soft tissue dissection and rib resection.

Combined approaches are being increasingly described in the literature. These approaches include simultaneous ventral and dorsal surgery for tumors and deformity.[20,26] Combined approaches may also refer to combining endoscopic and open techniques in "mini-open" or endoscopically assisted spine procedures to exploit the advantages of both techniques.[17,19]

Anatomic Considerations for the Video-Assisted Thoracoscopic Surgery Approach

The rib cage and chest wall form a rigid open space in which endoscopic surgery may be performed. Unlike the abdomen, CO_2 insufflation is not required to maintain a working space. Through most of the thoracic spine, ribs articulate at the disc space level. The rib number corresponds to the lower vertebral body at the disc space (e.g., the sixth rib comes off the T5-6 disc space). Because the rib comes directly off the disc space from demifacets arising on the vertebral body just above and below the disc, rib resection is required for adequate access to the posterolateral corner of the disc. In the lower thoracic region, T11 and T12, the rib head may be well caudal to the disc space, permitting unobstructed access.

The segmental vessels lie in the waist of the vertebral bodies, entering the epidural space via the foramina. When approaching the spine endoscopically, it is important not to inadvertently lacerate these vessels. Some spine procedures, including corpectomy and instrumentation, require unilateral and occasionally bilateral sacrifice of the segmental vessels. Discectomy and ventral release procedures, on the other hand, usually do not require vessel sacrifice. One cadaver study demonstrated adequate discectomy without sacrifice of the intercostal or segmental vessels once an adequate mobilization of the esophagus and azygos vein had been carried out. The authors concluded that the segmental vessels ought to be preserved to reduce the risk of spinal cord ischemia.[10] In a two-phase goat study, thoracoscopic discectomy and fusion were undertaken both with and without sacrifice of the segmentals.[27] In the first phase, the area of disc excision was slightly higher in the vessel-ligated group, but the investigators did not believe this to be significant. Operative times were the same. In the second phase, biomechanical testing of the resulting fusion was undertaken, and the vessel-spared group revealed less flexibility in lateral bending. The authors concluded that the segmental vessels in the thoracic spine can be effectively spared without injury during disc excision and fusion. They noted that while slightly more disc area was excised with ligation of the vessels, sparing the segmental vessels may provide a blood supply that aids in fusion. They recommended sparing the segmental vessels in patients with a higher risk for cord perfusion–related neurologic injury, such as revision surgery, severe kyphosis, paraparesis, and congenital anomalies.

These studies have been criticized for not adequately modeling the intraoperative conditions of spine deformity.[3] Many authors report that sacrificing the segmental vessels provides better visualization through improved pleural reflection and more complete discectomy.[21,22,28,29] In a report of 1197 procedures in which more than 6000 vessels were sacrificed, there were no adverse neurologic consequences.[30] It may be reasonable to use both vessel-sparing and vessel-sacrificing techniques as a function of the clinical situation. For example, in congenital deformity cases in which spinal cord blood supplies may be anomalous, vessel sparing may be more important.[21] Also, if the intervention requires the sacrifice of one or more segmental arteries in the mid to lower thoracic region, especially T9 to T11, a right-sided approach should be considered to avoid ligation of the artery of Adamkiewicz. The artery of Adamkiewicz can be visualized with either CT or MRI angiography, and this is recommended if a left-sided approach is being considered.

Other surgically important structures include the superior intercostal veins and the sympathetic chain. The veins empty into the azygos circulation at or about the T3-4 interspace.[1] Branches from the sympathetic chain run over the rib heads, just below the parietal pleura.[31] Over the 5th through 10th ribs, these coalesce as the greater splanchnic nerve that courses into the abdomen.

There are critical regional differences in thoracoscopic anatomy that dictate different exposure techniques. In the upper thoracic region, for example, the surgeon should elevate and support the ipsilateral arm to rotate the scapula away. Here, unless there are apical adhesions, the collapsed lung readily falls away from the spine, allowing excellent visualization.[32] In the midthorax, there is more available space that allows more variation in placement of the camera and retractor ports. On the other hand, a fan retractor or strategically placed sponges are typically needed to keep the collapsed lung out of the operative field. Similarly, a second retracting port may be needed to move aside a bullous or stiff lung.[32] Tilting the operating table forward may improve visualization with less forceful lung retraction. In the lower thoracic region, it may be necessary to retract the diaphragm, but here, as at the apices, lung retraction is not usually a problem.

Indications and Contraindications

Indications

The majority of endoscopic thoracic spine surgery is directed ventrally to avoid larger incisions and postthoracotomy pain. A traditional thoracotomy requires a large incision, division of the shoulder girdle musculature, rib resection, and forcible rib retraction. This approach can result in desiccation of the exposed lungs and vessels, measurable reduction in pulmonary and shoulder girdle function, postthoracotomy intercostal pain syndrome, and an unsightly scar.[2,20] On the other hand, thoracoscopic approaches visualize the ventral spinal elements from the T1-2 to L1-2 disc spaces from the side of approach to the midline.[14] VATS affords easier exposure of the extremes of the thoracic spine than open thoracotomy.[33] For example, a T12 corpectomy can be performed without diaphragmatic incision, and T3 can be accessed without mobilizing the scapula as would be required with an open technique. However, the great vessels, heart, and lungs remain major considerations for either open or endoscopic surgical egress.

Currently, VATS may be used for a number of pathologies affecting the anterior and middle columns of the thoracic spine (Box 127-2). These include infections of the vertebral bodies, paraspinal gutter, discs, and epidural space, which can be biopsied, debrided, or drained. Thoracoscopic access is also

BOX 127-2. Indications and Contraindications for Thoracoscopic Spine Surgery

Indications

Infections: biopsy, drainage, debridement

Tumor: biopsy, excision, cord decompression

Degenerative disease: thoracic discectomy

Trauma: canal decompression and stabilization

Deformity: ventral releases, stabilizations

Contraindications

Respiratory problems: insufficiency, inability to tolerate single-lung ventilation

Pleural symphysis

Prior ventral surgery: thoracotomy, tube thoracostomy

Bullous lung pathology

Empyema

highly suitable for tumor biopsy or piecemeal excision. A number of authors have also described the use of VATS in patients with degenerative conditions of the thoracic spine, including excision of herniated thoracic discs and fusion of painful degenerated segments. In trauma, corpectomy/decompression and stabilization procedures have been performed.[1] The largest early experience with VATS has been for the correction of deformity.[1] Here, a thoracoscope can be used to assist or perform ventral release surgery in moderate kyphotic or scoliotic deformities. VATS has included the pediatric patient population as well as those with neuromuscular scoliosis and adult degenerative scoliosis. Thoracic discectomy for ventral myelopathy has also become an established technique.

Contraindications

Contraindications to thoracoscopic spinal surgery include the inability to tolerate single-lung ventilation in patients with severe or acute respiratory insufficiency.[24] However, VATS should be considered as an alternative for patients who are at high pulmonary risk for thoracotomy.[24] VATS may decrease many of the detrimental physiologic sequelae of thoracotomy. For example, postthoracotomy rib splinting leads to atelectasis and decreased functional residual capacity.[34] Thus, although VATS is ideally avoided in patients with severe lung disease, its less deleterious effect on pulmonary mechanics may make it a better option than open thoracotomy. Typical patient groups include those with chronic obstructive pulmonary disease; pulmonary interstitial fibrosis; or significant restrictive lung disease from thoracic spinal deformity, such as children with neuromuscular scoliosis.

Other contraindications include difficulty visualizing and manipulating instruments due to a scarred chest cavity. Therefore, VATS should not be offered to patients with pleural symphysis, failed prior open ventral surgery, thoracic empyema, previous thoracotomy, previous tube thoracostomy, or bullous lung pathology with reduced lung function. A preoperative anesthetic and medical assessment is mandatory.

Anesthesia

Cooperation between the anesthesia team and a thoracoscopic spine surgeon begins with a careful preoperative evaluation, followed by meticulous room and intubation setup. An experienced anesthesiologist with expertise in thoracic surgery is strongly recommended. Selective double-lumen endotracheal intubation allows collapse of the lung on the operative side. The tube may easily migrate, and frequent bronchoscopic assessment of tube position is mandatory.[35] In small patients (<45 kg), even the smallest double-lumen endotracheal tube may not fit. In these cases, bronchial blockers are required.[3,21] Blockers are technically more difficult to use and have a higher rate of incomplete lung deflation, which may seriously impair visualization.[3] Prone positioning in deformity cases may allow single-lumen intubation.[36]

General anesthetic options include total intravenous technique, isolated volatile agent, or a combination of volatile and intravenous agents. Initially, intravenous technique was recommended because of the potential risk of hypoxic pulmonary vasoconstriction with inhalational agents during single-lung ventilation. Recently, however, a series of 85 patients found no difference among these techniques.[35] Hemodynamic monitoring includes a double-lumen central venous catheter. Alternatively, pulmonary artery catheterization may be undertaken.[35] Hypotensive anesthesia should be avoided in myelopathic patients or in those undergoing segmental artery sacrifice.[23]

Once the tube position has been confirmed, the ipsilateral lung is deflated by clamping the lumen of its endotracheal tube. Once the chest has been entered with the first portal, the lung should collapse. If inadequate collapse is noted, a short period of positive pressure CO_2 insufflation may assist in collapsing the lung. Usually, this insufflation is not necessary.[37]

Patient and Operating Room Positioning

A radiolucent operating frame is preferred for either lateral decubitus or prone positioning. Lateral decubitus, identical to open thoracotomy positioning, is most typical for VATS spine surgery. A beanbag or bolsters may be used to maintain laterality. If intraoperative imaging is to be used, it is necessary to assess the location and lucency of the positioning aids. The patient should be well padded, and an axillary roll is typically used.

The patient is belted into place so that the table may be tilted into the Trendelenburg or reverse Trendelenburg position or even tilted right or left as necessary to improve intraoperative visualization. It is important to ensure that the patient stays in a strict lateral position during the initial approach to the spine to maintain surgeon orientation. Some surgeons prefer to "airplane" the table up for portions of the procedure, but given the loss of tactile feedback and three-dimensional information associated with endoscopy, a strict knowledge of the patient's body position in space is necessary. In some settings, particularly in the lower thoracic spine, it may be useful to "jackknife" the table to improve access to the lateral body wall. However, in patients with significant spinal cord compression, excessive "jackknifing" may increase the risk of iatrogenic neurologic progression.[37]

Prone positioning may be used as part of a simultaneous ventral/dorsal approach.[20,36] Simultaneous surgery eliminates the need to stage the procedures, as well as the added time and costs for repositioning, redraping, and a new operating room setup. Prone position is particularly advantageous in cases of marked instability. For example, in ankylosing spondylitis or trauma, the spine may suddenly translate at the osteotomy site during repositioning. Prone position also allows a gravity reduction of hyperkyphosis.[36] Finally, prone positioning confers the additional advantage of allowing the lungs to fall away from the spine, decreasing the need for retraction.

A large operating room is typically needed to accommodate the special equipment required in VATS cases.[33] The gowned and sterile team typically includes two surgeons, one assistant, and one scrub nurse. Additional personnel include the anesthesia team, somatosensory-evoked potential monitoring personnel, cell saver transfusion technicians, and circulating nursing staff. Beyond the usual complement of anesthesia machines and back tables for instruments and implants, endoscopic spine surgery requires two video monitors, a fluoroscope, and neurologic monitoring equipment (usually sensory-evoked and motor-evoked potentials). The endoscopic surgeon and spine surgeon typically work on the same side of the patient (facing the patient in the lateral decubitus position). Alternatively, they can work opposite one another.

Video mixers can convert image orientation so that no mirror image instrument manipulation is required.[1] More and more frequently, voice-activated robotics are being used to replace the assistant surgeon in camera positioning. Robotics may improve visualization by providing a steady image.

Instruments for an open thoracotomy should be readily available for emergency use. In the prone position, open access can be achieved with an extended costotransversectomy approach. Because the lung has already been mobilized, it is easy to enter the chest. Once in, the surgeon is readily able to access, identify, and control the major vascular structures.[20] Immediate potential access to a thoracic surgeon is also recommended.

Equipment

The workhorse of spinal endoscopy is the video equipment. This begins with the endoscope itself. A number of standard 10-mm endoscopes are used, most commonly 0-degree and 30-degree scopes. Occasionally, 70-degree scopes are needed. The 0-degree scope is standard for thoracoscopy, but a 30-degree scope decreases instrument crowding and allows better visualization around bony corners.[24,38] Typically, a 10-mm, 15-inch end-viewing scope is used; however, in pediatric cases and, with increasing frequency in adults, a 5-mm scope may be preferred.[24] The smaller scope provides less illumination, but with improvements in high-resolution, three-chip technology is adequate in most cases. Three-dimensional endoscopes are becoming increasingly available and help visualize landmarks and render improved depth perception.[24]

Instruments are introduced into the chest through trocars. Initially, these trocars were hard. Hard trocars may protect the thoracoscope against the rigid fulcrum of the rib cage.[15] More recently, soft trocars have been developed that may be less traumatic to the neurovascular bundle on the inferior rib undersurface. Standard trocars are either 5 mm or 10 mm and are selected based on the size of instrument to be passed and the intercostal distance, which in adults is less than 12 mm.[37]

Typical spine instruments are customized for endoscopic applications by creating an extended shank of uniform diameter to match standard trocar sizes (Fig. 127-1). These include long-handled curets, Cobb elevators, pituitary rongeurs, disc shavers, nerve hooks, and Penfield dissectors. High-speed burs with long extenders are often required, as are more specialized types of endoscopic equipment such as Endo Shears, a bipolar endoscopic electrocautery, the harmonic scalpel, endovascular clips and loop ligatures, as well as endoscopic fan retractors.

A variety of spinal surgical implants are also available for the task required, including disc interbody cages, screw and rod combinations, and vertebrectomy cages.

Surgical Technique and Avoidance of Complications

A left-sided or right-sided approach to the thoracic spine may be used depending on the eccentricity of the pathology (Fig. 127-2). With a left-sided approach, the thick resilient aorta is less prone to injury than the large friable tortuous veins of the azygos system. Some authors prefer a right-sided approach when the pathology is not lateralized, because there is a greater spinal surface area lateral to the azygos vein than the aorta.[14]

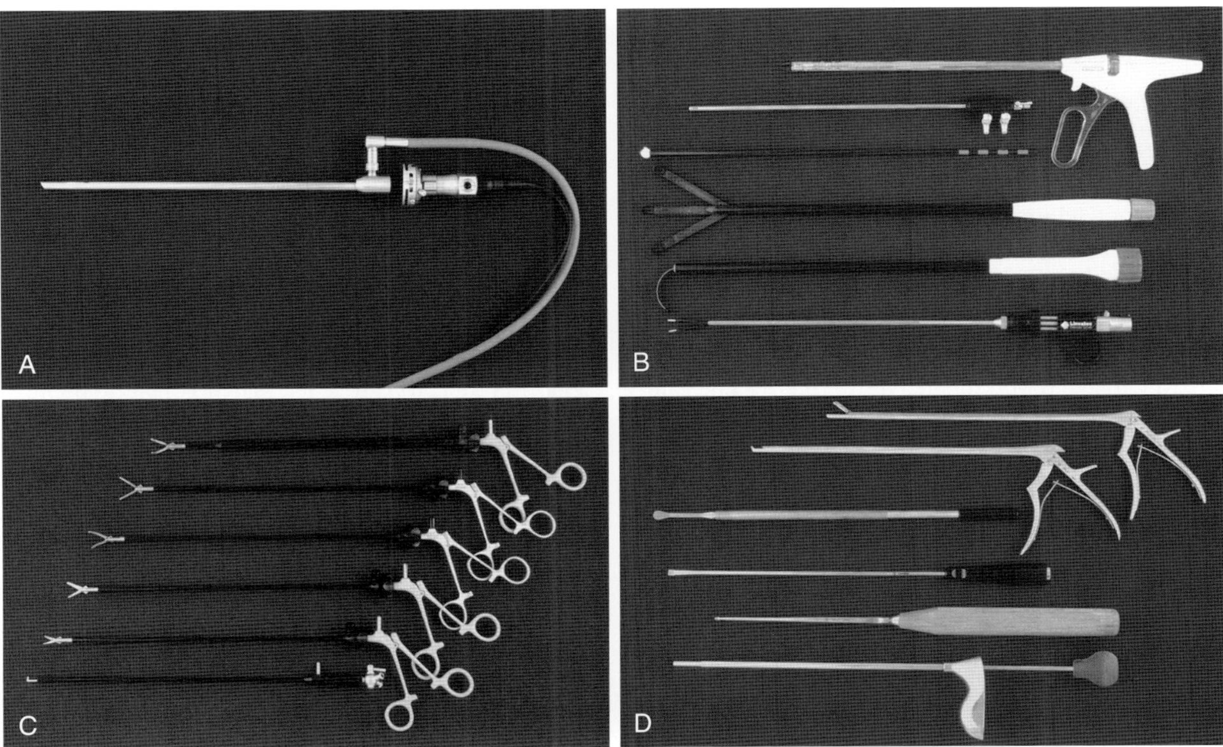

FIGURE 127-1. Spinal thoracoscopy benefits from an ever-increasing array of available instruments. Important among these are the endoscope itself (**A**); standard endoscopic instruments, including a fan retractor and autosuture device (**B**); endoscopic dissecting tools (**C**); and typical spine instruments modified for thoracoscopic use with long hands and uniform diameter shafts (**D**).

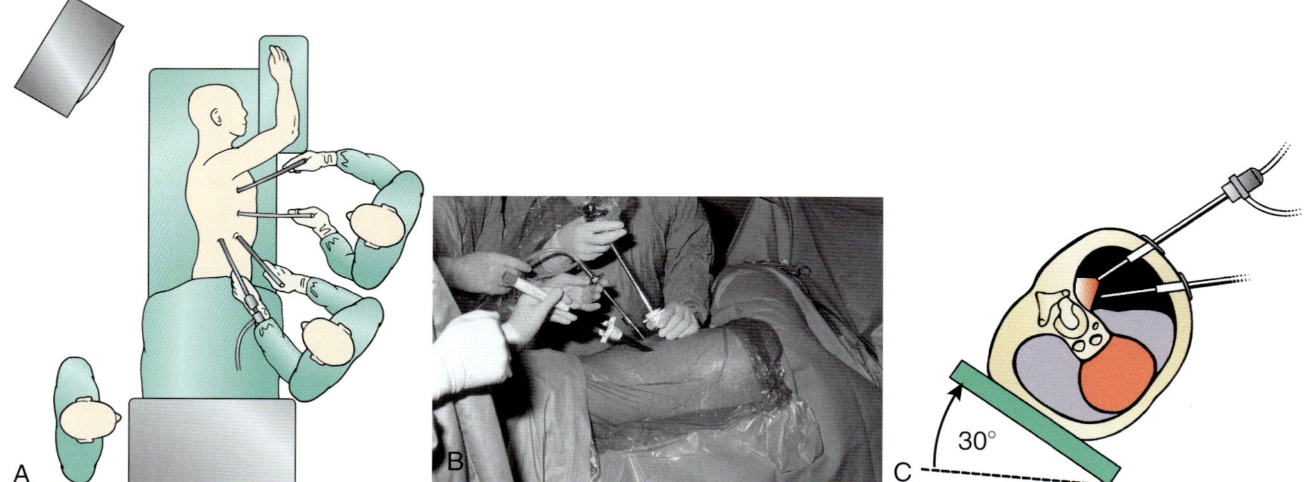

FIGURE 127-2. Lateral thoracoscopy. **A,** Operating room setup. **B,** Clinical photograph of lateral thoracoscopy. Note the assistant in the foreground holding the fan retractor. **C,** Visualization is improved when the lungs fall away from the spine with a ventral tilt of the operating room table of 20 to 30 degrees. (**C,** From Regan JJ, Jarolem KL: Thoracoscopy of the spine. In Herkowitz HN, Garfin SR, Balderston RA, et al, editors: *Rothman-Simeone: the spine*, ed 4, Philadelphia, 1999, WB Saunders, p 601.)

This difference can be assessed with preoperative axial CT or MRI images. Below T9, one may consider a left-sided approach to avoid the more cranial diaphragm reflection on the right.

The initial trocar creates the main viewing portal and is placed in the anterior axillary line at the sixth or seventh intercostal space, giving an unobstructed view of the entire hemithorax. The trocar is inserted in the manner of a tube thoracostomy with blunt dissection with a Kelly forceps just over the top of the rib to avoid damage to the neurovascular bundle or deep structures. A digital exploration is undertaken to exclude adhesions and avoid parenchymal lacerations of the lung. Some recommend Bovie dissection through the musculature to prevent bleeding around portals, which can obscure the camera image.[1]

This first portal is the only one to be inserted blindly. Once open to the atmosphere, the lung falls away from the thoracic wall, allowing insertion of the thoracoscope. The endoscope is inserted, and an exploratory thoracoscopy is performed. Minor lung adhesions are released. If complete atelectasis is not achieved, a brief period of CO_2 insufflation may help collapse the lung.

The camera assistant must maintain the camera orientation and keep the operative field centered in view with a steady hand. The camera and instruments should be in the same 180-degree arc to avoid working in a mirror image. The camera assistant and the operating surgeon should work in unison with small movements. The camera should be removed for cleaning at various intervals. It should be reinserted carefully, because the lung may have partially reinflated, and injury to the lung parenchyma is possible.[37] Self-cleaning and defogging arthroscopes are very helpful in this regard.[24]

It is necessary to manipulate only one object at a time. The camera operator zooms into the operative site. Then, as new instruments are introduced, the operator pans the camera out to follow the instrument into the operative field, preferably without changing the camera angle. Similarly, retractors and other instruments should be removed under direct visualization. Fan retractors should be removed in the fully closed position only. Levering instruments on the rib cage should be avoided to decrease pressure on the intercostal nerve.[39]

Once in the chest, surgical levels are identified. Operating at the wrong level is always a concern in the thoracic spine. It is important to screen for variant anatomy, such as accessory ribs, with preoperative radiographs, then find the level by counting down from the first rib. The first rib may be difficult to identify. It is necessary to mark the disc space and obtain radiographic confirmation. A Steinmann pin can be passed directly through the chest wall into the pathologic level.[33] A radiograph confirms level localization, and the pin also demonstrates the optimal location for the working portal. Only quality radiographic images are acceptable. Anteroposterior radiographs are typically more helpful than lateral radiographs.[31] In some centers, marking beads are placed at each spinal level, and radiographs or fluoroscopy are obtained prior to entering the operating suite. The appropriate level bead is maintained on the patient for intraoperative confirmation.[32]

To manipulate the spinal tissues, additional instruments need to be inserted into the chest through additional trocars. Typically, two working portals are created under direct video visualization with the lung protected. The chest is percussed, and by visualizing the percussions from within the chest, additional sites are chosen. As an alternative, 18-gauge spinal needles can be placed through the interspace to verify the level and trajectory. It is necessary to organize the remaining portals to center the instruments at the level of pathology. A number of portal patterns have been described and are covered in more detail in subsequent sections. Typically, an L or V shape at the dorsal axillary line two interspaces cephalad and caudad to the viewing portal is created, depending on the chest wall morphology and the intended spinal level. Portals should be spaced far enough apart that instruments do not "fence" with each other. The final viewing portal should be far enough away from the lesion to allow a panoramic view and to allow room to manipulate instruments.[3] During the procedure, the instruments and scope are interchanged between the portals to facilitate work at different levels. It is preferable to make another portal perpendicular to the operative level than to operate at an acute angle to the pathology.[32]

When the appropriate portals have been placed and the correct level identified, the surgeon incises the parietal pleura with monopolar cautery. Alternatively, he or she uses the harmonic scalpel to dissect with less smoke and char.[12,40] It is necessary to avoid monopolar cautery over the inferior margin of the rib head, where electrocautery injury to the intercostal nerve may occur.[37] The degree of pleural dissection depends on the extent of the intended surgery but may include longitudinal approaches parallel to the spine or transverse approaches parallel to each disc space. If the segmental vessels are to be preserved, smaller pleural incisions are created parallel to the disc space. Bluntly dissect the incised parietal pleura rostrally, caudally, and ventrally to expose as much of the vertebral margins as is necessary.

At each step, meticulous hemostasis is required. Methods to control bleeding include monopolar or bipolar electrocautery, harmonic scalpel, argon beam coagulation, and hemostatic packing. Uncontrolled bleeding may necessitate conversion to an open procedure.

At the conclusion of the procedure, it is necessary to irrigate out any disc or bony debris. Most authors do not attempt to close the parietal pleura. Some recommend an intercostal bupivacaine block to decrease postoperative pain.[9]

A chest tube is then selected—20F, 24F, or 28F—depending on the patient's chest size. One inserts the tube through the inferiormost portal and runs it cranially along the vertebral column. Rosenthal uses two chest tubes: one, an apical tube for air and second, a basilar tube for effusions.[41] Depending on the nature of the procedure, the tube can be maintained at water seal or at 20 cm of water suction. Typically, the tube can be removed 1 to 2 days postoperatively.

In the postoperative period, most patients are extubated immediately. A chest radiograph is obtained in the recovery room to verify full inflation of the lungs.[7] A brief period of postoperative ICU monitoring is recommended. Aggressive respiratory care and physical therapy are required to prevent "down lung" atelectasis and pneumonia.

Results and Complications

Anesthesia Issues

Liske et al.[35] described the anesthesia outcomes in their series of 82 patients who underwent thoracoscopic spine surgery under single-lung ventilation. The authors found that the anesthesia time was not significantly different than that for their series of patients who underwent open thoracotomy. They noted that VATS required extremely long single-lung ventilation times (mean, 270.2 minutes), a significantly longer period compared with open procedures. Also, the oxygenation index decreased significantly after initiation of single-lung ventilation. Despite these physiologic stressors, the authors concluded that VATS was a reasonable alternative to open thoracotomy from the anesthesia perspective because of the clinical benefits of accelerated return to activity as well as decreased ICU and hospital stays.

Other Complications

The types of complications associated with thoracoscopically assisted spine surgery in humans are essentially the same as with an open thoracotomy approach and can be categorized as incomplete operation, neurologic injury, lung injury, and vascular injury.[16,37,41] As in any spinal cord level procedure, dural laceration, cord injury, or ischemia is possible. Most common, however, is intercostal neuralgia. This may be seen in up to 21% of patients, but it is usually transient.[37] Flexible portals may reduce its incidence, but intercostal neuralgia still occurred in two cases in a series of 17 patients in which these portals were used.[16] Transection of the sympathetic chain causes little or no morbidity, but the surgeon should inform the patient and family of possible temperature and skin color changes below and ipsilateral to the level of surgery.

A variety of pulmonary complications have been reported. Longer periods of lung collapse increase pulmonary morbidity. To decrease the rate of prolonged atelectasis, the deflated lung should be reinflated for 5 to 10 minutes for every hour of operating time.[7] Trocars or instruments may cause direct trauma to the lungs. Larger air leaks should be repaired with an endoscopic suture ligature. Other common postoperative lung problems include pleural effusions and diaphragmatic injury.

More unusual pulmonary complications may stem from anesthesia or single-lung ventilation mishaps. Sucato and Girgis[42] reported a case of an 11-year-old patient with severe scoliosis who developed air in both chest cavities, mediastinum, peritoneum, retroperitoneum, and subcutaneous tissue after intubation with a double-lumen endotracheal tube. Although the patient remained hemodynamically stable, bilateral chest tubes were required. The authors note that just as for the surgeon, there is a significant learning curve for the anesthesiologist to become adept at obtaining and maintaining single-lung ventilation.

With any ventral thoracic procedure, devastating vascular injuries are possible. The trocars or other instruments may injure the heart, great vessels, azygos vein, esophagus, or segmental arteries. Thoracic duct injury with lymphatic leakage is uncommon and should be ligated with an endoscopic clip applier.

McAfee et al. reported their complications with VATS in a prospective series of 78 cases. Transient intercostal neuralgias were noted in six patients and atelectasis in five patients. One case was converted to an open procedure for extensive pleural adhesions. One case of partial spinal cord neurologic deficit was noted.[37] Huang et al.[39] reported their complications in a series of 90 consecutive patients treated with thoracoscopic techniques for a variety of pathologies, including infection, fracture, deformity, and degenerative disease. A total of 30 complications was noted in 22 patients (24.4%). Two of these complications were fatal, including one case of massive blood loss and another of pneumonia. One graft dislodgement required revision surgery. The other complications were transient and included four cases of intercostal neuralgia, three superficial wound infections, three cases of pharyngeal pain, two cases of atelectasis, and two cases of residual pneumothorax. Four cases were converted to open thoracotomy.

Video-Assisted Thoracoscopic Surgery in Deformity and Scoliosis Surgery

Indications and Contraindications

Endoscopic surgery may directly or indirectly address several of the goals of surgery for spine deformity, which include arrest

BOX 127-3. Indications and Contraindications to Thoracoscopic Spine Surgery in Deformity

Indications

The indications are the same as for thoracotomy:
- Curves greater than 60 degrees with less than 50% correction on bending
- Curves greater than 75 degrees
- Curves requiring rebalancing into the stable zone in either the coronal or sagittal plane
- Crankshaft prevention in skeletally immature patients with curves greater than 50 degrees
- Kyphotic deformities greater than 70 degrees
- Progressive congenital deformities requiring epiphysiodesis
- Patients at high risk for pseudarthrosis from dorsal fusion alone
- Patients for whom bone grafting will achieve an interbody fusion

Additional Indications
- Patients with compromised pulmonary mechanics

Contraindications*

Deformity-specific relative contraindications

Narrow anterior-posterior chest diameter or other anatomic variants that limit working space in the chest

Significant vertebral rotation at the apex

*See Box 127-2.

of curve progression, maximization and maintenance of curve correction, improvement in fusion rate, and decompression and protection of the neural elements[43-46] (Box 127-3). In scoliosis, morphologic studies demonstrate that the anterior longitudinal ligament migrates to the concavity of the curve. The anterior longitudinal ligament and costotransverse ligaments on the concave side form a structural tether that must be released to gain maximum mobility of the spine.[44] Typically, ventral approaches to the spine in deformity are indicated to release these tethers to allow correction of coronal and sagittal plane deformities.

Indications for endoscopic techniques in spine deformity are the same as those for thoracotomy.[1,47] The surgeon should consider ventral release in large scoliotic curves greater than 75 degrees and in rigid curves with less than 50% correction on bending films. Ventral epiphysiodesis is typically required to prevent the crankshaft phenomena in skeletally immature children with curves greater than 50 degrees or in those with progressive congenital deformities in the thorax. Patients with kyphotic deformities greater than 70 degrees or curves that require rebalancing into the stable zone in the coronal or sagittal plane are also candidates for ventral surgery. Interbody fusion techniques are often added to dorsal stabilization procedures to minimize pseudarthrosis risk.

Spine endoscopy should be given particular consideration in the patient with preexisting pulmonary mechanics compromise caused by the spine deformity or associated neurologic syndromes (e.g., polio). Here, endoscopic techniques may be indicated to minimize any thoracotomy-related pulmonary compromise. Finally, endoscopic techniques should be considered in any situation in which the cosmetic result is of particular concern to the patient.

Relative contraindications to the use of spinal endoscopy to treat patients with spine deformity include all of the contraindications to endoscopy in general.[20] Also, special consideration needs to be paid to the relationship of the spine to the thoracic cage. A narrow anterior-posterior chest diameter, significant vertebral rotation at the apex, or thoracic scoliosis curves greater than 75 degrees may preclude safe visualization and instrumentation of the spine. For example, in curves greater than 75 degrees, the chest cavity on the concave side and the rib interspaces are too small to accommodate the 10-mm-diameter endoscopic portals and instruments. Also, with spinal rotation, the mediastinal organs begin to obstruct exposure. In certain cases, these variables may be overcome by adding more working portals. However, for the novice spine endoscopist, formal open thoracotomy may be more prudent. Consultation with an experienced thoracic surgeon is usually helpful.

Operative Technique and Avoidance of Complications

During scoliosis correction, the spine may be exposed on the curve's convexity or concavity, depending on clinical circumstances or the surgeon's preference (Fig. 127-3). Historically, because the structural tether resides in the concavity, ventral releases through a concave side thoracotomy were recommended by Stagnara.[20] This approach has not gained popularity because of difficulty working deep in the concave portion of the deformity between the narrowed rib spaces. Moreover, the segmental vessels are clumped together and are more likely to be injured. The mediastinal structures, including the aorta, unfold into the concavity of the curve and must be meticulously dissected and mobilized. On the other hand, working in the concavity allows access to more disc spaces with fewer portals and a direct approach to the structural tether in the dorsolateral corner of the disc space.

Release of the convexity typically allows easier access to the apex of the curve and has become more common overall. However, complete release and exposure of the dorsolateral corner on the concave side is occasionally difficult at the most proximal and distal levels.[44] Working from the convexity may require more portals to gain parallel access to each disc space. If thoracoplasty is planned, a convex side approach is required. For kyphosis correction, the spine can be approached from either side at the surgeon's discretion.

The lateral decubitus position, mimicking open thoracotomy, is typically selected for spine deformity procedures.[1-3,12,24] However, if a subsequent dorsal stabilization is also required, lateral positioning requires repositioning and draping.[48] Simultaneous prone ventral thoracoscopic release with dorsal instrumentation[20,36] is another option (Fig. 127-4).

In gaining access to the spine, the first portal is created opposite the apex of deformity at the midaxillary line. The lung is retracted, and then the sympathetic chain is bluntly dissected out of the operative field. The surgeon incises the anterior longitudinal ligament and anulus. In scoliosis the aorta may need to be mobilized with blunt dissection, because it frequently lies in the acute angle between the rib head and the lateral vertebral body. Once it has been mobilized, a small sponge or peanut retractor is placed in the interval between the vertebral body and the aorta to protect the great vessels during the preparation of the disc space.

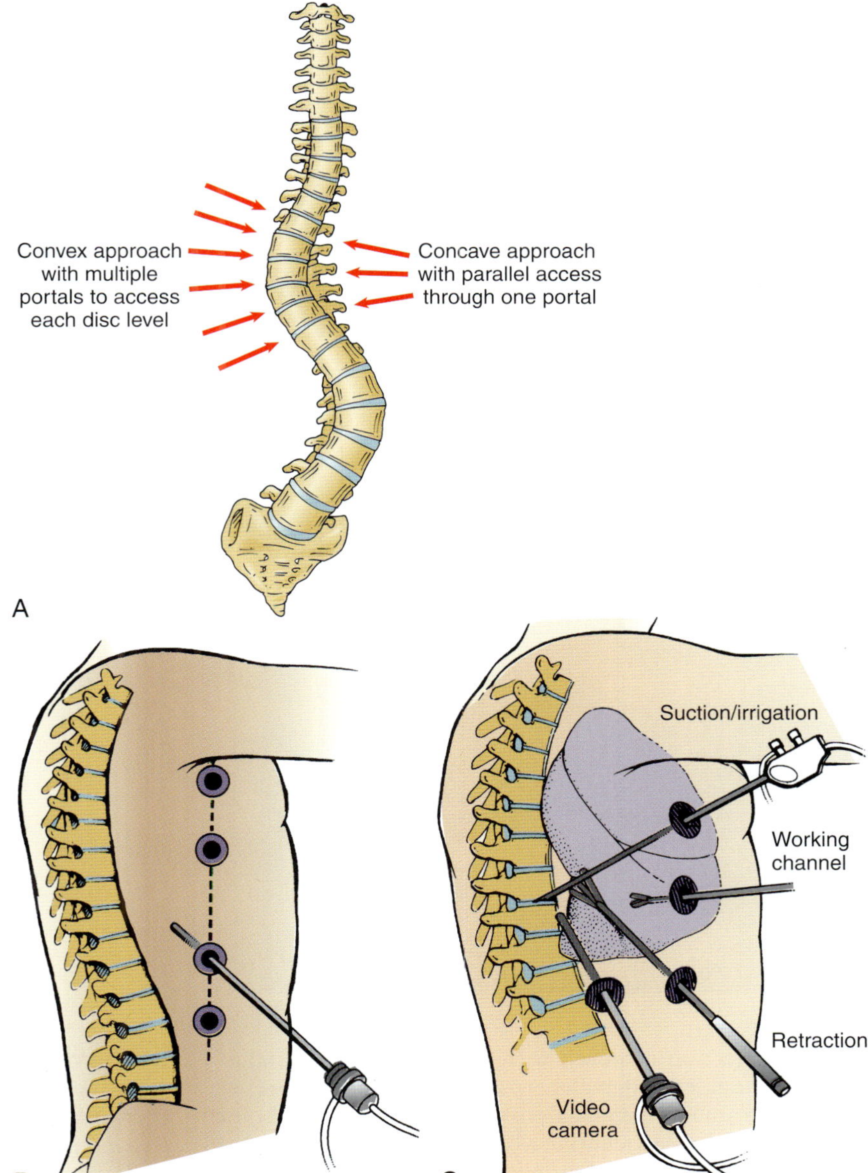

FIGURE 127-3. Portal placement for lateral thoracoscopy. **A,** Portal placement is affected by the presence of coronal plane deformity and the side of approach. **B,** Typically, in scoliosis cases, the portals are placed in the midaxillary line. **C,** For a thoracoscopic decompression, an L configuration is often used. (**A,** From Lieberman IH, Salo PT, Orr RD, Kraetschmer B: Prone position endoscopic transthoracic release with simultaneous posterior instrumentation for spinal deformity. *Spine* 25:2251–2257, 2000, Fig. 7. **B** and **C,** from Regan JJ, Jarolem KL: Thoracoscopy of the spine. In Herkowitz HN, Garfin SR, Balderston RA, et al, editors: *Rothman-Simeone: the spine*, ed 4, Philadelphia, 1999, WB Saunders, p 606.)

Unlike cord decompression procedures, formal resection of the pedicle is not necessary. Rather, the disc space is incised and the nucleus pulposus is evacuated with rongeurs and curets down to bleeding subchondral bone end plates to the posterior longitudinal ligament (Fig. 127-5). For the scoliosis cases approached from the concavity, the dorsolateral corner, costotransverse ligaments, and rib heads on the concave side are released under direct view to optimize correction. The convex lateral anulus is left intact as a pivot point to prevent overdistraction during the dorsal correction. If working on the convexity, the concave dorsolateral corner must be released to achieve a complete release. For kyphosis releases, the entire anterior longitudinal ligament and anulus must be incised. Once all levels are released, a periosteal elevator is inserted and rotated slightly to ensure that proper release has been achieved.[15]

Internal thoracoplasty can be performed just after ventral endoscopic release or as an independent procedure, as described by Mehlman et al.[49] The rib deformity associated with idiopathic scoliosis often represents a significant cosmetic concern to the patient but may not improve significantly after dorsal fusion.[50] Preoperatively, ribs to be resected are identified radiographically and by physical examination. From the lateral decubitus position, thoracoplasty is performed on the convex side (Fig. 127-6). Occasionally, ribs are cut but left in place to ensure adequate thoracic cage stability.[49]

Results

Wall et al.[51] and Newton et al.[52] independently reported their results with endoscopic discectomy in an animal model. These authors concluded that the extent of discectomy and quality of release are comparable to those of open techniques. Published studies describing results of open ventral releases by Kostuik et al.,[45] Simmons et al.,[46] and Byrd et al.[43] reveal that average curve correction ranged from 36% to 48%. The

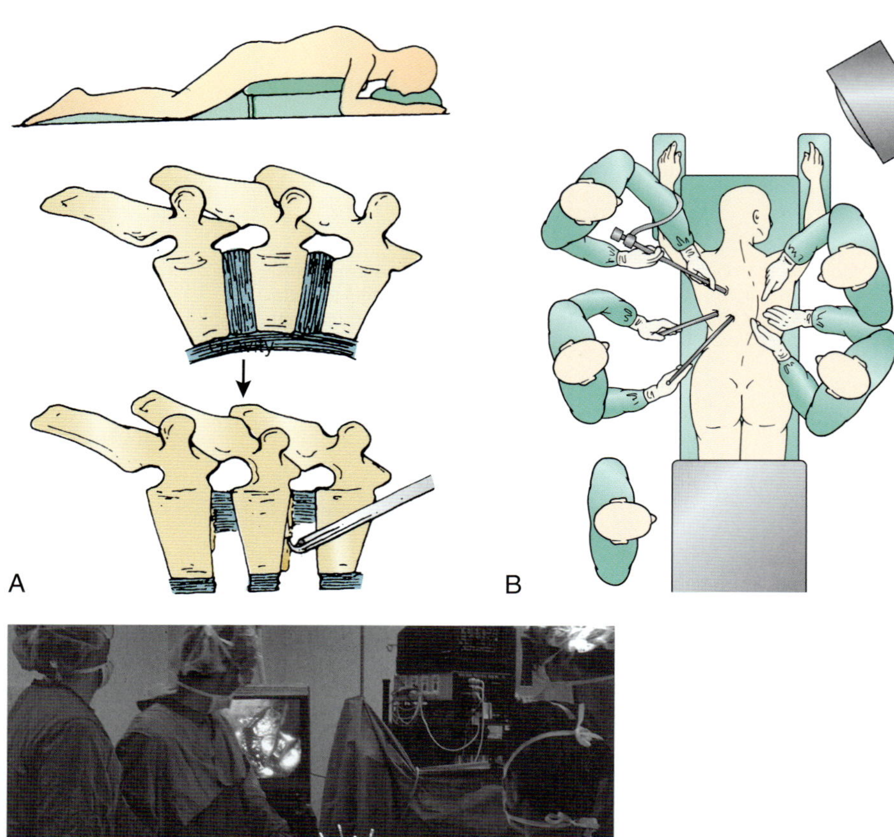

C

FIGURE 127-4. Prone thoracoscopy. **A,** Prone positioning is especially useful in the treatment of hyperkyphosis, in that gravity partially corrects the deformity. **B,** Operating room setup for prone thoracoscopy. **C,** Clinical photograph of a simultaneous ventral thoracoscopic release with dorsal fusion. (**A,** From King AG, Mills TE, Loe WA, et al: Video-assisted thoracoscopic surgery in the prone position. *Spine [Phila Pa 1976]* 25:2403–2406, 2000.)

average correction achieved with thoracoscopic techniques appears to be at least equivalent to those reports.[20,21] However, Arlet[28] performed a meta-analysis of the use of VATS in spine deformity surgery. He identified 10 articles that involved 151 procedures. He reported that most authors selected a convex side approach from a lateral decubitus position with four or more ports in the midaxillary line. Four to seven discs were excised and grafted over 2½ to 4 hours. Most procedures were followed by same-day dorsal stabilization. The mean scoliotic curve was corrected from 65 to 35 degrees, and the mean kyphosis was corrected from 78 to 44 degrees. He noted that 7 years after the first report, the literature still only showed 151 patients and no long-term follow-up or significant outcome data in terms of spinal balance, fusion rate, rib hump correction, cosmesis, pain, and satisfaction. Arlet concludes that a more complete discectomy is possible with open technique and that animal studies documenting equivalent discectomies do not account for the visualization difficulties encountered in deformity patients. In his view, the data do not yet support widespread implementation, and the individual surgeon must consider whether he or she treats enough of the relevant pathologies to make learning the technique worthwhile.

Alternatively, Niemeyer et al.[53] evaluated the 2-year clinical results, radiologic correction, and morbidity of ventral thoracoscopic surgery followed by dorsal instrumentation and fusion in their series of 29 patients with idiopathic scoliosis. A mean preoperative Cobb angle of 65.1 degrees was corrected to a mean 34.4 degrees at final follow-up. In nine hyperkyphotic patients, the mean preoperative Cobb angle of 81 degrees was corrected to 65 degrees. The average duration of the thoracoscopic procedure was 188 minutes, and this time decreased as the series progressed. No neurologic or vascular complications occurred. Postoperative complications included four recurrent pneumothoraces, one surgical emphysema, and one respiratory infection. The authors concluded that thoracoscopic ventral surgery is a safe and effective technique for the treatment of pediatric spine deformity but that a randomized controlled trial, comparing open with thoracoscopic methods, is required.

Newton et al.[21] reported a prospective series of 65 consecutive cases of thoracoscopic ventral release with discectomy and fusion performed by one surgeon for the treatment of pediatric spine deformity. This patient group was 14 ± 3 years of age and included patients with idiopathic scoliosis (13), Scheuermann kyphosis (9), neuromuscular spine deformity (35), congenital scoliosis (4), and tumor/syrinx (4). The average operative time for the thoracoscopic procedure was 161 ± 41 minutes (range, 50–240), with a slight decrease in the average operative time occurring as the series progressed. The average number of discs excised was 6.5 ± 1.5 (range, 3–10),

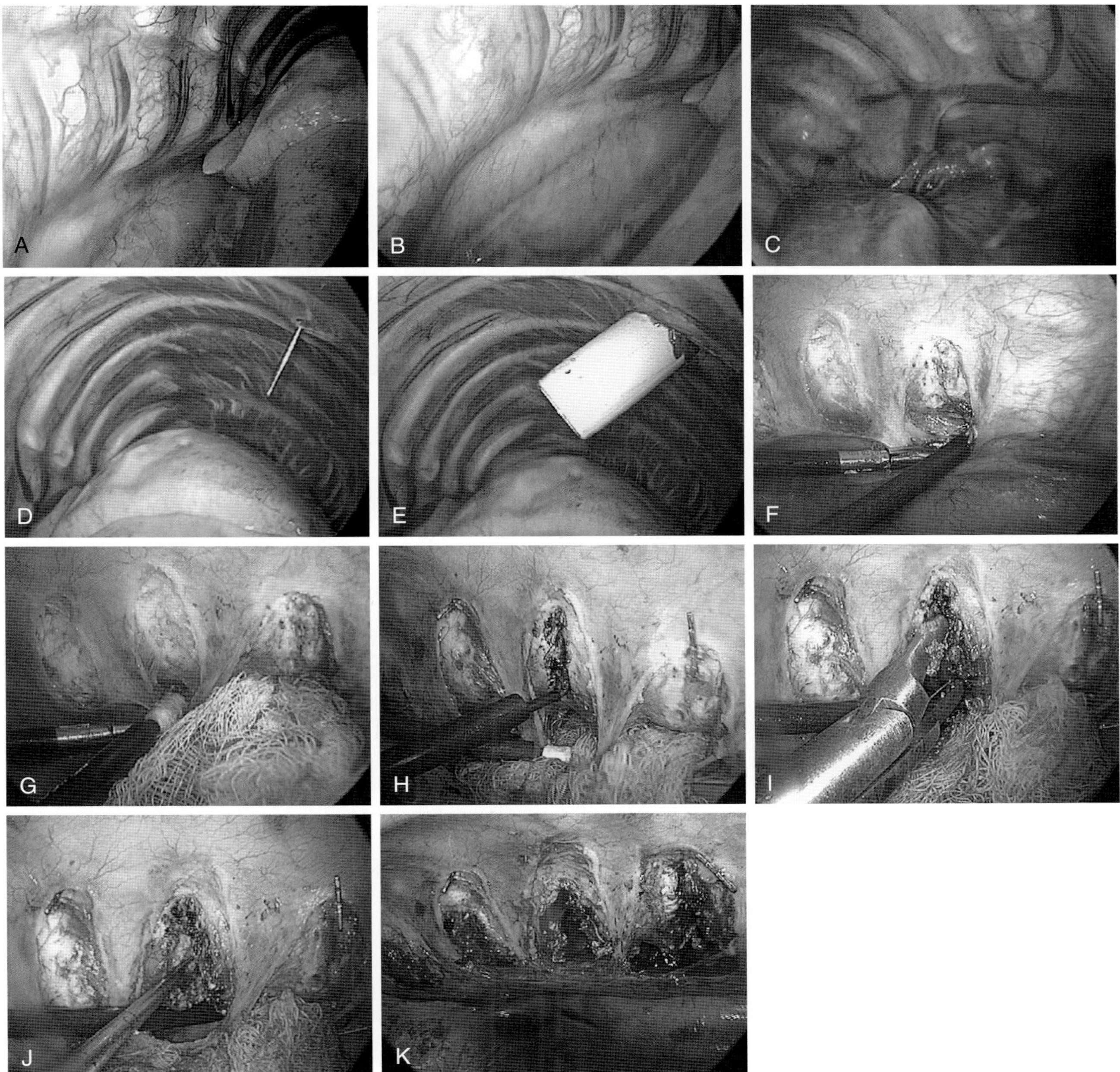

FIGURE 127-5. Multiple releases for scoliosis. **A,** Typical thoracoscopic anatomy. **B,** Further thoracoscopic exploration of the chest. Note the azygos vein and superior vena cava. **C,** Here, in the upper thoracic spine, the superior intercostal vein can be seen feeding into the azygos system. **D,** Further portal placement can be planned with a needle to ensure appropriate alignment. **E,** Next, the portal itself is inserted. **F,** An endoscopic dissector is used to take down a portion of the parietal pleura. This view shows three disc levels exposed without sacrifice of the segmental vessels. **G,** An endoscopic Kidner is used to further dissect the soft tissues from the disc space. **H,** An anulotomy is then performed. **I,** More disc material can be retrieved with a pituitary rongeur. **J,** A long, sharp Cobb elevator is used to dissect the remainder of the anulus and cartilaginous end plates. **K,** Completed discectomies are demonstrated. Structural or morselized graft can be inserted.

and this number increased as the series progressed. The average operative time per disc decreased as the series progressed. Initial postoperative scoliosis time was 29.3 ± 7.7 minutes in the first 30 patients, compared with 22.3 ± 4.7 minutes in the next 35 patients ($P < .01$). The average blood loss during the thoracoscopic procedure was 301 ± 322 mL (range, 25–2000) but it did not decrease as the series progressed. Initial postoperative scoliosis and kyphosis correction were 59% (from 62 to 25 degrees) and 92% (from 78 to 44 degrees), respectively. Complications occurred in six patients and were evenly distributed throughout the series. Complications included chest tube reinsertion for pleural effusion or chylothorax (three patients), conversion to thoracotomy (two patients), and incorrect levels of fusion (one patient). The authors concluded that the learning period for thoracoscopy is substantial but not prohibitive and that the technique provides a safe and effective alternative to thoracotomy in the treatment of pediatric spine deformity.

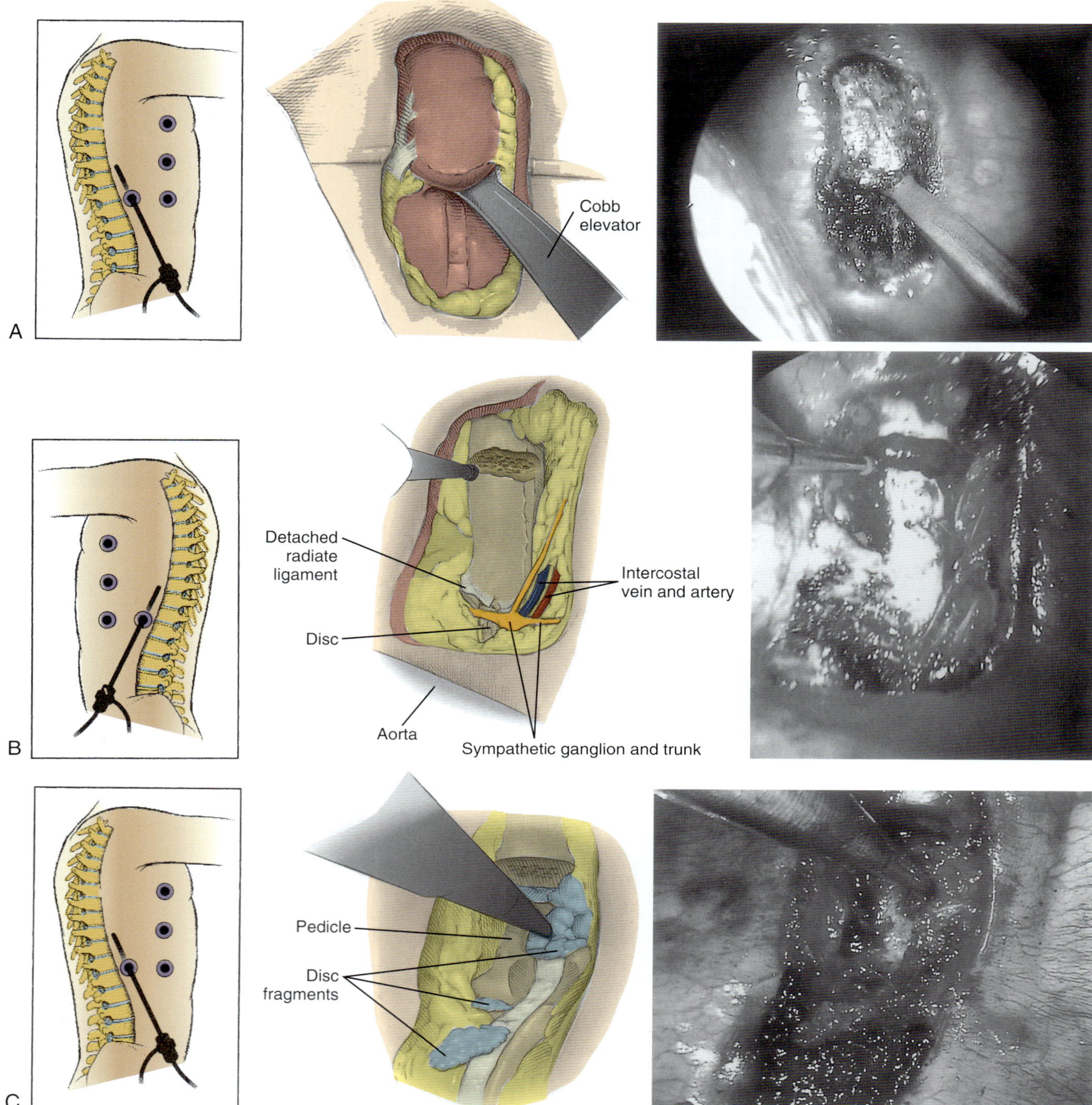

FIGURE 127-6. The endoscopic approach for canal decompression is different. Although typically performed at only one or two levels, more dissection of the rib head and pedicle is required to safely visualize the dura. **A,** After the pleura has been divided over the rib head, the proximal 2 to 3 cm of rib are exposed with a Cobb elevator. The radiate and costotransverse ligaments are cut away from the rib using the Cobb, curets, and special curved dissectors. **B,** A bur is used to divide the rib 3 cm from its head. The fragment is grasped with a pituitary rongeur and delivered through the port. **C,** The superior portion of the pedicle is identified and removed with an angled curet, bur, or Kerrison rongeur.

In another series, Newton et al.[22] compared their early outcomes and costs between a series of 14 consecutive thoracoscopic releases with 18 open thoracotomies performed the previous year. The percentage of curve correction was similar between the groups, with 56% correction in the thoracoscopic scoliosis group versus 60% in the open group and 88% in the thoracoscopic kyphosis group versus 94% in the open group. Blood loss and complication rates were the same in both groups, but chest tube output was greater in the thoracoscopic group. The length of hospital stay was not reduced in the open

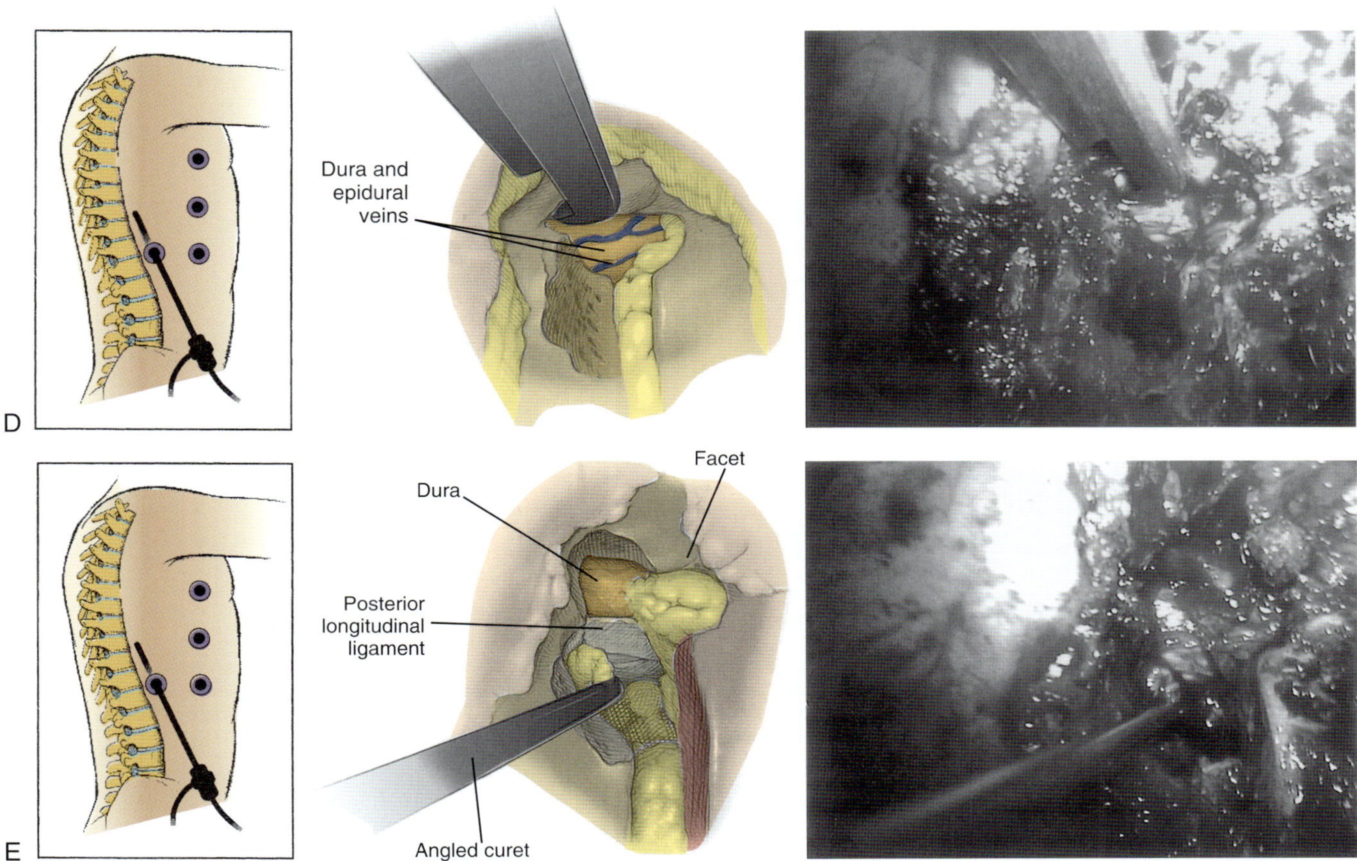

FIGURE 127-6, cont. D, Removal of this portion of the pedicle exposes the dura or epidural fat. Thoracic disc herniations can be identified at this point by following the pedicle back to the vertebral body. **E,** Disc or other compressive material is pulled ventrally with a pituitary or with a curet. (From Regan JJ, McAfee PJ, Mack MJ, et al: *Atlas of endoscopic spine surgery*, St Louis, 1995, Quality Medical Publishing, pp 168, 170, 173, 175, 177.)

group, and costs of the open procedure were 29% less than for the thoracoscopic procedure.

Holcomb and et al.[54] reported on their first seven patients with deformities undergoing ventral discectomy followed by dorsal fusion. These included patients with congenital deformities with hemivertebrae. They performed a mean of four discectomies in an average of 174 minutes. There was only one complication related to excessive bleeding from an intercostal vessel that was immediately controlled with vessel clips.

Rothenburg[34] reported a series of 20 ventral releases performed thoracoscopically in children from 8 to 17 years of age. The thoracoscopic portion of the procedure lasted a mean of 106 minutes. All patients underwent subsequent dorsal instrumentation and fusion. Corrections were noted to be acceptable and equivalent to those of the open technique. Earlier extubation, shorter ICU stays, and lower morbidity were reported.

Crawford and colleagues[1] reviewed their experience with VATS in the treatment of children with severe spine deformities. The authors noted that surgical time was reduced from that of open thoracotomy. More importantly, tissue damage, blood loss, postoperative pain, and ICU and hospital stays were all reduced. Respiratory and shoulder function were less affected. The authors list possible complications from the procedure, but these are not different from similar complications encountered in open procedures.

The prospective series of Lieberman et al.[20] followed 15 adult patients with spine deformity who underwent simultaneous ventral endoscopic and dorsal instrumentations for an average of 31 months (Fig. 127-7). There were no intraoperative technical problems with the endoscopic equipment or instruments, and visualization of the ventral spinal column was excellent. No vessel or organ injuries were encountered, and no cases were converted to open thoracotomy. No patient complained of postoperative radicular symptoms or chest pain consistent with a postthoracotomy syndrome, and there were no wound complications at the portal or dorsal incisions. There were no immediate, 6-month, or 2-year postoperative complications related to the endoscopic component of the procedure. In the scoliosis patients, the average correction was 60%. In the kyphosis patients, the average correction was 39%. Total operative time varied from 6 to 10 hours, depending primarily on the complexity of the dorsal instrumentation. Average time per disc space evacuation was 20 minutes, with a range of 15 to 35 minutes. Blood loss averaged 1200 mL for the entire series of ventral and dorsal procedures. Average hospital stay was 6.5 days (range, 5–8).

King et al.[36] describe 27 patients undergoing VATS in a prone position for scoliosis or kyphosis. No conversions to open technique were required. Only discs that did not correct to neutral or beyond on bending films were incised. A mean

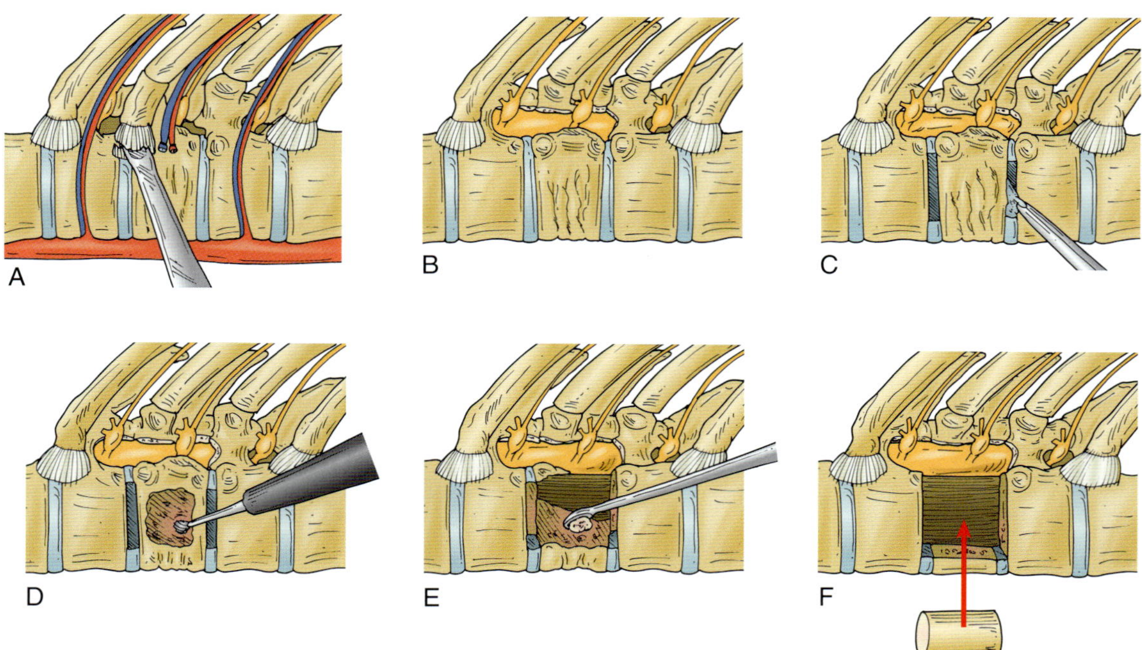

FIGURE 127-7. Thoracoscopic vertebrectomy is undertaken in a manner similar to discectomy. **A,** The ribs of the affected level and level below are removed to expose the pedicles. **B,** The pedicles are resected to expose the dura. **C,** With the dura in view, discectomies can be performed. **D,** A large cavity is created ventrally with burs, curets, and rongeurs. **E,** The remaining dorsal cortex is pulled ventrally into the defect. **F,** The defect is reconstructed with a strut graft or cage.

of 3.5 disc spaces were treated. In the scoliosis patients, the mean preoperative Cobb angle of 70.2 degrees was corrected to 22.9 degrees. For kyphosis patients, the mean Cobb angle improved from 82.3 to 48.1 degrees. Complications related to the ventral approach included one case of atelectasis and three persistent pneumothoraces after removal of the chest tube.

In summary, in experienced hands, this technique or combination appears to be at least equivalent in the short term to open surgery in terms of surgical outcome and deformity correction.

Video-Assisted Thoracoscopic Surgery for Thoracic Spinal Degenerative Disease

Although the majority of thoracoscopic procedures have been performed for deformity correction, implementation of this technique in patients with tumors or herniated thoracic discs is becoming increasingly common.[2,3,55,56] Overall, the incidence of clinical significant thoracic disc herniation is as low as 1 per million,[57] or 0.25% to 0.75% of all disc ruptures.[58]

For these uncommon lesions, a number of surgical approaches have been described, including laminectomy, pediculectomy, costotransversectomy, lateral extracavitary, transverse arthropediculectomy, and transthoracic approaches.[9] Laminectomy alone is ineffective for dorsal and dorsolateral canalicular disc herniations and may be associated with neurologic decline in up to 50% of patients.[59] Although costotransversectomy and lateral extracavitary approaches have the advantages of being able to decompress and stabilize the spine through a single incision in one stage, they are limited by their time-consuming and technically demanding nature.[60] Each of these has significant potential morbidity (Table 127-1). Moreover, they confer only a limited view of the ventral spinal cord. In one report, ventral approaches were found to have a complication rate ranging from 14% to 31%, whereas dorsal-approach–related complications ranged from 17% to 51%[7] (see Table 127-1). The first application of VATS to degenerative spinal disease was in 1993.[2]

When selecting a patient for endoscopic thoracic discectomy, the surgeon must remember that true radicular or myelopathic symptoms from thoracic disc herniations are rare. A more common scenario is the patient with diffuse midthoracic back pain with imaging showing multiple degenerative segments with or without herniations. This patient is typically not an ideal candidate for discectomy of any form, either open or endoscopic.

Operative Technique and Avoidance of Complications

Symptomatic thoracic disc herniations amenable to endoscopic transthoracic decompression are typically approached from the side of the herniation. In the context of previous surgery, a contralateral approach may be used. The first trocar is inserted at the sixth or seventh interspace toward the anterior axillary line. Then two to three additional portals are inserted under direct vision. Usually one to two portals are inserted at the anterior axillary line and one at the posterior axillary line. A 30-degree angled rigid scope may be used to see into the disc space and around the bony edges. It is necessary to identify the appropriate level and resect the proximal 2 cm of rib head if it is above T11 (Fig. 127-8). Resection of the superior part of the pedicle exposes the dura. Some authors excise the entire pedicle, particularly for larger and more central herniations.[56]

TABLE 127-1

Comparison of Approaches to Thoracic Disc Herniations

Note	Costotransversectomy	Thoracotomy	Thoracoscopy
Direction	Dorsolateral	Vertebrolateral	Vertebrolateral
View of cord	Oblique, indirect	Full, direct	Full, direct
Incision size	4–12 inches	6–15 inches	0.5–1.0 inches x 3–4 inches
Muscle transaction	Moderate to extensive	Extensive	Minimal
Relationship to pleura	Extrapleural	Intrapleural	Intrapleural
Chest tube	No	Yes	Yes
Access to post elements	Yes	No	No
Ventral fixation	No	Yes	Yes
Extent of rib resection	3–7 inches removed	6--2 inches	1 inch of rib head
Retraction	Moderate	Extensive	None
Postoperative intercostal neuralgia	Uncommon/transient	Common/prolonged	Uncommon/transient

From Dickman CA, Detweiler PW, Porter RW: Thoracoscopic spine surgery. *Clin Neurosurg* 43:396, 2000.

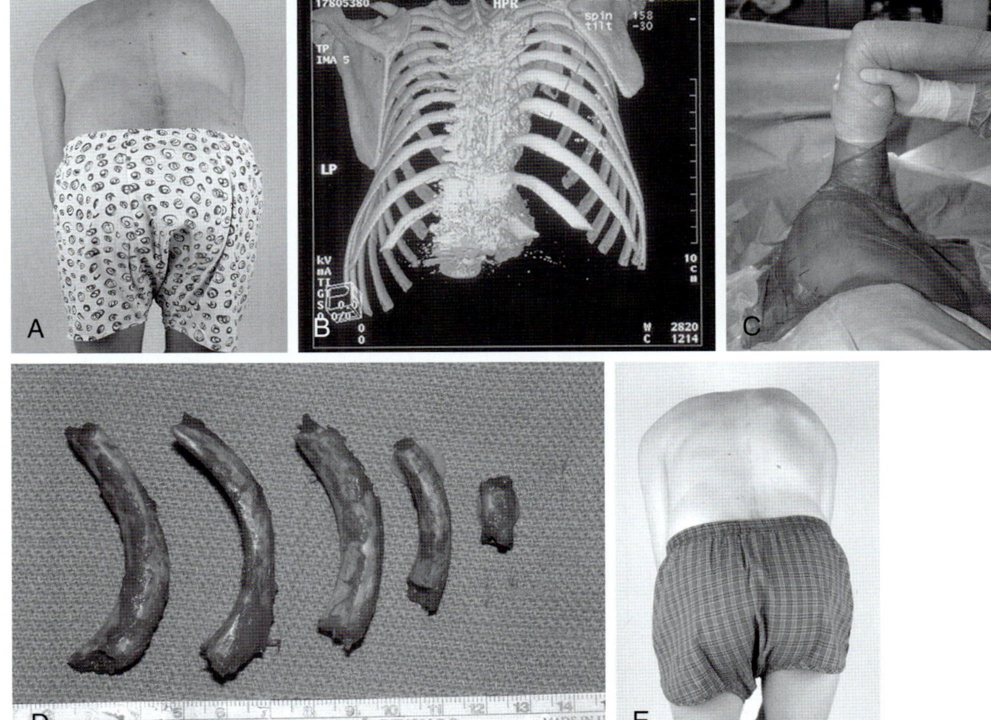

FIGURE 127-8. A, This patient had previously undergone dorsal spine fusion for scoliosis but continued to complain of a painful and unsightly rib hump. **B,** A three-dimensional CT reconstruction of the patient's chest was undertaken and planned rib resections marked. **C,** Here, the patient is positioned for thoracoplasty with the arm draped free. **D,** The removed rib sections. **E,** Postoperatively, the patient had significant improvement in pain and body contour.

Next, with the spinal cord continuously visualized to prevent inadvertent entry into the canal, a cavity is created in the disc space and vertebral bodies ventrally. The size of this space is increased for larger or more central herniations. The cavity should be wide enough that the surgeon can visualize normal dura above and below the herniation.[56] The cavity must be deep enough to expose the entire width of the ventral dura to the contralateral pedicle. A corpectomy may be required for larger or ossified herniations (Fig. 127-9).

The disc herniation is found by tracing the superior edge of the pedicle to the vertebral body and disc space. Fine instruments can then be used to pull the disc herniation into the created cavity. Once the decompression has been completed, its medial-lateral and cranial-caudal extent is documented by placing a Penfield dissector across the intervertebral space and using fluoroscopy or a radiograph. A portable CT scanner can also be used.

If a total corpectomy was required for adequate decompression, concomitant fusion should be considered. Typically, a trough is made with a side-cutting bur, and a rib fragment or iliac crest wedge is tamped into position across the disc space. Alternatively, Regan et al.[61] describe placement of an interbody cage into the disc space after decompression.

Results

Only a few centers are currently using endoscopic techniques to decompress thoracic disc herniations, and only a few clinical reports are published. In one series of thoracic endoscopic discectomies, the 14% complication rate was comparable

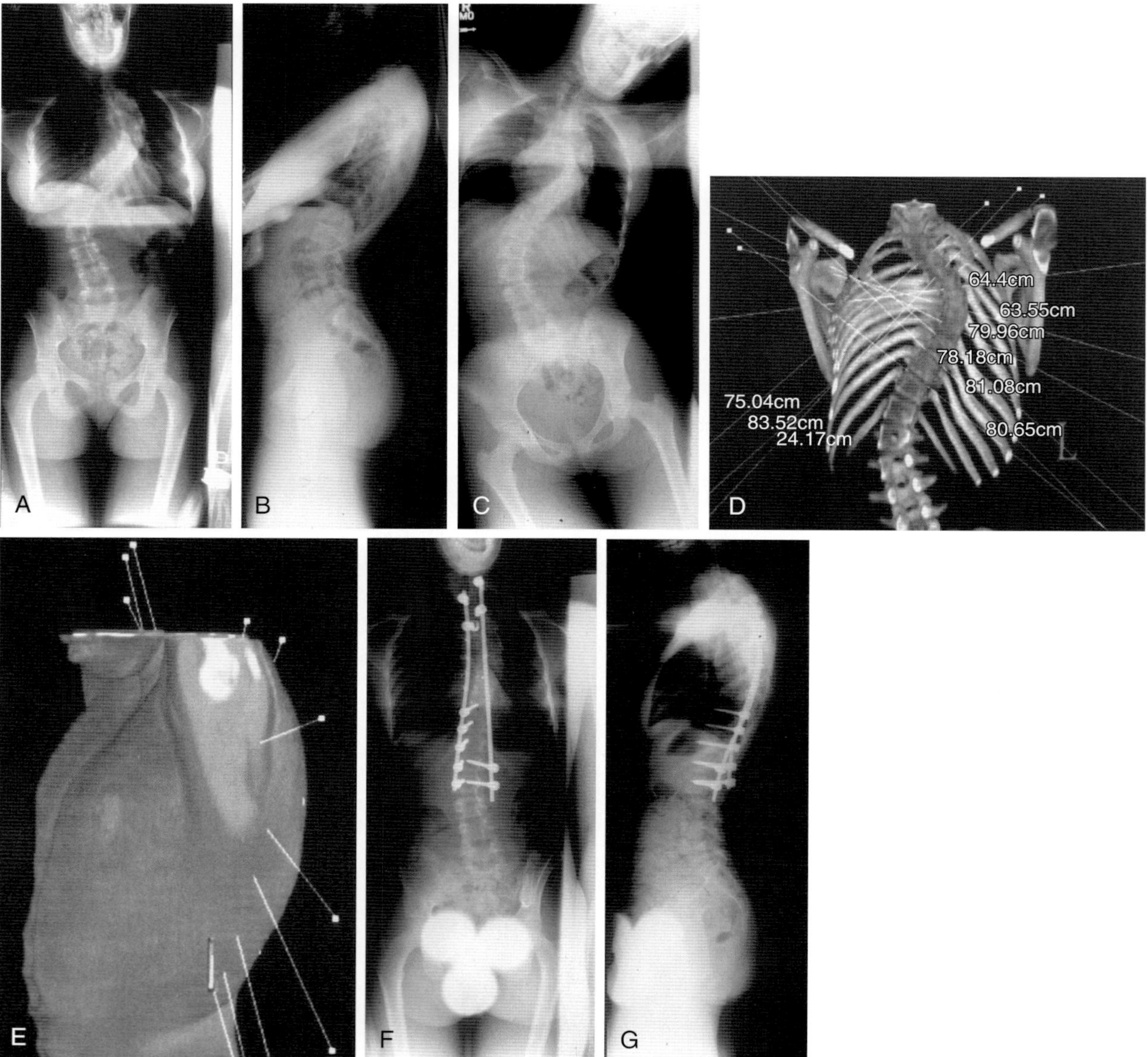

FIGURE 127-9. This patient presented with a progressive, rigid thoracic scoliosis. **A–C,** Anteroposterior, lateral, and side-bending films (respectively) are shown. **D** and **E,** Three-dimensional CT reconstructions are useful for surgical planning and portal preparation. **F** and **G,** Postoperative films are shown after a simultaneous ventral release and dorsal instrumented fusion.

with rates reported for open approaches.[3] Horowitz et al.[62] documented their experience with cadavers and a porcine model. At the time of their report, the authors were successful in decompressing the cord in five of seven cadaver disc spaces and two of three porcine spaces. One dural violation occurred. The authors thought that improvement in instrumentation would allow safer and more complete disc space access.

Rosenthal and Dickman[56] reported outcomes of 55 consecutive patients undergoing video-assisted thoracoscopic discectomy. In their group, 65% presented with myelopathic signs and symptoms caused by spinal cord compression and the remainder had severe thoracic radiculopathy. After surgery, 60% of the myelopathic patients recovered neurologically (22 completely and 5 with improvement but residual myelopathic symptoms). Seventy-nine percent of the radiculopathic patients recovered completely, and 21% improved. None worsened. The investigators compared their thoracoscopic patients with patients treated by costotransversectomy or thoracotomy and found that thoracoscopy was associated with 1 hour less time in the operating room and a reduction in blood loss by half. Postoperative chest tube output and narcotic usage were significantly lower in the thoracoscopic group.

Regan et al.[23] reported 1-year follow-up data on their first 29 patients undergoing video-assisted thoracoscopic excision of herniated discs at 32 levels. In this series, the mean operating time was 175 minutes and the estimated blood loss ranged from 75 to 2500 mL. The mean hospitalization time was 3.9 days. The investigators found that 75.8% of patients were satisfied with the procedure, 20.1% were unchanged, and 3.4% were worse. Significant improvements in Oswestry scores occurred in radiculopathic and myelopathic patients. There was a 13.8% complication rate but no long-term sequelae from any of the complications.

Subsequently, Anand and Regan[9] reported their results after 117 thoracoscopic discectomy procedures in 100 consecutive patients with an average follow-up of 4 years. Patient presentation ranged from pure axial pain to pure radiculopathy to pure myelopathy, with various combinations of these complaints. The mean operating time was 173 minutes, and blood loss averaged 259 mL. The average ICU stay was less than 1 day, and the average hospital stay was 4 days. Minor complications occurred in 21 patients, all of which resolved with no untoward effect. No patient's neurologic status worsened. Clinical success was defined as a modest 20% improvement in Oswestry score at final follow-up. Overall, objective clinical success was observed at final follow-up in 70% of these patients. The greatest gains were noted in myelopathic patients, followed by the radiculopathic patients. Axial pain patients exhibited the least postoperative improvement. The authors concluded that VATS appears to be a safe and efficacious method for the treatment of refractory symptomatic thoracic disc herniations.

McAfee[37] reported complications related to a thoracoscopic decompression, in a series of 77 patients, as excessive epidural bleeding in 1 patient and transient paraparesis in another. A number of other case reports and small series are also available with similar results.[63,64]

Video-Assisted Thoracoscopic Surgery in the Treatment of Spinal Tumors

Much as with thoracic disc herniations, the previous standard approach to cord compression from spinal tumors was laminectomy. However, for lesions ventral to the cord, the rate of neurologic improvement after surgery has been poor.[29] Over time, more aggressive and more highly morbid approaches such as costotransversectomy and thoracotomy have been espoused for more complete cord decompression. VATS techniques have been typically used in intralesional or "piecemeal" tumor debulking procedures, or for biopsy. Solitary tumor en bloc resections typically require open approaches.

The technique of decompression in patients with spinal tumors is similar to that in degenerative disease (Fig. 127-10). Preoperatively, it is necessary to consider the vascularity of the lesion. In many cases, preoperative embolization should be considered, particularly for vascular tumors such as renal cell carcinoma. Reconstruction techniques in malignancy may be liberalized depending on the anticipated life span of the patient. To avoid the morbidity of graft harvest and to achieve early stability, Rosenthal described reconstruction by injection of semiliquid polymethylmethacrylate (PMMA).[65] The PMMA is injected through a tube into the cavity and allowed to polymerize in situ. For patients with longer anticipated survival, a fusion should be performed. Ventral instrumentation options are improving. In Rosenthal's series, special equipment was used to dilate the skin incision to allow insertion of a ventral plate. Special instruments are used to handle the plates and screws in the chest cavity.

There are few published series describing the results of endoscopic decompression of spine tumors. Rosenthal et al. described outcomes in four patients with malignancies of the thoracic spine and progressive neurologic deficits treated with thoracoscopic decompression.[41] At an average of 11 months of follow-up, all patients were free of pain and neurologically improved. In this small series, there were no complications or hardware failures. All patients were also externally braced, and adjuvant chemotherapy or radiation therapy was used in several patients. Dickman et al.[16] reported on the outcomes of seven patients undergoing thoracoscopic vertebrectomy for tumor. They found that the operative time and blood loss were similar to that of a similar group undergoing open thoracotomy. Narcotic use,

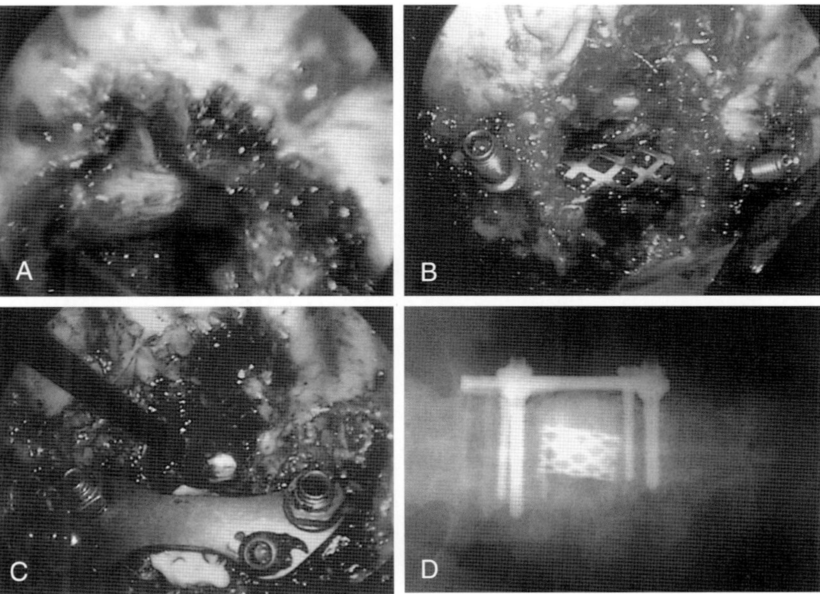

FIGURE 127-10. A patient with metastatic breast cancer and a pathologic fracture presented with impending paraplegia. **A,** A thoracoscopic corpectomy allowed complete decompression of the dura. The exiting nerve root is clearly visible. **B,** A Harms cage, in this case filled with polymethylmethacrylate (PMMA), is inserted into the defect. **C,** Further fixation is afforded by a plate applied over the cage. **D,** An intraoperative, cross-table anteroposterior radiograph demonstrates satisfactory positioning of the implants. (From Regan JJ, Jarolem KL: Thoracoscopy of the spine. In Herkowitz HN, Garfin SR, Balderston RA, et al, editors: *Rothman-Simeone: the spine*, ed 4, Philadelphia, 1999, WB Saunders, 1999, pp 608–609.)

ICU stay, and hospital length of stay were all dramatically reduced in the thoracoscopic group.

One subgroup of spinal tumors that has received special emphasis is the so-called dumbbell tumor groups. Up to 10% of neurogenic tumors in the dorsal mediastinum extend into the spinal canal.[26] These lesions have previously required resection through open thoracotomy, often with a staged laminectomy. Heltzer et al.[26] describe resection of such a dumbbell lesion through a staged laminectomy followed by a thoracoscopic approach. Subsequently, Konno et al.[66] reported on a series of five patients treated with a similar technique and followed for at least 3 years. In their series, postoperative instability did not develop in any patient.

Citow et al.[11] described a single-stage, combined laminectomy and thoracoscopic resection of a 4 × 5 × 5 cm mass filling 60% of the spinal canal at the T3 level. The lesion was first detached from the spinal cord by way of laminectomy with medial facetectomy. Then, a three-portal thoracoscopic approach was undertaken in which the parietal pleura was incised and the tumor bluntly dissected and removed through an expanded ventral portal in a specimen bag. The authors noted that a potential limitation to this approach was possible communication between the subarachnoid space with the low-pressure pleural cavity, which would increase the risk of cerebrospinal fluid fistula. They recommended an endoscopic suture of the parietal pleura. Further, because of the potential for malignant lesions to encase or invade the mediastinal structures, they suggested distinguishing between benign and malignant lesions prior to proceeding with the endoscopic approach.

Van Dijk et al.[67] described another combined technique for solitary spinal tumor resection in which thoracoscopically assisted ventral releases were followed by a dorsal en bloc spondylectomy and reconstruction. This approach allowed thoracoscopic access and release of the involved spinal segments to achieve surgical and histopathologic wide margins while avoiding the disadvantages inherent to thoracotomy.

McLain's technique for decompression of thoracic metastases is similar but is undertaken through a longitudinal incision.[8,68] The initial approach mimics costotransversectomy, wherein the proximal rib is removed with the entire pedicle. Here, too, a cavity is created ventrally, and ventral compressive pathology is collapsed into this cavity by using Epstein curets. After complete decompression, a corpectomy defect is created, and the space can be reconstructed by using titanium mesh cages followed by dorsal, segmental instrumentation (Fig. 127-11).

Video-Assisted Thoracoscopic Surgery in the Treatment of Thoracic Spine Trauma

The advantages of a thoracoscopic approach in trauma patients are similar to those in other etiologic groups. Thoracoscopic techniques may be particularly helpful in the decompression of burst fractures in elderly patients who may not tolerate a thoracotomy and possible diaphragmatic incision. Similarly, the decreased disruption of shoulder mechanics with the open approach to the upper thoracic spine may be helpful in patients with paraplegia or significant leg injuries to allow earlier rehabilitation and independent transfers.

Trauma applications typically require vertebral corpectomies or osteotomies, combined with internal fixation. These procedures may be performed in the lateral or prone position depending on subsequent procedures. For prone procedures, dorsal instrumentation can be manipulated to increase intervertebral exposure with kyphosis correction. The initial trocar is inserted at the seventh intercostal space in the midaxillary line, and the chest is explored.

Because a significant portion of thoracic trauma occurs at the thoracolumbar junction, the extended manipulating channel method described by Huang et al.[69] may be useful. For these injuries, an approach from the left is recommended because the aorta lies just left of the midline and there is more space available next to the vertebral surface. After the initial portal has been made at the seventh intercostal space, an extended portal 5 to 6 cm in length is made at the injured level or slightly behind the posterior axillary line at the T9-10 interspace. A similar length of underlying rib is removed, and a small, self-retaining rib spreader is then placed, allowing introduction of larger instruments and direct palpation of the spine. The diaphragm is pushed down with a sponge forceps introduced through the manipulating channel. The approach-side pedicles are key landmarks and are removed at the vertebrectomy level and the next caudal level.[7] The dura mater is exposed, and discectomy of the superior and inferior disc spaces is undertaken.

With the dura mater exposed and observed during the remainder of the procedure, damaged disc and bone fragments are carefully removed with a forceps and rongeurs. A defect in the ventral portion of the vertebral body is created with a high-speed bur or rongeur and then compressive pathologic structures, such as the dorsal cortex or retropulsed fragments, are pulled away from the dura. Complete decompressive corpectomy requires direct palpation of the contralateral pedicle.

Reconstruction after trauma also includes morselized or structural ventral grafting followed by ventral or dorsal instrumented stabilization. Morselized bone placed into partial corpectomy defects is typically stabilized dorsally with short-segment transpedicular instrumentation.[17] Alternatively, a corpectomy reconstruction can be completed by negotiating allograft struts, or mesh cages, into the defect, after inserting them into the chest through one of the portals. Then, either ventral or dorsal instrumentation is used to stabilize the construct to extension, rotation, and side flexion.

Hertlein et al.[17] describe eight cases of staged, ventral thoracic discectomy and bone grafting after dorsal transpedicular stabilization. Short-segment dorsal instrumentation is used to reduce the kyphotic deformity. Then tomograms or sagittal CT reconstructions are obtained to assess the size of the anterior column defect. If large, this ventral defect is directly bone grafted by using thoracoscopic means.

Dickman et al.[16] reported on the outcomes of six patients undergoing thoracoscopic vertebrectomy for fracture. They found that the operative time and blood loss were similar to that of a similar, open thoracotomy group. On the other hand, narcotic use, ICU stay, and hospital length of stay were all dramatically reduced in the thoracoscopic group.

Huang et al.[70] described their series of ventral decompressions and stabilization in eight elderly patients when

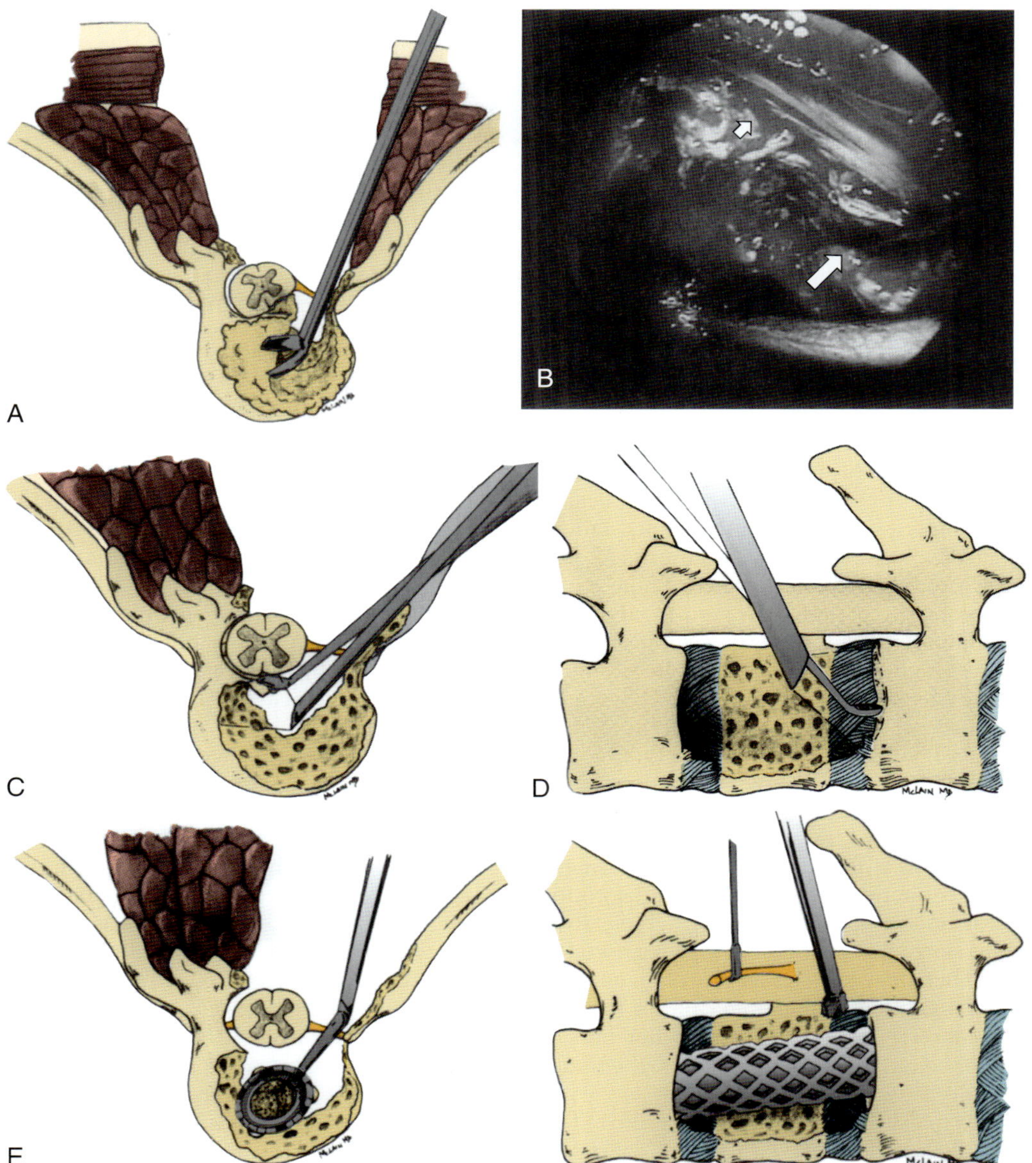

FIGURE 127-11. An endoscope may be used to assist dorsal spinal decompressions as well. **A,** The pedicle and medial rib are removed. This allows decompression of tumor or other compressive pathology to the vertebral midline. **B** and **C,** Then, a 70-degree endoscope can be used to visualize the posterior longitudinal ligament, and the remainder of the dorsal cortex can be collapsed into the vertebrectomy defect ventrally. In **B**, the *large arrow* indicates the interval between the dorsal vertebral cortex and dura, and the *small arrow* indicates the posterior longitudinal ligament. **D,** With the decompression completed, the vertebrectomy can be further prepared by removing the adjacent discs and end-plate cartilage with a curet or rongeur. **E,** Finally, the defect is reconstructed by using a strut graft or cage. (From McLain RF: Endoscopically assisted decompression for metastatic thoracic neoplasms. *Spine [Phila Pa 1976]* 23(10):1130–1135, 1998, Figs. 1–4.)

using a modified two-portal technique with a 5-cm minithoracotomy incision. Over the mean 30-month follow-up period, no injuries to the great vessels, internal organs, or spinal cord occurred. Complications included one screw migration with graft displacement and transient problems with iliac crest donor site pain and wound hypesthesias. Average neurologic recovery was 1.1 grade on the Frankel scale. The authors concluded that this minimal-access technique with thoracoscopic assistance is an ideal alternative in treating patients with osteoporotic vertebral fractures and neurologic deficits.

Video-Assisted Thoracoscopic Surgery in the Treatment of Spine Infection

Spine infections are typically divided anatomically into vertebral osteomyelitis, discitis, or epidural abscess.[33] Treatment decisions are based on the sensitivity of the organism, the response of the infection to antibiotic management, the presence of abscess, the presence of neurologic involvement, the progression of spinal instability or deformity, involved spinal levels, and host factors such as age and medical comorbidities. Increased age and cephalad level of infection predispose to neurologic decline and paralysis.[71]

Treatment begins with identification of the offending organism through blood culture or biopsy. When clear identification of the organism is not obtained with percutaneous biopsy, surgical biopsy can be considered. Endoscopic techniques are an ideal, less invasive means to obtain an adequate tissue sample. Tan et al.[72] reported the case of an 18-month-old infant with increasing back pain and gait difficulty. Low-grade fever was noted, as was irregularity of the end plates at T7-8. CT scan demonstrated a soft tissue mass, but attempts at percutaneous needle biopsy were unsuccessful. A standard thoracoscopic approach was undertaken, and a 4-mm pediatric biopsy forceps was used to take several samples from the affected site.

After the organism has been identified, appropriate antibiotic treatment can commence. Surgery is indicated in any patient with progressive neurologic deficits, failure to improve with medical management, or continued vertebral collapse and instability. In most cases, when spinal cord compression occurs, the pathology is ventral, and wide approaches such as thoracotomy or costotransversectomy are required. Unfortunately, these approaches are highly morbid in this compromised patient population.[33] VATS can be used in patients with spine infections in a manner similar to that of tumor patients. That is, VATS can be used for biopsy, debridement, cord decompression, and reconstruction.

The technical details of VATS for spine infection are similar to those of other indications. Surgical goals include confirmation of tissue diagnosis with biopsy, radical debridement of all necrotic debris, correction of any secondary deformity, and stabilization with autogenous bone grafting.[33] Typically, a four-portal technique starting with an initial viewing portal at the T7 level is used. There may be a higher rate of pleurodesis secondary to the inflammation that requires either meticulous thoracoscopic adhesion dissection or a higher rate of conversion to open procedures. For similar reasons, the risk of postoperative air leak is higher as well.

Frequently, a paraspinal subpleural mass is identified. The pleura is opened parallel to the spine with careful control of the segmentals at the midbody level. Extraspinal extension of necrotic material is debrided, and the disc levels above and below the infected segment are identified. Discectomies are performed, and the end plates are prepared for subsequent fusion. This process affords the surgeon excellent orientation to the spinal anatomy. The pedicles of the affected vertebral bodies are removed. Then the corpectomies themselves are undertaken from disc space to disc space, progressing in a cranial to caudal direction. As with trauma, it is necessary to begin by creating a hollow in the vertebral body ventrally. Then, dorsal cortex and compressive material can be delivered anteriorly with a curet or small Kerrison rongeur. The magnification and lighting afforded by the endoscope allows the decompressed dura to be inspected at close range to ensure adequate decompression.

Huang et al.[19] reported their experience with VATS in managing tuberculous spondylitis in 10 patients. At a mean 24-month follow-up, average neurologic recovery was 1.1 Frankel grade. Complications included one lung atelectasis, pleural adhesions requiring conversion to an open procedure in one case, and four transient postoperative air leaks. The authors concluded that thoracoscopic techniques were a useful adjunct in the management of patients with tuberculous spondylitis for either biopsy or formal decompression and reconstruction. For debridement and reconstruction, the authors recommended a combination of thoracoscopic visualization and minithoracotomy for debridement and instrumentation.

Dickman et al.[16] reported on the outcomes of three patients undergoing thoracoscopic vertebrectomy for infection. They found that the operative time and blood loss were similar to that of an open thoracotomy group. On the other hand, narcotic use, ICU stay, and hospital length of stay were all dramatically reduced in the thoracoscopic group.

Thoracoscopic Instrumentation

The next major step in endoscopic transthoracic spine surgery is the development and application of spinal implants capable of stabilization and correction. Interbody fusion cages have enjoyed widespread use in the lumbar spine, and this experience is now being applied to the thoracic spine. Cages can be applied in the coronal or oblique plane. Application in the thoracic spine may be technically less demanding, but the risks of malposition are clearly more significant. The fusion rates of single cages in the thoracic spine remain to be evaluated.

With some difficulty, existing rod and screw implant systems may be inserted in an endoscopic or endoscopically assisted fashion. These systems have also been modified by using, for example, cannulated screws and combinations of endoscopic and fluoroscopic insertion techniques.[73]

Hertlein et al.[18] described their first two cases of thoracoscopic osteosynthesis. After decompression and grafting as described previously, dynamic compression plates were brought into the wound through the working trocar. The plate was preliminarily fixed to the spine by using two Kirschner wires. A Cardan drill was then inserted into the trocar, and 3.2-mm holes of 2-cm depth were prepared. Next, 6-cm screws were inserted into the plate with a Cardan screwdriver. These patients were not braced postoperatively.

Crawford[1] and Picetti et al.[40] have described similar endoscopic instrumentation techniques in the deformity setting. The authors used circumferential C-arm access to the patient along with a tricannulated pitchfork. The tricannulated pitchfork was used to place guide pins and subsequently screws. The device allows the surgeon to line up the best coronal location for the screw and place a Steinmann pin through the cannula under image control. The pin is placed in the midcoronal plane of the vertebra and driven from slightly dorsal to ventral starting just ventral to the rib head. Starting at the rib head prevents the surgeon from starting the screw too far dorsally. The surgeon stands at the patient's back and places the instrumentation from back to front, aiming away from the spinal cord. Once the Steinmann pin has been placed, its external portion is secured to prevent penetration through the body into the opposite hemithorax. A cannulated tap prepares the site for a bone screw. When the screws have been placed, a measuring device for rod length is advanced through the inferior portal. The rod is inserted through the inferior portal and seated into the screw heads. Capture screws are seated into screw heads to secure the rod. The bottom screw is tightened first so that all compression projects superiorly toward the top of the thoracic cage rather than inferiorly toward the diaphragm. Once the rod has been fully seated, a compressor is introduced, each set of screws is individually compressed, and the capture screw is tightened and torqued. With present designs, a true rotational maneuver is not possible.

Recently, Assaker et al.[74,75] studied the feasibility of adding computer image guidance to endoscopic spine procedures. In this setting, three-dimensional assessment of instrumentation position would be possible through video monitors by using an extracorporeal fiducial and a CT-based navigational system. This may improve the speed and accuracy of endoscopically performed decompression and instrumentation.

Huang et al.[76] describe a combination thoracoscopic and "mini-open" approach to decompress and stabilize the spine in a series of four patients with thoracic myelopathy. A 3- to 4-cm manipulating channel is created for both endoscopic instrumentation and subsequent tumor removal and reconstruction. Standard reconstructive instrumentation may then be inserted.

These techniques are not without potential complications. The greatest of these is malposition of the instrumentation into the spinal canal or vascular structures because of the loss of three-dimensional vision and direct palpation. Roush et al.[73] also reported a case of tension pneumothorax during fluoroscopic guide pin placement for a video-assisted ventral scoliosis stabilization procedure.

Spine Endoscopy in the Thoracic Spine: Dorsal Approach

Direct dorsal approaches to midline neurocompressive thoracic pathology have largely been abandoned because laminectomy alone does not adequately decompress a kyphotic spinal segment. Moreover, attempts to indirectly decompress central pathologies have been unsuccessful, or worse, have resulted in neurologic decline.[77,78] On the other hand, costotransversectomy and lateral extracavitary approaches are associated with large incisions, increased postoperative morbidity, wound healing problems, and difficulty with visualization.[1,7] Smaller, transpedicular dorsal approaches can use small incisions and a 70-degree endoscope to better visualize the ventral dura and avoid the need for postoperative chest tube drainage required of either thoracoscopy or thoracotomy.

The role of endoscopic and minimally invasive techniques in treatment of metastatic and degenerative disease is evolving. Although ventral approaches to metastatic disease are favored overall, the use of an endoscope to assist dorsolateral decompression may obviate the need for a second, ventral surgery in patients undergoing dorsal stabilization. This approach is particularly useful in patients with radioresistant metastases of the upper thoracic spine, where thoracotomy is difficult and highly morbid.[8,68] Similarly, dorsal vertebrectomy and decompression techniques must be considered in patients unable to tolerate single-lung ventilation or thoracotomy. Contraindications to the currently available techniques include failed prior open surgery and large lesions. Dorsal transpedicular instrumentation is another area in which endoscopic assistance may allow for smaller incisions and decreased muscle injury. These resection techniques are intralesional and are therefore not indicated in patients with primary neoplasms.[8]

Anatomy and Technique

Osman and Marsolais[79] described a dorsal endoscopic approach to the thoracic disc space in a cadaver. The authors found that above T10, the rib neck was an ideal guide to the disc space and prevented lateral excursion into the lung. The shoulder girdle and transition from thoracic kyphosis to cervical lordosis made accurate insertion at the T1-2 and T2-3 levels difficult. They concluded that this approach would be technically feasible for soft lateral discs. With further development of endoscopic instrumentation, even calcified or adherent central discs could be approached in this manner.

Jho[80] described a minimally invasive dorsal approach to thoracic disc herniations using a 2-cm-long transverse paramedian incision at the pedicle level of the involved vertebra. Patients are positioned 60 degrees forward, inclined to keep the lesion side facing upward. The paraspinal muscles are dissected from the spinous process, lamina, and transverse processes by using a periosteal elevator. A tubular retractor is passed into the wound over the facet and lamina. The medial portion of the facet, the lateral portion of the lamina, and the rostral third of the pedicle are removed with a high-speed bur to gain access to the disc space and to expose the very lateral margin of the spinal cord dura. A 2-mm bur removes the bone spurs rostral and caudal to the herniated disc and creates a cavity into which material from the decompression is moved. When an appropriate 1.5-cm cavity has been created, a 4-mm-diameter rigid endoscope with a 70-degree lens is mounted to a custom-made endoscope holder. Surgical decompression of the ventral cord can then be performed by using 90-degree curved surgical instruments. For example, a down-biting curet can be used to push more osteophyte away from the cord and into the created cavity. Material can be removed from the cavity with a curved pituitary rongeur.

Results

Jho[80] reported on a consecutive series of 25 patients undergoing minimal-access thoracic discectomy. Seven patients were myelopathic, 6 presented with myeloradiculopathy, 10 presented with radicular complaints, and 2 were believed to have segmental pain. He reports the perioperative morbidity of this procedure to be similar to that of lumbar microdiscectomy, and radiculopathic patients are allowed to go home the same day. In his series, the 2 patients with segmental pain did not note relief of symptoms despite MRI documentation of complete decompression. Of the radiculopathic patients, 9 of 10 had complete relief of symptoms. Twelve of 13 myelopathic or myeloradiculopathic patients had significant relief of symptoms.

McLain[8] described the successful use of an endoscope to complete ventral decompression from a dorsal approach in five patients by using an endoscope to increase visualization. The mean operative time was 7.25 hours, and the mean blood loss was 1800 mL. Neurologic recovery was judged excellent.

Dorsal Spine Endoscopy in the Lumbar Spine

This phrase may refer to the tubular dilation/endoscopic camera system used for minimal access to the lumbar spine or to endoscopic laparoscopy used to gain an approach to the ventral lumbar region.

The ventral laparoscopic approach can be used for ventral fusion and stabilization procedures, resection of neoplasms, and spinal reconstruction.[81] Laparoscopic skills are not part of the repertoire of most neurosurgeons, and often a cosurgeon is necessary.

The dorsal spinal approach using a dilator is a tried, tested, and effective technique.[82] Robust clinical data suggest that the complication rates, length of stay, and cost are comparable to those of open techniques. The dorsal spinal endoscopic approach may be used for access for dorsal fusion and stabilization, nerve and canal decompression, tumor and infection removal, and intradural lesion surgery.[82]

Anatomy

The anatomy of the dorsal lumbar spine is familiar to most neurosurgeons. However, the endoscopic view is different from a traditional open approach and should be carefully studied. The endoscopic view does not use the midline as an anchor point, and the docking of the tubes is usually between lamina and facet depending on the lesion and approach.

Technique

Our technique was described by Khoo and Fessler in 2002.[83] The patient is usually positioned prone on a radiolucent spinal table (Jackson or similar). The level is confirmed on a lateral radiograph, and an incision is performed to allow access to the ipsilateral facet by a Steinmann pin, which is then followed by serial dilators and attachment of the dilators to a flexible arm retractor. The working tube is then docked and attached to a 30-degree endoscope, and the ipsilateral facet, interlaminar space, and caudal edge of the superior lamina are identified after removal of soft tissue. Access to the interlaminar space is gained with an angled curet, and the lamina is removed using a drill, punches, and rongeurs. The tube can then be angled to achieve medial, lateral, rostral, and caudal access. Ipsilateral or contralateral nerve decompression, disc access and sequestrectomy, canal decompression, and dural access can be achieved using this technique. The incision can be widened to achieve multilevel decompression or dural access as required.

Results

Khoo and Fessler[83] found a 68% improvement in symptoms following endoscopic decompression for lumbar canal stenosis, comparable to open techniques. Both endoscopic canal decompression and endoscopic microdiscectomy show statistically significant reduction in blood loss and hospital stay compared with open techniques.[83] Recent data show a comparable improvement in canal decompression area with endoscopic compared to open techniques.[84]

Lateral decompressions can also be combined with minimally invasive fusion and instrumentation, including dorsal osteotomies, dorsolateral vertebrectomy, and interbody cage fusion and combinations of these for tumor, trauma, infection, and degeneration.[83]

However, Sairyo et al.,[85] in an unselected series of 138 patients, suggest that the initial complication rates may be higher than in open procedures, highlighting the importance of appropriate training in these techniques. In a randomized multicenter trial of lumbar microdiscectomy, Arts et al.[86] propose that the rates of back pain and sciatica were higher in the endoscopy group compared with those of open techniques. Unfortunately, the experience of the treating surgeons in these techniques was not specifically mentioned. Three other randomized trials of microdiscectomy (Righesso et al.,[87] Ryang et al.,[88] and Mayer and Brock[89]) did not show a significant difference in complication rates. Recent papers also suggest a significant reduction in the incidence of postfusion infection rates.[90]

There has also been interest in recent years in endoscopic dorsal decompression of the cervical spine, which has also gradually become an established technique.[91,92]

Summary

Techniques for both ventral and dorsal endoscopically assisted access to the thoracic and lumbar spine are evolving rapidly. With this evolution, it is important to remember that endoscopic spine surgery refers only to a change in approach, not to a change in the operation itself. Therefore, the indications for operative intervention are not relaxed merely because these procedures may be performed through smaller incisions. As in any spine surgery, careful patient selection is the critical factor predicting successful outcomes.

Endoscopic spine surgery confers many proven and potential advantages to both the surgeon and patient, including improved surgical visualization through magnification and lighting, decreased perioperative morbidity, and shorter hospital stays. But these advantages must be counterbalanced with disadvantages of these approaches, including lack of familiarity, decreased three-dimensional perspective, and a loss of tactile sense. Initial experience with these procedures should include cadaveric and animal laboratory work, followed by visits to active centers or proctoring.[7] Every surgeon undertaking a VATS procedure should be able to convert to an open procedure or have a thoracic surgeon available. Early cases may be associated with higher complication rates and operating times. Ultimately, a less efficacious technique should not be used merely because it is endoscopic.

A second-approach surgeon, who may not be required in an open procedure, may be needed for a given endoscopic procedure. Specialized and often single-use instruments are required. These additional operating room costs may be recouped with earlier patient discharge. There is ample opportunity to study and improve on these techniques. A randomized clinical trial comparing open with endoscopic techniques is needed, and long-term outcome data are needed. Many of these procedures are promising, but significant advantages over previous techniques remain to be proven.

Lumbar endoscopic spine surgery is a more established field but also has a steep learning curve, and either fellowship training or proctoring is strongly recommended. The dorsal endoscopic approach to the thoracic and lumbar spine has a good experience and good safety profile.

KEY REFERENCES

Crawford AH, Wall EJ, Wolf R: Video-assisted thoracoscopy. *Orthop Clin North Am* 30(3):367–385, 1999.

Dickman CA, Karahalios DG: Thoracoscopic spine surgery. *Clin Neurosurg* 43:392–422, 2000.

Regan JJ: Percutaneous endoscopic thoracic discectomy. *Neurosurg Clin North Am* 7(1):87–98, 1996.

Rosenthal D, Marquardt G, Lorenz R, et al: Anterior decompression and stabilization using a microsurgical endoscopic technique for metastatic tumors of the thoracic spine. *J Neurosurg* 84:565–572, 1996.

REFERENCES

The complete reference list is available online at expertconsult.com.

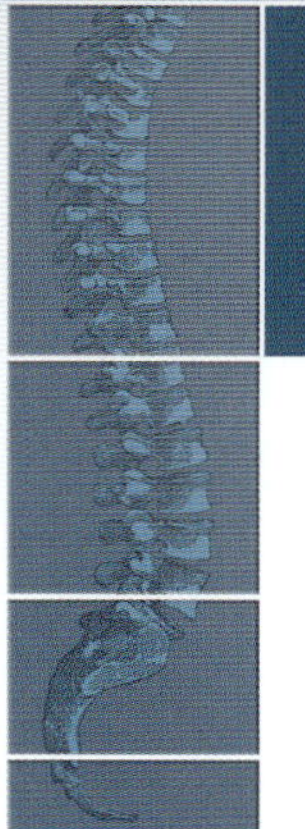

CHAPTER 128

Vertebroplasty and Kyphoplasty

Daisuke Togawa | Isador H. Lieberman

Osteoporotic Vertebral Compression Fractures

Osteoporosis and associated fragility fractures are major threats to the health of aging populations worldwide.[1] At 50 to 79 years of age, the incidence of a new vertebral compression fracture (VCF) in Europe is 1% per year in women and 0.6% per year in men, and at 75 to 79 years of age, the incidence is 2.9% per year in women and 1.4% per year in men.[2] In the United States, approximately 750,000 people are affected, and only one third receive treatment.[3] Despite nonsurgical management, including analgesia, bed rest, physiotherapy, and back bracing, pain sometimes resolves slowly and can persist.[4] The resulting vertebral deformity can cause height loss, kyphosis, reduced pulmonary function, and mobility and balance impairment. VCFs are associated with an increased incidence of mortality and morbidity, including back pain, loss of height, kyphotic deformity, increased risk of future fracture, and reduction in quality of life.[5] Osteoporotic VCFs are clearly a clinically significant health problem with continuously increasing economic and social ramifications. The National Osteoporosis Foundation predicts that the number of vertebral body compression fractures will double in the next 15 years due to the aging population and increasingly sedentary lifestyles.

Nonsurgical Treatment

In recent rears, various osteoporosis treatments have been developed to reduce the risk of fracture.[6,7] As a treatment for VCFs, traditional, nonoperative management includes bedrest, analgesics, and bracing. However, these types of medical management fail to restore spinal alignment, and the lack of mobility itself can result in secondary complications, including worsening osteoporosis, atelectasis, pneumonia, deep vein thrombosis, decubitus ulcer, and pulmonary embolism. An alternative approach is supervised ambulatory mobility by a physiotherapist plus hydrotherapy.[8] In one third of patients, severe pain, limited mobility, and poor quality of life persist despite appropriate nonoperative management. Whether the pain has or has not resolved, no patient after a VCF spontaneously achieves a realigned spine, corrected sagittal contour, or restoration of vertebral height.

Surgical Treatment

Historically, the only alternative to nonoperative management for symptomatic vertebral fractures was open surgical decompression (ventral or dorsal decompression and stabilization via internal fixation hardware and bone grafting), and this was usually reserved for those patients with gross spinal deformity or neurologic impairment (<0.5%).[9] The reason for this surgical caution was the adverse risk/benefit ratio in this elderly population with poor bone quality and multiple comorbid conditions.

Percutaneous vertebroplasty (PVP) is a minimally invasive method that involves the percutaneous injection of polymethylmethacrylate (PMMA) into a collapsed vertebral body to stabilize the vertebra. Originally developed for osteolytic metastasis, myeloma, and hemangioma, the procedure resulted in quick, effective pain relief and a low complication rate.[10-12] PVP is now also increasingly used for the treatment of osteoporotic vertebral fractures.[13] However, PVP does not expand the collapsed vertebra, potentially locking the spine in a kyphotic posture. In addition, the PMMA bone filler has associated problems (epidural leakage, thermal necrosis, inability to integrate with bone, handling difficulties, toxicity to patient and operator).[14,15]

Kyphoplasty is an advanced minimally invasive technique with a number of potential advantages over PVP, including lower risk of cement extravasation and better restoration of vertebral body height.[16] A cannula is introduced into the vertebral body, followed by insertion of an inflatable bone tamp, which when deployed, reduces the compression fracture and restores the vertebral body toward its original height, while creating a cavity to be filled with bone cement. The cement augmentation is therefore done with more control into the low-pressure environment of the preformed cavity with viscous, partially cured cement.

Vertebral Augmentation

Percutaneous Vertebroplasty

Background

Percutaneous vertebral augmentation (vertebroplasty, PVP) was first reported by Galibert et al. in 1984 and initially involved the augmentation of the vertebral body with PMMA to treat a hemangioma. PVP was reportedly not performed in the United States until 1994. Originally targeted for osteolytic metastasis, myeloma, and hemangioma, PVP resulted in early appreciable pain relief and a low complication rate.[12,17] Its indications subsequently expanded to osteoporotic vertebral collapse with chronic pain, further to include treatment of asymptomatic vertebral collapse and even prophylactic intervention for at-risk vertebral bodies.[18] Nevertheless, the treatment of acute fractures in ambulatory patients and prophylactic treatment remain controversial.[19] In fact, vertebral augmentation itself is somewhat controversial, with questions concerning a lack of defined indications, expected complications, outcome measures, and the need for long-term follow-up data.[14]

An open question in PVP is the mechanism of pain relief. The most intuitive explanation involves simple mechanical stabilization of the fracture. However, another possibility is the analgesic result from local chemical, vascular, or thermal effects of PMMA on nerve endings in surrounding tissue.[13,20] Supporting this concept is the lack of correlation between cement volume and pain relief.[21,22] Further evidence against an effect resulting solely from mechanical stabilization is the fact that PVP typically does not restore lost vertebral body height and therefore does not correct altered biomechanics.[19,23]

Technique

Injection of opacified PMMA is performed via a transpedicular or paravertebral approach under continuous fluoroscopic guidance to obtain adequate filling and to avoid PMMA leakage. For complex or high-risk cases, CT and fluoroscopic guidance are sometimes combined.[10,19] In routine cases, PVP can be performed under local anesthesia with slight sedation in less than 1 hour,[1] although general anesthesia is sometimes required because pain may intensify during cement injection.[13] Preceding PMMA injection, intraosseous venography is often used to determine the filling pattern and identify sites of potential PMMA leakage (outline the venous drainage pattern, confirm needle placement within the bony trabeculae, and delineate fractures in the bony cortex). However, others have dispensed with routine venography.[23]

Contraindications to vertebroplasty include coagulopathy, absence of facilities to perform emergency decompressive surgery in the event of a complication, and extreme vertebral collapse (>65–70% reduction in vertebral height).[13]

Results

Searching the literature with the term *percutaneous vertebroplasty* in PubMed, there are 766 papers found from 1987 to March 2010.[10,12,19,23-37] The first paper on vertebroplasty was published in 1987, treating C2 hemangioma in France.[17] Reportedly, pain has been reduced in 70% to 90% of patients.

There are several case control studies published recently. Alvarez et al. conducted a prospective, double-cohort study,[38] which consisted of 101 consecutive patients who underwent PVP and 27 patients who refused PVP treatment and were managed conservatively. The results showed that the patients elected for PVP had significantly more pain and functional impairment before the procedure than the patients in the group who did not have PVP ($P < .001$). The pain, functional, and general health scores of the PVP group were improved from the preoperative mean values ($P < .001$) in all postoperative periods. Compared with the conservative treatment group, there was a significant difference at 3 months. However, no statistical differences in function were observed between these groups at 6 months and 12 months postoperatively.

Diamond et al. designed a prospective, nonrandomized, "intention-to-treat" 2-year study.[39] Participants included 126 consecutive patients (39 men and 87 women, 51 to 95 years of age) with acute osteoporotic vertebral fractures. Of these patients, 88 received treatment by PVP and 38 by conservative therapy. Outcomes in the PVP-treated patients showed 60% reduction in visual analogue pain scores from 20 to 8 ($P < .001$); a rapid return to normal function (29% improvement in physical functioning from 14 to 18 ($P < .001$); and lower rates of hospitalization (43% reduction in the mean number of hospital bed-days occupied), which were better than those treated conservatively ($P < .001$ for the comparison of all variables at 24 hours). Lower pain scores persisted in the vertebroplasty-treated group at 6 weeks ($P < .001$), but no differences between the two groups were evident at 12 and 24 months. In the vertebroplasty-treated group compared with the control group, the rates of new vertebral fractures (clinically and by radiographic assessment: hazard ratio, 1.13; 95% confidence interval [CI], 0.52–2.46; $P = .76$) and death (hazard ratio, 1.07; 95% CI, 0.42–2.76; $P = .89$) showed no significant difference.

Voormolen et al. prospectively assessed the short-term clinical outcome of patients with subacute or chronic painful osteoporotic VCFs treated with PVP compared with optimal pain medication (OPM) (VERTOS study sponsored by Vertos Medical Inc.).[40] The investigators randomized the patients into two groups: treatment by PVP or OPM. After 2 weeks, patients from the OPM arm could change to the PVP arm. Patients were evaluated 1 day and 2 weeks after treatment. Their results showed that 18 patients treated with PVP, compared with 16 patients treated with OPM, had a significantly better Visual Analogue Scale (VAS) and used fewer analgesics 1 day after treatment. Two weeks after treatment, the mean VAS was less but not significantly different in patients treated with OPM, whereas these patients used significantly fewer analgesics and had better Quality of Life Questionnaire of the European Foundation for Osteoporosis (QUALEFO) and Roland-Morris Disability (RFD) scores. Scores in the PVP arm were influenced by occurrence of new VCF in two patients. After 2 weeks of OPM, 14 patients requested PVP treatment. All scores, 1 day and 2 weeks after PVP, were significantly better compared with scores during conservative treatment.

In Rousing's randomized controlled study, 50 patients (41 females) were included from January 2001 until January 2008. Patients with acute (<2 weeks) and subacute (2–8 weeks) osteoporotic fractures were included and randomized to either PVP or conservative treatment. Their results showed reduction in pain from initial visit to 3-month follow-up was comparable in the two groups ($P = .33$); for approximate VAS, 8.0 to 2.0, intragroup difference was significant ($P = .00$). Reduction in pain in the PVP group was immediate 12 to 24 hours after the procedure ($P = .00$). There was no significant difference in the other parameters when comparing the results at inclusion and after 3 months within both groups and between the groups after 3 months. This study found two adjacent fractures in the PVP group and none in the conservative group. The investigators' conclusions suggested that the majority of patients with acute or subacute painful osteoporotic compression fractures in the spine will recover after a few months of conservative treatment.

Recently, two new studies, reported in the *New England Journal of Medicine*,[41,42] were multicenter, randomized controlled trials that used sham procedure as a control. In the Buchbinder study,[41] the number of patients enrolled was 78, and 35 of 38 underwent PVP, and 36 of 40 underwent sham procedure in four Australian centers and completed the 6-month follow-up (91%). At 3 months, the mean reductions in the score for pain in the vertebroplasty and control groups were 2.6 ± 2.9 and 1.9 ± 3.3, respectively. Similar improvements were seen in both groups with respect to pain at night and at rest, physical functioning, quality of life, and perceived improvement. The researchers concluded that there was no beneficial effect of vertebroplasty compared with a sham procedure.

In another randomized, controlled trial, called the Investigational Vertebroplasty Safety and Efficacy Trial (INVEST) by Kallmes et al.,[42] 68 patients underwent PVP and 63 underwent sham procedure. Both groups had immediate improvement in disability and pain scores after the intervention. Although there was a trend toward a higher rate of clinically meaningful improvement in pain (a 30% decrease from baseline) in the vertebroplasty group (64% vs. 48%, P = .06), the two groups did not differ significantly on any secondary outcome measure at 1 month. The investigators also concluded that improvements in pain and pain-related disability associated with osteoporotic compression fractures in patients treated with vertebroplasty were similar to the improvements in a control group.

Complications

The principal risk of PVP, which involves the forced injection of low-viscosity PMMA cement into the closed space of the collapsed vertebral body, is cement extravasation. Extravasation rates are as high as 65% when cement is used to treat osteoporotic fractures.[12,30] The likelihood is greater when using cement with a liquid rather than paste consistency or with higher PMMA volume.[27] However, in most settings, the majority of extravasations have no clinical relevance, at least in the short term.[23]

The consequence of an extravasation depends on its location. In epidural or foraminal extravasation, nerve root compression and radiculopathy is the major risk. This occurred in 11 of 274 patients (4%) treated by Deramond.[10] Three of those patients required surgical nerve root decompression. Others have been described with a 5% rate of radiculopathy, as well.[9,21,43] Extravasation into perivertebral veins can cause cement embolism to the lungs; deaths attributed to cement embolism have been documented. However, two reported deaths attributed to pulmonary embolism were believed to be unrelated to the procedure; no cement material was detected by chest radiograph of the first patient,[13,44] and the second pulmonary embolism arose from deep venous lower extremity thrombosis.[10] On the other hand, extravasation into adjacent discs or paravertebral tissue, although common, generally produces no patient symptoms and carries little clinical significance; many such extravasations can be avoided by careful needle positioning.[10]

Other operative and long-term complications of PVP are specific to PMMA as a filler.[18,23,45] The physician may work with PMMA in large batches to keep it liquid and to extend the working time for vertebroplasty. However, its high polymerization temperature (86–107°C within cement core)[46] can damage adjacent tissue, including the spinal cord and nerve roots,[15] leading to an inflammatory reaction and transitory exacerbation of pain.[13] When injecting PMMA monomer, physician vigilance and caution are required. Absorption of PMMA monomer during the injection can induce hypotension by virtue of its cardiotoxic and dysrhythmogenic properties.[47] Keeping in mind that placing a material in the spine affords proximity and access to the chest and the heart, vertebral augmentation with PMMA demands meticulous attention to technique.

Overall, the risk of complications that carry clinical significance following PVP for osteoporotic vertebral fracture is thought to be 1% to 3%, and most potential complications can be avoided with good technique.[10]

Kyphoplasty

Background

Kyphoplasty is an advanced surgical technique having evolved from a marriage of vertebroplasty with balloon angioplasty. It has a number of potential advantages, including lower risk of cement extravasation and better restoration of vertebral body height. A cannula is introduced into the vertebral body, via a transpedicular (Fig. 128-1) or extrapedicular route (Fig. 128-2), followed by insertion of an

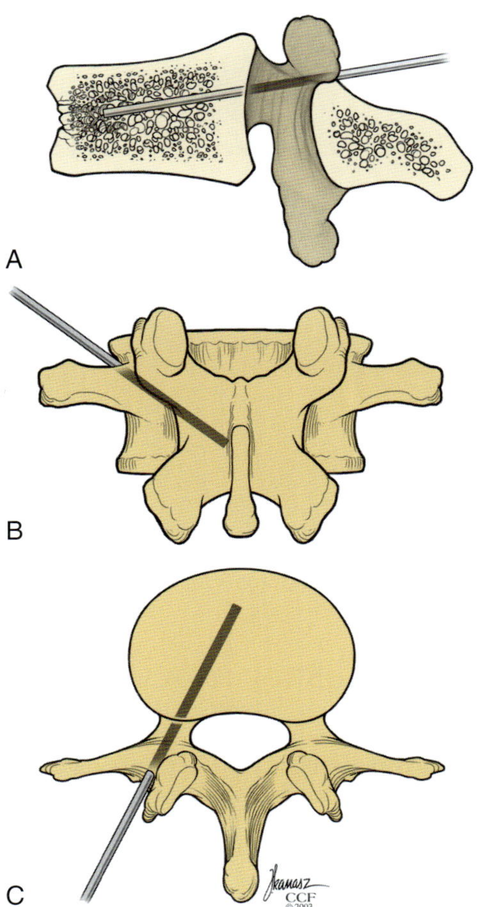

FIGURE 128-1. A–C, Transpedicular access.

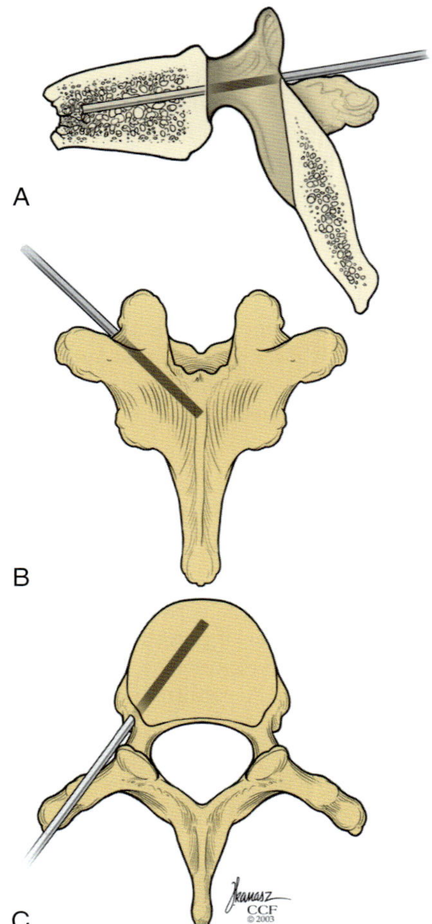

FIGURE 128-2. A–C, Extrapedicular access.

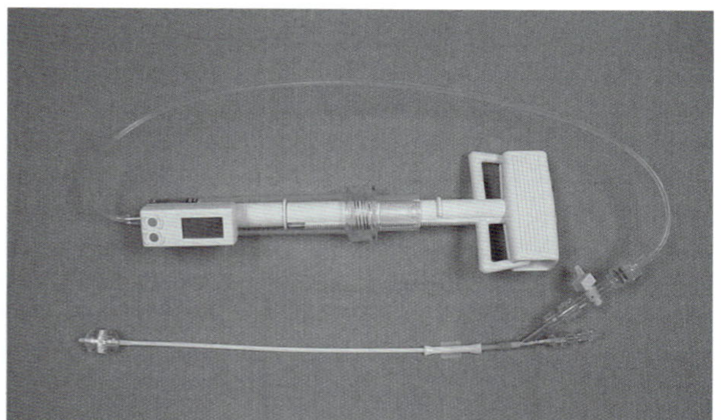

FIGURE 128-3. Inflatable bone tamp. (Courtesy of Kyphon, Inc., Sunnyvale, CA.)

inflatable bone tamp (IBT; Fig. 128-3), which when deployed, reduces the compression fracture and restores the vertebral body toward its original height. This then creates a cavity to be filled with bone cement. The cement augmentation can now be completed with more control into the low-pressure environment of the preformed cavity with viscous, partially cured cement. Using a cannula for bone filler with a steel stylet as a plunger enables the operator to apply cement at considerably higher viscosity than is possible with injection through a 5-mL syringe and 11-gauge needle. Both the higher cement viscosity and controlled fill reduce the risk of cement extravasation. Filling is performed under continuous lateral fluoroscopic guidance similar to vertebroplasty. The procedure can be performed under general anesthesia or local anesthesia with intravenous sedation, and most of the patients are able to return home the same day of procedure.

Technique

With the patient under general or local anesthesia in the prone position on a radiolucent spinal frame, two C-arms are positioned for anteroposterior and lateral fluoroscopic images. Once positioned the C-arms and patient are not moved, to ensure repeatable images throughout the case. Two 3-mm incisions are made at the vertebral level, parallel to the pedicles in both planes. Then a guidewire or biopsy needle is advanced into the vertebral body via a transpedicular or extrapedicular approach, depending on the fracture configuration and the patient's anatomy. The guidewire is then exchanged for the working cannula using a series of obturators. Once the working cannula is positioned, the surgeon reams out a corridor to accommodate the IBT and positions the IBT under the collapsed end plate (Fig. 128-4). To deploy the IBT, inflation proceeds slowly under fluoroscopy until maximum fracture reduction is achieved or the balloon reaches a cortical wall (Fig. 128-5). At this point, the surgeon deflates and removes the IBT, mixes the cement, prefills the cement cannulae, and allows the cement to partially cure in the cement cannulae. Once partially cured, PMMA is slowly extruded into the vertebral body through each pedicle under continuous lateral fluoroscopic guidance (Fig. 128-6). This technique permits a controlled fill. In most instances, the volume of cement can slightly exceed that of the bone cavity to interdigitate filler from the central bolus with the surrounding bone. Once filling is complete and the cement has hardened, the surgeon removes the cannula and closes the 3-mm incisions.

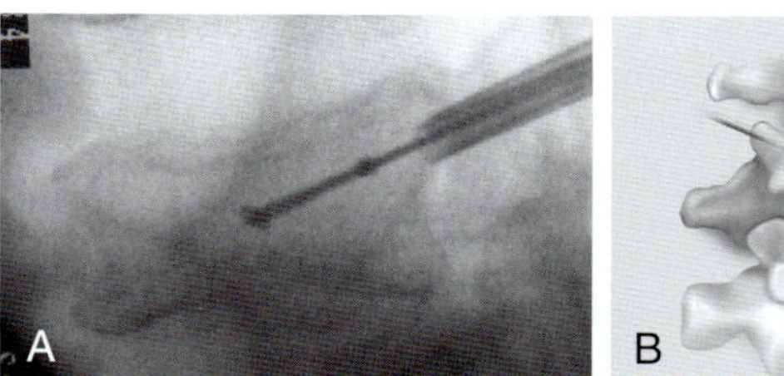

FIGURE 128-4. Radiograph (**A**) and drawing (**B**) of inflatable bone tamp in position.

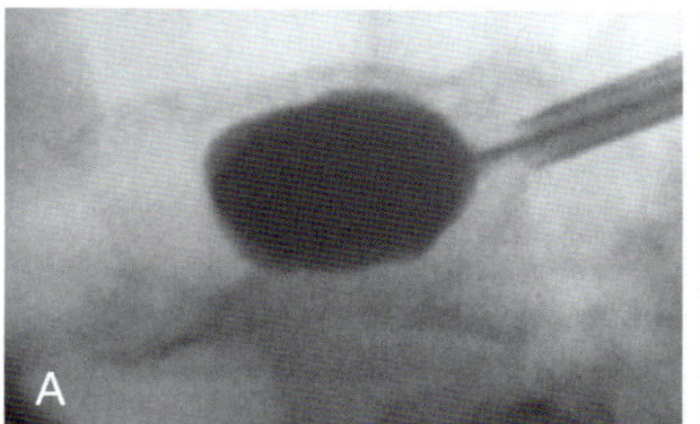

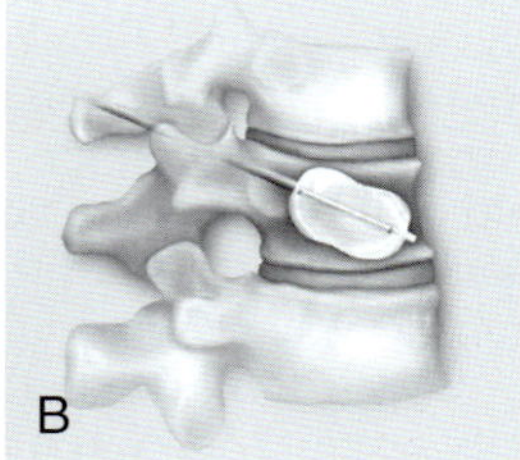

FIGURE 128-5. Radiograph (**A**) and drawing (**B**) of inflatable bone tamp inflated.

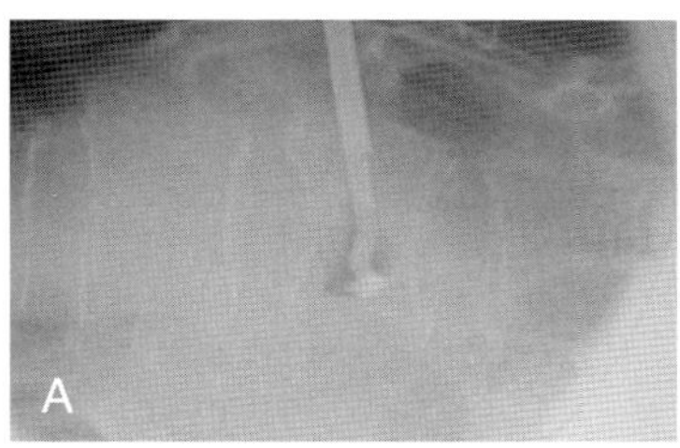

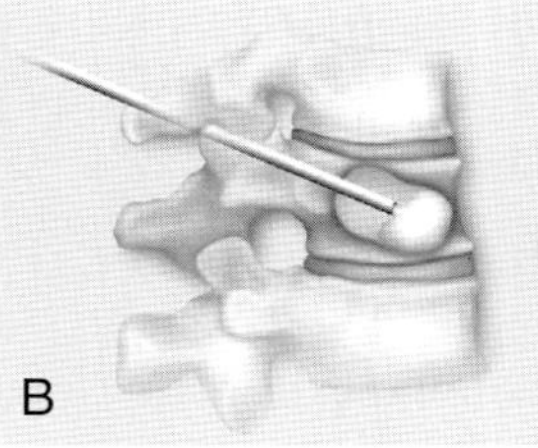

FIGURE 128-6. Radiograph (**A**) and drawing (**B**) of cement deposition.

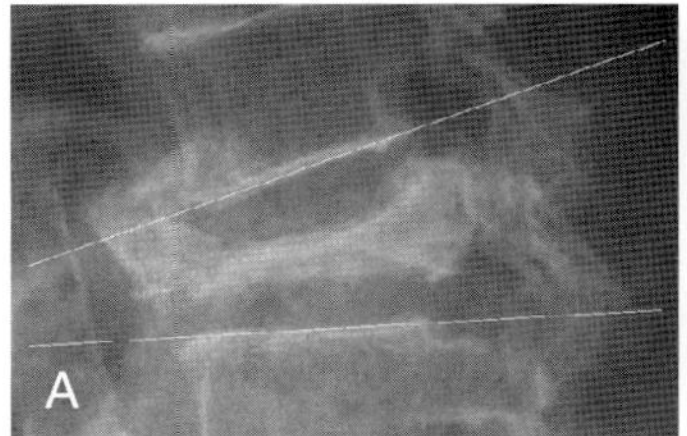

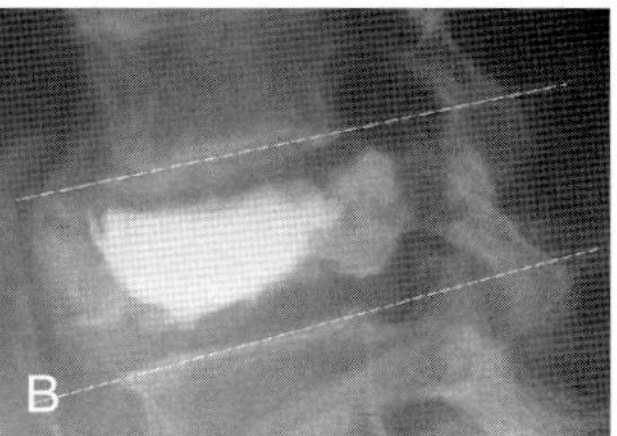

FIGURE 128-7. A and **B,** Radiographs from a representative case of height restoration. Vertebral height was restored by a kyphoplasty procedure. Segmental kyphosis was also corrected.

Results

Our published data from the Cleveland Clinic showed that kyphoplasty provided a safe and effective treatment for pain and disability in patients with vertebral compression fractures secondary to osteoporosis and multiple myeloma.[16,48-51] Outcome data were obtained by administering the 36-Item Short Form Health Survey (SF-36) and the VAS for pain rating; in addition, the patients underwent detailed neurologic and radiographic examinations preoperatively and postoperatively. In our experience, there were no clinically significant cement leaks and no perioperative complications attributable to the IBT or tools. Using SF-36 data (preoperative and postoperative), available on more than 210 patients with average follow-up periods of 10.8 months, SF-36 scores improved in every category, statistically significant in all but the General Health modality. Physical function improved from 15.0 to 30.0 ($P < .001$). Role physical improved from 9.3 to 27.3 ($P = .004$). Bodily pain improved from 22.0 to 32.0 (P □ .001). Vitality improved from 30.0 to 40.0 (P □ .001). Social function improved from 37.5 to 50.0 (P □ .001). Role emotional improved from 33.3 to 66.7 ($P = .39$). Mental health improved from 64.0 to 72.0 ($P < .001$). General health was unchanged from 52.0 to 55.0 ($P = .051$). The VAS scores improved from a preoperative level of 7.0 to an initial postoperative level of 3.2 ($P < .0001$). At the last follow-up examination, the value remained unchanged at 3.4 ($P < .0001$).

Ledlie et al. reported functional and radiographic outcomes in the first 117 consecutive patients with 151 fractures.[52] This report focused on the results for the subset of 77 patients completing follow-up. With regard to pain, rated by the patient using a 10-point VAS, the mean pain score decreased from 8.9 ± 1.5 before surgery to 2.8 ± 2.9 at 1 week postoperatively; this value remained low, at 1.5 ± 1.8 at 2 years postoperatively. The proportion of patients fully ambulatory increased from 45% before surgery to 85% at 1 week postoperatively and 88% at 2 years.

Garfin et al. reported clinical results of a total of 155 subjects with 214 VCFs who underwent balloon kyphoplasty at 19 study centers from August 2000 to June 2001.[53] Mean pain ratings decreased from 15.0 (maximum score, 20) before surgery to 6.0 within 7 days after kyphoplasty ($P < .001$), a 60% reduction, and remained decreased throughout follow-up to 24 months. The mean number of days of the previous 28 days spent in bed decreased from 8.8 at baseline to 1.9, 2.2, 0.7, and 1.4 at 1, 3, 12, and 24 months, respectively, after kyphoplasty.

Wardlaw et al. reported the results of their randomized controlled trial at 21 sites in eight countries.[54] In this report, 300 patients randomly assigned by a computer-generated sequence to receive kyphoplasty treatment (n = 149) or nonsurgical care (n = 151). Among them, 138 participants in the kyphoplasty group and 128 controls completed follow-up at 1 month. By use of repeated measures mixed effects modeling, all 300 randomized participants were included in the analysis. The mean SF-36 physical component summary score improved by 7.2 points (95% CI, 5.7–8.8), from 26.0 at baseline to 33.4 at 1 month, in the kyphoplasty group, and by 2.0 points (95% CI, 0.4–3.6), from 25.5 to 27.4, in the nonsurgical group (difference between groups 5.2 points, 95% CI, 2.9–7.4; $P < .0001$). The frequency of adverse events did not differ between groups. These results suggested that balloon kyphoplasty is an effective and safe procedure for patients with acute vertebral fractures and helps inform decisions regarding its use as an early treatment option.

In addition to good clinical results, height restoration by kyphoplasty has been reported in several studies (Fig. 128-7). Our initial results showed height restoration in 70% of 70 fractured vertebrae treated with kyphoplasty.[16] In patients in whom the vertebral fractures were reduced by kyphoplasty, vertebral height increased by a mean of 46.8%.

Ledlie et al. reported their radiographic measurement results for ventral and midline points of the fractured vertebrae using the two nearest normal vertebrae as reference points.[55] Pairs of preoperative and 2-year follow-up radiographs for 85 treated fractures were evaluated for vertebral height measurement. Mean preoperative ventral height (Ha), midheight (Hm), and dorsal height (Hp) were 61.3% ± 23.8%, 61.0% ± 20.1%, and 86.5% ± 18.4%, respectively. Compared to preoperative heights, mean Ha, Hm, and Hp were significantly higher ($P < .001$) at all postoperative intervals. Following kyphoplasty (1–6 weeks), mean Ha, Hm, and Hp were 81.2% ± 20.9%, 86.9% ± 17.9%, and 95.1% ± 10.1%, respectively. At 2-year follow-up, mean Ha, Hm, and Hp were 80.9% ± 19.8%, 88.1% ± 16.6%, and 91.4% ± 12.8%, respectively. There was no correlation between height increase and patient age, gender, fracture level, or fracture age.[52]

Garfin et al. reported the results of midline height restoration rates. The mean preoperative midvertebral height was 65% of the predicted height. Eighty-two percent of patients had at least 10% lost height restored during the pretreatment and post-treatment interval. The mean percent midvertebral lost height restored was 32% overall and 44% in those with measurable height restoration.[53]

Complications

Many kyphoplasty studies provided details on the number of cement leakage complications. In a meta-analysis, Taylor showed that a total of 189 (9%) cement leakages were reported in 2239 vertebrae that underwent kyphoplasty.[56] This corresponds to 81 cement leaks per 1000 fractures undergoing kyphoplasty per year. One leak (0.001%) was reported by Majd[57] to be symptomatic L1 radiculopathy. A few cases also reported inappropriate cement injection and needle placement in the early phase.[58] In our series of patients,[16,49] cement extravasation was seen in less than 10% of cases. No problems were identified clinically as a result of these extravasations immediately after surgery or at final follow-up. In one patient, a myocardial infarction occurred as a result of fluid overload during the procedure.

Ledlie et al. reported three complications in their series.[52] Two weeks after kyphoplasty, a patient with a history of deep vein thrombosis (no evidence of PMMA leakage to the lungs by CT) had a pulmonary embolism. A second patient with preexisting metastatic, cardiac, vascular, severe chronic obstructive pulmonary disease required mechanical ventilation and subsequently died 5 days postoperatively. A third patient had perioperative confusion and generalized weakness that gradually resolved (negative brain CT and neurologic workup). No complication was related to the kyphoplasty technique. Minor cement extravasations were observed in 11.3% (17/151) of treated fractures, but none of the leaks was associated with any clinical consequence.

Garfin et al. also reported that the extravasation of PMMA outside the vertebral body occurred in 21/214 (10%) of treated levels.[53] All PMMA extravasations were asymptomatic, the cement remained in the immediate area of the treated vertebrae, and no medical or surgical intervention was required to remove the extravasated PMMA.

Phillips et al. reported that asymptomatic cement leaks were observed in 6 of 61 vertebral fractures (9.8%).[59] In this series as well, there were no clinical consequences attributable to the bone tamp or cement deposition.

To date, no reports of primary or secondary infection of the cement mantle have been published. In our series of more 300 patients, there were no primary infections. However, we did encounter one hematogenous infection 2 years after the kyphoplasty in a patient receiving multiple blood and platelet transfusions for Waldenstrom macroglobulinemia.

Two papers reported "redo" vertebral augmentation in case the previous vertebral segmentation failed to relieve pain.[60,61] A report by Gaughen et al. concerned six patients whose initial vertebroplasty resulted in substantial improvement in pain. These six patients developed recurrent pain between 8 days and 167 days after initial vertebroplasty and underwent "redo" vertebroplasty. After repeat vertebroplasty, five of the six patients reported a reduction of at least 3 points in their pain rating, with a mean reduction of 6.5 points and a mean postoperative pain level of 3.5 points (11-point scale). Four of six patients reported impaired mobility before repeat vertebroplasty, and all four demonstrated a postoperative improvement in mobility. The mean increase in mobility was 1.50 points, and the mean postoperative mobility impairment was 0.25 points (5-point scale). The investigators concluded that the clinical outcomes of the patients within this case series suggest that repeat percutaneous vertebroplasty performed at previously treated vertebral levels for recurrent pain offers therapeutic benefit. Although the repeating of this procedure is technically demanding, "redo" vertebral augmentation could be performed over a previously treated kyphoplasty or vertebroplasty.

Mechanism of Pain Relief

The etiology of pain after an osteoporotic or an osteolytic vertebral collapse is multivariate (biomechanical, physiologic, or neurogenic). Although a number of reports describing clinical results of vertebral augmentation indicate good pain relief, the mechanism of this relief remains unclear. The most intuitive explanation involves simple mechanical stabilization of the fracture; the cement stabilizes the vertebral bodies and offloads the facet joints. However, another explanation is that analgesia results from local chemical, vascular, or thermal effects of PMMA on nerve endings in surrounding tissue. Supporting this concept is the lack of correlation between cement volume and pain relief. Further evidence against an effect resulting solely from mechanical stabilization is the fact that PVP typically does not restore lost vertebral body height and therefore does not correct altered biomechanics. Another potential mechanism of pain relief involves the normalization of strains through the centrum and away from the cortices of the vertebral body. It has been shown that with osteoporosis, the centrum of the vertebral body becomes deficient and the axial load is transmitted to the vertebral body walls. By augmenting the centrum with or without a sagittal realignment, the force transmission may now be normalized.[62] The contribution of metabolic bone disease such as osteomalacia to the pain remains unclear.

Biomechanics

The ability for organ systems to compensate for changes diminishes as humans age. The skeletal system and spinal column also become more vulnerable to fractures with increased age. There is a significant decrease in vertebral body strength with aging, resulting from the loss of cancellous bone support.[63,64] The compressive strength of any bone is dependent on numerous factors, including the species, site, health status, and quality of bone. The compressive strength of normal human cancellous bone shows great variation but typically resists 5 megapascals (MPa) or 725 pounds of load per square inch (psi).[65] Osteoporotic vertebral bone exhibits compressive strength in the lower region of this range (<2 MPa, or 290 psi), whereas younger, healthier, or cancellous bone from other sites may exhibit compressive strength in the upper region of this range. Carter and Hayes showed a strong correlation between bone density and the strength of cancellous bone.[66] The compressive strength of trabecular bone increases approximately with the square of its density. Therefore, doubling the density of a given bone results in a fourfold increase in compressive strength. In contrast, if the density of the bone decreases by 50%, the remaining compressive strength is only 25% of the original value.[67] Bell also reported a direct correlation between bone loss and strength, noting that a decrease of 25% in the osseous structure resulted in a 50% decrease in vertebral strength.[63] Rockoff et al. further characterized the effects of age on loss of bone strength by analyzing the cancellous or trabecular bone's ability to compensate for applied forces.[68] The cancellous vertebral body bone carries approximately 55% of axial loads in the adult spine before the age of 40 years, but this percentage declines to only 35% after the age of 40 years. These changes in bone density are directly responsible for the 4% annual incidence of VCFs in postmenopausal women (primary osteoporosis).[69] These fractures can result in functional limitations such as a decrease in gait velocity, an increase in muscle fatigue, and additional falls.

The thoracic and thoracolumbar regions of the spine have a natural kyphotic curvature. This curvature biomechanically places the ventral thoracic spine at an increased risk for developing compression fractures as a consequence of axial loads.[70-72] The kyphotic curvature concentrates the applied axial load on the ventral portion of the vertebral body. These axial loads cause all points ventral to the vertebral body (instantaneous axis of rotation; IAR) to come closer together, while simultaneously all points dorsal to the IAR are spread apart.[73] If the failure point of the vertebral body is exceeded, a compression fracture occurs. In younger patients, the forces required to produce a fracture are significant and typically result from high-energy trauma. However, as the vertebral body is weakened by osteoporosis, the amount of energy required to initiate a fracture significantly decreases. Once a VCF occurs, the transmission of forces through the vertebral column is altered. A VCF reduces the load-carrying capacity of the anterior column and causes the IAR to migrate dorsally to the region with intact supporting structures.[74] The dorsal migration of the IAR causes the previous mechanical advantage of a longer lever arm, from which the dorsal ligaments and muscles acted to maintain sagittal balance, to be shortened. The dorsal displacement of the IAR simultaneously causes the distance from the ventrally located center of gravity to the IAR to be greater, which places additional distraction on the posterior columns and compression on the anterior columns.[72,74]

Kayanja et al. investigated the distribution of ventral cortical strain at, above, and below an experimentally created index VCF to determine the vertebral body at risk of secondary fracture.[62] In this study, 17 human cadaveric thoracic vertebrae were divided into multilevel segments composed of three vertebrae (T1-3, T4-6, T7-9, and T10-12). Measurements of ventral cortical shear strain, applied moments, and applied flexion angle were made in compression and flexion. The results showed that the shear strain distribution was independent of the location of the multilevel segment level in the spine and was highest at the apex of a thoracic index VCF. The vertebra above the index VCF had increased ventral cortical shear strain and was therefore at greatest risk for secondary fracture. These results suggest that restoration of sagittal alignment minimizes strain on the vulnerable vertebral levels above an index VCF, preventing subsequent vertebral fractures. Kayanja et al. also determined the effects of load (compression and flexion) on the adjacent levels (above and below) an augmented VCF.[75] Six upper thoracic segments (T1-5) and six lower thoracic segments (T8-12) were biomechanically tested creating VCFs that were subsequently augmented in the intermediate vertebrae T3 and T10. Multilevel segment stiffness and adjacent vertebral strain at superior and inferior levels were measured before and after the vertebral augmentation. The results showed that VCF and augmentation reduced compressive and bending stiffness in the vertebral segment, while the adjacent vertebral strain increased. The augmentation also caused a greater amount of strain on the inferior adjacent level compared to the superior level. These results suggested that cement augmentation reduces stiffness while increasing adjacent level strain primarily on the inferior adjacent vertebra, and this alteration in strain distribution probably spares the superior adjacent vertebra from fracture.

Filler Materials

The filling materials that are used for vertebral augmentation require good biocompatibility, good biomechanical strength and stiffness, and good radiopacity for fluoroscopy-guided procedures.[76]

PMMA has been the material most commonly used during vertebral augmentation procedures.[77] In April 2004, the Food and Drug Administration approved the labeling of certain brands of PMMA for the treatment of pathologic fractures of the vertebral body due to osteoporosis and tumor using a kyphoplasty technique.[78] PMMA is reportedly bioinert and shows good biocompatibility over long-term follow-up. Several inherent advantages to PMMA include familiarity for orthopaedic surgeons, ease of handling, good biomechanical strength and stiffness, and cost effectiveness. Some disadvantages include no biologic potential to remodel or integrate into the surrounding bone, no direct bone apposition, excessive inherent stiffness, high polymerization temperature, and potential monomer toxicity. Although good clinical results have been reported in several series of both vertebroplasty and kyphoplasty procedures,[12,16,30,48,49,55,58,59,79] it is still unclear whether some component of the pain relief is secondary to the mechanical stabilization, chemical toxicity, or thermal necrosis of surrounding tissues and nerve ends. To date, the concern regarding thermal bone necrosis is still theoretical, and there has been no obvious evidence to support such a concern.[80,81]

Calcium phosphate cement offers the potential for resorption of the cement over time and replacement with new bone as a biologic method to restore vertebral body mass and avoid any potential thermal effects of PMMA.[82-86] This material is also expected to work as an optimum carrier for osteoinductive proteins.[87] Preclinical animal studies and human pilot studies have shown that these calcium phosphate cements are highly osteoconductive and undergo gradual remodeling with time.[88-93] There are only a few published manuscripts reporting histologic data with calcium phosphate cement in a vertebroplasty model.[82,94-96] In general, the cement undergoes resorption and remodeling, which was apparent as fragmentation with vascular invasion and bone ingrowth into the material. The reports also described evidence of osteoclastic resorption of the cement and direct bone apposition in a pattern that suggested remodeling similar to that of normal bone. Turner et al. tested both PMMA and calcium phosphate cement (BoneSource, Stryker Orthopaedics, Mahwah, NJ) in a canine vertebral body defect. In this study, both materials were well integrated histologically, but calcium phosphate underwent resorption and remodeling, and it demonstrated excellent biocompatibility and osteoconductivity.[95] Takikawa et al. also reported greater than 80% direct apposition to cancellous bone in postoperative osteopenic sheep vertebrae at 3, 6, 12, and 24 months.[96] A number of hydroxyapatite and calcium phosphate cements also have been biomechanically tested in vitro[45,97,98]; most are able to restore mechanical integrity to the vertebral body.[99-101]

Calcium sulfate, more commonly known as plaster of Paris, has a long clinical history for use as a bone graft substitute in various skeletal sites. This material is injectable, osteoconductive, and cures with a limited exothermic reaction.[102,103] Calcium sulfate paste has also been reported to significantly augment pull-out strength when used for augmentation of pedicle screw fixation.[104] However, this material is rapidly resorbed,[105-107] and it may not be able to support spinal alignment while it is remodeling; therefore, it would likely be inappropriate for use in a vertebral augmentation procedure.

These calcium phosphate and sulfate cements have some problems, including their low viscosity, handling characteristics different from those of PMMA, and high cost. These products are true cements—that is, ions in suspension. As such, they exhibit thixotropic properties in that when pressurized in a confined space such as a delivery tube, the suspension dewaters, leaving chalk that cannot move through a tube or even percolate through the interstices of the bone. Many synthetic bone substitute cements are currently being developed, but none are yet readily available for use in the spine.

Composite materials (acrylic cements in conjunction with ceramics) are bioactive, highly radiopaque, and feature excellent mechanical properties.[108,109] One such material, terpolymer resin reinforced with combeite glass-ceramic particles (Cortoss, Orthovita, Malvern, PA), is currently undergoing clinical trials for vertebroplasty and kyphoplasty in the United States and has been reported to be a potential alternative to PMMA. Cortoss was approved for vertebroplasty in Europe in January 2003 based on the results of a prospective clinical trial conducted in Europe.[110] Its osteoconductivity has been proven in several animal models,[109,111] but no human histology has been reported to date.

Biopsy Results

A diagnostic bone biopsy can be easily performed during a kyphoplasty procedure and does not affect the safety of the procedure if done appropriately. We histologically evaluated 178 biopsies obtained from 142 patients during 246 kyphoplasty procedures[112] (Figs. 128-8 and 128-9). These showed partially necrotic fragments of bone as well as areas of fibrosis and variable stages of woven bone, suggesting ongoing fracture healing. Specimens obtained from 30 patients (21%) showed markedly increased osteoid in undecalcified sections. These thickened osteoid seams may suggest a possible mineralization defect (osteomalacia). Osteoid can be increased either because of increased bone remodeling activity or a mineralization defect. Tetracycline labeling is the only way to distinguish between these two diagnoses. Careful administration of tetracycline labels may help identify any correlation between vertebral fracture and osteomalacia. Also in this series, four biopsies provided a definite diagnosis of plasma cell dyscrasia in otherwise unsuspected or unknown spinal lesions. These

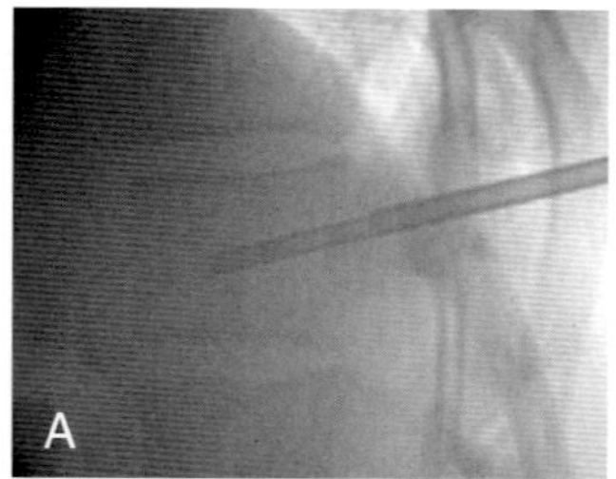

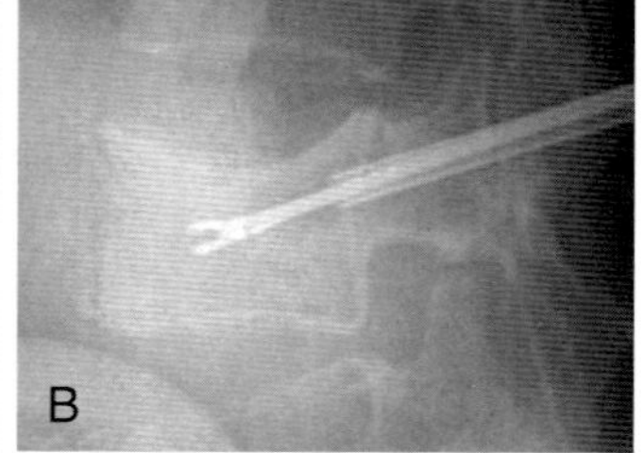

FIGURE 128-8. Intraoperative radiographs showing biopsy procedure. Biopsy trephine (**A**) and pituitary rongeur (**B**) can be used to take biopsy before vertebral augmentation.

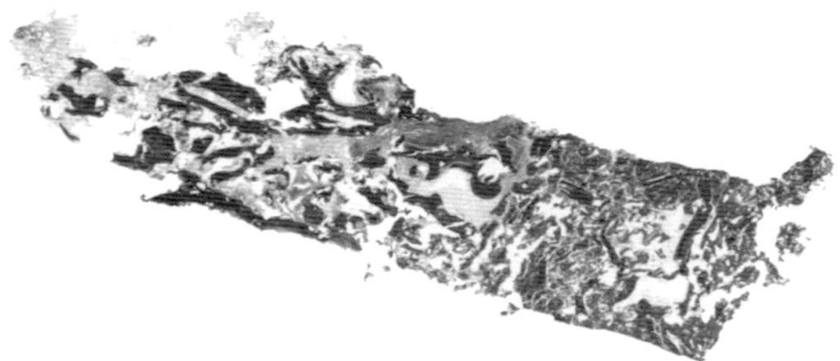

FIGURE 128-9. Biopsy specimen obtained from collapsed vertebra (stained with toluidine blue).

findings suggest that a biopsy is useful for all initial vertebral augmentation cases to rule out any occult lesions.

Histology of Vertebral Augmentation

In spite of reported good clinical results, several aspects of the vertebral augmentation procedure are controversial, including the optimum methods of mixing and depositing the cement, the potential importance of a foreign body reaction at the cement-bone interface, efficacy of bone tamp usage, the use of relatively high concentrations of radiopaque agents and antibiotics in the cement, and the clinical indications for the procedure. We were able to document histologically four vertebral bodies from two cases 1 month and 2 years after cement augmentation, after a surgical corpectomy and at an autopsy[80] (Fig. 128-10). In this study, the histology of vertebrae treated using the kyphoplasty technique revealed a dense cancellous shell around the cement mantle. This suggests that the tamping had displaced bone, essentially autografting the space around the cement. Bone immediately around the cement did not show extensive necrosis. However, foreign body giant cells contained material consistent with cement particles and/or barium sulfate. Particles were also identified within vascular spaces (Fig. 128-11).

In a baboon vertebral augmentation study, the same histologic features were observed in the vertebrae treated with both vertebroplasty and kyphoplasty.[81] There was evidence of a foreign body reaction to PMMA and a few necrotic

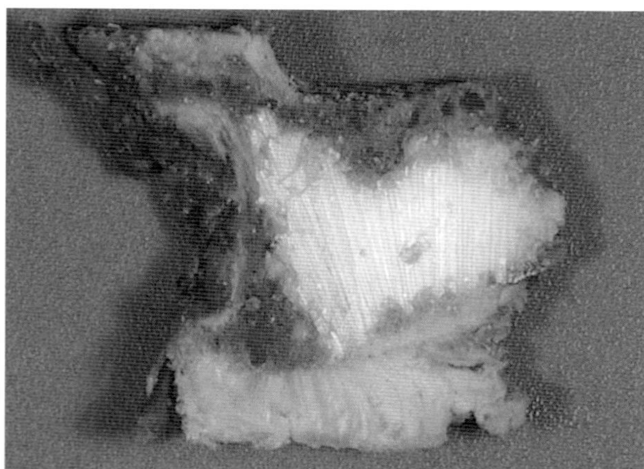

FIGURE 128-10. Photograph of a section of human vertebra retrieved during reconstructive surgery. Most of the vertebral body is occupied by polymethylmethacrylate.

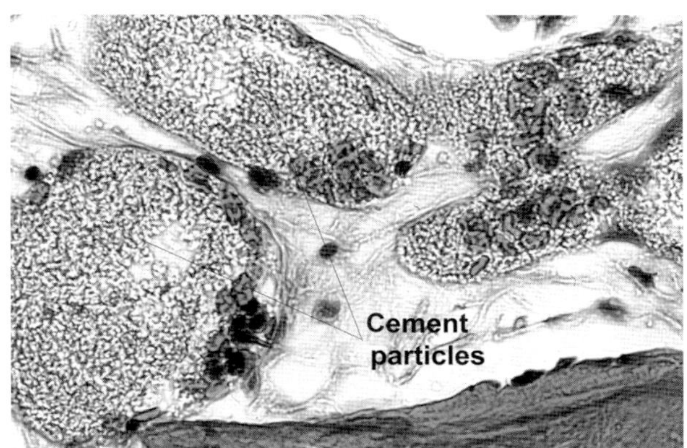

FIGURE 128-11. Cement particles and/or barium sulfate were found within vascular spaces of the vertebral body in an autopsy specimen.

segments of bone present in both the vertebroplasty and kyphoplasty vertebrae. However, it was not clear that the necrosis was caused by the PMMA polymerization process or bone tamping procedures. Further histologic evaluation may help clarify the safety and efficacy of vertebral augmentation.

Adjacent and Remote Fractures

One theoretical issue continuously raised by spine practitioners concerns the incidence of remote and adjacent-level vertebral compression fractures after an index VCF has been augmented by either vertebroplasty or kyphoplasty. Keller et al. investigated the biomechanics of age-related spine deformity using a sagittal plane biomechanical model and showed that postural forces were responsible for initiation and propagation of osteoporotic spine deformity in the elderly.[113] Kayanja et al. reported results of biomechanical tests for cadaveric thoracic wedge compression fractures and showed that ventral cortical strain was maximum at the apex of a thoracic kyphotic curve and that the vertebral body immediately above it had the next highest strain, with an increased risk of secondary fracture.[62] Moreover, in a 10-year Swedish population–based cohort study of 598 individuals, Hasserius et al. suggested that a prevalent vertebral deformity could predict both increased mortality and increased fracture incidence during the following decade in both men and women.[114] Left untreated, the incidence of subsequent vertebral fracture after an index fracture is reported in other studies as approximately 20%.[69,115]

There was no consistent rate of subsequent fracture after vertebroplasty. From the vertebroplasty literature, one study reported a 52% rate of remote or adjacent-level fractures after vertebroplasty.[33] A second study reported a 12% rate of remote fractures (one third) and adjacent-level fractures (two thirds).[116]

From the kyphoplasty literature, Harrop et al. reported that the incidence of postkyphoplasty VCF in primary osteoporotic patients was 11.25% (9 fractures/80 patients), whereas the incidence in steroid-induced osteoporotic patients was 48.6% (17 fractures/35 patients).[117] These results imply that the intervention, kyphoplasty, in primary osteoporotic patients does not increase the rate of remote or adjacent-level fractures compared with the published natural history reports. These results also imply that compared with primary osteoporotic patients, secondary osteoporotic patients are in fact at increased risk for subsequent VCFs, although there is no natural history benchmark to which we can compare this rate. Fribourg et al. also reported the results of retrospective review of charts and radiographs of patients who underwent kyphoplasty.[118] In 38 patients with 47 treated levels, 10 patients sustained 17 subsequent fractures in this study (9 above adjacent-level, 4 below adjacent-level, 4 at remote levels). Although this report is informative, 15 patients in this series had known oncologic disease, and 7 patients had steroid use, with known increased risk of subsequent fractures.

Osteolytic Vertebral Compression Fractures

Osteolytic destruction of the vertebral bodies secondary to metastatic disease or multiple myeloma affects up to 70% of cancer patients.[119,120] Pain is the initial complaint in up to 95% of patients despite the fact that more than 50% of spinal metastases are asymptomatic.[119,120] Only 10% of patients with spinal metastases present with neurologic signs or symptoms on initial presentation.[12] With modern advances in oncologic treatment, patient survival has improved to the point where disease that was once life-threatening can now be considered chronic. Unfortunately, the oncologic treatment itself also contributes to the already present osteolytic bone loss. With the increased survival and ongoing bone loss, osteolytic VCFs are becoming much more of a clinical and functional problem for affected patients. The indications for surgical intervention are reported as being progressive collapse, neurologic deterioration, and/or intractable pain. However, surgical intervention in this patient group is typically considered to be very difficult by virtue of comorbid conditions and poor bone quality. Similar to the scenario with osteoporotic compression fractures, possible complications associated with these osteolytic fractures include cord compression, urinary retention, ileus, intractable pain, and pulmonary compromise (9% loss in predicted forced vital capacity with each vertebral fracture).[121,122] Other chronic sequelae include deconditioning, deformity, insomnia, and depression, resulting in substantial physical, functional, and psychosocial impairment. Recently, to alleviate these issues, percutaneous minimally invasive vertebral augmentation techniques have evolved and show promising preliminary results for these debilitated patients.

Multiple Myeloma

Multiple myeloma is a monoclonal proliferation of malignant plasma cells that usually affects the bone marrow. Excessive bone resorption due to an increase of proinflammatory cytokines is a characteristic feature of the disease.[123] This tumor is grossly a very soft vascular tumor, as evidenced by the backflow of blood from the working cannulae during kyphoplasty. The near-fluid consistency of the tumor and the lytic nature of the bone make it easy for the IBT to displace tissue in the act of reducing the fracture and creating the cavity. This then results in impressive cement filling of the vertebra. Dudeney et al. reported satisfying results in the treatment of osteolytic VCFs due to multiple myeloma.[48] Fifty-five consecutive kyphoplasty procedures were performed over 27 sessions in 18 patients. The mean age of patients was 63.5 (48–79) years, the mean duration of symptoms was 11 months, and the mean follow-up was 7.4 months. There were no major complications related directly to use of this technique. On average, 34% of height loss at the time of fracture was restored. After stratifying for patients whose height was not restored, the remaining vertebral bodies showed an average of 56% height restoration. Asymptomatic cement leakage occurred at 2/55 levels (4%). Significant improvement in SF-36 scores occurred for bodily pain (23.2 to 55.4, $P = .0008$), physical function (21.3 to 50.6, $P = .0010$), vitality (31.3 to 47.5, $P = .010$), and social functioning (40.6 to 64.8, $P = .014$). The authors concluded that the kyphoplasty technique (1) was efficacious in the treatment of osteolytic VCFs due to multiple myeloma and (2) was associated with early clinical improvement of pain and function as well as some restoration of vertebral body height in these patients. The effects of potential tumor dissemination, in what is already widespread disease, are unknown. Any significant systemic effects are not suspected and have not been noted in the initial study group.[48] Lane et al. also prospectively evaluated 19 patients with multiple myeloma treated with kyphoplasty.[124] They reported significant improvement in functional status measured by the Oswestry Disability Index (ODI) score, with significant vertebral height restoration. In their comparison, there was no significant difference between the myeloma patient group and the osteoporotic compression fracture group in terms of either ODI score or vertebral height restoration.

Other Tumors

In an ongoing evaluation of nonmyelomatous osteolytic collapse, the results have remained very favorable. From April 1999 to April 2004, 21 patients with nonmyelomatous osteolytic vertebral collapse (9 breast, 4 leukemia/lymphoma, 3 lung, 1 pharyngeal basal cell, 4 unknown origin) underwent 42 kyphoplasty procedures over 24 sessions.[125] The procedure was successfully performed in all patients. The perioperative and clinical follow-up revealed that the procedure was well tolerated, with improvement in pain and early mobilization. The patients reported statistically significant improvements in their objective outcome scores (SF-36). Barr et al. also reported that the results with osteolytic metastatic vertebral collapse in eight patients revealed that only four patients experienced any pain relief. In this group of patients, there was a 6% complication rate.[19]

Other solid organ–type tumors and previously irradiated tumors may not be as amenable to the IBT while reducing the fracture or creating a cavity. Further investigation into various modalities of treatment need to be performed before a definitive recommendation on indications in other tumor types can be made.

Conclusions

Osteoporotic VCFs pose a significant clinical problem, including spine deformity, pain, reduced pulmonary function and mobility, as well as an overall increase in mortality in the elderly. Traditional medical and surgical options in many cases prove inadequate.

PVP is a relatively noninvasive technique that has gained increased acceptance over the past decade in the treatment of symptomatic osteoporotic vertebral fractures. The available clinical studies describe pain relief achieved in greater than 90% of symptomatic osteoporotic fractures, with only infrequent, mostly minor, complications. Some of the drawbacks of PVP stem from the use of PMMA, because of its toxicity and poor handling characteristics, rather than from the procedure itself.

Kyphoplasty is a modification of PVP that may add a margin of safety by virtue of a lower observed incidence of cement leakage. Kyphoplasty has been shown to be worthwhile in acute vertebral fractures to predictably restore vertebral height and to facilitate a controlled fill of the vertebral body. Favorable outcomes in early trials appear to imply that kyphoplasty permits early mobilization, which has the potential to decrease mortality. Considering the greater mortality that is associated with osteoporotic compression fractures, early mobilization in these patients is of prime importance.

Although these two minimally invasive techniques are shown to be quite beneficial for the VCF patients, controversy continues regarding the optimum timing of these surgeries and their true effectiveness and cost effectiveness over the long term, especially since the two randomized controlled studies were published in the *New England Journal of Medicine*.[41,42] Several ongoing randomized clinical trials would provide further information in the future.

KEY REFERENCES

Buchbinder R, Osborne RH, Ebeling PR, et al: A randomized trial of vertebroplasty for painful osteoporotic vertebral fractures. *N Engl J Med* 361:557–568, 2009.

Garfin SR, Buckley RA, Ledlie J: Balloon kyphoplasty for symptomatic vertebral body compression fractures results in rapid, significant, and sustained improvements in back pain, function, and quality of life for elderly patients. *Spine (Phila Pa 1976)* 31:2213–2220, 2006.

Kallmes DF, Comstock BA, Heagerty PJ, et al: A randomized trial of vertebroplasty for osteoporotic spinal fractures. *N Engl J Med* 361:569–579, 2009.

Lieberman IH, Dudeney S, Reinhardt MK, et al: Initial outcome and efficacy of "kyphoplasty" in the treatment of painful osteoporotic vertebral compression fractures. *Spine (Phila Pa 1976)* 26:1631–1638, 2001.

Lindsay R, Silverman SL, Cooper C, et al: Risk of new vertebral fracture in the year following a fracture. *JAMA* 285:320–323, 2001.

Wardlaw D, Cummings SR, Van Meirhaeghe J, et al: Efficacy and safety of balloon kyphoplasty compared with non-surgical care for vertebral compression fracture (FREE): a randomised controlled trial. *Lancet* 373:1016–1024, 2009.

REFERENCES

The complete reference list is available online at expertconsult.com.

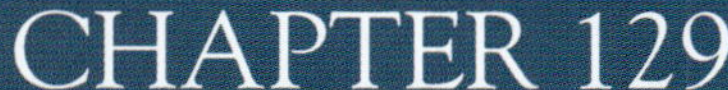
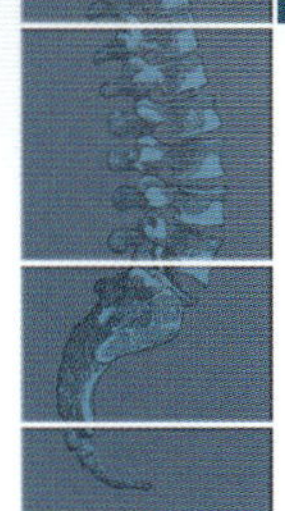

CHAPTER 129

The Obese Patient

Andrea L. Strayer | Gregory R. Trost

Obesity is a global issue. An estimated 300 million people throughout the world are obese, defined as having a body mass index (BMI) of 30 kg/m^2 or more and 1.5 billion are overweight (BMI ≥25 kg/m^2).[1] From 2007 to 2008, the prevalence of obesity in the United States was 32.2% among men and 35.5% among women.[2] Healthy People 2010 set a goal, in 2001, of lowering the percentage of people in the United States with obesity to 15%. In 2010, Colorado was the only state with an obesity rate below 22%. Thirty-six states had obesity rates of 25% or higher, with the rate in 12 of those 36 states being 30% or above.[3] The implications of obesity are far reaching. Medical costs related to obesity accounted for 9.1% of total U.S. medical expenditures in 1998, with total direct and indirect costs estimated to be $147 billion in 2000.[4] If the prevalence of obesity currently were the same as it was in 1987, health care spending in the United States would be 10% lower per person, or about $200 billion less each year.[5]

Obesity is a major risk factor for many diseases and conditions, including type 2 diabetes, hypertension, cardiovascular disease, pulmonary dysfunction, kidney disease, metabolic syndrome, and certain types of cancer. The prevalence of 11 chronic conditions, including those previously mentioned, associated with obesity grew 180% from 1997 to 2005, an increase equal to approximately 29 million additional cases of chronic conditions.[5] The implications for spine surgery are multifaceted, including poor wound healing, infection risk, caregiver safety, anesthesia considerations, intraoperative challenges, equipment needs, and biomechanical considerations.

Obesity and Overweight

BMI is defined as the weight in kilograms divided by the square of the height in meters (kg/m^2). A BMI over 25 kg/m^2 is defined as overweight, and a BMI greater than 30 kg/m^2 is defined as obese. Obesity rates, rising threefold or more since 1980 in some areas of North America, the United Kingdom, Eastern Europe, the Middle East, the Pacific Islands, Australasia, and China, is attributed to societal changes that have led to increased consumption of nutrient-poor and energy-dense foods combined with reduced physical activity.[1] These changes have dramatically affected children—worldwide it is estimated that 22 million children under age 5 and 18 million children between the ages of 6 to 13 years are overweight or obese. Approximately 30% of Australian, 25.5% of American, and 28.7% of Greek children are overweight or obese.[6] The ability to be outdoors is the strongest correlate with physical activity in children. Decreased physical activity and, consequently, decreased energy expenditure, coupled with increased caloric intake, is a major factor in childhood obesity throughout the world.[6]

Lumbar Spine Disease

Increasing weight causes increased axial loading on the spine. People with increased abdominal girth experience a ventral shift of the center of gravity, leading to loss of neutral position and sagittal alignment. As a result, the thorax is ventral to the pelvis, dramatically increasing the forces experienced by the spine. The repetitive, usual movements associated with activities of daily living are cumulative, subjecting the spine to excessive loads (Fig. 129-1).

The cumulative effect was demonstrated in a radiographic comparison of range of motion in obese and nonobese patients with chronic back pain. Reduced range of motion in obese participants was found to be due to reduced mobility at the pelvic and thoracic levels as well as an increased ventral pelvic tilt. Obesity in this study also was associated with increased lumbar lordosis.[7]

Repetitive axial loading and loss of sagittal balance in the obese population is known to lead to degenerative changes in the spine. Degenerative characteristics in the lumbar spine were evaluated in a sample of 187 individuals randomly selected from an ancillary project to the Framingham Study. There was a significantly higher prevalence of facet joint disease in obese subjects.[8]

Hangai et al. investigated factors associated with lumber intervertebral disc degeneration in the elderly. Aging, high BMI, high levels of low-density lipoprotein cholesterol, occupational lifting, and sport activities were all associated with degenerative disc disease in this group of 51- to 86-year-old subjects.[9] High BMI was associated with level 4 degenerative disc disease. Aortic calcification/atherosclerosis and lumbar artery stenosis/occlusion also have been associated with lumbar disc degeneration and low back pain.[10]

A recent meta-analysis of 33 studies evaluated the association between obesity and low back pain. A statistically significant association between BMI and low back pain was noted by Shiri et al., including seeking care for low back pain and chronic low back pain in persons who are overweight

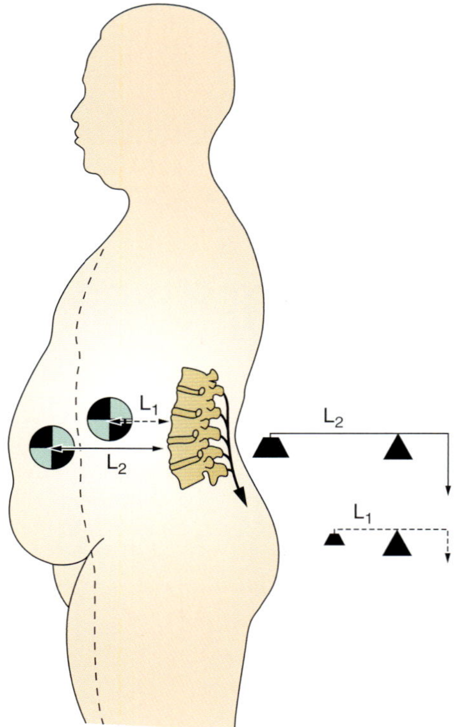

FIGURE 129-1. Spinal load effects of obesity. Vertical axial and ventral loads are increased with obesity, with larger joint reaction forces caused by the longer lever arm induced by the panniculus. (From White AA, Panjabi MM: *Clinical biomechanics of the spine*, ed 2, Philadelphia, 1990, JB Lippincott.)

or obese.[11] The association between excess weight and a higher prevalence of low back pain was stronger in women than men. Increased BMI was a risk factor for low back pain and low back pain–related disability in women.[12] A relationship has been reported between low back pain and obesity in women but not men. Waist circumference has been found to be a more significant factor than BMI.[13]

Thirty-eight patients (30 women, 8 men) were prospectively assessed for their axial low back pain before and after bariatric surgery. Study participants decreased their BMI from 52.25 ± 12.61 kg/m^2 to 38.32 ± 9.66 kg/m^2 ($P < .0001$). Twelve months after surgery, participants' VAS scale scores had decreased from 5.2 ± 3.35 to 2.9 ± 3.1 postoperatively ($P = .006$). Patients experienced increases in mean physical health and mental health components on the 36-Item Short Form Health Survey (SF-36). Low back pain disability demonstrated significant improvement postoperatively as noted on participants' Oswestry Disability Index scores.[14]

Obesity and Associated Comorbidities

Cardiovascular

The cardiovascular implications of obesity include altered metabolism as well as changes in cardiac structure and function. Risk factors associated with obesity include dyslipidemia, hypertension, glucose intolerance, elevated inflammatory markers, and sleep apnea. Adipose tissue is surrounded by an extensive capillary network and functions as an endocrine organ, synthesizing and releasing a variety of compounds. Approximately 30% of the total circulating concentrations of interleukin-6 (IL-6), which modulates C-reactive protein production, originates from adipose tissue.[15]

Hypervolemia from increased extracellular volume and increased cardiac output are evident in the hypertensive obese patient. Hypertension leads to left ventricular hypertrophy. As hypertension continues, the left ventricle becomes progressively noncompliant, increasing the risk of heart failure.[16]

Hemodynamically, obese individuals have an increased total blood volume and cardiac output caused by the metabolic demand of increased BMI. Left ventricular hypertrophy and diastolic dysfunction as well as cardiomyopathy are correlated with obesity, and may be predisposing factors to heart failure.[15] However, most of the extra volume is distributed to the adipose tissue, whereas renal and cerebral blood flow are normal.[16]

Diagnostic electrocardiogram interpretation also is influenced by obesity. Changes that may occur include increased heart rate, increased P-R interval, increased QRS interval, increased or decreased QRS voltage, increased Q-T interval, ST-T abnormalities, left axis deviation, flattening of the T wave in inferolateral leads, left atrial abnormalities, and false-positive criteria for inferior myocardial infarction.[15]

Hypertension is about six times more common in obese individuals. Cardiovascular dysmetabolic syndrome, also known as metabolic syndrome, associates hypertension with an increase in visceral fat. Additionally, a chronic inflammatory state, as evidenced by elevated C-reactive protein and IL-6 levels, may play a role in elevated blood pressure.[15]

Obese patients may be quite sedentary, with limited mobility, and may not have subjective complaints of cardiac impairment. Early symptoms usually are exertional dyspnea and orthopnea; however, severely obese individuals often do not sleep in bed, and sleep in a nonrecumbent position, such as in a reclining chair. Electrocardiograms may be low voltage and may underestimate right and left ventricular hypertrophy.[16] Careful preoperative assessment is necessary.

Diabetes

A recent meta-analysis found type II diabetes associated with overweight and obese individuals.[17] Diabetic patients who underwent cervical fusion secondary to myelopathy were found to be male, older, and have more levels fused. They also were more likely to have respiratory, cardiac, and peripheral vascular complications; hematoma or bleeding; transfusion; and dysphagia, with longer lengths of stay and more nonroutine discharges.[18]

Olsen et al. found diabetes to be the highest independent risk of spinal surgical site infection, and an elevated preoperative or postoperative serum glucose level was independently associated with increased risk of surgical site infection.[19]

Infection Risk

Obesity is associated with a number of changes in skin physiology, including larger skin folds and increased amount of sweating, which increase moisture and skin friction. Lymphedema can occur because of altered lymphatic flow. Lymphedema is associated with reduced tissue oxygenation and a chronic inflammatory state. Subcutaneous fat, made up almost entirely of white adipose tissue, plays a role in endocrine functions and metabolism of lipids and glucose[20] (Fig. 129-2).

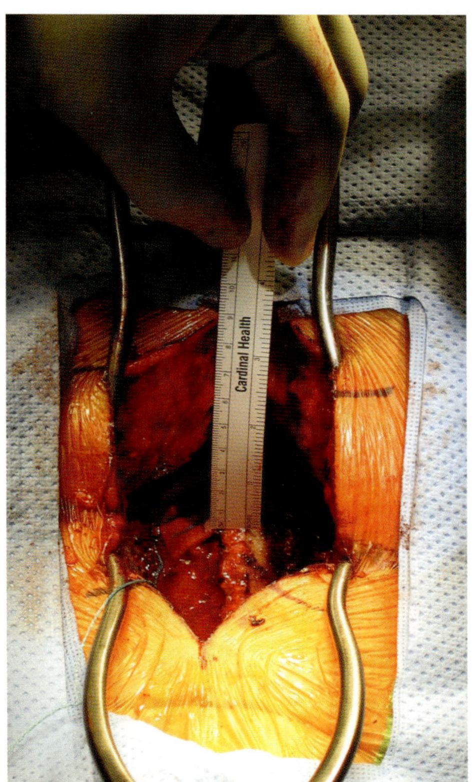

FIGURE 129-2. Intraoperative view of adipose tissue in a dorsal cervical exposure.

Obesity is a well-known risk factor for postoperative surgical site infection.[21-24] Watters et al. completed an evidence-based clinical guideline for the use of prophylactic antibiotics in spine surgery. Their conclusions were that while the obese patient population is at a higher risk for postoperative infection, the literature did not yield evidence that would support modification of standard therapy.[25]

In addition to antibiotic prophylaxis to prevent surgical site infection, thorough preoperative skin cleaning with antibacterial soap in the home preoperatively and adequate scrub prior to incision is of the utmost importance.

Pulmonary

The respiratory consequences of obesity include alterations in lung volumes, lung mechanics, gas exchange, and respiratory control. In short, reduced expiratory reserve volume, reduced functional residual capacity, reduced total lung capacity, and increased residual volume have significant implications for the anesthetized patient. Careful attention is needed during induction, because obese patients rapidly desaturate despite preoxygenation as a result of a smaller functional residual capacity and an increase in oxygen consumption.[16]

Mechanically, there is reduced lung and chest wall compliance, increased airway resistance and work of breathing, as well as respiratory muscle inefficiency. Total compliance can fall to 30% of predicted normal.[16]

Obstructive sleep apnea, difficult intubation, risk of aspiration, and positioning during induction can present unique anesthetic challenges.[26] Anatomic alterations associated with obesity include increased adipose tissue around the upper airway, and upper airway collapsibility is higher. Central obesity has been associated with reduced lung volumes. Structural alterations are further compounded by neuromuscular control disturbances, which also appear to play a role in sleep apnea.[27]

Obstructive sleep apnea occurs because the pharyngeal muscles relax, leading to upper airway collapse during inspiration during sleep. It is characterized by frequent episodes of apnea during sleep and recurrent episodes of hypoxemia and hypercapnea. Obstructive sleep apnea is more likely to lead to total obstruction if the pharyngeal muscle tone is reduced by drugs, as with surgery.

Because of the risks involved with intubation of the obese patient, awake fiberoptic intubation should be considered. Care must be taken to ensure that sufficient ventilation is being provided. During the postoperative period, effects of anesthetics, sedatives, and opioids can diminish ventilatory drive and upper airway control. Nursing staff must be educated on the potential of carbon dioxide retention.

Pharmacokinetics

Factors that affect drug dosing in obese patients include increased adipose tissue, renal blood flow, glomerular filtration rate, and total blood volume; elevated cardiac output; altered protein binding; and decreased total body water.[28] Both fat and lean masses are increased as compared with nonobese counterparts. The increase in lean body mass is 20% to 40% of total excess weight. However, the fat mass of total body weight increases more than lean mass, resulting in a decreased percentage of lean body mass and water as compared with otherwise similar nonobese patients, with the volume of drug distribution larger in obese individuals.[29]

Lipophilic drugs such as benzodiazepines, barbiturates, and propofol require larger loading doses in obese patients due to their elevated volume of distribution. However, maintenance dosing should be based on drug clearance. If the drug clearance is similar or reduced in the obese patient, the maintenance dose generally is based on ideal body weight. If drug clearance is increased in the obese person, then the dose is calculated on total body weight. Thus, midazolam used as a loading dose should be calculated on *total* body weight, whereas maintenance dosing should be calculated on *ideal* body weight.[30]

Diagnostic Considerations

As with any patient with a spinal disorder, a detailed history and thorough physical examination from the basis of the evaluation. In addition to completing a spinal disease-specific history, it is critical to obtain a comprehensive medical history in the obese patient. This will reveal known and potential medical comorbid conditions, as described previously. Preoperative assessment, a planned visit as an outpatient to assess surgical risk, by an anesthesist often is prudent, as is potential postoperative intensive care monitoring.

The physical examination may be less than optimal due to the patient's body habitus. Maneuvers such as the straight-leg raise and heel-toe walking may not be possible. Sensory disturbances such as stocking distribution peripheral neuropathy may be present. Diabetic neuropathy also can mask signs of myelopathy.

Diagnostic imaging in the obese patient can be challenging. Dynamic flexion and extension plain films can be limited and of poor quality. MRI and CT scanning can be difficult to perform because of size limitations. Although open MRI scans are an option for obese patients, image quality is compromised.

Caregiver Safety

Nurses' aides, orderlies, and attendants have the highest rates of work-acquired musculoskeletal disorders.[31] In one institution, the rate of work injuries attributed to obese patient handling was found to be 29.8%, and 27.9% of all lost work days and 37.2% of all restricted work days were attributed to bariatric patient handling.[32] Caregiver safety as well as patient safety is of the utmost importance in the context of obese spine patient handling. Ergonomically safe work environments that utilize state-of-the-art patient handling equipment must be a top priority for all health care organizations.[32-40]

Surgical Issues in Obesity

The surgical management of obese patients should follow the same individualized approach as that for nonobese persons, with special considerations taken when considering the operative approach, table and positioning, and equipment requirements.

Shamji et al. completed an analysis of 244,170 thoracolumbar and lumbar spinal fusions done in obese patients. They found that these patients had an increased number of blood transfusions and an increased likelihood of discharge to assisted living. Morbidly obese patients undergoing dorsal fusion were more likely to experience wound complications and postoperative wound infections.[41]

Operative Approach

The patient's specific body habitus, spinal disease process, and goals of the operative intervention are to be considered when planning the operative approach. For instance, an anterior cervical discectomy and fusion is less likely to be an option for a morbidly obese individual with a symptomatic cervical herniated disc that has failed conservative management. A dorsal decompressive approach is an alternative in this situation.

Operative Table and Positioning

The Jackson table is radiolucent and has a load-bearing capacity of up to 500 pounds. The Jackson table allows the abdomen to hang freely in the prone position, reducing epidural venous bleeding. Appropriate and ample padding as well as immobilization are especially necessary for patient safety. Gel pads are used to protect from pressure and subsequent skin breakdown. Skin is protected before the use of tape for immobilization. Peripheral nerve palsies from positioning and the increased patient body mass can cause traction stresses on the axillary and/or peripheral neurovascular bundles.[21] Operating table failure has been reported, so heightened attention to standard procedures should be followed.[42]

The goal of proper positioning is to obtain optimal exposure and visualization while optimizing cardiovascular and respiratory dynamics and avoiding blood loss, venous congestion, neurovascular compromise, and pressure point complications.[43] Supine, lateral decubitus, kneeling, and sitting positions all require the same preplanned, individualized approach to ensure patient safety. Additionally, preprocedure general medical conditions and anesthetic considerations should be included in preoperative planning.[44]

The supine position allows exposure for ventral cervical, transthoracic, and transabdominal approaches, as well as ventral iliac crest bone graft harvest. Arm boards, sleds, and draw sheets may be used to support the upper extremities. With substantial girth, care must be taken not to lean into the patient. Visualization for ventral cervical approaches can be adversely affected by a large submandibular panniculus. If ventral cervical exposure will be suboptimal due to the patient's body habitus, a dorsal approach should be contemplated.

The prone position poses a greater threat for respiratory compromise and abdominal compression, which may lead to increased venous congestion, more difficult hemostasis, and increased peak airway pressure. The Jackson table, previously described, aids in alleviating these issues. It is crucial to provide support to an excessive hanging abdominal panniculus.

The lateral decubitus position may used if the prone position is contraindicated or the operating table is insufficient, or for visualization of the ventral or lateral thoracolumbar spine. This position accommodates those patients with a large thoracoabdominal pannus that poses challenges in the supine position. However, dorsal midline dissections may be more difficult, especially in the cervical spine and in the case of spinal instability. Spinal alignment may be maintained with a pillow or other supports, but this position should be used with great caution in this setting.

Although the kneeling position may have the benefits of lowering intra-abdominal pressure and providing increased hemostasis, better visualization, and lower cardiac and respiratory pressures, it is more time consuming, increases susceptibility to pressure injuries, and may lead to potential difficulties by altering the lumbar curvature during surgery. These potential complications warrant careful consideration during preoperative planning.

The sitting position poses potential challenges due to the obese patient's large ventral mass along with limited flexibility. Additionally, the obese patient has the tendency to slip downward during the procedure, and shoulder immobilization may interfere with the operative field. Generally, the prone position provides adequate positioning for dorsal cervical approaches with fewer potential concerns.[43]

Preplanning is key, regardless of the patient positioning strategy used. Preplanning requires keen attention to available equipment, staffing, and what strategy is safest for the patient and care providers while still being able to meet the operative goals (Fig. 129-3).

Surgical Exposure

Optimal exposure depends directly on appropriate positioning and type of approach, appropriate incision size and configuration, adequate muscular relaxation, and the use of an appropriate retractor system. The approach and exposure must take into account the patient's specific body habitus. Additionally, intraoperative localization can be challenging with this patient population.[43]

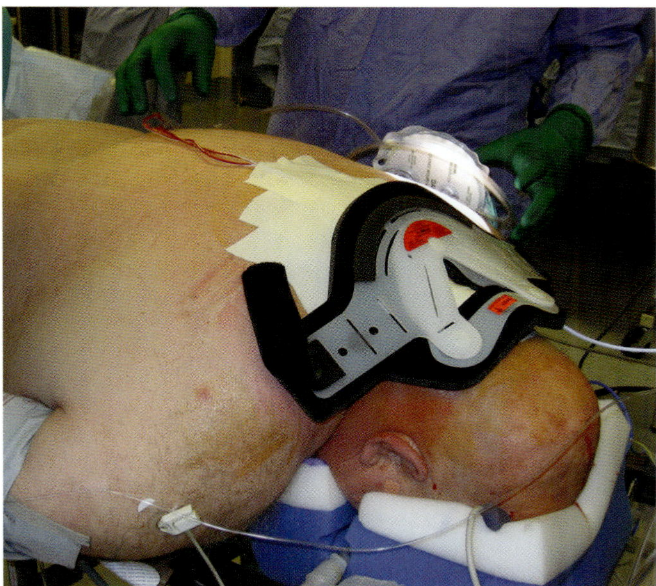

FIGURE 129-3. Immediate postoperative view, with the patient in the prone position on a Jackson table, following dorsal cervical procedure.

Wound Closure

Meticulous attention to tight wound closure will aid in the prevention of postoperative wound complications. The poor vascularity of adipose tissue and the overall thickness and lack of strength of the adipose layer for suture retention contribute to the morbidity associated with the wound in an obese patient. Dead space should be minimized with multilayered closure. Use of a closely spaced, interrupted dermal layer of suture, as well as approximation of the superficial fascia within the adipose layer, may add to the strength of the superficial approximation. Additionally, placement of a wound drain will prevent accumulation of blood and body fluid, which can be quite significant in the obese patient. Accumulation of blood and body fluid can lead to chronic wound leakage, a tense and painful wound area, hematoma formation, and potential for a large fluid-filled cavity in the surgical area and a nonhealing wound (Fig. 129-4).

Superficial drainage often is seen initially after surgery. Care providers must be taught to provide meticulous, frequent wound care. With persistent or recurrent drainage or dehiscence, general surgical techniques with superficial opening, debridement, and, if necessary, packing of the wound is warranted. Many wound-healing products are available, and consultation with a wound and skin care provider can be considered. Deeper subfascial infections usually require operative debridement and thorough irrigation followed by fascial reapproximation and layered drainage or suprafascial packing with healing by granulation. If debridement of the wound edges is required, large retention sutures or surgical undermining may be helpful for wound reapproximation.[43]

Aggressive surgical management is important when an infection has been identified. Antibiotic penetration into adipose tissue is poor. Only superficial infections should be treated by local debridement and antibiotic therapy. Deeper infections require intraoperative debridement and irrigation followed by a prolonged course of antibiotic therapy.

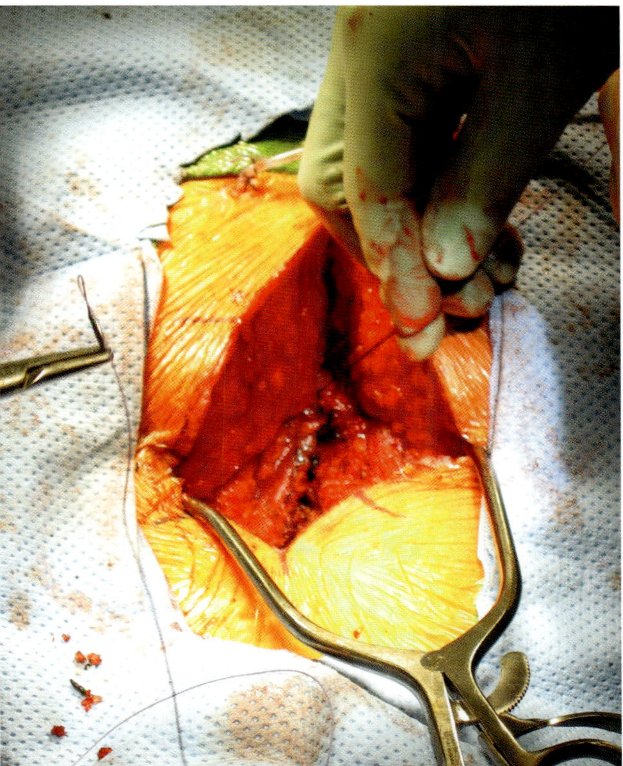

FIGURE 129-4. Intraoperative view of meticulous wound closure.

Postoperative Management and Complication Prevention

Recognition of the physiologic consequences of obesity and anticipation of potential postoperative complications are key to postoperative management. General medical considerations were discussed earlier in this chapter. Infection risk, as previously discussed, is higher than with nonobese patients. Meticulous wound care is essential, both as an inpatient and after discharge. Verbal and written instructions, as well as adequate dressing supplies, should be provided to the caregiver who will be responsible for wound care following discharge. Obese individuals have many skin folds and are prone to excessive perspiration, necessitating a high degree of wound monitoring vigilance. Patients and caregivers should be instructed to contact the appropriate clinic with any suspicion of healing delay or signs of infection, so that potential problems can be evaluated early.

The relationship of obesity to perioperative complications in spine surgery was evaluated by Patel et al. They found the risk of major complications increased with increasing BMI. In patients whose BMI was 25 to 29.9, the estimated chance of a major complication was 14%. Risk of major complication increased to 20% with a BMI of 30 to 39.9, and to 36% when the BMI was 40 or over.[21]

Summary

Obesity is a global health care issue affecting children and adults. The spine surgeon requires a heightened awareness of the associated comorbid conditions and potential challenges in caring for this patient population. Significant surgical preplanning, orchestration of personnel and appropriate equipment, and coordination with the patient's general medical providers are needed. Obesity itself is not a contraindication to surgery, but the patient must be well informed of his or her particular additional operative risks, and patient and physician expectations for the surgical intervention should be clearly communicated.

KEY REFERENCES

Patel N, Bagan B, Vadera S, et al: Obesity and spine surgery: relation to perioperative complications. *J Neurosurg Spine* 6:291–297, 2007.

Poirier P, Giles T, Bray G, et al: Obesity and cardiovascular disease: pathophysiology, evaluation, and effect of weight loss: an update of the 1997 American Heart Association Scientific Statement on Obesity and Heart Disease from the Obesity Committee of the Council on Nutrition, Physical Activity, and Metabolism. *Circulation* 113:898–918, 2006.

Shiri R, Karppinen J, Leno-Arjas P: The association between obesity and low back pain: a meta-analysis. *Am J Epidemiol* 171:135–154, 2009.

Sinha A: Some anesthetic aspects of morbid obesity. *Curr Opin Anaesthesiol* 22:442–446, 2009.

Thorp K, Ogden L, Galactionova K: *Weighty matters: how obesity drives poor health and health spending in the U.S. 2009*. www.businessgrouphealth.org/pdfs/NBGH%20WeightyMatters_Final.pdf. Accessed January 24, 2010.

U.S. Department of Veterans Affairs. *Safe bariatric patient handling toolkit*. www.visn8.va.gov/patientsafetycenter/safePtHandling/toolkitBariatrics.asp. Accessed November 24, 2009.

Yosipovitch G, DeVore A, Dawn A: Obesity and the skin: skin physiology and skin manifestation of obesity. *J Am Acad Dermatol* 6:901–916, 2007.

REFERENCES

The complete reference list is available online at expertconsult.com.

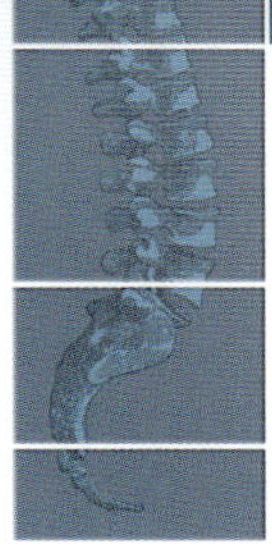

CHAPTER 130

Smoking and the Spine

David W. Schippert | Glenn R. Rechtine II

Tobacco is responsible for one in five deaths, and tobacco use is the single largest preventable cause of death and disability in the United States.[1] Smoking has been linked to numerous health conditions, including cancer, respiratory disease, cardiovascular disease, and peripheral vascular disease[1]; however, the delayed onset of these diseases makes it difficult for users to realize the potential consequences of tobacco use until significant damage has been done. The addictive properties of tobacco use, both chemical and psychological, make cessation difficult for even the most determined quitter. Despite numerous public health efforts, tobacco use continues to have significant adverse effects on the health of people everywhere.[2]

Tobacco use affects the entire body and has been identified as a risk factor for six of the eight leading causes of death in the world: malignancies, heart disease, cerebrovascular disease, lower respiratory infections, chronic obstructive pulmonary disease, and tuberculosis[2-5] (Table 130-1). Associated with increased osteoclast and decreased osteoblast activity, smoking has been implicated as a risk factor for osteoporosis, delayed fracture healing, and fusion pseudarthrosis. In general, multiple studies have indicated that spine-related disorders are more common in smokers, and spine surgeries are up to four times more frequent in cigarette smokers.[6] Symptomatic fusion pseudarthrosis is believed to be three to five times more common in smokers than nonsmokers.[6]

This chapter will highlight specific consequences of tobacco use on the spine, including contributions to disease development and effects on treatment outcomes. It will present the current prevalence of tobacco use in the United States and recent trends. The adverse effects of tobacco use on the entire body and the physiologic effects of nicotine will be discussed. Tobacco is a complex, variable substance composed of numerous chemicals; therefore, the compounds typically found in tobacco smoke will be identified and their adverse effects examined. The definitions of addiction and dependence and the roles they play in the perpetuation of tobacco use will be reviewed. Perhaps most importantly, current strategies for smoking cessation and their outcomes will be discussed.

Adverse Health Effects of Tobacco Use

Initially linked to lip, mouth, and throat cancers in the 18th and 19th centuries, tobacco use has been shown to result in significant damage throughout the body.[7] Typically associated with lung cancer, smoking actually results in more deaths from cardiovascular and respiratory diseases.[8] Lung diseases linked to smoking include cancer, bronchitis, emphysema, and a predisposition for pneumonia.[1] Injuries to the cardiovascular system resulting from smoking include coronary artery disease, myocardial infarction, cerebral vascular attack, aneurysm, and peripheral vascular disease.[1] Coronary artery disease is two to four times more common in smokers than nonsmokers.[1] In nonsmokers, exposure to secondhand smoke has been associated with a 25% to 30% increased risk for the development of coronary artery disease.[9] Smoking has also been associated with the development of insulin resistance, cataracts, and bacterial infections.[1,10,11] Smokeless tobacco

TABLE 130-1

Common Adverse Health Effects due to Tobacco Use

Adverse Effect	Signs
Cancer	Lung, trachea, bronchus, oral, esophageal, stomach, liver, pancreatic, bladder, kidney, and cervical cancers; leukemia
Cardiovascular	Atherosclerosis, cerebrovascular disease, coronary artery disease, abdominal aortic aneurysm
Dental	Implant complications and failure
Dermatologic	Advanced skin aging, wrinkles
Gastrointestinal	Peptic ulcer disease
Immunologic	Infectious disease susceptibility, tuberculosis
Ophthalmologic	Cataracts
Orthopaedic	Decreased bone mineral density, delayed fracture healing, increased fracture risk
Respiratory	Chronic obstructive pulmonary disease, pneumonia, impaired lung development
Reproductive	Maternal infertility, miscarriage, low birth weight, still birth, sudden infant death syndrome
Spinal	Back and neck pain, prolonged disability, poor surgical outcomes
Surgical	Surgical site infections, delayed healing

Data from Brunnhuber K, Cummings KM, Feit S, et al: Putting evidence into practice: smoking cessation, 2007. www.clinicalevidence.bmj.com/downloads/smoking-cessation.pdf; and Wipfli H, Samet JM: Global economic and health benefits of tobacco control: part 1. *Clin Pharmacol Ther* 86:263–271, 2009.

has been associated with increased risk of oral cancers, gingival recession, and oral leukoplakia.[5]

Spine-Specific Consequences of Tobacco Use

Although smoking has been the form of tobacco use most often studied, any type of tobacco use has been shown to affect the spine adversely in multiple ways (Table 130-2). Not only are tobacco users more likely to have back and neck pain or injuries, they are less likely to have significant improvement following treatment.

Back Pain

An estimated 15% to 20% of adults have at least one episode of low back pain every year, and 50% to 80% experience low back pain at least once in a lifetime.[12] Similarly, neck pain is experienced by approximately 20% of the adult population in one year and by 66% of the population in a lifetime.[12] A majority of evidence on the epidemiology of neck and back pain indicates that cigarette use is associated with higher rates of pain.[13-18] Although authorities have suggested the existence of a causal relationship between smoking and neck and back pain, a relative lack of prospective studies makes it difficult to confirm this theory.

Compared with nonsmokers, smokers who have back pain are often younger, report more severe symptoms, and indicate that the symptoms were present for a larger portion of the day.[16] Smokers are also more often extremely dissatisfied by their current health, more likely to report depression, more pessimistic regarding the resolution of their pain, and less likely to show a trend toward improvement following surgery.[16] Adolescent smokers are significantly more likely to develop back pain than nonsmokers, with evidence supporting a dose-response relationship.[17,18]

Disc Degeneration

Degeneration of the intervertebral disc is believed to be pivotal in the development of lower back pain. In addition to the effects of aging, variable dynamic and biologic stresses

TABLE 130-2

Adverse Effects of Tobacco Use on the Spine

Problem	Characteristics	Mechanism	References
Back and neck pain	Increased incidence in smokers Onset at younger age Symptoms more severe Symptoms more often present Attitude regarding improvement more pessimistic Dose-dependent relationship suggested	Accelerated disc degeneration Decreased blood flow to intervertebral disc due to vasoconstriction and atherosclerosis Decreased oxygen delivery due to elevated carboxyhemoglobin levels Increased levels of free radicals and toxic chemicals Decreased reparative capability of tissues Decreased production of collagen Osteoporosis-related fractures Chronic cough	13–22
Arthrodesis rates	Pseudarthrosis rates increased up to 40% in smokers Dose-dependent relationship suggested	Decreased expression of genes related to bone healing Decreased blood flow and oxygen delivery	23-32
Postoperative complications	Significantly increased in smokers Dose-dependent relationship suggested Smokers are more likely to require reoperation, up to 26%, with a relative risk of 2.59 Preoperative cessation significantly lowers complication rates	Decreased oxygen delivery, by up to 70% Less effective immune response Decreased collagen synthesis Increased adjacent-segment disease	11, 26, 33–39
Postoperative outcomes	Smokers less likely to return to work, more likely to be disabled, and less satisfied with outcomes	Multifactorial	27, 30, 40–42
Fractures	Increased risk of fractures in both males and females Dose-dependent relationship suggested Increased incidence of vertebral, hip, proximal humerus, and distal forearm fractures Earlier, by 5 years, occurrence of incident fragility fractures	Increased incidence of osteoporosis Smoking is an independent, dose-dependent risk factor Decreased body mass and altered body composition Decreased effective estrogen levels Decreased calcium absorption Decreased levels of 25-OH vitamin D Reduced bone size and decreased amounts of cancellous and cortical bone Decreased osteocyte function Increased fall risk due to physical and neuromuscular performance of someone 5 years older	50–63, 112

contribute to disc degeneration.[19] Following exposure to nicotine, catecholamine-mediated vasoconstriction results in decreased blood flow to the intervertebral discs.[19] Elevated carboxyhemoglobin levels in smokers and the expected presence of free radicals and toxic substances could further contribute to inadequate nutrition of intervertebral disc tissues. Alterations in cell morphology, increased levels of proinflammatory cytokines, decreased glycosaminoglycan levels, and decreased production of collagen with a shift toward production of type I collagen have been demonstrated following exposure of intervertebral disc cells to nicotine.[19,20]

Chronic cough has been linked to the development of back pain in the general population, and cigarette smokers are three times more likely to have a chronic cough than people who have never smoked or previous smokers.[21] Vertebral body or end-plate fractures resulting from smoking-induced decreased bone mineral density are also likely to lead to back pain.[22]

Fusion

Smoking has been associated with decreased fracture healing rates and increased incidence of nonunion; thus, it is not surprising that smokers also tend to have similar difficulties following arthrodesis procedures.[23-30] A rabbit model of intertransverse process fusion found reduced fusion rates in those receiving nicotine up to the day of surgery and a 0% fusion rate in those continuing to receive nicotine postoperatively.[31] Nicotine exposure resulted in decreased expression of genes for vascular endothelial growth factor, basic fibroblast growth factor, types I and II collagen, and bone morphogenetic protein (BMP)-2, BMP-4, and BMP-6.[32]

Following dorsal lumbar fusion procedures, smokers have been found to have pseudarthrosis rates increased up to 40% higher than nonsmokers.[26-29] Smokers able to stop prior to surgery and remain abstinent in the postoperative period have improved rates of fusion compared with people who continue to smoke.[27] The use of rhBMP-2 has been shown to significantly increase fusion rates in smokers.[28] Following surgery, smokers were less likely to return to full-time work, more likely to be disabled, and less satisfied with the outcome.[27]

Analysis of results from ventral cervical arthrodesis procedures indicate that there is an increased pseudarthrosis rate following multilevel discectomy and interbody grafting using autogenous grafts in smokers compared with nonsmokers.[30] The clinical outcome is significantly better for nonsmokers than smokers.[30]

Surgical Complications

Surgical site infections have been reported to be more common in smokers following spine surgery,[33] and chronic hypoxia decreases collagen synthesis and deposition in healing wounds.[34,35] Published results are mixed, but smoking has also been suggested as a risk factor for the development of deep venous thromboses following surgical procedures.[36]

Tissue oxygenation is compromised in smokers due to multiple factors, including increased levels of carboxyhemoglobin, atherosclerosis, and vasoconstriction. Subcutaneous tissue oxygen tension begins to decrease 10 minutes after initiation of cigarette smoking, reaches a low of 22% to 48% below baseline after approximately 30 minutes, and remains below normal for up to one hour.[35] The combination of nicotine-mediated vasoconstriction and increased levels of carbon monoxide in smokers results in an estimated 70% decrease in subcutaneous tissue oxygenation in regular smokers.[35]

The presence of oxygen is crucial for effective prevention of infection,[26,34] and smokers have demonstrated increased susceptibility to a number of bacterial infections, including meningitis, periodontitis, otitis media, and infection of the respiratory and urinary tracts.[11] Reactive oxygen species produced by neutrophils and monocytes are necessary for effective functioning of the immune system, and levels are decreased in smokers.[34] Increased subcutaneous oxygen levels postoperatively result in decreased surgical site infection rates, and smokers quitting smoking 4 to 8 weeks prior to surgery have shown a decreased incidence of surgical site infection.[34]

Following fusion with segmental fixation for adult spinal deformity, smoking was found to be a risk factor for adjacent-segment problems; the overall relative risk of reoperation for any reason was 2.59 in smokers, with 25.8% requiring another procedure.[37] Prior to elective general surgery or orthopaedic procedures, smokers randomized to receive smoking cessation counseling and offered nicotine replacement therapy had cessation rates significantly higher than the control group, up to 58%, and significantly lower postoperative complication rates.[38,39] Cessation had the largest effect on reducing surgical site complications.[39] The number needed to treat to prevent one complication has ranged from three to five patients.[38,39]

Overall Outcomes

After surgical procedures for isthmic lumbosacral spondylolisthesis or chronic low back pain, smokers were more likely to be dissatisfied and have worse results.[40-42] Patients actively serving in the military were significantly less likely to return to full-time work following a lumbar microdiscectomy if they were smokers.[43]

Musculoskeletal Consequences of Tobacco Use

General Adverse Effects

The remainder of the musculoskeletal system suffers similar consequences due to tobacco use. Smokers experience decreased rates of healing of fractures, fusions, and tissues, which results in poorer outcomes overall and an increased incidence of posttraumatic and postoperative infections. Postoperative smoking predicts failure of fingertip replantations[44] and reduced success of anterior cruciate ligament reconstruction.[45] Following tibial and femoral shaft fractures, smokers are more likely to experience delayed union or nonunion than nonsmokers.[46,47] Smokers are also at increased risk for rotator cuff tears[48] and are likely to have delayed tendon to bone healing following rotator cuff repair based on findings in a rat model.[49]

Osteoporosis

Smoking has long been associated with the development of osteoporosis and increased risk of fractures. Evidence indicates that smoking is an independent, dose-dependent risk factor for decreased bone density.[50,51] This finding is not limited to older patients. A study of young male military recruits found smoking to be a risk factor for decreased spine and hip bone mineral density.[52] Research has also shown that smokers have reduced bone size and amounts of cancellous and cortical bone. Estradiol activity is routinely decreased in smokers due to multiple mechanisms. This results in decreased intestinal absorption of calcium and increased risk of osteoporosis.[53,54] Smoking-related alterations in body mass and composition, estrogen metabolism, calcium absorption, and osteocyte function are thought to have important effects on bone health.[53,54]

Smoking is believed to increase fracture risk through multiple mechanisms; low bone mineral density cannot account for the entire increase in risk.[55] Effects are seen in both premenopausal and postmenopausal women, although effects are often more significant following menopause and in women with decreased body mass.[56,57] Men who smoke are also affected and have been found to have a 4% to 15.3% lower bone mineral density than men who had never smoked.[58] Twin studies of same-sex pairs discordant for smoking indicate a possible dose-dependent relationship.[56,59]

Smokers can have significantly reduced bone mineral density at the lumbar spine, forearm, and calcaneus, with more substantial deficits noted in the hip.[50] Smoking has been shown to increase the lifetime risk of vertebral and hip fractures in both men and women who smoke.[50,55,57,60-62] Current smoking has also been implicated as a risk factor for proximal humerus and distal forearm fractures.[63] Smokers have been shown to be at risk for sustaining fractures up to 5.2 years earlier than nonsmokers, and fracture risk increased as tobacco consumption increased.[63] Smoking cessation results in a rapid drop in fracture risk during the first 10 years, but the risk of fracture remains elevated for more than 30 years.[63]

There is also evidence that smokers may be more likely to fall than nonsmokers due to relative weakness, poorer balance, and impaired neuromuscular performance.[54] It has been estimated that smokers have the physical and neuromuscular function of someone 5 years older.[54]

Epidemiology of Tobacco Use

Worldwide

Tobacco use, which is linked to 100 million deaths in the 20th century and currently accounts for 5.4 million deaths a year, has been classified as an epidemic by the World Health Organization.[2] At current rates, tobacco use will result in over 8 million deaths a year by the year 2030 and an estimated 1 billion deaths in the 21st century.[64] *Tobacco kills one third to one half of all people who use it—one person every 6 seconds—resulting in death approximately 8 to 16 years prematurely.*[65] More than 40% of men and approximately 12% of women smoke tobacco worldwide.[4]

In the United States

In the United States, cigarette smoking kills an estimated 440,000 people each year. This is more than the number of people killed as a result of car accidents, alcohol abuse, illegal drug use, homicide, and AIDS combined.[1] In the 40 years between 1964 and 2004, more than 12 million Americans died prematurely due to smoking-related illnesses. At the current rate, 25 million smokers alive today will die due to the adverse effects of smoking.[1] Cigarette-related residential fires result in more than 1000 deaths each year, making cigarettes the number one cause of residential fire fatalities.[1]

TABLE 130-3

Current Tobacco Use among Americans 12 Years of Age and Older in 2007

	Number of People (in millions)	Percent of U.S. Population
Cigarette smokers	60.1	24.2
Cigar smokers	13.3	5.4
Smokeless tobacco users	8.1	3.2
Pipe smokers	2	0.8
Any tobacco use	70.9	28.6

Data from Substance Abuse and Mental Health Services Administration: *Results from the 2007 national survey on drug use and health: national findings,* Rockville, MD, 2008, Office of Applied Studies.

The 2007 National Survey on Drug Use and Health found that 70.9 million Americans 12 years of age and older were current tobacco users.[66] As shown in Table 130-3, a majority of these, 60.1 million, were current cigarette smokers.[66] The rate of tobacco use varies greatly between age groups, with people 18 to 25 years of age having the highest rate of tobacco use in the previous 30 days, 41.8%.[66] Of youths 12 to 17 years of age, 12.4% (3.1 million) had used a tobacco product in the past 30 days.[66]

Financial Costs

The financial burden of tobacco use on society is overwhelming. It is estimated that tobacco use is directly responsible for more than 96 billion dollars of the U.S. health care budget each year.[1] An additional burden of 97 billion dollars annually can be attributed to lost productivity due to tobacco use.[1] By not accounting for other costs associated with tobacco use, such as diseases due to secondhand smoke and burns related to tobacco use, the estimated annual cost associated with tobacco use of 193 billion dollars is likely a significant underestimate.[1]

Secondhand Smoke

Passive, or secondhand, smoke has also been shown to increase the risk of smoking-related illness. It is estimated that approximately 3000 lung cancer deaths and 46,000 deaths from coronary artery disease are due to passive smoke exposure each year.[67] Children exposed to tobacco smoke are at increased risk for sudden infant death syndrome and respiratory and ear infections. In addition, they are more likely to develop asthma and to have more severe symptoms.[1,9]

Recent Trends of Tobacco Use

As of 1960, approximately 50% of adult men in the United States were cigarette smokers.[4] Since the 1946 release of the Surgeon General's report on smoking and health, increased awareness of the harms of tobacco use have led to an almost

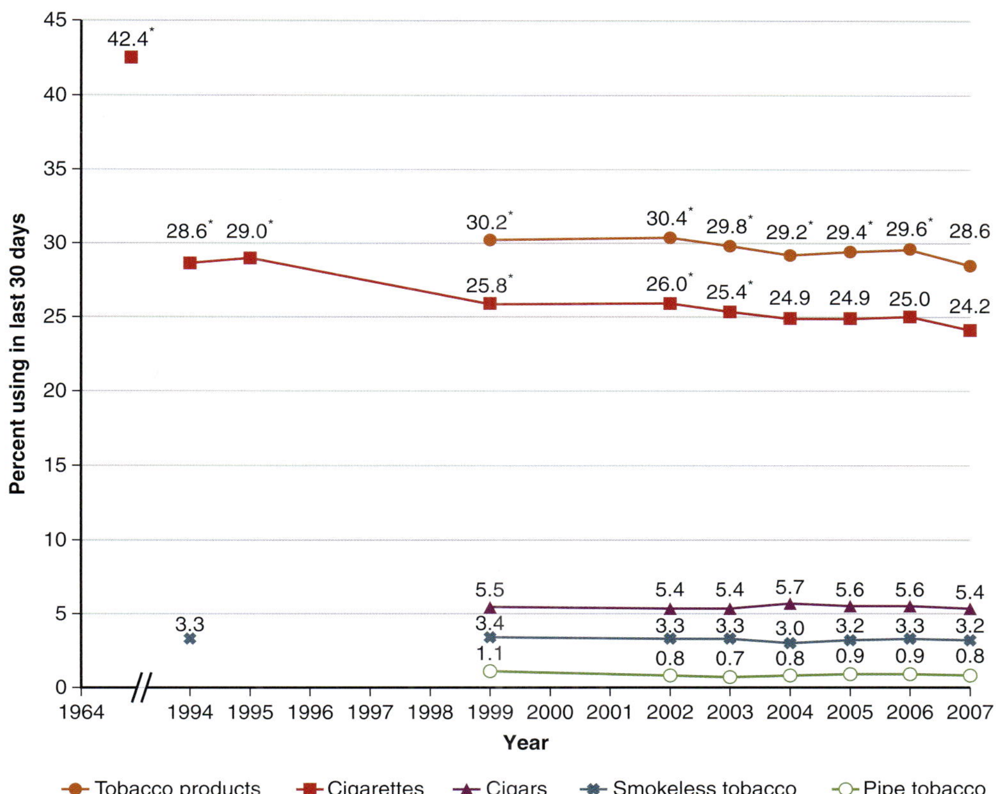

FIGURE 130-1. **Percent of U.S. population reporting current tobacco use, by type and year. *The difference between this estimate and the 2007 estimate is statistically significant at the 0.05 level.** (Data from 1965 represents users age 18 and above from the Centers for Disease Control and Prevention, Achievements in Public Health, 1900–1999: Tobacco use—United States, 1900–1999. *MMWR* 48(43):986–993, 1999. Data from 1994 to 2007 represents users age 12 and above from the Substance Abuse and Mental Health Services Administration: *Results from the 2007 national survey on drug use and health: national findings*, Rockville, MD, Office of Applied Studies, 2008.)

50% decrease in the number of Americans using tobacco[1,66] (Fig. 130-1). Between 2000 and 2007, there was an 18% decline in cigarette sales in the United States. The average price of a pack of cigarettes increased from $2.93 to $3.93 during the same period.[68] Although the rates of cigarette use and overall tobacco use by 18- to 25-year-olds decreased from 2002 to 2007, the rates of cigar and smokeless tobacco use slightly increased.[66]

In 2007, there were approximately 6100 new cigarette smokers 12 years of age and older every day, for a total of 2.2 million new smokers.[66] Of these, 59.7% were younger than 18 years of age.[66] In that same year, a higher percentage of males than females (53.2% vs. 22.4%) reported tobacco use during the previous 30 days.[66]

There is significant variability in the rate of tobacco use between the different ethnic groups in the United States. In 2007, the prevalence of past month tobacco use in those 12 years of age and older was 15.4% for Asians, 22.7% for Hispanics, 26.8% for blacks, 30.7% for whites, 35.2% for groups reporting two or more races, and 41.8% for American Indians or Alaska Natives.[66] Educational level inversely influences cigarette use, with use decreasing as education increases.[66]

As of 2006, Utah had the lowest smoking rates, with 10.4% of men and 9.3% of women 18 years of age or older reporting current cigarette use.[8] Kentucky had the highest smoking rates, with 29.1% of men and 28.0% of women, for the same period.[8]

People with mental illness compose one group that has not seen an appreciable decrease in smoking rates. Although smoking rates have been reported near 90% in people with schizophrenia, smoking rates are two to four times greater in people with bipolar disorder, major depression, posttraumatic stress disorder, and other mental illnesses than in the general population.[69] People with psychiatric disorders are believed to purchase more than 40% of cigarettes sold in the United States.[1]

Also associated with increased cigarette use, current illicit drug use was reported in 20.1% of smokers compared with 4.1% of those not currently using cigarettes.[66] Similarly, alcohol use was reported by 66.9% of cigarette smokers compared with 46.1% of nonsmokers.[66] Cigarette users were also more likely to be heavy drinkers and participate in binge drinking than those not currently using cigarettes.[66]

A corresponding increase in sales of other tobacco products negated approximately 30% of the decline in cigarette sales. For example, *cigar sales increased by 37% from 2000 to 2007*,[68] and use of noncigarette smoked tobacco products, including bidis, kreteks, and shisha, has also increased.[2]

Tobacco and Tobacco Smoke

The composition and behavior of tobacco smoke is a complex subject that is not fully understood. The identities, behaviors, and health consequences of many of the components of tobacco smoke have yet to be well defined. Tobacco and tobacco smoke contain approximately 6700 compounds, about 4000 of which have been identified. At least 63 of these compounds are known to be carcinogenic in mammals, and 11 are known to be human carcinogens.[70] An average commercially produced cigarette in the United States is filled with 700 mg of tobacco, which contains 10 to 14 mg of nicotine.[71,72] Nicotine ($C_{10}H_{14}N_2$, 1-methyl-2-(3-pyridyl)-pyrrolidine) is a naturally occurring plant alkaloid and is responsible for a majority of the addictive properties of tobacco.

Some compounds in tobacco smoke that are considered hazardous include formaldehyde, acetaldehyde, benzene, carbon monoxide, arsenic, isoprene, toluene, acetone, styrene, ammonia, hydrogen cyanide, and vinyl chloride.[73] Almost all of the common elements have been identified in tobacco, including a number of radioactive isotopes and free radicals.[73] Many, including cadmium, mercury, titanium, and lead, are also found in tobacco smoke. When inhaled, tobacco smoke is an aerosol with a gas phase containing approximately 8% particulate material on a weight basis.[74,75] There are approximately 10^9 to 10^{10} particles/cm^3 in tobacco smoke, with 50% to 90% being retained in the lungs after expiration.[73]

Although cigarettes are a roll of tobacco wrapped in a substance not containing tobacco, cigars consist of tobacco wrapped in leaf tobacco or in any substance containing tobacco.[70] Cigar tobacco is high in nitrate, and the fermenting process unique to cigars converts the nitrate to very high levels of carcinogenic nitrogen-containing compounds.[70] Cigar smoke also contains elevated levels of tar, ammonia, nitrosamines, and nitrogen oxides.[70] Having a higher pH than cigarette smoke, cigar smoke contains higher concentrations of free nicotine in the particulate and vapor phases.[70] This is absorbed through the oral mucosa and does not require the cigar to be lit. Some cigars contain as much tar and nicotine as a pack of cigarettes.

Nicotine

Cigarettes are very efficient means of drug delivery. With typical use, 10 puffs over a 5-minute period, an average smoker receives 1 to 2 mg of nicotine per cigarette.[1,76] When inhaled, nicotine is quickly absorbed into the venous circulation, avoiding first-pass metabolism and reaching peak concentrations within 10 seconds.[1,71,77] With smokeless tobacco and most cigar and pipe use, nicotine levels peak more slowly as the nicotine is absorbed through the mucosal membranes. To facilitate absorption of nicotine, a weak base, through the mucous membranes, chewing tobacco and snuff are buffered to an alkaline pH, near 7 or 8.[77,78] Peak nicotine concentrations following the use of chewing tobacco are reached in approximately 30 minutes and are maintained for about 2 hours.[71] Air-cured tobaccos, commonly used in pipes and cigars, produce smoke with a relatively alkaline pH, facilitating mucosal absorption of nicotine.[71]

Nicotine distributes throughout the body; plasma levels of nicotine in regular smokers range from 50 nmol/L in light smokers to 300 nmol/L in heavy smokers.[20,71] Nicotine concentrations in breast milk are approximately three times greater than maternal serum concentrations, and nicotine accumulates in amniotic fluid and fetal tissues.[71]

Specific Adverse Health Effects of Tobacco Use

Cancer

Approximately one third of all cancer deaths can be attributed to smoking, and rates of death from cancer are twice as high in smokers and four times as high in heavy smokers than in nonsmokers.[1,8] Smoking is linked to 90% of all lung cancer cases, and lung cancer accounts for 80% of cancer deaths attributed to smoking.[1,8] Other cancers associated with smoking include oropharyngeal, laryngeal, esophageal, stomach, pancreatic, cervical, renal, bladder, and acute myelogenous leukemia.[1,8] Of all possible carcinogens present in tobacco, the seven tobacco-specific nitrosamines have emerged as some of the most active based on rodent and preliminary human studies.[79] Nonsmoking adults living with a smoker have been found to have a 20% to 30% increased risk of lung cancer compared with the general population.[9]

Numerous rodent studies have confirmed the ability of oral snuff to cause oral cancers.[78] Many suspected carcinogens, including the tobacco-specific *N*-nitrosamines, are present in oral tobacco.[78] Snuff also contains the radioactive isotope polonium-210, formaldehyde, and acetaldehyde.[78]

Although nicotine investigators have not shown that smoking is a direct carcinogen, animal studies suggest that it acts as a tumor promoter by inhibiting apoptosis and preventing the killing of malignant cells.[77] Increased angiogenesis seen in animals receiving nicotine may contribute to tumor growth and eventual metastasis.[77]

Cardiovascular Effects

Cigarette smoking increases the risk of coronary artery disease by 80%. It also increases the incidence of stroke, angina, myocardial infarction, and fatal coronary artery disease.[10] Both primary and secondhand tobacco smoke are associated with the development of atherosclerosis. *Passive smoking increases the risk of coronary artery disease by 30%.*[10]

Proposed mechanisms leading to the increased incidence of acute myocardial infarction seen in smokers include increased coronary artery vascular resistance, stimulation of coronary vasospasm, increased risk of plaque rupture or erosion, and induction of thrombosis.[10] Cigarette smoking is associated with decreased availability of nitric oxide, a free radical responsible for initiating vasodilation, especially in the coronary arteries and microvascular beds.[10]

Cigarette smoke has been associated with an increased peripheral blood leukocyte count and increased markers of inflammation, including C-reactive protein, interleukin-6, and tumor necrosis factor alpha.[10] This results in increased leukocyte recruitment, adherence to the endovascular endothelium, and transendothelial migration of monocytes.[10] The lipid profiles of smokers traditionally show decreased levels of high-density lipoprotein with increased levels of low-density lipoprotein, serum cholesterol, and triglycerides.[10] Platelets from smokers have an increased propensity to aggregate, both spontaneously and following stimulation.[10]

Pulmonary Effects

Cigarette smoke leads to pulmonary emphysema through the initiation of inflammatory responses in lung tissues and impairment of repair processes.[80] Following exposure to cigarette smoke, appropriate recruitment and proliferation of lung fibroblasts and epithelial cells is inhibited.[80] Similarly, cigarette smoke inhibits lysyl oxidase, the enzyme responsible for cross-linking and polymerizing elastin.[80]

Pregnancy

Nicotine easily crosses the placenta and can reach fetal concentrations that are 15% higher than maternal levels.[1] Additionally, elevated levels of maternal and fetal carbon monoxide can decrease fetal oxygen delivery.[1] Adverse outcomes associated with smoking during pregnancy include fetal growth retardation, decreased birth weight, spontaneous abortion, and sudden infant death.[81] In addition to an estimated 910 infant deaths annually due to smoking,[1] costs due to smoking-related neonatal care are believed to be more than 350 million dollars a year.[82] As a later consequence, children of mothers who smoked more than one pack a day during pregnancy have almost twice the risk of developing nicotine dependence.[83]

Addiction and Dependence

The *Diagnostic and Statistic Manual of Mental Disorders-IV* (DSM-IV)[84] defines substance dependence as a maladaptive pattern of substance use leading to clinically significant impairment or distress (Box 130-1). Dependence on nicotine is more prevalent than on any other substance of abuse.[85] The most basic explanation of nicotine's addictive properties, like those of other drugs of abuse, is that it activates reward pathways[1] (Table 130-4).

BOX 130-1. Definition of Substance Dependence

Maladaptive pattern of substance use, leading to clinically significant impairment or distress, as manifested by three (or more) of the following, occurring at any time in the same 12-month period:

- Tolerance
- Withdrawal
- Substance is taken in larger amounts or over a longer period than was intended
- Persistent desire or unsuccessful efforts to decrease substance use
- Great deal of time spent in activities necessary to obtain the substance, use it, or recover from its effects
- Important social, occupational, or recreational activities that are given up or reduced because of substance use

From American Psychiatric Association Task Force on DSM-IV: *Diagnostic and statistical manual of mental disorders: DSM-IV-TR*, ed 4, Washington DC, 2000, American Psychiatric Association.

TABLE 130-4

Neurotransmitter Levels Increased through Activation of Nicotinic Receptors and Resulting Effects

Neurotransmitter	Effect(s)
Acetylcholine	Arousal, cognitive improvement
Beta-endorphin	Decreased anxiety, relaxation
Dopamine	Appetite suppression, enjoyment
Gamma-aminobutyric acid	Decreased anxiety, relaxation
Glutamate	Memory improvement
Norepinephrine	Appetite suppression, arousal
Serotonin	Appetite suppression, mood regulation

Data from Benowitz NL: Neurobiology of nicotine addiction: implications for smoking cessation treatment. *Am J Med* 121:S3–S10, 2008.

Rodent studies indicate that acetaldehyde, present in tobacco smoke and a metabolite of ethanol, increases the reinforcing properties of nicotine and has a more significant effect on adolescents than adults.[86] These findings may indicate why adolescents are more likely to become addicted to tobacco. Twin studies have found that up to 40% to 70% of the risk of nicotine addiction may be due to a genetic predisposition.[1] A number of genes, a majority located on chromosome 15, that may place people at increased risk for nicotine addiction have been identified.[87-90]

Tobacco users also commonly acquire a psychological addiction to tobacco use. Smokers frequently develop compulsive behavior, including the need to handle, light, feel, or smell cigarettes, and they associate certain behaviors, people, and situations with the pleasurable effects of tobacco use.[77] These conditioned cues are major factors preventing people from halting smoking and often lead to relapse.[77]

Certain populations appear to be more susceptible to tobacco addiction, including alcoholics and people with psychiatric disorders. Studies have shown that nicotinic acetylcholine receptors (nAChRs) play a role in regulating the effects of alcohol consumption, and 80% of alcoholics smoke regularly.[1,69] In tobacco users with psychiatric disorders, it is difficult to ascertain whether increased smoking rates in these people are due to self-medication with nicotine, an intrinsic predisposition to smoking, or, most likely, a combination of the two.

It is important to note that *nicotine is more addictive than alcohol, heroine, and cocaine*.

Withdrawal

Box 130-2 lists diagnostic criteria for nicotine withdrawal.[84] Often beginning within a few hours of the last nicotine use, common nicotine withdrawal symptoms include nicotine craving, anxiety, depression, cognitive and attention deficits, sleep disturbances, irritability, insomnia, and increased appetite.[1,77] Withdrawal symptoms are typically more significant in people who smoke cigarettes than in people using other forms of nicotine.[84] Peaking within a few days, withdrawal symptoms often decrease after a few weeks but may continue for months.[1]

BOX 130-2. Diagnostic Criteria for Nicotine Withdrawal

Daily use of nicotine for at least several weeks

Abrupt cessation of nicotine use, or reduction in the amount of nicotine used, followed within 24 hours by four (or more) of the following signs:

- Dysphoric or depressed mood
- Insomnia
- Irritability, frustration, or anger
- Anxiety
- Difficulty concentrating
- Restlessness
- Decreased heart rate
- Increased appetite or weight gain

Symptoms that cause clinically significant distress or impairment in social, occupational, or other important areas of functioning. (The symptoms are not due to a general medical condition and are not better accounted for by another mental disorder.)

From American Psychiatric Association Task Force on DSM-IV: *Diagnostic and statistical manual of mental disorders: DSM-IV-TR*, ed 4, Washington DC, 2000, American Psychiatric Association.

Cessation

Rates

A majority of tobacco users, approximately 35 million people in the United States, desire to quit each year.[1,91] Of those people who try to quit on their own, more than 85% relapse—most within 1 week—and only 3% are abstinent at 6 months.[1,92] Cessation studies have found that women are less likely to start the quitting process and, if they are able to quit, they are more likely to relapse than men.[1]

Benefits

A 35-year-old man who quits smoking increases his life expectancy by 5 years on average.[1] Surgeons have been found to significantly underestimate the potential benefits of preoperative smoking cessation, reported to be up to a 65% reduction in complications.[93] Blood pressure and myocardial infarction risk begin to decrease within 24 hours of smoking cessation, and the resting heart rate decreases by 5 to 12 beats per minute within the first few days.[1,84] Coughing and shortness of breath typically improve within the first 1 to 9 months. The excess risk for the development of cardiovascular disease drops by 50% within the first year of cessation and drops to approximately the same level as in a person who has never smoked after 5 years.[4] The risk of smoking-related cancers declines after cessation but never reaches that of people who have never smoked.[4] Weight increases 2 to 3 kg on average within the first year of cessation.[84]

Counseling

Limited time, frustration, uncertainty of available resources, fear of offending patients, and underestimation of the significant adverse effects of smoking are a few factors that may contribute to low rates of cessation counseling by health care providers. However, studies have shown that cessation rates improve significantly following physician-initiated interventions of less than 5 minutes. Patients are also more likely to attempt smoking cessation, and be successful, if they are aware of the direct impact smoking can have on their health. To cover tobacco cessation services, current procedural terminology (CPT) codes are available related to tobacco use assessment, cessation intervention, counseling, and use of pharmacologic therapy.

The American Cancer Society has identified four steps involved in smoking cessation: making the decision to quit, setting a quit date and choosing a quit plan, dealing with withdrawal, and continuing not to smoke.[1] Predictors of successful smoking cessation have been suggested to help providers effectively target counseling efforts[94] (Box 130-3).

BOX 130-3. Suggested Predictors of Successful Attempts at Smoking Cessation

Absence of excessive alcohol use

Absence of other smokers in the home or workplace

Elevated level of motivation

Lack of depression or anxiety

Lower nicotine dependence

Older age at initiation of cigarette smoking

Successful prior "quit" attempts of longer duration

From Caponnetto P, Polosa R: Common predictors of smoking cessation in clinical practice. *Respir Med* 102:1182–1192, 2008.

New patients presenting to a group of spine practitioners who were identified as smokers received either usual care, consisting of a suggestion that they should quit and a handout on the effects of smoking on spinal disorders, or aggressive treatment including the handout, education on the relationship between smoking and the patient's condition, and instruction that they must quit smoking.[95] This message was restated at every visit for members of the aggressive treatment group, and elective surgery was not completed if the patient was still smoking.[95] The effect of the practitioner's intervention was highly significant, with 35.6% of patients in the aggressive treatment group quitting smoking compared with only 19.5% in the usual care group.[95] Younger patients, patients with greater daily cigarette consumption, and patients smoking for a longer period of time were less likely to stop smoking.[95] There was not any difference in patients returning for follow-up care between the two groups, indicating that patients receiving aggressive treatment were not more likely to seek care elsewhere.[95] In addition to decreasing preoperative smoking rates, cessation counseling can have long-term effects on tobacco use.[29,96]

Approaches

The tobacco use status of each patient should be assessed at every opportunity. Once tobacco uses have been identified, they should be advised to quit, and their willingness to quit should be assessed. The "Five As" model guides clinicians in treating addiction and has been recommended as a

BOX 130-4. "Five As" Model for Treating Addiction

Ask about tobacco use at every visit
Advise all smokers to quit
Assess the patient's willingness to quit
Assist the patient in his or her "quit" attempt
Arrange for follow-up

From Tobacco Use and Dependence Guideline Panel: *Treating tobacco use and dependence: 2008 update*, Rockville, MD, 2008, U.S. Dept. of Health and Human Services, Public Health Service.

BOX 130-5. Stages of Change for Smoking Cessation Counseling

Precontemplation: not planning to quit within the next 6 months
Contemplation: considering quitting within the next 6 months
Preparation: planning on quitting within the next 30 days
Action: successfully quitting for less than 6 months
Maintenance: successfully quitting for at least 6 months

From Prochaska JO, DiClemente CC: Stages and processes of self-change of smoking: toward an integrative model of change. *J Consult Clin Psychol* 51:390–395, 1983.

component of smoking cessation counseling[97] (Box 130-4). The patient's willingness to quit using tobacco can then be categorized using the "stages of change" to follow the patient's progress and identify how efforts should be focused to best encourage cessation[98] (Box 130-5).

In the early stages of motivation, the negative effects of smoking and the benefits of cessation should be stressed. Once a patient is contemplating or planning to quit, assistance should be offered through counseling services, pharmacologic therapy, suggestions for dealing with cravings, and encouragement. During the action and maintenance phases, positive reinforcement should be provided and potential triggers for relapse should be addressed. Initial follow-up should occur within the first week after the quit date with a second appointment within the next month.

Behavioral Therapy

For many tobacco users, the most difficult things to overcome are the behavioral and social aspects associated with tobacco use. Triggers such as being around certain people, performing particular tasks, or consuming specific beverages or food items can often make cravings worse and reinforce any withdrawal symptoms. Behavioral therapies should be customized to each person to help recognize high-risk situations, improve problem-solving capabilities, identify social supports, and develop coping strategies.[1] Women having weight concerns addressed through cognitive-behavioral therapy have been found to be more successful at quitting than those not receiving therapy.[1]

Behavioral assistance is now available to most people over the telephone and Internet. Although typical intervention programs run from 1 to 3 months, 75% to 80% of smokers who quit relapse within 6 months.[1] Studies have found that extending the length of the smoking cessation program can result in cessation rates as high as 50% at 1 year.[1]

Pharmacologic Therapy

Pharmacologic agents currently used for tobacco use cessation include nicotine replacement therapies (NRTs) and medications with various mechanisms of action (Tables 130-5 and 130-6). NRTs are used to ease withdrawal symptoms and typically produce lower nicotine levels that do not result in the same pleasurable effects as tobacco products.[1] Although NRTs still contain nicotine, they do not contain the many other chemicals, including carcinogens, found in tobacco products.[1] The full nicotine content of NRT products is usually higher than that actually absorbed.[71] Transdermal nicotine patches provide sustained levels of nicotine throughout the day, and nicotine gums, nasal sprays, and inhalers provide more rapid increases in blood levels to help alleviate acute cravings.[77]

NRT is contraindicated for use by people concurrently using tobacco products due to concerns related to increased blood levels of nicotine. However, studies evaluating NRT use by people continuing to use tobacco products did not identify an increased risk of adverse cardiovascular events.[77,99,100] NRT also does not appear to increase the risk of adverse cardiovascular events in patients with a history of cardiovascular disease.[101]

All forms of NRT are effective and increase the long-term cessation rate by 50% to 70% when used by smokers motivated to quit who used more than 10 to 15 cigarettes a day.[101,102] There is not sufficient evidence to recommend one form of NRT over another, but therapy recommendations should be customized to meet each patient's needs.[101] Evidence does suggest that combining a nicotine patch with a more rapid-acting NRT may be more effective than either alone.[101]

The antidepressant bupropion (Wellbutrin) was approved in 1997 as a smoking cessation aid and is marketed for this indication under the trade name Zyban. Bupropion is believed to facilitate smoking cessation through two mechanisms. First, it may block some of the nAChRs and decrease the positive reinforcement received from tobacco use.[77] Second, it acts similarly to nicotine by increasing brain levels of norepinephrine and dopamine.[77,103]

More recently, varenicline tartrate (Chantix) has been approved for use in smoking cessation. An analogue of cytosine, varenicline is a selective nicotine receptor partial agonist targeted to the $\alpha_4\beta_2$ nAChR.[77] As a partial agonist, varenicline leads to less dopamine release than nicotine and is able to block the effects of additional nicotine consumption.[77] This action helps decrease withdrawal symptoms and prevent positive reinforcement associated with continued tobacco use.[77] Varenicline can reduce relapse rates in smokers who have been able to quit and was shown to have better cessation rates compared with placebo and bupropion.[77,102,104]

Nortriptyline is a tricyclic antidepressant that inhibits neuronal uptake of norepinephrine and acts as a weak nAChR antagonist.[102] Clinical trials indicate that when used with NRT, nortriptyline increases smoking cessation rates compared with NRT alone.[102] The α_2-adrenergic receptor agonist clonidine decreases sympathetic outflow from the brain and may work to decrease anxiety commonly experienced during cessation.[92]

TABLE 130-5

Commonly Used Nicotine Replacement Therapies

Nicotine Replacement Therapy	Availability	Potential Adverse Effects	Typical Dosing	Notes
Gum	Over the counter	Oral irritation, unpleasant taste, GI disturbance	1 piece every 1–2 hours for 6 weeks, 1 every 2–4 hours for weeks 7–9, 1 every 4–8 hours for weeks 10–12 2 mg if <25 cigarettes/day, 4 mg if ≥25 cigarettes/day	Maximum of 24 pieces per day
Patch	Over the counter	Skin irritation, sleep disturbances if used at night	>10 cigarettes/day; 21 mg per day for 4–6 weeks, 14 mg per day for 2 weeks, 7 mg per day for 2 weeks ≤10 cigarettes/day; 14 mg per day for 2 weeks, 7 mg per day for 2 weeks	
Lozenge	Over the counter	Oral irritation, unpleasant taste	1 lozenge every 1–2 hours for 6 weeks, 1 every 2–4 hours for weeks 7–9, 1 every 4–8 hours for weeks 10–12 2-mg lozenges if smokes first cigarette >30 minutes after waking, 4-mg lozenges if smokes first cigarette within 30 minutes of waking	Maximum of 5 lozenges in 6 hours or 20 per day
Nasal spray	Prescription	Nasal irritation, rhinorrhea	1 or 2 doses per hour for 6–8 weeks, at least 8 doses per day; reduce dosing over weeks 9–14 One dose consists of 1 spray in each nostril	Maximum of 5 doses per hour or 40 doses per day
Oral inhaler (buccal absorption)	Prescription	Throat irritation, cough, dyspepsia	6 to 16 cartridges per day for weeks 1–12, gradually reduce over next 6–12 weeks Each 10-mg cartridge contains 4 mg of nicotine	Maximum of 16 cartridges per day

Data from Brunnhuber K, Cummings KM, Feit S, et al: Putting evidence into practice: smoking cessation, 2007. www.clinicalevidence.bmj.com/downloads/smoking-cessation.pdf; and Okuyemi KS, Nollen NL, Ahluwalia JS: Interventions to facilitate smoking cessation. *Am Fam Physician* 74:262–271, 2006.

TABLE 130-6

Medications Commonly Used for Smoking Cessation

Medication	Class	Mechanism	Potential Adverse Effects	Typical Dosing	Notes
Bupropion SR	Atypical antidepressant	Uncertain, believed to block neuronal reuptake of dopamine and norepinephrine	Dry mouth, sedation, seizure	150 mg daily for 3 days, then 150 mg twice a day for 7–12 weeks	Quit date should be during second week of therapy Contraindicated in patients with a history of seizures, eating disorders, head trauma, or currently taking monoamine oxidase inhibitors
Clonidine	Antihypertensive	α_2 adrenergic receptor agonist, reduction of sympathetic activity	Constipation, dizziness, drowsiness, dry mouth, tiredness, weakness, altered blood pressure, drug interactions		Second-line therapy Dose should be tapered on cessation of therapy to avoid withdrawal effects and rebound hypertension
Nortriptyline	Tricyclic antidepressant	Inhibits neuronal uptake of norepinephrine, weak nAChR antagonist	Tachycardia, orthostatic hypotension, weight alterations, blurred vision, urinary retention, dry mouth, constipation	75–100 mg daily for 6–12 weeks	Second-line therapy
Varenicline	Tobacco cessation aid	Partial agonist of $\alpha_4\beta_2$ nAChRs and full agonist of α_7 nAChRs	Nausea, altered dreams, insomnia, questionable link to depression and altered behaviors	0.5 mg daily on days 1–3, 0.5 mg twice a day on days 4–7, 1 mg twice a day starting day 8 until 12 weeks completed	Recommend initiation 1 week prior to quit date; if successful, the 12-week course may be repeated to increase long-term abstinence rates

Data from references 3,103,105, and 113.

Self-reported smoking status has been found to be fairly accurate with the overall sensitivity and specificity for self-report near 90%.[105] To assess compliance with tobacco use cessation, levels of cotinine, the primary metabolite of nicotine, can be measured. Levels greater than 3.08 ng/mL are believed to indicate current tobacco use in adults living in the United States.[71] However, plasma levels of cotinine can be increased by exposure to secondhand smoke.

Resources

The availability of resources for tobacco use cessation varies from community to community. Numerous health organizations and government agencies provide a wealth of information on tobacco use and cessation appropriate for both health care providers and tobacco users (Table 130-7). Many have also developed cessation guidelines to help guide clinical interventions and provide support to those contemplating or attempting to halt tobacco use.

Telephone-based quitlines providing telephone-based cessation counseling are available to residents of all 50 states, the District of Columbia, U.S. territories, and all 10 Canadian provinces. Quitlines are operated by various vendors under contract from government organizations and are available to anyone with access to a telephone. In the United States, a quitline database is organized by the North American Quitline Consortium (www.naquitline.org). They also operate 1-800-QUIT-NOW, a toll-free number connecting callers in the United States to the appropriate local quitline. The database contains extensive information on each quitline and can help providers identify available resources. The National Cancer Institute operates another national quitline at 1-877-44U-QUIT.

The counseling format and schedule, as well as other provided services, vary from quitline to quitline. Additional services may include Internet-based resources, printed materials, and free or discounted medications. Free medications are available through 70% of quitlines in the United States. Many quitlines also offer referrals to local resources and provide education for health care providers.

Current Research

Nicotine vaccines have been developed to stimulate production of nicotine antibodies that bind to nicotine and delay or prevent its passage through the blood-brain barrier, decreasing nicotine's reinforcing effects.[1,77] Currently in clinical trials, early results are encouraging.[102] Early clinical trials of a cannabinoid receptor antagonist, Rimonabant (Acomplia), resulted in decreased smoking rates, but the trials were recently halted.[77] Oral nicotine formulations, including drops and ingestible beads, are currently undergoing testing. A nicotine-delivering pulmonary inhaler has yet to be developed.[102]

Taking advantage of already identified pathways, new selective nAChR agonists and antagonists are being investigated. Building on the finding that slow metabolizers of nicotine smoke less and are more likely to quit, inhibitors of cytochrome P450 (CYP) enzyme CYP2A6 have been developed. The CYP2A6 inhibitors developed thus far induce significant toxicity and have not been shown safe for human use.[77] Evidence supporting a genetic component to nicotine addiction has fueled research efforts to identify the specific genes involved and accurately predict a person's response to specific treatment plans.[1]

TABLE 130-7

Selected Organizations That Provide Tobacco-Related Resources

Organization	Web Address(es)
American Cancer Society	www.cancer.org
American Lung Association	www.lungusa.org
Centers for Disease Control and Prevention	www.cdc.gov/tobacco
National Cancer Institute	www.nci.nih.gov www.smokefree.gov
National Institute on Drug Abuse	www.nida.nih.gov
Office of the Surgeon General	www.surgeongeneral.gov
World Health Organization	www.who.int

Public Policy

Increasing the price of tobacco through higher taxes is one of the most effective ways to decrease consumption and encourage cessation.[106] In addition to discouraging tobacco use, tobacco taxes also raise revenue that can be used for tobacco control and cessation programs.[2] Increasing tobacco taxes by 10% has been found to decrease tobacco use by approximately 4% in high-income countries and 8% in low- and middle-income countries. This scenario still results in a 7% increase in tobacco tax revenue.[2] Increases in tobacco costs are especially effective in preventing and decreasing tobacco use by younger people.[107]

The largest federal cigarette excise tax increase on record in the United States went into effect on April 1, 2009, resulting in a combined federal and average state cigarette excise tax of $2.21 per pack.[108] This completed a 321% increase in the federal excise tax from $0.39 per pack in 1995 to $1.01 per pack in 2009.[108] Similarly, the average state excise tax on April 1, 2009, was $1.20 per pack, a 267% increase since 1995.[108] The state excise taxes in 2009 ranged from $0.07 per pack in South Carolina to $2.75 in New York.[108] Additional taxes applied by some local governments can significantly increase the cost of cigarettes, such as the additional $2.68 tax per pack of cigarettes assessed by Chicago-Cook County.[108]

As of July 2009, 17 states, plus Puerto Rico and the District of Columbia, had laws in effect that required workplaces, restaurants, and bars to be 100% smoke free.[109] An additional 14 states had laws in place that required workplaces, restaurants, and/or bars to be smoke free.[109] Eliminating smoking in the workplace has been associated with a 3.8% decrease in the number of smokers and a 29% decrease in cigarette consumption by people in the workplace.[110]

Implemented in 1989, California was the first state to have a comprehensive statewide tobacco control program consisting of antitobacco advertising, tobacco tax increases, and smoking cessation assistance.[111] This program rapidly expanded to include a smokers' help line and the first statewide workplace smoking ban.[111] As a result, California has made significant progress in reducing smoking rates and experienced the largest decrease in lung cancer death rates in the United States between 1975 and 2005.[8]

Summary

Tobacco use is the largest preventable cause of death and disability in the United States, and tobacco has been implicated in increased rates of osteoporosis, vertebral fracture, and back pain. Smokers have poorer outcomes following spine surgery and are prone to pseudarthrosis, surgical site infection, and continued disability. Brief interventions by health care providers can have a significant effect on increasing tobacco cessation rates. Tobacco use status should be assessed at each clinic visit, users should be instructed to stop, and the relationship between tobacco use and the patient's current health concern should be stressed. Current users should be referred to available tobacco use cessation resources and their primary care physicians for consideration of pharmacologic therapy. Elective surgical procedures should be postponed until at least 4 weeks after patients have ceased using tobacco.

Given the significant disease burden due to tobacco use, tobacco-related research continues to expand. A wealth of information on tobacco use and suggestions for tobacco use cessation are available from local, state, national, and international health organizations and government agencies. These groups should be used to help identify effective interventions and for patient reference.

KEY REFERENCES

American Cancer Society: *Guide to quitting smoking, 2009*. www.cancer.org/docroot/PED/content/PED_10_13X_Guide_for_Quitting_Smoking. Accessed October 17, 2009.

Hilibrand AS, Fye MA, Emery SE, et al: Impact of smoking on the outcome of anterior cervical arthrodesis with interbody or strut-grafting. *J Bone Joint Surg [Am]* 83:668–673, 2001.

Moller AM, Villebro N, Pedersen T, et al: Effect of preoperative smoking intervention on postoperative complications: a randomised clinical trial. *Lancet* 359:114–117, 2002.

Rechtine GR II, Frawley W, Castellvi A, et al: Effect of the spine practitioner on patient smoking status. *Spine (Phila Pa 1976)* 25:2229–2233, 2000.

Ward KD, Klesges RC: A meta-analysis of the effects of cigarette smoking on bone mineral density. *Calcif Tissue Int* 68:259–270, 2001.

REFERENCES

The complete reference list is available online at expertconsult.com.

CHAPTER 131

The Geriatric Patient

Robert A. Hart | Mark D. D'Alise | Edward C. Benzel

When planning either elective or emergent spinal surgery in elderly patients, the numerous physiologic changes associated with advanced age must be considered. Each organ system manifests specific changes that affect surgical decision making, preoperative evaluation, and intraoperative and postoperative management. This chapter addresses the unique aspects affecting spine care that must be considered in elderly patients.

Surgical morbidity and mortality have been shown to be greater in the elderly patient.[1] Although this subset of patients is very heterogeneous, the general decline in physiologic reserve and presence of coexistent disease are likely primarily responsible for this finding.[2,3] The spine surgeon should be able to recognize specific surgical risk factors and develop an appropriate treatment plan that accommodates the specific needs of elderly patients.

Organ Systems

Cardiovascular System

It has been reported that at autopsy 50% of patients older than 70 years of age have significant cardiovascular disease. The cardiac risk index, a commonly used assessment tool, incorporates myocardial infarction in the past 6 months, uncompensated congestive heart failure, aortic stenosis, nonsinus rhythm greater than five premature ventricular contractions per minute, diabetes mellitus, and age older than 70 years as major risk factors for postoperative cardiac complications of noncardiac surgery[4] (Box 131-1).

The basic cardiovascular workup in patients older than 65 years of age should include a thorough history and physical examination and a baseline electrocardiogram. Myocardial infarction, unaccompanied by recognized symptoms, occurs in as much as 10% of elderly patients.[5] Reports of syncope or dyspnea are the most suggestive symptoms of this event. Peripheral vascular disease is often present with coronary artery disease and may complicate the diagnosis of neurogenic claudication. Absent peripheral pulses or a history of transient ischemic attacks or stroke should lead to a more comprehensive cardiac workup.

In patients with unstable angina, elective spinal surgery is clearly contraindicated. Patients with well-controlled stable angina, however, have only a slightly increased risk for perioperative cardiac complications, and may therefore be considered for surgery.[6] Moderate to severe congestive heart failure is associated with a significant perioperative risk.[7-9] Jugular venous distention and peripheral edema are suggestive signs, whereas a history of dyspnea on exertion and orthopnea are symptoms of a more severe form of congestive heart failure.

BOX 131-1. Cardiac Risk Index (Major Risk Factors)

- Myocardial infarction in the past 6 months
- Uncompensated congestive heart failure
- Aortic stenosis
- Nonsinus rhythm greater than five premature ventricular contractions per minute
- Diabetes mellitus
- Age greater than 70 years

Respiratory System

Elderly patients are at particular risk for perioperative pulmonary complications for several reasons. Decline in pulmonary function and reserve, underlying chronic obstructive disease and bronchitis, lack of mobility or bed rest associated with spinal surgery, and airway obstruction all can lead to significant morbidity or mortality for these patients.[10,11] In a series of 100 patients older than 70 years of age, approximately 40% of those without a history of lung disease had abnormal pulmonary function.[12] Pulmonary function tests (spirometry) should be obtained for patients older than 65 years of age or with a history of obstructive lung disease if a ventral approach is being considered.[13]

A forced expiratory volume in 1 second of less than 50% of the predicted value does not suggest an increased risk of postoperative mechanical ventilation, but combined with dyspnea at rest and arterial hypoxemia, it is an established risk factor.[14] Room air arterial blood gas should be tested in elderly patients with lung disease, as well as those with a history of shortness of breath, poor exercise tolerance, orthopnea, or excessive smoking. Elevated partial pressure of carbon dioxide (P_{CO_2}) reflects a loss of pulmonary reserve. A preoperative P_{CO_2} of greater than 45 mm Hg is associated with an increased incidence of postoperative pulmonary complications,[15] and patients with a P_{CO_2} of greater than 50 mm Hg often require a period of postoperative mechanical ventilation.[16]

There is no well-defined lower limit of pulmonary function established by any criteria that strictly contraindicates surgery. Optimizing preoperative function certainly helps decrease the overall risks associated with lung disease. Equally important is an aggressive postoperative care plan, including early mobilization, incentive spirometry and coughing exercises, chest physiotherapy with postural drainage and nasotracheal suction, and use of bronchodilators and mucolytics as needed. Finally, an operative plan that avoids thoracotomy in patients with significant pulmonary compromise is well advised.

Renal System

Decline of renal function in the elderly is more consistent than that of other organ systems.[17] In geriatric patients, serum creatinine levels may be artificially low because of decreased production, caused by a shrinking muscle mass. For this reason, creatinine clearance is the preferred test for patients suspected of having significant renal disease. The effect of chronic nonsteroidal anti-inflammatory drug (NSAID) use on the kidney may also contribute to the decline in renal function with advancing age. These drugs can decrease renal blood flow, adding to an already diminished glomerular filtration rate.[18] This has clinical significance in the perioperative patient because water homeostasis may be difficult to achieve in elderly patients, leaving them prone to hyponatremia and volume overload. The use of isotonic fluids, restriction of free water, and careful administration of diuretics may be helpful.

Other Sources of Morbidity

Advanced age itself is a risk factor for deep venous thrombosis.[1] Given the risks associated with bleeding after spine surgery, many surgeons are hesitant to anticoagulate, even with deep venous thrombosis demonstrated by venous Doppler ultrasonography. Such patients can be considered for vena cava filter placement or delayed (5 to 7 days after surgery) anticoagulation. All patients should receive aggressive physical therapy with early ambulation and range-of-motion exercises. Pneumatic compression devices should be used on all patients during their period of bed rest.

Malnutrition is associated with increased morbidity and mortality in elderly surgical patients.[19] Dietary supplements should be added to the hospital diet of patients with reduced postoperative caloric intake to achieve a protein intake of 1 to 2 g/kg/day.

Advanced age is also a risk factor for wound infection. A sixfold increase in clean wound infections has been reported in patients older than 66 years compared with patients younger than 14 years of age.[20] The use of routine perioperative antibiotics, minimizing operative times, appropriate postoperative wound care, and attention to nutritional status all may decrease this risk.

Constipation can also be a major problem in elderly postoperative patients. Immobility, decreased gastrointestinal motility, narcotic medications, dehydration, and lack of privacy of the bedridden patient may all contribute to this problem. Stool softeners, fiber-enriched diets, gentle laxatives, and enemas should be used early in the postoperative patient. Perhaps the best method of avoiding postoperative constipation is simply early mobility and physical therapy.

Spinal Disorders in the Elderly Patient

Osteoporosis

Osteoporosis is a state of decreased density of mineralized bone. The biochemical makeup and structure of osteoporotic bone are normal, but the volume density of bone is below normal. Bone mass reaches its maximum in the third decade of life and then begins to decrease.[21] At its peak, the maximum surface area of bone crystals in an adult is estimated to be 100 acres.

Bone is a biphasic material consisting of an organic component, osteoid, which is a matrix of collagen and other proteins, and an inorganic component consisting of hydroxyapatite. The mineral component of bone accounts for the majority of its mechanical strength. Bone is constantly being remodeled by the opposing actions of osteoblasts and osteoclasts. When the balance falls in the direction of osteoclastic activity, net bone resorption occurs. Factors that are predisposed to bone resorption include loss of estrogen and androgens, corticosteroid use, alcohol and tobacco use, and poor nutrition. Bone mineral loss is also associated with increasing age in both men and women. These factors cause depletion of elemental calcium at a rate up to between 30 and 40 mg/day from a peak mass of 1000 g.

Loss of bone mineral content predominantly occurs from trabecular bone because of its increased baseline metabolic activity and greater surface area compared with cortical bone. Hence, structures formed of trabecular bone are more susceptible to osteoporosis.[22] In vertebral bodies, trabecular bone accounts for 90% of axial load-bearing resistance. As a result of primary osteoporosis, elderly people may sustain vertebral compression fractures with minimal trauma. Current recommendations for the medical management of osteoporosis are summarized in Box 131-2.

Bone densitometry has been shown to predict risk of osteoporosis.[23] Currently, two methods are used to evaluate bone density. Dual-energy radiography measures area density (g/cm^2) of the spine. This test is simple and accurate and carries a low radiation dose. It is also well tolerated, with a

BOX 131-2. Medical Treatment of Osteoporosis

Bisphosphonates*

Alendronate 10 mg daily or 70 mg weekly

Risedronate 5 mg daily or 35 mg weekly

Selective Estrogen Receptor Modulators

Raloxifene 60 mg daily

Recombinant Human Parathyroid Hormone 1-34

Teriparatide 40 IU SQ daily for 1 yr

Other Treatments

Conjugated estrogens (postmenopausal women) 0.625 mg daily

Calcium carbonate 400 mg twice daily

Calcitonin (salmon) nasal spray 200 IU daily

*Both with 1000 mg calcium plus 400 IU vitamin D.

procedure time of 10 to 15 minutes. Quantitative CT scanning is a measurement of true density (g/cm^3) through a cross-sectional view of the vertebral body. The precision of this test is excellent, but it can be compromised by patient positioning and movement. The small increase in accuracy provided by this test over dual-energy radiography may not justify the expense, discomfort, and added radiation dose.[24] A bone mineral density by dual-energy radiography of 1 g/cm^2 carries a fracture risk over time of 32%, whereas a density of less than 0.8 g/cm^2 carries a risk of 50%.[25,26]

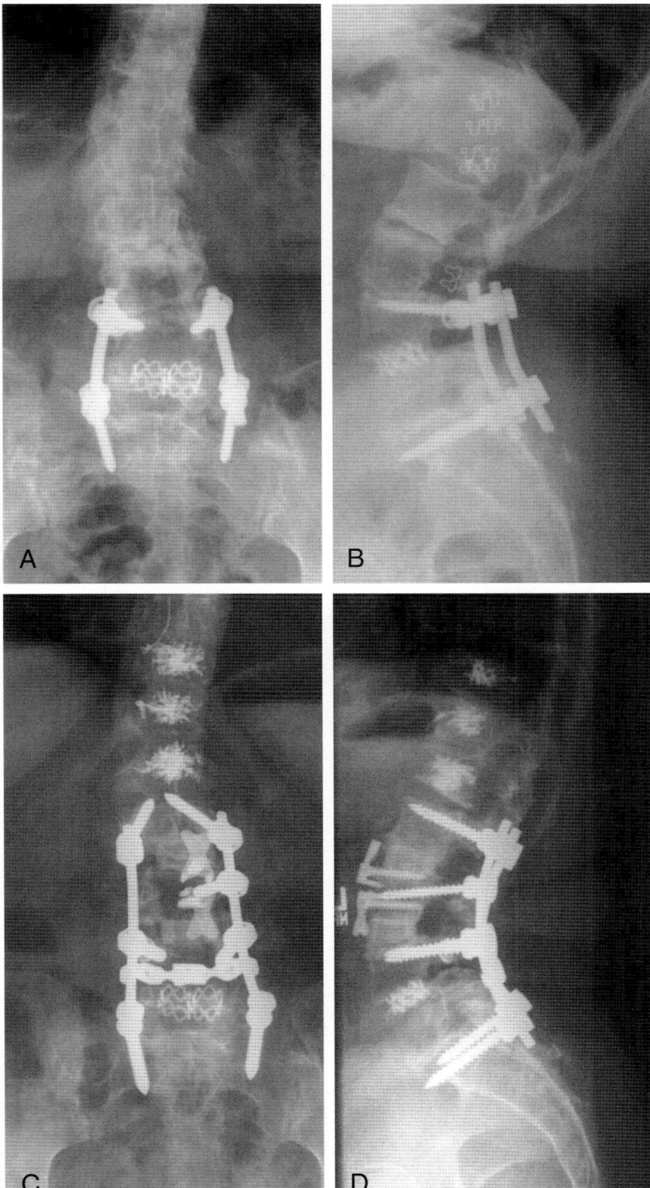

FIGURE 131-1. **A** and **B,** Myelograms of a 76-year-old woman who had undergone a prior fusion from L4 to the sacrum with clinical success. Adjacent-segment disease had led to a laminectomy above her fused segment at L2 and L3, with resulting segmental instability. At the time of her appearance, she suffered from intractable leg and back pain with severe functional limitations. **C** and **D,** Patient underwent a successful ventral/dorsal reconstruction with the revision laminectomies and fusion from L2 to the sacrum. Because of the patient's underlying osteoporosis and advanced age, adjacent vertebral levels were augmented with vertebroplasty. Note postoperative compression fracture of L1 vertebra on lateral view. This fracture did not collapse beyond the appearance shown and remained asymptomatic throughout the postoperative course.

Presence of osteoporosis may affect choices regarding instrumentation and fusion for patients indicated for spinal surgery. Obtaining adequate purchase in patients with significant osteoporosis may require using longer constructs to distribute forces and increase numbers of purchase points. On the other hand, some patients with osteoporosis may be more appropriately treated with uninstrumented spinal fusion or with operative approaches that avoid fusion entirely.

The effect of osteoporosis on vertebrae adjacent to areas of spinal fusion must also be considered. In elderly or osteoporotic patients in whom long fusion constructs are unavoidable, the long-term stability of adjacent vertebral segments is a significant concern. Particularly for areas of high mechanical stress, such as fusions stopping at the thoracolumbar junction, consideration should be given to prophylactic enhancement of the strength of vertebrae adjacent to long fusion constructs through procedures such as vertebroplasty[27] (Fig. 131-1).

Osteoporotic Compression Fractures

The most common type of spinal fracture in the elderly patient is the vertebral compression fracture. These fractures occur not only with higher-energy mechanisms but often with bending, lifting, or even during normal activity. Management should be directed primarily toward pain control. It should also be recognized that such low-energy fractures often are the first indication of underlying osteoporosis, and patients should be started on appropriate medical therapy (see Box 131-2).

Elderly patients with osteoporotic compression fractures who are requiring bed rest or significant narcotic analgesia, or for whom disabling pain has persisted over 4 to 6 weeks, may be candidates for percutaneous stabilization procedures, such as vertebroplasty or balloon-assisted vertebroplasty (kyphoplasty).[28] However, results of two randomized, controlled trials of vertebroplasty suggest limited benefit to such procedures.[29,30] This has led some insurers and academic organizations such as the American Academy of Orthopaedic Surgeons to recommend limits on the use of these procedures. At this time, evidence-based medicine guidelines for vertebroplasty must include the results of these studies, which represent the highest level of medical evidence available on this condition.

Degenerative Lumbar Spondylolisthesis

Degenerative spinal stenosis results from neurologic impingement by the disc, facet joints, and spinal ligaments. Kirkaldy-Willis et al.[24] proposed that biochemical and biomechanical changes associated with age cause increased mobility at a spinal segment, leading to osteophyte formation and joint hypertrophy that reduce spinal canal diameter and local stiffness. The increased joint laxity resulting from facet degeneration leads in some cases to spondylolisthesis between adjacent vertebrae.

Two prospective, randomized, controlled trials support treatment of patients with degenerative lumbar spondylolisthesis with laminectomy and dorsal fusion.[31,32] Several studies have demonstrated increased fusion rates with pedicle screw

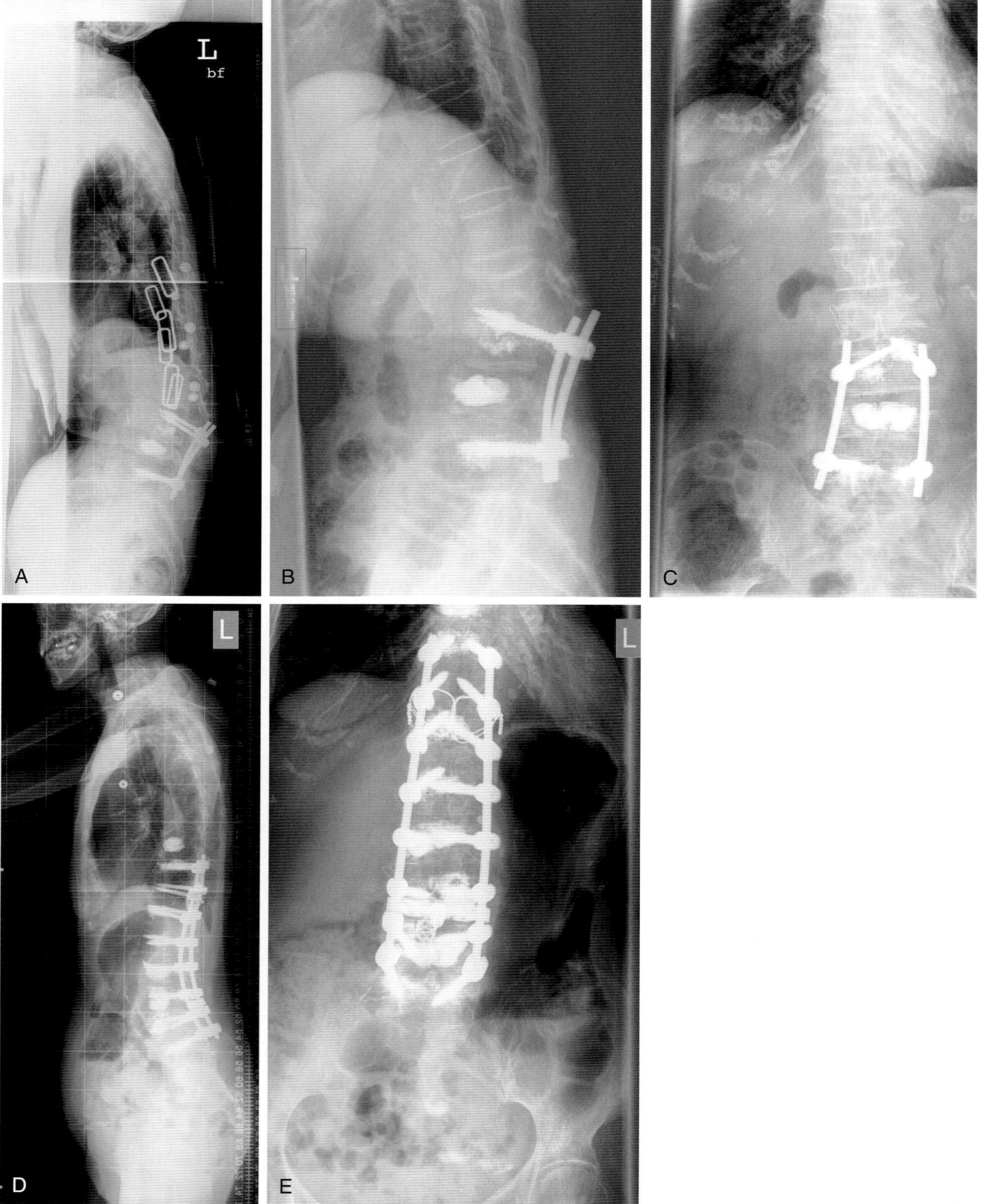

FIGURE 131-2. A–C, A 78-year-old woman with advanced osteoporosis reported after instrumentation and kyphoplasty with laminectomy for an osteoporotic burst fracture. She had an adjacent fracture of L2 with hardware failure at L3. **D** and **E,** After Smith-Petersen osteotomy and transforaminal lumbar interbody fusion at L3-4 and dorsal fusion from T10 to L5, the patient experienced significantly improved function and reduced pain. This result has been maintained at 4-year follow-up. Note augmentation of upper instrumented vertebra and first cranial level.

instrumentation, and further studies have shown better clinical outcomes in patients who achieve solid arthrodesis.[33-35]

Despite those results, use of instrumentation has not been convincingly shown to improve clinical outcomes after fusion for patients with degenerative spondylolisthesis.[32,36,37] Avoiding instrumentation when performing fusion in elderly, osteoporotic patients with degenerative spondylolisthesis may thus be a reasonable option, particularly when facets are oriented relatively in the coronal plane and segmental instability is not present.

Degenerative Scoliosis

Degenerative scoliosis, unlike idiopathic scoliosis, is an acquired disorder of adult patients. Patients often present with symptoms similar to those of degenerative lumbar stenosis, although for some patients the deformity itself becomes an issue. Nonoperative treatment modalities include physical therapy, muscle relaxants, and NSAIDs. Surgical options include neurologic decompression through laminotomy or laminectomy. Spinal fusion may or may not be appropriate, depending on the patient's presentation, health status, and expectations from surgery.[38-41] There are conflicting reports regarding the need for spinal stabilization after decompression for degenerative scoliosis.[38-40,42] Patients without lateral listhesis between adjacent vertebrae may be appropriately treated with laminectomy without fusion.

Patients of advanced age with significant scoliotic curves may not be appropriate candidates for the large reconstructive fusion procedures required to treat their spinal deformity. Judiciously selected nerve root blocks with isolated unilateral foraminotomies may be used to good effect in such patients with limited risk of deformity progression (Fig. 131-2). Elderly patients for whom stabilization is required will benefit from efforts to limit the extent of surgery, including use of dorsal (posterior) or transforaminal lumbar interbody fusions in favor of ventral approaches (Fig. 131-3).

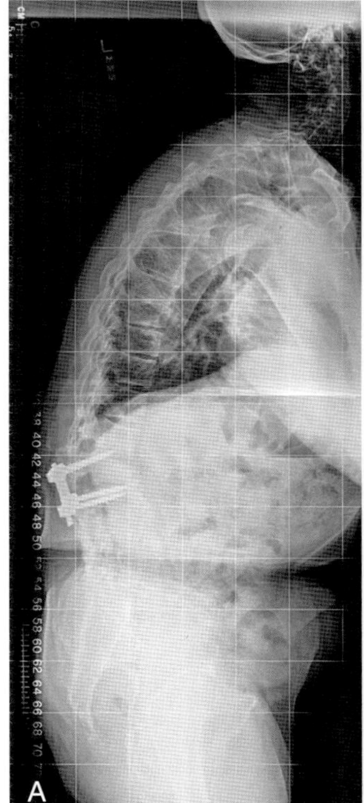

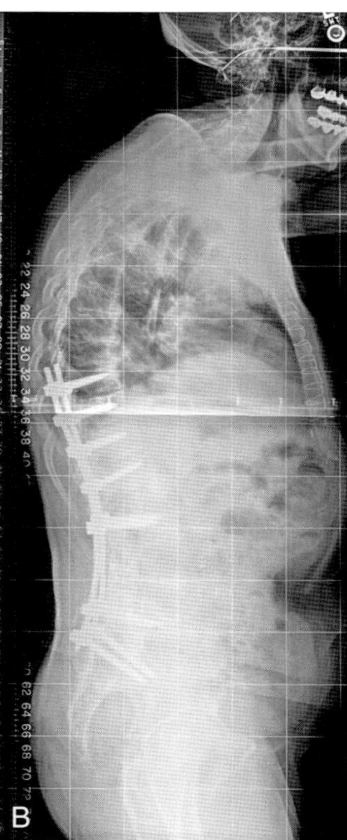

FIGURE 131-3. **A,** An 81-year-old man with a history of well-controlled Parkinson disease presented with rapid failure above a fusion from L2 to the sacrum. The fusion itself was healed. **B,** After pedicle subtraction osteotomy of L2, adequate sagittal balance is restored. Obtaining good sagittal alignment is a key element in achieving long-term success in longer fusions among older patients.

Cervical Degenerative Disease

Elderly patients with cervical degenerative disease and spinal stenosis also present a treatment problem significantly different than younger patients with similar conditions. Concerns over bone quality and physiologic ability to withstand large reconstructive surgery again play a significant role in decision making.

Ventral decompressive surgery by multilevel corpectomy may prove difficult in this patient population. Although ventral decompression may be appropriate on a neurologic basis because of kyphotic alignment of the cervical vertebrae,[42] reduced mechanical strength of vertebral bodies increases the risk of graft subsidence or dislodgement if an isolated ventral procedure is performed. In addition, the substantial surgery required to accomplish combined ventral-dorsal cervical reconstruction may not be well tolerated by elderly patients.

Patients with central stenosis and neutral or lordotic alignment may be treated via an isolated dorsal procedure, such as laminoplasty.[42] If ventral decompression is required, standard discectomy/corpectomy procedures with ventral plating may be performed for short segments (Fig. 131-4). Inclusion of dorsal instrumentation should be considered for patients requiring decompression over more than three disc spaces, and for those with significant kyphosis. These treatment approaches generally provide satisfactory clinical outcomes while reducing significant complications.

Spinal Trauma and Spinal Cord Injury

Numerous characteristics of spinal injury are unique in the elderly patient, including injury mechanisms, fracture types, incidence of neurologic deficits, and outcomes. The primary mechanism of injury in young patients is motor vehicle collisions, whereas the leading cause of spine fracture in patients older than 65 years of age is falls.[43,44] Significant neurologic deficits are also significantly more common in younger patients than in the elderly, possibly reflecting this difference in injury mechanisms.[43,45]

Outcomes from traumatic spinal injuries also differ significantly between elderly and nonelderly adult patients. Elderly patients have a significantly lower survival rate than nonelderly adults, both with and without neurologic injury. Neurologic injury is especially devastating in the elderly because the 60-day mortality rate for patients older than 65 years of age with traumatic paralysis approaches 30%.[43]

Understanding these issues may factor significantly in clinical decision making. Families of elderly patients with significant neurologic injuries should understand the high risk of poor outcomes in this age group. Given the significant risk of early mortality, as well as the likely disability resulting from profound neurologic deficits, patients and families may in some cases prefer withdrawal of support over aggressive interventional treatment.

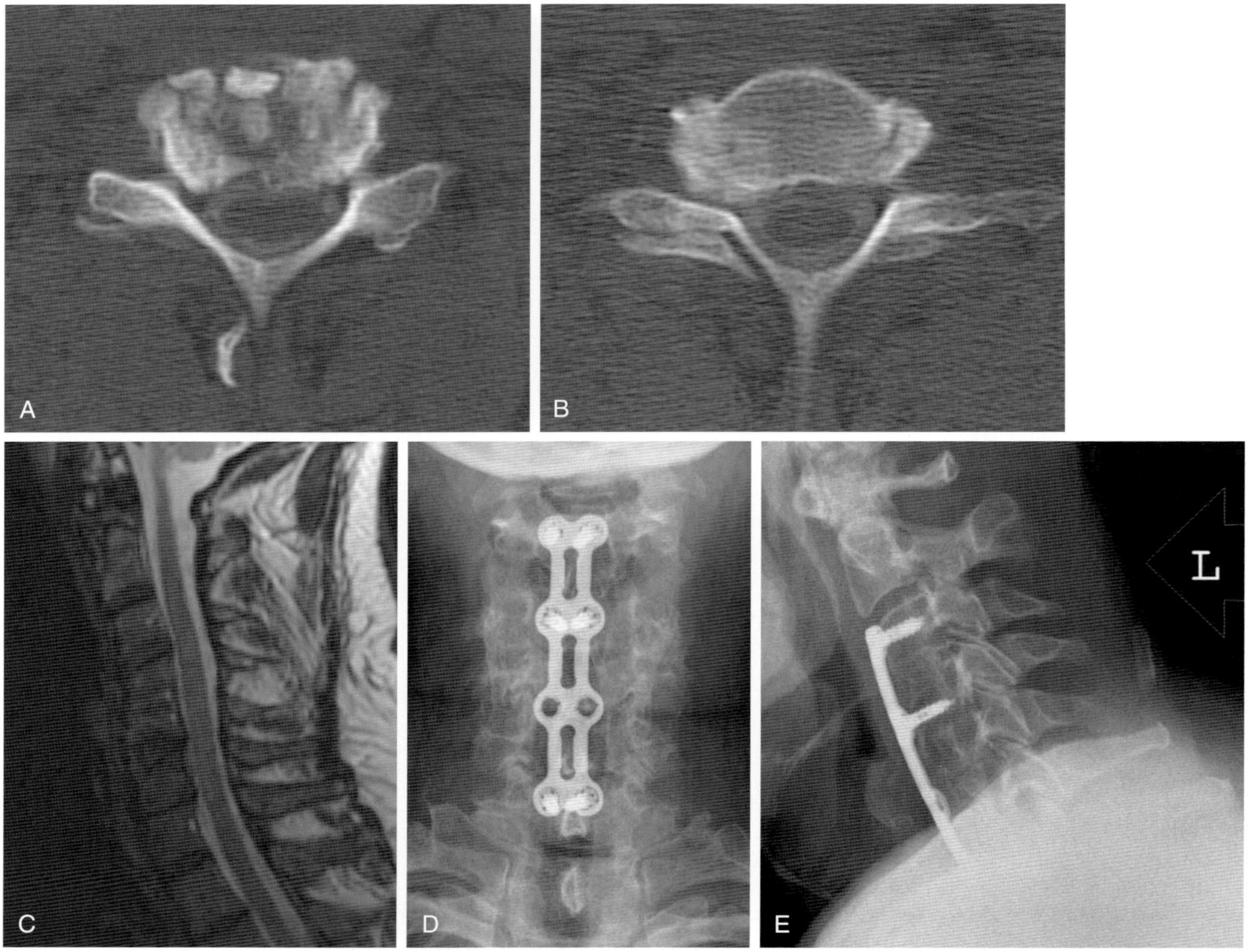

FIGURE 131-4. Myelograms (**A** and **B**) and MRI (**C**) of a 65-year-old man who developed recurrent symptoms of radiculopathy after a motor vehicle accident. He had undergone a prior two-level discectomy performed elsewhere with a solid fusion obtained at C4-5, but a nonunion had occurred at C5-6. A CT myelogram shows degenerative change and foraminal stenosis at C6-7 (**B**) and an MRI shows the same at the nonunion site at C5-6 (**C**). Note kyphosis across the C3-4 disc demonstrated on sagittal plane MRI. **D** and **E,** Anteroposterior and lateral views demonstrate solid consolidation after a corpectomy of the C6 vertebra, including resection of the C5-6 nonunion and a discectomy at the C3-4 level with structural iliac crest graft and spanning anterior cervical locking plate. Alternating levels of corpectomy and discectomy, as in this case, allow better anterior column support and segmental fixation with ventral instrumentation.

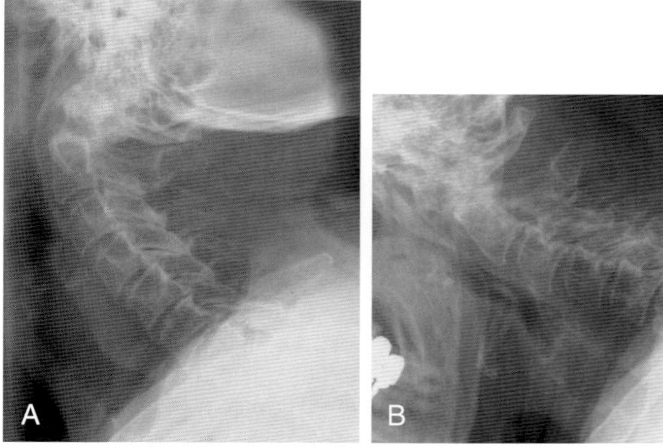

FIGURE 131-5. A, Myelogram of a 97-year-old woman discovered incidentally on admission to trauma service after a motor vehicle accident to have a mobile nonunion of a prior dens fracture. She was asymptomatic from this, both with respect to neck pain and neurologic symptoms. Workup included a CT scan with reconstructions at the time of injury. **B,** Space available for the spinal cord is 21 mm on the extension view. She was treated with observation, with no clinical incident at 6-month follow-up.

Finally, injuries appropriately treated with surgical intervention in younger patients may be treatable with minimal intervention in the elderly population. For example, risks associated with nonunion after dens fracture appear to be limited in elderly patients, and it is not clear that surgical stabilization of established nonunions is warranted.[28,46] Treatment decisions for these injuries are best decided on a case-by-case basis and depend on patient preferences, health, and mental status, and the nature of the injury (Fig. 131-5).

Summary

Elderly patients represent a distinct patient group when planning spine surgery. Disease and injury mechanisms, the ability to withstand significant surgical intervention, and the mechanical effects of osteoporosis all play a role in decision making and treatment outcomes. These issues must be considered on a case-by-case basis and discussed with patients and families when determining appropriate treatment approaches.

KEY REFERENCES

Fischgrund JS, Mackay M, Herkowitz HN, et al: 1997 Volvo Award winner in clinical studies. Degenerative lumbar spondylolisthesis with spinal stenosis: a prospective, randomized study comparing decompressive laminectomy and arthrodesis with and without spinal instrumentation. *Spine (Phila Pa 1976)* 22:2807–2812, 1997.

Hart RA, Prendergast M: Spine surgery for lumbar degenerative disease in the elderly and osteoporotic patient. *Instr Course Lect* 56:257–272, 2007.

Irwin ZN, Arthur MA, Mullins RJ, et al: Variations in injury patterns, treatment, and outcome for spinal fracture and paralysis in adult versus geriatric patients. *Spine (Phila Pa 1976)* 29:796–802, 2004.

Kornblum MB, Fischgrund JS, Herkowitz HN, et al: Degenerative lumbar spondylolisthesis with spinal stenosis: a prospective long-term study comparing fusion and pseudarthrosis. *Spine (Phila Pa 1976)* 29:726–733, 2004.

Weinstein JN, Lurie JD, Tosteson TD, et al: Surgical compared with nonoperative treatment for lumbar degenerative spondylolisthesis: four-year results in the Spine Patient Outcomes Research Trial (SPORT) randomized and observational cohorts. *J Bone Joint Surg [Am]* 91:1295–1304, 2009.

REFERENCES

The complete reference list is available online at expertconsult.com.

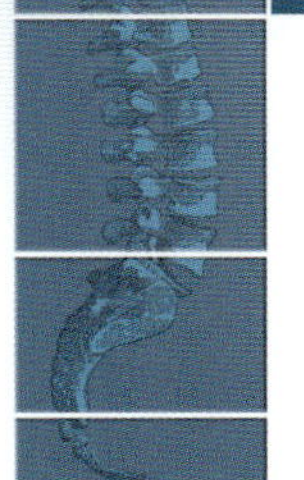

CHAPTER 132

Surgery of the Sympathetic Nervous System

J. Patrick Johnson | Saad Khairi | William C. Welch

Sympathectomy procedures involve interrupting thoracic or lumbar sympathetic pathways to provide relief from autonomically mediated syndromes. Currently the most common disorder treated is essential hyperhidrosis,[1,2] but sympathectomies have been used extensively in the past to treat various pain syndromes, including complex regional pain syndrome (CRPS; also known as reflex sympathetic dystrophy), causalgia, vascular insufficiency pain syndromes, and Raynaud phenomenon.[3-6] More recently, pain syndromes have been treated less frequently with ablative sympathectomy procedures because of the limited success with sympathectomy and potential improvement in outcomes with neurostimulation techniques.[7,8] This chapter reviews the history, relevant anatomy and physiology, surgical indications, and techniques of the open and closed sympathectomy procedures as well as the more recent endoscopic techniques, with particular regard to perioperative management, complications, and outcomes of the different sympathectomy procedures.

Historical Background

The earliest known investigations of sympathetic nervous system surgery were described by Francois Parfour du Petit in 1727, reporting on the results of sympathectomy in dogs, and Biffi reported similar findings in a doctoral thesis in 1846. Budge and Walker demonstrated the clinical effects of stimulation of the cervical sympathetic chain in humans in 1852. However, it was Claude Bernard, a French physiologist, in a series of articles published in the 1850s describing his observations after sectioning and stimulating the cervical sympathetic chain in rabbits, who provided a clearer understanding of clinical correlates. A well-recognized clinical correlate of Bernard's experimental observations is known as *Horner syndrome*, as described by Frederick T. Horner in 1869. However, the first clinical report of a sympathectomy causing the typical ocular changes was reported by Mitchell et al. in 1864, which actually predated Horner's description by 5 years. This book also coined the term *causalgia*, a condition that was treated primarily with sympathectomy for many years. Early surgical sympathectomy procedures were promoted by Jaboulay and Johnson, who stripped the periarterial sympathetics to treat exophthalmos, glaucoma, and tic douloureux, as well as vascular insufficiency. One of Jaboulay's students, Leriche, promoted the use of sympathectomy for ischemic vascular disease; sympathectomy was used frequently in the 1940s for soldiers sustaining nerve injuries in World War II. Subsequently, various sympathectomy procedures reviewed here were refined to treat hyperhidrosis and both ischemic and neuropathic pain syndromes.

Clinical Syndromes

Hyperhidrosis

Palmar and axillary hyperhidrosis are defined as excessive sweating in the upper extremities, particularly the hands and armpits, most often noted during periods of stress. The etiology is unknown, and the incidence is approximately 1% in Western populations but may be slightly higher in Asian populations. The sympathetic nervous system innervates the eccrine sweat glands by cholinergic fibers arising from the intermediolateral column of the thoracic and upper lumbar spinal cord segments. Sympathetic stimulation causes vasoconstriction to produce cooling of the skin and, when combined with sweating, exacerbates the symptoms. Anesthetic block of the stellate ganglion results in a dramatic drying and warming effect in the ipsilateral hand and armpit caused by decreasing sweating and increased blood flow through cutaneous vessels; similarly, resection of the sympathetic chain and ganglia in the upper thoracic region results in lasting relief from hyperhidrosis.

Neuropathic and Ischemic Pain

Chronic pain syndromes[9,10] such as causalgia and reflex sympathetic dystrophy (now referred to as CRPS) are thought to arise from peripheral nerve trauma that is usually ill defined. They also include several other related syndromes (e.g., phantom pain, shoulder-hand syndrome, posttraumatic neuralgia). Characteristic symptoms are burning pain, edema, and trophic skin changes in the extremity. Temperature changes are frequently noted in the affected extremity. Ischemic pain syndromes including Raynaud phenomenon and other vasculitic disorders typically have episodes of severe, painful skin blanching, primarily of the hands and fingertips.[11] Cold temperature or emotional response may exacerbate these episodes, and extreme cases may result in ischemia and gangrenous ulceration of the digits. The initial treatment is avoidance of cold and administration of α-adrenergic blocking agents, which are useful for less severe cases. Sympathectomy procedures have been used extensively in the past and can provide significant initial relief from severe pain and digital ulcers. However, the long-term outcomes of sympathectomy for relieving the episodic vasospasms associated with chronic pain syndromes and Raynaud phenomenon are less optimal.

Anatomy and Physiology

The autonomic nervous system includes both the sympathetic and the parasympathetic nervous systems. The sympathetic system mediates the "fight-or-flight" responses such as pupillary dilation, tachycardia, bronchial dilation, increased muscle blood flow, and the release of adrenergic agents from the adrenal glands. It is a two-neuron disynaptic system in which responses are mediated through autonomic ganglia, with the ultimate regulation occurring in the hypothalamus. Anatomically, the sympathetic nervous system has outflow in the thoracic and upper lumbar regions of the spinal cord. Preganglionic fibers from the intermediolateral cell column exit the spinal cord through the ventral nerve roots into spinal nerves and enter the paravertebral chain ganglia, coursing through the myelinated white rami communicantes.[3,4] Once in the ganglia, the presynaptic neuron can (1) synapse with a postganglionic neuron and exit as a gray ramus to the viscera, (2) synapse with a postganglionic neuron and exit as a gray ramus in a segmental nerve, (3) travel up or down the sympathetic chain, (4) stimulate the adrenal gland, or (5) exit the sympathetic chain in the splanchnic nerves and enter peripherally located ganglia such as the mesenteric ganglia. Postganglionic fibers travel in peripheral nerves or along arteries to reach their target organs. Afferent autonomic fibers travel from receptors though the dorsal spinal roots to enter the spinal cord, where they can trigger reflexes through spinal cord interneurons and efferent autonomic fibers.

The autonomic ganglia are variable in size, number, and location. There are generally three cervical ganglia (superior, middle, and inferior). The lowest cervical ganglia can fuse with the highest thoracic ganglia to form the stellate or cervicothoracic ganglion.[3,4] Pupillary dilation occurs as a result of sympathetic output from the spinal cord ciliospinal center of Budge. The preganglionic fibers exit the spinal cord at the T1 and T2 levels and travel through the thoracic, stellate, and middle cervical ganglia to synapse in the superior cervical ganglia; the postganglionic fibers then enter the sympathetic plexus surrounding the carotid artery and travel along the third, fifth, and sixth cranial nerves to enter the orbit and pass through the ciliary ganglion to the pupillary dilators via the long anterior ciliary nerves. A lesion anywhere along this course is manifested by pupillary miosis, anhidrosis (loss of sympathetic innervation to the sweat glands of the face), ptosis (loss of innervation of the superior tarsal musculature), and, occasionally, enophthalmos. The thoracic ganglia correlate with the corresponding thoracic level, as do the upper lumbar ganglia.

Sexual and urinary function are also influenced by the autonomic nervous system.[12] Sympathetic efferent innervation to the bladder arises from the lower thoracic and upper lumbar levels. The efferent nerves travel through a series of ganglia in the sacral region, and the postganglionic fibers travel to the vesicular plexus via the hypogastric nerves. There is also sympathetic stimulation involved in both erection and ejaculation in male patients.

Neurochemically, the presynaptic sympathetic neurons are believed to release acetylcholine and peptides that act on muscarinic, nicotinic, or peptidergic receptors of the postsynaptic neurons, which in turn release norepinephrine to achieve stimulatory responses in the innervated organs.

The effects of sympathetic denervation for the treatment of hyperhidrosis presumably arise from interruption of cutaneous sweating and vasoconstriction mediated by the sympathetic nervous system. The mechanisms of a sympathectomy for treating pain and ischemic syndromes are mediated through less well understood pathways from the denervated sympathetic ganglion into the central nervous system, and reducing sympathetic input by a sympathectomy will achieve at least temporary improvement in the pain symptoms.

Preoperative Evaluation

Patients with autonomically mediated syndromes require thorough diagnostic evaluation and aggressive medical treatment before being considered for surgical treatment. A thorough history and physical examination are necessary to begin the evaluation to consider possible underlying metabolic, infectious, or neoplastic disorders, and radiologic evaluation with plain radiographs and either CT or MRI of the thorax and brachial plexus may be needed. However, most preoperative diagnostic studies are limited, and imaging studies have not demonstrated any clear diagnostic information. Psychological evaluation should be considered, particularly in patients with chronic pain disorders.

Diagnostic sympathetic blocks with short-acting anesthetics provide temporary relief, but may cause transient Horner syndrome. Sympathetic blocks are useful indicators that a sympathectomy will be therapeutically successful. Occasionally, repeated blocks may provide temporary relief of pain syndromes that allow rehabilitation to proceed and preclude the need for a sympathectomy. Anesthetic lumbar blocks for diagnostic and therapeutic effects, particularly in lower extremity pain syndromes, may be quite useful.

Medical treatment of autonomically mediated syndromes is theoretically useful and may have potential in limited cases. Medications that produce systemic sympathetic blockade include phenoxybenzamine, which blocks the α-adrenergic receptors.[13,14] Alpha blockade is associated with frequent complications, including hypotension, miosis, and loss of ejaculatory function, but it is an effective test treatment for causalgia-type symptoms.

Neuromodulation

Spinal cord stimulation is increasingly being used to treat CRPS. The exact mechanisms by which it works require further study.[15] Broad reviews have found it to be both effective and cost effective.[16]

Open Sympathectomy Techniques

Open sympathectomy techniques have been used to treat hyperhidrosis effectively, but have less efficacy for treating pain syndromes, particularly given the need for highly invasive

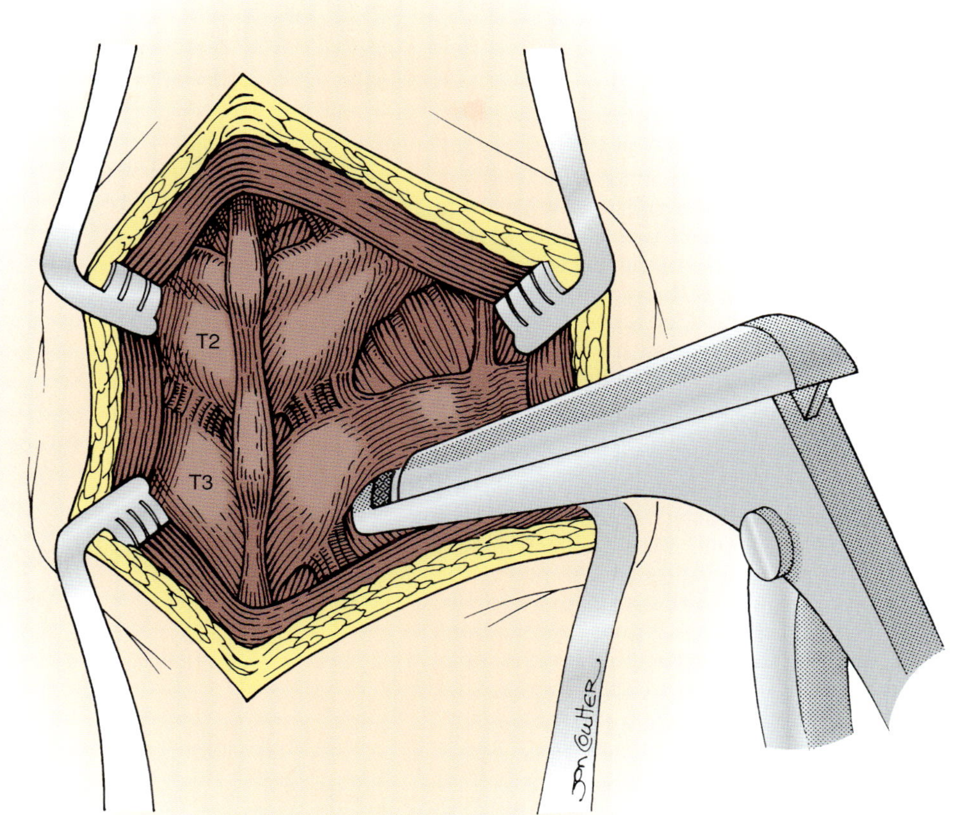

FIGURE 132-1. Dorsal T2 sympathectomy approach with removal of T2 transverse process and proximal T3 rib.

procedures. These approaches do not require specialized endoscopic equipment and techniques. The open techniques are generally known to most practicing physicians.

Cervical and Cervicothoracic Approaches

Operative Techniques

Cervical or cervicothoracic sympathectomy procedures can be performed using several techniques. These include ventral supraclavicular or transaxillary approaches or dorsal costotransversectomy approaches.[17,18] Ventral approaches provide good exposure of the sympathetic chain but carry risks of injury to the brachial plexus and pleural cavity.

The most common open approach for upper thoracic and stellate ganglionectomy is the dorsal approach, where a T2 ganglionectomy has been performed for hyperhidrosis and CRPS. The patient is placed in the prone position on the operating table after general anesthesia. A 4- to 5-cm midline incision over T2 and T3 and the paraspinal muscles is retracted to expose and remove the T2 transverse process and proximal rib of T3 (Fig. 132-1), with preservation of the intercostal nerves. The lateral surface of the vertebral body is then exposed by elevating the parietal pleura carefully to expose the sympathetic chain. The ganglia are usually clearly visible and easily dissected from the chain, which is then cauterized with bipolar electrocautery above and below the ganglia, and the ganglion is resected (Fig. 132-2). The ganglion can be sent to the pathology unit for histologic confirmation.

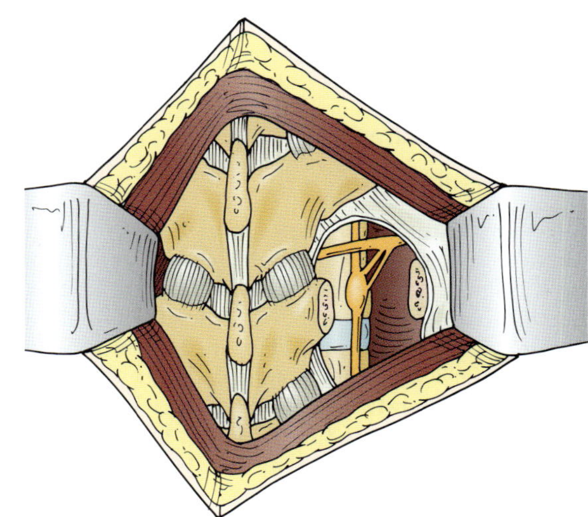

FIGURE 132-2. Dorsal sympathectomy and removal of the T2 ganglion.

A similar procedure is performed on the opposite side for patients with bilateral palmar hyperhidrosis.

In the transaxillary ventral approach described by Atkins,[17] the patient is in a lateral position with the arm extended forward. An incision is made in the second intercostal space from the latissimus dorsi to the pectoralis musculature. The pleural cavity is entered and the ribs slowly retracted. The lung is partially deflated, the sympathetic chain is located, and the appropriate ganglion is identified and removed. The transthoracic endoscopic approach developed in recent years has become the most frequently used method today.

The supraclavicular approach is performed with the patient in a supine position with the neck placed in hyperextension. An incision is made above the clavicle and the two heads of the sternocleidomastoid muscle are split. The phrenic nerve is identified and protected, after which the anterior scalene muscle is incised and arterial branches of the subclavian artery are sacrificed. The brachial plexus is then identified and the parietal pleura is dissected from the dorsal chest by blunt dissection. The parietal pleura and subclavian artery are retracted caudally, and the sympathetic ganglia are identified and incised.

Complications

The most common complications after ventral (or dorsal) cervical and thoracic sympathectomy include Horner syndrome, pneumothorax, pneumonia, wound infection and dehiscence, failure of the procedure adequately to relieve the preoperative symptoms, regrowth of the sympathetic chain, cerebrospinal fluid leak, and spinal cord injury. Horner syndrome is avoided by limiting the resection to the second thoracic ganglion and avoiding injury to the first thoracic and stellate ganglia.[19] Horner syndrome may be only a temporary effect caused by stretching of the chain. Pneumothorax is rare and requires placement of a small-tube thoracostomy. Hardy and Bay[3] recommend placement of a 12-Fr red rubber catheter in the pleural cavity if a pleural laceration is noted intraoperatively; negative suction is applied to the catheter with positive-pressure ventilation, and the catheter is then quickly removed and the wound closed. Postoperative chest radiographs should be obtained for all patients to ensure that pneumothorax has not occurred.

Lumbar Approaches

Operative Technique

The lumbar sympathectomy procedure[2,20] is performed with the patient in the supine position. A 10- to 12-cm incision is made in the flank from the tip of the 11th rib toward the anterior superior iliac spine (Fig. 132-3). The abdominal muscles are split longitudinally with the fibers into the retroperitoneal space and the fat is then bluntly divided with digital dissection to the ventrolateral aspect of the spine, where the lumbar sympathetic chain is located in the gutter between the psoas muscle and the spinal column (Fig. 132-4). The chain can be tethered by lumbar arterial branches on the left and lumbar veins on the right that must be mobilized and often divided to allow access to the lumbar sympathetic chain. The L2-4 ganglia can then be resected. Occasionally the vena cava must be partially mobilized to gain access to the sympathetic chain on the right side. Closure is obtained by reapproximating the fascia with absorbable suture and the subcutaneous layer and skin with absorbable sutures or staples.

Complications

Complications of open ventral lumbar sympathectomy include ileus, infection, injury to intraperitoneal contents, wound complications, impotence, ureteral injury, and vascular injury. Impotence can occur even with unilateral disruption or injury to the sympathetic chain and is difficult to predict or prevent; all male patients should be warned of this potential adverse outcome. The ureter is at risk during all retroperitoneal exposures; however, injury can be avoided by visualizing the ureter, which is usually on the psoas muscle lateral to the sympathetic chain. Injury to the ureter can be difficult to detect and may result in flank pain and tenderness. Some patients may

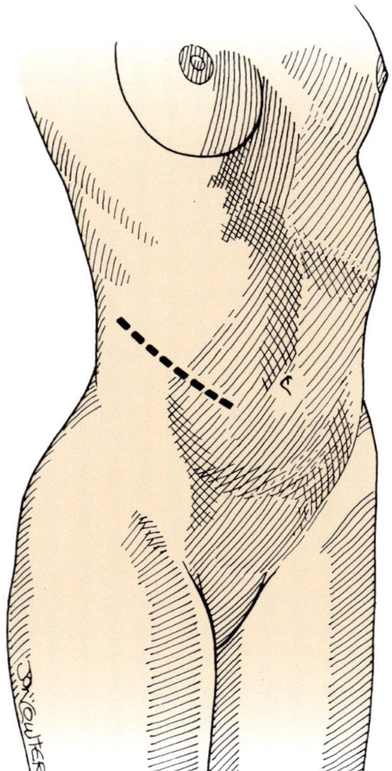

FIGURE 132-3. Lumbar flank incision for lumbar sympathectomy.

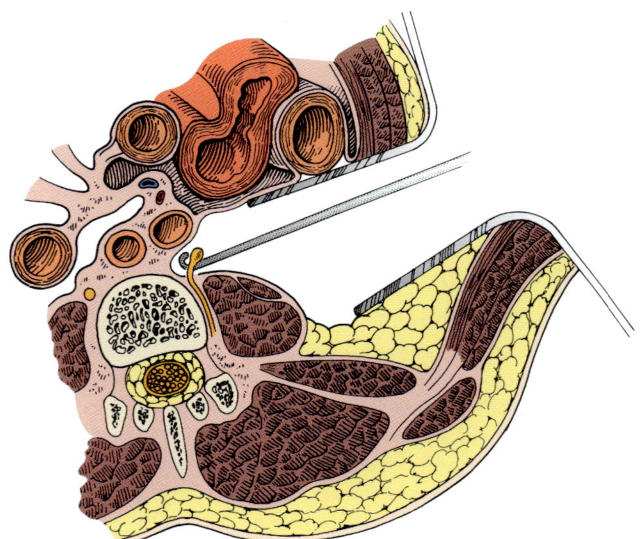

FIGURE 132-4. Approach into the lumbar retroperitoneum for lumbar sympathectomy.

experience thigh pain for several weeks after a lumbar sympathectomy, the etiology of which is unclear but may be due to muscle retraction.

Endoscopic Sympathectomy Techniques

Thoracoscopic Approach for Cervical and Thoracic Sympathectomy

Endoscopic thoracic sympathectomy for the upper extremity was originally reported in 1951 by Kux,[21] who described treatment of hyperhidrosis with excellent results. There has been significant recent interest in these minimally invasive procedures.[22] The attractiveness of minimally invasive treatment of autonomically mediated syndromes affecting the upper extremities is due to the development of endoscopic techniques. The most frequent indication for thoracic sympathectomy is hyperhidrosis.[23-27] Less frequently, CRPS, causalgia, Raynaud phenomenon, postamputation syndrome (phantom pain), and refractory cardiac tachyarrhythmias[28-30] are also treated with sympathectomy. Endoscopic techniques provide both a panoramic and magnified view for precise identification of the sympathetic chain and adjacent structures, allowing definition of the anatomy for resection of the sympathetic chain. This procedure has become the preferred method of thoracic sympathectomy, and extensive clinical experience has resulted in improvements in patient satisfaction and reduced hospital stays and costs. Because thoracoscopic procedures have a distinct learning curve, it is necessary to understand intrathoracic anatomy and gain initial endoscopic experience with a thoracoscopic surgeon.

Palmar hyperhidrosis is the main indication for thoracic sympathectomy with minimally invasive techniques. Severe axillary sweating (with or without palmar hyperhidrosis) has also been treated with good results. Some patients with facial hyperhidrosis have also been treated successfully with a sympathectomy procedure. The precise sympathectomy procedure for each of these clinical syndromes with regard to which ganglionic levels are to be resected remains somewhat speculative. Most authors agree that only a T2 and T3 sympathectomy will effectively treat palmar hyperhidrosis. However, some authors recommend either a T2 or T3 sympathectomy and cite a lowered incidence of compensatory sweating, but this has not been clearly substantiated. Axillary sweating is thought to be best treated with sympathectomy at T3, T4, and T5 for good results. Facial sweating is treated with a T2 sympathectomy just below the stellate ganglion.[31]

Patients with pain syndromes and vasculitis or Raynaud phenomenon may also respond to an endoscopic T2, T3, and/or T4 sympathectomy, but results are less optimal.[32] Spinal stimulation appears to have largely replaced sympathectomy for these indications, for several reasons[8]: (1) pain symptoms have a high incidence of recurrence after sympathectomy, (2) stimulation is a nonablative procedure, (3) stimulation is usually a technically less demanding procedure than a sympathectomy, (4) stimulation is a reversible procedure, and (5) stimulation can be modulated after the procedure is completed.

Recent reports also describe the utility and selective efficacy of pulsed radiofrequency for more selective ablation of the lumbar sympathetic chain.[33] However, the most recent (2010) Cochrane review found only one high-quality study directly comparing chemical with radiofrequency lumbar sympathectomy for CRPS, a study by Manjunath et al. in 2008 that demonstrated no difference in outcomes based on the technique of neural ablation.[34,35]

Patients with cardiac tachyarrhythmias have also been treated with sympathectomy procedures. Studies have demonstrated effectiveness in treating stress-related malignant tachyarrhythmias that may be related to disproportionate left and right sympathetic innervation. Patients treated inadequately with medical therapy can be considered for a left thoracoscopic sympathectomy; however, improved medical therapy has nearly eliminated the use of sympathectomy for this indication.[3-6]

Operative Technique

Anesthesia and Positioning

The patient requires general anesthesia and placement of a double-lumen endotracheal tube to allow collapse of the lung on the operated side. The supine position (Fig. 132-5) is used, and the head of the table can be elevated and rotated.

Instruments

The equipment and instruments needed for performing a thoracoscopic sympathectomy procedure are the same as those commonly used for laparoscopic surgery. A standard endoscopic video monitor system with either a 5- or 10-mm diameter rigid laparoscope (with either a 0- or 30-degree angled lens) is used. The essential endoscopic instruments are (1) 5-mm diameter blunt-tipped (mini-Metzenbaum-type) scissors with a monopolar electrocautery; (2) a 5-mm diameter curved grasper (a hemostat); and (3) a 5-mm diameter suction irrigator.

Ports and Port Placement

A soft, flexible thoracic endoscopic port is inserted through a 2-cm chest wall incision, similar to the placement of a chest tube. A single port (Fig. 132-6A), or occasionally two ports (Fig. 132-6B), can be used, and both the endoscope and other working instruments can be placed in the port.[36-39] The port is placed in the third or fourth intercostal space in

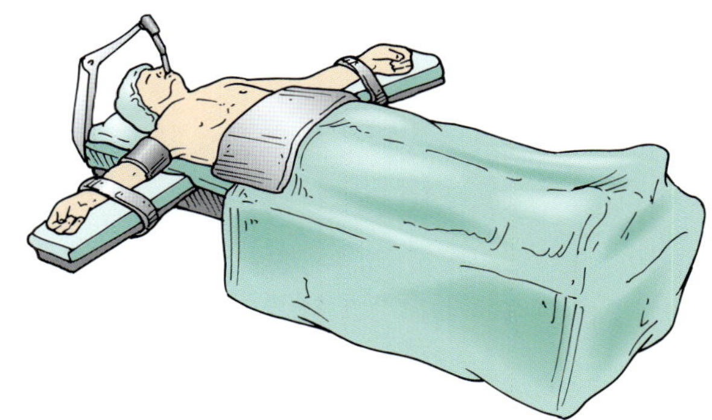

FIGURE 132-5. Supine position for bilateral thoracoscopic sympathectomy.

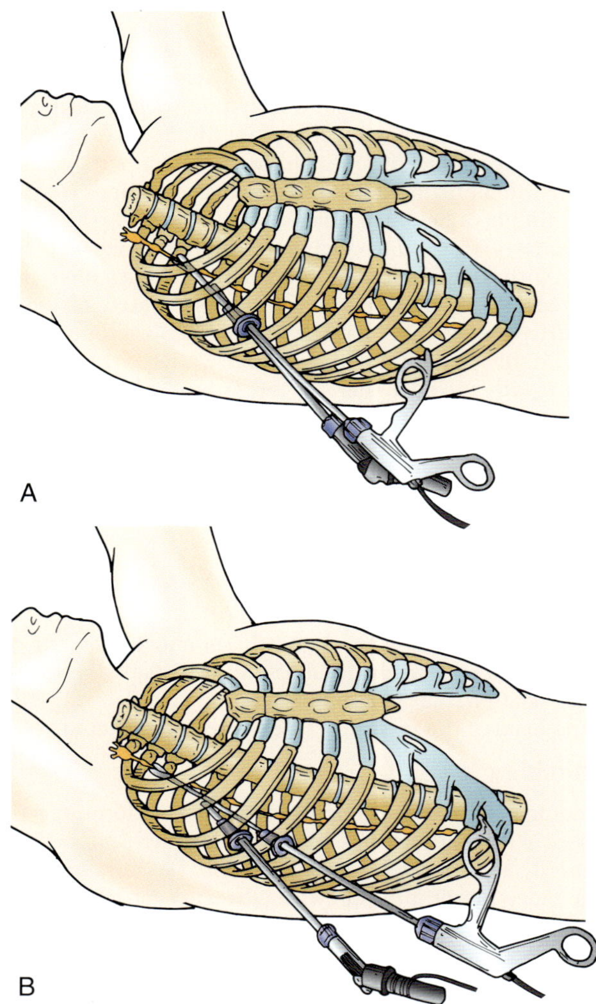

FIGURE 132-6. Single-portal (**A**) and double-portal (**B**) access for right thoracoscopic sympathectomy.

the midaxillary line while the anesthesiologist deflates the ipsilateral lung.

Operative Procedure

The endoscope is placed in the chest through the portal and the lung is retracted. The lung can be further retracted with a blunt instrument and rotation of the operating table, which allows the lung to fall forward and away from the vertebral column. The sympathetic chain is visualized overlying the rib heads in the upper thoracic region. The intercostal vessels course over the midportion of each vertebral body, usually beneath the sympathetic chain. The sympathetic chain appears as a pinkish-white, glistening, raised longitudinal structure. The rostral aspect of the sympathetic chain extends beneath a fat pad that envelops the subclavian artery and obscures the 1st rib and stellate ganglion.

The sympathectomy procedure begins with an incision in the pleura overlying the sympathetic chain at the T3 level, using the curved scissors (Fig. 132-7). The pleural incision is extended in a rostral direction over the sympathetic chain to T2 (Fig. 132-8), and the sympathetic ganglia and chain at T2 and T3 are then cauterized (Fig. 132-9). The nerve of Kuntz can often be identified as a large branch arising from the T2 ganglion and coursing laterally to the brachial plexus, likely providing much of the sympathetic innervation to the upper extremity. Thus, denervation of the T2 ganglion is important.[40] Horner syndrome is best prevented by avoiding injury or traction to the stellate ganglion, which can occur during the dissection and denervation of the T2 ganglion. Once the sympathectomy has been completed, a portion of the sympathetic ganglion can be sent for pathologic evaluation; the surgical site is then irrigated and hemostasis confirmed. A red rubber catheter is inserted through the port and aspirated while the lung is reinflated by the anesthesiologist; the port is then removed and the incision closed with absorbable sutures and Steri-Strips.

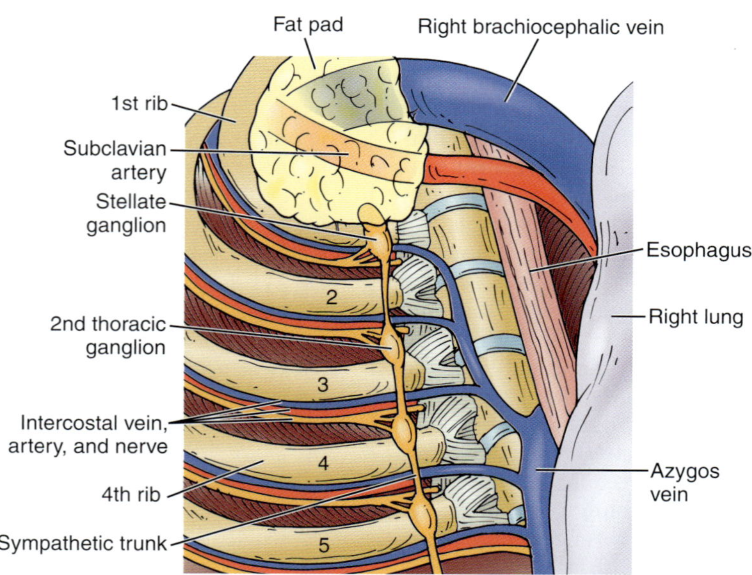

FIGURE 132-7. Anatomy of right thoracic sympathetic chain.

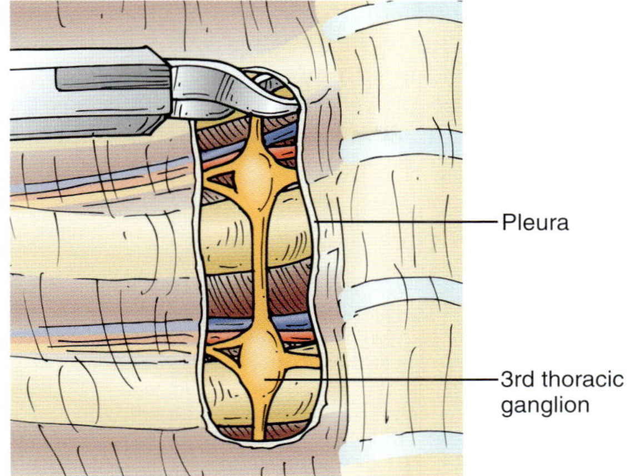

FIGURE 132-8. Pleural opening over right T2 and T3 ganglia.

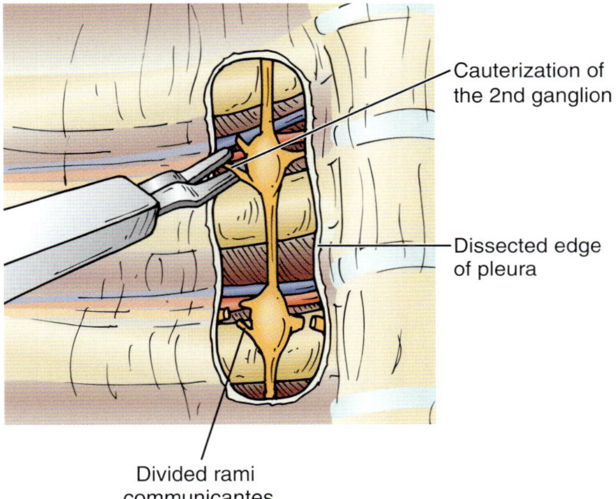

FIGURE 132-9. Cauterization and division of right T2 and T3 ganglia.

Postoperative Care

A postoperative chest radiograph is obtained in the operating room to ensure lung inflation. A small pneumothorax will resolve, but a large, persistent pneumothorax suggests a parenchymal lung leak that would require chest tube placement until the leak resolves. Oral analgesics are adequate, and the hospital stay is usually only 1 or 2 days.

Complications

Surgical complications[41-43] from thoracoscopic sympathectomy are few, and most do not require intervention. They include (1) pneumothorax, (2) Horner syndrome, (3) subcutaneous emphysema, (4) pleural effusions, (5) segmental atelectasis, and (6) intercostal neuralgia. Postoperative pneumothorax usually results from inadequate reinflation of the collapsed lung; however, a small apical pneumothorax can be observed and will spontaneously resolve. Horner syndrome results from injury to the stellate ganglion and is infrequent and usually transient. Injury to the intercostal nerves during port placement or pressure applied during the procedure may result in intercostal neuralgia. The incidence is minimized by using soft, flexible thoracic endoscopic ports rather than the rigid laparoscopic ports.

Compensatory hyperhidrosis is increased sweating, usually in the truncal area, that occurs after a sympathectomy procedure.[44] Facial anhidrosis can also occur.[45] The incidence is probably higher than previously recognized and has been reported to range from 10% to 90%. The severity is highly variable, ranging from mild to severe, and cannot be determined before surgery. Some authors suggest that a more limited sympathectomy of T2 alone may reduce the incidence of compensatory sweating, whereas others claim that only sympathectomy of T3 reduces the incidence.[46] Increasing data are emerging to indicate that more limited (i.e., T2) sympathectomy may have a lower incidence of compensatory hyperhidrosis.[47] Resympathectomy is also an option for both primary failure and recurrent hyperhidrosis, with success rates varying from 96% for unilateral primary failures to 50% for bilateral primary failure. Licht et al.'s study of 669 redo endoscopic sympathectomies found the reoperation to be 75% effective in recurrent palmar hyperhidrosis.[48] However, none of these theories and observations have been clearly substantiated. More recently, clipping of the sympathetic chain has been performed in hopes of creating a reversible lesion.[49,50] Reconstruction of the sympathetic chain has been reported, but no long-term data are available.[44]

Lumbar Endoscopic Sympathectomy

Endoscopic techniques have been used for sympathectomy in the lumbar region and are described by Onimus et al.[51] and others[52,53]; they are similar to an open lumbar sympathectomy except for being much less invasive (see Figs. 132-3 and 132-4). A 1- to 2-cm incision is made in the flank below the tip of the 11th rib, and the retroperitoneum is dissected by finger. Similar to the open procedure, a tissue expander or optical trocar can be used to dissect and expose the psoas and the lumbar sympathetic chain. An endoscopic portal is inserted, and CO_2 insufflation maintains the space for the procedure. A second portal is placed for instrumentation. The sympathectomy then proceeds as in the open procedure.

Radiofrequency and Chemical Destruction of the Sympathetic Chain

Percutaneous placement of a needle into or near a sympathetic ganglion allows destruction of the ganglion by injection of a neurolytic agent (i.e., alcohol, phenol), or a radiofrequency lesion can be created to achieve sympathectomy. Fluoroscopic or CT guidance can be used for localization.[54] These techniques can be performed without general anesthesia, with local anesthetics and mild sedation in older patients, and allow immediate evaluation of the results. They can often be performed on an outpatient basis and obviate the need for expensive and complicated endoscopic technology or large surgical incisions with open procedures. Although some authors report excellent results with these techniques, not all surgeons can achieve these outcomes, and in general the short- and long-term results have been less successful than with open or endoscopic procedures, presumably because of inadequate denervation.

The percutaneous radiofrequency thoracic sympathectomy technique has been well described and documented by Wilkinson.[55,56] The patient is positioned prone on a fluoroscopic table and a radiofrequency lesioning needle is placed in a paramedian location and directed between the ribs, with the needle tip at the rib head and the sympathetic ganglion at the T2-3 level. Stimulation is used to confirm the final needle position, and a radiofrequency pulse is generated to create a lesion. A success rate of more than 90% was noted at 3-year follow-up. Complications, including pneumothorax, occur at a low rate.

Chemical sympathectomy with phenol (6% to 10%) is described by Gybels and Sweet.[57] It has been used with fluoroscopic guidance primarily in the lumbar region to treat vaso-occlusive disease. Most patients obtain fair early relief of pain, but results deteriorate over time. Complications are infrequent and include groin pain and ureteral injuries.

Summary

The indications for sympathectomy have become clearer through 50 years of clinical research. Modern endoscopy creates less tissue disruption and provides a magnified and illuminated exposure, leading to precise, minimally invasive procedures. The technical challenges and complications of these procedures are now well understood and well defined, and the surgeon can customize the necessary procedure based on the individual patient's condition for optimal outcomes.

KEY REFERENCES

Bandyk DF, Johnson BL, Kirkpatrick AF, et al: Surgical sympathectomy for reflex sympathetic dystrophy syndromes. *J Vasc Surg* 35:269–277, 2002.

Barolat G, Schwartzman R, Woo R: Epidural spinal cord stimulation in the management of reflex sympathetic dystrophy. *Stereotact Funct Neurosurg* 53:29–39, 1989.

Johnson JP, Patel NP: Uniportal and biportal endoscopic thoracic sympathectomy. *Neurosurgery* 51(Suppl 5):79–83, 2002.

Singh B, Moodley J, Ramdial PK, et al: Pitfalls in thoracoscopic sympathectomy: mechanisms for failure. *Surg Laparosc Endosc Percutan Tech* 11:364–367, 2001.

Wang YC, Sun MH, Lin CW, et al: Anatomical location of T2-3 sympathetic trunk and Kuntz nerve determined by transthoracic endoscopy. *J Neurosurg* 96(Suppl 1):68–72, 2002.

REFERENCES

The complete reference list is available online at expertconsult.com.

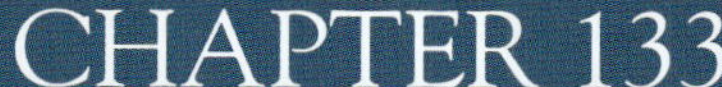

CHAPTER 133

Arachnoiditis and Syringomyelia

Ron Riesenburger | Steven Hwang | Edward C. Benzel

Syringomyelia can develop secondary to many pathologic processes such as Chiari malformations, spine tumors, cysts, traumatic events, spinal deformities, and arachnoiditis. All these conditions likely share a common pathophysiologic disruption of cerebrospinal fluid (CSF) flow regulation.[1,2] This chapter focuses solely on syringomyelia derived from spinal arachnoiditis, excluding traumatic etiologies. Spinal adhesive arachnoiditis has been associated most commonly with postsurgical inflammation, myelography, and infection. However, rare cases of idiopathic arachnoiditis, arachnoiditis after spinal subarachnoid hemorrhage, and familial arachnoiditis have also been reported.[3-5]

The first clinical presentation of syringomyelia was described by Portal in 1804.[6] However, the first case of cervical spinal cord cavitation secondary to arachnoiditis was probably described in 1861 by Vulpian from a necropsy.[7] The first treatment was performed by Abbe and Coley in 1892 as drainage of a postmeningitic syrinx.[8] Subsequently, more clinical cases attributed to postsyphilitic inflammation were published.[9] The first association between degenerative disc disease and arachnoiditis was largely attributed to French in 1946.[10] Although theories about the pathologic process and causative agents have evolved, treatment of arachnoiditis has improved little over the years.

Epidemiology and Definition

Spinal adhesive arachnoiditis (SAA) describes the scarring of pia and arachnoid membranes within the thecal sac. Although the pathophysiology remains elusive, thickening and adhesion of pia and arachnoid membranes are thought to arise secondarily from chronic inflammation. SAA can range from mild focal adhesions to severe scarring as is seen with arachnoid ossificans. SAA seems to have a predilection for the lumbar spine (up to 86% in some series), although this may simply reflect a predominance of postmyelographic arachnoiditis in the literature.[11] The diagnosis of arachnoiditis is confirmed radiographically by using MRI or myelography. The disease spectrum varies considerably from focal scarring or slight nerve root sheath changes to dense scarring throughout the spinal axis. Variations in defining the severity of arachnoiditis likely influence the reported incidence.

Risk factors are largely inherent in the varying underlying pathologic processes that cause inflammation (Box 133-1). Infection, subarachnoid hemorrhage, degenerative lumbar disease, history of myelography, prior lumbar anesthesia, prior spine surgery, transverse myelitis, prior baclofen pump insertion, and even intrathecal steroid injection have all been postulated as causative triggers leading to the development of spinal adhesive arachnoiditis.[12-18] Infectious etiologies include tuberculous meningitis, pyogenic infections, cysticercosis, candida tropicalis, chromoblastomycosis, cryptococcosis, listeriosis, and syphilis.[9,19-23] Some studies have suggested that the addition of blood products to contrast agents in myelography contributed to the increased risk of arachnoiditis. No study has evaluated whether durotomies or synthetic sealants used to reinforce durotomy closures influence the risk of developing arachnoiditis.

Several series have estimated the incidence of lumbar postmyelography arachnoiditis and symptomatic fibrosis to be near 1%.[24] However, published data on postmyelography arachnoiditis are limited by the use of varying contrast agents and a variable time to presentation. For example, one study reported the development of syringomyelia 44 years after myelography.[25] Some series have found asymptomatic but radiographic signs of arachnoiditis in 16.5% to 35% of patients after myelography.[26] However, other studies suggest a lower incidence in the absence of surgical intervention with myelography alone. Laitt et al. reported that 62.4% (68 of 109) of their patients had some degree of arachnoiditis after Myodil myelography, but 50 of their patients had prior lumbar surgery.[27] The incidence was only 3% in patients with myelography alone, whereas arachnoiditis was present in 88% of people who had prior lumbar surgery and myelography.

BOX 133-1. Etiologies of Arachnoiditis

- Infection (bacteria, tuberculosis, cysticercosis, candidiasis, chromoblastomycosis, cryptococcosis, listeriosis, syphilis)
- Subarachnoid hemorrhage
- Myelography
- Degenerative disc disease
- Prior spine surgery/prior lumbar anesthesia
- Transverse myelitis
- Intrathecal steroid injection
- Baclofen pump implantation

Failed back syndrome is an entity that is familiar to most surgeons. Some series have estimated that 6% to 16% of patients who have had prior spine surgery develop some degree of arachnoiditis contributing to persistent pain. Fitt and Stevens found 20% (26 of 129) of patients with a history of lumbar surgery to have some degree of arachnoiditis.[28] Many studies have grouped epidural scarring and intradural pathology such as arachnoiditis together in their evaluations; therefore, the incidence of arachnoiditis alone is likely overreported in the literature.[29] Burton reported that 11% of their failed back surgeries were due to arachnoiditis. Several studies have clearly associated an increased risk of arachnoiditis developing in patients who have undergone prior spine surgeries.[27,30] Certainly, arachnoiditis should be considered in managing postoperative patients with persistent or recurrent symptoms.

Pathophysiology of Arachnoiditis-Associated Syringomyelia

Although no definitive pathologic mechanism of arachnoiditis-associated syringomyelia has been elucidated thus far, several different theories have been postulated. One of these theories speculates that the blood products from myelography act as a catalyst coating oil drops in fibrin, thus emulsifying them and contributing to the development of severe arachnoiditis.[31] Several other authors propose that an initial minor trauma or local irritants such as contrast-myelography could serve as causative agents that trigger an inflammatory response.[17,25] McLean et al. hypothesize that tethering of the spinal cord from arachnoiditis causes repeated compression along the spinal cord with normal physiologic movements leading to pathologic injury.[32,33]

Another theory postulates that syringomyelia associated with arachnoiditis is secondary to formation of microcysts that develop within the spinal cord from ischemic injury. The impaired CSF flow from the arachnoiditis contributes to intramedullary cystic degeneration from ischemia due to circulatory disturbance in the pia-arachnoid, which would coalesce into a syrinx.[34,35]

Williams and Bentley created a syringomyelia model in dogs by injecting kaolin in the cisterna magna and causing significant arachnoiditis.[36] They noted that typical findings associated with ischemia were absent in their pathologic specimens. However, whether their model truly mimics the pathology that is seen in human arachnoiditis remains unclear, as all their specimens had a patent fourth ventricular communication with the syrinx.

Alternatively, other researchers argue that the increased CSF pressure differential from an obstruction leads to direct communication of CSF via Virchow-Robin spaces into the spinal cord that forms a syrinx.[37,38] Alternative drainage pathways that have been hypothesized include the dorsal root entry zone and perivascular channels.[39,40]

A more recent hypothesis that has growing support from various studies is that extracellular fluid from interstitial edema contributes to the formation of a syrinx secondary to the scarring of the pia-arachnoid. The scarring of the pia-arachnoid is thought to impair some degree of CSF absorption while increasing venous stasis, thus increasing the amount of interstitial fluid.[41] This theory has been supported by animal and mathematical models that obstruct the CSF space, leading to development of edema and possibly a "pre-syrinx" state.[42,43] Yet another hypothesis incorporates pressure dissociation above and below the obstruction with disruption along the blood–spinal cord barrier leading to ultrafiltration of protein-poor fluid into a syrinx.[44]

Hypotheses explaining the development of syringomyelia have ranged from hydrodynamic theories to pressure dissociation theories involving accumulation of extracellular fluid.[35,44,45] However, we still have an incomplete understanding of the pathophysiologic process that leads to syringomyelia formation.

Radiographic Findings of Arachnoiditis

With the advent of myelography, lumbar arachnoiditis has been described as nerve root clumping, contraction of the thecal sac, an appearance of an empty or thickened thecal sac, short/blunted perineural sheathes, or obliteration of nerve root sheathes.[46] Wilkinson further classified these findings into grades of severity[47]:

1. Unilateral defect on the nerve root exit pouch adjacent to the disc
2. Circumferential or anular defect with bilateral notch and filiform passage of contrast medium
3. Complete transverse obstruction with "stalagmites," candle-guttering, or paintbrush defects
4. Infundibulum cul-de-sac, loss of radicular striation, cutting off of root sleeves

In circumstances of complete obstruction, CT myelography from a cisternal injection may provide useful information delineating the rostral extent of obstruction for operative planning.

However, with the advent of MRI, less invasive imaging studies were available. Ross and Delamarter summarized their MRI findings into a classification with 92% sensitivity, 100% specificity, and 99% accuracy (Table 133-1). Classification of MRI findings associated with lumbar arachnoiditis[48,49]:

1. Conglomeration of nerve roots centrally located, no enhancement
2. Nerve roots attached laterally/clumped with meningeal thickening
3. "Empty thecal sac" appearance (Fig. 133-1)
4. Soft tissue mass within the canal obliterating subarachnoid space

Ross and Delamarter's definitions are commonly used, although other authors have further simplified their findings

TABLE 133-1

MRI Findings Associated with Lumbar Arachnoiditis

Grade	MRI Findings
1	Conglomeration of nerve roots centrally located, no enhancement
2	Nerve roots attached laterally, clumped with meningeal thickening, "empty thecal sac" appearance
3	Soft tissue mass within canal obliteration of subarachnoid space

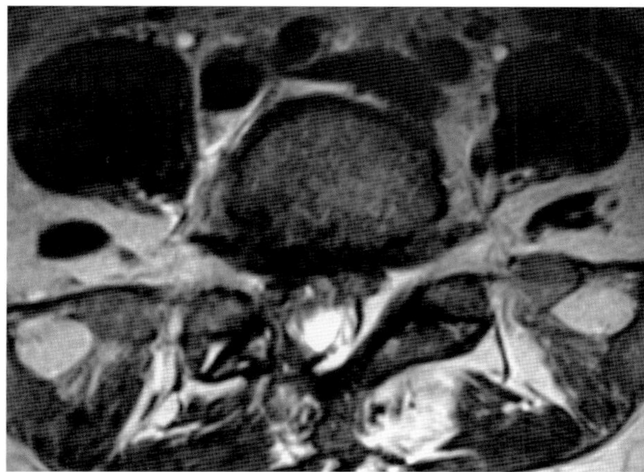

FIGURE 133-1. Axial T2-weighted MRI showing an "empty thecal sac" appearance with the nerve roots clumped laterally, Ross and Delamarter type 2.

into even fewer categories. Jorgensen et al. divided MRI findings into two categories[50]:

1. Adhesion of roots inside meninges, "sleeveless" appearance (Ross and Delamarter types 1 and 2)
2. Thecal sac changes, filling defects/narrowing/shortened/occlusion (Ross and Delamarter type 3)

Usually, MRI is adequate to confirm the diagnosis of arachnoiditis,[28,51] but some cases are quite subtle and might not be as evident on MRI. Brodbelt and Stoodley described three cases in which a mild, single arachnoid web was sufficient to cause CSF flow impairment.[14] Some authors have advocated that constructive interface steady state images are better suited to visualize dural thickening, syringomyelia, microcystic lesions, and deformity of the cord, but less adequate to identify "pre-syrinx" findings.[52] Myelography can be invaluable to identify small areas of CSF flow obstruction that are responsible for symptoms.

It is important to note that lumbar spinal stenosis in itself is often associated with radiographic findings that resemble Delamarter type 1 clumping of nerve roots and should be distinguished from arachnoiditis based on the clinical history.[53] These findings are likely due to mechanical pressures from the stenosis as opposed to arachnoid/pial fibrosis as seen in arachnoiditis.

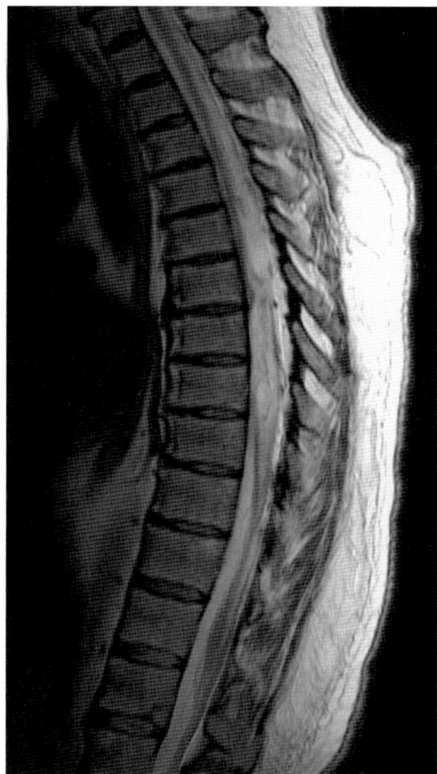

FIGURE 133-2. Sagittal T2-weighted MRI displaying thoracic postinflammatory syringomyelia after Pantopaque myelography 30 years previously. (Courtesy of Dr. Julian Wu.)

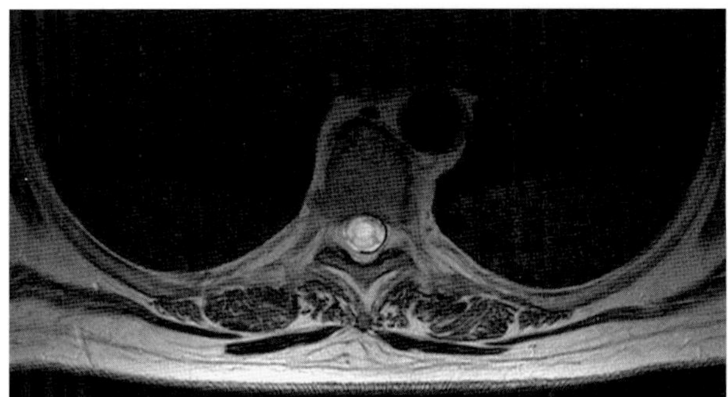

FIGURE 133-3. Axial T2-weighted MRI showing the syrinx. (Courtesy of Dr. Julian Wu.)

Clinical Presentation and Clinical Course

Patients typically present with slowly progressive, chronic symptoms. The symptomatology is largely defined by the anatomic location of the pathology. Given that lumbar arachnoiditis is more prevalent, a greater percentage of patients initially present with lumbar radiculopathy, sensory deficits, and back pain.[54,55] Eventually, patients develop more objective findings of decreased reflexes and motor deficits progressing to bowel and bladder dysfunction, essentially a cauda equina syndrome.[55] These patients often have a history of an invasive lumbar procedure, either myelography, surgery, or even a percutaneous injection for pain control. Alternatively, patients who develop cervicothoracic arachnoiditis present with myelopathy secondary to spinal cord compression (Figs. 133-2 to 133-5). Thoracic myelopathy is more commonly encountered, but cervical cases have been described.

In the absence of syringomyelia, many authors have stated that arachnoiditis is relatively stable with little clinical deterioration over time.[11,16] However, once the patient is symptomatic, the majority of cases progress clinically. Nevertheless, occasional cases of clinical stabilization for several years prior to deteriorating symptoms have been published.[56] The onset of symptoms can be quite variable and may range from 14 days to 44 years after an assumed cause such as myelography or infection.[11,25] The early onset of symptoms is atypical and most likely related to the initial causative event, such as vascular thrombosis associated with an infection. Most symptoms develop years after the inciting event.

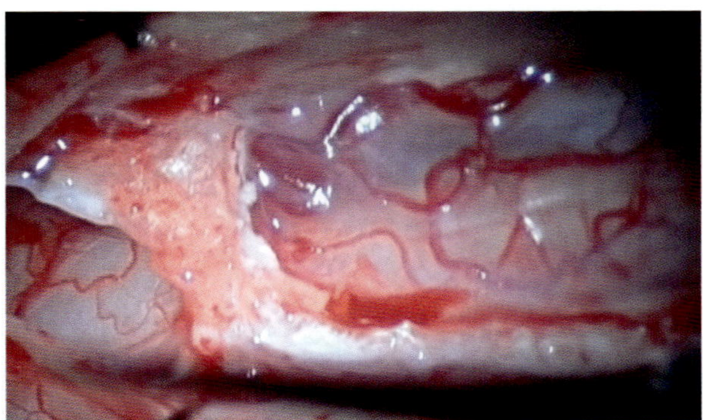

FIGURE 133-4. An intraoperative image of calcification/adhesions/syrinx. (Courtesy of Dr. Julian Wu.)

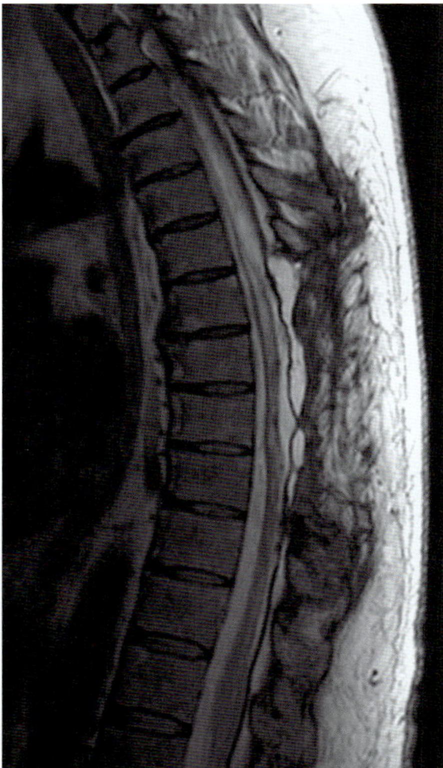

FIGURE 133-5. Sagittal T2-weighted follow-up MRI after decompression and duraplasty. (Courtesy of Dr. Julian Wu.)

Klekamp and Samii introduced a grading system to standardize the clinical examination and progression of patients with syringomyelia. Patients were divided into six categories (0–5) based on sensory, motor, gait ataxia, bladder function, and bowel function.[57]

Treatment and Outcomes

Nonsurgical Treatment

The clinical results of treating arachnoiditis have remained dismal. Generally, once symptoms appear, the course of the disease is progressive. Some authors have reported treating symptomatic syringomyelia from arachnoiditis conservatively with oral steroids.[58] This may transiently alleviate symptoms, but the clinical picture typically worsens over time. Trials of intrathecal steroids were conducted, but several reports of arachnoiditis developing from intrathecal steroid administration have tempered this approach.[13] Some mild success has been achieved by administering intrathecal hyaluronidase in attempts to minimize fibrin deposition, but this has not gained widespread practice.[59]

Surgical Techniques to Minimize Development of Arachnoiditis

Careful surgical technique to minimize the development of arachnoiditis is critical as a preventive measure. Historical contrast myelography agents (Thoratrast, Pantopaque, Myodil) that contributed to spinal arachnoiditis have largely been replaced by water-soluble nonionic agents such as Omnipaque. Intraoperatively, caution should be used to minimize trauma to the dura and avoid excessive blood product accumulation in the subarachnoid space. Surgical techniques of dural tacking sutures, use of hemostatic agents epidurally with neuro-patties, profuse irrigation, and suturing the arachnoid to the dura upon closure may theoretically reduce the likelihood of postoperative arachnoiditis. Furthermore, in cases of prior tethering, postoperative prone recumbency or pial sutures tethering the cord away from the dural closure may limit recurrent tethering and scarring.

Surgical Management of Lumbar Arachnoiditis

Primary lumbar arachnoiditis rarely extends beyond the lumbar spine, but treatment of this condition should be differentiated from treatment of cervicothoracic arachnoiditis leading to syringomyelia. Most commonly, treatment for lumbar arachnoiditis targets symptomatic pain relief. Unfortunately, outcomes for lumbar arachnoiditis have been equally disappointing. Roca et al. had "good" results (pain relief and only occasional medications) in 8 of 23 patients, fair outcomes in 9, and poor results in 6.[54] Intuitively, they had better results in patients with milder arachnoiditis (Wilkinson grade 1 and 2 as compared to grade 3 and 4), although most cases were reexplored for epidural fibrosis. Jorgensen et al. reported that 50% of patients in their series remained unemployed after repeat surgery, 20% worked full-time with intermittent symptoms, and only 10% to 15% were symptom free, but their study included extradural scarring as well.[50]

Johnston and Metheny compared 28 patients, of whom half were treated surgically with chymotrypsin intradurally as well as a postoperative oral regimen, and found long-term results comparable between their surgical and observational cohorts.[60] Patients did improve transiently, but the researchers concluded that until a method of limiting adhesive scar formation existed, surgery was not recommended for lumbar arachnoiditis. Wilkinson and Schuman treated 17 patients with arachnoidolysis and noted that 76% had initial improvement, which reduced to 50% after 1 year. They found that 71% of patients with neurologic deficits improved, but the study had only 1 year of follow-up.[61] Other authors have resorted to spinal cord stimulation, rhizotomies, or even cordotomies to treat unilateral pain, with mixed results.[16]

Surgical Management of Syringomyelia

Once symptomatic syringomyelia has developed, surgical intervention revolves between drainage such as syringocavitary, syringosubarachnoid, or lumboperitoneal shunting and direct adhesion lysis and duraplasty. Some authors favor syringoperitoneal shunting, while others prefer syringosubarachnoid shunts.[4,62] Many authors state that surgical lysis of adhesions is mandatory with consideration of duraplasty.[63-65]

Koyanagi et al. reported that 60% of their 15 patients treated surgically improved over a mean of 2.7 years of follow-up, but 8 patients required multiple procedures.[41] While all patients had decreased syrinx size on follow-up imaging, only 31% improved with a shunting procedure. Despite this low number, the authors concluded that there remains a role for shunting. Sgouros et al. placed 56 syringopleural shunts for varying etiologies and noted that initially 64.2% improved, but only 53.5% had sustained improvement with at least 1 year of follow-up.[65] Furthermore, shunting carries significant risks; 26.7% of their patients suffered clinical deterioration after placement of a shunt. In the subgroup of spinal adhesive arachnoiditis, 8 of 11 patients deteriorated even after multiple reoperations (two improved initially but then worsened), while three remained stable.

Batzdorf noted that 50% of their 42 patients with syringocavitary shunts experienced a complication or failure. In the subgroup of patients with postinflammatory syringomyelia, the rate was 36%.[66] This subset, however, had the greatest number of patients with postoperative deterioration. Sgouros and Williams have also advocated leaving the dura unopposed to create a meningocele, but others argue that this technique may promote more blood product accumulation and scarring.[67] Other complications of shunt placement include neurologic deficits from the myelotomy, shunt failure, shunting of a compartment within the syrinx, tethering of cord via the shunt, overdrainage of subarachnoid CSF, infection, CSF leak, aseptic meningitis, pneumothorax, and brachial plexus palsy.[66,68] A hemilaminectomy and placement of a syringosubarachnoid shunt have been advocated by some to minimize selective risks.[69]

Other researchers have also advocated that the primary goal of surgery should be to release adhesions and perform a duraplasty.[64,65] Shikata et al. reported good results using release of adhesions and duraplasty with or without spine fusion in 58.3% of patients. They encountered fair results in 19.4% of patients and deterioration in 22.2% of their sample. More recently four fifths of their patients with spine fusions had improved results.[55] Klekamp et al. reported that 67 patients treated for progressive symptoms all had scarring near the syrinx. Ninety-seven percent of patients who underwent shunting recurred symptomatically, whereas 78% of patients who underwent arachnoid release and duraplasty remained stable.[68] Klekamp and Samii reported far inferior results with either treatment in 154 patients; 11% of patients improved with shunting, while 31% had amelioration with arachnoidolysis. Complications were comparable between the two groups: 18% in the shunted group and 17% with arachnoidolysis.[70]

Klekamp et al. previously reported treating syringomyelic patients primarily with shunts but have subsequently adapted their algorithm to initially treat patients with arachnoidlysis and decompression. They do caution against overly aggressive arachnoidlysis with severe scarring that may contribute to further neurologic deterioration, and the most severe scarring tends to develop with postinflammatory arachnoiditis. Only 17% of patients with more severe scarring stabilized, whereas 83% of patients with mild arachnoiditis stabilized neurologically in their series. They found that the following correlated with a higher recurrence of symptoms: syrinx shunting, severe preoperative scarring, multiple prior surgeries, postoperative scarring, increase in syrinx size postoperatively, and severe neurologic deficits preoperatively.[68]

Parker et al. had equally tepid outcomes. In 12 patients with postinfectious etiologies, only 2 improved, while 4 worsened. In 11 patients with syringomyelia from cryptogenic, postoperative, or spinal subarachnoid hemorrhage etiologies, 4 patients improved and 3 worsened. Overall, drainage of the syrinx led to clinical deterioration in 60% of patients, while 40% remained stable or improved. With arachnoidolysis, 66% of patients remained stable, while 33% had poor outcomes. With infectious etiology, the outcomes were worse: 46.5% worsened clinically, 46.5% remained stable, and only 7% improved.[71]

In deciding on surgical approaches, consideration should be given to the extent of scarring. Certainly, focal areas can be treated with better results by arachnoidolysis and duraplasty. Extensive scarring may favor syringocavitary shunting provided that the syrinx is not loculated. Adjuvant treatment should also include management for spasticity and neuropathic pain.[72] Patients should be well informed of the risks and the often limited benefits.

Interpretation of published results needs to be tempered by the limited amount of long-term follow-up. Most series show initial success, but longer follow-up supports the concern that clinical deterioration is often encountered. In treating lumbar arachnoiditis, Wilkinson showed 75% initial improvement with 18% of patients worsening acutely. However, after 1 year, only 50% of patients had maintained that initial improvement.[73] Furthermore, most of the larger series with longer follow-up had worse outcomes, which may simply reflect the natural course of the disease even after intervention. Consideration should be given to weighing the considerable risk of iatrogenic clinical deterioration in these series against short-term gains. With our limited understanding of the pathophysiologic processes involved and our inability to reduce recurrent arachnoiditis after surgical intervention, surgical intervention should be recommended cautiously and only in patients with ongoing neurologic deterioration. If arachnoidolysis strategies are employed, the operative goal should be the establishment and maintenance of a patent subarachnoid space from rostral to caudal, spanning the entirety of the pathology. This often requires that the procedure include a duraplasty. Some surgeons have utilized the off-label use of DuraGen (Integra LifeSciences, Plainsboro, NJ) for this application. The senior author has applied DuraGen under a fascial graft (duraplasty) after arachnoidolysis. The DuraGen was used to create a DuraGen bridge from the rostral to caudal subarachnoid spaces.

It is certain that our ability to manage this difficult patient population will improve in the future. Advances in technique, with accompanying innovations, promise to help pave the way toward better outcomes.

Summary

Spinal adhesive arachnoiditis has been associated with varying inflammation-inducing factors that can lead to lumbar arachnoiditis or cervicothoracic syringomyelia. The clinical presentation of arachnoiditis is largely dependent on the location and anatomic structures that are affected, varying from radiculitis to myelopathy. Evaluation of arachnoiditis should include an entire spinal axis MRI and consideration of a CT myelogram if necessary. Unfortunately, both conservative and surgical treatment options have had limited results. Perhaps the most important concept in addressing arachnoiditis is prevention through careful surgical technique.

Lumbar arachnoidolysis has had very limited success, and patients should be counseled regarding recurrence of symptoms even after surgery. Syringomyelia associated with arachnoiditis typically progresses, and surgical intervention should be considered. Syringocavitary shunting is a useful treatment for arachnoiditis-related syringomyelia, especially if excessive adhesions are present. However, the literature suggests better outcomes and less iatrogenic risk with adhesion lysis and duraplasty.

KEY REFERENCES

Batzdorf U, Klekamp J, Johnson JP: A critical appraisal of syrinx cavity shunting procedures. *J Neurosurg* 89:382–388, 1998.

Delamarter RB, Ross JS, Masaryk TJ, et al: Diagnosis of lumbar arachnoiditis by magnetic resonance imaging. *Spine (Phila Pa 1976)* 15:304–310, 1990.

Klekamp J, Batzdorf U, Samii M, Bothe HW: Treatment of syringomyelia associated with arachnoid scarring caused by arachnoiditis or trauma. *J Neurosurg* 86:233–240, 1997.

Klekamp J, Samii M: Introduction of a score system for the clinical evaluation of patients with spinal processes. *Acta Neurochir (Wien)* 123:221–223, 1993.

Milhorat TH, Capocelli AL Jr, Anzil AP, et al: Pathological basis of spinal cord cavitation in syringomyelia: analysis of 105 autopsy cases. *J Neurosurg* 82:802–812, 1995.

Sgouros S, Williams B: A critical appraisal of drainage in syringomyelia. *J Neurosurg* 82:1–10, 1995.

Shikata J, Yamamuro T, Iida H, Sugimoto M: Surgical treatment for symptomatic spinal adhesive arachnoiditis. *Spine (Phila Pa 1976)* 14(8):870–875, 1989.

REFERENCES

The complete reference list is available online at expertconsult.com.

CHAPTER 134

Posttraumatic and Idiopathic Syringomyelia

Tarun Bhalla | Ajit A. Krishnaney

Syringomyelia denotes a collection of heterogeneous pathologic conditions characterized by abnormal, longitudinally oriented, fluid-filled cavities within the spinal cord (Fig. 134-1). Syringomyelia may be the result of congenital, traumatic, or neoplastic processes and therapy is directed at correcting the underlying pathology. However, in many cases the etiology of the condition remains unknown, and treatment results are usually unsatisfactory.[1] This chapter offers guidance for diagnosis and management of patients with posttraumatic and idiopathic syringomyelia and provides an update on current research.

Although Charles Estienne first described the condition in 1546, the term *syringomyelia* was suggested by Olivier d'Angers in 1827 from the Greek *syrinx*, meaning "pipe," "tube," or "channel," and *myelos*, meaning "marrow."[2,3] The term is restricted to this condition and should not be used to describe similar entities such as proteinaceous cysts or a terminal ventricle. The term *hydromyelia* refers to cystic dilation of the ependyma-lined central canal by cerebrospinal fluid (CSF; Fig. 134-2). However, the syrinx may dissect into the parenchyma of the spinal cord and its original connection with the central canal may disappear. Furthermore, the type of cellular lining is not a reliable criterion to distinguish between syringomyelia and hydromyelia. Because of these difficulties, the term *syringohydromyelia* has been used in the literature to refer to both entities.[4-7] In this chapter, *syringomyelia* is used to denote all abnormal fluid-filled cavities in the spinal cord.[8]

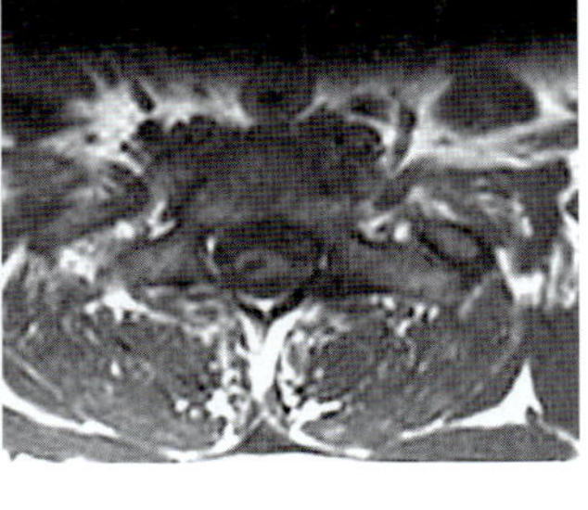

FIGURE 134-1. Sagittal T2-weighted MRI (*left*) demonstrates an idiopathic syrinx. Axial T1-weighted MRI (*right*) of the idiopathic syrinx shows irregular cord T1-weighted hypointensity.

Epidemiology

Syringomyelia affects primarily children and young adults, presenting on average before the third decade of life. Before the widespread availability of MRI, a prevalence of 9 per 100,000 and an incidence of approximately 0.44 cases per year were cited in the literature.[9-13] Approximately 50% of patients presenting with syringomyelia have a Chiari malformation, whereas 25% present with a history of spinal cord trauma or arachnoiditis.[9] The incidence of syringomyelia appears to be similar after quadriplegia or paraplegia. There is a statistically significant male preponderance in

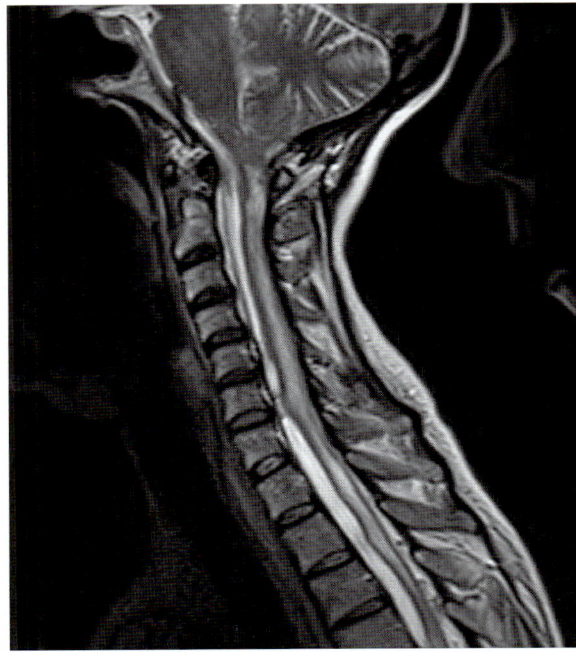

FIGURE 134-2. Sagittal T2-weighted MRI through cervical spine shows an extensive epidural collection with resultant cord expansion, hyperintense cerebrospinal fluid signal within the cord, and central canal dilation (hydromyelia).

posttraumatic syringomyelia (80%), which follows the gender distribution in spinal cord injury.[6,10,12] Of patients with a spinal cord injury investigated between 1 and 30 years after the initial insult, 21% to 28% have a syrinx and 30% to 50% have some degree of spinal cystic change. However, symptomatic syringomyelia is reported in only 1% to 9% of the spinal cord injury population.[8,14-18]

Classification

A distinction based on pathologic and MRI findings is made between communicating and noncommunicating syringomyelia.[19-21] Communicating syrinx cavities are central canal dilations in continuity with the fourth ventricle and are often associated with hydrocephalus. They occur in children and young adults with conditions that obstruct CSF outflow from the fourth ventricle, such as Chiari II malformations or Dandy-Walker cysts. Only 10% of the lesions are of the communicating type.[19]

Noncommunicating syringomyelia can be further classified into central canal and extracanalicular syringomyelia.[19,20] Noncommunicating central canal syrinx cavities are associated with Chiari I malformations, cervical spinal stenosis, spinal arachnoiditis, and basilar impression. The cavities are dilations of the central canal and are partially or completely lined by ependymal cells. Noncommunicating extracanalicular syrinx cavities are associated with spinal trauma, infarction, hemorrhage, or transverse myelitis. Most extracanalicular syrinx cavities are found in the vascular watershed zones of the central and dorsolateral gray matter. Extracanalicular syrinx cavities are irregular in shape and commonly have microglia, hemosiderin-containing macrophages, and gliosis of the cyst wall.[20] In addition, the perivascular spaces may be enlarged and direct communication with the subarachnoid space at the dorsal nerve root entry zones or the ventromedian fissure can occur.[20] Posttraumatic syrinx cavities are usually near the injury site and extend rostrally in 81%, caudally in 4%, and in both directions in 15% of cases.[8,20,21]

Etiology

The exact pathophysiologic process underlying posttraumatic syrinx formation is not clear, and various theories have been advanced. Two popular explanations are the hydrodynamic theory and a theory that assumes a differential between intracranial and spinal pressure caused by a valvelike effect at the foramen magnum.[8] The second of these theories does not adequately account for the occurrence of noncommunicating syrinx cavities. The hydrodynamic theory proposes that fluid flows into the central canal from the fourth ventricle because of a "water-hammer–like" transmission of arterial or respiratory pressure. These theories have concentrated on canalicular syringomyelia associated with Chiari malformations, frequently at the expense of ignoring posttraumatic cases.[22-24]

Historically, the explanation for syrinx cavities isolated from the fourth ventricle was a secondary obstruction of the rostral central canal. However, this conclusion is difficult to reconcile with the observation that the central canal in humans is obstructed by segmental occlusions by the end of the third decade of life, and that there is a clear anatomic distinction between the central canal and syrinx cavity in most cases of posttraumatic syringomyelia.[19,20,25] The initial formation of a spinal cord cavity may involve different mechanisms than the subsequent enlargement of the cavity to form a syrinx. Inflammatory responses to traumatic injury in the central nervous system result in localized edema and may lead to cyst formation.[26-28]

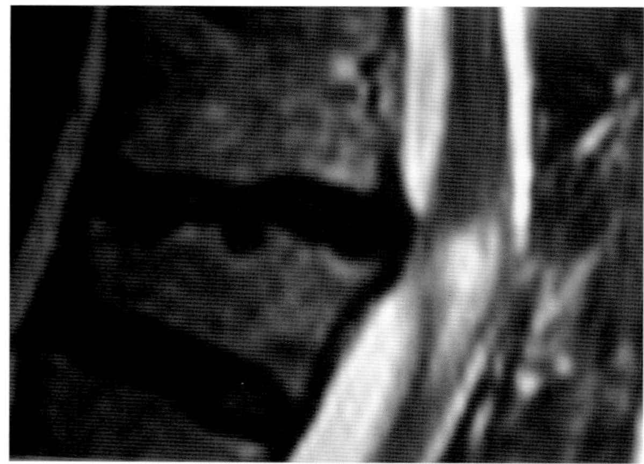

FIGURE 134-3. Sagittal T2-weighted MRI shows development of a syrinx after traumatic compression fracture.

It has been reported that an intramedullary hematoma after spinal cord trauma increases the likelihood of developing a syrinx.[6] Natural dissolution and absorption of the hematoma can leave a cystic cavity that can predispose the patient to syrinx formation. Furthermore, posttraumatic syrinx cavities are usually found in vascular watershed regions in the spinal cord.[6,19] This finding implicates ischemia during the primary injury or subsequent inflammatory response as a contributor to syrinx formation.[6,8,19]

Spinal cord injury results in multiple pathologic conditions that can disturb CSF flow and potentially contribute to syrinx enlargement. Subarachnoid adhesions, spinal deformity, or stenosis is often seen in patients with spinal cord injury who subsequently develop syringomyelia. It has been shown that the presence of uncorrected kyphosis correlates with syrinx formation and symptom severity and appears to correlate with disruption of CSF flow in the subarachnoid space[17,18,29-31] (Fig. 134-3). The pathophysiology of posttraumatic syringomyelia remains uncertain, but ongoing work with MRI and mathematical modeling supported by studies in animal models continues to shed light on this debilitating condition.

Clinical Presentation

Posttraumatic syringomyelia has been reported to develop anywhere between 3 months and 34 years after the initial injury to the spinal cord.[14,20,21,29,32] Although sudden neurologic decline due to hemorrhage into a syrinx cavity has been described, symptomatic progression is usually gradual.[6] Common initial symptoms include segmental pain and sensory loss. The pain is usually dull or burning, indicating injury to the spinothalamic tracts,[6,29] and is usually at or above the level of injury. It may be exacerbated by coughing, sneezing, straining, or sitting.[6,29] Characteristic dissociated pain and temperature sensation loss with preservation of light touch and proprioception in ascending segments are more common than is complete loss of sensation.[6,29] After the onset of sensory symptoms, patients generally report a gradual loss of motor function above the level of previous injury that is characterized by progressive asymmetrical weakness. Associated symptoms may include hyperhidrosis, autonomic dysreflexia, Horner syndrome, cardiorespiratory dysfunction, and an asymmetrical reduction in reflexes.[6,29,32] In rare cases, the syrinx cavity can extend rostrally into the brainstem and result in bulbar symptoms.[8]

Diagnosis

Syringomyelia was difficult to diagnose before the advent of modern neuroimaging. CT is at best unreliable for diagnostic purposes because of signal degradation by surrounding bony elements, and CT myelography misses approximately 50% of syrinx cavities.[33,34] MRI is the imaging modality of choice for the diagnosis of posttraumatic syringomyelia, and demonstration of a syrinx cavity in the spinal cord should prompt an MRI examination of the entire neuraxis.[33-35] However, MRI scans rarely enable differentiation of hydromyelia and syringomyelia because both entities are characterized on MRI by the presence of a longitudinally oriented fluid collection in the spinal cord. Congenital or posttraumatic syringohydromyelia does not show contrast enhancement.[33-35] Phase-contrast cine MRI may accurately localize subarachnoid space obstruction and demonstrate normalization of CSF flow after surgery, and may also be used to help confirm spinal cord tethering and communication of spinal cord cysts with the subarachnoid space.[8,33-35]

Management

Posttraumatic syringomyelia continues to be a difficult condition to manage because it is characterized by slow clinical progression, and the syrinx cavities may exist for years without becoming symptomatic.[8] Despite reports of neurologic recovery after surgery, in up to 80% of cases 5- and 10-year follow-up studies demonstrate stabilization of symptoms only regardless of the mode of treatment or degree of radiologic improvement achieved.[36] The goal of surgical management is to correct the assumed underlying mechanism. Surgical options include correction of deformity, alleviation of compression, shunting procedures, arachnolysis with or without duraplasty, and cord transection. When feasible, correction of a deformity or compressive lesion is usually preferable to a shunting procedure.[18] Syrinx cavities usually shrink after decompression of the spinal cord or correction of deformity. This has the added benefit of avoiding intradural surgery and, hence, postoperative arachnoid scarring.[18] Shunting of the syrinx to the subarachnoid space should be performed only in cases where these surgical measures fail or are not an option. Many authors advocate surgical treatment only for patients with progressive neurologic decline or extreme pain.[6,30,37,38] In patients managed nonoperatively, close clinical observation for progressive neurologic deficits is essential. Serial MRI studies for anatomic progression of the syrinx at regular intervals should be considered.

Surgical intervention should be considered in patients with progressive debilitating deficits. A number of surgical strategies have been suggested in the literature. These include cyst aspiration, fenestration and shunt placement, and intradural exploration and duraplasty. Currently, intradural exploration, lysis of subarachnoid adhesions, and duraplasty is recommended by many as the preferred primary treatment for posttraumatic syringomyelia. The goal of this intervention is to create a channel for CSF circulation extrinsic to the spinal cord itself. By creating this pathway, CSF is no longer forced into the parenchyma of the cord, thereby allowing the syrinx to collapse. In cases where duraplasty has failed, shunting of the syrinx may be considered. Syringosubarachnoid, syringoperitoneal, and syringopleural shunts have been described. In all cases, septations in the syrinx need to be lysed to allow for optimal decompression. Syrinx shunts, however, have a propensity to fail, which can limit their usefulness. Cyst aspiration by itself is a palliative procedure and as such has limited usefulness in this patient population.

Conclusions

Posttraumatic syringomyelia is a chronic, progressive, and debilitating condition. Because of the underlying neurologic deficits in patients with spinal cord injury, progressive syringomyelia is often missed and may be difficult to diagnose. Although current surgical therapies may offer only modest results in terms of return of function, they have been shown to halt progression in select cases. Clearly, there is a need for continued research to understand the underlying pathophysiologic process of the disease and to identify the most effective therapies.

KEY REFERENCES

Gardner WJ, Angel J: The cause of syringomyelia and its surgical treatment. *Cleve Clin Q* 25:4–8, 1958.

Milhorat TH, Johnson RW, Milhorat RH, et al: Clinicopathological correlations in syringomyelia using axial magnetic resonance imaging. *Neurosurgery* 37:206–213, 1995.

Oldfield EH, Muraszko K, Shawker TH, et al: Pathophysiology of syringomyelia associated with Chiari I malformation of the cerebellar tonsils: implications for diagnosis and treatment. *J Neurosurg* 80:3–15, 1994.

Perrouin-Verbe B, Lenne-Aurier K, Robert R, et al: Post-traumatic syringomyelia and post-traumatic spinal canal stenosis: a direct relationship: review of 75 patients with a spinal cord injury. *Spinal Cord* 36:137–143, 1998.

Sgouros S, Williams B: A critical appraisal of drainage in syringomyelia. *J Neurosurg* 82:1–10, 1995.

Tator CH, Fehlings MG: Review of the secondary injury theory of acute spinal cord trauma with emphasis on vascular mechanisms. *J Neurosurg* 75:15–26, 1991.

REFERENCES

The complete reference list is available online at expertconsult.com.

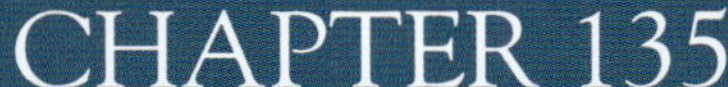

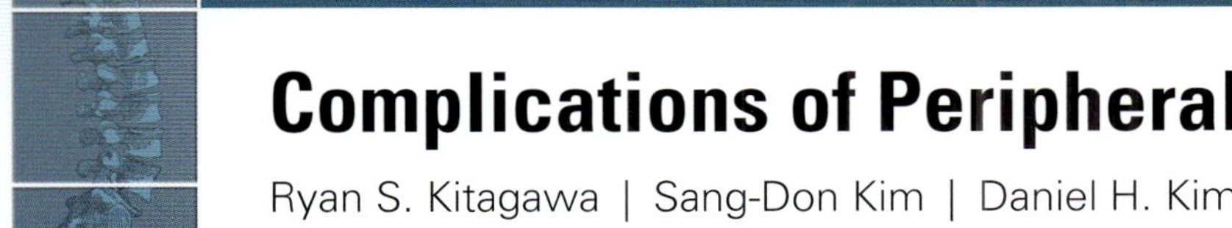

CHAPTER 135

Complications of Peripheral Nerve Surgery

Ryan S. Kitagawa | Sang-Don Kim | Daniel H. Kim

Complications involving the peripheral nerves are often difficult to assess and treat, and their consequences may be significant and irreversible. Because of sensory overlap and collateral motor control, even complete nerve lesions may go unrecognized. Before surgical intervention, a thorough clinical and radiologic evaluation is necessary to prevent future problems because injuries to surrounding anatomic structures such as bony fractures may complicate subsequent interventions. In addition, peripheral and central lesions can coexist. Other factors that can contribute to surgical complications include misdiagnosis, inappropriate or unskilled surgical technique, and poor infection control.

Accurate localization of the lesion in the damaged plexus or peripheral elements is essential, and differentiating between complete and partial lesions is also important. The etiology of the injury or disease process is equally important. Atypical clinical presentations can occur from anatomic variants, incomplete lesions, and other medical causes such as diabetes and renal disease. Nondiagnostic clinical findings warrant additional examinations with studies, such as electromyography and radiography.

This chapter summarizes two categories of peripheral nerve complications: (1) the complications that result from peripheral nerve surgery, and (2) the complications of other surgeries and injuries that directly cause peripheral nerve lesions.

Preoperative Assessment for Complication Avoidance

The goals of preoperative assessment include recognition of the pathology, identification of the disease etiology, and selection of an appropriate treatment plan. A number of considerations must be ruled out before any surgical intervention. These complicating factors include immunologic disorders, toxic polyneuropathies, metabolic processes, inflammatory diseases, nutritional deficiencies, drug-induced neuropathies, vasculitides, hormonal etiologies, and connective tissue disorders.[1,2]

Planning a successful surgery requires a thorough knowledge of normal and variant peripheral nerve anatomy, of the adjacent structures, and of the basic concepts of nerve regeneration and intraneural anatomy.[1,3-12] Thus, an inadequate or misinterpreted preoperative assessment can lead to improper surgical interventions and subsequent complications.[1,10,13-15]

Clinical Examination

Many variants of peripheral nerve anatomy exist, and misinterpretation of nonspecific sensory findings can lead to an inaccurate assessment of the nerve injury. For example, in the Riche-Cannieu anomaly, branches of both the median and ulnar nerves supply sensation to the thumb, instead of the normal anatomic splitting.[10,16] In the Martin-Gruber anastomosis there are median-to-ulnar crossover communications in the forearm.[10,16,17]

The clinical examination should begin with a visual and tactile examination for evidence of irregularities, tenderness, involuntary or voluntary movement, or atrophy. This examination should be followed by specific motor tasks to reveal a measurable neurologic deficit, and care is needed to differentiate between incongruous movements and legitimate pathologic processes. For example, muscle loss can be masked by compensatory adjacent muscle contractions.[1]

Medical Conditions

Investigation for other medical and nutritional conditions is necessary because unrecognized, organic conditions can lead to misdiagnosis and mismanagement. For example, alcoholic-nutritional neuropathy causes atrophy and weakness in the involved limb if left untreated. Other conditions include diabetes mellitus, peripheral vascular disease, hypothyroidism, hemophilia, and rheumatoid arthritis.

Electrodiagnostic Studies

Electrodiagnostic studies help determine the severity of the nerve injury and establish the baseline of the nerve's physiologic status and functional integrity.[18] In addition, sensory testing with electrophysiologic studies can confirm suspect findings, delineate the problem, or predict the possibility of spontaneous recovery.[10,14,19,20] These data can be influenced by a patient's adaptive response, temperature changes in the pain receptor area, thickness of the myelin sheath, or autonomic conditions.[21-27]

Nerve conduction velocity studies measure the velocity, intensity, and time that it takes an electrical signal to travel the length of the involved nerve. These studies are influenced by the type of instrument being used, the duration and intensity of the stimulation, and the relative distance of the internodes.[28-30] Conduction velocity normally decreases with age from myelin degeneration and changes in the internodal distances.[31] In addition, abnormal conduction test results do not necessarily correlate with a complete loss of sensation because a patient who has a sutured nerve may not fully display nerve conduction but can appreciate light touch.[32]

Nerve recordings are best measured directly proximal to a nerve lesion, and other interventions may hinder accurate recordings. For example, fluctuations in nerve waveforms can occur if a tourniquet is used or if a nerve is being dissected. Other confounding factors include extensive injuries, neurologic deficits, and the patient's age and associated medical conditions. Nerve conduction velocity is inconclusive and may demonstrate slow to below-normal values or fibrillations in neuropathies with wallerian degeneration or "dying back" in a portion of an axon.[33]

Many authors advise using nerve stimulation to ascertain if distal segments are innervated before surgical exploration.[34-37] However, in the absence of electrical conduction studies, surgical intervention within 3 months of the injury is warranted when there is loss of function in one or more neural elements.[10]

Imaging Studies

Frequently, peripheral nerve surgery is possible without any diagnostic imaging. A combination of a thorough history and physical examination with supplementary electrodiagnostic studies is often adequate. However, in cases where a mass lesion or tumor is suspected, MRI is necessary for a preoperative anatomic definition and for a differential diagnosis. Other imaging studies such as plain-film radiographs and CT scans play a role in diagnosing associated injuries that may complicate peripheral nerve surgery. When attempting to diagnose root avulsion, a CT scan with myelography is often helpful to visualize the pseudomeningocele.[16] However, even in the presence of a pseudomeningocele, the nerve rootlets may not be compromised.[38,39]

Timing of Surgery

Proper timing of surgery is crucial to restore neuronal function, to reverse end-organ dysfunction, and to facilitate recovery. Because neural regeneration occurs at the rate of approximately 1 inch per month, prompt reestablishment of neuronal connections is essential. In nonpenetrating, stretch, and compression injuries without evidence of transection, conservative management should be used for 3 months to allow for maximum recovery.[40]

In trauma or postsurgery, evidence of vascular injuries such as diminished extremity pulses, auscultation of bruits or thrills, or large pulsatile hemorrhage warrants immediate intervention.[41,42] A detailed clinical evaluation with careful documentation is needed, and further angiographic investigation may be used preoperatively or intraoperatively to outline the vascular anatomy and to rule out pseudoaneurysm. If available, MRI scans may be obtained to assess adjacent neurovascular structures, and a vascular surgeon should be consulted.

Immediate surgical intervention is also warranted when the patient presents with an acute neurologic deficit. If the nerve is nonviable and transected, nerve repair should be performed. Surgical exploration of gunshot wounds and other blunt transections can be delayed for 3 weeks when there is no evidence of neurovascular compromise.[40] However, if the neurologic function deteriorates, surgery should proceed without delay.

Techniques of Nerve Repair

Functional outcomes are significantly affected by proper procedure selection, and an understanding of axonal regeneration and neurotropic factors has led to advances in the treatment of these diseases.[43-47] Tube repair[13,48] (with silicone, collagen, and polyglycolic acid) and allograft nerve transplantation[49,50] are under investigation for restoring nerve continuity. The neurotropic factors produced by regenerating nerves are also being investigated for use in surgery or for implantation within the tubes.

Nerve allograft transplantation may be an alternative to autograft repair, but this technique requires immunosuppression to avoid graft rejection. The indications for and relative advantages and disadvantages of commonly used techniques of nerve repair are summarized in Table 135-1.

Postoperative Management

Postoperative care is essential for improving outcomes and avoiding complications, and monitoring for wound infections and neurologic improvement is important. Postoperative complications mainly arise in the surgical area and its adjacent structures. Routine wound cleansing with hydrogen peroxide followed by an application of an antibiotic ointment can reduce bacterial infection. Early mobilization is recommended because this measure improves circulation and prevents soft tissue adhesions, and physical and occupational therapy consultations are needed. Aggressive pain management is also important to recovery. Finally, prophylactic use of anticoagulants, such as intravenous dextran, intravenous or subcutaneous heparin, or oral aspirin, may prevent thrombosis at the microsurgical region.[51]

Rehabilitation

After a peripheral nerve injury or surgery, physical therapy and range-of-motion exercises will optimize the recovery of motor function and minimize tethering adhesion formation. The need for long-term rehabilitation is determined on an individual basis because functional recovery depends on the type and extent of injury, the capability of the nerve to regenerate, associated medical conditions, and the patient's motivation. The recovery process is slow and variable and may take as long as 5 years to complete. However, if functional recovery is not apparent after an appropriate rehabilitation period, other options such as arthrodesis and tendon transfers should be considered. Clearly, extensive injuries with

TABLE 135-1

Techniques of Nerve Repair

Technique	Indications	Advantages	Disadvantages
Epineural neurorrhaphy	Primary repair Proximal plexus lesion Polyfascicular nerve Monofascicular nerve	Simple technique Minimal intraneuronal scarring	Increased fascicular malalignment
Fascicular neurorrhaphy	Oligofascicular nerve Distal plexus lesion	More precise coaptation than epineural repair	Intraneuronal trauma Cannot resist tension
Interpositional graft	Primary coaptation cannot be achieved without tension	Establishes neuronal continuity without tension at suture line	"Suture line" delay at two sites
Free vascular graft	Recipient bed cannot maintain donor graft	Experimental evidence for faster axonal regeneration	Complex technique
Tube repair	Primary repair Alternative to nerve graft Painful neuroma	No donor site morbidity Simple technique Possible faster repair	Useful only for short nerve defect Extrusion of tube Kinking of tube
Nerve allograft transplantation	Severe extremity injury Composite tissue	Large nerve defect can be reconstructed	Limited clinical experience Need immunosuppression

multiple nerve lesions require a longer time to improve than isolated nerve injuries.

Complications of Peripheral Nerve Surgery

General Complications

Postoperative Wound Infections

Postoperative wound infections may occur and are particularly common in large exposures and lengthy operations. Meticulous sterile technique is the best preventative measure. In addition, preoperative prophylactic antibiotics and copious irrigation of the surgical site are recommended. The authors irrigate with a mixture of 500,000 U of polymyxin B with 50,000 U of bacitracin in 1 L of 0.9% NaCl.

To prevent infection, the dissection should be carried along intramuscular planes and along the nerve course, and wound closure should eliminate the dead spaces that can later become infected.[52] Postoperative wound care with an antibiotic ointment and daily inspections and dressing changes is needed. Postoperative antibiotic prophylaxis is used for 24 hours but should not be necessary beyond this point unless gross contamination was present.

Once an infection is present, culture-appropriate antibiotics are necessary. Surgical exploration of the infected wound may be needed for focal infections and abscesses; however, prevention is the best measure for this complication.

Postoperative Hematoma

Clinically significant postoperative hematoma is a rare but serious entity. This lesion may act as a nidus for infection, a source of postoperative scarring, and a compressive mass. Extensive and repetitive muscle dissection often creates fistulae, fascial planes, and bleeding points that can contribute to hematoma formation. Bipolar electrocautery is recommended for hemostasis because this modality minimizes thermal injury to the adjacent neurovascular structures and soft tissues.[10] Infected hematomas and adjacent tissues should be surgically excised and appropriate cultures and stains obtained.

Pulmonary Complications

Pulmonary complications can occur, especially if general anesthesia and lengthy operative time are necessary. These complications include atelectasis, pneumonia, pulmonary embolus, and acute respiratory distress syndrome.[53] Preoperative assessment of pulmonary risk factors aids in prevention, and postoperative pulmonary care assists in avoiding unnecessary complications. Specifically, pleural effusion, pneumothorax, hemothorax, and diaphragmatic paralysis can result from brachial plexus or thoracic outlet procedures. Each complication should be appropriately identified based on imaging and clinical judgment and should subsequently be treated appropriately.

Anatomic Variants

Anatomic variants of neural elements and non-neural structures are common and can be a source of iatrogenic injury (Table 135-2). These variations are usually encountered in certain areas, and a thorough knowledge of normal and aberrant anatomy is paramount.[1] For example, the nerve to the triceps commonly can arise off the dorsal spinal cord of the brachial plexus in the axilla. The subscapular nerve may arise from the posterior cord as part of a common trunk with the nerve to the subscapularis, or from the axillary nerve itself. The musculocutaneous nerve may arise from the median nerve or can be associated with the tendon of the pectoralis major muscle. Thus, when retracting, dividing, or reapproximating this tendon, the surgeon should pay close attention to preserving this nerve.

Complications of Surgery for Peripheral Nerve Tumors

Both benign and malignant tumors affect peripheral nerves.[54-57] These tumors cause motor and sensory symptoms through local mass effect with entrapment as well as compression of adjacent neurovascular structures. Before surgical

TABLE 135-2

Common Iatrogenic Nerve Injuries

Affected Nerve	Procedure
Spinal accessory	Lymph node biopsy
Transverse cervical or greater auricular	Lymph node biopsy
Brachial plexus	Radical neck dissection or mastectomy
Median	Carpal tunnel release or removal of ganglion
Radial	Arterial puncture or osteosynthesis
Ulnar	Removal of ganglion or wrist osteotomy
Superficial radial	Kirschner wire placement or removal of ganglion
Anterior interosseous	Internal fixation of forearm
Posterior interosseous	Osteosynthesis or cast
Sciatic	Hip arthroplasty
Femoral	Hip arthroplasty or femoral arterial graft
Genitofemoral or ilioinguinal	Hernia repair
Tibial	Injection or orthopedic procedure
Common peroneal	Surgery of the knee or removal of Baker cyst
Sural	Vein extirpation
Saphenous	Vein stripping

excision, it is prudent to consider all tumors malignant until confirmed by pathologic examination.

Patients with peripheral nerve tumors should be referred to specialized centers that have experience with peripheral nerve lesions. In general, nerve tumors should be removed when small to decrease the incidence of complications. Biopsies are not recommended in lesions likely to be benign because this may lead to nerve damage or hemorrhage.[58]

Intraoperative electrodiagnostic studies are mandatory to assess nerve viability and integrity and to determine if nerve grafting is necessary. During these studies, long-acting muscle relaxants should not be used, because these agents interfere with nerve conduction velocity and clinical findings.

Benign Peripheral Nerve Tumors

The most common benign peripheral nerve tumors are neurofibromas and schwannomas. Surgical management of schwannomas includes complete tumor excision, dissection beyond the entrapment site to release compression on adjacent structures, and minimization of postoperative edema. Using the surgical microscope, the tumor should be resected by gently separating it from the nerve bundles and neural elements with preservation of the uninvolved fascicles.

Neurofibromas can be multiple and fusiform, especially ones that arise from the nerve trunks, and surgery is needed for neurologic deterioration or intractable pain.[56,59] Resection typically does not result in loss of neurologic function or permanent disability. However, superficial neurofibroma resection may result in a temporary decrease in cutaneous sensation.[57]

Complications include infection, hematoma, and new neurologic deficits. The postoperative incision should be padded with soft wound dressings and inspected daily. Splint immobilization of the involved extremity for 1 to 2 weeks is recommended for nerve grafts to prevent stretching of the anastomosis. Postoperative pain management with appropriate pain medication minimizes discomfort. Finally, patient education is essential for proper medical care.

Malignant Peripheral Nerve Sheath Tumors

The appropriate diagnosis of malignant peripheral nerve sheath tumors is essential, and reliable clinical findings suggesting the presence of malignancy include a large tumor mass at initial presentation and rapid increase in size over a period of weeks to months.[56,60] Initial management should include a percutaneous nerve biopsy to provide histologic evidence of malignancy, because intraoperative frozen sections are frequently unreliable.[57] Once the diagnosis is established, radical resection of these lesions is recommended, and this resection needs to extend 5 to 10 cm beyond the tumor margin in a contiguous nerve if possible.

In tumor surgery, complications frequently result from a lack of surgical experience or understanding of tumor pathology. Successful excision depends on the origin and location of the tumor, and in many cases total resection is impossible to perform without causing severe functional loss. However, amputation is seldom warranted at the time of initial surgery.

Complications of Surgery for Entrapment Neuropathies

Entrapment syndromes are a diverse group of diseases with varying surgical interventions; although most surgical procedures are routine, complications can occur and can result in serious morbidity. For this reason, the specific cause should be determined before entrapment release.

Diagnostic Pitfalls

The preoperative assessment includes a thorough history and physical and electrophysiologic studies; misinterpretation of these findings may lead to delay in therapeutic or surgical interventions.[1,13,15] Associated medical conditions may include diabetes, hormonal diseases, connective tissue disorders, rheumatoid disease, arthritis, and metabolic deficiency. In addition, central nervous system pathologies such as syringomyelia, spinal cord lesions, and intracranial masses should be excluded before any surgical intervention.

Misinterpretation of physical signs can also lead to mismanagement. For example, the Hoffman-Tinel sign (a tingling sensation in the distribution of the median nerve over the hand) indicates axonal regeneration, but this sign may be absent in the early and late stages of nerve entrapment. Also, a negative Phalen sign may be due to a lack of pathology or to severe disruption of neural elements.

When a peripheral nerve is entrapped at more than one site such as would be present with carpal tunnel syndrome with cervical spine pathology, it is termed *double crush syndrome*. With this syndrome, the more distal compression is usually symptomatic. However, when the proximal compression is symptomatic, it is termed *reverse double crush syndrome*.

Electrodiagnostic studies are often used to confirm peripheral nerve entrapment neuropathies.[10,15] Inaccurate results may be due to anatomic variations, associated medical conditions, overlapping sensory innervation, errors in technical skill, and misinterpretation of the results. Examples of overlapping sensory innervation include the Riche-Cannieu anomaly (both branches of the median and ulnar nerves communicate) and the Martin-Gruber anastomosis (the median nerve or the anterior interosseous branch communicates with the ulnar nerve). Awareness of these pitfalls allows for correct interpretation and management.

Surgical Pitfalls

Meticulous surgical technique is essential to avoid complications, and complete decompression is necessary for a good outcome. Adequate surgical exposure includes a complete dissection along the course of the nerve distally and proximally until the lesion is well identified. Multiple or widespread dissections cause hemorrhaging, disrupt surrounding tissue, and create multiple, false fascial planes. In addition, careful hemostasis is essential because hemorrhage increases the risk of fibrous scar tissue formation and recurrent nerve compression.

Some lesions are unrecognizable or cannot be accurately localized with electrodiagnostic studies but will be detected intraoperatively. Aggressive radical decompression may carry more risks than benefits, and in many cases simple external or internal neurolysis is more beneficial to the patient.[61,62]

Cubital Tunnel Release

Cubital tunnel syndrome or so-called *tardy ulnar palsy* can have both traumatic and nontraumatic causes. The location of trauma is usually at the elbow, where the nerve is superficial. Nontraumatic palsies are caused by resting the elbow on hard surfaces for repetitive, prolonged periods or repetitively flexing or extending the elbow. In particular, elbow flexion elongates the nerve, accentuates the tethering effect, and ultimately increases intraneural pressure. Other nontraumatic causes include compression by aberrant bony structures or by space-occupying masses such as ganglia, synovial cysts, anomalous muscles, lipomas, or tumors.

Iatrogenic ulnar neuropathy may be caused by direct pressure on the nerve at the medial aspect of the elbow while positioning the patient, and thus appropriate cushioning is vital. Surgery on the ulnar nerve also can have significant complications. For example, nerve transposition procedures may exacerbate cubital tunnel syndrome because the recently transposed ulnar nerve can be compressed at the entry of the cubital tunnel, at the intermuscular septum, or by fascial slings.[10,15,63-65] This complication may be avoided by dissecting the nerve beyond the distal and proximal ends to permit relaxation of the nerve and to prevent kinking. Simple ulnar decompression is often preferred over transposition because it is relatively easy to perform and has fewer complications.[59,66,67]

Thoracic Outlet Syndrome

There are three approaches to thoracic outlet surgery: (1) supraclavicular, (2) dorsal scapular, and (3) transaxillary. The supraclavicular approach is preferred because it provides direct visualization of the brachial plexus roots and trunks, accessory ribs, neural structures, and fibromuscular bands. If the brachial plexus is tethered, the fibrous bands and accessory ribs should be released. Potential complications of this surgery include brachial plexus injury, hematoma, phrenic nerve palsy, pneumothorax, and scapular winging from a long thoracic nerve injury.

A dorsal subscapular approach is used for patients who have a large neck and large cervical ribs. The advantage of this technique is that it allows the surgeon to visualize the spinal nerves at their intervertebral foramina; however, this approach can cause damage to the long thoracic nerve, resulting in scapular winging. This approach may be used as a salvage procedure after failure of the transaxillary rib approach.[68]

The transaxillary approach is not recommended, because direct visualization of the plexus is not possible and removal of the first rib is required. In addition, the patient's arm has to be hyperabducted and the neurovascular structures retracted, which predisposes the brachial plexus to injury.

Standard Open Carpal Tunnel Release

Improper interpretation of the history and clinical examination is a common cause of inappropriate carpal tunnel release, and surgical intervention is difficult to justify without confirmation from electrodiagnostic studies. The Phalen maneuver and Tinel sign are consistent with carpal tunnel disorder, but abnormal nerve conduction velocity recordings and electromyography will confirm it.[10,15,69]

Iatrogenic injuries that result from anatomic variations are common in carpal tunnel surgeries. Caution should be taken not to injure the ulnar neurovascular bundle when retracting the retinaculum, or to damage the ulnar nerve and artery, which are located radial to the hook of the hamate. Injury to the superficial palmar arch during carpal tunnel release can also occur.[70,71] Beris et al. reported anatomic variations in the median nerve in 11 of 110 patients who underwent carpal tunnel release. The anomalous groups reported by these authors include variations of the thenar branch, accessory branches in the distal or proximal tunnel, and proximal division of the nerve.[72]

Persistent wrist pain after a carpal tunnel release indicates an incomplete resection of the transverse carpal ligament or an injury to the terminal branches of the anterior interosseous nerve.[13,71,73,74] These complications can be avoided by visualizing and inspecting the extended course of the transverse carpal ligament to ensure a complete ligamental transection. A small incision may be inadequate because the transverse carpal ligament may be located distally and is embedded in the palmar fascia. In addition, the distal edge of the ligament contains a ramus communicans located between the median and ulnar nerves that should be preserved.[75] The motor division of the median nerve also may course along the ligament and may come from a superficial or ulnar origin.[1,76] Thus, maintaining an extended incision along the ulnar aspect of the carpal ligament and an awareness of the motor branch during dissection are needed.[10] In rare cases, an anomalous ulnar nerve course can result in nerve transection as well.[77]

Minor or debilitating postoperative pain may be caused by the formation of a neuroma. Neuromas can occur with incisions at the thenar crease or transverse at the wrist.[71,76,78] When a neuroma is suspected, reexploration and resection of this lesion is indicated. Other causes of postoperative pain include injury to the dorsal sensory branch of the radial nerve, to the palmar branch of the digital nerve, or to the palmar cutaneous branch of the median nerve.[79] The palmar cutaneous branch is particularly at risk because of its inconsistent course.[1]

Postoperative carpal arch widening or flexor tendon bowstringing can occur, which may decrease grip strength.[71,74,80] Bony instability from ligamental transection also may compress the small cutaneous or periosteal nerves.[70,73,78] Although the free margins of the flexor tendon could be resutured, the risk of nerve injury is high.[10] The best preventive measure is early wrist splinting after surgery.[73]

Anterior interosseous nerve injury may result from retractor pressure beneath the distal antebrachial fascia, so careful placement is necessary.[13] In addition, a Colles fracture or forearm crush injury may significantly compress the distal antebrachial fascia.[1]

Keloid formation is a concern for both cosmetic reasons and its potential for nerve entrapment, and no particular incision reduces the risk of this complication. [73,74,81] Because keloid resection will likely lead to further keloid formation, other therapies such as cortisone cream, local anesthesia, analgesics, and reassurance are recommended.

Endoscopic Carpal Tunnel Release

Endoscopic techniques for carpal tunnel release are becoming increasingly popular because this procedure has a smaller incision, faster recovery, less pain, less scar tissue, and a shorter recovery time. However, the limited surgical exposure places additional risk on the neurovascular structures and may lead to incomplete resection of the transverse carpal ligament.

Ulnar neuropraxia due to pressure or retraction may result from the transbursal approach of the dual-portal Chow technique. In addition, a complete transection of the ulnar nerve may occur if the trocar is accidentally placed into the Guyon canal.[82] Thus, the endoscopic trocar should be inserted anterior to the superficial palmar arch and midpalmar digital nerve. Other complications of the Chow technique include tissue scarring, pseudoaneurysm and injury to the superficial palmar arch, median nerve injury, flexor digitorum superficialis laceration, and reflex sympathetic dystrophy (RSD).[83]

In the Brown dual-portal technique, common postoperative complications are superficial palmar arch injury, transient paresthesias, and RSD.[84-86] In the extrabursal approach (subligamentous dual-portal technique) developed by Resnick and Miller, the flexor tendon is dissected beneath the transverse ligament.[87] To avoid injuring the median nerve branches, an incision can be made at the ulnar margin and a Freer elevator used to delineate the median nerve from the carpal tunnel ligament before inserting the endoscopic trocar.

The single-portal Agee technique carries the risk of injury from blind sharp dissection through the carpal tunnel. The subsequent modified single-portal Agee endoscopic system allows blade visualization to reduce iatrogenic injury. The reported complication rate of this procedure is 1.83%, whereas the failure rate is 1.44%.[32,85,88-95] Other possible complications associated with the Agee technique include postoperative infection, hematoma, pillar causalgia, laceration of the flexor digitorum sublimis, and RSD.[93] The incidence of RSD can be as high as 5% and may be even higher with coexistent Dupuytren disease.[73,74,79,96]

A comprehensive review of 8068 endoscopic carpal tunnel release (ECTR) procedures by Jimenez et al.[93] demonstrated that complication, failure, and success rates are similar for both endoscopic and standard open procedures. The retrospective questionnaire revealed an overall complication rate of 2.6%.[93] Postoperative complications associated with artery, nerve, and tendon injuries were relatively higher in ECTR (1.6%) than in open carpal tunnel release (OCTR; 0.8%), and no statistically significant differences in persistent and recurrent symptoms were found in these two groups (ECTR 7.5% vs. OCTR 7.7%).

A successful outcome in ECTR depends on appropriate patient selection, proper identification of anatomic landmarks, and adequate endoscopic visualization. Contraindications to ECTR include previous fracture, cysts (ganglion or synovial), neuromas, aberrant anatomy, sepsis, and previously failed carpal tunnel release.[93] In addition, experience with these techniques plays a role in outcome. The option exists for conversion from ECTR to OCTR when encountering technical difficulty or poor visualization.

Brachial Plexus Surgery

Brachial plexus surgery may result in a variety of postoperative complications owing to the complex anatomy and close proximity of vital structures. A thorough knowledge of the relevant anatomy and familiarity with the procedures are needed. Complications may be divided into nerve, vascular, and orthopedic injuries as well as wound complications. Commonly reported nerve injuries include the phrenic nerve, the spinal accessory nerve, and the musculocutaneous nerve. Like other surgeries, postoperative infection and hematoma may result, but left supraclavicular brachial plexus exploration may also lead to damage to the thoracic duct and a lymphocele.

Vascular injuries include both venous and arterial sources. Most small veins may be sacrificed unless the patient had previous radiation or lymph node dissections, which may predispose the patient to lymphedema. The larger veins should be preserved to prevent upper extremity swelling. Any significant arterial injuries should be immediately repaired by a vascular surgeon, and these injuries are more likely with scarring from previous explorations.[40]

Other Peripheral Nerve Surgeries

Any peripheral nerve surgery carries the risk of nerve damage. Other such procedures include decompression of the sciatic, peroneal, tibial, femoral, and inguinal nerves. In sciatic nerve surgery, postoperative muscular atrophy, vascular injury, and nerve damage may occur. In particular, the superior and inferior gluteal arteries must be preserved because transection may lead to life-threatening hemorrhage from vessel retraction. Patients with peroneal and tibial nerve surgery also may have complicated postoperative courses because of pain and swelling for months after surgery. Procedures directed at the femoral, inguinal, and other associated groin nerves may also have surgery-related complications. In particular, the complex anatomy and frequent overlapping distributions in this region may lead to improper decompression, and the anatomic location is more prone to infection as well as lymphoceles.[58]

Pain of Peripheral Nerve Origin

Pain prevention is essential to the treatment of peripheral nerve problems.[15,36] Neuropathic pain results from neural injury in the central or peripheral nervous system and is characterized by paresthesia or numbness in a specific distribution. This pain may also lack an identifiable source.[97,98] Postoperative pain is a possible complication of peripheral nerve surgery and, as with other complications, the best method of treatment is prevention. Careful dissection and an anatomic awareness will prevent transection of the nerve, and electrocoagulation should be avoided to prevent neuroma formation.[99]

When a complete or partial cutaneous nerve laceration is the source of pain, immediate repair is necessary. When an intact nerve is the source of pain, neurolysis can successfully relieve symptoms.[100] Severe postoperative pain should be investigated immediately because it may be the source or sign of significant postoperative complications, and precise localization is necessary. For example, a stocking distribution of pain may be a sign of vascular injury.

Sympathetic involvement or "posttraumatic pain events" include paresthesia and intolerance.[101] These symptoms may progress to the pain syndrome of RSD, which is hypothesized to be related to impaired macrocirculatory and microcirculatory hemodynamics (nutritional deficiency).[101] Thus, the diagnosis is aided by evaluating the patient's hemodynamic and thermoregulatory components.[102-104] Nutritional homeostasis is reestablished by addressing the vascular injury.

Pain in the form of claudication may be a sign of vascular injury, and repair within 24 to 72 hours is necessary to prevent edema. Thrombosis also may produce segmental ischemia with subsequent neuropathic pain. However, these pathologies can be masked if adequate collateral circulation is present.[105]

Treatment of Peripheral Nerve Pain

Peripheral nerve pain may be treated by relieving a local trigger point and maintaining range of motion by therapy. This point may be identified by palpation and treated with 0.5% lidocaine hydrochloride using sterile technique. If the anesthetic block is ineffective a peripheral epineural infusion block can be considered, but this procedure can result in irritation or tissue necrosis of the injection site. Contraindications to upper extremity peripheral-epineural infusion are pain persisting for more than 3 months and contralateral pain involvement in an unaffected extremity.

The stellate ganglion is found in the neck region and supplies sympathetic innervation to the head, neck, and upper extremities. A nerve block in this area aids diagnosis and treatment for neuropathic pain in the head, neck, and upper extremities. However, complications of stellate ganglion block include respiratory depression and hypotension due to local anesthetic injection into a dural cuff. Furthermore, if local anesthetic is injected into a vertebral artery, it precipitates seizure and in some instances can cause loss of consciousness.[98]

Peripheral Nerve Biopsy

Nerve biopsy is used to diagnose a variety of peripheral nerve pathologies. The sural and popliteal nerves are commonly used for this purpose. Postoperative wound complications include infection, hematoma, and neuroma formation. Hilton et al. compiled their results with those of previous studies and found postoperative rates of 30% for pain, 40% for paresthesia, 33% for dysesthesia, and 8% for wound issues. These data highlight the importance of appropriate patient selection and indications for biopsy.[106]

Complications of Other Surgeries and Injuries Involving Peripheral Nerves

Many medical and surgical interventions place peripheral nerves at risk, and injury to these nerves can be a common complication. Common procedures that can injure the nerves include patient positioning, retraction during surgery, medication injection, local nerve blocks, and direct sectioning of the nerve during surgery. Postoperative hematomas are a potential source of peripheral nerve injury. Medical conditions such as diabetes, tobacco use, and hypertension can also contribute to poor outcomes. One study showed that the incidence of perioperative peripheral nerve injuries was 0.03%.[107]

Kömürcü et al. reported 82 cases of treatment of iatrogenic nerve injury and showed that nearly any nerve can be at risk. They treated their patients with a variety of conservative and surgical methods and emphasized the importance of timely diagnosis and an individualized, multidisciplinary approach.[108]

Complications of Surgery for Traumatic Nerve Injury

Traumatic peripheral nerve injuries can cause temporary or permanent nerve dysfunction as well as pain, and a prompt and accurate assessment is necessary. In many cases, immediate surgical intervention may be the most important strategy because nerve fiber damage can be irreversible when ischemia lasts more than 6 hours.[7,109] Until confirmed by intraoperative findings, it is prudent to diagnose traumatic peripheral nerve injuries as neurotmesis.

Most traumatic injuries fall into three categories: (1) laceration of the nerve, caused by knife wounds, motor vehicle accidents, or work-related injuries; (2) projectile injuries, such as gunshot wounds; and (3) dislocation, fracture, and traction injuries as can be found with sports injuries. Functional outcomes vary depending on the injury. For example, digital nerves are capable of regenerating and may recover sensory function to near-normal status.[27]

Laceration

In sharp nerve transections with avulsion, the current recommendation is to secure the nerve stumps to the adjacent soft tissues and return at 2 months for primary nerve repair. At that time, the normal and aberrant neural anatomy will be demarcated and the appropriate therapy may be selected. Laceration of the nerve (Seldon neurotmesis or Sunderland lesion V) can cause complete loss of nerve function and typically does not result in spontaneous recovery. Intraoperative nerve action potential recordings provide data on the functional status of the injured nerve and aid the surgeon in deciding whether to resect the injured nerve.

Complications after nerve repair may have several sources. For example, applying too much tension to the nerve ends may alter intracellular nutrition, change endoneural fluid pressurization, and cause scarring at the suture line.[9,110-112] Repair can be further compromised if the cross-sectional area of the nerve is diminished by high tension. Unsuccessful surgery may result from failure to resect the nerve stumps to normal, viable fascicular neural tissue or failure to recognize and resect a neuroma in continuity.

Projectile Injuries

Ballistic missile wounds cause crushing and laceration, shock waves, and cavitation.[113] Handguns typically create low-velocity shock waves, creating neurapraxia and axonotmesis, but shotgun wounds cause a higher percentage of peripheral nerve injuries because of the damage to neurovascular structures. These patients typically have a poor prognosis, but preventing further complications involves the four *Do Nots:*

1. Do not cut down both saphenous veins, because one saphenous vein may be needed for vascular grafting.
2. Do not insert intravenous lines into the injured limb.
3. Do not use a tourniquet on the injured limb.
4. Do not attempt to clamp the bleeding wound blindly, because of the risk of severing or lacerating the functioning neurovascular structures.

To avoid further complications and peripheral nerve injury, wound exploration and fasciotomy are necessary for ischemia greater than 4 hours or compartment pressures greater than 40 mm Hg. In addition, contact wounds, particularly shotgun injuries, are at high risk for infection, and intravenous antibiotics, usually a first-generation cephalosporin, should be administered and continued for 3 to 5 days.

With all appropriate interventions, spontaneous recovery has been observed in 90% of nerves 3 to 9 months after an injury, and in some cases has occurred as long as 11 months after an injury.[114] The functional recovery rate is faster in low-distal extremity injuries than it is in high-proximal extremity injuries, and the prognosis in low-velocity gunshot wounds is similar to that for high-velocity injuries, which is a 1- to 4-month recovery period for neurapraxia and 4 to 9 months for axonotmesis.[115]

Fracture and Dislocation

Patients presenting with an upper extremity fracture must be evaluated for nerve damage because 95% of upper extremity fractures have associated nerve injuries.[116] Humeral fractures frequently cause radial nerve damage, and complete medial nerve resection can rarely result from a Colles fracture.[117] The median nerve is also susceptible to pressure as it courses the carpal tunnel and may be entrapped by bony fractures, edema, or hemorrhage. This knowledge is important because surgical reduction can be complicated by further damage to the nerves.

The time frame for spontaneous recovery of clinical function after a fracture is 1 to 4 months, and 3 to 6 months after a traction injury.[21] The chance for spontaneous recovery is inversely related to the severity of the nerve injury.[25]

Iatrogenic Nerve Injuries

Iatrogenic injuries, those caused by surgical treatment, are the most common complications of peripheral nerve surgery, yet are frequently avoidable. Such injuries can be minor, in which case they may be resolved, or they can be severe and permanently debilitating.

Tourniquet Injury

Tourniquets are commonly used for hemostasis in severe extremity injuries and to improve visualization. However, tourniquet-induced peripheral nerve complications can result even with proper use because this device applies direct pressure on a nerve.[10,13,118] The most commonly injured nerve in the upper extremity is the radial nerve.[1,119]

The most important factor is tourniquet time because prolonged pressure creates considerable compression of the peripheral nerves. Although some surgeons advise releasing tourniquet pressure after 1 to 3 hours of surgery,[1,112,120] 30 minutes of high cuff pressure can produce palsies.[96,112] A tourniquet pressure not exceeding 70 mm Hg above the patient's systolic blood pressure should be sufficient to maintain hemostasis, and the risk of damage is significantly increased when the tourniquet is placed below the elbow or knee.[112] Electrophysiologic studies show changes in nerve action potentials and frequent fibrillations 5 to 10 minutes after pressure is applied, so deflation of the cuff for 10 minutes each hour is recommended to prevent nerve injury.

Tourniquet-induced peripheral nerve injuries are usually mild and spontaneously resolve within 3 to 6 months. Prognosis varies because these injuries are difficult to assess accurately and qualitatively.[1,13,82,112] Conservative management includes limb rest and appropriate physical therapy. Surgical exploration is necessary in cases of serious and irreversible damage or no evidence of functional improvement.

Patient Malpositioning

Malpositioning may result in peripheral nerve injury and even permanent neurologic deficits, but this complication is entirely avoidable. Malpositioning leads to peripheral nerve compression against rigid surfaces like aberrant joints or osseoligamentous structures.[112] However, no correlation has been found between the degree of compression damage and surgical duration; nerve compression injury has been reported in surgeries that lasted 1 hour, as well as those lasting up to 4 hours.[1,121-124] Nerve compression may range from a low-grade stretching that interrupts the blood supply to high-grade lesions with associated hemorrhage and necrosis, and the results of electrographic studies have varied from slowed conduction to complete block.[125]

High-risk patients include those who are thin and of small stature.[10] Several other factors can predispose a patient to nerve compression, including bony fractures, aberrant anatomy, compaction of the cervical ribs, associated medical conditions, a history of peripheral neuropathies, anticoagulant use, use of skeletal muscle relaxants during anesthesia, or physiologic hypothermia.[1,121-124]

Several sites and positions have an increased risk of nerve compression. For example, the superficial course of the radial and ulnar nerves in relationship to the shaft of the humerus is of concern, and when the arms are secured at the patient's sides, they should be fully padded with foam or soft towels. Improper arm positioning can also occur when the patient is placed in a lateral rotation position, internal rotation, external rotation, abduction, arm-shoulder distraction, pronation, or supination. The patient's arms should not be abducted further than the head for a long period and should never be crossed, because these positions can injure the upper brachial plexus.[10] Such injuries usually present as painless motor weakness.[125]

When the patient is placed in a lateral decubitus position, there is significant risk to the peripheral nerves in both the upper and lower extremities. The patient's legs should be placed on soft pillows and secured with a leg strap. The leg strap should be positioned away from the fibular head, where the peroneal nerve is superficially located. In addition, one must realize that the femoral cutaneous nerve is located adjacent to the pelvic protuberance and the sciatic nerve is confined within the pelvic outlet region. Injury to the saphenous and sciatic nerves has also been reported in patients who have been placed in a lithotomy position.[15] Nearly all peripheral nerves are vulnerable to injury, and a review by Winfree and Kline extensively details the many different nerve compressions.[125]

If a compressive neuropathy develops, recovery depends on the severity and extent of the injury. Complete recovery can be expected within 6 months in 90% of cases.[124] Mild forms of peripheral neuropathy, such as a first-degree conduction block, have better recovery rates than do severe forms. If the patient exhibits signs of compressive neuropathy, a careful history and physical examination in combination with electrodiagnostic studies are necessary, and if neurologic deficits fail to improve, surgical exploration is indicated.

Injection Injury

Various pharmacologic agents have been found to cause injection injury when inadvertently introduced into a nerve. A thorough knowledge of nerve anatomy and attention to needle trajectory are essential to avoid this complication. The highest risk of nerve damage comes from epineural, intraneural, and intrafascicular injections, and misdirected injections can have serious consequences.[1,13,126]

Specific nerve injury examples include radial nerve injury during arterial line placement, sciatic nerve damage from intramuscular injections, and brachial plexus injury from internal jugular vein cannulation. Other vulnerable structures include the cervical sympathetic trunk, the C5-8 nerve roots, cranial nerve XI, the phrenic nerve, and the recurrent laryngeal nerve.

Neurologic sequelae manifest within minutes of an injection, and the subsequent pain can be transient or permanently debilitating. A delayed onset implies an injury to the surrounding structures with subsequent swelling and nerve compression. If an injection injury results in an incomplete neurologic deficit, conservative management should be initiated for the first 2 months. Surgical intervention is indicated for persistent neurologic deficit, functional debilitation, and intractable pain. Intraoperative nerve conduction studies should be performed to determine if graft repair or neurolysis is indicated.

Injury from Regional Anesthesia

Local nerve blocks can have complications that cause injury to any peripheral nerve. In a review by Borgeat and Blumenthal, three types of injury were shown to occur: axonal sideration (neurapraxia), axonal interruption with sheath preservation (axonotmesis), and fascicular interruption (neurotmesis). The reported incidence of long-term complications was approximately 0.2%, but these complications may be a significant source of malpractice insurance claims. Any anesthetic agent is potentially neurotoxic if used without proper precautions.[127]

Newer studies have examined postoperative neurologic complications with the use of ultrasound. Fredrickson and Kilfoyle examined peripheral nerve complications in ultrasonography-guided local anesthetic nerve blocks for extremity orthopedic surgery in 911 patients. They found an immediate complication rate of 8.2% and a 6-month rate of 0.6%. The most common symptoms were numbness, tingling, and pain. Weakness was a rare complication.[128]

Misdirected Surgical Procedures

During surgical exploration, exposed nerves should be carefully protected to prevent iatrogenic stretching or tension injuries, nerve laceration, or intraneuronal physiologic damage. Most iatrogenic injuries are associated with orthopedic, trauma, or hand surgery.[129] For example, during open reduction of a fractured humerus, the radial nerve may be injured, and common procedures such as knee and hip arthroplasties and knee arthroscopy can place many of the lower extremity nerves at risk.[130] Minor surgical procedures such as lymph node biopsy in the dorsal triangle of the neck may transect or stretch the spinal accessory nerve.[29] In addition, cutaneous sensory nerves are often damaged during surgeries on wrist ganglions, operations at the elbow (antebrachial cutaneous nerves), decompression of the median nerve (palmar cutaneous branches of the median nerve), surgeries for varicose veins (saphenous nerve and branches), and surgeries to treat Dupuytren disease (digital nerves).[131]

Retractor blades are also a common cause of nerve injury.[123,132,133] For example, damage to the femoral nerve may be caused by the pelvic retractors used in gynecologic surgery.[129] Inexperience with peripheral nerve tumor surgery also can lead to significant complications. This is especially true for malignant tumor resections because of the more intrinsic nature of the lesion and its adherence to adjacent neural structures and other soft tissues.

Medicolegal Aspects of Iatrogenic Injuries

Iatrogenic peripheral nerve injuries may have medicolegal implications, and although many of these injuries are unavoidable, a few can result from negligence. To avoid further damage, appropriate management after injury is essential. This management begins with timely recognition and referral for the injury because outcome improves with prompt interventions.[134,135]

Despite aggressive management, functional recovery may be difficult to predict, but general trends can be identified. First, spontaneous recovery is more likely with incomplete lesions, but the recovery process is slow. Second, if operative intervention is necessary, a peripheral nerve specialist is most appropriate. Finally, repair should take place within the first 3 or 4 months after injury to produce optimal results.[134,135]

Summary

To avoid complications in peripheral nerve surgery, the peripheral nerve surgeon must

- Have a thorough understanding of normal and variant anatomy
- Perform a complete clinical assessment
- Correctly identify and localize lesions and interpret electrodiagnostic studies
- Anticipate complications that may arise during surgery and know how to manage them
- Position the patient properly during surgery
- Execute surgical techniques effectively

KEY REFERENCES

Kline DG, Hudson AR: *Nerve injuries: operative results for major nerve injuries, entrapments, and tumors*, Philadelphia, 1995, WB Saunders.

Kömürcü F, Zwolak P, Benditte-Klepetko H, et al: Management strategies for peripheral iatrogenic nerve lesions. *Ann Plast Surg* 54:135–142, 2005.

Reisner GG, Tindall SC: Complications of peripheral nerve surgery. In Benzel EC, editor: *Spine surgery*, Philadelphia, 1999, Churchill Livingstone, pp 947–959.

Russell SM, Kline DG: Complication avoidance in peripheral nerve surgery: preoperative evaluation of nerve injuries and brachial plexus exploration—part 1. *Neurosurgery* 59(4 Suppl 2):441–448, 2006.

Russell SM, Kline DG: Complication avoidance in peripheral nerve surgery: injuries, entrapments, and tumors of the extremities—part 2. *Neurosurgery* 59(4 Suppl 2):449–457, 2006.

Wilbourn AJ: Iatrogenic nerve injuries. *Neurol Clin* 16:55–82, 1998.

Winfree CJ, Kline DG: Intraoperative positioning nerve injuries. *Surg Neurol* 63:5–18, 2005.

REFERENCES

The complete reference list is available online at expertconsult.com.

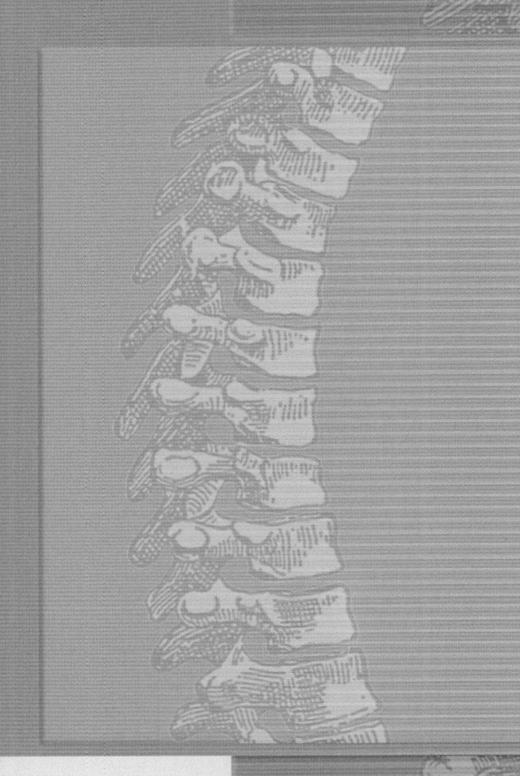

SECTION 5

Spinal Instrumentation

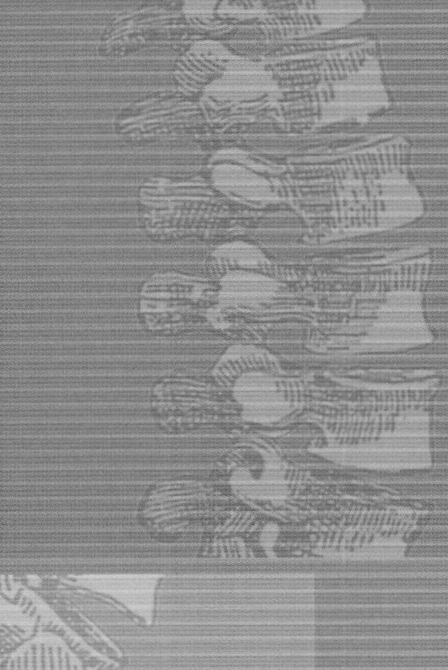

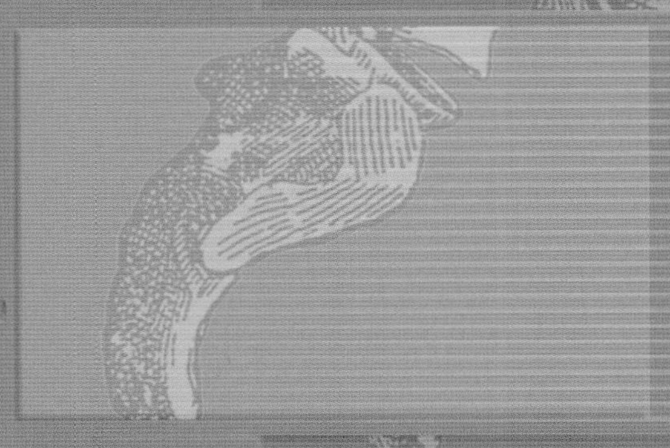

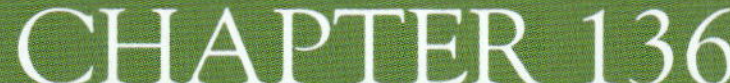
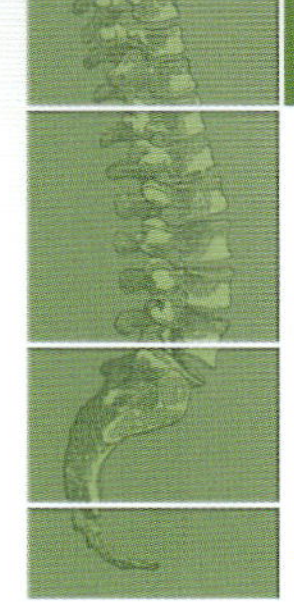

CHAPTER 136

Basic Biomechanically Relevant Anatomy

Eric Klineberg | Jeffrey C. Wang | John Butler |
Lisa A. Ferrara | Edward C. Benzel

Spinal instrumentation has led to many significant advances in how we treat our patients. This treatment may range from the early mobilization after operative treatment of spinal fractures to the prevention of late iatrogenic cervical kyphosis from laminectomy. Selecting the appropriate fixation techniques and instrumentation can be a complex problem. Often, the final surgical solution is one that balances the specific patient requirements, the spinal instrumentation available, and the biomechanics of the spinal pathology. Before we can begin to discuss the biomechanics of instrumentation, we must first understand the biomechanics of the relevant spinal anatomy.

Spine biomechanics is the application of basic engineering and physics principles to a biologic structure, the spinal column. It allows the surgeon to reduce the complex movement and forces on the spine to some basic concepts. The anatomy of the spine must be placed in biomechanical terms, such that the role of the each component is understood in relation to the overall structure and function of the spine. The spine is a complex load-bearing structure made up of bones, joints, ligaments, and muscles arranged to effectively dissipate forces and allow a physiologic range of motion, while at the same time protecting the spinal cord.

Stability may be compromised through trauma, tumor, degenerative disease, or iatrogenic artifacts. Spine surgery itself can often be a destabilizing process, and the surgeon must use instrumentation to restore stability. Spinal implants are designed to impart a force to the spine. To apply instrumentation appropriately, a thorough understanding of the basic biomechanics must be attained. Our goals in this chapter are to introduce the basic concepts of biomechanics and apply them to normal and pathologic spinal anatomy.

Biomechanics

Biomechanics involves the application of mechanical engineering principles to biologic problems. It is the science of the action of forces on the human body. It refers to the direction and quality of force as well as to the mechanical properties of the biologic material. It that way, it is possible to describe the force vector of a tendon as well as the plastic deformation of bone. Spine biomechanics is extremely complex, because it must deal with the local as well as global mechanics of the spine. This can be further complicated by any pathologic dysfunction of the spinal column. To appreciate the complexities, it is necessary to first consider some basics about biomechanics, including coordinates, vectors, and moduli.

Cartesian Coordinate System

The right-handed Cartesian coordinate system is routinely used in spine biomechanics as a system of reference. This system consists of three axes: the x-axis, the y-axis, and the z-axis. Translational and rotational movement can occur along or about these three axes. Translational movements are positive if they occur in the positive direction of the axis and negative if they occur in the negative direction. Rotational movements are considered positive in the clockwise direction when viewed from the origin and negative when counterclockwise from the same viewpoint. The right-handed Cartesian coordinate system as applied to the spine places the x-axis in the dorsal-to-ventral plane (axial plane), the y-axis in the right-to-left plane (sagittal plane), and the z-axis in the rostral-to-caudal plane (coronal plane). This placement results in positive moments with flexion, left-to-right lateral bending, and right axial rotation. Using these coordinates, any point can be defined by both its location and its rotation.

Vectors, Scalars, Bending Moments, and the Instantaneous Axis of Rotation

A vector is a force oriented in a fixed direction in three-dimensional space (as defined by the right-handed Cartesian coordinate system previously discussed). It possesses both magnitude and direction (i.e., force and velocity), and it may be broken down into its component vectors. A scalar is a quantity that is direction independent and possesses only magnitude (i.e., time, volume). A bending moment occurs when a force acts on a lever or moment arm. A bending moment, when applied to a point in space, results in a tendency to rotate about an axis. When these principles are applied to a vertebral body, the three-dimensional axis about which a bending moment causes the body to rotate; this is known as the *instantaneous axis of rotation* (IAR). The IAR is the axis about which a vertebral segment rotates at any given instant, and the IAR itself does not move during this instant of rotation or translation. It may be considered a fulcrum about which a segment moves. When a body moves in a plane, there is a point in the body or some extension of it that does not move, and the axis that passes perpendicular to the plane of motion and through this point is the IAR (as defined by White and Panjabi[1]). The IAR becomes the center of the Cartesian coordinate system used to define the motion. The IAR is dynamic, and as spinal movement occurs, the IAR of each involved segment moves. The location of the IAR depends on the manner in which it is determined and the theoretical foundation on which it is based, and it is therefore subject to error.

Free Body Analysis

Free body diagrams use the forces, moments, and IAR on various anatomic structures to isolate those forces and assign vectors, so that all the forces are represented. In that way, complex problems can be reduced to their component parts. It is then possible, for example, to determine the force necessary to stand upright or the increase in paraspinal and gluteal force required by leaning forward as in kyphosis. These diagrams help one to understand these complex problems. They also form the basis for understanding why tension band disruption may lead to kyphosis in either the cervical or lumbar spine. As the moment arm moves forward and increases, even small amounts of kyphosis (or loss of lordosis) can have large effects on the forces acting on the spine (Fig. 136-1).

Newton's Laws

Spine surgery involves the application of force to the spine. Fundamental to understanding the stresses withstood by the spine is the concept of action and reaction.[2] Newton's three laws of motion describe how objects respond to external forces.

1. The first law is the law of inertia, which states that if an object is subject to no net force, it maintains a constant velocity.
2. The second law is the law of superimposition of forces, which states that the momentum of an object is equal in magnitude and direction to the vector sum of the forces acting on it.
3. The third law is the law of conservation of momentum. which states that when two objects collide, the overall momentum is constant such that for every action there is an opposite but equal reaction.

As the spine is subject to various loads, force couples are created (based on the third law of motion), and the vertebral segments may fail. When applying forces to the spine, these same concepts need to be considered. All instrumentation will fail in time, and therefore the bony alignment must respect the body and gravitational forces or it will fail more quickly. The biomechanical environment must maintain a load balance between the implant and tissue environment to improve implant longevity.

Hooke's Law and Stress-Strain Curves

When external forces act on a solid at rest, the solid is deformed. According to Hooke's law, for small displacements, the size of the deformation is proportional to the deforming force. For solids within the elastic zone, the relationship between deformation and force is linear. To make sense of Hooke's law then as it applies to the spine, the concepts of stress-strain curves and deformation need to be expanded. Deformation of a solid can be either elastic or plastic. Elastic and plastic are defined by recovery once the deforming force is removed, and they exist on a spectrum that can be best illustrated with a deformation curve (Fig. 136-2). When a solid is subject to an external or deforming force, Hooke's law applies only when the load and deformation occur within the elastic zone of the solid. The elastic zone is defined by elastic deformation, when a solid totally recovers after removal of a stress. Deformation continues to be proportional to the deforming force until the

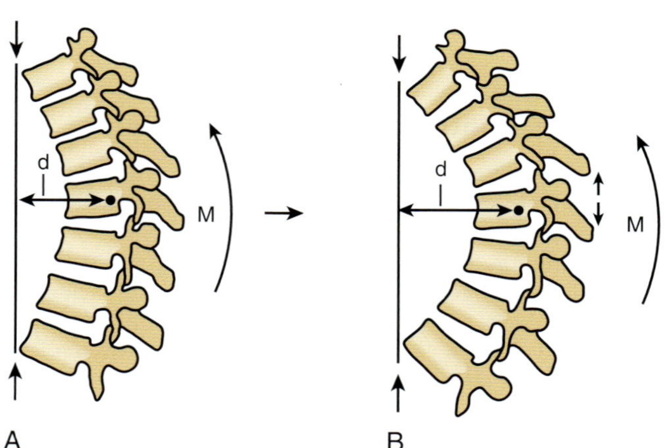

FIGURE 136-1. "Deformity begets deformity." A kyphotic deformity is pictured with moment arm (*d*). As an axial load is applied (*straight arrows*), a bending moment (*M*) is created (*curved arrow*) (**A**). As the kyphosis increases, the force is applied at a greater distance from the axis of rotation. This larger moment arm results in a larger bending moment and, ultimately, increased kyphosis (**B**). (From Benzel EC, editor: *Biomechanics of spine stabilization,* Rolling Meadows, IL, 2001, American Association of Neurological Surgeons.)

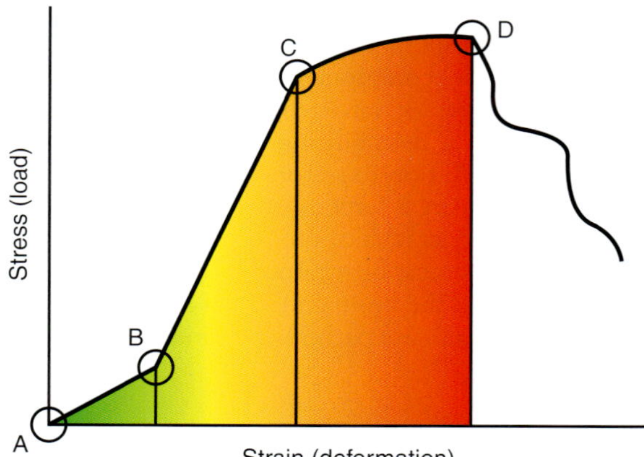

FIGURE 136-2. A typical stress-strain curve for a biologic tissue, such as a ligament. Between points A and B is the neutral zone. Between points B and C is the elastic zone. When the elastic limit (yield point) C is reached, permanent deformation can occur (permanent set). Between points C and D is the plastic zone, where a permanent set occurs. Past point D, failure occurs and the load diminishes. The colored portion under the curve (between points A and D) represents strength, whereas the orange-to-red portion (beneath the C to D portion of the curve) represents resilience. (From Benzel EC, editor: *Biomechanics of spine stabilization,* Rolling Meadows, IL, 2001, American Association of Neurological Surgeons.)

elastic limit of the solid is reached and the linear relationship between force and deformation no longer exists. Beyond the elastic limit of a material is the plastic zone, and this is the zone in which the solid acquires permanent deformation and does not completely recover once the stress is removed. As force continues to be applied, eventually the point of failure is reached. On a stress-strain curve (see Fig. 136-2), the area under the curve represents the amount of energy absorbed and the ultimate strength of a material (amount of energy required to reach failure). The neutral zone is an area of nonengagement where force is applied but deformation is minimal. It precedes the linear area of the curve.

Elastic Modulus

The elastic modulus is a constant that is defined by and characteristic of a given material. It is an indicator of deformability of a specific material. The modulus of elasticity is defined as stress-strain where stress is the force applied to an object and strain is the response of the object to the force. Strain is linear (normal) or angular (shear) and is manifest as a change in length or angle of an object subjected to a load. It reflects the force-resisting ability of a material, whether it is tensile or compressive forces in normal strain or angular deformation resistance in shear strain. Stress is defined as the force per unit area applied to an object (see the equation in Section Modulus and Moment of Inertia).

There are three types of elastic moduli:

1. Young's modulus, which measures the elastic properties of an object when it is stretched or compressed
2. Shear modulus, which measures the shear deformation that occurs when transverse forces of opposite direction are applied at opposing faces of an object
3. Bulk modulus, which measures the deformation that occurs when a solid is squeezed

Section Modulus and Moment of Inertia

The section modulus is a concept that is calculated and used to define the strength of an object. It is applicable here with regard to spinal implants and instrumentation as an indicator of the overall strength and, more importantly, potential failure of an implant. The section modulus or strength of a screw is exponentially related to the diameter of the screw. As this diameter increases, the strength increases by the power to the fourth. This concept is also applicable to plate design. The strategy for hole placement for screws must be carefully designed because the holes reduce the section modulus. This then causes failure of the plate at a lower load (Fig. 136-3).

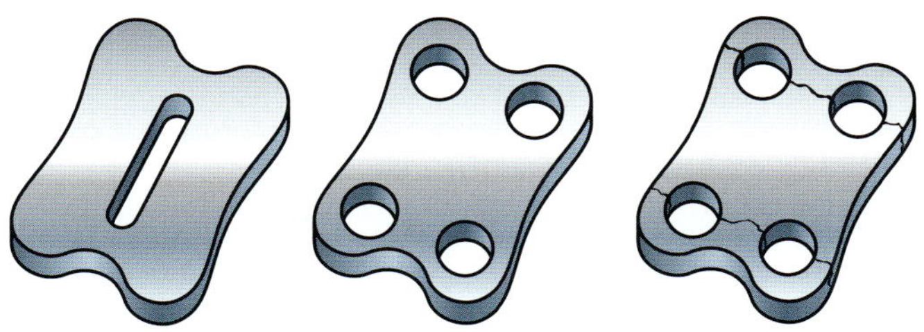

FIGURE 136-3. Cervical plate section modulus. Thicker plates have a high section modulus and therefore better fatigue strength. Holes or slots cut into the plate decrease this modulus (*left* and *center*), and if the plate is thin enough and with enough force, the plate may fail (*right*).

Other important factors relating to implant failure or potential failure that need to be considered are potential force applications (moment arms, loads, bending moments). Stress defines the relationship of section modulus and bending moment. It represents the force per unit area applied to an object and is defined as

$$T = M/Z$$

where T is stress, M is bending moment, and Z is section modulus. The bending moment (M) is also defined by an equation:

$$M = F \times D$$

where M is bending moment, F is the force applied, and D is the distance of the moment arm through which the force is applied.

The stiffness of an object (implant) is the resistance to deformability. It is also defined as the slope of the elastic or linear zone of a stress-strain curve. Therefore, the stiffness is affected to a greater extent by the diameter than the strength and increases more rapidly as diameter increases. This applies directly to screws and rods, which are often used in the spine.

Basic Biomechanics of Bone

Bone is composed of osteocytes, which account for 15% of the volume of bone; organic materials such as collagen; and nonorganic materials such as calcium and phosphate. The collagen has high tensile strength, and the nonorganic material resists compression. Because of the lattice orientation of the nonorganic material and the orientation of the cortex, bone is weakest in shear. This difference in strength is an example of an anisotropic material—that is, a material that has different mechanical properties depending on the direction the force is applied. These mechanical properties may also change with age. As people age, the mechanical properties of the bone decline as bone mineral is resorbed. As mentioned previously, this is the primary restraint to compression. This change may predispose older people to mechanical compression fractures.

Bone fractures and the fracture patterns also follow the magnitude and direction of the forces applied. Wolff's law, a theory developed by the German anatomist/surgeon Julius Wolff (1836–1902), states that bone adapts to imposed stress. If loading on a particular bone increases, the bone remodels itself over time to become stronger to compensate for greater load requirements.[3]

Rapidly applied loads to the spine may result in failure of the ligaments or bone, or both. The direction of force application, magnitude, and bony integrity all play a role in the fracture pattern and displacement. Several distinct failure patterns can be observed.

TABLE 136-1

Spinal Ligament Forces

Ligament	Cervical (N)	Lumbar (N)
ALL	112	450
PLL	75	324
ISL	240	125
SSL	36	150

ALL, anterior longitudinal ligament; ISL, interspinous ligament; PLL, posterior longitudinal ligament; SSL,supraspinous ligament.
From White AA, Panjabi MM: *Clinical biomechanics of the spine*, ed 2, Philadelphia, 1990, Lippincott, p 22.

Avulsion Fracture

These occur as a result of the strong ligamentous attachments to the spine. The ligaments, which are strongest in tension due to their high collagen content, can avulse bony fragments (Table 136-1). An example of this is the bony avulsion seen with Jefferson burst fractures, where the transverse ligament avulses a portion of the lateral mass of C1.

Anterior Wedge Compression Fractures

These occur with direct axial load to the spine, most commonly in osteoporotic cancellous bone. For these fractures, the force vector is anterior to the IAR and causes compression failure of the anterior aspect of the vertebral body. The result is a wedge-type fracture, often seen with low-energy injuries in osteoporotic bone.

Flexion-Distraction Fracture (Chance Fracture)

These fractures occur with a significant flexion moment, with the axis of rotation anterior to the spinal unit. This large moment (mass times acceleration times moment arm) results in a tremendous extension force to the spine. The mode of failure is tensile through the posterior elements and then progresses through the vertebral body. The classic example of this type of injury was described by Chance in 1948 and bears his name.[4] The bony or ligamentous component of the fracture is determined by the difference between the tensile strength of the bone and ligaments, and the force travels through the path of least resistance.

Burst Fracture

The burst fracture typically has both axial load components as well as a flexion moment. Comminution is a function of the magnitude of force that was transmitted to the bone. It can be graded on the amount of the vertebral body that is involved and the amount of displacement. These grades have been used to understand the ability of that bone to support the anterior spine. Gaines described this load-sharing classification and the necessity for long-segment fixation or supplemental anterior support based on the concept of vertebral body comminution and fracture displacement.[5] In healthy bone, this energy results in a burst pattern rather than a compression pattern. With failure of the anterior support, the spine falls into flexion with continued energy. The resultant disruption of the dorsal tension band or posterior bony fractures is usually the primary predictor of stability. Most classification systems recognize this, and posterior stability is a primary predictor of necessity of operative stabilization.[6]

Torsion

Complex fracture patterns often have a torsion component and can be responsible for fracture-dislocations with complete disruption of the anterior, middle, and posterior columns. Torsion injures are also common in the more flexible cervical spine. Typically, the failure is through the ligamentous structures because the oblique nature of the cervical facets allows for significant rotation. Torsional forces are the primary forces responsible for unilateral facet dislocations.[7]

Basic Anatomy of the Spine

The spine is made up of 33 separate vertebral segments that are interconnected by spinal ligaments, facet capsules, and intervertebral discs. Each bony segment is referred to as a vertebra, and each is numbered in a region-specific (i.e., cervical, thoracic) rostral to caudal fashion. Thus, there are 7 cervical vertebrae, 12 thoracic vertebrae, 5 lumbar vertebrae, 5 fused sacral vertebrae, and 3 to 4 fused coccygeal segments. All four normal curves of the spine occur in the sagittal plane. The cervical and lumbar spine is lordotic or concave posteriorly due to the wedge-shaped intervertebral discs. The thoracic and sacral regions are kyphotic or concave ventrally; at least in the thoracic spine where the segments are not fused, this is structural and due to the shape of the thoracic vertebral bodies. The anterior vertebral border height is less than the dorsal vertebral border height, resulting in a ventral or kyphotic curve.

These curves function to increase the flexibility and shock-absorbing capacity of the spine. The overall physiologic alignment must be maintained to prevent construct failure and accelerated degeneration. Sagittal balance is an indicator of physiologic alignment and is particularly important in lumbosacral procedures. In a normal spine, a plumb line called the sagittal vertical axis (SVA) can be dropped from the C7 vertebral body through the lumbosacral junction (Fig. 136-4). If the SVA is ventral to the lumbosacral junction, it is called positive sagittal balance; if the SVA is posterior to this junction, it is negative. Positive sagittal balance has significant implications for body mechanics and muscle work. Many authors describe a positive sagittal balance as an important factor in outcomes and muscle mechanics.[8,9] To compensate, the pelvis shifts posteriorly and allows the patient to continue to maintain his or her global balance even with a positive SVA.[10] The pelvis may also retrovert and move the center of gravity posterior to compensate for the positive SVA. Additionally, patients maximally extend their hips. Once this fails, they are forced to bend their knees and flex the hips in a biomechanically disadvantageous position.

Vertebral Body

The vertebral body is the bony cylinder that makes up the ventral aspect of each vertebra, except C1, which has no vertebral body. Each vertebral body consists of an outer rim of cortical bone surrounding a core of softer cancellous bone.

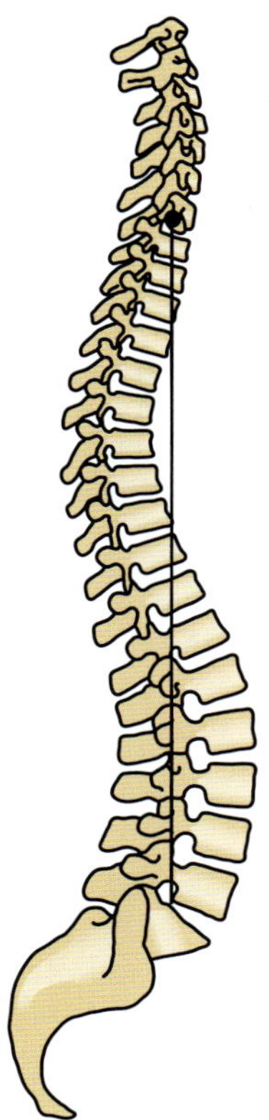

FIGURE 136-4. Sagittal balance. A plumb line dropped from the C7 vertebral body in the standing position should pass through the lumbosacral junction when normal sagittal balance is present, as depicted. (From Benzel EC, editor: *Biomechanics of spine stabilization,* Rolling Meadows, IL, 2001, American Association of Neurological Surgeons.)

The vertebral bodies resist much of the compressive loads placed on the spine in physiologic situations.

In general, the height, width, and depth of the vertebral bodies increase as the spine is descended, which seems to account for this increased strength at lower levels in the spine.[1] As previously alluded to, there is a regional variation to the shape of the vertebral body. In the thoracic spine, the anterior border is shorter than the posterior border, creating a structural kyphosis in the thoracic spine. The outer shell of cortical bone is more rigid than the softer cancellous core because it is arranged in vertical lamellae to resist compressive forces. The cancellous bone is made up of trabeculae that are arranged to resist a variety of loads. There is greater compressive deformation of the cancellous bone prior to failure than of the cortical bone because of the increased rigidity of the latter.[11,12] Numerous studies regarding the load-sharing properties of the cortical and cancellous bone have been performed showing that the load carried by the trabecular bone varies anywhere from 35% to 90%, depending on age and mineral content of the bone,[13,14] and that the strength of the vertebral body decreases with age. Bell et al.[15] have shown that there is a direct relationship between the mineral or ash content of the bone and the strength of the vertebral body. A 25% decrease in mineral content resulted in a greater than 50% decrease in vertebral strength due to loss of the trabecular columns that formed the core of the vertebral bodies. In osteoporosis, the mineral content of the bone is affected and results in loss of the horizontal trabeculae within the vertebral body core, thus lengthening the trabecular columns and compromising vertebral body strength.[1] In the thoracic spine, the vertebral bodies articulate with the ribs. This articulation with the rib cage significantly augments the strength of the thoracic spine. This articulation with the rib cage and the sternum significantly augments the stiffness of the thoracic spine by as much as 110% in extension and 30% to 45% in the other planes of motion.

The vertebral end plates are formed from the concave, 1- to 2-mm thick cortical bone at the rostral and caudal surface of the vertebral body. These are fused to the cartilaginous end plates of the intervertebral disc by a calcified layer of tissue known as the lamina cribrosa, which permits osmotic diffusion of nutrients for the intervertebral disc. In 1957, Perry[16] extensively studied failure of the end plates under compression and noted that one of three mechanisms of failure occurs, depending on the condition of the surrounding discs. Fractures occurred centrally or peripherally or encompassed the entire end plate. In specimens with nondegenerated discs, the fractures typically occurred centrally, and in specimens with degenerated discs, the fractures occurred peripherally. At high loads, the fractures encompassed the entire end plate regardless of degeneration. The strength of the end plate itself has been evaluated as well with regard to resistance to penetration by graft material (subsidence) or disc material (Schmorl node). Kumar et al.[17] determined the greatest resistance to penetration to be within the first 4 mm of depth and the end plate to be strongest at the periphery closer to the cortical margin. In fact, the weakest portion of the vertebral end plate is at the center, where it is the thinnest. With a nondegenerated nucleus, axial compression creates a central increase in pressure and deflection of the end plate. This leads to increasing bending stresses in the center of the vertebral end plate and ultimately results in its failure.[1] In contrast, in the degenerated disc, the nucleus lacks water content, and there is no build-up of central fluid pressure. The load is transmitted primarily through the anulus at the periphery of the disc and end plate, resulting in fracture in the same location or in the underlying vertebral body.[1]

Intervertebral Disc

The vertebral bodies are separated at each level by the intervertebral disc. This viscoelastic structure is made up of a central nucleus pulposus, peripheral anulus fibrosus, and cartilaginous end plate of the disc, which separates it from the vertebral bodies above and below. Viscoelasticity is defined as a property of a material that exhibits both viscous and elastic characteristics when undergoing deformation. The material then has different mechanical properties that vary depending on the different loading rates. That is, if a load is applied slowly, the disc can respond with greater deformation, whereas if a load is applied rapidly, less deformation occurs. This property also changes as people age; with increasing age, there is a corresponding decrease in the ability of the disc to deform. There are 23 intervertebral discs starting between C2 and C3 and ending at L5 and S1. They make up 20% to 33% of the total height of the vertebral column, and there are regional differences that seem to parallel those of the vertebrae. The cross-sectional area of the discs increases in the rostrocaudal direction.

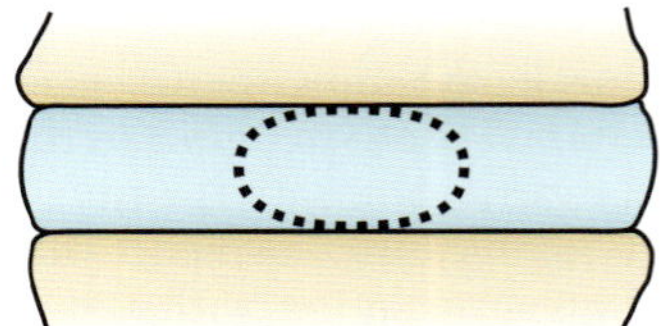

FIGURE 136-5. The intervertebral disc. The nucleus pulposus (*dashed circle*) is contained (in nonpathologic situations) by the anulus fibers. (From Benzel EC, editor: *Biomechanics of spine stabilization,* Rolling Meadows, IL, 2001, American Association of Neurological Surgeons.)

The central nucleus pulposus is composed of mucopolysaccharides and mucoprotein, forming a gel with water content ranging from 70% to 90%.[1] The water content is highest at birth and decreases with age.[18] The nucleus pulposus makes up approximately 30% to 50% of the cross-sectional area of the disc, and it seems to lie more posterior in the lumbar spine at the junction of the middle and posterior thirds of the disc in the sagittal plane.[1] The viscoelastic properties of the nucleus pulposus allow it to act as an effective shock absorber for the spine. Surrounding the nucleus pulposus is the anulus fibrosus, which is made up of collagenous fibers in concentric laminated bands, with each band oriented 90 degrees to the adjacent bands and 30 degrees to the disc plane (Fig. 136-5). The inner fibers of the anulus are attached to the cartilaginous end plates, and the outermost fibers, known as Sharpey fibers, are attached to the cortical bone of the vertebral body. Because of the orientation of the fibers, the intervertebral disc effectively resists rotational, tensile, and shear stresses. The anulus does not resist compressive forces.

With age, the water content of the nucleus pulposus decreases and the nucleus itself becomes less deformable. This desiccation results in an overall stiffer intervertebral disc that behaves differently under compressive loads. In a disc in a younger person, the nucleus is compressed, resulting in viscoelastic deformity at the central part of the end plate, but when the nucleus becomes less elastic and stiffer, the load is transmitted through the anular fibers around the periphery with very little deformation, leading to a higher load at the end plate. This can result in compression fractures, as are commonly observed in the elderly or osteoporotic population. The increased stiffness of the disc and bone results in a smaller elastic zone and lower threshold for failure.

Facet Joints

The vertebrae articulate with each other at the superior and inferior facet joints, which are diarthrodial joints with a loose synovial capsule located at the superior and inferior aspect of the pars interarticularis. In the cervical spine, the facet joints are oriented with an inclination of approximately 45 degrees from the horizontal, and this orientation changes in the thoracic and lumbar spine as the facets become larger and more vertical.[1] The shape, position, and orientation of these articulating surfaces largely determine the pattern of movements throughout the spine (Fig. 136-6). The cervical spine from C2 to C7 allows 8 to 12 degrees of rotation, whereas the entire lumbar spine only allows 2 to 5 degrees.

The coronally oriented cervical facet joints allow for supple flexion, extension, rotation, and lateral bending. In the thoracic spine, the inclination of the articulating surfaces is approximately 60 degrees, with an additional rotation about the *y*-axis of approximately 20 degrees toward the midline. This allows for limited flexion and extension but limits rotation. The facet surfaces in the lumbar spine are at an inclination of approximately 90 degrees, with approximately 45 degrees of rotation about the *y*-axis directed outward. This orientation allows for restricted rotation with greater flexion and extension. The orientations of the facet joints have a great deal of variation even within the specific regions of the spine.[1] The facets act as important stabilizing structures in the spine, with resultant instability following unilateral or bilateral excision.[19]

In the lumbar spine, the sagittal orientation of the facet joints allows for substantial resistance to rotation, which is well documented.[19-21] As the facet orientation begins to change from about T7 to L4, the torsional stiffness of the spine increases due to these changes in facet articulation, with the peak at T12-L1.[22] In the cervical spine, transection of the disc and longitudinal ligaments resulted in a 33% increase in horizontal translation with flexion. This increased by 140% following transection of the facets.[23] Removal of thoracic facets resulted in increased flexion and extension in the upper thoracic region and increased axial rotation in the lower thoracic–thoracolumbar region. The capsular ligaments also have a role in maintaining torsional strength.

The facets provide a load-bearing role when the spine is in extension. In dynamic studies with cadaver spines in various postures, the facets have been shown to carry anywhere from 0% to 33% of the load, depending on the force vector and position of the spine.[24]

Dorsal Elements

The remainder of the dorsal elements of the spine includes the pedicle, the lamina, the transverse processes, and the spinous process. Each of these elements varies significantly in morphology between regions of the spine. The pedicle serves as the bridge between the posterior elements and the vertebral body. The importance of pedicle anatomy is due to the major role pedicles now play in stabilization constructs. In the cervical spine, the pedicles are shorter with greater diameter. From the cervical to midthoracic region, the transverse pedicle width gradually decreases, and it then increases from the midthoracic to the lumbar region (Fig. 136-7).[25-27] Sagittal pedicle width increases from the cervical to the thoracolumbar region and then decreases in the lumbar region (Fig. 136-8).[25-27]

From the cervical to the thoracolumbar region, the transverse pedicle angle decreases, and it increases into the lumbar region (Fig. 136-9).[25-27] The sagittal pedicle angle is a final consideration with regard to pedicle anatomy; it becomes fairly steep in the thoracic and thoracolumbar regions (Fig. 136-10).[25-27]

The laminae form the dorsal aspect of the neural canal, which contains the spinal cord. They extend from the pedicles to the spinous process dorsally and form the foundation for the spinous processes, provide dorsal protection to the dural sac, and serve as the attachment site for one of the seven spinal ligaments, the ligamentum flavum.[2]

The spinous processes project dorsally and, for the most part, caudally. They form attachment sites for the interspinous

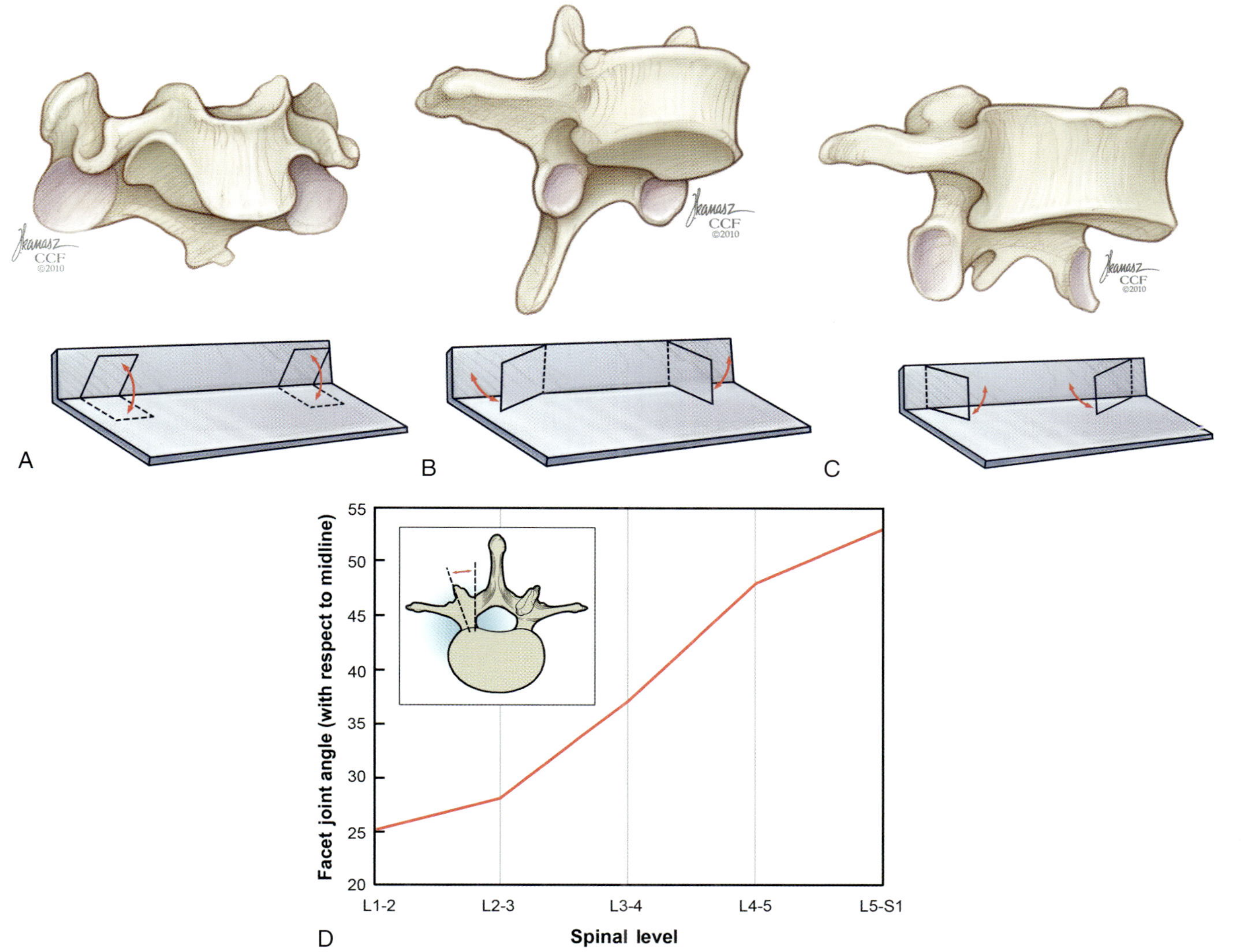

A B C D

FIGURE 136-6. Facet joint orientation. The relative coronal plane orientation in the cervical region (**A**), the intermediate orientation in the thoracic region (**B**), and the relative sagittal orientation in the lumbar region (**C**). The facet joint orientation changes substantially in the lumbar region; here the facet joint angle (with respect to midline) is depicted versus the spinal level (**D**). (**A–C,** Copyright Cleveland Clinic Foundation.)

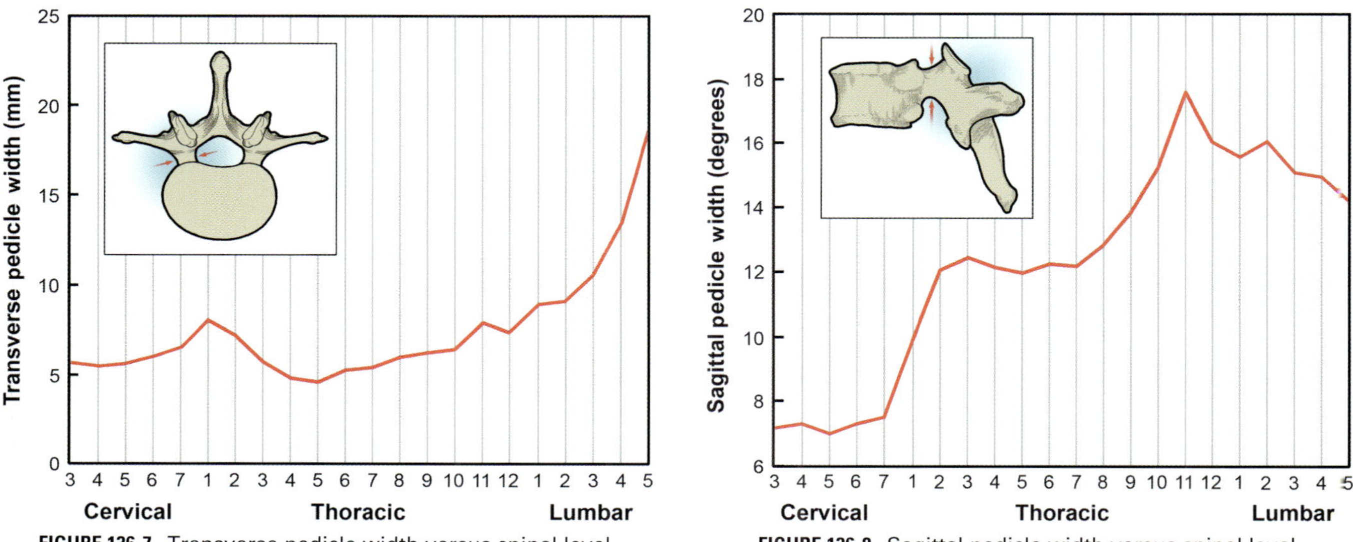

FIGURE 136-7. Transverse pedicle width versus spinal level.

FIGURE 136-8. Sagittal pedicle width versus spinal level.

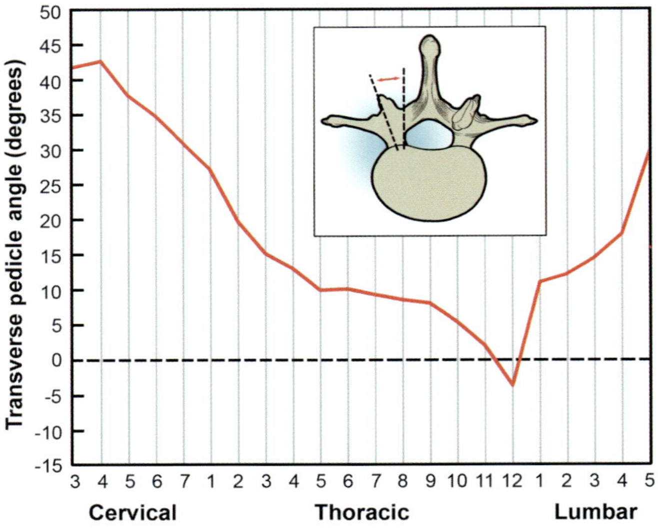

FIGURE 136-9. Transverse pedicle angle versus spinal level.

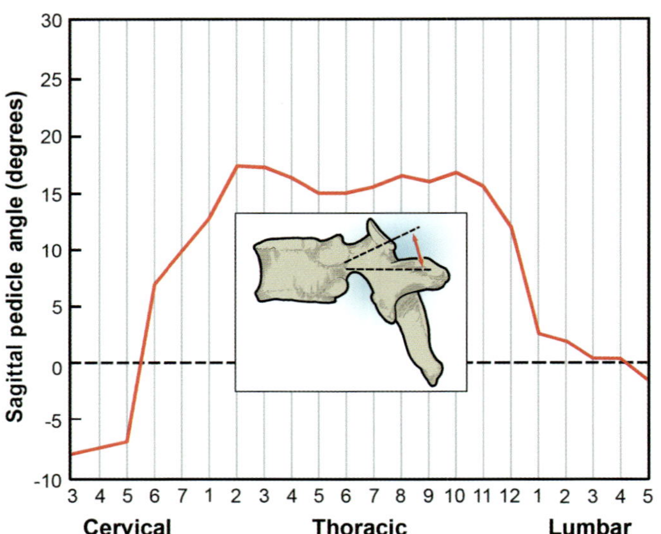

FIGURE 136-10. Sagittal pedicle angle versus spinal level.

ligaments and supraspinous ligaments. The spinous processes project more caudally as one descends to the midthoracic spine. In the thoracolumbar and lumbar regions, the spinous processes also project more dorsally.[2]

The transverse processes are located at the junction of the lamina and pedicle and in general extend laterally with some variation in the rostral-caudal dimension, depending on the region of the spine. They serve as sites of attachment for the paraspinal muscles. In the cervical spine, the transverse processes are smaller and transmit the vertebral artery through the foramen transversarium from C6 to C1. The transverse processes of the middle to lower thoracic spine become more substantial, projecting in a lateral and upward direction. The lower thoracic processes become smaller and more atretic, but those of the lumbar spine become more substantial, extending laterally and ventrally.

The transverse processes of the midthoracic and lumbar spine are sizable enough to serve as sites for hook placement and fusion, but they are limited by a poor blood supply and are easily fractured.[2]

Ligaments

The ligamentous complex from the occiput to C2 represents a continuation of ligaments of the subaxial spine (Figs. 136-11 and 136-12). The anterior longitudinal ligament begins at the occiput as the atlanto-occipital membrane, as it passes between the occiput and the anterior arch of C1. The posterior atlanto-occipital membrane passes from the posterior arch of C1 to the occiput. When intact, these ligaments offer some advantage in preventing anterior displacement of C1 on C2. The apical ligament stretches from the tip of the odontoid process of C2 to the basion of the skull. The alar ligaments run obliquely from the rostrolateral aspect of the odontoid to the occipital condyles. The cruciate ligament has a vertical and transverse portion. The transverse portion of the ligament attaches to the tubercles located at the lateral masses of C1 and runs dorsal to the dens. The vertical portion of the cruciate ligament attaches to the occiput immediately dorsal to the apical ligament and descends to intertwine with the transverse portion. The vertical portion then descends to attach to the dorsocaudal aspect of C2. The transverse ligament is the most important ligament of the occipitocervical complex because it prevents horizontal translation of C1 on C2. The tectorial membrane is a continuation of the posterior longitudinal ligament and runs from the body of C2 over the

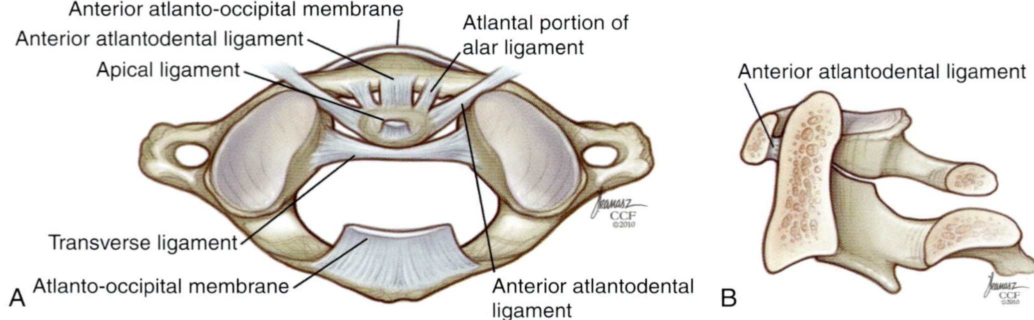

FIGURE 136-11. Axial (**A**) and midsagittal (**B**) schematic illustrations of the major ligaments involved in the clinical stability of the upper cervical spine. The anterior atlantodental ligament has been described recently. (Copyright Cleveland Clinic Foundation.)

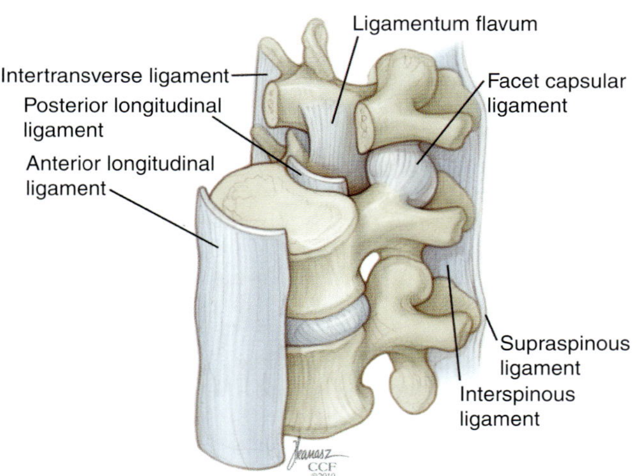

FIGURE 136-12. Ligaments of the spine. Besides the disc, seven ligaments connect one vertebra to the next. Contribution to the spine stability by an individual ligament is dependent on its cross section, its distance from the instantaneous axis of rotation, and its orientation in space. The anatomy of the ligaments is such as to collectively provide stability to the spine in its various physiologic motions. (Copyright Cleveland Clinic Foundation.)

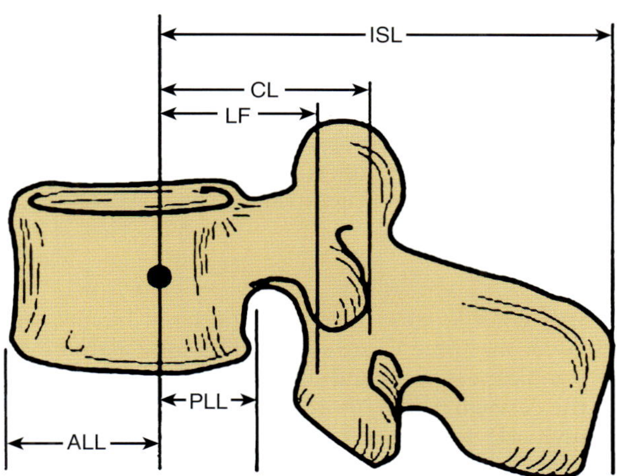

FIGURE 136-13. The ligaments and their effective moment arms. Note that this length depends on the location of the instantaneous axis of rotation (*dot*). An "average" location is used in this illustration. ALL, anterior longitudinal ligament; CL, capsular ligament; ISL, interspinous ligament; LF, ligamentum flavum; PLL, posterior longitudinal ligament. (From Benzel EC, editor: *Biomechanics of spine stabilization,* Rolling Meadows, IL, 2001, American Association of Neurological Surgeons.)

posterior portion of the dens to attach to the anterior foramen magnum (see Fig. 136-11).

Beyond the occiput-C1-C2 complex, there are seven major spinal ligaments that work to stabilize the subaxial spine in its physiologic range of motion. These ligaments also work to restrict the motion of the spine to well-defined limits while at the same time allowing adequate motion and fixed postures to protect the spinal cord. Starting anteriorly and moving posteriorly, the ligaments are the anterior longitudinal ligament, posterior longitudinal ligament, capsular ligaments, intertransverse process ligaments, ligamentum flavum, interspinous ligament, and supraspinous ligament (see Fig. 136-12). The strength characteristics of the ligaments vary, and the effectiveness of a ligament not only depends on the morphology but also on the length of the moment arm through which it works[28] (Fig. 136-13). A longer moment arm gives a relatively weak ligament a mechanical advantage so that it may contribute more to overall spinal stability.

The anterior longitudinal ligament spans the entire spinal column from the clivus, where it begins as the anterior atlanto-occipital membrane, to the sacrum. It covers the ventral one fourth to one third of the vertebral body circumference with interdigitizing layers of elastin and collagen fibers. The innermost layers bind to the intervertebral discs of adjacent vertebrae. The middle layer binds the vertebral bodies and discs over three levels, and the superficial layer extends over four to five levels. Because it is ventral to the IAR, it provides resistance to extension.

The posterior longitudinal ligament starts as the tectorial membrane and also spans the entire length of the spine. It also consists of several layers, with the deeper fibers spanning adjacent vertebrae and the more superficial fibers extending over several levels. The posterior longitudinal ligament only marginally attaches to the vertebral body compared with the anterior longitudinal ligament, which blends into the periosteum at times. The posterior longitudinal ligament is closely adherent to the anulus fibrosus, whereas the anterior longitudinal ligament is not. The posterior longitudinal ligament widens in the region of the disc space and narrows as it passes over the vertebral body. It is dorsal to the IAR and has a short moment arm, and, therefore, it is only able to weakly resist flexion forces.

The capsular ligaments are located at the facet joints. These fibers attach to the superior and inferior facets of adjacent vertebrae, and they act as significant stabilizers of the spine, particularly in the cervical spine. The fibers of the facet capsules run in a direction that is perpendicular to the plane of the facet joint. The moment arm (see Fig. 136-13) is not substantial, but the ligaments are strong enough for the stresses placed on them, which consist mainly of axial rotation, ventral shear loads, and axial loads under certain conditions. Other capsular ligaments in the thoracic spine attach the ribs to the vertebral bodies. These costochondral ligaments provide additional stability to the thoracic spine.

The ligamentum flavum has the highest percentage of elastic fibers of any tissue in the body. The ligamentum flavum is actually a pair of broad ligaments that connect the spinal laminae. They arise from the ventral surface of the caudal lamina and attach to the dorsal border of the adjacent rostral lamina, and they extend laterally to become confluent with the joint capsules. These ligaments begin at C1-2 and continue caudally to L5-S1. White and Panjabi noted that the ligament is in a state of resting "pretension" or tension, which is present with the spine in neutral position.[1] This is postulated to stabilize the spine by keeping the intervertebral discs under compression and keeping the ligament from impinging on the spinal cord when the spine is in extension.

The interspinous and supraspinous ligaments connect the adjacent spinous processes. The interspinous ligament extends from the base to the tip of each spinous process, and this ligament is present from C2 to S1. The supraspinous ligament begins at the dorsal aspect of C7, attaching to the tip of the spinous process, and extends to the lumbosacral region.

It is thought to be a continuation of the ligamentum nuchae associated with the dorsal cervical spine. These ligaments use the long moment arm of the spinous process to provide an effective resistance to flexion (see Fig. 136-13). These ligaments are extremely important in determining the stability of the spine, both for their importance in providing stability and for their inability to heal effectively.

Musculature

One final consideration regarding the basic biomechanical anatomy of the spine is the surrounding musculature, which lends significant support and stability to the spine.

In the cervical region, there is a fibrous intermuscular septum previously mentioned known as the ligamentum nuchae, which serves as an attachment to many of the occipitocervical muscles. The splenius capitis muscle arises from the lower ligamentum, cervical, and upper six thoracic transverse processes to attach to the occiput. The splenius cervicis muscle arises from the upper six thoracic transverse processes to insert on the posterior tubercles of C1-3. The semispinalis cervicis muscle occupies the next deeper layer and arises from the facets and transverse processes of the upper thoracic spine to insert on the spinous processes of the cervical spine. The semispinalis capitis muscle, occupying the same layer, is more lateral, arising from the transverse processes of C3-6 to insert on the occiput. Deeper muscles include the rectus capitis and the capitis obliquus, which serve as head extensors. Ventrally, the sternocleidomastoids arise bilaterally from the clavicles and insert on the mastoid processes of the occipital bone. The longus colli occupy a deeper layer in the anterior cervical region, arising from the atlas to insert on the transverse processes of C3 to C6.

In the thoracic region, the superficial musculature attaches to the thoracic spinous processes, and in the rostral thoracic region, it is made up principally of the trapezius muscle, which inserts laterally on the scapula and medially on the ligamentum nuchae. Lower in the lower thoracic and thoracolumbar region, the superficial musculature is made up principally of the latissimus dorsi muscle, which arises from the transverse processes of the lower thoracic spine and spreads ventrally to the axilla. The rib cage, which articulates with the thoracic spine and lends stability to this region, also possesses its own intrinsic musculature. The intercostal muscles and serratus posterior muscles run between ribs but in opposite directions. In the lower thoracic and thoracolumbar region, the lateral muscle groups include the psoas, intertransverse, and quadratus lumborum muscles. The psoas muscles arise from the lateral aspect of the vertebral bodies and insert on the femurs. The intertransverse muscles arise and insert between transverse processes throughout the spine, and the quadratus lumborum muscle arises from the transverse processes and inserts at the lateral ileum.

Ventrally, the lumbar spine is supported by those muscles surrounding the abdominal region, which include the internal and external oblique, transversus abdominis, and rectus abdominis muscles. Dorsally, lumbar support is principally from the very prominent paravertebral muscles. These make up the erector spinae muscle group, which begins as a broad tendon attached to the sacrum and iliac crest and extends the entire length of the spine. It is composed of three columns, each of which is composed of shorter fascicles. The lateral column is the iliocostalis muscle, the middle column is the longissimus muscle, and the medial column is the semispinalis muscle. The iliocostalis arises from the iliac crest to insert on the angles of each rib and the cervical transverse processes. The longissimus muscle is the largest and arises from the transverse processes at the lower spinal levels and inserts onto the transverse processes rostrally and onto the mastoid processes of the occipital bone. The semispinalis arises from the spinous processes of the sacrum and inserts onto the rostral spinous processes. Deeper to the erector spinae muscle group is the transverse muscle group, which principally arises from transverse processes and inserts onto the spinous processes. The multifidus muscle differs in the cervical and lumbar regions, where it arises from the articular joint as opposed to the transverse processes.

Weakness of the muscle groups that support the spine can lead to deformity or pain. The musculature plays a significant role in spine stability. Disuse or denervation atrophy can result in deformity, degeneration, or other painful pathology. Biomechancially, toned musculature can contribute to maintaining the load balance along the spinal column. Furthermore, in the degenerating spine, toned musculature aids in offloading the detrimental forces and disruption in load balance arising from the degeneration.

Application of Basic Principles to Instrumentation

Surgical implants must be designed with the basic biomechanical principles previously discussed in mind. A clear understanding of the complex forces applied to the spine is necessary when contemplating spinal instrumentation. Important considerations include implant materials, the implant-bone interface, and the various mechanisms of force application to the spine. Ultimately, the forces involved are complex, but they can be broken down into major vectors. By using vectors and basic biomechanical principles, spinal instrumentation can be systematically analyzed and the appropriate construct applied. Spinal instrumentation is applied for many reasons, and the pathology is beyond the scope of this chapter. Instrumentation and fusion are most often used to restore stability or prevent instability.

Implant Properties

Implants can be made of various materials, including metals, nonmetals (i.e., ceramic, glass), and bone. Each material has intrinsic properties that make it more useful for certain operations, and these specific properties must be kept in mind. An instrumented fusion is essentially a race between fusion formation and instrument failure, and, therefore, certain implants are more suited for this. Metallurgists have produced many alloys, which are now being used clinically in spinal implants.[2] Stainless steel alloys include 316L stainless steel and 22-13-5 stainless steel, which has the same modulus of elasticity and tensile strength as 316L but twice the ultimate tensile strength.[6] Titanium is available in pure, unalloyed forms, as well as various alloyed forms.

Pure titanium occurs in several grades (1–4) based on purity and degree of contaminants, and as the oxygen content increases, so does the strength of titanium.[2] The modulus of elasticity remains unaltered, but the ultimate strength and 0.2% tensile strength (stress that causes 0.2% deformation) increase with the grade.[29] Titanium has several advantages over other metals. Its modulus is very similar to bone, allowing for easy incorporation and limiting stress shielding.[2,30,31] In addition, it also is resistant to glycocalyx formation, which may prevent latent infections.[32] However, it is notch sensitive. This refers to the early fatigue failure of titanium with the addition of a notch or defect in its surface.[29] Care must be taken when bending these materials. Titanium may also be alloyed with other elements such as aluminum, vanadium, niobium, and zirconium in specific concentrations, resulting in specific properties such as increased resistance to wear.[2] The stainless steel alloys 316L and 22-13-5 are stiffer than titanium, resulting in a smaller transfer of stress from the implant to the bone, termed stress shielding. Cobalt chrome is now being used for spinal applications. It has the advantage of the imaging characteristics of titanium with the strength of stainless steel. Elements such as chromium and molybdenum present in these alloys provide resistance to corrosion.[2]

Deformability and the ability to resist fatigue are important characteristics of spinal implants. Implants do not fail because a static load exceeds the ultimate strength of the implant; they fail because of cyclical loading and fatigue. Fatigue refers to the cumulative damage of cyclical loading that occurs in the form of cracks and corrosion. Titanium performs better than steel at lower frequencies of loading.[33]

Other implant materials include synthetic nonmetals such as polymethylmethacrylate (PMMA), acrylics, ceramics, and glasses. PMMA is most commonly used but only in very specific situations. It has a high modulus of elasticity and is, therefore, very brittle. It has been shown that wire reinforcement, especially with the cobalt alloy Vitallium, yields a stronger construct.[34]

Finally, bone is commonly used as an implant. Bone graft harvested from the patient (i.e., fibula, iliac crest) is termed an *autologous graft*, whereas bone graft harvested from a cadaver is termed an *allograft*. It can be harvested as a strut graft with both cortical and cancellous bone, which can be cut and shaped to fit into a disc space or vertebrectomy cavity. Morselized bone chips may also be processed from cadavers and used as a graft extender. Bone is used to create a fusion, which ultimately lends stability to the spine, and instrumentation will ultimately fail unless fusion and stability are achieved.[2] Bone can be placed ventrally or dorsally in the spine to create a fusion. Ventrally, a bone graft is placed in the weight-bearing part of the spine as an interbody graft, which results in compression and load sharing by the graft. This leads to faster and better healing as dictated by Wolff's law. Wolff explained that internal and external changes in bone architecture occurred according to mathematical laws along with functional changes of bone.[2,3] It has also been shown that electrophysiologic changes occur when bone is placed under compression (i.e., a negative charge is generated).[35] Dorsally, bone is not exposed to the same fusion-enhancing forces as ventral weight-bearing grafts. The healing and fusion rates in dorsal fusions are less than in ventral fusions, probably because there is no compression that seems to encourage ventral, interbody fusion.[2,36] The dorsal fusion mass will diminish in volume with time, and it has been shown that a larger volume of initial graft is required for a larger fusion mass at 18 months.[37]

The interface between the implant and bone is important in ensuring stability. There are several ways in which implants and bone contact each other. According to Benzel,[2] these are (1) abutting, (2) penetrating, (3) gripping, (4) conforming, and (5) osseointegration. Abutting implants typically include the interbody bone. The role of the interbody implant is to resist axial loads, and this is done most effectively through a large surface area contact between the ends of the bone graft and the adjacent vertebral bodies. Placement of the graft in the IAR is ideal for resisting axial loads, and placement ventral to the IAR results in a moment arm and some degree of distraction.[2] Penetrating implants include nails, screws, and spikes. The role of the penetrating implant is that of an anchor, and important considerations with regard to these implants include pullout resistance and overall strength when they function as fixed-arm cantilevers.[2] Pullout resistance of screws is enhanced by engaging cortical bone, which markedly resists pullout, and through triangulation (Fig. 136-14) or placement of converging or diverging screws optimally at 90 degrees to one another.[38] As discussed previously, the bending strength is proportional to the cube of the inner diameter of the screw (section modulus). The outer diameter and thread depth are important in pullout resistance (Fig. 136-15). Hooks and wires are examples of the gripping implants. Wire may be looped around the laminae and spinous processes of adjacent vertebrae and secured via twisting the loops together, and hooks may be placed at the laminae, pedicles, or transverse processes to augment dorsal instrumentation, especially screws placed in osteoporotic bone.[2] They contact cortical bone over a greater surface area, and thus may perform

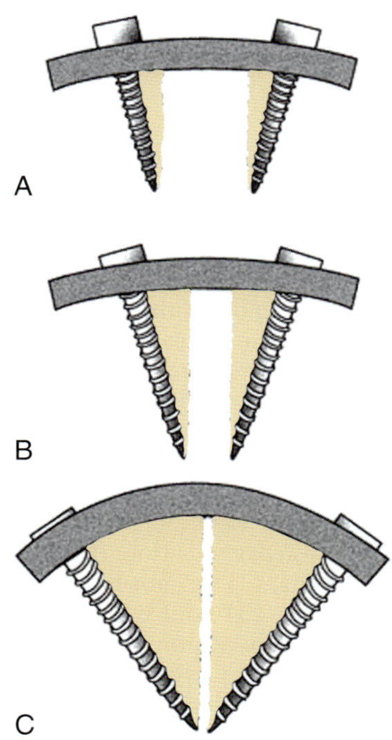

FIGURE 136-14. The triangulation effect is proportional to the shaded area subtended by the screw (**A**). The shaded area can be increased by lengthening the screws (**B**) or by altering the trajectory (**C**). (From Benzel EC, editor: *Biomechanics of spine stabilization,* Rolling Meadows, IL, 2001, American Association of Neurological Surgeons.)

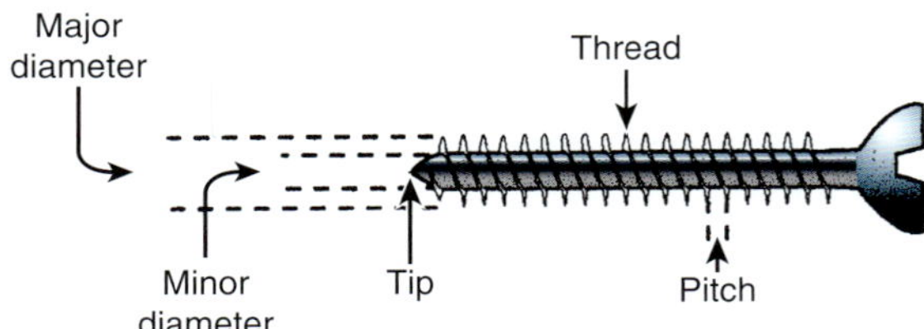

FIGURE 136-15. Screw core (minor) and outside (major) diameters, thread depth, and screw pitch. (From Benzel EC, editor: *Biomechanics of spine stabilization,* Rolling Meadows, IL, 2001, American Association of Neurological Surgeons.)

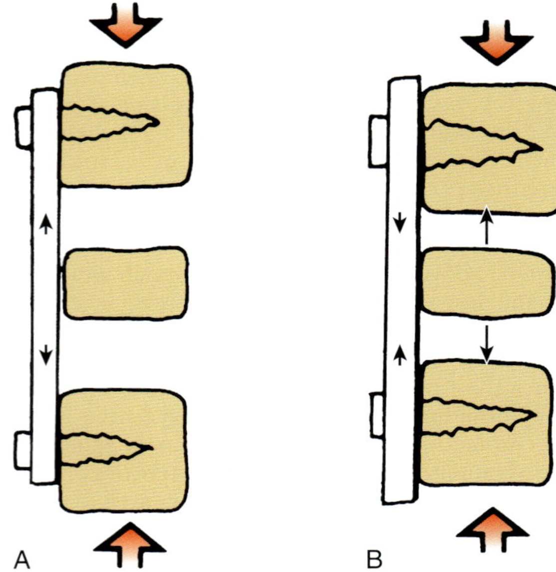

FIGURE 136-16. A, A spinal implant placed in distraction (*short arrows*). **B,** A spinal implant placed in compression (*short arrows*) shares the axial load (*orange arrows*) with intrinsic spinal elements (*long arrows*). The spinal implant is thus unloaded during weight bearing. If enough compression were applied, the spinal implant might conceivably bear no load compression if the force applied by the implant were equal to the weight of the torso above the implant itself; that is, the case of zero weight bearing. (From Benzel EC, editor: *Biomechanics of spine stabilization,* Rolling Meadows, IL, 2001, American Association of Neurological Surgeons.)

better in the setting of osteoporotic bone. Hooks may also be used to augment screw pullout resistance within the same construct.[2] Conforming implants have been mentioned briefly and at this point include PMMA and acrylics. These implants have the unique property of conforming to surrounding bone and are used by some surgeons to augment the screw-bone interface.[39-41] The bonding of bone to nonbiologic material is known as osseointegration, and when this occurs, the load transfer from implant to bone is distributed over a much larger surface area, reducing stress risers (focal concentrations of stress).[2] Titanium and a titanium alloy, Ti-13Nb-13Zr (niobium, zirconium), have exhibited potential for osseointegration.[2,30,31]

Application to Implants

Newton's third law of motion, which states that for every action there is an opposite but equal reaction, governs the placement of spinal implants. Because there is no net movement in the spine when the implant is placed, the forces applied to the spine must occur in pairs such that the net result is zero. No spinal implant is placed in a truly neutral mode because once upright posture is assumed, the implant is under some degree of stress, which it then must resist. Implants, when placed dorsally or ventrally, resist these loads dynamically, resulting in load sharing or rigidly resulting in stress shielding. The type of implant is determined by the surgeon when designing the construct, and the surgeon must take into account the region of the spine, the site of fusion (ventral or dorsal), and the forces that will be applied at the site of the implant when the spine is loaded.

Spinal implants impart complex forces on the spine that can be broken down into basic component vectors and that may be considered separately. Rarely is any one force applied in isolation, and spinal implants function through several of the basic mechanisms of force application. Benzel lists six basic mechanisms of force application: (1) simple distraction, (2) three-point bending, (3) tension-band fixation, (4) fixed moment arm cantilever, (5) nonfixed moment arm cantilever, and (6) applied moment arm cantilever.[2] These represent the basic mechanisms by which implants impart force to the spine, and a single implant often functions using several mechanisms at once.

Anterior spine surgery frequently incorporates simple distraction and tension band fixation through a nonfixed moment arm cantilever fixation. Three-point bending is also used in longer constructs to stabilize the plate and prevent translation. Because surgery in the anterior spine is located ventral to the IAR, a bending moment is applied to the instrumented segments. Simple distraction may be applied through ventral placement of an interbody graft (ventral to the neutral axis/IAR) or by placement of a fixed moment arm cantilever in the form of a plate and screws. Plates secured to the anterior spine by screws in distraction are more frequently applied in the cervical spine. Placement of ventral distraction results in extension of the spine, and implants placed in this manner resist axial loads (Fig. 136-16). Placement of an anterior graft allows for distraction of the vertebral bodies, although the graft is left in compression. Typically isolated distraction of implants is avoided because this places the implant in a load-bearing rather than load-sharing mode. These implants bear much of the axial load; thus, failure may occur typically at the screw-plate interface. These same implants resist extension of the spine, and, therefore, act as tension band fixators when the spine is placed in extension. Distraction and compression are forces applied perpendicular to IAR resulting in torque (Fig. 136-17). Three-point bending is applied parallel to the IAR and often is accompanied by distraction or compression forces[2] (Fig. 136-18). Three-point bending occurs when a fulcrum directs a force vector in a direction opposite to the two terminal force vectors. The force at the fulcrum is equal to the sum of the terminal forces.[2]

Three-point bending requires an intermediate point of fixation between the terminal points of fixation, and when used in a ventral construct will resist translational deformation (Fig. 136-19). Ventral compressive implants do not resist axial loads, and the axial load-resisting ability of the spine must be intact or augmented (usually by an interbody graft) when these implants are used. Dynamic ventral systems allow

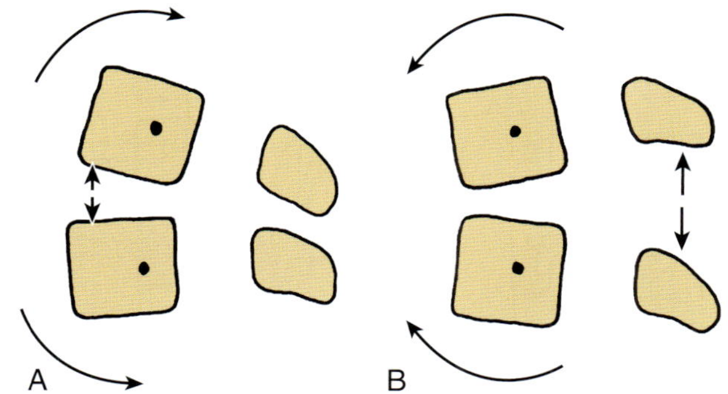

FIGURE 136-17. A, Ventral spinal distraction (*straight arrows*) can cause spinal extension (*curved arrows*) if the distraction forces area is applied ventral to the instantaneous axis of rotation (IAR) (neutral axis). **B,** Conversely, the application of distraction forces (*straight arrows*) dorsal to the IAR (neutral axis) results in spinal flexion (*curved arrows*) (i.e., in tension-band distraction). (From Benzel EC, editor: *Biomechanics of spine stabilization,* Rolling Meadows, IL, 2001, American Association of Neurological Surgeons.)

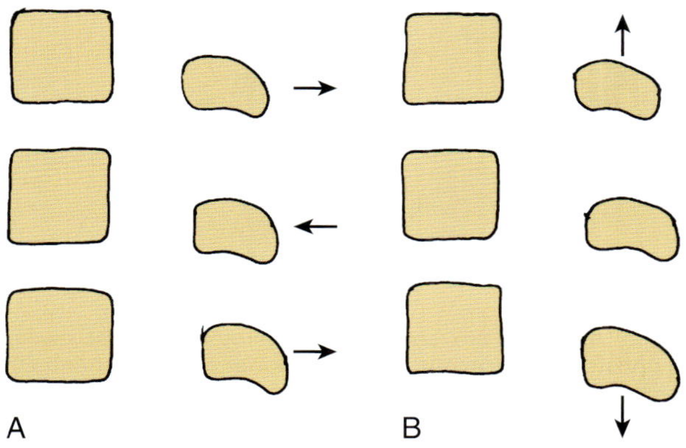

FIGURE 136-18. Three-point bending constructs are commonly applied in combination with distraction. These two components, three-point bending (**A**) and distraction (**B**), are independent of each other with respect to the forces they apply to the spine. (From Benzel EC, editor: *Biomechanics of spine stabilization,* Rolling Meadows, IL, 2001, American Association of Neurological Surgeons.)

controlled subsidence and therefore enhanced load sharing by the spine to augment bone healing and fusion of interbody grafts in the cervical spine.

Interbody grafts may be placed in the neutral axis of the spine or the IAR. These implants include autologous bone (i.e., rib, fibula, iliac crest), allograft, acrylic and wire constructs, and cages filled with morselized bone. These implants are usually placed to restore the axial load-bearing ability of the spine, and the principal forces are distraction and compression. Removal of a vertebral body (i.e., spondylectomy) or removal of a disc (i.e., discectomy), which incorporates the neutral or weight-bearing axis of the spine, usually requires placement of a graft to restore stability. There are several important considerations in placing interbody grafts. Migration of the bone graft into the adjacent vertebral body is known as subsidence. This can be avoided by ensuring that the abutting interbody graft occupies a large surface area and is able to withstand axial loads (Fig. 136-20). The cortical end plates of the vertebral body may be left intact to protect against subsidence as well. The cortical margins of the vertebral body are good buttresses for instrumentation and interbody grafts. Stress shielding occurs when the implant bears more of the axial load than the interbody graft, reducing compressive forces and the chance for fusion by increasing bone resorption. Stress shielding is avoided by placing the interbody graft under compression to incorporate load-sharing principles, which can be achieved by ventral tension band fixation. A final important consideration with regard to interbody grafts is that intact surrounding ligaments add stability when a graft that is sufficiently large is placed to distract the end plates and therefore ligaments are placed under tension.

Dorsal instrumentation incorporates distraction, tension band fixation, and three-point bending to reduce and stabilize the spine. Often dorsal instrumentation accompanies ventral instrumentation to augment the stability of the spine, especially in flexion. This is an important concept. Dorsal instrumentation must be very rigid and is load bearing in dorsal-only constructs. This consideration is critical when determining the need for additional fixation and the levels of fixation. Loss of anterior column support (i.e., fracture) leads to implant failure unless the anterior support is restored, or longer, more biomechanically rigid instrumentation is used.[5] The implants act as a cantilever beam in these dorsal-only constructs. Dorsal fixation techniques are numerous and include wires, hooks, screws, and rods. Cross fixation may be added to stabilize the construct and prevent a coronal

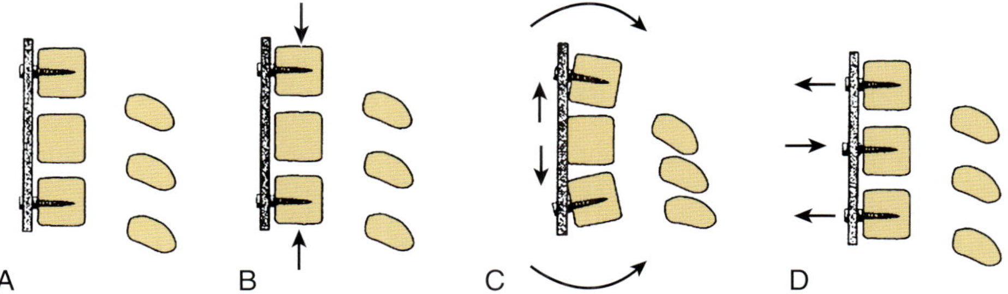

FIGURE 136-19. Versatile implants (i.e., implants that can resist a variety of deformations) are optimal. For example, a ventral cervical cantilever beam device (**A**) can resist axial loads (*straight arrows*) via distraction (**B**) and extension (*curved arrows*) via tension-band fixation (**C**). If an intermediate point of fixation is used, it can resist translation via a three-part bending mechanism (*straight arrows*) as well (**D**). (From Benzel EC, editor: *Biomechanics of spine stabilization,* Rolling Meadows, IL, 2001, American Association of Neurological Surgeons.)

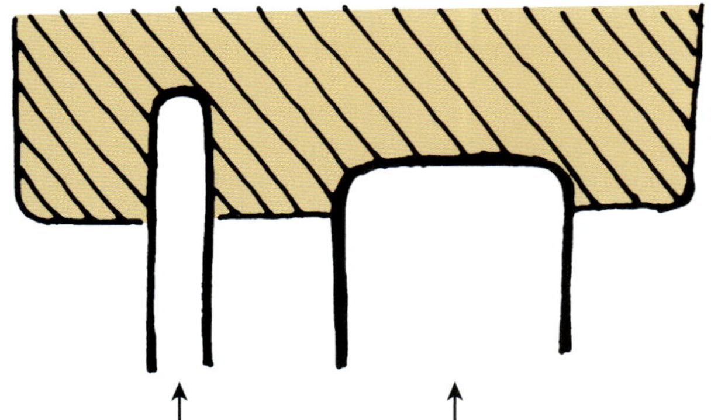

FIGURE 136-20. The surface area of the contact surface of interfaces between abutting implants and bone correlates with weight-bearing capacity. A smaller-diameter implant penetrates farther (*left*), whereas a larger-diameter implant withstands axial loading more effectively (*right*). *Arrows* depict load applied to bone (*hatched area*) by the implant. (From Benzel EC, editor: *Biomechanics of spine stabilization,* Rolling Meadows, IL, 2001, American Association of Neurological Surgeons.)

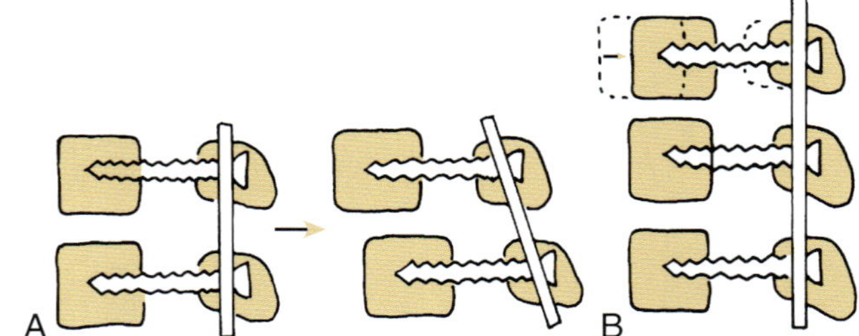

FIGURE 136-22. A parallelogram-like translational deformation of the spine in the sagittal plane can occur with nonfixed moment arm cantilever beam constructs (**A**). This untoward occurrence can be minimized by the use of more rigid constructs or the use of a nonfixed moment arm construct over additional caudal segments (**B**). (From Benzel EC, editor: *Biomechanics of spine stabilization,* Rolling Meadows, IL, 2001, American Association of Neurological Surgeons.)

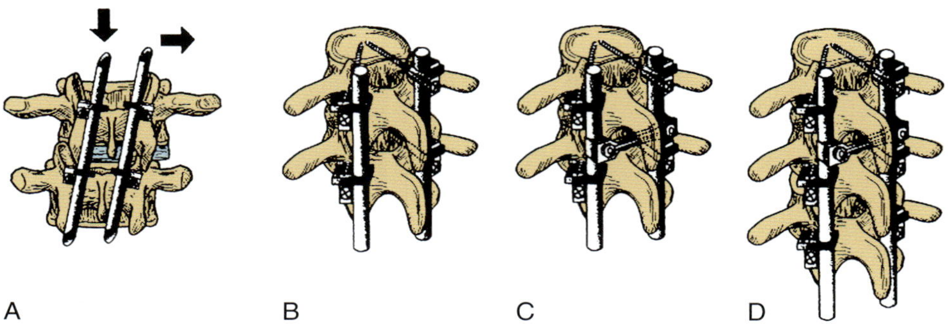

FIGURE 136-21. The parallelogram-like effect of lateral translational deformation (**A**) can be prevented by the toeing-in of the screws of the constructs (**B**), providing a cross-fixator (**C**), or increasing the length of the construct to incorporate an additional spine segment (**D**). The latter provides resistance to three-point bending fixation forces in a plane that is lateral to the spine (i.e., coronal plane), as well as in the sagittal plane. (From Benzel EC, editor: *Biomechanics of spine stabilization,* Rolling Meadows, IL, 2001, American Association of Neurological Surgeons.)

or sagittal parallelogram deformity (Fig. 136-21). Dorsal tension band fixation can be accomplished with laminar wires, clamps, springs, and rigid constructs consisting of lateral mass screws and rods in the cervical spine and pedicle screws, rods, laminar wires, hooks, and cross fixators in the thoracic and lumbar spine. Isolated dorsal compressive constructs are rare. Instrumentation over a number of segments often uses intermediate points of fixation and three-point bending to resist translational deformity (Fig. 136-22). Multisegmented instrumentation ensures that the load is distributed over a number of segments. Intact anatomy can be exploited such as in the cervical spine. Dorsal tension band fixation with engagement of the facets results in increased translational stability. At the same time, fusion of the cervical spine can be achieved ventrally and augmented by disruption of the facet joint and subsequent fusion of the lateral masses. As previously stated, axial load bearing by the facet joints is increased when the cervical spine is extended and the joints are engaged. The orientation of the facets resists translational deformity as well.

Pedicle screws are better able to control the vertebral body by virtue of the improved fixation. Often, the pedicle screw is at or beyond the IAR, giving it excellent three-dimensional control of the vertebral body. In this way, surgeons are able to perform derotation procedures in complex deformity cases and push the vertebral body to a more desirable position. Pedicle screws, however, are not the "be all and end all." Careful attention to spinal alignment and balance must be taken into account. The spine must be reduced properly, and the SVA must be returned to within 2 cm, to prevent increased stress on the vertebral levels. If residual imbalance remains, this may lead to pseudarthrosis[42] and worse clinical outcomes.[8,43] Patient factors are also critical; osteoporosis and obesity may also play a role in adjacent-level disease or fracture.[44] Often, posterior osteotomies must be performed, with or without anterior support, to shorten the posterior column and pull the spine to a more neutral alignment. In this way, the spinal instruments can change from load bearing to load shearing and support the spine while the fusion occurs.

Long moment arms may also play a role in adjacent-level degeneration and fracture. After long fusions, the fused spine imparts increased biomechanical loads to the adjacent segments. Long, rigid fusion constructs do not allow for adequate posterior elongation or stress dissipation; thus, the stress may be transferred to adjacent segments. This is particularly true at the distal segments. Several authors have advocated against long fusions ending at the L5 level, due to high revision rates at the

L5-S1 disc.[45-48] They noted high rates of degeneration and revision of that level. Additionally, for fusions to the sacrum, most authors recommend iliac fixation to prevent distal failure or sacral fracture.[49] The L5-S1 level, due to the high stress, is also the most likely level for pseudarthrosis. This can be prevented with iliac fixation and/or interbody grafting for structural anterior support.[50,51]

Summary

To effectively recreate normal spinal biomechanics and place appropriate spinal instrumentation, the biomechanical forces must be clearly understood. Although these concepts are complex, they can often be broken down into the most basic components. Often, the recreation of the normal spinal alignment and careful attention to bony carpentry can allow the instrumentation to serve as a static implant. A load-bearing implant with spinal misalignment often leads to increased rates of pseudarthrosis, hardware failure, and failure at the implant-bone interface. A clear understanding of the functional biomechanical anatomy of the spine and the mechanical properties of spinal implants will help surgeons select the appropriate intervention for their patients.

KEY REFERENCES

Benzel EC: *Biomechanics of spine stabilization*, Rolling Meadows, IL, 2001 American Association of Neurological Surgeons, pp 1–19.

Glassman SD, Bridwell K, Dimar JR, et al: The impact of positive sagittal balance in adult spinal deformity. *Spine (Phila Pa 1976)* 30(18):2024–2029, 2005.

Kim YJ, Bridwell KH, Lenke LG, et al: Pseudarthrosis in long adult spinal deformity instrumentation and fusion to the sacrum: prevalence and risk factor analysis of 144 cases. *Spine (Phila Pa 1976)* 31(20):2329–2336, 2006.

Kostuik JP, Valdevit A, Chang HG, et al: Biomechanical testing of the lumbosacral spine. *Spine (Phila Pa 1976)* 23(16):1721–1728, 1998.

White AA, Panjabi MM: *Clinical biomechanics of the spine*, ed 2, Philadelphia, 1990, Lippincott Williams & Wilkins, pp 1–125.

REFERENCES

The complete reference list is available online at expertconsult.com.

CHAPTER 137

Spinal Implant Attributes: Distraction, Compression, and Three-Point Bending

Fanor Manuel Saavedra | Vijay K. Goel | Edward C. Benzel

Surgeons and engineers who use and design spinal implants must understand the forces acting on the implant and the spine for successful application. These forces are quite complex and constantly change as the patient moves, the spine heals, and the spine-implant interface degrades.

Instrumentation techniques exert forces to the spine through six basic mechanisms: distraction, three-point bending, tension band fixation, fixed moment arm cantilever beam fixation, non–fixed moment arm cantilever beam fixation, and applied moment arm cantilever beam fixation.[1,2] All of these mechanisms can be used individually or in combination. This chapter discusses in detail how various types of distraction, compression, and three-point bending implants carry these forces and redistribute them to the remainder of the spine and related tissues. Strategies are presented that can help prevent overloading any portion of the spine-implant combination (construct) and subsequent failure. The information presented in this chapter is an overview; more in-depth information may be gleaned from numerous sources.[3-10] Implant-specific information is also available.[11-14]

Distraction Fixation

The use of distraction can be very effective in reestablishing spinal height. It can be applied from either a ventral interbody or a dorsal approach. However, it is uncommon to use distraction alone because it is difficult to apply forces directly in line of the instantaneous axis of rotation (IAR) or symmetrically around it. When distraction is applied away from the IAR, the resultant force develops a bending moment, as shown in Figure 137-1.

If we know the magnitude, the point and line of application of the distraction force, and the location of the IAR, we may predict the response of the spine segment.[15] In these cases, the bending moment results in compression of the spine on the opposite side of the IAR from the site of distraction force application (Fig. 137-2).

The ability to resist bending (originated by the distraction) is called *moment of inertia*[15]; this is usually derived from intrinsic spinal elements (e.g., ligaments). The moment of inertia can be increased by tensile structures (ligamentous or implant) that are farther from the IAR than the distraction forces. The bending moment can be eliminated by balancing the distraction and tensile forces as shown in the following equation:

$$F_d \times d_d + F_t \times d_t = 0 \qquad (1)$$

where F_d and d_d are the distraction force and lever arm length, and F_t and d_t are the tensile force and moment arm length (see Fig. 137-1).

The development of bending moments is particularly problematic when the isolated distraction forces are applied dorsal to the IAR. This difficulty is due to the propensity to exaggerate pathologically or cause a kyphotic deformity. Simple dorsal distraction is uncommonly applied, although it can be combined with three-point bending fixation to impart desirable results.

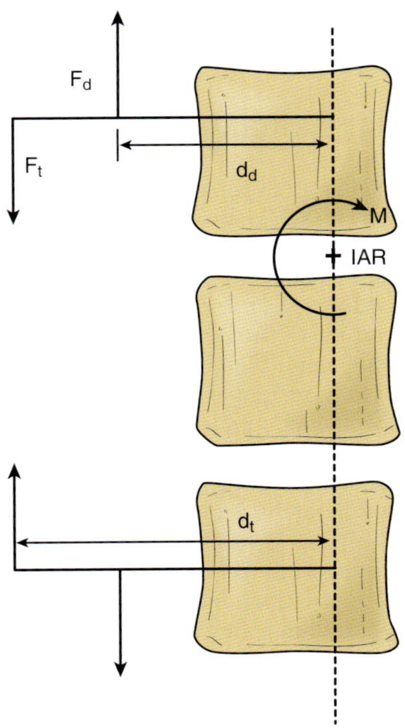

FIGURE 137-1. Bending moment (M) resulting from nonsymmetrical distraction forces (F_d). The negative moment shown results from the distraction bending moment being larger than the tensile bending moment (F_t, applied by interspinous and other ligaments). d_d, distraction moment arm; d_t, tensile moment arm; IAR, instantaneous axis of rotation.

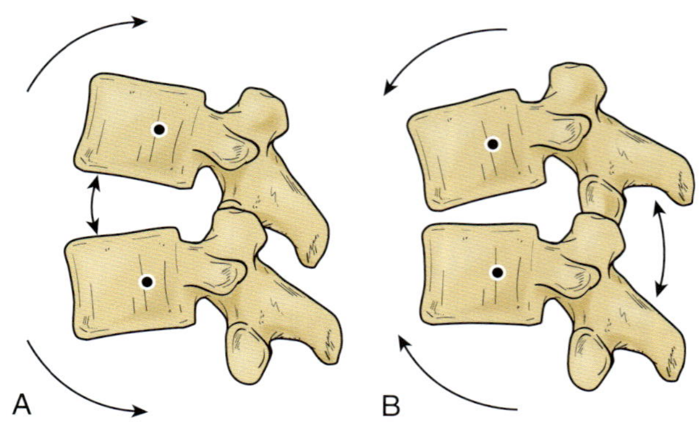

FIGURE 137-2. **A,** Ventral spinal distraction (*double-headed arrows*) can cause spinal extension (*curved arrows*) if the distraction forces are applied ventral to the instantaneous axis of rotation (IAR; neutral axis). **B,** Conversely, the application of distraction forces (*double-headed arrows*) dorsal to the IAR (neutral axis) results in spinal flexion (*curved arrows*) (i.e., in tension band distraction). (From Benzel EC: *Biomechanics of spine stabilization: principles and practice*, Rolling Meadows, IL, 2001, American Association of Neurological Surgeons.)

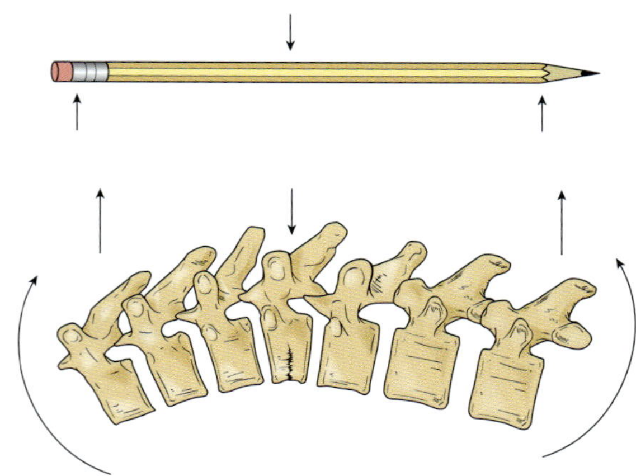

FIGURE 137-3. Three-point bending force application consists of a fulcrum that directs a force vector contralateral to the direction of the terminal force vectors. (Modified from Schlenk RP, Kowalski RJ, Benzel EC: Biomechanics of spinal deformity. *Neurosurg Focus* 14:e2, 2003.)

Ventral distraction constructs (interbody region) generally apply forces that are closer to or in line to the IAR. When applied in line to the IAR, they become very effective in resisting the bending moments caused by axial loads applied through the center of gravity. In addition, this application of forces results in less compression of the contralateral side of the IAR. When the interbody distraction force is applied ventral to the IAR, it generates a bending moment, which causes extension in the spine. These implants can be placed in either an active mode to decompress the fracture or in a neutral mode to resist recompression when the patient assumes an upright posture.

Three-Point Bending Fixation

A pencil can be placed in three-point bending by placing the thumbs together in the center and the fingers at the ends and pushing on the center of the pencil with the thumbs. The resulting fulcrum directs a force vector opposite the direction of the terminal force vectors.[1] The central force vector has twice the magnitude of the sum of the terminal force vectors and the opposite sign (Fig. 137-3).[16] Three-point bending spinal instrumentation applies similar force vectors. They are usually, but not always, applied with an accompanying distraction force by using instrumentation such as Harrington distraction rods or universal spinal instrumentation.

The bending moment generated by a three-point bending fixation construct is proportional to the length of the construct.[17] Three-point bending implants usually involve application of dorsal instrumentation over multiple spinal segments (five or more spinal segments). The forces at the rostral and caudal implant-bone interfaces are usually dorsally directed. The central force is usually in the ventral direction. This central force is equal to the sum of the two dorsally directed forces and is normally located over the dorsal surface of the vertebra that requires decompression (see Fig. 137-3). If the dorsal surface of this central vertebra is damaged so that it would not resist the application of the force, the location of ventral force application can be moved to the vertebrae above and below the damaged vertebra. The result is *four-point bending fixation*. The effects are very similar to three-point bending fixation, but larger forces or longer moment arms (more spinal segments) are required to obtain the same bending moment and decompression. Using the previous example with a pencil, this concept can be visualized by moving the thumbs apart while keeping the fingers in the same location when bending the pencil.

The maximum bending moment (M_{3pb}) in three-point bending fixation occurs at the location of the central force and is described by the following equation:

$$M_{3pb} = F_r \times l_r = F_c \times l_c \qquad (2)$$

The forces and lengths are as defined in Figure 137-4A, and the system is assumed to be at rest. The requirement that the sum of the three forces be zero can be used to derive the moment in terms of the central force,[11] as follows:

$$M_{3pb} = \frac{F_{cent} l_r l_c}{l_r + l_c\ l_t} = F_{cent} l_r l_c \qquad (3)$$

Examination of this equation shows that the largest moment is obtained when the lengths of the two moment arms—and hence the terminal forces—are the same, as follows:

$$\begin{aligned} F_r &= F_c = 0.5\ F_{cent} \\ L_r &= l_c = 0.5\ l_t \\ M_{3pb\ max} &= 0.25\ F_{cent}\ l_t \end{aligned} \qquad (4)$$

Figure 137-4B shows that the moment decreases linearly from the central loading point until it reaches a value of zero at the terminal loading points.

As discussed earlier, it is rare to apply isolated dorsal distraction forces; this is because dorsal distraction also results in flexion of the spine, as the IAR is ventral to the force application points. Because three-point bending fixation opposes this flexion, it is common to combine the two modes of force application. The application of sufficient dorsal distraction is needed so that the implant makes contact with the spine at the intermediate point along the construct (fulcrum), which is usually at the level of the pathology site; this can be accomplished by bending the rod so that it makes contact with the spine at the location at which the ventral force application

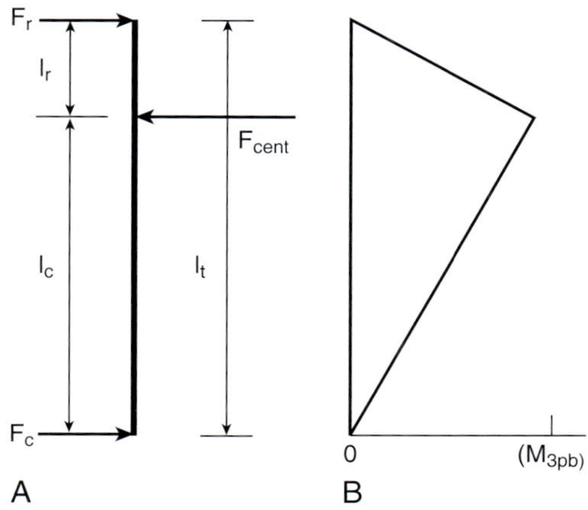

FIGURE 137-4. Three-point bending fixation showing forces and lengths (**A**) and bending moment as a function of position (**B**). F_c, caudally applied force; F_{cent}, centrally applied force; F_r, rostrally applied force; l_c, length of caudal portion of construct; l_r, length of rostral portion; l_t, length of construct; M_{3pb}, maximum bending moment in three-point bending fixation.

is desired or by using a sleeve to increase the diameter of the rod at this location.[14] Nevertheless, this technique has major disadvantages: (1) Achieving proper rod modeling is highly difficult; (2) multiple bends fatigue the rod and may result in failure; and (3) round rods can rotate at the hook interface so that the bend is no longer in the sagittal plane.

Terminal Three-Point Bending Fixation

The term *terminal three-point bending fixation* is used to define a three-point bending construct that corrects sagittal deformation situated at the rostral end of an implant. In this case, the fulcrum is situated near one end of the construct.[1] The moment arm attained by a terminal construct is less than the moment arm attained for a similar three-point bending construct where the fulcrum is in the midportion.

This type of construct may be useful in the clinical scenario of a sagittal deformation where the rostral segment is translated in a ventral direction with respect to the more caudal segment.[1,17] In this case, the use of a terminal three-point bending fixation construct results in reduction of translational deformation. It eliminates the pressure on the spinal cord by the dorsal surface of the spinal canal. Application of the ventral force by using the rostral terminus is much easier because the vertebra to be moved can be affixed to the rod, while the remainder of the rod is used as a lever (Fig. 137-5). In this application, the length of the rostral portion (l_r) is normally quite short (one segment), and the length of the caudal portion (l_c) is longer (two to four segments), which allows a large rostral force with application of a small caudal force.

Combined Distraction and Three-Point Bending Fixation

Combined distraction and three-point bending fixation creates a more complex loading state; this is particularly evident at the terminal rod hook, as shown in Figure 137-6 for the

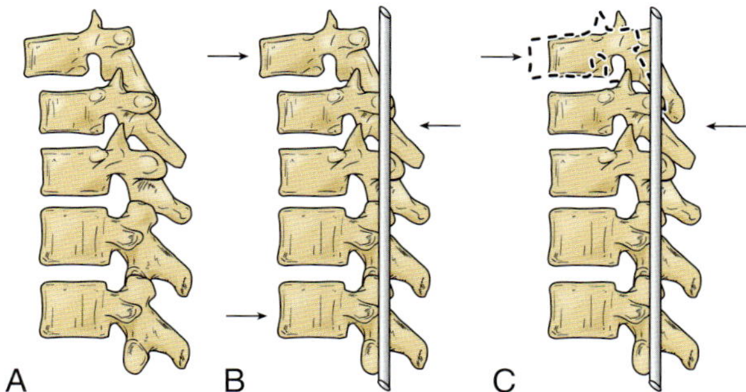

FIGURE 137-5. Terminal three-point bending. A ventral translational deformation relative to the next most caudal segment (**A**) can be corrected by the application of three-point bending forces to each of the three segments depicted (**B**), resulting in translational deformation reduction (**C**).

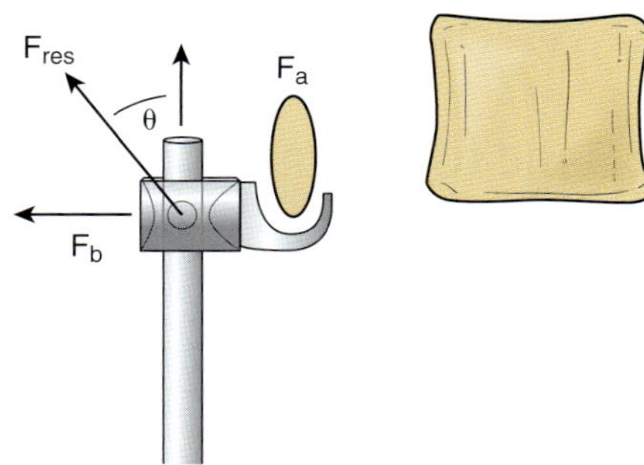

FIGURE 137-6. Forces at the rostral end of a combined distraction and three-point bending implant. F_a, distraction force; F_b, three-point bending force; F_{res}, resultant force.

rostral terminus. The resultant force at the hook is the vector sum of all of the distraction and dorsal bending forces and is described by the following equation:

$$F_{res} = F_a + F_b \tag{5}$$

where F_a and F_b are the distraction and three-point bending forces, and F_{res} is the resultant force. The magnitude and direction of this force are shown by the following equation:

$$\begin{aligned} F_{res} &= \sqrt{F_a^2 + F^2}\,(\text{magnitude}) \\ \theta &= \cos^{-1}\left(F_a/F_{res}\right)\,(\textit{direction}) \end{aligned} \tag{6}$$

where θ is the angle between the resultant and axial forces.

Combined distraction and three-point bending constructs result in the terminal force vectors being oriented at an angle with respect to the spinal axis. This may be a suboptimal orientation of the force vector for two reasons. First, the inclined force vector can result in loading of the lamina in a weak direction; this is particularly dramatic if the long axis of the lamina cross section is perpendicular to the loading direction, as shown in Figure 137-7. The lamina carries pure distraction or pure bending loads better than the combined load because its moment of inertia is higher in these directions. Second, when the rod terminus is being used to correct a kyphotic deformation, the inclined force vector distracts the rostral vertebra and rotates it dorsally. Both problems can be mitigated by clamping the rod to laminae between the center and the terminus, which divides the load between two or more laminae. Careful positioning of the clamps allows the

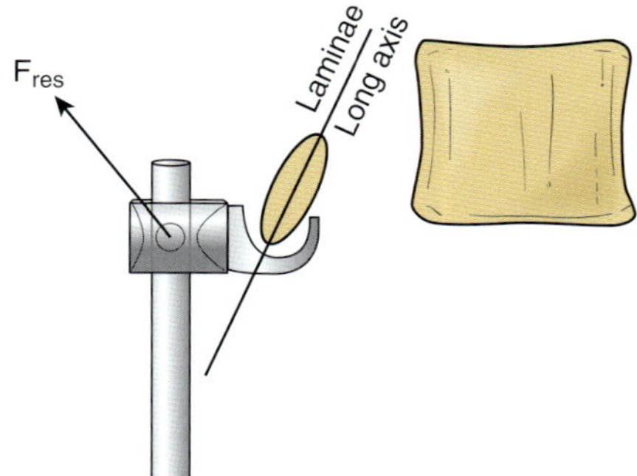

FIGURE 137-7. Inclined force at the terminus of a three-point bending construct loading the laminae in a weak direction. F_{res}, resultant force.

forces on the terminal vertebra to be almost entirely distraction forces or entirely bending forces.

Tension Band (Compression) Fixation

Tension band (compression) fixation applies spinal compression forces at their point of application. It can be used on the dorsal, ventral, or lateral surfaces of the spine. Different types of implants can be used applying this concept, including wires; springs; or rigid constructs such as Halifax clamps, Knodt rods (in compression), Harrington compression rods, or universal spinal instrumentation techniques applied in compression.

Tension band fixation develops bending moments in the compressed segments that can cause flexion or extension according to its location. The magnitude of the bending moment for the tension band fixation construct (M_{tbf}) is the result of the compression force applied by the tension band (F_{tbf}) by the perpendicular distance from the IAR to the applied force (d_{IARtbf}), as shown in Figure 137-8 and the following equation:

$$M_{tbf} = F_{tbf} d_{IARtbf} \quad (7)$$

The amount of flexion or extension that results from tension band fixation depends both on the distance from the IAR and on the flexural rigidity of the segment of the spine to be instrumented. Dorsal application of the tension band normally results in a larger moment than ventral application because the IAR is ventral to the spinal canal. Spinal segments are normally about twice as stiff in extension as in flexion. These factors essentially neutralize each other. The deformations are about the same for dorsal and ventral applications. However, the flexural rigidity of a damaged segment may be dramatically less than the flexural rigidity of a healthy segment; much larger extension and flexion deformations are possible for the same tension band force.

Normally, it is possible to fix only a few segments effectively with this technique primarily because of bending of the segments that is a consequence of the compressive force being offset from the IAR. When the segment bends, the distance between the anchor points is reduced, and a lower force is generated. For most implants, the generated force (F_i) depends linearly on the displacement in the implant, as follows:

$$F_i = S_i \Delta l_i \quad (8)$$

Where S_i is the stiffness of the implant, and l_i is the length of the implant. For rigid constructs and wires, the force reaches zero with very little decrease in the interanchor distance because the stiffness of the implant is so high, as in the following equation:

$$S_i = E_{i-l_i} A_i \quad (9)$$

The stiffness is due to the high elastic modulus (E_i) of most implant materials. Springs continue to apply a significant fraction of the initial force because the stiffness of the spring is much lower. Springs are designed to yield a linear force–displacement curve for large displacements.

One problem with tension band fixation is that extradural masses (bone or disc fragments) can be thrust into the spinal canal during application of instrumentation. Decompression procedures may be appropriate before the application of the implant. Another disadvantage for this type of construct is the inability to bear axial loads by themselves; if axial load bearing is inadequate, it must be restored (Fig. 137-9). Another drawback is the inability to control translational movements well, as shown in Figure 137-10. This motion

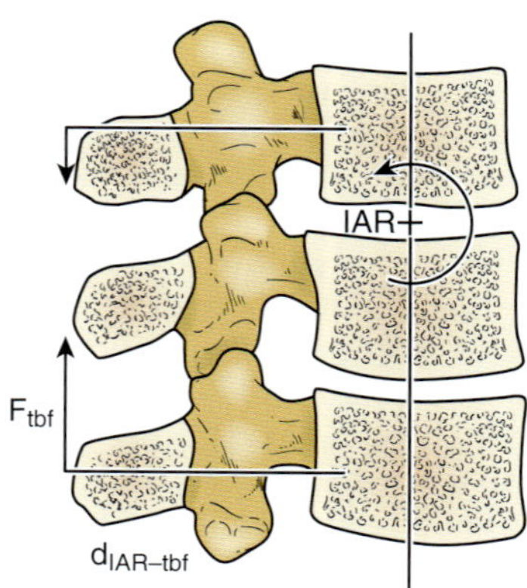

FIGURE 137-8. Dorsal tension band fixation showing the locations of the forces and the instantaneous axis of rotation (IAR). d_{IARtbf}, distance from the IAR to the applied force; F_{tbf}, force applied by the tension band.

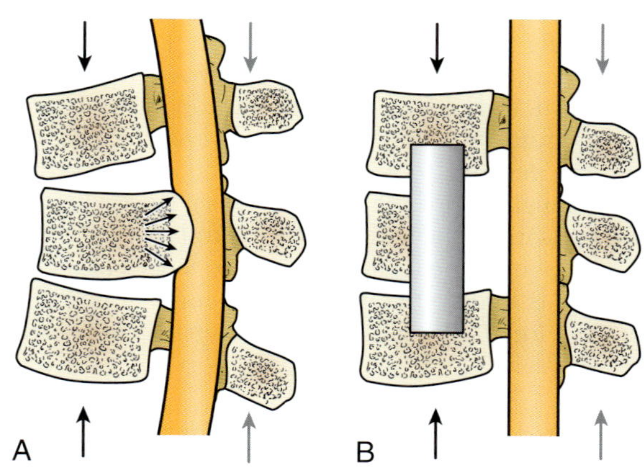

FIGURE 137-9. Application of dorsal compression (*gray arrows*) may result in retropulsion of the ventral disc or bone into the spinal canal (**A**). Decompression and restoration of axial load-bearing ability prevent retropulsion (**B**). Tension band fixators (*gray arrows*) do not, in and of themselves, bear axial loads. If axial load-bearing ability is not present, it must be restored (**B**).

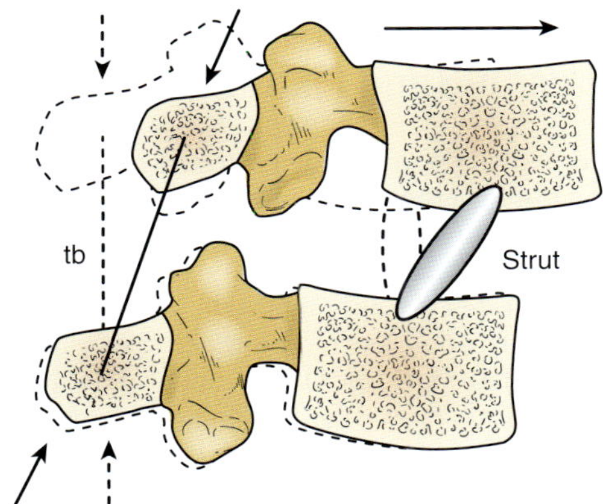

FIGURE 137-10. Translation instability of tension band fixation. *Arrows* depict applied tension band fixation forces. tb, tension band.

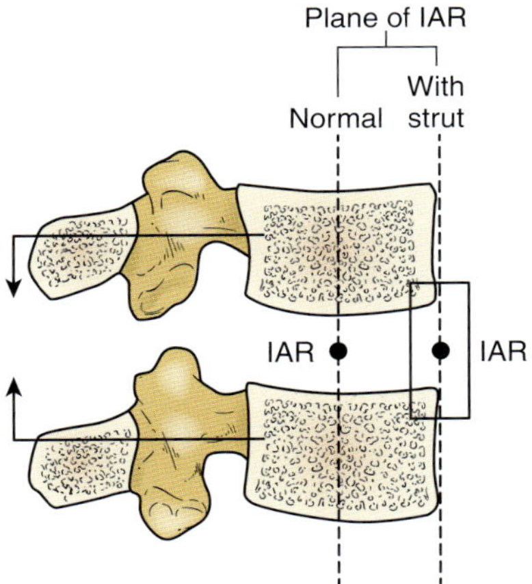

FIGURE 137-11. Effect of ventral strut on instantaneous axis of rotation (IAR) and forces resulting from physiologic loading.

may be accentuated if the distance between the insertion points of the tension band is decreased. Significant spinal integrity must be present when tension band fixation is used.

Loading of Rigid or Semirigid Distraction and Compression Constructs

The loading of a construct is much more complex than the simplified models used in the previous discussion. All implants are subjected to axial and transverse forces along with bending moments. These forces and bending moments change dramatically when the patient assumes an upright stance and during normal movement. The implant bears part of the load (load bearing) and shares the load with the spine and other structures (load sharing). The fractions of the load that are borne by the implant and shared with the anatomy must be considered each time a spinal implant is used. There is no usefulness for neutral constructs (zero loads) because the implant must bear loads to correct a spinal deformity or resist deformation. Even if the implant can be placed in a neutral mode during surgery, it bears a load when the patient assumes an upright posture or moves.

When the patient assumes an upright posture, the implant must bear a load approximately equal to the weight of the torso above it.[17] The nature of the forces that the implant has to bear depends on the mode of insertion (compression, neutral, or distraction) and on the location of the implant.

The center of gravity line of the body generally falls ahead of the lumbar spine, which creates a net forward bending moment.[18] Spinal structures ventral to the normal IAR (IAR_n) become compressed, and structures that are dorsal are tensioned during the assumption of the upright posture. For this reason, the physiologic loads on the implant depend on the location of the implant. The fact that any modification of the spinal structure during surgery changes the flexural rigidity of the functional spinal unit and the location of the IAR should also be considered.

In the case of disc or vertebral body replacement with a bone graft (strut), the IAR changes its location toward the position of the implant because the axial rigidity of the

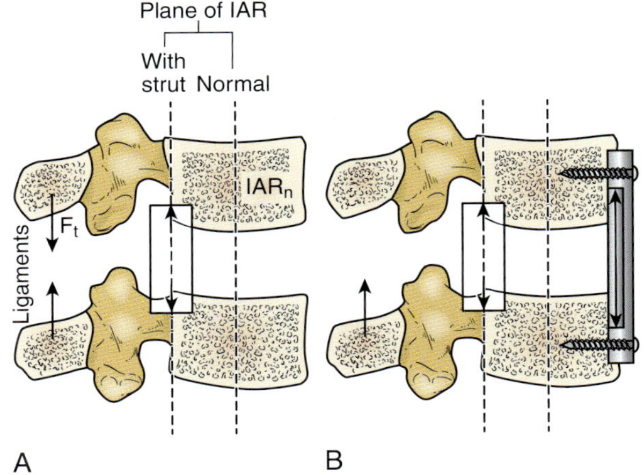

FIGURE 137-12. Effect of a dorsal strut on instantaneous axis of rotation (IAR) and forces resulting from physiologic loading. **A,** Without load sharing; **B,** with load sharing with a ventral implant. F_t, tensile force; IAR_n, normal IAR.

implant acts as a pivot point for intervertebral motion. It generates a bending moment, which causes extension in the spine. Forces that resist forward bending moment (moment of inertia) at the dorsal spine structures and implants located in this area are much lower than the forces applied to normal anatomy. This is because the moment arm available to resist the bending moment is longer (Fig. 137-11).

When the strut is located dorsally to the normal IAR, dorsal structures and any dorsal tension band construct are subjected to much larger forces that resist forward bending. This situation is the result of a longer moment arm for forward bending and shorter moment arm for the dorsal structures (Fig. 137-12A). To compensate this construct, a compressive implant can be installed on the ventral side of the normal IAR. It supports part of the compressive load and moves the IAR ventrally to alleviate these large loads as shown in Figure 137-12B.

The net forces on an implant during use are found by a vector summation of the forces resulting from physiologic and surgical loading. In the case of upright posture, the addition of axial loading to the construct increases or decreases the net forces according to the location of the implant.

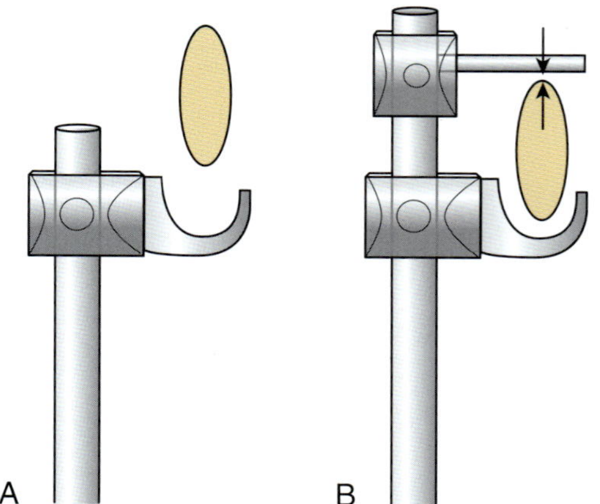

FIGURE 137-13. Reversal of loading for dorsal distractive constructs. **A,** Disengagement of hooks. **B,** Placement of opposed hooks to prevent disengagement.

The forces borne by distractive implants located dorsal to the IAR and compressive implants located ventral to the IAR are reduced or change the sign on application of the physiologic loads. This activity is due to the ventral location of the center of gravity of the spine with respect to the IAR. The resulting bending moment applies a tensile force to dorsal spinal elements and a compressive force to ventral spinal elements. Reduction of the forces borne by the implant is a form of load sharing. It minimizes complications because the deformation caused by physiologic loading is in the same orientation as that from the surgical loading (dorsal distraction or ventral compression). However, reversal of the forces borne by the implant may cause problems if the implant is normally designed to bear only one type of load. An excellent example is the disengagement of hooks from the laminae in Harrington distraction rods. This disengagement occurs when the distance between the laminae increases in response to the physiologic loading, as shown in Figure 137-13A. This problem can be prevented by placing opposing hooks (claw) around the laminae so that the implant becomes a compressive implant on load reversal (Fig. 137-13B). Screw-based implants do not produce this problem, because they are rigidly attached to both the vertebra and the rod.

The forces borne by distractive implants placed ventral to the IAR and compressive implants located dorsal to the IAR increase beyond the surgical loading after physiologic loading. The compressive forces applied to the ventral distractive implants increase dramatically when the patient assumes an upright posture. This increase is the result of the axial loading from the weight of the torso and the need to resist the bending moment caused by the offset center of gravity. However, the compressive forces resulting from the bending moment are not as large as for a normal spine, because the addition of the stiff implant moves the IAR ventrally. The tensile forces in the dorsal compressive implant increase to resist the bending moment associated with the center of gravity. However, this increase may be offset by settling of the spine as structures, such as the discs, undergo viscoelastic deformation. These additional forces may be large enough to cause failure of the implants or, more likely, of the interface between the implant and the bone.

Comparison of Three-Point Bending and Tension Band Fixation

Both three-point bending and tension band fixation can be used to generate therapeutic bending moments in the spine. However, the methods by which they generate these moments are significantly different. The three-point bending fixation technique generates bending moments that are proportional to the length of the construct. This technique usually requires a long construct to optimize its efficacy.[17] The moment arm applied by the three-point bending construct is parallel to the long axis of the spine (Fig. 137-14).

Tension band fixation techniques are independent of implant length. They may be used with only two segments. The moment arm applied by a tension band implant is perpendicular to the long axis of the spine (see Fig. 137-14).[17]

If the equations for three-point bending and tension band fixation are solved simultaneously, it can be proved mathematically that in achieving equal bending moments, the moment arm for three-point bending should be four times longer.[1,17] Three-point bending implants are usually employed over more spinal segments, typically five or more, compared with tension band fixation implants, which typically employ two or three segments.

A ventrally directed force is often desirable at the point of spine fracture to reduce the fractured vertebra ventrally. Tension band fixation constructs may be undesirable because the effective ventrally directed force applied at the fulcrum (fracture) decreases with increasing distance between the attachment points. This decrease is a result of either a progressive increase of the lever arm ($d_{IAR\text{-}ibf}$) as the spine extends or the spine buckling as the fracture site returns to a kyphotic orientation as shown in Figure 137-15. In addition, long constructs may cause hyperextension of the spine by creating terminal bending moments.[1]

The spine is a very inhomogeneous structure composed of stiff, rigid vertebrae connected through much more flexible discs. In addition, a damaged spine often contains regions with almost no stiffness and rigidity, where portions of one or more vertebrae have been removed. The ventral forces and resulting displacements for tension band constructs vary

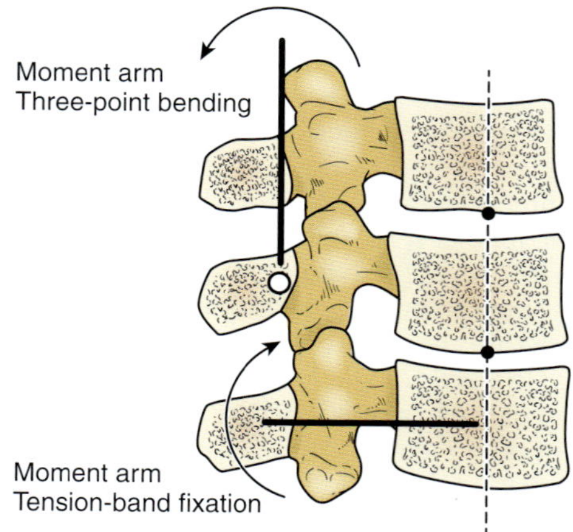

FIGURE 137-14. Moment arm for three-point bending construct is parallel to the long axis of the spine. Moment arm for tension band construct is perpendicular to the long axis of the spine.

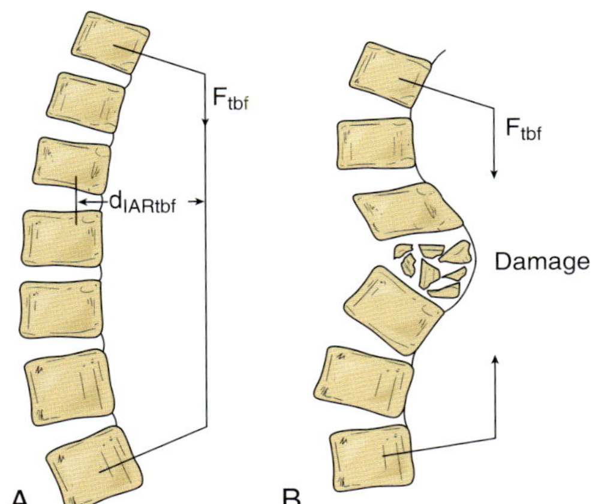

FIGURE 137-15. Exaggerated extension in a long tension fixation in an extended spine (**A**) and a "buckled" spine (**B**). d_{IARtbf}, distance from the IAR to the applied force; F_{tbf}, force applied by the tension band.

greatly along the construct and from installation to installation. If a ventral force is required in a specific location, it is better to use a three-point bending fixture to place this force precisely.

Three-point bending fixation techniques often incorporate distraction forces applied at the terminal (and intermediate) implant-bone interfaces. These distraction forces increase the stresses applied to the bone as discussed earlier. However, the bending moment is not changed if the central ventral force and the terminal dorsal forces are not changed. Some authors have advocated using exaggerated distraction forces in conjunction with three-point bending to accomplish spinal column reduction and spinal canal decompression.[4] However, this approach has not always met with success, because of the "sagittal bowstring" effect[11] and fracture of the dorsal fixation site.

Longer three-point bending implants (more than five spinal segments) can be used to spread the bending and distractive forces over more laminae. These implants often increase the stability of the construct with regard to physiologic forces because of the greater mechanical advantage and more numerous bone-implant junctures. In addition to increased resistance to the axial and sagittal plane loading discussed earlier, these constructs are also much more resistant to torsional and translational loads. This resistance is a consequence of connecting more segments, which stiffens the construct with respect to the out-of-plane stresses that create torsional and translational loads. However, such long constructs tend to increase patient discomfort and can result in spinal failure in the segments that are immediately rostral or caudal to the construct. Failure of the spine in these regions is a result of the concentration of the motion (rotation, flexion, and extension) just beyond the ends of the stiff construct.

KEY REFERENCES

Benzel EC: *Biomechanics of spine stabilization: principles and practice*, Rolling Meadows, IL, 2001, American Association of Neurological Surgeons.

Benzel EC, Kayanja M, Fleischman A, et al: Spine biomechanics: fundamentals and future. *Clin Neurosurg* 53:98–105, 2006.

Boos N, Aebi M: *Spinal disorders: fundamentals of diagnosis and treatment.* Berlin, 2008, Springer-Verlag.

Dickman CA, Fehlings MG, Gokaslan ZL: *Spinal cord and spinal column tumors: principles and practice.* New York, 2006, Thieme Medical.

Schlenk RP, Kowalski RJ, Benzel EC: Biomechanics of spinal deformity. *Neurosurg Focus* 14:e2, 2003.

White AA, Panjabi MM: *Clinical biomechanics of the spine*, ed 2, Philadelphia, 1990, Lippincott-Raven.

REFERENCES

The complete reference list is available online at expertconsult.com.

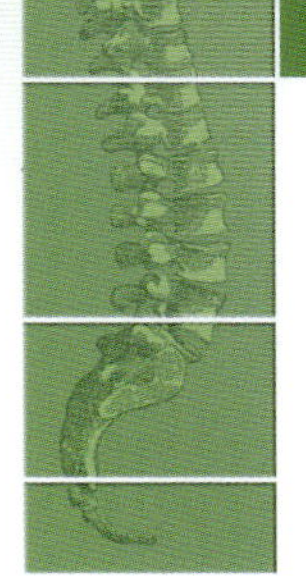

CHAPTER 138

Spinal Implant Attributes: Cantilever Beam Fixation

Christopher Wolfla | Narayan Yoganandan | Yabo Guan | Michael Martin

Cantilever

A *cantilever beam* is simply defined as a beam that is rigidly supported only at one end and carries a load. Examples of this commonly used engineering construct are numerous (Fig. 138-1). Spinal instrumentation constructs using cantilever beams are also common.[1,2] It is important to recognize, however, that spinal instrumentation constructs are rarely composed of pure cantilever beams and may function otherwise in different clinical scenarios and when challenged with other stresses or moments.

An idealized cantilever beam is shown in Figure 138-2. A load applied to the beam is resisted by shear stress and a moment at the point of attachment to the support. In this idealized situation, with axial loading, the beam experiences a shear stress parallel to the z-axis (vertical) and a moment. This moment consists of a force and an instantaneous axis of rotation about which the force is applied.[3]

Cantilevers in Spinal Instrumentation

Cantilevers are frequently used in modern constrained spinal instrumentation. Figure 138-3 depicts a simple idealized short-segment nonsegmental spinal instrumentation construct. Such a construct has been termed *cantilever beam fixation*.[1,2] Brief analysis reveals the presence of four potential cantilevers. Each screw is a cantilever beam supported by the vertebral body support. Each rod is a cantilever beam supported by a screw support. Analysis of such a complex system requires either significant simplification or separate analysis of each component before considering the properties of the entire system.

With regard to spinal fixation points, all screws function as cantilevers in response to vertical shear forces and y-plane (sagittal) moments. As discussed subsequently, screws may not function as cantilevers in response to other forces and moments. Hooks never function as cantilevers because they are not rigidly attached to a support. Although able to resist a shear force in certain circumstances, they are unable to resist a moment. Likewise, cables do not function as cantilevers because they function only when attached at both ends. When attached at only one end, cables resist neither shear force nor moment.

With regard to the longitudinal elements of spinal instrumentation constructs, a screw-rod interface functions as a cantilever only when the screw is rigidly attached to the longitudinal element. Nonconstrained plate and screw interfaces do not function as cantilevers because they are not rigidly attached to a support and are limited in their ability to resist an applied moment. Likewise, many "dynamic" stabilization systems incorporate a screw-rod interface that is very limited in its ability to resist a bending moment.

Bone-Screw Cantilever

In the clinical situation, a transpedicular or vertebral body screw often functions as a cantilever. In this situation, the vertebral bone acts as the support. Both a shear stress and a rotational moment are resisted at the bone-screw interface.

Resistance to Shear Stress

The shear stress resistance of a typical screw is typically much greater than the resistance of the bone in which is embedded. Resistance to shear stress at the bone-screw interface is primarily determined by the mechanical properties of the bone composing the vertebra. An idealized diagram of a vertebral body is shown in Figure 138-4. The screw traverses

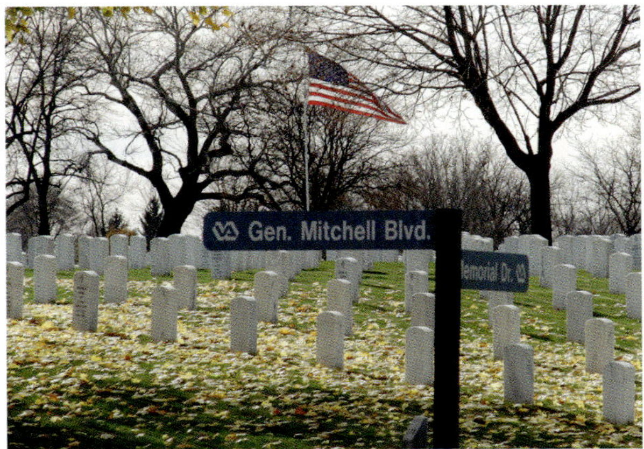

FIGURE 138-1. Cantilever street signs on the grounds of the Wood National Cemetery, Milwaukee, Wisconsin.

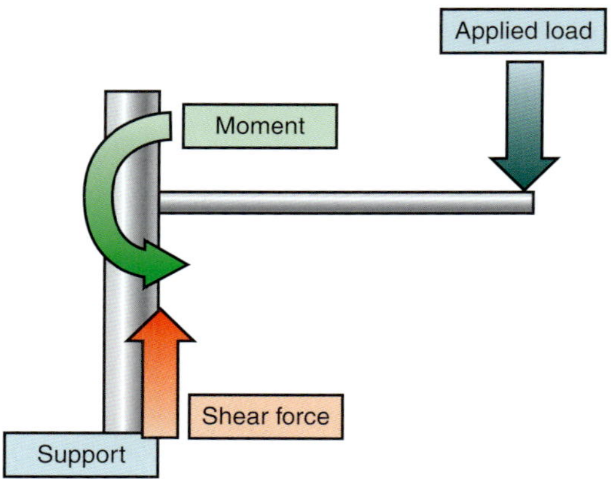

FIGURE 138-2. Idealized cantilever beam illustrating the applied load and the moment and shear forces.

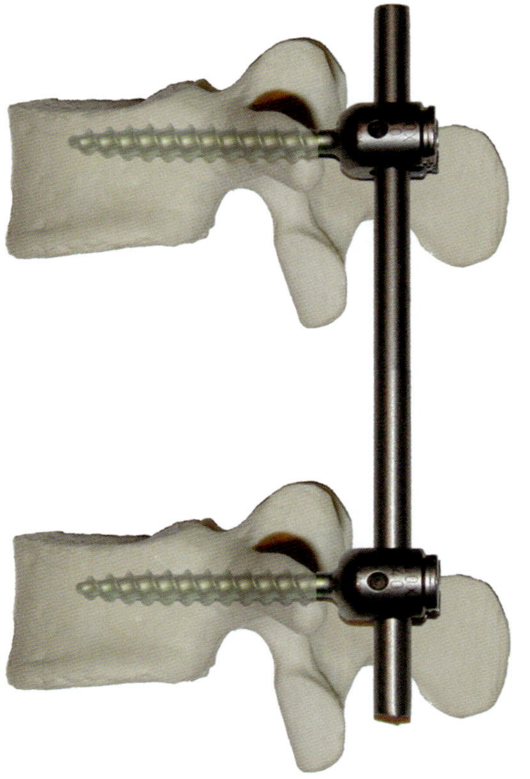

FIGURE 138-3. Diagram depicting a simple idealized short-segment nonsegmental spinal instrumentation construct consisting of two transpedicular screws and one rod.

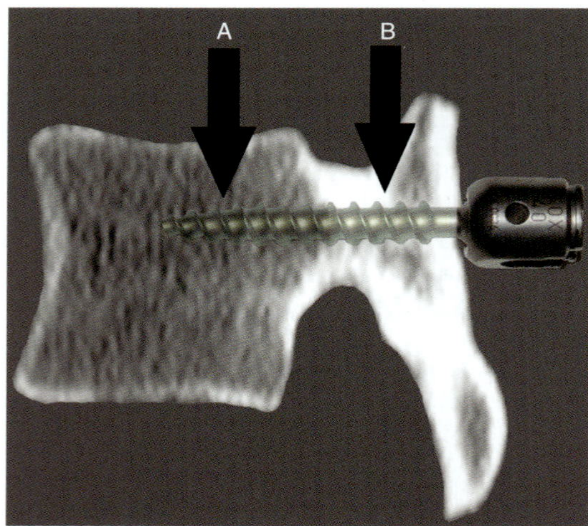

FIGURE 138-4. Composite representation of shear stresses at the cancellous (*A*) and cortical (*B*) regions of the bone-screw interface.

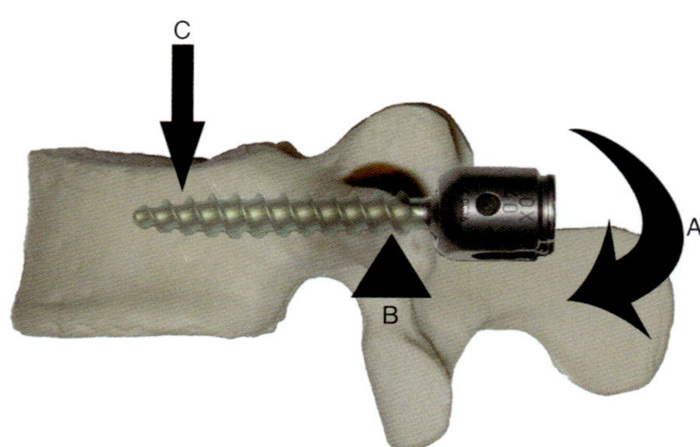

FIGURE 138-5. Representation of bending moment at the bone-screw interface. This moment (*A*) is applied across the fulcrum (*B*) and is resisted by a proportional force (*C*) within the cancellous region of the bone.

a finite thickness of cortical bone, entering the cancellous bone of the central vertebral body. Shear stress resistance is a function of the relative contributions of the bone-screw interfaces in these locations. This contribution is related to the yield strength of the material, the stress at which a material begins to deform plastically, and the area of contact. Although the cancellous bone has significantly lower yield strength, this property is mitigated by the larger area of the bone-screw interface. The total shear stress resistance is the sum of the values for the engaged areas of cortical and cancellous bone.

Resistance to Bending Moment

Resistance to y-plane bending moment is more complex. An idealized diagram of a screw and vertebral body is depicted in Figure 138-5. The effect of differing material properties between the screw, cortical bone, and cancellous bone produces a complex interaction.

A refined definition of a cantilever is a load-bearing member, such as a beam, that projects beyond a fulcrum and is supported by a balancing member or a downward force behind the fulcrum. This definition applies more accurately to resistance to bending moment at the bone-screw interface below the threshold for cortical bone failure—its yield strength. Because of the difference in yield strength of the two types of bone, the cortical bone at the entrance to the vertebral body, particularly in the region of the pedicle, can be regarded as a fulcrum. The screw functions as the load-bearing beam. A load is applied to the head of the screw across the instantaneous axis of rotation at the cortical fulcrum, creating a moment. The magnitude of this moment varies in accordance with the formula: moment = force × distance (from the fulcrum). The resisting moment is generated by downward stress applied by the body of the screw behind the fulcrum. With only the short screw head protruding beyond the cortex, the applied moment may be quite low because the length of the level arm is minimal unless extended by connection to other implants.

Failure at the bone-screw interface occurs in response to a bending moment if the yield strength of either the fulcrum (cortical bone) or the downward force (cancellous bone) behind the fulcrum is exceeded.[4] The yield strength for both regions is increased with increased contact area. This is a function of both screw diameter (cortical and cancellous) and screw length (relevant only for the cancellous portion). An increase in screw length increases contact area only in the cancellous region, whereas contact area is fixed for a given screw diameter and a given thickness of cortical bone at the entrance. In addition, longer screws increase resistance to a bending moment by increasing the distance between the cortical fulcrum and the distal tip of the screw, increasing the moment of the resistive force in the cancellous region.

In response to a bending moment, the mechanical properties of the screw shaft may also be relevant. The bending resistance of the screw is related to the area moment of inertia, determined primarily by the minor diameter of the screw. For a screw of circular cross section, elastic resistance to a bending moment is proportional to the fourth power of the minor diameter.[5] The bending moment is least at the proximal and distal end of the screw and is inversely proportional to the distance from the fulcrum. The bending moment reaches its maximum at the point of the cortical fulcrum. The advantage of a larger-diameter screw lies not only in the increased contact area between the screw and the bone behind the fulcrum but also in the larger area moment of inertia. The use of a longer screw increases both the area of bone-screw contact and the length of the lever arm in cancellous bone behind the fulcrum, although this effect occurs at the expense of increasing bending moment at the screw entry point.

Other Forces and Moments at the Bone-Screw Interface

The previous discussion does not take into account other potentially important loads and moments to which a single screw may be subjected. Pure axial (y-plane) pull-out, well described and modeled by numerous authors, is not included in the definition of a cantilever. If a screw were to experience this force, it would not be acting as a cantilever. Likewise, resistance to a coronal (x-axis) bending moment is not considered, minimal, and, for a cylindrical screw, related to the coefficient of static friction between the bone and screw. Axial (z-axis) bending moments and coronal (y-plane) shear forces, although not part of the definition of a cantilever, may be modeled in an idealized vertebra similarly to corresponding forces and moments in other planes.

Screw-Rod Interface

Under certain circumstances, the screw-rod interface may also function as a cantilever. In this case, the screw functions as the support and the rod as the beam. A simplified diagram is shown in Figure 138-6. When functioning as a cantilever, a shear stress is applied parallel to the long axis of the screw (the support), and a coplanar moment is applied to the rod (the beam) with an instantaneous axis of rotation near the

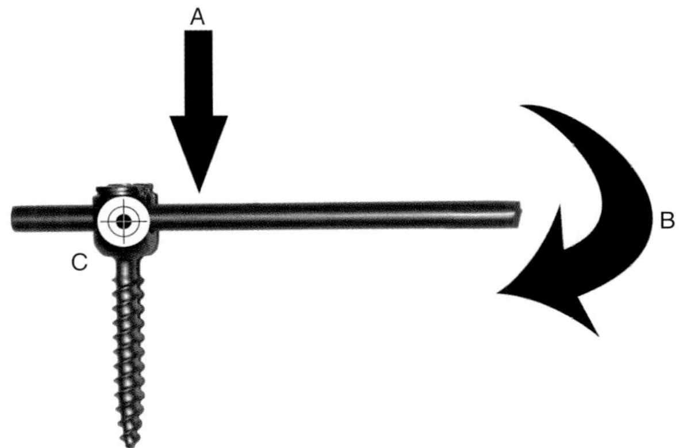

FIGURE 138-6. Representation of the shear stress (A) and bending moment (B) seen at the screw-rod interface (C) under certain conditions (see text).

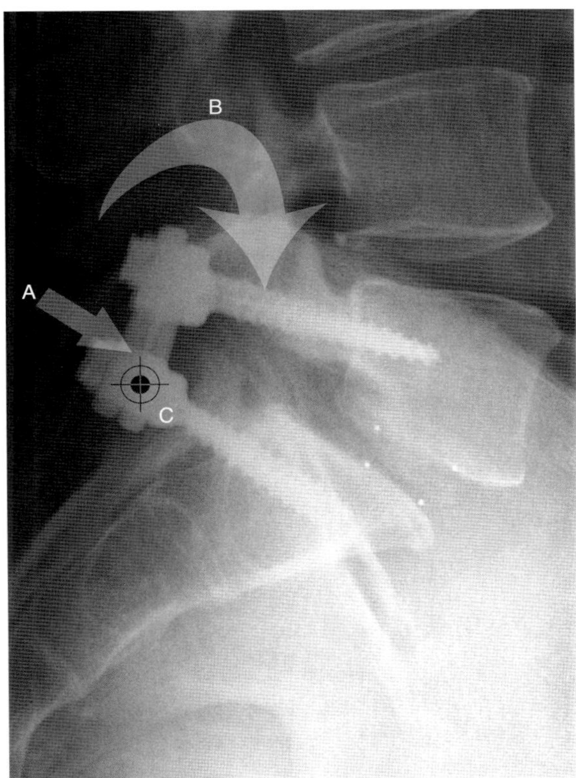

FIGURE 138-7. Annotated lateral radiograph depicting internal fixation and partial reduction of a spondylolisthesis at L5-S1. The caudal screw-rod interface (C) experiences shear stress (A) and moment (B) as the result of the application of reduction forces.

screw-rod junction. Certain clinical applications place significant cantilever stress on the screw-rod junction, most commonly reduction and internal fixation of a mobile spondylolisthesis (Fig. 138-7).

In the example of a construct such as depicted in Figure 138-3, this loading mode is unlikely to be encountered, and the screw-rod interface rarely functions as a cantilever. In most instances, including that depicted in Figure 138-3, the screw and rod frequently function as a single unit, with the rod acting as an extension of the beam (the screw) of the bone-screw cantilever. Lengthening of the rod significantly increases the moment applied across the cortical fulcrum at the entrance of the screw into the vertebral body. All elements of the beam experience a bending moment, although stress within the rod and screw increases toward the fulcrum. The maximum bending resistance of the unit is determined by the material properties of the components and the balance between the area moment of inertia and forces applied to each. Generally, however, thin components placed closest to the fulcrum are most subject to failure.

Clinical Modes of Failure and Strategies to Reduce Their Incidence

In the clinical environment, failures of cantilever-derived instrumentation do occur. Although many failure modes have been described, two predominate. The more common failure mode is loss of fixation at the proximal or distal end of a construct through failure of the bone-screw interface. A second, less common mode is failure of the instrumentation itself.

Bone-Screw Interface

Although failure at the bone-screw interface may occur catastrophically as the result of overwhelming shear stress, this is uncommon because the total shear stress resistance is the sum of the values for the cortical and cancellous bone. Failure occurs more commonly by either fracture of the cortical fulcrum or compaction of the cancellous bone behind the fulcrum as a result of the application of a moment. Of the two locations, failure of the cancellous bone is more frequent. Strategies to reduce the incidence of failure at the bone-screw interface generally can be divided into strategies designed to increase resistive moment behind the cortical fulcrum and strategies designed to decrease the moment applied to the beam.

Strategies to Increase the Resistive Moment

- The use of larger-diameter screws provides several advantages. First, larger-diameter screws increase the contact area between the screw and both the cortical and the cancellous bone. Increased contact area increases the yield strength in both regions.[6-8] Second, larger-diameter screws possess an increased area moment of inertia, also improving the bending resistance.[9] Disadvantages of this strategy include frequent anatomic constraints, in particular, with midthoracic transpedicular screws, where pedicle diameter may substantially limit screw diameter.
- Longer shaft screws also provide several advantages. The use of longer screws also increases the contact area between the screw and bone, although only in the cancellous region. For a given screw diameter and a given thickness of cortical bone, contact area in the cortical region is fixed. This increased contact area increases the yield strength of the cancellous region. Longer screws likewise increase the length of the lever arm behind the fulcrum; this produces an increase in bending resistance proportional to the increase in screw length. Much has been written about the relative merits of increased screw length, usually noting an increase in pull-out strength.[10] In the situation where screws are used as cantilevers, bending resistance is a more relevant consideration.
- The use of additional screws in a given vertebra has been shown to increase the bending resistance in certain instances. This strategy is primarily relevant for lateral vertebral body screws where the choice of one or two screws per vertebra is accompanied by significant technical limitations. Doubling the number of screws per level theoretically doubles the bending resistance of the parallel cantilevers. In practice, however, the use of additional screws is associated with only a modest increase in bending resistance, which is level-dependent and introduces a new failure mode—failure by fracture of the cortical bone.[11]
- Augmentation of cancellous bone with various types of bone cement has also been used in an effort to increase the yield strength. The disadvantages of this strategy are primarily technical and include cement extravasation, emboli, potential difficulty with revision, and permanence. This strategy has been tested primarily with regard to pure pull-out.[6,12-14]
- Augmentation of cortical bone by the use of a staple at the entry point of a cantilevered anterior vertebral body screw may increase the effective yield strength of the cortical bone in that region.[4,15] This technique may be particularly relevant at the rostral and caudal ends of the construct where deformational forces are predicted to be greatest.

Strategies to Decrease the Applied Moment

- The use of additional intervening screws (segmental fixation) has been examined in detail in the clinical and in the laboratory environment. For an otherwise mobile spine, the primary advantage of using intervening screws is related to the decrease in the length of the lever arm applied to the cantilever. Consider the diagram depicted in Figure 138-8. The rostral bone-screw interface experiences a moment proportional to the length of the lever arm, in this case determined primarily by the length of rod between fixation points. An intervening screw substantially decreases the length of this lever arm and proportionally decreases the magnitude of the applied moment. The addition of an intervening screw also changes the function of the other two screws, which function as a cantilever with the rod as the beam. The middle screw acts as a fulcrum, and the remote screw acts as an anchor. Also, these screws are subjected to a pure pull-out stress depending on the direction of the moment.
- Numerous strategies have been designed to modify the magnitude of the applied bending moment. Figure 138-9 is a simplified diagram of the forces acting on the beam of a bone-screw cantilever. At rest, the primary force acting on the lever arm is gravity. The length of the lever arm is the horizontal distance between the fulcrum and the distal end of the lever arm. When the distal end of the lever arm is in line vertically with the fulcrum, the

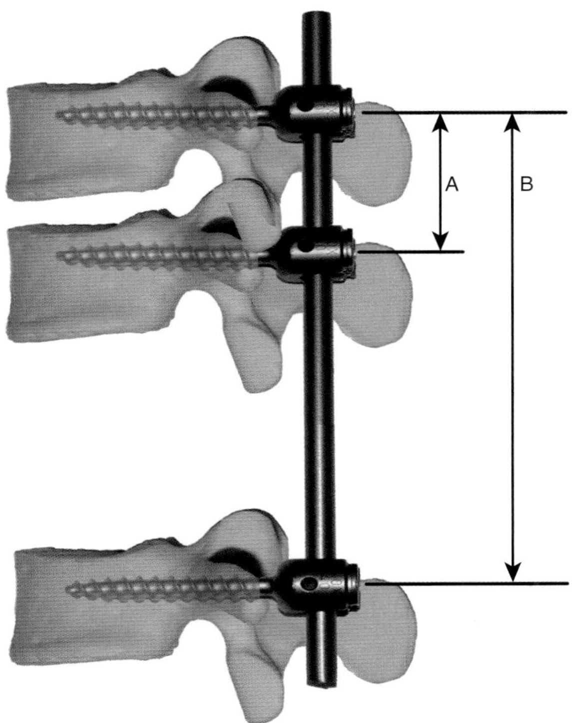

FIGURE 138-8. Diagram depicting the effect of adding an intervening fixation point to the construct depicted in Figure 138-3. Note reduction in length of the lever arm acting on the bone-screw interface of the rostral vertebra (A vs. B).

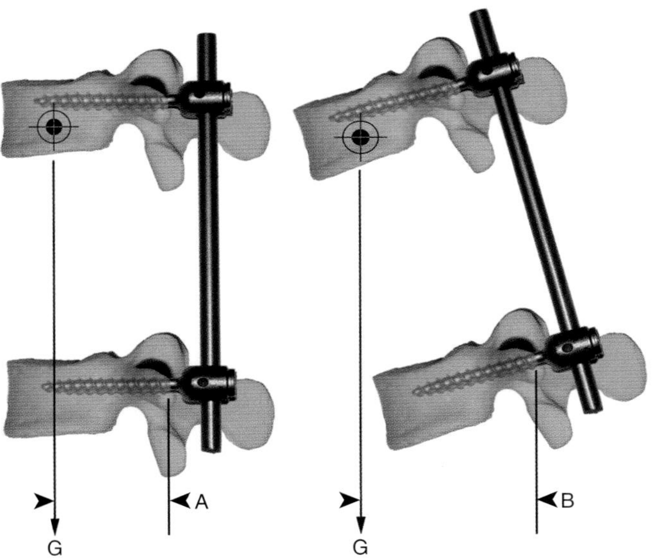

FIGURE 138-9. Diagram depicting the effect of alignment of bending moment. Note the increase in the length of the effective lever arm acting on the caudal bone-screw interface seen with only 15 degrees of kyphosis (A vs. B). G, gravity.

bone-screw interface experiences primary shear force, which it is better equipped to neutralize. Proper posture during the healing process helps protect the bone-screw interface from potentially excessive moments. Attention to sagittal balance, in particular, excessively positive (kyphotic) balance, may produce the same effect. A large study of surgical outcomes after adult scoliosis surgery confirmed that nonunion, loss of correction, and instrumentation failure all are more common when acceptable sagittal balance is not achieved.[16] Bracing, in addition to encouraging proper posture, decreases the magnitude of the moment by way of a buttressing effect.

- Many studies have confirmed the utility of anterior column reconstruction in cases where this is compromised.[17] Ventral column support has at least two potential effects on a dorsal nonsegmental instrumentation construct. First, provision of anterior column support decreases shear stress at the bone-screw interface through load sharing. Second, rigid anterior support in some instances may modify the function of the instrumentation. If the anterior column is bearing most of the axial stress, the instantaneous axis of rotation at an individual vertebral body may be shifted forward such that the construct functions as a tension band and the bone-screw interface experiences primarily shear stress.

Screw-Rod Interface

As discussed previously, the screw-rod interface rarely functions as a cantilever. Nevertheless, instrumentation failure often occurs in this vicinity. This failure occurs because the rod acts as an extension of the beam (the screw) of the bone-screw cantilever. Any applied bending moment reaches its maximum at the point of the fulcrum near the entrance into the cortical bone. Provided that neither the fulcrum nor the downward force behind the fulcrum fails and that a sufficient moment is applied, plastic (permanent) deformation or fracture may occur.

In a typical clinical situation where contemporary instrumentation systems are used, the bending resistances of the screw head, screw-rod coupler, and rod are rarely exceeded. However, cyclic loading of the metallic components occurs with activity. Over time, this cyclic loading results in the development of progressive and localized damage within the metallic components, and the bending resistance is reduced. With continued cyclic loading, the bending resistance may become less than the applied moment, and failure may occur.[1] There has been a trend in instrumentation design toward consideration of this degradation, which has seemingly decreased the incidence of failure in this region. Nevertheless, numerous strategies exist that are designed to reduce the incidence of failure at the screw-rod interface.

Strategies to Reduce the Incidence of Implant Failure at the Screw-Rod Interface

- Use of larger-diameter screws generally increases the bending resistance of the screw in response to an applied moment. This increased resistance is particularly important in the critical area adjacent the entry point of the screw into the bone where the bending moment is greatest.
- Formerly, many spinal instrumentation systems included components with particularly small diameter at the screw-rod interface. This deficiency has been largely corrected in modern implants.[1]

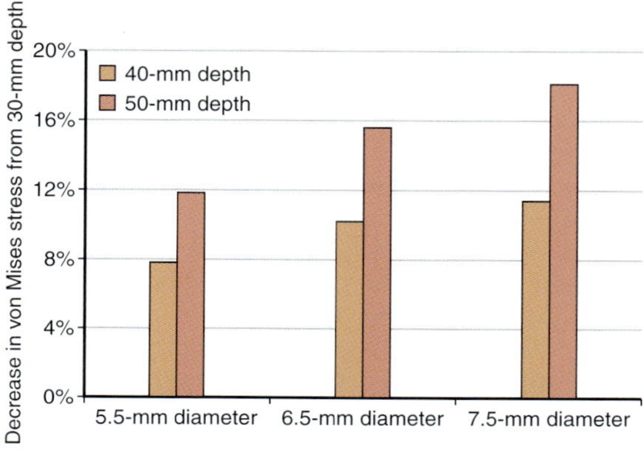

FIGURE 138-10. Bar chart showing the decrease in von Mises stress normalized with respect to the 30-mm depth. Note the percentage change as a function of increasing depth of insertion.

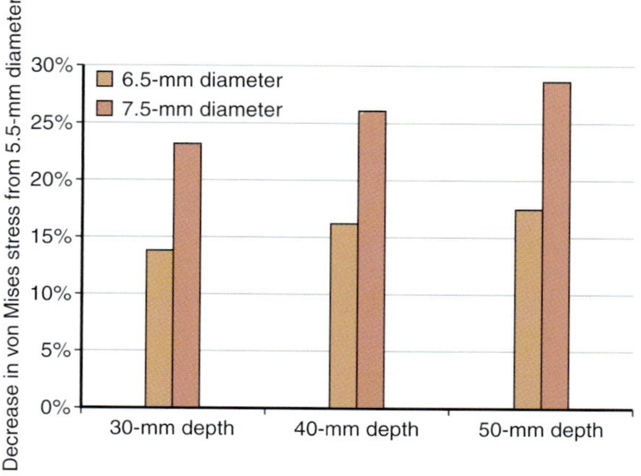

FIGURE 138-11. Bar chart showing the decrease in von Mises stress normalized with respect to the 5.5-mm diameter screw. Note the percentage change as a function of increasing screw diameter.

- Formerly, patients were subjected to long periods of bed rest to reduce the incidence of implant failure before the occurrence of fusion. It is now generally accepted that early mobilization decreases the incidence of complications and improves clinical outcomes. Bracing has been used to decrease the number and magnitude of load cycles applied to the instrumented spine. Although a detailed discussion of bracing techniques is beyond the scope of this chapter, it is important to consider that bracing primarily limits bending moments and must engage segments both above and below the instrumented segments to act as more than an "irritative reminder." Bracing of the L5-S1 segment requires extension to the thigh for optimal effectiveness.
- Application of reduction forces is often an integral part of the surgical procedure. When these forces are applied in the axial plane, as in the reduction of a spondylolisthesis, the screw-rod junction experiences a cantilever force. However, when application of these forces is not an integral portion of the procedure, every effort should be made to avoid prestressing of the instrumentation during placement. This situation is facilitated by careful contouring of the rod, judicious adjustment of screw head height, and avoidance of unnecessary use of rod reduction instruments ("persuaders").

To illustrate the preceding concepts, a simple two-dimensional finite element model of vertebra-screw-rod was developed, and parametric studies were conducted using the following variables: diameter of screw 5.5 mm, 6.5 mm, and 7.5 mm and depth of screw insertion into the cortical shell–cancellous core of the vertebra 30 mm, 40 mm, and 50 mm. Assuming linear elastic analysis, a vertical load of 50 N was applied on the screw end. The maximum von Mises stress occurred at the contact of the screw with the cortical shell. Stresses decreased with increased insertion depth for the same screw diameter and decreased with increased screw diameter for the same insertion depth (Figs. 138-10 and 138-11). Although the analysis was limited to illustrate the load-sharing concept between the bone and the screw, local principal stress and strain responses may approach or exceed the yield strain of a human vertebra.

Conclusion

Cantilevers are frequently used in spinal instrumentation constructs, in particular, at the bone-screw interface. Careful consideration of the anticipated stresses and moments at each cantilever facilitates construction of an effective and durable internal fixator.

KEY REFERENCES

Costanzo F, Plesha ME, Gray GL: *Engineering mechanics: statics and dynamics*, Boston, 2010, McGraw-Hill.

Hollowell JP, Yoganandan N, Benzel EC: Spinal implant attributes: cantilever beam fixation. In Benzel EC, editor: *Spine surgery. Techniques, complication avoidance, and management*, ed 2, Philadelphia, 2005, Churchill Livingstone, pp 1418–1429.

Kim YJ, Bridwell KH, Lenke LG, et al: Pseudarthrosis in long adult spinal deformity instrumentation and fusion to the sacrum: prevalence and risk factor analysis of 144 cases. *Spine (Phila Pa 1976)* 31:2329–2396, 2006.

Masaki T, Sasso Y, Miura T, et al: An experimental study on initial fixation strength in transpedicular screwing augmented with calcium phosphate cement. *Spine (Phila Pa 1976)* 34:E724–E728, 2009.

Rajpal S, Resnick DK: Rod cantilever techniques. *Neurosurgery* 63: A157–A162, 2008.

REFERENCES

The complete reference list is available online at expertconsult.com.

CHAPTER 139

Cervical Spine Fusion Using Dynamic Ventral Cervical Plating

Steven P. Leon | Denis DiAngelo | Edward C. Benzel | Hansen A. Yuan | Kevin T. Foley

The benefits of rigid implants (i.e., internal fixation) in the axial skeleton include rigid stabilization, maintenance of alignment, minimal postoperative immobilization, earlier return to function, and potentially enhanced fusion rates.[1] A potential shortcoming of rigid implants is that they may stress-shield the bone graft and result in nonunion or implant failure or both. *Stress-shielding* refers to an implant-induced reduction of bone healing–enhancing stresses and loads, resulting in stress reduction osteoporosis or nonunion (Fig. 139-1). This hypothesis is in keeping with Wolff's law, which postulates that the form and function of bone is a result of changes in the internal architecture according to "self-ordered" mathematical rules.[2] In contemporary terms, skeletal morphology is substantially controlled by mechanical function, and bone remodeling, both locally and throughout the skeleton, is influenced by the level and distribution of the functional strains within the bone.[3,4] A corollary to Wolff's law is that bone heals optimally under compressive, as opposed to tensile, forces. Experimental studies in the thoracolumbar spine show that a 70% or greater axial load should be transmitted through the spine, not the implant, optimally to enhance arthrodesis and provide acute stability.[5]

In an attempt to improve on the shortcomings of rigid implants, there has been a resurgence of interest in dynamic implants, in particular, for use in the cervical spine. The concept of dynamic implants is not new. Dynamic hip arthroplasties have been employed successfully for femoral neck fractures. These dynamic implants allow for the femoral neck to shorten or collapse along its axis so that the bone is subject to optimal bone-healing compressive forces.[6] Advocates of dynamic implants hypothesize that implants that permit a limited and controlled type of deformation may be desirable. Some experts have termed this *controlled dynamism*. In the spine, allowing for some axial deformation but not angular deformation (kyphosis) may be optimal. Occasionally, the failure of a rigid implant may permit fusion because the bone graft and vertebral bodies are subsequently exposed to the appropriate bone healing–enhancing forces. In this case, the implant has "dynamized by failing" (Fig. 139-2).

The first ventral cervical plate and screw system was introduced by Bohler[7] in 1964. This system ultimately culminated in the development of the Caspar (Aesculap, Center Valley, PA) and Orozco (Synthes, West Chester, PA) plate systems in the early 1980s. These early ventral cervical plates were dynamic implants and are classified as having unrestricted backout properties (i.e., nonlocking and nonrigid) because of a lack of fixation at the screw-plate interface. These implants permit a significant transfer of load through the bone graft, increasing the likelihood of fusion. The nonfixed moment arm nature of the screw causes degradation of the screw-bone interface with cyclic loading. This effect can be minimized with bicortical screw purchase, which requires C-arm fluoroscopy. The main disadvantage of these plates is that the nonlocking and nonrigid (i.e., variable angle) screws led to high rates of screw backout and screw breakage with graft subsidence (Fig. 139-3).

The next generation of ventral cervical plates included CSLP (Synthes) and Orion (Sofamor Danek, Memphis, TN). The CSLP was developed by Morscher in Europe in the early 1980s and introduced in the United States in the early 1990s. The major advantage of this generation of devices is that they do not require bicortical screw purchase. The CSLP uses a titanium expansion screw that rigidly secures the screw to the plate, greatly reducing the incidence of screw backout. In contrast to the Caspar plate where screw angulation could be

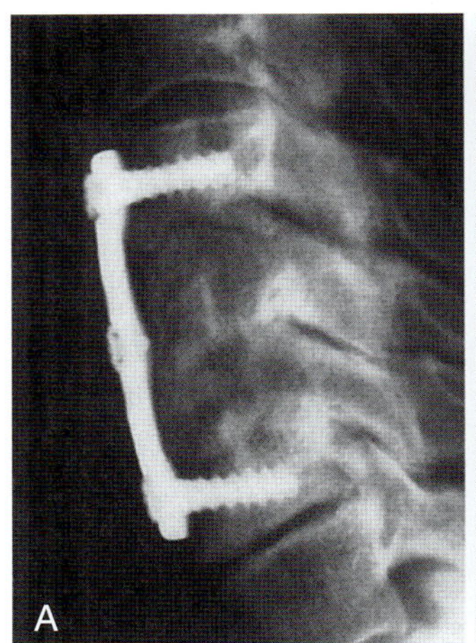

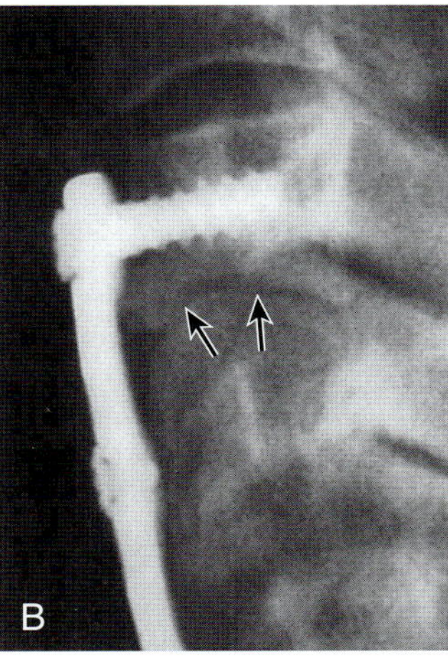

FIGURE 139-1. A ventral rigid cervical implant caused stress shielding. This resulted in nonunion (pseudarthrosis) in a patient with preexisting osteoporosis, as depicted. *Arrows* indicate the location of the nonunion (pseudarthrosis). **A**, Lateral radiograph; **B**, close-up. (From Benzel EC: *Biomechanics of spine stabilization,* Rolling Meadows, IL, 2001, American Association of Neurological Surgeons.)

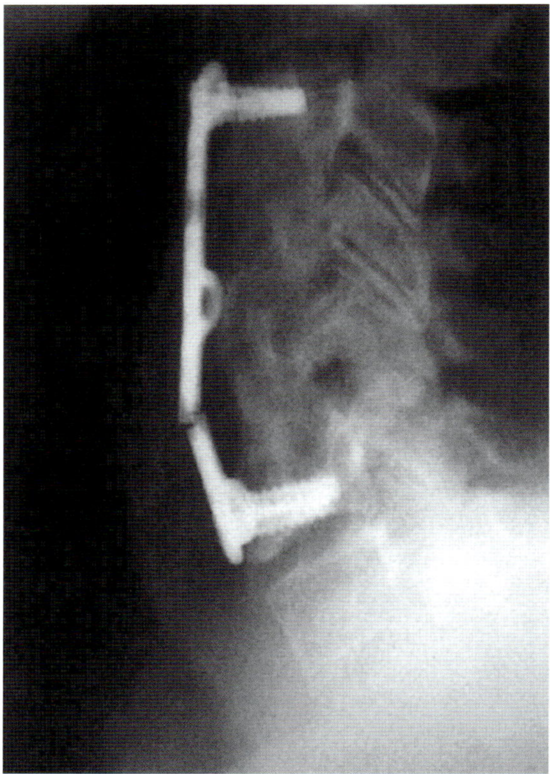

FIGURE 139-2. Failure of an implant (by fracture) may allow fusion to occur. In a sense this implant, dynamized by failure, as depicted, allows the bone graft to see bone healing enhancing compression forces. (From Benzel EC: *Biomechanics of spine stabilization,* Rolling Meadows, IL, 2001, American Association of Neurological Surgeons.)

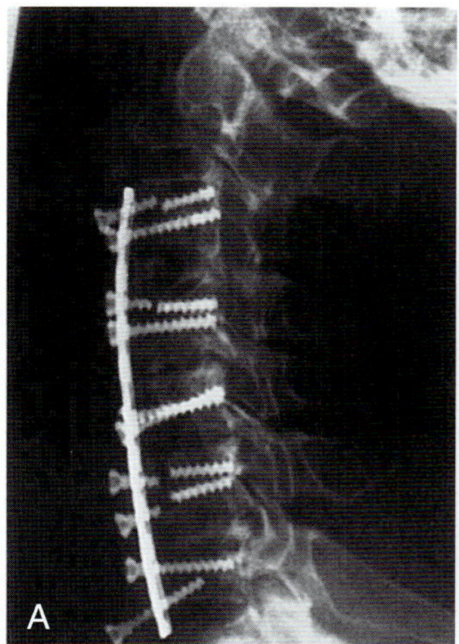

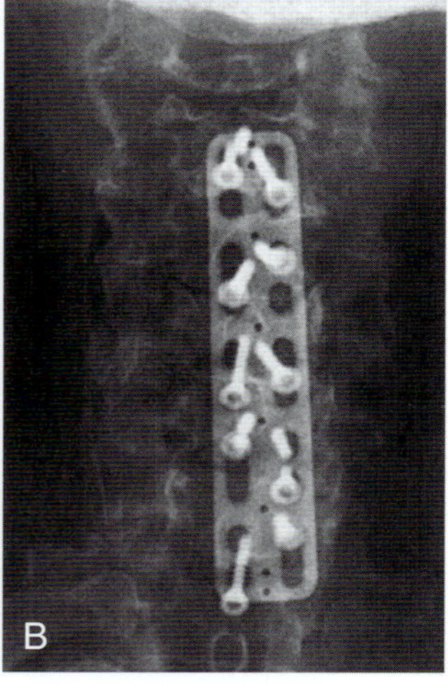

FIGURE 139-3. Screws may fracture as a result of excessive stresses placed on them by the subsiding spine, as depicted. **A**, Anteroposterior radiograph; **B**, lateral radiograph. The screws positioned in holes fractured; they could not axially subside. The screws positioned in slots maintained fixation while dynamizing, permitting, and encouraging fusion. (From Benzel EC: *Biomechanics of spine stabilization,* Rolling Meadows, IL, 2001, American Association of Neurological Surgeons.)

varied, the CSLP has a predetermined (rigid) screw trajectory: perpendicular at the caudal end and 12 degrees rostrally. It has been suggested that these types of restricted, constrained plate-screw configurations are preferable in trauma cases, in which obtaining immediate stability is desired; however, this concept remains unproven.

One concern with rigid plates such as CSLP and Orion is that they are thought to stress-shield the bone graft by reducing the compressive forces that the bone graft experiences and result in increased rates of nonunion (pseudarthrosis).[8] This concern led to interest in the design of dynamic implants. These newer-generation dynamic implants improved on the Caspar plate design by preventing screw backout, while allowing for some movement at the plate-screw interface. This dynamism allowed for compressive forces to be shared between the implant and the bone graft—so-called load sharing. Dynamic cervical plates can be classified into rotational or translational, depending on the type of movement that is permitted at the plate-screw interface. The translational dynamic plates also can be subdivided further into internally and externally dynamized plates.

Rotational Toggle Dynamic Plates

The original Codman plate system, now called Skyline (Depuy, Johnson & Johnson, Raynham, MA), uses screws that "toggle" at the screw-plate interface, increasing the load on the graft and allowing for controlled subsidence. As with the Caspar plate, variable screw trajectories can be used; however, a built-in cam-locking mechanism restricts the screws from backout.[9,10] The Atlantis cervical plating system (Medtronic, Memphis, TN) features a floating washer design that prevents screw backout. The Atlantis plate incorporates the most beneficial aspects of several types of cervical plate design. It uses either a variable (i.e., nonfixed) angle cantilever screw or a fixed-angle cantilever screw (Fig. 139-4). As a result of this flexibility, one can create a rigid construct (similar to CSLP or Orion) or a pivot rotational construct (similar to the Codman plate) or a hybrid construct with both fixed and rigid qualities. The fixed-angle screws using the Atlantis system are directed 12 degrees rostrally or caudally or both and 6 degrees medially. The hybrid Atlantis construct, with fixed-angle screws inferiorly and variable angle screws superiorly, may have the advantage of allowing for "controlled subsidence;" the rostral screws are allowed to pivot, while the caudal screws remain fixed. In this way, the graft is subjected to compressive forces as the construct settles.

Translational dynamic plates are believed to have some biomechanical advantages over rotational or screw toggle dynamic plates. Translational dynamic plates have shown decreased pseudarthrosis and revision surgery rates compared with screw toggle (fixed hole) dynamic plates.[11]

Translational Externally Dynamized Plates

The DOC (Depuy, Johnson & Johnson) cervical system represents an axial subsidence type of dynamic implant. The screws on the DOC system are not designed to pivot but

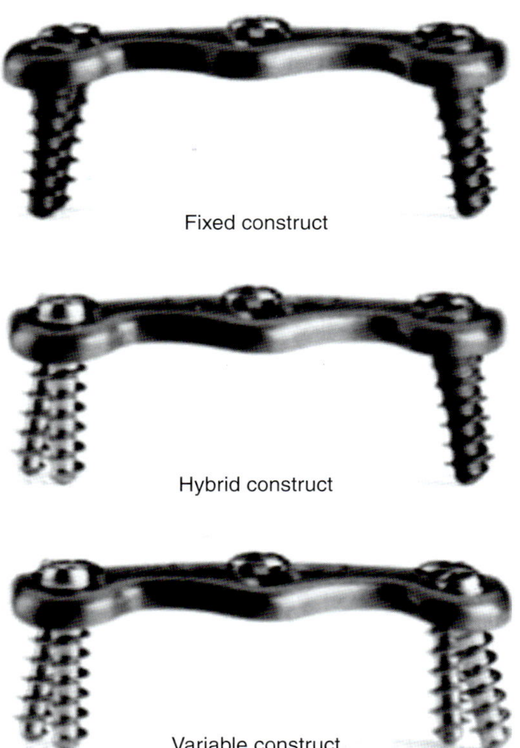

FIGURE 139-4. Lateral view of the three types (fixed, hybrid, and variable) of Atlantis constructs. The fixed screws at the caudal end of the hybrid plate act as a buttress, allowing for rotation only at the variable screws at the superior portion of the construct. Additionally, in the variable construct, rotation at both ends of the plate is allowed at the plate-screw interface. (From Haid RW, Foley KT, Rodts GE, et al: The Cervical Spine Study Group anterior cervical plate nomenclature. *Neurosurg Focus* 12:E15, 2002.)

instead translate, or "slide," along a rail. The screws are rigid at the caudal end, and all cephalad screws have the potential to slide along the rail. This design provides axial subsidence and load sharing with the graft, while minimizing angular subsidence (kyphosis). This configuration minimizes degradation of the bone-screw interface compared with a device in which screws toggle. This system also has been shown to be useful for ventral correction of postsurgical cervical kyphosis.

The ABC (Aesculap) and Premier (Medtronic Sofamor Danek) plates allow for both subsidence and pivoting motions at the screw-plate interface. Similar to the Caspar plate, the ABC and Premier plates allow for variable-angle screw placement but are able to restrict screw backout. With both plates, screws are allowed to subside in a slot and may then pivot after maximal translation. With the ABC plate, all screws can pivot and subside. As with the DOC system, the caudal screws of the Premier plate are rigid, and the rostral screws are dynamic, although a version in which caudal and rostral screws are dynamic is also available. These externally dynamized plates can potentially result in acceleration of adjacent segment degeneration because with subsidence the plate can translate up and impinge on the adjacent level.

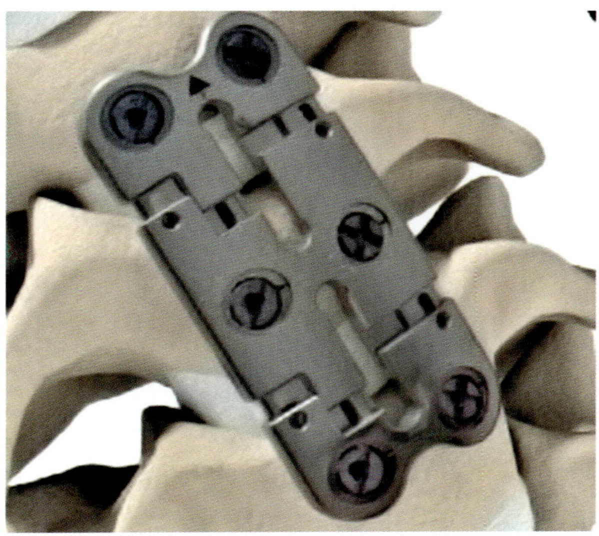

FIGURE 139-5. Dyna Tran translational internally dynamized plate manufactured by Stryker Spine. This construct allows for fixed position of screws in a vertebral body with dynamization of the plate. This prevents migration of the superior portion of the plate into the adjacent segment with subsidence and may provide for easier screw placement compared with externally dynamized translational systems. (From *Dyna Tran biomechanical review: dynamic anterior cervical plating system,* Stryker Spine, Allendale, NJ.)

Translational Internally Dynamized Plates

The Dyna Tran plate (Stryker Spine, Allendale, NJ) (Fig. 139-5) is a low-profile plate. It avoids the previously mentioned adjacent segment impingement that externally dynamized plates have. Screws remain fixed in the vertebral bodies while the plate can translate. There is no screw migration. It allows for 2 mm of subsidence per level. This plate allows for potentially easier screw placement and centering compared with externally dynamized plates and allows for graft visualization.

Summary

Despite the conceptual advantages provided by the use of dynamic cervical plates for cervical spine fusion, it is uncertain whether these are clinically more beneficial over other types of cervical plates. A few clinical studies have reported advantages of using dynamic cervical plates over static plates. Fewer implant complications and faster graft incorporation were noted when a translational dynamic plate was compared with a static plate.[12] Improved clinical and functional outcomes using Neck Disability Index and visual analogue scale were noted in multilevel fusions using dynamic cervical plating compared with static plates.[13] Loss of cervical alignment (lordosis) has been reported with dynamic cervical plates. However, the loss of lordosis, resulting from subsidence with dynamic plates, does not seem to affect clinical outcome.[14] At the present time, the role and clinical importance of dynamic cervical plating continue to be investigated.

KEY REFERENCES

Ghahreman A, Rao PJ, Ferch RD: Dynamic plates in anterior cervical fusion surgery: graft settling and cervical alignment. *Spine (Phila Pa 1976)* 34:1567–1571, 2009.

Hong SW, Lee SH, Khoo LT, et al: A comparison of fixed-hole and slotted-hole dynamic plates for anterior cervical discectomy and fusion. *J Spine Disord Tech* 23:22–26, 2010.

Nunley PD, Jawahar A, Kerr EJ 3rd, et al: Choice of plate may affect outcomes for single versus multilevel ACDF: results of a prospective randomized single-blind trial. *Spine J* 9:121–127, 2009.

Pitzen TR, Chrobok J, Stulik J, et al: Implant complications, fusion, loss of lordosis, and outcome after anterior cervical plating with dynamic or rigid plates: two-year results of a multi-centric, randomized, controlled study. *Spine (Phila Pa 1976)* 34:641–646, 2009.

Rubin CT, Hausman MR: The cellular basis of Wolff's law: transduction of physical stimuli to skeletal adaptation. *Rheum Dis Clin North Am* 14: 503–517, 1988.

Rubin CT, Lanyon LE: Regulation of bone formation by applied dynamic loads. *J Bone Joint Surg [Am]* 66:397–402, 1984.

REFERENCES

The complete reference list is available online at expertconsult.com.

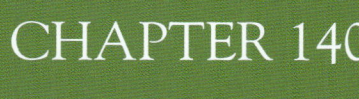

CHAPTER 140

Cervical Spine Construct Design

Ricardo Fontes | Paul D. Sawin | Vijay K. Goel | Vincent C. Traynelis

Fundamental Concepts

Successful cervical spine instrumentation depends on several factors, including the nature and extent of the disease process, bone quality, and technical expertise of the surgeon. One of the most important, but often overlooked, elements in this process is determined well before the surgical procedure is undertaken. This is construct design.

The term *construct* is a neologism that has become entrenched in the spine literature. For the purpose of this discussion, a construct denotes the aggregate of biologic and/or nonbiologic materials that are implanted for the purpose of providing stability to a mobile or an unstable region of the spine. Construct design, then, is the process of contriving such an implant. For the most part, this chapter addresses the design of constructs, composed of bone and instrumentation for application in the subaxial cervical spine.

Without a sound construct design strategy, cervical fixation systems are doomed to failure. The meticulous technical application of a poorly conceived construct is a futile exercise, as prone to failure as the correct system improperly applied. Despite its importance, relatively little emphasis has been placed on this element of the procedure. This chapter presents a strategy to aid in the selection of certain instrumentation systems designed for specific clinical problems of cervical spine instability. The advantages and shortcomings of each type of construct are also discussed.

Benzel[1] described an excellent method for preoperative mapping of thoracic and lumbar instrumentation procedures, using a "construct blueprint." This approach is practical in this region of the spine, because the choice of implant components that may be applied here is vast. The design of thoracolumbar constructs entails the selection of the longitudinal member, cross-fixation mechanism, and implant-bone junction fixators. Each element may be different at various levels of a long construct, adding to the complexity of the system.

Additionally, the modes of possible construct application for the thoracolumbar spine are extensive. This refers to the desired forces that are applied by the surgeon at the implant-bone junction. Constructs may be placed in compression, distraction, neutral, translation, flexion, extension, and lateral-bending modes.[2] In a single thoracolumbar construct, several modes of application may be required, depending on the structural demands at any given level. A systematic approach to the formulation of an operative plan is essential when designing constructs with this degree of complexity. The construct blueprint is a concise format capable of communicating complicated surgical strategies to all members of the surgical team.

The options concerning surgical approaches and types of fixation devices are more limited in the cervical region. The mode of application here is also less variable because most cervical constructs are applied in the neutral mode. Although this simplifies the cervical construct design scheme, the need for cogent preoperative planning is just as important. The format used to communicate the operative strategy is less important than the intellectual process of visualizing the biomechanical requirements of a given lesion and formulating an appropriate construct that satisfies these requirements.

The fundamental steps for appropriate construct design are (1) determine the need for instrumentation, (2) select the construct best suited to solve the instability problem, and (3) ascertain the need for postoperative orthotic stabilization to supplement the implant.

Indications for Cervical Construct Application

White and Hirsch[3] outline four general indications for spinal stabilization: (1) to restore clinical stability to a spine in which the structural integrity has been compromised, (2) to maintain alignment after correction of a deformity, (3) to prevent progression of a deformity, and (4) to alleviate pain. Cervical spinal instrumentation may be applied in conjunction with a bone fusion in all of these scenarios. In rare instances, instrumentation may replace bone fusion as the principal means of cervical stabilization.

Optimally, internal fixation provides immediate postoperative stability to the region before the development of osseous fusion. This is beneficial in two respects. Instrumentation protects the neural elements from trauma and the spine from deformity until the bony fusion matures and can assume this role. Internal fixation also obviates, or at least significantly reduces, the requirement for postoperative external immobilization while the fusion mass heals. This technique improves patient comfort, which encourages accelerated mobilization after surgery. Additionally, this may enhance the probability of attaining successful bone fusion by ensuring compliance with postoperative immobilization.

Internal fixation may allow a reduction in the number of levels that require fusion by adding intrinsic strength and load-sharing properties to the construct. A shorter fusion facilitates the preservation of cervical motion and limits the resultant moment arm created by the fusion mass.

Clinical Instability

The most frequent indication for cervical instrumentation is instability. To paraphrase an oft-quoted general definition, instability requires the loss of spinal biomechanical integrity such that the spine is unable to prevent initial or additional neurologic deficit, major deformity, or incapacitating pain under physiologic loads.[3] The precise definition of spinal instability is difficult to establish and may vary according to the specific clinical setting.

In practice, it is essential to precisely determine the nature and extent of spinal instability. The *nature of instability* refers to the status of specific structures that normally confer stability on each motion segment in the cervical region. This concern addresses the competency of the ligamentous structures, bony elements, and anulus fibrosus of the intervertebral disc. Identification of the incompetent elements allows the severity of segmental spinal instability to be estimated. The *extent of instability* denotes the number of unstable motion segments, as well as whether the instability is predominantly ventral, dorsal, or both. Defining these concepts precisely is of fundamental importance and affects the decision to instrument the spine and also dictates the selection of an appropriate construct.

The etiology of spinal instability is important. Symptomatic cervical instability may result from trauma, degenerative disease, neoplasia, or infection. Iatrogenic instability may also occur, particularly after cervical laminectomy for spondylotic disease. Construct design is influenced by the nature of the disease process that produced the instability. The long-term structural demands placed on a construct are often determined by the progression or remittance of the underlying disease. Posttraumatic instability may demand the least of a construct. Short-term immobilization is often all that is required to promote adequate healing. After the injury heals, the load-bearing and load-sharing properties of the construct are no longer required to maintain stability. Spondylotic and iatrogenic instability may require more from a construct, owing to the slowly progressive nature of the process. Instability arising from spinal neoplasia often mandates long-term instrumentation to maintain structural integrity. Bone fusion may not be attainable, because of the rapid progression of disease. In these situations, the instrumented construct must be designed to bear physiologic loads for the remainder of the patient's life.

Maintenance of Alignment

Cervical constructs are often required to maintain spinal alignment. Internal fixation may be indicated to prevent deformity or to preserve normal alignment after reduction. Unlike thoracolumbar instrumentation, cervical constructs are generally applied in the neutral mode. Thus, deformity reduction is essential before stabilization. This is often accomplished by applying axial skeletal traction. Many constructs designed for use in the thoracolumbar spine can apply significant compressive, distractive, translatory, and rotatory forces to a region of spinal deformity, thus affecting reduction. As a rule, most cervical instrumentation systems cannot apply the magnitude of force required to reduce a deformity. Internal cervical fixation may be used to maintain reduction, but application of reductive forces with these constructs should be avoided in most instances.

Prevention of spinal deformity may also be accomplished by the timely use of internal fixation. Progressive kyphosis or spondylolisthesis may result from spinal decompression procedures. If individuals at risk for this complication are identified preoperatively, cervical deformity may be preventable. Patients exhibiting a loss of the normal cervical lordotic configuration are prone to develop postlaminectomy kyphosis.[4] This complication may be avoided by proper internal stabilization at the time of decompression. Similarly, operative resections that compromise principal load-bearing elements may render the spine incompetent to withstand physiologic loads. Progressive postoperative deformity may be prevented by spinal reconstruction, using bone graft and instrumentation to reconstitute the axial spine.

Pain Management

Spinal stabilization may be indicated to relieve incapacitating pain by reducing motion between spinal segments. This concept has been applied more extensively in the lumbar spine, particularly for treatment of mechanical low back pain arising from spondylolysis and subsequent degenerative spondylolisthesis. Fusion of the cervical spine purely for amelioration of axial pain may benefit selected patients greatly. Such a procedure should be carefully considered and only be performed after conservative treatment measures have failed.

Construct Selection

Cervical constructs should be designed to solve case-specific problems of spinal instability. This requires an understanding of the nature, extent, and causes of instability; load-sharing and load-bearing demands; bone integrity; and biomechanical attributes of various internal fixation systems. Implant cost and facility of application are also important concerns. Constructs may fail as a result of poor design, usually because biomechanical expectations of the implant were unreasonable. Two general rules help guide the selection of a cervical construct and limit unrealistic expectations: (1) the graft and implant must correct the specific preoperative instability, and (2) the long-term success of a cervical construct ultimately relies on the quality of the osseous fusion.

General Considerations

In most cases cervical constructs are used to maintain clinical stability. This may be accomplished most efficiently by matching the implant with the major site of instability. That is, if the instability is primarily dorsal in location, a dorsal construct should be considered for stabilization. Similarly, ventral instability, created by incompetence of the anterior longitudinal ligament (ALL), vertebral body, or intervertebral disc complex, is most effectively treated by the application of a ventral construct. It is unreasonable to expect that a construct will function with optimal stability when implanted in a biomechanically disadvantageous position.

Internal fixation systems provide immediate postoperative stability to the instrumented region but do not provide long-term stability due to the "plastic" properties of bone at the implant-bone interface. As with most biologic materials, bone deforms and reforms in response to stress.[5] Eventually, even the most rigid construct allows a small degree of motion. Repetitive loading gradually increases the amount of movement and can ultimately lead to implant failure, unless bony fusion occurs. The long-term stability of all constructs thus depends on osseous fusion. No internal fixation system currently available can compensate for a poorly designed bone graft.[6]

Cervical spine implants may be considered as rigid, semirigid, or dynamic.[5] Rigid implants attempt to achieve complete immobilization of the instrumented motion segments. Ventral plate systems, with locking screws and dorsal screw-rod and hook-rod systems, provide rigid fixation. Luque rods and rectangles (Zimmer, Warsaw, IN), secured with segmental sublaminar or facet wires, and most lateral mass plate devices are examples of semirigid cervical implants. Rigid immobilization may be potentially detrimental to bone fusion because of stress shielding and stress-reduction osteopenia.[5,7] This concern has led to the development of dynamic instrumentation, such as nonfixed moment arm cantilever beam screw-plate implants and axially dynamic ventral fixators.[8]

Modes of Application

The modes of application available for cervical constructs are more limited than those available for use in other spinal regions. Thoracolumbar implants may be placed in distraction, compression, neutral, translation, flexion, extension, and lateral-bending modes. In contrast, cervical spine constructs are generally applied in the neutral mode. This is not universally true, because certain cervical plate systems and wire constructs may provide a modest degree of compression. Theoretically, cervical rod-hook devices can be placed in the compression or distraction modes as well. However, the vast majority of cervical constructs in clinical use are applied in the neutral mode at the time of surgery. Biomechanical conditions change as the spine is loaded after surgery. Most "neutral" implants must resist axial compression when the upright posture is assumed. These constructs then function in a distraction mode.[5]

Cervical construct designs are also more limited in their mechanism of load bearing than their thoracolumbar counterparts. Generally, cervical constructs conform to one of five fundamental load-bearing types: (1) distraction fixation, (2) tension band fixation, (3) three-point bending, (4) fixed moment arm cantilever beam, and (5) nonfixed moment arm cantilever beam fixation.[2] Applied moment arm cantilever beam fixation, a technique occasionally applied in the thoracolumbar spine, is not used in the cervical spine. Assigning an implant to one of these fundamental load-bearing types is somewhat artificial, because a given construct may exhibit features of several mechanical types. However, it permits classification of implants by their principal biomechanical attributes.

Simple Distraction

Simple distraction fixation occurs when a distraction force is applied by a cervical construct, usually from a ventral, interbody location.[2] Interbody strut grafts, with or without ventral plate instrumentation, are examples of this type of fixation. These devices principally resist axial loads. Dorsally applied distraction fixation is rarely used because it is prone to create a kyphotic deformity.

Tension Band Fixation

Tension band fixation is accomplished by any device that reconstitutes the ventral or dorsal tension band, thereby preventing distraction, and also possibly angulation, in the opposite direction. This type of fixation may be applied dorsally with interspinous wires or cables, sublaminar wires or cables, facet wires or cables, interlaminar clamps, or lateral mass plates. A hook-rod construct, applied in compression, also produces tension band fixation. These dorsal devices resist flexion most efficiently, because the flexion moment is coupled with dorsal distraction. Ventral tension band fixation is accomplished principally with ventral cervical plate systems. These implants reconstitute the ventral tension band, thereby resisting ventral distraction and providing sound biomechanical stabilization of extension injuries.[6]

Three-Point Bending

Three-point bending fixation occurs when forces are applied to the spine at three or more sites along the length of the construct.[2] Dorsally directed forces are applied at the rostral and caudal ends of the construct. An equal but opposite ventrally directed force is applied at the fulcrum, usually in the center of the construct. Three-point bending instrumentation is most often utilized dorsally in the cervical spine and includes fixation of multiple motion segments. Three-point bending forces may be applied with Luque rods and rectangles secured with sublaminar wires or cables, hook-rod implants, and, to a lesser degree, with lateral mass screw-plate or screw-rod instrumentation.

Cantilever Beam Fixation

A cantilever is formed by a projecting beam supported at one end only.[2] When the cantilever is rigidly attached to the supporting longitudinal member, a fixed moment arm cantilever beam is created. This variety of load bearing is accomplished by ventral cervical plate systems secured with locking screws and rigid lateral mass rod-screw instrumentation. A fixed moment arm cantilever beam device contributes some axial load-sharing properties to the construct. Nonfixed moment arm cantilever beam fixation employs a dynamic attachment of the cantilever to the longitudinal member. Lateral mass plates and nonfixed moment arm cantilever beam screw-plate implants and axially dynamic ventral fixators are representative of this type of load bearing.

The classification of spinal implants by a mechanism of load bearing is somewhat artificial. In practice a single implant may function by using several of the fundamental load-bearing mechanisms simultaneously. For example, the lateral mass plate is capable of stabilization by three such mechanisms. Dorsal tension band, three-point bending, and nonfixed moment arm cantilever beam fixation are all accomplished by this device.

Construct Materials

A variety of biologic and prosthetic materials have been used for cervical spine stabilization. Most constructs are composed of a bone graft, coupled with a metal prosthesis. Occasionally, bone and/or metal components may be supplemented or replaced by methyl methacrylate.

Bone Grafts

Autograft and allograft bone have both been used extensively in spinal stabilization. Some studies report that fusion rates with allograft bone are comparable to those obtained with autograft bone.[9-11] Other studies have maintained that autograft bone is superior.[3,12,13] This is particularly evident with dorsal cervical constructs, in which the bone graft is not placed under compression. Certainly, fusion rates with autograft bone meet or exceed those reported with allograft. The use of autograft bone eliminates the concern of infectious disease transmission (including HIV and hepatitis virus transmission) that may be associated with allograft bone.

The iliac crest provides a versatile and abundant source of bone graft material for incorporation into cervical spine constructs. Favorable attributes of this type of graft include ease of procurement in both the supine and prone positions, strength, and relative expendability of the donor site.[3,14] The tricortical structure of the iliac crest is responsible for much of the strength inherent in this graft, thereby providing excellent axial load-bearing capability. The abundant cancellous bone provides ample substrate for osseous remodeling. Although all commonly used configurations of iliac crest grafts can sustain high compressive loads, the Smith-Robinson–type graft is probably superior to other styles of grafts in this respect.[15] The principal disadvantage associated with iliac crest harvest is donor site morbidity, which may be substantial. Complications include pain, wound hematoma, infection, meralgia paresthetica, hip dislocation, and fracture of the anterior superior iliac spine.

Fibula is another commonly used site for graft material. It is particularly well suited for multilevel ventral reconstruction procedures, because the thick cortical bone in this graft resists high axial compressive loads. The relatively small amount of cancellous bone present in the fibula graft may delay bone remodeling, however. This may be partially overcome by packing additional cancellous bone in the center of the graft, as well as surrounding the outer cortical surface with the cancellous bone. Donor site morbidity arising from graft harvest may be significant, because one sixth of body weight is borne by the fibula.[5] This may be principally a theoretical concern, however, as fibular bone has been used quite successfully in many cases of spinal reconstruction.

Rib grafts have also been used, particularly with dorsal cervical constructs. The native configuration of rib is advantageous because it conforms well to the cervical lordotic curve. There is minimal morbidity in harvesting rib compared with iliac crest. This is an excellent graft to use for dorsal fusions.[16]

Many interbody allograft products are currently available. The overall fusion rate with these materials is similar to that of autograft, if instrumentation is used.

Implants

Currently most spinal implants are fashioned from metal. Stainless steel has been used extensively for the manufacture of wires, cables, plates, screws, hooks, and rods used in spinal constructs. This material possesses a relatively high tensile strength while retaining a reasonable degree of malleability. The latter permits custom implant modification, which is often required to tailor a component to a patient's individual anatomic specification. Recently, titanium alloys have replaced stainless steel for use as cervical spine implants. These alloys are strong and biocompatible and facilitate postoperative MRI and CT imaging.

Regardless of the material used, compatibility of the implanted components is essential. All metal implants should be made of the same material. This eliminates the theoretical possibility of internal current generation that may cause corrosion. The size of implanted components should also be compatible. Fixators at the implant-bone junction should be of appropriate diameter, length, and configuration to match the longitudinal member.[6]

Methyl methacrylate has been used to supplement or replace bone, metal components, or both. This material is simple to apply, relatively safe, and inexpensive. Long-term stability of any cervical construct requires osseous fusion. Therefore, the ultimate stability of a construct with methyl methacrylate cannot be guaranteed, because no provision is made for bone fusion.

The integrity of the patient's native bone is an important factor. Bone quality can affect construct selection, the biomechanical stability of a construct, and the need for postoperative external immobilization. Osteoporosis is detrimental to all forms of spinal fixation. It influences systems that rely on screw fixation most substantially. Hooks and sublaminar wires are less prone to pull-out than screws and thus may be more suited for use in the osteoporotic patient.[1] Poor bone quality may necessitate incorporation of additional levels into a construct to promote load sharing and enhance stability.

It is difficult to accurately assess bone quality. A general impression of bone mineralization may be gleaned from plain cervical radiographs. Dual-energy x-ray absorptiometry (DEXA) and quantitative CT provide an objective determination of bone mineral density. The clinical use of this technology is limited by the lack of cervical spine standards available for comparison. Also, the influence of bone mineral density on screw fixation biomechanics is poorly understood. Currently, it is not possible to predict the holding strength of fixators at the implant-bone junction from preoperative studies.

Construct Application

Cervical spine integrity may be restored by either ventral or dorsal stabilization techniques. The application of both may be indicated in cases of severe instability creating a "360-degree" construct. The rationale for selecting one approach over another is case dependent and relies on the degree and extent of instability. If the site of major instability is ventral, a ventral construct should be created to restore structural integrity to the ventral spine. Dorsal instability is treated most effectively through dorsal stabilization. This general rule is valid for all causes of cervical instability. The underlying disease process does influence the selection of specific construct components and the method by which they are applied.

Neural compression often accompanies cervical instability and must be alleviated before stabilization. Neurologic deficit may result from direct neural compression by the disease process itself or by attendant spinal instability. Decompressive procedures may exacerbate segmental instability as a result of key load-bearing structures. This is particularly important when disease involvement is extensive. The underlying pathology may predispose to postoperative instability by rendering other load-bearing elements incompetent.

The requirements of neural element decompression influence the approach that is selected for stabilization. Generally, ventral compressive or invasive pathology should be dealt with via a ventral approach. If dorsal neural compression is encountered, a dorsal decompressive procedure is indicated. Internal fixation techniques should attempt to restore the structural integrity of the elements made incompetent by the disease process or surgical resection.

The surgeon must be wary and avoid exacerbation of neural compromise by the process of spinal stabilization. For example, dorsal tension band fixation may increase ventral neural compression resulting from traumatic intervertebral disc herniation or neoplastic disease. This may produce additional neurologic deficit. Constructs must be designed with consideration for the structural alterations that they may induce and the effect that this may have on the neural elements. If this is not appreciated, disastrous consequences may follow.

Ventral Constructs

Ventral cervical spine constructs are designed to restore stability to the ventral spine when the osseous and/or ligamentous structures are incompetent. Intervertebral strut grafts without instrumentation have been used for more than 40 years to reconstitute the ventral load-bearing column of the cervical spine. Methyl methacrylate may be used as an alternative to bony fusion in this region.

Ventral stabilization is usually performed in conjunction with a ventral decompressive procedure. The corollary of this observation is also true. Ventral decompression is seldom undertaken without subsequent ventral stabilization. This differs from most dorsal decompression or stabilization procedures, which are often performed independently. Dorsal decompression (i.e., cervical laminectomy) is frequently undertaken without stabilization, and dorsal fixation may not require decompression.

A variety of cervical constructs may be applied via the ventral approach. The following review is not exhaustive but represents the majority of techniques currently used for ventral cervical stabilization.

Interbody Strut Graft

By definition, a simple interbody strut graft implanted after a ventral cervical discectomy constitutes a ventral cervical construct. Larger grafts are often used for vertebral body replacement after corpectomy for trauma, neoplasia, and spondylotic disease. Ventral strut grafts function predominantly in the simple distraction mode, reconstituting the ventral load-bearing column of the cervical spine. This construct offers excellent resistance to axial compressive loads (Fig. 140-1). It also imparts some stability in flexion, extension, axial rotation, and lateral bending.[13] In most cases, however, immediate postoperative stability is not provided with a simple strut graft.

Some means of fixation, whether external or internal, is usually required to provide temporary stability until osseous fusion occurs. The extent of supplemental fixation is dictated by the degree of instability that remains after placement of the bone graft. The instability created by a single-level ventral cervical discectomy may be managed adequately with interbody strut graft placement and immobilization in a cervical collar. More significant instability requires more rigid fixation while the fusion matures. This may be accomplished internally with instrumentation or externally with an orthosis. In the setting of multilevel corpectomy, some studies suggest that ventral corpectomy with instrumentation be supplemented with dorsal instrumentation to prevent postoperative

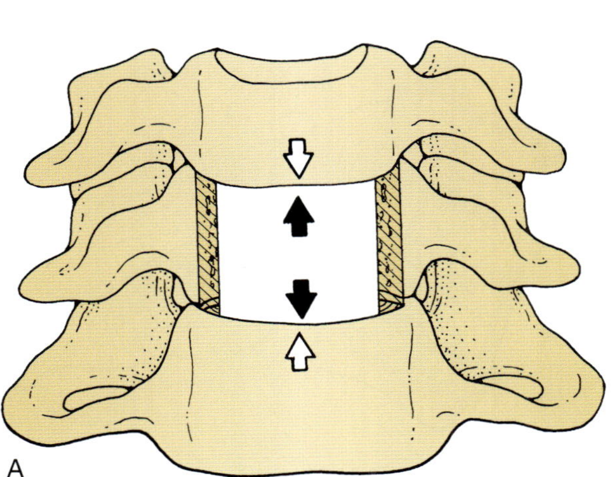

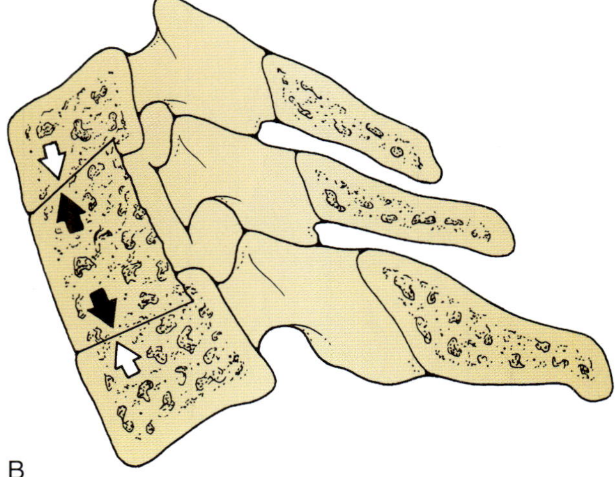

FIGURE 140-1. Coronal (**A**) and lateral (**B**) views of an osseous strut graft. This construct functions in a simple distraction mode (*black arrows*), providing resistance to axial compression (*white arrows*).

graft and instrumentation complications.[17,18] However, this is a point of controversy; others have advocated ventral cervical fixation as sufficient for multilevel corpectomy up to four levels.[19]

Ventral Cervical Plate and Screw Constructs

Ventral cervical plate and screw constructs were developed to provide immediate internal stability before osseous integration of a strut graft. When used in this context, these devices often eliminate the need for postoperative external bracing. All ventral plate constructs reconstitute the ventral tension band, thereby providing the most stabilization in extension.[20] Some of these devices also provide fixed moment arm cantilever beam fixation, thereby sharing some of the axial load with the strut graft. Rigid implants with fixed-angle locking screw mechanisms function in this capacity. Plating systems that use variable-angle screws or translationally mobile screws are more dynamic implants and provide less axial load sharing. These devices act as nonfixed moment arm cantilever beam fixators in addition to their tension band attributes (Fig. 140-2). Dynamic implants theoretically allow for the graft to be exposed to continuous axial loading, which may facilitate bone fusion.[8]

Biomechanical studies have demonstrated that ventral plates can restore stability to the injured spine in essentially all motion planes, although this is most significant in flexion and extension.[13,21] An interbody bone graft must supplement the instrumentation to effectively stabilize an injured motion segment. The load-bearing capacities of ventral cervical plates are temporary, so all plated segments must be fused to achieve long-term stability.

Ventral cervical plates are affixed with screws at the implant-bone junction. Some devices use screws with bicortical purchase, whereas others use unicortical fixation. Bicortical screw purchase confers greater holding strength to the construct.[11] Placement of bicortical screws is slightly more perilous than implantation of unicortical screws, because the dorsal cortex of the vertebral body must be drilled to accept these screws. To avoid drilling into the spinal canal and traumatizing the spinal cord, bicortical screw placement must be monitored using fluoroscopy.[22]

Unicortical screws may be applied with less hazardous results. Fluoroscopy is not mandatory, because the dorsal cortex is not violated. Imaging, however, is recommended as a confirmatory intraoperative study.

The indications for ventral cervical plating are extensive. Traumatic lesions that produce persistent instability may require surgical stabilization. Unstable injuries involving the vertebral body or intervertebral disc are managed most efficiently by ventral stabilization. This is particularly important when the ventral spinal canal is compromised by bone fragments or herniated intervertebral disc material. Cervical burst fractures may require ventral decompression and internal fixation. A strut graft for vertebral body replacement and a ventral plate for immediate internal stability are appropriate construct designs for this indication. Ventral plates should be applied to intact vertebral bodies above and below the involved levels, spanning the instability.

Other traumatic lesions may be stabilized ventrally. Irreducible facet dislocations are generally approached dorsally. However, when facet dislocation is complicated by concomitant disc herniation, decompression and reduction may be undertaken via a ventral approach. Stabilization is then accomplished with an interbody bone graft and a ventral plate. Neural decompression must precede reduction of the spinal deformity, thereby minimizing the risk of producing or exacerbating a neurologic deficit.

Spinal neoplasms often involve the vertebral body, potentially causing spinal instability and neurologic dysfunction. Ventral cervical plates may be applied after decompression to reconstruct the axial spine. In these instances, screw fixation must be performed in vertebrae that are free of disease.

Cervical spondylotic disease may also be treated by ventral decompression and stabilization, using ventral plates. Kyphotic deformities almost always require a ventral approach. Discectomy(ies) and/or corpectomy(ies), grafting, and ventral plate stabilization usually forms the first-line therapy for this type of spinal deformity.

Ventral cervical plate systems are extremely versatile. They provide substantial immediate postoperative stability, limit the extent of instrumentation, and facilitate aggressive reconstruction of the ventral spine. They enhance fusion rates and

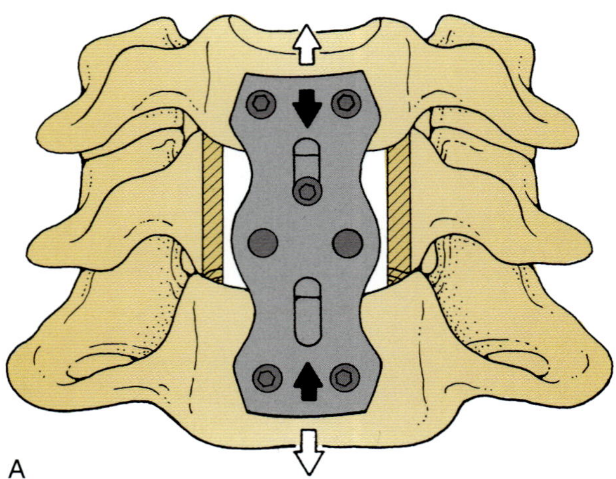

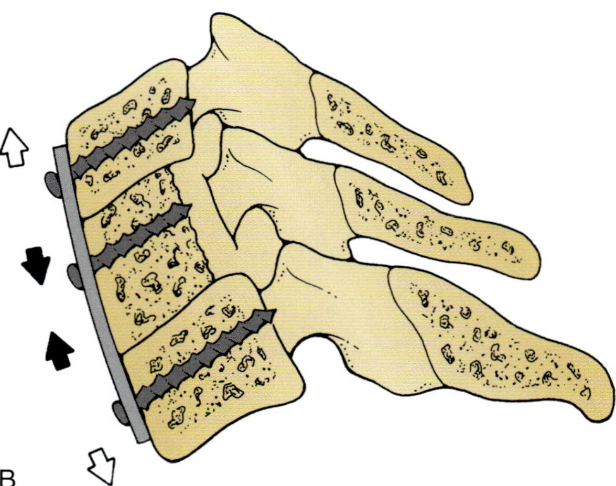

FIGURE 140-2. Coronal (**A**) and lateral (**B**) views of a ventral cervical plate (bicortical, unlocked) construct. The plate-screw device reconstitutes the ventral tension band (*black arrows*), thereby resisting ventral distraction and extension (*white arrows*). Axial compressive forces (not shown) are resisted by the strut graft, as depicted in Figure 140-1.

permit early patient mobilization. As with all devices that use screw fixation, the performance of ventral plating systems is Y-fixation. Supplemental fixation or additional bracing may be necessary in the setting of osteoporotic bone.

Cervical cages are another means of stabilizing the anterior column. These devices may be made of titanium, carbon, or other materials. Threaded cages appear to provide greater initial stiffness than the nonthreaded devices.[23-25] The results from acute biomechanical testing may be misleading since subsequent subsidence may lead to a subsequent decrease in stiffness.

Dorsal Constructs

Dorsal constructs are designed to restore stability to the spine when the dorsal osseous and/or ligamentous structures are incompetent. Several different constructs may be applied via this approach. Basic wiring techniques, incorporating the spinous processes, laminae, or articular facets with or without a bone graft, are time-tested methods used to treat spinal instability. Luque L-rods and rectangles have also been used with success in this region. Hook-rod devices and interlaminar clamps have also been used for specific applications in the posterior cervical spine. Lateral mass osteosynthetic plates gained widespread acceptance for dorsal cervical stabilization, but these semirigid fixators have been largely replaced by rigid screw-rod systems.

Wire Constructs

Dorsal stabilization with wire or braided cables usually entails incorporation of the spinous processes or articular facets, with or without bone autograft. These constructs function primarily by reconstituting the dorsal tension band (Fig. 140-3). Dorsal wire constructs provide some stability in flexion, minimal stability in extension, and add little to rotatory or translatory stability.[26] If translational instability exists, dorsal tension band fixation implants may be inadequate to prevent the "parallelogram effect."[3] This may result in translatory displacement and further spinal deformity. Wiring alone does not provide sufficient immediate internal stability in most cases. It must be supplemented with bone graft, methyl methacrylate, or external bracing to augment the construct until bony fusion occurs. Still, this is an inexpensive, rapid, and relatively safe method to reconstitute the dorsal tension band, particularly in cases of isolated dorsal ligamentous injury.

Wire constructs may be created with single-strand wire, twisted wire, or braided cables. The latter have the advantage of higher tensile strength, relatively uniform distribution of applied tension, and ease of application. Braided titanium alloy cables are available, and these produce less CT or MRI artifact. Titanium cables are more expensive than wire, although the aforementioned advantages may justify the added cost in many situations.

Interlaminar Clamps

The dorsal tension band may also be re-created by application of interlaminar clamps. These devices are used rarely because they are somewhat unwieldy to apply and may be hazardous.[5] These clamps function by reconstituting the dorsal tension band and may be adequate to restrict flexion. No stability is provided in extension or axial rotation. Extension is prevented by placing the bone graft between the spinous processes. Interlaminar clamps require intact laminae at the levels to be instrumented. They are also prone to experience the parallelogram effect if translatory instability is present.

Luque L-Rods and Rectangles

Originally used for thoracolumbar instability, Luque L-rods and rectangles may also be incorporated into dorsal cervical constructs. These devices are usually applied over multiple spinal segments and are secured with sublaminar or facet

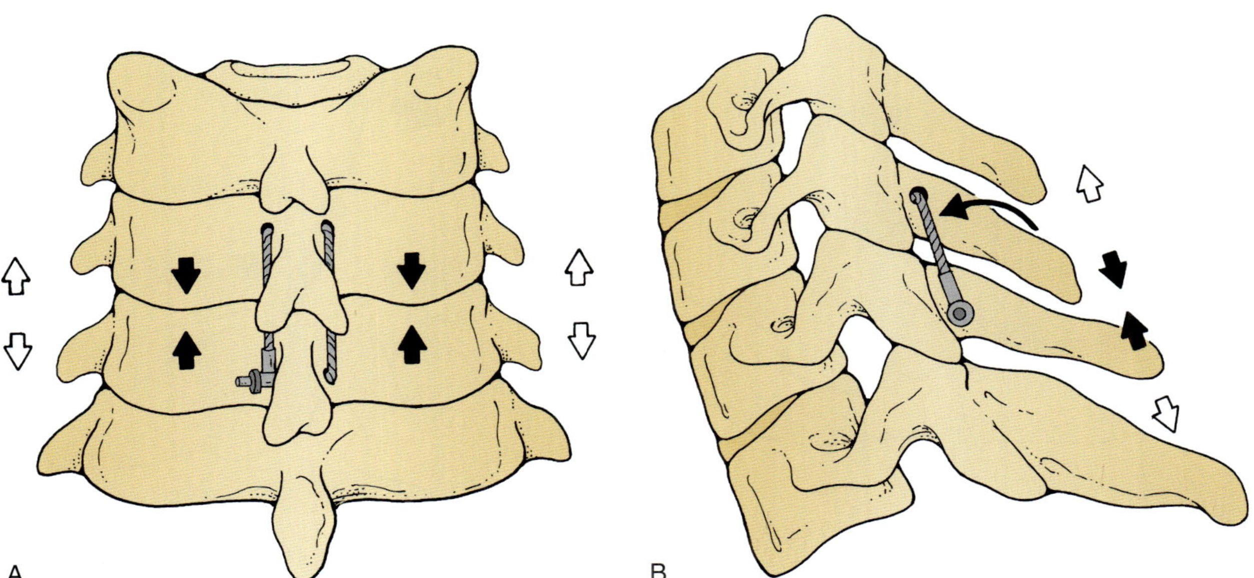

FIGURE 140-3. Coronal (**A**) and lateral (**B**) views of interspinous cable fixation. This construct reconstitutes the dorsal tension band (*black arrows*) and resists dorsal distraction (*white arrows*). As flexion and dorsal distraction are coupled the flexion moment (*curved arrow*) is resisted across the fixed level.

wires. Alternatively, braided cables may be used to affix the construct at the implant-bone junction. They act principally as semirigid implants, reconstructing the dorsal tension band. Additionally, they provide a significant degree of three-point bending fixation (Fig. 140-4). These implants stabilize in flexion, extension, and lateral bending modes.

The use of a rectangle rather than two L-rods is biomechanically advantageous because of the strong cross-fixation provided by the rectangle configuration. Torsional stability is enhanced by this design, and "telescoping" is less likely. These concerns may be partially alleviated by cross-fixation of L-rod constructs.

Luque L-rods and rectangles have been used for the treatment of instability from spinal neoplasia. After dorsal neural decompression, a Luque construct may be applied if instability or progressive spinal deformity is anticipated. Additionally, this type of construct may be advantageous in patients with poor bone quality because the construct has an extremely low profile, which may be important in thin patients. It is fairly simple to apply, inexpensive, and requires no special instrumentation to install. However, a Luque construct must often incorporate several motion segments to achieve an adequate biomechanical advantage, thus creating a long fusion. The risk of passing sublaminar wires in the subaxial cervical spine should not be underestimated, particularly if the canal diameter has been further compromised by spondylotic disease, traumatic injury, or neoplasm. In such cases, fixation to the spinous processes, facets, or lateral masses is preferable.

Lateral Mass Fixation

Dorsal cervical stabilization has been revolutionized by the development of lateral mass screw fixation systems. These include screws fixed to plates and screws fixed to rods. These devices provide a high degree of immediate internal stability, often eliminating the need for postoperative external immobilization or bracing. Lateral mass plates are dynamic implants and behave primarily as nonfixed moment arm cantilever beam fixators. They also provide some dorsal tension band fixation (Fig. 140-5). Biomechanical studies have demonstrated the ability of these devices to restore stiffness to the injured spine in flexion, extension, and torsion.[27,28] Similar to other constructs that restore the dorsal tension band, lateral mass plates are probably weakest in extension.[5,24] Lateral mass screw-rod systems are rigid devices and as such provide more stability than screw-plate systems.

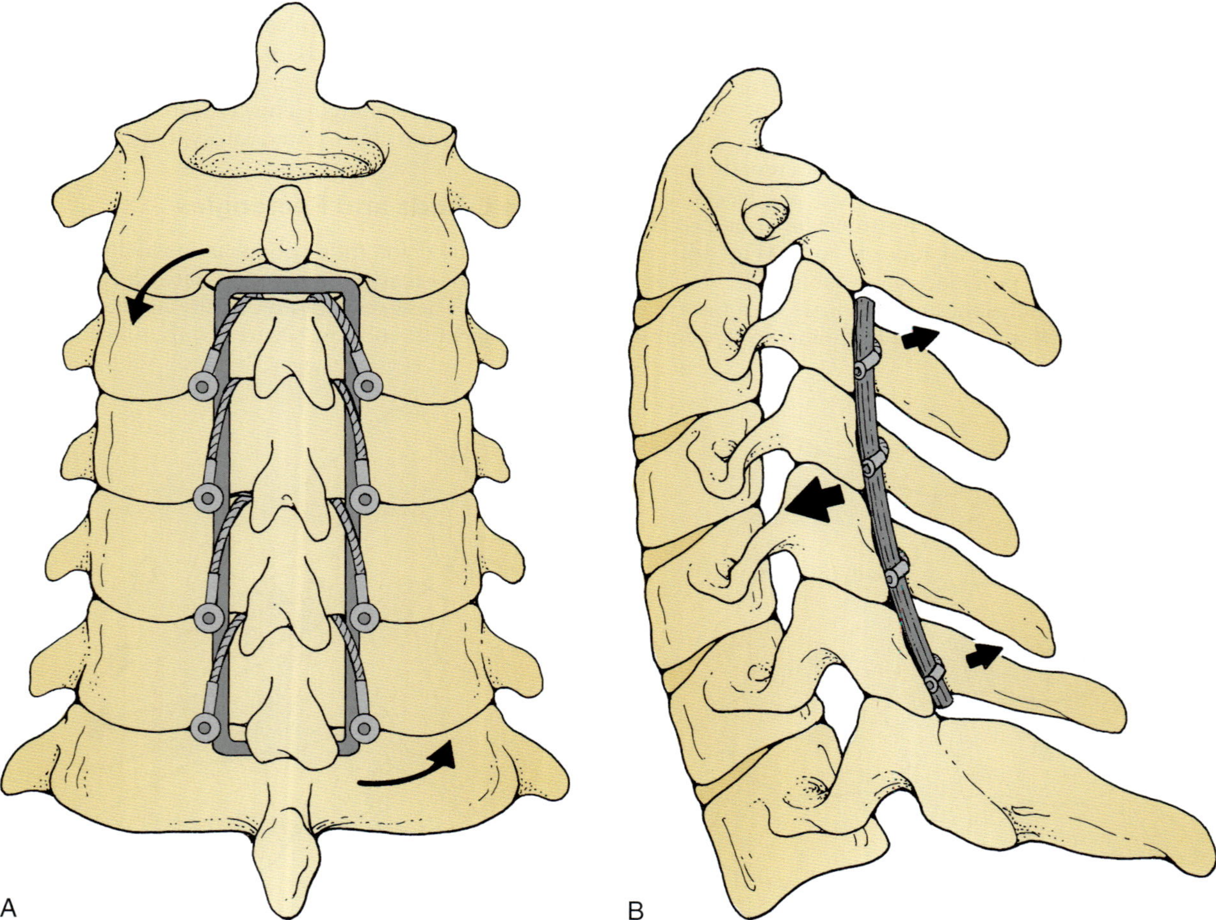

FIGURE 140-4. Coronal (**A**) and lateral (**B**) views of a Luque rectangle construct. This device provides three-point bending fixation. Dorsally directed forces are applied at both ends of the construct, with an equal but opposite force applied at the fulcrum (*straight arrows*). Torsional stability (*curved arrows*) is imparted by the strong cross-fixation of the rectangle. Distraction and flexion are also resisted, as this device reconstructs the dorsal tension band. Although the illustration depicts fixation with sublaminar cables, the authors do not recommend sublaminar cable passage in the midcervical spine.

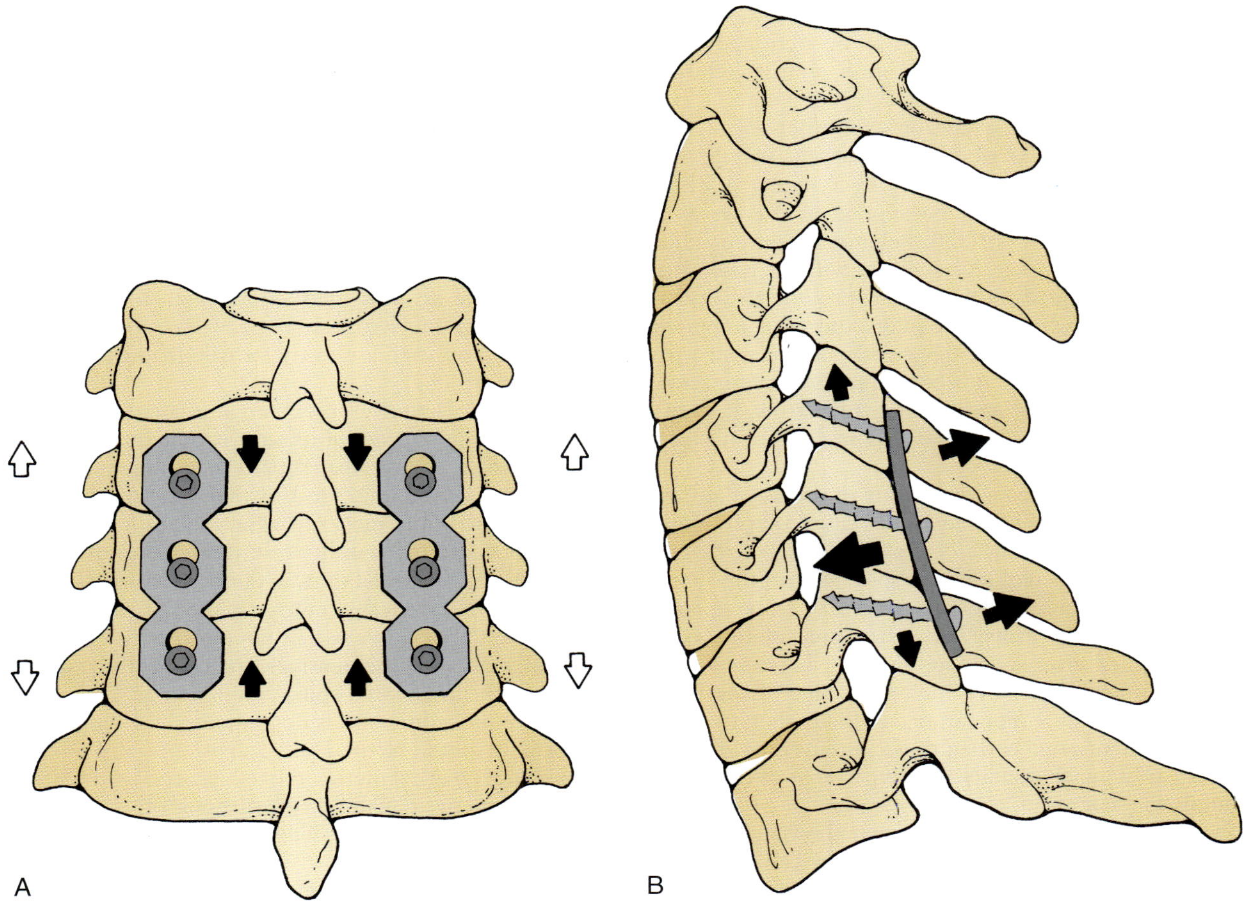

FIGURE 140-5. Coronal (**A**) and lateral (**B**) views of a lateral mass plate construct. This device provides stabilization in all motion planes, using tension band (*small, black vertical arrows* in **A**), three-point bending (*large, black horizontal arrows* in **B**), and cantilever beam fixation (*small, black vertical arrows* in **B**).

Lateral mass fixation may be used to treat instability from C2 to T1. Posttraumatic instability provides the most common indication for the use of lateral mass plates.[26,29] Dorsal ligamentous injury and irreducible unilateral or bilateral facet dislocations may be stabilized effectively with this type of construct after reduction of malalignment. In these cases instrumentation across the affected segment alone is usually adequate to restore stability. A longer construct may be required if instability of a single motion segment is severe, or if the dorsal elements at the level of instability are not intact. Multiple segments of instability may also mandate instrumentation of additional levels to achieve an adequate biomechanical advantage.

Unstable fractures of the dorsal cervical elements may be treated with lateral mass screw constructs. Fractures of the articular facet, pedicle, and/or lamina at a given level usually require a multilevel construct to restore stability. An intact level above and below the site of injury should be instrumented. Instability arising from vertebral body fractures has been successfully treated with lateral mass plates, usually incorporating multiple levels into the construct. This should only be attempted when the articular facets at that level are intact because they must contribute to axial load bearing in this situation. In most cases of vertebral body injury, a ventral approach is indicated. Certainly, if ventral spinal canal compromise is present, decompression and stabilization with a ventral construct should be considered.

Lateral mass fixation may also be used to reestablish stability after spinal tumor resection. The extent of instrumentation depends on the size and site of the tumor, but in general, several segments above and below the affected levels should be incorporated.[6] Lateral mass screws should be placed only in bone that is free of disease.

Instability created by degenerative disease may be treated with lateral mass fixation. This is particularly effective when the dorsal elements are incompetent. Additionally, these devices may be applied at the time of laminectomy to prevent progressive kyphotic deformity in patients who are deemed to be at risk. This is more effective than attempting to treat an established kyphotic deformity with dorsal instrumentation because constructs fixed to the articular pillars are at a mechanical disadvantage in the latter. Ventral decompression and stabilization should be considered in this situation.

Excellent results have been reported using lateral mass plates without fusion.[26,29] However, long-term structural stability is augmented by incorporating bone graft into the construct. This may be accomplished by denuding the articular processes at the unstable level(s) and packing cancellous bone graft into the joint space. Often, adequate material for bone autograft may be obtained from adjacent spinous processes or from bone removed during decompression.

Advantages of lateral mass fixation over other dorsal construct designs include superior biomechanical stability in essentially all planes and applicability to a variety of clinical settings. These devices may be applied in the presence of extensive laminectomies or dorsal element fracture. They provide immediate postoperative stability without passage of sublaminar wires. Their installation may prolong the operative procedure somewhat and requires special equipment and technical expertise. These devices should be used with caution in patients with inferior bone quality because screw fixation systems perform suboptimally in this setting. If screws are used in this situation, postoperative immobilization with a rigid orthotic should be considered.

Cervical hook-rod systems have many of the same advantages of lateral mass plates but may be less easy to apply. Hook constructs are probably not the best choice in the setting of stenosis since the hooks require some space within the canal. Polyaxial screws allow the lateral mass screws to be applied in the appropriate trajectory, with the appropriately conformed rod applied after screw application. This is in contrast to lateral mass plates, in which the shape of the plate and placement of screw holes can occasionally dictate screw placement. As mentioned earlier, these systems provide rigid fixation that is biomechanically superior to that of the semirigid lateral mass plates.[30]

Cervical pedicle fixation has also been shown to provide appropriate dorsal stabilization for the cervical spine.[31-33] However, cervical pedicle screws are significantly more difficult to place than lateral mass screws, and they carry a higher risk of injury to the nerve root and the vertebral artery. Lateral mass screws are probably equally effective in biomechanical stabilization and are safer in most situations.

360-Degree Constructs

Occasionally, cervical spinal instability is so severe that it warrants both ventral and dorsal stabilization, creating a "360-degree" construct. This approach is usually reserved for situations of ventral and dorsal instability. A 360-degree construct may also be indicated when extensive instability is anticipated from progression of underlying disease. This may be encountered in cases of advanced malignancy or extensive degenerative disease. To justify a 360-degree procedure, there must be a reasonable concern that instability will persist or recur, despite stabilization via an isolated ventral or dorsal approach.

Constructs that use wire-reinforced methyl methacrylate may be used for treatment of instability created by neoplastic disease. The biomechanical stability of methyl methacrylate reconstruction is optimized when a 360-degree construct is applied. Ventral stabilization is usually performed after decompression.

A methyl methacrylate strut may be used as a vertebral body replacement. More commonly, fibular strut grafts are used ventrally to span multiple vertebral levels. Struts function in a simple distraction mode, effectively resisting compressive axial loads (Fig. 140-6A). This can be supplemented by threaded Kirschner wires (K-wires), which are embedded into the vertebral bodies above and below the involved region. These devices prevent strut migration and provide some resistance to translatory forces.

A dorsal polymethylmethacrylate (PMMA) or fibular strut construct should be applied, in conjunction with ventral stabilization, which completes the 360-degree construct. Several techniques have been described for application of this material to the dorsal cervical spine. With one such method, K-wires are passed through the spinous processes, are bent, and then are encased in PMMA. These wires provide an increased surface area for interdigitation junction bonding between bone, wire, and cement.[3] The net result is an increase in the tensile load-bearing capacity of the construct.

The dorsal methyl methacrylate-wire construct functions primarily as a dorsal tension band fixator (Figs. 140-6B and 104-6C). Some three-point bending fixation is also provided. When applied in this manner, 360-degree methyl methacrylate constructs provide a substantial degree of immediate internal stability in virtually all motion planes.[34] It must be remembered that, in contrast to an osseous fusion, the strength of a methyl methacrylate construct is maximal initially and decreases over time. This type of construct is generally reserved for treatment of cervical instability associated with progressive spinal malignancy. This is a purely palliative procedure and is not intended for long-term stabilization. It should be used only in patients with a limited life expectancy. Methyl methacrylate has been used for the treatment of traumatic instability,[34] although this material probably should be avoided because other constructs are superior in this context.

Methyl methacrylate constructs are relatively simple and safe to apply. They provide significant immediate internal stability in multiple planes. Special instrumentation is not required, and the materials used are inexpensive. The major shortcoming of this construct is that its long-term stability is suspect. There is no attempt to create an osseous fusion. As a result, the full extent of load bearing must be assumed indefinitely by the cement-wire construct.

A 360-degree construct is occasionally used for treatment of instability created by benign disease. If the nature and extent of instability are such that a single approach would not adequately restore structural integrity, a 360-degree construct must be considered. This situation is occasionally encountered with multilevel procedures in which there is preexisting instability and/or deformity. When an osseous strut graft is internally stabilized with a ventral plate, only two motion segments are actually fixed. The intervening motion segments may require dorsal fixation to provide optimal stability to the construct in cases of extreme instability.

Ventral and dorsal cervical plating systems may be applied concurrently in conjunction with appropriate bone grafting. In most cases these devices should confer an optimal biomechanical advantage to the construct, providing immediate internal stability in all motion planes. Other constructs may be devised if screw fixation is contraindicated by poor bone quality. These situations are rare and necessitate individualized management. However, fundamental construct design concepts should guide the selection and application of hardware systems, just as in less complex problems of instability.

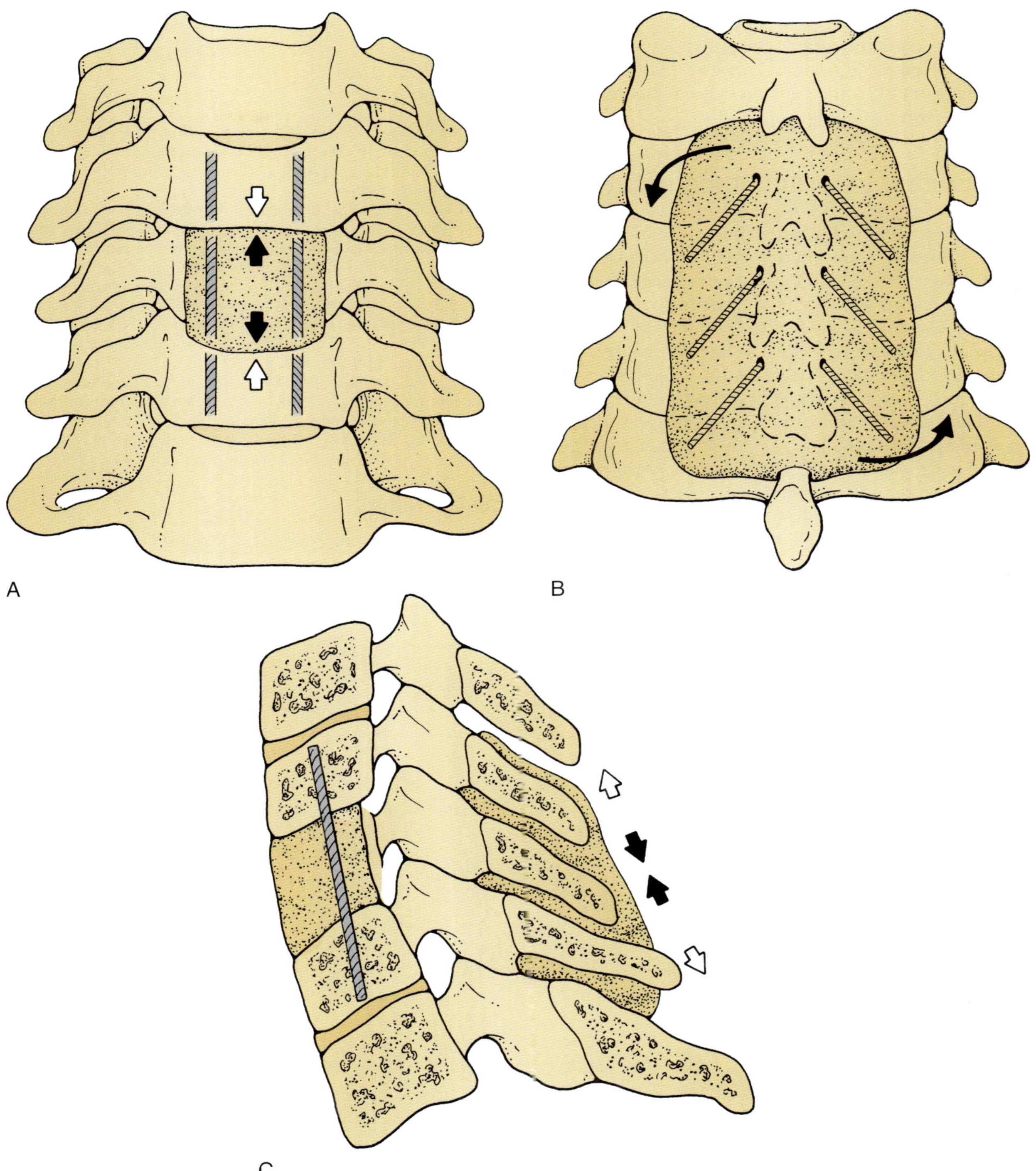

FIGURE 140-6. Ventral (**A**), dorsal coronal (**B**), and sagittal (**C**) views of a 360-degree wire-reinforced methyl methacrylate construct. The ventral strut provides simple distraction fixation (*black arrows*), resisting axial compressive loads (*white arrows* [**A**]). The dorsal construct imparts torsional stability (*curved arrows* [**B**]). It also functions as a dorsal tension band (*black arrows*), resisting distraction and flexion (*white arrows* [**C**]).

Economic Considerations

Historically, economic considerations have not been major determinants in the process of construct design. This is no longer true because rising health care costs and declining reimbursement mandate some fiscal responsibility. Material costs represent only a fraction of the expense accrued with spinal instrumentation. Surgeons' fees, operative time, anesthesia support, and fluoroscopy costs (if required) all reflect the complexity of a stabilization procedure. Thousands of dollars may be expended to apply a single construct. With this in mind, it is financially irresponsible to implant an elaborate, costly system when a less expensive alternative could suffice. However, the structural integrity of a construct should not be compromised for purely economic concerns. The spine surgeon must use restraint in the construct design process, minimizing expenses when possible.

Supplementary External Immobilization

The need for postoperative external immobilization may be reduced or eliminated when internal fixation provides immediate stability to a construct. Orthoses are selected in accordance with the nature and extent of preoperative instability, quality of the construct, cause of instability, and extent of residual disease. Young patients with isolated dorsal instability can be treated with a soft cervical collar for 4 weeks after most instrumentation procedures. Patients with more severe instability or residual disease require more aggressive postoperative bracing. A hard cervical collar is probably adequate in most cases. Those with osteoporosis, severe preoperative instability, and/or biomechanically inferior constructs that do not provide sufficient immediate internal stability require a postoperative halo vest or Minerva immobilization.[6] Regardless of the bracing method, all patients should be assessed often with serial examinations and radiographs until an osseous fusion is attained.

KEY REFERENCES

Albert TJ, Vacarro A: Postlaminectomy kyphosis. *Spine* 23:2738–2745, 1998.

Gill K, Paschal S, Corin J, et al: Posterior plating of the cervical spine. A biomechanical comparison of different posterior fusion techniques. *Spine* 13:813–816, 1988.

Roy-Camille R, Saillanr G, Mazel C: Internal fixation of the unstable cervical spine by posterior osteosynthesis with plates and screws. In The Cervical Spine Research Society Editorial Committee, editor: *The cervical spine*, ed 2, Philadelphia, 1989, Lippincott-Raven, pp 390–404.

Ryken TC, Goel VK, Clausen JD, et al: Assessment of unicortical and bicortical fixation in a quasistatic cadaveric model. Role of bone mineral density and screw torque. *Spine (Phila Pa 1976)* 20:1861–1867, 1995.

Traynelis VC: Anterior and posterior plate stabilization of the cervical spine. *Neurosurgery* 2:59–76, 1992.

Traynelis VC, Donaher PA, Roach RM, et al: Biomechanical comparison of anterior Caspar plate and three level posterior fixation techniques in a human cadaveric model. *J Neurosurg* 79:96–103, 1993.

Vaccaro AR, Falatyn SP, Scuderi GJ, et al: Early failure of long segment anterior cervical plate fixation. *J Spinal Disord* 11:410–415, 1998.

REFERENCES

The complete reference list is available online at expertconsult.com.

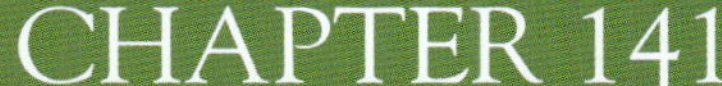

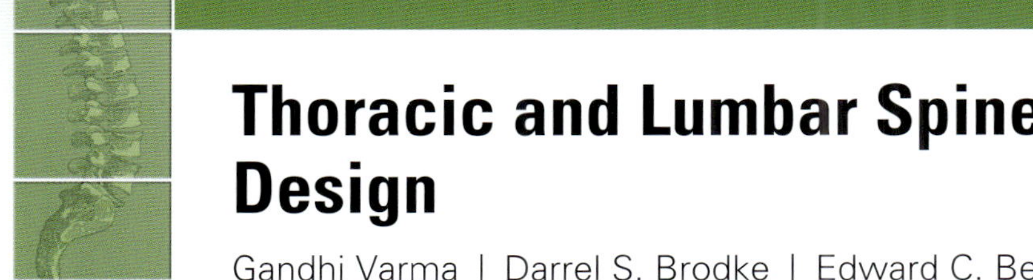

CHAPTER 141

Thoracic and Lumbar Spine Construct Design

Gandhi Varma | Darrel S. Brodke | Edward C. Benzel

Construct design is a process that formulates a specific blueprint for an orderly and thoughtful assembly of implantable spinal instrumentation, designed to correct instability or deformity or both of the spinal column.[1] Construct design requires specific understanding of the deformity or instability and the biomechanical forces acting on the pathologic alignment. An understanding of corrective forces and where they must be applied also is required. A keen knowledge of the anatomy and pathoanatomy is required to preserve neuralgic function and avoid adjacent segment injury. Although skillful assembly of the mechanical construct is a definite prerequisite, ultimate success is determined by the orderly thought process for designing the construct, based on personal experience, experience of others, and laboratory data. Creating a preoperative plan, or blueprint, can focus this design process. Spinal instrumentation surgery must not be assumed to be strictly "mechanical" or "routine"; rather, it requires serious and meticulous planning to ensure success.

Nomenclature

The nomenclature of spinal instrumentation is complex and often confusing at the outset. Factors that contribute to this complexity are the numerous components that constitute assembly, the numerous choices for purchase sites in the spine, and the variations in the mode of assembly of the hardware. There are four major categories: (1) *anchors*, devices that attach the construct to the bony spine (e.g., pedicle screws, cables, hooks); (2) *longitudinal members* (e.g., rods or plates); (3) *connectors*, devices that connect anchors to the longitudinal members or connect two longitudinal members (cross-connectors); and (4) accessories (e.g., washers or spacers). Most spinal instrumentation systems have all four of these components. The skill in designing a construct is reflected in the optimal choice of implants that result in biomechanically stable architecture.

Indications for Spinal Instrumentation

Spinal implants may be considered as internal supports that immobilize the spine until bony fusion occurs. In contrast to external orthoses that serve similar functions, spinal implants provide direct control of spinal segments and have a much broader scope.

The goals of spinal instrumentation are threefold. The first goal is the immediate restoration of stability so that the patient may be prepared for early rehabilitation efforts. Immediate stability often decreases pain and may improve early function. It may also increase the success of bone union or fusion. The second goal of instrumentation is indirect decompression of neural structures, often accomplished by controlled distraction. The instrumentation may also be used to restore or maintain physiologic alignment of the spine. The third goal of spinal instrumentation is the correction of deformity to prevent pain or neurologic compromise and the neutralization of pathologic, deforming forces. Surgeons designing spinal instrumentation constructs should clearly delineate which of the aforementioned goals, or which combination of goals, they are attempting to achieve.

Construct Types (Modes of Force Application)

The six fundamental construct types are simple distraction, three-point bending, tension band fixation, fixed-moment arm cantilever-beam fixation, non–fixed-moment arm cantilever-beam fixation, and applied-moment arm cantilever-beam fixation (Fig. 141-1).

Development of Construct Blueprint

The preoperative development of a blueprint for implant placement, based on the composite information obtained from clinical assessment and imaging studies, ensures a definitive plan and saves time in the operating room. Some flexibility in this plan may be required after surgical exposure of the bony spine because of unexpected findings. For instance, minor fractures at the implant-anchor site may necessitate deviation from the original plan.

A simple scheme should be used that provides (1) information about the level of the lesion or the level of the unstable segment or segments, (2) the types of implants to be used (anchors, longitudinal members, and cross-connectors), (3) the length of stabilization required on either side of the lesion, and (4) the mode of load bearing by the construct. The scheme guides selection of the appropriate implant

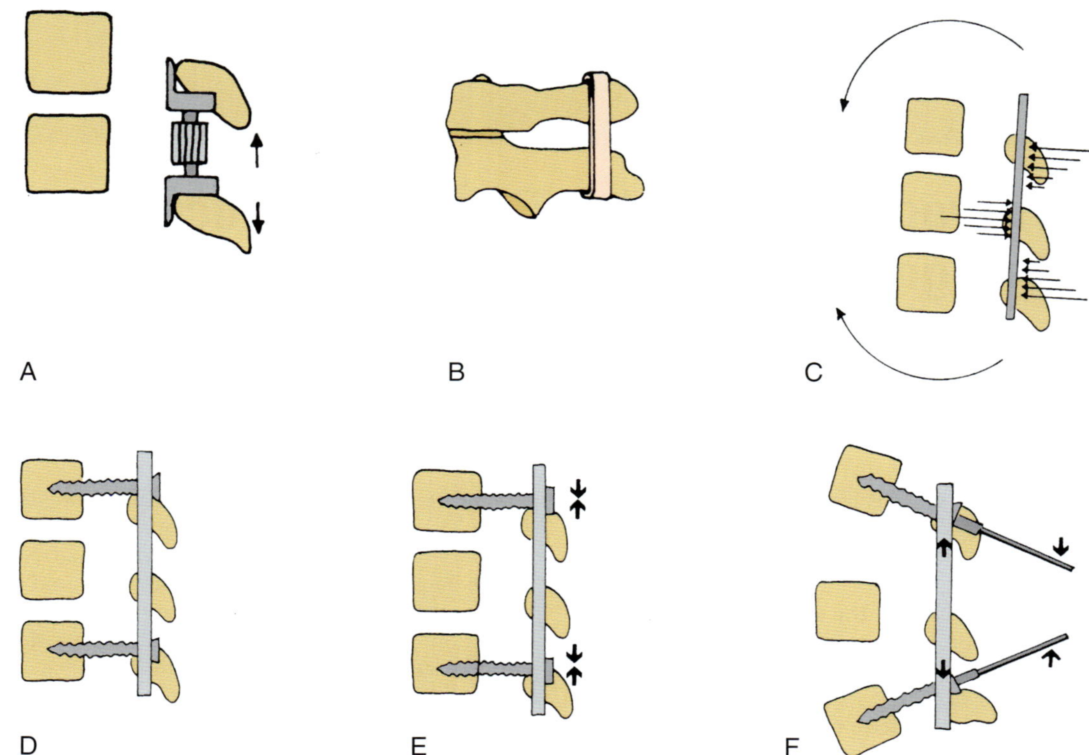

FIGURE 141-1. The application of forces to a construct can be broadly categorized into simple distraction (e.g., Knodt rod; **A**); tension band fixation (e.g., spinous process wiring; **B**); three-point bending using the middle point as a fulcrum (e.g., Harrington rods; **C**); non–fixed-moment arm cantilever beam design, in which axial load cannot be resisted because of nonrigid fixation between the screw and the longitudinal member (e.g., lateral mass plates; **D**); fixed-moment arm cantilever beam design, in which axial loading forces can be resisted because the screws are rigidly fixed to the longitudinal member (e.g., locking cervical plate systems; **E**); and applied-moment arm cantilever beam design, in which complex forces can be applied (e.g., universal spinal instrumentation; **F**).

components in advance, improves the intraoperative communication between surgeons and assistants, and enhances the chances of success.

Although the concept of construct design encompasses similar principles in all anatomic regions of the spine, designing a thoracolumbar construct poses more challenges than most cervical constructs. Various constructs, using a variety of anchors in different bony landmarks, each used in various mechanical modes (i.e., compression, distraction, neutralization, distraction followed by compression, or distraction and compression at different segmental levels), may be used in a successful strategy. In consideration of these complex decision-making dilemmas, this chapter focuses on thoracic and lumbar fixation design strategies.

Line Drawing of Proposed Construct

A simple dorsoventral or lateral line drawing of the spine provides a framework for the clear definition of the operative plan. Often only a dorsoventral drawing is necessary, although clear consideration of any sagittal plane deformity is vital. The line drawing provides the blueprint for surgery (Fig. 141-2).[2] This drawing can be easily obtained from a CT scan or from radiographs.

The convention used in this chapter, with regard to a dorsoventral line drawing, dictates that the left side of the drawing portrays the left side of the patient (i.e., the drawing portrays the patient as viewed from behind). This portrayal is in accordance with the most common surgical approaches for complex instrumentation constructs and decreases the chance for confusion.

Level of Lesion and Level of Fusion

The designation of the level of the lesion or location of instability, the levels to be fused, and the type of fusion should be placed next on the line drawing. The level of instability or lesion is designated by an "X," and the precise extent of proposed bony fusion is designated by a hatched outline. The number of unstable motion segments should be assessed carefully, as should associated deformity. These factors determine the number of levels to be spanned with the construct. The choice of implants also affects this decision.

Hook constructs, often used in the past throughout the spine and still used at the present time in the thoracic region, should incorporate three spinal levels above and two spinal segments below the limits of the lesion (*3A-2B rule*). For the past decade or so, hooks have mainly been reserved for situations in which the pedicles are very small or for additional support in osteoporotic patients along with pedicle screws. If the patient has a marked angular kyphotic deformity, and if three-point bending is considered in an attempt to reduce the deformity, inclusion of four or more spinal levels above the lesion is common (*4A-2B rule*) and may provide a more functional lever arm. Such long constructs are suited mostly for lesions in the middle and upper thoracic regions,

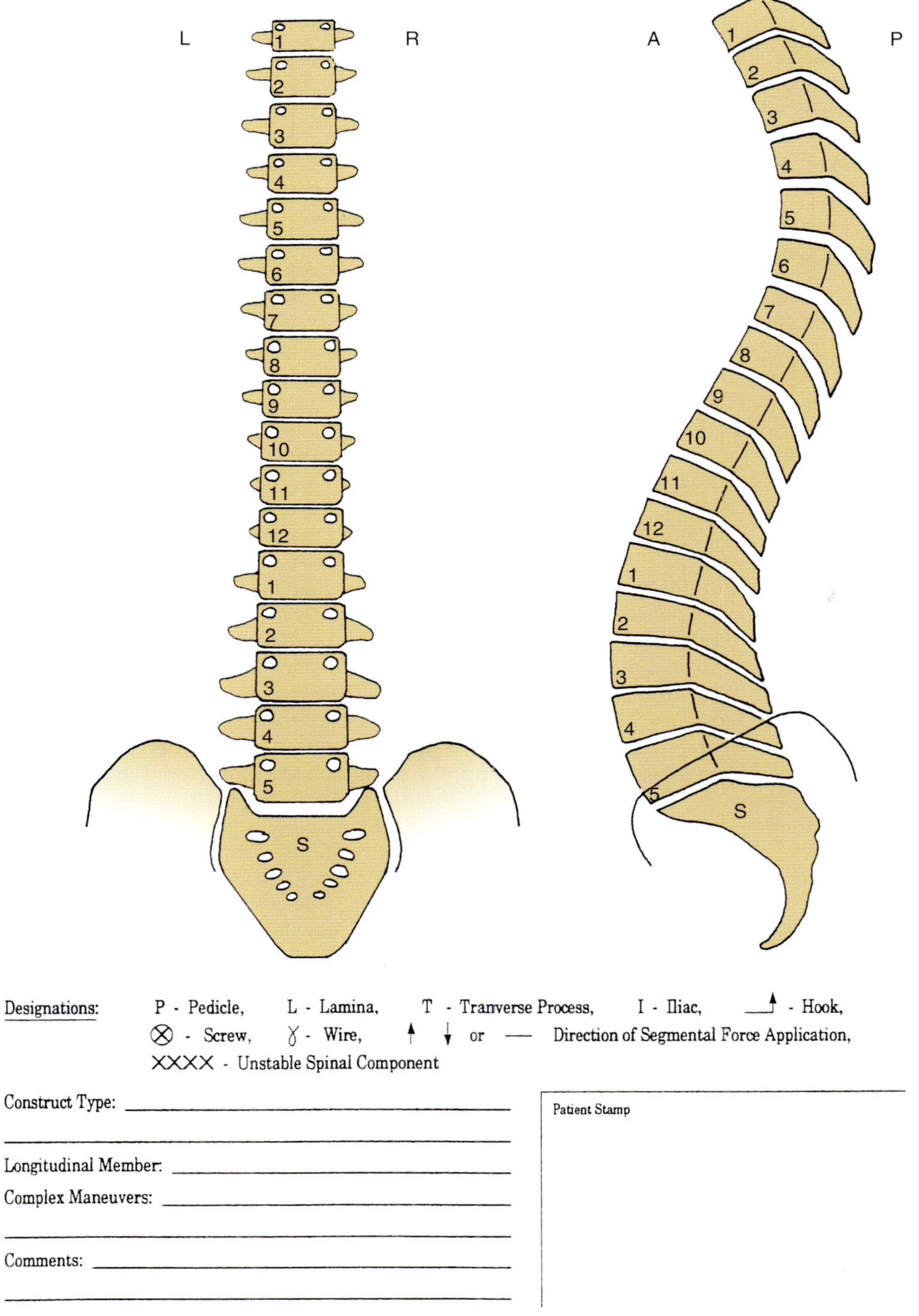

L
R
A
P
S
Designations: P - Pedicle, L - Lamina, T - Tranverse Process, I - Iliac, - Hook,
- Screw, - Wire, or — Direction of Segmental Force Application,
XXXX - Unstable Spinal Component
Construct Type:
Longitudinal Member:
Complex Maneuvers:
Comments:
Patient Stamp

FIGURE 141-2. A blueprint of the proposed surgery is helpful in clarifying the treatment plan for both the surgeon and the operating team. (From Benzel EC: Construct design. In Benzel EC, editor: *Spinal instrumentation,* Chicago, 1994, AANS Publications, pp 239–256.)

although thoracic pedicle screws are widely used even in these regions.

In the lower thoracic spine (T8-10), the thoracolumbar junction (T11-L1), and the lumbar region (L2-5), pedicle screw constructs are often preferred. The size of the pedicles and the increased stiffness these screws provide make them an ideal choice. Short-segment fixation, with the inclusion of only one vertebra immediately above and below the lesion, is appropriate if the anterior, load-bearing column is intact and kyphotic deformity is not present. The bone structure must also be of sufficient strength. With increasingly sophisticated fixation choices available, it must be remembered that a rigid, stable construct is the goal, and biology and biomechanics surrounding the implants must be taken into account.

Both segmental pedicle screw and hook instrumentation techniques are successful in obtaining global balance safely. Balance can be accomplished without neurologic injury, even in adolescent idiopathic scoliosis, where neurologic risk is greatest. Segmental pedicle screw instrumentation offers a significantly better overall major and minor coronal curve correction and maintenance without neurologic problems and slightly improved pulmonary function values for the operative treatment of adolescent idiopathic scoliosis. Pedicle screw constructs may also allow for a slightly shorter fusion length than segmental hook instrumentation.[3]

Depiction of Implant Components

The type of implant components used in the instrumentation construct should be delineated clearly on the blueprint. The implant component at each implant–bone juncture may be a cable, hook, or screw. The convention used is to designate hooks by a right-angled arrow, with the arrowhead pointing in the direction of the orientation of the hook. The purchase site—and the type of hook—is designated further by "P" (for pedicle), "L" (for laminar or sublaminar), or "T" (for transverse process). Screws are designated by an "X" surrounded by a circle and placed over pedicles. Cable (or wire) is depicted as a loop.

The mode of axial load application (distraction, compression, or neutral) at each implant–bone juncture is depicted as an arrow. The arrow points in the direction of force application for distraction and compression or a horizontal line for neutral. Bending moments are difficult to depict accurately on the line drawing and are described.

The modes of application of each segmental level are depicted with arrows and lines, as previously described. The arrows and lines are drawn lateral to the designations of implant types. If sagittal plane forces are to be applied, they are depicted on the lateral line drawing. Finally, cross-fixator locations can be designated by rectangles with circles.

Mechanical Attributes of Spinal Implants: Construct Type

The mechanism that the construct uses (types of construct) to bear loads is also designated. Six methods of load bearing are associated with the six construct types: distraction, three-point bending, tension band fixation, fixed-moment arm cantilever-beam, non–fixed-moment arm cantilever-beam, and applied-moment arm cantilever-beam. It is difficult to depict this information on the line drawing. This information may be recorded in the space provided at the bottom of the drawing.

Construct Design Strategies

Multiple factors should be taken into account in designing a spinal instrumentation construct.[4] Consideration should be given specifically to bony integrity, the location of the unstable spinal segment, the implant length with respect to the unstable segment, the need for cross-fixation, the need for dural decompression, the choice of ventral versus dorsal instrumentation, availability of specific instrumentation, metallic composition of instrumentation, and the familiarity of the surgeon with a particular technique. Each factor should be adequately addressed to achieve optimal outcome.

Bony Integrity

Osteoporosis poses a significant problem in spinal instrumentation. Hooks and cables may resist pull-out better than bone screws.[5,6] A longer construct is often required in osteoporotic bone. More anchors are needed to distribute the load over more segments, decreasing the load at any single site. Interbody stability, either from fully collapsed discs or interbody implants, may protect the dorsal construct from cantilever pull-out. If pedicle screws are required in a patient with marked osteoporosis, consideration should be given to filling the screw tracks with polymethylmethacrylate (PMMA). Addition of PMMA significantly increases screw pull-out strength and is accomplished by first placing and then removing the pedicle screw. The pedicle must be carefully assessed to ensure no cortical penetration has occurred that would allow the methyl methacrylate to leak. PMMA is placed using a large syringe under minimal pressure, and the pedicle screws are rapidly reinserted. The spinal canal should be inspected to ensure the methyl methacrylate has not inadvertently extruded into the canal with potential compression of neural elements. The instrumentation construct is then completed.

Biomechanical studies have shown that pedicle screw augmentation with PMMA using transpedicular and kyphoplasty techniques increased the pull-out failure load twofold to threefold in osteoporotic vertebrae.[7] Pedicle screws augmented using the kyphoplasty technique had significantly greater pull-out strength than screws augmented with the transpedicular augmentation technique.[7] Another option for osteoporotic spine fixation is use of expansive pedicle screws. The expansive pedicle screw can progressively compress bone at the screw-bone interface by the expansion of the ventral two thirds of the screw, which is thought to provide greater screw thread engagement of vertebral bone than a conventional pedicle screw of the same size. Biomechanical tests have shown that expansive pedicle screws can significantly improve the axial pull-out force compared with conventional screws in osteoporotic bones.[8-10]

Location of the Unstable Spinal Segment

The transition zones in the spine are key locations. These include the junctions of the occiput and cervical spine, the cervical and thoracic spine, the thoracic and lumbar spine, and the lumbar spine and sacrum. Each transition is associated with a change in anatomy, a change in the orientation of facets, and a change in inherent rigidity. Ideally, the construct should not end at an intermediate junction (e.g., cervicothoracic and thoracolumbar junctions). Ending the construct and the fusion at an intermediate junction may lead to higher loads on the implants, higher failure rates, and a greater likelihood of adjacent segment problems.

The closer the lesion or unstable segment is to the occiput or sacrum, the shorter the applied lever arm is to the terminal end of the construct. More rigid fixation is required at the terminal end of the construct.[11] Often, multiple points of fixation are used in the sacrum or occiput. Long constructs that end at the sacrum have a high rate of pseudarthrosis at the terminal end (L5-S1).[12] A very high flexion-extension bending moment exists on the S1 screws, which leads to loosening of the screws. The addition of iliac screws, alar screws, or S2 pedicle screws to the construct significantly decreases the bending moment on the S1 pedicle screws and increases the fusion rate.[12,13]

Implant Length

Generally, the shortest construct that provides adequate stability is preferred. Use of a short construct preserves as much motion as possible in the normal segments of the spine above and below the construct. Also, long constructs may place undue stress on the inferiormost aspect of the construct and the immediately adjacent motion segment. Although long constructs in the relatively immobile thoracic spine would not jeopardize physiologic motion, they should still be avoided if possible. A relative exception is the presence of gross instability.

A long construct may be required to provide greater purchase of adjacent segments and greater stability. In the treatment of gross spinal instability or long curvatures (scoliosis or kyphosis), longer constructs may apply greater force overall and less force at each individual segment. Adding bone anchors, rod diameters, or both can significantly increase overall stiffness.[14]

Specific issues arise regarding the length of instrumentation in circumstances in which it is desired to keep the fusion short. Two options are available: (1) use longer instrumentation—use a short fusion and remove the instrumentation later, or (2) keep the fusion and the construct short.

Instrumentation Fusion Mismatch ("Rod Long, Fuse Short")

Instrumentation fusion mismatch describes the discrepancy between the number of spinal levels incorporated within an instrumentation construct and the number of spinal levels undergoing bony fusion. This technique was particularly popular in the past, when only less rigid anchors were available. Consequently, construct length was increased to gain stability. Generally, only the spinal segments immediately adjacent to the unstable segment are fused.

The rationale for this approach is that a long instrumentation construct is used to achieve reduction and correction of deformity, while fusing only the minimum number of segments necessary. The hardware is later removed (after 1 year), when the fractures have healed, and the fusion has consolidated, releasing the instrumented, but not fused, segments from immobilization. There is some concern that the facet joints included within the instrumented nonfused segments may undergo degenerative arthropathy.[15] An additional disadvantage of the "rod long, fuse short" construct is the potential for the implants to loosen. Hooks and cables allow more movement at this juncture than screws and may not pose as great a problem. This design has generally fallen out of favor. If this mode of construct is desired, screws should not be used as anchors in the nonfused segments.

Short-Segment Fixation

Generally, hook and cable constructs require long constructs, three above and two below (3A-2B) the lesion. This design provides a longer and more efficient moment arm and a stronger construct.[16] The 3A-2B configuration is a logical compromise between the problems associated with longer constructs and the shorter moment arm achieved with the shorter constructs and has been shown to provide good stability. Pedicle screws may allow for shorter constructs and fewer fusion segments, a single level above and below the lesion (1A-1B). Short-segment fixation provides an increasingly popular alternative, particularly when applied in a compression mode. Reinforcement with fracture-level screw combinations in patients who underwent short-segment fixation can help to provide better kyphosis correction and offers improved biomechanical spinal stability in patients with thoracolumbar burst fracture.[17,18] Because of the limited fixation, there may be a higher rate of failure[19]; this is particularly true if the screw purchase is poor (osteoporosis) or if the loads are too great, secondary to a loss of anterior column stability. Long constructs have been shown to be reliable and effective in treating thoracic injuries, with or without ventral reconstruction. Short-segment pedicle instrumentation constructs have proved to be effective in stabilizing thoracolumbar and lumbar fractures, while limiting the disruption of lower lumbar motion segments. Loss of anterior column integrity leads to fixation failure when short constructs are not supplemented with further fixation or a ventral reconstruction.[20] In a very unstable spine, without significant anterior column loss and rotational and shear fractures, pedicle screw fixation with two above and two below should provide adequate stability in most circumstances.

Cross-Fixation

Cross-fixation between longitudinal members generally improves the torsional stability of longer constructs and the lateral bending stiffness (Fig. 141-3).[21-23] It is not as critical

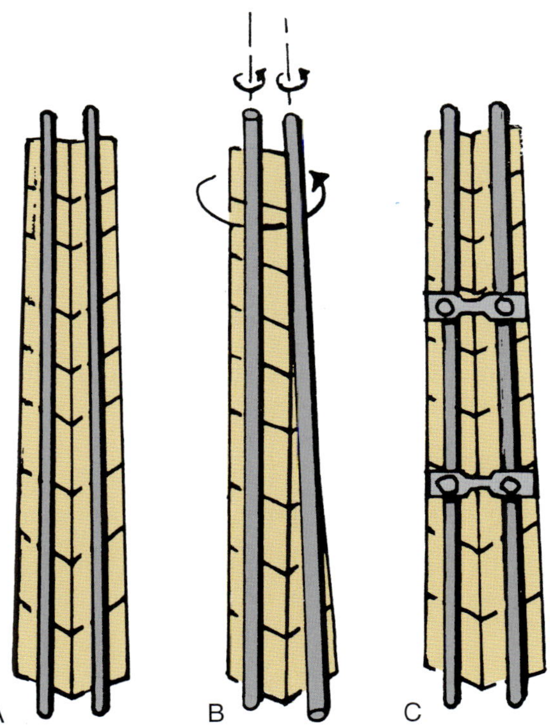

FIGURE 141-3. Cross-fixation can effectively resist torsional forces on the rods. **A** and **B,** Rods without cross-fixation are free to rotate with respect to one another. **C,** Cross-fixation prevents the rotation.

to use cross-fixation in short-segment constructs. For a short-segment rod construct with a skipped level (nonsegmental fixation), a cross-fixing device improves torsional stability to that of segmental fixation.[22] There is little effect of cross-links on flexion-extension stiffness.[21] When using long rod constructs with hook anchors, cross-fixation is essential to improve hook stability and torsional and lateral bending stiffness. Interconnecting the hooks on the two longitudinal members with cross-links significantly increases the fixation rigidity and decreases the failure rate. When the distal end is anchored by pedicle screws, the torsional and bending stiffness is much greater and not significantly different with cross-links.[24]

With long constructs, when cross-fixation is deemed necessary, two cross-fixators are optimal, creating a box construct. Further cross-links do not offer an advantage. Ideally, the links should be placed at the junction of the middle and terminal thirds of the construct.

Axial Load-Bearing Capacity of the Instrumented Spine

A major goal in the reconstruction of an injured spine is to restore its ability to carry axial loads. The construct should be designed so that the axial load is transmitted through the reconstituted bony spine, along the axis of the vertebral body rather than through the metallic implants inserted through the pedicles. The latter design may lead to stress risers within the implant, resulting in its ultimate failure.

Two clinical examples illustrate this point. In a case of grade 1 degenerative spondylolisthesis, there is a long-standing translational deformity (glacial instability) but no problem with axial load bearing. The role of instrumentation is to reduce the deformity, align the spine, and stabilize the motion segment rigidly to facilitate bony fusion. In a patient with a severe burst fracture of the L1 vertebral body with some loss of bone substance, axial load bearing is ineffective. This problem may be corrected by resection of the vertebral body, replacement with a strut graft, and short-segment stabilization with a locking plate or dual-rod device. The goal of spinal reconstruction in the latter case is to restore load-bearing ability and to decompress and stabilize the spine.[25] If a short-segment pedicle screw construct is used in such a case without vertebral body reconstruction, there may be significant axial loading of the screws, and they may fail.[19,26]

Regardless of the approach used, if a spinal implant is placed in a compression mode, the dural sac should be decompressed first. Potentially, doing otherwise would result in additional compression of neural elements.

Nature of Instability

A basic principle used for the correction of a deformity with instrumentation is to apply forces opposite of the forces that created the deformity. Specific maneuvers for the correction of some specific deformities are described in the following paragraphs.

Kyphotic Deformity

Kyphotic deformities of the spine may be corrected in one of two ways: (1) with a dorsal approach, using a three-point bending maneuver through a long rod construct, or (2) via a ventral approach, with the resection of a vertebral body, interbody grafting, and application of a plate or dual-rod device (Fig. 141-4). If the deficit is in the anterior column, such as with compression or burst fracture, the ventral approach may be more appropriate. If the dorsal tension band is lost, which leads to kyphosis, the dorsal approach may work best. Both approaches may be used if the bone quality is poor or if a fixed deformity requires both approaches.

Translational Deformity

Translational deformities (e.g., fracture-dislocation resulting from trauma) are generally corrected from a dorsal orientation (Fig. 141-5). Distraction and three-point bending with long hook-rod constructs often work well, as do shorter constructs (two above and two below) with pedicle screws. Translational deformity of a glacial type from degenerative spondylolisthesis is generally easily reducible by mere positioning or with a pull-back technique, using pedicle screws, although adding an interbody implant significantly improves the overall stability. Translational deformity resulting from isthmic spondylolisthesis is much more difficult to correct. It requires complete discectomy and intervertebral distraction, followed by pull-back with screws. Great care must be taken with any reduction maneuver, and monitoring of the exiting nerve roots with electromyography is recommended.

Axial Loading Deformity (Burst Fracture)

Saving motion segments by limiting the number of the fusion segments is a fundamental principle of spinal surgery. In milder forms of fracture, distraction and extension via pedicle screws restores the alignment. Some authors have used monosegmental pedicle instrumentation with placement of pedicle screws directly into the fractured vertebral body to treat thoracolumbar fractures. Controversy exists over whether monosegmental pedicle instrumentation is a more suitable method for thoracolumbar burst fractures than short-segment fixation. Data from the literature confirm that both monosegmental transpedicular fixation and short-segment transpedicular fixation are effective and reliable operative techniques for selected thoracolumbar burst fractures. The former technique shortened the operative time and decreased the amount of blood loss significantly.[27] In severe burst fractures with considerable bone loss, the preferred treatment is ventral excision of the vertebral body, strut grafting, and plating to reconstruct the anterior column.

Flexion-Distraction (Seat Belt) Deformity

Flexion-distraction injuries, accounting for 5% to 15% of all major vertebral trauma, are considered mechanically unstable because of the disruption and the separation of the dorsal elements, either ligaments or bones. The presence of severe dislocation indicates rupture of the anterior longitudinal ligament. This deformity is best corrected by compression followed by stabilization. This procedure may be performed via a dorsal approach and usually requires only short-segment fixation.

Scoliotic Deformity

Surgical goals when treating scoliosis include achieving a well-balanced spine in all planes, while working to preserve segments and maintain mobility. Multiple types of

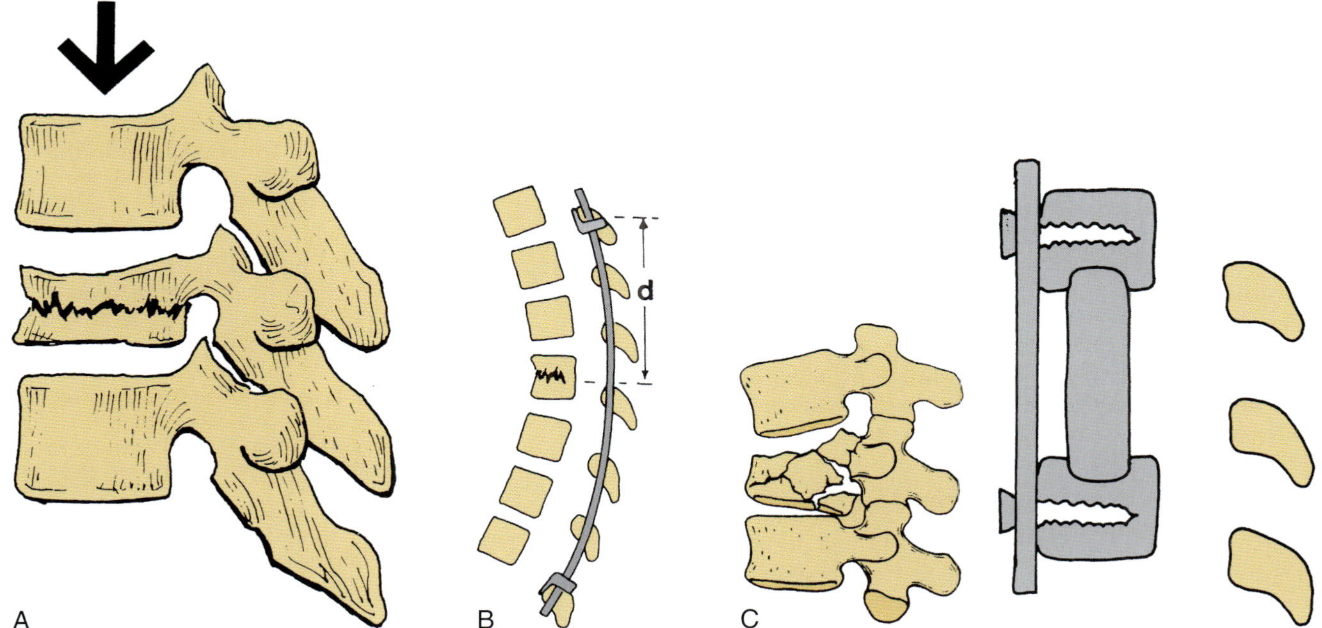

FIGURE 141-4. The best construct to use depends on various factors, and the choice must be individualized. Even a single fracture may require different constructs, depending on the severity of the injury. Mild burst fractures (**A**) can be treated with a dorsal construct (**B**), using a distraction combined with a three-point bending maneuver (**C**). A more severe burst fracture should be treated with a ventral construct, using a cantilever design.

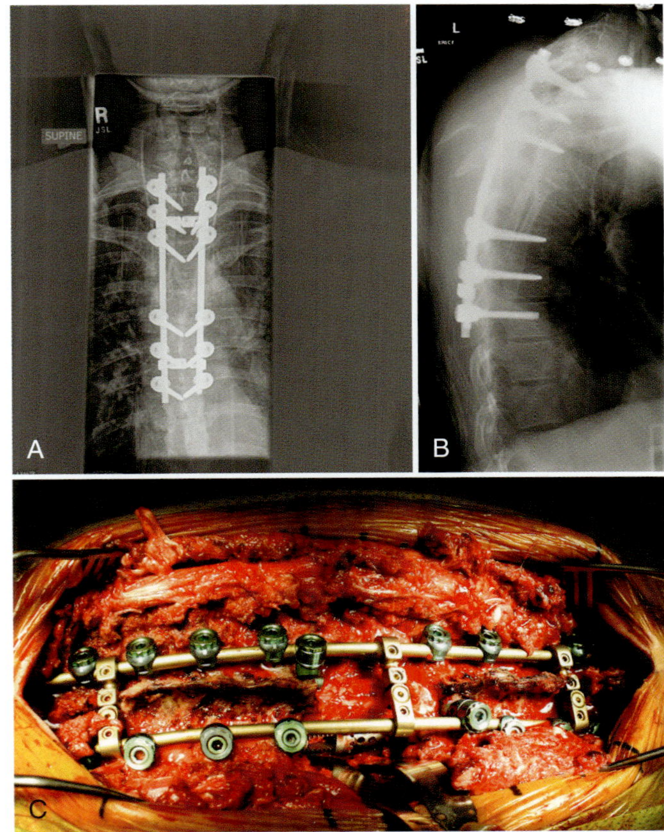

FIGURE 141-5. **A** and **B,** Radiographs show the pedicle screw construct for fracture of T5 and T6 with two cross-links. This is an example of a 3A-3B type of construct. **C,** Intraoperative picture shows a long pedicle screw construct reinforced with a sublaminar hook in an osteoporotic spine reconstruction.

instrumentation are available (hooks, sublaminar wires, and screws), although pedicle screws have gained in popularity because they offer superior multiplanar correction, the potential for shorter fusions, and a lower rate of implant failure or pull-out.[28] Generally, cantilever bending and rod rotation techniques are employed to reduce the curve magnitude, along with distractive force applied on the concave side of the deformity and compression applied on the convex side of the deformity. In addition, interbody fusions may help in correcting the scoliotic deformity. Spinal cord monitoring is essential because distraction may place the cord at risk. Attention should also be paid to the rotational malalignment, which can often be improved with segmental fixation, using screws, hooks, or wires. Constructs with rostral and caudal pedicle screws were statistically more rigid in torsion than constructs with hooks as distal anchors in scoliosis correction.[24]

Need for Dural Sac Decompression

As emphasized previously, adequate spinal canal decompression is essential before the placement of a compression instrumentation construct. Either ventral or dorsal decompressive operations, particularly in the setting of trauma, result in further destabilization of the spine and should always be followed by rigid internal stabilization.

Armamentarium of the Surgeon

The surgeon should be prepared to use alternative stable constructs when a primary (most desired) construct is not feasible for any specific region. The inability to decompress ventral compressive lesions dictates that a dorsal compression instrumentation construct not be applied; an inability to place pedicle screws because of an anatomic or pathologic state dictates that hooks or wires are required. These limitations force the surgeon to be versatile and thoughtful in the management of complex spinal disorders.

Acknowledgment. The authors thank Dr. Setti S. Rengachary, who coauthored prior editions of this chapter. His work laid the foundation for the present chapter.

KEY REFERENCES

Benzel EC: Construct design. In Benzel EC, editor: *Spinal instrumentation*, Chicago, 1994, AANS Publications, pp 239–256.

Brodke DS, Bachus KN, Mohr RA, Nguyen BK: Segmental pedicle screw fixation or cross-links in multilevel lumbar constructs: a biomechanical analysis. *Spine J* 1(5):373–379, 2001.

Cook SD, Salkeld SL, Stanley T, et al: Biomechanical study of pedicle screw fixation in severely osteoporotic bone. *Spine J* 4:402–408, 2004.

Krag MH: Biomechanics of thoracolumbar spinal fixation. *Spine (Phila Pa 1976)* 16:S84–S99, 1991.

McLain RF: The biomechanics of long versus short fixation for thoracolumbar spine fractures. *Spine (Phila Pa 1976)* 31(suppl 11):S70–S79, 2006.

Zindrick MR, Wiltse LL, Windell EH, et al: A biomechanical study of intrapeduncular screw fixation in the lumbosacral spine. *Clin Orthop Relat Res* 203:99–112, 1986.

REFERENCES

The complete reference list is available online at expertconsult.com.

CHAPTER 142

Upper Cervical Screw Fixation Techniques

Ronald I. Apfelbaum | Mehmet Zileli | Charles B. Stillerman

Internal fixation is often used to provide immediate stabilization to protect the vital neural and vascular elements rendered vulnerable by instability produced by trauma, disease processes such as rheumatoid arthritis or neoplasms, and surgical procedures such as transoral odontoidectomy. Immediate stabilization is especially important in the highly mobile cervical spine. The occipitocervical junction and atlantoaxial complex constitute a transitional region connecting the rest of the spinal column to the cranium. The vertebrae and joints in this area differ from the vertebrae and joints in the subaxial spine, with special modifications to allow unique degrees of motion. Possibly the most important of these are at the C1-2 complex, where the flat lateral articulations, absence of an intervertebral disc, and lax ligaments permit appreciable rotation at C1-2 (about 50% of total head rotation) (Fig. 142-1).[1] This motion is safely tolerated because the spinal canal is more generous, the instantaneous axis of rotation is located close to the spinal cord (minimizing distortion of that structure), and the vertebral arteries loop laterally (allowing for at least one to remain patent, even at the extremes of rotation). Potentially catastrophic translational movements, which would crush the spinal cord, are prevented by the very strong transverse component of the cruciate ligament (usually 8 to 10 mm in diameter in adults) that contains the odontoid process of the axis in the ventral compartment of the atlas. Disruption of this ligament, with or without bursting of the ring of C1 (Jefferson fracture), or disruption of the odontoid process results in gross instability. The remaining ligamentous structures, if intact, may provide some support, but they are too weak intrinsically to protect the spinal cord from even relatively minor trauma.

The restoration of structural integrity is critical. If the instability is caused by bone disruption, healing can occur with proper external immobilization. However, instability caused by ligamentous disruption requires surgery to achieve a bony fusion between previously hypermobile motion segments to protect the spinal cord. For bone healing or fusion to occur, two criteria must be met: (1) The bone graft (or bone fragments) must be touching or in proximity, and (2) motion must be eliminated or minimized.

Internal fixation can provide immediate stabilization to optimize bone graft and fragment healing. Internal fixation does this better than rigid external immobilization (e.g., a halo vest or Minerva jacket), while avoiding the cost, discomfort, and complications associated with these devices. Screw fixation offers biomechanical advantages to wiring in many instances and may minimize the demands on postoperative bracing.

General Considerations

Protection of the neural elements when instability exists is paramount. Before surgery, the patient must be properly immobilized. Depending on the degree of instability, immobilization may be achieved with a rigid cervical collar, or it may require skeletal traction, a halo vest, or a Minerva jacket. Ongoing spinal canal compromise, if present, should be corrected before fusion is attempted by restoring alignment with cervical traction via cranial tongs or by surgical removal of intraspinal masses. After the nature of the pathologic condition has been fully investigated and restoration of physiologic relationships between neural elements and the spinal column has been managed, surgical stabilization can be planned. The overall medical condition of the patient should be optimized, and other injuries should be evaluated and treated as appropriate.

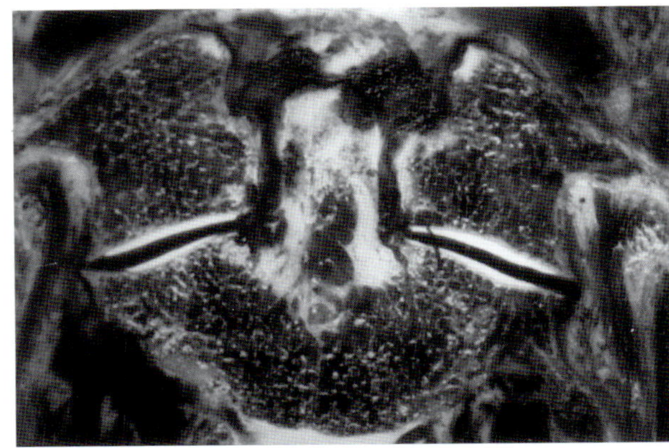

FIGURE 142-1. Coronal anatomic section through the atlantoaxial complex at the level of the odontoid process. Note the horizontal axis of the C1-2 articulation and absence of an intervertebral disc that contributes to the degree of rotatory motion at this joint. (Courtesy of Dr. Wolfgang Rauschning, Uppsala, Sweden.)

Anesthetic Considerations

The degree of cervical spine instability and direction of movement that produce subluxation can affect the choice of anesthesia. An odontoid process fracture is often unstable in both flexion and extension and requires an awake fiberoptic intubation, whereas a transverse ligament rupture may be unstable only in flexion, and routine laryngoscopic techniques can be used. If C-arm fluoroscopy is planned for intraoperative guidance, it can be set up before inducing anesthesia to monitor spinal alignment during intubation and positioning. Patients with spinal cord injury who have significantly reduced vasomotor tone may require substantial IV fluid volume replacement or vasopressors to maintain adequate circulatory volume and blood pressure.

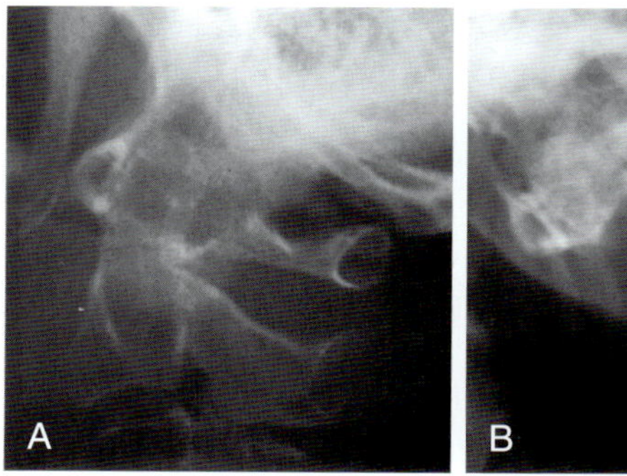

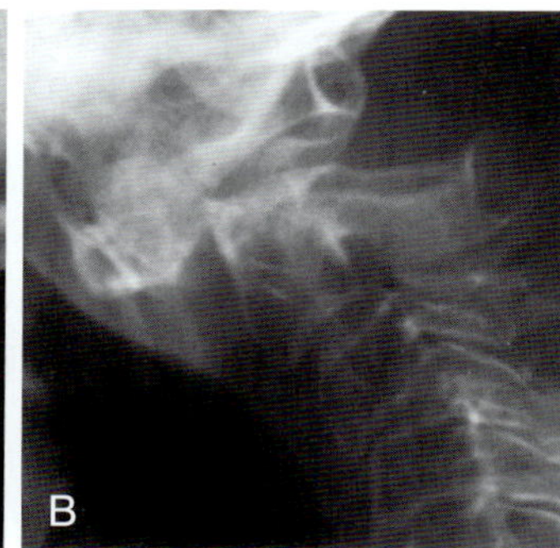

FIGURE 142-2. A, Patient with unrecognized odontoid process fracture after a fall. **B,** Flexion film shows severe instability with 100% anterolisthesis, showing the fallacy of relying on a single film to predict the degree of instability.

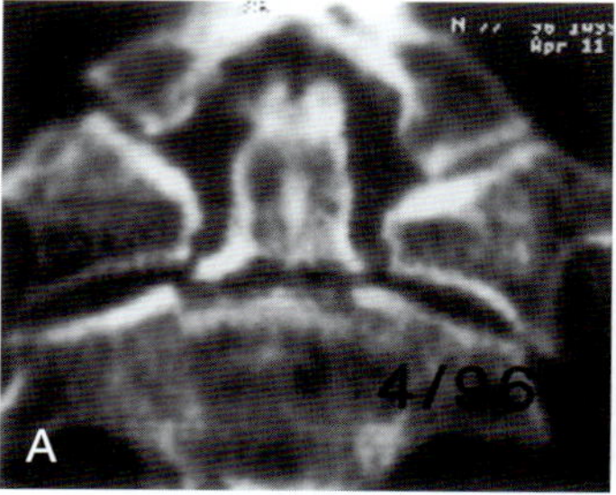

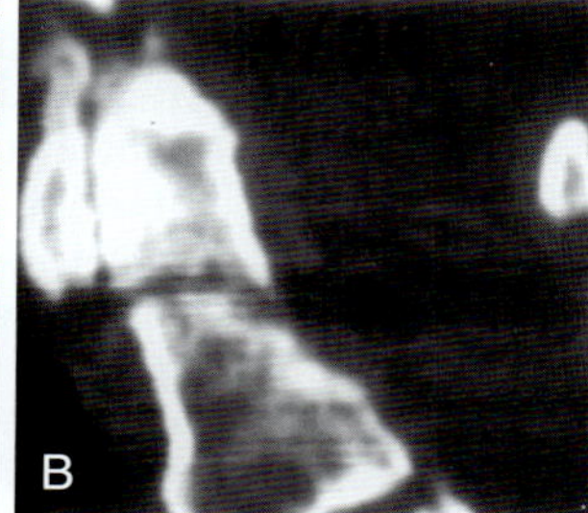

FIGURE 142-3. Anteroposterior (**A**) and lateral (**B**) CT images of a 78-year-old patient with a type II odontoid fracture sustained in a motor vehicle accident. At this juncture, he had been in a halo vest for 6 months and had no evidence of union despite being in good alignment.

Ventral Approaches

Indications

Ventral techniques are primarily indicated for direct screw fixation of odontoid process fractures. C2-3 ventral fusion and plating may be used for hangman's fracture.[2] It is no different from ventral cervical fusion and plating at lower levels other than the difficulty associated with the angle of approach to C2. The retractor system used for odontoid screw fixation sometimes may be useful in this regard.

Odontoid process fractures were classified by Anderson and D'Alonzo[3] as types I, II, and III. Type I fractures involve the apical part of the odontoid process, are quite rare, and are usually believed to be stable. However, one report suggested otherwise,[4] and dynamic imaging should be used to assess stability. Type II fractures involve the neck of the odontoid process and are the most common. Type III fractures extend into the body of C2 and generally heal well with immobilization. However, in a comprehensive review of fractures of the C2 vertebral body, Benzel et al.[5] noted that the type III fracture described by Anderson and D'Alonzo[3] is not an odontoid fracture at all. Benzel et al.[5] proposed a classification of C2 body fractures that is more comprehensive and more meaningful in regard to mechanisms of injury.

Debate continues regarding the optimal treatment of type II fractures. Reported nonunion rates range from 7%[6] to 100%.[7-12] A meta-analysis[13] found that halo vest immobilization produced a fusion rate of 65%. The variable success of immobilization led some authors to try to define parameters that would predict failure with external immobilization. Extent of dislocation (67% nonunion if dislocation is >6 mm,[14] 88% nonunion with dislocation >4 mm[15]), patient age (higher failure rate in older patients[15,16]), and direction of subluxation (higher failure rate with dorsal subluxation[16]) all have been suggested as predictors, as has a comminuted fragment of bone at the base of the odontoid process (type IIA).[17] Although these studies fail to agree on many points, they do emphasize the nature of the problem.

Degree and direction of offset may be misleading indicators because they have been identified based on single rather than dynamic radiographs (Fig. 142-2). However, age seems to be an important valid indicator of the propensity for nonunion. In a randomized controlled prospective study, Lennarson et al.[18] found the nonunion rate was 21 times greater in patients older than 50 years who were treated with halo immobilization than in younger patients. This study was a key factor leading to a recommendation for surgery in the guidelines for management of acute cervical spine and spinal cord injuries published by the Joint Section of Disorders of the Spine and Peripheral Nerves of the American Association of Neurological Surgeons and Congress of Neurological Surgeons.[19]

Because nonoperative treatment of type II odontoid fractures has a high nonunion rate (Fig. 142-3), several alternative methods of surgical fixation have been developed. The traditional operative technique for type II odontoid process fractures has been C1-2 dorsal wiring and arthrodesis. A relatively high fusion rate is associated with this technique; however, rigid postoperative bracing for at least 3 months is necessary, and successful fusion results in a significant reduction in head rotation. The dorsal approach also has an associated traumatic effect on cervical muscles. All these disadvantages can be obviated by using direct ventral odontoid screw fixation techniques.

Direct Ventral Odontoid Screw Fixation

Direct screw fixation of the odontoid process was first described in 1980 in the Japanese literature by Nakanishi,[20] who began using this technique in 1978. This description was followed in 1981 and in 1982 by publications from Böhler,[21,22] who reported his experience dating back to 1968. Although others[23-26] described their experiences with various approaches to achieve direct odontoid screw fixation, the procedure was not widely accepted. With the development of specialized instrumentation facilitating accurate screw placement and minimal trauma to the patient,[27-29] the procedure has gained in popularity. The technique has the advantages of (1) decreased postoperative pain resulting from lack of extensive muscle dissection, (2) avoidance of bone graft harvest, and (3) maintenance of normal anatomy and rotation at the C1-2 joint.[30] Many patients require no postoperative immobilization.

Direct ventral odontoid screw fixation can be used as the primary approach to treat acute type II fractures. Patients with type II dens fractures with concomitant C1 ring fracture may also be candidates for odontoid screw fixation. However, assessment of transverse ligament integrity by MRI preoperatively[31] and by flexion fluoroscopy postoperatively is essential. If the latter shows continued C1-2 instability, either a ventral or a dorsal C1-2 fusion is necessary. The direct screw fixation technique may also be used in some patients with chronic nonunion of type II odontoid fractures. Candidates should have a relatively small gap between the odontoid process and the C2 body and a reasonably sized odontoid fragment that has not autofused to C1 and does not have sclerosis of the surface opposing the body of C2. Chronic malunions that do not meet these criteria rarely fuse and ultimately fracture the hardware and become unstable. The chance of successful bony union in one small series of such patients with fractures of more than 18 months of age was only 25%[32]; this sharply contrasts with an 88% fusion rate for type II and high type III fractures of less than 6 months of age.[32] For this reason, we generally recommend posterior C1-2 fusion for chronically nonunited fractures. Unstable type III odontoid fractures that do not extend too far into the body of C2 are also potential candidates for direct screw fixation.

Contraindications

Absolute contraindications include comminuted fractures of the C2 body and transverse ligament disruption, as defined by MRI or suggested by a C1 lateral mass fracture with extensive lateral displacement (>7 mm total on anteroposterior radiographs)[33]; pathologic fractures; and nonunions of fractures that occurred more than 6 to 8 months previously that do not meet the aforementioned criteria. A relative contraindication is severe osteoporosis. In addition, an oblique fracture of the odontoid process, angled caudally and ventrally so that it is parallel to the planned screw trajectory, may not be as suitable for ventral screw fixation because the odontoid process may slide down the fracture plane as the screw is tightened. Although they account for only 16% of the cases in one published series,[32] these anterior oblique fractures had a significantly higher failure rate. By starting fixation in a position of slight retrolisthesis and augmenting the construct with a rigid cervical collar to restrict flexion, successful fusion has been achieved in patients with anterior oblique fractures.

A barrel-shaped chest and short neck or a neck that is immobile or kyphotic because of cervical spondylosis can render the surgical approach more difficult, but these are not usually contraindications to the procedure with the instrumentation described subsequently. Finally, using two quality C-arms is preferred, and the procedure should not be attempted without at least one.

Patient Positioning

The patient is placed supine with the neck extended for proper screw trajectory. A folded sheet or blanket is placed under the shoulders. If the neck cannot be initially extended, as judged by careful lateral fluoroscopic monitoring, the head is supported on folded towels in neutral neck alignment. Holter traction with a light weight (5 pounds) hung over the Mayfield U-bar attachment to the operative table is very useful for stabilizing the head.

For odontoid or ventral C1-2 screw placement, biplanar fluoroscopy is necessary. The anteroposterior view is obtained transorally. A wine bottle cork, notched for the teeth or gums, is an ideal radiolucent mouth prop. A single fluoroscope, swung back and forth frequently from the lateral to the anteroposterior position, can be used if necessary. A triangular space for one side of the C-arm can be walled off with drapes and IV poles to facilitate frequent positioning and minimize the need to redrape the C-arm. It is much easier, however, to use a second C-arm fluoroscope if one is available. One C-arm unit is placed laterally with the arc horizontally or up to 45 degrees above the horizon. The other can be brought in at a 45-degree angle from the head of the table and positioned for the transoral view (Fig. 142-4).

Some adjustments may be needed to optimize the views, but once the optimal view is achieved, the remainder of the procedure is greatly facilitated. The C-arm monitors should be positioned for optimal viewing by the surgeon, who stands on one side of the patient with the assistant on the opposite side. The anesthesiologist remains at the head of the table in the remaining quadrant. This setup provides optimal access to the patient's head and airway.

Operative Technique

Several screw systems have been used, but all ventral odontoid fixations begin with the same exposure. The initial approach to the spine is the same as for an anterior cervical discectomy. The spine is approached at about the C5 level through a unilateral natural skin crease incision (Fig. 142-5). We use a local injection with epinephrine (1:200,000) to minimize skin bleeding and complete hemostasis with bipolar

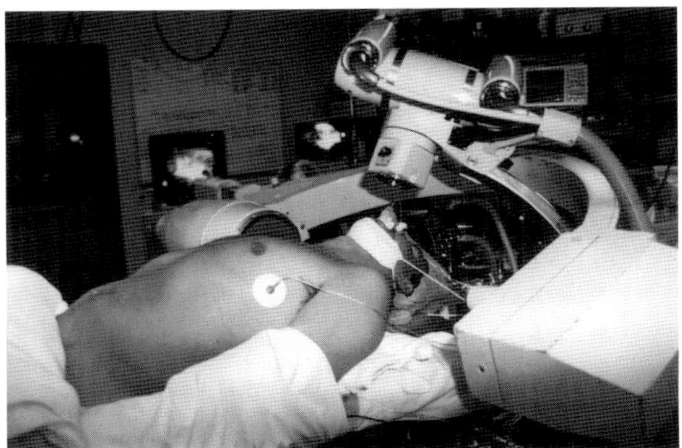

FIGURE 142-4. Patient positioned on operating table. Note the folded sheet placed under the shoulders to increase neck extension in this patient whose fracture reduced in extension. Note also the placement of two C-arm fluoroscopic units for anteroposterior (transoral) and lateral fluoroscopic control.

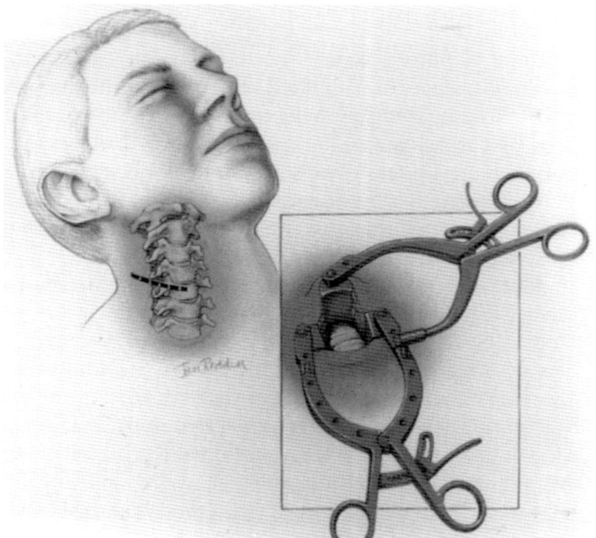

FIGURE 142-5. Skin incision in a natural skin crease at about the C5 level. *Inset* shows retractor in place.

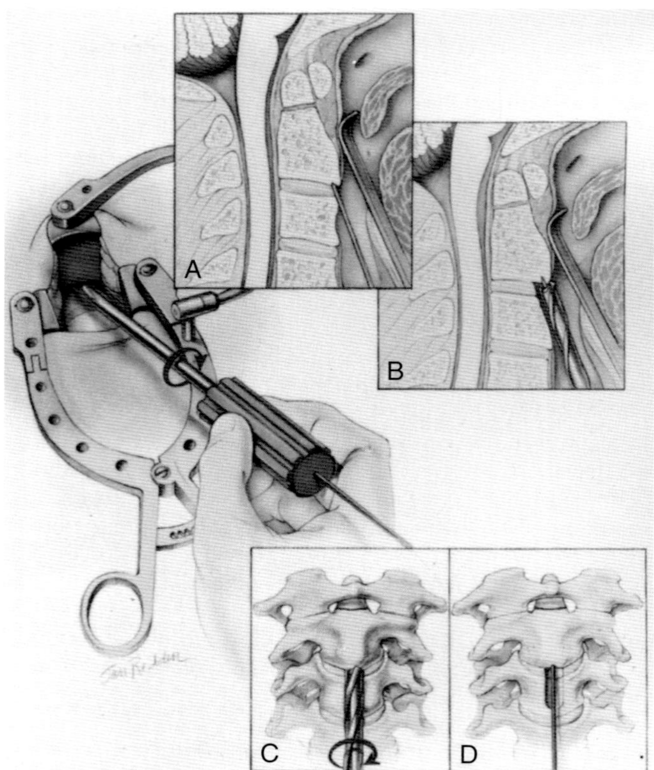

FIGURE 142-6. A, A guiding K-wire in place. **B–D,** Hollow hand drill creates a trough in the face of C3 and C2-3 anulus.

cautery. The platysma muscle is elevated and divided with monopolar cautery. The sternocleidomastoid muscle fascia is opened along the medial side of the muscle with sharp dissection. Blunt dissection opens the deeper tissue planes medial to the carotid sheath and lateral to the trachea and esophagus to expose the prevertebral space. Dividing the longus colli fascia and the anterior longitudinal ligament in the midline with electrocautery allows the bellies of the longus colli muscle to be elevated bilaterally over approximately 1.5 vertebral segments. Sharp-bladed Caspar retractor blades are set in place below the muscle and attached to the Caspar retractor.

The loose areolar tissue in the prevertebral space ventral to the longus colli muscles is easily opened with a Kittner or "peanut" dissector held in a curved tonsil clamp. It is swept from side to side while advancing up to the C1-2 level (monitored with lateral fluoroscopy). The Apfelbaum system (Aesculap Instrument Corporation, Center Valley, PA) has an angled retractor blade that reaches into this space under the mandible and holds open the working tunnel. It attaches to one side of the previously placed modified Caspar retractors (see Fig. 142-5). Other systems use different retractors, such as a curved hand-held retractor (Synthes) or small metal hook-shaped hand-held Hohmann retractors that lock over the shoulders of C2 bilaterally alongside the dens, as initially described by Böhler.[21] The key to the retraction is to create a working tunnel up to the caudal edge of C2, without having any device caudally in the wound that restricts the low trajectory needed for proper screw placement.

At this point, the various instrument systems use different approaches for placing the screws. The Apfelbaum system consists of an outer guide tube with spikes that anchor it to C3 and that can be used to optimize spinal alignment. An inner guide tube, within the outer tube, guides the drilling. After the pilot hole is drilled, the inner guide is removed, the hole is tapped, and the screws are placed through the outer guide tube. First, under biplanar fluoroscopic control, an entry site on the ventral caudal edge of C2 is selected, and a K-wire is impacted into C2 (Fig. 142-6A). If one screw is to be placed, a midline location is chosen. If two are to be placed, a paramedian location is selected 2 to 3 mm from the midline. Care and patience in selecting the entry site and setting the K-wire are rewarded by the remainder of the procedure being expedited. When the K-wire is set, a 7-mm hollow drill is placed over the K-wire and is rotated by hand to create a shallow trough in the face of C3 and in the C2-3 anulus (Fig. 142-6B–D).

No bone is removed from C2. The two guide tubes are mated together, passed over the K-wire, and walked up the ventral face of the spinal column until the spikes on the outer tube are over the body of C3. The inner guide tube is advanced in the trough to the ventral caudal edge of C2 (Fig. 142-7), and the K-wire is removed. Having the guide tube at the entry site prevents the drill from skipping off the edge of the bone and walking up the ventral face of C2. With the guide tube system firmly engaged in C3, the surgeon can optimize the C2 alignment on the fluoroscopic images by either pushing C2 and C3 dorsally relative to the odontoid-C1 complex or pulling C2 and C3 ventrally. In the case of a retrolisthesed odontoid process, this realignment can be performed while gradually extending the patient's head and removing the supporting towels beneath it to obtain an ideal working trajectory.

A pilot hole is drilled from the ventral caudal edge of C2 to the apex of the odontoid process, advancing the drill slowly under biplanar fluoroscopic control (Fig. 142-8). The dense cortical shell of the odontoid must be pierced to engage the screw properly and avoid splitting. Because the odontoid process is firmly held in position by its periosteum and attached supporting ligaments, it is not displaced as the drill enters from the soft cancellous fracture site. The angle of drilling is such that the drill can penetrate a substantial distance beyond the apex of the odontoid process into the apical ligaments

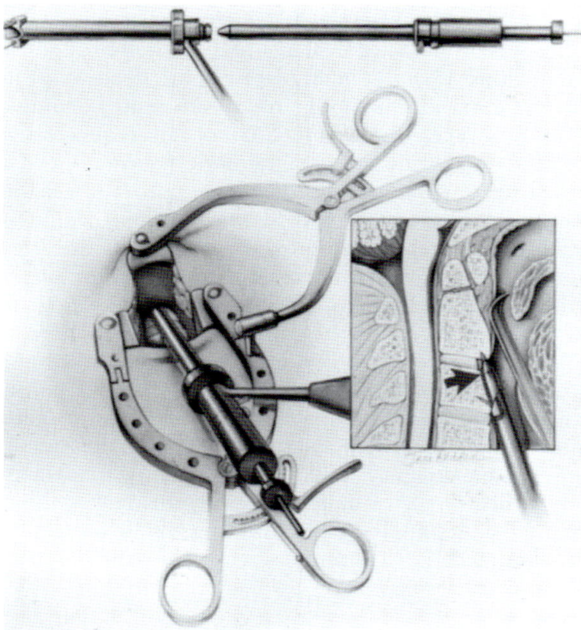

FIGURE 142-7. Drill guide system. Inner and outer guide tubes mate together and are placed over the K-wire. The spikes on the outer guide tube are impacted into C3, and the inner guide tube is advanced into the previously created trough (*arrow*) to the caudal edge of C2.

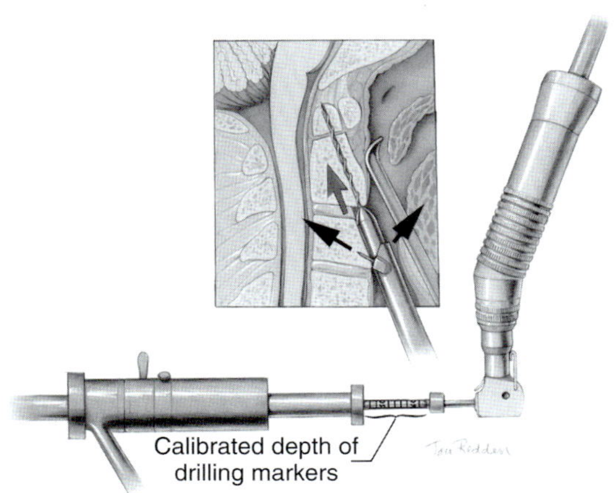

FIGURE 142-8. K-wire is removed and replaced with a drill, which is guided fluoroscopically to the apex of the odontoid process after reducing dislocation of the odontoid process. The guide tube is kept in place by steady upward pressure (*vertical arrow*) to keep the spikes engaged in C3. The alignment of C2 and C3 relative to the odontoid process and C1 is optimized and maintained by lifting up or pushing down on the retractor as appropriate, as indicated by the *oblique arrows,* before crossing the fracture site with the drill.

without threatening the dural or neural structures. However, if a more dorsal trajectory is needed, greater care must be taken not to penetrate too far into the spinal canal; this is controlled by visualizing the progress of the drill on the fluoroscope.

A right-angled (dental-type) drill hand piece can be used to avoid interference with the ventral chest wall when drilling; this allows the procedure to be performed even in barrel-chested patients. Once the drill is into the distal odontoid cortex, its depth of penetration is read on the calibrated

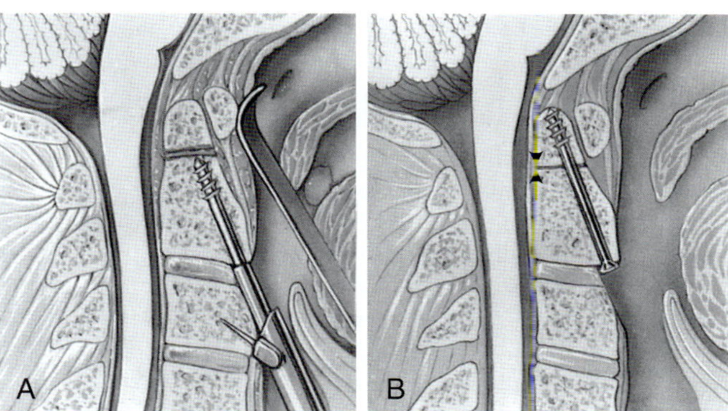

FIGURE 142-9. A lag screw is placed through the guide tube (**A**) and advanced through the tapped pilot hole to its final position (**B**). In fresh fractures, the gap at the fracture site is reduced (*arrows*) by the lag effect of the screw pulling the odontoid back toward the body of C2.

shaft, and the anteroposterior and lateral fluoroscopic images are saved on the monitor screens. Comparison of future live images with these saved images allows reestablishment of the identical alignment in successive steps.

The drill is withdrawn, and the inner guide tube is removed. A tap is placed through the outer guide tube, and the pilot hole is tapped. Threads are cut in the bone, allowing a more precise bone-screw junction that may reduce bone absorption around the screw caused by pressure necrosis if a self-tapping screw is used. The tap is removed, and a screw is placed through the guide tube (Fig. 142-9). A screw that is a few millimeters shorter than the measured drill depth may be chosen to allow for reduction at the fracture site, but it is important that the screw fully engages the apical cortex. Extending the screw a few millimeters beyond the cortex into the apical ligaments is safe and preferable to having one too short because the latter may (and has in our experience) back out. To achieve some fracture reduction, a partially threaded screw (lag screw) is used to pull the odontoid back toward the body of C2.

At each of these two steps, the odontoid process–C2 alignment that was achieved initially is easily restored by comparing the active fluoroscopic image with the stored image taken at the time of drilling. In practice, we have never had a problem reentering the same hole with the tap or screw, and improved modern fluoroscopes often show the drill track itself. If a second screw is to be placed, the identical series of steps is followed on the contralateral paramedian site except that either a partially threaded lag screw or a fully threaded screw can be used because no further lagging action would be expected to occur.

After removal of the guide tube, bleeding from C3 can be controlled with bone wax. Lateral fluoroscopy in flexion and extension confirms stability. Closure is routine and is performed in layers, closing the sternocleidomastoid fascia, platysma muscle, and subcutaneous tissue with absorbable sutures and the skin with sterile tape strips. No drains are placed. Unless concern exists regarding the patient's bone quality, external collars are not usually recommended, and patients are allowed to return to work and resume nontraumatic activities promptly.

Several alternative systems have been proposed that are often based on existing long bone screw fixation techniques. These systems use a K-wire to drill the pilot hole and pass a hollow overdrill over this, followed by a cannulated screw.[24] Theoretically, after the K-wire is placed, it does not have to be removed so that precise reentry into the same trajectory is assured; however, a drawback of these systems is that they do not appear to have any provision for optimizing alignment with the drill guide, as described earlier, except by trying to do this by repositioning the head or placing additional instruments beside the drill and pushing on C1 or C2. K-wires are suboptimal drills because they lack the torsional rigidity of drill bits and can be deflected by irregular densities within the bone. To redirect them, one must remove the K-wire and select a new starting point.[34] In addition, great care must be taken when drilling over the K-wire because the drill can bind to the K-wire and advance it into the spinal canal or cut the K-wire. This can also occur when placing the screw over the K-wire.

Controversies

One-Screw Constructs versus Two-Screw Constructs

Theoretically, with one screw, the odontoid process could rotate on C2, although with fresh fractures the interdigitation of the irregular fracture surfaces may prevent this; this may explain why both techniques have been reported to have similar clinical success.[35-37] Laboratory studies also show no greater resistance to screw fracture from bending with one-screw or two-screw constructs. However, a more recent clinical study by Dailey et al.[38] found a significant difference in fusion rates among 57 patients older than 70 years with odontoid fractures: a 56% success rate was achieved if one screw was placed, whereas a 95% fusion rate was achieved when two screws were placed. The different outcomes between this study and the previously mentioned ones are likely due to the fact that the earlier studies had a much younger patient population.

The demographics of patients with odontoid fractures are changing. The previous bimodal age distribution included a large number of younger patients who sustained this fracture when riding as an unrestrained passenger in a motor vehicle involved in an accident. With increased seat belt usage and air bag availability, this is a rare cause of this injury nowadays. Elderly patients who sustain odontoid fractures after relatively minor trauma, often a ground-level fall, constitute most patients with odontoid fractures, highlighting the importance of considering placement of two screws in older and possibly in middle-aged patients.

When two screws are placed, the entry site for each is located paramedially a few millimeters off the midline and the screws are angled toward each other at the odontoid apex. The diameter of the odontoid process should be assessed on the preoperative CT scan to ensure adequate bone volume for a second screw. Some patients may not have a sufficiently wide odontoid process to accommodate two screws side by side,[39] but the process may be deep enough that the screws can be placed in such a way that they end up in front of and behind each other to achieve the same fixation.

Screw Size and Type

Biomechanical data suggest that cannulated screws are only about 5% to 10% weaker than solid screws.[34] Various screw diameters have been used. These usually range from 3.5 to 4.0 mm and are occasionally larger. The initial experience was with cancellous threaded screws, which have a deeper thread (smaller minor diameter or core) and are better at resisting pull-out. However, pull-out forces on odontoid screws are minimal. An odontoid screw primarily has to resist bending and translational forces. Screw failure, if it occurs, is almost always due to fracture at the level of the bone fracture. Cortically threaded screws (4-mm outer diameter) with a larger minor diameter (2.9 mm vs. the previously used 2 mm) would seem optimal. Such screws have proven substantially stronger in laboratory tests, in which they fail to fracture after 1 million cycles at three times the load at which the older screws fractured at 33,100 cycles. In the experience of the senior author (R.I.A.), these screws are also more effective; no postoperative screw fractures were observed in more than 400 consecutive screw placements compared with a 5% fracture rate in odontoid fixation and 10% fracture rate in C1-2 fixation with the prior screw design. An additional benefit is that the pilot hole is drilled larger (3 mm vs. 2 mm); this makes the drill much more directionally stable, allowing precise correction of pilot hole trajectory to optimize screw placement.

Results

Type II odontoid fractures less than 6 months old treated with this technique have a high rate of fusion. The combined published series[32] of Veres in Hungary and Apfelbaum et al. in Salt Lake City, Utah, encompassed 147 patients whose ages ranged from 15 to 92 years. Successful bony union was achieved in 88% of patients, with an additional 3% achieving stability via fibrous union. These results agree with the results of other published series with fewer patients.[25,26,34,40,41] Failures usually occur in elderly patients with poor quality bone. In such circumstances, the screw may fail to hold in C2, in particular, if there is an associated fracture in the body of C2. If this complication is recognized early, manipulative realignment and external immobilization have been successful. If not, additional surgery was required. There was one late neurologic complication in which a patient became quadriplegic in the series from Hungary when the construct failed to hold and the fracture subsequently dislocated. There were no other neurologic complications, and other surgical complications are rare.

Other series have shown similar low complication rates; however, there has been a high incidence of dysphagia from the retropharyngeal approach in elderly patients, and some of these patients required temporary feeding tubes.[38] Although there are no published results detailing complications when using one of the cannulated systems, numerous serious and even fatal complications are known to result from the K-wire being driven in beyond the odontoid tip.

The high degree of success achieved by using this straightforward, easily mastered technique, usually with minimal complications, warrants its consideration as the primary treatment for many type II odontoid fractures. By allowing the patient to resume normal activity quickly while avoiding the cost and medical and social morbidity of a halo vest, screw fixation seems to be a very cost-effective treatment for this problem.

Ventral C1-2 Transarticular Screw Fixation

Ventral C1-2 transarticular screw fixation may provide an alternative if odontoid screw fixation is impossible or if successful odontoid screw fixation fails to stabilize C2 because of unrecognized concomitant transverse ligament incompetence. Stabilization is accomplished by inserting two screws through the lateral masses of C2 into the lateral mass of C1.[42] The entry site is just medial to the vertebral artery, which is placed at risk by this approach. The screws angle laterally about 20 degrees and dorsally at a similar angle. The entry site is selected by following the lateral edge of the vertebral body rostrally from the C2-3 interspace to its junction with the lateral mass, staying as medial as possible in that structure. The drill guide system used for odontoid screw fixation can be used for this as well, although the screw length is considerably shorter.

Although it achieves fixation, this technique does not permit placement of substantial bone graft. Rather, long-term stabilization is achieved by promoting arthrodesis of the C1-2 lateral articulation, primarily by immobilization. This stabilization may be enhanced by curetting the joint, but overall, the construct is less likely to succeed than dorsal screw fixation with dorsal grafting. Therefore, we believe it should be reserved for exceptional cases.

Other Ventral Techniques

There are a few reports of using plates and screws transorally.[43] Experience with these is limited because they do not appear to have been widely used. The risk of infection and, to a lesser extent, the limited working space seem to have deterred most surgeons from these approaches.

Dorsal Approaches

The dorsal approach is used to stabilize C1 to C2. Rather than providing stabilization and fixation of a fractured bone, it stabilizes what was previously a normal motion segment and provides an optimal environment for bone graft healing. However, bone grafting is almost always required for long-term stabilization because hardware in nonfused segments ultimately fatigues and fails.

Traditional techniques have used various C1-2 wiring strategies with interposed or onlay bone grafting (Gallie,[44] Brooks,[45] and interspinous [Sonntag][46] fusions). Because these impart limited stability that deteriorates significantly with cyclic loading,[47] an external rigid orthosis is usually necessary. Fractured or absent dorsal elements can preclude the use of these techniques. Even in optimal situations, nonunion rates of 30% are reported.[47]

Transarticular screw fixation, pioneered by Magerl in 1979, offers immediate stabilization, often without external orthosis.[48] By optimizing bone graft union with a high chance of success, transarticular screw fixation is a major advance in treating instability in this area. The construct can be extended with various devices to include the occiput and the subaxial spine if needed.

Indications

This procedure is indicated for atlantoaxial instability from almost any cause—traumatic disruption of the transverse ligament, rheumatoid or other degenerative diseases, iatrogenic instability after transoral decompression, congenital or acquired absence of a united odontoid process (os odontoideum), ligamentous incompetence associated with various genetic diseases (Down syndrome, Larsen disease), or chronic nonunited odontoid fractures. Occiput-C1 instability can occur from many of the same causes and, if present, can be treated by extending the stabilization and fusion up to the occiput.

Contraindications

Poor bone quality is always of concern during intraosseous fixation and must be evaluated carefully. It is not an absolute contraindication to surgery but may necessitate using both internal and external devices. Of paramount importance for transarticular screw fixation is an adequate pathway for the screw that traverses the pars interarticularis (isthmus) of C2 (not the pedicle) to the lateral C1-2 articulation before crossing that joint into the lateral mass of C1. Variations in anatomy and secondary effects of vascular elongation coupled with bone softening can result in the vertebral artery looping up into the pars of C2. This looping of the vertebral artery may occur to such an extent that an inadequate pathway remains for safe screw placement. Placing screws in such circumstances has resulted in vertebral artery injury with potentially serious neurologic sequelae. An alternative technique devised by Harms and Melcher[49] uses screws placed in the lateral masses of C1 and into the C2 pars or pedicle, which are connected posteriorly with rods. This technique is applicable in cases in which a safe pathway through the C2 pars to C1 does not exist. Another approach using translaminar screws in C2 that are then coupled to C1 screws has been proposed by Wright.[50]

Understanding the patient's anatomy and the availability of a safe bony pathway for screw placement before proceeding with the surgery is crucial. We obtain thin-section CT scans and build images that are not just in orthogonal planes but are also reconstructed along the planned screw pathways. This construction of images can be done on the consoles of most CT scanners. Alternatively, importing the images into a stereotaxic workstation allows the surgeon to look at various possible pathways and build a three-dimensional model that can be viewed in the operating room. This approach has been invaluable in evaluating whether screws can be passed safely (Fig. 142-10) and in assisting in achieving the desired pathway during surgery.

Patient Positioning

A Mayfield three-pin head holder and a cervical collar are placed. The patient is rolled into prone position on bolsters while the surgeon keeps the neck stable with axial traction and maintains it in a neutral position. Before the head clamp is secured to the table, final positioning is performed under lateral fluoroscopic guidance. The best reduction position is often with the neck in extension, but this may preclude C1-2 transarticular screw placement in many cases because lordosis would often dictate a screw trajectory starting within the thoracic cavity. The patient should be positioned with the chin slightly flexed but with the head pulled dorsally (Fig. 142-11). This position has been likened to the posture of military personnel standing at braced attention. This position usually reduces C1-2 dislocations via dorsal translation but leaves the rest of the cervical spine in a flattened or even slightly kyphotic posture so that the needed screw trajectory

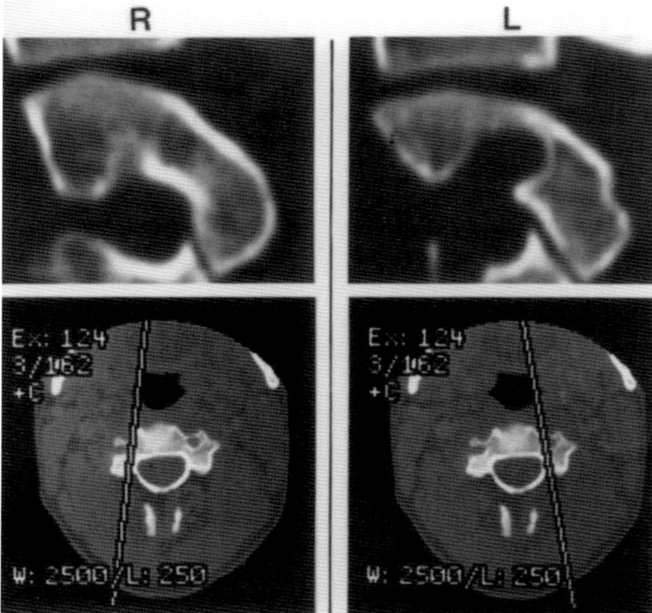

FIGURE 142-10. Upper views show CT reconstruction through the pars interarticularis of C2 on the right and left sides in trajectory shown on axial scout views in the lower two panels. Note the safe path for the screw on the patient's right side but abnormally large vertebral artery canal with inadequate bony dimensions for safe screw placement on the left. Only one screw was placed in this patient.

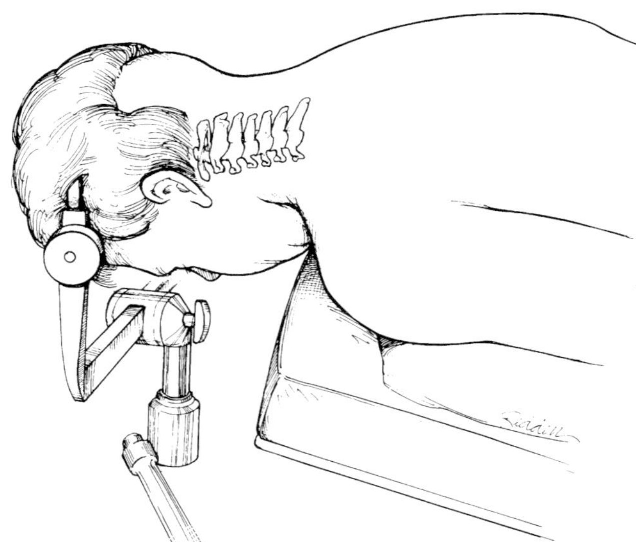

FIGURE 142-11. Patient positioning for transarticular screw fixation. The head is fixed in a three-pin head holder. Translating the head dorsally with the chin tucked reduces atlantoaxial dislocation and allows the lower spine to be kept in a straight or flexed position. This position facilitates the trajectory for C1-2 screw placement. The patient is positioned while vertebral alignment is monitored via lateral fluoroscopy.

can be achieved. The head should also be positioned so that it is not rotated; this can be judged by the symmetry of the ear canals relative to the table or floor. Careful monitoring of the fluoroscopic image facilitates safe positioning. An absolutely perfect position is unnecessary; minor residual translational movements are accepted because these can easily be corrected at the time of screw placement.

The low angle of screw trajectory needed to traverse the C2 pars interarticularis and enter C1 dictates a starting point at about the T1-3 level. Magerl's original technique called for an incision and paraspinal muscle retraction down to this level; however, percutaneous tunneling techniques make this unnecessary.

Operative Technique

A dorsal midline incision extending from just below the inion to C3 is usually adequate (Fig. 142-12A). The paraspinal muscles are dissected off the dorsal elements of C1, C2, and the occipital bone and are held back with angled Weitlaner retractors. The exposure may require sharp dissection assisted with electrocautery if the spine is unstable. The full extent of the dorsal elements of C1 and C2 should be exposed, with definition of the lateral aspect of the C2 dorsal elements and the C2-3 facet joint and of the C2 isthmus extending rostrally beneath the C2 nerve root and the associated venous complex (Fig. 142-12B). Bleeding can usually be arrested with small hemostatic gelatin (Gelfoam) pledgets soaked in thrombin or a slurry made with Gelfoam powder and thrombin. It is neither necessary nor desirable to disconnect the inferior midline attachments to the bifid C2 spinous process.

When the anatomic structures are fully exposed, fixation screws are placed. The entry site on each side is just rostral to the C2-3 facet joint and in line with the previously defined pars interarticularis. Standing back from the wound to reduce parallax, a line representing the inferior extension of the trajectory may be drawn on the drapes. A straight instrument such as a K-wire placed along the patient's neck and superimposed over the desired screw path on the fluoroscopic view provides the intersecting skin coordinates, usually at about T2.

A 1- to 1.5-cm skin transverse incision carried down through the dorsal fascia provides an entry for the drill apparatus (see Fig. 142-12A). As with odontoid fixation, a guide tube system (Aesculap Instrument Corporation) may be used. With this system, a smooth tube fitted with a conical tipped obturator is passed from the skin incision up to the drill entry site at the C2-3 junction by pressing firmly in a rostral direction and gently rotating the instrument back and forth to advance it into the surgical field (Fig. 142-12C). When the guide tube is in place, the obturator is removed, and an awl is used to make a starting hole in the C2 laminar bone. An inner drill guide is placed to support the drill (Fig. 142-13). The guide tube assembly allows precise control of the drilling direction.

The surgeon must visualize the dorsal lateral and medial borders of the pars interarticularis and direct the drill bit accurately between these limits. A tool, such as a small Penfield dissector held by an assistant, can help visualization of this area. Because it is placed on the dorsum of the pars, it serves as a fluoroscopic marker for that boundary. A low-angled trajectory to carry the drill bit just below the dorsum of the pars and across the C1-2 lateral articulation, as far dorsally as possible, engages the maximum amount of the lateral

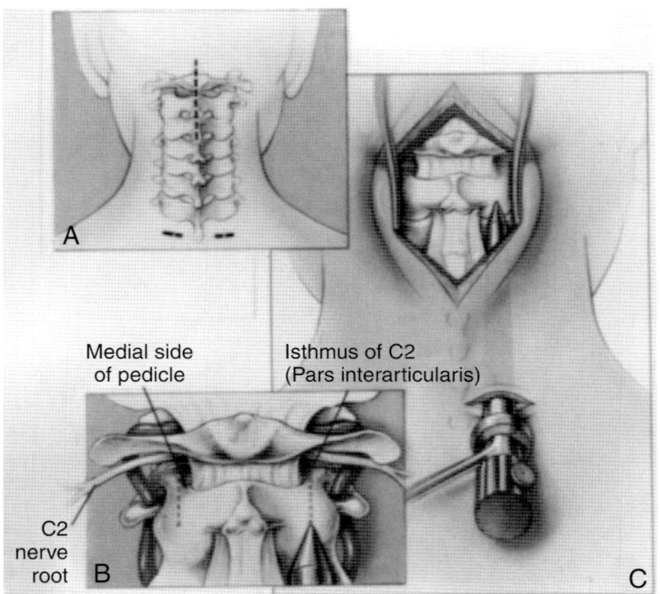

FIGURE 142-12. **A,** Site of surgical incisions. The level of the stab wound sites inferiorly for placement of the drill guide tube is determined fluoroscopically. **B,** Details of surgical anatomy. The desired screw placement is just lateral to the lateral edge of the spinal canal. It traverses the isthmus (pars) of C2 and the C1-2 articulation. The screw does not go down the pedicle, which would take it into the body of C2 and not across the C1-2 joint into C1. **C,** Placement of guide tube (with obturator) through stab wound and into the operative field.

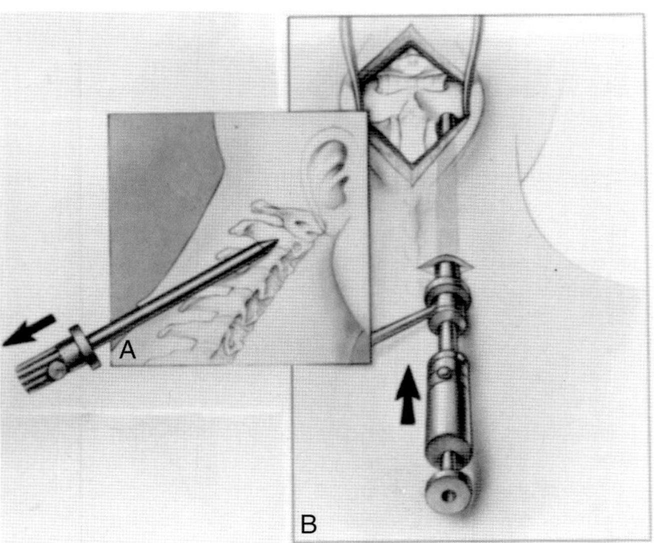

FIGURE 142-13. Guide tube in place as seen in sagittal (**A**) and dorsal (**B**) views. The obturator is removed (**A**) and replaced with an inner drill guide (**B**).

mass of C1 and keeps the drill above the vertebral artery. On the lateral fluoroscopic image (Fig. 142-14), the projection of the ventral arch of C1 is a helpful target to aim for, especially at its rostral margin. Generally, the screw trajectory should be in a straight paramedian direction or slightly medially as dictated by the bone anatomy and location of the vertebral artery foramen. Aiming too far medially results in a smaller area of C1 lateral mass engagement, whereas aiming laterally can jeopardize the vertebral artery.

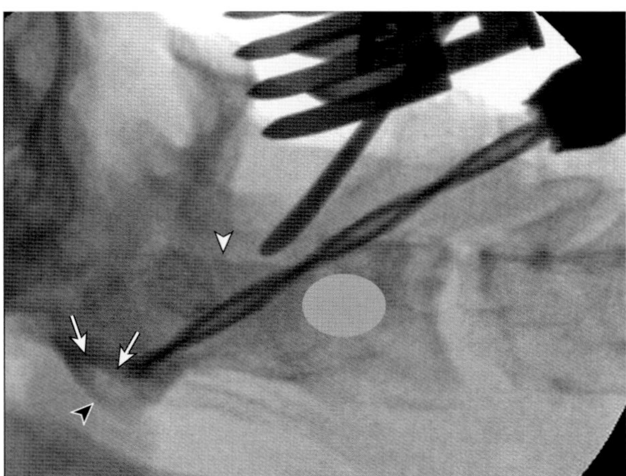

FIGURE 142-14. Lateral fluoroscopic view of drilling in process. The instrument, a Penfield dissector, is defining the dorsum of the pars, with the drill passing just ventral to this. The *white arrowhead* indicates the location of the C1-2 joint. The drill is aimed for the upper portion of the anterior tubercle of C1 (*black arrowhead*) but is not advanced beyond the anterior cortex of C1 (*white arrows*). The *gray oval* indicates the approximate position of the danger zone where the vertebral artery normally resides.

Attempts to adapt image-guided stereotactic systems to this procedure have met with mixed results. It is necessary to track C2 because the vulnerable anatomy is within C2 and because C2 is hypermobile in most of these cases. Tracking arrays placed on the skull clamp or on C1 would not compensate for this motion. However, tracking C2 is difficult because most tracking arrays are bulky and can obstruct the surgeon's access. They also are difficult to secure solidly to C2. It is also very hard to localize the C2 anatomy accurately to register it with the stereotaxic system. Fluoroscopic devices that obtain multiple images and generate a CT image from these may help in this regard. Despite these difficulties, using image guidance is a good way to evaluate and understand this complex anatomy and obtain the precision necessary to place screws safely. It is recommended to surgeons who lack experience with the technique.

When drilling, increased resistance is felt at the cortical margins of the C2 joint surface, and then at the C1 joint surface and at the ventral cortex of C1. If necessary, C2 can be translated ventrally or dorsally before drilling across the joint space by grasping the spinous process of C2 with a towel clamp, ensuring optimal alignment. When the pilot hole is drilled, the depth is noted on the calibrated drill shaft, and the images are stored. The drill and inner drill guide are replaced with a tap (Fig. 142-15) except in very soft bone. After the hole is tapped, a fully threaded screw is placed because no lag effect is needed. Vertebral alignment is reoptimized just before the C1-2 articulation is crossed by matching the active fluoroscopic image with its stored counterpart. If a polyaxial screw is being used, as in the Harms construct, for example, or to extend the construct to the occiput, a guide tube with an additional inner sleeve is used. Removal of the sleeve increases the inner diameter of the tube so that the polyaxial screw can be placed.

Bone bleeding may occur, in particular, in patients with inflammatory disease. However, if brisk arterial bleeding ensues from the drill hole, suggesting a vertebral artery injury, placement of one screw for fixation and tamponade is recommended, but a second screw should not be placed. If this occurs, it would be prudent to obtain postoperative angiographic

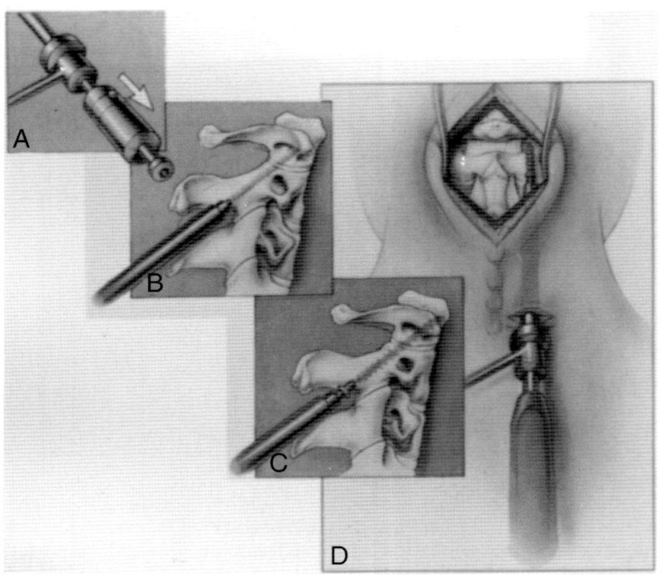

FIGURE 142-15. The inner drill guide tube is removed (**A**). Through the outer guide, the pilot hole is tapped (**B**), and the screw is placed (**C** and **D**).

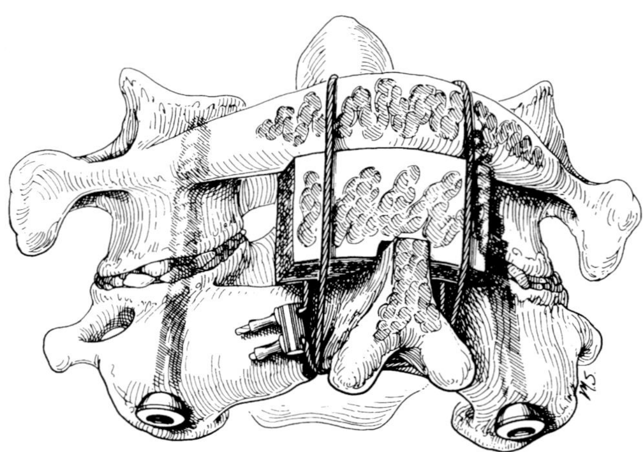

FIGURE 142-16. Illustration of completed screw fixation. This was the technique originally suggested by Sonntag's group and shows the cabling technique we prefer to use. In contrast to this illustration, however, we notch the graft to contact both the dorsal and the caudal edge of the C1 laminar arch (see Fig. 142-17) and extend it over and into the lamina of C2 to improve the fusion potential at this site. (From Marcotte P, Dickman CA, Sonntag VKH, et al: Posterior atlantoaxial facet screw fixation. *J Neurosurg* 79:234–237, 1993.)

images to ascertain the status of the vessel and to detect fistula formation.[51]

Immediately after the first screw is placed, significant improvement is observed in patients with gross instability. The same sequence of steps is repeated on the contralateral side.

If a safe pathway for transarticular screw fixation is not present, the Harms technique can be used. This technique involves placing a polyaxial screw directly into the lateral mass of C1 and coupling it with a rod to a separate C2 screw. The anatomy of the individual bones must be studied before placing these screws to avoid vascular or neural injury. The C1 lateral mass is accessed by depressing the C2 nerve root where it traverses over the posterior aspect of the lateral mass of C1 below its junction with the posterior arch of C1. The screw usually extends above the bone for 1 cm or more, so a partially threaded screw with a smooth shank proximally is recommended to avoid irritation of the C2 root by the screw threads. Depending on the patient's anatomy, the C2 screw can be a short pars screw that stops before a prominent vertebral artery foramen, a pars screw aimed anteriorly, a C2 pedicle screw, or a translaminar screw.

The Harms technique widens the options for screw fixation if the C2 pars is unsuitable for placing a transarticular screw, but the surgeon must be aware that the vertebral artery can also be (and has been) injured with the C1 screw, so a thorough understanding of its location and the bone anatomy of C1 is important. The procedure is more complex than transarticular screw placement because four polyaxial screws and the connecting rods must be placed. Using intralaminar screws in C2 also is an option, but this precludes using the lamina of C2 for the inferior end of the graft in the manner discussed in the next section.

Bone Grafting

Screw fixation functions as an internal splint. For long-term stability, bone fusion is required because all hardware ultimately fails without it. Magerl and Seeman[48] suggested curetting and then packing bone chips into the C1-2 articulation to encourage arthrodesis. Access to this joint is limited, however, and only a small portion of it can be treated in this manner even in ideal circumstances. We use a dorsal fusion construct if possible.

With intact dorsal elements, a modified construct consisting of a combined interpositional and onlay bicortical iliac crest graft was suggested by Sonntag's group.[46] The graft has ventral and dorsal cortices. After the mating surfaces have been denuded with a high-speed bur, the contact sites at the caudal surface of C1 and the laminar surface and rostral edge of the spinous process of C2 are to cancellous bone. The graft and donor surfaces are also contoured for maximum apposition (Fig. 142-16). The graft is secured with a braided titanium cable placed sublaminarly at C1 and around the spinous process of C2, so that the graft is sandwiched between the two layers of cable. This construct provides excellent three-dimensional stability. The screws resist translation and rotation, whereas the graft prevents extension, and the cable prevents flexion. Additional bone chips and curettings may be placed around the construct to enhance fusion.

There are significant advantages to being able to use allograft bone as the graft, including elimination of donor site pain and complications, reduced bleeding, and ability to select more optimal bone. Although allograft usually has been unsuccessful in onlay constructs, by modifying the C1-2 dorsal graft placement further so that the graft is notched to fit in close apposition to both the dorsal and the inferior edges of C1 and is mortised into the lamina of C2, we achieve a true interpositional graft (Fig. 142-17). Coupling this graft with internal screw fixation to eliminate all motion has allowed us to use bicortical iliac crest allograft bone with fusion results equal to autograft in this application and significantly reduced patient morbidity (Fig. 142-18).[52]

Alternative Systems

Drilling with a K-wire and placing hollow cannulated screws is an alternative technique used by some surgeons.[34] The K-wire may be drilled percutaneously or via a similarly placed

FIGURE 142-17. Lateral (**A**) and posterior (**B**) views showing the modified grafting technique to increase the graft contact along the inferior aspect of the C1 ring and its dorsal aspect (*small black arrows* in **A**). Both of these surfaces of C1 are decorticated and flattened to maximize graft contact. The bicortical graft is also mortised into the decorticated lamina of C2 (*large black arrow* in **A**) and contacts the decorticated spinous process of C2 (*arrows* in **B**). The artist has shown wiring, but braided titanium cable is used and placed as described by Dickman et al.,[46] enveloping the graft anteriorly and posteriorly with a cable that passes under the C1 posterior ring and behind the spinous process of C2. Leaving the interspinous ligaments intact on the spinous process of C2 (not shown) helps retain the cable. This graft modification improves grafting success with autograft and allows an equally good result with bicortical iliac crest allograft if desired.[52]

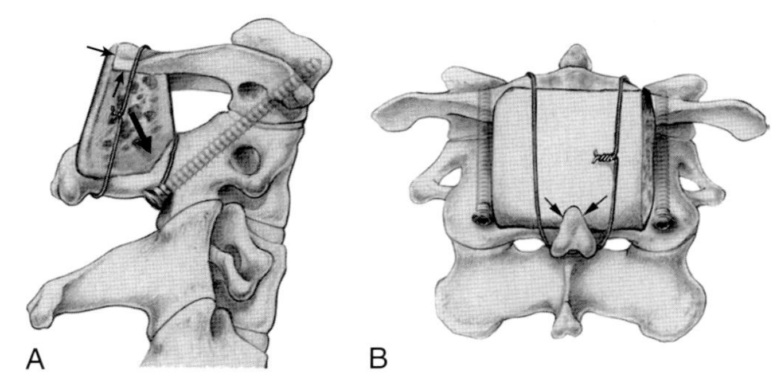

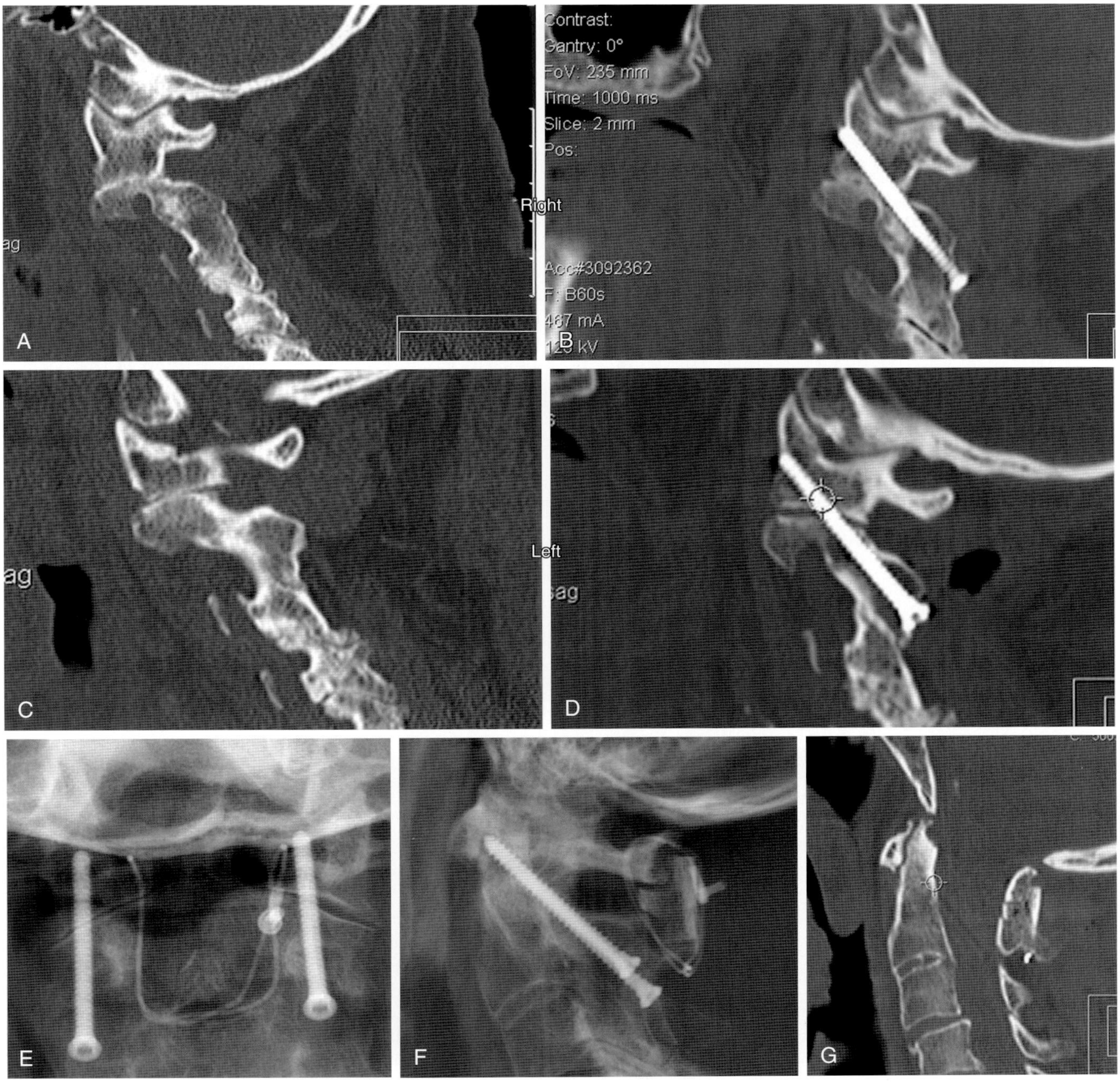

FIGURE 142-18. A–G, Preoperative and postoperative appearance of a patient with cortically threaded transarticular screws, which have a larger minor diameter. This patient had severe atlantoaxial joint degeneration on the right (**A**); however, the joint was still mobile. The left C1-2 joint had retrolisthesis (**C**). The alignment was restored to normal and held with the transarticular screws (**B** and **D**). The screw position is close to ideal crossing the C1-2 joints in their middle or slightly medially (**E**). Note also the interpositional location of the interspinous grafting (**F** and **G**). Allograft was used in this patient.

guide tube. The concerns expressed earlier with regard to lack of precise directional control and the risks of inadvertently advancing the K-wire with the drill and cutting the K-wire pertain here as well.

Screws

Screws measuring 3.5 to 4.0 mm or slightly larger in diameter have been used. As in odontoid screw fixation, there is little pull-out force but significant bending or translational forces. Cortical screws with a larger minor diameter, as described earlier in this chapter with regard to odontoid screws, have replaced the smaller minor diameter cancellous screws previously used. This has been a significant improvement that has eliminated screw breakage. The screw requires a larger drill (3 mm) because of its larger minor diameter. This drill provides more directional control and has resulted in the unexpected benefit of allowing more precise corrections to the trajectory as the drill is advanced.

Postoperative Care

Some surgeons prefer to use a cervical collar, but unless there is a question of bone quality, or if only one screw is placed, this is probably unnecessary. With the immediate elimination of motion, postoperative pain is significantly reduced, and most patients can be discharged from the hospital in about 2 days. Patients are monitored with serial radiographs until fusion is ensured. Nontraumatic activities, including driving, are allowed as soon as the patient is comfortable and no longer receiving narcotic medications.

Results and Complications

Numerous series report excellent stabilization and fusion rates. Magerl and Seeman's initial series[48] reported a 100% fusion rate; Grob et al.[53] reported a 99% success rate in 161 patients; Stillerman and Wilson[54] reported a 95% rate of successful fusion (21 out of 22 patients); and Marcotte et al.[55] had a 100% rate of fusion in 18 patients. Gluf et al.[56] reported successful fusion in 98% of 191 adult patients and had similar results in an additional 78 patients since that publication.

This procedure is particularly beneficial to patients with rheumatoid arthritis, who often present with significant pain and who cannot tolerate a halo vest orthosis well. Fusion in these patients also takes substantially longer, and the patients have a higher nonunion rate with conventional techniques. With internal screw fixation, they are stable and protected and have good pain relief and an optimal environment for bone healing.

The procedure is technically demanding. It requires a good knowledge of nuances in anatomy and thorough preoperative evaluation via high-resolution CT scans, preferably with reconstruction along the screw pathway. Neurologic complications from direct injury have not been reported; however, vertebral artery injuries have occurred, and in one case bilateral vertebral artery injuries resulted in a fatal brainstem infarction.[57] Unilateral injuries have not resulted in neurologic sequelae but have produced arteriovenous fistulae, one of which manifested as a delayed spinal cord compromise from epidural venous engorgement.[51]

Fusion of C1 to C2 restricts head rotation by about 50%. In a normal patient, this leaves a residual motion of ±45 degrees. Younger patients can regain some lost motion, often to a surprising degree, presumably by gaining extra motion at each of the subaxial facet joints. Less limber older patients must learn to compensate by torso rotation, and usually they do so without difficulty. Paradoxically, some patients have improved motion almost immediately after surgery because the pain-provoked cervical muscle spasm subsides. Occasionally, patients complain of occipital numbness. Numbness is presumably the result of C2 nerve root trauma during surgery and usually resolves within 3 to 6 months.

Occipitocervical Fusion

Instability or degeneration of the occiput-C1 joint or basilar invagination may require incorporation of the occiput into an upper cervical fusion. In the past, various plates or rod and plate devices were used to extend the hardware up from the C1-2 screws. The disadvantages with these systems have been resolved by using polyaxial screws at C1-2 (or individually at C1 and C2 if the Harms or Wright techniques are used). A contoured rod from these can be attached to a plate that is secured to the occiput (Fig. 142-19). Besides being easier to apply, the occipital plate can be fixed to the midline bone, which is the thickest and strongest portion of the occiput. A longer graft secured in the same manner as described for C1-2 fusions can be extended to the occiput and apposed to a denuded area to maximize incorporation potential. A small bone screw inserted through the graft into the occiput can enhance this contact.

For calvarial fixation, 4.5-mm to 5.5-mm screws can be used in a bicortical manner. In the midline, 10-mm to 12-mm (or longer) screws may be used, but often only 6-mm to 8-mm screws can be accommodated laterally. Screw depth is determined by a combination of sensation when drilling, using a special drill guide that allows advancing the drill bit in 0.5-mm increments, and probing the hole with a depth gauge. The construct can also be extended subaxially if needed, by using a longer contoured rod connected to lateral mass screws.

Summary

Screw fixation techniques have proven to be safe and extremely effective in the upper cervical spine. This highly mobile area has been difficult to stabilize reliably and effectively using other techniques. Previously used operative and nonoperative techniques have been only partially effective in addressing the problem of instability in this area. In addition, the techniques have often required prolonged rigid external immobilization resulting in prolonged inability to function normally or sacrifice of more normal motion than necessary to gain protection for the neural elements. The two major screw fixation techniques in this region—direct screw fixation of odontoid fractures and C1-2 screw fixation techniques—are extremely important additions to the surgeon's armamentarium. The available data suggest that these techniques are superior to other approaches.

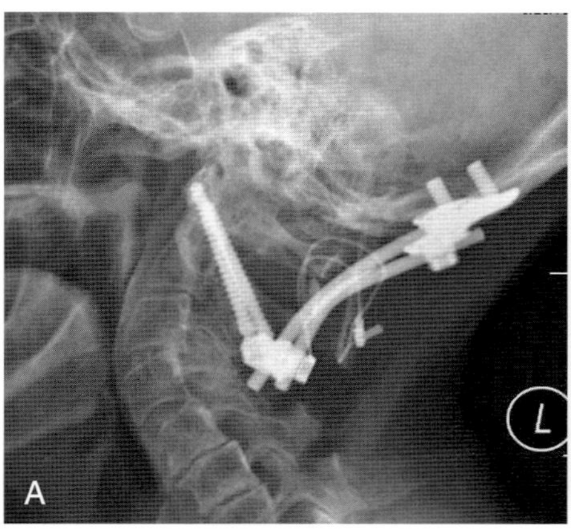

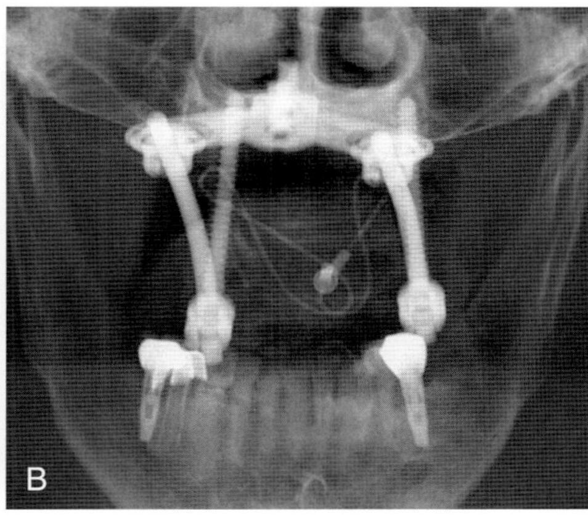

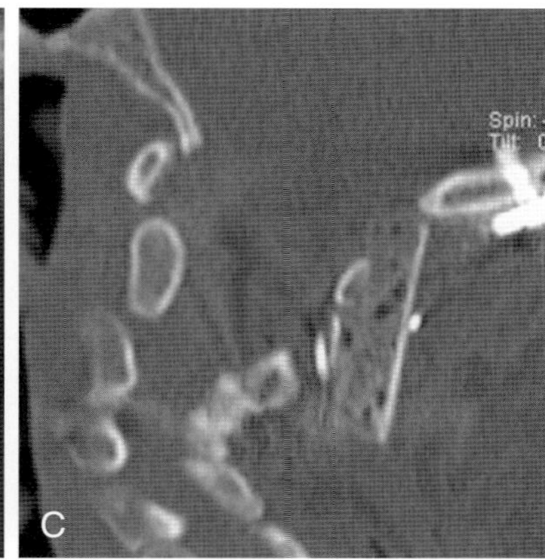

FIGURE 142-19. A, Occipitocervical fusion coupling C1-2 to the occiput with rods from polyaxial C1-2 screws to an occipital plate. **B** and **C,** Structural bicortical iliac crest bone is placed between the rods and held in apposition to the bone with the braided titanium cable.

Acknowledgment. The authors thank Kristin Kraus, MSc, for editorial assistance in preparing this chapter.

KEY REFERENCES

Apfelbaum RI, Lonser RR, Veres R, et al: Direct anterior screw fixation for recent and remote odontoid fractures. *J Neurosurg* 93(suppl 2):227–236, 2000.

Dailey A, Hart D, Finn M, et al: Anterior fixation of odontoid fractures in an aging population. *J Neurosurg Spine* 12:1–8, 2010.

Dickman CA, Sonntag VK, Papadopoulos SM, et al: The interspinous method of posterior atlantoaxial arthrodesis. *J Neurosurg* 74:190–198, 1991.

Gluf WM, Schmidt MH, Apfelbaum RI: Atlantoaxial transarticular screw fixation: a review of surgical indications, fusion rate, complications, and lessons learned in 191 adult patients. *J Neurosurg Spine* 2:155–163, 2005.

Grob D, Jeanneret B, Aebi M, et al: Atlanto-axial fusion with transarticular screw fixation. *J Bone Joint Surg [Br]* 73:972–976, 1991.

Harms J, Melcher RP: Posterior C1-C2 fusion with polyaxial screw and rod fixation. *Spine (Phila Pa 1976)* 26:2467–2471, 2001.

Hillard VH, Fassett DR, Finn MA, et al: Use of allograft bone for posterior C1-2 fusion. *J Neurosurg Spine* 11:396–401, 2009.

Lennarson PJ, Mostafavi H, Traynelis VC, et al: Management of type II dens fractures: a case-control study. *Spine (Phila Pa 1976)* 25:1234–1237, 2000.

Magerl F, Seeman PS: Stable posterior fusion of the atlas and axis by transarticular screw fixation. In Kehr P, Weidner A, editors: *Cervical spine i,* New York, 1987, Springer-Verlag, pp 322–327.

Stillerman CB, Wilson JA: Atlanto-axial stabilization with posterior transarticular screw fixation: technical description and report of 22 cases. *Neurosurgery* 32:948–954, 1993.

REFERENCES

The complete reference list is available online at expertconsult.com.

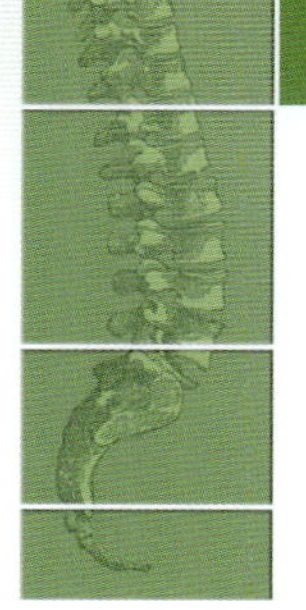

CHAPTER 143

High Cervical and Occipitocervical Plate, Rod, Wire, and Bone Techniques

Noel I. Perin | Nevan G. Baldwin | Paul R. Cooper

Abnormalities at the craniocervical junction were first reported in the early 19th century.[1] The craniocervical junction includes the occiput, atlas, and axis vertebrae. Numerous pathologic conditions can lead to instability at the craniocervical junction. Common mechanisms of injury include trauma, rheumatoid arthritis, inflammatory and infectious lesions, tumors, and congenital anomalies.

The occipitoatlantoaxial joints are complex, both anatomically and kinematically. Anatomically, two synovial joints are found between the condyles of the occiput and the atlas; four synovial joints are found between the atlas and the axis; and there is a synovial joint between the ventral arch of the atlas and the dens, a second between the dens and the transverse ligament, and two at the dorsolateral joints. The opposing surfaces of the dorsolateral joints are convex and facilitate the rotatory movement.

Stability of the occipitoatlantal joint is provided by the cup-shaped configuration of the occipitoatlantal joint and the thick articular capsule, along with the anterior and posterior atlanto-occipital membranes.[2-4] The fibrous capsule of the occipitoatlantal joint is usually thickest laterally and posteriorly and thin if not deficient medially. The tectorial membrane, which is a continuation of the posterior longitudinal ligament, attaches to the ventral foramen magnum and laterally to the medial aspects of the occipitoatlantal joints, playing an important role in the stability of the craniovertebral junction (CVJ).[5] The alar ligaments are paired and arise on either side of the dens and have two components: the atlantoalar and the occipitoalar ligaments. These two components connect the dens to the lateral mass of C1 and to the medial aspect of the ipsilateral occipital condyle, respectively.[6] These ligaments together with the cruciform and apical ligaments span from the axis vertebra to the occiput, and all provide some degree of stability to the occipitoatlantal joint.[7]

The occipitoatlantal joints allow 15 to 20 degrees of flexion-extension and 5 to 10 degrees of lateral bending. Head nodding occurs at the occipitoatlantal joint. The atlantoaxial joint allows 47 to 50 degrees of axial rotation, 15 to 20 degrees of flexion-extension, and 15 to 20 degrees of lateral bending coupled with axial rotation.

Causes of Instability in the Upper Cervical Spine

Instability of the upper cervical spine can be caused by congenital, traumatic, inflammatory, or neoplastic involvement.[8] Of the several congenital abnormalities that occur in the upper cervical spine, basilar impression (or cranial settling) is the most common. Basilar impression may be progressive and lead to cervicomedullary spinal cord compression. Congenital ligamentous laxity in the upper cervical spine (e.g., Down syndrome, Morquio syndrome) can cause instability and subluxation. Upper cervical spine involvement in patients with rheumatoid arthritis can also lead to atlantoaxial instability and cranial settling, both of which may require surgical decompression and stabilization. Trauma, however, is the most common cause of instability in the upper cervical spine. Most upper cervical spine injuries result from blows to the head (e.g., motor vehicle accidents and falls). The direction of the force vector determines the type of injury (i.e., blows to the head versus deceleration of the torso). Injuries of the occipitoatlantal junction are usually fatal and are only detected postmortem. Atlantoaxial instability, on the other hand, can result from disruption of the bony or ligamentous elements or both. Bony fractures often involve the dens. Fractures of the odontoid process of C2 are classified into three types: I, II, and III.[9] Type II odontoid fractures are unstable and notorious for nonunion with conservative management. Published reports of nonunion rates for conservatively managed type II odontoid fractures range from 30% to 60%. Type I fractures are always stable, and type III fractures may be unstable in 10% to 15% of cases.

Craniocervical instability can result from destructive tumors as well as iatrogenically, following resection of such craniocervical tumors. Instability may depend on the extent of condylar destruction or resection in these cases.

Instability at the Craniocervical Junction

Several definitions of instability at the craniocervical junction have been proposed. Craniocervical instability can be vertical or horizontal. Vertical instability or cranial settling usually occurs from a congenital or chronic inflammatory process. Destructive arthropathy of the occipital condyles and the lateral masses of the atlas and axis leads to progressive cranial settling in rheumatoid arthritis. Horizontal (ventrodorsal) instability usually results from acute traumatic situations that cause ligamentous disruption and/or bony disruption. A rotary component may or may not be present.

Common radiologic criteria used to document instability at the craniocervical junction include (1) predental distance greater than 5 mm in a child (<8 years of age) and greater than 3 mm in adults, (2) separation of more than 7 mm of the lateral masses of the atlas on the open mouth view, (3) greater than one third of the rostral dens above the ring of the foramen magnum, and (4) "bare occipital condyles," indicating an occipitoatlantal dislocation.

There is a paucity of reports in the literature regarding resection of the occipital condyle or the destruction of the condyle with tumors of the craniocervical junction causing instability and the necessity for stabilization in this group of patients. The recommendations to date have been to stabilize the occipitocervical junction when greater than 70% of the occipital condyle has been removed.[4,10]

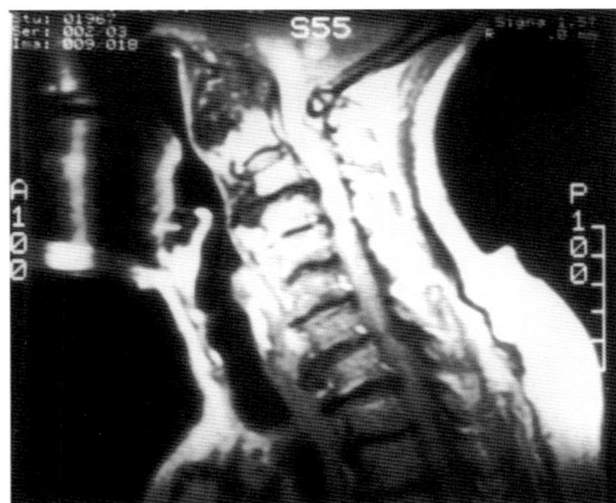

FIGURE 143-1. MRI of the cervical spine in a patient with rheumatoid arthritis showing atlantoaxial instability with pannus formation.

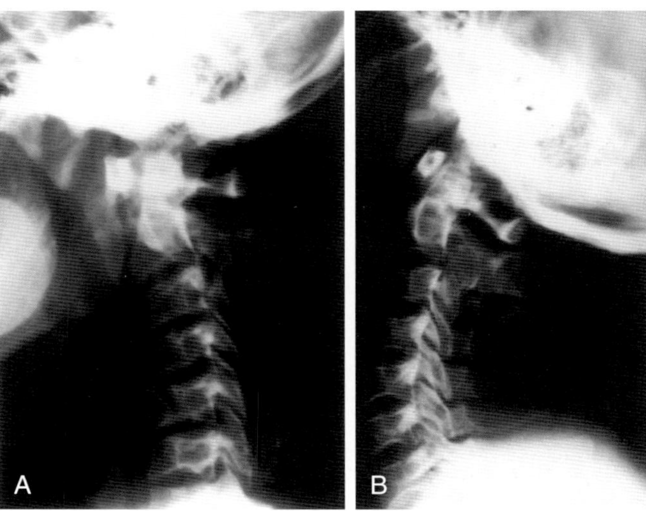

FIGURE 143-2. A, Plain lateral cervical spine radiograph in flexion showing ventrolisthesis of C1 on C2. **B,** Plain lateral cervical spine radiograph in extension showing reduction of the subluxation.

Management of Instability in the Upper Cervical Spine

Patients with instability of the upper cervical spine run the potential risk of fatal injury to the cervical spinal cord. Early recognition, reduction, immobilization, and stabilization are the goals of treatment.

Patients with upper cervical spine instability from congenital causes should be further evaluated for other associated congenital defects (e.g., Chiari malformation, spinal dysraphic lesions, and hydrocephalus). An MRI should be obtained to assess the soft tissue pathology. In addition, CT and plain radiographs (with or without flexion-extension views) should also be obtained when appropriate.

Patients with rheumatoid arthritis should have an MRI to ascertain the presence of inflammatory pannus and/or bony encroachment of the neural elements (Fig. 143-1). Patients who have evidence of neural compromise with occipitocervical instability should be considered for a ventral decompressive procedure before undergoing dorsal stabilization.[11]

Patients with radiologic evidence of subluxation on neutral radiographs should also be evaluated with dynamic, lateral flexion-extension radiographs to assess the reducibility of the subluxation. Patients with nonreduced subluxations should undergo a trial of cervical traction to reduce the dislocation before a decision is made about the appropriate surgical treatment. Patients with chronic instability should remain in traction for 4 to 5 days with muscle relaxation before being considered for surgical treatment. Patients with a reducible subluxation, reduction achieved with flexion-extension, or with axial traction (Fig. 143-2) and without compromise of the cervicomedullary cord, may be safely stabilized by a dorsal approach.[12] In contrast, patients who have a ventral spinal cord compression with a nonreducible subluxation may require a ventral transfacial decompression before undergoing occipitocervical stabilization. Usually, patients with instability related to rheumatoid arthritis or with pannus, but without neurologic deficit, can be stabilized from a dorsal approach without undergoing an initial ventral decompression.[13] The pannus typically resolves in 6 to 12 months after abnormal movement has been eliminated.

Indications for Instrumentation in Occipitoatlantal Instability

The majority of traumatic occipitoatlantal dislocations are fatal. Some patients who arrive in the emergency department are treated effectively in cervical traction followed by occipitocervical instrumentation and fusion. Chronic instability at the occipitoatlantal junction occurs with rheumatoid arthritis, with tumors, and following tumor resection.[14] Chronic instability at the craniocervical junction has been described as "glacial" instability in patients with chronic instability erosion of the occipitoatlantal articulation. This instability may result in cranial settling with associated rotary subluxation. In patients presenting with cranial settling with minimal or no neurologic deficits, reduction with cervical traction may be attempted, and if successful, dorsal occipitocervical instrumentation and fusion can be performed.[15,16] In patients with significant neurologic deficits, a ventral decompression may be necessary before dorsal stabilization and fusion. Patients with rheumatoid arthritis, atlantoaxial subluxation, and associated cranial settling are candidates for occipitocervical instrumentation and fusion.

Patients who have a traumatic atlantoaxial subluxation with fractured dorsal elements of C1 and C2 may also be candidates for an occipitocervical fusion because most of the current techniques require intact dorsal elements of C1 and C2 for stabilization.

The only scientific evidence for the assessment of instability at the craniocervical junction following tumor surgery comes from the biomechanical study by Shin et al.[17] Based on our clinical series, the biomechanical studies available, and new concepts of instability applied to the CVJ,[18] we recommend that occipitocervical stabilization and fusion be performed when 50% or more of one condyle is resected or noted to have been destroyed by the tumor. A strong argument supporting this guideline can be made when using the extreme lateral transcondylar approach[18] for the resection of these tumors. This approach removes the thickest parts of the capsule of the occipitoatlantal joint, and therefore renders the joint unstable (glacial instability). Thus, patients who have the condyle resected for surgical access and patients with tumor destruction of the condyle equal to or greater than 50% (but <70%) who do not undergo stabilization and fusion may progress to a glacial instability and eventually to overt instability with severe neck pain and torticollis.

Occipitocervical Techniques

Several techniques exist for upper cervical spine stabilization, with or without instrumentation. Bony arthrodesis usually is the long-term goal of these techniques. With occipitocervical junction arthrodesis, a bony ridge must be established between the occiput and the upper cervical spine. Techniques may be divided into those that use bone alone and those that use internal fixation with bone.

In 1959, Perry and Nickel described a simple onlay graft for neck fusion for instability after severe poliomyelitis. In 1969, Newman and Sweetnam[19] described the technique for occipitocervical fusion in atlantoaxial instability. Fusion was achieved by decortication and laying down strips of corticocancellous bone obtained from the iliac crest. Patients were kept in cervical traction for 6 weeks and then placed in a high plastic cervical collar until bone fusion was observed.

The combination of internal fixation with onlay bone grafting has reduced the need for postoperative traction and rigid immobilization. Pseudarthrosis rates in a series of 302 occipitocervical fusions and 98 atlantoaxial fusions have been reported to be as low as 1%.[7]

Perioperative Considerations

Patients placed in traction for traumatic instability or those in whom a reduction of cranial settling was attempted are brought to the operating room in their bed with the traction in place. Extension of the neck is usually the position of safety for most patients with upper cervical instability. Thus, oral endotracheal intubation that requires some extension of the neck is usually safe. Patients who achieve reduction when the neck is flexed or in a neutral position are at risk and should be intubated while awake with the aid of the fiberoptic scope, without extension of the neck. After intubation, a firm cervical collar is placed on the patient's neck. Traction on the cervical spine is applied manually by pulling the tongs while turning the patient to the prone position. The patient's head is maintained in a neutral to slightly extended position and supported in a horseshoe headrest or fixed in a three-pin head holder.

Exposure

A midline incision is made from the inion approximately to the C4 spinous process. The length of the exposure varies, depending on the length of subaxial spine to be fused. The suboccipital bone around the foramen magnum and the spinous processes and laminae of C1 to C3 are exposed subperiosteally.

Occipitocervical Fusion

In occipitocervical junction arthrodesis, a bony bridge is established between the occiput and the upper cervical spine. The techniques may be divided into those using bone alone versus internal fixation and bone grafting. A simple onlay graft alone in occipitocervical fusions was used first by Perry and Nickel and later by Newman and Sweetnam.[19] The technique entails decortication and laying down of strips of corticocancellous bone obtained from the iliac crest. The fusion extends from the occipital bone to the atlas and axis. Patients who underwent this procedure were placed postoperatively in a halo vest for 3 to 4 months until bony fusion was noted on radiologic studies. The authors reported good fusion rates; however, the patients in their series were young and healthy.

Occipitocervical Fusion with Internal Fixation

Rigid metallic implants to obtain immediate fixation with generous onlay bone graft have produced successful fusion without the need for postoperative halo-vest immobilization. Techniques with contoured rods, cables, plates, and screws have been described.

Contoured Rod and Cable Fixation

Different smooth and threaded rods have been used for internal fixation in occipitocervical fusions. We use a titanium rod, contoured similar to the "Ransford loop," with cross-linkage at the caudal end to conform to the craniocervical angle, with the patient's head in a neutral position (Fig. 143-3).

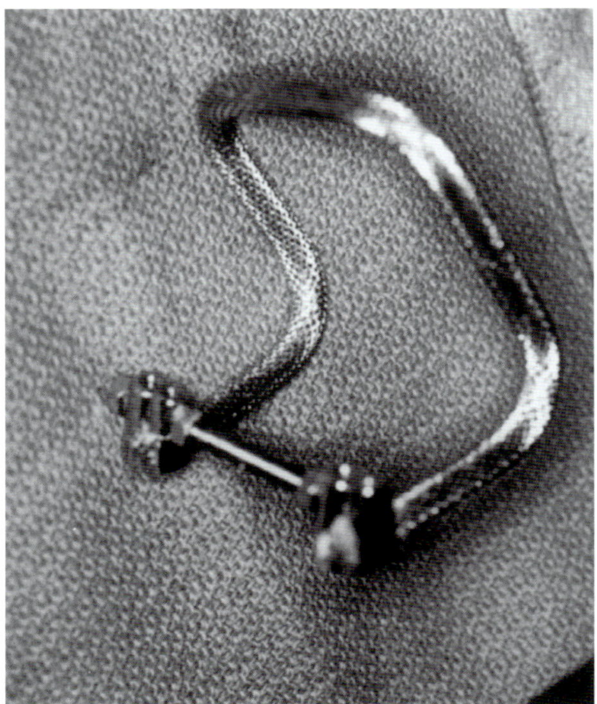

FIGURE 143-3. Contoured 5-mm Cotrel-Dubousset rod with cross-fixation linkage.

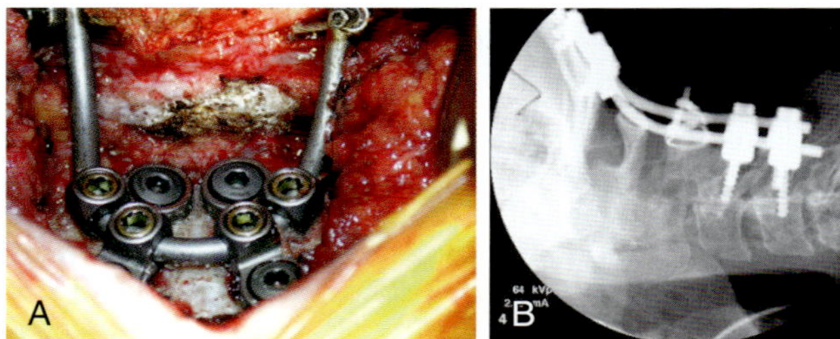

FIGURE 143-4. A case of occipitocervical fusion using a contoured rod, occipital screw fixation, and lateral mass and sublaminar wire fixation is depicted via an intraoperative photograph (**A**) and radiograph (**B**).

More recently, screw systems have become more popular and provide a more rigid fixation. Cortical screws are placed in the occiput close to the midline where the bone is thickest; this is combined with a rod and or plate system at the occiput and lateral mass and C2 pedicle screws (Figs. 143-4A and B).

Lateral cervical spine radiographs are obtained after the patient is positioned prone, as described previously. The head is maintained in a neutral position. The contoured rod is placed on the back of the occiput, and sites for the bur holes are marked on either side of the occipital portion of the contoured rod bilaterally. Four bur holes are thus made in the suboccipital bone—two on either side of the midline—ensuring an adequate bridge of bone between the bur holes.

The posterior fossa dura mater is separated from the inner table of the bridge of bone between the bur holes, and a double cable is passed from one bur hole to the other. This is repeated on the opposite side of the occiput. The use of a double cable on either side of the occiput provides two cables on either side to hold down the rod. Alternatively, a single

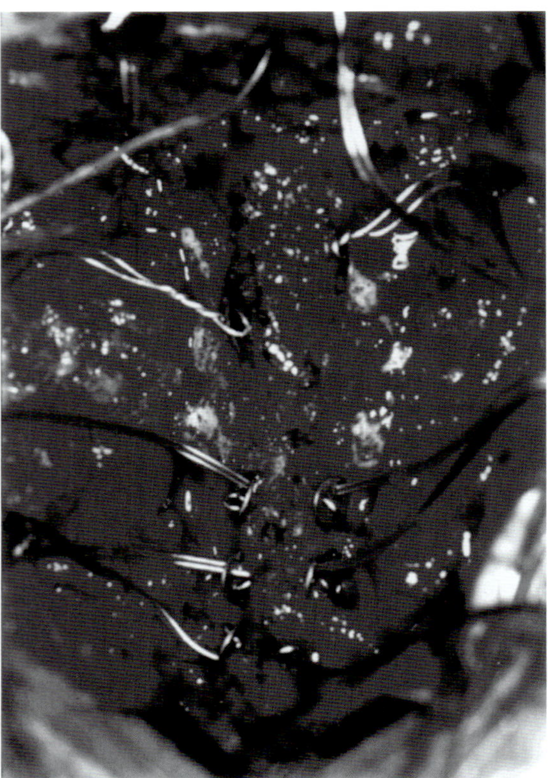

FIGURE 143-5. Operative photograph showing the spinolaminar junction wires in place. Note the use of Wisconsin wires and Drummond buttons.

bur hole on either side of the midline, with the cable passed around the rim of the foramen magnum, can be used.

After cable placement for cranial fixation, sublaminar placement for spinal fixation is achieved by passing a double cable under the dorsal arch of C1 and the lamina of C2. When separated, a single cable is available on either side of the dorsal arch of C1 and C2. At C3 and C4, a hole may be made at the spinolaminar junction using a right-angled drill. Single cables threaded through Drummond buttons are passed from either side of the spinolaminar junction (Fig. 143-5). Alternatively, sublaminar cables can be passed with due care under the subaxial cervical spine. The contoured rod is placed in the bed, and the cables are torqued sequentially. The distal end of the rod may be cross-fixed, just caudal to the C3 or C4 spinous process, to increase the rigidity of the construct (Fig. 143-6). After decortication, bone graft is obtained through a separate incision from the dorsal iliac crest and is laid as an onlay graft of corticocancellous bone. Care must be taken during head positioning before internal fixation and fusion to obtain the best subluxation reduction with optimal head and neck position, compatible with normal function. Care must be taken to avoid dural perforation during wire passage at the suboccipital bur holes and at C1 or C2. Bevelling the edges of the bur holes and meticulous dissection of the dura mater from the inner table should prevent dural laceration. The leader wire of the single cable should be bent back on itself to present a smooth surface during sublaminar passage. Monitoring the bony surfaces carefully during torquing can help prevent overtightening of the cable. Sequential cable tightening with torque not exceeding 4 to 5 inch-pounds with titanium cables

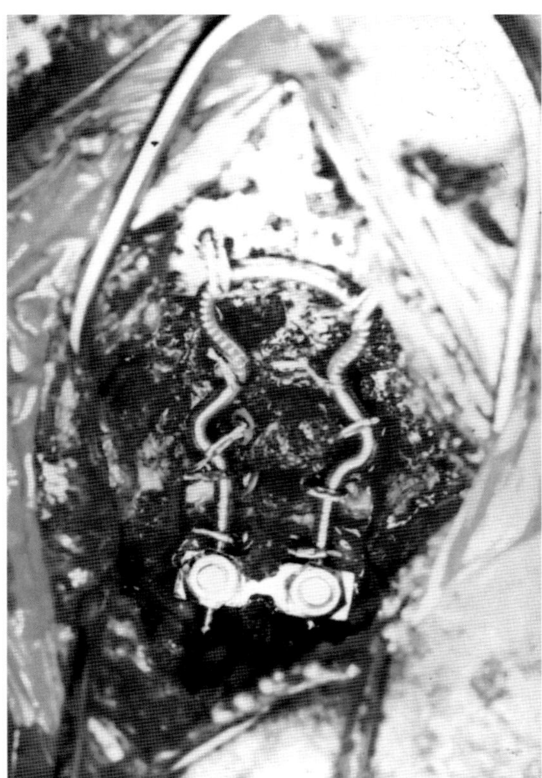

FIGURE 143-6. Intraoperative photograph of a contoured rod with occipital and sublaminar cables for occipitocervical stabilization.

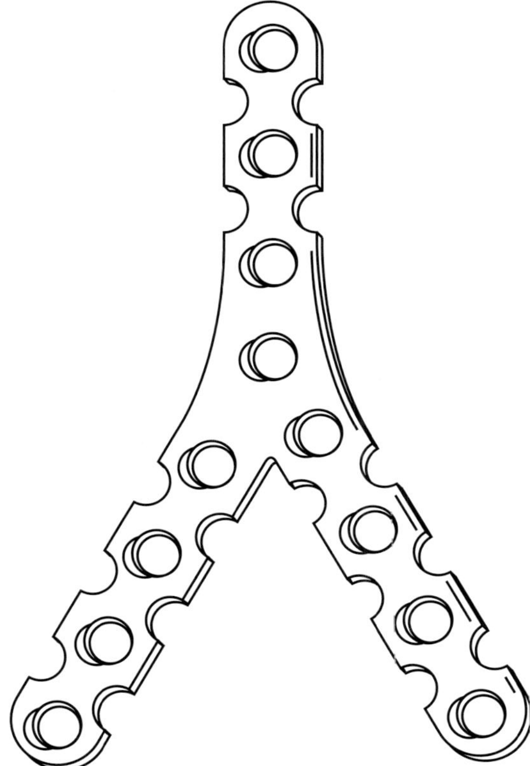

FIGURE 143-7. Illustration of a Y plate.

and 8 inch-pounds with stainless steel cables is appropriate in healthy adults. In patients with soft bones and in those with rheumatoid arthritis, the torque is reduced as appropriate (i.e., when cable begins to cut into the bone).

All patients are treated postoperatively in a Philadelphia collar for 6 to 12 weeks or until radiologic fusion is observed.

Plate Fixation

Plates and screws have been used for occipitocervical fixation; however, their limiting factor is the variable thickness of the occipital bone. Heywood et al.[1] reported that occipital bone thickness measured 9 to 16 mm in the midline and only 3 to 9 mm in the lateral suboccipital bone. No room exists between the dura mater and the cerebellum. Penetration of the inner table could lead to cerebellar injury. Therefore, it is possible that with bicortical purchase during plate fixation, especially laterally in the suboccipital bone, the tip of the screw could perforate the dura mater and the underlying cerebellum.

With the Y-plate system of plate and screws for occipitocervical fusion, the stem of the Y is laid over the midline of the occiput (Fig. 143-7). The occipital screws are 2.7 mm in diameter and 8 to 10 mm long. If subaxial fusion is necessary, transfacet screws are placed in the C1-2 facet joint (Magerl technique) and in the lateral masses of the subaxial spine.

Because of the risk of screws perforating the dura matter and the cerebellum, the use of the Y-plate and the lateral occipitocervical plate (see Fig. 143-4) is limited due to the need to place screws in the lateral suboccipital bone. Occipital plates with screws placed in the midline and connected to rod systems that connect to the screws placed in the C2 pedicle and lateral masses in the lower cervical spine are more rigid biomechanically than the wiring techniques.

Atlantoaxial Fusion

In 1910, Mixter and Osgood described the first atlantoaxial stabilization procedure using internal fixation. Gallie popularized wiring and bone grafting techniques for dorsal atlantoaxial arthrodesis.[20] A loop of wire is passed beneath the dorsal arch of the atlas from caudal to rostral. The loop of wire is then pulled caudally over the spinous process of C2. The free ends of the wire are run downward and around the spinous process of C2 and are twisted together. The dorsal surfaces of C1 and C2 are decorticated, and onlay bone graft from the iliac crest is placed to achieve bony union. This construct provides minimal rotational stability. In 1978, Brooks and Jenkins modified this technique.[10] They described passing two wires on either side, underneath the dorsal arch of C1 and the lamina of C2. Two unicortical wedges of iliac crest bone are placed between C1 and C2. This improves rotational stability. A modification of the Gallie technique described by Papadopoulos et al.[21] uses a bicortical H-graft placed between the dorsal arch of C1 and the spinous process and lamina of C2.

Preoperative evaluation and management for this technique is identical to that described with occipitocervical fusion. In the modified Gallie technique, a loop of cable is passed under the dorsal arch of C1 from caudal to rostral. The caudal edge of the dorsal arch of C1 and the rostral edge of the C2 lamina and spinous process are decorticated. A bicortical graft, notched on its caudal surface to hug the contour of the spinous process and lamina of C2, is placed between C1 and C2. The cancellous surfaces of the graft abut the decorticated areas of C1 and C2. The cable passes as with the Gallie technique. The loop is dorsal to the graft, and the free ends run ventral to the graft. This ensures that the graft does not migrate dorsally or ventrally while providing the necessary rotational stability. Further decortication and onlay bone grafting of the dorsal surfaces of C1 and C2 is carried out. Overtightening of the cable around the graft can lead to graft erosion and loosening. In the presence of dorsal subluxation of the dens, there is a risk of pulling the dens dorsally into the spinal cord during wire tightening. This risk is minimized by using a larger wedge of bone between the dorsal elements of C1 and C2. The tip of the leader wire should be doubled back to present a smooth surface during sublaminar wire passage to prevent dural laceration.

Several techniques have been described for wiring the atlas to the axis vertebra, with varying degrees of success. The disadvantage for patients undergoing wire and cable techniques alone is that in the presence of significant instability they must be placed in a halo body vest postoperatively for 3 to 4 months. The patient should undergo transfacet fixation of C1 to C2 when there is significant instability or fractured or absent dorsal elements of C1 or C2 or when a laminectomy of C1 and C2 is indicated.

Summary

Upper cervical spine stabilization can be achieved using a variety of techniques, depending on the surgical indications. Controversy still abounds regarding the use of occipitocervical fusion versus atlantoaxial fusion in the presence of atlantoaxial instability. Some surgeons continue to perform occipitocervical fusions in patients with instability at the atlantoaxial joint, arguing that the loss of 15 to 20 degrees in flexion-extension by including the occiput in the fusion is negligible. However, the 15 to 20 degrees of movement at the occipitoatlantal joint is responsible for the nodding or chin-tuck movement in the cervical spine, and the loss of this movement may be a cause of significant morbidity. We recommend that occipitocervical fusions be reserved for patients with occipitoatlantal instability or cranial settling with atlantoaxial instability. All other patients with instability at the atlantoaxial articulation alone should undergo the appropriate stabilization technique at C1-2. Rigid internal fixation techniques reduce the need for cumbersome and rigid external orthotics and increase the rate of bone fusion.

Guidelines for occipitocervical stabilization following resection of tumors at the CVJ have been based on anecdotal evidence with very little reported in the literature. Based on our clinical series[21] and the biomechanical studies available, we recommend that occipitocervical stabilization and fusion be performed where 50% or more of one condyle is resected or noted to have been destroyed by the tumor.

KEY REFERENCES

Bohlman HH: Acute fractures and dislocations of the cervical spine: an analysis of three hundred hospitalized patients and review of the literature. *J Bone Joint Surg [Am]* 61:1119–1142, 1979.

Menezes AH: Surgical approaches to the craniocervical junction. In Frymoyer J, editor: *The adult spine*, New York, 2003, Lippincott-Raven, pp 523–551.

Menezes AH, VanGilder JC: Transoral-transpharyngeal approach to the anterior craniocervical junction: 10-year experience with 72 patients. *J Neurosurg* 69:895–903, 1988.

Menezes AH, VanGilder JC: Abnormalities of the craniovertebral junction. In Youmans J, editor: *Neurological surgery*, ed 3, Philadelphia, 1990, WB Saunders, pp 1359–1420.

Menezes AH, VanGilder JC, Graf CJ, McDonnell DE: Craniocervical abnormalities: a comprehensive surgical approach. *J Neurosurg* 53:444–455, 1980.

Shin H, Barrenechea IJ, Lesser J, et al: Occipitocervical infusion after resection of craniovertebral junction tumors. *J Neurosurg Spine* 4:137–144, 2006.

REFERENCES

The complete reference list is available online at expertconsult.com.

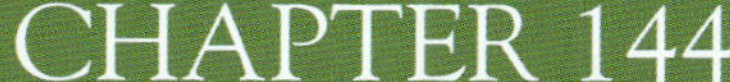

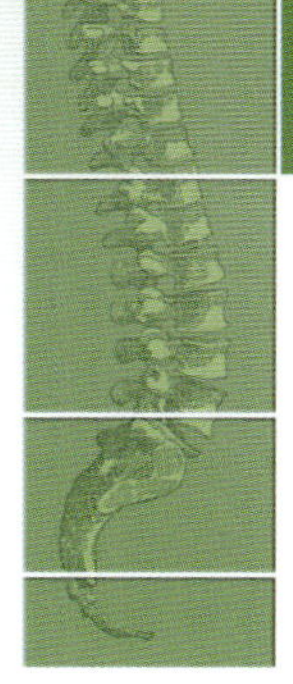

CHAPTER 144

Ventral Subaxial Cervical Fixation Techniques

Kene Ugokwe | Thomas E. Mroz | Gregory R. Trost

Cervical Spine Anatomy

The cervical spine can be subdivided into two regions: the upper (C1 and C2) and the lower (C3-7) cervical regions. The normal cervical spine is lordotic in alignment. The upper cervical spine is unique because of its distinct anatomic arrangements, compared with the rest of the cervical spine. C1 has no centrum, and as such, is a bony ring that allows for the intrusion of the dens of C2 between the lateral masses of C1. The dens articulates with the dorsal aspect of the ventral portion of the ring of C1. The lateral masses of C1 join with the occipital condyles and C2 by kidney-shaped articulations. The C2 vertebra has many attributes of the more caudal cervical vertebra. It also has a rostral extension known as the dens or odontoid process. The pars interarticularis is substantial and projects from the lamina to attach to the lateral mass. The atlanto-occipital joint allows flexion-extension (25 degrees), as well as a minimal degree of lateral flexion (5 degrees) and minimal rotation (5 degrees). The atlantoaxial joint allows 20 degrees of flexion-extension, 5 degrees of lateral bending, and 40 degrees of axial rotation.[1-3] The failure strength of the alar ligament is about 200 N, whereas that of the transverse ligament is 350 N.[4] The vertebrae of the middle and lower cervical spine are relatively uniform. A unique characteristic of this region is its lordotic alignment, which may aid in spinal cord injury prevention because most axial loads are imparted symmetrically to the spine rather than with a significant flexion component. Because the addition of a flexion component to an axial load greatly increases the chance of vertebral body failure and the retropulsion of bone and disc fragments into the spinal canal, the lordotic posture thereby helps to prevent catastrophic injury.

Ventral Instrumentation

Only relatively recently have ventral instrumentation constructs been applied to the cervical region. These constructs are used to treat a variety of abnormalities of the subaxial cervical spine, including degenerative, neoplastic, and infectious processes, and trauma-related injuries. These techniques involve cervical plating systems that are applied to the ventral cervical spine to promote fusion and to maintain graft position and spinal alignment. Caspar developed a semiconstrained (semirigid or dynamic) plate system that uses a bicortical screw purchase in the vertebral body.[5] Johnson et al. subsequently developed a rigid or constrained plate system that uses a screw-plate locking mechanism without bicortical purchase.[6] Several commercial ventral fixation systems are available, but prior to the placement of a single implant, a surgeon should ask these questions: Is a spinal implant indicated? Is a rigid or dynamic implant optimal? Is deformity reduction, correction, or prevention required? Which system is ideal for obtaining fusion and preventing subsidence? These questions are key and require a sound understanding of biomechanical principles as they apply to the cervical spine.

Biomechanics of Ventral Subaxial Spine Constructs

The implant types and biomechanical principles employed in ventral subaxial cervical fixation techniques include ventral distraction, ventral compression (tension band), and ventral cantilever beam fixation.

Ventral Distraction

Ventral distraction results from either the placement of distraction at the time of surgery or from the placement of a neutral construct with the expectation that the construct will bear the axial load and thereby distract the spine by resisting compression. Ventral distraction implants come in two fundamental types: interbody struts and cantilever beams. They both usually use screws in a fixed-moment arm, nonfixed-moment arm, applied-moment arm, or dynamic mode. The interbody struts may be composed of bone, acrylic, or metal implants; the cantilever beams are generally of a screw-plate construct type.

Ventral Compression (Tension Band) Fixation

Unlike ventral distraction techniques, ventral compression techniques do not employ interbody struts that apply compression forces to the spine. In general, it is difficult to use rods to provide significant compression or distraction in the ventral cervical spine as can be easily achieved in the thoracic and lumbar spine. However, with the development of implants such as the DOC VCSS (DePuy Spine, Raynham, MA; discussed later in this chapter), such use has been facilitated. This device allows the application of compression using a cantilevered screw-rod system, thereby enabling preloading of the bone graft and thus increasing bone healing.

Ventral Cantilever Beam Fixation

There are three types of cantilever beam fixation constructs: fixed-, nonfixed-, and applied-moment arm constructs. The fixed- and applied-moment arm constructs provide what has been termed constrained or rigid spinal fixation. The nonfixed-moment arm fixation provides what is termed as semiconstrained, semirigid, or dynamic fixation.

Multilevel Fixation

Multisegmental fixation is not used as extensively in the ventral as in the dorsal spine. Reasons include the often inadequate ventral longitudinal exposure and the relatively weak implant-vertebral body interface. The weak implant-vertebral body interface results from the fact that the vertebral body is primarily composed of cancellous bone. The utilization of bicortical screw purchase has been developed as a strategy to overcome this problem, but it is not without risk. Other problems encountered with multilevel constructs include subsidence—the process by which the interbody graft settles in the spine. This can be avoided when "good carpentry" techniques are employed in the preparation of the end plates and the interbody or strut graft. As previously discussed, a variety of commercial ventral plates are available on the market. These are usually classified as rigid or dynamic plates. It has been observed that dynamic plates load share more than rigid plates, thereby preventing the graft from absorbing most of the load applied to the spine.[7] With multilevel constructs, the caudal end of the construct is the most likely region to fail as a result of screw loosening or hardware failure, because there is a longer moment arm and increased forces at the caudal end of the construct.[8] The incidence of increased failure at the caudal end of a multilevel construct can be decreased by following a few key principles: (1) maximizing screw purchase at the caudal end of the construct, (2) using dynamic fixation, (3) using meticulous bone-grafting techniques, and (4) limiting postoperative spine motion with a rigid collar in the first few months after surgery.

First-Generation Plates

The first-generation plates were termed nonrigid implants. These implants allowed motion at the screw-plate interface. These constructs did not have a fixed-moment arm and had limited fixation at the screw-plate interface, leading to greater exposure of the graft to compressive forces and allowing for a higher chance of fusion. Examples of these plates include the Caspar plate (Aesculap, Center Valley, PA) and the Orozco plating system (Synthes, Paoli, PA). These plates were initially abandoned because they had unrestricted backout properties due to lack of fixation at the screw-plate interface. This leads to a high rate of screw backout and screw breakage. These unrestricted backout plates also required bicortical screw purchase, which is sometimes technically demanding since overpenetration could result in spinal cord injury and underpenetration could result in construct failure and screw pull-out.

Caspar Plate System

This titanium plate is nonconstrained, meaning that the screws are not locked to the plate (Fig. 144-1). The set comes with both unicortical and bicortical screws. The unicortical screws come in a variety of lengths from 10 to 28 mm. Screws have a constant outer diameter of 3.5 mm and an inner diameter of 2.2 mm. The bicortical screws are self-tapping and come in lengths from 14 to 19 mm. The outer diameter is 4 mm, and the inner diameter is 2.2 mm at the tip and 2.7 mm at the head. The screws are made of a titanium alloy with a corundum-blasted surface over a third of the length at the tip.

Techniques for Placing Caspar Ventral Cervical Plates

Prior to plate placement, distracting pins are placed in both the rostral and caudal vertebral bodies. The distracting pins are placed using a mallet and a screwdriver. The length of the plate to be used may be determined by reviewing preoperative imaging, which can be reconfirmed intraoperatively. It is important to place the plate in a manner that avoids the screw holes being placed in soft tissue or in the holes caused by the distracting pins. No screws should be placed within 2 mm of the vertebral end plates. The plate should be placed in the midline and should fit flush with the vertebral bodies. If the plate fits poorly, ventral osteophytes should be drilled off in order to ensure an adequate fit. If the curvature of the

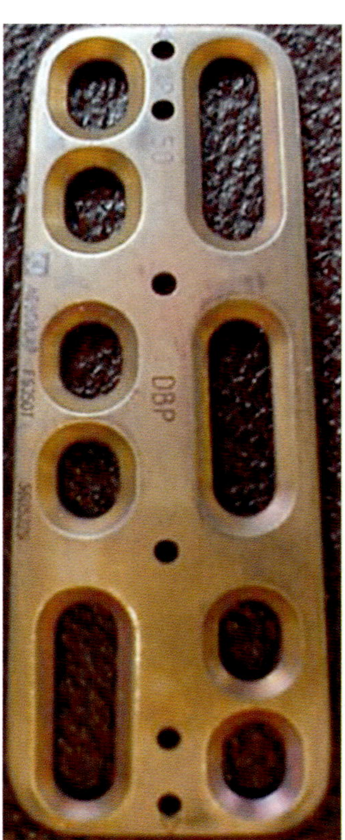

FIGURE 144-1. Caspar plate.

cervical spine does not allow for an adequate fit, the plate may be bent as a last resort. It is important to avoid multiple bends as this may weaken the plate. Next, the distance from the anterior to the posterior marginal line of the vertebral body is determined from the preoperative imaging, and the drill guide is set to 3 mm less than this distance. The plate is held in place with a temporary fixation pin or a plate holder. Next, the drill guide is placed into the screw holes, and the drill is used to drill the vertebral body to the preset length. Next, the screw holes are tapped and the first screw is placed. It is not fully tightened, and the rest of the screws are placed in a diagonal fashion.

Second-Generation Plates

The second-generation plates were rigid implants and have the benefits of providing rigid stabilization, maintenance of alignment, reduced need for postoperative immobilization, earlier return to function, and potentially enhanced fusion rates.[9] These implants were described as restricted and constrained. Their disadvantage is that they may stress shield the bone graft and result in nonunion or implant failure. Stress shielding, as the term implies, occurs when the implant reduces fusion-promoting stresses on the bone graft, thereby leading to a nonunion.

Cervical Spine Locking Plate

The Synthes Cervical Spine Locking Plate (Synthes CSLP, West Chester, PA) was developed and designed as a prelordosed plate. The bushings in plate holes allow for screw angulation and locking and come with a wide variety of screws, including self-drilling and self-tapping, as well as unicortical and bicortical screws. The screws vary in length from 12 to 20 mm (Fig. 144-2).

Techniques for Insertion of Cervical Spine Locking Plate

Once the discectomy is completed, the distraction pins are removed and the holes are sealed with wax. Plate selection is facilitated by using calipers that come in the set. Next, a Kirschner wire (K-wire) is placed approximately 1 cm into the vertebral body, and then the chosen plate is placed over the K-wire. A temporary fixation pin is then placed in the screw hole diagonal to the K-wire. Next, the screws are inserted. The screw holes are placed using a drill guide and drilled at the desired angle. In the upper vertebral body, the screws are angled superiorly and medially. In the lower vertebral body, the screws are angled medially. Once all the screws are serially tightened to engage the bushing, locking screws are then inserted into the permanent fixation screw.

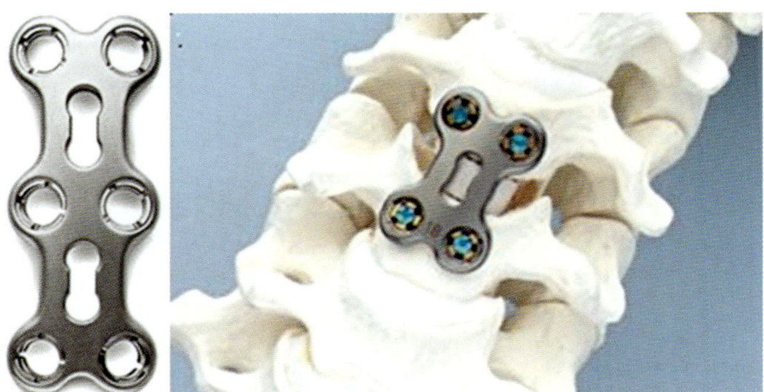

FIGURE 144-2. Synthes Cervical Spine Locking Plate. (Courtesy of Synthes, West Chester, PA).

Orion Anterior Cervical Plate System

The Orion plate (Medtronic, Sofamor-Danek, Memphis, TN) is highly constrained, and the screws are locked into the plate at a fixed angle. The Orion plate has a predetermined lordotic curvature. The fact that the cephalad and caudad screws are locked in place prevents screw migration if the screws break. The plate design also allows for convergent screw placement, thereby reducing the risk of injury to the vertebral artery. The superior screws are directed 15 degrees cephalad and 6 degrees medially, and the inferior screws are placed 15 degrees caudally and 6 degrees medially. Variable-length 4-mm cancellous screws are available ranging from 10 to 26 mm. The plates vary in size from 25 to 90 mm. The Orion plate is made of a titanium alloy with a titanium-anodized (Tiodized) surface coating, which increases the surface's resistance to wear and improves the fatigue life (Fig. 144-3).

Third-Generation Plates

Due to the problem of stress shielding encountered in the second-generation plates, the dynamic plates were again revisited. This improvement in the first-generation plates led to the development of a third generation of plates that improved on the original Caspar plate design by preventing screw back-out while allowing for some movement at the screw-plate interface, thereby enabling load sharing between the bone graft and the implant. These third-generation plates were described as dynamic plates. There are two subsets of dynamic plates: (1) rotational and (2) translational. The rotational dynamic plates allow screws to rotate or toggle at the screw-plate interface and include the Atlantis (Medtronic, Sofamor-Danek), Blackstone (Blackstone Medical, Inc., Springfield, MA), Aline (Surgical Dynamics, Inc., Norwalk, CT)

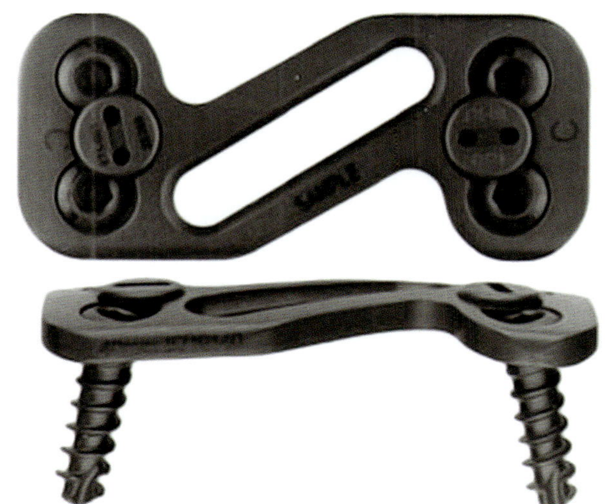

FIGURE 144-3. Orion Cervical Plate. (Courtesy of Medtronic, Sofamor-Danek, Memphis, TN).

Zephir (Medtronic, Sofamor-Danek), Slim-Loc (DePuy Spine, Raynham, MA) Acufix (Austin, TX) and Deltaloc (Alphatec Spine, Carlsbad, CA) plates. Translational dynamic plates allow for axial translation and rotation of the plate and include the Premier (Medtronic, Sofamor-Danek) ABC (Aesulap, Tuttlingen, Germany) and DOC (DePuy Spine) plates. Movement at the screw-plate interface was planned to avoid stress shielding so that, theoretically, fusion rates would increase and time to fusion would diminish.

Atlantis Anterior Cervical Fixation System

The Atlantis cervical plate (Medtronic, Sofamor-Danek, Memphis, TN) is made of titanium and has an integral locking mechanism that helps to reduce screw pull-out. The Atlantis plate was designed with the concepts of load sharing and load bearing in mind. The versatility of this plating system allows for different levels of fixation rigidity achieved by the design of the two types of fixation screws in the system. An Atlantis plate that is secured with fixed-angle screws is a relatively rigid load-bearing construct and is defined as a constrained construct with maximum stability at the graft site. The variable-angle screws, when used with the Atlantis plate, allows for transfer of axial load forces to the graft. Finally, a hybrid construct can be created by using fixed-angle screws at one end of the plate and variable-angle screws at the other end. This creates a semiconstrained construct that provides a moderate degree of fixation rigidity while allowing for some transfer of axial loading to the bone graft. The plates vary in size from 19 to 110 mm (Fig. 144-4).

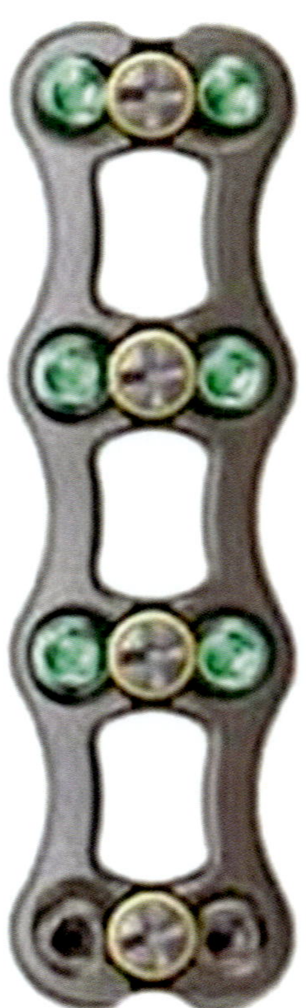

FIGURE 144-4. Atlantis Cervical Plate. (Courtesy of Medtronic, Sofamor-Danek, Memphis, TN).

Insertion Technique for the Atlantis Cervical Plate

The Atlantis plate can be secured with fixed-angle screws, variable-angle screws, or a combination of fixed-angle screws at one end or variable-angle screws at the other end. In placing the fixed-angle screws, the fixed-angle drill guide must be used. Screw holes are drilled using the adjustable drill bit and drill stop. There is also a fixed 13-mm drill bit. The screw holes are tapped, and the fixed-angle screws, which are usually 4.0 or 4.5 mm, are placed. Once all screws are placed, final tightening seats the plate firmly on the anterior vertebral body surface. The steps for the placement of variable-angle screws is the same as that for fixed-angle screws except for the fact that the insertion angle for the variable-angle screws has a range of 22 degrees in the sagittal plane and 17 degrees in the axial plane. If variable-angle screws are to be used, the surgeon has the option of using self-drilling, self-tapping variable-angle screws.

Premier Anterior Cervical Plate

The Premier is a dynamic plate designed by Medtronic that permits axial load sharing via translational movement of the screws at all levels except the most caudal end. The Premier plating system has screws that are either 4.0 mm or 4.5 mm in diameter. The 4-mm screws vary in length from 10 to 20 mm. The 4.5-mm screws come in 13-, 15-, and 17-mm sizes. The plate has fixed holes and slots, which can accept either diameter of screw. The caveat is that the 4.5-mm-diameter screws have less angle variability when placed in the slots. The plate comes in 32 different sizes, ranging from 23 to 110 mm (Fig. 144-5).

SLIM-LOC Anterior Cervical System

In 2002, DePuy Spine released the semiconstrained SLIM-LOC anterior cervical plate. The template for this new plate was the original Codman plate. The changes to the Codman plate that resulted in the development of the SLIM-LOC plate included reducing the plate's thickness to 2.1 mm and increasing the plate-screw bending rigidity by 40%. This was achieved by increasing the inner diameter

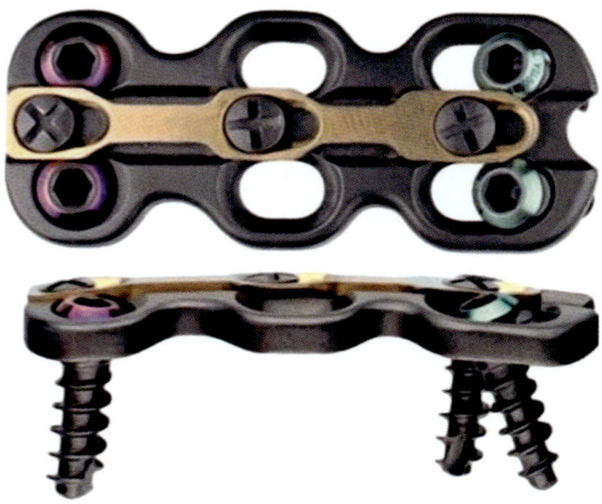

FIGURE 144-5. Premier Anterior Cervical Plate. (Courtesy of Medtronic, Sofamor-Danek, Memphis, TN).

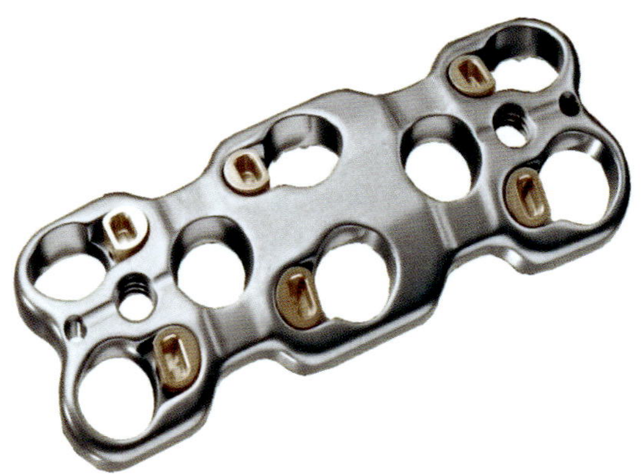

FIGURE 144-6. SLIM-LOC anterior cervical plate. (Courtesy of DePuy Spine, Raynham, MA).

of the screw in the direction of the screw head. The SLIM-LOC plate is a dynamic system that prevents screw backout using the cam-lock mechanism. The SLIM-LOC plate has a precontoured curvature, which is appropriate for the majority of cases. There is also a plate bender in the set if further curvature is required (Fig. 144-6).

Overall, the rationale behind using anterior cervical plates is that it helps maintain the bone graft in place, and it promotes fusion by providing stability between the bone graft and the adjacent vertebrae. It also helps maintain proper cervical alignment. The use of cervical plates has also allowed surgeons to more liberally use allograft since allograft success rates have been shown to equal those of autograft when ventral plating is used.[10]

General Guidelines for Plate Placement

Plate length is usually selected by visual inspection in the field and measurement on preoperative imaging. The plate should be long enough to extend beyond the graft-body junction both rostrally and caudally to avoid placing the plate screws into the graft. It is also important to ensure that the plate is placed at least 5 mm from the adjacent disc spaces that are not being fused in order to decrease the incidence of adjacent level ossification disease (ALOD) as reported by Riew et al.[11] ALOD is described as osteophyte formation and periplate ossification of the adjacent segments. The ventral vertebral bodies may need to have osteophytes drilled off in order to allow the plate to sit flush on the ventral aspect of the vertebral bodies. The plate should also be placed in the midline in order to prevent contact between the plate and vital structures such as the esophagus. If bicortical purchase is required, the dorsoventral vertebral body length should be measured on preoperative imaging and should be checked again in situ after the discectomy has been performed.

Corpectomy

Corpectomy is another method for achieving anterior spinal decompression by resecting part or all of a vertebral body. After completing the soft tissue exposure, the disc spaces above and beyond the vertebral body to be resected are incised, and, once the discectomies are completed, the anterior half of the vertebral body can then be resected with a rongeur. The use of a microscope might be helpful in completing the decompression during the corpectomy. The rest of the vertebral body can be removed using a high-speed drill. A diamond bur may be used when approaching the ventral aspect of the spinal dura. The spine may now be reconstructed using autograft, allograft, or synthetic cages.

Multilevel Anterior Cervical Discectomy and Fusion versus Corpectomy

A single-level anterior cervical discectomy and fusion (ACDF) with a plate is a very successful procedure, but as the number of levels increase, the fusion rates drop compared with those for a single-level operation. Wang et al. have postulated that a single-level corpectomy and strut graft may produce better fusion than two-level adjacent discectomies with multiple grafts.[12]

Bone Graft Options in Ventral Subaxial Cervical Fixation

BAK/C Interbody Fusion System

The BAK/C interbody system (Zimmer Spine, Minneapolis, MN) provides an alternative to either a tricortical structural autograft, which is associated with donor site morbidity, or allograft, which may be associated with a very small risk of disease transmission. The BAK/C is a threaded hollow device that is made of a titanium alloy (Ti-6Al-4V) and as such cannot collapse and is highly resistant to migration. It has a porous design, which allows bone growth through all sides. In comparison to anterior cervical plates, the BAK/C has a zero profile, and if adjacent segments need to be fused, it does not have to be removed. The device comes in five diameters (6, 7, 8, 10, and 12 mm) without factoring in the threads. The threads add an additional 2.5 mm to the outer diameter of the device. The BAK/C device allows for both unilateral and bilateral placement. It is important to note that the best fusion results are obtained when the BAK/C is packed with local bone graft and bone graft extenders (Fig. 144-7). Cauthen et al. described a 97% fusion rate with stand-alone BAK/C. Their study compared fusion rates between stand-alone BAK/C, ACDF without a plate, and ACDF with a plate.[13]

Bengal Carbon Fiber Interbody Cage

The Bengal (DePuy Spine, Raynham, MA) cervical cages are carbon fiber polymer cages that bear the mechanical forces of the spine to promote fusion. The modulus of elasticity of these carbon fiber cages is similar to that of cortical bone. This may help improve load sharing through the graft. The cages should be filled with cancellous autograft, which does not require as extensive a harvesting process as tricortical graft. As a result of the makeup of the interbody cage, it

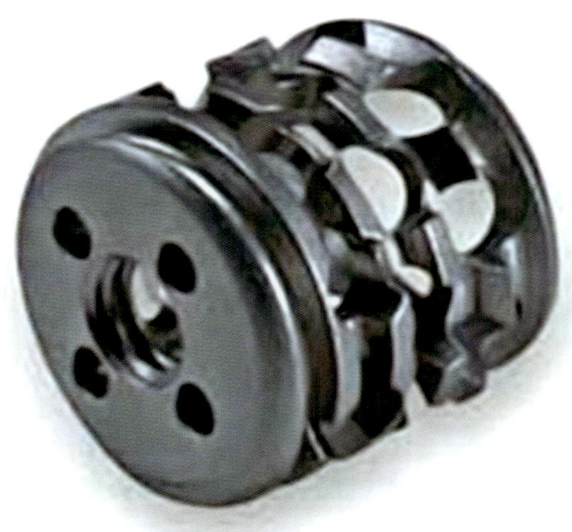

FIGURE 144-7. BAK/C interbody cage. (Courtesy of Zimmer Spine, Minneapolis, MN).

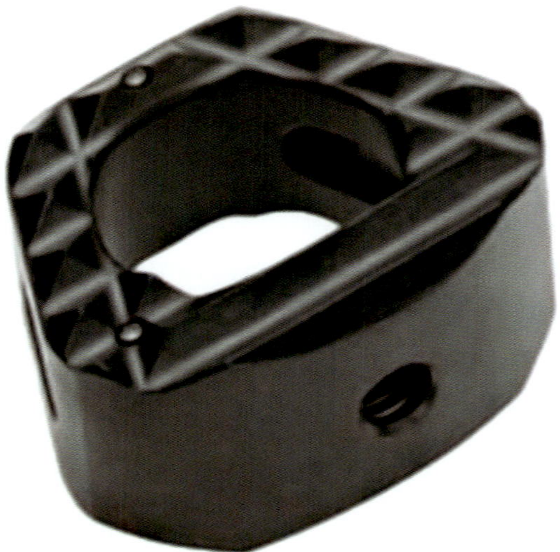

FIGURE 144-8. Bengal carbon fiber cage. (Courtesy of DePuy Spine, Raynham, MA).

is not susceptible to collapse and the inherent height results in indirect neuroforaminal decompression. The carbon fiber cages come in three sizes: standard (12 mm × 14.5 mm), large (14 mm × 17 mm), and extra large (16 mm × 20 mm) (Fig. 144-8).

Polyetheretherketone Spacer

Polyetheretherketone (PEEK) is a polymer with a modulus of elasticity within the range for cancellous bone. The modulus of elasticity is defined as stress divided by strain. The modulus of elasticity of cancellous bone ranges from 0.5 to 5, and the modulus of elasticity of PEEK is 3.7. These PEEK implants do not produce artifacts on plain films, CT, or MRI. The implant is identified on plain radiographs by a titanium wire that is inserted into the wall of the PEEK spacer. PEEK elicits a minimal inflammatory response and has excellent resistance to corrosion. PEEK is insoluble in most solvents and has long-term biocompatibility.[14,15] The use of PEEK spacers reduces graft subsidence that may be seen with titanium cages, and, as such, PEEK cages are a reasonable alternative to allograft for ACDF.[16] The center of the spacer may be filled with local autograft or other bone graft extenders with osteoinductive properties.

Summary

Although this chapter focuses on ventral cervical fixation techniques, it is important to note that the spinal instrumentation does not compensate for poor surgical technique. It is important for a spine surgeon to practice good carpentry technique without leaning too much on instrumentation. Also, the importance of an adequate decompression cannot be overemphasized. It is also important to note that although this chapter focuses on ventral techniques, some situations require supplemental posterior fixation techniques. These include situations in which a surgeon is considering doing an ACDF at four or more levels, corpectomy at three or more levels, significant cervical kyphosis, corpectomy required because of infection, or spinal reconstruction after tumor surgery.

KEY REFERENCES

Dvorak J, Schneider E, Saldinger P, et al: Biomechanics of the craniocervical region: the alar and transverse ligaments. *J Orthop Res* 6:452–461, 1988.

Johnsson H, Cesarini K, Petren-Mallmin M, et al: Locking screw-plate fixation of cervical fractures with and without ancillary posterior plating. *Arch Orthop Trauma Surg* 111:1–12, 1991.

Panjabi M, Dvorak J, Duranceau J, et al: Three dimensional movements of the upper cervical spine. *Spine (Phila Pa 1976)* 13:726–730, 1988.

Panjabi MM, Isomi T, Wand J: Loosening of the screw-vertebra junction in multilevel anterior cervical plate constructs. *Spine (Phila Pa 1976)* 24:2383–2388, 1999.

Tippets RH, Apfelbaum RI: Anterior cervical fusion with Caspar instrumentation system. *Neurosurgery* 22:1008–1013, 1988.

Wang JC, McDonough PW, Endow KK, Delamarter RB: A comparison of fusion rates between single-level cervical corpectomy and two-level discectomy and fusion. *J Spinal Disord* 14(3):222–225, 2001.

White AA, Panjabi MM: *Clinical biomechanics of the spine*, ed 2, Philadelphia, 1990, Lippincott, pp 1–125.

REFERENCES

The complete reference list is available online at expertconsult.com.

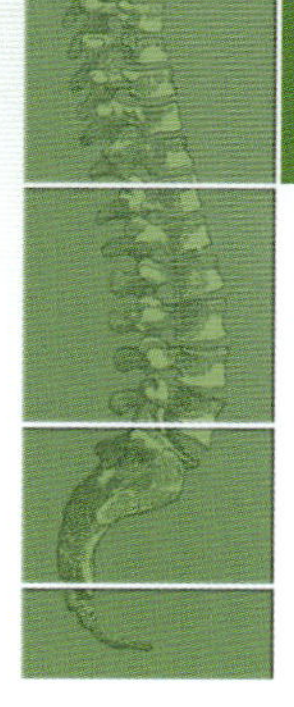

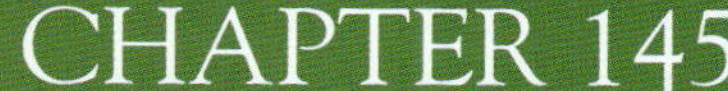

CHAPTER 145

Subsidence and Dynamic Cervical Spine Stabilization

Michael P. Steinmetz | Edward C. Benzel | Ronald I. Apfelbaum

Fundamental Concepts

The term *subsidence* has dual meanings and implications. It can refer to the loss of height that occurs normally with aging as the axial skeleton shortens. It can also refer to the loss of height at an operative site after surgery on the spine.

The loss of vertical height with aging has been observed for centuries. This process, resulting in humans losing height after the achievement of adult status, is multifactorial. It essentially involves the loss of disc height and vertebral body collapse.[1] Both of these processes may involve deformation along the neutral axis (axial deformation), but often deformation around an axis of rotation (angular deformation) is also involved. Both angular and axial deformities result in loss of vertical height. Gravity and repetitive axial loading contribute to the deformation. Angular deformation most often occurs in the sagittal plane, resulting in kyphosis. This kyphosis results in an applied moment arm. As kyphosis progresses, the moment arm is lengthened, and deformity progresses further.[1] This situation is portrayed by the phrase, "kyphosis begets kyphosis." Kyphosis is usually undesirable. In the cervical region, it places the cervical musculature at a biomechanical disadvantage and may lead to mechanical neck pain. It may also accelerate adjacent segment degenerative changes.[2,3] If kyphosis becomes severe, forward gaze and respiration may be adversely affected. Although subsidence occurs in all regions of the spine, subsidence after surgery is most evident in the cervical spine.

Angular and axial subsidence can occur during the normal aging process, and both may also occur after surgery. Postoperative subsidence can be caused by bone graft absorption with remodeling, graft collapse, or pistoning of the graft into the adjacent vertebral levels. Subsidence in these situations should be considered iatrogenic. Each of these mechanisms must be addressed.

Graft Resorption and Remodeling

Graft resorption and remodeling is a normal but complex biologic process. Bone healing occurs by a series of sequential steps that involve an inflammatory phase, with the arrival of inflammatory cells and bone progenitor cells accompanying vascular ingrowth into the graft. This phase is followed by a repair phase in which osteoclasts begin to absorb the graft, while osteoblasts lay down osteoid, and mineralization of the osteoid follows. This repair phase begins the process of new bone formation. The process continues into the remodeling phase as the bone is remodeled into new living mature bone, and necrotic bone is removed by creeping substitution.

Various humoral factors, proteins, growth factors, and mechanical forces mediate this process. Humoral factors include parathyroid hormone, vitamin D, and calcitonin. Proteins and growth factors include a large array of substances such as multiple bone morphogenetic proteins, insulin-like growth factor, transforming growth factor, platelet-derived growth factor, fibroblast growth factor, and nectins.

Mechanical forces are also crucial in this process. As defined by Wolff's law, bone remodeling (and bone strength) is determined by the load placed on it. This structural adaptation results in bone being formed where stresses engendered by compressive loading or tensile forces occur, and bone is reabsorbed where the stresses do not occur. Bone or bone graft placed in compression is exposed to "bone healing"–enhancing forces as defined by Wolff's law.

As a result of all of the aforementioned processes, bone grafts first partially resorb before being replaced by new living bone. The process results in subsidence of the bone graft after surgery. This subsidence is part of the normal biology of bone healing and not a pathologic process. It often is not appreciated in noninstrumented constructs. However, in studies that specifically measure construct height, subsidence is routinely observed.[4-6] The amount of subsidence varies with the type of graft used and number of levels fused. Bishop et al.[4] showed that in uninstrumented ventral cervical discectomies that used iliac crest autograft, the average settling was 1.4 mm for a single-level construct and 1.8 mm for two-level procedures. The amount of settling increased to 2.4 mm for single levels and 3.0 mm for two levels when iliac crest allograft was used.

Graft Collapse

A cervical interbody graft can collapse before its incorporation, also resulting in subsidence. Graft collapse occurs for numerous reasons. If the graft is inadequately sized to handle the loads placed on it, it may collapse. Collapse can occur if the graft is too narrow in width or depth with respect to the adjacent vertebrae. This size mismatch increases the load placed on a graft. A larger graft spreads the load over a larger area, reducing the load per unit of surface area, and the graft may be able to withstand axial loads more effectively. Finally, if there is a good match between the contours of the surface of the vertebrae and the graft (so-called gapless fusion), the weight-bearing forces are evenly distributed over the region of contact, diminishing the chance of graft collapse.

The choice of graft material is also important. The "gold standard" is bone because living structural bone can respond to stresses placed on it and strengthen itself via the aforementioned process and repair itself as needed. Synthetics and allograft bone do not have these properties. Allograft bone preparations are not equal. The techniques of bone handling and processing can affect the structural integrity and strength of bone and its suitability as a grafting material.

Allogeneic bone used for spine surgery must be sterile. The bone can be sterilely harvested. If sterility is maintained, it may not require further processing. If it is not culture negative or is not sterilely harvested and processed, it may be sterilized with gamma irradiation. Low-dose radiation (<1.5–2 megarads) has been shown to diminish graft strength nonsignificantly. However, high-dose radiation (≤4–5 megarads) used by some laboratories causes significant weakening of the bone. Such grafts have a high collapse rate and should be avoided.

The type of bone—cortical or cancellous—is also important. Cortical bone is significantly stronger than cancellous bone, but its density resists vascular ingrowth and the influx of osteoblasts. It is slower to become living bone via true incorporation. It is neither osteoinductive nor osteogenic. As such, osteoclastic activity predominates; this results in progressive weakening of grafts that are primarily of cortical consistency. Cortical bone provides significant early structural support compared with cancellous bone. Because of the aforementioned properties, true bony incorporation is slow, and the weakening of the graft may result in graft collapse or failure before the acquisition of solid fusion. Pseudarthrosis may also result.

Cancellous bone lacks the strength of cortical bone and alone is likely inadequate to support clinical loads. However, cancellous bone has many favorable properties, including significant osteoconductive activity and some osteoinductive capacity. Vascular ingrowth into its loose architecture readily occurs. Cancellous bone incorporates early and more completely. Instrumentation may be used to provide structural support until the cancellous bone fully incorporates and a solid arthrodesis is attained.

An optimal bone graft is one that has the structural integrity of cortical bone and the osteoconductive and osteoinductive properties of cancellous bone. The iliac crest has long been used as a graft source for cervical spine surgery and has both characteristics of an ideal bone graft. It seems to be an excellent choice because it contains a cortical shell that provides structural support and a cancellous core that incorporates quickly. If its size is chosen well, the axial load is shared by the cortical shells of the vertebrae by passing the load onto the cortical walls of the graft. Pistoning into the adjacent vertebrae can be minimized (see subsequent section).

Pistoning (Subsidence)

Pistoning refers to failure of the end plate of the vertebrae with impaction of the graft into the vertebral body above or below the graft. Factors that influence pistoning include graft density, graft/donor size mismatches, and donor site preparation. The density of the bone graft should be ideally matched to the vertebrae. Predominantly cortical implants such as fibula result in a significant graft-to-host density mismatch. Fibula (predominantly cortical graft) placed in an osteoporotic spine results in a significant graft/host density mismatch. This mismatch may result in pistoning of the graft into the vertebra if the stresses placed on the end plates exceed their load tolerance.

The weight or load on the graft is the same whether a small or a large graft is used. Greater forces per unit area of contact are applied to a small bone graft because the forces cannot be dispersed over a larger surface area. This load/surface area mismatch can result in end-plate failure and pistoning. With a larger graft, the load is dispersed over a large surface area, reducing the chance of graft collapse or pistoning. End-plate preparation can also influence this mismatch. Various types of end-plate preparation and various techniques for graft fitting have been described. The goals of end-plate preparation must include removal of the cartilaginous end plate to allow bone graft incorporation and the shaping of the end plate to maximize contact with the graft. Beyond these two considerations, considerable variation in techniques exists.

Some surgeons have attempted to devise methods of interlocking the grafts and vertebrae when fixation is not used. Other surgeons advocate mortising the graft into the vertebrae, that is, countersinking the graft into the cancellous region of the vertebrae beyond the end plates. This approach minimizes the chance of graft migration or expulsion but at the expense of increasing the chance of subsidence. Other surgeons perforate the end plate in various patterns to encourage vascular ingrowth. However, extensive violation of the end plate, especially when used with dense cortical bone, is likely to increase pistoning. Lim et al.[7] showed that it is important to preserve as much end plate as possible to prevent graft subsidence into the vertebral body. They found that making one central hole to increase vascular access to the graft rather than multiple smaller holes reduced stresses on the end plate.

Cervical Plating and Evolution of Dynamic Fixation

First-Generation Systems

The need to augment cervical spine stability after spine surgery, trauma, or other destructive pathologic processes led to the development of ventral cervical plating systems. The first generation of these devices included Orozco plates (Synthes, West Chester, PA), which were used primarily in Europe, and Caspar plates (Aesculap, Tuttlingen, Germany), which achieved significant acceptance worldwide. It became evident that such devices offered advantages to cervical spine surgeons and patients.

The use of such plates helps preserve or restore lordosis, reduces graft extrusion, and improves graft union rates. This use also facilitates the performance of more extensive procedures when indicated by the disease process.[8-13] Ventral cervical plating allows the surgeon to use allograft more liberally instead of autograft. Allograft success rates have been shown to equal success rates of autograft when ventral plating was used.[14] Use of allograft helped avoid donor site complications, which can be a significant source of patient morbidity (i.e., pain at the graft harvest site).

The initial ventral cervical implants were not perfect, and implant-related complications were observed. The initial Caspar plating system used parallel slots for the screws, which were not locked or constrained to the plate. This was a truly axially dynamic implant. The implant required bicortical screw placement for optimal stability. Despite bicortical placement, screw backout was observed sometimes. The dynamic nature of the implant permitted axial subsidence. However, this subsidence was not recognized at the time as part of the normal biology of bone healing (as already discussed) and was thought to be undesirable. The plate was modified so that holes replaced one half of the slots (Fig. 145-1). Rather than preventing subsidence, this modification led to screw breakage. The screw breakage virtually always involved the screws placed in the holes, which were subjected to excessive bending moments (Fig. 145-2). Fixed in the cortex dorsally and the hole in the plate ventrally, the screws typically fractured in the middle at the point of both the maximum bending moment application and the maximum stress application (stress = bending moment/strength). The screws placed into the slots were able to toggle or slide along the slots and did not fracture.

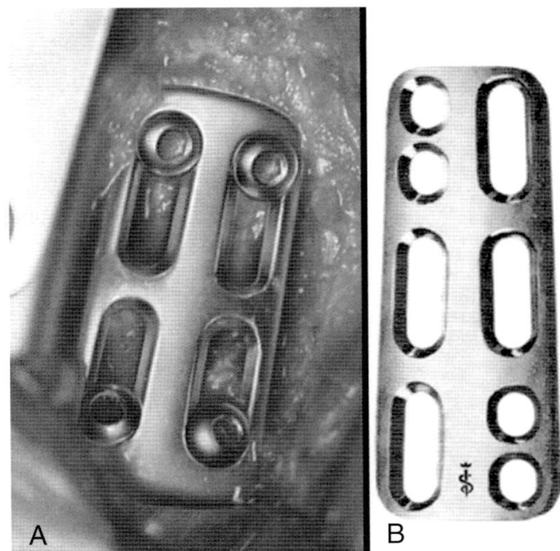

FIGURE 145-1. Original Caspar plate (Aesculap) with bilateral slots (**A**), which was modified to have slots alternating with screw holes (**B**) after settling was observed and thought to be undesirable.

Second-Generation Systems

In an attempt to prevent the aforementioned complications (presumed pathologic settling, screw backout, and screw fracture) and to avoid the need for bicortical screw purchase, a second generation of cervical fixation systems emerged. These devices featured screws fixed to the implant and permitted screw convergence on placement. The cervical spine locking plate (CSLP) from Synthes was the first such device. The ability to "toe-in" the screws secured the plate in part by triangulation and acted to reduce the chance of screw pull-out (Fig. 145-3). These devices were initially successful, but failures caused by plate or screw fracture, construct pull-out, and delayed union or nonunion were increasingly recognized. Attempts were made to remedy this situation by increasing the strength of the plate; examples are the Orion plate from Sofamor-Danek and the Codman plate (Fig. 145-4). These more rigid implants reduced hardware fracturing but may have increased the incidence of delayed union and pseudarthrosis caused by stress shielding (see later discussion).

Despite their shortcomings, second-generation plating systems have achieved better results than noninstrumented fusions, and they have become quite popular. Multiple variations on this basic theme have been developed as other manufacturers entered the market. Despite the popularity and ease of use of these systems, failures continued to occur. At the time (early 1990s), the spine community did not fully appreciate the reason for these nonunions and failures.

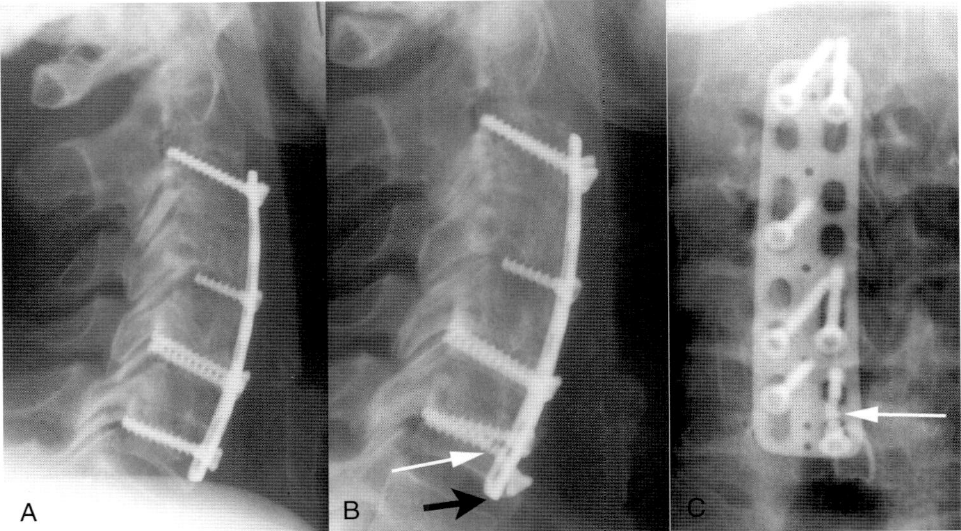

FIGURE 145-2. Caspar plate as initially placed (**A**) and with settling (**B** and **C**). Solid fusion occurred, but the screw in the holes (*white arrows*) fractured as settling occurred, as indicated by the plate overlapping the interspace (*black arrow*).

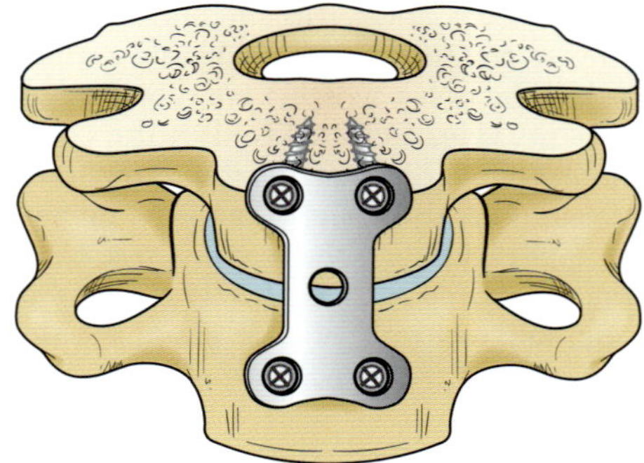

FIGURE 145-3. CSLP (Synthes). Triangulation of the locked unicortical screws was used to increase pull-out strength.

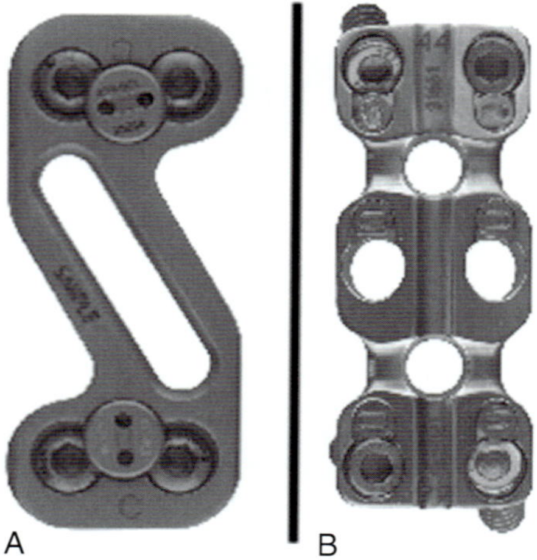

FIGURE 145-4. Orion plate (Sofamor-Danek) (**A**) and Codman plate (**B**) were made stronger to try to reduce hardware failures.

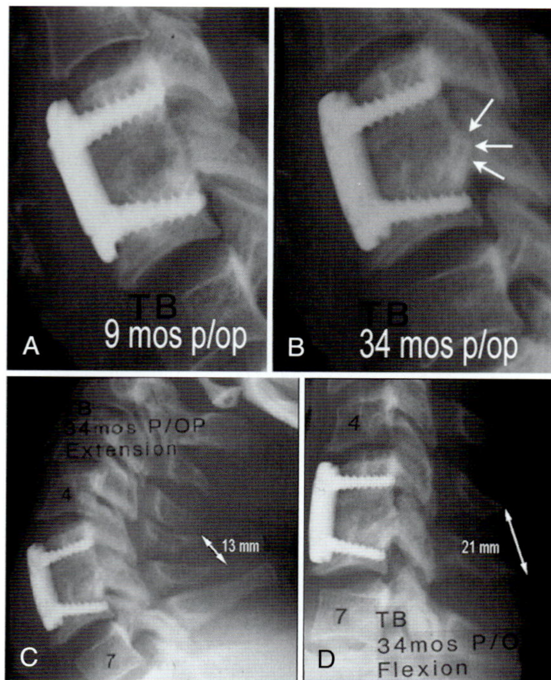

FIGURE 145-5. This patient appeared to have a solid fusion (**A**) at 9 months after an ACD/F with an Orion (Sofamor-Danek) plate. At 34 months (**B**), the growing osteophytes (*arrows*) indicate otherwise, and nonunion is confirmed by the motion between the spinous processes of the involved vertebrae comparing (**C**) and extension (**D**). This figure illustrates a late nonunion that could have been easily missed.

Because these were often late sequelae, many were not likely recognized or at least were underreported. Figure 145-5 illustrates such a case. This patient developed neck pain 3 years after an apparently successful fusion (see Fig. 145-5A). The growth of new osteophytes (shown by arrows on Fig. 145-5B) was the major clue that a nonunion was present. This nonunion was confirmed with flexion-extension films (see Figs. 145-5C and D), which showed 8 mm of motion at the tips of the spinous processes. No motion should have been present if a solid fusion was present.

It seemed that rigid implants were working against the biology of bone healing by stress shielding the graft, at least in some cases. Rather than becoming progressively stronger through bony fusion, these stress-shielded grafts either failed to incorporate fully or did so with suboptimal strength or with failure of fusion.

Third-Generation Systems

History and Rationale

Benzel et al.[15] focused attention on the problem of stress shielding. They used this knowledge to develop the first axially dynamic cervical implant. Although relatively new to the cervical spine (remember the slotted Caspar plates), the concept of dynamism has been used in other applications, in particular, orthopaedic surgery procedures involving the hip and long bones. Dynamic hip arthroplasties have been used for femoral neck fractures with significant success. This construct permits the femoral neck to deform along its axis so that the opposing fracture margins are exposed to optimal bone healing–enhancing forces. A meta-analysis of 2855 patients showed reductions in cutout (4% vs. 13%), nonunion (0.5% vs. 2%), breakage (0.7% vs. 14%), and reoperation (4% vs. 10%) when dynamic hip pinning was used.[16] The Weiss-spring, as modified by Larson, is also a dynamic implant with a spine application. When this implant is combined with interbody fusion in the thoracic or lumbar spine, subsidence is encouraged, and bone healing–enhancing forces are increased; this increases fusion success.[17]

Understanding the implications of Wolff's law, as applied to bone healing and specifically ventral cervical bone grafting, is crucial to understanding the rationale for and value of dynamic cervical spine stabilization. Wolff's law essentially states that every change in the function of a bone is followed by definite changes in its internal architecture and secondary alterations in its external configuration. The implication is that bone is formed where stresses require its presence and is resorbed where stresses do not require it. The load "seen" by a bone to some extent determines its shape and strength. In long bone fracture fixation with rigid plates, if the plate is not removed after initial healing, late fracture or pseudarthrosis may occur. If the plate is removed after the initial healing process has occurred, the bone is able to "see" normal weight-bearing forces with resultant maximal healing occurring. Cases of successful fusion after rigid cervical implant fracture provide a further illustration. Fracture of the plate permitted the bone grafts to "see" bone healing forces and encouraged fusion. If the plate had not fractured, a pseudarthrosis may have developed. This phenomenon has been referred to as *secondary dynamism by plate fracture* (Fig. 145-6).

This logical scenario described by Wolff's law follows the rules of evolution: "ontogeny recapitulates phylogeny." A quadruped requires, and has, larger and stronger forelimb bones than a biped. If bone growth were excessive or unchecked after fracture or grafting, exuberant overgrowth would occur that could compromise vital structures such as the contents of the spinal canal. Hence the wisdom of a system in which bone growth responds to the stresses placed on it, while regions of the fracture or graft that do not contribute to the stress sharing and load bearing are absorbed.

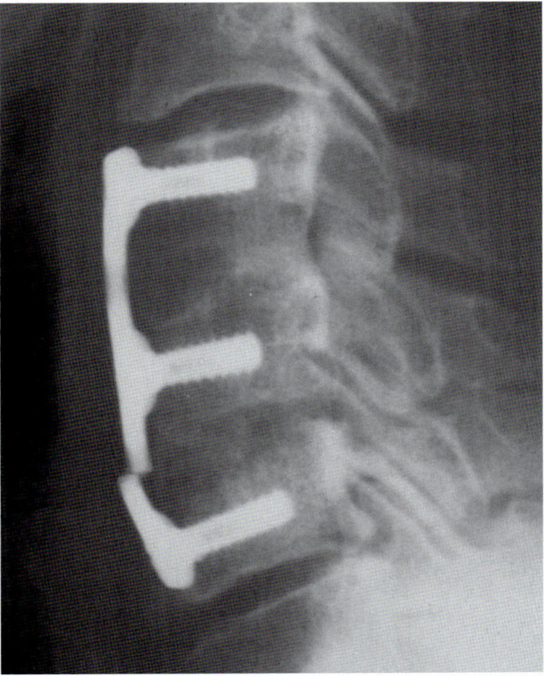

FIGURE 145-6. This plate fractured, and the pieces overlapped, allowing the graft to be loaded again and the dynamism principle to be applied again. This patient went on to solid fusion.

During the evolution of cervical fixation systems, it was recognized that a single fixed screw plate angle was not optimal for all patients. Variable screw angle designs were introduced. Some second-generation systems had the screw locked to the plate to prevent backout but did not lock the screw angulation when implanted, and this angle could change (i.e., toggle). Such designs theoretically could allow some settling as the graft absorbs or subsides. For this settling to occur, however, the screw must migrate or cut through the ventral cortex or toggle within the vertebrae (Fig. 145-7). That this activity can occur is clear; however, it is a slow process. This situation is in contrast to the early subsidence seen with true axially dynamic implants (see later disucssion). In some cases, the density of the vertebrae may prevent such screw migration, and screw fracture can occur (Fig. 145-8). In addition, such screw migration has the potential of weakening the screw-bone interface and may lead to implant failure by pull-out. In the series by Epstein,[18] failure occurred with a variable angled screw plate in 16% of cases.

System

The third-generation ventral cervical fixation systems, which provided true axial dynamic stabilization, were pioneered by Benzel and Yuan with the introduction of the DOC VCSS system from DePuy AcroMed (Raynham, MA). This plating system was developed after it was perceived that there was a need for a system that would enhance fusion rates, decrease deformity progression, improve deformity correction, and decrease the chance of construct failure. The observation that rigid plates could fracture in patients who were subsequently observed to have a solid arthrodesis provided some additional impetus for the development of an axially dynamic cervical implant. If the plate had not fractured, a pseudarthrosis may have resulted. These observations led researchers such as Benzel and Yuan to believe that implants that permitted subsidence may be superior for the attainment of cervical fusion.

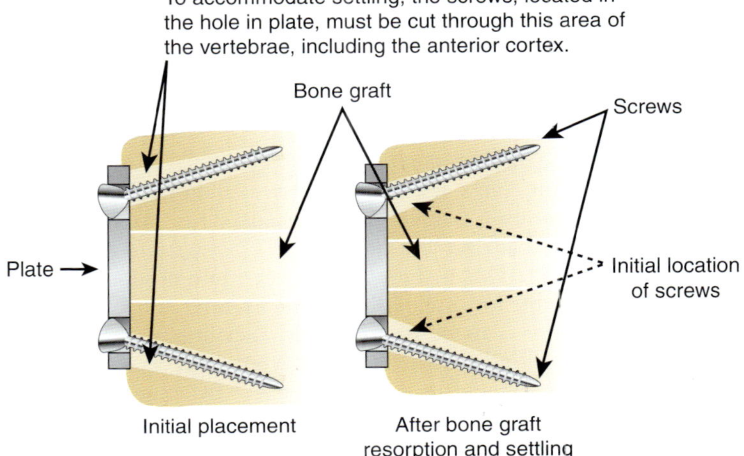
To accommodate settling, the screws, located in the hole in plate, must be cut through this area of the vertebrae, including the anterior cortex.
Bone graft
Screws
Plate
Initial location of screws
Initial placement
After bone graft resorption and settling

FIGURE 145-7. Diagram illustrating what occurs at the bone-screw interface to accommodate toggling of the screws. To change their angle to allow for graft settling, the screws must cut through the vertebrae as illustrated.

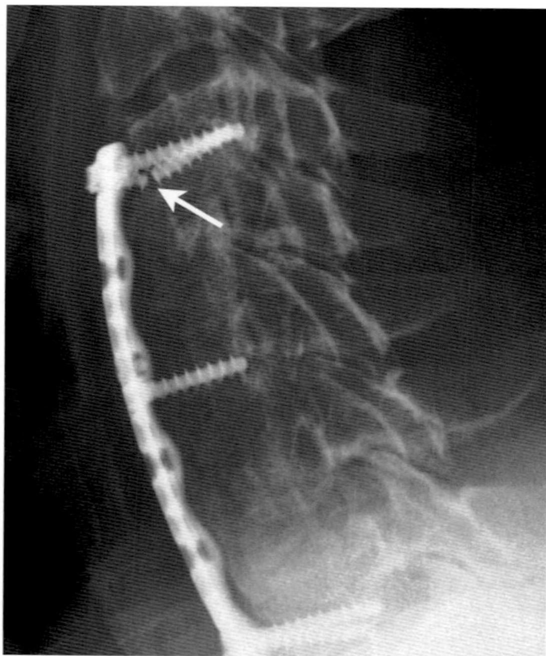

FIGURE 145-8. As subsidence occurs, screws may fracture (*arrow*) instead of toggling if the bone is strong enough to resist cut through, as this case illustrates.

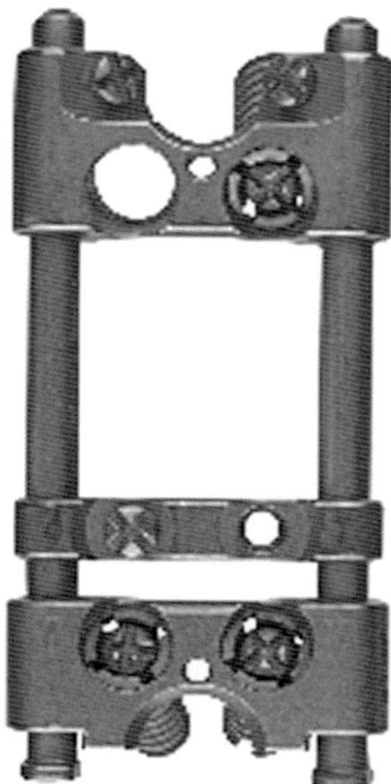

FIGURE 145-9. DOC VSS plate (DePuy AcroMed). The superior platform slides along the rods to achieve dynamism. The screws are locked to the platforms.

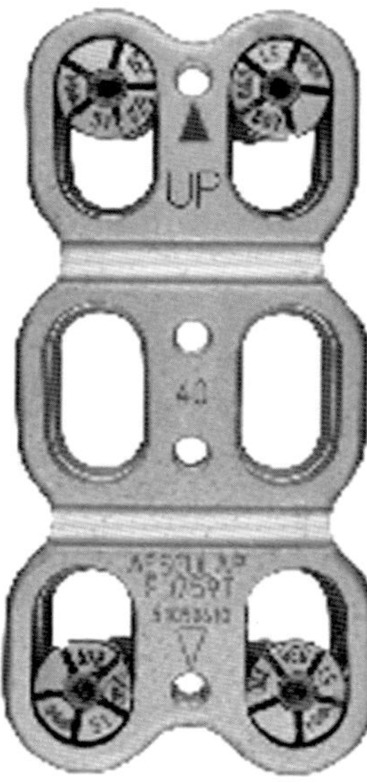

FIGURE 145-10. ABC plate (Aesculap). The screws are locked to the plate by a unique internal mechanism that prevents backout, but they are free to slide in the slots and toggle, achieving dynamism.

At the time of this writing, multiple axially dynamic ventral cervical plates are commercially available in the United States. The DOC VCSS (Depuy-Acromed), ABC plate (Aesculap), Premier plate (Sofamor-Danek), and C-Tek plate (Interpore Cross) were the early pioneers in this design. These systems differ regarding the method of implementation of the principle of dynamic spine stabilization and in their geometric and ergonomic design. The DOC plate is currently not commercially available but is discussed from a historical standpoint.

The DOC VCSS system consists of platforms that are rigidly affixed to the vertebral bodies via screws. Toggling the screws in the vertebral body is not permitted. The platforms slide along two rods, whereas a cross-fixator rigidly affixed to the rods limits the amount of sliding and the amount of subsidence permitted (Fig. 145-9). In this manner, axial deformation (subsidence) is controlled. The manufacturer sets this cross-fixator at 3 mm, but the surgeon may adjust it if deemed necessary. This system is not applicable to single-level constructs.

The ABC system (Aesculap Instrument Corp., Center Valley, PA) permits load sharing by allowing unrestricted subsidence. The plate has slots bilaterally at each level (Fig. 145-10). The screws are locked to the plate by a unique internal locking mechanism, which prevents backout but does not restrict either settling or screw rotation. This is the first implant with this unique design. It is available for single-level and multiple-level constructs. No attempt is made to limit the amount of subsidence, which occurs initially by the screws sliding in their respective slots. If more dynamism is required, screw angulation can occur. This situation is rarely seen. With true load sharing, early and more substantial graft incorporation and maturation is observed so that despite the absence of settling restriction, the extent of settling is not excessive, and often the full amount allowed by the slot does not occur. This situation has also been observed with the DOC VCSS system. Even with multiple-level discectomies, less than 3 mm of subsidence is the norm.

The Premier and C-Tek plates have similar slotted designs to allow settling, with a retaining band over the screw heads to prevent backout (Fig. 145-11). They differ functionally from the ABC plate in that they do not have a slot in the inferiormost (caudal) position but instead have a hole. It is unclear whether this restriction of caudal dynamism has a significant effect on outcomes, and no clinical series are yet available to answer such questions.

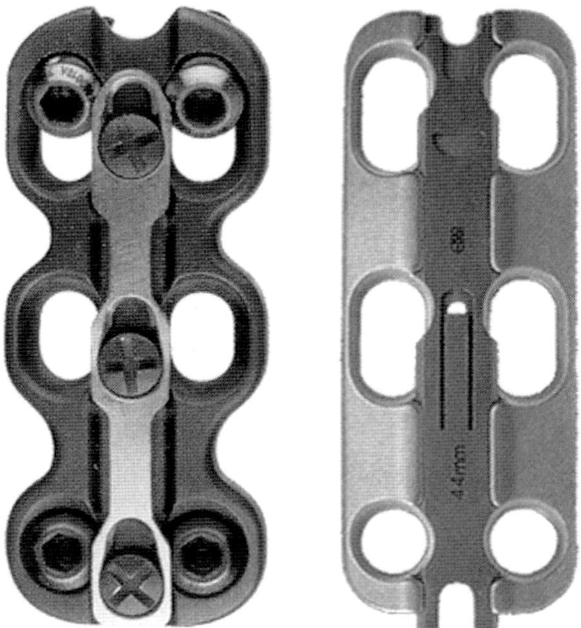

FIGURE 145-11. Premier plate (Medtronic Sofamor-Danek) on the left and C-Tek plate (Interpore Cross) on the right use similar mechanisms to prevent screw backout, while allowing the superior screws to slide in the slot to achieve dynamism.

Clinical Experience

Clinical series reported with these dynamic systems have shown that they do achieve their goals and offer advantages to spine surgeons and their patients. With the ABC system, early and more substantial graft incorporation has resulted in a very low nonunion rate. A review of nearly 500 patients involving more than 800 motion segments showed that the ABC system effectively stabilizes the spine in various conditions, including surgery for degenerative disease, herniated discs, and trauma.[19] This stabilization is achieved with both corpectomy and interbody approaches, with allograft and autograft iliac crest bone. Fusion was rigorously defined as absence of motion at the tips of the spinous processes between flexion and extension, in addition to the presence of bridging trabecular bone. When using this stringent definition, 67% of the levels (341 of 508) were fused at 3 months, 81% were fused at 6 months (310 of 384 levels), 93% were fused at 12 months (238 of 255 levels), and 100% (69 of 69 levels) were fused at 24 months. Essentially, early trabecular bridging and progressive graft maturation were observed. Measuring the deflection at the tips of the spinous processes magnifies the initial flexibility typically allowed by the weaker new bone. The amount of such movement progressively decreases as the bone graft matures. Most importantly, no regression with increasing motion is observed if the fusion is progressing.

Cobb angle measurements showed preservation of lordosis with minimal losses of 2 to 8 degrees in only 3% to 4% of patients. Kyphotic angulation corrections were maintained within 5 degrees. Dynamic fixation did not result in an increased angular deformation reported with uninstrumented fusion.[4,5] The amount of settling observed is consistent with uninstrumented fusions, averaging 1.5 to 2.0 mm per level, with slightly more settling observed with allograft. Most of the settling occurred within the first month of surgery, and virtually all occurred within 3 months. The unrestricted settling allowed by dynamic plating did not cause excessive settling but instead facilitated earlier and more substantial fusion.

Epstein[20] reported her experience with the ABC plate after single-level cervical corpectomy and fusion. Serial dynamic radiographs and two-dimensional CT scanning were used to analyze construct failure or nonunion, or both, up to 12 months after the procedure. Four patients developed postoperative plate or graft complications during the average of 34 months. One patient, with a plate and graft extrusion, required a second two-level corpectomy with posterior wiring and fusion. Two patients with nonunion and one with a delayed iliac crest strut fracture required secondary dorsal fusion. Epstein[20] concluded ". . . effective arthrodesis and a low incidence of complications following one level ACF performed utilizing dynamic ABC plates were attributed to reduced stress shielding and greater graft compression afforded by the unique plate design. Applying dynamic ABC plates for one level ACF was biomechanically advantageous with low morbidity."

Pitzen et al.[21] reported their experience treating cervical spondylosis using autograft and either a rigid or axially dynamic (ABC) plate. Patients were followed for 2 years. Four patients in the rigid plate group had implant complications, whereas no complications were seen in the ABC group. Mean segmental mobility before discharge for the ABC group was 1.7 mm, 1.4 mm after 3 months, 0.8 mm after 6 months, and 0.4 mm after 2 years. For the rigid plate group, these values were 1.0 mm, 1.8 mm, 1.6 mm, and 0.5 mm. The difference at 6 months between both groups was significant. The loss of segmental lordosis for the ABC group with respect to intraoperative radiograph was 1.3 degrees at discharge and 4.3 degrees after 2 years. For the rigid plate group, these values were 0.9 degrees and 0.7 degrees. The difference at 2 years was significant. No difference was seen in clinical outcomes at 2 years (visual analogue scale, Oswestry Disability Index). The authors concluded that an axially dynamic implant should be the implant of choice because of the significantly lower incidence of construct complications with equivalent outcomes.

Steinmetz et al.[22] reviewed their preliminary clinical experience with the DOC VCSS plate in the treatment of multiple-level cervical spondylosis. There were 34 patients with symptomatic multiple-level cervical spondylosis who underwent decompression and fusion with the DOC VCSS system. The operations included two-level, three-level, and four-level anterior cervical discectomy and fusions and one-level, two-level, and three-level corpectomies. Fusions included allograft (76%) and autograft (24%). Minimal follow-up was 6 months, with an average of 13 months. The DOC plate did permit subsidence, with an average of 1.7 mm of subsidence at 13 months after surgery. Most of this subsidence occurred within 3 months postoperatively, with 61% of patients showing 2 or more mm of subsidence in this early time period.

Lordosis was maintained after surgery in most patients, with an average of 14 degrees of lordosis observed in the entire patient population. This lordotic configuration was well maintained after surgery. An average change (postoperative compared with latest clinical follow-up) of 0.4 degrees of lordosis was shown at the latest clinical follow-up (13 months after surgery). These results show that the DOC plate permitted axial subsidence yet prevented angular deformation (kyphosis).

Most significantly, there were no instances of graft or implant failure, although one patient after a motor vehicle accident presented with a collapsed graft and displaced hardware. The overall fusion rate was 91%. A solid arthrodesis was determined if (1) there was no motion across the fusion site on flexion-extension radiographs, (2) trabeculae were observed across each fusion site, and (3) no lucency was observed at any of the fusion sites or around any of the screws.

Bose[23] reported experience using the DOC ventral cervical implant in the treatment of cervical spondylosis. Cervical discectomy or corpectomy, or both, were performed in 37 patients. At a mean follow-up time of 1.3 years, postoperative neck or arm pain was resolved in 52% of the patients, restriction on function was mild or absent in 88%, and fusion was successful in 80% of patients and 88% of the treated levels. There was one implant-related complication, one significant dysphagia complication, and a 10.8% donor graft site complication rate. Overall, the DOC implant resulted in excellent outcome, maintenance of sagittal angle, and controlled subsidence.

Saphier et al.[24] studied the clinical and radiographic results of the Premier plate or a rigid plate used during a one-level or two-level anterior cervical discectomy and fusion with allograft. Follow-up ranged from 12 to 35 months. The authors showed superior clinical results in the load-sharing Premier group along with a lower symptomatic pseudarthrosis rate. Vertical translation was found to be greater with the use of the Premier plate.

With the introduction of dynamic fixation systems, many authors have expressed concern that "too much dynamism" may be undesirable. In addition, these implants are nonrigid, so there has been concern as to whether they would be adequate to stabilize the spine in grossly unstable conditions. Initial (appropriately cautious) advice was to restrict use of these implants in cases with a significant instability, such as trauma, neoplasia, or multisegmental resections.

Laboratory studies have shown that dynamic systems actually are more stable than their more rigid counterparts. In an instrumented laboratory model, Brodke et al.[25] showed that DOC and ABC systems do load share with a simulated subsidence of 10% of the graft height in a corpectomy model. Compared with the CSLP and Atlantis systems, they provide equal initial stability in flexion and extension and lateral bending. Of great significance was the fact that they maintained a much higher level of stability after simulated subsidence. The CSLP and Atlantis systems lost 80% to 90% of their ability to resist flexion and extension, whereas ABC and DOC maintained most of their initial stiffness. Although perhaps counterintuitive, this result occurred because the construct was loaded axially, simulating the weight of the head and pull of the neck muscles.

With the dynamic systems, the graft-vertebra interface through load sharing participates in construct stabilization by remaining under axial load and imparting stability to the construct. With the more rigid systems, axial loading does not load the graft because of stress shielding. The axial forces are cantilevered through the screws to the plate and dorsal aspect of the spine (Fig. 145-12). The bone grafts are shielded from axial loads and are unable to participate in stabilizing the construct. Plate flexion or a degradation of the screw-bone interface can result. These data are supported by the laboratory report of DiAngelo et al.,[2] in which they observed a significant buffering of the loading and unloading of interbody grafts during flexion and extension when axially dynamic fixators were used.

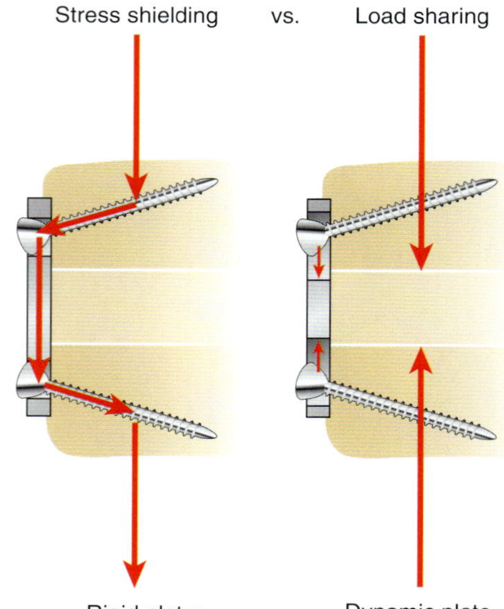

FIGURE 145-12. *Long red arrows* depict the pathway of the major axial loading forces in both static (rigid) and dynamic plating systems. In the rigid system, the load is cantilevered around the graft, traveling through the screws and plate. This shields the graft, which sees little of the axial loading forces. Dynamic systems transfer most of the axial load to the graft because the screws are free to slide in the slots in the plate (*small red arrows*). This keeps the graft loaded and allows the principle of Wolff's law to act, resulting in earlier and more substantial fusions.

More recent clinical data also support these data. Epstein[18] reviewed her series of multiple-level corpectomies performed for severe degenerative disease or ossification of the posterior longitudinal ligament with significant myelopathy. She used a ventral fibular strut graft and cervical plates augmented with dorsal wiring and grafting. In 56 consecutive cases, Epstein had a 10% ventral construct failure with Orion rigid plates, a 16% construct failure with Atlantis variable-angle plates, and no failures with the 18 ABC dynamic plates. Although not a pure ventral plating series, Epstein's series[18] shows that the dynamic systems are not weaker in these multiple-level constructs but rather appear superior.

Epstein[26] reported on her experience using the ABC plate for the stabilization of multiple-level anterior cervical corpectomies. No construct failures occurred in these two-level to four-level corpectomies with the inclusion of halo immobilization and posterior wiring. It seems that the gradual and controlled subsidence is beneficial in promoting stability and fusion in these complex cases.

Khoo et al.[27] reported a series of 61 patients with cervical trauma operated on at two large municipal trauma centers over a 5-year period. Four ventral cervical plates were used—CSLP, Atlantis, Codman, and ABC—representing a rigid plate, two variable-angle plates (one of which allowed more screw rotation [the Codman plate]), and a fully dynamic plate (the ABC plate) in conjunction with various constructs including interbody approaches in some and, more frequently, corpectomies. In some cases, supplemental dorsal fixation was also used. The follow-up was for a minimum of 12 months.

All images were scanned and analyzed by a computerized program, ensuring consistent operator-independent measurements. In these grossly unstable spinal injuries, the ABC system performed substantially better than the rigid and semiconstrained variable-angle screw systems with less settling, better preservation of lordosis, and no construct failures. Screw pull-out was observed in 13% of CSLP plates, 20% of Atlantis plates, 31% of Codman plates, and 0% of ABC plates. The construct failed in 13% of CSLP cases and 7% of Atlantis cases. The graft dislodged in 17% of CSLP cases, 7% of Atlantis cases, and 15% of Codman cases, but no such failures occurred with the ABC cases. The loss of graft height and lordosis was also measured. At 18 months after surgery, the cases in which the Codman plate was used averaged 37% loss of graft height compared with 32% with CSLP plates, 19% with Atlantis plates, and 10% with ABC plates. At 12 months, 7.31 degrees of lordosis was lost with the Codman system, 6.84 with CSLP, 4.3 with Atlantis, and 3.2 with ABC.

These results point to the advantage of load sharing by the graft, making it an integral part of the construct. The construct consists of the plate and screws and the graft and vertebral bodies sharing the load. This load sharing provides the stability needed to maintain alignment and protect the neural elements, while restoring and preserving lordosis. When load sharing does not occur, late failure of the construct is observed with an increasing amount of settling or lordosis, or both. True dynamic systems (axially dynamic) seem to offer substantial advantages over earlier-generation rigid plating systems.

Summary

Subsidence occurs naturally as part of the biology of aging. Subsidence after ventral cervical spine surgery may indicate construct failure caused by poor carpentry or suboptimal implant choices. Subsidence also refers to the normal graft absorption associated with osteoclastic activity, which is a major component of normal bone healing. This subsidence is a natural consequence of the normal biology of bone healing. It is a desirable effect that is seen in successful uninstrumented fusions. It cannot be prevented without interfering with successful fusion.

True dynamic fixation systems permit normal subsidence while stabilizing the spine. They essentially permit subsidence along an axis defined by the surgeon (via implant contouring), while preventing rotation, translation, and angular deformation. Axially dynamic implants are off-loaded axially, minimizing the chance of screw, plate, or rod fractures. These systems work with, rather than against, the biology of bone healing, resulting in earlier and more substantial fusions. As a result, fewer instrumentation or construct failures occur. No down side to their use has been reported. Dynamic fixation systems often seem to be the system of choice for ventral cervical stabilization after decompression.

KEY REFERENCES

Bishop RC, Moore KA, Weidner A, et al: Anterior cervical interbody fusion using autogeneic and allogeneic bone graft substrate: a prospective comparative analysis. *J Neurosurg* 85:206–210, 1996.

Brodke DS, Gollogly S, Alexander Mohr R, et al: Dynamic cervical plates: biomechanical evaluation of load sharing and stiffness. *Spine (Phila Pa 1976)* 26:1324–1329, 2001.

DiAngelo DF, Foley KT, Vossel KA, et al: Anterior cervical plating reverses load transfer through multilevel strut grafts. *Spine (Phila Pa 1976)* 25:783–795, 2000.

Pitzen TR, Chrobok J, Stulik J, et al: Implant complications, fusion, loss of lordosis, and outcome after anterior cervical plating with dynamic or rigid plates: two-year results of a multi-centric, randomized, controlled studies. *Spine (Phila Pa 1976)* 34:641–646, 2009.

REFERENCES

The complete reference list is available online at expertconsult.com.

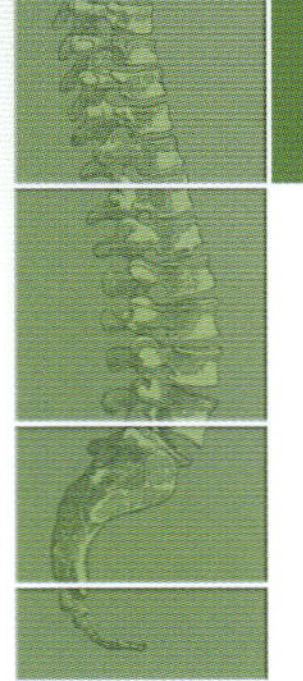

CHAPTER 146

Ventral and Lateral Thoracic and Lumbar Fixation Techniques

Daniel C. Lu | Gerald E. Rodts, Jr. | Regis W. Haid, Jr. | Kevin T. Foley | Praveen V. Mummaneni

Surgery on the ventral thoracic and lumbar spine began nearly 100 years ago. Ventral approaches for decompression of spinal pathology were first attempted in the early 1900s. Pioneers such as Royle[1] excised hemivertebrae for the treatment of scoliosis. Ito[2] as well as Hodgson and Stock[3] refined the ventral (transperitoneal) approach to the thoracolumbar spine for the treatment of Pott disease. These early efforts to decompress ventral spinal pathology were frequently complicated by postoperative mechanical instability and progressive deformity.

The first reports of ventral instrumentation of the spine were from Humphries,[4] who developed ventral interbody fusion with ventral plates and unicortical screws. These devices provided little biomechanical advantage. Most of these cases were transperitoneal approaches for debridement and stabilization in patients with Pott disease. The transperitoneal approach was eventually replaced by the retroperitoneal or extracavitary approaches for lesions of the lower thoracic and lumbar spine.

Throughout the 1970s, the preferred treatment for traumatic injuries was dorsal fusion and instrumentation, combined with ventral decompression and fusion. The Dwyer[5-7] and Zielke[8] devices were developed as ventrolateral implants that could augment or replace dorsal instrumentation. These consisted of screws that traversed the vertebral body that were interconnected with cable (Dwyer) or threaded rods (Zielke) that could be tightened in tension. These devices had limited ability to fixate two-column traumatic injuries. The Dunn device (developed in the late 1970s) represented a more rigid instrument for use in burst fractures. This double-screw, double-threaded rod device provided excellent strength but was removed from the market in 1986 after reports of great vessel erosion and rupture.[9]

It was not until the 1990s that numerous plate-screw and screw-rod systems were developed. Among the first were the Kaneda, Kostuik-Harrington, I-plate, and University plate systems. Later products included the anterior locking plate, the Z-plate, the Texas Scottish Rite Hospital system, the M-8 dual-rod system, the Expedium Anterior system, and others. Newer systems were developed for lower-profile, rigid ventral fixation of the spine. These systems have the added advantage of easier means of distraction and compression at the moment of plate or rod fixation. Furthermore, shorter segment fusions became more feasible. Some of the early generation ventral plating systems did not provide for a fully rigid screw-plate interface. Bicortical screw purchase was important but did not eliminate the possibility of screw toggle and possible mechanical failure in the early systems. However, most systems on the market by 2003 provided for a rigid screw-plate or screw-rod interface. To analyze the various systems critically, an appreciation of the biomechanics of the thoracolumbar spine is important. The reader is directed to other chapters outlining more detailed biomechanical information. It is also essential to understand some of the general indications for ventral instrumentation and fusion.

Biomechanical Considerations

A complex discussion of ventral thoracolumbar instrumentation is beyond the scope of this chapter; however, recognition of several basic concepts is essential to avoid complication. The anterior and middle columns provide the most resistance to axial loads. The ventral approach to spinal pathology has the distinct advantage of allowing for reconstruction of the vertebral body and intervertebral space with autologous or allogeneic bone or synthetic materials (e.g., methylmethacrylate, ceramic). The dorsal tension band—normally provided by the interspinous ligaments, ligamentum flavum, paraspinal musculature, and facet joints—must not be severely damaged if a ventral construct alone is to provide stability, because these devices cannot effectively withstand tremendous flexion forces. Complications arise when a posterior column injury has gone unrecognized or when too much is expected of a ventral construct. Plate and screw constructs can provide resistance against axial load, distraction, and extension. These implants have a higher success rate when axial loads are shared by a sturdy bone graft and the implant.

Certain biomechanical characteristics of implant systems are important to understand. Rigid implants (e.g., Z-plate, Kaneda systems, Expedium Anterior system, and M-8 dual-rod system) theoretically allow for greater immobilization of the spine. If the implant bears most of the stress, there is a risk of implant breakage or failure. Some plate systems have set screw holes rather than slots, thereby creating a static (nondynamic) condition beginning at the time of plate fixation. Also, stress shielding provided by the rigid fixation may prevent the beneficial compressive forces from enhancing bone fusion (Wolff's law). Because bone is a biologic, deformable material, repeated stress loading may cause bony erosion and failure at the metallic implant-bone interface.

Indications for Ventrolateral Instrumentation

A variety of infectious, neoplastic, congenital, and traumatic pathologic conditions are suitable for ventral thoracic or lumbar surgery. An initial step in complication avoidance is to determine whether a ventral approach truly provides the safest and most efficacious means of decompression of the neural structures, reconstruction of the anterior and middle column, application of corrective forces for realignment, and placement of an appropriate graft or spacer-implant construct. Conditions in which dorsal neural compression or posterior column bony/ligamentous damage are the predominant findings are best treated by a dorsal approach. Similarly, lesions with three-column pathology may possibly require circumferential treatment.

Anterior and middle column trauma (with preservation of the dorsal elements) may be treated adequately with a ventral approach (Fig. 146-1). Failure to recognize significant posterior column injury may result in delayed kyphotic deformity and neurologic deterioration. There are few clinical outcome data to encourage ventral decompression of trauma patients with complete neurologic loss below the level of the lesion. Ventral approaches, however, may be useful in paraplegic patients with a severe kyphotic deformity. Anterior reconstruction may provide better sagittal balance that could be important for long-term pulmonary function, independent transferring, and upper extremity function.

Patients with incomplete spinal cord injury, severe vertebral body collapse (≥40%) and kyphosis, and/or significant spinal canal compromise should be considered for ventral decompression and reconstruction. Intact patients with a myelographic block or ventral compression of the spinal cord on MRI may be considered for ventral decompression and stabilization. If the posterior longitudinal ligament (PLL) is intact on MRI and there is 30% or less loss in height of the anterior and middle column, a dorsal approach with reduction by ligamentotaxis could be considered in the intact or incomplete patient with a burst fracture.

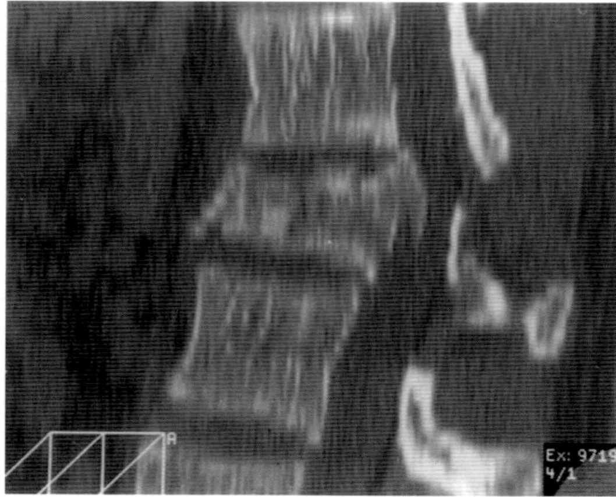

FIGURE 146-1. Thoracic burst fracture with retropulsed bone fragment and incomplete spinal cord injury suitable for anterior decompression.

Infection is another indication for ventral decompression, reconstruction, and instrumentation. The primary indication would be severe deformity of the spine, because most spinal infections can be treated without ventral instrumentation. Early ventral approaches for the treatment of Pott disease have been modified and are still very useful in debridement and stabilization of pyogenic, mycobacterial, or fungal infections. Reconstruction with autologous or allogeneic bone is feasible if a complete debridement of all necrotic tissue is accomplished. The risk of persistent infection or implant failure with instrumentation of infected cases is low if a prolonged course of antibiotics is given to these patients.

Metastatic neoplasms commonly affect the vertebral body before the posterior elements and therefore can be palliated with vertebrectomy. The cell kinetics of any malignancy, if known before surgery or determined by frozen section, must be considered when deciding on the material for reconstruction of the axial spine. In cases of a rapidly dividing carcinoma, synthetic spacers such as vertical titanium cages, methylmethacrylate, polyether ether, or carbon fiber cages can provide immediate stability of the vertebral column in patients with a short life expectancy. In more indolent neoplasms, such as breast or prostate cancer, longer survival can be expected, and autogenous or allogeneic bone can be expected to incorporate, thereby avoiding complications such as pseudarthrosis or implant migration. Use of titanium and other nonferromagnetic implants allows for long-term follow-up with MRI.

Treatment of other conditions, such as congenital or developmental scoliosis, iatrogenic lumbar kyphosis (flat back syndrome), and degenerative lumbar scoliosis may involve a ventral approach. Ventral procedures in adult scoliosis with curves greater than 40 to 50 degrees are associated with a higher rate of fusion than dorsal constructs alone. Ventral fusion and instrumentation may also be useful in patients with deficient laminae, facet joints, or pars interarticulari or extremely severe scarring from prior dorsal surgery.

Inadequate radiographic studies before surgery can lead to intraoperative or postoperative complications. Plain radiographs are essential and should include flexion and extension views when there is any suspicion of mechanical instability. In addition, attention should be paid to the density of bone as well as the sagittal and coronal alignment. Patients with scoliosis should have complete 36-inch standing films to assess overall spinal balance. The value of sagittal reconstruction of CT images is often overlooked, particularly after myelographic dye injection. Axial CT may be preferable over MRI to determine the amount of bony spinal canal compromise in trauma. Sagittal MRI often provides excellent views of the PLL. If intact, one may consider use of ligamentotaxis to reduce a burst fracture fragment. MRI has the added advantage of showing signs of soft dorsal tissue injury and hematoma that would commonly go unrecognized with plain radiographs and CT scan alone. Although cost-effectiveness is a primary concern, any patient with complex spinal pathology (and for whom aggressive surgery is contemplated) may require both CT and MRI as part of the workup.

Ventral Surgical Techniques

Positioning

Complication avoidance in the operating room begins with the simplest of steps. In positioning all patients, foam rubber padding is placed over ankles and elbows. For the prone position, gel pads are placed over the supports of the Wilson frame or chest rolls. The knees are flexed 45 to 90 degrees. Electrocardiography electrodes must not be on areas of the chest or trunk that contact the frame or rolls to prevent pressure necrosis. In females, the breasts must be tucked medially between the supports. Pillows are placed under the feet to provide knee flexion and relaxation of the sciatic nerve. Foam rubber rings are commonly used by anesthesiologists to protect the face and eyes, but care must be taken not to place the patient's neck in too much extension when in the prone position, particularly in one with diffuse spondylosis. It is necessary to double-check the eyes to ensure that there is no direct pressure on the globe. If the arms are not tucked at the patient's side but raised above the head, one should neither abduct the shoulders more than 90 degrees nor flex the elbow more than 90 degrees to prevent postoperative shoulder or elbow pain or even peripheral nerve ischemia.

Complications arising from the lateral decubitus position can also be averted with due diligence. We have all placed patients on a bean bag, but the bag must not extend into the axilla of the down arm. A roll (a liter bag of IV solution wrapped in a towel suffices) is placed above the edge of the bean bag just below the axilla. The peroneal nerve in the down leg must be protected with foam and/or gel padding over the fibular head. A pillow is placed between the legs, which are flexed 45 degrees at the hip and knees. The coronal plane of the patient's thorax must be perpendicular to the floor. Wide tape should be used to secure this position to allow rotation of the bed along its long axis ("airplaning"). Establishing this position assists the surgeon in remaining oriented throughout the procedure, especially during the critical steps of decompressing the spinal cord or placing a vertebral body screw. Some tables are equipped with a compass so that the desired neutral position can be recorded and reset by the anesthesiologist if an "airplane" maneuver is necessary. The perpendicular orientation of the coronal patient plane relative to the floor also allows for more efficient manual reduction of a kyphotic deformity by pressing on the back. The authors routinely "break" or flex the table at the level of the pathology to help open the disc spaces laterally and aid in the insertion of the bone graft (Fig. 146-2). Flexing the table also helps open the space between the 12th rib and the iliac crest. Once the bone graft is in place, the anesthesiologist is asked to return the table to the neutral, unflexed position.

We routinely administer suitable gram-positive antibiotic coverage (e.g., cefazolin 1 g or nafcillin 1 g). In cases of traumatic cord contusion or cord compression caused by tumor, we consider the use of methylprednisolone at least 1 hour before surgery. Using the spinal cord contusion protocol, the patient may receive a bolus of 30 mg/kg over 45 minutes followed by continuous infusion of 5.4 mg/kg per hour for 23 hours.[10,11]

Paralytic agents are not used after induction to allow for motor response in the event of inadvertent nerve or spinal cord stimulation. The role of somatosensory-evoked potential (SSEP) monitoring is debatable. A decrease in SSEP

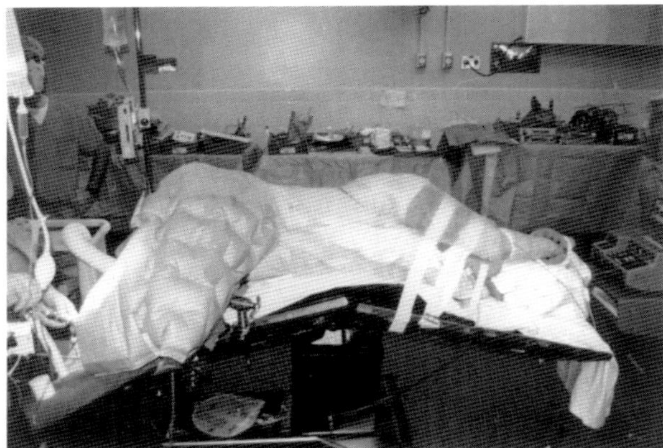

FIGURE 146-2. Lateral position for thoracoabdominal or thoracotomy approach with exposed iliac crest harvest site. (Note flexion of table at surgical site.)

amplitude of more than 50% and limited or absent intraoperative recovery of amplitude are predictors of a postoperative neurologic deficit.[12,13] Despite this reasonable sensitivity and low-false negative rate, SSEP monitoring measures only dorsal column function. False positives are common and often related to anesthetic considerations that can lead to a dangerous desensitization of the surgeon to warnings of intraoperative injury. SSEPs may be useful in deformity cases in which distractive or compressive forces are anticipated and could be reversed.

Motor-evoked potentials may be more accurate than SSEPs in monitoring spinal cord motor function during surgery.[14] This technique is extremely sensitive to anesthetics and requires expertise on the part of the anesthesiologist and monitoring team.

Approach and Exposure

The thoracic spine can be approached ventrally by the transmanubrial-transsternal approach, conventional thoracotomy, or thoracoscopic approach. The lumbar spine can be approached by the thoracoabdominal approach, transperitoneal approach, retroperitoneal approach, laparotomy, laparoscopy, balloon-assisted retroperitoneal endoscopy, or low pelvic approaches. These surgical approaches may be performed by the cardiothoracic, general, or vascular surgeon or by the spine surgeon. Detailed preoperative and intraoperative communication about the approach with an approach nonspine surgeon (if used) is important to ensure that not only is the pathologic level exposed but also that the exposure allows the spine surgeon to place instruments perpendicular to the axis of the spine for reconstructive and fixation techniques. Limited exposure may force a screw trajectory in an unsatisfactory cephalad or caudal direction.

Upper Thoracic Spine

Ventral exposure of the rostral levels of the thoracic spine is challenging. The first and second thoracic vertebrae usually can be approached ventrally with a low diagonal or transverse cervical incision. A vertical split of the manubrium often allows exposure down to T3 without sacrificing significant bone. A preoperative sagittal MRI should be obtained and inspected to ensure that the aortic arch does not block ventral access to the T2-3 area. Furthermore, one must be cognizant of the course of the recurrent laryngeal nerve as it emerges dorsal to the brachiocephalic arch to pass between the esophagus and trachea. Although its course is more constant on the left side, low-lying incisions to approach T1 and T2 on the left side put the thoracic duct at risk. This structure is intimately related to the subclavian vein off midline on the left and must be protected. Unrecognized pneumothorax is a complication of this approach because the pleura overlying the medial aspect of the cupola of the lung is adjacent to the spine. Filling the wound with saline and performing a positive pressure inspiration (Valsalva maneuver) at the close of the case is an essential step during closure. An oscillating saw or Gigli saw can be used to remove larger portions of the manubrium, but the retromanubrial space must be palpated to ensure that the brachiocephalic trunk is free. With the patient in the supine position, the upper thoracic spine slopes away from the surgeon, beginning at the T1-2 interspace. It can be difficult to place a ventral plate and screws in this region without a more aggressive removal or splitting of the manubrium or sternum.

Instead of sternotomy, lesions affecting the caudal aspect of T2 to T5 may be approached by a right-sided thoracotomy. The right-sided approach to the upper thoracic spine avoids the aortic arch. One must be cautious, however, to avoid injury to the superior vena cava and supreme intercostal vein. We have found instrumenting the T3-5 area to be easier with a high, right-sided thoracotomy than a midline sternotomy. This experience is particularly true with severe kyphosis (e.g., Scheuermann kyphosis) in this region.

The transaxillary approach is familiar to most vascular surgeons and can be considered for lesions affecting the upper thoracic levels. This approach, however, offers a limited exposure at the base of a cone-shaped cavity and should be reserved for small, more ventrolateral lesions not affecting the entire vertebral body and not requiring (complete) corpectomy or when only open biopsy is necessary. Ventrolateral instrumentation is very difficult because of the limited exposure. The transaxillary approach has associated risks to the lower brachial plexus, long thoracic nerve, and thoracodorsal nerve as well as to vascular structures in the axilla. Splitting of the pectoralis major muscle can also be a source of significant morbidity.

The ventral upper thoracic spine can also be accessed via a third-rib approach in which the patient is positioned in the lateral position with the arm elevated on a rest. The right side is preferable because of the straight course of the brachiocephalic artery. A curved incision is made beginning below the caudal angle of the scapula and ending between the medial scapula and the spinous process of C7. The trapezius and latissimus dorsi muscles are divided medially to minimize denervation, and the scapula is retracted laterally. The dorsal 10 cm of the 2nd, 3rd, and 4th ribs are resected, and the segmental vessels are ligated. The dorsal 3 cm of the 1st rib can also be dissected for additional exposure, but care must be taken not to injure the T1 motor root. The pleura and upper mediastinal structures can then be bluntly dissected for access to the vertebral bodies. Deflation of the lung with a double-lumen endotracheal tube can be very helpful. This approach requires tube thoracostomy placement at the end of the procedure because the parietal pleura is opened and the lung is exposed.

Midthoracic Spine

Lesions involving the midthoracic region are best approached via thoracotomy. Thoracic surgeons are very experienced with this approach. It is recommended that a thoracic surgeon perform the thoracotomy if the spine surgeon is not familiar with this approach. The patient is placed in the lateral decubitus position on a bean bag. The bean bag should not be higher than just below the axilla, and an IV bag or other suitable axillary pad should be placed to protect the brachial plexus and vessels. The area of break in the table should be determined before final positioning so that the desired thoracic level can be placed directly over this area to assist in exposure, opening of the disc spaces, and placement of the graft. Pillows may be placed under the down leg to protect the peroneal nerve and between the legs.

The left side is almost always used for the approach because it is safer and easier to visualize, dissect, and mobilize the aorta and segmental vessels than the vena cava or azygous venous system. It is easier to repair an injured aorta than the vena cava. One should consider obtaining a preoperative axial CT or MRI to assess the location of the aorta. If the aorta is lying very far lateral to the left (Fig. 146-3) or if the pathology is strictly right

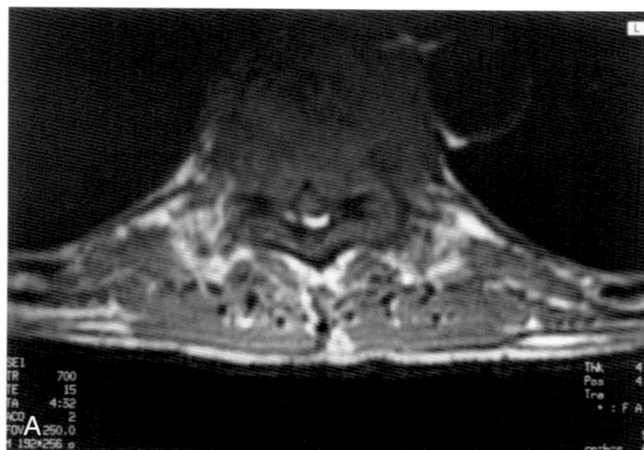

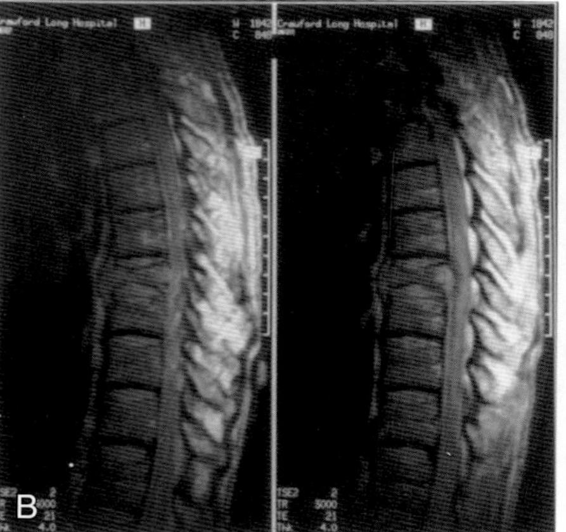

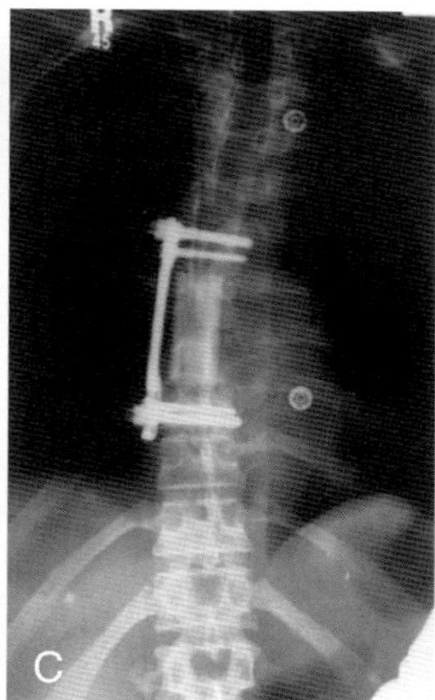

FIGURE 146-3. A, Laterally located aorta in which a right-sided approach was chosen. **B,** Sagittal view of the same metastatic tumor. **C,** Postoperative radiograph of this case instrumented with a Z-plate and humerus allograft packed with autologous cancellous bone harvested from the iliac crest.

sided, a right-sided approach can be performed. A standard thoracotomy incision is used beginning approximately two fingerbreadths below the angle of the scapula and coursing ventrally to the midaxillary line. One should select the intercostal space directly over the level of pathology to enter the pleural cavity. We have had satisfactory experience in performing a retropleural thoracotomy. In this procedure, the surgeon separates the endothoracic fascia from the parietal pleura, and the dissection is made down to the rib heads and spine extrapleurally. This is technically more difficult but can obtain a transthoracic approach without the need for a postoperative chest tube. A postoperative radiograph in the recovery room is essential to rule out a significant undetected pneumothorax.

In the lower thoracic spine, this usually corresponds to the rib two numbered levels rostral to the desired vertebral body. For instance, a T8 lesion usually corresponds to the horizontal segment of the 6th rib. Commonly, the rib need not be resected unless it is being harvested for bone graft or if unusually lengthy exposure of the spine is needed. Once the lung is deflated via a double-lumen endotracheal tube and the viscera are packed away with moist towels, the ribs are counted from inside the thoracic cavity. The rib identified as at the same level as the pathology is then exposed in a subpleural fashion down to its insertion on the pedicle. The segmental vessels are identified by blunt or scissor dissection in the midportion of each body. The disc spaces represent the "hills," and the midvertebral section (where the vessels are located) are the "valleys." The vessels are ligated with silk suture or metal clips in approximately the midbody. Taking the vessels too close to the aorta risks avulsion during this procedure. Conversely, sacrificing the vessels too close to the neural foramen may interfere with the collateral circulation of the spinal cord. Ligation of the vessels should be performed over the lateral aspect of the vertebral body between the aortic branch point and the neural foramen. Most surgeons and the scoliosis literature agree that up to three adjacent segmental arteries may be taken without neurologic sequelae, but the importance of the artery of Adamkiewicz (T10-L2) is still debated. Some surgeons advocate a preoperative spinal angiogram. Once the vessels are ligated and transected, a subperiosteal dissection of the vertebral body is carried out by using an elevator and unipolar cautery. The anterior longitudinal ligament (ALL) is elevated or incised if ventral release is necessary. If left intact during the exposure, the ALL can serve as a tissue barrier between the aorta and the operative site during the procedure. Some surgeons elevate the ALL sharply or use monopolar cautery from the bone and use that potential space to hold a malleable retractor for added safety.

In anticipation of instrumentation to the levels above and below the pathology, the segmental vessels should be taken here as well. Once this step is complete, a periosteal elevator or monopolar cautery is used to complete a subperiosteal exposure of the diseased level and other levels needed for instrumentation. Thus, the rostral end plate and disc space of the level above and the inferior end plate and disc space of the level below the pathologic levels must be clearly and completely visualized. Ventrally, the exposure is limited by the aorta, but with careful mobilization and retraction (i.e., with large malleable retractors) the cortical bone and disc can be dissected close to (but just short of) the midline. It is critical that a thorough exposure be completed dorsally. The dorsal 2 to 3 cm of each rib (level) involved must be removed with a ½- or ¾-inch osteotome. Rongeurs or a drill may also be useful. Once the heads of the ribs are disarticulated and removed, the pedicles at each level are exposed and the dorsolateral edge of the vertebral body is confirmed by palpation with a Penfield no. 4. Identification of the pedicle and dorsal vertebral body is essential for recognizing the location of the spinal canal and is necessary for safe and accurate identification of landmarks for placement of instrumentation. Frequently, there is a large mass of soft tissue, including the ligated ends of the segmental vessels, that has been swept into the area of the foramen. One should not attempt to cut away or use the monopolar to cauterize this tissue; the patent segments of the vessels often cause annoying bleeding. Shrinking the tissue near the foramen with the bipolar cautery and then placing a single silk suture through the cauterized mass and sewing it in traction to rib periosteum is often useful. This assists in identifying the spinal canal by moving this tissue in a more dorsal direction. Decompression should not be attempted until the limits of the spinal canal are clearly visualized. Catastrophic neurologic injury may result from initially not identifying accurately the borders of the pedicle, foramen, and dorsal vertebral body (i.e., the spinal canal).

Thoracolumbar Junction

For lesions affecting T10 through the upper lumbar spine (L1), a combined thoracoabdominal approach is necessary (Fig. 146-4). This may be true for lesions at L2 that require exposure to the T12-L1 disc space for instrumentation. During a standard thoracotomy, the patient is positioned in the right lateral decubitus position with a bend in the table to facilitate exposure. A double-lumen endotracheal tube is used for ipsilateral lung deflation. The incision is commonly made over the 10th rib and carried from the anterior axillary line to the posterior axillary line and extended as needed. The oblique and transversus abdominis muscles are incised, but care should be taken not to enter the peritoneal cavity. A subperiosteal dissection of the rib allows for efficient resection of the rib. The thoracic cavity is entered via the 10th or 11th rib space, and the diaphragm is immediately identified. The parietal pleura and peritoneal sac are bluntly mobilized by using finger- and sponge-stick dissection. Avoiding the monopolar cautery for most of this stage can prevent inadvertent entry into the peritoneal cavity, lung, or abdominal viscera. The diaphragm is mobilized from its peripheral attachment to the 11th rib. A 2- to 3-cm cuff of diaphragmatic tissue is maintained to allow for reapproximation during closure. The spinal attachments of the diaphragm are taken down sharply or with monopolar cautery. The medial attachment of the lateral arcuate ligament and the lateral attachment of the medial arcuate ligament are divided close to the tip of the transverse process of L1. The crus of the diaphragm is divided 2 to 3 cm away from the vertebral body and should be tagged. At this point, large self-retaining chest retractors can be placed to displace the peritoneal contents and diaphragm. Vessels that require sacrifice should be taken as close to the aorta or vena cava as possible to allow for maximal mobilization of these structures. Coagulation near the neuroforamen should be avoided to decrease the risk of compromising important radicular feeders to the spinal cord. The psoas muscle can be sharply

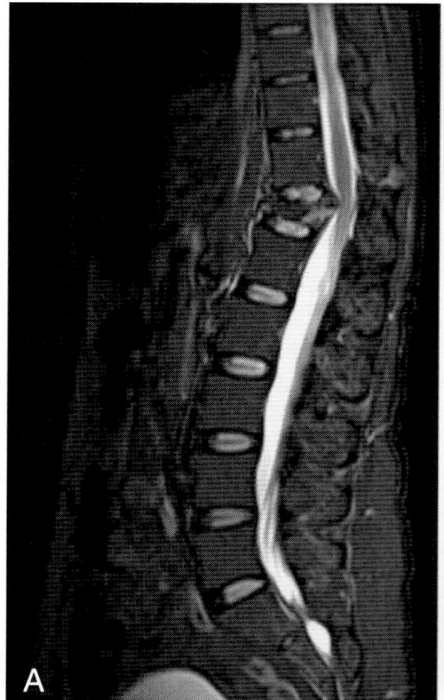

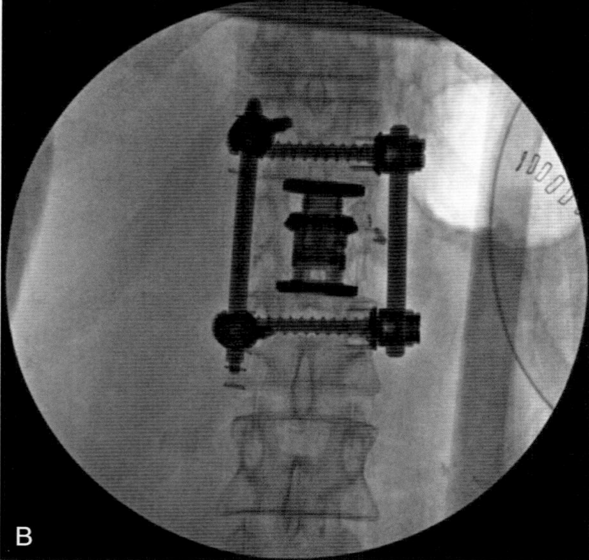

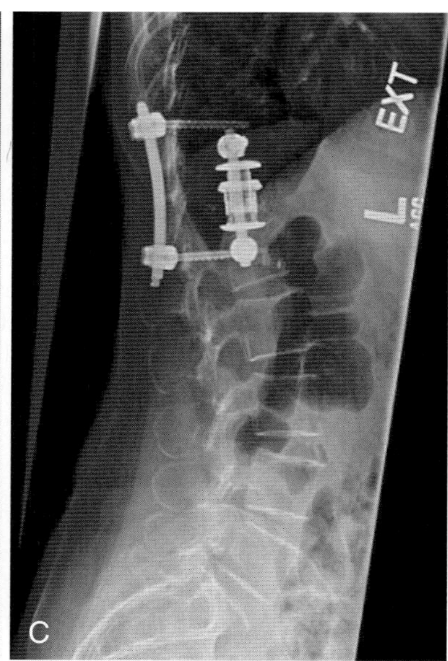

FIGURE 146-4. **A,** T12 burst fracture resulting in incomplete spinal cord injury. **B,** Decompression and reconstruction was performed with a Synex I expandable cage (Synthes Spine, Paoli, PA) filled with rib autograft and supplemented with the Expedium Anterior Spine (screw-rod) system (DePuy Spine, Raynham, MA) placed via a thoracoabdominal lateral approach. Further fixation was performed with a posterior percutaneous screw fixation (VIPER, DePuy Spine). **C,** Postoperative lateral radiograph demonstrates restoration of spinal alignment.

dissected with periosteal elevators or monopolar cautery back to the attachments to the pedicle to maximize exposure of the lumbar vertebral bodies. Gentle retraction can allow exposure from T9 through L3.

Although identification of severe fractures or tumor pathology is often easy, localization for less-obvious lesions at the thoracolumbar junction can be difficult. Although usually accurate, counting the ribs should not be relied on to identify the level. Plain radiographs are recommended and should be repeated with different orientation until the desired levels are confidently identified. With the patient in the lateral decubitus position, cross-table anteroposterior and lateral radiographs often are sufficient for accurate localization of the appropriate level.

Retroperitoneal Approach

The retroperitoneal approach is useful for lesions extending from the inferior surface of L1 to the superior surface of L5. It is necessary to keep in mind that instrumentation and fusion for pathology that actually extends to either the rostral or caudal limits of this exposure requires longer exposure that may not be provided by the retroperitoneal approach alone. As well, the iliac crest prevents true lateral access to the L5 vertebral body for transverse screw placement. To expose the vertebral body of L1 fully, dissection of some of the crural attachments may be necessary. A pneumothorax is a potential complication. At the caudal end, the L5-S1 interspace can be very difficult to expose fully (particularly in large male patients) because of the bulk of the psoas muscle.

Administration of cathartic agents before surgery and placement of a nasogastric tube during induction of anesthesia may facilitate easier retraction of the peritoneal contents during the case. Positioning for the retroperitoneal approach is similar to that for the thoracoabdominal exposure: the patient is in the lateral position with a break in the table at the level of the pathology. Upper lumbar exposure may require resection of the 12th rib. The incision is typically made from the lateral margin of the dorsal longitudinal paraspinal muscles (e.g., iliocostalis, sacrospinalis) and extends ventrally to the lateral border of the rectus abdominis muscles. The external and internal oblique and transversus abdominis muscles are divided with monopolar cautery. Clamp dissection and elevation of these muscles before incision can avoid entry into the peritoneal cavity. Blunt dissection with a sponge-on-a-stick can mobilize the peritoneum away from the spine. Great care must be taken to avoid damage to the ureter, although it is usually safely reflected ventrally with the peritoneal contents. Large, self-retaining table-mounted retractors (e.g., Omni, Thompson-Farley) are used over moist laparotomy sponges to maintain exposure. The transverse processes are palpable through the psoas muscle. This muscle can be dissected from its periosteal attachments by using monopolar cautery. This bovie technique results in less blood loss than a Cobb or periosteal elevator. Vigorous attempts at retraction with a Meyerding or similar retractor may cause laceration of the muscle and excessive bleeding. Careful "toeing-in" of the Meyerding or McElroy retractor is all that is usually necessary to put the psoas on stretch and facilitate subperiosteal exposure. Too much stretch, however, may cause postoperative psoas or iliopsoas weakness and pain. Mobilization of this muscle dorsally to the pedicle allows palpation and visualization of the ventral border of the spinal canal. Key points regarding closure of the retroperitoneal exposure include meticulous closure of the abdominal wall muscular layers to prevent hernia formation. We recommend leaving a large Hemovac drain in the retroperitoneal space for 24 to 48 hours, especially when decortication or resection of vertebral bone causes significant oozing of blood still seen at the time of closure. Another potential complication of this approach is intestinal ileus. Nasogastric suction is continued postoperatively until bowel activity is confirmed.

Transabdominal (Transperitoneal) Approach

Ventral decompression, reconstruction, and fixation of the lower lumbar spine and lumbosacral junction via the transperitoneal approach (open or laparoscopic) are possible.[15-17] Threaded interbody titanium cages, bone dowels, and other synthetic implants are available for interbody fusion and/or fixation. Typical thoracolumbar bone screws, plates, and rods are difficult to insert from this approach and have a high profile near vascular structures. The exposure tends to be triangular in shape because the field of view limited by the bifurcation of the iliac vessels and the L5-S1 disc space. Direct ventral screw fixation (e.g., buttress screw) of the upper sacrum is possible after a subperiosteal exposure of S1 immediately caudal to the disc space is performed. Use of Steinmann pins or a table-mounted vascular retractor is useful in retracting the iliac veins and arteries. Blunt dissection and avoidance of the monopolar cautery may avoid damage to the superior hypogastric plexus (and associated retrograde ejaculation). The L5-S1 disc space is readily evacuated, and bone graft and/or implants can be inserted.

Exposure of L4-5 is very feasible, but the surgeon must take extra care to immediately identify the iliolumbar vein. Although its origin is variable, this vein usually branches off the lateral aspect of the left iliac vein. Other times it originates directly from the vena cava. The vein courses to the region of the L5 pedicle and foramen. Heavy blood loss can occur if the left iliac vein is retracted to the patient's right before the iliolumbar vein is ligated. One may also consider low-dose heparin administration prior to retraction of the bifurcation and vena cava to help prevent thrombosis. Other helpful pearls include use of Steinmann pins to retract the iliac vessels laterally. The Trendelenburg position can facilitate the approach to the sacral angle. Currently, laparoscopic techniques are under investigation that may improve access to the L5-S1 level and allow for decompression, fusion, and instrumentation.

L5 vertebrectomy has been accomplished via the open, laparoscopic, or retroperitoneal approach, but the procedure is difficult and carries a higher risk of vascular injury than discectomy.[18,19] Furthermore, reconstruction of L5 from the direct anterior transperitoneal approach is also very difficult. Vertebrectomy of L4 is similarly very difficult from the anterior approach and can be more readily accomplished via the retroperitoneal approach. The midlumbar and upper lumbar levels (L3-4, L2-3, L1-2) are more difficult to expose via a transperitoneal approach because of the bulk of abdominal contents that must be retracted. The retroperitoneal approach should be considered.

Lateral Retroperitoneal Transpsoas Approach

This approach allows access to the lumbar spine via a lateral approach that passes through the retroperitoneal fat and psoas major muscle (Fig. 146-5). Variations of this approach include

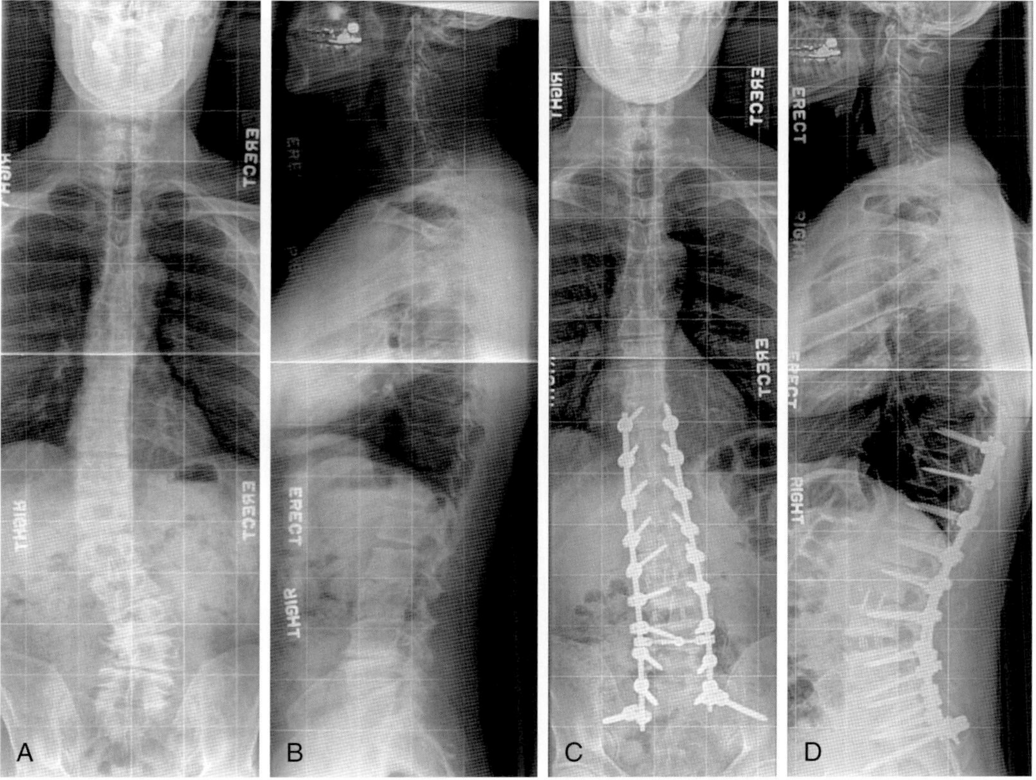

FIGURE 146-5. **A** and **B,** Preoperative radiographs demonstrating coronal plane deformity. **C** and **D,** Extreme lateral interbody fusion cages (NuVasive, Inc., San Diego, CA) were placed at L2-4 via a lateral retroperitoneal transpsoas approach. Subsequently, a transforaminal lumbar interbody fusion (Concorde cage, DePuy Spine, Raynham, MA) was performed at L5-S1 via a second-stage posterior open approach. In addition, posterior instrumentation at T10-S1 and ilium was performed with the Expedium Anterior Spine system (DePuy Spine).

the minimally invasive extreme lateral interbody fusion (XLIF) or direct lateral interbody fusion (DLIF) approaches.

Ideal patients for this procedure include those with low back pain or flat back syndrome without central canal stenosis. Relative contraindications include significant central canal stenosis, severe rotatory scoliosis, and high-grade spondylolisthesis. Although the XLIF/DLIF can create indirect foraminal decompression via interspace distraction, these approaches do not allow for central canal decompression. Furthermore, in severe rotatory scoliosis cases and high-grade spondylolisthesis cases, the normal anatomy may be skewed and surrounding structures (the iliac vessels or bowels) may be injured.

To prepare for XLIF or DLIF, the patient is placed in a 90-degree right lateral decubitus position with the left side elevated and laterally flexed by using a bump or a roll to increase the distance between the iliac crest and the rib cage. A lateral fluoroscopic image is taken with K-wires to demarcate the midpoint of the intended disc exposure. A small incision is created to encompass this location, and the retroperitoneal plane is dissected down to the psoas muscle. A second 2-cm incision may be made posterior to this initial incision between the erector spinae muscles and the abdominal obliques. This incision allows for the insertion of the surgeon's index finger to identify the retroperitoneal space and psoas muscle and by sweeping the peritoneum anteriorly; the direct lateral incision is palpated with the index finger. Tubular dilators and subsequently an expandable retractor is placed into the direct lateral incision with the assistance of the index finger guiding it safely from the direct lateral incision through the retroperitoneal space to the psoas muscle. The fibers of the psoas muscle are then separated by using dilators and blunt dissection with the concurrent use of electromyographic stimulation or neuromonitoring to assess the proximity of lumbar nerve roots from the advancing dilator. The dilator parts the psoas muscle centrally; therefore, the great vessels should remain anterior and the lumbosacral plexus nerves should be posterior to the retractor. Proper trajectory and position are assessed by fluoroscopy. Once the retractor is inserted over the dilators and its position is confirmed, the rigid articulating arm is attached to the retractor and the surgical table.

Discectomy is then performed using standard instruments. The posterior anulus is left intact, while an anulotomy centered over the anterior half of the disc space allows for discectomy. End-plate arthrodesis and interbody implant and bone graft placement are then completed. The retractor is removed after fluoroscopic confirmation of implant position. A layered closure is then performed.

Decompression

For a vertebrectomy, the discs above and below are incised with a knife blade, or a straight osteotome is used to separate the bulk of the disc from the end plates. One must keep in mind the concave curvature of the dorsal vertebral body in the thoracic spine to avoid the ventral spinal canal. If soft tumor is encountered, large scoop curets or the ultrasonic aspirator is an efficient tool for rapid tissue removal. For stronger bone, a 1- or 2-inch osteotome may be used to make two cuts to remove a large portion of the body. The first cut is 5 to 8 mm dorsal to the ventral-most cortex of the vertebral body in the vertical plane (perpendicular to the disc space) and is approximately 15 to 20 mm deep (toward the opposite side). The second cut is similarly perpendicular to the disc space and is approximately 8 mm ventral to the dorsal cortex of the vertebral body and spinal canal. A curved osteotome or large curet can then remove a large block of bone, leaving a barrier between the aorta and the decompression site and between the spinal canal and the decompression site. The remainder of bone is then removed either piecemeal with smaller curets or with a high-speed drill. Drilling may offer a less traumatic initial removal of bone compared with osteotomy, but blood loss may be less with the faster latter technique. The bone ventral to the canal is the last area to be removed. Once the dorsal cortex and PLL have been removed, the dura is decompressed from the ipsilateral pedicle to the contralateral pedicle. The ventral-most and far lateral cortex are preserved as much as possible to help secure the bone graft. One should be able to visually inspect the contralateral pedicle. The epidural space rostral and caudal is palpated with a double-ender (dental or Woodsen) instrument. One must decompress from pedicle to pedicle to fully ensure that there is no spinal cord compression.

The complication of neurologic injury is best avoided by clearly exposing the ventral spinal canal and dorsal body first. The next step is to create a cavity into which the critical bone fragments or tumor (compressing the spinal cord) can be safely reduced. Thus, one should first complete the bulk of the corpectomy or vertebrectomy (depending on the pathology), leaving the portion in the ventral epidural space last. Then the dorsal vertebral cortex, fracture fragments, or tumor in the epidural space is more safely removed via regular or reverse angle curettage. At times, a diamond bur may be useful. Instruments are best manipulated toward the vertebrectomy defect away from the spinal cord during epidural decompression.

Fracture Reduction

A pathologic or traumatic fracture-dislocation can be reduced with several maneuvers. The most direct technique is manipulation of vertebral bodies with a large Cobb elevator or curet. This can be difficult and runs the risk of having the instrument slip into the canal.

With the patient in the lateral position, the surgeon can push on the back at the apex of the kyphotic deformity. This technique is very effective, and the decompression site can be visualized during the manipulation. If the PLL is intact, then ligamentotaxis can aid to pull fracture fragments ventrally.

Several ventral thoracolumbar instrumentation systems have bolts that (once placed in the adjacent vertebral bodies) can be used with a distractor to accomplish reduction and distraction. Distraction is effective, but the distractor can obscure the surgeon's view and compromise access to the decompression site during placement of the bone graft. Interspace spreaders have the same limitation, although newer models are longer and more streamlined, allowing greater accessibility to the vertebrectomy site during distraction and reconstruction (Fig. 146-6). When combined with ligamentotaxis from the PLL, anterior distraction maneuvers can be an effective method to reduce posteriorly displaced fractures.

A fourth method to reduce posteriorly displaced fracture fragments is an eggshell osteotomy. The cancellous portion of the fractured vertebral body is removed with a high-speed drill, leaving the cortical remnants. The posteriorly displaced

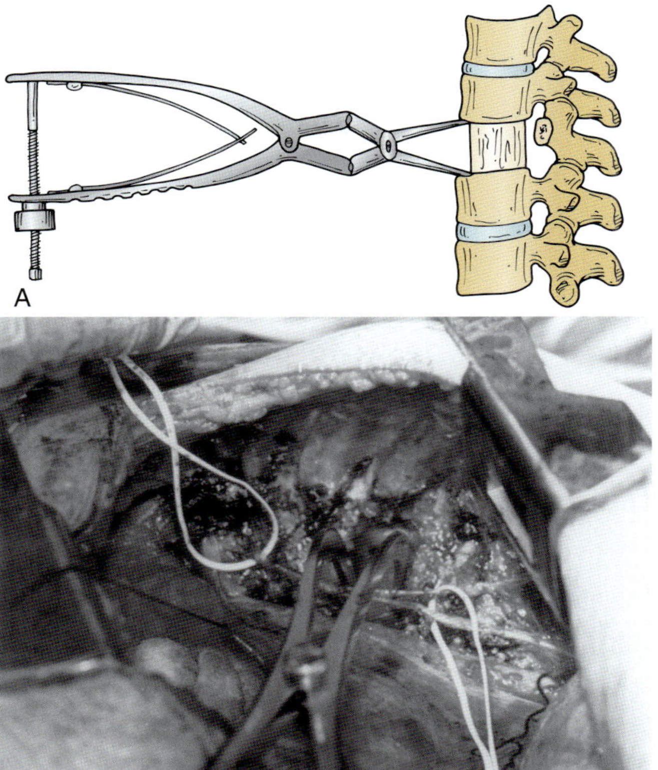

FIGURE 146-6. A, Diagram of intervertebral body spreader and bone graft reconstruction. **B,** Intervertebral body spreader (Synthes Spine, Paoli, PA) distracting the vertebrae prior to bone graft placement. The thoracic dura is visible posteriorly.

cortical fragments can then be pulled anteriorly by using reverse-angle and straight curets.

Bone Grafts and Vertebral Body Replacements

The choice of bone graft or reconstructive implant depends on the distance the anterior fusion needs to span. The location in the thoracolumbar spine and the patient's underlying pathology are also important. Factors such as the presence of osteopenia, tumor, previous radiation, diabetes, rheumatoid arthritis, and tobacco use are important. Grafts that span an entire vertebral body length or more must withstand greater axial loads. Allogeneic humerus, tibia, or femur can be used, and they are typically packed with autologous cancellous bone harvested during the vertebrectomy. Rib and iliac crest are also excellent sources of bone to use in and around allograft struts. One should keep in mind that allograft bone takes much longer to incorporate.

Portions of rib tied by suture or cable into a barrel-shaped cylinder can be used as a spacer fusion. Ribs are thought to be high in bone growth factors but provide less strength in resisting axial loads than some of the alternatives.

Autologous tricortical iliac crest provides satisfactory axial support. Harvest of large tricortical graft endangers the peritoneal contents. Great care should be taken during periosteal dissection. Significant morbidity can be associated with harvest of autologous iliac crest bone. We typically use a unipolar cautery with the tip angled ventrally to hug the dorsal cortex during stripping of the muscular and fascial attachments. A Cobb elevator is also useful, but it is necessary to take care to avoid plunging into the peritoneum. Vessels perforating the iliac crest must be coagulated or the emissary ostia treated with bone wax to help prevent accumulation of a hematoma. One should always stay one to two fingerbreadths dorsal to the anterior superior iliac spine to avoid injury to the lateral femoral cutaneous nerve. If one desires to reconstruct the defect in the iliac crest, both natural and artificial methods are possible. If rib is available, the ends can be impacted into the harvest site sides of the iliac crest to recreate the superior contour. Steinmann pins or screws (titanium or stainless steel) as a support for methylmethacrylate may be used.[20] If the latter technique is used, a postoperative drain is recommended, as the cement will elicit a collection of serous fluid.

Autologous fibula can also be used. In cases of infection, some surgeons also perform microvascular anastomosis to the intercostal arteries to preserve graft blood supply. Meticulous surgical technique must be used to avoid the peroneal nerve near the fibular head and to avoid the ankle joint (syndesmosis). A good rule of thumb is to stay 10 cm or more away from the ankle joint below and the fibular head above. A preoperative lower extremity arteriogram is useful to define the arterial supply to the fibula.

It is important to emphasize that regardless of the source of autologous bone, all soft tissue (e.g., muscular or tendinous attachments, cartilage, fascia) must be cleanly stripped off before implantation to maximize bone surface area for fusion. Leaving cartilaginous material adherent to the vertebral body end plate can result in pseudarthrosis; thus, the vertebral end plates should be meticulously stripped of all disc tissue. Scattered areas of decorticated end plate facilitate fusion, but significant amounts of cortical bone must be spared to allow strong purchase of the bone graft and to prevent impaction of the graft through the end plates during axial loading. Removing (decorticating) too much of the end plate may result in collapse of the bodies above and below with telescoping of the graft. This problem is encountered more often when rigid allograft tibia, fibula, or femur is used.

In addition to autograft or allograft bone, methylmethacrylate and artificial bone spacers are currently being marketed. Vertical mesh titanium cages (Pyramesh, Medtronic Sofamor Danek, Memphis, TN; Harms, DePuy Spine, Raynham, MA; SynMesh System, Synthes Spine, Paoli, PA), carbon fiber cages (Stackable Cage System, DePuy Spine), polyether ether blocks (PEEK, Medtronic Sofamor Danek), and expandable metallic implants (Synex System, Synthes Spine [Fig. 146-7]; VertiSpan, Medtronic Sofamor Danek [Fig. 146-8]) are available.

The benefit of having a break in the table can be enhanced with the use of an interspace spreader or by manual pressure on the dorsal spine to help open the disc space during distraction and bone impaction. When screw-rod systems are used, direct distraction of vertebral body screws allows for efficient placement of the graft. Once all graft material is in place, the table is returned to the neutral position to help lock in the graft. In addition, compression can be applied across the vertebral body screws and maintained by rod attachment.

The importance of meticulous shaping and "carpentry" with the graft during this step cannot be overemphasized.

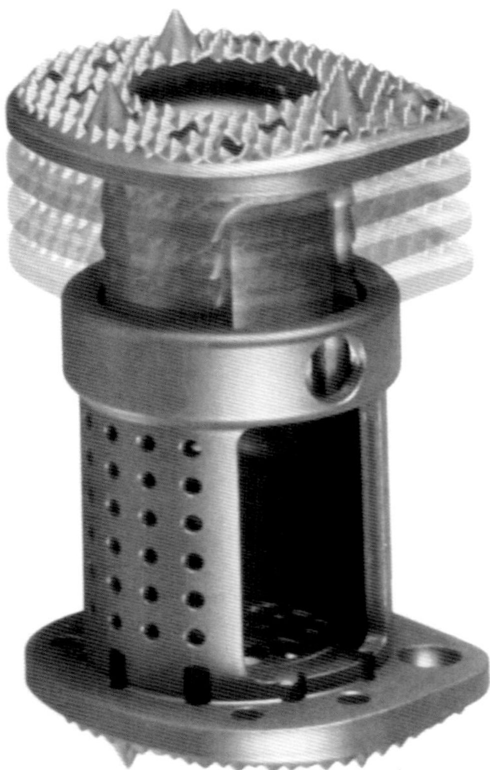

FIGURE 146-7. The expandable Synex I vertebral body implant demonstrating several possible ratcheted positions of the superior portion of the implant (Synthes Spine, Paoli, PA).

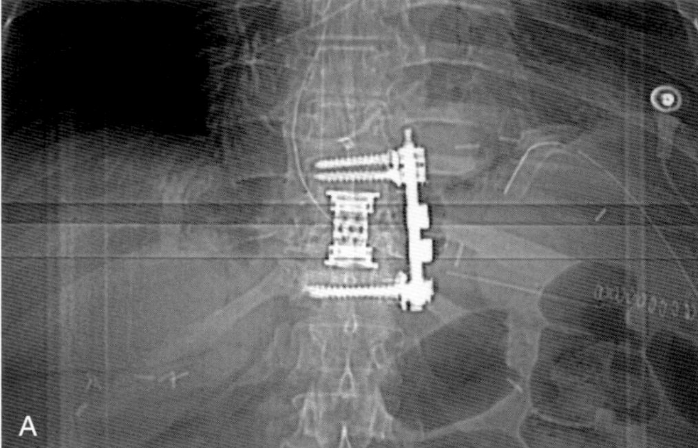

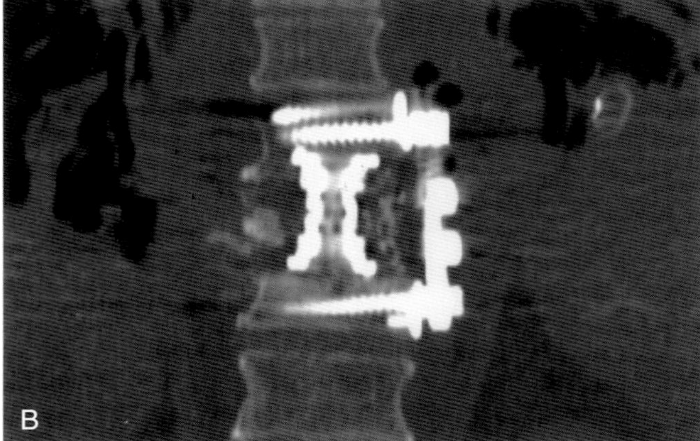

FIGURE 146-8. **A,** Immediate postoperative radiograph of the Verti-Span expandable cage system (Medtronic Sofamor Danek, Memphis, TN). **B,** Immediate postoperative coronal CT scan of the expandable cage. Note the central and peripheral placement of cancellous bone from the iliac crest.

A spinal metal implant is not a substitute or savior for a poorly shaped or fitted bone graft.

Instrumentation

Ventral or ventrolateral metal implants provide immediate rigidity, allow for compression of bone graft, and help maintain correction of a deformity. Based on individual experience, various amounts of time working with sawbone models or cadavers are needed before use in actual clinical situations. The three basic types of implants are rod, plate, and cable systems.

General Principles of Ventrolateral Instrumentation Systems

Whether rods, plates, or cables are being used, all implants in the thoracolumbar region should be placed on the lateral aspect of the vertebral body. The construct should have a low profile to avoid vascular or visceral injury. To avoid unequal strain and stress on the metallic implant, great care must be taken to maximize the total surface area of metal-to-bone contact. In a method commonly referred to as "gardening" the spine, rongeurs and drills should be used to flatten out the lips of the vertebral end plates, and the heads of the ribs should be removed at all levels to be instrumented. This is particularly important with plate implants.

The dorsal-most points of screw fixation in the vertebral body should be 8 to 10 mm ventral and caudal to the dorsal-rostral corner of the vertebral body at the rostral end of the construct or 8 to 10 mm ventral and rostral from the dorsocaudal corner of the caudal body in the construct. A minimum screw trajectory of 10 degrees ventrally away from the spinal canal is necessary to avoid injury. An awl should be used to begin screw or bolt holes to prevent skating of instruments near the spinal canal or the large vessels and viscera. Screw placement is dictated by the desired forces. To correct a kyphosis, the screws should be placed more ventrally with distraction/compression dual-rod systems (e.g., Kaneda, Expedium Anterior, or M-8 dual-rod systems). With dual-rod systems, the more ventral rod should be longer to correct the kyphosis. The longer segment is distracted initially. One must recognize that even minor distraction forces may cause spinal cord injury via stretch or vascular compromise. In general, when correcting scoliosis, tension forces should be applied on the convex side of the curve, starting at the apex and directed rostrally and caudally in sequential fashion. Bicortical screw penetration is preferred to provide the strongest purchase of the vertebral body, but care must be taken not to penetrate beyond 2 to 3 mm of the distant cortex of the vertebral body.

Cable Systems

The Dwyer cable system was first developed in the early 1960s for application to the convex side of thoracolumbar scoliotic curves. The basic principle of ventrolateral correction of scoliosis is to shorten the convexity by applying compressive forces. A screw with a staple (to maintain screw position and prevent movement) is placed on the convex side of a curve into the vertebral body on the lateral side. A titanium cable is then connected to the screws and tightened to create a compressive force. Excessive force, however, can produce undesirable thoracic kyphosis or, further caudally in the spine, the flattening of a normal lumbar lordosis. Dwyer reported a 43% complication rate, including screw pull-out and vascular or visceral injuries. This system can be used for degenerative lumbar curves, but it is not recommended in flat back or kyphotic deformities. This particular type of implant system has been abandoned by many surgeons in favor of rod and plate systems.

Rod Systems

Zielke Universal Spinal Instrumentation System

The Universal Spinal Instrumentation System (USIS), developed by Zielke, is a refinement of the Dwyer system and uses flexible rods instead of cables. This system allows for segmental compression or distraction via the ventrolateral approach and provides improved rotational control over scoliotic curves. A device is included that can derotate the scoliotic curve or produce lordosis. A correction of 10% to 15% per level fused can be obtained. This system is well suited for thoracolumbar and lumbar scoliosis but is somewhat limited for other applications because of the limited stability of a single point of fixation per vertebral body.

Kaneda Anterior Scoliosis System and Expedium Anterior Spine System

These screw-rod systems (DePuy Spine) correct scoliosis by securing each vertebral body in the curve with two screws inserted through a vertebral staple. Two contoured rods are placed into the heads of the screws. These systems are designed for the correction and stabilization of idiopathic thoracolumbar, lumbar, and thoracic scoliosis. The Frontier Anterior Deformity System is a similar system from DePuy Spine that is suited for thoracoscopic scoliosis surgery.

Kostuik-Harrington System

The Kostuik-Harrington system (Zimmer, Inc., Warsaw, IN) is a ventral modification of the dorsal Harrington distraction rod. Vertebral body screws and stabilizing staples are placed at each level ventrally, and a distraction rod is inserted through these screws and used for placement of the strut graft. Compression of the graft is then accomplished with placement of larger Kostuik spinal screws dorsally on the lateral aspect of the vertebral body. These screws hold a heavy ratcheted Harrington compression rod that, in concert with the ventral rod, also provides good rotational control. This system is useful for short segment fixation and allows for distraction to correct kyphotic deformity. Currently, this system is no longer in widespread use.

Kaneda System

A unique aspect of the Kaneda system (DePuy Spine; Fig. 146-9) is the tetra-plate with four corner spikes that is initially hammered into the center of the lateral aspect of the vertebral body. One should "garden" the spine to ensure flush contact between the staple plate and the bone. Two vertebral (preferably bicortical) screws are placed through each plate. The heads of the screws have a channel through which rods are placed. The design of the staple plate is such that the ventral screw holes are more rostral and caudal in the upper and lower plates, respectively. Thus, the ventral span of the rod is longer than the dorsal. The heads of these screws can be engaged by a distractor for placement of the strut graft. The Kaneda distraction system is very effective and allows ample working space through which the bone graft can be placed. Cross-fixators are available to enhance the rigidity of this implant. This device is very effective for short (one or two) segment fixation for a variety of pathologies. Sources of complication include failure to achieve maximal surface area contact between the staple plate and bone (by allowing rocking of the metal over a bony prominence) and placement of screws that are either too short or too long. Preoperative axial CT slices (bone windows) can be used to indirectly measure the length of screw needed. One can usually feel the screw engaging the opposite lateral cortex. Inadequate countersinking of the graft may make it difficult to apply a cross-link.

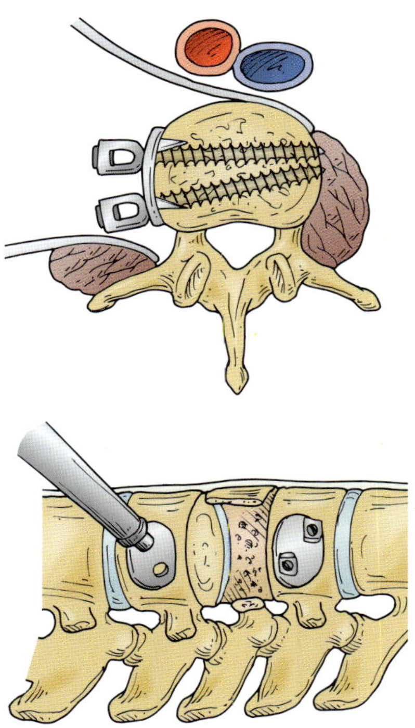

FIGURE 146-9. Tetra-plates and eye bolts of the Kaneda system (DePuy Spine, Raynham, MA). Smooth rods are placed through the eye bolts and tightened with a top-loading screw. The bolts can be used for distraction or compression.

Antares Dual-Rod System

The Antares dual-rod system (Medtronic Sofamor Danek) is very similar to the Kaneda system. An anchoring plate with cleats is inserted into the side of the vertebral bodies above and below. Bolts are then placed through holes in the plates and across the vertebral bodies. Rods are slid into the bolts and compressed, and locking screws are tightened. Cross-links are available.

VentroFix System

Also similar to the Kaneda device, the VentroFix system (Synthes Spine) uses plates that are screwed into the spine (as opposed to impacting cleats). Rods then slide through grooves and openings in the anchoring plates. Locking screws fix the rods to the anchoring plates.

Texas Scottish Rite System

The Texas Scottish Rite System (TSRH; Medtronic Sofamor Danek), an implant system of variable-angle screws and rods (connected by variable-width offset connectors or eye bolts), is most commonly applied to the dorsal spine but is easily adapted to ventrolateral fixation. Screws of 5.5-mm, 6.5-mm, 7.0-mm, and 7.5-mm diameter width and various lengths are available for bicortical purchase. Screws can be placed in a trapezoidal array similar to the Kaneda device so that the longer span is ventral. Rods of 3/16- or 1/4-inch or intermediate 5.5-mm diameter are (as with the screws) available in stainless steel and titanium. Distraction and compression forceps are available and connect to the rods below or above the screw-offset connection to apply the desired force. Use of the TSRH for ventrolateral fixation should be done with the knowledge that the heads of the variable-angle screws are somewhat higher in profile than those of other plate and rod systems. Side-tightening screws may be easier to apply than top-tightening ones.

Plate Systems

Z-Plate System

The Z-plate system (Medtronic Sofamor Danek), designed by Zdeblick (Figs. 146-10 to 146-12), combines the low-profile advantage of plates with the distraction and compression capability of vertebral body screws. Bicortical purchase is

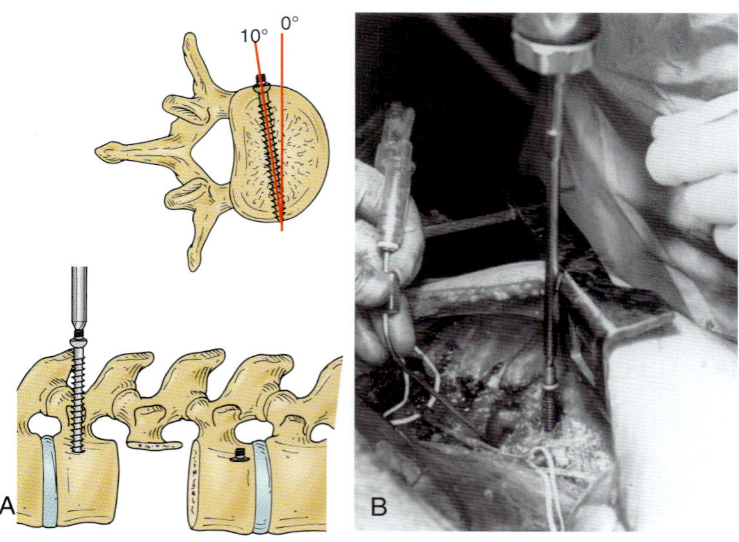

FIGURE 146-10. A, Diagram of the dorsal bolt trajectory (10 degrees away from the spinal canal). **B,** Placement of a Z-plate bolt (Medtronic Sofamor Danek, Memphis, TN) at the caudal, dorsal corner of the lower vertebral body. (Note dura mater visible through the corpectomy defect.)

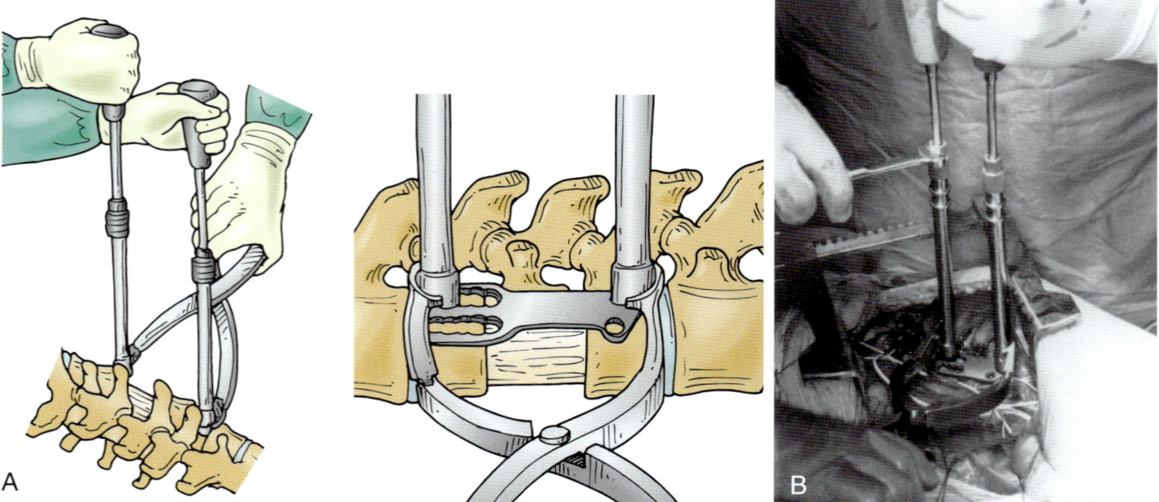

FIGURE 146-11. A, Diagram of simultaneous compression across and tightening of bolts in a top-loaded thoracic plate (Medtronic Sofamor Danek, Memphis, TN). **B,** Operative photograph of tightening of dorsal bolts in the Z-plate system with extended wrenches and long compressor (Medtronic Sofamor Danek).

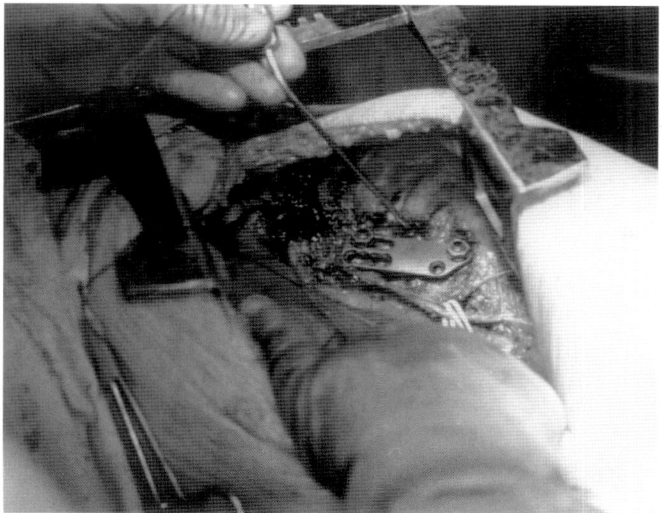

FIGURE 146-12. Ventral thoracic plate (Z-plate, Medtronic Sofamor Danek, Memphis, TN) with posterior bolts in place just before ventral screw placement. Plastic loops are around the sympathetic chain.

recommended, and a combination of bone screws and bolts is used to rigidly lock to the plate. Dorsally, screws are placed 10 degrees ventrally away from the canal. The starting point for the rostral body is 8 to 10 mm inferior and ventral to the upper dorsal corner of the vertebral body on lateral exposure. Conversely, the entry point for the caudal bolt is 8 to 10 mm superior and ventral to the lower dorsal corner of the vertebral body. An awl is used to pierce the cortex, but the bone is not tapped. These bolts can be used for distraction and allow for placement of a strut graft and correction of kyphosis. In patients with suboptimal bone strength, it is useful to use (initially) an intervertebral body spreader to apply force over a broader area. When the strut graft is in place, the bolts can be compressed and locked rigidly to the plate. As a last step, cancellous bone screws are placed through the ventral slots in the plate and angled 10 degrees dorsally. These screws are typically 5 mm longer than the dorsally placed bolts because of the configuration of the vertebral body. Complications can arise from placing a plate that is too long and that extends above or below, across, or into a disc space. This may accelerate degeneration at that motion segment. The usual risks of bicortical screw placement also apply. One must also make sure that the bolts, and especially the bone screws, are not angled down or up into the graft or adjacent disc. The latest version of the Z-plate allows for rigid fixation of the screw heads to the plate.

Anterior Thoracolumbar Locking Plate System

The Synthes plate system (Fig. 146-13) is also low profile and composed of titanium (MRI compatible). It differs from the Z-plate system in that distraction forces are not applied to the bolts or screws but are applied directly to the vertebral body end plates. Synthes makes a long-handled distractor with strong but thin blades that allows perhaps the best access to the graft site during placement of the strut. Once the graft is in place, angled screw hole trajectories in the plate cause up to 3 mm of compression as the screws are driven into the bone. This system uses wide, cancellous screws for unicortical

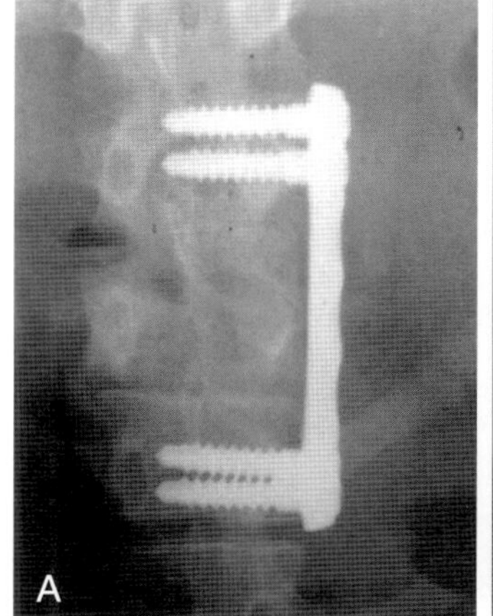

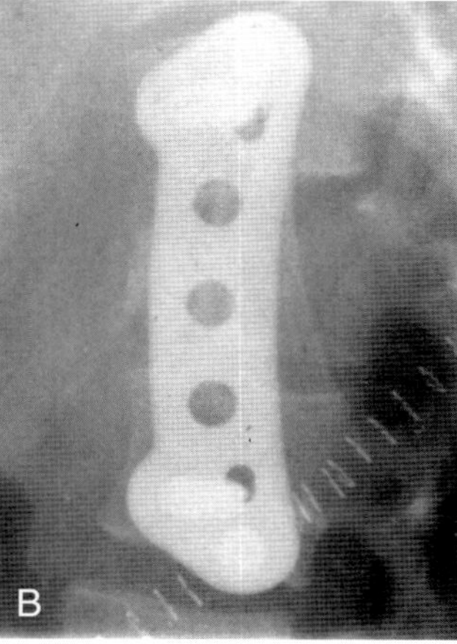

FIGURE 146-13. Ventral (**A**) and lateral (**B**) views of the anterior thoracolumbar locking plate (Synthes Spine, Paoli, PA), with iliac crest bone graft. (Note the convergent path of self-tapping, unicortical screws.)

purchase, although bicortical purchase is an option. Because placement is unicortical, equal-length screws are used dorsally and ventrally. This system has the advantage of being able to effectively provide distraction and compression, is low profile, and is perhaps the simplest in design. It is limited in the amount of compression (2 to 3 mm) provided by the dorsal compression screws. This system is no longer in widespread use.

Interbody (Disc Space) Metallic Devices

Implants have been developed to make interbody (disc space) fixation and fusion easier. These implants can be placed via the ventral approach and are used primarily in the lumbar spine. Either open or laparoscopic placement is possible ventrally. Generically referred to as cages, these cylindrical devices are usually threaded. Currently, implants are available in titanium (Ray cage [Surgical Dynamics]; Harms cage [Moss Systems]; Pyramesh cage, InterFix cage, lordotic LT cage [Medtronic Sofamor Danek]) or are cut from allograft femur (cortical bone dowels [Medtronic Sofamor Danek]). Others are available that are square-shaped and made from carbon fiber (Cougar cage [DePuy Spine]). All of these disc space or interbody implants can be packed with autologous bone to aid arthrodesis. In July 2002, a commercial form of recombinant human bone morphogenetic protein (rhBMP2; InFuse, Medtronic Sofamor Danek) was approved by the Food and Drug Administration for use in anterior lumbar interbody fusion.

Biomechanically, interbody implants offer resistance to axial forces across the ventral and middle columns of the spine and can resist flexion and extension. They are usually placed during distraction of the disc space, allowing for compression of the implant such as a screw. The Harms and the Pyramesh cages are not threaded. They are hollow titanium cages with teeth along both rostral and caudal surfaces that gain purchase into the end plates during placement into the disc space. Interbody implants may be used with or without ventral or dorsal segmental instrumentation (plates, pedicle screws, or hooks).

It may be difficult to assess fusion in the postoperative state because of the artifact from the implants. CT scans with sagittal reconstruction through the middle of the implants can be useful. Flexion and extension radiographs can determine whether pathologic motion is present but cannot directly assess the degree of arthrodesis. Despite these issues, long-term success has been reported.[21]

Summary

Ventral approaches to the thoracic and lumbar spine have advanced because of better understanding of the biomechanics of the spine, the importance of sagittal balance, the radiographic and clinical indications for any given approach, better appreciation of subtle anatomy, and improved implant technology. The recent introduction of commercially available rhBMP also ushers in an era of biologic advantage when performing anterior spinal reconstruction and fusion. Compared with more familiar or frequently practiced posterior approaches, there is significant potential for vascular and visceral injury. For surgeons inexperienced in performing thoracotomy, or thoracoabdominal, transperitoneal, retroperitoneal, or laparoscopic approaches, consideration of further training may be necessary. Alternatively, working with a thoracic, general, or vascular surgeon allows one to develop an experienced, efficient team for anterior thoracolumbar approaches. Recently, minimally invasive anterolateral approaches have also been introduced.

KEY REFERENCES

Alleyne CH, Rodts GE, Haid RW: Corpectomy and stabilization with methylmethacrylate in patients with metastatic disease of the spine. *J Spinal Disord* 8(6):439–443, 1995.

Muhlbauer M, Pfisterer W, Eyb R, et al: Minimally invasive retroperitoneal approach for lumbar corpectomy and anterior reconstruction. *J Neurosurg* 93(Suppl 1):161–167, 2000.

Rodts GE, McLaughlin MR, Zhang JY, et al: Laparoscopic anterior lumbar interbody fusion. *Clin Neurosurg* 47:541–556, 2000.

Rrajaraman V, Vingan R, Roth P, et al: Visceral and vascular complications resulting from anterior lumbar interbody fusion. *J Neurosurg* 91(Suppl 1): 60–64, 1999.

REFERENCES

The complete reference list is available online at expertconsult.com.

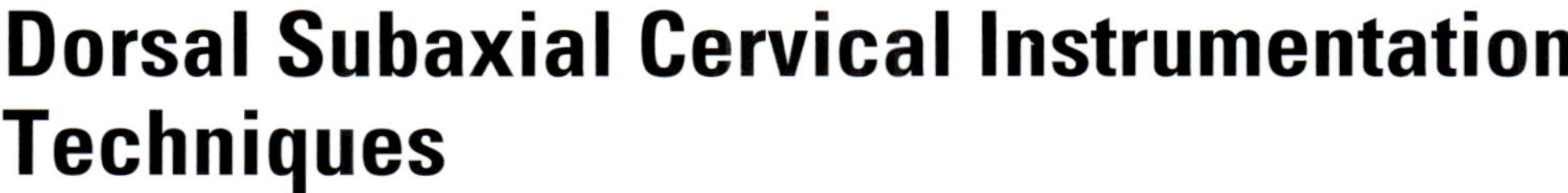

Dorsal Subaxial Cervical Instrumentation Techniques

Harel Deutsch | Kurt Eichholz | Regis W. Haid, Jr. | Vincent C. Traynelis

Subaxial cervical instability has many causes, including trauma, degenerative disease, neoplasm, and infection. Instability may also develop after spinal canal or foraminal decompression or in conjunction with tumor resection. Historically, the management of such instability first consisted of extended immobilization with traction or an orthosis to maintain proper alignment until bony and/or ligamentous healing transpired. Despite the usefulness of these treatment modalities, they predispose patients to a variety of medical complications. Furthermore, such management does not always result in long-term spinal stability. In 1891, Hadra[1] described the role of spinous process wiring to treat traumatic and inflammatory cervical instability. Subsequently a multitude of cervical fusion techniques were reported that used wires secured to the spinous processes, laminae, and/or facets. Cervical wiring techniques are important in the management of cervical instability.

Sophisticated cervical instrumentation has expanded the surgical capabilities for spinal reconstruction. Cervical fixation devices are particularly useful to treat multiplanar or multisegmental instability. Rigid internal stabilization usually provides excellent neural protection until fusion occurs, lessens the number of segments that require fusion, facilitates immediate postoperative mobilization, and minimizes the need for external orthoses. Several dorsal cervical fixation devices have been developed, and each has unique advantages and disadvantages.

This chapter discusses issues pertinent to the application of dorsal cervical instrumentation, including the indications for their use and operative implantation techniques. Specifically, wire fixation, Luque L-rod and rectangle constructs, laminar compression clamps, semirigid and rigid lateral mass fixation, hook-rod instrumentation, and pedicle screw fixation are reviewed. Concordant with the overall theme of this text, complication avoidance and management are emphasized here. Although biomechanical concerns are extremely important in the selection of the proper method of stabilization, they are discussed only briefly in this chapter.

Indications for Surgery

The decision to perform surgery, the operative approach, the need for fusion, and the method by which it is accomplished must be determined on an individual basis. Factors that influence the decision-making process include the patient's overall medical and neurologic condition, the particular pathologic process, the location of the pathology, the degree of instability, and the number of levels affected. These issues, as they pertain to trauma, neoplasia, and degenerative disease, are addressed briefly in this section.

Trauma

Trauma is a common indication for dorsal cervical stabilization.[2] The primary management of cervical spine injuries consists of realignment (when necessary), decompression of the neural elements (when indicated), and stabilization. In the setting of trauma, if the spine is in good alignment and no decompression is necessary, external immobilization may be all that is required to protect the neural elements while healing occurs. This is particularly true when the major cause of the instability is bony injury. Primary ligamentous instability is much less likely to resolve after immobilization; hence early surgical stabilization is often an appropriate consideration in the management of these injuries.

Instrumentation of the dorsal cervical spine should be considered seriously in all trauma victims who require an open reduction or a dorsal cervical decompression. Persistent dorsal ligamentous instability is most appropriately treated by dorsal surgical stabilization; in fact, it is not unreasonable to offer patients with severe ligamentous injuries internal fixation as an alternative to halo immobilization. Fixation across the afflicted level only is usually successful in achieving long-term stabilization in patients with dorsal ligamentous injuries; however, consideration should be given toward incorporating additional levels into the construct in the setting of severe instability[3] (Fig. 147-1). Bony cervical spinal injuries may also be stabilized by using dorsal instrumentation. In particular, cervical lateral mass instrumentation may be used in the presence of laminar and spinous process fractures that often preclude the use of many other types of dorsal fixation.

Extension instability and injuries of the ventral axial spine have been managed successfully by using multilevel dorsal fixation; however, a ventral approach is usually more appropriate. This is particularly true if the spinal canal is compromised from bone or disc fragments or when a burst fracture is associated with 25-degree or greater kyphosis.[3,4]

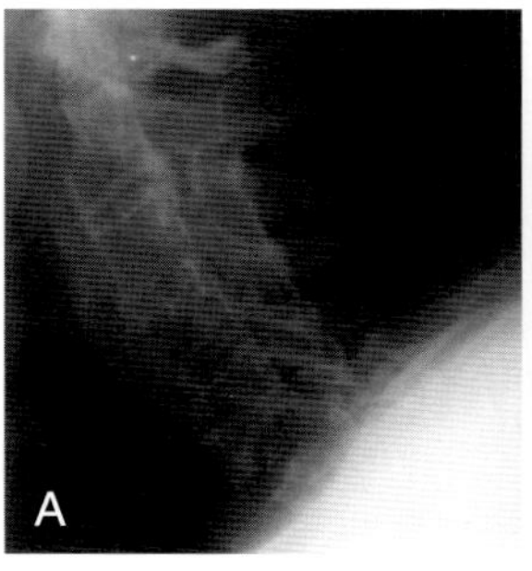
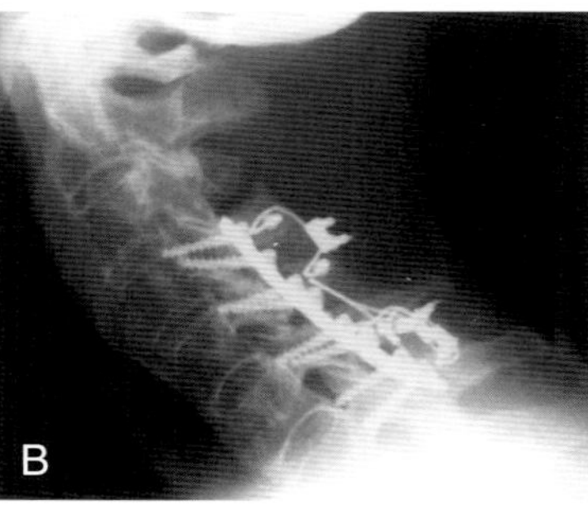

FIGURE 147-1. A, Lateral cervical radiograph demonstrating a C5-6 fracture in a patient with ankylosing spondylitis. **B,** Internal fixation was achieved with lateral mass plates and rib cabled to the spinous processes. The high degree of instability associated with this injury influenced the decision to obtain fixation two levels above and below the injury. Postoperatively the patient wore a rigid orthosis for 2 months. His fusion was noted to be solid 1 year postoperatively.

Neoplasia

Dorsal cervical instrumentation can be useful in the management of instability associated with neoplasia. If tumor resection is performed via an extensive laminectomy and/or a transpedicular approach, immediate internal stabilization may be accomplished with lateral mass plating. The number of motion segments to be instrumented depends on the location and magnitude of the tumor. In the setting of malignancy, the surgeon must be certain that solid fixation is achieved well above and below the affected levels. Significant tumor invasion of the vertebral bodies requires a ventral approach not only for decompression but also for stabilization. It should be remembered that the treatment of benign tumors may also result in cervical instability. This is particularly true when preoperative root and/or cord dysfunction is present and a wide exposure is necessary (e.g., with large neurofibromas).

Spondylosis

Dorsal cervical instrumentation is also useful in the management of spondylotic disease. Proper instrumentation at the time of initial decompression in patients with abnormal segmental motion or absent lordosis markedly decreases their risk of developing postlaminectomy kyphosis. In these cases, instrumentation and subsequent fusion are important to prevent further problems; when a kyphotic deformity has occurred, treatment with dorsal instrumentation alone does not usually provide the optimum result. Almost invariably, ventral spinal reconstruction is the necessary first step needed to correct or halt progressive postlaminectomy kyphotic deformities; dorsal fixation may then be considered as an adjunctive measure in select patients. Dorsal fusion may provide a more successful means of treating patients who experience symptoms from failed ventral arthrodesis than a second ventral surgery.[5,6] In highly selected cases of severe ventral and dorsal spinal incompetence, a combined or staged "360-degree" operation may be indicated.

Osteopenia

It is often difficult to maintain alignment and achieve fusion in severely osteopenic patients regardless of the fixation technique. Osteoporotic spines are also predisposed to screw pull-out, wire cutout, and instrumentation-associated laminar fractures. Increasing points of fixation may be necessary to offset poor bone quality. The use of rigid external orthotics in such patients aids in maintaining stability while fusion occurs.

General Considerations

Imaging

A complete radiographic workup is essential to properly plan and execute any spinal stabilization procedure. This does not mean that every imaging modality must be employed in every patient. MRI is extremely important in the evaluation of cervical pathology because of its excellent multiplanar visualization of the spinal cord, nerve roots, and surrounding soft tissue. Gadolinium contrast MRI studies should be used for imaging possible tumors and infections but have limited benefit in spondylosis. Static plain radiographs provide information concerning segmental and overall alignment and bone quality and should always be obtained. Considering the widespread use of MRI and CT, preoperative radiographs should still be ordered almost routinely. Preoperative radiographs serve as standards against which alignment can be judged after prone positioning and surgery.

Dynamic studies (i.e., flexion-extension lateral views) often provide valuable information, particularly in terms of assessing stability. Although dynamic films should be obtained in most patients, they are not universally appropriate, and judgment must be exercised before obtaining flexion-extension radiographs. Specifically, flexion-extension radiographs should not be obtained in the trauma patient until the potential for significant instability has been ruled out with static films and/or scans.

CT provides better bony detail than MRI and therefore is more useful to define fractures. MRI often complements CT in the trauma setting because of its ability to define ligamentous injury.[7] Both modalities are useful in assessing the extent of tumor involvement in patients with metastatic malignancies. CT myelograms should be considered in patients who are unable to have MRIs or when the MRI is equivocal, such as when a previous instrumentation artifact obscures adequate visualization. CT allows for evaluation of the transverse foramina and, by proxy, the vertebral artery. Localization of the vertebral artery is important in surgical planning for placement of screws in the cervical spine.

Intraoperative Monitoring

Neurophysiologic monitoring can be used to monitor the spinal cord integrity during surgery. Options include monitoring somatosensory-evoked potentials (SSEPs) and motor-evoked potentials (MEPs). SSEPs represent signal-averaged data often over several minutes and monitor the spinal cord dorsal columns. MEPs are usually associated with patient motion during recording and are therefore obtained episodically. Special anesthesia considerations exist with intraoperative monitoring. The usefulness of intraoperative monitoring is established for intradural tumors and vascular malformations but is unclear for other cervical spine surgeries. The authors rarely employ such monitoring (barring experimental protocols) in treating cervical pathology other than intrinsic tumors, vascular malformations, or severe deformities.

Tracheal Intubation

Awake fiberoptic intubations should be considered in patients with significant preoperative instability. Fiberoptic intubation allows for securing the airway with minimal manipulation and extension of the cervical spine. Awake intubation facilitates awake positioning of the patient. Careful intubation under general anesthesia is an alternative to an awake intubation. The head must be held in the neutral position or traction employed if there is a concern for preoperative instability. External orthoses, manual in-line immobilization, and/or axial traction may be used to limit the motion of unstable segments during intubation and positioning.[8-10]

Positioning

The prone position is most frequently used for posterior cervical operations, and positioning the patient is probably more dangerous than intubation because of the possibility of compromising spinal alignment. Awake positioning is a reasonable method of minimizing risk during turning; however, this technique is not advised for uncooperative patients. The surgeon should be responsible for maintaining proper cervical alignment while turning. Neurologic deterioration after positioning warrants prompt physical reappraisal of cervical alignment, evaluation of the amount and direction of axial traction, and radiographic examination. As always, the turn should be performed in a deliberate and controlled manner with care taken to maintain proper cervical alignment. Unstable patients positioned under general anesthesia should have lateral cervical spine films taken after positioning.

Surgical Exposure

The surgical opening should provide adequate visualization, but care should be taken to expose only the levels necessary to safely perform the procedure. Specifically, exposure of articular joints at additional segments should be avoided. The large ligamentous attachments to the spinous process of the axis are preserved when possible. The large ligaments are key in preventing postsurgical kyphosis. Any dorsal supporting structures, such as the interspinous and supraspinous ligaments, should be left intact whenever possible. Exposure should be carried out laterally up to the edge of the lateral mass.

Bony Fusion

Fusion is always part of a cervical instrumentation procedure, and the segments to be fused should be properly prepared. Complete removal of the soft tissues and periosteum from all bone surfaces is required for fusion. The cortex should be scraped with a curet or may be eburnated with a bur. If a drill technique is used, the bur should be of cutting design rather than a diamond. Copious irrigation should be employed while drilling to prevent scorching temperatures, which may inhibit bony fusion. The facet joint is frequently the site of fusion when using dorsal instrumentation. Each facet joint is prepared for fusion by removing all cartilage and scraping or using a bur on the bony joint surfaces. If a dorsal decompression is to be performed as part of the operative procedure, the facet joint is dissected and denuded of cartilage before the laminectomy (or laminectomies) is performed. Theoretically, the longer the spinal cord is protected by the bony and ligamentous dorsal elements, the less the chance of inadvertent intraoperative trauma. Approximation of the bony articular surfaces will result in a successful arthrodesis. Frequently, the lateral mass joint space is packed with autogenous bone to facilitate fusion.

Corticocancellous bone may be obtained from the cervical laminae if a laminectomy is performed. If spinal canal decompression is not warranted, adequate bone for a facet fusion may be obtained from the cervical or upper thoracic spinous processes. Another alternative is to harvest bone from the dorsal iliac crest or a rib.[11] Corticocancellous bone is placed over the dorsal elements.

Hemostasis

After the fusion construct (graft plus instrumentation) has been placed, intraoperative radiographs may be obtained to ensure proper alignment and document hardware position. Before closure, every reasonable effort should be made to achieve hemostasis. In lieu of bone wax, which inhibits bony fusion, thrombin-soaked hemostatic gelatin (Gelfoam [Upjohn, Kalamazoo, MI]) can be pressed into denuded bone surfaces. This maneuver can be a great aid for achieving hemostasis and may not decrease the likelihood of achieving a successful fusion. Epidural venous bleeding can be controlled with bipolar electrocautery. Thrombogenic substances such as oxidized cellulose (Surgicel), autogenous muscle, or thrombin-soaked Gelfoam may be placed in the epidural space, but care must be taken not to compress the neural elements.

Cerebrospinal Fluid Leak

If cerebrospinal fluid (CSF) is noted at any time during the procedure, the site of the leak should be determined. Ideally, all dural defects are closed primarily. If a dural violation cannot be directly repaired, such as may be the case if the defect is located laterally or ventrally, fibrin glue may help seal the leak.[12] If a watertight dural closure is not achieved, wound drains should be avoided. In some situations, lumbar CSF drainage will help decrease the risk of developing a CSF fistula or a pseudomeningocele.

Wound Closure

The wound should be closed in layers with interrupted suture. Removal of the dorsal portion of a prominent C7 and/or T1 spinous process can be extremely helpful for limiting wound tension in slender patients. If local irradiation has been performed or is anticipated, nonabsorbable suture should be considered, at least for the fascial closure. It may be wise to close the entire wound with such suture in these patients. Wound drain placement should be individualized. Some completely dry wounds need no drain; however, if there is oozing from the raw bone surfaces, it may be prudent to place a drain. This is particularly important if a laminectomy has been performed. All wound drains should be tunneled and exit via a separate stab incision.

Dorsal Subaxial Cervical Instrumentation Techniques

Luque Instrumentation

Stainless steel pediatric Luque L-rods and Luque rectangles (Zimmer, Warsaw, IN) may be used to stabilize the cervical spine.[13] The rectangular construct provides greater torsional stability than the L-rods and is therefore preferable. These devices are not indicated for one- or two-level fixation but rather multilevel stabilization procedures. Ideally, both the rods and the rectangles are segmentally secured to every level traversed; however, this is not always necessary. Luque instrumentation can be used to bridge dorsal element defects, such as may occur with metastatic malignancies; however, when using this technique, at least two levels of segmental fixation must be obtained above and below the incompetent region. These devices are most useful for fixation extending to the upper cervical spine or crossing the cervicothoracic junction.

For insertion, the majority of the facet should be exposed at each level one wishes to instrument. It is important to choose a rod or rectangle of correct length. The device should not extend above or below the segments at which arthrodesis is desired. When the proper size is selected, the instrumentation is bent to conform to the normal cervical lordotic curve. After contouring is performed, the surgeon should verify again that the length is appropriate. Luque instrumentation can be secured by using wires or braided cables. Cable is stronger and easier to work with than wire. An effort should be made to obtain segmental fixation at every level to undergo arthrodesis.

Laminar, facet, or spinous process purchase may be used. Cervical sublaminar cables are relatively easy to pass, but their use is associated with risk of neurologic injury. Sublaminar wires should be passed with trepidation in the region of the cervical enlargement of the cord; therefore, sublaminar fixation is often limited to the upper cervical segments (C1, C2), C7, and the upper thoracic spine. Spinal canal stenosis is an absolute contraindication to the use of sublaminar wires and cables. Safe passage of sublaminar wires requires opening the ligamentum flavum and directly visualizing the dura mater.

Sublaminar wires and cables should be passed very carefully by using two hands to push and pull simultaneously. When the wires or cables are passed, they should be held taut with heavy clamps hung over the side of the wound. These maneuvers minimize the risk of ventral displacement of the wire or cable. All wires and cables should be passed without the Luque rods or rectangle in the wound. Some epidural bleeding may occur with the dissection and passage of sublaminar wires and cables, but this often stops as the cables or wires are tightened. If the epidural bleeding persists, hemostatic agents such as thrombin-soaked Gelfoam should be employed.

If sublaminar fixation cannot be obtained, Luque instrumentation may be secured to the lateral masses or the spinous processes. Fixation of Luque instrumentation to an articular mass requires removal of the facet cartilage, entry into the joint space, and drilling of the lateral mass. After removal of the cartilage, a dissector such as a Penfield no. 1 or Freer dissector is inserted into the facet joint and a small drill hole made in the inferior articular process at each level to be instrumented. This hole should be placed at midposition of each inferior facet and be oriented perpendicular to the dorsal articular surface. A wire or cable is passed through this hole, and the ends are secured outside of the wound with a heavy clamp. Before the wires are tightened over the instrumentation, the facet joint is packed with cancellous bone chips. Alternatively, the instrumentation may be secured to the spinous processes with either wires or cables alone or in conjunction with Wisconsin buttons.

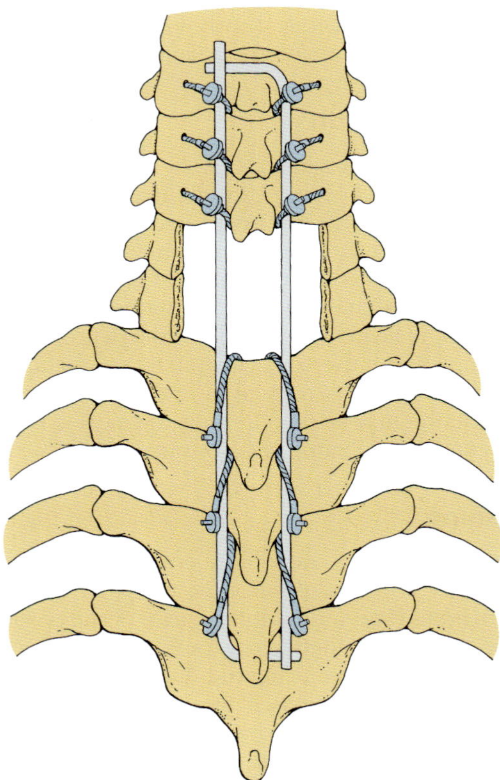

FIGURE 147-2. Illustration of the use of Luque L-rods for stabilization. This figure depicts a wide two-level laminectomy, as may be performed to remove a metastatic lesion, and subsequent stabilization with Luque L-rods. Note how the short arms of the rods are placed under the long arm to improve rotatory stability. Also note that the instrumentation extends several levels above and below the unstable segment and that sublaminar cables are used to secure the thoracic segments, whereas interfacet cable fixation is employed in the cervical region.

Securing the Luque instrumentation to the spine is performed in steps. First, the precontoured device is carefully introduced into the wound, and the previously placed cables or wires are positioned around it. L-rods are placed such that the short arm of each L lies beneath the end of the opposite long arm (Fig. 147-2). The wires or cables are tightened sequentially. Tightening is done gradually so that opposing levels are tightened concurrently, thereby minimizing torsional forces. Cables can generally be tightened to 6 to 8 inch-pounds of torque, but this value should be individualized. Excess wire or cable should be trimmed appropriately before closure to avoid future wound problems (Fig. 147-3). Before closure of the wound, bone grafts may be laid on the laminae and/or the lateral masses.

Compression Clamps

Another method of internal fixation that requires intact laminae to stabilize adjacent levels across one or two motion segments is the interlaminar compression clamp. These devices

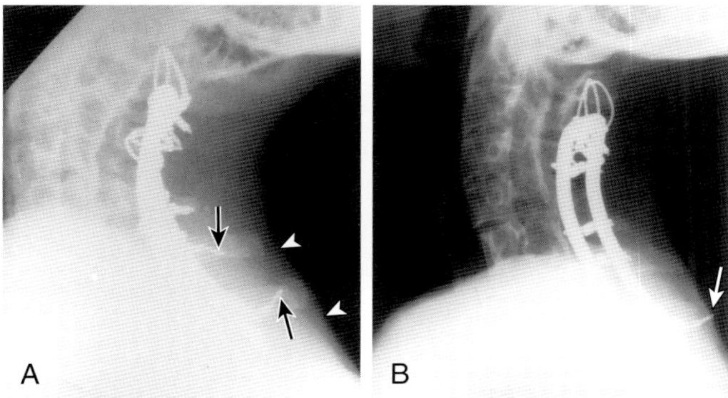

FIGURE 147-3. A, Immediate postoperative radiograph of a patient with ankylosing spondylitis and a fracture who was stabilized with a Luque rectangle. Note that the cables are not trimmed flush with the crimps (*arrows*) but they do not reach the surface of the skin (*arrowheads*). **B,** One year later the inferior cable eroded through to the skin (*arrow*), necessitating a second procedure to trim the cable ends.

include the Halifax clamp (American Medical Electronics, Inc., Richardson, TX) and Apofix (Medtronic Sofamor Danek, Memphis, TN).[14,15] One of the few indications for placement of this device is isolated dorsal ligamentous instability. Although their use in patients with facet injuries and even linear laminar fractures has been reported, they may not be indicated if there is any significant bony injury.[2] Other contraindications to placement of laminar compression clamps are the presence of significant vertebral body injury or facet fractures. Lack of ventral column support should be treated with ventral reconstruction, and loss of facet integrity will predispose the cervical spine to rotatory instability that this device is incapable of correcting.

Lateral exposure need only be carried to the medial or central portion of the facet. The pertinent laminae, spinous processes, and dorsal surface of the facets are denuded of periosteum and their bony surfaces prepared, as mentioned previously. The ligamentum flavum is detached from the laminae to be instrumented. For the Halifax instrumentation, appropriately sized clamps are selected and placed temporarily into the wound to estimate the minimal amount the jaws must be opened to pass over the laminae to be instrumented. The clamps are removed from the wound and adjusted accordingly. This maneuver saves time and decreases the amount of "fiddling" within the wound itself. A piece of corticocancellous bone is fashioned such that the dorsally placed clamps will tightly wedge it against the laminae. The clamps are tightened in a controlled, alternating fashion. Although unilateral implantation of cervical laminar compression clamps has been reported, optimum results can only be expected with bilateral fixation.[14]

The Apofix device is somewhat easier to implant. Each sublaminar hook extends into the tubular longitudinal member. The longitudinal tubes are of slightly different diameters, allowing one to telescope into the other. The hooks are set into position, and bone grafts are placed either between the Apofix instrumentation and the laminae or between the spinous processes. A compression instrument is applied, and the clamps are squeezed together. The tubes are secured in the compressed position by a crimper. The excess tube length is trimmed. The Apofix should be implanted bilaterally. Its design makes it less likely to rotate out of position than the Halifax clamp.

The bony implant is an extremely important part of the construct. It optimizes the chance of obtaining a successful fusion, which is necessary to avoid delayed instrumentation failure. Biomechanically, the interlaminar or interspinous position of the graft enables the entire construct to resist extension. Although compression clamps provide a resistance only to flexion (tension band fixation), if some effort is not made to limit extension at the instrumented segment, they can lose their purchase in extension. The graft also helps maintain proper alignment by acting as a "spacer" between the laminae as the clamps are tightened.

The complication rate for these devices is higher at the atlantoaxial level than in the subaxial cervical spine.[14] This difference is probably due to the large amount of axial rotation that occurs at this level. However, because of the risks of laminar fracture, device dislodgement, and screw loosening associated with laminar compression clamp fixation, the authors believe that if possible, other more effective methods for subaxial dorsal cervical instrumentation should be used.

Hook-Rod Systems

Immediate multilevel fixation may be achieved by using the hook-rod type systems that have been traditionally applied to the thoracolumbar spine. These devices may be used successfully in select cases of cervicothoracic instability.[16] Recently, rod systems have been developed specifically for the cervical spine. These systems primarily achieve rigid fixation by using lateral mass screws attached to the rods. These rods can also be attached to hooks sized to fit the cervical and upper thoracic laminae.[17,18] Avoidance of hook-rod construct complications in the cervical spine begins with a careful and thoughtful assessment of the true need to place such instrumentation.[19-21]

Unlike the thoracolumbar spine, hooks are not usually attached to the pedicles and transverse processes, and cervical fixation is therefore limited to the laminae. When used in the cervical region, these devices are most often applied in compression or as "claw"-type constructs. Pure distraction mode will predispose the cervical spine to kyphosis and is therefore not used.

The application of laminar hooks is described in detail elsewhere in this text. The laminar edge is prepared and a hook inserted. Rods bent to match the cervical lordotic curve are attached to the hooks. Whenever possible, the construct should be cross-linked to increase torsional stability. When instrumenting multiple segments, levels not secured with a hook should be fixed to the rods with sublaminar, facet, or spinous process wires. Care should be taken when designing a hook-rod construct for the cervical spine to avoid crowding the spinal canal significantly with the instrumentation.

Lateral Mass Instrumentation

Stabilization of the subaxial cervical spine with lateral mass instrumentation has gained popularity for a variety of reasons.[22-25] Lateral mass screws may be applied from C2 to the upper thoracic spine, and fixation does not depend on intact laminae or spinous processes. Lateral mass screws provide superb flexural stability and resist torsion and extension significantly better than wiring constructs.[25] In experienced hands, fusion with lateral mass plates requires significantly less operative time than segmentally wiring rib, iliac crest, or rods to the articular masses. The excellent stability achieved with lateral mass instrumentation can decrease or eliminate the need for postoperative orthotics. Lateral mass plates and screws are more expensive than wire, but this cost may be recouped in decreased operative time, diminished need for extensive orthotics, and improved outcomes.

The disadvantages of lateral mass stabilization include the potential for nerve root and vertebral artery injury. As with all cervical instrumentation, lateral mass screws must be used cautiously in osteoporotic patients, and adequate spinal alignment must be achieved before insertion. Lateral mass screws cannot correct kyphotic deformities, significant translation, or subluxation; therefore, normal lordosis or at least neutral alignment should be achieved before instrumentation with positioning or traction. The small screw sizes (on average 3.5-mm diameter × 14-mm length) are not capable of exerting sufficient force to correct spinal deformities or malalignments. Lateral mass instrumentation is also used to augment anterior decompression and kyphotic deformity reduction.

The standard midline approach described previously is expanded so that the entire lateral mass is exposed at each level to be plated. This is necessary to accurately determine proper screw trajectory and to facilitate surface area for arthrodesis. Dislocated facets must be reduced prior to application of instrumentation. The joint space is prepared for fusion as previously described. Occasionally, the facet joints may be lax and partly separated. Often, this occurs in conjunction with posttraumatic ligamentous instability. In these cases, simple interspinous process wiring approximates and preloads the facet joints, thereby rectifying this problem. If an interspinous process wire is used, it can be left after plating to augment flexural stability. If the dorsal elements are incompetent, approximation of separated facets should be attempted with positional adjustments, if possible.

Screw holes are drilled into the lateral masses. Several screw trajectories have been used. Based on anatomic, biomechanical, and clinical observations, we believe the best trajectory begins 1 mm medial to the midportion of the lateral mass and is oriented 15 degrees rostral and 20 to 30 degrees lateral (Fig. 147-4). Although a screw may be placed into C7 by using the angles mentioned, the lateral mass of this vertebra is very small. If C7 lateral mass fixation is desired, it may be more appropriate to drill by using trajectories that are slightly more rostral and lateral. It is often preferable to obtain pedicle fixation at C7 (as well as at T1). The pedicle may be entered 1 mm caudal to the facet joint. Drilling may continue in a directly ventral course, but a trajectory that angles medially 25 to 30 degrees is more consistent with the anatomic position of the pedicle. The orientation is perpendicular to the long axis of the spine at C7, T1, and T2[26,27] (Fig. 147-5). It is our practice to verify the position of the pedicle by palpation through a small laminoforaminotomy prior to drilling in all cases.

Screws may also be placed into the pars interarticularis of the axis. This technique is more difficult than placing lateral mass screws, and precision is required to avoid vertebral artery injury. The drill entry site is high and medial on the articular mass. The trajectory is as great as 15 degrees from the medial plane and is about 35 degrees from the long axis of the spine[6,28] (Fig. 147-6). Fluoroscopy is not necessary for

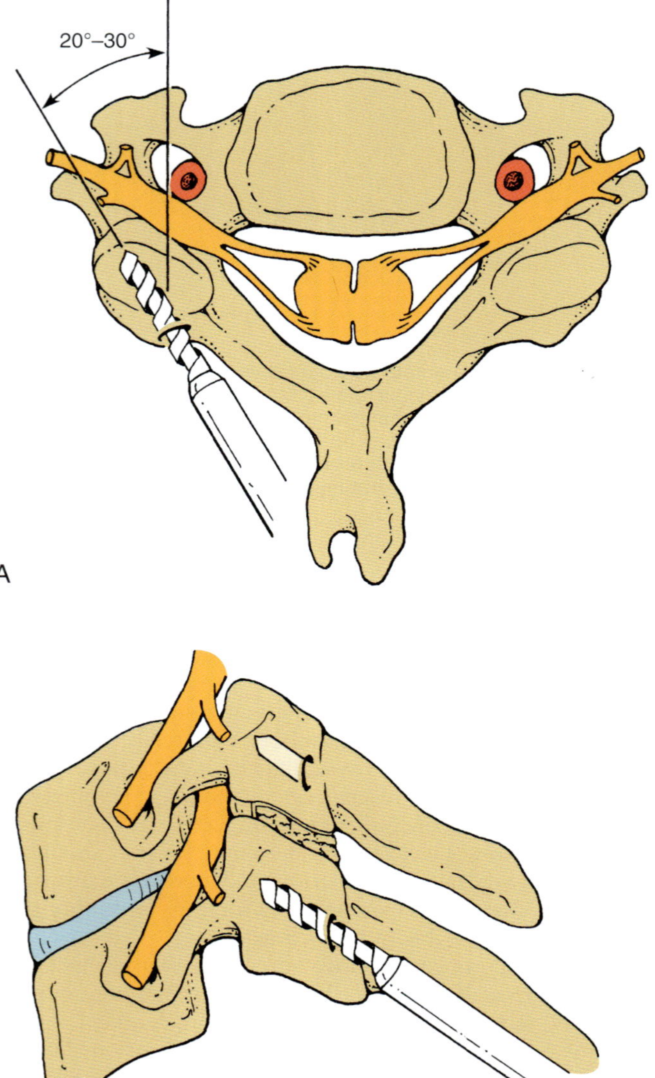

FIGURE 147-4. A, Lateral trajectory for subaxial articular mass drilling. **B,** Sagittal trajectory for articular mass drilling. Note that the facet joint is packed with autogenous bone.

subaxial lateral mass drilling and screw placement, but it should be used when instrumenting the C2 pars.

The dorsal cortex of the lateral mass is perpendicularly pierced with an awl or drill bit to facilitate initial drilling and limit the potential for deviation from the proposed trajectory. One should use a drill bit that incorporates a depth stop, usually at 14 mm. The diameter of the drill bit must comply with the manufacturer's recommendation for the particular screw to be implanted. Drilling is performed in a precise and steady manner to limit vibration and inadvertent creation of an irregular or oversized hole. Occasionally, the drill bit will be felt to penetrate the ventral cortex before its entire length is used. In this situation, drilling should stop. All of the holes on one side should be drilled and prepared and a plate or rod placed before drilling the opposite side. The screws used for lateral mass fixation are most frequently 3.5 mm in diameter. Cancellous screws provide better purchase than those with

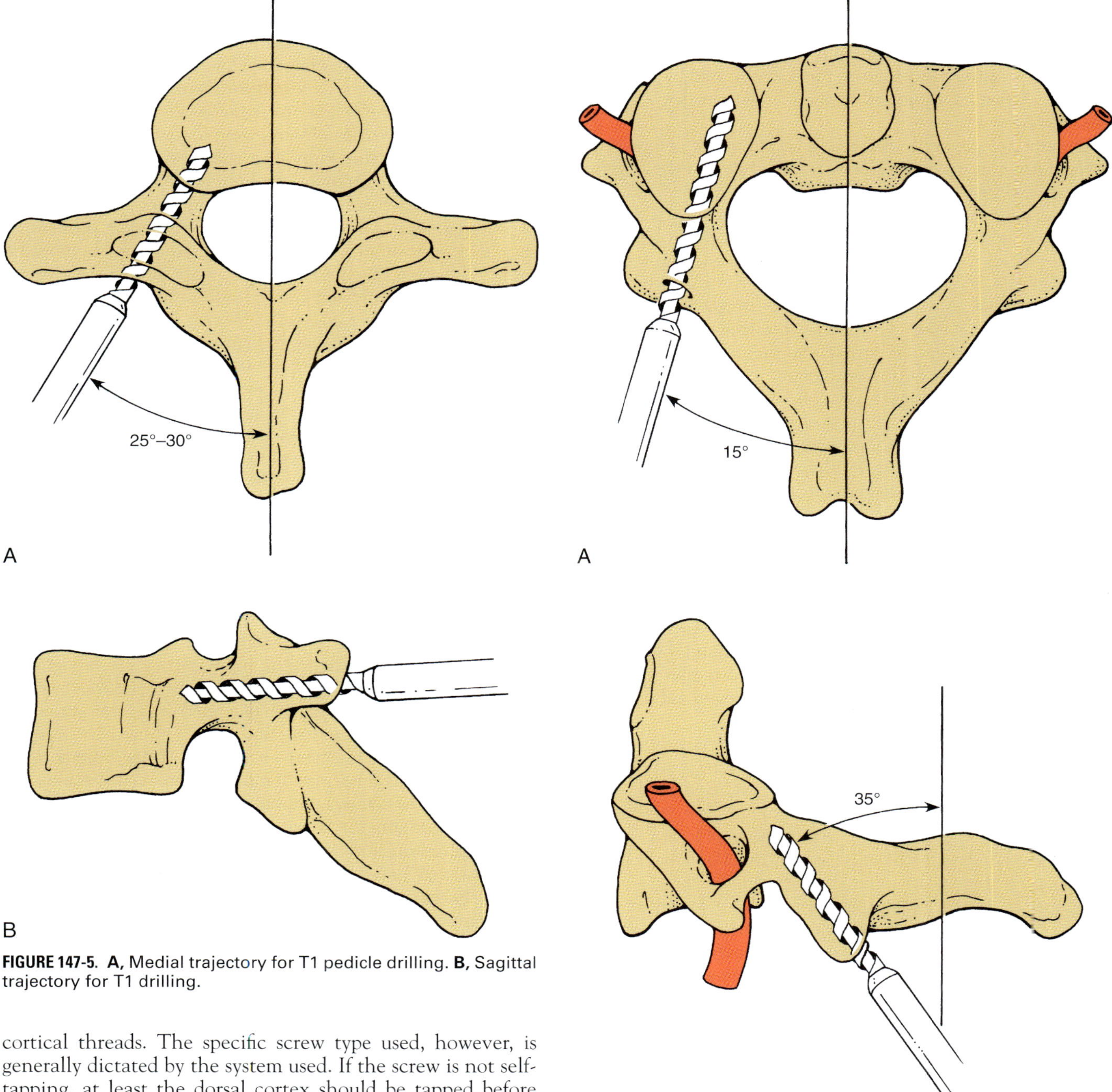

FIGURE 147-5. **A,** Medial trajectory for T1 pedicle drilling. **B,** Sagittal trajectory for T1 drilling.

FIGURE 147-6. **A,** Medial trajectory for drilling of the C2 pars interarticularis. **B,** Sagittal trajectory for drilling of the C2 pars interarticularis.

cortical threads. The specific screw type used, however, is generally dictated by the system used. If the screw is not self-tapping, at least the dorsal cortex should be tapped before screw insertion. Safe bicortical fixation is usually achieved with 14- to 16-mm screws. Only rarely are longer screws necessary, and shorter screws are appropriate for smaller patients. Although bicortical fixation is considered superior to unicortical fixation, it is not mandatory.[28,29] Primary pedicle fixation may be achieved with 4-mm diameter screws.

Inadequate screw purchase may result from osteoporosis, an excessively large hole secondary to inadvertent toggling during drilling, or stripping of threads in the corticocancellous bone during tapping or screw placement. Frequently, in these cases, a "rescue" screw of slightly larger diameter will improve bony purchase.[30] These are not placed without risk, however, because they may result in a fracture of the lateral mass. Alternatively, a small amount of polymethylmethacrylate may be placed in the hole before screw tightening. Cervical transfacet screws are an excellent choice for salvaging fixation if a lateral mass screw strips. The purchase achieved by these screws is excellent.[31] In selected cases, one may wish to place additional graft material over the dorsal elements after denuding their periosteum and burring the dorsal cortical surface.[18] Rods are then contoured and secured using set screws. Excessive force using a rod persuader in securing the screws to the rod should be avoided because the small lateral mass screws may dislodge from the lateral mass if force is applied to reduce the screw to the rod. Additionally, the close proximity to the cervical spinal cord can result in slippage and neurologic injury. Securing the rod is facilitated by the small 3.0- to 3.5-mm titanium rod diameters allowing for some rod flexibility.

Screws are generally polyaxial, allowing for greater freedom in orientation of the bone screw in relation the longitudinal rod. Some screws are "favored-angle screws," allowing for fewer angulations in certain planes and a bias in the way the screw saddle sits on the screw. Lateral offset connectors can be placed if a screw is significantly outside the rod longitudinal axis, as sometimes occurs with the transition from lateral mass screws to thoracic pedicle screws. Final tightening is often achieved using a torque-limiting screwdriver and antitorque instrument. Sets may also include occipital plates and mechanisms to transition to larger rod diameters used in the thoracic spine. Longer screws are often available for upper thoracic pedicle screw placement as well as for C1 placement. Because lateral mass fixation is successful in almost all patients and has little risk, we do not advocate pedicle fixation from C3 to C6 except in unusual circumstances.[32-34]

Postoperative Care

Thoughtful preoperative planning and strict adherence to meticulous surgical technique limit complications; however, complications invariably occur, even in the hands of the most careful and experienced surgeon. Some particular considerations are important to address complications in patients who undergo dorsal cervical fusion.

Immediate postoperative radiographs may be obtained to ensure proper cervical alignment and hardware position. Any deterioration in the patient's neurologic condition after surgery indicates the need for a complete workup. Although titanium alloy hardware is compatible with radiographic studies and MRI, these constructs still cause some artifact and may obscure pathology. If there is any question regarding postoperative spinal canal or neural foraminal compromise or hardware complication in a patient with neurologic deterioration, it may be prudent to obtain a myelogram or CT or reexplore the wound.

Postoperatively, patients should be mobilized. Radiographic assessment should be performed to ensure stability of the spinal construct. Appropriate external orthoses should supplement the internal fixation if there is preoperative instability or the bony purchase is suboptimal. If instability in a single plane of motion exists preoperatively and the surgeon is confident that the fixation is solid, then either no bracing or a soft cervical collar may be appropriate. A 360-degree procedure or more rigid external orthosis such as a halo vest may be needed when dealing with gross multiplanar instability or when the integrity of the construct is in question. The duration of external cervical immobilization is also individualized.

Complication Management

Postoperative complications may be subdivided into the following groups: general, neurologic, and spinal. Postoperative hematomas, CSF leaks, and wound infections are examples of general complications.

General Complications

Large postoperative wound hematomas can cause significant neurologic impairment. Smaller clots predispose the patient to infection by acting as a culture medium. Before closure, every effort must be made to achieve adequate hemostasis. Avoidance of hypertension and wound elevation and correction of coagulopathies help limit intraoperative hemorrhage. Thrombin-soaked Gelfoam can help decrease bone bleeding. Epidural venous hemorrhage may occur after a laminectomy or after passage of sublaminar wires. Whenever possible, it should be controlled with bipolar coagulation and hemostatic agents. Epidural bleeding associated with sublaminar instrumentation is usually self-limited and stops prior to wound closure. In very rare cases, such bleeding is brisk and does not cease, in which case one should consider exposing the spinal canal and directly attacking the source of hemorrhage.

Maintenance of a subperiosteal dissection plane minimizes muscle bleeding. Most significant muscular bleeding comes from violation of small and medium-sized veins. Bleeding from these vessels can be controlled by the pressure exerted by wound retractors. When the retractors are removed, the wound must be irrigated several times and a Valsalva maneuver performed by the anesthetist so these potential sources of postoperative hemorrhage may be identified and cauterized. Postoperative wound drainage is generally used routinely.

Frequent and regular wound inspection in the early postoperative period allows for the early identification of complications such as a wound infection or CSF fistula. Wound infections should be treated as soon as they are recognized. Wound infections typically manifest as persistent wound drainage. Antibiotic coverage is guided by Gram stain and culture results. Any fluid accumulations should be drained. Areas of loculated infection or regions of devitalized tissue should be treated surgically. If an infection occurs, it may not be necessary to remove implanted hardware, particularly if expeditious treatment is rendered. When an infection persists despite antibiotic coverage or if the construct integrity is threatened or compromised by significant osteomyelitis, it may be necessary to remove the instrumentation. If the instrumentation must be removed, immobilization, external orthosis, or traction may be used to manage instability. Rarely, a ventral stabilization procedure may be useful in these cases. It should be noted that metallic instrumentation may not be threatened by infection and does not usually need to be removed. This is particularly true when the infection remains superficial to the fascia.

The management of intraoperative CSF leaks has been discussed. Postoperative leakage of CSF from the wound should be treated aggressively with surgical reexploration accompanied by lumbar CSF drainage. The possibility of a wound infection must always be considered and definitively ruled out in these patients.

Neurologic Complications

Neurologic complications may be immediate or delayed. The workup of new postoperative neurologic deficits should proceed with great urgency. The possible causes of immediate deficits are numerous. Many instrumentation-related causes of neurologic deficit may be determined radiographically, but the evaluation of these patients must be individualized.

Delayed neurologic complications are more likely to be due to instrumentation failures, loss of reduction, or infection. Although evaluation of delayed deficits is dictated by the specific clinical presentation, all such cases should be promptly investigated and appropriate treatment instituted.

Placement of instrumentation may result directly in neurologic compromise. Lateral mass screws have the potential to compress or injure the nerve roots, spinal cord, and vertebral artery. Spinal cord injury secondary to lateral mass screws has not been reported to our knowledge. Anatomic studies support the concept that the spinal cord is not placed at any great risk from lateral mass screw placement. The direction of drill trajectory and screw placement is important for limiting the risk of arterial or root injury. Roy-Camille et al.[28] advocate a screw position that begins at the center of the lateral mass, is oriented perpendicular to the long axis of the spine, and is angled 10 degrees laterally. The Magerl technique involves placement of the screw 2 to 3 mm medial and rostral to the center of the lateral mass and a trajectory that runs parallel to the facet joint and is angled 25 degrees laterally.[35] Anderson et al.[22] suggest screw placement 1 mm medial to the center of the lateral articular mass with trajectory parallel to the facet joints and oriented 10 degrees laterally from the sagittal plane, whereas Cooper et al.[23] recommend placement of the screws 1 mm medial to the center of the lateral articular mass and oriented 10 degrees laterally but perpendicular to the long axis of the spine.

Overall, there seems to be a general agreement that the screw trajectory should be at least 10 degrees laterally and oriented no more rostral than the articular surface of the facet joint to minimize the risk of inadvertent injury to the nerve root or vertebral artery.[26,36] Cadaveric studies that use such a trajectory suggest that the predicted rates of injury to the nerve roots and vertebral artery would be 3.6% or less and 0%, respectively.[36] The actual clinical incidence of nerve root injury secondary to screw placement is much less. In a review of 704 lateral mass screw placements in 79 patients, Heller et al.[37] reported a 0.6% rate of nerve root injury. Patients with postoperative radiculopathy secondary to malpositioned screws usually improve significantly with removal of the offending screw.

Despite the fear of vertebral artery injury with lateral mass screw placement, vertebral artery injuries are very rare. Lateral angling of the screws is important to minimize the risk of vascular compromise. Vertebral artery injury may or may not be recognized at the time of surgery. There is usually bleeding from the drill hole in the lateral mass, and at times the flow may seem brisk; however, it should never be pulsatile or appear to be under high pressure. When arterial hemorrhage is noted after lateral mass drilling, an attempt may be made to control the hemorrhage by placement of thrombogenic substances and bone wax in the drill hole. A screw may be placed in the hole to control bleeding. Screw placement is not unreasonable if one assumes that (if vertebral artery injury has indeed occurred) the drill has already significantly lacerated the vertebral artery. If the bleeding is refractory to these measures, it may be necessary to expose the vertebral artery for primary repair or occlusion. No contralateral drilling or screw placement should be performed if a vertebral artery injury is suspected intraoperatively, and the patient must be examined immediately on conclusion of the procedure. Vertebral artery injury or occlusion may not be apparent immediately. The development of delayed posterior circulation deficits should alert the surgeon to this possibility. We recommend prompt angiographic evaluation of suspected vertebral artery injuries.

Spinal Complications

Postoperative spinal instrumentation complications usually, but not always, concern failure to maintain immediate or long-term stability. Poorly conceived stabilization procedures probably account for most dorsal cervical construct failures (Fig. 147-7). When a cervical kyphotic deformity is not adequately reduced, the instrumentation rate failure is increased. Instrumentation should be applied judiciously in osteoporotic patients, and in such individuals a 360-degree approach or postoperative external immobilization is very important. Preoperative evaluation and planning are important to ensure that the proposed construct is biomechanically appropriate for the clinical situation.

Instrumentation failure may occur without clinical consequence.[3] Heller et al.[37] observed a 1.3% rate of plate breakage over an average follow-up of 1.5 years. In the same review, the following incidences of screw complications were noted: breakage 0.1%, avulsion 0.1%, and loosening 0.9%. Minor instrumentation failures (i.e., 1-mm screw loosening) or those that occur many months after surgery (i.e., single wire breakage) often do not require treatment. Significant or early postoperative instrumentation failures and loss of reduction must be addressed. The management options include institution of rigid external immobilization, bedrest, and/or cervical traction during healing, or reoperation (either repeat dorsal approach or ventral instrumentation). The decision for appropriate treatment must be made on an individual basis, taking into consideration the patient's condition and prognosis, degree of bony union and instability, and rationale for initial choice of dorsal surgical stabilization.

Summary

Dorsal cervical instrumentation systems that are appropriately selected for the clinical problem, and properly implanted, generally produce excellent results and enjoy a low rate of complication. As with all surgical procedures, the complication rate is related to experience. Before using any of the techniques mentioned in this chapter, surgeons should acquaint themselves fully with the instrumentation and obtain adequate preoperative instruction if they are unfamiliar with the proposed procedure.

Some of the instrumentation systems described in this chapter are currently categorized as class III devices by the United States Food and Drug Administration. Surgeons should be aware of the classification of the instrumentation to be implanted and relay this information to the patient during the preoperative discussion. Most internal fixation devices are classified as temporary devices. *Temporary* is defined as a device intended to be implanted for more than 30 days but not intended to be implanted permanently. The Orthopedic Surgical Manufacturer's Association recommends that, whenever possible and practical, bone fixation devices should be removed when their service as an aid to healing is completed; however, the general clinical opinion is that cervical

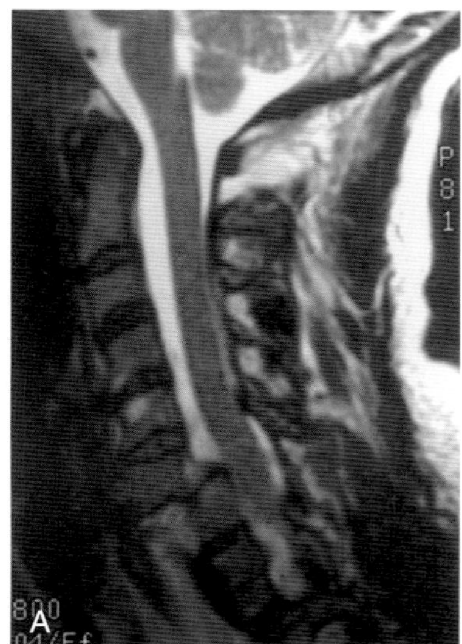

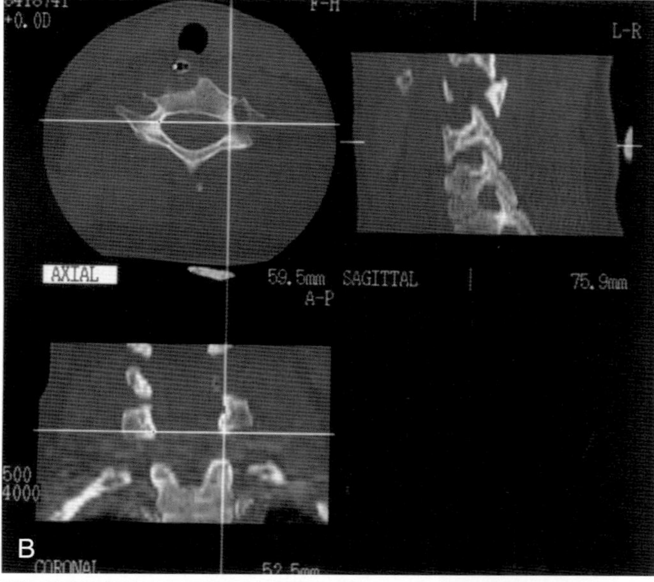

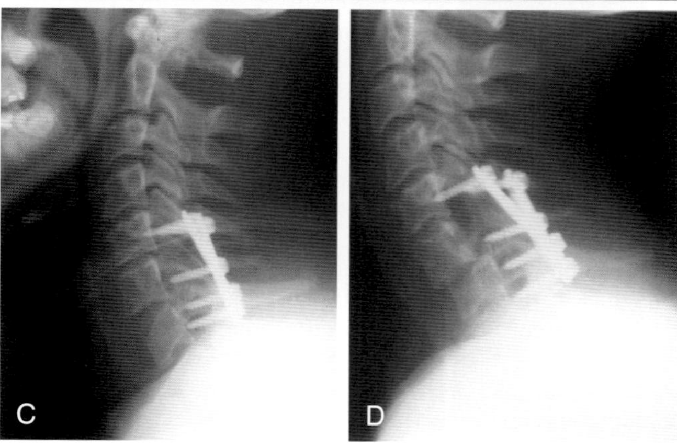

FIGURE 147-7. Severe C6-7 fracture-dislocation in a patient with only minor neurologic deficit. **A,** MRI on admission demonstrates significant ventral and dorsal injury. **B,** Reconstructed CT images demonstrate complete loss of left C6 facet integrity. **C,** After realignment, lateral mass plate stabilization was performed and the patient was immobilized in a halo for 3 months. **D,** Lateral radiograph after halo removal demonstrates resubluxation. This loss of reduction could probably have been prevented by either a 360-degree stabilization procedure or by extending the levels of dorsal fixation.

instrumentation that leads to successful fusion without complication does not need to be removed. Each patient should receive preoperative counseling concerning this difference of opinion. When patients understand the risks of repeat surgery yet request removal of hardware after bone fusion has occurred, every attempt should be made to comply with their wishes.

KEY REFERENCES

Abumi K, Shono Y, Ito M, et al: Complications of pedicle screw fixation in reconstructive surgery of the cervical spine. *Spine (Phila Pa 1976)* 25(8):962–969, 2000.

An HS, Gordin R, Renner K: Anatomic considerations for plate-screw fixation of the cervical spine. *Spine (Phila Pa 1976)* 16:S548–S551, 1991.

Heller JG, Silcox DH III, Sutterlin CE III: Complications of posterior cervical plating. *Spine (Phila Pa 1976)* 20:2442–2448, 1995.

Maurer PK, Ellenbogen RG, Ecklund J, et al: Cervical spondylotic myelopathy: treatment with posterior decompression and Luque rectangle bone fusion. *Neurosurgery* 28:680–683, 1991.

Mummaneni PV, Haid RW, Traynelis VC, et al: Posterior cervical fixation using a new polyaxial screw and rod system: technique and surgical results. *Neurosurg Focus* 12(1):E8, 2002.

Traynelis VC: Anterior and posterior plate stabilization of the cervical spine. *Neurosurg Q* 2:59–76, 1992.

Wellman BJ, Follett KA, Traynelis VC: Complications of posterior articular mass plate fixation of the subaxial cervical spine in 43 consecutive patients. *Spine (Phila Pa 1976)* 23:193–200, 1998.

REFERENCES

The complete reference list is available online at expertconsult.com.

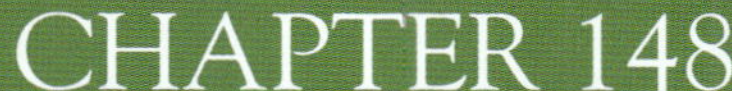

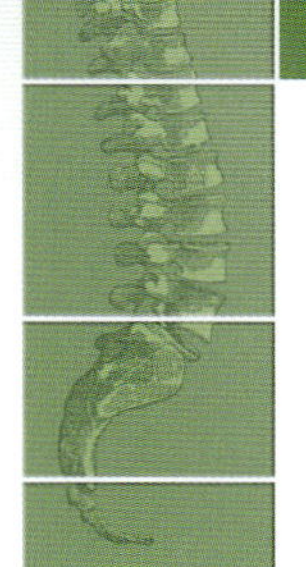

CHAPTER 148

Dorsal Thoracic and Lumbar Screw Fixation and Pedicle Fixation Techniques

Mehmet Zileli | Charles B. Stillerman | Edward C. Benzel

The popularity of pedicle-screw fixation has significantly increased in the past 2 decades. Pedicle-screw fixation is the only spinal fixation strategy that engages all three columns of the spine. The pedicle screw–bone junction provides the strongest point of attachment of instrumentation to the spine. Thus, pedicle-screw fixation systems can resist motion in all planes.[1] In addition, pedicle-screw systems do not require the presence of intact dorsal elements. A historic cohort study with the participation of 303 surgeons and 3498 patients has shown that the use of pedicle screws is a safe and effective form of treatment for spinal disorders.[2]

History

Toumey[3] in 1943 and King[4] in 1948 provided the first descriptions of the use of bone screws to obtain internal fixation at the time of fusion. Their techniques for lumbosacral fusion involved passing a screw from medial to lateral across the facet of the involved level bilaterally. Their screws were short and designed to cross the facet joint only. Pseudarthrosis rates were unacceptably high with this method of fixation.[5] For this reason, Boucher[6] modified their technique by using a longer screw that crossed the facet joint into the pedicle and body of the vertebra below. Boucher[6] was the first to use pedicle screws. The pseudarthrosis rate for this technique, including multilevel fusions, was 14% to 17%.[5,7] Magerl[8] introduced another variation of facet screws in which a screw was passed from one side of the spinous process into the opposite lamina between its two tables, across the facet joint to the base of the transverse process. One disadvantage of the Magerl technique was that it required intact laminae.

Harrington[9] initially used facet screws at multiple levels to correct scoliosis in patients with polio but found that this instrumentation eventually failed. This failure led to the development of Harrington instrumentation. Harrington[10] first used screws inserted into the pedicles of L5 attached to Harrington distraction rods by heavy stainless steel wire for the reduction and stabilization of spondylolisthesis. Roy-Camille[11] was the first to use pedicle screws connected to a dorsal plate. Beginning in 1963, Roy-Camille[11] used pedicle-screw fixation in the thoracic and lumbar spine for fractures, for instability after the resection of vertebral tumors, and in lumbosacral fusions. A biomechanical study by Panjabi et al.[12] demonstrated that facet-screw fixation stability was relatively low in flexion-extension and lateral bending compared with pedicle-screw fixation systems. Because pedicle fixation systems proved to be biomechanically superior for segmental fixation, numerous variations were developed. The first system that used both screws and hooks, connecting them with rods or plates (i.e., universal spinal instrumentation), was introduced by Cotrel and Dubousset.[13]

Pedicle-Screw Fixation

The pedicle is the sole bridge between the posterior column and the middle and the anterior columns. Hence, pedicle screws traverse all three columns and as such can rigidly stabilize both the ventral and dorsal aspects of the spine. However, hook-rod systems are affixed only to the posterior spinal elements. For these reasons, pedicle-screw fixation systems, at least in the lumbar spine, are more commonly used than hook-rod systems. Commonly used implant systems are listed in Box 148-1.

Advantages of Pedicle-Screw Fixation

The nature of the pedicle screw–bone junction is much more secure than the wire or hook-bone junction. A single screw provides stability in five planes of motion.[1] With transverse connection to the other side, stability is achieved in all six planes of motion.[1] The rigidity of pedicle fixation allows for the incorporation of fewer normal motion segments to achieve stabilization of an abnormal level. Because the pedicle represents the strongest point of attachment to the spine, significant forces can be applied to the spine without failure of the bone-metal junction.

BOX 148-1. **Commonly Used Implant Systems**

Cotrel-Dubousset (CD)
Texas Scottish Rite Hospital (TSRH)
Variable Screw Placement (VSP)
Isola
AO internal fixator
MOSS-MIAMI
Xia Spinal System
Synergy Variable Locking Screw (VLS)

Pedicle-screw fixation systems are superior in restoring and maintaining spinal alignment. Because they traverse all three columns of the spine, they provide a longer lever arm through which the longitudinal member can transmit greater corrective forces than are achieved with spine fixation systems that attach to the posterior elements alone. Just as pedicle fixation systems resist loads in multiple planes, they are able to apply multidirectional corrective forces.

Another advantage of pedicle fixation systems is that they do not require intact dorsal elements. Thus, they can be used after laminectomy or traumatic disruption of the laminae, spinous processes, or facets. Pedicle fixation systems also avoid placement of instrumentation in the spinal canal, unlike sublaminar wires and hooks. Additionally, postoperative bracing requirements may be less than with earlier, biomechanically inferior fixation devices. Finally, fusion rates are thought to be improved with the pedicle-screw systems compared with earlier devices,[14-16] as well as with noninstrumented fusions.[14-17]

Disadvantages of Pedicle-Screw Fixation

A steep learning curve is required for the safe implantation of pedicle screws. Caudal or medial penetration of the pedicle cortex can result in durotomy or neural injury. Implantation of pedicle screws requires extensive tissue dissection to expose the entry points and to provide the required lateral to medial orientation for optimal screw trajectory. Lengthy operations with significant blood loss and an increased risk of infection are not uncommon. Significant osteoporosis is a relative contraindication to the use of pedicle screws because a solid screw purchase is difficult to achieve. Postoperative imaging techniques (especially MRI) are, in part, obscured by the implant. Rigid fixation can accelerate adjacent motion segment degeneration. These are costly procedures.

Pedicle Anatomy

The pedicle is a very strong, cylindrical, anatomic bridge between the dorsal spinal elements and the vertebral body. It is composed of a strong shell of cortical bone and a core of cancellous bone.

Pedicle size and angulation varies throughout the spinal column. The transverse pedicle width is narrower than the sagittal pedicle width (pedicle height) except in the lower lumbar spine.[18] Pedicle width is more important than pedicle height for pedicle-screw placement (Fig. 148-1A). The transverse pedicle width increases from L1 to S1.[19] Most of the pedicles below T10 are greater than 7 mm in transverse diameter, and most below L1 are greater than 8 mm in diameter.[20] In a study measuring the pedicle diameters with CT, Bernard and Seibert[21] found that 20% of pedicles were less than 7 mm at L2, 15.6% at L3, and 1.9% at L4. There were no pedicles less than 7 mm in diameter at L5 and S1. They concluded that all surgeons should perform preoperative CT scans when instrumenting pedicles above L4.

The transverse pedicle angle or coronal plane angulation (Fig. 148-1B) decreases as one descends caudally in the spine until the lumbar region. The angle increases as the lumbar spine is descended. The sagittal pedicle angle (Fig. 148-1C) is steep throughout the midthoracic spine and in the upper lumbar spine.[18]

The intrathecal nerve roots course along the medial aspect of the pedicle. At T12, the dural sac is 0.2 to 0.3 mm away from the pedicle.[18] Below L1, the medial side of the pedicle

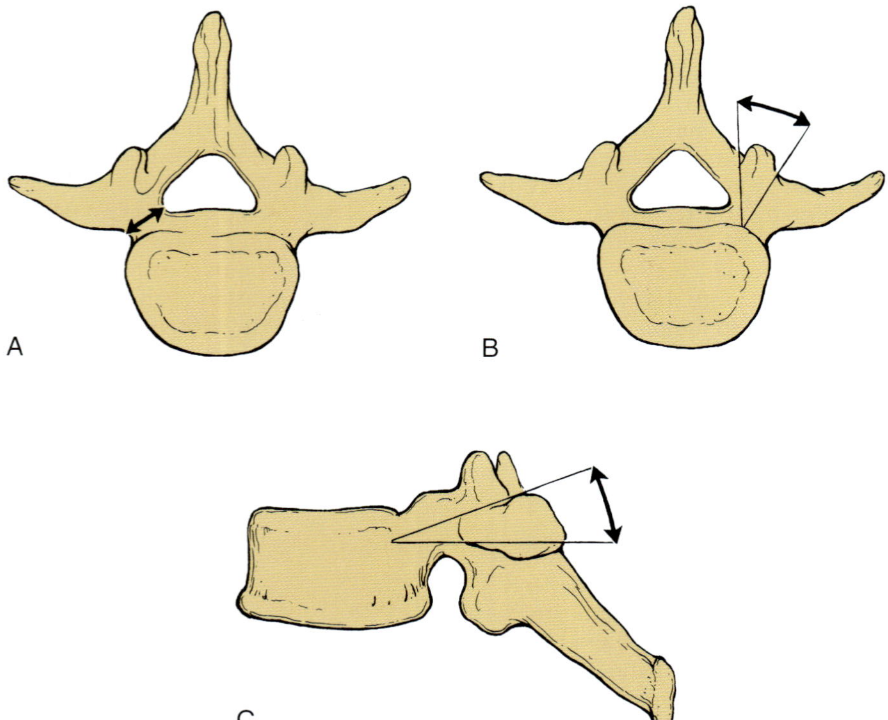

FIGURE 148-1. Diagram illustrating the pedicle width (**A**), the transverse or coronal pedicle angle (**B**), and the sagittal pedicle angle (**C**).

is almost touching the cauda equina. The nerve root occupies the ventral and rostral one third of the foramen. As a result, violation of the medial or caudal cortex of the pedicle risks injury to the nerve root.

Biomechanics

Rigid pedicle fixation techniques, such as rigid plate or screw-rod combinations, apply force to the spine by fixed moment arm cantilever beam fixation.[22] A cantilever is a projecting beam that is supported at one end only. It resists axial loads by rigidly buttressing the spine. In the absence of load sharing with the anterior column, significant stress occurs at the screw-plate or screw-rod junction. These constructs tend to fail by screw fracture at this junction.[23] However, modifications of the spinal implants (as discussed subsequently) have reduced the incidence of screw breakage.

Pedicle-screw fixation systems in which the screws are not rigidly affixed to the plate allow toggling of the screws (Fig. 148-2A). These systems constitute nonfixed moment arm cantilever beam fixation.[22] They are unable to resist axial loads without the assistance of an anterior column, which is capable of axial load bearing. Because these systems allow toggling of the screws, they may fail by screw pull-out (Fig. 148-2B).[22] For this reason, a fixed moment arm system more effectively resists sagittal translation.

Pedicle-screw fixation can be applied with either a flexion component or an extension component to the applied moment arm, which is usually a rigid pedicle fixator.[22] These constructs are used to reduce deformities. Extension moment arm application is their most common mode of application in this regard.

Pedicle fixation techniques may fail during axial loading. This is in part due to a tendency toward the development of a parallelogram-like translational deformity. Toeing-in of the screws and the use of transverse connectors help prevent this mechanism of construct failure.[24]

The most frequently encountered problems with pedicle-screw fixation are hardware failure or failure at the screw-bone junction. Screw pull-out, breakage, and toggle are often the result of biomechanically inappropriate applications.

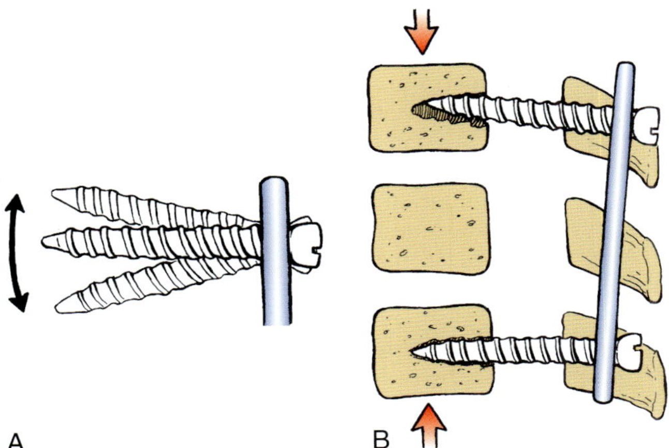

FIGURE 148-2. Pedicle fixation systems in which the screws are not rigidly affixed to the plate allow toggling of the pedicle screws (**A**). These systems may fail by screw pull-out (**B**).

Screw Characteristics

Most pedicle screws have a cancellous thread pattern. In general, screw outside diameters range from 4.5 to 7 mm. Screw lengths are measured from the tip of the screw to the base of the screw head. Pedicle-screw lengths range from 30 to 55 mm, with 5-mm increments. There are two predominant types of pedicle screws: self-tapping and nontapping screws. With nontapping screws, a separate tap is used to cut threads into the pedicle.

Screw strength is proportional to the cube of the core (minor) diameter.[25] The larger the minor diameter, the greater the resistance to screw bending or breakage. The outside (major) diameter is an important factor in screw pull-out resistance. Other important components of pull-out resistance are the thread depth, pitch, and shape. Thread pitch is the distance from one point on the screw thread to the corresponding point on the adjacent thread. Pull-out resistance is directly proportional to the volume of bone between the threads that is determined by the thread depth and pitch. The angle or shape of the thread can affect the interthread volume and hence the pull-out resistance.[25]

Some systems (e.g., compact Cotrel-Dubousset [CD]) have a smooth extended neck without threads. The diameter of this portion of the neck is greater than the tip and the body. This construction increases the strength of the neck of the screw where most breaks occur. Some systems use screws with a conical inner diameter. This conical shape minimizes screw fracture by increasing the diameter of the screw where it is most likely to fail.

Polyaxial heads have made the pedicle screw more versatile. Therefore, the screws may be easily connected to the rod. However, polyaxial pedicle screws have lower strength than conventional pedicle screws, and they are vulnerable to fatigue failure.[26] A biomechanical study has demonstrated that the polyaxial head coupling to the screw is the first to fail and may be a protective feature of the pedicle screw, preventing pedicle-screw breakage.[27]

Preoperative Planning and Surgery

Usually, preoperative plain radiographs and a CT scan should be examined to determine bone quality, pedicle transverse diameter, and screw trajectory. Because intraoperative radiographs are usually necessary, preoperative planning should include preparation for anteroposterior (AP) and lateral radiographs. Lateral radiographs can usually be obtained without difficulty whether either a table or frame is used. Special radiolucent spinal frames are useful, particularly for AP radiographs.

The patient is placed prone on rolls, a frame, or a table with the abdomen hanging as freely as possible to indirectly decompress the epidural venous plexus. A midline incision is used and carried down to the level of the spinous processes. An adequate incision length facilitates proper trajectory during screw hole preparation and screw placement. All soft tissue is dissected off subperiosteally to minimize blood loss. Muscle dissection should allow for a lateral exposure of the transverse processes on both sides, leaving the intertransverse membrane intact at all levels of the planned instrumentation. A crank retractor helps maintain the lateral exposure. Release of the retractor every 30 minutes reduces muscle necrosis and thereby decreases the risk of infection. The spinal level is identified either anatomically or radiographically, and a decompressive laminectomy is performed if appropriate.

After placement of the pedicle screws, the dorsolateral bone graft bed is prepared by decorticating the lateral aspect of the facet joints and the transverse processes with a combination of a high-speed drill with a cutting bur and sharp, cupped curets. The synovium can be removed from the facet joints that are included in the fusion and packed with cancellous bone. The importance of meticulous decortication to achieving bony fusion cannot be overstated.

Pedicle Screw Entry Sites and Trajectory

Every spine surgeon should have a thorough knowledge of pedicle anatomy, including the coronal and sagittal plane angulation of the pedicle (see Fig. 148-1). The sagittal pedicle angle increases in the thoracic spine from an average of 0 degrees at T1 to 10 degrees at T8 and then decreases to 0 degrees at T12.[28] Usually the L4 sagittal pedicle angle is 0 degrees, and subsequent rostral and caudal levels are associated with progressively greater sagittal angles. The lordotic curvature of the lumbar spine produces a rostral angulation for upper lumbar screws. The L5 pedicle is 5 to 10 degrees caudally inclined. Coronal plane angulation decreases from the cervical spine to the thoracolumbar region and then increases as the lumbar spine is descended. The coronal plane angulation at T1 is 10 to 15 degrees and at T12 is 5 degrees.[28] A 10-degree medial angulation is satisfactory at L1. A wider angle in the coronal plane is necessary to avoid lateral penetration of the pedicle in the lower lumbar spine. The coronal plane angle increases approximately 5 degrees per level from L1 to the sacrum.[24]

In the thoracic spine, the transverse process commonly does not align directly with the pedicle in the axial plane. For this reason, the anatomic landmarks that are used for lumbar pedicle-screw insertion cannot be used in the thoracic spine.[28] The transverse process is rostral to the pedicle in the upper thoracic spine and caudal to the pedicle in the lower thoracic spine. The crossover occurs at T6-7.[28] Because of the variability of the relationship of the pedicle to the transverse process, fluoroscopic guidance or direct vision and palpation of the pedicle via a laminotomy is recommended for insertion of thoracic pedicles. At the T1 to T3 levels, Louis suggests the use of 4.5-mm diameter screws that are 25 to 30 mm in length.[29] At the T4 to T10 levels, screws are usually 4.5 mm in diameter and 30 to 35 mm in length.[29]

The conventional entry site for pedicle-screw placement in the lumbar region is at the junction of the lateral facet and the transverse process (Fig. 148-3). Although the midline of the transverse process corresponds to the location of the pedicle at L4, this relationship does vary at different lumbar levels. Above L4, the midline of the transverse process is rostral to the pedicle, and at L5, it is an average of 1.5 mm caudal to the pedicle.[30]

Several nuances should be considered for accurate cannulation of the pedicle, as well as to enable proper screw trajectory. The muscle dissection is performed as lateral as possible to allow palpation of the transverse processes. The lateral aspect of the pedicle is palpated with a nerve hook over the transverse process. If a decompressive laminectomy is not

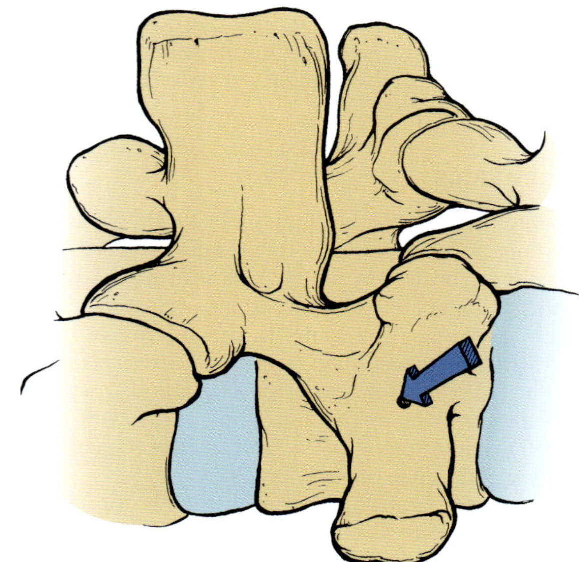

FIGURE 148-3. The junction of the lateral facet and the transverse process is the conventional pedicle-screw entry site (*arrow*) in the lumbar spine.

being performed as part of the operative procedure, a small laminotomy may be performed to palpate the medial aspect of the pedicle and its rostral and caudal borders. Palpation of the pedicle helps guide accurate placement of the screw into the pedicle and increases the safety of the placement. It is strongly recommended for placement of pedicle screws at the level of the conus medullaris and above.

Screw Insertion

The entry site is decorticated by using a bur and a high-speed drill or a rongeur. A bur or awl is also used to penetrate the dorsal cortex of the pedicle. A curved or straight pedicle probe is used to develop a path for the screw through the cancellous bone of the pedicle into the vertebral body. The advancement of the pedicle probe should be smooth and consistent. A sudden plunge suggests breaking out of the pedicle laterally. An increase in resistance indicates abutment against the pedicle or vertebral body cortex. After cannulation of the pedicle and vertebral body with the pedicle probe, the pedicle sounding probe is placed into the pedicle, which is then palpated from within to make sure there is not a medial, lateral, rostral, or caudal disruption in the cortex of the pedicle. The sounding probe should also be used to determine that there is bone at the bottom of the pilot hole, verifying that penetration of the ventral cortex of the vertebral body has not occurred.

After the pedicles have been probed, different-length Steinmann pins or K-wires are placed bilaterally into the pedicular hole at each level. Using different-length pins on each side helps distinguish right and left on the lateral plain radiograph in case the pedicle hole trajectory or depth needs to be corrected. A lateral and an AP radiograph or fluoroscopic image is used to verify the trajectory of the pins. This, however, does not guarantee accurate screw placement.[31] With slightly oblique AP views, a pin located in the middle of the pedicle has a characteristic "target sign." Direct AP views demonstrate the lateral-to-medial orientation of the screws. Excessive medial orientation of the screws seen on an AP film raises the concern of medial penetration of the pedicle by the screw. Lateral imaging is useful to view the depth of penetration into the vertebral body and the sagittal angulation of the trajectory. Ventral screw penetration is usually between 50% and 80% of the AP diameter of the vertebral body. Ventral screw penetration greater than 80% of the vertebral body on a lateral plain radiograph raises the concern of ventral penetration of the vertebral body cortex because of the convex shape of the vertebral bodies. To avoid vascular and visceral injury, the ventral cortex of the vertebral body is not penetrated, although this would enhance the overall strength of the construct.

After confirmation of correct placement of the K-wires or Steinmann pins, the pedicle screw path is tapped if non–self-tapping screws are used. Some tapping screws are hollow and are slid over K-wires into the pedicles. This helps guide the tap along the same trajectory that the pedicle was previously probed. The screw is then guided into the pedicle by its purchase of the threads tapped into the pedicle. However, tapping is less desirable in cancellous bone because tapping weakens the implant-bone junction.[25] It is of questionable value in the insertion of pedicle screws because pedicle screws rarely obtain cortical purchase within the pedicle.[32] To maximize the bone purchase of the permanent screws, a tap that is smaller in diameter than the screw is used. Tapping is usually not performed at a greater depth than the pedicle.

After tapping of the pedicles, the permanent screws with the largest diameter that will not fracture the pedicle are placed. The length of the screw is determined by measuring the length of the Steinmann pin or K-wire from the pedicle entry site to a depth of 50% to 80% of the vertebral body. Screws in the lumbar spine usually have a 4.5- to 7-mm diameter and a 35- to 50-mm length. Next, the transverse processes and lateral aspect of the facet joints are decorticated. The screws are connected to a longitudinal member, usually a rod. A bone graft is then placed on the previously prepared fusion bed.

Percutaneous Screw Placement

Percutaneous pedicle-screw placement to decrease the blood loss and muscle damage as well as to shorten the hospitalization time has increased in popularity. However, such screw placement may increase the operative time and radiation exposure.[33,34] The evolution of spinal navigation systems has also contributed to the widespread use of percutaneous screw fixations. Although most such techniques are predominantly used in lumbar spine, there are also reports of using them in the thoracic spine.[35]

Lehmann et al.[34] have compared open versus percutaneous pedicle-screw fixation in an animal model and concluded that percutaneous screw insertion can provide moderate advantages.

Measures for Correct Screw Placement

Although intraoperative fluoroscopy can demonstrate the proper position of the screws, CT provides even more information, but after the fact. Cadaveric studies have demonstrated rates of malpositioned screws to be as high as 21%.[36] A variety of techniques have been developed to detect pedicle wall violation and prevent pedicle screw misplacement intraoperatively.

Navigation and CT Guidance

Navigation systems have been created to enhance the surgical accuracy of pedicle-screw placement and to improve clinical outcomes. Computer-assisted fixation and conventional screw fixation have been compared in different studies, and the accuracy and safety of computer-assisted techniques were found to be superior to the conventional techniques.[37-41]

Modern computer-assisted techniques use frameless stereotaxy as a confirmation tool to identify the target. This may be enhanced by fluoroscopic navigation, the so-called FluoroNav,[42] and recently a robotic assistance has been implemented in these systems. A miniature robot has been designed to be mounted on bony landmarks to overcome the limitations of navigation systems.[43,44]

Fluoroscopically assisted thoracolumbar pedicle-screw placement exposes the spine surgeon to significantly greater radiation levels than other, nonspine procedures that involve the use of a fluoroscope. In fact dose rates are up to 10 to 12 times greater, primarily because of the increased energy required to image the lumbar spine fluoroscopically and the proximity of the surgeon's hands to the sources of radiation. Spine surgeons performing fluoroscopically assisted thoracolumbar procedures should monitor their annual radiation exposure. They also use measures to reduce radiation exposure, such as minimizing fluoroscopy time, lead shielding, pulsed image acquisition, and surgeon awareness of high-exposure body and hand positions.[45] Computer-navigated systems can reduce the radiation dose.[41]

Electromyographic Monitoring

Stimulus-evoked electromyographic (EMG) monitoring may be used for detecting a pedicle wall violation. Because the cortical bone has a higher resistivity (low conductivity) to electrical current flow than soft tissues, EMG responses are not elicited with low-stimulation currents in case there is no breakage of the pedicle wall.[47] If there is a break in the bony pedicle wall, sufficient electrical current flows through the soft tissue adjacent to the pedicle to cause depolarization of a nearby nerve root, which is easily recorded as a compound action potential by EMG.

False-negative responses occur with this technique. Applying neuromuscular blocking agents, chronically compressed nerve roots may fail to produce EMG activity within the standard stimulation voltages and high resistance of a pedicle-screw implant. For instance, polyaxial screws may have higher resistance values than monoaxial screws.[46]

Although lumbosacral pedicle-screw placement may be well monitored by lower extremity EMG recording, this has not been a routine for thoracic pedicle-screw fixation. Triggered EMG responses recorded from the rectus abdominis muscles have been successfully used to assess thoracic pedicle-screw placement from T6 to T12,[47] and recordings from intercostalis muscles have proved useful in the upper thoracic spine, from T3 to T6.[48]

Postoperative CT and MRI

MRI is associated with some distortion. CT provides more clinically relevant information regarding screw placement and fixation.

Two millimeters or less of medial pedicle perforation or 6 mm or less of lateral pedicle perforation is generally considered safe.[49] All neurologic deficits reported have been associated with medial pedicle perforation of greater than 4 mm.[50] It means that the safe zone for pedicle penetration is 4 mm.[51,52]

The malposition of a pedicle screw may be defined as screw placement that causes or has the potential to cause neurologic or vascular complications and/or is associated with suboptimal biomechanical strength due to the malposition. Xu et al. have graded the pedicle perforations: grade I, minimal penetration of the pedicle wall; grade II, less than half of the diameter outside; and grade III, more than half of the diameter outside.[52]

Screws in Osteoporotic Spine

In patients with osteoporosis, failures of implants can occur. These include screw loosening, pull-out, migration, and breakage.

Holding strength of screws in osteoporotic vertebral bone can be increased by a variety of means, such as by changing the geometric characteristics of the screw, by improving the bone-screw interface with polymethylmethacrylate,[53] or by biodegradable calcium phosphate bone substitute augmentation.[54] Application of vertebroplasty or kyphoplasty may also be a solution. Hydroxyapatite coating can improve fixation of pedicle screws, with increased pull-out resistance and reduced risk of loosening.[55]

Complications and Avoidance

Complication rates are as high as 25%. However, most are without permanent clinical consequence. Intraoperative complications occur at a 0.2% to 5% rate.[56] According to a cohort study, the complications are usually implant failures (approximately 7%), pedicle fractures (1%), vertebral body penetration (<0.5%), or neurologic deficit (<0.5%).[56]

In general, early complications after transpedicular stabilization of the spine are unusual and are infrequently associated with permanent morbidity. There is, however, a high proportion of postoperative radiographic failures. Ohlin et al.[57] have reported a 40% radiographic failure rate after surgery. Most of them involved screw loosening, angulation, or fracture. Implant removal was necessary within 1 year after operation in about 15% of the cases.

Misplaced Screws

Misplaced screws represent the most frequent pedicle screw complication. The misplacement rate ranges from 1.2% to 28.8% in different series.[11,50,58,59] A rostral breach of the pedicle cortex leads to penetration of the intervertebral disc with resultant poor screw fixation. A caudal misplaced screw risks injury to the dura mater and nerve root. Disruption of the medial cortex leads to violation of the spinal canal, which can cause injury to the dura, spinal cord, or nerve roots. Lateral screw placement risks injury to the segmental vessels and poor screw purchase.[59,60] A laterally placed screw hole can lead to possible retroperitoneal penetration by the pedicle probe because slippage of the probe off the side of the vertebral body occurs from the sudden lack of resistance to advancement of the probe. Although with postoperative CT approximately 15% of the screws have been reported to be suboptimal,[50] nerve root or spinal cord injury is uncommon because of the theoretical safe zones or spaces around the pedicle.

Intraoperative radiographic confirmation of correct screw placement, including the use of fluoroscopy, has still resulted in a high incidence of misplaced screws.[61] Therefore, other methods have been developed to ensure accurate placement of screws within the pedicle. Screw placement can be checked electrophysiologically with direct stimulation of the pedicle probe or screw, producing an EMG response peripherally. If this response occurs below the threshold expected for intact cortical bone, the screws may be redirected or removed. Stimulation can be intermittent[61-63] or continuous.[64,65] Spontaneous EMGs are also monitored, which may alert the surgeon to nerve root irritation from retraction during decompressive procedures, stretching during deformity reductions, or impingement by a pedicle screw.

Interactive frameless stereotaxy with surface reference landmarks has been successfully applied to pedicle fixation of the spine. Preoperative axial CT images of the appropriate spinal segments can be manipulated to assist the surgeon in determining the correct entry point, sagittal and coronal angulation, screw diameter, and length for each pedicle, thus reducing pedicle screw misplacement.[66] Frameless stereotactic guidance of pedicle-screw placement is particularly useful when the planned exposure does not allow for palpation of the pedicle at the time of screw insertion (e.g., when a lumbar decompression is not planned).

Nerve Root or Spinal Cord Injury

Neurologic injury during pedicular screw placement is reported to occur in about 2.5% to 7.5% of cases.[31] Nerve root injury may result either from improper screw placement or from correction of a deformity with traction on the nerve root or migration of the screw into the neuroforamen or spinal canal. If the symptoms caused by screw malpositioning do not resolve, the instrumentation should be removed or repositioned. In most cases, the radiculopathy improves after removal or repositioning of the misplaced screw.[57]

Pedicle Fracture

A break in the cortex of the pedicle can result from a misplaced screw, as discussed earlier, or the use of too large a screw. The transverse width of the pedicle is the narrowest dimension of the pedicle and determines the largest-diameter screw that can be used.[14,25]

Cerebrospinal Fluid Fistulae

The incidence of dural tears is less than 2.5%.[60] These are due to spinal canal or neuroforamen penetration. Primary repair of the durotomy, if possible, lessens the risk of a cerebrospinal fluid leak through the wound or pseudomeningocele formation.

Infection

In general, the infection rate after instrumentation is higher than with other spine operations because of longer operative times, extensive surgical exposures, and the placement of a foreign body. For these reasons, prophylactic antibiotic usage and vigorous irrigation of the wound with antibiotic solutions should be performed. Frequent relaxation of the paraspinous muscle retraction reduces the amount of muscle necrosis and lessens the risk of infection. Necrotic muscle should be debrided before closing the wound.

Damage to Retroperitoneal Structures

The retroperitoneal structures may be damaged as a result of ventral cortex penetration. In the upper lumbar spine, the aorta and vena cava lie ventral to the vertebral bodies. At L4-5 and caudally, the iliac vein and artery lie ventral (and ventrolateral) to the spine. Penetration of the ventral cortex is avoided by understanding that intraoperative imaging can be misleading regarding the distance from the tip of the pin to the ventral cortex because of the convex shape of the vertebral body. Penetration can also be avoided by sounding the anterior cortex with a probe and measuring this distance, which should not be exceeded by the length of the screw.

Hardware Failure

Mechanical failure has been reported to be between 5% and 31% in different series.[57]

Screw Breakage

The reported incidence of screw breakage is 0.8% to 24.6%. The incidence of screw breakage and bending is higher in patients in whom major deformity reduction and multilevel fusions were attempted.[57,67,68] Rostral screws are more prone to breakage than their caudal counterparts.[68] Matsuzaki et al.[69] have reported that rostral screw breakage is more common in multilevel fusions but that caudal screw breakage is more common in single-level fusions. Screw breakage after solid fusion is usually asymptomatic and may not require reoperation. However, screw breakage may indicate a pseudarthrosis.[29,60,67]

The following measures can be taken to avoid screw breakage: (1) choosing the largest-diameter screws that the pedicle can accept[20]; (2) making the upper portion of a construct longer if nonrigid fixation systems are used, and for fractures in the thoracolumbar junction, using fixation to two levels above the fracture site[58]; and (3) noting that if the anterior column is severely disrupted, the pedicle screw construct bears all of the load. Lack of anterior column support places significant stress at the screw-rod junction and can result in breakage of the screw at this point. In this situation, a ventral interbody fusion may be required to share the load with the pedicle-screw construct[69-71] (Fig. 148-4).

Removing broken pedicle screws is often not a simple task. One of the techniques is to create a groove on the broken head using a 2-mm diamond bur–equipped high-speed drill and a minus screwdriver.[72,73] Also, a friction technique has been described.[74]

Screw Pull-out

Screw pull-out increases with decreasing bone mineral density.[23,75] A solid screw purchase in osteoporotic bone is not easily achieved, and therefore osteoporotic bone is a relative contraindication to the use of pedicle screws. Hooks or wires provide superior pull-out resistance compared with pedicle screws in osteoporotic bone. This is due to the greater cortical bone-metal surface contact.[76] Instrumentation in patients with osteoporosis should include "extra" levels, with multiple points of fixation.

The length of the screw is important regarding screw pull-out. Lumbar screws should be placed approximately to a depth of two thirds of the vertebral body on the lateral radiographs.

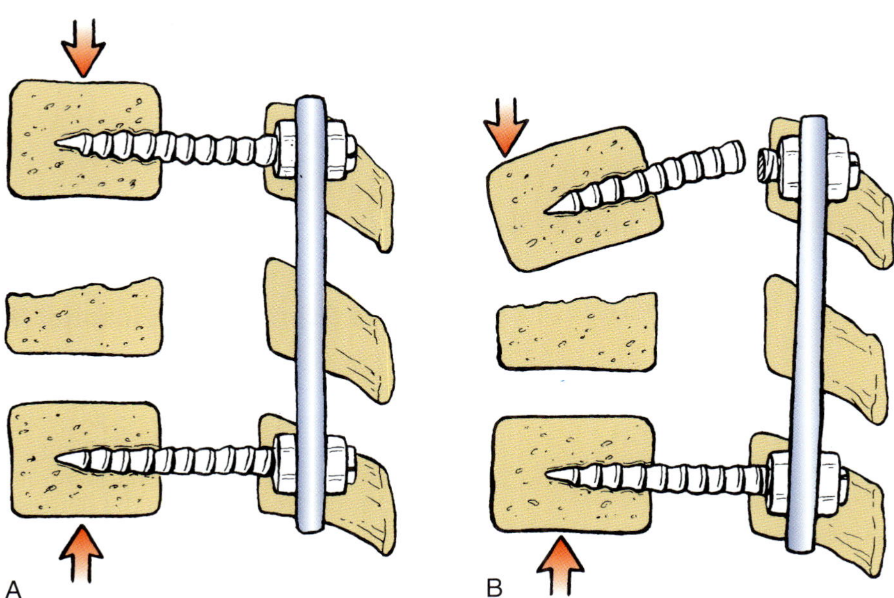

FIGURE 148-4. **A** and **B,** If the anterior column is severely disrupted, the pedicle-screw construct bears all of the load and rigid pedicle fixation systems may fail by screw breakage at the screw-rod interface.

This maximizes depth of penetration without risking bicortical purchase in the lumbar area.[77]

The outer diameter of a screw, particularly with an associated large thread depth and pitch (distance between threads), helps minimize the risk of pull-out. However, a larger-diameter screw may also cause the pedicle to fracture.

The use of pedicle-screw fixation systems that rigidly connect the screw to the plate or rod resist screw pull-out by not allowing toggling of the screws.[22] Screw toe-in results in greater pull-out resistance and translational deformity prevention if the two sides of the construct are rigidly affixed to each other. In this configuration, the screw pull-out is prohibited by its toed-in counterpart.[78]

Placement of a sublaminar hook caudal to a pedicle screw increases the pull-out resistance of the construct. This configuration is made possible by the location of the lamina approximately one-half segment below the pedicle. The pedicle screw–sublaminar hook construct resists pull-out while maintaining the rotation-, flexion-, and extension-resisting capabilities of the pedicle screw.[76,78] This is not appropriately applied at the most caudal segment of the construct.

Screw Loosening or Plate or Rod Breakage

Screw loosening is relatively rare and is often a delayed complication. It is diagnosed by the presence of a lucency seen around the screw on a lateral plain radiograph. It often indicates a fusion delay or pseudarthrosis. It may also be the result of inadequate screw purchase or diminished bone mineral density from osteoporosis.

Plate or rod breakage rarely occurs. It is often an indication of pseudarthrosis.

Loss of Correction

Loss of correction may occur after the reduction of a traumatic or congenital kyphosis, particularly if overdistraction or forceful correction was performed during the operation. The strength of the anterior column is important. If there is significant compromise of the anterior column, ventral grafting and fusion should be added. Otherwise, a loss of correction (kyphosis) may develop, resulting in screw angulation or breakage at the screw–longitudinal member junction (see Fig. 148-4).[70,77]

Wound Breakdown

In thin patients, bulky implants may be felt under the skin. They can cause wound breakdown, especially at the sacral level.[31,70] For this reason, low-profile constructs should be used in thin patients. A painful bursa may also develop over prominent parts of the instrumentation.

Universal Spinal Instrumentation Systems

Universal spinal instrumentation (USI) systems were developed for the treatment of scoliosis through application of multiple corrective forces at different points on a rod. These systems have proved readily adaptable to the treatment of a wide variety of spinal disorders. USI systems use both pedicle screws and hooks as anchors to the spine. The screws and hooks are connected by a rod. A major difference between the systems is the manner in which the rods are coupled to the anchors. The reasons for the selection of rods versus plates in modern systems are that (1) rods are more versatile than plates for connection with anchoring devices and (2) a larger area for grafting is available when rods are used.

The first USI prototype was the Cotrel-Dubousset (CD) device.[13] This was followed by the Texas Scottish Rite Hospital (TSRH)[79,80] and the Isola[5,81] systems. The CD system has been updated via the compact Cotrel-Dubousset (CCD)[82] and the CD Horizon spinal systems. The characteristics of the CD, TSRH, and Isola systems, and polyaxial screw systems as well as their advantages and disadvantages, are depicted in Tables 148-1 and 148-2.

Cotrel-Dubousset System

CD instrumentation is the oldest of the universal systems. It was designed by Cotrel and Dubousset in France between 1978 and 1982. It was first designed for correction of pediatric scoliosis.[13] This system provides a rigid three-dimensional short-segment fixation without the need for sublaminar wires in the spinal canal. It uses hooks and screws as anchors, coupled to a rod by a set screw. In the first version of the CD system, set screws of the closed-body type were broken (twisted off) at the end of the instrumentation. This makes the revision or removal of the instrumentation very difficult.[71] The CD system uses self-tapping pedicle screws, whereas the other systems use nontapping screws. The CD system has a lateral connector that facilitates the screw-rod connection in the presence of coronal plane deformities (Fig. 148-5).

Compact Cotrel-Dubousset System

The original CD instrumentation presented disadvantages such as an unnecessary number of implant components and a permanent implant locking system. Therefore, a new version, the CCD, was developed. The instrument set and the implants were streamlined, and an improved locking system enabled easy removal.[82]

Cotrel-Dubousset Horizon

The CD Horizon system is designed to be lower in profile. A recent addition to the CD Horizon system consists of polyaxial screws, which minimize rod contouring.

Texas Scottish Rite Hospital System

Perhaps the most important and unique feature of the TSRH system is the variable-angle screw that facilitates coupling to the rod regardless of the angle of screw insertion (Fig. 148-6A). The top-loading couplers are available with varying thickness, which accommodates coronal plane offsets and minimizes the need to contour the rod in this dimension (Fig. 148-6B).

Isola System

The Isola system is one of the newest of the USI fixators. A unique feature of the screws of the Isola system is a

TABLE 148-1

Specifications of Screws and Longitudinal Members of Universal Spinal Instrumentation Systems

	Cotrel-Dubousset	Texas Scottish Rite Hospital	Isola	Polyaxial New Systems
Screw diameters (mm)	6–7	5.5, 6.5, 7.5, 8.5	5.5, 6.25, 7	5.5–8
Screw length (mm)	30, 35, 40, 45, 50	25–75 (5-mm increments)	25–50 (5-mm increments)	25–50
Screw types	Closed Top-opening Side-opening	Fixed-angle head type Variable-angle head type Top-opening Side-opening	Closed Top-opening (machine-threaded portion with 23- to 33-mm lengths to aid sagittal plane disparity correction)	Open Top-opening with polyaxial flexibility
Titanium	—	+	+	+
Screw-tapping style	Self-tapping	Nontapping	Nontapping, with diameter of 8.5 mm and length of 30–35 mm (most are not threaded)	Self-tapping and nontapping types available
Sacral screws	NA	NA		
Iliac screws	NA	NA	Diameter: 6.25–7 mm Length: 60–80 mm	Diameter: 6.25–8 mm Length: 60–80 mm
Rods	Knurled rod (0.2 mm): diameters of 5 mm and 7 mm	Smooth rod ¼-inch rigid rod ¼-inch flex rod 3/16-inch flex rod	Smooth rod Diameter: 4.76, 6.35 mm Standard length: 46 cm	Smooth rod Diameter: 4.5, 6.5 mm Lengths: variable
Rod-screw Rod-hook anchorage	Blockers for open-body type screws Set screws for closed-body type screws	Eye bolt and nut assembly • For fixed screws, side-loading eye bolts • For variable screws, side-loading eye bolts • For variable screws, top-loading eye bolts	Slotted connector V-groove hollow ground (VHG) design allows maximal rod contact within hole Rod anchorage: set screws are loaded from top Screw anchorage: tapered nut and locking nut are tightened over pedicle screw over slotted connector	Variable in different designs
Transverse connector	Device for transverse traction (DTT) Threaded rod with nuts and set screws	DTT Small-diameter threaded rod with nuts and set screws	Transverse rod connectors Split connector jaws are connected with long threaded rod and fixed with hex nuts	Variable in different designs
Unique specifications		Radial serrated splines on variable-angle screw heads facilitate connection between screws oriented in different planes; this allows fixation without rod bending	Machine-threaded portion of screw that provides ability to correct sagittal plane disparities; they are cut at end of operation VHG design	

NA, not applicable.

machine-threaded portion that allows the correction of sagittal deformities by placing straight or angled washers over the threads.[82] Slotted plate connectors couple the rods to the screws. The connectors are first placed on the rods, and then the slotted portion of the plate is placed over the machine-threaded portion of the screw. Plate lengths vary. This minimizes the need to contour the rod to accommodate coronal plane deformities (Fig. 148-7).

Modern Polyaxial Systems

The versatility of fixation systems has increased in many ways. Also, low-profile systems for slim patients and for children have been developed. Stainless steel alloys essentially have been replaced by alloys, most commonly alloys of titanium. Reduced profile and implant volume, with greater ergonomy and ease of application, are the predominant features of the more modern systems.

TABLE 148-2

Main Advantages and Disadvantages of Universal Spinal Instrumentation Systems

	Cotrel-Dubousset	Texas Scottish Rite Hospital	Isola	Polyaxial New Systems
Main advantages	Knurled rod	Rod contouring is minimized Fewer parts Removal is easier Titanium available Top and side loading available	V-groove attachment is easy and strong construct Top loading is easy Titanium available	More flexible screw head–rod connection Top loading and titanium Some screws are cannulated to introduce bone cement
Main disadvantages	Extensive rod contouring is necessary Revision and removing is impossible without drilling or cutting implanted parts Multiple parts are confusing	Eye bolts should be preplanned and applied before connecting to screws and hooks Top-loading hooks are difficult to use	Adapters for connection can introduce points of movement	Multiple parts can cause confusion and may be associated with difficult assembly

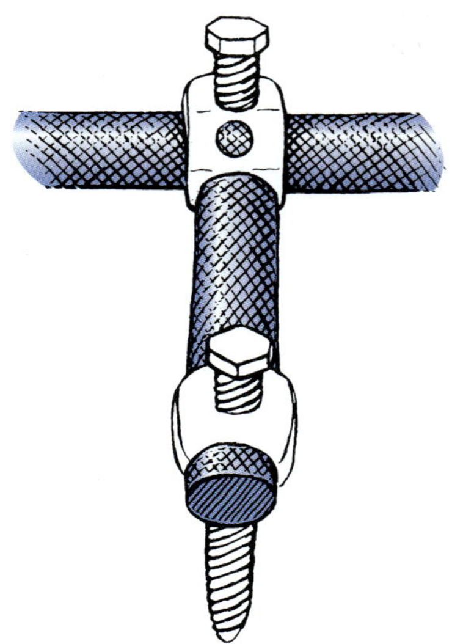

FIGURE 148-5. Diagram of the Cotrel-Dubousset lateral connector that facilitates coupling of the screw to the rod in the presence of coronal plane offsets.

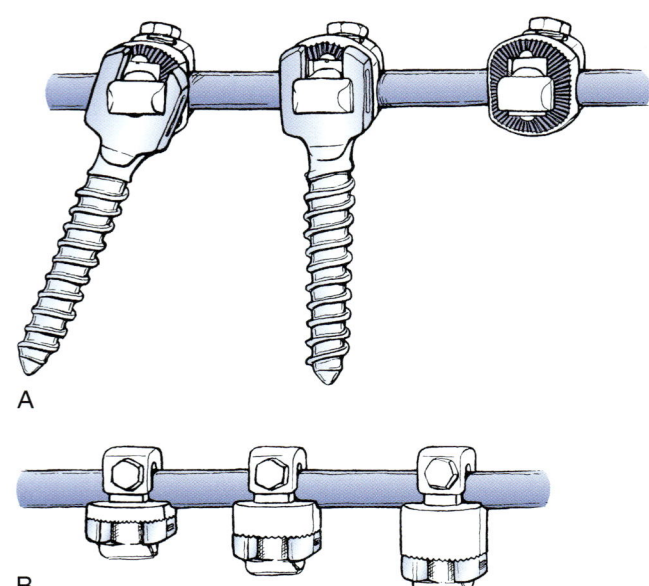

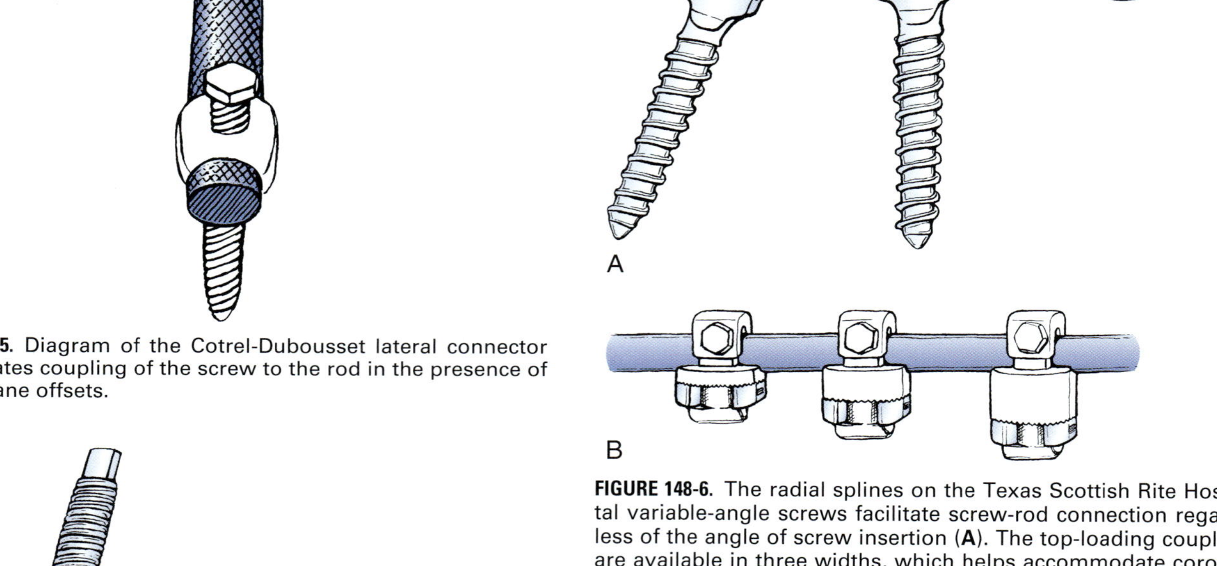

FIGURE 148-6. The radial splines on the Texas Scottish Rite Hospital variable-angle screws facilitate screw-rod connection regardless of the angle of screw insertion (**A**). The top-loading couplers are available in three widths, which helps accommodate coronal plane offsets (**B**).

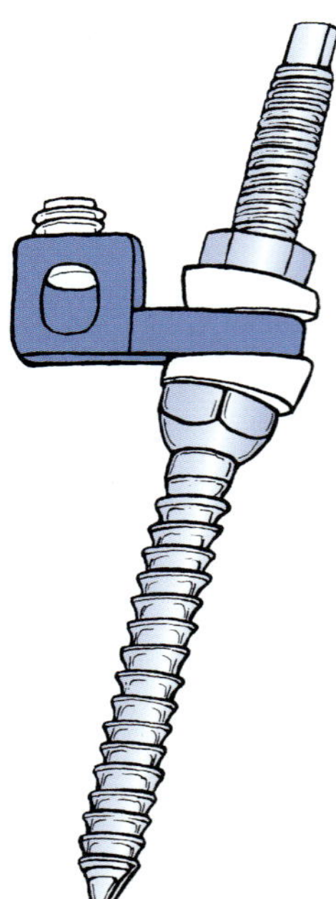

FIGURE 148-7. Coronal plane deformities are accommodated by slotted plate connectors of varying lengths that couple the rods to the screws.

Acknowledgment. Thank you to Dr. Andrea Halliday, who authored prior editions of this chapter. Her work laid the foundation for this third edition.

KEY REFERENCES

Bai B, Kummer FJ, Spivak J: Augmentation of anterior vertebral body screw fixation by an injectable, biodegradable calcium phosphate bone substitute. *Spine (Phila Pa 1976)* 26:2679–2683, 2001.

Darden BV II, Wood KE, Hatley MK, et al: Evaluation of pedicle screw insertion monitored by intraoperative evoked electromyography. *J Spinal Disord* 9:8–16, 1996.

Fessler RG, Sturgill M: Utilization of the Texas Scottish Rite Hospital Universal System for stabilization of the thoracic and lumbar spine. In Fessler RG, Haid RW, editors: *Current techniques in spinal stabilization*, New York, 1996, McGraw-Hill, pp 273–285.

Harrington PR, Dickson JH: Spinal instrumentation in the treatment of severe progressive spondylolisthesis. *Clin Orthop Relat Res* 117:157–163, 1976.

Kalfas IH, Kormos DW, Murphy MA, et al: Application of frameless stereotaxy to pedicle screw fixation of the spine. *J Neurosurg* 83:641–647, 1995.

Louis R: Fusion of the lumbar and sacral spine by internal fixation with screw plates. *Clin Orthop Relat Res* 203:18–33, 1986.

McCormack T, Karaikovic E, Gaines RW: The load sharing classification of spine fractures. *Spine (Phila Pa 1976)* 19:1741–1744, 1994.

Rengachary SS, Flores E: Segmental fixation of the lumbosacral spine using the Isola/VSP system. In Fessler RG, Haid RW, editors: *Current techniques in spinal stabilization*, New York, 1996, McGraw-Hill, pp 367–378.

Resnick DK: Prospective comparison of virtual fluoroscopy to fluoroscopy and plain radiographs for placement of lumbar pedicle screws. *J Spinal Disord Tech* 16:254–260, 2003.

Steffee AD: The variable screw placement system with posterior lumbar interbody fusion. In Zin PM, Gill K, editors: *Lumbar interbody fusion: principles and techniques in spine surgery*, Gaithersburg, MD, 1989, Aspen Press, pp 81–93.

Vaccaro AR, Garfin SR: Internal fixation (pedicle screw fixation) for fusion of the lumbar spine. *Spine (Phila Pa 1976)* 20(Suppl 24):157S–165S, 1995.

REFERENCES

The complete reference list is available online at expertconsult.com.

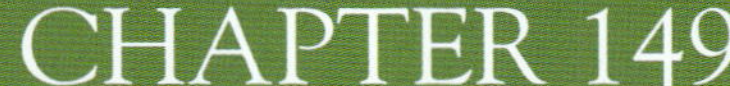
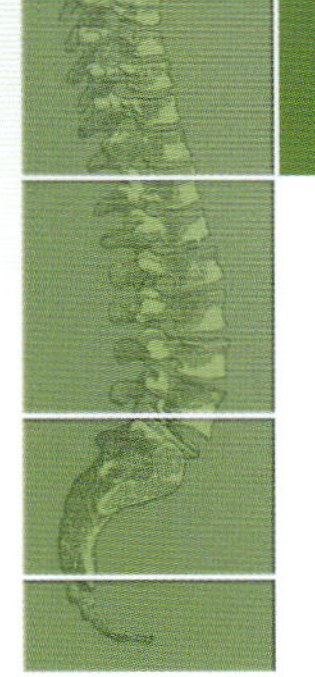

CHAPTER 149

Dorsal Thoracic and Lumbar Simple Hook-Rod, Wire, and Wire-Rod Techniques

Paul Kim | Bernardo Jose Ordonez

The first internal fixation device was designed by Harrington in 1947, a period in which the number of patients with poliomyelitis-induced scoliosis was growing, and there was dissatisfaction with the current management of corrective casting. The device was designed to correct scoliotic curvatures and halt progression of cardiopulmonary compromise in affected patients. Initial attempts consisted of screw fixation of facet joints in the corrected position. The results appeared promising, but early beneficial results were short-lived. Facet screw failure led to the development of a hook-and-rod construct, in which hooks were attached to the dorsal elements and held in place with a combination of distraction and compression forces. The clinical results of Harrington's new system were published in 1962.[1-3]

The Harrington system offered the first internal fixation device for the correction of scoliotic deformities. The system was quickly adopted by spine surgeons and applied to various conditions, including trauma, neoplastic disease, fixed deformities, and degenerative disorders.[2,4,5]

The Harrington system, although versatile, was plagued with inherent problems. The system was limited in its design, which allowed for only two points of fixation. Failure at any single hook site led to failure of the entire system.[6] However, the system has been modified over the years.

In the early 1970s, Luque was faced with an impoverished community in which postoperative bracing was impossible. From these circumstances arose the concept of segmental spinal instruumentation. The Luque system consisted of straight, L-shaped, or rectangular rods attached to lamina via sublaminar wires.[7] The advent of segmental spinal instrumentation addressed the main problem associated with the Harrington system that had only two points of fixation. Initially, sublaminar wires were used to supplement the Harrington system.[4-6] This innovation was followed by interspinous wiring techniques, such as Wisconsin wires and Dummond buttons. The original Harrington rod was rigid and difficult to contour, and the rounded caudal rigid tip failed to prevent rotation. This shortcoming led to the development of the square-ended Moe rod, which allowed rod contouring. The three-pointed bending force, which a contured rod provides, was enhanced further by the development of the Edward sleeve.[6,8] The Harrington system, although often replaced by newer universal spinal instrumentation systems, can be used to stabilize thoracic and lumbar fractures that result from axial loading and in which the anterior longitudinal ligament is intact.

Harrington Distraction Fixation

Technique

The patient is placed in the prone position, with a midline incision made to expose at least three levels above and two levels below the lesion. A subperiosteal dissection is performed and is carried laterally over the transverse process. The upper hook site is prepared after satisfactory exposure. Typically, this site is located three levels above the injury site, and the inferior facet is exposed at this level. The caudal tip is amputated with either a ¼-inch osteotome or a small Kerrison rongeur. The caudomedial margin of the lamina and underlying ligamentum flavum are excised.

The lamina is conformed to allow seating of the rostral ratcheted hook, typically a no. 1253 hook. A no. 1251 hook can be used as a starter hook, which can be replaced by a no. 1253 hook, a keeled hook, or a bifid no. 1262 hook. The hook is inserted to follow the angle of the facet joint and is gently tapped into position. A well-seated hook should lie orthogonal to the spine (Fig. 149-1). The caudal hook site is generally located two levels below the level of the injury. The interlaminar region at this level is enlarged with a Kerrison rongeur. The ligamentum flavum is excised, and the rostral margin of the lamina is conformed to accommodate the caudal hook, usually a no. 1254 round-hole hook or a no. 1201 square-hole hook (Fig. 149-2). Square-hole caudal hooks are most commonly used because they allow contouring of the rods and minimize rotation. A construct undergoing distraction is depicted in Figure 149-3.

Segmental Fixation

Segmental fixation of the Harrington system has been shown to increase stability.[5,6] Segmental fixation can be achieved with either sublaminar wires or cables or interspinous techniques.[5,9] When sublaminar fixation is chosen as a means of segmental fixation, use of the cables should be considered because they are stronger and more flexible, and the incidence of neurologic complications may be decreased. Placement of a sublaminar wire or cable can be accomplished by removing

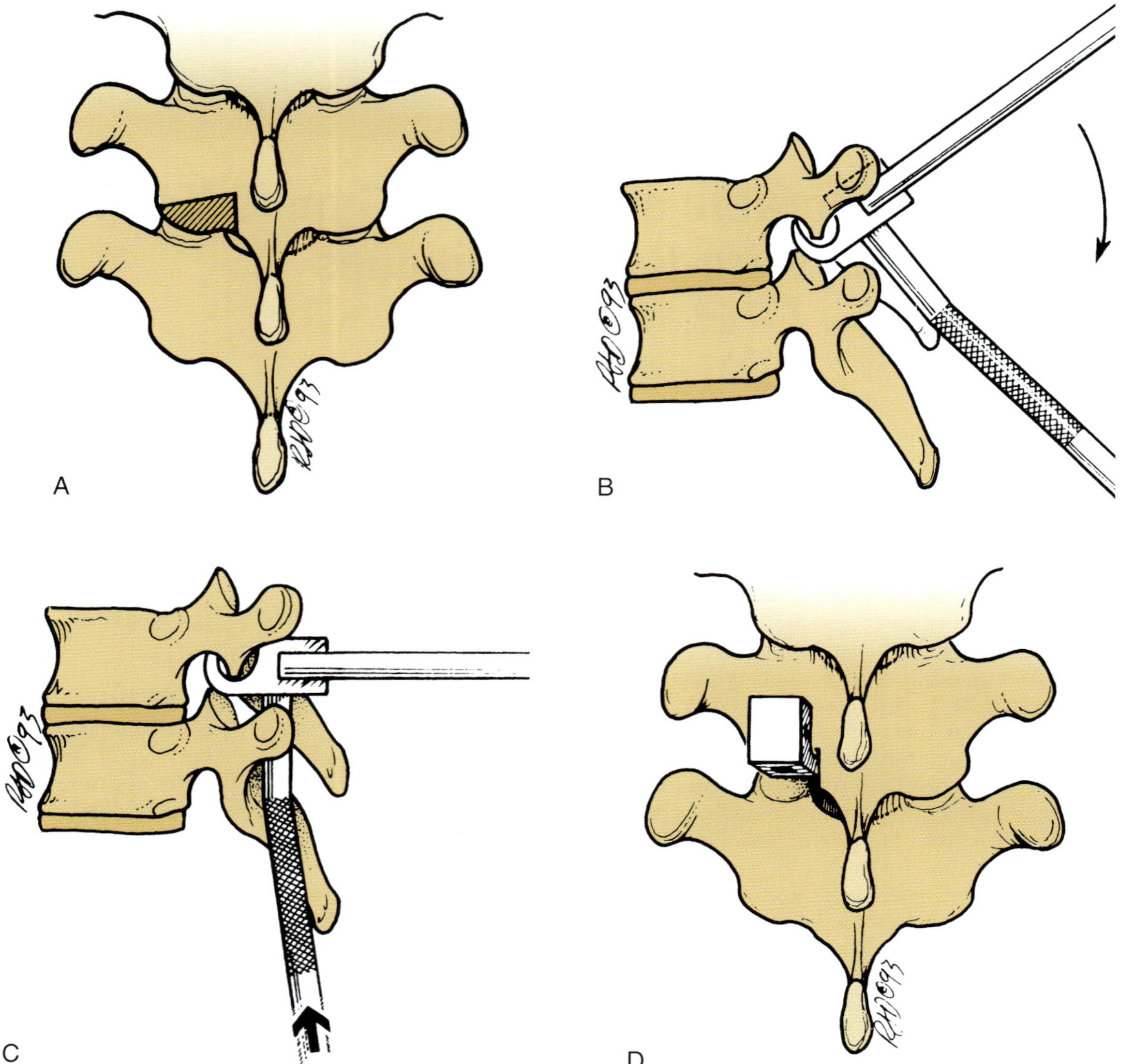

FIGURE 149-1. Harrington fixation, upper hook site. **A,** Preparation; **B–D,** insertion.

the interspinous ligament and performing an interlaminar laminotomy along the midline at each level that is to be instrumented. The ligamentum flavum is removed with a Kerrison rongeur, and the dura mater or epidural fat is visualized. Adequate removal of the ligamentum flavum ensures easy passage of the sublaminar wire or cable.

A 16-gauge or 18-gauge wire is doubled and formed into an S or a fishhook shape. Alternatively, a cable leader is bent into an S or fishhook shape. The leader or wire is passed beneath the caudal edge of the lamina gently, without any downward pressure to avoid injury to underlying neural elements. When the tip of the wire or leader is visualized, it is grasped with a clamp, and constant upward pressure is maintained on the wire or cable to minimize canal compromise. When the wire is passed, it is bent over the lamina to guard against inadvertently displacing the wire into the spinal canal. The cable leaders are cut at this point to create two single cables. Sublaminar wires or cables can be placed at each level to be stabilized.

Interspinous Segmental Instrumentation

Interspinous segmental instrumentation can also be used to supplement the strength of the construct.[3] A single hole is made at the base of each spinous process to be instrumented, with a curved awl, a bone tenaculum, or a drill. Beaded Wisconsin wires, with attached Drummond buttons, are passed through the base of the spinous process from each side. Once it is through the base of the spinous process, the beaded Wisconsin wire is passed through the contralateral Drummond button. The Wisconsin wires are pulled tight until the Drummond bottom fits snugly against the base of the spinous process. The beads are then cut. When the rods are in place, the wires are tightly secured to the rods, and the excess wire is removed. The free wire ends are bent to provide a low profile (Fig. 149-4).

A square-ended rod is chosen, with an appropriate length of rod that allows one ratchet to be visible beneath the rostral hook. The rod is contoured to maintain normal spinal

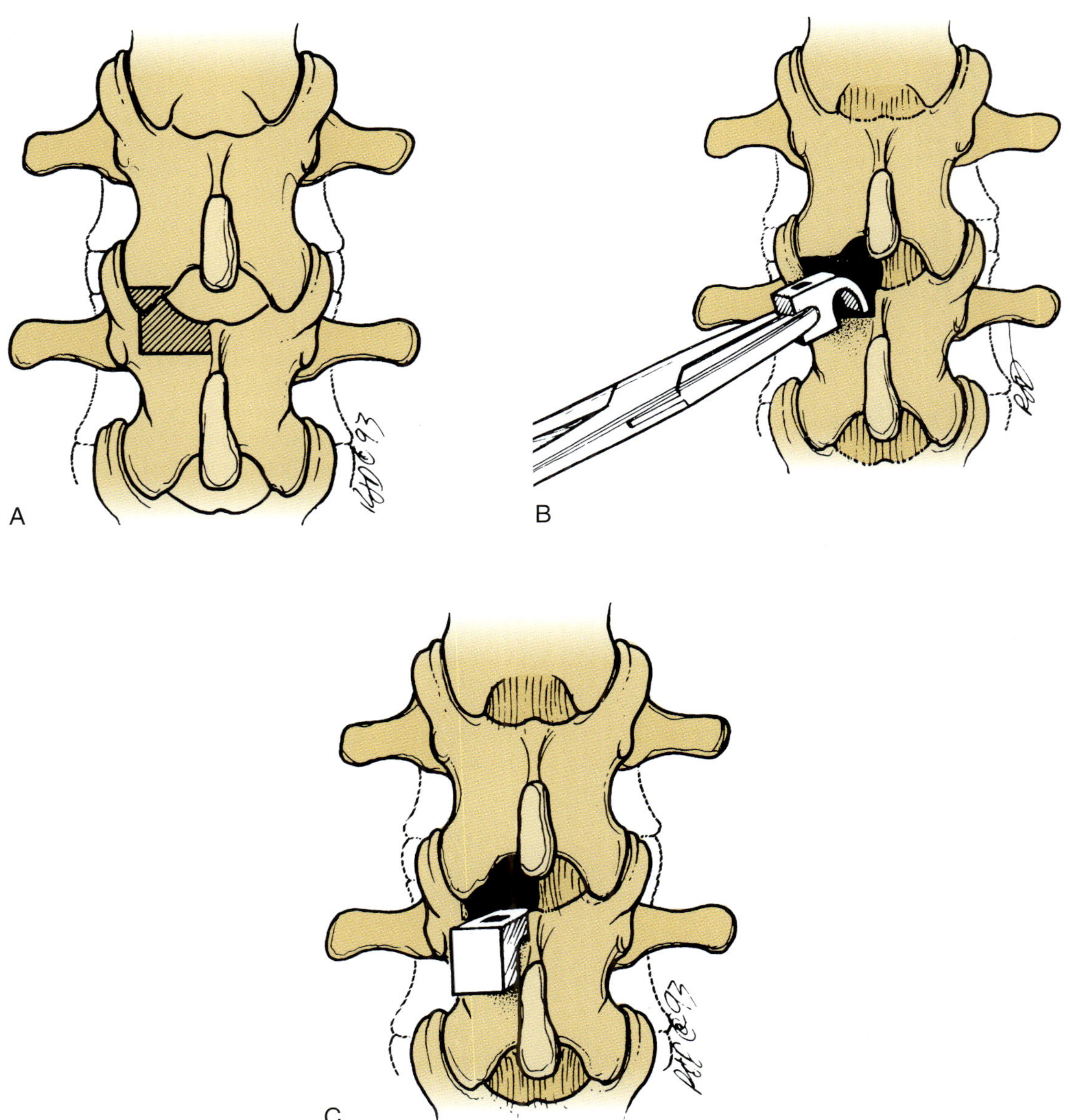

FIGURE 149-2. Harrington fixation, lower hook site. **A,** Preparation; **B** and **C,** insertion.

alignment. Edward sleeves can also be used to enhance reduction of kyphotic deformities.

Rod Sleeves

Rod sleeves are designed to provide reduction of kyphotic deformities.[5,6,8] They are made of high-density polyethylene with barium sulfate for radiodensity. Rod sleeves are made in various sizes: small 2-mm sleeves for use in the thoracic spine, medium 4-mm sleeves for use between T12 and L2, and elliptical sleeves for use in the lumbar region (Fig. 149-5). The rod is inserted into the rostral hook, and the rod sleeve is advanced along the rod until it overlies the apex of the deformity. The caudal end is grasped with a hook holder, and the distal rod is held with a rod holder. The deformity is reduced by applying constant ventral pressure. The rod is moved caudally until the distal tip engages the caudal hook, and distraction is applied with the rod distractor.

The second rod is placed in a similar fashion. Overdistraction is prevented by obtaining intraoperative radiographs. C-clamps are applied to the ratchet below the upper hook to avoid loss of distraction. Sublaminar wires or cables or interspinous wires are secured to the rods. Excess wire is cut, and the free ends are bent toward the midline to offer the construct a low profile.

Luque Segmental Wire Fixation

Luque instrumentation has been largely replaced by universal spinal instrumentation. Although the Luque system offers good stability against rotational and transitional forces, it provides less resistance to flexion-extension and little or

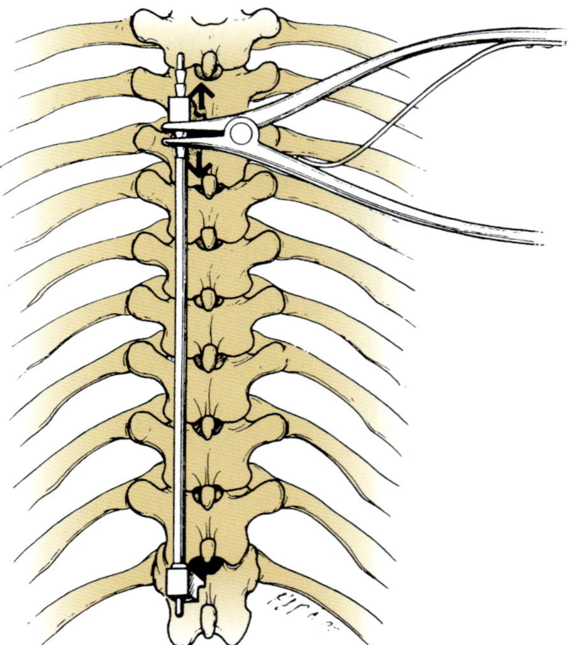

FIGURE 149-3. Distraction rod insertion.

no resistance to axial loading. The Luque system may still be used to treat slice fracture, in which the middle column fails because of shearing forces. It may also be useful in cases in which long fixation is required for correction of paralytic scoliotic deformities or in traumatic or neoplastic lesions that lead to flexion-compression fractures. The Luque system may be beneficial in patients with poor bone quality who require spinal stabilization.[4-7]

Technique

The technique for patient positioning and exposure is similar to the technique used for Harrington instrumentation. The technique for passage of wire or cable is as previously described for sublaminar wire or cable placement. An appropriate Luque rod is chosen and contoured to conform to the curvature of a normal spine. Alternatively, a Luque rectangle can be used.

Luque rectangles confer rotational and migrational stability to the construct. Sublaminar wires or cables are secured to the appropriately contoured Luque rod or rectangle (Figs. 149-6 to 149-8). The short limb of the L-shaped Luque rod should be secured beneath the long limb of the contralateral Luque L-rod (Fig. 149-9). Interspinous wiring techniques described for Harrington instrumentation can also be used with Luque L-rods. The interspinous wiring technique, although safer to perform than placement of sublaminar wires or cables, creates a weaker construct; also, it cannot be used with Luque rectangles, because the Luque rectangle cannot be adequately approximated to the spinous process.

Although originally designed for neutral fixation of the spine, the Luque system can be used to reduce kyphotic deformities. In this situation, the rostral end of one Luque L-rod and the caudal end of the contralateral Luque L-rod are attached and can be used to reduce kyphotic deformities. In this situation, the rostral end of one Luque L-rod is attached via sublaminar or interspinous wires or cables. The free ends of the rods are used as levers to reduce the existing kyphotic deformity (Fig. 149-10). After reduction, the wires or cables are sequentially tightened, ensuring lasting reduction. Excess wire or cable is cut, and the free ends are contoured to allow a low-profile construct. Closure is performed as described for Harrington instrumentation; postoperative care is also identical to Harrington instrumentation.

Universal Clamp

Although pedicle screw-rod systems largely predominate in thoracolumbar instrumentation at the present time, a more recent development has used the effectiveness of prior wire-hook constructs to achieve benefit in segmental fixation. The Zimmer Universal Clamp (Zimmer Spine, Minneapolis, MN) consists of a flat polyester band that can be used in sublaminar, transverse process, interspinous, or facet wiring techniques. Most often, it has been used in a Luque-type manner, in which the band is secured to a clamp. The clamp is placed onto the rod construct, where it is secured with a small locking screw. The band may be tightened with a reduction tool, which increases the tension on the band. Finally, the clamp is tightened to maintain the reduction. Purported benefits include a more optimal bone-implant interface strength, which has created complications in previous hook-wiring techniques. In addition, several titanium and stainless steel clamp diameters have been developed to accommodate the increasing number of rod sizes used.

Scott Wiring Technique

Few indications remain for the use of spinal wiring in the lumbar spine. One indication is symptomatic lumbar spondylolysis with or without grade I spondylolisthesis. This wiring technique for direct repair of spondylolysis was described by Nicol and Scott[10] and later modified by Johnson and Thompson.[11] The Scott wiring technique consists of wiring the transverse process to the spinous process.

Technique

The patient is positioned prone on the operating table. A subperiosteal dissection is performed and carried laterally, extending over the transverse processes. Bilateral pars interarticularis fractures are readily identified by the increased mobility of the affected segment. The defect is freed of any overlying or intervening fibrous tissue. The bony margins of the defect, base of the transverse process, and adjacent lamina are decorticated. Originally, a wire was passed around the transverse process bilaterally, and the free wire was passed beneath the subadjacent spinous process and was secured (Fig. 149-11). This technique was later modified to minimize the incidence of nerve root injury. With the modified technique, a hole is drilled at the base of the transverse process and the spinous process. A wire or, alternatively, a multistrand cable is passed through the hole at the base of the transverse process and then through the drill hole at the base of the spinous process, forming a figure-8 configuration. Autologous corticocancellous strips are placed over the pars interarticularis defect and decorticated transverse process and lamina. The bone grafts are secured into position by tightening the wire or cable.

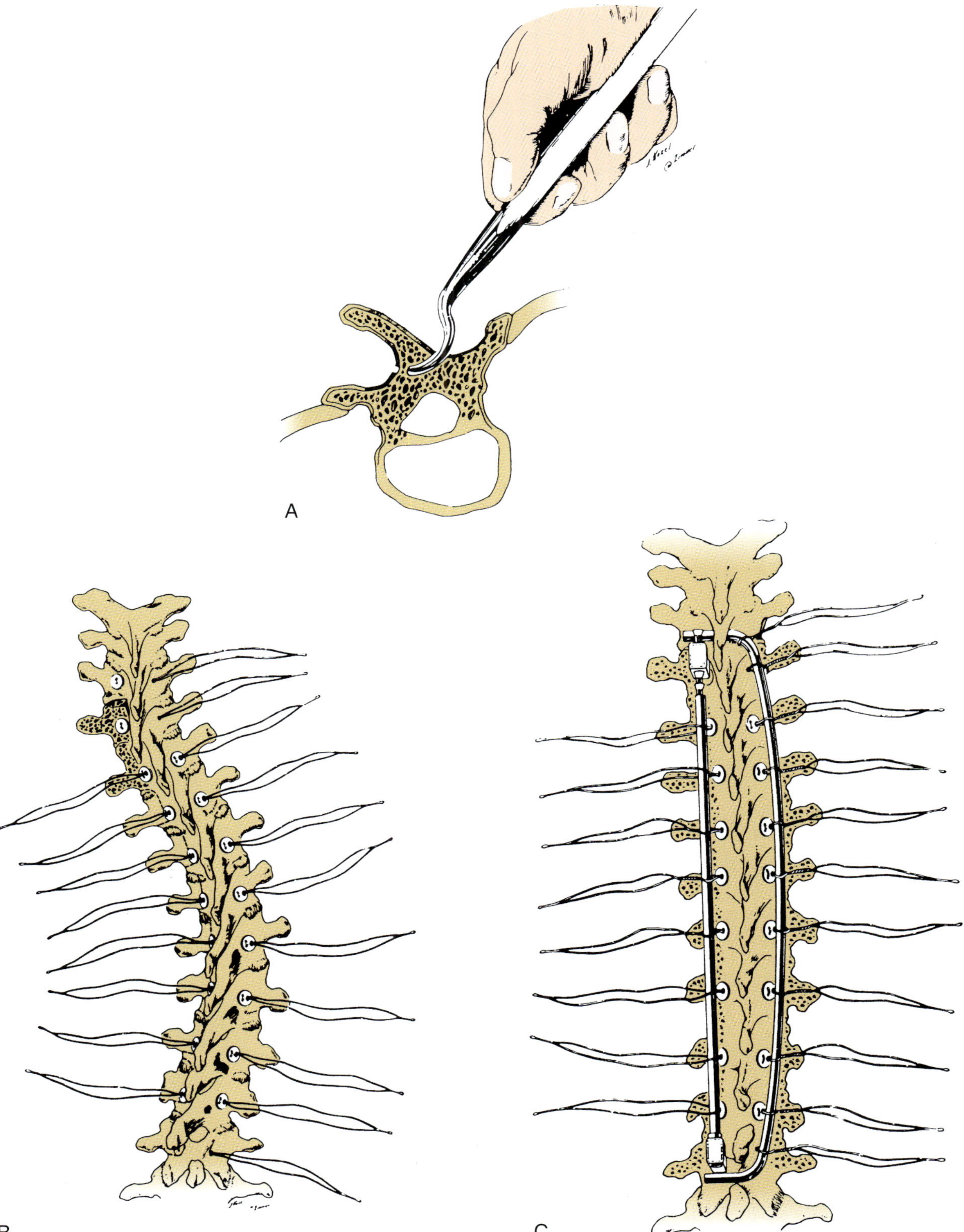

FIGURE 149-4. A–C, Placement of interspinous segmental instrumentation using Wisconsin wires and Drummond buttons.

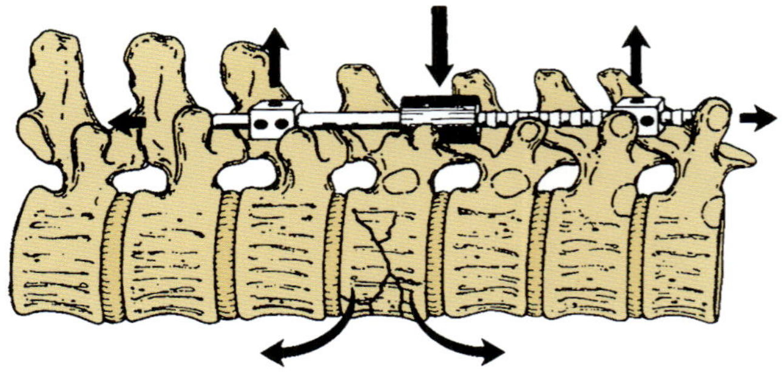

FIGURE 149-5. Placement of Edward sleeves.

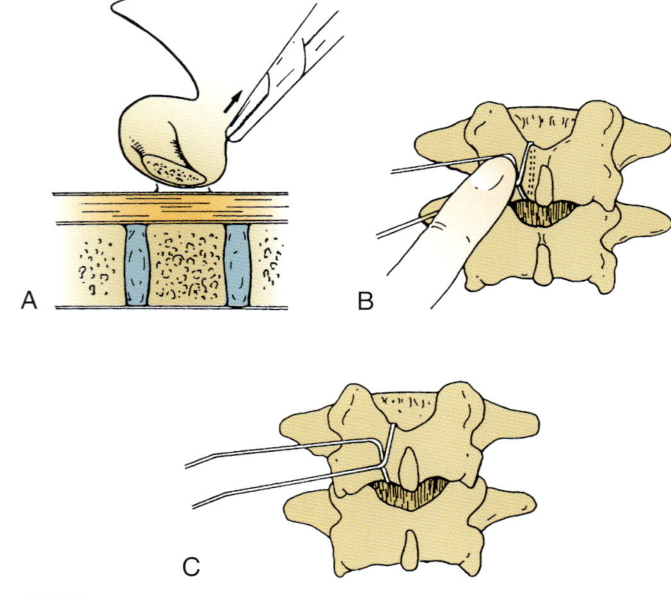

FIGURE 149-6. A, Placement of sublaminar wires via midline laminotomy. **B** and **C,** Crimping prevents spinal cord encroachment.

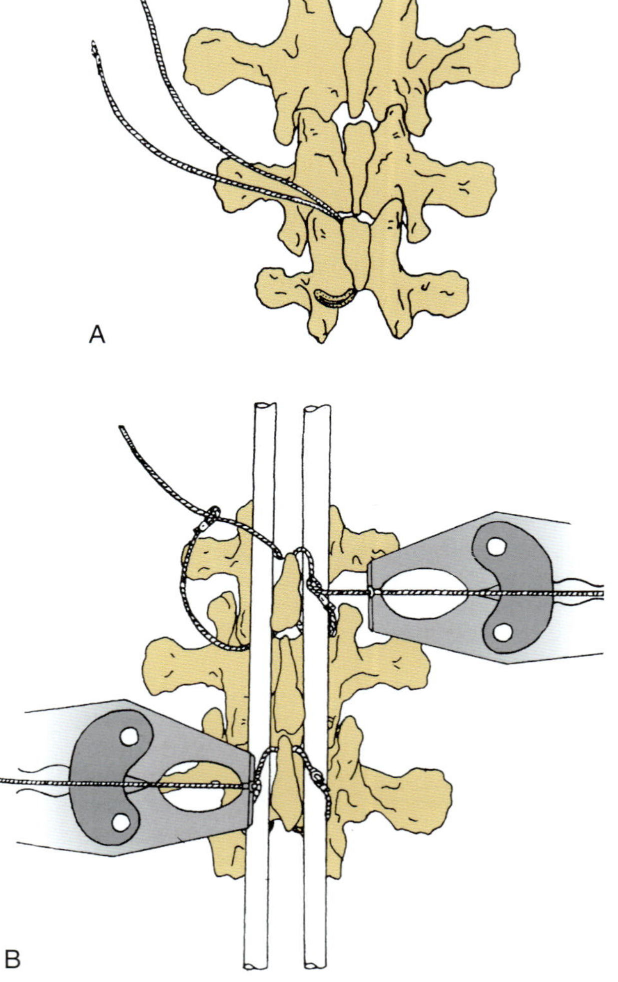

FIGURE 149-7. A and **B,** Placement of sublaminar multistrand cable via a midline laminotomy. (From Songer MN, Spencer DL, Meter PR, et al: The use of sublaminar cables to replace Luque wires. *Spine [Phila Pa 1976]* 16[suppl]:418–421, 1991.)

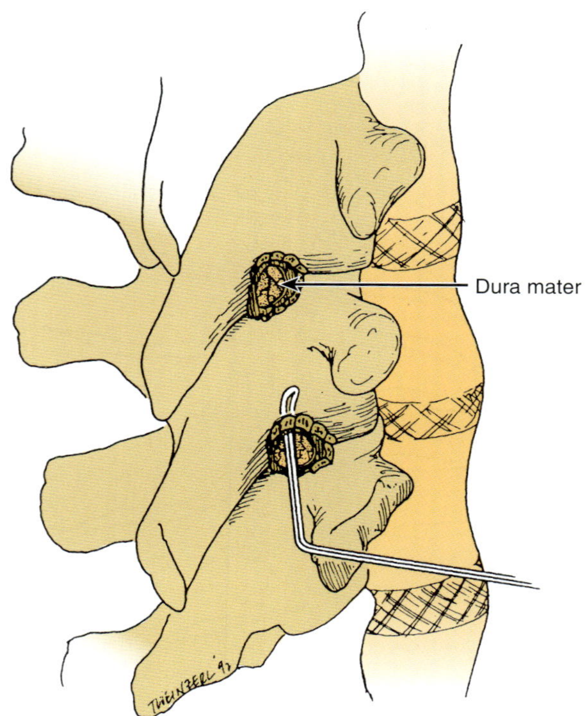

FIGURE 149-8. Placement of sublaminar wires via bilateral laminotomies.

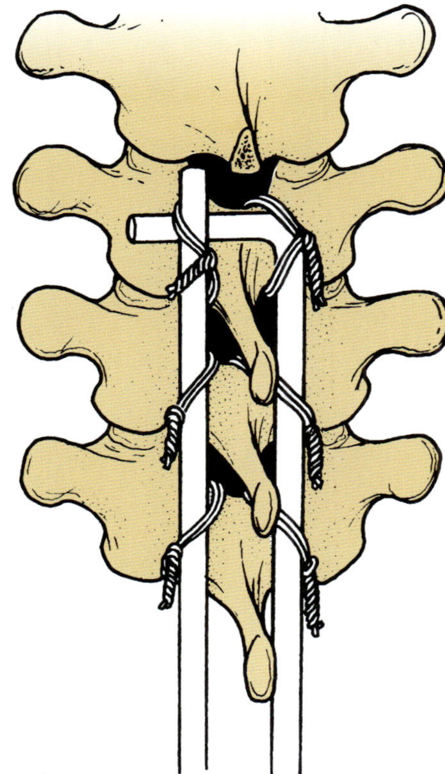

FIGURE 149-9. Luque L-rod configuration at termini of construct.

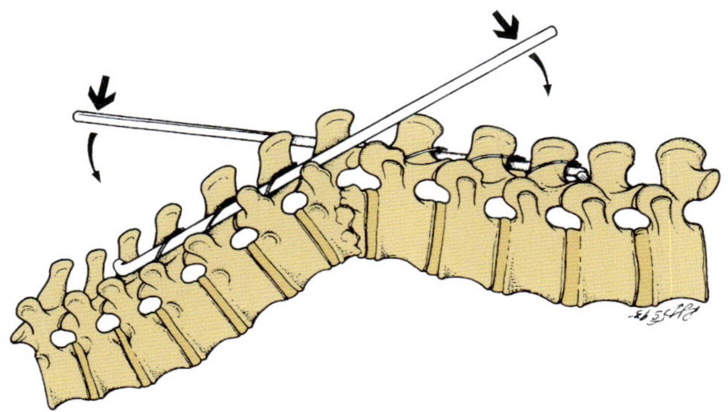

FIGURE 149-10. Harrington placement of Luque L-rods used in reduction of kyphotic deformities.

Summary

Simple hook-rod, wire, and wire-rod techniques for dorsal stabilization of the thoracic and lumbar spine have been available since the early 1960s. A testament to their utility is their longevity. These techniques provided the basic principles from which modern spinal instrumentation techniques have evolved, but they have been largely replaced by universal spinal instrumentation techniques. They are still used, however, for indications such as thoracic and lumbar instability, fixed deformities, neoplastic diseases, and degenerative disorders.

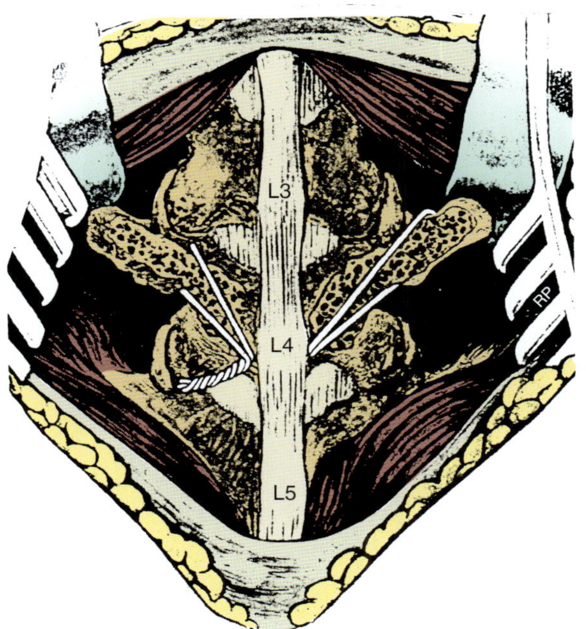

FIGURE 149-11. Scott wiring technique.

KEY REFERENCES

Drummond DS: Harrington instrumentation with spinous process wiring for idiopathic scoliosis. *Orthop Clin North Am* 19:281–289, 1998.

Harrington PR: Treatment of scoliosis: correction and internal fixation by spinal instrumentation. *J Bone Joint Surg [Am]* 44:591–610, 1962.

Harrington PR: Technical details in relation to the successful use of instrumentation in scoliosis. *Orthop Clin North Am* 3:49–67, 1972.

Harrington PR: The history and development of Harrington instrumentation. *Clin Orthop Relat Res* 93:110–112, 1973.

Luque ER: The anatomic basis and development of segmental spinal instrumentation. *Spine* 7:256–259, 1982.

McCormick PC: Dorsal distraction and neutral segmental fixation of the thoracic and lumbar spine: Harrington and Luque techniques. In Benzel EC, editor: *Spinal instrumentation*, Park Ridge, IL, 1994, Publications Committee of the North American Association of Neurological Surgeons, pp 125–141.

REFERENCES

The complete reference list is available online at expertconsult.com.

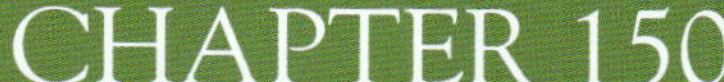
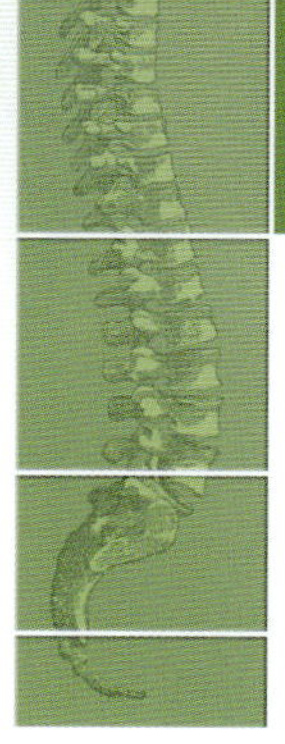

CHAPTER 150

Dorsal Thoracic and Lumbar Universal Spinal Instrumentation Techniques

Daniel K. Resnick | Basheal M. Agrawal | Sait Naderi

The treatment of traumatic, neoplastic, and degenerative disorders of the spine has evolved over the last several decades. A significant advance in the treatment of spinal disease has been the use of universal spinal instrumentation (USI). The term *universal* refers to the applicability of the construct throughout the thoracic and lumbar spine as well as to the variety of configurations with which it may be applied. These systems may be applied to the spine by using a variety of hooks and screws, alone or in combination. Multiple systems are currently available, and each has its own strengths and weaknesses of design. This chapter discusses the history of dorsal fixation techniques and the basic biomechanical principles used during the application of universal instrumentation systems. The techniques of implant insertion and the similarities and differences between several of the most commonly used systems are discussed.

History

Reports of wire and screw fixation of the thoracic and lumbar spine appeared in the medical literature in the late 1800s. In 1891, Hadra[1] described a procedure performed in 1887 in which Wilkins attempted fixation of T12-L1 in a neonate by using silver wire. Lange[2] contemporaneously described the (unsuccessful) use of nonfixed steel rods for the treatment of spinal deformity. Instrumentation of the thoracic and lumbar spine was restricted to wiring techniques and the occasional use of the facet screw until 1962, when Harrington introduced his spine instrumentation system. This system was the first that allowed for significant correction of spinal deformity and rigid fixation of the diseased spine.[3,4]

In the early 1970s, Luque[5] introduced segmental spinal instrumentation with sublaminar wires. The use of sublaminar wires provided multiple points of fixation, and when combined with closed loops instead of rods, or with the Harrington distraction system, provided significant resistance to flexion, extension, and lateral bending.[6] Continued modification of the Luque and Harrington systems through the 1970s laid the groundwork for the introduction of universal instrumentation in the early 1980s.

Pedicle screw fixation devices were introduced by Roy-Camille[7] in the 1980s. These devices use rods, plates, or fixators as longitudinal members. Pedicle screw fixation allows for the creation of rigid constructs. This rigidity has led to the advent of short-segment fixation. Because of the strength and the geometry of the systems, it is possible to allow for greater preservation of segmental motion at adjacent segments. Cotrel et al.[8] introduced the first "universal" spine fixation system in the late 1980s. This system used pedicle screws as well as multiple hooks. The latter were specifically designed to engage the pedicle, lamina, or transverse process. This allowed the application of the device throughout the thoracic and lumbar spine. Furthermore, the use of a combination of components allowed for the application of a variety of forces (compression, distraction, three-point bending). This in turn allowed for the efficacious correction of spinal deformities.[4,6] Recently the advent of frameless stereotaxic techniques has led to an increased popularity in the use of thoracic pedicle screws. The use of thoracic pedicle screws allows for rigid fixation of the thoracic spine without the need for intracanalicular instrumentation.

Surgical Indications

The indications for thoracic and lumbar dorsal instrumentation are evolving. Zdeblick,[9] Mardjetko et al.,[10] and others have demonstrated that instrumentation improves the rate of fusion in traumatic and degenerative conditions. In addition to increasing fusion rates, the stabilizing effect of dorsal universal instrumentation allows for earlier mobilization of patients with traumatic or neoplastic spinal instability. Although no benefit regarding neurologic outcome has been demonstrated, the ability to allow patients to ambulate soon after injury or surgery substantially lowers morbidity and allows for a more rapid rehabilitation.[11,12] The most common current use for thoracolumbar universal instrumentation systems is in the setting of degenerative lumbosacral instability.

Several current models and point systems are available to determine acute traumatic instability.[13,14] Subacute and glacial instability may be objectively demonstrated with serial and dynamic radiographs. Regrettably, the great majority of patients with back pain do not exhibit such clear-cut indications for surgery. The role of fusion and instrumentation for the treatment of "dysfunctional motion segments" remains somewhat controversial.[15,16] For nonradicular low back pain, fusion shows some benefit over standard conservative management, but is no better than intensive rehabilitation for improvement in pain or function.[17] The decision to use any of these systems for the treatment of back pain without clear radiographic evidence of instability is based solely on the clinical judgment of the surgeon.[6,18,19] Wide variation in surgical opinion due to the lack of consensus regarding indications for surgery has created a perception of overuse of instrumentation in many circles.[20]

Biomechanical Forces Imparted by Thoracic and Lumbar Spinal Implants

The human spine is daily subjected to a variety of stresses. The upright posture necessitates significant load bearing by the thoracic and lumbar spine. In addition, normal activity results in flexion, extension, lateral bending, and axial rotation of the spine. Each of these maneuvers results in the application of forces to the spinal elements. The intact spine, to paraphrase White and Panjabi,[14] resists these forces in such a manner as to avoid neural injury and deformation. When supraphysiologic forces are applied (e.g., in a motor vehicle accident), or when the integrity of the spinal elements is compromised (tumor or infection), deformation of the spine and possibly neural element damage results. A description of the forces acting on the spine is provided by clinical biomechanics. An understanding of these forces is helpful in planning corrective surgery.

Forces acting on the spine can be broken down into component vectors. A vector is a force that has both a magnitude and a fixed direction in three-dimensional space. A force vector may act directly on a point in space, causing translation (movement in the same plane as the vector). Alternatively, a force vector may act via a lever (moment arm), causing rotation about an axis. When a force vector acts via a moment arm, a bending moment is applied. The axis, or fulcrum, about which this bending moment causes rotation is termed the *instantaneous axis of rotation* (IAR). The IAR may be defined as the axis about which a given vertebral body rotates when acted on by a bending moment.[6,14] In the normal spine, the IAR is located in the region of the dorsal aspect of the vertebral body (middle column of Denis[13]). The bending moment (M) is defined as the product of the force (F) applied and the moment arm (D) or the perpendicular distance from the IAR ($M = F \times D$). The neutral axis is defined as the longitudinal axis that encompasses the IAR of adjacent vertebral bodies. Forces transmitted along the neutral axis cause no significant bending moment[14] (Fig. 150-1).

Newton's third law of motion, the law of conservation of momentum, states that interactions between objects result in no net change in momentum; thus for every action there is an equal (in magnitude) and opposite (in direction) reaction. In the present context, this implies that the spine (when at rest) exerts forces that are equal in magnitude and opposite in direction to the axial loads and bending moments applied. The ability of the normal spine to resist these forces depends on the material properties of the vertebral bodies and supporting bony, muscular, and ligamentous structures. When spinal instrumentation is applied, the construct may function simply as a replacement for a damaged spinal element (tension band fixation) or may apply forces to the spine in a relatively unusual and complex fashion (three-point bending).[6,14]

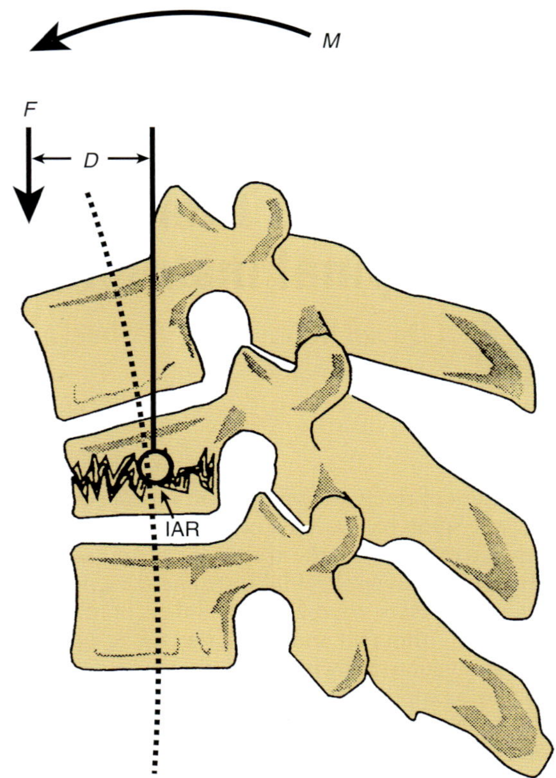

FIGURE 150-1. Biomechanical considerations. The forces acting on the thoracic and lumbar spine are depicted here as well as the effective kyphosis of the thoracic spine. An axial load (*F*) acts via a lever arm (*D*) to produce a bending moment (*M*) about the instantaneous axis of rotation (IAR). Forces that are transmitted within the neutral axis (*dotted line*) cause no bending moment. (Copyright University of New Mexico, Division of Neurosurgery.)

Distraction

Dorsal distraction fixation, usually applied with sublaminar hooks, has been used for short-segment distraction for deformity correction and foraminal stenosis. This mode of application has not found widespread use historically, however, because of a tendency for exaggeration of kyphotic deformity (Fig. 150-2).[6] Recently, Zucherman and others have introduced interspinous spacer devices that distract between the spinous processes of the lumbar spine.[21] Although these devices relieve symptoms of lumbar stenosis compared with nonsurgical treatment, they do induce kyphosis, which has generally been considered to be a contributor to failed back surgery syndrome and flat back syndrome.[22,23]

Tension Band Fixation

Dorsal compression fixation, applied with hooks, cables, or pedicle screws, is used for tension band fixation in the case of dorsal ligamentous insufficiency. This technique depends on the integrity of the load-supporting capacity of the ventral elements as well as the preservation of the relevant dorsal bony elements. This type of fixation should never be applied without adequate ventral spinal canal decompression. Tension band fixation may be used as a short-segment fixator, since the applied bending moment is independent of construct length (Fig. 150-3). Tension band constructs do

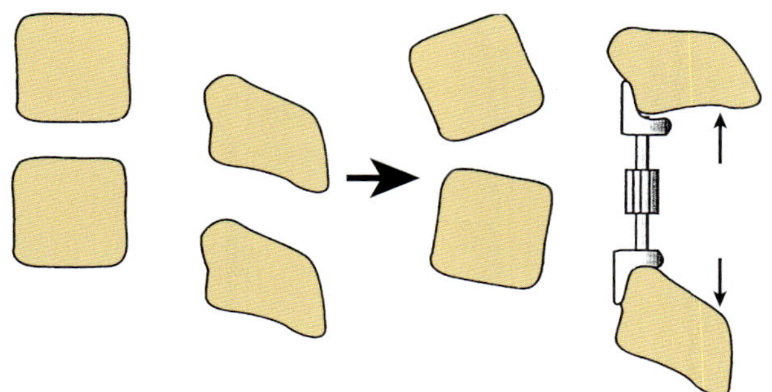

FIGURE 150-2. Dorsal distraction fixation may lead to kyphotic deformation, especially if used at or above the thoracolumbar junction. Use of distraction fixation in the lumbar spine may lead to a painful "flat back" syndrome. (Copyright University of New Mexico, Division of Neurosurgery.)

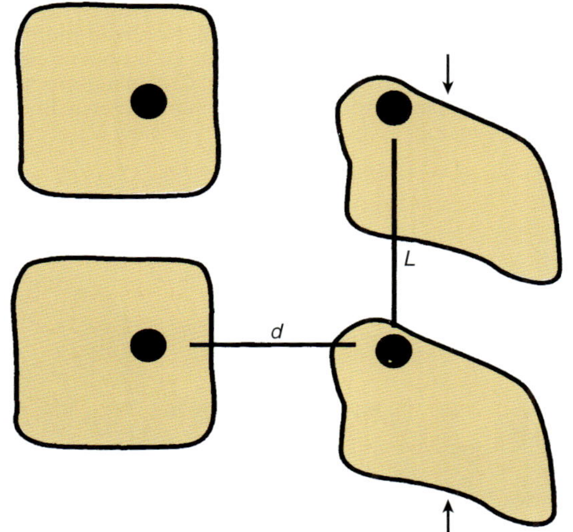

FIGURE 150-3. Tension band fixation of the dorsal spine is used most effectively when adequate ventral support is present. The bending moment applied is proportional to the distance between the implant and the instantaneous axis of rotation (*d*) and is independent of the length of the construct (*L*). Therefore, significant corrective forces may be applied with short-segment instrumentation. (Copyright University of New Mexico, Division of Neurosurgery.)

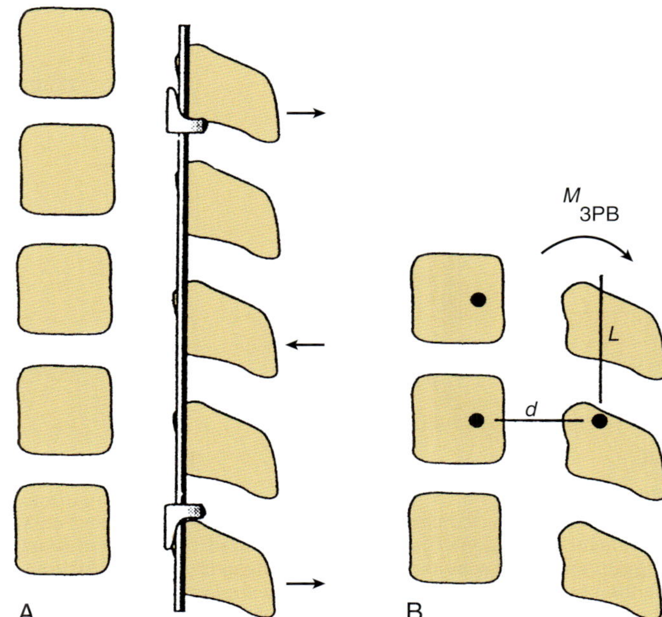

FIGURE 150-4. **A** and **B,** Three-point bending constructs rely on contact between the implant and the apex of a kyphotic curvature to produce forces perpendicular to the long axis of the spine. Forces are directed dorsally at the termini and ventrally in the center of the construct. These forces are equal in magnitude but opposite in direction. In the case of three-point bending implants, the bending moment (M_{3PB}) applied is directly proportional to the length of the construct (*L*). Therefore, since there is a limit to the dorsally directed forces that will be tolerated at the terminal implant-bone junctions, longer constructs are generally required for significant deformity correction. Alternatively, increasing the ability of the terminal interfaces to resist dorsally directed forces (e.g., using a claw configuration) allows for the application of greater corrective forces with shorter segment instrumentation. (Copyright University of New Mexico, Division of Neurosurgery.)

not, in general, resist translation and should not be relied on as stand-alone constructs when significant resistance to translation is required. When multiple segments are to be instrumented with this technique, multiple points of fixation should be used to prevent terminal bending moments.[6]

Three-Point Bending

Three-point bending forces are applied when translational forces are applied at both ends of a construct that are equal in magnitude but opposite in direction to a translational force applied to the fulcrum of a pathologic curvature. These constructs are usually applied in a distraction or neutral mode. The prototypical three-point bending construct is the Harrington distraction rod, especially when augmented with sleeves. The application of three-point bending forces depends on the physical contact between the longitudinal member and the fulcrum of the kyphotic deformity. These constructs, when placed dorsally, result in a dorsally directed force at both termini and a ventrally directed force at the fulcrum of the kyphotic curve (Fig. 150-4).[6] Three-point bending constructs must, by definition, traverse at least three spinal segments. Because the bending moments applied by a three-point bending implant are proportional to the length of the construct, multiple-segment instrumentation is frequently used to correct significant deformity. Because of the strong dorsally directed forces at the termini of the construct, three-point bending constructs are best applied by using multiple points of fixation. This maximizes the area of contact between the implant and bone. Laminar hooks are ideally designed to resist pull-out forces; however, sublaminar instrumentation placement carries a risk of injury to the neural elements. Pedicle hooks, transverse process hooks, and hook-screw combinations may be used in many cases to avoid sublaminar placement of hooks. A pedicle screw-hook construct at the same level provides substantial pull-out resistance and also contributes to load sharing (see later discussion) and is favored in many cases of significant instability. USI systems allow for the application of these constructs in a neutral mode by using hook "claws," which are able to engage the lamina without the significant distractive forces required by the Harrington rod system. Use of the claw technique allows for shorter segment fixation,

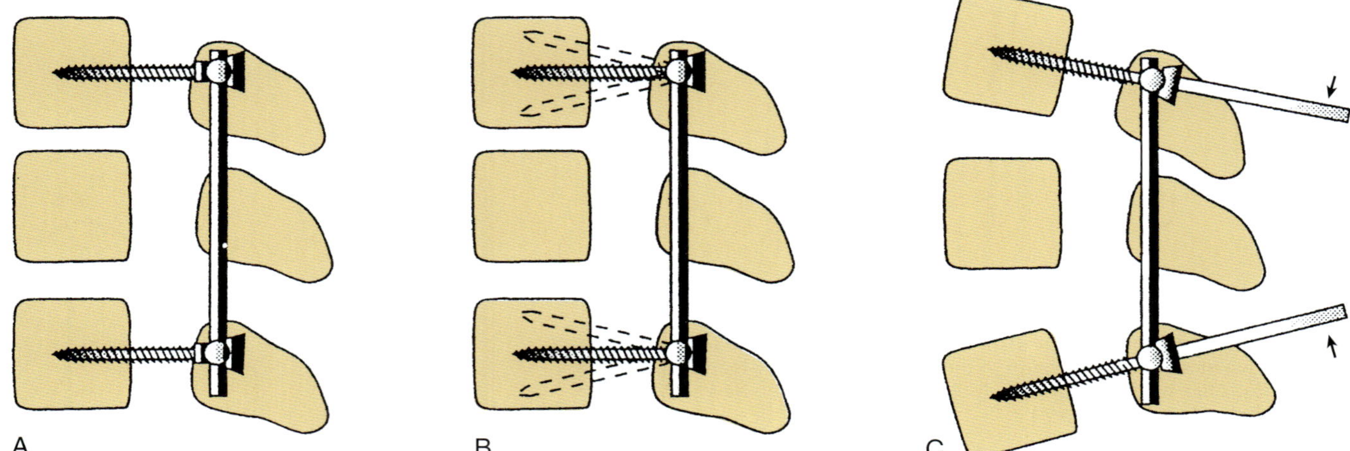

FIGURE 150-5. There are three types of cantilever-beam constructs. **A,** Fixed-moment arm cantilever-beam constructs employ constrained linkages between pedicle screws and longitudinal members and allow significant load bearing by the implant. **B,** Nonfixed-moment arm cantilever-beam constructs do not allow load bearing and function poorly as tension band constructs because of problems related to toggling and screw pull-out. Currently, these types of constructs are rarely used in the thoracic or lumbar spine. **C,** Applied-moment arm cantilever-beam constructs allow for the application of significant forces to the lumbar spine through the use of long screws. Because of the forces involved, screw breakage is likely to occur in the absence of strong bony fusion. (Copyright University of New Mexico, Division of Neurosurgery.)

since greater stresses may be borne at the hook-hook-lamina junction.[6]

Cantilever Beam Constructs

The final mode of application of dorsal universal instrumentation systems is cantilever beam fixation. A cantilever beam is simply a beam supported at one end, such as a balcony or awning support. These constructs are applied by using pedicle screws as the beams. Cantilever beams may be applied in one of three fashions. The great majority that are applied to the thoracic and lumbar spine are fixed-moment arm cantilever beams (Fig. 150-5A). A fixed-moment arm cantilever beam is one in which the pedicle screw is rigidly affixed to the longitudinal member. This type of construct allows for load bearing (when placed in a neutral or distractive mode) or load sharing (when placed in a compressive mode in conjunction with adequate ventral support).

Nonfixed cantilever beam constructs, in which the pedicle screw is not rigidly affixed to the longitudinal member, are rarely used in the thoracic and lumbar spine because of their inability to bear loads (like a hinged awning) and their poor performance as tension band constructs (caused by screw toggling and pull-out) (Fig. 150-5B). In the cervical spine, older lateral mass plate-screw systems are commonly applied nonfixed-moment arm cantilever beam constructs that work well. These systems take advantage of the anatomy of the cervical facet, which tends to resist translation. Due to recent tendencies to combine cervical and thoracic instrumentation systems and the extension of fixation techniques to the occipitocervical and atlantoaxial joints, fixed-moment arm cantilever beam systems have been developed for application in the cervical spine (Fig. 150-6). These systems allow for resistance to translation at C1-2 and seamless combination with thoracolumbar USI systems.[24]

The final cantilever beam construct is the applied-moment arm cantilever beam. This type of construct allows for the application of flexion or extension forces at the time of implant placement. Using long screws (Schanz type), a bending moment is applied to the spine. Once the desired corrective forces have been applied, the implant is fixed in place (Fig. 150-5C).[6] The application of these forces places great stress on the implant, which may result in failure of the implant, particularly if osseous union does not occur in a timely fashion.

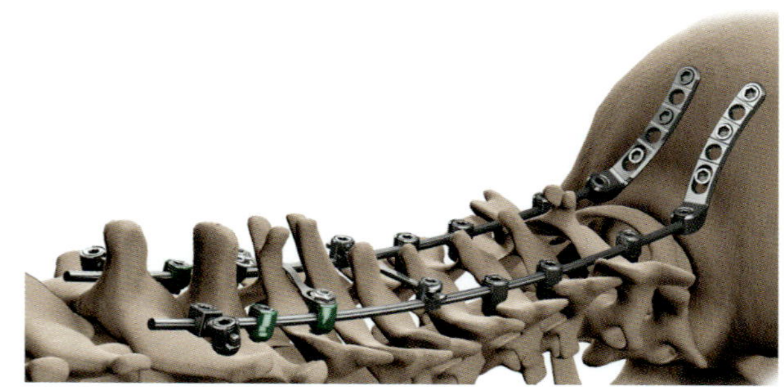

FIGURE 150-6. Combination of cervical and thoracic instrumentation systems with extension of fixation to the occipitocervical junction. (Courtesy of Stryker Spine.)

Biomechanical Properties of Universal Spinal Implant Systems

All universal spinal implant systems consist of screws, hooks, and longitudinal members. The composition, shape, and size of the implants vary to some extent. However, all conform to the constraints placed on them by the anatomic configuration of the bony spine. Some of the basic properties of the components and the effect that changes in these basic properties (e.g., the particular alloy of stainless steel used in a longitudinal member or the profile of the minor diameter of a screw) have on the performance of a given system are discussed in the following sections.

Metallurgy

USI systems are composed of stainless steel, titanium alloy, or pure titanium. Stainless steel implants are, in general, stronger than similarly sized titanium implants and have excellent corrosion resistance. The most commonly used alloy is 316L stainless steel, which contains 17% chromium, 13% nickel, and 2.25% molybdenum. A newer alloy, 22-13-5 (referring to percentages of chromium, nickel, and manganese, respectively) has even greater strength and surface hardness.[25] Stainless steel implants are ferromagnetic and thus interfere with MRI. Furthermore, osteointegration, or the ingrowth of bone into steel screws or rods, does not occur. A final caveat regarding the use of stainless steel is that it should not be used in patients with cutaneous nickel allergies. Dermal patch testing can rule out significant reaction to the alloy if there is a question regarding hypersensitivity.[25]

Titanium alloys have the advantages of being highly biocompatible and minimally interfering with MRI. The most common titanium alloy is Ti-6-4, a combination of titanium, aluminum, and vanadium. This particular alloy has tensile strength that approaches that of 316L stainless steel. It is quite brittle, however.[25] Titanium may also be used in its unalloyed, or "pure," form.[26] Pure titanium is available in several grades (1–4), depending on the amount of impurities found in the metal. The less-pure grades (2–4) have tensile and elastic properties that approach those of 316L stainless steel. Titanium is more resistant to corrosion than steel[6] and also allows for osteointegration, both of which should decrease the incidence of implant failure.[25]

In addition to the composition of the metal used to create a spinal implant, the processes used to forge the metal and the surface characteristics of the implant affect performance. For example, cold working of a metal implant produces a harder, stronger material than does annealing. Also, shot peening, a surface treatment in which the implant is hardened by firing small particles against it, increases fatigue resistance. Any surface irregularity will increase the rate of corrosion of any implant. Finally, metals in implant construction should not be mixed, to avoid creating a galvanic current between the implant components. Such a current could, theoretically, increase the rate of corrosion and weaken the implant.[6]

Polyetheretherketone

Polyetheretherketone (PEEK) is a carbon-based thermoplastic polymer that maintains stability at temperatures in excess of 300°C.[27] PEEK is biocompatible and inert, with few reports of cutaneous, muscular, or inflammatory reactions.[28] Biomechanically, PEEK rods have an elasticity, measured by Young's modulus, similar to cortical bone, unlike titanium rods, which are much stiffer.[29] PEEK rods may also have some biomechanical advantages in terms of resistance to static and fatigue angular displacements compared with their titanium counterparts; however, the clinical significance of this in the setting of a bony fusion is not established.[28] Few studies have been performed comparing PEEK and titanium instrumentation; however, potential advantages of PEEK include its radiolucency, load-sharing capacities, and resistance to pedicle fracture given a more favorable bone-screw interface.[30]

Hook Design

Hooks used for universal instrumentation may be placed in a variety of positions. Laminar hooks may be placed facing rostrally or caudally. Pedicle hooks are placed outside of the spinal canal and face rostrally, abutting the pedicle. Transverse process hooks are placed facing caudally over the transverse processes of the thoracic spine. Manufacturers have responded differently to the multiple locations and orientations of the hooks. Some systems, such as the Texas Scottish Rite Hospital (TSRH) system, provide a wide variety of hooks specially designed for placement at a specific site and with a specific orientation. Other systems, such as the Isola system, use similar hooks for all applications (Fig. 150-7). The choice of the system used depends on surgeon preference.

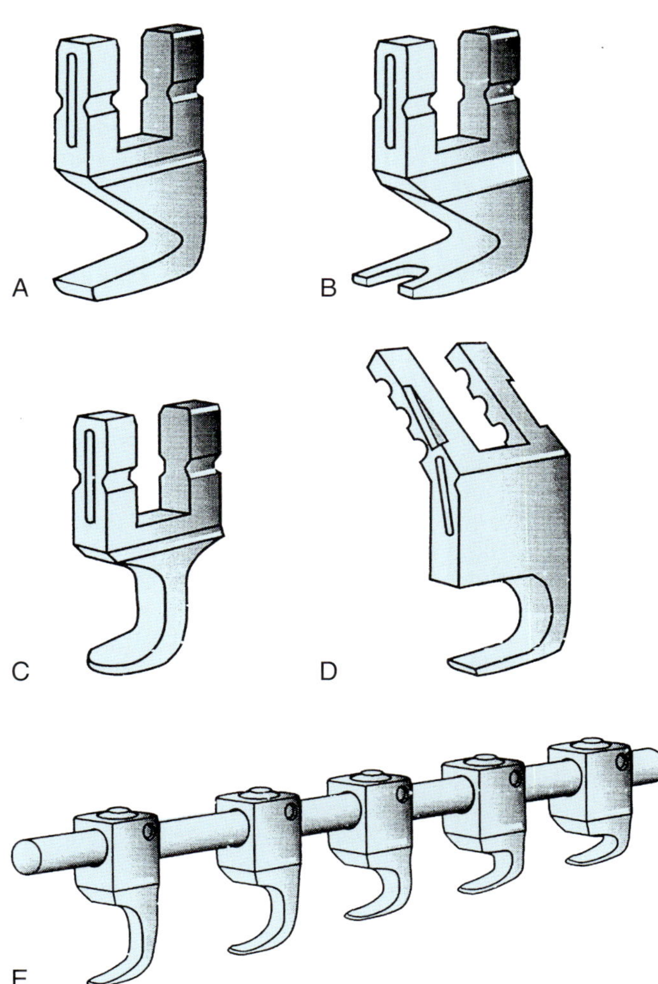

FIGURE 150-7. Hook design spinal hooks are available in a variety of configurations for placement under the lamina. TSRH laminar hook (**A**), abutting the pedicle (**B**, TSRH pedicle hook), or over the transverse process (**C**, TSRH transverse process hook). **D,** An offset hook allows for less rod contouring. Note the throat shape of the laminar hook (**A**), which causes dorsal movement of the hook away from the spinal canal when this caudal facing hook is compressed against the lamina. The bifid blade design of the TSRH pedicle hook (**B**) aids in engagement of the pedicle. **E,** The Isola System provides hooks that share a common design but vary in size. This variation may require more bone contouring but results in a more streamlined instrumentation set. (Copyright University of New Mexico, Division of Neurosurgery.)

More choices, in terms of hook configuration, require less bone contouring. However, more choices also require a more cumbersome instrumentation set.[31]

Hooks may be open ended, allowing top loading of the rod onto the hook, or alternatively, they may be closed so that the rod can slide through a circular aperture. Closed hooks are theoretically stronger and should in general be used at the terminus of a construct where applied forces are the greatest. Open-ended hooks are best used at sites of intermediate fixation, within the center of the construct, because of their ease of application.[31] In reality, the incidence of hook failure caused by failure of the hook-rod interface is extremely low in modern USI systems.

Pedicle Screws

Pedicle screws are used for fixation of spinal implants when the lamina or transverse processes are not present (after decompression or trauma) or when significant load bearing or resistance to rotation by the implant is desired. Pedicle screw design incorporates several biomechanical principles. The minor diameter of a screw is defined as the minimal (inner) diameter of the screw (base of one thread to the base of the opposite thread). The strength, or resistance to bending and breaking, of a screw is proportional to the third power of its minor diameter. Therefore, small increases in the minor diameter of a screw are associated with large increases in strength. Obviously, the anatomic configuration of the pedicle and the design constraints limit the minor diameter. Because the region of the screw subject to the greatest strain is the screw-plate or screw-rod junction, tapered screws have been developed to maximize strength where it is needed without sacrificing pull-out resistance.[25]

The pull-out resistance of a screw is related to the amount of bone that can be incorporated between the threads of the screw. The distance between the threads (pitch), major diameter, and thread shape all influence the pull-out resistance of a screw. Osteointegration should significantly increase resistance to screw pull-out. The most important factor in determining screw pull-out resistance is bone quality. Osteopenic bone and low-density medullary bone provide poor purchase for even the best designed screws. Severe osteopenia may be considered a contraindication for screw fixation. Augmentation of pedicles with polymethylmethacrylate or other cements has been described as a means to overcome the effects of osteoporosis; however, caution is advised when applying significant forces to the osteoporotic spine.[32,33] A screw diameter should be selected such that the relatively dense cortical bone of the pedicle walls is partially engaged by the threads of the screw to maximize pull-out resistance.

Screw length should be selected so that at least one half to two thirds of the vertebral body is engaged. This allows the screw to function as a load-bearing component in all three columns of the spine. Screws may be self-tapping, a property achieved through fluting of the first several threads to allow for the displacement of cut bone.

Like hooks, screws may be attached to longitudinal members in a variety of ways. The great majority of screw/longitudinal component junctions available for use in the thoracic and lumbar spine are constrained (rigid), allowing for the creation of fixed-moment arm cantilever beam constructs. End-loading, top-loading, side-loading, and through-the-plate connections are available. Multiaxial coupling systems may significantly simplify construct application. The ability to compensate for small discrepancies in sagittal and coronal alignment decreases the need for three-dimensional rod bending. However, the mechanical strength of these coupling mechanisms must be appreciated by the surgeon prior to application.

Longitudinal Members

The longitudinal components of USI systems consist of rods or plates. Surface characteristics of the rods vary to maximize component-component junction strength (e.g., the knurled surfaces of Cotrel-Dubousset [CD] rods) and/or implant corrosion resistance (smooth surfaces of the TSRH rods). Two factors that weaken any longitudinal member are stress risers and notching. Stress risers result from the application of focal stress, which usually occurs during contouring of the rods or plates. Notching is an injury to the surface of an implant that may result in significant alterations of structural integrity. A 1% notch (e.g., a 3.6-mm rod with a 36-μm-deep notch) reduces fatigue resistance of 316L stainless steel wire by 63%.[34] Titanium is known to be especially sensitive to the effects of notching.[6,35]

Component-Component Junctions

USI systems use different mechanisms for component-component junctions. The mechanism of engagement and the surface characteristics of the implants affect the durability and strength of the construct as a whole. The most commonly used mechanisms for attaching component hooks and screws to longitudinal members are the three-point shear clamp, lock screw connectors, circumferential grip connectors, constrained and semiconstrained screw-plate connectors, and semiconstrained hook-rod connectors.[6] Three-point shear clamp connectors use a three-point bending force applied to the longitudinal member (rod) to tightly approximate the components. The majority of TSRH connectors are of this type. A lock screw connector uses a screw to drive the rod into a contoured bed, as with the Isola V groove hollow ground system. Tangential application of the screw appears to have some mechanical advantage.[6]

Circumferential grip connectors provide both halves of a pincer to provide truly circumferential force application (e.g., Synthes locking screw-plate connector) or only half of the pincer (Isola VHG).[6] Constrained bolt-plate connectors do not allow toggling of the screw or hook at the component-component junction. The Steffee plate-pedicle screw connector is an example of this type of connection. The only example of a semiconstrained connector (that allows movement in at least one plane) used in the thoracic or lumbar spine is the Harrington rod-hook connection, which allows for rotation and some toggling of the hook about the rod.[6]

Surface characteristics of the component-component junction are important. Friction enhancers, such as knurled surfaces, radial spokes or grooves, or a grid pattern, increase friction between the components. Knurled surfaces should not be mixed with smooth surfaces, because this can result in poor surface contact.

Polyaxial Pedicle Screws

Traditionally, pedicle screw heads were fixed, necessitating adjustments to the depth of screw insertion so as to accommodate rod placement. Repositioning of pedicle screws, without increasing the diameter of the screw, decreases its purchase strength.[36]A polyaxial screw is designed with the screw head enclosed on a housing unit that allows for ball-joint motion of the screw head (Fig. 150-8).Variable-head screws minimize repositioning of pedicle screws and contouring of the rods, conferring a theoretical advantage to pull-out strength of pedicle screws and avoidance of "notching" due to contouring. Polyaxial screws do not significantly decrease construct stiffness, and there is a suggestion of increased resistance to torque conferred by better purchase of the intervertebral rod.[37] Biomechanical testing shows that the first failure point of polyaxial screws is the head-screw interface.[38]

Technical Aspects of Implant Application

USI placement techniques have been described.[6,7,31,39] What follows is a brief overview of the techniques used for the placement of dorsal spinal instrumentation.

Pedicle Screw Insertion

The pedicle is the strongest portion of the vertebra. It consists largely of cortical bone. The transverse width of the pedicle is the limiting factor in terms of screw size and may be determined by preoperative CT. The transverse pedicle angle increases from near 0 degrees (straight dorsal-ventral) at L1 to nearly 30 degrees (dorsolateral to ventromedial) at L5. The sagittal angle of the pedicle also varies somewhat, but in a narrower range (5 degrees craniocaudal at L1 to 15 degrees at L5).[14,39,40] Preoperative radiographic studies aid in the determination of optimal screw placement angles. Alternatively, recent advances in frameless stereotaxy allow facile comparison of surgical anatomy with preoperative axial imaging studies. A caveat to the use of these systems is that the images displayed are not real time. Therefore, the quality of the information provided to the surgeon depends completely on the accuracy of registration of the vertebral body involved. Alternatively, fluoroscopy or fluoroscopy-based frameless stereotactic systems may be used to provide feedback to the surgeon regarding hidden anatomy. The main limitation to the fluoroscopy-based frameless stereotactic systems is the quality of the source images. The use of frameless stereotaxy has been reported to improve the accuracy of pedicle screw placement in the lumbar and thoracic spine.[41-43] The use of such systems does not appear to degrade the fluoroscopic information and may in fact provide better feedback than live fluoroscopy because of the ability to use multiplanar imaging[44] (Fig. 150-9). Recent advances in imaging technology have allowed the use of real-time axial imaging in the operating room. These systems provide the advantages of axial imaging with real-time image acquisition.[45,46] Depending on surgical technique, the use of such systems may or may not be associated with improved outcomes. Intraoperative electrophysiologic stimulation has been used by some investigators for the purpose of increased sensitivity to cortical violation during pedicle preparation.[47,48] Although such systems can indicate a pedicle breach, no evidence has been reported that clinical outcomes are favorably influenced by the use of such systems.[49]

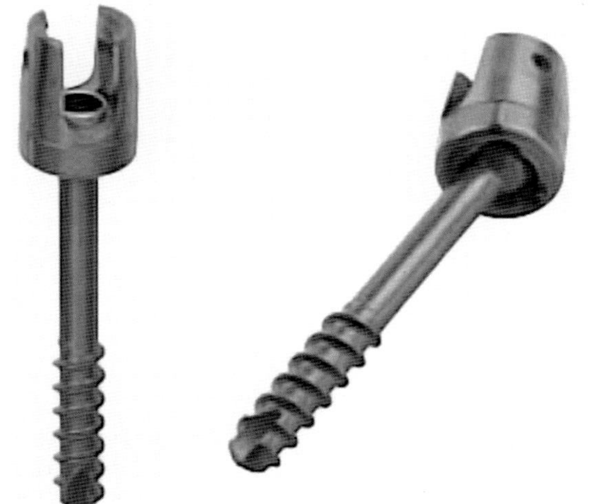

FIGURE 150-8. Polyaxial pedicle screws. Note that the screw head is mounted to allow for ball-joint maneuvering. (Images provided by Medtronic Sofamor Danek USA, Memphis, TN.)

The dorsal aspect of the lumbar pedicle is localized by using the junction of two lines. The first line is a straight rostrocaudal line drawn along the lateral border of the superior articular facet. The second line is a transverse line through the center of the transverse process (Fig. 150-10). The lateral aspect of the pedicle may be palpated with a dissector placed over the rostral border of the transverse process, and, when practical, the medial aspect of the pedicle may be exposed by laminectomy or laminotomy. The screw entrance site (dorsal aspect of the pedicle) is decorticated with a drill or rongeur, and the pedicle is probed with a blunt-tipped pin or small curet. Intraoperative radiographs are used to check the accuracy of pin placement and trajectory. Once adequate placement of the pins has been confirmed, the pins are removed and the holes prepared for screw placement. Alternatively, the pedicles may be cannulated with a 2.5-mm drill. This technique is largely used in conjunction with a frameless stereotactic system or with real-time fluoroscopy. Gentle pressure and a slight "tapping" motion help to keep the drill bit within the confines of the pedicle. This technique is especially useful in sclerotic pedicles (congenital spondylolisthesis) or in very small pedicles (e.g., in the thoracic spine, see later discussion). Hole locations are marked with radiopaque markers and verified with intraoperative radiographs or fluoroscopy.

Reliable anatomic landmarks used for the placement of thoracic pedicle screws probably do not exist. Unfortunately, there is a substantial amount of variability in pedicle location, size, and angle between individuals and between levels in the same individual.[50] As such, pedicle cortex violation is relatively common with blind insertion. One such series reported a 47% rate of pedicle breach.[51] Special aiming devices have been manufactured but have not been subject to critical review.[52] The use of frameless stereotactic techniques has improved accuracy of screw placement in several series.[41-43] An alternative technique, the performance of small laminotomies to directly palpate the pedicle for the placement of thoracic pedicle screws, has also been described as improving accuracy. The surgeon should choose the technique that

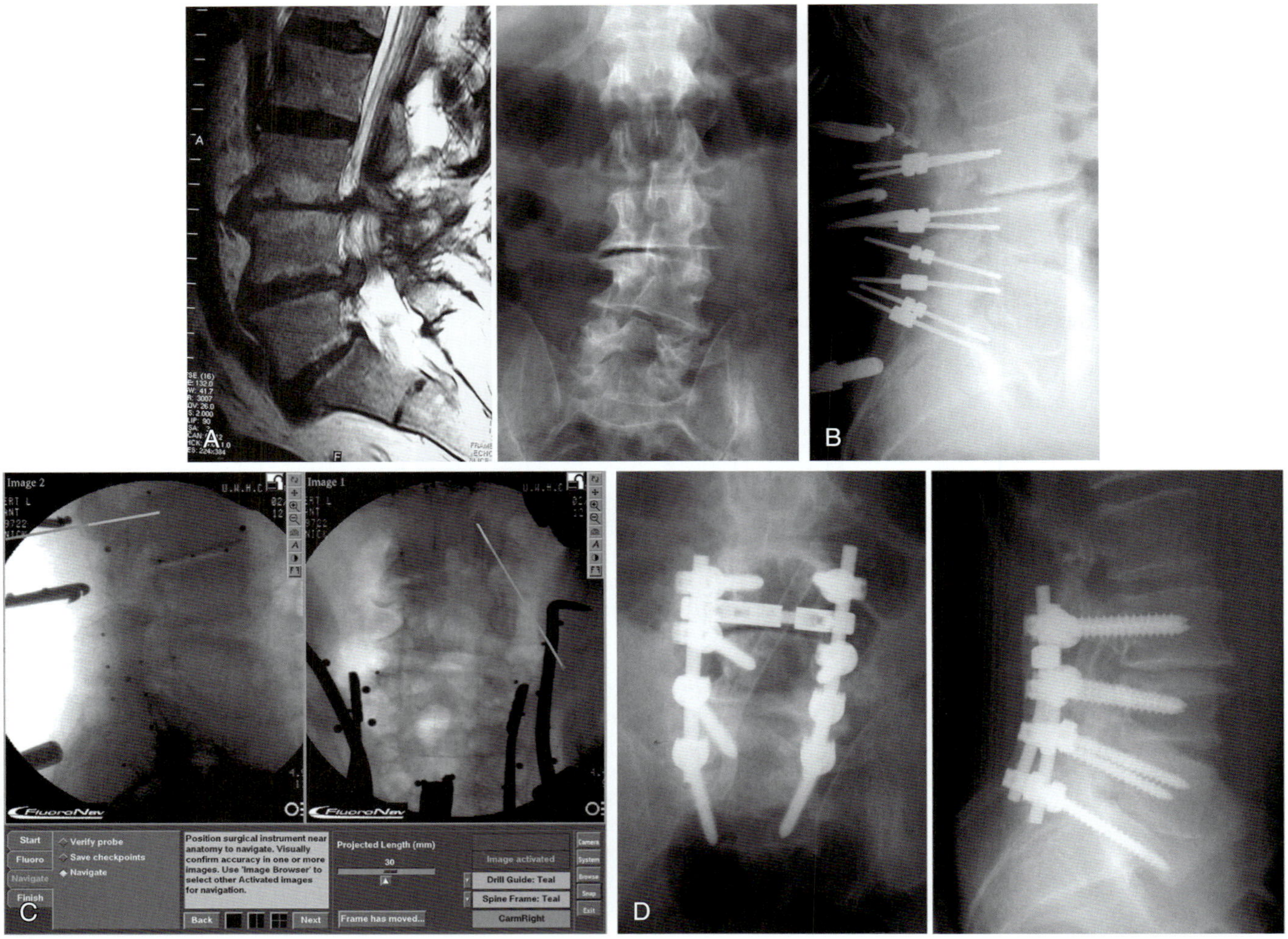

FIGURE 150-9. **A,** In this patient with degenerative stenosis instability of the lumbar spine, a significant coronal plane deformity exists. **B,** A lateral radiograph obtained after pin placement may or may not demonstrate optimal screw position. **C,** The use of frameless stereotaxy allows for multiplanar imaging. **D,** This ability greatly facilitated screw placement in this case.

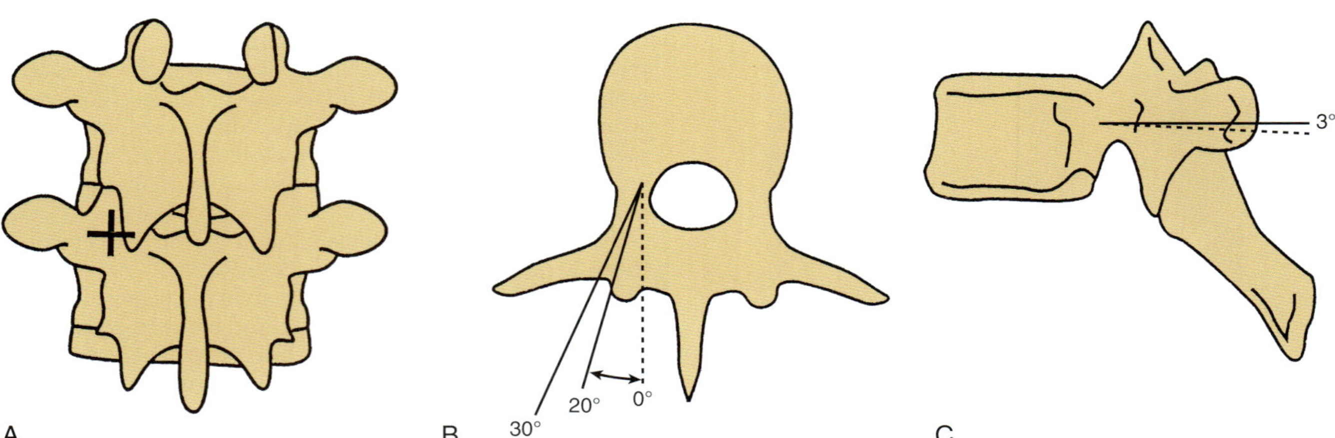

FIGURE 150-10. Pedicle screw placement. **A,** The entrance point for pedicle screw placement is at the junction of the rostrocaudal lateral facet line and the transverse midtransverse process line. **B,** Axial representations of pedicle screw placement in the L4 and L5 vertebrae. Note the difference in the angle of placement with the L4 screw oriented at a 20-degree angle from the sagittal plane and the L5 screw oriented at a near 30-degree angle from the sagittal plane.[12,14] **C,** Sagittal view of pedicle screw placement in L4 and L5. Differences in the sagittal angulation of the pedicles of the lumbar vertebrae are not as pronounced as in the axial plane. Note the slight difference in the angulation with the L4 screw placed parallel to the axial plane and the L5 screw placed at a 3-degree angle with respect to the axial plane.[12,14] (Copyright University of New Mexico, Division of Neurosurgery.)

works best in his or her hands and become a master at that particular technique.

Holes are tapped with successively larger taps until a desired diameter is reached. The walls of the pedicle should be palpated from within after each tap to verify the integrity of the cortical bone. Screws should be placed with as much lateral-to-medial angulation as possible so as to maximize the beneficial effects of triangulation on screw pull-out and parallelograming if cross-links are to be applied (see later discussion).[6] Screw placement lateral to the pedicle may allow for increased triangulation without significantly degrading pull-out resistance. We reserve this technique for salvage following pedicle stripping or fracture. Screw length should be selected such that the ventral two thirds of the vertebral body is engaged. Because of the constrained linkages between the screws and the longitudinal member in all thoracolumbar USI systems, no significant advantage is gained by penetration of the ventral cortex. A final intraoperative radiograph is obtained before linkage to the longitudinal member.

Laminar Hook Insertion

Laminar hooks are designed to be placed under the lamina, facing either rostrally or caudally. The use of laminar hooks in the lumbar and sacral spine is universally accepted, whereas use of such hooks above the level of the conus medullaris is more controversial. Preoperative imaging studies are useful for determining the adequacy of the spinal canal for sublaminar hook placement. If a relative stenosis exists at a particular level, that level should be avoided and fixation obtained at another level or by another means. In all cases, care must be taken to prevent the hooks from encroaching on neural elements. Laminotomies are performed, removing the caudal portion of the lamina above and the rostral portion of the lamina below the level of hook application (Fig. 150-11). The ligamentum flavum is removed, and in some cases, medial facetectomies are performed. A laminar tester is used to verify the adequacy of the sublaminar dissection. The largest hook that can be placed at a given level should be selected to maximize the bone-implant junction. It is often possible to "stagger" hooks from side to side so as to avoid placing two hooks under the same lamina. The hook must closely appose the laminar surface to avoid encroachment into the spinal canal. If an appropriately contoured hook is not available, the lamina should be contoured for an exact fit. Once a hook is placed, it should be compressed against its lamina to prevent migration into the spinal canal. Special care must be taken when hooks are used as intermediate points of fixation with three-point bending constructs (Fig. 150-12) because the hooks may be driven into the spinal canal by the application of such forces if they are not tightly apposed to their respective laminae.[6,31]

Pedicle Hooks

Pedicle hooks are placed beneath the caudal articulating surface of the thoracic facet. Pedicle hooks are placed outside of the spinal canal and therefore are used throughout the thoracic spine, with the exception of at the thoracolumbar junction. The more sagittal orientation of the lower thoracic facet joints makes hook application difficult at these levels. Most USI systems use bifid hooks, which make pedicle purchase more secure. However, placement of nonbifid hooks is aided by the "sandwiching" effect of the superior and inferior articulating surfaces of the facet joint.

Thoracic pedicle hooks are placed between the superior and inferior articulating surfaces of the facet. The caudal portion of the inferior articular process is removed by using a drill or osteotome. The amount of bone removed is critical,

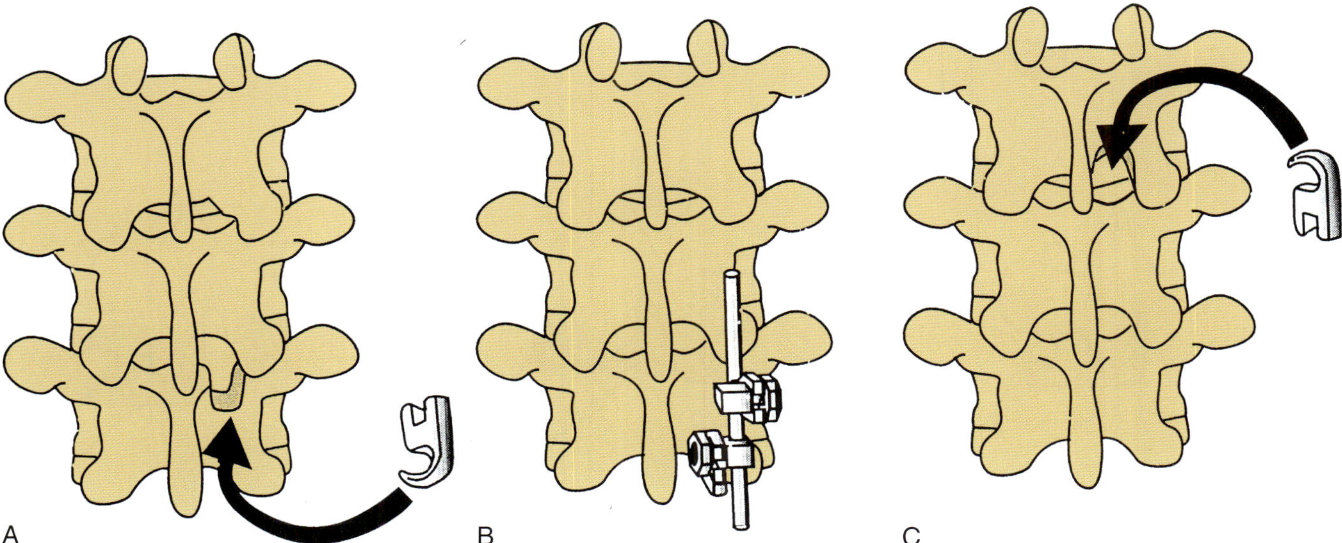

FIGURE 150-11. Laminar hook insertion. Laminar hooks may be placed facing rostrally or caudally. For placement of a rostral facing hook, a small laminotomy of the superior portion of the lamina below the level of fixation may be required (**A**). Because of the width of the lumbar laminae, it is often possible to affix a rostrally directed hook to the lamina of a vertebral body in conjunction with a pedicle screw (**B**). This configuration aids resistance to screw pull-out in cantilever beam constructs without incorporating additional motion segments (**C**). Caudally directed hooks are placed following a laminotomy of the inferior portion of the lamina above the level of fixation. Caudally facing hooks cannot be placed on the same vertebra as a pedicle screw because of the apposition of the screw and hook connectors. (Copyright University of New Mexico, Division of Neurosurgery.)

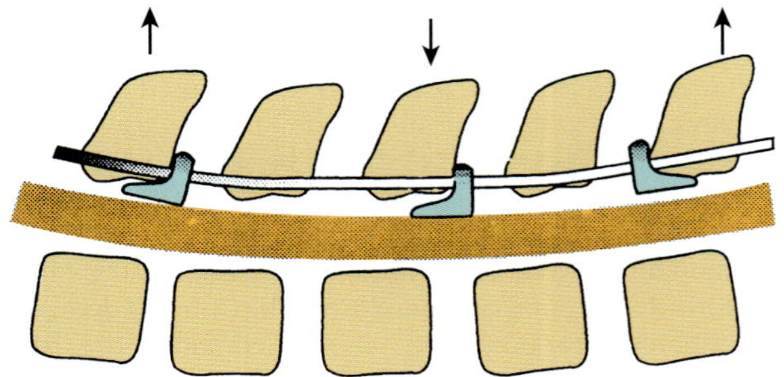

FIGURE 150-12. Hook use in three-point bending. Hooks are ideally suited for use as terminal components of three-point bending constructs because of the increased bone-implant contact surface area compared with screws. This increased surface area helps resist the dorsally directed forces at the termini. Because the forces generated at the apex of a kyphotic curvature are directed ventrally, caution must be exercised if hooks are used as intermediate points of fixation. The ventrally directed forces (*arrows*) may act to drive the blade of the hook into the spinal canal, as depicted. (Copyright University of New Mexico, Division of Neurosurgery.)

because if too little bone is removed, the hook does not engage the facet (Fig. 150-13). Transverse migration may not be prevented (with bifid hooks). Conversely, if too much bone is removed, the hook may cut into the pedicle, thus decreasing the strength of the pedicle/inferior articulating process connection. Frequent trial placements of the hook may be helpful in determining the optimal hook size and amount of bone removal necessary for good purchase.[6,31]

Transverse Process Hook Insertion

The transverse processes may be used for hook purchase in the thoracic spine. These hooks are usually placed facing caudally in conjunction with a rostrally facing pedicle hook. The costotransverse ligament is stripped off the transverse process by using a specially designed stripping tool, and the hook is placed over the rostral border of the transverse process. Offset hooks are frequently useful, as there is a substantial distance between the transverse process hook and pedicle hook fixation points in the coronal plane. Use of these hooks at the thoracolumbar junction is limited, since the transverse processes of T11 and T12 are usually too small to provide substantial purchase strength.[31]

Cross-Fixation

Cross-fixation increases the stability of a construct by preventing rotation or translation (coronal or sagittal) of the longitudinal members with respect to each other. The torsional stability of an implant is increased substantially by the use of a single cross-fixator (44%) and further increased with the use of two cross-fixators (an additional 26% gain in stability).[53] Screw pull-out resistance is also markedly improved with the use of rigid cross-links combined with toeing in of the screws. A lateral translational deformity caused by "parallelograming" is resisted by the use of cross-fixators.[6] Cross-fixators should be placed at the junctions of the middle third

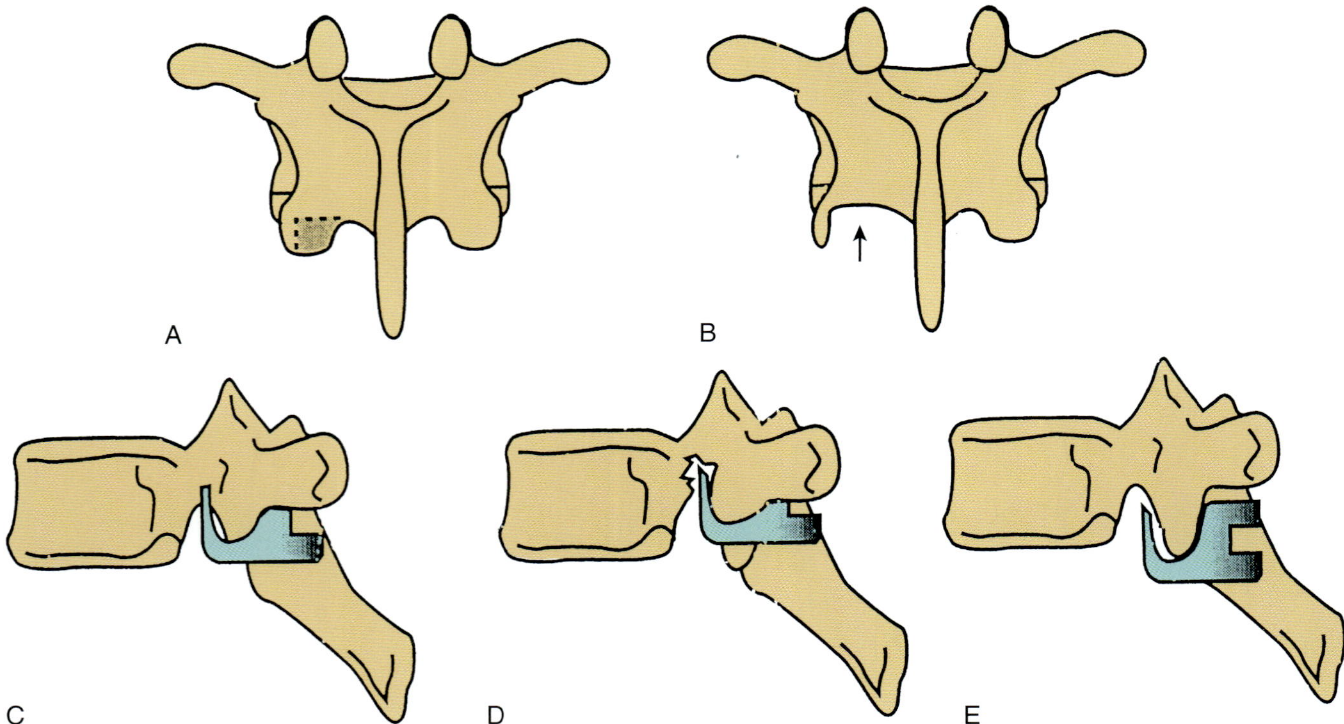

FIGURE 150-13. Pedicle hook insertion. Dorsal view of thoracic facet demonstrating the inferior articular process before (**A**) and after (**B**) bone removal (with an osteotome) for placement of a pedicle hook. **C,** Lateral view of pedicle hook in place, demonstrating appropriate bone removal. Note how the bifid hook properly engages the pedicle. **D,** If too much bone is removed, the pedicle may migrate rostrally and cut into the pedicle (if hook-rod connection is constrained) or toggle out of position (if hook-rod position is nonconstrained). **E,** If too little bone is removed, the hook will not engage the pedicle, and mediolateral hook migration may occur with manipulation of longitudinal members. The sandwiching effect of the facet joint will help hold the hooks in position to some extent. The stabilizing effect of pedicle purchase will be less significant with nonbifid hooks. (Copyright University of New Mexico, Division of Neurosurgery.)

of the implant with the rostral and caudal thirds. No significant biomechanical advantage is gained by the use of more than two cross-fixators. Although some USI cross-fixators are easier to apply than others, it is important, in general, not to mix sets or metals because of the potential for galvanically enhanced electrolytic corrosion.

Complication Avoidance and Management

The use of dorsal thoracic and lumbar USI systems is associated with a number of potential complications. The most significant short-term complications relate to loss of bony purchase, immediate implant failure, cerebrospinal fluid (CSF) fistula formation, and neural element injury.[26,54-56] Techniques for the prevention and management of these types of events are discussed in the following sections.

Complications of Hook Fixation

The use of three-point bending forces to reduce deformity may be associated with excessive force application at the terminal bone-implant junctions. This situation most commonly occurs with the use of the Harrington hook-rod system, in which substantial translational forces are borne by the terminal hook-bone junctions. Hook cutout at the rostral terminus is a common complication of these types of constructs. Use of a clawed construct lessens the risk of implant-bone junction failure by increasing the surface area of metal-bone contact. Furthermore, the use of clawed implants allows for the placement of the implant in a neutral mode (in contrast to distraction) with the immobilization of fewer motion segments.

Hooks placed in the spinal canal (laminar hooks) must tightly appose the ventral surface of the lamina to prevent neurologic injury. The use of such hooks above the level of the conus medullaris is possible but certainly carries with it a higher risk for neurologic injury. Great care must be taken with the use of laminar hooks as intermediate points of fixation in a three-point bending implant. The ventrally directed force at the center of such an implant may drive the hook blade into the spinal canal (see Fig. 150-12).

Pedicle hooks that are placed outside of the spinal canal may migrate during implant manipulation and may encroach on the spinal canal or neural foramina. Bifid hooks may lessen the risks of this complication. It is important to remove an appropriate amount of bone from the inferior articulating process of the facet before pedicle hook placement. Inadequate or overzealous bone removal may lead to malposition of pedicle hooks in the sagittal plane, which may lead to hook loosening or to pedicle fracture. Frequent use of hook testers will help to determine the correct amount of bone to be removed from the inferior articular process of the facet (see Fig. 150-13).

Complications of Transpedicular Fixation

Complications of pedicle fixation result from technical difficulties with implant application and from improper preoperative planning. The most common technical error in the placement of pedicle screws is malpositioning of the screw, resulting in pedicle fracture.[26,55,57,58] Pedicle fracture may occur if the pedicle screw entry site is inappropriate, the angle of screw placement is off, or the screw selected is too large in diameter. Depending on the location of the pedicle fracture, the consequence may be loss of purchase, CSF fistula, or neural injury. Preoperative studies must be obtained and reviewed to determine the correct size of the screw and angle of insertion (sagittal as well as coronal). Although intraoperative radiography is helpful, screw malposition in the axial plane may still occur despite radiographically acceptable positioning in the operating room.[58] The use of intraoperative electrophysiologic monitoring[47,48,59] and frameless stereotaxy may provide improved feedback to the surgeon for more accurate screw placement.[41-43]

We emphasize again that pedicle fracture can result in such sequelae as loss of purchase, CSF fistula, and neural injury. In the instance of loss of purchase, incorporation of an additional spinal segment may be necessary. CSF fistula should be repaired primarily when possible. When impossible or impractical, the pedicle defect may be packed with hemostatic gelatin (Gelfoam) soaked in thrombin or fibrin glue in an attempt to minimize CSF egress. Screws that are known to have perforated the medial cortex of the pedicle should be repositioned immediately. Screws that are found to be misplaced at the time of follow-up study may be well tolerated by the patient, as there may be up to 4 mm of a "safe" zone medial to the lumbar pedicle cortex.[60] This safe zone may not exist in the thoracic spine.[50] Patients with medial cortex fractures may develop late erosion of the screw threads into the neural foramina or spinal canal, which may cause nerve root injury. If the patient is symptomatic, such screws should be removed. Nerve root irritation may also result from caudal breaches of the pedicle cortex, where the exiting root is vulnerable to impingement or lateral pedicle breach, where the lumbosacral plexus may be irritated. Finally, perforation of the ventral cortex may result in significant vascular or visceral injury.

Postoperative complications related directly to implant failure may be avoided to some extent through proper preoperative planning and construct design. For example, application of three-point bending constructs should usually not be attempted with single screws as the terminal fixators. Although screw pull-out resistance may be maximized by the toeing-in of the screws (triangulation) and the use of cross-fixators, hooks still provide a greater resistance to translational forces. Similarly, when significant corrective forces are required, a sufficiently long construct should be used so as to avoid overly stressing the implant-bone or screw-rod junction.[22] Dorsal instrumentation cannot be relied on to replace the ventral load-bearing capacity of the spine, and attempts to do so are likely to fail.

Pedicle screw fracture may occur at the time of implant application, during attempted removal of instrumentation after fusion, or spontaneously in the months to years following implantation. The decision to remove implants in patients with persistent back pain after thoracic or lumbar fusion must be made on an individual basis. When there is evidence of implant failure, such as a broken rod or screw, medicolegal implications may prompt the surgeon to attempt removal. If a screw is fractured such that it cannot be removed by using standard techniques, a screw extractor kit may be used to remove distal screw fragments. A carbide-tipped drill is used to drill a hole in the screw fragment, and then a left-handed tap is inserted into the hole ("Easy-Out"). As the left-handed threads of the tap engage the screw, the screw begins to back out. Copious irrigation is required to remove fragments of metal, which will obscure postoperative imaging. We recommend using a hand drill instead of a pneumatic drill, as even a slight deviation from a coaxial trajectory may result in a violent removal with inadvertent pedicle fracture.

Summary

Dorsally applied USI increases the rate of bony fusion after surgery for traumatic, neoplastic, or degenerative conditions of the spine. By providing immediate stability to the spinal column, appropriately designed constructs allow for earlier mobilization and, hence, quicker rehabilitation of patients with spinal disorders. The safe and efficacious application of these systems is based on a clear understanding of the spinal anatomy and the particular pathology being addressed. Multiple systems are now available that differ in coupling mechanisms, metallurgic composition, screw and hook design, and cost. The surgeon must choose the appropriate system for a given patient and the associated pathology. This should be based on a clear understanding of the patient's pathology as well as an understanding of the strengths and limitations of USI systems.

KEY REFERENCES

Bennett GL: Materials and materials testing. In Benzel EC, editor: *Neurosurgical topics: spinal instrumentation*, Park Ridge, IL, 1994, American Association of Neurological Surgeons, pp 31–46.

Benzel EC: Construct design. In Benzel EC, editor: *Neurosurgical topics: spinal instrumentation*, Park Ridge, IL, 1994, American Association of Neurological Surgeons, pp 239–256.

Benzel EC: *Biomechanics of spine stabilization: principles and clinical practice*, New York, 1995, McGraw-Hill.

Chozick BS, Toselli R: Complications of spinal instrumentation. In Benzel EC, editor: *Neurosurgical topics: spinal instrumentation*, Park Ridge, IL, 1994, American Association of Neurological Surgeons, pp 257–274.

Stillerman CB, Gruen JP: Universal spinal instrumentation. In Benzel EC, editor: *Neurosurgical topics: spinal instrumentation*, Park Ridge, IL, 1994, American Association of Neurological Surgeons, pp 147–174.

White AA, Panjabi MM: *Clinical biomechanics of the spine*, ed 2, Philadelphia, 1990, Lippincott-Raven.

REFERENCES

The complete reference list is available online at expertconsult.com.

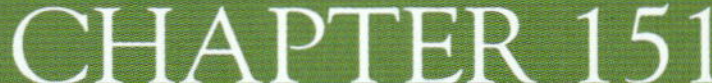
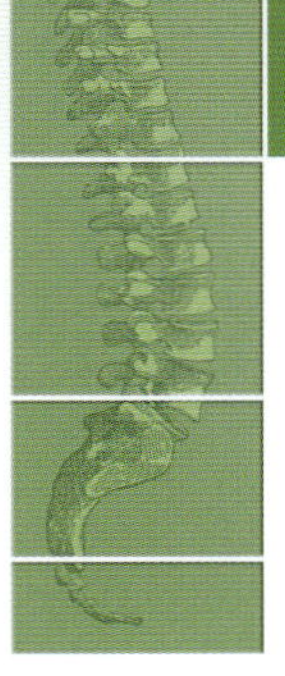

CHAPTER 151

Dorsal Thoracic and Lumbar Combined and Complex Techniques

Chris J. Neal | Tyler Koski

The goal of this chapter is to discuss the use of instrumentation and techniques required in complex or difficult cases from a dorsal approach. By the nature of the assignment, various components can be included under this heading. We have chosen to focus on concepts that are applicable not only to complex cases but those for which the rationale should be included in the preoperative planning phase of any instrumented spinal fusion. Behind each of the "complex" techniques are similar, although less involved, processes that occur in "noncomplex" spine cases. Typically, patients with severe osteoporosis, deformity, or spinal tumors or who require multilevel trauma surgery come to mind when we use the term "complex." More commonly, these ideas are practiced during revision spine surgery or as salvage techniques when other ideas have failed. The purpose of thinking about these "complex" techniques during the initial surgery, even if they are not put into practice, is so critical elements that can lead to failure can be identified and treated appropriately during the first surgery and revision surgery can be avoided.

Length of Construct

Although an appropriately sized construct for the pathology at hand is not exactly a complex technique, it is critical to optimizing patient outcome and avoiding revision surgery. Oversizing the construct means that the patient has undergone more surgery than is required and it has likely taken away normal motion and load sharing through the extrainstrumented segments. Undersizing the construct can place abnormal loads on the segments adjacent to the instrumentation and lead to adjacent segment failure. There are few rules to guide the surgeon in determining the length of the construct, but in general, the construct should include the Cobb angle of the curve and should not stop at the apex of a kyphosis. To put it a different way, instrumentation of spinal curves, whether in the coronal or sagittal plane, should include the entire curve so as not to place abnormal stress on a segment that is not normally acting in transition. Also, stopping an instrumented spine fusion at the junction between a mobile and a nonmobile segment should be done only with great thought and consideration of the stresses placed on the adjacent segment and the risk of a junctional kyphosis.

In adults, including the L5-S1 disc space in the fusion should be considered in any long construct that otherwise would have ended in the caudal lumbar spine. As outlined by Bridwell, indications for fusion to the sacrum in adults in a long construct include (1) L5-S1 spondylolisthesis, (2) previous L5-S1 laminectomy, (3) central or foraminal stenosis at L5-S1, (4) oblique takeoff of L5, and (5) "severe" degeneration of the disc.[1] Although fusing to the sacrum does decrease a significant amount of motion, there is a significant risk of adjacent segment degeneration when the construct is stopped at L5 in the adult degenerative deformity population. A retrospective study by Edwards et al. found that in a population of patients who had undergone a thoracolumbar construct that ended caudally at L5 who preoperatively had a "healthy" L5-S1 disc, 61% of patients had developed advanced degenerative disease at this level over a mean follow-up of 5.6 years.[2]

Because of the risk of pseudarthrosis at the L5-S1 space, many authorities have advocated for the use of interbody support at this level. Polly et al. found that L5-S1 interbody support increases biomechanical stability, restores junctional lordosis, improves the lumbosacral fusion rate, and increases disc and foraminal height, thus decreasing foraminal stenosis.[3] In the adult deformity patients undergoing spine fusion, the restoration or maintenance of sagittal balance has been found to have a significant impact on outcome.[4] Restoring junctional lordosis at L5-S1 through placement of an interbody graft is a powerful technique to correct sagittal imbalance. This is due to the long moment arm that occurs when the L5-S1 disc space angulation is altered relative to the C7 vertebral body on which sagittal balance is based. To maximize the footprint of the graft as well as the restoration of lordosis, an anterior lumbar interbody fusion (ALIF) is a better procedure than a transforaminal lumbar interbody fusion (TLIF) at L5-S1.[5] One must weigh the benefit of a larger interbody device against the morbidity of an anterior approach when selecting an anterior approach versus a TLIF or posterior lumbar interbody fusion (PLIF).

Long constructs that extend to the sacrum can be problematic from a fixation standpoint. Although the S1 pedicles are large, the sacrum is composed of primarily cancellous bone, resulting in a decreased pull-out strength compared with other pedicle screws. This has prompted many to attempt to place bicortical pedicle screws to capture the anterior and posterior cortical bone to increase the strength of the screw. Lehman et al. showed that the highest bone mineral density, and therefore the greatest insertional torque for pedicle screws, was in the anterior sacral promontory, so that from a biomechanical standpoint, the strongest S1 screws are the so-called "tricortical" screws. When screws are placed in this fashion, there is almost a 99% increase in the insertional torque.[6] In addition to an L5-S1 interbody and the placement of tricortical S1 pedicle screws, iliac screws have been advocated as another method to offload the S1 pedicles to allow for a solid arthrodesis at L5-S1. Indications for iliac screws include constructs greater than three levels that end in the sacrum, revision surgery for L5-S1 pseudarthorsis, high-grade spondylolisthesis, or trauma or pathology that does not allow for adequate sacral fixation.[7] Kuklo et al. evaluated 81 patients who underwent fusion procedures that included the L5-S1 space using S1 and iliac screws. Approximately 50% (n = 42) were for isthmic spondylolisthesis, whereas the remainder (n = 39) were for long constructs to the sacrum. The researchers found that even in patients who had previous iliac crest grafts taken, 94% (34/36) had iliac screws placed without screw loosening or iliac crest fracture. Overall, the fusion rate, to include revision surgeries, was 95.1%.[8]

Junctional Kyphosis

One of the reasons to plan and execute an appropriate-sized construct is to avoid proximal junctional kyphosis (PJK). In 1999, Lee et al. looked at 69 patients with adolescent idiopathic scoliosis (AIS) who underwent fusion up to T3. The investigators defined PJK as greater than 5 degrees above the summed normal of the angular segments from the proximal instrumented segment to T2. They found a 46% incidence of PJK. As would be expected, a predictor of postoperative PJK was preoperative kyphosis of more than 5 degrees above the proposed proximal instrumented level, indicating that these levels should be included in the construct to avoid this complication.[9]

In the adult deformity population, Kim et al. evaluated 161 patients with a minimum 5-year follow-up who had undergone long (more than five segments) dorsal constructs to determine the incidence and outcomes associated with PJK. The researchers found that at mean follow-up of 7.8 years, there was a 39% incidence of PJK defined either as a proximal junction sagittal Cobb angle of more than 10 degrees or as a proximal junction sagittal Cobb angle at least 10 degrees greater than the preoperative measurement. The time periods most notable for worsening of PJK were at 8 weeks postoperatively (59%) or after 2 years until final follow-up (35%). Scoliosis Research Society outcome measures did not show any significant difference in those with PJK as compared with those without except with self-image when PJK was more than 20 degrees. Age older than 55 years and combination anterior-posterior surgery were the only significant risk factors identified.[10] The time course between the identification of PJK suggests two different populations, given that one group was relatively close to surgery, whereas the other was more remote. Further understanding of the similarities and differences of the early and late group may lead to changes in treatment strategies to better prevent PJK.

Several methods can be used to reduce the risk of PJK in addition to how to determine an appropriately sized construct. Some experts have advocated the use of percutaneous screws in the proximal construct to avoid iatrogenic trauma associated with exposure of the soft tissues, specifically the proximal facet joint. This technique involves placing percutaneous pedicle screws, typically through the fascia layer of the most proximal screws and subcutaneously passing the rod through these proximal screws. Although theoretically this helps protect the soft tissue envelope, there have been no studies to demonstrate its effectiveness on reducing PJK.

Another technique used to avoid PJK as well as strengthen the screw pull-out strength is vertebroplasty. Recently there has been some controversy over the effectiveness of this procedure in the setting of compression fractures, but the concept is applied differently in deformity surgery. At the proximal and sometimes distal screws, polymethylmethacrylate (PMMA) is injected under fluoroscopy into the screw tracks or through the screws themselves if the screw design allows it. Care is taken that there are no pedicle wall breaches allowing the egress of PMMA into the spinal canal or the production of embolic material. Once the PMMA is in place, typically 1 to 2 mL per side, then the pedicle screw is placed. Another scenario is to perform vertebroplasty at the level cephalad to the proximal instrumented vertebrae to prevent compression fractures leading to PJK (Fig. 151-1). Alternatively, this procedure can be performed in a postoperative setting. Preoperative PMMA augmentation of the planned proximal instrumented bodies is not recommended because it increases the difficulty of placement of the instrumentation.

In a cadaveric study designed to look at effects of cement augmentation of pedicle screws compared with extension with a flexible rod, Tan et al. found that in a corpectomy model, cement augmentation significantly reduced the range of motion and resulted in a more stable construct.[11]

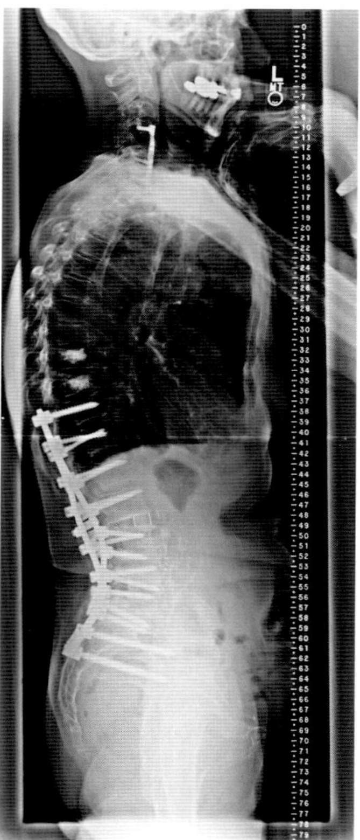

FIGURE 151-1. This is an example of vertebroplasty in the supra-adjacent segments of a T10 to the pelvis construct in a patient with osteoporosis.

In another cadaveric study, Becker et al. found that pedicle screws augmented with PMMA in an osteoporotic model had increased pull-out strength compared with non-PMMA augmented screws.[12] In a cost-effectiveness analysis published in 2008, Hart et al. evaluated 28 women older than 60 years of age who had undergone fusion to the thoracolumbar region. Fifteen of these patients had undergone vertebroplasty in the adjacent level cranial to the proximal instrumented vertebrae. Proximal collapse occurred in none of the patients who had PMMA augmentation and in two (15.3%) patients who did not. Assuming a 15% decrease in the incidence of this problem, the researchers determined that the cost to prevent a single proximal junctional collapse was $46,240 using vertebroplasty, whereas the cost of revising the instrumentation in a patient with proximal junctional collapse was $77,432.[13]

As with any spinal pathology, there is clinical and radiographic PJK. PJK seen on follow-up films that is not progressive and does not significantly alter the patient's sagittal balance can be followed radiographically. However, progressive PJK that results in alterations in sagittal balance, instability, or becomes painful should be addressed. If the PJK occurs in the upper lumbar or lower thoracic spine, then the revision strategy focuses on extension of the fusion to either the lower thoracic spine (T10) or upper thoracic spine (T4), respectively. By crossing the thoracolumbar junction and not stopping at the apex of a curve, the surgeon can minimize an additional junctional failure. However, the repair strategy becomes more involved when the PKJ occurs in a construct that already ends in the proximal thoracic spine. Often, this requires extension into the cervical spine. At our institution, this is often done in a staged setting. In the first stage, dissection of the proximal instrumented level to the appropriate level needed in the cervical spine occurs with placement of lateral mass screws in the cervical spine and pedicle screws placed in the remaining uninstrumented thoracic levels. Appropriately sized osteotomies are performed across the kyphosis. In some cases, osteotomies of the 1st and 2nd ribs are also completed in the first stage. A temporary rod is then placed across the cervical junction so that distractive forces are not placed across the cervical spine but instead across the kyphotic proximal thoracic spine. The wound is closed, and the patient is placed in halo traction while being monitored in the ICU. Serial radiographs and examinations are performed while weight is added to the traction until either there is reduction of the kyphosis, a change in the examination, or unwanted proximal distraction. The patient is then locked into position with a halo vest. The patient returns to the operating room where the osteotomies are enlarged or additional osteotomies are placed if needed. Permanent rods are then placed and the construct is compressed across the osteotomies to achieve final correction.

Interbody Fusion

Interbody fusions are achieved by removing the intervertebral disc and placing fusion material such as autograft, allograft, or osteobiologics. Achieving fusion across the disc space has been shown to provide a biomechanically stiffer construct.[3] But can interbody constructs stand alone? In 2006, Anjarwalla et al. evaluated their ALIF patients and divided them into four cohorts: stand-alone ALIF, ALIF with translaminar screws, ALIF with unilateral pedicle screws, and ALIF with bilateral pedicle screws. Using thin-section CT, the investigators reported a fusion rate of 51% in the stand-alone ALIF population, 58% in the ALIF population with translaminar screws, 89% in the ALIF population augmented by unilateral screws, and 88% fusion with ALIF augmented by bilateral pedicle screws.[14] Some studies have advocated the use of percutaneous pedicle screws to augment ALIF with good clinical and radiographic results.[15] Cadaveric studies have looked at the difference between stand-alone ALIF, ALIF with anterior plate, and ALIF with pedicle screws and found that augmentation of a stand-alone ALIF significantly reduced the range of motion and increased the stiffness of the construct. Overall, there was no consistent significant difference between an anterior plate and pedicle screws except that pedicle screws more effectively limited lateral bending.[16,17]

More recently, minimally invasive placement of lateral interbody support via a retroperitoneal approach has become more popular. The advantage to this approach is that it provides a graft with a large footprint to cover the end plate across the rim of cortical bone to provide maximal structural support. Conversely, great care should be taken to avoid the lumbar plexus and other critical retroperitoneal structures such as the kidney, ureter, aorta, and inferior vena cava. In general, the lumbar plexus is found in the dorsal aspect of the disc space, but as one descends more caudally, the nerves do appear more anterior. Therefore, this approach must be performed with neuromonitoring, stimulation, and direct visualization to determine the exact location of the lumbar nerves as they run through the psoas muscle. Although early reports have noted the utility of this approach and interbody support to change both coronal and sagittal alignment, we have found that a lateral interbody approach most consistently affects the coronal alignment of the spine and does not significantly affect sagittal alignment and hence sagittal balance. Of the current systems available, none recommend a stand-alone interbody from a lateral approach.

Connectors

When constructs need to be extended proximally or distally for problems such as a PJK or rod fracture, it is often difficult and frustrating to dissect out the fusion mass to remove the rod. A solution to this problem is the use of either in-line or domino connectors that allows for two rods to be connected. This allows two separate constructs to be joined as one. Depending on the situation, a pedicle screw or other fixation point may need to be removed to allow for the connector to be placed. Often, this requires the use of an in situ sagittal bending tool to bend the rod out of the previous pedicle screw so that the screw can be removed. Once there is space, the rod can be bent back into place and the connector placed over the rod. The new rod can then be placed into the contralateral end of the connector to allow the extension of the construct.

Osteotomies

From a spine perspective, osteotomies are cuts made through the spine to allow its mobilization and realignment—typically to correct kyphosis or to enhance lordosis. In general, there are three main types of osteotomies: Ponte or Smith-Petersen osteotomies (SPOs), pedicle subtraction osteotomies (PSOs), and vertebral column resections (VCRs). In ascending order, each of these osteotomies offers greater correctional power and can be used in combination to achieve optimal deformity correction. Prior to the application of osteotomies, one must have a firm understanding of why correction is important as well as the goals of correction.

Sagittal balance has been shown to be the single most important factor affecting outcome in adult deformity surgery.[4] Sagittal balance is measured by drawing a C7 plumb line and measuring the linear distance from this line to the posterior sacral promontory. Measurements greater than 5 cm correlate with poorer longer-term outcomes. Therefore, the goal is to correct the sagittal balance to within the normal range. However, osteotomies are measured in degrees, not centimeters of correction. Therefore, one must convert the degrees of correction achieved by an osteotomy to a linear distance to ensure successfully restoring sagittal balance.

Global sagittal plane correction is most reliably calculated using the tangent function as described by Ondra et al. (Figs. 151-2 and 151-3).[18] This technique allows the conversion of the distance of correction needed to an angle that can be used to determine the size of the osteotomies required. In most radiology systems, this can easily be performed by drawing a C7 plumb line and a sagittal vertical line from the posterior sacral promontory to the center of the C7 vertebral body. This angle represents the overall degree of sagittal plane correction needed for the patient to be in sagittal balance. Once this angle is known, preoperative planning of osteotomies can then be matched with the amount of correction needed. Placement of osteotomies more caudally has a greater effect on sagittal balance as opposed to those that are placed in a more cephalad fashion. The goal is to place the appropriate type, size, and number of osteotomies so that sagittal plane alignment can occur.

As discussed by Bridwell, SPOs, PSOs, and VCRs can be used to correct fixed sagittal and/or coronal imbalance.[19] Although it is beyond the scope of this chapter to discuss details in performing osteotomies, a general understanding is important. An SPO, also termed a chevron osteotomy because of its shape, is performed by removing the posterior column, bone, and ligament, between the facet joints at one or multiple levels while leaving the middle and anterior columns intact. With posterior compression, the anterior column opens through the disc space, providing increased lordosis. In general, an SPO can provide 5 to 10 degrees of lordosis. An important caveat in performing an SPO is to ensure complete removal of the superior facet so that compression does not entrap the exiting nerve root within the foramen.

A PSO is a V-shaped resection through the posterior elements, pedicles, and vertebral body that hinges through the bone. Dorsal compression results in bone on bone closure that

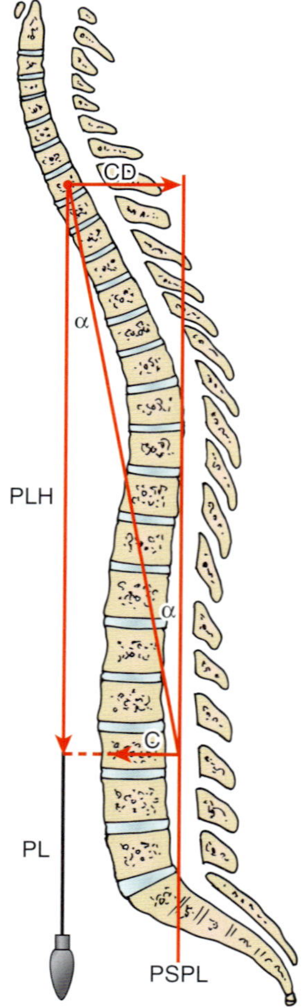

FIGURE 151-2. The tangent method uses simple geometry, where the length of the C7 plumb line (PL) and the distance from the pedicle to this line forms a right angle, allowing for the angle α to be solved. If the line *C* is measured at S1, then it is possible to solve for the degrees of global sagittal imbalance. Using this method allows for accurate determination of the degree of osteotomy needed at various levels to restore sagittal balance. PLH, plumb line height; PSPL, posterior sacral promontory line.

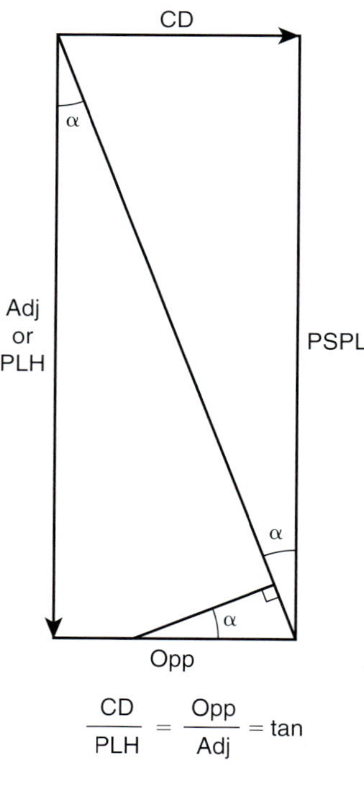

$$\frac{CD}{PLH} = \frac{Opp}{Adj} = \tan$$

$$\alpha = \tan^{-1}$$

FIGURE 151-3. Using basic geometry, the distance of sagittal imbalance or sagittal balance correction can be converted into an angle (α), which is more applicable to osteotomies. PLH, plumb line height ; PSPL, posterior sacral promontory line.

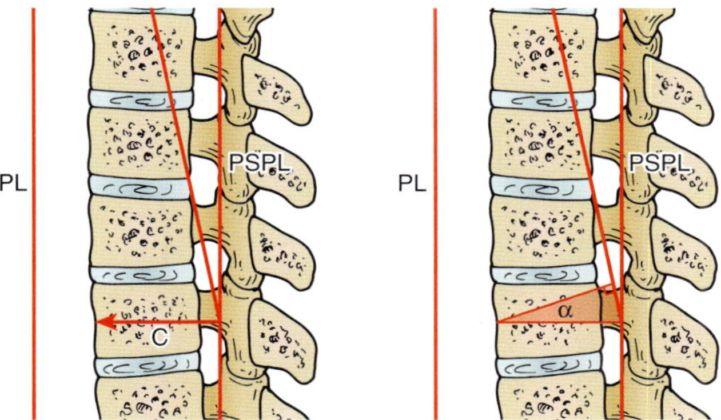

FIGURE 151-4. Applying the geometric proof illustrated in Figure 151-3 to the spine, the angle of correction (α) required is cut through the vertebral body. PL, plumb line; PSPL, posterior sacral promontory line .

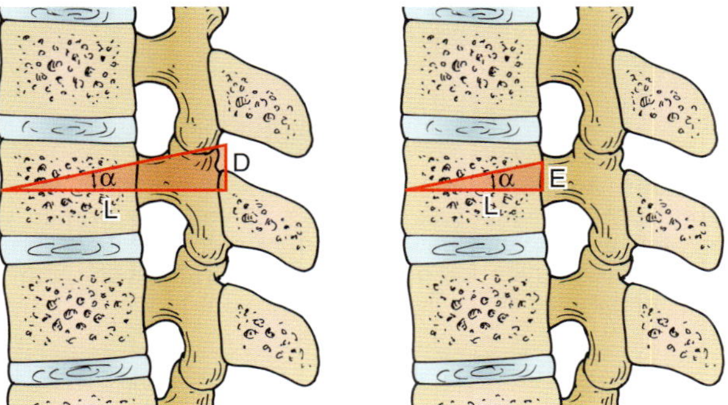

FIGURE 151-5. By knowing the angle of the pedicle subtraction osteotomy (α), the posterior height of the osteotomy (lines *D* and *E* in the diagram) can be calculated and measured intraoperatively to ensure an accurate cut. This is especially important with line *E*, because the height of this cut is critical to make sure the planned osteotomy is achieved.

can provide 25 to 35 degrees of lordosis. Including the disc space above can provide additional corrective forces and is sometimes referred to as a 1½ PSO or an extended PSO. PSOs are often used in the lumbar spine and are useful in correction of iatrogenic flat back deformity (Figs. 151-4 to 151-8).

A vertebral column resection is the most aggressive and powerful osteotomy, with complete removal of one or more vertebral bodies to include the cranial and caudal discs. Closure is usually not bone on bone, relying on a pivot such as a cage or bone graft. This technique can achieve up to 50 to 60 degrees of correction and is ideal for angular thoracic deformities.

When a pedicle subtraction osteotomy or vertebral column resection is performed, one side of the construct has a temporary rod to prevent spinal column translation. After the osteotomy is complete, compression is required to close the construct to gain the correction for which the osteotomy was performed. Often this is done by placing a permanent rod on the contralateral side and compressing against the pedicle screws. The potential problem with this is that the compression places an extra force on the pedicle screw, which may result in the screw breaking out of the pedicle, losing an important fixation point in the construct. An alternative method is to place two temporary rods on each side of the construct where the free ends of the rods meet at the

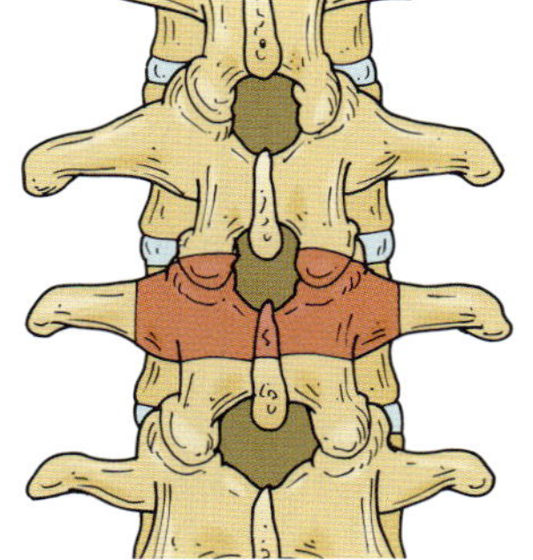
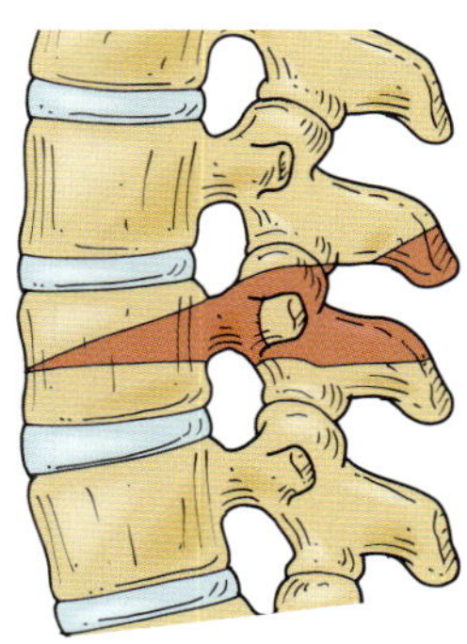

FIGURE 151-6. Anteroposterior and lateral views of the bony elements removed during a pedicle subtraction osteotomy. In order, this includes a laminectomy, complete facetectomies, complete pedicle resection, wedge resection of the vertebral body, and lateral wall resection, with the final element removed being the dorsal vertebral body wall.

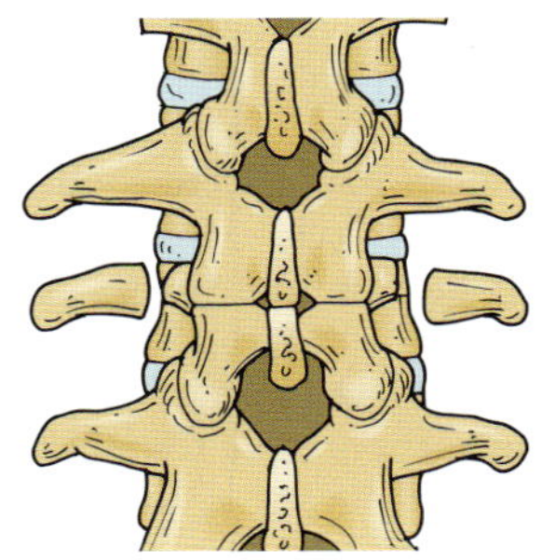
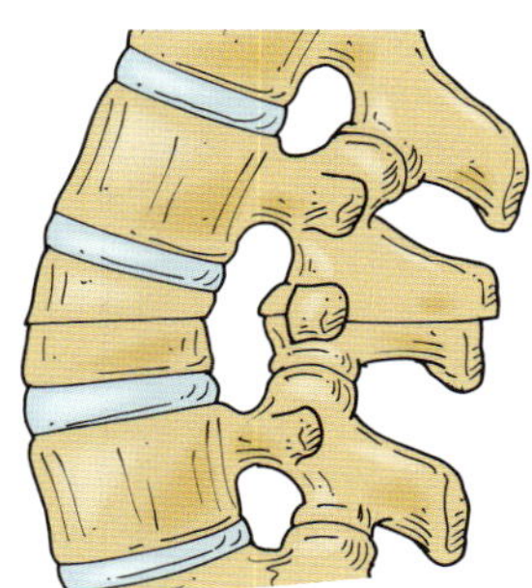

FIGURE 151-7. Anteroposterior and lateral views of a completed pedicle subtraction osteotomy. Note the creation of a superforamen where both nerve roots travel.

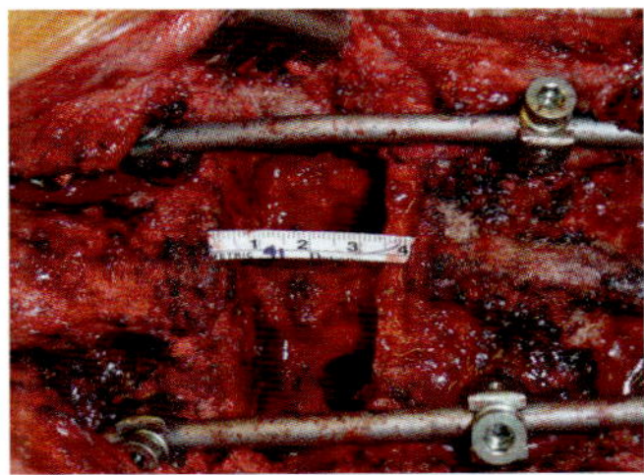
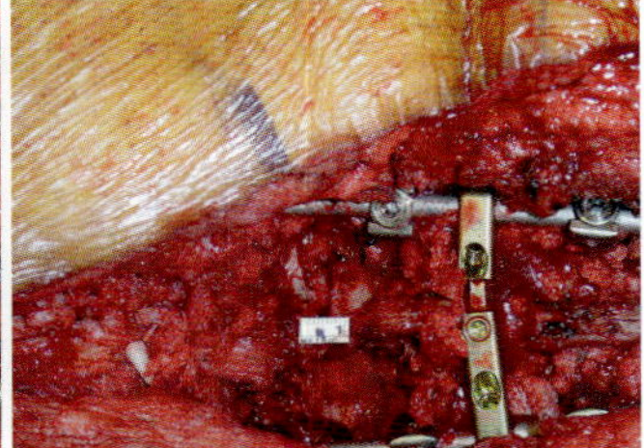

FIGURE 151-8. Intraoperative pictures showing a completed pedicle subtraction osteotomy before and after compression.

osteotomy site. Domino connectors are then placed across the rods and tightened. The same is performed on the other side, and the rod is secured to the pedicle screw heads. After gaining control of the construct with bilateral compression devices, the screws for either the cephalad or caudal rod are loosened. Compression can occur across the connector. It is important that with bilateral compression the same rod, either rostral or caudal, is chosen to be tightened so that symmetrical compression can occur. Although compression still occurs on one set of the pedicle screws, it can be alternated so smaller amounts of force are required for closure. Alternatively, others have described using laminar hooks rostral and caudal to the osteotomy site in a claw construct and closing the osteotomy with a temporary rod that spans the laminar hooks. This takes all force off of the pedicle screws until the permanent rod is placed.

Cross-Fixators

Cross-fixators are not an unusual component of instrumentation, and it is worth discussing their rationale and use. The purpose of placing cross-links, also termed transverse connectors, is to reduce rotational forces on the spine. Although cadaveric studies have shown that cross-fixators increase rotational, lateral bending, and flexion stiffness, resistance to rotation has been the most consistent finding.[20,21] In one such study by Kuklo et al., the authors found that a pedicle screw construct from T4-10 with 5.5-mm-diameter titanium pedicle screws with 5.5-mm titanium rods resulted in a 65% decrease in the range of motion compared with the uninstrumented spine. The addition of one cross-fixator anywhere along the construct resulted in decreased rotational motion, but it was the placement of a second cross-fixator, one at the rostral and one at the caudal portion of the construct, which provided the greatest stability with a 35% reduction in rotational motion compared with no cross-fixators. Flexion-extension and lateral bending were not significantly affected by the addition of cross-fixators. The authors concluded that in the thoracic spine, where the primary motion is rotation, the use of two cross-fixators provides superior resistance to that motion and therefore a more stable construct.[21]

Although cross-fixators are biomechanically favorable, there are caveats to their use. Some authors have found that there is a higher rate of pseudarthrosis at the site of the cross-fixator. Therefore, cross-fixators should not be placed over a junction, such as the thoracolumbar or lumbosacral junction. Along this same line of thought, a cross-fixator should not be placed at the level of an osteotomy. Others have criticized the concept of cross-fixators because it keeps the muscle pushed away from the decorticated bone surface, taking with it an important aspect of bone healing.

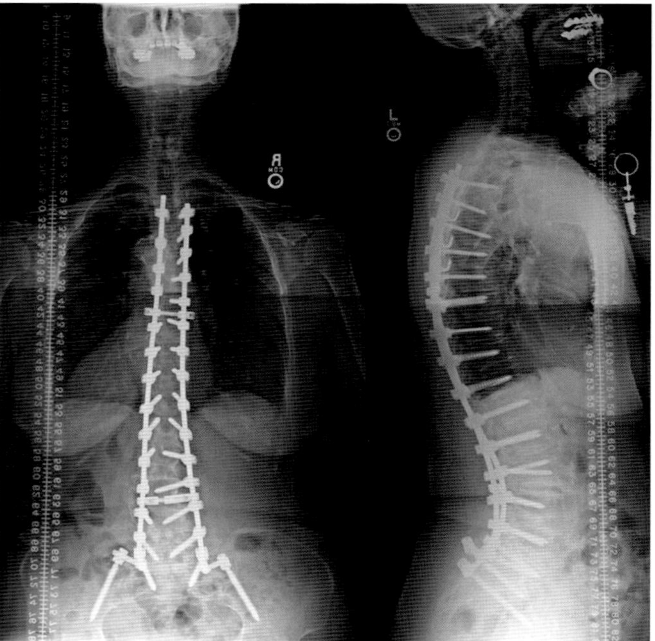

FIGURE 151-9. Anteroposterior and lateral scoliosis films showing a hybrid construct that was used in a 69-year-old woman who underwent a T4 to the pelvis construct with multilevel Smith-Petersen osteotomies for positive sagittal imbalance. Note the pedicle hooks used at T5, T6, and T7.

Hybrid Constructs

Pedicle screws provide for three-column control of the spine, allowing for greater forces to be imparted in order to achieve deformity correction. Currently, the role of hooks is often relegated as a revision strategy if placement of the pedicle screw fails. However, there is some thought that using hooks in combination with pedicle screws, a hybrid construct, theoretically provides a construct resistant to different modes of failure. When evaluating resistance to failure from dorsally directed forces in a cadaveric model, Coe et al. showed that laminar hooks were superior to spinous process wires and pedicle screws.[22] Hilibrand et al. showed that combining a supralaminar hook with a pedicle screw provided increased pull-out strength in models replicating osteoporotic or compromised pedicle. There was no difference, however, between the two when the pedicle was intact.[23] In the osteoporotic spine, where the cortical bone is spared relative to the cancellous bone, a fixation technique that relies more on the cortical bone, such as a hook, can be used. Typically, hooks are used in a hybrid fashion on one side of the cranial aspect of the construct (Fig. 151-9). Hooks do not have the same corrective power as pedicle screws and do not provide a construct as stiff as that of pedicle screws. Jones et al. evaluated whether a short-segment thoracic hybrid construct is equivalent to a pedicle screw construct. They found that there was a greater force required for construct failure in the pedicle screw group and that these constructs were significantly stiffer than the hybrid constructs.[24] In 2007, Lowenstein et al. looked at a cohort of 34 patients, comparing an all-pedicle-screw construct with a hybrid construct consisting of lumbar pedicle screws and thoracic hooks in a population with AIS. The investigators found that there were no statistically significant differences between the two constructs in coronal plane sagittal balance correction, although there was a significant differences in kyphosis correction.[25] Kuklo et al. looked at the revision rates of various constructs in patients with AIS. These researchers found that hybrid constructs had a statistically significant higher failure rate than pedicle constructs.[26] The population with AIS, with relatively healthy bone, likely would not see the benefits of a hybrid construct, compared with the osteoporotic spine where hooks can take advantage of the relatively stronger cortical bone.

Multirod Constructs

On rare occasions, revision cases sometimes require a multirod construct. These are constructs where the rods are placed in alternating pedicle screws. The rods are attached to each other with connectors and cross-fixators to make an integrated rod system. The focus of such a construct is to provide alternating stress points and to distribute the force along the construct more evenly. This concept has been described by Shen et al., where researchers used four rods to cross the lumbosacral junction.[27] By using four different anchoring points within the pelvis, the rods span the junction to the lumbar fixation points and are coupled using cross-fixators.

Summary

The goal of any instrumented spinal fusion is to stabilize the spine in sagittal and coronal balance and to provide a framework that allows a solid arthrodesis to occur with the least number of levels involved. Appropriate preoperative planning should take into account the specific pathology that needs to be addressed as well as potential revision strategies in case the original plan is unable to be executed. Understanding the capabilities of the instrumentation and how to overcome obstacles presented by either the patient's biology or pathology is critical to achieving optimal outcomes in what would otherwise be viewed as complex or high-risk patients.

KEY REFERENCES

Bridwell KH: Decision making regarding Smith-Petersen vs. pedicle subtraction osteotomy vs. vertebral column resection for spinal deformity. *Spine (Phila Pa 1976)* 31:S171–S178, 2006.

Bridwell KH: Selection of instrumentation and fusion levels for scoliosis: where to start and where to stop. Submission from the Joint Section Meeting on Disorders of the Spine and Peripheral Nerves, March 2004. *J Neurosurg Spine* 1:1–8, 2004.

Edwards CC II, Bridwell KH, Patel A, et al: Thoracolumbar deformity arthrodesis to L5 in adults: the fate of the L5-S1 disc. *Spine (Phila Pa 1976)* 28:2122–2131, 2003.

Glassman SD, Bridwell K, Dimar JR, et al: The impact of positive sagittal balance in adult spinal deformity. *Spine (Phila Pa 1976)* 30:2024–2029, 2005.

Ondra SL, Marzouk S, Koski T, et al: Mathematical calculation of pedicle subtraction osteotomy size to allow precision correction of fixed sagittal deformity. *Spine (Phila Pa 1976)* 31:E973–E979, 2006.

Polly DW Jr, Klemme WR, Cunningham BW, et al: The biomechanical significance of anterior column support in a simulated single-level spinal fusion. *J Spinal Disord* 13:58–62, 2000.

REFERENCES

The complete reference list is available online at expertconsult.com.

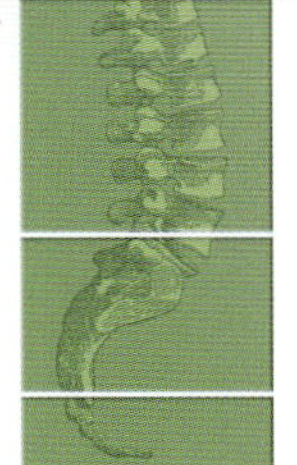

CHAPTER 152

Complex Lumbosacropelvic Fixation Techniques

Nevan G. Baldwin | Matthew B. Kern | David W. Cahill | Daniel M. Sciubba

Diseases of the sacrum and lumbosacral junction (LSJ) lead to clinically complex problems for surgical treatment and biomechanical stabilization. Trauma, infection, degenerative disease, and scoliosis (congenital or acquired) are among the common entities affecting the sacrum and LSJ. Although less common, neoplasms of this area often are especially challenging for postresection reconstruction. The sacrum and dorsal pelvis are also important points of fixation in the treatment of similar disorders at higher spinal regions in which long instrumentation constructs are required.

Anatomic and Biomechanical Considerations

The LSJ is a unique spinal level in several respects.[1] In the sagittal or flexion-extension axis, it has the largest range of motion of any thoracic or lumbar level, averaging 17 degrees of total movement. In the axial plane and during rotation and lateral (coronal plane) bending, the LSJ has the most limited range of motion of any spinal level, averaging 1 degree of rotation and 3 degrees of bending, respectively.[2] Because of the normal lordotic curvature of the lumbar spine, the slope of the lumbosacral intervertebral disc (L5-S1) is usually the steepest of any disc, with respect to the true horizontal. The summation of spinal load vectors results in exposure of the lumbosacral disc to the largest loads encountered throughout the spine. The large loads carried and the angular position of the disc at the LSJ produce unique load-bearing characteristics, including the highest level of translational shear force in the entire spine (Fig. 152-1).[1,3,4]

Sacrum

The sacrum is formed from five fused vertebrae in which the specially adapted and large transverse processes merge into thick lateral masses, the alae. The sacral spinal canal has four pairs of dorsal and ventral foramina. The subdural and subarachnoid spaces terminate as the thecal sac tapers at the caudal margin of S2. The filum terminale internum is an extension of the pia arachnoid of the conus medullaris, extending from the tip of the conus to the end of the subdural space. At the termination of the subdural space, the thecal sac tapers to invest the filum terminale internum and form the filum terminale externum. The filum terminale externum extends to the end of the sacral canal and attaches to the rostral portion of the coccyx.

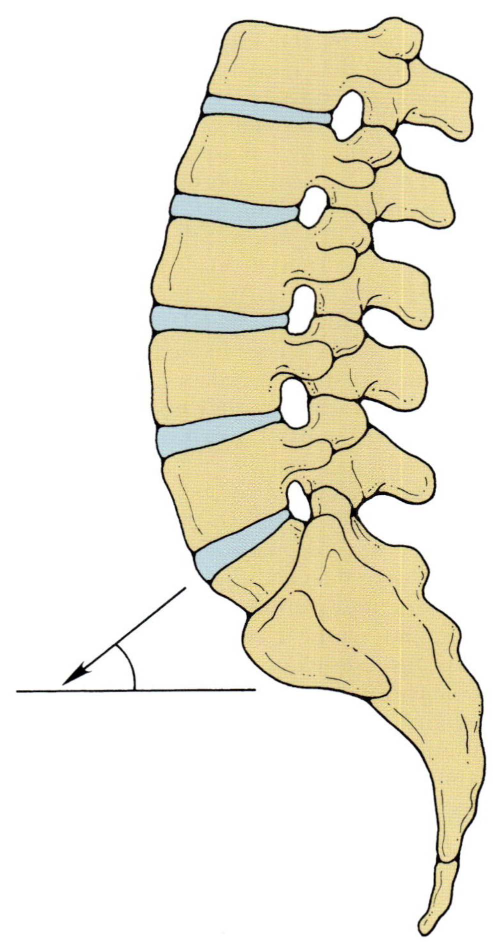

FIGURE 152-1. The L5-S1 disc space is the most vertically oriented of any disc space in the spine (*arrow* depicts approximate angle formed by the disc space). This predisposes the L5-S1 level to unique load-bearing characteristics.

Structures Adjacent to the Sacrum

For the safe placement and attachment of instrumentation constructs in the lumbosacralpelvic region, a thorough knowledge of the anatomic relationships of the neural, vascular, and visceral structures in the region is important. The common iliac arteries begin at the aortic bifurcation (L4 level) and pass along the lateral surface of the L5 vertebral body. They then bifurcate at the level of the LSJ, giving rise to the internal and external iliac arteries. The iliac arteries lie ventral and lateral to the iliac veins and therefore do not actually make contact with the spine. The internal and external iliac arteries pass ventral to the sacral alae. The internal iliac arteries pass close to the bony surface of the ala, whereas the external iliacs are separated from the bony surface by the psoas muscles. The lumbosacral trunk is formed by the ventral branches of the L4 and L5 nerve roots. It is joined by the sacral nerves located on the ventral surface of the alae between the iliac veins and the sacroiliac joint (SIJ). The sigmoid colon is also found in approximation to the ventral surface of the sacrum. It loses its mesentery and becomes far less mobile as it reaches the ventral aspect of the S3 vertebral body and becomes the rectum.

Sacroiliac Joint

The SIJ is formed by the interdigitating surfaces of the sacral alae and the iliac bones. It is predominantly a fibrocartilaginous amphiarthrodial (no synovial capsule) joint. There is a small diarthrodial (synovial capsule present) portion located at the ventral aspect of the SIJ. The interdigitation and matching contours of the iliac and sacral alar surfaces create an interlocking mechanism to help stabilize the joint. The wedgelike shape of the sacrum helps stabilize the SIJ and serves to transfer loads from the spine to the pelvis (Fig. 152-2).

The SIJ is essentially an immobile joint that functions as a shock absorber for the spine. In studies on fresh cadavers, there was minimal motion in pediatric specimens, and none in adults.[5] Another cadaveric study has demonstrated that in adults older than 50 years of age, autofusion of the joint is observed in 75% of specimens.[6]

The major biomechanical function of the pelvis is that of transferring loads from the SIJ to the hip joints. The stable transfer of these loads is dependent on the ligaments connecting the lumbar vertebrae and the sacrum to the pelvis. The ligamentous structures spanning the SIJ include the interosseous, dorsal, and ventral sacroiliac ligaments (Fig. 152-3). The interosseous, sacroiliac, and dorsal sacroiliac complex provides the major stabilization for the SIJ.

The iliolumbar ligament passes from the transverse process of the L5 vertebra to the iliac crests. A less substantial part of the ligament may span to the transverse process of L4 as well. The position of this ligament allows a wide range of motion in flexion and extension across the LSJ, but it severely restricts lateral bending and axial rotation.

The force vector of axial load from the spine is located ventral to the SIJ. This causes a ventral rotational tendency of the sacrum at the level of the SIJ. The center point of this rotational vector is located near the center of the S2 vertebral body (Fig. 152-4). The sacrospinous and sacrotuberous ligaments pass from the lower sacrum to the ischial bones.

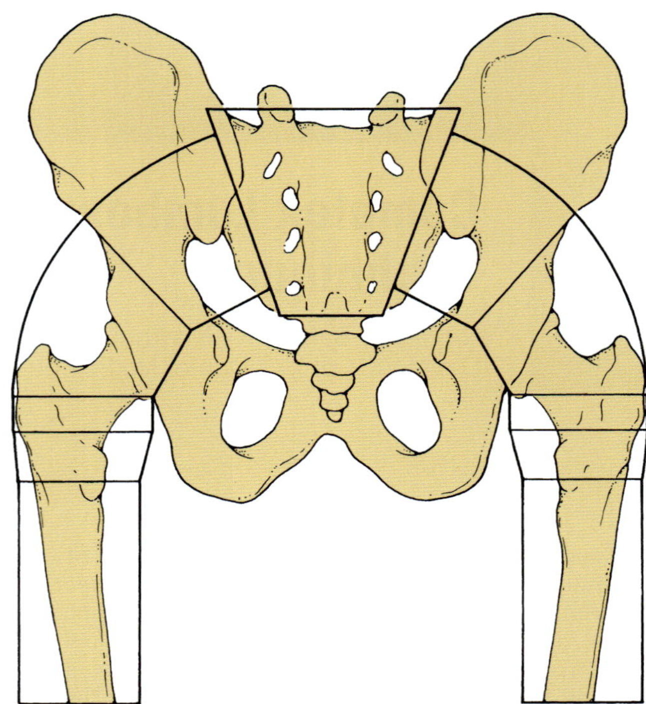

FIGURE 152-2. The keystone configuration of the pelvis allows the transfer of weight from the spine to the pelvis and ultimately to the lower extremities.

The position of these ligaments creates a long moment arm through which they are able to resist sacral rotation and are thereby able to maintain the lordotic lumbosacral posture despite the gravitational sagittal plane vector.

Muscular Interactions

The musculature of the lumbosacralpelvic region acts on the spine in a complex multidirectional fashion. The muscles and the weight of the upper body act in many instances via long moment arms and may place substantial forces on the spine. An example of such action is the force exerted on the spine by the rectus abdominis musculature. These muscles act by a moment arm extending from the pubic symphysis to the sternum, producing a spinal vector toward kyphosis. A pendulous abdomen does the same in providing a constant exaggerated spinal load in the upright position and to some extent during sitting.

In the resection of sacral tumors, stability of the sacropelvic region can be jeopardized because portions of the sacrum and possibly the SIJ are removed. Resection of the caudal portion of the sacrum up to the S1-2 interspace and removal of up to one third of the SIJ can be performed with only a 30% loss of weight-bearing capacity. The lower half of the S1 body and up to one half of the SIJ can be resected with a 50% loss of weight-bearing stability.[7] Preservation of 50% of weight-bearing capacity is adequate for early ambulation in the postoperative period, and further stabilization is not likely to be necessary. In general, in cases of tumor or other destructive lesions of the sacral (e.g., infection), the bilateral alae should be evaluated. If one ala or more than 50% of bilateral alae are destroyed, the patient will require lumbopelvic fixation.

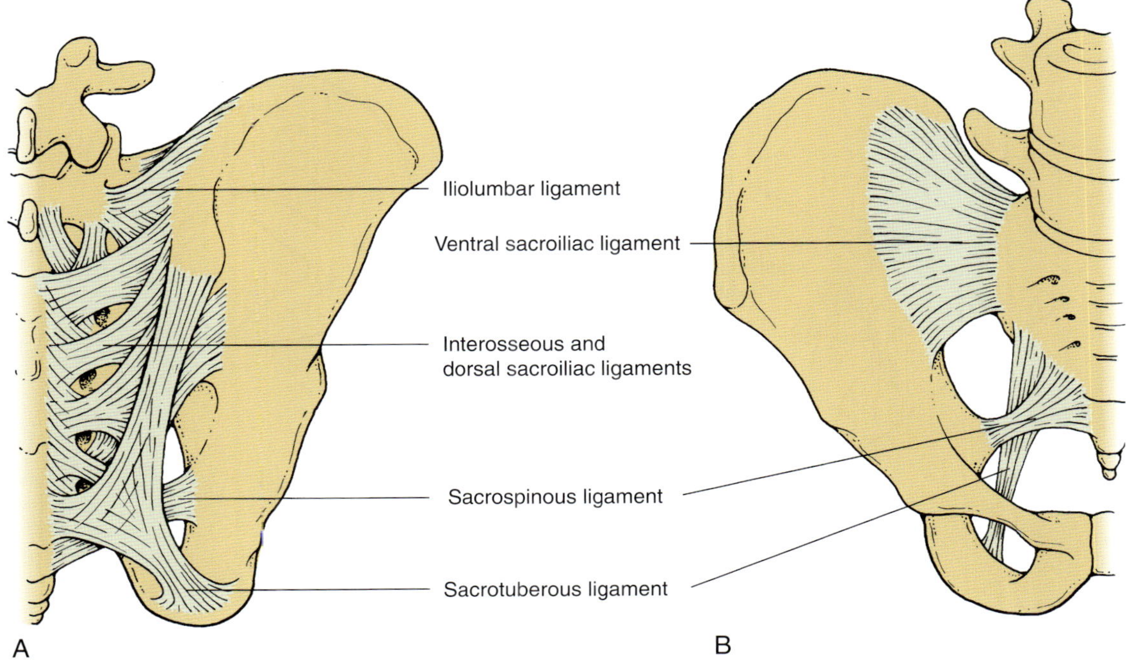

FIGURE 152-3. Dorsal (**A**) and ventral (**B**) views of the major ligamentous attachments of the sacroiliac joint.

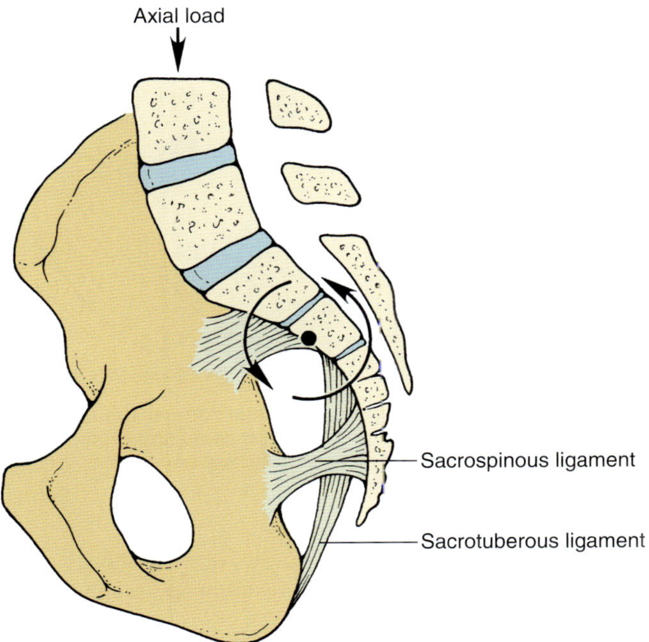

FIGURE 152-4. The center point of the rotational vector is located near the center of the S2 vertebral body. The diagram depicts the rotational tendency of the sacrum about this point. It is through the long lever arms created by the sacrospinous and sacrotuberous ligaments that this rotational tendency is counteracted and the sacrum is stabilized.

Indications for Lumbosacralpelvic Fixation

In short-segment cases and in the absence of osteopenia, sacral fixation with a single pair of bone screws is adequate. In longer-segment cases (e.g., scoliosis, postsacrectomy reconstruction, and multisegmental lumbosacral fusion) or with osteoporotic bone, more substantial segmental fixation is required to achieve rigidity. In addition, when high-grade lumbosacral spondylolistheses (grades III and above) are reduced, standard sacral screws may be inadequate and lead to loosening or sacral fracture. Rigidity is a crucial element in these constructs because fusion rates are directly related to use of rigid instrumentation, and better outcomes clearly correlate with the acquisition of a solid fusion.[8-15] If a long instrumentation construct is placed, the sacral attachment is usually subjected to large cantilevered forces that may lead to screw pull-out (Fig. 152-5). Additional points of sacral or sacropelvic fixation may prevent complications in such cases.

Instrumentation may be used in compression or distraction to reduce deformity. Distraction, in particular, may place a substantial stress on the implants, in addition to the physiologic loads that will be exerted by the daily activities and movements of the patient. This stress constitutes implant preload. Instrumentation that will bear a significant preload may require either further sacral fixation points or attachments that cross the SIJ. If the preload is not symmetrically distributed, as in the case of scoliosis correction, the additional instrumentation does not necessarily need to be placed bilaterally but should be included on the side that will bear the larger load. If significant pelvic obliquity is present, as occurs commonly with scoliosis of neuromuscular origin, the construct should cross the SIJ in most instances and should be symmetrical.

The SIJ is autofused in many adults older than 50 years of age. Long-term follow-up study of patients with instrumentation constructs crossing the SIJ has demonstrated no adverse effects relating to the presence of the implants.[16] Therefore, if it is necessary for additional security of fixation in the lumbosacropelvic

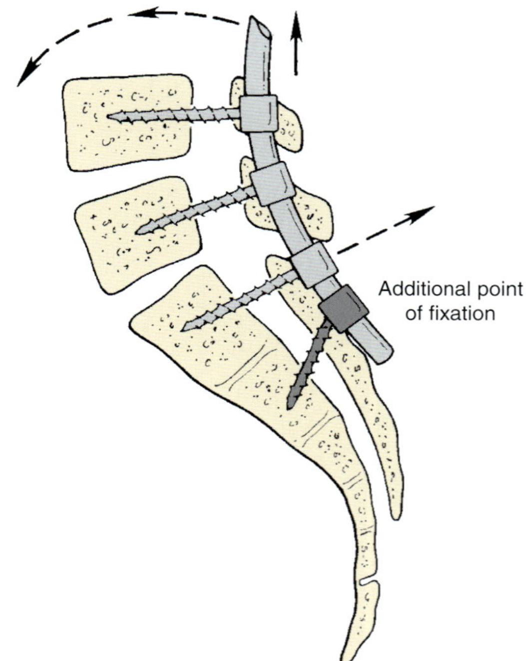

FIGURE 152-5. As the dorsal construct becomes longer, the potential cantilevered forces on the sacral attachment are increased (*dashed lines*). This predisposes to sacral screw pull-out. Additional points of fixation may thus be required (*shaded screw*).

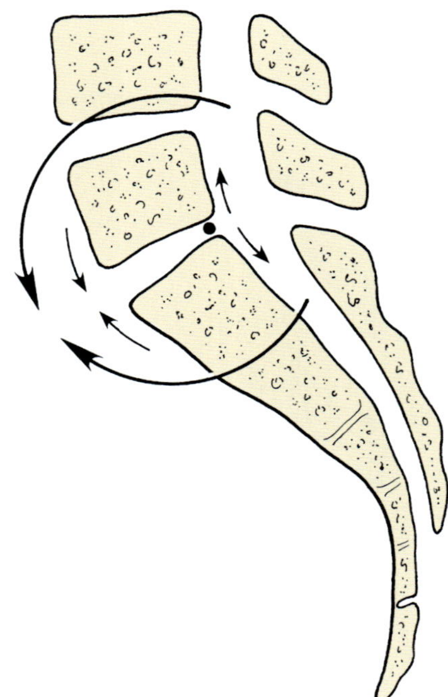

FIGURE 152-6. As the lumbosacral joint is flexed, those points located ventral to the pivot point (*dot*) move toward each other, whereas those dorsal to it separate.

region, placement of instrumentation across the SIJ is a rational approach for providing spinal stability.

Lumbosacral Pivot Point

In a study of the biomechanics of sacropelvic fixation, McCord et al. described the concept of the lumbosacral pivot point.[17] This is the axis of rotation at the lumbosacral junction. During flexion, the portions of L5 and the sacrum that are ventral to this pivot move toward one another. Likewise, the portions of L5 and the sacrum located dorsal to this pivot point will move apart during flexion (Fig. 152-6). Anatomically, the lumbosacral pivot point is marked by the intersection of the middle osteoligamentous column and the lumbosacral (L5-S1) disc. In constructs that cross the SIJ, only those devices that pass ventral to this point provide a significant biomechanical advantage regarding rigidity of fixation.

Complex Techniques of Sacral Fixation

Many lumbosacral fusions can be adequately immobilized with placement of bone screws into the sacral pedicles. These screws, however, obtain their thread purchase in the broad cancellous channel of the sacral pedicle. Therefore, bone screws in the sacral pedicles are subject to failure because of the relative porosity of the sacrum, the manner in which stress tends to be concentrated at the termini of a fusion construct, and the large flexion moments to which these constructs are subjected.[18,19] Sacral screws may fail by pull-out or by fracture.[18] In cases in which it is believed that

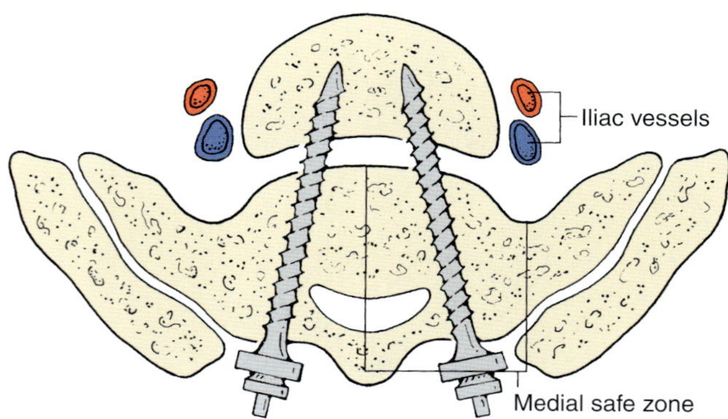

FIGURE 152-7. Depiction of the safe medial zone at the portion of the sacrum that lies lateral to the neural canal and medial to the iliac vessels. Therefore, sacral pedicle screws need to be "toed in" to avoid these vascular structures.

the use of a single pair of bone screws may not be adequate for stabilization, the use of more complex techniques is warranted.

With regard to injuring structures ventral to the sacrum, cadaveric studies have shown that the widest margin of safety is found at the medial safe zone (Fig. 152-7).[20] Therefore, placing the screws in a medial or toed-in direction is preferred at the S1 or promontory level. Some authors have advocated bicortical purchase of sacral screws to enhance pull-out resistance, which affords some pull-out strength advantage, although this involves additional risk.[20-25] Zindrick et al. found that bicortical purchase with a 6.5-mm diameter screw resulted in an increase in pull-out strength of about 30%.[25] Penetrating an excessive distance beyond the ventral cortex carries the risks of neurologic deficit, chronic pain from lumbosacral trunk injury, sympathetic chain injury, peritonitis, sepsis, and hemorrhage,[20,24] although these risks are minimal if the screw penetrates 1 cm or less.

Fixation with Sublaminar Devices

The addition of sublaminar devices such as hooks, wires, or cables at the sacrum is a simple means of enhancing fixation. It should be borne in mind that the sacral laminae are often quite thin and may not provide substantial strength to hold such devices. All of these devices, including hooks, are tension-band fixators. Dorsally placed tension-band constructs provide limitation of flexion but do not provide substantial torsional stability or resistance to extension. With fusions at the LSJ, it has been shown that fixation with sublaminar devices alone does not improve the fusion rate when this rate is compared with that of noninstrumented fusions.[26] Therefore, sublaminar devices should be used at the LSJ only in conjunction with other devices.

Although the bony thickness at the sacral lamina is meager, the bone stock is usually quite substantial at the nearby dorsal foramina. Thus, the dorsal foramina are excellent sites to place hooks for the purpose of enhancing construct strength. When added to a sacral pedicle screw construct, this technique has been shown to significantly increase rigidity.[27]

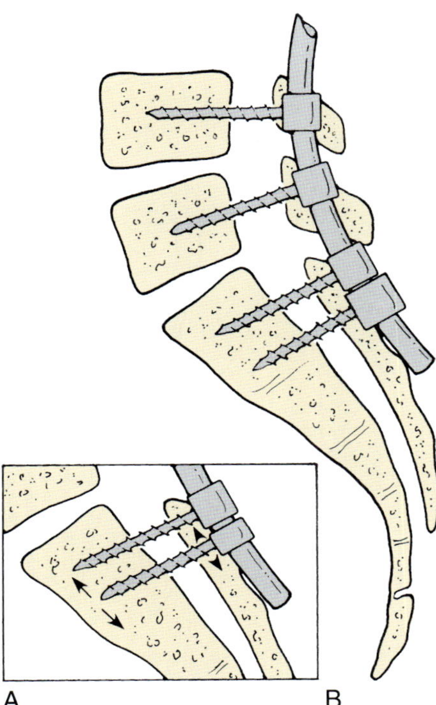

FIGURE 152-8. If the site of attachment of the second screw is narrow, sufficient latitude is present to allow proper trajectory (**A**). If the attachment is too broad, it impedes proper placement of the screw (**B**).

Fixation with Screws

A number of simple techniques use bone screws to enhance sacral fixation. Screws provide rigid three-dimensional stabilization and can be used for short-segment fixation at the LSJ. Shorter constructs provide a major advantage because immobilization of long segments of the spine increases the load, not only at the immediately adjacent segment but also at more distal segments.[28]

Directing screws medially (pedicular) or laterally (alar) and then rigidly attaching them to the rod or plate greatly enhances pull-out resistance. Studies are in conflict regarding which of these two methods is better, but both offer a substantial biomechanical advantage over a straight sagittal-plane trajectory.[25,29] Oblique trajectories dramatically increase the cross-sectional area of bone that resists screw dislodgement via the cantilevered forces applied by the spine in flexion. If the longitudinal members are then linked with cross-members, a triangulation effect is created. This enhances both the rigidity of the construct and its pull-out resistance.[25,30,31] Torsional stability is particularly enhanced by cross-fixation of the rods.[30,32,33]

Perhaps the easiest method for enhancing sacral fixation with screws is the placement of an additional pair of laterally directed bone screws into the sacral alae below the S1 level. This method provides a biomechanical advantage over a single pair of pedicle screws.[13,17] These screws are easily added to a construct without the need for preplanning or special devices, and fluoroscopy is not required. For this method, a type of screw whose attachment site to the rod is somewhat narrow is optimal. Screws with a broad attachment site may be difficult to place sufficiently close together for the optimal trajectory of the screws to be attained (Fig. 152-8).

The placement of screws into the S2 and even the S3 levels has been advocated to enhance the security of sacral fixation. Biomechanical testing has demonstrated that these screw placement sites do not add sufficiently to the security of fixation to warrant their use.[17,25] The thickness of the sacrum in the sagittal plane diminishes at the lower sacral levels. Therefore, inadvertent penetration of the ventral surface of the sacrum with such screws is more likely, and injury to the anatomic structures immediately adjacent to the ventral cortical surface may occur. However, such S2 alar screws can be used as more substantial anchor points if they are used as S2 sacroiliac screws, in which the screw transverses the SIJ and functions as an iliac screw in terms of longer length and iliac purchase.

The pedicular transvertebral screw fixation technique has been described for treatment of lumbosacral spondylolisthesis.[34] This technique involves placement of a long screw through the pedicle of S1, passing through the rostral end plate of S1 and into the caudal end plate of the L5 vertebral body. When combined with screws in the L4 pedicles, this provides a unique biomechanical construct. It appears to be a simple method for stabilizing high-grade spondylolisthesis. The simplicity of this technique is attractive, and the clinical results appear to be encouraging (Fig. 152-9).

Along with placement of screws spanning from vertebra to sacrum, fibular bone struts can be applied in a similar manner. Placement of fibular grafts to act as dowels can be performed from a dorsal or ventral approach.[35-39]

The procedure has been reported in use with autografts, allografts, and even with vascularized autografts.[36,37,40,41] Transvertebral fibular dowels should always be augmented with screw fixation.

Along with screw placement, sacral fixation can be supplemented by insertion of the rods directly into the lateral sacral bony masses. Jackson has described a method whereby screws

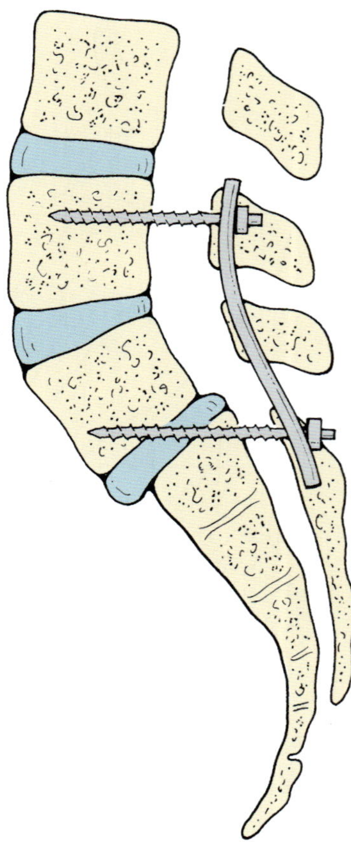

FIGURE 152-9. With the pedicular transvertebral screw fixation technique, the sacral screw passes through the pedicle of S1 and into the inferior portion of the end plate of the L5 vertebral body. The upper end of the construct consists of L4 pedicle screws.

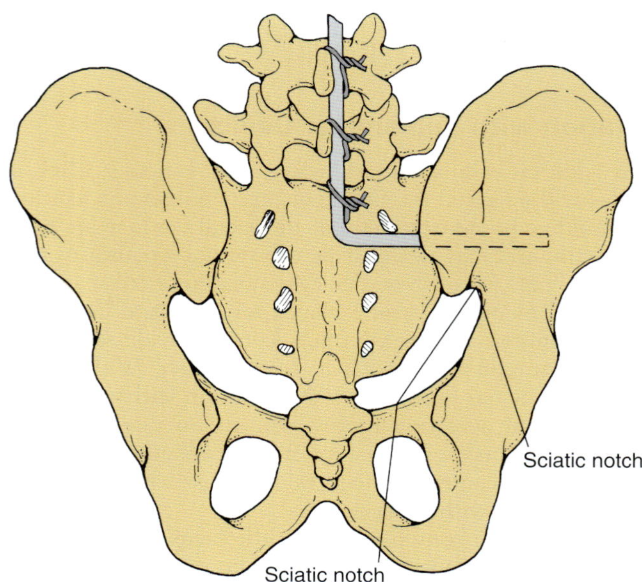

FIGURE 152-10. The Galveston technique for sacropelvic attachment uses angled rods that are placed into the iliac bones along the transverse bar of the ilium. The rods are passed into the cortical bone above the sciatic notch.

are directed through the S1 pedicle, and cortical purchase is obtained in the vertebral end plate of S1 as well. The rods are then passed into the lateral sacrum toward the SIJ and affixed rigidly to the screws.

Devices for Sacral Fixation with Multiple Screws

A number of devices especially designed for sacral and sacropelvic fixation have been marketed. The two basic types are those that cross the SIJ and those that affix directly to the sacrum only. The sacral fixation devices are generally platelike structures that are secured to the sacrum with screws. Asher and Strippgen described one early example of these.[42] It is called the Isola plate because of its butterfly shape (and is named after a species of Rocky Mountain butterfly). This design contained holes for the passage of multiple sacral screws. The position of the holes dictated placement of the screws, and anthropometric sacral measurements taken in male and female cadavers served as the basis for spacing of the holes.

The Tacoma plate (Medtronic Sofamor Danek, Memphis, TN) is designed to direct the additional screws to the sacral alae rather than to the pedicles. It is available in a two-screw and a three-screw model. Such devices are easily attached without special training beyond that required for pedicle screw placement.

Fixation across the Sacroiliac Joint

The most commonly used method for sacropelvic attachment is the Galveston technique or a variation of it. The procedure was originally described by Allen and Ferguson for the treatment of scoliosis.[43,44] It is accomplished by inserting angled rods into the iliac bones and passing them into the hard cortical bone above the sciatic notch (Fig. 152-10). This technique is useful for providing extremely rigid fixation in difficult cases, such as reconstruction after tumor resection or patients with lumbosacral agenesis.[45]

In conditions of large preload, such as the correction of pelvic obliquity in neuromuscular diseases, loss of correction can occur because of the slippage of one rod relative to the other. Several manufacturers have developed cross-fixation devices that attach to both rods and prevent such slippage and markedly enhance the rigidity of the constructs. Although the attachment mechanism, ease of use, and biomechanics of these devices differ substantially, they all enhance construct rigidity and lessen the risk of failure in multilevel constructs.

Placing Galveston rods into the ilium can be cumbersome and technically difficult. Therefore, specialized screws for iliac insertion have been developed (Isola iliac screws, DePuy AcroMed, Raynham, MA). Iliac screws are placed by using fluoroscopy, and the rods are then either directly attached or joined to the screw by a connector fitting. These devices markedly enhance the rigidity of lumbosacral instrumentation constructs. The increases in rigidity are similar for both the iliac screws and the Galveston rods.[17] Multiple studies have confirmed that iliac fixation provides the most effective means to supplement sacral screws.[46,47]

Bicortical Iliac Screw Fixation

A simple method of sacropelvic fixation is the placement of long, variable-angle bone screws obliquely through the iliac

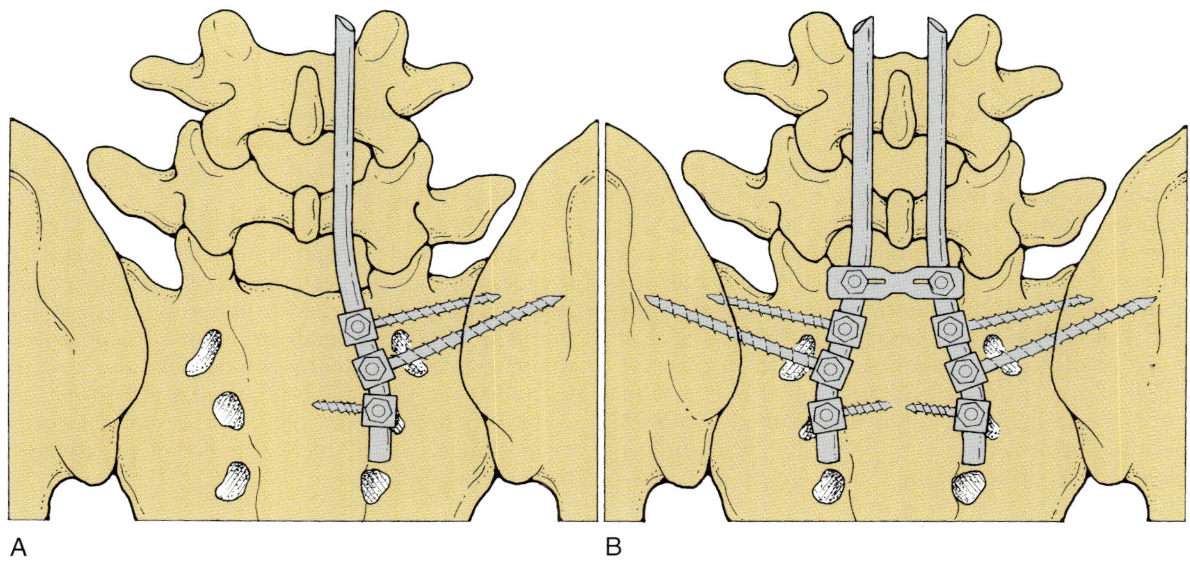

FIGURE 152-11. The tripod geometry of variable angle screws that are passed obliquely through the iliac bones as well as the sacrum provides an increased load-sharing capability of the implant (**A**). Adding a rigid cross-member increases the rigidity and stability of the construct (**B**).

bones (Fig. 152-11). When combined with additional sites of fixation at the sacrum, this technique creates a tripod effect for load sharing. This method has not been studied for its biomechanical characteristics, but early clinical results appear satisfactory.[48]

Bicortical iliac fixation is a simple technique to perform and does not require preplanning or specialized devices. It is important to pay strict attention to the screw trajectory and to ascertain that the screw tip will pass ventral to the lumbosacral pivot point. Also, a small section of the dorsal sacroiliac ligamentous complex must be removed to allow the screw to be placed in a low-profile configuration.

Complications of Complex Lumbopelvic Fixation

The majority of complications associated with complex instrumentation constructs are similar to those of any other spine fixation procedures. Infection remains a common adverse sequela of these operations, occurring in 3% to 5% of cases, even in experienced hands.[49] Problems such as blood loss, neurologic deficits, and poor bone quality should be managed with the same measures as would be used in any other implant case.

Accurate placement of sacropelvic instrumentation is crucial for optimal results. If difficulty is encountered in visualizing the necessary anatomy with fluoroscopy, further dissection should be undertaken to directly visualize the structures to be instrumented. Dissection along the lateral aspect of the ilium allows easy access for palpation of the sciatic notch, and placement of a Galveston rod above the notch is thereby simplified. Similarly, the sacral alae can be exposed for placement of alar screws. Screw sites should always be probed carefully before tapping or screw insertion. This aids in identifying inadvertent ventral cortical penetration or, if such penetration is desirable, in determining optimal screw length. Screw length can also be confirmed by measuring the appropriate region on a CT scan, although the obliquity of the placement may make this difficult.

Revision Surgery

One of the major complications of lumbosacropelvic instrumentation is loosening or failure of hardware. In some cases, however, such loosening or failure may not prevent solid bony fusion. Therefore, it is a matter of judgment about when these constructs should be revised. Patients with loosened hardware should be followed closely with serial radiographic studies. Reparation is recommended if evidence of either progressive unacceptable deformity or symptomatic pseudarthrosis is observed. Because late healing may occur, it is advisable to delay revision surgery until it is certain that an acceptable result does not occur without revision.

Revision surgery of instrumentation constructs should address the reason for the failure. If there is a fractured implant, more fixation points should be included to improve load sharing. If screw pull-out is observed, the use of larger-diameter or longer screws provides greater thread purchase. If the pull-out appears to be largely due to poor bone quality, pressurized injection of polymethylmethacrylate may improve screw pull-out resistance.[25]

In general, surgery for failed spinal instrumentation involves the implantation of more hardware. For failed sacral fixation, creation of a construct that spans the SIJ is advisable. Further bone grafting should always be performed by using autologous bone, if possible. Harvest of iliac crest bone may not be possible because many of these patients have had a previous harvest at the iliac sites. One limited alternative is the use of rib grafts. If iliac harvest is performed in patients with iliac fixation sites, the harvest sites should be placed as far ventrally as possible.

In cases of Galveston rod failure, additional fixation points can usually be secured. These rods tend to loosen by pull-out because they do not have purchase into the deep portion of the iliac bones. Further fixation should be attempted by placement of screws into the sacral pedicles or alae and attachment to the rod. Also, rigid cross-members should be added if these are not already present in the construct.

An alternative surgical approach may also be required for revision surgery. An interbody fusion is sometimes a reasonable alternative to augment a dorsolateral fusion. Ventral fusion at the lumbosacral junction may be accomplished by using interbody grafts after ventral discectomy or vertebrectomy for tumor, infection, or grade III or IV spondylolisthesis. Allograft bone is the usual substrate for grafting in cases of interbody fusion, but newer interbody cage devices that allow the use of autograft will soon be available. Because no rigid ventral stabilization device can be easily applied to the sacrum, either ventrally or laterally, such interbody grafts or cages should be supplemented with dorsal hardware, unless the decompression consisted of only simple lumbosacral discectomy in the absence of pathology in the posterior elements.

Screws may be placed through the sacral promontory retrograde into the S1 pedicles, but the bulk of the attached hardware usually produces risks of iliac vessel injury that outweigh any potential benefits. Because of this anatomic stumbling block, interbody cages should be viewed as supplemental devices rather than as primary stabilization hardware in any case of complex lumbosacral reconstruction. Many different types of interbody devices have been developed for placement via either open or endoscopic techniques (BAK cage, Ray cage, Brantigan device, Novus device, Harms cage). Some of these have received clearance from the Food and Drug Administration, and others are seeking clearance.

At the LSJ, it is far easier to place interbody grafts or devices via a true ventral (transperitoneal or extraperitoneal) approach or via a dorsal lumbar interbody approach than via a lateral (retroperitoneal) approach. The crossing iliac veins ventral to L5, the bony iliac wing that blocks the view, and the bulky psoas muscle at this level make the lateral approach to the lumbosacral junction uncomfortable at best. The ventral approach usually sacrifices the sympathetic plexus over the sacral promontory, sometimes producing ejaculatory dysfunction in males, and it may occasionally require sacrifice of one or both internal iliac vessels. The dorsal interbody approach usually involves the sacrifice of some or all of both facet complexes at L5-S1 and has a relatively high risk of nerve root injury. Regardless of which approach is chosen for interbody fusion at the lumbosacral junction, a good working knowledge of the pertinent anatomy and potential complications is critical.

Postoperatively, patients who have undergone revision surgery should be placed in thoracolumbosacral orthoses. The addition of a hip extension device to these orthoses has traditionally been recommended. However, it has been shown that spinal motion is not reduced by the addition of this cumbersome and uncomfortable attachment.[50]

In the management of sacral tumors, involvement of the S1 segment is often the only impediment to what might otherwise be a potential surgical cure. Particularly in chordomas, the most common of sacral tumors, complete surgical resection with margins is usually considered curative because the tumor is usually indolent, metastasizing beyond its site of origin only very late in its course. Many such tumors are detected only when they are quite large, although they are still localized. The ability to perform a total sacrectomy for cure is impaired by the difficulty of reestablishing spinopelvic stability in the absence of the sacrum.

In a few cases, such stability has been accomplished by attaching ventral allograft bone struts to transpelvic plates at the lower end and to the remaining lumbar vertebrae above.[51] Pelvic rim stabilization with transverse plates and stabilization with oblique allograft struts from the dorsal iliac wings to the telescoped lumbar vertebrae have also been attempted with some success.[52] Graft positioning oblique to the primary ventral rotational force vector in the upright posture is the main clinical and theoretical impediment to the success of these techniques.

Research continues regarding new techniques of lumbopelvic reconstruction after total sacrectomy. In cadavers, whole allograft sacral transplants may be plated between the iliac wings ventrally to reestablish anterior column support and pelvic ring integrity. The transplants are supplemented with iliolumbar rods (Galveston technique) dorsally and generous volumes of autograft bone. Much work remains, however, before this technique can be considered for clinical use. A number of manufacturers are also offering advanced plating and connector devices for enhancement of fixation in these very difficult cases.

Summary

Lumbosacralpelvic fixation methods are technically challenging and carry significant risk. Such techniques can, however, be used to manage a variety of complex spinal disorders. As with all surgery, strict attention to detail is the key to avoiding complications.

KEY REFERENCES

McCord DH, Cunningham BW, Shono Y, et al: Biomechanical analysis of lumbosacral fixation. *Spine (Phila Pa 1976)* 17:S235–S243, 1992.

Pintar FA, Maiman DJ, Yoganandan N, et al: Rotational stability of a spinal pedicle screw/rod system. *J Spinal Disord* 8:49–55, 1995.

Ruland CM, McAfee PC, Warden KE, et al: Triangulation of pedicular instrumentation. A biomechanical analysis. *Spine (Phila Pa 1976)* 16:S270–S276, 1991.

Tomita K, Tsuchiya H: Total sacrectomy and reconstruction for huge sacral tumors. *Spine (Phila Pa 1976)* 15:1223–1227, 1990.

White AA, Panjabi MM: *Clinical biomechanics of the spine*, Philadelphia, 1990, Lippincott-Raven.

Zindrick MR, Wiltse LL, Widell EH, et al: A biomechanical study of intrapeduncular screw fixation in the lumbosacral spine. *Clin Orthop Relat Res* 203:99–112, 1986.

REFERENCES

The complete reference list is available online at expertconsult.com.

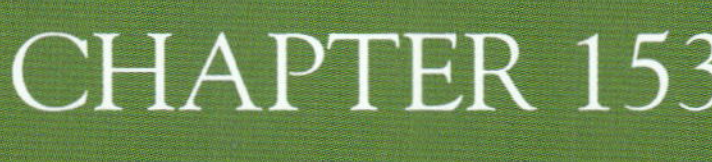

CHAPTER 153

Iatrogenic Spine Destabilization

Mehmet Zileli | Nevan G. Baldwin | Edward C. Benzel

An increased understanding of spinal mechanics, spinal cord physiology, anesthesia, critical care, and spinal instrumentation devices has allowed surgeons to approach the spine ventrally, dorsally, laterally, and circumferentially without excessive morbidity. However, these complex interventions often exaggerate spine instability.

The instability that exists after a spine operation may arise from pathologic (intrinsic) or iatrogenic (surgical) processes. Iatrogenic destabilization can result from a variety of sources, such as the destruction of ligaments, muscles, or bone, and the denervation of muscles (Table 153-1).[1]

Biomechanical Considerations

Spinal stability is often viewed in terms of support "columns" in the spine. Various systems for evaluating stability consider varying numbers of columns and the fact that the anatomic components of a given column, such as the anterior column, may differ from one system to the next. Also, a column may or may not have a true anatomic correlate.

One method that is commonly used for evaluating stability is the three-column method of Denis.[2] The anterior column is the ventral half of the vertebral body and the anterior longitudinal ligament (ALL). The dorsal half of the vertebral body and the posterior longitudinal ligament (PLL) constitute the middle column. The dorsal column consists of the facet joints and all ligaments dorsal to the spinal canal.

Using the method of Denis,[2] significant instability is considered highly likely if two or more columns have suffered substantial injury. The posterior column has true anatomic boundaries, whereas the anterior and middle columns arbitrarily consider halves of a single vertebral body. Many systems for evaluating stability have been devised, but the method of Denis is an example of such a system that is easy to use and widely accepted for clinical application.

Ligamentous Disruption

Iatrogenic ligamentous instability can be assessed by intraoperative traction and/or distraction maneuvers, such as distraction, application of vertebral body spreaders, and implant manipulation. These maneuvers may help determine whether an instrumented fusion is necessary.

Ventral Surgery

The ALL and the PLL, as well as the anulus fibrosus, contribute significantly to the stability of the spine.[3-5] The PLL is weaker than the ALL and is often intentionally destroyed during dorsal, ventral, or lateral spine surgery. However, the ALL is often not totally disrupted, even with a wide ventral exposure. A strong and wide ligament, the ALL provides a significant proportion of spinal stability in extension. This function may be considered as a tension band that limits extension. As a result, ventral decompressive spine surgery (e.g., corpectomy), which adequately decompresses the dural sac, generally causes a disruption of the PLL, with preservation of at least a portion of the ALL. The width of the PLL significantly narrows in the middle portions of the vertebral body, thus making it susceptible to surgical disruption. In conjunction with existing bony disruption, surgical decompression usually causes significant instability of the spine. The extent of this destabilization can be assessed via intraoperative manipulation, such as vertebral body distraction. If significant instability is iatrogenically created, an interbody strut graft is necessary, with or without supplementation by instrumentation. The PLL limits flexion and distraction.

Dorsal Surgery

Resection of the interspinous ligaments may lead to instability. Although the interspinous ligaments are relatively weak, their long moment arm (i.e., distance from the instantaneous axis of rotation to the ligament attachment site) provides a mechanical advantage with regard to their function as a tension band.[1] The capsular ligaments are strong. Although they function through a short moment arm, their relative strength allows them to provide a significant stabilizing effect, if they are intact.

Bone Destruction

Ventral Surgery

Bone destruction and additional surgical bone removal have a significant impact on spinal stability. Both the amount of vertebral body destruction and its location play an important role in the surgical destabilization process (Fig. 153-1). The first issue is the extent of ventral bony destruction. A

TABLE 153-1

Spine Destabilization: Etiology and Management

Surgery	Reason for Instability	Recommended Management
Extensive cervical laminectomy	Tension band destruction Facet joint destruction	Laminoplasty or lateral mass plating plus fusion
Extensive lumbar laminectomy	Tension band destruction Facet joint destruction	Controversial Possibly dorsolateral fusion Possibly dorsal instrumentation
Cervical corpectomy	Bony destruction ALL/PLL destruction	Ventral fusion Ventral instrumentation External orthosis
Thoracolumbar total corpectomy	Bony destruction ALL/PLL destruction	Ventral reconstruction plus ventral instrumentation or dorsal instrumentation
Corpectomy plus dorsal decompression or total spondylectomy	Extensive bony destruction plus ALL/PLL destruction Facet joint destruction	Circumferential fusion and instrumentation Equal ventral and dorsal instrumentation

ALL, anterior longitudinal ligament; PLL, posterior longitudinal ligament.

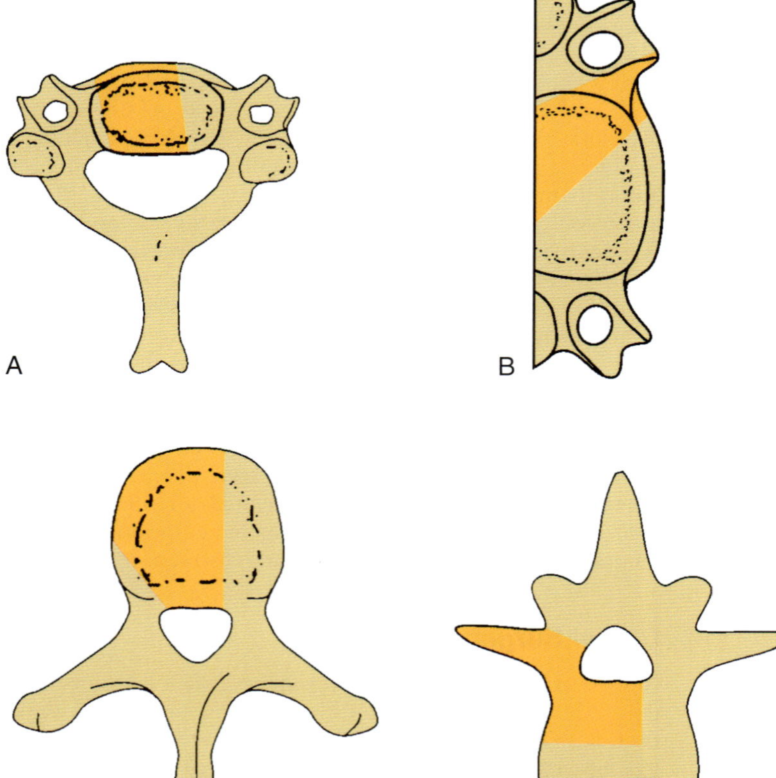

FIGURE 153-1. Resection portions of the ventral vertebral body in most frequently performed ventral spine surgeries. **A,** Cervical corpectomy—resection of the middle horizontal section of the body. **B,** Oblique cervical corpectomy, with resection of the lateral and dorsal sections of the vertebral body. **C,** Ventral thoracic or lumbar surgery. **D,** Lateral extracavitary surgery. In the latter two approaches, resection of the dorsolateral portion of the body is more extensive in ventral surgery. (Copyright Division of Neurosurgery, University of New Mexico.)

complete vertebrectomy causes an obvious instability (see Table 153-1). The extent of instability is closely related to the amount of bone removed.

White and Panjabi[5] used a three-column model to explain the effects of element disruption on spinal column stability. To determine the effect of a partial vertebral body resection on spinal stability, Benzel[1] used a hypothetical design that divides the vertebral body into 27 equal, small cubes (Fig. 153-2). In this regard, resection of the ventral portion of the vertebral body affects spinal stability more than a corresponding resection of the middle or dorsal portion of the vertebral body (Fig. 153-3), because the largest force to which the spine is subjected is that of flexion. The more ventral portion of the vertebral body is farther from the instantaneous axis of rotation, and it therefore exerts its resistance through a longer moment arm in resisting flexion. Also, resection of the middle horizontal section of the vertebral body affects stability more than does resection in the middle vertical sections (Fig. 153-4).

Minimizing bone removal helps decrease postoperative instability. To attain this goal, vertebral body resection in

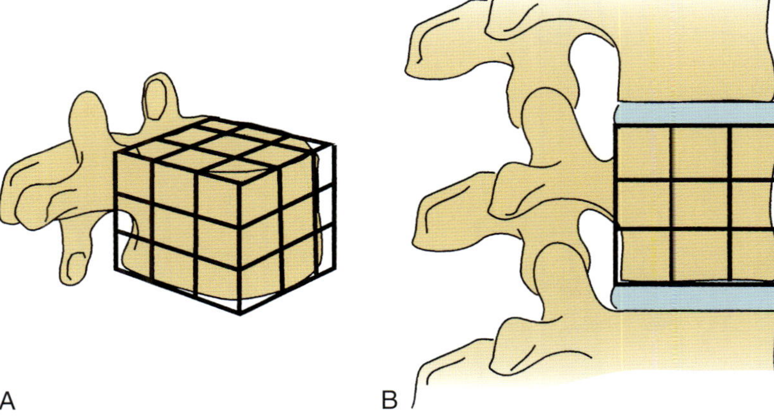

FIGURE 153-2. A vertebral body seen, for theoretical purposes, as a cube composed of 27 equal, small cubes (3 × 3 × 3). **A,** Oblique view; **B,** lateral view. (From Benzel EC: *Biomechanics of spine stabilization: principles and clinical practice,* New York, 1995, McGraw-Hill.)

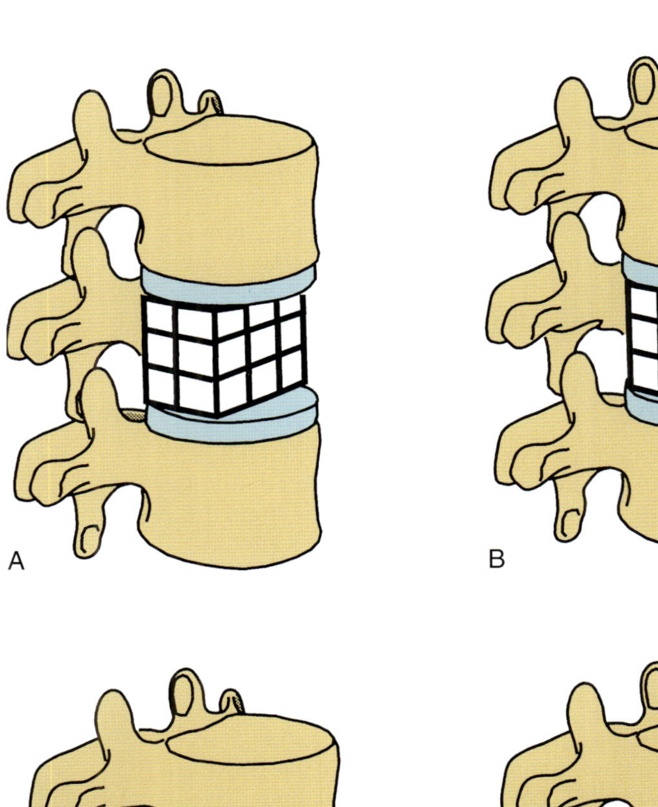

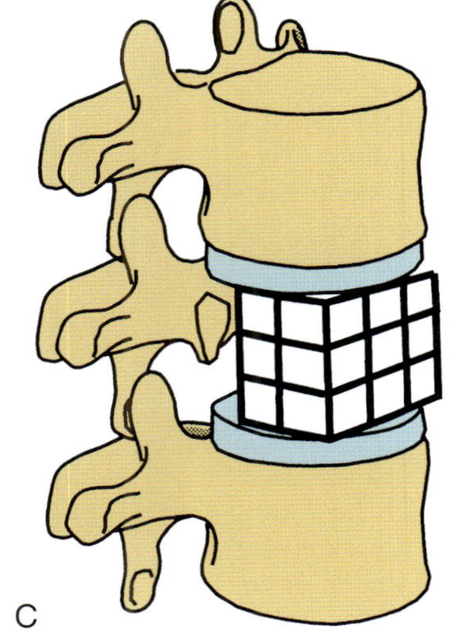

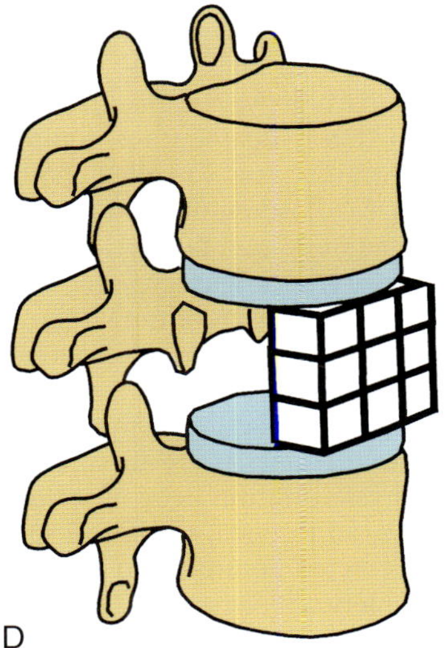

FIGURE 153-3. Resection of the components of the cubic vertebral body. Partial vertebrectomy involving removal of the ventral component in the coronal plane of the vertebral body (**A**) affects the stability more than resection of the middle (**B**) or dorsal portion (**C**) in the coronal plane. Resection of both the middle and the dorsal third of the vertebral body (in the presence of an intact posterior column and an intact ventral third of the vertebral body) may not significantly disrupt spinal integrity (**D**). (From Benzel EC: *Biomechanics of spine stabilization: principles and clinical practice,* New York, 1995, McGraw-Hill.)

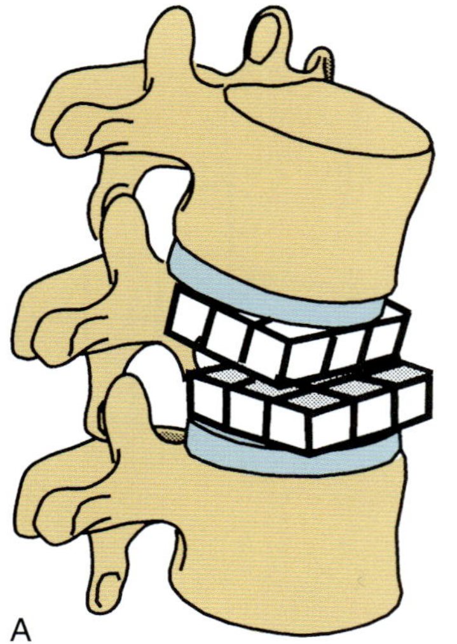

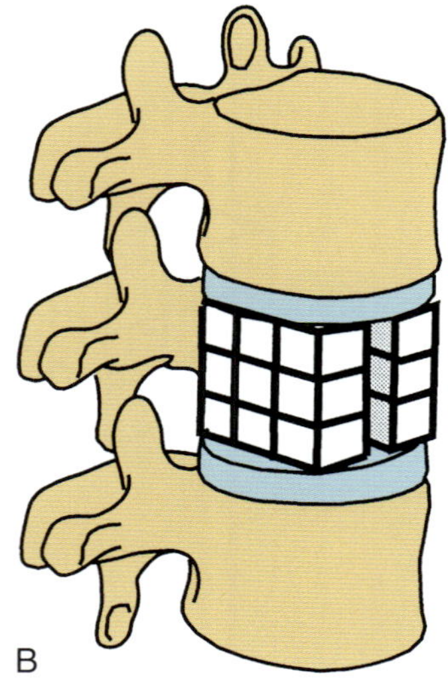

FIGURE 153-4. Resections of portions of the cubic vertebral body. **A,** Resection (or disruption) of the middle axial (horizontal) third of the vertebral body in its sagittal dimension, as may occur after trauma. **B,** Resection of the middle (vertical) third of the vertebral body. (From Benzel EC: *Biomechanics of spine stabilization: principles and clinical practice,* New York, 1995, McGraw-Hill.)

cervical corpectomy should be carefully determined. In this regard, oblique corpectomy is an approach that does not significantly interfere with the stability of the spine.[6,7] This approach protects the ventral portion of the vertebral body but sacrifices the dorsal and lateral aspects (see Fig. 153-1B).

As an aside, the uncovertebral joints add stability during extension, lateral bending, and torsion.[8] In general, if the (1) ALL, (2) ventral section of the vertebral body, (3) dorsal column integrity, and (4) dorsal column ligaments remain intact, a significant instability does not develop.

Dorsal Surgery

A laminectomy can cause instability because of destabilization of the spine. The frequency of iatrogenic instability is proportional to the width of the laminectomy.[9,10] Often, the extent of the injury is not readily apparent shortly after surgery. The prediction of its subsequent occurrence is even less obvious. If a ventral (vertebral body) lesion already exists, the incidence of postlaminectomy kyphosis is even higher.

Laminectomy often creates distortion of the dura mater and spinal cord, with flexion and distraction over the ventral fulcrum (Fig. 153-5). Even in the absence of the ventral pathology, the disruption of the laminae, facet joints, and dorsal ligamentous complex may result in progressive deformity, the so-called postlaminectomy kyphosis (Fig. 153-6). Postlaminectomy kyphosis occurs more commonly in the more mobile portion of the spine—the cervical spine. Laminoplasty may preserve a portion of the dorsal tension band and thereby diminish the instability observed after laminectomy.[11] Another alternative that minimizes the destabilizing effect of laminectomy is the addition of a stabilization strategy such as dorsal fusion or external orthosis.

In summary, there are three important issues that should be addressed during decompressive laminectomy: (1) the presence, or absence, of ventral spinal instability, (2) the extent of resected laminae and facet joints as well as the extent of ligamentous disruption, and (3) the location of the laminectomy (i.e., cervical, thoracic, or lumbar spine). The cervical spine is more prone to instability after laminectomy.

The contribution of the facet joints to dorsal column stability is very important. With axial loading, the anterior and

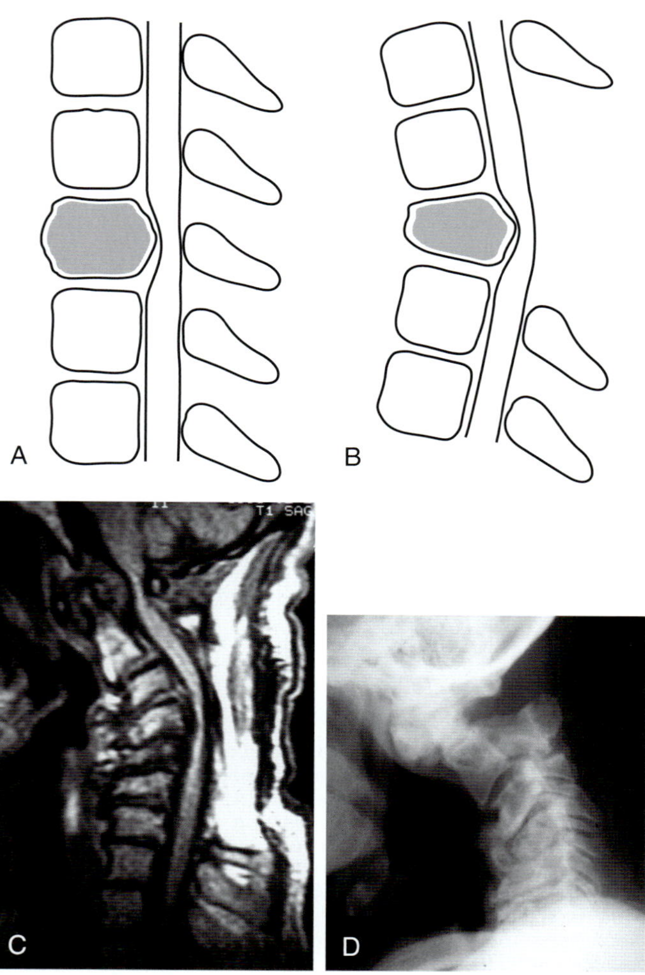

FIGURE 153-5. Development of postlaminectomy kyphosis. In the case of preexisting ventral pathology, laminectomy (**A**) can cause severe kyphotic deformity (**B**). In the cervical spine, even in the absence of ventral pathology, progressive kyphosis may develop (**C** and **D**).

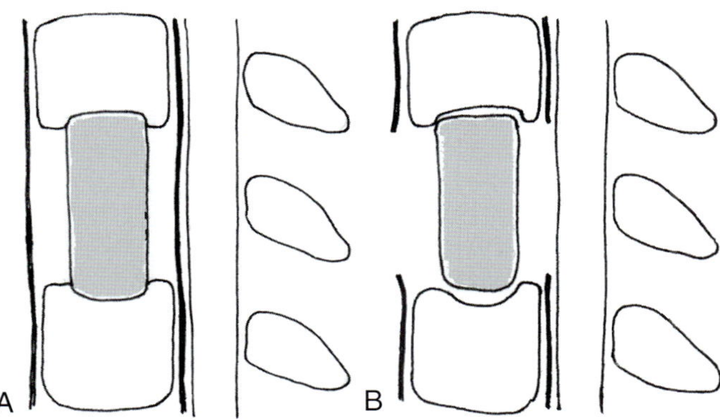

FIGURE 153-6. The "clamping down" phenomenon in the cervical spine. If the posterior longitudinal ligament and the anterior longitudinal ligament are intact, the graft firmly fits into the mortises of both end plates (**A**). If the ligaments are destroyed, their contribution to resisting distraction is lost, and the graft does not fit into the mortises firmly (**B**).

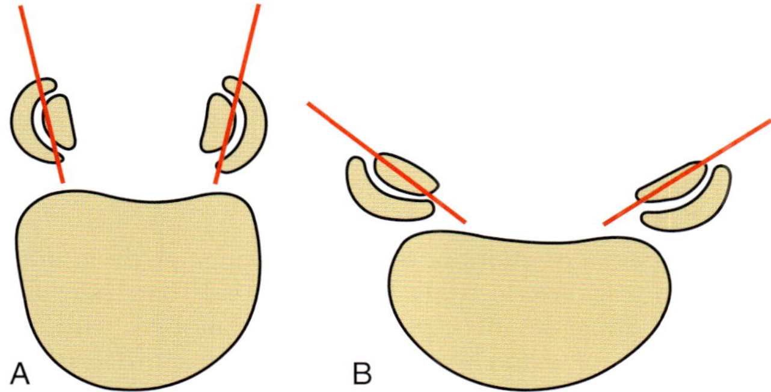

FIGURE 153-7. Facet joint angles at the L4-5 and L5-S1 levels. **A,** The L4-5 facet joints are sagittally oriented and do not resist translation. **B,** The L5-S1 facet joints are coronally oriented and resist translation well.

middle columns transmit only 36% of the applied load, whereas each pillar (facet) transmits 32% of the total applied load.[12] Therefore, regardless of the region of the spine involved, excessive facet joint resection can result in instability. In the cervical spine, the tolerable limit of resection is one third to one half of the facet joint.[10] In the lumbar spine, facet resection may often result in glacial instability. However, the value of fusion and instrumentation after partial facetectomies for spinal stenosis is controversial.[13]

The shape and angulation of the facet joints are also important. A ventral translational deformity is more likely to result if vertically oriented joints and a hyperlordotic posture are present. The L4 and L5 facet joints are sagittally oriented, whereas L5-S1 joints are coronally oriented (Fig. 153-7). Therefore, L5-S1 joints resist translational deformity, whereas L4-5 joints can easily glide on a sagittal plane. Degenerative listhesis frequently involves this level.

Clinical Considerations

The major indications for spine surgery are decompression and stabilization. Perhaps the most important indication is decompression. Whether the decompression is ventral or dorsal, it decreases spinal stability.

Trauma Surgery

Because trauma itself causes instability, additional iatrogenic instability caused by a decompression operation may be catastrophic. Therefore, most operations for spine trauma include a stabilization component.

The site of decompression (ventral vs. dorsal) is usually dictated by the type and location of the pathology. Spine stabilization can also be achieved from the same orientation.

Tumor Surgery

An important issue that the spine surgeon cannot avoid is the iatrogenic instability created by radical tumor surgery. Until recently, the surgical treatment of spinal tumors was accomplished predominantly via laminectomy, despite the fact that the neural compression was often ventral to the spinal cord. However, laminectomy was often ineffective. Ventral surgery is often the procedure of choice for treating most bone tumors of the spine.[14-16] Because the pathology in most patients with these bone tumors lies ventral to the spinal canal, attempts at tumor resection can cause loss of ventral spinal integrity.

Tumors involving both ventral and dorsal elements cause even greater instability. For oncologic tumor surgery, extramarginal resection of bone tumors of the spine is desirable. Although the spinal cord and nerve roots do not allow such a resection in many instances, there is an increasing trend toward accomplishing total spondylectomies by only a dorsal approach,[14,15,17,18] or by circumferential surgery.[19,20] Because the iatrogenic destabilization of the spine is so significant in these cases, radical measures to reconstruct and stabilize the spine are mandatory.

Preoperatively, the extent of tumor spread is the main determinant of stability. Instability is often not the sole reason for operation. The extent of neurologic deficit, the biology of the tumor, its radiosensitivity, and its sensitivity to chemotherapy are also important reasons. In selected cases, radiotherapy of a radiosensitive tumor and external bracing may be suitable.

Degenerative Spine Surgery

Cervical spondylotic myelopathy is often treated via a decompressive operation. Ventral and dorsal operations both may cause significant iatrogenic spine destabilization. This is similarly true for the thoracic and lumbar spine.

Ventral decompressive surgery of the cervical spine causes bony destruction and also some form of ligamentous disruption. The PLL is intentionally removed during ventral osteophyte excision for cervical spondylotic myelopathy. In this case, interbody strut graft stability, or "clamp down," a phenomenon that would have been provided by an intact ligament, is not realized.

Ventral cervical plates can help resist the distractive forces caused by the disruption of ligamentous resistance.

The anulus fibrosus contributes to the spinal stability in a similar manner on the PLL and ALL. Its disruption in degenerative conditions may cause transitional instability.

Adjacent-Level Spondylosis

It is common to observe degenerative changes above or below the level of a multilevel fusion. This type of instability is obviously iatrogenic. To avoid this, the use of more flexible (dynamic) fixation devices has been proposed.[1] Short-segment fixation and fusion may minimize the incidence of this complication. Another technique for dealing with this problem is to create a "transitional" level by using instrumentation that is less rigid at the first segment adjacent to the fused segments. For example, an L3 burst fracture might be treated by the use of rigid screw instrumentation, along with bony fusion from L2 to L4. The "transitional" segment might then be created by the use of laminar hooks (hooks are less rigid than screws) at L1.

Segmental fixation with the use of pedicle fixation systems can be very rigid. Although increasing rigidity may improve fusion rates, it also increases the rate of degeneration of adjacent segments.[21,22] Rahm and Hall[22] have reported an incidence of adjacent-segment degeneration of 35% in cases with lumbar fusion and internal fixation. They also noted that the degeneration was associated with increasing patient age, use of interbody fusion, and worsening of clinical results with time.

Lumbar spine fusion remains a pillar of degenerative lumbar spine surgical procedures. However, lumbar spine fusion surgery may increase the loads on the functional lumbar segments and cause advanced disc degeneration, facet joint arthritis, and an increase in intradiscal pressures in adjacent segments.

"Adjacent-level degeneration" and "adjacent-level disease" (both adjacent-segment degeneration [ASD]) are different entities. In a study by Sugawara et al.,[23] asymptomatic adjacent-disc degeneration was detected in 50% of the patients by their measurement methods. However, symptomatic adjacent-disc degeneration occurred in 5% of the patients, and only 2% required additional surgery. ASD may also cause a worsening of the clinical outcomes,[24] especially with the ASD after multiple-segment fusion. The most sensitive technique to evaluate ASD is MRI.[25]

Risk Factors for Adjacent-Segment Degeneration

Type of Surgery

Fusion surgery is associated with a greater incidence of adjacent-level problems than others. The location and extension of the fusion are also important. Patients who underwent fusions of the L5-S1 segment showed a significantly lower risk of ASD than patients with L4-5 fusions (20% vs. 46%). Compared with L4-5 fusions, bisegmental L4-S1 fusions showed a similar trend with a lower risk of ASD (24%).[26]

Because fusion may precipitate adjacent-level problems, the recommendation may be to not perform multiple-segment fusion in cases such as degenerative lumbar deformity.[24] In a retrospective study,[27] it was found that even a cervical posterior foraminotomy is associated with a low rate of same- and adjacent-segment disease (4.9%). Adjacent-segment disease following expansive lumbar laminoplasty was observed to occur in 11% of patients, who showed degeneration at the segment adjacent to the laminoplasty.[28]

Type of Fusion

It is not yet known whether the type of fusion affects adjacent-level degeneration. In a recent randomized study with very long follow-up,[29] there was no effect of anterior column support on the ASD after lumbar spinal fusion.

Similar adjacent-level degenerations happen after ventral cervical fusion. In a cadaveric study, a simulated C5-7 anterior cervical discectomy and fusion (ACDF) caused a significant increase in intradiscal pressure and segmental motion in the rostral adjacent-level during physiologic motion.[30] After ventral cervical plate fusion, adjacent-level degenerative changes commonly occur, and this may cause an ossification on the upper and lower ends of the plate.[31] Some of these postoperative radiographic changes may be related to the technique used. This ossification can be avoided by using the shortest possible plate so that extension of the plate into adjacent healthy discs does not occur.[32]

The so-called "adjacent-level ossification" after ventral cervical plating is a type of heterotopic ossification. With heterotopic ossification, the new bone forms in soft tissues that do not ossify under normal conditions. It may occur after total joint arthroplasty, trauma, and spinal cord injury. It starts to form 2 to 12 weeks after surgery and fully matures 1 to 2 years after its first appearance.

Osteoporosis

Adjacent-level degenerative changes may also occur in patients with osteoporotic vertebral body fractures after augmentation with vertebroplasty. As a long-term complication, failure of the adjacent vertebral body may develop. However, a biomechanical study has shown that there is no benefit of prophylactic vertebral reinforcement adjacent to vertebroplasty.[33]

Lordotic Angles

Adjacent-segment motion may also change with lordotic angles. In a cadaveric study,[34] it was found that there is a significant increase in adjacent-segment motion with the achievement of a modest increase in lordosis that is not observed with a greater increase in lordosis.

Avoiding Adjacent-Level Disease

There have been many implant designs to lower the risk of adjacent-level degeneration and related disease. Artificial discs, pedicle-based dynamic implants,[35] and ligamentoplasty[36] implants are the main groups of these devices, and they are known as motion preservation implants.

Artificial Discs

Because these discs have special complications[37] and require ventral surgery in the lumbar spine, their use has not increased in recent years.

Lumbar artificial discs have been shown to preserve the loads across the implanted and adjacent segments.[38] In a finite element analysis, Charité artificial disc placement slightly increased motion at the implanted level, with a resultant increase in facet loading when compared with the adjacent segments, whereas the motions and loads decreased at the adjacent levels.

In vitro investigation of cervical adjacent-level intradiscal pressures following a total disc replacement arthroplasty has shown that it did not change significantly after arthroplasty in accordance to the fusion.[39]

Pedicle-Based Systems and Ligamentoplasty

The Dynesys system (Zimmer, Warsaw, IN) is a prototype of these systems; it has reportedly provided substantial stability in cases of degenerative spinal pathologies.[40]

However, Rohlmann et al.[35] have used a finite element analysis to compare the effects of bilateral dorsal dynamic and rigid fixation devices on the loads in the lumbar spine. They have demonstrated that a dynamic implant does not necessarily reduce axial spinal loads compared to an uninstrumented spine. Hence, one might criticize pedicle-based dynamic systems as not truly dynamic.

In a retrospective study, ligamentoplasty, a motion-preserving surgery, has caused less ASD (9.2%) than posterior lumbar interbody fusion (14.1%) and dorsolateral fusion (13.3%).[36]

Postlaminectomy Instability

Although a dorsal approach is convenient and appropriate for most spine lesions, it causes a significant defect in the structural integrity of the posterior column as well as a loss of the dorsal tension band.

After cervical laminectomy in children, the incidence of kyphosis is very high.[41,42] The important factors that affect cervical instability after laminectomy are (1) patient's age, (2) number of laminae excised, (3) curvature of the cervical spine, and (4) degree of facet joint violation.[41] Although the relative incidence of instability after cervical laminectomy is controversial, there is a tendency to not perform multilevel laminectomies in pediatric patients and to provide additional stabilization measures in patients with cervical spondylotic myelopathy undergoing laminectomy.[6,41] In patients with cervical spondylotic myelopathy, these measures may either be a laminoplasty or fixation (e.g., lateral mass plating) and fusion after laminectomy.

Extensive lumbar laminectomy is often necessary for patients with spinal stenosis. Because of the nature of the compression, this procedure often includes a partial facetectomy. Although the exact incidence of instability after extensive lumbar laminectomy for lumbar stenosis is not well known, some surgeons have suggested the use of bilateral hemilaminectomies and partial facetectomies, without destruction of interspinous ligaments, while preserving the majority of the laminal and spinous process. Performing a fusion, with or without instrumentation, is controversial, however.[1,43,44]

Bone Graft Harvesting

Instability related to bone graft harvesting is a rare but important problem. It was first reported in 1962 by Lichtblau,[45] who observed that dorsal iliac crest graft harvesting can cause dislocation of the sacroiliac joint.

Prevention and Management of Iatrogenic Spinal Instability

For the management of spinal instability, one or a combination of the following three maneuvers is frequently performed: (1) external bracing with spinal splints, which provides time for healing of bone and ligaments; (2) ventral bone grafts or instrumentation; or (3) dorsal instrumentation or fusion.

Cervical Spine

Iatrogenic destabilization is most often caused by multilevel decompressions for spondylosis. This may be via a multilevel corpectomy or discectomy, or via laminectomy. Multilevel corpectomy or discectomy is usually accompanied by fusion. Therefore, stability is addressed by the fusion. A multilevel central corpectomy injures or destroys the ALL and the PLL, and it also affects bone integrity. In this circumstance, the destabilizing effect results from destruction of ligaments and bone.

Thoracic and Lumbar Spine

Because of the widespread use of ventral surgery for spinal tumors, more reconstruction materials and stabilization problems are discussed. In general, if the lesion is strictly ventral, and the operation has destroyed only the anterior column and part of the middle column, ventral reconstruction and stabilization would be adequate. For single- or two-level lesions in the upper and middle thoracic spine, only a ventral reconstruction can be used. However, for lesions below level T10, ventral instrumentation, in addition to reconstruction, may be necessary. If, however, two or three columns are involved in lesions below level T10, supplemental dorsal instrumentation may be used after ventral reconstruction and ventral stabilization.[46]

Some surgeons perform en bloc resections of the dorsal and ventral elements of the spine from a dorsal route.[14] Tomita et al.[17] have described this approach as "total en bloc spondylectomy." From an oncologic point of view, this method is superior to traditional spinal tumor surgery, curettage, and intralesional removal. The investigators have used a reconstruction material and additional dorsal fixation with instrumentation. It can be used in one stage and one position only. However, its disadvantage is the risk of spinal cord ischemia, resulting from bilateral occlusion of the segmental arteries.

Limiting the extent of dorsal element removal or disruption during laminectomy can minimize spine destabilization by limiting the disruption of the dorsal tension band (e.g., by performing multilevel laminotomies instead of laminectomy). Laminotomy, theoretically, restricts the amount of important bone and soft tissue removed. However, laminectomy provides a trajectory advantage that most likely outweighs the laminotomy advantage (Fig. 153-8).

Lumbosacral Spine

The sacrum is a transitory structure between the vertebral column and pelvis. The sacroiliac joint is the immobile joint that functions as a shock absorber for the spine. The pelvis itself transfers loads from the sacroiliac joints to the hip joints, with the help of strong ligamentous structures White and Panjabi examined the weight-bearing capacity of the sacroiliac joint. They found that, despite the lower half of the S1 vertebral body and half of the sacroiliac joint being resected, only 50% of weight-bearing capacity was lost. This, in fact, is adequate for ambulation, and there is no need for stabilization in most cases (Table 153-2).[5] If the sacral lesion is a primary tumor, and complete tumor removal with extra marginal resection is desired, combined ventral and dorsal approaches, with a significant amount of bone and ligamentous tissue destruction, is necessary. In this case, an adequate reconstruction is required.[18,47-49]

The key point for reconstruction is whether the sacroiliac joints are involved.[50,51] If the tumor is not large and the

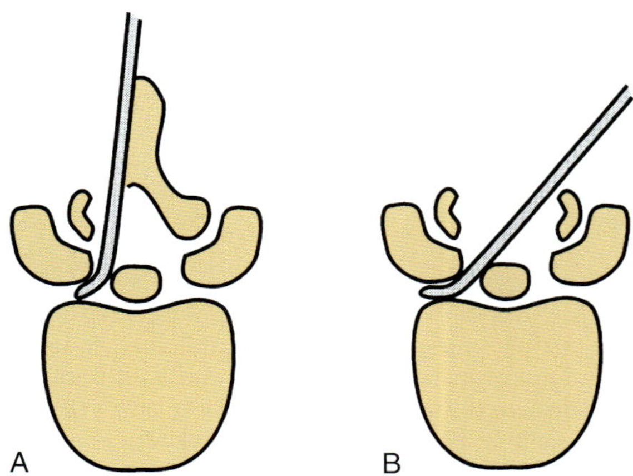

FIGURE 153-8. **A,** Trajectory to the lateral recess achieved via a laminotomy. Note that the Kerrison punch cannot adequately decompress the lateral recess without significant bone removal. **B,** Trajectory to the lateral recess achieved via a laminectomy. Note that a more optimal trajectory is achieved. An undermining of the lateral recess and foramina may thus be achieved without significant facet disruption. (Copyright Division of Neurosurgery, University of New Mexico.)

TABLE 153-2

Resection Levels and the Need for Reconstruction in Sacral Tumor Surgery

Resection Level	Reconstruction
One sacroiliac joint	Can usually compensate well with external support
Partial sacrectomy below S2 (most of the sacroiliac joints are preserved)	Not necessary
Total or subtotal sacrectomy above S2 (most of the sacroiliac joints are lacking)	Obviously necessary with instrumentation crossing the sacroiliac joint

sacroiliac joints are preserved, stability is not lost. However, involvement of one or both joints dictates the need for internal fixation and fusion. Kostuik and Esses[15] suggest surgical reconstruction if 50% or more of the sacroiliac joint is removed.

If the sacrum above the S2 segment is resected with some of the ilium, the L5 vertebral body drops into the pelvis.[18,52] In this case, an implant connecting the lumbar spine to both sides of the ilium is necessary. Three alternatives for the implant procedure are described in Box 153-1. Because the defect is so massive, the patient's own bones do not allow an autograft fusion, and allograft bone is usually used. The forces from the lumbar spine are distributed to both lower extremities via the sacrum and pelvis. This complicates the lumbopelvic instrumentation decision-making process.[53,54]

Because the sacrum is a transitory structure between the vertebral column and the pelvis and lower extremities, adding the sacrum into the long segment fixations for deformity correction is also an important point.[9,55] Achieving strong lumbosacral fixation and fusion poses unique problems because of the shape of the sacrum and the presence of a large amount of cancellous bone. For this reason, different adaptations, such as the use of larger-diameter screws, application of multiple screws, and insertion of the rod into the iliac cristae after significant bending (Galveston technique), have been recommended (Table 153-3).[3,9,55,56]

The modified Galveston L-rod technique is a reasonable reconstructive method after total sacrectomy.[53,57] It prevents caudal migration and axial rotation of the spinal column. Adding a threaded transiliac rod can prevent the open-book phenomenon and provide stability around the horizontal axis of the spinal column; at the same time, it also prevents rotation around this axis.

BOX 153-1. Indications for Reconstruction of the Sacroiliac Joints

- Resection of more than 50% of the sacroiliac joints
- Bilateral resection of the sacrum above S2
- Total resection of the sacroiliac joint on one side associated with ventral pelvic disruption or deficiency

From Bridwell KH: Management of tumors at the lumbosacral junction. In Marguiles JY, Floman Y, Farcy J-PC, et al, editors: *Lumbosacral and spinopelvic fixation*, Philadelphia, 1996, Lippincott-Raven, pp 109-122.

TABLE 153-3

Methods of Sacropelvic Fixation and Reconstruction

Technique	Reference
With Sacrum Preserved	
Isola plate	Asher and Strippgen[3]
Galveston technique	Allen and Ferguson[9]
Isola iliac screws	
With Sacrum Resected	
Fusion of L5 to the ilium	Shikata et al[47]
Autogenous grafting of residual lumbar vertebral bodies to residual pelvis and sacrum	Kostuik and Esses[15]
Massive structural allograft reconstruction (allograft sacropelvis)	

KEY REFERENCES

Cooper PR, Errico TJ, Martin R, et al: A systematic approach to spinal reconstruction after anterior decompression for neoplastic disease of the thoracic and lumbar spine. *Neurosurgery* 32:1–8, 1993.

Denis F: The three-column spine and its significance in the classification of acute thoracolumbar spine injuries. *Spine (Phila Pa 1976)* 8:817–831, 1983.

Heller JG, Whitecloud TS: Post-laminectomy instability of the cervical spine—etiology and stabilization technique. In Frymoyer JW, editor: *The adult spine: principles and practice*, vol. 2, New York, 1991, Raven Press, pp 1219–1240.

Hsu KY, Zucherman J, White AH, et al: Deterioration of motion segments adjacent to lumbar spine fusions. Presented at the Annual Meeting of the North American Spine Society, Colorado Springs, CO, 1988.

Kostuik JP, Esses SI: Sacral destabilization and restabilization—causes and treatment. In Frymoyer JW, editor: *The adult spine: principles and practice*, vol. 2, New York, 1991, Raven Press, pp 2172–2173.

Tomita K, Yoribatake Y, Kawahara N, et al: Total en bloc spondylectomy and circumspinal decompression for solitary spinal metastasis. *Paraplegia* 32:36–46, 1994.

REFERENCES

The complete reference list is available online at expertconsult.com.

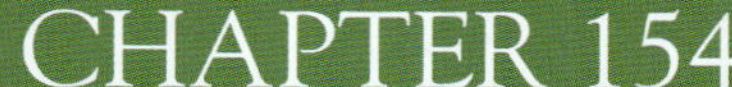

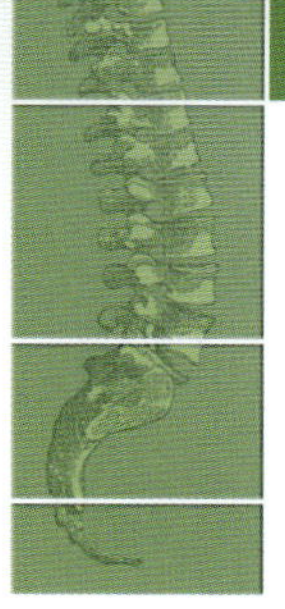

CHAPTER 154

Lumbar Facet Fixation Techniques

Marc Eichler | Jennifer Orning | Eldad Hadar

The concept of lumbar spine facet fixation has existed since 1948, with King's description of a novel method of internal fixation in the lumbosacral spine as an alternative to immobilization in plaster.[1] This was modified by Boucher in 1959 by using longer screws and slightly altered placement.[2] Translaminar placement was introduced in 1984 by Magerl in a paper describing its use as an adjunct to external spinal fixation.[3]

Despite the longevity of facet fixation as a method for spine immobilization, its use was largely usurped by pedicle screw fixation. Pedicle screws were believed to increase the stability and stiffness of the construct and do not require the presence of intact dorsal elements, as does the translaminar approach for facet screws. However, facet fixation is once again emerging as a viable alternative and useful maneuver in the field of lumbar stabilization.

Anatomy

Facet joints, or zygapophyseal joints, are the only truly mobile interfaces in the lumbar spine. They are described as either apophyseal or diarthrotic joints, consisting of sliding cartilaginous surface and capsules containing synovial fluid. Although situated dorsally, far from the instantaneous axis of rotation, their orientation can dictate the movement allowed in different areas of the spine. This orientation changes from the cervical to lumbar spine, and even within the lumbar spine itself.

The capsules of the facet joints are highly innervated. Medial branches from the dorsal rami of the same and often the upper level innervate them, emanating from the neuroforamina. Pain fibers, which are the smallest somatosensory neurons, innervate the capsule. The pain fibers are small myelinated A-delta fibers or unmyelinated C fibers with unencapsulated endings. Studies have demonstrated the presence of pacinian and Ruffini endings, which serve as mechanoreceptors for proprioception and movement sense.[4]

Wear and tear on the facet joints can cause remodeling consistent with arthritis in other mobile joints of the body. Perhaps meant to stabilize the joint, such remodeling also leads to enlargement of the overall facet interface and possible compression of the nerve roots.

Biomechanics

In direct axial loading, facet joints bear a relatively small amount of the overall load. However, with extension and hyperextension, they bear a larger portion of the load—approximately 30%, compared with 10% to 20% direct axial loading.[5] When flexed, they are reported to handle nearly 50% of the ventral shear load. Because of their motion and distance from the instantaneous axis of rotation, they, along with dorsal ligaments, facilitate the majority of movement in the flexed posture. This opens the joint and stretches the capsule. The capsule is viscoelastic. As such, the elastic zone may diminish over time. Without the ability to return to its neutral state, mobility may increase as the joint capsule is stretched.

The facet surface area of the articular surfaces increases as one descends the lumbar spine. The relatively sagittal orientation of the facet joints in most of the lumbar spine restricts rotational movements. Flexion and anteroposterior translation are not restricted by this portion of the vertebral column. The L5-S1 joint is the exception, with a more coronal orientation of the facet joint and its facet-facet interface. This is one of the main causes hypothesized to lead to the higher incidence of degenerative spondylolisthesis at L4-5, with translation contained by the facet interface at the lower level. Instead, pars defects occur at this level, causing a large percentage of the cases of subluxation. The lordosis at these levels also increases the shear forces at the lower levels as the orientation of the spine itself becomes more horizontal with respect to gravity in the upright posture. This places increased strain on the facet joints.

Tropism must also be considered. Tropism is manifested by asymmetry in the bilateral facet joints with respect to their angles, with one having a more coronal orientation than the other. The incidence of tropism is increased in degenerative disc disease—perhaps suggesting a contributory factor. The vertebral body rotates toward the more oblique facet with axial loading, possibly leading to increased stress on the anulus fibrosus and accelerated disc degeneration.[5]

Indications

Adjunct to Noninstrumented Fusions

Pseudarthrosis rates are reported at 10% with bone graft alone during fusion procedures for one level, and possibly greater than 30% with more than two or three levels.[6] Internal fixation has been used extensively to assist with fusion procedures in modern spine surgery.[7,8] Facet fixation specifically has been shown to decrease pseudarthrosis rates over noninstrumented fusion and to have a low incidence of complications.[9]

Dorsal fusions were largely supplanted by dorsolateral fusions in the 1980s owing to a decrease in pseudarthrosis rates. Kornblatt et al. also showed that internal fixation, specifically with facet fixation or pelvic rods, improved the rate of fusion (87% vs. 76% without fixation) and time to radiographic fusion (6.2 months vs. 10.5 months) significantly.[6] This was also shown by Jacobs et al., using translaminar facet fixation and judging fusion by oblique and flexion-extension films.[10] Both studies used patients who had a pseudarthrosis from a prior procedure. They demonstrated that facet fixation can promote fusion after failed procedures—with the caveat that outcomes deteriorate with each successive surgery in most spinal procedures.[11]

Adjunct to Anterior or Posterior Lumbar Interbody Fusion

Posterior lumbar fusion may be used for a variety of indications. Because facet fixation does not allow distraction or manipulation of alignment, the majority of uses involve restriction of movement to facilitate fusion, either because a discectomy has been performed or because the patient experiences painful symptoms with motion.

One of the uses that has caused a resurgence in facet screw popularity is as an adjunct to anterior lumbar interbody fusion (ALIF), when there is no need for posterior nerve root decompression. Failure of fusion with ALIF alone has been reported in up to 24% of cases.[12,13] Cadaveric studies have shown that ALIF alone allows more movement during extension with little preload than does the preoperative spine—a risk for graft displacement and poor fusion. Facet fixation with translaminar screws enhances stability, returning motion to the level allowed preoperatively.[14] Kandziora et al. showed the equivalence of ipsilateral facet screws to translaminar screws with regard to range of motion, neutral zone, and elastic zone.[15] However, they also demonstrated improved parameters in all test modes with pedicle screws.

For similar reasons, facet screws are also used as an adjunct to posterior lumbar interbody fusion; this was described as early as 1988, with only 1 complication in 35 patients and fusion apparent in all with the use of postoperative thoracolumbosacral orthosis immobilization.[16] This procedure is useful to enhance fusion acquisition and prevent motion that may lead to graft displacement. With posterior lumbar interbody fusion, no further surgical exposure is necessary to place the screws (Fig. 154-1).

Segmental Instability

Patients who have become unstable though degeneration or trauma may benefit from a dorsal arthrodesis. Although pedicle screw fixation with rods is increasingly used, facet fixation remains a viable alternative. However, the alignment must already be appropriate because facet fixation does not permit the application of enough leverage to mobilize spinal segments and alter the alignment.

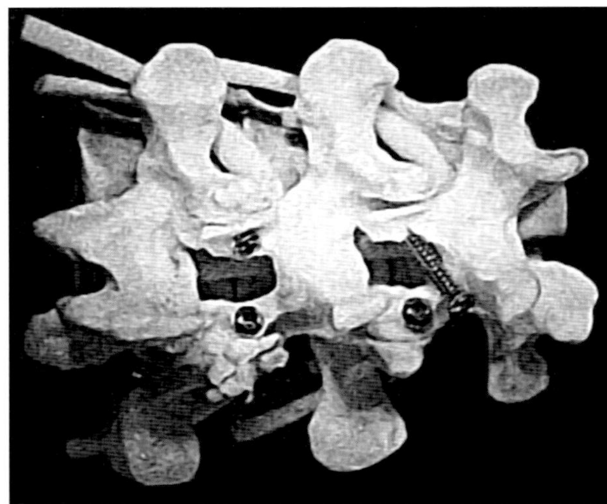

FIGURE 154-1. Model demonstrating orientation of cortical lag screws across inferior facet into superior facet and underlying pedicle.

Painful Disc Syndromes

The theory behind posterior lumbar fusion for degenerative disc disease is elimination of motion at the affected segment. Outcomes have been shown to be equivalent to interbody procedures in multiple studies.[17,18] It is thought that the painful portion of the segment is the disc as a whole or the anulus fibrosus and, therefore, dorsal fusion alone may yield poor outcomes unless the disc material is removed, such as with an interbody procedure (see earlier discussion). However, dorsal fusion alone has significant advantages, such as shorter operative time, less risk for complication, lower cost, preservation of the anterior column, and ease of procedure.

Painful Facet Syndrome

In the healthy spine, the nociceptors in the facet joint capsule fire only under supranormal physiologic conditions. However, it has been shown that with inflammation, chemical mediators can sensitize the pain sensors to fire excessively or spontaneously. One study suggested that 15% of patients with low back pain had pain of facet origin.[19] In patients with lumbar facet syndrome, Helbig and Lee demonstrated a positive response to facet block and facet rhizolysis in 50% to 60% of cases.[20]

The existence of the so-called facet syndrome is still rather controversial. In 1996, Cavanaugh et al. showed in rabbits that algesic chemicals, such as carrageenan or substance P, can sensitize pain receptors or induce persistent firing of these neurons with small movements.[4]

Results of studies examining the therapeutic potential of facet injections have been contradictory, with some showing significant improvement and others showing equivalent results with the injection of normal saline.[21] Once nonsurgical treatment has been exhausted, facet fixation can eliminate motion at the segment, thereby decreasing or eliminating pain.

Translaminar Facet Screws

Technique

The first description of the translaminar approach was by Magerl in 1984.[3] However, the topic of the paper was actually an external fixator and the method of placing facet screws was only vaguely referenced. Diagrams in the article clearly show the path of a translaminar facet screw: entering at the base of the spinous process, traveling the length of the contralateral lamina, crossing the facet joint, and ending at the base of the transverse process (Fig. 154-2). Multiple authors have described percutaneous translaminar screw placement using fluoroscopy.[22,23]

Comparison with Other Internal Fixation Techniques

Translaminar screws are thought to be more stable than the shorter construct associated with ipsilateral placement, but many studies have shown similar outcomes with both types. The ease of learning this technique and the limited time required to become facile make it a relatively convenient adjunct to many procedures. In addition, because both types of facet fixation can be performed percutaneously, they are in accord with the current trend toward minimally invasive spine procedures.

However, translaminar placement does require intact dorsal elements. Many surgeons have reported discectomy, lateral recess decompression, and even partial central decompression with preservation of sufficient lamina to perform the translaminar approach, according to Jacobs et al.[10] An isthmic spondylolisthesis with a pars defect is therefore an obvious contraindication to this procedure.

Because of the longer course of the translaminar screws, more muscle dissection must be performed and greater technical skill is required compared with the ipsilateral approach. The longer screw trajectory also makes canal intrusion more likely than with ipsilateral placement, which limits the path of the screw to the facet joint alone.

Concern also exists regarding the notion that a limited dorsal fusion has the potential for kyphosis over time, as the disc loses height. In addition, although improved pseudarthrosis rates are reported compared with uninstrumented fusion, the rate remains as high as 9% in some reports.[10]

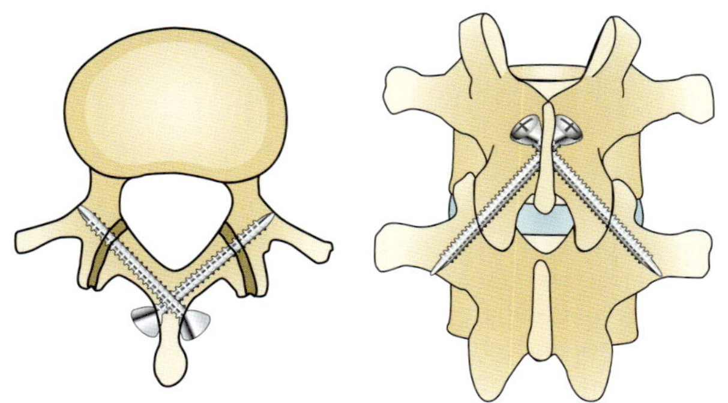

FIGURE 154-2. Translaminar screw fixation of facet joints at the thoracolumbar junction and the lumbar spine, where the joints are oriented toward the sagittal plane. To prevent splitting of the lamina, the screws should not be applied as lag screws.

Comparison with Pedicle Screws

There are some obvious advantages to the facet fixation technique over the more frequently used pedicle screw fixation technique: lower cost, less dissection, more room for bone graft, lower complication rates, and a lower rate of infection. The attraction of the pedicle screw technique is related to the prevailing notion that facet fixation is less stable. Studies have shown equivalence in biomechanics and stability between the two methods in objective tests, although most such studies have been performed in cadaver models.[23-25] In a prospective study of patients undergoing translaminar facet fixation versus pedicle fixation, Tuli et al. demonstrated a higher nonunion rate, as confirmed by radiographs, in patients undergoing facet fixation: 17.5% versus 2.7%. This finding correlated with symptoms. However, they also found a non–statistically significant difference in end-fusion degeneration, with pedicle screws having the higher rate (13.5% vs. 5%).[26]

Pedicle screw fixation requires the insertion of more hardware because of the presence of rods connecting the inserted screws, as well as cross bars. This bulk and higher profile may be one of the reasons that hardware removal is more common after pedicle screw than facet screw insertion. In a comparison with pedicle screws in circumferential interbody fusion, Best and Sasso found that less than 5% of the facet screw group had reoperations due to continued pain, whereas 37.5% of the pedicle screw group returned for another procedure.[27] As an aside, one of the facet screw patients who was found to have a pseudarthrosis underwent pedicle screw placement without removal of the facet screws.

Of note, the proximity of pedicle screws to the spinal cord causes significant imaging artifact that can make evaluation and diagnosis of complications difficult. The distance of facet screws from the canal reduces this artifact.

Ipsilateral Insertion of Facet Screws

The original literature by King and Boucher described the ipsilateral insertion of facet screws. The screw is initially inserted on the ipsilateral side, entering the caudal facet of the rostral lumbar level and crossing the joint, rather than being inserted from the contralateral base of the spinous process.

Technique

Ipsilateral insertion of facet screws has the advantage of not requiring an intact lamina and spinous process, as does the translaminar approach. In 2009, Su et al. analyzed 80 cadaveric facet joints from 37 spines in an anatomic study of appropriate screw placement.[28] The study was designed to determine the radiographic characteristics during percutaneous screw placement that would be expected to traverse the center of the facet joint without complications. They stated that the L2-3 segment could not be instrumented in this fashion because of the vertical orientation of the facet joint. For segments L3 through S1, they observed an appropriate orientation in the mediolateral and craniocaudal planes at each level. Rostrocaudally, the screw trajectory should begin over the caudal end plate of the rostral level.

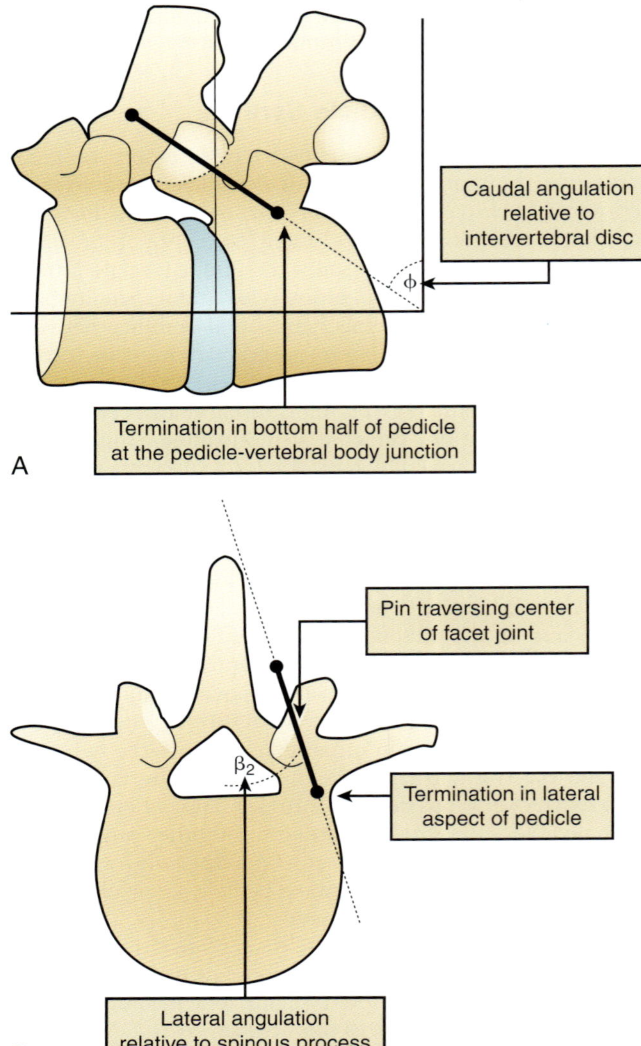

FIGURE 154-3. A, Caudal angulation (φ) of the pin in the sagittal plane relative to a line drawn parallel to the intervertebral disc of the instrumented level. Note that the pin terminates in the inferior half of the pedicle at the pedicle-vertebral body junction. **B,** Lateral angulation (β2) of the pin in the axial plane relative to the midline spinous process.

Mediolaterally, the view should show the screw's starting point to be located over the medial border of the pedicle.

The angle of the screw should be approximately 15 degrees in the axial plane and approximately 30 degrees in the sagittal plane—varying slightly depending on the levels being fused (Fig. 154-3). Another technique orients the screw such that it is parallel to the caudal edge of the lamina.[29] The tip of the screw should end up caudally and laterally in the caudal pedicle on the anteroposterior view, and in the caudal half of the pedicle on the lateral view. Su et al. also state that a 35-degree oblique angle on fluoroscopy is optimal for viewing final placement.[28]

Comparison with Translaminar Screws

The initial impetus for developing ipsilateral screws was to eliminate the long path of translaminar screws and the requirement for intact dorsal elements (spinous process and laminae). Multiple studies have shown equivalence between ipsilaterally placed screws and translaminar screws.[15]

The ipsilateral method of fixation requires a smaller exposure and can easily be added to a dorsal decompression with little or no additional dissection. Even when not placed percutaneously, ipsilateral facet screws require less retraction than translaminar placement.

There are significant limitations with ipsilateral placement, however, predominantly with regard to anatomy and biomechanics. First, certain levels do not lend themselves to the application (L2-3 and above) because of the orientation of the facets and the difficulty associated with obtaining the correct angle of insertion. The vertical and sagittal facet orientation dictates that the screw and driver be positioned in the space occupied by the spinous process, which could be accomplished only with dorsal element removal. This eliminates the percutaneous placement option and removes one of the advantages of ipsilateral placement over the translaminar approach. Therefore, translaminar fixation would be more appropriate at the upper lumbar levels.

Neither type of facet fixation permits the distraction and manipulation of spinal alignment, as can be accomplished with pedicle screws. This makes them less useful in the setting of traumatic fracture or malalignment from malignant or infectious etiologies, when correction of an angulation is required.

Comparison with Pedicle Screws

Although facet screws have always been considered inferior to traditional pedicle screw fixation in rigidity and stability, data suggest that ipsilateral facet screw placement may be equivalent biomechanically. In cadaveric models, Ferrara et al. conducted short- and long-term cyclical testing of facet screws and pedicle screws with flexion-compression and torsional loading. Although the two systems were equal in most parameters assessed, they found facet screws provided 30% more stiffness during flexion in short-term cycling. Agarwala et al. performed another cadaver model study showing that the Boucher method of facet screw placement demonstrated a trend toward reduced motion compared to pedicle screws in flexion extension, but not in lateral bending or axial rotation.[30] This trend was only shown in primary fusion procedures *without* ALIF, and did not meet statistical significance. Although performed in vitro, these studies provide support for the theory that facet fixation may be equivalent in stability to pedicle screw fixation and able to maintain its mechanical integrity over long-term cycling.[29]

Pins

Although no extensive investigation into the use of pins rather than screws to fixate lumbar facets has been performed, Deguchi et al. compared pedicle screw fixation, translaminar screw fixation, and a translaminar technique using bioabsorbable poly-L-lactide pin placement.[31] Sheep cadaveric spines were used. Pin placement resulted in restricted motion compared with the intact spine. However, both pedicle screw fixation and translaminar screw fixation provided greater stiffness and rigidity.

Conclusion

The concept of facet fixation is not new. It has been relatively usurped by the technique of pedicle fixation. However, pedicle screws do have serious drawbacks, including higher cost. Also, because of their trajectory and level of skill required for placement, risk of neurologic injury and the need for hardware removal are increased. Pedicle screws require more dissection and, therefore, longer operative times and increased risk for infection. However, although percutaneous pedicle screw insertion has been investigated,[32] the placement procedure of open cases is well known. Many spine surgeons are more familiar with this than placement of facet screws.

Overall, the outcomes for facet fixation compare favorably with other methods of fixation. At 10-year follow-up, Aepli et al. reported that 74% of patients stated that their translaminar facet fixation "helped" or "helped a lot"—results comparable with pedicle screw fixation outcomes.[33] There are some data showing that disc height significantly less than normal may be a positive predictor for a good outcome.[34] There are obvious advantages to this fixation technique and, although not suitable for all situations, it is a valuable technique in the armamentarium of spine surgeons.

KEY REFERENCES

Aebi M, Arlet V, Webb J: AO *spine manual*, Stuttgart, 2007, Thieme.

Kornblatt MD, Casey MP, Jacobs RR: Internal fixation in lumbosacral spine fusion: a biomechanical and clinical study. *Clin Orthop Relat Res* 203:141–150, 1986.

Prothero SR, Parkes JC, Stinchfield FE: Complications after low-back fusion in 1000 patients: a comparison of two series one decade apart. 1966. *Clin Orthop Relat Res* 306:5–11, 1994.

REFERENCES

The complete reference list is available online at expertconsult.com.

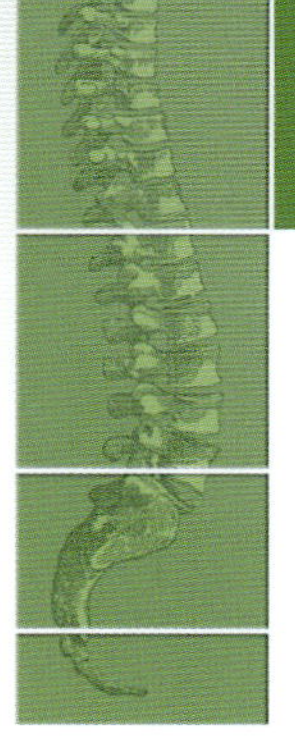

CHAPTER 155

Paracoccygeal Transsacral Approach to the Lumbosacral Junction for Interbody Fusion and Stabilization

Isador H. Lieberman | Krzysztof Siemionow

Over the past decade, we have seen an evolution of minimally disruptive surgical techniques. The goal of any minimally invasive procedure is to provide safe access to the pathology while minimizing collateral tissue morbidity. This surgical philosophy aims to preserve native function while promoting rapid recovery. In the development of minimally invasive surgical techniques, one requires a thorough understanding of the spinal anatomy, an appreciation of the pathology, and specialized tools to facilitate the intended intervention.

The interbody space can be approached from the ventral, dorsal, and direct lateral approaches. Each of these approaches has its limitations. Anterior interbody fusions allow for the instrumentation to be placed along the long axis of the spine, which has been shown to demonstrate favorable biomechanics, because the instrumentation is placed close to the instantaneous axis of rotation of the spine and perpendicular to the compressive moments of the vertebral bodies. The ventral exposure techniques to the lumbosacral segment have evolved from transperitoneal to retroperitoneal and even laparoscopic approaches. However, these exposures require mobilization of the abdominal contents and vascular structures, and this carries an element of risk and also frequently involves specialized expertise to perform the exposure safely. The use of interbody implants with these exposures necessitates partial resection of the anulus to place the implant. This, in turn, may contribute to a destabilizing effect on the spine despite the use of a specific implant. In response to the limitations of these contemporary exposures and techniques for lumbosacral fusions, Cragg et al.[1] recently described a novel percutaneous, fluoroscopically guided, access method to the lumbosacral junction. The access is gained through a paracoccygeal incision with blunt dissection through the presacral space, all while the patient is positioned prone. This approach allows for axial transsacral access to the lumbosacral junction. Along with this exposure, specially designed tools to evacuate the disc space, prepare the end plates, and introduce graft material, as well as a specialized axial stabilization rod, have all been developed to facilitate a minimally invasive fusion of the lumbosacral junction.

Presacral Anatomy

The paracoccygeal presacral access to the lumbosacral junction takes advantage of a well-defined anatomic potential space between the anterior surface of the sacrum and posterior surfaces of the sigmoid colon and rectum (Fig. 155-1). This presacral space is bounded by visceral fascia on the sigmoid colon and rectum and by parietal fascia on the anterior surface of the sacrum. The presacral space is filled with areolar tissue and fat. The rectum and sigmoid colon are not attached to any structures in the course of the presacral space; therefore, they can be easily mobilized with a blunt dissector. It is important to keep the dissection limited to the midline presacral space. The sacral nerve roots exit the foramina and course laterally and inferiorly, away from the midline presacral space. Because this space is devoid of any significant vascular or neurologic elements, there are no obstacles to establishing a corridor for access.

Yuan et al. studied the anatomic relationships of the presacral space.[2] These investigators reported that at the lumbosacral junction the iliac vessels and their accompanying sympathetic hypogastric nerves coursed laterally over the sacral ala. In the midline just beyond the lumbosacral junction, the midline sacral artery and vein follow a variable course and typically terminate in a fine reticular mesh. They defined the coronal safe zone at the S1-2 interspace as more than 6 cm wide in both males and females on the basis of CT and MRI measurements. Therefore, at the typical docking

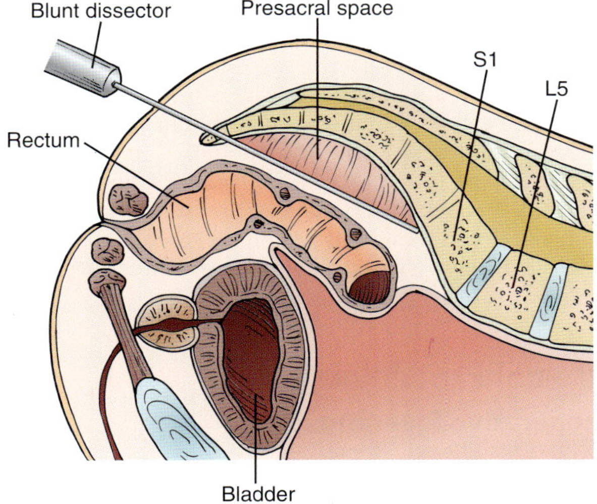

FIGURE 155-1. Schematic of the presacral anatomy.

and entry point into the sacral promontory, which is usually at the S1-2 junction, there are no significant obstructions.

Parke et al. described the variability of the middle sacral artery in 20 cadavers, reporting that in humans, it is only a minor contributor to any major segmental arteries, through bilateral segmental branches.[3] Furthermore, it was found to be absent in many specimens. Using 10 cadavers and MRI studies, Güvençer et al. measured the distances between the sacrum and the presacral structures (i.e., middle and lateral sacral arteries, sympathetic trunks, internal iliac arteries and veins, and colon/rectum).[4] This cadaver study showed that the middle sacral artery was located on the right side in 55.0% of cases, on the left side in 31.7%, and on the midline in the 13.3%. The distance between the sacral midline and middle sacral artery was 8.0 ± 5.4, 9.0 ± 4.9, 8.7 ± 6.0, 8.6 ± 6.4, and 4.7 ± 5.0 mm at the S1-2, S2-3, S3-4, S4-5, and S5-coccyx levels, respectively. The distance between the sacral midline and the sympathetic trunk ranged between 22.4 ± 5.8 and 9.5 ± 3.2 mm in different levels between the S1 and coccygeal levels. The study also showed that the distance between the posterior wall of the intestine (colon/rectum) and the ventral surface of the sacrum can be as close as 11.44 ± 7.69 mm on MRI. Because of the close relationships, as well as the potential for anatomic variations, the authors recommended the use of sacral and presacral imaging before a presacral approach. Oto et al.[5] described the sagittal width of the presacral space at the S1, S2, and S3 vertebral levels retrospectively on MRI in 193 patients. The researchers found that (1) the presacral width in males was significantly wider than in females and (2) in general, the presacral space was at least 1 cm wide in more than 60% of males and 40% of females.

Evolution of Technique

The paracoccygeal presacral access to the lumbosacral junction was validated in a series of cadaver, animal, and human trials. Cragg et al., in a series of 15 cadavers, refined the access technique and the necessary instruments.[1] The instruments evolved to include dissectors, cannulae, drills, discectomy tools, bone graft application tools, and axial rod implantation tools. The investigators validated the procedure with a fully percutaneous fluoroscopic approach through a single 2-cm paracoccygeal incision. Cragg et al. then assessed the safety of the access procedure in a series of six consecutive animals.[1] The access was performed without adverse events. Lumbosacral access in the animals was confirmed fluoroscopically by axial discography. Following the success of the preclinical studies, the researchers undertook a series of consecutive biopsies of the lumbosacral disc and vertebral body region for suspected pathologic lesions in three patients.[1] Again, the technique posed no significant issues.

Surgical Procedure

Preoperative Planning

In preparation for the surgical approach, the radiographic images, including a full sacral view, are analyzed to determine if the anatomy is suitable for the paracoccygeal transsacral approach to the lumbosacral junction. The standard field of view for a lumbar MRI scan should be expanded to include the entire sacrum and coccyx on the sagittal views. With the radiographs and MRI scans, one can plan and map the trajectory of the access and subsequent implantation of the axial rod (Fig. 155-2).

Patient Preparation

Typically, a standard bowel preparation the evening before surgery is advisable. In the operating room, the patient is positioned prone onto a radiolucent table with the lumbar spine in extension to facilitate lumbar lordosis. The lumbar and the sacrococcygeal regions are prepped and draped. The operative area should be isolated from the anus with an occlusive dressing (Fig. 155-3).

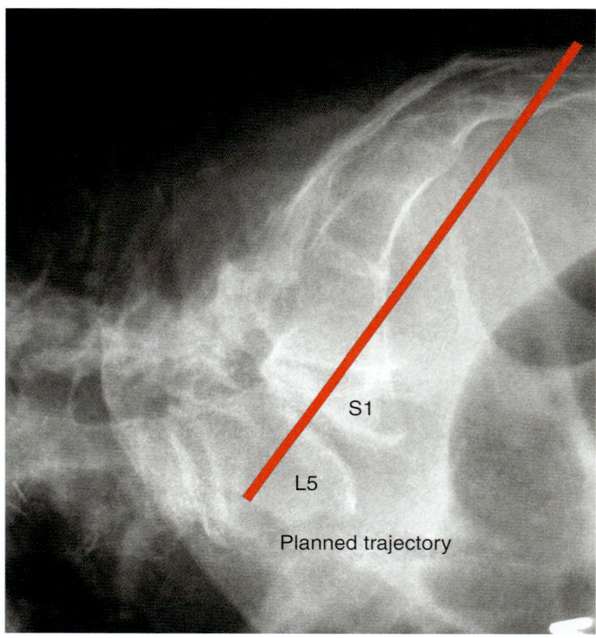

FIGURE 155-2. Preoperative planning.

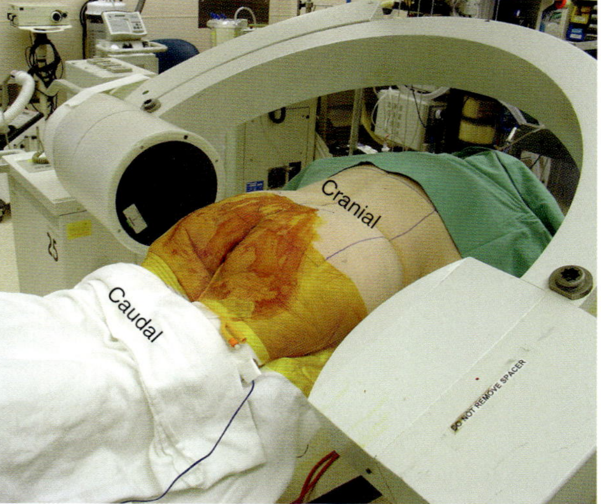

FIGURE 155-3. Isolation of the surgical site.

Operating Room Setup

Once the patient is positioned, two image intensifiers are positioned for simultaneous biplanar fluoroscopy. The posteroanterior C-arm should be adjusted to project a lordotic view of the lumbosacral junction. The lateral C-arm should be adjusted to achieve a true lateral view of the lumbosacral junction. The lateral and anteroposterior C-arms should be draped such that they can move in a parallel fashion from the tip of the coccyx to the lumbosacral junction freely as needed throughout the procedure (Fig. 155-4).

Access and Trajectory Planning

To begin, it is necessary to palpate the coccyx and sacrotuberous ligament arch and then create a 15- to 20-mm incision through the skin and superficial fascia 2 to 3 cm caudal to the paracoccygeal notch and left or right of the coccyx (Fig. 155-5). After making the initial 2-cm paracoccygeal skin incision, a Kelly clamp is used to bluntly dissect down to the parietal fascia. Penetrating the fascia is necessary to access the presacral space and the anterior face of the sacrum. Penetrating the fascia can be accomplished using finger dissection, blunt guide pin dissection, or a combination of the two. Once achieved, the blunt guide pin is then advanced in a cephalic direction under fluoroscopic guidance in the midline, keeping the tip engaged on the anterior cortex of sacrum to approximately the S1-2 junction (Fig. 155-6). This maneuver is accomplished with "fingertip" control on the handle of the guide pin introducer and should be completed using fluoroscopic guidance in both anteroposterior and lateral planes.

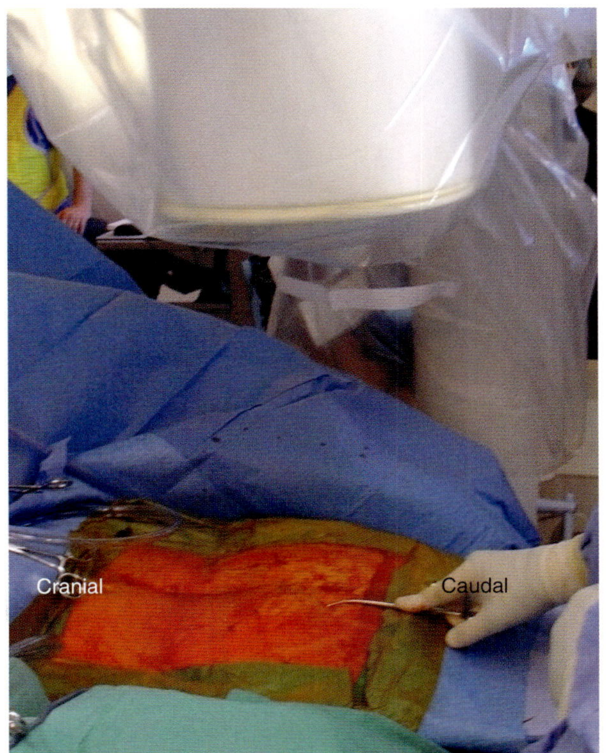

FIGURE 155-4. Setup of C-arms to facilitate posteroanterior and lateral images.

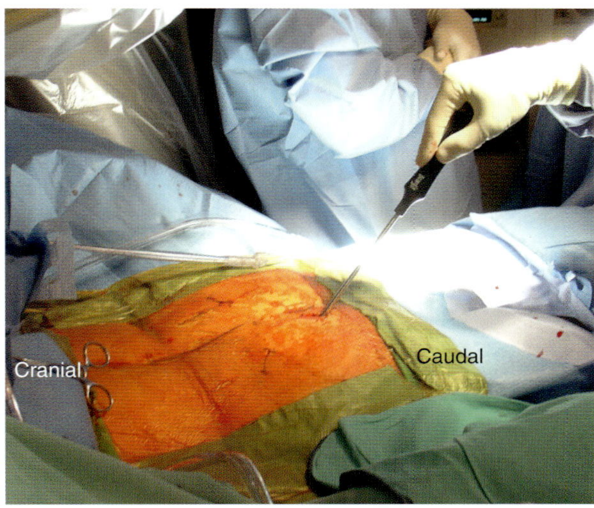

FIGURE 155-5. Paracoccygeal 2-cm incision.

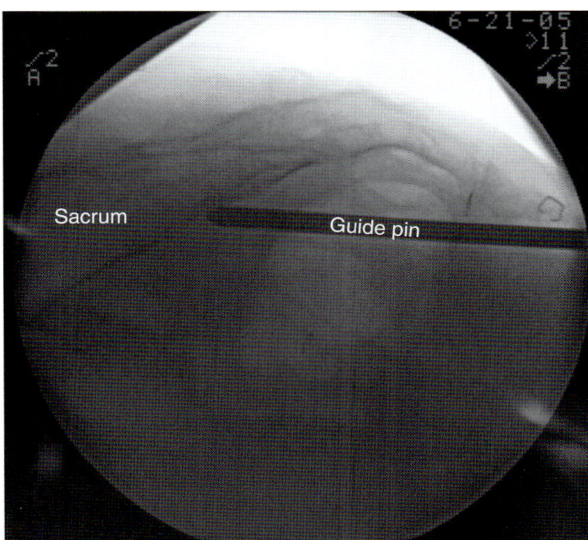

FIGURE 155-6. Intraoperative fluoroscopic image of a blunt guide pin.

Centerline Trajectory

Once the guide pin has reached the S1-2 junction, a midline trajectory for entry into and through the L5-S1 disc space is established by adjusting the angle of the guide pin. The aim is to traverse the L5-S1 disc space in its midpoint in both the posteroanterior and lateral planes. Once the trajectory is established, an exchange system is used to switch the blunt guide pin for a bevel tip extended K-wire. The bevel tip K-wire is then advanced across the disc space, keeping its predetermined trajectory (Fig. 155-7).

Working Cannula and Disc Space Preparation

Once the guidewire is situated, a series of instruments is used to dilate the soft tissue and sacral corticocancellous bone sequentially to create the working channel and to dock the working cannula (Fig. 155-8). Following this, several tools

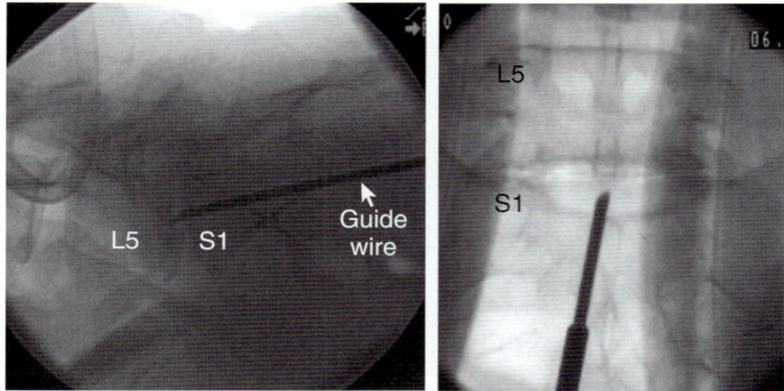

FIGURE 155-7. Intraoperative fluoroscopic image of a bevel tip K-wire across the lumbosacral junction.

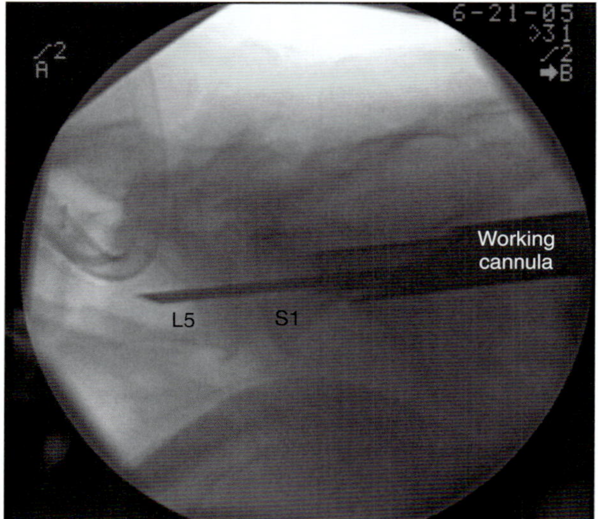

FIGURE 155-8. Intraoperative fluoroscopic image of a working cannula.

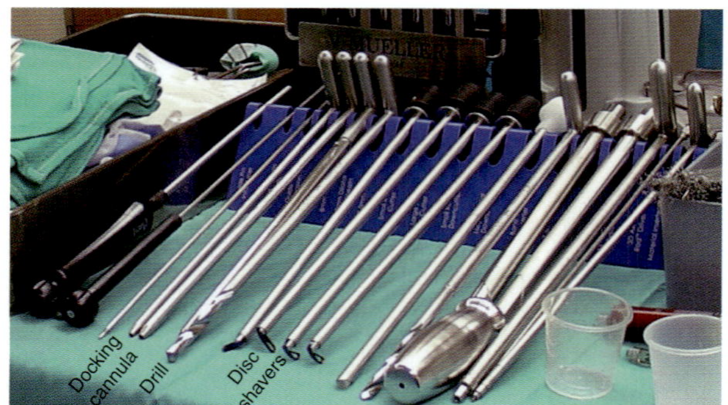

FIGURE 155-9. Instruments designed to evacuate disc space and prepare end plates for fusion.

are used to prepare the disc space for fusion. These include specially designed radial cutters and brushes (Fig. 155-9).

Bone Graft Application

After the disc space is evacuated and the end plates are denuded of cartilage, bone graft material is deposited into the disc space using the bone graft funnel. Approximately 10 to 15 mL of material is delivered into the disc space.

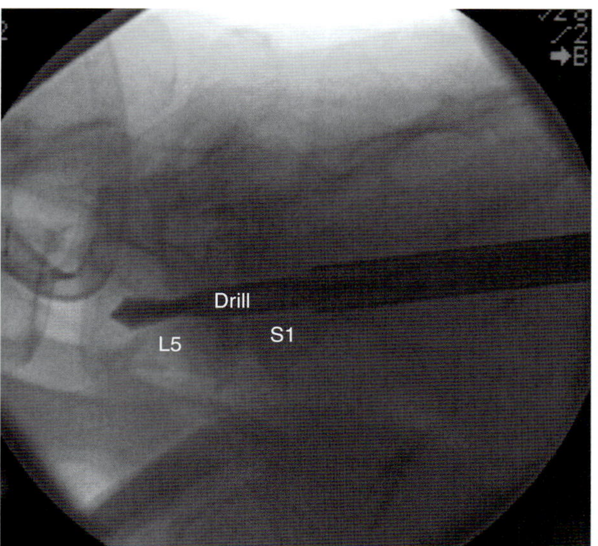

FIGURE 155-10. Intraoperative fluoroscopic image of a drill across the disc space into the L5 vertebra.

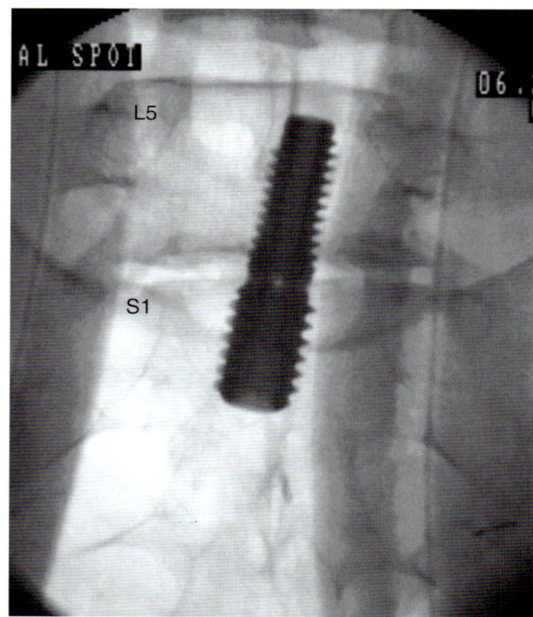

FIGURE 155-11. Final intraoperative fluoroscopic image of an implanted axial rod.

Preparing to Implant the Axial Rod

At this point, a drill is advanced across the disc space and into the L5 vertebral body to create a channel to accommodate the axial rod. The depth of the drilling is guided with the fluoroscopic views (Fig. 155-10).

Axial Rod Implantation

The final step involves the implantation of the axial stabilization rod over a guidewire. This frequently involves a significant torque force to advance the axial rod across the sacral promontory and disc space, into the L5 vertebra (Fig. 155-11).

Potential Complications

To date, more than 2000 cases using a paracoccygeal exposure have been performed worldwide.[6] Experience with this technique is still too limited to comment accurately on the magnitude of risk associated with it and the various potential complications. However, the possible complications that may be encountered as they relate to the surgical access include infection, injury to the presacral structures, fracture of the sacral promontory, and inaccurate trajectory or placement of the implants.

The presacral access tract traverses dorsal to the bowel and ventral to the sacrum. Possible access risks include infection due to bowel injury and bleeding due to injury to presacral veins or the middle sacral artery. Fluoroscopic monitoring, rectal air insufflation, blunt access instruments, and dilation rather than sharp dissection into the sacral face lessen these risks. The sacral entry site at S1-2 is a relatively bare area in the pelvis because the major neural and vascular structures are lateral to the midline at this point.

In the spine itself, there is a risk to spinal canal contents if the trajectory into the disc space is inappropriate or if rotational cutting tools used for discectomy are oversized. As with all image-guided operations, careful attention to landmarks is imperative to minimize the risk of complications. As with any lumbar fusion technique, inadequate disc space preparation can result in pseudarthrosis. In the event of a symptomatic nonunion, the surgeon should have a backup plan in place that addresses the pseudarthrosis. It is of paramount importance to ensure that patients are aware of this potential complication preoperatively.

The sympathetic plexus is usually situated across the L5-S1 interspace. Injury to this structure may lead to retrograde ejaculation. By virtue of the S1-2 anatomic entry point into the sacral promontory, risk of injury to the sympathetic plexus is minimized.

Outcomes

Both biomechanical and clinical investigations have been performed. A biomechanical study using human cadaveric lumbar spine designed to evaluate the biomechanics of paracoccygeal transsacral rod fixation has been performed by Akesen et al.[7] Unconstrained and nondestructive pure moments in axial torsion (AT), lateral bending (LB), and flexion-extension (FE) were applied to each specimen after applying a transsacral rod and after additional augmentation methods, including bilateral screws, facet screws, and a pedicle screw and rod system. Range of motion (ROM) was calculated for each surgical treatment. The mean ROM of the intact specimens was 3.5, 6.4, and 11.0 degrees in AT, LB, and FE, respectively. The stand-alone transsacral rod reduced ROM more than 40% compared with the intact condition (P = .002). Bilateral screws further reduced the ROM in AT (64%) and LB (70%) but not in FE (53%). Both facet screws and the pedicle screw and rod system achieved high construct stability under all loading conditions. The transsacral rod augmented with facet screws reduced ROM by 70%, 80%, and 90% in AT, LB, and FE, respectively, compared with the intact condition. When augmented with the pedicle screw and rod system, the transsacral rod reduced ROM by 73%, 87%, and 88% in AT, LB, and FE, respectively. There was no statistical difference between the two facet screws and the pedicle screw and rod system. The authors concluded that the transsacral rod fixation provides strong ligamentotaxis due to intact anulus. The stand-alone transsacral rod is able to reduce ROM significantly and achieve indirect decompression by distracting the L5-S1 disc space. However, additional posterior fixation, such as facet screws or pedicle screws, is required to achieve better construct stability.

The feasibility of a two-level transsacral rod has been evaluated by Erkan et al.[8] Unconstrained and nondestructive pure moments in AT, LB, and FE were applied to each specimen following intact, stand-alone transsacral rod, and transsacral rod with two posterior fixation options—facet screws and pedicle screws with rods. At the L4-5 level in AT and FE, none of the surgical treatments showed a statistically significant difference between the procedures, although facet screws and pedicle screws had higher stability on average. In LB, the two posterior fixation techniques had significantly higher construct stability than the stand-alone rod. No significant difference was found between facet screws and pedicle screws. At the L5-S1 level in AT and LB, none of the surgical treatments were found to be statistically significant. In FE, the stand-alone two-level transsacral rod had significantly higher ROM compared with the posterior fixation techniques. The authors concluded that the stand-alone rod reduced intact ROM significantly. However, they recommended supplementary fixations, including facet screws and pedicle screws, to increase construct stability.

In a prospective evaluation of 12 patients undergoing surgery for lumbar degenerative scoliosis, Anand et al. evaluated the feasibility of a transsacral rod placed at L5-S1 as an alternative to traditional anterior or posterior transsacral fixation.[9] Short-term follow-up demonstrated that this technique is a potential minimally invasive option for patients undergoing long instrumented fusions to the sacrum.

Aryan et al. reviewed these investigators' experience with the transsacral interbody fusion in 35 patients.[10] Average follow-up was 17.5 months. All patients had radiographic evidence of L5-S1 degeneration and underwent percutaneous paracoccygeal axial fluoroscopically guided interbody fusion with cage, local bone autograft, and recombinant human bone morphogenetic protein (rhBMP). Mean operative time for the L5-S1 paracoccygeal transsacral procedure was 42 minutes. Twenty-one patients underwent transsacral interbody fusion followed by percutaneous L5-S1 pedicle screw-rod fixation. Two patients underwent transsacral interbody fusion followed by percutaneous L4-5 lateral psoas splitting interbody fusion and posterior instrumentation. Ten patients had a stand-alone procedure. Unfavorable anatomy precluded access to the L5-S1 disc space during open lumbar interbody fusion in two patients who subsequently underwent transsacral rod instrumentation at this level as part of a large construct. Thirty-two patients (91%) had radiographic evidence of stable L5-S1 interbody cage placement and fusion at the last follow-up.

Asgarzadie et al. reported on 28 consecutive patients who underwent paracoccygeal transsacral interbody fusion.[11] Follow-up averaged 1 year. The operative time averaged 45 minutes, the estimated blood loss was minimal in all cases, and the hospital stay averaged 24 hours. There was an average 26-point decrease between preoperative and postoperative

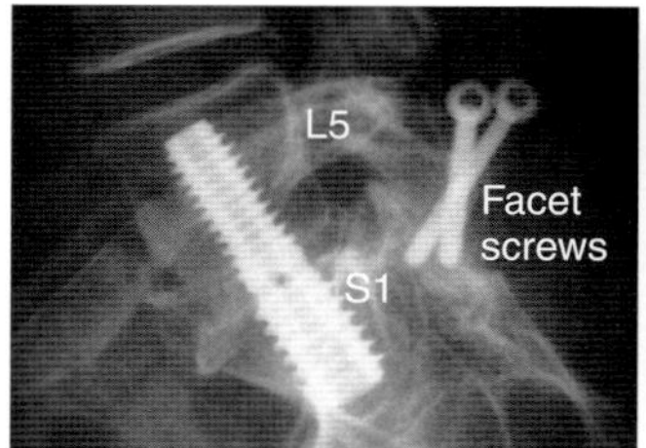

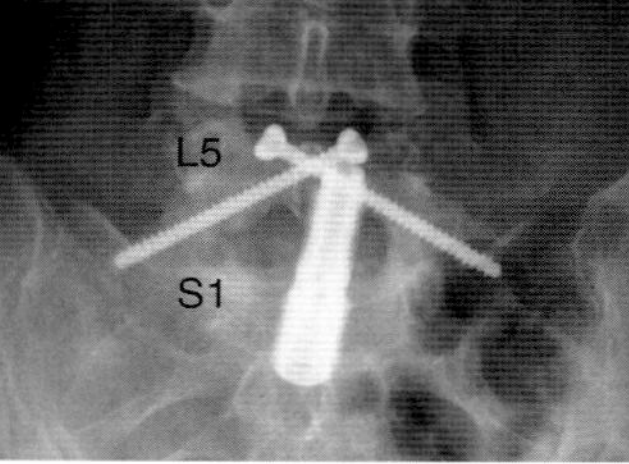

FIGURE 155-12. Example of a primary L5-S1 lumbar fusion.

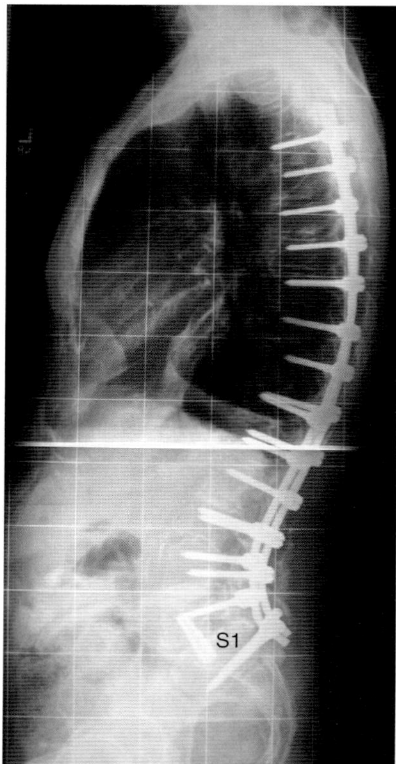

FIGURE 155-13. Example of an extension of previous long scoliosis fusion across the lumbosacral junction.

Oswestry Disability Index scores and a 7-point decrease in visual analogue scale scores at 1-year follow-up; these results were statistically significant. The rate of fusion was 90% at 1 year (16/16 patients with bone morphogenetic protein had radiologic fusion at 1 year). The investigators noted no complications.

Summary

The paracoccygeal transsacral exposure technique represents another option for minimally invasive access to the lumbosacral junction. This approach can be used either for primary lumbar fusions (Fig. 155-12) or as an extension of long fusions (Fig. 155-13) across the lumbosacral junction. The approach is associated with minimal soft tissue trauma, which could potentially result in faster postoperative recovery. It may serve as an alternative approach to the L5-S1 interspace in those patients who may have unfavorable anatomy or other contraindications to traditional open techniques. Currently, no randomized prospective studies exist that validate the advantages of this technique.

KEY REFERENCES

Akesen B, Wu C, Mehbod A, et al: Biomechanical evaluation of paracoccygeal transsacral fixation. *J Spinal Disord Tech* 21(1):39–44, 2008.

Anand N, Baron E, Thaiyananthan G, et al: Minimally invasive multilevel percutaneous correction and fusion for adult lumbar degenerative scoliosis: a technique and feasibility study. *J Spinal Disord Tech* 21(7):459–467, 2008.

Cragg A, Carl A, Casteneda F, et al: New percutaneous access method for minimally invasive anterior lumbar surgery. *J Spinal Disord Tech* 17(1):21–28, 2004.

Parke W, Whalen J, Van Demark R, et al: The infra-aortic arteries of the spine: their variability and clinical significance. *Spine (Phila Pa 1976)* 19(1):1–5, 1994.

Yuan P, Day T, Albert T, et al: Anatomy of the percutaneous presacral space for a novel fusion technique. *J Spinal Disord Tech* 19(4):237–241, 2006.

REFERENCES

The complete reference list is available online at expertconsult.com.

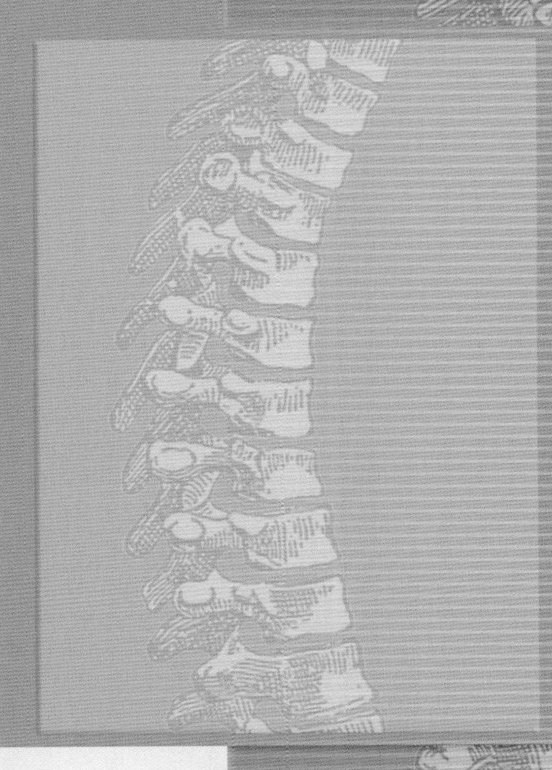

SECTION 6

Motion Preservation Strategies

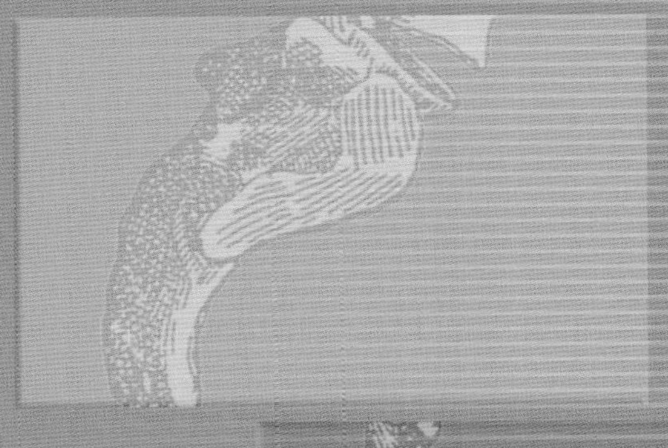

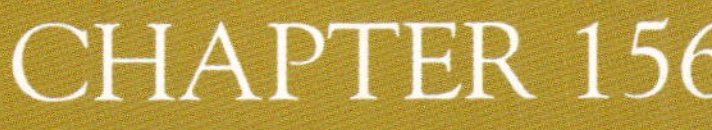

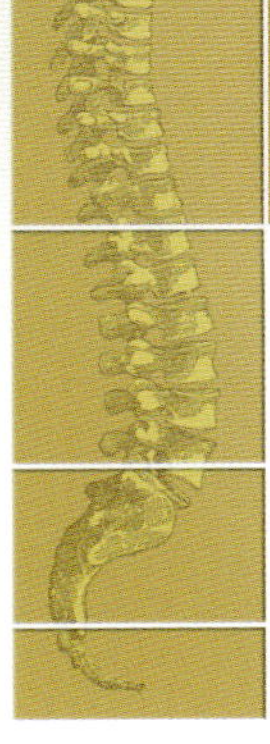

CHAPTER 156

To Not Operate

Ajit A. Krishnaney

The last 2 decades have seen the development of a number of "motion-sparing" implants to be used as an adjunct in spinal surgery. These implants are designed to obviate the need for fusion when one is indicated, thereby maintaining or restoring the normal multisegmental motion of the spine. In theory, maintenance of motion could lead to a smaller amount of adjacent-segment degeneration and, potentially, better outcomes.

A variety of motion-sparing implants have been developed. These include cervical and lumbar disc arthroplasties, nuclear replacements, facet replacements, and a variety of flexible rods and bands to be used with pedicle screws. Of these implants, only cervical and lumbar total disc arthroplasties (TDAs) have been approved by the U.S. Food and Drug Administration (FDA) for use as motion-sparing implants.

For any new device to become a valuable, viable addition to the surgeon's armamentarium, it must be either significantly "better" than what it is replacing in some way (e.g., safer, better outcomes, lower failure rate) or equivalent but less expensive.[1] Most of the studies published on disc arthroplasty to date have demonstrated equivalence to fusion. However, long-term results and cost analysis are still lacking.

Interestingly, few studies have been published comparing motion preservation surgery with nonoperative therapy. [2] As nonoperative management of spinal pathology maintains the spine's natural motion and has none of the operative risks of either fusion or disc arthroplasty, it may be the ultimate "motion-sparing" therapy for select spinal pathology.

Lumbar Spine

The major indication for lumbar disc arthroplasty is chronic back pain associated with degenerative disc disease. A number of studies have demonstrated that lumbar disc arthroplasty provides results equivalent to those of lumbar fusion. Three randomized controlled trials of fusion for chronic back pain, with mixed results, have been published in the last decade.[3-5] Fritzell et al. concluded that fusion was more effective than conservative therapy for chronic low back pain, when compared with the "usual therapy" directed by the patient's primary care physician.[5] Brox et al. observed no difference between fusion and a program of cognitive therapy and exercise.[4] Fairbank et al. found that fusion was only slightly more effective than a multidisciplinary rehabilitation program.[4] However, in both the Fritzell and Fairbank studies, the mean improvement in the Oswestry Disability Index (ODI) score, their primary outcome measure—11.6 and 12.5, respectively—failed to reach the threshold of 15 that the FDA considers the minimally clinically important change for the ODI.[1,6,7] Based on these trials, a number of authors have concluded that for nonradicular back pain, fusion is no more effective than an intensive rehabilitation program and is associated with only small to moderate benefit when compared with standard nonsurgical therapy.[6-9]

Only one study to date has compared lumbar disc arthroplasty directly with nonoperative management. Hellum et al.[2] conducted a multicenter prospective randomized trial comparing disc arthroplasty at L4-5 or L5-S1 with a 12- to 15-day outpatient multidisciplinary rehabilitation program. The study was powered to detect a 10-point difference on the ODI at 2 years, which was their primary outcome measure. Secondary outcome measures included low back pain, quality of life (36-Item Short Form Health Survey [SF-36], EuroQuol [EQ-5D]), Hopkins symptom check list (HSCL-25), fear avoidance beliefs (FABQ), work status, patients' satisfaction, and drug use. A total of 173 patients were enrolled, 86 with surgery and 87 with rehabilitation. Although the study did show a significant difference in ODI scores between the two groups, it was less than the 10 points the study was powered to detect. Moreover, there was no significant difference in any of the other outcome measures between the two groups.[2]

Cervical Spine

The published indications for TDA in the cervical spine are much broader than those for the lumbar spine. TDA has been shown to be equivalent to anterior cervical discectomy and fusion (ACDF) for management of myelopathy and radiculopathy.[10,11] Therefore, cervical TDA may be considered as an option in any case where a single-level ACDF may be indicated, including cervical radiculopathy, myelopathy, or neck pain secondary to single-disc-level pathology. Clearly, in cases of myelopathy or radiculopathy with progressive or severe neurologic deficit, surgery may be indicated for decompression of the neural elements. In those cases, TDA may be considered; however, it is still unclear whether TDA is any more beneficial than ACDF in either the short or long term.[10,11] As with discogenic low back pain, the literature does not seem to support surgery over nonoperative management for axial neck pain.[12] Furthermore, there is evidence to suggest that some patients with radiculopathy who had been considered surgical candidates may improve with epidural steroid injections alone, obviating the need for surgery.[13]

Summary

The advent of new "motion-sparing" implants in the last 2 decades has resulted in a renewed interest in surgery for back and neck pain. The literature has yet to show any clear advantage for this technology over fusion. Furthermore, the current literature fails to show any significant benefit to surgery for back or neck pain over a multidisciplinary rehabilitation program. Without further supportive studies in favor of TDA, one must conclude the best motion-sparing operation may be no operation at all.

KEY REFERENCES

Brox JI, Sorensen R, Friis A, et al: Randomized clinical trial of lumbar instrumented fusion and cognitive intervention and exercises in patients with chronic low back pain and disc degeneration. *Spine (Phila Pa 1976)* 28(17):1913–1921, 2003.

Chou R, Baisden J, Carragee EJ, et al: Surgery for low back pain. *Spine (Phila Pa 1976)* 34(10):1094–1109, 2009.

Fairbank J, Frost H, Wilson-MacDonald J, et al: Spine Stabilization Trial Group. Randomised controlled trial to compare surgical stabilisation of the lumbar spine with an intensive rehabilitation programme for patients with chronic low back pain: the MRC spine stabilisation trial. *BMJ* 330(7502):1233, 2005.

Fritzell P, Hagg O, Wessberg P, et al: 2001 Volvo Award Winner in Clinical Studies: Lumbar fusion versus nonsurgical treatment for chronic low back pain: a multicenter randomized controlled trial from the Swedish Lumbar Spine Study Group. *Spine (Phila Pa 1976)* 26(23):2521–2532, 2001.

Hellum C, Johnsen LG, Storheim K, et al: Surgery with disc prosthesis versus rehabilitation in patients with low back pain and degenerative disc: two year follow-up of randomised study. *BMJ* 342:d2786, 2011.

Mirza SK, Deyo RA: Systematic review of randomized trials comparing lumbar fusion surgery to nonoperative care for treatment of chronic back pain. *Spine (Phila Pa 1976)* 32(7):816–823, 2007.

REFERENCES

The complete reference list is available online at expertconsult.com.

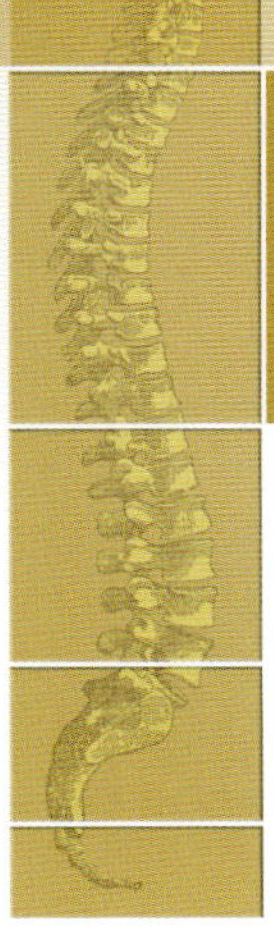

CHAPTER 157

Motion-Sparing, Nonimplant Surgery: Cervical Spine and Lumbar Spine

Ron Riesenburger | Paul Klimo | Edward C. Benzel

Motion-Sparing, Nonimplant Surgery: Cervical Spine

The last 20 years has seen an explosive increase in cervical spinal instrumentation development and use. However, there remain a number of motion-sparing procedures that do not require the use of a spinal implant. Such strategies eliminate the risk associated with the short- and long-term consequences of implants and spine stabilization. Motion-preserving surgery offers the patient relief of his or her neurologic symptoms while theoretically lessening spondylotic changes at adjacent levels. The disadvantage associated with motion-sparing surgery is that the spondylotic process may continue at the treated level(s). Fusion and instrumentation surgery, on the contrary, treats the symptomatic level definitively (assuming fusion is achieved).

The nonimplant, motion-sparing surgeries—laminectomy, laminoplasty, posterior laminoforaminotomy, and anterior foraminotomy—are discussed in this chapter. As with all spine procedures, outcomes are directly related to patient selection. Such is emphasized here.

Laminoforaminotomy

In 1946, Scoville presented the so-called keyhole foraminotomy technique at the annual Harvey Cushing Meeting. This was followed in 1951 by his report on 115 patients treated using this technique.[1] Despite its being developed several years before the now more common anterior cervical discectomy and fusion operations (Cloward[2,3] and Smith-Robinson types[4]), there are clear indications for and advantages to this approach.

The ideal patient for a posterior laminoforaminotomy is a patient with a single-level radicular syndrome, corresponding neurologic findings, and a concordant preoperative imaging study demonstrating foraminal stenosis. The nature of the foraminal stenosis can be adequately determined using a combination of plain radiographs, CT, and MRI. It can be due to a single or a combination of factors. The nerve root may be impinged by a soft disc herniation, typically seen as an extruded fragment that is hyperintense on T2-weighted imaging. This is usually the case in younger individuals. In older patients, the foramen is typically compromised by a disc-osteophyte complex that is a combination of disc material and uncovertebral osteophytes (hard disc). Foraminal stenosis, due to loss of disc height at the same level and osteophytes arising from the facet joint, may also coexist.

The keyhole foraminotomy typically provides a 3- to 5-mm exposure of the sensory root, which can then be retracted rostrally, thus facilitating the removal of the soft disc through the root's axilla.[5] It is difficult and risky to attempt removal of anterior uncovertebral osteophytes through this approach. In addition, this approach does not directly address foraminal stenosis due to a collapse of the disc space. However, as discussed later, numerous studies have shown excellent results in patients with hard discs. Webb et al. have described removing the superomedial aspect of the inferior pedicle using a drill to increase the foraminal volume in selected cases.[6]

The laminoforaminotomy has several advantages over the anterior discectomy and fusion. It preserves motion of the segment and therefore avoids the potential pitfalls associated with arthrodesis, namely, hardware complications, pseudarthrosis, graft subsidence, graft harvest complications, and the theoretical increased chance of accelerated adjacent-level degeneration. There are no issues with postoperative dysphagia or hoarseness and the decompression may be easily performed at multiple levels and bilaterally.

Because of the procedure's motion-sparing advantage, spondylotic changes may continue and further surgery may be necessary for recurrent or new symptoms at the same level. Clarke et al. calculated the 5- and 10-year risk rates for development of same-segment disease as 3.2% and 5.0%, respectively.[7] As previously mentioned, many patients have nerve root compromise as a result of bony growth into the foramen from the uncovertebral joint. The laminoforaminotomy allows an indirect decompression of the root but does not allow a direct decompression with removal of the anteriorly situated osteophytes, as would an anterior approach. Midline or collapsed disc pathology, kyphotic deformity, and disc herniation associated with unstable or traumatic cervical spine injury and the presence of significant axial neck pain are better treated with an anterior approach. The incision is typically more painful than a ventral approach for several days to weeks, and uses a midline approach and subperiosteal

TABLE 157-1

Summary of Recent Literature on Posterior Cervical Laminoforaminotomy

Author (Year)	Summary	Conclusions
Kim and Kim[9] (2009)	41 pts, 19 underwent midline approach (group 1), 22 paramedian tubular approach (group 2). Odom's criteria and VAS.	84% of group 1 and 86% of group 2 pts had good or excellent outcome using Odom's criteria. Group 2 had improved VAS for neck pain.
Jagannathan et al.[20] (2009)	162 pts followed for minimum of 5 yr. NDI and static/dynamic lateral radiographs.	NDI improved in 93% of pts, radiculopathy resolved in 95%. No significant changes in focal or overall sagittal balance.
Ruetten et al.[64] (2008)	86 pts underwent ACDF, 89 pts endoscopic paramedian tubular approach.	No difference in outcome between surgeries: 88% (ACDF) and 89% (foraminotomy) had resolution of arm symptoms after 2 yr. Recurrence rate of 3.4% in the foraminotomy group.
Cağlar et al.[65] (2007)	84 pts, 58% with soft discs and 42% with hard discs.	96% achieved resolution of radicular symptoms. Kyphosis developed in one patient (1.2%).
Hilton[66] (2007)	222 pts, 63% with soft discs and 37% with hard discs.	85% had complete relief of radicular pain. Three pts had no relief and required ACDF.
Korinth et al.[67] (2006)	124 pts underwent ACDF, 168 pts posterior foraminotomy. Odom's criteria used.	Excellent and good outcomes in 93.6% ACDF and 85.1% posterior foraminotomy (statistically significant). Pts with soft discs did better than pts with hard discs with both surgeries.
Fessler and Khoo[8] (2002)	51 pts, 26 underwent open midline approach, 25 microendoscopic approach.	Pts in both groups had 87% to 92% improvement with no difference between the groups. Endoscopic group had shorter hospital stay and less need for narcotics.

ACDF, anterior cervical discectomy and fusion; NDI, Neck Disability Index; pts, patients; VAS, visual analogue score; yr, years.

dissection of the paraspinal cervical musculature and lateral retraction. This may be improved with a paramedian muscle-splitting tubular approach.[8,9] No more than 50% of the facet should be resected to prevent instability and kyphosis.[10-18] Preoperative kyphosis at the symptomatic level, therefore, is a contraindication to this procedure.

A review of the recent literature is provided in Table 157-1. Typically, at least 80% to 90% of patients have good to excellent results. In the largest study, Henderson et al. reported resolution of radicular symptoms in 96% of 846 procedures performed in 736 patients, with 91.5% reporting good or excellent results.[19] Jagannathan et al. recently published their experience in 162 patients who underwent a unilateral, single-level posterior cervical foraminotomy with a minimum 5-year clinical and radiographic follow-up.[20] Resolution of radiculopathy and improvement in the Neck Disability Index occurred in 95% and 93% of patients, respectively. There were no statistically significant changes in focal or overall cervical kyphosis with time. Thirty patients (20%) experienced postoperative loss of lordosis (defined as a Cobb angle <10 degrees measured from C2 to C7). Factors found to be associated with worsening sagittal alignment included age greater than 60 years, the presence of a preoperative cervical lordosis of less than 10 degrees, and the need for posterior surgery after the initial foraminotomy.

Ventrolateral Foraminotomy

In 1996, Jho described a modified ventrolateral approach to the cervical foramen (ventral foraminotomy) to treat radiculopathy.[21] It was based on the previously described and more extensive lateral approach of Verbiest[22] and the transuncodiscal approach of Hakuba.[23] The key step in the procedure described by Jho is drilling and removal of the lateral uncovertebral joint (measuring approximately 5 to 8 mm transversely by 7 to 10 mm vertically) to expose the exiting nerve root as it passes under the vertebral artery. The surgical technique emphasizes preservation of the intervertebral disc as a functioning motion segment, while allowing direct access to the offending lesion (posterolateral disc herniation or uncovertebral osteophyte). Others, however, appear to have been using a similar technique before Jho's publication.[24] As in the posterior laminoforaminotomy, the ideal patient is one with one or more ipsilateral radiculopathies due to disc herniation or uncovertebral osteophytes. It cannot address foraminal stenosis due to loss of disc space height and would achieve only an indirect decompression of the root if the stenosis was due to facet arthropathy.

The ventrolateral approach has not found widespread acceptance among spine surgeons, with most publications coming from Europe and few centers in the United States. The reasons for this include fear of unnecessarily injuring the vertebral artery and sympathetic chain (Horner syndrome), inability to address bilateral symptoms, and the widespread use and teaching of the more common anterior (fusion and now arthroplasty) and posterior (laminoforaminotomy) approaches. Furthermore, a cadaveric study demonstrated a significant alteration in the mobility of the segment after unilateral uncoforaminotomy, with an increase in the range of motion in lateral bending and axial rotation.[25] The clinical implication is that with time this may lead to further disc degeneration and its sequelae (disc collapse, reherniation, development of osteophytes), requiring a reoperation. For example, a recent study by Yi et al. comparing 15 patients who underwent a total disc replacement with 13 patients who had an anterior foraminotomy found good clinical results in both groups, but the anterior cervical foraminotomy caused a significant loss of disc height after surgery.[26] Hacker and Miller found an unacceptably high revision rate of 30% (7 patients) in their series of 23 patients, with good or better outcomes using Odom's criteria in only 52% (12 patients).[27]

The revisions were performed between 2 weeks and 14 months from the index procedure and there were two patterns of failure that led to reoperation: recurrent radiculopathy or intractable neck pain. Six patients underwent anterior cervical discectomy and fusion, and one patient required a corpectomy. Nonetheless, multiple publications have indicated that anterior foraminotomy improves radicular symptoms and neck pain, with good or better outcomes using Odom's criteria in more than 80% of patients.[28] Some of this literature is summarized in Table 157-2. One of the largest series, by Jho et al., was published in 2002.[29] Of the more than 400 surgeries performed by the author and his team, 104 met the inclusion criteria for their study. Six weeks after surgery, 83 patients (79.8%) demonstrated excellent results, 20 patients (19.2%) demonstrated good results, and 1 patient (1%) experienced a fair outcome. No patient experienced a poor outcome or unchanged status. One patient required a reoperation to remove a persistent disc fragment, one patient developed discitis and had a spontaneous fusion with a slightly kyphotic angulation, one patient developed hemiparesis that resolved after 6 weeks (which the author believed was due to extended neck posture during surgery), and two patients developed transient Horner syndrome that resolved within 6 weeks. Dynamic cervical radiographs were obtained in 59 patients and all showed preservation of the motion segment.

A few surgeons, including Jho, have expanded the indications for the approach by treating myelopathic patients with partial oblique corpectomies while still preserving much of the disc space.[30-35] These results are not reviewed here, but good outcomes have been reported and a sheep cadaveric model has shown that the ventral oblique corpectomy does not result in instability.[36]

Laminectomy

Historically, cervical laminectomy has been a valuable motion-sparing, nonimplant surgery performed for the management of congenital or acquired multilevel cervical spinal stenosis associated with spondylosis, ossification of the posterior longitudinal ligament, and ossification or hypertrophy of the ligamentum flavum. The key factors in determining the optimal surgical candidate are the extent and nature of compression and the overall sagittal balance of the cervical spine.

Upright and dynamic (flexion-extension) MRI and CT are often recommended as preoperative imaging studies. The normal anteroposterior (AP) diameter of the spinal canal is approximately 17 mm. Stenosis is defined as a sagittal diameter of less than 12 to 13 mm. Congenital stenosis usually affects multiple levels and is readily apparent on a sagittal T2-weighted MRI. The Torg or Pavlov ratio, which is the AP diameter of the spinal canal divided by the AP diameter of the vertebral body at the same level, can be used as a guide in diagnosing congenital stenosis.[37] Stenosis is usually present if

TABLE 157-2

Summary of Literature on Anterior Foraminotomy

Author (Year)	Summary	Conclusions
Kotil and Bilge[68] (2008)	25 pts, VAS	A positive outcome at last follow-up examination was achieved in all patients. VAS pain rating was 6.36 pretreatment and 0.64 after 1 yr.
Balasubramanian et al.[69] (2008)	34 pts	94% achieved good to excellent outcomes. One patient required reoperation.
Cornelius et al.[70] (2007)	40 pts, average follow-up 4.3 yr. Odom's criteria.	85% of pts had no residual radicular pain, 94% had no more neck pain, 90% recovered their sensory deficits, and 83% recovered from their motor deficits. Good to excellent outcome in 95%. One patient had permanent Horner syndrome.
White et al.[71] (2007)	21 pts, follow-up 10 to 36 mo, VAS.	Mean VAS reduction in arm pain was 6.9, neck pain, 4.0. Arm strength improved 3.8, sensation by 3.8.
Lee et al.[72] (2006)	13 pts, average follow-up 19 mo.	All pts had resolution of their radicular pain. Motion preserved in each patient.
Koç et al.[73] (2004)	19 pts, average follow-up 23 mo. Odom's criteria and VAS.	Good or better outcome in 89.5%. One patient had developed contralateral foraminal stenosis at the level of the surgery and had undergone anterior discectomy and fusion.
Hacker and Miller[27] (2003)	23 pts, including 2 who had two-level procedures.	Good or better outcome in 52%. Seven pts (30%) required revision surgery.
Saringer et al.[74] (2003)	16 pts, average follow-up 18.3 mo. Endoscopic approach. NDI and VAS.	Average improvement of 44% in NDI and 96% in VAS for radicular pain. Overall subjective patient satisfaction rate 87.6%; return-to-work rate after 4 wk, 81.4%
Saringer et al.[75] (2002)	34 pts, average follow-up 8.2 mo.	100% relief of radicular neck pain. 97% of pts pleased with results of surgery. One patient suffered repeat herniation treated nonoperatively.
Jho et al.[29] (2002)	104 pts, average follow-up 36 mo. 52% soft disc herniations, 42% spondylotic spurs, 6% both.	79.8% experienced excellent results, 19.2% experienced good results, and one patient experienced fair results. Two pts developed transient Horner syndrome, one patient developed transient hemiparesis, and one patient developed discitis, resulting in spontaneous bone fusion.
Johnson et al.[76] (2000)	21 pts, follow-up 12 to 24 mo. Oswestry Pain Scale and VAS.	91% had improved or resolved radicular symptoms. Good or better outcome using VAS in 85%. Two pts required reoperations.

mo, months; NDI, Neck Disability Index; pts, patients; VAS, visual analogue score; wk, weeks; yr, years.

the ratio is less than 0.8. Another quick method to determine the presence of congenital stenosis is by assessment of plain lateral radiographs. If minimal space is present between the spinolaminar line and a line connecting the dorsal margin of the facet joints, significant canal stenosis is present.

Static and dynamic radiographs may provide information regarding instability. Concerning features, according to White and Panjabi,[38] include sagittal plane listhesis of greater than 3.5 mm on resting or dynamic radiographs, a sagittal plane rotation of greater than 20 degrees on flexion-extension radiographs, and a relative sagittal plane angulation of greater than 11 degrees on resting radiographs. It is critical to assess the overall sagittal balance of the cervical spine. Optimally, there should be approximately 14 degrees of lordosis from C2 to C7.

The optimal patient is one with single-level or multilevel circumferential central stenosis (i.e., congenital stenosis), or primarily dorsal impingement with preserved cervical lordosis. Preservation of lordosis is critical because maximal dorsal migration of the spinal cord takes place if the patient has an adequate cervical lordosis, typically 10 or more degrees, and 7 mm or less of ventral compression.[39] Those patients with a straight cervical spine or, of more concern, those with a kyphotic curve, may not be adequately decompressed through the dorsal approach and are at higher risk for development of a kyphotic deformity postoperatively. Decompression should be carried past the areas of focal stenosis to ensure that the transition areas from nonstenotic to stenotic regions do not themselves become compressed as the cord migrates dorsally. For example, if there is stenosis from C3 to C6, then the lamina of C2 should be undercut and the top of the C7 lamina should be resected.

Many reports since the 1970s have demonstrated the efficacy of laminectomy for the treatment of myelopathy. Ryken et al. recently provided an exhaustive review of this literature.[40] The surgery has numerous advantages; it can be performed relatively quickly and can address multiple levels, and it avoids the risks associated with anterior approaches, namely, hoarseness and dysphagia, which are significant risks in patients with advanced age and multilevel disease. There are disadvantages, however. The already compromised spinal cord may be damaged if instruments are placed under the midline lamina too aggressively. This has led some to recommend starting the decompression bilaterally at the laminofacet junction and then removing the central dorsal elements en bloc.[41] Postoperative C5 palsy is a complication associated with multilevel dorsal decompressive surgery (laminectomy or laminoplasty), occurring with a frequency of about 5% to 10%.[42] Its etiology continues to be a mystery and intraoperative monitoring has not been shown to prevent it.[43,44] Many believe that it may be due to the dorsal shift of the spinal cord, which is often maximal at the C5 level because it is usually at the midpoint in the laminectomy, causing tethering of the already short, less oblique C5 roots.[45,46] Some have advocated prophylactically performing foraminotomies at C4-5.[47,48] Recently, Sieh et al. have found that an average Pavlov ratio of less than 0.65 and compression at the C3-4 segment on preoperative MRI were reliable preoperative predictors for the development of this problem.[49]

The development of postlaminectomy spinal instability manifested by kyphosis is a concern that has garnered much attention and has led to the development of laminoplasty as an alternative technique (see next section). In their review, Ryken et al. found the risk ranged from 14% to 47%.[40] However, as stated by the authors, no study has clearly demonstrated a relationship between postlaminectomy kyphosis and deterioration in the patient's quality of life.

The trigger for the development of postoperative kyphosis is the denervation and weakening of the paraspinal musculature as a result of tissue dissection and bone removal. This alone may be enough to lead to kyphosis, such as in patients who already have a kyphotic cervical sagittal balance. On the other hand, in other patients, such as those with less cervical lordosis or straight spines, it may require the cumulative effect of other risk factors in addition to weakened muscles and lack of a bony scaffold to give rise to the kyphotic deformity. Not much can be done during surgery to limit the damage to the paraspinal musculature (other than possibly reducing the amount of electrocautery used and time under retraction), so it is the avoidance or limitation of other, more controllable factors that is of utmost importance in preventing this complication. One cannot overstress the importance of careful study of preoperative imaging, focusing on the presence of underlying instability and overall sagittal balance. The width and length of the laminectomy are important. If done for the treatment or prevention of myelopathy, the laminectomy should be taken to the lateral extent of the dural sac, which corresponds to the laminofacet junction. If further resection of the facets is required for decompression of the sac or individual nerve roots, this should be limited to 25% to 50% because numerous clinical, cadaveric, and finite element model studies have demonstrated that progressive facet resection produces increases in angular rotation and intervertebral disc stresses, leading to segmental hypermobility.[10-18] Laminectomies should be avoided at C2 and C7 because these laminae have been found to be relatively high load-bearing structures compared with C3 to C6, and the spinous process of C2 needs to be preserved because it is the insertion site of several key erector spinae muscles that are an integral part of the dorsal tension band.

The risk of postoperative kyphosis is greater in children for a number of anatomic reasons.[50] The child's cervical spine is hypermobile because the muscles and supporting ligamentous structures are less well developed, the orientation of the facets is more horizontal, the vertebral bodies are wedge shaped, and the head is disproportionately larger compared with the spine.[51]

Laminoplasty

Laminoplasty techniques arose as a result of concern over deterioration from the long-term effects of segmental instability and kyphosis that were being seen with laminectomy, as described in detail in the previous section. The first laminoplasty technique was described in the early 1970s, and this has spawned many different variations such as the "open-door," "French-door," and Z-plasty techniques, the technical details of which are beyond the scope of this chapter. Despite the multitude of different laminoplasty procedures, all share in the principles of enlarging the volume of the spinal canal while maintaining the bony neural arch and thus the reattachment site for the paraspinal muscles, and preserving segmental motion.

The indications for laminoplasty are the same as those for laminectomy. Laminoplasty has all the advantages of the laminectomy and has been shown to be as effective in ameliorating myelopathic symptoms as arthrodesis and other ventral approaches (e.g., discectomies, corpectomies).[52] Radiculopathy may be addressed by adding foraminotomies to the laminoplasty. As with laminectomy, laminoplasty allows indirect decompression of the cord by dorsal migration if there is ventral compression (e.g., disc-osteophyte complexes, ossification of the posterior longitudinal ligament) and direct decompression if there is dorsal compression (e.g., hypertrophied or calcified ligamentum flavum, shingling of the lamina, congenital stenosis). Dorsal migration depends on the presence of a neutral to lordotic sagittal alignment. Because laminectomy ideally should be reserved for patients with preserved cervical lordosis because of the risk for postlaminectomy kyphosis, laminoplasty offers the surgeon a greater degree of flexibility in that it may be performed on patients with a decreased lordotic to neutral cervical spinal curvature, but should also be avoided in patients with baseline kyphosis in the region that requires decompression. Again, careful analysis of preoperative imaging is required, as described in the laminectomy section.

Matz et al. have recently provided a comprehensive review of outcomes with the laminoplasty techniques.[53] Using the common Japanese Orthopedic Association scale for myelopathy, they found that the average recovery for patients was 55% to 65% and that this recovery was maintained in some studies for 5 years[54,55] and 10 years.[56-58] Despite the advantage of preserving segmental motion, many patients do experience a decrease in their range of motion and persistent axial neck pain.[53,59] A recent study did not show any benefit to preserving the muscles that attach to the spinous process of C7 in preventing or reducing postoperative neck pain.[60] As with laminectomy, C5 palsy can occur with this procedure, with the risk usually ranging from 5% to 10%. In some studies, it has been observed in up to 20%.[49,53,61] The incidence of kyphosis has been shown to be significantly less with laminoplasty (0% to 10%) than with laminectomy.[53,59,61] Unlike the situation with laminectomy, there is some evidence to support worse long-term neurologic outcomes if a kyphosis occurs following laminoplasty.[62,63]

KEY REFERENCES

Henderson CM, Hennessy RG, Shuey HM Jr, et al: Posterior-lateral foraminotomy as an exclusive operative technique for cervical radiculopathy: a review of 846 consecutively operated cases. *Neurosurgery* 13:504–512, 1983.

Jagannathan J, Sherman JH, Szabo T, et al: The posterior cervical foraminotomy in the treatment of cervical disc/osteophyte disease: a single-surgeon experience with a minimum of 5 years' clinical and radiographic follow-up. *J Neurosurg Spine* 10:347–356, 2009.

Jho HD, Kim WK, Kim MH: Anterior microforaminotomy for treatment of cervical radiculopathy. Part 1: disc-preserving "functional cervical disc surgery." *Neurosurgery* 51(Suppl 5):S46–S53, 2002.

Matz PG, Anderson PA, Groff MW, et al: Cervical laminoplasty for the treatment of cervical degenerative myelopathy. *J Neurosurg Spine* 11: 157–169, 2009.

Ratliff JK, Cooper PR: Cervical laminoplasty: a critical review. *J Neurosurg* 98:230–238, 2003.

Ryken TC, Heary RF, Matz PG, et al: Cervical laminectomy for the treatment of cervical degenerative myelopathy. *J Neurosurg Spine* 11:142–149, 2009.

Sakaura H, Hosono N, Mukai Y, et al: C5 palsy after decompression surgery for cervical myelopathy: review of the literature. *Spine (Phila Pa 1976)* 28:2447–2451, 2003.

REFERENCES

The complete reference list is available online at expertconsult.com.

Motion-Sparing, Nonimplant Surgery: Lumbar Spine

In the lumbar spine, motion-sparing, nonimplant operations such as laminectomy and discectomy have been used since the 1930s. The operating microscope and tubular retractor systems are new technologies that allow surgeons to perform these operations with smaller incisions but adequate visualization. However, long-term outcomes for these operations have not changed significantly over the past several decades, because the general principle of nerve root decompression has not changed. When indicated, these decompressive operations offer patients good clinical results while preserving motion and avoiding the costs and risks of implants.

Lumbar Discectomy

Lumbar discectomy is a motion-preserving operation that relieves lumbar radicular pain in 80% to 90% of patients.[1-4] The operation was popularized by Mixter and Barr in 1934.[5] The advent of the operating microscope in the 1970s has proved to be the main technologic advancement for this procedure over the past 75 years. Because the operation has otherwise not changed significantly over the past 40 years, very-long-term outcomes of the operation are relevant to patients currently being treated. A 90% patient satisfaction rate has been reported in a retrospective study of 201 patients with minimum 25-year follow-up.[3]

In most patients with lumbar disc herniations, instability is not present. Therefore, in most instances, fusion does not usually accompany discectomy, and segmental motion is preserved. Despite the excellent outcomes of discectomy, some authors have still questioned whether there may be a subgroup of patients who would benefit from fusion along with discectomy. Although fusion for lumbar disc herniation is rarely indicated, some studies suggest there are subgroups of patients that may have better outcomes with fusion than with motion preservation. Eie[6] reviewed a series of patients treated with surgery for a herniated disc. In this study, 119 patients underwent discectomy and 69 underwent

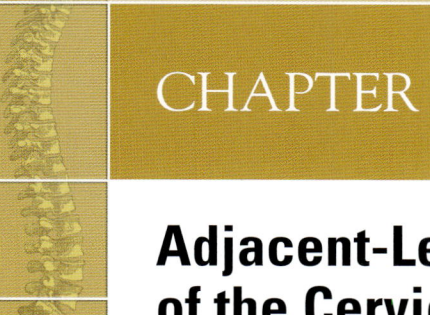

CHAPTER 158

Adjacent-Level Degeneration and Disease of the Cervical and Lumbar Spine

Kalil G. Abdullah | Thomas E. Mroz

Spondylosis is a natural and evolving process that occurs with aging, and it reflects the degeneration of intervertebral discs. Approximately 60% of asymptomatic persons older than 40 years of age have radiographic evidence of *cervical* spondylosis. By 60 years of age, 95% of men and 70% of women show similar radiographic findings.[1-3] In a separate study, Boden et al.[4] demonstrated that in patients younger than 60 years of age, the prevalence of abnormal results on *lumbar* MRIs averaged about 20%, whereas the prevalence was 57% in asymptomatic subjects older than 60 years of age.

Adjacent-level *degeneration* refers to radiographically apparent disc degeneration that occurs adjacent to interbody fusion. There is continued debate about whether this degeneration is a direct result of fusion or if it merely reflects the natural progression of spondylosis. Adjacent-level *disease*, on the other hand, refers to clinically relevant degeneration adjacent to a previous interbody fusion. This chapter considers adjacent-level degeneration and disease for both the cervical and lumbar spines.

Cervical Spine

Biomechanical Evidence

Nearly 50 years ago, cervical spine fusion was introduced by Cloward, Bailey, and Badgley, and Robinson and Smith.[5] Today, anterior cervical discectomy and fusion (ACDF) is a common surgical treatment for symptomatic cervical spondylosis. It is widely accepted, but it has been postulated that levels adjacent to a fused cervical segment(s) are prone to accelerated degenerative changes possibly owing to the significant forces transmitted to the adjacent levels after interbody fusion.

Certain biomechanical studies have generated data that lend credibility to the notion that fusion could cause degeneration of adjacent levels. Eck et al.[6] evaluated motion and intradiscal pressures at adjacent levels in a cadaveric C5-6 ventral fusion model. Compared with intact specimens, flexion at C4-5 and C6-7 both increased, with greater increases in motion at the rostral level. Extension also increased at both levels adjacent to the fused level; however, motion was greater at the caudal level. Intradiscal pressures increased by 73% at C4-5 and by 45% at C6-7 compared with control specimens, indicating that fusion causes a transfer of load to adjacent levels. Park et al.[7] reported similar findings in a cadaveric C5-7 ventral fusion model. The authors demonstrated that intradiscal pressures at C4-5 increased during physiologic range of motion. Cheng et al.[8] compared fluoroscopic imaging in patients with normal, degenerative, and fused (C5-6) cervical spines. Range of motion and estimated in vivo forces at levels adjacent (C4-5 and C6-7) to a C5-6 ventral fusion were both higher compared with normal and degenerative cervical spines. In contrast to these studies, Rao et al.[9] reported that intradiscal pressures and motion are not statistically different at adjacent levels after ventral fusion. Overall, most literature suggests that there is heightened loading and motion at levels adjacent to a fused segment(s).

Adjacent-Level Degeneration

Several authors have investigated adjacent-level degeneration radiographically. Baba et al.[10] retrospectively reviewed 133 patients who underwent ventral cervical fusion with an average follow-up of 8.5 years. The authors reported a 25% incidence of spinal stenosis and increased motion at the adjacent rostral level on dynamic radiographs. In another retrospective evaluation with an average 5-year follow-up of 121 patients who underwent ventral cervical fusion, Gore and Sepic[11] reported a 25% incidence of progression of spondylosis. In a radiographic review of 44 patients with a 4.5-year follow-up, Herkowitz et al.[12] reported rates of 41% and 50% of adjacent-level degeneration in patients who underwent ACDF and posterior foraminotomy, respectively. This would suggest that ACDF did not directly cause the adjacent-level degeneration, because foraminotomy is a not a fusion procedure. There was no correlation found in any of these studies between adjacent-level degeneration and clinical deterioration.

Adjacent-Level Disease

Attempts to define the incidence of adjacent-level disease, or clinically apparent adjacent-level degeneration, have been made by several authors. In 1968, Williams et al.[13] retrospectively studied 60 patients who underwent ACDF with an average follow-up of 4.5 years. Seventeen percent of these patients required additional surgery for progressive spondylosis after fusion. In a larger series with an average follow-up of 5 years, Gore and Sepic[2] reported that 14% of patients required further surgery after ACDF. In 1993, Bohlman et al.[14]

reported a 9% incidence of the adjacent-level degeneration in 122 patients after ACDF, with an average clinical and radiographic follow-up of 6 years; 81% (9 of 11) of patients with adjacent-level degeneration required further surgery at the adjacent level. Hilibrand et al.[15] performed a 10-year survivorship analysis of 409 ventral decompression and stabilization procedures. They reported a 2.9% annual incidence of adjacent-level disease, and an overall prevalence of 14% (follow-up, 2–21 years). Kaplan-Meier survivorship analysis predicted a prevalence of adjacent-level disease of 13.6% at 5 years and 25.6% at 10 years. The authors also concluded that the greatest risk of adjacent-level deterioration involved single-level fusions, particularly at C5-6 and C6-7. The authors could not determine from these results if degeneration was a result of the prior fusion or simply a manifestation of the natural progression of the spondylosis. These four studies indicate that there is 9% to 17% prevalence and an annual incidence of 1.5% to 4% of adjacent-level disease after ACDF.[16]

In addition, the control arms for the Investigational Device Exemptions trials for the various cervical artificial discs brought to market provide level I evidence and shed more light on the incidence of adjacent-level disease after one-level ACDF with allograft and plate. Mummaneni et al.[17] and Murrey et al.[18] reported a 3.2% and 1% incidence, respectively, of secondary surgeries for symptomatic adjacent-level degeneration at 2-year follow-up. Clearly, this refers to surgeries performed for adjacent-level disease and does not provide the absolute incidence. Presumably, there was a cohort of patients treated nonoperatively for adjacent-level symptoms.

Several authors have compared fusion and nonfusion procedures to further study adjacent-level disease. Lundsford et al.[19] reviewed 334 patients who underwent anterior discectomy, with and without fusion. They reported an annual prevalence of adjacent-level disease of 7% and an annual incidence of 2.5%. There was no difference in the development of adjacent-level disease between fusion and nonfusion procedures. In a review of 846 patients who underwent posterior foraminotomy without fusion, Henderson et al.[20] reported an overall prevalence of adjacent-level disease of 9% and an annual incidence of about 3%. Thus, these two reports provide evidence that suggests adjacent-level disease is not necessarily related to prior fusion procedures.

Prevention of Adjacent-Level Degeneration

As outlined previously, whether fusion causes adjacent-level degeneration remains a topic of debate. Regardless, there are steps the surgeon can attend to in order to minimize iatrogenic injury to adjacent levels. Needle level localization during ventral cervical surgery has been studied recently by Nassr et al.[21] They retrospectively followed 87 patients who underwent one- or two-level ACDF, 15 of whom had incorrect needle placement during level localization. In these patients, there was a threefold increase in adjacent-level degeneration compared with patients who had correct needle localization. Given these compelling data, it is very reasonable instead to place the needle into a vertebral body to avoid a potential disc injury. Surgeons should also avoid excessive subperiosteal dissection above or below the surgical levels. Typically, only 3 to 4 mm of the adjacent body needs to be exposed for plate placement. This minimizes the risk of injuring the adjacent level or compromising the integrity of the anterior longitudinal ligament and longus colli muscles.

Ventral plate placement has also been implicated in adjacent-level degeneration. Park et al.[22] retrospectively reviewed 118 patients with solid ventral plated fusion. The authors demonstrated a statistically significant higher incidence of adjacent-level ossification when the end of the cervical plate is less than 5 mm from the adjacent disc space. Sixty-seven percent of adjacent rostral levels and 45% of adjacent caudal levels developed ossification disease when the plate was less than 5 mm from the adjacent disc. To maintain an appropriate distance from the adjacent disc, the graft-vertebral body interface should be visible through the terminal screw holes of the plate when placing the screws. The rostral screws are placed in a superior trajectory and the caudal screws are placed in an inferior trajectory.

Lumbar Spine

Biomechanical Evidence

Similar to biomechanical studies in the cervical spine, lumbar data also support the notion that fusion results in higher biomechanical loads and more motion at adjacent, unfused levels. In an early cadaveric study, Lee and Langrana[23] demonstrated an increase in motion at unfused, adjacent levels after various forms of instrumented fusion. The authors also reported that loading of the cephalic adjacent facet joints increased with dorsal instrumentation compared with an anterior interbody fusion. Weinhoffer et al.[24] demonstrated in a cadaveric study that intradiscal pressures increased during flexion at the level adjacent to a pedicle screw construct. They also reported that the rise in pressure occurred earlier in flexion above two-level constructs versus one-level constructs. Other authors[25,26] have demonstrated biochemical degeneration of the lumbar intervertebral disc adjacent to fused segments in animal models.

Adjacent-Level Degeneration

Several authors have reported the association of adjacent-level degeneration and lumbar fusion, but the results are heterogeneous. The reasons for the variance in study outcomes likely include dissimilar end points (e.g., listhesis, loss of disc height, stenosis, signal change), different radiographic measures (e.g., radiography, CT, MRI), and different reporting methods across studies. Nonetheless, the available studies do consistently report an association between lumbar fusion and adjacent-level degeneration. However, one must also remember that this does not *prove* causality; that is, it may also reflect the natural history of spondylosis.

In 1987, Penta et al.[27] reported a 32% incidence of adjacent-level degeneration after anterior lumbar interbody fusion, and also noted that its evolution was independent of fusion achievement (vs. pseudarthrosis) and of length of fusion. These authors reported a 2.5% incidence of adjacent-level stenosis, which is in stark contrast to the study by Lehmann et al. (30%).[28] Leong et al.[29] also evaluated adjacent-level degeneration after anterior lumbar interbody fusion, but reported an incidence of 52%. Many other studies have reported a wide range (20–64%) of adjacent-level degeneration after dorsal fusion.[30-33]

Instability and listhesis (anteroposterior translation) at adjacent levels have been reported by several authors. Lehmann et al.[28] evaluated outcomes at long-term follow-up after dorsal lumbar fusion, and reported a 45% incidence of adjacent-level instability. Luk et al.[34] retrospectively reviewed a series of patients 12.8 years after fusion for idiopathic scoliosis and reported asymptomatic hypermobility of the adjacent level. In 1997, Wimmer et al.[35] reported a 10.8% incidence of asymptomatic adjacent-level listhesis after circumferential fusion. This was very similar to the 9.7% incidence of instability noted by Chen et al.[36] after dorsal instrumented fusion, but less than the 30% to 35% rate of listhesis reported by Guigui et al.[30] after dorsal instrumented fusion.

Radiographically apparent spinal stenosis as a consequence of adjacent-level degeneration has been reported less commonly. Like the reported rates of disc degeneration and listhesis/instability, the incidence range of stenosis is also quite wide, at 18% to 62%.[28] Overall, our ability to understand the magnitude of adjacent-level degeneration is limited. Again, this is due to the wide variety of reporting methods and study designs that have been used over the last several decades. Nonetheless, even the most conservative estimates of adjacent-level degeneration report a 20% rate of occurrence.

Adjacent-Level Disease

The literature suggests that most patients who develop radiographically apparent adjacent-level degeneration after lumbar fusion do not have symptoms referable to it. Etebar and Cahill[37] retrospectively reviewed 125 patients at 44-month follow-up after instrumented dorsal lumbar fusion for degenerative spondylolisthesis. They reported that 14% of patients required adjacent-level surgery. This is in contrast to another study[38] that reported only a 3% incidence of symptomatic L5-S1 degeneration after L4-5 fusion at 7-year follow-up. Throckmorton et al.[39] performed a retrospective review of 25 patients treated consecutively with a dorsal lumbar fusion ending adjacent to a degenerative disc (n = 20) or a normal one (n = 5). Surprisingly, at a minimum 2-year follow-up, patients with normal adjacent discs scored more poorly on the Short-Form Health Survey (SF-36), which suggests that radiographic degeneration alone is a poor indicator of future problems. In an important study, Ghiselli et al.[40] retrospectively reviewed 215 patients after lumbar fusion and reported a 27.4% incidence of second surgery at adjacent levels (decompression n = 15; fusion n = 45). Kaplan-Meier analysis predicted that the rate of secondary surgery at adjacent levels for either decompression or fusion was 16% at 5 years and 36% at 10 years.

Prevention of Adjacent-Level Degeneration

Several risk factors for adjacent-level degeneration after lumbar fusion have been identified. The addition of instrumentation to fusion has consistently been associated with faster appearance and higher rates of adjacent degeneration. Two separate studies demonstrated adjacent-level listhesis at 25 months[41] and 27 months[37] after dorsal lumbar instrumented fusion. This is in significant contrast to the studies of noninstrumented fusion by Schlegel et al.[42] and Lee[43] that reported adjacent-level breakdown at 8 and 13 years after surgery, respectively. The association of instrumentation and adjacent-level deterioration is likely multifactorial. Clearly, the instrumented segments are initially more rigid, particularly when an interbody fusion is added to the construct. This may accelerate the initial loading of the adjacent level and henceforth its degeneration. As mentioned in a previous section, the fusion itself is associated with increased loading of both the disc and the facet joints and, as such, it is possible that fusion really is a cause of accelerated degeneration at adjacent levels.

A very likely risk to the adjacent level is the index procedure itself. Exposure of the rostral facet with injury to the capsule or excessive denervation or stripping of the muscular insertions can predispose the adjacent level to degeneration. Also, in spite of their common use, pedicle screws clearly present a risk to the adjacent level. It is mandatory that a proper starting point be chosen for the rostral screws to avoid violation of the facet joint.

Although there is a paucity of data to corroborate the notion that sagittal alignment is important in terms of adjacent-level degeneration, it is at least plausible to assume that maintaining normal lordosis is ideal. Minimizing fusion segment length is also thought to be optimal in terms of maximizing normal kinematics at unfused lumbar levels. However, one must pay particular attention to long lumbar constructs that extend to L1 or L2. The thoracolumbar junction is unique biomechanically and anatomically. Ending a long lumbar fusion at L1 rather than crossing the junction with the fusion should be avoided if possible given the anticipated high risk of degeneration at the rostral end of the construct.

Conclusion

Adjacent-level disease is nearly ubiquitous after fusion in both the lumbar and cervical spine. However, it remains controversial whether it is a result of the fusion versus a progression of spondylosis. Although the clinical significance of degeneration may be negligible in most cases, adjacent-level disc disease after successful fusion likely will be encountered by the spine surgeon at some point in his or her career. An understanding of epidemiologic rates of occurrence and, perhaps most important, maintaining strict intraoperative vigilance may lead to a decrease in the incidence of these two common processes.

KEY REFERENCES

Eck JC, Humphreys SC, Lim TH, et al: Biomechanical study on the effect of cervical spine fusion on adjacent-level intradiscal pressure and segmental motion. *Spine (Phila Pa 1976)* 27:2431–2434, 2002.

Lee CK: Accelerated degeneration of the segment adjacent to a lumbar fusion. *Spine (Phila Pa 1976)* 13:375–377, 1988.

Lee CK, Langrana NA: Lumbosacral spinal fusion: a biomechanical study. *Spine (Phila Pa 1976)* 9:574–581, 1984.

Lehmann TR, Spratt KF, Tozzi JE, et al: Long-term follow-up of lower lumbar fusion patients. *Spine (Phila Pa 1976)* 12:97–104, 1987.

Rao RD, Wang M, McGrady LM, et al: Does anterior plating of the cervical spine predispose to adjacent segment changes?, *Spine (Phila Pa 1976)* 30:2788–2792, 2005; discussion 2793.

REFERENCES

The complete reference list is available online at expertconsult.com.

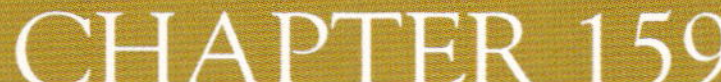

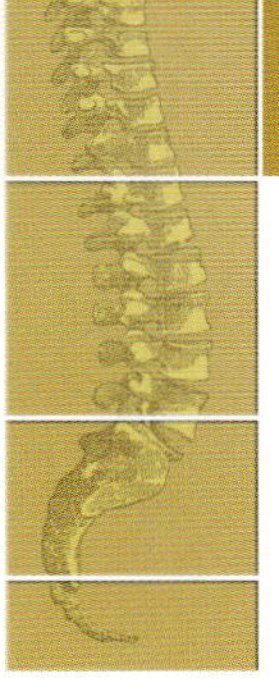

CHAPTER 159

Biomechanics of Motion Preservation Techniques

Todd B. Francis | Edward C. Benzel

For many years, cervical and lumbar arthrodesis has been the gold standard of treatment for a wide range of degenerative, traumatic, deformational, and oncologic spinal disorders. Although spinal arthrodesis has been used with great success, from a biomechanical perspective, it significantly alters the regional and global balance of physical forces and moments. As a consequence, several studies have demonstrated accelerated degenerative changes at levels directly adjacent to rigid spinal fusions.[1-3] This is commonly termed *adjacent-segment degeneration* (ASD). Specifically, it is thought that the stiffness imposed by a rigid fusion on an adjacent vertebral functional spinal unit (FSU) alters stress transfer between the vertebral segments and predisposes adjacent segments to accelerated degeneration. As a result of this, *motion-sparing technologies* have emerged in an attempt to preserve the native motion of the spinal unit, predominantly at the disc interspace. Theoretically, if a motion-sparing implant closely simulates the biomechanical properties of the intact FSU, the incidence of ASD would be expected to decrease.

The earliest and most traditional form of motion preservation surgery came in the form of laminectomy, laminoplasty, and laminoforaminotomy. These techniques were designed to treat underlying spinal pathology while preserving as much of the natural motion of the spine as possible. They involve a small amount of bone removal and preservation of the facets and many of the supporting ligaments, and do not violate the disc. In particular, the laminoforaminotomy has been shown to induce the least disruption in normal spinal mobility and stiffness compared with traditional laminectomy.[4] There is, however, a limited range of pathologic processes for which these techniques are indicated (and effective).

To best understand the biomechanics of motion preservation techniques, one must appreciate the biomechanical forces in play in and about the intervertebral disc, with particular attention to load transfer, intradiscal pressures, and the neutral zone. Biomechanical principles of the degenerating disc, including the concepts of dysfunctional motion and ASD, must also be considered. Once these concepts are understood, one can then examine the biomechanical principles behind motion preservation technologies.

Biomechanics of the Functional Spinal Unit

The FSU is defined as the smallest motion segment of the spine that exhibits biomechanical characteristics representative of the physiologic motion of the whole spine. Most authorities consider it to be synonymous with the spinal motion segment. It consists of two vertebrae, the intervertebral disc, the facet joints, and the associated supportive ligaments. A firm grasp of the biomechanics of the FSU is necessary to design implants aimed at replicating physiologic motion.

Physical Principles

A *vector* is a force oriented in a fixed direction in three-dimensional space. All forces acting on the spine can be described in terms of their component vectors. A vector may act on a lever (*moment arm*), resulting in a *bending moment*. A bending moment applied to a point in space causes rotation (or a tendency to rotate) about an axis, called the *instantaneous axis of rotation* (IAR). Movement about the IAR can be described in terms of the cartesian coordinate system (Fig. 159-1). The IAR

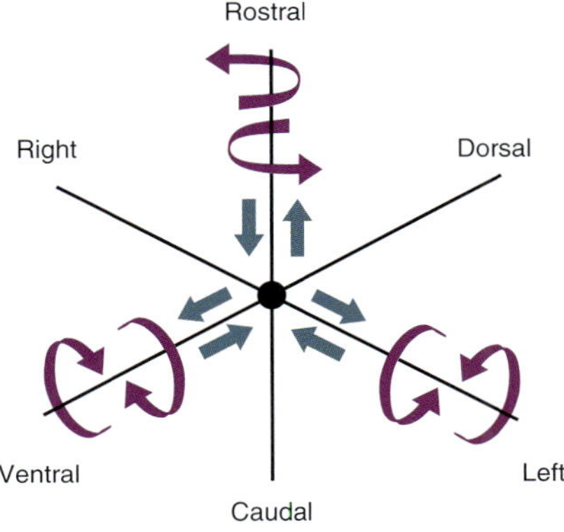

FIGURE 159-1. There are 12 potential movements about the instantaneous axis of rotation: 2 translational movements about the *x*, *y*, and *z* axes, and 2 rotational movements around each axis. (From Benzel EC: *Biomechanics of spine stabilization,* Rolling Meadows, IL, 2001, American Association of Neurological Surgeons, distributed by Thieme, New York, with permission.)

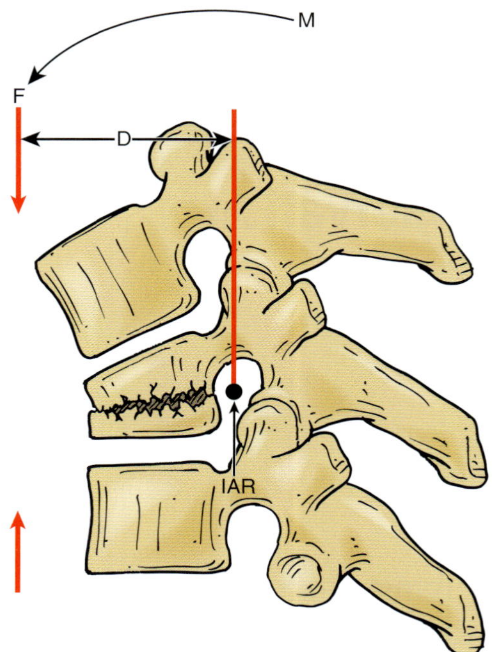

FIGURE 159-2. The bending moment (M) may be considered mathematically as the product of the distance (D) from the instantaneous axis of rotation (IAR) to the point of perpendicular application of force (F) and the magnitude of the force. (From Benzel EC: *Biomechanics of spine stabilization,* Rolling Meadows, IL, 2001, American Association of Neurological Surgeons, distributed by Thieme, New York, with permission.)

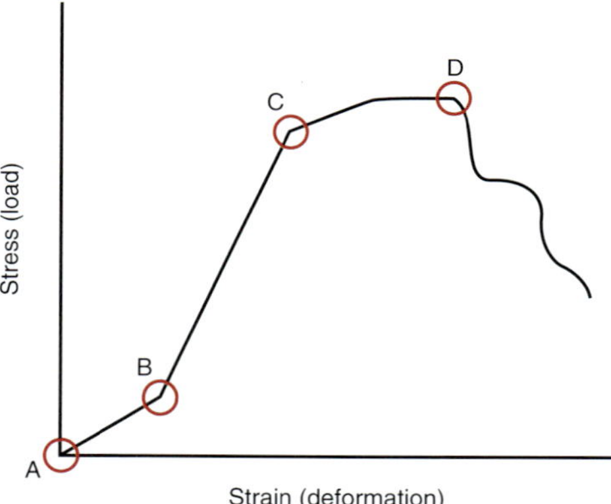

FIGURE 159-3. The neutral zone (AB) or zone of nonengagement describes the reaction of a solid to stress before deformation of that solid is realized. When the neutral zone is exceeded and stress continues, the solid enters into the elastic zone (BC). As the applied force increases, the *elastic limit* (C) is reached and the plastic zone is entered (CD). At this point, increased stress results in permanent deformation of the solid up to the *point of failure,* when the solid yields (D). (From Benzel EC: *Biomechanics of spine stabilization,* Rolling Meadows, IL, 2001, American Association of Neurological Surgeons, distributed by Thieme, New York, with permission.)

is the point or location in three-dimensional space about which each vertebral segment rotates at any given instant. The location of the IAR is not fixed, but rather is variable (mobile) depending on the intrinsic curvature of the spine and any other intrinsic or extrinsic forces that may act on the spine[5] (Fig. 159-2).

When several forces act on a solid with a resultant net force of zero, the solid is deformed. A *stress-strain curve* describes this relationship (Fig. 159-3). *Stress* is defined as the force applied to an object (load). *Strain* is defined as the response of the object to the force (deformation). The neutral zone or zone of nonengagement describes the reaction of a solid to stress before deformation of that solid is realized. When the neutral zone is exceeded and stress continues, the solid enters into the elastic zone. The elastic zone describes applied stress (usually of lower magnitude) that results in strain that is completely recoverable after removal of stress. As the applied force increases, the *elastic limit* is reached and the plastic zone is entered. At this point, increased stress results in permanent deformation of the solid up to the *point of failure*, when the solid yields.

Intervertebral Disc

The intervertebral discs contain a peripherally located anulus fibrosus and a centrally located nucleus pulposus. The cartilaginous end plates form the rostral and caudal limits of the intervertebral discs. The fibers of the anulus are arranged radially in opposite directions about the vertebral body interspace between the end plates, whereas the nucleus pulposus is contained within the anulus. The anulus contains two types of laminated (mostly collagenous) fibers: radial fibers that attach to the cartilaginous end plates (called *inner fibers*) and to the cortical bone on the edge of the vertebral bodies (called *Sharpey fibers*). These fibers are oriented roughly 30 degrees with respect to the end plate and opposite to each other, which gives the disc the ability to resist rotational forces (Fig. 159-4). The nucleus pulposus is a gel-like remnant of the embryonal notochord. It is composed of reticular bands surrounded by a thick mucoid ground substance.

The intervertebral disc can resist significant axial forces; however, this ability decreases with age. A pure (i.e., central) axial load causes symmetrical deformation of the disc because the intradiscal pressures are distributed symmetrically. In the presence of flexion, extension, or lateral bending (i.e., eccentric) forces, the intradiscal pressures are distributed asymmetrically and the normal disc will deform in a relatively predictable manner. The anulus bulges on the side of the deformation and stretches on the side opposite to the load, whereas the nucleus pulposus tends to move away from the area of applied force (in the opposite direction from the anular bulge)[5] (Fig. 159-5).

Studies of the nucleus pulposus in vitro demonstrate its importance in intervertebral disc biomechanics. Mechanical denucleation of intervertebral discs in cadaver lumbar spine segments results in increased range of motion and neutral zone compared with intact discs. Removal of the nucleus also results in decreased disc height and segment stiffness. Interestingly, the nucleus is most effective at lower loads, before the anulus has a chance to be engaged in a more effective tensile load-bearing state.[6]

Biomechanics of Intervertebral Disc Degeneration

Several in vitro and finite element analysis (FEA) studies have been conducted to examine the complex forces at play in the FSU and on the intervertebral disc. A complex state

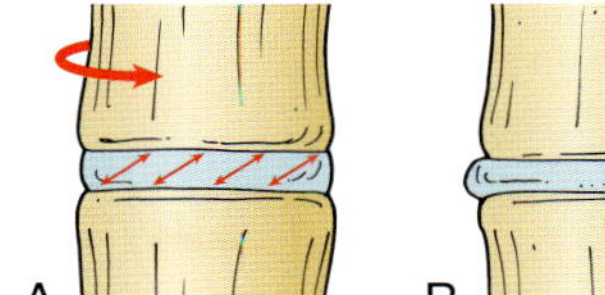

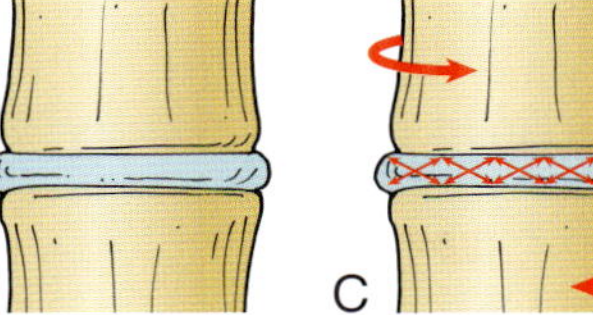

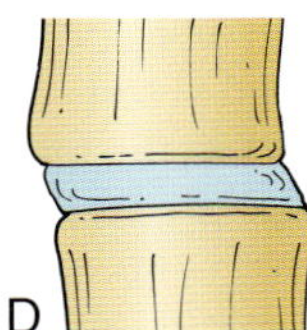

FIGURE 159-4. Anular fibers are oriented 30 degrees with respect to the end plate. This orientation resists torsion (**A**), but does not effectively resist compression (**B**) or distraction. If the anular fibers are lax, torsional resistance is lost (**C**) and subluxation may ensue (**D**). (From Benzel EC: *Biomechanics of spine stabilization,* Rolling Meadows, IL, 2001, American Association of Neurological Surgeons, distributed by Thieme, New York, with permission.)

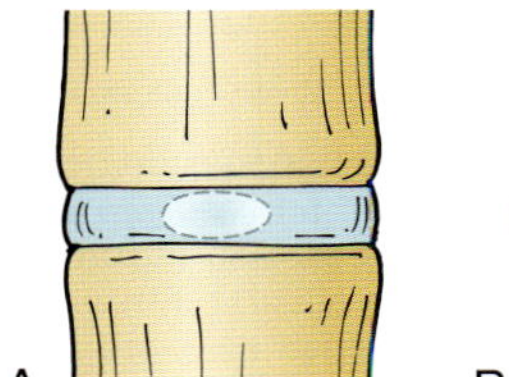

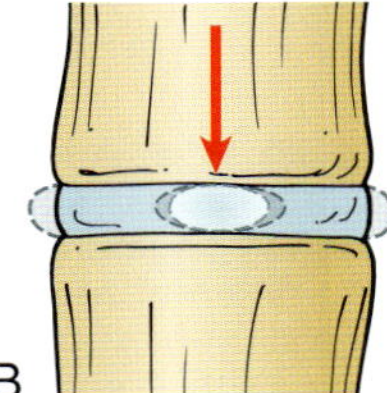

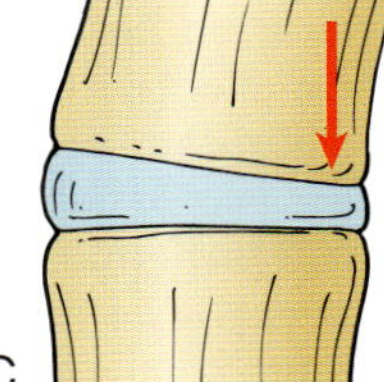

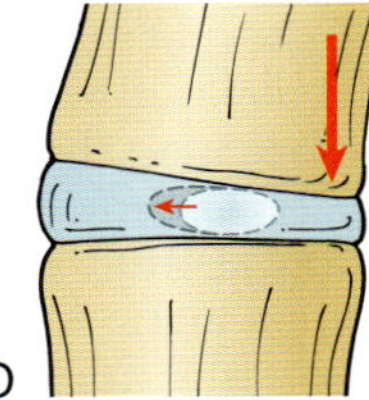

FIGURE 159-5. The normal intervertebral disc (**A**). Pure axial loads (**B**) cause an even distribution of force and symmetrical displacement of the nucleus pulposus and bulging of the anulus. Asymmetrical loading (**C**) causes the anulus to bulge on the same side as the force application. However, the nucleus pulposus will migrate in the opposite direction (**D**). (From Benzel EC: *Biomechanics of spine stabilization,* Rolling Meadows, IL, 2001, American Association of Neurological Surgeons, distributed by Thieme, New York, with permission.)

of loading exists in the physiologic scenario, and studies must strive to duplicate this. For example, the intervertebral disc rarely undergoes isolated axial loading but rather experiences a dynamic range of forces, usually in combination and varying from moment to moment. Many FEA studies have therefore measured a variety of combinations of forces applied to a given intervertebral disc and measured resultant intradiscal pressures and shear strains on the discs.

An FEA study of the L4-5 FSU demonstrated that the anulus fibrosus is strained maximally in the dorsolateral regions of the intervertebral disc.[7] This may explain why a disc prolapse occurs most commonly in this region. The shear and fiber strains on the anulus were greatest during combined movements such as rotation plus lateral bending or flexion and combined flexion or extension and lateral bending. These strains were also high in the dorsolateral regions of the disc. An in vitro study of human lumbar spine segments also supports these data.[8]

As the disc degenerates, a cascade of events ensues that eventually may result in symptomatic degenerative disc disease. In the early stages of disc degeneration, the disc gradually desiccates, losing water content and height in the process. Intradiscal pressures elevate as a result of this because the disc is no longer able to efficiently resist the forces placed on it. The disc interspace narrows, resulting in distortion and bulging of the anulus. The fibers of the anulus gradually break free of their bony attachments, and osteophytes form at these points because of subperiosteal bone formation. The patient may begin to experience pain of spinal origin. At this point, the FSU may become a *dysfunctional motion segment*, and its motion *mechanically unstable*. A dysfunctional motion segment is defined as a type of instability related to disc interspace or vertebral body abnormality that results in the potential for pain of spinal origin.[5] The patient may experience deep, agonizing back pain that worsens with activity and is relieved by rest; this symptom suggests the diagnosis.

The normal intervertebral disc, the fused intervertebral segment, and the dysfunctional motion segment all have characteristic stress-strain curves. For the fused segment, this curve is characterized by a straight line with a very steep slope. Because in this circumstance the disc has been effectively replaced by bone, the stress-strain curve resembles that of a relatively noncompressible substance (a large amount of load is required to provide a correspondingly small deformation in the material). The curve for the normal intervertebral disc is characterized by a shallow neutral zone and a steep elastic zone. When the healthy intervertebral disc is initially axially loaded (in the neutral zone), the disc undergoes a proportionally large deformation for a given load as the disc bulges. The nucleus pulposus absorbs this initial load. As the axial load increases (in the elastic zone), the anular fibers tighten and begin to resist and contain the bulging nucleus. There is, therefore, a proportionally smaller amount of deformation for a given load. The biomechanical equivalent of a dysfunctional motion segment is a widened neutral zone on the stress-strain curve. The disc is desiccated, the height is decreased, and the anular fibers are degenerated. The disc is less able to bear or resist axial loads effectively because it has become lax, and as a result the disc will readily deform to proportionally smaller loads. This creates a wide, shallow neutral zone. This also results in a shift of the IAR dorsally, which overloads the facets. In accordance with Wolff's law, the facets hypertrophy and the degenerative cascade continues.

Adjacent-Segment Degeneration

Vertebral arthrodesis has been used for many years as a treatment for the dysfunctional motion segment. A dysfunctional motion segment is defined as an FSU that, for one reason or another, can no longer bear and resist the loads placed on it during daily activity without exhibiting abnormal motion and often pain. By removing the dysfunctional joints and replacing them with a bony fusion, the abnormal motion of the motion segment is no longer present and the loads that were previously borne by that segment are now shared with the adjacent intact segments. This, many believe, is the driving force behind ASD.

Accelerated degeneration at vertebral levels immediately adjacent to a bony fusion has been observed for some time. ASD in the cervical spine was brought to the forefront in a landmark article by Hilibrand et al.[3] and was confirmed in many other studies.[9] Similar results have been noted in the lumbar spine.[10] Many biomechanical studies have demonstrated that there are significant increases in both intradiscal pressures and segmental spinal motion in segments immediately adjacent to a bony cervical spinal fusion.[11,12] Similar results have been shown in the lumbar spine.[13,14] Because most of these results were generated in a biomechanics laboratory with cadaver spines, the actual significance of these observations is unclear.

Despite these results, this phenomenon has been heavily debated. It remains difficult to distinguish the effect of the alteration of natural biomechanical forces in the spine after performance of a fusion on adjacent segments from the natural course of degeneration at those segments. Furthermore, the risk of developing symptomatic ASD in the cervical spine after single-level arthrodesis is actually greater than that after multilevel arthrodesis.[3] This is biomechanically contradictory because one would expect the larger lever arm and increased stiffness created by a multilevel fusion to have a stronger effect on adjacent segments. The same phenomenon appears to be true in the lumbar spine as well.[10] There is also evidence to suggest that the risk of developing ASD is not linked to the presence of spinal fusion. A retrospective study by Axelsson et al.[15] demonstrates that increased mobility of segments adjacent to a lumbar fusion is not a universal finding, and those patients in the study that did have adjacent-segment hypermobility did not experience accelerated ASD. In addition, there is a growing body of evidence suggesting that sagittal alignment plays a critical role in the development of ASD. In one study nearly half of the patients who presented with cervical ASD had cervical malalignment. Roughly 80% of patients whose cervical segments were fused in kyphosis developed ASD.[16] Similar results were shown to be true in the lumbar spine, where one study demonstrated that the incidence of ASD was approximately five times higher in patients with sagittal imbalance and/or vertical sacral inclination after lumbar fusion.[17] Nevertheless, the phenomenon of ASD has, in part, provided the impetus for the development of the field of motion preservation surgery.

Biomechanics of Motion-Sparing Implants

The ideal motion-sparing implant replicates the anatomy, motion, and mechanics of the intact, healthy FSU. Unfortunately, the theoretical ideal implant and the actual metal-on-poly or metal-on-metal implant curves are very dissimilar (Fig. 159-6). For example, an ideal intervertebral disc arthroplasty should replicate the form and function of a healthy intervertebral disc. The intact disc is akin to a radial tire, with a lamellated, firm but flexible outer shell and a soft, gelatinous core. This allows the disc both to accept and deform after the application of small loads and firm up and provide greater resistance to deformation as the load gradually increases.[18] The arthroplasty should not permanently alter the location of the IAR of the FSU so as not to place the dorsal ligaments and facets under undue stress. The implant must also be durable and able to stand up to decades of repetitive, cyclical motion and loading. To date, no spinal implant has successfully replicated normal spinal mechanics. However, many newer devices show promise.

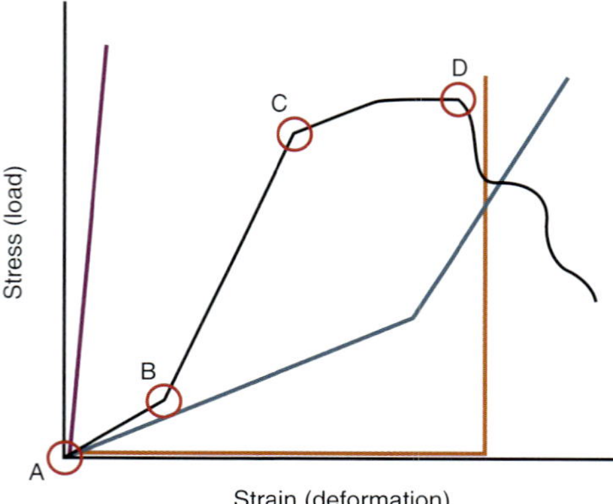

FIGURE 159-6. A stress-strain curve depicting a normal disc (*black line*), a fused spinal segment (*purple line*), and a dysfunctional motion segment (*blue line*). See Figure 159-3 for explanation of the different zones. Most current intervertebral metal-on-metal or metal-on-hard polymer prostheses are represented by the *orange line* (with a widened neutral zone until the limits of motion are reached.) Then the device reaches near infinite stiffness (vertical portion of curve). The most effective intervertebral prostheses should, perhaps, most closely approximate the black curve (A-B-C).

Nucleus Replacement Technologies

Nuclear implants are designed to replace the diseased nucleus pulposus. In theory, they restore disc height and anular tension, and assist in load transfer across the diseased disc.[18] From a biomechanical perspective, the restoration of disc height and intradiscal pressures should result in the normalization of intact disc mechanics in terms of range of motion, neutral zone width, and energy dissipation.[19] They are composed largely of viscoelastic materials and are either injected directly into the disc interspace or implanted through an open approach. Such devices require an intact anulus. Hence, large anular tears or defects are relative contraindications to this clinical strategy.

A limitation of this type of implant is the stress that it places on the end plate. Because most of these implants do not contact the entire end plate, they create end-plate contact pressure points that can lead to remodeling of the end plate. This can be associated with adverse outcomes. Furthermore, these implants may elevate shear strain in the anulus. These effects are related to the construction of the nuclear implant, where rigid nonconforming implants (e.g., polyetheretherketone [PEEK] devices) increase maximal shear strain and contact pressure points in the end plate, and conforming implants (e.g., viscoelastic hydrogel) do not.[20] Another significant limitation of this technology is the risk of extrusion of these devices from the disc after implantation.[21]

Pedicle-Based Dynamic Stabilization Devices

Pedicle-based dynamic stabilization systems such as the Dynesys Dynamic Stabilization System (Zimmer; Warsaw,

IN) are composed of "synthetic ligaments" suspended between pedicle screws with polyurethane sleeves incorporated over the ligaments. Dynesys is the only pedicle-based dynamic stabilization device approved for use today. The synthetic ligaments resist excessive flexion and the polyurethane sleeves limit extension. In extension, it unloads the intervertebral disc by a load-sharing mechanism. The FSU is stabilized in a relatively neutral alignment (as opposed to earlier designs, which induced lordosis). In theory, these devices are designed to add load-sharing ability to a diseased FSU. Several biomechanical studies have confirmed that implantation of these devices leads to reduced loading of the facets, decreased intradiscal pressures, and restoration of normal vertebral motion.[22] Other studies have shown a decrease in adjacent-segment hypermobility and intradiscal pressures.[23]

Despite the initial positive results from pedicle-based dynamic stabilization technologies, several problems have become evident. The polyurethane sleeve is rigid, and if the sleeve is loaded between excessively distracted pedicle screws, kyphosis can be induced. Furthermore, the sleeves place the pedicle screws under significant shear stress in axial loading, and a relatively high number of screw breakages and pull-outs have been observed.[24,25] It has been suggested that these devices actually may be a more effective adjunct to fusion rather than a motion-sparing strategy because several patients with these devices implanted went on to fuse at those segments.[25,26]

Other dorsal pedicle-based dynamic stabilization devices are in varying stages of development and clinical trials. Each uses unique mechanical strategies to overcome the known limitations of such FSU stiffening strategies. Each therefore harbors unique biomechanical nuances that diverge from those described for the Dynesys system. For example, an FEA of a new pedicle-based dynamic stabilization device called FlexPLUS (FlexSpine Pte Ltd.; Singapore) demonstrates a potential superior ability to offload the disc compared with Dynesys.[27] The Universal Clamp (Zimmer SAS; Bordeaux, France) is a non–pedicle-screw-based system that uses a sublaminar polyester band anchored to a supralaminar rod. A cadaveric biomechanical study showed that it effectively reduced total range of motion while preserving normal motion at adjacent levels.[28] This device would prevent the problems of screw loosening and breakage in the Dynesys system.

Total Disc Arthroplasty

Ideally, the clinical objectives of total disc arthroplasty (TDA) should be as follows: to preserve or restore normal biomechanical function, to preserve motion and the center of rotation of the FSU, to provide shock absorption for load transmission with shock attenuation, and to relieve stress on adjacent levels and structures. The implants should mimic the normal intervertebral disc in form and function.

Materials

Several materials are available for use with TDA technologies. Some models use a metal-on-metal interface (most commonly a titanium or cobalt-chromium alloy). This provides for the greatest amount of resistance to wear, but is associated with substantial axial load-related stiffness. Osteolysis from metal particulate debris may also be of concern in metal-on-metal implants.[29] Other devices have a metal-on-hard polymer (usually polyethylene) interface, and are less resistant to wear than their metal-on-metal counterparts. Finally, some devices are constructed of pliable polymers in combination with hard polymers and/or metals. These devices use elastomers that are situated between metal end caps that make contact with the rostral and caudal end plates. These devices typically have the least amount of wear resistance and may be susceptible to failure at the metal-soft polymer interface.[30]

Metals and hard polymers are relatively rigid, especially compared with the gelatinous nucleus pulposus of the healthy disc. The metals and hard polymers that compose the ball-and-socket devices are nearly infinitely stiff in axial loading because these materials have a very low compliance. When axially loaded they tend to act independently of the magnitude of the load and therefore produce a linear stress-strain curve with a uniform slope (see Fig. 159-6). They are not as rigid as a bony fusion. However, they are not nearly as pliable as soft polymers or the intact disc. Material stiffness plays a significant role in offloading of the facets and dorsal elements after implantation. Compared with stiff core implants, implants that use a soft core have a higher propensity to share loads with the facet joints during axial loading because of their greater allowed range of motion. This has been shown to closely resemble intact physiologic forces shared between the healthy disc and the facets.[31] Conversely, implants with high core rigidity bear the vast majority of the axial load alone, and do not share loads with the facets. This is concerning because it may produce a disuse osteopenia in the offloaded facets over time.[31,32] High core rigidity can also lead to high levels of contact stress at the interface between the end plate and metal end cap, especially if they are slightly malpositioned.[33] In general, implants that use soft polymer cores share axial loads with the facets but do not overload them, whereas rigid core implants nearly completely offload the facets. This may lead to higher stresses at the implant-bone interface and atrophy in the offloaded facets.

Design

Many current TDA models use a ball-and-socket design, very similar to prosthetic hips and shoulders. In some of these devices, the ball component is contained entirely within the socket and cannot be separated. This fixes the center of rotation of the implant (and the spinal segment in which it is implanted) in the center of the implant's ball. Many of these implants may be placed with the ball directed rostrally (rostral center) or caudally (caudal center). However, there is no difference in the resulting range of motion with either implant.[34] Unlike the IAR of a normal disc, this center of rotation does not move. Such a device should be placed as dorsally as possible within the disc space (to approximate closely the location of the normal IAR at rest); otherwise, significant stress will be placed on the dorsal osteoligamentous complex.[35] Other ball-and-socket devices use a (usually polymer) semispherical core that acts as the ball and fixed metal sockets that fuse to the end plates. These devices do not have an absolute immobile center of rotation because there is a very small amount of core translation allowed. However, this amount of translation is so small that they are nearly identical to fixed ball-and-socket devices in terms of resulting stress to

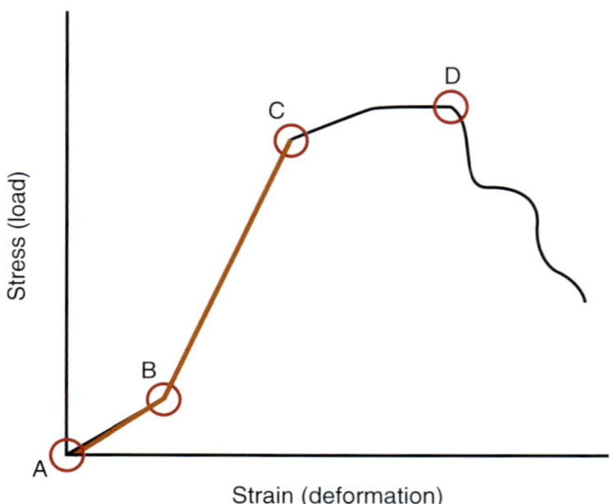

FIGURE 159-7. The stress-strain curve of the ideal total disc arthroplasty device (*orange line*). See Figure 159-3 for an explanation of the different zones (A-B-C).

adjacent structures. These devices are most successful when they use a ball with a large radius of curvature (allowing for more translation and less rotation about the axis of the ball) and are placed as dorsally as possible within the disc space (to better replicate the normal IAR).[18,36]

The most recently developed models of artificial disc use a pliable, soft, thermoplastic silicone polycarbonate urethane core bound by metal end caps that bond to the vertebral end plates. These devices are much more resistant to wear than their less successful polyurethane predecessors and closely replicate the range of motion, flexibility, and stiffness of a normal lumbar disc. Although more studies need to be performed on these devices, they show great promise.

Ideal Total Disc Arthroplasty

In an ideal world, the optimal TDA prosthesis will replicate nearly exactly the healthy intervertebral disc in form and function.

- Its structure will be nearly identical to that of a normal disc, in that it will contain a pliable, free-floating, soft core bound by a firm but flexible ring that both contains the gelatinous core and helps resist torsional forces. By these criteria, the ball-and-socket model does not replicate the anatomy of the normal disc.
- The stress-strain curve of this device will be nonlinear and will closely replicate that of a normal disc (Fig. 159-7). The device will accommodate the initial axial load through deformation, but as the load gradually increases so will the device's resistance to that load.
- The end caps of the device will readily bond with the end plates of the normal surrounding vertebrae.
- The device materials will have acceptable wear, fatigue, and failure resistance properties.
- The device will be constructed in such a manner as not to place undue stress on the surrounding intact spinal elements such as the facets and dorsal ligamentous complex. It will not excessively distract the disc space and will allow for the restoration of the normal variable IAR that moves in response to movement of the spinal unit. The device should restore disc height to a normal level, thereby taking stress off of the dorsal supporting elements.
- The normal range of motion of a healthy spinal unit will be restored by this device. It will not restrict movement of the spinal unit in any way, and it will preserve this motion for the life of the disc. It will not cause fusion at the disc space over time.
- In the unlikely case that the device fails, it should be easily removable and possibly replaceable.

Conclusions

The motion of the FSU is extremely complex. During daily activity the spine responds to a wide range of forces and reacts dynamically. In an attempt to minimize the incidence of accelerated degeneration of segments adjacent to a fused vertebral segment, the field of motion preservation surgery was born. Although early attempts have been suboptimally effective clinically, newer technologies are emerging that show promise. It stands to reason that optimal motion-sparing implants will preserve motion and the center of rotation, provide shock absorption, resist loads, restore biomechanical function, and offload stress on adjacent structures.

Disclaimer

Dr. Benzel is codeveloper of Freedom Lumbar Disc (AxioMed; Cleveland, OH).

KEY REFERENCES

Axelsson P, Johnsson R, Stromqvist B: Adjacent segment hypermobility after lumbar spine fusion: no association with progressive degeneration of the segment 5 years after surgery. *Acta Orthop* 78:834–839, 2007.

Benzel EC: *Biomechanics of spine stabilization*, Rolling Meadows, IL, 2001, American Association of Neurological Surgeons, distributed by Thieme New York.

Ghiselli G, Wang JC, Bhatia NN, et al: Adjacent segment degeneration in the lumbar spine. *J Bone Joint Surg [Am]* 86:1497–1503, 2004.

Huang RC, Wright TM, Panjabi MM, et al: Biomechanics of nonfusion implants. *Orthop Clin North Am* 36:271–280, 2005.

REFERENCES

The complete reference list is available online at expertconsult.com.

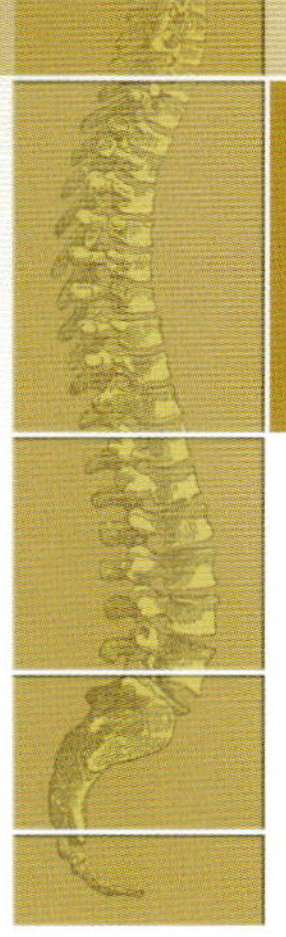

CHAPTER 160

Cervical Total Disc Arthroplasty

John H. Shin | Richard Schlenk

Anterior cervical discectomy and fusion (ACDF) has been routinely used for the treatment of degenerative disease of the cervical spine since the 1950s.[1] Interbody fusion has become the accepted method of treating cervical radiculopathy, myelopathy, segmental deformity, instability, and degenerative disc disease. With the evolution of technique and technology, fusion rates have exceeded 95%.[2] Despite these results, concern for the development of adjacent-level degeneration and disease after fusion has prompted interest in and development of implants designed to preserve motion and maintain anatomic disc space height and normal segmental lordosis. In this chapter, we review the indications for cervical total disc arthroplasty and discuss the preliminary data, with an emphasis on complications and their avoidance. A full discussion of each of the developed artificial discs is beyond the scope of this chapter. Implants for which U.S. Food and Drug Administration (FDA) Investigational Device Exemptions (IDE) studies have been completed are discussed herein.

Rationale for Arthroplasty

The long-term clinical success of ACDF has been limited by the development of adjacent-level degeneration, leading to further symptoms and possibly additional surgery. Adjacent-level degeneration is defined as radiographic changes at a segment adjacent to a fusion and is not necessarily associated with symptoms. Adjacent-level disease, however, is associated with pain, radiculopathy, or myelopathy.[3] Biomechanical studies have demonstrated that cervical fusion alters adjacent-level kinematics and that the loss of motion at the fused segment is compensated by an increase in motion and intradiscal pressure at adjacent levels.[4-6] Some clinical studies have supported these findings, giving weight to this theory of fusion-induced degeneration. Hilibrand et al.[7] reported that repeat surgical intervention was necessary for 2.9% of patients per year for symptomatic adjacent-segment disease after ACDF. They also found that 25% of patients reported symptoms from adjacent-segment disease 10 years after ACDF. In a comparative study, Goffin et al.[8] showed that 92% of fused patients demonstrated radiographic evidence of adjacent-segment degeneration 5 years after surgery for both cervical spondylosis and trauma, suggesting that adjacent-level degeneration is accelerated by fusion and not necessarily the natural history of preexisting degenerative disc disease. It has been postulated that adjacent-level degeneration may be attributable to higher shear strains at levels adjacent to fusions.[9]

Debate continues as to whether adjacent-level degeneration is truly due to increased loads after fusion or to the natural history of degenerative disc disease. In a retrospective study of 303 patients undergoing single-level dorsal cervical foraminotomy for cervical radiculopathy, Clarke et al.[10] showed that 15 (4.9%) of 303 developed symptomatic adjacent-level disease with a 0.7% annual rate for development of adjacent-level disease. The 10-year cumulative incidence of adjacent-level disease was 6.7%.

Biomechanical studies have suggested that cervical arthroplasty may allow for a more normal restoration of load transfer and kinematics at adjacent levels compared with fusion.[5] After disc replacement, stress profiles in specimens at adjacent-level discs were similar to those of intact, nontreated levels, with reduced stresses in the adjacent-level anulus compared with spines with simulated fusions.[11] Cervical disc arthroplasty may therefore be beneficial to patients because in theory it prevents the development of adjacent-segment disease by preserving normal neck motion.

Nomenclature and Design

With the development of numerous artificial discs in the last decade, the Cervical Spine Study Group developed a nomenclature system for cervical arthroplasty.[12] Artificial discs are categorized by material, articulation, fixation, design, and kinematics.[13] They can be classified as nonarticulating, uniarticulating, or biarticulating. Various designs include metal on metal (Prestige ST and LP; Medtronic Sofamor Danek, Memphis, TN), metal on polymer (Bryan, Medtronic Sofamor Danek; ProDisc-C, Synthes Spine, West Chester, PA), ceramic on polymer, or ceramic on ceramic. Discs are either modular with replaceable parts, or nonmodular. Some have points for vertebral body fixation and some have surfaces that promote bone ingrowth at the disc–end-plate interface. With regard to motion, they may be constrained, semiconstrained, or unconstrained. Constrained devices restrict motion to less than that seen physiologically, semiconstrained devices allow physiologic motion, and unconstrained devices rely on soft tissue and the inherent compression across the disc space to limit motion.[14] Each of these devices is available in a range of heights and depths to accommodate individual variances in anatomy.

The Prestige ST artificial disc is constructed of stainless steel and consists of two articulating components attached to the cervical vertebrae with screws (Fig. 160-1). The ball-and-trough design provides relatively unconstrained motion compared with that of a normal cervical spinal segment. The surfaces of the device contacting the end plates are grit-blasted to promote bone osseointegration.

The Prestige LP is the latest version of the Prestige artificial discs and differs from previous models in that fixation to the vertebral bodies is achieved by a set of rails that are imbedded in the vertebral end plates (Fig. 160-2). It is manufactured from a titanium-ceramic composite material that is highly durable and produces little artifact on CT and MRI. The ball-and-trough design is identical to that of the Prestige ST. A porous titanium plasma spray coating on the end-plate surface facilitates bone ingrowth and long-term fixation.

The Bryan cervical disc is designed to allow for motion similar to the normal cervical spine and resembles an actual disc (Fig. 160-3). It consists of two titanium alloy shells with a polyurethane nucleus. The bone-implant interface of each shell has an applied porous coating to facilitate ingrowth of bone and promote long-term stability. The nucleus is surrounded with a polyurethane sheath to establish a closed articulation. Sterile saline is injected into this sheath and functions as an initial lubricant. Titanium alloy seal plugs allow for retention of the saline lubricant. Small ventral flanges on the shells serve as handles to grasp the device for insertion.

The ProDisc-C cervical disc is a metal-on-polyethylene articulating device (Fig. 160-4). This modular implant consists of two cobalt-chromium-molybdenum end plates and an ultra-high molecular weight polyethylene inlay that is preassembled into the inferior. The end plates of the prosthesis are initially secured to the vertebral bodies with central keels and have a plasma-sprayed titanium coating for long-term fixation stability.

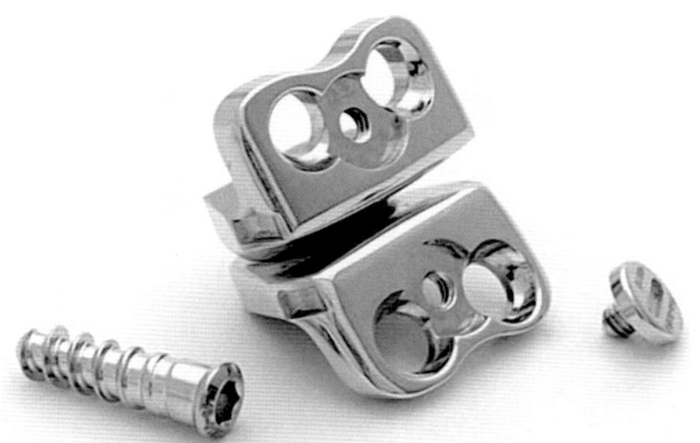

FIGURE 160-1. Prestige ST artificial cervical disc. (Courtesy of Medtronic Sofamor Danek, Memphis, TN.)

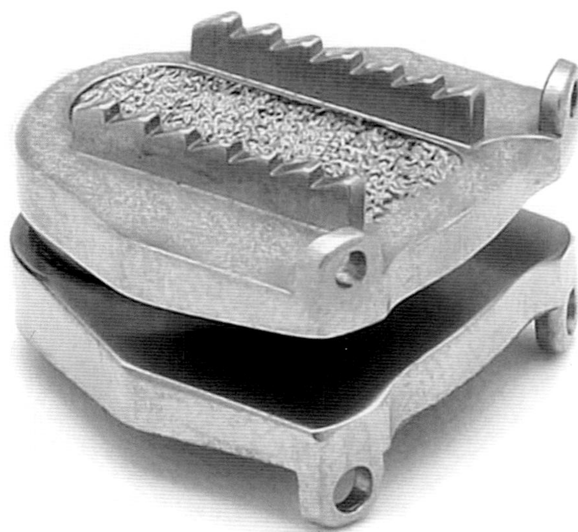

FIGURE 160-2. Prestige LP artificial cervical disc. (Courtesy of Medtronic Sofamor Danek, Memphis, TN.)

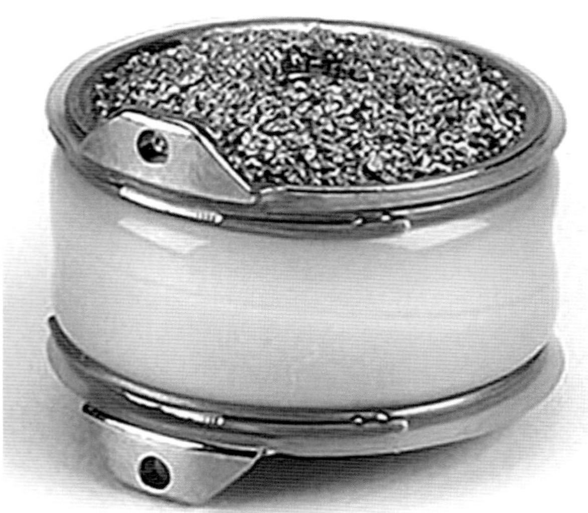

FIGURE 160-3. Bryan artificial cervical disc. (Courtesy of Medtronic Sofamor Danek, Memphis, TN.)

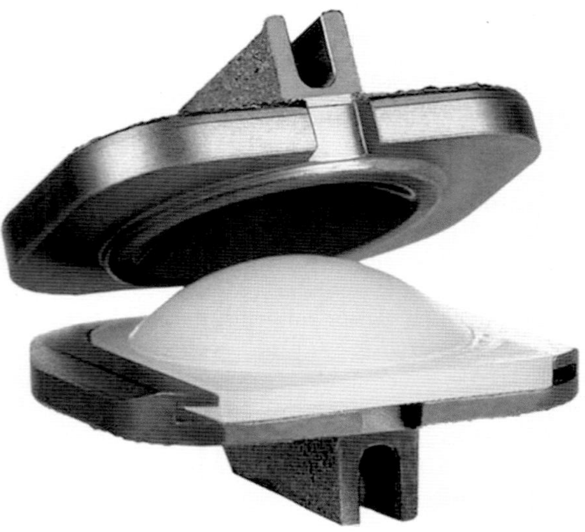

FIGURE 160-4. ProDisc-C artificial cervical disc. (Courtesy of Synthes Spine, West Chester, PA.)

Indications

Patients with cervical radiculopathy secondary to degenerative disc disease at one level with normal cervical spinal alignment and disc height who have failed conservative therapeutics are potential candidates for cervical arthroplasty.[15] Factors to consider when selecting suitable candidates for arthroplasty include the disc height at the level of degeneration, inherent range of motion, and cervical alignment. Arthroplasty requires the dorsal elements to be intact and functional, so patients with suspected ligamentous or facet disease are not suitable candidates. Those with radiographic instability should be treated with an arthrodesis. Those with cervical kyphosis, cervical spondylolisthesis, severe multilevel spondylosis, previous laminectomy, osteoporosis, metabolic bone disease, or cervical trauma are not ideal either.[16] Arthroplasty is contraindicated in the setting of significant segmental or global deformity. A recent history of infection or osteomyelitis precludes the use of a prosthetic disc device. Other relative contraindications include rheumatoid arthritis, renal failure, cancer, and chronic corticosteroid use. Multilevel cervical disc arthroplasty has not yet been evaluated prospectively.

Clinical Outcomes

There are currently seven artificial discs in the United States undergoing FDA IDE trials: Prestige ST, Prestige LP, Bryan, ProDisc-C, PCM (Cervitech, Inc., Rockaway, NJ), Kineflex (Spinal Motion, Inc., Mountain View, CA), and CerviCore (Stryker Spine, Allendale, NJ). To date, European and Australian clinical trials have demonstrated improved clinical outcomes with cervical arthroplasty compared with ACDF when using validated outcome measures such as the Neck Disability Index, an arm pain intensity visual analogue scale, and neurologic status.[15,17-19] No reports of excessive wear debris, material fatigue, fracture, or failure have been reported in any of these trials.[19-23] In the United States, published clinical data are available for the Prestige ST, Bryan, and ProDisc-C artificial discs.

The Prestige ST FDA IDE study was a prospective, multicenter, randomized trial comparing the Prestige ST artificial disc with an arthrodesis with allograft and ventral plate for symptomatic single-level cervical degenerative disc disease.[24] Clinical, radiographic, and outcome measures were followed for a minimum of 2 years. Two hundred seventy-six patients with cervical disc replacement were compared with 265 patients with ACDF. At 2 years, the arthroplasty group had better clinical results and neurologic function than the ACDF group. At 12 and 24 months, Neck Disability Index scores improved in both treatment groups; however, scores for the arthroplasty group were two points higher than for the arthrodesis group. The arthroplasty group had a statistically higher rate of neurologic improvement as well as a lower rate of revision surgery and supplemental fixation. Implant removal was required in five patients with arthroplasty for persistent radiculopathy and neck pain. In each of these cases, the arthroplasty was revised to ACDF. The removal rate was lower in the arthroplasty group, but the difference was not statistically significant. The mean improvement in 36-Item Short Form Health Survey (SF-36) scores was greater in the arthroplasty group at 12 and 24 months. The rate of adjacent-segment reoperation was significantly lower in the arthroplasty group. Three patients in the arthroplasty group required surgery for adjacent-level disease. There were no cases of hardware fracture or migration during the follow-up period for the arthroplasty group. Arthroplasty was able to maintain sagittal motion on average more than 7 degrees.

Similarly, the Bryan cervical disc FDA IDE study was a prospective, multicenter, randomized trial comparing the Bryan artificial disc with an arthrodesis with allograft and ventral plate for symptomatic single-level cervical degenerative disc disease.[25] In this study, 463 patients were randomized to arthroplasty (n = 242) or ACDF (n = 221). Clinical and radiographic evaluations were performed for 2 years after surgery. Pain and function were assessed using the Neck Disability Index, SF-36, and numeric rating scales for neck and arm pain. At 12 and 24 months, both groups showed improvement in all clinical outcome measures, although the arthroplasty group had a statistically greater improvement in the primary outcome measures, mainly the Neck Disability Index. Within the follow-up period, secondary surgical procedures at the treated level were performed in 2.5% of arthroplasty patients and 3.6% of ACDF patients. This difference was not statistically significant. In the arthroplasty group, there were three removals, two reoperations, and one revision. At 2 years after surgery, range of motion in the arthroplasty group was on average 8 degrees. No spontaneous fusions were noted in the arthroplasty group during the follow-up period. Fusion occurred in 94.3% of ACDF patients. Adjacent-level degeneration was not evaluated in this study.

Results from the prospective, randomized, multicenter ProDisc-C FDA IDE study were recently published.[26] Similar to the previously discussed studies, the artificial disc was compared with ACDF for single-level cervical degenerative disease and patients were followed for 2 years. A total of 209 patients were enrolled, with 106 randomized to ACDF and 103 to ProDisc-C. Outcome measures used included neck and arm pain and intensity scale, Neck Disability Index, neurologic status, device success, adverse event occurrence, and SF-36 standardized questionnaires. Neck Disability Index and SF-36 scores were significantly lower compared with presurgery scores at all follow-up visits for both the treatment groups. Neck and arm pain intensity were statistically lower than preoperative levels but not different between treatments. Neurologic success was achieved at 24 months in 90.9% of ProDisc-C and 88.0% of ACDF patients. At 24 months after surgery, 84.4% of ProDisc-C patients achieved at least 4 degrees of motion or maintained motion relative to preoperative baseline at the operated level. There was a statistically significant difference in the number of revisions between the two groups: 8.5% of the ACDF group and 1.8% of the arthroplasty group underwent revisions. The ProDisc-C was successful in 73.5% of patients, versus 60.5% for ACDF at 2 years. Adjacent-level degeneration was not evaluated in this study.

As more FDA IDE studies continue to report their findings of efficacy, safety, and equivalence of various artificial discs to ACDF for single-level degenerative disc disease, further long-term follow-up studies are required to evaluate and scrutinize the ability of these implants to prevent adjacent-level degeneration and preserve motion. In the only published series with long-term follow-up, Robertson and Metcalf[23] reported on the function of the Prestige I cervical disc after 4 years. The authors conducted clinical and radiographic examinations at 3 and 4 years after surgery to evaluate the long-term performance of the Prestige I device. Radiographic analysis in 14 patients showed that the Prestige I disc maintained motion at the treated segment at 3 and 4 years after surgery without the development of adjacent-level degeneration.

Avoidance of Complications

Complications of cervical disc arthroplasty can be attributed to patient selection, to surgical technique, or to the implant itself. Errors in patient selection can be avoided by selecting those patients who meet the previously discussed criteria. Patients with facet arthropathy, preoperative instability, osteoporosis, metabolic bone disease, previous dorsal cervical surgery, or sagittal deformity are not ideal candidates for arthroplasty.

Complications related to surgical technique include those related to surgical approach and implantation technique. Approach-related complications are well known and are the same as those for ACDF, including infection, vascular damage, and dysphagia. Specific implantation technique-related complications have been reported and include implant migration, subsidence, sagittal split fractures, and dorsal vertebral avulsion fractures.[27,28]

In general, when implanting artificial discs, strict attention to patient positioning is crucial to achieving the desired alignment. The neck should be in a neutral or lordotic position. Patients positioned in a kyphotic position will have implants sized inappropriately and this may worsen the overall sagittal alignment and increase the risk of implant migration and extrusion. Because cervical arthroplasty is not meant for sagittal deformity correction, the proper positioning of the patient is critical. Another key component to successful placement is wide, bilateral resection of the uncinate processes. Uncinate resection provides sufficient decompression of the exiting nerve roots to avoid nerve root impingement during extremes of flexion, extension, and rotation with the artificial disc. Proper end-plate preparation is also important to success. If the end plates are violated, subsidence of the implant may occur. This may lead to disc space collapse, causing nerve root compression and restricting the desired motion of the arthroplasty. Subsidence may also occur in osteoporotic patients whose end plates are not violated. Selection of the correct size of implant is also important. Small implants may migrate with repeated motion and large implants may limit range of motion because distraction of the facets and dorsal ligaments hinder the motion preservation mechanism.

Although published results of clinical trials have demonstrated and emphasized the clinical safety and efficacy of cervical arthroplasty, few reports have described complications associated with these implants. Few studies have shown heterotropic ossification as a potential complication of the artificial disc.[29,30] Although this phenomenon has been well described in the orthopedic literature in the context of artificial hip and knee replacements, the exact cause has yet to be determined. In a European multicenter study of the Bryan cervical disc, 16 (17.8%) of the 90 studied patients developed prevertebral ossification at 12 months after implantation.[29] Of these 16 patients, 6 developed heterotropic ossification extending across the vertebral end plate and eliminating motion at that segment. Less than 2 degrees of movement was shown in the other 10 patients. There was no association found between the development of these ossifications and clinical outcomes. It has been suggested that the amount of bone preparation involved with this implantation technique may predispose to heterotropic ossification. Although it has not been formally studied for cervical disc arthroplasty, the prophylactic use of nonsteroidal anti-inflammatory drugs has been suggested to reduce the incidence of heterotropic ossification.

Future Directions

The application of cervical arthroplasty continues to expand, with clinicians showing increasing interest in its use for the treatment of spondylotic myelopathy and multilevel degenerative disc disease. Novel applications for arthroplasty continue to be explored for an aging population with increasingly complex patterns of spinal degeneration. Reports have suggested a role for arthroplasty in treating adjacent-level disease for patients with previous multilevel anterior cervical fusions.[31] Hybrid constructs consisting of arthroplasty and arthrodesis performed in the same setting for multilevel degenerative disease have also been reported, with early results suggesting safety and efficacy.[32]

With regard to spondylotic myelopathy, there is concern that motion preservation may maintain and perpetuate microtrauma to the spinal cord, thus defeating the advantage of arthroplasty. To date, the majority of the literature on cervical arthroplasty has been focused on the outcomes in patients with both radiculopathy and myelopathy as a mixed cohort.[19,22,23] Although several studies have reported on the use of cervical arthroplasty for the treatment of myelopathy, these have been limited by a small number of patients and short follow-up.[15,33,34] Sekhon reported a series of 11 patients who presented with cervical myelopathy and underwent Bryan disc replacement.[33] Five patients were followed for 18 months or more and had improvements in Nurick grade by 1 and Neck Disability Index by 45%.

In a cross-sectional analysis of myelopathic patients who were enrolled in the FDA IDE prospective, randomized, multicenter trials of the Prestige ST and Bryan discs, myelopathic patients in both arthroplasty and arthrodesis groups had significant improvement after surgery, with no worsening myelopathy in the arthroplasty group.[35] Patients included in the study were those with myelopathy and spondylosis or disc herniation at a single level from C3 to C7. General exclusion criteria included the presence of infection, metabolic bone disease, osteoporosis, ankylosing spondylitis, rheumatoid arthritis, and previous cervical surgery. Those with moderate to advanced cervical spondylosis, bridging syndesmophytes, marked reduction or absence of segmental spinal motion, disc space collapse greater than 50%, moderate or severe facet arthropathy, cervical kyphosis or reversal of lordosis, and 2 mm or more of spondylolisthesis and/or 11 degrees or more of angular instability relative to an adjacent segment or segments were also excluded. At 24 months, there were no significant differences in neurologic function or improvement in gait between the arthroplasty and arthrodesis groups. The Neck Disability Index, SF-36, arm and neck pain scores, and gait function improved at all time points. There were no revisions or implant failures in the arthroplasty groups.

As with any emerging technology, the long-term outcomes of cervical arthroplasty will attest to its clinical usefulness and application. Further follow-up will provide useful data regarding arthroplasty and adjacent-level degeneration, material wear, maintenance of cervical lordosis, and motion preservation over time.

KEY REFERENCES

Clarke MJ, Ecker RD, Krauss WE, et al: Same-segment and adjacent-segment disease following posterior cervical foraminotomy. *J Neurosurg Spine* 6:5–9, 2007.

Eck JC, Humphreys SC, Lim TH, et al: Biomechanical study on the effect of cervical spine fusion on adjacent-level intradiscal pressure and segmental motion. *Spine (Phila Pa 1976)* 27:2431–2434, 2002.

Goffin J, Geusens E, Vantomme N, et al: Long-term follow-up after interbody fusion of the cervical spine. *J Spinal Disord Tech* 17:79–85, 2004.

Hilibrand AS, Carlson GD, Palumbo MA, et al: Radiculopathy and myelopathy at segments adjacent to the site of a previous anterior cervical arthrodesis. *J Bone Joint Surg [Am]* 81:519–528, 1999.

Maiman DJ, Kumaresan S, Yoganandan N, et al: Biomechanical effect of anterior cervical spine fusion on adjacent segments. *Biomed Mater Eng* 9:27–38, 1999.

Matsunaga S, Kabayama S, Yamamoto T, et al: Strain on intervertebral discs after anterior cervical decompression and fusion. *Spine (Phila Pa 1976)* 24:670–675, 1999.

Robertson JT, Metcalf NH: Long-term outcome after implantation of the Prestige I disc in an end-stage indication: 4-year results from a pilot study. *Neurosurg Focus* 17:E10, 2004.

REFERENCES

The complete reference list is available online at expertconsult.com.

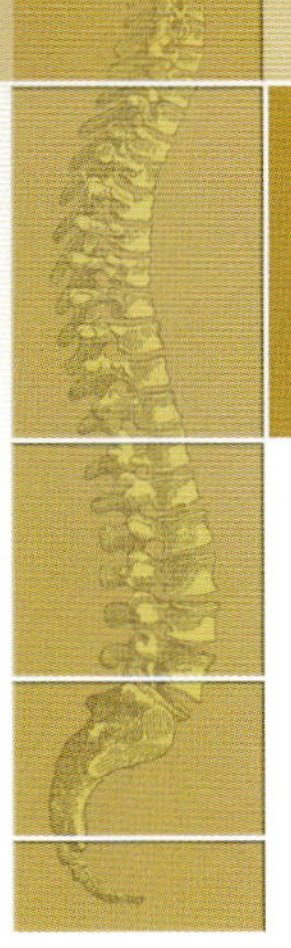

CHAPTER 161

Lumbar Total Disc Arthroplasty

Vladimir Sinkov | Paul C. McAfee

Lumbar degenerative disc disease (DDD) is a common cause of lower back pain—the most frequently encountered complaint in a primary care physician's office. In most cases DDD can be successfully treated nonoperatively with physical therapy, medications, and lifestyle modifications. Surgical treatment for refractory cases classically involves fusion of the affected spinal segment to eliminate motion and the pain that this motion generates. An alternative treatment to spinal fusion is replacement of the painful disc with an artificial prosthesis. Currently, there are two artificial lumbar disc replacement devices approved by the U.S. Food and Drug Administration (FDA): SB Charité (DePuy Spine, Johnson and Johnson, Raynham, MA) and ProDisc L (Synthes Spine, West Chester, PA). Multiple other designs are either in trial and development stages or being used in other countries. Extensive research is now under way into outcomes of lumbar disc replacement.

Background

The intervertebral disc is a complex structure that plays a key role in range of motion and load transfer in the lumbar spine. The nucleus pulposus absorbs compressive loads, whereas the anulus fibrosus resists shear forces and contains the nucleus. A disc in the normal lumbar spine bears 80% of compressive loads. It is subjected to 1 to 2.5 times body weight on ambulation and up to 10 times body weight when lifting a heavy load. The lumbar disc also allows for rotation and translation in three orthogonal planes. The characteristics of motion vary according to the level, with more rotation occurring in the upper lumbar spine and more flexion and extension in the lower lumbar spine. The center of rotation in the sagittal plane is usually located dorsal and caudal to the center of the distal end plate, but varies slightly with flexion and extension.[1]

With disc degeneration, the nucleus pulposus loses water content and becomes less compliant, leading to collagen degeneration and fissures in the anulus. Inflammatory cytokines are released from the nucleus and sensory nerve fibers proliferate deeper into the disc space, resulting in discogenic pain. The disc's biomechanical characteristics also become altered. As the disc becomes more rigid and loses height, more stress is transferred to the facet joints. The natural history of this process results in eventual disc space collapse, foraminal narrowing, facet degeneration, soft tissue hypertrophy, and compression of neural elements.

The gold standard of operative treatment for DDD in patients who fail conservative therapy is arthrodesis of the affected segment and decompression of stenosis, if needed. This may be accomplished through a dorsal approach, ventral approach, or a combination of the two with or without iliac crest autograft. The procedure has been performed since 1911 and carries success rates of between 60% and 90%. This treatment, however, has several significant drawbacks. Pseudarthrosis rates are reported at 14%.[2] Evidence of adjacent-segment degeneration is observed in 30% to 40% of fusions.[3,4] Iliac crest autograft harvesting results in significant rates of postoperative complications and donor site pain.[5]

Given the limitations of the established operative options for patients with DDD and considering the very high and reproducible success rates in arthroplasty of hip and knee joints, the need for an effective total disc replacement (TDR) alternative in the lumbar spine becomes obvious. The lumbar disc's structure and biomechanical characteristics are very complex. A successful TDR design must take into account multiple factors, including the multidirectional angular and translational range of motion, variable center of rotation, and need for ingrowth into vertebral end plates without significant subsidence. The implant materials must be durable enough to sustain approximately 8 million cycles per year without accruing significant wear.

Indications

As with many other spine operations, proper patient selection is one of the most important aspects of a successful TDR. The most common indications used in current disc replacement surgeries are listed in Box 161-1.[6] Typical indications are illustrated in Figure 161-1. The vast majority of patients who qualify for TDR are younger than 60 years of age. This excludes most patients with degenerative processes in dorsal spinal structures (e.g., facet degeneration, ligamentum flavum hypertrophy, disc herniation) and with inadequate bone stock. Bertagnoli et al. have shown that in a carefully selected group of patients older than 60 years of age, a TDR procedure resulted in equivalent patient satisfaction rates.[7] Even in this group of 22 patients, however, there were 2 cases

BOX 161-1. Common Indications and Contraindications for Lumbar Total Disc Arthroplasty

Indications

Age 18 to 60 years
Symptomatic DDD confirmed by discography
Failure of nonoperative therapy for at least 6 months
Ability to tolerate anterior approach

Absolute Contraindications

Poor bone quality (e.g., osteoporosis, osteopenia, metabolic bone disease, tumor)
Facet degeneration
Spondylolisthesis and spondylolysis
Circumferential stenosis
Herniated disc with radiculopathy not amenable to anterior indirect decompression
Scoliotic deformity greater than 11 degrees
Current or past trauma to involved vertebrae
Morbid obesity
Infection
Autoimmune disorder

Relative Contraindications

Age older than 60 years
Psychosocial disorder
Multiple DDD levels
Obesity

DDD, degenerative disc disease.

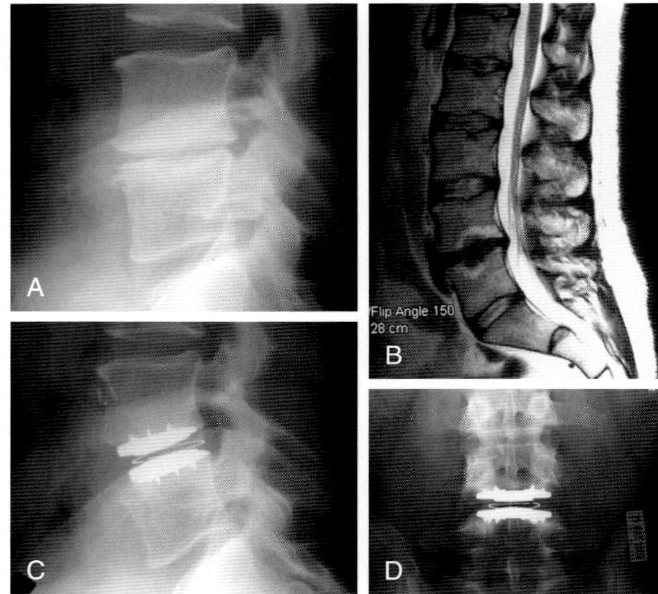

FIGURE 161-1. Indications for lumbar arthroplasty: typical case example. **A,** A 47-year-old male executive who has been disabled for 9 months due to lumbar spondylosis at L4-5, with mechanical back pain radiating down the posterolateral aspect of his right thigh and an Oswestry Disability Index (ODI) score of 55. **B,** Sagittal MRI shows single-level disc disease at L4-5, Modic type II changes. His discogram was also positive for concordant pain when his L4-5 disc was stimulated, but not when L3-4 or L5-S1 were injected. **C,** He underwent In Motion lumbar disc arthroplasty (the updated version of the Charité arthroplasty) with complete relief of his mechanical back pain (postoperative ODI = 5). He has returned to work full time. The lateral radiograph demonstrates good restoration of disc space height, which is uniformly successful with many types of arthroplasty. **D,** Anteroposterior radiograph of the In Motion Charité arthroplasty shows an ideal midline position of this nonkeeled type of lumbar disc replacement.

of radiculopathy due to circumferential stenosis and 2 cases of implant subsidence. DDD must be shown to be the main, if not the only, source of the back pain. Positive radiographic findings and a concordant discogram are currently thought to be the best ways to confirm DDD. Because most cases of low back pain from DDD resolve with nonoperative treatment, surgical candidates must have failed those options. They must have significant pain and disability to justify the potential risks and recovery period associated with operative intervention. Because current TDR implants are designed for a ventral surgical approach, patients must be able to tolerate such an approach from the standpoint of prior surgical interventions in that area and medical comorbidities.

TDR implants rely on fixation to vertebral end plates and ingrowth. Therefore, the patient's bone quality must be adequate. Osteoporosis, osteopenia due to a metabolic disorder, or tumor may cause implant failure by dislodgement or subsidence. Because lumbar TDR replaces only ventral elements of the spinal column, a good candidate for disc replacement should not have degeneration of dorsal structures, especially the facet joints. Radiographic studies and facet blocks may be used to diagnose facet arthropathy. Even though ventral insertion of a TDR device may offer some indirect decompression, circumferential stenosis is best treated by direct decompression of neural elements through a dorsal approach with fusion, if needed. Studies have shown that the disc space preparation necessary for insertion of a lumbar TDR increases the rotational instability of the spine. The currently available unconstrained disc replacement implants do not fully restore this stability.[8] Therefore, TDR in a spine with preexisting rotational instability (Cobb angle >11 degrees) might be expected to result in higher rates of failure.

Current Designs

Although only two TDR implants are currently approved by the FDA, there are multiple designs in various stages of testing and development. Charité is the oldest and one of the most extensively studied of the current-generation TDR designs. The first version, SB CHARITÉ I, was first implanted in 1984. The implant underwent two modifications and has been used in its current version, SB CHARITÉ III, since 1994. It consists of two cobalt-chromium end plates with a biconvex sliding central core of ultra-high molecular weight polyethylene (UHMWPE). This results in a floating center of rotation, allowing angular motion and translation. To encourage bony ingrowth, the end plates are covered with plasma-sprayed titanium and electrochemically coated with calcium phosphate. This has been shown in animal studies to result in 48% osseointegration, compared with the 10% to 30% ingrowth seen in successful hip and knee replacement prostheses.[9,10] The implant is inserted using a standard ventral retroperitoneal approach and is approved for single-level use.

TABLE 161-1

Current Lumbar Total Disk Replacement Designs

Implant	Manufacturer	Key Features	Approved Use
SB Charité	DePuy Spine (Raynham, MA)	Two metal end plates with biconvex mobile UHMWPE insert	Single-level lumbar disk replacement
ProDisc-L II	Synthes Spine (West Chester, PA)	Two metal end plates with fixed uniconvex UHMWPE insert	Single-level lumbar disk replacement
Maverick	Medtronic Sofamor Danek (Memphis, TN)	Two metal end plates with metal-on-metal articulation	In FDA IDE trial
FlexiCore	Stryker Spine (Allendale, NJ)	Two metal end plates with metal-on-metal articulation	In FDA IDE trial

FDA, U.S. Food and Drug Administration; IDE, Investigational Device Exemption; UHMWPE, ultra-high molecular weight polyethylene.

Another FDA-approved TDR implant, the ProDisc L, was originally developed in 1990 and has undergone one design revision since then. It also contains two cobalt-chromium end plates, but the UHMWPE insert is monoconvex and locked into the distal end plate. This results in a ball-and-socket joint that limits translation and allows rotation. A central keel on the end plates and plasma-sprayed titanium coating allow for bony fixation and ingrowth. Two other TDR implants designed for a ventral approach are currently in FDA Investigational Device Exemptions study stages: FlexiCore (Stryker Spine, Allendale, NJ) and Maverick (Medtronic Sofamor Danek, Memphis, TN). Both products have end plates with metal-on-metal, ball-and-socket articulations. Key features of current TDR designs are listed in Table 161-1.

Because of the known complications that have occurred during device implantation, including dislodgement and the need for revision surgery using the ventral approach, there is extensive work being done on TDR designs implanted by other means.[11] Among them is TRIUMPH (Globus Medical, Inc., Audubon, PA), which is inserted through a standard dorsolateral approach. It consists of two metal-on-metal articulating components of cobalt-chromium alloy with a titanium porous coating and multiple keels for bony ingrowth and fixation. The dorsal approach allows the surgeon to address any pathology in the dorsal structures, including facet overgrowth, disc herniation, and soft tissue hypertrophy. The smaller anulotomy and preservation of the anterior longitudinal ligament leaves the segment with greater stability. Such a design might greatly expand the surgical indications for TDR because most patients with DDD also have some pathologic processes in the dorsal structures. Another aspect of TDR research involves the search for alternative bearing surfaces. ORBIT (Globus Medical, Inc.) is an artificial disc that includes articulating polyetheretherketone (PEEK) units with a porous titanium coating for bony ingrowth. This results in nearly complete radiolucency, improved MRI compatibility, and excellent wear characteristics.

Nucleus Replacement

An alternative direction in disc replacement technology involves an artificial nucleus substitute, also known as *partial disc replacement*. The rationale behind this strategy is to remove the pain generator and restore the disc's biomechanical properties, while preserving more of the anulus and stability than in classic TDR.[12] The original designs by Fernstrom (stainless steel ball), Nachemson (injectable silicone), and Hamby and Glaser (bone cement) in the 1950s and 1960s failed to prevent further disc degeneration.[13-15] Better biomaterials have become available recently, prompting a new wave of nucleus replacement technologies. The earliest and most widely used of the current nucleus replacement designs is the Prosthetic Disc Nucleus (PDN, Raymedica Inc., Bloomington, MN). It consists of a hydrogel pellet in a polyurethane envelope. After implantation, the hydrogel absorbs water and expands to the limits of its outer liner, restoring disc height. An earlier design used two implants inserted into the disc space. In response to high rates of dislodgement, the implant was redesigned to a larger single pellet—the PDN-SOLO. New approaches are also being tested to lower dislodgement rates.[16] Other constrained, unconstrained, and injectable devices are being tested, but complication rates remain high. In addition, indications for nucleus replacement are more limited than those for TDR, and include at least 50% disc height preservation and an intact anulus.[12]

Outcomes

In a prospective, randomized, multicenter, FDA-regulated IDE clinical trial, the Charité disc was compared with the gold standard procedure of anterior interbody fusion using Bagby and Kuslich (BAK) threaded cages (Zimmer Spine, Minneapolis, MN) and iliac crest autograft.[6] Three hundred and four patients were enrolled, with approximately 95% follow-up at 12 months and 90% at 24 months. Data analysis demonstrated that the Charité implant was equivalent to the BAK cage regarding Oswestry Disability Index (ODI) scores and visual analogue scale (VAS) scores at 24-month follow-up. The TDR group had significantly shorter hospital stays (3.7 vs. 4.2 days), higher patient satisfaction rates (73.7% vs. 53.1%), and higher overall clinical success rates (57.1% vs. 46.5%). Index-level range of motion was preserved postoperatively, as illustrated in Figure 161-2. The conclusion of the study was that the Charité disc was at least as good as the control procedure in treatment of one-level DDD. Five-year follow-up to this study showed persistence of equivalent improvement in VAS and ODI scores between the two groups.[17] It also found that more patients in the TDR group were employed full time (65.6% vs. 46.5%) and fewer patients were on long-term disability (8% vs. 20.9%). Surgery for adjacent-level disease was performed on one Charité patient

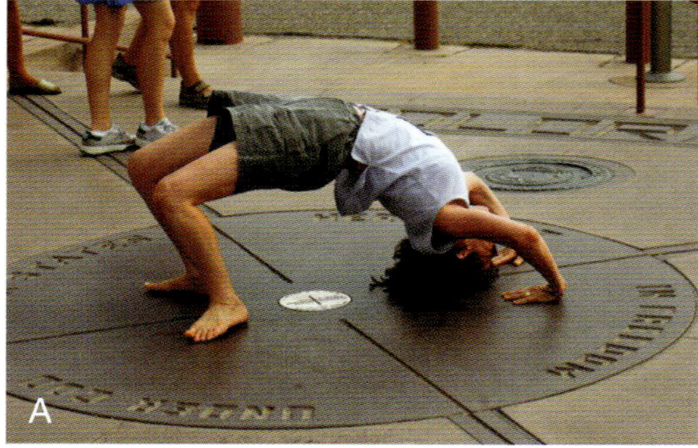
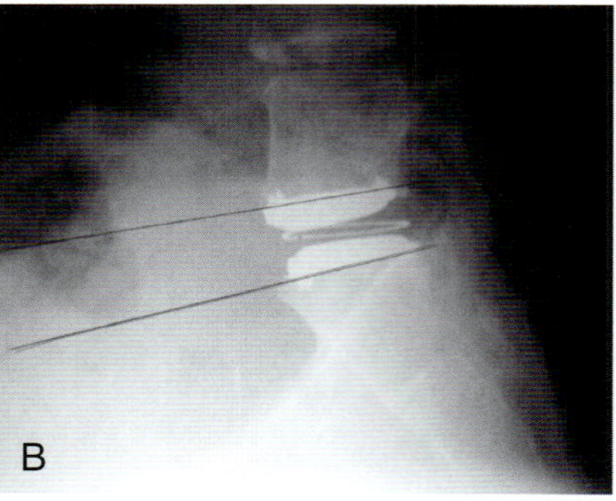
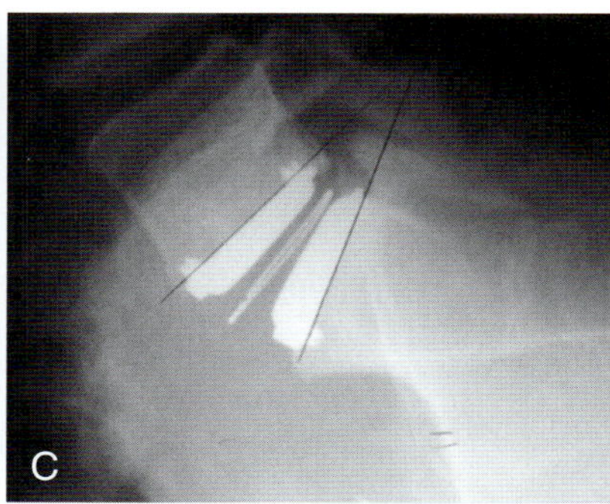

FIGURE 161-2. The average postoperative segmental mobility is more than 7 degrees of flexion-extension with lumbar arthroplasty. **A,** One year after lumbar disc replacement, this 52-year-old woman shows better global range of lumbar motion than before surgery because of resolution of pain and disability. She is performing a back bend with each extremity in a different state—"The Four Corners" of Utah, Arizona, Colorado, and New Mexico. **B,** Her lateral flexion radiograph 12 months after surgery. **C,** Accompanying lateral extension radiograph documents 18 degrees of flexion-extension range of motion.

and two BAK patients (1.1% vs. 4.7%), but these numbers were too small to show statistical significance. There was a significant patient dropout between years 2 and 5, with only 44% follow-up at 5 years. Comparison of the 5-year completers and the patients lost to follow-up showed that at 2 years the two groups were statistically similar in ODI and VAS scores. This demonstrates that the study's conclusion of the noninferiority of the Charité device to anterior fusion is still valid. Two recently published, nonrandomized, 10-year follow-up studies on the Charité arthroplasty demonstrated 80% to 90% good and excellent clinical outcomes, a 2% rate of adjacent-level degeneration, and close to a 90% return-to-work rate.[18,19]

Concurrently, a prospective, randomized, multicenter, FDA-regulated IDE clinical trial was conducted to compare the ProDisc L implant with circumferential fusion at one level in the lumbar spine.[20] At 24 months, the TDR group had similar improvement in VAS scores (41.6% vs. 36%), but a greater number of patients in the disc replacement group had improvements in ODI scores of more than 15 points (77.2% vs. 64.8%). The experimental group also had a statistically greater number of patients employed or enjoying recreational activities at 24 months after surgery than the control group. Index-level range of motion was preserved in 97% of patients. One limitation of this study was the fact that a ventral-only experimental surgery was compared with a front/back control surgery with an inherently greater operative time and risk of complications.

Leahy et al. used the data from this trial to evaluate whether the presence of prior decompressive surgery had any effect on outcomes of ProDisc L TDR.[21] Patients with prior microdiscectomy or traditional laminectomy and discectomy were compared with those without prior lumbar surgeries in the TDR cohort. The outcomes in both groups were similar, indicating that disc replacement is a viable option for patients with prior disc surgeries.

Tropiano et al. reported midterm results from a nonrandomized study on outcomes with the ProDisc I TDR.[22] They followed 64 patients with single- or multiple-level disc replacement for an average of 8.7 years. Approximately 75% of patients had good to excellent results in pain and functional improvement and 79% were satisfied or entirely satisfied with the outcome. The authors noted that small but significant negative effects on outcomes were seen in patients younger than 45 years of age and those with prior lumbar surgery. It should be noted that this study used an older ProDisc design that has since been improved.

Siepe et al. analyzed data from an ongoing, nonrandomized study on the ProDisc II to compare outcomes of TDR at different spinal segments.[23] Ninety-nine patients had TDR at L4-5, L5-S1, or both levels and were followed for an average of 25.8 months. All patients had significant improvement from baseline in ODI and VAS scores. The best results were achieved with L4-5 TDR, followed by L5-S1 TDR. TDR at both levels resulted in the worst outcomes. The incidence of facet or sacroiliac joint pain confirmed by injection was 9.1% in L4-5 TDR, 28.1% in L5-S1 TDR, and 60% in patients with both levels replaced. Bisegmental disc replacement also led to higher rates of complications and need for revision surgery.

Complications

Complications in TDR surgery can be divided into approach-related, device-related, and patient-related complications.[11] Currently available disc replacement devices are designed for the ventral approach. The most serious complications from this approach include injuries to the major vessels and ureters, as well as retrograde ejaculation. In current TDR studies, such complications are seen in up to 10% of patients, which is similar to the rates seen in anterior spinal fusions.[6]

Device-related complications include implant subsidence, migration or extrusion, malposition, and material wear. Subsidence is by far the most common issue, seen in up to 9% of TDRs in older studies and in 3% of patients in more recent trials.[3,5,6] Subsidence has also been observed in up to 56% of failed TDRs.[24] Of note, no clear clinical effect of subsidence on outcomes has yet been demonstrated. This complication may be minimized by screening patients with poor bone quality and seating the implants on the more cortical peripheral edges of the vertebral end plates. The risk of device migration or extrusion depends significantly on implant design, placement, and sizing. A TDR implant inserted in the midline that can be fixed to bone with spikes or keels, promotes bony ingrowth to the end plates, and is sized to provide good soft tissue tension would have a very low chance of migrating. In earlier studies, the rates of migration were up to 7%, but with improved designs and surgical experience, more recent studies have shown rates of 0% to 1%.[3,17,22] There are no reports of confirmed adverse reactions to particulate wear debris, and significant wear has been mostly associated with implant malpositioning.[24,25] Cunningham demonstrated, in an animal model, that only a local histiocytic reaction and no neuropathology or significant systemic or local response was observed in response to the wear particles generated by TDRs.[10] Most device-related complications are iatrogenic and can be minimized with proper patient selection, operative technique, and implant sizing.

Patient-related complications include adjacent-level disc degeneration, same-level facet degeneration, and heterotopic ossification. Successful motion preservation is the main mechanical goal of lumbar TDR. This has been well documented in recent studies.[17,20] The adjacent-segment degeneration seen after arthrodesis is thought to be related to increased stress at adjacent segments due to transfer of extra motion and loads from the fused segment. There are currently no long-term studies that definitively show that motion preservation using TDR avoids accelerated adjacent-segment degeneration. Intermediate-term data by Huang et al. using the ProDisc implant show that range of motion of at least 5 degrees is needed for improved clinical outcomes and reduction in degeneration of adjacent discs.[26]

The presence of degenerative disease in the facet joints is a contraindication to lumbar TDR. Early disease in the facets may be missed during initial screening, and patients may continue to experience pain after surgery from persistent motion in these degenerated dorsal structures. In a study assessing 175 patients complaining of persistent pain after ProDisc II implantation, facet joints were confirmed as a source by fluoroscopically guided blocks in 12.6% of patients, mostly at the index level (84%).[27] Van Ooij et al. reported facet joint arthrosis in 42% of patients with persistent pain after Charité TDR.[24] All 29 patients with failed TDRs in a study by Rosen et al. had evidence of facet distraction or compression on CT.[28] Facet distraction was also associated with radiculopathy, likely from capsular stretch.

TDR design may also affect the manner in which the facets are loaded. In the normal lumbar spine, the facets are loaded with ventral shear forces. TDR implants with a floating center of rotation, such as the Charité, maintain such a load on the facets, potentially accelerating degeneration. On the other hand, implants with a fixed center of rotation, such as the ProDisc, absorb anteroposterior shear forces, thus creating greater stress within the implant and at the implant-bone interface, while sparing the facets. The fixed center of rotation creates a greater arc of motion to compensate for the lack of translation. This changes the kinematics of a facet joint, causing greater stresses at the extremes of flexion and extension.[1]

Heterotopic ossification, limiting the TDR's range of motion, is of some concern. Although it was observed often with earlier implant designs, studies with modern TDRs show significantly lower rates. In addition, Tortolani et al. have reviewed the data from the Charité IDE study and evaluated the clinical significance of heterotopic ossification. Of 276 patients, 12 (4.3%) had radiographic evidence of new bone formation. All of these patients had ranges of motion and clinical outcomes similar to the rest of the study population.[29]

The rates of complications with TDR surgeries are relatively low. Nevertheless, strategies for revision have been developed. If additional surgery is necessary, either a ventral or a dorsal approach is used. Repeat ventral surgery carries a significantly higher risk of intraoperative complications. In the Charité IDE study, the incidence of vessel injury during reoperation was significantly greater than that with the index operation (16.7% vs. 3.6%), mostly because of scarring to the vertebral column.[30] Other structures at risk due to scarring and distorted anatomy are the ureters and the lumbosacral trunk. These complications may be minimized with use of preoperative angiography and the intraoperative placement of intravascular balloons and ureteral stents.

An alternative revision procedure involves dorsal fusion with dynamic or rigid instrumentation. This strategy avoids the area of previous surgery and solves problems of instability or persistent pain. Cunningham et al. performed an in vitro biomechanical analysis of such a construct. They found that augmentation of a ventrally placed TDR with dorsally placed pedicle screws provided stability similar to that of the combination of ventral cage and dorsal pedicle screws (circumferential fusion construct).[31] If TDR components must be removed because of dislodgement or malposition, however, the dorsal approach is inadequate. Alternative approaches, such as transperitoneal, contralateral retroperitoneal, and transpsoas (for levels L4-5 and above), have been described.

A prophylactic strategy involves placing an antiadhesive barrier over the vertebral column after TDR implantation to prevent scarring after a primary anterior approach. Various liquid and solid products are available and have been shown to be effective in adhesion prevention with abdominal and pelvic surgery.[32] These products are yet to be evaluated in the setting of lumbar TDR.

Future Direction

Lumbar TDR is a relatively new field with enormous potential for advancement. Long-term outcome studies are needed to show favorable results and TDR's ability to decrease the incidence of adjacent-level degeneration. Additional studies are also needed to evaluate the use of lumbar disc replacement in patients not included in current IDE trials. Potential benefits of TDR in a setting of disc herniation are illustrated in Figure 161-3.

Appropriate patient selection and proper surgical technique remain as the key aspects of successful arthroplasty. Future implant designs should improve biomechanics, possibly resulting in modular implants to address varying kinematics at different lumbar spine segments or the need for multiple-level surgery. Alternative approaches for TDR could eliminate risks associated with anterior retroperitoneal primary and revision surgery. Circumferential arthroplasty technology could allow for simultaneous disc and facet joint replacement, which would significantly broaden indications for lumbar joint replacement.

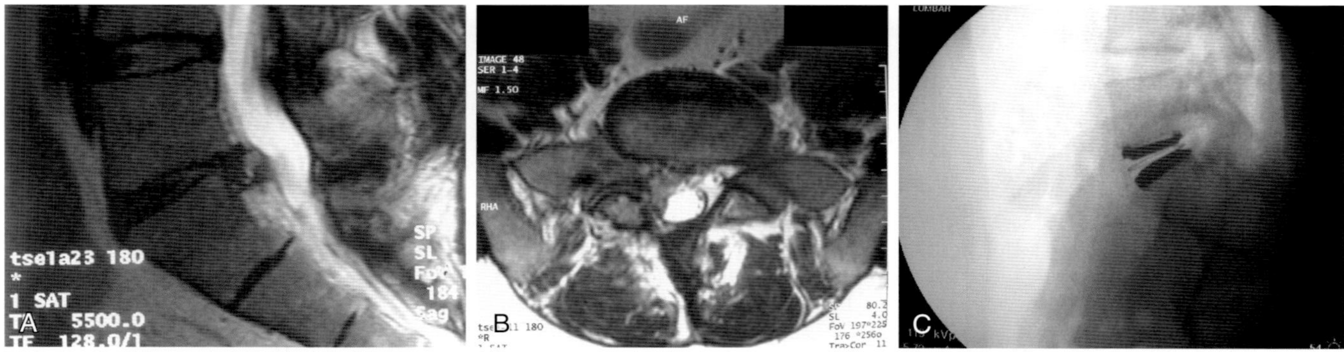

FIGURE 161-3. Indications for ventral lumbar discectomy and arthroplasty with recurrent lumbar disc herniation. **A,** This 27-year-old manual laborer has a right-sided recurrent lumbar herniated disc at L5-S1. He had already failed two lumbar posterior laminectomies. Sagittal MRI documents a posterior free fragment herniation, severe right S1 nerve root compression, and posterior fibrosis. **B,** Axial MRI confirms the severity of the lumbar disc herniation at L5-S1. **C,** Postoperative lateral radiograph after anterior retroperitoneal discectomy, removal of the herniated free fragment, and implantation of a lumbar disc replacement. Herniated lumbar disc disease was not included in the FDA studies for lumbar arthroplasty because this might have confounded the results with leg pain due to nerve root compression. There is no question, however, that the success rates of lumbar arthroplasty would have been improved if the FDA studies had included patients presenting with mechanical compression of neural elements and symptomatic radiculopathy. One should keep this fact in mind when interpreting "artificially pure" prospective FDA studies of lumbar arthroplasty.

KEY REFERENCES

Blumenthal S, McAfee PC, Guyer RD, et al: A prospective, randomized, multicenter Food and Drug Administration investigational device exemptions study of lumbar total disk replacement with the CHARITÉ™ artificial disc versus lumbar fusion. Part I: evaluation of clinical outcomes. *Spine (Phila Pa 1976)* 30:1565–1575, 2005.

Cunningham BW: Basic scientific considerations in total disc arthroplasty. *Spine J* 4(Suppl 6):219S–230S, 2004.

Guyer RD, McAfee PC, Banco RJ, et al: Prospective, randomized, multicenter Food and Drug Administration investigational device exemption study of lumbar total disc replacement fusion: five-year follow-up. *Spine J* 9:374–386, 2009.

Huang RC, Girardi FP, Cammisa FP Jr, et al: Correlation between range of motion and outcome after lumbar total disc replacement: 8.6-year follow-up. *Spine (Phila Pa 1976)* 30:1407–1411, 2005.

Patel AA, Brodge DS, Pimenta L, et al: Revision strategies in lumbar total disc arthroplasty. *Spine (Phila Pa 1976)* 33:1276–1283, 2008.

Siepe CJ, Korge A, Grochulla F, et al: Analysis of post-operative pain patterns following total lumbar disc replacement: results from fluoroscopically guided spine infiltrations. *Eur J Spine* 17:44–56, 2008.

Zigler J, Delamarter R, Spivak JM, et al: Results of the prospective, randomized, multicenter Food and Drug Administration investigational device exemption study of the ProDisc-L total disc replacement versus circumferential fusion for the treatment of 1-level degenerative disc disease. *Spine (Phila Pa 1976)* 32:1155–1162, 2007.

REFERENCES

The complete reference list is available online at expertconsult.com.

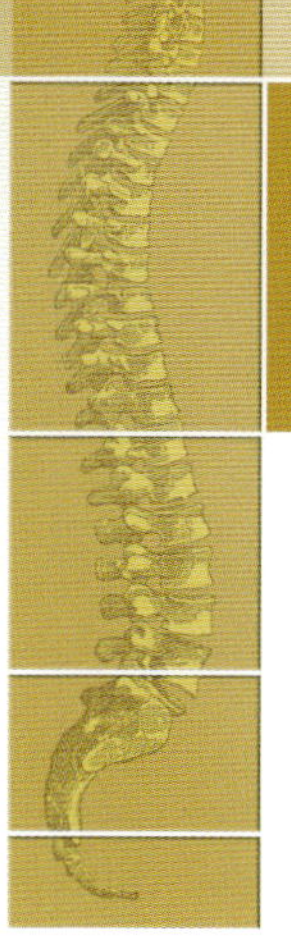

CHAPTER 162

Second-Generation Total Disc Arthroplasty

Krzysztof Siemionow | Isador H. Lieberman

The three basic functions of the spinal column are to allow movement, transmit loads, and protect the neural elements. The functional spinal unit (FSU) as defined by White and Panjabi[1] consists of a three-joint complex including the disc (end plate, anulus fibrosus, and nucleus pulposus) and the dorsal facet joints. More recently, the FSU has been redefined to include the passive and active constraints that are provided by the attached ligaments and muscles. The FSU performs as a continuous, semiconstrained joint, where complex three-dimensional movements occur. These movements, which occur through 6 degrees of freedom, include axial compression and distraction and anterior, posterior, and lateral bending, translation, and rotation. These movements are constrained by the need to protect neurologic elements and yet maintain the head balanced over the pelvis to facilitate interaction with the surrounding environment.

FSUs are typically subject to ongoing degenerative changes. These degenerative changes represent a continuum of mechanical deterioration, secondary to multiple etiologies (e.g., natural history, trauma, metabolic conditions), which may or may not be symptomatic (e.g., mechanical pain, inflammatory pain, radicular pain, stenotic symptoms). As the FSU degenerates, the normal biomechanical parameters are altered, and compensatory mechanisms (e.g., loss of lumbar lordosis, hip and knee flexion posture) are recruited to achieve the goals of spinal balance and motion.

The current surgical "gold standard" strategy for treating symptomatic degeneration of the FSU is to stabilize the degenerated segment by fusing the affected spinal level. The goal of fusion is to restore the native anatomic relationships including disc height, lordosis, and coronal alignment, while relieving the patient's painful symptoms. Surgical strategies have evolved from dorsal, dorsolateral, ventral, instrumented, and uninstrumented fusions to contemporary techniques involving interbody cages and synthetic and biologic bone substitutes. Despite this evolution, the results of fusion are less than perfect, with fusion rates ranging from 60% to 90% and clinical outcome improvement rates ranging from 60% to 70%.[2] Spinal fusion also is associated with the longer-term problem of increasing the strain at the adjacent levels, potentially contributing to premature degenerative changes.[3] To date, none of the increasingly complex implants and instruments has resulted in an improvement in the outcomes of fusion; with this in mind, similar to the evolution to arthroplasty from fusion of a peripheral joint, a philosophy of spine arthroplasty instead of spinal fusion is now evolving.

In the development of a spinal arthroplasty system, one must consider the following five principal issues: (1) an understanding of how the spine reacts to loading in the normal and degenerative state; (2) the ability of the device to replicate FSU mechanical properties including motion; (3) the clinical effectiveness of the arthroplasty device; (4) the ability of the device to prevent adjacent-level premature deterioration; and (5) the revisability of the implant in the event of infection, dislodgement, or device failure.

Spinal Biomechanics in the Normal and Degenerated Spine

Disc degeneration is part of the natural aging process, and it does not always result in painful conditions. Lee[4] compiled a critical literature review of spinal biomechanics for the lumbar spine, describing the significance of the individual spinal elements and their impact on maintaining a healthy, functioning spine. Analysis of the data Lee compiled shows that providing motion is not the primary function of the native disc, but that passive resistance to the forces during motion is the more important factor to be considered when designing a strategy for long-term restoration of the FSU. Likewise, Ito et al.[5] verified the notion of passive resistance by describing the nonlinear relationship between compressive load and disc stiffness. They reported low stiffness at lower loads (800 N/mm at 1000 N) and proportionately higher stiffness at higher loads (2000 N/mm at 4000 N). This differential allows for less resistance to motion at the lower loads of daily activities and more resistance to motion at the higher loads. This phenomenon presumably works to maintain spinal alignment and to protect the neurologic structures throughout the full range of motion.

Kimura et al.[6] illustrated and quantified the effect of loading on the lumbar spine in eight volunteers. These investigators described the functional response of the lumbar spine and the ability of the spine to adapt to normal loading. Their key finding was that the spine when loaded first responds by increasing the native lordotic or kyphotic curvature and subsequently responds by altering disc height. These changes in disc height and the differential stiffness described by Ito et al.[5] are reflections of the viscoelastic and biomechanical nature of the nucleus, anulus, and end-plate complex.

During development of the "follower load" biomechanical model, Patwardhan et al.[7] defined the mechanism by which the spinal system attempts to maintain and reduce the localized shear stress on each intervertebral disc at or near zero during body movements. The shear stress, if left unchecked, presumably can cause intradiscal disruption and injury, possibly contributing to degeneration and mechanical dysfunction. Clinically, any disruption of an index FSU either ventrally or dorsally by injury, aging, or surgery may exaggerate the degeneration observed at the adjacent levels, as a result of the spinal system attempting to compensate for a compromised index FSU.

Kirkaldy-Willis[8,9] schematically depicted the pathophysiology of degeneration of the lumbar spine as a degenerative cascade (Fig. 162-1). He described the three phases of degeneration as dysfunction, instability, and ultimately restabilization. Early degenerative events, such as disc herniation, lead to decreased stiffness of the spine. The natural response of the body is to resist abnormal stresses and strains with physiologic responses, such as osteophyte formation. Osteophytes are a manifestation of the body's attempt to reduce the shear stress toward zero and to restore the load-bearing capacity of the FSU. The fact that the restoration of stability and load bearing may lead to other clinical pathologies (e.g., nerve compression and loss of motion) emphasizes the critical importance of stability and load bearing even at the expense of neurologic compromise and loss of flexibility.

With the aforementioned in mind, any surgical intervention, especially disc arthroplasty, must take the biomechanical responses, the inherent disc function, and the degenerative cascade into account. Following the algorithm created by Kirkaldy-Willis,[8,9] the body's natural response to degenerative changes is to work toward stabilization, reducing motion through increased stiffness and osteophyte formation. It is imperative to match the proposed treatment to the stage of degeneration. If intervention on the degenerated disc uses a

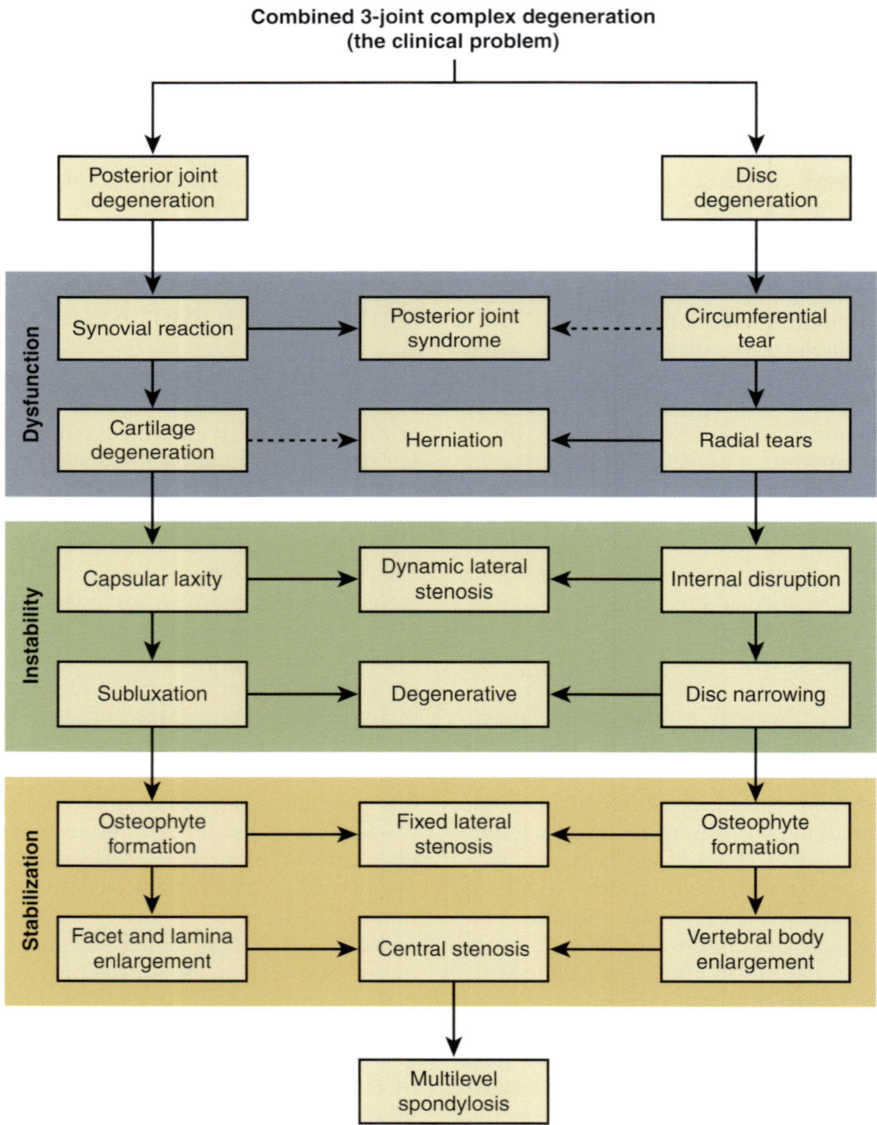

FIGURE 162-1. Kirkaldy-Willis degenerative cascade: pathophysiology of degenerative disease of the lumbar spine.

replacement prosthesis that introduces unnatural and unconstrained motion, it may reverse the process back toward the abnormally decreased stiffness phase.

First-Generation Artificial Discs

Over the last 3 decades, a considerable effort has been undertaken to develop alternatives to fusion. First-generation disc arthroplasty design evolved from experience with hip and knee replacement. These designs mimicked the ball-and-socket design used in artificial hips and knees. Although the first-generation devices may offer some benefit over fusion in that they reportedly preserve motion in the spinal segment, they do not function like the natural disc.[10] These devices force a fixed axis of rotation on the spine and do not allow for true coupled motion.[11] The natural disc provides for three-dimensional motion: flexion-extension, lateral bending, rotation, and compression. It is also viscoelastic, meaning that the stiffness varies with the loading rate and magnitude.[5] The first-generation discs restore only two-dimensional motion, providing no mechanism for axial compression, and they have no viscoelastic properties. Although they may prove successful in replacing a painful, degenerated disc with some motion, they cannot replicate the native function of the natural disc. These shortcomings are more than just theoretical limitations and are likely to lead to problems and disappointing long-term results.

Definition of the Ideal Artificial Lumbar Intervertebral Disc

Spinal motion does not rely solely on the intervertebral disc. Any prosthetic replacement should offer more than one dimension of function and should not act in isolation from the native biomechanics of the spine. Lemaire suggested that the ideal substitute for the lumbar disc "... should meet the following criteria: geometry, motion, deformability, inherent stiffness, and acoustics."[11]

The hallmark of a next-generation design is that it should replicate native function, embracing the four key biomechanical concepts: complex motion, viscoelasticity, load-bearing capacity, and passive resistance to loads. The load-bearing capability of the spine is also a function of anatomy and alignment. Kimura et al.[6] illustrated and quantified the effect of loading on the lumbar spine, describing the functional response of the spine and its ability to adapt to normal loading. The key finding was that the spinal system responds to loading first by increasing the native lordotic or kyphotic curvature and subsequently by altering disc height. This finding highlights the fact that the spinal response to motion is a system-wide response and not just local to the segments.

A prosthetic disc replacement should attempt to restore the natural curvature of the FSU. The ability of the disc to compress axially is fundamental to the load response and load-sharing function, so an artificial disc replacement must move in this dimension to act fully as a shock absorber. The concept of the next-generation design requires full replication of function. A biomechanical basis for an ideal prosthetic disc suggests that it must function in concert with the entire FSU, including the adjacent vertebral bodies, the surrounding ligaments, the facets, and the muscles. Additionally, it should replicate the viscoelasticity of the natural disc, responding with increasing stiffness at higher loads and higher rates of load application. It must compress axially, allowing changes in disc height required to respond to loads appropriately and naturally. It should also restore and maintain the proper angle of the spinal curve. Lastly, it should provide passive resistance to forces during motion.

To meet the aforementioned requirements, the implant must provide for short-term and long-term fixation. Short-term fixation is needed to allow for initial motion and preservation of biomechanics until long-term fixation is achieved. Long-term fixation, preferably by osteointegration, is required to maintain the motion and biomechanics and adapt to potential changes over time in bone and end-plate architecture. The fixation of the disc replacement to the bony end plates is also critical for the transmission of forces from one level to the next without creating artificial pathways of least resistance. These artificial pathways would have the propensity to become sites of wear between either the components of the disc replacement or the disc replacement and the vertebral body end plates.

Design of the Ideal Artificial Lumbar Intervertebral Disc

Material and Design Optimization

To satisfy the previously described requirements, the material chosen for the core of an artificial disc should possess the viscoelastic characteristics of a natural human disc so that it is capable of obtaining the geometry, motion, deformability, and inherent stiffness properties of the native disc. An ideal candidate for the design of next-generation technology is an elastomer-based artificial disc. At low loading rates, the elastomer material should be relatively flexible, and at accelerated loading rates, it should stiffen. This feature is useful for reducing the shock transmitted to the spine during normal day-to-day activities, while allowing the treated segment to function in a manner that is consistent with the rest of the spine. Fixation of the elastomeric core to the bony end plates may be achieved by metal or composite end plates. The bone-interface surface of the end plates must have an appropriate surface to promote osteointegration and long-term fixation. Fixation of the end plates to the elastomeric core is necessary to provide passive resistance to the forces applied to the spine.

Biomechanical Characterization

An artificial disc should be thoroughly biomechanically characterized to show its strength and durability. The device should have strength that exceeds the strength of the natural disc and surrounding anatomy in compression, rotation, shear, flexion, and extension. Because axial compression is the primary load-bearing mode in an artificial disc, compressive strength should be of the utmost importance. Durability evaluations include fatigue testing in compression, rotation, flexion-extension, and lateral bending to determine the endurance limits, failure modes, and potential for wear debris generation. Additionally, coupled motion fatigue testing may be used to predict more physiologically realistic loading scenarios and resulting failure modes. Device creep and resilience are also important properties to characterize to predict long-term performance. Device stiffness and range of motion should also be characterized and compared with a healthy natural disc. Stiffness and range of motion may be characterized statically and dynamically in compression, rotation, and flexion-extension. The propensity for subsidence of the device into the vertebral bodies or expulsion of the device from the disc space should be evaluated. Testing in simulated vertebral bodies made of polyurethane foam eliminates the variability associated with bone specimens. For multiple-component bonded devices, extensive bond strength and durability testing should be conducted. Evaluations of the bond should be a part of the testing described previously or, alternatively, done as separate investigations, using nonphysiologic tests designed to focus the stress on the bond.

Early Polymeric Total Disc Replacement Experience

Clinical experience with polymeric discs began with Steffee, the inventor of the AcroFlex lumbar disc. Three generations of the AcroFlex lumbar disc (DePuy Spine, a Johnson & Johnson company, Raynham, MA) were used in several pilot studies or custom implantations. All three generations of the device incorporated titanium alloy end plates and an elastomeric core bonded to the metal plates. The first-generation disc incorporated a hexane-based polyolefin rubber and adhesive system and was implanted in six patients.[12] Satisfactory results (one excellent, two good, and one fair) occurred in four of the six patients at 3 years of follow-up. The second-generation device, incorporating a silicone elastomer core, was approved by the U.S. Food and Drug Administration (FDA) in 1993 for implantation into 13 patients, but results have not been published.[13]

The third-generation AcroFlex lumbar artificial disc also used a hexane-based polyolefin rubber and adhesive. These discs had either flat end plates with a raised crescent or slightly domed end plates with six teeth for short-term fixation to bone.[14] Both third-generation discs had a sintered bead coating for bony ingrowth. Two prospective, nonrandomized pilot studies were conducted with the third-generation AcroFlex disc.[14] Although the overall clinical results up to 2 years appeared to be satisfactory, planned randomized studies were not carried out for the third-generation AcroFlex disc, because of the finding of mechanical failures in the elastomer cores.

Implants

All second-generation disc arthroplasty devices are elastomeric-based systems employing some form of compliant polymer. The characteristic of compression (compliance to loading) is the demonstrable difference between first-generation and second-generation total disc arthroplasty. The predominant lumbar next-generation devices include the following (Fig. 162-2):

- CADisc (Ranier, Cambridge, UK)
- eDisc (Integra Life Science, Plainsboro, NJ)
- Freedom (AxioMed Spine Corp, Cleveland, OH)

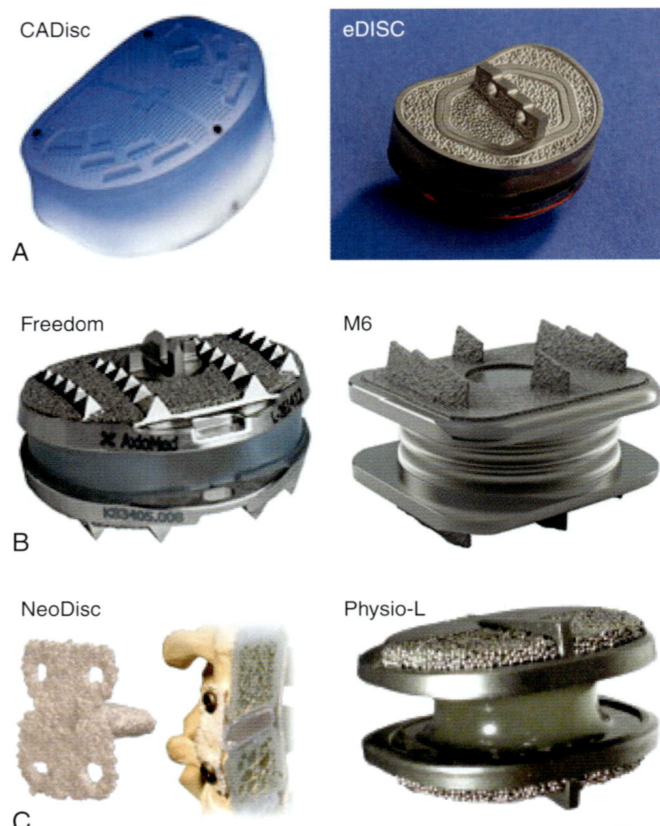

FIGURE 162-2. A–C, Lumbar next-generation devices. See text for manufacturers.

- M6 (Spinal Kinetics, Sunnyvale, CA)
- NeoDisc (NuVasive, San Diego, CA)
- Physio-L (NexGen, Whippany, NJ)

The design premise behind second-generation total disc arthroplasty is partly based on providing load compliance or compressibility. Compressibility is thought to be significant because the device can conform to the physiologic loading that occurs within the spinal system. The theory is that compressibility (shock absorption) plus motion is an improved approximation of natural disc function.

CAdisc

The CAdisc (Compliant Artificial Spinal Disc) has no articulating surfaces, and it is an entirely elastomeric, polyurethane polycarbonate graduated modulus device with integrated end plates. The "anulus" is harder (higher modulus), and the "nucleus" is softer (low modulus), with a region of continuously varying modulus joining the anulus and nucleus. The device is manufactured using proprietary technology, a computer-controlled polymerization of polycarbonate polyurethanes, integrated with the molding process to achieve the graduated modulus design. The disc is covalently bonded throughout, with "no regions of high stress concentration." A company-sponsored report in a baboon study showed that the implants did not migrate or subside after implantation for 6 months in baboons.[15] The disc left impressions in the vertebral end plates, and micro-CT showed "evidence suggestive of positive bone remodeling."

eDisc

The eDisc comprises a polycarbonate urethane core and titanium end plates, with a microelectronic module. The polymer, PH200, developed by Theken, is reported to have superior crack growth resistance, greater hydrolytic stability, and enhanced oxidation resistance.[16] The microelectronic module provides treating physicians with feedback allowing them to manage patients' postoperative courses.

Freedom Lumbar Disc

The Freedom disc is a one-piece viscoelastic artificial disc consisting of an elastomeric core bonded to titanium alloy retaining plates with end caps. The polymer core material is a silicone polycarbonate urethane thermoplastic elastomer. The polymer core is able to expand radially and axially. This axial feature, along with the mechanical characteristics of the polymer, is intended to allow the device to approximate the stiffness of a natural human disc. The manufacturer presented results of 50 patients with single-level, symptomatic lumbar degenerative disc disease at L4-5 or L5-S1, unresponsive to at least 6 months of nonoperative therapy.[17] Mean preoperative Oswestry Disability Index scores decreased from 48% preoperatively to 24% at 2-year follow-up. Mean visual analogue scale scores decreased from preoperative 7.1 to 2.7 cm at 2 years for back pain, 3.8 to 0.3 cm for right leg pain, and 3.7 to 1.7 cm for left leg pain.

M6

Spinal Kinetics developed the M6 cervical total disc replacement and M6 lumbar total disc replacement. The intent of M6 is to "replicate the anatomic and biomechanical attributes of a natural intervertebral disc" via an artificial nucleus and anulus. The nucleus allows axial compression, whereas the woven fiber anulus controls range of motion in all 6 degrees of freedom.[18]

A single-arm prospective feasibility study was conducted to evaluate the preliminary safety and effectiveness of the M6 disc in the treatment of patients with symptomatic cervical radiculopathy.[19] The study enrolled 32 cases, with 15 patients reaching 12 months of follow-up; 10 patients underwent artificial disc implantation at one level, and 5 patients had two levels treated. The mean Neck Disability Index (NDI) score improved from 48.1% before treatment to 20.4% at 12 months. The mean arm pain score improved from 6.8 before treatment to 3.2 at 12 months. The mean neck pain score improved from 7.2 before treatment to 3.5 at 12 months. The mean Physical Component Summary and Mental Component Summary scores of the 36-Item Short Form Health Survey improved from 34.7 and 43.6 before treatment to 44.6 and 50.4 at 12 months. All the improvements were statistically significant. Using dynamic flexion-extension radiographs, the mean range of motion at the treated level was 12.3 degrees before surgery and 9.7 degrees at 12 months. Mean global range of motion of the entire neck was approximately 47 degrees before treatment and returned to this value at 12 months. Disc height at the treated level was 3.4 mm before surgery, improved to approximately 6 mm, and remained constant through 12 months of follow-up. No cases of worsening neurologic status were reported, and there were no serious device-related adverse events; reoperations; or evidence of device migration, expulsion, or subsidence in this study group.

The implant is available in three heights (6 mm, 7 mm, and 8 mm) and two footprints (12.5 × 15 mm and 14 × 17 mm). A U.S. feasibility study is under way. The first M6 lumbar disc was implanted in Germany on February 18, 2009, marking the commencement of the system's initial commercial launch in Europe.

NeoDisc

The NeoDisc comprises an elastomeric nucleus contained within an embroidered polyester fabric, secured by four bone screws. The endurance limit of the NeoDisc implant under 500 N dynamic axial compression was determined to be at least 10 million cycles.[20] Static axial compression to half of the core height did not cause damage or failure of the NeoDisc implant. At 20 million cycles, the average volumetric loss of material from the NeoDisc device was 13.8 mg (approximately 11.2 mm^3); this corresponds to an average of 0.69 mg per 1 million cycles of testing (0.56 mm^3 per 1 million cycles). The 20 million–cycle test can be considered to be a worst-case test.[20] The investigators concluded that it is unlikely that any device in clinical use would experience this quantity of large, exaggerated motion. Animal trials provided macroscopic and histologic evidence of the tissue ingrowth.[20] There were no unforeseen causes of wear debris, and the tissue response to the wear debris generated was analogous to the tissue response of other medical devices.

Physio-L and Physio-C

The Physio-L (lumbar) and Physio-C (cervical) total disc replacements are intended to "functionally restore normal disc motion." The technology comprises polycarbonate urethane polymer core and titanium end plates. The polymer, ChronoFlex C, has been approved for use in an aortic graft and is intended to match closely the physiologic properties of the intact human intervertebral disc. The titanium plates are dome-shaped with a central keel. The Physio total disc replacement polymer is bonded to the titanium end plates via "perforated plate attachment (PPA)." The Physio-L device is available in three angles (0 degrees, 6 degrees, and 12 degrees) and three footprints (26 × 33 mm, 27 × 36 mm, and 30 × 40 mm). No wear or outcomes results have been reported to date.

Conclusion

The next generation of disc replacements must more closely replicate the biomechanical properties of the normal human disc. Elastomeric materials, by virtue of their viscoelastic properties, can closely approximate the native properties of the human disc. These next-generation materials must conform to toxicology and wear standards. Because these devices are mainly used in younger individuals, bonding between the viscoelastic material and the retaining plates has to withstand millions of cycles. Because implant displacement can result in early failure, it is of paramount importance to make the most adaptable design. Device insertion should be easy and reproducible, and catastrophic failure prevention and contingency management plans should be in place.

KEY REFERENCES

Cunningham B: Basic scientific considerations in total disc arthroplasty. *Spine J* 4(Suppl 6):219S–230S, 2004.

Eck J, Humphreys S, Hodges S: Adjacent-segment degeneration after lumbar fusion: a review of clinical, biomechanical and radiologic studies. *Am J Orthop* 28:336–340, 1999.

Enker P, Steffee A, Mcmillin C, et al: Artificial disc replacement: preliminary report with a 3-year minimum follow-up. *Spine (Phila Pa 1976)* 18:1061–1070, 1993.

Fritzell P, Hagg O, Wessberg P: Lumbar fusion versus nonsurgical treatment for chronic low back pain: a multicenter randomized controlled trial from the Swedish Lumbar Spine Study Group. *Spine (Phila Pa 1976)* 26:2521–2532, 2001.

Yong-Hing K, Kirkaldy-Willis W: The pathophysiology of degenerative disease of the lumbar spine. *Orthop Clin North Am* 14:491–504, 1983.

REFERENCES

The complete reference list is available online at expertconsult.com.

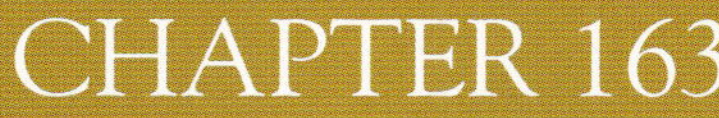
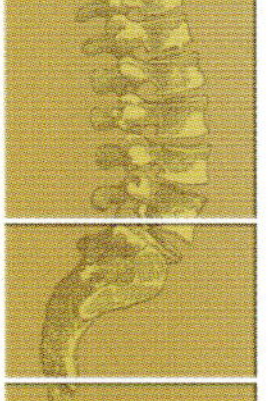

CHAPTER 163

Nuclear Replacement

Satyajit Marawar | William F. Lavelle | Richard Tallarico | Hansen A. Yuan

Spinal surgeons contend with back pain on a daily basis. Back pain has acquired epidemic proportions in industrialized nations. It has a prevalence of 60% to 90% and is second only to the common cold as a reason for a physician visit.[1,2] With the total costs associated with back pain ranging from 100 billion dollars to 200 billion dollars annually, back pain is a major health and socioeconomic burden.[3] Most episodes of back pain are short in duration. However, many cases have a recurrent course, and further acute episodes affect 20% to 44% of patients in the working population within 1 year. The lifetime recurrence rate can be 85%.[4]

Lumbar disc degeneration is the most common cause of back pain. Disc degeneration generally results from reduced proteoglycan content in the nucleus and reduced nuclear hydration. Resulting biomechanical changes in the disc lead to loss of disc height and increasing biomechanical demand on the anulus with imbalance in the stress distribution across the disc space.[5,6] When tension in the anulus is lost, ventral and dorsal instability of the motion segment can ensue. Increasing loads on the anulus can lead to anular tears with or without disc herniations. Continued loss of disc height can lead to osteophyte formation, facet arthrosis, and stiffness of the motion segment. Pain from disc degenerative disease (DDD) can occur at any stage of this degenerative cascade from early disc degeneration to instability and deformity.

Traditional treatment modalities for symptoms resulting from disc degeneration are focused on decompression with or without fusion. These treatment modalities do not attempt to halt the degenerative cascade and, in many instances, can lead to further progression of degeneration. Although short-term outcomes after lumbar discectomy have been shown to be superior compared with conservative care,[7,8] long-term outcomes have been compromised by persistent back pain and a high risk of reoperations with a significant number of reherniations.[9,10] Arthrodesis of the motion segment is still the "gold standard" for treatment of chronic disabling back pain of discogenic origin. However, it is difficult to predict the clinical response to arthrodesis. The outcome depends on multiple factors, such as the initial diagnosis, previous surgeries, prior fusion attempts, and the number of levels requiring fusion. Long-term studies have shown a fusion rate of 87% and clinical success rate of 76% for DDD.[11,12] There are several disadvantages inherent to arthrodesis. Most importantly, arthrodesis can change the biomechanical loading of the adjacent segment, leading to accelerated degeneration.

Treatment of discogenic pain is fraught with difficulty and unpredictable outcomes. Additionally, in patients with early disc degeneration with minimal or no loss of disc height, there are no reliable methods for the diagnosis of the origin of discogenic back pain. Discography has been used to aid in the diagnosis; however, its reliability has been questioned.[13-17]

Nucleus replacement and intradiscal electrothermal treatment has evolved as an option to treat discogenic back pain in patients with early nuclear degeneration with minimal or no collapse, no signs of instability, and arthrosis of the motion segment. Intradiscal electrothermal treatment can be used in patients with mild anular tears and early nuclear degeneration. However, it cannot be used in patients with more advanced disc degeneration and herniated nucleus pulposus. It is hoped that nucleus replacement can treat discogenic back pain in such patients and avoid fusion.

History of Nucleus Replacement

Early attempts at nuclear replacements consisted of injecting polymethylmethacrylate[18,19] or self-curing silicone[19] into the disc space after a nucleotomy. Clinical results were found to be similar to discectomy controls. Flow of the injected material and curing of the injected liquids were difficult to control. These variables led to abandonment of these procedures, but these initial attempts formed the theoretical basis of present-day preformed nuclear replacement systems.

Fernstrom[20] was the first to use stainless steel balls as nuclear replacement by inserting them into the central cavity created after a discectomy. He implanted these balls in 125 patients at 191 lumbar levels. In 1966, Fernstrom[20] reported that the outcome after this kind of nuclear replacement was better than discectomy alone and was similar to fusion. This procedure was largely abandoned owing to the subsidence of steel balls into the vertebral end plates. In 1995, McKenzie[21] reported long-term outcomes of the Fernstrom ball. At 17 years of follow-up of 67 patients implanted with Fernstrom balls, he reported an 83% success rate in patients with one or more disc protrusions and a 75% success rate in patients with DDD. Although the Fernstrom ball never found mainstream acceptance as a nuclear replacement device, it did suggest that nuclear replacement can be a viable alternative to either a stand-alone discectomy or a fusion.

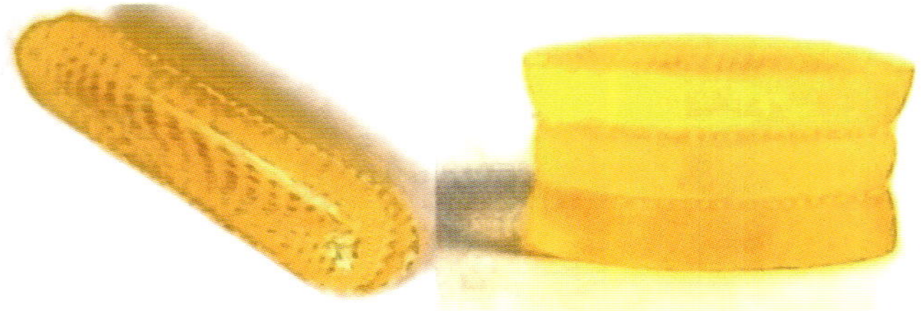

FIGURE 163-1. NeuDisc preformed hydrogel nucleus replacement. Before *(left)* and after *(right)* hydration images are shown. (Courtesy of Dr. James J. Yue.)

In 1981, Edeland[22] suggested a design for an elastodynamic disc replacement device that would mimic the native disc biomechanically and biologically. Such a device would allow influx or efflux of water molecules in response to the load applied to it. Finding an elastodynamic material remained the most limiting factor. Attempts at finding such material in the 1980s and 1990s focused on either silicone polymers or a hydrogel nucleus composed of polyvinyl alcohol that was used to make soft contact lenses. Hou et al.[23] designed a solid preformed silicone rubber horseshoe-shaped implant termed the *lumbar intervertebral replacement prosthesis*. Biomechanical cadaver studies and animal studies in monkeys showed restoration of the disc height and mechanical stability. Human studies with this implant have not been reported.

In 1991, Bao and Hingham patented a hydrogel nucleus made of polyvinyl alcohol that imbibed and extruded water and could replicate the biomechanical viscoelastic properties of the native nucleus. An animal study by Allen et al.[24] showed no evidence of systemic or local toxicity but a high incidence of implant extrusion. Despite this setback, proven preclinical benefits with hydrogel acted as a springboard for other nucleus replacement technologies. With its first clinical use in 1996, the prosthetic disc nucleus (PDN) is the most well-known nucleus replacement device made of hydrogel.[25] The device is made of hydrogel enclosed in a polyethylene terephthalate (PET) jacket to restrict expansion on hydration. Multiple design and material changes have followed after its first use (Fig. 163-1).

Current Nuclear Replacement Technology

Current nuclear replacement devices can be classified as either elastomeric or nonelastomeric. Elastomers can be subdivided into hydrogels and nonhydrogels that are either in situ cured or preformed. Preformed devices may be implanted in their final shapes or may take their final shape on expanding by hydration. Nonelastomers can be subdivided into articulating or nonarticulating based on the presence or absence of articulation as part of the implant design.

At the present time, there are several designs with active clinical or developmental activities. Most clinical activity is occurring outside of the United States. Such devices are elastomers such as Hydraflex, DASCOR, NuCore, NeuDisc, BioDisc, SINUX ANR and SINUX PNR, and Newcleus.

HydraFlex (Raymedica, Bloomington, IN) is the latest version of the PDN; it is inserted in a dehydrated form that rehydrates on implantation (Fig. 163-2). The hydrogel component is a block copolymer of polyacrylamide-polyacrylonitrile

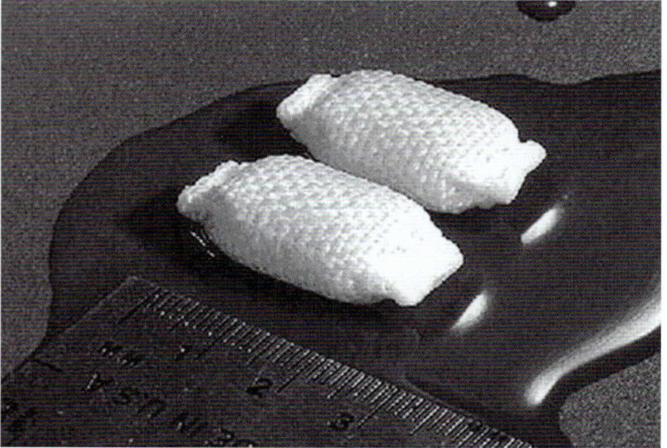

FIGURE 163-2. PDN replacement. (From Berlemann U, Schwarzenbach O: An injectable nucleus replacement as an adjunct to microdiscectomy: 2 year follow-up in a pilot clinical study. *Eur Spine J* 18:1706–1712, 2009.)

(Hypan, Lipo Technologies, Vandalia, OH) formed by solution casting. The jacket is formed of a dense woven circular tube of PET, which is a thermoplastic polymer. The PET jacket is inelastic but flexible, which helps the hydrogel core to maintain its shape when subject to compressive forces. The hydrogel core absorbs water on implantation. Hypan80, which is currently being used, absorbs 80% of its weight by water, which makes it softer and flexible. HydraFlex takes approximately 32 hours to reach hydration equilibrium.

DASCOR (Disc Dynamics, Eden Prairie, MN) is a two-part in situ curable polyurethane. It consists of a polyether polyurethane core encapsulated and adhered to a polycarbonate polyurethane balloon, which has cavity expansion and conforming capabilities. The device is fabricated by mixing a two-part, liquid, pre–polyether polyurethane reactive system and injecting a liquid mixture in a polycarbonate polyurethane balloon delivery catheter placed within the nucleus cavity (Fig. 163-3). A custom electromechanical injection system is used to apply a computer-controlled pressure profile designed to deliver the liquid polymer.[26]

NuCore Injectable Disc Nucleus (Spine Wave, Shelton, CT) is an in situ curing protein polymer hydrogel that mimics the properties of the natural nucleus. The polymer chain is composed of silk and elastin components designed for elasticity and toughness. The polymer (P27K) is mixed with a cross-linking agent at the time of implantation and is injected as a fluid through the anular defect where it adheres to the surrounding intradiscal tissue as it cures. There is no measurable temperature increase produced during the cure process. NuCore has been studied as an adjunct to discectomy[27] and is in the process of being studied for treatment of DDD (Fig. 163-4).

The NeuDisc device (Replication Medical, Cranbury, NJ) is composed of a material that is a hydrolyzed polyacrylonitrile hydrogel (Aquacryl). In the absence of mechanical restrictions, the hydrogel imbibes 90% volume as a liquid. When implanted in a dehydrated state, this hydrogel implant is substantially smaller than the volume of resected nucleus and is easily placed though an incision in the anulus. After hydration, it expands anisotropically, in the axial direction principally, and becomes substantially larger than the incision. The axial expansion is not constrained by a jacket and results from its structure of polymer layers tied together with an internal substructure[28] (Fig. 163-5; see also Fig. 163-1).

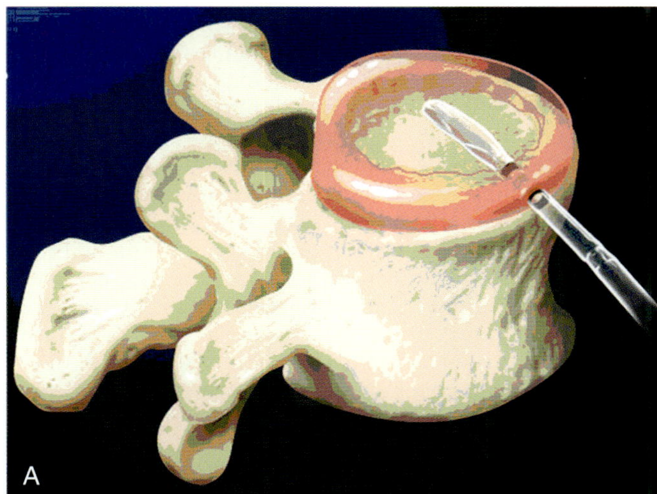

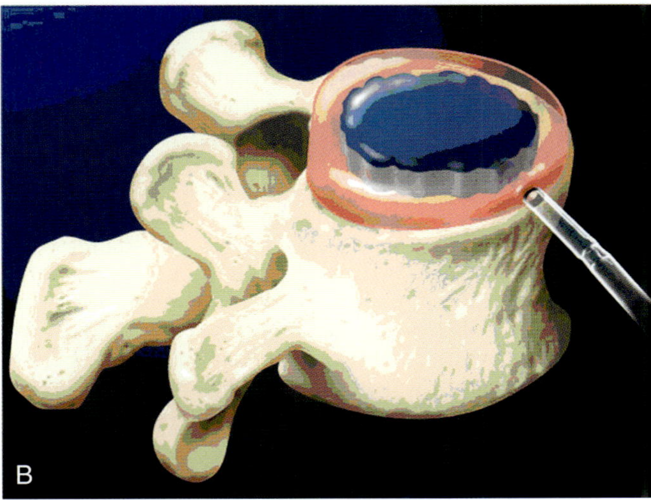

FIGURE 163-3. DASCOR nuclear replacement. Implant placement (**A**) and deployment (**B**). (From Ahrens M, Tsantrizos A, Donkersloot P, et al: Nucleus replacement with the DASCOR disc arthroplasty device: interim two-year efficacy and safety results from two prospective, non-randomized multicenter European studies. *Spine [Phila Pa 1976]* 34:1376–1384, 2009.)

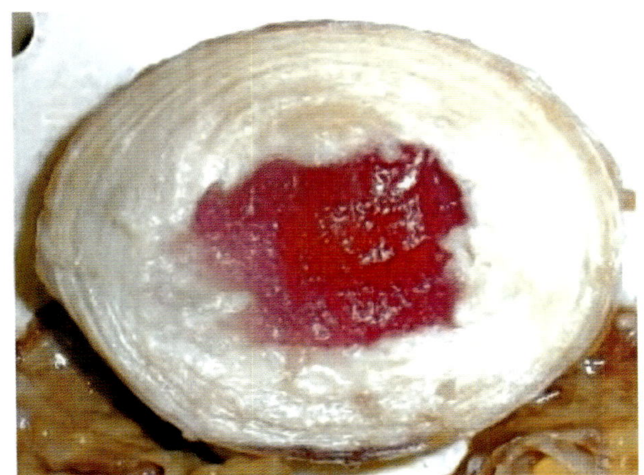

FIGURE 163-4. NuCore Injectable Disc Nucleus *(red)*, shown interdigitating with normal disc after injection into nucleotomy defect. (Used with permission of Spine Wave, Shelton, CT.)

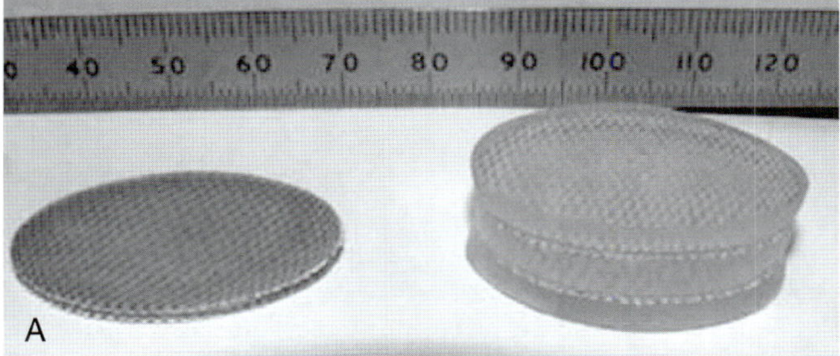

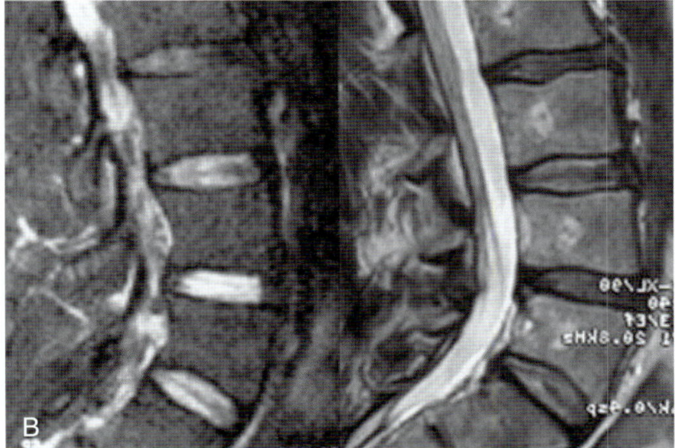

FIGURE 163-5. NeuDisc device shown clinically (preoperative and postoperative) (**A**) and on MRI (**B**). (From Bertagnoli R, Karg A, Voigt S: Lumbar partial disc replacement. Orthop Clin North Am 36:341–347, 2005.)

BioDisc is based on the CryoLife (Kennesaw, GA) BioGlue surgical adhesive with a formulation for spinal application. It comprises an in vivo mixture of serum albumin with gluteraldehyde as a cross-linking agent. Both substances mix and completely solidify within 2 minutes. SINUX ANR (DePuy Spine, Raynham, MA) is a liquid polymethylsiloxone (silicone) injectable polymer that cures within 15 minutes. PNR is an inflatable silicone device between threaded studs. The device is threaded into the vertebral bodies and inflated with silicone. It is implanted through the presacral approach and is the only nucleus replacement that is fixed to the vertebral end plates. Newcleus (Zimmer Spine, Warsaw, IN) is a memory coiling polycarbonate urethane that is coiled within the disc space. It absorbs 3% to 5% of its weight by water but does not have osmotic capabilities.

Among nonelastomeric devices, Regain (Biomet, Warsaw, IN) is a modified form of the Fernstrom ball with a larger radius for larger end-plate contact surface that is manufactured from pyrolytic carbon. NUBAC (Pioneer Surgical Technology, Marquette, MI) is the only articulating nonelastomeric implant and is made of PEEK-OPTIMA (Invibio, Greenville, NC), which is a proven biostable and biocompatible polymer widely used for spinal fusion and shown to generate minimal wear. NUBAC comprises two plates with a large contact surface area in an anatomic shape similar to the native nucleus with an inner ball-and-socket articulation[29] (Fig. 163-6).

Indications for Nucleus Replacement

The indications and contraindications for nucleus replacement are largely determined by the intended objectives

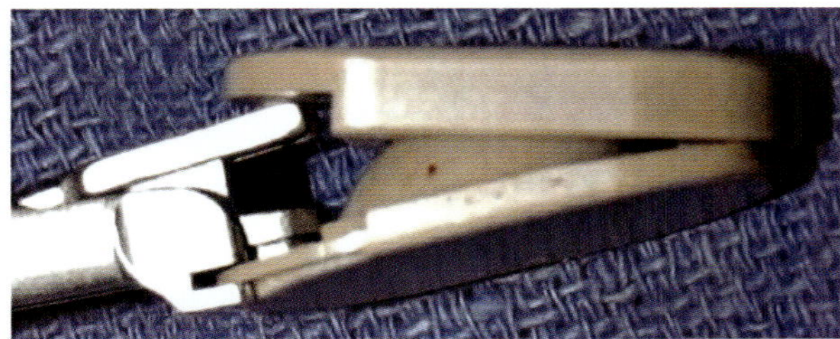

FIGURE 163-6. NUBAC two-piece mechanical nucleus. This is an articulated polyetheretherketone (PEEK)-on-PEEK device. (Used with permission from Pioneer Surgical, Marquette, MI.)

and the unique design of the nucleus replacement devices. Although the indications and contraindications for the initial clinical studies were determined a priori, a better idea of these criteria cannot be established until at least limited clinical follow-ups are performed. The criteria will then be based on the outcomes of such studies and the risk-to-benefit and cost-to-benefit ratios.

The primary indication for nucleus replacement is single-level discogenic pain caused by DDD with or without leg pain. Disc degeneration should be mild to moderate, and so disc height of 5 mm or more, or at least 50% of the adjacent level, is considered necessary. In the case of late DDD, the anulus may become biomechanically incompetent on distraction owing to secondary structural changes.

Nucleus replacement devices rely on the anulus and the end plates for biomechanical restraint and load sharing. It may be difficult for the nucleus replacement device to correct spinal deformities such as spondylolisthesis, scoliosis, or kyphosis because of morphologic and structural changes in the anulus that can lead to inappropriate load sharing and increased extrusion risk. Similarly, severe end-plate degeneration and the presence of Schmorl nodes would predispose to implant subsidence. End-plate geometry may have a further impact on clinical outcomes: Hyperconcave end plates pose the risk of scoliosis, whereas truly convex end plates pose the risk of implant extrusion.

Surgical Technique

The nucleus replacement device can be implanted via either a retroperitoneal approach or a posterior approach. The retroperitoneal approach is used more commonly. Although this approach is similar to the approach used for anterior fusion or a disc replacement, the amount of anular exposure required for nucleus replacement is less because of the smaller dimensions of the nucleus replacement implants. Also, because the size of the nucleus replacement device is smaller than a disc replacement prosthesis, it is possible to use the posterior or a direct lateral approach for placement of the device.

Careful surgical planning is required for effective placement of the device. Some general but critical surgical pearls are important. The size of the anulotomy window differs based on the approach and the size of the device to be inserted. The anulotomy window needs to be large enough for removal of the nucleus but small enough to reduce the risk of device extrusion.

With a dorsal approach, the anulus is thin or deficient if there is a disc herniation, so the approach should be from the side of disc herniation. Laminectomy and facetectomy should be done as required while trying to preserve as much of the posterior elements as possible. The anular defect caused by the disc herniation can be used, or a small anular slit or a box cut can be made if the anulus is intact. In the case of a larger implant, either a larger box cut is required or the window can be dilated to receive the implant. When performing a ventrolateral or direct lateral approach, because the anular wall is thick, a box cut or a circular cut by a trephine is necessary for nucleotomy. A ventrolateral anulotomy is usually better than a direct ventral anulotomy to reduce the risk of implant extrusion. The initial cut can be either dilated or enlarged to device dimension. Alternatively, an anular flap can be made for device insertion and can be sutured back later. A direct lateral approach is becoming more popular among spine surgeons and may become a preferred approach in the future for nucleus replacement.

The nucleotomy required for nucleus replacement involves removal of the entire nucleus to create a symmetrical cavity lined by the anulus and the end plates. The implant should be positioned in the center of this cavity. It is crucial to preserve the integrity of the end plates and the anulus.

Outcomes

Outcomes data for nucleus replacement technology are limited by the lack of large randomized prospective studies. Most of these devices have been used in limited Investigational Device Exemptions studies with short-term follow-up reported. None of these devices are approved for use in the United States by the Food and Drug Administration (FDA).

To date, the most widely studied device with the longest history is the PDN. The PDN has shown favorable biologic compatibility and biomechanical stability. Fatigue testing performed with loads of 200 N to 600 N for 50 million cycles showed that the device continues to function with maintained disc height and structural integrity. It has been shown not to form polyethylene wear debris.[30] Eysel et al.[31] analyzed the effect of the PDN on restoration of segmental mobility after a nucleotomy in human cadaver spines. These investigators found that there was a statistically significant ($P < .05$) increase in segmental mobility in all directions after nucleotomy with an increased mobility of the segment of 38% to 100%. After the introduction of two PDN implants, there was a restoration of segmental mobility for all movement directions with no statistically significant difference compared with the intact segment before nucleotomy.

In clinical studies, the major concerns with the PDN device have been the risk of implant migration and the potential for end-plate changes and subsidence. Schonmayr et al.[32] reported early clinical results with the PDN implant with a minimum 2-year follow-up in 10 patients with symptomatic lumbar DDD. They showed good functional outcomes with restoration of disc height and motion. However, three implants migrated, and one patient required a revision surgery for migration.

Multiple phases of implant trials following these early results involved changes made to the device shapes and to the surgical protocol to facilitate implantation and eliminate the high device migration rates. After these modifications, the success rate for the device improved significantly. Clinical data show excellent results with marked improvements in

Oswestry Disability Index (ODI) and Prolo scores with disc height measurements being well maintained within normal physiologic ranges. Klara and Ray[25] reported a cumulative 90% success rate with 10% of the patients requiring explantation. Following these early results, Bertagnoli and Vazquez[33] described implanting the PDN device through an anterolateral transpsoatic approach to reduce the risk of implant migration. They reported the results in eight patients after using this technique. Four of the first five patients developed a transient psoas neurapraxia. Ventral migration of the PDN was detected in three patients and was thought to be due to preexisting defects in the anterior anulus unrelated to surgery. Because the patients were asymptomatic, no revision was attempted. One patient required a revision surgery with fusion for implant subsidence. Of the remaining seven patients, significant improvements were noted in the mean ODI and Prolo scores at 6 months and 12 months with maintained disc heights.

In earlier studies, two PDN implants were used per disc level. It was suggested that using two implants per level may lead to overstuffing of the disc space and increased risk of implant migration. Manufacturers have advocated the use of a single larger implant sufficient to occupy the cavity after a nucleotomy. In 2002, 45 patients were implanted with a single PDN implant for lumbar disc herniation. Follow-up was reported by Jin et al.[34] for 33 patients at 6 months. Statistically significant improvements were noted in the ODI and Prolo scores with significant improvements in spinal mobility and disc heights. There were no cases of implant migration or failure in 6 months. Although Jin et al.[34] did not report any end-plate changes and subsidence at 6 months, these have been reported on longer follow-up after PDN implantation.

Shim et al.[35] followed 46 patients after PDN implantation for more than 6 months. Four patients (8.7%) showed device extrusion that needed revision surgery, and one patient had an infection. The investigators reported a 9.4% increase in the disc height at 1-year follow-up; 19.6% of patients showed some subsidence, 60.9% of patients showed end-plate sclerosis, and 82.8% of patients showed aggravation of Modic changes on MRI. Clinical results were excellent in 5 patients (10.9%), good in 31 (67.4%), fair in 3 (6.5%), and poor in 7 (15.1%), with an overall success rate of 78.3%.

Ma et al.[36] reported on the midterm to long-term follow-up of PDN. From March 2002 to October 2003, 34 patients who underwent PDN replacement were followed for an average of 52.6 months (range 48 to 66 months). Although initial clinical results were encouraging, the patients did not do as well over the longer term. At 12 months after operation, a significant proportion of patients recovered from low back pain or leg pain, with an ODI score that decreased an average of 18.2% and pain on the visual analogue scale (VAS) that decreased to 1.8. The average increase of the postoperative disc height was 17.6%, with a range of motion of 9.2 degrees. At the final follow-up, the ODI increased from 18.2% 12 months after operation to 31.2%, VAS increased from 1.8 to 3.1, disc height improvement averaged to 13.5%, and range of motion decreased to 6.8 degrees. The rate of degeneration or breakages of the end plates was 64.7% (22 of 34), and implant device migrations were observed in 25 patients.

Despite these complications, early clinical results with the PDN have been encouraging. With continuing changes in the implant structure and the use of suitable approaches such as the anterolateral transpsoatic approach and direct lateral approach, reduction in the complication rates can be expected.

Published clinical data are limited for other devices. For the DASCOR device, 2-year follow-up data have been reported from European centers for 85 patients implanted with the device for single-level DDD between February 2003 and July 31, 2007. Mean VAS and ODI scores improved significantly after 6 weeks and throughout the 2-year follow-up. Radiographic results showed, at a minimum, maintenance of disc height with no device expulsion and, despite Modic type 1 changes, no subsidence. Analgesic medication use decreased 84.6% by 24 months from the preoperative average. Seven patients required explants for various reasons, but the device was in its intradiscal implant position in all patients, and no expulsions of the device had been observed.[26]

Berlemann and Schwarzenbach[27] reported on the use of NuCore as an adjunct to discectomy to replace the loss of disc tissue after herniation and microdiscectomy. After a standard microdiscectomy procedure in 14 patients, the hydrogel material was injected into the nuclear void to replace what tissue had been lost to the herniation and surgery. Results showed significant improvement for leg and back pain and functional scores. No complications or device-related adverse events were observed. MRI controls confirmed stable position of the implants with no repeat herniations. Radiographic measurements indicated better maintenance of disc height compared with literature data on microdiscectomy alone.

A short follow-up has been reported after implantation of the NUBAC device. Ten patients in Mexico were implanted with NUBAC after discectomy and followed for 3 months. VAS score improved from 8.1 to 2.5 ($P < .05$), and the ODI improved from 58.2% to 24.2% ($P < .05$). Disc height before surgery was 9.4 mm and 3 months postoperatively was 12.5 mm with no complications, migration, or subsidence.[29]

Summary

As the population ages, the prevalence of DDD and its economic and social burden are expected to continue to increase. Current treatment modalities of discectomy and fusion do not slow down the degenerative cascade. It is hoped that nuclear replacement may bridge the gap between discectomy and fusion or a disc replacement procedure, while attempting to slow down the degenerative process. Nuclear replacement can be a minimally invasive, motion-preserving option with minimal risk of neurologic and vascular complications in contrast to a fusion or a disc replacement. Nuclear replacement strategies preserve the anulus and end plate, making it easier to be revised to a fusion or a disc replacement if required.

Over the years, attempts at nuclear replacement were limited by the lack of material technology and a suitable design. With more recent advances, it has been possible to use materials that replicate the native nucleus properties and are able to imbibe and hold water. Multiple designs are in the process of development and in clinical studies. Current outcome data have been encouraging in terms of improved VAS and ODI scores. However, owing to lack of randomized controlled trials, it is unclear if these results are better and more durable than stand-alone discectomy or fusion procedures. Longer-term studies are required to assess the effects of nuclear replacement on the progress of degenerative cascade.

Major clinical concerns with nuclear replacement have been the risk of implant extrusion and end-plate changes with subsidence. It is hoped that continuing improvements in material selection, design properties, and surgical techniques will address the issue of implant extrusion. Implant extrusion rates have been declining over the years with changes in technology. End-plate changes are thought of as precursors for subsidence. However, these are also common after most types of surgical procedures involving the disc, such as decompression, discectomy, and fusion. Subsidence seems to stabilize over time and, in most cases, leads to no clinical sequelae. Attempts at dorsal motion preservation systems such as dynamic rods and facet replacements in combination with a nuclear replacement are also ongoing. These technologies may provide options for 360 degrees of motion preservation.

KEY REFERENCES

Ahrens M, Tsantrizos A, Donkersloot P, et al: Nucleus replacement with the DASCOR disc arthroplasty device: interim two-year efficacy and safety results from two prospective, non-randomized multicenter European studies. *Spine (Phila Pa 1976)* 34:1376–1384, 2009.

Allen MJ, Schoonmaker JE, Bauer TW, et al: Preclinical evaluation of a poly (vinyl alcohol) hydrogel implant as a replacement for the nucleus pulposus. *Spine (Phila Pa 1976)* 29(5):515–523, 2004.

Fernstrom U: Arthroplasty with intercorporal endoprosthesis in herniated disc and in painful disc. *Acta Chir Scand Suppl* 357:154–159, 1966.

Hamby WB, Glaser HT: Replacement of spinal intervertebral discs with locally polymerizing methyl methacrylate: experimental study of effects upon tissues and report of a small clinical series. *J Neurosurg* 16:311–313, 1959.

Ray CD: The PDN prosthetic disc-nucleus device. *Eur Spine J* 11(Suppl 2):S137–S142, 2002.

Shim CS, Lee SH, Park CW, et al: Partial disc replacement with the PDN prosthetic disc nucleus device: early clinical results. *J Spinal Disord Tech* 16:324–330, 2003.

REFERENCES

The complete reference list is available online at expertconsult.com.

CHAPTER 164

Dorsal Dynamic Spine Stabilization

Lissa C. Baird | Anthony Sin | Anil Nanda

An estimated 1 million spine procedures are performed each year in the United States.[1,2] The primary strategies used in these procedures include decompression of neural elements or stabilization using rigid fusion techniques. Spine stabilization surgeries are performed to correct or prevent deformity, diminish pathologic motion, compensate for iatrogenic destabilization, or eliminate pain generators. The introduction of rigid instrumentation to these procedures dramatically improved the rate and success of fusion.[3,4] The use of rigid instrumentation provides an optimal environment for intervertebral or posterolateral fusion to occur by immobilizing two or more spinal segments. In addition, spinal instrumentation has allowed for more aggressive decompression and direct reduction or stabilization of spondylolisthesis.

The initial outcomes of fusion surgeries dramatically improved with rigid instrumentation, and long-term consequences have since been recognized.[4] Patients undergoing arthrodesis are exposed to numerous long-term morbidities, including pseudarthrosis, fixed sagittal alignment that cannot adapt to postural change, and adjacent-level degeneration. The risk to adjacent levels is the most concerning of these because the degenerative changes are noted to be significantly accelerated compared with the natural history.[5,6] Rigid titanium or stainless steel constructs have a supraphysiologic degree of stiffness that far exceeds normal bone or a noninstrumented fusion. This stiffness at the instrumented levels has a direct relationship to the stress load on the adjacent disc and facet joints.[4,7] Over time, this additional stress can result in segment hypermobility, osteophyte formation, facet hypertrophy, disc herniation, and stenosis.[4]

Although the reported findings of radiographically evident adjacent-level disease are widely variable in the literature, the incidence of symptomatic adjacent-level disease is higher in patients who have undergone an instrumented fusion (12.2–18.5%) than in patients who have undergone a noninstrumented fusion (5.2–5.6%) in the lumbosacral spine.[4,8,9] Other contributors to adjacent-level disease include muscular and ligamentous disruption, bone removal, and the underlying disease process; however, the supraphysiologic biomechanical stress created by rigid fixation seems to be the most influential factor.[3-5,7] Many patients subsequently need further surgery that may require an extension of their fusion.[10]

Posterior dynamic stabilization of the spine is a rapidly evolving technique in thoracolumbar spine procedures. The concept of dorsal dynamic stabilization was introduced as a potential alternative for treating spine disorders that would avoid the long-term morbidities associated with instrumented fusion constructs. These constructs are likely far more rigid than is necessary to augment a fusion. One objective of dynamic dorsal instrumentation is to move the construct toward a more optimal degree of stiffness that reduces the risk of developing adjacent-level disease, while still promoting fusion. This construct would provide sufficient immobilization for fusion, while diminishing the degree of supraphysiologic stress on adjacent joints. The ideal device would have an elastic modulus close to that of bone to replicate physiologic behavior best. The altered load transfer of the treated spinal segment theoretically would improve on the long-term results of rigid fusion.

An alternative goal of dynamic stabilization is to restore the function of segmental mobility by replicating the behavior and biomechanics of a healthy spinal segment. Intervertebral motion is maintained or restored, while restricting the extremes of movement or dampening the kinetic energy of motion.[2] Dynamic stabilization systems may help some pain syndromes by restricting movement to a range in which only normal loading may occur, preventing the spinal segment from reaching any position where abnormal loading generates pain.[11] In addition, a dynamic stabilizing device must withstand physiologic static and dynamic loads in any plane.[10]

Advantages of Dynamic Stabilization

The advantages associated with using dynamic constructs are primarily anticipated over the long term. Implantation of most dorsal dynamic stabilizing devices has similar immediate postoperative effects to a rigid construct. Both approaches have the capacity to restore lumbar lordosis, sacral tilt, and foraminal diameter in the immediate postoperative period, showing that dynamic devices have the potential for equally good short-term results regarding sagittal spine alignment and decompression of neural elements.[12] The only short-term advantage lies in the elimination of morbidities associated with harvesting autograft when the dynamic device is replacing a potential fusion construct.[13]

Pseudarthrosis is a significant factor associated with poor outcomes after surgical fusions. The incidence rate for pseudarthrosis varies widely depending on the location, surgical technique, and number of levels fused. A meta-analysis on pseudarthrosis after lumbar arthrodesis reported a rate of 14%.[14] Most reported incidence rates of pseudarthrosis after circumferential fusion are less than 10%.[13] Anterior cervical discectomy and fusion has a low rate of pseudarthrosis (<10%), although this is increased if multiple levels are involved. Regardless of this variability, pseudarthrosis is a clinically significant adverse outcome after spine fusion. Dynamic devices used in place of fusion constructs eliminate the potential adverse outcome of pseudarthrosis.

Although one postulated advantage of dynamic technology is the preservation of motion, the functional implications of this aspect are less relevant in the lumbosacral spine. However, retained mobility may contribute to the reduction of symptomatic adjacent-level disease—the most significant potential advantage of dynamic dorsal stabilization.

Because the prevalence of adjacent-level disease is so variable in the literature, it is difficult to make generalizations regarding its occurrence after fusion surgeries. The level, location, and length of the fusion all appear to have an impact on the likelihood of developing future degeneration at adjacent spinal levels. The reported incidence of the prevalence of adjacent-level disease during long-term follow-up after rigid spine fusion ranges from 32% to 36% in the lumbar spine.[13] Regardless of the exact etiology, a significant percentage of patients are affected by this problem after a successful spine fusion.

Several retrospective studies evaluating various posterior dynamic devices have shown lower rates of reoperation for and prevalence of adjacent-level disease. The theoretical reduction of this problem has yet to be definitively proven in the literature, however, and long-term follow-up of randomized controlled trials is necessary to determine absolutely the advantage of dynamic technology and the appropriate patient population for its application.[10,15,16]

Indications

The indications for dorsal dynamic stabilization vary depending on the device being considered and are likely to expand as this new technology evolves. The longest-standing indication has been for augmentation of interbody fusion. The typical adjunct to interbody fusion is rigid fixation with pedicle screws and rods. The supraphysiologic rigidity of these constructs creates stress shielding of the interbody graft and likely contributes to a certain portion of resulting pseudarthroses.[17] A dorsal dynamic stabilization device allows for an increase in anterior load sharing that augments fusion, while limiting any extremes of motion that could result in graft displacement.[2]

Dynamic devices may also be used in an iatrogenically destabilized spine to provide controlled motion. Decompressive surgeries that involve laminectomy and disruption of the facet joint are used to treat lumbar stenosis and lateral recess stenosis. If a significant amount of encroachment of the superior facet is involved, the decompression required may lead to iatrogenic destabilization. Typical management options for such a situation include primary fusion of the spine at the affected levels or observation for the development of sagittal plane imbalance or deformity.[2] Dorsal dynamic stabilization provides another option after a potentially destabilizing procedure and could allow for controlled mobility at the treated spinal levels, while avoiding the need for arthrodesis.[18]

At the present time, the most widely applied use of this technology is for prevention of fusion-related sequelae. Adjacent-level disease and pseudarthrosis are the most commonly considered problems; however, rigid arthrodesis may also lead to loss of lumbar lordosis if excessive distraction is used. The loss of lumbar lordosis can cause a fixed sagittal imbalance or flat-back deformity that may create symptoms of fatigue, gait disturbance, or construct failure. When applied for this indication, dynamic stabilization devices may avoid the need for reintervention from development of any of these adverse sequelae.

Patients with osteoporosis or osteopenia may benefit from dorsal dynamic stabilization. These patients are especially prone to construct failure when rigid stabilization devices are used because the bone-metal interface creates significant bony destruction. Using less rigid fixation may be ideal in these patients and reduce the incidence of construct failure.[2]

A controversial and poorly understood indication for the use of dorsal dynamic stabilization involves its use to protect and restore degenerated facet joints and intervertebral discs. Rather than attempting to remove or destroy the pain generators in the disc or facet joints via fusion, the placement of a dorsal dynamic device may shield the disc and facet joints from destructive motion, allowing for a reduction in inflammatory processes and permitting self-repair mechanisms to operate.[2] This application may become a more valid indication as understanding of the pathophysiology of back pain improves.

Finally, complete circumferential reconstruction of the motion segment may be possible with combined technologies. The presence of facet disease is a contraindication for total disc arthroplasty because this procedure alone is thought to accelerate facet degeneration. A dorsal dynamic stabilization device may be used in conjunction with a total disc replacement, allowing for reconstruction of all mobile joints in a spinal segment.[2]

Fundamental Concepts

The concept of dynamism involves controlled and limited deformation of the spine. An ideal dynamic implant prevents undesirable deformation, while allowing desirable deformation and controlling its extent.

Dynamic implants that are not intended for fusion need to bear substantial and repetitive loads for many decades. A thorough understanding of spinal biomechanics must be involved in the engineering of these implants. The vertebral motion segments are designed to provide stability, mobility, and load transmission to the spinal column. The primary joint responsible for load bearing and stability is the intervertebral disc. The secondary load-bearing and stabilizing structure is the facet joint. The anatomy of the facet joints varies depending on the region of the spine being considered.

The cervical spine facet joints are oriented in a plane that is midway between a coronal and an axial plane. They resist extension and anterior translation.[19,20] The facet joints are loaded by anterior shear forces during extension in the cervical spine. Facet joints in the lumbar spine are oriented in a plane that is midway between the sagittal and coronal planes with a slight anterior incline. Lumbar facet joints resist extension and bear large compressive loads while in extension. During flexion or axial compression, lumbar facets are unloaded.[20] Anterior shear forces load the lumbar facet joints, whereas posterior shear forces unload them. The prevalence of substantial and repetitive physiologic loads on the lumbar facets is clinically relevant given their source as major pain generators.[19] The posterior supraspinous and intraspinous ligaments resist posterior translation and bear tensile loads.

The biomechanics of dynamic posterior stabilization constructs vary among devices. Typically, the pain-generating tissue is left in situ, while the device restricts certain types of motion and alters load transfer.[19] Engineering of posterior dynamic stabilization devices must be done with the kinematics of a functional spinal unit in mind. The posterior and anterior elements of a motion segment move in harmony with each other, and a significant disruption of one could result in excessive loads being placed on the other. Dynamic implants should be constructed with the capacity to maintain range of motion similar to a healthy spinal segment. Excessive motion could lead to degeneration that may include facet arthrosis or hypertrophy, ligamentum flavum hypertrophy, or disc degeneration. Inadequate motion prevents the goals of the dynamic device from being met.[19]

Some applications of dynamism apply the phenomenon of Wolff's law to promote bone healing. Wolff's law states that bone remodels and becomes stronger under increased loads to resist those loads. The reverse is also true, and decreasing the load on a bone results in its weakening. When applied to spine fusions, this theory states that transmitting forces to an intervertebral graft and avoiding stress shielding increase the rate and success of arthrodesis.[18] Rigid posterior instrumentation may unload an intervertebral graft, resulting in fusion failure. However, a dynamic device loads the graft when used as a posterior tension band supplement, increasing the likelihood of fusion.

Avoiding adjacent-level disease is one of the driving goals behind the development of dynamic devices. The biomechanics behind this adverse effect have been studied in cadaver and animal models.[19,21,22] Fusion of a spinal segment increases the stress on the anulus and end plates of adjacent levels and increases intradiscal pressures. Restricted motion at the fused segment also leads to higher mobility at adjacent segments. In flexion and extension, the loss of mobility across a rigidly fused segment is compensated predominantly in the first rostral adjacent segment.[4] In a dynamic stabilization, the compensation is distributed across the first and second rostral segments and in the caudal adjacent segment.[23] Additionally, the fixed sagittal alignment prevents accommodation of regional alignment changes that occur with different postural positions. If a segment is fused with suboptimal sagittal alignment, degeneration of adjacent levels may be accelerated further.[19]

Dorsal Dynamic Devices

A wide variety of dorsal dynamic stabilization devices are in various stages of development and clinical investigation and use. Any implant that is not rigid and allows some motion provides some degree of dynamism. An absorbable implant could be considered dynamic because it permits delayed spine movement after its structural integrity is lost.[24] Absorbable implants in the posterior spine, in particular, the lumbosacral spine, are rare, and the focus of this classification is on deformable implants. Deformable implants may permit either angular deformation or axial deformation. The generalized objectives considered when designing these devices include avoidance of fatigue failure, maintenance of normal spine resting posture without excessive kyphosis or lordosis, prevention of abnormal load distributions, and easy salvage in case of construct failure.

Dorsal Dynamic Neutral Fixation

Some earlier dorsal dynamic implants that were used in the cervical spine include cerclage wiring with submaximal tension and lateral mass plates with nonfixed moment arm cantilevers. These types of constructs allowed for kyphotic deformation and encouraged fusion by permitting load sharing through the bone graft.

Available dorsal dynamic neutral fixation devices allow for limited movement to occur between the screw and the plate. The most common mechanism is a screw head that can pivot in a concave bed within the plate, allowing a "rocking" motion. Although this type of permissive motion may minimize the chance of failure at the screw-plate interface, the cyclic loading at the screw-bone interface causes degradation, and screws have the potential to pull out under flexion or axial loads. The weak point with this type of fixation is the screw-bone interface. In contrast, in rigid techniques, the weakest point is the screw-plate or screw-rod interface.[25] Considering this difference, a dynamic neutral plating technique in a patient with osteoporotic bone would lead to a high likelihood of construct failure given the poor screw pull-out resistance and the dynamic nature of the construct.[25] A dorsal dynamic neutral construct should always be coupled with sufficient axial load resistance to be stable in flexion. If either the intrinsic axial load-resisting abilities are insufficient or interbody support is not present, excessive flexion can lead to construct failure and potential spinal canal compromise.

Dorsal Dynamic Compressive Fixation

Different forms of dynamic spinal instrumentation allow for varying degrees of intersegmental movement. Although some degree of compressive motion augments bone healing according to Wolff's law, excessive intersegmental movement suppresses bony fusion. This concept can be applied to spine surgery in the form of dorsal compressive fixation. A dynamic dorsal tension band that supplements a ventral interbody fusion by providing compressive forces enhances bone healing by encouraging subsidence. When applying a dorsal dynamic compression device for axial loading, the presence of either a solid ventral interbody or intact spinal elements that would not allow excessive flexion is required. Given the substantial axial loads in the thoracic and lumbar portions of the spine, this concept has primarily been used for cervical fusions.[24]

Posterior Interspinous Devices

The purpose of this category of dorsal dynamic fixation device is to create neural decompression with only a minimal amount of tissue resection. The superficial location of these devices allows for implantation with minimal dissection and can be performed without general anesthesia if necessary. The decompression is indirect, and laminectomy is typically not performed, avoiding the risk of a cerebrospinal fluid leak or epidural scarring. The indication for placement of a posterior interspinous device is neurogenic claudication and pain associated with facet joint disease. The spine is kept in flexed position, allowing the device to distract the canal and vertebral foramen.[2] Extension is limited, unloading the facet joints and theoretically relieving any associated pain. Because of this limit in spine extension, however, there is some concern for the development of kyphotic deformity.

Wallis System

The Wallis system (Abbott Spine, Austin, TX), introduced in 1986, was the first interspinous device to be used clinically. The first version of the device consisted of a titanium spacer inserted between spinous processes and held in place by an artificial Dacron ligament wrapped around adjacent processes. The second-generation device changed the material to polyetheretherketone (PEEK), a polymer with an elastic modulus closer to bone, making the construct less rigid. Initial clinical studies showed the safety and efficacy of this device, and long-term follow-up in patients who had the Wallis device placed after initial plans to undergo decompression and fusion found that arthrodesis was avoided in 80% of patients.[26] A prospective controlled trial showed a lower incidence of adjacent-segment disease and need for reintervention when this device was placed at the spinal level rostral to a short fusion segment.[27]

X-Stop Device

The X-Stop device (Medtronic, Minneapolis, MN) was approved for use by the U.S. Food and Drug Administration (FDA) in 2005. It consists of an oval titanium spacer that fits between two adjacent spinous processes (Fig. 164-1). It is placed through a small midline incision after subperiosteal elevation of paraspinal muscles. The supraspinous ligament is left intact. Dilators expand a space between the spinous processes until the ligament is taut, and a sized X-Stop device is inserted. There is no rigid attachment; the implant is kept in place by the lamina, supraspinous ligament, caudal and rostral spinous processes, and device wings laterally.[28] Clinical studies have established the efficacy of the device for the treatment of neurogenic claudication secondary to lumbar stenosis and have shown improved outcomes compared with conservative management.[29] At 2-year follow-up of 175 patients selected for X-Stop implantation, only 4.6% of patients needed further surgical treatment.[30]

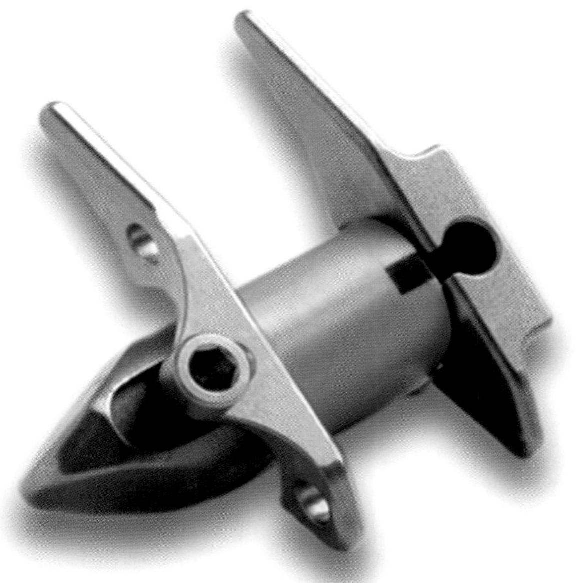

FIGURE 164-1. The X-Stop device comprises an oval titanium spacer that fits between two adjacent spinous processes. (Courtesy of Medtronic, Minneapolis, MN.)

DIAM System

The DIAM spine stabilization system (Medtronic) consists of a soft interspinous spacer created by a silicone core surrounded by polyethylene coating. In contrast to the X-Stop device, the interspinous ligament is removed before placement of the DIAM system directly above the ligamentum flavum. It is secured to the spinous processes. The goal of this implant is to reduce intradiscal pressure, retighten posterior elements, and reduce rotatory dislocation via posterior shock absorption of the implant; this theoretically protects the entire motion segment from excessive loads and slows the degenerative process.[31] The DIAM device has been used in Europe to treat foraminal stenosis and disc protrusions. Studies have shown efficacy and satisfaction among patients.[2,32] A prospective study following 68 patients who had the DIAM device placed after decompressive surgery found that none of the patients had recurrence of disease requiring further intervention, and all patients showed clinical improvement.[33] Controlled studies with this device have not been published yet.

Additional interspinous devices are in various stages of development, clinical trial, or clinical use outside of the United States. These include the Coflex device (Paradigm Spine, New York, NY), the ExtendSure and CoRoent devices (NuVasive, San Diego, CA), and the Aperius PercLID (Kyphon-Medtronic). Most of these devices are designed to treat neurogenic claudication and foraminal stenosis. Further information on the biomechanical properties and efficacy of these devices is needed before they become available for clinical application.

Pedicle Screw and Rod-Based Dynamic Devices

Pedicle screw and rod-based dynamic devices are designed to function by maintaining normal motion within a physiologic range, unloading degenerated discs and facet joints, and stabilizing the abnormal segment. The resultant decrease in load potentially alleviates any pain coming from degenerating joints. Another goal of these devices is the prevention of adjacent-segment disease. This goal can be approached either by placing a dynamic system as an entire construct or by using a dynamic device to extend a rigid construct across adjacent levels. When used as an adjunct to intervertebral fusion, these devices may provide an optimal environment by load sharing to the intervertebral implant and allowing micromovements across end plates. Another indication for their use is for stabilization after iatrogenic destabilizing procedures, such as wide laminectomies and facetectomies. Many of these implants have been approved for use with fusion, and many require further evidence of their efficacy as stand-alone constructs.

Graf System

The Graf ligamentoplasty system (Surgicraft, Redditch, UK) has a relatively long history of clinical application compared with other dynamic devices. Titanium pedicle screws are connected by prosthetic ligaments made of braided polyester bands. These bands are connected under a compressive force to hold the spinal segment in lordosis. The objective of this construct is to maintain a fixed lordosis of the lumbar spine, compress the posterior anulus to prevent anular tears, and splint the motion segment, allowing repair to damaged joints.[34] The posterior anulus acts as a fulcrum between the tensile forces of the construct and the compressive forces across the disc space. Load is transferred from the anterior disc to the posterior anulus and facet joints, limiting pathologic motion.

The device is indicated for the treatment of flexion instability, but it does not correct spondylolisthesis or scoliotic deformity. Over time, the bands relax, allowing for the return of some kyphotic motion. Although initially developed as a method of treating back pain from disc degeneration, this device has also been used to stabilize spondylolistheses after posterior decompression. The success of this procedure depends on appropriate patient selection, and its indication is restricted to patients with less than 25% of a vertebral slip, minimal disc space narrowing, and coronal facet tropism.[34] Long-term results have shown Graf ligamentoplasty to be an effective treatment option in appropriately selected patients. Concerns with this device include the development of iatrogenic lateral recess stenosis, overloading of the posterior anulus and facet joints, and some reports of high revision rates.[2,19,35,36]

Dynesys System

The Dynesys system (Zimmer Spine, Minneapolis, MN) consists of standard pedicle screws attached by polyester cords that pass through compression-resistant polycarbonate urethane spacers. This device has been in use since the early 1990s.[2] The Dynesys system is used to treat dynamic instability in the early stages of degeneration, degenerative disease causing low back pain, or iatrogenic instability after decompression.[10] This device realigns and stabilizes a spinal segment into its physiologic position, while neutralizing excessive loads. The dynamic relationship between the polyester cords and the spacers limits segmental mobility to a physiologic level and neutralizes bending, torsional, and shear forces.[37] The polyester cords resist flexion, whereas the spacers resist compressive forces and prevent excessive lordosis. The combination of these construct components limits the loading of the disc (Fig. 164-2).

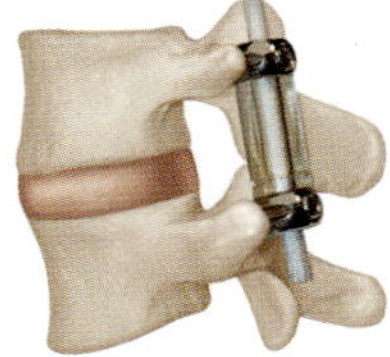

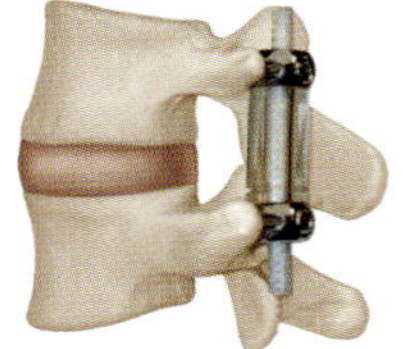

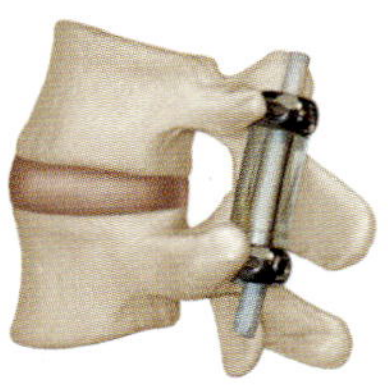

FIGURE 164-2. The Dynesys device is designed to neutralize excessive loads. The polyester cords resist flexion, and the spacers resist excessive extension and compressive forces on the intervertebral disc. (Courtesy of Zimmer Spine, Minneapolis, MN.)

Clinical studies have shown the efficacy of this device and shown improved outcome over conservative treatment. The short-term results are comparable to conventional rigid fixation.[38] Concerns with this system have focused on the high reported rate of construct failure (17% to 19%).[38] Excessive compressive loads on the spacers produce bending moments on the pedicle screws that can lead to breakage or loosening. Another concern is the potential for the compressive sleeves to become kyphogenic under excessive distraction. These sleeves also increase the rigidity of the construct and limit its ability to maintain physiologic motion.[19] Whether or not the Dynesys device decreases the development of adjacent-level disease remains to be seen. One study comparing range of motion after instrumented fusion and posterior dynamic stabilization using Dynesys at L4-5 analyzed preoperative and postoperative flexion-extension radiographs. Global and L4-5 segmental range of motion was reduced in the fusion group and unchanged in the Dynesys group. However, no significant changes in mobility at the rostral or caudal adjacent levels were seen in either group (Fig. 164-3).[39]

Semirigid Rods

Several indications exist for the use of semirigid rods. When attempting to treat spondylolisthesis, recurrent disc herniation, or degenerative disc disease with a solid osseous arthrodesis, semirigid rods may be used to create less potential stress on adjacent spinal segments. Another indication involves patients with a prior instrumented fusion. If symptomatic adjacent-level disease develops, an extension of the instrumentation to the newly affected level can be undertaken with semirigid rods to prevent a subsequent recurrence. Semirigid rods can be used to replace the entire construct length or as an adjunct extension over the adjacent level. A third indication for this type of construct involves patients with spondylolisthesis and stenosis. An osseous arthrodesis may be avoided in these cases if semirigid rods are placed after a facet-sparing laminectomy; this maintains the posterior tension band and limits any progression of the pathologic process.[4]

Dorsal rods made of the PEEK polymer (Medtronic) have semirigid characteristics. This polymer has a modulus of

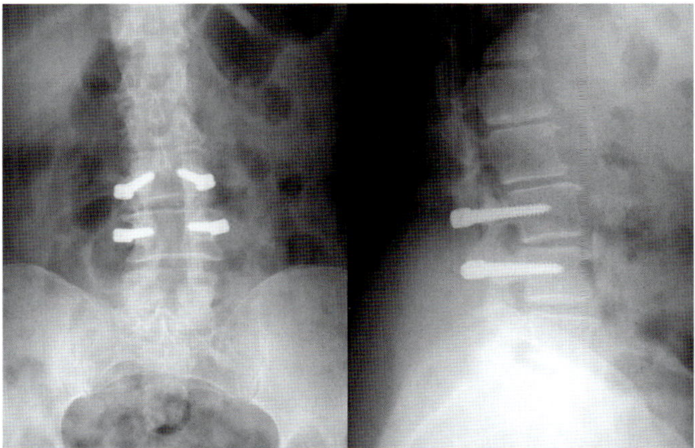

FIGURE 164-3. Anteroposterior and lateral spine radiographs obtained after implantation of the Dynesys system. (Courtesy of Zimmer Spine, Minneapolis, MN.)

elasticity between cortical and cancellous bone.[4] The rods allow some motion but resist any marked degree of flexion, extension, axial loading, or lateral rotation. Their use reduces stress and hypermobility at adjacent levels compared with rigid titanium constructs. PEEK rods can also reduce stress at the bone-screw interface, reducing the risk of construct failure.[4] Although these rods may address the causative factors of adjacent-segment disease, no studies establishing their long-term clinical outcomes have been reported.

The AccuFlex rods (Globus Medical, Audubon, PA) have helical cuts that allow for a limited range of motion, while providing a posterior tension band that unloads the intervertebral disc.[18] This system has been approved by the FDA for use in conjunction with an interbody graft, and studies have shown fusion rates and outcomes similar to rigid fixation. Further studies are needed to evaluate the impact on adjacent-level disease and its potential use as a standalone dynamic construct. Other semirigid dorsal rods are in development; however, limited clinical data are available on these devices.[2]

Total Facet Replacement Systems

The restoration of functional facet joints is a relatively new focus for dorsal dynamic stabilization devices. The facet joints can be potential pain generators whether associated disc degeneration is present or absent.[2] A primary indication for total facet arthroplasty is pain originating from degenerative facet joints. Another indication focuses on reconstructing an iatrogenically destabilized spine. Combining aggressive decompressive surgeries with total facet arthroplasty may reduce the likelihood of iatrogenic destabilization and the need for arthrodesis. A final application for this technology is for its use in combination with total disc replacement. Disease of the facet joints is currently a contraindication for total disc arthroplasty, but the combination of these technologies may allow for a circumferential motion segment reconstruction and a broader application of both devices (Fig. 164-4).[2]

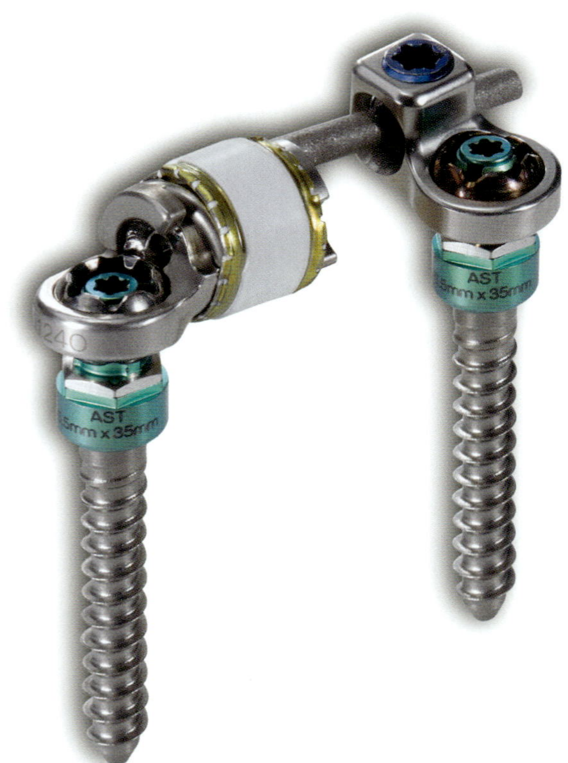

FIGURE 164-4. Total facet replacement systems are designed to treat destabilized or degenerating facet joints. The Stabilimax system uses a dual-spring mechanism to provide optimal stiffness, while allowing near-normal kinematics. The ball-and-socket pedicle screw connections minimize the load at the bone-screw interface during flexion and extension. (Courtesy of Applied Spine Technologies, Wellesley, MA.)

Stabilimax NZ Device

The Stabilimax NZ device (Applied Spine Technologies, Wellesley, MA) is designed to support a degenerating spinal segment while preserving normal mobility. This system potentially reduces pain associated with diseased joints and reduces adjacent-level disease. Removal of bony elements is not required to place this construct. Clinical trials are under way to establish its efficacy (Fig. 164-5).

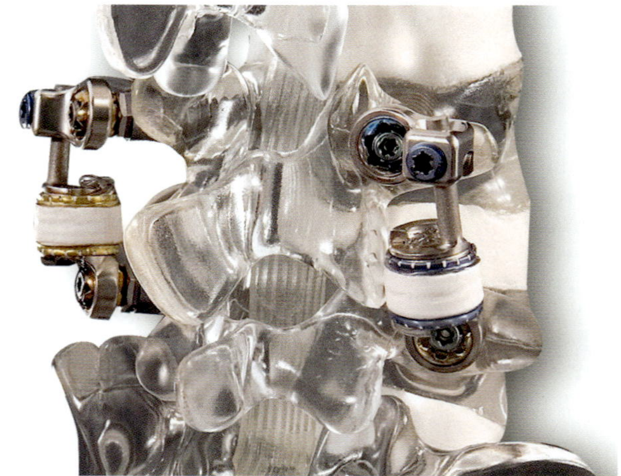

FIGURE 164-5. The Stabilimax NZ device can be placed with or without removal of bony elements to support a degenerating spinal segment, while preserving mobility. (Courtesy of Applied Spine Technologies, Wellesley, MA.)

TFAS Device

The TFAS device (Archus Orthopedics, Redmond, WA) can be used to restore motion after resection of diseased facet joints. It is typically used to treat patients with moderate to severe spinal stenosis. Biomechanical studies have verified restoration of physiologic mobility with movement of a sphere along the curved plate of the device. Clinical trials are under way to demonstrate effectiveness and safety compared with instrumented fusion for the treatment of lumbar stenosis after decompression and facetectomy.[2,40]

TOPS Device

The TOPS device (Impliant, Princeton, NJ) was designed to stabilize a motion segment after laminectomy and medial facetectomy. It shares axial loading with the intervertebral disc and controls lateral, axial, and lordotic mobility. Pedicle screws anchor the device, and an interlocking polyurethane core connects rostral and caudal titanium plates to create a construct that allows controlled physiologic motion. Clinical trials are under way with this device.

Other devices in development include the AFRS (Facet Solutions, Hopkinton, MA) system and the Zyre facet arthroplasty system (Quantum Orthopedics, Carlsbad, CA). The biomechanical function of implants in development is variable, and their introduction as effective devices awaits further clinical studies.

Disadvantages and Complications

The introduction of new technologies is likely to coincide with new methods of failure. Dynamic implants are subjected to biomechanical stressors that are minimal for rigid constructs, and associated complications vary. A dynamically stabilized motion segment is exposed to long-term cyclic loading and is susceptible to fatigue failure or migration of the construct over time. There have not been significant reports of mechanical implant failure in the literature so far; however, dynamic stabilization is a relatively new technology, and longer follow-up periods are needed to assess this risk accurately.

Pedicle screw fixation was initially designed to stabilize a spinal segment while the fusion completed and assumed the load-bearing function. In the setting of a dynamic implant, pedicle screws may be expected to anchor a device permanently. The extended cyclic loading of the pedicle screws can lead to loosening or fatigue fracture.[13] One study found a 10% incidence of radiographically evident pedicle screw loosening after placement of a dynamic device.[41] Loosening usually occurred within 6 months after implantation and was unlikely to occur after 1 year.

Compliance mismatch may become problematic in the setting of dynamic systems. Because a fusion mass loses bone mineral density along with global systemic loss, compliance mismatch is avoided in arthrodesis. A dynamic metallic device does not have the capacity to adjust its function in the setting of future development of osteoporosis or osteopenia.

A motion segment that has been successfully fused is typically stable over the long term. The absence of motion tends to prevent ligamentous or facet hypertrophy, disc herniation, or the recurrence of neural element compression. Preserving mobility at a spinal segment means preserving the possibility of future degeneration, a problem typically avoided with solid fusion. Degenerative changes can occur at the intervertebral disc, the facet joints, or the ligamentum flavum. The disc may herniate or develop pain generators, the facet joints may become arthritic or hypertrophic, and the ligamentum flavum may hypertrophy and contribute to stenosis. The prevalence of degeneration at dynamically stabilized spinal levels has not been established in the literature and may be difficult to distinguish from errors in patient selection.[13]

Conclusion

The biomechanical applications, appropriate indications, and long-term efficacy of dorsal dynamic stabilization are still being elucidated. Regardless, this technology is likely to be an important tool in the future management of degenerative spine disease. Developing dynamic constructs that are able to relieve pain, restore physiologic mobility, and endure repetitive loads is a tremendous challenge. Optimizing these devices requires a detailed understanding of the pathophysiology of spinal pain syndromes, spinal anatomy, motion segment kinematics, and applied loads, along with sound engineering principles and materials science.[19]

A wide variety of dorsal dynamic stabilization devices are available and in various stages of clinical investigation. Detailed evaluation and diagnosis of a patient's symptoms and pathology helps in selecting patients who may benefit from these devices. Well-designed clinical studies and long-term follow-up are needed to reveal which dynamic constructs are ideal for certain conditions and assist in guiding the evolution of this technology.

KEY REFERENCES

Ekman P, Moller H, Shalabi A, et al: A prospective randomised study on the long-term effect of lumbar fusion on adjacent disc degeneration. *Eur Spine J* 18:1175–1186, 2009.

Huang RC, Girardi FP, Moe RL, et al: Advantages and disadvantages of nonfusion technology in spine surgery. *Orthop Clin North Am* 36:263–269, 2005.

Kanayama M, Togawa D, Hashimoto T, et al: Motion-preserving surgery can prevent early breakdown of adjacent segments: comparison of posterior dynamic stabilization with spinal fusion. *J Spinal Disord Tech* 22:463–467, 2009.

Khoueir P, Kim KA, Wang MY: Classification of posterior dynamic stabilization devices. *Neurosurg Focus* 22:E3, 2007.

Park P, Garton HJ, Gala VC, et al: Adjacent segment disease after lumbar or lumbosacral fusion: review of the literature. *Spine (Phila Pa 1976)* 29: 1938–1944, 2004.

REFERENCES

The complete reference list is available online at expertconsult.com.

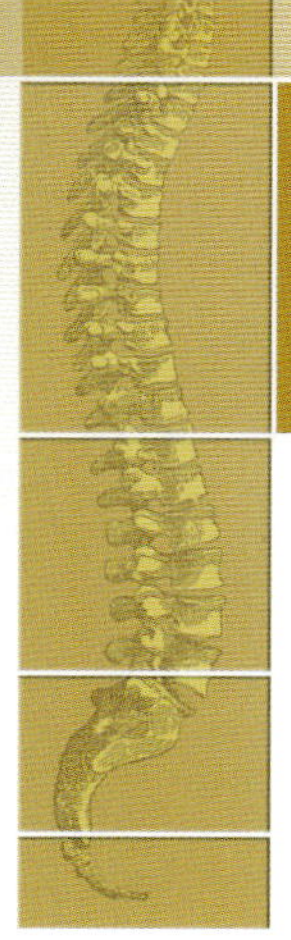

CHAPTER 165

Total Facet Arthroplasty

Vartan Tashjian | Michael Y. Wang

At the present time in the United States, there are four ongoing multicenter, prospective, randomized clinical trials analyzing the safety and comparative efficacy of four distinct total facet arthroplasty (TFA) devices. These studies are designed to compare these implants against control patients undergoing posterior instrumented fusion for management of degenerative lumbar stenosis. The overall common objective of these trials is to ascertain whether TFA can be performed safely in patients with degenerative lumbar stenosis and whether efficacy is at least equal to controls in terms of treating back pain and radiculopathy. As a secondary measure, these studies are likely to be used to assess the long-term effects of motion preservation on adjacent-level degeneration, which may be associated with rigid fixation constructs.

All of these studies were approved by the U.S. Food and Drug Administration (FDA) as Investigational Device Exemptions (IDE) studies; however, three of the four studies are still in the preliminary recruiting phase, with minimal published outcome data. The midterm results of the Total Facet Arthroplasty System (TFAS, Archus Orthopedics, Redmond, WA) U.S. IDE trial were published more recently and were promising.[1] Although the U.S. IDE trial for the Total Posterior-Element System (TOPS, Impliant, Ramat Poleg, Israel) has commenced only more recently, the potential efficacy and safety in the management of degenerative lumbar stenosis were recently underscored in a publication analyzing early clinical outcomes in 29 patients implanted with the device outside of the United States.[2]

Although it has been claimed that the preliminary results for TFA are promising with regard to both safety and efficacy, the relative paucity of published clinical outcome data and its current IDE status have served to limit application of TFA in the management of degenerative lumbar stenosis. This chapter focuses on the ample biomechanical data available for the two main facet replacement systems (TFAS and TOPS) in the context of both in vitro human cadaver and computer-generated finite element analysis models. The remaining two facet replacement systems (ACADIA Facet Replacement System [AFRS], Facet Solutions, Hopkinton, MA; and Stabilimax NZ; Applied Spine Technologies, New Haven, CT) are briefly described because comparatively few biomechanical and clinical data exist at this stage in their respective development. All available preliminary results from the associated clinical trials are presented.

Background

When surgical intervention was first advanced as a viable treatment option for lumbar degenerative disc disease by Dandy in 1929,[3] relatively little was understood with regard to spinal biomechanics. Since that time, as understanding of the underlying biomechanics of the spine has evolved, so too has the application of these principles to the surgical management of various disorders of the spine. Nowhere is this application more apparent than in nonpenetrating, blunt force trauma to the spine, in which management of the resultant stereotyped injury patterns produced in response to externally applied forces has become more intuitive through the application of biomechanical principles derived from anatomic (cadaver) and computer-assisted models. The relevance of biomechanics is not limited to trauma because the application of these same principles can also contribute to restoration of anatomic balance after iatrogenic destabilization of the spine.

The early history of lumbar surgery often involved midline, transdural approaches to the disc space. As surgical technique evolved to extradural discectomy and decompression, the surrounding ligamentous and articular structures began to represent greater barriers to adequate operative visualization. The introduction of the surgical microscope to lumbar discectomy by Yaşargil[4] and Caspar[5] in 1977 served to lateralize and decrease the size of the working surgical field, magnifying further the intimate anatomic relationship between the disc space, lateral recess, and facet complex. As a compensatory maneuver, partial facetectomy was eventually incorporated into the surgical technique to improve both visualization and access to the compressed neural elements. The degree of facetectomy required to achieve decompression safely varies, depending on both surgeon experience and facet joint size and orientation. In a prospective, nonrandomized study, Çelik et al.[6] showed that a facet angle of less than 35 degrees does not allow for a safe surgical corridor, resulting in the need for a more extensive facetectomy.

Over the past 20 years, the use of posterior instrumented fusion, primarily with pedicle screw fixation, has increased dramatically after iatrogenic destabilization of the facet joint in the context of surgical decompression for degenerative lumbar stenosis. In some cases, the facet complex represents the primary pathology, rather than a structural impediment to adequate decompression. This is typically seen in cases of

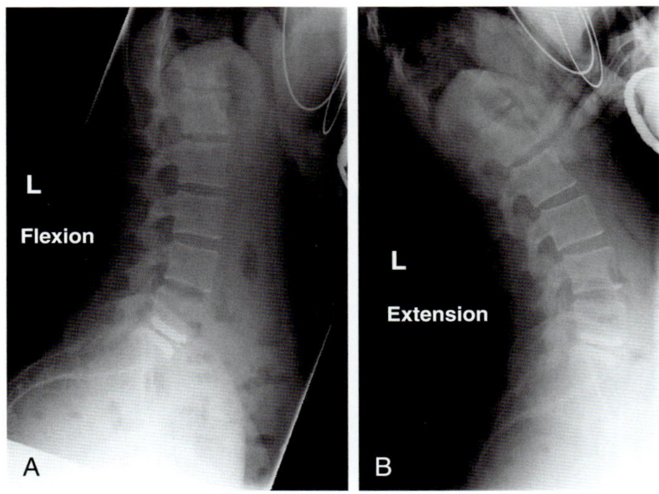

FIGURE 165-1. Flexion (**A**) and extension (**B**) radiographs showing the Charité artificial disc preserving motion at the L5-S1 motion segment.

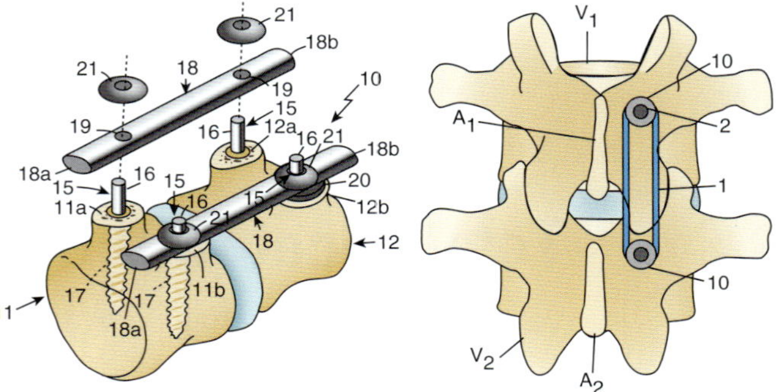

FIGURE 165-2. Early simple elastomeric tension band devices (Graf ligament).

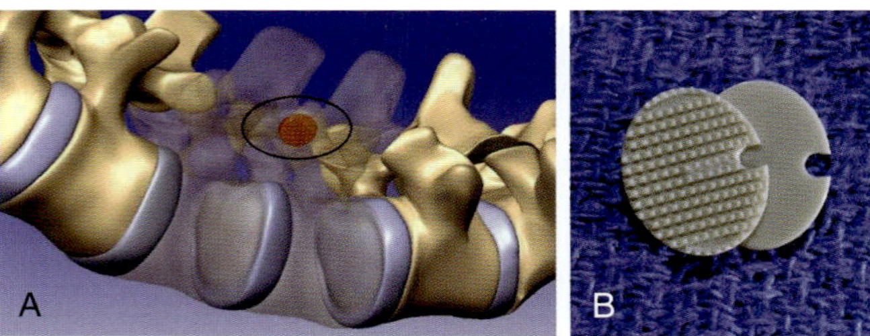

FIGURE 165-3. Facet resurfacing implant designed to replace the synovium, in place (**A**) and showing both sides of the implant (**B**). (From Zyga Technologies, Minneapolis, MN.)

severe facet arthropathy, resulting in significant lateral recess stenosis and nerve root impingement. The more recent, controversial concept of the degenerative facet joint as an independent pain generator has also contributed to the growing trend of combined aggressive facetectomy with posterior instrumented fusion as a common surgical practice.

Whatever the underlying pathology, it is generally accepted that rigid spinal fusion permanently alters both local and global spinal biomechanics. The resultant increased, compensatory range of motion (ROM) at neighboring spinal segments after instrumented fusion leads to accelerated rates of adjacent-level degeneration—25% to 40% over 5 years—often necessitating reoperation for decompression and extension of the fusion construct.[7,8] In this context, the emergence of motion preservation strategies and dynamic stabilization has garnered increasing interest in the both the neurosurgical and orthopedic literature.

Although the concept of motion preservation is not a novel one, the potential restoration of near-normal lumbar kinematics via facet replacement systems is a relatively recent development. Approved by the FDA for single-level disc disease with associated mechanical back pain, the lumbar artificial disc (e.g., Charité, DePuy Spine, Raynham, MA; ProDisc, Synthes Spine, West Chester, PA) has steadily gained acceptance despite limited surgical indications (Fig. 165-1). In contrast to facet arthroplasty, lumbar disc replacement does not allow for direct posterior decompression of neural structures and can accelerate facet degeneration, potentially exacerbating facetogenic pain symptoms. For this reason, its use is contraindicated in patients with radiographic evidence of moderate to severe facet arthropathy.

Dorsal dynamic stabilization (posterior dynamic stabilization [PDS]) devices are placed via a traditional posterior approach, allowing for direct surgical decompression before implantation. Early devices, such as the Graf ligament, were initially popular, but their popularity declined because of poor mechanical wear and issues with elastomeric material properties (Fig. 165-2). Khoueir et al.[9] described a useful classification scheme for PDS devices consisting of (1) interspinous spacer devices (i.e., X STOP, Medtronic, Minneapolis, MN; DIAM, Medtronic; Coflex, Paradigm Spine, New York, NY), (2) pedicle screw and rod–based devices (i.e., Dynesys, Zimmer Spine, Minneapolis, MN; Accuflex rod, Globus Medical, Audobon, PA; Isobar, Alphatec Spine, Carlsbad, CA), and (3) total facet replacement systems (i.e., TFAS, TOPS). Although more conventional pedicle screw and rod–based PDS devices were designed to reduce facet loads and preserve intersegmental kinematics, in vitro biomechanical studies have yielded mixed results. Niosi et al.[10] reported significantly increased peak facet contact forces in flexion-extension and lateral bending in cadaver human spines implanted with the Dynesys system. In theory, a facet arthroplasty system more accurately mirrors the anatomic facet joint, potentially restoring the intrinsic load-sharing properties of the intact facet complex.

Facet joint surgeries to treat the synovial surfaces without replacing the joint itself are being investigated as well. These joint "resurfacing" technologies are in their infancy, holding the promise of treating a dysfunctional synovial joint through less invasive approaches (Fig. 165-3). Because of the lack of scientific data on these devices, they are not discussed further in this chapter.

Facet Biomechanics

Because the biomechanics of the facet joints is rarely discussed, a brief review of facet kinematics in the context of their contribution to the functional spine unit (FSU) is appropriate. The FSU refers to the three-joint structural arrangement of a single spinal level and consists of the intervertebral disc, the two facet joints and their investing capsule, and the associated posterior musculoligamentous supporting structures. The vertebrae articulate with one another via the two diarthrodial encapsulated facet joints at the superior and inferior aspects of the pars interarticularis. By virtue of their bilateral and posterior location, the facets come into maximal contact with one another during extension and axial rotation, contributing more to overall load sharing under these conditions. Generally, the orientation of the facet joint changes at differing locations throughout the spine, from a more coronal orientation with approximately 45 degrees of inclination from the horizontal in the cervical spine to a more sagittal orientation in the lumbar spine.[11] These segment-specific differences in facet geometry and characteristics serve to impart differing patterns of movement at different spinal levels.

By virtue of their more sagittal orientation, the lumbar facet joints serve to provide greater resistance to axial rotation and significantly contribute to axial load bearing, in particular, with the spine in extension.[11-14] The articular surface area also increases from L1 to S1, mirroring the greater shear loads in the lower spine relative to the upper lumbar spine.[14] The application of eloquent computer-generated three-dimensional finite element analyses coupled with biomechanical data obtained from related in vitro human cadaver studies has furthered understanding of lumbosacral facet kinematics in response to iatrogenic destabilization. As anticipated, models replicating bilateral laminectomy and total facetectomy have shown marked increases in the angular ROM of the lumbar motion segment, under flexion-extension and axial rotation.[12,15-18] However, the relative preservation of angular ROM in the context of lateral bending underscores the greater role of the anterior column in load bearing during lateral bending.[19,20] Facet biomechanics also differ between individuals, by spinal level and laterality, making their biomechanics joint-specific.

Facetogenic Pain Syndrome

Although controversial, the concept of the facet joint as a potential pain generator has gained support in recent years. Hirsch et al.[21] first raised the possibility in 1963, when they reported the production of low back pain in subjects whose facet joints were injected with hypertonic saline. Since that time, various accounts in the literature have served both to validate and to refute this theory. Some accounts report a 50% to 60% success rate with facet blocks and rhizolysis procedures,[22] whereas others report a similar efficacy of pain relief in cases in which facet blocks were conducted with normal saline, suggesting a significant placebo effect.[23] Central to the theory of facetogenic pain syndrome is the innervation of the facet joint, which is derived from the medial branches of the dorsal rami originating at the same level and the cephalad spinal level.[24] The joint capsule itself is innervated by numerous mechanoreceptors, which can undergo extensive stretch under conditions of physiologic loading.

In their neuroanatomic and neurophysiologic analysis of the facet joint, Cavanaugh et al.[25] concluded that these nerves are activated by capsular stretch and by neurogenic and non-neurogenic modulators of inflammation, including substance P, bradykinin, and phospholipase A_2. This interplay of mechanical stretch and local inflammatory mediators may serve to propagate the cycle of chronic low back pain in a subset of patients with lumbago. In these patients, total facetectomy followed by facet arthroplasty may represent a viable alternative to rigid arthrodesis. Because facet arthropathy is often encountered concomitantly with advanced disc disease,

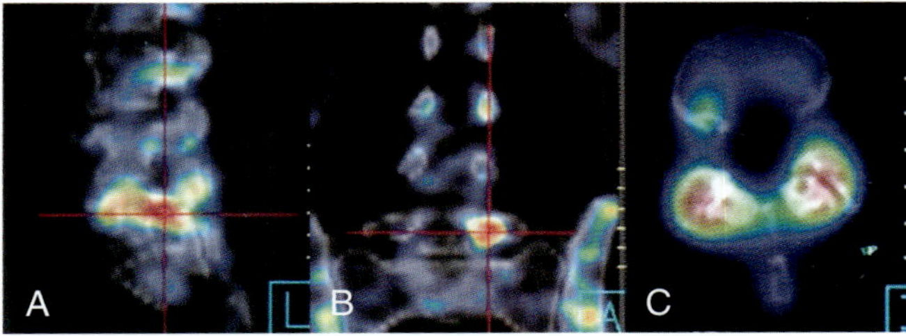

FIGURE 165-4. Single-photon emission computed tomography scan showing "hot" lumbar facets causing axial back pain in the sagittal (**A**), coronal (**B**), and axial (**C**) planes.

replacement of the entire three-joint FSU with combination disc and facet arthroplasty may also ultimately emerge as a future surgical treatment option in patients with severe lumbar degenerative disease.

Facetogenic pain can be diagnosed with imaging studies as well. Test injections, whether intra-articular or periarticular, can be useful for diagnosing facet pain. In addition, nuclear medicine bone scans showing "hot" facets can be useful for identifying inflamed synovial joints (Fig. 165-4).[26,27]

Facet Arthroplasty Devices

At the present time, four TFA devices have progressed to clinical trials: TFAS, TOPS, AFRS, and Stabilimax NZ. Although all of these systems are similar in motion preservation properties and surgical technique for implantation, they are vastly different with regard to their respective design technology and build material. To date, most published clinical outcome data have come from the TFAS U.S. IDE trial,[1] although limited clinical accounts regarding the relative efficacy and safety of the TOPS device in patients undergoing implantation outside of the United States can be found in the international spine literature.[2]

Total Facet Arthroplasty System

Implant Characteristics

The TFAS device consists of two rostral spherical bearings attached to stems implanted into the rostral pedicles, which articulate with two proportionately sized caudal bearing surfaces, affixed to the pedicles below (Fig. 165-5). The geometry of the caudal bearing surfaces is designed to provide a gradual resistance to motion, in an attempt to recapitulate the diarthrodial facet kinematics of the intact spinal segment.[15,16,18] Composed entirely of implantable grade metals, the TFAS device is placed via a standard open posterior surgical approach, following decompressive laminectomy and facetectomy. The implant-pedicle interface is augmented with polymethylmethacrylate, similar to the TOPS device, which uses hydroxyapatite to fortify the construct.[2,18]

Biomechanical Data

Several in vitro biomechanical studies analyzing linear and angular ROM in human cadaver lumbar spines under intact, injured (bilateral laminectomy and total facetectomy), and implanted (with TFAS) conditions, all have served to show

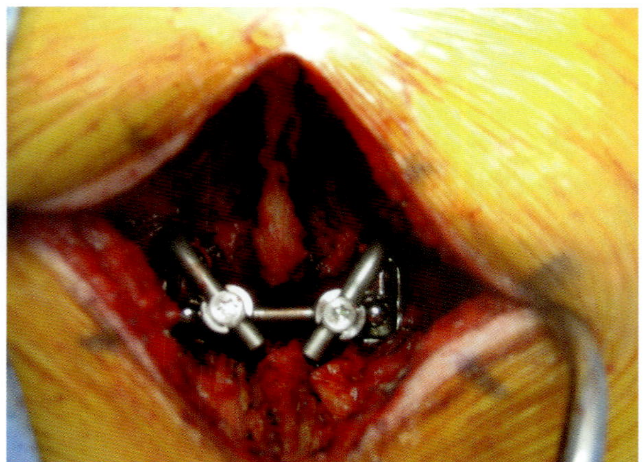

FIGURE 165-5. Intraoperative view of the Total Facet Arthroplasty System implant, with a cobalt-chrome ball riding within a metal "basket" during flexion and extension.

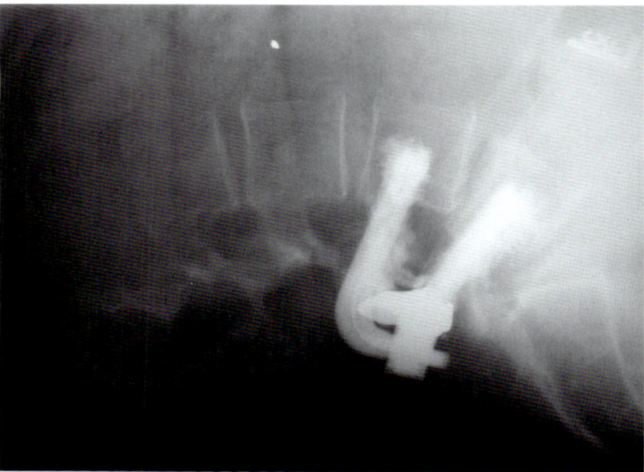

FIGURE 165-6. Lateral radiograph of the Total Facet Arthroplasty System implant with cemented pedicle stems.

a relative conservation of intact spinal biomechanics at implanted and adjacent levels in iatrogenically destabilized specimens.[14-16,18] Phillips et al.[15] assessed multidirectional flexibility in nine human cadaver spines under various conditions including intact, after L3-4 laminectomy and facetectomy (injured), after L3-4 pedicle screw fixation, and after stabilization with L3-4 TFAS implantation. The injured and rigidly stabilized models had increased (injured model) and decreased (rigidly stabilized model) flexion-extension, lateral bending, and axial rotation ROM at the intervened level, whereas TFAS implantation restored intact ROM in all directions and resulted in near-normal load displacement curves.[15] Additionally, the associated increase in ROM observed at adjacent spinal levels after L3-4 pedicle screw fixation was essentially restored to intact values after implantation of the TFAS device. Similar results have been published using in vitro models at L4-5 and L5-S1 and three-dimensional finite element analyses of the lumbosacral spine.[14,18,28]

Clinical Outcome Data

The midterm results of the TFAS U.S. IDE trial for the management of degenerative lumbar stenosis were released more recently; the longest clinical follow-up was 24 months.[1] This multicenter, prospective, randomized clinical trial with a concurrent surgical (pedicle screw fixation) control was designed to compare clinical outcomes between the two surgical cohorts as a primary end point, with relative safety and radiographic evaluation of ROM as important secondary end points. Of the 104 patients enrolled in the study to date, 96 had undergone TFAS implantation, whereas only 8 patients were randomly assigned to the instrumented fusion cohort. With regard to symptomatic improvement, 84% of the TFAS patients showed significant improvement in the Zurich Claudication Questionnaire (ZCQ) symptom scores, and 81% showed significant improvement in the ZCQ function scores. Visual analogue scale scores for leg and back pain improved in 95% and 85% of TFAS patients. Radiographic analysis revealed all implanted devices to be intact and functioning, with preserved ROM at the implanted level (Fig. 165-6). No device-specific complications were encountered. Although the preliminary results of this clinical trial suggest that the comparative efficacy and relative device safety of the TFAS implant in the management of degenerative lumbar stenosis appear to be at least equal to pedicle screw fixation, the data must be interpreted with caution given the small number of patients enrolled in the control group.

Total Posterior Element System

Implant Characteristics

In contrast to the diarthrodial, multicomponent structure of the TFAS implant, the TOPS device is unitary in design, composed of a titanium construct with an interlocking, flexible, articulating core, surrounded by a polyurethane elastomer cover that is capable of transmitting tensile and compressive loads, in addition to shear forces (Fig. 165-7). Surgical technique involves a standard open posterior approach for complete laminectomy and facetectomy, placement of cannulated polyaxial pedicle screws under direct fluoroscopic guidance, and attachment of the unitary TOPS implant to the pedicle screw heads with standard locking set-screw caps, which are ultimately counter-torqued to their final tightness. Finally, a small amount of sterile saline is injected through a port in the bottom of the implant to serve as a lubricant.

Biomechanical Data

Compared with the TFAS implant, fewer biomechanical data exist in the literature to support the TOPS device as a viable option for PDS in the surgical management of degenerative lumbar stenosis. The largest study, an in vitro analysis of six

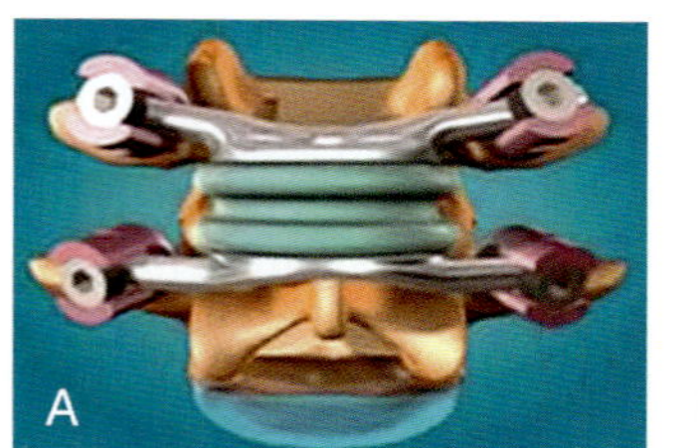

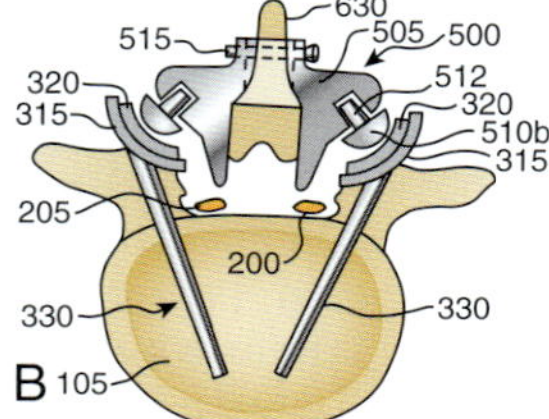

FIGURE 165-7. Photo (**A**) and schematic (**B**) of the Total Posterior-Element System device. (Courtesy of Impliant, Ramat Poleg, Israel.)

human cadaver spines implanted with the TOPS device at L4-5 after bilateral laminectomy and total facetectomy, showed restoration of near-normal motion behavior to the implanted spinal level in left and right lateral bending and axial rotation.[17] ROM in flexion-extension was 85% of that seen in an intact segment, which is higher than published results for both Dynesys and TFAS.[10,18] The spines implanted with the TOPS device did not show any significant increase in mobility at the adjacent spinal levels. Intradiscal pressure monitoring revealed a significant reduction in intradiscal forces at the implanted level, while still allowing the disc to participate in near-normal load sharing.[17]

Clinical Outcome Data

McAfee et al.[2] reported preliminary results of a prospective, multicenter, nonrandomized, clinical trial of 29 patients with degenerative lumbar stenosis implanted with the TOPS device, with longest clinical follow-up of 1 year. In this international trial, all 29 patients underwent surgery outside of the United States, with 28 of 29 having the device implanted at the L4-5 level. As a whole, the patients' clinical status seemed to improve after surgery. Of the 11 patients with 1-year follow-up, the mean Oswestry Disability Index score decreased by 41%, the mean visual analogue scale leg pain score decreased by 86%, and the mean ZCQ score decreased by 54%.[2] Radiographic analysis showed that both lumbar ROM and disc height at the implanted and adjacent levels were preserved at 1-year follow-up. Device-specific adverse events, including radiographic evidence of screw pull-out or device failure, were not observed during the brief follow-up period.

ACADIA Facet Replacement System and Stabilimax DZ

Implant Characteristics

The AFRS device is a pedicle screw and cross-link–based system that is similar to the TFAS device in design philosophy. Using surgical grade metals, this multicomponent implant most closely resembles the anatomic facet joint previously secured in situ. In contrast to the TFAS device, which employs a spherical bearing–bearing surface interface as a surrogate for the native facet joint, the AFRS implant uses an angulated metallic articular interface that is both spinal level–specific and patient-specific with regard to its implanted orientation and size.

The Stabilimax NZ implant is similarly anchored in place with pedicle screw fixation; however, motion preservation is achieved through bilateral independent concentric springs incorporated via connecting rods (Fig. 165-8). Panjabi and Timm[29] tested 70 bilateral assemblies of the Stabilimax NZ implant, which exceeded static, fatigue, wear resistance, and histologic requirements, resulting in permission to initiate an IDE trial for efficacy in the surgical management of degenerative lumbar stenosis. Although the IDE trials for both the AFRS and the Stabilimax NZ systems are in their relative infancy, preliminary results presented at national spine meetings have indicated safety and efficacy comparable to the other facet replacement systems.

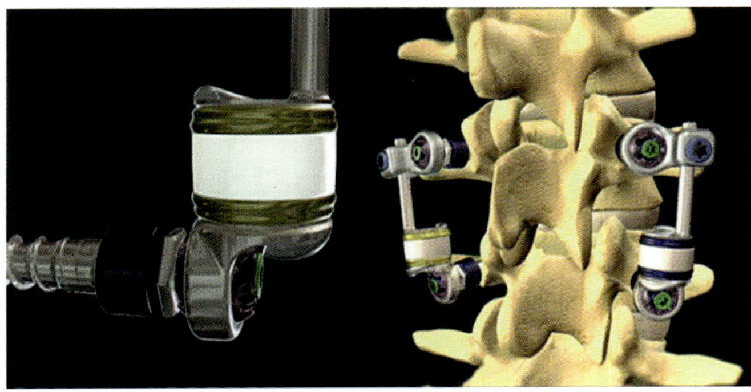

FIGURE 165-8. Stabilimax implant. (Courtesy of Applied Spine Technologies, New Haven, CT.)

Summary

Although the efficacy of spinal fusion as a surgical treatment for chronic low back pain is controversial, most clinicians would agree that the emergence of instrumented fusion after aggressive neural decompression for degenerative lumbar stenosis has served to reduce greatly the incidence of iatrogenic spinal instability. Rigid fixation of an iatrogenically destabilized spinal segment comes at the cost of increasing the multidirectional ROM at adjacent levels, accelerating breakdown. A better understanding of facet biomechanics and their relative contribution to axial and torsional load sharing in the FSU has led to the development of facet arthroplasty devices, which have shown at least equal efficacy and safety to traditional rigid pedicle screw constructs in limited, preliminary clinical trials. The greater questions surrounding facet arthroplasty center on device longevity and durability and whether their implementation will translate into lower rates of adjacent-level degeneration compared with pedicle screw fixation.

KEY REFERENCES

Butler J, Ferrara LA, Benzel EC: Basic biomechanically relevant anatomy. In Benzel EC, editor: *Spine surgery: techniques, complication avoidance, and management*, vol 2, Philadelphia, 2005, Saunders, pp 1397–1410.

Cavanaugh JM, Ozaktay AC, Yamashita HT, et al: Lumbar facet pain: biomechanics, neuroanatomy, and neurophysiology. *J Biomech* 29:1117–1129, 1996.

Lee KK, Teo EC: Effects of laminectomy and facetectomy on the stability of the lumbar motion segment. *Med Eng Physics* 26:183–192, 2004.

Panjabi MM, Oxland T, Takata K, et al: Articular facets of the human spine: quantitative three-dimensional anatomy. *Spine (Phila Pa 1976)* 18:1298–1310, 1993.

Schultz AB, Warwick DN, Berkson MH, et al: Mechanical properties of human lumbar spine motion segments—responses in flexion, extension, lateral bending, and torsion. *J Biomech Eng* 101:46–52, 1979.

Serhan HA, Varnavas G, Dooris AP, et al: Biomechanics of the posterior lumbar articulating elements. *Neurosurg Focus* 22:1E1, 2007.

REFERENCES

The complete reference list is available online at expertconsult.com.

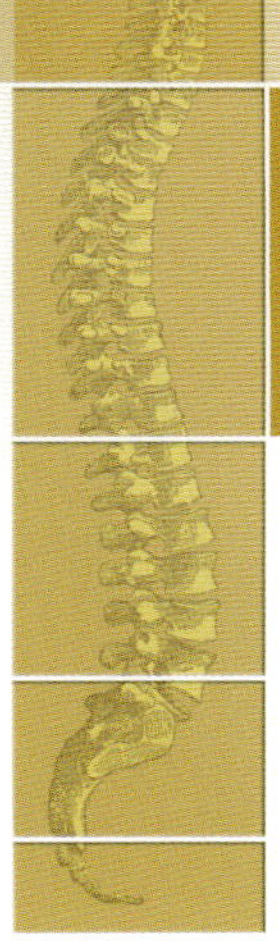

CHAPTER 166

Interspinous Bumpers

Basem I. Awad | Thomas E. Mroz | Michael P. Steinmetz

Lumbar stenosis is defined as the reduction in the diameter of the spinal canal, lateral recess, and/or neural foramina. Stenosis is most frequently a sequela of the degenerative process of aging, but recently genetic factors have been demonstrated to play a significant role.[1-3] The degenerative changes of disc desiccation with anular bulging, osteophyte formation, ligamentum hypertrophy, facet hypertrophy, and/or facet joint cyst all contribute to reducing the space available to the cauda equina and causing the classic symptoms of neurogenic claudications. In particular, compression and ischemia of nerve roots are the main source for this type of pain.[4-6]

Patients with the classic presentation of intermittent neurogenic claudication have buttock and leg pain when they stand and walk and have relief of symptoms when they flex forward, as when pushing a shopping cart, or when they sit or lie down (Figs. 166-1 and 166-2). This results mainly from the buckling of the ligamentum flavum and a decrease in the size of the central canal, subarticular region, and foraminal area with standing and walking.

The presence of canal stenosis on radiographic imaging does not itself define the syndrome, as there is a poor correlation between the degree of stenosis and the severity of symptoms.[7,8]

Surgery for lumbar spinal stenosis is generally accepted when conservative treatment has failed. The aim of surgery is to improve the quality of life and reduce claudication and its attendant radiating neurogenic pain. The use of wide decompression procedures for spinal stenosis, regardless of the integrity of the lamina and facet joints and without preservation of the spinous processes and interspinous ligaments, may lead to mechanical failure of the spine and chronic pain syndrome.

Recently, attention has been directed toward less aggressive surgical techniques. Options include fenestration, laminotomy, and selective decompression. These appear to provide adequate decompression with less postoperative morbidity. Moreover, these techniques may be done with minimal invasiveness. These considerations are mainly relevant for elderly patients.

The lumbar interspinous spacer devices provide a new minimally destructive alternative treatment for lumbar canal stenosis. These devices aim to unload the facet joints, restore foraminal height, and provide some stability, especially in extension, but still allow motion. The spacer is inserted between adjacent spinous processes and is placed dorsal to the neural elements. These techniques allow for the maintenance of spinal stability, minimal tissue disruption, and decompression. With some devices, there is no violation of the integrity of the lamina and/or facet joints.

This chapter reviews current concepts in the different types of interspinous spacer devices, Wallis, DIAM, and X-STOP.

Interspinous Spacers: Indications and Contraindications

Interspinous devices are generally indicated for patients age 50 years or older who have neurogenic intermittent claudication: buttock and/or leg pain relieved when the patient's spine is flexed or bending forward. The diagnosis must be confirmed via MRI and/or CT (myelography) evidence of a thickened ligamentum flavum, a narrowed lateral recess, and/or central canal narrowing. For most devices, stenosis must be limited to one or two levels. Low-grade spondylolisthesis (grade I) with neurogenic claudication is generally not a contraindication for device placement. The device is ideal for patients who have moderate to severe symptoms of neurogenic claudication and are not considered good candidates for decompressive surgery for whatever reason (e.g., excessive comorbities).

However, interspinous spacers are contraindicated in patients with spinal anatomy or disease that would prevent implantation of the device or cause the device to be unstable in situ. This includes significant instability of the lumbar spine, acute fracture of the spinous process or pars interarticularis, high-grade spondylolisthesis, an ankylosed segment at the affected level, significant scoliosis, or a diagnosis of severe osteoporosis by dual-energy x-ray absorptiometry (DEXA) scan, and/or active infection that is either systemic or localized to the site of implantation. In addition, patients with intermittent claudication associated with significant dermatomal weakness or cauda equina syndrome are not proper candidates for these procedures; they should have an open surgical decompression.

It should be noted that in the United States the primary use of these interspinous devices is for the treatment or stabilization of the lumbar spine to correct neurogenic claudication caused by canal stenosis. There is biomechanical evidence of unloading the facet joints and disc space,[9] which theoretically may limit back pain associated with a degenerative lumbar

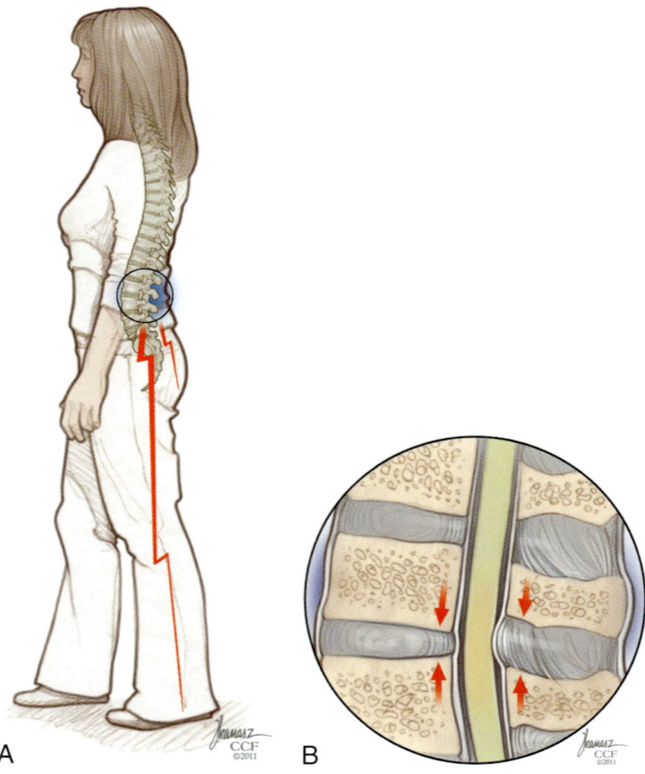

FIGURE 166-1. A, With upright posture, the spine is in extension, resulting in buckling of the ligamentum flavum and further narrowing of the spinal canal (**B**) with resultant symptoms. (Copyright Cleveland Clinic Foundation.)

segment. In other areas of the world, these devices are used primarily to treat lumbar axial pain, as opposed to neurogenic claudication.

Wallis Interspinous Spacer

In 1986 Sénégas[10] developed the first lumbar interspinous implant designed to stiffen unstable operated degenerative segments without eliminating mobility. At first called the Mechanical Normalization System, it included a titanium interspinous blocker and an artificial ligament made of Dacron.

This device was designed to stabilize the intervertebral axis of extension and flexion and reduce the mobility of the instrumented segment. The spacers placed between the dorsal arches produced an unloading effect, reducing pressure in the facet joints and dorsal portion of the intervertebral end plates in lordosis.

Between 1988 and 1993, more than 300 patients were treated for degenerative conditions with this first-generation device. It was concluded that many patients demonstrated significant resolution of residual low-back pain.[11]

The Wallis System (Abbott Spine, S.A., Bordeaux, France) was the second-generation interspinous spacer. The crucial change was in material properties. The Wallis spacer is made of polyetheretherketone (PEEK), a strong, completely radiolucent material compatible with MRI. This plastic-like polymer is more elastic, which reduces the risk of spinous process stress fractures. In addition, the Wallis device has notches that fit the physiologic shape of the lumbar spine, which minimizes the need for bone resection and avoids constraint on bone.

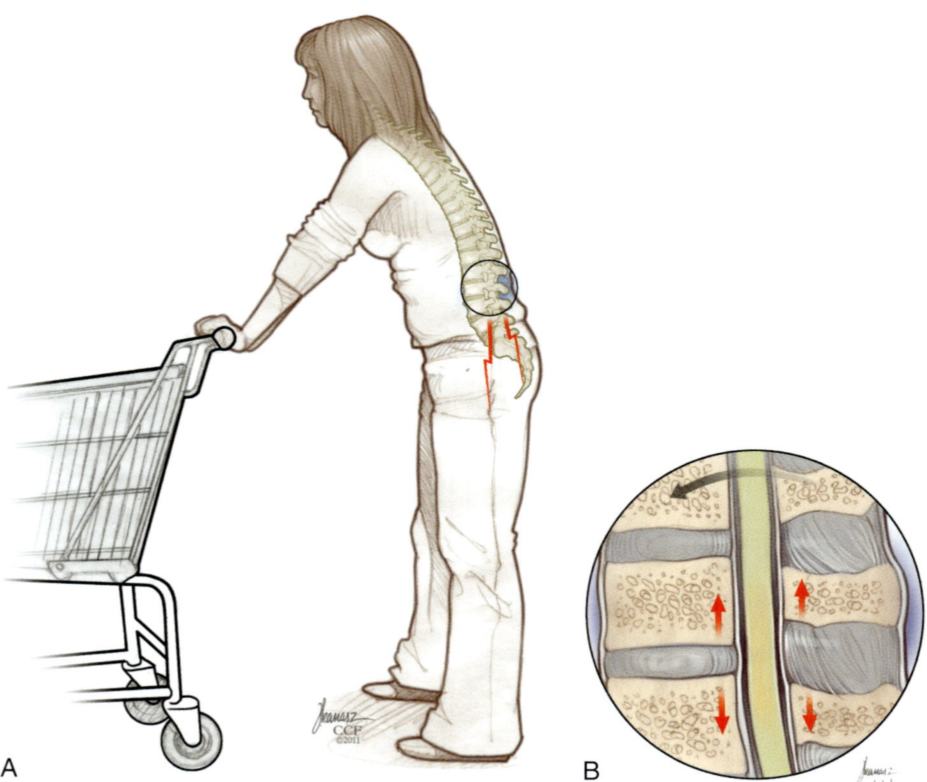

FIGURE 166-2. A, Bending forward, as with pushing a shopping cart, often relieves the symptoms of spinal stenosis. **B,** Flexion of the spine results in a tightening of the ligamentum flavum and an increase in the dimensions of the spinal canal. Symptoms are relieved in this position. (Copyright Cleveland Clinic Foundation.)

The Wallis interspinous device was designed as an alternative treatment for neurogenic claudication and the pain attributed to facet joint disease. By keeping the spine in a rather flexed position, the Wallis device increases the total canal and foraminal size and decompresses the cauda equina responsible for neurogenic claudication.

Surgical Technique

The surgical technique for the Wallis interspinous spacer was initially described by Sénégas.[12] The procedure is typically performed under general anesthesia with the patient in a prone position on a radiolucent operating table. The patient's lumbar midline should be marked before he or she is positioned. A neutral position of physiologic lumbar lordosis is best to optimize the effect of the implant.

Fluoroscopy is used to localize the affected level; localization is at the interspinous level, not the disc space level. A 4- to 6-cm midline skin incision is used, and the correct interspinous level is verified with fluoroscopy. A spinal needle may be used to aid in this identification. The paraspinal muscles are then separated from the spinous processes and the lamina of the treated level.

The supraspinous ligament is detached from the two spinous processes at the level involved and retracted laterally without sectioning. The interspinous ligament is then resected. An interlaminar distractor is used to facilitate insertion of the trial spacer, making sure that the gap between the spinous processes has not been enlarged to prevent local kyphosis.

The appropriately sized spacer is placed in the interspinous space; the bands are passed through the adjacent interspinous ligaments, as close as possible to the spinous process edges. A primary tension is then obtained with a forceps before inserting the bands in the clips.

Apply the clip holder and tab against the clip; both layers of the band are grasped and the clip is positioned next to its lodging in the spacer. The clipping forceps is inserted in the opening of the spacer closest to the clip being attached. The clipping forceps must be inserted in the spacer opening as deeply as possible to ensure introduction of all four clip stubs into the corresponding slots in the spacer. A snapping sound lets the surgeon know that the clip has been properly placed onto the spacer. Follow the same procedure for the other clip.

Primary tension ensures that the bands are optimally placed before the use of the final tightening device. The surgeon cuts the excess band with a scalpel, being careful not to damage the band that remains on the implant.

The supraspinous ligament is returned to its original position and reinserted onto each spinous process with a single silk suture passed through a hole made in the spinous process (Fig. 166-3).

X-STOP Interspinous Spacer

The X-STOP (Kyphon, Medtronic, Sunnyvale, CA) interspinous process decompression (IPD) device is a two-component oval titanium implant that fits between the spinous processes of the lumbar spine. A newer version has a PEEK sleeve over the titanium insert. Several clinical studies have shown the efficacy of the X-STOP device in treating neurogenic claudication secondary to lumbar stenosis.[13-16]

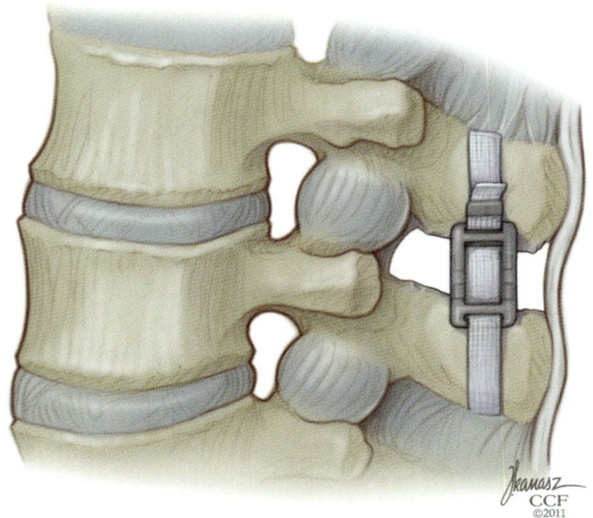

FIGURE 166-3. Depiction of the Wallis device placed in the interspinous space. The polyetheretherketone implant is held in position by notches in the implant and a strap placed around the spinous processes. The supraspinous ligament must be elevated to place the device; it may be reapproximated with suture after placement. (Copyright Cleveland Clinic Foundation.)

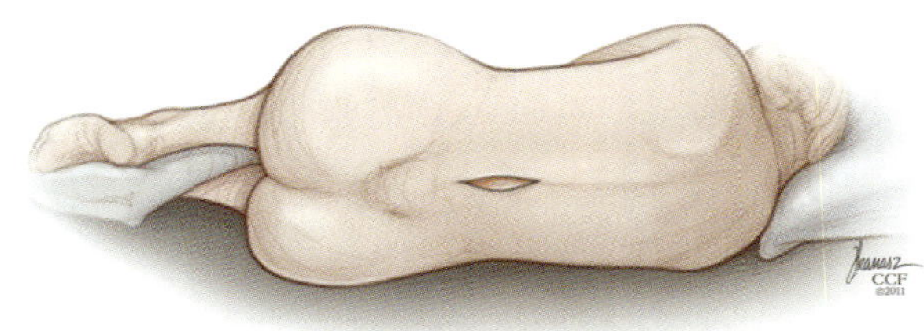

FIGURE 166-4. We prefer to place the implant with the patient positioned in the lateral decubitus position. (Copyright Cleveland Clinic Foundation.)

Surgical Technique

The implant procedure for this device can be done after induction of light sedation or general anesthesia. The patient is placed on a radiolucent table in a right lateral decubitus position; afterward the patient is asked to flex or assume a knee-chest position (Fig. 166-4). The level to be treated is identified by fluoroscopy; localization is at the interspinous level, not the disc space level.

After administration of a local anesthesia, a 4- to 6-cm midline skin incision is made over the spinous processes of the stenotic level. The incision is opened to the fascia, which is incised 2 cm to the right and to the left from the midline. The correct interspinous level is verified again with fluoroscopy.

The paraspinal muscles are lifted subperiosteally from the spinous processes using a Cobb retractor and/or electrocautery, and all midline structures are left intact. The small curved dilator is inserted across the interspinous space through the most ventral margin of the interspinous ligament (Fig. 166-5). The curved dilator is removed. A sizing distractor is then inserted between the spinous processes and expanded until the supraspinous ligament is taut, which is verified by palpation of the ligament (Fig. 166-6). The correct implant size is indicated on the sizing dilator.

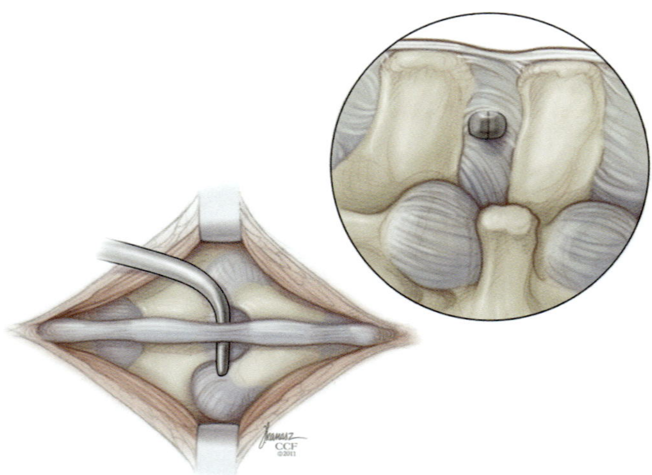

FIGURE 166-5. Following subperiosteal dissection, a dilator is first placed through the interspinous ligament between the spinous processes. The correct level is determined by fluoroscopy. (Copyright Cleveland Clinic Foundation.)

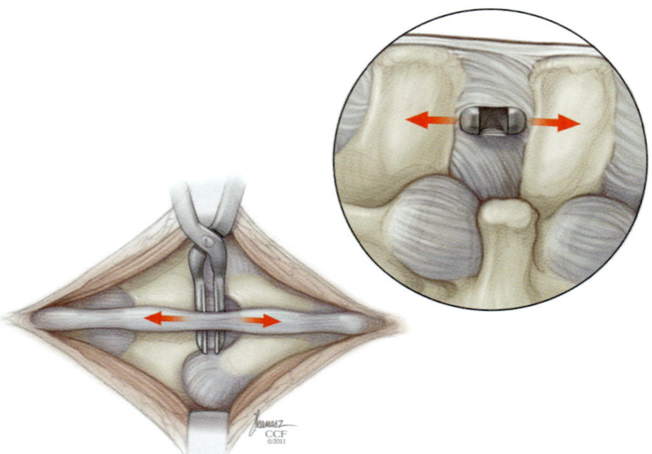

FIGURE 166-6. Following dilation, a sizing distractor is placed. Under fluoroscopic guidance, distraction is placed until the interspinous ligament is taut (*inset*). The size of the implant is determined at this step. (Copyright Cleveland Clinic Foundation.)

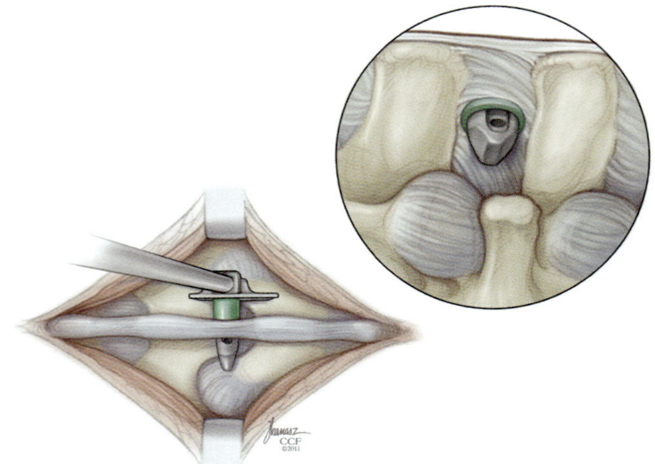

FIGURE 166-7. The correct-size implant is now placed between the spinous processes. The implant is placed until the wing is flush against the spinous process and the hole for the screw in the opposite wing is well visualized (*inset*). (Copyright Cleveland Clinic Foundation.)

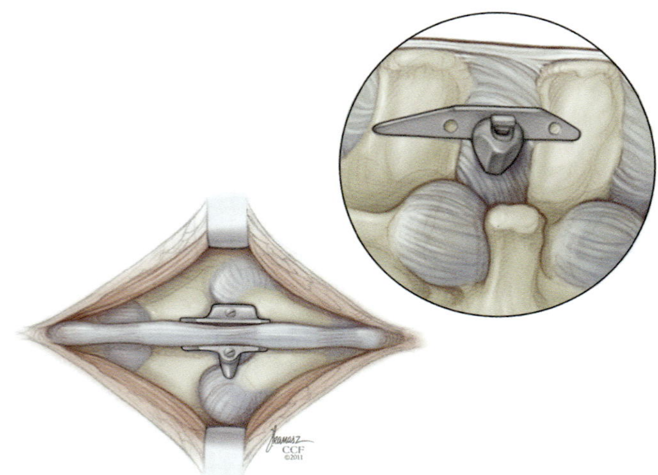

FIGURE 166-8. The opposite wing is placed. Compression may be placed against the wings, and the screw placed and torqued. (Copyright Cleveland Clinic Foundation.)

The appropriate X-STOP device is then placed between the spinous processes to the point where the wing is flush with the right side of the spinous process (Fig. 166-7). Fluoroscopy should verify the correct level and ventral placement. If the device appears to be placed too far dorsally, the facet will need to be trimmed. The two wings are approximated medially and the universal wing screw is secured (Fig. 166-8). The incision is then irrigated and closed in standard fashion (Fig. 166-9).

DIAM Interspinous Spacer

The DIAM Spinal Stabilization System (Medtronic, Sofamor Danek, Memphis, TN) is a soft interspinous spacer. The core is made of silicone, which is covered by a polyethylene coating. The DIAM implant was developed by Jean Taylor.[17] It is a dorsal interspinal dynamic stabilization or balancing device. The DIAM is thought to work by reducing loading of the disc, restoring the dorsal tension band, realigning the facet joint line, and increasing foraminal height. But, few articles on the efficacy of this product have appeared in the literature.[18,19]

Surgical Technique

The patient is placed prone, as is standard for interspinous spacer procedures. Fluoroscopic capability is indicated to detect the interspinous level of interest. There are two methods of implanting the DIAM; the first sacrifices the supraspinous and intraspinous ligaments and the second preserves them, which we prefer.

In the ligament-sacrificing procedure, the supraspinous and interspinous ligaments are removed at the level of interest for DIAM implantation. The interspinous space is then prepared by squaring it off with a rongeur. The space is then distracted, and measuring trials are used to determine the size of the DIAM. The implant is inserted and seated with a tamp and

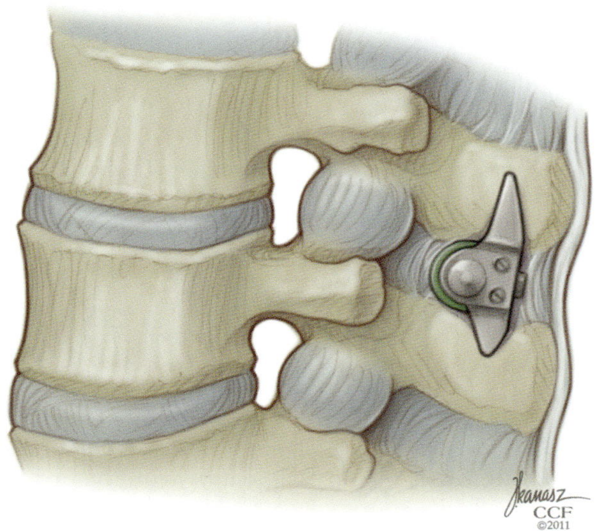

FIGURE 166-9. Final lateral view of the spine with the X-STOP implant in place. (Copyright Cleveland Clinic Foundation.)

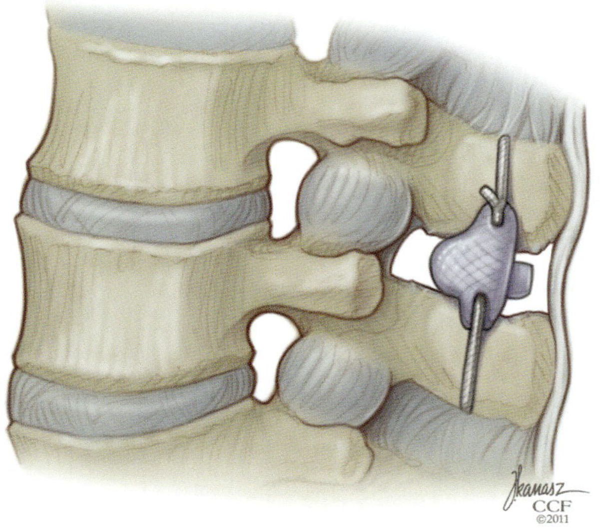

FIGURE 166-10. The DIAM implant is made of silicone that is covered by a polyethylene coating. The implant may be placed either by removing the supra- and intraspinous ligaments or by preserving them. The laces secure the device if the ligaments are removed. They do not need to be placed if the ligaments are preserved. (Copyright Cleveland Clinic Foundation.)

mallet. It is secured in place with two laces, one around the spinous process above, and another around the one below, the DIAM is then tightened and crimped. The wound is irrigated and closed in the standard fashion. No postoperative immobilization is required (Fig. 166-10).

In the ligament-sparing procedure, the supraspinous and interspinous ligaments are preserved. The exposure can be unilateral or bilateral. A space is created between the spinous processes. The distractor is then placed and the space is sized. The appropriately sized DIAM is folded and deposited. The DIAM cords are removed before insertion, because they are not necessary if the ligaments are preserved. The area is irrigated and closed in the standard fashion.

Outcomes

Anatomy and Biomechanics

Richards et al.[20] published the effect of the X-STOP spacer on the spinal canal, subarticular diameter, and foraminal height with and without the implant. With the device in place, the canal area was found to be increased by 18%, the diameter by 10%, and the subarticular diameter by 50%. The foraminal area was found to be increased by 25%, and the width increased by 41%.

Wilke et al.[21] evaluated in vitro the biomechanical segmental stability and intradiscal pressure achieved with the four different interspinous implants (i.e., Coflex, Wallis, DIAM, and X-STOP). Interestingly, the effect on the flexibility of all the treated segments is similar, despite the variations of implant design—referred to the neutral position of the intact segments, each device significantly stabilized and unloaded the disc in extension, but had little effect on range of motion (ROM) and intradiscal pressure in flexion, lateral bending, and axial rotation.

In 2008 Schulte et al.[22] studied biomechanically the effect of spinal decompression alone, as well as in conjugation with semirigid stabilizing implants (Wallis, Dynesys) on the ROM of lumbar spine segments. Undercutting decompression leads to a significant segmental instability in all planes. Implantation of Wallis or Dynesys spacers after decompression leads to a significant restriction of segmental ROM. The Wallis device limits only the flexion-extension plane; the Dynesys limits both flexion-extension and lateral bending. Axial rotation is minimally restricted by both implants. The observed effects on the neutral zone correspond well with the effects on ROM.

Clinical Outcomes

X-STOP

One- and 2-year outcomes utilizing the X-STOP device were published by Zucherman et al.[14,15] There were multicenter, randomized controlled studies for the treatment of lumbar canal stenosis with the X-STOP implant. The implant was directly compared with the best conservative care, usually involving epidural steroid injection. At 1 year, the success rate was 59% with X-STOP compared with 12% for nonoperative therapy. Six patients in the X-STOP group and 24 in the control cohort underwent decompressive laminectomy. Interestingly, the results following laminectomy were similar to those of the remainder of the X-STOP patients. At 2 years, 73.1% of patients were satisfied with their outcome compared with those who underwent conservative therapy (35.9%).

It also appears that the device is effective for treating spondylolisthesis. Anderson et al.[23] published a randomized controlled study in patients with neurogenic claudication secondary to degenerative spondylolisthesis. They concluded that the X-STOP device was more effective than nonoperative treatment. There was no increase in the degree of spondylolisthesis postoperatively. These data are appealing for the treatment of those patients who are not felt to be candidates for a fusion following decompression.

The durability of the X-STOP device has not been well defined. Kondrashov et al.[24] demonstrated the success rate among patients treated with X-STOP devices at one and two levels was 78% at a mean of 4.2 years postoperatively, which is consistent with the intermediate-term (1 and 2 years) results of Zucherman et al.[14,15] This indicates that the long-term durability is at least 4 years; unfortunately not many people were followed out to 4 years for the purpose of this study.

A recent study has shown slightly less promise than the aforementioned manuscripts.[25] Although 71% of patients reported satisfaction with the procedure, only 54% of patients reported clinically significant improvement in their symptoms. Twenty-nine percent of patients required caudal epidural steroid injection 12 months after surgery for recurrence of symptoms.

Wallis

The Wallis device has not been approved by the FDA for use in the United States. Despite this, long-term analysis has been reported regarding its use outside the United States. In 2009 Sénégas et al.[26] published a long-term retrospective clinical survey on 107 patients with canal stenosis or herniated disc, or both, who underwent lumbar dynamic stabilization with the Wallis system. One hundred thirty-three were alive at the time of analysis, but only 107 filled out the questionnaire. The average follow-up was 13.5 years. Twenty-three patients underwent a subsequent lumbar procedure, with 20 having the implant removed and fusion performed. The other three had surgery at adjacent levels. At an average of 13 years post-procedure, 95% of patients reported they were very satisfied or satisfied with the implant, and the same was seen in only 65% following fusion. There are many weaknesses of this manuscript, but it does lend credence to the long-term durability and clinical utility of the implant. It remains unclear, however, who is the most appropriate patient to utilize the device.

DIAM

Similar to the Wallis device, the DIAM implant is not currently FDA approved for use in the United States. It has been used extensively in other countries for the treatment of a variety of lumbar pathologies. One comparative study was published evaluating the use of DIAM following simple lumbar discecotmy.[27] Sixty-two patients underwent lumbar laminectomy and/or discectomy; 31 of these patients underwent concomitant placement of the DIAM device (33 devices total). At an average of 12 months following surgery no significant differences were noted between groups, using the VAS and McNab outcomes scales. There were three device failures noted in the DIAM group, two transverse process fractures and one infection. It appears that the device did not alter the sagittal alignment or disc height following placement; however, it did not improve outcome as well. What remains unclear in comparative studies is how the device may affect the treatment of other lumbar degenerative diseases, such as mechanical pain and pseudoclaudication. Certainly further research is warranted at this time.

Conclusion

The lumbar interspinous spacers provide a new minimally destructive alternative treatment for neurogenic claudication attributed to lumbar canal stenosis. Several interspinous implants are available on the market today, although only the X-STOP is available in the United States. They have different design strategies and are made of varying materials, but all have similar biomechanical effects. These devices permit neural decompression with only a minimal amount of tissue resection; also they make the procedure less invasive (destructive).

These devices may be implanted without a laminectomy and function through indirect decompression, thus avoiding the risk of epidural scarring and cerebrospinal fluid leakage. Of note, X-STOP cannot be placed following laminectomy as it requires intact supra- and infraspinous ligaments. Furthermore, these devices limit extension of the spine, unload the facet joints, and potentially relieve the pain attributed to facet disease.

In addition, it appears that they do not alter the mechanical behavior of the adjacent segment, possibly limiting the domino effect of degenerative disc disease.

KEY REFERENCES

Anderson PA, Tribus CB, Kitchel SH: Treatment of neurogenic claudication by interspinous decompression: application of the X-STOP device in patients with lumbar degeneration spondylolisthesis. *J Neurosurg Spine* 4:463–471, 2006.

Kirkaldy-Willis WH, Wedge JH, Yong-Hing K, et al: Pathology and pathogenesis of lumbar spondylosis and stenosis. *Spine (Phila Pa 1976)* 3:319–328, 1978.

Lindsey DP, Swanson KE, Fuchs P, et al: The effects of an interspinous implant on the kinematics of the instrumented and adjacent levels in the lumbar spine. *Spine (Phila Pa 1976)* 28:2192–2197, 2003.

Sénégas J, Vital JM, Pointillart V, et al: Long-term actuarial survivorship analysis of an interspinous stabilization system. *Eur Spine J* 16:1279–1287, 2007.

Sénégas J, Vital JM, Pointillart V, et al: Clinical evaluation of a lumbar interspinous dynamic stabilization device (the Wallis system) with a 13-year mean follow-up. *Neurosurg Rev* 32:335–342, 2009.

Zucherman JF, Hsu KY, Hartjen CA, et al: A prospective randomized multicenter study for the treatment of lumbar spinal stenosis with the X-STOP interspinous implant: 1-year results. *Eur Spine J* 13:22–31, 2004.

Zucherman JF, Hsu KY, Hartjen CA, et al: A multicenter, prospective, randomized trial evaluating the X-STOP interspinous process decompression system for the treatment of neurogenic intermitent claudication: two-year follow-up results. *Spine (Phila Pa 1976)* 30:1351–1358, 2005.

REFERENCES

The complete reference list is available online at expertconsult.com.

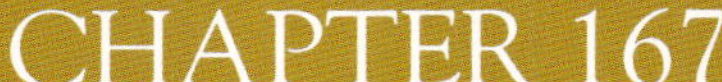

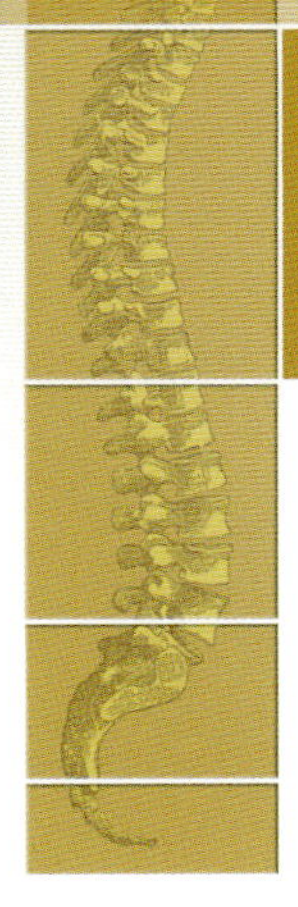

CHAPTER 167

Total Disc Arthroplasty: Associated Complications

Robert Talac

Surgical management of chronic low back pain remains challenging. Although lumbar fusion remains the gold standard, novel motion-sparing technologies are now available that offer several theoretical advantages over lumbar fusion. The use of intervertebral disc prostheses as an alternative to spinal fusion has been advocated to preserve segmental motion and prevent adjacent degeneration. As with any new technology, safety is a primary outcome measure.

Total disc replacement (TDR) is a relatively new procedure and thus reported complication rates are highly variable. Complications associated with TDR can be divided into three distinct groups. The first group involves surgical approach–related complications. These include vascular injuries, injuries to nerve roots, and retrograde ejaculation due to injury to the presacral sympathetic plexus. In general, the incidence of surgical approach–related complications ranges from 2.1% to 18.7%.[1] The second group includes implant-related complications. These may be divided further into short- and long-tem complications. Short-term complications include implant subsidence, migration, and displacement and vertebral end-plate fractures. There is a paucity of long-term data on the performance of TDR implants. In addition, these data reflect the first generation of implants that have since been replaced by newer, improved discs. Hence, many long-term complications are not well documented. These may include the effect of wear debris and of increased range of motion of the facet joint and adjacent segment. The overall incidence of short-term implant-related complications ranges from 2.9% to 39.3%.[1] The third group represents general complications such as infection, wound complications, persistent pain, and other adverse events related to surgical treatment. The incidence of these complications ranges from 1% to 14%.[1] Another method to assess the safety of the new procedure is to determine reoperation rates at the index level. Available literature suggests that reoperation rates for TDR range from 1% to 28.6%.[1]

The results of several randomized controlled trials have been published recently. In the Charité trial, Blumenthal et al. reported overall 2-year complication rates for patients undergoing TDR or fusion of 29.1% and 50.2%, respectively.[2] The authors also reported that 11 patients (5.4%) in the TDR group and 9 patients (9.1%) in the fusion group underwent reoperation at the index level. McAfee et al. reported similar findings for the Charité TDR. In their report, 6.3% of TDR patients and 10.1% of fusion patients required reoperation at the index level.[3] Van den Eerenbeemt et al. compared reported complication rates from Charité TDR studies with U.S. Food and Drug Administration (FDA) reports.[1] They found significant discrepancies in reported rates. In their report, 16 Charité patients (9.1%) experienced an approach-related complication (retrograde ejaculation), 8 patients (3.9%) had implant-related complications, and 33 patients (16.1%) had general surgery–related complications. In the fusion group, 9 patients (12.8%) reported retrograde ejaculation, 10 patients (10.1%) had implant-related complications, and 27 patients (27.2%) had general surgery–related complications. Geisler et al. analyzed a subgroup of patients from a Charité investigational device exemption study,[4] focusing on patients with neurologic complications. The incidence of neurologic complications was no higher in patients with the Charité TDR (16.6%) than in patients with Bagby and Kuslich (BAK) fusion (17.2%; $P = .3$). Zigler et al. reported the FDA randomized trial comparing the ProDisc-L artificial disc with circumferential fusion.[5] In this study, the overall complication rates were 7.3% for the ProDisc-L group and 6.3% for the circumferential fusion group. Reoperation at the index level was necessary for 3.7% of ProDisc-L patients and 5.4% of fusion patients. Van den Eerenbeemt et al. also analyzed the ProDisc-L trial and FDA reports.[1] Their findings suggest that 2.4% of ProDisc-L recipients experienced retrograde ejaculation, 3.1% reported implant-related complications, and 1.8% had general surgical complications. In the fusion group, two patients (2.5%) had retrograde ejaculation; there were no implant- or approach-related complications. Three patients (3.8%) reported general surgery–related complications. Most recently, Sasso et al. reported initial results from the FlexiCore randomized study. They reported an overall rate of complications of 22.7% in the TDR group and 43.5% in the fusion group.[6] Of 44 FlexiCore patients, 5 (11.4%) required reoperation. In the control group, 6 of 23 patients (26.1%) required reoperation.

In addition to recent randomized clinical trials, there are multiple case reports and retrospective studies addressing safety issues surrounding TDR. These studies have numerous shortcomings and limitations. Some of them provide important insight, however.

Van Ooij et al. reported their experience with 75 patients with suboptimal outcomes after implantation of the Charité prosthesis.[7-9] They found subsidence in 39 patients, an improperly sized prosthesis (too small) in 24 patients, adjacent disc degeneration in 36 patients, degenerative scoliosis in 11 patients, facet joint degeneration on CT scan in 25 patients, ventral implant migration in 6 patients, dorsal migration in 2 patients, metal wire breakage in 10 patients, wear and severe osteolysis in 6 patients, and subluxation of the device's polyethylene core in 1 patient. Of the 75 patients, 46 required one or more salvage surgeries to address these problems. Daxle et al. collected perioperative morbidity data for 66 patients after TDR.[10] They reported a 9% incidence of general surgical complications (e.g., urinary tract infection, wound infection). Four patients (6%) had significant blood loss (>1500 mL) during the surgery, one patient (1.5%) had major vascular injury, and one (1.5%) had a dural tear with subsequent epidural infection. Brau et al. analyzed the incidence of major vascular injury in 1315 consecutive patients undergoing ventral lumbar surgery.[11] Of these patients, 6 were identified with left iliac artery thrombosis (0.45%) and 19 (1.4%) had major vein laceration. The authors concluded that the incidence of major vascular injuries is relatively low (25/1315, or 1.9%).

In conclusion, there is a paucity of high-quality data regarding the true incidence of TDR-associated complications. The best available published evidence suggests that complication rates range from 7% to 29%. The procedure itself is relatively new and many factors affecting outcome are unknown. Revision surgeries for TDR have been described as very challenging as well.

KEY REFERENCES

Blumenthal S, McAfee PC, Guyer RD, et al: A prospective, randomized, multicenter Food and Drug Administration investigational device exemptions study of lumbar total disc replacement with the CHARITE artificial disc versus lumbar fusion. Part I: evaluation of clinical outcomes. *Spine (Phila Pa 1976)* 30:1565–1575, 2005.

Kurtz SM, van Ooij A, Ross R, et al: Polyethylene wear and rim fracture in total disc arthroplasty. *Spine J* 7:12–21, 2007.

Sasso RC, Foulk DM, Hahn M: Prospective, randomized trial of metal-on-metal artificial lumbar disc replacement: initial results for treatment of discogenic pain. *Spine (Phila Pa 1976)* 33:123–131, 2008.

van Ooij A, Schurink GW, Oner FC, et al: Findings in 67 patients with recurrent or persistent symptoms after implantation of a disc prosthesis for low back pain. *Ned Tijdschr Geneeskd* 151:1577–1584, 2007.

Zigler J, Delamarter R, Spivak JM, et al: Results of prospective randomized, multicenter Food and Drug Administration investigational device exemption study of the ProDisc-L total disc replacement versus circumferential fusion for the treatment of 1-level degenerative disc disease. *Spine (Phila Pa 1976)* 32:1155–1163, 2007.

REFERENCES

The complete reference list is available online at expertconsult.com.

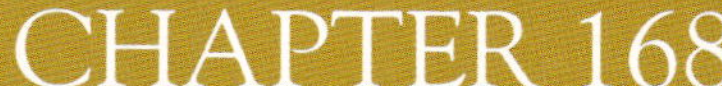

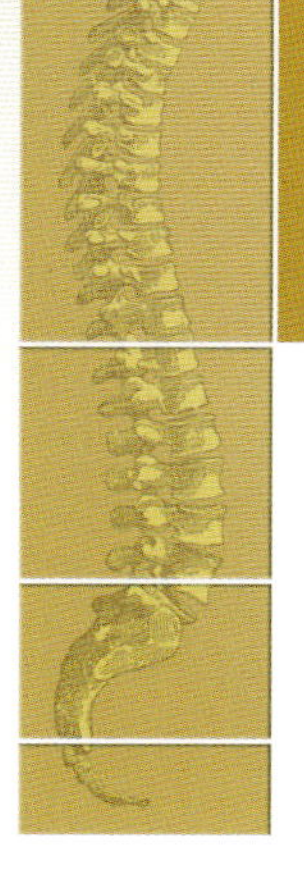

CHAPTER 168

Explant Analysis of Wear, Degradation, and Fatigue in Motion Preserving Spinal Implants

Allyson Ianuzzi | Steven M. Kurtz

Motion preserving spinal implants, including total disc replacements (TDRs), have emerged recently as a new technology for the treatment of a range of disorders in the cervical and lumbar spine. These implants must share load and also restore motion or stability, or both, to a diseased spinal joint. In contrast, the historical paradigm for spinal implants was predicated on static, load-sharing fusion devices. Because motion preservation treatment of the spine is in its infancy, the widespread practice of retrieval analysis elucidates mechanisms of failure, wear, corrosion, or fatigue that were unknown before clinical use of these devices.

Before clinical use of new motion preserving designs in humans, it is essential that the implants be exhaustively tested in the laboratory. However, because many motion preservation designs and their biomaterials are without clinical precedent, it may be challenging for bioengineers to develop test methods that accurately predict in vivo performance. Analysis of retrieved devices can serve to validate preclinical tests aimed at mimicking long-term use or failure modes. Before initiating a clinical trial, it is often impossible to anticipate the complete spectrum of clinical failure modes for a particular implant system. Experience gained by retrieval analysis can facilitate engineering judgment in designing clinically relevant tests. Although clinical failure of implant procedures may involve various factors related to the patient, surgeon, and implant, certain unusual clinical failure modes may occur as a result of a unique combination of these three factors.

Because of their rarity, certain failure modes may escape detection in a clinical trial. For this reason, the U.S. Food and Drug Administration (FDA) is keenly interested in the detailed analysis of explanted implants, as evidenced by the inquiry and recommendations of three FDA panels for cervical and lumbar artificial discs from 2004 to 2007. In the 2007 FDA panel meeting for the Bryan cervical disc (Medtronic, Memphis, TN), one of the conditions for approval was that the manufacturer conduct a 10-year postmarket retrieval analysis of the device (www.fda.gov/cdrh/meetings/071707-summary.html). Retrieval analysis is considered an absolutely essential companion activity not only for prospective, randomized clinical trials but also for the postmarket surveillance of new spinal implant designs.

Retrieval analysis is the study of explanted devices and tissues for the purposes of understanding the in vivo performance of the implant. The implants and tissues obtained during revision surgery are often helpful when attempting to determine the reasons underlying the failure of a particular surgical procedure. A detailed analysis of revision retrievals is essential to gain an understanding of clinical failure modes of a particular device and its biomaterials. However, the extrapolation of such findings to patients who have not undergone revision (i.e., with well-functioning implants) can be problematic. It may be desirable to study implants and surrounding tissues retrieved from autopsy specimens to obtain information that is applicable to patients with well-functioning implants. This approach is limited by the fact that motion preserving spinal implants have an elective patient population ranging in age from 18 to 60 years, which may result in a low yield of autopsy retrievals during an investigator's professional career.

Retrieval analysis has strong regulatory and societal implications and is performed by clinicians, engineers, and biologists. There are great advantages from their collaboration as a team, which allows for the relevant patient-related, surgeon-related, and implant-related factors to be considered in as broad a context as possible. When properly performed by experienced investigators, retrieval analysis can provide a definitive source of information on implant-related and biomaterial-related failure modes, biocompatibility, and their impact on the overall longevity of the surgical procedure. When compared with the findings of experimental or numerical studies, the results of retrieval analysis can help validate preclinical testing and computer-based methods that are essential when evaluating new designs. Taken one step further, when the aggregate results of retrieval analysis are integrated into the implant design process, the technique can provide feedback or motivation for adjusting implant designs or finding alternative biomaterials. As explained in a consensus statement from the National Institutes of Health,[1] "Technology progresses by facing its failures and learning from its successes. The goal of device research and development is to improve patient care through improvement of implants. A fundamental objective is to understand successful implants and assess failures through retrieval analysis."

There is also strong educational and ethical motivation for participating in retrieval analysis. When involving researchers, engineers, and clinicians in the early stages of their careers, retrieval analysis has a major educational component. Clinicians who are actively implanting motion preserving devices have an ethical responsibility to contribute to retrieval analysis to provide their patients with the best care possible. The removal of an implant, especially a lumbar artificial disc, exposes the patient to increased risk of serious, potentially life-threatening complications. The clinician has a responsibility to ensure that implanted and explanted devices and tissues are properly analyzed and the results disseminated to stakeholders. There are many scientific, educational, and ethical reasons why the research community, implant designers, and surgeons are motivated to participate in retrieval analyses. These reasons have been touched on in previous review articles and book chapters.[2] It is a testament to the varied and compelling motivations for retrieval analysis that it continues to play an important role in the evolution of implant technology.

In this chapter, we summarize the literature on retrieval analysis of motion preserving implants, including available information related to mechanisms of wear, corrosion, and fatigue. In addition, we provide support for combining these analyses with the evaluation of periprosthetic tissues to determine the biologic responses to the various implant designs. At our institution, we established an international repository for motion preserving spinal implants in 2004. Our repository is currently open to all spine surgeons and is intended to be inclusive of all cervical and lumbar implant designs, such as artificial discs and dorsal dynamic stabilization devices. Many of the examples in this chapter are drawn from our existing repository of metal-on-polyethylene and metal-on-metal lumbar TDRs and polyurethane-based dynamic motion preservation devices.

Practical Aspects of Retrieval Analysis

Retrieval Program

A retrieval program may be organized as the collection and analysis of implants from a single institution or from a multi-institutional study or independently as a more generalized retrieval repository. When a retrieval program is established as part of a clinical study, institutional review board approval or the equivalent should be obtained, which may require the informed consent of each patient to participate. A clinical study–type design is preferred when detailed clinical information, including protected health information, is being collected and analyzed as part of the study. Details on the design and establishment of a retrieval or repository program have been outlined previously.[3]

To ensure adequate receipt and processing of the retrieved implants, standard precautions should be used when handling the explanted components until they have completed a cleaning protocol. These precautions may include keeping the implant components in appropriate chemicals to preserve adhering tissue (e.g., formalin), provided that the preservative does not degrade the component itself. At our center, implants fabricated from titanium alloy, cobalt chromium (CoCr) alloy, and polyethylene are ultrasonically cleaned in soap and deionized water, rinsed, and sterilized using a 10% bleach solution. We omit the bleach solution for cleaning stainless steel implants because there is the potential for corrosion. Likewise, a mild cleanser is used for implant components composed of polymers that may be vulnerable to chemical changes from a bleach solution. Additional guidance for handling of retrieved implants and tissues may be found in American Society for Testing and Materials (ASTM) Standard F561.[4]

The analysis of retrieved implants and tissues may involve a broad range of test methods, which are comprehensively described in ASTM Standard F561.[4] This manual provides guidance for analysis of all implant components, including metallic, polymeric, and ceramic materials. Although a detailed summary of this standard is beyond the scope of this chapter, we highlight in subsequent sections specific test methods that have been particularly helpful in the characterization of retrieved metal-on-polyethylene and metal-on-metal disc replacements.

Wear and Damage Assessment

Because wear and damage of retrieved TDRs can occur at length scales that are invisible to the naked eye, microscopy may be necessary to identify damage modes. An optical stereomicroscope, with 10× to 40× magnification, is typically sufficient to identify worn regions of retrieved implants, but frequently it is helpful to analyze the wear surfaces using scanning electron microscopy (SEM), achieving magnifications of 5000× or greater. In addition to optical and SEM, micro-CT and white light interferometry (WLIR) are two methods that have proven particularly useful in our previous analyses of wear in retrieved TDR and dynamic stabilization components.[3,5-7] These novel wear assessment methods are highlighted in this section.

Micro-CT Analysis

We have used a micro-CT to detect nondestructively surface and internal voids and cracks within retrieved polyethylene TDR components[5] and polyurethane motion preserving spinal implants.[7] Depending on their thickness, CoCr alloy components produce substantial artifacts on micro-CT. Consequently, we have found it helpful to remove the wire marker before micro-CT analysis of rim wear in the Charité design. The removal of the wire marker for other analyses may be unnecessary because the artifact does not extend into the central core of the implant. For polymer components that do not incorporate wire markers (e.g., ProDisc [Synthes, Paoli, PA] or Dynesys [Zimmer Spine, Minneapolis, MN]), micro-CT artifacts are not an issue.

At the authors' institution, polymer components of motion preserving spinal implants are scanned at 18 μm voxel resolution using a commercial micro-CT scanner (μCT80, Scanco Medical, Bassersdorf, Switzerland).[5] The three-dimensional reconstructions of the component and two-dimensional sections taken through the component are evaluated for the presence of surface, through-thickness, and internal voids or cracks. Previously, we have observed the trajectory of cracks in polymer components of motion preserving spinal implants, including Dynesys.[7] Using optical microscopy, we have also characterized permanent deformation and wear patterns of polymer components from motion preserving spinal devices. Using these methods, we have been able to distinguish these forms of surface and subsurface damage from iatrogenic damage that occurs during implant removal.

Because of attenuation artifacts encountered with metallic components, micro-CT is useful only for polymeric components from TDRs. To measure the macroscopic surface geometry of metallic components, tools employed by the research community include coordinate measurement machines, laser profilometers, and optical profilometers. To measure microscopic changes in the implant surface, WLIR may be used. As discussed next, interferometry is applicable to both metallic and polymeric components of disc replacements.

White Light Interferometry

We use WLIR to characterize the microscopic surface morphology of retrieved disc arthroplasty components. WLIR is capable of detecting surface height changes that are on the nanometer length scale by measuring the interference of white light reflected off the component within a specified field of view compared with the light from a reference beam. We have successfully analyzed the wear surfaces of polyethylene and CoCr alloy TDRs at our institution using a NewView 5000 equipped with advanced texture analysis software (Zygo, Middlefield, CT).[6] We sample 5 to 10 square regions (typically 0.54 × 0.72 mm) of a component to obtain representative surface topography of the retrieved implant in both worn and unworn locations.

Figures 168-1A and B illustrate the surface topography obtained from unworn and worn surface regions of a retrieved polyethylene disc replacement component that was implanted for 12.7 years. The unworn polyethylene surface is dominated by machining marks that are on the order of several microns in amplitude (see Fig. 168-1A). Initially, microscopic evidence of adhesive and abrasive wear is detected by the erosion and removal of machining marks, along with the presence of fine scratches (see Fig. 168-1B).

The surface topography of a retrieved CoCr alloy disc replacement is shown in Figures 168-1C and D. The unworn CoCr surface is usually relatively flat and featureless, aside from microscopic scratches generated during the final polishing stage of the manufacturing process (see Fig. 168-1C). In a region of wear, the CoCr surface has evidence of localized, microscopic scratches with a characteristic length scale that is larger than the residual features from polishing (Fig. 168-1D).

As shown in Figure 168-1, surface characterization using WLIR provides useful information about the wear mechanisms in TDRs. In addition, by quantitatively analyzing the surface data, the roughness and waviness can be quantified and compared with as-manufactured components, providing insight into the magnitude of surface changes or wear that occur in vivo.[8-10] Ultimately, quantitative measurements of implant surfaces are used to validate in vitro and computational models that seek to simulate in vivo wear processes.

Wear and Damage Mechanisms

As discussed in the previous section, metal and polymeric components from retrieved motion preserving spinal devices should be evaluated macroscopically and microscopically for the presence of damage modes typically observed in large joint arthroplasty components (e.g., burnishing, abrasion, scratching, pitting, plastic deformation, fracture, fatigue damage, and embedded debris). A detailed description of wear and wear mechanisms is beyond the scope of this chapter and can be found in books dedicated to this subject.[11] A generic guide for the analysis of retrieved components is summarized in the Appendices for ASTM Standard F561.[4] This section provides a concise summary of the most relevant wear and fatigue damage modes that may be encountered when inspecting retrieved motion preserving spinal implant components.

Abrasion and Scratching

Abrasive wear is evidenced by scratching and is common to both metallic and polymeric components for TDR. Abrasion may be apparent macroscopically by the naked eye, or it may be apparent only when viewed using microscopy. Abrasive wear occurs when microscopic surface irregularities (also referred to as "asperities") in one implant scratch the surface of the opposing counterface. In the case of metal-on-polyethylene, the asperities on the metallic implant produce scratches in the softer polymeric implant. In the case of CoCr alloy metal-on-metal implants, abrasive wear is produced by locally stiffer asperities, such as carbides, plowing through the relatively softer cobalt alloy matrix. Abrasive wear can also occur when softer polymeric components of the implant contact surrounding bony structures (Fig. 168-2).

During retrieval analysis, the pattern of scratches on an implant, whether macroscopic or microscopic, provides clues to the kinematics (motion) of the surfaces while they were contact in vivo. The microscopic multidirectional scratches and crisscrossing wear paths at the dome of a retrieved

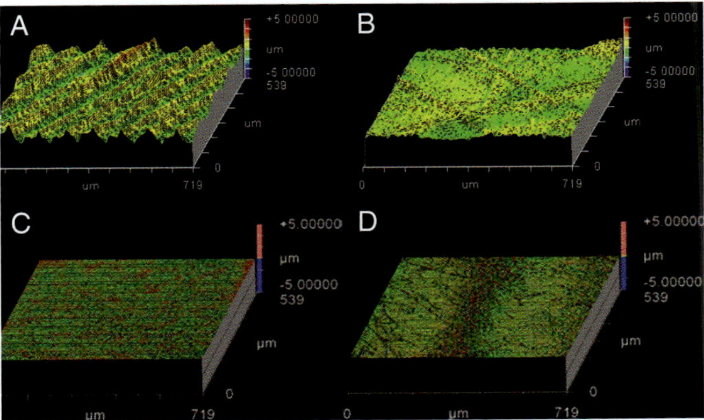

FIGURE 168-1. White light interferometry images of polyethylene unworn (**A**) and worn (**B**) implant surfaces compared with cobalt chromium implant unworn (**C**) and worn (**D**) surfaces.

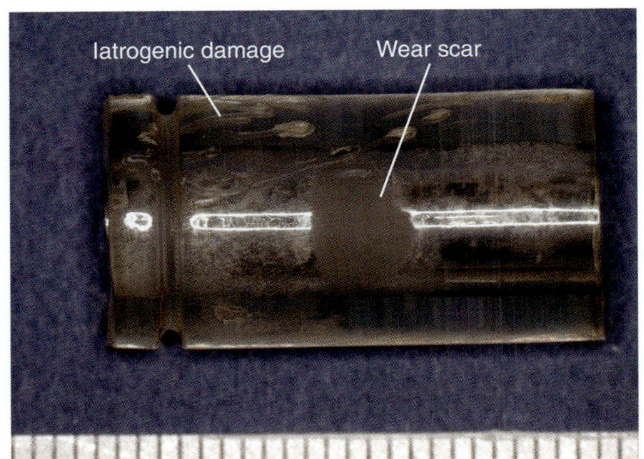

FIGURE 168-2. Abrasive wear observed on polymeric components from retrieved Dynesys systems, implanted 1.1 years.

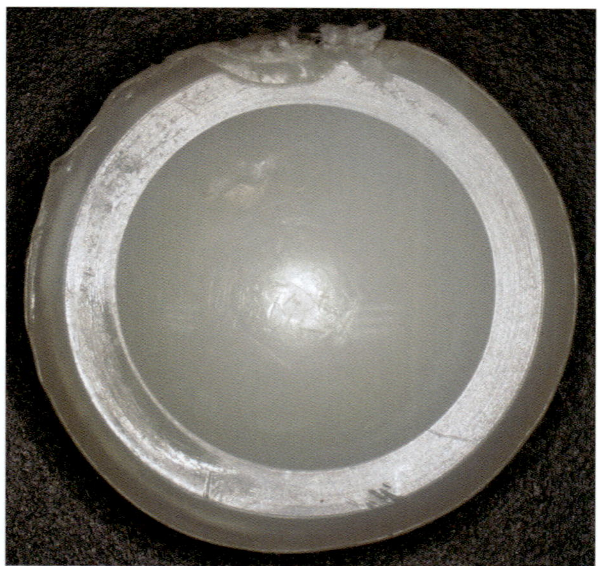

FIGURE 168-3. Microscopic, multidirectional scratches and crisscrossing wear paths at the dome of a retrieved polyethylene total disc replacement that was implanted 6.2 years.

polyethylene TDR (Fig. 168-3) are consistent with the type of microscopic abrasive wear mechanisms previously observed in retrieved hip replacement components.[12,13] By matching comparable regions of damage on two opposing bearing surfaces, it is further possible to infer the orientation of the components while they were in contact.

Burnishing

Typically encountered with polyethylene disc components, burnishing gives the polymer surface a polished, glossy appearance (Fig. 168-4). At a microscopic length scale, burnishing is associated with an adhesive wear mechanism, whereby the polyethylene surface wear occurs by adhesion to the metallic counterface. Magnified images of a burnished wear zone from a retrieved TDR are shown in Figure 168-4 and as noted also show evidence of scratching, which denotes the presence of abrasion. For this reason, the dominant wear mechanism in metal-on-polyethylene articulations is considered to be a combination of adhesion and abrasion, as seen in total joint replacements.[12,13]

Regions of burnishing on polyethylene retrievals may be appreciated with the naked eye under the proper lighting conditions. In contrast, the bearing surfaces of retrieved metallic components are typically highly polished after removal from the body. Burnishing on a metal-on-metal disc replacement that occurred in vivo is very difficult to discern without the aid of SEM.

Surface Deformation

Surface deformation, sometimes referred to as *plastic deformation* or *creep*, corresponds to permanent changes in the shape or geometry of a TDR, without the loss of material. Although surface deformation is not considered a wear mechanism, it could represent an undesirable damage mode. When permanent changes in the geometry of a device compromise the in vivo function or kinematics of the device, surface deformation is considered a failure mode for the implant.

In motion preserving spinal devices, macroscopic surface deformation has been observed in components that undergo compression in vivo. Polycarbonate urethane (PCU) spacers used in the Dynesys system undergo deformation owing to cold flow of the material, the compressive load applied during the surgery, and subsequent loading in vivo, which results in permanent bending of the implant and indentations from the supporting polyaxial screws (Fig. 168-5). Additional deformation of soft polymer components may occur from interaction with other components from the implant, for example, the cord component that passes through the center of the polyurethane spacer in the Dynesys system (see Fig. 168-5).

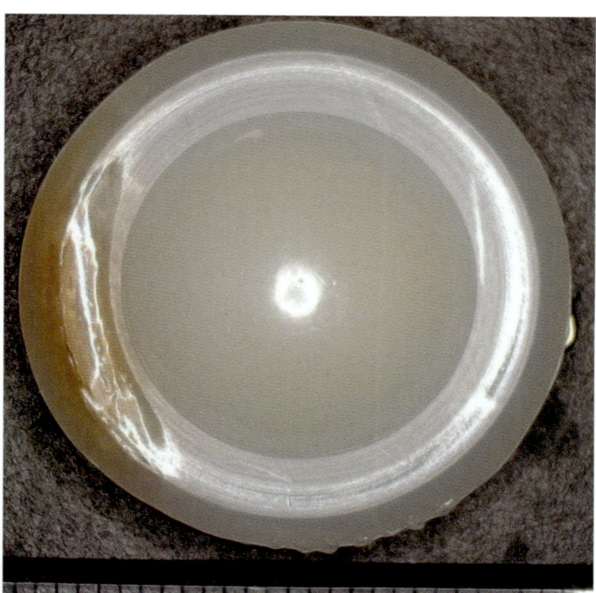

FIGURE 168-4. Burnishing observed on the dome of the polyethylene component of a retrieved total disc replacement.

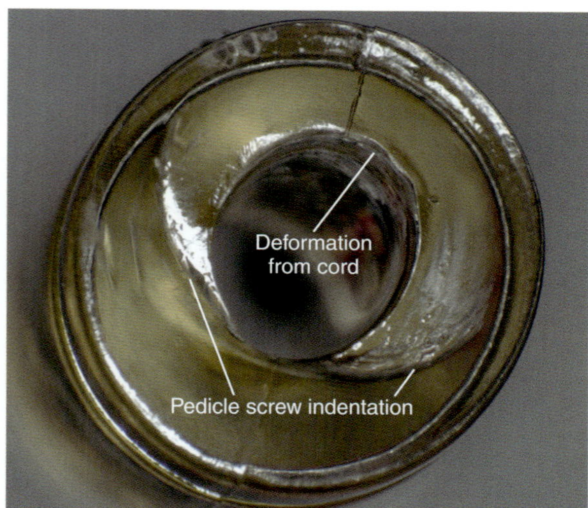

FIGURE 168-5. Polycarbonate urethane component of a retrieved Dynesys system that was implanted for 1 year, showing deformation from the polyester cord and the supporting pedicle screw.

Fatigue Wear and Fracture

Fatigue wear and fracture, especially of the rim, are a concern with polyethylene TDRs. David et al.[14] reported a case in which the entire rim of a disc replacement fractured from the central body of the core after 9.5 years in vivo. This case of rim failure was attributed to severe oxidation degradation after gamma sterilization in air.

The severity and clinical manifestation of fatigue-related rim damage in the Charité design varies widely, ranging from full-thickness transverse rim fracture (Fig. 168-6) to more benign radial crack formation (Fig. 168-7). In our retrieval studies of the Charité, radial cracks have been observed in 27 of 53 implants examined so far.[15] Similarly, transverse cracks have been observed in 17 of 53 retrieved implants.[15] In most cases, fatigue fracture is related to impingement by the metallic end plates. Fractures have also been observed in polymer components of dorsal devices such as the Dynesys (Fig. 168-8).

The etiology and incidence of fatigue wear and fracture in dynamic spinal systems are unclear because it may require many years for progressive fracture mechanisms in a particular design to result in clinical symptoms. It is further unknown what role gamma sterilization in air or in a low oxygen environment has on the fracture mechanisms in disc replacement. These research topics are currently under investigation at our institution.

There have been no reports of fracture of a metal-on-metal disc replacement component in the literature. Similarly, implant fracture has not been a clinical concern for contemporary metal-on-metal bearing surfaces in hip prostheses.

Embedded Debris

Embedded debris is an unusual but noteworthy damage mode for disc replacements. We have observed embedded debris in which a fractured radiographic wire marker became trapped between the rim and a metallic end plate of a TDR (Fig. 168-9). We have also observed embedded polymeric debris in dynamic systems with braided polymer cords (Fig. 168-10). The clinical significance of this wear mode is unknown at the present time. In large total joint replacements, embedded debris is a potential roughening mechanism for the metallic component, which can result in accelerated wear. Such a mechanism was not apparent in the retrieval shown in Figure 168-9, which appeared to be relatively stationary and resulted in only a faintly perceptible indentation of the metallic end plate. As a result, additional retrievals are necessary to understand better the incidence and clinical significance (if any) of embedded debris in TDRs. Although metallic surfaces are also theoretically susceptible to embedded debris, including third-body scratching by the radiopacifiers contained in

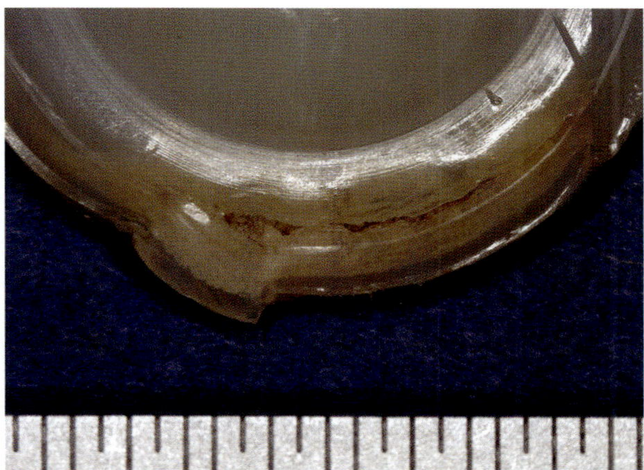

FIGURE 168-6. Fatigue-related rim fracture observed in a retrieved Charité implant that was implanted for 9.2 years.

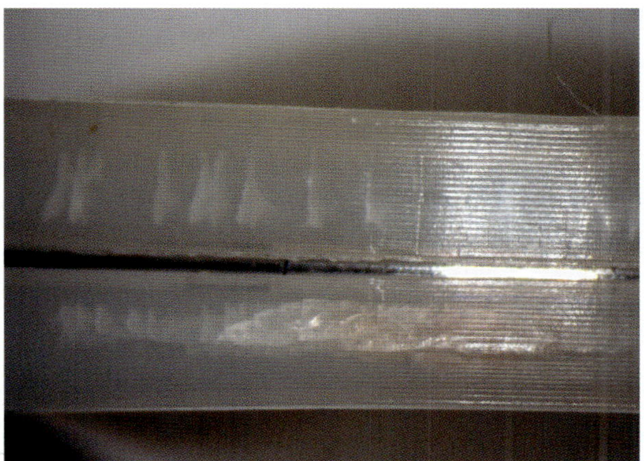

FIGURE 168-7. Fatigue-related radial rim cracking observed in a retrieved Charité prosthesis that was implanted for 3.1 years.

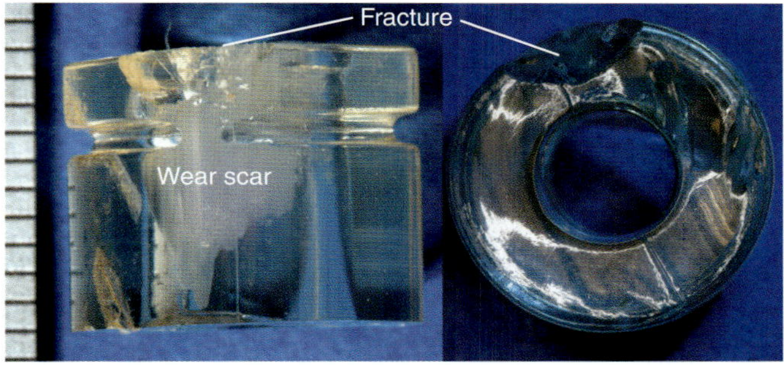

FIGURE 168-8. Optical microscopy of a fatigue-fractured spacer from a retrieved Dynesys system that was implanted for 1.1 years.

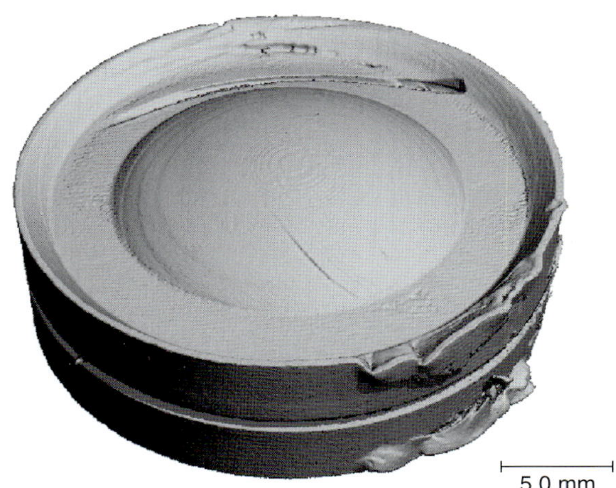

FIGURE 168-9. Micro-CT image of third-body damage caused by a fractured radiographic wire marker in a component implanted for 12.7 years.

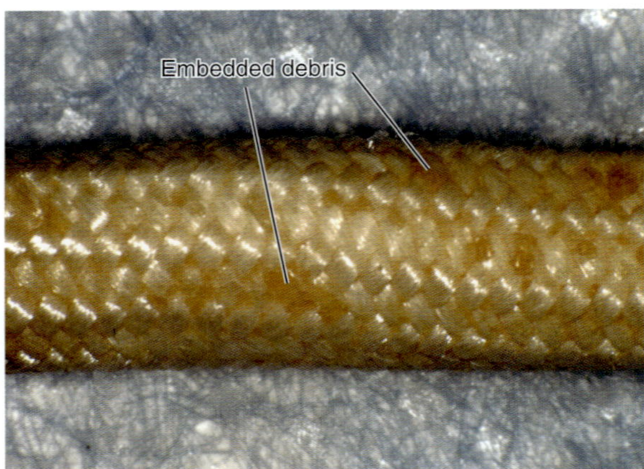

FIGURE 168-10. Explanted Dynesys polyethylene terethalate component with embedded debris observed within the braided cord.

bone cement for total joint applications, there are no reports yet in the literature of third-body wear being observed in metal-on-metal disc replacements.

Corrosion

Prior retrieval studies of dorsal instrumentation systems provide evidence that corrosion can occur in metallic spinal implants. Villarraga et al.[16] reported findings from retrieved posterior rod instrumentation systems. Wear and corrosion were not observed in any of the 21 titanium implants that were evaluated, but corrosion and wear were observed in 58% of stainless steel implants included in the study. A common location for corrosion was where the transverse connector interfaces with the rod, which can involve multiple surface-to-surface contact points and small cavities where no contact occurs.[16] These characteristics are inherently associated with micromotion, which can lead to wear, fretting corrosion, and wear particle formation. Corrosion of stainless steel components has also been reported in previous retrieval studies of spinal implants[17-19] to worsen the fatigue performance of orthopaedic implants,[20] and corrosion by-products are suspected to cause deleterious biologic tissue responses in the adjacent tissue surrounding the implant.[19,21]

Experience gained from dorsal spinal fusion instrumentation is important to keep in mind in evaluating TDR and other nonfusion spinal implant designs. Although retrieved motion preserving implant components from our laboratory and others[22] have not shown evidence of corrosion, the effects of wear or corrosion debris on local and systemic tissues remain clinical concerns.[23] Future long-term retrieval studies are needed to determine whether this remains a concern with contemporary motion preserving implant designs.

In Vivo Degradation

Although characterization of wear and damage mechanisms is perhaps one of the most fruitful goals of retrieval analysis, it is also equally important to investigate whether the biologic environment has resulted in any long-term chemical changes to the implant material, whether it be composed of polymer, metal, or ceramic. With polyethylene components, in vivo oxidation may be a potential long-term damage mechanism for artificial discs.[5] However, in vivo chemical changes to implants may be incidental and unrelated to clinical performance. For polyethylene acetabular components, severe rim oxidation has been shown to occur after 10 years in vivo,[24] but the clinical relevance is unclear because these implants do not normally articulate at the rim. With polyethylene TDR components, rim failure has been observed to occur in vivo, but it is unclear if oxidation is the driving mechanism in all of these cases, or whether impingement alone may be sufficient to generate the types of fractures that have been documented to occur clinically.[3] In PCU components, surface chemical changes associated with polyurethane degradation have been observed; these changes were associated only with implants that have been implanted for relatively long periods and primarily in regions where the implant was exposed to biologic fluid.[7] Trommsdorff et al.[25] reported that chemical changes in retrieved Dynesys PCU spacers were negligible at 100 μm below the surface. The clinical relevance of these surface chemical changes is unknown.

In vivo changes in chemistry may also occur with metallic components. In metal-on-metal hip implants fabricated from CoCr alloys, tribochemical deposits have been observed on the surface of retrieved implants.[26] These surface layers rich in carbon and oxygen, which have a smoky or hazy appearance, are attributed to joint fluids, which become fused to the bearing surface. The biofilms are thought to have a beneficial effect, by providing a solid lubricant for the articulating surface. We have observed comparable biofilms on retrieved CoCr alloy, metal-on-metal disc replacement components, suggesting that a similar mechanism may be occurring.[27]

A wide range of well-established techniques has been developed to assess chemical changes in polyethylene and metallic components for motion preserving spinal implants; a comprehensive list is provided by ASTM F561-05.[4] With polyethylene components, preferred methods include characterization of crystalline content using differential scanning calorimetry, measurement of oxidation using Fourier transform infrared spectroscopy (FTIR), and measurement of mechanical properties using the small punch test (ASTM F2183-02). In previous case studies of polyethylene disc replacements, both FTIR and the small punch test have been successfully employed.[5,14]

For metallic components, electron dispersive x-ray spectroscopy combined with SEM is useful for characterizing the chemistry of the alloys and biologic surface layers. As previously mentioned, we have successfully employed electron dispersive x-ray spectroscopy to analyze biofilms on the surface of retrieved metal-on-metal implants fabricated from CoCr alloys.[27] These electron dispersive x-ray spectroscopy analyses have enabled us to confirm that carbon-rich and oxygen-rich tribochemical reactions can occur on both the concave and the convex sides of metal-on-metal articulations in the spine. Further studies with an additional number of retrieved implants are necessary to determine the incidence of biofilms on CoCr alloy implants and for disc replacements produced from stainless steel or metalloceramic alloy composites.

Review of the Literature on Retrieval Analysis

At the present time, the literature regarding retrieval analysis of motion preserving spinal implants includes conference abstracts and individual case studies[5,14,28,29] but relatively few published journal articles with larger series.[6,15,30] In this section, we focus on studies that have included the analysis of a retrieval collection to seek commonalities in implant performance. We have included journal articles and more recent studies from conference proceedings in our review of retrieval analyses for motion preserving implants. Because the conference proceedings may not be readily available to all readers, we have also provided details about the findings from conference abstracts.

Cervical Spine Total Disc Replacements

The first published study in the field of artificial disc retrieval analysis was by Anderson et al.,[30] who examined short-term, retrieved cervical disc replacements of two designs: the Bryan and the Prestige designs (Medtronic). The Bryan artificial disc is a one-piece design consisting of two titanium alloy shells articulating against a mobile polyurethane core. The end plates are connected by a polyurethane sheath. The Prestige design consists of two stainless steel end plates that articulate with a ball-in-trough mechanism. Both the Bryan and the Prestige designs are fully described by Kurtz.[31] In the clinical study, the six Bryan retrievals were implanted on average 11.8 months (range, 4–16 months), and the two Prestige retrievals were implanted 18 months and 39 months.[30] Few details about the retrieval methodology are included in this study, but it appears that microscopic characterization and, in the case of the Bryan disc, FTIR and gel-permeation chromatography (GPC) were performed. No significant changes in FTIR or GPC results were detected relative to unimplanted controls, but this is not surprising given the generally short-term nature of the explants and the small sample size. As the first retrieval study of its kind in disc arthroplasty, the work of Anderson et al.[30] highlighted the importance of explant analysis for spine surgeons. However, because of the small numbers of retrievals and brief in vivo exposure, no conclusions can be drawn about generality of their findings.

Jensen et al.[32] reported bone ingrowth into the titanium shells of Bryan retrievals from two patients who were revised after 8 months and 10 months of implantation. New bone growth was observed into the porous coating of all four retrieved end plates. The mean bone ingrowth, quantified by histologic sectioning, was 30.1% (12% standard deviation), which compared favorably with bone ingrowth reported in the literature for hip and knee replacements.

A retrieval study was presented at the 2007 Spine Arthroplasty Society in which the wear patterns in the core and sheath of the Bryan artificial disc were characterized.[33] A secondary goal was to evaluate whether formalin storage could adversely affect the explants. Researchers tested the hypothesis that height loss of the core would increase with implantation time. Height loss was measured in the cores of 17 Bryan cervical TDRs that were retrieved from 14 patients (5 men, 7 women, 2 unknown) after 1.6 years in situ (range, 0.3–6.1 years). Implants were revised during 2003 to 2006 because of unresolved or recurring neck pain or radiculopathy (n = 15) and for infection or trauma (n = 1 each). Eight explants were stored in formalin for 1.4 to 3.3 years. Virgin, never-implanted sheaths and cores served as controls. SEM and WLIR were performed to identify wear mechanisms. The nominal height loss of the explanted cores (mean ± standard deviation) was 0.22 ± 0.09 mm (range, 0.04–0.35 mm). Although localized, microscopic evidence of adhesive and abrasive wear (confirmed by SEM and interferometry) was observed, researchers attributed most initial height loss to creep as opposed to material removal because the initial glossy surface finish of the cores was generally well preserved, even after 6.1 years in vivo. The sheaths typically showed evidence of folding or permanent deformation in regions where the core made repeated contact. No correlation was observed between core height loss and implantation time ($\rho = 0.4$, $P = .18$). No significant height difference was observed attributable to formalin storage. However, macroscopic changes in the explant surface, including cracking, occurred after 3 years of formalin storage; these findings were not present at the time of explanation. Researchers observed minimal wear and nominal changes in core height (approximately 0.2 mm) in this large series of polyurethane cervical disc explants. However, marked surface changes were noted after exposure of explants to formalin, and revising surgeons were cautioned to preserve polyurethane explants in a formalin-free environment.

The short-term in vivo wear performance of stainless steel Prestige cervical TDRs was characterized and compared with simulator results in two conference abstracts.[34,35] In a preliminary study, the early wear tests by Anderson et al.[30] were shown to produce similar wear mechanisms as retrievals; however, in the more recent study, the abrasion was more severe than what was observed in vivo.[34] Because available Prestige retrievals were implanted for the short term, researchers conducted a second study to characterize the short-term wear response within the first 1.0 million cycles.[35]

At the 2008 meeting of the Orthopedic Research Society, researchers presented the results of three Prestige ST cervical TDRs that were wear tested in accordance with ISO/FDIS 18192.[25] To evaluate the short-term in vitro wear behavior of the Prestige ST, the simulator was stopped after 0.05 million, 0.1 million, 0.2 million, 0.3 million, 0.4 million, 0.5 million, and 1.0 million cycles, and interval analyses were performed. These analyses consisted of photogrammetry and surface interferometry. The in vitro results from each interval analysis were compared with a Prestige ST retrieval collection analyzed from nine patients (two women and seven men). The artificial discs were Prestige I (n = 2), Prestige II (n = 2), or Prestige ST (n = 5), and all were of a stainless steel ball-and-trough design. The components had a range of implantation times from 0.7 to 3.3 years. Each component was previously characterized using the same methods as were used for in vitro interval analyses.

After 0.1 million cycles, the Prestige components exhibited a faint wear scar, produced by abrasive wear.[35] This wear mechanism was consistent with short-term explants. The average surface roughness of the worn regions for both the retrievals and in vitro tested components was measured to be 0.12 ± 0.08 μm and 0.16 ± 0.07 μm. The results of this Prestige retrieval study suggest that the ISO/FDIS 18192 standard test method replicates the in vivo wear patterns in TDRs after less than 1 million cycles of testing. Previous wear test methods have shown other in vitro methods with up to 20 million cycles, which generated much more severe abrasive scratches than seen in vivo.[30,34] The data also suggested that the same mechanism of abrasive wear is occurring at the bearing surface of both the retrievals and the components tested in vitro, although the greater worn surface area in the wear-tested components may indicate that the ranges of motion are more extensive than those experienced by TDRs in vivo.

Lumbar Spine Total Disc Replacements

Fixation, wear, and in vivo degradation are key functional aspects of lumbar TDRs that have been evaluated in more recent retrieval studies. Most of the retrieval research published to date for lumbar TDRs has been related to the historical Charité, manufactured by Link from 1989 to 2004 (this device is currently produced by DePuy Spine). A few retrieval studies have been published related to the ProDisc-L. Much less published retrieval data are currently available for metal-on-metal lumbar discs compared with metal-on-polyethylene discs.

With regard to fixation, bone ongrowth surfaces for TDRs have been tested in primate studies, but the fate of the bone-implant interface of lumbar TDRs in human patients has not yet been reported in the literature. Bone ongrowth could theoretically complicate revision. In an abstract presented at the 2006 Spine Arthroplasty Meeting,[36] researchers investigated the failure modes, bone-implant interface, and extent of remaining calcium phosphate (CaP) coating in retrieved Charité TDRs with textured end plates. Eight textured end plates from four explanted TDRs were studied after 3 to 6 years in vivo. In each case, the coated end plates were revised in straightforward fashion by an osteotomy adjacent to the implant. None of the end plates had evidence of residual CaP, and one end plate had adherent bone visible (<10% of the surface area) on optical microscopy. The bone ongrowth to the textured surfaces was judged to provide improved resistance of the prosthesis to shear forces, which can result in migration when the teeth are not securely engaged in this design. Based on their findings, the authors advocated the use of textured, coated end plates over smooth end plates for total disc arthroplasty. Bone ongrowth has also been visually observed on the titanium–plasma spray coating of retrieved ProDisc end plates.[29,37]

Analysis of wear and surface damage in long-term implanted Charité TDRs has been reported in a series of journal publications.[3,6,15] In the latest update of this multi-institutional series, 38 Charité components were retrieved with 16 years of implantation.[15] The components were revised for intractable pain or facet degeneration. Components were analyzed using optical microscopy and micro-CT. One-sided wear patterns were shown in 43% (15 of 35) of components analyzed using micro-CT.[15] Significant correlations were observed between implantation time and penetration and penetration rate. The dome of the components typically exhibited burnishing, which was consistent with the multidirectional wear observed in hip replacements, whereas the rim frequently showed evidence of radial and transverse cracking (19 of 38 and 14 of 38 retrievals), often produced by impingement. The rim damage modes of plastic deformation, delamination, and cracking were similar to those associated with knee components. The published Charité retrieval literature provides crucial long-term in vivo wear data for validation of spine wear simulators and for in vitro biomechanical testing.

Evidence of dome burnishing and rim impingement has also been noted in a more recent conference poster summarizing a collection of five short-term ProDisc-L prostheses implanted 2.2 years.[37] The bearing surface of the ProDisc-L showed burnishing (three of five implants), mild scratching, and pitting (three of five implants). Impingement was noted in three of five components and associated with burnishing and plastic deformation. The authors of the ProDisc retrieval study remarked that, "a potentially worrisome finding is the evidence of impingement. Whether caused by patients achieving a larger range of motion that the implant is designed to accommodate or by component positioning that allows impingement at even smaller range of motion, impingement can be problematic."[37] A detailed TDR retrieval study for the ProDisc-L, displaying mild anterior impingement, has been reported more recently as a case study by Choma et al.[29]

Although rim impingement has been observed in retrieved TDRs of different designs, the clinical consequences of chronic rim impingement are poorly understood. In a study presented at the 2008 Spine Arthroplasty Society meeting,[38] a retrieval collection of polyethylene mobile bearing TDRs was analyzed to determine whether rim impingement adversely affected dome penetration. Based on observations of plastic deformation, burnishing, or fracture of the rim, 28 of 40 (70%) of retrieved cores, implanted for 2 to 16 years (average, 7.9 years), were classified as exhibiting chronic rim impingement. Dome penetration was comparable in cores with chronic impingement (average, 0.3; range, 0.1–0.9 mm) compared with cores with no impingement (average, 0.3; range, 0.1–0.5 mm). Rim penetration was significantly greater in cores with chronic impingement ($P < .05$). Using linear regression, the dome penetration rate for cores with negligible impingement (0.036 mm/year, 95% confidence interval 0.012–0.061 mm/year) appeared slightly higher than for cores with chronic impingement (0.021 mm/year, 95% confidence interval 0.005–0.038 mm/year); however, the difference was not significant. The results of this study did not support the hypothesis that chronic rim impingement would be associated with greater dome penetration. However, the findings suggest that dome wear and impingement are effectively decoupled phenomena and may be studied independently of each other.

In addition to impingement, rim damage observed in polyethylene TDR retrievals has been associated with postirradiation oxidation.[39] Analysis of explanted Charité cores using FTIR spectroscopy has shown that the exposed rim experiences severe oxidation after 10 or more years.[39] These findings appear consistent for TDRs that were gamma irradiated in air and in first-generation polymeric barrier packaging.[40] However, the central dome appears to be protected from in vivo oxidation owing to contact with the metallic end plates. No correlation was observed between wear of the central dome and oxidation.[39] These observations are similar to the in vivo oxidation patterns noted in artificial hips, which exhibit rim embrittlement after 10 years in vivo but show reduced oxidation at the bearing surface where the femoral head contacts the polyethylene.[40] In contrast to hip replacement, the rim of a TDR core may be intended to support chronic loading for the lifetime of the patient. The findings of in vivo oxidation in gamma-sterilized polyethylene TDR components provide additional motivation for developing in vitro mechanical tests that incorporate accelerated aging or some other oxidative challenge to simulate changes in the bearing materials that may occur with long-term in vivo exposure.

A study presented at the 2008 Spineweek meeting was conducted to correlate better long-term clinical wear rates of the Charité with simulator wear rates.[41] It was hypothesized that the wear mechanisms of the retrievals would be more accurately simulated by International Standard of Organization (ISO) protocols with coupled motion compared with ASTM-type protocols that resulted in linear motion. Researchers analyzed dome wear rate and surface morphology of 41 Charité (SBIII) explants from 35 patients (71% female). The cores were implanted for 7.5 years (range, 1.8–16.3 years). Investigators also examined 12 Charité wear-tested cores and 6 controls. Six cores were tested according to an ASTM-type protocol for 10 million cycles[42]; three additional cores were unloaded and soaked. Six cores were tested according to the ISO protocol for 2 million cycles with three loaded and soaked controls. All of the cores in this study were produced by the same manufacturer (Link). The explanted cores typically exhibited burnishing or evidence of adhesive and abrasive dome wear, consistent with multidirectional motion. The wear rate of the explants, obtained by correlation of dome height with implantation time, was 0.023 mm/year. The ASTM-tested cores exhibited unidirectional abrasive wear at a rate of 0.007 mm/Mcycles (million cycles). The ISO-tested cores exhibited regional burnishing and wear at a rate of 0.124 mm/Mcycles. The ISO protocol generated wear surface morphology that was closer to the retrievals than the ASTM protocol, and 2 million cycles of the ISO protocol corresponded, on average, to about 5.6 years of clinical wear. The findings from this study further suggest that the ISO protocol provides a useful starting point for clinical validation of spine wear simulations incorporating lumbar polyethylene TDRs.

Because of its longer clinical history, more retrieval research has been published to date with metal-on-polyethylene lumbar discs than with metal-on-metal discs. At the present time, detailed results are available regarding the retrieval analysis of a single lumbar metal-on-metal TDR.[43] This implant was removed after 12 months in situ at L5-S1 from a 43-year-old woman because of nerve root impingement. The components generally exhibited highly polished surfaces, similar to the surfaces observed on explanted metal-on-metal hip implants. The primary wear mechanism was microabrasion, which was evident by microscopic scratching of the articulating surfaces. Focal microplasticity was also observed at the apex of the dome and the anterior and posterior vertices of the cupped component, suggesting that the primary motion in these locations was flexion-extension. Surface deposits, manifested as a smoky or hazy discoloration, were observed on both components, consistent with organic films previously observed in well-functioning metal-on-metal hip joints. The surface features of the Maverick retrieval were compared with wear-tested components in a study by Pare et al.[44] The surface topography of unidirectional tested components was found to be more severely abraded than the components that were tested under combined flexion-extension, lateral bending, and axial torsion. Although only a single retrieval was available for comparison at the time of the study, the retrieval results were more closely comparable to the wear test results with combined motion.

Dynamic Stabilization System Studies

Dynamic stabilization devices are nonfusion devices designed to stabilize the motion segment in lieu of fusion. Retrieval analysis for the Dynesys system (Zimmer Spine) has been reported. This system consists of fixed pedicle screws, PCU spacers that resist extension and compressive loads, and polyethylene terephthalate (PET) cords that resist flexion and tensile loading. Trommsdorff et al.[25,45,46] examined the biostability of retrieved spacer and cord components.

In a retrieval study of 12 cords retrieved from 10 different patients (implanted 2–5.5 years), changes in surface chemistry were evaluated using attenuated total reflectance Fourier transform infrared spectroscopy (ATR-FTIR).[45] Molecular weight distribution was evaluated using GPC. The retrieved cords were cleaned using an enzyme solution to remove biologic residue. The authors reported that the ATR-FTIR spectra obtained at different positions along the retrieved cords showed no signs of significant hydrolysis. Molecular weight analysis conducted on two retrieved cords (3.3 years and 5.5 years) did not show evidence of a significant change in molecular weight distribution. The authors concluded that the Dynesys PET cords showed good biostability at 5.5 years.

In a case study by Trommsdorff et al.,[46] a system that had been implanted for 5.5 years was retrieved from L3-4 in a 56-year-old patient who had an abscess in proximity to the left spacer, which was presumably caused by infection. The contralateral component was not infected. Both spacers were retrieved, and their chemical structure was compared with a control component using ATR-FTIR. SEM was also used to evaluate regions on the spacer surfaces. Compared with the control spacer, the left spacer that was adjacent to the abscess showed changes in the infrared peaks that could be attributed to hydrolysis of the soft and hard segments of the PCU. On the right spacer, there was no remarkable chemical degradation. No change in the chemical structure was observed in either spacer at a depth of 100 μ or in the bulk material. SEM showed microcracks on the left spacer, whereas the right spacer was described as "perfectly smooth." The authors concluded that the functionality of the implant was not impaired, because the degradation was limited to the surface layer (<2.5% of the wall thickness).

In a larger study of 50 retrieved Dynesys systems with implantation times ranging from a few months to 5.5 years, the investigators conducted optical microscopy, SEM, ATR-FTIR, and GPC analyses of the PCU spacers.[25] The PET cords were also inspected using optical microscopy. The PET cords showed minor damage to the outermost layers in the regions of fixation but were intact elsewhere. The PCU spacers typically showed minor deformation owing to cold flow of the material. Regions of wear were observed, which the authors concluded to have been from articulation of the spacer with the facet joint. No changes in molecular weight distribution were observed in 3.3-year and 5.1-year retrievals. At the surfaces of the PCU spacers, small changes in chemistry were observed, which the authors attributed to the absorption of biologic fluids and minor hydrolytic changes of the material. At a depth of 100 μ below the surface, no change in the chemistry of the PCU was found. The authors concluded that the PET cords and PCU spacers were biologically stable over an implantation time of 5.5 years.

In a more recent abstract by Trommsdorff et al.[47] summarizing the findings of 64 retrieved Dynesys systems, the results related to the PCU spacers were similar. The systems were implanted for up to 7 years. The authors also reported the incidence of screw loosening (20% of retrievals) and screw breakage (16% of retrievals). The screw breakages occurred at approximately one-third of the screw length from the tip of the screw and were apparently due to fatigue fracture. The authors reported that this rate was in the same range or lower than that of other comparable designs.

Ianuzzi et al.[7,48] have reported similar results from their collection of retrieved Dynesys systems, which consisted of 75 spacers from 17 patients with implantation an average of 2.3 years (range, 0.7–7 years). The systems were primarily revised for persistent pain (16 of 17 patients) and screw loosening (11 of 17 patients); 1 patient experienced complications secondary to implant migration. Optical microscopy was conducted to evaluate spacer deformation and wear. ATR-FTIR was used to evaluate changes in surface chemistry compared with two control components. Similar to the results of Trommsdorff et al.,[47] a focal region of abrasive wear was observed along the length of 51 of 75 spacers, which was likely due to impingement with surrounding bony structures. One spacer exhibited short surface cracks that extended from the center of the spacer to the outer surface. Changes in chemical structure were also observed on the surfaces of the spacers, although evidence of material degradation was observed in only 10 of 75 spacers. The findings from the spacers were determined to be incidental because the components from the short-term retrieval study were revised for reasons unrelated to wear, surface damage, or biostability.

The findings from two separate groups of researchers showed that components from Dynesys systems may undergo deformation, wear, and changes to surface chemistry. These findings are from short-term retrievals (up to 7 years). The long-term effects of these phenomena are unknown at this time and require further investigation as spinal implants composed of similar materials or design continue to be developed and used.

Recommendations for Future Testing and Research

Based on the body of retrieval evidence for Charité discs, wear simulators of the lumbar spine should be tuned to produce a similar extent of cross-shear as observed in hip replacements. This evidence suggests that the option for unidirectional wear testing currently offered in the recently approved ASTM Standards for wear testing of TDRs is inappropriate for the lumbar spine. In hip and knee simulator tests, 1 million cycles corresponds to about 1 year in vivo; little is known about the number of duty cycles cervical disc replacements experience in vivo. However, more recent comparisons between lumbar and cervical devices and simulator studies employing protocols detailed in ISO standards provide support for short-term intervals to be assessed when conducting a wear test. Based on simulator testing and retrieval analyses, we begin to see similar wear patterns (in the case of the Prestige cervical disc) at 100,000 to 200,000 cycles of wear testing using the ISO protocol. In the case of the Charité TDR, analysis of the penetration rates also suggests that 100,000 to 200,000 cycles corresponds, on average, to 1 year in vivo. It may be that the similarity in design and material explains the consistent results; validation testing with a greater number of designs and bearing materials is necessary. Current data support the hypothesis that wear mechanisms within the first 1 million cycles of testing in a simulator may be clinically relevant and provide important benchmarks for the validation of standard wear testing protocols for TDRs.

Because of the prevalence of impingement seen in the Charité retrievals, the authors recommend that impingement fatigue tests be developed to evaluate the performance of TDRs. In the Charité, impingement can occur during regular flexion or extension activities and has been shown with in vitro cadaver tests.[49] Impingement can also occur secondary to subsidence, subluxation, or migration of the end plates. Because resistance to chronic impingement damage is desirable, fatigue test methods should be developed to reproduce the rim fracture modes observed in the Charité retrievals presented in this study. Once validated, the protocol could be used to screen implant materials for fatigue resistance under clinically relevant loading conditions. Additionally, given the potential for component oxidation, it would be useful to precondition test specimens using accelerated aging before rim fatigue tests.

The recommendations for standardized wear testing and periprosthetic tissue analysis in this chapter are based on long-term wear findings of retrieved components of a single lumbar total disc design and short-term findings from other designs. These include evaluations in wear simulators, retrieval analysis of motion preserving spinal implants, and assessment of wear debris and biologic response in periprosthetic tissue. It remains to be seen how generalized these findings are to other lumbar TDR designs, in particular, designs with newer material couples, and to cervical spine designs.

KEY REFERENCES

Anderson PA, Kurtz SM, Toth JM: Explant analysis of total disc replacement. *Semin Spine Surg* 18:1–12, 2006.

ASTM F561–05ASTM F561–05: *Standard practice for retrieval and analysis of medical devices, and associated tissues and fluids*, West Conshohocken, PA, 2005, American Society for Testing and Materials.

Ianuzzi A, Kurtz S, Kane W, et al: In vivo deformation, surface damage, and biostability of retrieved Dynesys systems. *Spine (Phila Pa 1976)* 35:E1310–E1316, 2010.

Kurtz SM, MacDonald D, Ianuzzi A, et al: The natural history of polyethylene oxidation in total disc replacement. *Spine (Phila Pa 1976)* 34:2369–2377, 2009.

Kurtz S, Siskey R, Ciccarelli L, et al: Retrieval analysis of total disc replacements: implications for standardized wear testing. *J ASTM Int* 3:1–12, 2006.

Kurtz SM, van Ooij A, Ross ERS, et al: Polyethylene wear and rim fracture in total disc arthroplasty. *Spine J* 7:12–21, 2007.

REFERENCES

The complete reference list is available online at expertconsult.com.

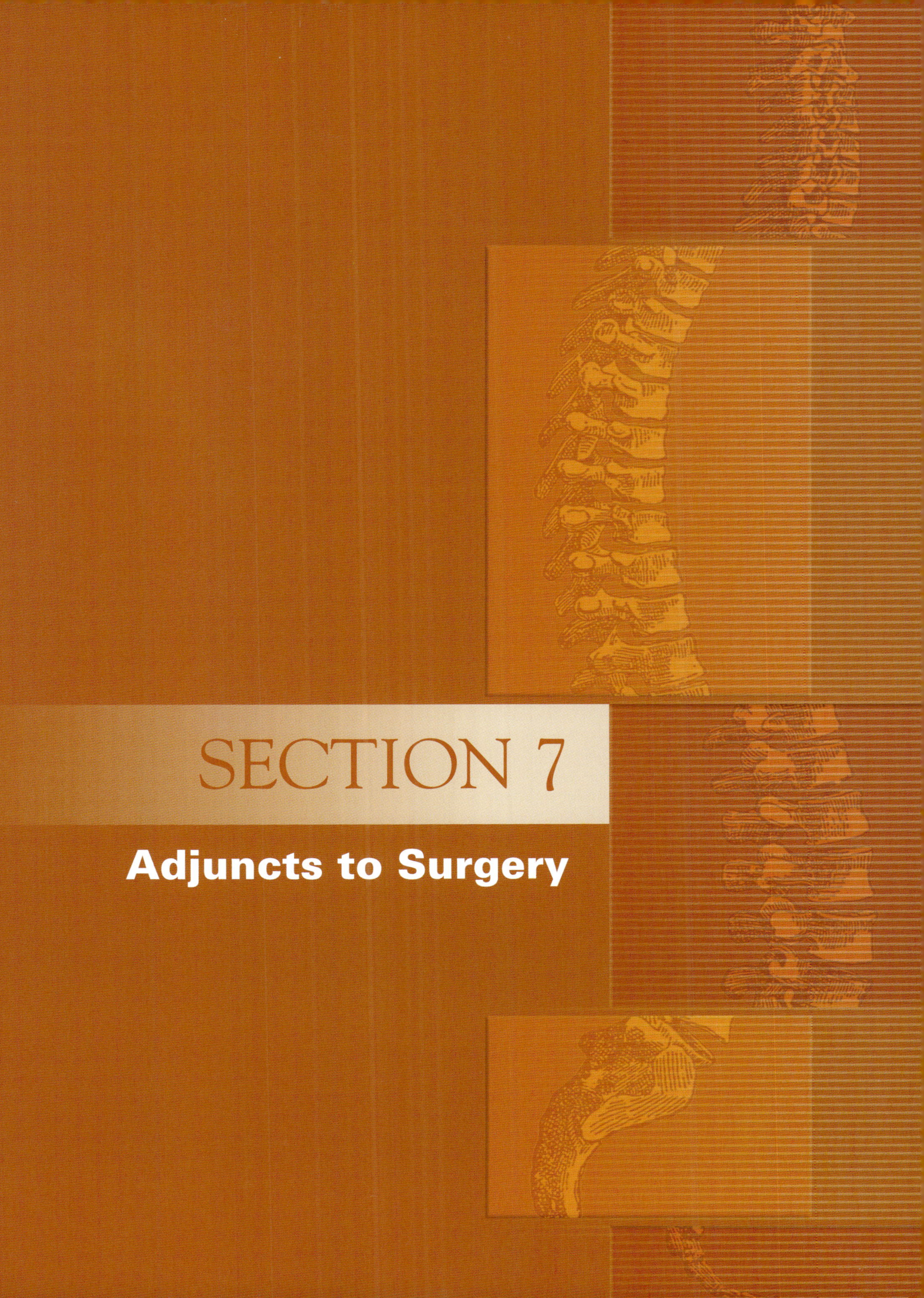

SECTION 7

Adjuncts to Surgery

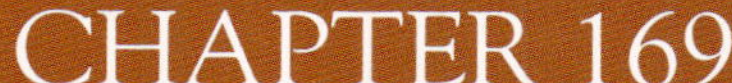

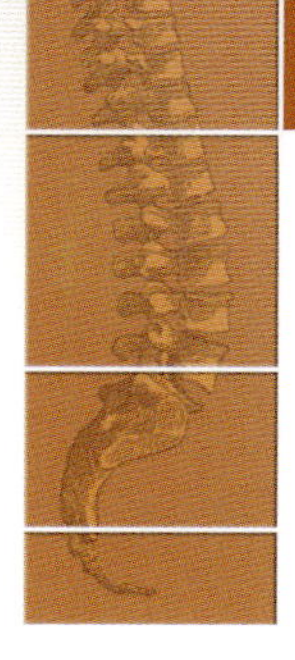

CHAPTER 169

Surgical Incisions, Positioning, and Retraction

Mehmet Zileli | Edward C. Benzel | Glenn R. Rechtine II

A variety of ventral and dorsal incisions are used to gain access from the upper cervical to the lower sacral spine. Appropriate positioning plays an important role in minimizing blood loss and providing adequate exposure of the spine. Tissue retraction plays an equally important role. Table 169-1 presents an overview of approaches and corresponding incisions. This chapter focuses on surgical decisions, patient positioning, and retraction techniques to avoid complications during surgery.

Patient Positioning

Appropriate patient positioning in the operating room is optimally determined by the combined efforts of the surgeon and the neuroanesthetist.

Sitting Position

An advantage of the sitting position is that it directs blood away from the surgical site (Fig. 169-1). The risk of air embolism, however, is a major disadvantage. Furthermore, if the patient is quadriplegic (with a decrease in sympathetic tone), the resulting hemodynamic changes and hypoperfusion associated with the sitting position may compromise the perfusion of the spinal cord. Therefore, the sitting position requires a competent anesthetist as well as right atrial and pulmonary artery catheterization, Doppler ultrasound heart monitoring, and end-tidal CO_2 monitoring.

Ventral Cervical Operations

A bolster beneath the neck and the interscapular region enhances cervical extension. Cervical distraction may be achieved by cervical traction or interbody distraction techniques.

Lateral Approaches

In the lateral decubitus position, the table may either be neutral or slightly extended to extend the rib cage. In this position, care should be taken to avoid compression of the brachial plexus; therefore, a roll should be placed under the axilla. The upper arm should be abducted no more than 90 degrees. The elbow must be properly padded (Fig. 169-2).

Retractors

Three major types of retractors are used in spinal surgery: hand-held retractors, patient-mounted self-retaining retractors, and table-mounted self-retaining retractors. Because intraoperative radiographs are commonly used in spinal surgery, radiolucent retractors may be very helpful.

Transoral Retractors

Self-retaining retractors are usually necessary to maintain an open mouth and to depress the tongue. Self-retaining retractor rings are fixed on the upper and lower teeth (Fig. 169-3). Table-mounted retractors are attached to the operating table to retract both the palate and the tongue. These retractors may also hold the neck in a fixed position; thus, they may eliminate the need for additional skeletal traction.

Ventral Cervical Retractors

Hand-held retractors with blunt tips are useful for the dissection phase of the operation. For subsequent phases of ventral cervical operations, the most commonly used self-retaining retractors are the Caspar (Aesculap, Tuftlingen, Germany; Fig. 169-4), Apfelbaum (Aesculap; Fig. 169-5), Cloward (Codman, Raynham, MA), and Farley-Thompson retractors (Thompson Surgical Instruments, Traverse City, MI; Fig. 169-6).

The transverse blades of self-retaining retractor systems often have teeth that should be placed under the longus colli muscles to avoid damage to the esophagus and carotid artery. The longitudinal blades are smooth.

A modified Caspar retractor has been recommended for ventrolateral foraminotomy; it enables retraction of the longus colli muscle laterally and facilitates vertebral artery retraction.[1]

Ventral Thoracic and Lumbar Retractors

A crank-type retractor is useful to distract the ribs. The lungs as well as the diaphragm or retroperitoneal organs are retracted with lung and abdominal hand-held retractors.

TABLE 169-1

Classification of Surgical Approaches and Commonly Used Incision Types

Region	Exposure	Incision
High Cervical Spine		
Dorsal approaches	Suboccipital craniectomy C1–2 laminectomy	Dorsal midline
	Lateral transcondylar approach	Hockey-stick, retromastoid
Ventral approaches	Transoral approach	Midline pharynx
	Median labiomandibular glossotomy	Median lower lip, mandible, tongue
	Transthyroidal approach	Transverse below hyoid bone
	Ventrolateral retropharyngeal approach	T-shaped submandibular or hockey-stick
Lateral approaches	SCM may be cut	L-shaped incision below mastoid process
Subaxial Cervical Spine (C3-T1)		
Dorsal approaches	Laminoforaminotomy for cervical disc disease	Dorsal paramedian
	Laminectomy	Dorsal midline
	Laminoplasty	Dorsal midline
Ventral approaches	Ventromedial approach	Parallel to skin crests or SCM
	Ventrolateral approach–medial to the carotid artery	Parallel to SCM
	Ventrolateral approach–lateral to the carotid artery	Parallel to SCM
Cervicothoracic Junction (C7-T3)		
Dorsal approaches	Laminectomy	Dorsal midline
Ventral approaches	Lower ventral-medial cervical approach	Parallel to SCM
	Transsternal approach	T-shaped; extending midsternum
	Transmanubrial approach	T-shaped; or parallel to SCM extending midsternum
	Transverse supraclavicular approach	Parallel to clavicle
	Transaxillary extrapleural approach	Subaxillary, parallel to T3 rib
	Transpleural-transthoracic approach	Parallel to T3 rib
Thoracic and Thoracolumbar Spine		
Dorsal approaches	Thoracic laminectomy	Dorsal midline
	Transpedicular approach	Dorsal midline
	Costotransversectomy	Curved to one side paramedian
	Lateral extracavitary approach	Curved to one side paramedian or hockey-stick
	Dorsal en bloc total spondylectomy	Dorsal midline
Ventral approaches	Transpleural thoracotomy	Parallel to rib
	Transdiaphragmatic approach	Flank incision
	Ventrolateral retroperitoneal approach	Flank incision
Lumbar and Lumbosacral Spine		
Dorsal approaches	Lumbar laminectomy	Dorsal midline
	Paraspinal approach	Paramedian
	Lateral extracavitary approach	Paramedian
Ventral approaches	Extreme lateral interbody fusion approach or ventrolateral transpsoatic approach	Lateral lumbar
	Pelvic brim extraperitoneal approach	Lower flank incision
	Transperitoneal approach	Midline/horizontal subumbilical laparotomy incision
Sacrum		
Dorsal approaches	Dorsal approach	Dorsal midline
Ventral approaches	Retroperitoneal approach	U-shaped suprapubic incision
	Transperitoneal approach	Midline subumbilical laparotomy incision

SCM, sternocleidomastoid muscle.

Although they may narrow the operating space, the placement of laparotomy sponges under retractor blades helps to prevent damage to the viscera. The disadvantages of handheld retractors include the risks of visceral organ damage and the difficulty of manually maintaining sufficient retraction force. Table-mounted systems retract both the rib cage and the lungs.

Dorsolateral Thoracic and Lumbar Retractors

The lateral extracavitary approach to the thoracic and lumbar spine requires significant retraction. A rostral and caudal self-retaining tissue-mounted retractor may be used to medially retract the paraspinous muscles. A wide-diameter, malleable

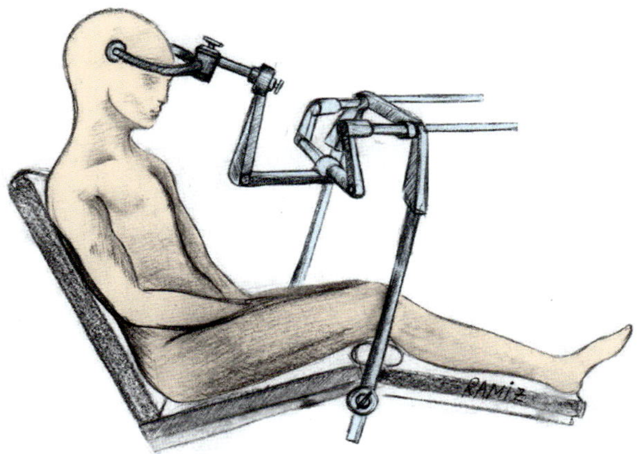

FIGURE 169-1. Sitting position.

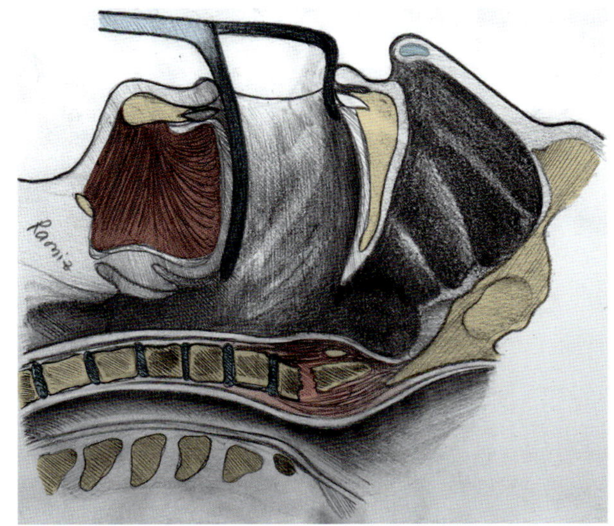

FIGURE 169-3. Retraction system used for transoral approach.

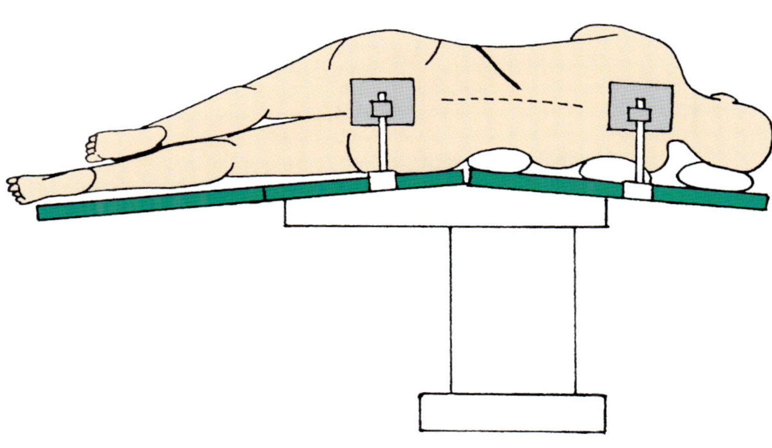

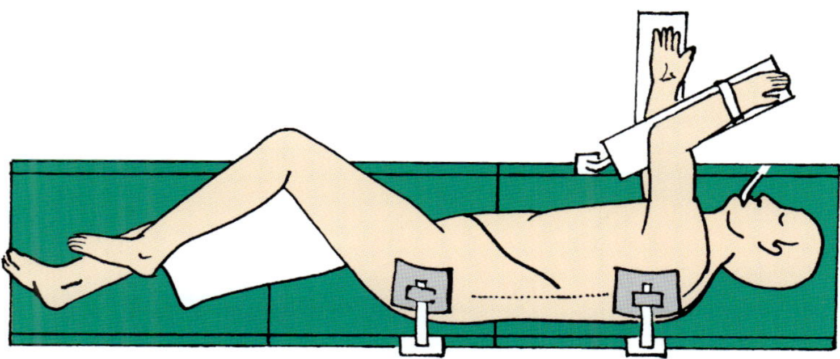

FIGURE 169-2. Lateral decubitus position used for thoracotomy or retroperitoneal approach. A pad under the desired vertebral level and another pad under the axilla are placed. Note that the ipsilateral hip is flexed.

retractor can be used to laterally retract the muscles of the chest wall or the lumbodorsal muscles. Either hand-held or table-mounted retractors may be used.[2]

Approaches

Dorsal Approaches to the Upper Cervical Spine

Midline Dorsal Approach

Either the sitting or the prone position can be used in a midline dorsal approach. If skull traction is required, the prone position with a horseshoe attachment should be considered (Figs. 169-7 and 169-8).

The dorsal scalp and cervical regions are prepared for incision. If a fusion is planned, the area for the bone harvest (usually the dorsal iliac crest) should also be prepared. A midline incision is made from the external occipital protuberance to the midcervical spinous processes (C5 or C6 or the most appropriate level). Avoid unnecessary dissection, especially of the interspine and ligaments.

Two deep-seated self-retaining retractors are usually satisfactory. Menezes recommends using two retractors placed at 90 degrees to each other to prevent motion of the occipitocervical and atlantoaxial joints.[3]

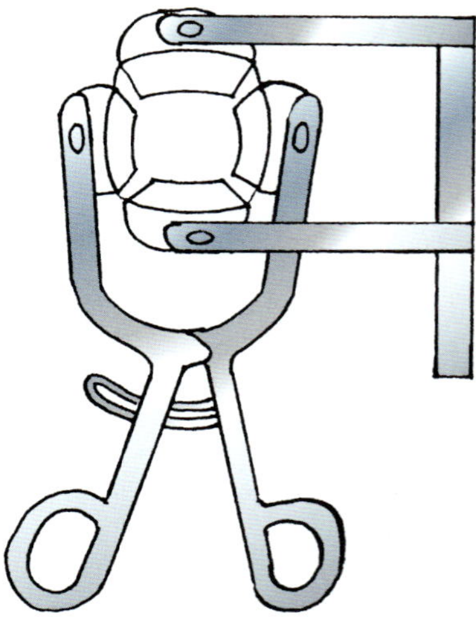

FIGURE 169-4. The Caspar retractor system for ventral cervical approaches (Aesculap).

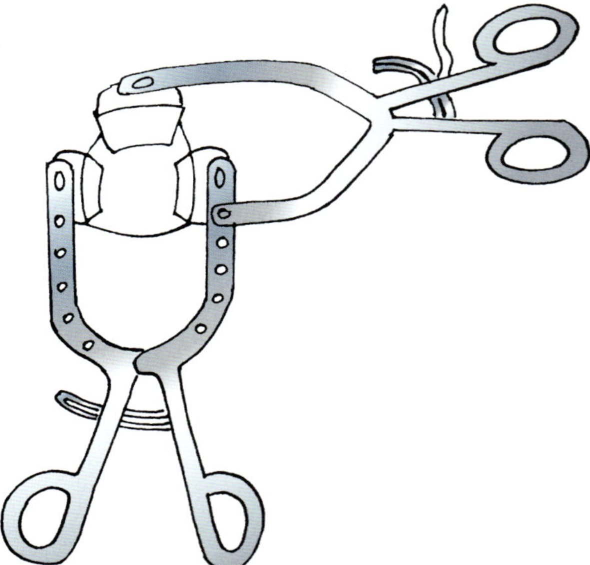

FIGURE 169-5. Apfelbaum self-retaining retractor for ventral odontoid screw fixation (Aesculap).

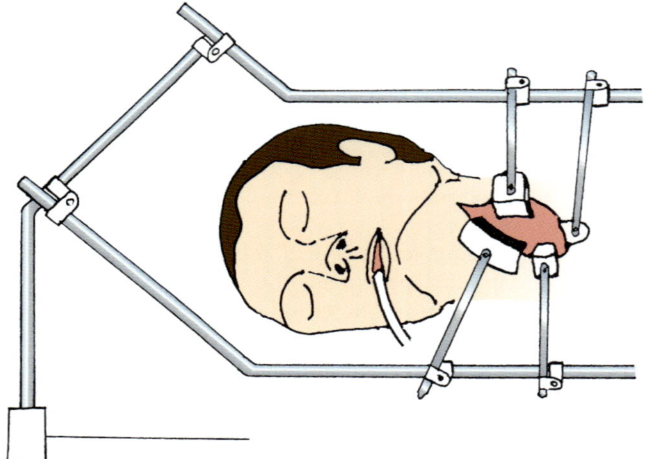

FIGURE 169-6. Table-mounted retractor system of the Thompson-Farley type.

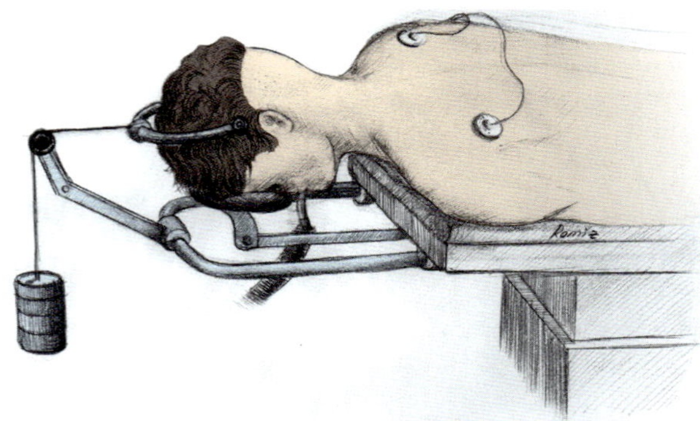

FIGURE 169-7. Dorsal midline cervical approach with horseshoe head holder and skeletal traction.

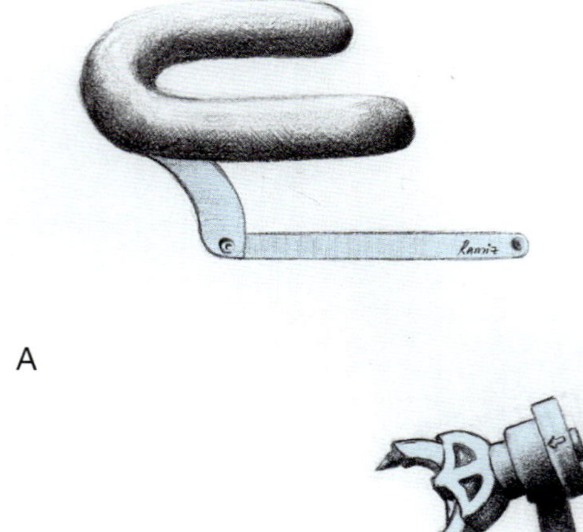

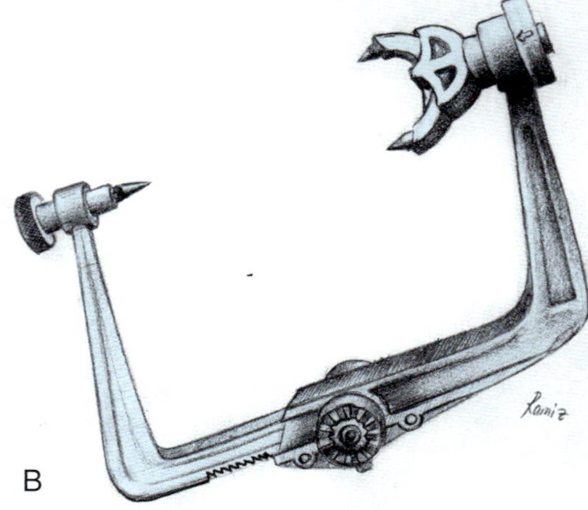

FIGURE 169-8. Two different fixation devices for dorsal cervical operations: horseshoe head holder (**A**) and Mayfield-type head clamp with three pins (**B**).

Lateral Transcondylar Approach

The lateral transcondylar approach is also termed the *extreme lateral transcondylar approach* or the *far lateral approach*. With this approach, it is possible to reach the lower clivus, the ventral foramen magnum, and the craniovertebral junction without significant retraction of the lower brainstem, the cervical spinal cord, or the cerebellum.

The sitting, lateral park-bench, or prone position may be used. In the prone position, the head should be turned to the side of the lesion (at least 20 degrees), and a rigid three-pin head holder should be used. The sitting position provides an excellent exposure, but it carries the risk of air embolism.

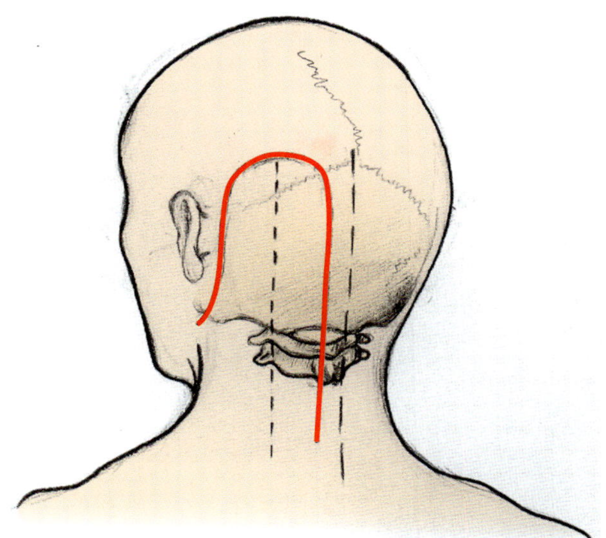

FIGURE 169-9. Various incisions used for dorsolateral transcondylar approach: inverted J-shaped incision (*red line*), midline dorsal incision (*dashed line*), and dorsolateral incision (*dotted line*).

The lateral position is a viable option, because the cerebellum falls away from the operating site and venous drainage is optimized. If a modified park-bench position is preferred, the head is rotated downward, flexed, and tilted away from the shoulder.

A straight dorsolateral incision may be used, although an inverted J-shaped incision is preferred (Fig. 169-9). This incision begins at the mastoid process, extends rostrally and medially, and then extends caudally in the midline to the level of C6. Because the occipital muscles cover the craniectomy after the use of an inverted J-shaped incision (compared with a linear incision placed over a craniectomy), this incision is useful in preventing postoperative cerebrospinal fluid leakage.

Hooks are useful for retracting the bulky cervical musculature. A self-retaining cerebellar retractor works well.

One of the most difficult aspects of this operation is the development of a dissection plane along the lateral aspect of C1 and C2 without causing injury to the vertebral artery or associated venous structures.

To avoid the introduction of occipitocervical instability, it is recommended not to remove more than one half of the occipital condyle. The roots of C2 may be sectioned. Only a slight retraction of the vertebral artery, if any, is usually necessary. The cerebellum and the brainstem should not be retracted.

Salas et al.[4] have defined four varieties of dorsolateral craniocervical approaches. The *transfacetal approach* is used to treat extradural and intradural lesions ventral to the upper cervical spinal cord. The *retrocondylar approach* is performed for intradural lesions that are located predominantly lateral or ventrolateral to the spinomedullary region or to expose the extradural portion of the vertebral artery. The *partial transcondylar approach* is performed to treat lesions that are located predominantly ventral to the spinomedullary junction. The *complete transcondylar approach* is performed to treat extradural lesions. The *extreme lateral transjugular approach* is performed to supplement the traditional lateral transtemporal approach for the treatment of jugular foramen lesions.

Ventral Approaches to the Upper Cervical Spine

Transoral Approach

A standard placement is to have the surgeon at the side and the anesthetic equipment and anesthetist at the head of the patient. Alternatively, the anesthetic equipment may be placed at the foot, and the surgeon may be at the head of the patient. The patient is positioned supine, and intubation is performed with a small endotracheal tube, which is securely fastened. Intubation when the patent is awake may be necessary if the spine is unstable. Slight extension facilitates the approach.

Although tracheotomy is not routinely used, an elective tracheotomy should be considered if the mouth does not allow adequate space for an endotracheal tube within the operating field.

Because the predominant difficulty with the transoral approach is the depth and narrowness of the operative field, a self-retaining retractor is imperative. Retraction of the uvula is also frequently necessary (see Fig. 169-3).

The soft palate may be held away from the surgical trajectory by a retractor or by suturing its border with the uvula to the dorsal palate. Alternatively, a rubber catheter may be passed through the nose and into the mouth. The distal tip of the catheter is sutured to the uvula, and upward traction is applied by gently pulling the catheter through the nose.

An incision is made in the midline of the dorsal pharynx after infiltration with a local anesthetic containing epinephrine to decrease oozing from the pharyngeal walls. The incision is carried along the tubercle of the atlas to the prominence of the C2-3 disc space. The incision may be extended, if needed, onto the soft palate and to one side of the uvula.

After dissection of the ventral surfaces of the atlas and axis laterally, a second self-retaining retractor is held to open the dorsal pharyngeal wall along the long axis of the spine. Stay sutures may be used to provide lateral retraction (see Fig. 169-1).

This surgery is relatively straightforward. Once the pharyngeal mucosa and prevertebral muscles have been cleared away, this approach offers an excellent view of the upper ventral cervical spine, which is relatively avascular.

Median Labiomandibular Glossotomy

Median labiomandibular glossotomy provides a wide ventral exposure from the clivus to the lower cervical spine.[5-7] A midline vertical incision starts from the lower lip, extends caudally, turns around the chin prominence, and again passes medially in the neck (Fig. 169-10). The mandible is cut in a stepwise configuration for subsequent approximation. The tongue is incised longitudinally from the central raphe, and the oropharyngeal mucosa is incised laterally.

When the mandible, mucosa, and tongue are divided, all the medial structures may be retracted laterally, and the dorsal structures, such as the epiglottis and the dorsal pharynx, are visualized.

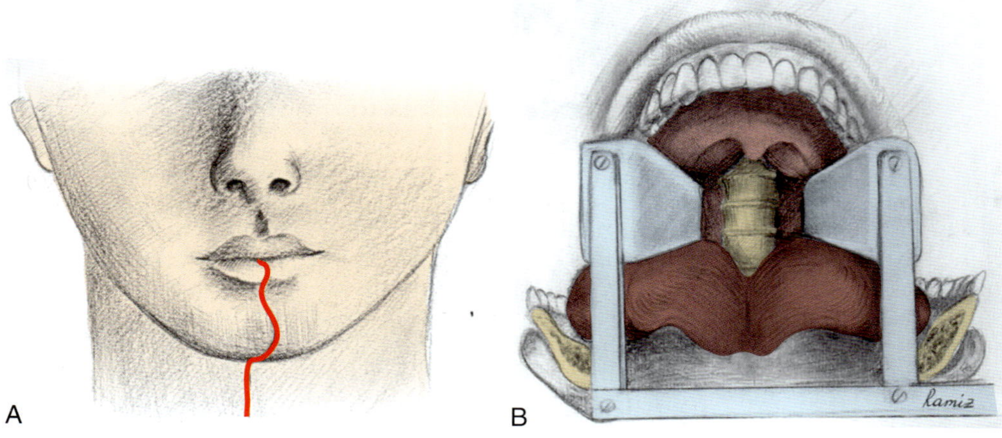

FIGURE 169-10. Mandible-splitting ventral approach to the upper cervical spine: incision line (A) and retraction and exposure following mandible and tongue splitting (B).

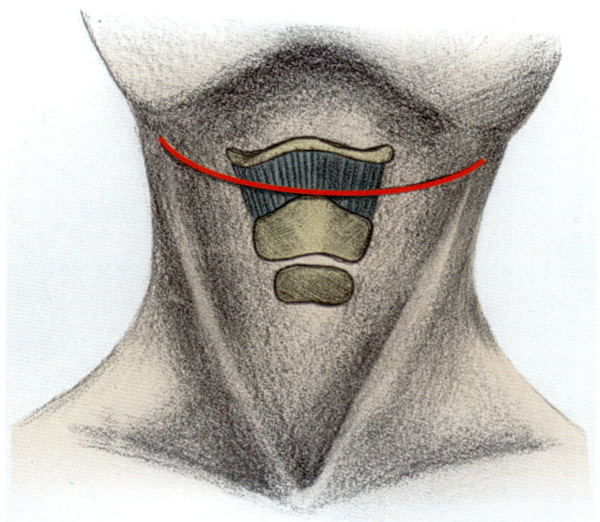

FIGURE 169-11. Incision line for transthyroid approach.

Because of high morbidity rates, this technique is preferred mostly in cases with primary malignant or aggressive benign tumors.[8]

Bilateral Sagittal Split Mandibular Osteotomies

This approach is performed in orthognathic surgery to repair a variety of facial and jaw deformities. Because all the incisions that are made in this approach are intraoral, they are not associated with the cosmetic deformities.[9] It is an adjunct to the transoral approach, and the retraction plane is rostrocaudal instead of lateral. Lingual or inferior alveolar nerve injuries are common complications.

Transthyroid Approach

The transthyroid approach may provide access to the first four cervical vertebrae.[10] A transverse incision is carried along the upper neck crease, between the hyoid bone and the thyroid cartilage, and is extended laterally (Fig. 169-11). The platysma and sternohyoid muscles are divided, and the thyrohyoid membrane is detached from the hyoid bone while the epiglottis is protected.

The internal laryngeal nerves are protected, and the ventral pharynx is entered. Rostral retraction of the hyoid bone and caudal retraction of the thyroid cartilage are performed. After incision of the dorsal pharyngeal wall, a self-retaining retractor exposes the vertebral bodies from C1 to C4. Because of the potential for significant morbidity, this approach is used infrequently. It has been associated with damage to the superior and internal laryngeal nerves and involves a significant risk of damaging the epiglottis.[10]

Ventrolateral Retropharyngeal Approach

The ventral retropharyngeal approach provides access to structures from the clivus to the third cervical vertebrae without entering the oral cavity.[3,11-14] The advantages of this approach are lowered risks of infection and more extensive exposure of the upper cervical spine.

The patient is positioned supine, and if the incision is on the right side, the head is turned to the left. Moderate extension of the head facilitates the approach to the upper cervical structures.

The upper transverse portion of a T-shaped incision is made just under the mandible. The vertical portion of the incision meets the sternocleidomastoid muscle caudally (Fig. 169-12A). Another option is a V-shaped incision (Fig. 169-12B).[13]

This ventral retropharyngeal approach may be called *retrovascular* or *prevascular* surgery (Fig. 169-13).[15] Prevascular surgery involves an access medial to the carotid sheath and traverses the same fascial planes as in the ventrolateral lower cervical spine surgery[12] (see Fig. 169-13B). It allows adequate spinal cord decompression up to the clivus and reconstruction of the anterior column of the spine with strut grafts and internal fixation.

The dissection is medial to the sternocleidomastoid muscle and the carotid artery. The submandibular gland may be resected. The facial, lingual, hypoglossal, and superior laryngeal nerves should be identified and protected. After rostral and lateral retraction of these nerves, the hyoid bone and hypopharynx may be retracted medially.

After the platysma muscle is incised, the inferior division of the facial nerve and submandibular gland may be divided. The carotid sheath is identified and protected. The dorsal belly of the digastric muscle is traced and transected near its tendon.

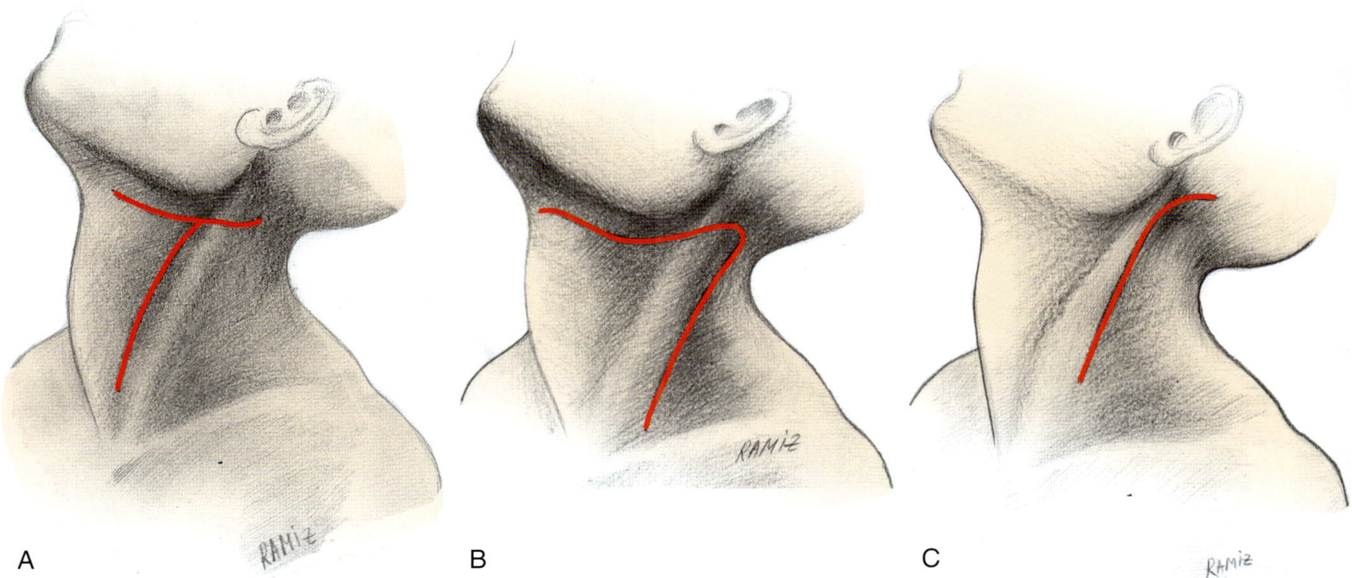

FIGURE 169-12. Incision lines used for ventral upper cervical approaches. Ventromedial retropharyngeal approaches: T-shaped incision of Schoerbringer (**A**); incision of Riley (**B**). Ventrolateral approach: incision of Whitesides (**C**).

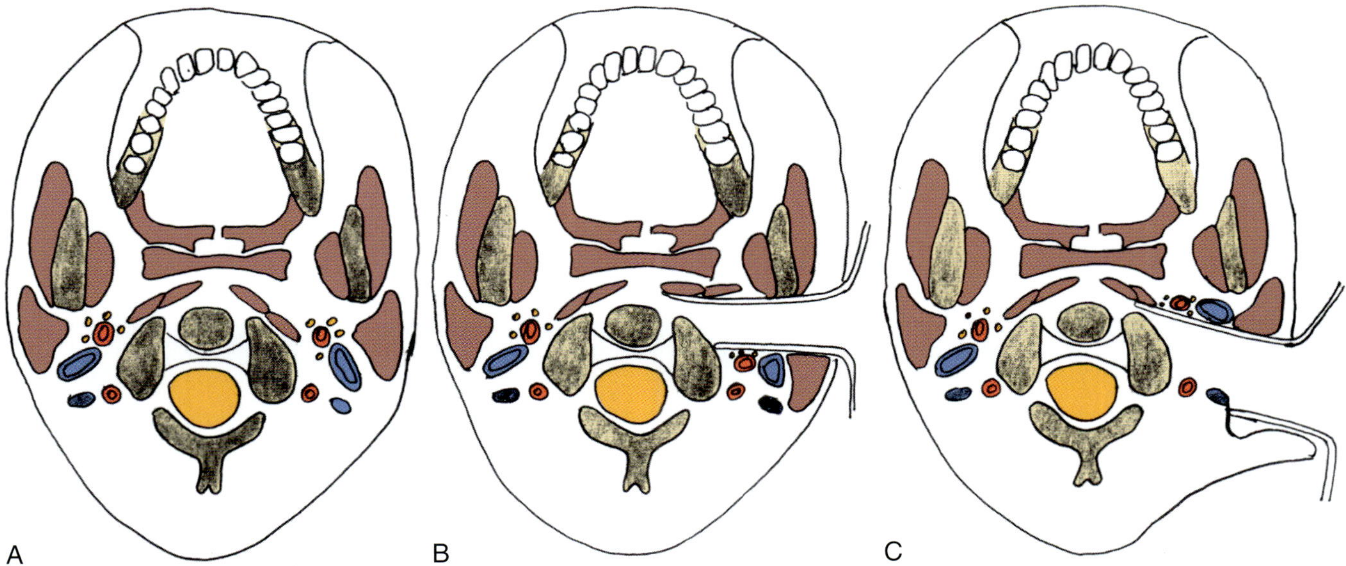

FIGURE 169-13. **A,** Ventromedial retropharyngeal approach may be accomplished by two different approaches. **B,** The prevascular route is taken medial to the carotid artery and internal jugular vein. **C,** Retrovascular surgery is performed lateral to these vascular structures. (Redrawn from Laus M, Pignatti G, Malaguti MC, et al: Anterior extraoral surgery to the upper cervical spine. *Spine [Phila Pa 1976]* 21:1687–1693, 1996.)

To retract the larynx, the stylohyoid muscle is transected. The hypoglossal nerve is identified and protected. The retropharyngeal space is opened and bluntly dissected. After retraction of the longus colli muscles, a self-retaining retractor is positioned.[1,13] It may be difficult to place a self-retaining retractor in this opening. A table-mounted system may be useful in this region.

Lateral Cervical Approach

Some authors refer to the lateral cervical approach as a retrovascular variant of the ventral retropharyngeal approach.[12] It is an anatomically complex access that requires sternocleidomastoid muscle eversion; exposition of the spinal accessory nerve and medial mobilization of the jugular vein, vagus nerve, carotid artery, vertebral artery, and cranial nerves XII, IX, VII[16] (Fig. 169-14). Although it provides a true lateral access to the upper cervical spine, only limited access is obtained, and neither grafting nor extensive bony decompression can be achieved. It is also noted to have a significant association with vertebral artery damage.[17]

The major difference between a ventrolateral retropharyngeal approach and a straight ventral retropharyngeal approach is that the exposure is lateral to the carotid sheath.[14,17,18]

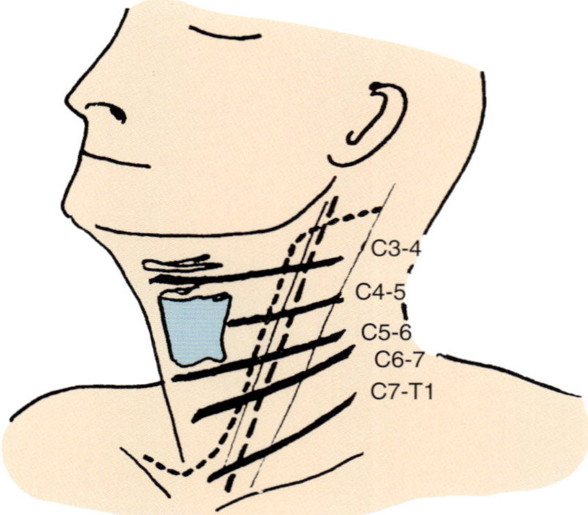

FIGURE 169-14. Incision lines used for ventral approaches to the midcervical and lower cervical spine. *Straight lines* are for transverse incision at different levels; the *oblique dashed line* is the longitudinal incision parallel to the sternocleidomastoid muscle; the *oblique small dashed line* is a curvilinear incision for wider exposure of the multisegmental disease.

The supine or lateral position is used. The neck is extended, and the head is turned maximally. Skeletal traction or a three-point head fixator may be used.

A hockey-stick incision is fashioned along the ventral border of the sternocleidomastoid muscle. The incision begins behind the ear, proceeds caudally over the mastoid process, and extends below the mandibular angle toward the midline (Fig. 169-12C).

The external jugular vein is ligated and divided. The sternocleidomastoid muscle is divided transversely below the mastoid process. The occipital artery is also ligated. The greater auricular and accessory nerves are identified and protected. A dissection plane is developed dorsal to the carotid sheath and the retropharyngeal space.[16]

This approach may be fashioned for primary tumors of the upper cervical spine (Fig. 169-15).

Dorsal Approaches to the Subaxial Cervical Spine

Laminectomy and Laminoplasty

The patient position for a midline dorsal cervical approach is similar to that used for posterior fossa approaches. Either the sitting position or a prone position may be used.

A longitudinal midline incision is centered over the vertebrae of interest. The occipital ridge must be exposed for occipital fusions.

A bilateral subperiosteal dissection is performed over the laminae with sharp elevators or electrocautery. If no fusion is anticipated, the facet capsules should be preserved. Avoid injury to supraspinous ligaments. To avoid postoperative swelling and excessive injury to the erector spinae muscles, self-retaining retractors should be released periodically.

To decrease the blood loss, packing with sponges may be helpful. Also, the dorsal branches of the segmental arteries that emerge lateral to the facet joints should be preserved to avoid excessive bleeding.

Laminoforaminotomy for Cervical Disc Disease

In laminoforaminotomy for cervical disc disease, three different positions may be used: the prone position, the sitting position, and the lateral or park-bench position.[19] Because

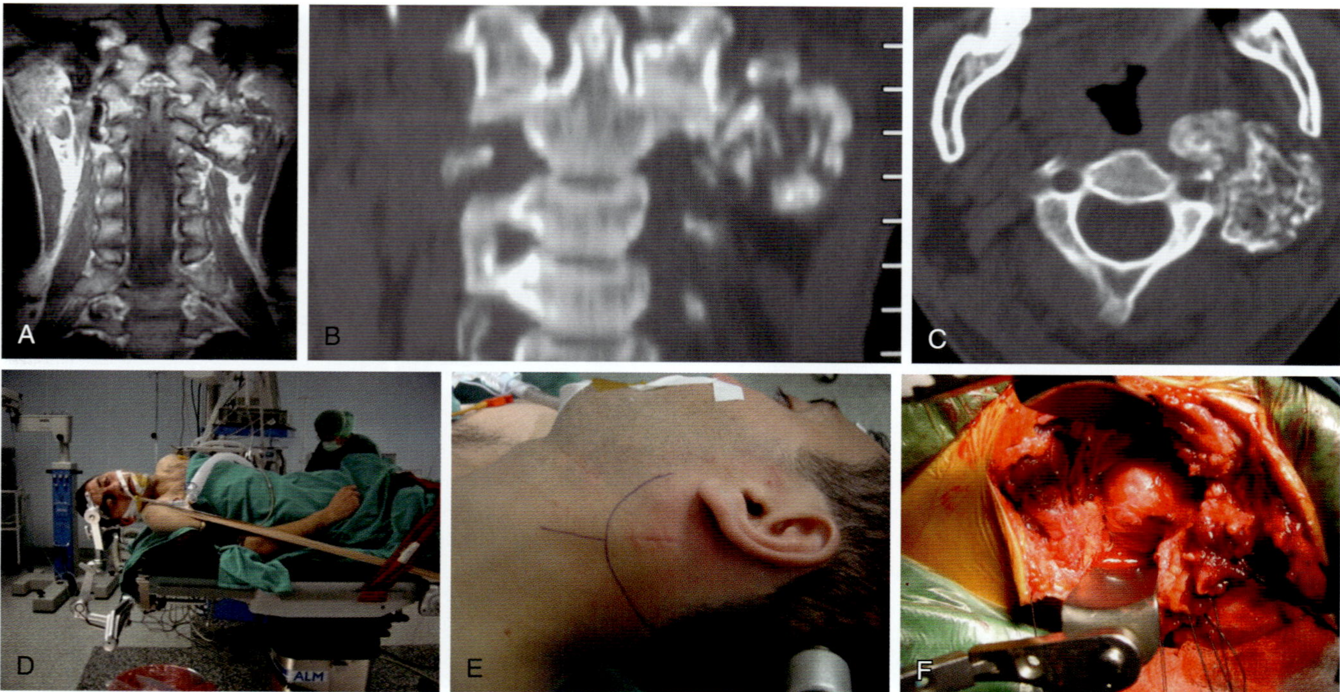

FIGURE 169-15. An osteochondroma of the C2 body (**A–C**) is removed totally by a lateral cervical approach and an incision line turned around the previous biopsy incision (**D–F**).

lateral muscle retraction is necessary for exposure, hyperflexion and hyperextension should be avoided. If the spine is hyperflexed, the tightened muscles and tendons make lateral retraction difficult. If the spine is hyperextended, the interlaminar spaces close, and interlaminar exposure is difficult.[19]

A midline dorsal or paramedian dorsal incision may be used. The dorsal paramedian incision is used only for single-level laminoforaminotomy.[19] This is a muscle-splitting approach, with only dissection of the muscles from the lamina and facet surfaces. This approach may be used for the keyhole foraminotomy.[20]

The classical midline dorsal approach requires the resection of the muscle attachments from the spinous processes to expose the facets and laminae.[21] Only strong lateral retraction is needed to retract the muscles.

Ventral Approaches to the Subaxial Cervical Spine

Ventromedial Approach

Exposure of the disc space and vertebral body is usually accomplished by a ventromedial approach.[22-25] The patient is positioned supine with the head and neck neutral or slightly extended. Extension of the upper cervical region, with chin retraction, is helpful to reach the C2-3 level. Extension of the midlower cervical region is helpful to reach the high thoracic region. The head is turned away from the surgeon. In the setting of severe cervical stenosis, extreme extension of the cervical spine may cause spinal cord damage and therefore should be avoided.

The sternocleidomastoid muscle is the surface incision landmark for the ventral approach. Either a transverse or a longitudinal incision is appropriate (see Fig. 169-14). Rengachary[26] suggests a longitudinal incision for patients with a short neck and kyphotic deformity. The incision begins below the angle of the mandible, extends forward toward the hyoid bone, extends caudally over the sternocleidomastoid muscle, and terminates in the suprasternal notch (see Fig. 169-14).[26]

A transverse incision may be used for patients with short necks and limited pathology, whereas a longitudinal incision parallel to the sternocleidomastoid muscle may be used for long thin necks with more extensive pathology. Right-handed surgeons may prefer to use right-sided incisions, although it is usually optimal to approach the patient from the side opposite the most prominent pathology. After the incision of the platysma muscle, the sternocleidomastoid muscle is freed from its attachments.

The carotid sheath is easily identified under the muscle. Both may be retracted laterally by the surgeon's fingers (Fig. 169-16A). Rostrally, the 12th cranial nerve and, caudally, the recurrent laryngeal nerve should be avoided. Other structures that cross the wound transversely may be sacrificed if necessary. These include the inferior and superior thyroid veins and arteries, the facial veins, and the inferior belly of the omohyoid muscle. Injury to the superior laryngeal and superior thyroid artery should be avoided.

The three main retraction systems that are available for ventral cervical surgery are hand-held retractors, self-retaining retractors, and table-fixed retractors (see Fig. 169-4). Saunders[16] prefers a table-fixed retraction system for both the ventromedial and ventrolateral approaches. Retractors themselves may cause injury to the lateral structures, such as the carotid artery, internal jugular vein, cranial nerves 10 and 12, nerve roots, sympathetic chain, thoracic duct, and lung apex. The medial structures, such as the esophagus and the trachea, are also at risk. Manual retraction is usually used at the beginning of the dissection until the deep cervical fascia is opened and the longus colli muscles are visualized.

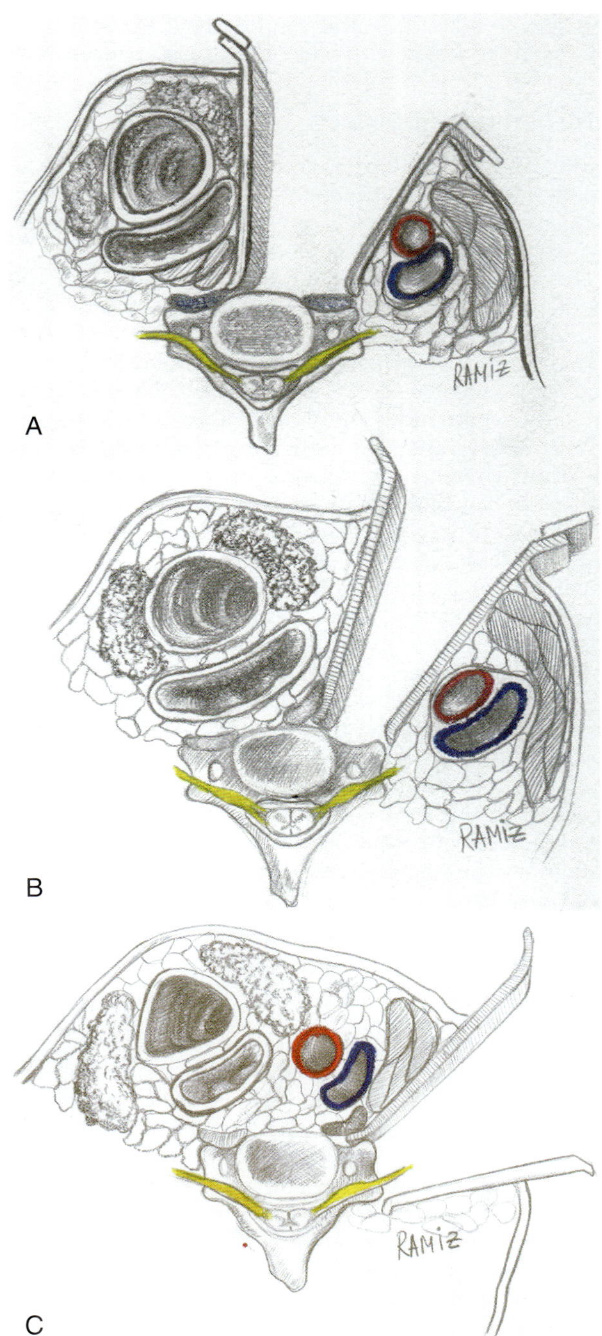

FIGURE 169-16. Three basic ventral approaches to the midcervical and lower cervical spine: ventral-medial approach (**A**); ventral-lateral approach, medial to the sternocleidomastoid muscle (**B**); and ventral-lateral approach, lateral to the sternocleidomastoid muscle and great vessels (**C**).

Soft tissue structures may be placed under significant tension with a self-retaining retractor. The positioning of the medial blades is particularly important. The most common retraction injury is caused by medial retraction of the esophagus; therefore, the retractor blade should be placed under the longus colli muscles. Careful attention must also be given to lateral retraction, which may cause compression of the carotid artery. The ipsilateral superficial temporal artery may be palpated by the anesthesiologist after placement of the retractor to assist with detection of occlusion of the carotid artery. It is prudent to relax the retraction hourly. If necessary, rostral and caudal retraction with blunt-tipped blades may be used.

Ventrolateral Approach

The lateral approach to the cervical spine from C3 to C7 can be performed via a ventrolateral exposure. However, the lateral exposure of C1 and C2 can only be performed with the dorsolateral transcondylar approach.[27]

The ventrolateral approach has two variations. The trajectory of one approach is medial to the carotid artery, whereas the trajectory of the other is lateral (Figs. 169-16B and C). In the latter approach, the sternocleidomastoid muscle is retracted medially with the carotid sheath. Therefore, retraction of the recurrent laryngeal nerve is avoided.

With either variation, the lateral retractor blade is positioned just lateral to the tubercle of the transverse process, and the medial retractor blade is positioned just medial to the uncinate process (see Figs. 169-16B and C). This exposes the ipsilateral longus colli muscle, which, together with the sympathetic chain, is mobilized medially. The muscle insertions to the transverse process are divided. Positioning and incision are the same in the ventrolateral approach as in the ventromedial approach.

For retraction, a medial exposure is made with blunt dissection. The tubercle of the transverse process is then palpated laterally. This tubercle is approximately 1 cm lateral to the foramen transversarium. Blunt dissection of the common carotid artery and jugular vein is carefully performed to allow retraction of these structures medially. Extreme care should be taken not to injure the vertebral artery or the sympathetic chain.

A ventrolateral approach medial to the carotid sheath is most frequently used to expose the vertebral artery and the nerve root foramen.[28,29] It is essentially a medial approach without midline exposure.[29,30] The carotid sheath is retracted laterally as with the ventromedial approach.

Decompression of lateral cervical disc herniations may be done via the same route. This approach may be termed the ventral cervical foraininotomy,[31] ventrolateral transpedicular foraminotomy,[1] or microsurgical ventral cervical foraminotomy-uncinatectomy.[32] The colli muscles are mobilized, allowing dissection around the lateral aspect of the vertebral body; a retractor between the vertebral body and the vertebral artery is placed; and the lateral portion of the uncovertebral joint is drilled. The herniated disc and uncovertebral osteophytes are removed to decompress the exiting nerve root (Fig. 169-17).

A ventrolateral approach lateral to the carotid sheath and sternocleidomastoid muscle is also termed the *oblique cervical approach*.[33] With this exposure, the incision may be fashioned lateral to the sternocleidomastoid muscle. Positioning is similar to that in the ventromedial approach. The head and neck may be slightly turned to the contralateral side. Both the sternocleidomastoid muscle and the great vessels are retracted medially, together with the trachea and the esophagus. A self-retaining retractor may be used, with care taken that the lateral blades do not cause severe retraction of the nerve roots.[33,34]

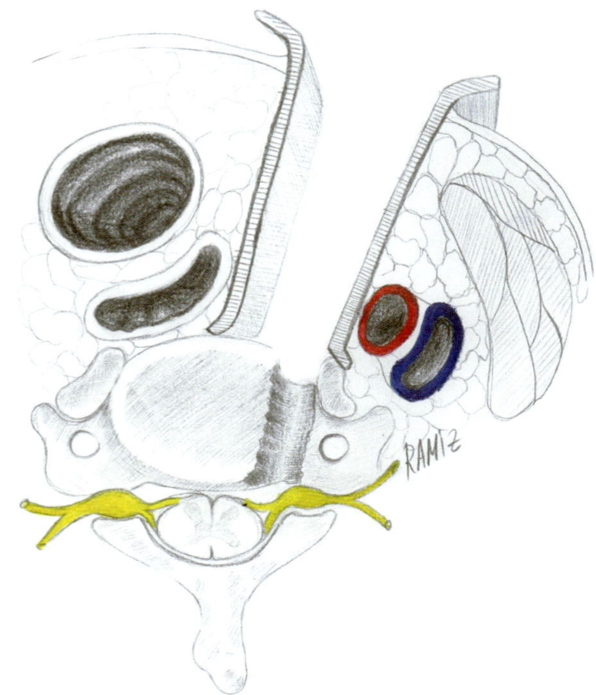

FIGURE 169-17. Ventral cervical foraminotomy-uncinatectomy and the amount of bone to be removed.

Oblique corpectomy is an effective alternative to other ventral cervical decompressions with advantages of no need for a graft or plate (Fig. 169-18).[33,35]

Dorsal and Ventral Approaches to the Cervicothoracic Junction

The dorsal approaches are similar to those used for lower cervical dorsal approaches.

The cervicothoracic junction is located between the cervical lordosis and the thoracic kyphosis. The brachial plexus, major vessels, and lung apex may obstruct approaches to this area. The thoracic cage narrows to reach the thoracic inlet. Therefore, the surgical approach to the ventral cervicothoracic junction is technically demanding. There are nine fundamental operative techniques in this region.

Lower Ventromedial Cervical Approach

The lower ventromedial cervical approach is indistinguishable from that used in the midcervical to lower cervical spine.[36]

Transsternal Approach

The transsternal approach provides a direct ventral route through a median sternotomy.[37] The morbidity and mortality are high. Hodgson and Yau[38] have reported a 40% mortality rate. Furthermore, this approach provides little advantage over

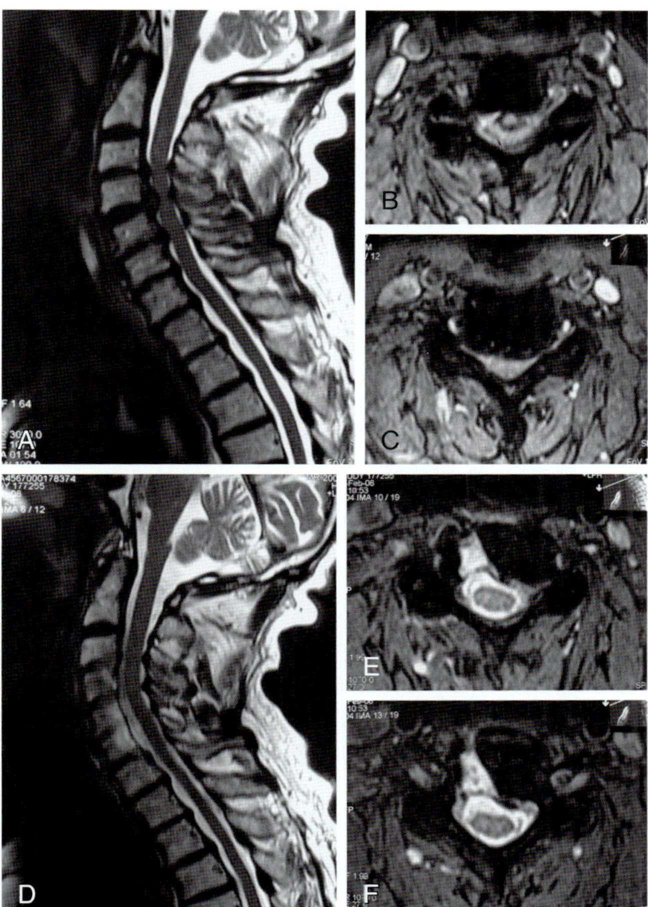

FIGURE 169-18. A 66-year-old man with quadriparesis had an oblique corpectomy at two levels: C4 and C5. Preoperative (**A–C**) and postoperative (**D–F**) MRIs show an effective ventral decompression.

the transmanubrial approach because the soft tissue structures are the predominant limiting factors.

Transmanubrial Approach

The transmanubrial approach is a variation of the transsternal approach.[39] It is performed by using an osteotomy of the manubrium, with or without a medial claviculotomy.[38-42] Sundaresan et al.[43] recommend resection of the medial third of the clavicle along with the creation of a window in the manubrium (Fig. 169-19).

The head is positioned slightly contralaterally in the supine position. Most authors recommend a left-sided approach.

Either of two incisions may be used: a T-shaped incision, with the transverse arm 2 cm above the clavicle and the midline vertical arm extending to the sternum, or a medial sternocleidomastoid incision extending to the sternum.[38,44] This incision permits a simultaneous ventromedial midcervical approach (Fig. 169-20).

The upper outer corner of the manubrium, the first costal cartilage, and the medial third of the clavicle are divided. With this exposure, the great vessels and the lower roots of the brachial plexus are retracted. If it is connected to a ventromedial cervical exposure, a generous exposure to the cervicothoracic vertebrae from C3 to T5 can be obtained.[45]

The sternocleidomastoid muscle and the omohyoid muscle are divided. The phrenic nerve, the 11th cranial nerve, the sympathetic chain, and, on the left side, the thoracic duct should be protected. If necessary, the left innominate vein may be divided.[44]

The manubrium and the clavicle may be reattached by using wires or miniplates. These bone fragments may be used as bone grafts without significant deformity or instability in a tumor patient. In a young healthy individual, the clavicle should be replaced.

Transverse Supraclavicular Approach

The transverse supraclavicular approach was originally described as an exposure for upper thoracic sympathectomy.[46] A transverse incision parallel to the clavicle and extending

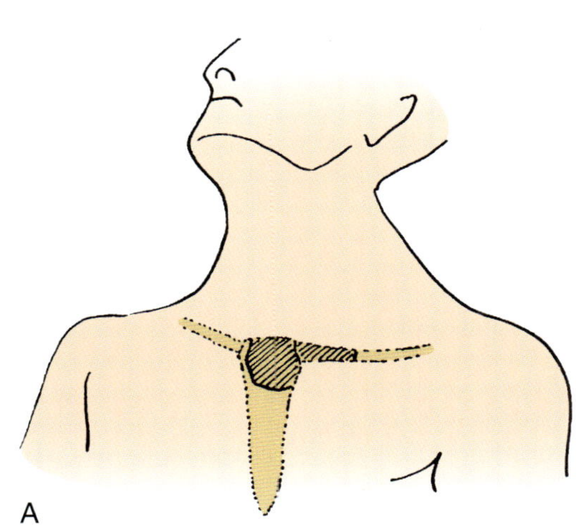

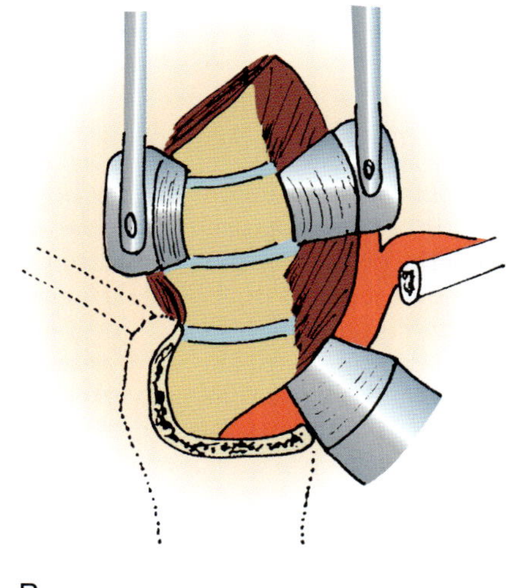

FIGURE 169-19. **A,** Transmanubrial exposure. **B,** Resection of the manubrium and the medial part of the clavicle.

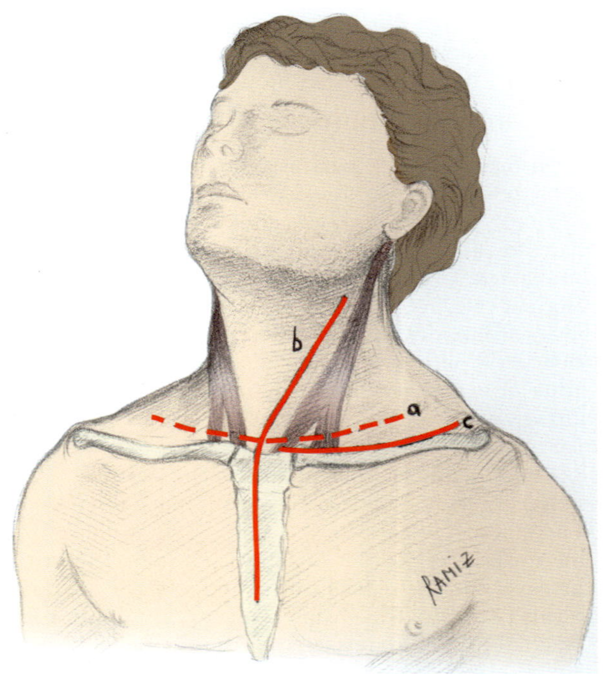

FIGURE 169-20. Incisions for ventral cervicothoracic approaches: *a*, T-shaped incision; *b*, ventromedial sternotomy incision; *c*, supraclavicular incision.

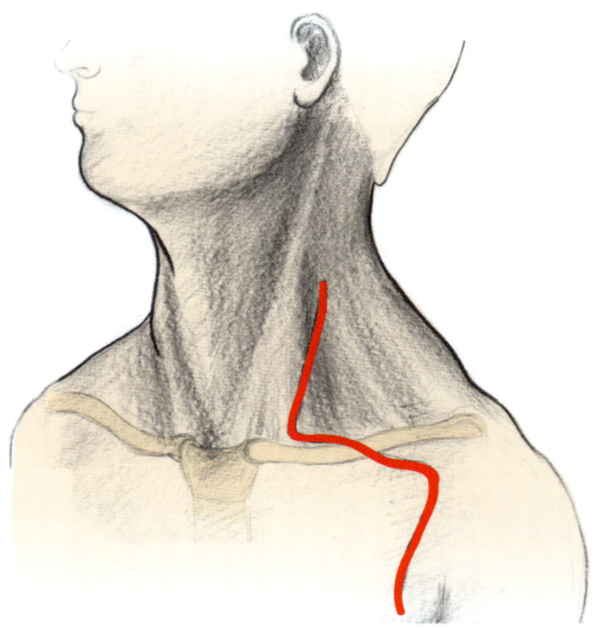

FIGURE 169-21. A zigzag-shaped incision for transclavicular approach to cervicothoracic spine tumors with paravertebral-plexus involvement. (Redrawn from Kuho T, Nakamura H, Yamano Y: Transclavicular approach for a large dumbbell tumor in the cervicothoracic junction. *J Spinal Disord* 14:79–83, 2001.)

beyond the lateral border of the sternocleidomastoid muscle is used.[18,42,47] The sternocleidomastoid muscle, the omohyoid muscle, and the strap muscles are divided. The carotid sheath, the internal jugular vein, and the phrenic nerve are identified and protected. Medial retraction of the neurovascular structures provides a limited exposure lateral to the C7 vertebral body.

Transclavicular Approach

The transclavicular approach (splitting the clavicle) provides an adequate access to the cervicothoracic junction. This approach is most useful for cervicothoracic spine tumors with paravertebral-plexus involvement. Dividing the clavicle assists in the separation of the intrathoracic components from the lung. A zigzag-shaped incision over the clavicle may be used[48] (Fig. 169-21).

Transaxillary Extrapleural Approach

The transaxillary extrapleural approach is a high thoracic variant of the transthoracic approach. Its advantage lies in the preservation of the pectoral and shoulder girdle muscles.[20] Its disadvantage is that it places the brachial plexus at risk for retraction and stretch injury.

A 60-degree semilateral position is used, with the ipsilateral shoulder and arm abducted. The arm may be fixed in a sling.

A transverse incision is made from the border of the pectoralis muscle to the border of the latissimus dorsi muscle. The third rib is resected, and the dissection is carried through the third rib bed.[39,47,49,50] Retraction is essentially an extrapleural approach. With blunt dissection, the apex of the lung is retracted caudally. A self-retaining retractor may be used.

Lateral Parascapular Extrapleural Approach

With this approach, the parascapular shoulder muscles are reflected off the spinous processes to the scapula with preservation of neurovascular structure.[51] The upper dorsal ribs are removed, the rami communicantes of C8 and T1 are transected, and the sympathetic chain is displaced ventrolaterally. This approach provides easy access to the T2-4 vertebrae.[51]

Transpleural Transthoracic Approach

With the transpleural transthoracic approach, the upper thoracic vertebrae can be adequately approached through the fourth rib.[52] The left-side-up position is preferred, because it is easier to mobilize the aorta than the vena cava. In the event of vascular injury, it is also easier to repair the aorta than the vena cava. It may be preferred over the extrapleural method, because lung retraction is easier. Unlike the extrapleural approach, however, a tube thoracostomy is required.

Segmental vessels are ligated two levels above and below the level of pathology. This allows retraction of the great vessels.

Trapdoor Approach

With the trapdoor approach, a partial median sternotomy and a ventrolateral approach are added to a standard ventral approach to the cervical spine along the medial border of the sternocleidomastoid muscle.[53] The sternoclavicular joint and clavicle itself are preserved. It provides a bilateral ventral approach from C4 to T3. Although it provides a wide exposure and proximal control of important vessels, it has a very high morbidity rate (Fig. 169-22).

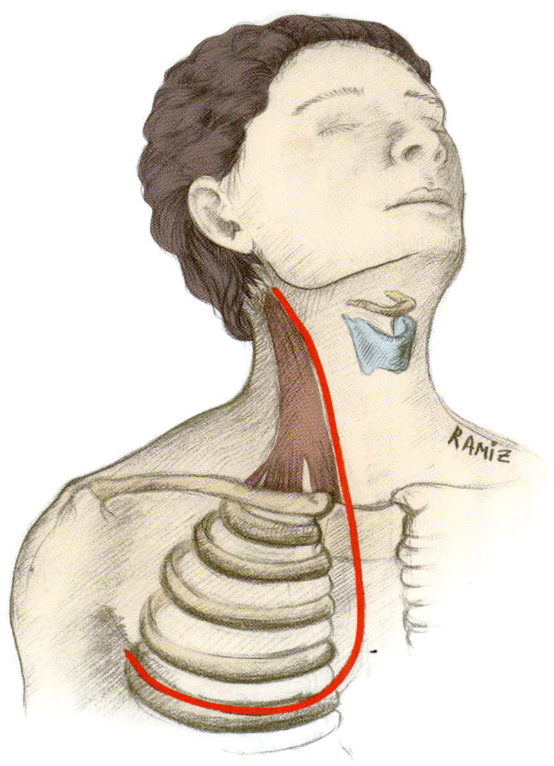

FIGURE 169-22. Trapdoor approach used for extensive cervicothoracic tumors. (Redrawn from Nazzaro JM, Arbit E, Burt M: Trap door exposure of the cervicothoracic junction: technical note. *J Neurosurg* 80:338–341, 1994.)

Dorsal Approaches to the Thoracic and Thoracolumbar Spine Junction

The most familiar of all approaches to the spine is the midline dorsal approach. Decompressive laminectomies and dorsal instrumentation procedures are most often accomplished via a midline dorsal incision.

Thoracic Laminectomy

The patient is positioned prone on a chest frame or on laminectomy rolls that allow the abdominal contents to be free of pressure, thereby reducing venous compression and decreasing blood loss during surgery. Both the pelvis and the knees are flexed to enhance the normal thoracic kyphosis (Fig. 169-23). Specialty tables and frames may be used to minimize abdominal pressure. These tables may also facilitate intraoperative radiography.

If an upper thoracic spine exposure is desired, the head should be fixed in the neutral position with either a Mayfield head holder or a horseshoe head holder. The patient's arms are positioned at the side.

If a midthoracic or lower thoracic spine exposure is desired, head fixation is not necessary, and the patient's arms may be fixed above the head. To avoid causing a brachial plexus stretch injury, care should be taken to not abduct the arms more than 90 degrees.

A few surgeons advocate the lateral position for thoracic laminectomy. This may be particularly useful in the obese patient. A dorsal midline incision is used (Fig. 169-24A).

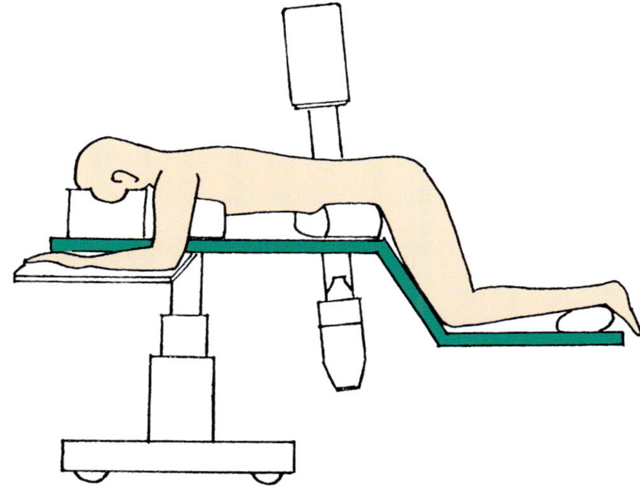

FIGURE 169-23. Prone position used for most thoracic, lumbar, and sacral dorsal approaches.

Several self-retaining retractors with blades of varying widths and depths are available (e.g., Weitlaner retractor, crank-type retractor, cerebellar retractor). Hemilaminectomy retractors and table-mounted retractors are also helpful in special situations.

Transpedicular Approach

The transpedicular approach may be used for thoracic disc removal and vertebral body biopsy.[54] It may also be performed in the cervicothoracic junction. The prone position is used with the transpedicular approach.

A midline vertical incision is performed (see Fig. 169-24A). The paraspinous muscles and the soft tissues are retracted to one side. The facet joint and the pedicle are removed by using a high-speed bur. The dorsal aspect of the vertebral body adjacent to the portion of the vertebral body near the rostral intervertebral disc space may be reached through the pedicle.

The exposure provided by the transpedicular approach, however, is limited. It allows only partial tumor or disc removal.

Costotransversectomy

This approach allows exposure of dorsal and dorsolateral structures, without violating the pleural cavity. It is different from the lateral extracavitary approach, because it involves a midline exposure and a plane of dissection that is medial to the erector spinae muscles. It was first described for drainage of tuberculous abscesses.[55]

The patient is placed in the prone position and a midline vertical incision is made (see Fig. 169-24A). A modified T-shaped incision has also been described[56] (Fig. 169-24E). After standard bilateral subperiosteal dissection, a plane of dissection on the ipsilateral side is extended to the tips of the transverse processes and proximal ribs. The 3- to 4-cm medial aspect of one or two ribs is then cut, disarticulated from its costotransverse and costovertebral articulations, and resected.

To find the ipsilateral pedicle, the neurovascular bundle is identified under the rib bed and followed proximally to the neural foramen. After the transverse process and the pedicle

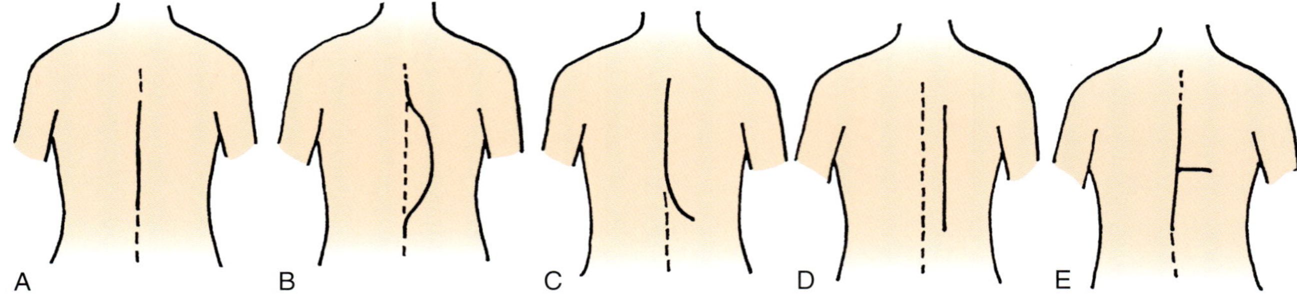

FIGURE 169-24. Different skin incisions for dorsolateral exposures of the thoracic and lumbar spine: Dorsal midline incision (**A**), semilunar incision (**B**), hockey-stick incision (**C**), straight paramedian incision (**D**), and T-shaped incision (**E**).

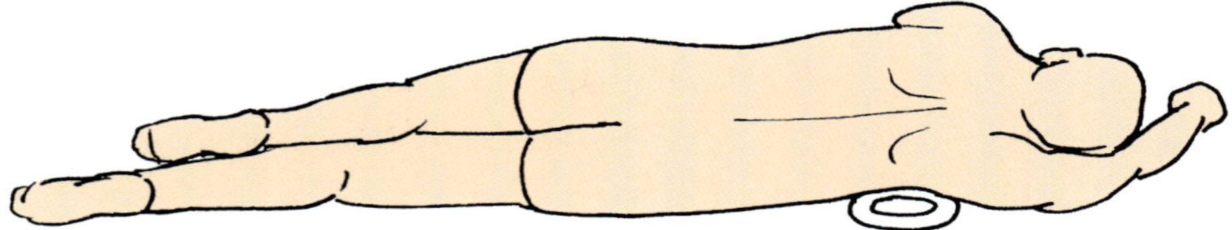

FIGURE 169-25. The three-quarter prone position used for lateral extracavitary approach.

have been removed, the lateral aspect of the thecal sac is visualized. Self-retaining retractors are used.

There is a controversy over the necessity of performing a rhizotomy of the associated nerve root during the procedure. Since the patients whose nerve roots were preserved can show late neuropathic pain, routine transection of the associated nerve root proximal to the ganglion may be desirable.[3]

Lateral Extracavitary Approach

The lateral extracavitary approach is a modification of costotransversectomy. It was introduced and popularized by Larson et al.[57] and then adopted by other surgeons.[47,58,59] The prone position is used frequently, although a three-quarter prone position has also been described (Fig. 169-25).[58] Several variations of a parasagittal incision are described (see Fig. 169-24).[23] Larson et al.[57] use a midline hockey-stick incision. This approach provides simultaneous access to both the dorsal and ventral aspects of the spine. Dorsal instrumentation may be placed via the same incision that is used for decompression.

Dissection is carried to the lateral border of the paraspinous muscles. The paraspinous muscles are mobilized in a lateral-to-medial direction. They may also be transected in a transverse fashion as was originally described by Capener.[60] The lateral exposure reaches 8 to 10 cm lateral to the midline. The remaining portion of the operation is similar to the costotransversectomy. It differs from the costotransversectomy, however, because an approximately 15% to 30% ventral angle of exposure is gained by the lateral extracavitary approach (Fig. 169-26).

The disadvantages of transpedicular, costotransversectomy, and lateral extracavitary approaches are that they cannot be used for directly ventrally located lesions. Removing the facet joint and pedicle may destabilize the spine.

Dorsal En Bloc Total Spondylectomy

En bloc total spondylectomy may be performed by bisecting the affected vertebrae through the pedicles and removing the vertebra en bloc.[27] This method was first introduced by Tomita et al.[61,62] and then used in other centers.[63,64] There are two variations described in the following paragraphs.[27]

Single Dorsal Approach: For Lesions from T1 to L2

Tomita et al.[27,61,62] proposed the removal of the dorsal component and lateral components of the spine en bloc by pediculotomy using a fine threadwire saw. If the unilateral pedicle is affected by the tumor, osteotomy may be performed through a neighboring healthy lamina. The involved nerve root occasionally had to be ligated and cut. If the affected pedicle or vertebral body markedly compressed the nerve root, the more severely affected side is sacrificed. Sacrificing both nerve roots in less important areas such as the thoracic spine is possible. After the dorsal bony column has been removed, the epidural venous bleeding is controlled (Fig. 169-27).

After resection of the neural arch, a Gigli saw is inserted to cut the upper and lower levels of the vertebral body or disc into two retractors protecting the ventral venous structure and two retractors protecting the spinal dura mater. During the operation, the spinal column is stabilized by connecting the unilateral rod to pedicle screws. Then the affected vertebra is removed dorsolaterally.

This operation is completed by using a long-segment dorsal instrumentation and placing a ventral vertebral body prosthesis (i.e., methylmethacrylate, bioactive ceramic, mesh cages, titanium mesh cylinder). Strut and cancellous bone grafts from the resected ribs or fibula are placed around the prosthesis and rods.

Combined En Bloc Total Spondylectomy: For Lesions from L3 to L5

In the case of large extravertebral tumor, extension or recurrence after radical excision combined with en bloc total spondylectomy is used regardless of the level.

The first step is a dorsal approach. The dorsal procedure is similar to the method of Tomita et al.[61,62] After removal of the dorsal bony column, the psoas muscles with segmental vessels are dissected as ventrally as possible on the contralateral side of the ventral approach. The posterior longitudinal

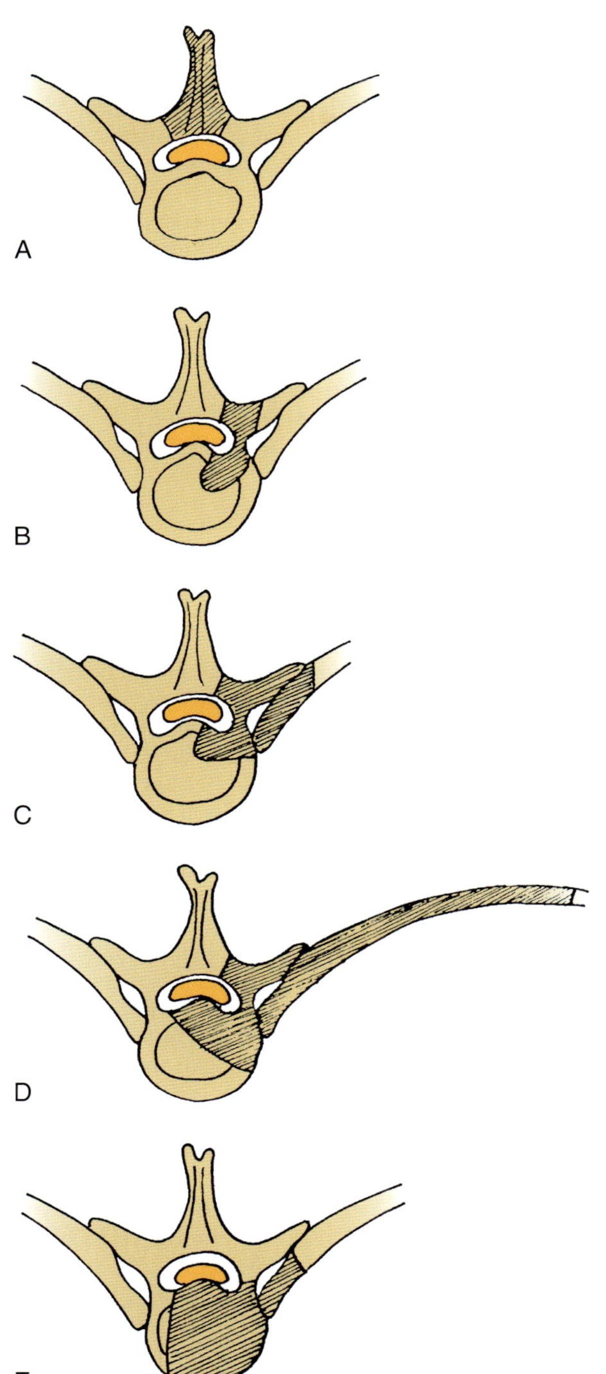

FIGURE 169-26. Alternative approaches to thoracic and lumbar spine: dorsal laminectomy (**A**), transpedicular approach (**B**), costotransversectomy (**C**), lateral extracavitary approach (**D**), and ventral intracavitary approach (**E**).

ligamentum and the dorsal and contralateral part of the adjacent intervertebral disks are cut through the dorsal approach. After dorsal stabilization according to the principle of "one above, one below" using a pedicle screw system, a ventral procedure, including en bloc corpectomy and reconstruction of the ventral column, is performed by replacing the affected vertebral body using a vertebral prosthesis or a titanium cage.

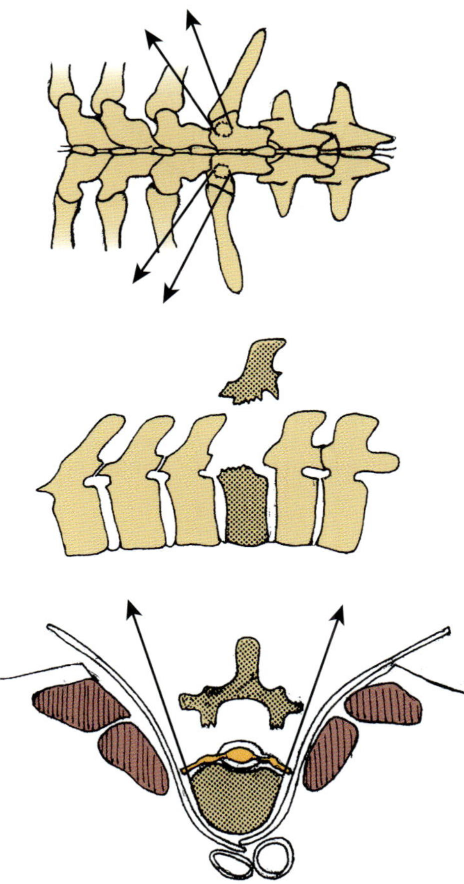

FIGURE 169-27. Dorsal en bloc total spondylectomy with single dorsal approach is suitable for lesions from T1 to L2. First, bilateral pediculotomy with the aid of a thin Gigli saw and resection of laminar arch is accomplished. After resection of the related nerve roots and dissection of ventral vascular structures, the vertebral body is removed by cutting through disc spaces. (Redrawn from Tomita K, Kawahara N, Baba H et al: Total en bloc spondylectomy for solitary spinal metastases. *Int Orthop* 18:291–298, 1994.)

This is supported by ventral spinal instrumentation. Bone is also placed around the prosthesis or inside the cages. The ventral fixation construct includes one vertebra above and one below the affected vertebra.

Ventral Approaches to the Thoracic and Thoracolumbar Spine Junction

For levels below T4 to the lower lumbar spine, a direct ventral approach is not possible. For anatomic reasons, a direct ventral approach is possible for the cervicothoracic junction and for the lower lumbar spine. Thoracotomy and retroperitoneal approaches provide a ventrolateral view of the spine.

Transpleural Thoracotomy

When a ventrolateral exposure of the spine is required for pathologic processes located rostral to the T12 vertebral body, a transthoracic approach is often appropriate.[23,36,65] It is most useful for the midthoracic segments between T3 and T11.

The main advantage of a thoracotomy is direct access to ventral pathology, multilevel exposure, and ease of ventral

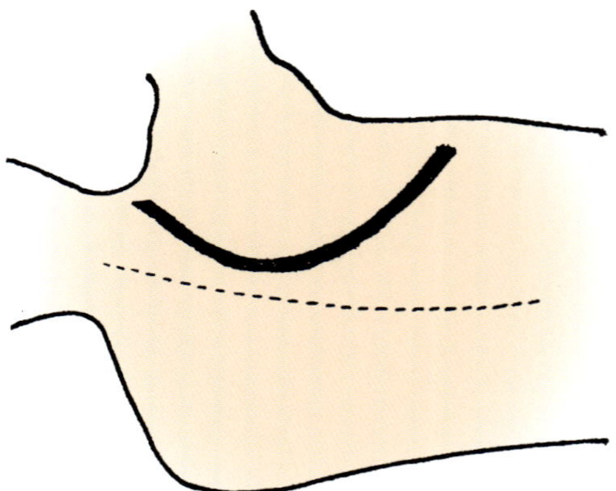

FIGURE 169-28. Skin incision for ventrolateral exposure of the upper thoracic spine. The right-side-up position and a curved incision around the scapula finishing at the C7 spinous process are used.

instrumentation. The disadvantages of this approach include violation of the thoracic cavity, the need for a tube thoracotomy, and a relatively weak instrumentation construct (short-segment fixation).

The patient is placed in the lateral decubitus position. Usually, the right lateral decubitus position is used. Most surgeons prefer a left-sided approach because it is easier to mobilize the aorta than the vena cava. To open the intercostal and intervertebral spaces on the operative side, a slight break in the table or cushions placed under the contralateral thorax is necessary. The lower arm should be protected by axillary rolls. The upper arm can rest on an arm table or over the cushions. The upper leg is flexed, and the lower leg is extended.

A curved incision is fashioned around the medial aspect of the scapula for a thoracotomy in the upper thoracic spine (T2-5) vertebral lesions (Fig. 169-28). For lesions between T5 and T10, a curvilinear incision is made along the designated rib, extending from the costochondral articulation ventrally to the lateral aspect of the paraspinous muscles dorsally (see Fig. 169-23A).

The optimal rib to be resected in the thoracic spine is the rib that is located at the level of the surgical pathology in the midaxillary line. Muscle and periosteum may be divided with monopolar cautery. The rib is then dissected subperiosteally with a small periosteal dissector. Resection of the rib is not essential. The pleura is then opened in the bed of the rib. After retraction of the lung, the spine is visualized. Segmental vessels in the desired area are ligated and divided. The periosteum on the ventrolateral spine is incised and retracted.

After the lung is collapsed, a self-retaining thoracotomy retractor is used. A malleable retractor with a reversed curve is placed on the ventral aspect of the vertebral body.[66]

Extrapleural Thoracotomy

An extrapleural thoracotomy approach provides a shorter route to the ventral thoracic spine. Its major advantage is avoidance of pleural cavity violation.[67] Postoperative morbidity, particularly pain and pulmonary complications, are thus reduced.

The patient is placed in the lateral decubitus position. As with a transpleural thoracotomy, a curved incision is fashioned around the medial aspect of the scapula.

Intercostal muscles are detached subperiosteally over an 8- to 10-cm rib segment.[67] Then, in the resected rib segment, the endothoracic fascia is incised in line with the rib bed. The parietal pleura is widely dissected from the undersurface of the endothoracic fascia with blunt dissectors. After adequate dissection and freeing the parietal pleura over the vertebral body is ensured, a self-retaining crank-type retractor facilitates the exposure.

Retropleural approaches are recommended to avoid direct lung trauma and to minimize the need for a tube thoracostomy. In the midthoracic spine, only limited lesions such as thoracic disc herniations may be approached via a retropleural thoracotomy. It is easier to perform an extrapleural operation at the thoracolumbar junction. The 11th or 12th rib extrapleural-retroperitoneal approach is a prototype for this.[68] The extrapleural space can be expanded to T10-L2. Some authors have advised resectimg the 12th rib to facilitate exposure.[67]

Transdiaphragmatic Approach

To approach the T11 or T12 vertebrae, either a supradiaphragmatic or infradiaphragmatic exposure may be possible. However, it is usually necessary to section the diaphragm to reach the L1 vertebral body.

The diaphragm is a key structure that should be taken into consideration for approaches to the thoracolumbar spine. Its limbs have attachments to the L1 transverse process and vertebral body. It extends laterally over the quadratus lumborum muscle to the tip of the 12th rib. Because its innervation from the phrenic nerve begins centrally, a peripheral incision is preferred. If a transdiaphragmatic approach to reach the ventral thoracolumbar junction is mandatory, the pleural and retroperitoneal cavities are violated. Because the morbidity of such an approach is higher than that of a retroperitoneal approach, which violates only one body cavity, it should be used only if absolutely necessary.

The patient is placed in the lateral decubitus position. For the thoracolumbar junction, the classical operation is the 9th or 10th rib transpleural-retroperitoneal thoracoabdominal approach. Most commonly, a T10 rib incision is made. The 10th rib may then be resected (Fig. 169-29). A self-retaining thoracotomy retractor is used as for thoracotomy. Care must be taken not to injure the spleen on the left side or the liver on the right side. The major disadvantage of this method is the division of the diaphragm and entering into two body cavities.

Kim et al.[68] have recommended using an 11th rib extrapleural-retroperitoneal approach (Fig. 169-30). Since it prevents entering the pleural cavity, thoracic complications should be minimal. However, it is technically demanding, it prolongs the operative time, and the operative exposure is limited.

Ventrolateral Retroperitoneal Approach

It is possible to reach the lumbar vertebrae from L1 to L5 with an extraperitoneal approach. Ventral instrumentation, however, is difficult below L4 because of the constraints of the iliac vessels and overlying iliac crest.

A supine position is appropriate for low ventrolateral lumbar exposure, using a log roll to elevate the operative side. For thoracolumbar approaches, however, a right lateral decubitus

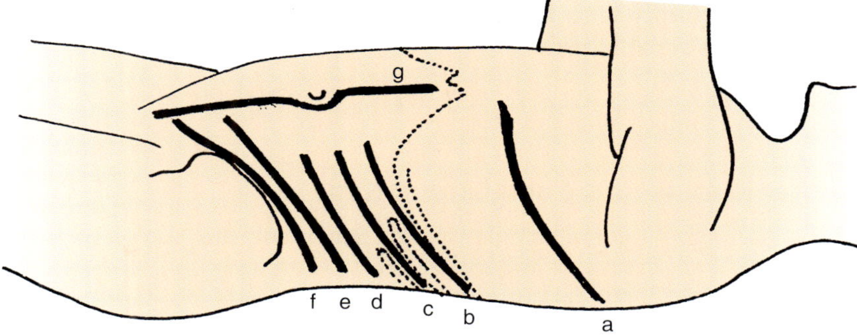

FIGURE 169-29. The incision lines for thoracotomy and lumbar ventrolateral retroperitoneal approaches: *a*, lower thoracotomy; *b*, T12-L1; *c*, L1-2; *d*, L2-3; *e*, L3-5; *f*, L5-S1 retroperitoneal approaches; and *g*, transperitoneal approach.

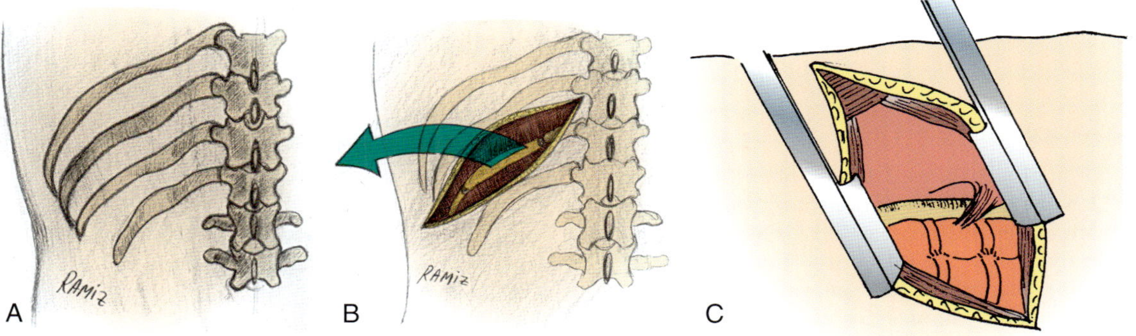

FIGURE 169-30. Eleventh rib extrapleural-retroperitoneal approach for lesions in the thoracolumbar spine. A left-sided approach is mostly preferred (**A**). After removing the 11th rib (**B**), a self-retaining retractor is placed, and with blunt dissection, ventral vertebral structures are shown (**C**). (Redrawn from Kim M, Nolan P, Finkelstein JA: Evaluation of 11th rib extrapleural-retroperitoneal approach to the thoracolumbar junction: technical note. *J Neurosurg* 93[1S]:168–174, 2000.)

position on an ordinary operating table is preferred. Table-mounted retractor systems may help to maintain this position during the operation.

The left-side-up position is preferred because it is easier to dissect, mobilize, or repair the aorta or iliac artery compared with the vena cava or iliac vein. The liver, because of its mass and location, is more difficult to retract and mobilize than the spleen is. Excessive splenic retraction may result in injury. An adjustable pad is placed at the level of the vertebra of interest.

The skin incision is run obliquely, caudally, and ventrally. This so-called flank incision can be made between the tip of the 12th rib and the anterior superior iliac spine. It begins dorsally at the edge of the paravertebral muscle and terminates at the lateral margin of the rectus abdominis muscle. However, the incision may vary on the basis of the spinal level and the surgical indication (see Fig. 169-29).[23]

For an infradiaphragmatic retroperitoneal exposure, subperiosteal dissection of the crus of the diaphragm from its vertebral attachments aids in the visualization of the higher lumbar and lower thoracic vertebral bodies. Resection of the 11th or 12th rib may be used to gain access to the thoracolumbar and upper lumbar spine via this approach.[69-71]

The exposure to the midlumbar spine is the same approach that is used for the lumbar sympathectomy. This exposure allows access to the ventrolateral spinal canal from L2 to below the pelvic brim. The advantages of this approach are its familiarity to all spine and vascular surgeons and its direct exposure of the midlumbar vertebral bodies. However, it provides a narrow longitudinal exposure that is limited rostrally by the crus of the diaphragm and caudally by the pelvic brim. The psoas muscle also limits the opening of neuroforamina.

It is very important to clearly conceptualize the pathologic levels. For example, if only the L1-2 disc space is to be surgically approached, a subcostal extrapleural, T12 rib resection approach without diaphragm incision should be considered. Excessive left-sided retraction may result in splenic injury. If an L1 corpectomy is needed, a transdiaphragmatic approach may be preferred, depending on the patient's anatomy.

The external oblique, internal oblique, and transversus abdominis muscles are split with cutting diathermy. Retraction of the peritoneal sac ventrally and medially away from the psoas muscle exposes the vessels located ventral to the spine. The attachments of the psoas muscle are dissected laterally and dorsally.

Ligature of the segmental lumbar vessels is necessary. After this ligation, the aorta and the inferior vena cava may be retracted ventrally and medially. Then a malleable retractor may be used to retract the peritoneal sac and the great vessels.

The vascular supply of the spinal cord is worthy of consideration. The most common location of the entrance of the radiculomedullary artery of Adamkiewicz into the spinal canal is on the left, in the midthoracic to lower thoracic region. Generally, the ventrolateral approach is not affected by the location of radiculomedullary arteries, because the angle of the approach does not violate terminal-end arteries. If the surgeon intends to disrupt the soft tissues at the level of the neuroforamina, terminal spinal cord blood flow may be endangered. In this circumstance, an alternative approach should be considered.

Dorsal Approaches to the Lumbar and Lumbosacral Spine

The dorsal approach to the lumbosacral spine is a standard exposure, and similar to the thoracic dorsal approaches.

Lumbar Laminectomy and Laminotomy

Because opening of the interlaminar space is important, the patient should not be in extreme lordosis. A standard dorsal midline incision is performed. If a single-level microdiscectomy is planned, the length of the incision may be as short as 2.5 cm. An intraoperative radiograph is necessary to confirm the correct level.

Hemilaminectomy retractors are used for two or more level single-sided discectomies. For microdiscectomy, specially designed retractors such as Caspar retractors may be used.

Paraspinal Approach

The paraspinal approach is used for far-lateral disc herniation[72] or for dorsolateral fusion of the transverse processes.[73] Its main advantage is the decrease in paraspinous muscle retraction.

The patient is placed in the prone position. Wiltse et al.[73] have described bilateral paramedian incisions and a muscle-splitting dissection between the erector spinae and multifidus muscles. If the operation is performed for an extraforaminal disc protrusion, a unilateral small incision is usually sufficient.

The paraspinal approach provides a direct exposure of the intertransverse region and the facet joint. A self-retaining retractor may be used between the muscles.

Jane et al.[72] have described a modification of this approach that makes it possible to expose the root both from medial and lateral to the facet joint. With this approach, the incision is extended from the midline, but the muscle fascia is incised as an arc, and the spaces first medial to the paraspinous muscles and then lateral to these are exposed.[72]

Lateral Extracavitary Approach

The lateral extracavitary approach in the lumbar spine is similar to the lateral extracavitary approach in the thoracic spine. However, it is more important to preserve the lumbar nerve roots. Because there is no rib in the lumbar region and because the nerve roots pass through the bulky iliopsoas muscle, the lateral extracavitary approach is technically demanding in the lumbosacral region. The obstacle of the iliac crest is another limitation of this approach.[5,49,50,57]

Ventral Approaches to the Lumbar and Lumbosacral Spine

Ventrolateral Transpsoatic Approach

Although this technique was used to implant prosthetic disc nucleus devices in patients with symptomatic degenerative disc disease,[74] it was then called an extreme lateral interbody fusion, and for the risks of iatrogenic injury to the lumbosacral plexus, electrophysiologic monitoring of the retracted roots inside the psoas muscle is recommended.[75]

Pelvic Brim Extraperitoneal Approach

The pelvic brim extraperitoneal approach provides a limited exposure of the L5 and S1 levels, because of the obstructing iliac vessels and the iliac crest. For this reason, only limited procedures, such as biopsy and simple resections, can be performed.

Usually, the supine position will suffice with slight elevation on the side of surgery with a log roll. An incision beginning lateral to, and slightly above, the anterior superior iliac spine can be carried medially and caudally. It must be parallel and rostral to the iliac crest and inguinal ligament.

The peritoneum and renal fascia are retracted medially, with great care taken not to injure the retroperitoneal nerves and ureters. This exposure provides a limited view of the vertebrae under the aorta and iliac arteries.

For a minimally invasive exposure of the L4-5 level, a 5- to 8-cm horizontal incision through the anterior rectus sheath has been described. The rectus abdominis muscle is then retracted medially. After incision of the posterior rectus sheath, the retroperitoneum is exposed.[23,58,70]

Transperitoneal Approach

It is possible to reach all the midlumbar and lower lumbar segments and the sacrum via the transperitoneal approach.[66,76,77] The transperitoneal approach provides a direct ventral exposure of the lumbar and sacral spine. It is most useful for L5-S1 pathology, when a wide exposure of this region is required.[78] The requirement of a laparotomy and the potential for neural and vascular injury are its disadvantages.

The patient is placed in the supine position. A midline or horizontal subumbilical laparotomy incision is made.

After entry into the peritoneal cavity, the small intestines are packed in the upper abdomen and retracted to the right. A break in the operating table to increase the lumbar lordosis is useful. Care is taken to avoid injury to the bladder. The sigmoid colon is retracted laterally, and a longitudinal incision is made in the dorsal peritoneum in the midline. The sacral promontory is an important landmark. The sigmoid colon limits the exposure on the left side, but caudal retroperitoneal structures on the right side are easily identified.

The bifurcation of the iliac arteries and veins does not allow exposure above the L5 vertebral body through the bifurcation. Instead, the approach is to the left of the vessels. Liberal use of epinephrine injection and, in males only, use of bipolar electrocautery decreases the risk of presacral plexus injury.

Dorsal Approaches to the Sacrum

The most common approach to the lumbosacral junction and the sacrum is via a dorsal midline incision. The ventral approach is difficult and requires vascular retraction. With dorsal approaches, there is adequate room for retraction of the cauda equina laterally to expose the ventral sacrum. However, the control of ventral vascular structures is not possible with the dorsal approach.

In case of a sacrectomy, it is suggested that the patient be prepared the day before surgery with repeated enemas. At the beginning of the operation, a vaginal pad is inserted into the rectum.

The patient is placed in the prone position. It is important to keep the abdomen free of pressure so that bleeding is minimized. If a lumbosacral fusion is to be undertaken and supplemented with internal fixation, the lumbosacral junction should be placed in extension. This can easily be achieved by placing pillows or bolsters under the hips. In the Krause position, the sacrum is prominent and constitutes the highest point of the table (Fig. 169-31).[79]

The incision varies according to the pathology and planned operation. A midline vertical incision, transverse incision, upward arched incision, or downward arched incision may be used (Fig. 169-32).

If a sacrectomy or excision of a large tumor is planned, a midline vertical incision is not suitable because of possible postoperative inflammatory processes and wound dehiscence due to major tissue defect. In addition, a vertical incision could injure the anal sphincter, and does not provide adequate exposure of the lateral sacrum.

Another problem during the sacrum tumor surgery is the necessity for inclusion of the biopsy scar into the excision material. In this case, a T-shaped incision may be most suitable (see Fig. 169-32C).

Wiltse et al.[73] introduced an incision and retraction technique using one or two incisions 5 cm lateral to the midline and medial to the posterior superior iliac spine (see Fig. 169-32A). The dissection is deepened to the sacrospinalis muscle and the transverse process of the fifth lumbar vertebra. Wiltse et al. have used this approach for lumbosacral fusions. Bone grafts from the dorsal iliac crest can easily be obtained with the same exposure.

For midline incisions with restricted operations in the sacrum, a self-retaining retractor is satisfactory. For operations such as sacrectomy, hand-held retractors are more convenient. In this case, skin flaps should be gently retracted.

The ligaments (sacroiliac and sacrotuberalis) and the gluteus maximus muscle are divided as near to the sacrum as possible, because their approximation before wound closure is necessary to avoid ventrodorsal postoperative wound problems.

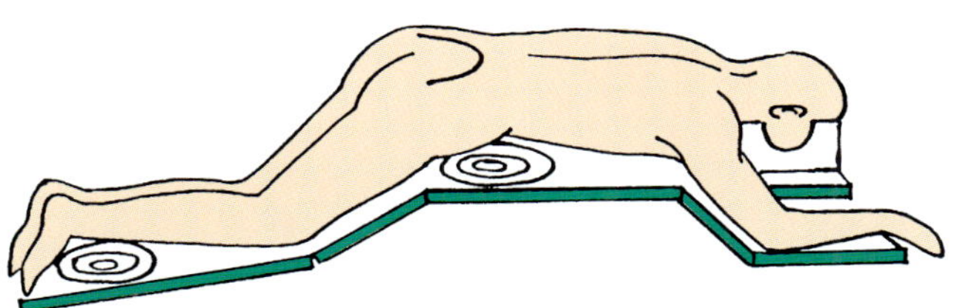

FIGURE 169-31. Krause position and inverted U-shaped incision for the exposure of the sacrum.

Ventral Approaches to the Sacrum

Retroperitoneal Approach

The retroperitoneal approach is restricted to the sacral pathologies without rectal invasion. Depending on the extent of the pathology, a unilateral or bilateral retroperitoneal dissection may be used.

A supine position with the legs elevated and partly separated (lithotomy position) is advised.[80] If a unilateral dissection is planned, one side of the pelvis may be elevated.

For bilateral retroperitoneal exposure, a large semicircular incision is performed through the skin on the lower abdomen (Fig. 169-33A). The rectus abdominis tendon is severed bilaterally just above the pubic bone. For unilateral exposure, a flank incision without violating the rectus abdominis muscle is satisfactory (Fig. 169-33B).

After dissection and medial retraction of the peritoneum, common iliac arteries and veins with external and internal branches are exposed. Then the dorsal parietal peritoneum is dissected medially together with the ureter and the superior hypogastric nerve plexus. The right and left dissections meet in the midline. Deep handheld abdominal retractors are used for retraction of the deep abdominal structures.

Transperitoneal Approach

The transperitoneal approach is primarily used for L5-S1 ventral fusion operations. It may also be used for the resection of sacral tumors, if the rectum has to be included in the specimen.

The patient is placed in the supine position, and an inferior midline abdominal incision is made (Fig. 169-33C). The median raphe of the rectus abdominis muscle is divided. A suprapubic transverse incision is not recommended, for it requires a rectus abdominis muscle section.

The peritoneum is cut in the midline, and after packing the bowel and small intestines rostrally and laterally, the rectum is released ventrally as far distally as possible.

Combined Abdominosacral Approach

Total resection of the major primary sacral tumors (i.e., chordoma, chondrosarcoma, giant cell tumor) requires a combined approach, both ventral and dorsal.[39,81] If the rectum can be preserved, the operation is begun ventrally

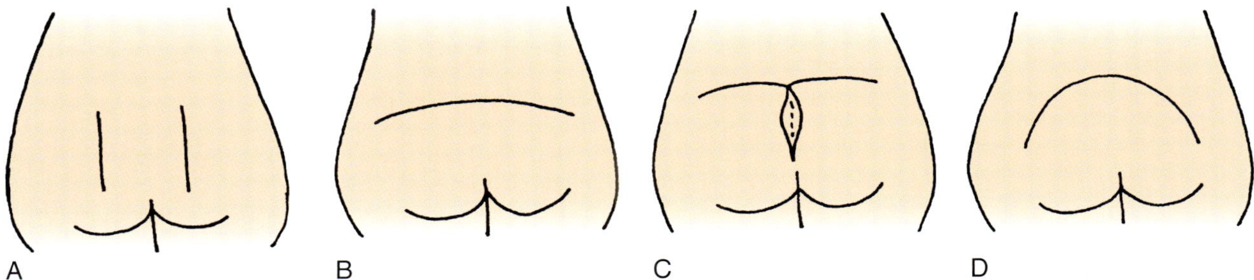

FIGURE 169-32. Different incisions used for dorsal sacral operations: **A,** dorsal sacrospinalis splitting approach (Wiltse); **B,** dorsal transversal incision; **C,** T-shaped incision including biopsy scar; **D,** inverted U-shaped incision.

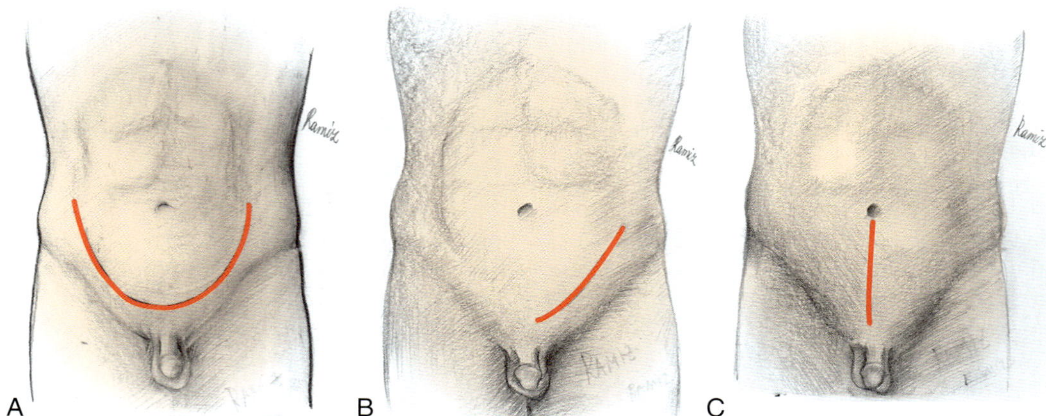

FIGURE 169-33. Different incisions used for ventral sacral operations: **A,** bilateral U-shaped retroperitoneal incision; **B,** unilateral flank retroperitoneal incision; **C,**ventral medial transperitoneal incision.

and finished dorsally. If not, a ventral, dorsal, and ventral approach sequence is advocated.[80]

Some surgeons prefer a dorsal exposure in the prone position. The patient is then placed in the lateral decubitus position so that a separation of tissue planes from both sides is possible.[43,82] In this case, two surgeons, one from the dorsal and the other from the ventral side, may operate simultaneously.

KEY REFERENCES

Abe E, Kobayashi T, Murai H, et al: Total spondylectomy for primary malignant, aggressive benign, and solitary metastatic bone tumors of the thoracolumbar spine. *J Spinal Disord* 14:237–246, 2001.

Benzel EC: *Surgical exposure of the spine: an extensile approach*, Rolling Meadows, IL, 1995, American Association of Neurological Surgeons.

Charles R, Govender S: Anterior approach to the upper thoracic vertebrae. *J Bone Joint Surg [Br]* 71:81–84, 1989.

Hall JE, Denis F, Murray J: Exposure of the upper cervical spine for spinal decompression by a mandible and tongue splitting approach. *J Bone Joint Surg [Am]* 59:121–123, 1977.

Hodgson AR, Yau ACMC: Anterior surgical approaches to the spinal column. In Apley AG, editor: *Recent advances in orthopaedics*, Baltimore, 1969, Williams & Wilkins, pp 289–323.

Woodard EJ: Indications, complications, and comparison of approaches. In Benzel EC, editor: *Surgical exposure of the spine: an extensile approach*, Rolling Meadows, IL, 1995, American Association of Neurological Surgeons, pp 157–178.

REFERENCES

The complete reference list is available online at expertconsult.com.

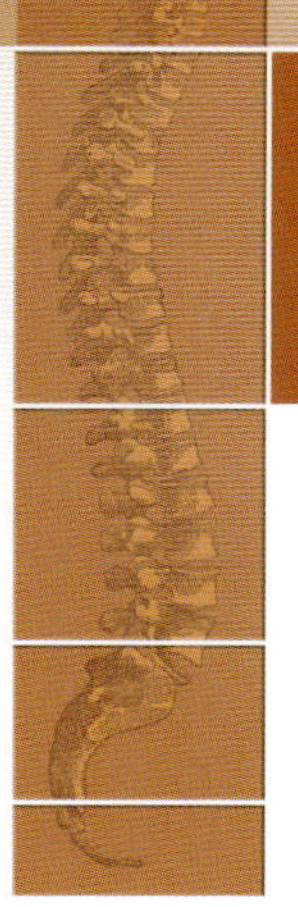

CHAPTER 170

Blood Loss Management

David G. Malone | Mitchell Martineau

Significant blood loss during spine surgery may occur for numerous reasons, including patient-related factors, dissection extending over multiple levels, bony decortication at the graft and fusion site, long duration of the procedure, and the release of a tamponade on the epidural veins. Blood loss and the resultant need for transfusion are largely affected by surgical techniques, including speed of surgery, hemostatic agents, positioning of the patient, and the adjunctive use of hypotension and pharmacologic agents during the procedure. Managing blood loss involves rational planning regarding transfusion needs, the use of antifibrinolytic drugs, replacement of blood through homologous or autologous blood transfusion, and intraoperative or even postoperative blood salvage.

Preoperative Evaluation

A key component of the patient evaluation for spinal surgery is the complete medical history, including medications and bleeding tendencies. If indicated, a hematologic profile with coagulation times, platelet counts, and, in some instances, platelet function testing should be obtained.

Medication History

Patients with a history of transient ischemic attack, stroke, deep venous thrombosis (DVT), heavy bleeding after minor trauma, alcoholism, hepatic dysfunction, neuromuscular scoliosis, cerebral palsy,[1] and cardiac disease have an increased risk of bleeding. Many patients who undergo spinal surgery take nonsteroidal anti-inflammatory drugs (NSAIDs). NSAIDs inhibit platelet function and may increase bleeding times. The bleeding time often returns to normal within 24 hours of cessation of some NSAIDs, whereas others require a full 18 days for the drug to be eliminated and normal platelet function restored. Antiplatelet drugs, such as ticlopidine hydrochloride (Ticlid), clopidogrel (Plavix), dipyridamole (Persantine), and aspirin may prolong the bleeding time and must be discontinued before surgery.[2] Patients who take warfarin (Coumadin) may require cessation or reversal of the anticoagulation (Table 170-1). Those rare patients with congenital coagulation deficits may undergo surgery after factor replacement and consultation with a hematologist.[3]

Patients treated with the anticonvulsant valproic acid (Depakote) appear to have increased blood loss during spinal surgery. This is thought to be related to an inhibition of platelet function. If possible, another antiepileptic drug should be used in the immediate preoperative and postoperative periods for such patients.[4]

Preoperative Estimation of Blood Loss

Factors associated with increased blood loss with spinal surgery include tumor, low preoperative hemoglobin level, numbers of levels fused, history of pulmonary disease, suboptimal autologous blood availability, the use of operating tables other than dedicated spine surgery tables, and antiplatelet drugs.[5-7] When surgery is contemplated for reconstruction in cases of spinal metastasis from renal cell carcinoma, preoperative embolization has been shown to significantly reduce intraoperative blood loss. Therefore, embolization should at least be considered as a preoperative adjunct in all vascular spinal tumors.[8]

The blood loss for a particular operation should be estimated and plans generated to ensure that such can be replaced if needed. An estimate of 200 mL of blood lost per fused segment can be made before surgery to plan the amount of blood that will be required for replacement.[8] Patients can usually tolerate a loss of 15% of the blood volume before transfusion.[9] In a 70-kg patient, estimating 70 mL blood/kg body weight, a volume of 735 mL would reflect a 15% blood loss.

Autologous Blood Use

Autologous blood donation can be instituted if the estimated blood loss exceeds 15% of the blood volume. Autologous blood can be obtained in three ways: preoperative donation, intraoperative salvage, and postoperative salvage. Although each requires expensive specialized equipment, a reduction in the potential for the development of chronic liver disease and infection transmission may be well worth the cost.[10] One unit of blood can be donated per week if the hematocrit remains above 34%.[11] Other guidelines for autologous donation include a patient age range of 12 to 70 years[11] and a hemoglobin of at least 11 mg/dL.[12] Full units can be taken from patients weighing more than 50 kg and half units from those between 25 and 50 kg. Supplemental iron should be administered when appropriate. In some instances, recombinant erythropoietin can be administered to facilitate increased blood volume for autologous donation.[13-16] This has been

TABLE 170-1

Drugs Affecting Coagulation

Drug	Plasma Half-Life	Platelet or Clotting Factor Completely or Partially Inhibited[64]	Days to Stop before Surgery
Aspirin	12 hr[65]	Complete platelet inhibition	7 d[71]
Ibuprofen	2 hr[65]	Complete platelet inhibition	1 d[72]
Naproxen	12–15 hr[66]	Complete platelet inhibition	2–3 d[72]
Celecoxib	11 hr[67]	Partial platelet inhibition	2–3 d[72]
Meloxicam	15–20 hr[68]	Partial platelet inhibition	10 d[72]
Warfarin	40 hr[69]	Partial clotting factor inhibition	6 d (check INR)[69]
Clopidogrel	8 hr[67]	Partial clotting factor inhibition	12–18 d[72]
Heparin	1–2 hr[70]	Complete clotting factor inhibition	4 d[70]
Enoxaparin	4.5 hr single dose, 7 hr repeated dose[70]	Complete clotting factor inhibition	1 d[70]
Ticlopidine HCL	12–13 hr[64]	Complete platelet inhibition	7 d[71]
Dipyridamole	10 hr[64]	Partial platelet inhibition	2–3 d[64]

INR, international normalized ratio.

shown to increase blood production significantly both in animal and clinical studies.[13,17]

Consideration should be given as to whether autologous packed red blood cells or whole blood should be transfused. The patient donates whole blood, and in autologous donation it may be best to return whole blood to the patient. Whole blood contains platelets, plasma, and cryoprecipitate, all of which are lacking in packed cells, and these components may help lessen bleeding.[13] Using autologous blood in a community hospital, 95% of the transfusion needs were met for 1600 patients who underwent major orthopaedic procedures.[18] Other studies have shown that autologous blood can supply approximately 70% to 80% of the transfusion needs.[10,12] Autologous blood may be cryopreserved or preserved with a storage solution.[19] Cryopreserved blood has a longer shelf life, and the in vitro survival of red blood cells is equivalent to that of fresh erythrocytes. Also, no preoperative effect on the hemodynamic status of the patient exists.[20] Oga et al.[19] used cryopreserved cells in patients who underwent scoliosis surgery and solution-stored blood for patients who underwent other spine procedures. More blood was collected for the scoliosis patients, and the less costly storage method was used for other patients.[19] There are risks to autologous blood transfusion, which include septicemia from bacterial contamination of the unit, nonimmune hemolytic transfusion reactions, febrile reactions, volume overload, and the possible risk of clerical error resulting in the administration of the wrong unit of blood.[21]

The criteria for returning autologous blood may vary. Albert et al.[22] found that the transfusion of blood during surgery was beneficial for the early postoperative hemoglobin and postoperative patient mobilization. There are different indications for homologous versus autologous blood return. Hemoglobin of less than 7 g/dL for homologous transfusions and less than 10 g/dL for autologous transfusions is a common indicator.[12,22]

Indications for transfusion of homologous blood include a hemoglobin of less than 7 g/dL in a medically healthy but symptomatic patient, a hemoglobin of less than 10 mg/dL in a critically ill patient, and a patient with medical risk factors such as cardiovascular disease, cerebrovascular disease, or active hemorrhage. Symptoms indicating hypovolemia, such as tachycardia, tachypnea, or low venous oxygenation, also indicate the need for transfusion.[12,22,23] Other transfusion requirements have been published. They include hemoglobin less than 8 g/dL in an otherwise healthy patient, hemoglobin less than 11 g/dL in patients with increased risk of ischemia, acute blood loss with 15% of blood volume lost, diastolic pressure less than 60 mm Hg, systolic blood pressure decrease of greater than 30 mm Hg, tachycardia, oliguria, symptomatic anemia with tachycardia, mental status changes, cardiac ischemia, and dyspnea. General transfusion requirements for coagulation products have been provided. Platelet transfusion for platelet dysfunction or thrombocytopenia is an effective strategy in such cases. Fresh-frozen plasma may be administered for evidence of coagulation factor deficiencies with prothrombin time or activated partial thromboplastin time greater than 1.5 times the upper limit of normal. Cryoprecipitate is administered for suspected specific factor deficiencies or fibrinogen less than 100 mg/dL.[5]

Homologous Blood Use

Since the early 1980s, there has been an increasing concern about the risks of blood transfusions. Although transmission of HIV has been the primary concern, allergic reactions, isosensitization, and the transmission of hepatitis are far more serious in terms of the number of patients affected. Hepatitis following transfusion has been reported to occur in as many as 10% of patients after homologous transfusion, with 3.3% developing chronic liver disease.[10]

The risks of allogeneic blood transfusion have decreased over the past several decades. Currently, transfusion-related acute lung injury (TRALI), hemolytic transfusion reactions (HTRs), and transfusion-associated sepsis are the leading causes of allogeneic blood transfusion–related fatalities. TRALI appears clinically similar to acute respiratory distress syndrome, but in TRALI the infiltrates typically clear in 96 hours, and the case fatality rate is only 5%. Fresh-frozen plasma is the most frequently implicated transfused component. White blood cell antibodies in the transfused component appear to be the most frequent trigger for TRALI. HTR occurred at a rate of 1 per 76,000 units transfused with a case fatality rate of 2% in a recent 10-year New York state study.

These cases of HTR are largely attributable to clerical error or undetected non-ABO antibodies.[24] Since the introduction of tests in 1990 for the detection of hepatitis C, the incidence of transfusion-acquired hepatitis has significantly decreased. The predominant risk is from donors in the "window period" of their infection who have donated blood before they have developed antibodies to the virus, rendering it impossible to detect the infection.

The current risk of hepatitis C transmission is 1 in one million units transfused, and the current risk of hepatitis B transmission is 1 in 100,000 units transfused. The current risk of HIV transmission in tested blood varies with the region of the United States, but is approximately 1 in one million units transfused.[24] This estimate of risk assumes a safe, plentiful, well-regulated, and tested blood supply; unfortunately, this is not universally the case in developing countries.[25]

Anesthetic Techniques for Lessening Intraoperative Blood Loss

Anesthetic techniques may affect operative blood loss. Specific medications, hemodilutional autotransfusion, and induced hypotension have all been used to decrease intraoperative bleeding.

Randomized, controlled trials have shown no difference in the amount of blood loss in patients who received desmopressin compared with those who did not.[26] Other studies have shown desmopressin to reduce blood loss in spine surgery by 32.5%.[23] It is administered immediately before surgery at a dose of 10 μg/m^2 of body surface area, up to a maximum dose of 20 μg. It is prepared by diluting it to a concentration of 0.5 μg/mL in normal saline and infusing over 20 minutes. Desmopressin does lessen bleeding in some subsets of patients, such as those with acquired platelet dysfunction from aspirin administration, von Willebrand disease, and uremia.[5,27] Desmopressin has been found to decrease the partial thromboplastin time, whereas factor VIII coagulant activity and von Willebrand antigen concentrations increased the partial thromboplastin time. A Cochrane review found no convincing evidence that desmopressin minimizes perioperative allogeneic red blood cell transfusion in patients who do not have congenital bleeding disorders.[28] Potential postoperative problems include oliguria, which usually responds to furosemide, and hyponatremia due to its potent antidiuretic hormone activity.[29]

Randomized, controlled trials of aprotinin (Trasylol) in dorsal spinal fusion reveal significant reductions in autologous but not homologous blood transfusion. Aprotinin has been shown to reduce blood transfusion requirements in cardiac surgery, liver resection, and some orthopaedic surgical procedures.[30] Aprotinin has been found to increase mortality in cardiac surgery patients and was relabeled by the U.S. Food and Drug Administration (FDA) for use only in high-risk cardiac patients. It was removed from the U.S. market in November 2007.[31]

ε-Aminocaproic acid (Amicar) is an antifibrinolytic agent that has been shown to reduce blood loss in cardiac surgery.[32] It has been tested in lumbar spinal fusion and has been shown to reduce autologous blood transfusion in a prospective, nonrandomized study by approximately 50%. No complications were noted, including thromboembolism or DVT. ε-Aminocaproic acid was given in an initial dose of 100 mg/kg, not to exceed 5 g over 15 minutes, followed by a continuous infusion of 10 mg/kg/hr over the remainder of the case, with the infusion terminating at skin closure.[33]

Tranexamic acid is a synthetic antifibrinolytic agent that has been studied as a means to reduce blood requirements in scoliosis surgery. In a double-blinded, prospective, placebo-controlled study, tranexamic acid, given in an initial dose of 10 mg/kg at the time of patient positioning and in a maintenance infusion of 1 mg/kg/hr, reduced blood transfusion requirements by 28%.[34] A recent study of tranexamic acid using a loading dose of 2 g, followed by a continuous infusion of 100 mg/hr in adults and 1 mg/kg/hr in children, resulted in a 49% reduction of blood loss.[35] Because tranexamic acid is an antifibrinolytic agent, it does not change the blood's intrinsic clotting ability but rather slows the breakdown of preexisting clots. Tranexamic acid has also been studied for use in reducing blood loss in metastatic spine tumor surgery and unfortunately did not significantly reduce blood loss in a retrospective study.[36]

Recombinant coagulation factor VIIa has shown promise in reducing blood loss in spinal surgery. Factor VIIa has been used in trauma management, craniotomy, and to reverse the effects of warfarin. Factor VIIa is approved by the FDA for use in patients with hemophilia with inhibitors to replacement factor VIII or IX. Use for hemostasis in other conditions is considered off-label at this time. The drug has a short half-life and is given as hourly bolus doses or by continuous infusion. Until more data are available, the drug should be used only as an agent of last resort in the event of bleeding when all other measures have failed. The drug is available in 1200-μg vials, and doses have been given in a wide range, from 16 μg/kg to 212 μg/kg, with no reported incidence of untoward events.[17,24,25,29,37,38] One multicenter, randomized, controlled trial of factor VIIa used in spine surgery demonstrated no adverse events and significantly reduced blood loss.[39]

Acute hemodilutional autotransfusion is another technique used to reduce the need for homologous blood transfusion. After the induction of anesthesia, a venesection is performed and 15% to 25% of the patient's blood volume is withdrawn into a sterile bag containing the anticoagulant citrate. The blood volume withdrawn is then replaced with colloid, on a milliliter-for-milliliter basis, or crystalloid, on a three-to-one basis. At the conclusion of surgery, the autologous blood is returned to the patient. The patient is then diuresed of excess fluid.[35,40] Patients with type O blood have lower concentrations of factor VIII and von Willebrand factor than patients with other blood types. Type O patients are at increased risk for development of disseminated intravascular coagulation (DIC) when blood is replaced with the colloid 6% hydroxyethyl starch.[41]

Hypotensive anesthesia has been evaluated in patients undergoing scoliosis surgery and fusion for degenerative disease.[15] Hypotension was induced with 25 mg of nitroprusside and 125 mg of trimethaphan in 500 mL of 5% dextrose, which was infused to maintain a systolic blood pressure between 60 and 70 mm Hg.[11,15] Enflurane can also be used as a supplement to the general anesthetic agents to induce hypotension. Both methods have been effective in decreasing blood loss in these patients with no adverse sequelae.[42]

thrombocytopenia, platelet dysfunction, heparin administration, DIC, impaired hepatic function, an undiagnosed hereditary coagulation disorder, or laboratory error failing to detect a coagulopathy. The source(s) of bleeding should be carefully ascertained (e.g., solely from the wound site, from intravenous cannula wounds and other puncture sites, and from occult or distant sites). Isolated bleeding from the surgical site may indicate a coagulation disorder or simply poor surgical hemostasis. Bleeding from multiple sites strongly suggests dysfunctional clotting mechanisms, in which case prothrombin time, partial thromboplastin time, fibrinogen, D-dimer, complete blood count, platelet count, fibrin split products, and bleeding time should be assessed.

While awaiting these laboratory results, the anesthesia record should be examined to determine if heparin, hypothermia, platelet washout, or dilution of clotting factors is a likely cause. Heparin may be reversed with protamine. If hypothermic, the patient should be warmed. Thrombocytopenia may be treated by platelet transfusion, and elevated prothrombin times and partial thromboplastin times may be treated with fresh-frozen plasma. Low fibrinogen levels may require cryoprecipitate transfusion.

DIC is a syndrome characterized by the generation of thrombin in the peripheral blood. The principal target protein of thrombin is fibrinogen. A delicate balance exists between the synthesis and catabolism of fibrinogen. In DIC, this balance is upset and greatly shifted toward catabolism. DIC can be caused by tissue damaged in spine surgery. The diagnosis can be confirmed by the observation of an elevated prothrombin time, an elevated partial thromboplastin time, a low fibrinogen, and a positive D-dimer test. Treatment is directed toward clotting factor replacement.[62,63]

The surgeon should be aware during the operation as to whether clot exists in the operative site. If there is no clotted blood in the operative site, a coagulopathy probably exists. At this point, coagulopathy screens should be performed. The greater the time the problem is left uncorrected, the worse it gets, and a vicious cycle begins.

Summary

The management of blood loss during spine surgery begins well before the patient enters the operating suite. A thorough medical history is obtained, with attention given to medications and those items indicating hemorrhagic tendencies. For elective surgery, an estimate of potential blood loss is made, and plans for collecting autologous blood are established. The procedure itself should be performed with controlled alacrity and with the use of appropriate hemostatic agents, pharmacologic agents, and surgical and anesthetic techniques.

The transfusion of homologous blood is performed only in patients who have no autologous blood available and who have symptoms of hypovolemia or a hemoglobin of less than 7 mg/dL. IAT can be used in those patients whose preoperatively estimated blood loss is 2 to 3 U or greater.

The use of hypotensive anesthesia may be considered relative to the individual patient's symptoms and neurologic condition. Patients with a history of hypertension, ischemic cerebral or cardiovascular disease, or other major medical problems should be evaluated carefully before using hypotensive anesthesia. Without the ability to monitor spinal cord function during surgery, hypotensive anesthesia should be very cautiously considered.

Thought is given to patient positioning, to avoiding abdominal compression, and to controlling blood loss at each stage of the operation. The surgical procedure is planned so that any available potential bone fusion material, such as laminectomy remnants or spinous process, can be used instead of or in addition to iliac crest. Intraoperative cell salvage and autotransfusion is extremely useful to avoid the use of homologous blood.

Diffuse postoperative and intraoperative bleeding should be aggressively investigated for its cause, and treated accordingly. With the use of the aforementioned surgical techniques and technical tools, the use of homologous blood can be significantly decreased.

KEY REFERENCES

Brenn BR, Theroux MC, Dabney KW, et al: Clotting parameters and thromboelastography in children with neuromuscular and idiopathic scoliosis undergoing posterior spinal fusion. *Spine (Phila Pa 1976)* 29:E310–E314, 2004.

Chambers HG, Weinstein CH, Mubarak SJ, et al: The effect of valproic acid on blood loss in patients with cerebral palsy. *J Pediatr Orthop* 19:792–800, 1999.

Kolban M, Balachowska-Kosciolek I, Chmielnicki M: Recombinant coagulation factor VIIa: a novel haemostatic agent in scoliosis surgery? *Eur Spine J* 15:944–952, 2006.

Vamvakas E, Blajchman MA: Transfusion related mortality: the ongoing risks of allogenic blood transfusion and the available strategies for their prevention. *Blood* 113:3406–3417, 2009.

REFERENCES

The complete reference list is available online at expertconsult.com.

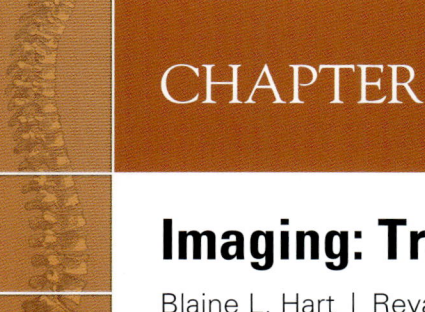

CHAPTER 171

Imaging: Trauma

Blaine L. Hart | Reyaad A. Hayek

Principles of Imaging Spine Trauma

It is essential to view the entire cervical spine and the junction with the thoracic spine and skull in cases of trauma. Incomplete visualization of the cervical spine through the C7-T1 junction is a well-recognized pitfall in acute trauma. If the shoulders obscure the C7-T1 junction on the lateral radiograph, additional imaging, which may include a swimmer's view or a CT, must be performed.

Multiple levels of spine injury are relatively common. Adjacent vertebrae are frequently fractured. In addition, noncontiguous injuries are also common following significant trauma. Detection of one fracture, therefore, should not end the search for spine injury. Especially with the widespread availability of spiral CT, evaluation of the entire cervical spine from the craniocervical junction through the cervicothoracic junction is very feasible.

Imaging complements the clinical examination. "Clearing" the spine is not a result of completing a set of radiographs or other imaging tests; it must come from a combination of clinical examination and appropriate imaging.

Integrity (stability) of the spine depends on both bone and soft tissue. Although uncommon, it is possible for a patient with no fractures, or seemingly insignificant fractures, to have an unstable spine because of severe ligamentous injury. Even with clearly demonstrated fractures, the outcome may be markedly affected by the extent of accompanying soft tissue injury. Alteration in alignment, worsening neurologic function, or persistent pain may be indications for MRI.

Techniques for Imaging Spine Trauma

Multiple imaging tools are available for the evaluation of traumatic spine injury. In order to utilize these tools appropriately, it is important to understand the strengths and limitations of the available techniques. The approach to imaging varies, depending on clinical circumstances, availability of imaging tests, and results of any previous imaging.

Radiographs

Radiographs ("plain films") of the spine have traditionally been the foundation of imaging acute spine trauma. However, this role is changing considerably with the wide availability of multidetector helical CT. Plain radiography should be readily available at any facility treating acute spine trauma. Radiographs can be obtained relatively quickly, and they are relatively inexpensive compared with CT and MRI. Spatial detail is excellent with good technique, although interpretation can be challenging with multiple overlapping structures. One of the strengths of plain radiography is its ability to quickly assess alignment.

There is no universal agreement on the views that should be obtained for acute cervical spine trauma. A lateral view is necessary, and often this is among the first radiographs (along with an anteroposterior [AP] chest radiograph), to be obtained in a patient with multiple trauma. As is discussed later, it is essential to view the entire cervical spine, including the junctions with the skull and thoracic spine. A swimmer's view may be useful, if needed, for visualizing the lower cervical spine. The lateral view is often followed by AP and odontoid views. The odontoid view, in particular, may be difficult with an uncooperative or intubated patient. Additional views may include oblique or pillar views. These can be particularly helpful in assessing the dorsal elements. The standard method of obtaining these views involves turning the patient's neck, which is not acceptable in the acute setting. Modified techniques can be used that involve angling the x-ray tube instead of turning the neck; these result in more distortion than a standard view but can still be useful.

AP and lateral views are usually obtained when acute thoracic or lumbar spine injury is suspected. Oblique views have little role in the evaluation of acute lumbar trauma. They add a considerable radiation dose with limited benefit.

Alignment is well assessed with plain films. Soft tissue injury can be inferred from prevertebral soft tissue swelling in the cervical spine. In the lumbar and thoracic spine, paraspinous swelling on the AP view is a sign of acute injury. Otherwise, however, radiographs are insensitive to the detection of significant soft tissue. The sensitivity of plain films to fracture varies depending on the location of the fracture. Vertebral body fractures are usually well visualized on radiographs, but fractures in the dorsal elements can be difficult. Sensitivity of radiographs to dorsal element fractures in the cervical spine has been found to be as low as 50%.[1-3] Fractures of the larger vertebrae of the thoracic and lumbar spine are usually well visualized on plain films.

Computed Tomography

CT has assumed a major role in imaging spine trauma because of the technological advances of the multidetector helical technique. It is possible to screen very rapidly for cervical spine trauma with the initial imaging evaluation of a patient with major trauma using a high-resolution technique that permits multiplanar reconstruction. Although not completely eliminated, the limitations of earlier CT technique, such as patient motion, lower resolution in reconstructed images, and relative insensitivity of CT for axially oriented fractures, are greatly diminished. Reformatted CT views in sagittal, coronal, or other planes are essential in such cases, as well as for viewing alignment. As CT increases in speed and technical capability, it has become feasible to incorporate it in a routine manner in the evaluation of major trauma, especially in cervical spine evaluation.[4-7]

In addition to planar (2D) reconstruction views, 3D projection views can be useful for evaluating the position of fractures. Considerable variation is possible in reconstruction techniques. The images can be created using surface reconstruction projection or varying degrees of apparent transparency of the reconstructed image. Each has advantages in specific situations, and the user of CT machines should become familiar with the options available.

Magnetic Resonance Imaging

The value of MRI for evaluating acute spine trauma may not be obvious. MRI is relatively insensitive to detection of fractures, since cortical bone provides very little signal and appears black on MRI. MRI has significant limitations in the acutely injured patient, including challenges in patient monitoring, longer imaging times than with radiography or CT, and difficulties in using standard coils in a patient with spine immobilization. For these practical reasons, MRI is often more suitable in the first few days than the first few hours after trauma. Nevertheless, MRI has unique advantages in assessing acute spine trauma.

MRI is highly sensitive to soft tissues, especially for edema.[8-10] MRI is the best method for visualizing the spinal cord. Compression or deformity of the spinal cord, edema, and hemorrhage are visualized well with MRI. It is also excellent for evaluating the intervertebral discs (Fig. 171-1). For example, detection of an acute disc disruption may alter plans for the surgical approach.[11] Cases have been reported in which the reduction of a dislocation worsened symptoms because of further herniation or displacement of disc material. MRI permits detection of such herniation before surgery. Ligament disruption can occasionally be directly visualized with MRI, especially the anterior and posterior longitudinal ligaments. Some evidence suggests that the extent of ligament disruption may correlate with the risk of instability in cervical spine dorsal element fractures.

The soft tissues around the vertebra are also visualized with MRI. Extensive edema can serve as a marker for acute injury and the need for further evaluation. Deep, interspinous edema in the setting of acute trauma may be an indication of high risk of instability due to flexion injury. Tears

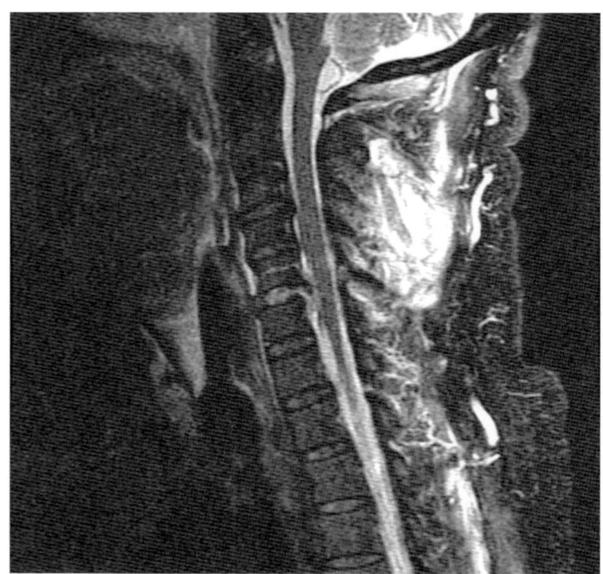

FIGURE 171-1. Traumatic disc and ligament disruption. Sagittal fast inversion-recovery MRI shows disruption of both anterior and posterior longitudinal ligaments at C5-6 and disc disruption with traumatic disc herniation and ventral and dorsal soft tissue edema. The findings were confirmed at surgery.

or stretching of the anterior and posterior longitudinal ligaments are especially concerning for instability. MRI can be helpful in a variety of clinical situations in which the combination of clinical and initial imaging findings is ambiguous or nondefinitive. For example, degenerative changes are very common in the cervical spine and can make detection of acute fractures difficult. Although CT can help to identify fractures, subluxation or chronic deformity can still be a challenge. A negative MRI in such situations, showing no evidence of any significant nearby soft tissue edema, makes acute injury unlikely as a cause of subluxation. MRI can be especially helpful when clinical assessment is limited, such as in the obtunded or intubated patient.[12]

Unexpected worsening of neurologic status after spine trauma can be due to a variety of factors. MRI may reveal such causes as epidural hematoma, disc herniation, or spinal cord edema from infarction.

The limitations of MRI mentioned earlier can be overcome in most cases. Monitoring is essential in the acutely injured patient. MRI-compatible monitoring equipment is available. The patient must be screened for the presence of metallic devices or metal within the body that would preclude MRI. Although standard spine coils may not be usable with a cervical collar, other coils can still permit diagnostic images. Faster imaging techniques continue to be developed for MRI, and it is often not necessary or appropriate to use the same sequences for acute trauma patients that would be used for evaluation of degenerative disc disease, for example. The specific sequences to be used can be tailored to the clinical situation.

Although it is impossible to specify MRI parameters that should be used because of the great variety of manufacturers, machines, and software available, some broad principles apply. A T2-weighted sequence is important for detecting edema. Fast-spin echo imaging, in which multiple echoes are acquired during each pulse sequence, is nearly always used in standard spine imaging. Such sequences are much faster than spin echo sequences and produce excellent signal-to-noise and high-quality images. Fast-spin echo sequences can be excellent for visualizing the spinal cord, for example. However, it is important to note that fat remains very bright on such sequences, even with T2-weighting. Therefore, if adjacent soft tissue edema is to be demonstrated, different sequences must be used that suppress the signal from fat (Fig. 171-2). A fat saturation pulse can be added to fast-spin echo imaging sequences. Alternatively, inversion recovery sequences (short-tau inversion recovery [STIR]) accomplish the same effect of heavy T2 weighting and fat suppression.

Edema within the bone marrow is also well demonstrated with MRI. This appears as low signal (dark) on T1-weighted images, replacing the normally bright signal from fat in the marrow and high signal on fat-suppressed T2-weighted images. Acute fractures, especially those that involve the vertebral body, cause marrow changes, but bone contusions that do not result in cortical bone disruption can also result in marrow edema. Over time, marrow signal intensity usually returns to an appearance close to that of normal vertebral body marrow. Thus, signal intensity in marrow of a compressed vertebral body that matches that of adjacent, normal vertebrae provides evidence for a chronic rather than an acute injury.

The sensitivity of MRI for acute soft tissue injury depends on several factors. Edema resolves over several days; the precise time course has not been defined but clearly depends on the severity of the original injury. In our experience, soft tissue edema associated with an acute cervical spine injury is likely to be less extensive on MRI in the setting of axial load injuries. Presumably, this is due to less stretching and tearing of the soft tissues. For example, a minimally displaced Jefferson burst fracture may result in very little soft tissue edema. When these limitations are understood, however, MRI can play a very useful adjunct role in assessing major acute cervical spine trauma.

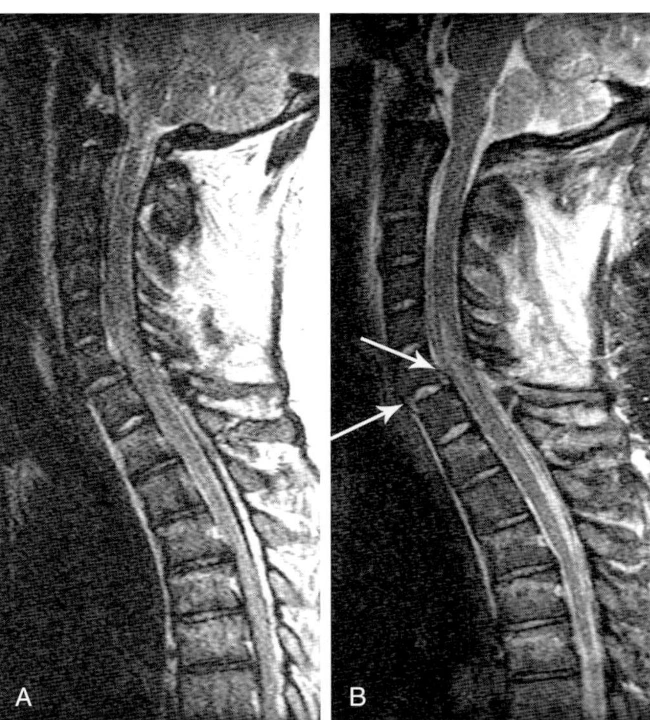

FIGURE 171-2. Fat suppression MRI for soft tissue evaluation. MRI was performed on a young man with myelopathic symptoms after a motor vehicle accident. **A,** Sagittal fast-spin echo T2-weighted image shows slight subluxation at C6-7, but edema from soft tissue injury is difficult to identify because fat also remains bright. **B,** On a sagittal fast-spin echo inversion-recovery image the fat is now dark, but edema in the dorsal soft tissues, the marrow space of upper thoracic vertebral bodies, and prevertebral space is very conspicuous. Anterior and posterior longitudinal ligaments at C6-7 are stretched (*arrows*).

Motion Radiography Studies

Radiographs of the spine in different positions (i.e., flexion and extension views in a lateral position) are excellent for evaluating the stability of the spine in a delayed or chronic setting (Fig. 171-3). Such studies have significant limitations in the acute setting, however. Most importantly, they pose major risks if the spine is in fact unstable. Complications of flexion-extension radiographs are rare but well known. If motion studies are to be undertaken, it is highly desirable that the patient be fully alert, cooperative, and capable of controlling or stopping the motion. If flexion and extension are performed on an obtunded or comatose patient, performing the study under fluoroscopy should improve the safety. The motion can be immediately stopped as soon as subluxation or abnormal movement is visualized. However, data on the safety and accuracy of performing motion radiography on an obtunded patient in the setting of acute injury are very limited. Such studies are often time-consuming, and visualization of the cervicothoracic junction is frequently difficult.

A second limitation in the acute setting is a high incidence of muscle spasm or guarding. From one quarter to one third of patients with acute cervical spine injury may have

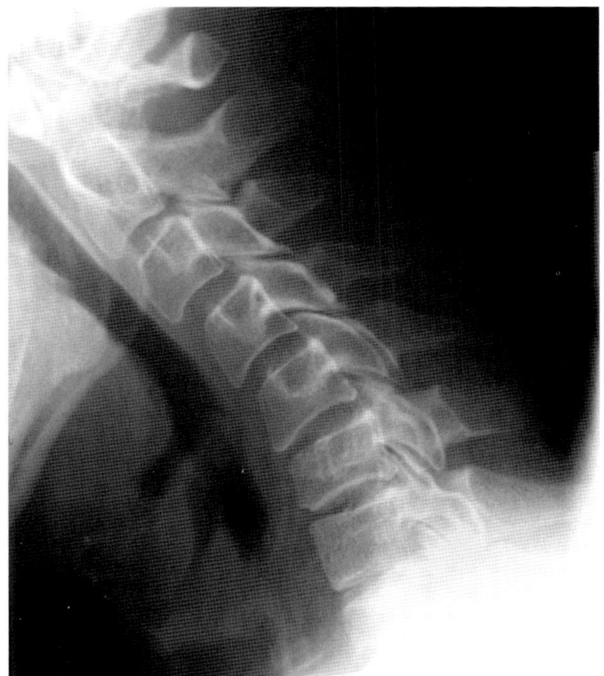

FIGURE 171-3. Instability on flexion film. Flexion lateral radiograph obtained on a delayed basis after cervical spine trauma shows focal kyphosis and dorsal widening. Alignment in neutral position was normal.

nondiagnostic results because there is inadequate movement of the neck to assess stability.[13] Delayed studies, several weeks after trauma and after muscle spasm has subsided, with the patient cooperative and in control of neck motion, remain the gold standard for evaluating the stability of the cervical spine.

Myelography

Because of the availability of MRI, myelography has a very limited role in the evaluation of spine trauma. There are occasional situations in which patency of the spinal canal must be assessed and MRI is not possible.

Imaging Findings

Cervicocranial Junction and Upper Cervical Spine

Upper cervical spine injuries can be multiple, complex, and difficult to identify on imaging.

C1 Fractures

The Jefferson burst fracture of C1 is a relatively common injury. CT can demonstrate the multiple fractures of the ring of C1 and the extent of displacement (Fig. 171-4). Plain films usually show prevertebral soft tissue swelling. Some components of the fractures can be visible on plain radiographs, more so if the fractures are displaced. The lateral masses of C1 are likely to be displaced laterally if the transverse ligament is disrupted. Total displacement of greater than 7 mm as seen on an odontoid view has been suggested as a guideline to the presence of transverse ligament rupture.[14] The transverse ligament can be visualized directly on MRI, and fluid signal in place of the expected low signal intensity of the ligament is evidence of rupture.[15]

The imaging findings just described apply to adults. In at least the first 4 years of life, the lateral masses of C1 often project lateral to the lateral margins of C2 on an AP view.[16] Because Jefferson fractures are uncommon in children, CT may be necessary to demonstrate such fractures in children.

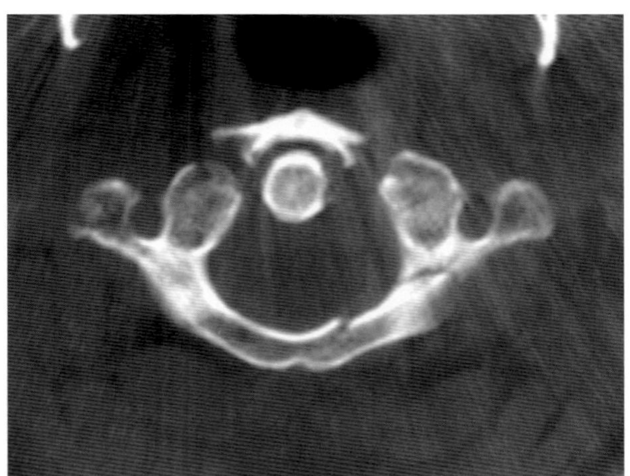

FIGURE 171-4. Jefferson fracture. Patient fell from a ladder onto the head. CT shows multiple fractures of the ring of C1.

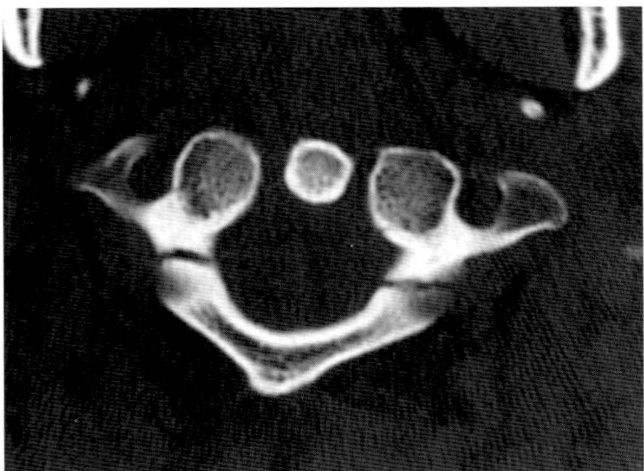

FIGURE 171-5. Dorsal arch C1 fracture. Extension mechanism: CT shows bilateral fractures through the dorsal arch of C1; the ventral arch was intact.

Isolated fractures of the dorsal arch of C1 can occur with hyperextension injuries (Fig. 171-5). In such cases, prevertebral soft tissue swelling would likely be absent, and the dorsal arch fracture can be seen on a lateral radiograph. Another type of hyperextension injury at C1 is an avulsion at the ventral caudal portion of the ventral arch, at the attachment of the atlantoaxial ligament. In this case, the fracture is visible on the lateral view, and focal prevertebral soft tissue swelling is usually present.

Transverse Ligament Injury

Transverse ligament rupture can be seen in association with a variety of upper cervical spine fractures, and this possibility should be considered in any such injury. In addition, transverse ligament injury uncommonly may occur without other fractures. Loss of integrity of the transverse ligament can result either from rupture in the midportion of the ligament or from avulsion of the ligament at one of the attachments to the lateral mass of C1. In the latter case, a small fracture is often visible at the tubercle where the ligament attaches (see Fig. 171-26). If the ventral atlantodental space is widened, transverse ligament rupture should be suspected. The ligament itself can be seen directly using MRI. In the case of rupture, fluid signal intensity (bright on T2-weighted images) can be seen in the expected location of the ligament, and fluid is also likely to be present between the dens and ventral arch of C1.

C2 Fractures

Odontoid fractures can occur from a variety of mechanisms. Anderson and D'Alonzo[17] described three types of odontoid fractures: type I, an oblique fracture near the apex of the dens; type II, a transverse fracture through the lower third of the dens but above the body of C2 (Fig. 171-6); and type III, which is a fracture below the base of the dens and through the body of C2 (Fig. 171-7). As with transversely oriented fractures elsewhere, odontoid fractures can be difficult to identify by CT. Axial images may show only a region of lucency or subtle gaps in the cortical margin. Reconstructed images from thin-slice axial images, especially from rapid spiral acquisitions, can be very helpful for identifying odontoid fractures on CT. Plain radiographs should be carefully inspected for signs

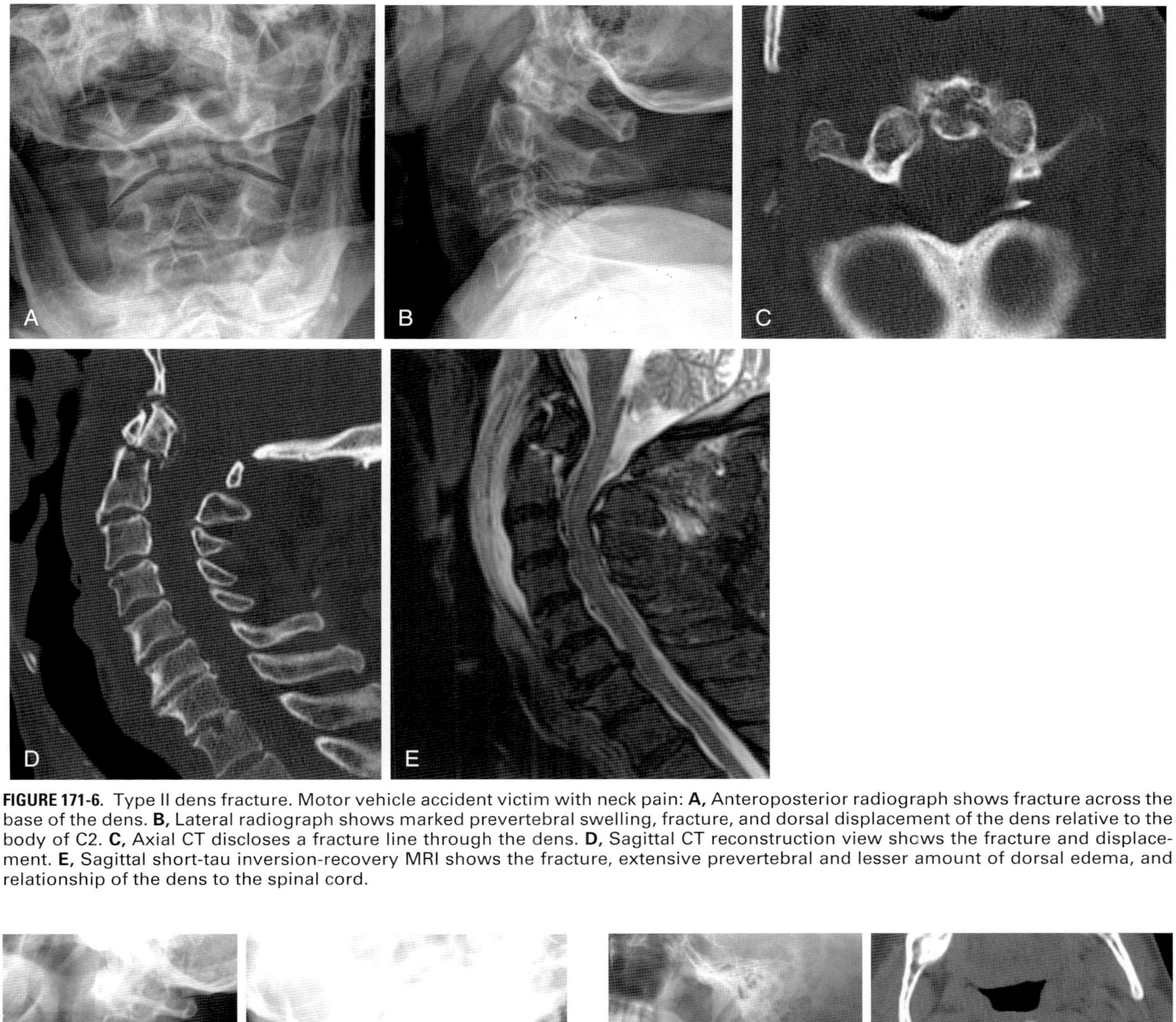

FIGURE 171-6. Type II dens fracture. Motor vehicle accident victim with neck pain: **A,** Anteroposterior radiograph shows fracture across the base of the dens. **B,** Lateral radiograph shows marked prevertebral swelling, fracture, and dorsal displacement of the dens relative to the body of C2. **C,** Axial CT discloses a fracture line through the dens. **D,** Sagittal CT reconstruction view shows the fracture and displacement. **E,** Sagittal short-tau inversion-recovery MRI shows the fracture, extensive prevertebral and lesser amount of dorsal edema, and relationship of the dens to the spinal cord.

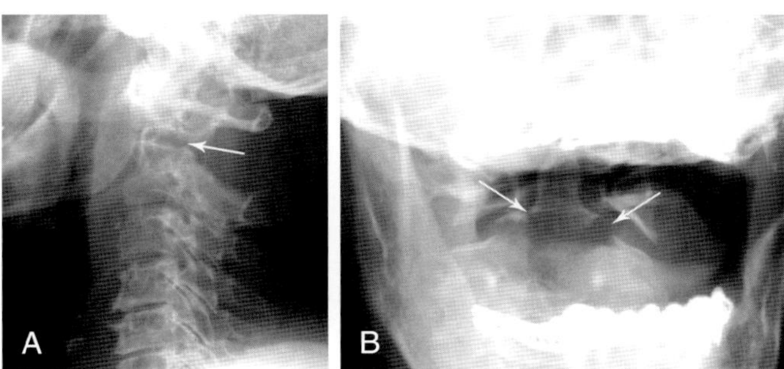

FIGURE 171-7. Low dens (type III) fracture. Motor vehicle accident patient: **A,** Lateral radiograph shows lucency that disrupts the ring appearance (*arrow*), unlike the type II fracture in Figure 171-6. **B,** The low fracture, actually a fracture through the rostral portion of the body of C2, is easily seen in the anteroposterior view (*arrows*).

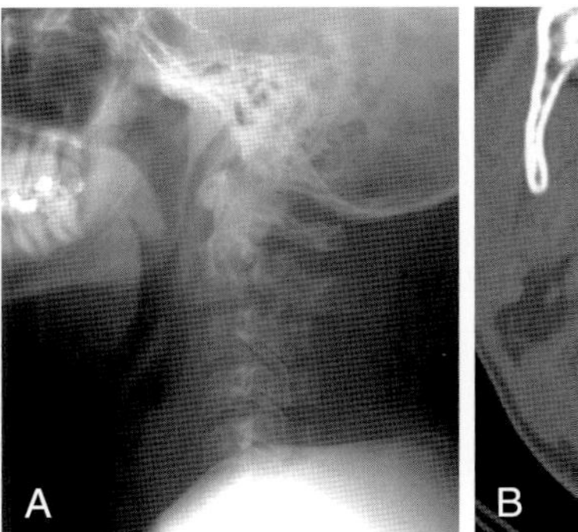

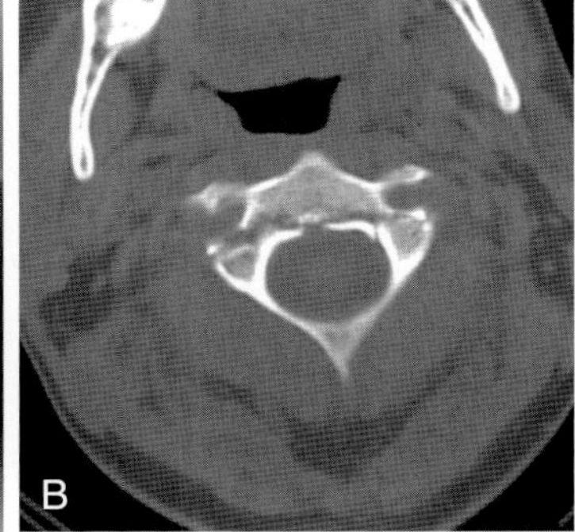

FIGURE 171-8. C2 body fracture, type I. **A,** Lateral radiograph shows lucency in the dorsal body of C2, with prevertebral soft tissue swelling. **B,** CT shows fractures through the dorsal portion of the C2 body.

of odontoid fractures, including prevertebral soft tissue swelling, abnormal angulation of the odontoid process, offset of the dens with respect to the body of C2, and disruption of the cortical margin. The type III fracture (or type 3 C2 body fracture) is a horizontally oriented, rostral fracture at the base of the dens. In such fractures, the lateral radiograph shows a break in the apparent ring that results from the superimposition of densities from the junction of the pedicle and body, dens and body, and dorsal cortex of the C2 body.[18] The AP or odontoid view usually shows a fracture with inferior convexity.

Fractures of the body of C2, which have received relatively little attention, include coronally oriented dorsal fractures (type 1), which are similar in some respects to the hangman's fracture through the pars interarticularis of C2 (Fig. 171-8);

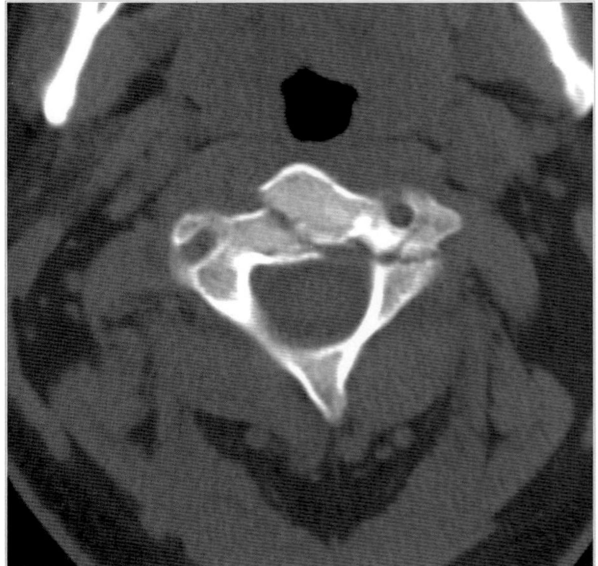

FIGURE 171-9. C2 body fracture, type 2. Axial CT of a patient who fell from a ladder onto his head shows an oblique fracture through the C2 body, with an additional fracture through the left lamina.

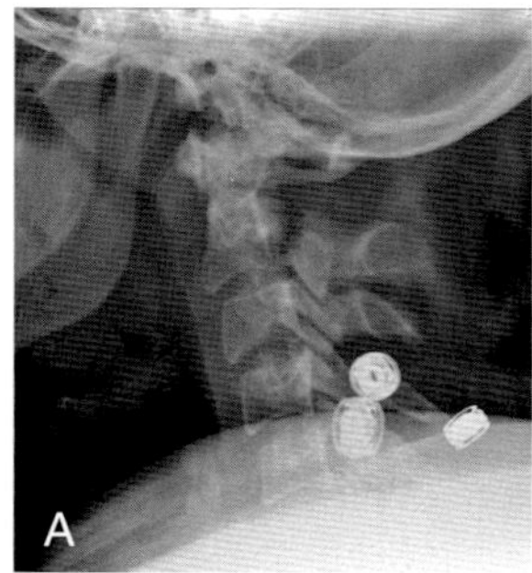

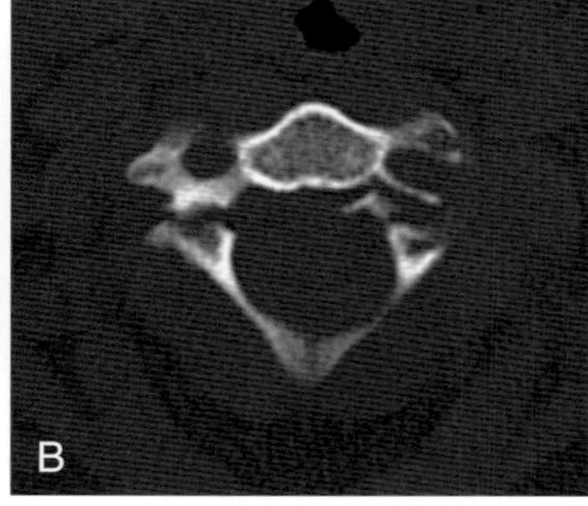

FIGURE 171-10. Traumatic spondylolisthesis (hangman's fracture). **A,** Lateral radiograph shows fractures through the pars interarticularis, with ventral displacement of the body of C2 relative to C3 in this case. **B,** Axial CT in this case shows bilateral fractures through the pars interarticularis.

oblique, sagittally oriented fractures (type 2), which result from axial loading (Fig. 171-9)[19]; and the horizontally oriented type 3 fracture described earlier (see Fig. 171-7). CT is particularly helpful in defining the location and extent of fractures in C2 body fractures.

The hangman's fracture, or traumatic spondylolisthesis, consists of bilateral fractures through the pars interarticularis (Fig. 171-10).[20,21] It is usually visible on lateral radiographs as a lucency, with prevertebral soft tissue swelling. The Effendi classification of these fractures is based on the extent of displacement: type I consists of minimal displacement; type II shows ventral displacement and an abnormal C2-3 disc; and type III is ventral displacement of the body of C2 in flexion, with bilateral facet dislocation of C2-3.[22]

The extension teardrop fracture of C2 consists of an avulsion of the ventral caudal corner of the C2 body at the attachment of the atlantoaxial ligament. A characteristic triangular shape is evident on lateral radiographs, usually with accompanying prevertebral soft tissue swelling.

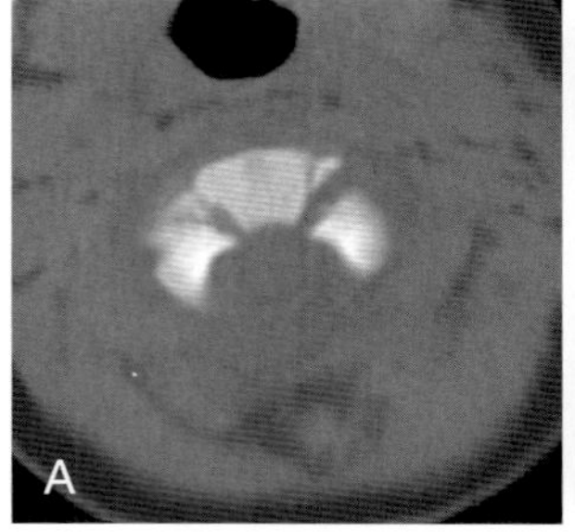

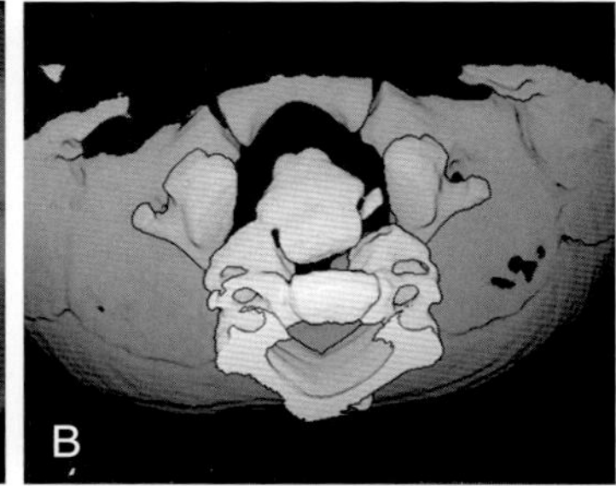

FIGURE 171-11. C2 synchondrosis fracture in an infant. An unrestrained infant in a motor vehicle crash had abnormalities at the C2 level on plain film. **A,** Axial CT shows fractures that mostly involve the neurocentral synchondrosis, separating the body and odontoid from the neural arch. **B,** 3D reconstruction from below shows the separation through the synchondrosis. The ventral aspect of the spine, including the ventral arch of C1, has been excluded to allow visualization of C2.

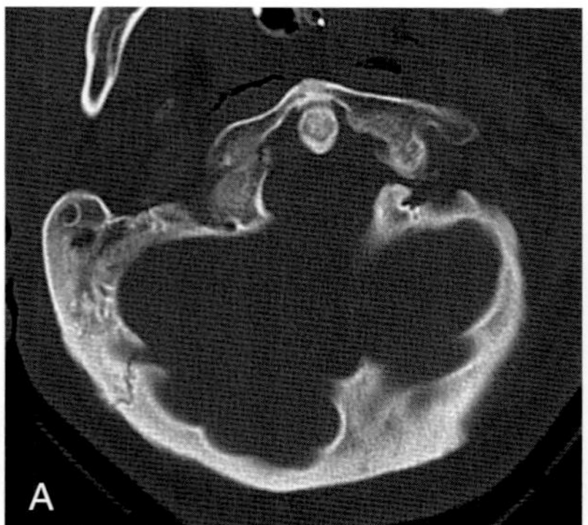

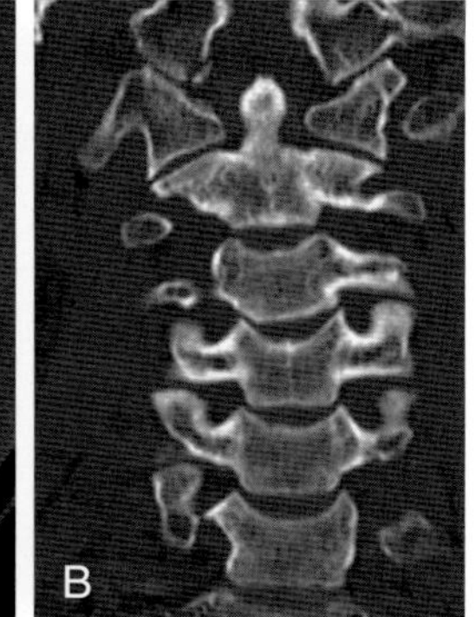

FIGURE 171-12. Occipital condyle fracture. **A,** Axial CT shows lucency in the right occipital condyle. **B,** Coronal reconstruction demonstrates more clearly the oblique right occipital condyle fracture.

Children can suffer a unique injury of C2, fracture through the subdental synchondrosis. The dens is separated in a sharp, geometric margin from the centrum of C2 below (Fig. 171-11).

Craniocervical Junction

Occipital condyle fractures are especially difficult to identify on plain radiographs. CT with thin-slice thickness and reconstruction images is the best imaging tool (Fig. 171-12). Occipital condyle fractures have also been classified in three groups. Type I fractures are compression fractures from axial loading. Type II fractures are basilar occiput fractures that extend into the occipital condyle. Type III fractures result from avulsion, a result of lateral bending and forced rotation. Because of ligamentous injury, type III are the condyle fractures most likely to be unstable.[23,24]

Atlanto-occipital dislocation is often a fatal injury, although less severe forms are increasingly being recognized. Prominent upper cervical prevertebral soft tissue hematoma is nearly always present (Fig. 171-13). Several methods of measuring atlanto-occipital dislocation have been proposed. The Powers ratio is the relationship of the distance from basion (*B*) to the dorsal arch of the atlas (*C*), compared with the distance from opisthion (*O*) to the midpoint of the dorsal surface of the ventral arch (*A*).[25] The ratio *BC*/*OA*, which is

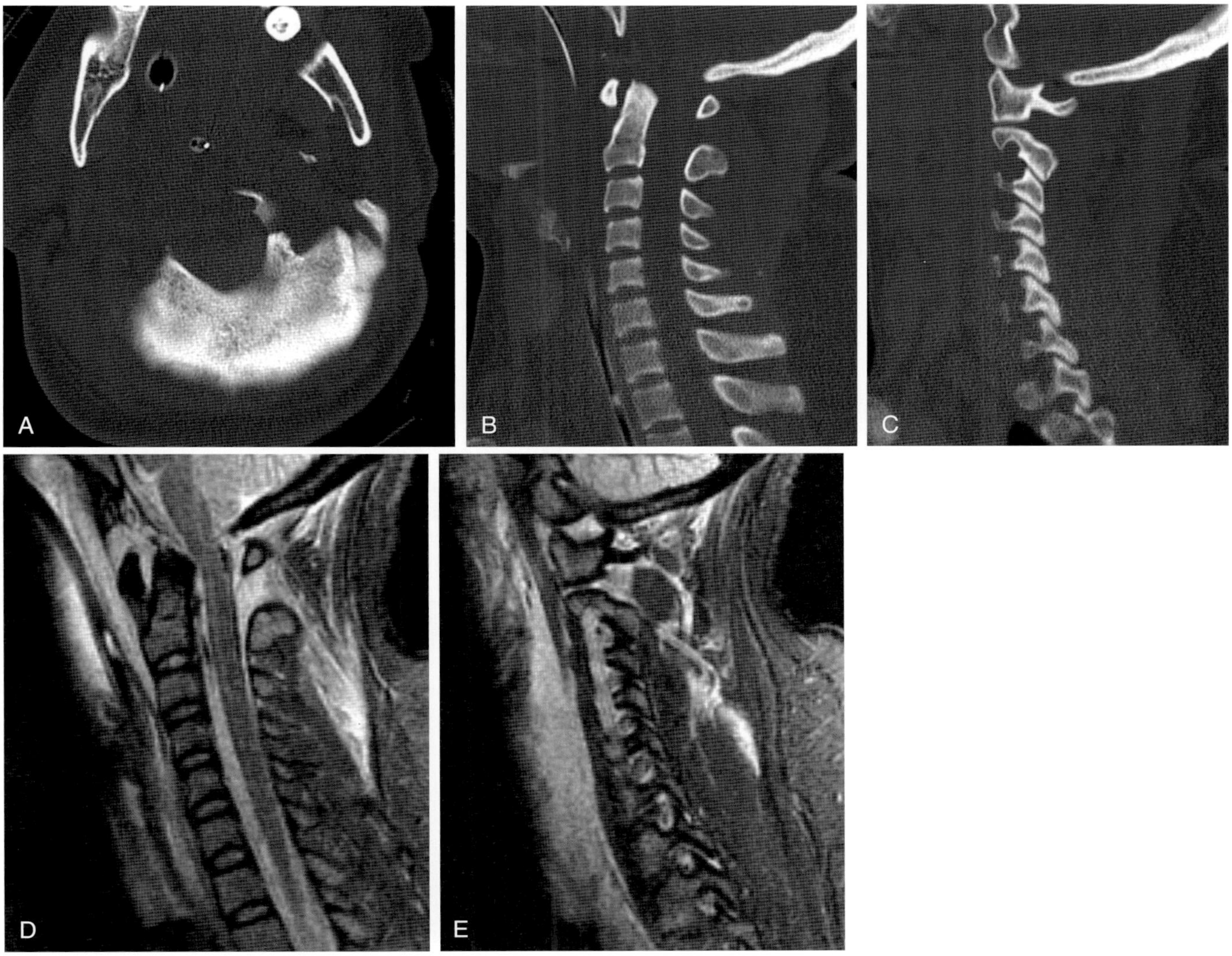

FIGURE 171-13. Atlanto-occipital dissociation. **A,** Axial CT through the cervicocranial junction is most remarkable for what is not present—little bone is visible at what should be the atlanto-occipital joint. **B,** Sagittal CT reconstruction demonstrates distraction between the tip of the clivus and the tip of the dens. **C,** Subluxation of the atlanto-occipital joint is demonstrated on a parasagittal view. **D,** Sagittal inversion-recovery MRI shows extensive ventral and dorsal soft tissue edema, disruption of the tectorial membrane, and the effect of the dissociation on the spinal cord. **E,** A parasagittal image from the same MRI sequence as part **D** demonstrates fluid in the disrupted joint space.

normally less than 1, increases with ventral dislocation. The bony landmarks to determine the Powers ratio can be difficult to identify, and Harris and colleagues have described two measurements that are easier to perform and less sensitive to the direction of dislocation.[26,27] Both measurements are performed on a lateral radiograph (Fig. 171-14). The first is between a dorsal axial line upward from the dorsal vertebral body of C2 and the basion. The basion-axial interval should be no less than 6 mm or more than 12 mm, in both adults and children. The second measurement is between the basion and the tip of the dens, the basion-dens interval. This distance should not be more than 12 mm. This basion-dens interval depends on complete ossification of the dens and therefore may not be obtainable in children younger than 13 years. Evaluation with multidetector CT is somewhat different.[28] The normal basion-dens interval is less than 8.5 mm in 95% of the normal adult population. The basion-axial interval is less reliable and useful on CT. The atlanto-occipital interval, or distance between

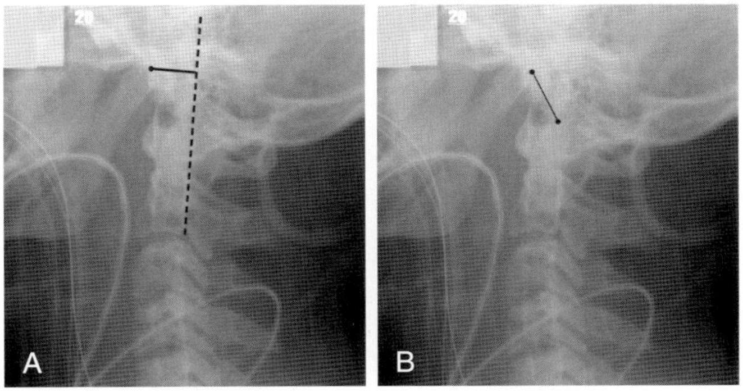

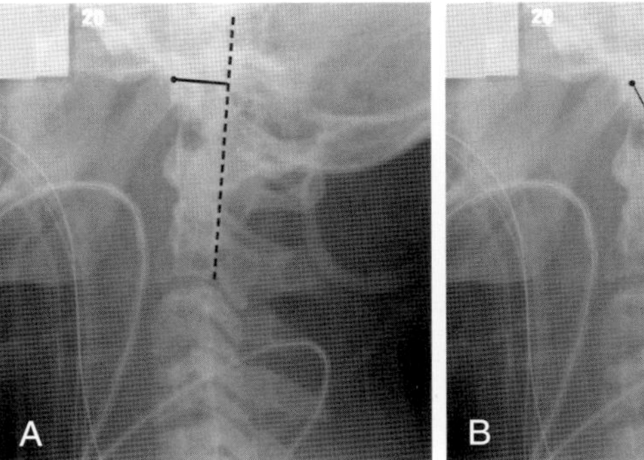

FIGURE 171-14. Craniocervical relationships and atlanto-occipital dissociation (AOD). Lateral radiograph of a patient who suffered AOD shows severe prevertebral soft tissue swelling and distraction of the cranium from the spine. Measurements described by Harris et al.[26,27] are illustrated: **A,** Basion-axial interval, distance from basion to a line extended upward from the dorsal margin of the body of C2. **B,** Basion-dens interval, distance from basion to the tip of the dens. (Copyright 2001, University of New Mexico Department of Radiology, Neuroradiology Section.)

the occipital condyle and C1 lateral mass at the midpoint of the joint, should be less than 1.5 mm. The relationship between the condyle and C1 lateral mass is readily assessed on parasagittal CT reconstructions and should be evaluated routinely (see Fig. 171-13C).

Subaxial Cervical Spine Injuries

Axial loading injuries in the lower cervical spine result in burst fractures. The basic pattern of the burst fracture is similar throughout the thoracic and lumbar spine, as well. The degree of comminution is variable, but there is usually a prominent sagittal component. Dorsal element fractures are common and variable. CT is very helpful in determining the extent of fractures (Fig. 171-15). Involvement of multiple vertebrae can occur with more severe injuries. MRI can directly demonstrate the relationship of displaced bone to the spinal cord, spinal cord compression, and spinal cord edema and hematoma, as well as disc disruption.

A variety of flexion injuries can occur in the subaxial cervical spine. Many of these injuries result in a pattern of dorsal widening or fanning of the facets and spinous processes at the level of injury (Fig. 171-16). This pattern of flexion injury is an important finding on lateral radiographs. Dorsal ligament injury without fracture can result in instability from flexion sprain. A simple ventral compression fracture results in loss of ventral height of a vertebral body. Dorsal ligament injury may or may not accompany a compression fracture. Focal kyphosis is often observed at the level of compression.[29-31] A fairly common pattern of flexion injury in the lower cervical spine is an avulsion fracture of the spinous process, or "clay-shoveler's fracture."

More serious flexion injuries can cause actual disruption of the facet joints and bilateral facet dislocation (Fig. 171-17). The vertebra above the level of dislocation is ventrally displaced relative to the vertebra below the level of dislocation. Dorsal widening and focal kyphosis are observed. CT often reveals small fractures of the articular processes at the level of dislocation. MRI shows a typical pattern of extensive dorsal soft tissue edema from the level of dislocation and above; and the relationship of the spinal cord to the narrowed spinal canal can be seen on MRI.

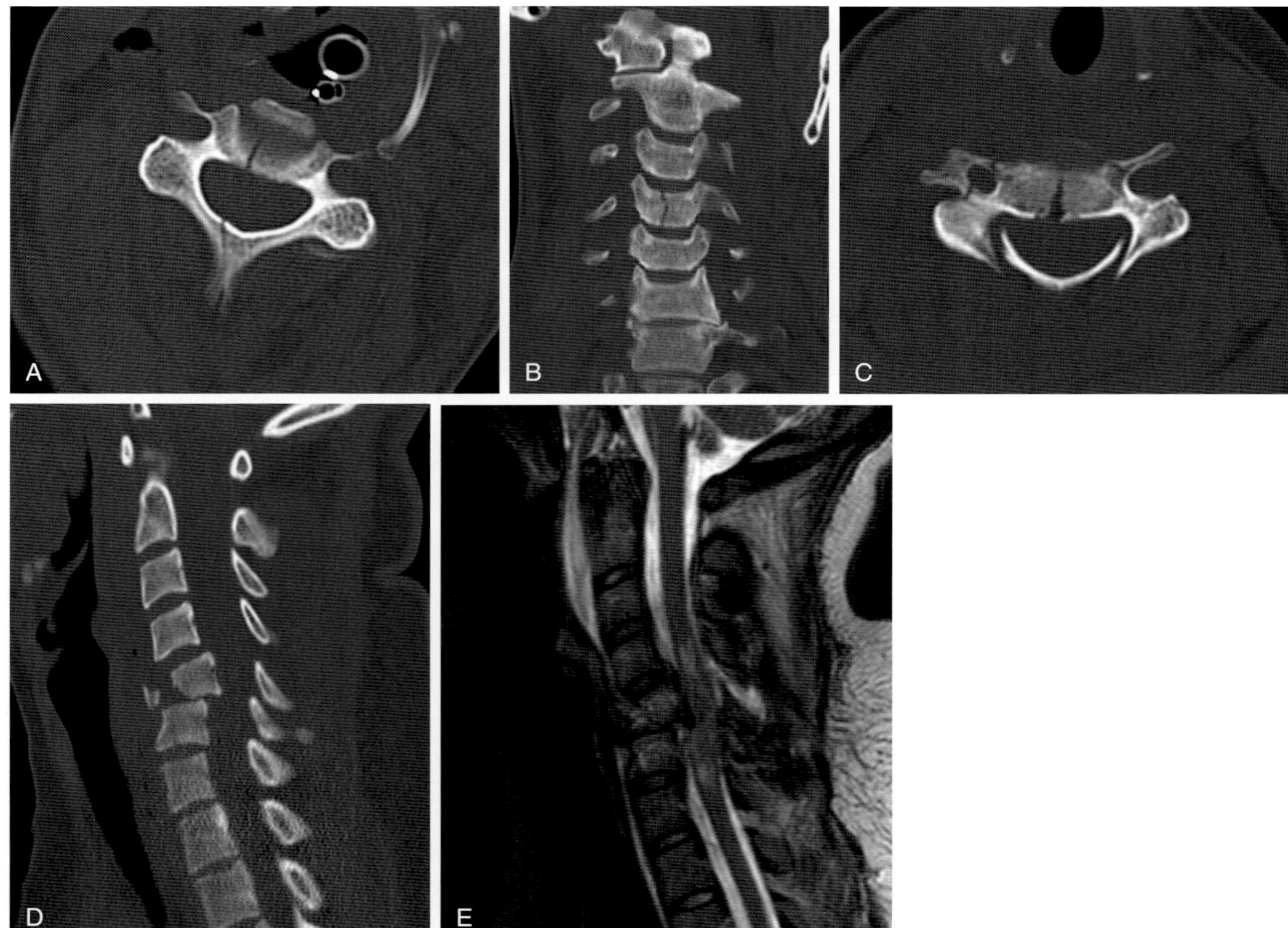

FIGURE 171-15. Burst fractures. **A,** CT of a patient in a motor vehicle accident through the C4 level reveals minimally displaced fractures, including sagittal fracture through the body and fracture of the right lamina. **B,** Coronal reconstruction shows the sagittally oriented fracture. **C,** CT at the C5 level of a different patient, who fell from a considerable height, shows much more comminuted and displaced pattern. **D,** Sagittal reconstruction shows displacement of bone into the spinal canal in this case. **E,** Sagittal fast-spin echo T2-weighted MRI of the second patient additionally shows the edema and possible hemorrhage within the spinal cord.

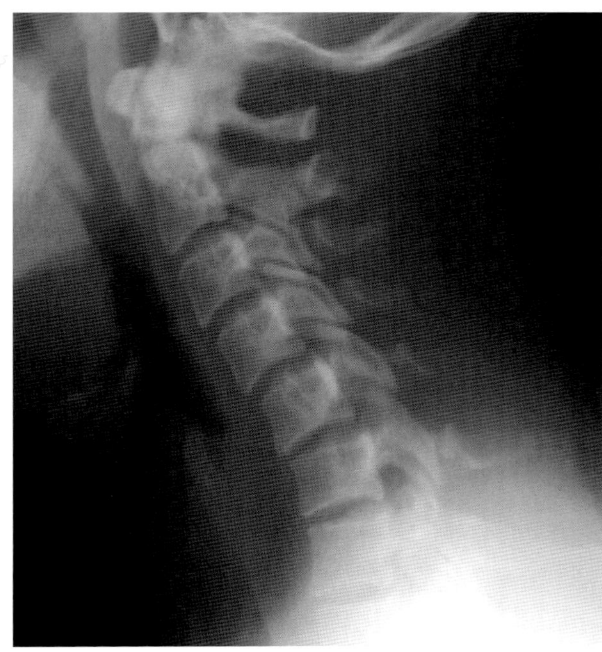

FIGURE 171-16. Flexion sprain. Lateral cervical spine radiograph demonstrates kyphosis and dorsal widening at C5-6, and to a lesser extent at C6-7.

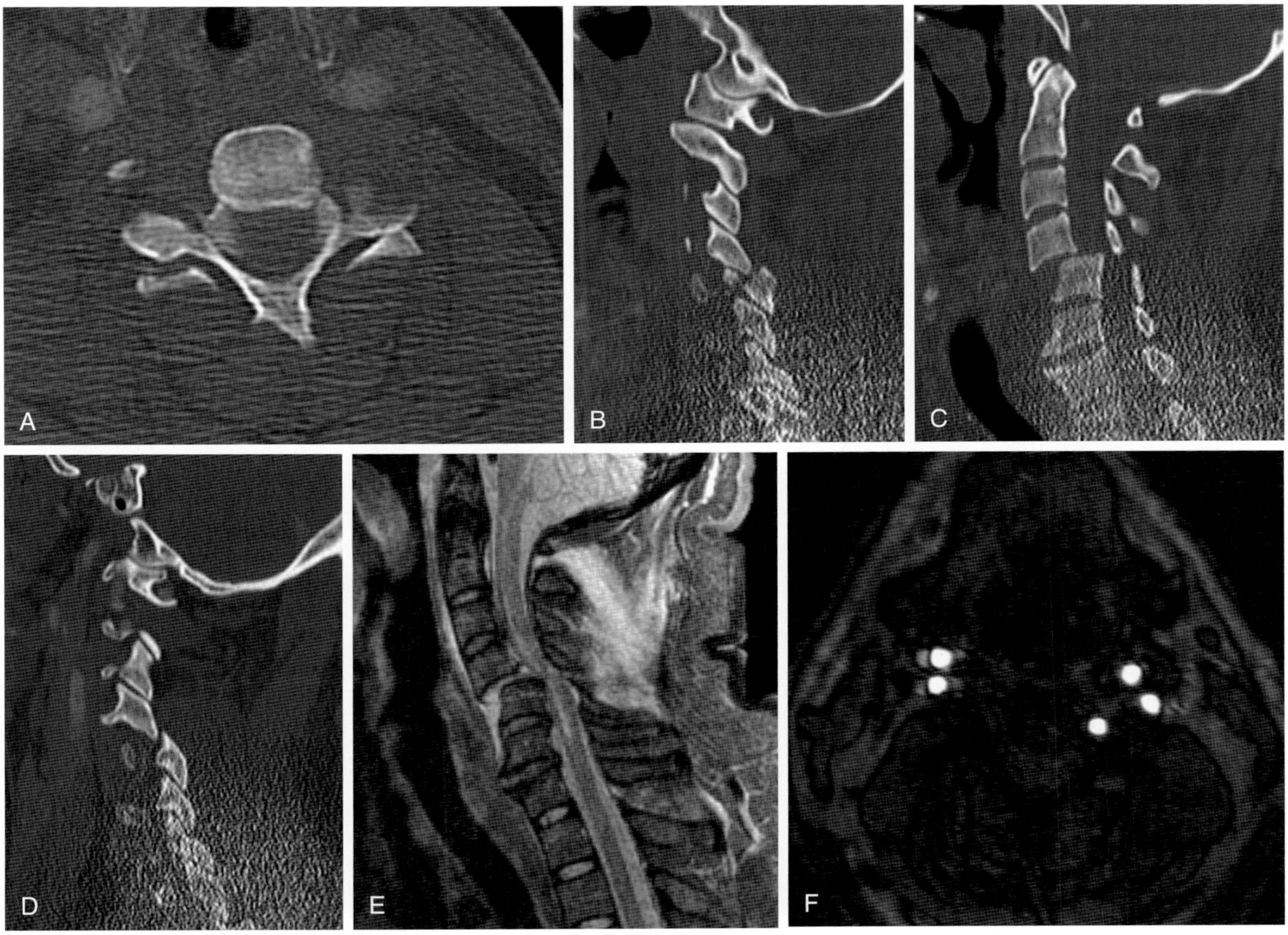

FIGURE 171-17. Bilateral facet dislocation. Patient was quadriplegic after motor vehicle accident. **A,** Axial CT shows reversal of the normal relationship of the facets bilaterally. **B–D,** Sagittal CT reconstruction views, (left, midline, and right, respectively) show greater than 50% subluxation of C4 on C5, bilateral facet dislocation, and fracture of the left C5 lateral mass. **E,** Sagittal inversion-recovery MRI shows spinal cord compression and edema and extensive soft tissue edema in addition to the subluxation and stretching of anterior and posterior longitudinal ligaments. **F,** Axial source image from magnetic resonance angiography of the same patient demonstrates no flow in the right vertebral artery, with intact flow in the left vertebral and bilateral carotid arteries.

A flexion teardrop fracture is one of the most severe flexion injuries of the cervical spine. Lateral radiographs show a large triangular fragment of bone from the ventral caudal corner of the fractured vertebra. Unlike the extension teardrop fracture, there is pronounced flexion of the spine at the level of injury. The typical clinical picture of anterior cord syndrome also distinguishes the flexion teardrop fracture.[32]

Extension mechanisms can cause a variety of cervical spine injuries. Compression of the lamina can cause laminar fractures, visible on lateral or oblique radiographs, and especially CT.

Hyperextension dislocation causes transient dislocation through a disc level and compression of the spinal cord. The usual clinical picture is a central cord syndrome. Radiographic signs are straightening of the cervical spine, diffuse prevertebral swelling, and often an avulsion fracture of the inferior end plate above the level of dislocation (Fig. 171-18). Such a fracture is horizontally oriented and is wider than it is tall. Disc space widening or gas within the disc space is less commonly seen.[33,34] MRI shows the prevertebral edema, abnormal signal in the affected disc space, and edema within the spinal cord. In the author's experience, MRI also often shows dorsal soft tissue edema. Another cause of central cord syndrome resulting from hyperextension was described by Taylor et al.[35,36] In such cases, preexisting osteophytes narrow the spinal canal and cause transient spinal cord compression. Diffuse prevertebral soft tissue swelling is lacking in such cases, but MRI shows edema within the spinal cord and the extent of spondylosis (Fig. 171-19).

Unilateral facet dislocation results from combined flexion and rotation. Such cases have a typical constellation of imaging findings (Fig. 171-20).[37,38] Lateral radiographs show an abrupt change from a typical lateral appearance below the dislocation to an appearance above that level of an oblique projection. The visualization of both facets on the lateral view just above the dislocation gives a "bow-tie" appearance.

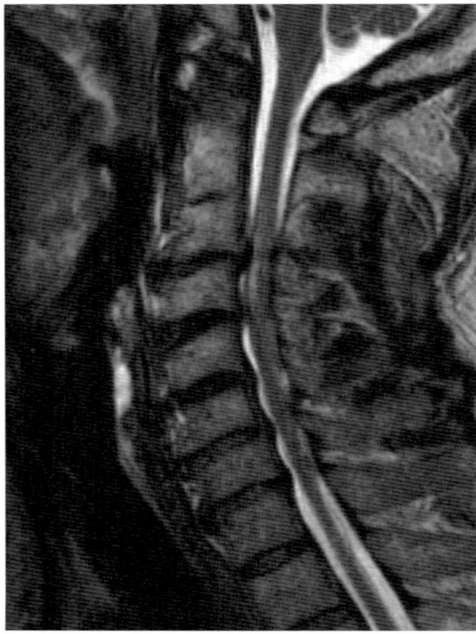

FIGURE 171-19. Central cord injury from Taylor mechanism. A man who fell and suffered a hyperextension injury with a central cord syndrome. Sagittal T2-weighted MRI shows spondylosis and spinal stenosis in the lower cervical spine and edema in the spinal cord.

On the AP view, there is an abrupt change in the line along the spinous processes. CT shows a reversal of the usual "clamshell" appearance of the facets where they are dislocated. In less severe cases, the facets may appear "perched" without frank dislocation, but this finding still implies major ligament and joint disruption.

Fractures involving the lateral masses, pedicles, and laminae can be very difficult to visualize on plain films. Close inspection of the lateral bony margins seen on AP views can

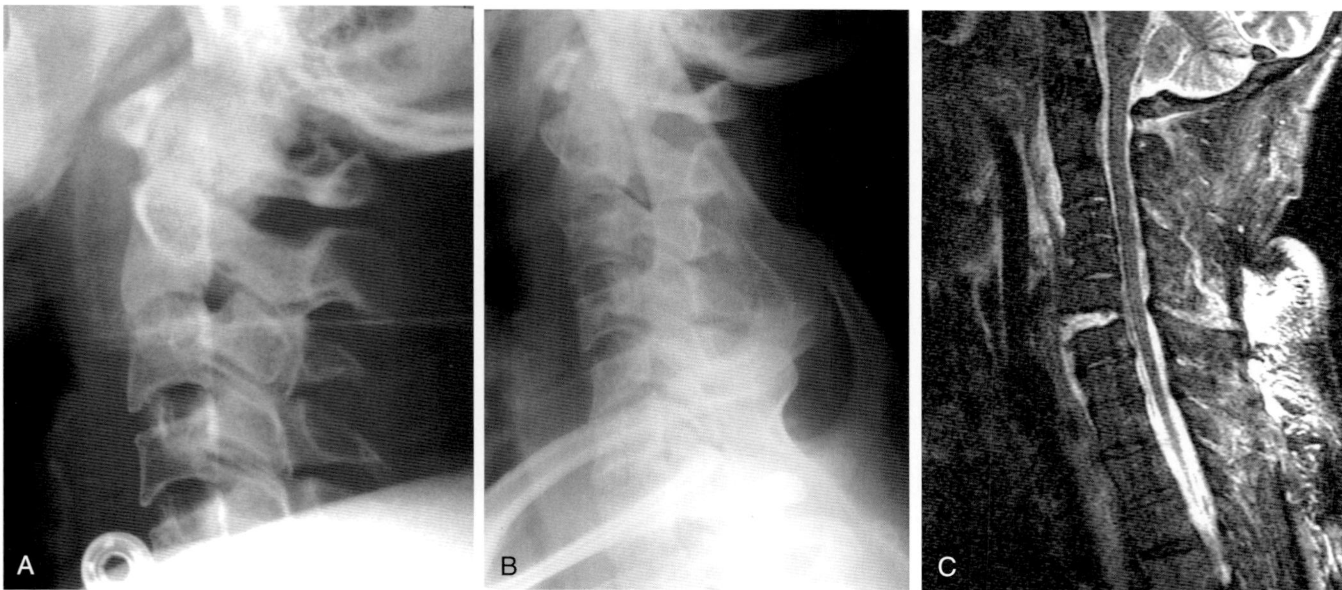

FIGURE 171-18. Hyperextension dislocation (hyperextension sprain). Lateral (**A**) and swimmer's (**B**) views of this patient who had a central cord syndrome after a motor vehicle accident show straightening of the cervical spine and diffuse prevertebral swelling. **C,** Sagittal inversion-recovery MRI of a different patient with hyperextension injury but no spinal cord injury shows disruption of the C6-7 disc space and anterior longitudinal ligament, with both prevertebral and dorsal edema.

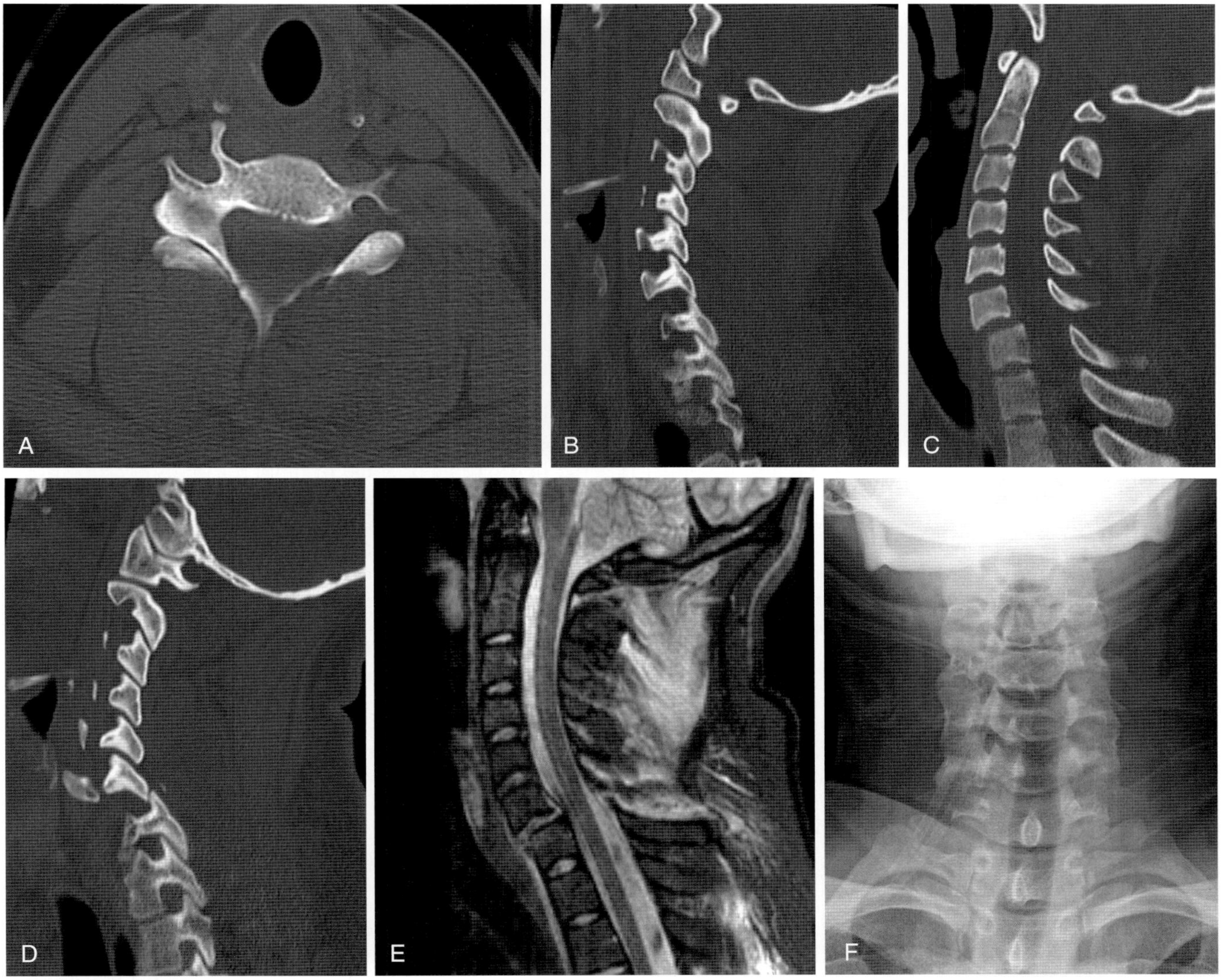

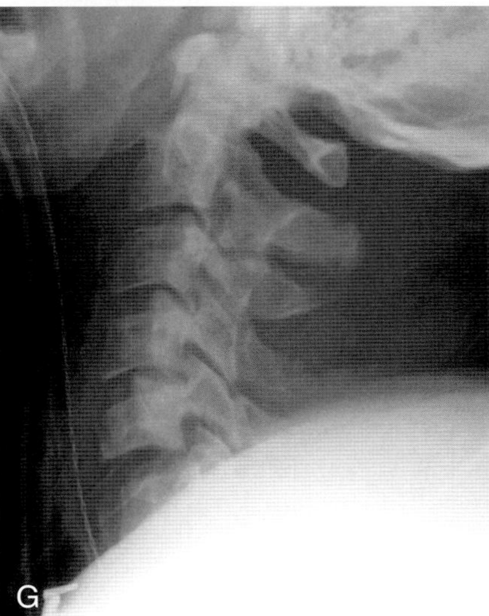

FIGURE 171-20. Unilateral facet dislocation. **A,** CT through the C6-7 level of a young man after a motor vehicle accident shows dislocation of the right facet joint, with reversal of the normal relationship of the facets. **B–D,** Sagittal CT reconstructions from left to right show mild subluxation on the left side (**B**), mild anterolisthesis in the midline with dorsal splaying (**C**), and facet dislocation on the right (**D**), with a small bone fragment dorsal to the dislocation. **E,** On sagittal inversion-recovery MRI the extent of ligamentous injury and edema is easily seen, with no evidence of spinal cord edema or compression. **F,** Anteroposterior radiograph shows a characteristic abrupt change in alignment of the spinous processes. The initial lateral radiograph (not shown) was obscured by the shoulders, but typical findings of unilateral facet dislocation are demonstrated on a different patient (**G**) who had dislocation at C5-6. There is an oblique orientation of the spine above this level and a straight lateral configuration below this level. Note the "bow-tie" shape of the articular processes above the level of dislocation.

show irregularity or overlap in some cases. If there is more extensive ligament injury and displacement, there may be rotational displacement that can simulate a unilateral facet dislocation on plain films. However, CT clearly demonstrates the location of fractures (Fig. 171-21). Fractures of both pedicle and lamina result in separation of the articular mass from the vertebral body and potential instability. MRI can be helpful in determining the extent of ligamentous injury, which may help predict the risk of instability.[39]

The injuries just described are those seen in some of the more common patterns of cervical spine injury. It is important to remember that fractures commonly occur at more than one level.

Identification of a fracture should not terminate the evaluation of the entire cervical spine.

Thoracic and Lumbar Spine

Indications for screening of the thoracic and lumbar spine in the setting of blunt trauma are not as clear-cut as in the cervical spine.[40,41] In the trauma patient with back pain, a good starting point for evaluation of thoracolumbar trauma is high-quality AP and lateral radiographs. However, if the patient is already getting chest/abdominal CT imaging, reconstructed axial bone windows with high-quality sagittal and coronal reformats are superior to plain radiography for the exclusion of trauma. In most cases, it suffices to obtain plain radiographs to screen the thoracolumbar spine in the obtunded or intoxicated patient and in the patient with unreliable clinical examinations.[40] Dedicated CT imaging of the thoracolumbar spine is usually reserved for patients with significant plain radiographic abnormalities, usually as a part of presurgical planning. In the setting of neurologic deficits, MRI is often indicated to exclude entities such as direct spinal cord injury, traumatic disc herniation, or epidural hematoma. In contrast to the cervical spine, MRI is not usually needed to exclude ligamentous injury if there is no associated fracture of the spine.

Along with more restricted movement in the thoracic and lumbar spine than in the cervical region, there exist fewer patterns of fracture. Compression fractures and burst fractures have features similar to those described for the cervical spine. Prevertebral soft tissue swelling is not a very useful plain film finding below the cervical spine, but paraspinal soft tissue hematoma can be visible on AP views, especially in the thoracic spine. With compression fractures, ventral loss of height and buckling of the superior end plate and ventral cortical margin occur (Fig. 171-22). In more severe cases, some dorsal buckling of the vertebral body is observed. There is usually focal kyphotic angulation. Mild compression fractures are often more obvious on lateral radiographs than on CT. CT may show only subtle lucency along the ventral, superior margin of the vertebral body in mild fractures. MRI or bone scan can be helpful in resolving any uncertainty about whether a fracture is acute or chronic. Edema will be seen in the marrow space on MRI in acute fractures; after a period of weeks to months, the marrow signal intensity returns to that similar to adjacent, normal marrow.

Burst fractures are usually visible on plain films, but CT can much more fully characterize the vertebral body fractures, degree of comminution and displacement, and dorsal element fractures (Fig. 171-23). Fractures of adjacent vertebrae are common, so CT should include enough of the nearby spine to ensure that all fractures near the obvious injury have been detected. This is of obvious value in planning instrumentation. MRI yields additional information about the integrity (or loss thereof) of discs and major ligaments as well as spinal cord damage.

Chance-type injuries are characterized by dorsal distraction in combination with flexion. The most common locations are around the thoracolumbar junction. The classic fracture described by Chance extends in a horizontal plane through a vertebral body into the pedicles (Fig. 171-24).[42] These fractures are often more easily appreciated on lateral radiographs than on the axial CT images. Since the fractures lie in the plane of imaging, axial images may be notable only for an absence of bone rather than distinct fracture lines. Sagittal and coronal reconstruction images show the fractures on CT more clearly than the axial images. However, the category of Chance-type injuries has been broadened to include other injuries that result from a similar mechanism.[43,44] Thus, the horizontally oriented disruption can also occur through an intervertebral disc, and the plane of dorsal distraction then typically extends through the facet joints. In any of these patterns, MRI demonstrates localized injury through the dorsal elements and soft tissues. In addition, a Chance injury should always suggest the possibility of associated abdominal injuries. Solid organ lacerations and perforations are present in up to half of patients with Chance-type injuries.

Fracture-dislocation of the thoracic or lumbar spine is the result of very severe injury mechanisms and carries a high risk of spinal cord injury. CT is especially helpful in such cases, and MRI is often also beneficial in evaluating the spinal cord (Fig. 171-25). As shown in Figure 171-26, CT is also helpful in evaluating ligament avulsion.

Nerve Root Injuries

Traction injuries can cause damage to the brachial plexus and/or avulsion of cervical nerve roots as they exit the spinal canal. MRI is especially helpful when such injuries are suspected. Imaging findings include absence of the nerve root in the foramen or lateral recess, a fluid collection (pseudomeningocele) in or lateral to the foramen, and displacement of the thecal sac to the opposite side. Myelography or CT can also demonstrate some of these findings (Fig. 171-27). The imaging findings, especially for fluid collections, are likely to evolve over time.

Penetrating Injuries

Plain films may be useful initially in assessing the location of bullet fragments. Once the level of injury is determined from the penetrating injury, CT is especially helpful for evaluating the precise nature of bone injuries and possible involvement of the spinal canal. After it is clear that no contraindications are present, such as metal in the spinal canal, MRI can be used to visualize the spinal cord and possible hematomas (Fig. 171-28).

Vascular Injuries

Vertebral artery injuries, ranging from intimal injury, dissection, and frank occlusion, are fairly common in cases of cervical spine injury, especially with fractures of the dorsal elements

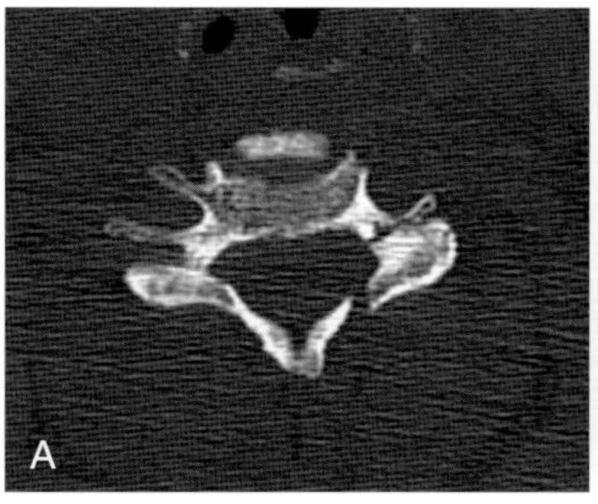

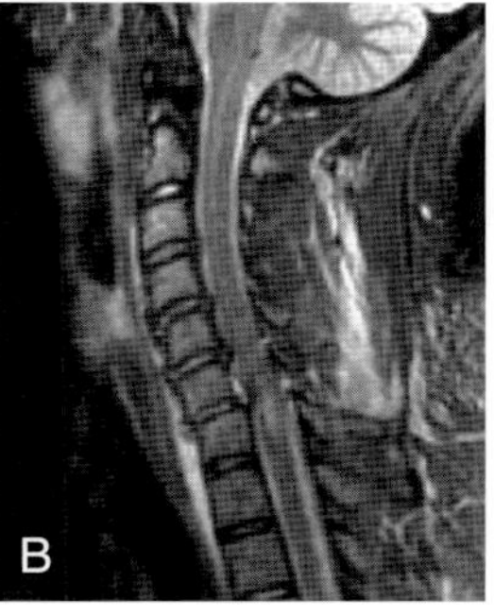

FIGURE 171-21. Pedicolaminar fractures. **A,** Axial CT of a motor vehicle accident patient shows fractures involving the pedicle and lamina on the patient's left side. There was spinal cord injury and rotational instability. **B,** Ligamentous injury and spinal cord edema are visible on sagittal inversion-recovery MRI.

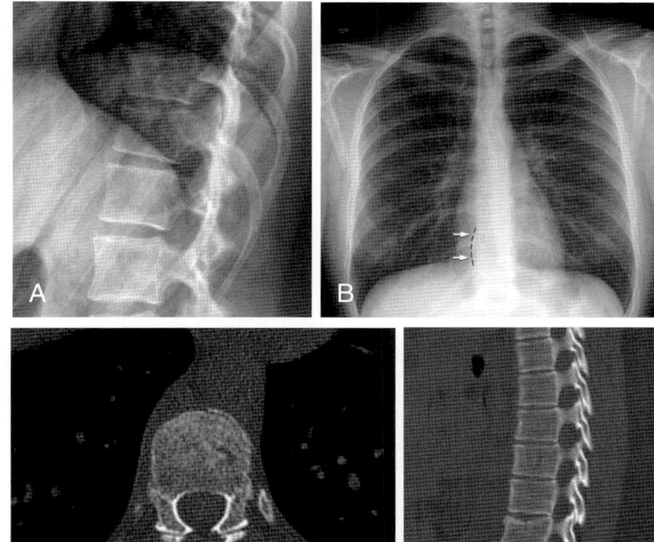

FIGURE 171-22. Thoracic compression fracture. **A,** Lateral radiograph of the lower thoracic spine shows mild ventral loss of height of T11 and buckling of the ventral cortical margin. **B,** Chest radiograph shows subtle paraspinous widening at T11 (*arrows*). **C,** Axial CT of T11 shows fractures only in the ventral body. **D,** Sagittal CT reconstruction shows mild ventral loss of height and superior end-plate and ventral rostral cortical disruption.

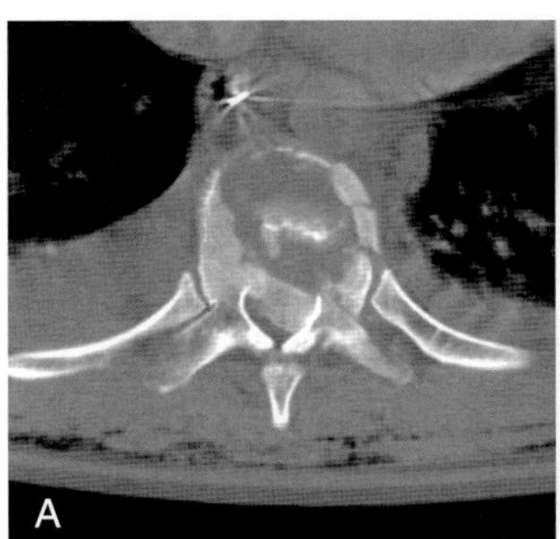

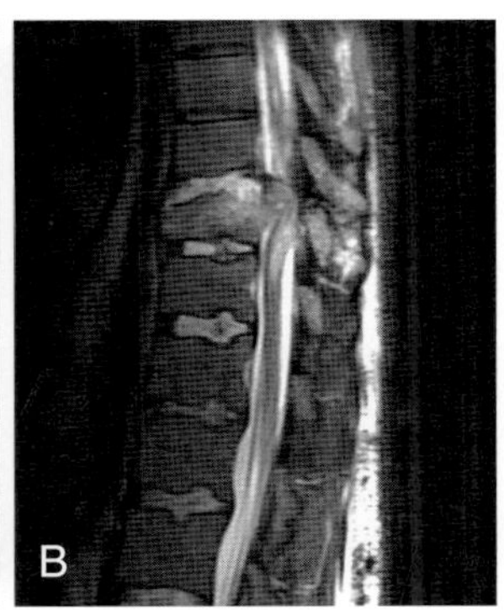

FIGURE 171-23. T10 burst fracture. **A,** CT of a paraplegic after motor vehicle accident shows burst fracture of T10, with severe narrowing of the spinal canal from a large bone fragment. **B,** Subsequent sagittal inversion-recovery MRI shows severe spinal cord compression and edema, with relatively little dorsal soft tissue edema. Note the alignment, without the kyphosis often accompanying compression fractures.

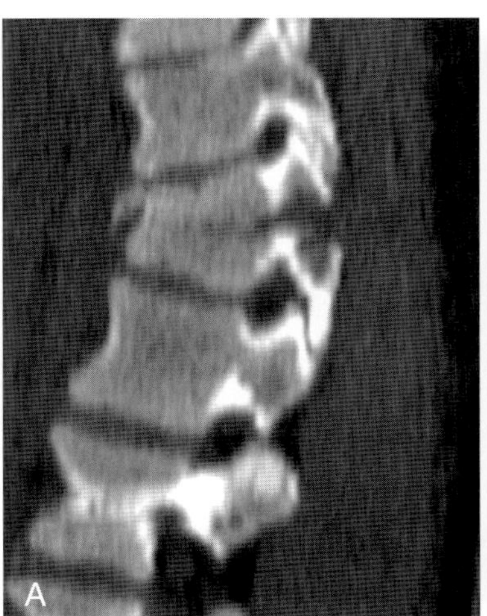

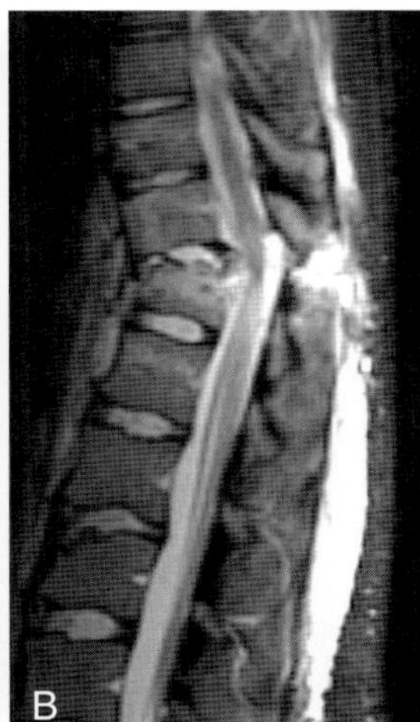

FIGURE 171-24. Severe flexion-distraction injury. **A,** CT sagittal 2D reconstruction shows T11 ventral compression with dorsal distraction and fracture component through a pedicle. **B,** Sagittal fast inversion-recovery MRI shows fractures, marrow edema within the T11 and T12 vertebral bodies, spinal cord compression, and focal dorsal soft tissue edema.

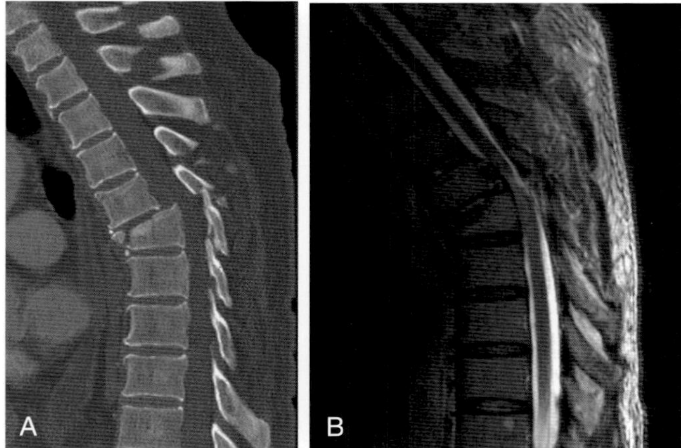

FIGURE 171-25. Thoracic fracture-dislocation. Patient fell from about 20 feet. **A,** Sagittal CT reconstruction shows kyphosis, compression of T6, subluxation, and dorsal element fractures. **B,** Fast-spin echo T2-weighted MRI shows the spinal cord edema.

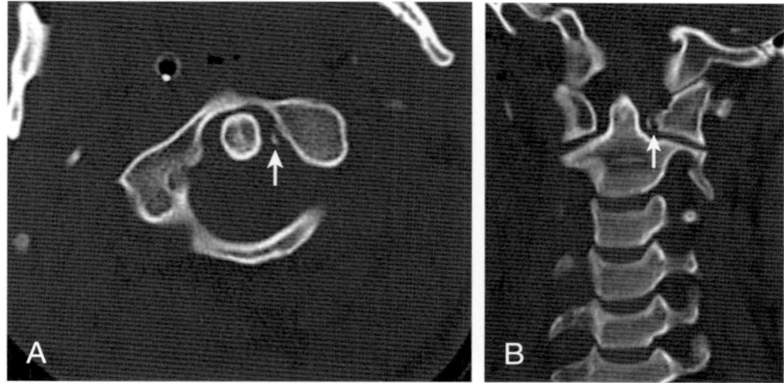

FIGURE 171-26. Transverse ligament avulsion. **A,** CT shows an avulsion fracture at the site of insertion of the transverse ligament on the left side (*arrow*). **B,** Coronal CT reconstruction demonstrates the displaced bone fragment (*arrow*).

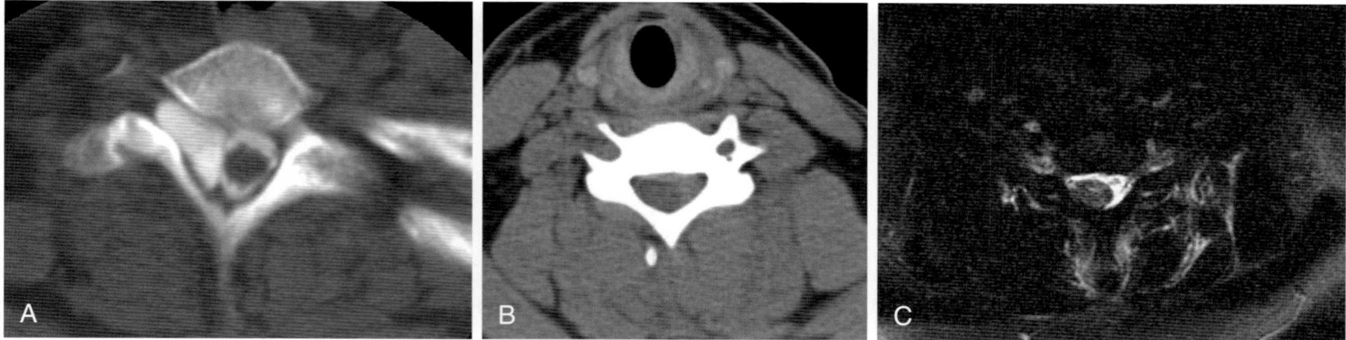

FIGURE 171-27. Nerve root avulsion. Patient had right upper extremity weakness after a motor vehicle accident. MRI could not be obtained because of orthopaedic external fixators. **A,** Axial CT after a myelogram demonstrates a collection of contrast material extending into the right neural foramen at the cervicothoracic junction and displacement of the thecal sac to the left. **B,** Axial CT through the lower cervical spine in a different patient in the acute setting after a motorcycle accident: soft tissue window shows displacement of the spinal cord to the right and probable blood in the left side of the spinal canal. **C,** Subsequent fast-spin echo T2-weighted MRI with fat saturation confirms spinal cord displacement to the right and accumulation of epidural fluid on the left side.

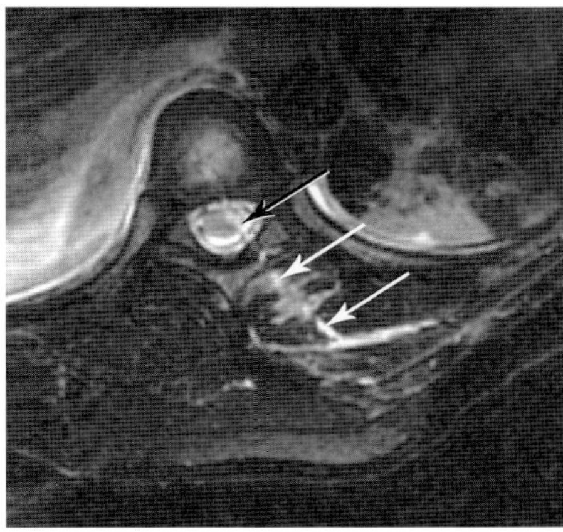

FIGURE 171-28. Stab injury to the spine. A young adult was stabbed in the back and suffered loss of sensation in left lower extremity; motor function was intact. Axial T2-weighted MRI with fat saturation demonstrates the path of the knife (*white arrows*) in the left lower thoracic spine into the spinal canal, with the knife injury visible in the ventral left side of the spinal cord (*black arrow*).

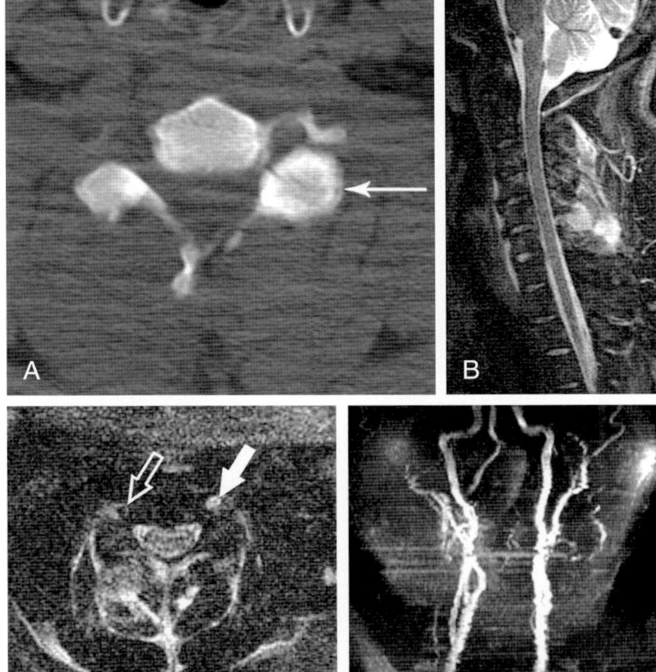

FIGURE 171-29. Vertebral artery occlusion. The patient had persistent neck pain after a motor vehicle accident. **A,** CT at the C5-6 level reveals a minimally displaced fracture through the lateral mass and articular processes on the left side (*arrow*). MRI shows deep, interspinous injury at C5-6 on sagittal inversion-recovery image (**B**), and an axial T2-weighted image with fat saturation (**C**) shows normal flow void from the right vertebral artery (*open arrow*) and bright signal from the left (*solid arrow*). **D,** Magnetic resonance angiography of the same patient confirms flow in the right vertebral artery and none in the left vertebral artery.

that involve the foramen transversarium. CT angiography can be obtained rapidly with multidetector CT (often during simultaneous acquisition of cervical spine CT) with multiplanar reconstructions possible. Magnetic resonance angiography (MRA) may be useful in some cases, especially if MRI is already being obtained. Routine axial MRI, for example, shows lack of signal ("flow void") in normal arteries. The normal black appearance of the artery is replaced by intermediate or high-signal intensity when there is no flow. Slow blood flow in an artery may give a similar appearance. MRA is a very useful tool for noninvasively evaluating normal and abnormal arteries in trauma patients. Axial MRIs and axial source images from MRA may also demonstrate a flap in cases of dissection or blood in the false lumen (Fig. 171-29). Catheter angiography is needed less often than in the past.

Spinal Cord Injury without Radiographic Abnormality

Spinal cord injury without radiographic abnormality (SCIWORA) can occur from a variety of mechanisms that result in neurologic injury without fractures. The term dates from earlier reliance on radiographs; MRI nearly always demonstrates imaging abnormalities when neurologic deficits occur.[45] Postulated mechanisms include flexion, transient distraction, compression of the spinal cord, and ischemia.

KEY REFERENCES

Benzel EC, Hart BL, Ball PA, et al: Magnetic resonance imaging for the evaluation of patients with occult cervical spine injury. *J Neurosurg* 85(5):824–829, 1996.

Como JJ, Diaz JJ, Dunham CM, et al: Practice management guidelines for identification of cervical spine injuries following trauma: update from the eastern association for the surgery of trauma practice management guidelines committee. *J Trauma*. 67(3):651–659, 2009.

Diaz JJ Jr, Cullinane DC, Altman DT, et al: Practice management guidelines for the screening of thoracolumbar spine fracture. *J Trauma* 63(3): 709–718, 2007.

Hanson JA, Blackmore CC, Mann FA, et al: Cervical spine injury: a clinical decision rule to identify high-risk patients for helical CT screening. *AJR Am J Roentgenol* 174(3):713–717, 2000.

Rojas CA, Bertozzi JC, Martinez CR, et al: Reassessment of the craniocervical junction: normal values on CT. *AJNR Am J Neuroradiol* 28(9): 1819–1823, 2007.

REFERENCES

The complete reference list is available online at expertconsult.com.

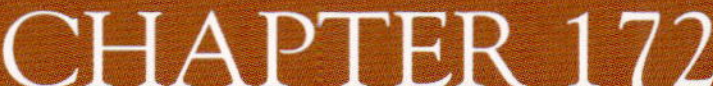

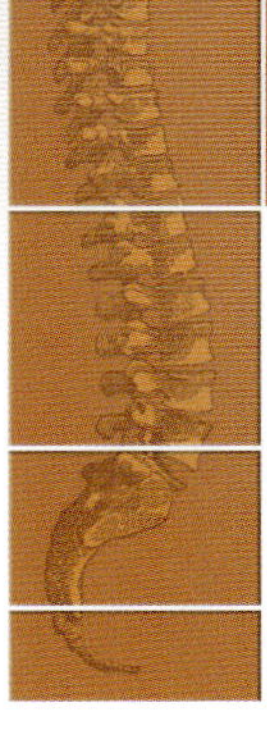

CHAPTER 172

Degenerative Disease and Infection: Role of Imaging

Manzoor Ahmed | Michael T. Modic

Imaging affects the management of disorders of the spine in both critical and confounding ways. The accurate depiction of morphologic abnormalities in conjunction with the history and physical examination is critical to therapeutic decision making. However, the significance of imaging findings in degenerative disease is strongly influenced by the wide range of normal variations, a high frequency of asymptomatic morphologic abnormalities, and the natural history of degenerative disease. The relationship of etiologic factors, the morphologic alterations, and the mechanism of symptom production are crucial to a better understanding of this relationship and require reproducible stratification of patient cohorts.

Degenerative disease and spinal infection illustrate the conundrum of what imaging method use and when to employ it. What follows is an effort to describe the advantages and limitations of the most commonly employed imaging tests for morphologic alterations in degenerative disease and spine infection in the thoracolumbar spine, integrated with what is known of the natural history of these disorders, the known confounding morphologic variations, and the clinical significance of morphologic alterations.

Degenerative Disease

The term *degeneration* is commonly applied to a variety of pathologic and imaging manifestations of spine morphology, reflecting the complexity of the process and gaps in our current knowledge. The distribution of axial load is responsible for the typical locations of spine degeneration. C5-6 and C6-7 levels are involved in most cases, because they are the sites of lordosis reversal. The thoracic spine, because of its lesser mobility, is less often affected by degeneration. L4-5 and L5-S1 are the most commonly affected levels because they are the sites of the highest dynamic and static loads.[1,2] Because degenerative spine sequelae are among the leading causes of functional incapacity and chronic disability, further research in the epidemiology, pathology, imaging, biomechanics, and therapeutics is warranted.

Generally, the purpose of a diagnostic test is twofold: (1) to provide reliable information about a patient's condition and (2) to influence a physician's plan for management. A necessary component that connects these two purposes is an accurate natural history. Only when this is understood can the results of a diagnostic test be integrated into therapeutic thinking. The relevance of an imaging finding requires knowledge relative to the spectrum of change, prevalence, significance, and behavior with time. This information is critical to developing effective case management guidelines that are based on well-controlled studies rather than on history or impression. Before one can assess the value of an imaging study, some type of perspective is needed in which to place the findings. Unfortunately, good natural history data are rarely available; only assumptions regarding the disease in question are found. If these assumptions are not accurate, one could be performing tests too soon or too late; both actions could have dramatically counterproductive effects on patient care and costs. Intervention in a disease condition requires that it be more beneficial, safer, and/or cost-effective than not intervening. In the case of thoracolumbar spine degenerative disease, most episodes of clinical symptoms are self-limited and can be divided into two major clinical groups.

Low Back Pain

The natural history of low back pain (LBP) with or without radiculopathy is not clearly understood. Traditional practice suggests that imaging has no role in evaluating back pain unless associated signs and symptoms are suggestive of a potentially treatable condition related to trauma, instability, infection, or malignancy. Foregoing imaging in these circumstances may not seriously affect the outcome in most patients and, in fact, may improve conservative management by avoiding the detection of confounding altered morphology. Because back pain is typically a recurrent problem, physicians and patients should benefit from information related to patient group stratification, prognosis for recovery from acute episodes, and likelihood of recurrence.[3]

Low Back Pain with Radiculopathy

Patients with LBP with radiculopathy constitute a relatively less diverse group in terms of etiology, and the symptoms usually suggest nerve root compression. Multiple authors[4-6] suggest that an imaging study is indicated for the evaluation of back pain and associated sciatica when (1) true radicular symptoms are present; (2) there is evidence of nerve root irritation on physical examination (i.e., positive straight-leg raise test); and/or (3) "conservative management" of 4 to 6 weeks' duration has failed. Earlier imaging is considered appropriate if clinical features raise concern regarding malignancy or infectious pathology or if neurologic findings worsen during observation. These recommendations are based on several studies of the successful nonoperative treatment of sciatica.[7-10] Thus, imaging is recommended only for the remaining minority of patients with persistent signs and symptoms who are felt to be surgical candidates or in whom diagnostic uncertainty remains.

Role of Early Imaging

The use of diagnostic imaging earlier in the course of a patient's symptoms is supported by the following evidence: (1) patients with herniated discs treated surgically have better short-term outcomes than those treated conservatively[10,11]; (2) the earlier the surgery the better the outcome[12]; and (3) surgery is cost-effective compared with conservative management (though this varies with the type of surgery).[13,14] However, the potential reduction in morbidity from early intervention requires the identification of accurate prognostic indicators, be they clinical or imaging based. Certainly, more than morphology is a factor. As has been suggested by Postacchini,[15] two needs likely require consideration: (1) protracted conservative treatment may lengthen the time off from work and reduce the chances of successful surgical treatment; and (2) surgery should be avoided in patients with a herniated disc that may become asymptomatic or even disappear within a few months of onset. Thus, the possible benefits of imaging for degenerative diseases of the spine, other than as a presurgical tool, have never been carefully documented and quantified. Predicting which patients will benefit from imaging is a complicated and controversial subject. Its use as a preintervention planning tool is critical, but its employment for diagnostic information per se is less well accepted and the subject of much debate. Nevertheless, if imaging could be employed to prospectively determine which patients will not do well with surgery or other types of therapy, it would be of great value. Conversely, its use to identify patients undergoing prolonged conservative treatment who require more aggressive therapy (e.g., surgery) might be equally beneficial. This would save the cost of lost work, medical expenses, and personal discomfort. Clearly, there is little consensus, either within or among specialties, on the use of diagnostic tests for patients with back pain.[16] The diagnostic evaluation depends heavily on individual physicians, their specialties, and patient socioeconomics, in addition to the patient's symptoms.[16,17] On the other hand, patients with underlying risk factors ("red flags"), mainly, infection, trauma, and malignancy, warrant early imaging for timely intervention.

Imaging Considerations

The major benefit of imaging is its ability to depict the presence or absence of anatomic derangement and, in the former case, its effect on adjacent structures. The contrast sensitivity and multiplanar imaging capability of proton magnetic resonance (MR) provides a unique noninvasive means of imaging the intervertebral disc, adjacent osseous structures, and associated soft tissues. From an anatomic perspective, it is important to be able to demonstrate the osseous, fluid, and soft tissue interfaces within the three traditional compartments: the intramedullary, extramedullary intradural, and extradural spaces. The potential combinations of pulse sequence parameters, imaging planes, and postprocessing techniques available are almost limitless, and they can be used to highlight different aspects of the discovertebral complex and adjacent spaces. The methods include, but are not limited to, surface coil technology, cardiac gating, gradient refocusing, paramagnetic contrast agents, saturation pulses, gradient echo volume imaging, Turbo (fast) T2-weighted spin echo, fat suppression, magnetization transfer, short-tau inversion recovery (STIR), and diffusion techniques (including diffusion tensor imaging). Other modalities certainly do have a role based on the cost-effectiveness, accessibility, individual unique characteristics of some modalities, and, more importantly, contraindications to MRI. The technical aspects, advantages, and disadvantages of conventional and new modalities are briefly discussed in the following sections.

Counting Reference

The topic is discussed in detail in Chapter 175. It is extremely important that counting reference is clearly stated in the spine imaging report. This is to avoid wrong level surgeries with potential medico-legal implications. The two major factors responsible for discrepancy are (1) a transitional vertebra, which can be a sacralized L5 or lumbarized S1, and (2) variations in the number of rib-bearing vertebrae. Lumbosacral transitional vertebra (LSTV) is a common finding in the general population. Identification of LSTV on imaging is the essential first step in the interpretation of lumbar and thoracic imaging.[18] The coronal MRI localizer image of the thoracic and lumbar spine can be useful because L4-5 is generally at the level of the iliac crest. Some prefer to use a vitamin E back-skin marker at an overlapping level in the thoracic spine, which, however, requires imaging of the entire spine. The iliolumbar ligament is easily identified on axial MRI and can be used as a marker of L5.[19] There is a greater tendency of counting the lowest lumbar-type intervertebral disc space as L5-S1. Nevertheless, it is crucial that these approaches and variations be specified and clearly communicated in the report.

Plain Radiography

Plain radiography (PR) is still a very useful and cost-effective diagnostic tool by virtue of its availability and efficiency.[20] PR is generally used in trauma, for screening of degenerative disease, and for evaluation of sagittal translation using flexion-extension views. PR can aid MRI in characterization of disc disease by better demonstration of vacuum phenomena, disc calcification, bridging osteophytosis, and dorsal longitudinal calcification (though less common in the thoracolumbar spine). Conventional screen-film imaging has been nearly completely replaced by digital acquisition modalities, using either imaging plates (computed radiography, CR) or flat-panel detectors (direct radiography, DR).

Routine Magnetic Resonance Imaging

Unlike CT and conventional radiography, which depend on information related to electron density, proton MR signals are influenced by the T1 and T2 relaxation time, proton density, and motion (both macro and micro) to provide greater tissue contrast. Thus, its role may go beyond gross anatomic appraisal to actual tissue characterization of pathology and biochemical change. The routine sequences and their significance are as follows: (1) sagittal T1 to evaluate bone marrow infiltration and end-plate bone marrow degenerative changes; (2) sagittal T2 to evaluate disc and end-plate degeneration, thecal sac extrinsic impression, the conus medullaris, and the cauda equina morphology; and (3) sagittal STIR to detect bone marrow and paraspinal soft tissue edema. Axial T1 and T2 basically confirm the findings on sagittal imaging and provide a better assessment of central canal/thecal sac narrowing, cauda equina abnormalities, facet disease, and lateral disc herniations. The major degrading factors are patients' gross motion, positioning, body habitus, and instrumentation.

Postcontrast Magnetic Resonance Imaging

The use of contrast agents is important for the improved depiction of reactive or inflammatory changes. Surgery results in reactive granulation tissue and scarring, typically in the epidural space. Noncontrast MRI is both sensitive and specific for the diagnosis of vertebral osteomyelitis. Contrast is helpful in the evaluation of paraspinal and epidural soft tissue involvement, including abscess formation. Contrast is not usually needed in the evaluation of bony neoplastic disease, unless epidural disease definition and diagnosis are required in selected cases. Contrast is essential in cases of malignant leptomeningeal disease.

Noncontrast Computed Tomography

Despite the preference for MRI in the evaluation of spinal canal stenosis, CT is essentially as accurate as MRI for the assessment of degenerative disease. Using bony and soft tissue algorithms and multiplanar reconstruction, CT is frequently used for preoperative planning.

Computed Tomography Myelography

Though still performed, conventional myelography has been significantly overshadowed by CT myelography. Because it is an invasive procedure, the CT myelogram is generally reserved for the following circumstances: (1) for instrumented spines, (2) as a problem-solving tool in clinically challenging cases supplementing or complementing MRI, and (3) for patients with contraindications to MRI. CT myelographic evaluation can be suboptimal if there is poor contrast mixing with the cerebrospinal fluid (CSF) or artifact from some of the instrumentations or the patient's gross motion. Multidetector-enabled CT acquisitions with thinner slices facilitate 3D multiplanar orthogonal and angular reconstructions of the CT myelogram.

Magnetic Resonance Myelography

MR myelography (MRM) is currently not practiced routinely in the United States for two major reasons: (1) Intrathecal gadolinium is not yet approved by the FDA, and (2) MRM has no significant added advantage compared with a CT myelogram or conventional MRI.[21,22] MRM is, however, comparably accurate in detecting CSF leaks in patients with intracranial hypotension compared with radioisotope cisternography.[23]

Open and Large-Bore Magnetic Resonance Imaging

The open-design MRI systems enable imaging of those who are claustrophobic and overweight and offer the potential of dynamic imaging. The major penalty is some compromise of the image quality due to decreased signal-to-noise ratio. However, the diagnostic information is satisfactory in most cases.[24,25] Closed high-magnetic-field scanners with short magnets and wide-bore tubes offer patients improved comfort and lessen anxiety.[26]

Dynamic Imaging and Upright Magnetic Resonance Imaging

Sagittal segmental lumbar motion is traditionally assessed with lateral flexion-extension radiographs. These dynamic studies often demonstrate a decrease in the slip percentage between the vertebral segments with extension and an increase with forward flexion. Ironically, the degree of spondylolisthesis can actually improve on the lateral film taken on the operating table in an anesthetized patient.[27] Somewhat analogous to the flexion-extension imaging, supine-prone imaging of the lumbar spine can also be more sensitive by showing a higher degree of listhesis in the prone position.[28] Position-dependent stenosis can be demonstrated on the lateral myelogram in flexion-extension postures, which would otherwise have been underestimated on the follow-up CT myelogram[29] (Fig. 172-1). Ben-Galim and Reitman in a study of a small group of patients showed position-dependent severe spinal canal stenosis on CT myelography with grade I or II spondylolisthesis. Additionally, they showed fluid-filled distended facet joints, a marker of positional translation.[30] Imaging findings on supine MRI may correlate poorly with clinical findings. This may be related to the positional dependence of spinal stenosis, which reflects dynamic changes in soft tissue structures. Therefore, it is potentially valuable to evaluate spinal disorders under mechanical loading. Hydraulic axial-loading devices have also been tried.[31] Upright MRI in different postures can reproduce the positions that bring about their symptoms and may unmask findings that are not visible with routine supine imaging. Small disc herniations and ventral spondylolisthesis can be unmasked, and disc

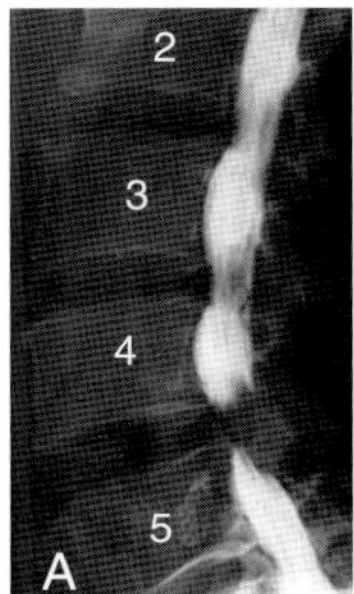

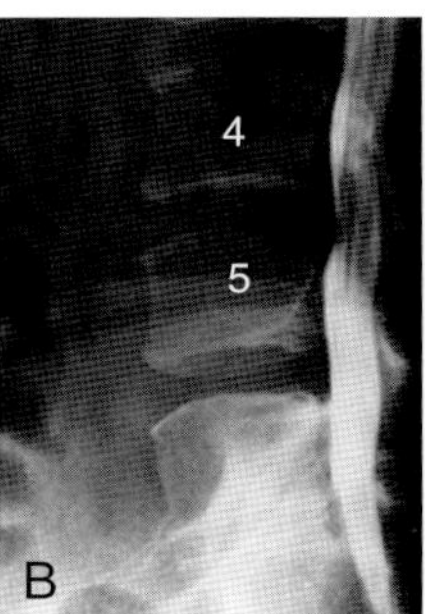

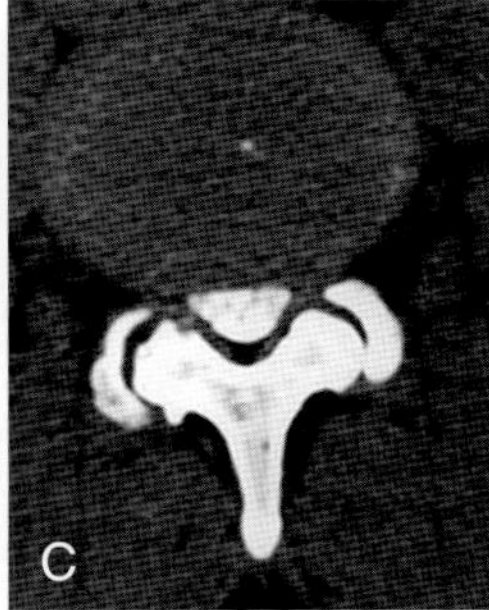

FIGURE 172-1. Dynamic imaging. Erect lateral views of a lumbar myelogram in the extended (**A**) and flexed (**B**) positions showing a subtotal block to the contrast column at the L4-5 level in extension that is relieved in flexion. **C,** Routine supine CT myelogram shows mild diffuse disc bulge without significant compression of the thecal sac. (From Saifuddin A: The imaging of lumbar spinal stenosis. *Clin Radiol* 55[8]:581–594, 2000, with permission.)

herniations can be increased in size on upright MRI compared with recumbent MRI.[32] Assessment of the degree of spinal stability in the degenerative and postoperative lumbar spine can also be performed.[33,34] Kinetic magnetic resonance images (kMRIs) in axially loaded, upright-neutral, flexion-extension positions can also accentuate the size of the disc herniations and play a potential problem-solving role in radiculopathy with negative supine static imaging.[35] Clearly, axial loading changes anatomic relations. The significance of the findings in terms of therapeutic decision making is not very clear.[36]

Morphologic Alterations on Imaging

Standardized reporting is a better means of communication and consistent reporting, as well as a useful source of database research. Given the complexity, inconsistency, and overlapping of terminology used to discuss the spine over the years, standardized report generation in spine imaging is needed the most to describe the morphologic alterations in the spine. A consensus-based terminology recommended by Millette et al.[37] is used in this chapter. It must be clearly understood that these terms are descriptive only and, in and of themselves, independent of the test. It cannot be overemphasized that these terms do not imply knowledge of etiology, symptoms, prognosis, or need for treatment. Recently, Carrinno et al.[38] showed moderate reliability in the interpretation of qualitative nondisc contour degenerative findings on lumbar MRI.

Degenerative morphologic changes are discussed in the following section as disc degeneration and end-plate bone marrow changes followed by facet joint degenerative alterations.

Disc Degeneration

The term *disc degeneration* is used for a variety of changes, including any or all of the following: real or apparent desiccation, fibrosis, narrowing of the disc space, bulging, fissuring or mucinous degeneration of the anulus, osteophytes of the vertebral apophyses, and end-plate/adjacent marrow changes. MRI and CT show disc space narrowing, T2-weighted signal intensity loss from the intervertebral disc, presence of fissures, fluid, vacuum changes and calcification within the intervertebral disc, ligamentous signal changes, marrow signal changes, and osteophytosis. These alterations result in disc herniation, malalignment, and spinal canal stenosis. Conventional theory suggests that aging and degeneration are very similar processes, albeit occurring at different rates. Historically, the two processes have been characterized morphologically and termed as *spondylosis deformans* and *spondylosis osteochondrosis* (deteriorated disc), respectively. The former affects the anulus fibrosus and adjacent apophyses, whereas the latter mainly affects the nucleus pulposus and the vertebral body end plates, particularly fissuring (numerous tears) of the anulus fibrosus. Scientific evidence suggests that spondylosis deformans is the consequence of normal aging, whereas intervertebral osteochondrosis represents a pathologic, though not necessarily symptomatic, process.[39] Anteriolateral osteophytosis is a reliable marker of spondylosis deformans, with a 100% incidence above 40 years.[39] Disc degeneration and aging are multifactorial processes that encompass a wide spectrum of changes and sequelae, of which the radial tear is but one. Disc degeneration may be explained primarily by genetic influences and complex unpredictable interactions of unidentified factors.

The nucleus pulposus is eccentrically located and more closely related to the dorsal surface of the intervertebral disc. With degeneration and aging, type II collagen increases outwardly in the anulus, and water loss from the nucleus pulposus is greater than from the anulus. This results in a loss of the hydrostatic properties of the disc, with an overall reduction of hydration in both areas to about 70%. In addition to water and collagen, the other important biochemical constituents of the intervertebral disc are the proteoglycans. It is not the individual composition but the relative composition of these constituents that in turn affects the hydrostatic properties and tensile strength of the intervertebral disc. The ratio of keratin sulfate to chondroitin sulfate increases. The disc becomes progressively more fibrous and disorganized, with the end stage represented by amorphous fibrocartilage and no clear distinction between nucleus and anulus. The degenerating disc manifests as diminishing T2 signal and loss of internal lamellation. T2 measurements also correlate with glycoaminoglycan concentration rather than absolute water content. So, it is not just the absolute concentration of water but also the state of water involved in the disc degeneration. The status of the proteoglycans is thus a major determinant of disc space T2 and T1 signal[39-41] (Fig. 172-2).

Anular Tears

Also called anular fissures, anular tears are separations between anular fibers, avulsion of fibers from their vertebral body insertions, or breaks through fibers that extend radially, transversely, or concentrically and involve one or many layers of the anular lamellae. The term *tear,* or *fissure*, describes the spectrum of such lesions and does not imply that the lesion is a consequence of trauma. Although it has certainly been verified that anular disruption is a sequela of degeneration and is often associated with it, its role as the causal agent of disc degeneration has certainly not been proved. Anular disruption initiates a reparative process as it is replaced by dense fibrous tissue and cystic spaces.[42-45] Fissuring, chondrocyte generation, and granulation tissue formation have been noted within the end plate, anulus fibrosus, and nucleus pulposus of degenerative discs, indicating attempts at healing.[39] Anular

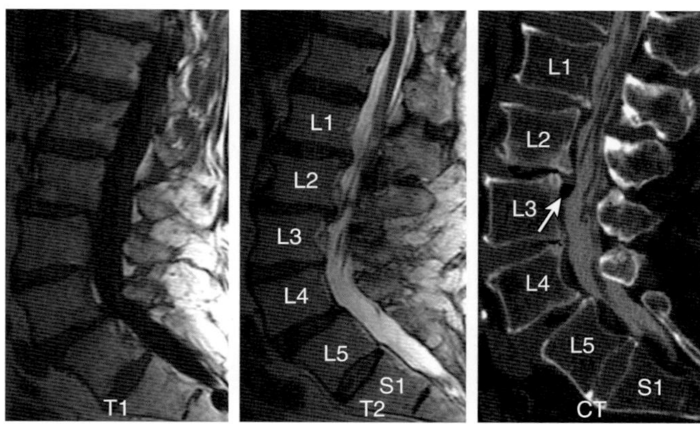

FIGURE 172-2. Degenerative disc changes. Anular disc bulges at L1-2 and L2-3. Disc space vacuum phenomena at L2-3 to L4-5, extending to the epidural space along the bulging disc at L2-3 (*arrow*). Mild degenerative spondylolisthesis, anterolisthesis at L4-5, and retrolisthesis at L2-3.

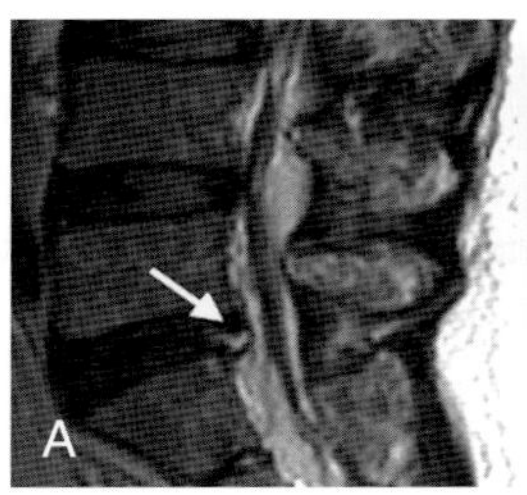

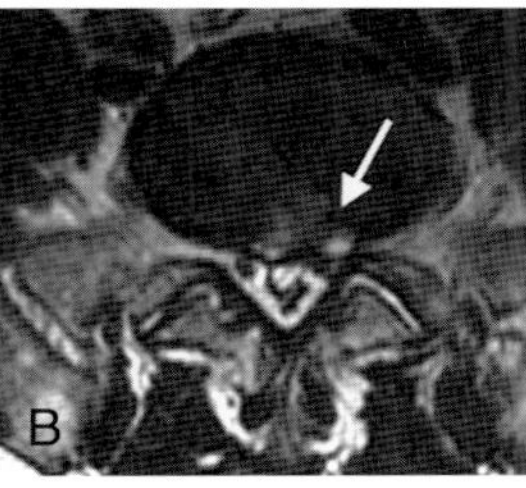

FIGURE 172-3. Anular tears. Sagittal (**A**) and axial (**B**) T2 images show typical posterior anular tear with hyperintense T2 signal (*arrows*) and associated small disc protrusion.

tears are commonly seen in the dorsal bulging discs as focal T2 hyperintensity on T2 and STIR imaging; there may be associated small disc protrusion. Anular tears consistently show focal contrast enhancement[46] (Fig. 172-3).

Disc Gas "Vacuum Phenomenon"

Radiolucent foci on CT or plain films representing gas, principally nitrogen, occur at sites of negative pressure produced by the abnormal spaces. The vacuum phenomenon within a degenerated disc is represented on spin echo images as areas of signal void. Whereas the presence of gas within the disc is usually suggestive of degenerative disease, spinal infection may (rarely) be accompanied by intradiscal or intraosseous gas.[47] A protruding disc with a vacuum phenomenon can present as epidural gas foci on CT and hypointensities on MRI (see Fig. 172-2).

Disc Calcification and T1 Hyperintensity

Patchy, partial, or complete calcification of the disc space can be seen either as an isolated finding without degenerative stigmata or as a chronic dystrophic change in a degenerated disc. The clinical significance of a calcified disc is unknown. The disc space on CT and plain films can appears as fused, perhaps "autofused." Calcification, depending on its biochemical status, can appear as hyperintense or hypointense on sagittal T1 imaging. Furthermore, the hyperintense T1 disc may represent an ossified disc, as can be proven by loss of signal on fat-suppressed MRIs due to lipid marrow. A calcified disc is easily demonstrable on CT (Fig. 172-4).

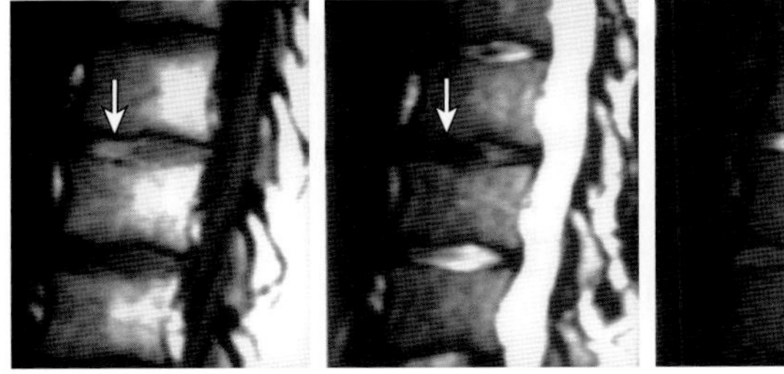

FIGURE 172-4. Disc space calcifications: Sagittal T1-, T2-, and fat-suppressed T1-weighted images of the upper lumbar spine. On the T1-weighted images, there is a focus of high signal (*arrow*). On the T2-weighted image, this same area has a decreased signal (*arrow*). On the fat-suppressed image, the region maintains its high signal, while areas which contain fat have a decreased signal (*arrow*). The high signal on T1, decreased signal on T2, and unaffected by fat suppression are indicative of calcification producing T1 shortening.

Degenerative Marrow Changes

The anulus fibrosus, vertebral end plate, and vertebral body have an interreactive relationship in the degenerative process, as is also evident from the model of chymopapain-treated discs.[48,49] Paradiscal MR signal changes in the end plate and vertebral bodies take three forms.

Type I Changes. Type I changes demonstrate decreased signal intensity on T1-weighted images and increased signal intensity on T2-weighted images. Type I change is found in about 4% of nonsurgical lumbar spines, 8% in postdiscectomy discs, and 40% to 50% of chymopapain-treated discs.[48-50] The last group can be used as a model of acute disc degeneration. Histopathology of type I changes demonstrates disruption and fissuring of the end plate and vascularized fibrous tissues within the adjacent marrow, accounting for prolonged T1 and T2 MR signal. Enhancement of type I vertebral body marrow changes is seen with administration of IV gadolinium. The enhancement may involve a portion of the disc itself and is presumably related to the vascularized fibrous change. The type I signal is expectedly accentuated on STIR, mimicking bone marrow edema, and may be very difficult in some cases to differentiate from discitis osteomyelitis (discussed later under the differential diagnosis of vertebral osteomyelitis; Fig. 172-5).

Type II Changes. Type II changes are represented by increased signal intensity on T1-weighted images and isointense or slightly hyperintense signal on T2-weighted images. Type II changes are identified in approximately 16% of patients on MRI.[48-50] Discs with type II changes, like type I, show evidence of end-plate disruption, with fat marrow in the end plate and adjacent vertebral body resulting in T1 hyperintensity due to T1 shortening (Fig. 172-6).

Type III Changes. Type III changes are represented by a decreased signal intensity on both T1- and T2-weighted images

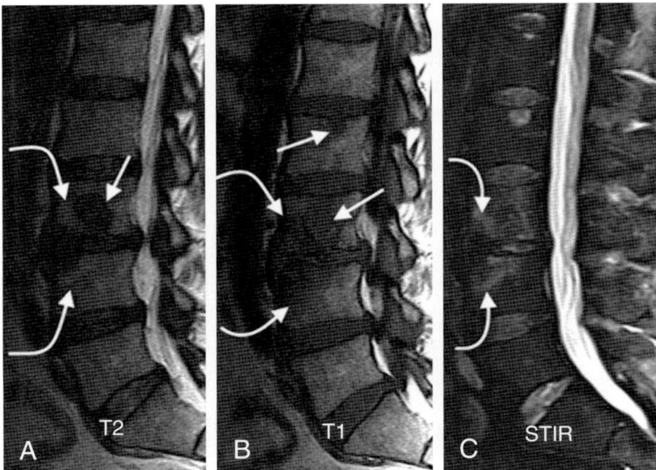

FIGURE 172-5. A–C, Type I end-plate changes. T1 hypointense and T2 hyperintense end-plate changes at L3-4 (*curved arrows*); the end-plate signal is accentuated on short-tau inversion recovery (STIR) image due to suppression of the fat in the surrounding marrow. Note that the same bone marrow changes also surround a large Schmorl node at L3 (*straight arrows*). Note a small Schmorl node at L2; however, there is no surrounding reactive change or hypointense rim.

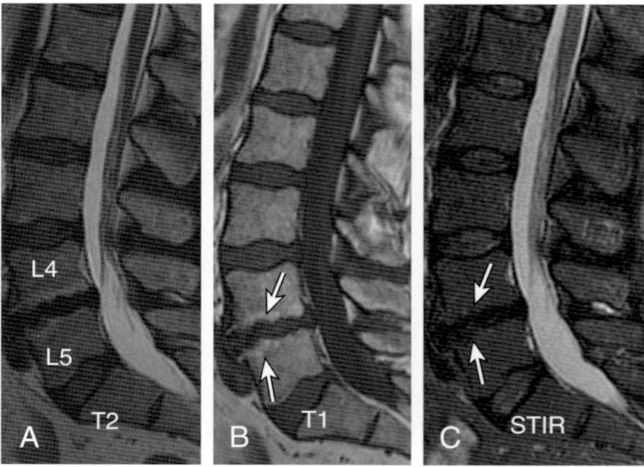

FIGURE 172-6. **A–C,** Type II end-plate changes. T1 and T2 hyperintense end-plate changes at L4-5 (*arrows*). Like the surrounding fatty marrow, the end-plate signal is suppressed on the short-tau inversion recovery (STIR) image.

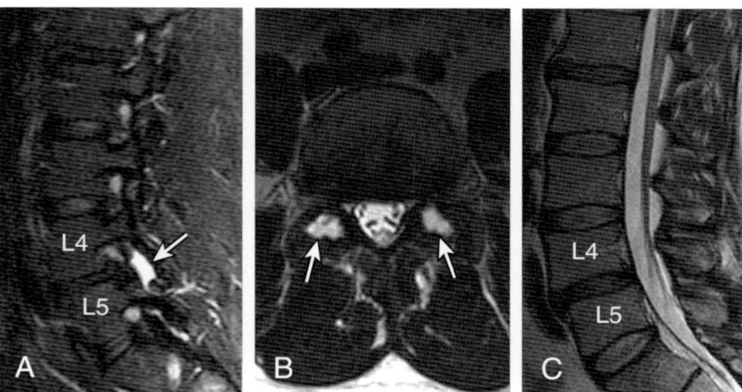

FIGURE 172-7. Facet effusions. Sagittal short-tau inversion recovery (**A**) and axial T2 (**B**) images showing facet joint effusions at L4-5 (*arrows*) and common associated finding of mild anterolisthesis at L4-5 (**C**).

due to extensive bony sclerosis, as evident on plain radiographs and CT. The first two types show no definite correlation with sclerosis seen at radiography, which is not surprising when one considers the histology. The sclerosis on plain radiographs is a reflection of dense woven bone within the vertebral body rather than of the marrow elements. The lack of signal in the type III change represents the relative absence of marrow in areas of advanced sclerosis (see Fig. 172-17B).

Facets, Pedicles, and Ligamentous Changes

The superior articulating process of one vertebra articulates with the inferior articulating process of the vertebra above by a synovium-lined articulation—the zygapophyseal joint. The lumbar facet joints are predisposed to arthropathy with alterations of the articular cartilage. Facet joint degeneration results in hypertrophic changes (osteophytosis), joint effusions, synovial cyst formation, and rostrocaudal subluxation. Mild to moderate facet joint osteophytosis is commonly seen in the lumbar spine at L4-5 and L5-S1 and is more suggestive of age-related change.[51,52] The important ligaments of the spine include the anterior longitudinal ligament, the posterior longitudinal ligament, the paired sets of ligamenta flava (connecting the laminae of adjacent vertebrae), the intertransverse ligaments (extending between transverse processes), and the unpaired supraspinous ligament (along the tips of the spinous processes). As these ligaments normally provide stability, any alteration in the vertebral articulations can lead to ligamentous laxity with subsequent deterioration. Loss of elastic tissue, calcification and ossification, and development of bone proliferation at sites of ligamentous attachment to bone are recognized manifestations of such degeneration.

Facet and Disc Degeneration

Generally, disc degeneration dominates facet arthropathy. Some degree of facet arthritic changes usually accompanies disc degeneration. Is facet disease a sequela of disc degeneration? The answer to this question is debatable, but at least it is clear that disc degeneration is more common and generally precedes facet joint arthropathy. Due to altered mechanics, disc degeneration probably accelerates facet joint arthropathy.[51-54] A systemic component is hypothesized to account for facet arthrosis since there is a high incidence of concurrent lumbar and cervical facet arthrosis.[55] Osteophytosis of the facet joints is, to a degree, a counterpart of end-plate osteophytosis and specifically contributes to lateral recess and foraminal stenosis. Facet arthrosis may occur independently and be a source of symptoms on its own.[56] A smaller group of lumbar spines in our experience show dominant facet and ligamentous degenerative hypertrophic changes with absent to minimal degenerative disc changes.

Facet Joint Effusions

Pencil-thin homogeneous bilateral facet joint effusion is a common and normal finding in the lower lumbar spine. In an arthritic facet joint, synovial villi may become entrapped within the joint, with resulting joint effusions. STIR is the best method for demonstrating joint effusions. Large joint effusions (>1.5 mm) are highly predictive of degenerative spondylolisthesis on dynamic imaging, particularly at L4-5[57] (Fig. 172-7).

Synovial Cysts

Herniation of the synovium through the facet joint capsule may result in synovial cysts. In a review of patients with degenerative facet disease, synovial cysts occurred at a ventral or intraspinal location in 2.3% of cases and dorsal or extraspinal location in 7.3%.[58] There is a more straightforward relationship of synovial cysts with osteoarthritis and the instability of the facet joints than degeneration of the intervertebral disc alone.[57] Intraspinal synovial cysts can be symptomatic, depending on their size. Typically, synovial cysts have T2 hyperintense cystic appearance, but signal intensity can vary due to debris, hemorrhage, gas, and superimposed infection. The cyst may exhibit rim enhancement (see Fig. 172-24). Distinguishing the synovial disc from the herniated disc is not usually difficult due to its location and MR characteristics. A dorsolateral extradural impression and associated juxtafacet asymmetrical soft tissue density on CT myelogram is a nonspecific finding; asymmetrical facet joint arthritis can be helpful in such cases.

Dorsal Elements and Paraspinal Edema

Routine use of STIR and similar sequences has resulted in increased detection of dorsal elements and paraspinal soft tissue edema.[59,60] Facet joint degenerative arthritis can result in para-articular and pedicular edema, joint effusion, and para-articular soft tissue edema. In patients at high risk, it may be

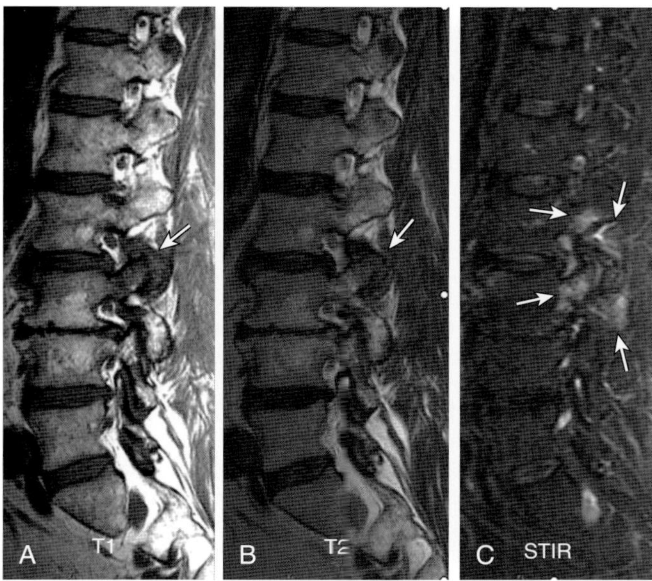

FIGURE 172-8. Facet edema. **A** and **B**, Hypertrophic facet arthropathy at L2-3 (*arrows*). **C,** Associated marrow and soft tissue edema (*arrows*). Also note L2 and L3 pedicles edema (*anterior arrows*).

difficult to differentiate from infected facet joints. The signal changes and sclerosis in the pedicles can be seen secondary to facet joint arthritis and underlying pedicle or pars fractures. The greatest mechanical stress is on the pars interarticularis, followed by pedicles as shown by Sairyo et al.[61] These stresses can result in a spectrum of reactive bone marrow changes in the pars and pedicles. T2 hyperintense signal in the pedicles has been shown as an early marker of spondylolysis.[61] There is evidence that categories of changes in MR signal intensity, similar to those described adjacent to degenerating discs, can be seen in lumbar pedicles adjacent to a spondylolytic defect of the pars interarticularis[62] (Figs. 172-8 and 172-9).

Morphologic and Functional Sequelae

Major sequelae of disc and dorsal elements degenerative changes are intervertebral disc displacement, malalignment, degenerative scoliosis, and spinal canal–foraminal

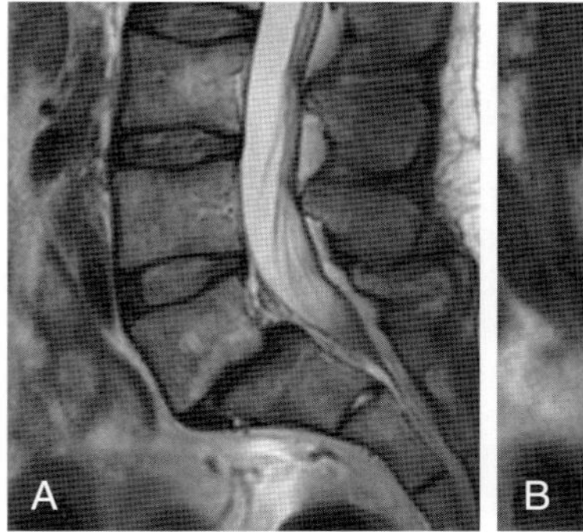

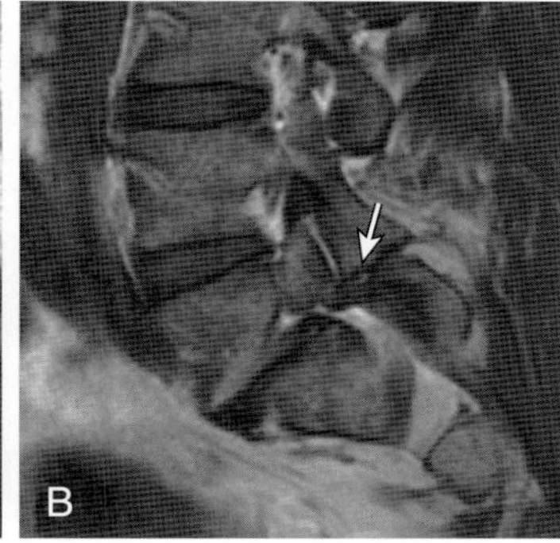

FIGURE 172-10. **A** and **B**, Isthmic spondylolisthesis. Sagittal T2 imaging showing grade I anterolisthesis due to L5 spondylolysis (*arrow*).

stenosis. Disc displacement can be found as an isolated finding. Otherwise, there is usually a combination of the sequelae mentioned before.

Segmental Instability

Each level in the thoracolumbar spine consists of three joints: intervertebral disc space and bilateral facet joints. Degeneration of these joints results in segmental instability replacing the normal spinal motion, which can be irregular, excessive, restricted, translational, and/or angular. Segmental instability, which can cause static and dynamic stenosis, is considered a cause of LBP but is poorly defined.[63] On flexion-extension plain radiography, generally about 3 mm or more of sagittal translation is equated with instability. *Spondylolisthesis* is a term used in static imaging and refers to intervertebral displacement—anterolisthesis, retrolisthesis, or lateral listhesis. The different types, based on etiology, include congenital, degenerative, isthmic, iatrogenic, pathologic, and traumatic (Fig. 172-10).

Grading of Spondylolisthesis

Spondylolisthesis in the sagittal plane can be graded by one of two methods, independent of the imaging modality and type of spondylolisthesis.[64] The first is the method described by Meyerding.[65] The anteroposterior (AP) diameter of the

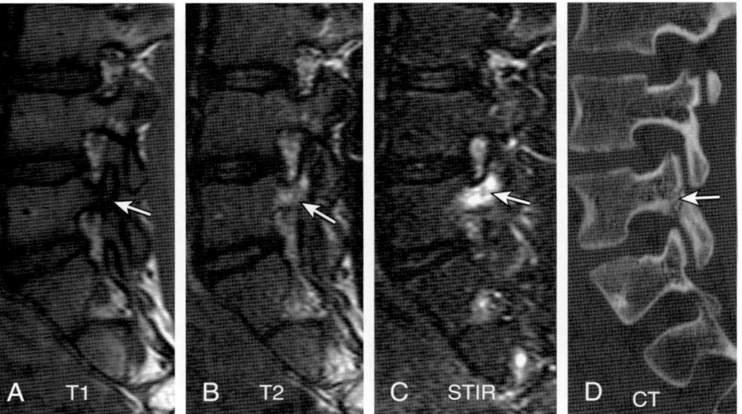

FIGURE 172-9. Pedicle edema. Hypointense T1 (**A**) and hyperintense T2 (**B**) pedicle signal (*arrow*) at L5. **C,** The T2 signal is accentuated on short-tau inversion recovery (STIR) image. **D,** CT shows pars interarticularis defect.

superior surface of the lower vertebral body is divided into quarters, and a grade of I to IV is assigned to slips of one, two, three, or four quarters of the superior vertebra, respectively. The second method, first described by Taillard,[66] expresses the degree of slip as a percentage of the AP diameter of the top of the lower vertebra. Complete slip of L5 on S1 is termed *spondyloptosis*. The second method is favored by most authors as it is more accurately reproducible.[67] Measurement of the slip and its apparent progression, however, should be viewed with caution. Studies have shown that inter- and intraobserver error of up to 15% is possible. This variation can increase if an element of rotation is present. Therefore, only a progression of greater than 20% slip can be reliably assessed.[68,69]

Degenerative Spondylolisthesis

Degenerative spondylolisthesis (DS), which is usually seen with an intact pars interarticularis, is related to degenerative changes of the apophyseal joints and/or intervertebral discs and is most common at the L4-5 and L5-S1 vertebral levels. Lumbar DS is a major cause of spinal canal stenosis and is often related to low back and leg pain.[70] Long-standing DS is almost invariably accompanied by disc and facet degenerative changes, which obscure the origin of the process. Discogenic DS and facetic DS cause secondary stress and stretch on the facet joints and disc spaces, respectively. The degree of sagittal listhesis is generally mild in DS relative to other types, particularly isthmic spondylolisthesis. There may be associated degenerative scoliosis and listhesis in nonsagittal planes. Type I end-plate changes, which may be more extensive and quite prominent on a STIR sequence, even without spondylolisthesis on static imaging, may represent segmental instability[71] and can mimic discitis osteomyelitis, as discussed later (Fig. 172-11).

Pseudarthrosis

Pseudarthrosis is more common in a postoperative spine and can occur at the fusion level (nonunion) or adjacent levels (transitional). The latter can also have noniatrogenic causes.

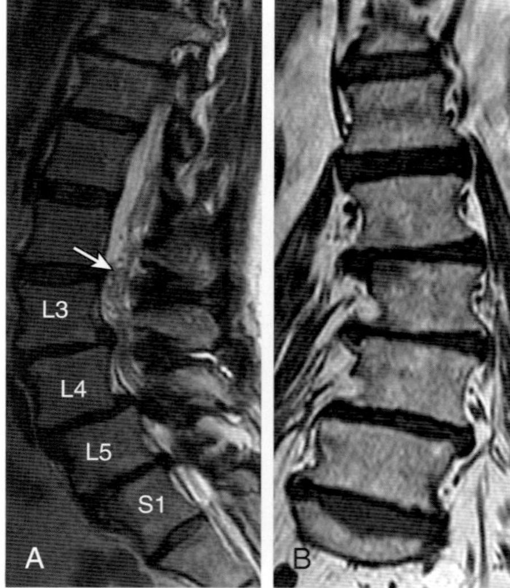

FIGURE 172-11. Degenerative spondylolisthesis and scoliosis. **A,** Grade I anterolisthesis at L3-4 and L4-5. Note high-grade stenosis at L4-5 with redundant nerve roots (*arrow*). **B,** Typical degenerative scoliosis with lateral listhesis.

Nonunion of Bone Fusion

Nonunion is the result of failed spinal fusion. The failed fusion typically manifests with axial or radicular pain months to years after surgery. The common causes of this complication are inadequate surgical technique, excessive stresses across the fusion site, insufficient internal or external stabilization, and unrecognized metabolic abnormalities.[72] Diagnosis is based on clinical presentation and imaging studies, after other causes of persistent pain are excluded.[73] The degree of fusion and associated motion seen on flexion-extension radiographs that is indicative of solid or failed fusion remains a point of controversy due to significant interobserver variations.[74] The choice of bone graft material can affect the radiographic assessment of interbody fusion. CT has higher contrast resolution and is therefore better than radiography for assessment of bone fusion. One of the main reasons for CT's superiority is that premineralized osteoid may be functionally fused but radiographically lucent, therefore leading to underestimation on plain radiography. Bony arthrodesis is usually evident by 6 months, with evidence of bridging trabecular bone. Bridging bone is usually seen lateral to the implant and may also be noted within the implant itself. Mature solid fusion is generally present at between 12 and 24 months[75,76] (Fig. 172-12).

Disc Space Failed Fusion. Failed fusion at the disc space manifests as lucency at the device margins or lucent lines through the fusion mass by about 18 to 24 months. Lucency around the fusion devices (e.g., cage or pedicular screws) represents abnormal motion and predicts delayed or failed fusion. Cystic change at the end plates adjacent to the implant is a reliable marker of failed fusion. Other signs include malpositioning and subsidence of the fusion devices[74-76] (see Fig. 172-12).

Posterolateral Failed Fusion. Posterolateral failed fusion is divided into three types: Type I shows atrophy and resorption of the grafted bone; type II shows a lack in trabecular continuity of the fusion mass; and type III shows a gap either cranially or caudally between the fusion mass and lumbar matrix (which includes the transverse process and superior facet). CT is better than PR for diagnosing all types of posterolateral failed fusion, particularly type III[77] (see Fig. 172-12).

Transitional or Segmental Pseudarthrosis

Segmental pseudarthrosis is usually secondary to transition of the mechanical loading to the adjacent level above the surgical fusion or fusion due to ankylosing spondyloarthropathies and advanced degenerative processes. Neuropathic spine (Charcot spine) can also result in segmental pseudarthrosis. The typical CT imaging pattern is lucency through the ventral and dorsal pillars in a transverse plane with or without associated spondylolisthesis. MRI shows corresponding hyperintense T2 (fluid) signal in the transverse plane defects and variable end-plate signal changes (see Fig. 172-12).

Intervertebral Disc Displacement (Disc Herniation)

Degeneration allows the disc to displace focally or diffusely in any direction beyond the end-plate margins of the disc space. The anulus fibrosus in a displaced disc tries to contain or limit the herniating nucleus pulposus. A variety of terms are used

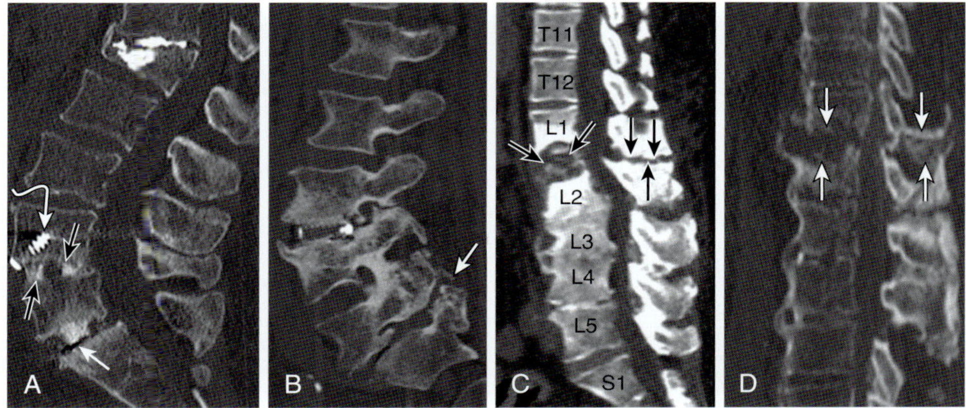

FIGURE 172-12. Pseudarthrosis. **A,** Postoperative spine with well-formed L4-5 interbody fusion (*black arrows*) but pseudarthrosis at L5-S1 interbody fusion (*white arrow*). Note anti-kickout screw at L4-5 (*curved arrow*). **B,** Posterolateral fusion mass at L5-S1 with gross defect due to pseudarthrosis (*arrow*). **C,** Segmental pseudarthrosis through anterior and dorsal columns at a level just above the L2-3 and L3-4 interbody fusion (*arrows*). **D,** Similar segmental pseudarthrosis due to neuroarthropathy (Charcot spine, *arrows*).

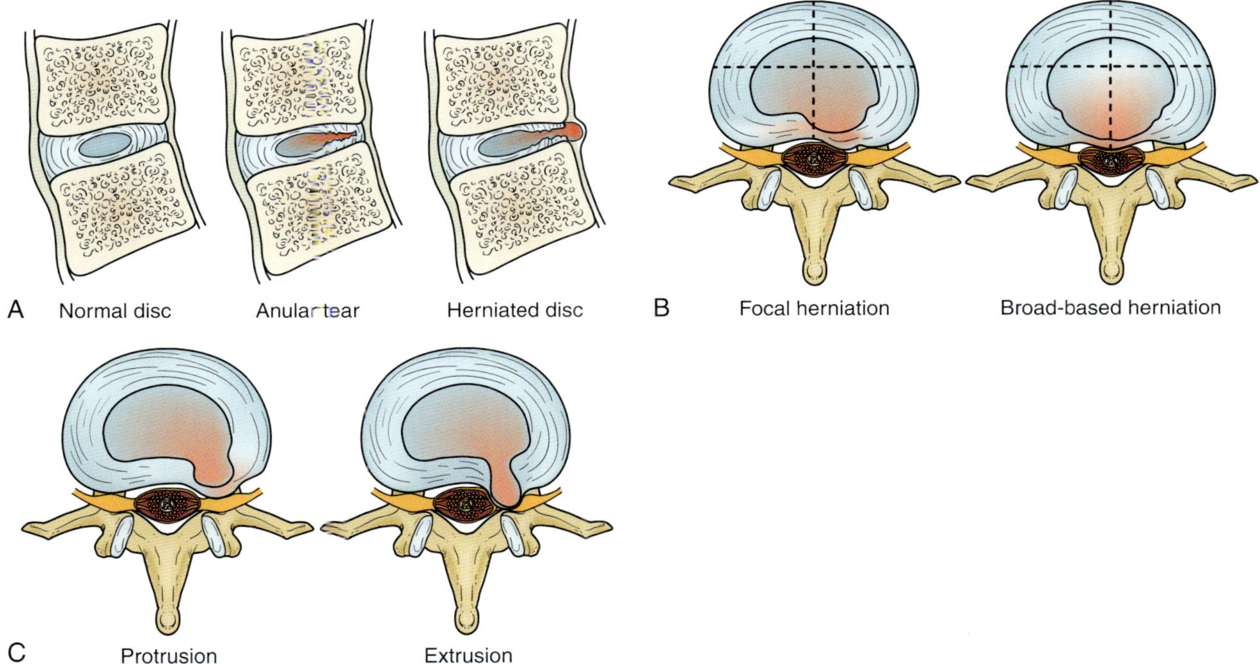

FIGURE 172-13. Schematics of disc herniations. Diagrammatic representation of disc herniations. **A,** Sagittal illustration of normal disc, anular tear, and herniation of the nucleus pulposus. **B,** Focal disc herniation (<25% of the disc margin) and broad-based herniation (>25% of the disc margin). **C,** Difference between protrusion and extrusion in the axial plane. Note that the base of the protrusion is broader than the extent of the disc herniation beyond the margins of the disc. The extrusion, on the other hand, shows a greater extension beyond the disc margins than the width of the base.

to describe disc displacement. See Figure 172-13 for diagrammatic representation of disc displacements.

Anular Disc Bulge

An anular bulge is a generalized extension, greater than 50% of the circumference of the disc tissues to a short distance (<3 mm) beyond the edges of the apophyses. A bulge is not a herniation; it is generally diffuse and may be asymmetrical. The latter usually occurs when associated lateral listhesis and scoliosis are present. The nucleus pulposus is contained by the anulus fibrosus. Grading of the disc bulging is subjective. Associated end-plate hypertrophy (spondylosis) may be present but is less prominent than in the cervical spine. Disc bulging may show crescentic calcification along its dorsal margin on sagittal CT (see Fig. 172-11A).

Intra-Anular Disc Displacement

Intra-anular disc displacement is the peripheral displacement of nuclear tissue into a fissure of the anulus. This is distinguished from disc herniation in that it does not extend beyond the disc space itself.

Protrusions

Protrusions are disc displacements in which the greatest distance in any plane between the edges of disc material beyond the disc space is less than the distance between the edges

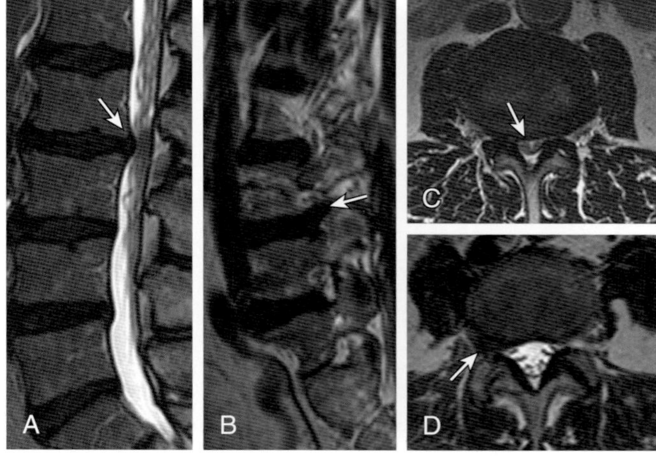

FIGURE 172-14. Disc protrusion. Mild broad-based disc protrusion at L2-3 with moderate thecal sac compression; there is underlying developmental shortened pedicles (*arrows,* **A** and **C**). Right foraminal L3-4 disc protrusion (*arrows,* **B** and **D**).

of the base in the same plane (neck is broader than dome). Protrusion is still contained by the anulus fibrosus fibers and therefore is not a true herniation. There may be an associated anular tear, which is usually evident on MRI as T2 hyperintensity, typically in the dorsal or dorsolateral disc protrusions. If the protrusion is less than 25% of the disc circumference, it is referred to as focal, and if between 25% and 50%, it is referred to as broad-based (Fig. 172-14).

Extrusions

Extrusions are disc displacements that are true herniations in which in at least one plane, any one distance between the edges of the disc material beyond the disc space, is greater than the distance between the edges of the base in the same plane (dome is broader than neck). Extrusions usually extend above or below into the suprapedicular or infrapedicular zone, resulting in further narrowing of the neck but still abutting the native disc. The signal intensity of the extruded portion may be increased on T2-weighted images. There may be associated curvilinear areas of decreased signal intensity on the T2-weighted images, which are related to torn portions of the anulus and posterior longitudinal ligament (Fig. 172-15).

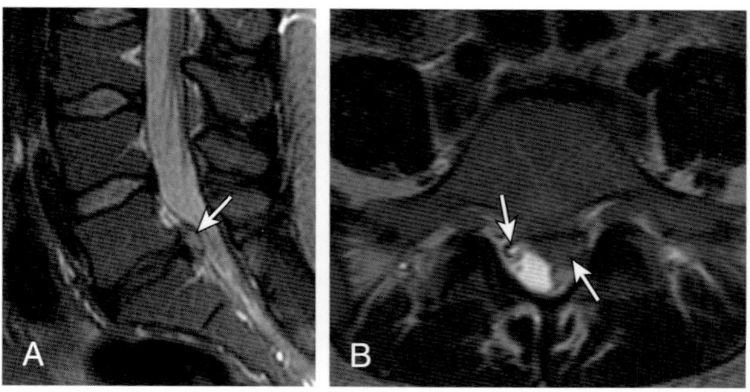

FIGURE 172-15. Disc extrusion. Sagittal (**A**) and axial (**B**) T2 imaging showing small left central disc extrusion (*arrows*) with compression of left S1 nerve root, which cannot be discretely identified (grade III compression). Note intact right S1 nerve root and its sheath (*arrow* on the right in **B**).

Sequestration

Sequestration is displaced disc material that has completely lost any continuity with the parent disc. The extrusion is referred to as "migrated" if it has displaced from the site of extrusion, regardless of whether it is sequestrated. Sequestrated fragments can lie ventral to the posterior longitudinal ligament (especially if they have migrated behind the vertebral bodies where the posterior longitudinal ligament is not in direct opposition), dorsal to the ligament, rarely in the intradural or intraradicular space, and even in the dorsal extradural space.[78] Nevertheless, penetration almost invariably occurs through the posterior longitudinal ligament; either dorsal, where it is fused with the anulus, or rostrally or caudally, where it fuses with the vertebral body margin. In the majority of patients in whom sequestrated fragments migrate behind the vertebral body, the sequestration usually lateralizes, with disc material pushing across the midline and the leading edge being smoothly capped. It has been postulated that this shape is imposed by a midline septum in the ventral epidural space. This space is largest in the lower lumbar region and is delineated dorsally by the posterior longitudinal ligament and laterally attached membranes and ventrally by the vertebral body. It is divided into two compartments by a sagittally aligned septum. Sequestrated fragments within the lateral recess and the neural foramen have been shown to produce eroded cortical bone and expansion of those spaces and, thus, should be considered in the differential diagnosis of a mass arising and expanding the neural foramen and lateral recess. Intradural disc herniation is very rare, with few cases reported.[79,80] It is most frequent in the lower lumbar spine. The mechanism is thought to be the development of chronic inflammation leading to adhesions between the dura mater and posterior longitudinal ligament. The appearance on axial MRI is described as a "hawk-beak sign."[81] As the herniated disc penetrates, the ligament extends through the dura instead of pushing it away. Other possible causes are congenital connections between the ligament and the dura or previous surgery (Fig. 172-16).

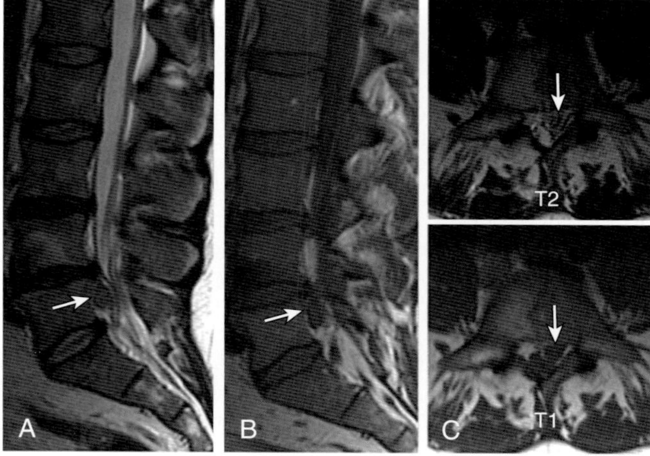

FIGURE 172-16. Sequestered disc. Sagittal T1 (**A**) and T2 (**B**) imaging shows left-sided sequestered disc with mild thecal sac compression. Note that extruded disc has lost contact with the bulging disc at L4-5 (*arrows*). **C,** Also note increased T2 signal in the herniated disc resulting in lesser conspicuity on axial T2 slice due to adjacent hyperintense fat (*arrows*).

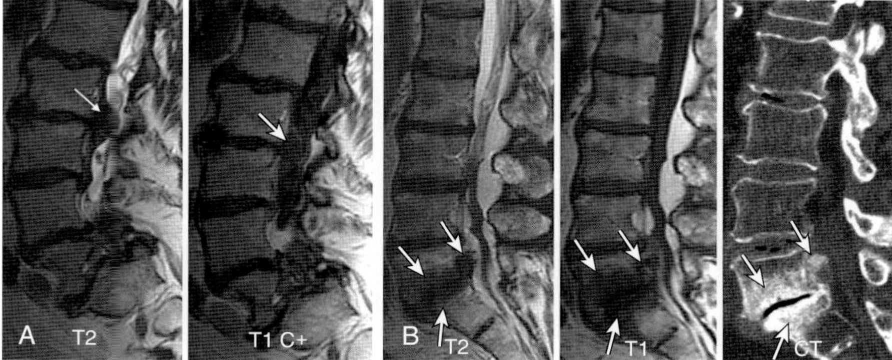

FIGURE 172-17. **A,** Calcified herniated disc. Large disc extrusion at L2-3 with severe central spinal canal stenosis. Note isointense T1 and T2 signal to the native disc and expected mild rim enhancement. Surgery revealed a calcified rocklike herniated disc material. MRI was not helpful in predicting the calcified nature of the herniated disc. **B,** Calcified herniated disc and type III end-plate change. Advanced disc degeneration at L5-S1 with type III end-plate changes, shown as hypointense T1 and T2 signal and sclerosis on CT (*anterior arrows*). CT also shows a calcified extruded disc as also predicted on MRI due to T1 hyperintense signal (*posterior arrow*). Surgery revealed an epidural perineural mass–like structure. Biopsy was negative for neoplasm.

Imaging Characterization of a Disc Herniation

Disc herniation is not always clear-cut on imaging, and it may appear as a protrusion in one plane and an extrusion in another. If there is displacement away from the disc space in craniocaudal plane, it should be referred to as an extrusion. In the transverse plane, the disc abnormality is usually described as central, right, or left central, lateral recess, foraminal, or extraforaminal (lateral and far lateral). In the sagittal plane, the terms *discal, infrapedicular,* and *suprapedicular* are most commonly employed.

Containment refers to the integrity of the outer anulus covering the disc herniation. Imaging is not accurate in delineating containment of the nucleus pulposus. One may view the continuum of herniated disc disease as starting with anular disruption, proceeding on to small focal herniation that is not broken completely through the anulus-ligamentous complex to frank herniation (extrusion), which has dissected through the anulus and dorsal ligamentous complex completely. Disc herniations may show variable degrees of containment, and a line of decreased signal intensity has been reported around sequestrated fragments and large extruded discs where disruption of the anulus and ligament is clearly evident. This is thought to be secondary to anular and ligamentous fibers, which are carried away with the disc herniation. The anulus fibrosus and posterior longitudinal ligament are so intertwined at the level of the disc that a distinction between the two structures may be impossible or, for that matter, irrelevant. Technical limitations of CT and MRI usually preclude the distinction of a contained from an uncontained disc herniation.

Contrast enhancement is commonly seen as rim enhancement along the dorsal margin of disc herniation. Rarely, the disc herniation is diffusely enhanced, and it may be difficult to differentiate from epidural scarring in a postoperative spine.

Hyperintense zone (HIZ) in a disc has been used in correlative studies of MR and provocative discography. This nonstandard term generally represents anular tears.[82,83]

Compression of the nerve root within its sleeve may not correlate with patient symptoms. A grading system by Pfirrmann et al.[84] had significant reliability and surgical correlation:

Grade 0 (normal): No contact of disc material with the nerve root.

Grade 1 (contact): Visible contact of disc material with the nerve root and loss of the epidural fat layer between the two.

Grade 2 (deviation): The nerve root is displaced dorsally by disc material.

Grade 3 (compression): The nerve root is compressed between disc material and the wall of the spinal canal; it may appear flattened or be indistinguishable from disc material (see Fig. 172-15B).

A herniated disc may be densely calcified, which may not be easily predictable on preoperative MRI. An isointense to hyperintense T1 signal can be helpful in such cases. CT clearly demonstrates calcification of disc herniation and ossification of the posterior longitudinal ligament (Fig. 172-17).

Intravertebral Disc Herniations (Also Known as Schmorl Nodes)

Nonacute Schmorl node (SN) intrabody herniations are common spinal abnormalities regarded as incidental observations. They have been reported in 38% to 75% of the population.[85,86] Most intrabody herniations probably form after axial loading trauma, with extrusion of nuclear material through the vertebral end plate, resulting in reactive bone marrow edema. Another theory is that Schmorl nodes are the end result of ischemic necrosis beneath the cartilaginous end plate, with secondary herniation into the body of the vertebra.[87] SNs are mostly well defined and have an isointense intrinsic T1/T2 signal to the disc.[88] SNs have been traced to episodes of significant, sudden-onset, localized, nonradiating back pain and tenderness. Wagner et al.[89] showed in symptomatic patients that 57% of cases on MRI had SNs surrounded by vertebral body marrow edema. The remaining nodes (43%) were not immediately apparent as SNs and manifested only as vertebral body edema, suggesting end-plate fracture, but did evolve into classical chronic SNs as revealed on follow-up imaging.[89] Contrast enhancement demonstrated vascularized SNs, with a higher incidence of surrounding edema. They are more common in symptomatic patients.[90,91] A concentric hypointense ring appearance has a high negative predictive value for the absence of underlying fracture, infection, or malignancy.[88] Giant cystic SNs have been described by Hauger et al.[92] as a clinicoimaging

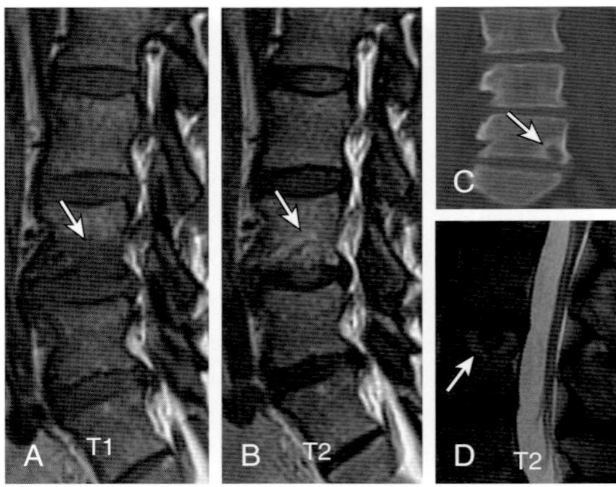

FIGURE 172-18. Schmorl node. Ill-defined hypointense T1 (**A**) and hyperintense T2 (**B**) reactive marrow changes (*arrows*) around Schmorl node at L4 inferior end plate. The signal alteration is similar to type I end-plate change. **C**, Note sclerosis along the margin of the Schmorl node. Also note hypointense rim of the node (**B**). **D**, Another patient with well-defined hyperintense T2 signal around the Schmorl node (*arrow*).

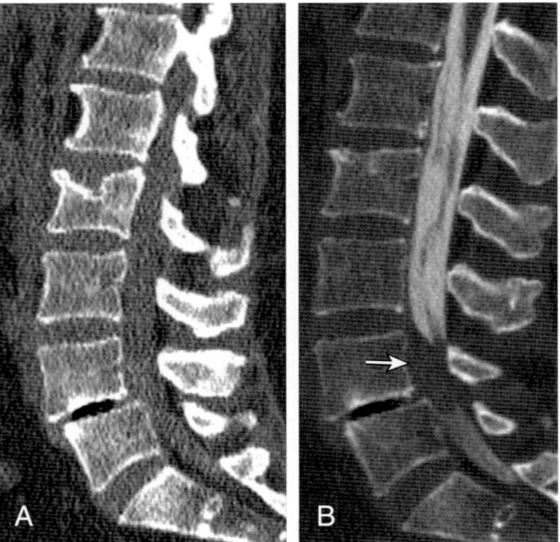

FIGURE 172-19. Degenerative spinal canal stenosis. **A,** Plain CT showing L4-5 disc degeneration and anterolisthesis. **B,** CT myelogram reveals severe central canal stenosis with large ventral extrinsic compression due to extruded disc (*arrow*). Note near-complete myelographic block with fainter opacification of the thecal sac caudal to the stenosis.

entity in a small series of six cases (Fig. 172-18; and see also Fig. 172-5).

Although consistent terminology is important for communication, it is not at all clear whether or not these categories of descriptive findings of disc herniations are clinically relevant. Although it has been proposed that it is critical to differentiate between various degrees of herniation, the reality is that disc herniation most likely represents a spectrum or continuum rather than discrete entities with specific clinical relationships. Therefore, the term *herniation* has been interchangeably used in the literature with protrusion, extrusion, and sequestration.

Spinal Canal and Foraminal Stenosis

Spinal stenosis refers to any type of narrowing of the spinal canal, nerve root canals, or intervertebral foramina.[93] Two broad groups have been defined: (1) acquired (usually related to degenerative changes) and (2) congenital or developmental. Developmental stenosis can be exacerbated by superimposed acquired degenerative changes. In the acquired type, there has been no association between the severity of pain and the degree of stenosis. The most common symptoms are sensory disturbances in the legs, LBP, neurogenic claudication, weakness, and relief of pain by bending forward. *Clinical stenosis* is perhaps a better term than spinal stenosis (as diagnosed on imaging studies). The imaging changes are in general more severe than expected from the clinical findings.[94] Although there does appear to be a correlation between cross-sectional area and midsagittal measurements in patients with symptomatic spinal stenosis, measurement of canal stenosis is not generally used.[39]

Acquired Lumbar Spinal Stenosis

Acquired lumbar spine stenosis (LSS) is typically a sequela of hypertrophic degenerative disc and facet/ligamentous changes that can be accentuated by static or dynamic degenerative DS. Anatomically, spinal stenosis is divided into central canal, lateral canal (subarticular and lateral recess), and foraminal stenosis. Subjective visual grading of the spinal stenosis is a routine practice in interpretation of the spine imaging. Quantitative evaluation by measuring the AP diameter or cross-sectional area of the central canal is used in research studies but is not commonly done in clinical practice.[95] Recent Framingham study data used a cut-off AP diameter of 12 mm for relative LSS, and 10 mm for absolute LSS.[96] There is tendency to subjectively grade central spinal canal stenosis as mild, moderate, and severe based on the effacement of the thecal sac due to a combination of anular disc bulging, end-plate osteophytosis, and dorsal ligamentum laxity. Nevertheless, spinal stenosis, even of a severe grade, is meaningless if it lacks a correlation to patient symptoms (Fig. 172-19).

Acquired Foraminal Stenosis

Acquired foraminal stenosis generally accompanies spinal canal stenosis and spondylolisthesis. Foraminal stenosis can be caused by asymmetrical anular disc bulges, associated end-plate osteophytosis, and/or facet joint changes (hypertrophy and rostrocaudal subluxation).

MRI (Conventional), CT (Plain), and CT Myelogram. These three imaging modalities are comparable in estimating the degree of stenosis but are limited by less perfect studies to really prove their difference in accuracy.[97,98] MRI is a study of choice in spines that have not undergone surgery, provided that the study is not motion degraded and axial imaging is parallel to the intervertebral disc planes and not hampered by angling or volume-averaging issues. Biplanar (sagittal and axial) evaluation is essential. Recently, Lurie et al.[99] showed moderate to substantial inter-reader agreement in assessment of central canal stenosis, foraminal stenosis, and nerve root impingement on MRI, whereas subarticular zone stenosis yielded the poorest agreement with marked variability. Plain CT alone is not a preferred preoperative modality and is usually supplemented by MRI or CT myelogram. Redundant nerve

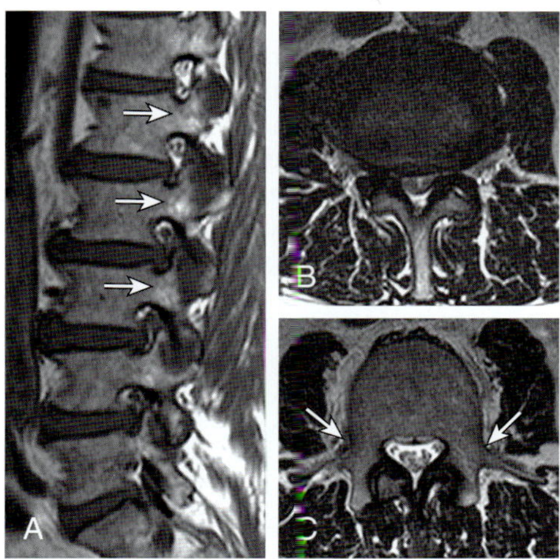

FIGURE 172-20. Congenital spinal stenosis. Sagittal (**A**) and axial (**C**) imaging shows developmentally shortened pedicles (*arrows*). Note slitlike narrowing of the foramina (**A**). Mild disc bulging causing relatively moderate central canal stenosis due to underlying limited reserve (**B**).

roots (RNRs) is a relatively common finding in association with spinal stenosis on MRI. Redundancy is caused by chronic constriction.[100] It tends to develop in patients of more advanced age[100] (see Figs. 172-11A and 172-22B).

Congenital Lumbar Stenosis

Congenital lumbar stenosis manifests at a relatively younger age with multiple levels of involvement. Relative milder degenerative changes can cause significant spinal and foraminal stenosis by virtue of developmentally compromised reserve. Radiographically, Dewing et al.[101] and Singh et al.[102] showed that these patients have a shorter pedicular length, resulting in a smaller cross-sectional spinal canal area (mean critical values of 6.5 mm and 213 mm^2, respectively). The AP pedicle:vertebral body length ratio was decreased (e.g., 0.36 in patients vs. 0.48 in controls at the L4 level). Recognizing congenital stenosis alerts the treating surgeon to the possibility of multilevel treatment. Subjective MR signs of congenital stenosis include elongated teardrop foramina in the sagittal plane and shortened pedicles with stubby dorsal elements and decreased AP diameter in the axial plane (Fig. 172-20).

Spinal Epidural Lipomatosis

A common incidental finding in the sacral and lower lumbar canal, spinal epidural lipomatosis (SEL) is typically of no clinical significance. Epidural lipomatosis is usually idiopathic and related to the patient's body habitus. Exogenous steroids can also result in SEL. There are reports of symptomatic epidural lipomatosis treated with decompression surgery.[103,104] SEL does reduce the reserve of the central canal in patients who have hypertrophic degenerative disease. Both CT and MRI demonstrate epidural lipomatosis well. Severe epidural lipomatosis compresses the thecal sac, resulting in a Y-shaped configuration[103,105] (Fig. 172-21).

Degenerative Adult Scoliosis

Degenerative scoliosis is the most common adult spinal deformity, typically developing after 50 years of age. Type 1 adult scoliosis is primarily degenerative. It is caused by disc degeneration and facet arthropathy. Type 2 is the progression of adolescent scoliosis in adulthood. Type 3 adult scoliosis is a secondary scoliosis mostly caused by osteoporosis.[106,107]

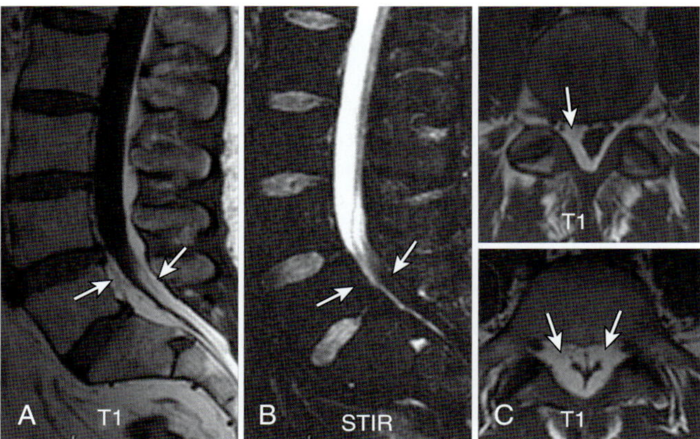

FIGURE 172-21. Epidural lipomatosis. Sagittal (**A** and **B**) and axial (**C**) imaging shows concentric epidural lipomatosis (*arrows*) with relatively small thecal sac; lipomatosis more prominent at L5-S1 and sacral canal.

Deformities of the spine in the sagittal or coronal plane considerably complicate the diagnosis and treatment of lumbar spinal stenosis. The deformities mainly consist of scoliosis, spondylolisthesis, and flatback deformity. Imaging may show listhesis in the sagittal and coronal planes in addition to angular deformities. There are associated asymmetrical changes of end-plate osteophytosis, disc bulges, facet joint hypertrophy, and foraminal encroachments. Coronal MRI is essential for characterizing and measuring scoliosis. The goals of surgery in complex stenosis are neural decompression and a well-balanced sagittal and coronal fusion.[108] As alluded to before, correction of deformity may be a relative indication for instrumented fusion in the setting of spinal stenosis[109] (see Fig. 172-11B).

Significance of Imaging Findings

Studies to date leave unanswered the question of the significance of morphologic abnormalities and do not adequately explain the role these changes play in the symptomatic population. There is no agreement on the prognostic value of morphologic changes detected by imaging.[110-112] It seems logical, therefore, to investigate the morphologic information available from modern imaging in an attempt to predict successful outcomes early in the clinical course of radiculopathy or LBP. Instead, investigators have mostly focused on epidemiologic variables such as gender, duration, litigation, compensation status, sociopsychosocial history, and so on. Any attempt to infer the prognosis from morphology will be confounded by the high prevalence of morphologic change in the asymptomatic population.

Why do some individuals without symptoms show the same morphologic abnormality as those with symptoms? Why do some individuals become symptom free without an obvious change in the morphology of the herniated disc thought to be responsible for the acute event? Why do some individuals show improving symptoms in the face of worsening morphologic changes? These questions still await clear answers. In the discussion that follows, we divide the subjects into three groups based on the presence and absence of symptoms and abnormal imaging findings.

Asymptomatic Subjects with Positive Imaging

There is a high prevalence of degenerative disc changes in asymptomatic patients. Irrespective of age, Wiesel et al.[113] found about 35% of spines to be abnormal in asymptomatic patients. Degenerative disc and/or facet disease, including spinal canal stenosis, was present in about 20% of patients younger than 40 years, whereas the prevalence rose to about 50% in patients older than 40 years. Other authors showed similar observations. The prevalence of morphologic alterations increases with advancing chronologic age. Boden et al.[114] showed that 57% of the scans were abnormal in a group of individuals older than 60 years of age (37% had disc herniations and 21% had spinal canal stenosis), whereas in the group younger than 60 years, 20% had disc herniations. Jensen et al.[115] evaluated MRI examinations of 98 asymptomatic patients and showed that 64% had disc space abnormalities, 52% anular disc bulges, 27% protrusions, 1% extrusions, 19% SNs, 14% anular defects, 7% central canal stenosis, and 38% had a disc abnormality at more than one level.

Boos et al.[116] showed a very high prevalence of disc herniation (i.e., 76% in age-, gender-, and occupation-matched asymptomatic cases), which was comparable to that of symptomatic patients (i.e., 96%); there was no statistical significance. Patients had more severe disc herniations (disc extrusions) than asymptomatic volunteers (35% vs. 13%). There were no significant differences regarding disc degeneration between both groups (96% vs. 85%). The only substantial imaging morphologic difference between the groups was the presence of a neural compromise (83% vs. 22%).

The preceding data emphasize the importance of correlating the clinical picture with the MRI examination when major surgical decisions are made. In fact, the findings on lumbar spine MRI may be meaningless when considered in isolation. In addition, with only 1% of the sample showing an extrusion in one of the larger studies by Jensen et al.,[115] subcategorizing herniations into protrusion and extrusion may be helpful for better characterizing asymptomatic versus symptomatic discs.

Symptomatic Patients with Negative Imaging

Back pain is thought to occur in some patients without evidence of such morphologic abnormalities as herniation or stenosis. The perplexing clinical scenario of patients who complain of incapacitating back pain but have no overt morphologic abnormality has given rise to the concept of the disc as a pain generator. This was classically described by Crock[117] as "chronic internal disc disruption syndrome." Many different names have been given to this idea, which becomes more confusing when combined with the various diagnostic tests that are used in an attempt to diagnose this confusing syndrome. Additional terms in the literature include internal anular tear, internal disc disruption, black disc disease, and discogenic pain. In a normal human lumbar disc, nerve endings can be found only in the periphery of the anulus, and the pain fibers are part of the sympathetic chain via the sinuvertebral nerve.[118,119] This innervates the outer layer of the anulus fibrosus. However, in very degenerated discs, nerves may even penetrate into the nucleus pulposus.[120] Potentially, stimulation of these fibers can occur not only from direct disruption and mechanical pressure on the anulus but also from various breakdown products of the nucleus pulposus or secondarily up-regulated inflammatory mediators. The normal disc acting as a source of pain is still a mystery. Provocative discography, as discussed in the following section under symptomatic patients, has been used in morphologically normal discs with an expected lack of pain reproduction.

Disc material leakage is hypothesized to cause back pain and radiculopathy through a chemoinflammatory mechanism. The nucleus pulposus can cause an inflammatory reaction with leukotaxis and increased vascular permeability.[121] A simple incision of the anulus fibrosus can produce morphologic and functional changes in the adjacent nerves, such as increased capillaries and reduced nerve conduction velocities,[122] with the presumed mechanism of disc material leakage into the epidural space. McCarron et al.,[123] using a dog model, demonstrated that autogenous placement of the nucleus pulposus into the epidural space caused acute and chronic inflammatory reactions, with influx of histiocytes and fibroblasts. Kayama et al.[122] and Olmarker et al.[124] demonstrated that the contents of the nucleus pulposus applied to spinal nerves induces a wide variety of functional, vascular, and morphologic abnormalities, often followed by intraradicular fibrosis and neural atrophy.

Symptomatic Patients with Positive Imaging

This group of patients may have positive scans, but the significance of these findings is rather confounding. The approach to positive findings from diagnostic imaging is threefold: (1) to determine the etiologic correlation to the patient's symptoms, (2) to stratify patients for conservative versus interventional treatment, and (3) to provide a patient prognosis. Unfortunately, diagnostic imaging produces no convincing, considerable, or consistent results on these three fronts.

Disc Space Degeneration

Treating the sequelae of disc degeneration (i.e., disc herniations, stenosis, and instability) is the goal of therapy and therefore the major focus in clinical and imaging trials rather than the disc degeneration itself. The intervertebral disc is considered to be the source of discogenic pain. Provocative discography has been used to identify one or more disc spaces as the source of pain. Weishaupt et al.,[125] however, showed a lower specificity (59%) and positive predictive value (PPV) (63%) for disc degeneration as a correlate of provocative pain, with mildly increased PPV for degenerated discs with HIZs. Their high negative predictive value (98%) in the normal-appearing discs at least indirectly suggests the origin of pain from other levels or causes. Recently, Kang et al.[83] demonstrated very high specificity (97.8%) and PPV (87%) for disc protrusion with HIZ in reproduction of pain. They classified the MR findings of the disc into four classes: (1) normal or bulging disc without HIZ; (2) normal or bulging disc with HIZ; (3) disc protrusion without HIZ; and (4) disc protrusion with HIZ. The first two classes had a less significant correlation to provocative pain. Disc protrusion without HIZ had a moderate correlation (specificity, 80.6%; PPV, 53.6%) to pain reproduction. As a note of caution, Carragee et al.[126] recently showed accelerated disc degeneration over 10 years in the discs that underwent discography using modern techniques.

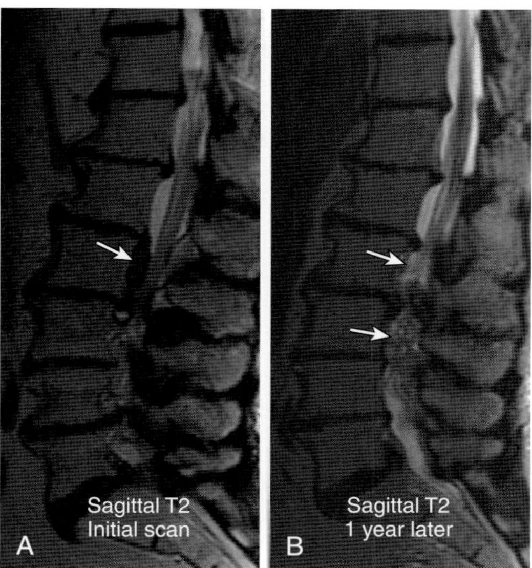

FIGURE 172-22. Spontaneous resolution of disc herniation. **A,** A large inferior disc extrusion at L1-2 (*arrow*). **B,** Follow-up imaging at about 1 year afterward shows complete spontaneous resolution of the herniated disc. Also note redundant nerve roots caudal to the degenerative central canal stenosis at L2-3 (*lower arrow*).

Disc Herniations

Anular disc bulges and larger disc herniations contribute to spinal canal stenosis. Smaller or lateralized herniations, on the other hand, can cause radiculopathy. Disc extrusions are more likely to correlate with patient symptoms than disc bulges and disc protrusions.[127] There is a high incidence of radiculopathy in patients with imaging findings of central canal stenosis and nerve root compression by disc herniation.[127,128] The presence of a disc herniation in a patient with radiculopathy is a positive prognostic marker.[127,129] Most of the available studies have shown that the size of disc herniation can reduce dramatically on conservative management; the larger herniation shows a more prominent decrease in size. Extrusion and sequestered discs are also more likely to show a reduction in size; protrusions are less likely to change. There was, however, no clear correlation of these alterations with patient symptoms.[9,8,130-132] The higher reduction and even disappearance of the extruded and sequestered discs is thought to be related to more vascular exposure.[131] As far as surgery is concerned, most surgeons believe that larger disc herniations do better after surgery than smaller disc herniations. By the same token, larger discectomy defects predict lower rates of reherniation.[133] Recently, Dewing et al.[101] showed significantly better outcomes in symptomatic patients after microdiscectomy in the following group of patients: younger, active, herniations at L5-S1 (compared with L4-5), and extrusions or sequestrations (compared with contained herniations). As far as patient preference for surgery is concerned, Lurie et al.[134] showed that younger patients having a lower level of education and higher disability/unemployment preferred the surgical option (Fig. 172-22).

End-Plate Marrow Changes

Type I and II changes are more common, whereas type III changes are relatively rare. The clinical significance is threefold: (1) correlation to back pain, (2) stability of end-plate changes, and (3) marker of segmental instability and fusion.

Back Pain

End-plate changes are less common in asymptomatic individuals. Degenerative disc disease is more likely to be associated with symptoms when end-plate changes are present.[135] Type I changes are more strongly associated with back pain.[136,137] Furthermore, conversion from type I to II is associated with clinical improvement of symptoms, and vice versa.[138] End-plate changes have a high correlation to pain production on discography compared with other disc degenerative changes; the correlation is much higher as the extent of the end-plate changes increases.[125,139] However, some authors have been unable to show a strong correlation of LBP to end-plate changes.[140,141] Albert and Manniche[136] showed that disc herniation is a strong risk factor for developing new end-plate changes, particularly type I.

Stability of End-Plate Changes

Type I changes are generally considered unstable, and type II are considered stable. Some studies have shown conversion of type II to type I changes.[136,142,143] Kuisma et al.[144] studied 60 patients with sciatica who did not undergo surgery and showed that 14% of end-plate changes evolved into another type within 3 years—80% of the conversions being from type II to either type I or mixed type I and type II. They also found that nonconverted end-plate changes increased in size and that new end-plate changes developed adjacent to degenerated discs in 6% of patients—77% of these new changes being either type I or mixed type I and type II. Basically, type I changes are a reflection of some type of biomechanical instability. On the other hand, type II changes are a reflection of stability, albeit associated with degeneration. Type II changes in the absence of superimposed accelerated degeneration or instability remain stable.

Segmental Instability

Type I changes have a higher correlation to segmental instability than type II changes do.[137] However, there is always a question about the methods for measuring instability. More convincing evidence of this correlation is shown by postfusion studies, which demonstrated a very high prevalence rather conversion into type II change in cases with solid fusion, whereas there was a higher type I change persistence in those with nonunion (pseudarthrosis)[145] (Fig. 172-23).

Facet Joint and Dorsal Elements

It is clinically important to identify pain originating from facet joints. Facet joint arthritis on imaging is a nonspecific finding usually accompanying disc degeneration. Dominant facet joint arthritis with or without effusion needs to be addressed in surgical planning. The relationship of joint effusions to spondylolisthesis and instability has already been discussed. Degenerative changes in the dorsal paraspinal structures on STIR are found in a higher percentage of subjects with LBP than in controls.[59] Lakadamyali et al.[59] showed a significantly increased incidence of facet joint effusions, para-articular soft tissue edema, and interspinous ligamentous edema in patients with LBP than in controls. Pedicle marrow changes are related to spondylolysis, as discussed earlier, but they are also

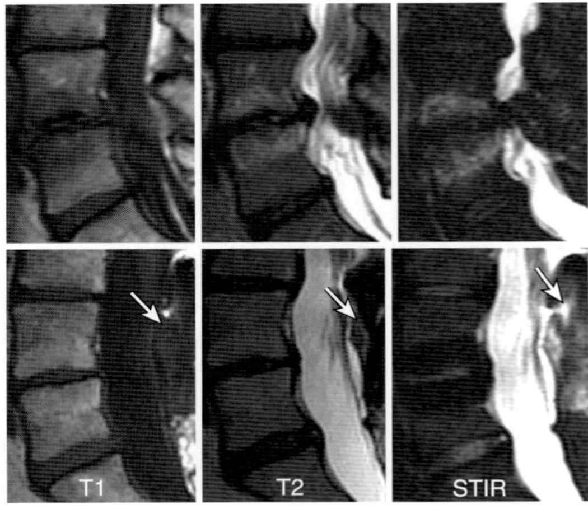

FIGURE 172-23. Postfusion type I to II end-plate conversion. Upper images demonstrate type I end-plate changes at L4-5. Patient underwent dorsal fusion (not shown) and decompression (*arrows, lower images*). Note conversion to type II end-plate change after surgery on follow-up imaging.

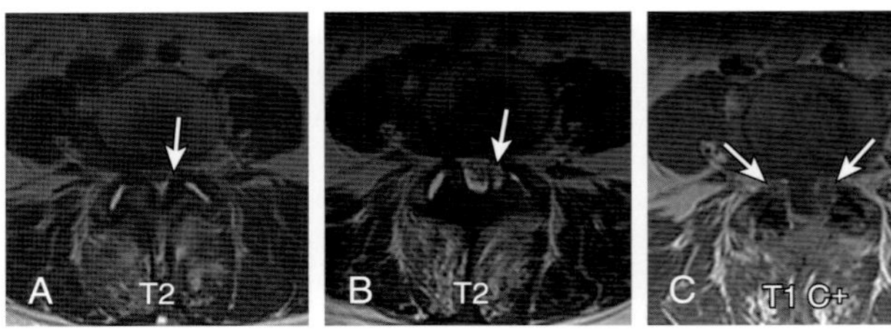

FIGURE 172-24. Facet joint instability and synovial cysts. **A,** Preoperative axial T2 image with moderate central canal stenosis at L4-5. Note bilateral facet joint effusions and small left ventral synovial cyst (*arrow*). **B** and **C**, Patient underwent decompression laminectomies at L4-5 without any fusion. Postoperative imaging showing progression of left-sided synovial cyst and development of a small ventral synovial cyst on the right side (*arrows*).

commonly seen with facet degenerative disease and reflect abnormal stresses related to abnormal motion or loading caused by the degenerative changes in the spinal segment[146] (Fig. 171-24; see also Figs. 172-8 and 172-9).

Degenerative Spondylolisthesis

The natural history of degenerative spondylolisthesis (DS) is generally favorable. About 15% to 25% of patients eventually need surgery.[147,148] Up to 35% of patients show progression of DS, but there is no clear relationship between DS progression and change in patient symptoms. Matsunaga et al.[148] studied the long-term (>10 years) nonsurgical natural course of DS. The intervertebral spaces of the slipped segments decreased significantly in size during follow-up examination in patients in whom no progression was found. LBP improved following a decrease in the total intervertebral space size. The development of osteoarthritic spurs, hypertrophy and ossification of the intervertebral ligaments, and facet arthrosis are thought to cause stabilization that prevents slip progression. About 75% of patients remained asymptomatic after 10 years of follow-up. However, most of the patients (83%) who had significant initial symptoms such as intermittent claudication or vesicorectal disorder and who refused surgery showed progressive worsening. Johnsson et al.,[149] in a study of symptomatic patients over 4 years, showed that about 75% of the patients had stable spinal claudication. Overall, symptoms in 70% of the cases were unchanged, 15% showed improvement, and 15% worsened. No proof of severe deterioration was found after 4 years. Therefore, DS is clinically significant in a small portion of the cases, and the majority of DS on imaging remains stable over a long period of time. DS is a relative indication for instrumented fusion in the setting of spinal stenosis. Other indications are correction of deformity, recurrent spinal stenosis with instability, adjacent segment stenosis with instability, and multiple-level fusions.[109]

Lumbar Spinal Stenosis

Lumbar canal stenosis is associated with a threefold higher risk of experiencing LBP.[96] However, the degree of lumbar spinal canal stenosis (LSS) on imaging is not strongly correlated with patient symptoms.[150,151] Also, imaging provides no clear means of management stratification and plays no prognostic role except in severe degrees of central canal stenosis, which has a fair correlation to functional disability and a favorable postoperative outcome.[150,152] Jonsson et al.[150] concluded that the "ideal patient for surgery" should have a pronounced constriction of the spinal canal, insignificant LBP, no concomitant disease affecting walking ability, and a symptom duration of less than 4 years. Regarding RNR in spinal canal stenosis, a recent study found a prevalence of about 33%; the longer the relative length of RNR, the better the outcome. Overall, the surgical outcomes in the RNR group were not statistically different from those in the non-RNR group.[153]

Thoracolumbar Spine Infection

Vertebral osteomyelitis, also referred to as "discitis osteomyelitis (DO)" or "spondylodiscitis" in the literature, is the most common infection of the spine. Facet joint infection is less common. Paraspinal and epidural soft tissue can be secondarily involved, resulting in phlegmon and abscess formation. Isolated epidural abscess is rare unless there has been previous intervention or a systemic source of septic embolism. The following discussion is mainly focused on vertebral osteomyelitis.

Vertebral Osteomyelitis

The single most important differential consideration to exclude when T2 hyperintense discal and adjacent marrow changes are noted is vertebral osteomyelitis. Vertebral osteomyelitis with discitis is seen in 2% to 4% of all cases of osteomyelitis.[154] Despite its low incidence, the potential morbidity and mortality from vertebral osteomyelitis are great. Accurate and specific imaging is required not only for diagnosis but also to guide biopsy for a microbiologic culture. MRI provides the best combination of sensitivity and specificity. Other imaging tests such as plain films, nuclear medicine imaging, and CT may provide additional information. In order to avoid a delayed diagnosis of vertebral osteomyelitis and the consequent devastating sequelae for the patient, keep in mind early discitis and osteomyelitis changes while interpreting spine imaging. Localized back pain is the most common presentation. In a series of 43 adult patients, Hitchon et al.[155] reported that 98% presented with local spine pain of longer than 6 weeks' duration, and 50% presented with fever. All had elevated sedimentation rates. In a review of 442 patients in all age groups with pyogenic infection of the spine, Malawski and Lukawski[156] showed that the disease seldom involved one vertebra, as usually both vertebral bodies were affected at the disc space. The lumbar spine was most commonly involved, followed by the thoracic and then the cervical spine. The sacrum rarely was involved.

Etiology and Risk Factors

The risk of vertebral osteomyelitis is increased in patients with IV drug abuse, endocarditis, sickle cell anemia, tuberculosis, malnutrition, alcoholism, diabetes mellitus, rheumatoid arthritis, as well as those undergoing hemodialysis and patients given steroids, due to compromise of host defenses.[157-159] The incidence of diabetes mellitus in patients with vertebral osteomyelitis is far out of proportion to that in the general population. Carragee et al. reported that up to 40% of patients had diabetes mellitus.[158]

Hematogenous vertebral osteomyelitis is caused predominantly by *Staphylococcus aureus*. Up to half of these infections can be caused by methicillin-resistant *S. aureus* (MRSA).[160] *S. aureus* is also a major cause of bacteremia and endocarditis in adults. In a series of 37 adult patients with vertebral osteomyelitis from the Cleveland Clinic,[161] *S. aureus* was the responsible organism in 68% of patients (25 of 37). *Staphylococcus epidermidis*, streptococci, gram-negative aerobic bacilli, and *Mycobacterium tuberculosis* were identified in 5% of the remaining patients. In IV drug abusers, *Pseudomonas aeruginosa*, other unusual gram-negative bacilli, and staphylococci cause spinal infection most frequently.[162,163] In elderly males with genitourinary tract infections, vertebral osteomyelitis is caused most often by *Escherichia coli* and *Proteus* spp.[162] Furthermore, pyogenic vertebral osteomyelitis may be caused by a different organism than the one isolated from blood, urine, or sputum culture, as reported by Velan et al. in a series of three older patients.[164]

Modes of Infection

There are three routes by which vertebral osteomyelitis can be established: (1) hematogenously, (2) iatrogenically, and (3) by contiguous spread.[165]

Hematogenous

Both the venous and arterial vessels have been proposed as possible routes for the development of vertebral osteomyelitis.

In 1940, Batson[166] described a valveless, low-pressure vertebral venous system. This is composed of tributaries from the vertebral body metaphyses that drain into a large channel that exits the vertebral body via the nutrient foramen into the plexus of veins lining the spinal canal in the extradural space. There are also connections through the vertebral body cortex to a plexus of veins on the ventral and lateral aspects of the spine.[167] Batson[166] demonstrated rich anastomoses of this vertebral venous system with the thoracic and abdominal cavities and with pelvic veins. Slight increases in pressure in the vena caval system resulted in a diversion of blood into the vertebral venous system.

Septic embolization via the arterial system has also been proposed as a route for vertebral osteomyelitis. The arterial system of the spine forms a ladder-like anastomosis on its surface. The horizontal components are segmental arteries (1–3 mm) arising from the abdominal aorta that lie at the equator of the vertebral body, and two metaphyseal (200 mm) anastomosing arteries at each vertebral metaphysis. The vertical components join the segmental arteries to the metaphyseal anastomosing arteries, the metaphyseal anastomosing arteries of adjacent vertebral arteries, as well as metaphyseal anastomosing arteries of the same vertebral body. The intraosseous arteries arise from the segmental and metaphyseal anastomosing arteries and parallel the disc surface. Children have rich anastomoses of the intraosseous arteries, which involute by adulthood. Thus, in an adult, infection of the disc cannot occur directly via hematogenous means. It can occur via contiguous spread from an adjacent infected vertebral body. Ratcliffe[168] has proposed that septic emboli were more likely to enter the greater number of arteries at the metaphysis and that the smaller caliber of the vessels allowed for the development of thrombosis with resultant infarction—a requirement for osteomyelitis to develop. These two observations explain the propensity for vertebral osteomyelitis to involve the subchondral aspect of the body with relative sparing of the central portion of the vertebral body. The vertical anastomoses among the metaphyseal anastomosing arteries allowed for the spread of infection across disc spaces as well as within the same vertebral body while sparing the central portion. The intraosseous anastomoses in children would prevent large foci of bony infarction, thus resulting in smaller foci of osteomyelitis.[168]

Whereas metastatic spread from the pelvic venous system to the vertebral bodies via the vertebral venous plexus has been shown in animals,[169,170] the spread of infection via the vertebral plexus could not be demonstrated experimentally. Further argument supporting arterial spread is that vertebral osteomyelitis is usually preceded by symptomatology compatible with bacteremia (sepsis). If spread is via the venous route, extradural thrombophlebitis with meningismus should be expected to represent a prominent feature of osteomyelitis.[171] This has not proven to be the case.

Iatrogenic or Posttraumatic

Organisms can be directly implanted secondary to surgical procedures or penetrating spinal trauma. Discitis has been reported as a complication of cervical and lumbar discography,[172,173] chemonucleolysis (chymopapain injection),[174,175] and laminectomy.[176,177] Discitis as a complication of discography is uncommon. Its incidence has been reported as 0.05% to 1.4% in various series. An aggravation or increase of neck and back pain and fever are typical presenting complaints.[172,173]

The diagnosis of disc space infection following discectomy is problematic. Patients typically present 2 to 6 weeks following surgery with recurrence of pain after initially having experienced the relief of symptoms. Patients are often febrile with muscle spasm and a positive straight-leg raising test.[176] The sedimentation rate is elevated. Roentgenographic findings appear several weeks after initial symptoms, with a decrease in the intervertebral disc space height and development of end-plate erosions.

Contiguous Spread

Vertebral osteomyelitis, or disc space infection, can result from contiguous spread from an adjacent infected source. It is the least common of the three mechanisms discussed here.[178] Contiguous spread requires the spread of a superlative soft tissue focus through the periosteum, cortex, and marrow of the vertebral body or through the longitudinal ligaments, anulus fibrosus, and nucleus pulposus of the disc. Contiguous spread of infection to the spine is encountered in the sacral region in association with infected decubitus ulcers, as well as genitourinary and intestinal processes.[178] Vertebral osteomyelitis and disc space infection have been reported as complications of colonic,[179] hypopharyngeal,[180] and esophageal[181,182] perforations or instrumentation, as well as pelvic abscesses.[183] Lesions of the aorta or of an aortic graft, such as mycotic aneurysm or pseudoaneurysm, may predispose to the development of vertebral osteomyelitis.[184] When considering vertebral osteomyelitis as a result of contiguous spread, the question often arises as to whether the infection was actually a result of hematogenous spread (either arterial or venous) rather than truly contiguous with direct invasion.[185-187] For example, the direct invasion of a vertebral body by a lung lesion is felt to be an unlikely sequence of events due to an effective barrier provided by the pleura.[185] Here it has been postulated that spread actually occurs via pleural veins communicating with the Batson plexus.

Imaging of Discitis Osteomyelitis

Conventional Radiography

Typically, the early findings of disc space infection on plain radiography are minimal disc space narrowing and erosions or indistinctness of the end plates. In addition to the bony changes, soft tissue swelling due to paraspinal phlegmon or abscess may also be evident. In the lumbar region, this presents as enlargement of the psoas shadows. In the thoracic region, disc space infection appears as a paraspinal soft tissue mass. In the cervical spine, prevertebral soft tissue swelling is evident. As the disease progresses, the disc space narrowing worsens. The destruction of the end plates becomes more obvious. In addition, sclerosis of the end plates and a periosteal reaction also become evident. In general, with healing, the disc space remains markedly narrowed or fuses, and there may be a concomitant loss of height of the vertebral body with resultant spinal deformity (see Fig. 172-31C).

Digby and Kersley[188] reported the following time sequence for the radiographic changes to correlate with the pathologic changes: at 2 weeks, decreased disc space height becomes evident; at 6 weeks, lytic vertebral body lesions are seen; reactive sclerosis is present at 8 weeks; and at 6 months, new bone formation and fusion are present. Malawski and Lukawski[156] also reported the time sequence of radiographic changes in a series of 150 cases of vertebral osteomyelitis. They found that radiologic changes became apparent after 4 to 6 weeks. In their series, an early sign was also a decrease in disc space height. After several weeks, lytic vertebral body lesions and end-plate disruption were evident.

Unique presentations of vertebral osteomyelitis have also been reported. McHenry et al.[189] reported a series of six patients with osteomyelitis who presented with underlying osteoporosis and compression fracture of a single vertebral body. On the initial plain radiographs, the end plates were intact. This unique presentation accounted for 13% of all hospitalized patients with vertebral osteomyelitis and 2.4% of inpatients with osteoporotic compression fractures over a 5-year period in our institution.

Nuclear Medicine

The role of nuclear medicine in vertebral osteomyelitis is diminishing. If MRI cannot be performed, nuclear medicine examinations have been used for diagnosis of vertebral osteomyelitis. Specificity is a major limiting factor with bone scans, which use the radionuclide technetium-99m. Gallium-67 is, however, a useful radionuclide with high specificity.[190] Both these tracers have significantly high specificity due to a complementary role. Indium-111 leukocyte imaging has little or no usefulness in detecting vertebral osteomyelitis and has been shown to be unreliable.[191]

Three-Phase and Total-Body Bone Scan

In the setting of vertebral osteomyelitis, the three-phase bone scan demonstrates increased uptake in flow and blood pool phases and in delayed images. Intense uptake in two adjacent vertebral bodies with loss of the disc space is seen in patients with vertebral osteomyelitis. The bone scan is sensitive for vertebral osteomyelitis. However, it lacks specificity. In the spine, it can be difficult to separate increased radionuclide uptake due to degenerative disc disease, benign compression fracture, or metastatic disease from that occurring as a result of vertebral osteomyelitis. Moreover, some investigators report bacteriologically proven vertebral osteomyelitis in patients who had a negative bone scan at 2 weeks following the onset of symptoms.[192,193] In addition, the increased uptake of tracer does not differentiate active from inactive osteomyelitis, since increased uptake can persist for long periods following resolution of the infection.[194]

Gallium-67

Gallium scan also demonstrates increased uptake in the setting of vertebral osteomyelitis. It also gives information about the surrounding soft tissues. The combination of gallium scanning and a three-phase bone scan may increase the specificity up to nearly 100%.[192] The sensitivity is approximately 90%. The two tests provide complementary information.[195] It is generally accepted that the combination of bone and gallium imaging can identify vertebral osteomyelitis when (1) the distribution of the two tracers is spatially incongruent or (2) their distribution is spatially congruent and the relative uptake of gallium exceeds that of technetium.[191] The combination of the two studies is currently the nuclear medicine study of choice for vertebral osteomyelitis. Gratz et al.[196] were able to demonstrate that gallium-67 (^{67}Ga)-citrate single-photon emission tomography (SPECT) activity correlated with the severity of infection in a small series of patients who had been receiving antibiotic treatment for an average of 7 weeks prior to scanning. The sensitivity in detecting vertebral osteomyelitis was 80% for individual foci and 100% for vertebral osteomyelitis. In addition, ^{67}Ga-citrate SPECT detected foci of infection outside

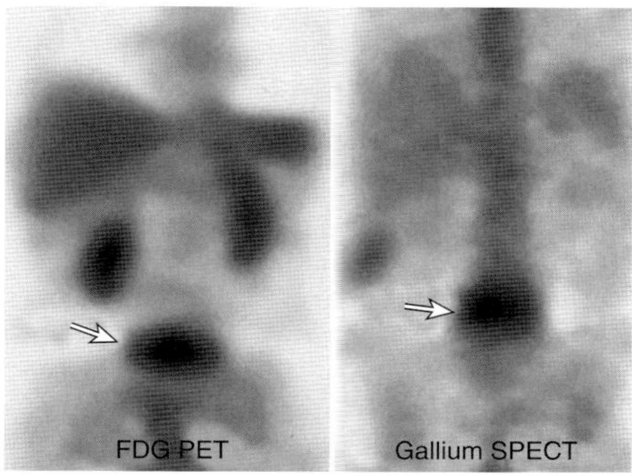

FIGURE 172-25. Vertebral osteomyelitis on gallium and 2-[18F] fluoro-2-deoxy-D-glucose/positron emission tomography (FDG-PET). Coronal images from FDG-PET and ^{67}Ga single-photon emission computed tomography (SPECT). Increased radiotracer accumulation (*white arrows*) at L5-S1 due to discitis osteomyelitis. (From Love C, Tomas MB, Tronco GG, et al: FDG PET of inflammation and infection. *Radiographics* 25(5):1357–1368, 2005, with permission.)

of the spine before other imaging techniques demonstrated these[196] (Fig. 172-25).

2-[18F] Fluoro-2-Deoxy-D-Glucose Positron Emission Tomography

With the exception of combined bone scan–gallium imaging, nuclear medicine imaging for vertebral osteomyelitis has been unsatisfactory. 2-[18F] fluoro-2-deoxy-D-glucose positron emission tomography (FDG-PET) has shown higher sensitivity and specificity in the diagnosis of vertebral osteomyelitis than has MRI.[197,198] FDG-PET has proven useful for differentiating degenerative and infectious end-plate abnormalities detected on MRI.[198] FDG imaging findings are likely due to increased glucose metabolism in inflammatory cells such as leukocytes, granulocytes, and macrophages. An additional advantage is that FDG-PET is not affected by metal implants. It may be useful in evaluating infection in patients with hardware. FDG-PET has better resolution than other nuclear medicine imaging techniques and can differentiate bone from soft tissue infection. Low FDG-PET uptake has been shown in fractures and pseudarthrosis. Hodges et al.[199] identified persistent disease on MRI as a sign of failure of conservative treatment. Recently, Kim et al.[200] showed the utility of FDG-PET in differentiating between residual and nonresidual disease based on standard uptake value measurements. FDG-PET may therefore be used in cases of vertebral osteomyelitis as a problem-solving tool in proper clinical settings (see Fig. 172-25).

Computed Tomography

CT can be used in the diagnosis of advanced vertebral osteomyelitis and discitis. Due to routine use of multiplanar reformats, vertebral osteomyelitis may be picked up as an incidental finding on CT of the abdomen and pelvis. CT allows detection of bony destruction and paraspinal swelling. CT demonstrates a decrease in the density of the affected vertebral body and disc.[178,200,201] The CT criteria for the diagnosis of pyogenic vertebral osteomyelitis include diffuse moth-eaten or permeative bone destruction, gas within the bone or adjacent soft tissues, and prevertebral soft tissue involvement.[178,202] Discal gas is generally considered a sign of degenerative change and excludes discitis, but rare exceptions have been reported.[47] Granulomatous vertebral osteomyelitis may manifest with fragmented end plates rather than as a purely lytic lesion, with paraspinal masses that extend for a greater length than the vertebral body itself and with paraspinal masses that may demonstrate calcifications.[203] With treatment and resolution of the infection, the density of the vertebral bodies increases and associated soft tissue masses decrease in size. At the Cleveland Clinic, CT is most often used for guiding needle biopsy for definitive diagnosis and microbiologic culture, rather than as a method of diagnosis (Figs. 172-26 and 172-27).

Magnetic Resonance Imaging

MRI has been found to have a sensitivity of 96%, a specificity of 92%, and an accuracy of 94% in the diagnosis of vertebral osteomyelitis.[204,205] This result is comparable to the

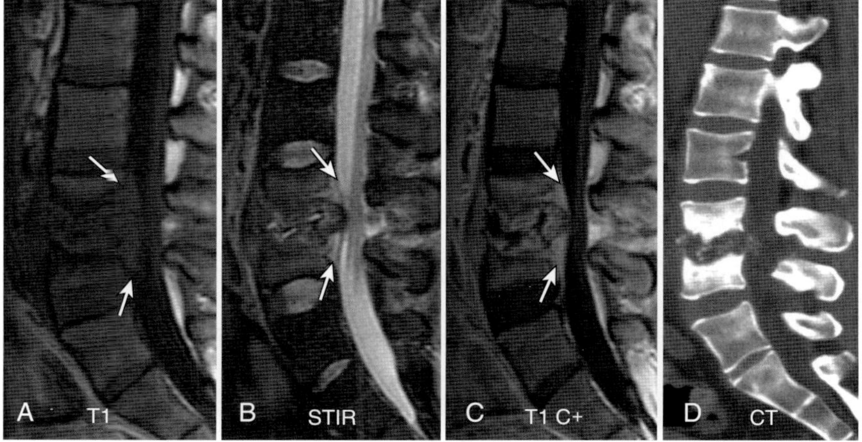

FIGURE 172-26. Pyogenic vertebral osteomyelitis and discitis. Typical imaging changes due to discitis and vertebral osteomyelitis at L3-4. Spondylodiscal hypointensity on T1 (**A**) and hyperintensity on T2 (**B**) images. Note ill-marginated end plates on the T1 image. **C,** Postcontrast image shows thick rind of soft tissue rim enhancement around fluid signal in the disc space. There is epidural phlegmon without epidural abscess (*arrows*). **D,** Note eroded end plates and sclerosis on CT.

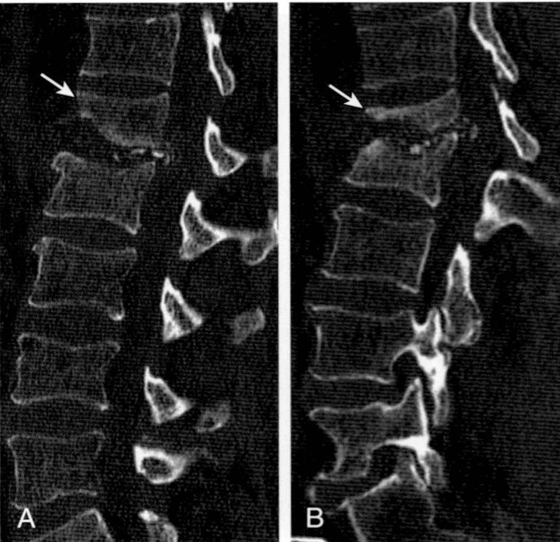

FIGURE 172-27. Progression of vertebral wedging in osteomyelitis. **A,** Initial CT imaging showed end-plate erosions at L1-2 due to pyogenic osteomyelitis. Note mild ventral wedging of L1 (*arrow*). **B,** Follow-up scan at about 6 months shows progression with severe loss of height of L1 body. No clinical or laboratory evidence of active infection was demonstrated.

combination of technetium-99m bone scanning and gallium scanning, as discussed previously. MRI is also more sensitive and specific for the diagnosis of vertebral osteomyelitis than is plain radiography.[204] It is superior to CT regarding its contrast resolution, its demonstration of epidural disease, and its detection of the effect of the infection on the spinal cord and thecal sac. The classic MRI changes of vertebral osteomyelitis are divided into *discal* and *paradiscal* (end-plate, paraspinal, and epidural soft tissue) spaces.[205] The findings on the sagittal imaging are as follows:

T1 imaging shows a confluent decreased signal intensity of the intervertebral disc and adjacent vertebral bodies with the inability to discern a margin between the two on T1-weighted images ("diffuse spondylodiscal darkening"). The typical MR findings of vertebral osteomyelitis are consistently seen on T1 sagittal imaging. A study from our institution showed typical T1 end-plate signal changes plus T2 disc hyperintensity in 95% cases of vertebral osteomyelitis.[161]

T2 imaging shows (1) corresponding end-plate and vertebral body hyperintensity on each side of the disc space, and (2) an abnormal configuration and hyperintense fluid signal intensity of the intervertebral disc with loss of the nuclear cleft[204,205] ("diffuse spondylodiscal brightening"). Conventional sagittal T2 imaging may not show the typical end-plate hyperintense signal, as occurs in about half of the cases in the study just mentioned.[161] However, STIR imaging is very helpful in such cases, not only illuminating the paradiscal end plates but also unequivocally showing the discal T2 hyperintense signal as well as paraspinal soft tissue edema. Disc space infection can originate in the soft tissue along the discs. The authors retrospectively noted few cases with early and subtle paradiscal soft tissue foci on STIR imaging later converting into full-blown cases of discitis and osteomyelitis. Isolated T2 discal hyperintensity itself is a nonspecific finding because a T2 hyperintense degenerated disc can have a similar appearance, as is discussed later in the differential diagnosis.

Contrast enhancement has been found to increase the accuracy of the diagnosis of vertebral osteomyelitis and discitis in cases with equivocal MRI scans.[206] The involved portions of the adjacent vertebral body and disc typically enhance following the administration of gadolinium. The typical enhancement pattern is rim enhancement of the inflamed disc space. Other patterns include homogeneous enhancement of the majority of the disc space and patchy nonconfluent areas of disc enhancement.[206] Absence of discal enhancement is rare in thoracolumbar spine discitis and osteomyelitis.[205,206] Post et al.[206] described abnormal enhancement of the vertebral bodies, disc, and paraspinal soft tissues that progressively decreased on follow-up imaging in patients successfully treated with antibiotics. Gillams et al.[207] also followed patients given antibiotic therapy with MRI. They saw both decreasing and stable, and even increasing enhancement patterns in patients who were improving clinically while taking medical therapy. They concluded that whereas decreasing spinal and soft tissue enhancement was a useful sign, persistent or increasing enhancement alone did not indicate treatment failure (see Figs. 172-26 and 172-27).

Follow-up MRI is generally used to monitor the response to therapy in combination with clinical and inflammatory markers. After 4 to 8 weeks of parenteral therapy, clinicians must decide whether to stop or continue parenteral therapy, begin oral therapy, or go for diagnostic imaging or ask for surgical intervention. Follow-up MRI at 4 to 8 weeks after the start of therapy may show variable imaging features indicating either improvement or equivocal or worsening of the findings. The bone marrow and disc space findings can be misleading and may not correlate with the clinical response.[208] However, paraspinal and epidural soft tissue changes (including abscess formation) are relatively reliable markers of response to therapy. Kowalski et al.[208] also showed some degree of vertebral body loss of height in all cases in the unfavorable group (however, it was a nonspecific finding). Most of the studies of vertebral osteomyelitis on follow-up MRI are limited due to the smaller size of the samples. Another major limitation is a marked bony and soft tissue vascularized response to the infection, which may remain for a long time. For example, gadolinium enhancement at the site of infection may not completely resolve even years after treatment.[208-211]

Specific Etiologies

Postoperative Discitis

Differentiating postoperative discitis from normal postoperative disc space change can be difficult. Boden et al.[212] reported postoperative MRI changes in 15 asymptomatic patients and 7 patients with proven postoperative discitis. They found gadolinium enhancement to be useful. The entire triad of vertebral bone marrow enhancement, disc space enhancement, and anulus fibrosus enhancement was not seen in any of the asymptomatic patients in their series. However, Ross et al.[213] showed similar results in 94 asymptomatic postoperative patients demonstrating anular enhancement (curet site), disc enhancement, and vertebral end-plate enhancement.

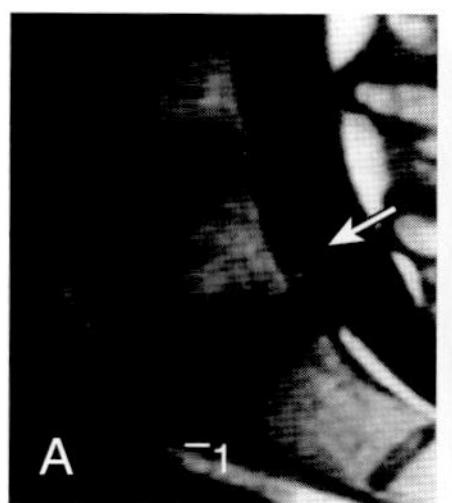

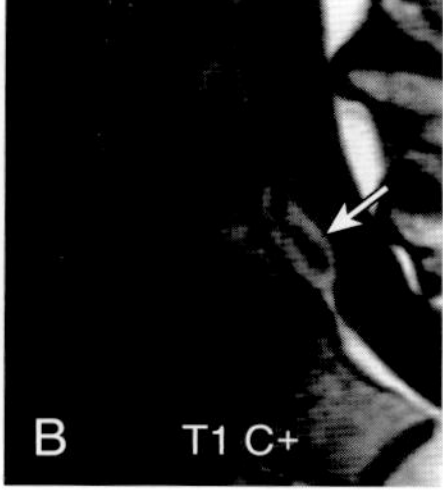

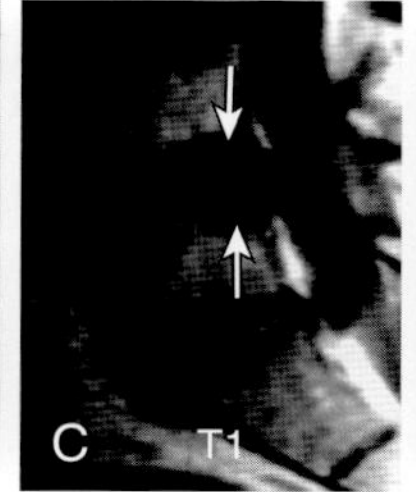

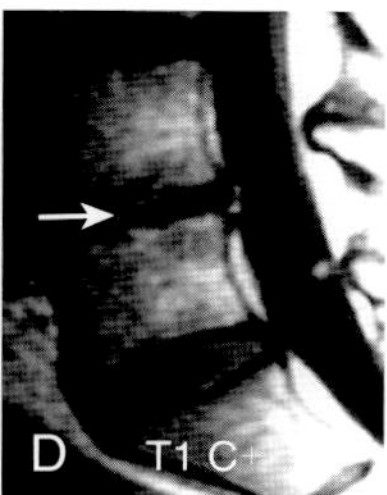

FIGURE 172-28. Postoperative spondylodiscal changes. **A,** Preoperative imaging shows caudally migrated free fragment (*arrow*) from the L4-5 disc level, which lies behind the body of L5. **B,** Following contrast, there is peripheral enhancement of the disc herniation (*arrow*). Postoperative pre- (**C**) and postcontrast (**D**) imaging shows successful removal of the disc fragment and typical type I marrow changes of decreased signal of the dorsal margins of L4 and L5 (*arrows,* **C**) and enhancement back to normal marrow signal following contrast. Note typical postoperative linear enhancement within the disc (*arrow,* **D**).

Approximately 20% (19 of 94) of the patients showed intervertebral disc enhancement at the surgical level 3 months after surgery. They also showed type I marrow changes at the surgical level that enhanced postoperatively. Type I marrow changes represent the conversion of normal marrow to fibrovascular marrow with low signal on T1-weighted images and high signal on T2-weighted images.[214] Some patients showed no marrow changes between preoperative and postoperative MRI scans, but others exhibited a change to type I enhancing marrow conversion on the postoperative scan. They emphasized the necessity of understanding normal asymptomatic postoperative changes, and that asymptomatic postoperative disc enhancement coupled with enhancing marrow changes can look similar to osteomyelitis but may be distinguished from infection by the smooth linear bands of enhancement within the disc (Fig. 172-28).

Spinal Epidural Abscess

Epidural soft tissue changes generally involve the ventral epidural space and abut the infected disc. The solid component is termed *epidural phlegmon* because no fluid is identified on MRI. Both epidural abscess and phlegmon cause mass effect on the thecal sac and spinal cord. Most of these epidural masses occur adjacent to the level of osteomyelitis and discitis and usually involve two to four vertebral segments.[215-218] Epidural abscesses can be extensive, noncontiguous, and even distant from the site of osteomyelitis. Spinal epidural abscess represents a significant complication of vertebral osteomyelitis.

Spontaneous epidural abscess is less common.[216] Karikari et al.,[219] in their 10-year experience of spontaneous epidural abscesses, divided them into two groups based on location: 65.4% of cases were ventral and 34.6% were dorsal abscesses. The patients with dorsal epidural abscesses had a higher rate of associated paraplegia or quadriplegia. MRI offers a distinct advantage in its ability to easily and noninvasively image the entire spinal column and therefore detect the presence of such distant foci of disease.

Postcontrast MRI exhibits enhancement of the epidural mass. This provides excellent distinction between the high signal enhancing epidural process and the lower signal of the cerebrospinal fluid and spine on T1-weighted images.[206] The administration of contrast aids in differentiating between epidural phlegmon versus abscess. Dense homogeneous enhancement of the mass suggests phlegmon, whereas peripheral or ring enhancement of the mass suggests an abscess.[160,220-222] The investigators have not found the unenhanced T1- and T2-weighted image signal characteristics to be helpful in differentiating phlegmon from abscess.[161] This distinction may be important clinically since an abscess usually requires surgical decompression and drainage but phlegmon does not (Fig. 172-29).

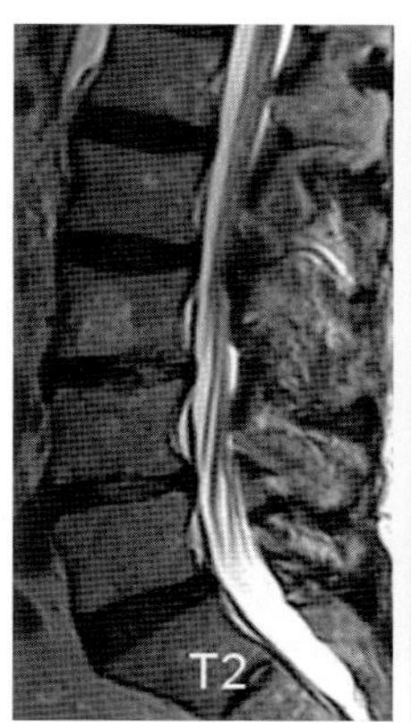

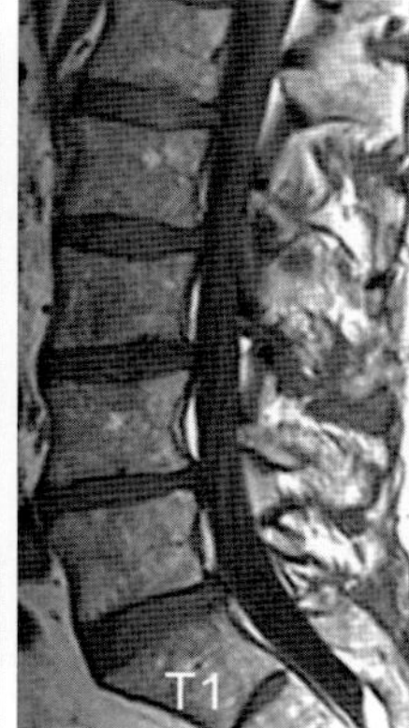

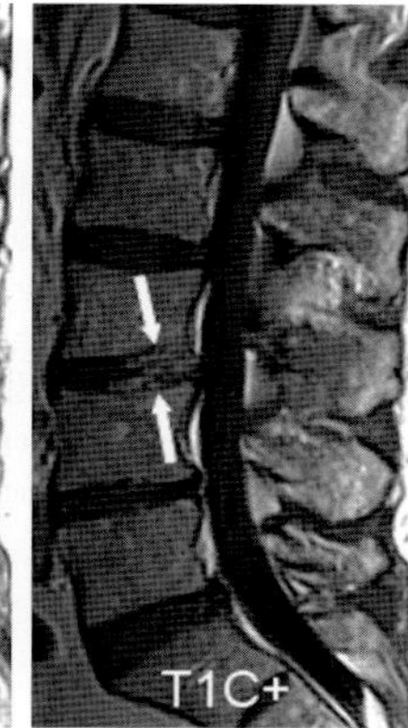

FIGURE 172-29. Postdiscectomy sagittal imaging shows dorsal linear and irregular region of T2 hyperintensity and enhancement in the intervertebral disc at L3-4 (*arrows*). The patient had a remote history of discectomy.

Nonpyogenic Discitis Osteomyelitis

Nonpyogenic discitis osteomyelitis mainly includes tuberculous and brucellar infections. Almost half of the skeletal tuberculosis is due to vertebral osteomyelitis.[223] Tuberculous spondylitis may be indistinguishable from pyogenic spondylitis. However, there are distinct imaging characteristics that, when present, should suggest the diagnosis of tuberculous rather than pyogenic spondylitis.[224] Tuberculous osteomyelitis tends to involve the ventral aspect of the vertebral body at the metaphysis. The infectious process tends to spread via the anterior longitudinal ligaments to adjacent vertebral bodies. Involvement of the intervertebral disc is relatively limited compared with the amount of vertebral body involvement. *Mycobacterium* requires a well-oxygenated environment to survive. It is able to infect the well-oxygenated, well-vascularized environment of the vertebral body but has difficulty invading the intervertebral disc.[225] The thoracic and lumbar spine are most commonly involved, with the organism having a predilection for the thoracolumbar junction.[203,226] Usually, more than one vertebral body level is involved, with more

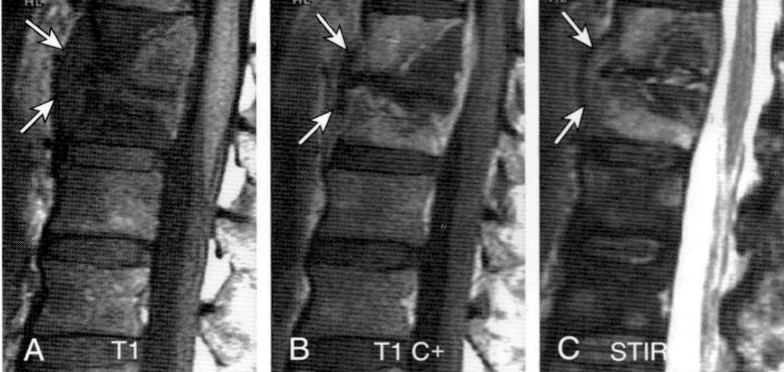

FIGURE 172-30. A–C, Tuberculous discitis and vertebral osteomyelitis. Predominant ventral inflammatory changes (*arrows*): prevertebral soft tissue thickening, ventral disc space involvement, and bone marrow changes. Bilateral psoas muscle large abscesses were present (not shown).

than 40% of cases involving disc spaces in one series.[226,227] Solitary and skip lesions can occur.[203,227,228] The ventral aspect of the vertebral body is most commonly involved, but dorsal elements can also be involved.[224,227] Isolated dorsal spinal tuberculosis is rare.[229] On plain films and CT, there is delay in destruction of the intervertebral discs; a large calcified paravertebral mass may be present (due to psoas abscess—highly suggestive of TB infection) and absent or less prominent reactive sclerosis[230] (Figs. 172-30 and 172-31).

Brucellosis is an insidious febrile illness with nonspecific signs and symptoms. Between 25% and 34% of cases have involvement of osteoarticular structures.[231] About 5% to 15% cases of patients with brucellosis can have spondylodiscitis.[232-234] One level of involvement is usually seen but, rarely, multilevel involvement may be seen.[235,236] Vertebral bodies, discs, and paraspinal soft tissues are involved. Specifically, ventral rostral vertebral body involvement and paraspinal soft tissue changes have been reported without abscess or dominant discal changes.[234]

Differential Diagnosis

Many disease entities (mostly benign) can mimic vertebral osteomyelitis on imaging. Even malignancies, both primary and metastatic, can sometimes be difficult to distinguish from infectious spondylitis. The diagnosis of vertebral osteomyelitis is critical due to its potential morbidity and mortality. Suspicion on the part of the physician is required in the appropriate clinical setting. Several imaging modalities are available to aid in diagnosis as well as to guide biopsy. In the correct clinical setting, these modalities and combinations of them can be very specific and sensitive for the establishment of the diagnosis of vertebral osteomyelitis.

Type I Degenerative Marrow Changes

Type I degenerative marrow changes may mimic vertebral osteomyelitis. Type I marrow signal intensity change may enhance following the administration of gadolinium, and enhancement of the central portion of the cervical and lumbar intervertebral discs in patients who have not undergone surgery does occur in the setting of degenerative disc disease.[237] In advanced disc degeneration, blood vessels once again can be seen within the disc. Usually, the signal intensity of the disc on T2-weighted images helps differentiate the two entities. The disc is usually decreased in signal on T2-weighted images in degenerative disc disease. On occasion in degenerative disc disease, the intervertebral discs may show increased T2 signal, as discussed in the following section. In infectious spondylitis, the distribution of the increased signal intensity on T2-weighted images does not conform to the anatomic configuration of the disc. The clinical history and the presence or absence of increased sedimentary rate help to differentiate the two entities. Only 4% of patients in a series of 474 patients with degenerative disc disease demonstrated the type I pattern[215] (Fig. 172-32).

T2 Hyperintense Degenerated Disc

A T2 hyperintense degenerated disc is not an uncommon presentation. Typically, a diffuse T2 hyperintense disc, disc space narrowing, variable end-plate changes, and degenerative disc disease are evident at other levels. Generally, this does not represent a major challenge, but in a high-risk patient for whom there is strong clinical suspicion for vertebral osteomyelitis, contrast enhancement may be needed to further characterize the disc space. Lack of paraspinal soft tissue edema strongly argues against infection (see Fig. 172-32).

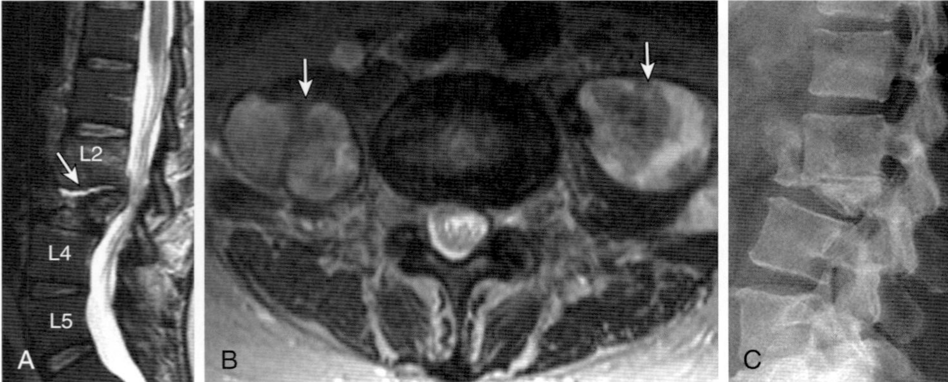

FIGURE 172-31. A–C, Tuberculous discitis and vertebral osteomyelitis. Long-standing treated case of tuberculous vertebral osteomyelitis at L2-3. Note ventral L3 wedge deformity (**A** and **C**) with dominant disc space T2 hyperintensity (*arrow,* **A**) and less prominent bone marrow T2 hyperintensity evident on fast-spin echo T2 imaging. **B,** Bilateral large psoas muscle abscesses are also present (*arrows*).

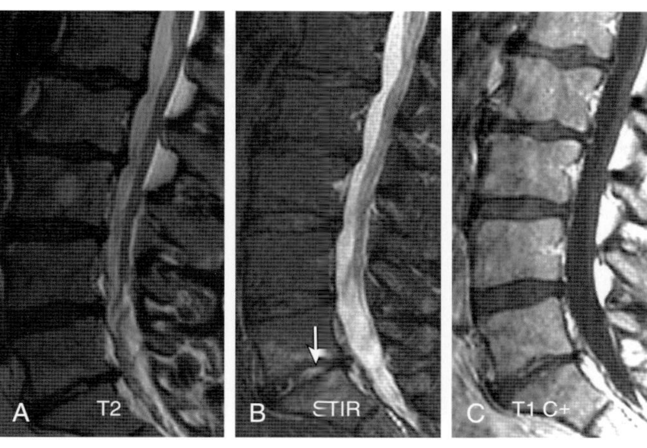

FIGURE 172-32. **A,** T2 hyperintense degenerative disc. Patient presented with intractable back pain. **B,** Hyperintense T2 signal in the L5-S1 disc space (*arrow*), better demonstrated on short-tau inversion recovery imaging (STIR), represents disc hydration. Note type I end-plate changes and disc space narrowing (noncontrast T1 image not shown). **C,** The type I end plates enhance after contrast administration.

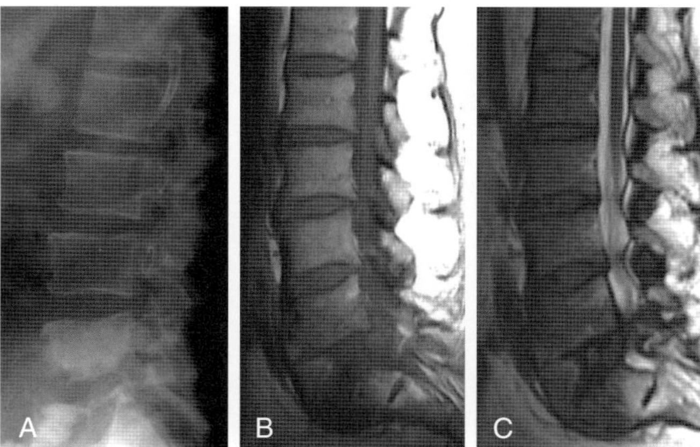

FIGURE 172-33. Charcot spine. Patient with long-standing spinal cord injury. L5-S1 erosive and hypertrophic sclerotic changes on plain film (**A**) with corresponding hypointense T1 (**B**) and T2 (**C**) spondylodiscal signal change.

Metastatic Disease

Metastatic disease can be differentiated from vertebral osteomyelitis by its sparing of the intervertebral disc space. Disc involvement with metastatic disease is rare.[238,239] In addition, metastatic disease commonly involves the pedicles of the vertebral body, whereas osteomyelitic foci tend to be subchondral and do not affect the pedicle.

Primary Tumors of the Spine

Primary tumors of the spine are rare compared with metastatic tumors. There are, however, primary tumors of the spine that involve contiguous vertebral body levels and may therefore have disc involvement. Such tumors include plasmacytoma,[240] aneurysmal bone cysts,[241] giant-cell tumors,[242] and chordoma.[243] Eosinophilic granuloma presents with lytic vertebral body lesions that can progress to nearly complete destruction of the vertebral body or vertebral plana. Despite this, the adjacent intervertebral discs usually remain intact, allowing for differentiation from disc space infection. Aneurysmal bone cysts and giant-cell tumors of the spine can be characterized by lytic lesions that can span vertebral body levels. However, these tumors usually involve the dorsal elements. These tumors may be more difficult to distinguish from tuberculous spondylitis than from pyogenic spondylitis. Chordomas are uncommon tumors derived from notochordal elements. They can be found throughout the spinal column with a marked propensity for the clivus and sacrococcygeal regions. They are isointense or hypointense in signal on T1-weighted images and increased in signal on T2-weighted images. The intervertebral disc and adjacent vertebral bodies are commonly affected. A paraspinal soft tissue mass is often present.[243]

Spinal Neuroarthropathy (Charcot Spine)

Spinal neuropathy, or Charcot spine, is most commonly related to tabes dorsalis, syringomyelia, or diabetes mellitus and can be difficult to differentiate from infectious spondylitis on plain films and CT. Park et al.[244] found MRI to be useful for distinguishing between the two entities. MRI in neuropathy demonstrated hypointensity in the abnormal disc and adjacent vertebral bodies on both T1- and T2-weighted sequences. In neuroarthropathy, the disc space and surrounding marrow were of lower signal intensity on T2-weighted images than that seen in spinal osteomyelitis. Wagner et al.[245] evaluated the plain film, CT, and MRI findings in 14 patients with spinal neuroarthropathy versus 19 patients with disc space infection. They found that facet involvement with narrowing or erosions and vacuum disc were more common in spinal neuroarthropathy on imaging studies and rare in disc space infection. Vertebral body spondylolisthesis, osseous joint debris, joint disorganization, disc rim enhancement, and diffuse vertebral body enhancement were more frequent imaging findings in spinal neuroarthropathy (Fig. 172-33).

Destructive Spondyloarthropathy

Destructive spondyloarthropathy (DSA) has been described in patients undergoing long-term hemodialysis and, more commonly, in the lower cervical spine.[246-248] Plain film changes include disc space narrowing and irregular end-plate destruction. CT images reveal osteolytic areas, with bone sclerosis of adjacent vertebral end plates and minimal osteophytosis.[249] This entity typically demonstrates decreased signal in the disc on T2-weighted images and absence of an associated soft tissue mass that helps to distinguish it from vertebral osteomyelitis.[250] With progression of the disease, collapse of a vertebral body and spinal instability may occur.[249] Distinction between these two entities may be difficult since the sedimentation rate is typically elevated in both groups. Intervertebral disc biopsy may be required in some cases (Fig. 172-34).

Ankylosing Spondylitis

Ankylosing spondylitis (AS) can mimic discitis osteomyelitis due to inflammatory and noninflammatory processes. Ventral and dorsal end-plate focal inflammatory changes (Romanus

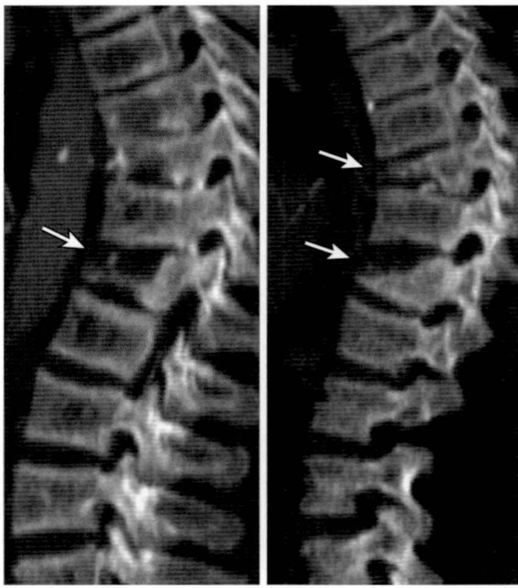

FIGURE 172-34. Destructive spondyloarthropathy. Patient with chronic renal disease and long history of hemodialysis. There was no clinical evidence for spine infection. Sagittal reconstructed images from CT abdomen and pelvis; no further imaging was needed. Note osteolysis of the end plates at two levels in thoracic spine resulting in vertebral plana (*arrows*) with no evidence of hypertrophic sclerotic changes. Also note typical bandlike end-plate sclerosis ("rugger-jersey appearance").

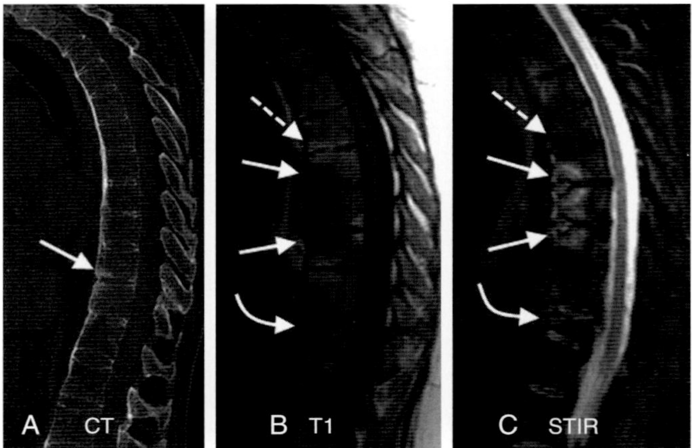

FIGURE 172-35. Ankylosing spondylitis. **A,** Ventral and dorsal margins spondylotic ankylosing changes on CT with ventral sclerotic ("shiny") corner (*arrow*). **B** and **C,** Follow-up MRIs show anterior Romanus lesions of different stages: T1 hypointense (**B;** *straight arrows*), T2 hyperintense (**C;** *straight arrows*), and T1 hyperintense, which demonstrate fat-suppressed hypointense signal on short-tau inversion recovery (**C;** *dashed arrows*). Note ventral compression deformity (*curved arrows*). No Andersson lesions are present.

lesions) are multifocal and limited to the bones. Imaging shows focal changes at the ventral and dorsal end-plate margins. Andersson lesions represent rheumatic spondylodiscitis. The imaging features depend on the stage of the process. Early findings include end-plate erosion and hypointense T1 and hyperintense T2 signals. Later on, there is development of sclerosis and hyperintense T1 signal due to fatty marrow change. Differentiation from discitis osteomyelitis is usually not difficult in these lesions due to multilevel involvement, localized nature of the lesions, and lack of paraspinal soft tissue thickening.[251-253] Segmental pseudarthrosis can develop in AS following fracture of the spine and can better mimic disc space infection.[254] It is usually seen at the thoracolumbar junction. On MRI, the segmental pseudarthrosis exhibits an increased signal on T2-weighted images. Shih et al.[253] showed both T2 hyperintense and T2 hypointense discovertebral changes in fractures and pseudofractures in AS. Associated segmental dorsal element involvement and disruption of the thickened anterior longitudinal ligament (ALL) are specific features of AS (Fig. 172-35).

KEY REFERENCES

al-Mulhim FA, Ibrahim EM, el-Hassan AY, et al: Magnetic resonance imaging of tuberculous spondylitis. *Spine (Phila Pa 1976)* 20:2287–2292, 1995.

Alyas F, Connell D, Saifuddin A: Upright positional MRI of the lumbar spine. *Clin Radiol* 63:1035–1048, 2008.

Gallucci M, Puglielli E, Splendiani A, et al: Degenerative disorders of the spine. *Eur Radiol* 15:591–598, 2005.

Gilbert FJ, Grant AM, Gillan MG, et al: Low back pain: influence of early MR imaging or CT on treatment and outcome–multicenter randomized trial. *Radiology* 231:343–351, 2004.

Kowalski TJ, Layton KF, Berbari EF, et al: Follow-up MR imaging in patients with pyogenic spine infections: lack of correlation with clinical features. *AJNR Am J Neuroradiol* 28:693–699, 2007.

Lakadamyali H, Tarhan NC, Ergun T, et al: STIR sequence for depiction of degenerative changes in posterior stabilizing elements in patients with lower back pain. *AJR Am J Roentgenol* 191:973–979, 2008.

Modic MT, Feiglin DH, Piraino DW, et al: Vertebral osteomyelitis: assessment using MR. *Radiology* 157:157–166, 1985.

Modic MT, Ross JS: Lumbar degenerative disc disease. *Radiology* 245:43–61, 2007.

REFERENCES

The complete reference list is available online at expertconsult.com.

CHAPTER 173

Overview of Imaging Procedures Available for Spinal Diagnosis

Ryan D. Murtagh | F. Reed Murtagh | Glenn R. Rechtine II

Imagine practicing medicine today—especially while attempting to sort out the multiple overlapping causes of back and neck pain—with no imaging guidance. That is what it was like before Wilhelm Roentgen produced the first x-ray image (of his own hand, as it turned out) at the turn of the last century. Physicians engaged in a lot of guesswork. When the senior author of this chapter had his radius fracture set circa 1954, plain radiography and fluoroscopy were the only available means to view the osseous structures. The dosage to the patient and to the operators must have been huge. Spine imaging likewise was severely limited to depiction of osseous structures only until the introduction of the plain x-ray myelogram, which permitted visualization of the subarachnoid spaces, spinal cord, and nerve roots directly.

Plain-film radiography and fluoroscopy remain the mainstays of spinal imaging over 100 years after the discovery of x-rays, even though radiography often does not prove as alluring as some of the newer techniques, including CT myelography, nuclear medicine scans, CT, and MRI. Plain radiography today "gets less respect" than do any of its more expensive kin, but it is still essential. This chapter provides a critical overview of these and other available techniques, along with a bit of a historical perspective and a little editorializing.

Plain-Film Radiography

For basic anatomic depiction of the entire spinal column, plain films are optimal (Fig. 173-1). The images are relatively easy to obtain, the machines and film are readily available, and the images are mostly straightforward to interpret with a basic knowledge of spinal anatomy. Although actual hardcopy x-ray film is now replaced in many practices by direct digital images, there are still some older clinicians who insist on preserving the tactile experience of holding an x-ray film in their hands to aid in diagnosis. This will fade eventually, mostly because of cost factors (film is still fairly expensive, whereas digital images are not), but also because the benefits of going digital include the ability to change window widths, enlarge an area of interest, and store images on a central server and transmit them.[1]

One drawback is that proper radiographic technique must be used at all times and someone must ensure the dosages are correct and the images are diagnostic and satisfactory, or have them repeated. One must be cautious about the total ionizing radiation exposure to the patient, taking into account the number of repeated exposures endured, the part of the body being exposed, and the age of the patient.[2] For instance, the total exposure of a newborn with hip dysplasia undergoing a plain radiographic examination every few weeks to determine if the therapeutic harness is working must be weighed against the fact that a superior method that does not involve ionizing radiation, ultrasonography, is available to accomplish the same end.

For evaluating the spine, plain radiographs have one distinct advantage over other imaging techniques: they observe the spine in a position of function, specifically, with the patient upright and bearing weight.[3] This is not true of any other modality, with the exception of upright MRI (which has its own drawbacks). In addition, the spine can be imaged from a lateral viewpoint, with the patient engaging in flexion and extension, or with ventral views of the patient bending from side to side (Fig. 173-2; see Fig. 173-1). This can be performed using fluoroscopy as well, but plain radiographs are less expensive to produce and result in lower doses of radiation to the patient. Either technique is acceptable, provided the images are properly obtained and interpreted.

Plain radiographs can show excellent bony detail, assuming they are done correctly, and any fracture or misalignment is usually obvious. Instability is even more obvious if flexion and extension views are obtained.[3] Congenital osseous

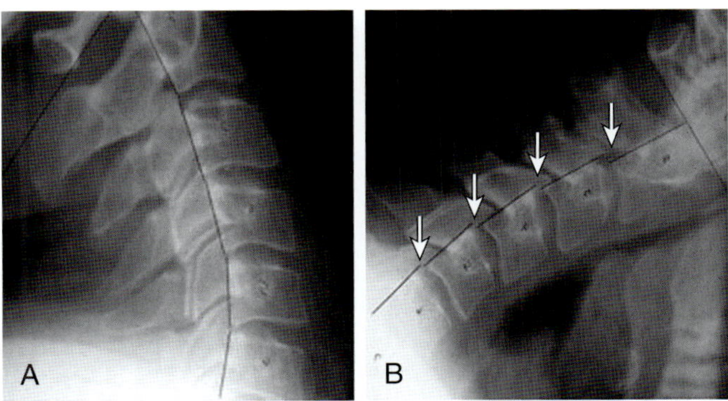

FIGURE 173-1. Extension (**A**) and flexion (**B**) plain radiographs of the cervical spine are relatively easy to obtain, demonstrate alignment in different positions, are less expensive than other imaging methods, and expose the patient to less ionizing radiation than does fluoroscopy.

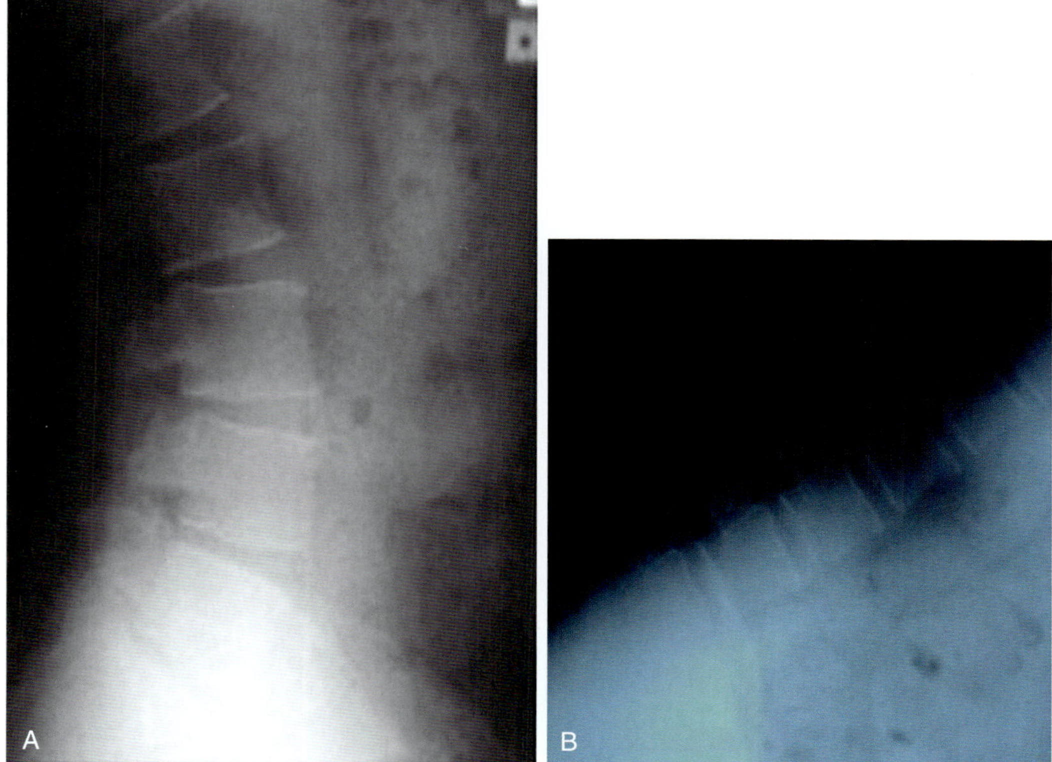

FIGURE 173-2. These lateral upright plain radiographs show some of the technical difficulties inherent in obtaining an extension (**A**) and then a flexion (**B**) plain film on a large patient.

abnormalities can be diagnosed and the normal curvatures of the spine assessed. Bearing in mind that not every individual naturally has the expected amounts of cervical and lumbar lordosis and thoracic kyphosis, observers should refrain from stating that loss of any of the spinal curvatures automatically means that the patient has muscle spasms in that region because that diagnosis can be made only by physical examination. Assessment of postural curves can be done only on upright images; otherwise, scoliosis, kyphosis, and lordosis are modified by the shape of the backboard or bed.

Very little can be said about soft tissues in and around the spine because plain-film radiography cannot differentiate tissue densities; all it can differentiate is bone from soft tissue, fat, and air. As such, contrast agents play an essential role in plain radiography, particularly in myelography. Today, the most commonly used contrast agents for spinal imaging are any of a number of brands of nonionic, iodine-containing myelographic media.

Myelography

Iodine attenuates the x-ray beam to the same extent as bone and, as a result, shows up white on x-ray film. When compounded into a nonionic liquid, iodine can safely be injected into the spinal canal, specifically into the cerebrospinal fluid of the subarachnoid space, to outline that part of the spinal anatomy. After injection and imaging, the contrast is absorbed into the bloodstream and ultimately excreted by the kidneys. This is a relatively safe and well-tolerated procedure with the most significant side effect the occasional spinal headache. Arachnoiditis or spinal abscesses are very rare with today's techniques and contrast agents. Pantopaque, an oily iodinated contrast medium used for myelography in the latter half of the 20th century, is no longer the standard of care because it was not reabsorbed readily, had to be physically removed after myelography, and has been implicated in cases of arachnoiditis.

The most useful modern role of myelography is to reveal the details of the subarachnoid spaces in conjunction with anatomic detail provided by CT (Fig. 173-3). The myelogram/CT combination is the current gold standard of spinal imaging, but is used only as a last resort because it is, after all, an invasive procedure that requires a lumbar puncture and intrathecal injection.[4]

Fluoroscopy

This technique is essentially continuous, real-time radiography. Consequently, the dosages of radiation to the patient and to the operator can be very large if the physician is not aware of the fact that the longer the activation pedal is depressed, the more radiation is delivered.[5] Although fluoroscopy can effectively evaluate motion of the spine in real time, with or without intrathecal contrast, flexion and extension plain films serve the same purpose, depict exactly the same anatomy, involve less radiation, and are less expensive to produce. The most frequent use of fluoroscopy today is in the form of the ubiquitous operating room C-arm used with every spinal surgical procedure for direction, localization, and documentation during and after surgery. It is very important that the

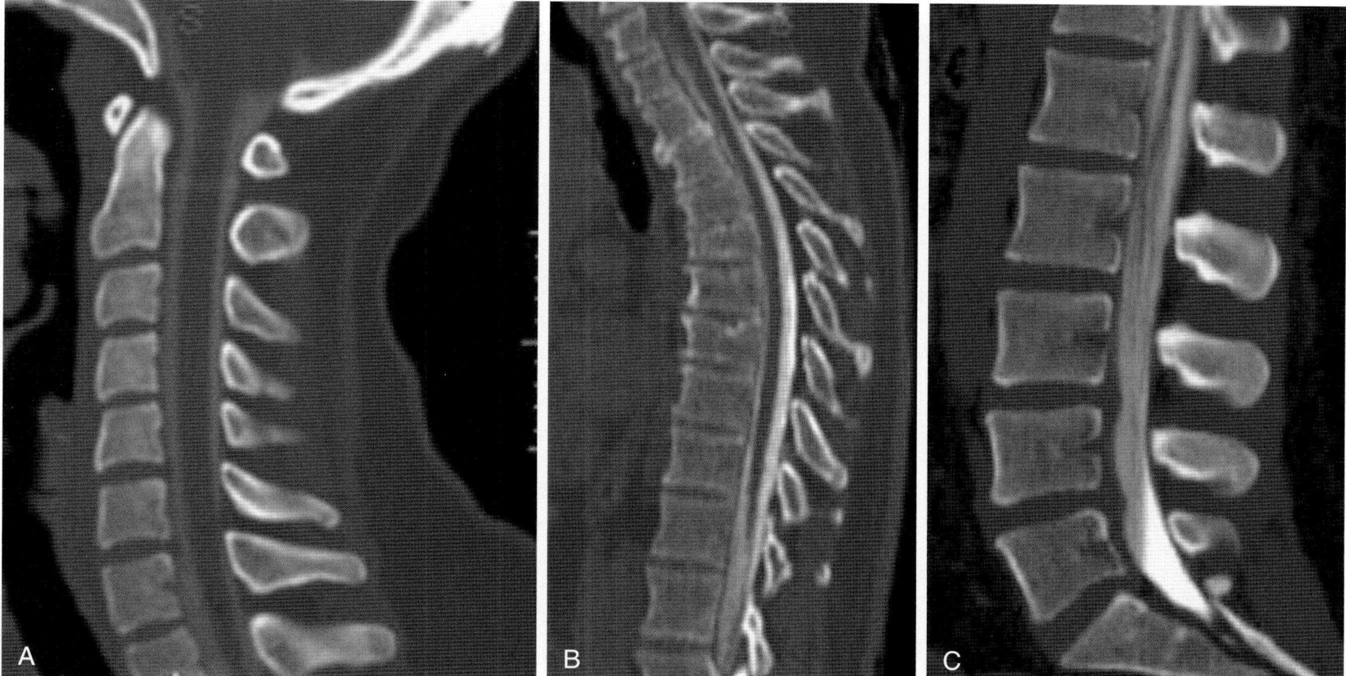

FIGURE 173-3. Sagittal reformatted images from a CT myelogram of the cervical (**A**), thoracic (**B**), and lumbar spine (**C**). This method is still considered the gold standard of spinal imaging techniques.

operating physician be cognizant of the dose delivery curves for the specific machine that is being used, because they do vary according to manufacturer. Also, common sense dictates that the operator should not "keep their foot on the pedal" continually during usage, but instead develop the habit of taking "snapshots" of the target organ/structure as needed during the surgical procedure.

Computed Tomography

Computed tomography is an x-ray technique capable of producing images of the inside of the body using ionizing radiation (Fig. 173-4). As a result, CT carries the same risks and benefits as plain-film radiography. The x-ray source in the CT scanner is housed in a doughnut-shaped device that is capable of rotating circumferentially around the patient. Early-generation devices consisted of a single x-ray source and a single 180-degree detection device. In these devices, the x-ray beam passes through the body part of interest and exposes the detector on the opposite side in exactly the same manner as the plain radiograph is generated. Unlike plain radiographs, however, the CT x-ray source and detection device are capable of moving in tandem. After an image is created, the source and the detector move in parallel inside the cowling and another exposure is made, followed by another and then another. After the acquisition of multiple consecutive images, a computer compiles the image data and displays it according to complex algorithms as an axial image of the inside of the body part being imaged. This was a revolution—clearly as large a step forward as was Roentgen's original hand x-ray image.

The early, single-row technique for CT scanning is a slow and cumbersome process. Since then, the CT scanner has evolved through at least eight additional generations to become the ultrafast, ultra-detailed diagnostic machine that it is today. Up to 256 x-ray sources and 256 corresponding detectors now image the body part at incredible speeds, producing excellent images in time frames that rarely exceed a few minutes. Although image resolution is significantly better and scan times markedly shorter, the dosage of ionizing radiation

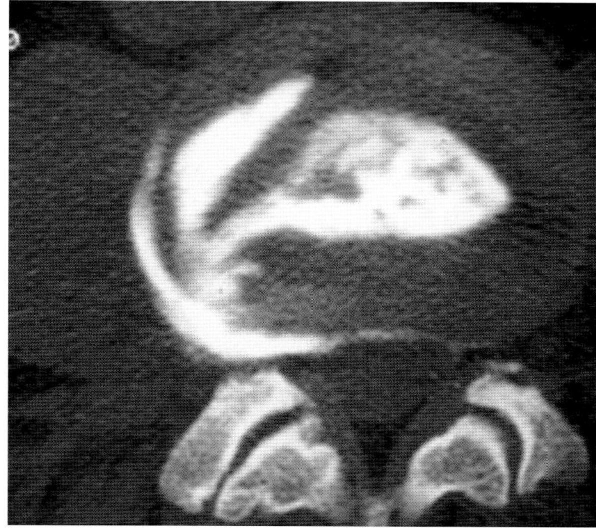

FIGURE 173-4. Axial CT image taken after injection of iodinated contrast material into the center of the nucleus pulposus. This was a positive anatomic CT-discogram, in that it shows a complete full-thickness tear of all of the anular fibers of the disc. Another important discographic observation was the fact that the injection reproduced the patient's pain symptoms, and hence the disc could be designated a "pain generator."

increases with every additional source/detector added and the radiation dosage to the patient can be massive. The 64-slice option is generally used only when imaging the beating heart. Most, if not all, of the fine imaging produced today, particularly when imaging the spine, is performed with the 16- or 32-slice options, which produce excellent images with much less radiation dosage.

There is no question that the anatomic detail of osseous structures such as the vertebral bodies and motion segments is best depicted with the CT scanner.[6] Even though a CT scanner is capable of acquiring images only in the axial plane, powerful computer algorithms routinely allow extremely detailed sagittal and coronal images to be reconstructed during postprocessing, with very little effort. Surface algorithms are also available to build a three-dimensional representation of the surface of the spine that can then be rotated on the computer screen into any orientation the clinician requires. CT myelography provides an excellent in vivo demonstration of spinal anatomy and, as noted previously, is the gold standard of spine imaging, beating even the highest-quality MRI scan for detail of osseous and soft tissue anatomy on the same study (see Fig. 173-3).

Ultrasonography

Ultrasonography does not use ionizing radiation at all to generate images of the inside of the body. Anyone who fishes for a hobby is familiar with an ultrasound machine, except that they call it a "fish-finder" instead. Sound waves are transmitted into the body part in much the same way that sound waves are directed into the depths with the fish-finder. Anything that is not water-density reflects the sound back to a detector. Unfortunately for spinal imaging, the tissue that reflects sound waves most effectively is bone and, as a result, there is very little usefulness in this area. Once the laminae of the spine have been removed during surgery, however, ultrasonography has some use, mostly in establishing the exact location and extent of intradural, extra-axial or intradural, intra-axial spinal cord pathology. Ultrasonography for diagnosis of soft tissue injuries of the paraspinal muscles has been attempted in the past, but has never been fully accepted as a diagnostic modality worth the trouble or the cost.

Discography

The old-fashioned discogram has made a resurgence (see Fig. 173-4). Direct injection of contrast material into the nucleus pulposus has always been an effective, if extremely painful, invasive procedure with the potential to yield valuable clinical information on the effect of pressure loading on an intervertebral disc.[7] This procedure had limited usefulness until recently because of its invasiveness. There has always been the potential for development of discitis as an adverse outcome, and until recently the discogram technique has been difficult to master. With the advent of better C-arm fluoroscopy and fluoroscopy-like guidance applications for CT, direction of a needle into the exact center of a disc has become much easier and less painful for the patient, at least until the injection into the disc itself takes place. When a normal disc is pressure loaded with 1 mL or more of contrast material, it typically does *not* respond by duplicating or significantly worsening the patient's pain. However, when the material is injected into a disc that is responsible for the patient's symptoms, those symptoms are typically made much worse, and the disc can then be labeled a "pain generator."[7,8] Axial CT images of the disc may then be acquired that often adequately demonstrate the internal architecture of the disc and the extent of anular tearing that is present. The modern discogram, properly performed, has definite value as an adjunct to other routine diagnostic procedures, but because it is still an invasive procedure it is reserved for the most difficult diagnostic problems. Carragee et al. received a prize at the 2009 meeting of the International Society for the Study of the Lumbar Spine for their review of 10 years of follow-up from discography. They showed that there was "accelerated disc degeneration, disc herniation, loss of disc height and signal and the development of reactive end plate changes compared to match-controls."[9] Therefore, when MRI or CT myelography does not yield a clear diagnosis, one may consider discography.[8]

Diagnostic Spinal Anesthetic and Steroid Injections

These are anesthesia procedures that have been adapted to the imaging realm by adding image guidance to aid proper performance and improve outcomes. Whether that guidance is with fluoroscopy or CT makes no difference, as long as proper protocol is followed. The target is either a facet joint or a dorsal root ganglion as it exits the nerve root foramen. In either case, care must be taken in the cervical and thoracic spine to avoid injection into a vascular structure, such as a radicular artery or vein, which might supply/drain into the spinal cord and cause a cord infarct. If the injection is into a nerve root or a nerve root sleeve, it is technically a localized epidural steroid injection. If the injection is into a facet joint, it is an intra-articular injection into a synovial joint. In either case, temporary relief of the patient's specific pain sensations is good diagnostic information that the injected structure is anatomically either entirely or partially responsible for the patient's pain syndrome. These minimally invasive procedures are also reserved for cases in which there is still some question of diagnosis after exhausting all other noninvasive diagnostic modalities.[8]

Magnetic Resonance Imaging

Magnetic resonance imaging provides visualization of the vertebral bodies, thecal sac and intradural structures, disc spaces, and adjacent soft tissue structures of the spine with startling clarity, and without resorting to invasive maneuvers (Fig. 173-5). MRI was so revolutionary when it appeared in the mid-1980s that everyone wanted their own machine. Despite the immense setup costs involved, the new technique was so well reimbursed and so lucrative that even a businessman without any medical experience knew that he could buy a scanner, hire a radiologist, and be profitable.[10] As a direct result of those initial economic conditions, which lasted well into the turn of the century, there are now many more MRI scanners than are necessary in the United States. A legitimate

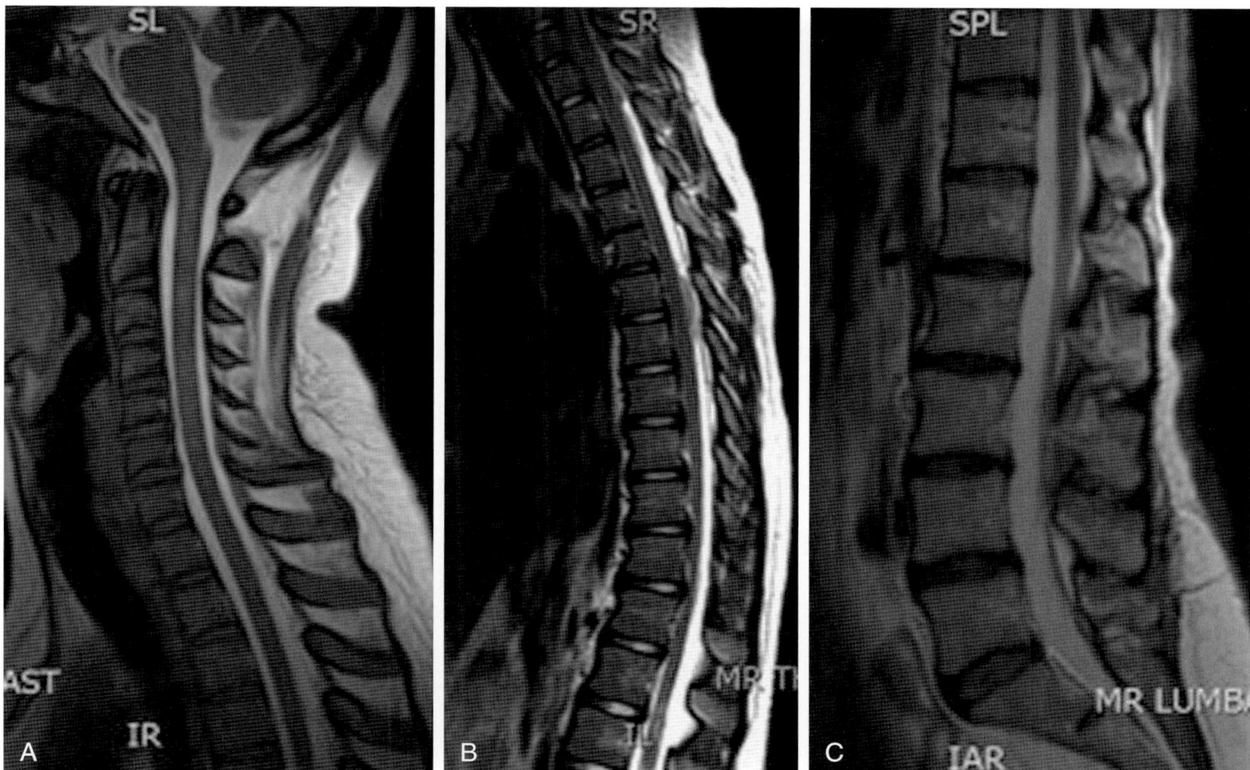

FIGURE 173-5. Sagittal T2-weighted MRIs of the cervical (**A**), thoracic (**B**), and lumbar spine (**C**). Excellent images are obtained noninvasively with appropriate technique and a cooperative patient.

argument can be made that the ultimate cost of MRI scanner proliferation to the American medical bottom line was at least partly responsible for today's medical insurance crisis.[11]

MRI scanners are available in an open or a closed general configuration. Open scanners are, by necessity, low field-strength magnets, whereas any scanner over 1.0 Tesla is a closed configuration. In fact, "open" scanners are not truly open, because the bore must be partially encased by large flat magnets on both sides of the patient. They do not, however, have the long, narrow bore of the closed scanner that may cause some patients consternation. Because of the length of time required to acquire images, it is essential that the patient be cooperative and able to hold completely still during the examination. The length of time required is particularly problematic in open scanners, where a single series of images constituting a single image sequence can take up to twice as long to obtain as in a closed machine.

The differences in image quality between open and closed systems is directly related to field strength.[12] Faster MRI scanners in the 1.5- to 3-Tesla field-strength range are routinely capable of producing superior anatomic detail compared with lower field-strength machines. On the other hand, there is the minor downside of the enclosed magnet bore (uncomfortable for those claustrophobic and/or very large patients) and the problem of core heating (referred to as *SAR*, the specific absorption rate). As a result, one must consider the trade-off between image quality and speed of acquisition versus patient comfort when ordering MRI studies. Unlike the hazards of ionizing radiation in x-ray techniques, the downsides of long-term exposure to high magnetic fields are not well known at this time and may be nonexistent other than core heating.

The only absolute contraindication to MRI today appears to be the presence of a cardiac pacemaker, implantable defibrillator, or spinal cord stimulator. Virtually all other modern devices, including stents, aneurysm clips, surgical clips, orthopaedic implants, spinal fixation screws, and fusion constructs, are thought to be safe because no manufacturer today makes surgically implanted devices from ferromagnetic materials. MRI compatibility should, however, be confirmed with a reliable source before imaging.[13] Pregnant women should not be imaged in the first trimester unless the risk-benefit ratio indicates otherwise. Contrast administration with gadolinium carries a very rare but specific risk of systemic fibrosis and should be used only in patients with suitable renal function.[14] Fortunately, there are not many instances in which contrast is warranted when imaging the spine for anything but tumors and postoperative examination of the lumbar spine.

Axial and sagittal T1- (T1WIs) and T2-weighted images (T2WIs) are typically all that is required for imaging of the cervical, thoracic, and lumbar spine. If there is a question of congenital vertebral body abnormality, as in children with scoliosis, a sequence in the coronal plane is also indicated. T2WIs can be either T2* (gradient echo) images or fast-spin echo T2. If there is a question of metastatic disease, or acute fracture, a sagittal short-tau inversion recovery (STIR) sequence can be added to evaluate for marrow edema. At least one series of axial T2WIs is necessary, and it is helpful if a gradient echo sequence is added as well. The axial images should be 3 to 4 mm thick and contiguous. Some 3-Tesla scanners are capable of excellent 1- and 2-mm thick, contiguous axial T2WIs, which are ideal for spinal cord anatomy. A series of axial T1WIs can also be added.

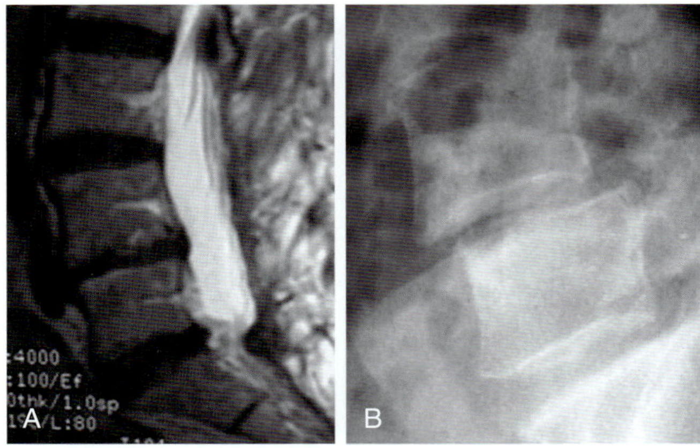

FIGURE 173-6. Sagittal conventional lateral MRI scan (**A**) with the patient recumbent in the MRI scanner shows all vertebral elements well aligned. Upright plain radiograph (**B**) shows the grade I degenerative, and presumably biomechanically unstable, spondylolisthesis that could not be seen with the patient supine.

One drawback with conventional MRI is that the patient is not in a position of function when the spine is being studied.[15] The patient must be supine to fit into the bore of the high-field machine and into the image volume of most of the open MRI scanners. Because the spine is not weight bearing in such a position, some information may be lost, as in the case of a 65-year-old man who had a perfectly aligned spine while recumbent in the scanner (with a few degenerative discs) but who clearly exhibited instability when the upright, weight-bearing plain radiograph was obtained (Fig. 173-6). Open upright MRI scanners have been developed and are in the community, but they are available only as low-field scanners, which are less technically optimal than high-field systems.

Nomenclature

One of the more Sisyphean projects of all time has been the American Society of Spine Radiology's (ASSR) Nomenclature Project, an attempt to bring consistency to the naming of disc abnormalities.[16] The project was initiated in 1994 and was not formalized until the year 2000. The ASSR initially saw a need to bring consensus to the chaotic nomenclature of disc abnormalities, as first proposed in the seminal article by Jensen et al.[17] The resultant 54-plus-page document earned the stamp of approval of all of the major spine organizations, yet is still not widely used even today. The entire document is very accessible and appears in its entirety online at www.asnr.org/spine_nomenclature.

Historically, nearly everyone involved in diagnosing and treating spinal diseases had an unfortunate tendency to refer to every disc abnormality, no matter what it looked like, as a "herniation." With the superior routine ability to visualize spine anatomy that came with the advent of MRI, it was clear that there were multiple variations. "Herniations" are now subdivided into "protrusions" and "extrusions," depending on morphology, and neither one should be confused with a degenerative disc "bulge" (Figs. 173-7 to 173-9). As defined by the Nomenclature Project, a disc bulge is a deformity of the circumference of a disc margin between 90 and 360 degrees, whereas a protrusion is a deformity of less than 90 degrees.

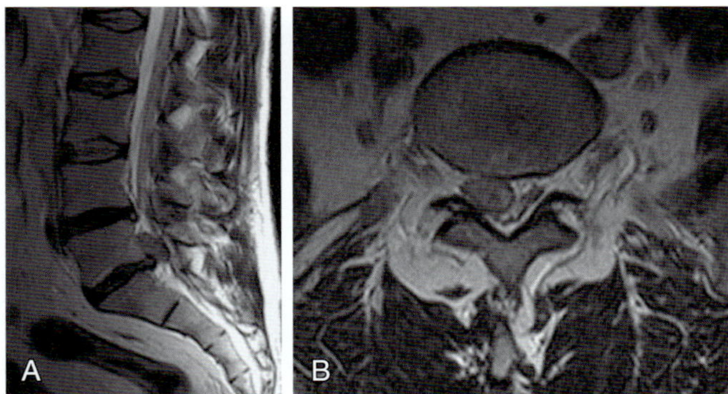

FIGURE 173-7. A, Sagittal MRI of an extruded lumbar disc. Note the "collar-button" appearance of the extruded material. **B,** Axial MRI of the extruded lumbar disc.

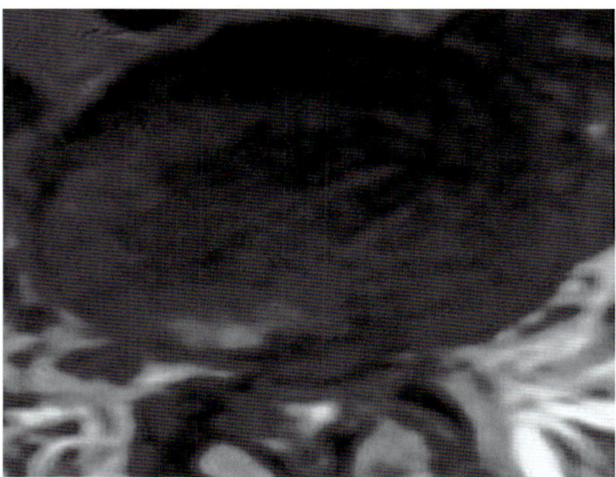

FIGURE 173-8. Axial MRI of a diffusely bulging disc. The disc material extends beyond the border of the vertebral bodies on either side of the motion segment for 360 degrees in this instance.

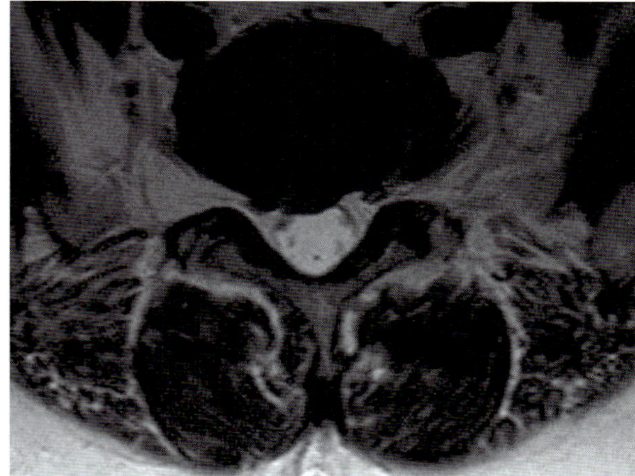

FIGURE 173-9. Axial MRI of a disc protrusion, in this case a focal deformity of the dorsal disc margin that extends over less than 90 degrees of the circumference.

An extrusion is a true "herniated nucleus pulposus" in which nuclear material extrudes through a full-thickness defect of the anulus. The project is currently limited to describing only lumbar discs, but may be applied empirically to thoracic and cervical discs. However, it is important to take into account anatomic differences among the three regions, which probably are not significant when considering thoracic discs, but can cause problems when viewing cervical discs because of their morphology, particularly the presence of lateral limitation afforded by zygapophyseal joints.

KEY REFERENCES

Fardon DF, Milette PC, et al, for the combined task forces: *Nomenclature and classification of lumbar disc pathology: recommendations of the combined task forces of the North American Spine Society, American Society of Spine Radiology, and American Society of Neuroradiology*. American Society of Neuroradiology website, http://www.asnr.org/spine_nomenclature/ Updated February 2003. Accessed September 10, 2011.

Leone A, Gugliemi G, Cassar-Pullicino VN, et al: Lumbar intervertebral instability: a review. *Radiology* 245:62–77, 2007.

Jensen MC, Brant-Zawadzki MN, Obuchowski N, et al: MRI of the lumbar spine in people without back pain. *N Engl J Med* 331:69–73, 1994.

Walker J, El Adb O, Isaac Z, et al: Discography in practice: a clinical and historic review. *Curr Rev Musculoskelet Med* 1:69–83, 2008.

Williams AL, Murtagh FR: *Handbook of diagnostic and therapeutic spine procedures*, St. Louis, 2002, Mosby.

REFERENCES

The complete reference list is available online at expertconsult.com.

CHAPTER 174

Postoperative Imaging

Robert G. Whitmore | Zoher Ghogawala | William T. Curry, Jr. | Sohrab Gollogly | Darrel S. Brodke

Postoperative images of the spine are obtained for a wide variety of indications and require several radiographic modalities. Proper selection of studies and appropriate interpretation of the results depend on a thorough understanding of spinal anatomy, the mechanics of the procedure being used and its attendant risks, and foresight about expected pathologies. Postoperative spinal imaging may explain unexpected symptoms, verify implant positioning or correct spinal level, evaluate fusion or healing of fractures, or confirm the extent of resection of a tumor or vascular malformation. Depending on the original pathology, imaging may focus on any of the anatomic structures of the spine, including bone, ligament, muscle, and neural elements.

The management of chronic degenerative spinal conditions in the United States is estimated to cost nearly $85 billion annually.[1] Spine surgery to treat degenerative disease represents a large portion of this expenditure, and procedures such as lumbar fusion have increased dramatically over the last 20 years.[2] In the past, routine fusion procedures for common indications such as spondylolisthesis did not necessarily require postoperative imaging, especially with the widespread use of fluoroscopy for intraoperative placement of instrumentation. Imaging was reserved for those situations in which preoperative symptoms did not resolve or new symptoms arose postoperatively. However, the margin for error in instrumentation position is now much narrower, despite a lack of evidence of neurologic injury. In addition, determining the correct level of surgery is paramount, and when anatomic abnormalities such as transitional vertebral segments raise doubt about the precise level of pathology, imaging is increasingly utilized. Increasingly, 3D intraoperative imaging, with real-time navigation, is being used to confirm the correct level and instrumentation position.

This chapter addresses common uses of postoperative imaging and correct interpretation of radiographic studies in the postoperative setting. It also focuses on the use of radiology for prospective assessment of surrogate outcomes, such as bony fusion or tumor growth. Finally, the increasing use of intraoperative radiographic modalities beyond plain films is discussed.

Normal Postoperative Spine

Analysis of the postoperative image requires understanding not only the anatomy but also the surgical approach, the goals of surgery, and any potential complications. Imaging abnormalities in the spine related to surgical trauma persist typically through the first 6 to 8 weeks. The extent of bony removal at surgery greatly influences the postoperative imaging appearance. The removal of bone may allow dorsal expansion of the dura through defects, which can resemble a pseudomeningocele, seroma, or postoperative hematoma. Additionally, asymmetry in the paraspinal muscle-fat planes related to surgical dissection is a normal finding. Edema may obscure muscular margins. MRI T2-weighted images, particularly fast spin-echo sequences, provide excellent resolution of water content, allowing visualization of edema or fluid collections.[3]

When the intervertebral disc has been violated or partially excised, distinction between epidural tissue edema and the disrupted anulus fibrosus and recurrent disc herniation or residual disc material can be complex.[4] Well-vascularized granulation tissue usually enhances homogeneously with gadolinium administration, whereas disc material typically enhances poorly or, at best, heterogeneously. Nonenhanced MRI is approximately 85% accurate in achieving this distinction,[5] whereas enhanced MRI is 95% to 100% accurate.[6] Both fibrosus and disc can be hyperintense relative to bone on T2-weighted images. An important technical point for these evaluations is the timing of imaging following contrast administration. If imaging is delayed more than several minutes beyond the administration of the contrast medium, gadolinium seeps across the disc, which is then seen to enhance more homogeneously. To avoid this phenomenon and to increase the specificity for detecting fibrosus, imaging should commence within 2 minutes of gadolinium injection.

Epidural fibrosus is present in all patients following spine surgery to some degree. In some patients, formation of epidural granulation tissue is excessive and has been reported to contribute to residual pain and radiculopathy after surgery.[7,8] However, other reports have contested this claim because granulation tissue is not thought to exert a compressive force.[9] In the setting of recent discectomy and residual postoperative pain, enhancement of the epidural fibrosus, as well as the end plates and anulus fibrosus, may be easily mistaken for early signs of infection (Fig. 174-1).

Van Goethem et al. prospectively studied 34 patients with excellent outcomes following lumbar discectomy and obtained MRIs at 6 weeks and 6 months.[10] Imaging findings

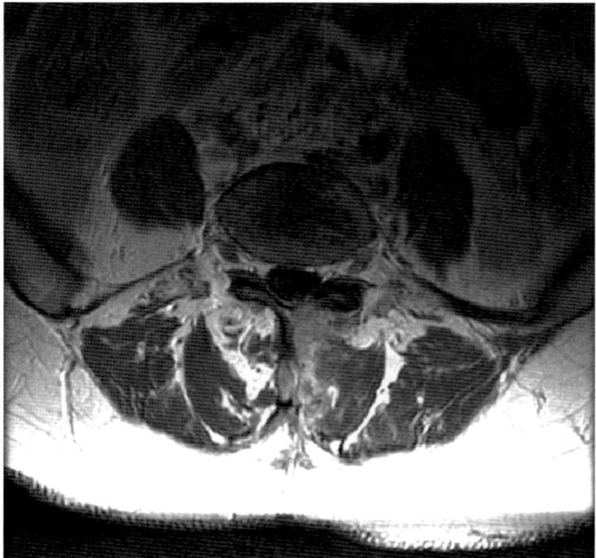

FIGURE 174-1. Normal postoperative axial T1-weighted MRI with gadolinium of the lumbar spine 3 months after the patient underwent lumbar microdiscectomy on the left.

in these asymptomatic patients mimicked diagnostic findings in patients with complications. Twenty percent of patients had recurrent disc herniation, and an additional 20% demonstrated nerve root enhancement at 6 weeks. At 6 months, contrast enhancement was seen along the surgical tract in all patients. Likewise, facet joint enhancement was also seen bilaterally and was attributed to mechanical stress during laminectomy.

A similar study reported MRI findings on 15 patients who had undergone anterior cervical discectomy and fusion (ACDF) immediately postoperatively, at 6 weeks, and at 6 months.[11] Foraminal narrowing persisted in 66% of the first postoperative scans and did not resolve in the follow-up scans up to 6 months, despite symptomatic improvement. Nearly all cases demonstrated persistent edema, with high T2 signal, in the operative disc space at 6 weeks. In addition, all cases showed enhancement in this disc space at 6 weeks, and 50% persisted at 6 months.

Therefore, in clinically successful cases, postoperative spinal imaging demonstrates pathologic changes. Edema, shifting and compression of the thecal sac, epidural fibrosus, and enhancement at almost any portion of the operative field or tract may be noted. It is particularly important to maintain direct communication with the interpreting radiologist so that the clinical history and reasons for the study are understood.

Unresolved or Recurrent Symptoms

In the immediate postoperative period, the causes of symptoms that are of most concern are compressive hematoma, retained or recurrent disc, or problems with instrumentation with or without spinal instability. The appropriate imaging modality depends on the procedure performed and the suggested diagnosis. In cases of rapid neurologic deterioration, prompt return to the operating room (sometimes without postoperative imaging) for urgent surgical exploration is warranted.

Recurrent Disc Herniation

The incidence of recurrent disc herniation in the immediate postoperative period is unknown. In addition, for the reasons discussed earlier, small fragments of retained disc are difficult to identify on imaging. The appearances of recurrent or residual disc are low signal intensity on T1-weighted MRI without enhancement after the administration of IV gadolinium in contrast with epidural fibrosus that typically does enhance. A large sequestered disc may have central high signal intensity on T2-weighted images (Fig. 174-2). In contrast to scar, disc fragments tend to have a smooth margin.

Approximately 10% of discectomy patients experience recurrent lumbar disc herniation requiring revision discectomy. The mean time for this complication in one study was 10.5 months.[12] Patients with a larger preoperative anular defect and with a smaller percentage of disc volume removed had a significantly greater chance of recurrent disc herniation. Common hemostatic agents used in lumbar discectomy, such as oxidized cellulose (Surgicel), have been reported to cause immediate postoperative radiculopathy.[13] The increasing use of minimally invasive techniques, with less direct visualization of the disc and nerve roots, may eventually result in a higher incidence of retained disc fragments. However, at present, the literature suggests that the rate of complications is the same for minimally invasive techniques as for traditional open surgery.[14]

Postoperative Hematoma

One of the most critical immediate postoperative complications to look for after spine surgery is a compressive hematoma, usually in an extradural location (Fig. 174-3). Fortunately, new onset of a major neurologic deficit in the lumbar spine is rare, due to canal space and mobility of nerve roots. However, in the cervical and thoracic spine, neural compression by a postoperative hematoma can have devastating neurologic consequences. Of nearly 12,000 adult spine operations performed over 10 years, the incidence of a major neurologic deficit immediately after surgery was 0.178%; in the cervical spine 0.293%, thoracic spine 0.488%, and lumbosacral spine 0.0745%.[15] Epidural hematoma accounted for 38% of these complications, and it was the most common cause of immediate neurologic deficit. Other reasons for new deficit included inadequate decompression, presumed vascular compromise, graft or cage dislodgement, and presumed surgical trauma.

When a compressive hematoma is suspected, T2-weighted MRI is most sensitive for the detection of blood products in the spine.[4] Instrumentation caused artifact on MRI and may obscure a subtle compressive lesion. It is sometimes necessary to also perform fine-cut CT with sagittal and coronal reconstructions to visualize hardware and bony anatomy. However, choice of imaging modality depends on the clinical scenario, since prompt reexploration is required with severe neurologic deficit.

The chances of a successful outcome following spine surgery depend on the initial indications, but generally are greater than 90% for common procedures such as microdiscectomy. However, a significant number of patients do not clinically improve following surgery, with estimates varying

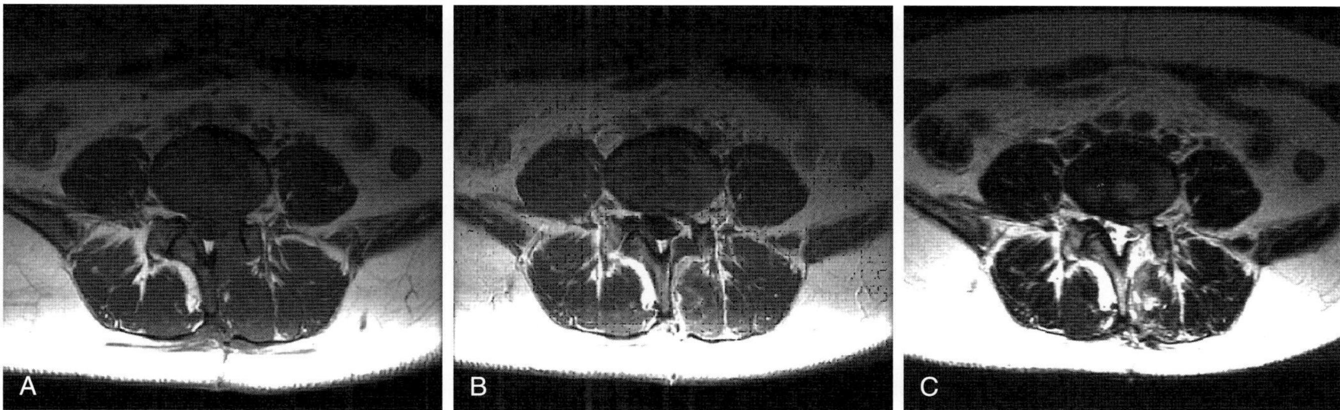

FIGURE 174-2. Axial MRIs of a patient with a recurrent left-sided disc herniation causing symptoms. A, Axial T1-weighted MRI without gadolinium. B, Axial T1-weighted MRI with gadolinium. C, Axial T2-weighted MRI.

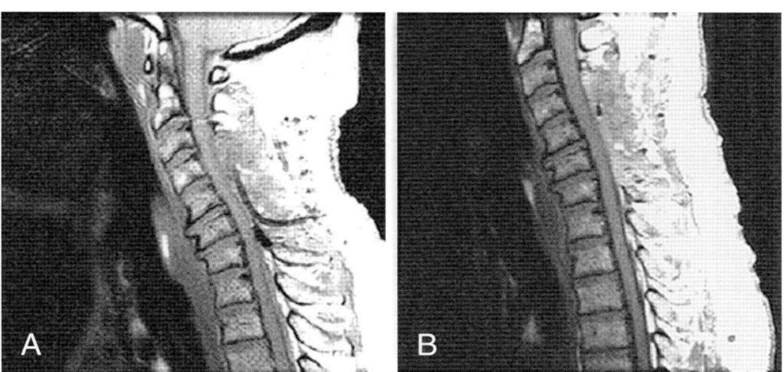

FIGURE 174-3. Quadriparesis was observed in this patient following uneventful C3-5 laminectomies for spinal stenosis. A, An isointense epidural hematoma is seen compressing the thecal sac and spinal cord. B, Following evacuation of the clot, the patient's weakness improved.

from 10% to 30%.[16] In these instances, careful imaging of the operative site and spine is warranted.[17] Several etiologies of continued pain and their imaging characteristics are discussed in the following sections.

Postoperative Infection

Radiographic diagnosis of postoperative spine infection is complicated—the time course of normal postoperative findings such as anular enhancement also mirrors when the same imaging characteristics represent pathologic infection. Postoperative infection may vary in its presentation, including spondylodiscitis, superficial cellulites or infected fluid collection, and paravertebral or epidural abscess (Fig. 174-4). Postprocedural discitis is relatively uncommon, with an incidence of less than 1%, although some studies reported an incidence as high as 3% of patients.[18,19] Early in the infection, radiographs are not sensitive at detecting spondylodiscitis. CT may demonstrate destructive lesions and erosions in the vertebral end plates, as well as collapse of disc height. MRI is the best imaging modality for diagnosing discitis, with sensitivity and specificity of 93% and 97%, respectively.[20] MRI may be supplemented with radionuclide scintigraphy, which has been reported to improve the specificity of MRI.[21] The reported sensitivity and specificity of gallium scanning in detecting postoperative discitis is 89%

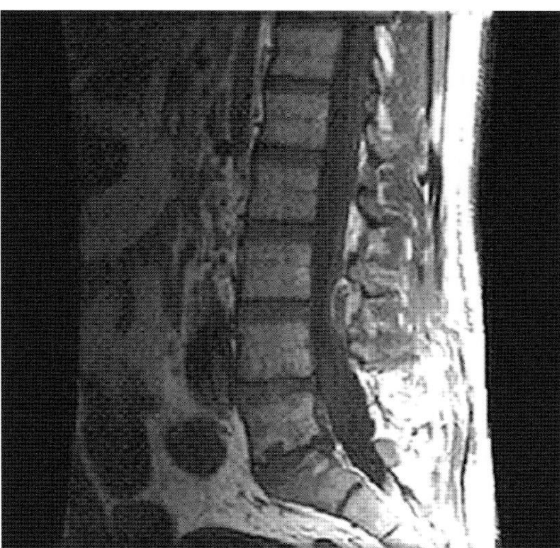

FIGURE 174-4. Postoperative epidural abscess. A rim-enhancing epidural collection is apparent dorsal to the thecal sac, opposite the L3-4 disc.

and 85%, respectively.[22] The MRI findings of postoperative spondylodiscitis include[4,18]

- Vertebral end-plate or marrow changes (low signal on T1- and high signal on T2-weighted images)
- Enhancing bone marrow adjacent to disc
- Enhancing spinal canal tissue
- Enhancing paravertebral soft tissue mass: rim (abscess) or homogeneous (phlegmon) enhancement

Although some of the aforementioned signal changes can occur normally after surgery (including disc enhancement), extensive contiguous enhancement of the disc and adjacent marrow is more consistent with infection. However, severe Modic changes from degenerative disease and aseptic discitis may appear indistinguishable from infection on MRI.[23] Laboratory evaluations including serum white blood cell count, erythrocyte sedimentation rate (ESR), and C-reactive protein (CRP) are often more helpful in diagnosing infection than is imaging.[24] Both ESR and CRP are nonspecific inflammatory markers and demonstrate a postoperative peak from the trauma of surgery. Nevertheless, a second rise or a persisting elevation of CRP levels after surgery has a sensitivity and specificity of 82% and 48%, respectively, for infectious complications.[24] In addition, when following documented spine infection to ascertain clinical improvement after long-term antibiotic administration, ESR and CRP levels are crucial as measures of infection clearance and responsiveness to antibiotics. Administration of gadolinium in serial MRI has also been reported to assist in the conservative management of nonspecific spondylodiscitis.[25]

Although epidural abscess is a rare postoperative complication, the overall incidence of this condition has been increasing to 2 cases per 100,000 people annually.[25] An infected epidural collection may either enhance homogeneously, if phlegmonous, or in a rim fashion, as with abscesses. An epidural collection may cause neurologic symptoms from mass effect or thrombosis of spinal draining veins, and in either case, emergent decompression is required. Recently, limited surgical approaches have been advocated to prevent the spread of infection to other anatomic structures such as vertebral bodies or discs.[26]

Postoperative Arachnoiditis

Chronic arachnoiditis is another potential cause of the failed back surgery syndrome (FBSS).[27,28] The potential causes of arachnoiditis are protean, but not proven. The inflammatory response may be to blood, infection, trauma, contrast medium, or any other intrathecally injected substance. The incidence of arachnoiditis after spinal surgery is approximately 3%.[29] Clinical findings of radiculopathy do not necessarily correlate with the severity of the arachnoiditis as appreciated on imaging.[30]

Myelography, with and without CT, and MRI (particularly T2-weighted fast-spin echo sequencing) both depict arachnoiditis with high accuracy, and classical findings on each correlate well with each other (Fig. 174-5).[29] MRI can detect arachnoiditis with 92% sensitivity, 100% specificity, and 99% accuracy.[31] There are three typical imaging patterns of arachnoiditis:[32]

1. Nerve roots are conglomerated in the center of the thecal sac, representing mild disease.
2. An "empty" thecal sac caused by adhesions of the nerve roots to the walls of the dura, representing moderate disease.
3. An intrathecal soft tissue mass with a broad dural base that may obstruct the cerebrospinal (CSF) pathway. The mass has intermediate signal intensity and may show varying degrees of enhancement.

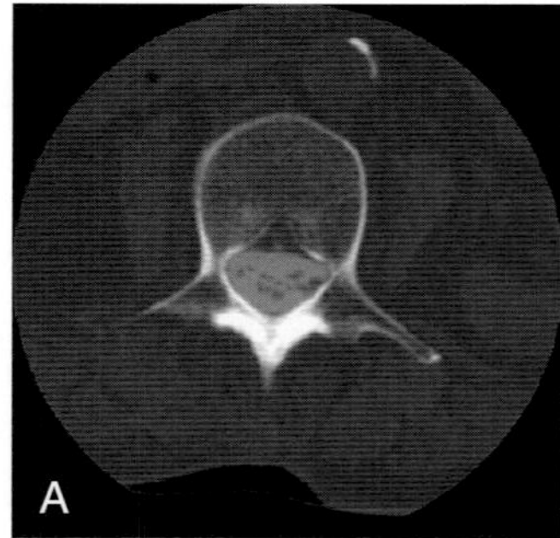

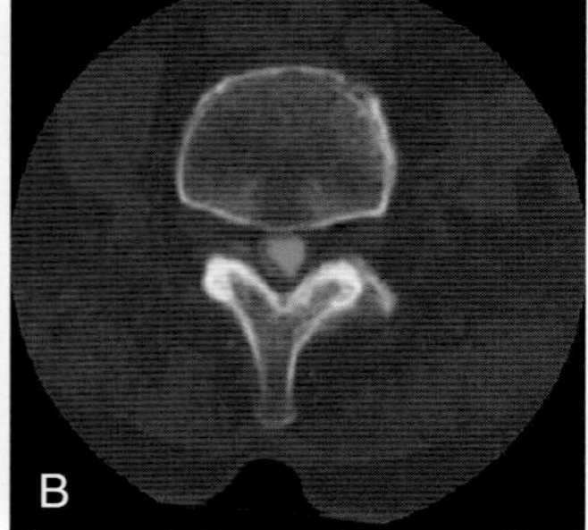

FIGURE 174-5. A, Axial CT-myelogram demonstrates normal appearance of the nerve roots. **B,** The nerve roots are clumped on one side, consistent with arachnoiditis.

Postoperative Radiculitis

Enhancement of nerve roots is a common finding in a normal postoperative spine but may also represent a source of ongoing symptoms. The enhancement is caused by disruption of the blood-nerve barrier, either after surgery or from chronic or severe compression by a herniated disc. Root enhancement can be seen in asymptomatic patients for 6 to 8 months postoperatively, after which it usually resolves.[33] Thereafter, root enhancement correlates well with radiculopathy.[34]

A recent study correlated patient symptoms after lumbar discectomy with MRI findings.[35] A total of 120 postoperative patients underwent MRI to evaluate their nerve roots for enhancement, thickening, and displacement. The incidence of nerve root enhancement was 65.7%, and this MRI finding was associated with symptoms in the offending nerve root distribution, with sensitivity of 91.7%, specificity of 73.2%, and a positive predictive value of 83.7%. When all three imaging findings were present (enhancement, thickening, and displacement), the positive predictive value increased to 94.1%.

Pseudomeningocele

A pseudomeningocele is a collection of CSF that is not lined by arachnoid or dura. Intraoperatively, a dural violation is either not recognized or is inadequately repaired, resulting in a persistent opening. Back pain or radiculopathy can ensue.[36] Most commonly, the imaging characteristics of CSF are identified (Fig. 174-6); in the immediate postoperative period, blood products may be mixed in. It is difficult to distinguish between a normal postoperative fluid collection that is not in communication with the thecal sac and a true pseudomeningocele that requires surgical repair. Serial imaging may reveal continued expansion of the collection, indicating that a

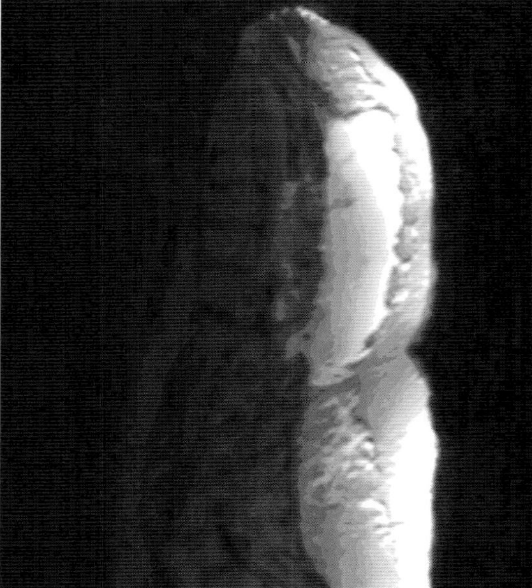

FIGURE 174-6. Pseudomeningocele. Laminectomy and successful removal of a thoracic schwannoma were complicated by formation of this massive posterior thoracic pseudomeningocele, here demonstrated by the dorsal hyperintensity on sagittal T2-weighted MRI.

communication exists. Recently, digital subtraction myelography has been used successfully to detect small dural leaks associated with pseudomeningoceles.[37,38]

Instrumentation

In 2004, more than 300,000 spinal fusions were performed in the United States, accounting for more than $16 billion in hospital charges alone.[39] The widespread use of instrumentation in spinal procedures raises unique challenges for imaging, both intraoperatively and postoperatively. Although implanted hardware is composed of a variety of composite materials, the vast majority are radiopaque, causing MRI artifact and signal scatter. Titanium has the advantage of being nonferromagnetic and therefore MRI compatible. However, a 360-degree spinal construct greatly diminishes the resolution of neural elements within the canal on MRI. Polyetheretherketone (PEEK) hardware is increasingly employed because of its radiolucent characteristics. Despite radiopaque markers, migration of PEEK cages is more difficult to detect on postoperative plain radiography.

Preoperative Use of Imaging

Preoperative imaging, CT or MRI, not only confirms the indication for placement of instrumentation, but also allows for important planning for hardware dimensions, trajectory, and fine bony anatomy. Although plain radiographs may provide some measurement of such details as pedicle diameter, fine-cut CT with sagittal and coronal reconstructions is increasingly being used for preoperative planning. The equivalent mineral density (EMD), calculated from quantitative CT, has been correlated with the ability of cancellous bone to hold screws.[40] Recently, dual-energy x-ray absorptiometry (DEXA) is used to determine preoperative bone mineral density. Those patients with bone mineral density less than 0.45 g/cm^2 required a significantly lower number of loading cycles to induce screw loosening.[41]

Fusion

Intraoperative Imaging for Fusion Procedures

Intraoperative imaging for instrumented fusion procedures is rapidly changing both in radiographic modality and in its purpose. Traditionally, instrumentation such as pedicle screws were placed using an intricate knowledge of bony anatomic landmarks, supplemented with either plain radiography or fluoroscopy. For minimally invasive procedures or kyphoplasty, in which direct visualization of the pedicle was not possible, biplanar fluoroscopy was employed. Neuromonitoring using electromyography can often help detect an instrumentation breech in the pedicle or nerve root irritation, but many surgeons routinely obtain a fine-cut postoperative CT with reconstructions to verify correct level and position of the hardware construct.

Unfortunately, it is relatively common to detect misplaced instrumentation on postoperative imaging. The accuracy of screw placement varies widely, with some reporting a misplacement rate as high as 41%, even in the hands of experienced spine surgeons working with the benefits of intraoperative fluoroscopic guidance.[42] The rate of misplacement differs depending on the type of radiography used to measure screw position, by plain film or CT, as well as the definition of misplacement.[43-45] Using postoperative CT and defining accurate screw placement as "within 2 mm of the medial border of the pedicle," one study reported a misplacement rate of 19%.[46] Placement of pedicle screws in the thoracic spine is more technically difficult because of the small pedicle diameter and vital structures nearby. A recent review found a 20.3% rate of misplacement for upper-middle thoracic pedicle screws as determined by CT.[47] It is now accepted that the rate of detection for misplaced screws is greater with high-resolution CT imaging, which allows excellent bony detail, compared with either plain radiographs or MRI.[43,48-50]

Detection of a misplaced screw postoperatively usually occurs in an asymptomatic patient. In 50 patients who underwent 360-degree lumbar fusion, 41% of pedicle screws breached.[42] Of these, 32% breached medially and were associated with displacement of the dura. However, only one patient presented with symptoms related to a misplaced screw, in this case, an S1 radiculopathy. In addition, all patients in this study were reported to have achieved normal fusion. In the lumbar spine, a breach of 4 mm or less has been reported as safe, due to the large epidural space.[51] Minimally invasive techniques, such as percutaneous pedicle screw placement, have a similar rate of instrumentation misplacement and clinical consequences. In a study of 51 patients, 27 screws (6.6%) were misplaced, and only 1 misplaced screw resulted in an injury to the L4 nerve root.[52]

As more fusion procedures are performed, surgeons routinely face the dilemma of whether to reoperate for an asymptomatic misplaced screw, especially if neurologic compromise could theoretically occur at a later time. In addition, the changing medicolegal climate has led to a policy among some spine surgeons requiring that all instrumentation be documented as correctly positioned. In this atmosphere, the role of intraoperative imaging is taking on new importance. The use of fine-cut CT and 3D guidance, such as the O-arm Imaging System (Medtronic, Minneapolis, MN), is increasingly being employed for routine elective degenerative spine cases. Using such navigation systems can improve the accuracy of even upper thoracic pedicle screws to greater than 90%.[53] In surgeries to correct scoliosis deformity, use of intraoperative navigation for screw placement can decrease the breach rate to only 2%.[54] The sensitivity and specificity of 3D guidance systems for placement of pedicle screws has been reported as 91.3% and 98.2%, respectively.[55] Intraoperative evaluation of the reconstructed fine-cut CTs resulted in a revision rate of 2.7% of pedicle screws and lowered the secondary reoperation rate to 0.5%.[55] After careful review of an intraoperative CT, many surgeons do not obtain additional postoperative imaging.

Postoperative Imaging after Fusion

Patients who develop new pain or neurologic deficits postoperatively should receive expeditious imaging in order to detect any reversible hardware-related complications. Depending on the urgency of the symptom, many surgeons still begin with conventional radiographs to evaluate the primary instrumentation. The use of at least two perpendicular planes (anteroposterior and lateral) greatly enhances the ability to detect complications such as bony fracture or misplaced screws. However, plain

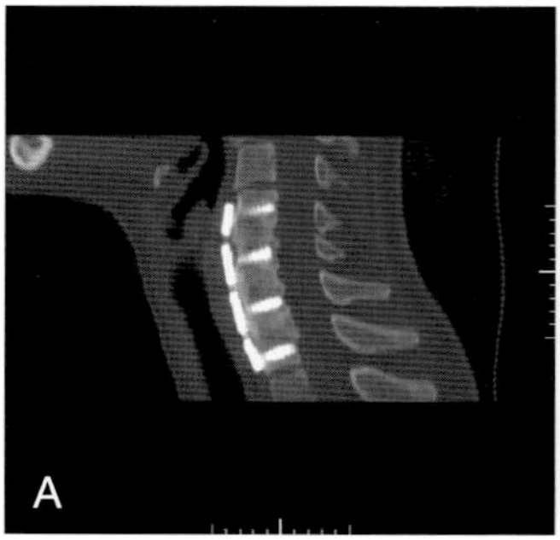

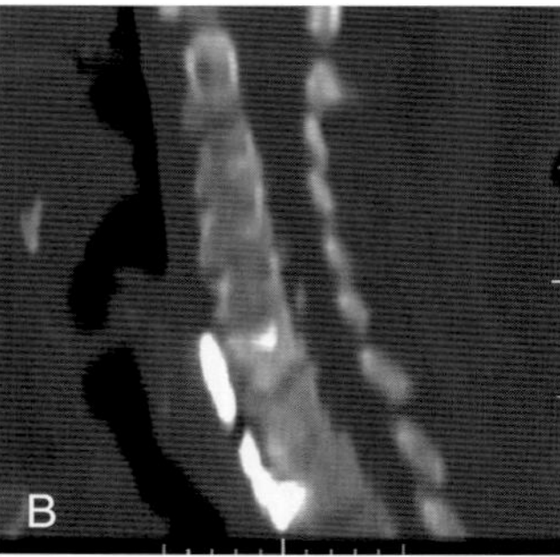

FIGURE 174-7. CT sagittal reconstruction imaging of the cervical spine. **A,** The image demonstrates solid fusion 3 months after surgery at three levels, with ventral cervical plating. **B,** The patient had neck pain with movement 1 year after surgery. A pseudarthrosis is evident at the upper level, whereas fusion is shown at the lower level. Flexion-extension images demonstrated movement at that level.

radiographs are reported to correlate with intraoperative findings in fusion cases less than 70% of the time.[56,57]

Fine-cut, high-resolution CT with coronal and sagittal reconstruction is generally accepted to provide the greatest level of instrumentation detail. Precise information regarding cortical bone is provided.[58] Evidence of fusion, bridging bony trabeculation around cages, was detected in 90% of patients by CT compared with only 7% of patients by plain radiograph, as confirmed by surgical reexploration.[59] CT also shows subtle lucencies surrounding instrumentation, either cages or pedicle screws, earlier and with a higher sensitivity and specificity than plain radiographs (Fig. 174-7).[59-61] Finally, fine-cut CTs with reconstructions have a significantly greater degree of interobserver and intraobserver agreement regarding fusion status than do flexion-extension and anteroposterior plain radiographs.[62]

However, evaluation for a new neurologic symptom following a fusion procedure should not only include CT but also another modality to assess the nerve roots and spinal cord. As discussed earlier, MRI has its limitations due to artifact signal that may obscure detail within the spinal canal. Although more invasive and time intensive, CT myelography provides fine detail of both instrumentation and neural structures.[63] A recent study compared CT-myelogram with MRI in patients who had previously undergone anterior cervical discectomy and fusion.[64] Despite the presence of the ventral titanium plate, MRI was more useful for detecting disc abnormalities or nerve root compression. However, CT-myelogram provided better detail of foraminal stenosis and bony lesions in the cervical canal. CT-myelogram, particularly in the cervical spine, requires an experienced interventional radiologist for injection of contrast medium into the subarachnoid space. The risks inherent with the CT-myelogram procedure may reduce its utility; especially as new, less-invasive technology is developed. 3D MRI/CT fusion imaging allows for construction of colored images that combine both imaging modalities. This technique also shows promise for depicting lumbar instrumentation in relation to neural architecture.[65]

Assessment of Fusion

The chief goal of any stabilizing spinal procedure—with or without instrumentation—is fusion of bony elements. Although successful fusion does not necessarily lead to good outcome, documentation of arthrodesis is an essential component of patient follow-up.[57,66,67] It is well-established that pseudarthrosis, a leading complication associated with thoracolumbar spinal arthrodesis, can contribute greatly to persistent postoperative pain.[68,69]

Successful fusion depends on the establishment of a continuous mass of bone across a motion segment, preventing movement in any plane across that segment. A spinal pseudarthrosis is defined as an absence of bridging bone between adjacent vertebrae.[68] Assessment of fusion depends on the time of postoperative imaging and the imaging modality. Either iliac crest bone graft or cadaveric bone, placed into the dorsolateral gutters during spinal fusion, shows high-density characteristics on immediate postoperative CT but exhibits decreased density at 6-week follow-up. The physiologic process of bone fusion, with extensive remodeling and surrounding tissue edema, obscures the presence of the dorsolateral bone. In addition, before solid fusion occurs, the bone is a trabecular network bridging different spinal levels. High-density cortical bone is not typically visible until at least 3 months after surgery and thereafter continues to increase in density beyond 1 year. Radiolucent zones around pedicle screws often indicate delayed union or pseudarthrosis. However, these radiolucent zones may be present in up to 40% of postoperative patients as evidenced by plain radiograph at 6 months.[70] At 3 years, 15% of patients still showed radiolucent zones by plain radiograph, but only 53% of these patients actually had pseudarthrosis on reexploration.[70]

Many imaging characteristics have been studied to determine whether the evidence of radiographic fusion truly equates with solid bone fusion in an actual patient. Using fine-cut CT, one study reported that evidence of bone fusion in dorsolateral gutters represented actual fusion in 89% of cases, compared with only 74% of cases when both facets were fused.[71] When both facets and dorsolateral gutters were fused on CT, the probability of a solid fusion on exploration is 96%. Another study specified that determination of fusion involves a multistep approach.[60] First, spinal alignment should be assessed over a 6-month period, by plain radiographs in the standing position. Progressive subsidence or change in spinal alignment represents a fusion failure. Second, dynamic flexion-extension radiographs should demonstrate no significant motion across the fusion segment. Third, close evaluation of the host bone reaction to instrumentation, as shown by CT, is required. Cystic or sclerotic changes within subchondral bone of the vertebral end plates and progressive radiographic lucencies around pedicle screws are suggestive of pseudarthrosis. Fourth, radiographic evidence of the formation of new bone, in dorsolateral gutters and across the disc space, is the most reliable finding of solid fusion.

There are several published grading systems for fusion. Brantigan describes radiographic criteria for fusion:[72]

1. Radiographic pseudarthrosis: Collapse of construct, vertebral slip, broken screws, resorption of bone graft, or major lucency or gap visible in the fusion area.
2. Uncertain fusion: Bone graft visible, but it has not increased in density, or a small lucency or gap is visible in the fusion area.
3. Radiographic fusion: Graft shows a higher density, and there is no interface between graft bone and vertebral bone. Mature bony trabeculae bridge the fusion area, ventral vertebral traction spurs are minimal, facet joints are

fused, and there is ventral progression of the graft within the disc space.

Molinari et al. specified five categories of fusion:[73]

1. Definite—Solid trabeculated transverse process and facet fusion
2. Probable—Thick fusion mass on one side, difficult to visualize on other side
3. Probably not—Possible lucency or defect in the fusion mass
4. Not fused—Definite resorption of graft with fatigue of instrumentation
5. Unable to assess

Glassman et al. performed a prospective, randomized study of iliac crest bone graft versus recombinant human bone morphogenetic protein-2 in dorsolateral instrumented fusion.[74] Using CT at 6 and 12 months, they employed a five-part grading system to evaluate the fusion mass:

1. No fusion—evidence of radiolucencies around instrumentation and no evidence of bone graft cortication
2. Partial or limited unilateral fusion—Some bone formation, although with possible lucencies or sclerotic margins
3. Partial or limited bilateral fusion—The same imaging characteristics bilaterally
4. Solid unilateral fusion—Corticated bone spanning the disc space, dorsolateral gutter, and facet
5. Solid bilateral fusion—The same imaging characteristics bilaterally

For pseudarthrosis of Glassman grade I/II or Molinari grade III/IV, plain radiographs may suffice for diagnosis and surgical decision to reoperate. A recent study demonstrated a sensitivity of 100%, specificity of almost 90%, and negative predictive value of 100% for healed fusion, for plain x-ray films.[75]

The radiographic diagnosis of failed fusion and pseudarthrosis is best achieved through multiple imaging modalities and over different time points. Despite the increased sensitivity of fine-cut CT, surgical reexploration remains the gold standard in cases of radiographic ambiguity.

Postoperative Imaging for Tumor

In most instances, postoperative imaging after spinal tumor resection is done to confirm the extent of resection and serve as a baseline for subsequent follow-up studies. In benign intradural extramedullary tumors such as meningioma or schwannoma, gross total excision is often achieved. However, yearly follow-up imaging is generally recommended to identify recurrence prior to the onset of symptoms. The recurrence rate for spinal meningioma is approximately 7.5% at 10 years and 9.3% at 20 years.[76]

The frequency of imaging is determined by the tumor pathology. A biologically aggressive intraspinal neoplasm requires close follow-up imaging after surgery, usually at 6 months and then annually until the chance of recurrence is remote. In addition, atypical spinal tumors may exhibit drop metastases or leptomeningeal spread, requiring full craniospinal imaging. MRI with and without administration of gadolinium is the most common imaging modality for following tumor regrowth. During initial surgical planning and after obtaining frozen pathology, careful consideration must be given to the type of instrumented construct that may be required after tumor resection. At the very least, the instrumentation must be MRI compatible, but efforts should also be made to limit the amount of hardware implanted, so that future MRI studies have minimal artifact. Laminoplasty with nonmetallic points of fixation allows for nondistorted imaging and should be considered during resection.

Summary

Advances in different modalities of imaging technology have improved the surgeon's ability to diagnose and treat disorders of the spine even when the anatomy has been altered by previous surgery. The recent availability of intraoperative navigation and immediate axial imaging techniques in the operating room can potentially increase the surgeon's ability to make a diagnosis that might alter treatment and improve patient care. Further studies are needed to study the cost effectiveness of the increased use of postoperative imaging for patients with spinal disorders.

KEY REFERENCES

Carreon LY, Djurasovic M, Glassman SD, et al: Diagnostic accuracy and reliability of fine-cut CT scans with reconstructions to determine the status of an instrumented posterolateral fusion with surgical exploration as reference standard. *Spine (Phila Pa 1976)* 32(8):892–895, 2007.

Jinkins JR, Van Goethem JW: The postsurgical lumbosacral spine. Magnetic resonance imaging evaluation following intervertebral disk surgery, surgical decompression, intervertebral bony fusion, and spinal instrumentation. *Radiol Clin North Am* 39(1):1–29, 2001.

Lee YS, Choi ES, Song CJ: Symptomatic nerve root changes on contrast-enhanced MR imaging after surgery for lumbar disk herniation. *AJNR Am J Neuroradiol* 30(5):1062–1067, 2009.

McGirt MJ, Eustacchio S, Varga P, et al: A prospective cohort study of close interval computed tomography and magnetic resonance imaging after primary lumbar discectomy: factors associated with recurrent disc herniation and disc height loss. *Spine (Phila Pa 1976)* 34(19):2044–2051, 2009.

Molinari RW, Bridwell KH, Klepps SJ, et al: Minimum 5-year follow-up of anterior column structural allografts in the thoracic and lumbar spine. *Spine (Phila Pa 1976)* 24(10):967–972, 1999.

Rajasekaran S, Vidyadhara S, Ramesh P, Shetty AP: Randomized clinical study to compare the accuracy of navigated and non-navigated thoracic pedicle screws in deformity correction surgeries. *Spine (Phila Pa 1976)* 32(2):E56–E64, 2007.

Van Goethem JW, Parizel PM, van den Hauwe L, De Schepper AM: Imaging findings in patients with failed back surgery syndrome. *J Belge Radiol* 80(2):81–84, 1997.

REFERENCES

The complete reference list is available online at expertconsult.com.

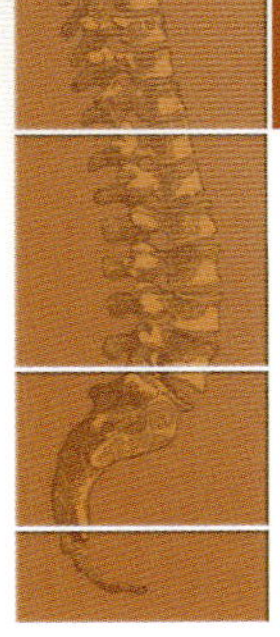

CHAPTER 175

Intraoperative Imaging

Iain H. Kalfas | Bruce M. McCormack | Hansen A. Yuan

Few surgical specialties are as dependent on intraoperative imaging as is the field of spine surgery. Whether it involves obtaining a lateral radiograph to confirm the level of a lumbar disc herniation or using ultrasonography to localize an intramedullary syrinx, intraoperative imaging provides information that can significantly affect the course of surgery.

The most commonly used intraoperative imaging techniques are plain film radiography, fluoroscopy, and, to a lesser degree, ultrasonography. These techniques each have their own advantages and disadvantages, but when used appropriately, each can provide valuable information. In addition to these standard intraoperative imaging techniques, image-guided spinal navigation (IGSN) and intraoperative CT have evolved into proven and versatile tools for orienting the spine surgeon to the complex 3D anatomy of the spinal column. This chapter reviews each imaging technique as well as the indications for their use.

Plain Film Radiography

Plain film radiography was the first imaging technique applied to spine surgery. The segmented bony anatomy of the spinal column lends itself readily to this form of imaging. Images are easily obtained, relatively inexpensive, and generally reliable. Differential attenuation of x-rays by the various tissues provides the image contrast seen in a radiograph. Bone attenuates x-rays the most, followed by muscle, fat, and air, which attenuate very few x-rays. Soft tissue structures such as the spinal cord, nerve roots, or intervertebral discs are not well visualized by plain film radiography.

In spine surgery, plain radiography is typically used to localize a specific spinal level. During the surgical exposure of the cervical, lumbar, or thoracic spine, a radiopaque marker (e.g., clamp, probe, spinal needle) is positioned in the surgical field. For the lumbar or cervical spine, a lateral radiograph is obtained with the lumbosacral or occipitocervical junction at one end and the inserted marker at the other end. The number of vertebral levels between the imaged junction and the marker can be determined and the appropriate spinal level easily localized. In general, the range of view from the occipitocervical junction extends caudally to the cervicothoracic junction, depending on the prominence of the patient's neck and shoulders. The range of view from the lumbosacral junction extends rostrally to the lower thoracic region.

Spinal levels in the mid- and upper thoracic spine can be more difficult to precisely localize because of their distance from a reliable anatomic reference point. In this case, an alternative to the conventional method of radiographic localization is to obtain two adjacent lateral images. The first film is positioned to include the lumbosacral or occipitocervical junction at one end and an instrument marker attached to the spinal anatomy at the other end. A second film can then be positioned to include the first instrument marker and a second instrument marker centered in the operative field. The location of the first instrument marker can be determined on the first film by its relationship to the lumbosacral or occipitocervical junction. The location of the appropriate spinal level can then be determined on the second film by determining its relationship to the localized first instrument marker.

Radiographic imaging of the upper thoracic spine can be difficult because the patient's shoulders may obstruct the view on a lateral radiograph. An alternative to the lateral radiograph is the anteroposterior (AP) view. This view can be obtained by positioning the patient on a radiolucent operating table. The film cassette can then be placed immediately below the table and an AP view obtained. With this view, either the T1 or T12 vertebra and its associated ribs serve as the reference point for spinal level identification.

When intraoperative localization involves exposure of the spinal column at the level of a collapsed or fractured vertebra, the relationship of the operative field to the lumbosacral or occipitocervical junction is not as critical. A film that centers over the operative field can approximate the appropriate level. The abnormal vertebrae can usually be identified on a lateral radiograph and the appropriate exposure confirmed.

The most common error related to the use of intraoperative plain radiography is incorrectly identifying the appropriate spinal level. This can be due to inadequate image quality that obscures the appropriate spinal anatomy. This can lead the surgeon to misinterpret the radiograph and incorrectly count the number of spinal levels from the lumbosacral or occipitocervical junction to the operative field. Suboptimal imaging should not be accepted. If satisfactory localization cannot be obtained, the radiograph should be repeated until correct localization is confirmed.

Even when the correct level is identified, localization errors may occur. For example, localization in the lumbar spine typically involves placing a marker on a spinous process and obtaining a lateral radiograph. Although the correct spinous process may be visualized on the film, continued surgical dissection down to the level of the lumbar canal may cause the surgeon to easily drift to an adjacent lumbar segment above or below the desired level. Placement of a marker at the level of the lumbar lamina in addition to the marker on the spinous process can help prevent this error.

In addition to localization of the spinal level, plain radiography can be used in isolated instances to assess the extent of neural decompression. This technique is particularly useful during transoral decompressive procedures. It involves placing a radiopaque contrast medium into the decompressed site and obtaining a lateral radiograph. The radiograph will show the extent of the decompression and can be compared with a preoperative study demonstrating the neural compression. If the configuration and location of the contained contrast medium does not approximate the configuration and location of the epidural compression on the preoperative studies, the surgical site can be modified until a satisfactory decompression of the neural elements is achieved (Fig. 175-1).

Plain radiography can also be used in conjunction with intraoperative myelography to determine the extent of canal decompression.[1] In the setting of a thoracolumbar burst fracture decompressed through a dorsolateral approach, radiopaque dye can be placed in the subarachnoid space by a small-gauge spinal needle to assess the adequacy of the surgical decompression. A lateral radiograph is taken and the relationship of the dye to the ventral spinal cord can be assessed (Fig. 175-2).

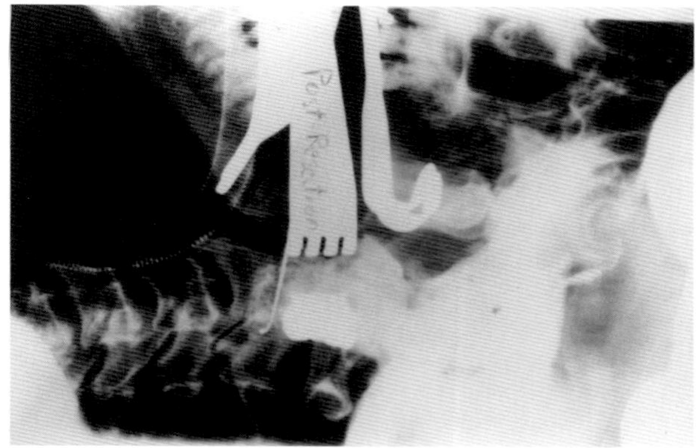

FIGURE 175-1. Lateral radiograph after a transoral odontoidectomy. Radiopaque contrast media has been placed into the decompressed site. The position and configuration of the contrast media can be compared to the preoperative studies to confirm a satisfactory decompression.

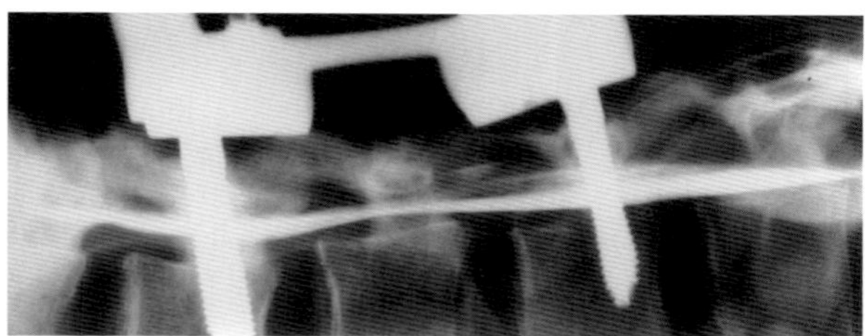

FIGURE 175-2. Intraoperative lateral myelography after lumbar decompression and fixation.

Fluoroscopy

Fluoroscopy is used when real-time imaging or multiple images of the spine are required during surgery. Fluoroscopic images are generated with a lower radiation dose than that for standard radiography. A camera records the image and displays it on a television monitor. The images can be recorded on x-ray film, cinefluoradiography film, or videotape.[2]

The primary use of fluoroscopy in spine surgery is to facilitate the optimal placement and positioning of spine fixation screws, interbody cages, or arthroplasty devices and to monitor the injection of methyl methacrylate into osteoporotic vertebral body fractures. Fluoroscopy can provide the surgeon with real-time imaging of the spinal column in several planes depending on the positioning of the fluoroscope's C-arm. When used for the insertion of pedicle screws, the C-arm can be positioned to provide a lateral view of the spinal column. This shows the sagittal (rostrocaudal) orientation of a pedicle marker or screw (Fig. 175-3). By rotating the C-arm from the lateral position toward the AP position, an oblique view of the spinal column can be obtained. This view demonstrates the position of a pedicle marker or screw in relationship to a cross-sectional view of each pedicle. If the correct entry point and trajectory in both the sagittal and axial planes has been properly selected, the oblique fluoroscopic view will demonstrate these markers within the cortical margins of the individual pedicles (Fig. 175-4). When the correct entry point and trajectories have been confirmed, the markers can be removed and the pedicle screws inserted along the same path.

When used for cervical screw fixation (e.g., ventral odontoid screw fixation), an AP as well as a lateral view may be required. This can be obtained by alternating the position of a single C-arm unit from the lateral to the AP position or by using two separate fluoroscopy machines with arms positioned 90 degrees with respect to each other.[3]

Fluoroscopy has also been used for ventral cervical plate instrumentation procedures to assist in the positioning and placement of the fixation plates and screws.[4] However, the

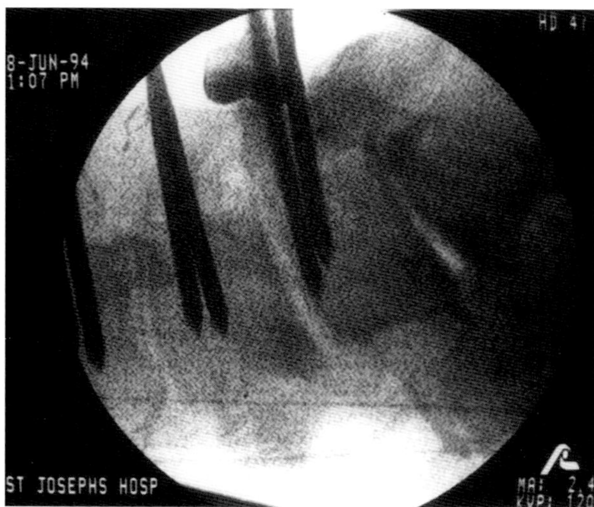

FIGURE 175-3. Lateral fluoroscopic view of the lower lumbar spine showing the sagittal orientation of Steinmann pins placed within the pedicles of L3, L4, and L5.

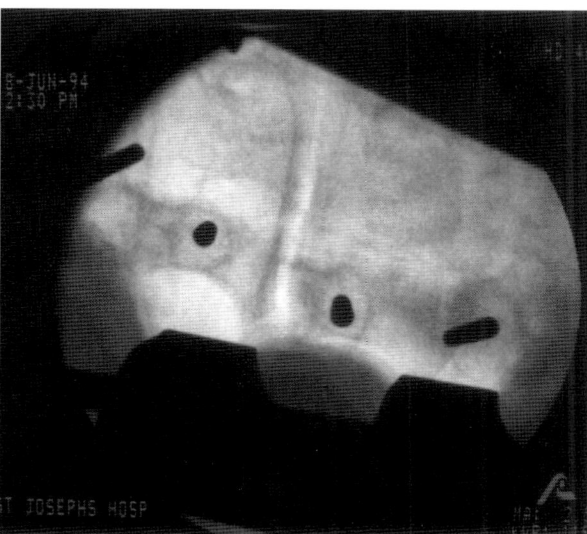

FIGURE 175-4. Oblique fluoroscopic view of the lumbar spine showing the pedicles in cross section. Three Steinmann pins have been placed within the pedicles and are noted to be lying within the cortical margins of the pedicles.

lower cervical and upper thoracic regions can frequently be difficult to visualize because of image obstruction by the patient's shoulders. This problem can be addressed by placing an interscapular roll beneath the patient and taping the shoulders down to the table or by using wrist slings to pull down on the patient's arms during imaging.

A potential problem with fluoroscopic imaging is difficulty in obtaining a true lateral image of the spinal anatomy. This can produce a parallax effect that can result in the suboptimal positioning of fixation screws. In the cervical spine, this problem can be addressed by ensuring that the angle of one mandible viewed on the fluoroscopy screen overlaps the angle of the other mandible. In the thoracic and lumbosacral spine, the superior and inferior cortical margins of the vertebrae can be used to ensure a true lateral image. If two cortical margins are seen at one end of a vertebral body, a true lateral image has not been obtained and an adjustment of the C-arm is needed.

The recent development of minimally invasive techniques for spine surgery has led to a significantly increased use of intraoperative fluoroscopy. The limited exposure of soft tissue in these procedures reduces the ability of the surgeon to directly visualize the pertinent surgical anatomy. This makes fluoroscopy a critical component of any minimally invasive procedure.

The primary disadvantage of intraoperative fluoroscopy is the exposure of the surgical team to repeated amounts of low-dose ionizing radiation. Several studies have attempted to quantify the amount of occupational radiation exposure to health-care professionals under different and real clinical scenarios.[5-9] These studies have typically demonstrated that the radiation exposure to hands, eyes, head and neck, and body during fluoroscopically assisted procedures is well below the recommended values for annual allowable occupational radiation exposure as outlined by the International Commission on Radiological Protection.[10] However, the health-related risks of this chronic exposure to radiation remains relatively unknown and may not be realized for years.

Unlike other fluoroscopically assisted musculoskeletal procedures (e.g., intramedullary femoral nailing), the techniques and instruments used for pedicle fixation bring the surgeon's hands very close to the primary area of exposure.[11,12] The amount of radiation exposure needed to achieve adequate visualization of the lumbar spine is greater than that for other anatomic sites.[13] Rampersaud et al. reported on the radiation exposure occurring during the placement of thoracolumbar pedicle screws.[14] Pedicle screws were placed into six cadaver specimens using fluoroscopy. Dosimeter badges and rings were placed on the surgeon's neck, torso, and dominant hand. Radiation exposure to these sites was quantified.

Ninety-six pedicle screws were placed with an average of 8.5 fluoroscopic images taken per screw. The average exposure time per screw was 9.3 seconds. The results of this study demonstrated that fluoroscopically assisted pedicle screw fixation exposes the spine surgeon to significantly greater radiation levels than other, nonspinal musculoskeletal procedures involving the use of fluoroscopy. The radiation exposure to the dominant hand was noted to be as high as 10 to 12 times the amount of hand exposure experienced in other procedures. The greatest level of exposure was noted on the side ipsilateral to the beam source due to backscatter radiation. This study emphasizes the need for appropriate lead shielding, including the use of a thyroid shield and leaded glasses. The use of radiation attenuation gloves resulted in a 33% decrease in dose rate to the hand. Using limited, pulsed-image acquisition and maintaining a safe distance (3–4 feet) from the radiation source also helped reduce the dosage to negligible levels.[14] This study confirmed that spine surgeons who regularly use fluoroscopy should monitor their annual radiation dose.

Ultrasonography

The application of ultrasonography to spine surgery was first reported in 1982.[15] Like fluoroscopy, ultrasonography provides continuous and real-time imaging. However, unlike fluoroscopy, which only provides images of the bony spinal column, ultrasonography can image the adjacent neural and soft tissue structures as well.

Diagnostic ultrasound scanners consist of a scan head containing transducers that convert electrical energy to mechanical or sound energy. To obtain a sonogram the scan head of the ultrasound probe is placed against a contact surface. A short ultrasonic pulse is generated by the transducers and transmitted into the contact surface. This pulse travels continuously into the medium until it strikes another surface or encounters a change in acoustic impedance. Acoustic impedance, the product of the density of a material and the velocity of the sound wave, depends not only on tissue density but also on the actual composition and internal structure of a tissue substance.[16]

When the ultrasound pulse strikes a surface, some of the energy is reflected back to the transducer and some of the energy continues forward. Structures that reflect most or all of the ultrasound pulses striking them, specifically air and bone, prevent the imaging of structures behind them. A reflected ultrasonic pulse returns to the scan head and hits the transducer. The shape of the crystal in the transducer is changed, inducing a voltage across it. This voltage is recorded—its amplitude dependent on the strength of the reflection that contacts the transducer face. The location within the tissue from which the reflection came can easily be calculated once the speed of sound in the tissue being scanned and the interval of time between the generation of the impulse and the reception of the reflected wave are known.

The spinal canal can be imaged with ultrasonography during surgery by filling the wound with saline after a laminectomy has been performed. The tip of the transducer is immersed in the saline and manipulated in several directions to give the surgeon an orientation to the specific anatomy. By rotating the scan head 90 degrees, the images can be changed from a longitudinal to a cross-sectional image of the structure.

Dense anatomic structures capable of reflecting ultrasonic pulses are termed *echogenic* and appear white on the ultrasound images. These structures include the spinal cord, the vertebral body, and any solid intramedullary or extramedullary lesion. The nonechogenic black layers consist of the saline immediately beneath the transducer tip, the subarachnoid space on either side of the spinal cord, and any intramedullary syrinx or cystic lesion.

Ultrasonography can be used to localize a variety of lesions within the spinal canal. It is effective for localizing and characterizing intramedullary spinal cord tumors as well as intradural and extramedullary tumors. Ultrasonography can be used before opening the dura to visualize the extent of the tumor and to localize specific areas of interest such as a cyst within the tumor. The images guide the opening of the dura and can often direct the surgeon to a particular location to start the myelotomy and exploration.[17] When a cystic tumor such as a hemangioma is present, ultrasonography can help identify the specific mural nodule of the tumor.[18]

Edema proximal or distal to the tumor also causes widening of the cord seen on ultrasonography and can create confusion in determining the absolute limits of the tumor. However, in most cases, the tumor border is well defined and the edema is less echogenic than the tumor.[19]

In the setting of syringomyelia, ultrasonography can be used to localize the maximal extent of the syrinx as well as to identify any small septae present (Fig. 175-5).[18] If a drainage catheter is placed into the syrinx, ultrasonography can be used to assess the degree of collapse of the cavity and determine whether additional catheters are needed.

Ultrasonography has also been used in the setting of vertebral body fractures or dislocations to assess the spinal canal following a decompressive procedure. This is particularly useful in the thoracic and thoracolumbar areas when a dorsolateral approach is used to access ventral and ventrolateral epidural compression. Following removal of the lamina, the ultrasound probe can be placed over the dorsal dura and the extent of the ventral decompression assessed.[20,21]

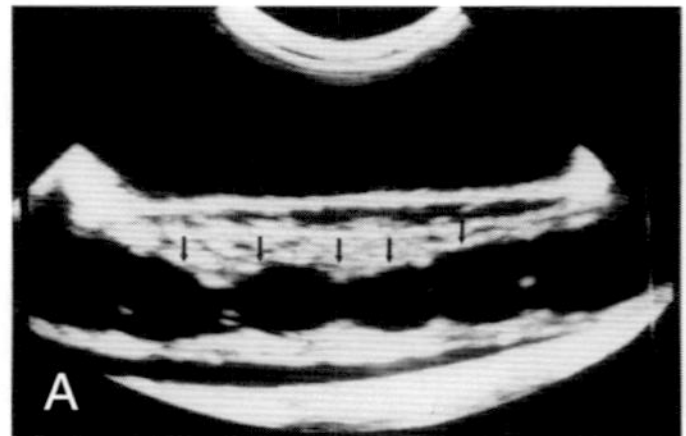

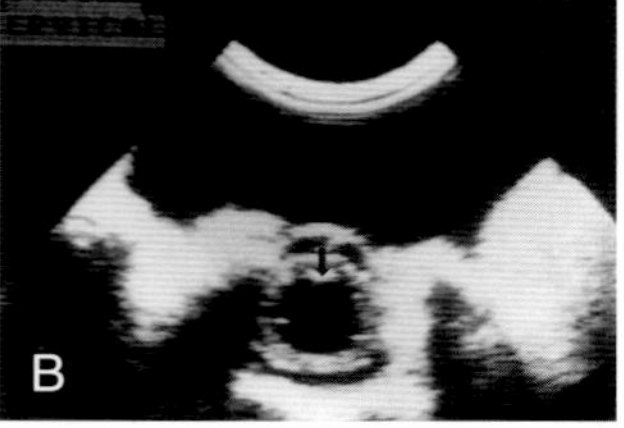

FIGURE 175-5. A, Sagittal ultrasound image of the cervical spinal cord demonstrating a large syrinx (*arrows*). **B,** Axial ultrasound image of the same patient demonstrating the syrinx (*arrow*).

Image-Guided Spinal Navigation

Image-guided spinal navigation (IGSN) involves the use of an image-processing workstation coupled with a digitized localizer system to virtually link preoperative CT images of the spine to the corresponding surgical anatomy. By enabling the manipulation of multiplanar images through any surgical point, IGSN gives the surgeon a greater degree of orientation to the unexposed, and therefore nonvisualized, spinal anatomy.

The development of image-guided technology for spine surgery was influenced by the difficulties of intraoperative spatial orientation associated with surgery for complex spine disorders.[22,23] The 3D anatomy of the spinal column can present challenges for even the most experienced surgeon. Standard dorsal surgical approaches expose only a portion of the spinal column at a given level. Although this partial exposure is not problematic for most laminectomy or discectomy procedures, it can be limiting in the setting of complex spinal column disorders such as fractures, neoplasms, or deformities.

The placement of spine fixation devices such as pedicle screws requires an accurate orientation to the unexposed spinal anatomy. Although intraoperative fluoroscopy and serial radiography have proven useful, they are both limited because they provide only 2D imaging of a complex 3D structure. Consequently, the surgeon is required to extrapolate the third dimension based on an interpretation of the images and knowledge of the pertinent anatomy. This so called "dead reckoning" of the anatomy can result in varying degrees of inaccuracy when placing screws into the unexposed portions of the spinal column.

Several studies have shown the unreliability of routine radiography in assessing pedicle screw placement in the lumbosacral spine. The rate of penetration of the pedicle cortex by an inserted screw ranges from 21% to 31% in these studies.[24-26] However, Steinmann et al., using an image-based technique for pedicle screw placement that combined axial CT of cadaver spine specimens with fluoroscopy, was able to demonstrate a reduction of this screw insertion error rate to 5.5%.[27]

The application of image-guided navigational technology to spine surgery provides 3D and multiplanar views of image data to improve the surgeon's "visualization" of the spinal anatomy. This image data is provided in near-real time and can be manipulated to show every aspect of the intraoperative spinal anatomy through any selected point in the surgical field.[22,23,28-30]

Navigational Technique

The primary components of an IGSN include an image-processing computer workstation interfaced with a two-camera optical localizer (Fig. 175-6). Customized navigational probes with three to four small reflective spheres attached in a known arrangement serve as the tools that link the surgeon to the navigational system (Fig. 175-7). The optical localizer camera system emits infrared energy toward the surgical field, where it is captured by the spheres on the probe and reflected

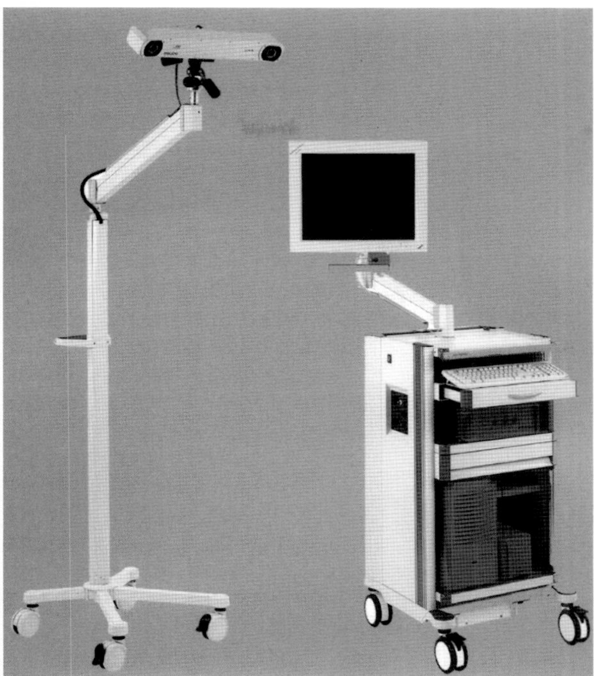

FIGURE 175-6. Image-guided navigation system. Image-processing computer workstation (*right)* and an infrared camera (*left*).

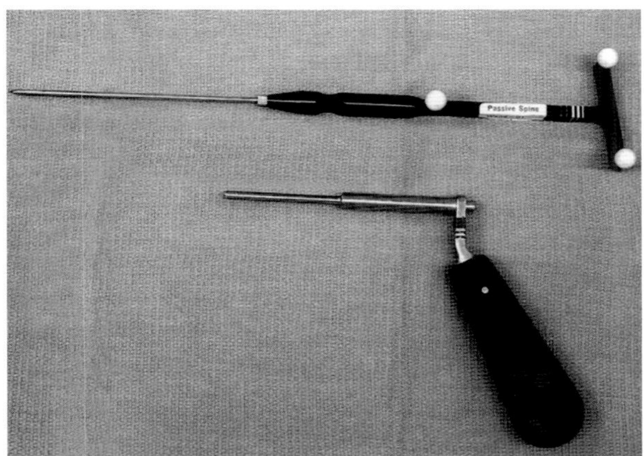

FIGURE 175-7. Navigational probe (with passive reflectors) and hand-held drill guide.

back to the camera. The spatial orientation of the reflected light is passed on to the computer workstation, which can then use mathematical principles of localization by triangulation to localize and track not only the exact position of the probe's tip but also the position of any anatomic structure in the surgical field on which the probe tip rests.

Bone landmarks on the exposed surface of the spinal column provide the frame of reference necessary for image-guided navigation. Specifically, any anatomic landmark that can be identified during surgery and in the preoperative image data set can be used as a reference point. Typically, for spine surgery, the reference points are the tips of the spinous process and transverse processes at each spinal level to be instrumented, although other bony landmarks such as facet joints or prominent osteophytes can also be used.[22,23,28-30]

After a surgical exposure, each selected reference point in the image data set is mapped onto its corresponding point in the exposed surgical anatomy by a process termed *registration*. This process involves highlighting one of the selected reference points in the image data set while placing the navigational probe on the corresponding point in the surgical field. As the camera localizer system tracks the position of the probe, the spatial location of the probe tip is relayed to the computer workstation and the selected anatomic point in the surgical field is linked spatially to its corresponding image data point. This paired point registration step is then repeated for each of the three to five reference points required for accurate registration.

Alternatively, the surgeon can perform the registration process by creating a surface map of the exposed spinal anatomy. This technique involves placing the probe on multiple nondiscreet points on the exposed and debrided surface in the surgical field. The positional information of these points is transferred to the workstation, and a topographic map of the selected anatomy is created and "matched" to the patient's CT data set. This surface mapping technique is typically more time-consuming and inherently less accurate than the paired point registration technique.[30]

Registration can have the greatest effect on navigational accuracy. Registration accuracy depends on the surgeon carefully selecting the correct reference points or performing the contour mapping process. If properly performed, registration will allow for the display of reformatted, multiplanar CT or MRI images to assist the surgeon with orientation to the unexposed spinal anatomy.[23]

The registration process establishes a precise spatial relationship between the image data and the spinal anatomy. If the patient is inadvertently moved after registration, the spatial relationship is distorted and the navigational information is inaccurate. This problem can be minimized by the optional use of a spinal tracking device, which consists of a separate set of passive reflectors attached to a spinous process in the surgical field. It alerts the system if the spine is inadvertently moved and provides for the necessary correction within the navigation data set to keep the registration process accurate and to eliminate the need to repeat registration.

Once the registration process is completed, the surgeon can place the navigational probe on any exposed point in the operative field and the workstation will automatically generate three reformatted images through the selected point. The three planar images are oriented perpendicular to each other in relationship to the long axis of the probe. For pedicle screw fixation, these three reformatted images will be the corresponding axial, coronal, and sagittal images through a selected point. On each reformatted image, a cursor or trajectory line marks the position of the navigational probe in the surgical field. The diameter of the cursor and the width of the trajectory line can be adjusted in proportion to the selected screw diameter. The length of the trajectory line relative to the imaged spine is displayed in millimeters, providing for accurate screw length selection (Fig. 175-8). As the surgeon moves the probe through the surgical field, each planar image updates immediately to show the probe's orientation to the spinal column and provides the surgeon with an optimal orientation to the pertinent spinal anatomy and to the precise screw entry point and trajectory.

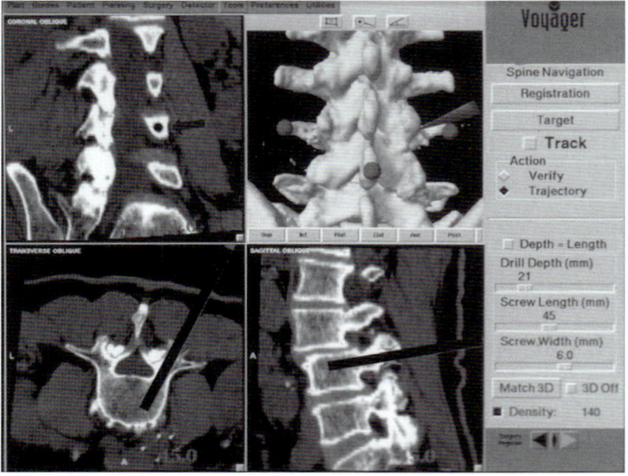

FIGURE 175-8. Screen from image-guided workstation demonstrating a satisfactory trajectory selection through the L4 pedicle. The upper left quadrant displays the coronal image with the computer cursor positioned within the cross section of the pedicle (*arrow*). The left and right lower quadrants show the selected trajectory in the axial and sagittal planes, respectively. The length of the trajectory line is set at 45 mm and its diameter set at 6 mm. The upper right quadrant displays a surface-rendered image of the spinal anatomy.

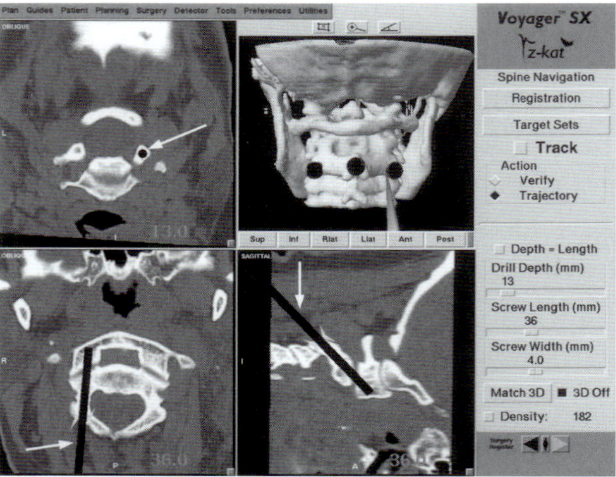

FIGURE 175-9. Screen from image-guided workstation demonstrating screw entry point and trajectory for C1-2 transarticular screw fixation. The left upper quadrant displays the virtual position of a screw tip placed along the selected trajectory (*arrow*). The two lower quadrants display the selected screw trajectory in the sagittal plane (*right lower quadrant*) and in a plane that is perpendicular to the long axis of the navigational probe (*left lower quadrant*). This latter view represents an oblique plane that is midway between a coronal and an axial plane. The length of the trajectory line is set at 36 mm, and its diameter set to 4 mm. The right upper quadrant shows a surface-rendered image of the cervical anatomy.

At each level to be instrumented, the surgeon identifies standard bony landmarks used for selection of a screw's entry point and trajectory. The navigational probe is placed through a drill guide onto the selected entry point. The navigational images are generated, and the surgeon can then make subtle modifications to the selected entry point and trajectory as needed by simply changing the angle or location of the drill guide-probe assembly. When the appropriate entry point and trajectory have been determined, the navigational probe is removed from the drill guide and a 3-mm pilot hole is drilled along the selected trajectory. The process is then repeated for the contralateral side. Each level to be instrumented undergoes a separate registration process. This segmental registration eliminates the potential error that can occur with changes of vertebral body position between the preoperative scanned position and the intraoperative position. Because each vertebra is a rigid body, the spatial relationship of registration points at a single vertebral level to the pedicles of the same vertebrae remains unchanged regardless of changes in patient positioning.

At any point during the orientation procedure, the accuracy of the system can be tested by placing the probe on a known bony landmark and confirming its location on the workstation screen. If there is any discrepancy between the position of the probe and the corresponding position of the cursor on the workstation screen, the registration process can easily be repeated.

When applied to screw fixation of the spinal column, IGSN reduces or eliminates the need for intraoperative imaging.[22,23,28-30] It can facilitate the optimal placement of screws within the spinal column. However, unlike intraoperative fluoroscopy, IGSN does not provide true real-time imaging. It does not show changes in the spinal anatomy as they occur. The system functions as a confirmation tool to assist the surgeon in identifying the pedicle and relating its position and orientation to the exposed spinal anatomy. It is an alternative method to the more conventional means of interpreting 2D images of the spine, relating them to the surgeon's knowledge of the pertinent anatomy, and estimating the location of the pedicle. It is not intended to function as a substitute for an understanding of the appropriate spinal anatomy and the indications and techniques for insertion of pedicle screws.

Applications of this technology to spine surgery have proven IGSN to be a practical and extremely useful alternative and adjunct to conventional intraoperative imaging. It has been used routinely for pedicle screw fixation in the lumbosacral as well as the thoracic spine. It is very useful for placing transarticular screws at the C1-2 level (Fig. 175-9) and for providing optimal orientation to spinal anatomy during transoral surgery and during ventral thoracolumbar surgery.[22,23,28-30] Additionally, it serves as a highly effective image manipulation system allowing the surgeon to scroll through CT images in any selected plane prior to and during surgery. This feature allows the surgeon to better conceptualize the complex 3D anatomy of the spinal column than is possible by the standard method of viewing multiple 2D image sheets.

Fluoroscopic Navigation

Fluoroscopic navigation is the combination of standard fluoroscopy with image-guided navigational technology. It was developed to address the difficulties of some earlier image-guided systems that typically took much longer to use than standard fluoroscopy.[31] Although standard fluoroscopy is employed with this technique, the amount of fluoroscopic time is significantly reduced.

With the patient in position prior to surgery, an AP and lateral fluoroscopic view of the pertinent spinal anatomy

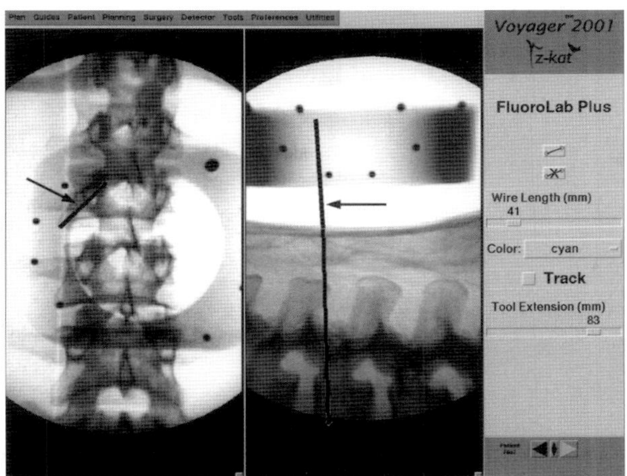

FIGURE 175-10. Screen from fluoroscopic workstation demonstrating selected trajectory through the L2 pedicle in the coronal (*arrow, left panel*) and sagittal (*arrow, right panel*) planes. An image in the axial plane is not available with fluoroscopic navigation.

is obtained. This is done with a customized reference frame attached to the C-arm. The frame serves to superimpose a specific reference grid on the two images obtained. The navigational workstation can then take the two images with the superimposed grid and relate the spatial position of the imaged anatomy to a navigational probe. As the navigational probe is placed on the patient's anatomy, a corresponding trajectory line and cursor can then be superimposed on the lateral and AP images, respectively (Fig. 175-10).

Despite the advantages of fluoroscopic navigation, it still presents some of the same difficulties experienced with standard fluoroscopy. Although the radiation dosage to the patient and surgical team is reduced, it is not eliminated. Positioning difficulties are the same in the upper thoracic region. Both the upper thoracic region as well as the lumbosacral region in obese individuals can be difficult to adequately visualize with fluoroscopic imaging.

The primary disadvantage of fluoroscopic navigation compared with CT-based navigation is the limitation of the image plane. As with conventional fluoroscopy, fluoroscopic navigation provides the surgeon with only AP and lateral planar images. Unlike CT-based navigation, it does not provide an axial image, which, in most spinal screw fixation procedures, is the critical plane for identifying intrusion into the spinal canal by a medially displaced screw.

A variation of conventional fluoroscopy, isocentric fluoroscopy, offers some improvements to the limitations of fluoroscopic navigation. This device acquires images intraoperatively by rotating the C-arm in a 180-degree arc around the patient. As with conventional CT imaging, the acquired images can then be reconstructed into multiplanar images, including images in the axial plane. Although the images are not of the same quality as standard CT scans, they are sufficient for navigational purposes. Image acquisition can also be repeated during surgery if needed to assess the adequacy of decompression or screw positioning.

The most recent advancement in intraoperative imaging involves the use of flat panel detector technology to improve intraoperative CT image acquisition and quality. A flat panel detector can be mounted onto a mobile imaging unit similar to a conventional C-arm fluoroscope. While this unit can be used to acquire standard anteroposterior and lateral images, its C-arm configuration can be "closed" to completely encircle the patient. This allows the flat panel detector to be swept in a 360-degree arc around the patient, thereby significantly improving the acquired image quality. The reformatted images are similar in quality to conventional CT imaging and superior to isocentric C-arm imaging. This ability to acquire high-quality planar images in addition to reformatted CT images makes this technology ideal for minimally invasive spine surgery. It is also easily adaptable to IGSN technology.

Summary

Intraoperative imaging of the spinal column is an important aspect of spine surgery. Although the primary role of intraoperative imaging is to facilitate correct spinal localization, recent technologic advancements in imaging and image processing allow for a greater degree of orientation to the unexposed spinal anatomy. The appropriate use and interpretation of intraoperative imaging enhance the accuracy, precision, and safety of spine surgery.

KEY REFERENCES

Brunberg JA, Gabrielsen T, Rubin J, et al: Diagnostic imaging technology. In Crockard H, Hayward R, Hoff JT, editors: *Neurosurgery: the scientific basis of clinical practice*, ed 2, Boston, 1992, Blackwell Scientific, pp 758–786.

Chandler WF, Knake JE, McGillicuddy JE, et al: Intraoperative use of real-time ultrasonography in neurosurgery. *J Neurosurg* 57:157–163, 1982.

Foley KT, Simon DA, Rampersaud YR: Virtual fluoroscopy: computer-assisted fluoroscopic navigation. *Spine (Phila Pa 1976)* 26(4):347–351, 2001.

Kalfas IH: Image-guided spinal navigation: principles and clinical applications. In Ozgur B, Benzel E, Garfin S, editors: *Minimally invasive approaches to the spine*, St Louis, 2009, Springer, pp 7–22.

Murphy MA, McKenzie RL, Kormos DW, Kalfas IH: Frameless stereotaxis for the insertion of lumbar pedicle screws: a technical note. *J Clin Neurosci* 1(4):257–260, 1994.

Rampersaud YR, Foley KT, Shen AC, et al: Radiation exposure to the spine surgeon during fluoroscopically assisted pedicle screw insertion. *Spine (Phila Pa 1976)* 25:2637–2645, 2000.

REFERENCES

The complete reference list is available online at expertconsult.com.

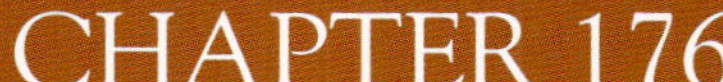

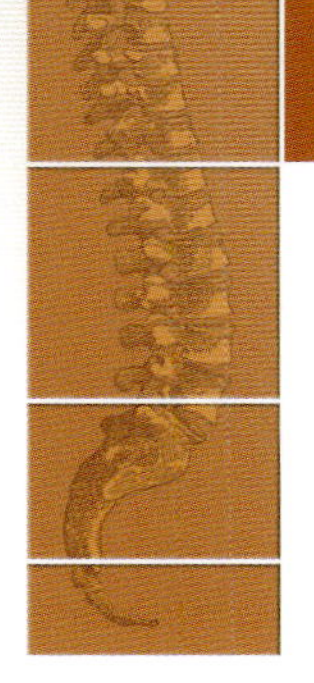

CHAPTER 176

Stereotactic Radiosurgery for the Treatment of Spinal Metastases

John H. Shin | Lilyana Angelov

Metastatic tumors are the most common tumors affecting the spinal column and are the cause of significant pain and disability in cancer patients. The management of symptomatic spinal metastases presents unique challenges to surgeons. A number of considerations specific to the underlying tumor histology, extent of disease, and the patient's functional status and response to systemic therapy often affect the role, timing, and effectiveness of any surgical intervention. As surgical techniques have evolved, attention has shifted toward minimizing the morbidity associated with treating patients in whom limited nutrition and functional reserve affect their overall survival. As such, stereotactic spinal radiosurgery (SRS) has emerged as a powerful adjunct to surgery as well as a standalone treatment option for patients with metastatic disease.

Spinal metastases are estimated to be 20 times more common than primary spine tumors affecting the spine.[1] They are reported in as many as 50% of cancer patients and can result in devastating sequelae in 5% to 14%.[2-4] Patients with spinal metastases often present with disabling pain, as well as neurologic deficits, as a result of epidural spinal cord compression. Whereas the surgical goal for primary spine tumors such as chordoma and chondrosarcoma is en bloc resection for potential cure, the role of surgery in spinal metastases is generally palliative.[3,5] With this in mind, treatment decisions for spinal metastases are made with the intent of resuming systemic therapy as soon as possible for overall disease control or improving quality of life in the final stages of disease.

In North America, over 200,000 new cases of spinal metastases are diagnosed each year, with 20,000 clinical cases of spinal cord compression.[6-8] This number is expected to rise as patients live longer with improved response to systemic therapy. These patients have a median overall survival of 7 months, with a range of 3 to 16 months.[9-11] Both early detection and appropriate intervention are essential to minimize the sequelae of spinal metastases and maximize patient function and quality of life.[12]

The principle treatment modalities for solid tumor spinal metastases are surgery and radiation.[3,4,13-17] These treatments are generally considered palliative in nature. Typically, most patients have concurrent systemic visceral and/or bone disease at presentation with spinal metastases. Even in the presence of solitary spinal lesions, it is unclear when systemic metastases will develop, providing reason for caution when considering "curative resections" for solitary spinal metastasis.[18-20] In terms of other therapeutic options, with few exceptions (e.g., multiple myeloma, lymphoma, breast, and prostate carcinoma), chemotherapy, hormonal therapy, and immunotherapy play a limited role in the treatment of metastatic spine tumors.

With the development of SRS in the past decade, a novel, noninvasive, and very effective addition to the treatment options for patients with metastatic spine tumors has become available. Herein, the indications, limitations, and application of SRS to clinical practice are discussed after a brief overview of the role of surgery and conventional external-beam radiation therapy in the management of spinal metastases.

Characterization of Pain

Metastatic involvement of the spine can occur anywhere along its axis. These tumors, however, most frequently involve the thoracic spine (70%), followed by the lumbar spine (20%) and cervical spine (10%).[5,21] Pain is the most common symptom and can be characterized as either oncologic or mechanical, or a combination of both.[19] It is essential to determine which type of pain patients are experiencing as this plays a major role in determining the most effective treatment. Pain that is oncologic or biologic in nature is described as dull, constant, and responsive to steroids. It is often worse at night and in the morning but typically does not worsen during the day with activity. As such, patients often complain of pain during sleep. The diurnal variation is thought to be related to the variable secretion of endogenous steroids, which is why this type of pain is responsive to oral steroid administration in the early stages.[19] Though the pathophysiology is uncertain, it is thought to be related to inflammation of tumor within the vertebral body and stretching of the periosteum with tumor growth.

Mechanical pain is associated with activity and worsens with movement.[22] In the cervical spine, neck pain that worsens with flexion, extension, and rotation is common and is related to progressive bony destruction. Pain of this type is often suggestive of underlying instability, deformity, or fracture. Rotational pain is suggestive of atlantoaxial instability, whereas pain with flexion and extension is indicative of subaxial pathology. In the thoracic spine, pain is often worse with extension as patients attempt to lie on their back during sleep. Mechanical pain in the lumbar spine is also associated with flexion, extension, and axial loading. Painful radiculopathies may occur as a result of loss of vertebral height and neuroforaminal compression of exiting nerve roots due to either tumor or loss of height with axial loading.

Pain, whether oncologic or mechanical, may be severe enough to make ambulation impossible. Though these patients may have preserved strength in their legs and appear comfortable while supine or on their side, pain may make any movement unbearable. Though a full discussion of the numerous treatment options available for metastatic disease is beyond the scope of this chapter, a number of treatments, including vertebral cement augmentation, surgery, radiation therapy, or SRS, or a combination of these, may play a role in the multimodality treatment of these patients.[12] Each patient requires a specifically tailored treatment plan based on clinical and radiographic findings.

Role of Surgery

To fully appreciate the role of SRS in the management of metastatic spine tumors, an understanding of the current role of surgery for metastatic spine disease is required. In 2005, Patchell et al.[4] published a prospective randomized trial comparing surgery and conventional external-beam radiation therapy to radiation therapy alone for high-grade spinal cord compression. This study showed that surgery followed by conventional radiation resulted in significant advantages in terms of overall maintenance and recovery of ambulation, continence, narcotic requirements, and survival.

Patients who did not undergo surgery but had radiation upfront had worse outcomes overall than did the surgical group. Fifty-seven percent of ambulatory patients in the radiation arm maintained ambulation for only 13 days compared with 122 days in the surgical arm.[4] Nonambulatory patients in the radiation group recovered ambulation in 19% (3/16); however, these patients all recovered ambulation only after crossing over to the surgical arm.[4] Essentially no patient recovered ambulation without surgery due to the radiation insensitivity of solid tumor malignancies. Although the study demonstrated the superiority of surgery and conventional radiation therapy to radiation alone in terms of neurologic function, it did not address the durability of tumor control given the relatively short survival of the patients studied.

Despite the study's limitations, the current recommendation for optimal functional outcomes in patients with high-grade spinal cord compression resulting from solid tumor malignancies or in situations where gross spinal instability exists, is that surgery should be the first-line treatment when possible.[4,18]

Limitations of Conventional External-Beam Radiation Therapy

Many patients with spinal metastases may have significant medical comorbidities that preclude aggressive surgical treatment when otherwise indicated. For this reason, radiation continues to be the mainstay of treatment for many of these patients. The historical benefits of conventional radiation therapy for treating spinal metastases have been demonstrated in numerous retrospective studies showing improvement or maintenance of neurologic function.[11,13-16] Although the Patchell study demonstrated the superiority of surgery, radiation is essential for achieving postoperative local tumor control.[23] In a recent review of the literature, Gerszten et al.[23] found that the ambulatory rate after conventional radiation was 60% to 80%, pain control was achieved in 50% to 70%, and local tumor control was achieved in 20% to 89% of patients. However, though conventional radiation (usually 30 Gy, in 3 Gy/fraction) provides durable control for the hematologic malignancies and breast carcinoma, the majority of solid tumors demonstrate radioresistance or nondurable long-term tumor control when it is used as either a primary or a postoperative treatment.[24] In addition, because treatment plans with conventional radiation often include a margin of one healthy vertebral body above and below the area of concern, this results in a large volume of normal tissue being irradiated.[8,25]

The variable responsiveness of spinal metastases to radiation was originally reported in a series by Greenberg et al.,[26] comparing outcomes of surgery and radiation to radiation alone. Though the surgical approach in this series was mainly laminectomy, thus rendering the surgical results less applicable today with the facile use of advanced decompression and instrumentation techniques, the authors demonstrated marked differences in the response to radiation based on tumor histology. Patients with breast carcinoma and hematologic malignancies showed improved outcomes compared with those with radioresistant tumors such as renal and lung carcinomas.

Maranzano and Latini[16] also demonstrated significant differences in the sensitivity of various tumor types to conventional radiation when used as initial treatment. In a study of 275 patients, those with radioresistant tumors such as non–small-cell lung, bladder, and renal cell carcinoma demonstrated significantly less recovery than those with typically radiosensitive tumors, such as breast and hematologic malignancies. Patients with gross instability were excluded from the study. Overall, 98% of patients maintained ambulation but only 60% recovered. Of those who regained ambulation, 70% had radiosensitive tumors. For example, breast carcinoma demonstrated an 80% response rate compared with hepatocellular carcinoma with a 20% response rate. Furthermore, the durability of the response was 10 to 16 months for radiosensitive tumors compared with 1 to 3 months in radioresistant tumors. A number of other studies have also demonstrated this variable response based on tumor histology.[27-29]

Limited surgical studies have evaluated the utility of conventional radiation as a postoperative adjuvant. Klekamp and Samii[30] reported on 101 surgeries, of which 91% were aggressive subtotal or complete resections. All patients underwent postoperative radiation therapy. Local recurrences were 57.9% at 6 months, 69.3% at 1 year, and 96% at 4 years. The primary factor predictive of recurrence was tumor histology.

Although surgery and conventional radiation therapy are the current mainstays of treatment for spinal metastases, the major drawback to this approach is the relatively low radiation tolerance of the spinal cord.[31-33] This is particularly relevant in cases of progression or recurrence of metastatic disease following standard radiation therapy. Further conventional radiation at recurrence is typically not an option, and patients who undergo surgery after having previously had radiation are known to do poorly and have increased risk of wound complications and worse functional outcomes.[23,33-35]

Issues related to tumor radiosensitivity and the need for higher dosing to achieve effective and durable tumor control as well as limited spinal cord radiation tolerance has fueled the development of advanced radiation delivery systems such as SRS to achieve conformal high-dose radiation delivery and durable tumor control.[8,23,25,36,37]

Stereotactic Radiosurgery

The failure of conventional radiation to achieve long-standing tumor control for radioresistant tumors has limited its modern day application. Though earlier studies have demonstrated success with pain reduction, local disease control, and neurologic improvement in select tumor types, these results do not apply across all histologies.[2,23,27,38] As mentioned earlier, one of the main limitations to achieving local tumor control with conventional radiation therapy is the high dose required. However, the ability to deliver this dose is limited due to the adjacent spinal cord, where standard radiation tolerance is considered to be 45 to 50 Gy.[31] Though clinical studies continue to improve our understanding of spinal cord tolerance to radiation, the therapeutic index of radiotherapy limits the radiation dose near the spinal cord to such an extent that tumor control is compromised.[33,34]

SRS has emerged as an advanced image-guided technology, allowing for more targeted and higher radiation dosing to tumors adjacent to organs at risk (OAR) such as the spinal cord. With technological advances in image guidance and radiation delivery platforms, it is now possible to deliver SRS in a highly conformal manner with a steep dose fall-off gradient either as a single fraction or as a hypofractionated regimen (two to five fractions).[8,39-44] Such a gradient allows for delivering high doses of radiation within millimeters of vital OAR such as the spinal cord, kidney, and esophagus. This enables the very focused delivery of a potentially cytotoxic tumoral dose that can spare nearby normal tissue.

SRS is increasingly being applied to primary malignant and benign spine tumors; however, its application to spinal metastases represents the largest experience to date.[36,42,45,46] The increased application of SRS is further redefining the term *radioresistant* as tumors traditionally regarded as radioresistant, such as renal cell carcinoma and melanoma, have demonstrated marked responses with durable tumor control following SRS.[37] These improved tumor control rates are seen whether used as stand-alone therapy or as a postoperative adjuvant.[37,47,48]

The emergence and effectiveness of SRS as an instrument to achieve durable local control has also fueled the debate regarding the optimal management strategy for solitary metastatic lesions to the spine, which by some investigators have been considered ideal candidates for en bloc resection for potential cure.[17,49,50]

Indications and Treatment Planning

The indications for treatment with SRS are not rigidly defined in the literature and are currently evolving based on the experience of several high-volume centers.[25,37,43] The most common indication for spine radiosurgery is pain, with 70% to 90% of all patients presenting with severe oncologic pain referable to a corresponding lesion involving one to three levels on imaging. Other indications include upfront treatment for radioresistant histologies, treatment after surgery for residual tumor, impending spinal cord compression, and local disease progression either during observation or after other treatment modalities such as surgery, radiation, and chemotherapy have failed.

In a prospective series evaluating pain and quality of life in 154 cases of spinal metastases treated at the Cleveland Clinic, pain scores improved over baseline in 77% of patients ($P < .001$) as early as week 1 after treatment. At 12 months after treatment, 89% of patients had continued pain improvement ($P < .008$) over baseline, indicating that early and durable pain relief is achievable with SRS (Angelov L, Cleveland Clinic, unpublished data). In this way, whether applied in the short term preterminal palliative setting or in patients with a longer prognosis, there is an overall meaningful enhancement of the patient's quality of life with SRS.

Patients who are unsuitable candidates for treatment are those with evidence of diffuse spinal metastases, spinal instability, progressive deformity due to pathologic fracture, and extensive epidural spinal cord compression.

The overall workflow is divided into four general components: (1) target identification, (2) treatment planning, (3) patient immobilization and isocenter verification, and (4) dose delivery. The treatment planning and delivery are typically coordinated in a multidisciplinary fashion among neurosurgeons, radiation oncologists, and radiation physicists. Once treatment volumes have been identified, treatment doses and beam delivery are based on inverse treatment planning. This planning takes into account the therapeutic dose to the tumor, as well as constraints of normal tissue tolerance.

The prescribed dose normally takes into account the point maximum dose and volume of spinal cord being irradiated as well as previous radiation exposure to normal tissue. However, there are currently no guidelines for optimal dose and dose constraints. Common dose regimens range from 14 to 24 Gy in a single fraction, or hypofractionated regimens such as 5 Gy in six fractions or 9 Gy in three fractions.[25,36,38,40,44,51]

Spine Radiosurgery as Monotherapy

The utilization of SRS as monotherapy has several advantages over conventional radiation therapy. With the conformal nature of dose delivery with SRS, vertebral levels adjacent to the treated target are spared from ionizing radiation. This limits the deleterious effect of radiation on whatever viable bone marrow remains. This is particularly important for patients whose hematologic cell counts often decrease as a result of systemic chemotherapy. SRS also allows patients to resume systemic treatments quickly as radiation is usually given in one fraction versus multiple fractions for conventional radiation therapy.[12]

In one of the largest series to date, Gerszten et al.[37] reported on 500 tumors of various histologies treated with high-dose single-fraction radiation at a median dose of 20 Gy (range 12.5–25 Gy) throughout the spine. Pain and radiographic tumor control were achieved in 86% and 90% of cases, respectively. Radiographic tumor control differed based on primary pathology, with breast and lung carcinomas showing 100% radiographic tumor control, compared with renal cell tumors (87%) and melanoma (75%).

The role of SRS is currently being evaluated in a prospective randomized trial by the Radiation Therapy Oncology Group (RTOG, protocol 0631) for patients with significant pain and no history of surgery or radiation. The goal of the trial is to compare pain response after delivery of 16 Gy in a single radiosurgical fraction to delivery of 8 Gy in a single fraction with conventional radiation. Though this trial seeks to validate the effectiveness of SRS for pain palliation, it does not address the role of SRS for postoperative patients or those with previously irradiated spinal metastases.

SRS allows for the delivery of tumoricidal radiation doses to tumors historically radioresistant to conventional radiation. This response appears to be histology independent. For instance, renal cell carcinoma has traditionally been considered resistant to conventional radiation therapy. Gerszten et al.[46] reported 60 cases of renal cell carcinoma treated with single-fraction SRS. The majority (48/60) had progressed despite previous conventional radiation. Treatment doses ranged from 14 to 21 Gy with a mean maximum tumoral dose of 20 Gy, and the median follow-up was 37 months. Pain improved in 34/38 (89%) of patients who presented with oncologic pain, and tumor control was achieved in 7/8 patients who presented with tumor progression. Only 6/60 patients (10%) required surgery for progressive neurologic symptoms after SRS. Despite the high number of reirradiated patients undergoing single-fraction SRS for salvage, no radiation myelopathy or other toxicity was seen in the follow-up period.

Yamada et al.[43] reported 101 cases treated with single-fraction SRS predominantly to radioresistant histologies, with the exception of six breast cancer patients. No patient had prior radiation or surgery to the treated area. The treatment paradigm was a dose escalation of 18 to 24 Gy, with the maximum dose to the spinal cord set to 14 Gy. At a median follow-up of 16 months, the overall radiographic control rates were 90%. Seven failures occurred at a median time of 9 months. A statistically significant dose response was demonstrated at 24 Gy compared with 18 Gy. Yamada reanalyzed the data in 248 patients receiving single-fraction radiation, and this dose response difference was maintained at 5-year follow-up. Toxicity was limited to grade 1 and 2 esophageal and skin cancers. No patient experienced myelopathy or functional radiculopathy.

A representative case of a patient with radioresistant histology (renal cell carcinoma) from our own center is illustrated in Figure 176-1. As illustrated in this case, excellent pain control and control of tumor growth by SRS can ensure acceptable quality of life and functional performance in patients with metastases and would avoid the unnecessary morbidity and risk associated with extensive spinal surgery. SRS also allows patients to return home the same day and avoid lengthy hospitalizations.

Radiosurgery and Surgery

The decision to use SRS as part of a multimodality treatment plan needs to be tailored to the individual patient and take into consideration all of the previously discussed factors. It should be emphasized that SRS is not necessarily an alternative to surgery but is a component of a multifaceted treatment plan that may or may not include surgery at some point. Though the merits of surgery for high-grade epidural spinal cord compression and spinal instability followed by conventional radiation therapy are supported by the Patchell et al.[4] study, the role of SRS as a postoperative adjunct continues to be debated and explored. It is clear that surgery cannot provide durable local tumor control and that postoperative radiation is essential for this purpose.[24] Though SRS has been shown to achieve high rates of local tumor control for radioresistant pathologies, no studies to date have compared SRS versus conventional radiotherapy as a planned postoperative adjunct.

The current state of the literature is limited to three retrospective series, each with small patient numbers, limited clinical follow-up, varying treatment algorithms, and no comparative control group. Two of these report on SRS after surgery, and the third focuses on SRS after kyphoplasty.[47,48,52]

Due to the poor local control rates of conventional radiation therapy for classically radioresistant tumors such as renal cell carcinoma and melanoma, the application of SRS as a postoperative adjunct has been advocated. It is not known if local control is better than conventional radiation in the postoperative setting, given the lack of randomized data comparing the two. Local control data based on imaging studies are also not typically reported for palliative conventional radiation therapy used to treat spinal metastases. Furthermore, it is unclear if postoperative SRS yields superior, inferior, or equivalent local control to postoperative conventional radiation therapy for specific histology due to the lack of comparative data.

One challenge to this treatment paradigm is the difficulty in delineating and identifying residual tumor and the spinal cord due to imaging artifact from spine hardware.[24,53] Particularly for cases in which vertebral column reconstruction has been performed using titanium cages following corpectomy, the proximity of the cage to the spinal cord often precludes appreciation of the extent of decompression due to the imaging artifact generated. Despite the use of CT and MRI fusion, this can pose significant challenges to accurately identifying key anatomic structures. For this reason, CT myelography can be used to better visualize the spinal cord in relation to the surgical hardware in these cases.

Rock et al.[48] at the Henry Ford Hospital specifically evaluated the combination of open surgery followed by adjuvant SRS in a series of 18 patients for a wide variety of histopathologies, including metastases, sarcoma, multiple myeloma, and giant-cell tumor. Patients underwent a broad range of surgical interventions for epidural spinal cord compression, including laminectomy and corpectomy with instrumented fusion. SRS with a dose of 6 to 16 Gy prescribed to the 90% isodose line was delivered in a single fraction 2 to 4 weeks after surgery. Ninety-two percent of patients remained neurologically stable or improved, and only one patient became worse due to tumor progression within 1 month of treatment. There were no wound complications following either surgery or SRS. Despite the small number of patients, this is the first study that demonstrated the feasibility and safety of performing SRS postoperatively for spinal metastases.

Moulding et al.[47] subsequently reviewed 21 patients who underwent surgical decompression and instrumentation for high-grade epidural spinal cord compression from metastatic tumor at the Memorial Sloan-Kettering Cancer Center followed by single-fraction SRS dosed between 18 and 24 Gy. The mean time from surgery to SRS was 43.9 days (range, 26–63 days), and none of the patients previously received radiation.

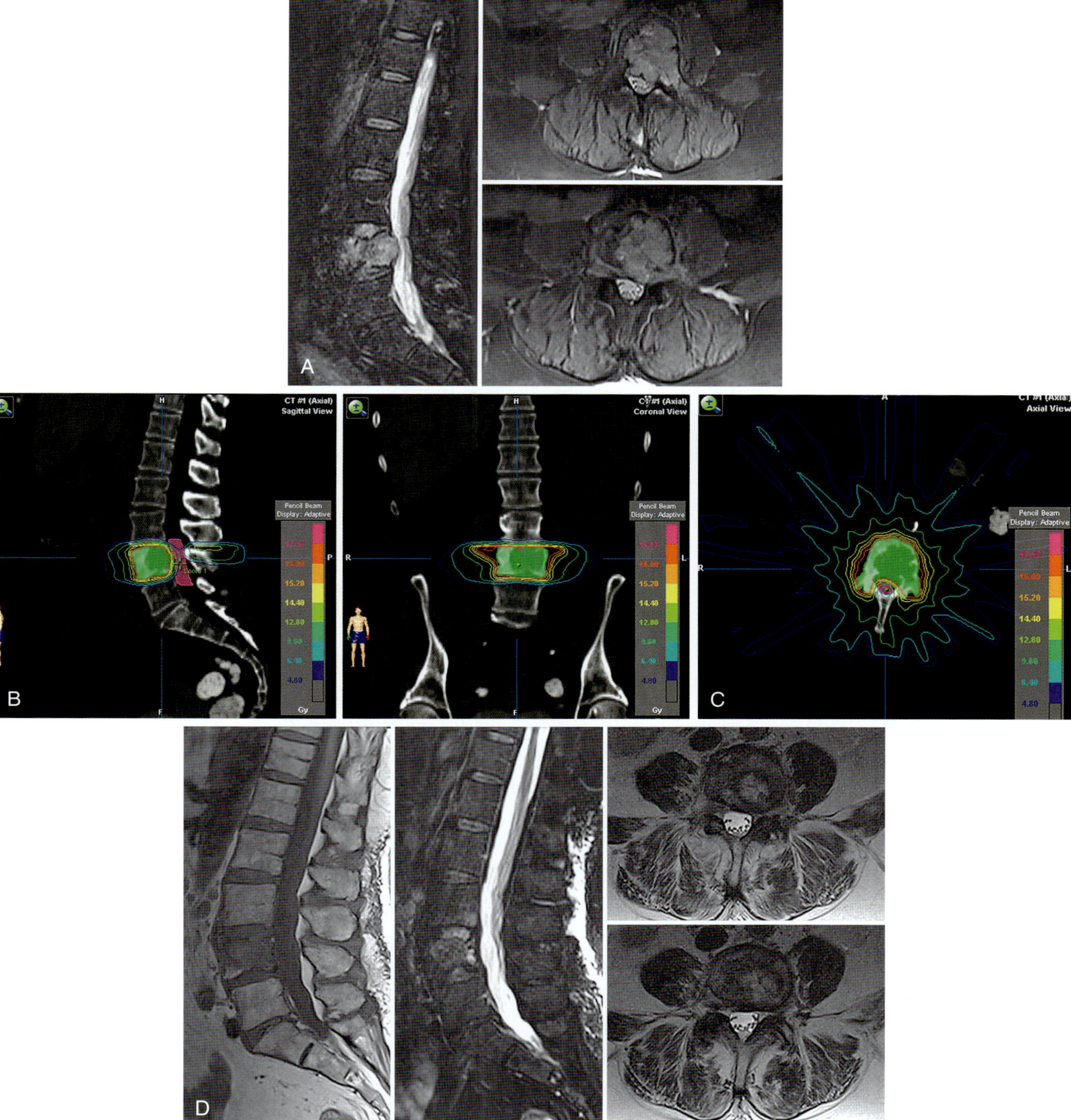

FIGURE 176-1. Sixty-eight-year-old woman with solitary renal cell carcinoma at L4 presented with 6 months of back and left leg pain. **A,** Sagittal (*left*) and axial (*right*) short-tau inversion recovery MRIs demonstrate near-complete replacement of the L4 vertebral body with tumor, minimal epidural disease, and extension of tumor into neural foramen on the left. **B,** Stereotactic radiosurgery (SRS) contours. The thecal sac is outlined in magenta, and the vertebral body in green. **C,** SRS plan: 16 Gy to the 100% local isodose line over one fraction was administered. **D,** MRIs 20 months after treatment show decrease in tumor size and no tumor within the left neural foramen. Pain symptoms resolved within 3 months of treatment with no signs or symptoms of subsequent vertebral body fracture.

Ninety-five percent of the treated tumors were radioresistant pathologies, consisting mostly of melanoma, renal cell carcinoma, and sarcoma. Tumor volume was delineated using CT myelography based on the preoperative tumor volume rather than the postoperative residual tumor.

The overall local control was 81%, with an estimated 1-year failure of 9.5%. The authors found that local control was significantly better in the group receiving 24 Gy (94%) than for those receiving less than 18 Gy (60%). Although there were no wound complications after either surgery or

SRS, acute grade 1 skin reactions were observed in three patients. One patient experienced acute neuritic pain requiring hospitalization, and esophagitis was seen in three patients, one of whom eventually required surgical repair of a fistula.

Another consideration in the postoperative setting is the effect of radiation dose on instrumentation failure and fusion. Though the surgical bed in cancer patients provides a poor substrate for fusion due to previous or planned radiation, poor nutrition, and limited bone quality, the structural integrity of any instrumented construct is vital for continued pain palliation as patients undergo systemic therapies until death. In a study by Harel et al.,[53] 43% of patients treated with conventional radiation had evidence of instrumentation failure compared with 0% in the SRS group. Furthermore, fusion rates were 50% in the SRS group versus 17% in the conventional radiation group. Data such as these indicate that like other OARs, the surgical site, in particular the bone-screw interface, may also be subject to a dose-related effect.

Overall, details specific to the definition of tumor treatment volume, total dose, and fractionation vary significantly among postoperative series. There are no dedicated phase I dose-escalation studies, nor are there any randomized studies testing various SRS dose schemes. Therefore, the optimal practice is unknown, making the widespread application of these principles difficult. Yamada et al.[43] reported their retrospective experience in which the dose was escalated over time. Based on their institutional experience, greater rates of local control were observed with a higher single-fraction dose. This has led to their current practice of prescribing 24 Gy in a single fraction. In the three postoperative studies totaling 65 tumors treated with single-fraction SRS with doses between 14 and 24 Gy, local control rates of 81% to 94% were reported without major complications. An example of how SRS is applied in the postoperative setting is illustrated in Figure 176-2.

Concept of "Separation Surgery"

The application of SRS following surgery for spinal metastases is emerging as a new treatment paradigm that challenges previous concepts of palliative postoperative radiation.[12] It is also changing how surgery is being approached for these patients. Though the tenets of decompression and stabilization have not changed, the extent of decompression and reconstruction of the vertebral column is now being redefined as the focus has shifted toward performing less morbid surgeries for metastatic disease. Though aggressive surgical strategies including en bloc resections are often utilized to manage primary spinal tumors where there is a chance for cure, surgery for spinal metastases is palliative and directed toward minimizing morbidity and improving function.

Whereas extensive and aggressive vertebrectomies were being performed in the past for fear of local tumor recurrence, particularly with radioresistant tumors, surgery now often entails decompression of epidural tumor away from the dura, sufficient tumor debulking, and stabilization in order to provide an adequate window for SRS. By providing several millimeters of space between the dura and metastatic tumor, sufficient room for dose fall-off is provided, allowing for highly precise single-fraction SRS dose administration. At the Cleveland Clinic, this concept of "separation surgery" has been championed as a treatment philosophy by which surgery is performed to sufficiently decompress the spinal cord in order to permit definitive local tumor control by postoperative SRS.

En Bloc Resection versus Radiosurgery

With data showing improved rates of tumor control for radioresistant tumors, SRS has since challenged a shift in the treatment paradigm for solitary renal cell metastases without epidural disease.[9,10,17,18,49,50] Though the role of en bloc resection for solitary metastases has long been debated among surgeons, largely due to questionable long-term survival and local tumor control following these operations, the application of SRS for upfront treatment of these lesions has introduced a less morbid and arguably just as effective (if not more effective) method of treatment for solitary metastatic spinal lesions.

Because there are no accurate predictors of the propensity for systemic metastases to develop despite aggressive local treatment with either en bloc resection or SRS, a strong argument can be made for not operating on these patients because the likelihood of cure is small.[18]

Analysis of local tumor control rates after en bloc resection of solitary renal metastases and after SRS reveals similar results. Although there is a paucity of published outcomes reporting local control following en bloc resection, analysis of 40 patients reported in the literature reveals a 7.5% recurrence rate at a median follow-up of 16 months.[18] The reported symptomatic and radiographic tumor control failures after SRS range between 6% and 13% with comparable follow-up periods.[18] As en bloc tumor resection and SRS appear to have comparable tumor control rates, the less invasive and less morbid option may be the preferred upfront treatment, with surgery reserved for long-term survivors who progress despite SRS.

Complications Avoidance and Management

Despite being a noninvasive treatment, SRS has a potential for spinal cord, cauda equina, or nerve root injury, just as occurs with conventional radiation therapy. Though the incidence of damage to these neural structures is low in published series, considerable effort is made during contouring and dose planning to take advantage of the steep dose fall-off gradient and minimize radiation injury to the spinal cord.[32,54] Likewise, the dose of radiation given to nearby organs such as the skin, esophagus, kidneys, and bowel must also be taken into consideration. Though the complications of radiation injury to these tissues are not different from the effect of conventional radiotherapy, the acute effect may be more severe because a larger single dose is given during SRS.

Neurologic Complications

The maximum dose constraint for the spinal cord varies in the literature and is reflective of various institutional practices.

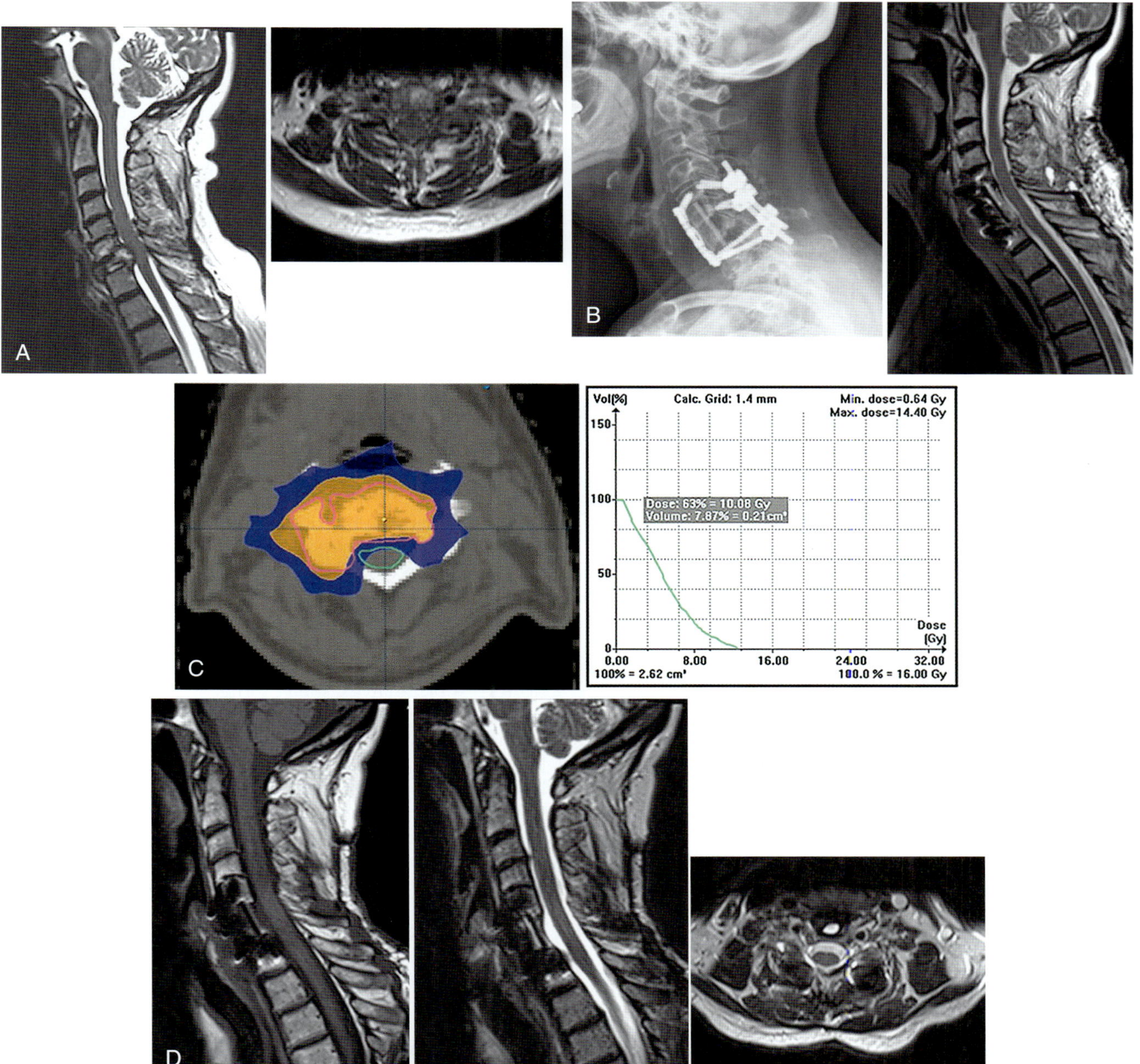

FIGURE 176-2. Sixty-four-year-old woman with large-cell lung adenocarcinoma presented with 3 months of progressively worsening neck and left arm pain. **A,** MRI revealed a pathologic vertebral fracture at C7 with severe spinal cord compression. Sagittal (*left*) and axial (*right*) T2-weighted images show absent cerebrospinal fluid (CSF) dorsal and ventral to the spinal cord. **B,** C6-7 corpectomy followed by dorsal C5-T1 instrumented fusion was performed. Lateral radiograph (*left*) and postoperative MRI (*right*). Sagittal T2-weighted image shows restoration of CSF around the spinal cord and separation of tumor away from the dural surface. **C,** Stereotactic radiosurgery plan: 16 Gy to the 100% local isodose line over one fraction was given 3 weeks after surgery. Dose volume histogram for the spinal cord shows 10 Gy delivered to <10% of the spinal cord volume. **D,** MRI after 2 years. No evidence of local recurrence or instrumentation failure.

Spinal cord constraints are usually set as either a percentage of the spinal cord or a maximum dose to a single voxel on the spinal cord (D_{max}). Ryu et al.[32] defines spinal cord tolerance as a maximum of 10 Gy to 10% of the spinal cord, whereas Yamada[43] reports safely treating to a cord D_{max} of 14 Gy. At the Cleveland Clinic, spinal cord tolerance is set as a maximum of 10 Gy to 10% of the spinal cord.

In the largest published series, Gibbs et al.[54] reported 6 cases of delayed radiation-induced myelopathy after SRS in 1075 patients. Six patients developed myelopathy at a mean of 6.3 months (range, 2–9 months) after SRS. Three tumors were metastatic in the mid- to upper thoracic spine, and the other three were benign cervical lesions. Two of these cases had been previously irradiated 70 and 80 months prior to SRS at doses of 50.4 and 39.6 Gy in 1.8-Gy fractions. Both of these patients also received an antiangiogenic or epidermal growth factor inhibitor–targeted therapy within 2 months of developing myelopathy, which may have had a radiosensitizing effect. Specific dosimetric factors contributing to this complication could not be identified, but all patients received spinal cord equivalent doses greater than 8 Gy, ranging from 8.5 to 29.9 Gy.

Strategies for treatment of radiation-induced myelopathy include corticosteroids, vitamin E, pentoxifylline, hyperbaric oxygen, or gabapentin.[54] Of the six patients in this series, three improved after treatment, two stayed the same, and one progressed to paraplegia. All three patients who showed clinical improvement had complete radiographic resolution of their spinal cord edema on MRI.

Recent human studies have investigated spinal cord tolerance to radiation in the context of conventional radiotherapy, reirradiation, and stereotactic radiosurgery.[33,34] With conventional fractionation of 2 Gy per day, total doses of 50 Gy, 60 Gy, and 69 Gy are associated with a 0.2%, 6%, and 50% rate of myelopathy, respectively.[34] For reirradiation of the spinal cord after previously fractionated treatment, spinal cord tolerance appears to increase by 25% 6 months after initial treatment.[34] With regard to radiosurgery, a maximum cord dose of 13 Gy in a single fraction or 20 Gy in three fractions is associated with a less than 1% risk of myelopathy.[34]

With increased use of SRS, it is anticipated that further reporting of long-term outcomes will provide greater insight into the factors predictive of developing such a potentially devastating and irreversible injury. However, such reporting continues to present a challenge. The limited survivial time for patients with metastatic disease makes toxicity less likely to manifest as radiation-induced damage and it may occur later than the median survival time for these patients.

Organs at Risk

Though other organs are at risk for radiation injury, no significant toxicity has been reported other than grade 1 to 2 skin and esophageal toxicity. The skin may be susceptible to injury in thin patients whose targeted lesions involve the dorsal elements (Fig. 176-3). In previously irradiated patients or patients who recently underwent surgery, a careful examination of the skin or surgical incision is critical prior to treatment planning. Mucositis of the pharynx and esophagus may also occur after treatment of cervical or thoracic lesions. Because these structures are within millimeters of the targeted treatment area, odynophagia, dysphagia, nausea, and even emesis may occur. Most symptoms resolve within days to weeks with appropriate treatment. Renal toxicity must also be considered because careful dosing is important for those patients who have preexisting renal disease or those who have undergone nephrectomy for renal cell cancer or renal transplantation.

In a recent series (Rahmatulla G, Angelov L, Cleveland Clinic, unpublished series), the dosimetry and acute and delayed effects of cervical and thoracic SRS on the larynx, trachea, esophagus, and brachial plexus were evaluated. Clinically, no patient developed any evidence of toxicity such as hoarseness, dysphagia, strictures, esophagitis, or evidence of a brachial plexopathy at a median follow-up time of 9.3 months when treated with a single-fraction dose of 13 to 16 Gy to the cervicothoracic spine.

Vertebral Body Fracture

Another complication observed following SRS is delayed vertebral body fracture. Rose et al.[55] reviewed 62 patients undergoing single-fraction SRS with the planned treatment volume receiving 18 to 24 Gy for solid tumor malignancies at 71 sites and noted a 39% delayed fracture risk of the vertebral body at a median time of 25 months. Patients with prior surgery or radiation therapy were excluded. Multivariate logistic regression analysis showed that CT appearance, lesion location, and percentage of vertebral body involvement by tumor independently predicted fracture progression. Lesions located between T10 and the sacrum were 4.6 times more likely to fracture than were lesions above T10. Lytic lesions were also 6.8 times more likely to fracture than were sclerotic and mixed lesions.

Overall, lytic disease involving more than 40% of the vertebral body and location below T10 led to a high risk of fracture. Other factors such as obesity, dorsal element involvement, bisphosphonate use, and local kyphosis were not associated with increased risk for fracture. The authors suggest that patients at high risk for fracture may benefit from

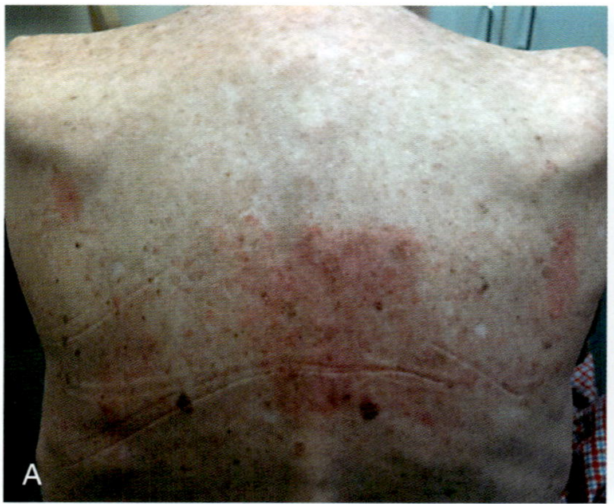

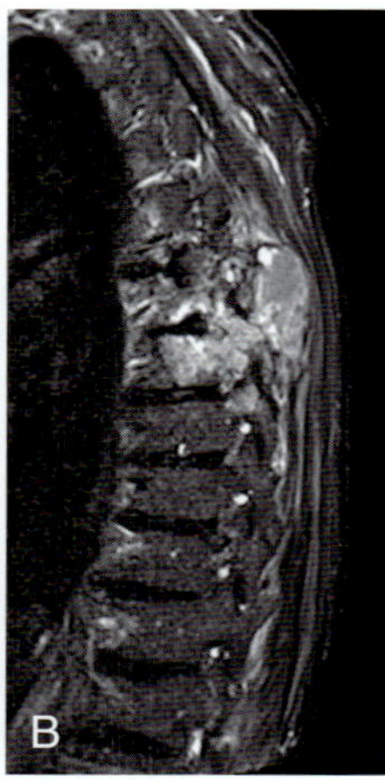

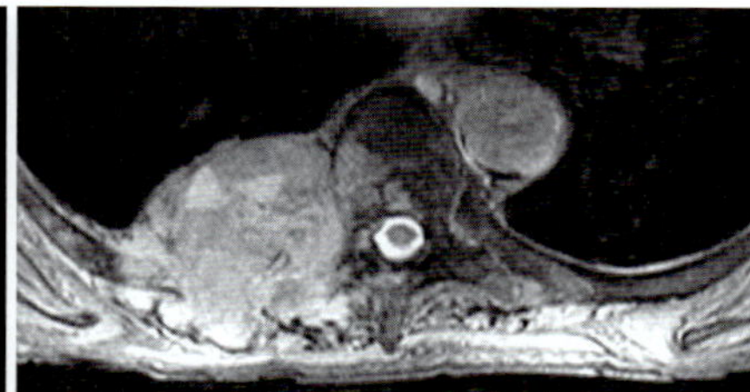

FIGURE 176-3. Skin complications. **A,** An example of a grade 2 skin reaction following stereotactic radiosurgery to the thoracic spine. This 86-year-old patient with metastatic pancreatic cancer received 16 Gy in one fraction to a paraspinal mass at T6 and T7 for palliation of severe back pain. **B,** Sagittal (*left*) and axial (*right*) short-tau inversion recovery MRIs demonstrate a large right side paraspinal mass at T6 and T7. Note the proximity of the dorsal extent of the tumor to the skin in this cachectic patient.

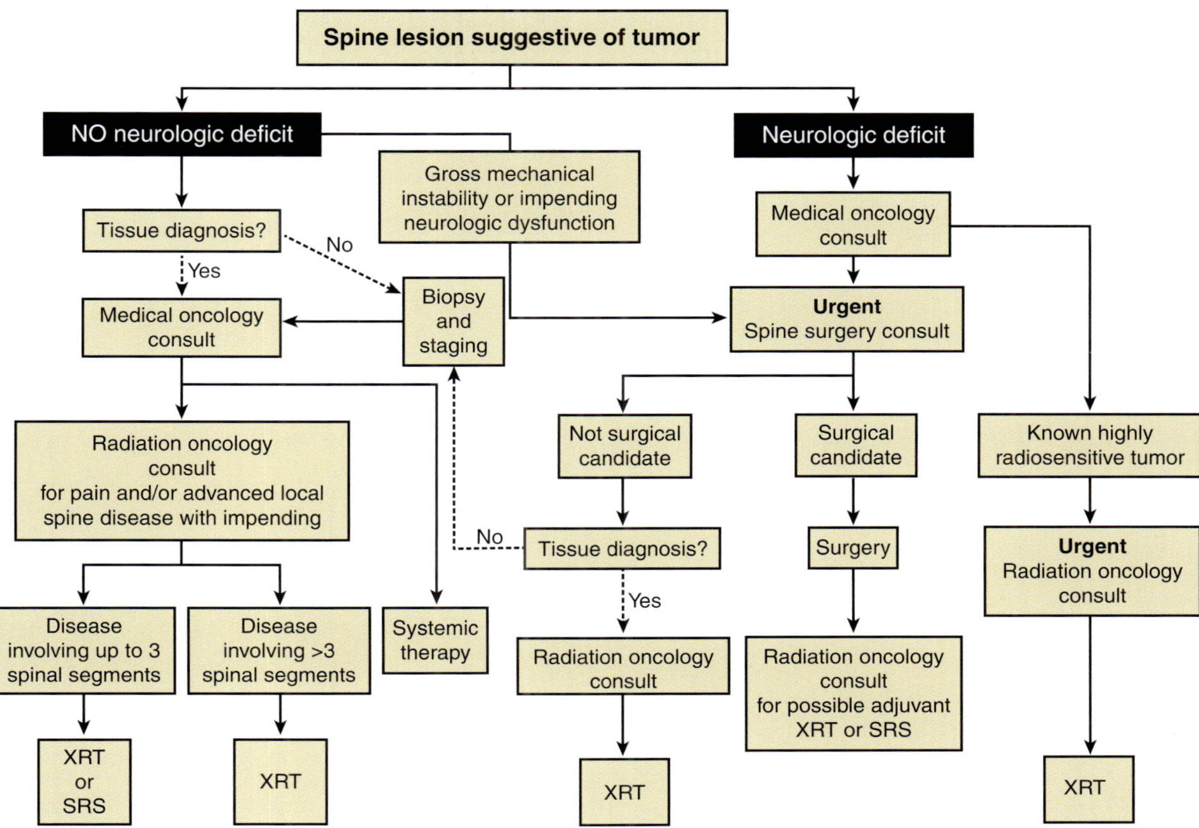

FIGURE 176-4. Proposed treatment algorithm for the management of metastatic spine tumors. The presence or absence of neurologic deficits, confirmation of pathology, and multidisciplinary integration of current adjuvant therapies are essential to treatment of these patients. SRS, stereotactic radiosurgery; XRT, radiotherapy. (Adapted with permission from Harel R, Angelov L: Spine metastases: current treatments and future directions. *Eur J Cancer* 46:2696-2707, 2010.)

prophylactic cement augmentation of the body involved, though it could be argued that augmentation should be performed following SRS only if a symptomatic fracture develops since 39% of patients in this study developed fractures, of which the number that were symptomatic with worsening pain was not provided.[55]

Conclusion

Although SRS is a relatively new treatment modality, it offers a promising and powerful treatment option for managing metastatic spine tumors. The overall effectiveness of SRS for achieving palliation of pain and local tumor control are still being studied; however, evidence from retrospective series suggests that local control rates with SRS are better than those with conventional radiation therapy. Though the toxicity profile of normal tissue tolerance has not been clearly defined, the conformal nature of radiosurgical dose administration theoretically poses less risk to vital nearby organs. This is evident by the low rate of radiation-induced myelopathy and other organ damage in published series.

As the treatment of metastatic spine tumors continues to evolve with the development of new interventions such as SRS, previously published algorithms that have attempted to define which patients would potentially benefit from surgery have become outdated since none of these account for newer treatments such as vertebral augmentation and SRS.[12,18] Despite these antiquated algorithms, patients with epidural compression from radioresistant tumors or spinal instability will continue to require surgery. Because high-grade epidural compression requires that the marginal dose at the spinal cord be reduced, this potentially underdoses the epidural tumor, with resultant continued compression or progression.

Nonetheless, the paradigm for the treatment of metastatic spine tumors has shifted, and it is imperative that further treatment algorithms and management decision schemes for metastatic disease incorporate SRS as an option for either stand-alone or postoperative treatment[12] (Fig. 176-4). With a better understanding of the safety profile and clinical effectiveness of SRS, patient-specific treatment programs can then be tailored with the overall goal of minimizing morbidity, alleviating pain, and improving function and quality of life.

KEY REFERENCES

Bilsky MH, Laufer I, Burch S: Shifting paradigms in the treatment of metastatic spine disease. *Spine (Phila Pa 1976)* 34:S101–S107, 2009.

Gerszten PC, Burton SA, Ozhasoglu C, et al: Radiosurgery for spinal metastases: clinical experience in 500 cases from a single institution. *Spine (Phila Pa 1976)* 32:193–199, 2007.

Gerszten PC, Mendel E, Yamada Y: Radiotherapy and radiosurgery for metastatic spine disease: what are the options, indications, and outcomes? *Spine (Phila Pa 1976)* 34:S78–S92, 2009.

Harel R, Angelov L: Spine metastases: current treatments and future directions. *Eur J Cancer* 46:2696–2707, 2010.

Moulding HD, Elder JB, Lis E, et al. Local disease control after decompressive surgery and adjuvant high-dose single-fraction radiosurgery for spine metastases. *J Neurosurg Spine* 13:87–93, 2010.

Patchell RA, Tibbs PA, Regine WF, et al: Direct decompressive surgical resection in the treatment of spinal cord compression caused by metastatic cancer: a randomised trial. *Lancet* 366:643–648, 2005.

Sahgal A, Bilsky M, Chang EL, et al: Stereotactic body radiotherapy for spinal metastases: current status, with a focus on its application in the postoperative patient. *J Neurosurg Spine* 14:151–166, 2011.

REFERENCES

The complete reference list is available online at expertconsult.com.

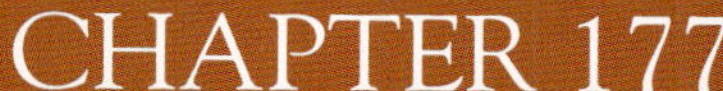

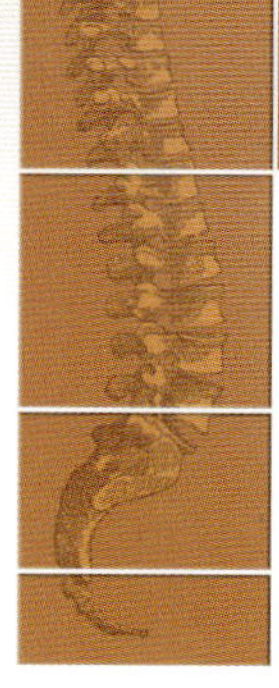

CHAPTER 177

Somatosensory-Evoked Potential for Spine Surgery

Virgilio Matheus | Jorge A. Gonzalez-Martinez | Dileep Nair

Because degenerative spinal conditions and deformities are relatively prevalent, surgical procedures for the spine are common. Furthermore, the evolution and understanding of spinal mechanics and physiology have allowed the introduction of many newer spinal surgical techniques. Nevertheless, a small proportion, less than 0.5%, of patients may develop a persistent neurologic deficit immediately after surgery. Careful surgical techniques, including stabilization of the spine during surgery, have helped reduce this complication somewhat. However, it is apparent that a neurologic injury related to such an intervention can be disabling. For this reason, the monitoring of somatosensory-evoked potentials (SSEPs) from peripheral nerve stimulation (posterior tibial, peroneal, or median nerves) during spinal column or spinal cord surgery is common.[1-31]

The spinal cord and nerve roots are at risk during a variety of surgical procedures performed on the spinal cord and surrounding structures. The risk varies with the underlying disease, as well as the type and location of surgery.[32-35] Patients with intramedullary tumors, syringomyelia, spinal arteriovenous malformation, thoracoabdominal aneurysms, and any other disorder associated with a baseline neurologic deficit are at greatest risk. The frequency of neurologic injury following scoliosis surgery, correction of congenital spinal deformities, and decompression (with and without spinal fusion) is low, but when damage to the spinal cord occurs, the resulting deficits are often severe, permanent, and devastating.[35-37] The detection of significant changes in the monitored-evoked potentials (MEPs) can indicate damage to the motor pathway and may permit appropriate intervention to prevent spinal cord damage.

The "wake-up test" was developed in an attempt to reduce the risk of spinal cord injury in patients undergoing scoliosis surgery. This technique rapidly became the standard against which other monitoring techniques were compared. Although helpful, the wake-up test disrupts the surgical procedure, can be performed only intermittently, and is associated with considerable risks (e.g., extubation, pulmonary embolism). Furthermore, it is not applicable to patients undergoing surgical procedures in which no period of major risk is defined, as in resections of spinal neoplasms.

In the 1970s, SSEP monitoring was developed as an alternative to the wake-up test. SSEP recordings provided the means of monitoring spinal cord function continuously without interfering with surgery or producing additional risk. A large body of data, including clinical experience in thousands of patients, has provided significant information regarding the utility and limitation of SSEP monitoring during spinal surgery, but no prospective controlled trial of SSEP monitoring has ever been published.[1,2,5,7,11,14,15,36,38]

More recently, several studies from different institutes around the world have proven that a single method of potential recording usually carries a high incidence of misdiagnosing an injury. Based on this, the growing tendency has been to establish a multimodal intraoperative monitoring (MIOM) system that usually combines SSEPs with MEPs and sometimes other varieties. The use of MIOM has documented benefits on specificity and sensitivity as well as for clinical experience and outcome measurements during different spinal surgical procedures.[39]

Neuroanatomic and Functional Basis

SSEP monitoring evaluates the integrity of the dorsal column. Consequently, if the dorsal columns are preserved, injury to other important pathways could occur without a change in the SSEP.[16,40,41]

Specifically, SSEPs are used to assess whether the lemniscal somatosensory system is intact. Impulses generated from the median nerve at the wrist (radial aspect) are transmitted through the sensory fibers to the dorsal horn of the cervical spinal cord. Next, impulses follow the dorsal tract (fasciculus cuneatus) to the ipsilateral posterior tract nuclei (nucleus cuneatus) located in the dorsal medulla. Conduction then leaves the medullary nuclei through the medial lemniscus, which, after crossing the midline, terminates in the ventrobasal nucleus of the thalamus. From the thalamus, multiple radiations connect to the primary sensory cortex. When received at the level of the cortex, afferent volleys are processed, both in the somatosensory cortex and in the parietal association fields.

In addition, SSEPs recorded from upper-extremity stimulation do not reflect lower-extremity abnormalities. Posterior tiblial SSEP monitoring must also be recorded if there is concern for damage during surgery to the spinal cord below the midcervical level. Stimulation at the level of the medial malleolus generates afferent volleys that are transmitted by sensory fibers to the dorsal horn at the conus medullaris and then carried by the dorsal tract (fasciculus gracilis) to the dorsal medullary nucleus (nucleus gracilis). Cortical conduction is then achieved via the medial lemniscus and thalamus.

MEP monitoring is typically performed by transcranial electrical stimulation of the scalp. The electrical stimulation is typically a multipulse electrical stimulus applied to the scalp overlying the motor cortex. Motor-evoked responses are recorded by EMG electrodes placed over the limbs. These responses do not require averaging but can result in movement of the patient during stimulation.

Methods of Monitoring

The two basic types of spinal cord monitoring currently used in surgery use noninvasive and invasive techniques.

Noninvasive Techniques

The noninvasive techniques involve the monitoring of potentials generated by spinal, subcortical (brainstem), or cortical pathways from the skin surface or from subdermal needle electrodes. In all the noninvasive studies, peripheral nerves in the upper extremity (median or ulnar nerve) or lower extremity (posterior tiblial or peroneal nerve) are stimulated. Recordings outside the operating field (noninvasive technique) are by far the simplest and can be performed without disturbing the surgeon's attention from the surgical field. Recordings are most commonly made from standard scalp derivations, usually Cz-Fz (International 10-20 System)[42] with leg stimulation, and C3 (C4)-Fz with arm stimulation. Other reference electrodes, such as the ears, are also used. Most of the early studies of surgical monitoring used peripheral stimulation with scalp recording, which generally gives a well-defined, although unstable, response.

The technique of monitoring potentials from a single recording site (i.e., cortical potentials) has some criticisms that must be mentioned. At times technical problems could result in loss of potentials. This result requires that both the technical and professional staff have the expertise to identify significant changes versus technical problems. Another criticism of recording only cortical potentials is that they are very sensitive to the effects of changing levels of anesthesia and decreases in blood pressure as opposed to the subcortical or spinal cord potentials.

Invasive Techniques

A number of methods of recording in the operating field have been developed to facilitate recording closer to the neural tissue.[4,12,17,25,43-45] These methods include subarachnoid, epidural, spinous process, and intraspinous ligament recordings. The spinal cord recording (not cortical potentials) facilitates direct evaluation of segmental changes that occur above and below the operative site. Dinner et al.[4] assessed 70 of 100 scoliotic patients who were monitored with interspinous electrodes and confirmed that the spinal-evoked potentials were both reliable and reproducible, whereas the wires posed little risk to neurologic function. Lüders et al.[17] successfully used spinal-evoked responses during 40 spinal procedures, 32 for scoliosis and Harrington rod placement and 8 for syrinx drainage and resection of tumors and arteriovenous malformations.

Although recordings in the surgical field can yield a much larger response, they are associated with technical problems (including disturbing the surgeon's attention and adding to the risk of infection), with mechanical artifact, and with being limited to those surgical procedures in which the spine is opened to expose the dura. In general, such recordings require considerable technical expertise for satisfactory recordings and require that the surgeon be familiar and cooperative with the procedure. Recordings in the surgical field are most useful for spinal cord surgery (e.g., for tumors or arteriovenous malformations), in which recorded potentials can localize the area of damage or record responses that are too small to detect with other methods.

Spinal cord–evoked potential monitoring, another method of invasive recording, can be achieved by direct, segmental spinal cord stimulation using subdural electrodes. Polyphasic action potentials produced by these subdural electrodes are larger in amplitude and less likely to deteriorate or vary with minimal adjustments in anesthetic concentrations than is the case with those noted during cortical monitoring. Simultaneous ascending and descending signals are generated and can be assessed in shorter periods of time. Recordings are made over 1- to 2-minute intervals with the interspinous ligament or spinous process devices, whereas longer 10- to 230-second intervals are required when extradural or subarachnoid thoracolumbar potentials are followed. Spinal potentials may also be used in conjunction with other monitoring modalities such as the MEP or cortical-evoked responses. Limitations of this technique include intraoperative displacement of monitoring electrodes, which results in unreliable recordings and/or inadvertent neurologic injury.

Monitoring Techniques

SSEPs are recorded from the cortex with only two of the many electrodes composing the cortical array used by the International 10-20 System.[42] One electrode is placed in the midsagittal plane (Cz1), and the second is applied more ventrally in the midline. A third ground is always added (Fz). Placing an additional cervical needle electrode (at C2) helps confirm whether cortical changes reflect true spinal cord changes, as opposed to local cortical variations that may occur in response to alterations in anesthetic administration. Such needle electrodes may also be placed over a lumbar spinous process (L5) to differentiate between similar alterations. SSEP skin and surface electrodes are noninvasive and are applied far away from the operative field, and monitoring may begin before induction and continue through closing.

The large mixed peripheral nerves (median, ulnar, peroneal, or posterior tiblial nerves) receive short 200-msec pulses at rates of 3 to 5 per second. The larger-diameter peripheral sensory A alpha and A beta fast-conducting fibers are stimulated with intensities set at two or three times the motor threshold, sufficient to produce a motor twitch.[46] Two hundred recordings are then averaged and passed through band-pass filters of 30 Hz to 3 kHz to improve signal-to-noise ratio. Alternate stimulation of the right and left sides allows both waveforms to be simultaneously monitored with a split-screen array. This requires 50 seconds (means of 200 recordings) for two extremities and 100 seconds for all four extremities. Findings may be reproduced by repeating stimulation of one or both sides, enabling the surgeon to be alerted to significant changes in any of the four extremities within minutes (Fig. 177-1).

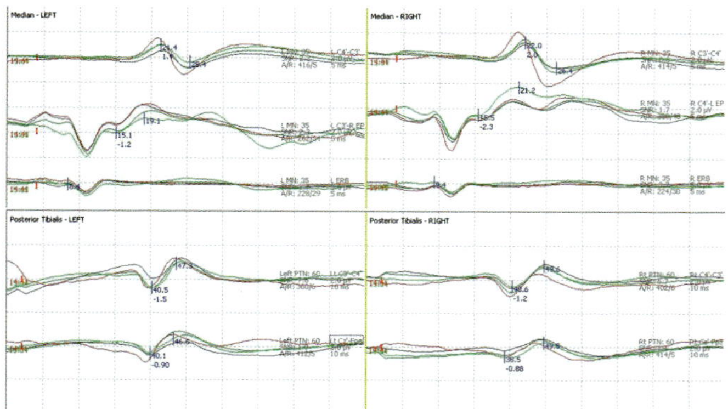

FIGURE 177-1. Example of a somatosensory-evoked potential recording at baseline. The upper boxes show the median nerves recordings; lower boxes show the posterior tiblial nerves recordings.

The most reliable SSEP recordings are produced by electrical stimulation of large mixed nerves in the limbs. Stimulation is applied to distal nerves (e.g., ulnar, median, tiblial) with surface electrodes or to proximal nerves (e.g., sciatic, cauda equina, brachial plexus). Each nerve is stimulated unilaterally in a consecutive fashion so that those pathways carrying information from all potentially affected limbs are monitored. Bilateral simultaneous stimulation may miss a unilateral injury and therefore is performed only when an adequate response cannot be obtained with unilateral stimulation. Stimulation duration and intensity are adjusted (0.2–0.5 msec, 5–90 mA) to produce maximal stimulation of sensory axons. The rate of stimulation is kept under 5 Hz to minimize rate-dependent attenuation of the SSEP, which is accentuated by anesthetics. Rates less than 2 Hz are sometimes required to record cerebral potentials in children and adolescents, especially at deeper levels of anesthesia. Stimulation rates that are even fractions of 60 Hz are avoided to prevent averaging of 60-cycle interference into the recording. The number of stimuli required for averaging varies with the amount of background noise, as well as with the size and reproducibility of the SSEP. In the absence of a preoperative deficit or excessive artifact, 200 to 300 stimuli are usually necessary for recordings made from surface electrodes. The number of stimuli averaged should be kept to a minimum so that the surgeon receives feedback as rapidly as possible.

The type of electrode recording used depends on the location of recording sites and the type of surgery. Typically, needle electrodes are used; they are held in place by staples or taped in place with steri-drape. This allows for rapid placement of electrodes and low impedance during long surgical procedures. Esophageal or nasopharyngeal electrodes are used to record cervical cord potentials outside the surgical field in cervical spine surgery. Needle electrodes inserted between spinous processes or over the laminae of the spine can be used to record spinal cord activity. Needle electrodes placed in the interspinous ligaments can be used within the operative field if the dorsal vertebral elements are left intact. Small cotton-tipped electrodes or platinum electrodes are used to record directly from the surface of the spinal cord or cerebral cortex.

For each of these active electrodes, an appropriate reference must be chosen. Nearby electrodes reduce noise, but distant electrodes enhance signal amplitude. In general, active and reference electrodes should be of the same material to minimize impedance mismatch, which increases noise. Recordings can be made at multiple peripheral and central sites along the sensory pathways. Adherence to this important principle minimizes the incidence of false-positive changes and makes troubleshooting for technical errors more efficient.

Signal amplification and filter settings are similar to those used for diagnostic outpatient SSEP recordings, although at times the sensitivity must be reduced or the band-pass restricted because of the amount of noise in the surgical environment. Amplification of 5 to 10 μV/cm, sweep speed of 2 to 10 msec/cm, low-frequency filters of 30 to 100 Hz, and high-frequency filters of 2000 to 3000 Hz are generally satisfactory. The equipment used for intraoperative SSEP recordings must be versatile and easily tailored to the specific type of procedure being monitored. The ability to record other modalities (e.g., electromyogram [EMG], MEP) concurrently with SSEP may be essential. Preamplifiers need to tolerate high current loads caused by cautery and other sources of electrical interference. Automatic cautery suppression; artifact rejection; and software for digital filtering, trend analysis, data reproduction, and storage are desirable features.

MEPs can be obtained reliably and are useful for monitoring the motor pathway function. They are elicited by either electrical or magnetic stimulation of the cortex or the spinal cord itself. Recordings are obtained as neurogenic potentials in the distal spinal cord or peripheral nerves. They also can be recorded as myogenic potentials from the innervated muscle. Contraindications for MEPs include history of seizures, past surgical skull defects, and/or metal implants in the head.[47] Electrical stimulation also can be applied directly over the cord with distal neurogenic potentials recordings if a surgical decompression has been performed.

Anesthesia

Anesthesia reduces the amplitude and increases the latency of cortical SSEP recordings. This is especially true in the presence of disease and in children and adolescents. Because the reduction of amplitude is directly related to depth of anesthesia, the level of anesthetic agents should be kept as light as possible. Anesthetic effect varies with the agent used, with halogenated anesthetics producing the greatest effects, followed by moderate changes with IV barbiturates and nitrous oxide, and the least with narcotics and benzodiazepines. Etomidate and ketamine have been shown to enhance the amplitude of the cortical SSEP potentials. All volatile anesthetics, as well as nitrous oxide, produce a dose-dependent reduction in MEP signal amplitude. Because the signal amplitudes of MEP recordings are already quite small, the effect of these inhalational agents can limit the practitioner's ability to detect significant changes intraoperatively. These drugs can be used occasionally to record cortical potentials during surgery when responses are absent with standard anesthetics. Alterations in blood pressure can also reduce the amplitude of the evoked response, especially with mean blood pressures lower than 70 mm Hg. Similar effects can be found with hypothermia, which increases latency and decreases conduction velocity.

To further limit perioperative morbidity, a consistent anesthesia protocol should accompany SSEP monitoring. In cervical spine surgery, the risk of spinal cord injury related to intubation led to the adoption of the awake, nasotracheal, fiberoptic intubation protocol, with patients at times immobilized in hard cervical collars. Often, when patients with severe cervical spinal cord compromise are being positioned, the neutral position is not the optimal position. SSEP changes may indicate that a greater or lesser degree of flexion or extension may be warranted. Induction of anesthesia proceeds only after the SSEPs return to baseline levels, because bolus injections of barbiturates transiently compromise the SSEP response for 5 to 10 minutes.

The anesthesia protocol uses preoperative and intraoperative medications. Premedications include hydroxyzine (1 mg/kg), meperidine (1 mg/kg), and atropine (0.2–0.4 mg). Numbing of the nasopharyngeal passageways is achieved with either 4% cocaine applied with cotton swabs to the nasopharynx or 10 mL of 2% lidocaine jelly applied with a no. 14-Fr nasotracheal catheter to the same area. Both regimens include a transtracheal injection with 5 mL (100 mg) of 2% lidocaine (Xylocaine). Next, a 7- to 8-mm anode tube, placed over an adult fiberoptic bronchoscope, is introduced through the nares into the larynx and trachea, with the patient receiving midazolam 1 to 5 mg as needed.

Although patients who undergo ventral surgery remain supine, those who undergo dorsal procedures may be brought to the sitting position. In this case, while the patient is still awake, a Mayfield head holder is applied using 15 mL of 1% Xylocaine and 1:200,000 epinephrine to locally anesthetize the pin sites. Careful attention must be given to positioning the arms. They should be elevated, gently flexed, and padded at the elbows to reduce traction of nerve roots or the brachial plexus.

When bringing a patient to the sitting position, it may be preferable to keep him or her awake to avoid hypotension as well as preserving intact barometric reflexes. However, even with these precautions, some awake patients demonstrate declines in both amplitudes and latency responses. These changes are attributed to a relative drop in spinal cord perfusion despite systemic normotension (relative hypotension). This may readily be reversed by the pharmacologic induction of hypertension.

During induction, infusing a bolus of thiopental (2–3 mg/kg) or propofol (Diprivan, 1–2 mg/kg) results in a transient 5- to 10-minute decline in SSEP responses. As an option, remifentanil (0.2–0.9 μg/kg/min) can be used. Inhalation anesthetic concentrations are kept between 0.2% and 0.4%, and nitrous oxide is maintained below 60% to 70%. Vecuronium is given in a loading dose of 0.1 mg/kg and then administered repeatedly as required. Alternatively, recuronium can be given, but only for intubation. Local anesthetic infiltrated into the operative wound may allow the anesthesiologist to use lower doses of anesthetic throughout surgery, which may be desirable for monitoring. Patients are immediately awakened and neurologically assessed on the operating table after surgery. Only then are the patients brought to the recovery room.

Interpretation

Animal and human studies have shown that SSEP changes can occur when there is injury to adjacent motor pathways at the spinal and brainstem levels.[3,35,37,40] Assuming that appropriate stimulation and recording can be achieved, a major issue to be resolved is what constitutes a significant change and how reliably this can be detected. To further complicate matters, the primary disease often produces an SSEP abnormality that can be recognized in baseline recordings.[4,12,17,25,43-45] Recording methods may have to be modified. Despite averaging, multiple sources of artifacts may result in unstable potentials that are different for each patient. It is essential to determine the limits of SSEP amplitude and latency variation with repeated samples during the early part of the surgery. Significance criteria can be determined that are beyond the baseline limits of variability. In patients with high-amplitude, well-defined potentials at peripheral, spinal, and cortical levels, a reproducible drop in amplitude of 50% or greater or an increase in latency of 2 msec or greater (or >5–10% prolongation of latency), or both, is considered significant. Equally, a complete loss of waveform not explainable by technical malfunction is considered significant.

SSEPs rely on the recording of amplitude and latency values elicited from median and posterior tiblial nerve stimulation. The responses are recorded from the postcentral sulcus (noninvasive technique). Amplitude is measured, in microvolts, from the wave's height to its trough. The amplitude reflects the integrity of a number of fibers being simultaneously stimulated to form an action potential. Amplitude varies from patient to patient according to age, height, temperature, and integrity of the system being tested. Comparison of right and left sides and assessment of changes compared with the patient's preoperative baseline are important.

If baseline recordings with the patient under anesthesia show highly variable, low-amplitude cortical or spinal potentials, then all potentials recorded rostral to the area at risk might be required to disappear for the change to be considered significant. Implicit in these judgments is the understanding that effects of a change in physiologic variable, limb position, artifacts, and technical failures be identified and either corrected or accounted for before a final decision is made regarding the significance of a change in the SSEP.

Early in the procedure, an effort is made to identify and eliminate all sources of noise, especially 60-cycle interference. Care must be taken to avoid ground loops. Any conductor in contact with the patient (including IV lines) or electrical equipment in the room can be a source of interference. The recording system should suppress input during cautery and reject high-amplitude artifact. EMG activity from surrounding muscle can also produce unwanted artifact if neuromuscular activity is not blocked. Especially with the patient under light anesthesia, EMG activity can obscure the SSEP. A short, constant, controlled level of short-acting neuromuscular blocking agent or intermittent doses of benzodiazepines can be used to control muscle artifact in cases that require simultaneous monitoring of SSEP and EMG.

In the upper extremities, although the entire waveform from N10 (brachial plexus), N12a/N12b (segmental ascending dorsal column), N13a/N13b (dorsal horn/cuneate nucleus), and P14 (medial lemniscus) is recorded, the final cortical median N20 proves to be the most clinically relevant. Similarly, N22/P22 (dorsal horn T10 to L1), N29 (cervical gracile nucleus), P31 (medial lemniscus), and N34 (thalamus/brainstem) are noted, but the P38/N38 and P40 constitute the most used cortical potentials.

The cortical potential recorded from median nerve stimulation shows three positive peaks before the final negative trough of N20. The first of the waves at P15 indicates the afferent volley arriving at the thalamic level, whereas P16 and P18 indicate transmission via the thalamocortical tract to the primary sensory cortex. Once as the volley arrives at the cortex, additional positive peaks up to P25 indicate additional volley transmission to the surrounding sensory cortical regions.

Cortical responses noted after tibial nerve stimulation follow a similar but more prolonged pattern. The mean latency for the posterior tiblial response P40 is typically 38.8 msec.

TABLE 177-1

Some of the Common Responses Seen during Stimulation of the Median and Tiblial Nerves

Name	Recording Site	Latency (msec)	Location
Median Nerve			
Erb point	Erb point	9	Brachial plexus
N11	Cervical	11	DREZ of cervical roots
N13	Cervical	13	Posterior columns
P14	Scalp to extracephalic	14	Nucleus cuneatus
N18	Scalp to extracephalic	18	Subcortical structures
N20	Scalp	20	Somatosensory cortex
Tiblial Nerve			
N20	Lumbar	20	Conus
P31	Scalp to extracephalic	31	Nucleus gracilis/ medial lamniscus
N34	Scalp to extracephalic	34	Thalamus
P37/P40	Scalp	37	Somatosensory cortex

DREZ, dorsal root entry zone.

Multiple initial negative peaks may also be visualized with these responses. These varied responses reflect the different anatomic locations along the somatosensory pathway of the posterior tiblial nerve to the cauda equina, lumbosacral spinal cord, gracile nucleus, thalamus, and cortex (Table 177-1).

Somatosensory cortical-evoked responses (compared with invasive spinal-evoked responses) have the disadvantage of being more vulnerable to changes in anesthetic techniques and are susceptible to changes in peripheral skin conditions (i.e., temperature). Cortical responses are also smaller in amplitude, and they more readily deteriorate, particularly in the presence of excessive electroencephalographic (EEG) activity or environmental noise. Averaging 200 responses per recording enhances the response, largely by eliminating random noise.

Resuscitative Measures

Anesthetic and surgical resuscitative measures may be instituted as soon as significant SSEP deterioration is detected. This measure may take place either during the first 50 seconds or after findings have been reproduced at 100 seconds. The more rapid the adoption of these techniques in response to imminent tissue damage, the faster the potentials return to baseline.

Medical causes of SSEP changes include hypotension, hypothermia, increased levels of halogenated inhalation anesthetics (>0.4% fluorane), and IV sedation. These may be reversed by inducing hypertension and hyperthermia artificially and by hyperoxygenating the wound with peroxide irrigation while increasing systemic oxygenation. The reduction or elimination of inhalation anesthesia by switching to a barbiturate "balanced" technique may also foster recovery. High-dose methylprednisolone may be emergently administered to limit neurologic injury signaled by persistent SSEP abnormalities.

Surgical maneuvers may require cessation of surgical manipulation, release or elimination of distraction, removal of excessively large grafts resulting in overdistraction, and removal of instrumentation. An example of cortical SSEP changes during spine surgery for scoliosis in shown in Figure 177-2.

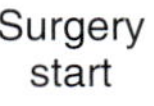

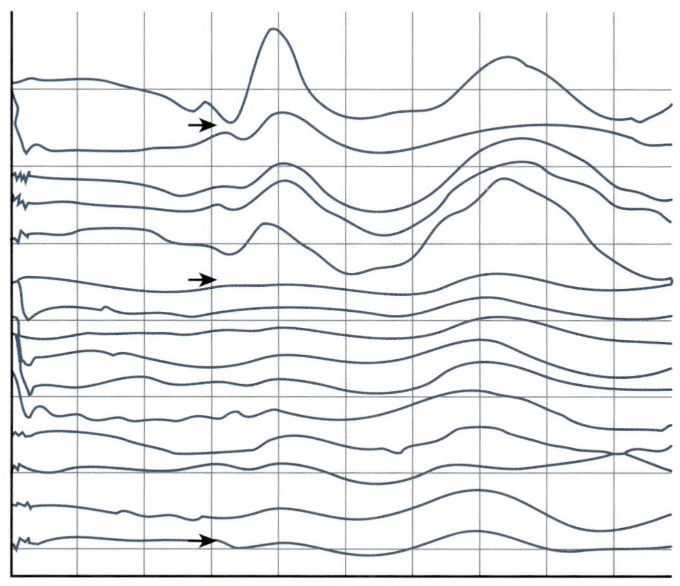

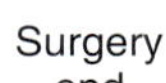

FIGURE 177-2. Example of intraoperative somatosensory-evoked potentials recording (tiblial nerve stimuli) during spine surgery for a scoliosis procedure. During the first stage of surgery, the P32 potential is clearly evidenced (*top arrow*), but soon after surgical distraction, the potential almost disappears (*middle arrow*). The surgeon was informed, and the distraction was reversed. The potential returned at the end of the procedure, but with smaller amplitude (*bottom arrow*).

For patients with ossification of the posterior longitudinal ligament, changes in SSEP responses are common. For these individuals, distraction is therefore avoided until the pathologic abnormality has been fully excised.

Summary

SSEP monitoring is a relatively new form of monitoring compared with other techniques such as ECG or even blood pressure monitoring. Despite its relatively recent introduction, SSEP monitoring has already contributed much to the ability of the spine surgeon to deal with difficult problems that only a few years ago were considered too risky to even consider. SSEP plays a valuable role during spine surgery by decreasing patient risk and improving outcome. It is essential that spine surgeons continue to improve intraoperative monitoring techniques to provide optimal care for their patients. Further information regarding this topic and future updates can be obtained from the web page of the recently created International Society of Intraoperative Neurophysiology (www.neurophysiology.org).

KEY REFERENCES

Allison T: Recovery functions of somatosensory evoked responses in man. *Electroencephalogr Clin Neurophysiol* 14:331, 1962.

Dinner DS, Lüders H, Lesser RP, et al: Intraoperative spinal somatosensory evoked potentials monitoring. *J Neurosurg* 65:807, 1986.

Giblin DR: Somatosensory evoked potentials in healthy subjects and in patients with lesions of the nervous system. *Ann NY Acad Sci* 112:93, 1964.

Grundy BL: Monitoring of sensory evoked potentials during neurosurgical operations: methods and applications. *Neurosurgery* 11:556, 1982.

Macon JB, Poletti CE, Sweet WH, et al: Conducted somatosensory evoked potentials during spinal surgery. Part 2: Clinical applications. *J Neurosurg* 57:354, 1982.

Sutter M, Deletis V, Dvorak J, et al: Current opinions and recommendations on multimodal intraoperative monitoring during spine surgeries. *Eur Spine J* 16(Suppl 2):S232, 2007.

REFERENCES

The complete reference list is available online at expertconsult.com.

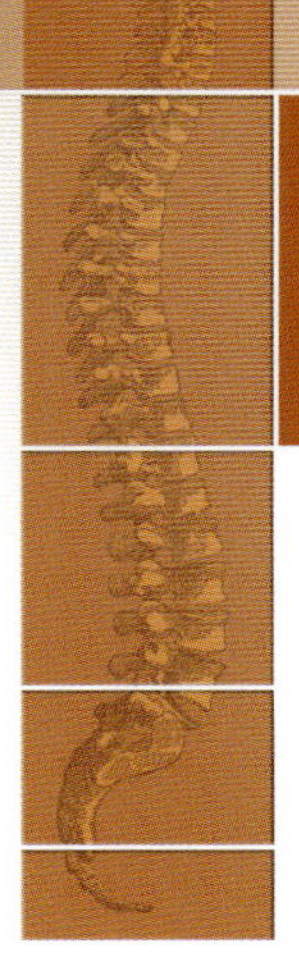

CHAPTER 178

Electrodiagnostic Studies

Steven Shook

The electrodiagnostic (EDX) is an important adjunct to the neurologic examination for diagnosis and management of disorders affecting the peripheral nervous system. Components of the EDX examination include (1) nerve conduction studies (NCSs), (2) needle electrode examination (NEE, or electromyogram), and (3) special studies (e.g., H reflexes, F waves). Each part of the examination has specific advantages and limitations. Diagnosis is best facilitated when these components are used in combination. Although all complete studies include at least an NCS and NEE, the relative value of each test varies depending on the goal of the examination.

A well-designed EDX study should be individualized to address a specific clinical question. Although many EDX laboratories have routine NCS/NEE protocols established by suspected pathology (e.g., cervical radiculopathy protocol, lumbosacral plexopathy protocol, peripheral polyneuropathy protocol), the patient's history and examination should influence selection of motor and sensory NCSs and specific muscles to be sampled by NEE. Moreover, the study is often modified as it is being conducted based on important and occasionally unexpected findings. When performed in this manner, the EDX examination can facilitate localization, focus differential diagnosis, estimate lesion severity, and provide information useful for estimating prognosis in neuromuscular disorders.

Key Anatomy for Electrodiagnosis

An understanding of key aspects of peripheral nervous system (PNS) anatomy is required for planning and interpreting the results of an EDX study. The motor division of the PNS begins at the anterior horn cell within the spinal cord, whose axon projects outward into the ventral root. The sensory division begins distally along the dorsal root at the dorsal root ganglion, which is typically found within the ostium of the intervertebral foramen.[1] Thus, the dorsal (sensory) roots within the spinal canal are preganglionic. For this reason a lesion within the intraspinal canal (e.g., compression by an intervertebral disc) may damage the sensory fibers and cause clinical sensory symptoms, but the postganglionic fibers remain intact and unaffected for the purposes of sensory NCSs. By contrast, an intraspinal canal injury causing ventral (motor) root axon loss is postganglionic, and thus loss of sufficient motor fibers is measurable by motor NCSs and NEEs. This arrangement is of considerable value in localizing intraspinal canal injury electrodiagnostically.

The dorsal and ventral roots merge segmentally to form mixed spinal nerves, including 8 cervical, 12 thoracic, 5 lumbar, 5 sacral, and 1 coccygeal.[2] Once the spinal nerves emerge from the intervertebral foramen, they divide into the posterior primary rami, which supply the skin and intrinsic muscles of the posterior neck and back (including the *paraspinal* muscles) and the anterior primary rami. The anterior primary rami supply the brachial plexus and peripheral nerves of the arm at the cervical segment (Fig. 178-1), the anterolateral aspect of the trunk and the thoracic level, and the lumbosacral plexus and nerves of the leg at the lumbosacral level. Muscles supplied by a given spinal segment are referred to as a *myotome*, and sensory regions supplied by each spinal segment are referred to as *dermatomes*.

The motor unit is the basic functional element of the motor PNS. It consists of the anterior horn cell, its axon, and all of the muscle fibers it innervates via neuromuscular junctions. The number of muscles fibers innervated by one motor neuron varies (e.g., 10:1 in the extraocular muscles and 2000:1 in the gastrocnemius muscle) and depends on the degree of fine-motor control required. Muscle is organized into fascicles, with the fibers of a single motor unit distributed randomly over as many as 100 different fascicles. Thus, a skeletal muscle consists of a mosaic fiber from 20 to 50 overlapping motor units.[3] Analysis of the electrical activity of the motor units and their muscle fibers is the objective of the NEE.

Nerve Fiber Injury Types and Relevance

The EDX examination tests large myelinated nerve fibers, which can be subject to a range of injury. Regardless of whether nerve fibers are compressed, stretched, mechanically deformed, or lacerated, the damage manifests as either axon loss or demyelination, or a combination of the two. Axon loss produces conduction failure along the affected fibers. Of note, for several days after a focal axon loss lesion (2–3 days for motor fibers and 5–6 days for sensory fibers), the nerve fibers distal to the lesion can conduct an action potential when tested by NCSs, after which wallerian degeneration ultimately results in failure of the entire axon segment distal to the lesion site (5–7 days for motor fibers and 10–11 days for sensory fibers).[4] In contrast, focal demyelination remains restricted to the injury site

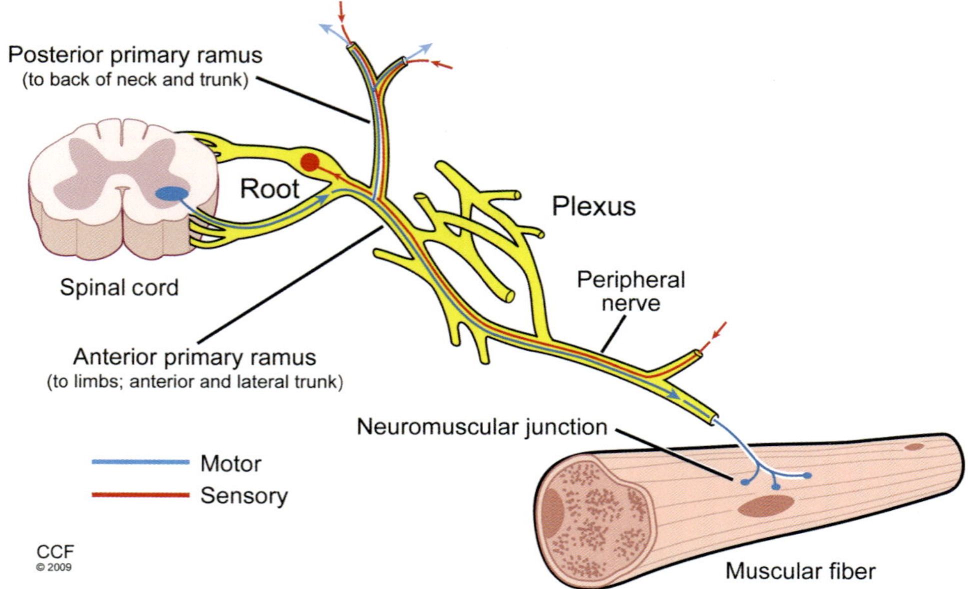

FIGURE 178-1. Basic anatomy of the peripheral nervous system. (Illustration by David Schumick, BS, CMI. Reprinted with the permission of the Cleveland Clinic Center for Medical Art & Photography © 2009. All rights reserved.)

and only affects the largest myelinated nerve fibers, including motor fibers, and sensory fibers mediating vibration and proprioception. Focal demyelinating conduction block thus can only be demonstrated with NCS by stimulation proximal to the area of injury.[5]

When nerves are injured, the type and degree of axon loss or demyelination affects prognosis. Clinically useful scales rating the degree of nerve injury have been developed by Seddon[6] and Sunderland.[7] Seddon divides focal nerve injuries into three broad categories by severity: neurapraxia, axonotmesis, and neurotmesis. *Neurapraxia*, the mildest injury type with the best prognosis, is transient and does not involve loss of nerve continuity. Underlying pathophysiology may include functional conduction block (without demyelination), mild demyelinating lesions, and demyelinating conduction block. *Axonotmesis* occurs when the nerve axon and myelin sheath are completely interrupted, while the surrounding endoneurium, perineurium, and epineurium remain intact. Prognosis in axonotmesis is better than in neurotmesis (loss of the axon and severance of its supporting connective tissue). Axon regeneration in *neurotmesis* is limited due to disruption of the conduit through which regenerating axons might extend to reinnervate their target organ. Sunderland's classification system further divides these injury types, particularly with respect to the degree of supporting structure damage in neurotmesis. EDX testing can differentiate between neurapraxia and axonotmesis, providing useful prognostic information. However, axonotmesis and neurotmesis cannot be differentiated, because they appear identical electrodiagnostically.[3]

Components of the Electrodiagnostic Examination

Nerve Conduction Studies

NCSs can be divided into motor, sensory, and mixed studies (Fig. 178-2). Motor and sensory NCSs are considered part of

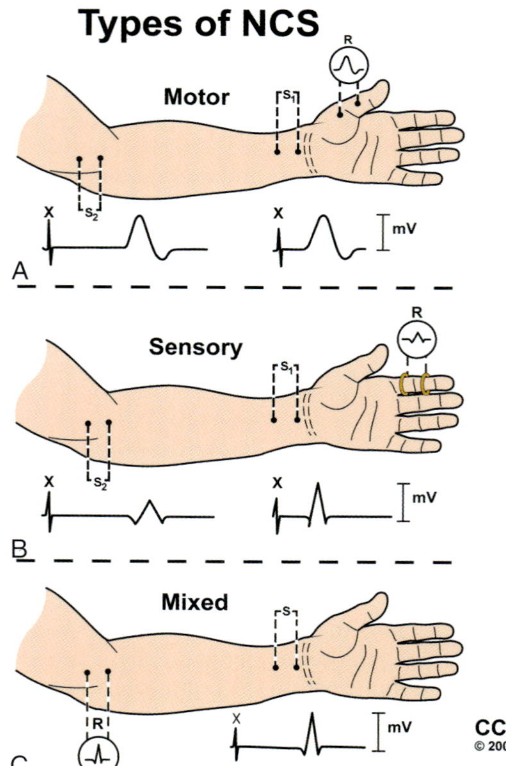

FIGURE 178-2. Basic nerve conduction studies performed on the median nerve. **A,** Motor nerve conduction studies, measured at the abductor pollicis brevis muscle. **B,** Sensory nerve conduction study measured at the second digit. **C,** Mixed study. R, recording site; S_1 and S_2, stimulation sites; X, stimulus artifact on each response tracing. (Illustration by David Schumick, BS, CMI. Reprinted with the permission of the Cleveland Clinic Center for Medical Art & Photography © 2009. All rights reserved.)

a routine EDX evaluation, whereas mixed studies are typically used only in special situations (e.g., median, ulnar, or tibial nerve entrapment). Although both surface and needle electrodes can be used for stimulating and recording, most EDX laboratories select noninvasive surface electrodes for NCSs.

Motor Conduction Studies

Motor NCSs are typically performed using an "active" recording electrode over the center of a muscle belly and reference electrode distally over the tendon of the muscle ("the belly-tendon montage"). A two-pronged (anode-cathode) stimulator is placed over the nerve supplying the muscle, with the cathode oriented closer to the recording electrode. Current is applied over the nerve to induce an action potential in the underlying nerve fibers. As the current is gradually increased with each subsequent stimulation, action potentials are triggered in more nerve fibers, and in turn more muscle fiber action potentials are generated and recorded distally as a single compound muscle action potential (CMAP). When increases in amperage no longer augment the size of the CMAP (i.e., all axons within the nerve are being stimulated), one final increase in current by 20% is performed to achieve a "supramaximal stimulation," and the resulting CMAP is recorded for analysis.[8]

Several key aspects of the CMAP waveform are analyzed (Fig. 178-3). First, the distal latency is measured in milliseconds from the stimulus artifact to the initial baseline deflection. This measurement combines the action potential travel time from the stimulus site to the neuromuscular junction (NMJ), time across the NMJ, and time required for the muscle fibers to depolarize. Note that this measurement only reflects the fastest conducting fibers (i.e., those that reach the recording electrode earliest and produce the initial baseline deflection). Second, the duration of the negative phase is assessed as a measure of muscle fiber discharge synchrony in response to the stimulus. Demyelinating lesions not severe enough to cause conduction block may slow motor fiber conduction to varying degrees within a stimulated nerve, resulting in *dyssynchrony* or "temporal dispersion," increasing the CMAP duration. Third, the amplitude and area of the negative phase are measured, providing an index of the number of muscle fibers depolarizing within the range of the recording electrode. Although a reduction in CMAP amplitude (and area) is most often attributed to axon loss, demyelinating conduction block between the stimulus and recording site has the same effect.

Further analysis of motor nerve conduction requires a second, more proximal stimulus over the nerve recording at the same location, using the technique just described. The more proximal stimulation is performed at a measured distance from the first. The difference between the proximal latency (PL) and distal latency (DL) in milliseconds reflects the conduction time along the fastest nerve fibers between the sites, eliminating the travel time from the distal site and across the NMJ, as well as muscle fiber depolarization time. The distance between the sites in millimeters divided by the nerve conduction time (i.e., PL minus DL) is known as the conduction velocity (Fig. 178-4). The configuration of the CMAP generated by the proximal stimulation is also compared with that of the distal CMAP. Assuming supramaximal stimulus at both sites, the CMAPs should be essentially identical. A proximal stimulation CMAP amplitude less than 50% of the distal CMAP amplitude is consistent with conduction block, or a very early focal axon loss lesion in which wallerian degeneration has not yet occurred.

In most electrodiagnostic laboratories, routine motor NCSs of the arm include median nerve (recording the abductor pollicis brevis muscle) and ulnar nerve (recording the abductor digiti minimi muscle), and in the leg, the tibial nerve (recording the abductor hallucis muscle) and peroneal nerve (recording the extensor digitorum brevis muscle). Proximal stimulation sites can be added to address specific clinical questions (e.g., stimulating the ulnar nerve above and below the elbow, or common peroneal nerve above and below the fibular head to assess for evidence of demyelination). In many cases

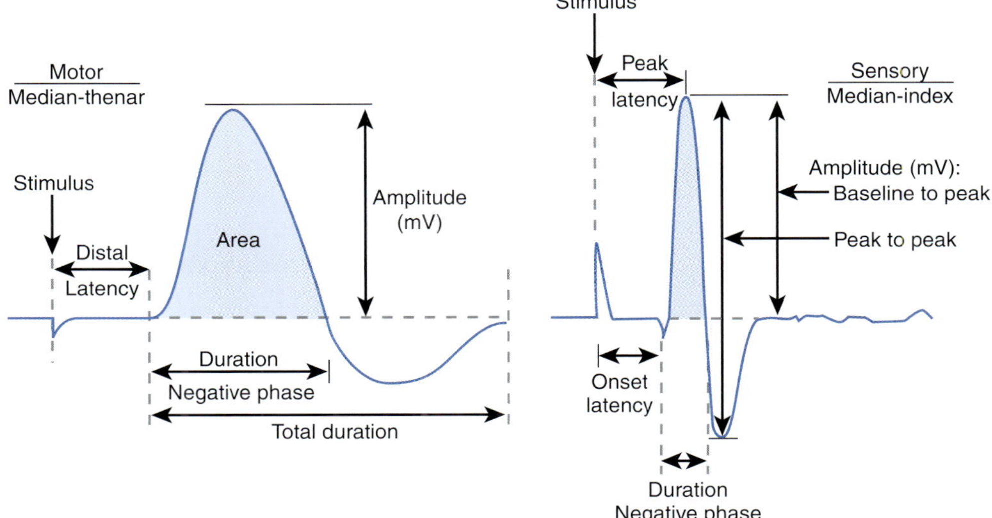

FIGURE 178-3. Compound muscle action potential (*left*) and sensory nerve action potential (*right*) examples, both obtained from the median nerve. Note that by convention, deflection above the line is referred to as the "negative" phase and below the line as "positive." (Illustration by David Schumick, BS, CMI. Reprinted with the permission of the Cleveland Clinic Center for Medical Art & Photography © 2009. All rights reserved.)

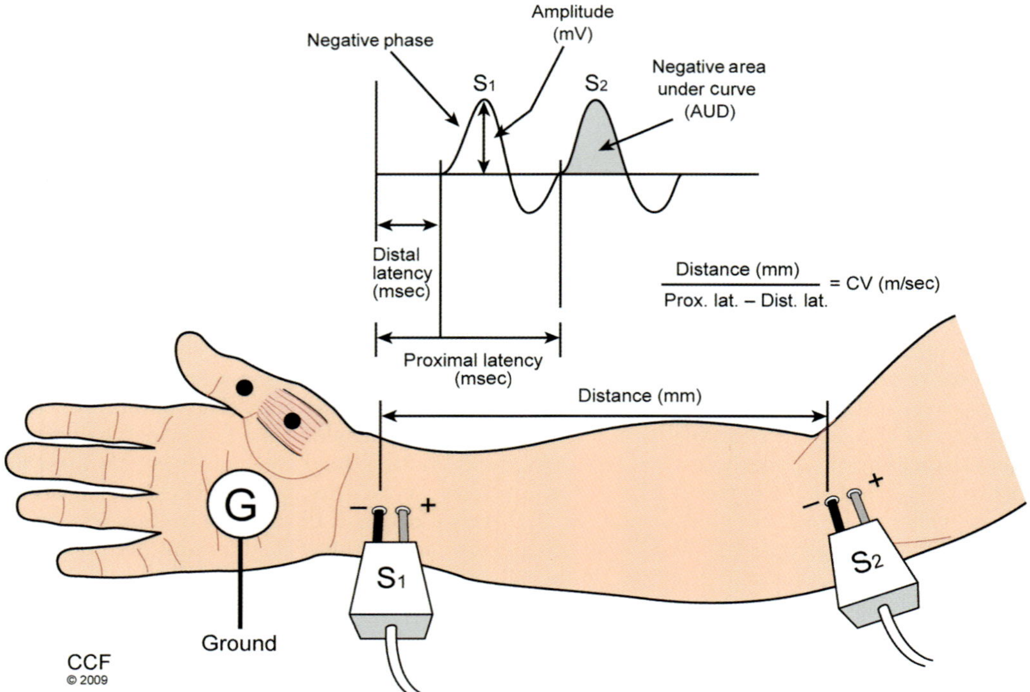

FIGURE 178-4. Motor conduction velocity calculation example, performed on the median nerve. S_1 (distal) and S_2 (proximal) are stimulation sites, (–) is cathode and (+) is anode of the stimulator. (Illustration by David Schumick, BS, CMI. Reprinted with the permission of the Cleveland Clinic Center for Medical Art & Photography © 2009. All rights reserved.)

these routine studies must be supplemented to adequately assess an area of potential injury. In the arm, motor studies of the radial nerve (recording the brachioradialis, extensor digitorum communis, or extensor indicis proprius muscles), ulnar nerve (recording the first dorsal interosseous muscle), musculocutaneous nerve (recording the biceps muscle), or axillary nerve (recording the deltoid muscle) may be indicated.[5]

Sensory Conduction Studies

Sensory NCSs are performed with the two-pronged stimulator and pair of recording electrodes over the nerve. These studies may performed antidromically (stimulating proximally and recording adjacent to the sensory receptor) or orthodromically (stimulating distally and recording proximally). These responses are relatively small and are measured in microvolts (μV, 1/1000 of the unit used to measure a CMAP). As with motor NCSs, current is applied over the nerve to induce an action potential and is gradually increased with subsequent stimulations. At supramaximal stimulation, the combined action potentials of the sensory fibers are recorded as a sensory nerve action potential (SNAP). SNAP latency, duration, and amplitude are measured. Latency is measured to onset (representing the conduction of the fastest fibers) or, more commonly, to the peak of the negative deflection (see Fig. 178-3).[8]

Routine sensory NCSs in most laboratories include the median nerve (recorded over digit 2) and ulnar nerve (recorded over digit 5) in the arm and are supplemented by studies of the radial, dorsal ulnar cutaneous, lateral antebrachial cutaneous, medial antebrachial cutaneous, and median sensory responses recorded over digit 1 or 3, as indicated. In the leg the sural sensory response (recorded over the lateral ankle) is routine, and supplemented by the lateral/medial plantar, superficial peroneal, saphenous, and lateral femoral cutaneous sensory responses, depending on the clinical indication for the study. For example, the superficial peroneal SNAP is of particular importance when differentiating between an intraspinal canal lesion affecting the L5 root and a common peroneal mononeuropathy.

Particular advantages of NCSs compared with the NEEs include the ability to perform these studies with minimal patient cooperation (e.g., patients under anesthesia), provide key localizing information with regard to the sensory nerve fibers, and superior potential for identifying demyelinating lesions. It is, however, important to appreciate that NCSs only assess the large myelinated nerve fibers of the PNS, and thus disorders affecting only the smallest nerve fibers (e.g., small sensory fiber peripheral polyneuropathies) will not be demonstrated. NCSs are also relatively insensitive to motor axon loss compared with NEEs, underscoring the complementary nature of NCSs and NEEs.[5]

Needle Electrode Examination

The NEE allows rapid, widespread assessment of the motor component of the PNS. The procedure involves inserting an electrode into individual muscles and evaluating the insertional, spontaneous, and volitional electrical activity present, both visually on an oscilloscope, which displays voltage as a function of time, and aurally. NEE is particularly sensitive for identifying axon loss when compared with a motor NCS. Importantly, an optimal NEE requires patient cooperation and can be uncomfortable for patients, occasionally limiting its usefulness due to poor patient tolerance.

The first step of the NEE of a muscle is to evaluate "insertional activity," which is generated by needle movement within a muscle at rest. When an electrode is quickly moved through normal muscle, the fibers depolarize, generating a brief burst of electrical activity lasting 100 to 200 msec. This finding confirms that the electrode is in viable muscle. Although increased insertional activity lasting more than 300 msec is nonspecific, it is the earliest NEE finding in a partially denervated muscle, typically consisting of unsustained trains of positive sharp waves. These spontaneous electrical potentials have a characteristic initial positive phase followed by a long negative phase. Conversely, insertional activity may be decreased or absent in chronic neuromuscular conditions because the muscle has been replaced by electrically silent fat and fibrous tissue.

Next, the examiner assesses for spontaneous electrical activity with the needle electrode at rest within the muscle. Normal muscle should be electrically silent during this phase. *Fibrillation potentials* are an important electrophysiologic marker of denervation. This form of spontaneous activity is characterized by regularly firing potentials, most commonly of a brief sharp spike configuration, derived from a single denervated muscle fiber. Larger-amplitude potentials are observed in acute disease[9] and are present in greater density in more severe disorders. Fibrillation potentials are sensitive to denervation because disruption of a single motor axon results in fibrillation of all muscle fibers within that motor unit. They can thus be seen when motor axon loss is insufficient to cause clinical weakness. Although these potentials are most commonly associated with injury to motor axons, they may also be found in inflammatory myopathies and rarely in other neuromuscular disorders. Importantly, in the setting of denervation, fibrillation potentials require an average of 21 days to appear after injury and persist until reinnervation occurs or the muscle fibers degenerate at around 18 to 24 months after axon loss.[10]

Other forms of spontaneous activity can be observed during the resting phase. *Fasciculation potentials*, which are irregularly firing spontaneous discharges of an entire motor unit, are a marker of nerve fiber irritation as opposed to denervation. Complex repetitive discharges, which are recurrent, cyclic discharges of a series of muscle fibers, are a marker of chronicity, typically seen in neurogenic or myopathic disorders of at least 6 months' duration.[3]

During the *activation phase* of the NEE, the muscle is contracted in order to analyze the firing pattern and morphology of voluntarily generated motor unit action potentials (MUAPs). A *MUAP* represents the summed electrical activity produced by depolarization of the muscle fibers of a single motor unit within the range of the recording electrode. The force generated by a muscle is a function of the number of different MUAPs firing and the rate at which they fire. At minimal contraction, a single MUAP may be observed firing in a semirhythmic pattern at a basal rate of approximately 5 to 10 Hz. As the patient is asked to gradually contract the muscle with greater force, a second MUAP is "recruited," and the firing rates of both MUAPs are increased until a third MUAP is recruited, and so on. A normal ratio of firing frequency to the number of different MUAPs firing is approximately 5:1 (e.g., when the MUAP firing rate reaches 20 Hz, four different MUAPs should be identifiable).[8] At maximal contraction, MUAPs overlap and create an *interference pattern*, in which no single motor unit can be distinguished.

The interference pattern is reduced at maximal patient effort when either MUAP activation (ability to increase the firing rate) or recruitment (ability to add motor units as the firing rate increases) is diminished. Reduced activation occurs when MUAPs fire in equally decreased numbers at a slow to moderate rate and is indicative of either suboptimal patient effort (e.g., intentional, or due to pain) or a disease state of the CNS (e.g., stroke, multiple sclerosis, or other upper motor neuron lesion). Conversely, abnormal recruitment is consistent with a lower motor neuron disorder. Reduced MUAP recruitment (i.e., a neurogenic firing pattern) is observed when motor units cannot be activated due to conduction block or axon loss. With fewer MUAPs capable of firing, the intact potentials fire at a faster rate in order to generate the force intended. When a sufficiently large number of motor axons are damaged, reduced recruitment is immediately apparent, unlike fibrillation potentials, which appear after an average of 3 weeks.

Finally, the morphology of the MUAPs is analyzed. In partial or gradual axon loss disorders, chronic neurogenic changes in the MUAP configuration can be appreciated after a period of 4 to 6 months. These changes occur due to collateral sprouting of the surviving motor axons, resulting in a greater number of muscle fibers belonging to each remaining motor unit. As more adjacent muscle fibers join the motor unit, the MUAP increases in duration and amplitude and appears more complex (*polyphasic*). Once present, these changes persist indefinitely and may be the sole evidence of a remote neurogenic injury.[3]

Late Responses

H Reflex

The H reflex is the electrophysiologic equivalent of the Achilles tendon muscle stretch reflex ("ankle jerk") and is unique in its ability to assess the preganglionic sensory fibers of the S1 nerve root. The reflex is elicited by stimulating the tibial nerve within the popliteal fossa at a progressively greater stimulus intensity, while recording the soleus muscle. Beginning at a submaximal stimulus intensity, lower-threshold sensory fibers are discharged first, resulting in an afferent (proximally directed) action potential, which synapses at the anterior horn cells of the S1 root. This initiates an efferent (distally directed) motor action potential, which is recordable as an H response at the soleus muscle. As the strength of the stimulus intensity is increased by the examiner, the tibial motor fibers at the stimulation site are depolarized, directly resulting in a measurable direct motor response, the M *wave*. Further increases in stimulus intensity depolarize additional motor fibers and thus result in a progressively higher-amplitude M wave. Direct discharge of these motor fibers results in a lower-amplitude H response because the orthodromic H response is blocked by an antidromic motor fiber discharge from the stimulation site. At supramaximal stimulus, only the M wave is apparent.

The H response amplitude and latency can be compared contralaterally and to values in normal controls adjusted for age and height, providing evidence of nerve fiber injury within the S1 reflex arc. Although H reflex abnormalities are considered sensitive for root impingement caused by S1 radiculopathy, the finding lacks specificity, also being found in patients with polyneuropathy, proximal tibial or sciatic mononeuropathies, and lumbosacral plexopathy. Absent H reflexes are also commonly observed in patients older than age 65 and in patients with a history of lumbar laminectomy and are thus of unclear clinical significance in this context.[11] Overall, the usefulness of an absent H reflex is limited when the remainder of the EDX examination is within normal limits.

F waves

F waves[12] are produced after a distal motor nerve stimulation. They can be measured during routine distal motor nerve conduction after reversing the stimulator orientation (the cathode is positioned proximal and the anode distal) and adjusting recording equipment settings to account for the low amplitude and long latency of these responses. F waves are different from H reflexes because they are conducted solely along motor axons, do not synapse within the spinal cord, and are thus not a measure of a true reflex arc. They are produced when some of the antidromic impulses cause a subpopulation of anterior horn cells to "backfire." The resulting impulses travel back down the motor axons, and the latency of these late responses can be measured. These can be compared contralaterally and with height-adjusted normal values. A prolonged F wave latency is consistent with demyelination of the motor axon between the stimulus site and the recording muscle, as might be observed in acquired demyelinating polyradiculoneuropathy or demyelination in other causes or radiculopathy.[5]

TABLE 178-1

Sensory Nerve Action Potentials (by Root)

Root	Sensory Response	Recording Site
C5 and C6	Lateral antebrachial cutaneous	Lateral forearm
C6	Radial	Thumb
C6	Median	Thumb
C6 and C7	Radial	Anatomic snuffbox
C6 and C7	Median	Index finger
C7	Median	Middle finger
C7 and C8	Median	Ring finger
C7 and C8	Ulnar	Ring finger
C8	Ulnar	Fifth digit
C8	Dorsal ulnar cutaneous	Dorsal forearm
T1	Medial antebrachial cutaneous	Medial forearm
L4	Saphenous	Medial ankle
L5	Superficial peroneal	Lateral ankle
S1	Sural	Posterior ankle

A lesion affecting the nerve root within the intraspinal canal will not affect the postganglionic sensory nerve action potential.

TABLE 178-2

Typically Affected Muscles in Cervical Radioculopathy (by Root)

Root	Abnormal Muscle	Nerve
C5 (or C6)	Supraspinatus	Suprascapular
	Infraspinatus	Suprascapular
	Deltoid	Axillary
	Biceps brachii	Musculocutaneous
	Brachioradialis	Radial
C7 (or C6)	Triceps	Radial
	Anconeus	Radial
	Pronator teres	Median
	Flexor carpi radialis	Median
C8	Extensor indicis proprius	Radial
	Flexor pollicis longus	Median
	First dorsal interosseous	Ulnar
	Abductor digiti minimi	Ulnar
T1 (or C8)	Abductor pollicis brevis	Median

Electrodiagnostic Localization of Spinal Disorders

Radiculopathy

Assessment for nerve root injury in patients with back pain radiating to a limb is a common reason for referral to EDX laboratories. Whereas imaging studies visualize the nerve roots and their relationship to the intervertebral discs, neuroforamina, and other associated structures, EDX studies provide important functional information, including the presence, severity, and acuity of axon loss and evidence of compensatory reinnervation. Moreover, structural causes of radiculopathy (e.g., a herniated intervertebral disc, impingement from spondylosis, epidural abscess, neoplasm) are most common, but imaging may be normal when the cause is infection, ischemia, inflammation, or microscopic neoplastic infiltration, and thus more effectively demonstrated by EDX studies.

Injury to a single spinal nerve root within the intraspinal canal usually results in normal sensory and motor NCSs. Since the lesion occurs proximal to the dorsal root ganglion (DRG), intact distal sensory fibers yield normal sensory conductions within the distribution of the suspected nerve root injury (Table 178-1). One important exception to this rule can occur at the L5 root, whose DRG can be found within the intraspinal canal in between 10% and 40% of patients.[13] In these cases, an intraspinal canal lesion affecting the L5 level root (and DRG residing within the canal) causes loss of the superficial peroneal SNAP, complicating localization. Using the NEE to identify denervation changes within non-peroneal-innervated L5 muscles (e.g., gluteus medius, tensor fascia lata, semitendinosus, flexor digitorum longus, and tibialis posterior muscles) is required for proper localization in these cases. Motor NCSs are usually also normal, unless damage to a nerve root supplying the recording muscle results in sufficient axon loss to reduce the CMAP amplitude. Thus, the most important role of NCSs in radiculopathy evaluation is often to exclude mimicking causes, including plexopathy and mononeuropathy.

Abnormalities on NEE are identified in muscles innervated by the same spinal root, or myotome. Finding evidence of neurogenic injury in more than one muscle (ideally both proximal and distal muscles) supplied by different nerves sharing the same spinal root is central to NEE localization. However, only a subset of motor fibers within the nerve root undergoes axon degeneration in all but the most severe radiculopathies, and thus findings on NEE may be limited to a few muscles within the affected myotome. A myotomal map based on systematic studies of the various NEE patterns occurring with single cervical root lesions, as defined by surgical localization for the upper (Table 178-2)[14] and lower (Table 178-3)[15] extremity, is provided, arranged by root. Note that due to overlap, particularly between the C5 and C6, C6 and C7, and L3 and L4

TABLE 178-3

Typically Affected Muscles in Lumbosacral Radiculopathy (by Root)

Root	Abnormal Muscle	Nerve
L3-4	Iliopsoas	Femoral
	Adductor longus	Obturator
	Rectus femoris	Femoral
	Vastus lateralis	Femoral
	Vastus medialis	Femoral
L5	Gluteus medius	Superior gluteal nerve
	Tensor fascia lata	Superior gluteal nerve
	Semitendinosus	Sciatic (tibial division)
	Flexor digitorum longus	Tibial
	Tibialis posterior	Tibial
	Tibialis anterior	Peroneal (deep branch)
	Peroneus longus	Peroneal (superficial branch)
	Extensor hallucis longus	Peroneal (deep branch)
	Extensor digitorum brevis	Peroneal (deep branch)
S1	Gluteus maximus	Inferior gluteal nerve
	Biceps femoris, long head	Sciatic (tibial division)
	Biceps femoris, short head	Sciatic (peroneal division)
	Medial gastrocnemius	Tibial
	Lateral gastrocnemius	Tibial
	Abductor hallucis	Tibial
	Abductor digiti quinti	Tibial

myotomes, the ability to differentiate root lesions at these levels from one another is limited.

NEE of the paraspinal muscles is also a routine component of the radiculopathy EDX assessment. Fibrillation potentials in the paraspinal muscles indicate axon loss affecting the posterior primary ramus of the spinal root, consistent with a lesion within or adjacent to the intraspinal canal (i.e., proximal to the brachial or lumbosacral plexus with regard to the arm or leg, respectively).[10] However, due to the overlapping innervation of the paraspinal muscles, findings are not reliably segmental, often occurring caudal to the affected root. They are also not specific for radiculopathy, occurring in patients who have undergone prior spinal surgery via a posterior approach, motor neuron disease, or myopathy and in a portion of normal patients older than age 40. Thus, paraspinal fibrillation potentials cannot be interpreted in isolation and must be considered within the context of the rest of the EDX.[11]

The specific pattern of neurogenic injury on NEE depends on the lesion duration and severity. During the first 3 weeks after nerve root injury, active motor axon loss changes (i.e., fibrillation potentials) are likely to be absent, particularly in distal limb muscles, resulting in false-negative studies in patients studied too early. Within a few months after localizing changes from active motor axon loss, the process of reinnervation begins. Early compensatory reinnervation is accomplished by collateral sprouting of the remaining intact fibers within a partially affected root and from adjacent nerve roots supplying the same myotome. In the earliest stages, the process is more effective proximally and progresses in a centrifugal fashion, beginning in the most proximal (e.g., paraspinal) muscles and gradually progressing to the distal limb muscles. As muscle fibers are reinnervated, fibrillation potentials cease, unless ongoing axon loss occurs. Thus, in a static radiculopathy (i.e., no additional axon loss), only the most distal muscles of the myotome may appear abnormal after several months. In mild nerve root injuries, the EDX findings may normalize with time. When more severe axon loss has occurred, reinnervation via collateral sprouting results in a larger number of muscle fibers within each motor unit and, in turn, longer-duration, increased-amplitude neurogenic MUAPs within the affected myotome.

Overall, the presence of fibrillation potentials in proximal and distal muscles of a myotome in the absence of chronic neurogenic MUAP changes is most consistent with a recent nerve root lesion. When chronic neurogenic MUAP changes and fibrillation potentials are both prominent within a myotome, either chronic progressive radiculopathy or an acute form superimposed on a more remote root lesion is likely. In contrast, chronic neurogenic motor unit potential changes limited to distal muscles of the myotome are supportive of a static, remote lesion.[11]

Late responses can also be abnormal in patients with injury to a single nerve root. Since F responses assess conduction both distally and proximally, an abnormal F wave latency in combination with a normal standard distal NCS suggests proximal demyelination affecting the proximal portion of the nerve, plexus, or root supplying the recording muscle. The H reflex can be abnormal in a lesion affecting the S1 nerve root and may be prolonged in latency in demyelinating lesions or absent in patients with demyelinating conduction block or axon loss affecting this level. Importantly, an absent H reflex should not be interpreted in isolation, as this findings may be present in other disorders, including sacral plexopathy and polyneuropathy.

Case Examples

Case 1

A 49-year-old, right-handed woman presented with dysesthesias and weakness in the right upper extremity, starting immediately after a fall onto her outstretched arm 8 weeks prior. No fractures were discerned at the time of the injury. She had pain in the right side of her neck and shoulder, particularly when trying to raise the arm up over her head, and numbness in the right index finger and thumb. Her examination revealed mild weakness of shoulder abduction, elbow extension, and forearm pronation. Triceps reflex was lower on the right. The patient was referred for EDX testing to evaluate for cervical root injury versus brachial plexopathy. See Table 178-4 for EDX results.

Impression

Acute right C6-7 radiculopathy was present.

Notes

The NCSs are within normal limits. Additional sensory NCSs were performed for exclusion of a brachial plexus lesion, including the lateral and medial antebrachial cutaneous SNAPs. Changes in the sensory NCS are the most sensitive indicator of

TABLE 178-4

Electrodiagnostic Examination: 49-Year-Old, Right-Handed Woman

SENSORY SIDE-TO-SIDE COMPARISON TABLE

			B-P Amp (μV)		LatNPk (msec)		CV (m/s)		Dist (mm)				Temp (°C)	
Nerve	Stimulus	Recording	L	R	L	R	L	R	L	R	Norm B-P Amp	Norm LatNPk	L	R
Median	Wrist	Index	—	18.17	—	2.93	—	60.0	—	130	>15 μV	<3.6 ms	—	32.0
		Thumb	—	24.69	—	2.83	—	58.2	—	130	—	—	—	31.8
Ulnar	Wrist	5th digit	—	26.66	—	3.03	—	46.5	—	110	>10 μV	<3.1 ms	—	31.3
Radial	Forearm	Thumb	—	27.88	—	2.00	—	68.2	—	100	>14 μV	<2.7 ms	—	31.0
Lat. ante. cut.	Elbow	Forearm	11.50	11.14	2.90	2.83	—	—	—	—	>12 μV	—	32.5	30.3
Med. ante. cut.	Elbow	Forearm	6.22	8.52	2.73	2.63	—	—	—	—	>5 μV	—	31.5	29.9

MOTOR SIDE-TO-SIDE COMPARISON TABLE

			B-P Amp (mV)		LatOn (msec)		CV (m/s)		Dist (mm)			
Nerve	Stimulus	Recording	L	R	L	R	L	R	L	R	Norm B-P Amp	Norm LatOn
Median	Wrist	Thenar	—	6.55	—	3.17	—	—	—	50	>6 mV	<4 msec
Median	Elbow	APB	—	6.42	—	8.92	—	51.3	—	295	—	—
Ulnar	Wrist	Hypothenar	—	7.32	—	2.67	—	—	—	50	>7 mV	<3.1 msec
Ulnar	Below elbow	Hypothenar	—	6.21	—	6.50	—	53.5	—	205	—	—
Ulnar	Above elbow	Hypothenar	—	6.00	—	8.75	—	50.1	—	305	—	—

F-WAVE SIDE-TO-SIDE COMPARISON TABLE

			Latency (msec)	
Nerve	Stimulus	Recording	L	R
Ulnar	Wrist	Abductor digiti minimi	—	30.00

NEEDLE ELECTRODE EXAMINATION SUMMARY

			Spontaneous Activity					Motor Unit Action Potentials		
Side	**Muscle**	**InsAct**	**Fib**	**PW**	**Fasc**	**Activation**	**Recruitment**	**Dur**	**Amp**	**Poly**
Right	Cervical PSP—mid	Norm	+	0	0	NE	NE	Norm	Norm	Norm
	Cervical PSP—low	Norm	+	0	0	NE	NE	Norm	Norm	Norm
	Deltoid	Norm	0	0	0	Norm	Norm	Norm	Norm	Norm
	Biceps brachii	Norm	0	+	0	Norm	Decreased	Norm	Norm	Norm
	Brachioradialis	Norm	0	0	0	Norm	Norm	Norm	Norm	Norm
	Pronator teres	Norm	+	+	0	Norm	Decreased	Norm	Norm	Norm
	Flex. carpi radialis	Norm	+	0	0	Norm	Decreased	Norm	Norm	Norm
	Triceps (lateral)	Norm	+	+	0	Norm	Decreased	Norm	Norm	Norm
	Ext. indicis proprius	Norm	0	0	0	Norm	Norm	Norm	Norm	Norm
	Flex. pollicis, long	Norm	0	0	0	Norm	Norm	Norm	Norm	Norm
	First dorsal, int.	Norm	0	0	0	Norm	Norm	Norm	Norm	Norm
	Abd. pol. brevis	Norm	0	0	0	Norm	Norm	Norm	Norm	Norm
Left	Cervical PSP	Norm	0	0	0	NE	NE	Norm	Norm	Norm
	Low deltoid	Norm	0	0	0	Norm	Norm	Norm	Norm	Norm
	Brachioradialis	Norm	0	0	0	Norm	Norm	Norm	Norm	Norm
	Triceps (lateral)	Norm	0	0	0	Norm	Norm	Norm	Norm	Norm
	Flex. carpi. radialis	Norm	0	0	0	Norm	Norm	Norm	Norm	Norm
	First dorsal, int.	Norm	0	0	0	Norm	Norm	Norm	Norm	Norm

+, present; –, absent; Amp, amplitude; B-P Amp, baseline-to-peak amplitude; CV, conduction velocity (meters/second); Dist, distance (millimeters); Dur, duration; Faso, fasciculation potentials; Fib, fibrillation potentials; InsAct, insertional activity; L, left; LatNPeak, latency-to-negative peak; LatOn, latency to onset; NE, not examined; Norm, normal; Poly, polyphasic; PSP, paraspinal; PW, positive waves; R; right; Temp, temperature.

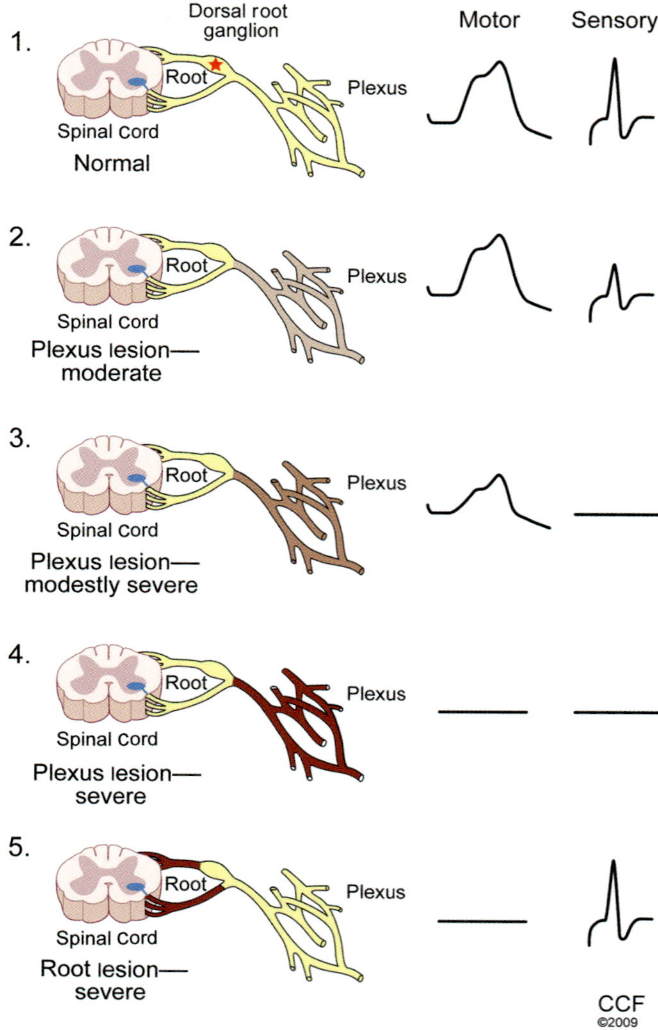

FIGURE 178-5. Variations in compound muscle action potentials and sensory nerve action potentials. Comparing normal findings (1) with axon loss lesions of varying severity affecting the brachial plexus (2–4) and the roots within the intraspinal canal lesion (5). (Illustration by David Schumick, BS, CMI. Reprinted with the permission of the Cleveland Clinic Center for Medical Art & Photography © 2009. All rights reserved.)

axon loss affecting the brachial plexus (Fig. 178-5) and are useful for differentiating a brachial plexopathy from a radiculopathy. The NEE revealed fibrillation potentials and decreased recruitment throughout the proximal and distal C6 and C7 myotome, consistent with an acute lesion. There is no evidence of early compensatory reinnervation (i.e., increased duration MUAPs), consistent with a lesion of less than 3 months in duration.

Case 2

A 68-year-old, right-handed man presented with long-standing low back pain and more recent numbness of the top of the left foot of 4 weeks' duration. Examination revealed mild weakness of the left ankle dorsiflexion, eversion, and toe extension and sensory loss over the dorsum of the left foot. The gait appeared normal, but the patient had some difficulty walking on his heels. The patient was referred for EDX testing to evaluate for lumbar root injury versus peroneal mononeuropathy. See Table 178-5 for the EDX results.

Impression

Subacute left L5 radiculopathy (bilateral chronic L5 radiculopathy) was present.

Notes

Superficial peroneal and sural sensory responses are within normal limits, the former reducing the odds of a significant axon loss lesion affecting the postganglionic fibers of the peroneal nerve on either side. The left peroneal CMAP (measured at both the extensor digitorum brevis and tibialis anterior muscles) is comparable to the right with regard to amplitude, and there is no evidence of conduction block or slowing across the fibular head, suggestive of a peroneal mononeuropathy at the knee segment. The NEE revealed decreased MUAP recruitment and neurogenic MUAPs in the L5 myotome bilaterally. There are fibrillation potentials in the distal left L5 myotome. These findings are consistent with long-standing bilateral L5 radiculopathies, with a more subacute lesion affecting the left L5 root.

Polyradiculopathy

Injury to multiple nerve roots within the intraspinal canal is associated with extensive degenerative changes affecting multiple spinal levels, as well as diabetes mellitus, infection (e.g., cytomegalovirus infection), or spinal root infiltration by a neoplastic process, among other causes. The pattern of abnormality is similar to that described for single-level radiculopathies; most importantly, the sensory NCSs are expected to be normal. However, motor NCSs are more likely to be reduced in amplitude when contiguous roots are injured, proportionate to the severity of axon loss to the root supplying the recording muscle. NEE reveals neurogenic changes in the affected myotomes.

Cervical Root Avulsion

Root avulsions in which the nerve root is severed from the spinal cord at one or more levels typically affect the cervical region and are associated with violent trauma in adults. Motor NCSs are severely reduced in amplitude or absent within the distribution of the avulsion. Similarly, the NEE reveals profuse fibrillation potentials and reduced to absent motor unit potential recruitment. Sensory NCSs from the same segment are normal in a "pure avulsion" because the injury occurs proximal to the dorsal root ganglia. However, relatively reduced sensory responses can occur due to presumed coincident damage to the postganglionic sensory fibers resulting from stretch injury. In these cases, precise localization is complex; however, complete segmental motor fiber axon loss and relatively mild or absent sensory fiber involvement are suggestive of avulsion within the proper clinical context.

Lumbar Canal Stenosis

There is no characteristic EDX finding indicative of stenosis of the lumbar canal. Abnormalities depend entirely on the severity and duration of axon loss present. Findings can range

TABLE 178-5

Electrodiagnostic Examination: 68-Year-Old, Right-Handed Man

SENSORY SIDE-TO-SIDE COMPARISON TABLE

			B-P Amp (μV)		LatNPk (msec)		CV (m/s)		Dist (mm)		Norm B-P	Norm	Temp (°C)	
Nerve	**Stimulus**	**Recording**	**L**	**R**	**L**	**R**	**L**	**R**	**L**	**R**	**Amp**	**LatNPk**	**L**	**R**
Sural	Mid-calf	Ankle	3.50	4.25	3.03	3.57	57.5	48.3	140	140	>3 mV	<4.4 msec	33.0	33.6
Peroneal	Lower leg	Ankle	4.09	4.19	2.33	2.80	54.5	49.2	100	100	>3 mV	<4.5 msec	32.9	33.1

MOTOR SIDE-TO-SIDE COMPARISON TABLE

			B-P Amp (mV)		LatOn (msec)		CV (m/s)		Dist (mm)		Norm B-P	Norm	Temp (°C)	
Nerve	**Stimulus**	**Recording**	**L**	**R**	**L**	**R**	**L**	**R**	**L**	**R**	**Amp**	**LatOn**	**L**	**R**
	Ankle		2.83	3.01	4.83	3.50	n/a	n/a	70	70	>2.5 mV	<6 msec	32.8	33.1
	Popliteal fossa		2.63	2.60	10.75	10.42	54.9	49.2	325	340	—	—	32.7	33.1
	Post exercise		2.74	—	4.67	—	—	—	—	—	—	—	33.4	—
Tibial	Ankle	AH	10.16	—	4.42	—	—	—	80	—	>4 mV	<6 msec	33.1	—
	Popliteal fossa		6.88	—	11.58	—	47.4	—	340	—	—	—	33.0	—
Pero-neal/TA	Fibular head	Tibialis anterior	3.61	5.49	2.58	2.25	—	—	—	—	—	—	32.3	32.8
	Popliteal fossa		3.56	5.03	4.17	3.92	56.8	60.0	90	100	—	—	32.3	32.7

F-WAVE SIDE-TO-SIDE COMPARISON TABLE

			Latency (msec)	
Nerve	**Stimulus**	**Recording**	**L**	**R**
Tibial	Ankle	Abd. hallus brevis	45.17	—

H REFLEX SUMMARY TABLE

					M Wave		H Reflexes	
Nerve	**Stimulus**	**Recording**	**Side**	**Wave**	**Lat (msec)**	**Amp (mV)**	**Lat (msec)**	**Amp (mV)**
Tibial	Popliteal fossa	Soleus	Left	All	5.00	4.77	30.83	1.20
			Right		5.33	6.25	27.50	1.03

Table continues on following page

TABLE 178-5

Electrodiagnostic Examination: 68-Year-Old, Right-Handed Man—cont.

NEEDLE ELECTRODE EXAMINATION SUMMARY										
			Spontaneous Activity			Motor Unit Action Potentials				
Side	**Muscle**	**InsAct**	**Fib**	**PW**	**Fasc**	**Activation**	**Recruitment**	**Dur**	**Amp**	**Poly**
Left	Lumbar PSP—low	Norm	0	0	0	NE	NE	Norm	Norm	Norm
	Sacral PSP—high	Norm	0	0	0	NE	NE	Norm	Norm	Norm
	Iliacus	Norm	0	0	0	Norm	Norm	Norm	Norm	Norm
	Vastus lateralis	Norm	0	0	0	Norm	Norm	Norm	Norm	Norm
	Tensor fascia lata	Norm	0	0	0	Norm	Decreased	Inc	Norm	Inc
	Gluteus medius	Norm	0	0	0	Norm	Decreased	Inc	Norm	Inc
	Gluteus maximus	Norm	0	0	0	Norm	Norm	Norm	Norm	Norm
	Semitendinosus	Norm	0	0	0	Norm	Decreased	Inc	Norm	Inc
	Peroneus longus	Norm	0	+	0	Norm	Decreased	Inc	Norm	Inc
	Tibialis anterior	Norm	+	+	0	Norm	Decreased	Inc	Norm	Inc
	Flex. digitorum longus	Norm	+	+	0	Norm	Decreased	Inc	Norm	Inc
	Ext. digitorum brevis	Norm	+	0	0	Norm	Decreased	Inc	Norm	Inc
	Gastrocnemius md.	Norm	0	0	0	Norm	Norm	Norm	Norm	Norm
	Abd. hallus brevis	Norm	0	0	0	Norm	Norm	Norm	Norm	Norm
Right	Vastus lateralis	Norm	0	0	0	Norm	Norm	Norm	Norm	Norm
	Gluteus medius	Norm	0	0	0	Norm	Decreased	Inc	Norm	Inc
	Tibialis anterior	Norm	0	0	0	Norm	Decreased	Inc	Norm	Inc
	Flex. digitorum longus	Norm	0	0	0	Norm	Decreased	Inc	Norm	Inc
	Ext. digitorum brevis	Norm	0	0	0	Norm	Decreased	Inc	Norm	Inc
	Abd. hallus brevis	Norm	0	0	0	Norm	Norm	Norm	Norm	Norm

+, present; –, absent; Amp, amplitude; B-P Amp, baseline-to-peak amplitude; CV, conduction velocity (meters/second); Dist, distance (millimeters); Dur, duration; Fasc, fasciculation potentials; Fib, fibrillation potentials; Inc, increased; InsAct, insertional activity; L, left; LatNPk, latency-to-negative peak; LatOn, latency to onset; NE, not examined; Norm, normal; Poly, polyphasic; PSP, paraspinal; PW, positive waves; R, right; Temp, temperature.

from evidence of severe bilateral (most often asymmetrical) lumbosacral radiculopathies to a relatively normal study. Due to potential involvement of the cauda equina, H reflex recordings and lower-extremity NEE should be performed bilaterally in cases of suspected lumbar canal stenosis.[11]

Postoperative Electrodignostic Examination

EDX examinations are often obtained in patients who have already undergone spine surgery. When using the EDX examination in the postoperative setting, it is important to keep in mind that the diagnostic utility of an NCS and NEE changes with time from surgery.

Immediately after surgery (10–14 days), a new, severe axon loss lesion can be evidenced by an absent or significantly reduced amplitude motor response (ideally with a preoperative study comparison). A normal CMAP amplitude recorded from a clinically weak muscle (e.g., the tibialis anterior muscle in a patient with footdrop) can exclude motor axon loss as the cause. The remaining possibilities at this stage include proximal conduction block, a lesion affecting the CNS, and nonorganic causes. Active motor axon loss changes identified on NEE during this period must be attributed to lesions predating surgery because sufficient time has not passed for new changes to become apparent.

In the 3-week to 4-month postoperative period, evidence of new perioperative motor axon loss changes becomes apparent on NEE. This may not address whether a nerve root decompression was "successful," because the typical EDX abnormalities caused by the preoperative root compression, including fibrillation potentials, may still be present during this period. However, any conduction block at the root level may resolve after decompression, resulting in a more normal MUAP recruitment pattern on NEE. In the case of an S1 radiculopathy, a previously absent H reflex may be found during this period.

In the remote postoperative period, active motor axon loss changes and their distribution in a given myotome can provide some helpful information. In particular, abundant fibrillation potentials within proximal and distal muscles of a myotome suggest the presence of ongoing or recurrent radiculopathy. As a general principle, the longer the time that has passed since surgery, the more likely that fibrillation potentials are caused by a progressive or postsurgical lesion. In contrast, chronic neurogenic motor unit potential changes may be permanent, particularly within the distal muscles, and may be the manifestation of a root injury 6 months to years prior.[11]

Recommendations for the Referring Physician

To get the most out of an EDX examination, the following recommendations are offered for referring physicians:

1. *Refer with a specific question in mind.* A patient should be referred after a complete history and neurologic examination. The EDX examination can then be focused to facilitate localization and attempt to answer the clinical question of interest. Referring for a general survey of a limb may result in more extensive testing than is required and is less likely to yield useful results.
2. *Keep the limitations of the test in mind.* In particular, with regard to radiculopathies, the EDX examination cannot detect all compressive radiculopathies and therefore cannot be used to exclude the diagnosis. In this context, the examination is more useful for establishing the presence of a radiculopathy, estimating its acuity/severity, and excluding other potential localizations as described earlier.

Other important limitations apply to patients with extensive peripheral edema and morbid obesity. In these cases, an NCS may be unelicitable due to increased distance between the recording electrode and the target muscle or nerve, and ability to access certain muscles may not be possible even with the longest-needle electrode. In these cases, the diagnostic utility of the EDX examination is limited.

Finally, EDX localization can be more difficult in elderly patients. In particular, a portion of normal individuals older than age 60 have bilaterally unelicitable sural and superficial peroneal SNAPs.[3] In these cases, differentiation between an intraspinal and extraspinal canal localization can be challenging, particularly in the absence of localizing active motor axon loss changes (e.g., fibrillation potentials) throughout a particular myotome. Thus, in older patients, normal aging, a mild chronic peripheral polyneuropathy, and mild bilateral chronic L5 and S1 radiculopathies may appear electrodiagnostically similar, even with contralateral comparison and evaluation of an upper extremity to assess for evidence of a gradient (i.e., suggestive of a length-dependent polyneuropathy).

3. *Consider the onset of symptoms and timing of the examination.* A 3-week waiting period after symptom onset is recommended prior to EDX examination in order to allow fibrillation potentials to develop, maximizing the localizing value of the test. Studying the patient as soon as feasible after the initial waiting period is also advisable, due to the tendency for the EDX examination to normalize with time.
4. *Prepare patients for the test.* Although testing is generally well tolerated by most patients, some degree of discomfort is inherent to both NCSs and NEEs. Patients should be made aware of this prior to their arrival at the EDX testing site. Also, the EDX laboratory should be contacted in advance to determine their procedures for managing special situations such as coagulation abnormalities, use of the medication warfarin, and patients with implantable electronic devices (e.g., spinal cord stimulators), as protocols vary.

KEY REFERENCES

Levin KH: Electrodiagnostic approach to the patient with suspected radiculopathy. *Neurol Clin* 20:397–421, vi, 2002.

Levin KH, Lüders H: *Comprehensive clinical neurophysiology*, Philadelphia, 2000, WB Saunders.

Levin KH, Maggiano HJ, Wilbourn AJ: Cervical radiculopathies: comparison of surgical and EMG localization of single-root lesions. *Neurology* 46:1022–1025, 1996.

Preston DC, Shapiro BE: *Electromyography and neuromuscular disorders: clinical-electrophysiologic correlations*, ed 2, Philadelphia, 2005, Butterworth-Heinemann.

Wilbourn AJ: AAEE case report #12: Common peroneal mononeuropathy at the fibular head. *Muscle Nerve* 9:825–836, 1986.

Wilbourn AJ: Nerve conduction studies. Types, components, abnormalities, and value in localization. *Neurol Clin* 20(305):38, 2002.
Wilbourn AJ, Aminoff MJ: AAEM minimonograph 32: the electrodiagnostic examination in patients with radiculopathies. American Association of Electrodiagnostic Medicine. *Muscle Nerve* 21:1612–1631, 1998.

REFERENCES

The complete reference list is available online at expertconsult.com.

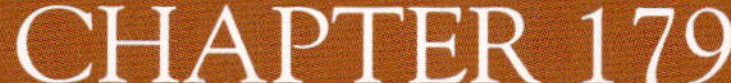
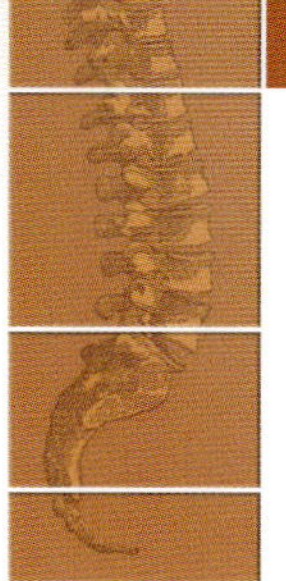

CHAPTER 179

Intraoperative Nonparalytic Monitoring

Robert F. McLain | Fanor Manuel Saavedra

Spinal surgery is continuously evolving and becoming increasingly complex. Surgeons are routinely tackling more difficult pathologies. Technical and material advancements have made this possible. Adjunctive measures such as a myriad of monitoring techniques have been present and available for some time but have varied in their usage and proven effectiveness. To understand the role of intraoperative monitoring and the techniques used, the available information is presented.

Current Techniques

Currently available techniques for intraoperative neurophysiologic monitoring of the spinal cord include somatosensory-evoked potential (SSEP), motor-evoked potential (MEP), and electromyography (EMG). In addition, some institutions use other methodologies, including neurogenic MEP, also known as spinally elicited MEP and dermatomal SSEP. Continuous neurophysiologic monitoring is an important tool that may reduce intraoperative neurologic morbidity. The principles, advantages, and disadvantages are discussed.

Although objective evidence for efficacy of electrophysiologic monitoring techniques is sparse, improvements in monitoring and advances in technique have made their use routine. Reliance on electrodiagnostic techniques remains solely at the discretion of the surgeon, and there are some instances where external monitoring is either not necessary or not helpful. Alternative monitoring techniques, such as nonparalytic monitoring techniques, may provide an alternative approach in these cases. This chapter discusses such a strategy.

Wake-Up Test

A number of methods have been developed for the intraoperative monitoring of spinal cord function. The earliest documented systematic approach to the intraoperative monitoring of spinal cord function was the wake-up test.[1] Commonly referred to as the Stagnara wake-up test, this technique often provides an unequivocal demonstration of the integrity of long motor tract function. However, it provides this information for one point in time and, in fact, is observed after any potentially harmful surgical manipulation has already taken place. The ability to monitor evoked potentials accurately has made the need for this test less common.[1-4]

In 1973, Vauzelle et al.[5] described the intraoperative wake-up test, which is still considered the gold standard by some centers. It enables the surgeon to perform a brief neurologic examination to the sedated but arousable patient and to directly evaluate the functional integrity of the neuronal structures. The patient is awoken from general anesthesia prior to wound closure, allowing the surgeon to assess for any neurologic deficits that may have resulted from surgical manipulation or instrumentation. If there is a neurologic deficit, the deformity correction and/or instrumentation can be revised immediately.

The requirements of the intraoperative wake-up test are simple. The patient must be told that the test may be performed. If the test is anticipated, a full explanation must ensue, describing the procedure and expected conditions on awakening (i.e., intubation, confusion, levels of discomfort).[6]

The anesthetic technique is critical for managing patient wakefulness and limiting the degree of discomfort. Introduction of local anesthetic to the pharynx and larynx, either by transcutaneous injection or spray, ensures patient comfort on awakening. An initial loading dose of a narcotic with continuous infusion is the preferred anesthetic regimen, because concomitant electrophysiologic monitoring may be affected by halogenated anesthesia. Narcotics and halogenated anesthesia, typically fentanyl and isoflurane, are discontinued 30 minutes prior to awakening the patient. Approximately 10 minutes prior to awakening, paralytic agents are reversed and nitrous oxide is discontinued. This regimen should provide a wakeful patient who is able to follow commands in approximately 5 more minutes.

Once awakened, the patient is asked to appropriately move the arms and legs (e.g., "squeeze my hand," "wiggle your toes"). Discovered deficits require reevaluation of the patient's position, the instrumentation, and consideration of vascular compromise. Therefore, both the surgeon and anesthesia team must be prepared for reawakening following their initial assessment. The use of the intraoperative wake-up test is limited by patient tolerance, additional operative time, and a limited assessment of the neurologic status during the test only. Modern neurophysiologic monitoring provides the benefit of patient comfort with the indirect continuous assessment of neurologic status during surgery.

Although electrophysiologic monitoring may obviate the need for the intraoperative wake-up test in most patients, technical difficulties or potentially misleading results of the neurophysiologic monitoring may warrant a wake-up test. It is particularly useful when electrophysiologic changes suggest a progressive deterioration with no apparent cause—the test can either confirm or refute the concern that a clinically relevant problem exists. For instance, in a case of scoliosis correction, 2 hours after a ventral correction with limited vessel ligation and no related change in monitoring at that time, and 30 minutes after completion of dorsal instrumentation and curve correction, a change in amplitudes and latencies was noted on neural monitoring. The implants were checked, and no apparent compression at any level could be seen. Because the monitoring had been inconsistent during the case, a Stagnara wake-up test was performed. The test confirmed a dense paresis of the lower extremities in the face of normal upper extremity function. Medical management was optimized and steroids given. Hemodynamic support was optimized to increase cord perfusion, and imaging was performed to rule out a compressive lesion along the extent of the constructs. Reduction was relaxed to a modest degree. The patient recovered normal function within 1 hour of the observation and recovered completely. The ability to confirm the suspected deficit supported the use of all medical means to increase cord perfusion in this case.

There are two fundamental disadvantages associated with the Stagnara wake-up test: (1) it provides only momentary information about the integrity of the nervous system, and (2) the information pertains to voluntary movements only. However, this test should remain a tool in the surgeon's armamentarium.

Other Monitoring Methods

Some surgeons believe that the data acquired from intraoperative evoked potential monitoring most often are less helpful than the immediate surgical feedback provided by observation of unparalyzed muscles. However, the ability to perform monitoring in the face of partial paralysis allows surgeons to follow both electrodiagnostic input and direct motor responses to intraoperative spinal cord or nerve root manipulation. The spine surgeon, therefore, must determine the relative benefits and risks associated with these alternative techniques of intraoperative monitoring.

Deficiencies of Electrophysiologic Monitoring

In the past, authors have argued that electrophysiologic monitoring was flawed and unreliable, by virtue of its nature, because the observation of an electrophysiologic response becomes manifest after the adverse event occurs. There is a real-time lag associated with monitoring, either due to the time required for signal averaging or the need to stop for triggered motor stimulation. This time lag could mean that injury might not be recognized or minimized for some time after it occurs in the paralyzed patient.

SSEPs monitor sensory function that is transmitted through the posterior columns of the spinal cord,[2,7,8] whereas the majority of pathologic compressive lesions are ventrally located. The posterior columns monitored by SSEPs are, therefore, positioned farthest from the operative site of all spinal tracts. In the days before this vulnerability was recognized, and before MEPs were widely available, failure to detect injury was reported.[4,9,10]

SSEPs monitor the dorsal column function within the spinal cord via stimulation of peripheral nerves in the arms and in the legs. False-negative and false-positive recordings have been reported. Although reported rates vary, a large series of 50,000 patients demonstrated a 0.067% false-negative rate.[11] On average, the false-negative rate is reported to be less than 2%, and the false-positive rate is less than 3%.[12-16]

One must be aware of the technical limitations of SSEP to avoid misinterpretation. Securing both peripheral and central recording sites for the afferent volley helps differentiate technical failure from neurologic injury. A technical failure affects changes in the latencies or amplitude in both the peripheral and central recorded responses; neurologic injury affects only central responses. Moreover, following significant spinal cord injury, changes in SSEP signals may be delayed for up to 30 minutes.[14]

An undetermined fraction of monitoring errors results from unrecorded injury to the ventral spinal cord.[17,18] Deformation of the ventral spinal cord may have a limited effect on dorsal column function, thereby accounting for the false-negative rate of SSEP. Monitoring with MEP enables the assessment of the ventral spinal cord and is associated with a shorter delay between injury and changes.

Transcranial electrical stimulation must overcome the resistance of the skull. As such, current requirements are higher and associated with a significant degree of discomfort in the awake state.[19,20] Preinduction baseline recording of MEPs is therefore not possible.

MEPs can be elicited without averaging, unlike SSEP, which offers a significant advantage in terms of assessing spinal cord function in real time. In addition, it enables direct assessment of the motor function. But the interpreter must select the time to trigger and record the MEPs and must sometimes interrupt the procedure to obtain a reading.

EMG has been increasingly used during lumbar pedicle screw placement, when free-run EMG is continuously monitored for mechanical responses. The presence of neurotonic discharges or continuously discharging EMG activity may indicate nerve root irritation. The data can be confusing at times, especially with a fractured pedicle, because the clinical impact of a fractured pedicle is unknown, and the changes in capacitance associated with cortical fracture do not correlate with actual nerve injury or irritation. Because the patient is not fully paralyzed during this form of monitoring, the direct observation of nerve root stimulation and muscle contraction is still possible.

Rationale for Nonparalytic Intraoperative Monitoring

The principal argument in favor of nonparalytic intraoperative monitoring revolves around the use of intraoperative observation of motor responses evoked by surgical manipulation as a monitoring technique. The point is made that the majority of surgical procedures during which electrodiagnostic monitoring

TABLE 179-1

Effectiveness of Electrodiagnostic Testing

	SSEPs		MEPs		EMG	
Area or Condition	**Sensitivity (%)**	**Specificity (%)**	**Sensitivity (%)**	**Specificity (%)**	**Sensitivity (%)**	**Specificity (%)**
Scoliosis	92	98.9				
Cervical-thoracic	52	100	100	96	46	73
Lumbar	28.6	98.7			100	23.7

	Multimodality Monitoring (SSEPs, MEPs, EMG)	
	Sensitivity (%)	**Specificity (%)**
All spine	89–100	84.3–99

EMG, electromyography; MEP, motor-evoked potential; SSEP, somatosensory-evoked potential.

might be beneficial involve neural decompression.[21] The surgeon is able to directly observe the neural elements during the critical components of laminectomy and decompression, and this "direct observation" type of monitoring is, therefore, the most useful to the surgeon. For example, the observation of the dural sac and its relationship to surrounding and confining bony and soft tissue structures affords the skilled and alert surgeon the opportunity to monitor the extent of neural distortion and compression in real time. Some might argue that this is not so much monitoring as just careful surgical technique.

Direct observation can play little or no role in scoliosis surgery, however. In scoliosis surgery, the spinal cord is threatened indirectly by ischemia associated with stretching or tethering, brought on by curve correction or ligation of segmental vessels. There is no way to predict the degree of cord stress by observing the magnitude of curve correction achieved during instrumentation. Similarly, in situations where the cord has been chronically stressed, as in thoracic kyphosis and chronic stenosis, there is no way to predict the effect of additional stresses imparted during surgical exposure or fluctuations in perfusion pressure. In these circumstances, electrophysiologic monitoring clearly provides insight that cannot be gained otherwise.

A purported advantage of immediate intraoperative feedback provided by a motor response "felt" by the surgeon during a particular maneuver is that there is no delay; the patient's movement is indeed so frightening that one stops reflexively whatever action evoked the response. Even if minuscule, the delays inherent in electrophysiologic monitoring of the fully paralyzed patient are deemed unacceptable when compared with the immediacy of clinical monitoring of the unparalyzed patient. Proponents of observational monitoring note that motor responses triggered by nerve root stimulation have been noted frequently with bipolar or unipolar coagulation on the lateral vertebral body and the posterior longitudinal ligament. Patients experiencing surgical maneuvers that have caused a more global, total body movement, demonstrate a spinal cord response to inadvertent percussion or pressure. Unfortunately, even real-time feedback may not prevent permanent injury in this kind of event. Any device or instrument that triggers this sort of response should be removed from the canal immediately.

Using current electrodiagnostic monitoring methodologies, full paralysis is unnecessary, and almost any case can be carried out with some residual capacity for neural response. In these cases, inadvertent stimulation of a nerve root with a probe or cautery triggers a motor response that the surgeon will recognize immediately. Intrusion into the spinal canal or shift in spinal structures that impinge the cord itself still results in a sudden, profound total body "jump." The surgical effort is reflexively stopped even before the monitoring personnel can sound a warning. With monitoring in place, however, the surgeon and staff can assess the clinical relevance of that "jump" and the possibility of injury and weigh the need for medical or further surgical treatment based on data as opposed to clinical suspicions (Table 179-1).

Summary

If inadvertent neural trauma occurs from heating, compression, distraction, or trauma, a motor response in affected nonparalyzed muscles usually occurs. This, in a sense, is the equivalent of a real-time MEP. Immediate surgical feedback is provided by observation of the motor response to a specific intraoperative neural manipulation. Immediate feedback to the surgeon makes this an effective method of preventing or limiting neurologic injury.

Technologic advances, such as electrophysiologic monitoring, cannot be used to replace intelligent surgeon input into the intraoperative decision-making process. However, common sense suggests that electrophysiologic monitoring should be used as an intraoperative decision-making tool alongside classic observational techniques of nonparalytic monitoring.

KEY REFERENCES

Lesser RP, Raudzens P, Luders H, et al: Postoperative neurological deficits may occur despite unchanged intraoperative somatosensory evoked potentials. *Ann Neurol* 19:22–25, 1986.

Minahan RE, Sepkuty JP, Lesser RP, et al: Anterior spinal cord injury with preserved neurogenic "motor" evoked potentials. *Clin Neurophysiol* 112:1442–1450, 2001.

Nuwer MR, Dawson EG, Carlson LG, et al: Somatosensory evoked potential spinal cord monitoring reduces neurological deficits after scoliosis surgery: results of a large multicenter survey. *EEG Clin Neurophysiol* 96:6–11, 1995.

Powers SK, Bolger CA, Edwards MS: Spinal cord pathways mediating somatosensory evoked potentials. *J Neurosurg* 57:472–482, 1982.

Vauzelle C, Stagnara P, Jouvinroux P: Functional monitoring of spinal cord activity during spinal surgery. *Clin Orthop Relat Res* 93:173–178, 1973.

REFERENCES

The complete reference list is available online at expert.consult.com.

SECTION 8

Nonsurgical Management

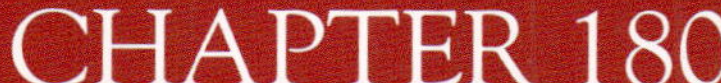

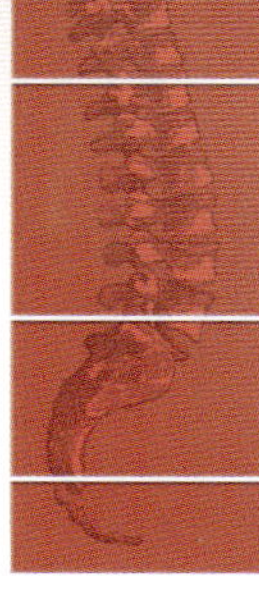

CHAPTER 180

Anesthesia

Marc L. Bertrand | Lisabeth L. Maloney

Historically, spine surgery has played "second fiddle" to intracranial neurosurgery in the minds of many anesthesiologists. With advances in surgical technique and concomitant improvements in anesthetic management, however, surgical spine procedures are performed increasingly on elderly and medically compromised patients. Spine surgeons are now able to perform procedures once considered impossible, providing anesthesiologists with some of their most significant clinical challenges. This chapter acquaints spine surgeons with anesthetic concerns and with techniques used during anesthesia for spine surgery.

Preoperative Assessment

Preoperative evaluation allows the anesthesiologist to become familiar with the spine surgery patient's functional status, coexisting medical diseases, medications, allergies, and anesthetic concerns. It also provides the opportunity to obtain informed consent for anesthesia. A thorough review of symptoms attributable to cardiac or respiratory dysfunction is especially important during the preoperative interview, given that these two systems contribute most to postoperative morbidity. Anesthesiologists can assess airway anatomy and cervical spine mobility to identify patients who may require specialized airway management.

Laboratory Studies

Routine laboratory screening tests, including coagulation studies, rarely reveal abnormalities that were not apparent from the history and physical examination. It is reasonable to obtain a preoperative hemoglobin and hematocrit in patients with coexisting disease or a history of anemia and serum electrolytes in patients being treated with diuretics. Chronic hypokalemia, to a serum potassium of 3 mmol/L, is not a contraindication to elective surgery in the absence of cardiac comorbidity, symptomatic arrhythmias, or digitalis therapy.[1] Symptomatic chronic hypokalemia in the perioperative period requires oral replacement on an outpatient basis because rapid IV supplementation may increase morbidity and mortality.[2] Preoperative electrocardiograms and chest radiographs should be limited to elderly patients or to those with known or suspected cardiopulmonary disease.

Considerations in Patients with Spinal Cord Injury

Preoperative considerations in spinal cord injury (SCI) patients vary with the timing of surgery in relation to the time of and the anatomic level of injury. Patients who show symptoms of neurologic deficits secondary to acute SCI are the most challenging. SCI patients must have sufficient respiratory muscle strength to oxygenate and ventilate effectively. They may have impaired coughing ability and significant ventilation-perfusion mismatch.[3] Pneumonias are common in patients with acute or chronic SCIs due to the high incidence of aspiration and pulmonary dysfunction with lesions above T7.[4] The potential for associated injuries related to trauma, including rib fractures, pneumothoraces, closed-head injuries, and pelvic fractures, must be considered. Most of these patients show symptoms of varying degrees of hypotension as well as impaired myocardial contractility resulting from acute sympathetic denervation. They require judicious volume loading and, often, vasopressors and/or inotropes to maintain adequate organ perfusion pressure. Depolarizing muscle relaxants may result in fatal hyperkalemia.

In the patient with chronic SCI, a history of autonomic hyper-reflexia usually portends an intraoperative exacerbation. Autonomic hyper-reflexia is most often seen in patients with sensory levels at or above T4-7. Distention of the stomach, bladder, or rectum is the most common precipitating factor, and removal of the inciting stimulus is the primary treatment. Both spinal anesthesia and deep general anesthesia assist in blocking this reflex response.

Considerations in Patients with Scoliosis

It is important to evaluate the degree of preoperative pulmonary compromise in the patient with scoliosis. Pulmonary function tests are quite useful in this patient population. The forced vital capacity (FVC) and forced expiratory volume in 1 second (FEV_1) are the best indicators of the extent of restrictive lung disease caused by the thoracic deformity. Baseline arterial blood gas measurement or preoperative oximetry may also be helpful in guiding postoperative care.

Considerations in Patients with Rheumatoid Arthritis

Patients with rheumatoid arthritis must be carefully evaluated for the extent of their systemic disease so that the risks of surgery and anesthesia may be minimized. Deformities produced by articular involvement may make intravascular catheter placement difficult and increase the risk of positioning-related injury. Cervical spine films should be obtained because up to 30% of these patients may have asymptomatic cervical instability.[5] Cervical spine instability or significant temporomandibular joint disease may require awake fiberoptic airway management and strict attention to positioning. The electrocardiogram should be examined for the presence of conduction abnormalities, and an echocardiogram should be obtained if there are any history or physical examination findings compatible with valvular dysfunction. The serum blood urea nitrogen (BUN) and creatinine should be checked to assess renal function in patients taking high doses of nonsteroidal anti-inflammatory drugs. Liver function tests are useful in patients taking cytotoxic drugs. Finally, stress-dose steroids should be ordered for all patients with a recent history of steroid use.

Other Disorders

A variety of other disorders affect spine surgery patients in the preoperative period. Patients with mass lesions of the cervical spine require preoperative assessment to determine whether specialized airway management is necessary. Patients with primary vascular spinal cord tumors require preoperative preparation for massive transfusion. Those with a history of myelomeningocele, SCI, or other disorders that require chronic catheterization may be sensitive to latex. A latex-free environment should be ensured at the time of surgery for all patients with a history of latex sensitivity. Consideration should also be given to preoperative prophylaxis with H_1- and H_2-receptor blockers and steroids in patients with a documented history of significant reaction to latex.

Pharmacology

Preoperative medications serve a variety of functions, including sedation, amnesia, anxiolysis, and aspiration prophylaxis. The goal of premedication in the neurosurgical patient is to provide anxiolysis with minimal sedation at the termination of surgery. Benzodiazepines have largely supplanted barbiturates and anticholinergics for this purpose. The reliability of midazolam in the immediate preoperative period has greatly reduced the need for longer-acting premedicants. H_2 blockers raise the pH of gastric fluid[6] and usually decrease gastric volume in patients at risk for aspiration. However, the routine use of histamine blockers for aspiration prophylaxis in patients not at risk is difficult to justify, given their cost.

Ideal Agent

The ideal anesthetic agent for spine surgery provides stable hemodynamics with rapid awakening to permit prompt postoperative neurologic assessment. In addition, it would be beneficial if such an agent conferred some neurologic protection against ischemic injury. Most anesthetic agents in current use have been studied extensively in relation to these goals for intracranial procedures. Few studies, however, have examined their effects specifically on the spinal cord. The following pharmacologic descriptions are based on studies that examined cerebral physiology and cerebral protection primarily.

Induction

Agents used to induce anesthesia include barbiturates, narcotics, benzodiazepines, and a variety of other unclassified drugs. Since the early 1940s, the barbiturates have been used for this purpose and reliably decrease cerebral blood flow, cerebral metabolic rate of oxygen ($CMRO_2$), and intracranial pressure (ICP). Treatment with barbiturates after a global ischemic event does not appear to provide neuronal protection. Barbiturate administration after focal or partial ischemic events, however, seems to provide some protection from neurologic injury.[7] These agents have limited use in maintaining anesthesia secondary to their prolonged effects. Most of them depress cardiac output and systemic vascular resistance, so care must be taken when they are given to a hypovolemic or traumatized patient.

Propofol

Propofol, a sedative-hypnotic agent, possesses all the benefits of the barbiturates with regard to reduction of cerebral blood flow and $CMRO_2$.[8] Propofol is cleared rapidly and produces prompt awakening in patients shortly after an infusion is discontinued. The autoregulatory capacity of the cerebral circulation remains intact during propofol anesthesia.[9] To date, there is little experimental evidence indicating that propofol provides a significant degree of neurologic protection in temporary focal ischemia models. The only animal study suggesting a protective benefit of propofol in burst-suppressive doses failed to measure or control cerebral perfusion pressure.[10]

Ketamine

Ketamine, a phencyclidine derivative, differs from most induction drugs in that it raises $CMRO_2$, blood flow, and ICP.[11] It is thus less ideal for neuroanesthesia, but these are desirable properties for use in the hypovolemic patient. Ketamine preserves central circulating volume and afterload in patients with traumatic spinal cord lesions secondary to the release of endogenous catecholamines. However, in severely hypovolemic patients who have exhausted their sympathetic reserve, the bolus administration of ketamine may result in hemodynamic collapse because of its unopposed direct myocardial depressant effects.

Inhalation Agents

Inhalation anesthetics are the agents used most commonly for the maintenance of general anesthesia. Their mode of delivery and pharmacokinetics allow for controlled, predictable action and easy reversal. They are typically mixed with inspired gases via vaporizers, which are devices that make adjustments for temperature, flow rate, and anesthetic vapor pressure so that a known quantity can be delivered over a wide range of conditions. The inhalation agents act on the brain via an unknown mechanism. Hypothesized mechanisms include membrane protein inhibition and membrane depolarization through membrane swelling or carrier protein inhibition.[12] Anesthetic potency parallels the lipid solubility of the agent. A standard known as the minimum alveolar concentration (MAC) is used as a guide to compare anesthetics of different potency. One MAC of any anesthetic is the end-tidal concentration that will render 50% of patients immobile to the surgical incision. The MAC for different anesthetic agents is additive; 0.5 MAC of nitrous oxide mixed with 1 MAC of isoflurane yields 1.5 MAC of anesthetic.

A number of factors determine the rate of increase of the partial pressure of an anesthetic in the brain, and hence its speed of onset. These factors include the concentration of the anesthetic delivered, solubility of the anesthetic in both the blood and the brain, alveolar ventilation, cardiac output, and presence of intrapulmonary or intracardiac shunts.[13] For example, nitrous oxide is a poorly soluble gas with a MAC of 105% that is routinely delivered in high concentrations (50–70%) and has the most rapid onset of action. Isoflurane has intermediate solubility, a MAC of 1.2%, and a slower onset.

The inhalation anesthetics currently in common use include isoflurane, desflurane, and sevoflurane. They all possess cerebral vasodilator properties and decrease blood pressure by reducing either cardiac output or systemic vascular resistance. The increased cerebral blood flow seen with isoflurane can be attenuated by hyperventilation and a reduction in the partial pressure of carbon dioxide (P_{CO_2}).[14] Desflurane and sevoflurane are both less soluble in blood than isoflurane and possess the theoretic advantage of more rapid emergence. Their effects on the cerebral vasculature parallel those of isoflurane,[15] although sevoflurane appears to preserve the autoregulatory ability of the cerebral vasculature at higher MAC levels than either isoflurane or desflurane. Nitrous oxide is the least potent and most used inhalation agent and exhibits a favorable safety profile in spine surgery. It causes a mild rise in blood pressure and ICP when used alone. It is not clear if any inhalation agent confers specific advantages in spinal cord surgery, and agent choice should be dictated by the overall anesthetic plan.

Narcotics

Narcotics are used frequently in conjunction with other agents as part of a balanced anesthetic. They provide reliable suppression of the catecholamine response to surgical stimulation and superior analgesia without appreciable changes in spinal cord blood flow. Narcotics also provide a stable background for intraoperative neurophysiologic monitoring. The use of continuous-infusion techniques for narcotic administration allows for predictable pharmacokinetics and reliable termination of action at the termination of surgery.

Remifentanil, one of our newest narcotic agents, is unique in that it does not demonstrate any significant accumulation over prolonged periods of infusion. Recovery from remifentanil is essentially dose-independent because of its rapid esterase metabolism.[16] Remifentanil is particularly useful in cases involving somatosensory-evoked potential (SSEP) or motor-evoked potential (MEP) monitoring as well as any case requiring a total intravenous anesthetic (TIVA). Because of the rapid offset of remifentanil, which is faster than the onset of most other analgesics, care must be taken to provide supplemental analgesics prior to stopping remifentanil in cases where substantial postoperative pain is anticipated.[17]

Muscle Relaxants

The use of muscle relaxants in spine surgery optimizes the conditions for intubation, provides an immobile surgical field, and reduces the risk of patient coughing and straining. Muscle relaxants may be broadly classified into two groups: depolarizing and nondepolarizing. Succinylcholine, the only depolarizing agent approved for use in the United States, has a rapid onset and short duration, qualities that make it useful when rapid intubation conditions are desired. This agent actively depolarizes the muscle at the myoneural junction until it becomes refractory to further stimulation. Typically, the administration of succinylcholine produces a 0.5-mEq/L rise in serum potassium.[18] Succinylcholine also depolarizes extrajunctional acetylcholine receptors in patients with burns or denervation injuries. These receptors are more numerous and have a greater ionic permeability, leading to acute, profound hyperkalemia when stimulated.[19] The risk of hyperkalemia is greatest after 3 to 7 days after injury and may persist for several years.[20] Life-threatening succinylcholine-induced hyperkalemia has been hypothesized but not reported after immobilization or disuse atrophy in the absence of other causal factors.[21] Succinylcholine is also a triggering agent for malignant hyperthermia and is contraindicated in any patient with a family history of malignant hyperthermia or a history of degenerative muscular disease. The routine use of succinylcholine is also contraindicated in children based on several reports of postadministration hyperkalemic cardiac arrest presumed secondary to unrecognized or undiagnosed muscular dystrophy.

The nondepolarizing muscle relaxants, including pancuronium, vecuronium, rocuronium, and cisatracurium, differ from one another primarily in onset and duration of action. These agents all bind to the myoneural junction and competitively inhibit the binding of acetylcholine. The extent of neuromuscular blockade is monitored intraoperatively in a number of ways. The most reliable method is with the use of a train-of-four (TOF) monitor. This device allows for subjective or objective comparison of the ratio of the first and fourth muscle stimuli, which correlates well with the density of receptor occupation. A ratio less than 0.25 correlates with dense paralysis, and a ratio greater than 0.75 correlates well with the patient's ability to maintain protective airway reflexes after extubation.[22]

Muscle relaxants provide both optimal intubation conditions during induction of anesthesia and maintenance of muscle relaxation intraoperatively. Paralysis is preferred by some spine surgeons and ensures a "quiet" operative field. Other surgeons prefer to avoid muscle relaxation so that any direct stimulation of peripheral nerves will be readily apparent (nonparalytic anesthetic intraoperative monitoring).

Muscle relaxation is reversed by the administration of anticholinesterase agents. These agents reliably reverse a blockade when the effects of the nondepolarizing muscle relaxant have begun to fade. Because these compounds increase acetylcholine levels at all cholinergic receptors, they are usually given in conjunction with a muscarinic anticholinergic drug (e.g., atropine or glycopyrrolate) to prevent unwanted bradycardia, salivation, and bronchial secretions.

The most important factors that affect the ability to reverse muscle relaxation are the depth of block at the time of reversal, choice and method of administration of relaxant, and dose of reversal agent. Other factors that may antagonize the ability to reverse a nondepolarizing blockade include hypothermia, metabolic acidosis, respiratory alkalosis, and the administration of certain antibiotics.[23] As previously mentioned, reversal is followed with the TOF monitor. The best clinical assessment of adequate reversal is the ability of the patient to sustain an unassisted head lift for at least 5 seconds. The assessment of less cooperative patients can be carried out by observing the negative inspiratory force generated during spontaneous ventilation. A negative inspiratory force of at least –25 cm H_2O correlates well with adequate reversal but not airway protection.[24]

Monitoring

General Monitoring

The single most important monitor in the operating room is the anesthesia provider. This person is responsible for collecting and analyzing both subjective and objective data about the patient's vital organ function. The perioperative use of monitoring equipment greatly enhances the ability to perform this vital function. Routine monitoring during spine surgery includes electrocardiography, noninvasive blood pressure measurement, pulse oximetry, end-tidal CO_2 levels, temperature, urine output, neuromuscular blockade, and auscultation of breath and heart sounds. More invasive forms of hemodynamic monitoring may be indicated based on the complexity of the operative procedure or the severity of coexisting disease. Electrocardiographic monitoring is useful in detecting myocardial ischemia and cardiac conduction disturbances and in the analysis of arrhythmias.

Patients with both acute and chronic cervical spine injuries may show symptoms of a variety of specific electrocardiographic abnormalities. These abnormalities have been attributed to the autonomic imbalance created by disruption of sympathetic pathways located in the cervical cord. Severe acute cervical spine injury is frequently associated with marked sinus bradycardia. It also carries an increased incidence of ventricular and supraventricular arrhythmias, as well as cardiac arrest, when compared with injury of the thoracolumbar spine.[25] Multilead ST-segment elevation has been noted in a significant percentage of patients with chronic, complete SCI. These alterations in ventricular repolarization are hypothesized to be manifestations of central sympathetic dysfunction and, indeed, resolve with low-dose isoproterenol infusion.[26]

Systemic blood pressure is used as an indirect monitor of organ perfusion. For the majority of elective spine procedures, noninvasive blood pressure monitoring is adequate and sufficient. Invasive monitoring of arterial blood pressure is recommended for patients with a history of significant cardiopulmonary disease, those with preoperative hemodynamic instability, those at risk for significant blood loss, and those who may require a period of postoperative ventilatory support when frequent blood gas measurements are anticipated.

Central monitoring of venous or pulmonary artery pressure may be indicated in patients with a history of ischemic heart disease or left ventricular dysfunction, particularly in the setting of anticipated large blood loss or fluid shifts. In patients with normal cardiac function, central venous pressures provide an adequate estimate of left ventricular end-diastolic volume. A pulmonary artery catheter, however, may more accurately assess left ventricular volume in patients with ventricular dysfunction. Acute cervical spine injury with spinal shock is associated with substantial hemodynamic lability and a high incidence of left ventricular dysfunction.[27] Spinal shock patients are less tolerant of aggressive fluid replacement and more prone to develop pulmonary edema. The acutely quadriplegic patient qualified for surgery should be monitored with both an arterial line and either a central venous or pulmonary artery catheter.

In the majority of spine surgery patients, intravascular volume status can be monitored without invasive central monitoring techniques. For those patients in whom central monitoring is necessary, two practical points should be considered. First, long-arm placement of central lines is the preferred approach to cervical spine procedures because it allows for optimal field avoidance. Second, the absolute accuracy of central monitoring in general, and pulmonary wedge pressures in particular, is questionable in positions other than supine. Thus, patient position for surgery may influence the decision of whether central monitoring is employed.

Neurophysiologic Monitoring

Awake Patient

The awake patient is the ultimate spinal cord monitor. Several case reports describe the use of local anesthesia for spine surgery in the awake patient, although it is not a common means of neurologic monitoring. Chang[28] and Drummond et al.[29] both describe the use of anesthesia by local infiltration for dorsal cervical osteotomy. From these descriptions it appears that at least a short period of unconsciousness may be required because of significant discomfort associated with the fracturing of the anterior longitudinal ligament. Zigler et al.[30] presented a series of 34 consecutive cases of dorsal cervical stabilization and fusion in patients with unstable cervical spines and variable degrees of neurologic injury using local anesthesia in conjunction with light sedation. They encountered no untoward complications and found that the technique was well tolerated by patients, although occasionally bone graft harvesting under local anesthesia was uncomfortable.

Wake-Up Test

In 1973, Vauzelle et al.[31] described their use of an intraoperative "wake-up" with observation of limb movement for the assessment of spinal cord function. This simple test is an excellent monitor of gross motor function and is used most commonly during surgical procedures involving spinal column instrumentation and distraction. Its use is based on clinical evidence that neural impairment resulting from distraction is reversible when the distracting forces are modified during its early phase.[29,32] Currently, an awake patient is the only available monitoring modality to provide unequivocal intraoperative documentation of intact motor function.

An advantage of the wake-up test over more highly technical forms of neurophysiologic monitoring is that specialized equipment or ancillary monitoring personnel are unnecessary. Two limitations are (1) that the patient can only be awakened intermittently and, therefore, the anesthesiologist and surgeon are restricted to a few spot checks of the integrity of motor pathways; and (2) it is possible that neurologic impairment may occur despite a successful wake-up test. Diaz and Lockhart[33] reported one case of unresolved paraplegia after a normal wake-up test. This test may be difficult or impossible to perform in young children, patients with cognitive difficulties, and those with significant hearing impairment. A number of complications of this technique have been described, including dislodgement of spinal hardware, displacement of IV lines and monitors, accidental extubation, air embolism, and the possibility of intraoperative recall. These complications appear to be uncommon in the clinical setting, although they are always a reason for concern.[32,34]

The most important factors contributing to the successful performance of an intraoperative wake-up include adequate preoperative rehearsal with the patient and good intraoperative communication between the surgeon and anesthesiologist about the timing of the wake-up. A wide variety of anesthetic techniques can provide suitable conditions, namely a patient who is free of discomfort, is able to follow commands, and has amnesia for the event. A common technique is a nitrous oxide/narcotic/relaxant-based anesthetic with the addition of a low-dose volatile agent as needed. Frequently, a narcotic infusion provides better control of analgesia and timing of the wake-up. Other possibilities include the use of a nitrous oxide/narcotic/relaxant technique in conjunction with a propofol infusion or a total IV anesthetic using propofol and remifentanil infusions. The choice of anesthetic may be influenced and/or limited by the concurrent use of evoked-potential monitoring.

The general procedure for an intraoperative wake-up is as follows. The wake-up protocol is reviewed in detail with the patient preoperatively. If a nitrous oxide/narcotic/relaxant technique is used, the narcotics, relaxant, and any background volatile agent are discontinued approximately 30 minutes before the anticipated wake-up. The muscle relaxation is monitored using a nerve stimulator, and, if necessary, reversal agents may be given. As a rule, patients become responsive shortly after the discontinuation of the nitrous oxide. Patients are first asked to grip the anesthesiologist's hand to assess their ability to respond to commands, and then to flex and extend their feet within the direct vision of the surgical team. It is helpful to provide some gentle restraint of their head and arms in case struggling should occur. One should always be prepared to administer a bolus dose of a sedative-hypnotic agent immediately if struggling becomes problematic. The risk of air embolism may be minimized if the wound is packed and flooded with irrigating solution. Generally, the choice of anesthetic matters far less than the skill and attention with which it is administered.

Nonparalytic Anesthesia and Intraoperative Monitoring

The provision of anesthesia without the use of muscle relaxants has become increasingly popular during spine surgery. This technique provides the surgical team with a real-time means of monitoring the effects of electrocautery and surgical manipulation on neural tissues. However, the lack of muscle relaxation may pose a challenge for the anesthesiologist. Without paralysis, anesthesiologists lose their "safety net" for preventing patient movement during periods of mismatch between the level of anesthesia and the level of surgical stimulation. In other words, a greater degree of vigilance is required to maintain a quiet surgical field when muscle relaxants are not used.

Somatosensory Spinal-Evoked Potentials

SSEPs are the electrophysiologic responses of the CNS to stimulation of a peripheral nerve. SSEPs may be categorized as peripheral, spinal, subcortical, or cortical, based on the location of the recording site. Clinically, cortical SSEPs are the most commonly used, with the stimulus applied to either the posterior tibial, peroneal, and/or median nerves.

Interpretation of SSEP data is based on changes in response amplitude and latency. Amplitude is defined as the vertical dimension of the waveform and can be measured as the difference between two peaks of opposite polarity or between a specific peak and a reference point of zero potential. Latency is defined as the elapsed time between the stimulus and the response. Apel et al.[35] considered a clinically significant change in SSEPs to have occurred if latency was increased by 10% or amplitude was reduced by at least 50%. Owen,[36] however, believes that an interpretation criterion of 50% for amplitude reduction may be too sensitive and may result in unnecessary false-positive findings. He recommends that the surgeon be informed of degraded data if latency increases more than 10% or amplitude decreases more than 60% relative to baseline.

The clinical utility of SSEPs lies in their ability to demonstrate the functional integrity of neural pathways in an anesthetized and presumably unresponsive patient. Grundy et al.[37,38] have shown that intraoperative SSEPs are very sensitive indicators of hypoxia and ischemia associated with spine manipulation. Numerous cases have been reported in which early recognition of SSEP changes appeared to have prevented permanent neurologic damage by alerting the surgeon to the need for appropriate corrective action. There are also several case reports of false-negative SSEPs in which postoperative neurologic deficits occurred with preserved intraoperative waveforms.[39,40]

SSEP monitoring may not always be reliable for several reasons. Because SSEPs primarily assess posterior column function, false-negative results may occur if the neural injury is located outside the tract being monitored, that is, the anterior motor tracts. Technical problems may result in suboptimal recordings, leading to undetected changes, or a deficit may be a result of a slowly progressive structural change that began, but was not detectable, intraoperatively. Lastly, the anesthetic agents used may degrade the signal quality to such an extent that they are no longer a reliable diagnostic tool. As with many monitoring modalities, SSEPs appear to be reasonably reliable but not perfect.

In the operating room, baseline SSEPs should be recorded after the induction of anesthesia and skin incision. Serial intraoperative recordings are obtained and should always be interpreted relative to these baseline measurements. If significant changes are noted in the SSEPs, a review of the monitoring

TABLE 180-1

Effects of Anesthetic Agents on Somatosensory Spinal-Evoked Potentials

Agent	Amplitude	Latency
Isoflurane	Decrease	Increase
Nitrous oxide	Decrease	Minimal change
Propofol	Minimal change	Increase
Pentothal	Mild decrease	Increase
Ketamine	Increase	Increase
Etomidate	Marked increase	Increase
Fentanyl	Minimal increase	Mild increase
Midazolam	Decrease	Minimal increase

equipment and all temporally related surgical and anesthetic events should ensue. Physiologic alterations that may affect SSEPs include hypotension, hypothermia, anemia, hypoxemia, and changes in arterial P_{CO_2}. Changes in the depth of anesthesia may have profound effects on evoked potential waveforms. Every effort should be made to avoid alterations in the inhaled gas concentration and/or bolus injection of hypnotic agents during periods of risk. If the SSEP changes persist without adequate explanation, the possibility of injury to neural tissues exists and a wake-up test should be performed.

The preferred anesthetic for SSEP monitoring is one that allows for the recording of adequate baseline waveforms and avoids rapid alterations in anesthetic depth during the course of the surgical procedure. Many techniques satisfy these requirements but a commonly used anesthetic is a balanced O_2/N_2O/narcotic technique with low-dose volatile anesthetic supplementation ($\leq$1%). Although this regimen decreases the amplitude of SSEPs, most believe that it is compatible with effective monitoring. The use of a continuous narcotic infusion will have the least effect on evoked potential monitoring and provides additional hemodynamic stability to any anesthetic regimen. As noted in Table 180-1, IV agents generally have only modest effects on SSEPs, whereas volatile agents, such as isoflurane, attenuate the SSEP waveforms in a dose-dependent fashion. Care must be taken to maintain isoflurane concentrations at the lowest practical level.

SSEP monitoring has been associated with several unique complications. Legatt and Frost[41] reported electrocardiogram artifact produced by the triggering of the pacer enhancement circuitry in the electrocardiogram monitor by the somatosensory stimuli. Merritt et al.[42] described a case of pacemaker-mediated tachycardia induced by intraoperative SSEP stimuli. The tachycardia and associated hypotension were a result of mistaken interpretation by the programmable pacemaker of the SSEP stimulus as its own intrinsic atrial event.

Motor-Evoked Potentials

MEPs are the electrical activity measured in peripheral nerves and muscles after cortical or spinal stimulation. MEPs appear to provide a useful measure of the functional integrity of motor pathways. Theoretically, when used in conjunction with SSEPs, they allow for the monitoring of both motor and sensory pathways in the anesthetized patient and may provide more complete information about neural integrity.

MEPs may be categorized as either transcranial or spinal, depending on the location of the stimulating electrode. The stimulus may be either electrical or magnetic, with electrical stimulation being the most commonly used. The same interpretation criteria used for SSEPs of 60% loss of amplitude and 10% prolongation of latency may also be used for MEPs.[43]

MEPs are extraordinarily sensitive to anesthetic agents, with transcranial MEPs being more sensitive than spinal cord MEPs. The anesthetic techniques normally used during the monitoring of SSEPs are not compatible with MEP monitoring. Volatile anesthetics, nitrous oxide, and sodium pentothal all cause significant depression of MEPs.[44-47] Ketamine, etomidate, propofol, and narcotic agents appear to produce less significant changes.[48] The bolus injection of any of these agents during MEP monitoring may cause a transient decrease in amplitude, suggesting that continuous infusion techniques are preferable to repeated boluses.[49] The most common anesthetic currently used at our institution to provide optimal monitoring conditions for MEPs is a total IV anesthetic technique using propofol and remifentanil infusions.

A controlled level of neuromuscular blockade (90% reduction in twitch), as provided by an infusion of a neuromuscular blocking agent, permits recording of compound muscle action potentials while eliminating motor activity that could interfere with surgery.[50] However, our neuromonitoring team feels that the complete avoidance of neuromuscular blockade provides the best conditions for monitoring MEPs.

Anesthetic Techniques

With increasing numbers of diagnostic and therapeutic procedures performed in an outpatient setting, demands for safe, short-acting analgesia from the anesthesia care team have increased. The concepts of monitored anesthesia care and conscious sedation have developed from these needs. Many drugs or techniques may be used. The most common drugs for sedation are IV narcotics, benzodiazepines, or an infusion of propofol. The essential aspects of care dictate that ventilation, oxygenation, and sedation be properly monitored and that an anesthetist skilled in airway management be given the sole task of monitoring the patient during the procedure.

Regional Anesthesia

Regional anesthesia may be used for spine procedures, including lumbar discectomy. Advantages include an awake patient at the end of surgery, a lower incidence of postoperative nausea and vomiting, and more complete suppression of the stress response to surgery. Typically, with spinal anesthesia, an intermediate-acting local anesthetic such as bupivacaine is used. The disadvantage of using spinal anesthesia for spine procedures is the discomfort some patients may experience with a prolonged prone positioning. The anesthesiologist may also be concerned about emergent airway management in a prone patient, should problems arise during surgery. However, when spine surgeons and anesthesia personnel are knowledgeable in this technique they use regional anesthesia with great safety and patient satisfaction.

Regional analgesia is a useful adjunct for the management of postoperative pain after thoracic or lumbar spine surgery. Epidural or intrathecal morphine provides long-lasting analgesia and improved pulmonary mechanics with fewer systemic side effects than if given intravenously. Patients receiving neuraxial opioids require some sort of monitoring for respiratory depression, a rare but potentially fatal side effect.

General Anesthesia

Given the location and positioning requirements, most procedures that involve the spine are performed under general anesthesia. Following application of routine monitors, the patient is given an IV induction agent such as propofol Narcotics may be added to further blunt the hemodynamic response to laryngoscopy. A muscle relaxant is then administered to facilitate placement of an endotracheal tube. If the patient has a history of gastroesophageal reflux, symptomatic hiatal hernia, prior gastric surgery, gastroparesis, or recent food ingestion, a rapid sequence induction may be selected. In this case, the induction agent and rapid-onset muscle relaxant are given simultaneously without bag-mask ventilation. Endotracheal intubation can usually be accomplished within 60 seconds in patients losing their airway reflexes. Accurate endotracheal tube position is then confirmed by auscultation of breath sounds and documenting the presence of end-tidal carbon dioxide in the expired gases. The endotracheal tube is secured, the eyes are protected, and the patient is positioned for surgery.

After induction, the patient is usually given an inhalation agent or continuous IV infusion for the maintenance of anesthesia with or without further muscle relaxation. Gas exchange, systemic perfusion, and body temperature are monitored frequently throughout the procedure. At the end of it, the maintenance agents are discontinued, muscle relaxation is reversed, and the patient is extubated after adequate strength and responsiveness can be demonstrated. The patient is transported to the recovery room for continued monitoring of vital signs.

Airway Management

The inability to manage a patient's airway successfully has resulted in as many as 30% of intraoperative deaths attributable to anesthesia.[51] Effective airway management in the patient undergoing spine surgery must account for any abnormalities in airway anatomy as well as any potential or known instability in the cervical spine.

Preoperative Evaluation

Preoperative evaluation of the airway can be accomplished using three relatively simple tests that predict the difficulty of orotracheal intubation. How well the examiner can visualize the dorsal pharynx when the patient is facing the examiner in a neutral position with tongue protruded predicts the difficulty of visualization of the airway during laryngoscopy.[52,53] In addition, if the distance between the thyroid cartilage and the end of the mandible is greater than 7 cm, adequate space is usually available for ventral displacement of the tongue during visualization.[54] The third parameter is an assessment of atlanto-occipital mobility. Adequate neck extension ensures that proper alignment of the oral, pharyngeal, and laryngeal axes can be obtained.

Difficult Intubation

The probability that it will be difficult, if not impossible, to intubate a patient increases with some disease states. The most common of these are (1) congenital facial and upper airway deformities, (2) maxillofacial trauma, (3) airway tumors, (4) any known or suspected cervical spine immobility secondary to prior surgery or radiation therapy, and (5) degenerative disease or trauma to the cervical spine. When patients appear difficult to intubate, it is advisable to further evaluate the airway while they are still awake. Using topical anesthesia, with or without minimal sedation, one may perform gentle laryngoscopy to determine whether the laryngeal view will be adequate. If any uncertainty remains at this juncture, awake fiberoptic intubation should be used.

The American Society of Anesthesiologists has developed an algorithm that is designed to facilitate appropriate airway management during rapidly evolving clinical situations[55](Fig. 180-1). Patients who are known to be difficult to intubate are much less likely to suffer morbidity due to airway management if proper preparations can be made before the induction of anesthesia. Awake fiberoptic intubation under light sedation and administration of topical local anesthetic to the airway allows the anesthesiologist to definitively secure the airway while the patient is spontaneously ventilating. In addition, retrograde intubation via a guidewire fed through the cricothyroid membrane and threaded through the mouth or naris may be used as a guide for intubation during spontaneous ventilation. The retrograde technique is most useful in patients with significant maxillofacial trauma in whom visualization of the airway with a fiberoptic scope may be quite difficult because of the presence of blood and secretions.

Sometimes a difficult airway is not recognized in advance and general anesthesia is induced in the usual fashion. An immediate decision for the best management strategy centers on the ability to maintain oxygenation and ventilation through a mask airway. If the patient can be ventilated with ease using a mask and positive pressure, there is obviously more time to allow for positioning and gathering of personnel and equipment to facilitate intubation. When the patient cannot be ventilated with a mask or intubated from above, a laryngeal mask airway (LMA) can be utilized as a rescue device. The advantage of this device as an adjunct in the management of the difficult airway is that it may be inserted blindly and rapidly into the posterior pharynx, producing acceptable gas exchange in most instances. It may then be used to facilitate fiberoptic or blind endotracheal intubation. If intubation remains impossible, one must quickly provide oxygenation from a site below the oral aperture. This is accomplished most easily by the placement of a large-bore IV catheter into the trachea via the cricothyroid membrane. The catheter is then connected to a high-flow gas injection system, such as a jet ventilator. Jet ventilation may provide oxygenation until the patient is intubated or a cricothyroidotomy can be performed.

One potential disadvantage of the LMA in patients qualified for spine surgery is the need for cervical spine extension during placement, although in experienced hands the success rate of placement of the device with the head in a neutral position has been reported to be as high as 95%.[56] The LMA does not provide protection against the aspiration of stomach contents and is, therefore, contraindicated

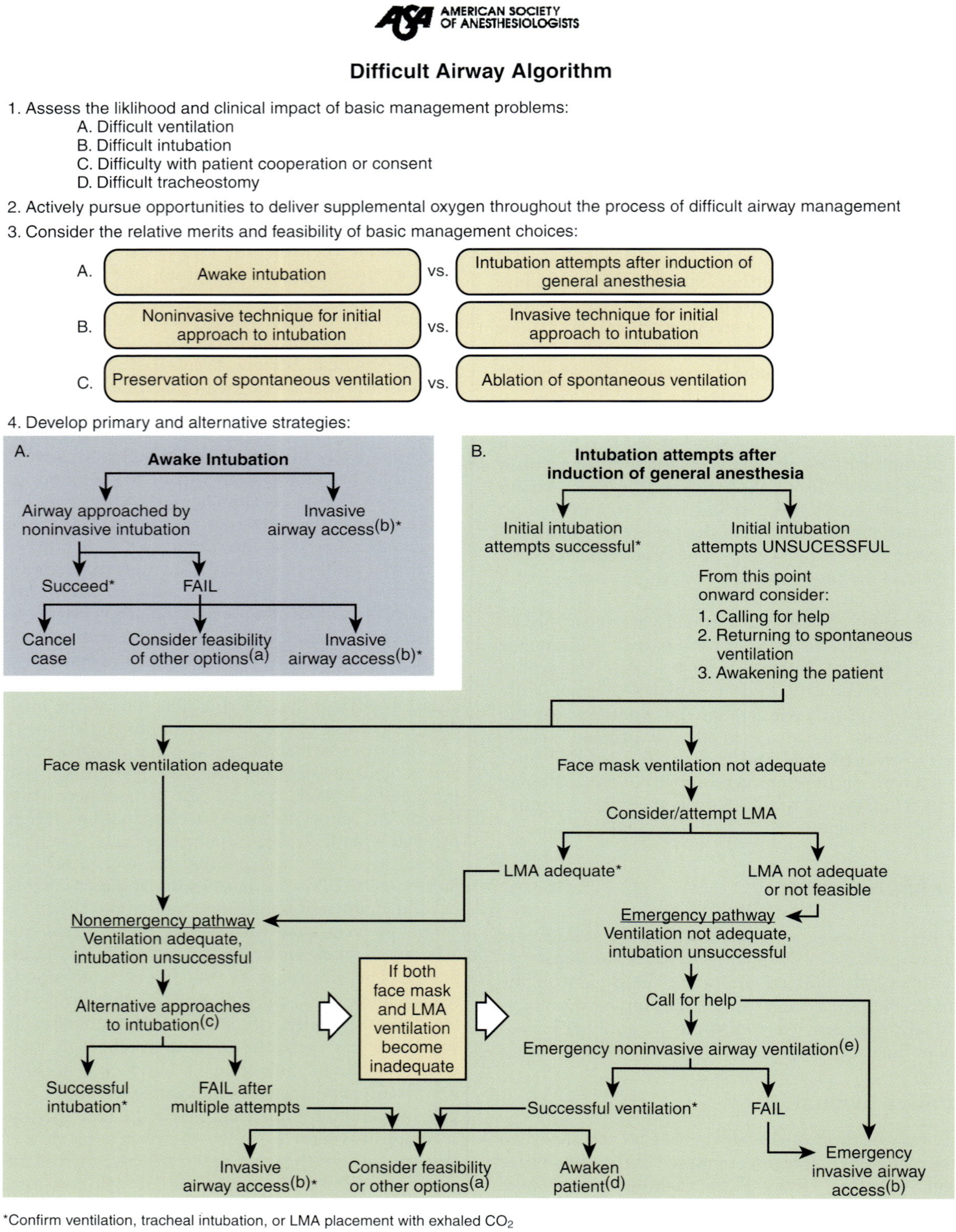

Difficult Airway Algorithm

1. Assess the liklihood and clinical impact of basic management problems:
    - A. Difficult ventilation
    - B. Difficult intubation
    - C. Difficulty with patient cooperation or consent
    - D. Difficult tracheostomy
2. Actively pursue opportunities to deliver supplemental oxygen throughout the process of difficult airway management
3. Consider the relative merits and feasibility of basic management choices:

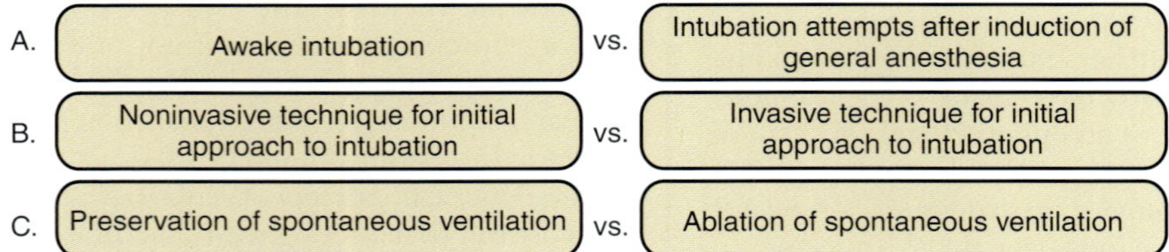

4. Develop primary and alternative strategies:

A. **Awake Intubation**

Airway approached by noninvasive intubation
Invasive airway access(b)*

Succeed*
FAIL

Cancel case
Consider feasibility of other options(a)
Invasive airway access(b)*

B. **Intubation attempts after induction of general anesthesia**

Initial intubation attempts successful*
Initial intubation attempts UNSUCESSFUL

From this point onward consider:
1. Calling for help
2. Returning to spontaneous ventilation
3. Awakening the patient

Face mask ventilation adequate
Face mask ventilation not adequate

Consider/attempt LMA

LMA adequate*
LMA not adequate or not feasible

Nonemergency pathway
Ventilation adequate, intubation unsuccessful

Emergency pathway
Ventilation not adequate, intubation unsuccessful

Alternative approaches to intubation(c)

If both face mask and LMA ventilation become inadequate

Call for help

Emergency noninvasive airway ventilation(e)

Successful intubation*
FAIL after multiple attempts
Successful ventilation*
FAIL

Invasive airway access(b)*
Consider feasibility or other options(a)
Awaken patient(d)
Emergency invasive airway access(b)

*Confirm ventilation, tracheal intubation, or LMA placement with exhaled CO_2

a. Other options include (but are not limited to): surgery utilizing face mask or LMA anesthesia, local anesthesia infiltration or regional nerve blockade. Pursuit of these option usually implies that mask ventilation will not be problematic. Therefore, these options may be of limited value if this step in the algorithm has been reached via the emergency pathway.

b. Invasive airway access includes surgical or percutaneous tracheostomy or cricothyrotomy.

c. Alternative noninvasive approaches to difficult intubation include (but are not limited to): use of different laryngoscope blades, LMA as an intubation conduit (with or without fiberoptic guidance), fiberoptic intubation, intubating stylet or tube changer, light wand, retrograde intubation, and blind oral or nasal intubation.

d. Consider re-preparation of the patient for awake intubation or canceling surgery.

e. Options for emergency noninvasive airway ventilation include (but are not limited to): rigid bronchoscope, esophageal-tracheal combitube ventilation, or transtracheal jet ventilation.

FIGURE 180-1. American Society of Anesthesiologists' difficult airway algorithm. LMA, laryngeal mask airway.

in elective airway management for the patient at risk for aspiration.

Patient with Cervical Spine Injury

In patients with potential or known cervical spine injury, airway management must be dictated by the acuity of the situation. Patients who require immediate intervention secondary to hemodynamic instability, acute respiratory failure, inability to protect their airway, or elevated intracranial pressure probably are best treated with bag-mask assisted ventilation followed by tracheal intubation with direct laryngoscopy. Usually, this can be safely accomplished with in-line stabilization of the neck in a neutral position. The risk of neurologic complications from direct laryngoscopy in patients with unstable cervical spines has not been quantified, but is probably quite low. Atlantoaxial extension with minimal movement of the lower cervical spine has been demonstrated during laryngoscopy in anesthetized patients.[57] Movement of the cervical spine is also significantly reduced when in-line stabilization is performed during laryngoscopy.[58] Several studies in the literature have shown no neurologic deterioration in patients with known cervical spine injuries after direct laryngoscopy with stabilization of the cervical spine,[59-62] and Holly and Jordon[63] reported similar safety with nasotracheal intubation. Although the risk of neurologic injury secondary to direct laryngoscopy is low, it is not zero. Recent studies of different intubation strategies on cervical spine motion suggest potential advantages with the use of fiberoptic bronchoscopy as well as the Bullard laryngoscope.[64-66]

Patient with Rheumatoid Arthritis

Airway abnormalities in patients with rheumatoid arthritis deserve special mention. In addition to having atlanto-occipital instability, these patients may exhibit scoliotic deformities of the larynx and trachea, making intubation difficult even with a fiberoptic bronchoscope.[67] Arthritic changes of the cricoarytenoid joint associated with this disease have been reported as a source of upper airway obstruction after extubation.[68]

Extubation

Extubation of the patient with a difficult airway should proceed with caution. Extra care must be taken to ensure that the effects of all respiratory depressant anesthetics are eliminated and that the patient has fully recovered from any neuromuscular blockade. This can be assessed most effectively by examining the patient's ability to maintain a voluntary head lift for greater than 5 seconds. This maneuver correlates well with the ability to maintain protective airway reflexes after extubation and to cough effectively.[24] When in doubt about the integrity of the airway resulting from surgical trauma, altered anatomy, hematoma formation, facial edema, or neurologic injury, prudence would dictate a period of postoperative mechanical ventilation with the patient in a head-elevated position until recovery is complete. Then it is possible to anesthetize the trachea with the topical administration of local anesthetic and extubate the patient under direct vision using the fiberoptic bronchoscope to assess airway integrity. A guidewire or intubating stylet may be left in place in the patient's airway after extubation to facilitate reintubation, if needed.[55]

There are several case reports of upper airway obstruction after multilevel cervical corpectomies.[69] The cause of the airway compromise is unclear but may relate to severe hypopharyngeal and supraglottic swelling secondary to either disruption of lymphatic drainage during the operative dissection, inflammation, and/or venous obstruction from small blood clots. Some centers have developed guidelines for minimizing postoperative airway complications in these patients. This includes 48 hours of postoperative intubation if a multilevel corpectomy is performed, or if operative time exceeds 5 hours.[70] Intermittent retractor release throughout the surgical procedure may help prevent this complication.

Positioning

Surgery on the spine may be performed with the patient in a variety of positions including, but not limited to, the lateral, prone, knee-chest, Concorde, or sitting position. Proper positioning and careful padding of the patient is of utmost importance and may occupy a significant period of time after the induction of anesthesia. When the patient is moved out of the supine position, the risk of positioning related nerve and soft tissue injury increases dramatically. The time spent padding and checking all pressure points is time well spent and should be a priority for all those in the operating room. Attention must be paid to the potential for hemodynamic changes and the loss of airway patency during patient positioning.

Peripheral Nerve Injury

Brachial plexus injury accounts for the greatest number of positioning-related peripheral nerve injuries. The brachial plexus is very susceptible to both excessive compression and stretch injury. Arms should not be abducted more than 90 degrees, and care should be taken to keep supports and axillary rolls well away from the axilla. Injury to the ulnar nerve is the most common nerve injury of the upper extremity, and the ulnar groove should be well padded and protected at all times. Injury to the peroneal nerve is the most common nerve injury of the lower extremity because of its vulnerable course as it wraps around the head of the fibula. Care should be taken to avoid any pressure over this area with patients in the lateral position.

Cranial Nerve Injury

Recurrent laryngeal nerve injury remains an important cause of postoperative morbidity following anterior cervical spine procedures and is generally felt to be related to retractor-mediated injury. The reported incidence of paresis and paralysis is 15% to 20%, whereas the incidence of paralysis alone is 3%.[71] Failure to perform direct laryngoscopy on asymptomatic patients in some studies may contribute to underestimation in cases of mild paresis. A predilection for injury during right-sided procedures has been noted and may be related to the anatomic pathway of the right recurrent laryngeal nerve lying outside the tracheoesophageal groove. A commonly used maneuver to help mitigate injury to the nerve (i.e., deflation and reinflation of the endotracheal tube cuff following retractor placement) does not appear to significantly affect the frequency of recurrent laryngeal nerve injury.[71]

Postoperative Visual Loss

Postoperative visual loss (POVL) after spine surgery is a relatively rare event that has been reported with increasing frequency over the past decade.[72-74] Concern regarding the apparent increased reporting frequency of this event led the ASA Committee on Professional Liability to establish the ASA Postoperative Visual Loss Registry in July 1999. The registry collects detailed information on cases of POVL in an effort to better define intraoperative risk factors and patient characteristics that may predispose to this perioperative complication.[72] Anonymous reporting is encouraged, and the standardized, anonymous case report form can be accessed via the Internet at www.asaclosedclaims.org under the POVL Registry subheading.[72]

The precise cause of POVL is not completely defined but is most likely a multifactorial phenomenon. Suggested contributing factors include hypotension, large blood loss, high-volume fluid resuscitation, anemia, direct ocular pressure, head-dependent position, long operative time, and the presence of vascular disease. Review of the POVL Registry data as of Winter 2001[72] shows that the majority of cases reported involved patients in the prone position for spine procedures (Fig. 180-2). The most common type of ophthalmic lesion associated with POVL is ischemic optic neuropathy (89%), with only 6% of cases being associated with central retinal artery occlusion. Based on registry data, the incidence of ischemic optic neuropathy appears to increase when time spent in the prone position exceeds 6 hours in duration (Fig. 180-3). Blood loss of 1 L or more was associated with ischemic optic neuropathy in 86% of spine cases in the registry (Fig. 180-4). Ischemic optic neuropathy occurs across all age ranges, and younger age does not appear to guarantee protection against it. It should be noted that the registry does not contain denominator data of all cases of prone spine surgery; therefore, definitive conclusions regarding risk cannot be made.[72]

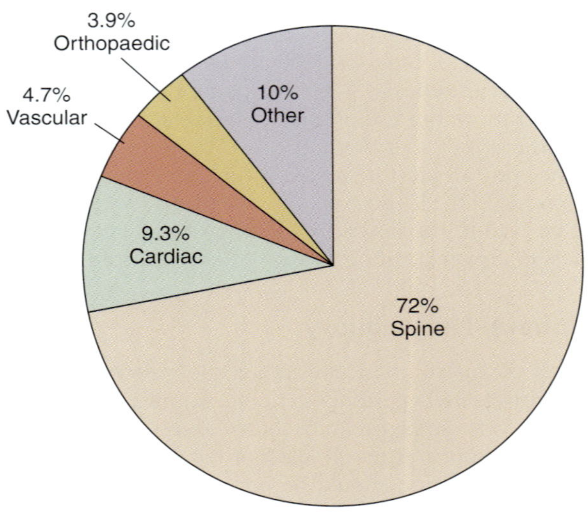

FIGURE 180-2. Percentage of cases in the American Society of Anesthesiologists' Postoperative Visual Loss Registry associated with a particular operation. (Data from Lee L: The ASA postoperative visual loss [POVL] registry. *Anesthesiology* 105:652–659, 2006.)

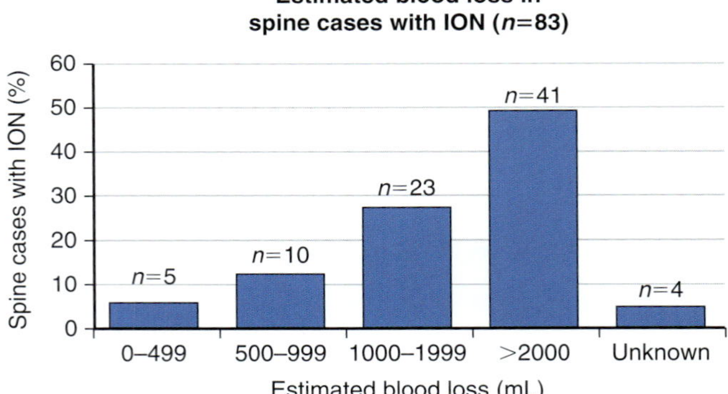

FIGURE 180-4. American Society of Anesthesiologists Postoperative Visual Loss Registry data: Estimated blood loss for 83 spine cases associated with ischemic optic neuropathy (ION). (From Lee LA, Roth S, Posner KL, et al: The American Society of Anesthesiologists postoperative visual loss registry: Analysis of 93 spine surgery cases with postoperative visual loss. *Anesthesiology* 105:652–659, 2008.)

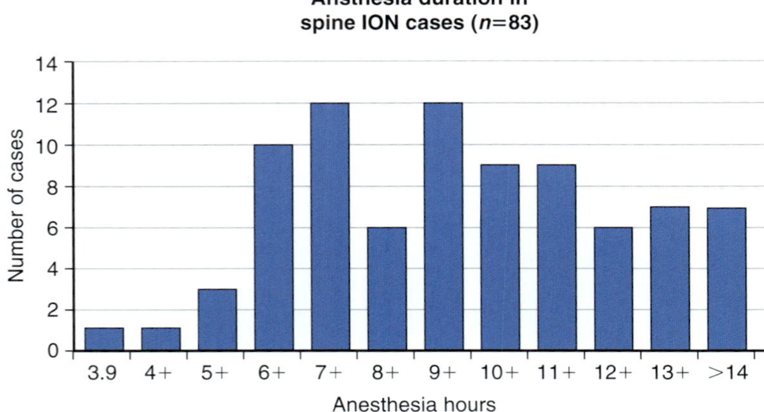

FIGURE 180-3. American Society of Anesthesiologists' Postoperative Visual Loss Registry data: Anesthetic duration for 83 spine cases associated with ischemic optic neuropathy (ION). (From Lee LA, Roth S, Posner KL, et al: The American Society of Anesthesiologists postoperative visual loss registry: analysis of 93 spine surgery cases with postoperative visual loss. *Anesthesiology* 105:652–659, 2008.)

Sitting Position

The sitting position provides the anesthesiologist with unique challenges. It provides distinct advantages for the surgeon but poses some risk to the patient, including cardiac instability, venous air embolism, and quadriplegia. The sitting position can induce significant venous pooling, which may lead to severe hypotension. This problem may be attenuated by judicious fluid administration, the use of compressive stockings, the slow assumption of the sitting position, and maintenance of the knees at the chest level. Contraindications to the sitting position include (1) documented patent foramen ovale or right-to-left shunt, (2) cerebral ischemia in the upright position while awake, and (3) cardiac instability.

Venous air embolism is one of the most feared complications of the sitting position. The incidence of air embolism during spine surgery in the sitting position appears to be substantially less than that during intracranial procedures in the sitting position (7% vs. 43%).[75] The most sensitive monitors for venous air embolism include end-tidal partial pressure of carbon dioxide (ET_{CO_2}), end-tidal nitrogen concentration (ET_{N_2}), the precordial Doppler sonogram, and, most sensitive of all, the transesophageal echocardiogram. A long-arm central venous line is routinely placed for aspiration of air should an embolus occur. It may be accurately positioned just below the junction of the superior vena cava and the right atrium under electrocardiographic guidance within a matter of minutes.[76] Treatment of an air embolus involves the identification of the source, flooding the field to prevent further influx of air, aspiration of air through the central venous line, discontinuation of nitrous oxide to avoid expansion of the air bubbles, and supportive therapy with fluids and pressors.

Cervical spinal cord infarction associated with the sitting position is a rare injury but may occur secondary to extreme flexion or inadequate spinal cord perfusion. Overly aggressive flexion may also result in facial swelling and macroglossia requiring postoperative intubation for airway control. Confirmation that two fingers fit between the chin and the chest once the patient has been positioned will help to avoid these complications.

Fluid and Blood Therapy

Goals of fluid management in anesthesia for spine surgery include the maintenance of adequate plasma volume to preserve spinal cord perfusion while avoiding decreases in plasma oncotic pressure and interstitial fluid accumulation. Fluid replacement can be accomplished with isotonic crystalloid solutions, colloid preparations, or blood products to satisfy these goals. Glucose-containing solutions should be avoided in the absence of documented hypoglycemia because of their demonstrated ability to worsen neurologic outcome following temporary focal ischemia.[77] Hypertonic saline has been used with a safety record similar to isotonic fluids and provides more rapid restoration of intravascular volume after trauma.[78]

Blood Loss and Replacement

When blood losses become greater than one blood volume, many patients develop a progressive increase in bleeding. Presumably, this occurs due to dilution of circulating procoagulants and platelets. At a 1984 National Institutes of Health (NIH) consensus conference, the committee concluded that during massive transfusion, the component required most frequently when increased bleeding occurred was not fresh-frozen plasma but platelets.[79] Thrombocytopenia, or a qualitative platelet dysfunction, is probably the most likely cause of bleeding even in the presence of elevated prothrombin and partial thromboplastin times.[80] With the exception of surgical hemostasis, disseminated intravascular coagulation is the most common unanticipated cause for major bleeding in patients without an underlying coagulopathy.

Given the worldwide concern over the risks of transfusion-related infectious disease transmission, alternative modalities to minimize the need for the administration of donated blood products should be considered. Currently, only 2% to 5% of transfusions in the United States are of autologous blood. Blood donated and preserved with adenine, dextrose, sorbitol, sodium chloride, and mannitol (ADSOL) has a shelf life of 42 days, allowing time for the treatment of possible postoperative anemia. The aggressive preoperative administration of adequate iron supplements and erythropoietin along with autologous donation could greatly reduce requirements for allogeneic blood.

There is debate over the optimal hematocrit for surgical procedures,[81] and this mystical value has drifted downward over time.[82] Acute normovolemic hemodilution remains a safe and effective means of intraoperative blood conservation in those patients expected to have blood losses of 1 to 2 L. Reduction in hematocrit reduces the oxygen-carrying capacity of blood, thus decreasing the "margin of safety" of effective oxygen transport. However, this reduction in hematocrit also causes a reduction in viscosity and an increase in cardiac output. A normovolemic decrease in hematocrit from 40% to 20% induces a 50% drop in oxygen-carrying capacity, but only a 10% drop in oxygen delivery secondary to increased cardiac output. This change parallels the decrease in oxygen consumption seen with the institution of general anesthesia or mild hypothermia. This form of therapy should be reserved for moderately healthy patients without preexisting cardiac, cerebrovascular, or pulmonary disease. There is no evidence that hemodilution has adverse effects on wound healing, infection rates, or immunologic status. Conversely, hemoconcentration may have detrimental effects based on animal studies of focal ischemia.[83]

Replacement of blood losses during surgery with the patient's own shed blood is also an attractive conservation option. Most cell-saving devices currently in use mix salvaged blood with an anticoagulant, then wash and concentrate it to a hematocrit of about 50%. The effluent, which contains plasma fractions, platelets, leukocytes, free hemoglobin, anticoagulant, saline, and other debris, is discarded. Induction of disseminated intravascular coagulation does not appear to be a problem with these devices.[84] Their use is contraindicated in the presence of tumor cells or bacterial contamination. Residual anticoagulation is not a problem with sufficient washing.

Induced Hypotension

Induced hypotension may be useful in helping to minimize blood loss and transfusion therapy during spine surgery, although its efficacy has not been consistently demonstrated.[85] With the use of high concentrations of volatile anesthetics or direct-acting vasodilators such as nitroprusside or nicardipine, the mean arterial pressure may be dropped to the lower limits of autoregulatory control of blood flow, thereby reducing capillary venous pressure and blood loss. Obviously, this technique should be reserved for the otherwise healthy patient.

Pharmacologic Aids

Agents that attempt to reduce bleeding pharmacologically have also been used. Desmopressin (DDAVP), an analogue of the natural hormone vasopressin, induces endothelial cells to release von Willebrand factor, tissue-type plasminogen activator, and certain prostaglandins.[86] With these effects in mind, DDAVP has been used in two human trials during scoliosis surgery with variable results.[87,88] Aprotinin is a serine protease inhibitor that preserves platelet integrity and adhesiveness. It has shown promise as an agent for the prevention of blood loss during cardiac surgery in multiple studies and appears to reduce blood loss and transfusion requirements in spine fusion procedures as well.[89] However, recent studies have suggested an increased risk of long-term mortality following cardiac surgery in patients treated with aprotinin.[90]

A meta-analysis was conducted in 2008 to determine if antifibrinolytic agents reduced blood transfusions in patients undergoing spine surgery and to compare their effects.[91] Aprotinin, tranexamic acid, and ε-aminocaproic acid were all found to be effective in reducing blood loss and the need for transfusions. With the exception of aprotinin, side effects of these agents have not been shown to cause substantial morbidity or to increase the rate of thromboembolic events. Their use should be considered for patients undergoing spinal procedures in which significant blood loss is anticipated. Note, however, that this is not an FDA-approved indication for these agents.[91]

KEY REFERENCES

Audu P, Artz G, Scheid S, et al: Recurrent laryngeal nerve palsy after anterior cervical spine surgery. *Anesthesiology* 105:898–901, 2008.

Benumof JL: Practice guidelines for management of the difficult airway. *Anesthesiology* 98:1269–1277, 2003.

Caldwell MW, O'Hara RC, Bloom MJ, et al: Postoperative airway complications in patients undergoing anterior cervical corpectomy with graft placement: a review of the Pittsburgh experience. *J Neurosurg Anesthesiol* 6:311, 1994.

Gill JB, Chin Y, Levin A, et al: The use of antifibrinlytic agents in spine surgery. *J Bone Joint Surg [Am]* 90:2399–2407, 2008.

Guay J, Reinberg C, Poitras B, et al: A trial of desmopressin to reduce blood loss in patients undergoing spinal fusion for idiopathic scoliosis. *Anesth Analg* 75:405–410, 1992.

Keenan MA, Stiles CM, Kaufman RL: Acquired laryngeal deviation associated with cervical spine disease in erosive polyarticular arthritis. *Anesthesiology* 58:441–449, 1983.

Lee LA, Roth S, Posner KL, et al: The American Society of Anesthesiologists postoperative visual loss registry—analysis of 93 spine surgery cases with postoperative visual loss. *Anesthesiology* 105:652–659, 2008.

REFERENCES

The complete reference list is available online at expertconsult.com.SECTION 8 | Nonsurgical Management

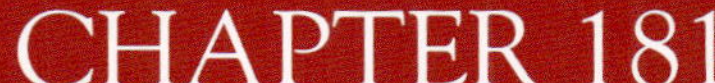

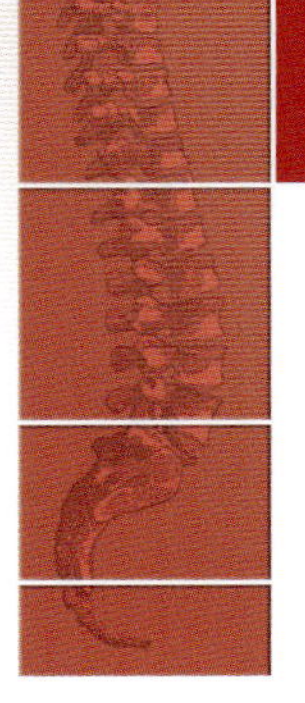

CHAPTER 181

Advances in Anesthesia for Spine Surgery and the Prevention of Complications

Ehab Farag | John Doyle

The anesthetic management of spine surgery has advanced considerably in the last decade. The aim of this chapter is to highlight a number of recent advances in the anesthetic management of spine surgery. Recent developments in understanding postoperative visual loss after spine surgery and recent advances in airway management for cervical spine surgery also are discussed. Finally, the pathophysiology of the prone position and recent advances in fluid management for spine surgery are covered in detail.

Anesthesia for Cervical Spine Surgery

Movement of Cervical Spine with Intubation

The primary force applied by the laryngoscopist is upward lift with a little bit of angular force. This force can be as high as 50 to 70 N (40 N is enough to lift 10 pounds). The more difficult the exposure, the greater the force usually applied. Intubation needs extension at occiput-C1, combined with flexion at lower vertebrae (the fulcrum is probably at C7-T1).[1] Direct laryngoscopy with a Macintosh size 3 blade results in near-maximal extension at occiput-C1 (with the posterior arch of C1 touching the skull).[1,2]

To identify an ideal method for intubation,[3] Sahin et al. studied upper cervical vertebral motion with three intubation devices. Comparisons were made between direct laryngoscopy, the intubating laryngeal mask airway (ILMA), and fiberoptic intubation. In their study, the mean motion at the C1-2 level was 10.2 ± 7.3, 5.0 ± 6.3, and 1.6 ± 3.2 degrees, respectively. The fiberoptic method was found to produce the least motion in the upper cervical spine. The authors concluded that fiberoptic laryngoscopy is the most suitable intubation technique when cervical spine movement is not desired.

There are a few degrees less extension at C1-2 with use of a straight blade.[4] It is unlikely that this difference is clinically meaningful. During intubation under general anesthesia with neuromuscular blockade and manual in-line stabilization, the use of the GlideScope video laryngoscope (Verathon, Inc., Bothell, WA) produced better glottic visualization, but did not significantly decrease movement of the nonpathologic cervical spine compared with direct laryngoscopy.[5]

Cervical Spine Movement and Laryngeal Mask Airways

Keller et al.[6] implanted microchip sensors into the pharyngeal surfaces of C2 and C3 in 20 cadavers to determine the pressures exerted against the cervical spine by the laryngeal mask airway (LMA) and ILMA. The authors concluded that these devices exert high pressures against the upper cervical vertebrae during insertion, during inflation, and in situ. These pressures could produce posterior displacement of the upper cervical spine.

Manual In-line Stabilization and Cricoid Pressure

The goal of manual in-line stabilization is to apply forces to the head and neck equal in magnitude and opposite in direction to those generated by the laryngoscopist so as to limit the movement that might result during airway management; traction forces should be avoided. Manual in-line stabilization failed to reduce movement at the site of instability in cadaver models.[7,8] Cricoid pressure (as long as it is not excessive) did not result in movement in a cadaver model of an injured upper cervical spine.[9]

Maintaining the head in neutral or near-neutral position can be very important in maintaining proper cervical cord blood supply. Flexion of the spine causes elongation of the cord with narrowing of the diameter of the longitudinal vessels.[10] Extension causes an increase in diameter of the cervical cord and folding of the ligamentum flavum, which may exert pressure on the cord and posterior longitudinal vessels.[11] Rau et al.[12] described a case of quadriplegia in a patient who underwent posterior fossa surgery in the prone position. The authors state that during a prolonged period in which the neck was in hyperflexion, overstretching of the cervical spinal cord and compromise to its blood supply likely caused this devastating complication.

Practical Points to Remember

- Awake fiberoptic intubation is the gold standard for patients with *unstable* neck injuries.
- Surveys indicate that the majority of U.S. anesthesiologists would prefer to use a fiberoptic bronchoscope to intubate at-risk patients and to do so with the patient awake.[13]
- Induction of anesthesia diminishes the protective stabilization of the neck musculature. Neck motion during this phase can be substantial, sometimes producing dynamic cord compression that could result in cervical cord injury.
- If the cervical spine is grossly unstable, consideration should be given to both intubating the trachea and positioning the patient while he or she is still awake.

If new neurologic symptoms developed during positioning, repositioning should be attempted. During that period, tight control of the patient's blood pressure and even inducing hypertension can help resolve these new symptoms.

- Airway complications are common after anterior cervical spine surgery and may range from acute airway obstruction to chronic vocal cord dysfunction. Recurrent laryngeal nerve injury after anterior cervical spine surgery could be due to direct nerve injury at the time of neck dissection, surgical retractor placement, and endotracheal balloon insufflation pressure.[14,15]
- Cervical spine surgery in the prone position could result in laryngeal edema and macroglossia.[7,16]
- The use of fiberoptic intubation was shown to result in fewer airway complications after cervical spine surgery, thought to be due to a reduction in soft tissue trauma.[17]
- For patients with subaxial spondylotic myelopathy, neck extension can narrow the diameter of the spinal cord, whereas in patients with atlantoaxial subluxation, such as those with rheumatoid arthritis or Down syndrome, neck flexion will widen the atlantodental interval, narrowing the spinal canal.
- Maintaining adequate spinal cord perfusion is crucial during cervical spine surgery in patients with spondylitic myelopathy. Chronic mechanical compression inhibiting the spinal cord blood supply leads to gradual, intermittent microinfarction of the cord. In this setting, invasive blood pressure monitoring using an arterial line and close attention to maintaining adequate perfusion pressure are very important.[14]

Physiologic Changes in the Prone Position

The prone position is the most important and frequently used position in spine surgery. However, it is associated with major physiologic changes. Understanding these changes allows one to reduce the incidence of complications associated with the prone position.

Cardiovascular Changes

Using a noninvasive cardiac output monitor, both cardiac index (CI) and venous return[18] decreased in unanesthetized, healthy volunteers in the prone position. CI decreased compared with the supine position as follows: knee-chest position (20%); on pelvic props from a modified Relton-Hall frame under the anterior superior iliac spines and padded support under the chest (17%); on an evacuatable mattress (11%); and on pillows (3%; one pillow under the thorax and one under the abdomen, leaving the abdomen free to move). Toyota and Amaki[19] studied transesophageal echocardiograms in 15 healthy patients undergoing prone-position lumbar laminectomy. The prone position caused left ventricular volume and compliance to decrease. These changes were attributed to a decrease in the venous return due to inferior vena caval compression, and decreased left ventricular compliance due to increased intrathoracic pressure in the prone position. These results had been confirmed by other studies using thermodilution pulmonary artery catheters to measure the cardiac index when transferring from the supine to the prone position. Cardiac output in these studies decreased by 17% to 24%.[14] The reduction in cardiac output in the prone position also leads to a decrease in the metabolism of propofol.[20] A reduction in propofol metabolism while in the prone position could also explain the results of Sudheer et al.,[21] who showed a significant reduction in cardiac output in the prone position during maintenance of anesthesia using propofol compared with isoflurane. Pearce[22] observed vena caval pressures to be 0 to 40 mm H_2O in patients in the prone position with the abdomen hanging free. In contrast, patients with abdominal compression had vena caval pressures greater than 300 mm H_2O. Increased venous pressure not only increases bleeding during spine surgery owing to congestion of vertebral veins but can impair spinal cord perfusion.

The use of the prone position with abdominal compression was identified as a plausible cause of spinal cord ischemia leading to neurologic deficits after cervical laminectomy. The authors of this case series recommended the avoidance of abdominal compression and hypotension, especially in myelopathic patients for whom maintenance of spinal cord perfusion pressure is of paramount importance.[23]

Changes in Respiratory Physiology

In an elegant study, Nyren et al.[24] studied the regional distribution of pulmonary blood flow in 10 healthy volunteers. The subjects were studied in both prone and supine positions with and without lung distention caused by 10 cm H_2O of continuous positive airway pressure. The results demonstrated that ventilation-perfusion matching during both normal breathing and positive pressure is more favorable in the prone than in the supine position. Because perfusion is more evenly distributed in the prone position, the recruitment of dorsal airways results in an increase in lung units and consequently increased functional residual capacity, with near-normal ventilation-perfusion matching and a reduction in shunt.[25] By turning the patient prone and recruiting airways in the dorsal lung, prone positioning achieves similar beneficial effects as positive end-expiratory pressure ventilation but without the risks of barotrauma or interference with cardiac function. Of note, the prone position is sometimes used in patients with acute respiratory distress syndrome to improve oxygenation and decrease shunt.[25] Similar findings were confirmed by Pelosi et al.[26] during general anesthesia. Prone positioning during general anesthesia did not negatively affect respiratory mechanisms, and it improved lung volumes and oxygenation.

Estimating Intravascular Volume Status and Predicting Fluid Responsiveness

Although unquestionably useful, the traditional clinical findings in hypovolemia often lack sensitivity and specificity. This fact has led to a decades-long program of ongoing research to improve the clinical monitoring of volume status. Earlier expectations that cardiac filling pressure data (e.g., central venous pressure, pulmonary capillary wedge pressure) would be helpful in guiding fluid therapy were not fully realized when it became apparent that cardiac filling pressures are often influenced by factors other than blood volume. Later experience with transesophageal echocardiography showed that this technique can be especially helpful in assessing right- and left-sided ventricular filling, but the technique is intermittent in nature, requires extensive training to use and interpret, and entails a very high equipment cost. Consequently, the search for practical and reliable means of monitoring blood volume and related parameters continues. Approaches to this search fall into one of three broad areas: identifying occult hypoperfusion (e.g., by tissue oxygen and carbon dioxide levels), assessing preload responsiveness (e.g., by systolic pressure variation, pulse pressure variation, or stroke volume variation), and identifying end points for fluid resuscitation (e.g., seeking a specific cardiac output or aortic flow velocity value rather than a specific blood pressure). The following is a brief description of some of the methods that show particular promise in this regard.

Arterial pressure variation as a consequence of respiration has been advocated as a relatively simple technique that requires only an arterial line. Clinically, one can "eyeball" the degree of pressure variation with mechanical ventilation to get a rough indication of the degree of hypovolemia. However, more quantitative measures such as measurements of pulse pressure (systolic−diastolic) variation, systolic blood pressure variation, and delta down (decrease in systolic blood pressure from the value during apnea) have all been advocated as more appropriate alternatives to simple visual inspection.[27-29]

In a similar manner, respiratory variation of stroke volume has been demonstrated to predict fluid responsiveness in mechanically ventilated patients.[28,30,31] Methods using either pulse pressure variation or aortic blood flow variation have been advocated. The mechanisms involved in producing this variation have been explained by Mahjoub et al.[32]

Four mechanisms participate in the cyclic changes of stroke volume observed during mechanical ventilation. First, during insufflation, venous return decreases because of an increase in pleural pressure. This decrease in right ventricular preload leads to a decrease in right ventricular output, which subsequently leads to a decrease in left ventricular output. Second, right ventricular afterload increases during inspiration because the increase in alveolar pressure is greater than the increase in pleural pressure. However, left ventricular preload increases during insufflation, because blood is expelled from the capillaries toward the left atrium. Finally, left ventricular afterload decreases during inspiration because positive pleural pressure decreases the intracardiac systolic pressure and the transmural pressure of the intrathoracic aorta. In clinical practice, the use of pulse pressure variation is based on the fact that the first mechanism is the prevailing mechanism.

Developments in Pulse Oximetry Technology

Recent advances in pulse oximetry technology have led to developments that should be of special interest to clinicians dealing with complex surgical cases such as major spine surgery. For example, existing and pending developments from Masimo Corporation (Irvine, CA), a major vendor of pulse oximeters, will allow clinicians continuously to measure oxyhemoglobin, oxygen content, carboxyhemoglobin, methemoglobin, and total hemoglobin by simple, noninvasive means. Perhaps even more important, respiratory variations in the pulse oximeter waveform can be used to predict fluid responsiveness in mechanically ventilated patients. As noted earlier, this can be helpful in discerning which hypotensive patients will respond to a fluid challenge. Masimo makes a pulse oximeter that provides a measurement known as the *Pleth Variability Index* (PVI) that has been shown to be useful in predicting fluid responsiveness. In a 25-patient study by Cannesson et al.,[33] a ventilated patient was defined as a "responder" if his or her cardiac output increased by 15% or more after administration of 500 mL of hetastarch 6%; otherwise, the patient was considered to be a "nonresponder." Of the patients evaluated, 16 were responders and 9 were nonresponders. In this study, a PVI greater than 14% before volume expansion discriminated between responders and nonresponders with 81% sensitivity and 100% specificity. In addition, the noninvasive PVI was as accurate at predicting fluid responsiveness as was analysis of pulse pressure variation from an invasive arterial catheter. Finally, the PVI had superior predictive accuracy compared with traditional central venous pressure and pulmonary capillary wedge pressure indicators of intravascular volume. Figure 181-1 shows sample waveforms from a responder and a nonresponder.

Automating the Delivery of Intravenous Fluids in Hypovolemic Patients

For some time there has been interest in developing methods to automate the delivery of intravenous fluids in hypovolemic patients, such as patients undergoing major spine surgery or those with severe trauma. Although a number of hemodynamic parameters have been suggested as end points to guide plasma volume expansion, simple measurements of systemic blood pressure (e.g., data obtained from an arterial line) are used most commonly for the initial assessment of hypovolemic shock and the need for plasma volume expansion. However, many other hemodynamic parameters (e.g., central venous pressure, pulmonary artery pressures, systolic pressure variation, cardiac output) may also be useful in such a setting. Although this technology is still very much in its infancy, closed-loop systems are slowly undergoing the transition from experimental animal studies to clinical application.[34,35] An example of the state of the art is a series of systems described by Kramer et al.,[36] who studied algorithms based on proportional-integral, fuzzy logic, and nonlinear decision table methods. They studied three sets of sheep that were subjected to a 25 mL/kg hemorrhage. In each case, closed-loop resuscitation with a target mean arterial pressure of 80 mm Hg began 30 minutes from the beginning of the hemorrhage, with two additional hemorrhages of 5 mL/kg being carried out during the resuscitation. The authors noted that all three algorithms were equally effective in restoring mean arterial pressure and cardiac output. Future systems of this genre may benefit from new noninvasive technologies for monitoring volume status and from continuing developments in computer-controlled infusion pumps.

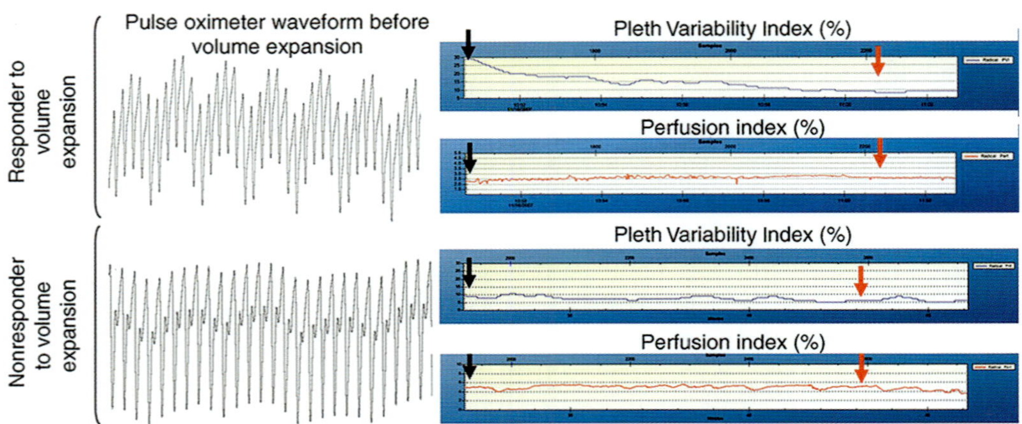

FIGURE 181-1. Pleth Variability Index (PVI) and perfusion index (PI) evolutions during volume expansion in a responder to volume expansion and in a nonresponder to volume expansion. PVI (*blue line*) and PI (*red line*) evolutions during volume expansion are shown. The *black arrows* show volume expansion beginning and the *red arrows* show volume expansion ending. Volume expansion was performed over a 10-minute period. The authors observed a PVI value of 21% at baseline in the responder patient. This value decreased progressively to 9% after volume expansion. In the nonresponder patient, baseline PVI was 9% and after volume expansion, 6%. A steady PI value was observed in both patients. (From Cannesson M, Desebbe O, Rosamel P, et al: Pleth variability index to monitor the respiratory variations in the pulse oximeter plethysmographic waveform amplitude and predict fluid responsiveness in the operating theatre. *Br J Anaesth* 101:200–206, 2008. Reprinted with permission from Oxford University Press.)

Voluven

A recent important entry in the colloid scene in the United States is Voluven (6% hydroxyethyl starch, 130/0.4), which is produced by Fresenius Kabi (Bad Homburg, Germany). This new colloid was approved by the U.S. Food and Drug Administration in late 2007. Voluven has characteristics such as a smaller molecular weight that suggest it may have improved pharmacokinetic properties and better effects on coagulation parameters compared with older hydroxyethyl starch (HES) products. Because Voluven is more rapidly degraded than older HESs with higher molecular weights, it is eliminated more quickly by the kidneys, has a shorter volume effect, and (perhaps most importantly) has fewer adverse effects on coagulation. Experience in the settings of orthopaedic and other forms of surgery has been favorable.[37-39]

Postoperative Visual Loss after Spine Surgery

Vision loss or impairment after spine surgery is a devastating problem with an incidence of 0.1% to 1%.[40] The causes remain poorly understood, but appear to be multifactorial and may include impaired perfusion of the eye or occlusion of retinal vessels from improper positioning.

Retinal Perfusion Pressure

The main source of blood supply to the optic nerve head is the posterior ciliary circulation by way of the pericapillary choroids and the short posterior ciliary arteries. The blood supply in the optic nerve head has a sectorial distribution, which helps to explain why visual loss is usually segmental in anterior ischemic optic neuropathy. The blood supply to the optic nerve head shows marked interindividual variation, and even varies within an individual from eye to eye. This anatomic variability may explain why vision loss or impairment develops in some people after spine surgery but not in others despite exposure to similar conditions. Posterior ciliary arteries in vivo behave as end arteries. They also have watershed zones between their distributions (i.e., no anastomoses between the arteries in these areas). These areas are most vulnerable to ischemia when perfusion pressure is inadequate.[41]

Perfusion pressure of the eye is defined as the difference between mean systemic arterial pressure and intraocular pressure (IOP).[41] Either decreased mean arterial pressure or elevated IOP will thus decrease ocular perfusion pressure. Most commonly, perfusion pressure is impaired by a combination of decreased mean arterial pressure and increased IOP.[41]

Arterial Blood Pressure

Arterial hypertension, as well as arterial hypotension, may influence blood flow in the optic nerve head. In hypertensive individuals, autoregulation of ocular blood vessels usually shifts to higher levels to maintain constant blood flow. Although this improves the patients' tolerance to high blood pressure, this upward shift in the autoregulation range makes hypertensive patients less tolerant to low blood pressures. In the optic nerve head, reduction in blood pressure below the critical autoregulatory level decreases blood flow.[41] Hence, hypotension is associated with perioperative vision loss.[42-44]

Intraocular Pressure

Intraocular pressure is the other factor that determines ocular perfusion pressure. IOP usually increases over time in the prone position. Cheng et al.[45] showed that IOP can reach up to 40 mm Hg (normal is 8–20 mm Hg) after 6 hours in the prone position. Hunt et al.[46] confirmed that IOP increases in the prone position. However, they could not find a relationship between an increase in IOP and duration of the procedure, as did Cheng et al.[45] The causes for increased IOP during prone positioning might include increased episcleral venous pressure,[47] but also might be related to positive intraoperative fluid balance. In healthy volunteers, acute water loading (14 mL/kg) increased IOP,[48] whereas exercise-induced dehydration reduced IOP.[49]

Types of Visual Loss and Impairment Associated with Spine Surgery

The principal visual defects associated with spine surgery are ischemic optic neuropathy, cortical blindness, central retinal artery occlusion, and central retinal vein occlusion.

Ischemic Optic Neuropathy

Ischemic optic neuropathy occurs either in the anterior part of the optic nerve where the nerve enters the globe or the posterior part where the nerve lies within the orbit. Blood flow to the optic nerve is autoregulated[41] to maintain a nearly constant supply despite changes in perfusion pressure. However, autoregulation operates effectively only over a particular range of perfusion pressures. Above and below this range, blood flow depends directly on perfusion pressure, so ischemic damage can result. Anterior ischemic optic neuropathy can also result from a low hematocrit because choroidal blood flow decreases with hemodilution, whereas the blood flow to the retina increases.[50] A small increase in IOP can lead to a decrease in perfusion pressure and in anterior ischemic optic neuropathy, especially in the presence of arterial hypotension and defective autoregulation. Anterior ischemic optic neuropathy is frequently first noticed immediately on awakening from normal sleep, which corresponds to a diurnal peak of IOP.[51] The true incidence of postoperative anterior ischemic optic neuropathy may be underestimated because small areas of anterior optic nerve infarction may produce only small visual defects that pass unnoticed during the postoperative period. These patients present later with low-pressure glaucoma with multiple areas of optic atrophy.[52]

Posterior ischemic optic neuropathy is relatively rare, and presents clinically as a retrobulbar optic neuropathy. It is believed to result from infarction of the intraorbital portion of the optic nerve. Visual impairment is often severe because the optic nerve swells as a consequence of ischemia. Posterior extension of swelling along the nerve involves the portion of the nerve within the sphenoidal optic canals, where it is encased in bony, nonelastic structures.

Diagnostic criteria for posterior ischemic optic neuropathy include the following:

- An acute deficit in visual acuity, visual field, or both
- An ipsilateral relative afferent papillary defect with unilateral disease and sluggish or nonreactive pupils with bilateral symmetric involvement
- Visual deficit in the presence of a normal optic disc and funduscopic examination
- Normal electroretinogram
- Abnormal visual evoked response
- Development of optic atrophy within 4 to 8 weeks of the onset of visual loss

The main causes of posterior ischemic optic neuropathy are hypotension, anemia, and facial edema. Facial edema can lead to increased IOP and accumulation of fluid in the orbit, which jeopardizes perfusion of the optic nerve. Posterior ischemic optic neuropathy has been described after bilateral neck dissection due to bilateral ligation of the internal jugular veins, which led to facial edema, venous congestion, and increased intraorbital pressure.[44,53,54]

Cortical Blindness

Cortical blindness results from damage to the occipital cortex or optic radiation; the main causes for cortical blindness are ischemic or traumatic. Clinically, loss of visual sensation is accompanied by retention of pupillary reaction to light and a normal funduscopic examination.[55] Cortical blindness is usually best diagnosed by CT or MRI, which helps identify infarcted areas in the occipital lobe. Cortical blindness has been described after cardiopulmonary bypass due to generalized hypoperfusion or emboli. It also has been described after craniotomy and laryngectomy surgery due to hypoperfusion caused by hemorrhagic hypotension.[55,56] Cortical blindness has been reported during spine surgery due to hypotension, anemia, and abnormal head position jeopardizing the vertebrobasilar circulation.[57,58]

Central Retinal Artery Occlusion

Central retinal artery occlusion is often caused by an embolic ulcerated plaque from the ipsilateral carotid artery.[56] The main cause of central retinal artery occlusion after spine surgery is external ocular pressure from a head rest combined with arterial hypotension, resulting in obstruction to flow in the retinal artery.[59] Central retinal artery occlusion typically presents as a complete loss of vision in one eye that usually improves with time. Funduscopic examination reveals pallor and edema of the retina, with a cherry-red spot at the fovea.

Central Retinal Vein Occlusion

Central retinal vein occlusion has been reported after spine surgery due to external pressure on the globe from a head rest in the prone position.[60] Funduscopic findings usually include retinal hemorrhages in all quadrants, cotton-wool spots, and dilated, tortuous retinal veins.[61]

Factors Contributing to Vision Loss and Impairment after Spine Surgery

Case reports and studies of postoperative vision loss after spine surgery suggest that hypotension and anemia are major culprits in the development of ischemic vision loss. This results from the end-arterial nature of the posterior ciliary arteries, with no collaterals to compensate for low perfusion pressure.[42,43,62]

This is consistent with findings by Lee et al.,[63] who used a porcine optic nerve model to show that the optic nerve has a limited compensatory mechanism to maintain blood flow and oxygen delivery in the presence of anemia and hypotension. Also, in the presence of severe anemia and hypotension, there is a "steal" from the ophthalmic artery to the brain to maintain perfusion of the brain in preference to the eye.[63]

Increased resistance to blood flow can also decrease ocular perfusion pressure. As mentioned previously, increased IOP during spine surgery in the prone position can lead to decreased ocular perfusion pressure.[40,64] The other interesting finding is that blindness has been observed after bilateral ligation of the internal jugular veins. Blindness in these patients was attributed to increased IOP due to impaired drainage of the orbital venous plexus into the ophthalmic veins.[54,65]

During extensive spine surgery, the excessive use of crystalloids to maintain the intravascular compartment and replace blood loss has been suggested as a cause of vision loss after surgery.[43] Roughly two thirds of administered crystalloid volume distributes to the extravascular compartment; the eye socket is part of this compartment. Accumulation of fluid in the eye socket can thus lead to increased IOP, along with facial edema, and therefore development of eye compartment syndrome, which compromises the retinal blood supply.[66] It has been shown that a decrease in plasma oncotic pressure results from using crystalloid as the primary solution for cardiopulmonary bypass rather than colloid.[67] The American Society of Anesthesiologists practice advisory for perioperative vision loss associated with spine surgery thus recommends the increased use of colloids to maintain intravascular volume in patients who have substantial blood loss.[68]

Effect of the Type of Fluid Replacement on Facial Edema, Chemosis, and Intraocular Pressure

Fluid management during spine surgery in the prone position plays a crucial role in determining the degree of facial edema, accumulation of fluid in the eye socket, chemosis, and IOP. It has been shown that large amounts of intravenous fluids and prolonged duration of the prone position can result in fluid collection in the face, and especially the globe, during the prone position because of venous stasis in the dependent soft tissues.[53] Furthermore, a recent report of vision loss after spine surgery attributed the defect to excessive use of crystalloids leading to massive facial edema with severe chemosis, which could have increased the IOP to such a degree that eye perfusion was jeopardized despite the patient's blood pressure and hematocrit being kept within normal limits.[69] Jeon et al. have demonstrated that patient position, intraoperative fluid balance, and duration of surgery all influence the severity of postoperative chemosis.[70]

The type of fluid used in prone-position spine surgery is likely to determine the extent to which facial edema and chemosis develop. After crystalloid infusion, only one third remains in the intravascular compartment, whereas two thirds distributes to the extravascular compartment and to soft tissues. This leads to tissue edema and aggravates facial swelling, accumulation of the fluid in the globe, and chemosis, and increases the IOP. The potential for edema is aggravated by the fact that blood loss is usually replaced at a three-to-one ratio with crystalloid. In contrast, a major advantage of using colloids is that they stay mainly in the intravascular compartment, thus potentially decreasing facial edema, chemosis, and accumulation of fluid in the eye socket that can lead to an increased IOP. Consistent with this theory, use of crystalloid for priming bypass machines increases IOP by decreasing the colloid oncotic pressure, whereas priming with colloid solutions does not increase the colloid oncotic pressure.[67]

Head Position and Compartment Syndrome

Ocular chemosis (i.e., conjunctival edema) can cause short-term decreased visual acuity, patient discomfort, and an increased risk for bacterial keratitis.[71] The risk factors for chemosis after prone spine surgery are the following[70]:

1. Head-down position (odds ratio [OR] = 8.8 [confidence interval (CI) = 2.3–33.5]; P = .001, vs. neutral position)
2. Positive fluid balance >700 mL (OR = 6.3 [CI = 1.6–24.1]; P = .007, for <700 mL vs. 700–1399 mL; and OR = 32.8 [CI = 2.7–403]; P = .006, for <700 mL vs. >1400 mL)
3. Surgery lasting 180 minutes or longer

In a recent case report, a patient underwent a 4-hour L3-4 decompression with fusion in the prone position.[72] His head was positioned on a C-shaped head rest on a soft bed with the left side of the face up. After surgery. the patient developed ischemic orbital compartment syndrome, manifested in his right eye with proptosis, ptosis, loss of light perception and visual acuity, and complete ophthalmoplegia. The right eye IOP was 33 mm Hg, which reached 40 mm Hg 24 hours after surgery despite emergency administration of mannitol and acetazolamide. The apparent reason for the development of compartment syndrome in this case was that the patient's face was turned to one side, which occluded the right internal jugular vein and resulted in impaired venous drainage and increased IOP in the right eye.[72]

This case highlights the importance of keeping the head in the neutral position and elevated to avoid the development of an ocular compartment syndrome. In a French survey of ophthalmic complications after spine surgery, the authors proposed two preventive measures to avoid vision loss after spine surgery in the prone position. The first was to avoid eye compression when using a horseshoe-shaped head rest, and the second was to avoid lateral rotation of the head in patients with suspected carotid atheroma.[73]

Effect of α_2-Adrenergic Agonists on the Eye during Spine Surgery

α_2-Adrenergic agonists decrease IOP. After several hours of use, the topical α_2 agonist brimonidine decreased aqueous production by 29%. After days of use, uveoscleral outflow was increased by 60%.[74] As might thus be expected, brimonidine has been used successfully as monotherapy for glaucoma. α_2-Adrenergic agonists have also been shown to have a neuroprotective effect on retinal ganglion cells, the mechanisms of which can be summarized as follows:

- α_2-Adrenergic agonists increase basic fibroblast growth factor in retinal photoreceptors but not in the brain.[75]
- α_2-Adrenergic receptor stimulation activates the antiapoptotic phosphatidyl inositol-3 kinase and protein kinase/AKt pathways. These are major pathways in the promotion of cell survival, and they block apoptosis by phosphorylation-dependent inhibition of proapoptotic signaling molecules, including BAD and capsase-9, and activation of antiapoptotic molecules such NF-κB.[72] α_2-Adrenergic stimulation also leads to activation of extracellular signal-regulated kinase and increased synthesis of survival factors, such as basic fibroblast growth factor and Bcl-2.[76,77]
- α_2-Adrenergic receptor stimulation may reduce ischemic retinal injury by preventing accumulation of extracellular glutamate and asparate.[78]

- Brimonidine 0.2% is a commonly used ocular α_2-adrenergic agonist. It has a peak effect 2 hours after administration and its effect lasts at least 8 hours.[75]

Conclusion

Advances in perioperative fluid management—in upper airway management and in our understanding of the pathophysiology of vision loss after spine surgery in prone position—will ensure better perioperative management and outcome after spine surgery.

KEY REFERENCES

Cannesson M, Desebbe O, Rosamel P, et al: Pleth variability index to monitor the respiratory variations in the pulse oximeter plethysmographic waveform amplitude and predict fluid responsiveness in the operating theatre. *Br J Anaesth* 101:200–206, 2008.

Cheng MA, Sigurdson W, Tempelhoff R, et al: Visual loss after spine surgery: a survey. *Neurosurgery* 46:625–630, 2000.

Crosby ET: Airway management in adults after cervical spine trauma. *Anesthesiology* 104:1293–1318, 2006.

Hayreh SS: Anterior ischemic optic neuropathy. *Clin Neurosci* 4:251–263, 1997.

Toyota S, Amaki Y: Hemodynamic evaluation of the prone position by transesophageal echocardiography. *J Clin Anesth* 10:32–35, 1998.

REFERENCES

The complete reference list is available online at expertconsult.com.

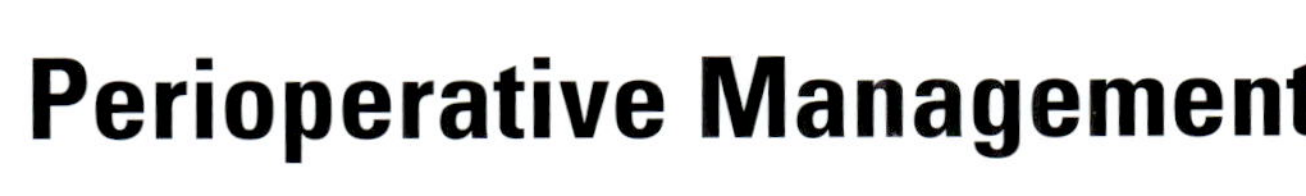

CHAPTER 182

Perioperative Management

Basheal M. Agrawal | Seth M. Zeidman | Laurence Rhines | Nathan H. Lebwohl | Gregory R. Trost

The spectrum of spine surgery ranges from straightforward cervical procedures in healthy, young adults to emergent fixation of unstable thoracolumbar spine fractures in clinically unstable patients with multiple traumatic injuries. Preoperative evaluation and postoperative care share equal importance with the surgical procedure. The continuum of care begins at the initial meeting of the surgeon and patient and continues long after surgery. The clinician should be cognizant of coexisting medical problems and their implications, commonly used anesthetic and surgical techniques, potential postoperative complications, and prophylactic measures that can minimize postoperative morbidity. This chapter provides an overview of these issues.

The purpose of preoperative evaluation is to identify problems affecting surgical risk and, in so doing, reduce perioperative morbidity and mortality. Preoperative evaluation often uncovers other health problems that need attention, regardless of whether they directly affect the proposed operation. A complete health history should be obtained, including the present illness, past illnesses, and associated diseases. One should inquire about bleeding tendencies, current medications, and allergies. Coexisting medical problems are common in spine surgery patients and can be associated with an increased incidence of postoperative complications and a lengthy hospital stay.

General Conditions Affecting Surgical Risk

Age

Patients at either extreme of the life span are at risk for complications or death from operation because of their narrower margin of safety. Small errors that are well tolerated by young, healthy adults are quickly compounded in children or geriatric patients, sometimes with catastrophic results.

Infants and young children have a relatively low tolerance for infection, trauma, blood loss, and nutritional and fluid disturbances.[1] The management of these disorders in infants and children differs from their treatment in adults. Particular aspects of surgical care deserving special attention include fluid and electrolyte management, nutrition, and temperature maintenance.[1,2]

Advanced age is an independent risk factor for postoperative morbidity, and the prevalence of coexisting medical problems increases with age.[3] As a result, elderly patients who undergo spine procedures have higher rates of postoperative complications, including excessive bleeding, postoperative confusion, and urinary tract infections.[4] They tend to recuperate more slowly than do their younger counterparts. A recent study has shown that age is a positive risk factor for postoperative complications in multilevel thoracolumbar spine fusion surgery. Furthermore, it is correlative with higher rates of reoperation.[5]

It is safe to consider every patient older than 65 years of age to be at high risk for generalized atherosclerosis and for potential limitation of myocardial and renal reserve. Elderly patients often develop cardiac failure if they are fluid overloaded. Close monitoring of vital signs, intake, output, body weight, and serum electrolytes is mandatory. Elderly patients generally require smaller doses of narcotics, sedatives, and anesthetics than do younger patients. Barbiturates, sedatives, and steroids may cause confusion, and narcotics can produce respiratory depression.[6]

Osteoporosis and falls are common in the geriatric population and result in an increased incidence of spine fractures with advancing age. Elderly patients with spine fractures after a fall pose special problems. In addition to assessing the overall medical condition, the clinician should evaluate the cause of the fall because it may uncover an important coexisting medical condition and, in turn, help to prevent future injury. Nonoperative measures may be more appropriate in the elderly patient with a spine fracture if he or she is unable to tolerate the rigors of a prescribed treatment. Furthermore, bracing of the elderly patient is different from that of younger patients. For example, use of a halo vest in the geriatric population is fraught with morbidity.

Although most falls are results of accidents or environmental factors, they can also be caused by important cardiovascular or neurologic disorders, including arrhythmia, orthostatic hypotension, and cerebral ischemia. Special consideration should also be given to alcohol and drug use as possible causes. The incidence of falls in the elderly has been correlated with use of benzodiazepines, antidepressants, and diuretics.

Finally, advanced age is an important independent risk factor for postoperative deep venous thrombosis and pulmonary embolism, which are major causes of morbidity and mortality after surgical procedures.

Obesity

Obesity increases the technical difficulty of surgery and anesthesia. Obese surgical patients have a greater incidence of serious concomitant disease and higher rates of postoperative wound breakdown, thromboembolic complications, and pulmonary disease. Early patient mobilization, aggressive pulmonary toilet, and appropriate prophylaxis against deep venous thrombosis are all necessary adjuncts to good perioperative care. Occasionally, it may be advisable to delay elective surgery until the patient loses weight by appropriate dietary measures. There are increasing data to suggest that minimally invasive techniques, including tubular surgery, diminish the risks incurred by obesity.[7]

Coagulation Abnormalities

Spine procedures may result in substantial blood loss. Excessive bleeding at the surgical site increases the chances of wound infection and impaired wound healing. Although the prevalence of underlying coagulopathies is no higher in patients undergoing spine surgery, many regularly take nonsteroidal anti-inflammatory drugs (NSAIDs). Because NSAIDs are reversible inhibitors of platelet aggregation, their use can increase postoperative bleeding. NSAIDs should be discontinued at least 1 week before a major spine procedure. NSAIDs have also been shown to inhibit the healing of spine fusions. In patients undergoing spine fusion, NSAIDs should be avoided in the postoperative period as well.[8,9]

Malnutrition

Increasing evidence suggests that many surgical patients are moderately to severely malnourished.[10] The increased metabolic demands of patients undergoing or recovering from spine surgery are often unmet because of insufficient caloric intake. With inadequate caloric intake, the hypercatabolic state induced by trauma or surgery results in significant visceral and skeletal protein depletion. Malnourished patients have increased rates of mortality and morbidity from sepsis, wound complications, impaired healing, and protracted rehabilitation. Although no single test demonstrates malnutrition conclusively, a variety of laboratory studies and physical measurements can help reveal nutritional inadequacies.[11] These include preoperative weight loss of more than 10 pounds, a serum albumin level of less than 3.5 g/dL, and a total lymphocyte count less than 1500 to 2000 cells/μL.[12]

If malnutrition is identified, a vigorous regimen of nutritional supplementation should begin, preferably before surgery, and the patient should be monitored throughout the perioperative period.[11] Total or peripheral parenteral nutrition should be considered in patients who either cannot tolerate or cannot meet their caloric needs with enteral nutrition alone.[13-16]

Smoking

The harmful effects of smoking tobacco on the rate of postoperative pulmonary, cardiac, and thromboembolic complications are well known. In a recent study of 875 patients undergoing orthopaedic reconstructive surgery, the incidence of cardiopulmonary complications in smokers was double that of nonsmokers. In that study, smoking was identified as the single most important risk factor for the development of complications after elective hip or knee arthroplasty. Similarly increased rates of pulmonary complications were identified in a multicenter review of 400 patients undergoing abdominal surgery.[17-20]

A review of wound infections after dorsal spine operations involving instrumentation implicated smoking as a significant risk factor for development of an infection.[21]

Wound complications in soft tissue procedures have also been reported to occur much more frequently in smokers. In a study of 425 patients undergoing reconstruction after breast cancer surgery, the risk of skin flap necrosis was nine times as high in heavy smokers as in nonsmokers. Similarly, in a review of patients undergoing face lift, the risk of skin slough was 12.5 times as high in smokers compared with nonsmokers.[22,23] In spine surgery, current smoking increases the rate of postoperative wound infection and subsequently increases hospital stay and 30-day mortality rates.[24]

Stopping smoking before surgery has been shown to decrease the rate of postoperative complications, but only if a significant amount of time elapses between smoking cessation and surgery. A 2-week smoke-free period in a study of 60 patients before colorectal surgery did not decrease the rate of postoperative complications. In contrast, 4 weeks of smoking cessation significantly reduced the rate of wound infections in a randomized, controlled trial of minor dermatologic procedures. In another randomized trial of 120 patients scheduled to undergo hip or knee replacement, enrollment in a smoking cessation program at least 6 weeks before surgery resulted in a substantial decrease in complication rates. The rate of wound complications decreased from 31% to 5%, and of cardiovascular complications from 10% to 0%.[25-27]

In addition to the aforementioned general postoperative problems, tobacco smoking has been associated with unique complications after spine surgery. Smoking was identified as a significant risk factor in the development of postoperative airway obstruction after cervical corpectomy. In a review of 133 patients undergoing cervical corpectomy, 6 of 7 patients who developed airway obstruction were smokers. Two of these patients died as a result of this complication. Other risk factors were myelopathy and multilevel surgery. In patients with these risk factors, the authors recommend delayed extubation and careful assessment of the airway for swelling before extubation.[28]

Smoking has been shown to inhibit the healing of spine fusions in many clinical reviews. This effect has been well documented in patients undergoing spine fusion surgery and in animal models. In a randomly selected retrospective study of 50 smokers and 50 nonsmokers undergoing uninstrumented lumbar dorsolateral fusion, the pseudarthrosis rate was 40% for smokers and 8% for nonsmokers. A corresponding diminution in resting oxygen saturation was identified. The authors theorized that this relative hypoxia was responsible for the failure of the arthrodesis to heal.[29]

Animal studies, however, have shown that the inhibition of fusion can be attributed directly to the pharmacologic effects of systemically administered nicotine, without hypoxia.[30] Inhibition of bone graft vascularization has been shown in animal models. Cytokine expression is decreased, suggesting that the inhibitory effects of nicotine involve more than just local vasoconstriction.[31,32]

Although the effect of hypoxia has not been studied independently, these observations suggest that the negative effects of smoking on arthrodesis cannot be avoided by switching from inhaled tobacco to oral or transdermal nicotine.

Smoking has been demonstrated to be a risk factor for nonunion after thoracic and cervical fusion surgery as well. In a review of 90 patients undergoing ventral instrumented spine fusion for adolescent scoliosis, 4 of 5 patients who developed a nonunion were smokers.[33]

A retrospective review of 131 patients who had multilevel cervical discectomies and fusions with autogenous interbody graft without instrumentation found a pseudarthrosis rate of 50% in smokers compared with 24% in nonsmokers.[34]

In animal models, bone morphogenetic protein was effective in reversing the inhibitory effects of nicotine on spine fusion.[35]

In some clinical series, the use of instrumentation and electrical stimulation has been reported to help overcome the inhibitory effects of smoking on spine fusion.[36,37]

Two studies have assessed whether the negative effects on fusion can be reversed by smoking cessation, with conflicting results. Glassman et al.[9] reported that whereas smokers had a nonunion rate of 26.5% after lumbar fusion surgery, those who stopped smoking for more than 6 months after surgery had a successful arthrodesis rate of 82.9%. This was not significantly different than the union rate of 85.8% in nonsmokers. However, Deguchi et al.[8] found no improvement in arthrodesis rate in their patients who stopped smoking.

Infection

Urinary tract infections are frequent in patients undergoing spine surgery. When associated with bacteremia, these infections are of particular concern because of the possibility of bacterial seeding of hardware. Thus, it is important to identify and treat established urinary tract infections before spinal instrumentation is applied.[38]

Compromised Host

The capacity of a compromised host to respond to infection or trauma is significantly impaired by disease or medication. Increased susceptibility to infection and delayed wound healing are the major postoperative problems in these patients and may arise from drugs such as corticosteroids, immunosuppressive agents, or cytotoxic agents and from prolonged antibiotic therapy. Infections in these patients can be caused by either common or opportunistic organisms. Malnutrition, renal failure, diabetes mellitus, and other immunocompromising diseases, including acquired immunodeficiency syndrome, significantly increase susceptibility to infection.

Multiple Trauma

Many spine surgery patients are the victims of severe accidents and have sustained multiple concomitant traumatic injuries. In such cases, urgent repair of spine injuries almost always takes precedence over assessment and treatment of chronic medical problems because acute spine stabilization dramatically reduces mortality, incidence of acute respiratory distress syndrome, length of hospital stay, and need for mechanical ventilation. Nonetheless, it is important to realize that the severity of neurologic injury, number of comorbidities, and use of high-dose steroids increase the risk of complication after thoracolumbar spine fracutrues.[39]

Patients with multiple trauma are often in their best state of health on admission. Efforts to delay spine stabilization may not be in their best interest.

After surgery, it is important to search for factors contributing to the accident, including alcohol and drug abuse, and unrecognized or untreated conditions such as liver disease, withdrawal syndromes, myocardial infarction (MI), arrhythmias, seizures, and hypoglycemia. All these conditions have postoperative implications and may require specific diagnostic and therapeutic interventions.

Rheumatologic Conditions

Patients with rheumatoid arthritis undergo a variety of spine procedures, particularly cervical fusion. These patients experience high complication rates for all surgical procedures. Wound breakdown, infection, loosening of instrumentation, and pseudarthrosis occur more frequently in patients with rheumatoid arthritis and can be attributed to poor tissue integrity, compromised vascular status, and the use of immunosuppressive drugs.[40,41]

Patients with rheumatoid arthritis should be examined for cervical spine involvement. Dynamic flexion and extension radiographs should be obtained to exclude occult instability before the administration of general endotracheal anesthesia. A variety of other problems, including anemia, pulmonary fibrosis, and pleural effusions, may be present. Chronic steroid use often results in adrenal suppression, requiring administration of perioperative stress-dose steroids. Similarly, patients with systemic lupus erythematosus and other rheumatologic conditions require thorough preoperative evaluation and may prove difficult to manage.[42]

Particular attention should be paid to patients with ankylosing spondylitis. These patients warrant very different management than the typical spine surgery patient with degenerative disease, especially with regard to positioning, traction, and orthoses.

Nonsurgical Diseases Affecting Surgical Risk

Cardiac Disease

Preoperative Evaluation

The most common symptoms of heart disease are dyspnea, fatigue, chest pain, and palpitation. It is important to inquire about exercise tolerance, paroxysmal nocturnal dyspnea, orthopnea, peripheral edema, irregular heartbeat, and chest pain. One should document significant past illnesses such as congenital heart disease, rheumatic fever, MI, atherosclerotic cerebrovascular and peripheral vascular disease, diabetes mellitus, hypertension, and autoimmune disease. Also, use of cardiac pacemakers, previous cardiac surgery, and past or present use of diuretics, digitalis, coronary vasodilators, antihypertensive drugs, and antiarrhythmic drugs should be noted. A history of angina pectoris, MI, Adams-Stokes attacks, stroke, cerebral ischemic attacks, intermittent claudication, or previous treatment for heart disease or hypertension should alert the surgeon to the possibility of a cardiac abnormality requiring further evaluation.

Conditions contraindicating elective surgery because of increased risk are acute MI, recent or crescendo angina pectoris, aortic stenosis, and atrioventricular block.

Physical Examination

The heart rate and rhythm must be recorded and any cyanosis, clubbing, petechiae, neck vein distention, and peripheral edema noted. The lungs should be auscultated for rales or wheezes. Auscultation permits evaluation of the first and second heart sounds, as well as of gallops and murmurs.

Radiologic Examination

Most preoperative patients require an anteroposterior chest radiograph to exclude cardiac enlargement, pulmonary vessel distention, and pulmonary infiltrates. Lateral views permit diagnosis of individual chamber enlargement.

Electrocardiography

An electrocardiogram (ECG) can help detect arrhythmias, conduction defects, chamber enlargement, and myocardial ischemia. Routine preoperative ECGs are obtained on all adult patients undergoing spine surgery. The ECG is useful diagnostically and also as a baseline measurement to evaluate subsequent changes in the myocardium and conduction system. In general, a stable abnormality on the ECG, in the absence of cardiac failure or angina pectoris, is indicative of only slightly increased perioperative risk.

Laboratory Tests

Serum concentrations of hemoglobin, sodium, potassium, and calcium may be relevant in the assessment of cardiac function. Arterial blood gas and pH studies indicate the adequacy of oxygenation.

Hemodynamic Studies

Pulse rate and cuff blood pressure are useful indicators of cardiac function. Monitoring arterial pressure with an intra-arterial line provides a more accurate value and permits waveform analysis. Central venous pressure (CVP) and pulmonary capillary wedge pressure (PCWP) indicate cardiac preload. PCWP reflects left ventricular filling pressure and left ventricular performance, whereas CVP reflects right ventricular function.

Elevations of CVP above 10 mm Hg suggest right ventricular failure. In most patients, left heart function correlates with right heart function. CVP exceeding PCWP by greater than 5 mm Hg indicates pulmonary artery hypertension; PCWP exceeding CVP by more than 5 mm Hg indicates isolated left ventricular failure. However, presence of a normal CVP does not exclude left ventricular failure. A PCWP below 10 mm Hg may be associated with shock and a PCWP above 25 mm Hg, with pulmonary edema.

For patients with cardiac or pulmonary disease, monitoring of PCWP with a Swan-Ganz catheter provides the best indication of left ventricular preload. Cardiac output can be measured by thermodilution using a Swan-Ganz catheter. Serial measurements can guide fluid therapy, even in the presence of left ventricular failure.

Echocardiography is a noninvasive method of studying cardiac anatomy and function. Cardiac catheterization with coronary angiography remains the most definitive cardiac diagnostic study, showing the vascular supply to different areas of the myocardium. This type of study is not without inherent risks.

Preoperative Preparation

The cardiac status of a spine surgery patient with cardiac dysfunction should be optimized before surgery. Special attention should be paid to correction of electrolyte imbalance, fluid excess, and anemia. It is important to avoid hypotension, hypoxia, fluid overload, and undue pain or excitement.

Cardiac Contraindications

Relative cardiac contraindications to operation are recent MI, uncontrolled congestive heart failure (CHF), unstable angina pectoris, intractable cardiac arrhythmias and conduction defects, and uncontrolled hypertension. Preoperative evaluation is directed toward detecting and treating these conditions.

The mortality rate after a major operation is 25% if the surgery is within 3 weeks of MI, 10% if within 3 months, and 5% if within 6 months. A patient with a healed MI has an added mortality risk of about 3%. Only emergent and urgent operations are indicated within 3 months; only semiurgent procedures are indicated from 3 to 6 months. Elective operations should be postponed until 6 to 12 months after MI.

Treatable causes of CHF include myocardial ischemia and its sequelae, valvular disease, bacterial endocarditis, sepsis, arrhythmias, hyperthyroidism, and hypertension. Careful perioperative management of these conditions will certainly decrease morbidity. Anginal chest pain may reflect severe coronary artery disease. Symptoms and signs denoting severe angina include associated sweating and nausea, poor response to coronary vasodilators (nitroglycerin), no relief with rest, frequent attacks, prolonged pain, and ECG evidence of ischemia.

High-risk coronary artery lesions include left main coronary artery occlusion, high left anterior descending artery lesions, and lesions in multiple vessels. Elective procedures should be postponed in patients with such lesions. Nonelective procedures may necessitate preliminary or coincident coronary artery bypass surgery. Patients who need urgent or emergent procedures require intensive perioperative management.

In hypertensive patients the blood pressure should be normalized before surgery. There is a linear correlation between preoperative blood pressure and postoperative myocardial ischemia.[34]

Postoperative Management

Patients with significant cardiac disease require close postoperative monitoring. Monitoring typically includes treatment in an intensive care setting for the first 24 hours after surgery.

Most postoperative MIs occur on the second or third postoperative day, and hence serial ECGs for 3 days are indicated in patients with known coronary artery disease. Chest pain is often difficult to evaluate in the postoperative period, and an MI may become apparent only because of hypotension or arrhythmia. Serial cardiac isoenzyme studies are especially useful for identifying postoperative infarcts, and should be obtained as well. Postoperative treatment for MI entails vigorous support and monitoring. Arrhythmias and cardiac failure should be treated as they arise.

Typically, cardiac failure shows symptoms of hypotension or oliguria and is most often a result of hypovolemia in the postoperative patient. If hypotension or oliguria persists after IV fluids are administered, the patient must undergo complete evaluation. When cardiac failure results from hypertensive crisis, blood pressure can be reduced with nitroprusside.

Cardiac failure unresponsive to other measures may respond to afterload reduction. Judicious use of drugs with a positive inotropic effect (e.g., dopamine, dobutamine, isoproterenol, and digitalis) may also prove to be beneficial. Heart performance is most efficient at a rate of 100 to 120 beats/min.

Pericardial restriction resulting from constrictive pericarditis or pericardial effusion is suggested by a decreased cardiac output with a high CVP. Typically, jugular veins are distended, and a paradoxical pulse may be present. Echocardiography may assist in making the diagnosis. Treatment consists of pericardiocentesis or pericardiotomy.

In the presence of bradycardia, one should look for anesthetic excess, hypoxia, atrioventricular block, or vagal stimulation by visceral traction, carotid sinus compression, or traction on extraocular muscles.

In the presence of falling blood pressure, one should look for anesthetic excess, myocardial ischemia, or inadequate preload caused by blood or fluid losses, obstruction of venous return, or vasodilation. Absence of blood pressure, carotid pulse, or respiration is an ominous sign. Treatment should include identification of the underlying cause and immediate correction of the abnormality (e.g., for ventricular fibrillation, electrical defibrillation should be used; for asystole, cardiac massage, vagolytic or sympathomimetic drugs, or cardiac pacing should be used). Cardiopulmonary resuscitation should be initiated immediately and continued until the underlying problem has been corrected. Four minutes without blood flow to the brain results in a fatal ischemic injury. Preexisting inadequacy of cerebral blood flow and oxygenation shortens the time available for correction. Closed chest cardiopulmonary resuscitation is the initial method of resuscitation. Open chest cardiac massage should be undertaken only as a last resort.

Treatment of the major arrhythmias is a complex problem requiring close collaboration of the internist and surgeon. If the surgeon is required to provide emergency treatment until the internist arrives, a general knowledge of cardiac arrhythmias and their treatment is important. Diagnosis of the arrhythmia is made from the ECG.

Atrial fibrillation decreases cardiac efficiency and may cause congestive failure. Treatment involves slowing the rate by adequate digitalization. Calcium channel blockers can be used in patients with no history of heart failure or cardiomyopathy. Conversion to normal sinus rhythm by quinidine or direct current (DC) countershock may be required if shock or pulmonary edema is noted.

Atrial flutter often causes congestive failure. Digitalization will slow the rate, either by increasing the degree of block or converting the flutter to sinus rhythm or atrial fibrillation. DC countershock is the treatment of choice, especially if the rhythm is poorly tolerated.

Paroxysmal supraventricular tachycardia often occurs in patients with otherwise normal hearts. In the absence of heart disease, serious effects are rare. Digitalis toxicity must be excluded as a cause. Vagal stimulation (carotid sinus massage, Valsalva maneuver) should be tried initially. If mechanical measures fail, pharmacotherapy is indicated. There is, however, no unanimity on the most effective medical therapy. Digitalis, vasopressors, procainamide, and propranolol can all be tried. Continuous ECG and blood pressure monitoring are essential. DC cardioversion may be indicated if the patient's condition deteriorates.

Ventricular tachycardia and ventricular fibrillation are usually associated with myocardial damage, especially MI. Lidocaine is the drug of choice for emergency treatment because of its short duration of action. If the arrhythmia recurs, an IV infusion may be given or the IV injection repeated. If lidocaine has no effect, DC cardioversion is preferable to additional pharmacotherapy.

Ventricular fibrillation produces cardiac arrest and requires defibrillation and cardiopulmonary resuscitation. DC cardioversion is often effective in converting patients back to sinus rhythm. If the initial attempt at cardioversion is unsuccessful, repetition with sequentially higher energy levels is indicated.

Pulmonary Disease

Preoperative Evaluation

The most common symptoms of pulmonary disease are dyspnea at rest or after minor exertion, cough, sputum production, wheezing, chest pain, and hemoptysis. It is important to document any history of tuberculosis, recent upper respiratory infection, chronic pulmonary disease, or asthma. One must determine the degree of tobacco and alcohol use as well as previous occupational exposures to coal dust, asbestos, and silica dusts. Establishment of a medication history, particularly regarding the use of corticosteroids, is especially important.

Physical Examination

The examiner must look for physical signs of pulmonary disease such as cyanosis or nail clubbing. It is important to observe the respiratory rate and respiratory effort as well as to percuss the chest for dullness or hyperresonance and to determine inspiratory diaphragm excursion. Auscultation of the chest allows the examiner to hear rales, rhonchi, wheezes, and decreased breath sounds.

Radiologic Examination

The chest radiograph may demonstrate pulmonary infiltrates, granulomas, atelectasis, hyperlucency, pneumothorax, abnormalities of pulmonary vasculature, or a mass. A negative radiograph does not exclude pulmonary disease. If any question exists, a CT scan of the chest may be obtained.

Laboratory Examination

Yellow, green, or brown sputum suggests active infection. Sputum culture is indicated to identify specific organisms and to determine antibiotic sensitivities. Arterial blood gas measurements help evaluate pulmonary gas exchange. The arterial partial pressure of oxygen (PaO_2) is an indicator of oxygen uptake by the blood in its passage through the lungs. PaO_2 is affected by the fraction of inspired oxygen, right-to-left shunting, and diffusion capacity across the alveolocapillary membrane. Normally, PaO_2 is 70 mm Hg or greater. A PaO_2

of 60 mm Hg indicates mild respiratory failure; a PaO_2 of 50 mm Hg or less indicates severe pulmonary disease. The oxygen saturation (SaO_2) reflects the percentage of hemoglobin actually bound by oxygen. Normally, SaO_2 is 93% or more; an SaO_2 of 90% indicates mild respiratory failure; an SaO_2 of 84% or less indicates severe pulmonary disease. The arterial partial pressure of carbon dioxide ($PaCO_2$) reflects the adequacy of ventilation. Normally, $PaCO_2$ is 38 to 43 mm Hg. A $PaCO_2$ of 44 to 54 mm Hg indicates mild impairment of ventilation; a $PaCO_2$ of 55 mm Hg or greater indicates severely impaired ventilation. Arterial blood pH is affected by both metabolic and respiratory factors. Normally, the arterial blood pH is 7.38 to 7.42.

Spirometry

The vital capacity (VC) is the maximum volume expired after a maximum inspiration. VC is decreased in restrictive disease but is usually normal in obstructive disease. A VC that is 50% or less of predicted indicates severe disease. The forced expiratory volume is the maximum volume expired after a maximum inspiration. Forced expiratory volume equals VC in restrictive disease but is less than VC in obstructive disease.

Preoperative Preparation

Patients without pulmonary symptoms can be expected to tolerate surgery from a respiratory standpoint. If a patient can climb two flights of stairs without shortness of breath, further evaluation of respiratory status is generally unnecessary. Factors that can predispose a patient to postoperative pulmonary complications are long-term cigarette smoking, chronic obstructive pulmonary disease, upper abdominal and thoracic procedures, acute respiratory infections, and restrictive disorders such as obesity, pulmonary fibrosis, and neuromuscular and skeletal disease. Patients with one or more of these factors require careful preoperative preparation, and most should undergo complete pulmonary evaluation. Elective procedures should be postponed until maximum pulmonary function has been achieved. All patients should stop smoking at least 2 weeks before any elective operation. Overweight patients should try to achieve ideal body weight. All patients should receive preoperative instruction in coughing, deep breathing, and use of the incentive spirometer.

Respiratory infections should be treated before elective operations. Viral infections resolve with symptomatic treatment; bacterial infections can be treated with the appropriate antibiotics. Whenever possible, preoperative preparation and treatment should be performed on an outpatient basis to avoid superinfection with hospital-acquired antibiotic-resistant organisms. Adequate hydration, humidified air, and expectorants can help liquefy sputum. Postural drainage and chest percussion can help clear these secretions. Bronchodilators are often helpful for patients with chronic obstructive pulmonary disease. In addition, patients with bronchospasm or asthma may benefit from the administration of bronchodilators either by aerosol or by intermittent positive-pressure ventilation. Corticosteroids may be necessary for patients with severe asthma or pulmonary fibrosis.

If aspiration is observed, endotracheal intubation, airway suctioning, and saline lavage should be performed immediately. Bronchorrhea will neutralize the acidic gastric juices within 10 minutes so lavage after this interval is of no benefit. Moreover, steroid treatment has no objective benefit. Antibiotics should be reserved to treat specific organisms and should not be used prophylactically.

No patient should be denied operation for emergent and urgent conditions because of pulmonary disease. Whenever possible, the risks should be recognized and pulmonary function optimized.

Postoperative Management

The postoperative effects of major procedures under general anesthesia include decreases in total lung capacity, vital capacity, functional residual volume, and compliance. Aggressive postoperative care minimizes these effects. Administering low doses of analgesics at frequent intervals promotes improved respiration by controlling pain without compromising respiratory drive. Frequent change of position and early ambulation are also beneficial. Changing the volume of ventilation prevents atelectasis. Incentive spirometry promotes deep inspiration that can also help prevent atelectasis.

Oxygen administration should be used when necessary but with judiciousness; 100% oxygen promotes atelectasis and may result in oxygen toxicity. Administering oxygen to patients with chronic hypercapnia may depress respiratory drive. The elderly and patients with acutely impaired respiratory function may require ventilatory support over the first postoperative night. Arterial blood gases and fluid therapy should be closely monitored; administration of both insufficient and excessive fluid impairs respiratory function. Patients with bronchospasm may benefit from bronchodilator therapy.

Pulmonary Complications

Ventilatory impairment is typical after ventral thoracic and lumbar approaches to the spine. In most instances, the impairment does not prevent spontaneous breathing. However, if the operative procedures are extensive, if there has been massive trauma, if the patient is elderly, or if the patient has preexisting chronic disease or malnutrition, ventilatory impairment may be so great that a period of assisted ventilation is necessary.

The first postoperative hours are critical because this is when acute ventilatory failure most commonly occurs. The effects of muscle relaxants may not have worn off completely, and muscle weakness can cause reduced vital capacity. If a respiratory complication develops, decreased lung compliance may also contribute to inadequate ventilatory function.

Pneumothorax is an uncommon complication in elective surgical procedures, but it should be considered in any patient who develops acute respiratory distress or intraoperative deterioration. The principal cause of pneumothorax in hospitalized patients is iatrogenic lung puncture during percutaneous central venous catheter placement. It can also occur in a patient who coughs and thereby ruptures a pulmonary bleb or bulla. Diagnosis is made on the basis of decreased or absent breath sounds on the affected side, with hyperresonance to percussion. When a tension pneumothorax develops there may also be a lateral shift of the trachea away from the affected side. Any patient who develops respiratory distress after insertion of a central venous catheter should be presumed to have a pneumothorax, and a chest tube should be inserted immediately and not delayed for the radiograph.

If pneumothorax is suspected but the patient is comfortable, one should first obtain the chest radiograph and insert a chest tube if indicated.

Atelectasis is the most common complication in the first 2 to 3 postoperative days. It results from collapse of the most dependent portions of the lung. Clinical signs include fever, tachypnea, and tachycardia that typically develop within the first 2 postoperative days. Chest radiographs usually show linear densities in dependent segments of the lungs or frank areas of collapse. There is often radiographic evidence of volume loss in the affected lung. Treatment entails deep breathing and coughing to expand underventilated lung segments. The patient should be mobilized if there are no contraindications. Mechanical devices, including the incentive spirometer and devices to maintain positive airway pressure, help achieve adequate ventilation.

If the preceding methods fail to reverse atelectasis, bronchoscopy may be indicated for suctioning secretions out of the atelectatic segment. This is rarely necessary and should be used only when the atelectasis is severe and involves an entire lobe, if the patient is developing respiratory distress, or if blood gas levels are deteriorating.

Acute pulmonary edema is common in elderly patients with compromised cardiac function or in patients with significant cardiac disease. Typically, it develops on the second or third postoperative day as third-space fluid is mobilized. Alternatively, it can occur with excessive administration of fluid during surgery or immediately after surgery if cardiac or renal function is compromised. Healthy patients with normal cardiac and renal function usually tolerate fluid overload with prompt diuresis and no pulmonary symptoms.

The diagnosis of acute pulmonary edema is made by the presence of tachypnea, tachycardia, shortness of breath, and orthopnea. These symptoms are often coupled with elevated CVP, distended neck veins, and wet rales bilaterally in the basilar lung segments. These rales may extend two thirds of the way up the lungs. In addition, the sputum is often frothy and pink. Chest radiographs show symmetrical perihilar fluffy infiltrates, cardiac enlargement, prominent pulmonary vascular shadows, and lymphatic congestion in the costophrenic angles (Kerley B lines).

Pneumonia in the postoperative patient usually results from inadequately treated atelectasis, airway contamination, or preexistent pulmonary disease, most commonly a consequence of cigarette smoking. Pneumonia rarely develops earlier than 4 to 5 days after operation unless an unusual event, such as aspiration, occurs. The source is almost always bacterial, and if the patient has been given prophylactic or therapeutic antibiotics from the time of surgery, one may assume that the organism causing the pneumonia is resistant to the antibiotics.

The diagnosis is made by the presence of fever, leukocytosis, increased sputum production, decreased breath sounds or rales on physical examination, and a localized or diffuse infiltrate on radiographs. Gram staining of the sputum usually reveals heavy colonization by a single organism, and a large number of polymorphonuclear leukocytes are present. If pneumonia is diagnosed, antibiotic therapy should be started immediately, on the basis of the Gram stain. Confirmatory cultures must be obtained, and the antibiotic sensitivities checked. Antibiotic therapy can then be guided by these sensitivities. Therapy should include supportive care as well as measures directed at the underlying cause of the pneumonia. Blood gases should be monitored and endotracheal intubation and ventilation carried out if the patient's status deteriorates.

Acute Respiratory Distress Syndrome

In rare instances after extensive surgery or massive trauma, patients develop tachypnea, hypoxemia, diffuse pulmonary infiltrates, and decreased compliance of the lungs. Physical examination does not reveal rales, bronchospasm, or evidence of alveolar edema. In these situations, the diagnosis of acute respiratory distress syndrome (ARDS) is made. In many cases, ARDS appears to be related to pulmonary microembolism, and the findings are similar to those described for fat embolism. Evidence of intravascular coagulation is common with this syndrome, but the role of intravascular coagulation as a specific cause has not been proved. ARDS normally does not develop until 3 days after surgery, and it is often associated with sepsis.

When the disease is mild, supportive care with oxygen administration may be sufficient. In most cases, the symptoms are severe and hypoxemia mandates intubation and mechanical ventilation. In severe cases, positive end-expiratory pressure must be used to improve oxygenation.

A pulmonary artery catheter to monitor PCWP is mandatory for careful titration of fluid therapy. Because of the high mortality associated with the development of renal failure in patients with ARDS, attempts must be made to preserve renal function by adequate hydration. At the same time, one must avoid overhydration, which can increase pulmonary interstitial edema. PCWP should be kept as low as possible, while adequate peripheral perfusion and a urine output of 0.5 mL/kg/hr are maintained. PCWP should not exceed 15 mm Hg. Steroids and diuretics have not been shown to be of benefit.

Fat embolism syndrome may occur after extensive trauma. Although the true etiology of this syndrome is poorly defined, it was initially postulated to result from embolization of marrow fat to the pulmonary capillaries, producing symptoms by mechanical obstruction and inflammation. Arguing against this mechanism are the pathologic findings of fat in pulmonary, renal, and cerebral capillaries in traumatized patients without fractures or evidence of bony injury. The symptoms are nearly indistinguishable from those of ARDS: tachypnea, hypoxemia, pulmonary infiltrates, and decreased lung compliance. The only clinical difference is a higher incidence of cerebral symptoms, including disorientation, confusion, and progressive obtundation without localizing signs.

Pulmonary Embolism

Dyspnea, pleuritic chest pain, and hemoptysis are the classic symptoms of pulmonary embolism. Physical examination may reveal decreased breath sounds, pleural rub, or pleural effusion. Moreover, chest radiographs may demonstrate a wedge-shaped density and the ECG may show evidence of right ventricular strain. Ventilation-perfusion scan of the lungs often reveals areas of decreased perfusion. Pulmonary angiography, the gold standard for diagnosis, occasionally shows obstruction of large pulmonary arteries.

Pulmonary embolism accompanied by circulatory and respiratory instability mandates treatment with high-dose IV heparin. Placement of a Greenfield filter or ligation of the inferior vena cava may be required if anticoagulants are contraindicated, if bleeding complications develop in a patient receiving anticoagulants, or if pulmonary embolism recurs in a fully anticoagulated patient.

Renal Disease

Preoperative Evaluation

Urinary frequency and volume, dysuria, nocturia, poor stream, incontinence, and hematuria must be checked. It is important to note any history of renal disease, calculi, diabetes mellitus, or hypertension and to establish whether there has been any use of diuretics or nephrotoxins.

A history of the use of acetaminophen, a potential nephrotoxin, is particularly revealing in patients who undergo spine surgery. Often, patients with low back pain consume substantial quantities of acetaminophen without recognizing its potential harm. Symptoms and signs of renal disease frequently reflect the degree of renal failure; however, it is not uncommon for patients with marked impairment of renal function to be asymptomatic.

Urinary tract obstruction should be suspected in any anuric patient. Upper tract obstruction must be bilateral for azotemia to occur. A renal hippurate scan, infusion IV pyelography, renal ultrasonography, and retrograde ureteral catheterization are important diagnostic tests. Renal scans are very useful for detecting acute obstruction. Sonography, infusion IV pyelography, and retrograde catheterization are indicated in patients with chronic obstruction. Obstruction of the lower tract is recognized by the inability to insert a Foley catheter.

Physical Examination

The patient must be carefully checked for edema or dehydration. Metabolic acidosis may result in hyperventilation, and pericardial effusions can sometimes produce a friction rub.

Laboratory Examination

Blood urea nitrogen (BUN), serum creatinine measurements, and routine urinalysis are adequate screening tests for renal disease. A freshly voided urine sample yields much information about renal status.

Hematuria may be secondary to glomerular disease or to a lesion in the collecting system. In addition, the finding of different types of casts in the urine may be a sign of advancing renal disease. Red cell casts are suggestive of acute glomerular dysfunction, whereas white cell casts are indicative of acute pyelonephritis. It must be kept in mind that in patients with reduced muscle mass, serum creatinine levels can remain within the normal range even though creatinine clearance is no more than 20% of normal values. BUN-to-creatinine ratios greater than 10:1 may reflect prerenal azotemia, gastrointestinal bleeding, or enhanced catabolic states or may be secondary to catabolic drug effects.

Random urine samples usually have a specific gravity of 1.012 to 1.015. A higher specific gravity reflects dehydration or the presence of solutes, such as radiograph contrast medium, glucose, or mannitol. Dilute urine (specific gravity <1.007) reflects overhydration, diuretic therapy, water intoxication, or diabetes insipidus. A fixed specific gravity of 1.010 to 1.014 (isosthenuria) signifies a lack of renal tubular concentrating ability and occurs in renal parenchymal disease, congenital tubular defects, and acute tubular necrosis (ATN).

The normal pH range of the urine is 4.3 to 5.0. This range can be affected by diet and other factors. Aciduria may result from metabolic or respiratory acidosis, potassium depletion, starvation, or fever. Alkaline urine results from metabolic or respiratory alkalosis, certain urinary infections, and carbonic anhydrase-B–inhibiting diuretics.

Transient proteinuria may result from fever, cold exposure, strenuous exercise, and acute stress. Persistent proteinuria may signify true renal disease. Proteinuria is the earliest sign of aminoglycoside toxicity. Glucosuria usually signifies diabetes mellitus but may result from benign renal glucosuria, renal tubular disorders, pregnancy, or glucose infusion. The presence of reducing agents in the urine may also yield significant information about the patient's status. Ketonuria occurs with diabetic ketoacidosis, excessive vomiting, starvation, or cachexia and after strenuous exercise and cold exposure. One must keep in mind that ascorbic acid, cephalosporins, salicylates, paraldehyde, and chloral hydrate can alter reactions that measure urinary reducing agents. The dipstick test for occult blood is a useful screening test. It is positive with more than 10 red blood cells per high-power field in a spun urine sediment. However, myoglobinuria and hemoglobinuria can also give a positive reaction.

BUN concentration varies with dietary nitrogen consumption, hepatic urea production, and endogenous protein catabolism. It is increased by dehydration, gastrointestinal hemorrhage, hemolysis, corticosteroid therapy, and the tissue breakdown associated with trauma, shock, or sepsis.

Finally, the serum creatinine concentration is an important value because it reflects glomerular filtration. Creatinine production is correlated to muscle mass and, in a given individual, remains nearly constant in the absence of muscle destruction. Creatinine clearance (CLcr) is a more exact indicator of glomerular filtration and is defined by the equation

$$Clcr = (U[cr] \times V)\ P[cr]$$

where U[cr] = urine creatinine concentration in mg/dL, P[cr] = serum creatinine concentration in mg/dL, and V = urine volume in mL/min. Normal creatinine clearance is 125 ± 25 mL/min/1.73 m^2. A minimum clearance of 10 mL/min/1.73 m^2 is needed to maintain life without dialysis. Serum creatinine level may remain normal until the clearance is reduced by more than half.

Preoperative Preparation

In the preoperative period, it is important to assess renal function carefully and correct any electrolyte abnormalities. Anephric patients, if managed carefully, tolerate operations well. Preoperative preparation should maximize renal function and is important for preventing postoperative failure. Urinary tract infection should be treated preoperatively with appropriate antibiotics as determined by urine culture and sensitivity tests.

Obstructive lesions of the urinary tract should be removed or corrected, if possible, before other major operations are planned. Dehydration, hypovolemia, and electrolyte imbalance should be corrected, and adequate urine volume should be ensured before surgery. Metabolic acidosis, even though compensated, should be corrected with sodium bicarbonate.

Anemia is a frequent finding in patients with renal disease and should be evaluated preoperatively. A hemoglobin level of 9 g/dL and a hematocrit of 25% are satisfactory for patients with chronic renal insufficiency. Patients on hemodialysis adapt to hematocrits in the range of 20% and do not need transfusions unless there is significant blood loss. Blood transfusion should be used cautiously to avoid cardiac decompensation.

Coagulation defects in patients with chronic renal disease should be identified and corrected. Patients with severe renal failure often have platelet dysfunction that can cause bleeding. Elective procedures should be delayed until platelet dysfunction is corrected with hemodialysis on the day before surgery. Follow-up hemodialysis, with its attendant anticoagulation and fluid shifts, can be delayed until the second or third postoperative day.

It is important to maintain all antihypertensive medications, including beta-blockers and catecholamine-depleting drugs, until the night before surgery. Discontinuation of clonidine may result in paroxysmal hypertension, and abrupt withdrawal of certain beta-blockers can produce cardiac dysrhythmia. Patients who take diuretics may require correction of volume contraction and hypokalemia. When possible, one should avoid nephrotoxic drugs and be on the alert for medications that accumulate because of decreased renal excretion. Use of nephrotoxic IV contrast media should be limited.

Postoperative Management

The diseased kidney is unable to concentrate urine and must excrete a urine volume greater than normal to rid the body of metabolic end products. At the same time, the kidney may be unable to excrete water and electrolytes. There is a slim margin between further renal insufficiency from dehydration and CHF secondary to excess salt and water retention. Effective management requires monitoring of body weight, intake and output, serum electrolytes, pH, CVP, and PCWP. Keeping track of urine electrolyte concentrations and of all measurable fluid losses helps guide appropriate fluid therapy. By themselves, however, urine output and specific gravity do not reliably reflect the state of hydration.

Nephrotoxic drugs must be administered carefully and in reduced doses to patients with impaired renal function. These agents include aminoglycoside antibiotics, cephaloridine, colistin, polymyxin B, and amphotericin B. Spot checks for urine protein are useful for detecting early aminoglycoside toxicity. Drugs requiring major dose modification in the renally impaired patient include allopurinol, digoxin, methotrexate, phenobarbital, procainamide, quinidine, and tolbutamide.

Postoperative urine output less than 25 mL/hr requires immediate evaluation. Oliguria suggests prerenal or renal parenchymal failure. Anuria suggests vascular obstruction, cortical necrosis, or urinary tract obstruction.

Acute Renal Failure

The hallmark of acute renal failure is rapidly progressive azotemia, generally accompanied by oliguria (urine output <400 mL/24 hr). Prerenal azotemia results from renal hypoperfusion caused by volume depletion (dehydration or blood loss) or decreased cardiac output from pump failure (CHF). An expeditious diagnosis of prerenal azotemia is essential because the condition is easily reversible and persistent renal hypoperfusion results in ATN.

The physician must assess the patient's volume status frequently (i.e., fullness of neck veins, skin turgor, orthostatic changes in blood pressure and heart rate, and peripheral perfusion). Examination of the heart and lungs may reveal signs of CHF.

Bladder catheterization can be helpful for obtaining urine specimens and monitoring urine output carefully. Measurements of serum BUN, creatinine, electrolytes, and osmolality, as well as of urine electrolytes and osmolality, can also be of diagnostic value.

Following the aforementioned suggestions should help distinguish whether prerenal azotemia is secondary to hypovolemia or CHF. In patients with tenuous cardiac function, measurement of CVP or even PCWP may be necessary before therapy is instituted.

Hypovolemic patients should be given normal saline solution at a rate of 100 to 500 mL/hr depending on the severity of volume depletion. Diuretics should not be administered before hypovolemia is corrected.

If there is no improvement in urine output after blood volume has been replenished, a bolus of furosemide or mannitol may be administered. Mannitol should be infused carefully because if oliguria persists, failure to excrete mannitol will produce volume expansion and pulmonary edema. If there is no response to these diuretics, ATN or obstructive uropathy is probably present.

The clinical setting and the laboratory tests, especially the results of urinalysis, are generally sufficient to establish the diagnosis of ATN. ATN may be a consequence of ischemia, nephrotoxins, or unknown mechanisms. The course of ATN is divided into three phases: pre-ATN, oliguric, and diuretic phases. As the kidneys recover, the urine output gradually increases. Occasionally, this postoliguric diuresis is massive. The severity of renal damage varies. In mild cases, there may be high urinary output rather than oliguria (nonoliguric ATN). Anuria (urine output <50 mL/24 hr) is rare in ATN. Bilateral cortical necrosis, acute glomerulonephritis, urinary obstruction, and thrombosis of the major renal vessels are more likely to produce anuria.

The abnormalities described in chronic renal failure also occur in acute renal failure, frequently with greater severity because of the acuteness of renal dysfunction. Fluid and electrolyte abnormalities are invariably present, and profound acidosis and severe hyperkalemia are common. In ATN, infection and gastrointestinal bleeding are the major associated complications. Infection is the principal cause of death.

Treatment of ATN is supportive and is directed at preventing or treating complications until renal function returns to normal. There is no evidence that the course of established ATN is modified by the administration of furosemide or mannitol. Diuretics should not be given.

Measurable fluid losses and insensible losses should be replaced. Fluid intake, fluid output, and body weight should be meticulously assessed. In addition, sodium losses from urine or other measurable sources should be replaced. Hyponatremia developing in the course of ATN is usually indicative of fluid excess rather than of sodium deficit and is best treated by fluid restriction. In addition, hyperkalemia frequently occurs in these patients. A variety of factors contribute to hyperkalemia, including acidosis and potassium release from tissues secondary to excessive catabolism, trauma, or hemolysis. The serum potassium concentration and the ECG must be monitored.

Severe hyperkalemia (serum potassium level >7 mEq/L) requires more urgent therapy, including administration of sodium bicarbonate or hypertonic glucose solution and an insulin drip. Life-threatening cardiac arrhythmias due to hyperkalemia should be treated by IV calcium gluconate, or calcium chloride dialysis may be required to remove excess potassium. It is advisable to restrict magnesium and check for hypocalcemia. Acidosis in ATN may be treated cautiously with sodium bicarbonate, but this may result in hypernatremia and heart failure. Acidosis associated with volume overload is best treated by dialysis.

Adequate nutrition is fundamental in the treatment of ATN. Dosages of drugs, including antibiotics, digoxin, and magnesium-containing antacids, must be modified. If a nephrotoxin may have caused the ATN, it should be discontinued.

As suggested previously, the indications for dialysis include uncontrollable hyperkalemia or acidosis, overhydration, and the development of uremic symptoms. Peritoneal dialysis and hemodialysis are equally effective. Early and aggressive dialysis seems to result in improved survival in patients with ATN.

ATN has an overall mortality rate of 50%. Mortality is approximately 80% in patients with burns, trauma, or surgical procedures and only 30% with medical ATN. This is presumably because there are more complications of the underlying condition in the surgical group.

Urinary Retention

Inability to urinate after surgery is a frequent problem and may be seen after any operation. Causes include reflex spasm of the voluntary sphincter because of pain or anxiety, medications (usually anticholinergics and narcotics), preexisting partial bladder outlet obstruction (e.g., enlarged prostate), and intraoperative overdistention.

Preoperative voiding patterns should be evaluated if a bladder outlet obstruction is suspected. Obstruction can be corrected before operation, or catheter drainage may be instituted immediately after surgery. Excessive use of narcotics and parasympatholytic drugs should be avoided. Patients scheduled for lengthy operations should be catheterized preoperatively and the bladder drained throughout the procedure.

If a patient is unable to pass urine for several hours after surgery, and there is no urge to urinate, one must explore the possibility of oliguria as a consequence of diminished volume status. Occasionally, a heavily sedated patient does not recognize the sensation of fullness and does not urinate for that reason.

A palpable bladder in the midline above the symphysis pubis is highly suggestive of acute urinary retention. Any patient who does not urinate for 6 hours after operation should be evaluated carefully. In this way, overdistention of the bladder, which may induce bladder atony and even myogenic damage to the bladder wall, can be avoided.

Urinary retention can be relieved in a variety of ways. Narcotics or sedatives may help relieve local pain. Moreover, if the condition permits, the patient can be positioned in the standing or sitting position instead of the supine position for urination. Cholinergic drugs such as bethanechol chloride may be administered.

When all other measures fail, if the bladder is markedly distended and severe bladder contractions occur without voiding, single-pass, straight catheterization should be performed so that patients can void on their own. A preoperative history of any voiding difficulty is very important to help decide on the duration of catheter drainage. If there was minimal preoperative obstruction, the patient should be able to resume normal voiding spontaneously. Under no circumstances should the bladder be allowed to overdistend. If the patient cannot void spontaneously after two catheterizations and there is evidence of overstretching or mild mechanical obstruction, a Foley catheter should be left in place for 2 to 3 days before testing for spontaneous voiding again. It is of note that men after middle age often have mechanical obstruction secondary to prostatic enlargement. Women are more susceptible to detrusor atony after overstretching, especially if the period of overstretching is prolonged.

Gastrointestinal Complications

Gastric Distention and Dilation

The stomach frequently becomes distended with gas during anesthesia induction, and further quantities of air are swallowed in the postoperative period. Gastric juices and duodenal secretions that reflux into the stomach contribute to this distention. Marked gastric distention can result in nausea and vomiting. Moreover, the distended stomach may impair diaphragmatic excursion and cause tachypnea. Nasogastric intubation for 12 to 24 hours is usually sufficient treatment; however, intubation for longer periods is occasionally necessary.

Vomiting immediately after an operation may be the result of a direct anesthetic effect or the result of gastric distention. Regardless of the cause, the best management is nasogastric intubation and suction to maintain an empty stomach for 12 to 24 hours. Medications that suppress nausea are less effective and can have untoward side effects, including vasodilation. Vomiting later in the postoperative period may be the result of drugs, ileus, mechanical obstruction of the gut, or other problems and should be investigated. Gastric stress ulcers and acid reflux must be considered in patients with multiple traumas, ICU patients, and patients who were in the prone position for an extended period of time. Appropriate prophylaxis against gastrointestinal bleeding should be considered in these patients. Agents include a low-dose proton pump inhibitor or a histamine type 2 receptor antagonist.

Gastric dilation occurs when the stomach becomes massively distended. Hemorrhage from the gastric mucosa can develop. This uncommon surgical complication is an occult cause of shock in the first few hours after operation. If the fluid is vomited, aspiration may occur. The distended, tympanitic stomach may be visible in the epigastrium or on a radiograph. Typically, nasogastric intubation yields dark, bloody fluid. Fluid and electrolyte losses must be replaced. Acute gastric dilation can be fatal if it is unrecognized, and prompt treatment usually results in dramatic improvement.

Paralytic ileus is the cessation of effective gastrointestinal motility after trauma, severe illness, or surgery. Ileus is primarily a gastric phenomenon because the remainder of the gut can usually handle fluids earlier than the stomach. Vomiting and abdominal distention are the main manifestations. Decreased bowel sounds are an unreliable finding. Abdominal radiographs show gas in the stomach, small bowel, and colon. Mechanical bowel obstruction must be excluded in such patients. Any patient with ileus should be given bowel rest (given nothing by mouth) and should have a nasogastric tube inserted and left in place until the ileus resolves.

Another potential gastrointestinal complication is constipation. Several factors contribute to postoperative constipation. First, taking nothing by mouth eliminates gastrocolic reflexes and reduces fecal bulk. Second, dehydration encourages fluid absorption from the colonic contents, desiccating the stool. Third, ileus has a component of impaired colonic motility. Finally, incisional pain makes patients unwilling to increase intra-abdominal pressure, eliminating an important force contributing to defecation. Physical inactivity removes stimuli to movement of feces through the colon. Furthermore, opiates and antacids containing calcium or aluminum exacerbate constipation. Often, attempts to defecate on a bedpan are unsuccessful because the patient is semirecumbent. The normal sitting or squatting position raises abdominal pressure and helps evacuate the rectum.

Hiccups are another potential complication. Typically, they are self-limited; however, they can be sufficiently persistent and exhausting to endanger life in a severely debilitated patient. They are produced by any process that stimulates the afferent or efferent phrenic nerve pathways. Therefore, the causes are quite varied and include central nervous system, cardiopulmonary, and gastrointestinal conditions, as well as renal failure, infectious diseases, and steroid therapy.

Treatment should be directed at the cause when possible, but therapy is frequently only symptomatic. Breath holding, drinking a large glass of water, or gastric lavage with a warm 1% solution of sodium bicarbonate may be effective. Rebreathing into a paper bag or administration of 10% to 15% carbon dioxide by face mask induces hyperventilation and may interrupt the reflex. Tranquilizing drugs such as chlorpromazine hydrochloride or other phenothiazine preparations are worth trying in patients with prolonged hiccups. Barbiturate sedation may be effective.

Disorders of Hemostasis

Patients with preexisting hemostatic disorders undergo operations more frequently than in the past. Because specific replacement therapies are available, it is essential to identify the exact defect before surgery whenever possible. Occasionally, the first sign of a hemostatic defect is excessive bleeding at operation. This distressing situation will seldom arise from a preexisting disorder if a bleeding history and screening laboratory tests are obtained before surgery.

Screening Procedures

Blood is potentially the most dangerous substance prescribed by most physicians. Complications are common and may be fatal. Transmission of syphilis, malaria, bacteria, and viruses is infrequent with current blood banking practices. Hepatitis, however, remains a problem. Blood products carry a hepatitis risk proportional to the number of donors contributing to the blood pool. Recently, available assays for hepatitis have greatly reduced the potential of distributing blood from hepatitis carriers, but most cases of hepatitis that occur after transfusion in the United States are not a result of hepatitis B or other known viruses. The statistical risk of hepatitis is unknown because the majority of cases are subclinical. Blood is an allograft, and the recipient may become immunized against human leukocyte antigens, platelet antigens, and red cell antigens. Reactions to leukocyte antigens are the probable cause of many febrile responses to transfusions. Reactions to transfusions of proteins, especially immunoglobulin A, are frequently severe and may be hemolytic in nature.

Administration of blood to the wrong recipient is the most common error and is usually the result of a clerical error such as incorrect specimen labeling. Such an error can cause serious immunologic complication. Massive hemolysis may occur, leading to renal failure and death. Symptoms of early hemolysis are chills, fever, back pains, circulatory collapse, and hemorrhage. Delayed hemolysis occurs from several days to 1 month after transfusion and is manifested by anemia or mild jaundice.

Transfusion Reactions

In the case of a transfusion reaction, the transfusion should be immediately halted and the remaining blood returned to the bank for investigation of the appropriateness of the cross-match, the Rh compatibility, and the Coombs test. The patient should be adequately hydrated. Samples of plasma and urine should be tested for hemoglobin. The presence of hemoglobin in these fluids implies hemolysis. Cultures should be obtained of the recipient's blood and the donor's blood. If a severe reaction has occurred, renal function should be evaluated and protected by administration of mannitol and bicarbonate. Febrile reactions, without hemolysis, should be treated with antihistamines and acetaminophen. Isoimmunized patients who require subsequent transfusions should receive washed red cells.

Surgical patients usually receive blood transfusions for the restoration of red cell mass or blood volume. Anemic patients who are asymptomatic are able to tolerate operations of almost any magnitude if operative blood loss is minimal. If a surgical procedure commonly associated with substantial blood loss is planned, anemia should be corrected 1 to 2 days before operation so that the storage-related defects of transfused blood can be normalized. Moreover, preoperative transfusion permits preoperative detection of transfusion reactions. Red cell concentrates are preferred for correction of preoperative anemia in stable patients.

The need for transfusion to correct mild postoperative anemia is assessed by measurement of the reticulocyte count. If the count is elevated and the patient does not have postural hypotension or dyspnea, transfusion is not indicated. If the reticulocyte count is low, the response to oral or parenteral iron should be determined before giving blood. Chronically ill patients frequently have a regenerative anemia and may require serial blood transfusions.

Banked blood lacks functioning platelets. Platelets lose their aggregability in cold storage, and preservatives do not maintain platelet viability beyond 72 hours. In addition, most banks with component programs routinely remove the platelets from donated blood. Absent or nonfunctioning platelets contribute to posttransfusion bleeding, and the magnitude of the problem is proportional to the number of units of blood administered. Platelet concentrates (or platelet packs) should be given to patients receiving 10 or more units of blood within 1 hour.

Whole blood is preferable for patients with exsanguinating hemorrhage because red cell concentrates cannot be rapidly administered.

Prophylaxis

Autologous Blood Donation

Autologous blood transfusion avoids most of the complications associated with transfusion of homologous blood, including transmission of disease, hemolytic transfusion reactions, and other immune phenomena. Despite existing medical problems, most patients are able to donate at least two units of autologous blood before surgery. This could potentially enable over 90% of patients to avoid homologous transfusion during major spine procedures. Autologous blood can normally be stored for up to 40 days (longer storage requires an expensive and complex freezing process). One unit of autologous blood can be processed from a given patient every 3 days up to 3 days before surgery, provided the hematocrit remains at least 34%. Iron supplementation is recommended. Treatment with erythropoietin can increase the patient's hematocrit and allow more blood to be stored in advance of surgery. It can also be used without predonation to minimize the need for transfusion at the time of surgery.[43]

There are two forms of autotransfusion. In one type, a patient donates blood in advance of elective operation, and this blood is stored for transfusion back into the donor, should it be required. This practice permits stimulation of erythropoiesis and results in restoration of red cell mass to near-normal levels by the time of operation. A further advantage is the availability of the safest possible blood, should the patient require it.

The other type of autotransfusion is useful in emergencies. Blood lost by the patient is collected into an apparatus designed for this purpose (e.g., the cell-saver), anticoagulated, and immediately returned to the circulation. This type of autotransfusion is most useful in cases of massive bleeding. It may be life saving when compatible blood is unavailable. Reinfusion of large amounts of blood, however, can cause coagulopathies.

Antibiotic Prophylaxis

Prophylactic antibiotics are administered routinely to patients undergoing spine surgery, particularly those undergoing spinal instrumentation, because of the severe consequences of infected prostheses. Short courses of antibiotics are safe and effective. Longer courses have been associated with *Clostridium difficile* colitis. Prophylaxis for endocarditis is not necessary for clean spine procedures, because the risk of bacteremia is low.

Prophylaxis for Thromboembolism

The most important prophylaxis issue in patients undergoing spine surgery is the prevention of deep venous thrombosis and pulmonary embolism. The incidence of deep venous thrombosis in spine surgery is not known. Estimates as high as 60% have been made. Prophylaxis for thromboembolism should therefore be considered in all patients undergoing major spine procedures, especially if patients are not immediately ambulatory. Thigh-length sequential compression devices, thromboembolic stockings, and low-dose heparin serve as prophylaxis for deep venous thrombosis in elective spine surgery. Initial studies suggest that low-molecular-weight heparin and heparinoids may be effective and safe in these patients. The benefits of prophylactic anticoagulation must be balanced against the risk. Cain et al.[44] reported a high rate of complications due to therapeutic heparinization after pulmonary embolus in spine surgery patients. In a poll of Scoliosis Research Society members representing more than 13,000 thoracic and lumbar fusions, they identified 9 patients who were treated with heparin anticoagulation. Complications attributable to anticoagulation were reported in two thirds of these patients.

Anticoagulation

Anticoagulation is defined as suppression of the coagulation mechanism. The term is used loosely in clinical practice, however, and it may refer to the suppression of clotting or the inhibition of platelet aggregation.

The only absolute anticoagulant is heparin, a physiologic substance present in mast cells that suppresses thrombin formation. Oral anticoagulant agents are less effective. They block coagulation indirectly by depressing certain factors in the clotting cascade. Antiplatelet agents interfere with platelet aggregation and thus inhibit coagulation.

Venous clots are composed of fibrin. As a result, anticoagulants are effective for preventing and treating venous thrombosis. Arterial clots are composed mainly of platelets. Therefore, antiplatelet medications are useful for preventing arterial thrombosis.

Heparin can be administered either subcutaneously or intravenously. Subcutaneous heparin is used only when small amounts of heparin are required, most often for prophylaxis against clotting. Larger doses of heparin required to treat thrombotic states should be administered intravenously.

In general, for clotting prophylaxis, sufficient heparin is administered to decrease the coagulation tendency without altering coagulation parameters. This avoids the complications inherent in systemic anticoagulation. Clotting measures such as the Lee-White clotting time, the activated partial thromboplastin time, or the prothrombin time are all used for this purpose. These tests help to quantify the effect of a given dose of anticoagulant.

A dose of heparin is metabolized in 4 to 8 hours. In the presence of bleeding complications, it may be necessary to reverse the heparin immediately by infusing protamine sulfate. Not more than 1 mg of protamine should be given for every 100 units of heparin. Administration of too much protamine can produce hypotension or bleeding complications. Protamine, therefore, should be administered slowly and carefully.

Anaphylactic reactions to heparin are very rare. Hemorrhage is the primary complication. Patients at risk should have their hematocrit checked frequently (at least twice daily). Typically, bleeding occurs into wounds or into the retroperitoneum and is not serious if the problem is promptly recognized and appropriately treated. Cerebral hemorrhage is a rare but serious complication.

Depression of platelet function occurs in some patients after 3 to 4 days of heparin therapy. The risk of hemorrhage is greatest in these patients. This complication can often be anticipated, however, because it is usually preceded by a decrease in the platelet count to below 100,000/mm^3.

Heparin should be given in adequate doses. The rate of heparin infusion should be adjusted to maintain a partial thromboplastin time that is 1.5 to 2 times the control value. Enoxaparin, a low-molecular-weight heparin, is an alternative that does not require continuous infusion or such careful monitoring and regulation of laboratory values. The usual dose for prophylaxis is 40 mg given subcutaneously once daily. The dose for treatment of deep venous thrombosis is 1 mg/kg body weight given subcutaneously every 12 hours. Special caution is necessary when treating the elderly, those with renal impairment, or patients weighing less than 45 kg.

Warfarin is less effective than heparin but is practical for prophylaxis, especially in outpatients, because it is administered orally. The dosage required in individual patients varies considerably. The preferred regimen for initiation of oral anticoagulation is 10 mg of warfarin orally each day until anticoagulation is obtained. The dose is then adjusted to maintain a prothrombin time that is 1.5 to 2 times the normal value. The average maintenance dose is 5 mg/day.

The prothrombin time returns to normal within 3 to 4 days after warfarin is discontinued. Rapid reversal is obtained by administering 5 to 10 mg of IV vitamin K. Immediate reversal can be obtained by the administration of fresh-frozen plasma IV.

The most common complication of oral anticoagulation is hemorrhage, frequently into the retroperitoneum or into the urinary or gastrointestinal tract. The urine and stool should be monitored for the presence of blood. Abdominal pain suggests retroperitoneal hemorrhage.

Antiplatelet agents are used to treat arterial thrombotic conditions. These agents carry less risk of hemorrhage than do anticoagulants, but they are not as effective. Aspirin, dipyridamole, and related drugs depress platelet aggregation for the life span of the platelet. Reversal of drug effect therefore depends on generation of new platelets. The half-life of platelets is approximately 4 days; therefore, these agents are effective for 1 to 2 days.

Plasma volume expanders can also depress platelet aggregation. Low-molecular-weight dextran reduces viscosity, increases microcirculatory flow, and decreases the tendency toward platelet aggregation. This agent is often used postoperatively.

Postoperative Complications

Nonspecific Complications

Fever

Pulmonary atelectasis is the most common cause of fever during the first 2 days after major spine procedures. Typically, the pulse and respiratory rates are elevated along with the temperature (the "triple response"). Pneumonia seldom develops before the third postoperative day unless pulmonary disease was present at the time of operation or unless the patient aspirates.

Wound infection caused by beta-hemolytic streptococci or clostridia can develop within hours of operation. Other bacterial wound infections require several days before they progress sufficiently to cause fever.

In general, cystitis alone does not cause fever, but infection of the upper urinary tract does. Infection in the operative site (deep to the incision) can also cause fever. Examples include epidural abscess, empyema, meningitis, and graft infection. IV catheters can become infected quickly unless rigid aseptic precautions are used during and after insertion.

Reactions to drugs, notably antibiotics, may cause fever. The extent to which fever is investigated by laboratory tests and radiographs depends on the interval between operation and the appearance of fever, the severity of fever, and the physician's certainty about the cause on the basis of the history and physical examination. The patient must be questioned about symptoms (e.g., dysuria, unusual pain) that may be clues to the source of fever. Physical examination, including auscultation of the chest, inspection of the wound, and examination of IV sites, is essential.

Leukocyte count and urinalysis are ordered in nearly every case. Cultures of urine, sputum, blood, and drainage fluid may be indicated. Chest radiographs are not necessary for patients with a clinical diagnosis of atelectasis in the first day or two after operation. Persistent fever of suspected pulmonary origin, however, requires a chest radiograph. Radiographs of other areas (e.g., the abdomen) are obtained as indicated. The search for deep infections may require special tests such as gallium scan, liver scan, ultrasonography, CT, or MRI scans.

Postoperative fever is treated best by correction of the underlying cause. Because high fever (temperature >38.5°C) is itself debilitating, antipyretic drugs (e.g., acetaminophen or aspirin) can be given by mouth or rectal suppository while the cause is being investigated. Application of ice packs or 70% alcohol to the skin surface or placement of the patient on a refrigerated blanket are other methods of lowering body temperature.

If the cause of fever remains undefined, IV catheters and central lines should be removed and new ones placed. Potentially fever-causing drugs should be changed or discontinued.

Confusion and Delirium

Elderly patients and those who are acutely and severely ill may experience postoperative psychosis. Causative factors include pain, sleep deprivation, isolation, and unfamiliar surroundings. The patients may become disoriented, hallucinatory, agitated, combative, and fearful of personnel who are caring for them, particularly at night. The derangements are transient, and patients usually regain their former mental status as the recovery from the operation progresses. It is essential to determine whether a patient with these symptoms is hypoxemic. Hypoxemia is a common cause of postoperative restlessness and mental status alteration, and the administration of analgesics or sedatives to a hypoxic patient may be lethal.

Simple helpful measures include keeping a light on in the room and providing a companion. Efforts should be made to reorient confused patients as often as possible. Mechanical restraints should be avoided unless the patient is at risk of self-injury or injury to others. Tranquilizers should be used cautiously, especially in elderly patients.

Delayed Wound Healing and Dehiscence

Many systemic factors contribute to wound healing failure by altering collagen metabolism or impairing oxygen delivery to the wound. Local and technical problems may cause impaired blood supply or inadequate resistance to mechanical forces.

Infection, corticosteroid or cytotoxic drug use, malnutrition, hypovolemia, hypoxemia, increased blood viscosity, tissue irradiation, and errors in technique may all contribute to impaired wound healing.

Wounds may dehisce because tissue is devitalized by dissection or strangulated by placement of too many sutures or by tying sutures too tightly. The latter is a common technical cause of dehiscence, which is confirmed when intact sutures are found to have cut through the tissue on one side of the wound. Inadequate suture strength or number or premature suture removal may also lead to similar complications. Absorbable sutures may not maintain their tensile strength long enough for secure healing, especially in debilitated patients.

Dehiscence of the skin is apparent on inspection. Fascial dehiscence is manifested by spontaneous serosanguineous fluid drainage from the wound. One must assume that fascia has dehisced when this type of drainage appears, especially when it persists. Fluid from a seroma or hematoma is not serosanguineous, and it usually does not continue to drain.

Obvious major dehiscence of the fascia should be treated by resuture under anesthesia in the operating room. Minor disruptions of fascia may be managed without resuture; however, the extent of fascial disruption is often underestimated until the skin is opened and the wound is explored. It is best to do this under aseptic conditions in the operating room.

Bleeding from the incision is apparent within minutes to hours after the operation is completed. Bleeding vessels may be in the skin, in the cutaneous fat, or at the fascial level.

Decubitus Ulcers

Decubitus ulcers are caused by sustained pressure on the skin, usually over bony prominences such as the sacrum, ischium, trochanter, and heel. Poor nutrition is the most important factor leading to decubitus formation. The ulcers occur in bedridden patients who are weak, aged, malnourished, or paralyzed and who are receiving inadequate nursing care. Soiling of the bed because of bowel or urinary incontinence frequently leads to skin irritation, which in turn increases the risk of ulcer development. Unrelieved pressure of only a few hours may be sufficient to produce a decubitus ulcer in a susceptible individual. Usually, decubitus ulcers begin as small areas of erythema and tenderness that soon break down to form indolent ulcers, unless they are protected from further pressure. In neglected cases, large defects in skin and soft tissues may result from the combined effects of pressure, infection, and poor healing capability. Osteomyelitis of underlying bone may occur.

The most important elements in prevention of decubitus ulcers are vigilant nursing care, mobilization, and nutrition. Bedridden patients should be inspected frequently for areas of skin damage that may progress to ulcer formation. Soiling of the bed by incontinent patients should be prevented as much as possible. An alternating pressure or foam rubber mattress may be used to decrease pressure on the skin. Washable sponge pads under pressure points are also protective.

It is essential to change patient position frequently and protect involved skin areas by pillows and pads. The clothing and skin must be kept clean and dry. Correction of malnutrition and anemia and control of infection are often critical to healing.

Decubitus ulcers should be kept clean and well debrided. They may be exposed to air or covered with dry sterile dressings. Topical applications have little value. Invasive local infection should be treated with drainage, saline compresses, and systemic antibiotics, as indicated.

Surgical treatment of large, resistant lesions consists of complete debridement, including removal of any bony prominences or sequestra, and closure of the wound with a local myocutaneous flap. This provides an adequate pad over the bone and avoids suture lines over the critical area of pressure. The donor area may be closed frequently by direct approximation, but a split-thickness skin graft may be required.

Postoperative Complications Specific to Spine Surgery

Infection

Spine Surgical Wound Infection

Spangfort[45] reviewed more than 10,000 laminectomy cases and reported an operative infection rate of approximately 2.9%. More recent series indicate that preoperative antibiotic prophylaxis may lower the incidence of infection.[46,47]

In 1980, Ramirez and Thisted[48] reported an incidence of infection of 0.3% in an analysis of 28,395 patients who underwent lumbar laminectomy for radiculopathy in the United States.

The clinical and radiographic characteristics of interspace infection were described first by Milward,[49] in 1936, after the inadvertent introduction of microorganisms into a disc space during lumbar puncture. Gieseking[50] reported the first postoperative interspace infection in 1951. Typically, patients with aseptic necrosis or interspace infection are asymptomatic immediately after surgery but begin to experience excruciating spasms in the lower back, with or without radiation into the legs, within 2 weeks. Typically, the white blood cell count and temperature are normal but the erythrocyte sedimentation rate is elevated, often to more than 100 mm/hr. Lumbosacral radiographs may reveal erosion of the cartilaginous plates as the disease progresses. Needle aspirations of the interspace may reveal the offending organisms but are often negative.[51] Patients with a clear-cut syndrome should be placed on IV antibiotics.

Wound infection should be suspected when persistent temperature elevation occurs several days after surgery. The wound should be examined for erythema, swelling, tenderness, and drainage. Management should include a Gram stain and culture, with antibiotic treatment if the clinical suspicion is strong. In the presence of probable infection or persistent infection despite antibiotic treatment, the patient should be returned to the operating room and the wound reopened, thoroughly debrided, and irrigated. Hardware should not be removed. If there is substantial tissue necrosis, the wound can be managed open, with frequent dressing changes. If the tissues look healthy and well vascularized, the wound can be closed over drains.

Discitis

The incidence of postoperative intervertebral disc space infection (discitis) is 0.75%. Disc space infection rates vary from 0.1% to 3.8%.[45,52-55] The higher incidence of disc space infection with microsurgery has been attributed to the presence of the microscope over the open wound.[56] Postoperative discitis produces persistent, intense back pain with unremarkable associated physical findings 2 weeks to 3 months after discectomy.

Elevated erythrocyte sedimentation rates are typical. Bone scan, CT, and MRI are quite sensitive for detecting discitis and can identify changes associated with discitis earlier than can plain radiographs. CT is effective in the early diagnosis of discitis, with hypodensity of the affected disc space being detected as early as 10 days after surgery. The responsible bacteria are identified in less than 50% of cases, with *Staphylococcus* species the most common organisms cultured.[51] Early diagnosis and immediate treatment are important for preventing chronic infection. Immobilization is often effective for pain relief, and 4 to 6 weeks of IV antibiotic therapy is recommended. Uncomplicated discitis should not require surgery, and most patients undergo spontaneous interbody fusion. Occasionally, lumbar epidural abscesses may develop that produce paresis. Under these circumstances, immediate decompressive laminectomy is indicated.

Postoperative Osteomyelitis

Infection may be introduced directly into the intervertebral disc space during surgery and can spread to the adjacent vertebral bodies, producing osteomyelitis. Surgery for protruding or herniated discs is the most frequent factor in the direct introduction of infection into the intervertebral disc space. This complication occurs in less than 1% of patients who undergo disc surgery. Organisms may be inadvertently inoculated at the time of surgery, and residual hematoma, necrotic tissue, and foreign bodies provide an environment conducive to bacterial proliferation. Weeks, months, or even years may elapse before the diagnosis of a disc space infection is established. Symptoms may not be apparent immediately after operation. Often there is initial pain relief followed by recurrence several days to weeks later. Fever may be transient, intermittent, or absent, and there is often no evidence of infection when symptoms develop. The degree of pain may appear to be out of proportion to the objective findings and may be attributed erroneously to malingering or even psychoneurosis.

The typical radiologic changes of vertebral osteomyelitis may not be apparent for months. Radionuclide bone scans are quite sensitive and often demonstrate evidence of infection before plain films of the spine show any changes. However, they are not specific; surgical edema and disc changes may yield false-positive results.[57] Furthermore, early in the course of disc space infection, the bone scan may be negative in a significant proportion of patients.[58] CT scans may show destructive changes of the vertebral bodies before these are evident on plain films. End-plate irregularities on CT scan, however, are not specific for discitis, and normal curettage changes in vertebral end plates may mimic erosions of discitis.[59] MRI may show changes of discitis long before any changes are apparent radiologically.[60] It is, however, important to note that MRI and CT studies may be negative early in the course of postoperative or posttraumatic discitis,[58] and a high index of suspicion is necessary. Any patient with increasing back pain more than 2 weeks after surgery and an erythrocyte sedimentation rate greater than 50 mm/hr should be considered to have discitis until proven otherwise.[60] Percutaneous disc biopsy can be helpful in the diagnosis of postoperative discitis,[61] but this often produces false-negative results.

In a study comparing MRI, plain radiographs, and radionuclide studies in the evaluation of vertebral osteomyelitis, MRI was judged to be as accurate and sensitive as combined bone and gallium scanning and more sensitive than plain radiography.[60] The MRI appearance of pyogenic infection is characteristic, making MRI a rapid, noninvasive method for the detection of vertebral osteomyelitis and its complications, including epidural abscess. On T1-weighted images, infected disc material shows decreased signal intensity from the intervertebral disc space and contiguous vertebral bodies relative to the normal vertebral signal. On T2-weighted images, these tissues show increased signal. MRI provides more anatomic detail than radionuclide scanning and allows differentiation of neoplasm and degenerative disease from osteomyelitis. The disc space is nearly always spared in neoplastic disease, whereas degenerative disease with nucleus desiccation produces decreased disc signal on T2-weighted images. Gallium scans may show positive results earlier than MRI in the course of infection, and this technique is more sensitive to changes arising from treatment and decreasing inflammation.

In many patients, postoperative discitis and vertebral osteomyelitis resolve spontaneously, and a diagnosis is never made.[62] In some patients with postoperative vertebral osteomyelitis, intermittent antibiotic therapy obscures the diagnosis and permits the illness to go undetected for years.[63,64] Kern[63] reported a patient in whom vertebral osteomyelitis and meningitis became manifest 2.5 years after lumbar spine surgery. The ability of infections to remain dormant and recur after long periods is illustrated by a patient in whom postoperative staphylococcal lumbar vertebral osteomyelitis developed and cleared after 3 years of treatment. Thirty-four years later, after 30 years without symptoms, the patient developed a staphylococcal psoas abscess.[64]

Epidural Abscess

Spinal epidural abscess (SEA) is an uncommon entity, but its clinical importance overshadows its rarity. Although SEA is rare, it should be considered in any patient with increasing neurologic symptoms and signs in the early postoperative period. It may be difficult to differentiate from an expanding hematoma in the absence of systemic evidence of infection.

The importance of early diagnosis of SEA was emphasized by Heusner as early as 1948. Several studies have emphasized the frequently rapid deterioration and substantial permanent morbidity associated with this infection. Despite the recognition of SEA as a potential neurosurgical emergency and the increased sophistication of diagnostic studies, the morbidity and mortality associated with SEA remain significant. Advances in imaging have made the diagnosis of SEA less elusive and the options for therapeutic intervention more rational.[65]

SEAs are categorized as acute lesions (gross pus in the epidural space), usually with accompanying sepsis, or chronic lesions (granulation tissue in the epidural space) that may persist for months. The clinical presentation of an acute SEA is often stereotypical, but it can be difficult to appreciate in its earliest stages. The classic triad is intense localized back pain, progressive neurologic deficit, and fever. The initial complaint is almost uniformly axial pain. Paresthesias are also very common. Fever or other symptoms of infection are present about 50% of the time. Without treatment, the progression and time course of symptoms beyond this point are astoundingly uniform. Within 3 days, patients generally note radicular symptomatology, followed within 36 hours by weakness. Rapid deterioration to paralysis occurs typically over the next 24 hours. This pattern of symptoms is so uniform that some authors suggest that this establishes the diagnosis until proven otherwise.[65]

Laboratory findings are often unhelpful. Fever and leukocytosis are useful markers when present but are absent in more than 50% of the cases. Leukocytosis is common in the acute group (average white blood cell count of <16,000/mm^3). The erythrocyte sedimentation rate is almost universally elevated but is a nonspecific indicator.

Plain radiographs are typically unremarkable in the absence of concomitant osteomyelitic involvement of adjacent vertebral bodies. The vertebral end plates directly adjacent to the disc space may show erosion. This often develops as late as 4 to 6 weeks after the onset of infection. The degree of local bone destruction from associated osteomyelitis is best appreciated by CT, and this information is often essential to formulation of the optimal management strategy.

CT myelography is an excellent technique that is often diagnostic. Lateral C1-2 puncture is our preferred method. This identifies the upper limit of any epidural mass but may not define the lower edge, and a second puncture below the block is required occasionally. Myelography has the added benefit of providing a cerebrospinal fluid sample for a cell count with differential, protein and glucose levels, Gram stain, and culture. The cerebrospinal fluid profile is generally consistent with parameningeal inflammation, although up to 15% of patients have concurrent meningitis. Myelography, however, carries the risk of converting an epidural process into a subdural empyema by subarachnoid contamination from puncture of the thecal sac during traversal of an unsuspected focus of epidural infection. Because of this potential morbidity, MRI is used as a first-line diagnostic imaging modality.

MRI is indispensable for diagnosing SEA and is extremely valuable in guiding the patient's management. MRI is considered the diagnostic test of choice, and it is diagnostic in nearly every case. MRI rapidly and accurately identifies inflammatory foci, defines the degree of spinal cord compression, and shows the predominant location of the abscess; in addition, it will often dictate the surgical approach. MRI provides more information than does CT about the extent of abscess involvement and degree of cord compromise.

The traditional therapy for SEA has been immediate surgical spinal cord decompression. Early studies of SEA recommended this policy and warned of patients who had deteriorated before delayed surgical decompression could be performed. The fundamental principles of surgical management are drainage of pus, debridement of granulation tissue, copious irrigation, and postoperative drainage.

Summary

The perioperative management of the spine surgery patient is both straightforward and potentially complex. It is critical to evaluate patients carefully, both before surgery, to avoid intraoperative catastrophes, and after surgery, to eliminate development of preventable associated morbidities. Perfect surgical procedures are often negated by suboptimal perioperative care. Spine surgery should never be considered potentially less morbid than other areas of neurosurgery.

KEY REFERENCES

Brooks-Brunn JA: Predictors of postoperative pulmonary complications following abdominal surgery. *Chest* 111:564–571, 1997.

Brown MD, Seltzer DG: Perioperative care in lumbar spine surgery. *Orthop Clin North Am* 22:353–358, 1991.

Forrest JB, Rehder K, Cahalan MK, et al: Multicenter study of general anesthesia: III. Predictors of severe perioperative adverse outcomes. *Anesthesiology* 76:3–15, 1992.

Glassman SD, Rose SM, Dimar JR, et al: The effect of postoperative nonsteroidal anti-inflammatory drug administration on spinal fusion. *Spine (Phila Pa 1976)* 23:834–838, 1998.

Hilibrand AS, Fye MA, Emery SE, et al: Impact of smoking on the outcome of anterior cervical arthrodesis with interbody or strut-grafting. *J Bone Joint Surg [Am]* 83:668–673, 2001.

Howell SJ, Hemming AE, Allman KG, et al: Predictors of postoperative myocardial ischaemia: the role of intercurrent arterial hypertension and other cardiovascular risk factors. *Anaesthesia* 52:107–111, 1997.

Lapp MA, Bridwell KH, Lenke LG, et al: Prospective randomization of parenteral hyperalimentation for long fusions with spinal deformity, its effect on complications and recovery from postoperative malnutrition. *Spine (Phila Pa 1976)* 26:809–817, 2001.

Moller AM, Villebro N, Pedersen T, et al: Effect of preoperative smoking intervention on postoperative complications: a randomised clinical trial. *Lancet* 359:114–117, 2002.

Rubinstein E, Findler G, Amit P, et al: Perioperative prophylactic cephazolin in spinal surgery: a double-blind placebo-controlled trial. *J Bone Joint Surg [Br]* 76:99–102, 1994.

REFERENCES

The complete reference list is available online at expertconsult.com.

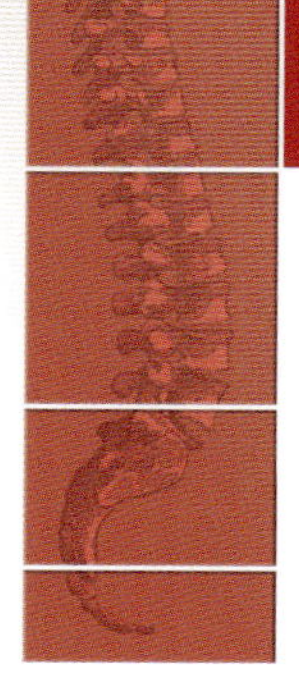

CHAPTER 183

Medical Management of the Patient with Acute Spinal Cord Injury

S. Scott Lollis | Perry A. Ball

Epidemiology

Spinal cord injury (SCI) has an incidence of approximately 40 cases per million population per year, which in the United States translates to approximately 12,000 cases per year.[1] In 2008, there were an estimated 259,000 people in the United States living with SCI. In addition to being one of the most profoundly disabling and psychologically devastating injuries, SCI has a substantial societal cost: the lifetime cost of caring for a patient who becomes paraplegic at 25 years of age is $1,055,869, and for a tetraplegic patient, $3,160,137.[1] One 1994 estimate put the annual cost of caring for all SCIs in the United States at $4 billion.[2]

With the exception of age at injury, the epidemiology of SCI has remained fairly constant over time. In the United States, the most common cause of SCI is motor vehicle accidents (42.1%), followed by falls (26.7%) and violence (15.1%). Mean age at the time of injury has increased in recent decades, from 28 years in the late 1970s to 40 years from 2005 to 2009.[1]

The mortality rate of patients with traumatic SCI is high. An estimated 79% of patients die at the scene of the accident or on arrival at the hospital; for survivors at hospital admission, reported hospital mortality rates range from 4.4% to 16.7%.[3] Predictably, long-term survival is lower than the general population; however, advances in medical care, and in urologic care in particular, have improved long-term survival considerably over the last half-century.[4] Today, a person who becomes paraplegic at age 20 years has a mean life expectancy (years remaining) of 45.5 years; using the same age at injury, a person with a low tetraplegia (C5-8) has a mean life expectancy of 40.8 years, and a person with a high tetraplegia (C1-4) has a mean life expectancy of 36.9 years.[1] A greater-than-expected number of deaths is found for virtually all causes, except ischemic heart disease. The greatest excess mortality occurs as a result of septicemia, deep venous thrombosis (DVT) and pulmonary embolism (PE), and pneumonia; compared with someone without SCI, an SCI patient between the ages of 25 and 54 years is 170 times more likely to die of septicemia, 63 times more likely to die of DVT/PE, and 50 times more likely to die of pneumonia.[5,6] For those who survive the initial injury, medical management and the prevention of secondary complications will dictate long-term survival.

Medical care of the patient with acute SCI requires an understanding of the far-reaching pathophysiologic effects of the injury and an attention to detail. As with any traumatic injury, initial management focuses on maintaining adequate ventilation and ensuring adequate tissue perfusion. For injuries above the T6 level, this may be complicated by autonomic derangements and neurogenic shock. Physicians must be aware of the susceptibility of the injured or compressed spinal cord to ischemic damage and remain vigilant so that even brief periods of hypotension or hypoxia are avoided. Early consideration should be given to pharmacologic and surgical interventions to maximize neurologic recovery. Surgical considerations, such as the timing of decompression and strategies of spine stabilization, which have been the subject of extensive research and ongoing debate, are beyond the scope of this chapter and are discussed elsewhere.

After acute stabilization, attention is focused on preventing and treating the myriad secondary complications of SCI. A systems-based approach is essential because these complications may involve virtually every organ system. Broadly speaking, they can be divided into pulmonary complications, complications of autonomic disruption (sympathectomy), complications of immobility, and psychiatric complications.

This chapter is intended for the clinician caring for patients with SCI in the acute and subacute phases of their injury (i.e., during the first hospitalization). Although many of the management principles described here are also applicable to the chronic care of these patients, detailed discussion of subspecialty long-term care is beyond the scope of this chapter.

Neuroprotection

Acute SCI is really a two-stage process, consisting of a primary mechanical insult and a secondary cascade defined by tissue hypoxia and ischemia, edema, excitotoxicity, free radical activation, caspase activation, and, ultimately, cell death by apoptosis and necrosis.[7] Despite ongoing research into neural regeneration and brain-machine interfaces, there is at present no therapy to reverse or circumvent the effects of the primary injury. Attention has therefore been focused on interventions to mitigate the deleterious effects of the secondary cascade.

The only pharmacologic intervention for acute SCI that is supported by randomized human trials is the administration of intravenous methylprednisolone. This was the subject of three National Acute Spinal Cord Injury Study (NASCIS) trials. NASCIS I was a negative study comparing methylprednisolone 1000 mg/day versus 100 mg/day for 11 days; there was no treatment effect seen at 6 weeks or 6 months postinjury.[8] NASCIS II was a three-armed trial comparing a higher dose of methylprednisolone (30 mg/kg bolus followed by infusion of 5.4 mg/kg/hr for 23 hours), naloxone (5.4 mg/kg followed by 4.0 mg/kg/hr for 23 hours), and placebo.[9] It found statistically significant improvements in motor score, pinprick sensation, and light touch at 6 months postinjury for the methylprednisolone group, when methylprednisolone was given within 8 hours of injury; benefit was seen in patients with complete as well as incomplete injuries. A 1-year follow-up of the same cohort found benefit for motor scores only.[10] NASCIS III was another three-armed study in which all patients received a methylprednisolone bolus followed by a 24-hour infusion (5.4 mg/kg/hr NASCIS II protocol), or a 48-hour methylprednisolone infusion (5.4 mg/kg/hr), or tirilazad mesylate (2.5 mg/kg bolus every 6 hours for 48 hours); it did not include a placebo control. NASCIS III found comparable outcomes between the 24-hour and 48-hour infusions when therapy was initiated less than 3 hours after injury; when therapy was initiated between 3 and 8 hours after injury, patients receiving 48-hour infusions demonstrated improved motor scores and functional independence at 6 weeks and 6 months postinjury.[11] Tirilazad mesylate resulted in outcomes comparable with the 24-hour methylprednisolone infusion, but because all patients had received a methylprednisolone bolus on presentation, it is unclear whether this outcome was the result of tirilazad or steroid administration. A 1-year follow-up of the NASCIS III cohort using intention-to-treat analysis did not demonstrate a statistical difference in motor scores between the 24-hour and 48-hour groups for the 3- to 8-hour treatment window; however, an analysis limited to compliant patients did demonstrate a small benefit for the 48-hour regimen over the 24-hour regimen.[12] No difference in functional independence between the groups was seen at 1 year.

Despite their status as class 1 evidence, the NASCIS trials have been extensively criticized in the medical literature. Because NASCIS II is the basis for the use of methylprednisolone in SCI, it has been the subject of the most vigorous debate. The most common concern is that the authors' choice of an 8-hour window is the result of a post hoc analysis rather than a prospectively defined end point. Others have questioned the inclusion of patients with minimal neurologic deficit, the use of right-sided motor scores only, the lack of a functional outcome measure, the lack of standardized medical or surgical therapies and the failure to control such variability, the small size of subgroups that formed the basis for the study's determination of efficacy, the poor neurologic status of the control subgroup, and the medical risks associated with high-dose steroid therapy.[13-15] Reflecting this controversy, current guidelines from the American Association of Neurological Surgeons (AANS) and Congress of Neurological Surgeons (CNS) Joint Section on Disorders of the Spine and Peripheral Nerves conclude that administration of methylprednisolone can be recommended only at the level of a treatment option.[13]

Further, the use of methylprednisolone for SCI appears to be diminishing, according to a number of recent physician polls and studies.[16,17] Nevertheless, it remains the only therapy with evidentiary support of large-scale human trials.

A number of other candidate neuroprotective agents have undergone randomized, controlled trials in human subjects but have failed to show efficacy. Monosialotetrahexosylganglioside (GM-1) showed promise in animal models as an antiexcitotoxic, antiapoptotic, and proregenerative agent; it was the subject of two human trials. The first was a small study involving 37 patients who were randomized to receive either a test protocol of 100 mg of GM-1 intravenously per day for 18 to 32 doses, or placebo.[18] Study subjects demonstrated significantly greater improvement in both Frankel grade and American Spinal Injury Association (ASIA) motor score at 1-year follow-up. This was the basis for a second, larger study involving 797 patients, the Sygen Multicenter Acute Spinal Cord Injury Study.[19] In this study, all patients received methylprednisolone according to the NASCIS II regimen; after completion of the methylprednisolone infusion, patients were randomized to high-dose GM-1 (600-mg load followed by 56 days of 200 mg/day), low-dose GM-1 (300-mg load followed by 56 days of 100 mg/day), or placebo. The Sygen study failed to meet its primary end point; there was no difference in the proportion of patients with "marked recovery" (two-point improvement in the Modified Benzel Classification over baseline ASIA Impairment Scale) at 26 weeks postinjury. Current guidelines from the AANS/CNS Joint Section on Disorders of the Spine and Peripheral Nerves list GM-1 as a treatment option without demonstrated clinical benefit.[13] The *N*-methyl-D-aspartate (NMDA) glutamate receptor blocker gacyclidine was also the subject of a randomized, double-blind phase II clinical trial of over 200 patients.[20] Outcome at 1 year failed to demonstrate improvement, and further development was halted. Because of the central role of calcium in both neuronal excitotoxicity and vasospasm-induced ischemia, calcium channel blockers have also received attention as candidate neuroprotectants. Nimodipine was the subject of a randomized clinical trial involving 106 patients split into four arms (nimodipine, methylprednisolone, both, or placebo).[21] No benefit of nimodipine was demonstrated at 1-year follow-up.

Other therapies have shown promise in laboratory studies but have not yet been the subject of clinical trials. Polyethylene glycol is thought to confer neuroprotection through preservation of axonal cytoskeletal proteins, stabilization of the cell membrane, and preservation of mitochondria; multiple animal studies have shown reduction in cellular injury and modest improvement in functional outcome.[22-24] Magnesium sulfate has also shown significant improvement in motor scores and reductions in myelin loss and overall lesion size in rat models of SCI.[25-27] Finally, the resurgence of therapeutic hypothermia as a neuroprotectant after cardiac arrest has rekindled interest in potential application to SCI.[28,29] Despite multiple animal studies showing therapeutic benefit,[30-33] human trials to date have been limited to small, noncontrolled case series,[34-39] from which it is difficult to draw any conclusions of efficacy. Indeed, widespread application of these experimental therapies to the patient with acute SCI will have to await positive results from well-designed human trials.

Pulmonary Management and Complications

Spinal cord injury is often accompanied by acute changes in respiratory function, and approximately one third of patients with acute cervical SCIs will require mechanical ventilatory support during the acute phase of injury.[40]

Respiratory Physiology

The process of inspiration involves the contraction and descent of the diaphragm and the expansion of the chest wall by the intercostal muscles. The action of these muscles creates a negative pressure so that air is drawn into the thoracic cavity. Expiration is mostly passive, but forced expiration and coughing are aided by the contraction of the abdominal muscles.

A complete injury above C3 usually results in apnea due to loss of innervation of the diaphragm. Lesions below this level will usually have retained diaphragm function but there will still be a significant reduction in ventilatory function. During the acute phase of SCI, there is flaccid paralysis of the muscles below the level of injury, and in cervical SCIs this paralysis results in loss of muscle tone in the intercostal muscles, which are innervated by the motor roots at each level of the thoracic spine. Thus, when the diaphragm contracts, the chest wall collapses instead of expanding. What is commonly observed, therefore, in a patient with an acute cervical SCI is paradoxical breathing: with each inspiration the chest wall collapses inward and the abdominal wall distends outward. There is a marked decrease in the ability to generate the negative intrathoracic pressure necessary to draw air into the lungs and vital capacity is reduced to about one third of the preinjury level.[41] This reduction results in shallow breathing, and the respiratory rate is often elevated in an attempt to compensate for this. Shallow breathing is inefficient because a larger part of the air moved during each inspiration stays within the trachea and bronchi and does not reach the alveoli to participate in gas exchange. This in turn promotes alveolar collapse with progressive atelectasis and respiratory fatigue. The loss of function of the abdominal muscles results in a decreased ability to cough and clear secretions. Thus, some patients with an acute cervical SCI will appear to be breathing satisfactorily shortly after injury but over the next 24 to 48 hours develop progressive respiratory failure; therefore, careful sequential monitoring of respiratory function is important in the early phase of injury. It is preferable to perform intubation under controlled circumstances when personnel and equipment can be assembled, so it is best to make the decision to proceed with intubation before respiratory failure occurs.

Intubation

During intubation of the patient with an acute cervical SCI, care should be taken to prevent further injury to the spinal cord. Intubation can be performed using direct laryngoscopy assisted by manual in-line traction, or fiberoptic laryngoscopy. Either option can be performed safely in the setting of SCI by experienced practitioners.[42] The use of muscle relaxants is often a helpful adjunct to intubation; succinylcholine is an excellent choice in the acute period after injury but should not be used after the fourth postinjury day because of the risk of precipitating hyperkalemia.

Ventilator Management

More than half of patients with acute SCI will need mechanical ventilator support for more than 2 weeks.[40] This is because improvement in respiratory function depends on the progression from flaccid to spastic paralysis: once the intercostal muscles become spastic, the chest wall becomes rigid and no longer collapses with inspiratory effort, and progressive improvement in negative inspiratory force and forced vital capacity occurs. This usually begins at about 3 to 5 weeks after injury.[41] The management of the intubated patient with an acute cervical SCI is directed at preventing and treating complications while waiting for respiratory function to improve.

Ventilator-Associated Pneumonia

Prevention

The development of pneumonia is a major source of morbidity in mechanically ventilated patients, and strategies to attempt prevention are important. The Society for Healthcare Epidemiology and the Infectious Diseases Society of America have published recommendations for the prevention of ventilator-associated pneumonia (VAP).[43] The core recommendations are directed at the three most common mechanisms that lead to VAP: aspiration of secretions, colonization of the aerodigestive tract, and contamination of respiratory equipment. Elevation of the head of the bed to 30 degrees appears to reduce aspiration. Regular decontamination of the oral cavity with antiseptic solution should be used to prevent bacterial colonization of the upper airway. There is evidence that acid-suppressive therapy such as histamine receptor blocking agents or proton pump inhibitors used to prevent gastrointestinal bleeding may increase the colonization of the digestive tract with pathologic organisms, so the risk-benefit ratio must be individualized for each patient. Measures to prevent contamination of the respiratory circuit, such as removal of condensate and changing the ventilator circuit only when soiled or malfunctioning, are recommended.

Diagnosis

The diagnosis of VAP can be challenging: fever is common in ventilated patients and may not be due to infection, and distinguishing pneumonia from bacterial colonization of the respiratory tract is often difficult. The process of establishing the diagnosis of VAP should begin with a chest radiograph and sampling of secretions from the lower respiratory tract. Sampling of secretions can be done with either bronchoscopy or endotracheal suctioning. There is some controversy about which method is preferable, but it is not clear that there is a difference in clinical outcome.[44] If the chest radiograph reveals no infiltrates or the Gram stain of the sputum shows no organisms, it is unlikely that pneumonia is present.[45] If there are new or progressive infiltrates on the chest radiograph along with two of the following, fever, leukocytosis, or purulent secretions, there is a strong likelihood of VAP.[46]

Treatment

Timely selection of appropriate antibiotic therapy is important in decreasing mortality from VAP. The American Thoracic Society and Infectious Diseases Society of America have issued guidelines for the treatment of VAP.[47] While awaiting the results of sputum culture, the first step is to determine whether there is a likelihood of multidrug-resistant (MDR) organism involvement. The risk factors for this are recent exposure to antibiotics, hospitalization for greater than 5 days, immunosuppression, or a high incidence of MDR pathogens in the particular hospital or unit. If no risk factors are present, monotherapy with ceftriaxone, levofloxacin, moxifloxacin, ciprofloxacin, ampicillin/sulbactam, or ertapenem is acceptable. If risk factors for MDR pathogens are present, then combination therapy with three agents is appropriate. This includes the use of either vancomycin or linezolid to cover for methicillin-resistant *Staphylococcus aureus*; either an antipseudomonal cephalosporin, carbapenem, or piperacillin-tazobactam; and either ciprofloxacin, levofloxacin, or an aminoglycoside. Once the culture results are available, the antibiotics can be narrowed to cover the identified organism.

Tracheostomy

If a patient is mechanically ventilated for more than 2 weeks, strong consideration should be given to performing a tracheostomy. A tracheostomy is more comfortable for the patient because the endotracheal tube does not irritate the dorsal pharynx and it is easier for the nursing and respiratory staff to suction secretions from the tracheobronchial tree. The other advantage of tracheostomy is that it makes the process of weaning from mechanical ventilation easier because the patient can be allowed to alternate periods of spontaneous breathing with rest periods on mechanical ventilator support.

Complications of Autonomic Disruption

Autonomic Physiology and Pathophysiology

Autonomic effects of SCI have both immediate and long-term relevance. Understanding the effect of autonomic dysregulation on the cardiovascular, gastrointestinal, and urinary systems, in particular, requires an understanding of autonomic anatomy and physiology.

The parasympathetic nervous system is sometimes referred to as a *craniosacral* system. The cranial portion of this system, the vagus nerve, is unaffected by SCI; parasympathetic innervation to the heart and most abdominal visceral organs (pancreas, kidneys, liver, gallbladder, stomach, and intestine up to the splenic flexure) will be spared. However, outflow through the pelvic splanchnic nerves (S2-4) may be partially or completely disrupted by an SCI at any level; thus, parasympathetic innervation to the ureters, urinary bladder, urinary sphincter, anal sphincter, uterus, prostate, vagina, and penis are at risk. This distinction between the extraspinal cranial portion and the intraspinal sacral portion is central to the cardiovascular, urologic, and gastrointestinal phenomena that follow acute SCI.

The degree of sympathetic system disruption largely depends on the level and severity of injury. The sympathetic outflow to the body emanates from the spinal cord at levels T1 through L3. Preganglionic axons then enter the sympathetic chain, where they synapse on postganglionic neurons that are distributed among target organs, including the heart (cardiac accelerator nerves), blood vessels, skin, bronchial tree, esophagus, and large intestine, as well as papillary dilators and various glands in the head. Because of the anatomic differences between the sympathetic and parasympathetic systems, the effect of SCI on autonomic function and autonomic balance depends entirely on the level of the injury.

Cardiovascular Complications

Hypotension

Injuries above T6 may disrupt sympathetic cardiac and vascular control but leave parasympathetic (vagal) tone intact, often resulting in hypotension. In this setting, hypotension (systolic blood pressure <90 mm Hg) may be the result of bradyarrhythmia or distributive pathophysiology, or both.

The term *neurogenic shock* is applied when hypotension is accompanied by impaired tissue perfusion and other causes of shock have been addressed or ruled out. The latter point is important: internal hemorrhage, tension pneumothorax, cardiac tamponade, and other causes of hypotension in the trauma patient can have disastrous consequences if not detected in a timely fashion. Clinically, neurogenic shock has a more varied presentation than other forms of shock. Distributive/hypovolemic pathophysiology is belied by a normal or low heart rate and warm skin. Above the level of the injury the patient will often be diaphoretic, whereas below the injury the skin may be dry. This confusing clinical picture, combined with a high probability of other, concurrent shock physiology, makes neurogenic shock a diagnosis of exclusion.

It is worth distinguishing between the terms *neurogenic shock* and *spinal shock*, which are often confused in the literature. The term *neurogenic shock* refers to a distributive and/or cardiogenic hypotension as a result of acute sympathectomy in SCI; it is a cardiovascular phenomenon and lasts for a mean of 4 to 6 weeks after injury. The term *spinal shock* refers to a flaccid, areflexic period after acute SCI that precedes the gradual transition to spasticity; it is a neurologic phenomenon and its end is heralded by the return of various spinal reflexes (bulbocavernosus reflex after approximately 2 days, deep tendon reflexes after approximately 2 weeks, bladder reflex after 2 months).

Initial management of hypotension resulting from acute SCI should be directed toward volume resuscitation of the expanded intravascular volume and correcting bradycardia. If 1 to 2 L of intravenous fluid fails to normalize blood pressure, consideration should be given to vasopressor and chronotropic support. A mixed α- and β-adrenergic agonist is recommended because of the need to restore both peripheral arteriolar tone and heart rate. A pulmonary artery catheter may be useful in directing therapy. As with any shock state, the restoration of tissue perfusion may be assessed by examination of the extremities, mental status, and urine output.

It is not known whether a higher blood pressure target should be sought in the setting of SCI. Because of the exquisite sensitivity of the injured spinal cord to ischemia, some authors have recommended using fluids and pressor support to maintain higher-than-usual target mean arterial pressures (MAPs) in the acute phase of injury. Although the avoidance of hypotension in acute SCI is supported by animal research,[48-50] there is a dearth of evidence to support any particular target. Of the uncontrolled case series in the current literature, strategies have included target MAPs greater than 85 mm Hg[51,52] and greater than 90 mm Hg.[53] Reflecting the lack of rigorous human studies, the AANS/CNS Joint Section currently lists the avoidance of hypotension and maintenance of MAP at 85 to 90 mm Hg for 7 days after injury as options for treatment.[54]

In the subacute and chronic phase of injury, orthostatic hypotension (OH) may be a persistent problem. It is defined as a decrease in systolic blood pressure of 20 mm Hg or more or a decrease in diastolic blood pressure of 10 mm Hg or more upon transition from a supine to an upright position. Using this definition, the prevalence of OH after SCI is 82% in tetraplegia and 50% in paraplegia.[55] It results from venous pooling in the lower extremities with secondary loss of preload and reduction in end-diastolic volume. In cervical SCI, this is exacerbated by sympathetic denervation of the heart and difficulty compensating with increased heart rate. OH is associated with light-headedness or other symptoms in over half of the SCI population.[55] Treatment may include volume expansion, pressure devices, functional electrical stimulation, exercise, and pharmacologic therapy. Volume expansion may be accomplished with increased dietary salt and oral fluids, or with sodium-retaining drugs such as fludrocortisone. It should not be undertaken in patients with a history of congestive heart failure. Pressure devices include abdominal binders and compression stockings; success from these measures alone has been limited.[56] Functional electrical stimulation uses direct electrical stimulation of the lower extremity musculature to promote venous return. Its efficacy is supported by three small-scale, randomized, controlled trials.[57-59] The most commonly used drug to treat OH is midodrine, an α-adrenergic agonist that has been tested in the SCI population in a number of small trials.[60-62] Other medications that have been used to treat symptomatic OH, with varying success, include fludrocortisone, ephedrine, and dihydroergotamine.[56]

Arrhythmia

Sinus bradycardia is the most common arrhythmia after cervical and upper thoracic SCI, again because of unopposed parasympathetic outflow to the heart; however, supraventricular tachycardia and ventricular arrhythmias can also occur.[63] Sinus bradycardia with hemodynamic compromise should be treated with atropine 0.5 mg IV. If it is ineffective or episodes are recurrent, aminophylline may be given as a bolus injection, followed by infusion.[64,65] Aminophylline may be substituted with oral theophylline if chronotropic support is needed for a more prolonged period.[61] Occasionally, the bradycardia can result in asystole. For severe or refractory bradyarrhythmias and ones that persist longer than 2 weeks, consideration should be given to pacemaker placement.[66,67] Tachyarrhythmias are less common in the patient with acute SCI; when supraventricular tachycardia or ventricular tachycardia occurs, it is usually in the context of a midthoracic lesion.[68] Treatment is governed by the specific electrophysiologic derangement involved, but will commonly include beta blockade, antiarrhythmic drugs, and, in the case of unstable, sustained ventricular tachycardia or ventricular fibrillation, defibrillation.

Autonomic Dysreflexia

Injuries above T6 may produce life-threatening episodes of autonomic dysreflexia, in which a stimulus below the level of the injury causes an increase in sympathetic activity. The most common triggers are sacral-level stimuli, such as bladder distention, bowel distention, and manual disimpaction, although mild cutaneous stimuli at any level below the injury may also cause this response. By definition, a dysreflexic episode is characterized by a minimum increase in systolic blood pressure of 20 to 30 mm Hg; blood pressure often becomes out of control, reaching the level of hypertensive emergency. In addition to hypertension, dysreflexic episodes are characterized by bradycardia and arrhythmia, diaphoresis above the level of the lesion, flushing, muscle spasm, and paresthesias. Although most episodes are short-lived, there are reports of dysreflexic episodes lasting for weeks.[69]

Dysreflexia is thought to result from changes in spinal and extraspinal autonomic circuits. Up-regulation of peripheral alpha receptors, in particular, is thought to play a role.[70] It is more severe with more rostrally located lesions and with neurologically complete injuries. Autonomic dysreflexia is observed in 91% of patients with neurologically complete tetraplegia, but in only 27% of patients with incomplete tetraplegia.[71]

Autonomic dysreflexia is a medical emergency. Prompt treatment is essential to preventing hypertensive emergency and secondary intracranial hemorrhage, retinal hemorrhage, seizure, and death. The inciting stimulus should be identified and alleviated. If a stimulus is not immediately apparent, physical examination or bladder ultrasonography should be used to ensure that the bladder is adequately drained. The head of the bed should be elevated to an upright posture and clothing should be loosened. Multiple medications have been used to truncate dysreflexic episodes, including nitrates,[72] prostaglandin E_2,[73] and sublingual captopril.[74] Dysreflexic episodes may be prevented through mitigation of stimuli as well as prophylactic antihypertensive therapy. Current literature supports the use of prazosin[75] and terazosin[76] for prophylaxis. The use of nifedipine for prophylaxis also has evidentiary support, but its use has declined substantially in the wake of increased reports of adverse events and premature death associated with this medication.[72,77]

Genitourinary Complications

For SCI severe enough to cause urinary dysfunction, the initial stage of injury is that of an areflexic or acontractile bladder and loss of external urethral sphincter tone. This correlates with the period of spinal shock. For injuries located above the sacral cord level (i.e., upper motor neuron lesions), bladder contractions usually return within 6 to 8 weeks after injury[4]; conus and cauda equina lesions will remain in this acontractile state indefinitely. Typically, electromyographic activity and contractile function return first in the external urethral sphincter, followed some time later by the bladder. Once bladder reflexes have been restored, typically in the rehabilitation stage of treatment, patients should be followed by a urologist for urodynamic studies, consideration of anticholinergic therapy and restoration of voiding function, and management of chronic issues such as urinary tract infection and urolithiasis.

For the physician treating acute SCI, the central urologic question is when to transition from an indwelling urinary catheter to intermittent catheterization. An indwelling catheter is helpful during the period of acute management, when monitoring and treating hemodynamic instability or impaired tissue perfusion. Once this period has passed, there are multiple benefits to replacement of the indwelling catheter with a regimen of intermittent catheterization. First, periodic distention of the bladder wall may promote the early return of bladder reflex contractions, hastening recovery of voiding function.[4] Second, the incidence of urinary tract infection, particularly upper urinary tract infection with secondary renal failure, is lower with intermittent catheterization.[78,79] Third, other complications related to indwelling urinary catheters, such as urethritis, prostatitis, epididymo-orchitis, fistulae, and strictures may be reduced or avoided.[4,80] It is believed that a substantial reduction in mortality related to SCI in the last half-century is due to a reduction in the use of indwelling catheters in the chronic SCI population.[81] Thus, intermittent catheterization should be adopted as soon as is practically feasible.

Intermittent catheterization should be carried out every 4 hours, with bladder volumes kept to less than 400 mL to prevent overdistention. Once patients start to void, intermittent catheterization may be changed to every 6 to 8 hours, and the acceptable volume may be increased to 500 mL.[82] If possible, fluid intake should be restricted to 1.5 L/24 hours; when urine volumes are greater than 500 mL/6 hours, the aforementioned regimen becomes impractical, and unless intake can be further restricted, intermittent catheterization should be delayed.[82] While patients are in the hospital, sterile technique is recommended. Once out of the hospital, patients may use clean technique, in which the patient washes his or her hands, but does not don sterile gloves, and uses a clean, rather than sterile, catheter.[4,79] No antiseptic preparation is required for clean catheterization. For patients unable to perform clean intermittent self-catheterization, a suprapubic cystostomy tube, combined with anticholinergic medication, frequent catheter changes, bladder washing, and volume maintenance procedures, may provide a morbidity profile comparable with clean intermittent catheterization.[83]

In the long term, the goals of urologic management include reduction of voiding pressure to less than 40 cm H_2O, prompt treatment of urinary tract infection, prevention and treatment of urinary stones, and, when possible, attaining a catheter-free state. Elevated bladder pressures may be the result of hyper-reflexia and detrusor sphincter dyssynergia and, if prolonged, can lead to hydronephrosis and chronic renal failure. Treatment options include anticholinergic medication as well as transurethral sphincterotomy. Urinary tract infection results from upper and lower urinary tract stasis, vesicoureteral reflux, and chronic catheterization and is a significant cause of long-term morbidity. Complicating management is the difficulty of distinguishing between true infection and colonization. Undertreatment may result in upper tract infection and kidney damage, whereas overtreatment may lead to MDR bacteria. At present, most clinicians advocate treatment in the presence of fever, flank pain, hematuria, or pyuria (>10,000 leukocytes/mL urine).[4,84] Recurrent infections should prompt evaluation with an intravenous urogram and urodynamic studies. Prophylactic antibiotics are ineffective in reducing the frequency of urinary tract infections and cause the emergence of antibiotic-resistant bacteria.[85] Recent approaches to reduce the incidence of urinary tract infection have included the use of hydrophilic-coated catheters and bacterial interference.[86,87] Urinary stones are another common complication with significant secondary renal morbidity. The incidence of stone disease is greatest during the first 3 months after injury. This early peak of "immobilization hypercalciuria" corresponds to a period of relative immobility and the development of nonoxalate calcium stones.[88] Stone disease presenting after 3 months is more commonly the result of chronic infection and should prompt a search for such.

Gastrointestinal Complications: Ileus and Nutrition

Ileus may result from SCI, regardless of spinal level. Although parasympathetic input is the primary driver of peristalsis, sympathetic input is required to organize peristalsis into an effective motile force. The preservation of vagal input to the upper gut may result in bowel sounds in the face of significant upper gastrointestinal dysfunction. Distal to the splenic flexure, visceral function may be rendered atonic as a result of injury to sacral parasympathetic outflow. It is therefore judicious to defer enteral feeding of a patient with SCI until after the passage of flatus. If prolonged ileus precludes enteral feeding, parenteral nutrition should be undertaken.

Protein intake should be modulated with the understanding that muscle paralysis will inevitably result in catabolism and negative nitrogen balance; this cannot be reversed with nutritional supplementation.[89,90] Protein requirements for the patient with acute SCI are typically estimated at 1.0 to 1.3 g/kg.[91] In the acute phase, overall energy expenditure is also substantially less than that of other traumatically injured patients.[92] The Harris-Benedict equation is a standardized means of assessing energy requirements and has been independently validated for this purpose in the SCI population.[89] Nevertheless, indirect calorimetry remains the most accurate means of assessing nutritional needs and should be used whenever possible.[93] For short-term, practical purposes, a reasonable shorthand estimate of caloric requirement is 20 kcal/kg ideal body weight.

It should be noted that early nutritional support of the trauma patient is supported by substantial medical literature.[94,95] Though tempered by at least one report of increased incidence of infection among patients receiving early enteral nutrition, early feeding has become a common theme in trauma critical care.[96] Whether this benefit accrues to the patient with SCI, given the specific metabolic concerns outlined previously, remains uncertain; however, studies are ongoing.[91]

Disorders of Thermoregulation and Sweating

Post-SCI sympathectomy results in loss of vasomotor and sudomotor effectors below the level of the lesion. Acutely, this may be evident as a "sweat line"—a dermatomal transition from diaphoresis above the lesion to dry skin below the lesion. Skin may be markedly cooler below the level of the lesion than above. With time, the return of local reflexes may permit some sweating and vasoreactivity below the level of the lesion, but the effectiveness of these reflexes is substantially less than that of centrally mediated pathways.

Autonomic innervation to cutaneous blood vessels, sweat glands, and piloerectors is exclusively sympathetic. There is no opposing parasympathetic input. Hence, both vasodilation and vasoconstriction are lost, and the patient is rendered susceptible to thermal derangements in both directions. For lesions below T6, compensation by the trunk and upper limbs prevents significant hyperthermia or hypothermia except in conditions of strenuous exercise or extreme ambient temperatures.[97,98] For patients with injuries above T6, particularly middle and high cervical injuries, attention must be paid to even moderate changes in ambient temperature; these patients are sometimes referred to as "partially poikilothermic."[98]

In the hospital, this phenomenon usually manifests as fever of unknown origin, although hypothermia also occurs. Given their high risk for infection and DVT, the presence of elevated body temperature or hypothermia in patients with SCI should prompt a careful clinical investigation. Only after repeated negative workups should an autonomic cause be invoked. The converse concern of sympathetic denervation eliminating the febrile response, and thus masking infection, has not been borne out in clinical practice. This may be due to some heretofore-undefined humoral factor or pyrogen that is capable of transmitting hypothalamic signals to thermal effectors in the body, without neural transmission.[98]

Complications of Immobility

Deep Venous Thrombosis and Pulmonary Embolism

Deep venous thrombosis and PE represent a significant mortality risk for the patient with SCI, particularly in the period immediately after the injury. Within the first month after injury, a patient with SCI is 500 times more likely to die of DVT/PE than an age-matched control subject; between 1 and 6 months postinjury, the relative risk is 116, and for 6 months postinjury and beyond, it is reduced further to 20.[5] Studies with routine screening for DVT have found a 60% to 100% prevalence of DVT in patients with SCI.[99,100] Because of this risk and the level of evidence supporting prophylactic measures, the American College of Chest Physicians recommends routine thromboprophylaxis in the form of low-molecular-weight heparin (LMWH) or unfractionated heparin with compression stockings, recognizing that pharmacologic prophylaxis may be postponed because of epidural hematoma or other bleeding risk.[101,102] Similarly, the AANS/CNS Joint Section currently recommends low-dose heparin and pneumatic compression devices as a standard of care in the cervical SCI population.[13]

Mechanical prophylaxis alone is not an adequate long-term strategy in the patient with SCI. The incidence of DVT when sequential compression devices are used in lieu of pharmacologic prophylaxis may be as high as 40%.[103] Sequential compression devices and graded compression stockings represent a low-cost, low-risk adjunct to other measures of prevention, and in the patient with high bleeding risks, may be a useful short-term strategy while pharmacologic prophylaxis is withheld.

There is evidence to suggest that LMWH is more effective than unfractionated heparin in preventing venous thromboembolism. One randomized, controlled study comparing unfractionated heparin plus intermittent pneumatic compression stockings versus enoxaparin found a statistically significant reduction in pulmonary embolism from 18.4% in the unfractionated heparin group to 5.2% in the enoxaparin group.[99] Superior efficacy of LMWH is also reflected in the trauma literature; one randomized, controlled study found relative risk reductions of 30% for DVT and 58% for proximal DVT when enoxaparin was used instead of unfractionated heparin after major trauma.[53] In the chronic phase of treatment, LMWH may be continued or patients may be transitioned to an oral vitamin K antagonist (warfarin) with a target international normalized ratio of 2 to 3.[101] The latter requires active management of dosing but is significantly less expensive than LMWH.

The presence of traumatic intracranial bleeding, spinal epidural hematoma, or other bleeding concern complicates the issue of pharmacologic prophylaxis. The most common concern is concomitant cerebral contusion or other intracranial hematoma, and at present no adequate studies have been done to address the questions of timing and choice of agent in this population. Studies of DVT prophylaxis after elective brain tumor resection suggest a higher incidence of postoperative bleeding with LMWH, but not with unfractionated heparin.[104,105] Therefore, in this subpopulation, the use of unfractionated heparin combined with mechanical compression devices may be a reasonable choice in the short term.

Some have suggested the routine use of prophylactic inferior vena cava filters in patients with significant motor deficit after SCI.[106] This practice is currently not supported by the American College of Chest Physicians because of the risk of major complications and cost-ineffectiveness.[101] In the only randomized, controlled study of permanent inferior vena cava filter placement in patients with DVT and high risk of PE, the addition of filter placement to appropriate anticoagulation therapy reduced, but did not eliminate, the risk of PE (4.8% vs. 1.1% at 12 days and 6.2% vs. 15% at 8 years); there was no associated reduction in mortality risk, and filter placement was associated with a significantly higher risk of recurrent DVT (35.7% vs. 27.5% at 8 years).[107,108] When bleeding concerns preclude appropriate pharmacologic prophylaxis during the acute phase of injury, there may be a limited role for filter placement. Retrievable filters, in particular, may be useful for this purpose.

There is no high-quality evidence to support or refute the use of screening tests to identify asymptomatic DVT in the SCI population. Screening methods include Doppler ultrasonography, compressed ultrasound, D-dimer assay, 125-I fibrinogen scanning, impedance plethysmography, or a combination of methods. A recent literature review and meta-analysis of nine small trials and case series found no differences among these methods in their ability to detect asymptomatic DVT in the SCI population.[109] The mean pooled frequency of DVT detected by these methods was 16.9%, with all patients receiving pharmacologic thromboprophylaxis at the time. The noninvasive nature and relative ease of Doppler ultrasonography has made it the most common screening tool, but its sensitivity for proximal and distal DVT has been estimated at only 29%.[99] Taking into account the imperfect sensitivities of screening tests and the relative infrequency of fatal and nonfatal PE, it is unlikely that a large enough trial will be undertaken to definitively establish the efficacy of DVT screening in reducing risk. The American College of Chest Physicians describes screening ultrasonography as a "reasonable consideration."[101] Because of the diminishing frequency of DVT/PE after SCI, any benefit of this practice will erode with time, and it is probably reasonable that screening, if undertaken, be discontinued 3 months after injury.[109]

PE may present with acute deterioration, characterized by hypotension, tachycardia, and hypoxemia, or it may present more insidiously, with one or more of these signs present only to a mild degree. The clinician should have a low threshold of suspicion because early identification and treatment of a small PE may stave off a second, more catastrophic event. When there is clinical suspicion for PE, a helical CT scan of the chest with contrast should be performed. Ventilation-perfusion scans have limited sensitivity and specificity and are used only when there is a contraindication to the administration of intravenous contrast. As noted earlier, ultrasonography of the legs is a relatively insensitive test and is incapable of identifying intrapelvic thrombus. When a diagnosis of PE is being entertained, a negative lower extremity duplex examination provides a false sense of security and should not be used for this purpose. Treatment of PE requires prompt heparinization and, in some cases, inferior vena cava filter placement. Long-term management typically involves transition to warfarin or continuation of a therapeutic-dose LMWH for 3 to 6 months.

Integumentary Complications

Decubitus ulcers result from tissue ischemia. In the patient with SCI, this ischemia is primarily the result of the patient's inability periodically to shift pressure points and restore circulation to previously compressed areas of skin and soft tissue. In the acute phase of injury, tissue ischemia may be exacerbated by hypotension and diminished cardiac output stemming from sympathetic denervation. The persistence and progression of decubitus ulcers result from impaired nutritional status, inadequate local hygiene, and a failure to restore adequate local tissue perfusion.

Multiple studies have attempted to establish risk factors for decubitus ulcer formation; a recent review and meta-analysis synthesized this disparate literature and found the following risk factors to be significant: neurologically complete lesion, hypotension on presentation, degree of mobility deficit, decreasing albumin level, and duration of stay on a neurosurgical ward.[110] The following variables were found not to be associated with increased risk: tetraplegia versus paraplegia, smoking status, complete blood count, pulse oximetry measurements, and arterial blood gas measurements.[110] The Braden, Norton, and Waterlow scales are all established instruments for decubitus ulcer risk assessment; the Spinal Cord Injury Pressure Ulcer Scale (SCIPUS) and SCIPUS-A are newer instruments devised specifically for SCI, but they have yet to be independently validated.[111] The incorporation of one of these instruments into standard nursing documentation focuses attention on this pivotal aspect of nursing care for the patient with SCI.

Minimization of pressure effects is the mainstay of preventing decubitus ulcer development. After injury, the patient should be removed from the spine board as soon as it is safe to do so; ulcers can develop after as little as 6 hours on a hard surface. Thereafter, patients should be repositioned frequently, although how frequently is a question not addressed in the current literature. Log-roll technique with in-line cervical stabilization should be used until spinal stability is ensured. At this stage, pneumatic, rotating, and oscillating beds are useful adjuncts that reduce the burden on nursing personnel. The placement of a pillow under the calf is a simple, effective way to reduce heel pressure.

Data supporting specific hemodynamic or metabolic goals in prevention of decubitus ulcers are lacking in the literature. However, it is reasonable to expect that timely correction of hypotension and hypoxemia, the avoidance of severe anemia, tight control of serum glucose in diabetic patients, and early attention to nutritional status would all be beneficial in the prevention and treatment of decubitus ulcers in the SCI population.

Heterotopic Ossification

Heterotopic ossification (HO) is the presence of lamellar bone in soft tissue structures where bone is not normally present. It is distinct from metastatic calcification, which results from hypercalcemia, and dystrophic calcification as a result of tumor. The precise mechanism of HO is unknown. Current evidence suggests that it results from the differentiation of pluripotential mesenchymal stem cells into osteoblasts.[112] Factors believed to play a role in this process include a permissive HLA genotype, overexpression of bone morphogenetic proteins (BMP; particularly BMP-4), tissue hypoxia, changes in sympathetic tone, as well as immobility.[113]

The prevalence of HO in the SCI population is approximately 25%.[114] It typically becomes manifest about 4 months after injury, with increased joint stiffness, decreased range of motion, warmth, swelling, and erythema. The early inflammatory phase is often confused with phlebitis/DVT, septic arthritis, or tumor.[113] Joint stiffness may be difficult to detect with the onset of spasticity. Radiographic workup of HO includes serum alkaline phosphatase levels and three-phase bone scintigraphy. CT and MRI have little role early in the course of the disease. Treatment includes nonsteroidal anti-inflammatory medications, local radiation, and, in severe cases, surgical excision.

For the physician treating acute SCI, preventative strategies are the most relevant. The efficacy of range-of-motion exercises in HO continues to be debated. Data on the subject are sparse and divergent. Some authors recommend that once early signs of HO are evident, an aggressive regimen of passive, progressive range-of-motion exercises may mitigate its ultimate effects,[115] whereas others believe such a regimen exacerbates the underlying pathophysiology.[116] Recent evidence suggests that passive range-of-motion exercises are also ineffective in preventing flexion contracture after SCI[117-119]; however, abandonment of this practice in the early stage after injury should await further, confirmatory study.

Psychiatric Complications

Spinal cord injury prompts a grief reaction very similar to that experienced by terminally ill patients. The grieving process of denial, anger, sadness, and, it is hoped, acceptance is experienced not only by the patient but by his or her family. These monumental emotional issues must be recognized and addressed by the physicians and nurses caring for the patient. Unfortunately, this is often difficult and unnatural. Because SCI victims are often young and previously healthy, the psychological barrier between "us" and "them" is diminished; this proximity, combined with the horrible nature of the injury (particularly with cervical SCI) makes empathy and forthrightness emotionally taxing for the physician. Clinicians may find themselves fighting the urge to avoid the patient or the family, or else focusing discussion solely on medical issues, without addressing the "elephant in the room." However, ignoring the long-term significance of the injury and its emotional toll comes with a significant price. The patient and family are deprived of a shepherd during a period of severe psychological trauma. Nurses and staff may feel victimized as the patient and family externalize their anger on them. And, at the most practical level, patient care may be compromised by the interpersonal conflicts that result. Recognizing the stages of grief and their manifestations is an important first step toward overcoming our natural aversions in this regard.

KEY REFERENCES

American Thoracic Society, Infectious Diseases Society of America: Guidelines for the management of adults with hospital-acquired, ventilator-associated, and healthcare-associated pneumonia. *Am J Respir Crit Care Med* 171:388–416, 2005.

Ball PA: Critical care of spinal cord injury. *Spine (Phila Pa 1976)* 26(Suppl 24):S27–S30, 2001.

Crosby ET: Airway management in adults after cervical spine trauma. *Anesthesiology* 104:1293–1318, 2006.

Frankel HL, Mathias CJ: Severe hypertension in patients with high spinal cord lesions undergoing electro-ejaculation: management with prostaglandin E2. *Paraplegia* 18:293–299, 1980.

Perkash I: Long-term urologic management of the patient with spinal cord injury. *Urol Clin North Am* 20:423–434, 1993.

Tator CH, Fehlings MG: Review of clinical trials of neuroprotection in acute spinal cord injury. *Neurosurg Focus* 6:e8, 1999.

REFERENCES

The complete reference list is available online at expertconsult.com.

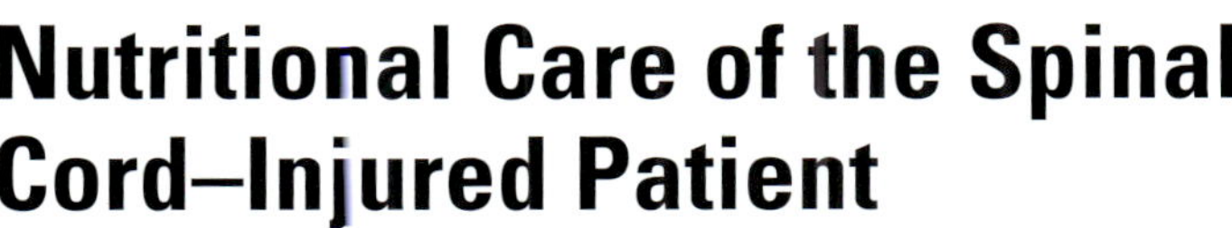

CHAPTER 184

Nutritional Care of the Spinal Cord–Injured Patient

Stavropoula Tjoumakaris | Edward C. Benzel | James S. Harrop

Spinal cord injury (SCI) is a devastating and life-changing event that often results in significant morbidity and potential mortality. A multidisciplinary team approach consisting of surgeons, critical care intensivists, rehabilitation physicians, nurses, therapists, and dietitians is helpful to both the initial and long-term management of these challenging patients. In addition to recent advances in technology and surgical techniques, there have been significant medical advances in the management of patients with SCI. Nutritional optimization of these patients is one such critical element because malnourishment increases the risk of infection and potentially limits the recovery of the affected individual. This chapter provides an overview of the unique metabolic demands and nutritional support strategies in the SCI population.

Estimation of Nutritional Requirements

Prediction of Calorie Requirements

An accurate determination of the metabolic profile of each patient is necessary in the initial evaluation of patients with SCI. A variety of factors such as age, sex, level of injury, and medical comorbidities must be considered.[1] Inaccuracy in calculating patient metabolic requirements could lead to either underfeeding or overfeeding, both of which can be detrimental to the patient. Underfeeding results in muscle wasting, decreased immunocompetence, and poor wound healing. Overfeeding, however, is associated with fluid overload, hyperglycemia, elevated blood urea nitrogen (BUN), elevated triglyceride levels, abnormal hepatic enzyme levels, respiratory distress caused by increased CO_2 production, and ventilator weaning difficulties.

Standard Nutritional Requirement Formulas

The energy required to fuel basic life processes in healthy, resting, fasting individuals is defined as the basal energy expenditure (BEE). A variety of factors, including age, sex, body surface area, and fasting versus fed states, directly affect BEE.[1] The Harris-Benedict equation is the most common method used to estimate this energy requirement. This formula requires weight to be measured in kilograms, height in centimeters, and age in years.[2] As shown in the following equations, BEE is calculated differently for men (BEE_m) and women (BEE_w):

$$\begin{aligned} BEE_m &= 66 + (13.7 \times \text{weight}) + (5 \times \text{height}) - (6.8 \times \text{age}) \\ BEE_w &= 655 + (9.6 \times \text{weight}) + (1.7 \times \text{height}) - (4.7 \times \text{age}) \end{aligned} \tag{1}$$

As previously mentioned, critically ill patients require more energy than indicated by their BEE. This additional energy requirement is termed the *predicted energy expenditure* and is estimated by multiplying the BEE by either an activity factor (1.2 for bedrest) or a stress/injury factor (1.6 to 1.75 for major trauma).[3,4] In the patient with SCI, this posttraumatic hypermetabolic and hypercatabolic state is superimposed on a state of muscle inactivity caused by paralysis. Therefore, the use of the usual activity factor of 1.2 for bedrest may overestimate caloric needs and result in excessive delivery of calories.[3,5-7]

Factors That May Escalate Energy Expenditure

Major traumatic injury such as SCI increases the metabolic rate and has been described as "sudden stimuli to which the organism is not quantitatively or qualitatively adapted."[6] The extensive multisystem trauma and long bone fractures that commonly occur in association with SCI can augment this hypermetabolic response.[8]

Postinjury hypermetabolism is a cascade response caused by the hormonal effects of increased glucagon, cortisol, and catecholamine levels. There is a small decrease in plasma thyroxine with SCI, but this does not appear to influence the metabolic rate.[9] However, some conditions such as pancreatitis, a relatively common complication of SCI,[10,11] can significantly increase energy expenditure.

Increase in body temperature after SCI is a common phenomenon and frequently the result of a pulmonary or urinary tract infection. However, the loss of sympathetic innervation and the inability of muscles to shiver can lead to wide changes in basal metabolic rates.[12-14] The degree of temperature regulation impairment is also proportional to the extent and spinal level of the paralysis. In addition, greater fluid retention and subsequent increased body weight result in falsely elevated predictions. Ventilated patients do not require as much energy because they are not performing spontaneous breathing. Critically ill patients who are sedated and relatively motionless exhibit an even lower energy state.[15]

Although the Harris-Benedict equation does account for activity and the metabolic stress/injury response, there are certain deficiencies in its use. For instance, other critical factors such as infection, body temperature, nutritional support regimens, clinical procedures, surgical operations, and medications are omitted. Patient variability regarding these factors can complicate the use of predictive equations for energy expenditures. Therefore, the more complicated the patient, the poorer the ability to predict metabolic rates based on these equations and formulas. Actual energy expenditure measurements represent a more sophisticated and complete assessment of the patient with SCI.

Calorimetry: Measurement of Energy Expenditures

Calorimetry is a more accurate technique to determine energy expenditure. Unfortunately, it is more expensive and requires precision equipment and appropriately trained personnel. Nevertheless, energy expenditures can be accurately determined by using either direct or indirect calorimetry.

Direct calorimetry measures heat production or heat loss by the body.[16] To obtain these measurements, a subject is placed in a sealed chamber with a supply of oxygen. Because the chamber is well insulated, the heat produced by the body is absorbed by a known volume of water that circulates through pipes located in the chamber. The change in water temperature reflects the person's heat loss and represents expended metabolic energy. Although this method is very precise, it is neither practical nor feasible for acutely traumatized patients with SCI. However, the commonly used equations to predict resting metabolic rate overestimate this rate in patients with SCI by 5% to 32%.[17] Specifically, measurements of resting metabolic rates in patients with SCI are 14% to 27% lower than their healthy counterparts because of decreased fat-free body mass and baseline sympathetic activity.

Indirect calorimetry is a more useful and accurate alternative to the direct method. This technique is used to measure energy expenditure in critically ill patients. Heat production or resting energy expenditure (REE) is determined with a metabolic cart (Critical Care Monitor, Medical Graphics Corporation, St. Paul, MN) by measuring respiratory gas exchange between the inspired and expired samples.[16] The basis for this calculation is that oxygen consumption ($\dot{V}_{O_2}$) and carbon dioxide production ($\dot{V}_{CO_2}$) accurately reflect a significant portion of systemic intracellular metabolism. The REE is determined from the data obtained by the metabolic cart study and the Weir equation,[18] as explained in the following equation:

$$REE = (3.9 \times \dot{V}_{O_2} + 1.1 \times \dot{V}_{CO_2}) \times 1.44 \quad (2)$$

An additional feature of the metabolic cart is the ability to calculate not only the REE, but the respiratory quotient (RQ) from the measured $\dot{V}_{O_2}$ and $\dot{V}_{CO_2}$. The RQ is the ratio of $\dot{V}_{CO_2}/\dot{V}_{O_2}$, and can be used as an indicator of substrate use.[16] Each energy source (carbohydrate, protein, and fat) is oxidized at a known RQ, ranging from 0.7 to 1 (Table 184-1). Therefore, the RQ can be used occasionally to determine the predominant substrate used. For example, when the measured RQ is greater than 1, lipogenesis is assumed to occur.

TABLE 184-1

Respiratory Quotient (RQ) Depending on Substrate Used

Substrate Used	RQ
Ethanol	0.67
Fat	0.71
Protein	0.82
Mixed substrate oxidation	0.85
Carbohydrate	1
Ketone bodies	1
Lipogenesis	>1

Substrate adjustments can be made in the nutritional support regimen based on the useful information acquired from the metabolic cart study.

Overview of the Metabolic Stress Response

Major Trauma, Surgery, and Sepsis

After acute SCI, the patient enters a hypermetabolic and hypercatabolic state. This phenomenon is similar to that seen after trauma, major surgical interventions, and sepsis. This hypermetabolic and hypercatabolic state results in a remarkable increase in energy expenditure, total-body protein catabolism, and nitrogen excretions.[19-26] The energy requirements of the trauma patient, often in excess of 200% of BEE, are necessary to maintain lean body mass. If the nutritional requirements are not met from exogenous sources, the body will use internal sources, such as body fat and muscle reserves. For example, increased protein turnover indicates that postinjury caloric requirements are much higher than maintenance levels. This accelerated protein breakdown results in a supply of amino acids for the gluconeogenesis that is needed to fuel anaerobic glycolysis in the injured tissues.

There are numerous metabolic variables in the critically ill patient that deserve close scrutiny. Hypervigilance to the nutritional status of these patients helps prevent the detrimental consequences of depleted muscle mass, increased susceptibility to infections, and impaired wound healing. The patient with SCI differs from other patients in that the neuronal disconnection of the muscles causes a decrease in muscle use and compensatory atrophy, thus lowering the energy expenditure. In addition, there are two unique metabolic responses to SCI superimposed on this already complex pathophysiologic process: an acute nutritional response and a delayed nutritional response.

Acute Nutritional Response to Spinal Cord Injury

In the acute period after SCI, which we define as less than 4 weeks postinjury, the patient's metabolic response is influenced by the hypermetabolism related to the traumatic injury, as well as by the decreased energy requirements related to the muscle paralysis. The degree of neuronal injury resulting in loss of muscle stimulation and atrophy has been directly correlated with REE.[5,20,27-33] Therefore, a quadriplegic patient has a lower energy expenditure than a paraplegic patient, whose energy expenditure in turn is less than that of a patient without SCI.[34]

Actual REEs, measured by indirect calorimetry during the first and second weeks after SCI, have demonstrated that calorie needs are overestimated when the Harris-Benedict equation for BEE (see Equation 1) is used in conjunction with injury and activity factors.[3] Kearns et al.[29] also reported that the average REE after acute SCI was lower than predicted by the Harris-Benedict equation for BEE. They hypothesized that nonspecific changes in neurogenic stimuli and decreased oxygen consumption by flaccid muscles contributed to these findings. Their hypothesis was further supported by the observation that the REE increased by 5% as muscle tone returned.[29] Young et al.[35] excluded the injury and activity factors used in the Harris-Benedict equation for predicted energy expenditure in four patients with acute SCI, despite their traumatic injuries. The result of this calculation, which was significantly lower because of the loss of activity and trauma factors, and additional factor adjustments, was determined to be 97% of the predicted value using indirect calorimetry.[35] This emphasizes the inaccuracy and elevation of the predicted energy expenditure obtained using standard formulas and equations for the patient with acute SCI. These patients also have persistent negative nitrogen balance during the first 3 weeks after injury despite aggressive nutritional replacement.[3,32,36] This obligatory negative nitrogen balance is not corrected with increased caloric intake.[32]

Delayed Nutritional Response to Spinal Cord Injury

Resolution of the hypermetabolic and hypercatabolic states after SCI occurs between the third and fourth weeks postinjury. The patient then enters the delayed nutritional response to SCI. This change in metabolism is indicated by resolution of the negative nitrogen balance.[3,28,29,32,37] Several investigators have reported that the delayed metabolic response to SCI is marked by a reduction in energy expenditure of up to 67% and is associated with a progressive loss in lean body mass. Agarwal et al.,[38] in a study of 15 quadriplegic patients at a mean of 9.2 years after injury, found that measured energy expenditures were markedly lower than calculated expenditures based on the Harris-Benedict BEE. The results of this study illustrated that the delivery of calories based on the Harris-Benedict formula leads to overfeeding. This was further demonstrated by Kearns et al.,[30] whose five chronic quadriplegic patients showed that the BEE as calculated using the Harris-Benedict equation exceeded energy expenditure by a factor of 1.5. Although the time frame of this study in relation to injury was not specified, they suggested reducing the estimated number of calories by 20% in the patient with chronic SCI.[30]

The reduced caloric needs of patients with SCI appear to be proportional to the spinal level of the neurologic lesion or the mass of denervated muscle.[5,7,20,27,33] By studying 22 patients with SCI at more than 2 months after injury, Cox et al.[20] showed that quadriplegic patients required 22.7 kcal/kg/day, whereas paraplegic patients required 27.9 kcal/kg/day. They further noted that upon allowing uncontrolled diets, patients gained on average 1.7 kg per week.[20] Mollinger et al.[7] also confirmed the lower caloric needs of patients with SCI compared with the calculated BEE, as well as a significant correlation of energy expenditure with the level of the spinal cord lesion. Clarke[5] concluded that metabolic data obtained from healthy subjects could not be used to predict caloric expenditures in paraplegic patients, even when allowances were made for body weight. Sedlock and Laventure[33] attributed this discrepancy to the loss of lean body mass after paralysis.

Total calorie intake, nutrient consumption, and body mass index (BMI) were investigated in a cross-sectional study of 73 patients with SCI with respect to sex and level of injury.[1] Female sex and lower levels of injury were both associated with lower calorie intake and BMI. Using the SCI-adjusted BMI (recommended <22 kg/m^2, overweight 22–25 kg/m^2, and obese >25 kg/m^2), 74% of the patients were overweight or obese. Therefore, clinicians should consider adjusting BMI for the SCI population to better determine the risk of obesity and associated comorbidities in these patients.

Basic Nutritional Requirements

Carbohydrate Requirements

Glucose is the preferred energy substrate for CNS tissue, blood cells, granulation tissue, testes, and renal medulla. A minimum of 100 to 150 g/day of glucose is required for their basic function as well as for the prevention of excessive protein breakdown.[39] The rate at which the body oxidizes carbohydrate or glucose is approximately 2 to 4 mg/kg/min under normal conditions. During severe stress, the oxidation rate of glucose is elevated to 3 to 5 mg/kg/min. In most patients, the provision of more than 400 to 500 g/day of glucose exceeds the body's ability to oxidize it and use it for energy. The excess glucose is converted to fat and can be measured by calorimetry as an increased $\dot{V}_{CO_2}/\dot{V}_{O_2}$ ratio (increased RQ).[19] Despite the CNS's need for glucose, patients with chronic SCI have been shown to have glucose intolerance due to insulin resistance.[40]

The relationship between derangements in glucose metabolism and neural injury has been studied extensively, especially with regard to ischemia.[41-45] The results of these studies suggest that hyperglycemia at the time of, and immediately after, neurotrauma (including SCI) may worsen outcome. High serum glucose levels increase the substrate available for anaerobic glycolysis, and thus for the production of lactic acid.[46] CNS lactic acid production may have an adverse effect on the recovery from neurologic injury.[47] Control of serum glucose levels (i.e., prevention of hyperglycemia), especially during the first 2 to 8 hours postinjury, appears to be crucial for optimal recovery. However, increased glucose availability may be advantageous after 2 to 8 hours postinjury, and early calorie supplementation can then be implemented.[47]

Lipid Requirements

After glucose is stored, the body preferentially resorts to lipid metabolism rather than depleting protein stores.[48] Provision of lipid as a concentrated source of calories can facilitate protein sparing, decrease the risk of carbohydrate overfeeding, and help limit total fluid volume. Fat should generally constitute 30% of the total calorie delivery. In the acute postinjury stage, large amounts of fat (>30%), especially linoleic or omega-6 fatty acids, can have an immunosuppressive effect by stimulating the release of arachidonic acid.[39] This precursor leads to prostaglandin formation and subsequently depresses cell-mediated hypersensitivity, lymphocyte proliferation, and natural killer cell function. High serum triglyceride levels also indicate fat intolerance and the need to reduce the amount of intravenous lipid emulsions delivered. A minimum of 4% of total energy needs should be provided as essential fatty acids to avoid deficiency.[39]

Protein Requirements

Proteins are essential for tissue growth, maintenance, and repair, and for the synthesis of hormones, enzymes, antibodies, and transport molecules. All amino acids serve important functions. When excess protein is ingested, it is either metabolized into energy or stored as fat. The recommended dietary allowance for healthy adults is 0.8 g of protein per kilogram of ideal body weight daily (ideal body weight for males is estimated to be 106 pounds for the first 5 feet in height plus 6 pounds for every inch taller; for females, it is 100 pounds for the first 5 feet plus 5 pounds for every inch taller).[49] Protein requirements increase dramatically to 2 g/kg of ideal body weight after multiple trauma, major burns, or severe sepsis. Increased levels of protein are also recommended after acute SCI.[50]

After glycogen stores are depleted in the muscles and liver through glycogenolysis, the body protein is catabolized by gluconeogenesis. As a part of this process, for every 6.25 g of protein broken down, 1 g of nitrogen is excreted.[51]

Micronutrients

Calcium

Alterations in calcium metabolism after acute SCI have been well documented.[8,52,53] Bone homeostasis represents a balance between bone destruction and building. After SCI, the skeleton is often no longer capable of carrying and supporting the body. This state of effective immobilization causes bone reabsorption below the level of injury beginning within 10 days of injury and lasting for at least 6 months.[54,55] This may lead to high serum and urine calcium levels. Adults are susceptible to hypercalcemia because of impaired renal function and excretion difficulties, whereas children may have hypercalcemia because of increased bone turnover rates.[40,56] Although rare after SCI, symptoms of hypercalcemia include anorexia, nausea and vomiting, abdominal cramps, constipation, headache, and lethargy.

A low-calcium diet does not appear to be effective in decreasing serum calcium levels.[57] Ultimately, this negative calcium balance leads to osteoporosis in all skeletal structures below the lesion. Ragnarsson and Sell[58] showed, in a retrospective study, that the incidence of lower extremity fractures is greater in paraplegic patients than in quadriplegic patients. This is believed to be due to higher activity levels in the former group. Most of these fractures occurred in osteoporotic bones, without known trauma or after trivial injuries.[58]

Women with SCI have decreased bone density and increased fracture risk compared with healthy control subjects.[59] Increased bone resorption rate, low parathyroid hormone levels, and low vitamin D levels are some contributing factors. Aggressive therapies to treat and prevent osteoporosis in patients with SCI include adequate nutritional supplementation (especially calcium and vitamin D intake), bisphosphonates, estrogen (in postmenopausal women), weight bearing, and functional electrical stimulation.

Iron

Anemia is a common complication of acute SCI, even in the absence of significant blood loss.[50,60] Huang et al.,[60] in a study of 28 patients with acute SCI, found normochromic, normocytic anemia in 71% and normochromic, microcytic anemia in 14%. They speculated that iron deficiencies, immune system changes that alter bone marrow maturation, and the effects of stress were causative factors. The process of erythropoiesis was not found to be altered in patients with SCI.[60]

Anemia associated with chronic disorders, such as decubitus ulcers or urinary tract infections, was the most common type discovered in patients with chronic SCI studied by Perkash and Brown.[61] Anemia has also been identified as a factor related to increased length of stay for patients admitted to rehabilitation centers.[62] Recognition of the potential causes of anemia might speed the rehabilitation process.

Sodium

The prevalence of hyponatremia in patients with acute SCI is reportedly much higher than in general surgical populations.[63,64] The strongest predictor of the development of hyponatremia is the extent of neurologic injury. The highest risk is observed in patients with complete motor and sensory SCI. Low serum sodium levels (<135 mM/L after correction for hyperglycemia) usually occur within the first week postinjury. Possible mechanisms include increased fluid intake, intrarenal defects in water excretion, resetting of the osmostat, and excessive sodium losses.[65]

Vitamins

Evidence of inadequate vitamin intake in patients with SCI has been well documented in recent studies.[66-68] In a cross-sectional study by Walters et al.,[66] the vitamin intake of 77 patients was followed at baseline and at 6 months after SCI. Inadequate intake based on nationally accepted dietary references was documented in all patients for vitamins A, B_6, B_{12}, and C, thiamine, folate, and riboflavin. Moussavi et al.[67] measured serum levels of vitamins A and E in 110 adults with chronic SCI (>2 years) and correlated the results with injury-related data and overall patient health status. Their results showed that many of the participants (16–37%) had serum levels below the reference value for each vitamin. Older age at injury onset and a lesser degree of impairment were both associated with higher vitamin levels. Furthermore, higher levels of serum vitamin A were related to improved patient function and health status and absence of pressure ulcers in the previous 12 months. Recent education programs on nutritional support in the SCI population have raised patient awareness. In 2009, a Canadian study of community-dwelling adults with chronic SCI showed that vitamin supplementation was prevalent in 71% of the studied patient sample.[69]

Feeding Modalities

After the patient is admitted to the intensive care unit, a number of critical and acute life-saving interventions occur, beginning with resuscitative efforts that culminate in reduction and stabilization of the initial spine fractures. It is unfortunate, yet common, that nutritional optimization is overlooked. Feeding the patient with acute SCI is further complicated by issues such as mechanical ventilation, traction, immobilization, and abdominal distention.[70] Cooper et al.[6] stated "it is not a rare occurrence to see a patient who is paraplegic ... literally die of starvation, despite vigorous attempts to supply adequate nutrients." Many factors hinder adequate nutrient intake in patients undergoing spine surgery, or those with spine trauma or SCI.

GI function in patients with acute and chronic SCI is compromised as a result of posttraumatic ileus and neuronal motility dysfunction.[71] This lack of nutritional support during a time of hypermetabolism can result in malnutrition if not addressed immediately. Although many patients with SCI present with paralytic ileus, bowel activity commonly returns within the first postinjury week.[8] Patients with SCI commonly experience dysphagia caused by cervical fractures, retropharyngeal hematomas, and immobilization devices, but nutritional intake can be improved with puréed or mechanical soft diets and supplemental tube feedings.[72] Constipation may be mitigated by adequate dietary intake of fiber and fluids and an appropriately aggressive bowel regimen.

Oral Intake

Oral intake is the preferred route of nutrition support. Paraplegic patients with SCI can typically partake of adequate nutrition if they do not have multiorgan injuries. Unlike quadriplegic patients, they have full use of their hands and arms and often do not require ventilatory support. The use of oral nutritional supplements can be tailored to the individual patient to meet his or her needs (Table 184-2).

Successful nutritional management often includes assistance in meal selection, change of meal patterns to smaller, more frequent meals (six to eight times per day), high-nutrient-density commercial supplements, and nocturnal tube feedings. Laven et al.,[73] in a study of 51 patients with acute SCI, reported that anorexia was present in 57% of the patients 2 weeks after injury, and continued until 8 weeks postinjury in 33%. Depression and the sensation of early satiety are common causes of decreased appetite in these patients. Assistance by nursing staff at mealtimes may be necessary in the acute stages. Patients may become more independent by using assistive eating devices.

Patients with chronic SCI require increased vitamin, mineral, and complex carbohydrate intake and decreased fat intake.[31] High levels of fat intake, low intake of dietary fiber, nominal activity levels, and a predisposition to the development of cardiovascular disease place patients with SCI at an increased risk for cardiopulmonary morbidity and mortality.

Parenteral Nutrition

Indications

Because of the common complications of GI dysfunction and prolonged ileus after SCI, total parenteral nutrition (TPN) is essential if an optimal nutritional status cannot be maintained by the enteral route.[35] The combination of TPN (which provides nutrient needs) and small volumes of enteral feedings (which maintain gut integrity) provides added benefit in selected situations. If the GI tract is not provided with a minimum amount of nutritional support (i.e., 10–20 mL/hr of enteral feeds), the mucosal villi will atrophy.[74] Villous atrophy impairs the natural immunogenic barrier and allows bacteria to translocate across the mucosa and invade the bloodstream, leading to bacteremia or sepsis.

Administration

Specialized nutritional support techniques using either central or peripheral veins can deliver TPN and are available to prevent malnutrition (Fig. 184-1). Concentrated TPN formulas should be infused only through a central venous catheter to prevent thrombophlebitis of the smaller peripheral veins.[75] Central venous access is appropriate if TPN delivery is needed for more than 5 to 7 days. TPN solutions with osmolarities of less than 900 mOsm can be administered by peripheral venous access. However, peripheral access is difficult to maintain and should be used only if nutritional supplementation is anticipated for no longer than 5 to 7 days.

Most institutions have standard TPN solutions that can be ordered from stock. Information about these formulas can be obtained from the institutions' pharmacies. Patient-specific formulas can also be designed to meet individual calorie, protein, and fluid requirements. The energy substrates in TPN are dextrose solutions in concentrations of 5% to 70%, and lipid emulsions in concentrations of 10% (1.1 kcal/mL) to 20% (2 kcal/mL).[75] Protein is provided by commercial crystalline L-amino acid solutions in concentrations of 3% to 15%. Electrolyte additives, multivitamins, trace element preparations, and medications can also be administered in TPN solutions according to each patient's needs.

Complications

Complications of TPN include mineral and electrolyte imbalances, acid-base disorders, substrate intolerances (hyperglycemia, hypertriglyceridemia, elevated BUN levels), and catheter-related infections.[75] In the acute postinjury stage, daily monitoring of serum electrolytes, glucose, BUN, and creatinine is necessary to detect and minimize excesses or deficiencies. Changes in sodium, potassium, magnesium, and phosphorus deliveries are frequent in critically ill patients. Careful evaluation of fluid balance by daily weights and intake and output records is necessary to prevent volume depletion or overload. Meticulous line care is essential for reducing catheter-related infections. As stated previously, loss of the intestinal barrier due to mucosal atrophy during TPN has been shown to promote bacterial translocation from the intestine to the bloodstream.[74] Trophic tube feeds (10–20 mL/hr) while using parenteral nutrition can prevent disuse atrophy and bacterial translocation. This flow rate is minimal and well tolerated in most posttraumatic ileus states.

Enteral Nutrition (Tube Feeding)

Indications

When adequate dietary intake cannot be achieved orally but the GI tract is functional, enteral nutrition by tube is the

TABLE 184-2

A Guide to Enteral Feeding Formulas

	Calories/mL	Protein (g/L)	Fat (g/L)	Carbohydrate (g/L)	mOsm/kg H_2O	Special Features
Oral Supplements						
Boost	1	43	18	173	640	Multiflavor
Boost with Fiber	1	43	18	178	480	Fiber
Boost Plus	1.5	59	58	200	720	High calorie
Boost HP	1	61	23	210	540	High protein
Choice	1	39	43	101	380	Diabetes
Ensure	1	37	25	165	470	Multiflavor
Ensure Plus	1.5	55	47	210	690	Multiflavor
Kindercal	1.1	30	44	135	440	Ages 1–10 yr
Resource 1.5	1.5	67	67	230	600	—
Resource Shake	1.7	55	74	240	600	—
Resource 2.0	2	108	103	270	600	—
Sustacal	1	61	22	132	650	High protein
Standard Tube Feeds						
Comply	1.5	60	61	180	460	Restricted fluids
Isocal	1	34	44	135	270	—
Isosource	1	51	35	142	240	—
Osmolite	1	37	34	151	300	Isotonic
Nutren	1	40	38	128	300	—
Ultracal	1	45	39	142	360	Moderate nitrogen
Kindercal TF	1.1	30	44	135	345	Ages 1–10 yr
Fiber-Containing Supplements						
Ensure Fiber with FOS	1.1	38	25	169	470	—
Glucerna	1	42	59	96	355	Diabetes
Jevity	1	44	35	155	300	—
Jevity Plus	1.2	55	39	173	365	—
Isosource Fiber	1	38	34	138	275	—
Nutren 1.0 with Fiber	1	40	38	128	300	Vanilla
Ultracal HN Plus	1.2	54	40	156	370	—
High-Calorie-Density Formulas						
Comply	1.5	60	61	180	460	Restricted fluids
Deliver 2.0	2	75	101	200	640	Restricted fluids
Ensure Plus HN	1.5	63	49	202	650	—
Isocal HN Plus	1.2	54	40	156	400	—
Isosource Energy	1.6	57	62	200	390	—
Magnacal Renal	2	75	101	200	570	Renal dialysis
Nepro	2	70	96	333	665	Renal dialysis
Nutren 1.5	1.5	60	68	170	430	—
Nutren 2.0	2	80	106	196	710	—
Probalance	1.2	54	41	156	350	Elderly
Pulmocare	1.5	63	93	106	475	Ventilated patient
Suplena	2	30	96	255	600	Renal dialysis
TwoCal HN	2	84	91	219	690	High nitrogen
High-Protein Formulas						
Ensure High Protein	1	50	25	130	470	—
Isocal HN	1.1	44	45	124	270	—
Isosource Protein	1.2	66	40	148	300	—
Osmolite HN	1	44	45	144	300	—
Osmolite HN Plus	1.2	55	39	158	360	—
TwoCal HN	2	84	91	219	690	—
Ultracal HN Plus	1.2	54	40	156	370	—
Special Disease State Formulas						
ChoiceDM	1	45	51	119	300	Diabetics
Deliver 2.0	2	75	101	200	640	Restricted fluids

TABLE 184-2

A Guide to Enteral Feeding Formulas—cont.

	Calories/mL	Protein (g/L)	Fat (g/L)	Carbohydrate (g/L)	mOsm/kg H_2O	Special Features
Glucerna	1	42	59	96	355	Diabetes
Introlyte	0.5	22	18	71	200	Starting tube feeds
Lipisorb	1.4	57	57	161	630	Fat malabsorption
Magnacal Renal	2	75	101	200	570	Renal dialysis
Oxepa	1.5	63	94	106	493	Lung injured, ventilated
Probalance	1.2	54	41	156	350	Elderly
Protain XL	1	57	30	145	340	Wound healing
Pulmocare	1.5	63	93	106	475	Ventilated patient
Respalor	1.5	75	68	145	400	Limited respiratory function
Subdue	1	50	34	130	450	Impaired GI function
Suplena	2	30	96	255	600	Renal dialysis
TraumaCal	1.5	82	68	142	560	Trauma
Elemental Formulas						
AlitraQ	1	16	165	575	575	Impaired GI tract
Peptamen	1	40	39	127	260	Ready to feed
Peptamen VHP	1	63	39	105	300	Ready to feed
Perative	1.3	67	37	177	385	—
Subdue	1	50	34	130	330	Malabsorption
Subdue Plus	1.5	76	51	127	400	Calorically dense
Optimental	1	51	28	139	540	Malabsorption
Criticare HN	1	38	5	220	650	Malabsorption
Modular Supplements						
Casec powder	3.8	90	2	—	—	Protein powder
Moducal powder	3.8	—	—	—	—	Glucose polymers
Microlipid	4.5	—	45	—	80	Fat emulsion
MCT oil	7.7	0	0	—	—	MCT
Polycose powder	2 cal/mL	—	—	—	—	Glucose polymers
ProMod powder	12 cal/T	3 g/L	—	—	—	Protein powder
Pediatric Formulas						
Isosource Jr	1.2	54	94	340	346	Ages 1–12 yr
Kindercal TF	1.1	30	44	135	345	Ages 1–10 yr
Pediasure Enteral	1	30	48	110	—	Ages 1–10 yr
Pediasure Enteral with fiber	1	30	44	114	—	Ages 1–10 yr

GI, gastrointestinal; MCT, medium-chain triglycerides.

preferred method for nutritional support. The enteral route for nutrient administration is always preferable to parenteral feedings. In a study by Rowan et al.,[76] 33 patients with acute SCI were started on enteral feedings within 2 days of injury. The feeds were delivered by nasogastric or nasojejunal tubes. High gastric aspiration was the most common cause of feeding interruption, but was temporary and reversible. No major complications were noted in this study and the authors concluded that early commencement of enteral feedings is a safe technique of nutrient delivery to the patient with SCI even in the acute stages.

The benefits of enteral feedings include more physiologic metabolism and use of nutrients, maintenance of gut integrity, decreased risk of bacterial translocation lower cost of nutrient delivery, and decreased risk of catheter-related infections.[77] Use of the enteral route is contraindicated in the presence of mechanical obstruction of the GI tract, prolonged ileus, severe GI hemorrhage, severe diarrhea, intractable vomiting, and high-output GI tract fistula.

Administration

The decision regarding the type of enteral access depends on the anticipated duration of tube feeding and the risk of pulmonary aspiration of gastric contents (see Fig. 184-1). Short-term (<6 weeks) enteral access is possible by the nasogastric, nasoduodenal, or nasojejunal routes. Surgical or percutaneous endoscopic gastrostomy and jejunostomy tubes can be inserted for long-term (>6 weeks) nutritional support.[78] Gastric feedings should not be instituted in patients without an intact gag reflex or with gastroesophageal reflux, gastroparesis, gastric outlet obstruction, or gastric atony.[77] Jejunal feedings can usually be initiated immediately after injury and potentially reduce the risk of aspiration.

A wide variety of specialized commercial formulas is available for both oral and tube feeding supplementation (see Table 184-2). These supplements differ by calorie and protein densities, fiber contents, form of nutrients, and the amount of micronutrients.[77] Selection of the appropriate formula is

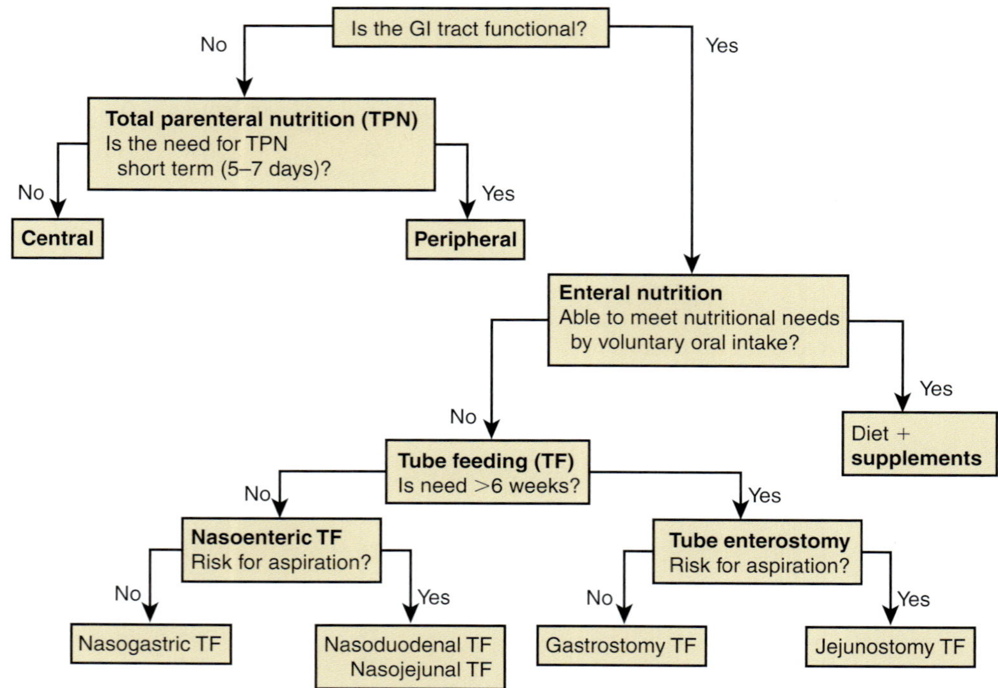

FIGURE 184-1. The decision-making process for nutritional support.

based on the individual's digestive and absorptive capacity and the specific characteristics and indications for the product. Most commercial formulas provide the recommended dietary allowances for vitamins and minerals in approximately 1 to 1.5 L.

Formulas can be administered by bolus, intermittent, or continuous methods. Bolus feedings involve the rapid delivery of 300 to 400 mL of formula over 10 minutes several times daily. Intermittent feedings are also given several times daily, but over at least 30 minutes. The bolus and intermittent methods are especially suited for gastric feedings. Small-volume, continuous-drip feedings over 10 to 24 hours are recommended for intestinal delivery of nutrients. Continuous feedings are usually better tolerated than bolus feedings in critically ill patients.[77]

The final goal of delivered formula depends on the product's nutrient density and the individual's estimated daily calorie and protein requirements. Bolus or intermittent feedings can be initiated with 100 mL of formula. The bolus volume can be advanced by 50 mL every 4 hours to the goal amount if gastric residuals are not significant (<100 mL or half the volume previously delivered) when aspirated before each feeding.[79] Continuous tube feeding is initiated at rates ranging from 20 to 40 mL/hr. Rates are then advanced by 10 to 25 mL/hr every 6 hours to the goal amount as the patient tolerates.

Complications

Complications of enteral feedings interrupt adequate nutrient delivery (Table 184-3). Diarrhea and tube obstruction are the most common problems associated with tube feedings. Recognition of the causes and solutions to these complications can improve formula tolerance and increase nutrient delivery.[77]

Monitoring of Nutritional Status

There is little documentation of the effectiveness of early aggressive nutritional support in terms of improved outcome or decreased incidence of complications for SCI.[28,73] However, there is a large body of evidence supporting improved outcomes in other neurologic injuries, such as head trauma.[23,35,80,81] Applying these data to the SCI population supports the notion that hospitalized patients with SCI should be maintained at optimal nutritional status. Two thirds of the patients with SCI admitted to rehabilitation units are reportedly malnourished.[82] In addition, quadriplegic patients are at a higher risk for malnutrition than are paraplegic patients and should be nutritionally supported even more aggressively.[83]

Body Composition

Patients with serious injuries, such as major fractures, will often lose 10% to 25% of their body weight during recovery from injury.[25] Studies of tissue composition show that protein accounts for 8% to 12% of the total weight loss and fat accounts for 15% to 30%. However, in patients with SCI, early weight loss consists primarily of muscle rather than fat.[73]

Several studies have demonstrated that the loss of muscle tissue and body cell mass (BCM) after SCI is a progressive process that occurs over a prolonged period.[33,63,84,85] Body composition studies by Sedlock and Laventure[33] indicate that although their subjects with SCI were not overweight, they had an increased proportion of body fat with a decreased lean body mass. Nuhlicek et al.[86] also compared control subjects to patients with SCI and showed no difference in body weight or extracellular water, but an increase in the ratio of extracellular to total body water, along with an increased fat mass in higher-level injuries. Claus-Walker

TABLE 184-3

Complications of Enteral Feeding

Complications	Possible Causes	Suggestions for Prevention or Treatment
Gastrointestinal		
Diarrhea	Formula hyperosmolarity	Initiate feeding at slow rate (10–20 mL/hr); advance rate gradually as patient tolerates
	Bolus feedings	Change to continuous-drip feedings
	Low-residue formulas	Use fiber-containing formulas
	Gut atrophy (prolonged NPO status)	Deliver peptide-based formulas or initiate slow rates of feeding and gradually advance
	Concurrent drug therapy	Evaluate medication regimen (antibiotics, magnesium-containing antacids, oral potassium supplements, sorbitol); adjust as possible
	Bacterial contamination	Limit formula hang-time to no more than 8 hr; change tube feeding bag and extension tubing every 24 hr
	Bacterial overgrowth	If stool culture for *Clostridium difficile* is positive, treat with vancomycin; Lactinex granules, 1 package tid
	Lactose intolerance	Use lactose-free formulas
Gastric residuals	Delayed gastric emptying	Confirm placement of feeding tube distal to the ligament of Treitz; trial metoclopramide (10 mg IV q6h)
	Bolus feedings	Change to continuous-drip feedings
Mechanical		
Tube obstruction	Medications given by tube	Use crushed medications or elixirs only; irrigate tube before and after each medication; use nasogastric tube (instead of nasoduodenal) for delivery of medications
	Irregular irrigation of tube	Irrigate tube with 30–50 mL of water every 4 hr for continuous feeding or before and after each bolus feeding
Tube displacement	Removal by patient	Consider use of feeding tube bridle or modified nasal cannula

and Halstead[63] demonstrated that connective tissue, lipids, and water replace the atrophied muscle. Greenway et al.[84] noted no consistent trends in body composition changes in patients with long-term SCI. They commented that caloric restriction compensates for reduced muscle activity and that it can control increases in body fat. Shizgal et al. stated that in well-nourished quadriplegic patients, the loss of BCM is accompanied by a similar loss of extracellular mass as body size decreases.[63,85] In malnourished patients with SCI, however, body weight may actually increase as a result of expansion in the extracellular mass, even in the presence of a corresponding loss of BCM. Therefore it was concluded that body weight is a poor predictor of nutritional status.

Anthropometric Measurements

Anthropometric measurements are an inexpensive and easily applied tool to access and follow nutritional status in the healthy individual. The values consist of direct measurements of height, weight, triceps skinfold thickness, midarm circumference, and midarm muscle circumference. Unfortunately, patients with SCI typically undergo water shifts, denervation muscle atrophy, an increase in the percentage of body fat, and unavoidable weight and body compositional changes, which diminish the accuracy and validity of these nutritional gauges.[7,50,83] The Metropolitan Life Insurance guidelines for ideal body weight for a given height and frame size for patients with long-term SCI illustrate these changes.[12] Paraplegic patients are approximately 10 to 15 pounds (and quadriplegic patients are approximately 15–20 pounds) below the recommended guideline weights for patients with long-term SCI.[12]

Serum Protein Markers

Serum total protein and albumin levels do not represent useful nutritional assessment parameters for patients with acute SCI. Albumin levels are often distorted by fluid shifts and acute blood loss. Hepatic transport proteins respond as acute-phase reactants and serum levels decline after acute stress.[6] Also, patients with SCI have an extremely high elimination rate of serum albumin.[50,83] With its long half-life of 18 to 21 days, serum albumin is an insensitive marker for adequacy of nutritional support. In fact, serum albumin may be a better indicator of severity of illness than of nutritional status. Serum prealbumin is a more appropriate parameter, with its half-life of 1 to 2 days.[22]

Creatinine-Height Index

The creatinine-height index is based on the amount of creatinine excreted in the urine over 24 hours. This index is typically compared with standard values to assess nutritional status. However, denervation muscle atrophy after SCI causes a dramatic increase in creatinine excretion, regardless of dietary intake or nutritional status. Thus, the creatinine-height index does not truly reflect the nutritional status of the patient with acute SCI.[12] Despite this measurement flaw, a standard index of less than 60% has been established as an indicator of nutritional risk in patients with SCI.[83]

Nitrogen Balance and Nitrogen Turnover

Nitrogen balance (NB), or nitrogen equilibrium, occurs when nitrogen intake equals nitrogen output (NB = 0).[22] A positive NB or anabolic state exists when nitrogen intake exceeds nitrogen output. A net 24-hour positive NB of 2 to 4 g is optimal for anabolism. When nitrogen excretion is greater than nitrogen intake, a negative NB or catabolic state exists.

NB can be calculated by subtracting the total nitrogen output from the total nitrogen intake. The total nitrogen intake is determined by dividing the daily protein intake (grams) from both enteral and parenteral sources by 6.25.[79] Nitrogen output consists primarily of urine urea nitrogen (UUN). An aliquot of a 24-hour urine collection is assayed for its urea nitrogen content by a standard enzymatic laboratory technique (Beckman Astra; Beckman Instruments, Fullerton, CA).[3] This value, plus 4 (the constant used for nitrogen losses from the skin and feces), is subtracted from the grams of nitrogen intake during the same 24-hour period to calculate the NB, as demonstrated in the following equation:

$$NB = (\text{protein intake [g]} / 6.25) - (\text{24-hour UUN} + 4) \quad (3)$$

The provision of inadequate calories forces the body to break down muscle mass to meet energy demands. This muscle breakdown results in the nitrogenous byproducts urea, creatinine, and 3-methylhistidine, which are excreted in the urine.[29] Endogenous protein stores are also used as an amino acid supply when insufficient exogenous protein is provided; therefore, increasing calorie and protein deliveries can minimize net protein losses. Glucocorticoid administration also can increase the catabolism of protein. In this situation, the catabolized protein fuels gluconeogenesis.[28]

After non-SCI major trauma and surgery, REE and nitrogen excretion levels are parallel. However, in patients with SCI, calorie needs decrease, whereas urinary nitrogen losses, primarily from muscle tissue,[6] increase in proportion to the severity of the SCI.[6] This negative NB arises in the spinal cord–injured population despite more-than-adequate calorie and protein administration.[3,28] The phenomenon has also been observed in severe cases of botulism poisoning that have resulted in muscle paralysis.[87]

Nitrogen losses after SCI are obligatory and persist for at least 7 weeks.[3,6,37] Peak negative NB has been previously observed in patients with SCI during the third week after injury, despite adequate delivery of predicted and measured calories.[32] Cooper and Hoen[6] reported that urinary nitrogen excretion of greater than 25 g/day during the first 2 postinjury weeks is a poor prognostic sign for the eventual functional return of paralyzed muscles. In some patients the administration of growth hormone has reduced nitrogen loss.[88] Growth hormone studies after SCI, however, have not been conducted.

During the first week after injury, many patients with SCI have been observed to experience a transiently positive NB.[3] This observation may reflect a delay in protein losses. Dietrick and Shorr[89] evaluated four conscientious objectors who were immobilized in pelvic girdles and leg casts for 6 to 7 weeks on a metabolism ward. All four subjects showed an increase in nitrogen excretion and negative NBs. This, however, took 4 to 5 days to develop. From the data they presented, it is concluded that acute immobilization could contribute to the increased nitrogen excretion observed in paralyzed patients that begins approximately 1 week after injury. Rodriguez et al.[32] showed an obligatory negative NB in 11 of 12 patients with SCI, despite excessive feedings, and the only patient who did not have a negative NB had an incomplete myelopathy. They concluded that relying on NB determinations to calculate nutritional requirements in patients with SCI resulted in overfeeding.

Nutritional Deficiency–Related Wound Complications

Patients with SCI are at increased risk of developing wound-related or skin breakdown problems. In the perioperative period, patients with SCI are typically insensate over the operative region. This results in prolonged pressure and decreased blood supply and nutrition in an already nutritionally compromised patient. Klein et al.[90] showed that even without SCI, a spine patient's preoperative nutritional status was an independent predictor of postoperative infectious complications.

Decubitus ulcers can also develop acutely or in the patient with chronic SCI; their development is associated with the prolonged application of focal pressure and completeness of the SCI.[91] Other factors include anemia, immobility, hypoproteinemia, and systemic infections. After SCI, increased degradation of integument collagen results in the excretion of hydroxyproline, hydroxylysine, and glucosyl-galactosyl hydroxylysine in the urine.[53,92] This leads to a decreased amino acid content per unit weight of skin in patients with SCI, and may account for its decreased tensile strength and increased susceptibility to decubitus ulcer formation. Decubitus ulcers may lead to protein depletion at a rate of up to 50 g/day.[73] The larger the pressure ulcer, the greater the protein loss from the wound, which further augments protein deficiencies.

Lack of weight bearing results in collagen degradation, as does weightlessness in astronauts.[93] Poor circulation below the level of injury can reduce nutrient and oxygen delivery to the tissues, further increasing the risk of decubitus ulcer formation.[92] Defective wound healing has also been reported in nondecubitus wounds below the level of the spinal lesion.[94] Notably, growth hormone levels have been observed to be elevated in patients with SCI. This may in fact be related to an overall increase in collagen turnover.[9]

Obesity and Associated Comorbidities

The prevalence of obesity has reached epidemic proportions worldwide. Inherently, the SCI population is predisposed to obesity because of reduced physical activity, REE, and total lean body mass. Nelson et al.[95] demonstrated the presence of metabolic syndrome in 55% of an SCI population sample. Metabolic syndrome is a constellation of findings such as abdominal obesity, hypertension, hyperlipidemia, and increased glucose tolerance levels. It has been closely associated with the development of cardiovascular disease, diabetes, and certain cancer types. BMI adjusted to the SCI population can be used to determine patient risk for obesity and cardiovascular disease. Patient waist circumference has been reported as a potential surrogate measure of visceral adipose tissue; however, further studies are pending for validation of this parameter.[96]

Hyperlipidemia in the SCI population has been linked to nontraditional cardiovascular disease risk factors, such as elevated C-reactive protein (CRP). The American Heart Association has recognized the inflammatory effect of CRP and recommends its measurement as a cardiovascular risk assessment in certain patient populations.[97] A cross-sectional study of 129 infection-free patients with SCI showed that these patients were more likely to have high CRP levels than normal control subjects.[98] CRP levels were higher in patients with complete injuries as opposed to their incompletely injured counterparts. This elevation was independent of age, smoking status, physical activity, waist circumference, and weight. It was, however, associated with a decrease in the protective cardiovascular levels of high-density lipoprotein cholesterol.

Patient Nutrition and Fitness Education

To maximize the nutritional and overall health status of patients with SCI, a systematic program of nutrition education, exercise, and behavioral intervention needs to be implemented. A recent study of the special requirements of this patient population developed a pilot intervention called the BENEfit program (Behavioral intervention, Exercise, and Nutrition Education to improve health and fitness).[99] Twenty patients with SCI received weekly nutrition education, aerobic and strengthening exercise routines, and behavior modification sessions over a 4-month period. Individuals who participated in the program showed a significant increase in lean body mass, maximum power output, work efficacy, and strength measurements. The BENEfit and similar programs show tremendous promise as methods of improving the nutritional fitness of patients with mobility impairments secondary to SCI.

Summary

A thorough understanding and appreciation of nutritional status is a critical element in the management of patients with SCI. Because of a variety of physical and metabolic changes postinjury, patients with SCI represent a delicate subset of patients whose nutritional needs must be addressed to obtain an optimal outcome. Recent advances in nutrition, including the analysis of basic metabolic needs, noninvasive measurements, and improved nutritional delivery, represent progress in our ability to manage all the issues that relate to the care of these patients.

Methods for estimating caloric and nutritional needs provide the most accurate information during the initial nutritional assessment. Actual metabolic measurements with indirect calorimetry represent advanced techniques in subsequent nutrient delivery. Adjustments can be made based on the patient's clinical condition, available feeding routes, and tolerance of substrates and the modification of requirements as his or her hospital course progresses. Coupled with available assessment techniques and the use of appropriate nutritional supplements, health care providers may further optimize nutritional management and the outcomes of patients with SCI. Dietitians and nutritionists represent an integral piece of the SCI team and their expertise benefits those for whom they care.

KEY REFERENCES

Barboriak JJ, Rooney CB, El Ghatit AZ, et al: Nutrition in spinal cord injury patients. *J Am Paraplegia Soc* 6:32–36, 1983.

Blissitt PA: Nutrition in acute spinal cord injury. *Crit Care Nurs Clin North Am* 2:375–384, 1990.

Chin KP: Nutrition in the spinal-injured patient. *Nutr Clin Pract* 6:213–222, 1991.

Harris JA, Benedict FG: *A biometric study of basal metabolism in man, Carnegie Institute of Washington Publication No. 279*, Philadelphia, 1919, JB Lippincott, pp 190–227.

Kearns PJ, Thompson JD, Werner PC, et al: Nutritional and metabolic response to acute spinal-cord injury. *JPEN J Parenter Enteral Nutr* 16:11–15, 1992.

Mollinger LA, Spurr GB, el Ghatit AZ, et al: Daily energy expenditure and basal metabolic rates of patients with spinal cord injury. *Arch Phys Med Rehabil* 66:420–426, 1985.

Sedlock DA, Laventure SJ: Body composition and resting energy expenditure in long term spinal cord injury. *Paraplegia* 28:448–454, 1990.

REFERENCES

The complete reference list is available online at expertconsult.com.

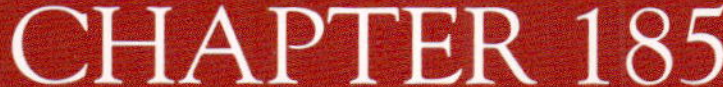

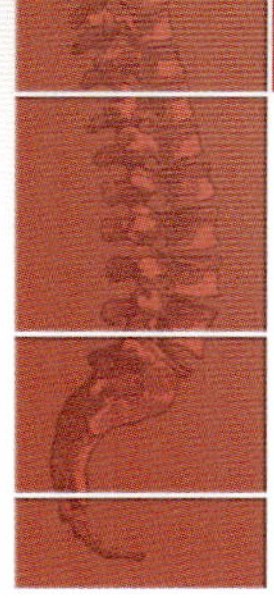

CHAPTER 185

Skin and Wound Care

Ann M. Henwood | Sait Naderi | Edward C. Benzel

A multidisciplinary approach to skin care can effectively minimize the unnecessary morbidity and mortality secondary to pressure ulcers (PUs). In addition to contributing to patient morbidity and negatively affecting quality of life, PUs also result in considerable expense. It has been reported that 1.6 million PUs develop in U.S. hospitals every year. The total cost to treat PUs has been estimated to be between $2.2 billion and $3.6 billion annually. In 2006, adult hospital stays noting a diagnosis of PUs totaled $11 billion.[1] Approximately $125 to $200 is spent for each stage I and stage II PU that develops, and $14,000 to $23,000 is spent for each stage III and stage IV PU. Seventy-five percent of acute care acquired ulcers occur in patients who have undergone a surgical procedure that lasted 3 hours or longer. This same group accounts for 30% to 40% of the total cost associated with PUs.[2] Hospitalizations involving patients with PUs developed either before or after admission increased by nearly 80% between 1993 and 2006. [1]

It has been estimated that 25% of the medical costs associated with spinal cord injuries (SCIs) are incurred as a result of PUs. Overall, the average cost of treating a single PU can range from $5000 to $50,000[3,4]; 1 to 6 months of additional hospital stay is often required. Infectious complications of PUs, such as cellulitis, osteomyelitis, sepsis, and endocarditis, account for more than 60,000 deaths annually.[5-7]

The skin is the largest organ of the body and is composed of a sequence of layers (epidermis, dermis, and subcutaneous fat) that together provide its varied features. The outermost layers provide protection from the elements. These layers permit secretion, excretion, insulation, sensation, and thermoregulation.

A PU (also known as a *pressure sore, decubitus ulcer,* or *bedsore*) is an area of damaged skin and underlying soft tissues resulting from prolonged unrelieved pressure between a bony prominence and an external surface. In a patient, pressure ulcer injury can occur over the scapula, occiput, sacrum, and heels when placed in the supine position; the ear, shoulder, greater trochanter, medial knee, malleolus, and foot edge when laterally positioned; and the nose, forehead, chest, iliac crests, foot edge, and toes when placed in the prone position.[8]

Incidence and Prevalence

The incidence of PUs occurring in postoperative patients varies from 12% to 45%[9]; others report an incidence of 12% to 66%.[9,10,11] In one study the prevalence of ulcer development within 4 days of surgery, by stage, ranged from 0.65% (unstageable) to 6.44% (stage I). The total number of intraoperatively acquired PUs is 23% of the total number of ulcers developed in hospitals.[2]

PUs occur in 28% of SCI patients. According to the National Spinal Cord Injury Statistical Center, the incidence of PUs during the initial hospital stay is 32%.[12] Another study reported a PU rate of 30% to 85% during the first month after injury.[13-19] In a retrospective study of SCI the PU rate was found to be 60% and 50% in quadriplegic and paraplegic patients, respectively; also, multiple PUs developed in most quadriplegic patients.[20-24]

Etiology

Although various factors are involved in determining the incidence of PUs, it is clear that the main cause of PUs is pressure over a bony prominence.

Historically, PUs have been blamed on poor nursing care and have been used as outcome indicators to quantify good versus poor nursing care.[11,25] In fact, PUs are acute injuries that develop rapidly when compression of tissues causes ischemia and necrosis during serious illness and trauma, including surgery.[26] The primary factor contributing to PU formation is constant pressure for extended periods. Pressure induces ischemia and causes reactive hyperemia. Because muscles and subcutaneous tissues are more susceptible than epidermis to pressure-induced injury, PUs are usually worse than they initially appear. The visible portion of a PU is not truly indicative of the extent of the problem.[27]

The mean skin capillary pressure in healthy persons is approximately 25 mm Hg.[28] External compression with a pressure of more than 30 mm Hg occludes the blood vessels, so that the surrounding tissue becomes anoxic and cell death occurs. Tissue pressure, however, depends on the patient's health. In addition, the amount of tissue damage is proportional to the magnitude and length of application of the pressure. PUs can develop within 24 hours of the insult but can take as long as 5 days to manifest themselves.[27] Kosiak[28] demonstrated that applying a constant pressure of 70 mm Hg to the skin caused irreversible changes in less than 2 hours. He also demonstrated an inverse relationship between time and pressure. Intense pressure for short periods was tolerated by patients as well as low pressure for long periods of time without sustaining tissue injury. Even a brief period of pressure relief can reduce the likelihood of PUs.

Risk Factors and Their Assessments

Most hospitals use a standardized risk assessment tool to predict the likelihood of an individual developing a PU. An individual prevention plan will be created and implemented based on the patient's risk assessment/score. Several tools for risk assessment of PU prevention are available. The most commonly used validated and reliable tool for predicting patients at risk for pressure ulcer development is the Braden Scale for Predicting Pressure Sore Risk. Full risk assessment includes determining a person's risk for pressure ulcer development and inspection of skin condition, particularly of pressure points.[29] Recommendations for culturally sensitive early assessment for stage I pressure ulcers in patients with darkly pigmented skin include the use of a halogen light to look for skin color changes, which may occur in blue hues, and to compare skin over bony prominences to surrounding skin, which may be boggy or stiff, warm or cooler.[30]

Numerous factors that influence PU formation have been documented. Both intrinsic and extrinsic factors contribute to the risk of the development of a PU.

Intrinsic Risk Factors

Age

Several changes that occur in normal skin with aging may predispose older persons to PU development. These factors include decreased epidermal turnover, flattening of the dermoepidermal junction, and decreased number of dermal blood vessels. Bridel[31] reported gradual reduction in collagen formation between ages 20 and 60. A marked drop in collagen synthesis with concurrent loss of its protective mechanism occurs after age 60. In general, the risk of PU development doubles after age 40 and triples after age 70.

Pattern of Spinal Cord Injury

Each year 25% of SCI patients will develop a PU. Regardless of the type of treatment of these PUs, they will recur in 5% to 91% of SCI patients.[27] The pattern of SCI (completeness of neurologic deficit, level of injury [quadriplegia vs. paraplegia], and muscle tone [spastic vs. flaccid]) can affect skin care and PU formation. Richardson and Meyer[18] examined variables related to PU formation in acutely injured SCI patients and found that quadriplegic patients with complete injuries were more likely to develop PUs than were those with lower level or incomplete injuries. However, Curry and Casady[14] reported that cervical injuries were not associated with an increased rate of PU formation. They reported PUs in 22.2% and 28.5% of patients with cervical and thoracolumbar injuries, respectively. Spasticity can contribute to PU development. Shearing forces in SCI are increased threefold, partly as a result of lower limb spasticity.

Immobility

Immobility has been found to be the most significant risk factor for PU development.[32] Immobility may be caused by mental status changes, physical deficit, or neurologic deficit, or may occur during surgery.

Malnutrition

Increased PU risk occurs in malnourished patients by the reduction of tissue tolerance.[33] Integrity of the skin and support structures is influenced by nutritional status. Low serum albumin levels have been shown to predict injury from pressure.[12] Collagen and elastin can diminish the ability of soft tissue to absorb pressure. Lack of vitamins and trace elements necessary for collagen formation and cell metabolism can predispose the patient to increased risk of pressure damage.[34]

Decreased fluid intake in the malnourished patient can lead to increased risk for dehydration. Dehydration can affect tissue perfusion, resulting in reduced pliability and dry, flaky, or scaling skin associated with fissuring and cracking of the stratum corneum. This ultimately places the patient at an increased risk for PU formation.[27]

The patient's nutritional status has an important effect on the maintenance of tissue vitality. Wound healing can be affected by several variables, such as a negative nitrogen balance, anorexia, obesity, and repeated infections. Negative nitrogen balance and anorexia after SCI frequently contribute to weight loss and tissue wasting. Thus, bony areas become more prominent, resulting in an increase in the applied force per unit area. Obesity can also contribute to the formation of PUs by decreasing mobility.

Body Weight

The emaciated patient has little padding over bony prominences and is vulnerable to pressure injury. The obese patient may be malnourished with poor tissue perfusion and may be difficult to move while avoiding shearing and frictional forces. Patients are at risk of pressure damage if they are less than 90%, or more than 120%, of their ideal body weight.[9]

Cardiovascular Changes

Some cardiovascular changes secondary to SCI can diminish tolerance to pressure and pressure-induced ischemia. The loss of sympathetic innervation and unopposed parasympathetic activity contribute to vascular stasis and tissue hypoxia in SCI patients. The loss of vasomotor tone produces vasodilation, bradycardia, and an increased cardiac index. This results in an increased stroke volume and a decreased venous return. The reduction in venous return is further accentuated by decreased muscle tone and the absence of the muscle pump. Gravity, acting mainly when the patient is in the sitting position, and a decreased negative inspiratory force, resulting from pulmonary insufficiency, may also diminish venous return. In the SCI patient, soft tissue blood flow below the level of injury is reduced to 33% of its normal value. A decrease in transcutaneous oxygen tension is observed in the SCI patient, even in the absence of pressure.[17] All of these factors contribute to the formation of PUs. In summary, poor tissue oxygenation, poor cell nutrition, and a decrease in venous return may accentuate the process of PU formation.

Extrinsic Risk Factors

Extrinsic risk factors are those elements that may be manipulated through interventions and help to prevent PUs.

Shearing

Shear forces are the second key factor in the development of PUs. *Shear forces* are defined as forces created by sliding adjacent structures, which cause a relative displacement of tissue and, in turn, occlusion of capillaries. Shear forces can be more significant than pressure itself in the dermis (where capillaries run perpendicular to the skin) and near the bone (where nutrient vessels pierce the fascia, also in a perpendicular manner) (Fig. 185-1). Shear forces, alone or in combination with pressure, significantly compromise circulation in tissues, whereas the skin may remain stationary. The elevation of the head of the bed by more than 30 degrees may increase shear forces.

Friction

Another important external force that acts directly on the epidermis is friction. Friction between skin and stationary surfaces, such as bedclothes, results in the loss of stratum corneum and, in turn, causes intraepidermal blisters and superficial erosions. Lack of this protective layer leads to further breakdown.

Frictional forces indirectly underlie shearing, and like shear forces, friction alters the critical pressure–time relationship affecting skin ischemia. Because friction contributes to PU formation, SCI patients should not be dragged across the bed; rather they should be lifted and moved, with a bed sheet used as a drag sheet.

Moisture

Contact of skin with moisture, resulting from urinary or fecal incontinence, leads to skin maceration and edema. This makes the epidermis more susceptible to abrasion. The likelihood of further tissue breakdown thus increases. The effect of moisture on PU formation is well known. One study demonstrated that incontinence caused a 5.5-fold increase in the incidence of PUs.[35] Fecal incontinence is a greater risk factor for PU development than urinary incontinence, because stool contains bacteria and enzymes that are caustic to the skin.[11,27]

Surgery

Preoperative factors that place patients at risk for PUs include the following comorbidities: diabetes, underlying respiratory disease, hypertension, and vascular disease. Low preoperative hemoglobin and hematocrit, as well as a preoperative serum albumin level lower than 3 g/dL, also have been shown to place patients at greater risk for PU.[12,36,37]

Surgical patients are at an increased risk because of forced immobility during surgery.[12] The amount of time on the operating room (OR) table is the most statistically significant risk factor associated with PU injury in perisurgical patients.[9] Studies have shown variable amounts of time before PU injury occurs. Hoshowsky and Schramm[38] found that PU injury can occur in as little as 2.5 hours on the OR table. Surgery lasting more than 4 hours can triple the risk of skin changes and quadruple the risk of PU formation. Hicks[39] found that PU injury was twice as likely to occur if time on the OR table was more than 4 hours.

Not only does the amount of time on the OR table contribute to PU formation, but anesthetic agents lower blood pressure and alter tissue perfusion, which also contributes to tissue damage.[40] Surgical patients' skin may be made more susceptible to PUs because of pooled prep solution, causing skin maceration, change in skin pH, and the removal of protective oils.[9,11] In addition, one study showed that 75% of patients placed on a hyperthermia blanket during surgery went on to develop PUs.[9,10,41]

Firm positioning devices in the OR are used to hold patients in place by exerting pressure on bony prominences, retractors increase pressure on internal tissues, and OR personnel increase

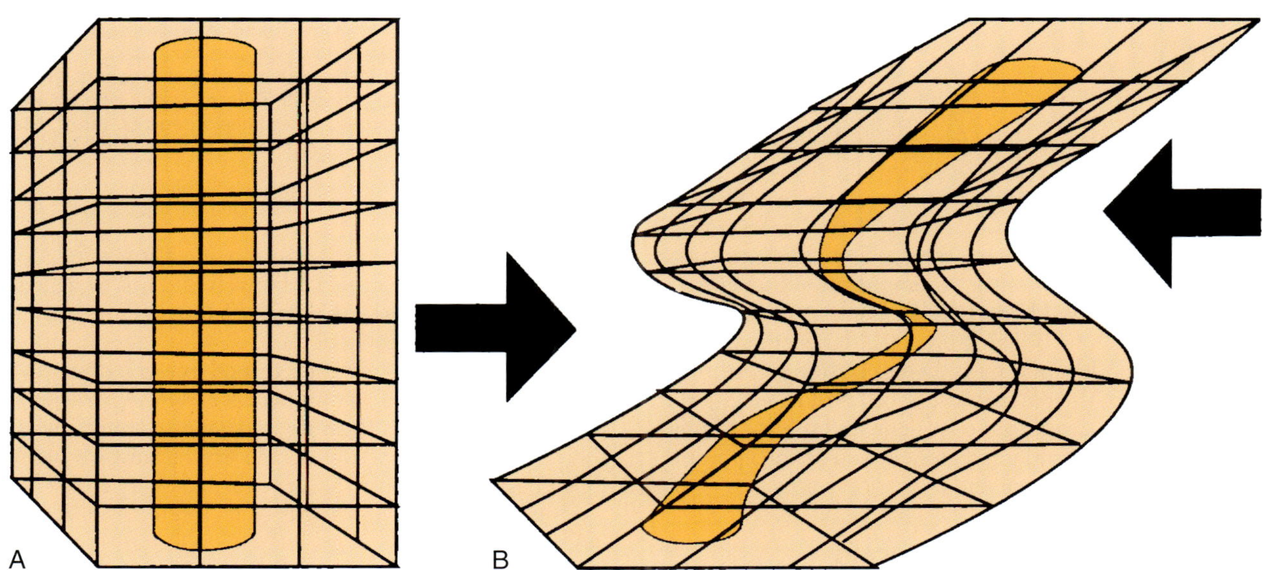

FIGURE 185-1. A, Appearance of the skin and relationship between a perpendicular capillary and skin. **B,** Application of a shear force can lead to obstruction of the capillary and result in pressure ulcer formation.

pressure on external tissues by leaning on the patient.[11] All of these events can cause pressure over bony prominences, eventually leading to PU injury.

Assessment and Staging of Pressure Sores

Routine skin inspection is customarily included in any skin care program because it provides important information regarding the formulation and evaluation of skin care plans. At least once daily the skin should be examined from head to toe, and high-risk areas should be assessed more frequently, with special attention paid to bony prominences. Assessment involves the entire integument, not just the ulcer, and is the basis for a treatment plan and its evaluation. PU assessment should include location, size (length, width, and depth), the extent of sinus tract undermining or tunneling, exudate, color of wound bed, epithelialization, and staging.[11] Photographs can document PU status better than hand-drawn diagrams.

Although several different staging and classification systems have been developed for PU classification, the Agency for Healthcare Research and Quality (AHRQ) (formerly the Agency for Healthcare Policy and Research) has adopted the National Pressure Ulcer Advisory Panel's PU classification system as part of the PU clinical practice guidelines. PUs are staged to classify the degree of observed tissue damage. The use of this classification tool permits universal assessment and consistent communication of the severity of tissue damage among health care personnel (Fig. 185-2).[19,36]

Skin inspection should be followed by laboratory investigations, such as culture and assessment for infection markers. In the case of a chronic nonhealing PU and underlying osteomyelitis, a triad of a white blood cell count higher than 15,000/μL, plain radiographic signs, and a high sedimentation rate (>100 mm/hr) provides a sensitivity and specificity of 90% for diagnostic screening of this complication.[4]

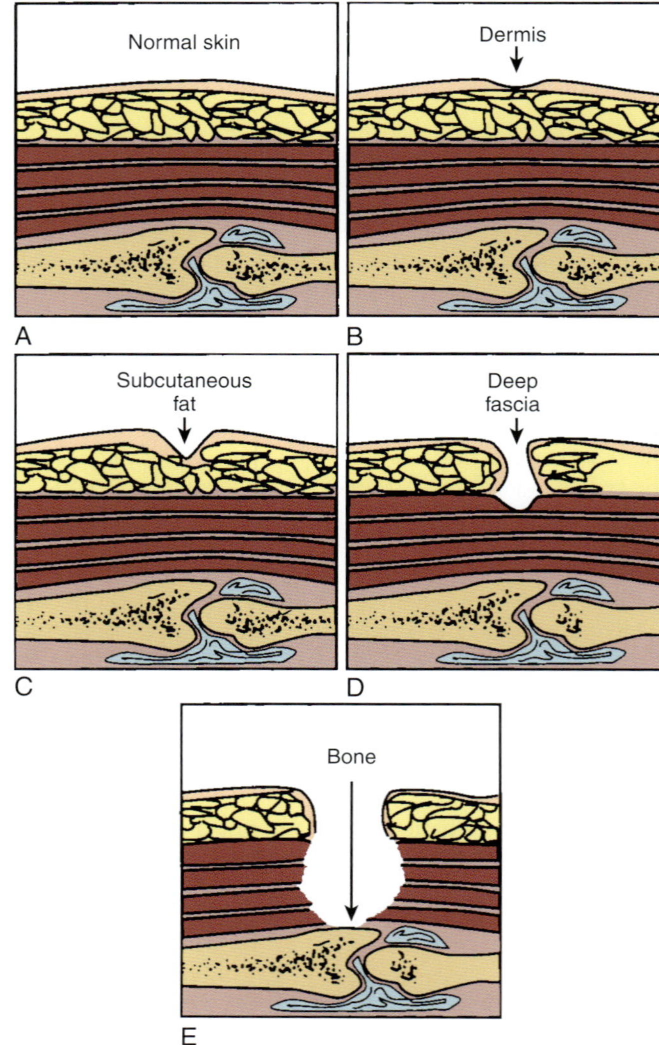

FIGURE 185-2. Normal gross anatomy of the skin and its changes in the different stages of the pressure ulcer. **A,** Normal anatomy. **B,** Stage I: An observable pressure-related alteration of intact skin compared with adjacent skin. Observable changes may include skin temperature, tissue consistency, and skin sensation. **C,** Stage II: Superficial, partial-thickness skin loss that presents clinically as a blister or abrasion. **D,** Stage III: Full-thickness skin loss extending down to the fascia that presents as a deep crater. **E,** Stage IV: Full-thickness skin loss with extensive destruction or damage to muscle, bone, or supporting structures.

Prevention

The foundation for the prevention of PUs is based on the elimination of risk factors. The first step in PU prevention is to be knowledgeable of risk factors, specifically which ones place the patient at high risk for PU development. The second step in prevention is to be aware of the interventions that reduce the risk of pressure injury. The third step is to evaluate the effectiveness of the intervention.[27] Proper measures can minimize the PU rate by as much as 59%.[4,23,42-44] Prevention is a 24-hour, ongoing process. Management of PU risk includes an understanding of body positioning, turning, and mobilization of the patient in the bed and wheelchair. It also includes paying attention to hygiene and the use of pressure reduction devices and strategies, as well as the appropriate monitoring of nutritional and hydration status.

Mobilization and Turning Program

The primary goal of this program is to relieve pressure, which is achieved by regular turning. The patient should be placed in the full lateral decubitus position when it is safe. A patient with a very unstable spine perhaps should not be aggressively turned until the spine is surgically fixated. This restriction is uncommon.

At-risk patients should be turned every 2 hours to minimize pressure on bony prominences.[15,45,46] A written schedule for systematically turning and repositioning the patient should be used. Norton et al. reported a lower incidence of PUs in at-risk patients who were turned every 2 to 3 hours.[47]

The goal of repositioning is to facilitate tissue reperfusion before the tissue becomes ischemic. Repositioning should involve a sustained relief of pressure. As skin tolerance improves, the amount of time spent in one position may be increased gradually.

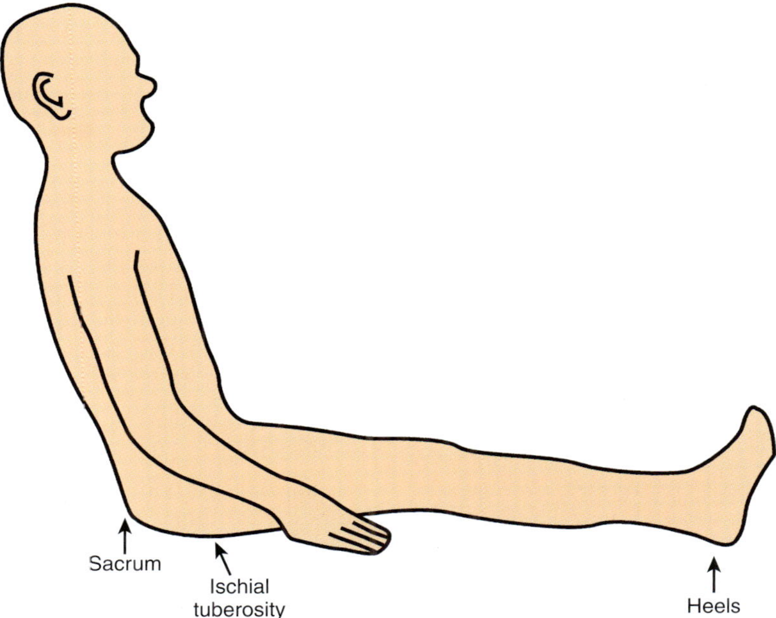

FIGURE 185-3. Potential sites for pressure in the sitting position.

After the acute phase of care, when the SCI patient is able to tolerate wheelchair activities, continuation of pressure relief techniques in the wheelchair is equally important. These activities serve to relieve pressure and maintain (and increase) the strength in the upper extremities. Wheelchair pushups, lateral weight shifts to each side, and forward over-the-knees positioning are some of the effective pressure relief techniques used.[48]

Improper transport of the patient increases the incidence of PUs. When transferring patients, care should be taken to not slide or drag the skin across the bed surface.[49] The patient may also help prevent friction injuries by taking an active role and using the trapeze during turning and repositioning (if the spine is stable).

Ischial PUs are a manifestation of prolonged sitting without focal pressure reduction. Appropriate care, patient education, and patient diligence should minimize incidence of this complication (Fig. 185-3). Sacral PUs also may be caused by sitting, particularly if an inappropriate or worn-out chair is used or if the patient sits with the pelvis excessively flexed.

Uninterrupted sitting in a chair or wheelchair is a common cause of PU. When in a wheelchair, SCI patients should reposition themselves at least once every hour and shift their weight every 15 minutes. If the patient needs assistance, simply standing the patient and reseating in the chair may minimize the risk of tissue injury. Small shifts in weight such as elevating the legs can help to reduce the risk of tissue injury.[27]

General Hygiene

Proper patient hygiene can help to prevent or at least minimize the likelihood of PUs. Bathing programs should include washing with mild soap and water to avoid excessive skin drying and cracking. The skin should be kept clean and free of moisture from urinary and fecal incontinence, perspiration, and wound drainage. However, it is important to keep the skin well lubricated with a simple standard hospital skin moisturizer. Studies have shown that petrolatum is more effective than lanolin on dry skin.[50]

The type of material next to the skin may either diminish or increase moisture retention. Cotton disperses moisture, whereas nylon and plastic materials cause moisture to be retained. Clothes should fit properly without causing excessive focal pressure or friction. Tight clothes make dressing difficult and may also cause localized pressure and vasomotor changes. Similarly, the patient's shoes should be one half or one full size larger than normal.

Nutrition

Proper nutrition is an important factor in maintaining the vitality of intact tissues. Nutritional needs are based on the patient's age, gender, body mass index, anorexia or obesity, current disease state, severity of illness, and presence and severity of wounds. A through nutritional assessment is an important component of the initial evaluation of a patient with a PU.[51]

A high-protein diet, with an increased caloric intake, is initially needed to replace weight loss and to prevent protein deficiency and anemia. If necessary consult a dietitian and correct nutritional deficiencies. Monitor and order vitamins A, C, and E supplementation as needed.[30] Normal albumin is 3.5 to 5.5 g/dL and prealbumin is 15 to 25 mg/dL.[51]

Adequate fluid intake is 30 to 35 mL/kg of body weight. Patients on air-fluidized beds for the prevention of PUs must have their fluid intake increased an additional 10 to 15 mL/kg of body weight to prevent dehydration.[52]

The nutritional state of the patient is also affected by drugs, alcohol, nicotine, and caffeine. Nicotine and caffeine are vasoconstrictive, leading to a decrease in tissue oxygenation that, in turn, affects tissue healing. Smokers have a higher rate of extensive PUs than do nonsmokers.[44,53-55]

Patient Support Surfaces

Patients with an unstable spine, who cannot tolerate frequent turning, may require a pressure support surface that can lower the surface pressure below capillary filling pressure (32 mm Hg). Thick foam mattresses, water mattresses, alternating-pressure air mattresses, and static multilayered air mattresses have been found useful in preventing PUs. Air-fluidized beds and low-air-loss beds, which have elaborate support surfaces, probably provide the most effective surface for functionally dependent patients with large, deep, or multiple PUs.

Beds

A variety of beds can be used to prevent PUs, with some being appropriate for patients with unstable spines. For patients with a stable spine, low-air-loss beds, oscillating low-air-loss beds, or air-fluidized beds can be used alternatively. The patient, the caregiver, and the family may develop a false sense of security with use of these beds. Specialized beds do not prevent PUs but can minimize their likelihood. However, skin care may be difficult when using these beds.

In general, studies comparing several specialized beds show no statistical significance in the prevention or healing of PUs from one bed to another. However, studies do show that PUs heal more quickly on specialized beds when compared to foam overlays or standard hospital mattresses.[56]

Rotating Beds

A patient with an unstable spine can be placed on a rotating bed that rocks side to side in a continuous motion or on an oscillating support surface or kinetic treatment table to prevent PUs. These beds are often used in trauma or intensive care units but are usually not practical for rehabilitation units. A rotating bed must be adjusted properly; otherwise it slides the patient back and forth as it rocks. This sliding, in turn, subjects the skin to shear forces, causing, rather than preventing, skin breakdown.

Air-fluidized Beds

An air-fluidized bed is an oval space with up to 2000 pounds of glass beads covered by a polyester sheet. The beads are fluidized by a flow of warm, pressurized air that floats the polyester cover on which the patient is placed. Feces and body fluids are able to flow through the polyester sheet; thus the skin is kept dry. Most studies have demonstrated a rapid rate of wound healing using these beds, compared with conventional treatment.[5,43,57,58] These beds have a bactericidal effect because of sequestration and desiccation of micro-organisms by the ceramic beads. Adverse effects include fluid loss, dehydration, dry skin, scaly skin, and epistaxis from the flow of the dry air. Turning and repositioning may be difficult.

Low-Air-Loss Beds

Low-air-loss beds consist of multiple inflatable fabric pillows that are attached to a modified hospital bed frame. An electric fan maintains the buoyancy of the pillows. The head and foot of the bed can be elevated. They are cooler and more portable than air-fluidized beds; however, urine and feces cannot pass through the fabric. Their use has been found to be associated with a threefold increase in tissue healing.[43]

Cushions

Several different forms of gel- or water-filled mattresses and cushions are used with beds or wheelchairs. These mattresses and cushions may aid or inhibit patient mobility, particularly during transfer. Smooth surface cushions provide less resistance to sliding and aid in board placement during transfer. However, they do not optimally eliminate pressure. Furthermore, the patient cannot perform meticulous skin care and inspection. Cushions and mattresses may increase local tissue temperature, which, in turn, causes an additional rise in tissue metabolism and greater oxygen demand.

Patient Positioning

Perhaps the most important anatomic and soft tissue bony prominences in the bedridden patient are the sacrum and the heels.[59] The importance of these pressure points is diminished when the patient assumes positions other than the supine position.

The sacrum is located superficially at its dorsal aspect, with very little soft tissue separating the bone from the integument. When the supine position is assumed, significant pressure is applied to this point. Although the sacrum is a common site for PU formation related to supine positioning, the scapula and occiput are also potential points of pressure (Fig. 185-4). Both regions have bony prominences with minimal overlying soft tissue. The prevention of sacral, scapular, and occipital PUs is predicated on limiting the time spent in the supine position.

Evidence suggests that when the side-lying position is used, pressure on the greater trochanter should be minimized; the patient should be placed at a 30-degree laterally

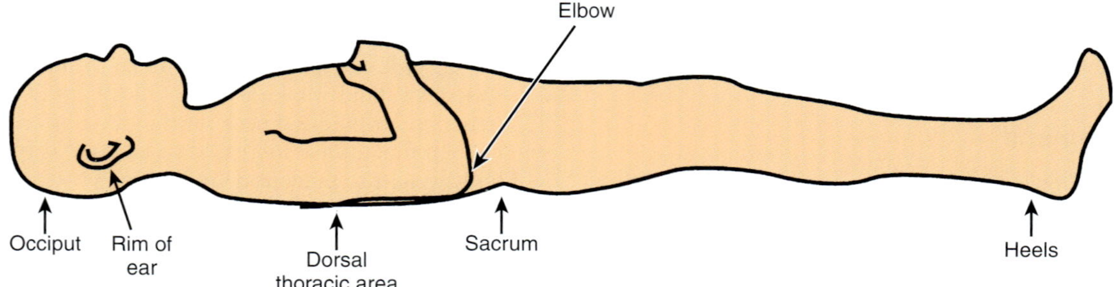

FIGURE 185-4. The supine position can lead to pressure application predominantly on sacrum, scapula, heels, and occiput.

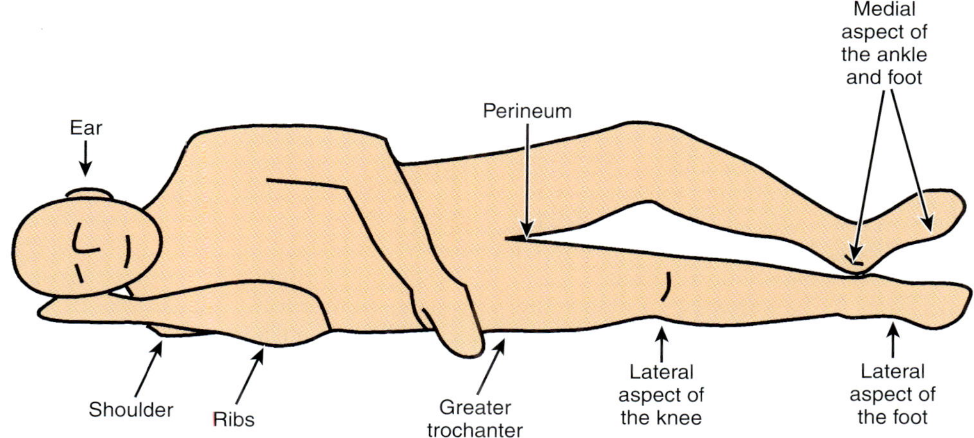

FIGURE 185-5. The lateral position can lead to pressure application on the greater trochanter, ribs, shoulder, and lateral aspect of the knee and foot. Note that the perineum and medial aspect of the foot and ankle may also be exposed to increased focal pressure.

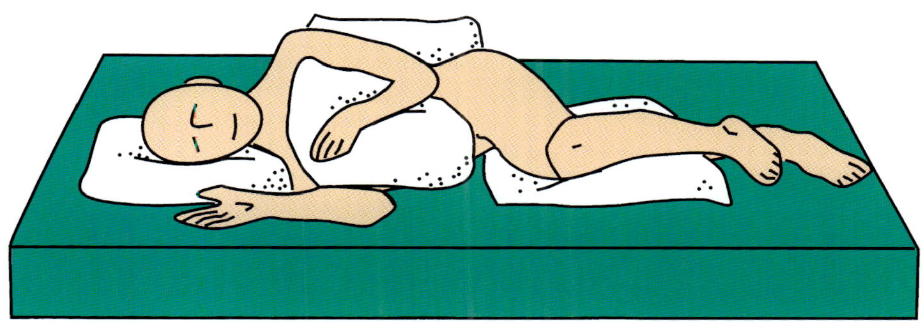

FIGURE 185-6. The lateral decubitus position, using pillows, may reduce the pressure applied to the body surface, particularly the greater trochanter.

inclined angle rather than a 90-degree angle to avoid direct pressure on the greater trochanter.[11] Placing a patient in a position that is intermediate between the full lateral decubitus and the supine position perhaps applies significant pressure to the downside scapula while lessening pressure on the sacrum. Dorsolateral buttock pressure is also increased. This, however, is usually tolerated well because of the significant soft tissue mass overlying this region. This position, for the reasons listed, is a reasonable alternative intermittent position. No single position should be maintained for any significant length of time, however. The full lateral decubitus position exposes the downside greater trochanteric region to significant focal pressure, if proper technique is not used. The anatomic arrangement of the greater trochanter and surrounding soft tissues is of great importance in this regard. One must keep in mind the dynamic relationship between the overlying soft tissues and the bony prominence (greater trochanter).[11]

In the hip-flexed position the greater trochanter is more superficial (exposed) relative to the immediately overlying soft tissue surrounding the trochanter itself. The latter is composed of the gluteus maximus and the lateral thigh muscles. When the hip is extended (leg straightened), the greater trochanter retracts relative to the surrounding soft tissue. This extended position results in a distribution of pressure over a significantly wider surface area, thereby minimizing focal trochanteric pressure (Fig. 185-5). It would therefore seem prudent to straighten the downside leg in the full lateral decubitus position. This essentially eliminates the negative effects of the lateral decubitus position (Fig. 185-6).[11]

Heels are at an increased risk of PU development because they have higher tissue interface pressures than other tissues covering bony prominences. Heels must be elevated off the bed surface by some protective mechanism. A common practice is to use pillows under the calves to prevent heels from bearing pressure loads, which prevents them from resting on the surface of the bed.[27]

Treatment of Pressure Sores

When a PU occurs it can be treated either medically or surgically, depending on the chronicity, position, and size. When developing a plan of care for treatment, the treatment goal must first be determined. The care will be healing, palliative, or maintenance; the treatment goal will help to determine the plan of care.[51]

Knowledge of comorbidities and chronic conditions and how they affect the healing process by reducing available oxygen, amino acids, vitamins, and minerals at the wound site determines the appropriate interventions for optimal

PU healing.[51] Many of the components used in prevention of PUs are also used in their treatment, but at a more intense level of management. The extrinsic and intrinsic contributing factors of PU formation must be identified. Eliminating the cause of pressure should improve the course of treatment.

The stage of a PU determines its treatment. A stage I PU most often heals spontaneously, simply following relief of pressure. Depending on the source of the trauma to the skin, pressure relief may be easily attained by adjusting an orthosis or, with multiple PUs, by avoiding a certain posture. A special bed may occasionally be necessary to reduce the pressure.

Treatment of an open wound (stages II, III, and IV), however, is more complex. Prevention or elimination of infection facilitates healing. Local treatment combined with systemic antibiotic and supportive therapy often heals a PU. Chronic PUs, however, are more resistant to therapy.

With respect to wound care, the goal is to achieve a clean wound with a low level of bacteria that is kept moist with a nonadherent dressing until complete wound healing has occurred.[11]

Systemic Therapy

In some circumstances, oral antibiotics and vitamin C may be indicated. Vitamin C has been found to help in chronic nonhealing PUs.[60]

With osteomyelitis, cellulitis, and sepsis, and also as prophylaxis for endocarditis, systemic antibiotic therapy may be indicated.[61] Sepsis secondary to PU infections is associated with 50% mortality in the hospital setting (Fig. 185-7). Gentamicin and clindamycin are antibiotics of choice in patients with good renal function. In older patients cefotetan disodium or ticarcillin-clavulanic acid and fleroxacin are reasonable alternatives.[4,62] First-generation cephalosporins do not penetrate PU wounds well and should not be used.

Topical Therapies

Topical therapies for PUs include a variety of cleaning and open-air wound care regimens; antibiotics; topical surface materials; biologic, mechanical, and chemical debridement; electrical stimulation; laser therapy; whirlpools; and hyperbaric oxygen strategies.

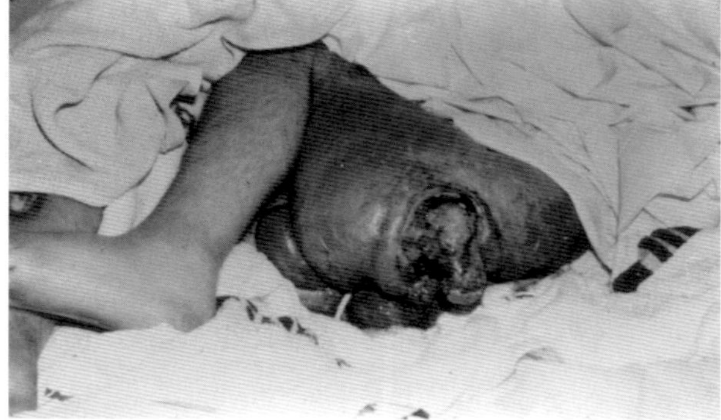

FIGURE 185-7. Macroscopic appearance of a stage IV pressure ulcer in a patient who developed osteomyelitis and deep soft tissue infection. He ultimately died of these complications.

Wound Dressings

The main goal when using moist PU wound dressings is to keep the wound moist and the surrounding skin intact and dry.[51] Traditional wound dressings are considered to be passive products because they protect the wound from further injury while healing occurs. However, many new wound dressings are interactive in that they act to alter the local wound environment. Regardless of the type of dressing selected, the main purpose is to absorb exudates, provide thermal insulation, allow gaseous exchange, protect the wound from infection, maintain a moist wound environment, and relieve pain. Interactive dressings have a varying number of properties and are currently undergoing research.[27,63]

Gauze

Currently most gauze dressings are inexpensive. They must be changed two or three times daily. Maintaining moistness may be difficult with gauze dressings. If they become dry, they may adhere to the wound. Their removal may then be painful and the risk of removing healthy granulation tissue will be increased. Gauze dressings must be fixed with a cover dressing or wrap.

Films

Semipermeable polyurethane films allow gases to pass through but are impermeable to water. They are believed to mimic the function of the skin and may enhance healing by sequestering wound fluids. Because the films are transparent, the wound can be directly visualized with the dressing in place. Such a dressing can remain in place as long as 7 days. This type of dressing, if used, is appropriate for stage I PUs.

Foams

Semipermeable polyurethane foams are transparent and waterproof. They absorb excessive wound exudate. A moist environment is maintained, and excessive autolysis or maceration is avoided. Because these foams do not adhere to the wound, they must be fixed with a cover dressing or tape; hence, direct visualization of the wound is obscured. Foams can be used for stage I and stage II PUs. They should not be used for deep PUs extending into the underlying muscle, sores covered by eschar, infected sores, or heavily exuding PUs.

Hydrocolloid

Hydrocolloids contain an adhesive material that physically interacts with wound fluid. These occlusive or semiocclusive dressings encourage wound cleaning and debridement through the process of autolysis. They promote the development of granulation tissue by stimulating angiogenesis. They may not adhere to highly exudative wounds. They can be used for stage II and stage III PUs.[43,64] Currently, hydrocolloids are cost effective and require changing every 3 to 7 days.

Hydrogel

Hydrogels are three-dimensional hydrophilic polymers that interact with aqueous solutions by swelling and maintaining water in their structure. They are nonadhesive and conform to the wound surface. Hydrogels are very absorbent and dehydrate easily. They can be used in stage IV PUs.

Alginate Dressings

Alginate dressings, derived from seaweed, are highly absorbent. They have been used for PUs with copious drainage. They should not be used for dry wounds and must be fixed with a cover dressing or tape.

Amino Acid Copolymer Membrane

Amino acid copolymer membranes are moderately permeable to water vapor and impermeable to bacteria. Early results have shown that they are helpful for tissue healing.[65]

Cleaning Agents

AHRQ guidelines recommend cleaning PUs at each dressing change. Techniques should be chosen that use the least amount of chemical and mechanical trauma necessary to clean the wound adequately. Traumatized wounds have a higher rate of infection and slower healing time.[51] For some wounds isotonic saline irrigation is a sufficient cleanser. Extremely dirty wounds may need a stronger cleanser and more mechanical force. As the wound heals and becomes cleaner, less mechanical force and a gentler cleanser should be used.[11,66]

It has been shown that whirlpool therapy results in faster wound healing than standard treatment. Pulsatile irrigation and lavage of PUs has been shown to be more effective than whirlpool therapy, especially in the presence of slough and necrotic tissue.[11,51]

Normal saline solution is a safe and effective cleanser for all wounds because it is physiologic and will not harm tissue. New guidelines recommend against the use povidone-iodine, acetic acid, hydrogen peroxide, and sodium hypochlorite because they are cytotoxic and may impair wound healing by damaging granulation tissue.[51] Some antimicrobial agents, such as mupirocin ointment and silver sulfadiazine, may decrease the bacterial count. In general, topically applied antibiotics do not penetrate deeply into the ulcer, and their use is not recommended. They can lead to a resistance to antibiotics, as well as cause hypersensitivity reactions, contact dermatitis, and drug toxicity from drug absorption.[67] A 2007 Cochrane Review of wound cleaning for pressure ulcers determined that there is no good evidence that cleaning PUs or cleaning with a particular solution helps healing. Very little research has studied the cleaning of PUs; therefore, conclusions cannot be drawn.[68]

Negative Pressure Wound Therapy

Negative pressure wound therapy creates a controlled negative pressure in an attempt to provide evacuation of wound fluid, stimulate granulation tissue, decrease bacterial colonization, and enhance the body's natural capacity to heal.[51]

Vacuum-assisted closure uses an open-celled foam that can be cut to the size of the PU and placed on top of or inside the PU. It is then secured with a transparent film. Negative pressure is applied to the wound by means of flexible tubing that is embedded in the foam and attached to a vacuum pump. Constant tension approximation uses a device to place tension traction on the wound margins.[66] Although this is a new PU wound treatment, the literature is equivocal. Studies do not show that it is inferior to other treatments, and it may increase patient comfort and decrease nurse staff hours for fewer dressing changes.[51] A patient must have an overall physiologic capacity of heal to be an appropriate candidate for negative pressure wound therapy.[51] Currently, negative pressure therapy is recommended for patients with stage III or IV nonhealing PUs in whom other conventional treatments have failed. Contraindications for negative pressure dressings include necrotic tissue with eschar, untreated osteomyelitis, or malignancy in the wound. Precautions to consider include active bleeding, anticoagulation use, and difficult wound hemostasis.[51]

Adjunctive Therapies

The role of several adjunctive therapies in PUs has been investigated. These therapies include electrotherapy, infrared therapy, ultraviolet therapy, low-energy laser irradiation therapy, ultrasound therapy, hyperbaric oxygen therapy, vacuum-assisted closure, constant tension approximation, normothermia, use of miscellaneous topical agents (e.g., sugar, vitamins, hormones, cytokine growth factors, skin equivalents), and systemic drugs other than antibiotics, such as vasodilators, hemorheologics, serotonin inhibitors, and fibrinolytic agents.

Electrical Stimulation

Low-voltage direct current and high-voltage pulsed galvanic stimulation has been used successfully in treating PUs. During treatment, the negative electrode is placed directly on the wound and the positive electrode is placed at some point distally. In a randomized, double-blind, multicenter study, electrical stimulation has been shown to increase the rate of healing of PUs. The Pressure Ulcer Guideline Panel recommended the use of electrotherapy in stage III and stage IV PUs that have proven to be unresponsive to conventional therapy. Electrical stimulation may also be useful for recalcitrant stage II PUs.[43,66,69]

Hyperbaric Oxygen Therapy

Hyperbaric oxygen therapy is defined here as the use of high-pressure, pure, humidified oxygen applied by a portable chamber to either the entire body or to an extremity. The chamber forces 100% oxygen into superficial tissue and assists with wound healing. This modality has been found helpful in SCI patients, because they have an underlying intact arterial supply.[44,70] However, the AHRQ does not recommend this therapy, because its effectiveness has not been established.[66]

Ultrasound

The use of ultrasound for healing of PUs has produced equivocal results, with some studies demonstrating efficacy but more series finding it ineffective.[27,71]

Laser

Laser therapy has been used effectively in animal models for the treatment of PUs. Studies have demonstrated healing of PUs using the helium-neon laser in one third of cases, compared with nonlaser-treated wounds.[44] Research on the use of lasers for human PUs is still in the early stages.

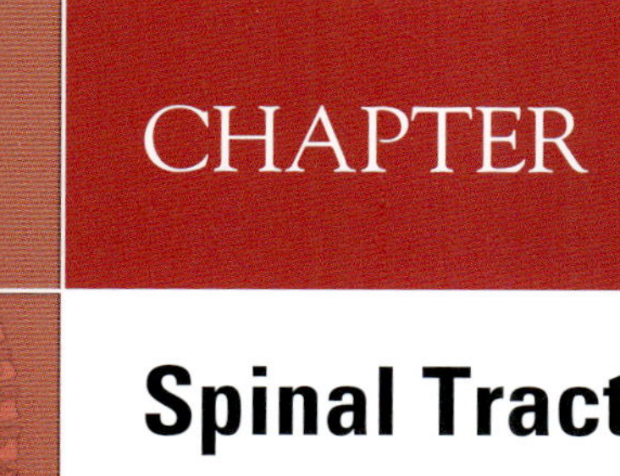

CHAPTER 186

Spinal Traction

Perry A. Ball | Michael A. Morone

Spinal traction produces a longitudinal force along the spine that can aid in the stabilization of the spine, and in the reduction of deformity. Spinal traction is most commonly used for cervical pathology because there is little evidence to support the use of traction for lumbar pathology.[1]

History

Hippocrates described the use of traction for the reduction of vertebral dislocation more than 2000 years ago,[2] but the modern era of traction started with the use of a halter device by Taylor in 1929 to reduce a cervical dislocation.[3] In 1933, Crutchfield introduced the use of tongs inserted into the skull, and this method forms the basis for the current practice of skeletal traction.[4] Crutchfield's tongs were placed near the vertex of the skull and thus were prone to dislodgement if greater than 30 pounds of weight was applied. In 1973 the Gardner-Wells tongs were introduced, which are designed so that pins are placed below the equator of the skull and thus have greater resistance to pull-out.[5] The halo device, which uses four pins for skull fixation, was described for use in skeletal traction by Nickel et al.[6]

Head Halter Traction

Head halter systems usually consist of two pads, one placed under the chin and one placed under the occiput. The pads should be fitted so that pressure is applied evenly to both pads and a metal spreader connects the pads to a rope to which weight is applied.

Head halter traction is often used as a component of nonsurgical treatment of painful manifestations of cervical spondylosis, including neck pain and radiculopathy. This is usually done on an outpatient basis and often as part of a home program. The patient typically uses up to 10 pounds of weight attached for several sessions per day. The effectiveness of this treatment is uncertain: a systematic review of published series found some evidence to suggest a benefit, but the methodological quality of the studies was felt to be poor.[7]

Head halter traction has been used for the reduction of atlantoaxial rotatory subluxation in pediatric patients. Subach et al. used halter traction to reduce atlantoaxial subluxation in a series of patients ranging in age from 3 to 11 years. They were able to achieve reduction in over 90% of patients; the mean amount of weight used was 4 pounds and the mean length of time necessary to achieve reduction was 4 days.[8]

Skeletal Traction

Skeletal traction involves the attachment of a "clamp" to the bony calvarium, which allows a greater amount of weight to be used to generate the distraction force. The most common use of this type of traction is to stabilize or reduce traumatic deformities such as cervical fractures and dislocations. This type of traction can also be used to correct deformities that have a degenerative, neoplastic, or infectious etiology. Skeletal cervical traction has the benefit of allowing the gradual and regulated realignment of the spinal column while the neurologic status of the patient is closely monitored.

Before traction is applied to the cervical spine, it is important that the patient's hemodynamic and pulmonary status be stabilized, including the placement of intravascular catheters and intubation if necessary. A baseline neurologic examination should be documented, and a lateral cervical spine radiograph should be obtained.

Gardner-Wells Tongs

The Gardner-Wells tongs consist of a C-shaped rectangular rod with an S-shaped link in the center to which the application rope is applied. At each end of the C that arches over the head are threaded bolts with sharp, pointed tips. The pins should be placed through the outer table of the calvarium but should not penetrate the inner table. On one pin is a spring device that protrudes 1 mm when the appropriate amount of tension is applied to penetrate the outer table of the calvarium (Fig. 186-1).

The pins of the tongs are placed below the equator of the calvarium and 2 to 3 cm above the ears. The location of the pins varies, depending on whether traction is desired with the cervical spine in the neutral, flexed, or extended position. A fixation point that is on a line from the tip of the mastoid process to the tip of the pinna results in traction in the neutral orientation. If a site is selected ventral to this point, traction will be applied in extension; conversely, if the site selected

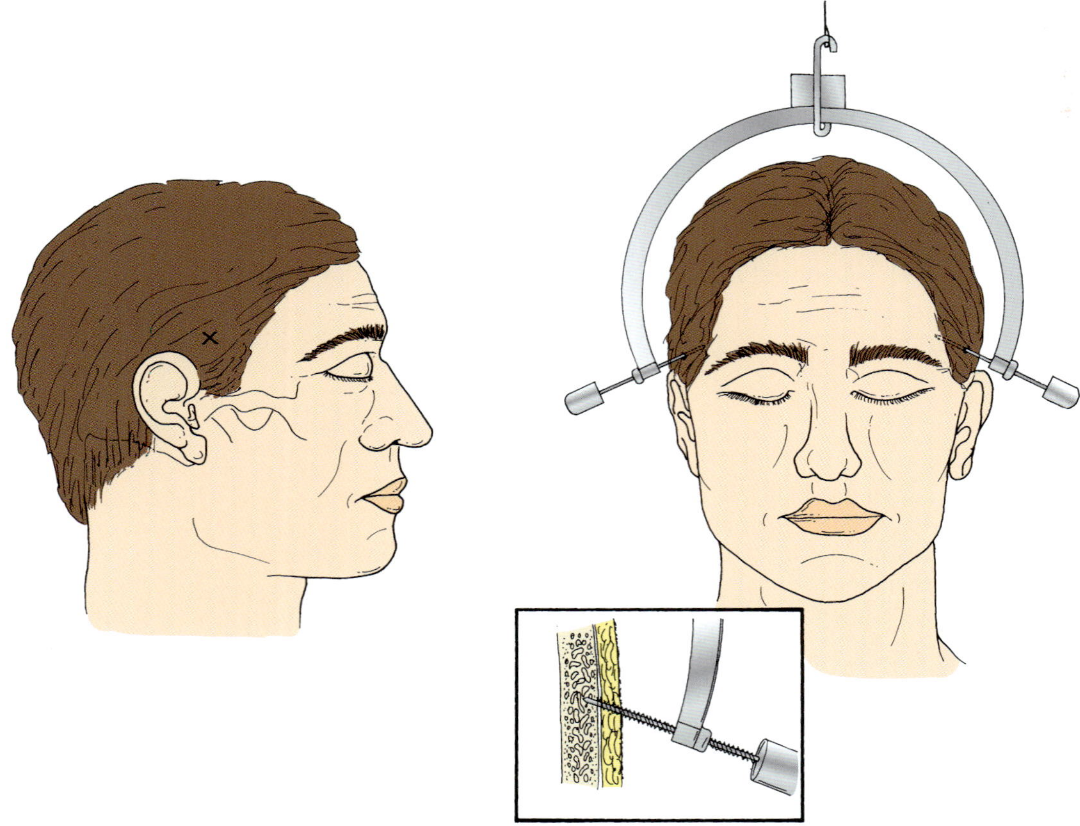

FIGURE 186-1. Gardner-Wells tongs may be applied without shaving the head. The regions over the ears are thoroughly prepared with a sterilizing solution, and a local anesthetic is instilled into the skin, subcutaneous tissue, and periosteum. Once the device is properly aligned, the screws are tightened until the pressure indicator (*inset*) appears.

is dorsal, the result will be traction with the spine in flexion. Alternatively, the amount of extension or flexion can be changed by altering the height of the pulley, which will alter the angle of the traction line: if the pulley is raised, flexion is usually achieved, and if the pulley is lowered, extension usually results.

Once the site of pin placement has been selected, the area is shaved and skin cleansed with povidone-iodine solution. It is important to anesthetize the skin, subcutaneous tissue, and periosteum by infiltrating with 1% lidocaine since inadequate anesthesia may cause the patient to move, resulting in movement of an unstable cervical spine. The pins are twisted into place at the selected entry point by hand simultaneously by tightening the curled knobs until the spring device pushes out 1 mm. This indicates that 25 pounds of force is applied; tightening beyond this point could lead to penetration of the inner table. At this point the tongs are tilted back and forth to set the pins. Nuts on the threaded pins allow the depth of position to be precisely fixed. Traction can now be applied. Within 12 to 24 hours a slight tightening should be attempted; after this the pins should not be disturbed.

Cranial Halo

Cranial halo traction provides four-point skeletal fixation via a circumferential metal ring. This ring can be attached to a rope and weights much like Gardner-Wells tongs or may be attached through metal uprights to a rigid vest that can be used for stabilization during mobilization. The halo vest has been used for stabilization of fractures or other unstable conditions of the cervical spine. If it is planned that a halo vest or jacket is to be subsequently used for ambulatory stabilization, the use of the halo ring for the initial traction may obviate the need to switch from tongs to a halo ring once the desired degree of reduction has been achieved and the patient is to be mobilized.

For application of the halo ring, the patient is positioned supine. The use of a mild sedative can be helpful to minimize patient anxiety during the procedure. Halo rings are available in several sizes, and the head circumference should be measured; ideally there should be about 1 to 1.5 cm of clearance between the skull and the halo ring. The halo pins have a broad base and a narrow tip to prevent penetration beyond the outer table of the skull. Four proposed pin sites are chosen. The ventral pin sites are located approximately 1 cm above the lateral third of the eyebrows to avoid injury to the supraorbital nerve (Figs. 186-2 and 186-3). The dorsal pins are diagonally opposite the ventral pins, approximately 1.5 cm above the ears. The selected areas are shaved and prepped with povidine-iodine, and 1% lidocaine is infiltrated into the skin, subcutaneous tissue, and periosteum. It is helpful to have an assistant available to hold the halo ring in position while the pins are inserted. Hexagonal lock nuts should be placed outside the ring before advancing the pin. The pins are threaded through the ring and advanced until the outer

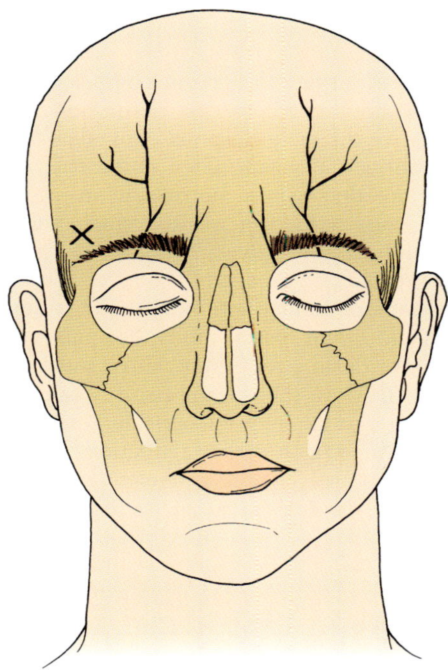

FIGURE 186-2. The safe area for anterior pin placement is over the lateral eyebrow (X). Care must be taken to avoid the nerves and frontal sinus medially, and the thin temporal bone and the temporalis muscle laterally.

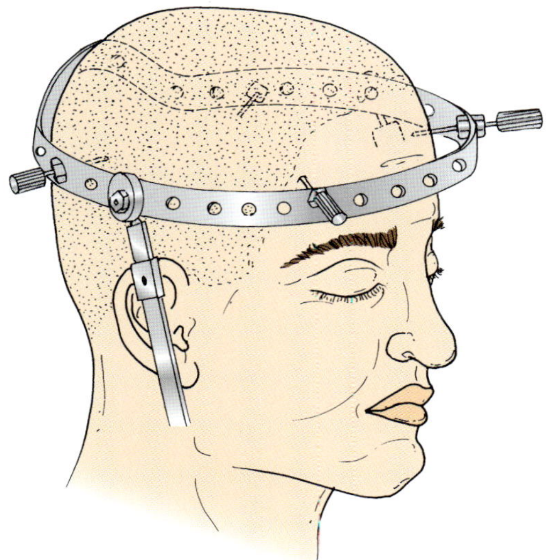

FIGURE 186-3. The halo traction ring provides four-point skeletal fixation using pins that pierce the outer table of the skull. These pins are attached by threads to a circumferential steel or titanium ring. The pins are locked to the ring by hexagonal nuts.

layer of the dermis is penetrated; the pins should be perpendicular to the skull. To prevent the halo from shifting during insertion, one ventral pin and the diagonally opposite dorsal pin are tightened simultaneously, followed by simultaneous tightening of the remaining ventral and dorsal pins. Once the pins have engaged the outer table of the skull, the diametrically opposite pins are tightened alternately with a torque wrench to 8 inch-pounds. The hexagonal nuts are then tightened against the halo ring, securing the position of the pins and preventing backing out of the pins. Twenty-four hours later, the hexagonal nuts should be loosened and the skull pins retorqued to 8 inch-pounds using the torque wrench, and then the hexagonal nuts are retightened. Daily pin care is important in preventing infection; this can be done with daily swabbing of the pin sites with dilute hydrogen peroxide.

The two most common problems with the halo pin sites are loosening and infection.[9] Pin loosening has been postulated to be due to bone restoration underneath the pin.[10] The pin can be retorqued to 8 inch-pounds as long as resistance is felt as the pin is being tightened[11]; if there is no resistance, the pin should be removed and a new pin placed in a new site. Infection at the pin site can present as erythema, swelling, or drainage at the pin site. Minor degrees of erythema can be treated with antibiotics and the pin left in place. If the erythema fails to respond or worsens, the pin should be removed and a new pin placed in a new site.

Reduction of Fracture-Dislocations

The most common use of cervical traction is for reduction of cervical facet dislocations. Unilateral facet dislocations, due to flexion and rotation, have the characteristic radiographic appearance of subluxation of less than 50% of the width of the vertebral body, whereas bilateral facet dislocations, due to flexion and distraction, appear as subluxation of greater than 50% of the width of the vertebral body.

The reduction of these injuries can be achieved through the application of skeletal traction (Fig. 186-4) or alternatively by open reduction through either a ventral or dorsal approach. There have been several large case series of patients with facet dislocations reduced with traction.[12-16] The advantage of traction is that reduction can be achieved relatively rapidly with the patient awake so that neurologic function can be monitored as the reduction is achieved. It should be noted, however, that some patients with facet dislocations are not able to participate in a careful neurologic examination due to intoxication or other injuries, and some facet dislocations simply cannot be reduced with closed techniques.

A baseline neurologic examination and lateral radiograph should be obtained before traction is applied. Because facet dislocations are principally flexion injuries, application of the tongs with the pins dorsal to the line between the mastoid and the pinna results in flexion of the neck as the force is applied, which may make reduction easier. Application of weight

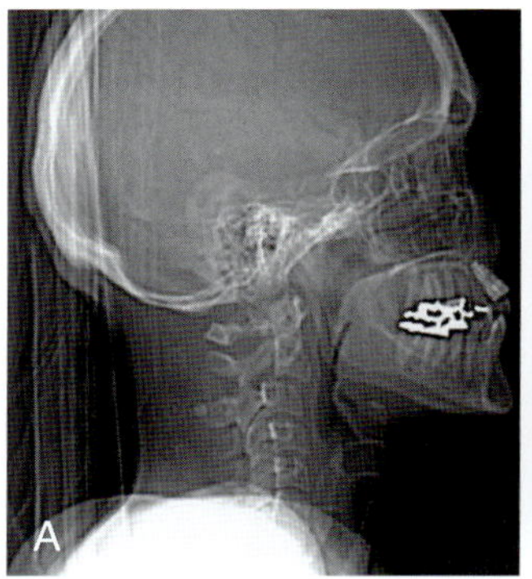

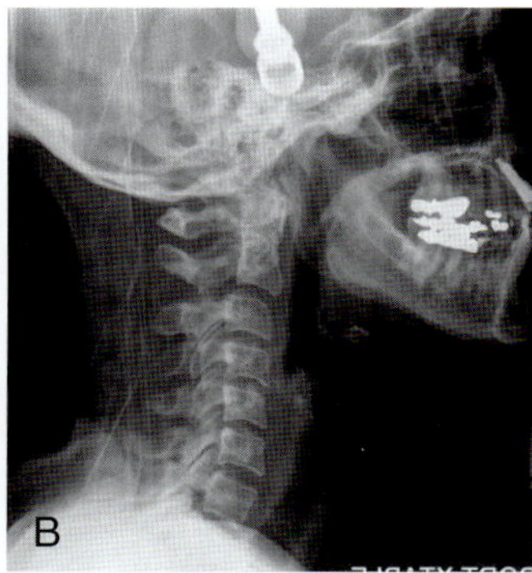

FIGURE 186-4. Unilateral facet dislocation before (**A**) and after (**B**) 15 pounds of traction.

should begin with 5 pounds, and a repeat examination and lateral radiograph should be obtained; the radiograph should be examined for alignment as well as evidence for distraction. Distraction can cause neurologic injury, especially if there is an unrecognized more rostral injury. An indication of distraction is the presence of widening of the disc space by more than 5 mm. If this is detected, the weight should be removed and further attempts at closed reduction should be abandoned. If the neurologic examination is stable and there is no distraction on the radiograph, weight is added in 10-pound increments, repeating the examination and radiograph after each increase in weight. The examination should evaluate motor and sensory function but also pain level. The total amount of weight that should be used is uncertain. Crutchfield's original recommendation was for no more than 5 pounds per vertebral level, but some authors have advocated higher weights, even up to 150 pounds of total traction.[15] Traction tongs tolerate a large amount of weight: cadaver studies suggest that stainless steel Gardner-Wells tongs can tolerate up to 200 pounds before pulling out and titanium tongs up to 75 pounds.[17] Careful, sequential examination of the patient and the radiograph is probably preferable to an arbitrary choice of weight. Once reduction has been achieved, all but 5 pounds of weight can be removed to maintain alignment.

Neurologic deterioration has been reported during or following the use of traction for reduction of these injuries. This has generated controversy. The principal issues are the possibility of disc herniation at the level of the dislocation and whether MRI should be obtained prior to attempts at closed reduction. There have been reports of patients who have undergone reduction of facet dislocations and then suffered neurologic deterioration. These patients were found to have a disc herniation.[18,19] This has led to the argument that open reduction from a ventral approach that addresses the disc pathology at the same time might be a preferable strategy to closed reduction.[20] Conversely, a significant percentage of patients with facet dislocations have disc herniations on prereduction[21] or postreduction[22] MRI scans. An evidence-based review of closed reduction of facet dislocations was undertaken by the American Association of Neurological Surgeons/Congress of Neurological Surgeons Joint Section on Spinal Disorders.[23] The authors found that the literature on this subject consists of class III evidence. Hence, no standards or guidelines could be recommended. The reported case series that they reviewed involved more than 1200 patients. They found an overall success rate of traction achieving reduction of 80% and a permanent neurologic complication rate of 1%, with a 2% rate of transient neurologic deterioration. They found that the causes of deterioration were not limited to disc herniation. Such causes also included overdistraction, spinal cord edema, and a more rostral noncontiguous injury. They noted that the number of deteriorations due to disc herniation in awake patients undergoing closed reduction was extremely small. On the basis of the literature reviewed, the authors proposed a set of treatment recommendations at the level of options. They recommend early closed reduction in awake patients who do not have an additional rostral injury. For patients who cannot be examined during traction or whose injuries cannot be reduced with traction, they recommend obtaining an MRI, and if a disc herniation is found, consideration can be given to ventral decompression before reduction. They conclude that a prereduction MRI in the awake patient is of uncertain benefit. As these recommendations are options and, hence, are made on the basis of level III evidence, there is latitude for judgment based on the particular clinical situation. If a prereduction MRI demonstrates a significant disc herniation, an argument could be made that even if the patient is no worse following closed reduction, the spinal cord will not have been fully decompressed by reduction of the dislocation and a ventral discectomy and fusion would ultimately be needed to achieve complete decompression. Thus, a ventral decompression and open reduction can be considered as an initial treatment that achieves both restoration of alignment and stabilization at the same time.

KEY REFERENCES

Fleming BC, Krag MH, Huston DR, et al: Pin loosening in the halo-vest orthosis. *Spine (Phila Pa 1976)* 25:1325–1331, 2000.

Graham N, Gross A, Goldsmith C: Mechanical traction for mechanical neck disorders: a systematic review. *J Rehab Med* 38:145–152, 2006.

Grant GA, Mirza SK, Chapman JR, et al: Risk of early closed reduction in cervical spine subluxation injuries. *J Neurosurg* 90(Suppl 1):13–18, 1999.

Hadley MN, Walters BC, Grabb PA, et al: Initial closed reduction of cervical spine fracture-dislocation injuries. *Neurosurgery* 50(Suppl 3):S44–S50, 2002.

Subach BR, McLaughlin MR, Albright AL, et al: Current management of pediatric atlantoaxial rotator subluxation. *Spine (Phila Pa 1976)* 23:2174–2179, 1998.

REFERENCES

The complete reference list is available online at expertconsult.com.

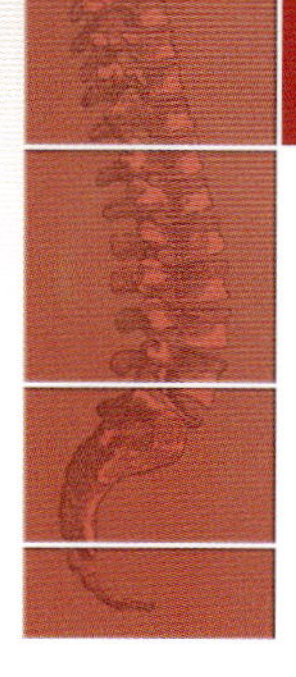

CHAPTER 187

Orthoses: Complication Prevention and Management

Eric J. Woodard | Robert J. Kowalski | Nicolas Marcotte | Edward C. Benzel

Spinal bracing encompasses a variety of time-honored techniques that provide external support to injured or diseased segments of the vertebral column. The practice of bracing is as old as medicine itself, having appeared throughout history in the medical and surgical writings of Hippocrates, Galen, Pare, Levacher, and Andry.[1-4] In more modern times, Frankel et al.[5] showed that bedrest and immobilization can be effective means of achieving bony fusion. The pressures of modern medicine, however, require early mobilization both to decrease hospital length of stay and to minimize medical complications.

Although many of the basic principles the ancients used have not changed significantly, great strides have been made in understanding both the art and the science of orthotics in the era of modern medicine. This mainly reflects interval advances in materials technology and development of the field of spinal biomechanics.

A spinal orthotic or brace is a unique type of spinal instrumentation, with principles of application and complications of use similar to those of its internally fixed counterparts. For the modern spine surgeon prescribing an appropriate orthosis, the avoidance of device-related complications requires thorough consideration of the intended purpose of the device. The biomechanics of the spinal pathology of interest, the biomechanics of the appliances available, and a variety of patient-specific factors are key elements in orthotic decision making. This chapter emphasizes the principles of spinal bracing and device classification, reviews the complications of spinal bracing, and concludes with some of the new advances and developments.

Principles of Spinal Bracing

By definition, all orthoses are externally applied devices that apply indirect forces to the spine for correcting or preventing deformity, stabilization, unloading, and/or supportive effects (e.g., massage, warmth, psychological comfort).[6] The most common element among these goals is motion restriction.

The Spine as a Column

The manner by which orthoses exert restrictive effects is perhaps best understood in terms of column mechanics. Several authors have described the spine as a complex variant of an ideal column with a fixed base and free upper end.[2,7] As a theoretical structure, this "ideal" column is considered a homogeneous rod of constant composition, length, and cross-sectional area. Its behavior when loaded by a balanced axial force has been described mathematically by Euler's relationship for long-segment column dynamics:

$$P > \frac{E(A)^2}{L^2}$$

where P is the magnitude of the applied axial load, E is related to the modulus of elasticity of the column material, A is the cross-sectional area of the column, and L is the length[8] (Fig. 187-1A). As the structure is progressively loaded, it initially shortens along its longitudinal axis. Once the axial load P exceeds a critical load specific for the column, failure occurs by elastic buckling.[7] Methods for stabilizing or increasing the column axial load-bearing capacity involve altering one or more of three variables: column elasticity (E), cross-sectional area (A), or length (L).

Prototypical spinal orthoses consist of two end-fixation elements and a connecting longitudinal member (Fig. 187-1B). An example is the chairback, thoracolumbosacral orthosis (TLSO), which purchases the rib cage with a thoracic band and the hips with a pelvic band. Uprights interconnect the thoracic and pelvic bands.[3] Sleeve-type orthoses, such as the clamshell TLSO (see later discussion), incorporate these elements into their circumferential design.[1] In terms of column mechanics, braces add to the relative cross-sectional area and the total modulus of elasticity of the spine, thus creating a heterogeneous composite structure that shares the axial load.

Internal segmental fixation applies direct immobilization to spinal segments, while most spinal orthoses apply their forces at some distance from the spine. There is an inverse relationship between the thickness of the soft tissue separating the spine from the inner surface of the orthosis and the resulting effectiveness of immobilization. Conformation of the brace to the body helps to maintain the cylindrical body shell, thereby increasing the stability of the spine.[9-12] Also, longer braces provide more stability than shorter ones do; therefore, the length-to-width ratio of the orthotic significantly affects efficacy (see Fig. 187-1A).

Orthoses may also apply balanced transverse forces in a three-point bending arrangement that resists bending forces and thus contributes to axial load bearing.[1,8,13] The Jewett brace utilizes the aforementioned biomechanical advantage

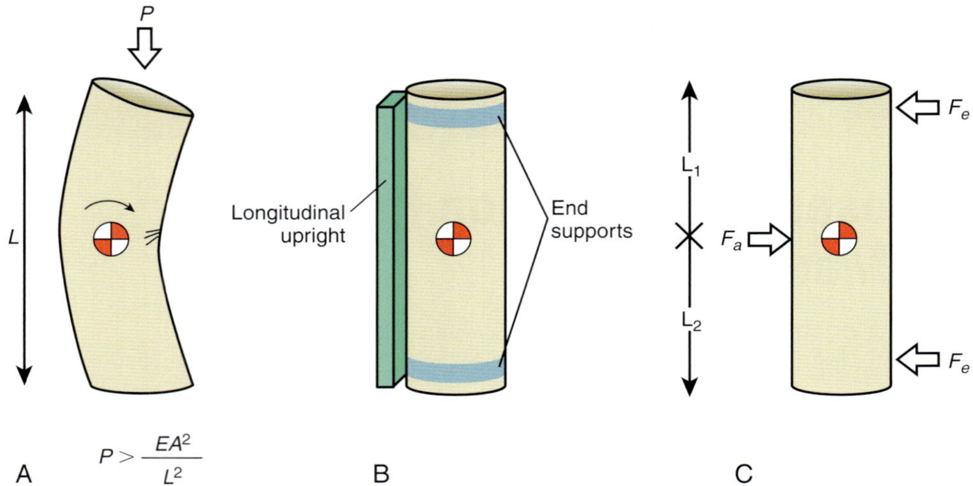

FIGURE 187-1. **A,** Elastic buckling of an ideal column of length *L* under an axial load *P*. This column has failed by buckling because *P* exceeds the critical load for this column as given by Euler's relationship, where *E* is the modulus of elasticity for the column material, *A* is the cross-sectional area of the column, and *L* is the length. **B,** Prototype spinal orthosis consisting of at least two end-stabilizing elements, such as circumferential bands, and an interconnecting longitudinal upright. **C,** Three-point bending strategies of orthoses utilize two horizontal end forces: F_e, which are balanced by a third oppositely directed force and F_a, at or near the axis of rotation for the column. This effectively segments the column into two shorter columns, increasing their respective axial load-bearing capacities.

of a three-point bending force application produced by applying dorsal forces at the sternum and pubis in combination with a ventral force at the affected thoracic or lumbar vertebra.[4,11] The long lever arms minimize the force required to produce a sufficient bending moment. Three-point bending also effectively divides the column functionally into two portions of smaller length, increasing the critical failure load of the whole column to that of each segment (Fig. 187-1C).

An underlying principle in long bone splinting is the immobilization of the fractured bone from one joint above to one joint below the site of injury. Extrapolating this concept to the axial skeleton, one may consider it to be composed of five segments, each of which may be considered a long bone (cranial, cervical, thoracic, lumbar, and sacropelvic) (see Figs. 187-1A and B). Therefore, one segment above and one segment below the unstable motion segment would be included in the brace.

Although the in vivo spine differs considerably from an ideal column in its specific composition and mechanical behavior, this model can serve as a useful paradigm for thinking about the mechanisms underlying the beneficial effects of orthoses.

Dynamic and Passive Control

All orthoses control spinal motion by a combination of dynamic and passive mechanisms. Dynamic control describes the significant role of intrinsic musculature in actively stabilizing the spine and is the major component in the action of most orthoses. It has been demonstrated experimentally that opposing muscular forces significantly stiffen the spinal column, increasing its load-bearing capacity.[9] If isolated from its muscular support, the osseous and ligamentous spinal column holds only 2 kg of axial load before failure by buckling.[2] In terms of a column model, muscular action directly affects the modulus of elasticity and relative cross-sectional area of the composite spinal column. Orthoses promote this muscular stabilization by tactile feedback that guides the patient to maintain proper positioning of the body. Pressure at the orthosis-skin contact site creates a reminder to maintain a safe position and limit unwanted gross body motion.[4,13-16] The patient therefore is able to prevent undesirable motion of the spine by using only intrinsic muscular support guided by the orthosis. A stiffer, more securely worn appliance is more effective at limiting motion than is a flexible brace because of the heightened sensation of resistance that the stiffer appliance produces. Sypert and others have noted that the effectiveness of an appliance is directly related to the level of its discomfort.[3,4] However, this discomfort may also contribute to higher levels of noncompliance.

Passive mechanisms for motion control are important in three-point bending mechanisms and are derived from intrinsic properties of the orthosis itself such as design, size, and material composition. The two common design elements of all orthoses are similar in principle to internal fixation constructs and include end-stabilizing elements (e.g., thoracic bands, pelvic bands) and longitudinal members or uprights that interconnect the end elements.[1] Passive mechanisms apply reactive forces to the body that oppose forces resulting from physiologic movements of the head or trunk; viscoelastic forces of ligaments, discs, and muscles; and gravitational force.[17] As summarized by White and Panjabi,[8] passive mechanical strategies form the basis for most orthotic techniques and include spinal distraction, fluid compression, balanced transverse force application, and skeletal fixation. Most appliances use a combination of techniques for spinal motion control.

Distraction

Distracting the ends of a column is a useful means of correcting or preventing deformity. Its effectiveness depends on the efficiency of transmitting the distracting force directly to the column. Spinal distraction is a major strategy of internal fixation devices used for spine correction and stabilization. This is best illustrated by the Harrington apparatus.[7] Distraction is also the technique that is used to reduce acutely unstable spine fractures with tong or halo traction. A braced column in distraction can be considered a composite of an externally applied distracting force plus the axial supporting properties of the original structure.

Distraction orthoses typically act on the head and thorax and cannot directly affect individual vertebral segments. Purchase of the head is either indirect, with pads located at the mandible and the occiput (conventional orthoses), or direct by means of skull pins (halo-skeletal fixation). Thoracic purchase is obtained at the sternum and rib cage through a combination of pads, straps, or vest attachment. The effectiveness of a distraction orthosis depends on the efficiency of force transmission to the vertebral segment of interest and the mechanical rigidity of the orthosis material itself.[13] Inefficiency in transmitting external force to the spine has been termed "the transmitter problem" by White and Panjabi[8] and represents the loss of energy that occurs when force is applied to "low stiffness, viscoelastic" structures such as overlying soft tissues, intervening normal joints, and ligaments. In the cervical area, distraction applied to the mandible is compromised by cushioning effects of soft tissue under the chin, the temporomandibular joint, cervical muscle tone, the C0-1 articulation, and each successive segmental articulation above the level at which the force is to have its effect (level of pathology). A more rigid brace with a tighter fit improves the efficiency of transmitting force by compressing intervening soft tissue.[17] These factors paradoxically increase the risk of pressure injury to overlying soft tissues.[18] Skeletal fixation improves the effectiveness of force transmission by directly purchasing the skull, minimizing the risk of pressure injury in the head and neck region.

Point-of-contact problems also exist with thoracolumbar braces that involve the shoulder girdle, pectoral muscles, rib cage, and upper abdomen. The shoulders have a significant amount of overlying skin, fat, and muscle and are by definition highly mobile structures involved in arm movement. Because of this mobility, orthoses that rely on shoulder straps or pads to apply a counterforce cannot consistently distract the spine.[13] Changes in body position from sitting to supine also produce shoulder movement contributing to the difficulty of spinal distraction. Koch and Nickel[19] studied this effect in six patients wearing the halo apparatus by measuring the forces of distraction and compression exerted through the device with an attached strain gauge. Distraction force varied by more than 20 pounds in a halo vest and 30 pounds in a halo cast when patients changed from supine to sitting positions. Similar variations in distraction with the halo device were noted during shoulder shrugging, coughing, sneezing, and deep breathing. Shoulder purchase is thus a highly variable means of anchoring the caudal end of a distraction orthosis.

Appliances with pads overlying the pectoral areas are compromised by the energy-absorbing effects of fat, muscle, and breast tissue. Movement of the chest occurs with arm motion in a manner similar to that of the shoulders. Although the rib cage is generally a stable structure, deep breathing, coughing, and sneezing produce significant motion that is directly transmitted by all devices purchasing the thorax. Orthoses extending below the thorax to the upper and lower abdomen are at an even greater disadvantage because of the highly elastic nature of this fluid- and air-filled region.[8]

Therefore, all orthoses are limited in their ability to distract the spine because of inherent inefficiencies in force transmission at both the rostral and caudal ends of the devices and because of limitations in exerting pressure through soft tissues. Because distraction is poorly maintained by an orthosis, even when combined with halo fixation, bracing alone is generally not recommended if distraction is required to maintain reduction or to prevent dangerous instability.

Fluid Compression

Fluid compression refers to the ability of a tight circumferential binder, such as a corset, to compress partially fluid-filled soft tissues surrounding the spine, thus creating a fluid cylinder.[6,8] Because of its mechanical incompressibility, a fluid-filled cylinder has axial load-bearing capacity. For a column model, this technique increases the aggregate cross-sectional area by converting soft tissues into load-bearing structures. Several studies have directly measured the effect of abdominal and thoracic cavity compression, noting little effect of compression on intra-abdominal pressure.[6,9,12] In Nachemson and Morris's[20] classic report, however, a 25% reduction in intradiscal pressure was observed in lumbar segments that were braced with an inflatable abdominal corset. The true unloading effect of fluid compression is thought to be a minor factor for orthotic thoracolumbar stabilization and is beneficial only for restricting sagittal plane motion.[6] Fluid compression is a strategy that is not applicable for the cervical spine, in which airway, vascular, and muscular tissues make up a relatively large proportion of the cross-sectional area of the neck and do not tolerate significant compression.[4]

Transverse Loading

Balanced transverse loading describes a common and effective strategy for restricting spinal rotation and translation. Orthoses typically use a three-point bending force application arrangement with two horizontal reactive forces applied at the ends of the column in one direction and a third balancing force in the opposite direction at the fulcrum of the deformity[8,13] (see Fig. 187-1C). Because the system is in equilibrium, the sum of all horizontal forces is zero. This prevents translation. Similarly, bending moments generated by the applied forces acting at the axis of rotation for the injured segment also equal zero if rotational motion is adequately controlled.[13] Keys to an effective transverse loading strategy include (1) identifying the axis of rotation at the level of injury or point of instability by using an appliance that is centered at or near this axis of rotation and (2) using an adequately long appliance that maximizes the length of the applied moment arm to control the spinal segment of interest.[13]

Classification

Spinal orthoses are generally considered either conventional orthotics or skeletal fixators. Conventional devices are contact-type orthoses that control spinal motion through direct contact with the skin and soft tissues of the head, neck, thorax, abdomen, or pelvis. A contact orthosis may have only limited skin contact through discrete pads and straps or extensive surface area coverage (e.g., total contact orthosis).

TABLE 187-1
Classification of Orthoses

Appliance Category	Examples
Cervical orthoses	
Cervical collars	Foam collar
Occipital-mandibular-cervical	Thomas collar, Queen Anne collar
Occipital-mandibular-high thoracic	Philadelphia collar, Miami J collar, Guilford two-poster brace, four-poster brace
Cervicothoracic orthoses	Yale brace, Minerva brace, SOMI (sternal-occipital-mandibular immobilizer) brace
Thoracolumbosacral orthoses	Clamshell thermoplastic body jacket, Jewett extension brace, Boston overlap brace
Lumbosacral orthoses	Lumbosacral corset, chairback orthosis, Knight brace
Sacroiliac orthoses	Sacroiliac corset with perineal straps
Halo devices	Vest halo, four-pad halo, thermoplastic Minerva body jacket

Examples of total contact devices are the Yale brace[21] and the molded clamshell TLSO (see later discussion). Advantages of newer contact orthoses that use thermoplastic materials include ease of application, light weight, warmth, ventilation, ability to be removed for optimal hygiene, and patient acceptance.[22,23] All conventional devices provide some control of flexion and extension but are more limited in reducing lateral bending and rotation.[24] Additional drawbacks include poor patient compliance, excessive warmth causing sweating, variability of fit, and complications of skin or soft tissue contact. All devices have limitations that must be balanced with their advantages. Each segment of the spine must be considered individually because of the variability of anatomy, mobility, and applicability of an orthosis.

Harris[25] reported the results of a consensus task force of orthotists, spine surgeons, and other health officials who set forth a common nomenclature for conventional spinal orthoses with the intent of standardizing communication among spine professionals and avoiding the plethora of eponyms describing individual appliances (Table 187-1). In this scheme, devices are classified as cervical orthoses (CO), cervicothoracic orthoses (CTO), TLSO, lumbosacral orthoses (LSO), or sacroiliac orthoses (SIO). This classification, which was intended to reflect the region of the spine that is immobilized by the device, has become the standard nomenclature of spinal orthotics since 1973. Krag[16] has recently expanded the cervical classification into four subcategories based on the specific anatomy of the region: cervical (CO), occipital-mandibular-cervical (OMC), occipital-mandibular-high thoracic (OMHT), and occipital-mandibular-low thoracic (OMLT).

Cervical Orthoses

COs are basically soft foam or felt collars with minimal purchase of the mandible or occiput[16] (Fig. 187-2A). These collars are light, inexpensive, easy to use, and relatively comfortable to wear. Regrettably, they offer negligible resistance to cervical motion in any plane of motion, functioning only to remind patients to limit voluntary extremes of neck movement.[26-28] Because they are only supportive, cervical collars are inappropriate for patients with bony instability. They can provide tactile generated support of cervical musculature and psychological comfort in cases of myofascial strain or sprain or in straightforward postoperative patients without instability.[23]

Occipital-Mandibular-Cervical Orthoses

OMC orthoses are hard plastic collars that are more rigid than foam collars and offer slightly better purchase of the mandible or occiput[16] (Fig. 187-2B). Most usage is as a prophylactic measure, in conjunction with a backboard, in acute trauma situations. They have no thoracic extension; therefore, while offering an improved cranial point of fixation, they lack a true caudal one. The addition of an adjustable chin or occipital piece increases resistance to flexion or extension to a mild degree.[26] Lateral bending and rotation are poorly controlled with these braces.[24] Like the soft collars, OMC orthoses do not provide significant immobilization to the cervical spine and are not recommended for patients with instability.

Occipital-Mandibular-High Thoracic Orthoses

When the brace is extended caudally to the shoulders and a more rigid material is used (e.g., the Philadelphia collar), movement is restricted. As with previous devices, flexion and extension are the motions that are most effectively limited, and there is a general trend of decreased motion at all levels with further extension of the caudal fixation point. However, this limitation of motion can produce a parallelogram effect. The ends remain fixed along the spinal axis, but motion can occur by the rostral segment translating ventrally and the caudal segment translating dorsally, or vice versa.

Examples of OMHT orthoses are the widely used Philadelphia collar, the four-poster brace, the two-poster brace (e.g., Guilford, Duke), and several newly available hard plastic collars[16] (Figs. 187-2C–F). All OMHT appliances control head movement with occipital and mandibular supports and have better upper thoracic purchase than collars because of longer length. Like the collars, they are relatively easy to apply, are lightweight, and are relatively inexpensive.

The popular Philadelphia collar is a Plastazote foam device reinforced with hard plastic. It is available in different sizes and consists of front and back halves connected by Velcro straps.[3] Although generally well tolerated, it can be quite hot to wear, causing significant sweating and secondary skin maceration. The Plastazote material is less rigid than other OMHT appliances such as the poster orthoses.[29] Despite its limitations, Johnson et al.[24] found this device to be as effective in controlling upper (C0-3) flexion-extension as the rigid OMHT orthoses. It was less effective in restricting flexion-extension in the midcervical and lower cervical segments (Fig. 187-3) and poor in controlled rotation and lateral bending at all levels. The device is frequently used for patients with mild cervical injuries and in postoperative patients with minor instability. Polin et al.[30] evaluated the use of the Philadelphia collar and the halo device in odontoid fractures. Their findings indicated no significant difference in the rate of fracture healing between

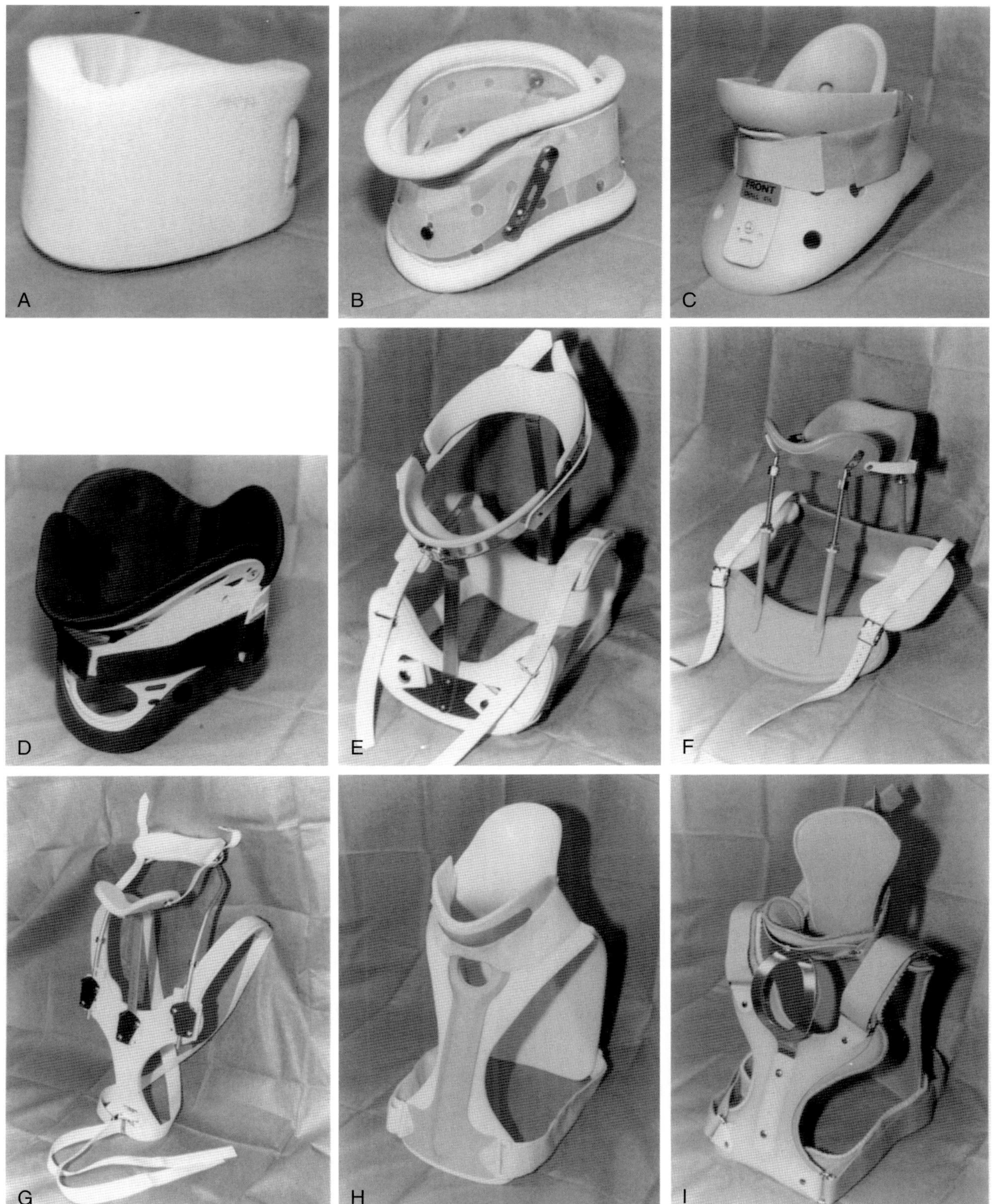

FIGURE 187-2. Cervical and cervicothoracic orthoses. **A,** Foam collar. **B,** Thomas collar. **C,** Philadelphia collar. **D,** Miami J collar. **E,** Two-poster Guilford brace. **F,** Four-poster brace. **G,** Sternal-occipital-mandibular immobilizer (SOMI). **H,** Yale orthosis. **I,** Minerva brace.

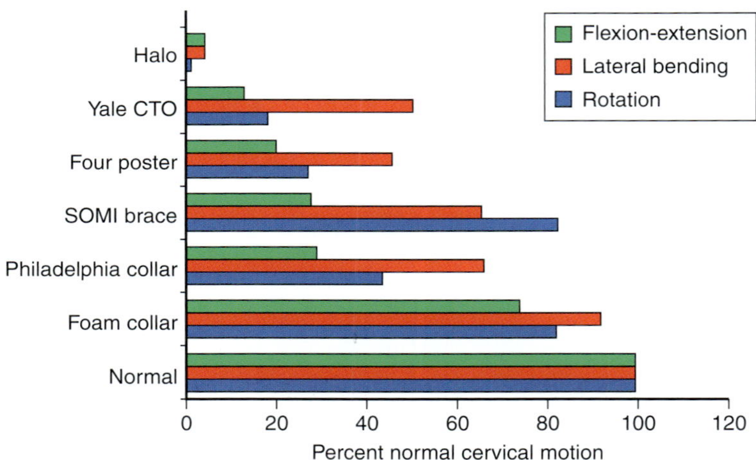

FIGURE 187-3. Overall motion allowed in cervical orthoses. (From Johnson RM, Hart DL, Simmons EF, et al: Cervical orthoses: a study comparing their effectiveness in restricting cervical motion in normal subjects. *J Bone Joint Surg [Am]* 59:332–339, 1977.)

the two orthoses for both type II and type III fractures and suggested that the less invasive collar may be adequate in this setting. Modifications of the Philadelphia collar have been developed that maintain cervical immobilization yet improve the comfort and convenience of a plastic removable collar. In 2009, Koller et al.[31] did an in vivo analysis of atlantoaxial motion in 20 healthy volunteers, comparing the halo thoracic vest and the Philadelphia collar. They found that, as expected, the absolute range of motion of the subaxial spine was more restricted by the halo vest than that of the Philadelphia collar. However, they found that the atlantoaxial complex had a tendency to be more restricted in sagittal motion between extreme flexion and extension in the Philadelphia collar (mean, 1.3 degrees) than in the halo vest (mean, 3.3 degrees). The author subsequently suggested that a Philadelphia collar might be sufficient in the conservative treatment of stable odontoid fractures.

The Miami J collar is an example that is more rigid than the Philadelphia collar at all cervical levels and has the added benefit of removable chin and occipital pads for improved comfort and hygiene.

Schneider et al.[32] did a biomechanical evaluation of common cervical orthoses. They looked at reduction in head and intervertebral motion provided by seven contemporary cervical orthoses in 45 individuals. They evaluated the overall range of motion of the head in three planes as well as intervertebral motion in the sagittal plane. The tested subjects also reported comfort for each brace being tested.

The seven cervical orthoses were the Philadelphia collar (Philadelphia Cervical Collar Co., Thorofare, NJ), Aspen cervical collar (Aspen Medical Products, Irvine, CA), PMT cervical collar (PMT Corp., Chanhassen, MN), Miami J cervical collar (Jerome Medical, Moorestown, NJ), Minerva cervicothoracic orthosis (Seattle Systems, Poulsbo, WA), Lerman noninvasive halo (Seattle Systems), and Sternal-Occipital-Mandibular-Immobilizer (SOMI) (U.S. Manufacturing Corp., Pasadena, CA). The first four were considered to be cervical braces; the last three were cervicothoracic orthoses. All collars were tested in their original configuration without any modifications.

With respect to patient-reported comfort, there was a significant association between the type of brace and patient-reported brace comfort score. The most comfortable orthoses were the Miami J and the Aspen. In general, the cervical collars were more comfortable than the cervicothoracic orthoses[32] (Fig. 187-4A).

With respect to the motion restriction of the head, all cervical braces significantly reduced overall sagittal plane flexion-extension motion of the head as well as axial rotation and coronal plane side-to-side bending. As was expected, however, some braces reduced motion significantly more than others did[32] (Fig. 187-4B).

The intervertebral motion was measured from the fluoroscopic images of maximum flexion and extension; all braces significantly reduced intervertebral rotation at all levels. Some of the braces reduced rotation more than others, and the differences between braces were more pronounced at the midcervical than the upper or lower cervical levels[32] (Fig. 187-4C).

Occipital-Mandibular-Low Thoracic Orthoses

Extending the orthotic further caudally to include the thorax adds a three-point bending moment, which provides a significant biomechanical advantage. Such devices (e.g., SOMI, four-poster, and cervicothoracic brace) substantially restrict motion in the midcervical to lower cervical spine.

The OMLT orthoses are represented by the sternal-occipital-mandibular immobilizer (SOMI), the extended Philadelphia collar (Yale brace), and the Minerva brace (Figs. 187-2G–I). These devices are essentially longer versions of the OMHT appliances with the addition of circumferential chest straps. In general, they are the most rigid of the conventional orthoses because of their increased length and better thoracic purchase[24,29] (see Figs. 187-3 and 187-4). Advantages of the OMHT orthoses include best immobilization of flexion-extension and rotation of the conventional braces, noninvasiveness, and ease of application. However, they are more cumbersome and uncomfortable to wear than the smaller appliances. With the exception of the Yale brace, they are moderately expensive and still have limited control of lateral bending.[21,24]

Thoracolumbosacral Orthoses

Representative TLSOs include the clamshell thermoplastic body jacket and the thoracolumbar extension orthosis or Jewett brace (Figs. 187-5A–C). There are a number of modifications of these two basic designs. By definition, these

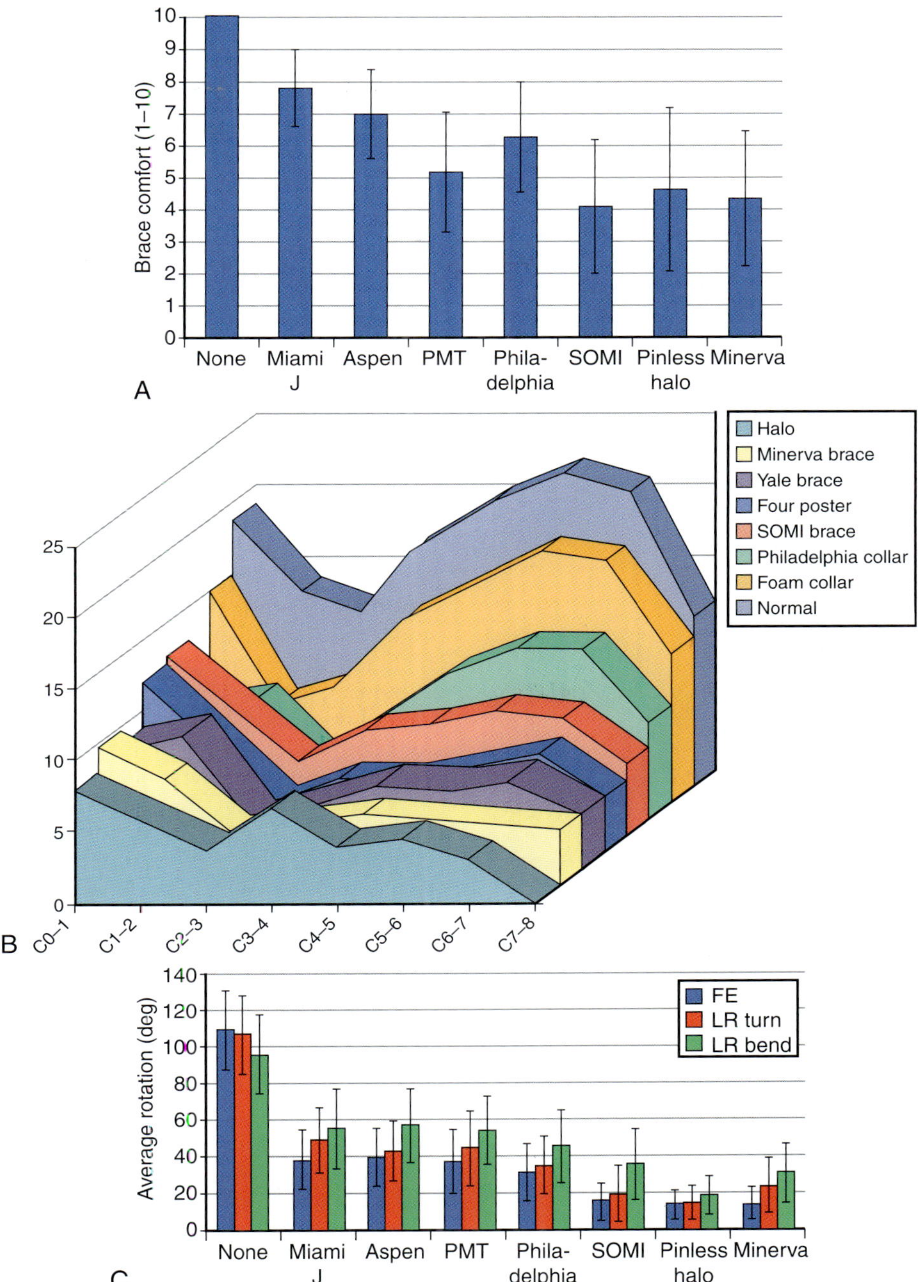

FIGURE 187-4. **A,** Mean brace comfort score for the different braces. The error bars show one standard deviation. **B,** Sagittal plane intervertebral rotation by level and brace. **C,** The mean sagittal plane rotation of the head from maximum flexion to maximum extension, the mean axial head rotation from maximum left to maximum right turn, and mean coronal plane tilt of the head from maximum left to maximum right tilt of the head toward the shoulders while wearing no brace and while wearing each of the seven braces. (Adapted from Johnson RM, Owen JR, Hart DL, Callahan RA: Cervical orthoses: a guide to their selection and use. *Clin Orthop Rel Res* 154:34–45,1988.)

appliances apply three-point bending forces at the upper thorax and pelvis and at the midportion of the brace across the thoracolumbar junction.[1] This class of orthotic is best suited for restricting thoracolumbar and lumbar gross-body motion[33] and poorly controls low lumbar and sacral segments.[14] Molded appliances are particularly useful for thoracolumbar junction trauma in which the total contact feature helps to control lateral bending and rotation. Velcro straps and thermoplastic materials have greatly improved the ease of wear and comfort of TLSOs in recent years, improving both compliance and effectiveness.

Jewett braces primarily control flexion-extension and are therefore often used for minor flexion compression injuries such as stable compression fractures.[3] More severe thoracolumbar injuries were recently studied by Patwardhan et al.[34] with a finite element computer model. The Jewett brace was effective at preventing deformity under physiologic flexion loading with injuries that resulted in less than 50% normal

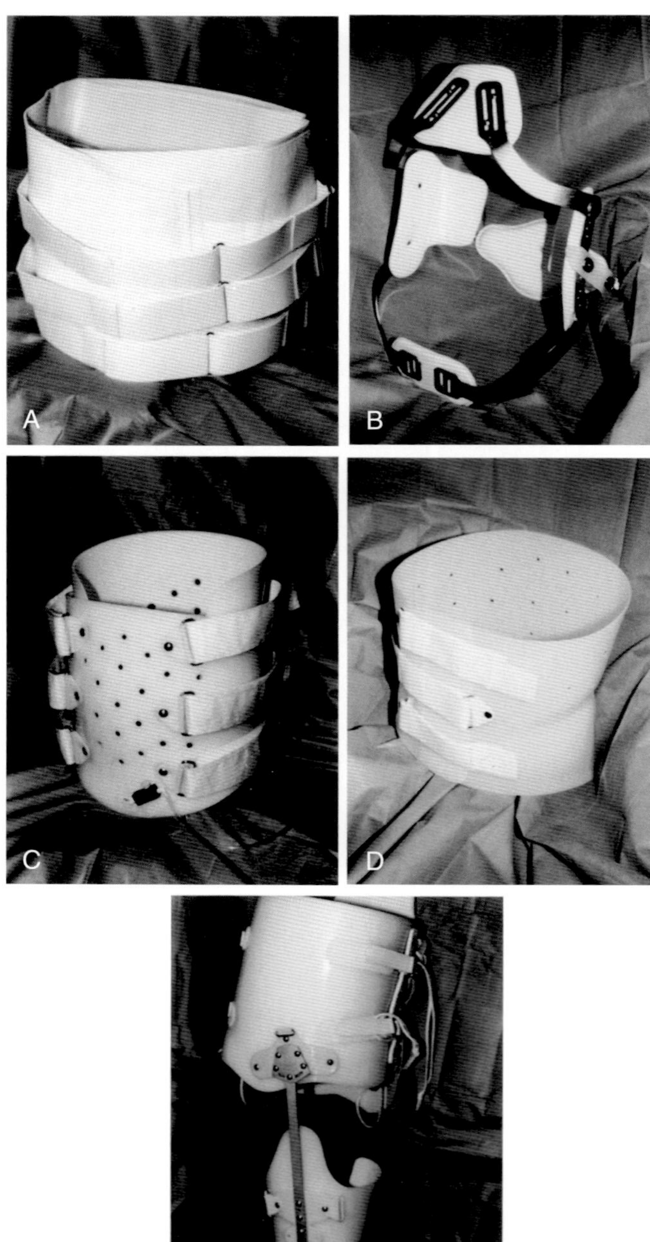

FIGURE 187-5. Thoracolumbar orthoses. **A,** Lumbosacral corset. **B,** Jewett hyperextension brace. **C,** Clamshell-type molded thoracolumbosacral orthosis. **D,** Boston overlap brace. **E,** Clamshell TLSO with thigh extension.

spinal stiffness (single-column injuries). With injuries that reduced stiffness to between 50% and 85% (two-column injuries) and those greater than 85% (three-column injuries), the brace was ineffective for resisting spinal deformation.[34]

Lumbosacral Orthoses

Perhaps the most frequently prescribed appliances, LSOs are also the most controversial because of their questionable effectiveness.[6] Lumbosacral corsets with or without stays, chairback braces, and the Knight brace are representative[3] (Fig. 187-5D). LSOs stabilize the lumbar and sacral regions by encircling the upper abdomen and rib cage and the pelvis. Because of the difficulty in firmly purchasing these areas, three-point bending is probably not a major mechanism in the action of this class of orthosis. Fluid compression likely has a role, although measurements of intra-abdominal pressure while wearing the devices have been inconsistent.[9]

To quantify the effect of bracing on segmental motion, Norton and Brown[11] measured lumbar motion in volunteers by following the motion of K-wires inserted into the spinous processes. Movement at the lumbosacral junction was paradoxically greater while sitting with an LSO than without the brace. The effect was thought to be secondary to stress concentration at the caudal end of the supported segment. Waters and Morris[12] studied lumbosacral stabilization in orthoses by monitoring paraspinal muscle electromyography. Although back muscle activity during standing was reduced with an LSO, activity during fast walking was greater, possibly because of altered pelvis rotation. Lantz and Schultz[33] measured gross trunk motion and myoelectric activity in five volunteers wearing the lumbosacral corset, a chairback brace, and a molded TLSO during standing and sitting. Gross upper body motion was reduced up to 20% in flexion and 45% in extension, lateral bending, and rotation. The TLSO was overall the most effective device tested. Myoelectrical activity varied widely, however, ranging from a 9% reduction to a 44% increase.[35] Axelsson et al.[14] used stereophotogrammetry in seven patients to analyze the effects of the LSO and the molded TLSO on intersegmental lumbar spine movement. Neither device had any effect in restricting segmental translation in sagittal, vertical, or transverse planes. They concluded that the orthoses serve only as a reminder to the patient to restrict gross trunk movements.[14]

These observations substantiate clinical experience that the LSO and TLSO do not adequately stabilize segmental motion of the lower lumbar spine and lumbosacral junction. They do appear to limit gross trunk movement, which is thought to be their major mechanism of action.[33]

Consistent with the principles of long bone splinting discussed earlier, control of the pelvis may be necessary to restrict movement at the lumbosacral junction.[4,13] Fidler and Plasmans[36] have shown that including the thigh with an extension (thigh spica) reduces gross pelvis motion more significantly than a conventional LSO does. Segmental translation with axial loading, however, is not affected by this device.[37] In clinical practice, patient acceptance of thigh spica orthoses is limited because of severe restriction of walking and sitting (Fig. 187-5E).

Sacroiliac Orthoses

Rarely used today, sacroiliac orthoses were developed for pelvic instability after traumatic or postpartum pelvic disruption.[14] They are not effective at reducing motion but rather serve as a kinesthetic device to remind the patient to maintain proper pelvic posture.

Halo Skeletal Fixation

Halo fixation is currently the most effective method of externally immobilizing the cervical spine.[16] Its basic components

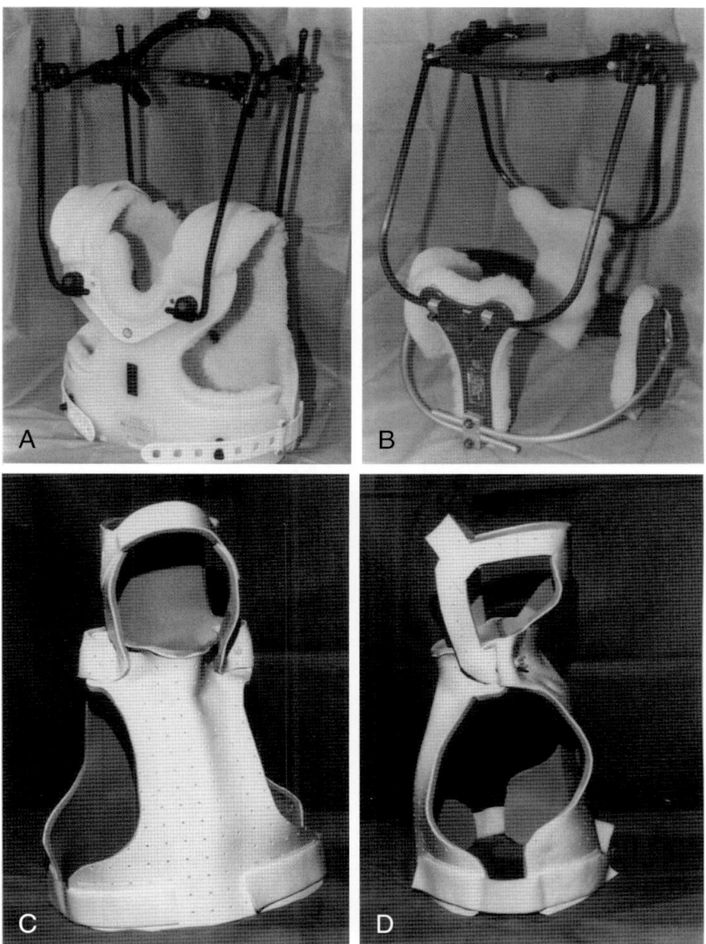

FIGURE 187-6. Halo-type orthoses. **A,** Standard halo vest. **B,** Four-pad halo vest. **C** and **D,** Thermoplastic Minerva body jackets.

consist of a halo ring (or crown) for pin fixation of the skull, a plastic vest or pads secured with straps that encircle the thorax, and two or more upright connecting posts. A variety of commercial products are available that incorporate design features that reflect clinical experience and advances in metal and plastic technology[38] (Fig. 187-6).

Halo bracing has several advantages over the conventional orthoses. The skin and soft tissues of the mandible and occiput are unencumbered, so it is cooler about the head and neck. The jaw is free, which allows easier eating and speaking as well as prevention of temporomandibular joint pain. Skin irritation and breakdown are avoided in the head and neck area. In difficult cases, the device may also encourage compliance for both reducing excessive activity and keeping the orthosis in place. Halo use has been credited with enabling earlier ambulation of patients with severe cervical instability, thereby allowing a more rapid entry into rehabilitation and decreasing secondary complications of immobility.

Clearly, the major advantage to the use of the halo is the degree of stabilization that can be achieved. Johnson et al.[24] demonstrated a reduction of lateral bending and axial rotation in five patients to 1% of that of normal volunteers. Whole cervical spine flexion-extension was similarly reduced to 4% of normal (see Fig. 187-4). Although the halo affords a high degree of stability, persistent significant motion does occur. Koch and Nickel[19] studied halo immobilization in six patients with fractures, demonstrating an average of 31% normal motion for cervical spine flexion and extension at each motion segment. The greatest movement occurred between C2 and C3, with the least at C7-T1. They emphasized the importance of body position or activity such as lying, bending, or sitting in transmitting undesirable force to the cervical spine through the halo itself.

Although distraction is frequently useful to maintain reduction of highly unstable spines, the ability of the halo to provide fixed distraction is limited because of this significant effect of trunk position and patient activity.[19] It should not be used as a principal distraction device.

Paradoxical spinal motion described as snaking accounts for most of the undesirable movement that occurs with the halo.[13,15,39] It is the segmental motion that occurs while the end points of the braced region remain relatively fixed along the spinal axis and involves simultaneous capital protraction and flexion of the upper cervical spine with extension of lower cervical segments (e.g., C0-3 flexion with C5-T1 extension on attempted neck flexion). The measured whole cervical spine movement from C0 to T1 may be minimal, yet individual midcervical segments move significantly without effective fixation[13] (Fig. 187-7). Increasing the

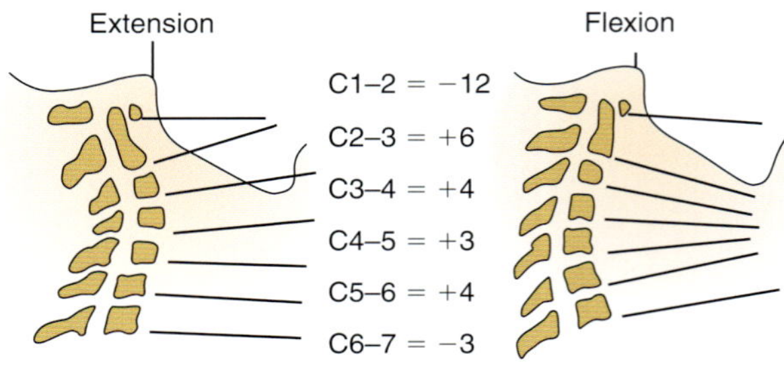

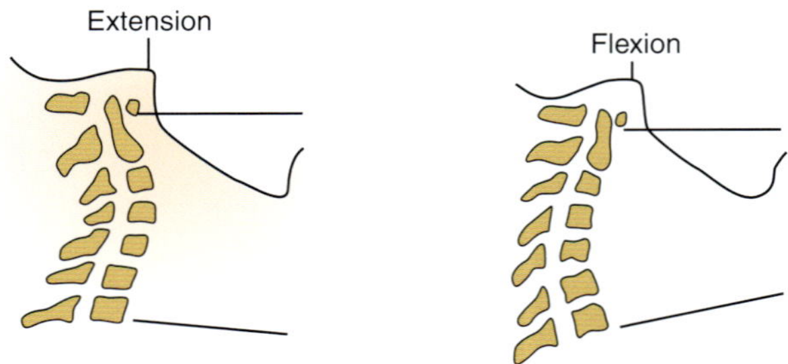

FIGURE 187-7. Paradoxical motion ("snaking") induced by the halo device. Capital flexion with simultaneous lower cervical extension produces significant absolute motion at each segment despite minimal overall motion measured between C0 and T1. (Adapted from Benzel EC: Spinal orthotics. In Menezes AH, Sonntag VKH, editors: *Principles of spinal surgery*, New York, 1996, McGraw-Hill, pp 181–190.)

length and the conformation of a brace minimizes the parallelogram deformation of the spine and the snaking phenomenon. This also maximizes the biomechanical effect of the brace.

The thermoplastic Minerva body jacket (TMBJ)[22] is an alternative to halo bracing (see Fig. 187-6). This device consists of a bivalved molded plastic shell that has contact-type purchase of the thorax like that of a standard halo vest and lateral extensions that incorporate a mandibular support, an occipital support, and a circumferential headband.[23] Benzel et al.[22] compared its effectiveness with the halo in 10 patients with cervical spine injuries. Each patient was tested in whole cervical spine flexion-extension with both the halo and the TMBJ. Their results indicate improved control of individual vertebral angulation at all levels except C1-2 with the TMBJ versus the halo. There was less paradoxical movement with the molded device, indicating a higher overall level of immobilization. Eight of 10 patients reported improved comfort.[22] Maiman et al.[40] also studied the TMBJ in 20 normal volunteers for controlling flexion-extension, lateral bending, and axial rotation. The TMBJ significantly reduced motion as compared with unrestricted controls in all planes except rotation. It was more effective than the halo in restricting flexion-extension and lateral bending when compared with the historical data of Johnson et al.[24] and Wang et al.[41] In practice, the effectiveness of the device depends on the ability to achieve an excellent fit, which requires an expert orthotist who is familiar with its use. The TMBJ also suffers the disadvantages of any contact orthosis, such as skin irritation, mandible obstruction, discomfort, and warmth.

BOX 187-1. Complications of Orthoses

Skin and Soft Tissue Injury
Pain
Skin/wound breakdown
Muscle atrophy, contracture formation
Ineffective Stabilization
Inappropriate orthotic for spinal level
Loss of reduction—halo
Distraction, paradoxical movement ("snaking")
Miscellaneous
Halo pin site complications
Overdistraction
Dysphagia
Cardiopulmonary complications
Pulmonary edema, reduced vital capacity
Venous hypertension
Varicose veins, hemorrhoids, extremity edema
Gastrointestinal dysfunction
Superior mesenteric artery syndrome
Psychological dysfunction
Secondary gain, adjustment disorders

Complications of Spinal Bracing

Complications of bracing can be organized into three general categories: skin and soft tissue injuries, ineffective stabilization, and a variety of miscellaneous complications, largely related to halo skeletal fixation (Box 187-1).

Skin and Soft Tissue Injury

All orthoses require some degree of skin-appliance connection to apply forces indirectly to the vertebral column. Excessive pressure on the skin causes ischemia with resulting pain, breakdown, and/or frank ulceration. Pressure is defined as force per unit area and is the major cause of decubitus ulcers occurring over bony prominences in patients with poor mobility and prolonged recumbency.[17] Tissue breakdown is normally avoided because of painful exteroceptive feedback that occurs when skin pressure is prolonged. Discomfort stimulates subconscious shifting of position to unload the dependent body part. Altered sensation (Fig. 187-8), consciousness, or mobility impairs normal protective mechanisms[13,42] and can lead to a variety of possible injuries, depending on the severity of the ischemic deficit[43] (Table 187-2). Careful and frequent inspection of skin contact areas beneath braces is mandatory to identify the earliest stages of injury and allow intervention before irreversible skin damage occurs.[42]

Because of their significant effect on patient management and the economic impact of treatment, decubitus ulcers have been the focus of a number of clinical and basic science investigations.[18] Important factors identified experimentally for developing pressure sores include the magnitude and duration of the applied pressure, associated shear or friction of the skin, tissue distribution, skin moisture, hydration, and general nutrition.[17,18,42] Tissue damage from pressure occurs by microvessel occlusion that impairs perfusion and leads to

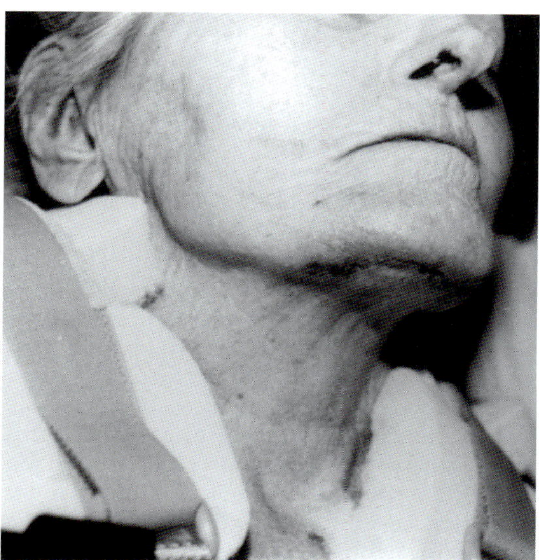

FIGURE 187-8. Soft tissue breakdown beneath the mandible in a 72-year-old woman with multiple myeloma after using the Minerva brace. Predisposing factors included pressure being applied over the prominent bony mandible, thin skin and subcutaneous tissue in this area, and poor nutrition from chronic disease.

TABLE 187-2

Stages of Pressure Sore Development

Stage I	Hyperemia	Nonblanching erythema appearing within 30 minutes of pressure that disappears within 1 hour
Stage II	Ischemia	Seen after 2–6 hours of continuous pressure; erythema requires 36 hours to resolve
Stage III	Necrosis	Skin appears blue and firm after 6 hours of pressure; skin changes do not resolve
Stage IV	Ulceration	Occurs 2 weeks after stage III injury appearing as ulcer formation and infection; may involve underlying bone

Adapted from Edberg EL, Cerny K, Stauffer ES: Prevention and treatment of pressure sores. *Phys Ther* 53:246–252, 1973, with permission.

secondary ischemia. External pressures exceeding normal tissue capillary perfusion pressure (32 mm Hg)[44] will interrupt blood flow, leading to ischemia and permanent tissue death if unrelieved. The duration of application is inversely related to the absolute pressure.[18] Kosiak[45] has reported the relationship between duration and the risk of pressure sores in a series of studies that used a canine model. Pressures of 500 mm Hg applied to the skin surface for only 2 hours produced ulceration, whereas 150 mm Hg was tolerated for up to 12 hours. Pressure as low as 70 mm Hg, however, was sufficient to produce microscopic ischemic changes after only 2 hours. Thus, a continuum of injury may be seen that is related to increasing pressure magnitude and duration.

Surface friction potentiates the risk of ulceration by creating shear in deeper soft tissues. Shear leads to capillary occlusion by kinking, stretching, and tearing and produces ischemia at lower absolute externally applied pressures.[17,42] A study in a porcine model compared the threshold for skin damage from a force applied with and without linear shear.[46] Ulceration occurred at less than one sixth the external pressure (45 mm Hg) when combined with shear than without added shearing forces (290 mm Hg). Surface friction also can abrade outer layers of skin, especially if the subcutaneous tissues are very firm or tightly tethered to the underlying bone.[17] Friction abrasions then further contribute to decubitus ulcer formation. Adequate systemic hydration can mitigate the effects of shear by increasing the mechanical resilience of skin.[42]

An important consequence of pressure in advanced-stage injuries is the effect on muscle. Muscle is more vulnerable to ischemia than is skin, because it typically develops necrosis earlier and more extensively.[18] Pressure distribution between the skin surface and the underlying bone concentrates force at the deep bone-muscle junction because of the abrupt tissue transition from bone to muscle. Necrosis tends to be maximal at the level of the underlying bone and decreases gradually outward toward more superficial layers.[47] External skin ulceration is usually only the external manifestation of a more extensive soft tissue injury.[42] Although vulnerable to ischemia, muscle and fat layers paradoxically are important for dissipating force through the energy-absorbing process of elastic deformation. Thus, poorly covered bony prominences such as the sacrum, greater trochanter, and heels that are without significant soft tissue layers are particularly vulnerable to skin breakdown. Pressure dissipation plays a major role in the beneficial effects of muscle flap transfers used to cover ulcerated bony prominences.[48]

The barrier function of skin is compromised by prolonged exposure of its surface to moisture. Moisture from incontinence or sweating overhydrates the outer layer of the stratum corneum, reducing its mechanical strength and resistance to bacterial permeation.[42] Increased temperature caused by impaired heat convection further allows microflora to proliferate and reduces the tissue pH. These changes result in epidermal sloughing, deep layer exposure, and microbial invasion of the underlying dermis, all of which promote ulceration.

Similar conditions frequently threaten skin integrity beneath occlusive spinal orthoses. Braces that poorly dissipate pressure, impair proper hygiene, create significant shear, and allow moisture buildup are most likely to promote tissue injury. Regrettably, little data for the frequency of skin ulceration exist for conventional orthoses other than that noted in anecdotal reports. For the halo device, pressure sores have been observed in 4% to 11% of patients and usually occur over the scapulae or rib cage.[49-52] Practical means to prevent these complications include optimizing the orthotic fit, maximizing the applied surface area of the brace to dissipate pressure, and avoiding appliances with sharp or uneven edges.[17] As was stated, areas over bony prominences have minimal overlying soft tissue to distribute pressure by elastic energy absorption and are most vulnerable to ischemic injury under an orthosis. Adding special padding or cutting out a hole immediately over a prominence may avoid breakdown by shifting pressure away from high-risk areas to more tolerant tissues.

Hygiene is a function of patient education and proper nursing and is greatly facilitated by modern, removable appliances.[42] Patients should be fully educated as to the risks and warning signs of early skin ulceration and should participate actively in its prevention. Special problems occur with anesthetic skin that does not produce noxious feedback to warn of excessive or prolonged pressure[13] (Fig. 187-9). This can also occur in obtunded or comatose patients. Shear under an orthosis can be avoided by a properly fitted brace and by maintaining a moisture-absorbing layer between the skin and appliance at all times. A cotton undergarment that can be changed daily is useful in this regard both for hygiene and moisture reduction.

In the nutritionally depleted patient, general protein wasting may lead to tissue edema, altered tissue repair, and compromised antimicrobial mechanisms. Edema impairs tissue oxygenation, decreases elasticity, and reduces skin resistance to mechanical deformation. Marker serum proteins such as transferrin and albumin and anergy to injected antigens are common and useful indicators of nutritional status. Assessment of nutritional status and correction if inadequate may prevent or delay developing pressure sores associated with orthoses.[42]

To determine the incidence and risk factors associated with the development of cervical collar-related decubitus ulceration (CRU) in trauma patients immobilized in Philadelphia cervical collars, Ackland et al. did an exploratory study from a trauma registry database at a level 1 trauma center; 299 major trauma patients admitted over a 6-month period were identified. Predictors of CRU were retrospectively examined and assessed for relative importance by using medical records and prospective infection control and radiology databases. Using logistic regression analysis, they found that significant predictors of CRU were ICU admission (P = .007), mechanical ventilation (P = .005), the necessity for cervical MRI ($P \leq .001$), and time to cervical spine clearance ($P \leq .001$). Time to cervical spine clearance was the major indicator, such that the risk of CRU increased by 66% for every 1-day increase in cervical collar time.[53]

Postoperative wounds are especially prone to skin edge maceration and secondary bacterial invasion if covered by occlusive orthoses, because of the combined negative effects of sweating, external pressure, and shearing forces.[54]

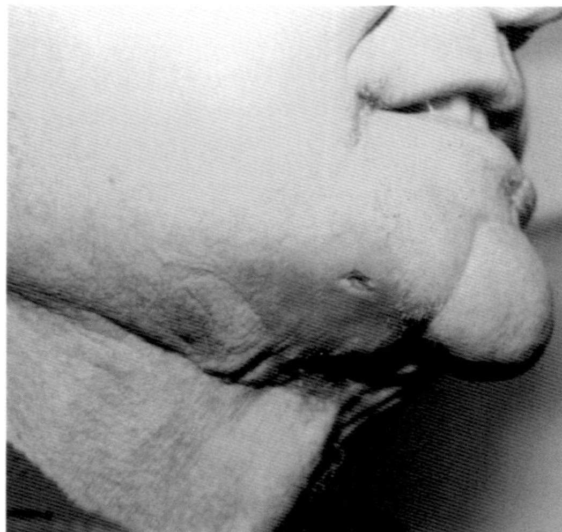

FIGURE 187-9. Soft tissue ulceration beneath the mandible in a 56-year-old man using a Philadelphia collar. The skin over this area was anesthetic because of a prior radical neck dissection for laryngeal carcinoma. Anesthetic areas of skin under braces are at significant risk for breakdown, especially for patients with limited mobility.

Frequently changed, dry dressings over the wound reduce these effects and prevent most orthosis-associated wound infections. Alternatively, a noncontact or ventilated device may reduce this risk.

Other soft tissue complications of spinal bracing include muscle atrophy and contracture formation.[4,6] Atrophy occurs rapidly after even brief periods of disuse because of a lack of normal motion and tone. Resulting loss of bulk and weakness may be profound, requiring progressive weaning from the appliance and active rehabilitation after bony healing is established. Although commonly observed in this setting, atrophy associated with spinal bracing has not been thoroughly quantified. Contractures are rigid deformities of a joint caused by immobilization or unbalanced effector forces across the joint. With time, the associated muscles can become painful and permanently fibrotic. Contractures are occasionally observed with long-term cervical bracing or halo use and primarily involve limited cervical rotation. Lind et al.[52] have reported up to 80% residual neck pain and stiffness after halo bracing, which probably represents minor cervical contracture formation.

Korovessis et al.[55] recently reported an interesting soft tissue complication associated with long-term use of a modified Boston brace in young women braced for scoliosis. The appliance uses a rigid pelvic band that covers the dorsolateral hips over the greater trochanters and is open over the lower flank region. Prolonged use (>6 months) led to upward migration of the lateral trochanteric fat pads in 23% of 300 subjects, resulting in significant cosmetic deformity. Suction lipoplasty was required in 74% of this group. Pressure atrophy of developing fat deposits with local redistribution appears to account for this phenomenon.[55]

Ineffective Stabilization

As was previously discussed, most conventional braces poorly transmit force directly to the spine and are limited in their ability to restrict segmental motion and/or unload the vertebral column. Long conventional appliances spanning many segments across the level of interest are most effective for controlling gross body movement because of significant three-point bending.[33] Mismatch between the point of spinal instability and the optimal effective range for a particular brace (typically at its midpoint) accounts for a common cause of ineffective brace selection. Similarly, extensive instability or injuries that are only reduced by axial distraction are not usually amenable to conventional bracing. Most studies of orthotic effects involve kinematic evaluation of stability in single trials of spine motion, usually in healthy subjects. The questions of clinical effectiveness are less well answered because of limited availability of longitudinal outcome data for various devices.

Despite its limited effect on segmental motion, the TLSO may improve fusion success by restricting gross trunk motion. Johnsson et al.[56] recently studied the effect of a molded TLSO in 22 patients undergoing dorsolateral fusions. One group of 11 patients was braced for 3 months, and the other group was braced for 5 months. Segmental motion was evaluated by stereophotogrammetry. Fusions became progressively more rigid beginning at 3 months in both groups. By 1 year, however, patients who had been immobilized for 5 months showed a higher rate of fusion than the 3-month group, indicating a direct benefit of longer immobilization.[56]

Although the halo is the most rigid cervical appliance in kinematic testing, success in clinical application varies, especially with ligamentous instability. Cooper et al.[57] reviewed their experience with halo bracing of unstable injuries in 33 patients. They reported few minor complications and restored stability in 85%. In only four patients did therapy fail. Patients with ligamentous subluxation or angulation were most prone to lose halo reduction. Whitehill et al.[58] also reported five patients with unstable ligamentous facet dislocations or subluxations who failed to maintain reduction with the halo. Of 36 patients with facet dislocations or fracture-dislocations reviewed by Beyer et al.,[59] 19 underwent halo immobilization. Only one third achieved proper alignment, and one fourth achieved anatomic reduction. Half of the halo group lost reduction during bracing. They recommended open reduction and fixation of facet dislocations for better alignment and fusion results. Rockswold[60] reviewed 604 patients in five studies from the literature who were treated with halo stabilization for a variety of cervical injuries. Failed reduction and/or fusion occurred in 12% to 23% of patients. Hyperflexion ligamentous injuries had the highest failure rate. From these and other observations, it appears that the halo is an effective means for stabilizing many cervical injuries unless primary ligamentous instability exists. Paradoxical motion, or snaking, of the spine with associated midcervical angulation may account for the inadequate stability in ligamentous injuries.[13]

Noncompliance

As was previously stated, it was shown that the effectiveness of an appliance is directly related to the level of its discomfort.[3,4] This also contributes to higher levels of noncompliance.

Regardless of the patient population, a limitation to studies assessing the effectiveness of bracing is the lack of objective data on how long a brace is actually worn. The majority of available literature regarding brace compliance is based on the assumption that subjective reports of brace compliance are accurate. Diaries, logs, and self-reporting have all been used as means of recording compliance with bracing. DiRaimondio and Green[61] reported, on the basis of patient interviews, that fewer than 15% of their patients were highly compliant with the prescribed wearing schedule. Compliance rates as high as 64% and 88% have been reported with subject self-reporting.[62,63] Subjective reports should not be considered the most accurate measurement of brace compliance. According to a recent study, Helfenstein et al.[64] found that subjective reporting does not appear as accurate as using an objective measure of brace compliance. The investigators in this study used a temperature data logger to monitor the brace wear of nine women with idiopathic adolescent scoliosis up to 3 months. A questionnaire to measure self-reported compliance was used. The average objective compliance was 68% (subjects were recommended to wear the brace 23 hours per day), and the subjective self-reported compliance average was 94%.

Over the last several years, sensors that can be attached to braces have been designed to measure wearing time objectively. Takemitsu et al.[65] used a temperature sensor embedded in the TLSO of children with idiopathic scoliosis. Havey et al.[66] developed a force-sensitive resistor that was placed in TLSOs to assess wear time in normal volunteers and found it to be accurate and reliable.

Miscellaneous Complications of Spinal Bracing

Halo-vest immobilization (HVI), developed by Koch and Nickel,[19] is the gold standard for providing maximal, externally mediated immobilization of the cervical spine. However, studies citing high complication rates and low success rates have called its clinical usefulness into question.[19,67]

Bransford et al.[68] evaluated the survival of the halo vest to full completion of the originally prescribed treatment plan, as well as failure and complication rates. It was found that the intended duration of HVI was completed in 74% of patients. Also, the desired clinical outcome of avoiding surgical intervention was achieved in 85% of patients in whom the intent had been definitive halo treatment. This success rate is identical to the ones reported by Bucholz and Cheung[69] and by Cooper et al.,[57] in previous similar series.

Other than pin site infection, Bransford et al.[68] found that the primary complications were instability or failure of the halo to maintain acceptable alignment, which consisted of approximately one third of all complications. In fact, failure to maintain acceptable stability of the spine was the leading cause of cessation of HVI. Other studies have shown similar secondary loss of reduction or persistent spinal column instability, with a previously reported incidence ranging from 9% to 15%.[51,52,69-71] Two thirds of all failures occurred within the first 3 weeks of halo application, suggesting that this early phase is critical in determining the likelihood of success.

Halo Pin Site Complications

Pin site complications are among the most common limitations of halo bracing and have been studied extensively[49,50,52,68,72] (Table 187-3).

Pin Loosening

Pin loosening is seen in 36% to 60% of patients and is usually heralded by pain in the absence of associated infection.[52,71] Occasionally, a fall or blunt trauma to the halo ring will result in acute loosening.[50] Current pin tip designs use a broad pin

TABLE 187-3

Complication Frequency of Halo Pin Fixation

Complication	Percentage
Loosening	36–60*†
Pin site infection	20–22*†
Local pain	18†
Ring migration	13*†
Scarring	9–30*†
Nerve injury	2*
Pin site bleeding	1*
Intracranial puncture	1*

*Data from Garfin SR, Botte MJ, Waters RL, et al: Complications in the use of the halo fixation device. *J Bone Joint Surg [Am]* 68:320–325, 1986.

†Data from Lind B, Sihlbom H, Nordwall A: Halo-vest treatment of unstable traumatic cervical spine injuries. *Spine (Phila Pa 1976)* 13:425–432, 1988.

Adapted from Botte MJ, Byrne TP, Abrams RA, Garfin SR: Halo skeletal fixation: techniques of application and prevention of complications. *J Am Acad Orthop Surg* 4:44–53, 1996, with permission.

shoulder to maximize skull contact and help to limit loosening or perforation.[73] Ballock et al.[74] evaluated optimal pin site placement in a cadaver model, noting that pins inserted lower on the skull above the supraorbital ridge were more rigidly affixed than were more superiorly placed pins. The lower pins were more perpendicular in orientation, which reportedly accounts for their improved rigidity. Botte et al.[71] studied the effect of pin insertion torque on subsequent pin loosening and reported improved mechanical characteristics of the pin-bone junction at 8 inch-pounds versus 6 inch-pounds. Loosening was reduced to 7% from 36%, respectively.[13] Rizzolo et al.[75] also addressed pin insertion torque, randomizing two groups with pins inserted to torques of 8 or 6 inch-pounds. No significant difference between groups was noted, although a trend toward higher rates of loosening (26% vs. 20%) and infection (13% vs. 7%) occurred with the 8-inch-pound insertion torque. Currently, 6 to 8 inch-pounds are recommended for initial insertion torque, which is subsequently checked at 24 to 48 hours.[72] If remote loosening occurs without infection, the pins should be tightened once as long as resistance is encountered. Garfin et al.[50] found that 16% of loosened pins reloosened after tightening. Pins that were moved also loosened in 17%, suggesting that loosened pins compromise the balance of the other pins in the halo ring.[50] Repeated tightening leads to cranial perforation, because local bone erodes rapidly under pressure from the pin.

The actual force that is applied through the pin at the pin-skull junction appears to vary considerably for a given torque, depending on the method of insertion and the size and type of halo ring used. Whitesides et al.[76] measured force exerted through the pin for different insertion torques in several types of halo rings. They noted a wide variation in force among rings of different size and material composition. Flexibility of the ring and its effect on the coefficient of friction at the pin-ring junction reportedly accounted for the variation. Lubrication of the junction with saline significantly reduced friction between the pin and the ring. They recommended using an insertion torque specific for the type of halo used to standardize the force applied to the skull.[76] Kerwin et al.[77] also found wide variation of pin force with different ring sizes and materials. Friction between the ring and pin threads increased with ring flexibility. Addition of a locking nut paradoxically reduced pin force by either backing out the pin or altering the ring shape.

Infection

Skeletal fixation by definition violates the integrity of the scalp, risking local infection. Pin sites require continuous daily inspection and cleaning with hydrogen peroxide and application of a topical antibiotic such as polymyxin ointment. Despite excellent pin site care, local infection will occur in between 13%[68] and 22% of patients.[49] Increasing erythema and purulent drainage around the pin indicate early soft tissue involvement and can usually be treated with a culture-specific oral antibiotic and close follow-up.

In 2009, Bransford et al.[68] published a retrospective study of 490 cases of traumatic cervical fractures treated with HVI. The author classified the infection type in three categories (Fig. 187-10).[68] Overall, 38% of infections were limited locally and required only local wound care and PO antibiotics (class I). Fifty-six percent were considered class II infections and required pin removal and local debridement. Finally, 5% were considered complicated infections such as brain abscess or major craniofacial abscess and required surgical debridement and IV antibiotics.

Staphylococcus aureus is the most commonly involved organism. If extensive cellulitis or abscess occurs, the pin must be removed, and a new pin must be inserted at an adjacent site. Infected pin site care follows standard principles of local wound care, including appropriate debridement and intravenous antibiotic therapy.

Brain abscess is a rare but serious result of cranial pin fixation that is typically associated with overlying soft tissue infection and/or secondary osteomyelitis. Of five cases reviewed by Goodman and Nelson,[78] three had associated osteomyelitis, and all involved tightening of a loosened pin. Rosenblum and Ehrlich[79] described a patient who presented with acute psychosis as an initial manifestation of an intracranial abscess. His halo pin had been tightened twice because of loosening, the second time 1 week before presentation. These reports underscore the danger of repeatedly tightening loose pins. A pin that becomes loose should be retightened only once in the absence of frank scalp infection. Further loosening after initial retightening is an indication for insertion at another site.

A

Class I	Focal irritation or infection; no pin loosening; responsive to local measures; responsive to local pin tract care, oral antibiotics, retightening of pin
Class II	Pin loosening, productive purulent drainage; requires pin removal and debridement
Class III	Intracranial abscess, craniofacial abscess, requires surgical debridement/reconstruction, IV antibiotics

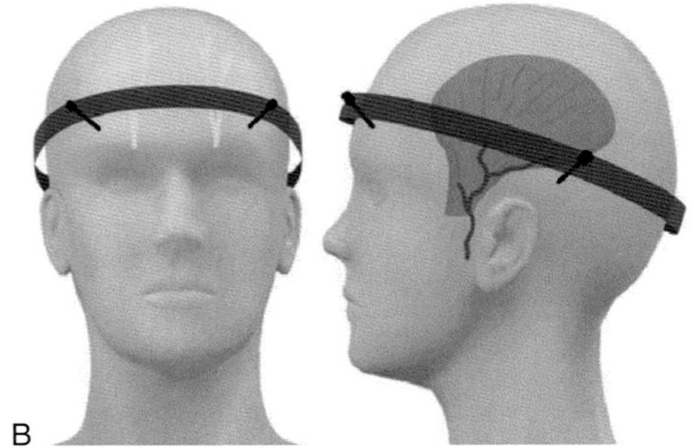

FIGURE 187-10. A, Distinction of pin-tract infections. **B,** Recommended halo pin placement. Temporal pins should avoid the frontal sinus and supraorbital nerve medially and the temporal artery and fossa laterally. Posterior pins should avoid the mastoids. (Adapted from Bransford RJ, Stevens DW, Uyeji S, et al: Halo vest treatment of cervical spine injuries: a success and survivorship analysis. *Spine [Phila Pa 1976]* 34[15]:1561–1566, 2009.)

Less frequent halo complications include frontal scarring, nerve injury, bleeding, and cranial puncture.[72] Scars from frontal pin sites are usually cosmetically acceptable for most patients. However, up to 30% of patients develop severe scarring that may require further treatment.[52] Local infection, pin migration, and keloid formation may contribute to this problem. Incising the skin before insertion does not improve cosmetic outcome.[72] Garfin et al.[50] reported continuous local pain at pin sites in 17% of 180 patients who were treated in halos. Repeated periosteal irritation was thought to be the basis for chronic pin site pain.[50] Alternatively, pins that are mistakenly positioned through the temporalis muscle in the temporal fossa are also painful because of muscle trauma and continued irritation during jaw movement.[72] Paradoxically, newly developed pin site pain often indicates a loosening pin. Nerve injury with pain and paresthesias may occur with pin trauma to the supraorbital or supratrochlear nerves as they course superiorly from their foramina to innervate the frontal scalp. Pin movement is often required because of the severity of symptoms. Avoiding medial pin placement should prevent this complication.[72] By placing frontal pins into the fronto-orbital crest, obvious scars, nerve injuries, and temporalis muscle pain may be avoided. Bleeding from pin sites has been reported in patients receiving chronic anticoagulants.[50] Discontinuing anticoagulation resolves this rare and unusual complication. Intracranial puncture has been discussed in association with repeated pin tightening or frank trauma to the halo ring such as with a fall. Although rarely reported, this can lead to serious intracranial infection and loss of fixation[72] (see Table 187-3). Figure 187-10B depicts the appropriate halo ring positioning to avoid nerve as well as cosmetic complications.

Overdistraction

Because the thoracic vest of the halo transmits significant force through the device to the cranium, distraction and compression forces vary widely with different patient positions and activities.[19] Overly vigorous attempts to maintain axial traction in a halo can result in overdistraction and cause associated swallowing difficulties or neck discomfort. Dysphagia has been noted in up to 2% of patients[50] and results from impaired larynx movement required for coordinated swallowing. Avoiding excessive distraction and head extension will usually prevent this complication.

Cardiopulmonary Complications

Cardiopulmonary complications of bracing mainly involve changes in venous pressures of the trunk, abdomen, and lower extremities. Kaplan et al.[80] described acute pulmonary edema occurring in an obese 63-year-old trauma victim after removal of a halo that had been in place for 14 weeks. Occult mitral stenosis was subsequently diagnosed. They postulated that removal of the halo vest resulted in a loss of the mechanical impediment to venous return, resulting in rapid volume loading of the heart, which was not compensated because of occult mitral stenosis. Improved ventilatory mechanics after halo removal also increased venous return, worsening pulmonary edema. Lower-extremity venous hypertension is an additional concern for developing varicose veins, venous stasis with thrombosis, or hemorrhoids.[4] This is most commonly seen with the TLSO, although it has not specifically been reported or quantified.

Conventional orthoses and halo vests may compromise respiratory function by restricting expansion of the chest and abdomen. To measure this effect, Lind et al.[81] studied spirometry of 20 trauma patients in halos at 1 week of treatment, at 3 months, and after removal of the appliance. The halo reduced vital capacity by 8% to 9%. With prolonged wearing, vital capacity increased by 10% because of adjustment of the vest, reduction in acute pain, loss of cautiousness, and respiratory training. Levels remained at all times more than adequate to support normal respiratory function.[81] Although this study demonstrates only a minimal reduction in vital capacity, the effect on patients with chronic obstructive pulmonary disease is unknown and may be more functionally significant.

Gastrointestinal Dysfunction

Compression of the abdomen, especially combined with extension, may occasionally stretch the superior mesenteric artery across the ventral aspect of the distal duodenum, compressing it against the aorta.[13] The superior mesenteric artery syndrome or cast syndrome results in postprandial bilious emesis, epigastric pain, and distention from partial duodenal obstruction.[82] A barium study typically shows duodenal compression with delayed passage into the small bowel. Contributing factors include acute weight loss, recumbency, posturing, and spasticity.[83] Treatment is expectant with discontinued bracing, gastric decompression, parenteral alimentation, or enteral feeding through a tube passed beyond the duodenum. Refractory cases may require surgical exploration. Dysphagia is a frequent complaint related to the use of the halo. Mechanical changes in swallowing, with subsequent dysphagia, were noted with the application of the halo vest in overdistraction or hyperextention in healthy volunteers.[84]

Psychosocial Dysfunction

A number of authors have noted severe psychological problems associated with spinal bracing in up to 3% of patients.[6,50,85] Scoliosis bracing typically involves female adolescents with a significantly intrusive appliance that markedly affects body image. Initial adjustment disorders have been described, ranging from varying degrees of depression to noncompliance and eating disorders.[86-88] Similar adjustment problems with other conventional devices have not been quantified, although concerns about appearance, complaints of claustrophobia, and anxiety over lost independence are commonly expressed. Orthoses are very visible symbols of infirmity, which may foster adoption of a sick role. Psychological dependence and secondary gain are not uncommon among chronic collar users because of this change in body image and its connotation of legitimate injury.[4] Bracing should therefore be used only when indicated for specific stabilization goals that have defined end points.

New Advances and Developments

Recent developments in materials and techniques have led to many improvements in older orthoses as well as the invention of some new strategies. Advances have sought to both

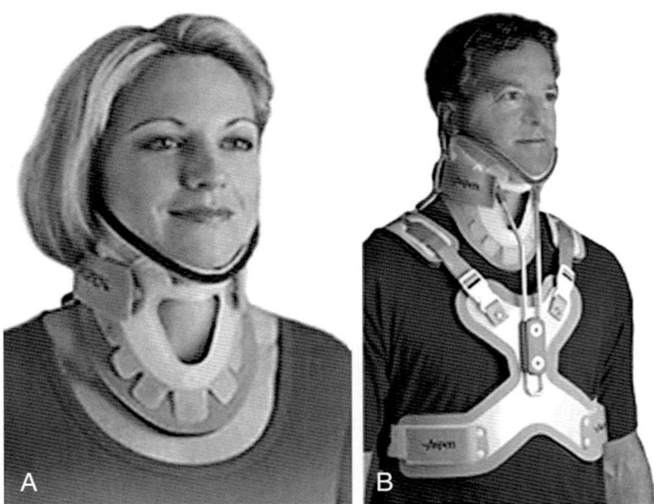

FIGURE 187-11. A, The Aspen Cervical Collar (Aspen Medical Products, Long Beach, CA) incorporates large anterior and posterior openings to promote better airflow, which increases patient comfort. **B,** The Aspen CTO incorporates the cervical collar into an integrated system, allowing the flexibility of stepping down from a four-poster brace to a two-poster brace and finally to a stand-alone cervical collar. (From http://www.aspenmp.com.)

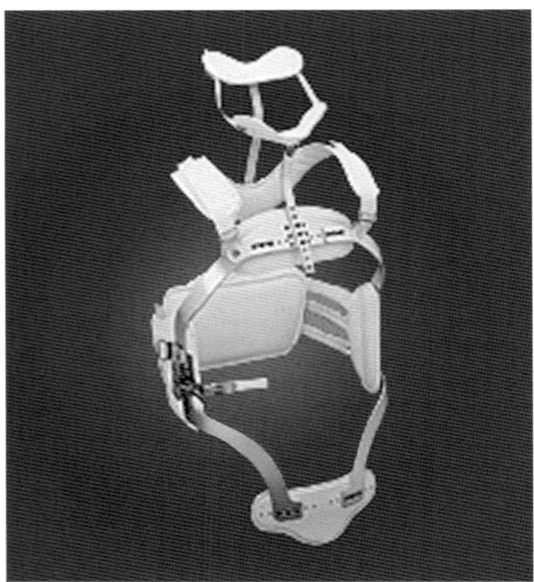

FIGURE 187-12. The original Jewett Brace (Florida Brace Corporation, Winter Park, FL) is now available with a full cervical extension. (From http://www.flabrace.com.)

simplify their application and to increase patient comfort, in turn delivering greater compliance. Specifically, new strap and closure configurations have made some devices easier to apply, adjust, and remove. Further front adjustments allow additional customization to follow body contour variations from the top of the torso to the waist and hips. Additional options include male and female liners, pendulous fronts, and adjustable lumbar control permitting custom curvatures from 0 degrees to 40 degrees. These advances have led some companies to claim the ability to fit 98% of the adult population (ComfAlign, The Bremer Group Company, Jacksonville, FL).

Some companies have adopted novel techniques to increase support while decreasing the incidence of skin breakdown. The Aspen cervical collar (Aspen Medical Products, Inc., Long Beach, CA) utilizes a three-layered system to achieve effective motion restriction. Two stiff inner layers of plastic provide the majority of support, while an outer, more flexible layer is slotted along its edges, allowing better conformation with the patient's anatomy. The resultant better fit reduces the pressure points that are commonly found at the mandible, sternum, and clavicles. Studies have documented that the reduced pressure from an improved fit is significantly less than capillary closing pressure, an underlying cause of skin breakdown.[5] The advent of cleanable and replaceable liners also results in better skin care without the need for multiple collars. Large anterior and posterior openings promote better airflow, increasing patient comfort (Fig. 187-11A). The Aspen CTO (Fig. 187-11B), which incorporates the Aspen cervical collar, gives the practitioner the flexibility of stepping down the level of motion restriction as the patient progresses. The integrated system allows one to go from a four-poster brace to a two-poster brace and finally to a stand-alone cervical collar. Other manufacturers have also developed options and attachments to increase their available applications, such as the Jewett brace (Florida Brace Corporation, Winter Park, FL) anterior and full cervical extensions to the company's original hyperextension orthosis (Fig. 187-12).

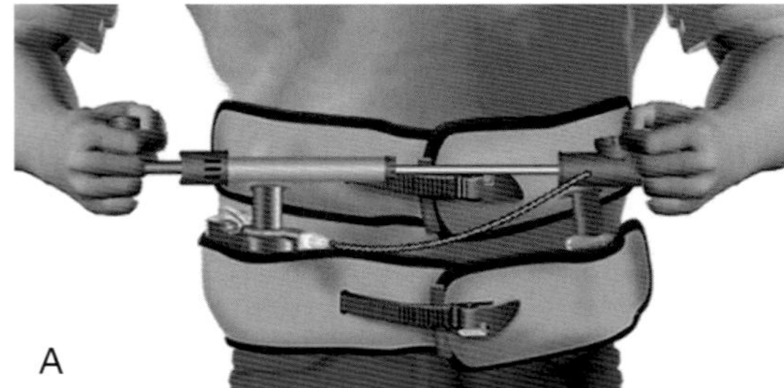

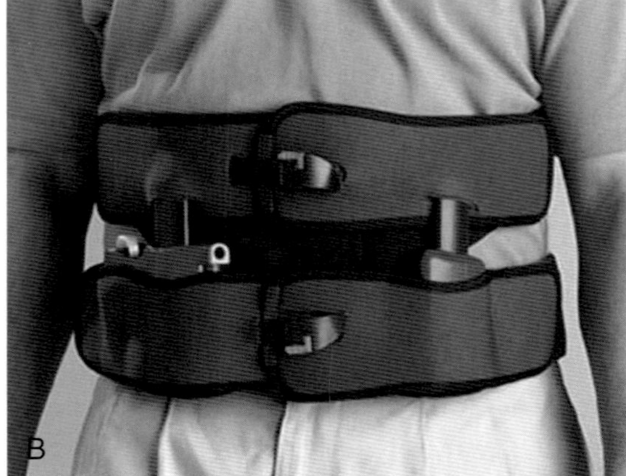

FIGURE 187-13. The Orthotrac Pneumatic Vest (Orthofix, Inc.) utilizes a hand pump (**A**) to activate pneumatic lifters that tie into two custom-fitted belts, which shift body weight from the lumbar spine onto the iliac crests (**B**). The vest is designed to shift up to 30% to 50% of the body weight off of the spine. (From http://www.treatmyback.com.)

The Orthotrac Pneumatic Vest (Orthofix, Inc., Lewisville, TX) represents a unique, noninvasive approach to low back pain. Utilizing a hand pump, the patient activates pneumatic lifters that tie into two custom-fitted belts that shift body weight from the lumbar spine onto the iliac crests (Fig. 187-13). Company literature claims the vest is designed

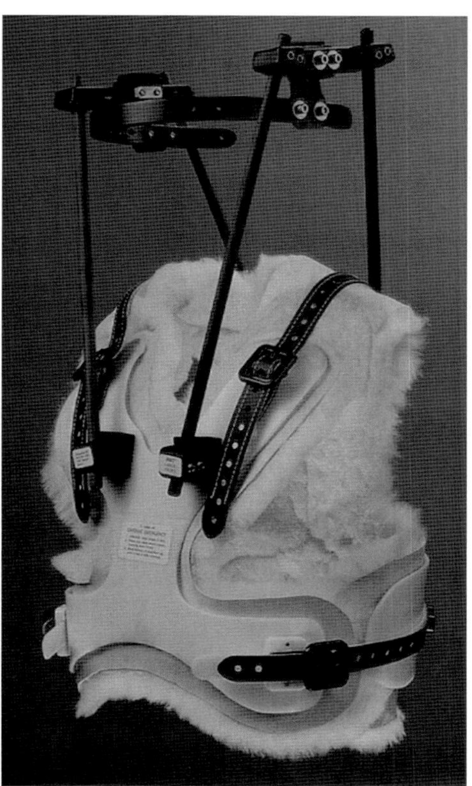

FIGURE 187-14. The latest model of the Halo System (PMT Corporation, Chanhassen, MN) has incorporated several changes, including displaced buckles for cleaner lateral radiographs, the use of carbon graphite and titanium materials to provide clear MRI or CT scans, new nylon ball joints to make assembly quicker and easier, and adjustable headblocks that can be independently adjusted in three ways, allowing anterior-posterior positioning, flexion-extension, and traction-distraction. (From http://www.pmtcorp.com.)

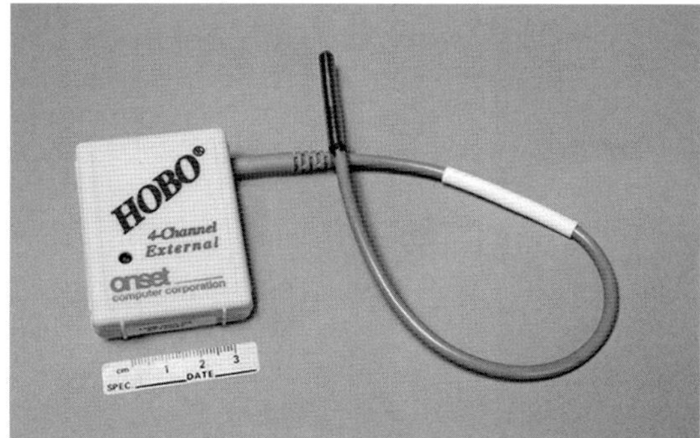

FIGURE 187-15. HOBO H8 4-channel external monitor. (From Hunter LN, Sison-Williamson M, Mendoza MM, et al: The validity of compliance monitors to assess wearing time of thoracic-lumbar-sacral orthoses in children with spinal cord injury. *Spine [Phila Pa 1976]* 33[14]:1554–1561, 2008.)

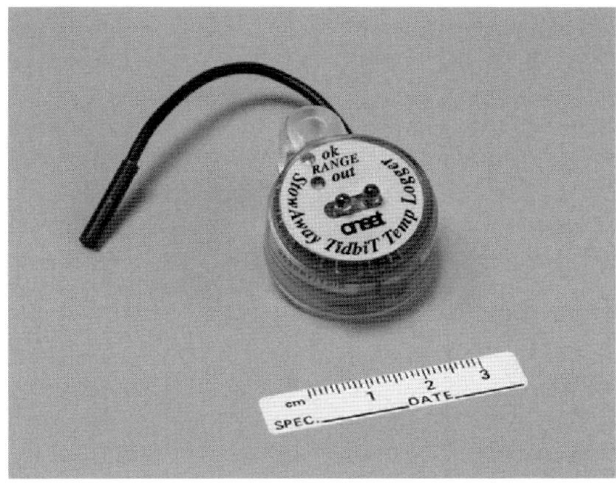

FIGURE 187-16. StowAway TidbiT. (From Hunter LN, Sison-Williamson M, Mendoza MM, et al: The validity of compliance monitors to assess wearing time of thoracic-lumbar-sacral orthoses in children with spinal cord injury. *Spine [Phila Pa 1976]* 33[14]:1554–1561, 2008.)

to shift up to 30% to 50% of the body weight off of the spine and distract adjoining vertebral bodies up to 1 mm, which appears sufficient to off-load the spine in most cases.

Many older companies have spent much time and effort to improve their product line. Jerome Medical (Morristown, NJ), maker of the Miami J, has developed a proprietary material, Sorbatek. The company claims that it breathes better and dries more quickly. It is also antibacterial and exhibits good thermal conductivity.

The latest model of the Halo System (PMT Corporation, Chanhassen, MN) has incorporated several changes to keep up with the times (Fig. 187-14). Simply displacing the buckles yields cleaner lateral radiographs. The use of carbon graphite and titanium materials provides clear MRI or CT scans. New nylon ball joints make assembly quicker and easier. Adjustable headblocks can be independently adjusted to allow anterior-posterior positioning, flexion-extension, and traction-distraction.

Compliance monitors have been developed to objectively assess and optimize patient compliance to prescribed orthoses. Three devices are currently commercially available: the HOBO H8 4-Channel External device, the StowAway TidbiT data logger and temperature sensor, and the IntelliBRACE force sensor system.[89]

The HOBO H8 4-Channel External device consists of a data logger and a temperature sensor (Fig. 187-15) and is manufactured by Onset Computer Corporation (Bourne, MA). This compliance monitor weighs approximately 1 oz. Data obtained by the HOBO may be uploaded by using Onset Computer Corporation's BoxCar Pro software and personal computer (PC) interface cable.[89]

The commercially available StowAway TidbiT consists of a data logger and an internal temperature sensor (Fig. 187-16). This device was adapted for this study by Onset Computer Corporation, the manufacturer, with a permanently attached external temperature sensor. The TidbiT weighs 0.8 ounces and may be mounted to a brace, such as a TLSO, with Velcro. To upload data to a PC also requires the use of Onset Computer Corporation's BoxCar Pro software. For launching and readout purposes, the StowAway TidbiT uses an Optic Base Station connected to the PC.[89]

The IntelliBRACE System consists of a data logger and a force sensor that detects pressure (Fig. 187-17). This compliance monitor is manufactured by X3 Technologies (Edmonton, Canada). Data obtained from this compliance monitor were read by using IntelliBRACE Clinical Analysis Software and a PC interface cable.[89]

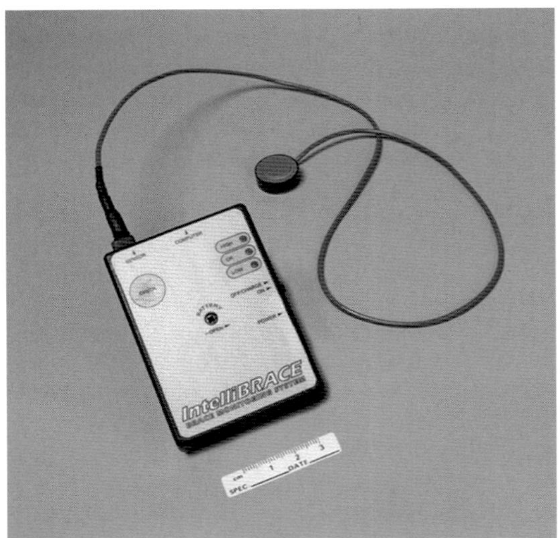

FIGURE 187-17. IntelliBRACE system. (From Hunter LN, Sison-Williamson M, Mendoza MM, et al: The validity of compliance monitors to assess wearing time of thoracic-lumbar-sacral orthoses in children with spinal cord injury. *Spine [Phila Pa 1976]* 33[14]:1554–1561, 2008.)

KEY REFERENCES

Benzel EC: Spinal orthotics. In Menezes AH, Sonntag VKH, editors: *Principles of spinal surgery*, New York, 1996, McGraw-Hill, pp 181–190.

Benzel EC, Hadden TA, Saulsbery CM: A comparison of the Minerva and halo jackets for stabilization of the cervical spine. *J Neurosurg* 70:411–414, 1989.

Johnson RM, Hart DL, Simmons EF, et al: Cervical orthoses: a study comparing their effectiveness in restricting cervical motion in normal subjects. *J Bone Joint Surg [Am]* 59:332–339, 1977.

Krag MH: Biomechanics of the cervical spine: orthoses. In Frymoyer JW, editor: *The adult spine: principles and practice*, ed 2, Philadelphia, 1997, Lippincott-Raven, pp 1110–1117.

Patwardhan AG, Li SP, Gavin T, et al: Orthotic stabilization of thoracolumbar injuries: a biomechanical analysis of the Jewett hyperextension orthosis. *Spine (Phila Pa 1976)* 15:654–661, 1990.

Sypert GW: External spinal orthotics. *Neurosurgery* 20:642–649, 1987.

White AA, Panjabi MM: *Clinical biomechanics of the spine*, Philadelphia, 1978, Lippincott-Raven.

REFERENCES

The complete reference list is available online at expertconsult.com.

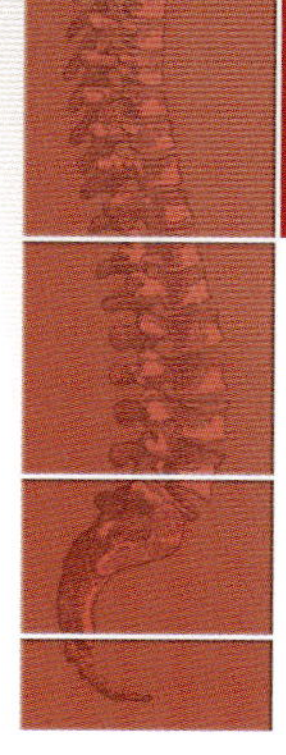

CHAPTER 188

Medical Management of Neck and Low Back Pain

Daniel J. Mazanec | Russell C. DeMicco

Back pain is common and costly. It was the most frequent type of pain reported by U.S. respondents in the 2002 National Health Information Survey (NHIS), with more than one fourth of adults reporting an episode of low back pain lasting at least 1 day in the preceding 3 months.[1] In the NHIS survey, neck pain ranked third, with 13.8% of persons reporting at least a 1-day episode. Back pain ranks in the top five reasons for visits to primary care physicians in the United States.[1,2] Up to 71% of the adult population may experience a significant episode of neck pain in their lifetimes.[3] Approximately 2% of the U.S. workforce sustains a compensable back injury each year.[4] The direct cost of health care attributed for low back pain exceeds $25 billion dollars in the United States.[5] The largest proportion of direct medical costs for back pain is spent on physical therapy (17%), followed by pharmacy (13%) and primary care physician visits (13%).[6] Indirect costs related to lost productivity in the workplace or homes are substantially higher than the direct costs of back pain.[6]

An appreciation of the benign short-term prognosis of acute nonradicular low back pain is fundamental to the management of these patients. Most patients recover within 1 month and more than 90% of patients have returned to work by 3 months.[7] However, about one fourth of patients have persistent symptoms at 3 months and about 20% have substantial limitations of activity at 1 year.[8,9] Clearly, an important objective of medical treatment should be to reduce the likelihood of progression from acute symptoms to chronic pain and functional impairment. The primary determinants of persistent disability at 12 months are psychosocial in nature.[8,10] In fact, psychosocial variables have been shown to be superior to structural findings or discography as predictors of both long- and short-term disability, duration of symptoms, and health care visits for back pain.[11] High levels of psychological distress, depressive mood, and somatization are well established as risk factors for transition from acute back pain to chronicity.[8,12] Coping styles characterized by catastrophizing or fear avoidance are suspected but less well established as predisposing to the development of chronic symptoms. Failure to recognize these psychosocial issues in patients with low back pain will frustrate even the most well-conceived medical management strategy.

Etiology of Back and Neck Pain

The specific anatomic etiology of nonradicular spinal pain is often ambiguous. Up to 85% of patients have pain that cannot be assigned to a particular pain generator.[13] "Abnormal" findings on plain radiographs, including spondylolysis, spondylolisthesis, facet joint degenerative changes, Schmorl nodes, and mild scoliosis, are common in asymptomatic persons.[14] Radiography of the lumbar spine in patients with back pain of at least 6 weeks' duration (mean, 10 weeks) has been shown to increase patient satisfaction without any improvement in functional outcome or severity of pain.[15] The addition of lateral dynamic flexion-extension radiographs to the initial evaluation of patients with low back pain rarely provides information that alters clinical management, at the expense of significant additional cost and radiation exposure.[16] Disc abnormalities are found on MRI in more than 50% of asymptomatic persons by age 40 years and include degenerative disc bulging and protrusions as well as Schmorl nodes.[17] The lack of specificity of clinical symptoms and signs for the multiple potential sources of spinal pain—ligaments, facet joints, discs, paravertebral musculature—confounds the attempt to attribute symptoms to radiographic findings. In some patients previously categorized as having nonspecific pain, interventional diagnostic techniques, including discography, facet joint medial branch block or injection, and sacroiliac joint injection, may suggest a specific pathoanatomic etiology. However, these studies have high false-positive rates, particularly in patients with psychosocial issues, and fail to reliably predict the success of specific surgical or interventional treatments.[11,14]

Cancer and infection are serious but fortunately uncommon specific causes of back pain found in 0.7% and 0.01%, respectively, of patients presenting in a primary care setting.[13] The spine is one of the most common sites of metastasis, most commonly arising from breast, lung, prostate, or kidney primary tumors.[18] Ankylosing spondylitis is identified in about 0.3% of patients with low back pain, typically younger men.[14] Acute or subacute vertebral compression fractures are identified in about 4% of patients. A variety of nonspinal conditions may present with symptoms that mimic spine disorders. These include common musculoskeletal problems such as greater trochanteric bursitis and osteoarthritis of the hip, as well as visceral problems such as kidney stones, aortic aneurysms, and peptic ulcers.

The American College of Physicians and American Pain Society's recently published evidence-based clinical practice guideline for the management of back pain suggests a focused history and physical examination should permit placement of patients with back pain into one of three broad categories: nonspecific low back pain, back pain with radicular symptoms including lumbar spinal stenosis, and back pain associated with another specific spinal cause.[13] Diagnostic imaging is

BOX 188-1. American College of Physicians and the American Pain Society: Recommendations for the Evaluation of Low Back Pain

Recommendation 1: Conduct a focused history and physical examination to categorize patients into one of three categories: nonspecific low back pain, back pain potentially associated with radiculopathy or spinal stenosis, or back pain potentially associated with another specific spine cause. Evaluate for psychosocial risk factors which predict risk for chronic, disabling low back pain.

Recommendation 2: Imaging or other diagnostic tests should not be obtained routinely in patients with nonspecific low back pain.

Recommendation 3: Perform diagnostic imaging and testing for patients with low back pain when severe or progressive neurologic deficits are present or when serious underlying conditions are suspected on the basis of history and physical examination.

Recommendation 4: Evaluate patients with persistent low back pain and signs or symptoms of radiculopathy or stenosis with MR (preferred) or CT only if they are potential candidates for surgery or epidural steroid injection.

From Chou R, Qaseem A, Snow V, et al: Diagnosis and treatment of low back pain: a joint clinical practice guideline from the American College of Physicians and the American Pain Society. *Ann Intern Med* 147:478–491, 2007.

recommended only when a serious etiology (cancer or infection) is suspected or when surgical or other interventional treatment is imminent (Box 188-1). For patients with nonspecific, nonradicular back pain, the guideline incorporates education, activity, physical therapy, medications, and a range of nonpharmacologic therapies.

Medical Treatment Options

Prevention

In view of the enormous personal, societal, and financial burden of back pain, numerous preventive approaches have been investigated. A recent systematic review of prospective, controlled trials of interventions to prevent back pain in working-age adults identified 20 trials that met inclusion criteria.[19] Only exercise, in seven of eight trials, was found effective in preventing self-reported episodes of back pain. A variety of exercise approaches were used, including stretching, strengthening of abdominal, back, and leg muscles, and general conditioning. Interventions found ineffective in reducing back pain episodes included stress management, shoe inserts, back supports, ergonomic and back education, and reduced lifting programs. Although evidence for efficacy in prevention of back pain is lacking, smoking cessation and reduction to appropriate weight for height should be encouraged because both smoking and obesity have been associated with increased severity of back symptoms.[20,21]

Exercise and Physical Therapy

For patients with acute (<4 weeks) back or neck pain, there is little evidence that formal physical therapy is necessary.[22] The best advice for such patients is probably to continue with their usual activities as tolerated. In fact, early referral to physical therapy prolonged duration of symptoms compared with patients simply advised to stay active.[23] For patients with persistent chronic neck or back symptoms, however, exercise therapy is the cornerstone of medical treatment to decrease pain and restore function and mobility. An impairment-based manual physical therapy and exercise program resulted in clinically and statistically significant short- and long-term improvements in pain, disability, and patient-perceived recovery in patients with mechanical neck pain compared with a program comprising advice, mobility exercise, and subtherapeutic ultrasonography.[24] Similarly, a recent meta-analysis found that exercise therapy was effective at decreasing pain and improving function in adults with chronic low back pain and may improve work absenteeism in patients with subacute symptoms.[22] Unfortunately, studies comparing different exercise approaches, including stabilization, McKenzie, Pilates, and general aerobic conditioning, are insufficient to strongly recommend a single approach in a particular subset of patients. However, two recent studies have suggested that selection of a physical therapy approach based on diagnosis or mechanical assessment is more effective than general nonspecific exercise advice.[25,26]

General aerobic conditioning is often recommended for patients with chronic neck or back pain. The sense of well-being and accomplishment acquired from a planned aerobic exercise program such as walking, running, cycling, or swimming creates a positive treatment milieu and further establishes the extent of patient motivation and commitment to the overall treatment plan. Patients participating in an aerobic exercise program have been shown to receive fewer prescriptions for pain, were given fewer physical therapy referrals, and had improved mood states and lessened depression.[27]

Evidence suggests the superiority of neck stabilization exercises, with some advantages in pain and disability outcomes, compared with isometric and stretching exercises in combination with physical therapy agents (transcutaneous electrical nerve stimulation, continuous ultrasonography, and infrared irradiation) for the management of neck pain.[28] There is moderate evidence that lumbar stabilization exercises are effective in improving pain and function in a heterogeneous group of patients with chronic low back pain.[29] Unfortunately, available studies are unable to define a specific subgroup of patients with chronic low back pain most suitable for this exercise approach. The current evidence suggests that in the short term, lumbar extensor strengthening exercise administered alone or with cointerventions is more effective than no treatment and most passive modalities in improving pain, disability, and other patient-reported outcomes in chronic low back pain.[30]

Yoga and Pilates exercises have grown in popularity over the last decade and represent two mind-body exercise interventions that address both the physical and mental aspects of pain with core strengthening, flexibility, and relaxation. There has been a gradual trend toward inclusion of these nontraditional exercise regimens into treatment paradigms for back pain, although few studies critically examining their effects have been published.[31] A retrospective analysis of two randomized, controlled trials and one case-controlled series found significant improvement in general function and pain with the Pilates approach in treating nonspecific chronic low back pain in adults. However, as with other exercise paradigms, currently available data do not predict which groups of patients might be best managed with this approach.[32]

The McKenzie method is a unique and comprehensive approach to neck or low back pain that includes both assessment and intervention. The assessment is designed to detect a directional preference, which refers to a particular direction of movement or sustained posture that causes symptoms to centralize, decrease, or be abolished. *Centralization* is defined as the sequential and lasting abolition of all distal referred symptoms and subsequent abolition of any remaining spinal pain in response to a single direction of repeated movements or sustained postures. The finding of centralization has positive prognostic value, provided treatment is guided by assessment findings. Noncentralization is a strong predictor of poor prognosis and correlates well with "nonorganic" signs.[33] In limited clinical trials, McKenzie-based therapy produces results comparable with those of stabilization or strengthening programs.[34,35]

Aquatic exercise is potentially beneficial to patients suffering from chronic low back pain and pregnancy-related low back pain.[36] Patients with barriers to land-based programs, including lower extremity joint disorders and obesity, are often able to exercise actively in the pool.

Medication

In addition to passage of time, participation in an active exercise program, and use of nonpharmacologic treatments, medicinal treatment is an important component of medical management of neck and back pain. Medications with reasonable evidence of short-term effectiveness for low back pain include nonsteroidal anti-inflammatory drugs (NSAIDs), acetaminophen, skeletal muscle relaxants (for acute low back pain), and tricyclic antidepressants (for chronic low back pain).[37] Evidence suggests that NSAIDs are no more effective than pure analgesics for low back pain.[33]

Acetaminophen

Acetaminophen (acetyl-para-aminophenol [APAP]) has analgesic and antipyretic properties comparable with aspirin, but its anti-inflammatory effects are weak. APAP's analgesic effects and excellent safety profile make it a reasonable first-line medication for acute back and neck pain. Peak analgesic effects are typically noted from 30 to 60 minutes after ingestion. APAP is relatively inexpensive and produces fewer adverse reactions than NSAIDs. Although recent systematic reviews have found APAP as effective as NSAIDs in the treatment of back pain, in other musculoskeletal disorders, particularly osteoarthritis of the hip or knee, NSAIDs provide better pain relief.[39] The accepted oral dose of acetaminophen is 325 to 1000 mg every 4 to 6 hours, not to exceed 4000 mg in 24 hours. The most serious adverse effect of acute acetaminophen overdosage is hepatotoxicity. Risk of hepatotoxicity is increased in patients with known liver disease, heavy alcohol use, or severe fasting states due to vomiting, diarrhea, or severe flu. A major current concern is accidental overdosage in patients who take APAP in addition to a prescription analgesic containing APAP. In adults, serious hepatotoxicity may occur from a single dose of 10 to 15 g.

Nonsteroidal Anti-Inflammatory Drugs

The NSAIDs relieve both pain and inflammation and are a reasonable choice as a first-line agent for the control of acute low back or neck pain in patients without significant risk factors for adverse effects. A recent systematic review of randomized, controlled trials found NSAIDs were effective for short-term relief of acute and chronic back pain, but no more effective than acetaminophen.[40] This review and others have concluded that all NSAIDs, including cyclooxygenase-2 (COX-2) inhibitors, are equally effective in treating low back pain.[41] Because efficacy among these drugs is comparable, the choice of a particular NSAID is based on cost and safety, particularly in patients at higher risk for adverse effects. GI toxicity is the major limiting factor to NSAID therapy, with serious ulcer complications (bleeding or perforation) seen in about 1.5% of treated patients. All NSAIDs may increase the risk of a cardiovascular event in patients at risk. The American Heart Association recommendations for drug therapy for musculoskeletal pain in patients at cardiovascular risk favor pure analgesics as the drugs of first choice, with nonacetylated salicylates such as salsalate or non-COX-2–selective drugs (particularly naproxen) as alternative choices.[42] Other potential side effects include renal failure, tinnitus, fluid retention, and high blood pressure. Although some variability with regard to adverse effects has been recognized, all NSAIDs can cause central nervous system side effects such as drowsiness, dizziness, and confusion. If an NSAID is used, frequent clinical and laboratory monitoring for adverse renal or GI reactions is mandatory. Risk factors for NSAID toxicity include age older than 65 years, known or suspected cardiovascular disease, history of congestive heart failure, history of recent GI bleed or ulcer, kidney disease, hepatic cirrhosis, and history of aspirin-induced respiratory disease. NSAIDs should also be avoided in patients in the third trimester of pregnancy. Acetaminophen is relatively inexpensive with a superior safety profile to NSAIDs and is the first choice in such high-risk patients.[43]

Oral Steroids

Medications such as prednisone and methylprednisolone are potent corticosteroids with strong anti-inflammatory properties. Corticosteroids are effective in the treatment of inflammatory reactions associated with allergic states, rheumatic and autoimmune diseases, and respiratory disorders. Studies designed to investigate the use of oral steroids in the setting of low back or neck pain are limited. A placebo-controlled trial of a single dose of intravenous methylprednisolone in acute low back pain demonstrated no significant improvement in the steroid-treated group.[44] Despite lack of any published evidence for efficacy, oral corticosteroids are widely prescribed to treat acute back or neck pain, particularly with radicular symptoms. Dosage schedules vary, but 7 to 14 days of tapering from a prednisone equivalent dose of 40 to 60 mg is typical. Patients with diabetes should be warned about steroid-induced hyperglycemia. The risk of steroid-induced osteonecrosis is a concern, but the risk appears low.

Antidepressant Medications

Antidepressants are often used in the treatment of chronic musculoskeletal pain as well as in neuropathic pain syndromes.

Although there is no evidence to support their use in acute pain, the efficacy of antidepressants in patients with chronic low back pain is reasonably well established. Antidepressant drug therapy may be beneficial in these patients because up to one third of them also experience depression. However, treating nondepressed patients with tricyclic antidepressants has been shown to significantly improve neuropathic-type pain compared with placebo, but without an improvement in functional status.[45] In contrast to tricyclic antidepressants, newer selective serotonin reuptake inhibitors have not been demonstrated to be effective in treating back or neck pain.

Opioids

Since the initial report of Portenoy and Foley describing the use of long-term opioid analgesics in treating nonmalignant pain, opioids have gained increasing acceptance as an appropriate therapy for carefully selected patients with spinal pain.[46] A recent study found 66% of patients treated in an orthopaedic spine practice received opioids, 25% for longer than 3 months.[47] Despite increasing use, concerns about long-term opioid use in chronic nonmalignant pain remain, including risk of abuse, tolerance, and dependence as well as fear of disciplinary action by medical boards for prescribing physicians. In addition, studies of opioids in chronic back pain have inconsistently demonstrated improvement in functional status in addition to pain. Furthermore, long-term trials demonstrating sustained benefit with acceptable toxicity are few.

Opioids are available in sustained-release (sustained release [SR], controlled release [CR], extended release [ER]) forms with prolonged analgesic effect lasting up to 72 hours (fentanyl transdermal), or short-acting immediate-release preparations with analgesic effect for 2 to 6 hours.[48] Most opioids undergo first-pass metabolism in the liver, by oxidation involving cytochrome P-450 enzymes (fentanyl, oxycodone) and/or by glucuronidation (morphine, oxymorphone).[49] Differences in opioid efficacy are partially related to genetic factors involving cytochrome P-450 alleles. Other clinically important differences in opioid metabolism are related to age, sex, and ethnicity.

Although most opioids share common pharmacologic properties and mechanisms of action, unique properties of selected agents are clinically relevant. Methadone is an effective and relatively inexpensive, long-acting opioid analgesic with unique pharmacokinetics and mechanism of action. In addition to activity at the mu-opioid receptor like other agents, methadone inhibits serotonin uptake and antagonizes the *N*-methyl-D-aspartate (NMDA) receptor, potentially offering superior efficacy for neuropathic pain. However, because of a disparity between duration of analgesic effect (8 hours) and drug half-life (24–26 hours), initiating treatment with methadone must be done cautiously, with increments in the dose at 5- to 7-day intervals.[50] Tramadol and its active metabolite exert their analgesic effect as both mu receptor agonists and by nonopioid inhibition of serotonin and norepinephrine reuptake.[49] Coadministration of tramadol with antidepressants of the selective serotonin reuptake inhibitor class risks development of a "serotonin syndrome" manifested by hyperactivity, agitation, fever, seizures, and even death.[51] Finally, meperidine has a half-life of 3 hours, but the half-life of its inactive metabolite normeperidine is about 20 hours. Repeated administration of meperidine for pain relief may result in toxic levels of normeperidine, particularly in elderly patients. Clinical manifestations of normeperidine toxicity include tremors, hallucinations, and seizures.[52]

Several recent reviews of both short- and long-acting opioids in chronic low back pain have concluded that opioids are safe and effective, at least in the short term, in reducing symptoms.[48,53,54] In general, among patients able to tolerate opioid therapy, about one third can be classified as excellent responders, one third as "fair" responders, and one third as nonresponders.[48] Magnitude of pain reduction in these trials as assessed by visual analogue scale ranges from 2.0 to 3.8. In most studies approximately one third of opioid-treated patients withdraw because of intolerable adverse effects. Significant improvement in pain and function, assessed by the Oswestry Disability Index (ODI) for low back pain, was sustained up to 1 year in a case series of patients with refractory chronic low back pain treated with opioids.[55] Two recent trials found little evidence of tolerance or addiction and abusive behavior in patients with back pain treated with long-term opioids.[47,56] However, another recent systematic review of opioid treatment in patients with chronic low back pain found "aberrant medication-taking behavior" in 5% to 24% of patients.[53] However, the authors noted that the studies reviewed failed to control for aberrant behavior related to inadequate pain control ("pseudoaddictive behavior").

Unlike other analgesics, including acetaminophen or NSAIDs, opioids are not toxic to the liver, kidneys, brain, or other organs. Common adverse effects include constipation, nausea, vomiting, dry mouth, sedation, and sweating.[48] Unlike most other adverse effects, tolerance does not develop to opioid-induced constipation. Prophylactic treatment with laxatives and stool softeners should be considered in all patients beginning opioid therapy. Although concerns have been raised whether opioid-treated patients can drive safely, a systematic review found no impairment of psychomotor abilities of opioid-dependent patients.[57] The best approach is probably to counsel patients to be aware of possible transient cognitive impairment and not to drive or engage in dangerous work situations, particularly when initiating opioid treatment or increasing the dose. In men, androgen deficiency manifested by low libido, erectile dysfunction, and lack of energy is a concern because opioids suppress gonadotropin-releasing hormone.[58] Whether long-term opioid therapy with gonadotropin-releasing hormone suppression results in bone loss ("opioid osteoporosis") is uncertain.

Tolerance, the need to increase opioid dosage to maintain the same therapeutic effect, appears to be uncommon in patients with low back pain treated with opioids.[47,55] Physical dependence on opioids and addictive behavior are often confused. Dependence is a state of physiologic adaption characterized by withdrawal symptoms when the drug is abruptly discontinued. Most opioid-treated patients become dependent within a few weeks of initiating treatment. Addiction, on the other hand, represents a maladaptive disorder characterized by compulsive use of an opioid despite biologic psychological, or social harm.[48] In the absence of a prior history of substance abuse, the risk of addiction in opioid-treated patients with low back pain appears low. When opioid therapy is considered in patients with chronic spinal pain, a careful assessment of risk for abuse, misuse, or diversion should be performed. This assessment should include evaluation for known risk factors, including smoking, psychiatric disorders, and personal history or family history of substance abuse.[59] In patients on long-term opioid therapy, risk management for abuse should include use of a prescription monitoring program as is available in most states, an opioid treatment agreement outlining risk, benefits, and behavior expectations to the patient beginning therapy, compliance monitoring with urine drug screens or pill counts, and regular assessment of the "Four A's" of pain treatment: analgesia, activities of daily living, adverse events, and aberrant drug-taking behavior.[59]

Muscle Relaxants

Muscle relaxants are widely used to treat low back and neck pain, presumably to address muscle spasm as the primary source of spinal pain or as a secondary phenomenon superimposed on underlying spine pathology. These drugs, which include benzodiazepine and nonbenzodiazepine antispasmodics and antispasticity agents, are believed to act centrally at the brainstem or spinal cord level.[60] Systematic reviews of muscle relaxants for nonspecific low back pain have concluded that all are comparably effective in providing early, short-term pain relief compared with placebo, but with significant risk of side effects. In acute back pain, the treatment benefit appears greatest in the first few days and declines rapidly after the first week of symptoms. There is limited evidence that combination of an NSAID and a muscle relaxant is modestly more effective than either agent alone.[61] No studies have demonstrated benefit of muscle relaxants in chronic low back pain.[62,63]

Approximately 50% of persons treated with muscle relaxants experience an adverse effect, most commonly dizziness and sedation.[60] Benzodiazepines, cyclobenzaprine, and tizanidine tend to be more sedating than metaxalone or methocarbamol. However, alertness and cognitive acuity may be impaired by any muscle relaxant. Carisoprodol is metabolized to meprobamate, a highly addictive barbiturate. Because carisoprodol is not more effective than alternative muscle relaxants, it should be avoided. Cyclobenzaprine is chemically in the same class as tricyclic antidepressants and should not be used in patients with significant cardiac arrhythmias.

The selection of a muscle relaxant is based primarily on the risk of adverse effects, abuse potential, and drug interactions because efficacy is comparable for all of the agents. In patients with insomnia or disrupted sleep, a sedating agent such as cyclobenzaprine or tizanidine may be preferable. For patients intolerant of sedative effects, a trial of metaxalone or methocarbamol is appropriate.

Anticonvulsants, Antiepileptics, and Membrane Stabilizers

There is limited evidence directly evaluating the efficacy of antiepileptic medications for chronic low back, radicular, or neuropathic pain. However, use of these medications may be reasonable for patients with persistent back or neck pain despite treatment with simple analgesics, NSAIDs, or tricyclic antidepressants.[64] Gabapentin has U.S. Food and Drug Administration (FDA)–approved labeling for trigeminal neuralgia, but is widely used to treat neuropathic pain of other sources. Dose-related sedation is a limiting factor with gabapentin. Pregabalin is one of the newer membrane stabilizers used in painful neuropathic and musculoskeletal conditions, including fibromyalgia. Carbamazepine is an older anticonvulsant that has FDA-approved labeling for trigeminal neuralgia and is sometimes used for other types of neuropathic pain. Oxcarbamazepine, topiramate, lamotrigine, tiagabine, and valproate have been reported in case studies to offer relief from neuropathic discomfort. These agents are typically used at their anticonvulsant dosages. Antiepileptic drugs act at several sites that may be relevant to pain, but the precise mechanism of their analgesic effect remains unclear. They may limit neuronal excitation and enhance inhibition. Transmission of painful stimuli through the spinal column and central nervous system is modulated by excitatory and inhibitory neurotransmitters, as well as actions at sodium and calcium channels. Antidepressants and antiepileptic drugs are also thought to diminish neuropathic pain through interaction with specific neurotransmitters and ion channels.

Topicals

Topical pain-relieving medications are preparations applied to the skin as a cream, ointment, gel, patch, or spray. Although widely used by patients with spinal pain, evidence of significant benefit for pain and function is minimal. Common types of topical pain relievers include local anesthetics, analgesics, and anti-inflammatories, including salicylates. Another readily available, somewhat unusual, and widely used topical medication is capsaicin, which is derived from hot peppers. Capsaicin's therapeutic effect is attributed to reduction of the pain neurotransmitter, substance P.

Acupuncture

Acupuncture is based on Chinese traditions and concepts dating to more than 2000 years ago. Illness in classical Chinese medicine is defined by disharmony or imbalance in *yin* and *yang*, with resultant disruption in the flow of *qi* in the various meridians or channels through which it flows. In this paradigm, treatment requires insertion of needles in specific points to influence movement of *qi*, tonify deficient *yin* or *yang*, or disperse excess *yang*.

As acupuncture has become established in the West, studies investigating its physiologic effects have found several potential explanations for the analgesic effect of the procedure. Because acupuncture stimulates A delta fibers entering the dorsal horn of the spinal cord, potentially inhibiting unmyelinated C-fiber pain impulses, a gate theory mechanism of analgesia has been suggested. Acupuncture needling increases cerebrospinal fluid levels of various neuropeptides, including serotonin, endorphins, and enkephalins, an effect that can be blocked by naloxone.[65] An anti-inflammatory effect of acupuncture has been proposed based on elevated adrenocorticotropic hormone levels noted after needling. Functional MRI of the brain has demonstrated that acupuncture activates central antinociceptive pathways while decreasing activity in limbic areas involved in pain processing.[66] Evidence that acupuncture meridians and points correspond to intermuscular or intramuscular fascia has led to the hypothesis that needling may stimulate bioelectrical or biochemical signaling along these connective tissue planes.[67]

Acupuncture has been increasingly accepted as a useful modality in the treatment of back and neck pain.

Approximately two thirds of pain specialists and rheumatologists report referrals to practitioners of acupuncture.[68,69] A National Institutes of Health consensus conference in 1998 concluded that acupuncture might be useful as an adjunct treatment for low back pain or an acceptable alternative to be included in a comprehensive management program.[70] Ten years later, the recently published American College of Physicians and American Pain Society guideline on the diagnosis and treatment of low back pain recommends acupuncture be considered as a nonpharmacologic treatment with proven benefits for patients with chronic or subacute, nonspecific low back pain.[13] A recent systematic review of the effectiveness of acupuncture for back pain found 23 randomized, controlled trials including more than 6000 patients.[71] This analysis concluded that there is moderate evidence that acupuncture is more effective than no treatment and strong evidence of no significant difference between acupuncture and sham acupuncture for short-term pain relief. The authors also concluded that there is strong evidence that acupuncture can be a useful supplement to other forms of conventional treatment for nonspecific low back pain. Another recent systematic review of acupuncture in patients with chronic low back pain included 19 studies with more than 5000 patients and concluded that the most consistent evidence demonstrated that the addition of acupuncture to other therapies was superior in pain relief and functional improvement compared with the same therapies without acupuncture.[72] A variant of acupuncture, percutaneous electrical nerve stimulation (PENS), has been demonstrated to be significantly more effective than sham-PENS, transcutaneous electrical nerve stimulation (TENS), and exercise in treating back pain attributed to degenerative disc disease.[73] This technique uses electrical stimulation of acupuncture needles that have been placed in soft tissue or muscular points arrayed to stimulate peripheral sensory nerves in a dermatomal distribution corresponding to the local pathologic process.

A systematic review of acupuncture for neck pain found 10 randomized, controlled trials of variable quality and concluded there was moderate evidence that acupuncture was more effective for pain relief than sham procedures immediately after treatment and at short-term follow-up.[3] For chronic neck pain, acupuncture has been shown to be superior to massage.[74] In this study, however, no difference was found between "real" and "sham" acupuncture.

A reasonable trial of acupuncture in most patients requires 6 to 10 treatments, perhaps more in older patients. Acupuncture is contraindicated in patients with severe bleeding disorders or systemic infection. Electroacupuncture should be avoided in patients with pacemakers, defibrillators, implanted medication pumps, and implanted neuromodulating devices. In pregnant patients, acupuncture points that may stimulate labor are "forbidden." Opioid-dependent patients may be less responsive to acupuncture. Serious complications of acupuncture such as organ or vascular puncture are extremely rare. Minor adverse effects, including local bleeding or pain, are seen in about 5% of patients.[72]

Manipulation

Spinal manipulation is defined as the application of high-velocity, low-amplitude manual thrusts to the spinal joints with movement beyond the passive range of motion.[75] Although the use of spinal manipulation for healing was described in the writings of Galen and Hippocrates, the "modern era" of manipulation dates to the late 19th century, when both chiropractic treatment and osteopathy emerged as medical disciplines.[76] Chiropractors perform more than 90% of all manipulations in the United States, but other practitioners include osteopathic physicians and physical therapists.[77] Almost 90% of visits to chiropractors are for neck or back pain.[78]

Manipulation techniques vary considerably based on the training of the practitioner. In general, osteopathic manipulation uses a long-lever, lower-velocity technique using a long bone such as the femur to apply force to one or more joints.[77] Short-lever, higher-velocity manipulation of a specific joint represents the more commonly performed chiropractic spinal "adjustment." More recently, medicine-assisted manipulation has been reintroduced, primarily in the chiropractic community. This technique involves spinal manipulation after local anesthesia (epidural or facet) or with deep conscious sedation.[79] To date, medicine assisted–manipulation has not been evaluated in a controlled trial.

The precise mechanism of action for any effects attributed to manipulation remains unknown. Current hypotheses focus on either direct effects on the facet joints themselves or secondary neurologic effects of facet and myofascial manipulation. Manipulation may release trapped synovial plica, alter orientation of the joint, relax periarticular hypertonic muscles, disrupt adhesions, or unbuckle abnormal motion segments.[75,77] There is some evidence that manipulation may affect afferent nerves in the paraspinal musculature, inhibiting excessive reflex activity and potentially affecting central pain processing.[80,81]

For patients with acute or subacute low back pain, manipulation has been shown to be superior to sham manipulation but not statistically or clinically superior to general care, analgesics, physical therapy, exercises, or back schools.[82] In a randomized clinical trial, patients with acute and subacute back pain treated with osteopathic manipulation required significantly less medication than the standard care group, however.[83] In another large, prospective, randomized trial comparing chiropractic manipulation with medical care, including physical therapy, similar outcomes were noted in pain and disability, but patients treated with manipulation had a greater likelihood of perceived improvement.[84] For patients with chronic low back pain, a recent systematic review of 11 trials including approximately 1200 patients found moderate evidence that manipulation was superior to usual medical care or placebo for patient-rated improvement.[75] Manipulation with strengthening exercises was comparable to prescription NSAIDs for pain relief. For mechanical neck pain, manipulation in addition to exercise was found superior to waiting list controls for pain reduction in a systematic review of 33 trials.[85]

Mild adverse effects of spinal manipulation occur in 30% to 61% of all patients.[86] Most of these effects occur within 4 hours of treatment and resolve the same day. The most common symptoms reported include local discomfort (53%), headache (12%), tiredness (11%), radiating discomfort (10%), and dizziness (5%).[87] Serious adverse affects of lumbar manipulation such as disc herniation or cauda equina syndrome are rare, estimated at 1 event per 3.72 million manipulations.[88] Risk of serious injury from cervical manipulation, particularly vertebral artery dissection, is well described, but the frequency is unknown. Although likely rare, the consequences of this complication are potentially catastrophic, such that some have suggested avoidance of cervical manipulation in patients with known atherosclerotic cardiovascular disease.[86]

Massage

Massage, defined as manipulation of muscle and fascia using one's hands or a mechanical device, is a widely used adjunctive treatment in patients with neck and back pain. Common variations of massage include Rolfing, Swedish massage, acupuncture massage, myofascial release, and craniosacral therapy. Therapeutic benefits of massage have been attributed to local effects, including increased blood flow and oxygenation of tissues and relaxation of tight muscles.[89,90] Other proposed mechanisms include stimulation of serotonin or endorphin release, as well as effects on pain transmission at the spinal segmental level.

Recent systematic reviews of massage therapy have concluded that massage is effective for subacute and chronic low back pain.[89,90] Although limited in number and mixed in quality, clinical trials have shown massage is more effective than exercise, acupuncture, and self-care education in improving symptoms and function in patients with nonspecific low back pain.[91,92] Several trials have suggested that the addition of massage to exercise improves outcome in patients with low back pain compared with exercise alone.[90] These studies also suggest that the experience of the massage therapist influences outcome. The optimal number and frequency of treatments are not known.

Studies of massage for chronic neck pain are less definitive. A recent review of 19 trials of massage for "mechanical" neck pain found 12 were of low quality.[93] The remaining studies of massage for neck pain as a stand-alone treatment or as part of a multimodality treatment approach were inconclusive.

Traction

Theoretically, the objective of spinal traction is to distract the vertebrae, potentially reducing protrusion of a bulging or herniated disc. Approximately 1.5 times a patient's body weight is needed to develop distraction of the vertebral bodies. This is rarely achieved in clinical practice because patient tolerance is poor. No specific effect of traction over standard physiotherapeutic interventions was observed in adults with chronic neck pain. Conceptually, traction may be useful as an adjunct to active exercise therapy to assist in releasing muscle spasm and facilitating active therapy, but evidence for benefit is lacking.[94] The current literature does not support or refute the effectiveness of continuous or intermittent traction for pain reduction, improved function, or global perceived effect compared with placebo traction, tablet or heat, or other conservative treatments in patients with chronic neck disorders.[95] Only limited evidence is available to warrant the routine use of nonsurgical spinal decompression, particularly when many other well-investigated, less expensive alternatives are available.[96]

Summary: An Aggressive, Evidence-Informed Approach to Nonsurgical Management of Back and Neck Pain

Acute Pain (<4 Weeks)

If a focused history and physical examination, carefully assessing risk factors for underlying serious causes ("red flags") and psychosocial risk factors for prolonged recovery and disability ("yellow flags") is unrevealing, initial treatment should include a simple, age-appropriate analgesic or NSAID for symptom control and emphasize the importance of maintaining physical activities as tolerated (Box 188-2). For patients with significant muscle spasm, the addition of a muscle relaxant for up to 1 week is appropriate. Perhaps the most important feature of early treatment is education of the patient about the favorable natural history of low back or neck pain, the benefits of early appropriate physical activity, and the importance of general health measures in promoting spine wellness, including smoking cessation, aerobic exercise, and weight management.

Subacute Pain (4 to 12 Weeks)

Patients with nonspecific back or neck pain who have persistent significant symptoms and impaired function after 4 weeks of appropriate medical therapy must be reevaluated. Repeating a careful history and physical examination is required, including another search for previously unrecognized serious causes (infection, malignancy, or fracture) of pain as well as psychosocial barriers to recovery. Some patients may be identified whose clinical picture has now evolved from a purely axial pain syndrome to a radicular pattern, requiring a different approach. If indicated, and particularly in older

BOX 188-2. American College of Physicians and the American Pain Society: Recommendations for the Treatment of Low Back Pain

Recommendation: Provide patients with evidence-based information on low back pain with regard to expected course, advise patients to remain active, and provide information about effective self-care options.

Recommendation: Consider the use of medications with proven benefits in conjunction with back care information and self-care. Assess severity of pain and functional deficits, potential benefits, risks, and relative lack of long-term efficacy and safety data before initiating therapy. For most patients, first-line medication options are acetaminophen or NSAIDs.

Recommendation: For patients who do not improve with self-care options, clinicians should consider addition of nonpharmacologic therapy with proven benefits:

- For acute low back pain: manipulation
- For chronic low back pain: intensive interdisciplinary rehabilitation, exercise therapy, acupuncture, massage, manipulation, yoga, cognitive behavioral therapy, or progressive relaxation

From Chou R, Qaseem A, Snow V, et al: Diagnosis and treatment of low back pain: a joint clinical practice guideline from the American College of Physicians and the American Pain Society. *Ann Intern Med* 147:478–491, 2007.

patients, appropriate laboratory and imaging studies may be required. If this evaluation fails to identify new findings, more aggressive medical treatment is indicated, including referral for formal physical therapy, emphasizing an active exercise approach with education. Additional nonpharmacologic modalities, including acupuncture, manipulation, and massage therapy may be used to provide additional analgesic benefit and facilitate rehabilitation. Patients manifesting "yellow flags" may be referred for more formal psychosocial assessment and treatment. In the case of work-related back pain, vocational rehabilitation and active job-specific rehabilitation ("work hardening") may be indicated.

Chronic Pain (>3 Months)

When back or neck pain has persisted despite appropriate pharmacologic and nonpharmacologic treatment beyond 12 weeks, consideration should be given to more aggressive evaluation to identify a specific "pain generator," at least in certain subsets of patients. Patients younger than 50 years of age with persistent, severe, functionally limiting axial back pain and without apparent psychosocial barriers should have MRI to identify discrete potential anatomic sources of pain, including single-level degenerative disc disease and facet joint changes. If significant degenerative disease is found, interventional diagnostic testing with discography or facet joint block may be considered if the patient would consider interventional or surgical treatment if the diagnostic findings are positive. Unfortunately, the size of this subset of patients is unclear and clinical features purported to suggest discogenic or facet-mediated back pain are not reliable in predicting the results of interventional diagnostic studies. Clearly, therapeutic decisions require a shared decision-making approach based on a frank discussion with the patient about the limitations and uncertainties of these diagnostic studies. For most patients with chronic back and neck pain, the precise etiology remains ambiguous. Medical management should include aggressive active exercise as well as pharmacologic and nonpharmacologic symptom management, as discussed earlier. Pure nonopioid analgesics are appropriate for most patients and probably safer than long-term NSAID therapy. Adjunctive agents, including tricyclic antidepressants and newer mixed serotonin and norepinephrine reuptake inhibitors such as duloxetine, should be considered. For carefully selected patients with a clear structural source of pain, long-term opioid therapy may be considered. Regular monitoring for efficacy (pain and function) and abuse is mandatory. There is limited evidence that massage, acupuncture, yoga, and manipulation may also have an adjunctive role in some patients. In patients with significant functional impairment despite appropriate therapy, referral to a multidisciplinary center should be considered.

KEY REFERENCES

Carragee EJ, Alamin TF, Miller JL, et al: Discographic, MRI and psychosocial determinants of low back pain disability and remission: a prospective study in subjects with benign persistent back pain. *Spine J* 5:24–35, 2005.

Chang V, Gonzalez P, Akuthota V: Evidence-informed management of chronic low back pain with adjunctive analgesics. *Spine J* 8:21–27, 2008.

Chou R, Huffman LH: Medications for acute and chronic low back pain: a review of evidence for an American Pain Society/American College of Physicians clinical practice guideline. *Ann Intern Med* 147:505–514, 2007.

Chou R, Qaseem A, Snow V, et al: Diagnosis and treatment of low back pain: a joint clinical practice guideline from the American College of Physicians and the American Pain Society. *Ann Intern Med* 147:478–491, 2007.

Malanga G, Wolff E: Evidence-informed management of chronic low back pain with nonsteroidal anti-inflammatory drugs, muscle relaxants, and simple analgesics. *Spine J* 8:173–184, 2008.

May S, Donelson R: Evidence-informed management of chronic low back pain with the McKenzie method. *Spine J* 8:134–141, 2008.

Schofferman J, Mazanec D: Evidence-informed management of chronic low back pain with opioid analgesics. *Spine J* 8:185–194, 2008.

REFERENCES

The complete reference list is available online at expertconsult.com.

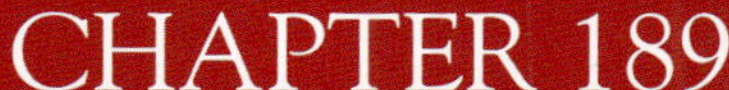
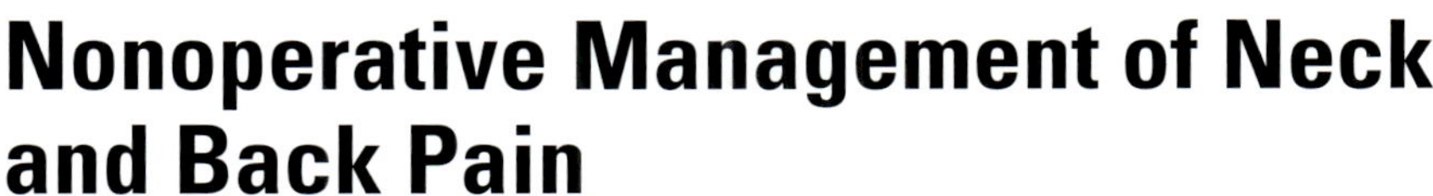

CHAPTER 189

Nonoperative Management of Neck and Back Pain

Ann M. Henwood | Edward C. Benzel

Low back pain (LBP) usually is benign and self-limiting. Health care providers are in a position to improve patient response to back symptoms greatly by providing reassurance, encouraging activity, and emphasizing that more than 90% of LBP complaints resolve without any specific therapies.[1]

LBP is second only to upper respiratory problems as the reason why patients visit a primary care provider.[2] Pain of spinal origin will affect 70% to 85% of the population at some point in their lives and is the most common cause of disability in patients younger than 45 years of age.[3] It accounts for a large fraction of the health care budget. LBP treatment costs increased from $4.6 billion in 1977 to $11.4 billion in 1997. In 2005, an estimated $85.9 billion was spent in the United States.[4] Annually, $20 to $50 billion is spent on workers' compensation claims, with 10% of patients with back pain accounting for 85% to 90% of the costs.[3,5,6] Although most adults experience low back and neck pain, only a small percentage (~1%) require surgery.

In 2005, 15% of adults in the United States reported back problems, compared with 12% in 1997.[4] As more people seek treatment for back pain, the cost per individual is rising. One study[4] found that the inflation-adjusted cost per study subject rose from $4695 in 1997 to $6096 in 2005. The natural history of LBP suggests that the passing of time is the best treatment, as 90% of cases resolve spontaneously within 2 weeks to 3 months of onset.[3,7] LBP affects men and women equally, and the onset most often occurs between the ages of 30 and 50 years. Eighty percent of the population will experience acute LBP at least once, and 30% of this group will become chronic sufferers. The annual prevalence ranges from 14% to 45%.

Nonoperative management can be complex and time consuming because of the need to determine the most appropriate management scheme for each patient individually. The data on the effectiveness of the variety of management schemes are sometimes misleading. Even establishment of the etiology of back pain is not consistent in the literature. This complicates the interpretation of outcome data. Unlike most drug treatments, it is difficult to blind clinical trials of physical treatments. Many studies have grouped pain syndromes into single treatment groups, which, in turn, degrades the meaningfulness of the results. Even though a particular pain syndrome may respond well to a particular management scheme, a statistically significant result may not be observed because of such a grouping. Given the natural history of these pain syndromes, most patients recover rapidly; therefore it is difficult to know whether the therapeutic interventions are efficacious or if the passing of time played a larger role.

Etiology

The etiology of spine pain is multifactorial. The cause of LBP may originate within spinal structures such as ligaments, facet joints, vertebral periosteum, paravertebral musculature and fascia, blood vessels, the anulus fibrosus, and spinal nerve roots. Disease states or processes such as cancer, infection, or musculoligamentous injuries also are causes of spinal pain, as are degenerative processes of the spine such as spinal canal stenosis, foraminal stenosis, and disc disease. No pathoanatomic diagnosis can be given to 85% of patients with isolated spine/LBP because of the poor association between symptoms and imaging results.[6] "Strain" and "sprain" are commonly used as catch-all diagnoses for generalized LBP in the absence of major red flags.

Classification of Spinal Pain

Mechanical Pain

Mechanical spinal pain is generally described as deep and agonizing. It is worsened with loading of the spine during activity and relieved or alleviated by unloading of the spine with rest. Mechanical pain has a deep and aching quality. It usually is associated with degenerative conditions seen in older adults or the development of a pseudarthrosis after a failed fusion. It also may be present with tumor.[8]

Myofascial Pain

Myofascial pain is consistent with "muscle spasm." Patients with significant trapezius spasm will describe tension-type headaches. Myofascial pain usually is self limiting and responds well to stretching exercise and muscle relaxants. Patients with underlying instability or mechanical pain often describe associated myofascial pain. "Strains" and "sprains" of the neck or low back are catchall terms used for nonspecific spine pain and usually are grouped within this category.[8]

Risk Factors

Adults are at risk of an episode of back pain regardless of timing, activity, or environment. However, many factors may make one patient's risk comparatively higher than another. Risk factors for low back and neck pain include advancing age up to 55 years, Caucasian race, living in the western United States, prolonged driving of a motor vehicle, heavy lifting and twisting, overexertion, prolonged sitting or standing, trauma, obesity, poor conditioning, and smoking.[9-12] In addition, there is a high prevalence of major depression in patients with chronic pain.[13]

Special attention should be given to the definite link between psychological variables and pain of spinal origin that has been discussed in the literature. Recognition of psychological variables emphasizes the need to highlight the multidimensional approach needed for caring for individuals with spine pain. Psychological distress can more than double the risk of low back pain.[14] Stress, distress, anxiety, mood, emotion, cognitive functioning, personality factors, and abuse have been shown to be linked to the onset of back and neck pain. Psychological variables may play a role not only in chronic pain but also in the etiology of the onset of acute pain.[15] Resultant disability caused by LBP may be a psychological stress-related disorder.[16] A complex pathway of physical work demands, the patient's reaction to the psychosocial environment, and the unique attributes of the person may affect physical loading on the spine, increasing the risk of LBP.[17]

Prevention

Ultimately, the best way to prevent LBP is to reduce risk factors. Patient education focusing on the prevention of episodes of LBP should include participation in an exercise program consisting of aerobic exercise, stretching, and strengthening exercise.[18] Exercises showed strong positive results as an effective preventive measure against back and neck pain.[19] Stretching and strengthening exercises may be done at home, thereby helping to reduce the monumental financial burden on the health care system. Smokers should be instructed to quit, because smokers have more severe symptoms that are present a greater portion of the day compared with nonsmokers.[20] Another preventive intervention includes maintaining weight appropriate to height, because obesity is positively linked to LBP.[12] Linton and van Tulder[19] reviewed 27 controlled trials regarding interventions for the prevention of back and neck pain. Their review found that back schools were not effective for prevention. Evidence showed that lumbar supports were consistently negative, and there is strong evidence that they are not effective. Neither ergonomic interventions nor risk factor modification could be considered because of a lack of quality controlled trials and subsequent evidence.

Current Treatment Therapies

Points for Patient Education

The first step in management of spine pain is educating the patient with regard to the probable cause of his or her pain, including a brief explanation of the anatomic pain generators. By understanding the cause of the pain, patients are more likely to become active participants in their treatment plan. Patients should be encouraged to accept responsibility for managing their recovery rather than expecting the provider to provide an easy fix. The patient recovery process is then directed by activity level rather than level of pain as a limitation.[1] The second step is to discuss the process of eliminating or reducing risk factors for future episodes of LB or neck pain and to reinforce the patient's lifetime commitment to working toward this goal. Third, the patient must be reassured that LBP is a normal and common occurrence, has an excellent prognosis, and, in most cases, abates with the passage of time. Fourth, the patient should be informed that because LBP has a multifactorial etiology, more than one intervention or treatment method probably will be necessary. Finally, whichever treatment methods are chosen, follow-up care is essential, whether the doctor initiates the treatment or refers the patient to another physician or health care provider.

Patients should be encouraged to return to work as soon possible, because this is a predictor for positive outcomes and relief of back pain and helps to reassure patients that they will be able to resume their usual activities/lifestyle.[1] Although many invasive and noninvasive therapies are intended to cure or manage LBP, no strong evidence exists to suggest that any single therapy is able to accomplish this as successfully as a therapy that focuses on restoring functional ability without focusing on pain. Patients should be aware that returning to normal activities usually aids functional recovery.[1]

The following sections discuss acute pain syndromes, defined as those lasting 6 weeks or less from onset, and chronic pain symptoms, defined as lasting 12 weeks or more from onset. It is also important to recognize that patients may have acute exacerbations of a chronic pain syndrome.

Medication Therapy

Nonsteroidal anti-inflammatory drugs (NSAIDs) have been shown to be effective for short-term improvement in patients with LBP.[1] No single type of NSAID is more effective than any other.[21] Evidence suggests analgesics are not more effective than NSAIDs.[22] Evidence has shown that muscle relaxants reduce pain intensity and that the different types are equally effective. Evidence for the use of muscle relaxants for LBP lasting longer than 3 months is lacking. However, the results show symptom relief when compared with a placebo.[22] Evidence shows more effective symptom relief when medications are used in conjunction with NSAIDs and are prescribed around the clock rather than on an as-needed basis.[6,23]

Antidepressant drug therapy may be beneficial, because one third of patients who suffer from chronic LBP also have depression and may benefit. Antidepressants may decrease the patient's perception of pain by treating underlying depression and improving sleep.[1,24] Hypotheses of similarities between the physiology of pain and depression exist; therefore, there may be beneficial effects of antidepressant drug therapy on pain separate from the drug's antidepressant effects.[25] Treating patients who do not have signs and symptoms of clinical depression is controversial. However, tricyclic antidepressants have been shown to be effective in the treatment of nondepressed patients with neuropathic-type pain and significantly increased pain relief over placebo without a significant difference in functioning.[26,27]

Exercise Therapy

Stretching and strengthening exercises have mixed results, with studies nearly equally divided between positive and negative results. Overall, evidence suggests that exercise improved pain and functional status more than other treatments for LBP.

Aerobic Activity

Recently, aerobic exercise has shown the best evidence of efficacy among the exercise regimens, whether for acute, subacute, or chronic LBP.[1] Benefits of aerobic exercise include weight loss and psychological effects of improved mood and lessened anxiety. The sense of well-being and accomplishment achieved from a planned aerobic exercise program creates a positive self-image and increases the level of motivation and commitment to the prescribed therapy. Some researchers have suggested that particular types of high-impact exercise should be avoided because of the potential for raising intradiscal pressure.[28] This stance, however, has not been backed by objective data. It has been shown that patients participating in an aerobic exercise program received few prescriptions for pain, were given fewer physical therapy referrals, and had improved mood states and lessened depression.[29]

Stretching Exercises

The literature is inconclusive as to whether or not aggressive stretching exercises help to reduce low back pain.[1] Stretching exercises help to improve the extensibility of muscles and other soft tissues, and to reestablish normal joint range of motion. Pain commonly limits mobility. Muscle spasm, or sprain, also may be present. Stretching is thought to maintain mobility and reduce spasm. Kraus et al.,[30] in a study of the effects of stretching exercises on back pain, found that nearly 80% of people with chronic back pain who entered the program reported improvement at the end of a 6-week training session.[31] More recent investigations have found that unless the exercises are continued, the benefit of stretching exercise may be lost.[32] Patient compliance is, again, a large determinant in the outcome.

Isometric Exercises

Isometric exercises and exercise regimens have enjoyed significant popularity. Several studies[33,34] suggest that isometric flexion offers the best relief of pain and improved function for LBP and neck pain. With regard to LBP, the rationale in these studies was that flexion (1) widened intervertebral foramina and facet joints, reducing nerve compression; (2) stretched hip flexors and back extensors; (3) strengthened abdominal and gluteus muscles; and (4) reduced dorsal fixation of the lumbosacral junction. Concerns have been raised over the use of flexion exercises, specifically regarding substantial increases in intradiscal pressure that may aggravate bulging or herniation of an intervertebral disc. Randomized controlled trials have shown conflicting results.[35-37] However, core strengthening exercises are recommended after the acute pain has diminished.[1]

McKenzie advocated extension exercises, because they limit the risk of aggravating nerve root compression from extrusion of a disc fragment. This program is complicated and is individualized according to the patient's symptoms. However, there is a very high noncompliance rate. McKenzie exercises are helpful for pain radiating below the knee.[38]

Mounting evidence indicates that weak muscles are associated with back and neck pain.[31,39,40] Therefore, strengthening exercises may reduce or eliminate back and neck pain. The supporting muscles of the spinal column provide support and prevent excessive or abnormal spinal movement. Activities that stress the spine without simultaneously strengthening muscles that support the spine (i.e., the ventral and dorsal support muscles) could result in stress/muscle strength imbalance. This could result in an application of excessive stress to the spine, thus accelerating degenerative changes and worsening pain.

Bed Rest

Bed rest for the treatment of acute episodes of LBP is controversial. Contrary to what was once recommended, bed rest is not effective in the treatment of LBP and may actually be harmful as treatment for an acute episode of nonspecific LBP.[21,41-43]

Bed rest has significant disadvantages, including its psychological association with a severe illness that requires many days in bed. This may lead to depression, exacerbation of pain, and a predisposition to diminished effort in an exercise program. Deconditioning, with muscle atrophy (1–1.5% per day[44]), cardiopulmonary function loss (15% in 10 days),[45] and bone mineral loss, occurs relatively rapidly. In addition, medical complications, including deep venous thrombosis and pneumonia, are more common with bed rest.

Smoking Cessation

Smokers have been found to have more severe pain that is present for longer periods during the day when compared with nonsmokers, and smoking may exacerbate episodes of pain.[20,46] Smokers should be encouraged to quit, because this may reduce the severity as well as duration of LBP.[10,11]

Appropriate Weight for Height

Obesity has a modest positive association with the chronicity as well as the recurrence of LBP.[12] Obese patients have been shown to have more severe pain symptoms than nonobese patients.[47]

Bracing

Bracing does diminish and may alleviate acute LBP because it supports the muscles of the spine. However, long-term use of bracing may lead to atrophy of these supporting muscles, ultimately resulting in a chronic pain syndrome. Wearing a brace may lead to weakening the supportive muscles of the spine.[48] Lumbar braces in the workplace have been shown to have no effect on muscle fatigue or lifting.[49] There is little evidence in the literature for the effectiveness of orthoses in the treatment of LBP.[21] Ultimately, lumbar braces probably serve best as a reminder to the patient to use correct spine mechanics when performing activities such as lifting and bending.[23]

Traction

Theoretically, traction is used to stretch the back and neck, distracting the vertebrae, and thereby potentially reducing protrusion of a bulging or herniated disc. Approximately 1.5 times a patient's body weight is needed to develop distraction of the vertebral bodies. This may cause compliance issues, because it may be burdensome and time consuming. Conventional traction has not been shown to be efficacious for either acute or chronic back or neck pain,[34,50] and, therefore, the use of traction is not recommended for the treatment of back or neck pain symptoms.

Adjunct Therapies

The etiology of LBP is multifactorial, as is its treatment. Patients in a passive modality-intensive program have poor functional outcomes when compared with patients in an exercise-based program.[51] Therefore, adjunct therapies should be used in conjunction with conservative treatment therapies and not as a sole treatment for pain of spinal origin.

Injection Therapy

The types of injection therapy most commonly used for LBP and radiculopathy include trigger point injections (TPIs) and nerve root, epidural, and facet joint injections (FJIs). All injection therapy should be used in conjunction with stretching and strengthening exercises to maximize the benefit of the effect of reduced pain, thereby increasing function. Multiple reviews of controlled trials show that the evidence for use of epidural steroid injections is conflicting, and they probably should not be used for acute or chronic LBP.[22,23,34] Limited evidence supports trigger point therapy as a therapeutic treatment for LBP. TPI should be prescribed for muscle spasm only when a patient has not responded to 4 to 6 weeks of medication and exercise therapy.[23] FJIs are not indicated during the first 4 to 6 weeks of treatment of LBP. FJI therapy is controversial, and, once again, evidence for its use is lacking. When compared with placebo, no significant difference in pain relief was noted.[27] If FJI therapy is prescribed, it should be used in patients for whom surgery is not an option. FJIs may help patients who complain of LBP with walking, standing, and extension activities and have an otherwise normal neurologic examination.[23]

Ice and Heat Therapy

Within the first 24 hours of the back or neck pain caused by a benign injury, alternating treatments of ice and heat for 20-minute periods can be effective in reducing inflammation.[7] When used in conjunction with home exercise therapy, patients may be instructed to use heat to warm the affected muscles prior to home exercise and ice packs after home exercise therapy for symptomatic relief. Insufficient data exist for the treatment of acute and chronic neck pain with thermotherapy.[34]

Continuous Low-Level Heat Wrap Therapy

Heat wrap therapy has been shown to be effective in LBP. It also has been shown to be superior to ibuprofen or acetaminophen for relief of LBP. The heat wrap is worn around the lumbar region and secured with Velcro. It heats the area to 104°F for up to 8 hours.[52]

Ultrasound

Ultrasound is used as a deep-heating modality because it reaches tissue depths that superficial heat cannot reach. Its use is not recommended for acute inflammatory conditions, because it may only increase the inflammatory response.[23] The literature lacks reports of any controlled research trials on its use for or against the treatment of LBP. Reviews of the literature found no clinical benefit for the use of ultrasound for chronic neck pain and no evidence for acute neck pain.[34]

Massage Therapy

Pennick and Sinclair found that massage therapy improved symptoms and function and was more effective when used in combination with a program for the treatment of LBP.[27] Further studies are needed to confirm these findings.[53]

Transcutaneous Electrical Nerve Stimulation

Several studies have shown no clinically or statistically significant effect of transcutaneous electrical nerve stimulation (TENS) in the treatment of acute or chronic LBP or of acute neck pain.[22,27]

Percutaneous Electrical Nerve Stimulation

Percutaneous electrical nerve stimulation (PENS) is a combination of acupuncture and TENS therapy. The evidence is insufficient to support its effectiveness for relief from LBP.[1]

Chiropractic or Manual Therapy

Modest evidence shows that chiropractic/manual therapy is more effective than placebo but not more effective than other forms of therapies for patients with acute LBP.[21,54] For the treatment of chronic LBP, chiropractic/manual therapy has been shown to be more effective than traditional therapies.[21]

Acupuncture

Limited discussion with regard to acupuncture has been published in the spine literature. However, it has been shown to have positive effects on LBP and return to work.[55,56]

Bipolar Permanent Magnet Therapy

Bipolar permanent magnet therapy has been shown to have no effect on LBP.[57]

Whole-Body Vibration Exercise

Whole-body vibration exercise significantly reduced pain sensation in a study group of patients experiencing LBP. This new type of exercise elicits muscular activity through stretch reflexes.[58] At one time, continuous vibration was considered a cause of LBP; now, however, it is considered to be helpful in the treatment of LBP.

Intradiscal Electrothermal Anuloplasty

Intradiscal electrothermal anuloplasty (IDET) is a minimally invasive procedure that has received mixed reviews because of its uncertain mechanism of action and is not yet widely accepted. IDET is recommended for patients who have discogenic pain, in whom other conservative treatment therapies or modalities have failed, and who may be candidates for lumbar fusion surgery.[59] Provocative discography must be performed prior to the IDET procedure itself to determine whether or not an intervertebral disc is the source of LBP. Discography is yet another cause of controversy. Evidence for the reliability of discography as a diagnostic method for degenerative disc disease is mixed.[60,61] In addition, there have been several reports of previously asymptomatic patients developing long-term back symptoms after diagnostic provocative discography.[59,62]

Overall, patients should be encouraged to return to their normal lifestyle as quickly as possible, taking into consideration the type of work the person performs. Light multidisciplinary treatment for LBP is a cost-effective treatment for LBP. This type of treatment includes evaluation by a physical therapist, a nurse, and a psychologist, if necessary. The patient is then instructed on exercise, lifestyle, and ways to overcome the fear that the pain will recur.[63]

Components for Aggressive Nonsurgical Management of Back Pain

An ideal exercise program should be efficacious and associated with a high level of compliance, as well as cost effective. Similarly, it should incorporate a lifestyle alteration component (i.e., active rather than passive participation in the program). Patient motivation should be assessed by monitoring compliance with exercises.

In most cases, regardless of the type of spine-related pain, the nonoperative management scheme is similar.

Four management components (a four-point program), a grouping referred to as GASS, are integral to the nonsurgical management process associated with mechanical back pain: (1) ***g***eneral health promotion, (2) ***a***erobic exercise, (3) ***s***tretching exercises, and (4) ***s***trengthening exercises. Each component requires patient education as an integral component of the pain management process, on the part of either the surgeon or the midlevel health care providers, or, more appropriately, both. This four-point management scheme may be individualized to individual patient syndromes (e.g., flexion exercise may be eliminated from the regimen of patients with acute sciatica, to prevent further herniation of disc fragments).

General Health Promotion

Augmentation of well-being causes the patient to simultaneously become a better surgical candidate (if surgery is deemed appropriate) and assists in a physiologically and biomechanically improved clinical status, all by improving attitude. This process includes a program for the cessation of smoking and weight loss. Tobacco use and obesity are associated with back and neck pain. Both can and should be assessed objectively and recorded on a periodic basis. If the patient cannot demonstrate progress in these areas, his or her motivation may be insufficient to warrant surgery or even further nonoperative care.

Aerobic Exercise

Aerobic exercise progress also can be quantified (at least by patient history) and recorded. The sense of well-being and accomplishment derived from a planned aerobic exercise program (e.g., walking, running, swimming, cycling) creates a positive internal milieu and further establishes the level of the patient's commitment.

Stretching Exercise

The augmentation of flexibility is an integral component of the program. The spine of a patient with mechanical instability should be thought of as akin to a frozen joint associated with immobilization. Flexibility can be improved with stretching, and progress can be quantitatively monitored. Toe touching can be monitored by asking patients to reach for their toes with knees locked and to hold the lowest position achievable for 20 seconds. The distance from the floor is measured and recorded. Bouncing is discouraged. Documentation is mandatory. Progress is encouraged. In fact, lack of progress may very well be a manifestation of a lack of adequate motivation. Other exercises include extension; however, they are not as easily quantified and monitored (Fig. 189-1). Less aggressive exercises may be more appropriate initially.

Strengthening Exercise

For many patients, much of the pain of spinal origin associated with mechanical instability can be reduced by an appropriate strengthening program. The supporting muscles of the spinal column can be thought of as exactly that, supporting muscles. These muscles assist in activities of daily living, provide support, and prevent excessive spinal movement. If an asymmetry of muscle strength exists, excessive stresses may be placed on either the spine or its supporting muscles. In such a case, strengthening the muscles that stress the spine (e.g., by weight lifting or by running) without strengthening the muscles that support the spine (i.e., the abdominal and paraspinous muscles) could result in an excessive spinal stress application-to-spinal support muscle strength ratio. This disparity may augment the dysfunctional nature of a dysfunctional motion segment.

The specific muscle groups to be exercised include the dorsal paraspinous muscles and the abdominal muscles. Specific exercises include supine leg lifts progressing to sit-ups for abdominal muscle strengthening and prone leg lifts progressing to the airplane or rocking chair exercise for paraspinous muscle strengthening (see Fig. 189-1). Initially, less aggressive exercises may be more appropriate. Similarly, strengthening exercises may be used for cervical pain (Fig. 189-2).

Spine surgeons cannot divorce their work from exercise and educational programs. Without active participation by both the patient and the surgeon, the chance that the management plan will not succeed assuredly increases.

Patient Education

An essential component of the program is patient education. If patients understand the importance of their active

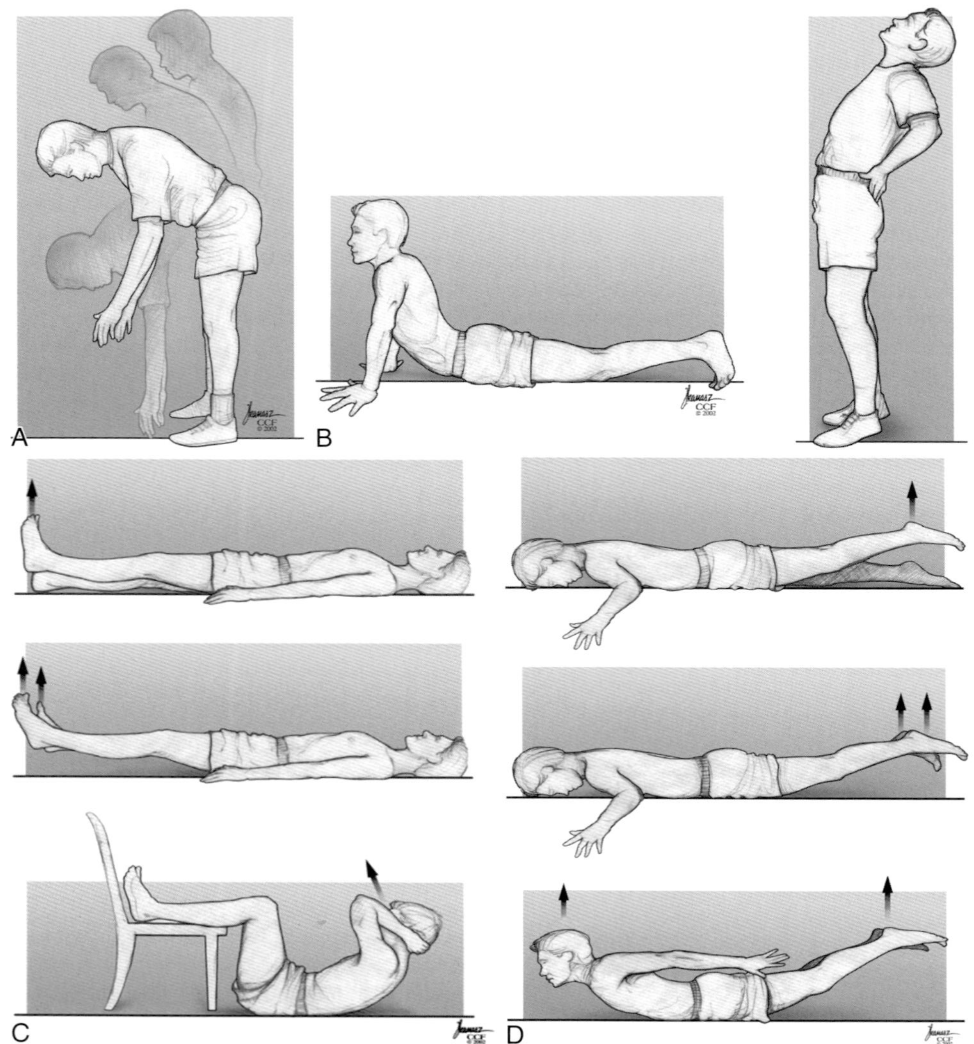

FIGURE 189-1. Progressive degrees of stretching and strengthening exercises are depicted. For stretching exercises (**A** and **B**), the patient must hold the position for 10 to 20 seconds. For strengthening exercises, strength imbalances may increase pain. Both abdominal (**C**) and paraspinous (**D**) muscle strengthening are recommended, therefore. Progress may be measured in terms of duration and progression of complexity of exercises. (Courtesy of the Cleveland Clinic Foundation.)

participation, it is more likely that they will achieve the goal of the program. Documentation of patient progress also is imperative for longitudinal monitoring purposes. If patients cannot or refuse to participate, they have demonstrated their relative inability to succeed in a program such as that just outlined and should, perhaps, seek relief elsewhere.

In conclusion, due to the multifactorial etiology of LBP and neck pain, the treatment therapies and modalities also should be multiple. The natural history of LBP shows that most patients will recover from their symptoms within a relatively short period of time; patients must be reassured that this is the case. Early identification of risk factors and implementation of preventive measures seem to be the most effective methods to avoid future episodes of LBP and neck pain and would greatly affect the huge financial strain on the health care system. Interestingly, research has provided evidence that LBP and neck pain often are manifestations of psychological stressors. Psychological variables cause patients to have more severe pain. Bed rest is not recommended for episodes of acute or chronic LBP. Return to normal daily activities is the best treatment, along with the appropriate use and management of NSAIDs for acute episodes of LBP. Isometric exercises are the best treatment for neck pain. Aerobic activity has been shown to be the best exercise regimen for LBP. Weight control, smoking cessation, and back exercises have been shown to reduce pain level and duration as well as aid in the treatment of chronic LBP. Many therapies and modalities in the treatment of back and neck pain exist; many have been shown to be effective and others not effective at all. However, many of the effective methods may have benefited, as the patient has, from the passing of time, and the symptoms may have improved in spite of the prescribed therapy. Larger and repeated studies are necessary to further the advancement of appropriate prevention and treatment of episodes of LBP and neck pain. Extensive patient education campaigns are needed to reduce risk factors.

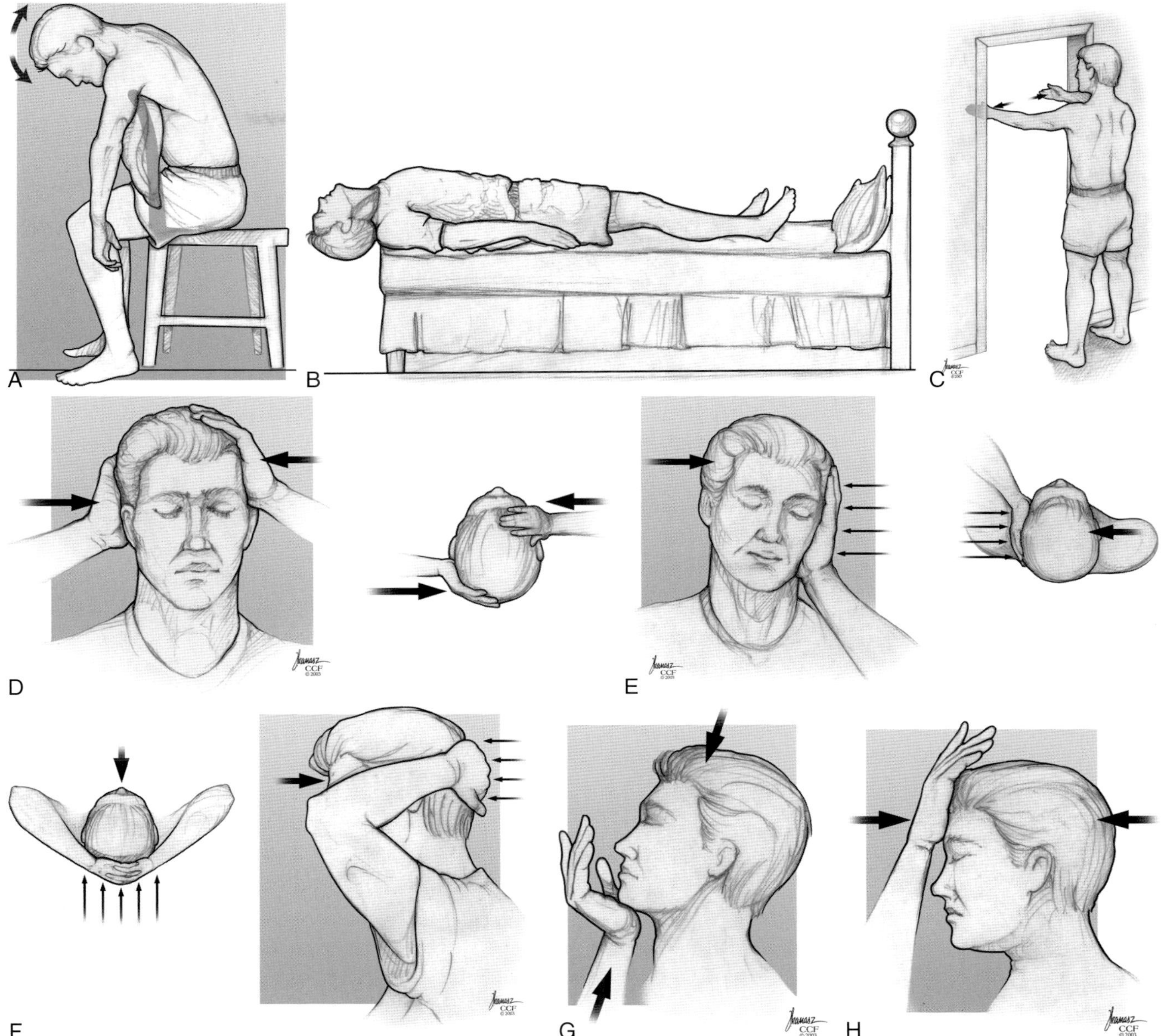

FIGURE 189-2. **A** and **B**, Stretching exercises. Each position should be held for 10 to 20 seconds. **C–E,** Resistance exercises. The goal of each position is to hold resistance for 1 minute. **C,** The backs of the arms are pushing against the door frame. **D,** Rotational resistance (mirror and bird's-eye views are depicted). **E,** Resistance to left lateral bending is shown; however, both right and left resistance should be practiced. **F,** Resistance in forward and backward motion. **G,** Resistance in downward motion. **H,** Resistance in right and left rotation (Courtesy of the Cleveland Clinic Foundation.)

KEY REFERENCES

Hegmann KT: Low back disorders. In Glass LS, editor: *Occupational medicine practice guidelines: evaluation and management of common health problems and functional recovery in workers*, ed 2, Elk Grove Village, IL, 2007, American College of Occupational and Environmental Medicine (ACOEM), p 366.

Martin BI, Deyo RA, Mirza SK, et al: Expenditures and health status among adults with back and neck problems. *JAMA* 299(6):656–664, 2008.

Michigan Quality Improvement Consortium: *Management of acute low back pain*, Southfield, MI, 2008, Michigan Quality Improvement Consortium, p 1.

REFERENCES

The complete reference list is available online at expertconsult.com.

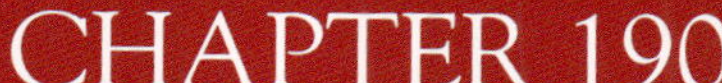
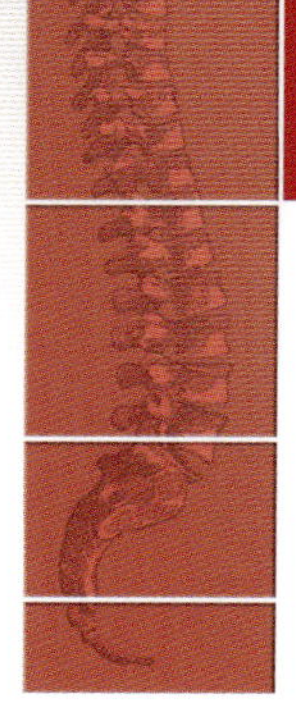

CHAPTER 190

Psychosocial Aspects and Work-Related Issues Regarding Lumbar Degenerative Disc Disease

Andrew M. Bauer | Daniel K. Resnick

There are few diseases that are so pervasive, yet so difficult to treat satisfactorily, as low back pain. Physicians are scientists first. Therefore, they look to treat diseases by making logical assumptions based on a group of clinical signs and symptoms combined with clinical tools such as imaging and laboratory tests. This is called the disease model of illness: the progression from signs and symptoms, to diagnosis, to treatment, to cure. Why then, is the diagnosis and treatment of low back pain so difficult? Few other disease processes have provided as much clinical material to the biopsychosocial model of disease as low back pain.

Over previous centuries, back pain was poorly understood, and the affected, unfortunate patients were left to go about life and deal with their pain. More recently, it was proposed that pain was a direct indication of tissue injury and that repair of the injuring mechanism would relieve the pain. It is now understood that some components of low back disability may be a manifestation of actual physical pain, but the vast majority of this may be due to the psychological reaction to pain. In his review in 1991, Waddell[1] considered the history of low back pain and disability. Interestingly, the first reported case of low back pain was from the Edwin Smith papyrus in 1500 BCE, and not much has changed about back pain since then. The first idea that back pain came from spine and nervous system dysfunction came from Brown in 1828.[2] After the industrial revolution, the concept of back pain due to injury became quite popular.[3] Changes in the law allowed individuals to benefit from compensation due to work injuries. By 1915, King[4] declared that "pain in the back as a result of injury is the most frequent affection for which compensation is demanded from the casualty company." This has certainly been expanded since that time, and low back pain continues to be one of the most common reasons for loss of work today.

The history of the development of various specialties in the medical profession also tells an interesting story with regard to low back pain. Development of the fields of orthopaedics and neurosurgery in the early 20th century has had a great impact on the role of back pain as a disease process today. As orthopaedics advanced as a specialty, the concept of rest for treatment of back pain came about. Prior to this, patients who had pain remained at work, and the concept of pain as a disability was unheard of. This was followed by the discovery of the ruptured disc by Mixter and Barr[5] in 1934, which led to the revolutionary treatment of low back pain and sciatica with surgery. This trend has remained today with much controversy surrounding the treatment of back pain and discogenic disease by surgical means.

Epidemiology and Risk Factors

Studies regarding the epidemiology of low back pain are highly variable. This is not surprising—it is a condition that is highly specific to each individual patient. Survey studies are difficult because one patient's perception of pain may be quite different than that of another. The incidence of developing a new episode of back pain has been estimated as low as 4% and as high as 93%.[6-9] On the basis of larger longitudinal studies, this incidence has been estimated to be much lower, between 3% and 5% for episodes where patients sought medical attention. The incidence of back pain that did not require professional medical care was much higher, at 30%.[7] Prevalence is difficult to study due to variance among study populations and the different factors that may affect the development of low back pain. Studies estimate that 15% to 20% of adults experience memorable low back pain within 1 year and up to 80% experience such pain over a lifetime.[10-13]

In terms of age, back problems do not necessarily occur more frequently during the third to fifth decades. When they do, however, they are certainly more often related to claimed disability during this period. These are the prime working years, where low back pain leads to the greatest disability and days off work. Interestingly, the symptoms of low back pain do not become worse with age-related degeneration of intervertebral discs.[1,14-17] Back pain in the elderly is thought to be one of the most important factors to affect the individual state of health.[18] Similar to younger adults, the prevalence of back pain in patients older than 65 years of age is 13% to 49%,[19] but this pain seems to be more episodic and intermittent with a lesser occurrence of chronic pain.[20] Despite the relatively high prevalence of abnormal curvature of the spine in adolescents, the chance of these children presenting with low back pain is quite low. Some studies suggest that the peak age for development of back pain in children is 13 to 14 years and that beyond this age, the risk factors for developing back pain in adults also apply in children.[21-23]

Risk factors for the development of low back pain are demographic, physical, socioeconomic, psychological, and occupational factors. Many studies of these risk factors are small and include only self-reports of the variables. A review by Hildebrandt discusses 55 personal factors and 24 occupational factors that have been linked to low back pain.[24] Many studies have looked at the relationship between socioeconomic status and level of education and the development of back pain. The association seems to be not so much with the incidence of pain but with the ability to adjust to pain. The incidence of disability from back pain appears to be 22 to 25 times higher in patients with less than 7 years of education compared with those with college degrees.[25]

Observations Regarding Low Back Pain and Disability

First, it is important to differentiate between pain and disability. Both are related in that they are generally subjectively relayed by the patient and are not viewed the same in any two patients. There is no objective measure for either of these disorders. Disability is related to the patient's perceptions and attitudes about pain[26,27] and may be based on avoidance based on previous painful experiences.[1,28,29] Many people live with low back pain, and few patients view this condition as a disability.

It is also useful to discuss the difference between acute and chronic pain. Acute pain often bears a close relationship to an inciting event and may be thought to stem directly from tissue injury. Chronic pain, on the other hand, is often a behavioral adaptation of an individual who may or may not have had an initial injury. This bears very little relationship to physical injury and is very difficult to treat by medical and surgical means. The failed back syndrome is indeed closely related to this concept. Chronic pain becomes a syndrome of emotional distress, depression, and disease conviction.[1] If these patients are taken to surgery under the misconception that their pain is actually related to tissue injury, they are virtually never cured and are often made worse. Surgery in these patients also plays into the "sick role" and gives them further reason to take time off work and to claim that they are disabled. These patients often clog pain clinics and spine clinics and place a heavy burden on the health-care system.

Despite low back pain and sciatica taking center stage in many medical circles today, there is no evidence that the biology of the problem has changed at all over the years. Back pain is the same as it always has been. It is low back disability that is a new concept. Ninety percent of patients with low back pain become better within 6 weeks in spite of technologically advanced medical and surgical care, or interestingly, no care at all.[1,15,30,31] This is likely a product of the explosion in the size and complexity of the health-care systems of Western countries and individuals' perceptions that the abilities of modern health care should be able to end pain. Physicians bear some responsibility in this regard because it is they who certify patients with pain to be excused from work, thereby feeding into the concept of low back disability.

Perhaps the most referenced expert to publish on low back pain and disability is Gordon Waddell. In his book *The Back Pain Revolution*,[32] he discusses his time spent in Oman. At the time of his writing, Oman was an emerging, primarily developing country. In the mid-1980s, new oil money soon brought modern medical treatments to this country. At the time, patients with back pain flooded into the newly established clinics seeking treatment for their pain. These patients had very similar problems with similar etiology to patients in developed Western countries. The interesting part is that nearly none of them were off work or "disabled" as a result of their pain. Waddell's observation was that the patients who were able to escape the confines of their country to have "modern" medical procedures in other countries became disabled after surgery at a much higher rate than those who did not have access to modern medical care. This is another illustration that suggests that low back pain is nothing new but that low back disability is largely a product of modern Western medicine.

Breakdown of the Disease Model of Illness

As mentioned earlier, modern medicine now largely depends on the disease model of illness. This model, which has been adapted over the years from roots in the 16th and 17th centuries, follows a progression from physical signs and symptoms, to diagnosis, to treatment, to cure. This depends directly on the fact the "disease" (pain, in this case) comes from physical pathology and excludes factors such as psychogenic and social issues. As this model breaks down, one can easily see that a prospective therapy does not lead to cure unless there is a true link between a presumed tissue injury and the physical signs of pain. This is probably not the case in the vast majority of patients with low back disability.

Chronic low back pain probably is better considered in the context of a different disease model, the biopsychosocial model. This model stresses the integration of the mind-body continuum, which has been proposed by philosophers since before science was born. This suggests that it is not only the responsibility of the physician to treat the body but also to assist the patient in adjusting to their illness and coping with it mentally. The gate theory of pain and experience with psychosurgery both support the assertion that pain perception requires both sensory and emotional components and can be modified by mental, emotional, or sensory mechanisms.[33]

These concepts are very solidly related to the diagnosis and treatment of low back pain. As it turns out, many patients are not satisfied with an office visit without the establishment of a diagnosis based on real pathology. Disc disease has become so popular and common, and patients may be given the nominal diagnosis of disc prolapse without any signs of nerve root compression or radiographic evidence. It is not long until this nominal diagnosis is confused with real disease pathology, and the patient receives the label of discogenic low back pain. These patients may eventually end up being treated with surgery and then bouncing from clinic to clinic when this operation fails. Clinics are clogged with these patients, making it difficult to care for patients with real pathology. Making matters worse, patients often go from clinic to clinic until a diagnosis is made, leaving an incentive for physicians to make nominal diagnoses or risk losing patients. Indeed, a large study of the indications for spinal surgery in the mid-1980s showed that surgical decision making was often driven by duration and severity of pain and disability, patients' illness behavior, and failure of conservative treatment.[34] As might be expected, the success rate for surgical treatment based on a nominal diagnosis is at best 30% to 40%. Interestingly, nearly every study in the past 50 years has shown that the presence of a psychiatric disease as an extremely poor predictor for good surgical outcome.[1,35-43] Thus, the responsible surgeon must use the history and physical examination to tease out signs of psychiatric imbalance and consider this carefully prior to proceeding with surgery.

Work-Related Issues

Since complaints of low back pain hit a peak during the working years, it is essential to discuss this process as it relates to time off work. First, this problem is most prominent in the group of patients with chronic low back pain. In a study by Volinn et al., 2% of workers eligible for industrial insurance filed a claim for back pain in 1 year. Of those, 12% were off work for 90 days or more, consuming more than 88% of the wage and medical compensation paid by insurance.[44] This same study found that the complaints of back sprain and pain were closely related to workplace dissatisfaction and monotonous job tasks. The medical costs largely involved surgery and hospital stays for "medical back problems." One study of Medicare patients found that 71% of these "medical back" hospitalizations were inappropriate.[45] In a review of low back pain and health care utilization, Volinn et al. suggest that the level of both cognitive and economic investment in low back pain drives therapy.[46] Only when further knowledge and education of outcomes regarding the treatment of low back pain become available, and third party payers invoke more stringent guidelines for what will and will not be reimbursed, will the trends in surgical and medical management change.

The historical and still common practice of "therapeutic rest" appears to be based on multiple fallacies. First, pain is related to tissue injury and inflammation in the spine, and rest will help reverse or alleviate this process. Second, if the pain does not come from inflammation of the spine, it must come from degenerative disc disease, and the only way to allow the disc to heal is with rest. By the disease model of illness, this seems to be a logical progression, but as previously discussed, the disease model of illness does not translate well into the world of low back pain. Considering the biopsychosocial model and assuming that chronic pain is not due to significant injury to or instability of the spine, this treatment does not make sense at all. It aims to treat a process that likely is not active and fails to treat and may actually *worsen* the psychological aspects of the disease and help the patients fit into the sick role.

Indeed, there is no good evidence in the literature that rest improves low back pain or even sciatica. This is a somewhat difficult area to study without a high degree of bias, and as one might expect, the major studies are methodologically flawed. Even in the majority of these studies, it was found that shorter periods of rest were more beneficial (or less harmful) than longer periods.[1] Along with these findings, there have been no studies to suggest that activity worsens pain or tissue injury in the absence of a known lesion. Many of these patients continue to complain of the same degree of pain whether or not they are performing their daily activities. It is clear that prolonged rest is harmful to both body (bone demineralization,[47] cardiac deconditioning,[48,49] and loss of muscle strength) and mind (depression and anhedonia).[50,51] The physician who prescribes to the patients with low back pain has clearly done them no favors.

Similarly to the notion that an individual's back pain can affect his or her job, the characteristics of the job can affect the back pain. A study by Boos et al. showed that the characteristics of one's job (listlessness, job satisfaction, working in shifts) were more likely than MRI to identify disc abnormalities and to predict whether one would seek medical treatment.[52] Similarly, these factors also are useful in predicting which patients are likely not to be working at follow-up.

All of these issues have opened up much controversy and academic thought to litigation and workers compensation in the current health-care system. In the present system, compensation is largely tied to the presence of physical examination findings and imaging confirmation of disc herniation. Some studies suggest that psychological factors may also be tied in to the selection of patients for workers compensation benefits and that patients with emotional instability may be less likely to receive compensation.[53] There is decent evidence to suggest that patients who receive time-limited workers compensation as opposed to long-term disability are more likely to return to work and have a good outcome.[54] Another study by Atlas et al. also revealed that patients who were receiving workers compensation at baseline prior to their low back disability were more likely to be receiving long-term disability benefits than those who were not (27% vs. 7%), and they were also slightly less likely to be working at 4-year follow-up.[55] This correlates with the earlier assertion that time off work and prolonged compensation benefits allow patients to more easily adopt the sick role.

Summary

It is clear that low back pain and disability are epidemic in virtually all parts of the industrialized world today. The main differences among countries are the way back pain is viewed and treated. In Western society, the expectation from patients is generally that they will benefit from surgery, and if not, rest and time off work are the best treatment options. It is also clear that low back pain does not fit into the classic treatment paradigm of the disease model of illness. In this case, the biopsychosocial factors may be more at work than actual physical tissue injury. These patients place a large burden on the medical system and often bounce from clinic to clinic until they find a physician who will treat them. They then are often the victims of unindicated surgery and fall into the category of failed back syndrome. It is clear that only when surgical candidates are chosen carefully and selectively, surgical therapy can lead to the best and most efficient outcomes, with early return to work and relief of symptoms. It is also apparent that the traditional method of therapeutic rest is inadequate and may actually lead to a decline in the patient's functional status. The exact roles of workers compensation and disability are still somewhat unclear, but it is likely that these only reinforce sick behavior.

We advocate a multidisciplinary approach in the spine clinic that involves spine surgeons, occupational therapists, physical therapists, mental health professionals, sports medicine specialists, and social workers. Using this method, appropriate surgical candidates can be selected, and the remainder of patients can be funneled into a low back training program. This program allows them to become empowered and take control and initiative in their disease and avoids their "shopping" around to other clinics. Only by addressing all of these issues can care for patients with low back pain be adequate and efficient.

KEY REFERENCES

Jamison RN, Matt DA, Parris WC: Effects of time-limited vs. unlimited compensation on pain behavior and treatment outcome in low back pain patients. *J Psychosom Res* 32:277–283, 1988.

Melzack R, Wall PD: Pain mechanisms: a new theory. *Science* 150:971–979, 1965.

Volinn E, Turczyn KM, Loeser JD: Theories of back pain and health care utilization. *Neurosurg Clin North Am* 2:739–748, 1991.

Volinn E, Van Koevering D, Loeser JD: Back sprain in industry. The role of socioeconomic factors in chronicity. *Spine (Phila Pa 1976)* 16:542–548, 1991.

Waddell G, Morris EW, Di Paola MP, et al: A concept of illness tested as an improved basis for surgical decisions in low-back disorders. *Spine (Phila Pa 1976)* 11:712–719, 1986.

Waddell G: Low back disability. A syndrome of Western civilization. *Neurosurg Clin North Am* 2:719–738, 1991.

Waddell G: *The back pain revolution*, ed 2, London, 2004, Elsevier.

REFERENCES

The complete reference list is available online at expertconsult.com.

CHAPTER 191

Interventional Nonoperative Management of Neck and Back Pain

Eric A.K. Mayer | Adrian M. Zachary

Throughout the 1990s, interest in spine procedures increased with anecdotal success in reducing morbidity from spinal pain. Reimbursement issues, complications, and the failure to publish adequate outcome research have led to increasing scrutiny and the formulation of prejudicial opinions by physicians and insurers regarding the utility of spine procedures. This chapter briefly describes available spine procedures, explains when their benefit may be seen, and provides evidence for or against use of interventional procedures in specific clinical instances.

Pain and disability from spine pathology are usually benign, temporally limited occurrences that may be accompanied by anxiety and hypervigilance on the part of the sufferer. Occasionally, symptoms of pain are caused by tumor, infection, or trauma, requiring aggressive and often morbid interventions. On the other hand, most acute episodes of spinal pain improve substantially within 90 days.[1,2] When the complaint of spinal pain is accompanied by minor/mild neurologic deficit and ample evidence of degenerative change, the answer may become confounded by contradictory evidence. In such cases, interventional procedures are increasingly utilized to relieve symptoms, ameliorate disability, and reduce surgical risk.[3,4] This chapter presents an overview of available interventional spine procedures, their indications, and the best available evidence for efficacy within a continuum of clinical care.

Conservative Care Progression

When discussing treatment options with patients in acute distress, it is important to keep in mind the first tenet of Western medicine: "first, do no harm." This is best accomplished by following a progression of conservative care that first presents strategies that provide the least risk with the highest likelihood of success. In the rush to ameliorate pain, experienced physicians occasionally forget that any intervention should have patient function as the primary goal and pain relief as a laudable, but secondary, goal (Fig. 191-1). Moreover, it has been shown that people will accept a degree of chronic pain if they are able to participate in desired activities.[5] The decoupling of symptoms and radiologic/anatomic findings can lead similarly well-trained professionals to vastly different opinions. In the end, the patient is best served when the treatment modality with the least risk is applied to relieve a given pathology. Following the "do not harm" tenet, efficacious, timely applied spinal injections may allow enough time for the body to heal and return to function without the need for further invasive procedures.

Overview of Selective Spinal Procedures

As stated previously, selective spine procedures are being used with increasing frequency to manage acute and chronic pain syndromes.[3] The implied societal benefit of a greater number of procedures is more robustly measurable functional improvements. To the contrary, literature states that increasing expenditures for interventional and surgical procedures have not translated into improved health status for spinal pain sufferers.[6,7] Moreover, disability from spine-related pain is increasing in the United States.[8] Overutilization of procedures is a problem that undermines the fundamental doctor-patient relationship as well as the collegial doctor-doctor relationship. Failure to live up to the promise of increased function leads to a rapid erosion of the trust that underlies everything physicians do. Therefore, this chapter follows the principles of Edward Benzel, MD, when discussing and describing indications and evidence for selective spine procedures. These principles enable increasing trust: Wisdom has foremost importance, but should be combined with evidence, and statements of risk/efficacy should be based on what one would do to their own mother, spouse, or child.[9]

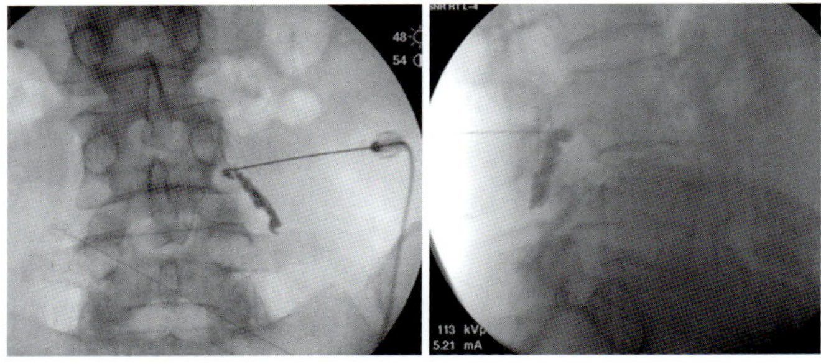

FIGURE 191-1. Right L4 selective nerve root blockade with dye pattern lateral to foramen.

The *pain generator*, the Holy Grail of clinical and diagnostic medicine, is often illusory in spinal pain patients. Multiple studies by Boden, Wiesel, Mayer, Rainville, and Carragee[10-14] have shown the discordance between pain and anatomic or physiologic abnormalities. Given that pain is as much a cognitive as it is a nocioceptive phenomenon, if pain response is the sole outcome measure, the selection bias will always trend toward failure. This chapter, therefore, attempts to utilize evidence that has a functional component (sparse in spine literature) accompanying the usual visual analogue scale (VAS) when discussing the various procedures available to spine surgeons to improve their outcomes.

One must also understand the *masquerade*, or the concept of pain referral. Often a lumbar issue can masquerade as or coincide with a hip problem.[15,16] This concept applies to the neck and shoulder as well as to various nerve entrapment syndromes in the upper or lower extremity.[17] Acumen to unlock the masquerade is found in the office and not in the operating suite. Therefore, a skilled interventionist who performs a thorough physical examination can accrue good internally valid, reproducible diagnostic information to keep a surgeon from making a hasty, unwise decision.

The inflammatory basis for pain's relation to the degenerative changes in spinal structures and diarthrodial joints is an additional concept to critically consider. Although concepts of legal indemnity and political policy lag behind, there is substantial evidence that degenerative changes to intervertebral discs, cartilage, and joints begin with inflammatory changes and not with mechanical stress/injury (cumulative or otherwise). This subtle concept is important for two reasons. First, the radiologic appearance of the structure is less important than its functional range and strength, which may recover through a combination of aggressive treatment of acute-phase inflammation with maintenance of functional range of motion over the same time. Second and more importantly, physician advocacy of inactivity to prevent further injury undermines the ultimate benefit of any proposed intervention. Specifically, patients who have been advised by physicians that activity (not inflammation) causes injury have higher pain scores and trends to disability.[18] Physician advice that worsens the cognitive aspect of pain begin a self-fulfilling pain/disability cycle that rarely ends well.

The final concept is a surgeon's understanding of quality control for diagnostic or therapeutic procedures if performed by another physician (interventionist). A common tip-off of inferior quality is when every patient you refer receives a series of three injections, or when every patient with predominant axial pain is given an epidural injection first, or when patients report that spinal procedures are done without imaging/fluoroscopic guidance. There are many other red flags to inferior quality; quality only improves when the referring physician demands such improvement.

Spinal pain is a widely prevalent, usually self-limited condition. Physicians are coming under increasing scrutiny to produce functional outcomes that demonstrate the efficacy of expensive interventions for such pain. The spine procedures described in the remainder of this chapter can assist in creating functional outcomes by adding to the volume of information available when deciding to proceed with surgery.

Radicular Nerve Pain and Therapeutic versus Diagnostic Injections

Radiculopathy is a pathologic process affecting a spinal nerve root in which sensory and/or motor symptoms present distant from the pathology. Whether the process is mechanical/compressive, inflammatory, or both remains poorly elucidated. What is clear is that the sodium-channel blocking effects of local amide or ester anesthetics provide relief from pain but do not improve any functional deficits. Due to the pharmacokinetics of existing local anesthetics, this benefit is temporary but can (when applied discreetly and correctly) provide excellent diagnostic information. Synthetic glucocorticoids act to suppress production of inflammatory mediators, stabilize membrane irritability, and enhance macrophage demargination to the site of injury. Due to the complexity of the interactions, there is often a delay before the benefit from locally or remotely administered glucocorticoid is perceived by the patient.[19] Depending on the nature of the nerve irritation/injury, the benefit of the glucocorticoid can often be long-lived. A tapering dose of medication that up-regulates systemic circulating glucocorticoid is still in common use for suspected radiculopathy; however, rapid steroid metabolism and intolerable systemic side effects occasionally make systemic use impractical or too short-lived for functional improvement. For this patient, treatment targeted to the pathology is often beneficial.

Epidural steroid injection for radiculopathy was first described in the United States in 1960 in the *Cleveland Clinic Quarterly* and was expanded upon thereafter.[20,21] In the years since that time, its efficacy has been enhanced by use of imaging guidance as well as training programs that ensure a physician's safe delivery of medication closest to the site of pathology. The intent of delivery of glucocorticoid medication to the site of pathology is the deposition of fat-soluble steroid in a nearby plane of epidural fat. Glucocorticoid steroids will release from this adipose tissue in a prolonged fashion to reduce pain by down-regulating pro-anti-inflammatory, acute-phase chemical mediators from inflamed/reactive tissue. Broadly, the three ways of accessing the epidural fat are through the sacral hiatus (*caudal injection*), between the bony lamina and traversing the ligamentum flavum (*interlaminar injection*), and through the neural foramina near the bifurcation of the nerve root from the spinal cord or dural sac (*transforaminal injection*). Each method has its utility, with research showing a trend toward greater efficacy, fewer systemic effects, and increased cost utility when the injection delivers medicine closest to the pathologic process responsible for pain and functional inhibition. In general, all of these types of injections should be assisted by imaging guidance. The studied rate of misapplication of medication with resultant complications varies from 22% to 69%. Therefore, an interventionist's failure to use imaging guidance should be a red flag to the referring physician (Fig. 191-2).

Caudal Epidural Steroid Injection

The starting needle placement for a caudal injection can be guided by palpable anatomic landmarks or by imaging. With this in mind, there is a greater than 25% rate of needle-tip misadventure without imaging guidance.[22] The procedure is

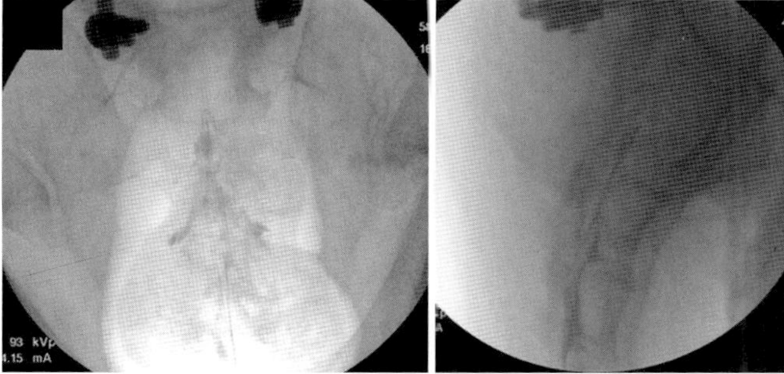

FIGURE 191-2. Caudal injection: dye flow in epidural space craniad of needle tip at midbody of S3.

fairly simple, with a blunt-tipped needle directed through the sacral hiatus assisted by a simple two-picture confirmation in anteroposterior and lateral views. The needle is advanced along the dorsal bony elements of the sacrum to approximately the S3-4 space. The thecal sac typically ends around S2, but may extend as low as S4. Nonionic contrast material is used to confirm that the needle is placed within the epidural space and outside the thecal sac. Violation of the dura mater results in a spinal headache. Injection of a steroid and anesthetic solution into the caudal epidural space may result in urine retention. Additionally, delivery of the medicine through the caudal approach is often remote from the location of pathology. Finally, the concentration of corticosteroid is significantly less well distributed in the sacral epidural fat, with a concentration decrement of tenfold or more of the injectate reaching the site of pathology (Fig. 191-3).

Interlaminar Epidural Steroid Injection

Accessing the epidural space between the lamina is common both for pain procedures and for regional anesthesia for surgical procedures or childbirth. The common usage of this technique may have led some to overlook some of the hazards of steroid delivery. The goal of this procedure is defined by the name: to deliver steroids to the epidural space,which is often a potential space whose upper volume boundary is defined by the volume of cerebrospinal fluid (CSF) in the subarachnoid space. Specifically, if stenosis is present and no CSF is visible at a particular level on axial cuts of advanced imaging, this would be a poor location to depot steroid medication. Common use of the interlaminar technique has resulted in people underestimating the risk associated with it.

The steps for getting good results from interlaminar epidural steroid injections are similar to those for other techniques. First, the physician should plan the procedure by taking a history, performing a thorough physical examination, and correlating that information to appropriate imaging. If the predominant complaint is axial back pain, the chances of a medium or long-term, nonplacebo, beneficial result from depot of steroid in the epidural space is low. Alternatively, when the pain presentation is predominantly in the limb and subjective complaints correlate with discreet pathology on radiology, the chance of injection benefit and avoiding surgery is high.[23]

Preprocedure planning for an interlaminar approach should include seeing that there is adequate CSF (or epidural fat) at the level of approach and judging the thickness of the ligamentum flavum. Additionally, knowledge of operative

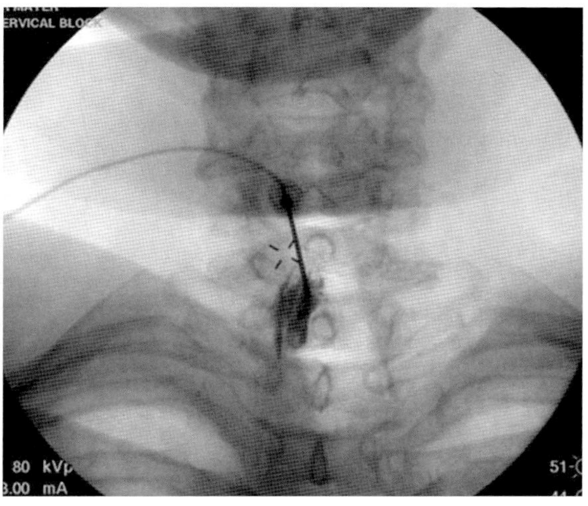

FIGURE 191-3. Cervical intralaminar epidural steriod injection: C7-T1 perimedian dye flow.

sites, of other causes of dural ectasia, and of underlying causes of bleeding diathesis are critical planning steps that will help reduce the rate of needle-tip misadventures or other harms to patients.

Once planning is complete, the procedure is straightforward. Fluoroscopic guidance facilitates the localization of the desired level in the lumbar, thoracic, or cervical spine. The skin overlying the interspace between the spinous processes is anesthetized, and most commonly a blunt-tipped needle is passed through the skin and directed midline. The needle is advanced using a combination of direct, fluoroscopic visualization and "loss of resistance" technique with a syringe containing water or air. Skillful completion of these techniques is important in reducing the incidence of spinal headache by dural puncture. A sound understanding of anatomy is vital for this procedure, because the spinous processes are oriented differently in the cervical, thoracic, and lumbar spinal divisions. Additionally, the thickness of ligaments, depth of lateral recesses, and location of vascular anatomy changes over the course of the spine. To obtain an efficacious result, medication needs to be placed in the epidural space only. To ensure proper placement, it is strongly recommended that a form of nonionic contrast be used to verify placement once loss of resistance is encountered. Frequently, even in the most experienced hands, a false loss of resistance may be encountered between the interspinous ligament and the ligamentum flavum or, more problematically, tissue may become lodged in the bevel of the needle, resulting in a failure to perceive loss of resistance. This failure often results in dural puncture and in the contrast flow pattern appearing identical to a myelogram. Finally, knowledge of anatomy allows one to understand that the epidural space is not uniform in shape but is pyramidal in cross section, meaning that if the needle tip is directed away from midline, the likelihood of dural puncture increases in proportion to the decreased epidural space laterally. McGoldrick expanded on the cryomicrotome dissection work of Hogan to show that failure of ligamentum fusion in the dorsal midline occurs in the cervical and high thoracic space in 51% to 74% of dissections.[24,25] Additionally, controversy persists about whether a "fat pad" exists dorsally above the dura mater at a level above C7.[24] The lack of landmarks for traditional loss of resistance technique make dural puncture in the cervical and high thoracic spine more likely. The consequence of dural puncture with intrathecal infusion of anesthetic can range from slow-onset respiratory depression (~30 minutes) to seizure to cardiovascular collapse.[26]

Finally, Cluff et al. noted a disturbing trend: that only 39% of academic institutions used fluoroscopy for epidural injections, whereas 74% of private practices used fluoroscopy.[27] In light of the compelling data that only 26% of blind attempts (without fluoroscopic guidance) by experienced anesthesiologists placed medication at the site of pathology, this trend may account for the jaundiced view held by many referrers with regard to the efficacy of injections.[28] This jaundiced view is seen at its most extreme in the oft-cited study by Valat that, in attempting to demonstrate the efficacy of epidural steroid injection versus placebo merely showed that blind epidural steroid injection is no better than placebo even when delivered three times.[29] In conclusion, the prosaic use of the interlaminar technique has bred contempt that can only be improved if referring physicians demand excellence; one may consider the oft-quoted Edward Benzel aphorism: "A fool with a tool is still a fool."

Transforaminal Epidural Steroid Injection

The transforaminal epidural steroid injection technique (Fig. 191-4) has been used with increasing favor owing to beliefs around the selectivity, proximity (to the pathology), and longevity of benefit with this technique. These assumptions have proven difficult to substantiate in the literature. Riew et al. published two very persuasive studies that were shrewdly designed to eliminate the winner's bias seen in many studies examining injection versus surgery.[30] The authors took all patients who were scheduled for surgery and randomized them to receive a transforaminal injection of either anesthetic alone or anesthetic plus steroid. Of those receiving steroid via transforaminal delivery, 71% elected to not have surgery at end points ranging from 13 to 27 months. This was a statistically significant difference compared to the anesthetic-alone group, in which only 33% elected not to have surgery by the end point ($P < .004$). This finding held at 5-year analysis, with 3 of 4 patients requiring late surgery (between 27 and 73 months) with progression of symptomatic spinal stenosis.[23]

The transforaminal technique is highly dependent on imaging guidance and on bony landmarks. The proximity of vasculature, neural elements, and dura mater require proprioception, skill, and experience to obtain the best results. Readers of this chapter intending to refer these procedures to an interventionist should be aware of what constitutes quality. Use of fluoroscopy and documentation of outcomes (usually with use of a pain diary) between injections should be self-explanatory. Consistent repetition of the same injection at the same site with a less than 30-day interval, or consistent use of a series-of-three may be tipoffs of inferior quality. Finally, different ways of accessing the epidural space should be employed, depending on whether neuritis is caused by disc herniation, stenosis, metallic instrumentation, or deformity. The three main transforaminal approaches to keep in mind are the subpedicular route, the retroneural route, and the preganglionic route. It is beyond the scope of this chapter to fully explore these routes, but they are well described in the literature.

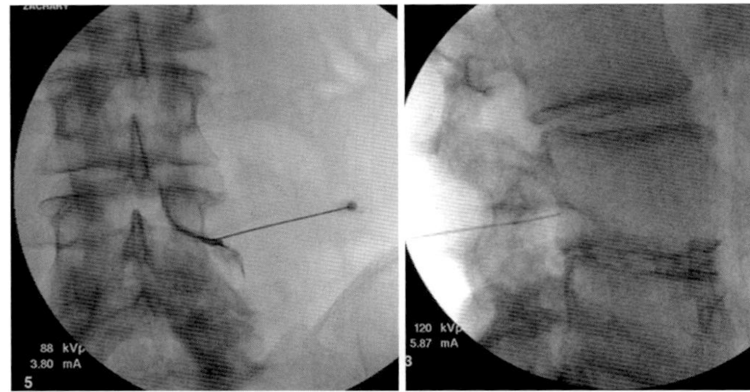

FIGURE 191-4. Right L4 transforaminal epidural steroid injection: anteroposterior (*left*) and lateral (*right*).

Recently, there has been a proliferation of expert opinion about the risks associated with cervical epidural steroid injections in general and cervical transforaminal injections specifically. The main concerns originate from case reports of catastrophic complications, including death, persistent vegetative state, stroke, spinal cord infarction, and high anesthesia-related cardiorespiratory collapse. For the most part, the culprit is injection of medication into the arterial circulation supplying the brain or spinal cord. Several safeguards exist and should be known by a fellowship-trained interventionalist—including use of contrast enhancement to confirm needle-tip placement, use of "live" fluoroscopic visualization to confirm arterial uptake, use of test-dose anesthetic medication, and use of digital subtraction technology. Each of these recommendations has its benefits; however, the most convincing evidence to recommend modifying current practice comes from an animal study that demonstratied zero infarction rate with administration of nonparticulate steroid in two different formulations; 100% of the particulate steroid group suffered neurologic damage that correlated with hypoxic and ischemic damage.[31]

In conclusion, epidural steroid injections show benefit when performed for the correct reason (radicular, not axial, pain) and when medicine is delivered to the correct location (using fluoroscopic guidance and contrast confirmation). These injections have been shown to help reduce surgical rate, allow for earlier return to function, and save $12,666 per responder (in 1999 dollars).[30,32,33] Therefore, referring physicians should insist on the highest clinician acumen and the highest-quality training for proper delivery of medication to the site of pathology.

Joint-Mediated Pain

The joints of the spine include a three-part joint that combines the disc and a matched pair of dorsal joints at each spinal segment colloquially called the *facet joints*. Additionally, the cervical spine has accessory joints that aid with shear forces; these are named after the anatomist Luschka, or are commonly called the *uncovertebral joints*. A separate joint comprises the skull, first vertebra, dens, and second vertebra and allows for complex head movement in relation to the neck and the rest of the body. Finally, a pair of complex joints that transmit/disperse rotational force applied through the pelvis are called the *sacroiliac joints*. All of these joints are diarthrodial joints of the spine, and each one can produce pain. Briefly we discuss the role of injection procedures in diagnosis and treatment of pain syndromes involving the various spinal joints.

Facet Joints of Cervical, Thoracic, and Lumbar Spine

The facet joints are paired diarthrodial joints on the dorsal aspect of the vertebral bodies. These joints provide stability and are a key component to ensuring accommodation of a neutral zone in the three-joint complex model of the vertebral motion segment. As early as 1911, Goldthwait postulated that the facet joints, specifically the zygapophyseal joints (Z joints) of the lumbar spine, could be a potential pain generator in the spine.[34] Anatomic studies have verified the presence of nociceptive structures and mechanoreceptors in the capsule and synovial folds of the facet joints.[35-37] Additionally, Mooney and Hirsch et al. identified the zygapophyseal joint as a source of pseudoradicular pain in both a control hypertonic saline group and in study patients.[38-40] And why wouldn't high-stress joint complexes be a potential source of pain? It stands to reason that like the knee, the shoulder, or any diarthrodial joint, the facet joint is subject to the ravages of time, inflammation, and apoptosis, giving it the ability to act as a pain generator in the spine.

Statistical methodology varies, but epidemiologic studies note that facet-mediated pain may account for between 4%[41] and 45%[42] of chronic spine pain.[43] The large variance in these statistics may be due to study inclusion criteria and the lack of adherence to exacting standards. Although proof for the existence of facet joint–mediated pain is debated, the ubiquity of facet joint arthropathy is undeniable. Cadaveric studies have shown facet joint arthropathy to be present in 100% of cadaveric spines over 60 years old.[44] Although clues to facet-mediated pain may be obtained from a thorough history, physical examination findings, and imaging, no pathognomonic test/maneuver exists. Facet joint pain is currently diagnosed by a preponderance of evidence because we lack a single test for facet pain that combines high sensitivity and specificity. The lack of any test with a high positive prognostic value is likely due to known compensatory mechanisms that are associated with joint pain/inflammation, such as muscle spasm, altered movement mechanics, and pain referral patterns. Facet joints present more of the prerequisites to be a pain generator than pain associated with the more amorphous construct of discogenic pain. Facet joints have a robust nerve supply and are capable of causing pain similar to that seen in peripheral joints, as in overuse injuries elsewhere in the body. Articular joints possess a known pattern of disease/injury susceptibility, and their pain can be ameliorated using well-described diagnostic techniques with acceptable reliability and validity (Fig. 191-5).[45]

Unfortunately, today there is no "gold standard" criterion to confirm with high positive predictive value the presence of facet-mediated pain. The accepted standard combines clinical judgment with a diagnostic or therapeutic facet joint injection. Early studies performed by Hirsch et al. and Mooney not only supported the existence of facet joint pain but also seemed to show improvement when injections of anesthetic or glucocorticoids were combined with exercise. Similar results were seen with provocative injections to the medial branch nerves that supply the facet joints.[46] Though prone to operator error, these studies show that wise use of facet joint injections can serve dual diagnostic and therapeutic goals in returning patients to function. Currently two techniques are employed to block pain from facet joints: intra-articular injection of the facet joint capsule and blockade of the medial branch nerves transmitting pain signals from the joint to the spinal cord/brain. Both techniques have been shown to possess variable, operator-dependent accuracy/efficacy when combined with appropriate clinical judgment.[47,48]

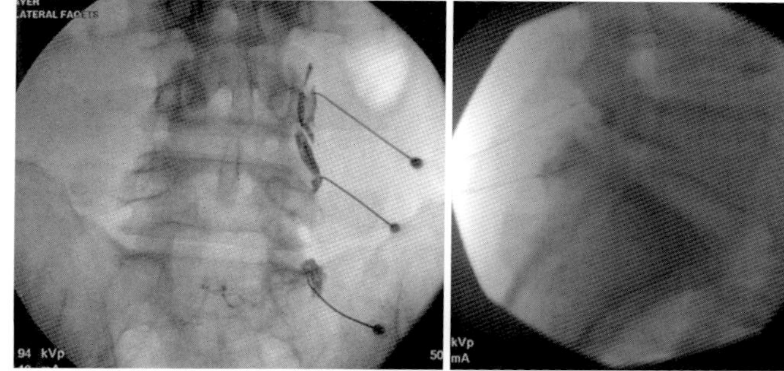

FIGURE 191-5. Right L3, L4, and L5 medial branch/dorsal rami nerve blocks.

The early standard for the diagnosis of facet joint pain was to seek mitigation of pain with a single facet joint injection. However, this methodology produced an unacceptably high false-positive rate of up to 38%,[49] meaning results showed poor prognostic value. Coupled with a known/accepted positive placebo response rate of up to 32% with many interventional procedures, this result significantly reduced the validity of this treatment protocol.[50] It has therefore been advocated that a reliable control be employed in the form of the double-block protocol, in which anesthetics of varying durations of effect are administered on subsequent injections and the patient maintains two accurate postinjection pain diaries. If the duration of pain relief is concordant with the half-life of the diagnostic anesthetic, the injection is considered diagnostic for facet pain. In addition, many of the best-performed postoperative studies advocate the use of a cut-off score of 75%, 80%,[51] or even 100%[52] pain relief to indicate a positive response, as opposed to the earlier practices of 50% pain relief.[51-54] Furthermore, the importance of outcome measures cannot be stressed enough. As was alluded to earlier in this chapter, the focus of diagnostic and therapeutic injections should be functional improvement rather than mitigation on VAS scores. Therefore, evaluation with validated functional measures such as the Pain Disability Questionaire (PDQ), Pain Disability Index (PDI), Euro-Qual, SF-18, or even the old standard Oswestry Disability Index should be utilized when interpreting the effectiveness of any of the interventional procedures discussed in this chapter.

Much debate has arisen regarding the selectivity of intra-articular injection versus medial branch blocks. Cadaveric studies by Dreyfuss et al. suggest that volume control is important in limiting spread of local anesthetic to nearby structures to avoid anesthetizing other nociceptive structures and providing a false-positive result by exerting pain relief and functional benefit to structures other than the facet joint.[53] This research has led many clinicians to follow the "less is more" axiom and to use less than 1 mL of anesthetic for their diagnostic blockade. This small aliquot of anesthetic medication seems to have the best postprocedure positive predictive value, correlating to prospective successful outcomes.[51]

Understanding the myriad of variables that complicate all clinical research, many functional outcome studies have been performed with questionable enrollment criteria. Meta-analyses utilizing stringent compliance with Agency for Healthcare Research and Quality (AHRQ) and Quality Assessment of Diagnostic Accuracy Studies (QUADAS) criteria for evaluation of diagnostic tests suggest that there is strong evidence that controlled diagnostic facet joint blocks establish a diagnosis of facet joint pain in chronic cervical and lumbar spinal pain and moderate evidence for diagnosing thoracic facet joint pain.[55-57] A review by Boswell et al. and another by van Tulder have supported the diagnostic efficacy of facet joint blockade.[58,59] Some reviews still conclude that the multifactorial nature of degenerative joint-associated pain means that there is insufficient evidence to support the use of facet joint injections to diagnose or treat facet joint pain.[7,60]

As with epidural injections, it is important that the reader note that the use of fluoroscopy or CT imaging guidance is critical to success when performing any diagnostic spinal procedure. Significant care should be taken when selecting an interventionist to perform diagnostic injections on patients who you may ultimately be taking to surgery. These procedures cannot be performed with any degree of accuracy without the use of imaging to verify appropriate needle placement and ensure patient safety. Most interventional societies also advocate the additional use of nonionic contrast to verify placement of injectate. This has additional benefit if the interventionalist and/or the referring physician need to review the procedure at a later date. In preparation for an injection, prior review of available advanced imaging studies (CT or MRI) is important to understand the three-dimensional anatomy of the target joints. This is especially true with intra-articular facet joint injections because there can be considerable variability in joint morphology among individuals. The C arm is usually aligned in a slightly oblique fashion to afford the physician access to a portion of the facet joint capsule. The facet joint capsule can be accessed at various locations along the joint line or at the superior or inferior recess. The amount of subcutaneous anesthetic required to keep a particular patient comfortable varies from practitioner to practitioner and from patient to patient. Overinjection of large amounts of anesthetic into the subcutaneous structures and paraspinal musculature has been criticized as a likely contributor to the false-positive rates seen in some studies.[61] Yet another reason to follow the "less is more" dictum, with use of a 25G needle smaller amounts of subcutaneous anesthetic are required. The needle is advanced under fluoroscopic guidance and is often felt piercing the joint and capsule. Confirmation of intra-articular needle placement is made with a small amount of contrast material. The resulting arthrogram will typically reveal retained contrast material in the superior and inferior capsular recesses of the facet joint. At times, a well-demarcated plane of contrast will be seen between the two articular surfaces. Fluoroscopic confirmation is best made in at least two planes, preferably 90 degrees from each other. As stated previously, retention of fluoroscopic images can be critical for future evaluation of the efficacy of the injection and for quality control by the referring surgeon. Once intra-articular flow of contrast is confirmed, a small amount of anesthetic or a solution of anesthetic and long-acting glucocorticoid is injected into the joint before the needle is removed. Typically the amount of this solution is less than 1.25 mL.

The medial branch block is performed in a similar fashion, with the target being the mammillary process, seen fluoroscopically at the osseous junction of the superior articular process and the transverse process in the lower thoracic and lumbar spine. The nerve courses below the mammillary ligament; contrast is often used to outline the ligament and the nerve before placement of anesthetic. In the cervical spine, the target points are located along the waist of the cervical articular pillars. This target is approached from a slightly lateral oblique view with confirmation of needle placement in at least the anteroposterior and lateral planes before injection of contrast. Then the anesthetic is injected and the needle is removed. The most important aspect of a facet joint or medial branch block is not the injection itself but the pain diary recorded by the patient after the procedure has been completed. The diagnostic efficacy of the injection cannot be determined until the duration and degree of pain relief have been recorded and evaluated by the physician on subsequent follow-up 2 to 3 weeks after the injection.

When performing these procedures, a thorough understanding of anatomy is critical. In the cervical spine, the proximity of the dorsal rami, nerve root, radicular arteries, and vertebral artery increase the risk profile of these injections when compared to the relative capaciousness of the lumbar spine. The thoracic spine is very challenging due to the variable location of the medial branch nerves, some of which do not overlie the thoracic transverse process; ventral misadventures can result in a pleural puncture and pneumothorax. These procedures have been proven safe in countless studies, but they are not risk-free. Risks should be discussed before subjecting patients to any interventional procedures.

An additional confounding issue surrounds the routine use of moderate or deep sedation by anesthesiologists during interventional procedures; this may have unintended consequences and can worsen the predictive value of these procedures. Manchikanti et al. studied the effects of IV midazolam and/or fentanyl during cervical and lumbar facet joint injections and showed that with strict criteria the effects of sedation may be minimized to a 10% false-positive rate.[61]

We do not advocate consideration of medial branch nerve radiofrequency ablation (or rhizotomy) unless suspicion of facet joint–mediated pain is supported by clear clinical suspicion, imaging evidence, and two successful diagnostic blocks. This literature-supported opinion has been brought into question by a recent paper by Cohen et al., who contend that the cost of blocks to increase the positive predictive value exceeds the cost utility from pain relief and increased function seen when one proceeds straight to radiofrequency rhizotomy of medical branches.[62] First described by Shealy, this procedure denervates the neural pathways (medial branch nerves) that supply the afferent pain information from the facet joint to the central nervous system.[63] This procedure has been shown to offer longer relief than intra-articular facet joint injections and medial branch blocks.[51] The consistent locations of the medial branch nerves in the lumbar and cervical spine, reported by many anatomists, make these excellent locations for dorsal rami radiofrequency rhizotomy. However, one must recall the redundant nature of the medial branch innervation of the facet joints. Namely, each joint receives innervation from two different dorsal rami levels. For example, the L4-5 facet joint receives its innervation from the L3 medial branch from above and the L4 medial branch at that level. The innervation of the cervical facet joints is somewhat different. The cervical facet joint is innervated by the medial branch nerve of that level and the level below. The reason for this variance lies in the presence of the C8 nerve, which innervates the T1-2 facet joint in conjunction with the T1 medial branch. This consistency of location explains the favorable success rates with cervical and lumbar medial branch blocks and radiofrequency procedures. On the other hand, the location of the thoracic medial branch nerves is known to be quite variable along the length of the thoracic transverse process, which makes effective lesioning of these nerves quite challenging technically. There is ongoing debate as to the most effective techniques to effectively denervate the thoracic facet joints. Directing the radiofrequency rhizotomy probe to its target is performed in much the same manner as in the medial branch block procedure. The major difference is considerations of cross-sectional area in placing a maximal amount of the uninsulated tip of the special insulated radiofrequency needle in the area where the nerve resides. Care is taken to avoid adjacent structures such as nerve roots and deep muscles that were partially lesioned and can cause a new and persistent pain.[64] Again, placement of these needles is performed using fluoroscopy and radiopaque contrast. A lesion is created using either a continuous or pulsed radiofrequency apparatus at 80 to 90 degrees for 80 to 90 seconds. Some practitioners repeat this procedure with slight adjustment to the location of the active tip to create several lesions along the same nerve.

A review by Slipman et al. reports moderately strong evidence (level III) in accordance with the guidelines described by the AHCPR that radiofrequency ablation of the medial branch nerves is an effective treatment for facet joint pain.[65] Other reviews have supported the presence of only moderately weak evidence or conflicting evidence regarding the efficacy of a radiofrequency rhizotomy of medial branch nerves for facet-mediated pain.[66-68] The goal again is increased function and avoidance of the surgical alternative, which is often a fusion. Many continue to argue that the studies reviewed showed poor efficacy due to the authors' failure to employ the double-block criteria that are advocated to identify patients with facet joint–related pain. Therefore, many studies that refute the efficacy of radiofrequency rhizotomy of the medial branch nerves for facet joint pain may have not been treating facet joint pain. In a study by Dreyfuss et al. that employed strict standards and double-block techniques, 60% of patients experienced at least a 90% pain reduction, and 87% of patients experienced at least a 60% reduction in pain after a radiofrequency ablation procedure for low back pain, lasting at 12-month follow-up.[51] Patient safety and efficacy of procedure should remain stronger considerations than cost despite ongoing pressure from insurers. It is the authors' opinion that double-block protocol to determine the injection location and pain generator remains the standard of care.

Despite the continuing debate regarding the efficacy of these procedures, there is a consensus that facet joint injections, medial branch blocks, and radiofrequency ablation are safe, reliable, and minimally invasive options to diagnose and treat patients with facet joint pain (Fig. 191-6).

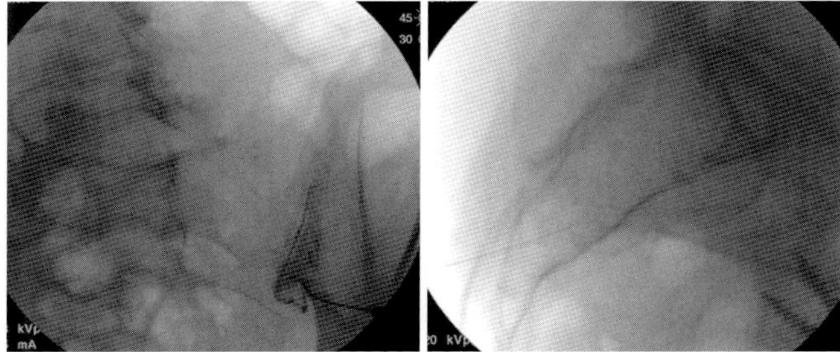

FIGURE 191-6. Sacroiliac joint injection with sacroiliac arthrogram illustrating intra-articular placement.

Sacroiliac Joint Injections

The sacroiliac (SI) joint is a well-accepted source of low back, upper buttock, and leg pain.[69] Much like the facet joint, the SI joint is a true diarthodial joint, receiving its innervation via nerve branches from the lumbar and sacral nerve roots.[70] Debate still remains as to whether the innervation of the SI joint arises primarily from the sacral dorsal rami[71] or from a combination of dorsal and ventral rami.[72] Studies support the presence of neural structures and mechanoreceptors within the SI joint capsule and intra-articularly.[71-73] SI joint pain has been attributed to numerous pathologic processes, including autoimmune inflammation (e.g., spondyloarthropathies), trauma, pregnancy, SI joint dysfunction, and chronic degenerative changes. Studies on asymptomatic individuals who underwent provocative SI joint injections have defined the common pain referral patterns of this joint.[69,74]

The diagnosis of SI joint pain has historically been accomplished through examination findings and pain elicited with provocative maneuvers. Some physicians have advocated a battery of maneuvers, including Gaenslen's, Patrick's, and Gillet's maneuvers, as well as distraction, compression, and thigh thrust tests, as a fairly reliable method to determine the presence or absence of SI joint pain.[75] Others suggest a simpler approach of having the patient point to the area of greatest pain. If the patient points just medial to the dorsal rostral iliac spine, there is a high likelihood of SI joint pain; this simple but effective test is known colloquially as the *Fortin finger test*.[76]

The efficacy of imaging studies to accurately diagnose SI joint pain has been shown to be poor. Despite some reviews that suggest certain physical examination findings or tests as effective in localizing SI joint nociception, SI joint pain remains bereft of a diagnostic "gold standard." Unfortunately, SI joint anesthetic injection has been held by some to be a "pyrite" standard.[7,77] Although there are significant limitations with regard to specificity, many physicians believe this procedure provides the best method of differentiating a clinical suspicion of SI joint pathology from other etiologies of low back pain.[78]

If patients have failed a conservative treatment course that includes medications, physical modalities, stretching, core strengthening, and/or an "SI belt," diagnostic/therapeutic SI joint injection remains a reasonable consideration. Reproducing a patient's pain by distention of the suspect SI joint or mitigating the pain with SI joint injection clearly helps to define a problem isolated to this complex diarthrodial joint, which is innervated in a more redundant/complex fashion than many other diarthrodial joints. Diagnosis of SI joint pain through SI joint injection serves two purposes: (1) to diagnose and treat SI joint pain and (2) to rule out other structures as the possible etiology for back pain. The latter may prevent unnecessary interventions or surgery to nearby structures (i.e., hip and spine).

Similar to other injections, SI joint injections are best performed with the assistance of fluoroscopic or CT imaging guidance. The patient is positioned in the prone position and imaging is adjusted to view an accessible portion of the dorsal SI joint. Due to its tortuous architecture, the joint is typically approached at the most caudal and dorsal location or even at the inferior recess, where the joint capsule is most accessible. Once the spinal needle has entered the joint capsule and imaging has verified the intra-articular location of the needle tip, nonionic contrast material is injected to verify the adequacy of the SI joint arthrogram. After verification of intra-articular flow, an anesthetic or combination of anesthetic and steroid is injected into the joint. Typically this volume will be 1.5 to 2 mL. If while reviewing a patient's interventional procedure note, a physician learns that the injectionist endorses introducing 4 to 6 mL of injectate, this is an indication of poor quality control. This type of injection is often a near-SI joint injection, colloquially known as the *Hail Mary*. This is a negative quality indicator and possibly a reason to seek out a new interventional practice to perform diagnostic injections.

Radiofrequency rhizotomy of dorsal rami nerves has been shown to offer long-term relief of facet-mediated pain. As of the publication of this chapter, radiofrequency technology remains an investigational option to treat SI joint pain. No level I, II, or III studies were found in Medline to support radiofrequency ablation of lumbar or sacral nerves as an effective way of ameliorating SI joint pain. The negative studies to date are likely the result of the variable and circuitous routes of the sacral dorsal rami branches and co-innervation by select ventral rami innervating the SI joint. Needless to say, the paucity of high-quality literature belies the strong support for this procedure among entrepreneurs advocating for novel devices to treat SI pain.

McKenzie-Brown et al. evaluated the specificity and validity of SI joint injections and found there to be moderate evidence to support this procedure using AHRQ, Cochrane Review Group, and QUADAS criteria for diagnostic studies.[79,80] The authors also concluded that the evidence for moderate to long-term therapeutic value from SI joint injections and/or radiofrequency denervation of nerves innervating the SI joint was limited.

Sympathetic Blockade

The sympathetic nervous system plays an important role in certain chronic pain states that can be relieved by sympathetic blockade.[81] The pathways and mechanisms by which the sympathetic nervous system facilitates a persistently painful pathologic state remain poorly understood. Techniques for lumbar sympathetic and cervical sympathetic (stellate ganglion) blockade are primarily used to diagnose and occasionally assist in treatment of sympathetically mediated complex regional pain syndrome (CRPS).

Lumbar sympathetic blocks have been performed since the early 1900s to treat such conditions as circulatory insufficiency, Raynaud phenomenon, diabetic/vascular gangrene, reflex sympathetic dystrophy, CRPS types I and II, phantom-limb pain, and stump pain, as well as select painless conditions such as hyperhydrosis. The anatomy of the lumbar sympathetic ganglia is variable in location and in number, but they tend to be aggregated at the L1 through L4 levels (often ventral to L2 or L3 vertebral bodies). Originally the procedure involved a three-needle technique; however, many practitioners today utilize a two- or one-needle technique. The procedure is performed using fluoroscopy to navigate the needle. The trajectory involves oblique navigation to arrive ventral to the vertebral body in the lateral quarter of either the L2 or L3 vertebral body, approximating the great vessels. A loss of resistance syringe is occasionally used to identify when the needle has entered the retroperitoneal space. Nonionic contrast material is injected to identify the cranial-caudal spread of contrast material along the sympathetic chain dorsal and lateral to the great vessels in the retroperitoneal space. Successful blockade is noted with vasodilation, increased limb temperature (>3°C), or immediate reduction of edema. Complications include bleeding, vascular injury, infection, hypotension, renal injury, impotence, failure to ejaculate, and genitofemoral nerve injury.

The stellate ganglion block remains a commonly performed injection for pain management, although the injection should be referred to as a lower cervical or upper thoracic sympathetic block because the stellate ganglion is present in only about 80% of the population.[82] The conditions commonly treated with this block include CRPS of the upper limb, Raynaud phenomenon, arterial embolism, postherpetic neuralgia, phantom limb pain, and stump pain. The stellate ganglion is formed by the fusion of the inferior cervical ganglion and the first thoracic ganglion. The stellate ganglion is approached ventrally by palpating the landmark at the lateral aspect of the ventral C6 vertebral body (known as the *Chaussignac tubercle*). This landmark can occasionally be seen radiographically. When performing this procedure, a combination of palpatory and fluoroscopic guidance is helpful. One must manually retract the carotid artery while palpating the Chaussignac tubercle to avoid inadvertent vascular puncture. Fluoroscopic guidance helps one to avoid advancing the needle past the C6 tubercle where the vertebral artery lies. Once the needle is positioned correctly, it is withdrawn slightly from the periostium; contrast is injected and should be observed spreading evenly in a rostral-caudal fashion (as with the lumbar sympathetic chain). Failure to observe spread of contrast in both the cranial and caudal directions may indicate intramuscular injection. The needle should be repositioned so a wispy, rostral-caudal spread is visualized. A small test dose of anesthetic is usually administered; barring any untoward effects, the remainder of the solution (up to 8 mL) is injected. The total injectate needed depends on the desired block. Sympathetic block of the ganglion can be easily documented with the presence of Horner syndrome: miosis, ptosis, enophthalmos, conjunctival injection, nasal congestion, and facial anhidrosis. Successful sympathetic blockade to the upper limb can be determined by venous engorgement, psychogalvanic reflex, positive sweat test, and rise in skin temperature. Complications from this procedure have included tracheal trauma, injury to the brachial plexus, injury to the pleura and lung, diaphragmatic paralysis, intraspinal injection, and seizures from intravascular injection (Figs. 191-7 and 191-8).[82]

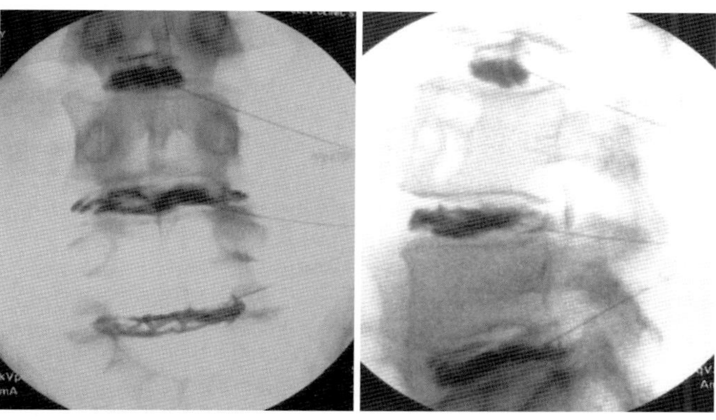

FIGURE 191-7. Three-level discogram; L3-4, L4-5, and L5-S1, with L3-4 as the control level.

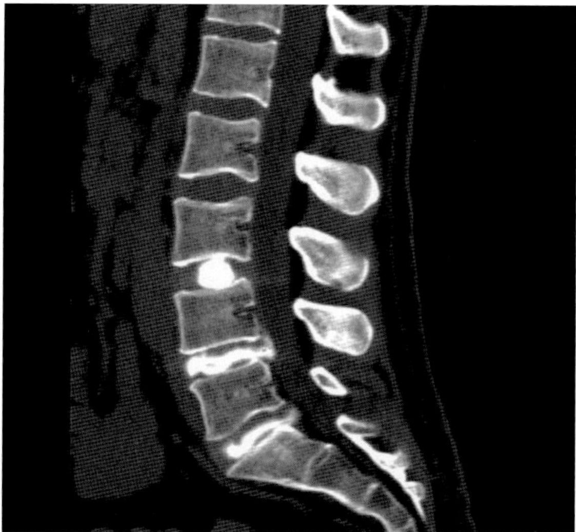

FIGURE 191-8. Postdiscogram CT sagittal image.

Discogenic Pain

Discogenic pain is a topic that has warranted multiple chapters and even books. For those readers who do not believe that the disc is a source of pain and disability, it may be best to skip to the next section. For those of you still reading out of either loyalty to the disc or equipoise, this section is fraught. At the publication of this chapter the state of discography as a diagnostic technique still remains in flux. The crux of the argument lies in the paradox of spinal pain. If a plurality of the asymptomatic population share a similar radiologic appearance (disc dessication, herniations, anular tears, osteophytes, degenerative changes.), why do some hurt so much and why are they seemingly refractory to treatment? This question is not answered here, but the debate centered on diagnosing discogenic pain is discussed.

For much of the latter half of the 20th century, provocative discography and a host of scoring criteria were the mainstays of algorithmic decisions for or against fusion surgery.[83,84] In 2006, Carragee et al. presented the first of a series of high-level, prospective collected evidence showing high false-positive rates, poor specificity, and false sensitivity and questioning the safety of discography's role in confirming discogenic pain.[85,86] The final coffin nails appeared with data from multiple prospective studies showing outcomes of lumbar fusion remaining poor even when discography was utilized to supplement the clinical decision making. These outcomes look especially poor when outcomes such as return to work are employed (rather than the usual soft outcomes such as VAS scores alone or combined with Oswestry scores).[87-90] The system of remuneration continues to shift toward evidence-based recommendations. Both the Official Disability Guidelines (ODG) and American College of Occupational and Environmental Medicine (ACOEM) guidelines now recommend against discography. Does the continuing poor outcome data for lumbar fusions (as opposed to much better outcome data for cervical fusions) mean that the diagnostic test is a poor test?[91] Alternatively, does poor lumbar fusion data mean that lumbar fusion is an overutilized procedure,[4] while saying nothing about the positive predictive value of discography? These questions remain unanswered. As it stands in 2011, the raw numbers of discographies requested by surgeons has fallen in the authors' practice by more than 90%. The seeming final nail in discography's coffin is an as-yet unpublished paper presented at a national meeting that purports to show 10-year data with advanced radiologic visualized degenerative changes to the normal, control-level disc used in prior discography tests.[92] Should this paper pass peer review, showing that discography is both inaccurate at improving outcomes and has the additional component of harm, causing degeneration and eventual symptomatic herniation in otherwise healthy discs, that would likely eliminate the use of discography as a reasonable test.

An emerging technology that remains under study is anesthetic discography. The principle is quite simple: irritate (either mechanically or chemically) the disc of interest (the assumed source of nociception). If concordant pain is reproduced, infuse the disc percutaneously with anesthetic to see if the pain resolves. At the moment, one product is available in the United States, but prospective data remain unconvincing that use of this diagnostic test will improve results on hard outcomes such as return to work.[93]

A number of minimally invasive disc procedures focusing on treatment of the painful disc have emerged in recent years. These procedures target one of three mechanisms of disc action (specifically, hydraulic performance): reducing the intradiscal pressure, remodeling the anulus (by coagulation), or denervating the neural structures (believed to transmit the afferent pain from the anulus).

Heat-modulated disruption of the "degenerative cascade" is the stand-alone mechanism of action. The thought of "annealing" the proteoglycan structure of the nucleus via thermocoagulation seems to be a dead end. Placing a straight radiofrequency probe in the center of the disc nucleus and creating lesions at varying duration and varying temperatures has failed to show benefit despite the initial hope/hype. Only two studies have emerged, with neither showing any significant improvement in discogenic back pain.[94,95]

Another "orphan" intradiscal procedure that enjoyed the limelight as the original minimally invasive procedure is chemonucleolysis. This procedure involves the injection of chymopapain (a derivative of the papaya fruit) into the nucleus pulposus to dissolve nuclear material. Additionally, the chemical digestion of the nuclear material often causes a robust inflammatory response that occasionally resulted in interbody fusion of the treated level. Although the risks of severe complications from this procedure are relatively rare, the inability to control spread of the chymopapain injectate through anular fissures likely results in irritation of nearby neural, arthrodial, and vascular structures. Although still performed by some physicians, this procedure has fallen out of favor in light of lack of supporting evidence of its effectiveness and the pain patients experienced in the first 6 to 8 weeks postprocedure.

One prominent and briefly popular method focused on modulating pain nerve innervation of the anulus by heating this area of the disc. This modality, known as *intradiscal electrothermal therapy*, or IDET, had initial strength of evidence to receive a category I Current Procedural Terminology (CPT) code. One prospective trial demonstrating the procedure's effectiveness won a national "best paper" award from *The Spine Journal*.[96] This procedure utilizes a percutaneous catheter that allows deployment of a 5-cm active tip wire. The wire is wound along the curved, dorsal aspect of the nucleus–anulus junction.[94,97] Once in place, the wire is heated to 90°C. The resulting effect is believed to promote thermal coagulation of the anular nerve endings, remodeling of the degenerating anulus, and possibly structural reinforcement near weak areas of the anulus, spilling nuclear material. In their review, Derby et al. proposed several mechanisms by which heat may reduce disc-related pain, including changes in disc biomechanics, anular contraction, thermally induced healing response, sealing of anular tears, and anular denervation. After a thorough biomechanical analysis, the authors concluded that the mechanism of pain relief remains unclear.[98] Early studies by Saal and Saal demonstrated 24-month outcomes with mean improvement in VAS of 3.16 points, improved sitting times on average by 52.7 minutes, mean improvements in SF-36 of 31.33 points, and at least a 7-point improvement on a bodily pain scale in 78% of subjects.[99]

Although IDET has been the most frequently performed anuloplasty procedure in recent times, much debate remains regarding the efficacy of the procedure and its mechanism of pain relief. The two available randomized, prospectively collected, sham-control studies have had conflicting results and conclusions. Pauza's award-winning paper demonstrated significantly better improvement in pain severity (36% vs. 17%, $P = .045$) and back function (35% vs. 12%, $P < .05$) among patients treated with the IDET procedure compared to patients randomly assigned to sham control.[96] Freeman et al., on the other hand, demonstrated failure to improve at any of the outcome end points in either the treatment or sham subjects. Numerous issues have been raised regarding the conflicting results. The issues mostly center around aspects of patient selection, including severity of degenerative disc changes, patient comorbidities, duration of pain, and lack of *any* response to treatment (in the Freeman paper), which seems to contradict the accepted internal control for the placebo.[100] Andersson et al. compared 18 IDET studies and 33 published studies of spine fusion for treatment of discogenic pain, which seemed to show comparable outcomes with regard to pain severity and quality of life.[101] However, complications were far more common in the fusion studies compared to the IDET studies.

Two other percutaneous anuloplasty procedures are currently being reported: percutaneous intradiscal radiofrequency thermocoagulation and biacuplasty. The first procedure involves the placement of a unipolar radiofrequency probe into the nucleus–anulus junction. The literature regarding the success of this procedure to date has been equivocal; no significant improvements have been shown in patients suffering from discogenic pain. Kapural et al. published a study regarding the efficacy of unipolar anuloplasty compared to IDET and found that at 12-month follow-up, those who underwent IDET experienced significantly better improvement and significantly greater reductions in pain severity (81% vs. 33%, $P = .001$).[102] Biacuplasty is a newer version of the same anuloplasty procedure that utilizes two radiofrequency probes introduced into the dorsal anulus that create a radiofrequency lesion across the dorsal anulus. Six-month follow-up data from this procedure have reported improvements in several pain assessment scales (e.g., VAS) without associated improvement in functional scales. Further prospective, randomized studies are clearly needed given the mixed record with IDET.[103]

Other minimally invasive intradiscal procedures focus on reduction of disc pressure by removal of disc material. These procedures employ various devices that use either mechanical means or thermal energy to remove disc material. One procedure, known as *nucleoplasty*, utilizes a radiofrequency probe to create small channels in the nuclear material to attempt to decrease the nuclear volume. Based on U.S. Preventive Services Task Force (USPSTF) criteria, Manchikanti et al. maintain that level II-3 evidence exists that favors an indication that nucleoplasty decreases lower extremity pain due to disc herniation.[104] However, evidence of efficacy is lacking for relief of back pain. Techniques to manually remove disc material go by several names. One, the automated percutaneous lumbar discectomy device, utilizes a modified vitrectomy instrument with a reciprocating suction-cutter to aspirate, cut, circulate, and remove fluid and extruded disc material. Although initial studies were promising, a subsequent randomized, controlled study shows a 29% success rate; this evidence has caused this procedure to fall out of favor.[105] Another mechanical device utilizes a high-RPM Archimedes screw to remove nuclear material through the cannula of the device. Level III evidence (by AHRQ criteria) was cited to support relief of pain, with functional data notably missing from the review.[106] Finally, percutaneous laser discectomy utilizes a high-powered visible-spectrum laser to vaporize nuclear material, thereby reducing intradiscal pressure. Recent review for this procedure purports to show level II-2 evidence of efficacy based on USPSTF criteria.[107]

The success of these procedures and published evidence relies largely on patient selection. The goal is to harness/enhance the body's natural, self-healing processes, but the evidence of true mechanism of action for functional improvement remains sparse for these techniques. Enrollment criteria for all of the aforementioned safety procedures state that the disc space should be preserved. Loss of more than 50% of the disc space excluded patients from most studies. Unfortunately, patients with concomitant pain, functional loss, and disc degenerative changes still represent the majority of our patient population. Does this fact make many of the studies of efficacy nongeneralizable? Patients studied also had normal neurologic examination results, imaging supporting/concordant with pain at the degenerative disc levels, positive disc pain on provocative discography, and lack of significant confounding psychosocial issues.

Does this represent the standard patient? Although these procedures are performed percutaneously, they still have a substantial risk profile. Complications from these procedures have included both aseptic and septic spondylodiscitis, bleeding, nerve root injury, vascular injury, sigmoid artery injury, worsening pain, and failure of the mechanical device requiring surgical removal. Contraindications to these procedures include chronic radiculopathy, large fragmented or sequestered disc fragments, equivocal results from diagnostic discography, severe spinal canal stenosis, uncontrolled coagulopathy and bleeding disorders, cauda equina syndrome, and infection.

Diagnostic Tests

In the authors' experience spine injection procedures are used for diagnostic as well as therapeutic purposes. Multiple studies have shown that abnormalities seen on MRI or CT do not necessarily correlate with symptoms.[10,12,108,109] Moreover, even a first episode of pain may not correspond to new MRI pathology.[110] With these complicating factors, injections serve a purpose to improve surgical outcomes. Several authors of recent meta-analyses have opined that evidence is insufficient to recommend diagnostic injections.[111,112] As discussed in the facet joint portion of this chapter, the relevance of a diagnostic test lies in the acceptance of false-positive and false-negative rates. Diagnostic injections are used frequently in clinical practice, and many surgeons find them clinically helpful. Most physicians understand that no test is perfect. The crux of a test's utility lies in the rigor of the person interpreting the test. Therefore, if there is incentive to shade diagnostic results, the test loses all value in the eyes of the public. The lack of rigor in so-called meta-analyses does not allow for good recommendations regarding positive predictive value.[111] Instead, diagnostic and prognostic tests should be evaluated in prospectively controlled trials with hard outcomes.[112]

Diagnostic nerve root blockade is one of the mainstays of diagnostic injections. The approach is similar to the transforaminal epidural steroid injection described in this chapter, with several important differences; these include lateral placement of the needle tip, rigorous contrast confirmation of no epidural or intravascular flow, confirmation of extraneural placement of the needle tip, and limiting of the volume of infused medication. Violation of any of these principles may lead to unintended propinquity anesthesia.

Yeom et al. elegantly demonstrated with blocks of affected and unaffected nerve roots that the diagnostic predictive value of selective nerve blocks approaches 80% when the best practice principles are adopted.[113] These tests, like virtually all diagnostic tests in medicine, should be used in conjunction with other information to maximize benefit for the patient.[114,115] In this chapter, we have discussed reliability issues surrounding diagnostic techniques for facet joint pain, SI joint pain, articular hip pain, and articular shoulder pain, as well as the maelstrom of controversy surrounding the diagnosis of discogenic pain. The arguments are not repeated here, with the exception of stating that if this information improves surgical outcomes and prevents even one catastrophic failure, it probably has shown its worth (Fig. 191-9).

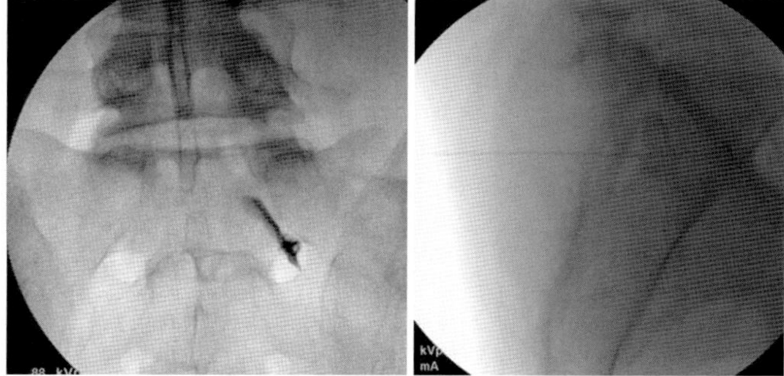

FIGURE 191-9. Diagnostic selective nerve root block of right S1 nerve root (anteroposterior [*left*] and lateral [*right*] images).

Intrathecal Drug Delivery

Since the late 1980s, the use of intrathecal analgesia for the treatment of severe chronic cancer pain and neuropathic and chronic nonmalignant pain has been growing in popularity. Delivery of intrathecal analgesics is not a new concept. As early as 1885, Leonard Corning reported on intrathecal anesthetic administration.[116] Intrathecal morphine administration in the treatment of cancer pain was reported in 1979 by Wang et al.[117]

Over the past 20 years, continuous infusion of intrathecal baclofen via a subcutaneously implanted pump has become a powerful tool in the management of spasticity in various neurologic conditions. Baclofen (Lioresal), the *p*-chlorophenyl derivative of GABA, possesses poor lipid solubility and therefore crosses the blood-brain barrier poorly. The resulting positive evidence, safe management, and increased function for spinal cord–injured patients demonstrates a safety profile that allowed pumps to be applied for narcotic infusions.[118] Originally introduced as a treatment modality for patients suffering severe pain from malignancy, intrathecal administration of morphine directly to the site of therapeutic action provided better analgesia at a lower dose with fewer adverse effects than oral medications. Morphine is the current gold standard in intrathecally delivered pain medications and is the only opiate approved by the Food and Drug Administration for spinal administration. Because the typical life expectancy of the pump outlasts the typical life expectancy of the patient, this offers a pain management modality that has been deemed very effective. Strong disagreement still surrounds the use of intrathecal morphine pumps for chronic nonmalignant pain. Although administration of opiate medications is common practice in treating chronic nonmalignant pain, the systemic adverse effects of these medications often limit their use.[119] In light of longer life expectancy in patients with nonmalignant pain, these patients are much more likely to experience the adverse physiologic and psychosocial effects of long-term opiate therapy. Early studies suggested that intrathecal delivery of morphine was effective in about 60% of patients with chronic pain of nonmalignant origin.[120] Neuraxial morphine administration has been found to be safe and efficacious in the short term in palliating chronic, intractable malignant, and nonmalignant pain.[120-122] Despite its relative safety, adverse effects from intrathecal morphine include nausea, vomiting, drowsiness, pruritus, weakness, diaphoresis, urine retention, respiratory depression, weight gain, impotence, amenorrhea, hypothyroidism, paranoia, nystagmus, polyarthralgia, myoclonus, peripheral edema, and failure to sustain benefit.[119,123]

Another rare side effect that has been receiving much attention in recent years is the development of granulomatous tissue near the tip of the infusion catheter. Although reported symptomatic cases are still relatively rare, this complication has resulted in some significant neurologic sequela. There is much debate as to the cause of these granulomas, but their development is believed to be related to the concentration of morphine administered.[124] Although morphine is the most common medication administered through the intrathecal route, other medications, such as fentanyl, sufentanil, clonidine, and bupivacaine, have been employed as well. Due to each drug's pharmacokinetics and lipophilic or lipophobic characteristics, each has its own set of positive and negative qualities. Newer medications, including N-type calcium channel blockers, have shown a high side effect profile with relatively modest benefits over opioid infusion.

Neuromodulation

Spinal cord stimulation has been evolving as a treatment modality since the 1970s. Advances in technology around spinal cord stimulators or dorsal column stimulation have tracked with good short-term and medium-term evidence of efficacy. Since the 1960s, this technology has been considered a clinical application of Melzack and Wall's "gate-control theory."[125] First reports of spinal cord stimulation clinical use in patients were published in 1975.[126] Over the years, this modality has been applied to the treatment of peripheral ischemia, cardiac ischemia, complex regional pain syndrome, diabetic neuropathy, postherpetic neuralgia, phantom limb pain, postamputation stump pain, and chronic pain resulting from postlaminectomy syndrome. The exact mechanism of action underlying the sustained efficacy of spinal cord stimulation is unknown.

The sympatholytic effect is still postulated to be the major underlying property behind the success of spinal cord stimulation. While recent research around the plasticity of the neuron-axis has called into question some of the original theories, spinal cord stimulation has recently gained greater acceptance in the treatment of both neuropathic pain and axial spine pain resulting from chronic radiculopathy and postlaminectomy syndrome.[127] In light of its growing clinical significance and advancements in stimulator and electrode design, an entire chapter of this text has been dedicated to the discussion of this technology and its applications. The rigor of recent research and protocols for reasonable use has allowed for evidence-based acceptance of neurostimulation and the inclusion in guidelines as an adjunct to return patients to function (Figs. 191-10 and 191-11).

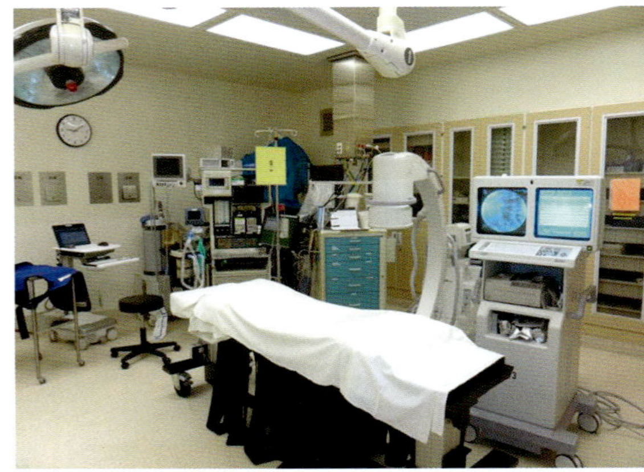

FIGURE 191-10. Standard injection suite with fluoroscopy, noninvasive monitoring, and clean conditions.

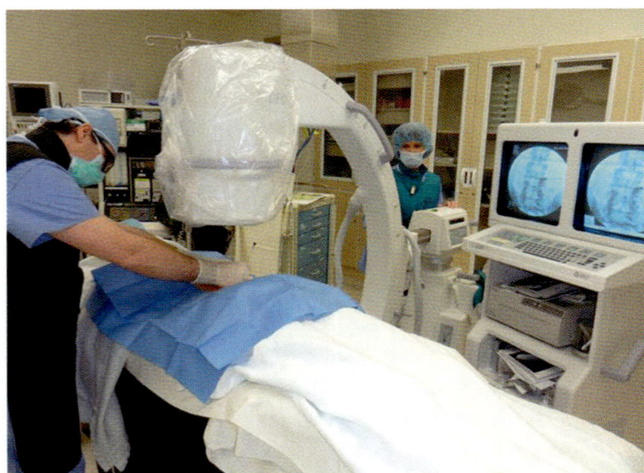

FIGURE 191-11. Fluoroscopically guided injections to maximize safety and minimize risk of infection or needle misadventure. The radiation technologist and nurse are present with physician.

Radiation Safety

As stated multiple times throughout this chapter, the procedures enumerated previously should only be performed using image guidance. For the most part, fluoroscopy remains the imagery modality of choice. The fundamentals of x-ray generation and harm are beyond the scope of this chapter, but the fundamentals of radiation safety apply to the surgeon and the interventionist alike. The main principle is that dose effects of x-rays are cumulative over a lifetime. As such, controlling for proximity and distance from the x-ray source, minimizing scatter, shielding, pulse dosing, and positioning can add up, varying dose-equivalent by more than a factor of 10. Appropriate fluoroscopic training to minimize the dose is mandatory to avoid dermatologic, ophthalmic, or oncologic complications. Experience with fluoroscopy is important to avoid self-inflicted complications with greater consequence than those listed in the next section.

Complications

The side-effect profile for injections is relatively benign when compared with surgery. However, it should not be counted as a risk-free procedure and the surgeon must advocate for the safest performance of these procedures. Safety and quality control should clearly include the use of fluoroscopy and the performance of these procedures in a procedure room using sterile equipment in a sterile environment.

The most common risk both in terms of frequency of occurrence and potentially catastrophic effects (as with surgery) is bleeding inside the spinal canal. This risk is minimized by avoiding patients with bleeding diathesis, avoiding patients actively using anticoagulation, knowing the location of the vascular anatomy under fluoroscopy/CT, and utilizing nonionic contrast dye to avoid misadventure.

The second major risk is infection. Published infection rates vary between 0.1% and 2.0%. In the office environment, use of sterile technique with appropriately thorough patient scrub and draping keeps infection rates to a minimum. The routine use of preoperative antibiotics for these procedures may carry more risk than benefit—unless the planned procedure includes long-term, indwelling, externalized devices or entry into an avascular environment such as the intervertebral disc.

Examples of other potential complications involve steroid reactions, vasovagal stress reactions, arrhythmia, hyperglycemic response to steroids, spinal headache, exacerbation of pain, intraneural injection, and anaphylaxis.

The final risk that should be strongly taken into consideration is intravascular injection of particulate steroid medication. Is the risk of using a (possibly riskier) medication that may have a longer half-life outweighed by the risk of repeated procedures to achieve the same length of benefit? This question is not satisfactorily answered. The interventionist performing the injection should explain the risk-benefit ratio to the patient to maximize both degree and time of benefit with the low likelihood of intravascular injection with good technique. The authors of this chapter strongly recommend adequate training before starting to perform these injections on patients.

KEY REFERENCES

Carragee E, Alamin T, Cheng I, et al: Are first-time episodes of serious LBP associated with new MRI findings? *Spine J* 6(6):624–635, 2006.

Dreyfuss P, Halbrook B, Pauza K, et al: Efficacy and validity of radiofrequency neurotomy for chronic lumbar zygapophysial joint pain. *Spine* 25:1270–1277, 2000.

Mooney V, Robertson J: The facet syndrome. *Clin Orthop Relat Res* 115: 149–156, 1976.

Okubadejo GO, Talcott MR, Schmidt RE, et al: Perils of intravascular methylprednisolone injection into the vertebral artery. An animal study. *J Bone Joint Surg [Am]* 90(9):1932–1938, 2008.

Rainville J, Pransky G, Indahl A, Mayer EK: The physician as disability advisor for patients with musculoskeletal complaints. *Spine* 30(22):2579–2584, 2005.

Riew KD, Yin Y, Gilula L, et al: The effect of nerve-root injections on the need for operative treatment of lumbar radicular pain. A prospective, randomized, controlled, double-blind study. *J Bone Joint Surg [Am]* 82(11):1589–1593, 2000.

Rubinstein SM, van Tulder M: A best-evidence review of diagnostic procedures for neck and low-back pain. *Best Pract Res Clin Rheumatol* 22:471–482, 2008.

Tachihara H, Sekiguchi M, Kikuchi S, Konno S: Do corticosteroids produce additional benefit in nerve root infiltration for lumbar disc herniation? *Spine* 33(7):743–747, 2008.

REFERENCES

The complete reference list is available online at expertconsult.com.

CHAPTER 192

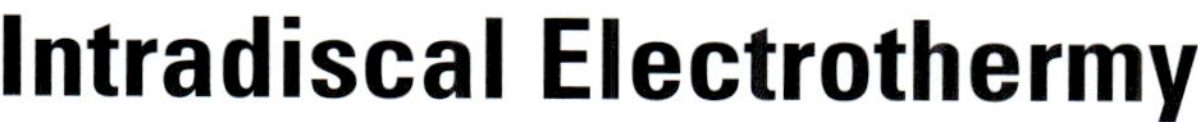

Intradiscal Electrothermy

Christopher Baggott | Nirav J. Patel | Gregory R. Trost

Low back pain affects up to 80% of the U.S. population at least once in their lifetime.[1-3] Although many cases of acute low back pain are self-limiting, resolving within 12 weeks, there is a recurrence rate of 20% within 6 months and an overall recurrence rate of 70% to 90%.[1,4] In approximately 5% of patients, low back pain becomes chronic and disabling.[5] Thus, chronic low back pain is the most common cause of disability between the ages of 45 and 65.[3,6]

Low back pain presents a diagnostic challenge, as only 10% to 20% of cases are attributable to a precise anatomic cause.[7] There is poor correlation between symptoms, imaging findings, and physiologic changes. However, it has been estimated that about 40% of chronic low back pain originates from the intervertebral disc.[8] Kuslich et al. demonstrated concordant pain on direct stimulation of the outer anulus of in vivo intervertebral discs, supporting the role of the disc as a "pain generator."[9] With degeneration theorized to be the underlying cause, the mechanism of discogenic pain has been pursued recently in clinical and basic research. Pathologic neoinnervation, nociceptive sensitization, biomechanical alteration, and internal anular fissuring/disruption have been implicated as possible mechanisms.

Treating chronic discogenic low back pain has been difficult. Medication and aggressive nonoperative treatment, such as physical therapy, often fail to improve function or to reduce pain significantly. In the past, individuals with continued pain and disability after initial therapy were treated with conservative pain management therapy or surgical intervention. Discectomy and fusion can have a 40% failure rate, particularly with multiple degenerative disc levels, in addition to the risk of complications, surgical morbidity, and prolonged recovery.[10,11] As another option, less invasive intradiscal interventions have been the subject of much clinical and basic research since 1997, when Saal and Saal proposed intradiscal electrothermal therapy (IDET).[12]

IDET targets the intervertebral disc that is thought to be the pain generator, often aided by provocative discography. Under conscious sedation, a thermal coil is introduced into the dorsal aspect of the anulus fibrosus, and an amount of thermal energy is delivered. Though the mechanism of action is unclear, it has been proposed that the heat applied may alter the collagen organization in the anulus and coagulate nociceptive fibers to improve biomechanical function and reduce pain.[13]

Discogenic Low Back Pain

Intervertebral discs are bordered by thin hyaline cartilage end plates of the superior and an inferior vertebral body. The nucleus pulposus is the core of the disc, consisting of type II collagen and elastin embedded in the gelatinous substance aggrecan, which is rich in hydrated proteoglycans.[3] Encasing the nucleus is a dense ring of type I collagen known as the anulus fibrosus; it is highly organized into lamellae and maintained by fibroblast-like cells. The disc is avascular, though nutrients can diffuse from the marrow cavity of the adjacent vertebrae across the cartilaginous end plates. In the lumbar spine, intervertebral discs are about 40 mm in diameter and 7 to 10 mm in height.[3]

Degeneration of the intervertebral disc seems to be intimately linked to the loss of nuclear hydrostatic pressure. Fragmentation of proteoglycans in the nucleus leads to reduced hydrostatic pressure, fewer proteoglycans in the nucleus, and fewer proteoglycans adjacent to the cartilaginous end plates. End-plate subchondral sclerosis and calcification will occur and further reduce the nutrient flow to the disc.[14] It has been proposed that the anulus delaminates and buckles inward when the nuclear hydrostatic pressure is lost, leading to collapse of the normal anular organization.[13] Resultant internal mobility and shear stress can lead to fissuring of the anular wall.[15]

Fissuring of the anulus can be assessed by CT discography. Although CT discography is not generally the diagnostic test of choice for discogenic low back pain, provoked pain concordant with chronic symptoms and CT evidence of internal disc disruption can be helpful in determining the benefit of possible operative intervention.[3] However, no class I studies exist that compare outcomes in patients with and without positive discography for either spine fusion or IDET.

MR imaging demonstrating a high-intensity zone on T2-weighted images correlates with painful fissured discs in 65% to 95% of individuals; however, MR has a sensitivity of less than 50% for predicting the presence of anular fissures.[13,16-18]

Pain resulting from degeneration may arise from the disc, the mechanical effect of the disc on an adjacent structure, and the inflammatory mediators that are present in the setting of a degenerated disc.[3] The anterior aspect of the disc is sparsely innervated by perivascular nerve plexuses joining branches of the sympathetic trunk. The posterior aspect is innervated more densely, with nociceptive nerve endings containing substance P primarily arising from the sinovertebral nerve endings with contributions from the sympathetic trunk.[13,19,20] Discogenic pain is primarily axial, though referred leg pain can occur from converging nociceptive fibers from the leg and from the sinovertebral nerve.[21]

Nociceptive fibers are generally present in the outer third of the anulus fibrosus, the posterior longitudinal ligament, and the cartilaginous end plates.[22] In vivo studies have shown that the two most common pain generators are the posterior longitudinal ligament and the dorsal anulus fibrosus.[20] However, a degenerated disc may undergo neoinnervation with small, unmyelinated nociceptive fibers growing deep into the anulus fibrosus and even into the nucleus pulposus.[23,24] Furthermore, nociceptors undergo presensitization from granulation tissue and inflammatory substances, including phospholipase A2, interleukin-1, nitrous oxide, and metalloproteinase.[25-27]

The complex interplay between continued mechanical loading and neural properties, including neoinnervation and presensitization, underlies the development of chronic discogenic low back pain.[13] This entity is distinct from pain due to nerve compression from protruding or herniated discs; it is the disc that is the pain generator owing to an internal derangement.[13] Therefore, the target of intervention is the disc itself.

Intradiscal Electrothermal Therapy

Given the suboptimal results of surgical treatment, the difficulties of chronic pain management, and the widespread prevalence of degenerative disc disease, a minimally invasive treatment for chronic discogenic low back pain is appealing. Saal and Saal developed IDET in 1997, theorizing that the clinical benefits that are observed from heat-induced collagen alteration as performed in joint stabilization procedures could translate to the degenerated, painful intervertebral disc.[12]

Briefly, the IDET procedure targets a painful disc as identified on provocative discography. IDET can be performed under conscious sedation. With fluoroscopic guidance, a navigable thermal resistive heating coil is introduced into the outer portion of the anulus fibrosus in the region of an anular fissure as noted by imaging, typically in the dorsal anulus. The catheter should lie about 5 mm from the outer edge of the anulus for adequate heating of the inner and outer anulus.[28] In practice, the final position of the catheter is generally the contralateral posterolateral outer anulus, then passing anteriorly parallel to the anular lamellae.[28] The coil is heated gradually to achieve tissue temperatures that are adequate to disrupt hydrogen cross-linking in the collagen triple helix, 60°C to 65°C, and coagulate nerve endings more than 42°C.[5,29] Saal and Saal give 60°C to 75°C as a target tissue temperature.[13] Up to 40% of the time, a bilateral approach is necessary to address the entire posterior anulus. Intradiscal antibiotics are given as discitis prophylaxis.[13]

Course of Recovery

IDET typically causes a transient increase in pain that lasts 1 to 2 weeks. Within 6 to 12 weeks, significant pain improvement and reduced disability are reported (Fig. 192-1). Benefits seem to be enduring, with progressive improvement 1 to 2 years postprocedure.[30,31] However, some reports suggest that a significant population that will revert to baseline after initial improvement (Fig. 192-2).[32]

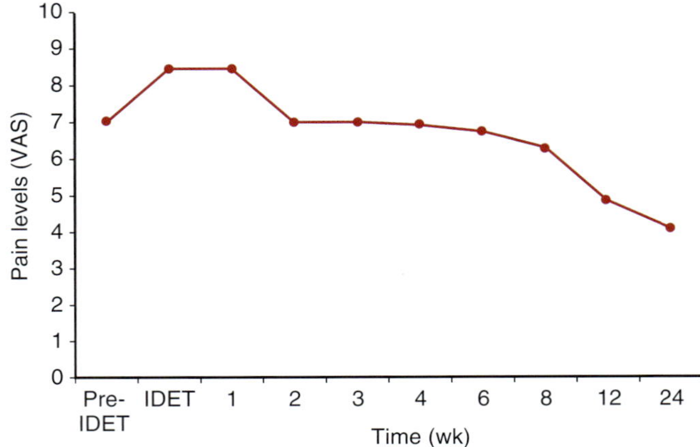

FIGURE 192-1. Typical recovery curve as presented by Saal and Saal, based on their first 100 treated patients. (Redrawn from Saal JA, Saal JS: Intradiscal electrothermal therapy for the treatment of chronic discogenic low back pain. *Clin Sports Med* 21[1]:167–187, 2002.)

Postprocedure Rehabilitation

Transient worsening of symptoms is expected after IDET. Avoiding bending, lifting, and prolonged sitting should be recommended initially postprocedure. A corset is recommended for 6 to 8 weeks. Patients can gradually increase activities to include low-intensity stretching and walking over the first 4 weeks. Floor stabilization exercises at 4 weeks can be encouraged. Waiting 6 months postprocedure is recommended for athletic activity. Box 192-1 lists guidelines for patients following the procedure.

Selection Criteria

Pain reduction and functional improvement from IDET are observed in 23% to 86% of individuals, but it is widely accepted that stringent inclusion criteria are necessary, given the large number of nonresponders that has been observed.[30,33-35] Studies suggest that individuals with multilevel degenerative disc disease respond poorly to IDET, on the basis of improved study outcomes with selection criteria excluding severe multilevel disease.[31,33,36] Another group presents a study demonstrating poor outcomes correlated to obesity, with only 10% benefiting from IDET.[37]

Kloth et al. recently published a review of IDET selection criteria and indications for use to achieve clinical benefit in 75% of patients.[38] Criteria that may be used include the following:

- Persistent axial low back pain with or without leg pain and nonresponsiveness to 6 or more weeks of conservative care
- History consistent with discogenic low back pain (e.g., pain with lumbar motion, decreased sitting duration and tolerance) with a normal lower-extremity neurologic examination

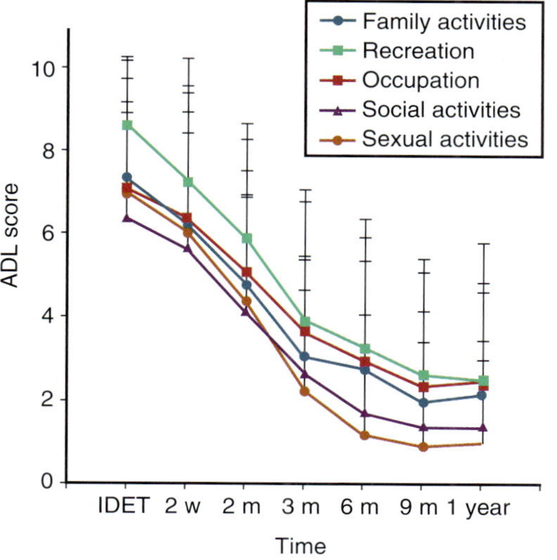

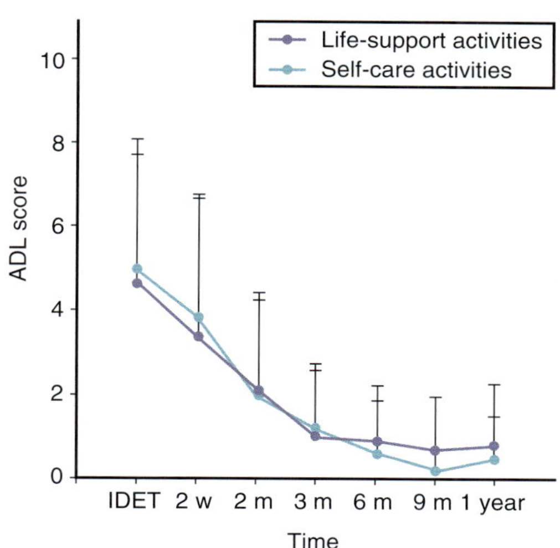

FIGURE 192-2. Activities of daily living after intradiscal thermal anuloplasty according to the Pain Disability Index, based on 32 patients presented by Mekhail and Kapural. (Redrawn from Mekhail N, Kapural L: Intradiscal thermal annuloplasty for discogenic pain: an outcome study. *Pain Pract* 4[2]:84–90, 2004.)

- One to three desiccated discs seen on T2-weighted MRI with or without a high-intensity zone, with or without small, contained disc protrusion, with at least 50% remaining disc height
- Concordant pain with low-pressure provocative discography (<50 psi above opening pressure) without discordant pain at pressures greater than 50 psi
- Posterior anular disruption (radial or concentric fissuring) on postdiscography CT images[38]

Exclusion Criteria

Contraindications presented by Kloth et al. include the following[38]:

- Severe disc degeneration at the affected lumbar level(s) as evidenced by greater than 50% disc height loss on plain anteroposterior and lateral lumbar radiographs and/or sectional imaging
- Extruded or sequestered herniated nucleus pulposus at the affected level(s)
- Previous lumbar back surgery (e.g., laminectomy, discectomy, or fusion) at the affected level(s)
- IDET performed within the last 6 months at the same level
- Nerve root impingement and/or compression with chronic lower extremity radiculopathy causing new-onset motor deficit
- Moderate to severe spinal stenosis (i.e., central, lateral, or foraminal) due to osteophyte and/or ligamentous overgrowth as evidenced by MRI or CT, provided that stenosis is the cause of pain
- Moderate to severe end-plate degenerative changes (e.g., spondylosis) at the affected level(s)
- Spondylolisthesis with motion on flexion-extension radiographs or any translational instability at the affected level(s)
- Cervical degenerated disc(s)
- Pregnancy
- Major psychological impairment

Relative contraindications presented in the same review include (1) moderate spinal stenosis (i.e., central, lateral, or foraminal) due to soft disc bulging, protrusion, or herniation with claudication; (2) grade I spondylolisthesis with no or minimal motion on flexion-extension radiographs; (3) previous discectomy at the affected level(s); and (4) thoracic degenerated disc(s).[38]

Risks

IDET is a minimally invasive procedure, but it is not without risks. Cohen reports a 10% complication rate, though most of the complications in this study were transient and self-limiting.[37] Severe complications have been infrequent.[28] Cauda equina syndrome after IDET has been reported several times.[39-41] Osteonecrosis of the vertebral body and giant herniation of the disc have been associated with IDET.[42-44] Derby reports end-plate damage post-IDET leading to disc space collapse in two patients.[45] A case of intradural catheter migration has also been reported.[46]

At the 16th North American Spine Society Meeting, Saal and Saal presented a review of 1675 IDET procedures and 35,000 SpineCATH devices from five centers. Six nerve root injuries, 6 cases of disc herniation (4 resolved nonoperatively), 19 catheter breakages, 8 superficial skin burns, and 1 case of bladder dysfunction post-IDET were reported.[47]

Proposed Mechanisms

Targeting the disrupted and degenerated anulus fibrosus is the basis of the IDET procedure. The proposed mechanisms underlying observed clinical benefits of IDET are compelling though widely speculative. Collagen denaturation and contraction may increase disc stability, heating-induced fibroblast activation may lead to reduced mobility and pain, and coagulation of granulation tissue may reduce inflammatory mediators responsible for presensitizing nerve fibers. Furthermore, the direct effect of coagulating nociceptive fibers in the anulus

BOX 192-1. Guidelines for Patients

Plan to rest for 1 to 3 days after your intradiscal electrothermal therapy (IDET) in a comfortable position (i.e., lying down or reclining); limit sitting or walking to 10 to 20 minutes at a time.

Return to work: You may return to sedentary work in roughly 1 week; however, you may still be sore after your IDET. Be aware of sitting restrictions listed below. For other jobs, the decision will be made by your physician.

Driving: None for the first 1 to 5 days; then limit your driving to 20 to 30 minutes for the first 6 weeks after your IDET. Make sure your vehicle has good lumbar support. You may need a pillow to help maintain your lumbar lordosis (normal low back curve). As a passenger, recline the seat and try to limit driving times to under 45 minutes for the first 6 weeks. It is okay to recline and be driven home the day of your procedure or to lie down in the back seat.

Sitting: Limit to 30 to 45 minutes at any one time in a chair with good support for the first 6 weeks. Avoid sitting on soft couches or chairs. Use a pillow or towel to maintain your lumbar curve when sitting. Standing and walking about in between sitting periods or short periods of lying down are helpful.

Lifting: Limit 5 to 10 lb for the first 6 weeks.

No bending or twisting of the low back.

Housework: No bending or twisting for the first 6 weeks.

No chiropractic, manipulation, massage (unless otherwise instructed), inversion traction, or traction for the first 12 weeks.

Exercise: Walk daily, beginning at the end of the first week, for approximately 20 minutes. Increase to 20 minutes twice per day, if tolerated; then progressively increase to 1 hour a day by the end of the fourth week. If back or leg symptoms increase at any point, decrease walking time. You may do gentle leg stretches (hamstring, pyriformis) with your back flat on the floor (be sure you know how to do these properly). Abdominal brace exercises can be begun at 2 to 3 weeks, with your back flat on the floor. No swimming for the first 6 weeks. Formal physical therapy will usually begin at 6 to 8 weeks after IDET. Do not use a treadmill or a stairmaster for the first 6 weeks, unless otherwise instructed.

You will be wearing a lumbar corset for the first 6 to 8 weeks after your IDET.

Saal JA, Saal JS: Intradiscal electrothermal therapy for the treatment of chronic discogenic low back pain. *Clin Sports Med* 21(1):167–187, 2002.

may reduce pain; however, the postprocedure pain flare that is observed clinically suggests that neural coagulation is not wholly responsible for any observed benefits. Though neural coagulation often is cited as a primary mechanism for IDET, convincing evidence does not currently exist.[48-51]

Much of the debate in the literature scrutinizes the thermal distribution in the anulus during IDET. Clearly, temperatures less than 45°C are necessary at the posterior longitudinal ligament and the neural foramina to prevent iatrogenic neurologic impairment. Closer to the catheter, temperatures of 60°C to 65°C are theoretically optimal to disrupt hydrogen cross-linking in the collagen triple helix, causing collagen contraction. Southern et al. describe collagen fibrillar disorganization on histology and evidence of collagen denaturation on quantitative spectroscopy with IDET.[50] Despite evidence of functional and histologic changes in cadaver models, attempts to map the thermal distribution of IDET in cadaveric discs have demonstrated contradictory results.[29,49,50]

Also theorized, heating to temperatures that do not cause irreversible cellular damage will lead to fibroblast activation, anular thickening, and stabilization in the intervertebral disc following IDET.[28] In vivo models in sheep, though, have not been encouraging. One such study presented by Bass et al. showed that high-dose thermal treatments led to biomechanical degradation, while low-dose and sham intervention led to little biomechanical change at 180 days post IDET.[52]

Pollintine et al. found that IDET has a significant but inconsistent effect on compressive stress distribution in 18 cadaveric motion segments of the lumbar spine. Twelve "responders" showed a 78% mean reduction in anular peak pressure; two discs demonstrated increases in anular peak pressure; four discs demonstrated no change. These outcomes did not correspond to degeneration grade or fissuring present in the disc.[53] Lee et al. found no significant difference in the stability of five cadaveric motion segments after IDET ($P > .05$).[54] However, another study demonstrated a 10% mean increase in motion at 5 Nm torque.[49]

Despite great scientific effort, the mechanism by which IDET imparts any clinical benefit is unknown. Certainly, this pursuit is of importance, given the clinical uncertainties in patient selection and optimal procedure to achieve the best result.

Subgroups of Intradiscal Electrothermal Therapy

Variations on the theme of intradiscal thermal anuloplasty-type procedures have been reported. Saal and Saal performed their IDET procedure with the SpineCATH (ORATEC Interventions, Inc., Menlo Park, CA) with a 5-cm active thermal tip. Also available is the Decompression catheter (Smith & Nephew, Memphis, TN), with a 1.5-cm active thermal tip. Differences in the heating protocol may lead to tissue temperature increases of 13°C to 15°C compared to those with the 5-cm catheter. [28] However, any benefit of increased temperature remains unproven, as a retrospective analysis by Derby et al. found that procedures achieving higher temperature via SpineCATH showed no correlation with improved outcomes at 16 months; in fact, a correlation with negative outcomes at 8 months was observed.[55]

Higher temperatures appear to increase the postprocedure pain flare without significantly affecting outcomes.[55] A cadaveric study performed by Southern et al. comparing the SpineCATH and the Decompression catheters demonstrated temperatures sufficient to denature collagen using both instruments, though the clinical importance of collagen alteration has not been established.[51]

Clearly, study of the optimal device and temperature to achieve clinical benefit would be greatly aided by the precise mechanism of action, which is not available currently.

It is important to distinguish intradiscal anuloplasty-type procedures from the broad category of percutaneous intradiscal intervention. For example, radiofrequency intradiscal interventions with either unipolar or bipolar electrodes are commonly employed.[28] Barendse et al. performed a randomized, controlled trial demonstrating no effect from radiofrequency thermocoagulation at the *center* of the disc.[56] It is inappropriate to use this and other studies in reference therapies targeting the anular pathology specifically.

Another common variation uses radiofrequency energy targeted at disruptions in the posterior anulus (DiscTRODE, Radionics, Burlington, MA). One study demonstrated benefit compared to conservative therapy only in a subgroup of individuals studied.[57] However, a recent randomized, double-blind controlled trial demonstrated no benefit at 12 months and increased pain in some patients following radiofrequency intra-anular thermal therapy.[58] Furthermore, Kapural et al. present a comparison between radiofrequency intradiscal anuloplasty and thermal intradiscal anuloplasty. Radiofrequency treatment led to no observed improvement, while thermal treatment showed significant improvement in pain and self-reported function.[59] Therefore, generalization between thermal and radiofrequency intradiscal anuloplasty-type procedures may not be possible.

Bipolar radiofrequency therapy, known as biacuplasty, has been performed with the Trans-Discal system (Baylis Medical, Montreal, Canada). This new technology delivers a bipolar current through the posterior anulus. This has been studied with a porcine model, a cadaveric application, and a 12-month, 15-patient prospective pilot study demonstrating sufficient temperatures for neural ablation, safe temperatures near neural structures, and clinical benefits enduring up to one year in about half the patients treated.[60-62] More research is needed to comment on the usefulness of biacuplasty in the treatment of chronic discogenic back pain.

Outcomes

Pauza et al. in 2004 conducted the first randomized, placebo-controlled, prospective trial to address IDET. The study presents the 6-month follow-up of 64 patients randomized to either IDET or sham IDET procedure, though eight patients were excluded or lost. The group found more than 50% pain relief in 40% of those who had undergone IDET; however, 50% of those in the IDET group reported no significant pain relief. To achieve 75% pain relief, the number needed to treat was five. The group that had undergone sham treatment did demonstrate improvements, but the IDET group demonstrated significantly less pain on visual analogue scale (VAS) scoring ($P = .045$) and better function outcome on the Oswestry Disability Scale ($P = .050$). The authors concluded that the efficacy of IDET cannot be entirely attributed to a placebo effect.[63]

Freeman et al. in 2005 presented contradictory results from a prospective, randomized, double-blind, placebo-controlled trial of 57 patients followed for 6 months, though 2 patients were excluded or lost. No significant improvement compared to placebo was observed. The authors attributed this difference to methodologic differences as well as to more significant disability in the present study when compared to Pauza et al.[64]

Though Freeman et al. argue that the statistical significance observed by Pauza et al. does not necessarily represent clinical significance, proponents of IDET point out that the benefits observed by Pauza et al. are the result of more stringent selection criteria.[64,65] For example, Freeman et al. included individuals with multilevel disc degeneration, full-thickness anular tears, and up to 50% loss in disc height.[65] Freeman et al. state that secondary analysis of patients with single-level disease yielded no statistically significant or clinically important benefits.[64]

It is difficult to reconcile the data from the two randomized, controlled trials on the matter. The majority of prospective controlled and observational trials have demonstrated significant benefit in highly selected patient groups.[66]

Saal and Saal presented their own prospective 2-year follow-up data for 58 patients; 27 had undergone single-level treatment, and 28 had undergone multilevel treatment.[30] At 24 months, 72% reached at least a two-point reduction in pain based on the VAS score, and 50% reached at least a four-point pain reduction. Similarly, 59% reached at least a 14-point improvement in the SF-36. No significant difference was observed in single-level or multilevel IDET.

In an observational study of 35 IDET-treated individuals with a "convenience control" of 17 individuals who were denied IDET by their insurance provider, Bogduk and Karasek reported the 2-year follow-up, with about 54% experiencing more than 50% improvement in pain and 20% of patients treated with IDET experiencing complete relief; only 1 control patient partially improved.[31]

Kapural et al. compared a group with multilevel disc degeneration to a group with one- or two-level disc degeneration. The two groups started out with a difference in VAS pain scores of .353 ($P = .6673$) that was not significant; 12 months post-IDET, a significant difference in VAS pain scores of 2.412 ($P = .0037$) was observed. Twelve of 17 from the one- or two-level group maintained more than 50% pain improvement at 12 months. Seven of 17 in the multilevel group maintained more than 50% pain improvement at 12 months. Improvement in Pain Disability Index–based assessment of function was also significantly different between the groups at 6 and 12 months ($P = .455$, $P = .410$, respectively).[36] The results of this comparative study are augmented by a prospective study from the same authors, which includes patients with only mild one- or two-level degenerative disc disease. This study demonstrates an average 78% pain decrease based on VAS at 12 months.[33]

Because of almost universally poor outcomes among workers' compensation claimants, a number of studies have investigated the utility of IDET in this population. Among 53 claimants, Nunley et al. found a mean 63% reduction in VAS score and 69% reduction in Oswestry scores at 12 months; 19 patients halted consumption of narcotic pain medications.[67] This does correlate with the outcome study by Mekhail and Kapural, which demonstrated a difference in the IDET outcome of workers' compensation claimants compared to nonclaimants, although both groups did benefit from treatment.[33]

In a recent review of the literature, Kloth et al. state that with proper inclusion criteria clinicians may expect benefit from IDET in 3 out of 4 patients treated.[38] A meta-analysis by Appleby et al. in 2006 concludes that there is compelling evidence for the relative efficacy of IDET.[68] Derby et al., in a systematic review, support IDET as treatment more for pain than for disability in a highly selected group.[28] However, in a critical appraisal of the evidence, Freeman states that evidence of efficacy has not yet passed the standard of scientific proof.[69]

A systematic review by Helm et al. and the American Society of Intervention Pain Physicians–Intervention Pain Management guidelines grade the available evidence at level II-2 according to the U.S. Preventive Services Task Force grading of evidence.[66,70] A 2A/weak recommendation for IDET was given in both publications, with the conclusion that the benefits are closely balanced by the risks and burdens of the procedure.[70]

Summary

As in all medical diseases that have no obvious cure, chronic discogenic pain has many treatment options, each with proponents that base their opinion on technical comfort, reimbursement, and theory but lack class I data to support one course of therapy overwhelmingly over all others. IDET is no different. It provides significant pain relief and functional improvement in a highly selected population of individuals suffering with chronic discogenic low back pain but not without controversy, and future research is required. Advances in published selection criteria and research into risk factors contributing to treatment failure are important steps as clinicians attempt to deliver beneficial treatment without causing undue morbidity. A precise mechanism of action must be defined. Understanding the beneficial effects of IDET will optimize technique and patient selection. Continued debate and critical appraisal of the literature will advance the clinical utility of IDET as one of many options to treat chronic discogenic pain.

KEY REFERENCES

Freeman BJ, Fraser RD, Cain CM, et al: A randomized, double-blind, controlled trial: intradiscal electrothermal therapy versus placebo for the treatment of chronic discogenic low back pain, *Spine (Phila Pa 1976)* 30(21):2369–2377, 2005; discussion 2378.

Kapural L, Hayek S, Malak O, et al: Intradiscal thermal annuloplasty versus intradiscal radiofrequency ablation for the treatment of discogenic pain: a prospective matched control trial. *Pain Med* 6(6):425–431, 2005.

Kloth DS, Fenton DS, Andersson GB: Block JE: Intradiscal electrothermal therapy (IDET) for the treatment of discogenic low back pain: patient selection and indications for use. *Pain Physician* 11(5):659–668, 2008.

Manchikanti L, Boswell MV, Singh V, et al: Comprehensive evidence-based guidelines for interventional techniques in the management of chronic spinal pain. *Pain Physician* 12(4):699–802, 2009.

Mekhail N, Kapural L: Intradiscal thermal annuloplasty for discogenic pain: an outcome study. *Pain Pract* 4(2):84–90, 2004.

Pauza KJ, Howell S, Dreyfull P, et al: A randomized, placebo-controlled trial of intradiscal electrothermal therapy for the treatment of discogenic low back pain. *Spine J* 4(1):27–35, 2004.

Saal JA, Saal JS: Intradiscal electrothermal therapy for the treatment of chronic discogenic low back pain. *Clin Sports Med* 21(1):167–187, 2002.

REFERENCES

The complete reference list is available online at expertconsult.com.

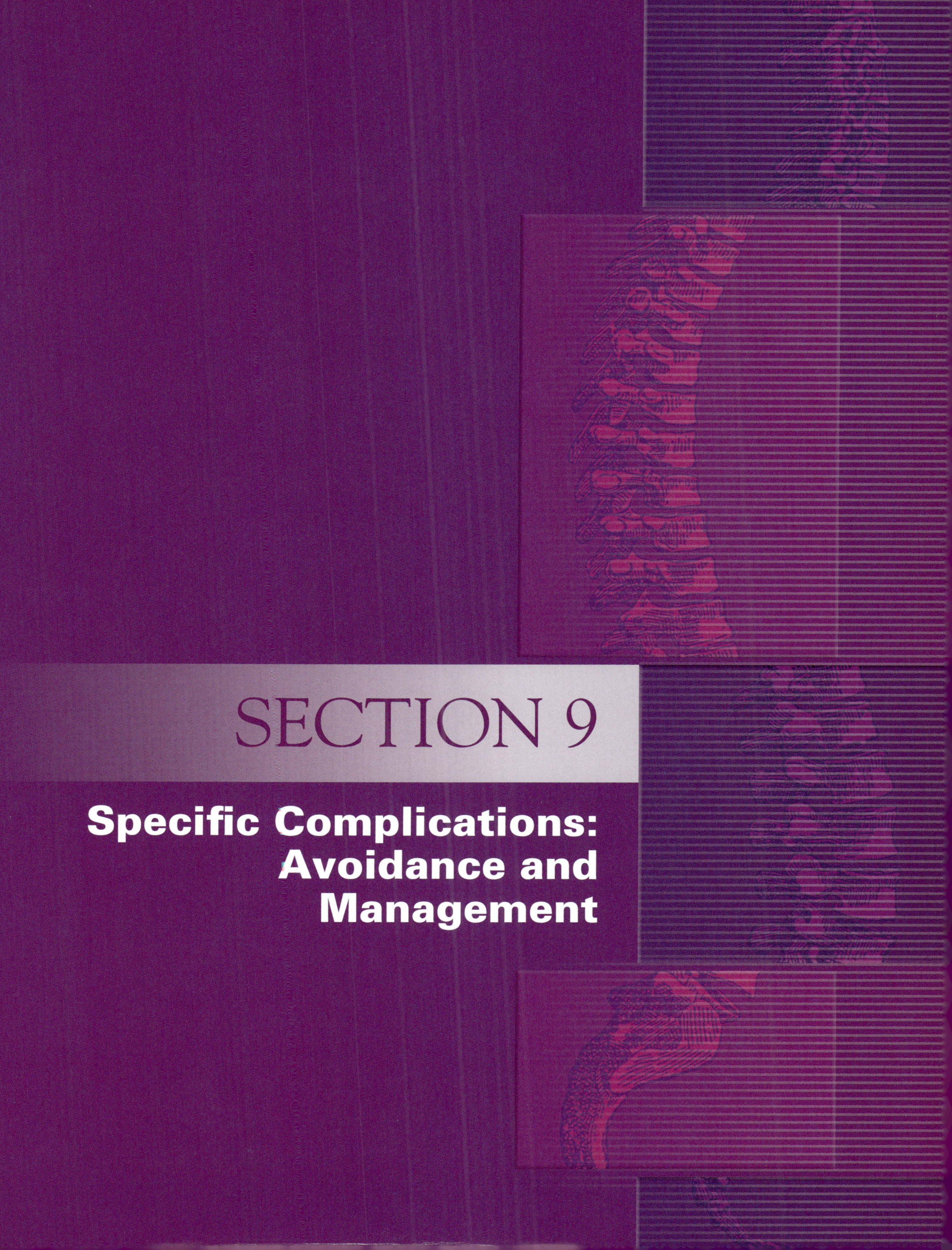

SECTION 9

Specific Complications: Avoidance and Management

CHAPTER 193

Neurologic Complications of Common Spine Operations

David G. Malone | John R. Caruso | Robert F. McLain

Whether the result of surgical or treatment errors, or anatomic or physiologic conditions beyond the surgeon's control, neurologic injury or impairment ranks at the very top of the concerns harbored by both patients and physicians during spine surgery. Proper planning and meticulous technique can reduce the risk of some types of complications. Early recognition and intervention can limit the impact of other types of injury that the surgeon cannot reliably prevent.

Ventral Cervical Surgery

Ventral cervical surgery, whether for discectomy or corpectomy, has many potential neurologic complications, but devastating neurologic injuries are a rarity.[1]

Specific complication types and rates vary with the side selected for the approach. Injury to the cervical sympathetic chain can occur during dissection of the longus colli muscles from the ventral cervical spine.[2] The cervical sympathetic chain ascends on the lateral border of the longus colli muscles and has three ganglionic enlargements. The superior cervical ganglion is at the level of C2-3, the middle ganglion is at the level of C6, and the stellate ganglion is at the level of C7-T1. Injury to the sympathetic chain can be prevented by limiting dissection of the longus colli muscles to their medial aspect only and by careful positioning of the self-retaining retractor blades on the medial side only of the dissected muscle. The stellate ganglion may occasionally be observed during low dissection in the neck. If it is observed, injury may be avoided by repositioning the retractor to move this structure out of the operating field. Injury to the cervical sympathetic nerves is manifested clinically by Horner syndrome (miosis, anhydrosis, and ptosis). Injury of the cervical sympathetic chain is seldom of any clinical significance, and recovery is usually spontaneous. Injury to the superior laryngeal nerve can occur during ventral cervical discectomy. This usually occurs during dissection in the deep cervical fascia because the superior laryngeal nerve is in close proximity to the superior and inferior thyroidal vessels.[3]

Injury to the recurrent laryngeal nerve may occur during ventral cervical discectomy, resulting in vocal cord paralysis.[2] The nerve is more often injured during a right-sided operative approach because of the anatomic course of the nerve. In some instances, the right recurrent laryngeal nerve does not loop around the subclavian artery and takes a more direct course, making the nerve more vulnerable to surgical injury. For this reason, some surgeons prefer a left-sided approach because the left recurrent laryngeal nerve has a more predictable course and has a more medial position between the trachea and the esophagus. However, the left nerve has a higher incidence of idiopathic palsy.[3] Vocal cord paralysis from recurrent laryngeal nerve palsy is usually the result of a stretch injury from retraction and usually resolves spontaneously within 6 months after injury. In some patients with vocal cord paralysis, the opposite vocal cord hypertrophies, allowing normal phonation. In any patient who has repeat ventral surgery to the cervical spine, either the approach should be through the previously operated side or the patient should have an otolaryngologic evaluation to confirm normal vocal cord function on both sides before surgery. If vocal cord paralysis is noted, the operative approach should be on the side of the paralyzed vocal cord. Voice hoarseness is often attributable to swelling and does not reflect recurrent laryngeal nerve injury. The incidence of postoperative hoarseness may be lessened by placing a closed suction drain.[4] Direct injury to the spinal cord and nerve roots has been reported with an incidence of approximately 2% after ventral cervical operations for myelopathy. These can be avoided only by meticulous operating technique and proper visualization.[5]

Dural tear is an uncommon intraoperative complication during ventral cervical surgery, more common when the posterior longitudinal ligament is taken down to complete a neural decompression or when corpectomy is carried out. Direct trauma caused by cutting instruments such as the bur or Kerrison rongeurs is the most common cause, but dural defect can be caused by cautery and even by focused application of the bipolar. Dural repair is desirable whenever possible, but access to the site of the leak and consideration for the dangers of retracting and manipulating the cord itself make many repairs unfeasible. In a large series of cervical surgeries that was reviewed for incidence and care of durotomies, laterally located leaks and those occurring behind the vertebral body were found to be unrepairable. Fibrin glue, mobilization precautions, bedrest in a partially seated position, and occasional use of a subarachnoid drain were required to obtain closure in these patients. While successful resolution was inevitably accomplished, additional care and prolonged hospitalization had a significant cost.[6]

Late postoperative complications of radiculopathy and myelopathy have been reported after ventral cervical discectomy and fusion. Five percent of patients developed myelopathy or radiculopathy an average of 5.5 years after ventral cervical discectomy and fusion, with myelography revealing pathology one level above or below the site of previous fusion. No compression was found at the previously operated site, and only 2.5% of these patients required reoperation at a second level.[7] Other researchers have obtained different statistics. Deterioration within the first year after ventral decompression from advancing osteophytic spurring at adjacent levels occurred in 5% of cases, and deterioration in the second and third years after ventral decompressive surgery occurred in another 5% of cases because of osteophytic processes, for a total deterioration rate of 10% within 3 years of surgery.[5] This deterioration may be preventable only by postoperative surveillance, reoperating on symptomatic patients, and considering the inclusion of all spondylotic levels in the fusion.[5] Complications caused by bone grafts have an incidence of 13%. Nonunion of bone graft was also noted in 7% of patients as an early cause of deterioration and in 4% of patients in the second and third years, for a combined total of 11% for deterioration caused by nonunion.[5,8] Nonunion rates may be lowered by paying meticulous attention to bone grafting and by adding ventral cervical instrumentation in multilevel decompressions. Spinal cord compression from malpositioning of the bone graft occurs less often. Bilateral brachial paresis has been reported after ventral cervical surgery for spondylosis. This occurred in a delayed fashion and was associated with angulation at the surgical site, with extrusion of the bone graft.[9] Worsening of neurologic function has been reported after ventral cervical fusion from cord compression by the bone graft. Neurologic function improved after removal of the offending graft.[5] Proper morticing of the graft bed is key to preventing compression of the spinal cord during graft placement. Precise measurements must be obtained of the depth of the decompression at the superior, inferior, and both lateral walls, as well as the length and width of the graft bed, because these measurements are not uniform. A minimum buffer of 3 mm must be preserved between the decompressed spinal cord and the bone graft, with the mortices cut to provide a dorsal shelf that will prevent the graft from compressing the spinal cord.

Dorsal Cervical Surgery

Central cord syndrome has been reported as a delayed complication that occurs several days after dorsal cervical decompressive laminectomy for cervical stenosis. Central cord syndrome occurred after a period of hypotension and was often associated with abnormal neck position. It is recommended that laminectomy be avoided in patients with abnormal cervical lordosis; that hypotension be avoided, especially when the patient is mobilized for the first time postoperatively; and that a cervical collar be used in the immediate postoperative period.[10] Jackson and Simmons[11] have reported a case of cervical laminectomy in a markedly kyphotic patient who had local anesthesia, with the patient serving as his own monitor. During the operation, the patient lost neurologic function. This rapidly reversed when the dura was opened. Other reported complications of dorsal cervical surgery include death from air embolism when the sitting position was used, neurologic deterioration from poor positioning of the cervical spine during operation, and tetraplegia from epidural hematoma.[12] Neurologic worsening has been noted in myelopathic patients if a laminectomy of inadequate length or width is performed. Laminectomy should extend to the lateral margin of the thecal sac, and if more than 50% of the medial facet is resected, fusion should be considered to lessen the risk of instability. Laminectomy should extend one level higher and one level lower than the highest and lowest compressive lesions.[13] Syringomyelia has become symptomatic after cervical decompressive laminectomies for cervical stenosis in patients with an unrecognized syrinx. It is postulated that decompression changes the transmural pressures across the syrinx wall, causing an increase in syrinx size and the appearance of symptoms. This is a rare complication that is lessened by obtaining preoperative MRI to differentiate between syrinx and cervical stenosis.[14]

Cervical laminectomy may cause instability if more than one half of the medial facet is removed. Other risk factors for postlaminectomy kyphosis include young age and preoperative kyphosis.[5] Kyphosis may result in progressive angulation with pain and cervical spondylotic myelopathy. This complication can be lessened by restricting decompression to less than one half of the medial facet or, when more lateral decompression is needed, by performing a fusion.[15] During dorsal cervical fusion, spinal cord injury has been reported in a case in which the dorsal bone graft loosened, compressing the spinal cord and causing Brown-Séquard syndrome.[15]

Dorsal cervical foraminotomy may worsen radiculopathy.[15] Care must be taken not to place any instruments into the narrowed foramen because this will further compress the nerve root, and the nerve root should not be retracted until the foramen is opened, allowing easy retraction of the nerve root.

Thoracic Spine Surgery

Ventral approaches to the thoracic and lumbar spine can cause ischemia to the spinal cord by interrupting the blood supply to the cord. Approaches to the ventral thoracic spine at levels T4-9 are especially dangerous. The risk of causing spinal cord ischemia can be lessened by performing preoperative angiography to localize the artery of Adamkiewicz and then planning surgery to avoid this artery. In addition, temporary segmental artery occlusion with somatosensory-evoked potential (SSEP) monitoring has been advocated to help identify key intersegmental arteries supplying the cord. The segmental arteries are identified and temporarily occluded during a ventral approach to the thoracic spine while SSEP monitoring is carried out. If the SSEP waveform deteriorates, the occlusion is released, and that segmental vessel is spared.[16] Thoracic disc herniations may be operated on via a variety of approaches. Neurologic complications are highest with central thoracic disc herniations approached from a dorsal laminectomy. In this setting, the paraplegia rate approaches 18% and is due to excessive spinal cord retraction. Complications may be lessened by a lateral extracavitary approach, costotransversectomy approach, or transthoracic approach.[17] Complications may be lessened further by performing preoperative spine angiography to avoid damage to the radiculomedullary artery of the spinal cord.

Lumbar Spine Surgery

Injuries to the dura mater and nerve roots may occur during lumbar disc surgery. Nerve root injury may occur from laceration, thermal injury, and excessive retraction. Lacerations to the nerve root most commonly occur because of lack of identification of the nerve root or because of failure to recognize a flattened root spread over the top of a herniated disc. Adequate illumination and magnification are extremely helpful in locating lumbar nerve roots. The anulus should never be cut until the nerve root has been positively identified. Bone and ligament should be removed until the root can be easily retracted. Further dissection of bone is often needed in the lateral direction to accomplish this goal. Bipolar electrocautery is useful for providing hemostasis, but no cauterization should be attempted until the nerve root is identified to avoid electrical or thermal injury to the nerve root.[18] Dural tears may occur during lumbar surgery with an incidence of approximately 4%. Care must be taken to avoid aspirating multiple nerve roots into the suction device and thereby causing neurologic deficit. The dural tear should be covered with a cottonoid, a smaller-diameter suction device should be inserted into the field, and exposure should be improved until the dural tear is fully exposed and then closed, if possible, in a watertight fashion.[18]

Lumbar discectomy in patients with cauda equina syndrome requires rapid evaluation and treatment. Some authors have found that persistent urinary incontinence is common in patients who are operated on 48 hours or more after presentation of symptoms but is uncommon in those who are operated on within 48 hours.[19] Kostuik et al. found two separate modes of presentation in patients with cauda equina syndrome to an acute mode with rapid onset, more severe symptoms, and a poorer prognosis after decompression and a mode with more gradual onset of symptoms. In both groups of patients, those with complete perineal anesthesia tended to have permanent bladder paralysis. Kostuik et al. also found no correlation between timing of surgery and extent of recovery. Despite this lack of correlation, they recommend early surgery for patients with cauda equina syndrome.[20]

Acute postdiscectomy cauda equina syndrome occurs at a rate of approximately 0.2%.[21] The majority of these patients develop symptoms of perineal numbness, urinary retention, motor weakness, and multidermatomal numbness in the recovery room. Stenosis of the lumbar spinal canal at the operative level with anteroposterior dimension of 13 mm or less was the most common factor found in postdiscectomy cauda equina syndrome, with swelling, hematoma, retained disc fragments, and hemostatic gelatin (Gelfoam) contributing to the compression. A large epidural fat graft has also been a reported cause of cauda equina syndrome after lumbar discectomy.[22] In this case, a large fat graft herniated into the spinal canal on the first postoperative day, causing cauda equina syndrome. These complications may be avoided by limiting the size of the fat graft to between 5 and 8 mm and by suturing the graft to adjacent paraspinous muscle tissue, by measuring the lumbar canal preoperatively, and, if stenosis is present, by avoiding use of keyhole laminotomy to provide the approach to the disc space. Additionally, hemostasis should be obtained to avoid hematoma formation.[23] The operation for lumbar disc herniation causing cauda equina syndrome differs from the usual lumbar discectomy in that a much wider bony exposure is required. Complete hemilaminectomy is recommended to provide space to remove the disc herniation while lessening retraction that could cause permanent deficit. Microdiscectomy should be avoided in these patients because it provides less bony exposure.[24]

Cauda equina syndrome has also been reported after surgery for lumbar spinal stenosis. Compressive hematoma has been implicated as a cause of cauda equina syndrome after decompressive laminectomy. Cauda equina syndrome has been reported to occur after application of large epidural fat grafts in lumbar decompressive laminectomies.[25] This may occur by the fat graft acting to seal a hematoma against the thecal sac or by compression of the large fat graft by the paraspinal muscles. This complication may be prevented by limiting the size of the fat graft to a thickness of 0.5 to 1.0 cm and to a height less than the height of the spinous processes.[25] Several cases of cauda equina syndrome have resulted after decompressive laminectomies in which a higher lesion, such as a herniated disc, was later identified. To minimize these complications, the following steps should be taken: Hemostasis should be obtained before closure, or a closed suction drain should be placed if hemostasis cannot be obtained. The entire lumbar spine and thoracolumbar junction should be visualized by MRI or myelography preoperatively so that pathology in the upper portions of the spinal canal is not overlooked. Lumbar decompression should have sufficient length to include all compressed elements. Cauda equina syndrome may also occur on a vascular basis, as the artery of Adamkiewicz may enter at the upper lumbar segments and may be damaged during operation at the thoracolumbar junction. Preoperative spine arteriography should be considered carefully to verify the presence or absence of vascular supply to the spinal cord in the area of the proposed operation if the operation is to be performed in the regions from T4 to L2. In postoperative cauda equina syndrome, mechanical causes must be ruled out and, if present, removed in an urgent fashion. Only after all mechanical causes have been included should a vascular etiology be diagnosed.[21]

Automated percutaneous discectomy carries risk. The most severe reported complication is one of cauda equina syndrome caused by improper placement of the nucleotome probe in the thecal sac. In animal tests, the device could pierce dura, amputate nerve roots, and make holes in intravascular structures. Complications with the nucleotome probe can be minimized by the following procedures: The nucleotome should never be placed outside the disc space; once properly positioned, the device cannot incise the anulus and therefore cannot exit the disc space. The thecal sac is outlined by the line of the dorsal vertebral bodies ventrally, the line of the junction of the lamina and spinous processes dorsally, and the medial borders of the pedicles laterally; therefore, the probe should be placed under radiographic guidance using these landmarks to avoid the thecal sac. The device should be used only by an operator who has been trained in its proper usage. The procedure should be performed only under local anesthesia, as patient discomfort will alert the operator to any potential injury.[26-28]

Surgery for lumbosacral spondylolisthesis may also cause cauda equina syndrome even with no attempt at reduction of alignment.[29] Paresis of proximal roots after reduction of lumbosacral spondylolisthesis has also been reported and is caused by stretching of proximal nerve roots after reduction of the spine.[30] The L5 nerve root is the most often damaged during reduction of lumbosacral spondylolisthesis, followed in frequency by the S1 and S2 nerve roots.[30,31] To lessen these complications, SSEP monitoring and prereduction decompression of the nerve roots should be performed. When the patient awakens from surgery, a thorough neurologic examination should be performed on the lumbosacral nerve roots, and if new deficit is found, the patient should be returned to the operating room for decompression of the involved root.[29]

Surgery at the Cervicomedullary Junction

Operation at the level of the cervicomedullary junction for tumor carries risk. Three approaches are commonly used: the transoral, the dorsolateral, and the lateral suboccipital. The neurologic complications associated with surgery in this area include lower cranial nerve palsy, brainstem infarction from vertebral artery damage, and direct injury to the medulla. These complications may be lessened by the choice of surgical approach. Some surgeons have recommended the lateral suboccipital approach for lesions in this region because it provides direct visualization of the ventral surface of the brainstem and spinal cord and provides a sterile approach with the ability to close the dura in a watertight fashion, and neither mastoidectomy nor transposition of the vertebral artery is required.[32]

Trauma

Cervical fractures with malalignment may have associated disc herniation. Neurologic deterioration has been reported at a rate of 6 per 68 cases for patients with cervical dislocation undergoing reduction. The preferred management of reduction of cervical dislocation remains controversial. One school of thought advocates closed reduction with emergent ventral cervical discectomy if the patient worsens from disc herniation. Another group recommends MRI to rule out cervical disc herniation before closed reduction to eliminate the risk of neurologic deterioration from herniated disc fragments.[33]

Gunshot wounds to the spinal cord are the third most common cause of spinal cord injury. Complications of these injuries include osteomyelitis, meningitis, spine instability, cerebrospinal fluid leak, and delayed paraspinal infection. Neurologic recovery is less than 1% in injuries above the T10 level, but as many as 47% of patients with injury to the terminal spinal cord or cauda equina have some degree of recovery with surgical management. Complications may be minimized in patients with transperitoneal gunshot wounds to the spine by vigorous irrigation of the spinal missile track during laparotomy, with rapid closure of any bowel perforations. Debridement and laminectomy are advocated as soon as the patient is stable for gunshot wounds to the spine to provide dural closure, debride bone and missile fragments, and cleanse latent infection.[34,35]

Neoplastic Disease

Five percent of cancer patients develop neurologic deficits because of spinal metastases.[36,37] The majority of metastases occur in the lower thoracic and upper lumbar spine, and 80% of metastases occur ventral to the thecal sac.[19] Treatment of these lesions with laminectomy alone often causes instability with resultant paraplegia, especially when there is vertebral body involvement.[36] Vertebral body collapse is a particularly ominous finding.[38] Treatment in these cases should involve either a ventral approach or a dorsal approach with transpedicular decompression of the ventral thecal sac, reconstruction of the vertebral body with a ventral strut, instrument, or methylmethacrylate and dorsal instrumentation.[19,36-39]

Spine Instrumentation

Spine instrumentation may cause neurologic injury at the time of implant placement because of neural trauma, ischemia, or hemorrhage or even years after placement from compression by fibrosis or implant loosening. Harrington rods can cause nerve and thecal sac compression in a delayed fashion. Hooks placed on the L5 lamina and attached to Harrington rods have been reported to cut through the lamina over time, causing thecal sac compression. In all these reported cases, the problems resolved after removal of the hardware.[40,41]

Overdistraction of the spine with spine fixation systems can cause spinal cord injury from ischemia, because distraction stretches the segmental and intrinsic vessels feeding the cord, lessening their cross-sectional area. Intraoperative SSEP monitoring has been useful but not infallible in detecting overdistraction.[42] If SSEP waveforms degrade during distraction, the implant should be removed. If postoperative deficit is noted, even if SSEP waveforms are preserved, consideration should be given to removing the distraction system.[42,43] Care must be taken at sites at which the spine is predisposed to injury during distraction. Distraction over a fixed mass, during systolic hypotension, in multicolumn spine injury, and in a kyphotic spine, increases the chance for spinal cord injury.[42-44]

Malpositioning of pedicle screws can cause radiculopathy, with a reported incidence as high as 7%.[45,46] Damage to the nerve root may be caused by the screw itself or by bone fragments from fracture of the pedicle wall. The nerve root travels along the medial border of the pedicle and exits around the inferior border of the pedicle. During placement of pedicle screws, the nerve root is at risk if the medial or inferior border is violated. After the pedicle has been localized and the center of the pedicle has been dissected into the vertebral body, the channel should be probed to detect any breaches into the medial or lateral wall of the pedicle. If no wall defects are found, the channel should be tapped and should be probed after tapping to determine whether any breaches occurred during tapping of the channel. If a defect in the wall is detected, a decision must be made as to whether the channel can be redirected in the same pedicle to avoid the breach or whether an alternative site of fixation must be used. Screw depth should be chosen to penetrate 50% to 75% of the vertebral body, and no attempt should be made to routinely gain bicortical purchase, because neurologic injury to the sympathetic chain in the sacrum and to the presacral plexus at L5 may rarely result. Intraoperative and preoperative imaging with plain films or fluoroscopy is extremely useful for placing pedicle screws.

If a new radiculopathy is noted postoperatively in a patient who has undergone pedicle screw placement at the level of the radiculopathy, radiologic studies should be immediately performed to evaluate screw position. If malpositioning is found, the offending screw should be removed. While placement of the pedicle screw outside of the pedicle wall can cause direct irritation of the nerve root, placement through the neural foramen can result in actual transection or penetration of the nerve or the dorsal root ganglion. The neural function loss and pain experienced in either circumstance can be crippling. Another less common error can occur when the surgeon fails to recognize that the screw is fully inserted and continues to advance the screw down the pedicle. The head of the screw will then advance down the pedicle shaft, trapping and compressing the exiting nerve root under the combination of fractured bone and the base of the screw head as it approaches the back of the vertebral body. Early recognition and revision are the keys to symptom relief if recovery is a possibility.

Ventral cervical fixation devices rarely cause hardware complications that result in neurologic injury. The most common theoretical complication causing neurologic injury is excessive screw length in a ventral cervical plate that compresses or impales the spinal cord. This complication may be avoided by using intraoperative fluoroscopy or plain radiographs while placing these screws. The proper length of screw may be estimated by measuring the adjacent disc space, and the screw should be measured by the surgeon personally before implantation to ensure that the desired screw will be implanted. By using the operative technique described in Chapter 144, this complication may be avoided. Dorsal cervical fixation devices can lead to hardware complications that cause neurologic injury. Dorsal spinous wiring in traumatic injuries to the cervical spine has been associated with worsening of neurologic function by causing retropulsion of herniated disc fragments into the spinal canal.[33,47] Nerve root injuries during placement of lateral mass plates are possible and can be avoided by using the technique of placing the screw starting 1 mm medial to the center of the facet and at an angle of 25 to 30 degrees rostrally and 20 degrees laterally to avoid the nerve root and vertebral artery.[48]

Sublaminar wiring techniques for segmental fixation are associated with a 1% to 17% incidence of neurologic injury.[45] Nerve root injuries occur more frequently than do spinal cord injuries with this technique. Acute injuries caused by excessive depth of passage, attempt at passage in an acquired or congenitally narrow canal, and epidural hemorrhage are the most common causes of defects after segmental fixation. Placement of sublaminar wires through the sacral foramina has been noted to cause sacral radiculopathy. Passage of wires medially instead of laterally, thinning of the lamina to lessen length of passage, immediately crimping the wires around the lamina after passage to prevent dislodgement into the canal, and using smaller-gauge double-twisted wires or cables all decrease the incidence of neurologic injury with sublaminar wiring techniques.[9] Removal of sublaminar wires may also cause neurologic injury. The wire should be cut as close to the lamina as possible to minimize the radius of arc that the wire will travel during removal. Single wires and double-independent wires should be removed individually in a direction parallel to the thecal sac. Double-twisted wires should be removed with the aid of a wire extractor guide.[45]

Neurologic complications caused by reducing malalignment of the spine in cases of scoliosis and spondylolisthesis are numerous in the literature. Cases of L5 radiculopathy have occurred during reduction of L5-S1 spondylolisthesis.[31] This complication may be avoided by decompression before reduction or by fusion in situ. There are reports of neurologic injury with in situ fusion for spondylolisthesis.[29]

Surgical Technique

Neurologic complications may be caused by poor surgical technique. The unipolar electrocautery, if used improperly, can cause neurologic damage and should never be used in the vicinity of neural tissue without extreme caution being exercised. Spinal cord damage has been reported from the use of unipolar cautery on the posterior longitudinal ligament.[49] Dissection of dorsal structures with electrocautery may result in dissection through the ligamentum flavum and dura with cord or root injury. Care must be used to ensure that dissection is taking place over bone and not over interspace.

High-speed burs and drills can also cause neurologic injury in spine surgery.[49] Drills should never be used around unprotected neural structures. Appropriate bit selection is important because a diamond-tipped drill is less likely to wrap up adjacent tissue than is a fluted bit. The drill should be started near the region of its intended use, and a spinning drill bit should never be moved into or out of the operating field. Direct damage to dura mater or nerve root by the fluted bit occurs, but more commonly, damage occurs when loose soft tissue becomes wrapped up in the spinning bur, either pulling the neural tissue into the bit or pulling the bit into the important tissues. Keeping the working area free of loose fronds of soft tissue is important. Likewise, paddies or other elements that are placed in the canal to protect the dura can become destructive weapons if they become engaged in the bur and are allowed to whip against the neural tissues as the bur spins.

Neurologic damage has also been reported by incorrect identification of anatomic structures. Sectioning of the hypoglossal nerve has been reported in ventral cervical surgery in which the nerve was mistakenly identified as the superior laryngeal artery.[49]

KEY REFERENCES

Allen BL, Ferguson RL: Neurologic injuries with the Galveston technique of L-rod instrumentation for scoliosis. *Spine (Phila Pa 1976)* 11:14–17, 1986.

Boccanera L, Laus M: Cauda equina syndrome following lumbar spinal stenosis surgery. *Spine (Phila Pa 1976)* 12:712–715, 1987.

Cloward RB: Complications of ventral cervical disc operation and their treatment. *Surgery* 69:175–182, 1971.

Levy WJ, Dohn DF, Hardy RW: Central cord syndrome as a delayed postoperative complication of decompressive laminectomy. *Neurosurgery* 11:491–495, 1982.

Schoenecker PL, Cole HO, Herring JA, et al: Cauda equina syndrome after in situ arthrodesis for severe spondylolisthesis at the lumbosacral junction. *J Bone Joint Surg [Am]* 72:369–377, 1990.

Transfeldt EE, Dendrinos GK, Bradford DS: Paresis of proximal lumbar roots after reduction of L5-S1 spondylolisthesis. *Spine (Phila Pa 1976)* 14:884–887, 1989.

West CG: Bilateral brachial paresis following ventral decompression for cervical spondylosis. *Spine (Phila Pa 1976)* 11:176–178, 1985.

REFERENCES

The complete reference list is available online at expertconsult.com.

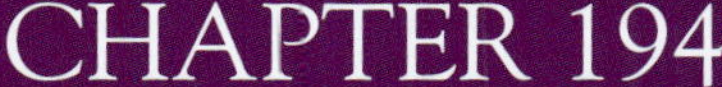

CHAPTER 194

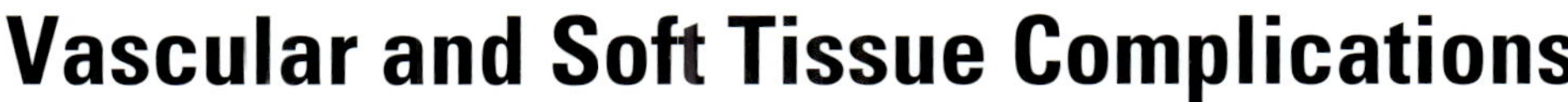

Vascular and Soft Tissue Complications

Neel Anand | Eli M. Baron | Donald A. Smith | David W. Cahill

Complications at the Craniovertebral Junction

The simplest and most direct ventral access to the craniovertebral junction is the transoral/transpharyngeal approach. Many different variations of this operation have been described, including combined resection of the hard palate, median labiomandibular glossotomy, maxillectomy, and LeFort osteotomies to expand the exposure from the midclivus to the C3 level. The main limitation of these procedures is the inevitable contamination of the wound by mouth flora. Additionally, the location of the vertebral arteries limits the lateral extent of these procedures.[1] By reserving these approaches for extradural pathologic conditions and by using perioperative antibiotics, many of the septic complications that were initially encountered with this operation have been overcome. Airway management in transoral procedures demands special attention. Significant tongue swelling is often encountered, and this can easily lead to obstruction of the oropharynx. In cases of major resections or those in which the patient has any preoperative difficulty with swallowing or aspiration, a tracheotomy is routinely performed. In more limited operations at the C1-2 level and without concurrent lower cranial neuropathy, the patient may be left intubated for 48 to 72 hours postoperatively or until glossal swelling has abated. Periodic relaxation of the intraoral retractors during surgery may mitigate the problem. Additionally, precautions should be taken to ensure that the tongue is not trapped between the retractor blade and the lower teeth. Steroids are often invoked as well, but they are no substitute for controlled extubation in an intensive care unit setting by someone who is skilled in airway management. Close observation with a bedside tracheostomy setup is mandatory. Although intradural procedures and bone grafting can be successfully performed through this route, these maneuvers carry a heightened risk and can be the source of significant morbidity. A layered, tensionless reapproximation of the dorsal pharyngeal musculature and mucosa with resorbable sutures is important, especially if the dura mater has been violated. In this case, reinforcement of the dural repair with a fascial graft and fibrin glue and placement of a spine drain postoperatively are advised. If bone grafts or reconstructive cages have been inserted, they should have a low profile, without protrusion into the pharynx and resultant compromise of the soft tissue closure. Because the retropharyngeal soft tissues are well vascularized, surgeons tend to use electrocautery to divide and reflect these structures off the bone. This can result in significant retraction of the wound margins, which becomes most apparent at the time of closure. Infiltration of the retropharyngeal tissues with a dilute epinephrine solution before sharp incision and blunt reflection with the use of bipolar cautery for direct hemostasis minimizes this problem. If a primary closure cannot be obtained (or if one should subsequently break down), satisfactory repair can usually be achieved with either a pharyngeal or a septal flap reconstruction. When the soft palate has been divided, a similar degree of attention should be devoted to the tensionless anatomic reapproximation of its edges, so that a cleft or fistula does not result. In the immediate postoperative period, oral feedings should be avoided for the first 5 days to minimize risk of fascial dehiscence.

Vertebral artery injury is always a theoretical risk during these procedures. At the arch of C1, the vertebral arteries are located approximately 24 mm laterally from the midline; at the level of the foramen magnum and the level of the C2-3 disc space, the arteries are approximately 11 mm from the midline. Pathology such as rotatory subluxation can significantly distort the relationship of these structures to the midline. Identification of the midline structures such as the anterior tubercle of C1 and the pharyngeal tubercle on the clivus are the most important steps in establishing orientation for these approaches. Furthermore, the anatomic midline can be identified by the symmetry of the anterior longitudinal ligament and longus colli muscles.[1] Fluoroscopy is also useful in establishing the midline, as may be intraoperative neuronavigation. Regarding management of vertebral artery injury, please see the next section.

Complications in the Subaxial Spine

The ventrolateral approach to the subaxial spine as popularized by Robinson and Smith[2] is among the most commonly performed spine surgeries. The esophagus, larynx, and trachea are mobilized medially as a unit, and the carotid sheath is retracted laterally. The incidence of clinically significant injuries to these structures is low during primary surgeries. When an injury does occur, sharp-toothed retractors are often implicated. Hand-held blunt retractors are used exclusively until the musculus longus colli have been reflected off the vertebral bodies ventrolaterally to create two soft tissue leaves into which a self-retaining retractor system can be anchored. Great care is taken with the initial placement of retractors, because this permits safe, stable, and sustained exposure that sets the stage for the remainder of the case. Toothed blades are inserted accurately under the musculus longus colli under direct vision. Proper engagement of the muscles usually requires the use of asymmetrical blade lengths, the medial blade being a bit longer.

The cervical sympathetic chain overlies the musculus longus colli more laterally. Occasionally, Horner syndrome ensues after reflection of these muscles or because of heat transmission from electrocautery. This is usually transient and is not functionally disabling. Other structures that are at potential risk are the recurrent laryngeal nerve and the vertebral arteries. Injuries to the thoracic duct are occasionally incurred in left-sided approaches at the C6-7 and C7-T1 levels; these are reviewed separately in the following sections.

Recurrent Laryngeal Nerve Injury

Vocal cord paresis is a complication in anterior cervical surgery that is probably underappreciated. In patients who have undergone the anterior cervical approach to the spine for discectomy or corpectomy, the reported rate of injury varies from 0% to 16%.[3] Nevertheless, a prospective study looking at 120 patients undergoing anterior cervical spine surgery who underwent preoperative and postoperative laryngoscopy revealed a clinically symptomatic recurrent laryngeal nerve palsy rate of 8.3%, and the incidence of recurrent laryngeal nerve palsy not associated with hoarseness (i.e., clinically unapparent without laryngoscopy) was 15.9% (overall incidence, 24.2%). At 3-month follow-up evaluation, the rate had decreased to 2.5% in cases with hoarseness and 10.8% without hoarseness.[4] Most of these are blunt injuries, believed to have resulted from retractor pressure against the recurrent laryngeal nerve within the tracheoesophageal groove. The left recurrent laryngeal nerve has a longer course, swinging around the aortic arch before ascending in the relatively protected cleft between the trachea and esophagus, whereas the right recurrent laryngeal nerve loops around the subclavian artery, and thus has a correspondingly shorter course. The extra length of nerve available on the left allegedly renders it less vulnerable to stretch injury than its counterpart on the right is, but the evidence for this is scant. A recent prospective study assessed 242 patients undergoing anterior cervical spine surgery postoperatively with laryngoscopy. All patients underwent a left-sided approach, but one group (149 patients) was operated on with an additional reduction of endotracheal cuff pressure to below 20 mmHg. Ninety-three patients underwent a left-sided approach without reduction in cuff pressure. In the group with the left-sided approach and the low cuff pressures, the total rate of persisting (at 3 months) symptomatic and asymptomatic recurrent laryngeal nerve palsy was 1.3%. In the group with the left-sided approach without the reduced cuff pressures, the total rate of persisting (at 3 months) symptomatic and asymptomatic recurrent laryngeal nerve palsy was 6.5%. The authors noted that this compared favorably with their historic data, in which they noted a total rate of persisting recurrent laryngeal nerve palsy of 13.3% in patients undergoing the right-sided approach without reduction of cuff pressure.[5]

In cases of suspected vocal fold motion impairment, an otorhinolaryngology consult should be obtained. Initial evaluation should include a detailed history with the patient relating symptoms and their time of onset, followed by a physical examination, in which particularly close attention is paid to the neck, and a neurologic examination of the lower cranial nerves.[6] This should be followed by visualization of the vocal cords with a fiberoptic laryngoscope.[7] Also very valuable is a videofluoroscopic swallowing evaluation. This can show signs of pharyngeal plexus injury such as disruption of velar movement, cricopharyngeal spasm, and other patterns of swallowing dysfunction.[6] If there is an immobile vocal cord, a useful examination tool is laryngeal electromyography. Laryngeal electromyography can help in determining the site of a peripheral vagal lesion (high cervical vs. low cervical), as it allows separate testing of laryngeal muscles supplied by the recurrent laryngeal and superior laryngeal nerves. Laryngeal electromyography also allows for differentiation between vocal cord paralysis and vocal cord fixation.[8]

As a rule, functional recovery occurs over a period of weeks to months. Nevertheless, injury may be permanent or slow to heal, and surgical intervention may be required. Various options exist for the treatment of unilateral vocal fold paresis and paralysis. These include injection laryngoplasty, medialization laryngoplasty, arytenoid adduction, and nerve-muscle transfer. Injection laryngoplasty may be done with hemostatic gelatin (Gelfoam), fat, collagen, or Teflon (El Du Pont de Nemours & Co., Inc., Wilmington, DE). Medialization laryngoplasty is usually done with silicone elastomer (Silastic) or hydroxylapatite. More recently, novel materials such as titanium, GORE-TEX (W. L. Gore and Associates, Inc., Flagstaff, AZ), and polylactic/polyglycolic acid have been used. Arytenoid adduction uses a permanent suture to relocate the arytenoid into a more physiologically sound position.[7,9]

Esophageal Injury

Transient swallowing disorders are commonly recorded after even uncomplicated primary anterior cervical surgeries. This may be seen in up to 80% of patients who undergo anterior cervical spine surgery.[10] Symptoms usually resolve within a few weeks but may persist in up to 10% of patients, although only rarely at a level that is functionally disabling.[11] Refractory cases should be evaluated with videofluoroscopic swallowing evaluation (modified barium swallow) to determine the integrity of the swallowing mechanism and whether the patient will safely tolerate oral intake. This then can expedite appropriate swallowing therapy and an appropriate route for nutrition.[12,13] Though many patients will do well, recovery, presumably through reinnervation of pharyngeal musculature, does not always occur.[14] The speech pathologist can be of tremendous help here in determining the patient's potential for recovery. If the dysphagia is related to cricopharyngeal spasm and lasts several months and follow-up study does not show improvement with conservative therapy, surgical intervention such as cricopharyngeal myotomy may be considered.[6]

Esophageal perforation is a much more serious problem. It is in the context of reoperative surgery or surgery performed for infection, for tumor, or after irradiation that most of these injuries occur. Tissues are fibrotic and sometimes friable, and tissue planes are often scarred, distorted, and unyielding. Blunt mobilization of the esophagus off the prevertebral fascia might not be successful, and sharp dissection can be equally hazardous. Passage of a nasogastric tube that can be palpated within the esophageal lumen serves as a further point of orientation and as an aid to dissection. A combination of blunt and sharp techniques may be useful for dissecting the junction between the ventral aspect of the vertebral bodies and the overlying soft tissue structures as precisely as possible. If normal planes of dissection are not apparent, exposure is extended rostrally and caudally in search of recognizable anatomy in more virginal tissues. This may enable definition of the lateral margin of the vertebral corpus concealed beneath swollen musculus longus colli. The prevertebral fascia can then be incised in a paramedian plane down to bone, and the fascia and overlying laryngotracheal esophageal bundle can be mobilized as an undissected unit. Depending on the quality of the tissue planes that are developed in this fashion, the use of any form of toothed retractor should be avoided. In reoperative cases, some of these difficulties may be averted altogether simply by approaching from the side opposite the initial procedure. In this case, direct laryngoscopy should be performed preoperatively or at intubation to confirm preserved vocal cord function on the initially operated side, thereby precluding the catastrophic outcome of bilateral vocal cord paralysis at the second procedure.

Esophageal perforation is also encountered as a delayed complication associated with ventral graft extrusion and hardware failure. This occurs most commonly because of infection, poor carpentry, a technical error in the method of instrumentation, or application of instrumentation in softened osteoporotic bone. This can also occur in the setting of pseudarthrosis (Fig. 194-1). When screws are observed to back out in follow-up radiographs, their elective removal should be considered. There are now abundant reports of esophageal injury secondary to screw migration.[15-20] Screw heads should be flush with the plate to minimize their profile and allow their locking mechanism to function properly to prevent backout. Plate length must be selected carefully so that there is no overhang over adjacent disc spaces, and unfused segments should not be instrumented, because these circumstances promote hardware loosening. If the quality of the bone stock is poor, bicortical screw fixation should be used. If this is not feasible, posterior segmental instrumentation should be performed.

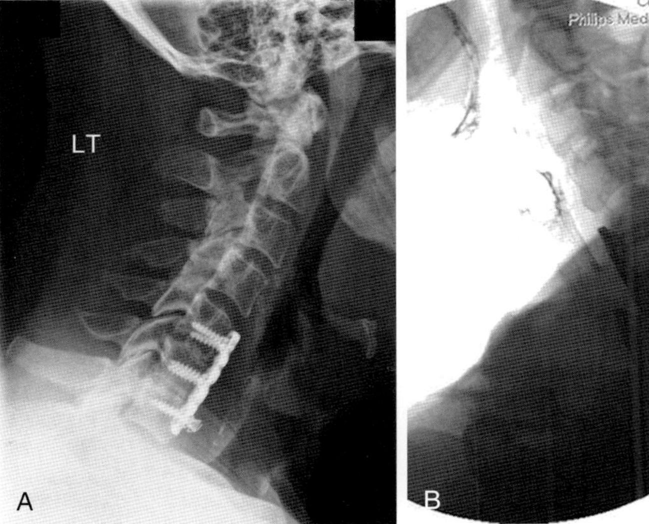

FIGURE 194-1. **A,** Lateral radiograph in a patient 2 years status post anterior cervical discectomy and fusion showing backing out of an inferior screw in the setting of pseudarthrosis where the patient presented with dysphagia. **B,** Esophagram shows an intact esophagus without penetration of the screw into the esophagus. Note the close relationship of the plate to the esophagus.

Esophageal Repair

Esophageal perforation may be apparent intraoperatively, but more often it presents postoperatively with deep wound infection, severe dysphagia, and mediastinitis.[19,20] Perforation related to hardware failure might not occur until years after the operative procedure.[21,22] Intraoperative tears may be either partial or full thickness. A partial-thickness injury to the esophagus is readily repaired with resorbable sutures and should not cause modification of the primary procedure. To ensure that a transmural injury has not occurred, the surgeon may instill indigo carmine dye into the hypopharynx and monitor for dye egress within the wound. Transmural injuries are repaired primarily, again with the surgeon observing the principles of a layered, tensionless closure using resorbable sutures. The wound is irrigated copiously with antibiotic-containing solution, and systemic antibiotic coverage is broadened to include anaerobic organisms. Assuming an absence of gross contamination and a satisfactory repair, the surgeon can proceed with the intended decompression and fusion in most instances. In these circumstances, any form of spine instrumentation should be used with caution. The patient is fed through a Silastic feeding tube during the first postoperative week. Intravenous antibiotics are continued for 2 to 6 weeks postoperatively. A further course of oral antibiotics thereafter is discretionary.

More complicated injuries with longer segments of tissue loss that no longer allow for tensionless reapproximation require longitudinal mobilization of the midesophagus and a reinforced repair backed by a pedicled sternocleidomastoid muscle flap. Extensive injuries that do not lend themselves to repair in this fashion should be diverted proximally and distally to the skin surface and then reconstructed later. Primary reanastomosis may still be achievable after mobilization of the esophagus at the diaphragmatic hiatus to gain additional length. Although lacking in intrinsic coordinated propulsive activity, colonic and jejunal interpositions are yet other reconstruction options.

Delayed perforation may present with similar though less fulminant symptoms or with spinal osteomyelitis. In most cases, the original site of injury will have sealed over, although this should be evaluated with a swallowing study using a water-soluble contrast agent. Subsequent procedures depend on several factors. Any sign of contrast extravasation mandates operative repair; any deep abscess requires drainage. Grossly infected or collapsed bone grafts or vertebrae should be thoroughly debrided and regrafted after a vigorous washout. Long-term (6 weeks), organism-specific intravenous antibiotics should be administered. In less fulminant infections with good anatomic and neurologic preservation, a more conservative approach with drainage of superficial pus and administration of systemic antibiotics may be elected initially. Close clinical and radiographic follow-up is extremely important. If the patient is without signs of deep infection, nonoperative management may be a viable option, even in the presence of spine instrumentation. The erythrocyte sedimentation rate and C-reactive protein level are useful laboratory parameters to monitor. Clinical or radiographic progression would then mandate operative management.

Laryngotracheal Injuries

Sore throat and hoarseness are common and mostly transient complaints after anterior cervical surgery. Some researchers have sought to relate this phenomenon to increased pressure exerted on the laryngotracheal lumen by the endotracheal tube cuff following insertion of deep retractors. Venting enough air from the cuff to create a small air leak around the endotracheal tube may alleviate at least some of this problem.[23]

Fortunately, serious injury to the trachea is rare. Minor lacerations that are observed intraoperatively are repaired primarily, leaving the patient intubated for 48 to 72 hours to allow the wound to seal. More severe injuries and those that are detected in a delayed fashion because of pneumomediastinum or neck emphysema may be more appropriately managed with primary repair and tracheostomy. Occasionally, the parietal pleura is violated during low anterior or upper thoracic discectomy. This requires no specific treatment as long as the visceral pleura has not been violated to cause a persistent air leak. This possibility can be assessed by flooding the wound with saline and observing for a bubble stream during positive-pressure ventilation. This bubble stream implies an ongoing air leak and indicates tube thoracostomy.

Carotid and Vertebral Artery Injury

Carotid artery injury is unusual in the midcervical spine if care is taken during placement of toothed retractor blades. At this level, the artery is sufficiently removed from its tether points at the skull base and the aortic arch that the required degree of lateral mobilization is easily achieved. If the carotid sheath is scarred by previous radiation or operation, it should be freed longitudinally until the vessel can be displaced laterally without undue force or distortion.

Direct suture repair of carotid injuries is straightforward in virginal cases, because good proximal and distal control is readily achieved and the arterial wall willingly accepts suture. Unfortunately, this complication is most likely to occur in the reoperated case and/or history of irradiated wound. Exposure is more difficult, the vessels can be very friable, and the repair is challenging.

Vertebral artery injury is an unusual complication for cervical spine surgery, with an overall estimated incidence of 0.14%.[24] The vertebral artery is not routinely encountered in routine anterior cervical approaches. It may be injured by lateral exploration of the neural foramen in pursuit of uncovertebral joint osteophytes. This type of injury is usually minor and is controlled with small amounts of hemostatic packing. Most commonly, the vertebral artery is injured in anterior cervical spine surgery in the V2 segment (extending from the C6-1 transverse foramina) by using the drill off the midline, excessive lateral foraminal decompression/bone disc removal, or pathologic softening of the bone of the lateral part of the spinal canal caused by infection or tumor. Additionally, the artery runs between the transverse process of C7 and the longus colli musculature. Thus, extensive lateral dissection at C7 should be avoided.[25] More significant injury to the vertebral artery can result during cervical corpectomy if the decompression is taken too far laterally.[26] These injuries are usually incurred by overly aggressive drilling. They can be avoided if all dissection is performed under magnification and if the drill is not permitted to penetrate the deep bony cortex. The vertebra is "eggshelled out" by the drill, leaving only a thin bony cortex to be avulsed with a fine curet or thin-footed Kerrison rongeur. The ventral aspect of the transverse processes of C3-6 is also marked by a small bony tubercle that alerts the operator to the laterality of the exposure. More often, however, the point of injury occurs on the medial side of the artery, where the drill has broken through the vertebral cortex.

Vertebral artery injury with posterior cervical surgery has been most commonly associated with C1-2 transarticular screw insertion with a reported incidence of 1.3%.[24] The artery may be injured if the screw trajectory is too low or too lateral. C1 lateral mass and C2 pedicle constructs may reduce the risk of vertebral artery injury. Nevertheless, lateral perforation of the C2 pedicle may result in vertebral artery injury. Also, too far lateral exposure of the posterior or superior ring of C1 may predispose to vertebral artery injury.[27] Subaxial lateral mass screw insertion may result in vertebral artery injury, but such an injury is most unusual.[28]

When a vertebral artery injury occurs intraoperatively, there is usually sudden, nonpulsatile, copious bright red bleeding, although it may appear dark because of injury to the surrounding venous plexus. Injury is dangerous, as hemorrhage may be massive and cerebral ischemia/embolic phenomena may result.[25]

Strategies to manage a vertebral artery intraoperatively include tamponade, repair, and ligation. Tamponade includes use of hemostatic agents such as Gelfoam and oxidized cellulose (Surgicel).[25] Should this fail to control hemorrhage, the surgeon must enlarge the exposure, including deliberate resection of the ventral lip of the transverse process to uncover more of the artery proximally and distally as localized pressure is applied over a cottonoid at the point of hemorrhage. The surgeon must then weigh the options of vertebral ligation versus repair. Most patients, especially youths, tolerate unilateral vertebral ligation well.[26] However, a small number of patients will have an isolated vertebral artery terminating in the posterior inferior cerebellar artery or a compromised contralateral vertebral artery. Ligation of a vertebral artery in these circumstances could result in cerebellar or brainstem infarction. Because the status of the vertebral artery anatomy might not be known preoperatively, significant effort should be made to preserve vascular patency whenever possible. In this setting, intraoperative angiography should be considered.[25] If injury occurs at C1-2 during transarticular screw insertion, many surgeons advocated placement of a screw into the drilled hole to reduce bleeding.[24,25]

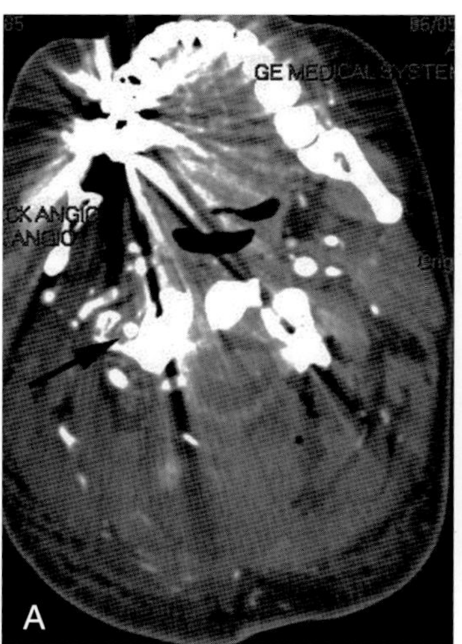
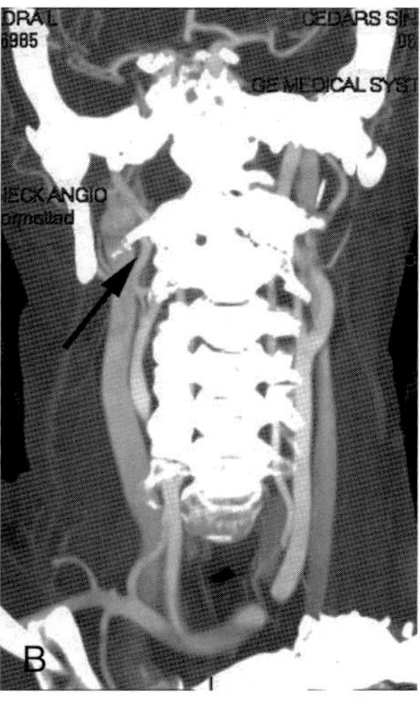

FIGURE 194-2. **A,** Axial CT angiogram image demonstrating a vertebral artery injury in a patient who underwent C1-2 arthrodesis. Note the patent vertebral artery at the level of C1 on the right (*arrow*) and its absence on the left. **B,** Coronal reconstruction in the same patient showing normal vertebral artery by C1 on the right (*arrow*) and its absence on the left.

Postoperative management remains controversial. Some surgeons advocate that the patient be observed and any postoperative intervention be dictated by the patient's clinical course. Others recommend that a postoperative angiogram be obtained to rule out significant injury, stenosis, pseudoaneurysm, or arteriovenous (AV) fistula (Fig. 194-2). This may allow for endovascular intervention or vessel sacrifice, if need be. Additionally, the postoperative neurologic examination should be followed as anticoagulation and antiplatelet therapy may be needed to prevent vertebrobasilar thromboembolism. Complications of vertebral artery injury include AV fistulae, late-onset hemorrhage, pseudoaneurysm and thrombosis with embolic incidents, cerebral ischemia, stroke, and even death. The vascular complications might occur days to years later. Thus, after identifying an injury, serial imaging with magnetic resonance angiography or CT angiography should be considered to rule out development of a pseudoaneurysm.[25]

Studying preoperative CT and MRI scans and noting the possibility of ectatic, tortuous, or aberrant vasculature can reduce the risk of vertebral artery injury. Additionally, these studies are useful for tumor surgery.[25]

Complications at the Cervicothoracic Junction and in the Thoracic Spine

Ventral exposure of the cervicothoracic junction remains problematic. The standard ventrolateral cervical exposure can be extended through division of the sternocleidomastoid and anterior scalene muscles, but working angles within the narrowing confines of the thoracic inlet, along with convergence of the common carotid arteries toward the innominate artery and aortic arch, often make this an awkward endeavor. The potential for esophageal injury is probably heightened somewhat by the difficulty in applying conventional self-retaining retractor systems stably at this depth and orientation. An increased risk for pneumothorax and recurrent laryngeal nerve injury also exists at the thoracic inlet. A deliberate effort to identify the recurrent laryngeal nerve at the base of the neck before its ascent into the tracheoesophageal groove may help to avert a stretch injury through injudicious placement of the retractor blades.

Between T1 and T4, transsternal approaches yield favorable working angles to the ventral spine through enlargement of the thoracic inlet. Ventral access caudal to T4 remains limited by the aortic arch and the innominate artery, which cannot be readily mobilized. Excessive spreading of the sternal retractor can cause a brachial plexus injury. Transaxillary thoracotomy centered on the 3rd rib provides an alternative access route to this region. This yields a lateral view up to the T1-2 level, working behind and to the side of the subclavian and innominate arteries. A left-sided thoracotomy is attended with a lower frequency of recurrent laryngeal nerve palsy, but the aortic knob is rather prominent in the field at this level. Because of this prominence and to lessen the risk of thoracic duct injury, transaxillary thoracotomy is usually performed from the right side.

Thoracic Duct Injuries

Although the thoracic duct is highly vulnerable to injury during operations at the level of the thoracic inlet, it is not a source of lingering morbidity. The thoracic duct ascends as an indistinct plexus behind the esophagus to join the left jugular and subclavian veins. The anatomy of the thoracic duct is variable, and ramifying branches and a right-sided confluence with the veins are not uncommon. The duct may be made visible if the patient ingests Federal Food, Drug and Cosmetic Act (FD&C) no. 6 dye preoperatively. This dye is taken up by lymphatics into the chyle, thereby aiding in the duct's intraoperative detection. If the duct is injured, the damaged segment is securely oversewn, and a low-fat diet is implemented postoperatively. Thoracic duct injuries that go unrecognized intraoperatively may result in chylous effusions in the wound or chest cavity. These injuries usually resolve without treatment, but large effusions may be a source of discomfort, wound irritation, respiratory embarrassment, and significant caloric loss. Simple aspiration is usually successful as an interim measure while the point of leakage scars over. Uncontrolled leaks are reexplored (after ingestion of FD&C no. 6 dye) to assist with the intraoperative delineation of the ductal system. If the precise point of leakage can be defined, it is simply ligated. Often, only a region of leakage can be identified. In this case, multiple "stick-tie" sutures are used to imbricate the suspect tissues. This can then be backed with a buttress of fascia or muscle and a film of fibrin glue.

Vascular Injuries

One of the principal concerns during the conduct of any transthoracic procedure is the avoidance of injury to major arterial and venous structures. The aortic arch is usually located at the T4 level. Rostral to this, the esophagus and the trachea lie immediately ventral to the spine; however, they are tethered by the brachiocephalic trunk and cannot be readily mobilized. Below the level of the arch, the descending aorta lies closely applied to the lateral aspect of the thoracic vertebrae on the left side. The thoracic duct swings dorsal to the esophagus to lie nearly in the midline, interposed between the esophagus and spine. Paired azygos veins flank the spine and anastomose extensively with each other and with the vena cava. Crossing transversely at each midvertebral body level are paired segmental arteries and veins. These are branches of the aorta and azygos systems, respectively, and they divide into an intercostal vessel and a radiculomedullary branch at the level of the neural foramen.

Vascular complications are best avoided through careful preoperative planning and exacting surgical technique. Selection of the most appropriate side for surgical approach is fundamental for a safe and effective procedure. Sometimes the lesion itself dictates this choice, as in the case of a lung tumor with direct spinal extension. However, concurrent pathologic abnormalities in the access route, such as pleural scarring from prior surgery, may sometimes indicate a contralateral approach. All else being equal, a left-sided exposure of the spine below the T6 level is preferred. Although the aorta presents ventrolaterally on the left side of the spine, it is a robust and thick-walled vessel that lends itself to mobilization; if injured, the aorta readily accepts suture for direct repair. The heart can be easily reflected ventrally out of the way, although the surgeon must be alert to altered hemodynamics because this maneuver occasionally interferes with venous return to the right and left atria, a problem that is compounded by hypovolemia. The advantage of the left-sided thoracotomy increases in the lower thoracic spine, where the right hemidiaphragm is elevated into the line of sight by the underlying liver. The liver does not easily lend itself to caudal displacement, because it is tethered by the hepatic ligament and the inferior vena cava. The esophagus, which is applied to the ventral aspect of the thoracic spine, is relatively less vulnerable during transthoracic approaches, because it is flanked on either side by major vascular structures. In primary transthoracic or thoracoscopic procedures, injury to the great vessels is usually avoidable by using sound surgical technique. Segmental vessels crossing the involved vertebra are secured at the level of the midbody. Interruption at this level may enhance the probability of continued patency of the radiculomedullary branches to the spinal cord through retrograde flow from the intercostal artery. A wide flap of mediastinal pleura is then developed, one leaf of which is reflected laterally toward the pedicles and foramina, and the opposite leaf is reflected medially. Dissection proceeds in a strictly subperiosteal plane, with all instruments kept firmly applied to bone lest the aorta be inadvertently entered as the flap is developed medially. Once the edge of the anterior longitudinal ligament is reached, malleable self-retaining retractors are inserted to maintain exposure and to protect the aorta. Division of the segmental arteries and veins untethers the great vessels and permits mobilization of the mediastinal contents to the midline. Taking the segmental vessels adjacent to the rostral and caudal disc spaces to be resected assists in this mobilization and is required in patients who undergo ventral instrumentation. Major vascular injury appears to be exceedingly uncommon during primary ventral thoracic spine operations.

Oskouian and Johnson reviewed an institutional experience of 207 patients who underwent anterior reconstructive procedures in the thoracic and lumbar spine. Direct vascular injuries were identified in seven patients, including one thoracic aortic dissection ascribed to retraction, one torn intercostal artery, and five venous injuries.[29] Injuries that are recognized intraoperatively obviously mandate immediate repair. The exact technique that is required depends on the size and anatomy of the injury. Branch avulsions are simply ligated. Small tears in the aorta proper or the vena cava are oversewn directly with fine vascular suture technique. Larger and more complex tears require placement of vascular clamps proximally and distally to isolate the injured segment for repair. Intraoperative consultation with an experienced cardiothoracic or vascular surgeon is appropriately sought. In cases of reoperation, prior infection, or irradiation, the possibility of scarification or friability of tissues in the mediastinum may be anticipated. These dissections can be tedious, and occasionally, it may be advisable to place umbilical tapes about the aorta preemptively or to prepare sites for cross-clamping in cases that are deemed high risk.

Pulmonary Complications

Atelectasis and pulmonary contusion with attendant potential for AV shunting and hypoxemia are minimized by periodic reexpansion of the lung and by accurate positioning and padding of any retractors. The opportunity to reinspect the lung parenchyma at these intervals discloses evolving surface contusions that may prompt alteration in retractor placement or technique. If a rib has been removed, sharp edges should be smoothed and waxed to avoid lung impalement. Pneumothorax is an inevitable consequence of thoracotomy, and a chest tube is always placed at the time of closure to encourage lung reexpansion, to control any air leak, and to evacuate blood from the wound. Thin, opalescent drainage postoperatively is suggestive of a chyle leak. Persistent or increasing volumes of chylous output may require operative reexploration as described previously.

Thoracolumbar Junction and Lumbar Spine

The thoracolumbar junction and lumbar spine are usually approached from the left side. On the right side, access is impeded by the liver and inferior vena cava, which can be difficult to mobilize. The bifurcation of the great vessels and the width of the psoas muscles make lateral exposure through the retroperitoneum awkward below L4. The peritoneal envelope containing the stomach and spleen in the left upper quadrant is reflected ventrally and caudally, together with the retroperitoneal structures, including the kidney and ureter. Although standard operative descriptions of this approach always caution about potential injury to abdominal viscera, in practice, injuries of a clinically significant magnitude appear to be extremely uncommon.

Splenic and Vascular Injury

Splenic injury has rarely been reported in the literature and should not present a problem as long as it is recognized promptly.[30] Recent abdominal trauma, splenomegaly, and venous hypertension may be predisposing factors. Presumably, these injuries are most often caused by overzealous mobilization or retraction. General surgical self-retaining retractor systems provide a significant advantage over hand-held instruments. The smooth blades that are used with these systems can be placed accurately and maintained without the trauma of repeated readjustments that are the inevitable outgrowth of the fatigue of prolonged manual retraction. A large moistened laparotomy pad is placed under the retractor to minimize the risk of injury. If a splenic injury occurs, consultation with a general surgeon should be sought. Brisk bleeding from the hilum necessitates splenectomy. However, in many cases of lesser injury, the spleen can be salvaged. When it is feasible, splenorrhaphy is preferable to splenectomy because of the increased incidence of overwhelming sepsis in patients who have been splenectomized. Surgeons should bear in mind the possibility of an occult splenic injury in cases of otherwise unexplained hypotension intraoperatively or postoperatively.

The aorta lies almost directly ventral to the spine in the lumbar region. Anatomy is inconstant, but the bifurcation into the common iliac arteries usually occurs at the level of the caudal L4 body. Aortic mobilization and methods to address aortic injury have been discussed previously. The inferior vena cava lies to the right of the midline. It is thin walled and has an extensive and variable network of tributaries and anastomoses that are easily torn and that are less readily repaired than are arterial structures. The level of confluence of the common iliac veins to form the vena cava is variable but typically occurs opposite the L4-5 disc space, just dorsal to the proximal portion of the right common iliac artery.

Ureteral Injury

The ureters lie in loose areolar tissue on the psoas muscles. They cross ventrally over the iliac arteries to descend into the pelvis. They can be distinguished by observing peristalsis after a momentary pinch with an atraumatic forceps. The risk of ureteral injury in primary surgeries is exceedingly small. However, if normal tissue planes have been obscured by previous surgery, retroperitoneal fibrosis, tumor, or irradiation, dissection must proceed with utmost caution. During reoperations, sponge and Kittner dissection is advantageous. Intraoperative identification of the ureter may be facilitated by retrograde placement of a stent at the outset of the procedure. If a ureteral injury is incurred, immediate repair is undertaken. The exact nature of the repair is dictated by the type of injury. Clean lacerations may be simply reanastomosed end to end, whereas a segmental injury, as may be caused by a drill or rongeur, requires segmental resection and reanastomosis with ureteral mobilization to allow for a tensionless repair. In either case, the reconstruction should be accomplished over a stent that can be subsequently retrieved cystoscopically. Injuries over segments that are too lengthy to permit primary repair are uncommon; however, they demand more sophisticated reconstructive techniques such as appendiceal interposition or ureteroureteral anastomosis. Obviously, the input of a urologic surgeon should be sought. Not all ureteral injuries are recognized during surgery. The postoperative development of hydronephrosis, a urinoma, or a retroperitoneal abscess should prompt investigation of the upper urinary tract by CT scan with contrast injection with delayed scans.[31] Two instances of delayed ureteral obstruction attributed to retroperitoneal fibrosis after scoliosis surgery with Dwyer instrumentation have been reported.[32,33]

Bowel Injury

Because the bowel is mobilized ventrally within the peritoneal envelope during a retroperitoneal approach, the possibility of an iatrogenic perforation exists. Obviously, such an event is a cause for grave concern because of the high potential for wound contamination. If a surgeon recognizes a bowel perforation intraoperatively, it is advisable to establish barrier isolation of the spinal exposure to minimize the risk of further wound contamination. The perforation should be repaired primarily, and the prophylactic antibiotic coverage should be expanded to include anaerobic organisms. Once the repair is complete, the wound is thoroughly irrigated with an antibiotic-containing solution. The decision whether to proceed with decompression, fusion, and instrumentation is individualized according to the phase of the procedure at which soilage occurred, its magnitude, and the relative penalty for not proceeding with a definitive procedure as planned. In most cases, the surgeon should be most reluctant to instrument a wound that he or she knows is contaminated. An extended course of antibiotics is advised postoperatively.

Transabdominal Approaches to the Lumbosacral Spine

Ventral exposure from the L4-5 level to the sacrum can be a surgical challenge. Retroperitoneal approaches through the flank to this level are limited by the caudolaterally coursing iliac veins, by the large mass of the psoas muscles, and by the obliquity of the working angle caused by the iliac crest. The latter two difficulties can be circumvented by midline transperitoneal or retroperitoneal approaches through the hypogastrium. The overlying great vessels are still a considerable impediment to this exposure and are the major source of morbidity. Foreknowledge of advanced atherosclerotic occlusive disease or of the presence of an abdominal aortic aneurysm may temper enthusiasm for a ventral operation. Dedicated vascular studies are not routinely obtained preoperatively unless clinical circumstances warrant concern. Excellent information about the condition of the aorta and its bifurcation can usually be gleaned from the preoperative spine imaging studies or sonography.

Vascular Injury

Arterial anatomy is more consistent than is venous anatomy. The level of the aortic bifurcation can be anticipated at L4; therefore, a direct ventral approach to the lumbosacral junction necessitates dissection within the limbs of the bifurcation. Typically, the right iliac artery has to be mobilized to uncover the L4-5 disc, and great care must be taken with insertion and removal of interbody retractors to minimize the possibility of blunt or sharp vascular injury. It is wise to confirm the presence of the femoral and pedal pulses periodically throughout the surgery. Loss of pulses should prompt an intraoperative angiogram and any indicated repair.

The venous anatomy is the more problematic aspect of these exposures. The level of confluence of the iliac veins to form the vena cava is at the L4-5 disc level in approximately 70% to 80% of patients. A more caudally situated confluence is often associated with unusually large common iliac veins. They may then directly overlie the L5 body or the L5-S1 disc space, sometimes precluding ventral access at this level entirely. These anatomic variations may be discerned in close inspection of the preoperative MRI or CT examinations.[34] In patients who are more typical, the left common iliac vein requires the greatest mobilization. Depending on the scope and level of the surgery, this vein may have to be retracted medially, laterally, or in both directions. In inflammatory or degenerative conditions, the left common iliac vein can easily become scarred down in the soft tissues immediately ventral to the disc. Successful collapse and mediolateral retraction are possible in this case only if the vein is carefully dissected longitudinally along its axis. The middle sacral vessels originate from either the common or the internal iliac vessels, and they overlie the L5-S1 disc space. They often can be retracted with ease, although no harm attends their sacrifice. The surgeon should take care to clearly identify all major vascular structures in the field before incising the disc space. The use of monopolar cautery over the disc space should be minimized to spare the hypogastric (sympathetic) plexus. Bipolar cautery is used to secure smaller vessels, and clips or ligatures are used to occlude larger vessels. Injuries to the common iliac veins or the vena cava are encountered in 1.9% to 15% of transabdominal approaches to the lumbosacral junction.[35-41] Additionally, complication rates for revision anterior lumbar surgery may be three to five times higher than those reported for primary exposures.[42] If a major vein is injured, venorrhaphy is preferred over ligation if at all possible. Hemorrhage is initially controlled by direct pressure at the point of injury until the vessel can be isolated proximally and distally. Particularly challenging are "backside" repairs brought on through avulsion of unseen tributaries into the dorsal wall of the common iliac veins or vena cava during blunt dissection. The largest and anatomically most consistent of these tributaries are the lateral lumbar veins and the iliolumbar vein. Because the inferior vena cava lies slightly to the right of midline, the most efficient strategy is to mobilize it farther rightward if it is in the way. Special effort must be taken to clearly identify, doubly ligate, and divide the lumbar and iliolumbar veins on the left side before retracting the inferior vena cava in this manner, in case the veins are avulsed or the vena cava is ruptured. Regrettably, efforts to graft veins using either autologous or prosthetic materials have been fraught with a high incidence of occlusion.

Lymphocele after the Anterior Approach to the Spine

Lymphocele is a complication after anterior lumbar spine surgery that may occur as often as 1% of the time after retroperitoneal approaches.[43] They may relate to surgical disruption of the lymphatics surrounding the iliac artery and vein. In performing retroperitoneal approaches to the lumbosacral spine, fluid may be sequestered in the retroperitoneal space and subsequently compress the peritoneum. Clinical presentation includes abdominal mass, wound drainage, fever, and weight gain. CT scanning is used for the diagnosis of an uncomplicated lymphocele that shows a low-attenuation mass. The differential for such a mass includes a complicated lymphocele (infected), urinoma, and cerebrospinal fluid collection. Though conservative treatment options exist, typical treatment involves drainage, open or laparoscopic marsupialization of the cyst to the peritoneal cavity, or sclerotherapy.[43-46]

Complications of Minimally Invasive Thoracolumbar Discectomy and Fusion

Minimally invasive spine procedures have grown in popularity. Theoretical benefits include less tissue trauma, less blood loss, and possibly reduced medical complications.[47,48] This is most apparent in minimally invasive deformity correction and fusion. Recently, the transsacral approach for discectomy and fusion and the transpsoas approach have increased in popularity. However, these access corridors have a unique set of complications associated with them, somewhat different than those of traditional anterior lumbar surgery.

The transsacral approach has been used for L5-S1 discectomy and interbody fusion but also, more recently, for L4-5 and L5-S1 discectomy and fusion.[47,49-51] This approach relies on a normal presacral space, which exists between the anterior sacral margin and the mesorectum.[52,53] The complication rate with the technique has been noted to be low. A retrospective analysis of complications noted, per the U.S. Food and Drug Administration medical device reported data (in 5300 cases of transsacral fusion), that this technique was associated with a 0.7% complication rate. A 0.47% bowel injury rate was noted.[54]

Preoperative imaging should confirm no midline vessels at the level of the S1-2 junction to minimize risk of vascular injury with this procedure. Additionally, when doing this procedure, the operator should keep the probe in continuous contact with the sacrum. If at any point the working channel loses contact with the bone, the procedure should be started from the beginning. Contraindications to transsacral surgery that could result in a theoretically higher rate of soft tissue or vascular injury include high-grade spondylolisthesis, previous surgery in this region, and a history of prior colostomies or pathology in the region of the rectum, such as fistulas.

If a bowel injury is suspected after such a procedure, rigid proctosigmoidoscopy, flexible sigmoidoscopy, or Gastrografin (Bayer AG, Germany) enema can be performed to identify injury. Alternatively, if a patient presents in a delayed manner, CT of the abdomen and pelvis with rectal Gastrografin contrast should be performed. Venous bleeding tends to tamponade in the presacral space. Arterial bleeding is unusual in this situation. For a stable hematoma, observation is recommended. Any expanding pelvic hematoma requires emergency resuscitation and angiography/embolization.[55]

The transpsoas approach to the lumbar spine is a strictly retroperitoneal approach to the disc space. Complications commonly seen, such as thigh paresthesias or hip flexor and quadriceps weakness, are typically related to the neural structures that have a close relationship to this muscle.

Nevertheless, retroperitoneal structures such as the ureter and kidney can be injured, in addition to bowel and vasculature, although the rates of these injuries are probably significantly lower than those in traditional abdominal approaches.[56-58] If at any point there is excessive bleeding from this approach, the exposure can be readily converted to a laparotomy and/or thoracotomy.

Positioning of the patient for the transpsoas approach is critical in complication avoidance, as the surgeon should be working at a 90-degree angle toward the disc space. We prefer to work with a left-sided approach to avoid a potentially catastrophic venous injury. Care should be taken to avoid violation of the anterior longitudinal ligament, as this provides a safeguard against intraperitoneal injuries. Instruments' depth should be checked under strict fluoroscopic control. Retractors should be secured to the bed with an articulating arm after serial soft tissue dilatation. We also prefer to secure the retractor to the vertebrae, thereby minimizing the risk of soft tissue creep and subsequent injury. In working near the thoracolumbar junction, the diaphragm is pushed out of the way while a targeting probe or percutaneous access kit needle targets the disc space. In entering the chest cavity, expiration is held to minimize the risk of pulmonary injury. A red rubber catheter (with a watertight closure) can be used to evacuate intrapleural air while the anesthesiologist has the patient perform a Valsalva maneuver. A chest tube can also be considered to avoid pneumothorax in cases in which the chest cavity is entered.

Complications of Posterior Lumbar Discectomy

Lumbar discectomy is among the most commonly performed spine operations. Complications are few and usually relate to infection, instability, cerebrospinal fluid leak, and neurologic events. Although vascular injuries are uncommon, the potential for bowel, ureteral, and catastrophic vascular injury is now well documented. The shared mechanism of these injuries is violation of the anulus ventrally with some type of biting instrument. A review of the literature in English since 1965 identified 98 cases of vascular injury associated with posterior lumbar discectomy and estimated an incidence of one to five events per 10,000 procedures.[59] Goodkin and Laska noted a rate of symptomatic anular perforation (with vascular or viscus injury) of 1.6 to 6 per 10,000 cases.[60] Nevertheless in another series, the incidence was noted at 17 per 10,000.[61] It is likely that these complications are considerably more common than is generally appreciated.

Bleeding from the disc space that is not caused by epidural or bone bleeding; findings of fat, viscera, or vessel wall in the specimen; and unexplained hypotension during surgery should lead the surgeon to suspect a vascular or visceral injury. Should this occur, a general or vascular surgeon should be immediately consulted, the wound should be packed or closed, and laparotomy or additional appropriate testing should be performed. Delay of treatment after injury was associated with a 40% mortality rate, while early operation was associated with a 24% mortality rate in one series.[60]

Vascular Injury

Vascular injury during posterior lumbar surgery may take several forms. The most dramatic are lacerations or partial wall avulsions in large-caliber retroperitoneal arteries or veins that result in massive, acute retroperitoneal hemorrhage. Bleeding is manifested through the disc space itself in fewer than half of these cases. Often, the injury is first suspected because of unexplained hypotension and tachycardia, either in the operating room or during postanesthetic recovery.[59,62,63] Lesser injuries may tamponade themselves in a contained retroperitoneal hematoma, later giving rise to a pseudoaneurysm, which can present with delayed rupture or distal embolization. Venous injuries are probably more common, but their diagnosis is less obvious. They may be a source of retroperitoneal hemorrhage, venous thrombosis, leg swelling, and pulmonary embolism. The presence of an expanding lower abdominal mass, unexplained anemia, an unexpected degree of back or leg pain, and lower-extremity swelling or thromboembolism should prompt consideration of a vascular injury. If an artery and a vein are injured in proximity to each other, the potential for the development of an AV fistula exists.[59,63] These fistulas are recognized by the presence of a thrill, symptoms of limb claudication, and cardiac overload secondary to a left-to-right shunt. Although AV fistulas may present in the first days postoperatively, full symptomatic maturation is more typically delayed by weeks to months. Violation of the ventral anulus with curets and rongeurs may be a much more common occurrence than is generally realized. Three of 25 patients undergoing follow-up lumbar discography were shown to have new, but asymptomatic, ventral anular defects at the operated levels.[64] The L4-5 and L5-S1 levels have been implicated with equal frequency. The anatomy of the aortic bifurcation and the more variable confluence of the common iliac veins have been reviewed. Because the aorta usually terminates opposite the L4 vertebra, aortic injury per se is rare. The common iliac veins usually join at the level of the L4-5 disc space to the right of midline to form the inferior vena cava. Injuries on the lateral aspect of the disc on the right side are expected to involve the terminal inferior vena cava (at L4-5) or the proximal right common iliac vein. In paramedian injuries, the right common iliac artery and the right or left common iliac vein are vulnerable. With left lateral injuries, the left common iliac artery is at risk. With rostral bifurcation of the common iliac arteries, occasional instances of isolated internal iliac injury have been reported during L5-S1 discectomy. The likelihood of breach of the ventral anulus is increased by the vigor with which disc space evacuation is pursued. Prevention of such an injury involves the surgeon's consciously attempting to avoid breach of the anterior longitudinal ligament. Nevertheless, this often occurs without appreciation of the surgeon. Other risk factors for anterior longitudinal ligament violation may also be present, such as preexisting fissures and peridiscal fibrosis.[60]

The diameter of the targeted disc space along the projected axis of the discectomy can be accurately measured from preoperative MRI or CT studies acquired in axial planes oriented parallel to the disc space. Ordinarily, this varies from 37 to 48 mm from L3 to the sacrum and is somewhat larger in men than in women.[61] The shafts of instruments that are to be introduced into the disc space may then be appropriately marked with a small adhesive strip as a caution against overly deep insertion. The disc rongeur should enter the disc space with the jaws in a closed position to discourage engagement of the thecal sac or a nerve root; however, once within the disc space, the jaws are opened while the rongeur is advanced to its working depth. This distributes any applied forces over two contact points and makes unintended breach of the ventral anulus more difficult. The management of vascular complications is context specific. In the face of acute hemodynamic instability, the prone patient must be quickly returned to the supine position to aid resuscitation and enable exploratory laparotomy. Swift diagnosis and appropriate action are of paramount importance if a catastrophic outcome is to be avoided. Skin edges can be swiftly reapproximated with a whipstitch closure or staples while the anesthetic is lightened and volume resuscitation is begun. The assistance of a general or vascular surgeon should be sought immediately. The area of injury will lie beneath a bulging retroperitoneal hematoma. Arterial hemorrhage may be controlled with manual compression of the distal aorta until desired personnel and equipment can be mobilized. The retroperitoneal hematoma must be explored carefully to delineate the site of injury precisely and to obtain proximal and distal control. It may then be repaired primarily or grafted according to circumstances. Although retroperitoneal hematoma remains an uncommon complication of lumbar discectomy, mortality approaches 50%, in part because of delayed diagnosis. Only through early recognition of such injuries and prompt institution of corrective action can these patients be salvaged. Less calamitous vascular injuries present in a delayed fashion in hemodynamically stable individuals.[63] Typically, such injuries are initially evaluated by an abdominal CT scan. If a retroperitoneal mass is defined adjacent to a discectomy site, it should be further evaluated angiographically. In some institutions, magnetic resonance angiography and CT angiography can obviate the need for invasive examination in select settings. Color flow Doppler studies may also be appropriate in patients with significant lower-limb swelling that is suggestive of proximal venous injury or thrombosis. Arterial injuries such as AV fistulas or pseudoaneurysms are repaired or reconstructed as open procedures, usually on an elective basis. Evolving reconstructive endovascular techniques may soon allow for percutaneous management of some of these conditions. Partial or complete thrombosis of an iliac vein or inferior vena cava may require either systemic anticoagulation or placement of an infrarenal caval filter, depending on the circumstances.

Other Visceral Injury

Ureteral injury after lumbar discectomy appears to be an even rarer complication than vascular injury.[65] The ureters are located more laterally in the retroperitoneum than are the great vessels, lying in the cleft between the psoas muscles and the spine, within a bed of periureteral fat. Therefore, they are somewhat more mobile than the great vessels and are less vulnerable to injury. In cases in which the ureter is not recognized as part of the operative specimen, diagnosis is usually delayed by several weeks and is announced by abdominal pain, distention, hematuria, and urinary or systemic sepsis. A urinoma may be visualized sonographically or on abdominal CT. Abdominal CT with contrast injection and delayed scans is the gold standard for staging such injuries.[31] It is postulated that an aberrantly medial course of the ureters or a thin body habitus allowing compression of the retroperitoneal structures against the spine in the prone position is a factor that contributes to this unusual complication. Treatment includes proximal diversion by nephrostomy followed by a definitive urologic reconstruction according to principles already discussed.[66] The possibility of concomitant vascular injury must be excluded by vascular imaging studies and through thorough intraoperative assessment. Another rare but serious complication resulting from ventral penetration of the disc space is bowel perforation.[67,68] Most were injuries to the ileum after L5-S1 discectomy. The mesenteric root attaches to the retroperitoneum obliquely, crossing the midline at the L5-S1 interspace as it courses toward the right sacroiliac joint. Because the great vessels bifurcate above this level, it is postulated that a narrow window is thereby created in the midline through which instruments may be passed into the mesentery. It has also been postulated that air-filled loops of bowel tend to float upward and apply themselves ventrally against the spine in the prone position. Intraoperative diagnosis is obvious if the rongeur retrieves intestinal mucosa. Otherwise, in the early postoperative period, patients have an acute abdomen or, in a delayed fashion, chronic wound infections attributable to intestinal flora. Patients with a bowel injury may also present with discitis.[60] Treatment is usually surgical, especially when a walled-off abscess is suspected.

Instrumentation Complications

The use of instrumentation has introduced a new level of complexity and complications to spine surgery. Apart from issues related to biomechanical failure, the various forms of dorsal instrumentation, including assorted types of pedicle screws, claws, hooks, and sublaminar wires, mainly pose a threat of neurologic injury or cerebrospinal fluid leak. Placement of transarticular C1-2 screws must be technically exact to avoid vertebral artery injury. Consideration of placing C1-2 instrumentation first on the side with the safer trajectory (considering the artery) should be made. For transarticular screws, the safest trajectory involves placing the screw through the most dorsal and medial part of the isthmus.[25] If an initial C1-2 screw placement results in arterial injury, a pars screw may be a preferable option on the contralateral side rather than risking bilateral vertebral artery occlusion. It is conceivable that overly long pedicle screws could penetrate far enough through the vertebral cortex ventrally to transfix the esophagus or great vessels.

Bicortical screw fixation at the S1 level raises concern for internal iliac vein or lumbosacral trunk injury. Both of these structures lie in close apposition to the sacrum just medial to the sacroiliac joint. On the basis of anatomic studies in cadavers, the potential for injury to these structures seems to be increased with screws that are placed laterally.[69] Screws that are directed medially through the S1 pedicles to engage the ventral sacral cortex have only a remote chance of causing visceral injury. Major vascular structures are located more laterally, and the sigmoid colon is still attached on a short mesentery at this level. It is possible that the preparatory drilling, probing, and tapping of the pilot holes are more likely to produce injury than is the placement of the screw itself. These maneuvers must be performed with extreme caution to minimize the risk of overdrilling or overtapping of the holes, which could easily puncture a vessel or viscus. Clinically relevant injuries appear to be extremely uncommon thus far, but continued strict attention to the technical details of instrumentation insertion is mandatory if these untoward events are to be avoided. Presumably, the expanding use of image-guidance technologies will add an extra margin of safety to these endeavors. Ventral thoracic and thoracolumbar spine instrumentation has demonstrated its potential to cause serious vascular complications. The Dunn device was withdrawn from clinical use after it was associated with the development of abdominal aneurysms in three cases. Whether this was caused by the device's design or by the method of its application in these particular individuals remains unclear. Contemporary ventral fixation systems for use in the thoracic and lumbar spine, using rod or plate constructs, have been free of vascular complications thus far. This is attributed to design parameters that emphasize a low profile and that demand an exactly lateral application on the vertebral bodies with an orthogonal screw trajectory dorsal to all major vessels. If care is taken to apply the instrumentation as intended, with screws of appropriate length, the potential for significant vascular or soft tissue injury should be exceedingly small. Aortic injury at the T6 level may result from screw penetration during ventral spine fixation.[70] Delayed aortic rupture has been attributed to erosion by a mesh cage placed for ventral reconstruction in the thoracic spine.[71] Complications such as these underscore the need for careful correlation of the field as viewed intraoperatively with preoperative and intraoperative imaging to reconfirm that spine instrumentation is applied as intended. Such cross-checking is especially advisable in cases of deformity correction, in which normal anatomic relations can be highly distorted. The use of screws with a blunt tip and a tapered run out to the threads may mitigate the possibility of engagement of a major vessel. Above all, surgeons must adhere to proper operative technique and pay close attention to screw length and trajectory. The width of the vertebral body and the exact location of the great vessels relative to the projected screw path can be ascertained through inspection of the axial CT or MRI scans at the levels to be instrumented.

Summary

Contemporary surgical techniques enable both ventral and dorsal exposure of the entire spine from occiput to sacrum. This allows any pathologic condition to be addressed in an anatomically appropriate fashion. As a group, the ventral approaches are more likely to have soft tissue or vascular complications because of the need to reflect these structures that overlie the spine. This inevitably subjects the patient to heightened risks of exposure-related complications compared with the simpler midline dorsal approaches.[72] This risk is justified only if it is kept acceptably low and if patient outcomes are significantly improved in relation to the natural history of the disease and to safer but possibly less definitive procedures. Sound case selection and excellent surgical technique are the keys to avoiding or minimizing these complications.

Acknowledgment. Drs. Neel Anand, Eli M. Baron, and Donald A. Smith updated this chapter on *Vascular and Soft Tissue Complications* originally authored by David W. Cahill for the first and second editions of this textbook. Dr. Cahill perished tragically in 2003 at the height of his career. He had extensive personal acquaintance both with the successes of surgery and with its complications. Ambitious, brilliant, and unapologetically self-confident, he bootstrapped himself to become a largely self-created neurosurgical pioneer in the evolving field of complex and reconstructive spine surgery. He only half-jokingly referred to himself as a "maximally invasive surgeon," content not merely to perform cutting-edge deformity corrections, but ultimately coming to do all his own retroperitoneal and transcavitary approaches as well.

Dr. Cahill held himself and others to the highest personal and technical standards. He was bluntly honest in dispensing his opinions and rarely in doubt. While this habit was not endearing to all, it was refreshing to hear such plain talk from someone in the know. David's knack for critical thought and openness to challenge have been fittingly memorialized in the highly popular *Cahill Controversies in Spine Surgery* debates featured annually at meetings of the Joint Section.

Above all else, David was a devoted husband and parent. Within the professional arena his proudest professional achievements were the establishment of a Neurosurgical Spine Fellowship and a fully accredited Neurosurgical Residency at the University of South Florida, where he was also the founding chair for the Department of Neurosurgery. He personally graduated over 20 fellows and residents who are the daily renewal of his legacy to our profession.

—*Donald A. Smith*

KEY REFERENCES

Baron EM, Soliman AM, Gaughan JP, et al: Dysphagia, hoarseness, and unilateral true vocal fold motion impairment following anterior cervical diskectomy and fusion. *Ann Otol Rhinol Laryngol* 112:921, 2003.

Faciszewski T, Winter RB, Lonstein JE, et al: The surgical and medical perioperative complications of anterior spinal fusion surgery in the thoracic and lumbar spine in adults: a review of 1223 procedures. *Spine (Phila Pa 1976)* 20:1592, 1995.

Goodkin R, Laska LL: Vascular and visceral injuries associated with lumbar disc surgery: medicolegal implications. *Surg Neurol* 49:358, 1998.

Jung A, Schramm J: How to reduce recurrent laryngeal nerve palsy in anterior cervical spine surgery: a prospective observational study. *Neurosurgery* 67:10, 2010.

Oskouian RJ Jr, Johnson JP: Vascular complications in anterior thoracolumbar spinal reconstruction. *J Neurosurg* 96:1, 2002.

Peng CW, Chou BT, Bendo JA, et al: Vertebral artery injury in cervical spine surgery: anatomical considerations, management, and preventive measures. *Spine J* 9:70, 2009.

Tormenti MJ, Maserati MB, Bonfield CM, et al: Complications and radiographic correction in adult scoliosis following combined transpsoas extreme lateral interbody fusion and posterior pedicle screw instrumentation. *Neurosurg Focus* 28:E7, 2010.

REFERENCES

The complete reference list is available online at expertconsult.com.

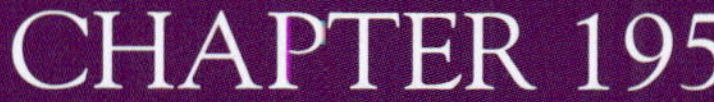

Postoperative Spinal Deformities

Sigurd Berven | Eijiro Okada

Definition

Deformity of the spine encompasses malalignment in the coronal, sagittal, and axial planes. Spinal deformity may result from either pathologies that are intrinsic to the development and aging of the spine, including congenital failures of formation or segmentation, developmental conditions, and degenerative pathologies, or the influence of extrinsic factors acting on the spine, including trauma, infection, and surgical intervention. Postoperative spinal deformity encompasses a spectrum of spinal disorders that includes initial fixation of the spine in a position of malalignment, decompensation of the spine in the sagittal or coronal plane after surgery, and adjacent-segment kyphosis.

Postoperative deformity is an important complication, and a major reason for revision spine surgery. Revision rates in spine surgery have been reported variably, and the rates depend on the primary pathology treated, patient factors, methods of treatment, and choice of levels for arthrodesis.[1-4] Postoperative deformity with adjacent-segment pathology is associated with significant disability and is one of the most common reasons for revision surgery.[5-9] This chapter addresses the etiologies of postoperative spinal deformity and provides guidance for both avoiding and managing deformities after spine surgery.

Fusion of the Spine in Malalignment

Initial fusion of the spine in a malaligned position is a common cause of postoperative deformity. Malalignment of the spine at the time of initial surgery may be the result of inadequate correction of deformity, asymmetrical correction of deformity, or failure to recognize deformity in preoperative surgical planning or intraoperatively. Importantly, malalignment of the spine may occur after fusion for degenerative pathology as well as after fusion for deformity. Careful attention to segmental alignment of the spine, even in short-segment arthrodeses, is important, especially at the lumbosacral junction and at the lower lumbar spine. Fusion of the spine in malalignment is apparent immediately after surgery but may be recognized only after the patient is observed standing after surgery. Awareness of patterns of immediate postoperative deformity is important for avoiding malalignment.

Fusion of the spine with inadequate correction in the sagittal plane is a common cause of immediate postoperative deformity. Neutral sagittal alignment follows a vertical axis from C2, in front of T7, behind L3, and within 3 cm of the dorsal margin of the sacrum.[10] There is significant normal variation of lumbar lordosis and thoracic kyphosis in maintaining overall sagittal balance.[11,12] Sagittal balance is important for biomechanical optimization of forces at segmental interspaces. Sagittal plane malalignment is most often clinically significant when there is loss of normal lordosis of the lumbar and cervical spine. Excessive kyphosis across these mobile, unsupported segments increases intradiscal pressures and compromises the mechanical advantage of the erector spinae musculature.[13,14] Clinically, the patient with fixed sagittal deformity presents with intractable pain, early fatigue, and a subjective sense of imbalance and leaning forward and difficulty with horizontal gaze. Compensation can be gained with extension of the hips, increased positive tilt (retroversion) of the pelvis, and flexion of the knees, although at the expense of increased fatigue.[15]

Flatback deformity or *syndrome* is the term commonly applied to postoperative malalignment of the spine. Flatback syndrome first was recognized by Doherty in 1973 as a postural disorder of the spine caused specifically by distraction instrumentation in the correction of scoliosis. Doherty recognized the loss of normal lordosis that occurred as a result of distraction across the lumbar spine and the thoracolumbar junction with the use of Harrington instrumentation for correction of coronal deformity in adolescent idiopathic deformity.[16] *Kyphotic decompensation syndrome* is a more general term for postoperative kyphosis that is caused by immediate malalignment of the spine.[17] Kyphotic decompensation may occur at a single segment of the spine or, more commonly, in fusion of the spine over multiple segments.

Fixation of the spine in coronal plane malalignment also is an important cause of immediate postoperative malalignment. Coronal plane malalignment after surgery may result in significant truncal shift, shoulder asymmetry, apparent leg-length discrepancy, pelvic obliquity with imbalance, rib-on-pelvis deformity, and complaints regarding appearance.[18] A small malalignment or coronal tilt at the lumbosacral segments may cause a significant truncal shift and imbalance. A common cause of postoperative coronal malalignment is asymmetrical correction of balanced curves in a double major deformity or in a thoracolumbar scoliosis with a fixed lumbosacral obliquity.

Avoiding Fusion of the Spine in Malalignment

Preoperative planning and recognition of global sagittal and coronal plane alignment are important for avoiding postoperative malalignment of the spine.[19] On physical examination, evaluation of the patient with knees fully extended is essential to assess the sagittal plane. Recognition of pelvic tilt (version of the pelvis) is important to determine whether a patient may be compensating for sagittal deformity in the spine with hyperextension of the hips and increase in pelvic tilt. In the coronal plane, correction of pelvic obliquity during the examination is important to assess coronal alignment of the spine prior to surgery. Leg-length discrepancy or apparent pelvic obliquity may be corrected with standing blocks to evaluate the spine with a level pelvis. Standing 36-inch radiographs are important in the evaluation of preoperative deformity and for identifying goals of surgical correction. Preoperative planning is based on calculations of sagittal and coronal changes needed for spinal realignment and may include digital image manipulation or modeling of the spine.[20] Preoperative planning in deformity surgery may be characterized by significant variability within and between observers.[21]

During the procedure, patient positioning and intraoperative radiographs are critical for obtaining optimal alignment of the spine and for avoiding immediate postoperative deformity. Patient positioning has a significant impact on spinal alignment in the coronal and sagittal planes, and use of an appropriate operative frame to optimize passive correction of deformity and to avoid generation of deformity is important.[22,23] Positioning the patient in a flexed posture may be useful for decompressive procedures, but arthrodesis of the spine with the patient in a knee-chest position, or in a flexed posture, is an important cause of postoperative deformity in even short-segment fusions.[24,25] Intraoperative radiology is useful in assessing alignment of the spine after placement of fixation. Full-length, 36-inch radiographs obtained in the sagittal and coronal planes are most useful for assessment of global balance.

Treatment of Postoperative Malalignment of the Spine

Recognition of postoperative deformity is the most important first step in planning the treatment of postoperative spinal malalignment. Immediately after surgery, deformity may be difficult to recognize due to antalgic stance and use of support, including a walker. A careful assessment of the patient's alignment with the knees extended and the pelvis neutral is critical for recognizing immediate postoperative deformity. Treatment of postoperative deformity is significantly easier in the immediate postoperative period than it is in the patient who develops a solid arthrodesis in fixed malalignment.

When postoperative malalignment is recognized immediately after surgery, the patient may be treated with early revision and may not require osteotomies to correct a fixed deformity. Early revision may include improving segmental or regional sagittal alignment in a mobile spine with facetectomies or, more significantly, with Ponte osteotomies.[26] In a patient with coronal imbalance due to asymmetrical correction of double curves, revision surgery may include improving the correction of the curve contralateral to the coronal offset or reducing the correction of the curve ipsilateral to the coronal offset Early detection of immediate postoperative deformity facilitates correction in a mobile spine.

The patient in whom postoperative deformity is recognized late, or after solid arthrodesis of the spine in a malaligned position, can present a difficult challenge for realignment. Osteotomies of the spine are the most commonly used technique for correction of postoperative malalignment.[27] Surgical correction of fixed sagittal deformity was first reported by Smith-Petersen et al. in 1945.[28] This osteotomy pivots on the posterior longitudinal ligament, with consequent lengthening of the anterior column through the disc space.[29] The technique is well suited for patients with flexible discs ventrally and dorsal pseudarthrosis at multiple levels. Combined ventral and dorsal surgery offers the advantage of a controlled manipulation of the anterior column and fusion with structural graft. LaChapelle described a combined ventral and dorsal osteotomy for the management of ankylosing spondylitis that involved cutting the anterior column directly, followed by grafting to avoid risks of a ventral opening wedge.[30] The combined ventral and dorsal osteotomy for the correction of iatrogenic lumbar kyphosis has led to good restoration of lumbar lordosis, maintained at more than 2 years' follow-up.[31]

A dorsal-only approach to correction of sagittal deformity offers several advantages, including single-stage surgery, reduced morbidity compared with combined surgery, addressing the deformity at the apex, creation of compressive forces at the osteotomy site, and maximal correction with a minimal number of osteotomies.[32] Dorsal surgical options can be categorized by the fulcrum across which correction is achieved. Dorsal osteotomies that hinge on the posterior longitudinal ligament (e.g., Smith-Petersen) cause opening of the anterior column. Spinal shortening osteotomies gain sagittal plane correction without distraction of the anterior column. Heinig's eggshell decancellation procedure includes a controlled compression fracture of the anterior column with differentially more closure dorsally.[33] In contrast, the Thomasen osteotomy maintains the height of the anterior column and hinges on the anterior longitudinal ligament.[34] Asymmetrical closure of the pedicle subtraction osteotomy may permit up to 6 cm correction of coronal plane deformity as well as sagittal plane deformity.[35] Larger corrections of trunk translation or coronal deformity may require a vertebral column resection.[18,36,37]

Case Examples: Immediate Postoperative Deformity

Case 1

A 54-year-old woman presented with a double major scoliosis. Asymmetrical flexibility of the lumbar and thoracic curves resulted in overcorrection of the lumbar curve relative to the thoracic curve and postoperative coronal decompensation. Realignment of the spine with an asymmetrical pedicle subtraction osteotomy (PSO) at L3 resulted in improvement of sagittal and coronal plane alignment (Fig. 195-1).

Case 2

A 41-year-old woman was treated with combined ventral and dorsal surgery for lumbar adult scoliosis. The patient was fused in a fixed kyphotic and coronal plane decompensation. An

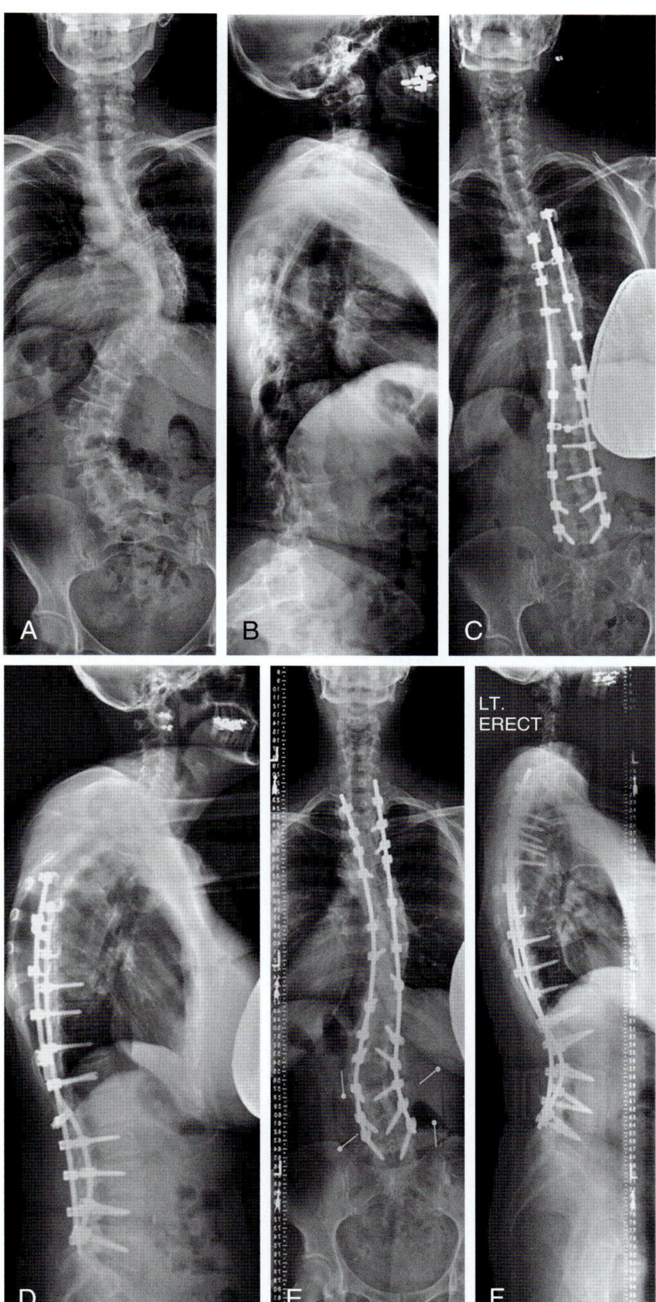

FIGURE 195-1. Preoperative standing anteroposterior (**A**) and lateral (**B**) radiographs. **C** and **D**, Initial postoperative appearance with asymmetrical curve correction. **E** and **F**, Final postoperative appearance with restoration of coronal and sagittal imbalance using an asymmetrical pedicle subtraction osteotomy.

asymmetrical PSO provided correction of deformity in the sagittal and coronal planes (Fig. 195-2).

Case 3

A 67-year-old man with degenerative spondylosis was fused in kyphotic malalignment from L3-S1. The patient developed adjacent-segment kyphosis and fixed sagittal plane decompensation. Use of a PSO resulted in sagittal plane realignment (Fig. 195-3).

Postoperative Decompensation

Even when the spine has adequate alignment immediately after surgery, it may decompensate over time. Late decompensation of the spine may result in progressive postoperative deformity and the need for revision surgery. Late decompensation may occur within the fused segments of the spine or may occur at adjacent segments, including compensatory curves that were not included in the initial levels of arthrodesis. Patients with late onset of postoperative deformity may present with progressive loss of correction, loss of height, and new onset of pain of spinal origin. Long-term clinical and radiographic follow-up of patients is required to identify late postoperative deformity.

Late decompensation within the fused segments is most characteristic of incomplete fusion, or pseudarthrosis of the spine. Failure to achieve solid arthrodesis of the spine may lead to symptoms including progressive deformity, pain, dyspnea, and neurologic deficit. Pseudarthrosis of the spine is a contributing factor in as many as 80% of reoperations in failed spinal fusions.[38-40] Symptomatic pseudarthroses are most common in the thoracolumbar and lumbosacral regions. Because revision surgery for symptomatic pseudarthrosis is characterized by high rates of recurrent pseudarthrosis and clinical failure,[41,42] obtaining solid arthrodesis of the spine at the time of initial surgery is valuable because this may help avoid revision for pseudarthrosis. The role of biologics in improving arthrodesis in ventral dorsal spinal fusion surgery may reduce the burden of revision surgery for late postoperative deformity due to pseudarthrosis.[43-45]

Postoperative deformity due to pseudarthrosis may occur in both instrumented and noninstrumented fusions. Recognition and detection of pseudarthrosis may be challenging. The reported rates of pseudarthrosis are highly variable, and an important cause of observed variability in published rates is the difficulty of making a radiographic diagnosis of pseudarthrosis.[46,47] In an instrumented fusion, pseudarthrosis may be apparent by implant loosening with osteolysis around screws, or by rod breakage. In noninstrumented fusions, identification of a pseudarthrosis may be more challenging. In a study correlating radiographic findings with intraoperative findings, Dawson et al. reported that plain anteroposterior and lateral views of the spine accurately identified a pseudarthrosis in only 48% of cases.[48] The authors identified CT in the coronal plane as the most accurate study for identifying pseudarthrosis, with a 96% correlation with findings at surgery. Deckey et al. reported a finding of progressive deformity in 4 of 14 patients (28%) who underwent removal of instrumentation with an apparently solid fusion.[49] This finding brings into question the effectiveness of even second-look surgery. DePalma and Rothman reported that the condition of pseudarthrosis is iatrogenic and responsibility for it lies entirely within the hands of the surgeon.[50] Although surgical technique is an important consideration in the generation of a successful arthrodesis, other factors also have an important influence on the occurrence of nonunion in the spine, including the region of the spine fused, surgical approach, underlying diagnosis, implant stiffness, local conditions for bone formation, smoking, infection, and bone graft choices.[7, 51-57]

Crankshaft deformity of the spine is an important example of postoperative deformity within a fused region of the spine.

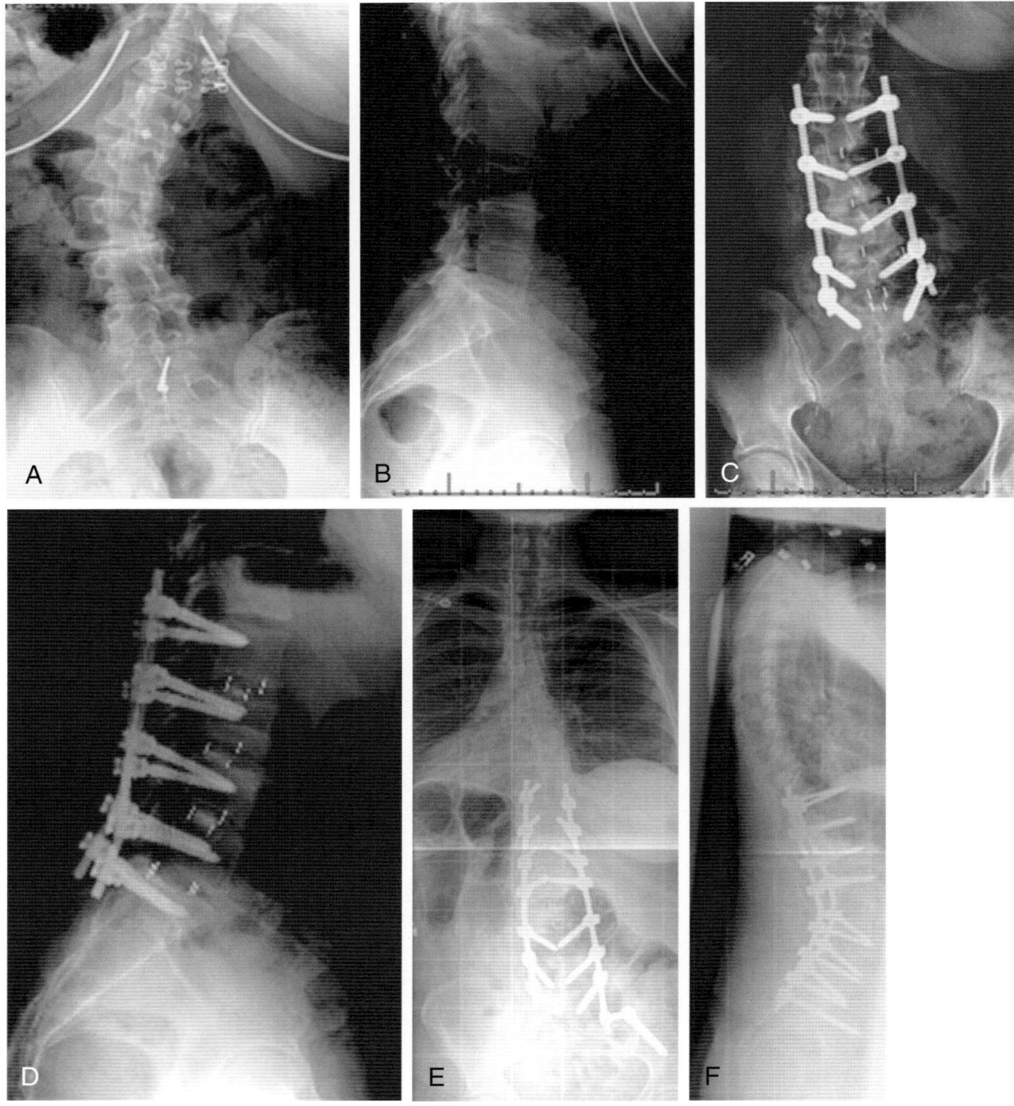

FIGURE 195-2. Preoperative anteroposterior (**A**) and lateral (**B**) radiographs of the lumbar spine. Postoperative coronal (**C**) and sagittal (**D**) views of malalignment. **E** and **F,** Postoperative views after asymmetrical pedicle subtraction osteotomy for restoration of sagittal and coronal balance.

In children with spinal deformity, progressive curvature, vertebral rotation, and rib prominence after a dorsal fusion may be due to continued anterior column growth of the spine despite a solid dorsal arthrodesis. This pattern of deformity progression was first identified by Hefti and McMaster.[58] Duboisset et al. introduced the term "crankshaft phenomenon" as a descriptive term for this type of progressive deformity, making the analogy with an automotive crankshaft rotating around a center arm.[59] Young patients who have significant ventral growth remaining at the time of a dorsal spine fusion are at risk of postoperative deformity progression, and incidences of 37% to 43% have been reported in patients who are Risser 0 and have open triradiate cartilages at the time of dorsal fusion.[60,61] A more accurate radiographic parameter for predicting the risk of the crankshaft phenomenon after dorsal surgery may be the assessment of peak height velocity. Saunders et al. reported a high incidence (8/8) of crankshaft phenomenon in patients fused before reaching peak height velocity, and a low incidence (2/15) in patients fused after reaching peak height velocity.[62] The risk of crankshaft phenomenon causing progressive deformity in children may be limited in the setting of contemporary rigid segmental instrumentation systems. Burton et al. reported only one case of progressive deformity after dorsal-only surgery in a cohort of skeletally immature patients, suggesting that ventral surgery may be unnecessary to prevent crankshaft deformity.[63]

Late decompensation of the unfused segments of the spine in patients undergoing selective thoracic or lumbar fusions for deformity is another important cause of postoperative deformity. It may lead to deformity in the sagittal or coronal plane. Late decompensation of the unfused segments in the sagittal plane is commonly due to proximal junctional kyphosis, a cause of postoperative deformity that is addressed in the next section of this chapter. Late decompensation in the coronal plane most commonly is due to progression of scoliosis in the unfused region of the spine. The choice of fusion levels at the

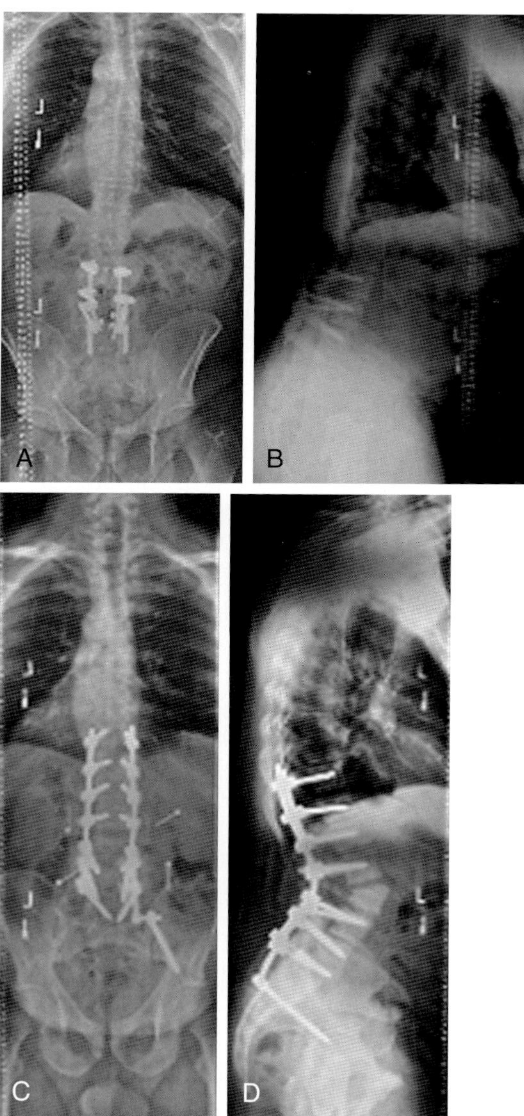

FIGURE 195-3. Preoperative anteroposterior (AP) (**A**) and lateral (**B**) radiographs showing deformity in a spine with degenerative pathology. Postoperative AP (**C**) and lateral (**D**) views after L3 pedicle subtraction osteotomy.

time of initial surgery, and the techniques of correction used in the initial surgery are important determinants of the rate of late coronal plane decompensation in spine surgery.

In the coronal plane, decompensation after surgical correction of deformity may occur due to either deformity progression in the mobile lumbar spine or the exclusion of a structural curve from the segments chosen for arthrodesis. The development of progressive lumbar deformity after selective thoracic fusion, or fusion to the mobile lumbar spine, is an important cause of postoperative degenerative changes, pain, and decompensation in the coronal plane.[64-66] Spontaneous correction of lumbar deformity may be reliably expected to occur in some cases of selective thoracic fusion with compensatory lumbar deformity.[67] However, Miller et. al demonstrated an incidence of coronal decompensation after selective thoracic fusion of nearly 17% at 2 years in patients with adolescent scoliosis.[68] Newton et al. demonstrated that factors determining the surgical choice to include a nonstructural lumbar curve in the fusion levels include the magnitude of the curve, the apical displacement, and the ratio of the size of the lumbar curve to the thoracic curve.[69] Late decompensation of the lumbar unfused segments may occur secondary to degenerative changes. Cochran et al. reported a high incidence of retrolisthesis, facet joint changes, and disc degeneration subjacent to the fused levels in patients fused below L3 with Harrington instrumentation.[70] Correction of thoracic deformity using derotation of the thoracic spine may increase rotation of the unfused lumbar segments.[64,65,71] The choice of an appropriate lower-end vertebra for deformity surgery is important in limiting the occurrence of early or late coronal decompensation in scoliosis surgery. Accurate and reproducible recognition of the stable, end, and neutral vertebrae is important in choosing a lowest instrumented segment. Similarly, recognizing whether a curve within a deformity is structural or nonstructural and classifying the type of curve are critical to surgical strategies in scoliosis surgery.[72]

The choice of fusion levels in the upper end of a spinal deformity construct may also have a significant impact upon coronal decompensation. Recognition and inclusion of a structural upper thoracic curve is important in the preoperative planning of the cephalad extent of spinal arthrodesis for deformity. Lenke et al. demonstrated that the failure to identify and include a structural upper thoracic curve may lead to shoulder asymmetry and postoperative coronal plane decompensation.[73] The authors recommend extending a dorsal fusion to the level of T2 when preoperative criteria are present, including a proximal thoracic curve measuring more than 30 degrees and correcting to more than 20 degrees on side-bending films, the presence of rotation or translation at the apex of the thoracic curve, and preoperative shoulder elevation on the concave side or T1 tilt toward the concave side. Subsequently, Kuklo et al. demonstrated that spontaneous curve correction of the unfused upper thoracic curve occurs more reliably after ventral fusion of the main thoracic curve than after dorsal fusion.[74] The authors identify T1 tilt toward the convexity of more than 5 degrees, shoulder asymmetry with elevation of the concave-sided shoulder, and bending correction to more than 25 degrees as factors that may predict postoperative shoulder asymmetry and coronal decompensation after selective thoracic ventral spine fusion. Overall, careful radiographic assessment of the thoracic spine is useful in predicting postoperative decompensation in the upper thoracic region.

Avoiding Postoperative Deformity Due to Late Decompensation

Pseudarthrosis and late decompensation of unfused segments of the spine are the two major causes of postoperative deformity due to late decompensation. Avoiding these complications is challenging, and a reasonable goal may be to minimize the rate of late decompensation rather than expecting to avoid it completely.

Regarding pseudarthrosis, the lumbosacral junction is especially susceptible due to strain on the S1 screws, especially in fusions above L2 to the sacrum.[75] Supplementing lumbosacral fixation with instrumentation to the pelvis is a useful technique for avoiding loss of fixation to the sacrum and progressive loss of sagittal or coronal balance.[76-78] Circumferential arthrodesis of the spine also may be useful in avoiding late revision surgery due to nonunion or progressive deformity.[79,80] The role of biologics and bone graft substitutes in reducing postoperative deformity due to pseudarthrosis remains to be demonstrated in a prospective clinical study.[43]

Avoiding late postoperative deformity in the coronal plane may be difficult, because progressive deformity of the unfused segments may be part of the natural history of spinal deformity rather than an avoidable complication. Accurate identification of structural and nonstructural deformity in the lumbar spine is important in determining when the lumbar curve may correct spontaneously after a selective thoracic fusion, and when the lumbar curve is likely to progress. Lenke et al. demonstrated that in King II deformity, spontaneous correction of the lumbar curve was predictable after selective thoracic fusion using either a ventral or a dorsal approach, with a ventral approach resulting in improved thoracic and lumbar curve correction.[67] Behensky et. al demonstrated that fixed apical vertebral rotation in Lenke 3C curve type is predictive of progressive deformity and spinal decompensation after surgery.[81] Differentiation between a King type II and type III or a Lenke 1 and Lenke 3 deformity is essential in determining the risk of decompensation through progressive deformity in the lumbar mobile segments. Overall, the maintenance of mobile segments in the lumbar spine remains an important goal of deformity correction surgery in both children and adults, and an accurate assessment of symptomatic changes of the lumbosacral spine and of the mobility of the lumbar compensatory curve is important in choosing to end a fusion in the mobile lumbar spine. Moderating surgical correction of the thoracic spine in patients with compensatory or structural lumbar deformity also may be useful for the avoidance of progressive lumbar deformity after selective thoracic fusion.[82]

Treatment of Postoperative Decompensation of the Spine

The treatment of symptomatic late postoperative deformity of the spine often is surgical. Operative management of postoperative deformity due to pseudarthrosis is challenging, and is characterized by high rates of failure and recurrent pseudarthrosis. In lumbar and lumbosacral pseudarthrosis, circumferential fusion with combined ventral and dorsal surgery is the most reliable technique for treating a symptomatic pseudarthrosis.[83] In the thoracic spine, progressive deformity due to pseudarthrosis may be treated effectively with dorsal-based osteotomies and dorsal-only fusion (see Case 4).[84] Biologics, including recombinant bone morphogenetic proteins, may have a role in improving union rates after revision surgery for pseudarthrosis, but in patients with deformity due to pseudarthrosis, realignment of the spine will still be required.

Patients with coronal decompensation of the spine due to progression of unfused regions of the spine may require revision surgery with extension of the fusion to include the region that was not fused originally (see Case 5). Bracing a compensatory curve after selection of a structural curve may be useful in preventing curve progression but will not be useful in treating symptomatic decompensation Arlet et. al described two cases in which they released the overcorrection of the main thoracic curve in patients with postoperative coronal plane decompensation and observed a spontaneous correction of the lumbar compensatory curve.[85] They proposed that the derotation of the main thoracic curve directly caused decompensation of the contralateral lumbar curve. Late symptomatic degeneration below a fusion to the mobile lumbar spine may require extension of fusion to the pelvis (see Case 6).

Case Examples: Scoliosis and Kyphosis

Case 4

A 14-year-old girl presented with adolescent idiopathic scoliosis and a Lenke 1CN deformity. Fusion was performed at levels from T3 to L1. The patient's lumbar deformity progressed over the 2 years following surgery, requiring extension of fusion to L4 (Fig. 195-4).

Case 5

A 26-year-old man presented with Scheuermann kyphosis. Dorsal spine fusion was attempted, with implant failure at the apex of the patient's kyphosis followed by removal of apical implants for prominence. Progressive deformity developed due to nonunion. The patient was treated with dorsal-only deformity correction with Smith-Petersen osteotomies across the apex of the deformity (Fig. 195-5).

Case 6

A 62-year-old woman had undergone prior spinal fusion to L5 15 years earlier. She presented with progressive kyphotic decompensation due to advanced degenerative changes at L5-S1. Revision surgery with a combined ventral and dorsal approach with extension of fusion to the pelvis resulted in improvement of her sagittal malalignment (Fig. 195-6).

Postoperative Deformity Due to Adjacent-Segment Pathology

Postoperative deformity due to sagittal decompensation adjacent to a fused section is an important pathology in both degenerative and deformity surgery. Adjacent-segment pathology encompasses degenerative changes adjacent to a fusion, including disc degeneration and stenosis, and deformity adjacent to a fusion, including spondylolisthesis and kyphosis. Adjacent-segment degeneration is defined radiographically, and there is significant variability in the criteria used to define the pathology.[86] Adjacent-segment disease is defined by the need for revision surgery due to adjacent-level pathology. There is significant variability in the indications for revision surgery among and between surgeons and patients, resulting in imprecise outcome measures. This section of the chapter focuses on adjacent-segment kyphosis, with or without spondylolisthesis.

Proximal junctional kyphosis is a postoperative deformity that is defined radiographically as segmental kyphosis of more than 5 degrees greater than the summed normal angular segments.[87] Postoperative proximal junctional kyphosis is common after long spinal fusions, and the rates of proximal junctional kyphosis have been reported variably in adolescents and adults. In adolescent patients with scoliosis, proximal junctional kyphosis has been reported in up to 46% of patients postoperatively.[88] In adult patients with long fusions, the postoperative prevalence of proximal junctional kyphosis was up to 39% of patients.[89,90] The association between

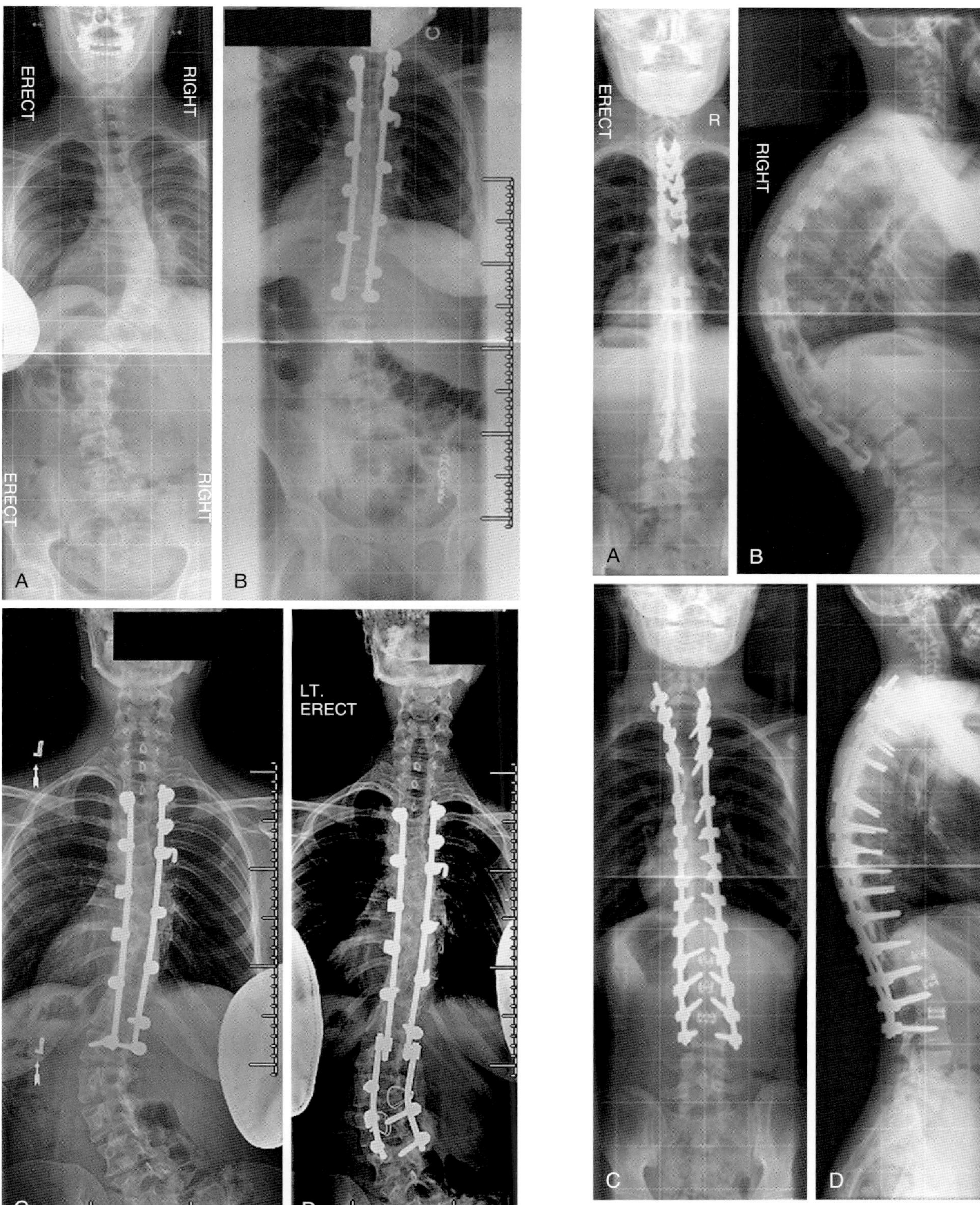

FIGURE 195-4. **A,** Preoperative posteroanterior view of a Lenke 1CN curve. **B,** Immediate postoperative lateral view. **C,** Radiograph shows progression of lumbar deformity. **D,** Extension of deformity to include lumbar curve, which has become structural.

FIGURE 195-5. **A** and **B,** Radiographs showing Scheuermann kyphosis with progression of deformity after limited correction. Postoperative anteroposterior (**C**) and lateral (**D**) radiographs after correction with Smith-Petersen osteotomies.

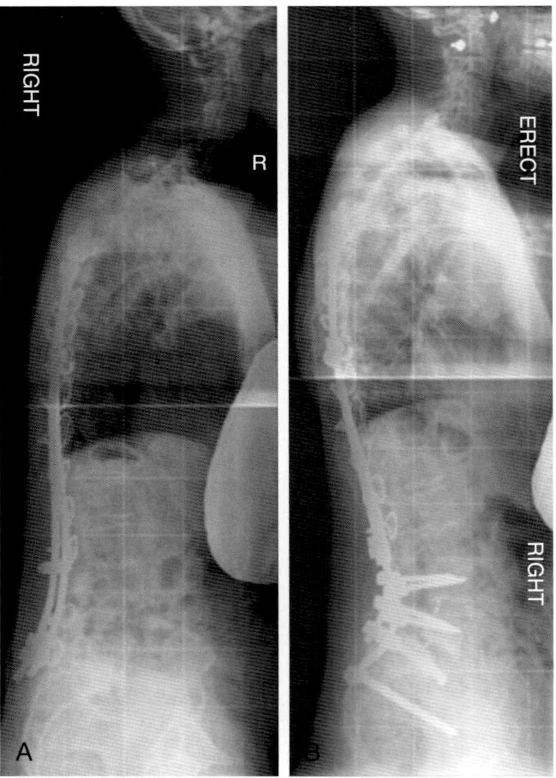

FIGURE 195-6. **A,** Long dorsal fusion to L5 in malalignment. **B,** Postoperative correction with ventral interbody grafts followed by dorsal Smith-Petersen osteotomies.

proximal junctional kyphosis and clinical symptoms has been variable, and Kim et al. reported that SRS outcome scores were not adversely affected by the presence of proximal junctional kyphosis radiographically.[90] However, proximal junctional kyphosis often is a clinically significant pathology. Mok and Pichelmann, in separate studies, both recognized proximal junctional kyphosis as an important cause of reoperation after surgery for spinal deformity.[5,8] Sagittal thoracic decompensation is a progressive kyphotic deformity of the thoracic spine that results in a global sagittal imbalance of more than 8 cm from C7 plumb relative to the dorsal aspect of the sacrum. Sagittal thoracic decompensation is associated with significant disability and poor outcomes.[91] Proximal junctional kyphosis and sagittal decompensation may be associated with significant pain, disability, and neural compromise.

The cause of proximal junctional kyphosis is not well defined. Lee et al. described sagittal decompensation in the thoracic spine in 11 of 23 cases (48%) after osteotomies for lumbar degenerative kyphosis.[92] The authors proposed that atrophy of the thoracic extensor muscles after surgery and postural habits may account for the predominance of thoracic decompensation. Yagi et al. proposed a classification of proximal junctional kyphosis into three types: ligamentous and disc failure, bone failure, and bone/implant interface failure.[93] The authors identified most cases in their series as ligamentous and disc failure with little clinical consequence. However, Watanabe et al. described two mechanisms for proximal junctional kyphosis: upper instrumented vertebra fracture with subluxation of the adjacent vertebra, and fracture above the instrumented vertebra.[94] Patients with fracture of the upper instrumented vertebra with subluxation of the adjacent vertebra presented early, on average within 3 months of surgery, and two of the five patients with fracture at the upper instrumented vertebra and subluxation presented with severe neural impairment. The authors identified marked correction of preoperative sagittal malalignment as a risk factor for upper instrumented vertebra fracture with adjacent vertebral subluxation. Lowe and Kasten confirm an increased risk of proximal junctional kyphosis with correction of kyphotic deformity greater than 50%.[95]

Avoiding Postoperative Adjacent-Segment Kyphosis

Surgical strategies to avoid proximal junctional kyphosis include preoperative planning and intraoperative techniques. The choice of an upper instrumented vertebra may be important in avoiding proximal junctional kyphosis. Lee et al. demonstrated that fusion and instrumentation ending below a segment with more than 5 degrees of kyphosis was a significant risk factor for the development of progressive adjacent-segment kyphosis.[92] There is no reliable difference in the occurrence of proximal junctional kyphosis in fusion to the structural thoracic spine (T9-10) compared with the mobile thoracolumbar junction (T11-12, L1- 2).[96]

Implant rigidity may have a role in the development of proximal junctional kyphosis. The pathology was relatively rare when less rigid implants were used, including Harrington instrumentation of the spine. The stress gradient between rigid internal fixation and the adjacent unfused and uninstrumented spine may be a risk factor for developing proximal junctional pathology.[97-100] The role of a more gradual transition in stiffness from the instrumented spine to the noninstrumented spine with dynamic implants or with implants of variable stiffness has not been defined.[101,102] Augmentation of the adjacent segments of the spine with ligamentoplasty to prevent dorsal ligamentous failure, or with cement augmentation to prevent fracture of the upper instrumented vertebra, or above the upper instrumented vertebra also may be useful strategies, but their effectiveness has not been well demonstrated in a prospective study.[103,104]

Treatment of Postoperative Adjacent-Segment Kyphosis

Proximal junctional kyphosis may be radiographically apparent with limited clinical impact. However, proximal sagittal decompensation, or fracture of an upper instrumented vertebra with adjacent subluxation, may be associated with significant disability and possible neural deterioration. Extension of fusion and instrumentation above the junctional kyphosis is the most reliable technique for correcting postoperative kyphotic deformity and for stabilizing the spine above an unstable subluxation (see Cases 7 and 8). The choice of proximal levels in revision surgery may help to avoid recurrence of junctional pathology, and principles including avoiding cantilever forces to gain large corrections and avoiding fusion below a kyphotic segment will be useful in revision surgery as well as primary approaches. In a series of 26 patients undergoing revision surgery for thoracic proximal junctional kyphosis and postoperative sagittal decompensation, significant improvement in sagittal alignment and in SRS-30 scores was obtained with dorsal-based osteotomy and extension of fusion and instrumentation to a proximal lordotic or neutral segment.[105]

Case Examples: Scoliosis and Kyphosis

Case 7

A 73-year-old woman presented with adult scoliosis. She was treated with a combined ventral and dorsal approach to the deformity. Three months after surgery she developed progressive sagittal plane decompensation due to fracture above the fusion. Revision surgery with dorsal Smith-Petersen osteotomies and extension of fixation to T3 resulted in improvement of deformity and clinical symptoms (Fig. 195-7).

Case 8

A 67-year-old woman presented with systemic lupus erythematosus and steroid-dependent osteoporosis. She complained of progressive thoracolumbar kyphosis and pain. She underwent a dorsal spine fusion from T3 to L4 with greater than 50% correction of thoracic kyphosis. Six weeks after surgery, she developed adjacent-segment kyphosis at T3-4 with fracture of the upper instrumented vertebra and subluxation of the adjacent segment. Revision surgery involved extension of fusion to T1 with hybrid fixation (Fig. 195-8).

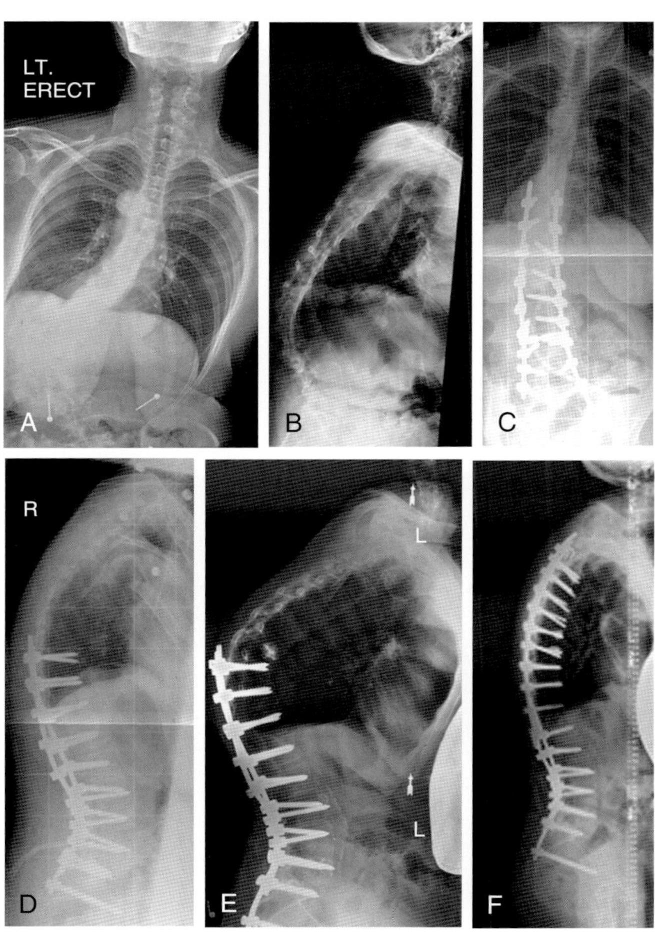

FIGURE 195-7. Preoperative anteroposterior (**A**) and lateral (**B**) radiographs of progressive adult deformity. **C** and **D,** Immediate postoperative standing radiographs demonstrating residual upper thoracic kyphosis. **E,** Progressive proximal junctional kyphosis despite augmentation of T9 above the upper instrumented vertebra. **F,** Realignment achieved with Smith-Petersen osteotomies across the thoracolumbar junction.

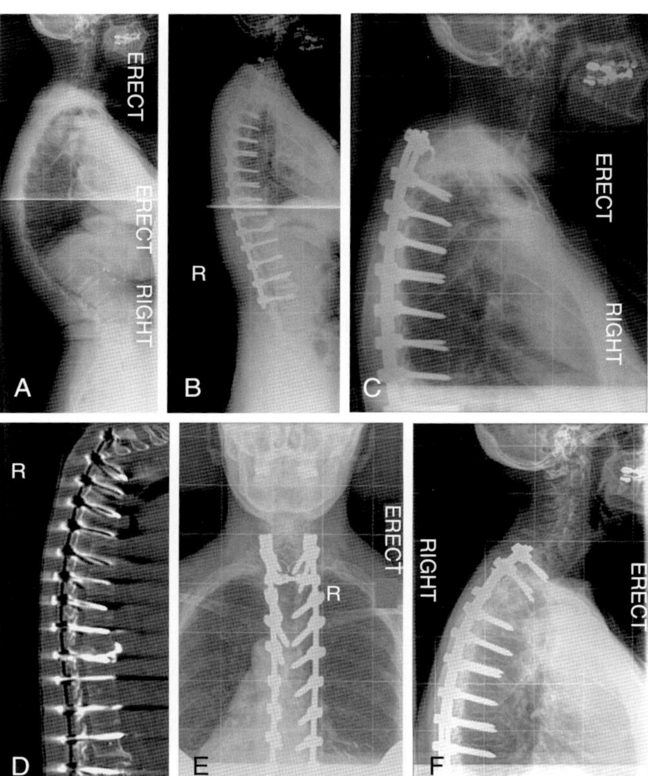

FIGURE 195-8. **A,** Preoperative lateral radiograph shows thoracic kyphosis. **B,** Postoperative lateral view at discharge (4 days) shows instrumentation from T2-L3. **C,** Proximal junctional kyphosis with fracture at T3 and hook pullout at T2. **D,** CT scan shows proximal junctional kyphosis. **E** and **F,** Revision with extension of instrumentation to T1.

Summary

Postoperative deformity is an important and significant sequela of surgery for spinal disorders including degenerative pathologies and deformity. Postoperative deformity includes malalignment of the spine at the time of initial surgery, and progressive deformity of the spine over time due to curve progression within the fused region of the spine or adjacent to the fused region. The occurrence and prevalence of postoperative deformity may be managed and minimized with strategies that include preoperative planning and choice of levels for instrumentation and fusion, with attention to sagittal and coronal alignment prior to surgery. Intraoperative strategies including optimizing patient position on the operating frame and modifying corrective forces to minimize adjacent-segment decompensation in the sagittal and coronal planes are useful to avoid postoperative deformity. Surgical techniques to achieve effective arthrodesis and minimize the risk of nonunion or implant migration will reduce the incidence of late deformity due to pseudarthrosis or subsidence of fixation. Prevention is the most valuable and cost-effective technique for avoiding clinical consequences of postoperative deformity, and the most effective way to avoid the need for revision surgery. However, in many cases, late decompensation and deformity progression may be unavoidable, and represent the natural history of disease progression. Ongoing and critical clinical and radiographic follow-up is most important for identifying postoperative deformity, and for guiding subsequent care.

KEY REFERENCES

Bridwell KH: Decision making regarding Smith-Petersen vs. pedicle subtraction osteotomy vs. vertebral column resection for spinal deformity. *Spine (Phila Pa 1976)* 31(Suppl 19):S171–S178, 2006.

Glassman SD, Bridwell K, Dimar JR, et al: The impact of positive sagittal balance in adult spinal deformity. *Spine (Phila Pa 1976)* 30(18): 2024–2029, 2005.

Kim YJ, Bridwell KH, Lenke LG, et al: Sagittal thoracic decompensation following long adult lumbar spinal instrumentation and fusion to L5 or S1: causes, prevalence, and risk factor analysis. *Spine (Phila Pa 1976)* 31(20):2359–2366, 2006.

Luhmann SJ, Lenke LG, Bridwell KH, Schootman M: Revision surgery after primary spine fusion for idiopathic scoliosis. *Spine (Phila Pa 1976)* 34(20):2191–2197, 2009.

Mok JM, Cloyd JM, Bradford DS, et al: Reoperation after primary fusion for adult spinal deformity: rate, reason, and timing. *Spine (Phila Pa 1976)* 34(8):832–839, 2009.

Park P, Garton HJ, Gala VC, et al: Adjacent segment disease after lumbar or lumbosacral fusion: review of the literature. *Spine (Phila Pa 1976)* 29(17):1938–1944, 2004.

REFERENCES

The complete reference list is available online at expertconsult.com.

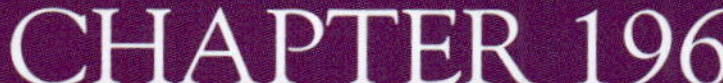

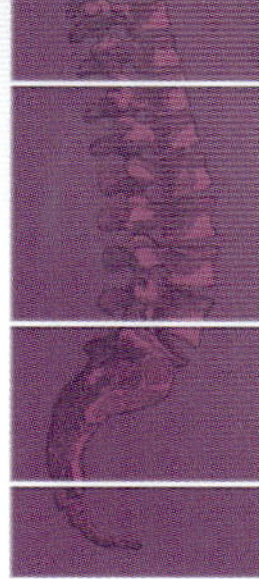

CHAPTER 196

Arachnoiditis

Robert F. Heary | Antonios Mammis

Spinal arachnoiditis is a nonspecific inflammatory process of the arachnoid layer of the spinal cord or cauda equina. Arachnoiditis was first described by Victor Horsley in 1909.[1] Since Horsley, numerous authors have described this condition with a variety of terms, including chronic spinal arachnoiditis, adhesive spinal arachnoiditis, meningitis serosa circumscripta spinalis, chronic spinal meningitis, spinal meningitides with radiculomyelopathy, lumbar adhesive arachnoiditis, spinal arachnoiditis, spinal fibrosis, and lumbosacral adhesive arachnoiditis. Furthermore, on the basis of the specific radiographic or pathologic findings, arachnoiditis can be termed arachnoiditis ossificans, calcific arachnoiditis, or pachymeningitis.[1]

Anatomy

The arachnoid mater is an avascular membrane that lies between two vascularized membranes: the pia mater and the dura mater. The arachnoid is attached to the underlying pia by numerous arachnoid trabeculae, which create a space between the arachnoid and the pia.[2] This space, or potential space in some instances, transmits arterioles and is referred to as the subarachnoid space. The arachnoid is composed of layers of squamous cells held together by a network of connective tissue. The arachnoid contains intercellular pores that allow for the passage of molecules.[3]

Pathogenesis

A chronic infection or irritation can cause the arachnoid membrane to become thickened and adherent to both the overlying dura mater and the subjacent pia mater.[4] The pia-arachnoid carries the blood vessels to the spinal cord, and this layer contains mesenchymal cells. In 1951, Smolik and Nash recognized that when the outer arachnoid layer is injured, both the blood vessels and mesenchymal cells lend themselves to extensive proliferation. The ensuing reaction between the pia-arachnoid and the dura mater leads to obliterative arachnoiditis.[5]

When the arachnoid membrane is exposed to an insult, an inflammatory response ensues, which is characterized by fibrinous exudates, neovascularization, and a relative paucity of inflammatory cellular exudates.[6,7] Vascular occlusive changes can occur, which can lead to spinal cord ischemia.[4,8-11] The small perforating blood vessels that supply the portions of the white matter may be obliterated, with resultant necrosis and cavitation of the spinal cord parenchyma.[8,9,11] In addition to ischemia, blockage of venous return from the spinal cord or occlusion of cerebrospinal fluid (CSF) pathways may occur.[8]

Burton described the stages of progressive inflammation of the arachnoid that occur in lumbosacral arachnoiditis. The initial stage, radiculitis, consists of an inflamed pia-arachnoid with associated hyperemia and swelling of the nerve roots. The second stage, arachnoiditis, is characterized by fibroblast proliferation and collagen deposition. During this stage, nerve root swelling decreases, and the nerve roots adhere to each other and to the pia-arachnoid. The final stage, adhesive arachnoiditis, is the resolution of the inflammatory process and is characterized by dense collagen deposition. There is marked proliferation of the pia-arachnoid as well as complete nerve root encapsulation, hypoxemia, and progressive atrophy.[12] For reasons that are not fully understood, the adhesions occur preferentially on the dorsal segments.[1] The exact time course of these three phases has not been elucidated. Furthermore, it is not known how the specific causative insult for the development of arachnoiditis might affect the time course of each of the three phases.

Yamagami et al. postulated that the pathologic changes in arachnoiditis may be secondary to diminished nutritional supply. They found that in an experimental rat model, the development of arachnoiditis and neural degeneration directly corresponded to the magnitude of extradural inflammation and wound-healing processes that occurred after laminectomy, with or without foreign bodies. Furthermore, adhesions of the arachnoid cause the nerve roots to lump together, and in the process, these nerve roots are isolated from contact with the CSF, with resultant nutritional compromise.[13]

Etiology

In the first half of the 20th century, arachnoiditis was most often attributed to infectious causes.[8] Furthermore, arachnoiditis had been described mainly in the cervical and thoracic regions.[1] Since the 1950s, there has been a trend toward a higher incidence of arachnoiditis of noninfectious origin affecting the lumbar region.[1,8] The precise causes of spinal arachnoiditis are not clear; likewise, the incidence and

TABLE 196-1

Causes of Spinal Arachnoiditis

Infectious	Noninfectious
Tuberculosis Bacterial infections Syphilis Parasitic diseases Viral meningitis	Trauma Postsurgery Myelographic contrast media (oil-based > water-soluble; water-soluble ionic > water-soluble nonionic) Intrathecal medications Steroids Anesthesia Epidural injections Neoplasms Arthritis (especially ankylosing spondylitis) Spinal stenosis Herniated intervertebral disc Intrathecal hemorrhage Foreign materials

prevalence of spinal arachnoiditis in the general population are unknown[8] (Table 196-1).

As was stated previously, arachnoiditis was mainly of infectious origin in the first half of the 20th century. Syphilis, tuberculosis, and gonorrhea were the most prevalent causes.[1,14] Less common infectious causes include parasitic diseases and viral meningitis.[15,16] These infectious causes are important to differentiate from noninfectious causes of arachnoiditis because, in most cases, effective treatment is available for arachnoiditis of infectious origin. However, despite adequate treatment of the causative agent, scarring of the arachnoid membrane may lead to permanent damage.

Arachnoiditis has a number of important noninfectious etiologies. In the 1940s, blood in the CSF following subarachnoid hemorrhage or surgery became the most prevalent cause of arachnoiditis.[1] Spinal arachnoiditis following subarachnoid hemorrhage continues to be common and is usually treated in a conservative fashion.[17] The breakdown products of hemoglobin form free radicals, and it has been postulated that these cause damage to nerves.[18,19] In experiments on dogs, it has been shown that injecting blood breakdown products into the subarachnoid space causes more meningeal inflammation than does the injection of fresh blood.[18] Cases of patients who have received epidural blood patches have given controversial results. Digiovanni et al. described that the placement of an autologous blood patch into the epidural space produced no more inflammation than a standard lumbar puncture.[20] Other authors, though, have described cases in which an epidural blood patch had allegedly been responsible for arachnoiditis.[21] Abouleish et al. described 118 cases of epidural blood patches over a 2-year period. This group found 19 cases of axial back pain, 2 cases of radiculopathy, and no cases of arachnoiditis.[22]

Oil-based contrast media have been an historically important cause of arachnoiditis. Iophendylate (Myodil, Pantopaque) is an oil-based contrast medium used in diagnostic myelograms. It was first used in the United States in 1944, and its usage continued for 40 years. In Sweden, iophendylate was banned from clinical use in 1948 because of animal studies that identified it as a causative agent for arachnoiditis.[23] The incidence of arachnoiditis after the use of iophendylate is dose dependent and is quoted as 1%.[24] Iophendylate has a very long half–life, so it is usually removed from the thecal space by aspiration at the conclusion of the myelogram.[8] Often, this removal process is not entirely successful; in fact, incomplete removal of the contrast dye may produce further trauma and cause bleeding into the CSF.[25]

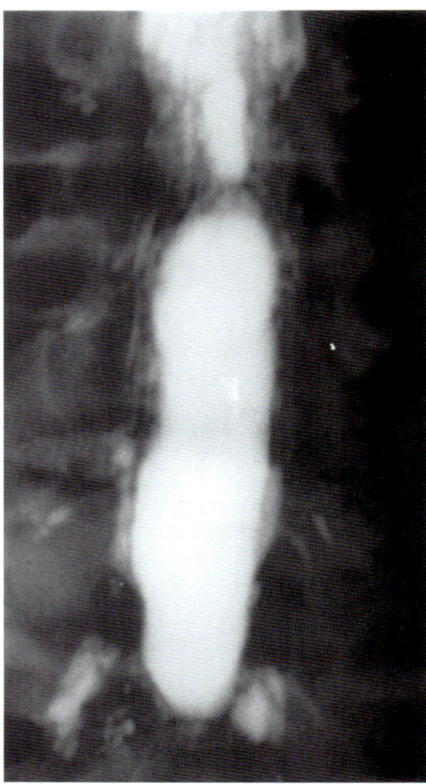

FIGURE 196-1. Myelogram (anteroposterior view, oil-based contrast medium [Pantopaque]) of severe adhesive arachnoiditis. This myelogram demonstrates marked lack of filling of the nerve roots throughout the lumbar spine with blunting of the thecal sac.

Guyer et al. listed the following factors as influencing the development of arachnoiditis after myelography: the type of contrast agent used (the risk is greater with oil-based than with water-soluble media and greater with ionic than with nonionic media), the dosage of contrast medium, and the observation time after myelography[25] (Fig. 196-1).

The use of intrathecal medications, either steroids or anesthetic agents, has been implicated as a cause of arachnoiditis. Intrathecal injection of corticosteroids was previously used for multiple sclerosis.[8] Epidural injection of corticosteroids for back pain is a common practice. One of the most commonly used agents is methylprednisolone acetate (MPA), which has been reported to cause arachnoiditis.[26-28] MPA is suspended in polyethylene glycol, which can cause arachnoiditis.[26-28] Furthermore, MPA is known to easily cross the intrathecal space, thus causing arachnoiditis.[28] However, animal studies have not shown MPA to cause significant meningeal inflammation after epidural injections.[29-31]

The use of intrathecal bupivacaine, with or without epinephrine, has also been reported to cause arachnoiditis.

Boiardi et al. described several cases of arachnoiditis after administration of bupivacaine with epinephrine.[32] Gemma et al. described a case of arachnoiditis after intrathecal administration of bupivacaine without epinephrine.[33] It is unclear in these cases whether the arachnoiditis was triggered by the bupivacaine or other preservatives. Furthermore, it is unclear whether epinephrine plays a role in the pathogenesis of arachnoiditis.

A history of spine surgery is a risk factor for arachnoiditis.[8] In particular, some investigators have specifically stated that surgery for a herniated intervertebral disc may lead to arachnoiditis.[5,7,25] Carroll and Wiesel showed that a postoperative pain-free interval lasting between 1 and 6 months, followed by the gradual onset of leg pain, increases the likelihood that some scar tissue is responsible for the symptoms.[34] Smolik and Nash showed that simple dural retraction for the visualization of a ruptured intervertebral disc may trigger arachnoiditis.[5] Haughton et al. showed that in monkeys, the nucleus pulposus of an intervertebral disc was able to cause focal arachnoiditis.[35]

Clinical Features

The diagnosis of arachnoiditis requires a detailed medical history and physical examination as well as a review of confirmatory radiographic imaging studies. In obtaining a medical history from a patient with arachnoiditis, the clinician should seek three major characteristics of the pain. Pain of arachnoiditis is typically described as a burning pain that is constant and worsened by activity.[12] The pain of arachnoiditis may be located in the back, the lower limbs, or both. The symptoms of arachnoiditis can vary from nonspecific back pain to radiculopathy and myelopathy.[36] Intractable pain that occurs secondary to arachnoiditis has a diffuse, poorly localized pain pattern. In many patients, arachnoiditis is asymptomatic and is discovered as an incidental radiographic finding.[37] The pain symptoms of chronic arachnoiditis may be similar to those of other chronic pain syndromes, such as complex regional pain syndrome. The exact relationship of these pain syndromes has not been fully elucidated.

The physical examination findings in patients with arachnoiditis have been reviewed in two large clinical series. Burton followed 100 patients with arachnoiditis and found little motor weakness to be present. These patients were commonly found to have a positive straight-leg raise sign, a tender sciatic notch, limited range of motion of the trunk, and paravertebral muscle spasms.[12] Guyer et al. followed 51 patients over more than 10 years and found that a decreased range of motion of the trunk was the most common finding on physical examination.[25] In cases of chronic arachnoiditis with resultant syrinx formation, physical examination findings of syringomyelia are present. These include dissociative sensory loss and variable long tract signs.[8]

Radiographic Features

After a history and physical examination, radiographic imaging studies are used to confirm the clinical impression of arachnoiditis. Plain radiographs are not a useful diagnostic tool for detecting or confirming the presence of arachnoiditis.

On myelography, two distinct patterns of radiographic arachnoiditis can be differentiated. In type I arachnoiditis, there is pure adhesion of the nerve roots to the meninges with a homogeneous contrast pattern. No nerve root shadows are seen, and there is a rounded shortening of the nerve root pocket. In type II arachnoiditis, some proliferation is added inside the dural sac that may be localized or diffuse.[38] The filling defects, narrowing, shortening, or occlusion of the spinal canal are also seen in this type of arachnoiditis. In early arachnoiditis, there is central nerve root clumping and thickening. As the arachnoiditis progresses, the nerve roots become adherent peripherally to the thecal sac and the terminal thecal sac appears "sleeveless," when the nerve roots do not fill it out in the normal pattern.[8] This finding can cause the thecal sac to appear empty.

On MRI, one of three patterns is commonly found.[39] The first pattern is characterized by conglomerations of nerve roots, which are located centrally within the thecal sac. The second pattern is characterized by nerve roots that are clumped and attached peripherally to the meninges (Fig. 196-2). This appearance is similar to the empty sac appearance of myelography. The third pattern demonstrates increased soft tissue signal within the thecal sac with central obliteration of the subarachnoid space (Fig. 196-3).

There are times when CT or MRI reveals calcification or ossification of the spinal arachnoid in an entity called arachnoiditis ossificans. There are several subtypes of spinal arachnoiditis ossificans based on imaging characteristics. Type I has a semicircular arrangement, type II is circular, and type III demonstrates englobing of the caudal fibers.[40-42]

Spinal Epidural Fibrosis

Spinal epidural fibrosis is an entity observed after spine surgery that contributes to up to 14% of cases of failed back syndrome. Spinal epidural fibrosis is caused when fibroblasts from damaged paraspinal muscles enter the vertebral canal and proliferate, forming extensive epidural scarring.[43] This entity has been most typically described after cases of discectomy, whether open or percutaneous, as well as cases of implantation of spine-stimulating electrodes.[43,44]

Treatment

There are a number of therapies aimed at preventing or treating arachnoiditis or epidural fibrosis. Much of the research aimed at preventing failed back syndrome has dealt with strategies to prevent epidural fibrosis.

In a rat model of spinal epidural fibrosis, the administration of tissue plasminogen activator helped to prevent postlaminectomy epidural fibrosis. The presence of arachnoiditis was also less in the treatment group (P = .01).[45] Lee et al. showed that in a rat model, the administration of 0.1 mg/mL of mitomycin C reduced epidural fibrosis after lumbar laminectomy. This group made macroscopic, histologic, and MRI evaluations of the animals.[46] Epidural scarring was significantly reduced and dural adhesions were absent, while wound healing was not affected.

In a dog postlaminectomy model, it has been shown that a single fraction of 700-cGy external-beam radiation helped to

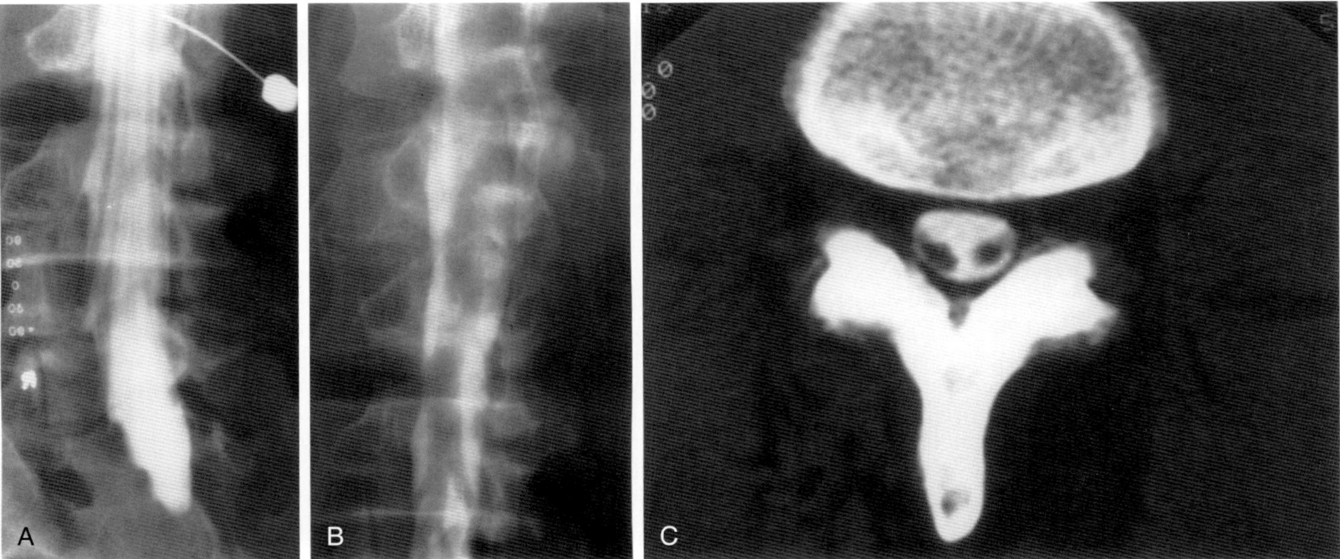

FIGURE 196-2. **A,** Myelogram (oblique view, water-soluble contrast medium [metrizamide (Amipaque)]) demonstrates normal nerve root filling throughout the cauda equina region. **B,** Myelogram (oblique view, water-soluble contrast medium [iohexol (Omnipaque)]) of the same patient 7 years later. Clear evidence of arachnoiditis is shown by the thickened, "clumped" nerve roots that no longer show the normal filling of the nerve root sleeves. **C,** CT scan after water-soluble myelogram demonstrates the clumping of nerve roots in the thecal sac. This study was performed in the same patient immediately after the myelogram in **B**.

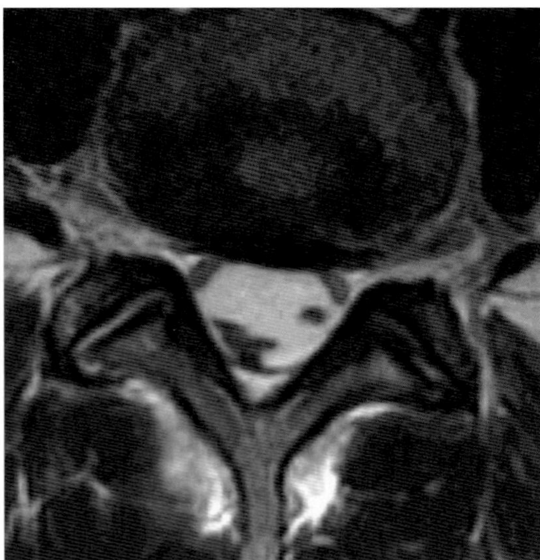

FIGURE 196-3. T2-weighted MRI demonstrates peripheral location of nerve roots in a patient with arachnoiditis. No nerve roots are seen in the central region of the thecal sac. This MRI scan is the correlate to the classic empty sac appearance seen on standard myelography.

prevent epidural fibrosis as well as arachnoiditis. The authors demonstrated statistically significant reductions in the extent of fibrosis and density of fibroblasts. MRI confirmation of the efficaciousness of the therapy was also demonstrated.[47]

A recent study, in humans, aimed to evaluate the role of epidural steroids in preventing epidural fibrosis. Eighty-five of 178 patients received epidural steroids following discectomy. Patients were followed for 1 year and were assessed by questionnaire containing the pain scale. Application of epidural steroids resulted in less pain on the first and third days after surgery and resulted in shorter hospital stays but did not prevent failed back syndrome or prevent epidural scar formation.[48]

The role of surgery in the treatment of arachnoiditis and epidural fibrosis is controversial. Surgical procedures that have been used to treat arachnoiditis include spine fusion procedures, decompressive spine procedures without fusion, neuroablative procedures, and implantation of spinal cord stimulators.[8]

A substantial body of literature exists that suggests that open surgical procedures are not useful in the treatment of arachnoiditis. Carroll and Wiesel found that no open surgical technique could eliminate the pathologic scar or significantly reduce the pain of arachnoiditis.[34] Grahame et al. also found that open surgical procedures had little or no effect on the long-term course of arachnoiditis.[37]

Some groups argue for aggressive open surgical intervention for arachnoiditis and spinal epidural fibrosis. Shikata et al. compared microlysis for arachnoiditis with and without spine fusion.[49] They found significant improvement in the clinical results when fusion was performed.

Spinal cord stimulation has been shown to have some benefit in patients with arachnoiditis. North et al. have shown that with proper patient selection, spinal cord stimulation can be a successful therapy. North et al. used temporary percutaneous electrodes as a screening technique before implantation of a permanent stimulator. A minimum of 50% pain relief with temporary electrodes over a 2- to 3-day course, as well as evidence of improved activity level and stable or decreased use of analgesics, was deemed satisfactory pain relief.[50-54]

Recent work has focused on minimally invasive techniques to treat arachnoiditis and spinal epidural fibrosis. A number of endoscopic techniques for adhesiolysis and promotion of CSF flow pathways have been developed, with promising results.[55,56] Manchikanti et al. demonstrated, in a recent randomized controlled trial of spinal endoscopic adhesiolysis in chronic, refractory, low back pain and lower-extremity pain, that adhesiolysis with targeted delivery of local anesthesia and steroids is a successful technique in the treatment of arachnoiditis. This study demonstrated significant improvement in pain in 48% of subjects at 1 year follow-up.[57]

Summary

Arachnoiditis and epidural fibrosis are chronic conditions that result in significant morbidity. The long-term prognosis of these conditions is poor, and there is no optimal management strategy that has been proven or widely accepted. Prevention of these conditions is ideal and is achieved by avoiding agents that have been shown to lead to fibrosis as well as by handling neural elements with care at surgery. In recent years, there has been a renewed interest in the management of arachnoiditis and spinal epidural fibrosis. and we have seen a number of promising experimental therapies. Pharmacologic therapy has shifted toward prevention, and surgical therapy has shifted toward minimally invasive techniques. Although some surgeons advocate open surgical treatments to attempt to treat the cause of pain, we have found the best treatment results, as a whole, with the utilization of dorsal column stimulation to treat the effects of pain. Alternative treatments of the effects, including long-term use of narcotic medications, have been less effective in our hands. As these therapies and techniques are developed, there will be a need for more randomized, prospective, placebo-controlled, double-blind studies to determine the optimal methods for preventing and managing these devastating problems.

KEY REFERENCES

Burton CV: Lumbosacral arachnoiditis. *Spine (Phila Pa 1976)* 3(1):24–30, 1978.

Delamarter RB, Ross JS, Masaryk TJ, et al: Diagnosis of lumbar arachnoiditis by magnetic resonance imaging. *Spine (Phila Pa 1976)* 5(4):304–310, 1990.

Manchikanti L, Boswell MV, Rivera JJ, et al: A randomized, controlled trial of spinal endoscopic adhesiolysis in chronic refractory low back and lower extremity pain. *BMC Anesthesiol* 5:10, 2005.

North RB, Kidd DH, Piantadosi S: Spinal cord stimulation versus reoperation for failed back surgery syndrome: a prospective, randomized study design. *Acta Neurochir Suppl* 64:106–108, 1995.

Smolik EA, Nash FP: Lumbar spinal arachnoiditis: a complication of the intervertebral disc operation. *Ann Surg* 133(4):490–495, 1951.

REFERENCES

The complete reference list is available online at expertconsult.com.

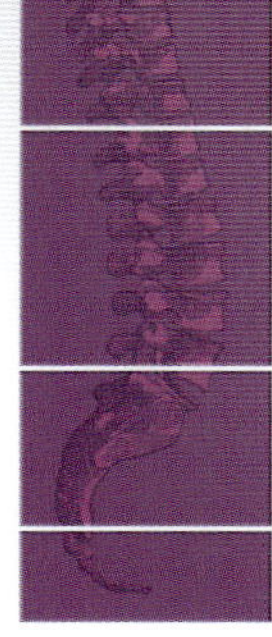

CHAPTER 197

Spine Infection

Kyle I. Swanson | Kene Ugokwe | Seth M. Zeidman | Thomas B. Ducker | Gregory R. Trost

Postoperative Spine Infection

Infectious complications of spine surgery are not uncommon and occur in 0.5% to 12% of patients.[1-9] Infections can range from limited superficial wound infections or isolated discitis to more serious deep subfascial wound infections, osteomyelitis, epidural abscess, or meningitis. Postoperative infection results in an increase in health-care costs and increases the risk of poor outcomes, including persistent pain, permanent neurologic deficit, and death.[1-11] Some of the risk factors associated with surgical site infections include patient age,[12,13] obesity,[9,14-18] diabetes,[18-20] urinary incontinence,[9] alcoholism, extended steroid use, tobacco use,[18] poor nutritional status,[12] prior infection, prior surgery, prolonged hospitalization prior to surgery,[18] complete neurologic deficit,[21,22] trauma,[23] tumor resection,[9] prior radiation therapy,[24] and the presence of more than three comorbid diseases.[9]

The rate of postoperative infection is in large part determined by the type of operation. Surgeries without bone grafting or instrumentation have a lower rate of infection. The incidence of infection after intervertebral disc procedures is between 0.5% and 1%.[25,26] There is uncertainty whether microdiscectomy with the use of an operative microscope increases the infection rate.[27] The rate of infection with laminectomy without fusion is estimated to be around 1.5% to 2%.[16,26] The incidence of infection is higher when grafting and instrumentation are used,[28] which was first documented in a case series involving the use of Harrington instrumentation for fusion in scoliosis surgery.[5] The increased risk has many components, including addition of a foreign body; lengthier, more complicated surgeries; increased blood loss; and the use of prolonged retraction. Instrumented fusion of the lumbar spine carries an infection risk of approximately 2.8% to 6%.[16,18,26,29] Surgery after spine trauma carries a 10% risk of postoperative infection.[23]

Ventral operations have a markedly lower incidence of infection than dorsal approaches, likely due in part to the injury caused by the use of prolonged retraction in dorsal approaches. The addition of a combined anterior and dorsal approach does not seem to increase the risk of infection over that for a dorsal approach alone.[23,30] Other surgical factors that have been shown to increase the risk of postoperative infection include increased blood loss (>1 L),[18] use of blood transfusion,[19] prolonged surgical time (>3 hours),[31] multilevel surgical fusions extending to the sacrum,[32] and spinal fluid leak.[18] The use of drains has not been shown to increase the risk of infection.[33] Participation of residents or fellows in the surgical team is not associated with an increased risk of infection.[34]

The optimal method of dealing with surgical site infections is prevention. Prophylactic antibiotics have been shown convincingly to decrease the rate of postoperative infection, and their use is recommended by published clinical guidelines for all spine operations.[35,36] A large meta-analysis found a statistically significant decrease in the rate of postoperative spine infection in those patients given preoperative antibiotics versus controls (2.2% vs. 5.9%).[37] Prophylactic antibiotics should be given prior to the start of incision, should be redosed for prolonged procedures, and should not be continued for more than 24 hours. First- or second-generation cephalosporins, such as cefazolin or cefuroxime, adequately cover the most common causes of surgical site infection and are recommended for most patients. Patients with cephalosporin allergies can be given vancomycin or clindamycin. Vancomycin should be used for patients colonized with methicillin-resistant *Staphylococcus aureus* (MRSA).[29,35]

One large prospective case-controlled study found that the rate of discitis after microdiscectomy was significantly decreased when a gentamicin-soaked collagen sponge was placed in the cleared disc space versus the rate for historical controls (0% vs. 3.7%).[38] The benefit of prophylactic local antibiotics for discectomy procedures is in part due to the poor penetration of IV antibiotics into the relatively avascular intervertebral disc.[39] The use of irrigation solution with antibiotics such as bacitracin and gentamycin, or dilute iodine, is widespread, but there is not good evidence demonstrating additional benefit over irrigation with just saline.[35,40] Use of chlorhexidine-alcohol instead of povidone-iodine for preoperative skin cleansing has been shown to decrease surgical site infections in randomized controlled trials.[41] In a Cochrane review, alcohol-based rubs were found to be equivalent to aqueous chlorhexidine-based scrubs for preoperative hand antisepsis, with aqueous povidone-iodine–based scrubs being inferior.[42] Operating rooms with vertical laminar airflow have been demonstrated to decrease infections in dorsal spine fusion surgery.[43] Double-gloving; frequent release of retractors to prevent ischemia; and copious, frequent irrigation are reasonable, though unproven, strategies for also minimizing postoperative infection.[29,44]

Postoperative wound infections can be classified as early onset (occurring <1 month after surgery) or late onset (occurring >1 month after surgery). Late-onset infections include isolated discitis and infections of instrumented fusions by indolent organisms. *Staphylococcus aureus* is responsible for approximately 50% to 75% of infections, followed by *S. epidermidis*, gram-negative organisms, and multimicrobrial infections.[16,26] Late-onset infections associated with instrumentation are more likely to be caused by more fastidious organisms such as *S. epidermidis*, *Priopionibacterium acnes*, or *Corynebacterium*.[44,45]

One of the chief symptoms of a surgical site infection is pain, which is often initially attributed to the surgery itself. Pain that continues to worsen days after the surgery or returns after initial relief of symptoms should raise suspicion for infection. Patients with an infection frequently, but certainly not always, have fever. A careful evaluation of other causes of fever should be undertaken, including a chest radiograph to evaluate for pneumonia or atelectasis, urinalysis to check for urinary tract infection, and possibly a lower extremity Doppler ultrasound to rule out deep vein thrombosis. The possibility of drug fever should also be explored. Other constitutional signs of infection include chills, sweating, malaise, and anorexia. Frank sepsis with hypotension and organ failure warrants emergent exploration if there is any concern for wound infection.

The most frequent sign of postoperative spine infection is wound drainage, which in one series was present in 93% of cases.[26] Often patients with infection are discharged home after an apparently normal recovery and return because of drainage and associated swelling, tenderness, erythema, and wound dehiscence. The average time of presentation for a postoperative spine infection is 2 weeks, though it can be days for aggressive organisms, such as *Clostridium perfringens*, or years for indolent infections.[26]

New or worsening neurologic deficits, such as numbness, urinary or bowel dysfunction, weakness, or paralysis, are ominous signs and should raise suspicion for epidural hematoma or abscess. Postoperative spinal epidural abscess is a neurosurgical emergency that can lead to rapid decline if not promptly diagnosed and treated with antibiotics and surgical drainage.[46]

Late-onset infections often provide fewer clinical signs or symptoms, with worsening pain generally being the only complaint. Discitis frequently manifests more than a month after discectomy as increasing pain in an afebrile patient with a normal-appearing incision. Symptoms of infection of the disc space can be misdiagnosed as recurrent disc herniation, or patients may be dismissed as hysterical or malingering. Worsening pain in a patient with a history of spine surgery should be evaluated for possible infection.

Laboratory studies are an important adjunct in diagnosing infection, especially when the wound site does not show obvious signs. Patients often demonstrate leukocytosis, with or without associated neutrophilia, but a large portion of cases will have a normal white blood cell count and differential. Erythrocyte sedimentation rate (ESR) and C-reactive protein (CRP) levels are much more sensitive, though nonspecific, markers of inflammation and are almost always significantly elevated with infection. Care must be taken in interpreting these levels since they are initially elevated after any surgery. In uninfected postoperative patients, CRP typically peaks on postoperative day 2 and returns to normal levels between days 5 and 14. ESR peaks around day 5 and can remain elevated for weeks after surgery.[47,48] ESR and CRP levels are particularly helpful in diagnosing late-onset infections in patients with minimal signs or symptoms besides worsening or persistent pain, such as postoperative discitis.

Blood cultures should be obtained in all patients in whom a surgical site infection is suspected. Cultures of the skin or drainage site are rarely helpful because they culture normal skin flora. Needle aspiration cultures are much more reliable, and intraoperative cultures are the best option. Since most patients will need surgical debridement, the best course of action is to wait for the results of intraoperative cultures before starting antibiotics. For late-onset infections, it is especially important to continue cultures for at least 7 to 15 days to increase the chance of growing indolent organisms such a *P. acnes*.[45] When surgery is not indicated, as in suspected isolated discitis, and blood cultures are negative, then a percutaneous biopsy should usually be obtained to confirm the diagnosis and guide treatment.

Plain radiography, CT, and MRI can be useful in diagnosing postoperative infection, but their utility is often clouded by the similarities in imaging findings between infection and normal postoperative inflammation. Radiographs can demonstrate retained foreign bodies, disc space narrowing that develops with discitis after 7 to 10 days, erosion of vertebral end plates, or vertebral collapse.[49] Loosening of implants can also be revealed, which is often a sign of late-onset infection.[50] CT reveals many of these same features but with superior anatomic detail.

Contrasted CT and MRI both have excellent sensitivity for identifying fluid collections, but it can sometimes be difficult to differentiate between abscess and postoperative seroma or hematoma. Either modality helps differentiate superficial from subfascial infections. Contrasted MRI is the best study for determining postoperative epidural abscess.[51] MRI with contrast is also the study of choice for diagnosing discitis and osteomyelitis. T1-weighted images reveal hypointensity of the disc and vertebral body. On T2-weighted images, the involved bone and disc are hyperintense due to edema and the involved disc demonstrates a loss of the intranuclear cleft.[52] Areas of inflammation enhance with contrast administration.[49] Unfortunately, many of the same MRI signal findings are seen with normal postoperative changes.[53] Radionuclide studies, such as gallium/bone (technetium) scintigraphy, can be useful when MRI is contraindicated or nondiagnostic due to artifact from implants.[49,54]

Treatment consists of targeted antibiotics and surgery in nearly all cases, though there are a few exceptions. There is a significant difference between the treatment of spine infections in the presence of grafting and instrumentation versus simple decompression procedures. The treatment is also different for early-onset infections versus that for late-onset infections in the setting of instrumentation. Some very superficial wound infections or stitch abscesses can be treated with empirical antibiotics alone, but there must be no evidence of deeper infection or significant systemic signs of infection. Ensuring adequate nutrition is vital for the successful treatment of all postoperative infections.[12,50]

Isolated postoperative discitis often presents later than other postsurgical infections with worsening back pain, elevated ESR/CRP, and characteristic findings on radiograph and MRI. Discitis can frequently be treated successfully with 4 to 6 weeks of IV antibiotics alone. This requires obtaining bacterial diagnosis via blood cultures or percutaneous biopsy. Spontaneous fusion across the disc space usually occurs after resolution of the infection. Many surgeons recommend bracing to minimize pain. Surgery for debridement of the disc space is indicated in the setting of new or worsening neurologic deficits, significant associated infection (especially epidural abscess), and progression of infection and bony involvement or worsening pain despite antibiotics.

Surgical debridement is warranted for most other surgeries that do not involve bone graft or instrumentation. This is especially true for subfascial infections. Exploring below the fascia is recommended for all but the most superficial of infections. All necrotic, infected, and foreign material, such as sutures, must be completely debrided. Cultures should be obtained and sent for Gram stain and aerobic, anaerobic, and fungal cultures. Once culture specimens have been sent, empirical broad-spectrum antibiotics, such as vancomycin and a third-generation cephalosporin, can be started. The wound should be copiously irrigated with large volumes, with many institutions using 9 L of bacitracin-containing irrigation.[26,50] Pulse-lavage irrigation may improve debridement.

Primary closure over a drain can frequently be used for more superficial infections; however, deeper infections should usually be left open to heal via secondary intention or with a delayed closure. Vacuum-assisted closure (VAC) dressings have been increasing in popularity and are purported to decrease nursing requirements and aid in healing, but no good trials have yet proved their benefit over traditional gauze packing.[55-57] Repeat debridement at 48 to 72 hours can be beneficial for treating septic or immunocompromised patients or in the setting of infections caused by multiple organisms or those associated with extensive myonecrosis.[26,29,50] Tailored IV antibiotics are continued for 4 to 6 weeks.

Infections after instrumented spine fusions require the same aggressive debridement and irrigation. For early infections, almost all published reports advocate leaving the spinal instrumentation and viable bone graft in place in order to maximize the chance of fusion.[1-3,24,26,29,30,32,50,58,59] Loose instrumentation and nonviable bone graft should be removed. Surgical wounds should usually be left open to heal by secondary intention or with delayed closure. Repeat irrigation and debridement is occasionally needed for reasons listed earlier. Levi et al. reported success using an irrigation-suction system for postoperative care.[30] IV antibiotics selected based on culture and sensitivies are continued for at least 6 weeks. In addition, Kowalski et al. found a significant decrease in the late recurrence of infection in patients treated with oral suppression therapy for at least 6 months after an initial course of IV antibiotics.[24]

Late infections after instrumented fusion are usually the result of more fastidious organisms that are capable of creating a glycocalyx covering on implanted hardware that is resistant to antibiotics and the normal immune response.[60] Surgical treatment involves debridement, irrigation, and removal of hardware.[24,60,61] Fortunately, in most cases bony fusion has already occurred, as assessed on CT or intraoperatively, and the hardware is no longer needed for stabilization. Patients with late infections who have implants left in place have a significantly higher risk of treatment failure.[24] Postoperatively, patients should be monitored closely for evidence of pseudarthosis or deformity that would warrant repeat instrumented fusion. After removal of hardware, debridement, and irrigation, the wound can typically be closed over a drain, and appropriate antibiotics are continued for 6 weeks,[24,61] although one group reported good outcomes with just 2 days of IV antibiotics followed by 7 days of oral antibiotics.[60]

Spontaneous Spinal Infections

Discitis

Pyogenic discitis is a bacterial infection of the intervertebral disc that is frequently associated with involvement of the adjacent vertebral end plates (spondylodiscitis). Incidence is estimated to be between 0.2 and 2.4/100,000 each year, with two peaks in age distribution: one in early childhood and another between ages 60 and 70 years.[62,63] The relatively high proportion of children with pyogenic discitis is likely related to the anatomy of the disc space during development. Children still have a vascular supply into the nucleus pulposus of the disc, which allows septic emboli to lodge with the disc. The vascular supply in adults only reaches the anulus fibrosus. In the adult population, more men are affected than women.[64] Risk factors for developing discitis include invasive procedures, diabetes (11–31%), malignancy, IV drug use (IVDU), immunosuppression, alcoholism, renal failure, and cirrhosis.[62,63,65]

The majority of cases are caused by *S. aureus*, with gram-negative rods, *Streptococcus*, and *Enterococcus* being the next most frequently involved organisms.[63,64] Gram-negative organisms are more common when associated with diabetes, immunocompromise, infections of the genitourinary or gastrointestinal tracts, or IVDU.[65] Tuberculosis (TB) and brucellosis are atypical bacterial infections that can cause discitis in endemic regions and in at-risk populations. Fungal discitis is rare but should be considered in patients who are critically ill, immunosuppressed, taking multiple antibiotics, or have an indwelling catheter.[66] The most frequent location is the lumbar spine (60%), followed by the thoracic (30%) spine and the cervical spine (10%).[62,64]

In 1936, Milward and Grout were the first to describe the clinical and radiographic characteristics of interspace infection after the inadvertent introduction of microorganisms into a disc space during a lumbar puncture.[67] More than 90% of patients complain of back or neck pain.[62] This pain often is not relieved by medications or recumbency. Radicular pain symptoms are not uncommon. Guarding against movement and a positive straight-leg raise may be present. Fever is present in approximately 60% to 70%.[63] Neurologic deficits, especially weakness, should raise concern for more a extensive infection such as an epidural abscess. In children, discitis often presents as a refusal to bear weight or walk.[68] The time from onset to diagnosis is often months. ESR and CRP are elevated in most patients, but leukocytosis is present in less than half of cases.[69]

The differential diagnosis for discitis includes other infections of the spine and adjacent structures, trauma, osteoporotic fracture, degenerative disc disease or acute herniation, metastatic disease, and inflammatory spondyloarthopathies. Discitis is often also associated with bacterial endocarditis (3.7–15%). Echocardiography is recommended for patients with spontaneous discitis. Back pain in the setting of endocarditis or bacteremia should lead to an evaluation for discitis.[70]

MRI with contrast is the image modality of choice for diagnosing spontaneous discitis, with a sensitivity and specificity greater than 90%. If an MRI is not possible, the next most sensitive studies are radioisotope scans followed by CT with contrast. Radiographs also show typical changes such as disc space narrowing and end-plate erosion, but these changes usually take several weeks to develop.[49] CT is particularly helpful for guiding percutaneous biopsy.

If possible, antibiotics should be held until cultures can be obtained. Blood cultures are positive in approximately half of discitis cases.[64] To maximize yield, three culture specimens taken at different times and locations should be obtained, ideally when the patient is febrile. If after 48 hours there is no growth, a CT-guided percutaneous biopsy should be obtained, which increases the yield to between 60% and 70%.[64] Samples should be taken from both adjacent vertebral end plates and the disc itself, and the disc space should be rinsed and aspirated. Biopsy samples are sent for histopathologic studies, aerobic, anaerobic, fungal, and mycobacterial cultures, and stains.[62] A second percutaneous biopsy has been shown to increase yield when the first biopsy is negative.[69] Occasionally open biopsy is required to obtain a diagnosis.

Approximately three-quarters of spontaneous pyogenic discitis cases can be treated nonoperatively with IV antibiotics tailored according to the results of the cultures and sensitivities.[62] There are no good studies comparing various antibiotic regimens, duration of antibiotic therapy, or the role of oral antibiotics after administration of IV antibiotics. Traditionally 4 to 6 weeks of IV antibiotics was recommended, but recent reports suggest there is a decreased risk of recurrence if antibiotics are used for 12 weeks, often with a switch to oral antibiotics after 6 weeks.[62,65] Spinal immobilization for pain control, using bracing or short-term bed rest, is recommended by most surgeons.

Response to therapy is demonstrated by diminishing pain, resolution of fever, and progressive decrease in CRP levels.[48] Radiographs should be obtained at regular intervals after initiation of treatment and should show sclerosis and osteophyte formation by 3 months if healing is occurring.[65] Patients generally progress to fusion over 6 to 12 months. Repeat MRI is generally not helpful and often initially appears worse than pretreatment scans.[71] MRI should usually be reserved for patients with new or worsening neurologic symptoms to rule out expanding abscess.

Surgery is reserved for patients with neurologic deficits, especially those with associated epidural abscess and spinal cord compression, for clinical failure after conservative treatment, for treatment of spinal instability or correction of deformities, for obtaining a diagnosis by open biopsy after failed percutaneous biopsy, and occasionally for persistent pain.[72]

Recurrence rates after a course of antibiotics are generally around 10% (0–16%).[62,69] Chronic pain is the most common residual complication. Functional impairment and neurologic deficits occur in a minority.[64] Mortality is generally low and usually related to associated sepsis, endocarditis, or underlying disease.[63,69]

Vertebral Osteomyelitis

Infection of the bones of the spinal column—vertebral osteomyelitis—can occur after trauma, as a result of direct manipulation during surgery, via contiguous spread from adjacent structures, or via hematogenous spread from distant sources.[73] Vertebral osteomyelitis is relatively rare, with an estimated incidence of 2.4/100,000 people. Older adults are more likely to be affected, with the incidence increasing from 0.3/100,000 for those younger than 20 years of age to 6.5/100,000 for those older than 70.[74] There is a male predominance that also increases with age.[74,75]

Patients with vertebral osteomyelitis usually have predisposing factors, with the most common being diabetes mellitus, end-stage renal disease requiring dialysis, sepsis, endocarditis, cancer, HIV infection, immunosuppression, alcoholism, and IVDU.[73,75,76] Urinary tract infections followed by skin infections were the most common sources of infection.[75]

A vast majority of cases of pyogenic spine osteomyelitis involve the vertebral body, with only 3% to 12% involving the dorsal elements of the spine.[77] Infection generally begins at the highly vascular end plates. Most cases involve two or more contiguous vertebral bodies and the intervening disc. Vertebral osteomyelitis occasionally manifests as the collapse of an isolated vertebral body. The lumbar spine is the most commonly involved (58%), followed by the thoracic spine (30%) and cervical spine (11%).[75] Associated epidural abscesses (17%), paravertebral abscesses (26%), and disc space abscesses (5%) are frequent.[73]

The most common causative organism is *S. aureus*. *Escherichia coli* is the most commonly reported gram-negative organism and is especially associated in cases when genitourinary or gastrointestinal infections are the source.[75] *S. aureus* is the most frequent organism in IV drug users, but they also have an increased frequency of *Pseudomonas aeruginosa*.[76] In many developing regions of the world TB is a frequent cause of chronic vertebral osteomyelitis.

There is often a substantial delay in the diagnosis of vertebral osteomyelitis due to the nonspecific nature of its presenting symptoms. In one large series the mean time to diagnosis was 1.8 months, with only a quarter of cases being diagnosed in less than a month. The same study revealed that on initial presentation only a quarter of the patients had vertebral osteomyelitis considered in the differential diagnosis. The majority of patients (86%) present with several weeks of worsening back or neck pain.[73] Fever has been reported in 35% to 60% of patients.[73,78] Neurologic deficits are present in approximately a third of cases, and only around one fifth of patients have localized tenderness.[78] Rapidly worsening neurologic deficits and paralysis should raise the concern for associated spinal epidural abscess. Acute worsening of pain is often associated with vertebral collapse. Back pain in the setting of bacteremia, such as with endocarditis, should always lead to an evaluation for vertebral osteomyelitis. The differential diagnosis for vertebral osteomyelitis includes other localized spine infections, osteoporotic or traumatic fractures, spondyloarthopathies, degenerative disc disease, herniated disc, metastasis, and infections such as pancreatitis and pyelonephritis.[79]

Leukocytosis is present in approximately two thirds of cases, and there is an associated neutrophilia in about a third of cases.[80] ESR and CRP measurements are much more sensitive to the presence of inflammation and are elevated in almost all cases of vertebral osteomyelitis.[48,80] Serial CRP is more accurate than ESR for gauging response to therapy.[48] Blood cultures should be obtained in all patients with suspected vertebral osteomyelitis because 58% (range, 30–78%) of cultures will be positive.[75] Identifying the organism via blood cultures often obviates the need for more invasive procedures.

MRI is the best imaging modality for evaluating for vertebral osteomyelitis, with a sensitivity of nearly 100% and accuracy over 90%.[81] Findings associated with osteomyelitis include a low intensity on T1-weighted images with loss of the usual hyperintense signal of fat in the bone marrow, hyperintensity on T2-weighted images in the bone or adjacent disc and soft tissues indicative of edema, and enhancement with contrast of the end plates and associated abscesses. There is usually a loss of the intranuclear cleft of involved discs. End-plate destruction is a late finding.[81]

Radiographs and CT are beneficial in the delineation of bony destruction. Radiographs often reveal narrowing of intervertebral disc spaces, rarefaction of the vertebral body, loss of trabeculations near the end plate, or frank vertebral body collapse. Besides providing more accurate anatomic details of the bony involvement for assessment of stability, CT with IV contrast can be used for guiding percutaneous biopsy.

Combined gallium/bone scintigraphy is the most useful radionuclide study for diagnosing vertebral osteoarthritis in patients unable to have MRI due to incompatible implants or in whom MRI imaging is nondiagnostic. 2-[^{18}F] Flouro-2-deoxy-D-glucose positron emission tomography (FDG-PET) is a promising new modality that also has a high reported accuracy. In contrast, labeled leukocyte imaging is not considered useful in the diagnosis of vertebral osteomyelitis.[54,81]

The overall goal of treatment of vertebral osteomyelitis is to eliminate the infection while maintaining neurologic function and spinal stability. A majority of patients are able to obtain this goal without surgical intervention with antibiotics and spine immobilization via bracing or bed rest. The overall rate of surgery has likely been rising, and a recent systematic review found that 42% of patients had some form of surgical intervention. The reasons for surgery include open biopsy, spine stabilization (23%), drainage of associated abscess (21%), decompression of the spinal cord (13%), and correction of deformity after infection had been cleared (2%).[75] The use of instrumentation for stabilization in patients with acute infection does not appear to increase the risk of relapse when the patient has an appropriate course of antibiotics.[82]

Antibiotics are chosen based on the results of culturing a causative organism and should be withheld prior to obtaining the culture results if possible. If blood cultures are negative, CT-guided percutaneous biopsy or open biopsy should be obtained. Aerobic, anaerobic, fungal, and mycobacterial culture specimens should be sent. Histopathology is useful in identifying granulomas that might be indicative of tuberculosis or brucellosis.[79] Antibiotics are usually continued for at least 6 weeks, but recommended courses ranging from 4 weeks to 3 months have been reported.[83] Longer courses should be considered in patients with complicated infections or implanted hardware. Antibiotic courses of less than 4 weeks have a higher incidence of relapse.[84] In certain instances oral regimens have been used successfully after a course of IV antibiotics. One randomized trial found similar outcomes in patients treated with a combination of an oral fluoroquinolone and rifampin and in those treated with IV antibiotics.[85]

Patients should be monitored closely for failure of therapy. Failure of symptoms to improve and persistent CRP elevations at 4 weeks indicate likely treatment failure.[48] MRI obtained after starting treatment is a poor predictor of treatment outcome and should be reserved for patients in whom a change in symptoms occurs that might suggest new or worsening abscess.[79] Relapse occurs in 1% to 22% of cases and is more likely in patients with recurrent bacteremia, a chronically draining sinus, or a paravertebral abscess.[73]

The systematic review by Mylona et al. found a mortality rate of 6%, with most deaths attributable to associated sepsis. Approximately a quarter of patients had a significant decrease in quality of life. The most common complications reported were chronic pain (28%), weakness (16%), and dysfunction of the bowels or bladder (7%).[75] Predictors of worse outcome include motor weakness or paralysis at presentation, delayed diagnosis (>2 months), and acquisition of the infection in the hospital.[73]

Spinal Epidural Abscess

Spinal epidural abscess (SEA) is a relatively rare but extremely important clinical condition involving supportive infection in the epidural space of the spinal canal. SEA is considered a neurosurgical emergency because severe neurologic decline or death may become unavoidable if diagnosis and treatment are delayed. The mortality rate from SEA has been reported to be between 4.6% and 31%.[86]

Incidence reports from longer than 2 decades ago estimated that 0.18 to 1.96 cases of SEA occur per 10,000 hospital admissions.[87,88] However, evidence suggests that the incidence has increased as the number of susceptible patients with known risk factors, such as IVDU and HIV infection, has increased.[46,86,89] This apparent increase in incidence may in part be due to the fact that the diagnosis of SEA is also made easier due to the advances in medical imaging. The male-to-female ratio was previously reported to be approximately 1:1,[87,88] but a large meta-analysis in 2000 revealed a ratio of 1:0.56.[90] This predominance is likely related to the higher incidence of trauma, alcoholism, IVDU, and other risk factors in men. SEA is more common in adults, with the majority of cases occurring from ages 30 to 60, but it can occur with any age group, with the youngest reported case being a 10-day-old patient.[90] The most common location for SEA is the thoracic spine, followed by the lumbar and lumbosacral regions.

Most patients with SEA have an underlying predisposing condition such as diabetes, end-stage renal disease with dialysis,[91] cirrhosis, medical immunosuppression for transplant, chronic steroid therapy, HIV, malignancy and related chemotherapy, alcoholism, or previous trauma or spine intervention.[86,88,90,92] Approximately half of SEA cases are caused by hematogenous spread from a focus of infection, which can be either arterial or via the paravertebral venous plexus.[93] The most common source of infection is skin abscesses.[90] Other commonly reported sources include IVDU, indwelling venous or arterial catheters, dental abscesses, bacterial endocarditis, urinary tract infections, and respiratory infections. Iatrogenic introduction of disease via surgery, epidural anesthesia, or corticosteroid injection, among other causes, is another important source for the introduction of bacteria. Finally, contiguous spread to the epidural space can occur and has been reported from such sources as adjacent psoas abscesses, decubitus ulcers, abdominal infections, pyelonephritis, mediastinitis, and pharyngeal abscesses.

The most common microbial agent in SEA is *S. aureus*, which causes two-thirds to three-quarters of all cases.[46,90,94] Of concern is the increasing prevalence of MRSA, which in some reports represents almost 40% of abscesses.[95] Overall, aerobic gram-positive organisms, such as *S. epidermidis*, *Streptococcus viridans*, *Enterococcus*, and *Propionibacterium*, among others, account for nearly 80% of SEA cases.

Coagulase-negative staphylococci, such as *S. epidermidis*, are more common in patients who have undergone invasive spine procedures or who have implanted foreign bodies. Gram-negative organisms, such as *E. coli*, *Enterobacter*, *Salmonella*, *Proteus*, *Serratia*, and *Pseudomonas*, among others, are more likely to be involved when the source of the infection is gastrointestinal infection or urinary tract infection. *Pseudomonas* is more likely in patients with IVDU.[96] Multiple organisms can be found in up to 10% of abscesses. Anaerobic cultures should always be obtained since anaerobic bacteria, such as *Bacteroides* and *Peptostreptococcus* species, also rarely cause SEA.[87,97] Other causes of SEA include atypical bacterial infections, such as TB, brucellosis, and actinomycosis, for which acid-fast bacillus staining and extended cultures may be necessary; fungal infections, such as aspergillosis, in patients who are immunocompromised; and even parasitic infections, such as echinococcosis and dracunculiasis.[90]

SEA can present acutely over the course of days, with gross pus in the epidural space and signs of sepsis, or in a more chronic presentation of symptoms that develop over months, with granulation tissue in the epidural space. The organism responsible for the infection often determines the time course of presentation.

Diagnosis begins with recognition of the clinical presentation. Heusner's classic description of the presentation of SEA in 1948 describes four stages: (1) severe back pain, local tenderness and fever; (2) signs of spinal irritation such as Kernig sign, neck stiffness, and radicular pain; (3) development of neurologic deficits such as weakness, fecal or urinary incontinence, and sensory deficits; and (4) progression of weakness to paralysis.[98] Most patients with SEA do not present with such a characteristic course and often initially present with only complaints of isolated back pain. For this reason it is very common for the diagnosis of SEA to be initially missed. The most common signs and symptoms are back pain (71%) and fever (66%),[90] and the combination should always raise the possibility of SEA. Atypical signs and symptoms such as localized tenderness to percussion, thoracic radicular pain, and pain with recumbency should also raise red flags. Symptoms of systemic infection such as chills, night sweats, or sepsis may be present.[99] New-onset neurologic deficits are more common with cervical and thoracic SEA and need to be rapidly evaluated due to the possibility of progression. Approximately one third of patients present with some degree of paralysis.[90]

In a patient with back pain, the addition of laboratory tests to identify systemic signs of inflammation can greatly enhance screening for pyogenic spine infection. The leukocyte count, ESR, and CRP are often elevated, though a normal lab value by itself should never be used to rule out the possibility of SEA. The incidence of leukocytosis is approximately 68% to 78%.[100,101] Approximately 94% to 100% of patients have an elevated ESR.[90,100] Leukocytosis and an elevated ESR are relatively nonspecific symptoms and must be interpreted in the setting of the patient's condition as a whole. All patients thought to have SEA should also have blood cultures drawn as this can help with the diagnosis of SEA as well as identifying the offending pathogen.

After the history, clinical examination, and laboratory markers have raised the possibility of SEA, the next step is to identify or rule out the diagnosis with radiologic imaging. The most sensitive and specific imaging modality is MRI with gadolinium contrast. Plain-film radiographs, CT, and CT-myelography may be useful as adjuncts or when MRI is not possible.

MRI findings in SEA reveal an epidural mass that is hypointense to isointense on T1-weighted images and hyperintense on T2-weighted images. The abscess usually enhances with contrast administration, often as a linear rim enhancement surrounding a nonenhancing core that represents purulent material.[102] More heterogeneous enhancement may be present if the abscess has more of a phlegmon consistency as opposed to liquid pus.[44] MRI is also excellent for identifying other conditions that may mimic SEA, such as spinal tumors, transverse myelitis, spinal cord infarction, or intervertebral disc herniation.

Radiographs and CT are useful for evaluating for adjacent osteomyelitis. Bony erosion or destruction may be seen on radiographs after 4 to 6 weeks of infection; however, delineation of bone involvement is appreciated much better with CT imaging. CT may show evidence of inflammation, such as stranding in the paravertebral soft tissues. After contrast administration, SEA may be identified as an enhancing epidural mass. However, there are reports of CT imaging alone missing a relatively high proportion of SEAs.[103] CT imaging can be useful for surgical planning, especially in deciding whether fusion and instrumentation will be needed after surgical debridement.

If MRI is not possible, CT-myelography can be a very useful diagnostic substitute. Prior to widespread availability of MRI, myelography and then CT-myelography were the gold standards for radiologic diagnosis of SEA. With CT-myelography contrast is directly injected into the thecal sac and an epidural mass can be identified as blockage of flow from above or below, depending on where the puncture was performed. In a direct comparison study, MRI and CT-myelography were found to be equally sensitive (91% vs. 92%).[104] CT-myelography is less specific than MRI and provides less information about the characteristics of the epidural mass. Moreover, CT-myelography requires an invasive procedure that can introduce infection or spread an epidural infection to a subdural space, causing a subdural empyema or meningitis.[105] Since SEA in the upper cervical spine is relatively rare, a lateral C1-2 puncture is often recommended to limit the chance of traversing the epidural collection during the myelogram. A myelogram also allows for the evaluation of CSF, which reveals associated meningitis in up to 15% of patients. However, most authors recommend against lumbar puncture for the purpose of CSF examination alone in the evaluation of suspected SEA due to the low specificity and risk of seeding infection.[51,90,104-106]

Many conditions can present with back pain and signs and symptoms of inflammation in a manner similar to SEA. A large percentage of SEA cases are still initially misdiagnosed, leading to a delay in treatment. In a large meta-analysis, the most common initial misdiagnosis was intervertebral disc herniation, followed by meningitis, vertebral osteomyelitis, sepsis, endocarditis, and spinal tumors.[90] The differential diagnosis for SEA should also include epidural metastasis, acute transverse myelitis, subdural empyema, intramedullary abscess, epidural hematoma, autoimmune spondylitis, discitis, infections of adjacent structures (pyelonephritis, psoas abscess, etc.), vascular malformations, subarachnoid hemorrhage, and lymphoma. Acute transverse myelitis is more common than SEA and typically presents with rapidly progressing neurologic deficits without significant back pain. A history of a recent viral illness would also make acute transverse myelitis more likely.

The next step in the diagnosis of SEA after obtaining radiologic imaging is to obtain a culture of the organism causing the infection. Obtaining cultures prior to starting antibiotics is imperative to ensure the highest yield; however, this is not always possible when the patient is frankly septic. Antibiotics given prior to culture or biopsy can result in a failure to isolate a bacterial source and lead to the patient being unnecessarily treated with broad-spectrum antibiotics. The easiest method for isolation of the bacterial source involves obtaining blood culture specimens, which should be obtained from multiple sites and at different time points. Ideally, at least three separate blood specimens are obtained while the patient has spiking fevers. The yield from blood samples in the setting of SEA is between 30% and 60%.[44]

If blood cultures are negative, then percutaneous needle biopsy with either fluoroscopic or CT guidance should be performed.[107] If the biopsy is unrevealing, a repeat percutaneous biopsy or open biopsy may be necessary. Antibiotics should be withheld, even in a patient with rapidly progressing neurologic symptoms, until an adequate sample can be obtained at the time of surgery. All biopsy samples should be sent for aerobic, anaerobic, mycobacterial, and fungal stains and cultures. Occasionally extended periods of incubation are necessary for fastidious organisms.

All patients with SEA need antibacterial treatment. After obtaining appropriate cultures or biopsy specimens, the patient is usually started on broad-spectrum antibiotics that are tailored once the species and antibiotic sensitivities are known. The initial antibiotic regimen should have activity against *S. aureus*, the most common organism, should be tolerable for weeks of therapy, and should have good bone penetration due to the frequency of adjacent osteomyelitis.[108] Many regimens of empiric antibiotics have been reported in the literature.[90] The combination of a synthetic penicillin with activity against *Staphylococcus*, such as nafcillin, with a third- or fourth-generation cephalosporin for gram-negative rod coverage is one option. Vancomycin should be substituted for nafcillin in areas with a high prevalence of MRSA or if the patient is allergic to penicillin.[109] Antipseudomonal coverage should be considered in patients with a history of IVDU.[96] Duration of antibiotic treatment is usually at least 6 weeks and sometimes longer in patients with extensive bony involvement or immunocompromise. Consultation with an infectious disease specialist is highly recommended for determining the best antibiotic regimen and the length of treatment and for monitoring for adverse effects of the antibiotics selected.

Surgical decompression with debridement and drainage of infected material is the other cornerstone of treatment of SEA. Traditionally, the recommendation was that all patients with SEA should undergo urgent surgical decompression and drainage. The guiding principle was "ubi pus, ibi evacua."[110] There are numerous reports of deterioration when surgical decompression was delayed. This principle still holds for most patients; however, there have been a number of reports of good outcomes in carefully selected patients who have received antibiotics or antibiotics plus percutaneous drainage without surgical decompression. Rigomonti et al. described the use of nonoperative treatment in patients in whom the causative organism had been identified and who had minimal or no neurologic symptoms, medical comorbidities precluding surgery, extensive spine involvement, or stable paraplegia. Overall they found that two thirds of these patients had a good outcome without surgical intervention.[46] Since then, a number of other nonrandomized comparisons have been conducted of nonoperative versus operative management in similarly selected groups of patients that have found conflicting data, with some groups finding that nonoperative management can provide equivalent results as long as close monitoring is performed,[111-113] as opposed to a report by Curry et al. that indicated worse outcomes in patients treated conservatively.[114] The most important determinant of the need for surgery is the presence of neurologic deficits, which if present, and not long standing, warrant urgent decompression. Any patient being treated nonoperatively needs to be monitored extremely closely for the development of neurologic deficits, which occur in approximately 20% of patients,[115] that would require urgent surgical intervention.

Surgical approach is dictated by the location of the abscess either ventral or dorsal to the spinal cord. The majority of SEAs are located dorsally[88] and are managed with laminectomy, drainage of pus, debridement of infected material, and copious irrigation, with the option of postoperative drainage or suction-irrigation.[116] Care must be taken not to cause instability by extending the laminectomy too far laterally. The possibility of concomitant subdural abscess should be considered if the dura appears tense and nonpulsatile after evacuation of the epidural pus.[117] Laminotomy for the drainage of dorsal abscesses has also been described, which may be especially beneficial in children to minimize the risk of future spinal instability.[118,119] Monofilament suture is recommended for closure.

An SEA located ventrally to the thecal sac usually requires an anterior approach, especially since concomitant discitis or osteomyelitis is often present and requires debridement as well. A ventral liquid pus collection, as opposed to a more solid, granulomatous collection, can sometimes be drained via a dorsal approach, especially below the conus medullaris; however, the great majority of cases require an anterior approach to achieve adequate decompression and drainage. Anterior approaches require graft with or without placement of instrumentation. The risk of infection of graft material or instrumentation is minimized with adequate debridement of infected bone and tissue. Numerous studies have shown that infection does not preclude the use of autograft, allograft, or instrumentation when combined with adequate debridement and appropriate courses of antibiotics.[120-123]

Cervical SEAs tend to become symptomatic more rapidly, have a higher risk of severe neurologic deficits, and an overall higher mortality rate.[124] The severity of presentation is due to the smaller epidural space in the cervical region. Cervical SEAs are more likely to be ventrally located and have associated discitis and osteomyelitis for which an anterior approach with resection of disc and bone and reconstruction with graft with or without instrumentation is warranted.

Thoracic epidural abscesses also often present with significant neurologic compromise and present a technical challenge due to the difficulty of approach to a ventral SEA. The region involved dictates the approach. The cervicothoracic junction is particularly difficult to access. Partial sternotomy or manubrial resection[44] and transpedicular, lateral extracavitary,[125,126] or parascapular extrapleural[127] approaches have all been used to access this region. Anterior approaches in this region often necessitate concurrent dorsal instrumentation and fusion to prevent instability.[122,128] Anterior approaches to the midthoracic spine include thoracotomy,[44] lateral extracavitary,[125,126] or the retropleural approach.[129] Anterior approaches to the lower thoracic spine can be accomplished via a thoracoabdominal approach.

Lumbar and lumbosacral epidural abscesses are more likely to present without neurologic deficits and are more likely to have a favorable outcome, due to the increased size of the subarachnoid space below the conus medullaris. Ventral abscesses in this region are more likely to be accessible from a dorsal approach, though a ventral approach, such as a retroperitoneal approach, should be used if there is significant bony involvement or the purulent material does not appear to be liquid.

Extremely large SEAs involving the entire length of the spine have been reported. Medical management is often recommended for multisegmental SEA; however, there are case reports of good outcomes with extended laminectomy and surgical debridement of cervicothoracolumbar SEAs.[127]

All patients with SEAs should be followed closely for changes in clinical condition. Serial monitoring of white blood cell count and ESR can be beneficial in determining the response to therapy. Most patients benefit from use of an orthosis and a course of rehabilitation.

Outcomes for patients with SEA have been improving since Walter Dandy's 1926 review, which reported an 81% mortality rate.[130] A comprehensive meta-analysis found that mortality has decreased from around 34% during the period of 1954 to 1960 to 15% between 1991 and 1997. Moreover, the number of patients experiencing complete recovery has improved from 28% to 41% in the same time periods.[90] Mortality from SEA is likely now closer to 5% to 10%, usually caused by sepsis, meningitis, or underlying disease.[95] The best predictors of outcome are neurologic status at presentation and duration of neurologic deficits.[88,103,104,131] Patients with paralysis of more than 48 to 36 hours' duration have very little chance of recovery. Permanent paralysis still occurs in approximately 4% to 22% of patients.[95] Location of the SEA in the cervical or thoracic region, older age, significant cord compression, and delay of diagnosis also negatively affect the overall prognosis.[115] Unfortunately, an estimated one half of cases of SEA are still initially misdiagnosed, emphasizing the importance of clinical suspicion to aid in the early diagnosis of SEA prior to permanent neurologic injury.[95]

Spinal Subdural Empyema

Spinal subdural abscesses are localized infections inside the dura surrounding the spinal cord with or without associated meningitis. No estimate of incidence is available, and the total number of patients presented in case reports is less than a hundred.[115,117,132] The vast majority of reported cases are caused by *S. aureus*, although a number of other gram-positive cocci, gram-negative rods, anaerobes, and tuberculosis microbes have been reported as causative agents. The lumbar region is the area most likely to be involved, followed by the thoracic and cervical regions.[132] Cases of simultaneous spinal and cranial subdural empyemas have been reported.[133] The reported cases reveal an approximately equal distribution between men and women, with the most common age range being between 50 and 70, though all ages can be affected.[132]

Patients with spinal subdural abscesses have many of the same predisposing factors as patients with SEA. The pathogenesis is thought to be most commonly hematogenous spread from a distant source, such as a skin abscess. Other sources include direct extension from infected CSF, introduction of infection during surgery, direct inoculation during lumbar puncture or spinal anesthesia, and occasionally via a dermal sinus tract.[134,135] Injury to the spinal cord can be caused by direct compression, associated meningitis, or inflammation of the vessels of the spinal cord, causing thrombosis or hemorrhagic infarction.

Clinical signs and symptoms, as well as progression of neurologic deficits, are similar to SEAs except that subdural abscesses are more likely to present with signs of meningeal irritation and are less likely to demonstrate localized tenderness. The most common symptoms are of back pain and fever, followed by neurologic deficits. Most reported cases presented with symptoms developing in a subacute fashion (1–8 weeks).[117] Spinal subdural empyema is often initially misdiagnosed for one of the more common conditions on the differential diagnosis, including transverse myelitis, epidural hematoma or abscess, vertebral osteomyelitis, discitis, or intradural tumor.

As with SEA, patients with subdural empyemas often have a leukocytosis with a left shift as well as elevations of ESR and CRP; however, normal values do not rule out the condition. Blood cultures may be useful for identifying the causative organism faster if the abscess has a hematogenous origin.

The best radiologic tool for diagnosing a subdural empyema is MRI with contrast because of its sensitivity, noninvasiveness, and ability to clearly identify the location and extent of the abscess.[136] CT-myelography may be useful when the patient is unable to undergo an MRI, but there are reports of difficulty in differentiating a subdural abscess from an epidural abscess with a CT-myelogram.[137,138] There is often minimal or no involvement of bone, making radiographs and noncontrasted CT less useful.

The management of subdural empyemas involves urgent surgical drainage and IV antibiotics. The surgery usually involves laminectomy, durotomy, drainage of pus and debridement of infected tissue, and copious irrigation. The dura is often found to be tense and nonpulsatile. If an extended area is involved, multiple separate laminectomies might be used to minimize the risk of future instability. Aerobic, anaerobic, and mycobacterial cultures should be obtained to guide antibiotic treatment. Though spinal subdural empyemas caused by fungal infection have not been reported, fungal cultures should probably also be obtained. Antibiotics should only be started after obtaining cultures, unless the patient is frankly septic. Intraoperative ultrasound can aid in identifying the true extent of the abscess and ensuring complete drainage.[139] Associated epidural abscess or osteomyelitis should also be debrided, and, if such an infection is present, the dermal sinuses should be excised. Most patients are found to have frank pus at surgery, even if they presented with chronic symptoms (>8 weeks of symptoms).[117]

The importance of surgical drainage is illustrated in the review by Bartels et al. of 44 patients, in which only one of five patients treated conservatively survived, in contrast to the 81% survival rate of patients treated with surgery in addition to antibiotics. Moreover, in the surgical group, approximately 30% of patients made a complete recovery, with the remainder of survivors showing improvement.[117] Broad-spectrum IV antibiotics, similar to the regimen used for SEA, are started once cultures are obtained and narrowed appropriately once species and sensitivities are known. Antibiotics are continued for at least 6 weeks. Spinal subdural empyemas have a high mortality rate if not properly managed but with prompt diagnosis, surgical drainage, and appropriate IV antibiotics, a majority of patients should survive and have a good recovery.[117,140]

Intramedullary Pyogenic Spinal Cord Abscess

Intramedullary spinal cord abscess (ISCA) is a rare lesion involving infection contained within the spinal cord parenchyma. Slightly more than a hundred cases have been reported in the literature.[141] Only one case of ISCA was found in a series of 40,000 autopsies.[142] The proportion of pediatric cases is much higher for ISCA than epidural or subdural spinal abscesses, with approximately 40% of all cases presenting prior to age 20 and 25% of cases occurring in children younger than age 10.[143] The increased preponderance of pediatric patients is a result of the role played by congenital spine lesions in the pathophysiology of the disease, especially dermal sinuses, which are responsible for approximately a quarter of infections.[144] Overall, the thoracolumbar and lumbrosacral regions are the most commonly involved, especially in patients with midline deformities. In ISCA patients without midline deformities, the cervical region was more likely to be involved.[141] These patients were also more likely to be adults. Most cases of ISCA are solitary, but some have multiple foci of infection and a number of cases of holocord ISCA have been documented.[145-147]

The majority of currently diagnosed ISCAs have a cryptogenic source, likely from transient bacteremia from breaks in the mucosa or skin. Other sources include contiguous spread from congenital defects, surgery, or trauma, and hematogenous spread from known sources including IVDU.[144] Many of the patients, especially in the adult population, have comorbid conditions that impair the immune response (e.g., HIV), similar to those seen in the SEA population.[92]

Staphylococcus species are the most common causative organisms, followed by *Streptococcus* species. However, the proportion of ISCAs caused by *S. aureus* is much lower than in other types of spinal abscess. ISCAs caused by *Listeria, Brucella, Actinomyces,* gram-negative rods including *Pseudomonas,* anaerobes, *Mycobacterium tuberculosis, Histoplasma, Toxoplasma, Candida,* and parasites have been reported.[141,148] Unfortunately, around 30% of cases strongly suggestive of ISCA have negative cultures.[148]

Clinically, ISCAs have been categorized by duration of symptoms as acute (<1 week), subacute (1–6 weeks), or chronic (>6 weeks).[149] Acute cases often present with pain, fever, leukocytosis, elevated ESR, and progressive neurologic defects similar to acute transverse myelitis, though, like SEAs, presentation can be quite varied. Chronic ISCA often presents in a fashion similar to intramedullary spinal cord tumors, with a predominance of neurologic deficits occurring in the absence of fever or systemic signs of inflammation.[150] Patients can also have concurrent meningitis or brain abscesses.

MRI with contrast is the most useful diagnostic test for identifying ISCA and delineating its location and extent. Most lesions are hypointense on T1-weighted imaging, hyperintense on T2-weighted imaging, and demonstrate nodular or rim enhancement on postcontrast T1 imaging. The areas of T2 signal abnormality are usually more extensive than that seen with the postcontrast T1 sequences and likely represent adjacent edema. The differential diagnosis for ISCA includes intramedullary spinal cord tumors, acute transverse myelitis, multiple sclerosis, Guillain-Barré syndrome, and spinal cord infarct.[151] Increased diffusion restriction on diffusion-weighted imaging at the center of the lesion may help differentiate ISCA from intramedullary tumors. CT-myelography can be used to diagnose an intramedullary enlargement and is useful when MRI is not possible, but its specificity and ability to delineate anatomic details is limited.

Treatment entails surgical drainage and IV antibiotics. The surgical approach involves laminectomy, dorsal myelotomy centered at the site of maximal thickness of the abscess, drainage of the abscess with collection of specimen for cultures, and copious irrigation.[152] The specimen should be sent for Gram stain and aerobic, anaerobic, mycobacterial, and fungal cultures. The use of a limited laminectomy and myelotomy to allow a drainage catheter to be passed rostrally has been described for holocord ICSAs.[146] Excision of any associated dermal sinus should also occur. The risk of ISCA in patients with dermal sinuses is one of the reasons children should be screened for midline back abnormalities and why dermal sinuses should be prophylactically excised at the earliest possible time.[146]

Broad-spectrum IV antibiotics are started after obtaining cultures and are narrowed as speciation and specificities become available. The choice of empiric antibiotics is similar to those used for SEA except that high-dose ampicillin should be added because of the relative frequency of *Listeria monocytogenes* in reported cases of ISCA.[141] The duration of IV antibiotics should be at least 4 to 6 weeks, with follow-up neurologic examinations, laboratory studies, and imaging to demonstrate successful response to therapy and resolution of the lesion.[144] A few case reports and reviews discuss successful treatment of ISCA with antibiotics alone, but the role of medical management alone has yet to be defined.[141]

ISCA mortality rates have been progressively improving from the reported 90% mortality rate in cases in the preantibiotic era (1830–1944).[153] A recent review of cases from 1977 to 1997 reported a mortality rate of 8%.[144] Rapidly progressive deficits increase the likelihood of a poor outcome.[149] Most survivors have an improvement in neurologic status after treatment with surgery and antibiotics, but a substantial proportion, approximately 70%, have persistent neurologic deficits.[144]

Atypical Bacterial Infections

Tuberculosis

Tuberculosis may involve the vertebral column, the epidural space, the dura mater, the arachnoid, or the spinal cord itself. Tuberculous spinal infection most commonly involves the vertebral body. However, in up to 10% of patients the neural arch, transverse processes, or spinous processes may be affected. Tuberculous spondylitis most commonly involves the lower thoracic and upper lumbar vertebrae and most commonly affects the vertebral body. It is usually confined to a single level. Tuberculous spondylitis, with subsequent spinal cord compression, continues to be a major public health problem throughout much of the world.

Neurologic complications occur in 10% to 25% of cases, particularly if the thoracic spine is involved. Neurologic impairment may be caused by direct spinal cord compression or may be secondary to collapse of infected vertebrae, with subsequent spinal cord compression.

No distinctive pattern of neurologic signs or symptoms exists with Pott paraplegia. However, pain and local spine tenderness occur in an overwhelming number of patients. Radicular pain is common.

Radiographically, early vertebral body decalcification is observed about the disc, with slight diminution of the height of the disc space. Later, frank vertebral erosion and collapse occur, and paravertebral or psoas abscesses may appear. Sclerotic changes also may be present because of concomitant bone regeneration and fusion of vertebral bodies. Caseation beneath the anterior longitudinal ligament causes scalloping of the ventral vertebral border.

CT shows the expected vertebral body involvement. However, CT can also depict paraspinal abscess and an epidural tuberculous collection. Contrast enhancement may be useful for further delineation.

Spinal tuberculosis can be treated either medically or surgically. Treatment objectives include healing the disease, preventing or minimizing neurologic dysfunction, and preventing any further gibbus deformity. Treatment with pharmacologic agents has been shown to be successful in multiple series. The current recommendations for the first-line antibiotic treatment of spinal tuberculosis involve 6 to 9 months of isoniazid and rifampin with ethambutol and pyrazinamide added for the first 2 months.[154] This shorter 6- to 9-month course was equivalent to longer 18-month regimens involving isoniazid and *para*-aminosalicylic acid or ethambutol in clinical trials.[155,156] *M. tuberculosis* isolates should be tested for drug susceptibilities to guide therapy.

When the spine is stable and neurologic signs are absent or minimal, initial therapy should be pharmacologic rather than surgical. More than 85% of patients with Pott paraplegia make an excellent recovery with pharmacotherapy. Routine focal debridement and abscess evacuation in addition to antibiotics has not been shown to provide major benefit over antibiotics alone.[156] In general, surgery should be reserved for diagnostic biopsy, spinal instability, severe deformity, significant abscesses, open draining sinuses, or myelopathy.[157] Surgery often requires ventral decompression and stabilization. These ventral procedures in the thoracic spine are extensive and are often dangerous, fraught with the potential for catastrophe. In addition, any deformity correction obtained with surgery may subsequently recede with time.

Brucellosis

The causative agents in brucellosis are small, nonmotile, non–spore-forming, aerobic gram-negative coccobacilli that are commonly found in domestic animals, including *Brucella melitensis* (goats), *Brucella abortus* (cattle), *B. canis* (dogs), and *B. suis* (swine). The organism is usually transmitted to humans by ingestion of contaminated products, skin wound contamination from infected animal tissues, and inhalation of aerosols. The disease affects approximately 500,000 people per year worldwide.[158] Increasing use of milk pasteurization has resulted in a decreasing incidence of brucellosis in the United States. Likewise, brucellosis is also uncommon in other developed countries because of milk pasteurization.

Brucella infections are often asymptomatic. Initial infection leads to immunity in more than 90% of cases. After an incubation period of 10 days to 3 weeks, the patient typically develops a low-grade fever, malaise, lymphadenopathy, hepatosplenomegaly, and diffuse arthralgias. The infection spreads through the lymphatic system, resulting in acute systemic infection and chronic relapsing disease (undulant fever). However, a classic undulant fever rarely occurs in patients.[159]

Failure to provide adequate treatment at this stage can result in involvement of almost any organ system. After the initial illness, which may last for several days to weeks, relapse occurs in approximately 5% of patients. Relapses seldom occur in appropriately treated patients and often are the result of focal suppurative lesions. Musculoskeletal involvement is the most common complication of brucellosis. The spine is most commonly affected. Brucellar spondylitis typically develops secondary to chronic brucellosis and occurs in 10% to 50% of patients with brucellosis.[160] Brucellosis is one of the major causes of spondylitis in the Mediterranean basin. Of those patients with spinal brucellosis, approximately 12% have some degree of spinal cord compromise.

Brucellar spondylitis should be part of the differential diagnosis of any patient with back and radicular pain in a region where brucellosis is endemic. Lumbar involvement is most common. Localized back pain is the most common symptom. It may be present even at rest. In most cases, radiating pelvic and girdle pains are often noted, along with restriction of movement, muscle spasms, tenderness, and signs of nerve root involvement. Neurologic deficits occur in approximately 20% of patients. Formation of a paraspinal or epidural abscess is uncommon but can occur with severe infections.[161]

Pathologic studies suggest the infection originates within the body of the vertebra, particularly in the more vascularized ventral portion, and only later extends to the intervertebral disc. The infected disc then may become necrotic and subsequently degenerate. As it bulges, the disc may press on adjacent neural structures. Usually, only one or two vertebrae are involved in brucellar infections. Infective organisms can be recovered from the infected disc or bony material in approximately 20% of cases. Serologic tests may be required to diagnose a brucellar spine infection.

Involvement of the spine can be either focal or diffuse, with a predilection to the lumbar region. Hallmarks of focal brucellar spondylitis include vertebral end-plate erosion and sclerosis, inflammatory changes, and intact discs. Features of diffuse brucellar spondylitis include osteomyelitis of neighboring vertebrae, involvement of the intervening disc, and epidural extension.[162] Radiographic changes occur relatively late in the course of the disease and are similar to but less severe than those observed with tuberculosis. Plain radiographs demonstrate disc space involvement with erosion of the adjacent cortical bone, preservation of relatively intact vertebral architecture despite the amount of infection present, and absence of gibbus formations. Plain radiographs demonstrate a thinning of the disc space and erosion of the vertebral body adjacent to the involved disc. This epiphysitis usually occurs in the ventral-rostral angle and may be the main sign of bone destruction. Osteophytic bridging occurs across the infected disc interspace. CT demonstrates destruction of both cortical and cancellous bone. MRI and CT findings are similar for tuberculosis and brucellosis, except that tuberculosis produces more kyphosis and paraspinal abscess formation.

The mainstay of treatment for brucellosis is antibiotic therapy. A recent systematic review recommends that the first-line treatment for brucellosis should be combination therapy with doxycycline for 6 weeks and gentamicin for the initial 2 weeks, with the optional addition of rifampin for a total of 6 weeks.[163] Spinal brucellosis appears to have a higher incidence of recurrence, which leads some authors to recommend an antibiotic course of 6 months.[164]

Although surgery is rarely necessary, the indications for surgery for brucellar spondylitis are similar to those for tuberculosis. The role of stabilization of the spine, or decompression of the spinal cord with stabilization, is determined by the clinical condition. Disc excision may be required for an infected, bulging disc causing neurologic symptoms, and laminectomy may be indicated for an epidural infection producing neural decompensation. The use of a spine orthosis should be considered if there is spinal involvement, but surgical intervention is not warranted.

Brucellosis is a completely curable infection. The primary pitfall is a delay of more than 1 month in diagnosis and treatment, which can lead to multisystem involvement and severe sequelae. Many patients with brucellar spondylitis recover spontaneously, which differentiates this entity from spinal tuberculosis, which is progressive.

Actinomycosis

The actinomycetes are a heterogeneous group whose morphology suggests fungus; however, they are classified as bacteria because of their small size, primitive nuclear organization, and cell wall composition. The usual infective organism for most cases of actinomycosis is *Actinomyces israelii*. Once known as *ray fungus*, *A. israelii* is now recognized as a gram-positive, non-acid–fast anaerobic bacterium that is intermediate between classic bacteria and higher fungi. The bacteria are present in the oral cavity, both on carious teeth and on tonsillar crypts. Endogenous organisms gain entry to the body via breaks in mucous membranes.

Actinomycosis is a noncontagious, suppurative, bacterial infection characterized by chronic inflammatory induration, sinus tract formation, fever, and leukocytosis. The pathologic reaction of the body to actinomycetes is typically suppuration. Acute and chronic inflammatory tissue is reminiscent of staphylococcal infections. Areas of infection are most characteristic for their gross appearance of sulfur granules, which are actually collections of foamy macrophages.

The common sites of involvement are the face, thorax, and abdomen. Involvement of the spine is rare (<1% of all patients with actinomycosis) and is usually the result of contiguous spread from nearby structures (e.g., thoracic infection). Early in the disease there may be vertebral body destruction, with new bone formation leading to a honeycomb appearance that may involve the pedicles, transverse processes, and ribs. After treatment, increasing sclerosis occurs, along with bone bridging and fusion between involved vertebrae. Unlike tuberculosis, from which this infection must be differentiated, actinomycosis rarely destroys the intervertebral disc.

Involvement of the CNS occurs by hematogenous spread from a pulmonary focus or by direct spread from lesions involving the skull, face, and throat, possibly via the lymphatics. Diagnosis is generally made by percutaneous needle biopsy and culture.

Most patients can be treated nonoperatively with antibiotics and spinal immobilization. Before the advent of penicillin, approximately 75% of cases were diagnosed postmortem. The disease involves the vertebrae and ribs in less than 1% of patients who have actinomycosis. Isolated vertebral body infections can be adequately treated nonoperatively with aggressive antibiotic therapy, usually IV penicillin G for 6 weeks followed by 6 to 12 months of oral penicillin or amoxicillin.[165] Tetracycline, doxycycline, and clindamycin have all been used successfully in patients with penicillin allergies. Indications for operative intervention include epidural infection with spinal cord compression, large abscesses, and progressive spinal deformity.

Mortality is high in untreated or improperly treated cases. Thus it is important to distinguish actinomycosis from other vertebral infections, such as pyogenic osteomyelitis or tuberculosis. Even today, an accurate diagnosis often is not made until a late stage; therefore, assiduous efforts must be made to obtain bacterial specimens from the infected site.

Nocardiosis

Nocardia asteroides is the most common human pathogen in this family of aerobic, weakly gram-positive bacteria. It is a natural soil saprophyte, often found in decaying organic matter. Infection most often occurs through the respiratory tract, although other modes of infection may occur. The infection is most commonly observed in immunocompromised hosts.

Nocardiosis may imitate a chronic granulomatous response, but more commonly the histologic features are suppurative necrosis and abscess formation, which are typical of pyogenic infections.

The most common primary site is the pulmonary system, but dissemination to nearly any organ occurs in 45% of cases. Dissemination to the brain, meninges, and spinal cord occurs in 23% of patients, but hematogenous involvement of the vertebrae is uncommon. Epidural spinal cord compression from vertebral osteomyelitis has been reported.

If there is no spinal cord compression or large abscess, medical therapy alone is often sufficient. Sulfonamides, in conjunction with appropriate surgery, have been the mainstay of treatment since the 1940s. The use of trimethoprim-sulfamethoxazole (TMP-SMX) for 6 or more months has been described for the treatment of systemic nocardiosis.[166] Many other antibiotics have been used, either alone or in combination. The optimal duration of therapy is uncertain, but because of the possibility of relapse, treatment is often continued for many months after apparent cure. A poor response to treatment may be related to the presence of a second pathogen.

Syphilis

Syphilitic spinal involvement was common at the beginning of the 20th century but is now quite rare due to the availability of antibiotics. The spirochete *Treponema pallidum* is responsible for syphilis. Syphilis is often referred to as *the great imitator*, because it can present and resemble many other diseases. Spinal involvement typically occurs with tertiary syphilis and presents as either Charcot arthropathy or intraosseous gumma formation.

Neuropathic (Charcot) arthropathy of the axial skeleton occurs in approximately 10% to 20% of patients with tabes dorsalis. Charcot arthropathy is a neuropathic disorder producing spinal degenerative changes. Tabes dorsalis causes posterior column degeneration with consequent loss of protective proprioceptive sensation; consequently, there is subluxation and traumatization of the intervertebral joints, destruction of the discs, and fragmentation of the articular cartilage and the subchondral bone. This produces excessive bone formation within and around the joint, as well as reactive bony sclerosis and spinal deformity. These changes occur most commonly in the lumbar and thoracic spine and are identifiable on plain radiographs. Charcot arthropathy may be detected coincidentally or may produce low back pain or nerve root involvement if destruction and hypertrophic changes are severe. Characteristically, the radiographic changes are out of proportion to the severity of the patient's complaints.

Charcot arthropathy affecting the spine is notoriously difficult to treat. Treatment includes an orthosis to limit excessive movement and to minimize further injury. The role of fusion is undetermined.

The syphilitic gumma lesion is composed of microorganisms and the local tissue reaction to the organisms. Gummas are rare, destructive, and usually symptomatic, causing collapse and neurologic deficits. The clinical features of spinal gumma are often difficult to distinguish from those of coincident neuropathy, which is often present, and biopsy is necessary for the diagnosis of spinal gumma. The indications for surgically treating syphilitic gummas are similar to those for treating tuberculous spondylitis. The treatment of choice for syphilis is penicillin, though the dosing depends on the specific manifestation of the disease.[167]

Fungal Infections

Fungal infections of the spine are rare and generally occur in debilitated, diabetic, or immunocompromised patients. Patients with acute leukemia, patients with lymphoma, recipients of organ transplants, and those receiving chemotherapy are particularly susceptible.[168] Accurate diagnosis is often delayed because other medical conditions mask the diagnosis and because fungal spondylitides are often indolent in nature. Notably, sporadic cases of fungal osteomyelitis have been reported in immunocompetent patients.[169]

Although certain radiographic features are characteristic for each type of infection, the diagnosis ultimately depends on a tissue specimen. Evaluation of specimens with fungal stains and cultures is mandated because the latter may be negative or may take several weeks before identification is possible. Percutaneous biopsy is positive in less than 50% of cases, whereas open biopsy is positive in most cases.

The management of the different fungal infections is similar. The cornerstone of treatment is correction of those host factors that compromise wound healing or immune defense mechanisms. Antifungal agents are the mainstays of treatment, but surgery is occasionally necessary.

Surgery is generally reserved for patients with neurologic deterioration secondary to instability or progressive deformity. The selected operative approach should address the specific pathologic features encountered. Dorsal segmental instrumentation and fusion may be necessary in the face of spinal instability. However, in general, ventral debridement with stabilization is preferred.

The prognosis for patients with fungal osteomyelitis depends on the organism involved, as well as on the host. As with bacterial infections, patients with diabetes mellitus or neurologic deficits have a worse prognosis. Mortality rates following fungal infection are often high, reflecting both the severity of the fungal infection and the patient's underlying disease.

Aspergillosis

Aspergillus is a saprophytic mold that is ubiquitous in the environment. Although *Aspergillus* involvement of the CNS does occasionally occur in otherwise healthy individuals, it is more commonly associated with IV drug abusers and severely immunocompromised patients.

Infection typically is acquired by inhaling small spores (conidia). Although uncommon, spine involvement nearly always results from hematogenous spread from the lungs; though postoperative *Aspergillus* discitis has been reported after lumbar discectomy.[170] Vertebral involvement can also result from contiguous spread from the lungs to the vertebral bodies. Vascular invasion is common in immunocompromised patients, and it leads to tissue necrosis with abundant hyphal proliferation.[171] In patients with chronic granulomatous disease, vascular invasion is uncommon and hyphae are sparse.

The radiographic findings of aspergillosis are similar to those for tuberculous spondylitis. Destruction of adjacent disc plates with subsequent collapse leads to severe pain and neurologic deficits. Disc space narrowing, involvement of adjacent vertebrae, and the presence of paraspinal abscesses are common. Dense new bone formation with small lytic lesions without sequestration may be observed. Spinal CT scans are extremely useful in delineating the extent of spinal involvement, but the radiographic picture is not specific for *Aspergillus*.

Clinically, sinus tract formation is characteristic, though often not present. The incidence of epidural abscess formation, in association with neurologic deficits, is high. Diagnosis is established by percutaneous or open biopsy. Voriconazole has been demonstrated to be superior to amphotericin B for the treatment of invasive aspergillosis. Liposomal amphotericin, posaconazole, itraconazole, caspofungin, or micofungin are all possibilities for salvage therapy in cases refractory to voriconazole therapy. Treatment duration is usually 6 to 8 weeks minimum for patients with normal immune systems. Immunocompromised patients likely require longer treatment and usually warrant chronic suppression therapy.[172]

In addition to antibiotics, surgical debridement with resection of devitalized bone and cartilage is important to achieve cure in most cases. With *Aspergillus* discitis, early surgery with vigorous surgical debridement combined with antifungal treatment, yields a good outcome in most cases.[170,173] There are rare reports of successful treatment with antifungal agents alone.[174,175] The prognosis of patients with *Aspergillus* spondylitis overall is guarded, in large part due to the patient's usually poor condition and numerous comorbities.

Blastomycosis

Blastomycosis is caused by *Blastomyces dermatitidis*, a dimorphic fungus that is endemic to the midwestern, southeastern, and south central United States. Primary infection in humans occurs by inhalation of conidia, which then convert to the yeast phase in the lung. The incubation period for acute pulmonary infection is 30 to 45 days. The symptoms are nonspecific, and acute pulmonary infection may occasionally be undetected. Extrapulmonary disease involving the skin, bones, genitourinary system, or CNS occurs in approximately 25% to 40% of cases and is much more common in immunocompromised patients. The organism spreads hematogenously from the lungs to the spine.[176] Men are affected nine times more commonly than women, particularly those with a history of alcohol abuse.

Thoracic and lumbar lesions are more common than cervical lesions. The radiographic findings resemble those of tuberculous spondylitis, with disc space narrowing, ventral vertebral body involvement, and the development of large paraspinal abscesses. Unlike lesions in tuberculosis, thoracic and lumbar lesions often invade adjacent ribs, involve the dorsal elements, and produce draining sinuses. Collapse and gibbus deformity are more common with blastomycosis than with any of the other fungal diseases. Diagnosis usually requires biopsy, unless blastomycosis has been reliably detected elsewhere in the body either via culture of respiratory secretions or antigen testing. Serologic testing generally has low sensitivity and specificity.

Before the availability of effective antimicrobial therapy, the mortality rate exceeded 60%.[177] CNS blastomycosis should be treated with IV liposomal amphotericin B for 4 to 6 weeks followed by oral azole therapy (fluconazole, itraconazole, or voriconazole) for at least 12 months. Though mild pulmonary blastomycosis often resolves without treatment, antibiotic therapy should be considered to prevent dissemination to extrapulmonary sites.[178] Surgery is generally reserved for patients with severe infections, such as epidural abscesses, that are causing neurologic deficits.

Coccidioidomycosis

Coccidioidomycosis is caused by *Coccidioides immitis*, a fungus that is endemic to the southwestern United States, Central America, South America, and central California, where the infection is often referred to as *San Joaquin Valley fever*.

The primary focus of disease is the lungs, but the disease becomes disseminated in 0.5% of cases, and the rate of extrapulmonary disease is much higher in immunocompromised hosts.[179] The organism enters the body when arthroconidia are inhaled into the lungs and can secondarily disseminate via hematogenous spread. Osseous lesions are found in 20% of those with disseminated disease. Vertebral lesions are most common in the thoracic and lumbar spine. Multicentric disease is common. Radiographic studies usually reveal that the intervertebral disc is relatively uninvolved compared with the vertebral body, pedicles, and transverse processes. Contiguous rib involvement is also common. Paraspinal abscesses and skin tracts are common.

Extrapulmonary coccidioidomycosis is usually treated with oral ketoconazole, itraconazole, or fluconazole. IV amphotericin B is indicated for rapidly progressive infections or with infections not responsive to initial therapy. Surgical debridement is indicated for large abscesses, neurologic compromise, spinal instability, or failure of medical therapy.[180]

Cryptococcosis

Cryptococcosis is a subacute or chronic infection caused by a yeastlike fungus surrounded by a gelatinous capsule, *Cryptococcus neoformans*. Infection is acquired by inhalation of the aerosolized organism. Because many cases of cryptococcal osteomyelitis occur in normal hosts, it should be considered in the differential diagnosis even in a normal host.[181] Osseous involvement occurs in less than 5% of all cases and resembles cold abscesses. Sinus tracts and abscess formation are rare.

The onset of cryptococcosis is usually insidious. The bone infection typically has an indolent course. Both serum and CSF agglutination tests are available. Testing for cryptococcal antigen in the serum should be done prior to invasive diagnostic procedures.[181] Radiographic studies show lucent lesions of the vertebral bodies with sharply scalloped margins and little, if any, reactive sclerosis or periosteal new bone formation. The disc spaces are typically unaffected.

Treatment for cryptococcosis consists of a 4- to 6-week combined induction regimen of IV amphotericin B and oral flucytosine followed by an 8-week course of high-dose oral fluconazole for consolidation. A lower maintenance dose of fluconazole is then continued for 6 to 12 months. A high relapse rate is common, particularly in patients with AIDS, whose disease is usually controlled rather than cured. All patients with cryptococcosis should be screened for HIV.

Parasite Infections

Cysticercosis

Cysticercosis is caused by the pork tapeworm *Taenia solium*. This disease is rare in developed areas such as the United States and Western Europe; however, it remains a significant problem for many economically deprived regions, including Central and South America, Africa, India, and Asia. This disease should be considered when treating patients who have recently emigrated from these areas.

Humans usually become infected by ingesting infected undercooked pork. For disseminated disease to occur, gravid proglottids or eggs must be digested by gastric juices before they hatch and liberate oncospheres, which penetrate the intestinal wall and spread widely.

Spinal cysticercosis occurs in 2% to 5% of all neurocysticercosis cases, usually as a result of intracranial parasites migrating caudally into the subarachnoid space, where they may settle at any level within the spinal canal. The presentation is variable. Backache, radiculopathy, and slowly progressive paraparesis are all possible.

Cysticercosis is suggested by a history of infection with an adult worm, multiple subcutaneous nodules, typical symptoms, previous residence in highly endemic regions where undercooked pork may have been eaten, and eosinophilia.

Indirect hemagglutination tests may be positive in the blood or spinal fluid; however, a negative result does not rule out cysticercosis.

MRI is superior to CT for recognition of the subarachnoid cyst, the contained lesion, and adjacent spinal cord edema. Intramedullary inflammatory changes associated with those cysts may also be demonstrated.

Both albendazole and praziquantel have proven effective in the treatment of both cerebral and spinal cysticercosis. Recent analysis favors albendazole over praziquantel.[182] Because of the CNS's inflammatory reaction to dying parasites, concomitant administration of steroids to minimize this inflammatory reaction has been recommended. Excision of the cyst has produced significant improvement in patients with neurologic deficits secondary to neural compression.

Echinococcosis

Echinococcosis (also known as hydatidosis) is a rare disease in developed countries. It is caused by either *Echinococcus granulosus* or *E. multilocularis*. It is more commonly seen in the sheep-rearing areas of South America, the southern and central parts of the former Soviet Union, Australia, and parts of Africa. Humans become infected after the ingestion of raw meat containing viable parasites. Under the action of gastric juices, the oncosphere is released and penetrates the intestinal wall, where it is transported to the liver and other organs. The skeleton is affected in approximately 2.4% of patients with echinococcosis. Of those cases, approximately 50% involve the spine.

Once the oncosphere reaches the vertebral body, it develops into its larval stage, commonly known as the hydatid cyst. The organism grows within the intratrabecular space, destroying the bone like a tumor. Unlike other organisms, it does not elicit a large inflammatory response. Adjacent bones such as ribs or the ilium may also be invaded. The organism spreads beneath the periosteum and ligaments. Spinal cord compression occurs once the bony center has been perforated.

The clinical manifestations and duration of symptoms vary considerably. Back and radicular pain is common. Paraparesis or paraplegia is a common symptom.

Plain radiographs demonstrate an expansile lytic mass that is poorly delineated and that appears multiloculated. A complete blockage of flow is a common finding with myelography. The disease is usually confined to a single vertebra with predilection to the thoracic spine. The cyst appears as a well-defined area in the vertebral body, which may be apparent only on tomography. The articular cartilage and the intervertebral disc are usually resistant to the cyst. However, in untreated and advanced cases, the articular surfaces and discs may be destroyed, vertebral collapse may occur, and the cyst may spread into the paravertebral tissues or beneath the psoas sheath, simulating an abscess caused by tuberculosis. In an endemic area, the findings suggestive of hydatid disease are ring-shaped calcification in the cyst wall, eosinophilia, and specific enzyme-linked immunosorbant assay (ELISA) or Western blot serology. CT of hydatid disease reveals more specific findings than does conventional radiography. It may show cysts within the paraspinal muscles. In addition to bone destruction, the presence of daughter cysts is pathognomonic. Arachnoiditis may be demonstrated on CT or myelography.

All patients with echinococcosis should undergo surgical debridement if possible, with complete excision of the cyst and affected bone and stabilization, as needed. Unfortunately the relatively high risk of cyst rupture (up to 44% in extradural cases) can cause anaphylaxis or seed the surgical site, leading to future recurrence.[183] A hyperosmolar saline solution washout is recommended intraoperatively to prevent cyst recurrence. Although its value remains to be established, presumably, the hypertonic saline solution disrupts any residual cysts osmotically. Albendazole and mebendazole have both been used to treat echinococcosis, with most evidence favoring albendazole as the primary agent. Treatment with albendazole should be continued for a minimum of 3 to 4 months, with one report suggesting 1 year of treatment after neural decompression.[184]

Recent studies have observed an improved prognosis for what was once thought to be a uniformly fatal disease. However, for spinal echinococcosis, reports of recurrence rates range from 30% to 100%, and mortality rates range from 5% to 50%.[185] Response to therapy should be monitored with serial imaging, given the high incidence of recurrence.

Schistosomiasis

The parasitic flukes (trematodes) of the *Schistosoma* genus can rarely involve the CNS, including the spinal cord. Three species have been implicated in causing diseases of the spinal cord: *Schistosoma mansoni*, *S. haematobium*, and *S. japonicum*.[186] The trematode larvae gain access to humans by piercing the skin of people exposed to infected waters. Once the larvae penetrate the skin, they gain access to the vascular system, develop into adults, and produce eggs, which are passed out of the urine (*S. haematobium)* or feces (*S. mansoni* and *S. japonicum)*. Their natural hosts are freshwater snails.

Injury to the spinal cord in schistosomal infections is caused by an inflammatory response to the schistosomal eggs that have been deposited in the spinal cord parenchyma or subarachnoid space. These eggs reach the area either via direct deposition or by embolus from anastomosis of the pelvic veins with the paravertebral vascular plexus. The vertebrae and intervertebral discs are not usually involved in schistosomiasis.

The most typical clinical picture is that of transverse myelitis or myeloradiculopathy. The lumbosacral region is the most commonly affected region, though all regions of the spinal cord, including the cervical spine,[186] can be affected. In the acute stage of lumbosacral myeloradiculopathy the patient presents with lumbar pain, lower extremity sensory changes, and bladder dysfunction, followed by lower extremity weakness, sexual dysfunction, or bowel dysmotility.

Diagnosis is based largely on a high index of suspicion in patients with exposures to regions of the world, including South America, Asia, and Africa, where schistosomiasis is endemic. Diagnosis is aided by either positive parasitic stool examination or positive antischistosomal immune reaction in serum or CSF in the presence of MRI findings of inflammatory myelopathy, myeloradiculopathy, or intramedullary mass. Serum and CSF eosinophilia are also usually present. The gold standard of diagnosis is demonstration of *Schistosoma* eggs from biopsy, but the risk of biopsy often outweighs the benefits in a disease that is usually treated medically.

Treatment involves the use of schistosomicidal drugs, such as praziquantel, to kill the adult worms and stop the production of eggs. Treatment with corticosteroids has been recommended as an adjuvant to praziquantel to stop the inflammatory response to the eggs that have already been deposited, though length of treatment has not been defined, with some groups recommending up to 6 months of steroid treatment.[187] Surgical intervention is reserved for acute paraplegia or evidence of medullary compression, medically refractory cases, or biopsy when the diagnosis is unclear. Surgery usually involves laminectomy for decompression and possible release of spinal nerve roots with biopsy if diagnosis is uncertain.[188] Resection of focal lesions has also been described.[186]

KEY REFERENCES

Cottle L, Riordan T: Infectious spondylodiscitis. *J Infect* 56(6):401–412, 2008.

Khoo LT, Mikawa K, Fessler RG: A surgical revisitation of Pott distemper of the spine. *Spine J* 3(2):130–145, 2003.

Kowalski TJ, Berbari EF, Huddleston PM, et al: The management and outcome of spinal implant infections: contemporary retrospective cohort study. *Clin Infect Dis* 44(7):913–920, 2007.

McHenry MC, Easley KA, Locker GA: Vertebral osteomyelitis: long-term outcome for 253 patients from 7 Cleveland-area hospitals. *Clin Infect Dis* 34(10):1342–1350, 2002.

Reihsaus E, Waldbaur H, Seeling W: Spinal epidural abscess: a meta-analysis of 915 patients. *Neurosurg Rev* 23(4):175–204, 2000; discussion 205.

Watters WC, Baisden J, Bono CM, et al: Antibiotic prophylaxis in spine surgery: an evidence-based clinical guideline for the use of prophylactic antibiotics in spine surgery. *Spine J* 9(2):142–146, 2009.

Weinstein MA, McCabe JP, Cammisa FP Jr: Postoperative spinal wound infection: a review of 2,391 consecutive index procedures. *J Spinal Disord* 13(5):422–426, 2000.

REFERENCES

The complete reference list is available online at expertconsult.com.

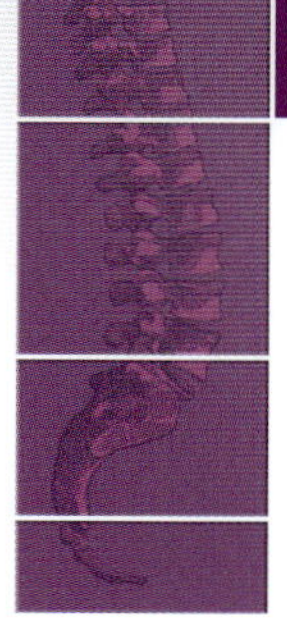

CHAPTER 198

Prevention of Operative Infections: An Evidence-Based Approach

G. Alexander Jones | Vincent Miele | Edward C. Benzel

Surgical site infections (SSIs) are a known problem in spinal surgery. According to the National Nosocomial Infections Surveillance Survey (NNISS), they complicate up to 2.46% of laminectomies and 6.35% of fusion operations.[1] These rates vary, depending on patient risk factors and hospital-related factors. They may even be higher in some circumstances. In general, an SSI is associated with a twofold increase in mortality rate, as well as an increase in the likelihood that a patient will require readmission to the hospital or treatment in the intensive care unit.[2] The length and cost of the hospital stay are increased, as well.

Clearly, the best treatment for SSIs is prevention. Although most surgeons first think of sterile technique, other factors must be optimized as well, including those intrinsic to the patient, anesthetic factors, and perioperative medical management.

Most SSIs are caused by the patient's normal skin flora (*Staphylococcus* species being the most common). This is true for spinal surgery as well,[3,4] and is an important concept in prevention of SSIs. The keys to prevention include reduction of the bacterial burden in the wound, minimization of patient-related factors that contribute to SSIs (e.g., hyperglycemia, hypothermia), and optimization of patient nutrition and baseline health status preoperatively.

This review is structured in a chronological order, with emphasis at steps that can be taken preoperatively, during the procedure, and postoperatively.

Preoperative Factors

Several factors can influence the risk of SSIs long before the patient enters the operating room. They warrant careful attention in the office.

Nutrition

More has been reported about the relationship between infection and nutrition in the general surgery and critical care literature than the spine literature.[5-9] Often such studies involve polytrauma and burn victims in severe catabolic states. However, the principles involved apply to elective spine surgery as well.

A study by Klein et al.[10] followed three groups of patients and analyzed infections and other complications against markers of nutritional status. Patients were deemed nutritionally replete if they had a serum albumin of at least 3.5 g/dL and an absolute lymphocyte count (a stable immune marker) of at least 1500 cells/mm^3. Patients falling below either or both of these cutoffs were considered malnourished.

In a group of 114 patients undergoing elective spinal procedures, a total of 85 were found to be replete prior to surgery, and 29 malnourished. The former group had a total of 2 complications, and the latter 11, a difference that is even more dramatic considering the disparate sizes of the groups. Of note, they found that 40% of patients older than 60 years were malnourished. They found similar results among patients who were operated on for spondylodiscitis, as well as spinal cord injury.

Considering the aforementioned, a reasonable nutrition assessment and management approach would be to check serum albumin and absolute lymphocyte counts preoperatively, especially in older patients. If abnormal, surgery should be deferred until a nutrition consult is obtained and the patient is nutritionally replete.

Antiseptic Shower

The use of antiseptic showers, either with povidone-iodine (Betadine) or chlorhexidine gluconate (CHG), has been advocated by some. A study of 700 surgical patients demonstrated a reduction of bacterial skin colonization with either soap, by a factor of 1.3-fold with iodine and 9-fold with CHG.[11] Similar results have been found elsewhere.[12] Although evidence to support a clear reduction in SSIs is lacking,[13] a bottle of CHG solution sufficient for two preoperative showers costs about $9 US at the time of this writing, and its use is likely of great enough benefit to offset that minor cost. Thus, the practice is recommended.

Mupirocin Nasal Ointment

Staphylococcus aureus is the leading cause of SSIs in clean surgical procedures, including spinal operations. An association has been noted between nasal carriage of *S. aureus* in patients and the occurrence of SSIs. Twenty-five percent to 30% of the U.S. population are nasal carriers of *S. aureus* at any given time.[14] A short course of treatment with mupirocin (Bactroban) ointment has been shown to eliminate *S. aureus* in many of these carriers.

To date, two randomized, controlled trials (RCTs) have been conducted to evaluate the efficacy of preoperative mupirocin ointment usage in reducing SSI rates.[14,15] Both studies showed a trend toward efficacy, but neither was significant. A later analysis showed that pooling of the results showed a nearly significant decrease in the infection rate.[16] However, when all nosocomial *S. aureus* infections (not just SSIs) among patients with nasal *S. aureus* were considered, the study from Perl et al. did show a statistically significant decrease in incidence with the use of mupirocin ointment.[14]

At this point, it is difficult to advocate the widespread use of mupirocin ointment preoperatively, considering the lack of convincing evidence showing benefit, as well as the cost (about $40 US). However, a rapid screening test for *S. aureus* that uses polymerase chain reaction (PCR) technology has been developed[17] and has shown excellent sensitivity and specificity. This has allowed treatment targeted only toward carriers, which shows promise.[18] It is reasonable to expect that within the next several years this technology will be more widely accessible. If so, it could allow for the selective treatment of carriers, which would be expected to demonstrate a beneficial effect.

Hair Removal

Possibly one of the most ingrained practices in all of surgery is shaving the skin prior to an operation. Unfortunately, it is probably also detrimental. Removing hair by shaving with a razor has been compared with the use of electric clippers in three RCTs.[19-21] These trials were similar in design and focused on clean operations (general and cardiac procedures), so their results were pooled in a recent Cochrane review.[22] This yielded a total of 3193 patients, divided nearly evenly between shaving (1627) and clipping (1566). The infection rate was 2.8% for the former group, and 1.4% for the latter, yielding a relative risk (RR) of 2.02, which surpassed statistical significance.

In addition to this strong evidence against shaving, two other points can be made. First, there is no good evidence to show that hair removal lowers the infection rate. The step may be omitted entirely. Second, depilatory creams have been associated with a lower infection rate than shaving in several trials[22]; this provides another alternative to razors should complete hair removal be desired.

Razors should only be used for hair removal with the clear understanding that their use has been associated with higher infection rates in several large, well-designed trials.

Skin Preparation

The rationale for preparing the skin prior to incision is twofold. First, the mechanical scrubbing of the skin removes dirt, as well as some bacteria and dead skin cells. Second, the prep solution should have an intrinsic bactericidal and/or bacteriostatic effect.

Commonly employed agents contain alcohol (isopropyl or ethyl), CHG, or iodine/iodophors. Alcohol has excellent activity against bacteria and good activity against mycobacteria, fungi, and viruses.[23] However, it cannot be used alone because it has essentially no residual activity once allowed to evaporate. Prior to evaporation it is flammable, which makes it incompatible with electrocautery.

CHG has good to excellent activity against bacteria and viruses. It is fair at eliminating fungi and has little activity against mycobacteria.[23] Its residual activity is excellent; however, it can cause keratitis and ototoxicity with serious consequences.

Triclosan (the active ingredient in dishwashing detergent) and parachlorometaxylenol (PCMX) are less efficacious and are not generally considered suitable for use in skin preparation or as surgical hand scrubs.

Given the clinical limitations of other preparations, CHG and iodophor solutions are most commonly used as surgical skin preps. CHG has been shown to reduce bacterial skin colonization to a greater degree than iodophors (see prior section), but no evidence yet demonstrates a lower SSI rate when using CHG.

Nevertheless, in a large RCT, CHG has been shown to reduce the line infection rate when compared with iodophor prep in the placement of central venous catheters.[24] A similar level of evidence does not yet exist for CHG as a surgical skin prep, but it is logical to expect that the superiority of CHG would hold true here as well. Thus, favoring CHG as a skin prep is advisable, provided that there is no risk of the solution entering the eyes or ears.

Handwashing

Several options exist here as well. Iodophor and CHG solutions are available and are commonly used with scrub brushes for a specified period of time. Ten minutes has been traditional, but there is no evidence to support this ritual; the U.S. Centers for Disease Control and Prevention (CDC) recommends a duration of 2 to 5 minutes.[23]

In addition, waterless hand cleansers have recently come into more widespread use. Typical of these is Avagard (3M, St. Paul, MN). It consists of ethyl alcohol 61% w/w, CHG 1%, and a mixture of skin conditioners and fragrances.

Another category of hand cleaners includes water-aided, brushless formulations. Triseptin (Healthpoint Ltd., Fort Worth, TX) is one of these. It also contains ethyl alcohol 61% w/w, as well as a proprietary formulation of conditioners and fragrances. A large RCT has demonstrated equivalence of an aqueous alcohol-based hand rub with traditional handwashing techniques[25]; the results of this trial can safely be extrapolated to the products available on the U.S. market.

Because most SSIs arise from the patient's skin flora, the use of one type of hand cleanser over another is largely left to individual preference. If there is a difference amongst the different agents available, it is likely quite small and has yet to be proven. Guidelines from the CDC regarding this are available.[23]

First, artificial nails should be avoided. They can harbor micro-organisms and predispose gloves to tearing. A series of *Serratia marcescens* wound infections have been traced to a surgical team member with artificial nails.[26] Second, fingernails should be kept short and neat. Third, cleaning under the nails is recommended, as is removal of jewelry on the hands and arms, but the scientific support for this is overshadowed by the clear theoretical basis on which these recommendations are founded.

Surgical Gowns

The U.S. Occupational Safety and Health Administration (OSHA) requires that gowns have a minimum level of strikethrough resistance. All of the commercially available, disposable surgical gowns in the United States meet this standard. Porous cloth gowns have generally been eliminated because they do not offer this protection to the patient or to the surgeon.

Some have recommended that gowns and gloves be changed every 1.5 to 2 hours during lengthy cases.[27] Although this recommendation is sensible, the cost of this practice must also be considered.

Double-Gloving

The practice of double-gloving has been advocated as a protection to both the medical staff and the patient. For the staff, the risk of transmission of a communicable disease, such as HIV or hepatitis, is likely reduced, as is the risk of gross contamination through a compromised glove. Not only is perforation of two gloves more difficult than one, but in the event of a needlestick, the "squeegee effect" of the second glove has been shown as well.[28]

Double-gloving may reduce the risk of SSI as well. Perforation rates of greater than 20% have been reported for the primary operator.[29,30] This puts the surgeon's skin in direct contact with the surgical bed, increasing the chance of bacterial contamination for the patient and creating a hazardous exposure for the surgeon.

Although the superiority of double-gloving in prevention of SSI has not been shown, a perusal of a recent Cochrane review reinforces the theoretical benefit of double-gloving to the patient.[31] When studying the risk of perforation of the inner glove (which is the only glove for single-gloved surgeons, and the inner for those double-gloving), there is a clear trend across the 18 studies reviewed toward a lower likelihood of perforation for those who were double-gloved.[31]

It is important to remember here the axiom that the *absence of proof* of a benefit is not *proof of absence* of said effect. In addition to middling clinical evidence, there is a strong theoretical rationale for double-gloving to protect the surgeon and the patient. The cost is minimal, and the potential benefits to all parties are significant.

Intraoperative Factors

Antimicrobial Adhesive Drapes

Antimicrobial adhesive drapes, such as Ioban (3M), are commonly used. These consist of an adhesive-backed plastic film that is impregnated with an iodine-containing compound. They have been shown to reduce bacterial contamination of wounds[32] but have not reduced SSI rates in a prospective trial.[33] However, because of their insignificant cost (about $7 US), their use remains at the discretion of the surgeon.

Antibiotic Prophylaxis

The cornerstone for antibiotic prophylaxis is the assumption that every wound will be contaminated by skin flora. The goal is to reduce bacterial contamination to levels that can more easily be eradicated by host defenses. Although debate continues regarding the role of antibiotic prophylaxis in clean soft tissue surgery, there is general agreement that it is indicated whenever bone is incised or hardware is implanted, or when SSI would pose catastrophic risk; these criteria neatly circumscribe spinal surgery.

Timing and route of administration should follow the tenet of providing a tissue concentration of antibiotic that is greater than the minimum bactericidal concentration (MBC) of the organisms most likely to cause infection (i.e., *Staphylococcus* spp.) at the time of incision and maintaining same until the skin is closed. A first-generation cephalosporin (usually cefazolin) is most often given. Peak serum concentration of cefazolin, when given intravenously, is achieved within 5 minutes. The half-life is 1.5 to 2.5 hours; however, with doses commonly given (1 g), the MBC is generally maintained for 4 hours or more. Based on this, redosing cefazolin every 4 hours during the operation is indicated. This regimen also provides for adequate concentrations of cefazolin in clotted blood that remains in the surgical bed postoperatively. Patients allergic to penicillins may require vancomycin or clindamycin for prophylaxis. Vancomycin is also recommended by the CDC if a cluster of infections due to methicillin-resistant organisms is detected; however, no scientific cutoff has been determined for this, and its routine use as prophylaxis is discouraged.[23]

Antibiotic prophylaxis, according to the guidelines of the CDC and others,[23,34] should be continued throughout the operation, but should be terminated not more than 24 hours postoperatively. It is important to remember that the use of prophylactic antibiotics can be associated with infectious complications and *Clostridium difficile* colitis.[35,36] There is no good evidence to support the practice of "drain prophylaxis" or the continuation of antibiotics until surgical drains have been removed.

Core Body Temperature

Maintenance of normothermia during a surgical procedure is perhaps one of the most important tools in preventing SSI. Hypothermia is easily caused by the combination of general anesthesia, patient exposure, and a cold operating room.

Hypothermia can cause impaired immune function, including reduced antibody production, decreased chemotaxis, and phagocytosis. Kurz et al. conducted an RCT of 200 patients undergoing major colon surgery.[37] Core body temperature was allowed to trend downward in the control group (n = 96; mean, 34.7°C) and maintained with warmed fluids and forced warm air heating blankets in the experimental group (n = 104; mean, 36.6°C). The infection rate in the former was 18.8% compared with 5.8% in the latter, a significant difference. Additionally, the normothermic patients tolerated solid food sooner, were discharged earlier, and had greater collagen deposition in the wound. Several other studies were not nearly as well-designed but showed similar results.[38,39]

It is incumbent on the surgical team to assist the anesthesiologist in maintenance of normothermia throughout the case. Anecdotally, it seems easier to maintain temperature than it is to warm up an anesthetized patient who has been allowed to become hypothermic. This can generally be accomplished by keeping the patient covered until skin prep and the operating room warm until the drapes and warm air blankets are applied.

Intraoperative Hyperoxygenation

Providing hyperoxygenation during an operation has recently gained attention as a possible means of reducing SSIs. The theoretical backing is strong; however, the clinical evidence is mixed, and prolonged hyperoxia is known to have detrimental effects.

The rationale for hyperoxygenation is based on the positive role of oxygen in both the immune system and wound healing. Superoxide radicals are generated by neutrophils to carry out nonspecific killing, which is the body's first line of defense against micro-organisms. An increase in the arterial partial pressure of oxygen, P_aO_2, should lead to a subsequent increase in the tissue partial pressure of oxygen, P_tO_2. Furthermore, an increase of P_tO_2 should lead to optimal collagen formation via the increased activity of prolyl hydroxylase.

In experimental studies the role of operative hyperoxia has proven uncertain. Greif et al. studied 500 patients undergoing major colorectal procedures.[40] Oxygen was administered at the fraction of inspired oxygen, F_iO_2 = 0.3 (control) or 0.8 (experimental). This was continued throughout the procedure and for 2 hours postoperatively. The infection rate in the hyperoxic group was 5.2%, compared with 11.2% in the control group.

These results have yet to be repeated in a study of similar size and design. In another study of 160 patients, Pryor et al. found the infection rate of the hyperoxic group to be 25%, compared with 11% in the control group.[41] This is the opposite of what the earlier study showed, and what would be predicted theoretically. However, this study's design has been criticized on several grounds, including the small sample size and some significant differences between the control and experimental groups. Finally, Belda et al., in a study of 300 patients, found results similar to those of Greif et al.[42]

This is an area of study that shows some promise, and hopefully further studies will be published. Nevertheless, the results are far from consistent at this point, and with the known risks of hyperoxia, it is difficult to justify the routine use of this technique for the prevention of infection.

Surgical Drains

Few subjects spark as much controversy among surgeons as the use of surgical drains. Advocates point out the theoretical basis that drains remove blood (itself an excellent culture medium), remove bacteria, and prevent hematoma formation. Opponents cite local immunosuppression and the role of drains as a conduit for bacteria.

At all events, no convincing evidence proves that drains alter the infection rate, one way or the other, in spinal surgery. There is some argument from other disciplines that drains can increase the infection rate, at least drains of the open (i.e., Penrose) variety.[27,43-45] However, this must be taken with a grain of salt, as direct interdisciplinary comparisons cannot necessarily be made.

General surgeons and others who work in the abdomen and pelvis are afforded several luxuries that are not available to spine surgeons. First, they generally work in well-defined tissue planes. This is not the case with dorsal approaches to the spine, which involve a subperiosteal dissection. Second, their dissections along clean tissue planes allow for optimal hemostasis. In the case of spine surgery, incised bone always bleeds, and muscle often does. And third, a hematoma of 200 mL in the peritoneum or retroperitoneum is a nonevent. This is hardly the case for a hematoma of similar size in a subfascial laminectomy bed.

Because of the inherently low infection rate in spinal surgery, and the likely minimal impact of drains on the infection rate, the number of patients needed for an RCT are substantial. Illustrative of this point is an article by Brown and Brookfield.[46] Eighty-three patients were enrolled and underwent lumbar procedures "larger than single-level unilateral decompressions." Drain placement was randomized. However, there were no infections. In fact, the only significant result was a higher temperature on postoperative day 1 in the drained group. The significance of this is unclear. In their discussion, the investigators eloquently summarized the reason definitive evidence for or against the use of drains in spinal surgery is unlikely: "We used data on rates of infection from previously published drain studies to estimate the sample size necessary to achieve a power of 0.80. Based on these numbers, it was determined that 9,539 patients would have to be randomized into two groups to determine a true statistically significant difference. We discontinued the study after enrolling a more realistic sample size of 83 patients."

The most reasonable alternative, and the place where the spine community should look for answers to this question, is probably the orthopaedic literature, especially that related to total joint arthroplasty. Similarities include the need to dissect through muscle, the necessary incision of bone in every case, similar blood loss, and the implantation of hardware.

In a meta-analysis of RCTs in the orthopaedic literature, 3689 wounds were studied in 3495 patients.[47] All patients underwent total hip or knee arthroplasty, and the groups were evenly divided with regard to drain placement. Although there was a trend toward lower infection rates in the group with drains, it was not significant. What was significant, however, was an increased transfusion requirement in the drained patients.

Any good evidence for or against drains is offset by the evidence on the other side of the argument. However, general words of caution always apply. Drains are not a substitute for good hemostasis. They should not be left as a matter of routine, but should be used when indicated. And if drains are employed, one should realize that the studies cited here all utilized closed-suction–type drains, and the results likely do not apply to open (i.e., Penrose) drains.

Operating Room Hygiene

In the United States, the design of operating rooms, including size, layout, and air-handling systems, is dictated by the recommendations of the American Institute of Architects. Surgeons have little control over these factors. They can, however, control what happens inside the operating room, and they can empower the operating room staff to exert such control as well. Much of what we do is dictated by expert opinion and tradition. We should not expect any more solid evidence to support this, as the ethical justification for such scientific trials would be suspect, at best. Summarized here are some of the protocols that are violated most frequently.

Traffic should be kept to a minimum during a procedure. Although the surgeons are generally present in a case for the duration, this is not true of the others in the room. Allowing breaks for the scrub and circulating nurses and the anesthetist is a matter of established routine, but it still increases traffic flow into and out of the operating room. To be avoided is the practice of a person entering the room to ask if breaks are desired. This can be accomplished by use of the telephone. Certainly the restocking of surgical and anesthetic supplies should not take place during a case.

The Association of periOperative Registered Nurses (AORN) maintains a list of operating room standards and recommendations.[48] This set of clear, straightforward guidelines should be familiar to all practicing surgeons. Among other things, they advise against covering sterile fields. This is because the cover can create air currents during removal, which could carry bacteria or contaminants onto the field and also because nonsterile parts of the cover may brush against the field during removal.

One of the most important aspects is maintenance of the sterile field. AORN recommends a boundary of 12 inches between nonsterile personnel and the sterile field; asking for a greater distance in order to achieve the specified 12 inches seems a perfectly reasonable approach.

Postoperative Factors

Glucose Control

The importance of tight glucose control in the postoperative period cannot be overstated. Although most of the evidence here comes from the critical care, general, and cardiothoracic literature, it clearly shows that poor control of serum glucose levels is associated with infectious complications.

In a landmark study, 1548 ICU patients (mostly postsurgical) were randomized to one of two regimens of glucose control.[49] In the control group, patients were started on an insulin drip if the serum glucose measured 215 mg/dL or higher, and the same was adjusted to maintain serum glucose of 180 to 200 mg/dL. The study group was started on an insulin drip for any reading greater than 110 mg/dL and titrated to maintain 80 to 110 mg/dL.

The amount of insulin administered to the study group was over twice what was given to the controls, and 98.7% of the study group received insulin at some point. (It is noteworthy that this study looked at all ICU patients, and not just diabetics.) Compared with the control group, the patients receiving intensive insulin therapy had a decreased chance of requiring ventilator support or hemodialysis; a 46% reduction in the number of patients who became bacteremic at any point; and a lower mortality rate if the ICU stay extended beyond 5 days.

A dose-response–type relationship between postoperative blood glucose levels and deep sternal wound infections has been reported in several studies of cardiac surgery patients.[50,51] These levels seem to be most important in the first 48 hours postoperatively.

Summary

SSIs are one of the greatest challenges that we face in spinal surgery. Considering the devastating effect on patients, emphasis must be on prevention rather than treatment. A certain proportion of infections occur regardless of the preventative measures employed; however, spine surgeons must be vigilant in modifying the many variables within our control. It is important to remember that the process of preventing infections extends well beyond the operating room, to the clinic preoperatively and the ICU and ward postoperatively.

KEY REFERENCES

Klein JD, Hey LA, Yu CS, et al: Perioperative nutrition and postoperative complications in patients undergoing spinal surgery. *Spine (Phila Pa 1976)* 21(22):2676–2682, 1996.

Kurz A, Sessler DI, Lenhardt R: Perioperative normothermia to reduce the incidence of surgical-wound infection and shorten hospitalization. Study of Wound Infection and Temperature Group. *N Engl J Med* 334(19):1209–1215, 1996.

Maki DG, Ringer M, Alvarado CJ: Prospective randomised trial of povidone-iodine, alcohol, and chlorhexidine for prevention of infection associated with central venous and arterial catheters. *Lancet* 338(8763):339–343, 1991.

National Nosocomial Infections Surveillance (NNIS) System Report, data summary from January 1992 through June 2004, issued October 2004. *Am J Infect Control* 32(8):470–485, 2004.

Tanner J, Woodings D, Moncaster K: Preoperative hair removal to reduce surgical site infection. *Cochrane Database Syst Rev* 3:CD004122, 2006.

van den Berghe G, Wouters P, Weekers F, et al: Intensive insulin therapy in the critically ill patients. *N Engl J Med* 345(19):1359–1367, 2001.

REFERENCES

The complete reference list is available online at expertconsult.com.

CHAPTER 199

Medical Complications

Robert G. Louis | Monir N. Tabbosha | Mark E. Shaffrey

The morbidity and mortality that result from medical complications of complex spine surgery have been extensively documented. The rate and severity of these complications vary widely depending on a number of factors, including age, medical comorbidities, length and complexity of the operation, and acuity of the inciting problem. The range of complications is wide and can include thromboembolic disease, pneumonia, cardiac-related events, ileus, renal failure, infection, paralysis, and blindness. Although preventive measures can help to minimize the risks, a high index of suspicion is imperative for early recognition and timely management. Even with the most comprehensive prophylactic standards in place, medical complications can and do occur. However, by employing an evidence-based approach to preventing, diagnosing, and treating these complications, we can hope to continue to increase the safety and cost-effectiveness of complex spine surgery.

Thromboembolic Disease

Incidence

Thromboembolic disease is one of the most significant potential complications after spine surgery, with rates of acute deep venous thrombosis (DVT) ranging from 0.3% to 31%, with an overall DVT incidence of 2.2%.[1] These rates vary substantially depending on a number of factors. Overall, as expected, the lowest rates occur in younger patients undergoing simple elective procedures, whereas the highest reported rates are those in patients with preexisting risk factors that predispose them to DVT.

Risk Factors

Virchow's triad of venous stasis, endothelial injury, and hypercoagulability is the classic description of the combination of factors that may predispose a person to DVT. In addition, general clinical risk factors include advanced age, trauma, previous DVT, stroke, malignancy, smoking, and exogenous estrogen replacement. While numerous systems have been developed to attempt stratification of DVT risk in surgical patients, many are cumbersome and therefore not of practical utility for most surgeons. However, one of the simpler systems involves assignment of a patient into one of four categories on the basis of complexity of procedure (major vs. minor), age, and additional risk factors such as prior DVT, hypercoagulability, and malignancy.[2] In general, spine surgery patients are at a higher risk than general surgery patients secondary to the postoperative immobility that may occur due to pain or neurologic deficits.[3,4] Conversely, the risk is significantly lower than that for patients undergoing lower-extremity surgery such as total hip or knee replacement, which can be associated with DVT rates as high as 50%.[2] While the overall risk of DVT in spine surgery patients can be described as moderate, the degree of immobility, and thus the risk of DVT, can be directly correlated with the type of spine procedure being performed. For example, patients undergoing a single-level anterior cervical discectomy and fusion are often treated in outpatient surgical centers and discharged home the same day, thereby minimizing the amount of postoperative bedrest and risk of DVT. Patients undergoing more extensive and complex surgery, particularly those with traumatic spinal cord injury (SCI), are at the highest risk. With regard to acute SCI, the incidence of DVT has been reported as ranging from 10% to 100% without prophylaxis and from 0% to 7% with prophylaxis. Interestingly, no correlation has been observed between level of injury, American Spinal Injury Association (ASIA) grade, or spasticity and the incidence of DVT.[1]

Unfortunately, there is a limited amount of evidence regarding the specific risks of DVT in spine surgery patients. One study that used routine venography in patients undergoing spine surgery who did not receive any prophylaxis reported an incidence of 15.5%.[4] It is important to note that none of these patients had any clinical evidence of DVT, underscoring the low sensitivity of physical signs in the diagnosis of DVT. Furthermore, the same authors found that lumbar surgery carries a much higher risk of DVT (21%) as compared to cervical surgery (6%).[4] As was previously noted, the risk of DVT may also increase with the complexity of the procedure because more complex operations have longer operative times and often increased postoperative immobility. The use of ventral and lateral approaches further elevates the risk by requiring manipulation of vessels, particularly major veins, and thus increasing the chance for endothelial disruption. Dearborn et al. reported an incidence of 6% in patients undergoing combined ventral/dorsal approaches compared to 0.5% in patients in whom only a dorsal approach was employed.[5]

Prevention

Recommendations for DVT prophylaxis for patients undergoing spine procedures are varied and inconsistent. This inconsistency stems largely from the lack of rigorous supporting evidence for many of the prophylactic measures that are employed. Available prophylactic modalities include the use of gradient compression stockings (GCSs) or intermittent pneumatic compression devices (ICDs), administration of low-dose unfractionated heparin (LDUH) or low-molecular-weight heparin (LMWH), and the placement of a caval filter. The first step in determining appropriate DVT prophylaxis for an individual patient is assessing the risk of DVT using the criteria described previously. This risk depends heavily on the procedure being performed and the patient's age and comorbid conditions. In 2004, the American College of Chest Physicians published guidelines for prevention of venous thromboembolism.[2] These recommendations are summarized in Box 199-1.

While these guidelines may serve as a foundation on which clinical decisions may be based, the decision on when and how to appropriately administer DVT prophylaxis for spine surgery patients remains a subject of significant controversy. The risks of each prophylactic intervention must be compared to the risks of DVT in each individual patient. Most spine surgeons routinely prescribe some form of DVT prophylaxis in almost all patients. As was previously mentioned, the evidence to support these policies is far from unequivocal. At baseline, most spine patients will be fitted with ICDs or GCSs as a primary method of DVT prophylaxis, as the effectiveness of mechanical prophylaxis has been demonstrated and the risks associated with their use is extremely low. One caveat of ICD use is that their effectiveness depends on perioperative and postoperative employment, as the highest risk for DVT development occurs at induction of anesthesia.

While the risk of DVT may be further decreased with the use of pharmacologic anticoagulation, the controversy surrounding its use is significant. Several small studies have demonstrated the effectiveness of LDUH and LMWH in spine surgery patients. In a double-blind randomized controlled trial, Agnelli and Becattini demonstrated a reduction in DVT incidence from 30% in patients treated with ICD alone to 17% in patients treated with ICD plus LMWH.[6] The paucity of sufficient evidence to definitively support the use of medical anticoagulation combined with concerns for increased intraoperative blood loss and postoperative epidural hematoma formation has led to a lack of standardized guidelines for DVT prophylaxis in spine surgery patients.[1]

We adjust the prophylactic regimen according to the neurologic condition, ambulatory status, age, procedure performed, and medical comorbidities of each patient. Preoperatively, hospitalized patients on bedrest or patients with neurologic deficits that affect the lower extremities are treated with ICDs. Intraoperatively, all patients receive continuous treatments with ICDs. It is also customary during prolonged ventral approaches to provide periodic release of retraction to decrease tension of the great vessels. Postoperatively, ICDs alone are continued if the patient will be ambulatory within the first 24 hours. If there are significant neurologic deficits or pain control issues that limit mobility within the first 24 hours, LDUH (given as 5000 IU subcutaneously every 8 hours) is started on the morning of postoperative day 1. If ICDs cannot be tolerated owing to injury of the lower extremities, LDUH is administered perioperatively. For long-term prophylaxis in an outpatient or rehabilitation setting, LMWH is used, the higher cost being traded for improvement of patient compliance and reduction in the need for laboratory monitoring.

BOX 199-1. Recommendations for Deep Venous Thrombosis Prophylaxis in Patients Undergoing Spine Surgery

- For spine surgery patients with no additional risk factors, the routine use of any thromboprophylaxis modality, apart from early and persistent mobilization, is not recommended.
- Some form of prophylaxis may be used in patients undergoing spinal surgery who exhibit additional risk factors, such as advanced age, known malignancy, presence of a neurologic deficit, previous venous thromboembolism (VTE), or a ventral surgical approach.
- For patients with additional risk factors, any of the following prophylaxis options is recommended: postoperative low-dose unfractionated heparin (LDUH) alone, postoperative low-molecular-weight heparin (LMWH) alone, or perioperative intermittent pneumatic compression devices (ICDs) alone.
- In patients with multiple risk factors for VTE, combining LDUH or LMWH with gradient compression stockings (GCSs) and/or ICDs is recommended.
- Thromboprophylaxis should be provided for all patients with acute spinal cord injury (SCI).
- The use of LDUH, GCSs, or ICDs as single prophylaxis modalities in patients with acute SCI is not recommended.
- In patients with acute SCI, we recommend prophylaxis with LMWH, to be commenced once primary hemostasis is evident. The combined use of ICDs and either LDUH or LWMH as alternatives to LMWH is recommended.
- The use of ICDs and/or GCSs when anticoagulant prophylaxis is contraindicated early after injury is recommended.
- The use of an inferior vena cava filter as primary prophylaxis against pulmonary embolism is not recommended.
- During the rehabilitation phase following acute SCI, the continuation of LMWH prophylaxis or conversion to an oral anticoagulant agent (international normalized ratio [INR] target, 2.5; INR range, 2–3) is recommended.

Based on 2004 American College of Chest Physicians Guidelines.

Screening and Diagnosis

Clinical diagnosis of DVT remains a concern as less than 50% of patients will exhibit clinical signs.[1,7] This raises the question of whether routine screening should be employed as a method of early detection. While there are some authors who advocate routine screening, there does seem to be at least a majority consensus that routine screening for DVT with ultrasound or venography is not clinically indicated after spine surgery. Similarly, a comprehensive review by Furlan and Fehlings concluded that there is insufficient evidence to support routine screening for DVT in patients with acute SCI.[7]

If routine screening is not indicated, the question arises as to the most sensitive and cost-effective method for diagnosis of DVT in patients in whom DVT is suspected. Lower-extremity pain and tenderness, leg edema, and low-grade fevers can be nonspecific indicators of DVT. While DVT is confirmed in only 10% to 25% of patients in whom it is suspected clinically, clinical suspicion remains an important first step in the initiation of more accurate diagnostic testing.[8]

Beyond clinical suspicion, objective confirmatory tests remain mandatory for accurate diagnosis of DVT. Contrast venography continues to be the gold standard for diagnosis of DVT against which other tests are measured. No other modality is as sensitive and specific for both proximal and distal DVT. However, high cost, limited availability, patient discomfort, and contrast reactions have led to the increased use of less invasive diagnostic modalities. By using a pressurized cuff, impedance plethysmography measures the change in electrical impedance of the lower extremity in response to occlusion of the deep venous system. The sensitivity and specificity are high for proximal DVT and lower for distal DVT on single examinations. The accuracy can therefore be increased with serial examinations. By comparison, B-mode ultrasonography is as sensitive as plethysmography for proximal DVT and more sensitive for distal DVT. The addition of Doppler flow analysis in conjunction with ultrasonography has demonstrated sensitivity and specificity of 95% to 100% and has therefore become the diagnostic modality of choice in most clinical settings.[9-11]

Treatment

Management of acute DVT is directed toward reducing both the short-term (pulmonary embolism [PE], clot propagation) and long-term (postphlebitic syndrome) complications. General management includes bedrest, elevation of edematous extremities, and administration of appropriate analgesics (non–platelet-active agents). Definitive management of acute proximal DVT requires a decision regarding risk of anticoagulation to the patient. If the risk for systemic anticoagulation is acceptable, treatment of established DVT may be initiated in several ways. Because the risks of using oral anticoagulation agents alone have been well documented, a safe and effective treatment strategy must include an initial course of continuous intravenous unfractionated heparin (IVUH), subcutaneous LMWH, or subcutaneous fondaparinux. The need for an initial course of heparin has been demonstrated in a double-blind, randomized trial with a threefold reduction in recurrent venous thromboembolic events compared with oral anticoagulants alone.[12] This is thought to be the result of the long half-life of factor II (compared to proteins C and S), which results in an initial hypercoagulable state at the onset of oral anticoagulant therapy. Recommendations for treatment of acute DVT, summarized in Box 199-2, are based on the ACCP guidelines for patients with DVT.[13]

The aforementioned regimen remains our preferred means of managing thromboembolism. It does, however, carry risks of morbidity. The medical and surgical literature contains numerous reports of complications related to heparin therapy. These complications include thrombocytopenia and thrombotic disorders, skin necrosis, priapism, spontaneous hemorrhage, gastrointestinal bleeding, and epidural hematoma formation.[14,15] Decortication of portions of the vertebral column and the creation of large potential dead space during exposure predisposes the spine surgery patient to an even higher risk of hemorrhagic complications and hematoma formation.[16] Furthermore, following decompressive surgery, hematomas are often in direct continuity with the thecal sac, placing neural structures at risk of injury, thus necessitating further surgical intervention and its additional risks.

BOX 199-2. Recommendations for Treatment of Deep Venous Thrombosis

Anticoagulation

- Treatment should begin simultaneously (day 1) with both oral anticoagulants and intravenous unfractionated heparin (IVUH), low-molecular-weight heparin (LMWH), or fondaparinux.
- IVUH, LMWH, or fondaparinux should continue until the international normalized ratio (INR) is ≥2 for 24 hours.
- IVUH, LMWH, or fondaparinux should continue for a minimum of 5 days.
- For both inpatients and outpatients, LMWH is preferred over IVUH.
- For patients treated with LMWH, routine monitoring of antifactor Xa levels is not recommended.
- Target INR of 2–3 should be maintained throughout the duration of treatment.

Inferior Vena Cava Filter

- The routine use of an inferior vena cava filter (IVCF) in addition to anticoagulation is not recommended.
- If anticoagulation is contraindicated due to risk of bleeding, an IVCF should be placed for the prevention of pulmonary embolism. In these patients, anticoagulation therapy should be initiated once the risk of bleeding resolves.

Duration of Treatment

- For patients with first-time deep venous thrombosis (DVT) and known transient risk factors, anticoagulation should be continued for 3 months.
- For recurrent DVT or in patients for whom risk factors cannot be identified or have not resolved, long-term anticoagulation is recommended, with reassessment at periodic intervals.
- Graduated compression stocking should be initiated as soon as possible after initiation of anticoagulation and should be continued for at least 2 years.

Based on 2004 American College of Chest Physicians Guidelines.

Pulmonary Embolism

The diagnosis and treatment of DVT and PE are often discussed separately, but there is increasing evidence that these two entities should be considered the same disease process. The incidence of PE in spine surgery has been reported as ranging from 0% to 13%, with a mean incidence of 2.5%.[17] As with DVT, the risk of development of PE is lowest in patients undergoing simple elective surgery (i.e., microdiscectomy) and highest with ventral or combined thoracolumbar/lumbar procedures.[17]

Initial Evaluation

Common clinical manifestations of PE include tachypnea, dyspnea, and pleuritic chest pain. The initial evaluation for clinical suspicion of PE includes chest radiograph, arterial blood gas measurements, and electrocardiogram. The arterial blood gas measurement is useful to demonstrate alterations of oxygen transfer that accompany the ventilation of lungs that have a reduction of pulmonary vascular inflow (ventilation/perfusion mismatch). Arterial blood gases typically reveal respiratory alkalosis, variable reduction in partial arterial oxygen pressure, and widening of the alveolar-arterial oxygen pressure gradient. Chest radiographs and electrocardiograms are more important and are used to rule out other diagnoses, such as pneumonia, pneumothorax, myocardial infarction, or pulmonary edema. Occasionally, the electrocardiogram may reveal right axis deviation or a right bundle branch block that may aid in the diagnosis of PE. Most commonly, chest radiographs reveal nonspecific findings such as pleural effusion, infiltrate, atelectasis, or elevation of the hemidiaphragm or are negative. Measurement of brain natriuretic peptide (BNP) is sensitive but not specific for diagnosis of PE.[18] Similarly, measurements of serum D-dimer (by enzyme-linked immunosorbent assay) have a high sensitivity but low specificity, particularly in postoperative patients, as the D-dimer may be elevated from the procedure.[19] However, the utility of D-dimer assays remain in that the negative predictive value of levels below threshold (<500 ng/mL) are sufficient to exclude PE in patients with low or moderate pretest probability.

Diagnostic Modalities

If suspicion remains high for PE after initial evaluation, further diagnostic workup is recommended. The choice of diagnostic tests depends on multiple factors, including clinical probability of PE, availability of modality, patient condition, and cost. While pulmonary angiography remains the gold standard for diagnosis of PE, its invasive nature and the development of modern imaging techniques have dramatically decreased its utility. The widespread availability of spiral CT scanners has allowed for the increasing use of a CT pulmonary angiogram in the diagnosis of PE. The diagnostic sensitivity and specificity of a CT pulmonary angiogram are 83% and 96%, respectively.[20] In patients who are intolerant to IV contrast or those with prohibitively poor renal function, a ventilation/perfusion scan remains an option for the diagnosis of PE. The diagnostic accuracy of the ventilation/perfusion scan appears to be similar to that of the CT pulmonary angiogram both in overall sensitivity and in the observation that results must be correlated with clinical suspicion. Specifically, a negative scan in a patient with low pretest probability virtually excludes the diagnosis of PE.

Treatment

The treatment of patients with "nonmassive" PE is exactly the same as that previously described for DVT. However, IVUH is recommended over LMWH for the treatment of massive PE and in patients with significant renal impairment.[21] Massive PE with significant hemodynamic compromise requires urgent intervention with acute thrombolysis, surgical embolectomy, or, more recently, percutaneous transvenous fragmentation or removal of emboli.

Disseminated Intravascular Coagulation

Spine surgery and, in particular, deformity surgery have been associated with an increased incidence of disseminated intravascular coagulation. Several mechanisms may contribute to this, including injury to soft tissue, muscle, and bone, which releases tissue thromboplastin and may lead to disseminated intravascular coagulation.[22] Disseminated intravascular coagulation is a consumptive coagulopathy in which microvascular thrombosis results in end-organ damage and depletion of clotting factors and platelets. The result is a mixed picture of organ ischemia and hemorrhage. Laboratory findings included depletion of platelets, prolongations in both prothrombin time and partial thromboplastin time, and increased D-dimer. However, many of these may be nonspecific, as they can arise from surgical blood loss with inadequate repletion. Treatment involves replacement of platelets and clotting factors with both fresh-frozen plasma and cryoprecipitate. Transfusion of platelets should be based on bleeding or a high risk of bleeding. Included in this group are postoperative patients with a platelet count of less than 50,000 μL. In patients with a predominantly thrombotic picture, anticoagulation with IVUH should be considered. As with DVT and PE, the benefits of anticoagulation must be carefully weighed against the risks of significant bleeding.[23]

Other Pulmonary Complications

Pneumonias, respiratory failure, and prolonged intubation are all common in patients undergoing major spine procedures, especially those with SCI. Immobility, particularly when combined with neurologic injury, can lead to atelectasis, stasis of respiratory secretions, and pneumonia. Bacterial pneumonia may be either an early-onset (within 4 days) or a late-onset complication. Organisms associated with early-onset pneumonia are similar to those found in community-acquired pneumonia, mainly *Streptococcus pneumoniae*, *Haemophilus influenzae*, and methicillin-sensitive *Staphylococcus aureus*. Late-onset pneumonia is often more severe and associated with more virulent and resistant organisms, including *Pseudomonas* and *Acinetobacter*.[24]

Severe and diffuse lung injury has also been documented following spine surgery, including acute respiratory distress syndrome (ARDS) and transfusion-related acute lung injury. Risk factors for ARDS in patients undergoing spine surgery include aspiration, pulmonary contusion, hypotension, multiple transfusions, infection, and sepsis.[25] Clinically, ARDS presents with hypoxemia that is resistant to increasing oxygen therapy. The diagnosis of ARDS is established by the following criteria: chest radiograph demonstrating multiple diffuse infiltrates, pulmonary capillary wedge pressure greater than 18 mmHg, and PaO_2 to FiO_2 ratio of 200 or less. ARDS is treated with mechanical ventilation that trades increased positive end expiratory pressure to decrease FiO_2 requirements and uses low tidal volumes and plateau pressures of 30 mm H_2O or less. Additional measures include frequent changes in body/bed position, bronchodilators, and sufficient sedation to prevent asynchronous ventilation.[26] Even with aggressive treatment, the mortality associated with ARDS is greater than 30%.[27]

In patients with a complete SCI above C4, phrenic nerve function is lost; therefore, diaphragmatic function is typically absent. These patients require mechanical ventilation. With injury at C4 and C5, the patient has compromise of diaphragm function and may require short-term ventilatory support (long-term support if there is preexisting pulmonary disease). At lower cervical and thoracic levels, the loss of innervation to the accessory muscles of respiration and to the intercostal muscles can impair respiratory function. Because of the recumbent position in postoperative patients and patients with unstable spines, the respiratory capacity is decreased.

To decrease the pulmonary complications associated with these factors, clinicians should immediately institute aggressive pulmonary toilet, including aerosol treatments, chest physiotherapy, and frequent turning (either by logrolling or preferably by using rotational beds). Shifting the body position prevents any portion of the lung from remaining chronically dependent. In mechanically ventilated patients, frequent suctioning is essential. Instillation of normal saline (5 mL) or acetylcysteine often helps to mobilize viscous secretions. Bronchoscopy may become necessary for refractory atelectasis or mucous plugging, especially in quadriplegic patients who are unable to cough and clear their own secretions. In patients who are not intubated, incentive spirometry should be encouraged hourly while they are awake. In patients with SCI, stabilization of the spinal column should be carried out as soon as the patient's medical condition permits. Early mobilization is important. Postoperatively, patients should be mobilized as soon as their condition permits, and early, aggressive physical and occupational therapy should be initiated.

Cardiac and Vascular Complications

Cardiac complications, including myocardial infarction, are the most common cause of perioperative death in spine surgery patients. The overall incidence of myocardial infarction in patients without known coronary artery disease who are undergoing lumbar fusion procedures is 0.8%.[28] It is important to consider that these complications can occur in patients with no history of coronary artery disease and that the incidence of silent myocardial ischemia is estimated to be as high as 15%. The specific risks for development of perioperative myocardial infarction include age over 60 years, male gender, abdominal obesity, smoking, hypertension, diabetes mellitus, reduced high-density lipoprotein, and calcified atherosclerosis in the aorta or common iliac vessels. Asymptomatic myocardial ischemia can be identified with dobutamine echocardiography, thallium perfusion scintigraphy, or continuous 24-hour electrocardiographic monitoring.[29] In patients with multiple risk factors, we recommend preoperative screening with one of these modalities. Interestingly, one study of lumbar fusions found no correlation between cardiac complications and factors related to surgery, including approach, type of surgery, operating time, and blood loss.[30]

Neurogenic Shock

Neurogenic shock can occur in patients with SCI at T6 or above because of the loss of thoracic sympathetic outflow. This results in decreased venous tone, causing pooling of the blood volume in the extremities and hypotension. The decreased sympathetic tone to the heart may result in bradycardia, exacerbating hypotension. Peripheral vasculature dilation results in core hypothermia, although the skin temperature remains warm. Hypotension should be treated with pressor agents such as dopamine (which also increases the heart rate at higher doses); if there is a component of hypovolemic shock, fluid resuscitation is also necessary, but hypervolemia should be avoided.

Gastrointestinal Complications

Stress Ulcerations

The stress resulting from a complicated surgery, traumatic injury, and mechanical ventilation as well as preoperative use of steroidal and nonsteroidal anti-inflammatory drugs can predispose a patient to ulcer formation. Stress ulcerations appear to be related to ischemia of gastric capillary beds, resulting in diminished resistance of the gastric lining to the digestive secretions of the stomach. The incidences of gastritis and ulcer formation in spine surgery patients are 0.33% and 0.08%, respectively.[31] There has been a gradual reduction in the incidence of severe bleeding from stress ulcerations. This is thought to result from a combination of routine prophylaxis (antacids, H_2 blockers, proton pump inhibitors, or sucralfate) and improved attention to tissue oxygenation.[32] We advocate standard administration of either an H_2 blocker or a proton pump inhibitor for all patients undergoing spine surgery.

Adynamic Ileus

Adynamic ileus is a well-known complication of spine surgery, with an incidence of 5% to 12%.[33] Ileus is characterized by abdominal distention and absent bowel sounds. Nausea and vomiting, respiratory distress, a feeling of constipation, or abdominal tenderness may be present. Copious gas is diffusely distributed through the intestine and colon, often with fluid levels. The diaphragm may be elevated and have diminished motion. If the clinical picture and plain radiography provide an inconclusive diagnosis, contrast medium can be given orally. In adynamic ileus, some contrast medium should reach the cecum in 4 hours; a stationary column for 3 to 4 hours indicates complete obstruction. Ileus usually persists for 36 to 48 hours, and treatment includes restriction of oral intake and administration of bowel stimulants, enemas, or laxatives. In some cases, nasogastric suction and replacement of electrolytes may be required.

In SCI, patients rapidly become catabolic, and parenteral nutrition should begin early, often with total parenteral nutrition within 24 to 48 hours of admission. Metoclopramide, a dopamine antagonist, can increase intestinal motility without inducing spasm and can be used for postoperative ileus. In rare instances, adynamic ileus does not respond to conservative treatment, and operative intervention is needed. If no mechanical obstruction is found, a long nasogastric suction tube is fed into the small bowel, and tube cecostomy may be indicated. This initially exacerbates the ileus. However, the bowel can now be adequately decompressed.

Ogilvie Syndrome

Ogilvie syndrome, or pseudo-obstruction of the colon, is characterized by massive abdominal distention with a cecal diameter greater than 9 cm. Nausea and vomiting, constipation, diarrhea, and pain are all more common in Ogilvie syndrome than in adynamic ileus. The diagnosis is made by the clinical findings, including high-pitched bowel sounds, and radiographic findings of marked distention of the proximal colon with distal cutoff of colonic gas. The radiographic findings may be difficult to distinguish from those of cecal volvulus.

Colonic pseudo-obstruction is a major contributor to morbidity and lengthened hospital stays, occurring in as many as 12% of all spine surgery patients.[34] Delayed diagnosis can result in serious complications, including spontaneous perforation in up to 3%, with an attendant mortality rate of 50%.[35] Patients at increased risk are those who have had previous abdominal surgeries, more extensive dissections, retroperitoneal hematomas, major intraoperative fluid shifts, and excessive narcotic use.[33] Initial treatment for Ogilvie syndrome includes nasogastric suction, insertion of rectal tubes, cessation of oral intake, and cessation of narcotics. Patients who fail to respond to these measures may undergo pharmacologic interventions, if they are not contraindicated, before the clinician considers colonoscopic decompression. Numerous studies have reported the use of the acetylcholinesterase inhibitor neostigmine for treatment of refractory postoperative spine surgery ileus.[36,37] The obstruction is thought to result from an imbalance in the autonomic motor system via excess parasympathetic suppression. Thus, neostigmine acts to increase parasympathetic stimulation, thereby normalizing autonomic stability. Cure rates have been reported to range from 86% to 94% following a single 2-mg IV bolus infusion in appropriately selected patients.[37-40] Side effects following infusion have been reported to occur in fewer than 5% of patients; however, it is essential to note the contraindications to using parasympathetic agents, which includes patients with bradyarrhythmias and bronchospasm. Patients must be monitored by experienced personnel and with telemetry during neostigmine infusion, and atropine must be readily available at the bedside. At our institution, patients are transferred to the intensive-care unit for monitoring if neostigmine is administered.

If pharmacologic means fail or are contraindicated, endoscopic decompression may be performed, though undoubtedly under suboptimal conditions in an unprepared and distended colon, further complicating and increasing the morbidity and mortality of the procedure.[41] Endoscopic decompression is reported to be successful in approximately 70% of cases, although approximately one third of patients require multiple endoscopic procedures for complete resolution.[42] Failure of colonoscopic decompression requires surgical laparotomy and tube cecostomy with a concomitant mortality rate reported as high as 26%.[43]

Preventive measures for both adynamic ileus and Ogilvie syndrome include minimizing bedrest, returning to ambulation as rapidly as possible, and limiting the use of narcotics. Early recognition and treatment of these conditions are essential to reducing morbidity and mortality.

Superior Mesenteric Artery Syndrome

Superior mesenteric artery syndrome has been described in patients undergoing correction of kyphotic deformity, with an incidence of 0.5% to 1%.[44,45] While more common in adolescents, superior mesenteric artery syndrome has also been described in adults.[46] Crowther et al. proposed two possible mechanisms: disruption of autonomic supply to the bowel from retroperitoneal dissection and compression of the duodenum between the aorta and the superior mesenteric artery after gain of height (resulting in reduction of the angle between the aorta and the superior mesenteric artery).[47] The onset of superior mesenteric artery syndrome is usually more than 1 week after surgery, and it presents with epigastric distention and tenderness accompanied by present bowel sounds and tympanic percussion. The administration of oral contrast will demonstrate a blockage at the level of the third part of the duodenum. Conservative management is similar to that for ileus, including restriction of oral intact, nasogastric suction, and intravenous alimentation. Failure of these measures warrants a general surgery consultation and may require surgical mobilization or division of the ligament of Treitz.

Pancreatitis

Acute pancreatitis has been reported in patients who have undergone spine surgery. Leichtner et al. reported elevated pancreatic enzymes in 14% of adolescents who had undergone surgery for correction of scoliosis.[48] Up to 70% of these may have associated signs or symptoms. Risk factors include both significant blood loss and intraoperative hypotension. Clinical presentation includes abdominal and back pain, nausea, vomiting and fever, accompanied by tachycardia and leukocytosis. Because these symptoms are relatively nonspecific, a high index of suspicion is necessary for diagnosis. Specific laboratory abnormalities include elevation of amylase and lipase. As isolated elevation of amylase is somewhat common, a diagnosis of clinical pancreatitis requires that the signs and symptoms should be present as well as elevations in both amylase and lipase. While the mechanism of pancreatitis associated with spine surgery remains unknown, treatment is mostly conservative. If pancreatitis is suspected, a consultation from general surgery is recommended along with observation in the intensive care unit.[22] Initial management includes nothing by mouth (NPO) status, aggressive IV fluid resuscitation, and, if necessary, total or partial parenteral nutrition. It is important to differentiate patients with pancreatitis from the more common postoperative ileus; in general, the diagnosis of pancreatitis should be considered in patients with prolonged or severe abdominal pain. If pancreatitis is undiagnosed, the resulting morbidity can be significant. Bragg et al. reported a 50% incidence of subsequent complications, including pancreatic pseudocyst, abscess, or fistula. Furthermore, the same authors reported mortality from pancreatitis in 2 of 15 patients.[49]

Genitourinary Complications

Urinary complications related to retention, infections, and acute renal failure continue to be significant sources of morbidity after spine surgery. The most common genitourinary complication in spine surgery patients is postoperative urinary retention, with an incidence of 38%.[50] Risk factors include advanced age and preoperative use of beta-blockers, while preoperative administration of NSAIDs and narcotic analgesics may reduce the risk. SCI patients are at a particularly high risk, as SCI usually results in a period of spinal shock resulting in the absence of detrusor motor function and bladder sensation, as well as compromise of sphincteric activity. Incomplete emptying of the bladder is common, and elevated bladder pressures may result. This can lead to renal damage from hydroureteronephrosis or vesicoureteral reflux if an appropriate bladder routine is not followed. Initially, placement of a Foley catheter is recommended. If voluntary control of urination is not established at the time the Foley catheter is removed, intermittent clean catheterization is instituted every 4 hours, with the goal of keeping the bladder volume to less than 500 mL.

The overall incidence of urinary tract infection (UTI) in spine surgery patients is 9%.[51] In addition to their importance in increasing cost and length of hospital stay, UTIs are the most common source of sepsis in the postoperative patient. The majority of these UTIs are due to *Escherichia coli* and other gram-negative rods such as *Proteus*, *Enterobacter*, and *Klebsiella*. Fungal UTIs with *Candida* species are also common. Although routine surveillance cultures are not recommended, fever or other signs, including dysuria and urgency, should prompt a diagnostic workup.[52] Urine must be sampled by using aseptic technique and should be sent for laboratory analysis. According to the Centers for Disease Control and Prevention, diagnostic criteria include positive nitrites, positive leukocyte esterase, pyuria, or positive Gram stain.[53] Upon diagnosis, the Foley catheter should be removed or exchanged, and antibiotic therapy should be initiated. Initial therapy should provide broad-spectrum coverage with an antibiotic such as a fluoroquinolone or third-generation cephalosporin. Antibiotic coverage may be narrowed according to culture and sensitivity results. Prevention of UTIs is extremely important, including hand washing prior to insertion and early removal of Foley catheters.

Acute renal failure (ARF) has been reported in up to 1.2% of spine surgery patients and usually results from either prerenal failure or acute tubular necrosis (ATN).[54] Hypotension and hypovolemia that result from long operative times and significant blood loss can often lead to prerenal ARF following spine surgery. Risk factors for prerenal ARF include age, diabetes mellitus, and preexisting chronic renal failure. ARF is defined by an increase in creatinine to 1.65 mg/dL in previously normal patients or a doubling of creatinine in patients with a baseline of more than 2 mg/dL. Adequate volume resuscitation and maintenance of normotension can significantly decrease the risks even in predisposed patients. Similarly, prerenal ARF is readily treated with volume resuscitation and restoration of renal perfusion. Delay in treatment can result in acute tubular necrosis.[55] Additional causes of acute tubular necrosis in spine surgery patients include exposure to nephrotoxins, rhabdomyolysis, and intravenous contrast administration. The treatment of ARF involves reversal or removal of inciting causes, including restoration of normovolemia and discontinuation of nephrotoxic agents. In severe cases, hemodialysis may be required.

Sexual dysfunction is well recognized as a complication following complex spine surgery particularly with ventral approaches. The reported incidence varies by author but has been found to account for as many as 20% of spine surgery–related complications.[33,56] Retrograde ejaculation in particular has been reported by numerous studies, with an incidence ranging from 9% to 24% following anterior lumbar interbody fusion procedures.[33] This is conceivably the result of injury to the superior hypogastric plexus of the sympathetic chain located ventral to the L5-S1 vertebrae.[56] The incidence appears to be higher following transperitoneal and laparoscopic as opposed to retroperitoneal approaches.[57] With regard to complications related to great vessel manipulation and DVT formation secondary to retraction injuries, periodic release of pressure cannot be overemphasized to help minimize the incidence of neural injury. Interestingly, Hagg et al. reported an increase in sexual performance and pleasure in both men and women who had undergone dorsal spine surgery.[57]

Miscellaneous Complications

Delirium

Alterations in mental status are known to occur following spine surgery, particularly in older patients undergoing larger procedures. This is compounded by administration of narcotics and muscle relaxants. One study reported an incidence of delirium of 12.5% in spine surgery patients over 70 years old.[58] Risk factors associated with postoperative delirium include anemia, hypercarbia, hypoxemia, hypoglycemia, UTI, and sepsis.[59] Accordingly, prevention includes maintenance of hematocrit greater than 30%, avoidance of benzodiazepines and anticholinergics, administration of supplemental oxygen, and normalization of glucose and electrolyte balance.[60]

Perioperative Blindness

Acute visual loss is a rare but significant complication following spine surgery. Proposed mechanisms include central retinal artery occlusion, ischemic optic neuropathy, and occipital stroke. Being in a prone position for a long time may result in central retinal artery occlusion by direct compression.[22,61] Risk factors for ischemic optic neuropathy include anemia, dehydration, and hypotension. Prevention is essential; this is achieved by avoiding pressure on the eyes while in the prone position (proper padding around the orbits and placing the table in some reverse Trendelenburg position), maintenance of euvolemia and normotension by anesthetists, and mindfulness concerning the length of the operative procedure.[61] Should visual loss occur, an urgent neuro-ophthalmology consultation is indicated.

Decubitus Ulceration

Sacral and other pressure ulcerations may occur with increased frequency in spine surgery patients. These ulcerations result from prolonged immobility, especially in patients with SCI. Avoidance requires constant vigilance, frequent changes in position, early stabilization and mobilization, and specialized mattresses or air beds that decrease pressure on vulnerable sites. Consultation from a wound care specialist may aid in treatment, including cleansing, prevention of infection, maintenance of adequate nutrition, and protection of adjacent skin.[62]

Conclusions

Medical complications following spine surgery are common and span the entire spectrum of organ systems. More lengthy and complicated procedures place patients at higher risk of suffering these complications and threaten patients' well-being. High clinical suspicion and knowledge of the literature are the keys to early recognition and treatment. Through increased awareness of the possible range of complications, we must work toward minimizing these problems to effect better outcomes for our patients and to control the increasing medical expenditures associated with spine procedures.

KEY REFERENCES

Baron EM, Albert TJ: Medical complications of surgical treatment of adult spinal deformity and how to avoid them. *Spine (Phila Pa 1976)* 31:S106–S118, 2006.

Harmanci A, Harmanci O, Akova M: Hospital-acquired pneumonia: challenges and options for diagnosis and treatment. *J Hosp Infect* 51:160–167, 2002.

Lee DY, Lee SH, Jang JS: Risk factors for perioperative cardiac complications after lumbar fusion surgery. *Neurol Med Chir (Tokyo)* 47:495–500, 2007.

O'Grady NP, Barie PS, Bartlett J, et al: Practice parameters for evaluating new fever in critically ill adult patients: Task Force of the American College of Critical Care Medicine of the Society of Critical Care Medicine in Collaboration with the Infectious Disease Society of America. *Crit Care Med* 26:392–408, 1998.

Stein PD, Woodard PK, Weg JG, et al: Diagnostic pathways in acute pulmonary embolism: recommendations of the PIOPED II investigators. *Radiology* 242:15–21, 2007.

REFERENCES

The complete reference list is available online at expertconsult.com.

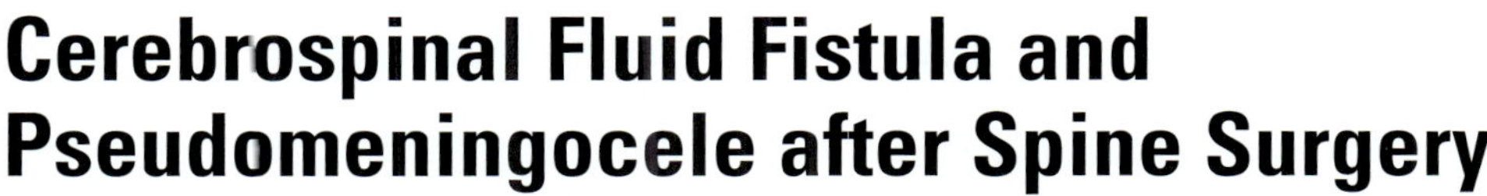

CHAPTER 200

Cerebrospinal Fluid Fistula and Pseudomeningocele after Spine Surgery

Iain H. Kalfas | Bjorn Lobo | Bruce M. McCormack | Barry M. Zide

Cerebrospinal fluid (CSF) fistulas and pseudomeningoceles are relatively rare complications of spine surgery.[1] Although durotomies encountered during spinal surgery are not uncommon, most heal uneventfully after primary suture closure. If a watertight dural closure is not possible, CSF may drain through the surgical tract to form a cutaneous CSF fistula. The presence of CSF leakage requires that immediate measures be taken to stop the leak due to the potential for infection.[2-5] CSF leakage contributes to increased perioperative morbidity, prolonged hospitalization, and increased cost of care. These factors are further compounded when additional surgery is needed to manage the leakage.

CSF leakage that occurs after satisfactory wound healing can lead to the development of a pseudomeningocele in the paraspinal tissues. This typically develops slowly into an encapsulated CSF-filled mass that may be confined to the subfascial region or, with greater pressure, may extend through the fascia into the paraspinal tissues. As they enlarge, pseudomeningoceles may contribute to chronic back pain, persistent headache, and, less commonly, nerve root entrapment.[6-9]

Most cases of CSF leakage can be successfully managed by nonoperative methods, but some may require additional surgical repair. The appropriate treatment depends on the timing, size, symptoms, and location of the leak. Small, localized leaks may be resolved by placing additional sutures to close the cutaneous tract. Persistent leakage may require the insertion of a subarachnoid drain for temporary CSF diversion or placement of an epidural blood patch. Surgical reexploration of the wound is indicated when these measures are unsuccessful or when the patient presents with significant symptoms due to a pseudomeningocele.

Incidence

The incidence of CSF fistula is relatively rare because most dural tears heal spontaneously and only a small percentage of patients develop symptoms. In a study of 3038 spinal surgeries, the incidence of dural tears during the course of bone removal or during dural sac or root retraction was noted to be 5.9%.[10] In Mayfield's review of 1408 laminectomies, the incidence of CSF fistula requiring reoperation was 0.3% and the incidence of pseudomeningocele was 0.8%.[1]

The incidence of pseudomeningoceles is difficult to determine because most cases are asymptomatic. Swanson and Fincher reported a 0.068% incidence of pseudomeningocele in a review of 1700 exploratory laminectomies.[9] Schumacher et al. reported the incidence of pseudomeningoceles to be less than 0.1% in 3000 patients who had undergone a lumbar discectomy.[11] Teplick et al.[12] reported a 2% incidence of pseudomeningocele in a series of 400 symptomatic postlaminectomy patients examined with CT. None of these patients required reoperation.

The relatively low incidence of CSF wound complications in these series may be because a majority of the patients underwent uncomplicated laminectomy for discectomy.[1,9-12] The incidence is much higher and has not been well reported in patients who have undergone laminectomy for spinal dysraphism or in patients with a history of prior spinal irradiation or surgery. Zide et al. reported that 43% of patients with intramedullary spinal cord neoplasms previously treated with radiation developed a CSF fistula or pseudomeningocele after surgery.[13] They also found a high incidence of pseudomeningocele (43%) and CSF fistula (13%) in patients after surgical correction of the tethered spinal cord.[14]

Shapiro and Scully reviewed 39 patients with CSF fistula after spinal surgery.[5] Sixteen leaks occurred after intradural procedures, despite a primary closure or dural patch graft. Of the remaining 23 cases, 19 occurred in lumbar surgeries. In 6 out of 19 lumbar cases (33%), a dural tear was identified and repaired at the time of surgery. In 13 of the lumbar cases (66%), no tear or leak was identified at the time of surgery. A myelogram was performed the day before surgery in 5 out of these 13 cases (38%). Three cases occurred after cervical spine surgery.

Pathophysiology

A dural tear, either occult or recognized, is the initial event that leads to postoperative CSF cutaneous fistula and pseudomeningocele.[15] Tears may result from excessive traction or inadvertent disruption during surgical decompression. A myelography needle puncture performed shortly before lumbar surgery can also be the cause of postoperative CSF leaks.[5] Durotomies that are recognized and repaired may still result in postoperative CSF leakage due to inadequate closure, particularly of tears that are difficult to access (i.e., ventral and lateral dura). Resection of dural-based tumors may create dural defects that are impossible to close in a watertight manner.

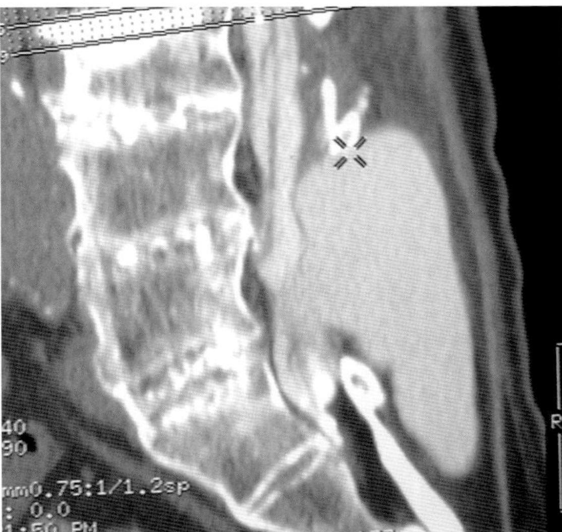

FIGURE 200-1. Lumbar postmyelogram CT demonstrating a postoperative pseudomeningocele.

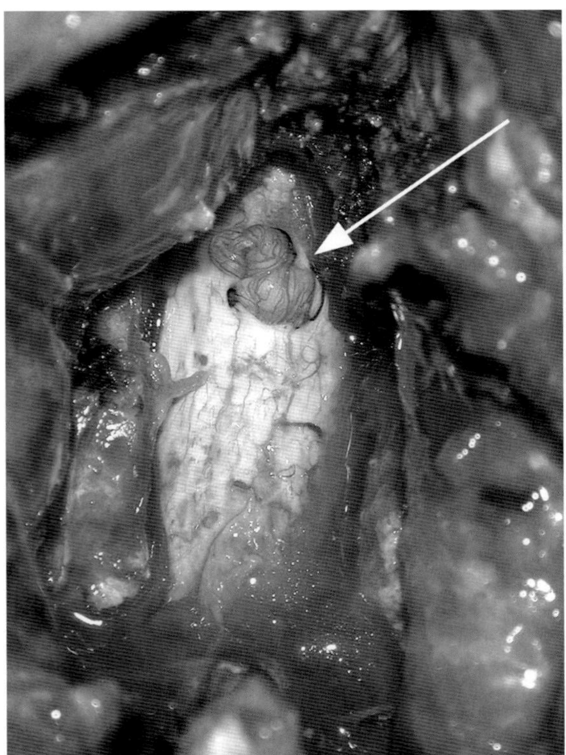

FIGURE 200-2. Intraoperative photograph during lumbar surgery demonstrating herniation of nerve rootlets (*arrow*) through a dural defect.

Cutaneous CSF fistulas most commonly occur in the immediate postoperative period (1–7 days). CSF typically passes through an incompletely healed area of the surgical wound or through a drainage tract. Fistulas may be aggravated by an upright posture, coughing, sneezing, or straining during bowel movement.

Pseudomeningoceles are caused either by herniation of the arachnoid through a dural tear, which subsequently forms an arachnoid-lined sac filled with CSF,[8] or by direct extravasation of CSF into the soft tissues, with eventual development of a fibrous capsule.[8,12] CSF pulsations force the fluid into the muscular and superficial subcutaneous tissues (Fig. 200-1). The size, shape, and location of the sac depend on the nature of the soft tissue into which the fluid is forced. In rare cases the capsule may ossify.[16] Entrapment of nerve roots in the pseudomeningocele may be a barrier to dural healing[6,7] (Fig. 200-2).

The majority of dural tears heal uneventfully after primary repair. Although the most likely cause of a CSF fistula or pseudomeningocele is an inadequate repair at the time of the durotomy, other factors may contribute to persistent CSF leakage. These include factors that delay or prevent healing of the dura mater and overlying soft tissue.[15] Dural and wound healing may be compromised by scar tissue, irradiation, localized infection, or foreign body reaction. Systemic factors that impair healing include nutritional deficits, endocrine disorders (e.g., diabetes), chronic disease, and steroid administration.

CSF leakage through a repaired dural tear may be exacerbated by elevated CSF pressure. Cutaneous CSF fistula after myelomeningocele repair is often caused by hydrocephalus (CSF pressure 350–450 mm H_2O) and is typically treated with ventricular shunting to correct the abnormal CSF dynamics. Excessive straining can transiently elevate CSF pressure (to >400 mm H_2O) and should be avoided in the perioperative period.[17] Lumbar intradural pressure is markedly elevated with an erect posture (350–450 mm H_2O), compared with supine recordings (70–170 mm H_2O).[18,19] For this reason, patients at risk for CSF leakage are kept flat in bed in the immediate postoperative period. Less commonly, CSF leakage following a durotomy can be exacerbated by the lowering of paraspinal tissue pressure created by the placement of drains under suction adjacent to the dura.

Diagnosis

The diagnosis of a cutaneous CSF fistula is most often established by inspection of the patient's wound. A watery discharge is assumed to be CSF, particularly if leakage is augmented by upright posture or Valsalva maneuver or is associated with postural headaches. When headaches occur, they are typically more severe with an erect posture and are relieved in a recumbent position. Headaches are secondary to the reduction of the CSF volume when CSF loss through the fistula exceeds its production. The lowered intracranial pressure induces traction on pain-sensitive structures, such as meninges and blood vessels. In the recumbent position, traction is reduced and the pain is relieved.[20] Fever or evidence of meningismus suggests bacterial meningitis. When leakage is profuse and clear at the incision site, the diagnosis is unmistakable. Small and intermittent leaks may be overlooked or misinterpreted, especially if they are mixed with blood. If the leaking fluid produces a clear halo that surrounds a central pink stain on an absorbent surface (e.g., sheets or cotton gauze), the fluid is most likely CSF.

Laboratory analysis of the fluid may be helpful in making a diagnosis. Although determining the glucose content of the fluid has been described as a potentially helpful diagnostic test, it is not consistently reliable in being able to identify CSF.[21] A more specific test is immunofixation of β_2-transferrin.[22] A high proportion of transferrin in CSF exists as a carbohydrate-free isoform (β_2-transferrin) that is not present in sweat or serous fluid. Detection of β_2-transferrin in such fluids is indicative of CSF leakage. Only a small sample (<1 mL) is required, and no special handling or refrigeration is required.

Pseudomeningoceles may present clinically with localized back pain and postural headaches. Localized nerve root entrapment or adhesions of roots to the dural edges of the pseudomeningocele can produce radicular symptoms.[6] Symptoms may occur several weeks to months after surgery. The clinical syndrome in the lumbar region may mimic the symptoms of lumbar disc herniation. Cervical and thoracic pseudomeningoceles may be palpable as boggy masses. Lumbar pseudomeningoceles are usually not palpable on physical examination, but occasionally the collections track into the subcutaneous tissues, producing a noticeable swelling of the wound site.

Imaging Studies

MRI and CT will adequately localize the CSF fistula tract or pseudomeningocele.[7] MRI is the study of choice because of its superior imaging of soft tissue compared with CT. To best define the fistula tract for operative planning, iopamidol is injected into the subarachnoid space, followed by CT scanning. Suspected pleural CSF fistula[23-25] or slow and intermittent leaks, such as those occurring after a lumbar puncture, are often best evaluated with radionuclide myelography.[23,26]

Conservative Management

Cerebrospinal Fluid Fistula

Several options are available for the initial treatment of postoperative CSF fistula. Successful treatment has been reported with simple measures, including bedrest, oversewing of the wound,[19] closed subarachnoid drainage,[2-5,27] and percutaneous injection of an epidural blood patch.[28] Others have recommended reoperation for repair of the dura mater as an initial treatment.[21]

A trial of CSF diversion through a subarachnoid drain can predictably stop most CSF cutaneous fistulas that occur through small durotomies. After percutaneous insertion of the subarachnoid drain, CSF is drained (120–360 mL/day) for 3 to 5 days. Spinal headaches occur in approximately 60% of patients,[1,3,5] and treatment consists of IV hydration, adjustment of the rate of drainage, and medication, particularly caffeine. The risk of infection is approximately 10% and includes meningitis (2.5%), discitis (5%), and wound infection (2.5%).[5] Transient lumbar nerve root irritation occurs in 24% of patients and resolves after drain removal. Catheter blockage has been reported in up to 10% of patients,[2] but this is less common with the relatively recent development of Teflon or silicone catheters.[5] CSF diversion is successful at alleviating the cutaneous fistula in 90% to 100% of cases.[3-5]

A percutaneous blood patch, commonly used for headaches following lumbar punctures,[29] has also been reported to be effective in treating postoperative CSF fistula.[28] Advocates for the procedure cite a theoretically smaller risk of infection and earlier mobilization compared with a trial of CSF diversion. Approximately 10 to 25 mL of fresh autologous blood is injected into the epidural space near the dural puncture or laminectomy site.[28] Injected blood stops the leak by forming an occlusive clot over the dural breach and increasing extradural tissue pressure.

The use of prophylactic antibiotics for patients with cutaneous fistula is controversial. Most of the literature reviewing the use of prophylactic antibiotics for CSF fistula pertains to rhinorrhea and otorrhea. The evidence does not appear to favor their administration.[30] If antibiotics are administered, a broad-spectrum antibiotic is recommended.[31]

Pseudomeningocele

Symptomatic pseudomeningoceles may be observed for progression or, in many cases, spontaneous resolution of symptoms. Those that are associated with subcutaneous swelling at the wound site may be managed with a compressive dressing, liposuction garments, or abdominal binders. Children and infants can be fitted for Jobst garments.[13,14,32] Serial aspirations of the pseudomeningocele may also be helpful, although this may increase the potential for infection. A 3- to 5-day period of subarachnoid drainage is another reasonable treatment option to consider.

Surgical Management

Indications

Surgical reexploration should be considered in those patients with profuse CSF leakage and in all patients in whom conservative management has failed. Patients who have significant symptoms due to a pseudomeningocele should also be considered for surgical reexploration and repair. This surgery may be delayed for several weeks or months, as opposed to surgery for persistent CSF cutaneous fistula, which should be performed more acutely.

Some patients may have impaired CSF absorption with elevated intradural pressures that will compromise any attempts at direct surgical repair of a durotomy. These patients may be considered for a ventricular shunt before any attempted surgical repair. Shunts have also been successfully used to treat leaks in which wound exploration and dural repair may be complicated (e.g., pleural fistulas)[24] and fistulas at the occipitocervical junction.[27] Postlaminectomy cutaneous fistulas have also been successfully managed with the insertion of a lumboperitoneal shunt. This option has been promoted as the initial management option in preference to a trial of temporary CSF diversion.[33] The rationale is that lumboperitoneal shunting minimizes the risk of infection and does not require prolonged bedrest.

Surgical Principles

In most cases of persistent CSF leakage, a successful outcome can be achieved by accurately identifying the dural opening, obtaining a satisfactory watertight closure, and performing a sufficient reapproximation of the three layers of the surgical wound. In some complex cases, this approach may not be adequate. Novel wound closure techniques have been developed from experience with wound complications after resection of intramedullary spinal cord neoplasms in patients with a history of multiple surgeries and postoperative radiation and in children following tethered cord surgery.[13,14] In some complex cases, plastic surgery consultation for the use of myofascial flaps and other innovative wound closure techniques may be necessary to successfully obliterate the leakage of CSF.[13,14,32]

Dural Closure

Most durotomies can be repaired with interrupted or running 4-0 or 5-0 Nurolon or polypropylene (Prolene) suture. For an additional barrier to CSF leakage, a small piece of paraspinal muscle or fat can be harvested and secured to the suture line. Larger dural defects may be more difficult to close primarily. In this setting it may be necessary to use a patch of fascia or cadaver dura mater to achieve satisfactory closure. After closure, the dural suture line should be tested by observing for CSF leakage while the anesthesia team performs a Valsalva maneuver to increase intrathecal pressure. Alternatively, saline can be injected into the lumbar thecal sac through a small-gauge needle. Any sites of observed leakage can be further reinforced.

In addition to primary suture repair and tissue patch application, the use of sealant materials for dural repair has been investigated. Jankowitz et al. evaluated the use of fibrin glue in the repair of incidental durotomies following lumbar laminectomies.[34] Fibrin glue was not found to have any benefit compared to primary closure alone in preventing percutaneous CSF leaks. However, Shaffrey et al. noted a 90% success rate with the use of fibrin glue as an adjunct to dural closure.[35]

Polyethylene glycol hydrogel (PEG) glue (DuraSeal Spine Sealant, Covidien, Bedford, MA) is a synthetic, biocompatible material. Unlike fibrin glue, it is nonbiologic, eliminating any risk of disease transmission. Flexible, absorbable, and adherent to tissue, it has been approved by the U.S. Food and Drug Administration for use as a dural sealant. It is sprayed directly onto the primary suture line and surrounding dura after satisfactory suture closure. Due to a potential for swelling of the hydrogel material, it should be used on dura that is exposed in the surgical field rather than on dura in confined areas (i.e., intraforaminal).[36]

Than et al. compared PEG glue to fibrin glue for dural repair following posterior fossa surgery. A statistically significant reduction in CSF leaks was found when PEG glue was used compared to fibrin glue.[37] A prospective multicenter study found that PEG glue had a higher success rate of watertight closure at the time of initial dural repair when compared with standard treatment (more sutures, fibrin glue). However, no statistically significant reduction in postoperative CSF leaks was observed.[38]

The use of collagen matrix overlays (DuraGen Dural Graft matrix, Integra LifeSciences, Plainsboro, NJ) to facilitate dural repair has also been investigated. This bovine-derived material is biodegradable and serves as a scaffold for the regrowth of natural tissue. It is typically placed over the primary suture line without the need to suture it into place. The material is safe and effective and has been demonstrated to be a satisfactory adjunct for dural repair.[5,39]

When CSF leakage persists despite all of the primary closure and dural sealant measures attempted, a subarachnoid catheter can be placed intraoperatively through the partially closed durotomy and brought out through a separate stab incision (Fig. 200-3). After catheter placement, dural sealant is placed over the dura around the catheter. The wound is closed and CSF is drained for several days. When sufficient wound healing has occurred, the drain can be removed. The dural sealant placed around the catheter's site of dural entry helps prevent any further leakage. If CSF continues to leak through the drainage tract, it can be managed with one or two sutures to close the tract.

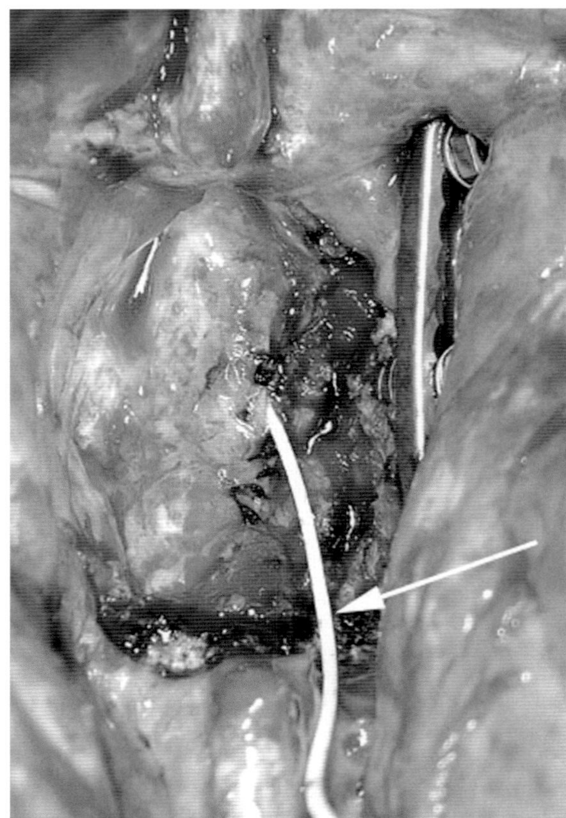

FIGURE 200-3. Intraoperative photograph during lumbar surgery demonstrating placement of a subarachnoid catheter (*arrow*) through a durotomy defect. The catheter is brought out through a separate stab incision for several days of cerebrospinal fluid diversion.

Pseudomeningocele Repair

The repair of clinically significant pseudomeningoceles may take place several weeks or months after the index procedure. The delay allows for the development of a well-defined capsule that may be incorporated into the repair. After the wound is reopened, the residual CSF is evacuated and the field is inspected for a fistulous tract. The tract is dissected free of any confining bone, scar, or ligamentous tissue that may interfere with a primary repair. If a rootlet is found to be herniated through the defect, it should be dissected free and placed back into the thecal sac. The durotomy is then closed with suture, patch graft, and sealant. The capsule of the pseudomeningocele does not need to be removed but instead can be incorporated into a multilayered closure.

Wound Closure

Once a watertight dural closure or pseudomeningocele repair has been achieved, wound closure is performed using a standard multilayered technique. Nonabsorbable sutures are used to obtain a tight fascial closure. The fascia may be reinforced with a second embricated running suture closure over the first suture line. In cases of irradiated or scarred tissue it may be necessary to adequately mobilize the fascia and paraspinal muscles before attempted closure. If sufficient fascial closure cannot be achieved, it may be necessary to obtain plastic surgery assistance to create a myofascial flap for adequate coverage. The subcutaneous fat and dermis are then closed in single or multiple layers depending on the depth of the wound. The skin is then closed with sutures as opposed to staples, using either an interrupted mattress or running technique.

The use of tissue expanders to create adequate soft tissue coverage has been described as another alternative for assistance with complex wound closures.[40] Deflated silicone elastomer (Silastic) tissue expander reservoirs are inserted into the paraspinal region through a small incision several weeks before the anticipated spinal surgery. Periodic expansion is performed by injections of sterile saline solution into the expander reservoir. The expanders, removed at the time of definitive spine surgery, provide sufficient midline soft tissue coverage without undue tension.

The use of a subfascial drain in the setting of a durotomy repair is controversial. Concerns about drain placement include promotion of CSF leakage due to the suction placed on the drain, as well as the potential for infection. Alternatively, drain placement allows for removal of postoperative serosanguineous fluid from the surgical site, facilitating the obliteration of any dead space and local approximation of tissue onto the dura for additional CSF leakage control. The drain can be placed on low suction to limit the potential for promotion of a CSF leak.

The presence of CSF in the drainage fluid does not necessarily call for immediate drain removal.[41] In this setting, CSF diversion from the wound provides more time for sufficient wound healing. Once the drain is removed, the drainage tract typically collapses. Any persistent CSF drainage through the tract can be managed by placement of a single suture as opposed to the multiple sutures frequently necessary to manage CSF leakage through a surgical wound.

Conclusion

CSF cutaneous fistulas and pseudomeningoceles are relatively uncommon complications of spine surgery that, when present, increase morbidity, hospitalization, and cost of care. Most dural tears can be successfully managed with a primary suture repair. Supplemental use of a muscle patch, dural sealants, or collagen matrix material can increase the success of primary suture repair. If a CSF cutaneous fistula develops, early recognition and management are critical. Treatment includes additional sutures at the site of the leakage, epidural blood patching, or insertion of a subarachnoid drain for several days of CSF diversion. When pseudomeningoceles develop, they are usually asymptomatic and most resolve spontaneously. Those that present with limited symptoms can be managed conservatively. If symptoms worsen, surgical reexploration for closure of the durotomy and obliteration of the pseudomeningocele is indicated.

KEY REFERENCES

Hadani M, Findler G, Knoler N, et al: Entrapped lumbar nerve root in pseudomeningocele after laminectomy: report of three cases. *Neurosurgery* 19:405–407, 1986.

Kim KD, Wright NM: Polyethylene glycol hydrogel spinal sealant (Durseal Spinal Sealant) as an adjunct to sutured dural repair in the spine: results of a prospective, multicenter, randomized control study. *Spine (Phila Pa 1976)* 36(23):1906–1912, 2011.

Kitchel S, Eismont F, Green B: Closed subarachnoid drainage for management of cerebrospinal fluid leakage after an operation on the spine. *J Bone Joint Surg [Am]* 71:984–987, 1989.

McCallum J, Maroon J, Jannetta P: Treatment of postoperative cerebrospinal fluid fistulas by subarachnoid drainage. *J Neurosurg* 42:434–437, 1975.

Schumacher H-W, Wassman H, Podlinski C: Pseudomeningocele of the lumbar spine. *Surg Neurol* 29:77–78, 1988.

Waisman M, Schweppe Y: Postoperative cerebrospinal fluid leakage after lumbar spine operations: conservative treatment. *Spine (Phila Pa 1976)* 16:52–53, 1991.

REFERENCES

The complete reference list is available online at expertconsult.com.

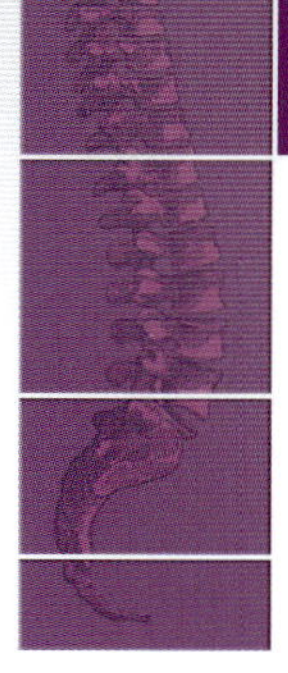

CHAPTER 201

Nonunion

Fernando Techy

Recent advances and refinements in instrumentation have greatly expanded the capacity of surgeons to successfully treat complicated problems over the entire spine (Fig. 201-1). These systems aid the reestablishment of normal or near-normal alignment, may apply complex multidirectional force vectors, and may allow immediate immobilization over multiple spinal segments. As important as the meticulous and thoughtful use of this instrumentation is, careful consideration must be given to the material that will, for a lifetime, bear the stresses that instrumentation supports only temporarily. Solid bony union alone provides enduring spinal stability, and failure to achieve this goal can have consequences ranging from a benign radiographic finding to persistent pain or catastrophic construct failure. The nonunion rate varies with the type of operation performed, being higher when multiple-level fusions are attempted. A pseudarthrosis is defined as a documented failure of continuous bone formation over time that leads to a definitive absence of bone healing through a fracture or new bone formation at an intended arthrodesis site. From a practical standpoint, a nonunion in spine surgery has been defined as the absence of solid fusion 1 year after the operation with concomitant symptoms and signs.[1] A large, population-based, prospective review of lumbar spine revisions showed that 23.6% of the indications were for pseudarthrosis.[2] Overall, the true incidence of post–spine surgery nonunion is probably underestimated, because many cases are asymptomatic and require no treatment.

This chapter reviews the basic principles of bony fusion, clinically relevant factors influencing fusion, and specific principles designed to minimize the incidence of nonunion. As in every other surgical arena, an understanding of basic principles, coupled with common sense, best equips surgeons to deal with the variety of problems they encounter.

Biology of Bone Healing

Bone is a dynamic living tissue that undergoes constant remodeling.[3] It is unique in its capacity to repair and regenerate after disruption.[4] The amazing qualities of bone are derived from its unique composite structure of organic and inorganic materials. The organic component, chiefly a strongly cross-linked (type I) collagen, gives bone plasticity that allows substantial deformation without fracture and tolerates stress in tension.[5] The inorganic component, chiefly in the form of hydroxyapatite, precipitates around the collagen fibers in a process of nucleation and maturation of mineral crystals.[6] The inorganic-mineral component of bone gives the tissue tremendous strength in compression and bending.[7]

The cellular components of bone include osteoblasts, osteocytes, and osteoclasts, connected through an intricate and well-organized system of canals.[8]

Osteoblasts are derived from mesenchymal stem cells from the bone marrow and periosteum.[9-12] They are responsible for bone formation. Osteoblasts fabricate bone in response to many stimuli and under different conditions such as growth, physiologic remodeling, fracture healing, and heterotopic ossification.[13-15] Researchers have shown that new bone is formed in response to tumors and infections.[16] An investigation has shown that osteoblasts have the ability to form bone during distraction osteogenesis,[17] when substituting the void initially filled by autologous or allogeneic bone graft, demineralized bone matrix, or synthetic bone substitutes. When performing anterior cervical discectomy and fusion (ACDF) and plating, 97.5% of fusion with new bone formation has been achieved with either autograft or allograft.[18] In a recent study, Jensen showed an 86% union rate after single- and multiple-level ACDF using patella allograft and plating.[19] In a study from Japan, Momma has reported complete bone remodeling after 6 to 12 months on CT scan, after the use of B-tricalcium phosphate to fill a partial ventral vertebrectomy defect done for cervical decompression surgery.[20]

Osteoclasts are derived from hematopoietic stem cells. They exit the circulation close to the site to be remodeled.[6,21] They are responsible for the bone resorption.

The mature osteoblast produces proteins such as type I collagen, osteocalcin, and alkaline phosphatase, a key enzyme in bone mineralization. Osteoblasts become entrapped in their own osteoid matrix and develop long cytoplasmic processes to remain in contact with surrounding cells.[22] They then begin expressing a whole new set of genes to continue bone turnover and mineral homeostasis. These cells are now considered osteocytes (mature bone cells).[6]

The process of bone healing after injury is an indistinct continuous sequence of inflammation, repair, and remodeling.[10,12] The inflammatory response to injury includes vascular dilatation with exudate and edema, as well as inflammatory cell (polymorphonuclear lymphocytes, macrophages, and lymphocytes) infiltration. A variety of hormones, cytokines,

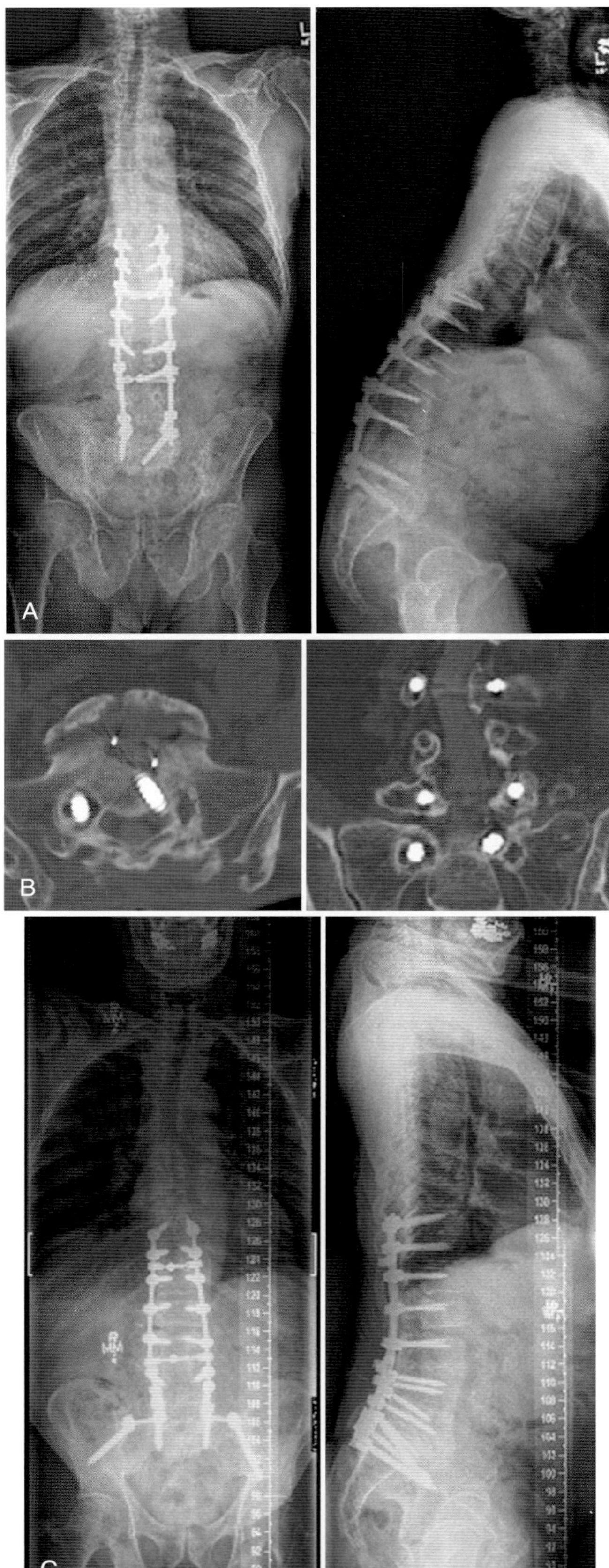

FIGURE 201-1. A 74-year-old man with multiple previous spine surgeries and a chief complaint of back pain. Severe positive sagittal imbalance and nonunion at L1-2 and L5-S1 is diagnosed through intersegmental motion during surgery. **A,** Instrumentation failure at L1-2, suggestive of pseudarthrosis. **B,** Bone reabsorption on the CT scan around the sacral screws, indicating segmental motion and possible nonunion at L5-S1. **C,** Postoperative radiographs of the patient treated with revision of the posterolateral fusion and instrumentation from T9 with extension to the ilium. Iliac crest bone graft and bone morphogenetic protein. Smith-Petersen osteotomy and transforaminal lumbar interbody fusion at L1-2 and pedicle subtraction osteotomy at L3. (Courtesy of Richard Schlenk, MD, Program Director, Neurosurgery Residency at the Cleveland Clinic, Cleveland, OH.)

growth factors, and matrix proteins (e.g., bone morphogenetic protein [BMP]) is involved throughout the healing process. Nonsteroidal anti-inflammatory drugs (NSAIDs), steroids, or chemotherapeutic agents given during the first week of healing may blunt the inflammatory response and impair bone healing.[10,12,23] As the debris of the inflammatory phase is removed, fibroblasts begin laying down new matrix in the early phases of the repair. Initially, a fracture callus that is composed of fibrous tissue, cartilage, and woven bone may form to bridge the bony defect. This is then replaced by woven bone and, ultimately, by mature cortical or cancellous bone. This process may take 3 to 6 months or longer, depending on age and other factors.[10,23] Although the general sequence of inflammation, repair, and remodeling that occurs in long bone fracture healing also occurs with bone graft repair, there are some distinct differences. Autograft bone used in spinal fusion is initially deprived of blood supply, although a robust nonspecific inflammatory response occurs as a result of preparation of the graft recipient bed. The collection of coagulated blood around the graft is somewhat analogous to the hematoma of an acute fracture, with the complex processes of inflammation ongoing within this milieu. Although some of the periosteum, endosteum, mesenchymal cells, and osteocytes within 0.2 to 0.3 mm of the borders survive transplant, most of the transplanted bone cells, separated from their blood supply, die.[24] The cancellous portion of the bone graft may be revascularized within 2 weeks, and cortical bone is revascularized within 1 to 2 months. Cancellous bone is more rapidly remodeled and is initially strengthened during the remodeling phase, because osteoblasts are first laid down over the trabeculae.[5]

Cortical bone is weakened during initial remodeling, and the process is slower than in cancellous bone. Bone graft is gradually replaced with new bone in a process called *creeping substitution*.[24] Osteoclasts that act as cutting cones bore into the graft from the margins of host bone, followed by osteoblasts that lay down new bone. This process of healing and remodeling may leave as much as 50% to 90% of the original matrix, even after many years.[25,26] The strength of cortical autograft is halved during the first 6 months after fusion but is gradually restored over 1 to 2 years. Autograft bone provides some living bone cells with the ability to make bone (i.e., osteogenic properties). It contains BMP and other substances capable of inducing cellular differentiation (i.e., it has osteoinductive properties), and it provides a scaffolding for bone growth (i.e., osteoconductive properties).[27]

Harvesting and Handling of the Bone Graft

An effort to maximize the advantages of autograft bone as graft material begins with a plan to harvest sufficient quantity of bone for the planned application. Preoperative discussions with the patient about the potential need for multiple bone harvest sites helps avoid the problem of insufficient graft in most situations. Routinely preparing and draping both iliac crests allows ready access to alternative graft material when needed. On occasion, harvesting ventral iliac crest for a dorsal application may be performed before turning the patient into the prone position. In a situation with a high risk of nonunion or with failed prior fusion, a sufficient quantity of autogenous bone is desired. Occasionally, unconventional graft sources should be considered and planned for in advance. Reliance on a single source for graft material, with a less than anticipated volume yield of harvested bone, may increase morbidity at that harvest site, as a result of overzealous harvest and extension of the harvest beyond safe and reasonable boundaries.

Surgical exposure of the donor site should be performed to maximize the viability of the graft. Heating of bone with the electric cautery, although frequently unavoidable, has the potential of destroying those surface osteocytes most capable of surviving via diffusion of nutrients. A sharp periosteum elevator can be used to open the subperiosteal plane in a remarkably atraumatic fashion, with minimal blood loss. For tricortical bone grafts placed in compression, harvesting with an oscillating saw provides a graft that is better at resisting compressive loads than a graft harvested with an osteotome.[28,29] The clinical significance of this is unknown. For bone used purely for onlay, one should bear in mind that 5 mm is the maximal thickness that can be nourished by diffusion of nutrients.[30,31] If possible, the bone graft should be harvested within 30 minutes of planned use. The graft should be kept moist in a saline- or blood-soaked sponge before use. The graft should not be allowed to dry or come into contact with toxic chemicals (e.g., antibiotic solutions).[32]

Preparation of Recipient Bed

Because few graft osteoblasts and osteocytes survive the transplant, it is imperative that preparation of the recipient bed be undertaken with utmost care and that the bed protects the viability of the tissues that will serve as the primary source of the cellular components required for bony fusion. This process begins with meticulous subperiosteal dissection of the donor site, with complete removal of all soft tissue capable of interposition between planned fusion sites. Soft tissue should be removed to minimize thermal injury, and the use of the bipolar cautery should be emphasized when possible. Areas of planned fusion should be decorticated, allowing contact of graft with cancellous bone, while avoiding weakening the structure of the recipient bed with overzealous destruction of the cortical bone. Drilling and burring should perhaps be performed with a self-irrigating drill or with aggressive irrigation from an assistant to avoid thermal injury to the recipient bed. Bone wax should not be used in the recipient bed.

Grafts should be well fitted into the recipient site. Meticulous crafting of the graft to the recipient site cannot be overemphasized, because direct bone-to-bone contact facilitates union. In some situations, cancellous bone can be packed into gaps when a perfect fit is simply not possible. The sequence of preparation of the recipient bed, decortication, and application of the bone graft must be considered relative to application of instrumentation, because access to the recipient bed may be compromised by the implant. This is particularly the case with pedicle screw fixation in which complete assembly of all of the components limits access to the transverse processes and lateral aspects of the articular surfaces. Thorough irrigation of the recipient site before placement of the graft avoids inadvertent loss of onlay graft material.

Selection of Graft Material and Instrumentation

Ideally, graft material should have the capacity to form bone (i.e., osteogenic properties), induce undifferentiated mesenchymal cells to mature into osteoblasts (i.e., osteoinductive properties), serve as scaffolding for bone healing (i.e., osteoconductive properties), harbor no risk of infection, and be genetically identical to the patient. It should also be mechanically strong, durable, potentially viable, nonreactive to the host tissue, sterile, anatomic, and cost effective.[33] Currently, the material that comes closest to these requirements is the patient's own (autograft) bone. The most common choices for autograft in spine surgery include iliac crest, local bone, or rib. The disadvantages of an autograft include the potential for inadequate bone graft volume or quality, risk of wound hernia, pelvic fracture for iliac crest grafts, blood loss, infection, nerve injury, and, most commonly and bothersome at the iliac crest, chronic graft harvest site pain. The incidence of major complications with autograft harvesting can be as high as 10%[33] or even 17.9% when using the same skin incision for iliac crest harvest and the primary spine procedure.[34] Chronic persistent pain at the donor site ranges from 2.8% to 70% of patients,[35-39] with most series reporting it to be about 20% to 30%.[35-37]

Allograft bone has the advantage of being readily available in multiple structural forms and without donor site morbidity. Allograft has some osteoinductive and osteoconductive, but no osteogenic, properties. Vascular ingrowth and new bone formation are delayed with allografts.[40-42] The mode of preparation of allograft may have an impact on its success as a graft material. Allograft bone may be treated with freezing, freeze drying, or ethylene oxide to reduce its immunogenicity; however, because it is genetically dissimilar to the patient, an inflammatory response similar to graft rejection noted in other tissue transplants may occur.[43,44] Fresh-frozen allograft appears to have a superior fusion rate to freeze-dried graft, with ethylene oxide–sterilized grafts demonstrating uniformly poor results.[45]

Cervical Spine

The reported outcomes of noninstrumented single-level ACDF procedures with the use of autologous ventral iliac crest bone graft (ICBG) include fusion rates between 83% and 100%.[46-52] The use of allograft bone for single-level ACDF appears to yield results that are approximately

TABLE 201-1

Rate of Successful Fusion by Different Surgical Techniques

No. of levels	ACDF (%)	ACDFP (%)	Corp (%)	CorpP (%)	Statistical Significance
1	92.1	97.1	NA	NA	.0002
2	79.9	94.6	95.9	92.9	.0001
3	65	82.5	85.8	96.2	.0001

ACDF, anterior cervical discectomy and fusion; ACDFP, anterior cervical discectomy and fusion with plating; Corp, anterior cervical corpectomy and fusion; CorpP, anterior cervical corpectomy and fusion with plating; NA, not applicable.

From Fraser JF, Härtl R: Anterior approaches to fusion of the cervical spine: a meta-analysis of fusion rates. *J Neurosurg Spine* 6:298–303, 2007.

equivalent to use of autograft bone.[47,53-60] For multilevel ventral procedures, autograft classically appears to be superior.[58,61-63] A recent study, however, shows equal fusion rates of 97.5% using either autograft or allograft and ventral plating for multilevel ACDF.[18] For bone struts used over multiple segments, pseudarthrosis rates with allograft are higher (41%) than with autograft (27%).[64] When supplemented with dorsal fusion, the pseudarthrosis rate falls to 26%.[65]

A separate study using notched fibular struts and a halo orthosis demonstrated delayed fusion, but seven of eight patients had good or excellent results.[53] In fusions unsupplemented with dorsal instrumentation or a halo orthosis, autograft bone appears to be the favored graft material. For dorsal cervical fusions, autograft bone appears to be superior in some studies.[4,66] Ventral plating to add stability to the ACDF construct, especially if multilevel, has clearly increased the union rate of the procedure.[48,51,52,67-69] In a recent meta-analysis, the authors concluded that plating significantly increases the fusion rate of ACDF regardless of the number of levels. They also noted that corpectomies had higher fusion rates than multilevel ACDFs and that the use of plates improved the fusion rate of three-level but not two-level corpectomy surgery[70] (Table 201-1).

The use of a cylindrical titanium mesh cage packed with bone salvaged from the corpectomy may avoid the need for harvesting a separate graft. Fusion rates using this method of reconstruction have been reported to be greater than 90%.[71,72]

Lumbar Spine

It is well established that instrumentation in the lumbar spine increases fusion rates. In 1997, Fischgrund et al.[73] published a prospective, randomized trial comparing decompression and dorsolateral fusion with and without instrumentation in patients with degenerative spondylolisthesis and spinal stenosis. The average follow-up was 2 years. The fusion rate was significantly better with instrumentation than without (82% vs. 45%, respectively; $P = .0015$); however, no significant difference was found in clinical outcome. In 2004, Kornblum et al.[74] analyzed the patients from the 1997 Fischgrund study (now with a follow-up of 5–14 years) and noted that the patients with a solid fusion did significantly better than patients with a nonunion. Other authors have also conducted prospective, randomized studies looking at the same issue. Whereas Zdeblick's results also support rigid instrumentation,[75] Thomsen et al.[76] reported fusion in 68% of instrumented cases and in 85% of noninstrumented cases.

In the only randomized trial comparing circumferential fusion with dorsolateral fusion alone (to our knowledge), a significantly higher fusion rate was found with circumferential fusion (92% vs. 80%; $P < .04$).[77] In a meta-analysis looking at different lumbar fusion procedures, Bono et al. concluded that the highest rate of fusion was obtained with a circumferential technique (91%; $P = .06$), followed by posterior interbody (89%; $P = .05$), anterior interbody (86%), and finally posterolateral (85%) techniques.[78] The clinical relevance and cost of the circumferential procedure for fusion in the lumbar spine is still open to debate.

In a study of long-segment fusion to the sacrum (mean of 11.9 vertebrae) for adult spinal deformity, the pseudarthrosis rate was 24% (much higher than for short constructs). Half of these pseudarthroses occurred through the thoracolumbar junction and one fourth through the lumbosacral junction. Risk factors were kyphosis of 20 degrees or higher, positive sagittal balance of 5 cm, hip osteoarthritis, a thoracoabdominal approach, age older than 55 years, and incomplete lumbopelvic fixation (complete lumbopelvic fixation defined as L5-S1 interbody fusion and iliac screw fixation). Augmenting the number of fused levels into the upper thoracic spine did not improve the fusion rates.[79]

In the lumbar spine, allograft bone plays a limited role with dorsolateral fusion. However, its use as a ventral interbody strut (particularly femoral shaft allograft packed with cancellous autograft) when used with dorsal segmental instrumentation has been substantiated.[80-82]

Pediatric Spine Surgery

The use of allograft versus autograft bone has been well studied for scoliosis.[83-86] In uninstrumented cases, autograft performed superiorly. Instrumented dorsal fusions supplemented with allograft bone performed comparably in a pediatric population (although it took a long time to achieve fusion). Ventral allograft struts supplemented with autologous bone (packed into the hollowed marrow space of the allograft), in conjunction with dorsal fusion and segmental instrumentation, yielded better results than allograft fusion without ventral graft supplementation.[86] When treating high-grade pediatric isthmic spondylolisthesis, Molinari et al. performed a very interesting study. He divided patients in three groups with the following results:

Group 1: uninstrumented in situ fusion (45% nonunion/0% neurologic compromise)

Group 2: posterior decompression and instrumented fusion (30% nonunion/0% neurologic compromise)

Group 3: reduction with 360-degree fusion (0% nonunion/5% extensor hallucis longus partial weakness)[87]

Bone Graft Substitutes

Demineralized Bone Matrix

Demineralized bone matrix (DBM) facilitates bone fusion through osteoinduction and, to a lesser degree, through osteoconductive properties. During the fabrication of DBM, the demineralization of allograft reduces its antigenicity and may uncover osteoinductive factors, including BMP.

However, BMP-2 and BMP-7 exist in nanogram concentrations in DBM, which is one million times less than the concentration of BMP required to produce a lumbar fusion clinically.[88-90] DBM may vary in its osteoinductive capabilities, based on the cadaveric bone from which it is derived, by vendor, and even among batches of the same brand. Several animal studies favor DBM when compared with autogenous bone in achieving spinal fusion.[91-93] Clinically, the data are more limited. A prospective trial comparing allograft and DBM with autograft in ventral cervical fusion demonstrated only a higher rate of graft collapse and pseudarthrosis in the allograft group.[94] In the lumbar spine, the use of DBM plus local bone achieved the same fusion rates as ICBG for a single-level posterolateral fusion.[95]

Synthetic Bone Substitutes (Ceramics)

Numerous calcium-based synthetic products have emerged as bone graft substitutes and/or extenders in spine fusion. These products serve as scaffolds that support new bone ingrowth. During manufacturing, the porosity of these materials can be optimized for bony ingrowth.[96] Calcium sulfate is not sufficient for use as an osteoconductive material, because it absorbs in only a few weeks, much before new bone has formed in a fusion.[97] Hydroxyapatite takes several years to be reabsorbed, and its radiopacity makes the radiographic diagnosis of fusion difficult. Beta tricalcium phosphate absorbs in months, thus lasting an adequate period to conduct bone growth during fusion.[97] For this reason, most ceramic products used in spine fusion these days are made of beta tricalcium phosphate and/or hydroxyapatite in combination with bovine collagen in varying ratios. Collagen affects the workability and reabsorption rate of the ceramic and may also serve as a carrier for osteoinductive agents, such as BMP.[98]

Animal studies show excellent fusion rates (superior to the control group with autologous bone) when ceramics are used in combination with bone marrow aspirate (osteoinductive and osteogenic) and very poor results when ceramics are used alone. The authors concluded that the association of bone marrow aspirate is paramount to the success of the procedure.[99,100]

In prospective case-controlled clinical series, the fusion rates for lumbar posterolateral fusion and transforaminal lumbar interbody fusion using ceramics in conjunction with bone marrow aspirate and/or local autograft yield similar good results as with ICBG (fusion rate from 92% to 100% for a single-level instrumented fusion).[101-104] In the cervical spine, Momma has reported complete bone remodeling, after 6 to 12 months, on CT scan, after the use of beta tricalcium phosphate to fill a partial anterior vertebrectomy defect done for cervical decompression.[20]

Bone Morphogenetic Protein

BMPs are a group of growth factors originally discovered because of their ability to induce the formation of bone and cartilage. Originally, seven proteins from this group were discovered. Of these, six (BMP-2 through BMP-7) belong to the transforming growth factor-beta superfamily of proteins, whereas BMP-1 is a metalloprotease, involved in cartilage development. Since then more BMPs have been discovered, making a total of approximately 20 today.[105] BMP bone induction is a sequential cascade. The key steps in this process are chemotaxis, mitosis, and differentiation as shown on early studies by Reddi.[106] They are known to stimulate osteoblasts and inhibit osteoclasts.[107,108] Currently, the Food and Drug Administration (FDA) has approved two BMPs for use in humans as bone growth inducers—BMP-2 and BMP-7. BMP-2 is the BMP used in almost the totality of current spinal fusion cases because of FDA regulation issues with BMP-7. Multiple preclinical animal studies have shown that the use of BMP results in similar, if not superior, fusion rates with biomechanically stronger fusion masses when compared with autogenous bone graft.[109-111]

Prospective, randomized clinical studies have shown that BMPs have at least comparable fusion rates and clinical outcomes when compared with ICBG in both interbody and posterolateral lumbar fusions.[112-114]

One prospective nonrandomized study in the ventral cervical spine reports that fusion rates of allograft and recombinant human bone morphogenetic protein (rhBMP-2; 0.9 mg per level) were slightly better than those of ICBG. However, 50% of the patients receiving the BMP had significant neck swelling.[115] Another study reported 27.5% clinically significant neck swelling after ACDF with BMP.[116] The safe dose of BMP and the best method for delivery are yet to be determined in the cervical spine. In 2008, the FDA issued a warning concerning its use in cervical surgery.[117]

Recently discovered bone morphogenetic protein-binding peptide (BBP) is a 19–amino acid peptide that has been shown to bind BMP and potentiate its effect of bone healing in animal studies. BBP may provide for improved fusion rates with a smaller dose of BMP required, potentially reducing cost, as well as potential side effects of BMP such as inflammation and ectopic bone formation.[118]

Influence of Electromagnetic Stimulation on Bone Healing

Direct current stimulation was first proposed in 1972 as a modality for improving fusion.[119,120] Application of pulsed electromagnetic fields for nonunion in long bone fractures appears to have no hazardous side effects. Areas of tension are associated with a net positive charge, and compressive stresses are associated with a net negative charge (10–100 mV) and osteogenesis.[120] Electromagnetic stimulation is believed to promote osteogenesis as a result of more rapid angiogenesis and decreased osteoclastic activity.[121] The effect of improved osteogenesis may be mediated by growth factors.[122] More recent evidence also suggests the activation of a second messenger system involved in bone remodeling. Three broad types of electromagnetic fields are used: implantable direct current, pulsed electromagnetic fields, and capacitively coupled electrical energy. Pulsed electromagnetic fields and capacitively coupled electrical energy are examples of external electromagnetic fields. These are delivered via external electrodes attached to a corset. Implantable direct current requires surgical placement of the electrodes and has been shown to be the most effective.[123] Direct current may be more effective than external electrodes secondary to its increased precision in the distribution of current.[124] The cost of these devices is not insignificant. Although some investigators have noted no significant benefit of electrical stimulation for canine spinal fusions,[125,126] one randomized blinded study in 195 patients demonstrated a significant difference in fusion rates between stimulated (92%) and unstimulated (65%) groups.[127] In a study of 59 patients who underwent reoperation for failed lumbar fusions, there was an 81% fusion rate in stimulated patients versus a 54% fusion rate in unstimulated patients.[128] Another contemporary series found a 96% fusion rate with implanted stimulators versus 85% with no stimulation.[129] Clinical trials have been faulted for having a high degree of variation in electrical stimulation protocols, surgical intervention, and disease-treated patient populations.[123] Strong, consistent, and clear evidence supporting the effects of electrical stimulation on long-term fusion rates is yet to be published.

Factors Affecting Bone Healing

Smoking

Studies have shown a threefold to fourfold increase in the occurrence of nonunion of spinal fusions in smokers over that in nonsmokers.[56,130,131] Smoking interferes with osteoblastic function,[132] leads to increased bone resorption at fracture sites,[133] and interferes with normal bone metabolism.[134] Smoking has also been associated with bone mineral loss in several studies.[135,136] Nicotine, the chemical most responsible for physical dependency, also has deleterious effects on spine fusion rates and revascularization of bone graft, as shown in animal studies.[137] One particular article demonstrated decreased intertransverse fusion rates in rabbits receiving systemic nicotine and also suggested that the bone formed during nicotine use has inferior biomechanical properties.[60] These studies strongly indicate that the use of nicotine patches or gums, in an effort to curb patient smoking perioperatively and during bone healing, may be ill advised. It is likely, however, that other components of cigarette smoke also have a deleterious effect on fusion, although this is less documented. Even the pulmonary compromise associated with smoking, as reflected in a decreased arterial partial oxygen pressure, has been suggested as a potential explanation for increased nonunion rates in smokers.[61]

A case-control study of two-level lumbar laminectomy and fusion demonstrated a nonunion rate of 40% in smokers and 8% in nonsmokers.[131] Similarly, in a study of anterior cervical fusion with allograft, the authors found a higher rate of fusion in nonsmokers than in smokers (81% vs. 62%).[138]

Although there is consensus that smoking inhibits bony fusion, there is considerable disagreement over the management of the smoker facing spine fusion.

In our opinion, an intermediate approach should be used in an attempt to avoid an excessively fatalistic or autocratic view. The decision should always be based on the urgency and severity of the disease.

Radiation Therapy

Radiation impairs bone healing,[139-141] inhibiting cell proliferation and producing a vasculitic reaction that limits vessel ingrowth. Radiation delivered before long bone fracture in animals results in delayed fracture healing.[142] In a canine model, bone healing was superior when radiation was given either preoperatively or only after 21 days postoperatively. The worst bone healing results were seen when radiation was administered on postoperative day 3.[143] The total radiation dose, delivered preoperatively or postoperatively, has been shown to correlate well with reduction in strength of healing bone in an animal model.[144] A total radiation dose exceeding 4000 cGy has been proposed as a risk factor for nonfusion in patients undergoing perioperative radiation for neoplasm.

Delaying radiation, at least until after the first or second postoperative week, appears well founded because the untoward effects of radiation seem maximal during that interval (both on bone and soft tissue healing). The total dose of radiation should be customized to the indication, with consideration given to delivering a minimal effective dose. With the recent advent of stereotactic radiosurgery, we have been able to deliver higher doses of radiation to tumors, with fewer deleterious effects to the surrounding tissues.

Nutrition

Malnutrition has a negative impact on fracture healing,[144] blunts the immune response, and impairs wound healing. A nutritional support team can provide vital preoperative evaluation and education to optimize nutritional status preoperatively and postoperatively.

Rheumatoid Arthritis and Ankylosing Spondylitis

Rheumatoid arthritis affects 1% of the world's population, with 60% to 70% of patients with the disease eventually suffering cervical spine symptoms.[145] In patients requiring fusion, bone healing is often compromised by osteoporosis,[146] and the direct immunosuppressive effects of the disease itself (coupled with the effects of steroid medications)[147] can lead to osteomyelitis.[148] Despite these factors, the use of contemporary instrumentation and arthrodesis techniques in patients with rheumatoid arthritis has resulted in spine surgery fusion rates of 90% or higher in multiple centers.[149-152]

Nonunion does not seem to be a problem when operating on patients with ankylosing spondylitis. Bony union is usually the rule in patients with ankylosing spondylitis after surgery, and fusion rates exceeding 95% have been reported after the correction of spinal deformity.[153-159]

Age

Generally, skeletally immature patients have the greatest healing potential and heal more quickly.[160] It is hypothesized that children may have a greater number of undifferentiated mesenchymal cells, and that these cells may be capable of more rapid differentiation when necessary.[161,162] In one study looking at long thoracolumbar constructs, age greater than 55 years was a risk factor for nonunion.[79]

Nonsteroidal Anti-Inflammatory Drugs

There is clearly a negative association between spine fusion and use of NSAIDs in animal models.[111,163-165] In the clinical setting, a recent meta-analysis looking at the use of NSAIDs and spine fusion rates found that the odds ratio of a nonunion was higher (3.0) in the anti-inflammatory use group only in lower-quality studies. The better-quality articles failed to show an association of NSAID use and nonunion. The authors conclude that higher-quality, prospective, controlled, randomized studies are needed to further elucidate this issue.[166]

Diagnosis of Nonunion

The diagnosis of pseudarthrosis remains a challenging endeavor that in most instances requires a high index of suspicion. It has classically been based on the triad of persistent pain, radiographic evidence of instability, and loss of correction/fixation. Diagnosis by imaging is often difficult and may require multiple modalities. Results may be misrepresented, not only by the limitations of technique but by the prejudgment of the surgeon. A study comparing radiographic analysis of ACDF fusion at 6 months between the surgeon and an independent panel had a correlation of k = 0.308. The correlation was even poorer when the surgeon noticed favorable clinical results.[167]

Flexion-Extension Radiographic Studies

There is controversy concerning the angular amount of motion accepted in a segment to correlate with a solid fusion. Most studies range from 0 to 5 degrees.[168]

One study developed a finite element model to simulate different types of lumbar fusion and concluded that, overall, a solid fusion should have less than 4.1 degrees of motion between the segments of interest. This study, however, did not account for instrumentation.[169] Simmons considers a nonunion when more than 2 degrees of difference is seen between the flexion and extension films.[170] One should keep in mind that with the advent of rigid instrumentation, pseudarthrosis may be present even without motion of the segment on dynamic radiographs.[168]

Computed Tomography

CT has become widely used for the diagnosis of nonunion after spine surgery. A recent prospective study of intraoperative evaluation (gold standard) versus imaging evaluation of pseudarthrosis after anterior cervical fusion found that CT most closely agrees with intraoperative findings ($P < .05$) compared with plain radiography and MRI.[171] Another study comparing thin-slice CT and dynamic radiography for the diagnosis of nonunion found pour correlation between the two methods.[172]

Magnetic Resonance Imaging

Due to its cost and metal artifact on imaging after instrumentation, MRI is not a good choice for assessing bone union after fusion.[168]

Nuclear Medicine and Ultrasound

Bone scans have a low sensitivity and positive predictive value for identifying pseudarthrosis and are considered to be ineffective for the reliable diagnosis of nonunion after spinal fusion.[168] Single-photon emission CT scans have a sensitivity and a specificity of about 50% and therefore cannot be used reliably for the diagnosis of pseudarthrosis.[173] The use of ultrasound in detecting pseudarthroses has been explored in the past. In a series by Jacobson et al., it was used to evaluate pseudarthrosis after posterolateral spinal fusion. There was a reported sensitivity of 100%, but the specificity was only 60%.[174] In conclusion, ultrasound and nuclear medicine modalities do not seem to play a major role in modern intervertebral pseudarthrosis investigation.

No single modality has shown perfect accuracy. A high index of suspicion and possibly a combination of tests may be necessary to consolidate the indication for revision surgery. In the end, surgical exploration, aggressive curettage, and intraoperative stress testing remain the most accurate means of diagnosing a nonunion.

Technical Aspects and Results

Ultimately, an understanding of the basic principles of bone fusion must be coupled with technical execution in the operating room. Although a well-crafted arthrodesis does not guarantee success, a poorly performed one can virtually ensure failure. Also, before any treatment of spinal pseudarthroses, one should proceed with identification of the factors that lead to failure (e.g., segmental motion or shear stresses, underlying metabolic/medical causes, smoking/NSAIDs) and correct them in the revision surgery.

Cervical Spine

Ventral cervical interbody fusion, using the Smith-Robinson technique, is one of the most common procedures performed by spine surgeons. Although this technique provides a high rate of solid arthrodesis, attention to some details can optimize the likelihood of solid success. Meticulous preparation of the recipient site, including the complete removal of the cartilaginous end plates, is required. Widening the exposure to the width of the uncovertebral joints helps provide a broad surface for fusion and helps localize the midline. Very often it is helpful to remove the overhanging ventral caudal lip of the rostral vertebral body. Performed early in the decompression, this phase allows for a better view of the dorsal interspace while also allowing for a smooth fit of the interbody graft. The final preparation of the recipient surfaces involves smoothing any irregular contours that may leave gaps in the interface between the graft and the recipient site. After the recipient site is prepared, the graft may be precisely contoured to just exceed the height of the recipient site. The graft should be impacted into the interspace, with great care taken to avoid driving it into the spinal canal. Controlled cervical traction, applied by the anesthesiologist, or an interspace spreader can provide the additional interspace height that is required to allow gentle tamping of the bone graft into position with only moderate force. Excess force, poor fit of the graft, or use of a small impactor may result in fragmentation of the graft, necessitating replacement. The implant should seat securely in the interspace, and the surgeon should be able to feel it settling solidly into position. Grafts that freely spin or move within the space after the release of cervical traction, or grafts that splinter, crack, or fray are suboptimal and should be replaced. Long interbody grafts require special consideration. A variety of strategies have been used that are largely based on the preference of the surgeon.

Symptomatic nonunion after ventral procedures can be managed in many ways. One option, when there is no overt ventral instrumentation failure and no symptomatic ventral compressive pathology, is simply a dorsal fusion, usually using instrumentation. A dorsal fusion that incorporates all levels included by the ventral procedure avoids reoperating through distorted anatomy. If overt hardware failure or residual ventral pathology demands reoperation, one may proceed from the side opposite the initial procedure. The decision to operate through a previous exposure is largely one of personal preference, unless a recurrent laryngeal nerve injury was sustained with the initial surgery (as documented by laryngoscopy), in which case the same-side incision is clearly indicated. Although the procedure is generally straightforward, a few points deserve mention with regard to ventral cervical operations.[175] First, on exposure of the ventral spine, it may be difficult to precisely localize the level of suspected pseudarthrosis on gross inspection. Identifying adjacent disc space levels provides some guidance, as does an aggressive mobilization of the longus colli musculature, which provides lateral bony exposure that may reveal some preserved interspace laterally at the operated level. Second, the actual removal of graft from a previously operated level may be challenging. Usually a high-speed pneumatic drill is used to remove it. When ventral instrumentation is planned, particular care must be taken to avoid overzealous vertebral body resection adjacent to the graft site. Excessive straying into an adjacent vertebral body can quickly result in the loss of a suitable anchor point for the implant, necessitating inclusion of another level in the construct. Fluoroscopy can provide a helpful gauge of depth during drilling. One may drill down the old graft just slightly beyond its rostral and caudal margins, staying near the midline. This provides exposure of the posterior longitudinal ligament remote from previous surgical exposure. In this fashion, the surgeon can easily broaden the dural exposure and extend it rostrally and caudally, beginning on tissue away from the initial surgery. The technique of beginning far laterally and drilling on either side of the graft should be used with caution, because as the exposure deepens, one may inadvertently encounter a nerve root with little warning from normal anatomic landmarks.

In a series of 120 patients with post-ACDF pseudarthrosis, the union rates for revision surgery were 56% if a ventral approach was chosen for the revision, as opposed to 98% if the fusion was done from a dorsal approach.[176] Two other studies corroborate the same findings.[177,178] Others, however, have successfully achieved 100% of fusion when revising ACDF nonunion from the front.[175,179]

Thoracic Spine

The rigidity of the thoracic spine, afforded by the articulation of the ribs, enhances the integrity of most midthoracic constructs.[180] The tremendous loads concentrated at both ends of the thoracic spine, by virtue of the leverage of the craniocervical and lumbosacral lever arms, stress constructs at these locations.

Failed dorsal instrumentation constructs are frequently the result of suboptimal placement of hardware. This is particularly true when addressing the cervicothoracic junction, an area between the mobile cervical and fixed thoracic spine, submitted to enormous stresses and prone to instability.

Berven published on the revision of 10 cases of thoracic nonunion treated with extension osteotomy, rigid dorsal-only instrumentation, and autograft. His results show 100% of fusion and 70% of patient satisfaction.[181]

Lumbar Spine

The management of failed lumbar fusion remains a source of great controversy. Every effort should be made to optimize the chance for successful union by analyzing the mechanism of previous failure and thoughtfully tailoring the planned procedure to the patient's individual situation.

In a study treating dorsal surgery lumbar pseudarthrosis with anterior lumbar interbody fusion, the authors achieved solid fusion in 52 of 53 cases. Despite the excellent fusion rates, the functional results were dismal, with only approximately 30% of patients being able to return to work.[182] Gertzbein et al. retrospectively reviewed 25 patients treated with circumferential fusion after pseudarthrosis following attempted dorsolateral fusion surgery. Besides a 100% fusion rate, only 52% of patients had considerable pain relief.[183]

It is well determined in lumbar nonunion history that even if fusion is achieved in the revision surgery, the clinical outcomes are usually not as good.[184-187] On the other hand, it is also known that patients with successful fusion after revision surgery are far more likely to have a satisfactory outcome than are those who remain unfused.[188-190]

Summary

It is fundamental to understand the symptoms and expectations of the patient when surgically treating spine pseudarthrosis. Successful bony fusion requires consideration of the patient's general physiologic state, with attention paid to metabolic derangements, comorbidities, age, or habits likely to have a negative impact on bone healing. An attempt must be made to modify those factors prior to surgery because most spine arthrodesis surgeries are elective procedures. The basic principles of biomechanics, as they apply to the patient's situation, should be used in the surgery plan. The location of the operation, number of levels, type of bone graft, and kind of instrumentation are important variables in the procedure success. Meticulous attention is essential to technical details. Even with the best efforts of an excellent surgeon and a compliant patient, successful bony union is occasionally not attained. In those situations in which there are persistent symptoms related to nonunion, another attempt to provide successful fusion may be considered. In these circumstances, every possible effort must be made to optimize the chance for successful bony union, beginning with a critical review of the previous failure. Every phase of the procedure must be thoughtfully optimized. Recent advances in instrumentation and biologics should be carefully analyzed and, if appropriately applied, are considered of great help in the current treatment of nonunions.

As in every other surgical arena, an understanding of the basic principles, coupled with common sense, best equips the surgeon to deal with adversity and achieve optimal results. Finally, it is important to always keep in mind that even though patients who attain fusion generally do better than those who go into a nonunion, achieving a firm arthrodesis between segments is not a guarantee of clinical improvement.

Acknowledgments. Thank you to Drs. Vinay Deshmukh, Arnold B. Vardiman, and Howard W. Morgan, Jr., who authored prior editions of this chapter. Their work laid the foundation for this third edition.

KEY REFERENCES

Bono CM, Lee CK: Critical analysis of trends in fusion for degenerative disc disease over the past 20 years: influence of technique on fusion rate and clinical outcome. *Spine* 29:455–463, 2004.

Burkus JK, Gornet MF, Dickman CA, et al: Anterior lumbar interbody fusion using rhBMP-2 with tapered interbody cages. *J Spinal Disord Tech* 15:337–349, 2002.

Buttermann GR: Prospective nonrandomized comparison of an allograft with bone morphogenic protein versus an iliac-crest autograft in anterior cervical discectomy and fusion. *Spine J* 8:426–435, 2008.

Kim YJ, Bridwell KH, Lenke LG, et al: Pseudarthrosis in long adult spinal deformity instrumentation and fusion to the sacrum: prevalence and risk factor analysis of 144 cases. *Spine* 31:2329–2336, 2006.

Kornblum MB, Fischgrund JS, Herkowitz HN, et al: Degenerative lumbar spondylolisthesis with spinal stenosis: a prospective long-term study comparing fusion and pseudarthrosis. *Spine* 29:726–733, 2004.

Wang JC, McDough PW, Endow K, et al: The effect of cervical plating on one-level anterior cervical discectomy and fusion. *J Spinal Disord* 12:467–471, 1999.

Zdeblick TA, Hughes SS, Riew KD, et al: Failed anterior cervical discectomy and arthrodesis: analysis and treatment of thirty-five patients. *J Bone Joint Surg [Am]* 79:523–532, 1997.

REFERENCES

The complete reference list is available online at expertconsult.com.

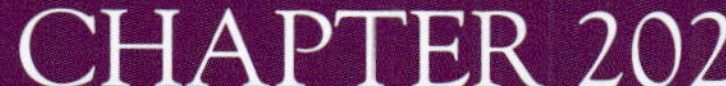

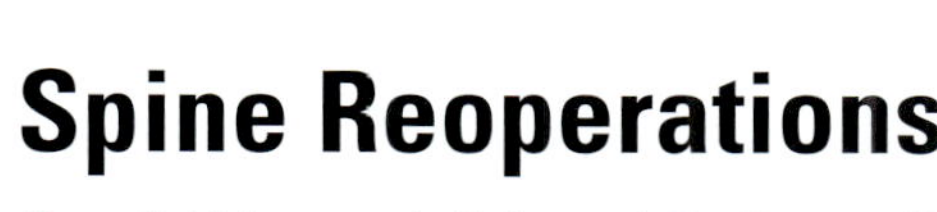

CHAPTER 202

Spine Reoperations

Gandhi Varma | Edward S. Connolly | Donlin M. Long

Preventing repeat spine surgery is an important goal for surgeons and their patients. Reoperation is generally an undesirable outcome, implying persistent symptoms, progression of the underlying disease, or complications related to the initial operation. A higher risk of reoperation was observed among patients covered by workers' compensation insurance compared with those with other types of insurance. Patients under age 60 were more likely than those age 60 years and older to have second operations. Males had a slightly lower risk of reoperation than females, and having any comorbidity resulted in a higher risk of reoperation.[1]

Often reoperations on the spinal column are more technically difficult than the first operations, and the risk of surgical complications is potentially greater. In addition to the technical problems of reoperation, clinical and radiographic evaluation of the patient is more difficult. Because normal anatomic relationships and normal tissue planes have been altered, imaging is less accurate and the surgical pathology is more difficult to recognize.

Patients undergoing surgery for degenerative spine disease may require further surgery for disease progression at the original operative level or at adjacent levels or for instability. Reoperation has proven to be much less effective than initial surgery, and it is estimated that only 30% to 50% of patients benefit from this second surgical procedure. Reoperation rate varies with the region of the spinal column, type of disease, and type of previous surgery. Reoperations are performed at the rate of 2.5% per year at the cervical spine level and range from 8.9% to 10.2% at the lumbar level. Reoperations are more expensive; a recent study found that the average hospital charge for a cervical spine reoperation is $57,205.[2] Identifying modifiable factors, such as the choice of approach, might reduce the need for spine reoperations and might improve public health and curb health care expenditures.

MRI remains the most valuable imaging study, but it may not be adequate for examination of bony detail. Plain films are of great importance for determining exactly what was done previously, and CT scanning with two- and three-dimensional reconstruction can provide bony detail that is useful during reoperation. These techniques are particularly useful for recognizing failed fusion or instability. CT myelography is still useful when there is question about pathology definition.

Some general principles of wound healing should be kept in mind when reoperating on the spine. If the reoperation is being performed through the same approach as previous surgical interventions, the scar in the skin may be excised so that fresh skin edges are approximated. This may reduce the chance of superficial wound infection, wound dehiscence, and a poor cosmetic outcome. The surgical field in reoperation should be exposed beyond the scar tissue and into normal surgical planes, so that the surgeon is working from normal anatomy on either side of the scar. Foreign material in the wound, which could be a source for bacterial contamination, should be removed unless doing so would create excessive tissue destruction or unacceptable instability.

Usually, reoperations on the spinal column are performed for the following reasons: (1) recurrent or persistent neural compression; (2) development of, or persistence of, instability; (3) CSF leak; (4) hematomas; and (5) infection.

Neural Compression

The most common reason for reoperation on the spine is recurrent or persistent neural compression. Of all the indications for reoperation for neural compression, recurrent or persistent radiculopathy (radiculitis secondary to disc or scar) is by far the most common.[3-11] Persistent symptoms with neural compression are seen in patients with a recurrent disc herniation, large foraminal osteophyte, thickened ligamentum flavum, facet joint hypertrophy causing root compression and inadequate decompression of the spinal cord or cauda equina in spinal stenosis, calcified nerve, ossification of the posterior longitudinal ligament, recurrent disc herniation, or neoplasia.[12,13]

Lumbar Radiculopathy or Radiculitis

The reported incidence of symptomatic recurrent disc herniation after lumbar discectomy varies between 3% and 18% in retrospective studies.[14] Subjects with larger anular defects and those in whom a smaller proportion of disc volume was removed during the first surgery were associated with an increased risk of symptomatic recurrent disc herniation. Carragee et al. demonstrated that the reherniation rate varied from 1.1% with small fissure-like anular defects to 27.3% for large open anular defects.[15] Recurrent disc herniation or progressive disc space loss after discectomy often leads to increased pain and disability, which necessitates repeat surgery. Revision surgery, however, does not always improve symptoms.[16] The differentiation of a recurrent disc herniation from an epidural scar presents a dilemma. Characteristics associated with recurrent disc herniation include a nonenhanced or rim-enhanced abnormality surrounding a low-signal-intensity lesion on MRI and extension of contrast into the epidural space and an enhancing abnormality on CT/discography.[17] However, the discovery of a focal mass of scar that is obviously compressing a nerve root may still be an indication for surgery. Diffuse epidural scar without nerve root compression, however, is not.

Reoperation for a recurrent lumbar disc herniation often requires lengthening the surgical incision to expose the normal laminae above and below the interspace and freeing of the scar from the previous laminotomy using sharp dissection with a tool such as a sharp curet or a no. 15 knife. A high-speed drill or angled punch is used to obtain further bony decompression and to allow visualization of normal epidural tissue. Residual ligamentum flavum from previous surgery should be removed and the disc space approached from normal epidural tissue rostrally toward the disc space and nerve root. It is important to completely dissect out the nerve root, with good exposure of the axilla of the nerve root and its entire course in the lateral recess. If the dura mater or the nerve root is firmly attached to a recurrent disc fragment, sharp dissection and magnification should be used to free it so that no dural tear occurs during manipulation of the disc fragment. Utmost care should be taken to visualize the paramedian aspect of the disc, which is frequently the site of residual or persistent compressive disc herniations. Exploration, both above and below the disc space, should be carried out to ensure that at the conclusion of the second procedure, no extruded fragment has migrated over the body of the vertebra above or below the disc space. Using a microinstrument, the surgeon should circumferentially feel around the nerve root as it passes through the lateral recess and along its course in the neural foramen. Any dural tears that occur during the dissection should be repaired, if possible, before further dissection is performed. Repairing the dura mater prevents significant CSF fluid loss, with resultant decompression of the dural sac and increased risk of epidural venous bleeding. Primary closure of the dural defect with microsurgical technique or a dural patch graft gives a better result in preventing postoperative CSF leak. If the dura mater cannot be repaired primarily, it can be covered with absorbable gelatin sponge or muscle with fibrin tissue adhesive. A subcutaneous or epidural fat graft covering the dural defect is an effective alternative seal.

Reoperation for Thoracic Disc Herniation

Between 7% and 15% of patients with thoracic disc herniations are asymptomatic; symptomatic herniation is very rare, accounting for only 0.25% to 0.57% of herniated discs in the whole spine. The true incidence for recurrent thoracic disc herniation is not known. An accurate diagnosis may be difficult to determine and therefore may be delayed, resulting in either progressive or occasionally relapsing and remitting neurologic impairment. Reoperation at the thoracic spine level is usually due to persistent or inadequately removed centrally located calcified discs. Thoracotomy for treatment of centrally located recurrent thoracic disc herniations is associated with improvement in or stabilization of myelopathic symptoms in the majority of patients, with an acceptable rate of complications. Modified transfacet pedicle-sparing decompression and fusion is also an alternative. Other indications for reoperation for thoracic disc herniation are missed level at the first operation, missed intradural herniation, and CSF leaks.

Inadequate Decompression of the Nerve Root in Patients with a Large Foraminal Osteophyte

Vertebral osteophytes are a common radiologic finding, affecting 20% to 30% of the elderly population. A number of factors are responsible for the local osteogenesis, notably mechanical factors.

Reoperation for persistent cervical nerve root compression can usually be undertaken via one of several options. In a patient with a previous ventral cervical discectomy and fusion and with a persistent large osteophyte in the neural foramen, correction may be accomplished by performing a simple cervical foraminotomy from a dorsal approach, with or without drilling off the osteophyte. This procedure is probably easier than reoperating from the ventral approach and drilling out the previous fusion and decompressing the foramen. If, however, the osteophyte is ventral and medial in location and cannot be decompressed adequately from a dorsal approach, a reoperation from the ventral approach should be performed. The soft tissue planes may be scarred, but the tissue plane between the carotid sheath and the esophagus and trachea is usually maintained and easily dissected. If the soft tissue scarring is due to previous infection or radiation therapy, the operation may be simplified by operating from the opposite, or virgin, side. An operation being performed from the ventral approach for inadequate neural decompression requires increased bone resection, at least a minicorpectomy, to remove 7 or 8 mm of each vertebral body rostrally and caudally to the disc space and to allow definitive visualization of both nerve roots with magnification. This is often best accomplished by using a high-speed drill and an operating microscope. If the problem is a persistent central osteophyte or ossification of the posterior longitudinal ligament, corpectomy is the safest ventral approach, allowing complete decompression of the spinal cord. The corpectomy is followed by a ventral interbody fusion.

Inadequate Decompression of the Cauda Equina in Spinal Stenosis

Cauda equina syndrome (CES) is a complex of clinical symptoms and signs most commonly secondary to a massive prolapsed intervertebral disc, accounting for 2% to 6% of all lumbar disc herniations. Less common causes of CES are epidural hematoma, infections, primary and metastatic neoplasms, trauma, and prolapse after manipulation, chemonucleolysis, or spinal anesthesia. Meta-analysis of surgically treated CES suggests benefit if decompression is undertaken within 48 hours from symptom onset[18] in pooled data from retrospective studies. However, not all studies support this argument, which has raised the notion that the principal determinant of outcome may be not timing, but the extent of the neurologic deficit before surgery.[19]

Recurrent symptoms of CES occur not only from inadequate previous decompression but also from progression of the disease. The most common radiographic findings are disc herniation and hypertrophic facet arthritis, whereas other features, such as acquired spondylolisthesis, osteophyte formation, stenosis, and scoliosis, are observed less frequently. The pathophysiology remains unclear but may be related to damage to the nerve roots composing the cauda equina from direct mechanical compression and venous congestion or ischemia. A high index of suspicion is necessary in the postoperative spine patient with back or leg pain refractory to analgesia, especially in the setting of urine retention. Regardless of the setting, when CES is diagnosed, the treatment is urgent surgical decompression of the spinal canal.

Recurrence and Inadequate Decompression of the Spinal Cord in Neoplasia

Spinal cord compression from neoplasms is characterized based on location as intramedullary, intradural extramedullary, and extradural. Reoperation represents a viable option in patients with high-grade epidural spinal cord compression who have recurrent metastatic tumors at previously operated spinal levels. In carefully selected patients, reoperation can prolong ambulation and result in good functional and neurologic outcomes. Treatment is palliative, with the goals of achieving pain control and improving or maintaining neurologic function. Reoperation should be considered as a treatment option in patients with tumor recurrences who are no longer candidates for radiotherapy or those who have high-grade spinal cord compression.

A reoperation for persistent spinal cord compression secondary to epidural tumor usually results from a dorsal decompression that was performed on a ventrally or ventrolaterally situated tumor. A different surgical approach, either a lateral extracavitary or a ventral approach, is required for resection of tumor and decompression of the spinal cord, as well as for appropriate stabilization of the spinal column. Reexposure of the dorsal spine may also be necessary for performing dorsal arthrodesis and segmental instrumentation to supplement the ventral arthrodesis.

Reoperation for intramedullary tumors needs a special mention. With advances in microsurgical technology, management of these tumors has shifted toward aggressive treatment with radical resection. This approach is associated with increased long-term survival and improved quality of life for both intramedullary and extramedullary tumors. Spine deformity, a well-documented complication after intradural spinal tumor resection, has been reported in up to 10% of cases in adults and 22% to 100% of cases in children.[20,21] Laminoplasty for the resection of intradural spinal tumors is not associated with a decreased incidence of short-term progressive spinal deformity or improved neurologic function. However, laminoplasty may be associated with a reduction in incisional CSF leak.[22]

Reoperation for intradural tumors requires exposing the dura mater. Intraoperative real-time ultrasound is extremely helpful for planning the dural opening and its extent. If a previous dural incision with retained suture material is present, the dura mater should be opened above and below the previous dural closure, and a small blunt dissector should be used to free the underlying spinal cord or arachnoid from the dura mater. When the dura mater has been opened a second time, placing a dural patch graft on the closure is usually prudent, both to reduce the chances of the dura mater adhering to the spinal cord and to provide increased room for the spinal cord.

Dissection of recurrent tumor from nerve roots and the spinal cord needs to be accomplished under high magnification. Great care regarding hemostasis is necessary to allow good visualization. Dissection is obtained best by using sharp dissection with two-point microcoagulation. If no neurologic structures are deep to the tumor, a laser may be used. The laser is particularly effective in removing ventrally based dural tumors.

Instability

Extrusion of a bone graft, failure of fusion, the development of instability, or failure of instrumentation is an indication for reoperation.[12,13,23-35]

Extrusion of a Bone Graft

Extrusion of a cervical interbody bone graft with persistent pain, cervical deformity, or swallowing difficulty is an indication for reoperation. The graft extrusion is more common in C2-3, C6-7, and C7-T1 levels due to the anatomic variation in the bony spine. The extrusion of a strut graft associated with a corpectomy may have been caused either by a poorly fitting graft or by fracture of the vertebral body into which the graft is fixed. This allows for the caudal portion of the graft to extrude ventrally. The dislocation of the graft may be associated with collapse of the disc spaces, which, in turn, may cause nerve root irritation and pain. Furthermore, the extruded graft may result in adjacent structure compression, causing symptoms such as dysphagia and hoarseness of voice.

The extruded bone fragment is removed, the graft site is freshened, usually by use of a high-speed drill to accomplish good preparation of the end plates, and a new graft is inserted. A ventral plate-and-screw construct provides further assurance of retention of the bone graft. High reoperation rates for extruded grafts and symptomatic pseudarthrosis have been associated with nonplated two-level anterior discectomy and fusion (ADF) and single-level anterior corpectomy with fusion (ACF) procedures. However, comparison of single-level ACF performed with and without plates showed that plating did not appear to reduce pseudarthrosis or graft extrusion rates.[36] If the vertebral body is fractured as well, partial corpectomy of the fractured segment must be performed and the graft refitted. This necessitates a longer graft. Ventral plating with screw fixation may add to the stability of the new construct. A supplement to fixation via a dorsal approach should often be considered.

Failure of Fusion

The ultimate goal of spinal hardware is to provide temporary stability allowing for bony fusion, usually requiring 6 to 9 months. Failure of fusion and the development of pseudarthrosis or fibrous union are the sequelae of ongoing low-grade mobility. Pseudarthrosis is defined as an absence of bridging bone between grafted bone and vertebral bodies and the presence of a radiolucent defect, a halo sign, or a loss of grafted bone. Despite advances in the technologies and instrumentation of spine surgery, pseudarthrosis still occurs in 10% to

15% of all patients.[37] Pseudarthrosis itself can be a source of pain, or it may provide a lead point for ongoing mobility leading to increased stress on hardware and inevitable failure, one of the indications for reoperation. Revision spinal arthrodesis for pseudarthrosis and loose instrumentation with widely dilated screw tracts is a difficult clinical problem.

The optimal revision strategy in cases of lumbar pseudarthrosis depends on the specific clinical scenario, and multiple techniques have been described. If stable fixation cannot be achieved in these cases, revision fusion may fail, or adjacent normal levels may need to be fused to gain stable fixation. According to the latest Cochrane review,[38] pedicle screw instrumentation produces a higher fusion rate, but any improvement in clinical outcome is probably marginal as compared to fusion without instrumentation.

Single-level anterior cervical discectomy and fusion (ACDF) is a highly successful procedure yielding high reported fusion rates, ranging from 83% to 97% for autograft and 82% to 94% for allograft, respectively. However, in multilevel ACDF, as the number of grafts increases, the cervical spine is predisposed to decreased fusion rates as contact stress increases between the graft–body interface, further contributing to unacceptable micromotion. Pseudarthrosis after ACDF has been recognized as a cause of continued cervical pain and unsatisfactory outcomes. Debate continues as to whether a revision ventral approach or a dorsal fusion procedure is the best treatment for symptomatic cervical pseudarthrosis. Patients with symptomatic cervical pseudarthrosis that develops after ACDF may be managed successfully with dorsal lateral mass screw fixation and fusion. The rationale for the dorsal approach includes the advantages of avoiding the scar tissue and potentially difficult tissue planes encountered in a revision ventral approach, as well as encountering a fresh fusion bed when a dorsal approach is used. Contraindications to the dorsal approach include those problems that can only be addressed through a ventral approach, such as graft migration or kyphosis. Advocates for a revision ventral approach suggest that patients experience more stiffness and pain after a dorsal approach secondary to disruption of the dorsal musculature.[39]

Since it became clinically available in 2002, bone morphogenetic protein (BMP) has been widely used as an adjunct to promote fusion in lumbar spine surgery, especially in the setting of established pseudarthrosis or a limited availability of autograft. Use of BMP has demonstrated comparable fusion rates and clinical outcomes while avoiding iliac graft harvest site morbidity when compared with iliac bone graft in both interbody and dorsolateral fusions in prospective, randomized clinical studies.

Development of Instability

Kyphosis may develop in up to 21% of patients who have undergone laminectomy for cervical spondylotic myelopathy. Progression of the deformity appears to be more than twice as likely if preoperative radiologic studies demonstrate a straight spine. The incidence of progressive deformity and instability after cervical laminectomy was highest in the pediatric population and in those with a malignant intramedullary lesion, adjuvant radiotherapy, or preoperative findings of kyphosis or instability. Other intraoperative factors, including resection of the C2 lamina, multilevel laminectomies (>3 levels removed), and removal of greater than 25% of the facet joint, have also been correlated with an increased risk for subsequent development of deformity, instability, and neurologic sequelae. Although cervical laminoplasty has been proposed to reduce the risk of postsurgical deformity, recent reports suggest no significant reduction in the incidence of spine deformity, especially in the setting of intradural spinal tumor resection.[22,40]

Late failures in lumbar spinal stenosis may be due to persistent or acquired instability, recurrence of stenosis at operated levels, new stenosis at adjacent levels, epidural fibrosis, or arachnoiditis. Degenerative discogenic pain and reports of narrowing of the intervertebral disc space, reactive changes in adjacent vertebral bodies, vacuum disc phenomenon, spondylolisthesis (ventral or dorsal), and abnormal motion of 3 mm or more on flexion-extension radiographs are all indicative of lumbar instability.[41] The development of postoperative intraspinal facet cysts has been related to the presence of postoperative segmental spinal instability, including a progression of spondylolisthesis and disc degeneration. Pedicle screw fixation fusion with interbody fusion gives better results in postoperative spinal instability. Dorsal closing wedge osteotomy is suitable to treat kyphosis of less than 40 degrees. Ventral release and dorsal spinal osteotomy is effective, especially in patients with severe kyphotic deformity or with previous surgery.

Failure of Instrumentation

Assessment of spinal hardware often involves a multimodality approach, including nuclear medicine, CT, and MRI, but plain radiographs are an essential component that can provide information other modalities cannot. Changes in component position, bony alignment, hardware fractures, and changes in the implant–bone interface (e.g., screw loosening with haloing) can be first identified and sometimes best appreciated on serial radiographs.[42] Hardware fracture generally occurs secondary to metal fatigue from repetitive stress. The presence of a fracture is frequently associated with regional motion and instability, which may lead to or result from pseudarthrosis.[43] Hardware failure includes hardware fracture, loosening of the screws, and screw pullout leading to junctional failure. Hardware loosening can be caused by osseous resorption surrounding screws and implants. Loosening in turn allows for movement, which causes further osseous resorption, increased mobility, and eventually catastrophic screw pullout or vertebral fractures.[44,45] Serial radiographs, starting from the earliest postoperative study, should be evaluated for any evidence of hardware migration or fracture. Identification of a change in sagittal or coronal balance is often a valuable initial step. Set-screw loosening, rod fatigue bending without frank fracture, and sacral screw subsidence are subtle abnormalities that should also be carefully examined in patients with late postoperative loss of sagittal alignment.[46]

A review of the literature noted a 28.1% to 39.9% rate of pedicle screw malposition in clinical studies and a 5.5% to 31.3% malposition rate in cadaver studies. However, meta-analysis shows that only 0.6% to 4.3% of patients need reoperations for device malposition.[47] The percentage of malpositioned screws may be higher when normal anatomic landmarks have been obscured, as with revision surgery in the setting of a dorsolateral fusion.[48] Minor violations of the cortex are not uncommon and may be asymptomatic. In these cases, the screw position may be acceptable. Screw malposition with related clinical symptoms needs revision surgery. Pedicle screw loosening has been recorded as being caused mainly by cyclic caudocephalad toggling at the bone–screw interface. To prevent pedicle screw loosening, a meticulous screw insertion technique to prohibit the toggling effect that could be occurring during screw insertion is needed. On reoperation, a larger-diameter screw or augmentation with polymethylmethylacrylate (PMMA) gives a better result.

Reoperation to remove instrumentation that has either failed or has eroded through the skin requires full exposure of the instrumentation and construct, with care taken to not create fracture of the bone grafts or vertebral column when removing the implant. Large metal shears and rod cutters may create enough torque to actually fracture the dorsal elements of the vertebra and should be used with great caution. A high-speed carbide bur may be used to cut the rods, but all exposed soft tissue should be covered to prevent the small metal filings from being spread throughout the wound. Otherwise, these filings cause a great deal of artifactual change on future imaging studies.

Cerebrospinal Fluid Leak

CSF leakage may occur at the dural suture line postoperatively or may be caused by inadvertent dural tears during extradural spinal approaches for disc surgery or decompressive laminectomy. Prior surgery, with subsequent development of scar tissue, altered anatomy, poor dissection planes, and adherence of tissue to the dura, all have been demonstrated to increase the risk of incidental durotomy. Possible sequelae of incidental durotomy include the formation of a pseudomeningocele, a CSF cutaneous fistula, arachnoiditis, meningitis, epidural abscess, or deterioration in neurologic status. A persistent CSF leak may result in a chronic pain disorder associated with radiculopathy or postural headaches. A CSF leak also predisposes the patient to poor wound healing and possible wound dehiscence.

Reoperation for CSF leak requires adequate exposure of the dural defect, which may require further bone removal. Primary closure is attempted whenever possible. A patch of autologous fascia or artificial dura material with fibrin tissue adhesive is useful if primary closure is not possible.[49-51] Black[52] used a large sheet of fat to cover not only the dural tears but also all of the exposed dura with good results. A randomized, controlled trial concluded that the PEG hydrogel spinal sealant (DuraSeal) is safe and effective for providing watertight closure when used as an adjunct to sutured dural repair during spinal surgery.[53] Placement of a CSF drain for 5 days may be used for dural repair if primary dural closure fails. Good muscle and fascia closure will prevent dead space and prevent CSF collection and postoperative pseudomeningocele. In recurrent CSF leak, myocutaneous muscle flaps can be considered an option with good results.

Infection

Surgical site infection in the setting of spine fusion is associated with significant morbidity and medical resource utilization. The reported rate of spinal surgical site infection in the literature ranges from 0.7% to 16 %.[54,55] Risk factors include smoking, diabetes, prolonged operative time, large-volume blood loss, previous surgery, use of nonautograft bone graft alternatives, and number of levels affected. Spinal surgical site infections can be challenging to manage and often require prolonged hospitalizations, extended antibiotic therapy, repeated surgery for wound debridement, instrumentation removal, or delayed complications of deep infection. It is often difficult to diagnose postoperative spine infection before clinical symptoms become apparent. In the early stages, plain film radiography is often normal. In this setting, nuclear scintigraphy with either gallium-labeled bone scan or indium-111-labeled white blood cells or MRI can be useful. MRI can help to diagnose the soft tissue change but is expensive to use as a screening tool. Although inflammatory markers, such as C-reactive protein (CRP), white blood cell count, erythrocyte sedimentation rate, and body temperature are easily measured, their specificities are not high. Elevated serum procalcitonin levels of greater than 0.5 ng/mL may serve as a useful tool for evaluating fevers of unknown origin after spine surgery.[56]

Reoperation for wound infection is best handled by reopening the complete length of the incision to the depth of infectious involvement. After all suture material is removed, along with any dead tissue, the wound is debrided to bleeding tissue. The wound should then be irrigated thoroughly with antibiotic solution. If the infection is superficial, the wound is closed in layers, and the patient is given appropriate intravenous antibiotics to which the organism is susceptible. For deep infections and for infections in the presence of instrumentation or bone grafts, a similar procedure is carried out, or staged closure with wound vacuum is helpful. If osteomyelitis or discitis is present, debridement of the involved bone and disc is performed via a retroperitoneal or dorsal-only approach in the lumbar spine, a lateral extracavitary approach in the thoracic spine, and a ventral or dorsal approach in the cervical spine. A fresh autologous cortical bone graft is inserted for ventral stabilization. Unlike in joint arthroplasty, hardware removal is not mandatory to eradicate most infections, although removal of the hardware may be indicated in certain cases in which medical treatment has failed, especially if the infection is delayed and fusion is solid.[42,57] The antibiotics are usually continued for 6 weeks or even longer if the CRP level has not returned to normal by that time.

Hematomas

Spinal epidural hematoma is a known complication of spine surgery. Most surgical procedures involving the spine will result in a small, clinically insignificant epidural hematoma. However, some spinal epidural hematomas are significant enough to cause spinal cord compression and neurologic symptoms requiring surgical intervention. Postoperative epidural hematomas should be suspected in the patient who either demonstrates a new postoperative neurologic deficit or develops deficits in the immediate postoperative period. Lawton et al.[58] reported the incidence rate of spinal epidural hematomas to be 0.1%. Spinal epidural hematoma is a significant cause of morbidity and needs to be diagnosed as early as possible because the timing of decompression and evacuation of the hematoma is critical. Extra precautions for meticulous hemostasis during the surgical procedure should be considered in patients who require multilevel decompressions or have a preoperative coagulopathy. Placement of a postoperative wound drain to prevent epidural hematoma is still controversial.

Compared with virgin spine operations, reoperations require more extensive exposures. Therefore, the risk of spine instability, neural damage, and infection is increased. The same techniques as used in the virgin operation are used in reoperations, but limitations created by scar tissue and the loss of bone and ligamentous structures that aid in spine stability are present. When undertaking any reoperation on the spine, the surgeon must keep in mind that with each succeeding operation, the challenge is increased and the chance of a good result is reduced. Pain alone is not an indication for reoperation. Correctable anatomic abnormalities must be present to warrant repeat surgery. It is always worthwhile to remember that the most common cause of failure of spine surgery is not a technical error or complication but failure of appropriate patient selection. When patients have been improperly chosen for surgery in the first place, it is not likely that repair of an unintended consequence of the first operation will be beneficial. On the other hand, it is unfair to leave patients with an uncorrected abnormality that is producing symptoms. Repair of the demonstrated problem in such patients is reasonable. All patients with failed spine surgery should, however, be carefully assessed for the presence of important comorbidities that may exaggerate the complaint of pain. These should be addressed simultaneously with reparative surgery.

Acknowledgements. Thank you to Edward S. Connolly and Donlin M. Long, who authored prior editions of this chapter. Their work laid the foundation for this third edition.

KEY REFERENCES

Ahn UM, Ahn NU, Buchowski MS, et al: Cauda equina syndrome secondary to lumbar disc herniation. A meta-analysis of surgical outcomes. *Spine (Phila Pa 1976)* 25:1515–1522, 2000.

Berquist TH: Imaging of the postoperative spine. *Radiol Clin North Am* 44(3):407–418, 2006.

Carragee EJ, Han MY, Suen PW, et al: Clinical outcomes after lumbar discectomy for sciatica: the effects of fragment type and anular competence. *J Bone Joint Surg [Am]* 85:102–108, 2003.

Lawton MT, Porter RW, Heiserman JE, et al: Surgical management of spinal epidural hematoma: relationship between surgical timing and neurological outcome. *J Neurosurg* 83:1–7, 1995.

Martin BI, Mirza SK, Comstock BA, et al: Are lumbar spine reoperation rates falling with greater use of fusion surgery and new surgical technology? *Spine (Phila Pa 1976)* 32(19):2119–2126, 2007.

McGirt MJ, Ambrossi GL, Datoo G, et al: Recurrent disc herniation and long-term back pain after primary lumbar discectomy: review of outcomes reported for limited versus aggressive disc removal. *Neurosurgery* 64(2):338–345, 2009.

McGirt MJ, Garces-Ambrossi GL, B.S., Parker SL, et al: Short-term progressive spinal deformity following laminoplasty versus laminectomy for resection of intradural spinal tumors: analysis of 238 patients. *Neurosurgery* 66(5):1005–1012, 2010.

REFERENCES

The complete reference list is available online at expertconsult.com.

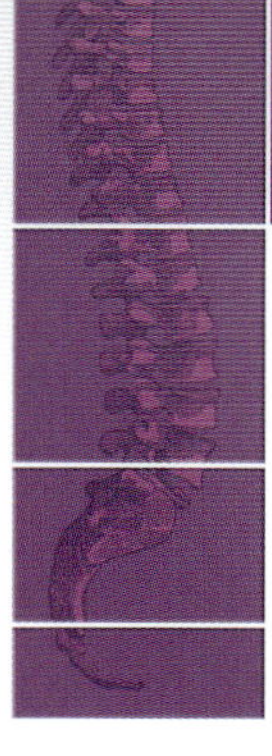

CHAPTER 203

Intraoperative Crisis Management in Spine Surgery: What to Do When Things Go Bad

Kalil G. Abdullah | Eve C. Tsai | Edward C. Benzel | Michael P. Steinmetz

Complications in spine surgery may occur in spite of the surgeon's best attempts at prevention. The previous chapters of this text addressed the prevention and management of complications. This chapter addresses the management of catastrophic intraoperative and perioperative complications.

Many types of complications in spine surgery have been reported, but most are not crises. A crisis requires swift and decisive action by the health-care team. The crises outlined in the following discussion refer to those in which action must be taken intraoperatively or during the immediate postoperative period. We do not discuss complications that do not require immediate action (e.g., while a nerve root avulsion is a major complication, it does not require immediate action). Here, we divide crisis management into four sections: (1) anesthesia-related crises, (2) surgical crises, (3) electrophysiologic spinal cord monitoring issues, and (4) neurologic injuries.

Anesthetic Crises

Prone Cardiopulmonary Arrest

Most spine operations are carried out in the prone position. However, this position may present some difficulty for the anesthesiologist by interfering with monitoring techniques, altering respiratory function, and limiting airway and vascular access.[1] Cardiac arrest in patients who undergo surgery in the prone position is very uncommon. The major preoperative risk factor is understandably cardiac disease, while intraoperative factors include hemorrhage, gas embolism, and diminished venous return.[2] The rare occurrence of cardiac arrest during spine surgery and modern anesthetic techniques nearly obviate the need for cardiopulmonary resuscitation (CPR) in the operating room. Nevertheless, it may be necessary in some circumstances. The prone position substantially complicates cardiopulmonary arrest management for several reasons. First, the time necessary to procure a stretcher and turn the patient to the supine position to perform CPR may delay therapy. The wound must be closed quickly, risking infection and costing valuable time. Interruption of the surgical procedure may also leave the spine unstable, risking further injury. Additionally, spinal implants may not be fully attached or may protrude from the wound.

Turning the patient might not be feasible in some situations, owing to the risk of neurologic injury. In these situations, the resuscitation begins with the anesthesiologist, while the wound is being closed. However, the surgeon must initiate CPR. Two options are available in these situations. Closed CPR in the prone position has been described and is typically used first.[1-3] If sternal support is present, the surgeon may place his or her hands on either side of the incision at the midthoracic level with the palms placed over the patient's scapulae[1] (Fig. 203-1). Compression is then initiated. The arterial wave form, blood pressure, and end-tidal CO_2 should be observed to monitor cardiac output and adequacy of resuscitation. If there is no sternal support (e.g., the patient is placed on chest rolls), the surgeon may clench a fist and place it under the patient's chest over the lower third of the sternum[3] (Fig. 203-2). This requires a break in sterility. The surgeon's other hand (or an associate's) then compresses at the midthoracic level.

If the aforementioned techniques are not feasible or are unsuccessful owing to lack of adequate cardiac output or in the presence of spine instability, the surgeon has the option to perform a left dorsal thoracotomy.[3] This procedure provides direct access to the heart. Following exposure, open internal cardiac massage or defibrillation may be performed (Fig. 203-3).

Air Embolism

Intraoperative venous air embolism (VAE) occurs most commonly when patients are in the sitting position. For this reason, surgeons often avoid the sitting position. Negative pressures are greater in the sitting position, owing to the elevation of the head. However, it should be noted that VAE can occur in any position in which the head is elevated at a higher level than the heart. Depending on the type of monitoring technique that is used, the overall incidence of air embolism has been reported to be anywhere between 25% and 50% in surgeries involving the posterior fossa.[4] The incidence during cervical laminectomy has been estimated at 25%.[5] In one study in which transesophageal echocardiography was used, 100% of patients in the sitting position demonstrated VAE.[6] While the occurrence of VAE may be high, its sequelae remain low as long as appropriate measures to treat the embolism are carried out rapidly. During surgery in the sitting position, appropriate monitoring should be used. This includes the use of the electrocardiograph, arterial catheter, right atrial or pulmonary artery catheter, end-tidal CO_2 monitor, and a precordial Doppler (the most sensitive and practical monitor for VAE).

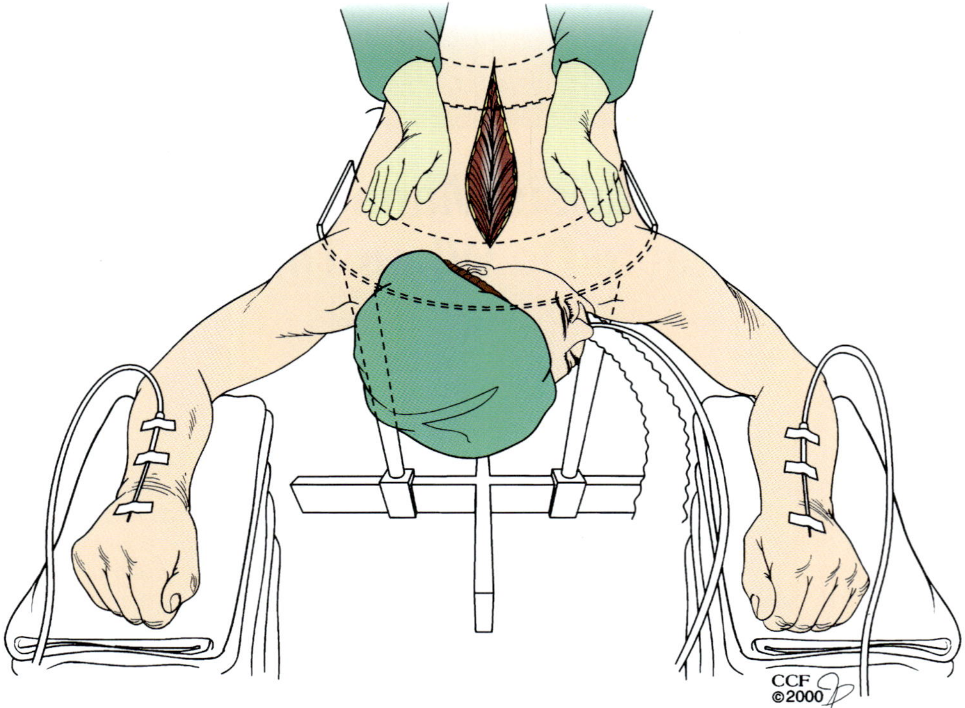

FIGURE 203-1. When sternal support is available, the surgeon may place his or her hands on either side of the spine at the midthoracic level for compressions during CPR. (Copyright Cleveland Clinic Foundation.)

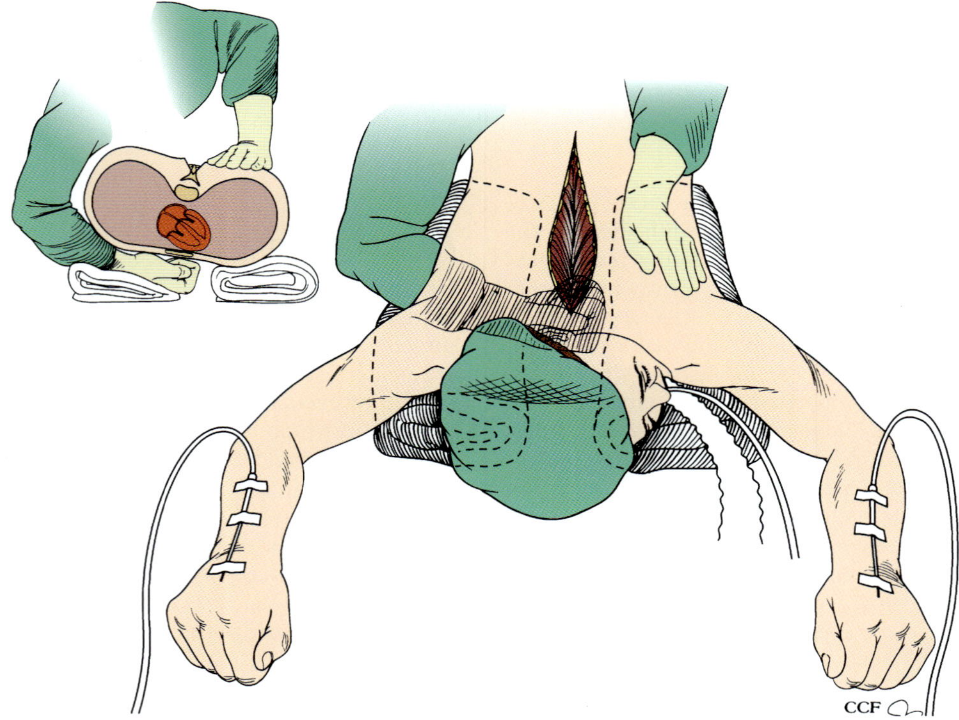

FIGURE 203-2. When there is lack of sternal support, the surgeon or assistant may place a clenched fist on the lower sternum, and the other hand may compress at the midthoracic level during CPR. (Copyright Cleveland Clinic Foundation.)

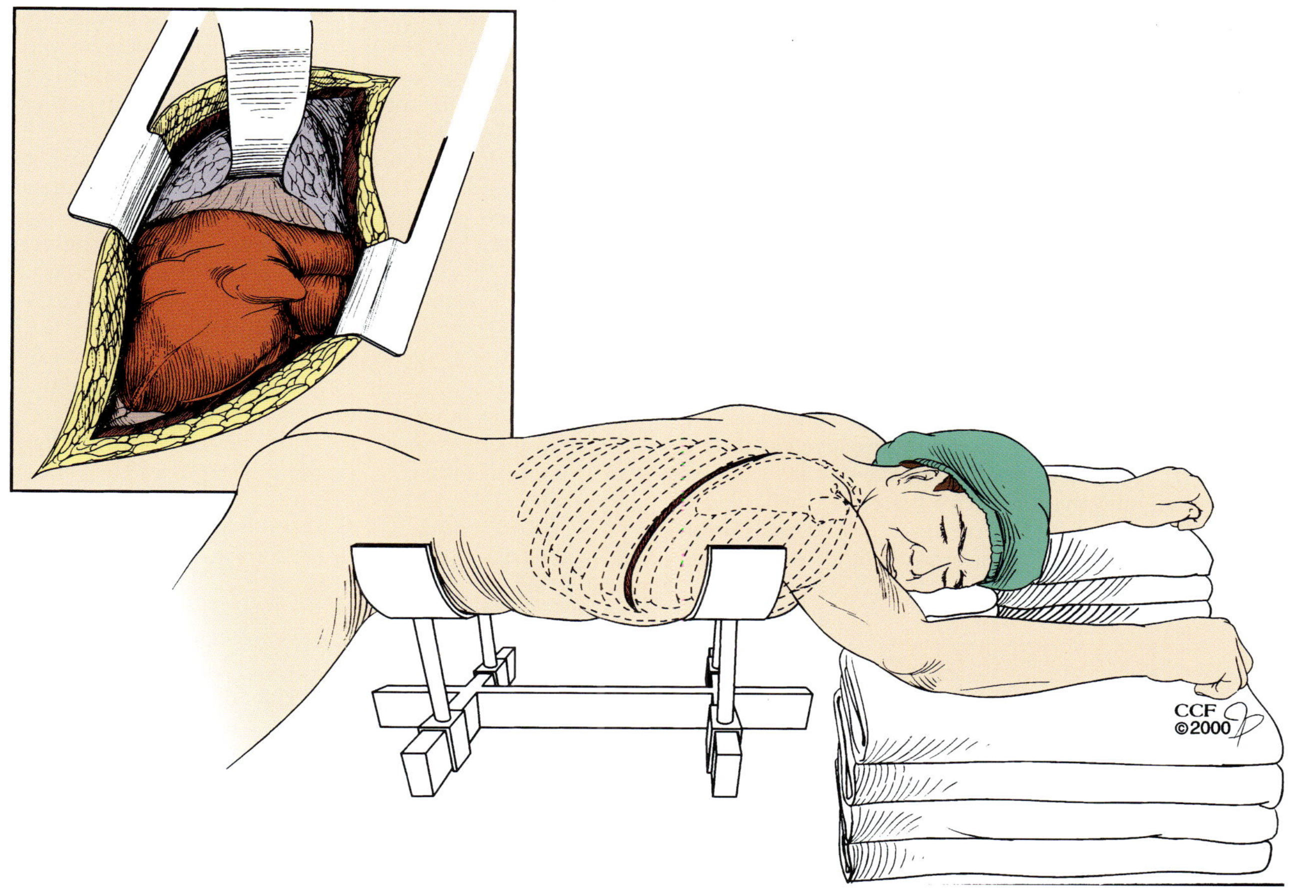

FIGURE 203-3. Left dorsal thoracotomy. An incision is made between the ribs. The dissection is taken down to and through the intercostal muscles. The parietal pleura is incised. The heart may now be visualized, and internal cardiac massage may be undertaken. (Copyright Cleveland Clinic Foundation.)

These devices allow for the early detection and treatment of VAE prior to paradoxical air embolism or cardiopulmonary incident. Most frequently, the initial indication of the presence of VAE is the precordial Doppler. A significant VAE elicits audible Doppler indicators and possibly a decrease in end-tidal CO_2, ventricular arrhythmias, and hypotension and/or an increase in pulmonary artery pressure. At the first indication of VAE, the surgeon should flood the operative field with saline, wax all bleeding bone edges, and occlude any visual sources of venous bleeding. Bilateral jugular venous compression by the anesthesiologist increases the central venous pressure and may help in identifying the venous source. If only one jugular vein can be compressed, the right one should be chosen. The anesthesiologist should discontinue nitrous oxide infusion, as this has been shown to enlarge the gas volume of air-containing cavities.[7,8] Positive end-expiratory pressure should be discontinued (it may alter right-to-left atrial pressure gradients and facilitate the passage of air across an existing patent foramen ovale), and air should be aspirated by using a right atrial catheter if one is available.[9,10] These steps should lead to the resolution of VAE-related symptoms. The patient may also be placed in a head-down position with the patient's right side up in order to trap air in the right atrium to aid in aspiration of the air bolus and minimize pulmonary and cerebral ischemic complications, but this is rarely required.[11]

If the aforementioned maneuvers resolve the symptoms, the procedure may be completed as planned. If the VAE is severe and does not respond to therapy or continues to progress, then the procedure should be terminated. Surgery may be completed at a later date, with modification of position such as utilizing a prone position rather than a sitting position.

Surgical Crises

Vascular Injuries

Cervical Approaches

Vertebral artery injuries in the cervical spine are uncommon but potentially catastrophic. The ventral approach places both the carotid and vertebral arteries at risk for injury, but the carotid artery is fully visualized during ventral exposure and therefore is rarely injured.[12] If injury does occur, it can be readily identified and controlled with direct pressure, with or without primary vascular repair. Shunting or temporary clamping of the carotid artery may be performed while a primary or patch repair of the artery is performed.

The ventral and dorsal cervical approaches both place the vertebral artery at risk for injury. In the anterior approach, the rate of injury has been estimated to be between 0.3% and 0.5%.[13-17] Injury during the ventral approach can occur because of excessive lateral bone–disc removal, drill use too far off midline into the uncinate processes, subperiosteal elevation of the longus colli muscles, vertebral artery anatomic anomalies, or the softening of bone of the lateral part of the spinal cord owing to pathologic processes.[17] Injury to the vertebral arteries during posterior cervical screw placement in the subaxial spine is considered to be rare and generally due to improper drilling and poor trajectories during placement.[18]

The vertebral artery is hidden within the foramen transversarium, and initial injury to the artery is usually announced by the presence of brisk, bright red arterial bleeding. Occasionally, darker venous bleeding may be seen if damage has been done to the neighboring venous plexus. The management of vertebral artery damage in the subaxial spine is diagrammed in Fig. 203-4. First, manual pressure and the use of a hemostatic agent should be employed at the site of suspected injury. When bleeding is under control, time is available for the anesthesiologist to "catch up" with regard to volume replacement and, if necessary, blood transfusion. Proximal and distal control of the artery should be attempted.

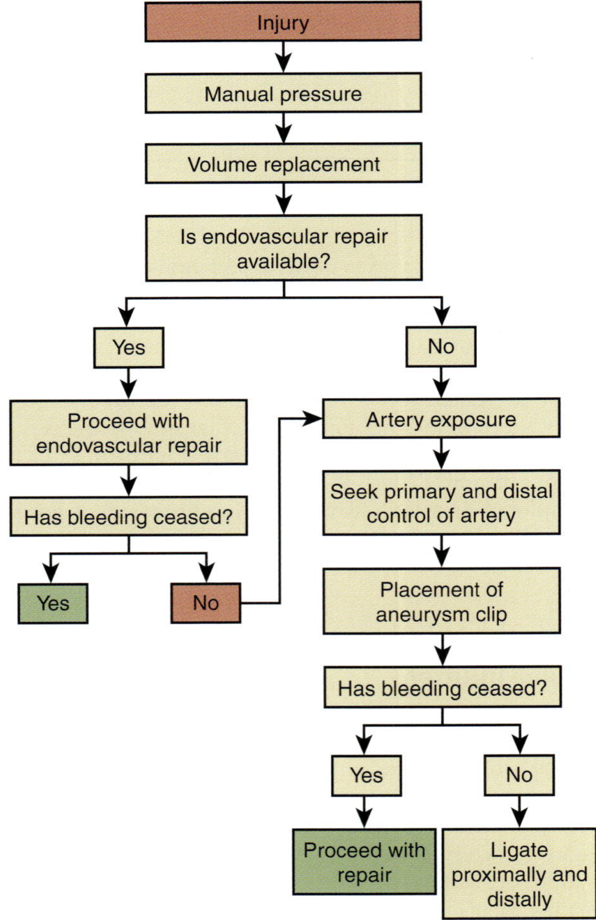

FIGURE 203-4. Algorithm for the treatment of iatrogenic injury to the vertebral artery during cervical spine surgery. Note this should be viewed in the setting of an inability to control bleeding from an injured vertebral artery. If the bleeding can be stopped with packing and hemostatic agents, a clinical decision may be made to either manage expectantly if the patient remains stable clinically or proceed to angiography for potential endovascular repair or occlusion.

In either a ventral or a dorsal approach, the transverse process should be dissected to expose the artery one level above and below the injury. A high-speed drill with a diamond tip bur may be used to open the foramen transversarium and expose the artery. An aneurysm clip may be placed to achieve temporary control of bleeding during injury repair.[14] Primary repair of the artery should be considered. If reconstruction of the artery cannot be achieved, it should be ligated proximally and distally.

If bleeding can be controlled with packing or hemostatic agents, consideration should be given to completion of the operation. Instrumentation should be placed on the side contralateral to the side of injury with great care, if at all. Consideration must be given to the chance of occlusion or damage of the contralateral vertebral artery and the morbidity and/or mortality that may occur as a result.

Intraoperative angiography may be considered.[17] Once primary control of the bleeding has been attained, the patient can be taken to the endovascular suite and the vertebral artery can be stented or occluded. Perioperative management remains controversial, with some surgeons choosing immediate postoperative angiography while others reserve further intervention to be based on the patient's observed clinical course.[19]

Injury during C1-2 transarticular screw placement has been reported to be as high as 2.2% per screw.[19] As in the subaxial spine, injury to the vertebral artery is often heralded by brisk arterial bleeding seen during drilling or K-wire placement. Control of the hemorrhage can be obtained by placing the transarticular screw into the drill hole or by packing the hole with bone wax. Placing the screw into the drill hole is preferred, as it both plugs the hole and provides stability. The opposite screw should not be drilled or placed. Doing so invites a high risk of disastrous sequelae associated with bilateral vertebral artery injury.

Dorsal Thoracic and Lumbar Approaches

Vascular injury during dorsal thoracic surgery is rare. Therefore, the following discussion is limited to dorsal lumbar approaches. Lumbar disc surgery is one of the most commonly performed spine operations. The incidence of vascular complication has been recently estimated to be 0.14% at the most.[20-23] The most commonly injured vessels are the common iliac arteries.[24] Other potentially injured vessels are the left common iliac vein, median sacral artery, aorta, and inferior vena cava.

Vascular injury is typically caused by aggressive use of a pituitary rongeur that penetrates the ventral anulus fibrosus and causes breach of the vessel wall.[25] Neither surgeon experience[26] nor amount of disc material removed[25] has been demonstrated to affect the incidence of this injury. Brisk bleeding into the interspace is observed in only 25% of these injuries, and so may not be immediately evident to the surgeon.[25] When brisk bleeding is observed, it may actually be due to damage to extradural veins and not an arterial injury.[26]

The injury is usually recognized in the recovery room, although with venous injuries, the symptoms and signs of injury can be delayed. The patient is most often hypotensive and tachycardic and has abdominal distention and pain. Pallor and weak pulses are also usually present. The patient should immediately be taken back to the operating room for laparotomy. Cross-clamping of the aorta can facilitate resuscitation.[25] All vessels should be carefully inspected. A tear in a vein may be primarily repaired with suture. The iliac artery may be divided to gain access to an injured vein and then must be reanastomosed. Arterial injuries may be repaired primarily or with an interposition graft. Damage to an internal iliac vessel (artery or vein) may be repaired by ligation if primary repair is not possible.

Ventral Thoracic and Lumbar Approaches

The incidence of vascular injury during the ventral approach to the lumbar spine has recently been estimated to be between 11% and 12%.[27,28] However, the majority of injuries are venous and require only simple suture or clip repair. Major crises occur at a rate of only 2%.[27] Injury usually occurs during exposure and is more likely to occur with exposure of L4-5.[27] Chances of injury increase with use of preoperative radiation therapy or if osteomyelitis is present. Vessels that potentially can be injured include the left iliac vein, the iliolumbar vein, the middle sacral vessels, and the left iliac artery. During ventral exposure and dissection, the middle sacral vessels (Fig. 203-5A) and iliolumbar vein (Fig. 203-5B) should be identified and ligated. If sudden hemorrhage occurs, direct pressure is applied to the vena cava, and identification of the injured vessel is attempted. A torn lumbar or iliolumbar vein may be clamped and ligated. If an iliac vein injury is suspected, direct pressure should be applied, and then proximal and distal control of the vein should be achieved. The perforation can then be repaired primarily.[29] If an artery is injured, proximal and distal control must be attained, and the injury is repaired either primarily or with an interposition graft.

Injury to the aorta is rare in the upper lumbar and thoracic region. This injury should be treated immediately with thoracotomy and/or laparotomy to repair the vessel. If injury is suspected in the recovery room and the patient is stable, angiography may be performed to identify the injury prior to attempted repair.[11]

Iliac Crest Graft Harvest

Injury to the superior gluteal artery is a reported but uncommon occurrence during iliac graft harvest.[30,31] Injury usually occurs during exposure of the iliac crest with inadvertent placement of a sharp self-retaining retractor into the sciatic notch. If the vessel is encountered and identified, it should be ligated. This is usually not possible, owing to vessel retraction; in this case, the operative site should be packed, and the patient should be taken to the angiography suite for embolization. The primary operation may be completed the following day. While direct surgical approach and ligation are possible, they require a retroperitoneal approach because the vessel usually retracts to an intrapelvic location.[30]

Visceral Injuries

The majority of visceral injuries (such as ureteral and intestinal) are not considered crises to the spine surgeon; they are discovered and dealt with postoperatively. The exception is esophageal injury. Estimates of esophageal injury have been placed as high as 3.4% in some series, but it is thought that the true incidence is underreported.[32,33] These injuries can be divided into those that are noticed intraoperatively, those that are discovered in the immediate postoperative period, and delayed cases that are brought to light only days, weeks, or even months after discharge from the hospital. The last type is not discussed here. Should an injury be identified intraoperatively, the tear should be primarily repaired with interrupted resorbable sutures in two layers. It may be advantageous to reinforce the repair with muscle (strap) as well. Timing of antibiotics and nasogastric tube drainage will be variable depending on surgeon and institutional preferences.[32] An esophagram should be obtained at or around day 7; if it is normal, oral feeding may be started.

Identification of esophageal perforation in the postoperative period has been shown to reduce mortality from nearly 50% to 20% if the perforation is noticed within 24 hours of surgery.[33] Therefore, vigilance should be maintained. Warning signs may include dyspnea, dysphagia, dysphonia, swelling, fever, leukocytosis, or consistent unexplained tachycardia.[32,33] Plain radiographs may show subcutaneous emphysema, widening of the retropharyngeal space, or displacement or migration of hardware. Imaging and endoscopic tests can have a false-negative rate of 10% to 46%.[32] If there is high clinical suspicion of an esophageal perforation, the patient should be taken back to the operating room immediately for exploration. Repair of the perforation may be performed as previously described for intraoperative perforations. Because of contamination, the wound may be left open, and consideration should be given to placing a tissue layer between the fresh suture line and the bone graft. The sternal head of the sternocleidomastoid muscle may be reflected and sutured to the contralateral paravertebral muscles to accomplish this.[34] If a ventral spinal implant was placed, the surgeon should strongly consider its removal. Prolonged diversion of the salivary flow and oral intake through the use of gastric feeding or parenteral nutrition should also be considered, should there be any concern about the esophageal repair.

Durotomy

Unintended durotomy is one of the most common complications of spine surgery. While unintended durotomy occurs in anywhere between 1% and 17% of surgeries, the vast majority can be repaired with simple primary repair.[35-39] Controversy surrounds the management of dural tears. Differing opinions can be found regarding whether or not a subfascial drain should be placed and the number of days of postoperative bedrest necessary to facilitate healing.[39] It is important to note that unintended durotomy, if recognized and repaired, has repeatedly been shown not to influence the final clinical outcome of procedures on the lumbar spine.[36,38]

As has already been stated, unintended durotomy should be repaired primarily. The type of suture and suture technique are the surgeon's choice. We favor #4-0 Neurolon (Ethicon, Summerville, NJ) suture, using a running locking technique. Adequate exposure of the tear must be achieved prior to suturing. Proper illumination and often magnification (loupe/microscope) can assist in repair. After exposure, a surgical patty is used over the tear, and a smaller sucker tip is used. If the surgeon believes that the primary closure may lead to excessive tension on the nerve roots, a patch may be used. Many patch varieties are available, including synthetic, cadaveric, and autologous (we prefer autologous tissue). In cases of small defects, the lumbar fascia may be secured to the dura mater with interrupted sutures. A large defect may

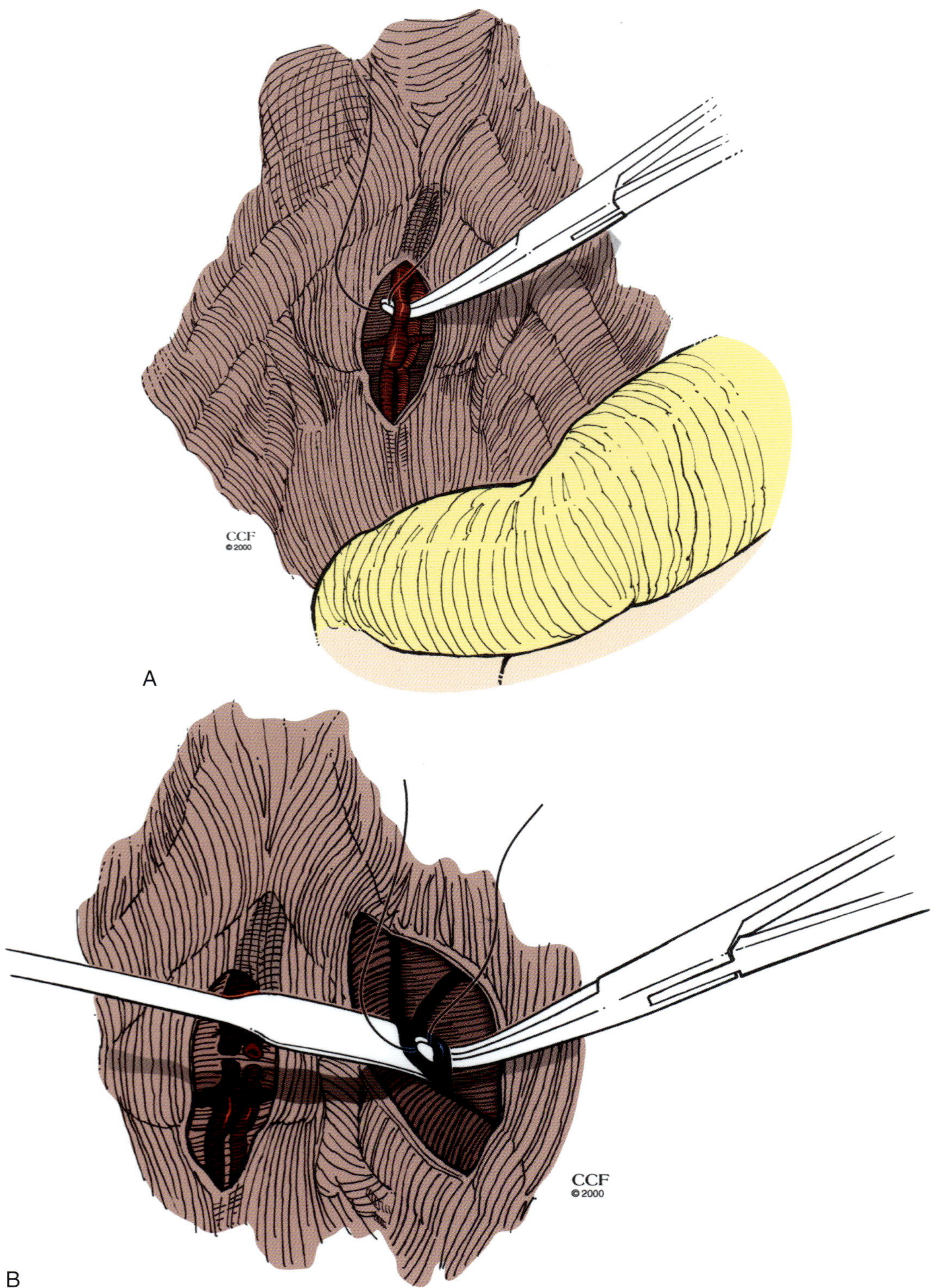

FIGURE 203-5. During dissection for a ventral lumbar approach, the middle sacral vessels (**A**) and iliolumbar vein (**B**) should be identified and ligated. (Copyright Cleveland Clinic Foundation.)

necessitate the use of fascia lata. Very large dural defects may require patch placement and the use of fibrin glue.

After repair, a Valsalva maneuver should be performed to check for leaks. Any leak that is present should be oversewn. A dry piece of hemostatic gelatin (Gelfoam) or DuraGen (Integra, Plainsboro, NJ) may be placed over the suture line. The more superficial tissues should then be tightly and meticulously closed in layers. A few muscle sutures using nonabsorbable O-gauge braided suture may be placed. The fascia is then closed with the same suture in a watertight manner by using an interrupted stitch that is reinforced with a running locking stitch. Next, #2-0 absorbable suture may be used to close as many layers as possible, including Scarpa's fascia and dermis. The skin should be carefully closed, usually with sutures. Interrupted vertical mattress closure should be considered because of its excellent skin approximation characteristics. The use of a subfascial drain is controversial because of concerns about cerebrospinal fluid fistula formation.[35] Significant recent evidence now exists showing that drain placement can be used with very low rates of complication.[36] Khan et al. demonstrated that removal of a subfascial drain the morning following surgery resulted in no cases of fistula in any of their 388 patients who experienced unintended durotomy.[38] This is the second large study to report no increased incidence of myelocutaneous fistula with this type of drain.[36] The use of a subarachnoid drain during surgery may be considered as well, but no conclusive evidence exists regarding its efficacy.

Facet Reduction

Facet reduction is included in this chapter as a "crisis" because it may be necessary to take immediate action in the case of exacerbation of neurologic symptoms during closed reduction. In brief, closed reduction followed by an external orthosis is a frequently performed procedure but may, in the presence of a previously unknown disc herniation, cause catastrophic neurologic deterioration. Open reduction avoids this complication and in small case series has been successful in treating unilateral or bilateral locked facets. Discussion here is limited to open reduction.

For a ventral approach to reduction and stabilization, the patient is positioned in the supine position, and a standard approach for anterior cervical discectomy is performed. After discectomy is complete, vertebral body posts are placed at 10- to 20-degree diverging angles to each other (Fig. 203-6A). Distraction is applied, and the locked facets are disengaged (Fig. 203-6B). A dorsally directed force is applied to the rostral body by manual pressure (Fig. 203-6C) or curet (Fig. 203-6D), facilitating reduction. Interbody disc spreaders that are placed at an angle and then rotated rostrally may also be used for the reduction (Fig. 203-7). A plain radiograph may then be taken to visualize reduction. If reduction is not accomplished, the procedure should be repeated. In cases such as those involving commuted facet fractures, reduction might not be possible using the aforementioned technique. Instead, the patient should undergo dorsal reduction and arthrodesis followed by ventral arthrodesis. After reduction has been obtained, standard iliac crest harvesting and strut placement are performed. Finally, a ventral cervical fixation device is placed.

Level Identification

Level localization in spine surgery can be challenging. However, it is of obvious importance. Wrong-level spine surgery is an adverse but preventable event. A recent anonymous survey of 415 spine surgeons reported that half had performed at least one wrong-level surgery during their careers.[40] It is likely that the incidence of wrong-level surgery is underreported; studies have estimated a rate of 0.4% to 4.3%.[41-43] Despite poor reporting, wrong-level surgery is widely recognized as a preventable cause of patient morbidity.

Generally, level identification is accomplished by performing a lateral intraoperative radiograph with a marker in place. In the lumbar spine, an Alice clamp or sharp towel clip may be placed on the presumed most appropriate spinous process along with a Penfield no. 4 or Woodson elevator under the same lamina, both being directed perpendicular to the spine. A lateral radiograph is obtained. We choose to count up from the lumbosacral junction and assume five lumbar vertebrae. The most caudal normal disc space is labeled as L5-S1, with the iliac crest serving as a secondary internal landmark to identify the L4-5 level to reduce any confusion about the L5-S1 position in patients with transitional lumbar vertebrae at the lumbosacral junction.

Localization in the thoracic spine presents more difficulty. Often, anterior posterior radiographs are obtained, and ribs are counted to the desired level. We believe that this is frequently misleading. Localization with lateral radiographs may be used as in the lumbar or cervical spine. Marking may be performed as in the lumbar spine, but care must be taken in placing an instrument under the lamina owing to the narrow spinal canal dimensions at this level. A marker may be placed on the transverse process. A large-plate radiograph is then performed that includes the sacrum. Counting is performed from the sacrum. At times, there is inadequate visualization using this technique; in these cases, a marker (Alice clamp) may be placed at the most rostral or caudal level (spinous or transverse process) that is exposed. A lateral cervical or lumbar radiograph is then obtained, which includes the occiput or sacrum, respectively. Levels are then counted to this marker. A lateral radiograph of the thoracic spine is then performed, and levels are counted from the prior marked level to the pathology (which has also been marked with an Alice clamp).

Marking of the pathologic level after it has been identified must be performed with care. Some surgeons mark the lamina and interspinous ligament with a marking pen, but this may be washed off with blood or irrigation. The level may also be marked with a small bite off the spinous process, a rongeur, or a suture placed through the spinous process. If the expected pathology is not found at the expected level, the appropriate location should be confirmed by radiologic localization with a radiopaque instrument placed to identify the level. Lateral radiographs should continue to be performed with different marking techniques until the surgeon is satisfied that he or she is operating at the appropriate level.

Radiographs can help to identify pathologic levels, but they are helpful only if the radiographs can be correlated with preoperatively acquired images that identify the pathology. Fluoroscopy may assist in expediting localization, as the time required to develop the radiograph plates will be eliminated. In relying on an MRI to demonstrate thoracic pathology, it is essential that the radiographic localization correspond to the MRI localization, as the number of cervical, thoracic, and lumbar levels can be variable. For example, suppose the MRI demonstrates that there is a thoracic vertebra pathology that is 14 vertebral bodies rostral to the sacrum. If the patient has the normal 5 lumbar vertebrae and 12 thoracic vertebrae, then the thoracic vertebral pathology would be at T3. However, if the patient has 4 or 6 lumbar vertebrae and 12 thoracic vertebrae, then the pathology would be at T2 or T4, respectively.

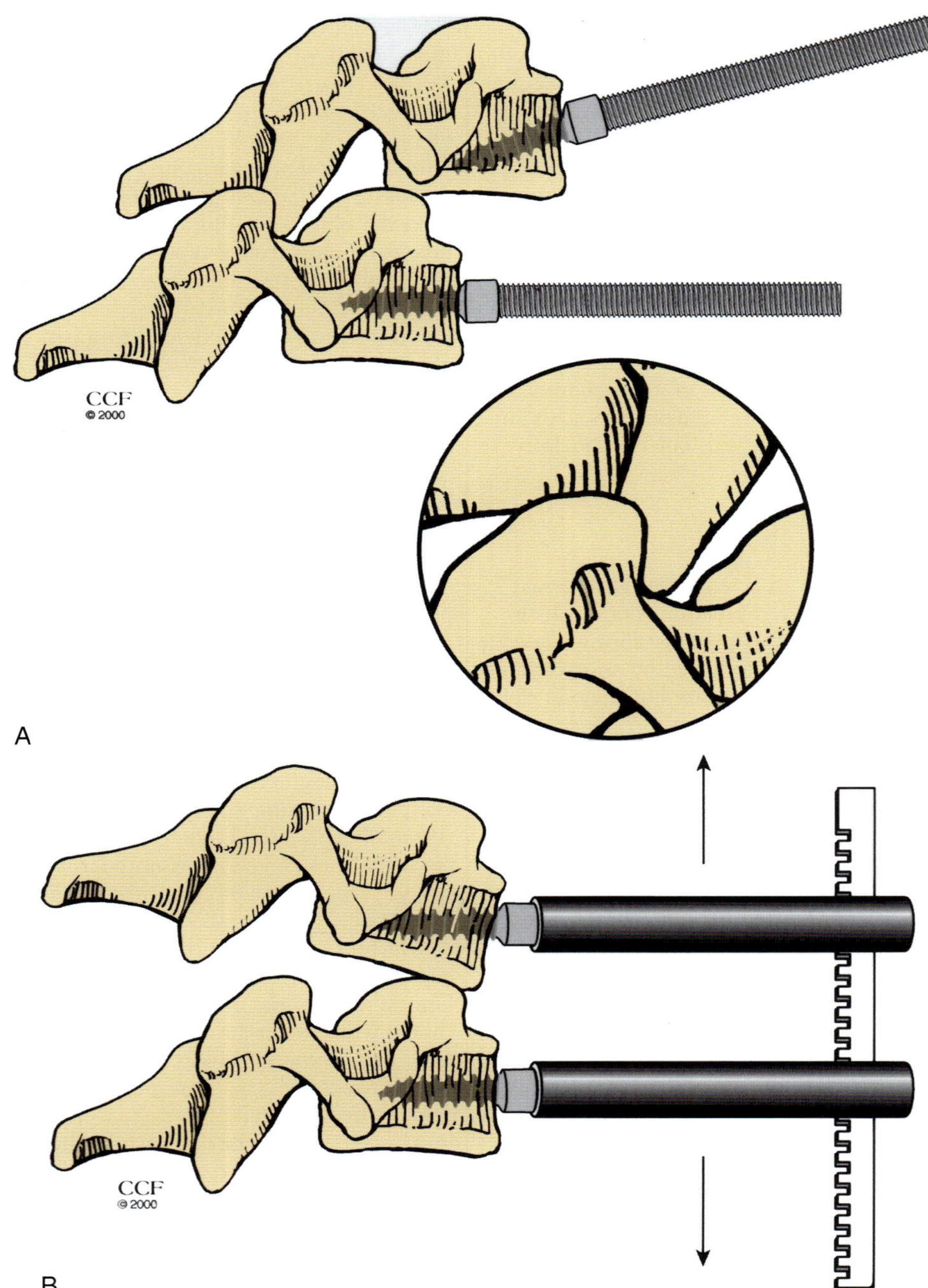

FIGURE 203-6. Cervical facet dislocation management via the ventral approach. **A,** The vertebral posts may be placed at 10- to 20-degree diverging angles to each other. When distraction is applied, this will allow disengagement of the facets. **B,** When distraction is applied, the facets become disengaged.

If the surgeon then uses a radiologic localization using the C7 spinous process to count down to the pathology relying solely on the MRI that did not include the corresponding cervical levels, then the identification of the pathologic level could be erroneous if the patient had anomalous segmentation. If the surgeon used a radiologic localization corresponding to the MRI localization and counted from the sacrum up, then this error in identifying that pathologic level could be avoided. In some cases, myelography may be helpful in the thoracic spine by providing a radiographic correlate that "relates anatomically" to the pathology. Ribs may then be used as markers with confidence, as this eliminates errors related to discrepancies between radiographs and MRI. Wide anteroposterior myelographic views should be obtained so that ribs can be visualized (particularly the lowest rib) and counted.

Beam trajectory should be considered during interpretation of intraoperative radiographs. Beam trajectory error can be minimized by placing the marker as close to the pathology in the sagittal plane as possible (Fig. 203-8).

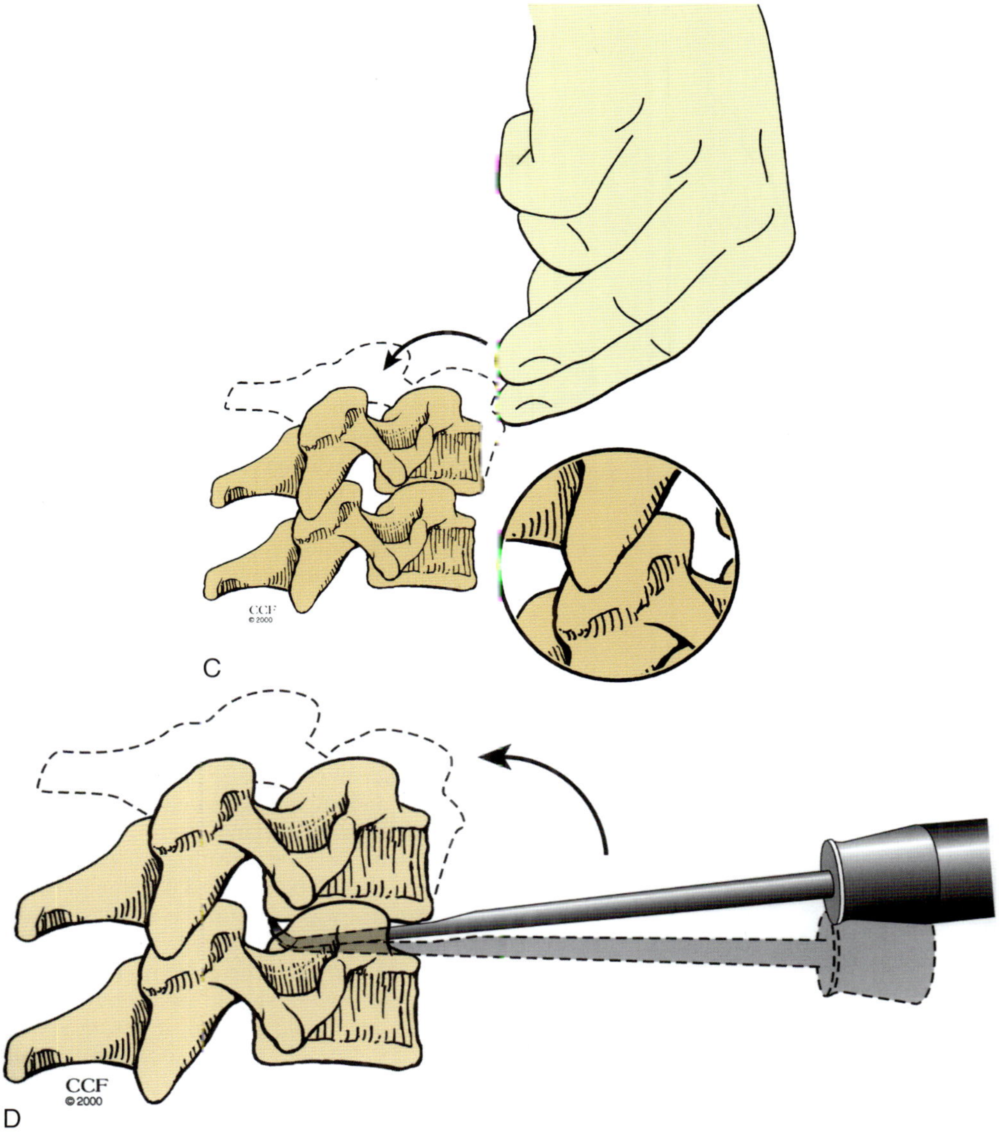

FIGURE 203-6, cont. C, The rostral body may be reduced by manual pressure. **D,** The rostral body may be reduced by placing an osteotome into the disc space and rotating it rostrally. (Copyright Cleveland Clinic Foundation.)

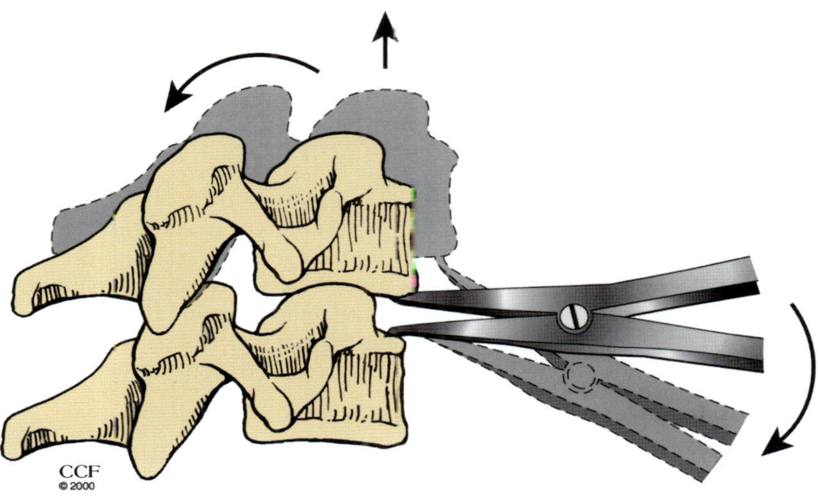

FIGURE 203-7. An alternative technique for ventral cervical facet dislocation management. Disc interspace spreaders may be placed into the disc space once the facets are disengaged. Rotating the spreaders rostrally facilitates reduction. (Copyright Cleveland Clinic Foundation.)

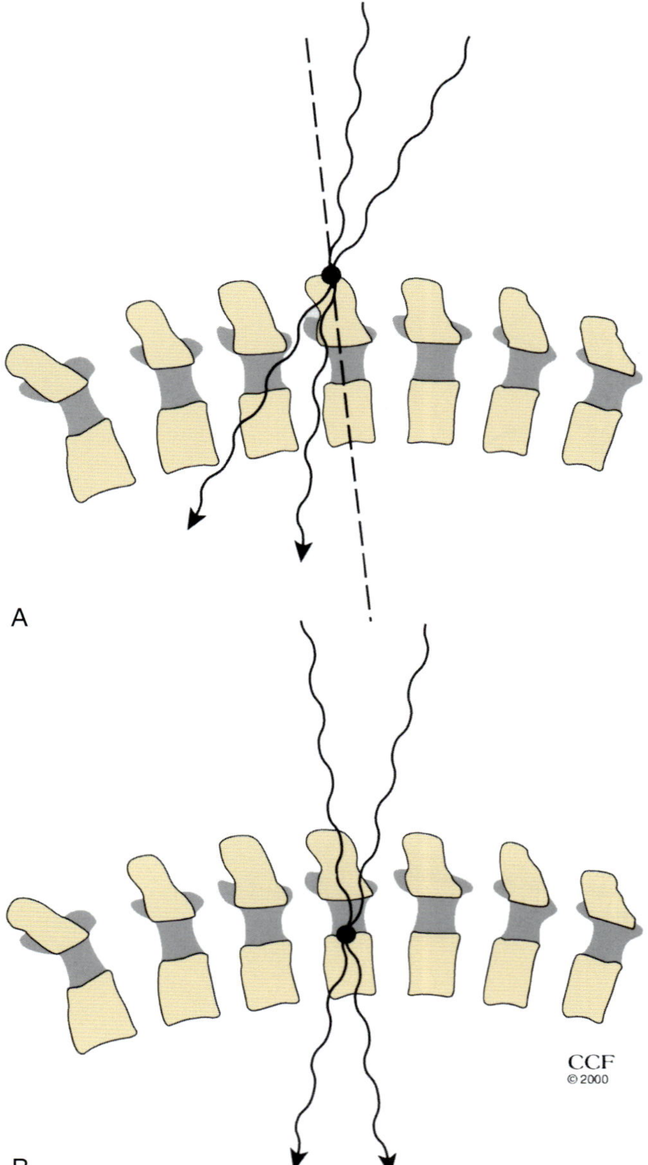

FIGURE 203-8. **A**, With the marker placed on the spinous process (*black dot*), an alteration in the radiograph beam trajectory may result in misinterpretation of the spinal level. The dashed line is the ideal radiograph beam trajectory. Altering the beam angle in a more rostral direction (*wavy lines*) can lead to misinterpretation. In this case, a level or two below the marked level will be interpreted as the marked level. **B**, When the marker is placed near the vertebral body, altering the beam trajectory will not be nearly as misleading. Note: Both wavy lines (representing different radiograph trajectories) pass through the marked level. (Copyright Cleveland Clinic Foundation.)

Electrophysiologic Spinal Cord Monitoring

Intraoperative spinal cord monitoring has become popular, especially for deformity correction. The goal of monitoring in these cases is to ensure that neural element injury has not occurred secondary to deformity correction maneuvers. Multiple techniques are available, and each is measured against the gold standard of the wake-up test (performed by lessening the level of anesthesia until the patient is able to follow commands, allowing for a gross assessment of motor function). These monitoring techniques include somatosensory-evoked potential (SSEP), motor-evoked potential, spinal-evoked potential, and electromyographic monitoring. SSEP and spinal-evoked potential are intended to monitor dorsal column integrity, while motor-evoked potential is intended for ventral column integrity. Electromyography monitors nerve root integrity and may be used continuously[45] or be stimulus evoked.[39] It is also possible to utilize multimodality monitoring, which includes the use of ventral and dorsal spinal cord interrogation as well as the nerve roots.

These techniques have not been demonstrated to be without error. False-positive and false-negative test findings for each technique have been documented.[40] False-negative results can be due to the failure to detect minor injury, the temporal difference between the actual injury and the observed change on the monitor, and the discrepancy between the area of the spinal cord injured and the region assessed by the monitoring technique.[39] Of even greater concern is the lack of a recognized standard for the assessment of injury during electrophysiologic monitoring.[39]

Nevertheless, if electrophysiologic monitoring is used, the surgeon must have a plan (strategy) for dealing with intraoperative electrophysiologic abnormalities. SSEP monitoring is the most commonly used technique, and there is substantial experience in treating SSEP changes; therefore, it is discussed here. If a change is observed (e.g., a 10% change in latency or a 50% change in amplitude), it is prudent to alter parameters that could be causing the change. The patient's blood pressure should be elevated if low, and the temperature of the patient and room should be increased. Infused blood or IV solutions should be warmed. The electrodes should be examined to ensure that there are no technical problems. Inhaled anesthetic agents should be discontinued, and barbiturates and opioids should be used. If low, the patient's oxygen saturation level should be increased. The placement of hydrogen peroxide in the wound may increase local oxygen saturation. If these actions do not return the tracing to baseline, mechanical factors should be considered next. Sublaminar wires or hooks may be removed, or their position may be critically assessed. A bone graft that was placed in proximity in time with the SSEP change should be removed and remeasured or reassessed. Distraction forces should be relaxed. Consideration should then be given to performing a wake-up test.

Time should be given for observation of the tracing to return to baseline. This period of observation may be up to 60 minutes. A re-formed bone graft should be replaced (if it was removed), and forces should be reapplied to the construct (but not in excess). If evoked potentials do not return to baseline, only enough force should be placed on the implant to maintain its position. Postoperatively, serial neurologic examinations are in order. Repeat radiography and/or myelography should be considered to document the position of the construct. Any aberrantly placed implants should be explored in the operating room.

Neurologic Injuries

New and unexpected neurologic deficits that appear following surgery are indeed a crisis. They are most commonly observed in the recovery room immediately following emergence from anesthesia. Early assessment of these injuries is imperative.

In some cases, an irreversible neural injury may already have occurred. When the surgeon cannot rule out an intraoperative event that might have caused such a deficit, an aggressive approach to diagnosis and identification of reversible causes of injury should be considered immediately. Bone graft misplacement, instrumentation encroachment on neural elements, and postoperative hemorrhage should be ruled out. Emergent imaging is often indicated and may include radiography, CT, and/or MRI. If appropriate, any abnormality that is found should be surgically rectified immediately. If there is a profound or progressive neurologic deficit, imaging is often not performed, and the patient is taken back to the operating room immediately for exploration of the previous site of surgery. The offending culprit (e.g., epidural hematoma) is most often evident and removed and/or repaired. If no hematoma is found, the construct should be inspected. As was previously described, the grafts should be removed, and hooks, wires, screws, and rods should be addressed. If encroachment on neural elements is identified, the construct, including the bone graft, may be removed, resized, and replaced. If no apparent abnormality is demonstrated at the time of surgical exploration, the patient should be taken for emergent MRI. The MRI should include the region of the spine rostral and caudal to the surgical site, which may disclose a distant epidural hematoma.

Ischemia caused by radicular artery injury can be diagnosed only on an exclusionary basis. Anterior spinal cord syndrome is often preceded by surgical obliteration of the contents of the neuroforamen that includes a radicular artery such as the artery of Adamkiewicz and may be untreatable. Angiography is usually not helpful because of the variable presence of vital radicular arteries in the normal situation. Treatment of these cases should consist of maintenance of normotension (or slight hypertension), the establishment of a euvolemic state, and the elimination of external neural element compression.

Complete pharmacologic reversal of anesthesia is imperative in situations in which a new neurologic deficit is suspected. Naloxone should be administered in sufficient doses to ensure reversal of opioids given during surgery. As an aside, narcotic antagonists have been shown to reverse ischemic neurologic deficits.[46,47] Therefore, the administration of naloxone should perhaps be considered more liberally under such circumstances.

Summary

Crises in spine surgery are not common. When they do occur, the surgeon must have the knowledge to deal with them effectively. Many spine "emergencies" are identified not in the operating room but in the recovery room. The period for crisis management extends beyond the operating room and into the perioperative period, and this requires continued vigilance by the surgeon. These issues should be dealt with in an expedient and thorough manner to treat and prevent further complications.

KEY REFERENCES

Bingol H, Cingoz F, Yilmaz AT, et al: Vascular complications related to lumbar disc surgery. *J Neurosurg* 100:249–253, 2004.

Golfinos JG, Dickman CA, Zabramski JM, et al: Repair of vertebral artery injury during anterior cervical decompression. *Spine (Phila Pa 1976)* 19:2552–2556, 1994.

Mody MG, Nourbakhsh A, Stahl DL, et al: The prevalence of wrong level surgery among spine surgeons. *Spine (Phila Pa 1976)* 33:194–198, 2008.

Orlando ER, Caroli E, Ferrante L: Management of the cervical esophagus and hypofarinx perforations complicating anterior cervical spine surgery. *Spine (Phila Pa 1976)* 28:E290–E295, 2003.

Porter JM, Pidgeon C, Cunningham AJ: The sitting position in neurosurgery: a critical appraisal. *Br J Anaesth* 82:117–128, 1999.

Smith MD, Emery SE, Dudley A, et al: Vertebral artery injury during anterior decompression of the cervical spine: a retrospective review of ten patients. *J Bone Joint Surg [Br]* 75:410–415, 1993.

REFERENCES

The complete reference list is available online at expertconsult.com.

Chapters 204 to 234 are available online only at expertconsult.com. See inside front cover for details.

INDEX

Page numbers followed by b, f, or t indicate boxes, figures, or tables, respectively. "E" pages appear online only on Expert Consult.

B

C

D

E

G

H

J

K

M

O

P

Q

R

T

U

Spine Surgery

Techniques, Complication Avoidance, and Management

THIRD EDITION

VOLUME ONE

EDITOR

Edward C. Benzel, MD

Chair
Department of Neurosurgery
Neurological Institute
Cleveland Clinic
Cleveland, OH

VIDEO EDITOR

Todd B. Francis, MD, PhD

Clinical Spine Fellow
Center for Spine Health
Neurological Institute
Cleveland Clinic
Cleveland, OH

ELSEVIER
SAUNDERS

ELSEVIER
SAUNDERS

1600 John F. Kennedy Blvd.
Ste 1800
Philadelphia, PA 19103-2899

SPINE SURGERY: TECHNIQUES, COMPLICATION AVOIDANCE, AND MANAGEMENT, THIRD EDITION

ISBN: 978-1-4377-0587-4

Notices

Knowledge and best practice in this field are constantly changing. As new research and experience broaden our understanding, changes in research methods, professional practices, or medical treatment may become necessary.

Practitioners and researchers must always rely on their own experience and knowledge in evaluating and using any information, methods, compounds, or experiments described herein. In using such information or methods they should be mindful of their own safety and the safety of others, including parties for whom they have a professional responsibility.

With respect to any drug or pharmaceutical products identified, readers are advised to check the most current information provided (i) on procedures featured or (ii) by the manufacturer of each product to be administered, to verify the recommended dose or formula, the method and duration of administration, and contraindications. It is the responsibility of practitioners, relying on their own experience and knowledge of their patients, to make diagnoses, to determine dosages and the best treatment for each individual patient, and to take all appropriate safety precautions.

To the fullest extent of the law, neither the Publisher nor the authors, contributors, or editors assume any liability for any injury and/or damage to persons or property as a matter of products liability, negligence or otherwise, or from any use or operation of any methods, products, instructions, or ideas contained in the material herein.

Spine surgery : techniques, complication avoidance, and management / editor, Edward C. Benzel ;
video editor, Todd B. Francis. — 3rd ed.
p. ; cm.
Includes bibliographical references and index.
ISBN 978-1-4377-0587-4 (hardcover : set : alk. paper)
I. Benzel, Edward C. II. Francis, Todd B.
[DNLM: 1. Spinal Diseases—surgery. 2. Intraoperative Complications—prevention & control.
3. Spine—surgery. WE 725]
617.5'6059—dc23 2012004307

Content Strategist: Charlotta Kryhl
Content Development Specialist: Taylor Ball
Publishing Services Manager: Pat Joiner-Myers
Senior Project Manager: Joy Moore
Design Direction: Ellen Zanolle

Printed in China.

Last digit is the print number: 9 8 7 6 5 4 3 2 1

This book is dedicated to my wife, Mary, and to those whose shoulders upon which I have stood while assimilating the wherewithal to complete this book. They include present and past partners, collaborators, fellows, residents, and assistants. Finally, it goes without saying that this book would not have come to fruition without the constant vigilance of Christine Moore. She indeed represents all things to all people.

—Edward C. Benzel, MD

CONTRIBUTORS

Khalid M. Abbed, MD
Chief
Yale Spine Institute;
Director
Minimally Invasive Spine Surgery
Department of Neurosurgery
Yale University School of Medicine
New Haven, CT

Kalil G. Abdullah, BS
Cleveland Clinic Lerner College of Medicine
Cleveland, OH

Steven S. Agabegi, MD
Michigan Orthopaedic Institute
Southfield, MI

Basheal M. Agrawal, MD
Associate Professor and Vice Chair
Department of Neurosurgery
University of Wisconsin
Madison, WI

Manzoor Ahmed, MBBS
Staff Radiologist
Imaging Institute
Neuroradiology Section
Cleveland Clinic
Cleveland, OH

Michael Ahrens, MD
Consultant (Oberarzt)
Spinecenter
Roland Klinik
Bremen, Germany

Yunus Alapan, BS
Research Assistant
Yildiz Technical University
Istanbul, Turkey

Rodolfo E. Alcedo-Guardia, MD
Neurosurgery Resident
University of Puerto Rico Medical Sciences Campus
San Juan, Puerto Rico

Joseph T. Alexander, MD
Assistant Professor
Department of Neurosurgery
Wake Forest University School of Medicine
Winston-Salem, NC

Neel Anand, MD
Professor and Chair
Department of Neurosurgery
Louisiana State University Health Science Center
Shreveport, LA

D. Greg Anderson, MD
Professor
Departments of Orthopaedic Surgery and Neurological Surgery
Thomas Jefferson University
Philadelphia, PA

Lilyana Angelov, MD, FRCS(C)
Staff
Brain Tumor and Neuro-Oncology;
Gamma Knife Center;
Center for Spine Health;
Taussig Cancer Institute;
Section Head
Spinal Radiosurgery and Neurological Surgery
Neurological Institute
Cleveland Clinic
Cleveland, OH

John A. Anson, MD
Las Vegas, NV

Ronald I. Apfelbaum, MD
Professor Emeritus
Department of Neurosurgery
University of Utah
Salt Lake City, UT

Paul M. Arnold, MD, FACS
Professor of Neurosurgery
University of Kansas Medical Center;
Attending Neurosurgeon
University of Kansas Hospital
Kansas City, KS

Harel Arzi, MD
Spine Fellow
Department of Neurosurgery
University of Kansas Medical Center
Kansas City, KS;
Chaim Sheba Medical Center
Ramat Gan, Israel

Ferhan A. Asghar, MD
Assistant Professor
Department of Orthopaedic Surgery
University of Cincinnati
Cincinnati, OH

Michelle Aubin, MD
Resident
University of Massachusetts School of Medicine
Worcester, MA

Basem I. Awad, MD
Department of Neurosurgery
Mansoura University Hospital
Mansoura, Egypt

Christopher Baggot, MD
Resident
Department of Neurological Surgery
School of Medicine and Public Health
University of Wisconsin–Madison
Madison, WI

Lissa C. Baird, MD
Chief Resident
Division of Neurosurgery
University of California–San Diego Medical Center
San Diego, CA

Jamie Baisden, MD
Associate Professor
Department of Neurosurgery
Medical College of Wisconsin
Milwaukee, WI

Nevan G. Baldwin, MD, FACS
Clinical Associate Professor
Texas Tech University
Lubbock, TX

Perry A. Ball, MD
Associate Professor
Departments of Surgery and Anesthesiology
Dartmouth Medical School
Hanover, NH;
Staff Neurosurgeon
Dartmouth-Hitchcock Medical Center
Lebanon, NH

Eli M. Baron, MD
Neurosurgeon and Spine Surgeon
Cedars-Sinai Medical Center
Los Angeles, CA

H. Hunt Batjer, MD
Professor and Chair
Northwestern University Feinberg School of Medicine;
Chair
Department of Neurological Surgery
Northwestern Memorial Hospital
Chicago, IL

Andrew M. Bauer, MD
Resident Physician
University of Wisconsin
Madison, WI

Thomas W. Bauer, MD, PhD
Departments of Orthopaedic Surgery and Pathology
Cleveland Clinic
Cleveland, OH

James R. Bean, MD
Neurosurgical Associates at Central Baptist
Lexington, KY

Gordon R. Bell, MD
Director
Center for Spine Health
Neurological Institute
Cleveland Clinic
Cleveland, OH

J. Brad Bellotte, MD
Chief
Department of Neurosurgery
Hamot Medical Center
Erie, PA

David M. Benglis, Jr., MD
Complex Spine Fellow
Department of Neurosurgery
University of Miami
Miami, FL

Gregory Bennett, MD
Clinical Director
Neurosurgery
Erie County Medical Center
Buffalo, NY

Edward C. Benzel, MD
Chair
Department of Neurosurgery
Neurological Institute
Cleveland Clinic
Cleveland, OH

Darren L. Bergey, MD
Loma Linda University Medical Center
Loma Linda, CA

Marc L. Bertrand, MD
Associate Professor
Department of Anesthesiology
Dartmouth Medical School
Hanover, NH;
Director
Graduate Medical Education
Dartmouth-Hitchcock Medical Center
Lebanon, NH

Sigurd Berven, MD
Associate Professor in Residence;
Co-Director
Spine Fellowship;
Director
Resident Education Program
University of California–San Francisco
San Francisco, CA

Tarun Bhalla, MD
Resident
Department of Neurosurgery
Neurological Institute
Cleveland Clinic
Cleveland, OH

Aaron J. Bianco, MD
Spine Fellow
Warren Alpert Medical School
Brown University
Providence, RI

Dani S. Bidros, MD
Resident
Department of Neurosurgery
Neurological Institute
Cleveland Clinic
Cleveland, OH

Mark H. Bilsky, MD
Professor
Weill Medical College of Cornell University;
Memorial Sloan-Kettering Cancer Center;
Attending Surgeon;
Chief
Multi-Disciplinary Spine Tumor Center
Memorial Hospital for Cancer and Allied Diseases
New York, NY

Barry D. Birch, MD
Department of Neurosurgery
Mayo Clinic Scottsdale
Scottsdale, AZ

Frank S. Bishop, MD
Director
Comprehensive Spine Center
Neuroscience & Spine Institute
Kalispell Regional Medical Center
Kalispell, MT

Kevin Blaylock, CPA
Oklahoma Spine Hospital
Oklahoma City, OK

Maxwell Boakye, MD, FACS
Assistant Professor
Department of Neurosurgery
Stanford School of Medicine
Stanford, CA

Scott D. Boden, MD
Professor of Orthopaedics and Director
Emory Orthopaedics & Spine Center
Emory University;
Staff Physician
Department of Orthopaedic Surgery
Atlanta VA Medical Center
Atlanta, GA

Christopher Bono, MD
Assistant Professor
Orthopaedic Surgery
Harvard Medical School;
Chief
Orthopaedic Spine Service
Brigham and Women's Hospital
Boston, MA

Charles L. Branch, Jr., MD
Professor
Wake Forest School of Medicine;
Chair
Neuroscience Service Line
Wake Forest Baptist Medical Center
Winston-Salem, NC

Darrel S. Brodke, MD
Professor and Vice Chair
Department of Orthopaedics
University of Utah
Salt Lake City, UT

Nathaniel Brooks, MD
Fellow
Center for Spine Health
Neurological Institute
Cleveland Clinic
Cleveland, OH

Cristian Brotea, MD
Clinical Instructor
New York Medical College;
Associate Director
Spine Service
Westchester Medical Center
Valhalla, NY;
Sound Shore Medical Center
New Rochelle, NY;
White Plains Hospital
White Plains, NY

Samuel R. Browd, MD, PhD
Assistant Professor of Neurological Surgery
University of Washington;
Attending Neurological Surgeon
Seattle Children's Hospital
Seattle, WA

Harlan Bruner, MD
Assistant Professor
Department of Neurosurgery
University of Minnesota
Minneapolis, MN

John Butler, MD
Coastal Neurosurgical Associates
Wilmington, NC

David W. Cadotte, MD
Department of Surgery
Division of Neurosurgery
University of Toronto;
Resident
Division of Neurosurgery
Toronto Western Hospital
Toronto, Ontario, Canada

David W. Cahill, MD*
Department of Neurosurgery
College of Medicine
University of South Florida
Tampa, FL

John R. Caruso, MD
Neurological Specialists, LLC
Hagerstown, MD

Jeroen Ceuppens, MD
Department of Neurosurgery
University Hospital Gasthuisberg
Leuven, Belgium

Saad B. Chaudhary, MD
Assistant Professor
Department of Orthopaedic Surgery
New Jersey Medical School–University of Medicine and Dentistry of New Jersey
Newark, NJ

Morgan N. Chen, MD
Assistant Clinical Professor of Orthopaedics
Mount Sinai School of Medicine
New York, NY;
Attending Surgeon
Saint Charles Hospital
Port Jefferson, NY

Thomas C. Chen, MD PhD
Associate Professor
Departments of Neurosurgery and Pathology
Keck School of Medicine;
Director
Surgical Neuro-oncology;
Co-Director
University of Southern California Neuro Spine Program
Los Angeles, CA

Tanvir Choudhri, MD
Assistant Professor and Director
Neurosurgery Spine Program
Department of Neurosurgery
Mount Sinai Medical Center
New York, NY

Adam Conley, MD
Resident
Department of Neurosurgery
Virginia Commonwealth University Medical Center
Richmond, VA

Camille Connelly, MD
Resident
Department of Orthopaedic Surgery
University of Cincinnati College of Medicine
Cincinnati, OH

Edward S. Connolly, MD
Professor
Department of Neurosurgery
Ochsner Clinic Foundation
Louisiana State University School of Medicine
New Orleans, LA

Kevin Cooper, MD
Spine Medical Center of Pascagoula
Pascagoula, MS

Paul R. Cooper, MD
Professor of Neurosurgery
New York University School of Medicine
New York, NY

Domagoj Coric, MD
Chief of Neurosurgery
Carolinas Medical Center
Charlotte, NC;
President
North Carolina Spine Society
Raleigh, NC

Jean-Valery C.E. Coumans, MD
Assistant Professor
Department of Neurosurgery
Massachusetts General Hospital
Boston, MA

Sorin Craciunas, MD
Staff Neurosurgeon
Bagdasar-Arseni Hospital
Bucharest, Romania

Albert E. Cram, MD, FACS
Professor Emeritus
Department of Surgery
University of Iowa
Iowa City, IA

*Deceased.

Charles H. Crawford III, MD
Assitant Professor
Department of Orthopaedic Surgery
University of Louisville;
Adult and Pediatric Spine Surgeon
Norton Leatherman Spine Center
Louisville, KY

H. Alan Crockard, MD
The National Hospital for Neurology and Neurosurgery
London, United Kingdom

William T. Curry, Jr., MD
Assistant Professor
Department of Surgery
Harvard Medical School;
Attending Neurosurgeon
Massachusetts General Hospital
Boston, MA

Joseph F. Cusick, MD
Professor
Medical College of Wisconsin
Madison, WI

Scott D. Daffner, MD
Assistant Professor
Department of Orthopaedics
Robert C. Byrd Health Sciences Center
University of West Virginia School of Medicine
Morgantown, WV

Nader S. Dahdaleh, MD
Fellow Associate
Department of Neurosurgery
University of Iowa
Iowa City, IA

Sedat Dalbayrak, MD
Chair
Department of Neurosurgery
Trabzon Numune Teaching and Research Hospital
Trabzon, Turkey

Mark D. D'Alise, MD, FACS
Neurosurgical Associates
Complex Reconstructive Spinal Surgery
Lubbock, TX

Russell C. DeMicco, DO
Staff Physician
Center for Spine Health
Neurological Institute
Cleveland Clinic
Cleveland, OH

Michael DePalma, MD
President and Director of Research
Virginia Spine Research Institute, Inc.;
Medical Director
Interventional Spine Care Fellowship
Virginia Spine Physicians, PC
Richmond, VA

Harel Deutsch, MD
Assistant Professor
Department of Neurosurgery
Rush University Medical Center
Chicago, IL

Denis DiAngelo, MD
Associate Professor
School of Biomechanical Engineering
University of Tennessee Health Science Center
Memphis, TN

Curtis A. Dickman, MD
Associate Chief
Spine Section;
Director
Spinal Research
Division of Neurological Surgery
Barrow Neurological Associates
Phoenix, AZ

Christian P. DiPaola, MD
Assistant Professor
Memorial Medical Center
University of Massachusetts
Worcester, MA

Gary A. Dix, MD, FRSC(C)
Clinical Professor of Neurosurgery
George Washington University Hospital
Washington, DC;
Attending Neurosurgeon
Anne Arundel Medical Center
Annapolis, MD

John Doyle, MD
Associate Professor
Department of Neurology;
Chief
General Neurology Division
University of Pittsburgh
Pittsburgh, PA

Thomas B. Ducker, MD
Professor of Neurosurgery (retired)
Johns Hopkins Hospital;
University of Maryland Medical Center
Baltimore, MD;
Anne Arundel Medical Center
Annapolis, MD

Michael Ebersold, MD
Professor of Neurosurgery
Mayo Clinic College of Medicine;
Department of Neurological Surgery
Luther Middlefort Clinic–Mayo Health System
Eau Claire, WI

Bruce L. Ehni, MD
Associate Professor
Department of Neurosurgery
Baylor College of Medicine;
Neurosurgery Section Chief
Operative Care Line
DeBakey VA Medical Center
Houston, TX

Kurt Eichholz, MD
Resident
Department of Neurosurgery
University of Iowa
Iowa City, IA

Marc Eichler, MD, FACS
Chief of Neurological Surgery
Trinity Medical Center
Newton Centre, MA

John P. Eickman, MD
Wake Forest School of Medicine;
Resident
Wake Forest Baptist Medical Center
Winston-Salem, NC

Samer K. Elbabaa, MD, FAANS
Director
Division of Pediatric Neurosurgery;
Assistant Professor
Department of Neurosurgery
St. Louis University School of Medicine
St. Louis, MO

J. Bradley Elder, MD
Assistant Professor
Department of Neurological Surgery
The Ohio State University Medical Center
Columbus, OH

Richard Ellenbogen, MD, FACS
Professor and Chair
Department of Neurological Surgery
University of Washington School of Medicine
Seattle, WA

Sanford E. Emery, MD
Professor and Chair
Department of Orthopaedics
West Virginia University
Morgantown, WV

Nancy E. Epstein, MD
Clinical Professor
Department of Neurological Surgery
Albert Einstein College of Medicine
Bronx, NY;
Chief
Neurological Spine and Education
Winthrop University Hospital
Mineola, NY;
President
Long Island Neurological Associates, PC
Long Island, NY

Thomas J. Errico, MD
Professor
Department of Orthopaedic Surgery and Neurosurgery;
Director
Spine Surgery Fellowship Program;
Director
International Spine Surgery Fellowship Program
NYU Medical Center Hospital for Joint Diseases
New York, NY

Malik Fakhar, BS
Cleveland Clinic
Cleveland, OH

Steven M. Falowski, MD
Fellow
Department of Neurosurgery
Rush University Medical Center
Chicago, IL

Ehab Farag, MD, FRCA
Staff Anesthesiologist;
Assistant Professor of Anesthesiology
Cleveland Clinic
Cleveland, OH

Chad W. Farley, MD
Deparment of Neurosurgery
University of Cinncinnati
Cincinnati, OH

Michael G. Fehlings, MD, PhD
Department of Surgery
Division of Neurosurgery
University of Toronto;
Krembil Chair in Neural Repair and Regeneration
Division of Neurosurgery
Toronto Western Hospital
Toronto, Ontario, Canada

Frank Feigenbaum, MD, FAANS
Midwest Neurosurgery Associates
Kansas City, MO

Lisa A. Ferrara, PhD
President and CEO
OrthoKinetic Technologies, LLC
Southport, NC;
President and CEO
OrthoKinetic Testing Technologies, LLC
Shallotte, NC

Richard G. Fessler, MD, PhD
Professor
Department of Neurosurgery
Northwestern University Feinberg School of Medicine
Chicago, IL

David Fiorella, MD, PhD
Professor
Clinical Radiology and Neurosurgery
Cerebrovascular Center
Stony Book University Medical Center
Stony Brook, NY

Jeffrey S. Fischgrund, MD
Professor
Department of Orthopaedics
Oakland University School of Medicine
Rochester, MI;
Director
Spine Surgery Fellowship
William Beaumont Hospital
Royal Oak, MI

Kevin T. Foley, MD
Professor
Neurological Surgery
Semmes-Murphey Neurologic and Spine Institute
Memphis, TN

Ricardo Fontes, MD
Department of Neurosurgery
Rush University Medical Center
Chicago, IL

Todd B. Francis, MD, PhD
Clinical Spine Fellow
Center for Spine Health
Neurological Institute
Cleveland Clinic
Cleveland, OH

Kai-Ming G. Fu, MD, PhD
Department of Neurosurgery
University of Virginia
Charlottesville, VA

Brian R. Gantwerker, MD
The Craniospinal Center of Los Angeles
Los Angeles, CA

Mark Garrett, MD
Chief Resident
Department of Neurosurgery
Barrow Neurological Institute
St. Joseph's Hospital and Medical Center
Phoenix, AZ

Rasha Germain, MD
Chief Resident
Department of Neurosurgery
Barrow Neurological Institute
St. Joseph's Hospital and Medical Center
Phoenix, AZ

John W. German, MD
Associate Professor
Division of Neurosurgery
Albany Medical College
Albany, NY

Alexander J. Ghanayem, MD
Associate Professor and Chief
Department of Orthopaedic Surgery
Division of Spine Surgery
Loyola University Medical Center
Maywood, IL

George M. Ghobrial, MD
Resident
Neurological Surgery
Thomas Jefferson University Hospital
Philadelphia, PA

Zoher Ghogawala, MD
Clinical Assistant Professor
Department of Neurosurgery
Yale University;
Attending Physician
Department of Neurosurgery
Yale–New Haven Hospital
New Haven, CT;
Lecturer in Neurosurgery
Tufts University
Boston, MA;
Attending Physician
Department Neurosurgery;
Director
Wallace Clinical Trials Center
Greenwich Hospital
Greenwich, CT;
Attending Physician and Chair of Neurosurgery
Lahey Clinic
Burlington, MA

Paul A. Glazer, MD
Assistant Clinical Professor
Department of Orthopedic Surgery
Harvard University;
Spine Surgeon
Beth Israel Deaconess Medical Center
Boston, MA

Vijay K. Goel, PhD
Distinguished University Professor
Departments of Bioengineering and Orthopaedic Surgery;
Endowed Chair and McMaster-Gardner Professor of Orthopaedic Bioengineering;
Co-Director
Engineering Center for Orthopaedic Research Excellence
Univeristy of Toledo
Toledo, OH

Jan Goffin, MD, PhD
Professor
Catholic University of Leuven;
Chair
Department of Neurosurgery
University Hospital Gasthuisberg
Leuven, Belgium

Ziya Gokaslan, MD
Donlin M. Long Professor of Neurosurgery, Oncology, and Orthopedic Surgery;
Vice Chair
Department of Neurosurgery;
Director
Spine Division
Johns Hopkins University Hospital
Baltimore, MD

Harry S. Goldsmith, MD, FACS
Clincal Professor
Department of Neurosurgery
University of California–Davis School of Medicine
Sacramento, CA

Sohrab Gollogly
University of Utah
Salt Lake City, UT

L. Fernando Gonzalez, MD
Assistant Professor
Department of Neurological Surgery
Division of Neurovascular Surgery and Endovascular Neurosurgery
Jefferson Medical College
Thomas Jefferson University
Philadelphia, PA

Jorge A. Gonzalez-Martinez, MD
Associate Staff
Epilepsy Center;
Department of Neurosurgery
Neurological Institute
Cleveland Clinic
Cleveland, OH

Jeffrey D. Gross, MD
Medical Director
O.A.S.I.S. Wellness Center
Laguna Niguel, CA

Yabo Guan, PhD
Department of Neurosurgery
Medical College of Wisconsin
Milwaukee, WI

İlker Gulec, MD
Vice Chief
Department of Neurosurgery
Antalya Teaching and Research Hospital
Antalya, Turkey

David Gwinn, MD
Staff Orthopaedic Spine Surgeon
Department of Orthopaedics and Rehabilitation
Walter Reed Army Medical Center
Washington, DC

Elad Hadar, MD
Associate Professor
Department of Neurosurgery
University of North Carolina School of Medicine
Chapel Hill, NC

Alexander Hadjipavlou, MD, MSc, FACS, FRCS(C)
Professor
Orthopaedic Surgery and Rehabilitaton
University of Crete
Heraklion, Crete, Greece

Mark N. Hadley, MD, FACS
Charles A. and Patsy W. Collat Professor of Neurological Surgery;
Program Director
Neurosurgery Residency Training Program
University of Alabama
Birmingham, AL

Regis W. Haid, Jr., MD
Atlanta Brain and Spine Care
Atlanta, GA

Fadi Hanbali, MD, FACS
Clinical Associate Professor
Department of Neurosurgery
Texas Tech University HSC;
Faculty Neurosurgeon
Sierra Medical Center;
Providence Memorial Hospital;
University Medical Center of El Paso
El Paso, TX

Ran Harel, MD
Faculty
Spine Surgery Unit
Sheba Medical Center
Ramat-Gan, Israel

Jurgen Harms, MD
Center for Spine Surgery;
Department of Orthopedics and Traumatology
Klinikum Karlsbad-Langensteinbach
Karlsbad-Langensteinbach, Germany

Colin B. Harris, MD
Spine Fellow
Department of Orthopedics
Rush University
Chicago, IL

James S. Harrop, MD
Associate Professor of Neurologic and Orthopedic Surgery
Jefferson Medical College
Philadelphia, PA

Blaine L. Hart, MD
Professor
Department of Radiology
University of New Mexico School of Medicine
Albuquerque, NM

Robert A. Hart, MD
Professor and Spine Fellowship Director
Oregon Health & Science University
Portland, OR

Reyaad A. Hayek, MD
Associate Professor
Department of Radiology
University of New Mexico School of Medicine
Albuquerque, NM

Robert F. Heary, MD
Professor
Department of Neurological Surgery
New Jersey Medical School–University of Medicine and Dentistry of New Jersey
Newark, NJ

Joshua E. Heller, MD
Assistant Professor
Neurological Surgery
Thomas Jefferson University
Philadelphia, PA

Fraser C. Henderson, MD
Chief
Division of Neurosurgery
Doctors Community Hospital
Lanham, MD

Ann M. Henwood, MSN, CNS, RN
Department of Neurosurgery;
Advanced Practice Nurse
Center for Spine Health
Neurological Institute
Cleveland Clinic
Cleveland, OH

Yoshitaka Hirano, MD
Center for Spine and Spinal Cord Disorders
Southern Tohoku General Hospital
Iwanuma, Miyagi, Japan

Girish K. Hiremath, MD
Staff Neurosurgeon
Riverside Methodist Hospital
Columbus, OH

Patrick W. Hitchon, MD
Professor
Departments of Neurosurgery and Bioengineering;
Director of Spine Surgery
University of Iowa College of Medicine;
Department of Neurosurgery
University of Iowa Hospitals and Clinics
Iowa City, IA

Daniel J. Hoh, MD
Assistant Professor
Department of Neurological Surgery;
Joint Assistant Professor
Department of Neuroscience
University of Florida
Gainesville, FL

Paul J. Holman, MD
Assistant Professor
Department of Neurosurgery
Weill-Cornell Medical College
New York, NY;
Staff Neurosurgeon
Methodist Neurological Institute;
Department of Neurosurgery
Methodist Hospital
Houston, TX

Noboru Hosono, MD, PhD
Chief
Spine Surgery
Osaka Kosei-nenkin Hospital
Osaka, Japan

John K. Houton, MD
Associate Professor
Department of Neurological Surgery
Montefiore Hospital;
Albert Einstein/Jaboni Hospital
Bronx, NY

Augusto T. Hsia, Jr., MD
Staff
Center for Spine Health
Neurological Institute
Cleveland Clinic
Cleveland, OH

Steven Hwang, MD
Department of Neurosurgery
Tufts Medical Center
Boston, MA

Christopher A. Iannotti, MD
Chief Resident
Department of Neurosurgery
Neurological Institute
Cleveland Clinic
Cleveland, OH

Allyson Ianuzzi, PhD
Visiting Research Assistant Professor
Biomedical Engineering
Drexel University;
Senior Scientist
Exponent
Philadelphia, PA

Serkan İnceoğlu, PhD
Assistant Professor
Department of Orthopedic Surgery
Loma Linda University
Loma Linda, CA

Robert E. Isaacs, MD
Head
Section of Minimally Invasive Spine Surgery
Cleveland Clinic Florida Spine Institute
Weston, FL

Yasunobu Itoh, MD
Neurosurgical Service
Akita University Hospital
Akita, Japan

Adam W. Jackson, MD
Fellow Associate
Department of Neurosurgery
University of Iowa
Iowa City, IA

Pinakin R. Jethwa, MD
Resident
Neurological Surgery
New Jersey Medical School–University of Medicine and Dentistry of New Jersey
Newark, NJ

Neilank Jha, MD
Division of Neurosurgery
McMaster University
Hamilton, Ontario, Canada

J. Patrick Johnson, MD
Director
Academic Research and Fellowship Programs
Cedars-Sinai Institute for Spinal Disorders
Los Angeles, CA

G. Alexander Jones, MD
Assistant Clinical Professor
Department of Neurosurgery
New York Medical College
Valhalla, NY;
Medical Director
Spine Care
Orange Regional Medical Center
Middletown, NY

Christopher D. Kager, MD
Lancaster Neuroscience and Spine Association
Lancaster, PA

Udaya K. Kakarla, MD
Department of Neurological Surgery
Barrow Neurological Institution
St. Joseph's Hospital and Medical Center
Phoenix, AZ

Kyriakos Kakavelakis, MD
University Hospital of Heraklion
Heraklion, Crete, Greece

M. Yashar S. Kalani, MD, PhD
Resident
Department of Neurological Surgery
Barrow Neurological Institute
Phoenix, AZ

Iain H. Kalfas, MD
Staff Physician
Department of Neurosurgery
Neurological Institute
Cleveland Clinic
Cleveland, OH

Tara Kamali-Nejad, MD
Resident
Department of Family Medicine
Hennepin County Medical Center
Minneapolis, MN

Youssef R. Karam, MD
Department of Neurosurgery
University of Iowa
Iowa City, IA;
Instructor
Clinical Surgery
Lebanese University;
Department of Neurosurgery/Spine
Clemenceau Medical Center
Lebanese Hospital;
Middle East Institute of Health
Beirut, Lebanon

Reza J. Karimi, MD
Resident
Department of Neurological Surgery
New Jersey Medical School–University of Medicine and Dentistry of New Jersey
Newark, NJ

Irene Katzan, MD
Director
Primary Stroke Center;
Director
Center for Outcomes Research and Evaluation
Cleveland Clinic
Cleveland, OH

Vikas Kaul, MS
Research Assistant
Department of Bioengineering
University of Toledo
Toledo, OH

Michael Kelly, MD
Resident
Department of Neurosurgery
Neurological Institute
Cleveland Clinic
Cleveland, OH

James A. Kenning, MD
Chestmont Neurosurgical
Main Line Health Center
Newtown Square, PA

Tyler J. Kenning, MD
Fellow
Department of Neurological Surgery
Jefferson Medical College
Thomas Jefferson University
Philadelphia, PA

Matthew B. Kern, MD
Neurological Surgery, PC
Great Neck, NY

Saad Khairi, MD
Volunteer Clinical Assistant Professor
Department of Neurological Surgery
Indiana University School of Medicine;
Partner
Goodman Campbell Brain & Spine
Indianapolis, IN

Tagreed Khalaf, MD
Center for Spine Health
Neurological Institute
Cleveland Clinic
Cleveland, OH

Ali Kiapour, PhD
Postdoctoral Associate
Department of Bioengineering
University of Toledo
Toledo, OH

Brendan Killory, MD
Director
Epilepsy and Functional Neurosurgery
Department of Neurosurgery
Hartford Neurosurgery & Spine Specialists
Hartford Hospital
Hartford, CT

Daniel H. Kim, MD
Professor
Department of Neurosurgery;
Director
Neurological and Orthopedic Spine Fellowship;
Co-Director
Spine Stem Cell Program
Cedars-Sinai Institute for Spinal Disorders;
Director
California Association of Neurological Surgeons
Los Angeles, CA

David H. Kim, MD
Harvard University
Cambridge, MA

Paul Kim, MD
Carolina Neurosurgery and Spine Associates
Charlotte, NC

Sang-Don Kim, MD
Department of Neurosurgery
Holy Family Hospital;
College of Medicine
The Catholic University
Bucheon, Korea

Brian J. Kistler, MD
Resident
Department of Orthopedic Surgery
SUNY Upstate Medical University Hospital
Syracuse, NY

Sameer A. Kitab, MD

Ryan S. Kitagawa, MD
Resident
Department of Neurosurgery
Baylor College of Medicine
Houston, TX

Paul Klimo, MD
Semmes-Murphey Neurologic & Spine Institute
Memphis, TN

Eric Klineberg, MD
Assistant Professor
Department of Orthopaedics;
Fellowship Director
Spine Program;
Assistant Director
Residency Program for Orthopaedics
University of California–Davis
Sacramento, CA

Thomas A. Kopitnik, MD
University of Texas Southwestern Medical Center
Dallas, TX

Panagiotis Korovessis, MD
Department of Pathology
General Hospital "Agios Andreas"
Achaia, Greece

Tyler Koski, MD
Assistant Professor
Department of Neurological Surgery
Northwestern University
Chicago, IL

Robert J. Kowalski, MD
Clearwater, FL

Chandan Krishna, MD
Resident Neurosurgeon
Department of Neurosurgery
Methodist Neurological Institute;
Methodist Hospital
Houston, TX

Ajit A. Krishnaney, MD
Staff
Center for Spine Health
Cerebrovascular Center
Department of Neurosurgery
Neurological Institute
Cleveland Clinic
Cleveland, OH

Varun R. Kshettry, MD
Resident
Department of Neurosurgery
Neurological Institute
Cleveland Clinic
Cleveland, OH

Charles Kuntz IV, MD
Associate Professor and Vice Chair
University of Cincinnati College of Medicine;
Mayfield Clinic and Spine Institute
Cincinnati, OH

Steven M. Kurtz, PhD
Research Professor
Biomedical Engineering
Drexel University;
Corporate Vice President
Exponent
Philadelphia, PA

John A. Lancon, MD, FAAP, FACS, FAANS
Affiliate Faculty
University of Mississippi Medical Center;
Chief of Neurosurgery
St. Dominic Jackson Memorial Hospital;
Consultant
Regency Hospital of Jackson;
Mississippi Methodist Rehabilitation Hospital
Jackson, MS

Jorge Lastra-Power, MD
Assistant Professor
Neurosurgery Section
University of Puerto Rico
San Juan, Puerto Rico

Elizabeth Demers Lavelle, MD
Assistant Professor of Anesthesiology
SUNY Upstate Medical University
Syracuse, NY

William F. Lavelle, MD
Assistant Professor;
Orthopaedic Spine Surgeon
SUNY Upstate Medical University
Syracuse, NY

Nathan H. Lebwohl, MD
Chief of Spinal Deformity Surgery
Department of Orthopaedics
University of Miami Miller School of Medicine
Miami, FL

Joon Y. Lee, MD
Associate Professor
Department of Orthopaedic Surgery
University of Pittsburgh Medical Center
Pittsburgh, PA

Lawrence G. Lenke, MD
Jerome J. Gilden Professor of Orthopaedic Surgery;
Professor of Neurological Surgery;
Co-Chief Adult/Pediatric Scoliosis and Reconstructive Spinal Surgery
Washington University School of Medicine;
Chief
Spinal Service
Orthopaedic Surgery
Shriners Hospital for Children
St. Louis, MO

Steven P. Leon, MD, FACS
Clinical Assistant Professor
Weill–Cornell Medical College
New York, NY;
Brookhaven Memorial Hospital Medical Center
Patchogue, NY;
St. Charles Hospital and Rehabilitation Center
Port Jefferson, NY

Allan D. Levi, MD, PhD, FACS
Professor of Neurosurgery
University of Miami;
Chief of Neurosurgery
University of Miami Hospital;
Chief of Neurospine
Jackson Memorial Hospital
Miami, FL

Isador H. Lieberman, MD, FRCSC
Director
Scoliosis and Spine Tumor Program
Texas Back Institute;
Texas Health Hospital
Plano, TX

Timothy Lindley, MD, PhD
Fellow Associate
Department of Neurosurgery
University of Iowa Hospitals and Clinics
Iowa City, IA

James K.C. Liu, MD
Resident
Department of Neurosurgery
Neurological Institute
Cleveland Clinic
Cleveland, OH

Andrew D. Livingston, MD
Resident Neurosurgeon
Department of Neurosurgery
Methodist Neurological Institute;
Methodist Hospital
Houston, TX

Bjorn Lobo, MD
Resident
Department of Neurosurgery
Neurological Institute
Cleveland Clinic
Cleveland, OH

S. Scott Lollis, MD
Assistant Professor of Surgery
Department of Neurosurgery
Dartmouth Medical School
Hanover, NH;
Attending Neurosurgeon
Dartmouth-Hitchcock Medical Center
Lebanon, NH

Donlin M. Long, MD
John Hopkins University Medical School
Baltimore, MD

Miguel Lopez-Gonzalez, MD
Chief Resident
Department of Neurosurgery
Neurological Institute
Cleveland Clinic
Cleveland, OH

Robert G. Louis, MD
Department of Neurosurgery
University of Virginia
Charlottesville, VA

Daniel C. Lu, MD, PhD
Assistant Professor
Department of Neurosurgery
University of California–Los Angeles
Los Angeles, CA

Mark G. Luciano, MD
Staff
Pediatric Surgery and Neurosciences
Department of Neurosurgery
Neurological Institute
Cleveland Clinic
Cleveland, OH

Andre Machado, MD, PhD
Director
Center for Neurological Restoration;
Staff
Center for Spine Health and Pain Management
Department of Neurosurgery
Neurological Institute
Cleveland Clinic
Cleveland, OH

Dennis J. Maiman, MD, PhD
Professor and Chair
Department of Neurosurgery
Medical College of Wisconsin;
Attending Neurosurgeon
Children's Hospital of Wisconsin;
Froedtert Memorial Lutheran Hospital
Milwaukee, WI

David G. Malone, MD
Oklahoma Spine and Brain Institute
Tulsa, OK

Lisabeth L. Maloney, MD
Associate Professor of Anesthesiology
Dartmouth Medical School
Hanover, NH;
Director
Anesthesiology Residency Program
Dartmouth-Hitchcock Medical Center
Lebanon, NH

Antonios Mammis, MD
Resident
Department of Neurological Surgery
New Jersey Medical School–University of Medicine and Dentistry of New Jersey
Newark, NJ

Satyajit Marawar, MD

Edward Marchan, MD
Resident Physician
Department of Radiation Oncology
Emory University
Atlanta, GA

Nicolas Marcotte, MD
Staff Neurosurgeon
New England Baptist Hospital
Boston, MA

Joseph Maroon, MD
Clinical Professor and Vice Chair
Department of Neurosurgery
University of Pittsburgh Medical Center
Pittsburgh, PA

Michael Martin, MD
Assistant Professor
Department of Neurosurgery
University of Oklahoma
Oklahoma City, OK

Mitchell Martineau, MSN
Oklahoma Spine and Brain Institute
Tulsa, OK

Eric M. Massicotte, MD
Associate Professor
University of Toronto;
Coordinator of Spine Fellowship;
Director
Undergraduate Studies for Neurosurgery
University Health Network
Toronto, Ontario, Canada

Virgilio Matheus, MD
Resident
Department of Neurosurgery
Neurological Institute
Cleveland Clinic
Cleveland, OH

Hidenori Matsuoka, MD
Southern Tohoku General Hospital
Koriyama, Japan

Paul K. Maurer, MD
Professor
Department of Neurosurgery
University of Rochester;
Chief
Department of Neurosurgery
Unity Health System
Rochester, NY

Eric A.K. Mayer, MD
Staff
Center for Spine Health;
Center for Neurological Restoration
Neurological Institute
Cleveland Clinic
Cleveland, OH

Daniel J. Mazanec, MD
Associate Professor
Cleveland Clinic Lerner College of Medicine of Case Western Reserve University;
Associate Director
Center for Spine Health
Neurological Institute
Cleveland Clinic
Cleveland, OH

Paul C. McAfee, MD
Part-time Associate Professor
Departments of Orthopedic Surgery and Neurosurgery
Johns Hopkins Hospital;
Chief of Spinal Surgery
St. Joseph Hospital
Baltimore, MD

Bruce M. McCormack, MD
Clinical Faculty
University of California–San Francisco Medical Center
San Francisco, CA

Paul C. McCormick, MD, MPH
Herbert and Linda Gallen Professor of Neurological Surgery
Columbia University College of Physicians and Surgeons
New York, NY

William McCormick, MD
Schwartzapfel Novick
West Islip, NY

Robert A. McGuire, Jr., MD
Professor and Chair
Department of Orthopaedic Surgery and Rehabilitation
University of Mississippi Medical Center
Jackson, MS

Michael D. McKibben, JD
Bradley Arant Boult Cummings, LLP
Birmingham, AL

Robert F. McLain, MD
Professor of Surgery
Cleveland Clinic Lerner College of Medicine at Case Western Reserve University;
CCF Adjunct Professor
Department of Chemical and Biomedical Engineering
Cleveland State University;
Staff Spine Surgeon
Center for Spine Health
Neurological Institute
Cleveland Clinic
Cleveland, OH

D. Mark Melton, MD
Resident
Department of Neurosurgery
University of South Florida College of Medicine
Tampa, FL

Muhammad Zeeshan Memon, MD
Department of Neurosurgery
Neurological Institute
Cleveland Clinic
Cleveland, OH

Umesh S. Metkar, MD
Spine Surgeon
Department of Orthopedics
Carolina Pines Regional Medical Center
Hartsville, SC

Vincent Miele, MD
Assistant Professor of Neurological Surgery and Orthopaedic Surgery
Department of Neurosurgery;
Chief
Neurosurgery Spine Section;
Director
WVU Neurosurgery Southern Division
West Virginia University
Morgantown, WV;
Faculty
Cleveland Clinic Spine Research Lab
Cleveland, OH

Amrendra S. Miranpuri, MD
Resident
University of Wisconsin School of Medicine and Public Health;
Resident
University of Wisconsin Hospital and Clinics
Madison, WI

Junichi Mizuno, MD
Associate Professor
Department of Neurological Surgery
Aichi Medical University School of Medicine
Aichi, Japan

Sergey Mlyavykh, MD
Institute of Traumatology and Orthopaedics
Nizhni Novgorod, Russia

Michael T. Modic, MD
Chair
Neurological Institute;
Staff
Diagnostic Radiology
Cleveland Clinic
Cleveland, OH

Hikaru Morisue, MD, PhD
Instructor
Department of Orthopaedic Surgery
Kawasaki Municipal Hospital
Kawasaki-shi, Kanagawa-ken, Japan

Michael A. Morone, MD
Deaconess Billings Clinic
Billings, MT

Thomas E. Mroz, MD
Assistant Professor
Cleveland Clinic Lerner College of Medicine;
Director
Spine Surgery Fellowship;
Neurological Instititute
Center for Spine Health
Cleveland Clinic
Cleveland, OH

Jeffrey P. Mullin, MD
Resident
Department of Neurosurgery
Neurological Institute
Cleveland Clinic
Cleveland, OH

Praveen V. Mummaneni, MD
Associate Professor and Vice Chair
Department of Neurosurgery
University of California–San Francisco
San Francisco, CA

F. Reed Murtagh, MD
Professor
Department of Radiology
University of South Florida;
Department of Diagnostic Imaging
Moffitt Cancer Center
Tampa, FL

Ryan D. Murtagh, MD
Assistant Professor
Department of Radiology
University of South Florida;
Department of Diagnostic Imaging
Moffitt Cancer Center
Tampa, FL

John S. Myseros, MD
Associate Professor
Departments of Pediatrics and Neurosurgery
George Washington University School of Medicine;
Attending Neurosurgeon
Children's National Medical Center
Washington, DC;
Attending Neurosurgeon
Inova Fairfax Hospital for Children
Fall Church, VA

Sait Naderi, MD
Professor and Chair
Department of Neurosurgery
Umraniye Teaching and Research Hospital
Istanbul, Turkey

Dileep Nair, MD
Director
Intraoperative Monitoring;
Section Head
Adult Epilepsy
Department of Neurology
Cleveland Clinic
Cleveland, OH

Hiroshi Nakagawa, MD, DMSc
Professor Emeritus
Aichi Medical University Nagakute
Aichi-gun, Aichi, Japan;
Director
Spine Center
Kushiro Kojinkai Memorial Hospital
Kushiro City, Japan

Anil Nanda, MD, FACS
Professor and Chair
Department of Neurosurgery
Louisiana State University Health Science Center
Shreveport, LA

Chris J. Neal, MD
Department of Neurosurgery
National Naval Medical Center
Bethesda, MD

Russ P. Nockels, MD
Professor
Departments of Neurosurgery and Orthopedics;
Vice Chair
Department of Neurosurgery;
Director
Complex Spinal Surgery
Loyola University Medical Center
Maywood, IL

Chima Ohaegbulam, MD
Resident
Department of Neurosurgery
Brigham and Women's Hospital
Boston, MA

Eijiro Okada, MD, PhD
Assistant Professor
Department of Orthopaedic Surgery
Keio University School of Medicine
Tokyo, Japan

Bernardo Jose Ordonez, MD
Neurosurgical Associates
Norfolk, VA

Jennifer Orning, MD
Resident Physician
University of North Carolina Hospitals
Chapel Hill, NC

R. Douglas Orr, MD
Attending Staff
Center for Spine Health
Neurological Institute
Cleveland Clinic;
Chair of Surgery
Lutheran Hospital
Cleveland, OH

John O'Toole, MD
Assistant Professor
Department of Neurosurgery
Rush University Medical Center
Chicago, IL

A. Fahir Ozer, MD
Professor
Department of Neurosurgery
Koe University;
American Hospital
Istanbul, Turkey

Richard J. Parkinson, MD
Visiting Neurosurgeon
Department of Neurosurgery
St. Vincent's Clinic
Darlinghurst, New South Wales, Australia

Robert S. Pashman, MD
Director of Scoliosis and Spinal Deformities
Cedars-Sinai Institute for Spinal Disorders
Los Angeles, CA

Nirav J. Patel, MD
Cerebrovascular and Skull Base Fellow
Macquarie University
Sydney, New South Wales, Australia

Vishal C. Patel, MD

Stanley Pelofsky, MD
Oklahoma Spine Hospital
Oklahoma City, OK

Noel I. Perin, MD, FRCS
Professor
Department of Neurosurgery;
Director
Minimally Invasive Spine Section
NYU Medical Center
New York, NY

Olga Perlmutter, MD
Leading Scientific Fellow
Neurosurgery Department
Research Institute of Trauma and Orthopaedics
Novgorod, Russia

Frank M. Phillips, MD
Professor
Department of Orthopaedic Surgery;
Co-Director
Spine Fellowship
Rush University Medical Center
Chicago, IL

Rick Placide, MD, PT
Assistant Clinical Professor
Department of Physical Medicine and Rehabilitation
Virginia Commonwealth University;
Spine and Orthopaedic Surgeon
OrthoVirginia;
Chief
Orthopaedic Surgery
Chippenham Medical Center
Richmond, VA

Paul Porensky, MD
Neurosurgical Resident
Department of Neurological Surgery
The Ohio State University Medical Center
Columbus, OH

Srinivas Prasad, MD
Assistant Professor
Departments of Orthopaedic Surgery and Neurosurgery
Thomas Jefferson University
Philadelphia, PA

Mark L. Prasarn, MD
Assistant Professor
Division of Orthopaedic Surgery
University of Texas;
Memorial Hermann Hospital
Houston, TX

Gregory J. Przybylski, MD
Professor of Neuroscience
Seton Hall University
South Orange, NJ;
Director of Neurosurgery
New Jersey Neuroscience Institute at JFK Medical Center
Edison, NJ

Doron Rabin, MD
St. Luke's University Health Network
Fountain Hill, PA

Ashraf A. Ragab, MD
University of Mississippi Medical Center
Jackson, MS

Sharad Rajpal, MD
Staff Neurosurgeon
Boulder Neurological and Spine Associates
Boulder, CO

Y. Raja Rampersaud, MD, FRCSC
Assistant Professor
Division of Orthopedic Surgery
University of Toronto;
Spinal Program
Krambil Neuroscience Center
Toronto Western Hospital
University Health Network
Toronto, Ontario, Canada

Peter A. Rasmussen, MD
Director
Cerebrovascular Center
Neurological Institute
Cleveland Clinic
Cleveland, OH

Wolfgang Rausching, MD
Research Professor
Clinical and Applied Anatomy and Pathology
Uppsala University Hospital
Uppsala, Sweden

Gary L. Rea, MD, PhD
Assistant Professor
Department of Neurosurgery
The Ohio State University
Columbus, OH

Davis L. Reames, MD
Chief Resident
Department of Neurosurgery
University of Virginia
Charlottesville, VA

Glenn R. Rechtine II, MD
Professor
Department of Orthopaedic Surgery
University of South Florida
Tampa, FL;
Professor
Department of Orthopaedic Surgery
Univerity of Rochester
Rochester, NY;
Associate Chief of Staff
Bay Pines Veterans Administration Health Care System
Bay Pines, FL

John Regan, MD
Medical Director
Institute for Spinal Disorders
Cedars-Sinai Medical Center
Los Angeles, CA

Daniel K. Resnick, MD
Associate Professor and Vice Chair
Department of Neurosurgery
University of Wisconsin
Madison, WI

Laurence Rhines, MD
Assistant Professor and Director
Spine Program
Department of Neurosurgery
Universitiy of Texas M.D. Anderson Cancer Center
Houston, TX

Ron Riesenburger, MD
Assistant Professor
Department of Neurosurgery
Tufts University School of Medicine
Boston, MA

K. Daniel Riew, MD
Mildred B. Simon Distinguished Professor of Orthopedic Surgery;
Chief
Cervical Spine Surgery;
Professor of Neurosurgery;
Co-Director
Spine Fellowship;
Director
Ortho-Rehab Cervical Spine Institute
Orthopaedic Surgery Section
Washington University School of Medicine
St. Louis, MO

Gerald E. Rodts, Jr., MD
Associate Professor and Director of Neurosurgery Spine
Department of Neurological Surgery
Emory University
Atlanta, GA

Andrew C. Roeser, MD
Department of Neurosurgery
Methodist Hospital
Houston, TX

Eric Roger, MD
Assistant Professor
Department of Neurosurgery
State University of New York
Buffalo, NY

Eloy Rusafa, MD
Cleveland Clinic
Cleveland, OH

Fanor Manuel Saavedra, MD
Chief Resident
Department of Neurosurgery
University of Puerto Rico
San Juan, Puerto Rico

Krishna Satyan, MD

Paul D. Sawin, MD
Orlando Neurosurgery
Orlando, FL

Amirali Sayadipour, MD
Department of Orthopaedics
Thomas Jefferson University
Philadelphia, PA

Edward H. Scheid, Jr., MD
Senior Resident
Department of Neurosurgery
Thomas Jefferson University
Philadelphia, PA

David W. Schippert, MD
Orthopaedic Surgery Resident
Department of Orthopaedics and Rehabilitation
University of Rochester Medical Center
Rochester, NY

Richard Schlenk, MD
Director
Neurosurgery Training Program;
Staff
Department of Neurosurgery
Neurological Institute
Cleveland Clinic
Cleveland, OH

Meic H. Schmidt, MD
Associate Professor
Department of Neurosurgery
University of Utah
Salt Lake City, UT

Daniel M. Sciubba, MD
Assistant Professor of Neurosurgery, Oncology, and Orthopedic Surgery;
Director of Spine Research;
Director of Minimally Invasive Spine Surgery
Johns Hopkins University Hospital
Baltimore, MD

Meryl Severson, MD
Staff Neurosurgeon
Walter Reed National Military Medical Center
Bethesda, MD

Christopher I. Shaffrey, MD
Harrison Distinguished Teaching Professor
Departments of Neurosurgery and Orthopaedic Surgery
University of Virginia;
University of Virginia Medical Center
Charlottesville, VA

Mark E. Shaffrey, MD
Professor and Chair
Department of Neurological Surgery
Univeristy of Virginia
Charlottesville, VA

Alok D. Sharan, MD
Chief
Orthopedic Spine Service
Orthopaedic Surgery Section
Montefiore Medical Center
Bronx, NY

Ashwini D. Sharan, MD
Assistant Professor
Department of Neurosurgery
Thomas Jefferson University
Philadelphia, PA

Daniel Shedid, MD, FRCS(C), FABN
Assistant Professor
Division of Neurosurgery
University of Montreal;
Assistant Professor
Centre Hospitalier de l'Université de Montreal
Montreal, Quebec, Canada

Christopher B. Shields, MD, FRCS(C)
President
Norton Neuroscience Institute
Louisville, KY

John H. Shin, MD
Instructor
Department of Neurosurgery
Harvard Medical School;
Attending Neurosurgeon
Massachusetts General Hospital
Boston, MA

Steven Shook, MD
Staff
Neuromuscular Center
Neurological Institute
Cleveland Clinic
Cleveland, OH

Krzysztof Siemionow, MD
Assistant Professor
Department of Orthopaedic Surgery
University of Illinois
Chicago, IL

Fredrick A. Simeone, MD
Department of Neurosurgery
Thomas Jefferson University
Philadelphia, PA

James W. Simmons II, MD
Clinical Professor
Department of Orthopaedics and Rehabilitation
University of Texas Medical Branch
Galveston, TX;
Director
South Texas Orthopaedic Fellowship;
Baptist Health System
San Antonio, TX

Anthony Sin, MD
Department of Neurosurgery
Louisiana State University–Shreveport
Shreveport, LA

George L. Sinclair III, MD
Resident
Department of Neurosurgery
University of Medicine and Dentistry of New Jersey
Newark, NJ

Harminder Singh, MD
Department of Neurosurgery
Stanford University
Stanford, CA

Vladimir Sinkov, MD
Physician
New Hampshire Orthopaedic Center
Manchester, NH

Donald A. Smith, MD
Associate Professor
Department of Neurosurgery and Brain Repair
University of South Florida College of Medicine
Tampa, FL

Justin S. Smith, MD, PhD
Assistant Professor of Neurological Surgery
Department of Neurosurgery
University of Virginia
Charlottesville, VA

Maurice M. Smith, MD
Semmes-Murphey Clinic
Germantown, TN

Sean R. Smith, MD
Fellow in Spine Surgery
University of Toronto;
Division of Neurosurgery and Spinal Program
Toronto Western Hospital
Toronto, Ontario, Canada

Zachary A. Smith, MD
Assistant Professor
Department of Neurosurgery
Northwestern University
Chicago, IL

Volker K.H. Sonntag, MD
Emeritus
Barrow Neurological Institute
Phoenix, AZ;
Professor
Clinical Surgery
University of Arizona Medical School
Tucson, AZ

Micheal J. Speck, BS
Liaison
Information Technology Institute
Cleveland Clinic
Cleveland, OH

Robert F. Spetzler, MD
Director and J.N. Harber Chair of Neurological Surgery
Barrow Neurological Institute
Phoenix, AZ;
Professor
Department of Surgery
Section of Neurosurgery
University of Arizona College of Medicine
Tucson, AZ

Alejandro Spiotta, MD
Chief Resident
Department of Neurosurgery
Neurological Institute
Cleveland Clinic
Cleveland, OH

Robert M. Starke, MD
Department of Neurological Surgery
University of Virginia
Charlottesville, VA

Peter Steenland, MD
Department of Neurosurgery
University of North Carolina
Chapel Hill, NC

Michael P. Steinmetz, MD
Associate Professor
Case Western Reserve School of Medicine;
Chair
Department of Neuroscience
MetroHealth Medical Center
Cleveland, OH

Charles B. Stillerman, MD
Attending Neurosurgeon
Trinity Health Hospital
Minot, ND

Andrea L. Strayer, MS, A/GNP
Neurosurgery Nurse Practitioner
University of Wisconsin School of Medicine and Public Health
Madison, WI

Brian J. Sullivan, MD
Clinical Professor of Neurosurgery
George Washington University Hospital
Washington, DC;
Attending Neurosurgeon
Anne Arundel Medical Center
Annapolis, MD

Kyle I. Swanson, MD
Department of Neurosurgery
University of Wisconsin
Madison, WI

Monir N. Tabbosha, MD
Department of Neurosurgery
University of Arkansas–Little Rock
Little Rock, AR

Robert Talac, MD, PhD
Orthopaedic Spine Surgeon
Advanced Spine Institute
Jackson, TN

Richard Tallarico, MD
Assistant Professor of Orthopaedic Surgery
SUNY Upstate Medical University;
Division Chief
Orthopaedic Surgery Clinic
Upstate Bone and Joint Center
Syracuse, NY

Vartan Tashjian, MD
Kaiser Permanente Fontana Medical Center
Fontana, CA

Charles H. Tator, MD, PhD, FRCSC
Professor of Neurosurgery
University of Toronto;
Division of Neurosurgery
Toronto Western Hospital
Toronto, Ontario, Canada

Fernando Techy, MD
Assistant Professor of Clinical Orthopaedics and Spine Surgery
Department of Orthopaedic Surgery
University of Illinois–Chicago;
Spine Surgery Specialist
Illinois Bone and Joint Institute;
University of Illinois Medical Center
Chicago, IL

Sonia G. Teufack, MD
Department of Neurological Surgery
Jefferson Medical College
Thomas Jefferson University
Philadelphia, PA

Nicholas Theodore, MD
Chief
Spine Section
Division of Neurological Surgery
Barrow Neurological Institute
Phoenix, AZ;
Professor
Department of Surgery
Creighton University School of Medicine
Omaha, NE

Nicholas W.M. Thomas, MD
Department of Neurosurgery
Kings College Hospital
London, United Kingdom

James D. Thompson, BS
Medical Student
Drexel Univesity College of Medicine
Philadelphia, PA

Steven W. Thorpe, MD
Resident
Department of Orthopaedic Surgery
University of Pittsburgh Medical Center
Pittsburgh, PA

Robert E. Tibbs, Jr., MD
Oklahoma Spine Hospital
Oklahoma City, OK

Scott Tintle, MD

Stavropoula Tjoumakaris, MD
Instructor
Department of Neurosurgery
Thomas Jefferson University Hospital
Philadelphia, PA

Daisuke Togawa, MD, PhD
Assistant Professor
Department of Orthopaedic Surgery
Hamamatsu University School of Medicine
Hamamatsu, Shizuoka, Japan

C. Philip Toussaint, MD
Assistant Professor
Clinical Neurosurgery
University of South Carolina School of Medicine
Columbia, SC

Vincent C. Traynelis, MD
Professor and Vice Chair
Department of Neurosurgery;
Director of Spinal Surgery
Rush University Medical Center
Chicago, IL

Gregory R. Trost, MD
Professor
Departments of Neurological Surgery and Orthopaedics and Rehabilitation Medicine;
Vice Chair
Department of Neurosurgery
University of Wisconsin School of Medicine and Public Health
Madison, WI

Eve C. Tsai, MD
Neurosciences Unit
Ottawa Hospital
Ottawa, Ontario, Canada

Luis M. Tumialán, MD
Neurosurgical Faculty
Barrow Neurological Institute
St. Joseph's Hospital and Medical Center
Phoenix, AZ

Michael Turner, MD

Gary W. Tye, MD
Assistant Professor
Departments of Neurosurgery and Pediatrics;
Chief
Department of Pediatric Neurology
Virginia Commonwealth University Health Systems
Richmond, VA

Kene Ugokwe, MD
Chief Resident
Department of Neurosurgery
Neurological Institute
Cleveland Clinic
Cleveland, OH

Timothy Uschold, MD
Senior Resident
Department of Neurosurgery
Barrow Neurological Institute
Phoenix, AZ

Andrew Utter, MD
Clinical Associate Professor
Department of Orthopaedic Surgery
Louisiana State University Health Sciences Center;
Spine Surgeon
Spine Institute of Louisiana
Shreveport, LA

Alexander R. Vaccaro, MD, PhD
Professor and Attending Surgeon
Departments of Orthopaedics and Neurosurgery
Thomas Jefferson University Hospital/Rothman Institute
Philadelphia, PA

Alex Valadka, MD
Baylor College of Medicine
Texas Medical Center
Houston, TX

Gandhi Varma, MD
Fellow
Center for Spine Health
Department of Neurosurgery
Cleveland Clinic
Cleveland, OH

Shoshanna Vaynman, MD

Kushagra Verma, MD
Resident
Department of Orthopaedic Surgery
Thomas Jefferson University Hospital
Philadelphia, PA

Anthony A. Virella, MD, FACS
Director
Virella Neurosurgery
Westlake Village, CA

Elizabeth Vitarbo, MD
University of Miami
Miami, FL

Todd W. Vitaz, MD
Director
Neurosurgical Oncology;
Co-Director
Brain Tumor Center
Norton Healthcare
Louisville, KY

Tatiana von Hertwig Fernandes de Oliveira, MD
Staff
Division of Neurosurgery
Hospital Universitario Cajuru;
Hospital Pequeno Principe
Curitiba, Parana, Brazil

Jean-Marc Voyadzis, MD
Resident
Department of Neurosurgery
Georgetown University Hospital
Washington, DC

Kevin M. Walsh, MD
Department of Neurosurgery
Cleveland Clinic
Cleveland, OH

Sharon Walton, MD
Resident
Department of Orthopedic Surgery
University of Illinois–Chicago
Chicago, IL

Jeffrey C. Wang, MD
Professor
Departments of Orthopaedic Surgery and Neurosurgery
UCLA Spine Center
UCLA School of Medicine
Los Angeles, CA

Michael Y. Wang, MD
Associate Professor
University of Miami
Miami, FL

John D. Ward, MD, MSHA
Chief of Pediatric Neurosurgery
Department of Neurosurgery
Medical College of Virginia
Virginia Commonwealth University
Richmond, VA

Zabi Wardak, MD
Department of General Surgery
Loma Linda University Medical Center
Loma Linda, CA

Joseph Watson, MD
Associate Professor
Department of Neurosurgery
Virginia Common Wealth University Inova Campus;
Director
Inova Regional Neruosurgery Service;
Department of Neuroscience
Inova Health System
Falls Church, VA

Philip R. Weinstein, MD
Department of Neurosurgery
University of California–San Francisco School of Medicine
San Francisco, CA

Michael Weisman, MD

William C. Welch, MD, FACS
Associate Professor
Department of Neurological Surgery
University of Pittsburgh Medical Center
Pittsburgh, PA

Simcha J. Weller, MD
Director
Neurosurgery Spinal Disorders Program
Beth Israel Deaconess Medical Center
Boston, MA

L. Erik Westerlund, MD
Attending Orthopaedic Surgeon
St. Francis Spine and Neurosurgery Center
Columbus, GA

Andrew P. White, MD
Instructor in Orthopaedic Surgery
Harvard Medical School;
The Spine Center at Beth Israel Deaconess
Boston, MA

Jonathan A. White, MD
Birsner Family Professorship in Neurological Surgery
UT Southwestern Medical Center
Dallas, TX

Robert G. Whitmore, MD
Department of Neurosurgery
University of Pennsylvania Health System
Philadelphia, PA

Robert J. Wienecke, MD
Oklahoma Spine Hospital
Oklahoma City, OK

Jack E. Wilberger, MD
Professor and Chair of Neurosurgery;
Vice President of Graduate Medical Education
Drexel University College of Medicine
Philadelphia, PA;
Allegheny General Hospital–West Penn Allegheny Health System
Pittsburgh, PA

Brian J. Williams, MD
Resident
Department of Neurosurgery
University of Virginia
Charlottesville, VA

William A. Wilson IV, MD
Computational Biodynamics, LLC
Alexandria, VA

Christopher Wolfla, MD
Professor
Department of Neurosurgery
Medical College of Wisconsin
Milwaukee, WI

Jean-Paul Wolinsky, MD
Associate Professor
Departments of Neurosurgery and Oncology
Johns Hopkins University;
Clinical Director of Spine Service
Johns Hopkins Hospital
Baltimore, MD

Eric J. Woodard, MD
Chief of Neurosurgery
New England Baptist Hospital
Boston, MA

Sarah I. Woodrow, MD, FRCSC
Spine Fellow
Department of Neurosurgery
University of Miami
Miami, FL

Daniel S. Yanni, MD
Assistant Professor
Clinical Neurosurgery and Minimally Invasive and Complex Spine Surgery;
Surgical Director
Neuro-Intensive Care Unit
Department of Neurological Surgery
University of California–Irvine School of Medicine
Irvine, CA

Philip A. Yazbak, MD
Neuroscience Group of Northeast Wisconsin
Neenah, WI

Anthony T. Yeung, MD
Medical Director
Squaw Peak Surgical Facility
Phoenix, AZ

Mesut Yilmaz, MD
Chief Resident
Department of Neurosurgery
Kartal Dr. Lutfu Kirdar Teaching and Research Hospital
Istanbul, Turkey

Narayan Yoganandan, PhD
Professor of Neurosurgery and Orthopaedic Surgery
Department of Neurosurgery;
Chair of Biomedical Engineering
Medical College of Wisconsin
Milwaukee, WI

Kenneth S. Yonemura, MD
Wasatch Neurological Surgery
Bountiful, UT

Kazuo Yonenobu, MD, DMs
Director of Hospital
National Hospital Organization
Osaka Minami Medical Center
Kawachinagano, Osaka, Japan

Hansen A. Yuan, MD
Professor Emeritus
SUNY Upstate Medical University
Syracuse, NY

Adrian M. Zachary, MD
Staff
Center for Spine Health
Neurological Institute
Cleveland Clinic
Cleveland, OH

Seth M. Zeidman, MD
University of Rochester Medical Center
Rochester, NY

Barry M. Zide, MD
Professor
Department of Plastic Surgery
New York University Medical Center
New York, NY

Mehmet Zileli, MD
Professor of Neurosurgery
Faculty of Medicine
Department of Neurosurgery
Ege University
Izmir, Turkey

PREFACE

I stated in the front matter of the second edition of this book that "[it] was bigger and better than the first." The same is true for this third edition: It is without question much bigger and better than its predecessors.

The purpose of this book (to assist the spine surgeon with the avoidance, identification, and management of complications) has not changed. Its presentation, however, has: It is more colorful; the contributors are more seasoned—and, hence, they have refined the information transmission process, as well as the dialogue employed. This edition is easier to read, more organized, and much more user friendly. In this third edition good contributions from the prior editions were made better. Some have been eliminated; others have been added; new topics are addressed; and antiquated topics have been dropped.

This edition remains a *techniques* book but provides much, much more. In addition to the "*how* tos," it provides significant discussion regarding the "*when* tos," the "when *not* tos," and the "*whys*" associated with the decision-making process.

Decision making is, indeed, the central focus of this text. Decision making is facilited by understanding both the triumphs and the mistakes made by our predecessors. This book liberally provides such understanding. In addition to technique, it focuses on ethics, logic, nonoperative management, and controversies. Perhaps more important than any other factor, it focuses on the fundamentals. The fundamental disciplines of anatomy, biomechanics, and physiology provide the foundation for all we do as spine surgeons. I am perpetually compelled to focus on this foundation and have striven to do so in the pages that follow.

Risk Taking

Surgeons are risk takers and surgery is a risk-taking process. The patient places himself or herself in the hands of the surgeon, and the ensuing decision-making process involves the resolution (or the attempts at such) of many technical and quality-of-life–related issues and dilemmas. A surgical procedure may be warranted if the sum of the costs (both financial and personal) and risks is less than the sum of the benefits. This risk/benefit analysis should be of paramount concern and should be emphasized by the surgeon and realized by the patient. This book is designed to help surgeons achieve these goals, by minimizing the *risk-taking* component and by maximizing the *benefit* component of this "equation."

Repetition

We learn most effectively by having data presented in a repetitive manner, often from different perspectives, using differing techniques (e.g., written, mathematical, or visual).

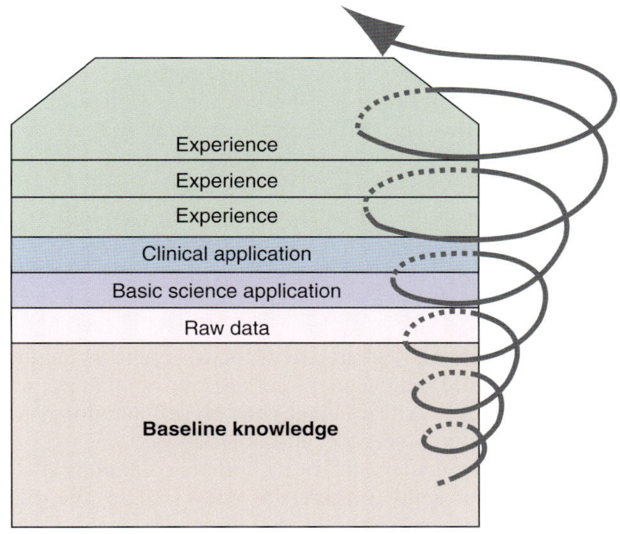

FIGURE 1. The spiral of learning.

The true understanding of a concept or body of knowledge involves the *spiral of learning*, which often involves multiple exposures to information so that a solid database (foundation of knowledge) is acquired. New (raw) data are then added and assimilated. This "expanded" knowledge base can then be applied to, and enhanced by, additional basic science, clinical input, and applications. This entire process is perpetually refined and reshaped by new experiences, such as clinical encounters or through reading and other sources of learning (Fig. 1). Repetition is the mother of learning. Repetition is, indeed, good—very good.

What Is a Complication?

The definition of what constitutes a complication is usually unclear and often argued. In a way, it's like pornography: "I cannot define it, but I know it when I see it."

> *I shall not today attempt further to define the kinds of material I understand to be embraced within that shorthand description ["hard-core pornography"]; and perhaps I could never succeed in intelligibly doing so. But* I know it when I see it, *and the motion picture involved in this case is not that.* [Emphasis added.]
>
> —Justice Potter Stewart, concurring opinion in *Jacobellis v. Ohio 378 U.S. 184 (1964)*, regarding possible obscenity in *The Lovers*.

Perhaps complications and pornography alike do not require strict definition, which may be too confining and, in the case of complications, detract from the purpose of focusing on its mitigation—i.e., *doing what's right*!

In the first and second editions of this book, I made reference to the Canadian Thistle as both a weed and a flower. To some it is a weed and to others it is considered a flower. To the spine surgeon, the patient, and the attorney, a complication has different meanings, and often different consequences. Postoperative pain (as subjective as it may be) may not be considered a complication by the surgeon. It may be perceived as annoying or even as a source of substantial distress to the patient. Conversely, it may be viewed as a source of revenue, and, therefore, joy by a plaintiff attorney. Beauty is clearly in the eye of the beholder, and without question, *ugly* is indeed a matter of perception and perspective.

Thus, the definition of a complication is not as clear as *outsiders* (e.g., the lay public and the legal system) often believe, or want to believe, is the case (as is the case with the definition of pornography). With all this in mind, and in the best interest of our patients, we should attain and maintain objectivity. We should not be swayed by uneducated or undeserved accolades from the medically naive, or by threats from entrepreneurs or the devious. Complications must be defined to the best of our ability, avoided when possible, and aggressively managed when they occur. Their avoidance, identification, and management should not be charged with emotion and anger but attacked with an armamentarium of logic, thoughtfulness, science, and objectivity.

The avoidance, identification, and management of the complications of spine surgery are addressed in the pages that follow by experts in the field. These experts themselves are not infallible. They address complications with which they have had first-hand experience. We must seize the opportunity to benefit from their wisdom and experience. A wise person can learn from the observations and mistakes of others.

Like a Canadian Thistle, a complication (and, yes, pornography) implies different things to different people. We must put complications in their appropriate perspective by clarifying their definition as they pertain to the situation at hand. We should then actively avoid them and aggressively identify and manage them when they do occur.

Bias and Conflict of Interest

Bias and conflicts of interest can skew and pervert objectivity. Please remember as you read the pages that follow that all of us (including the contributors to this book) are biased and conflicted. It is literally impossible not to harbor such biases. Some are more obvious than others. Nevertheless, as with the definition of complications and pornography, the definition of bias and conflict of interest is often unclear. I, in an attempt to inform our readership regarding the more obvious biases and conflicts of interests, have had each contributor disclose such conflicts as they pertain to the subject matter presented herein. They were asked to fill out the form depicted in Figure 2. Please remember that we all have bias and conflicts of interest. Those listed here represent but a scratching of the surface. Like so many other aspects of interpersonal communications—it's a start.

—*Edward C. Benzel, MD*

The Components and Factors Involved with the Definition of a Complication of Spinal Surgery: A Survey

1. Does your service have an explicit written (or "understood") definition of what constitutes a surgical complication? If so, could you append it to this questionnaire? If not, would you briefly describe your own concept of a complication under comments below?
   Yes 9% *No 88%* *No response 3%*
2. How do you decide what will be presented at a Morbidity and Mortality conference?
   Residents decide 31% *Faculty decides 24%*
   Faculty/residents decide 35% *Other 10%*
3. Do you consider a complication as an adverse event occurring (check all that apply):
   a. *Within 48 hours of surgery 45%*
   b. *Within a week of surgery 46%*
   c. *Within a month of surgery 75%*
   d. *While the patient was in the hospital 43%*
   e. *With reasonable assurance as a result of the surgical manipulation 75%*
   f. *None 23%*
4. Do you consider recurrent sciatica that is identical to the preoperative lumbar laminotomy pain pattern to be a complication if it occurs (check all that apply):
   a. *Within 48 hours of surgery 35%*
   b. *Within a week of surgery 36%*
   c. *Within a month of surgery 41%*
   d. *Within 2 months of surgery 25%*
   e. *Within 6 months of surgery 35%*
   f. *None 1%*
5. Do you consider the occurrence of pneumonia to be a complication if it occurs (check all that apply):
   a. *In a 25-year-old postoperative ventilated cervical quadriplegic patient 57%*
   b. *In a 65-year-old postoperative lumbar fusion patient with chronic obstructive pulmonary disease 13%*
   c. *In a 25-year-old nonoperated ventilated cervical quadriplegic patient 45%*
   d. *In a 40-year-old healthy nonsmoker on day 2 following a routine lumbar discectomy 96%*

6a. Do you consider a dural tear that is successfully repaired during surgery and that has no adverse sequelae to be a complication of surgery?
   Yes 43% *No 57%*

6b. Do you consider this same dural tear to be a complication of surgery if (check all that apply):
   a. *It is associated with 2 days of severe positional headaches 74%*
   b. *It is associated with CSF leakage through the wound and requires lumbar drainage to manage successfully 96%*
   c. *It requires reoperation to manage 96%*

7. Do you consider pedicle screw fracture at 6 months following surgery to be a complication if (check all that apply):
   a. *It is asymptomatic and associated with a solid fusion 24%*
   b. *It is asymptomatic and associated with a pseudarthrosis 65%*
   c. *It is associated with persistent back pain and a solid fusion 38%*
   d. *It is associated with persistent back pain and a pseudarthrosis 86%*
   e. *None of the above 13%*
8. In a patient who has undergone an anterior cervical discectomy with fusion, do you consider a pseudarthrosis (without excessive movement on flexion/extension x-rays) to be a complication if (check all that apply):
   a. *It is asymptomatic 24%*
   b. *It is associated with neck pain 80%*
   c. *It is associated with radicular pain 80%*
   d. *None 15%*
9. One year following a fusion and the placement of a hook-rod system for an unstable LI fracture in a patient without neurologic deficit, the patient complains of back pain at the rostral implant insertion site. Do you consider this a complication if (check all that apply):
   a. *You successfully manage the pain with an exercise program 12%*
   b. *Narcotic analgesics are required to manage the pain 30%*
   c. *The pain is managed successfully by surgical removal of the spinal implant 40%*
   d. *None 52%*
10. If we as surgeons could more accurately define what constitutes a complication (check all that apply):
   a. *Would the quality of our practices be improved?*
   Yes 63% *No 28%* *No response 9%*
   b. *Would medical reporting in the literature be enhanced?*
   Yes 92% *No 6%* *No response 2%*
   c. *Would quality assurance be enhanced?*
   Yes 76% *No 14%* *No response 10%*
   d. *Would the medico-legal climate be:*
   Worsened 29% *Improved 38%* *No effect 29%* *No response 4%*
   e. *And if we could simultaneously standardize which complications were the result of negligence, would the medico-legal climate be:*
   Worsened 20% *Improved 50%* *No effect 23%* *No response 7%*

FIGURE 2. Bias and conflict of interest survey.

CONTENTS

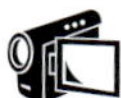

To view corresponding videos, please visit the Spine Surgery video collection online at expertconsult.com.

VOLUME ONE

SECTION 1 History

SECTION 2 The Fundamentals

SECTION 3 Extraspinal Anatomy and Surgical Approaches and Exposures of the Vertebral Column

SECTION 4 Surgical Procedures

4.1 Decompression and Arthrodesis of the Cervical Spine

4.2 Decompression and Arthodesis of the Thoracic and Lumbar Spine

VOLUME TWO

SECTION 5 **Spinal Instrumentation**

SECTION 6 **Motion Preservation Strategies**

SECTION 9 Specific Complications: Avoidance and Management

SECTION 10 Postscript

SECTION 11 Controversies

Chapters in this section are available online only at expertconsult.com. See inside front cover for details.

CONFLICT OF INTEREST

In order to minimize bias, the disclosure of potential conflicts of interest is imperative. The following contributors to this book have disclosed financial relationships with industrial partners. These relationships could bias the author's opinion and, therefore, should be considered accordingly.

Author	Industrial Partner
Lilyana Angelov	BrainLab
Edward C. Benzel	AxioMed, Cervical Spine Research Society, Computational Biodynamics, DePuy, Elsevier Publishing, OrthoMEMS, Rawlings, Stryker, Thieme Publishing, Turning Point
Christopher Bono	Deputy Editor of Journal of the American Academy of Orthopedic Surgeons
Darrel S. Brodke	Amedica, DePuy, Medtronic, Pioneer, Vertiflek
Charles H. Crawford III	Alphatec, Medtronic, Synthes
Gary A. Dix	Alphatec, Biomet, DePuy Spine, Globus, ISTO, Pioneer, Spine Wave
Ehab Farag	Hospira
David Fiorella	Codman & Shurtleff, Cordis, Covidien EV3, Microvention, Micrus Endovascular, Nfocus Medical, Siemens
Jeffrey S. Fischgrund	Baxter, Cervical Spine Research Society, Lumbar Spine Research Society, Relievant, Salient, Smith & Nephew, Stryker, Trans1
Jan Goffin	Medtronic
Regis W. Haid, Jr.	Globus Medical, Medtronic, Nuvasive
Fraser C. Henderson	Computational BioDynamics
Patrick W. Hitchon	DePuy Spine
Brian J. Kistler	Synthes
Joon Y. Lee	Stryker
Isador H. Lieberman	Alphatec Spine, Axiomed Spine Corporation, Collplant, CrossTrees Medical, Mazor Surgical Technologies, Merlot OrthopediX, NOC2 Healthcare, Orthofix, Pearl Diver, Stryker Spine, Synthes Spine, Trans1, Zyga
Eric M. Massicotte	DePuy Canada, Medtronic
Junichi Mizuno	Ammtec
Thomas E. Mroz	Globus Medical, PearlDiver
Praveen V. Mummaneni	DePuy Spine, Quality Medical Publishers
Hiroshi Nakagawa	Stryker
R. Douglas Orr	Medtronic
Frank M. Phillips	Nuvasive
K. Daniel Riew	Amedica, Benvenue Medical, Biomet, Cervical Spine Research Society, Expanding Orthopedics, Korean American Spine Society, Medtronic Sofamor Danek, Nexgen Spine, Osprey, Paradigm Spine, PSD, Spinal Kinetics, Spineology, Vertiflex

Meic H. Schmidt	Aesculap, NREF
Christopher I. Shaffrey	AO, Biomet, Department of Defense, DePuy, Medtronic, National Institutes of Health, North American Clinical Trials Network
Daniel Shedid	Baxano, DePuy Spine
Justin S. Smith	Biomet, DePuy Spine, Globus, Medtronic
Volker K.H. Sonntag	Medtronic
Robert F. Spetzler	Boston Scientific, Dicom Grid, EmergeMD, iCO Therpeutics, Katalyst/Kogent, Neurovasc, RSB Spine, Stereotaxis, Synergetics, Zeiss
Michael P. Steinmetz	Biomet Spine, Medtronic Power Division
Brian J. Sullivan	Globus Medical
Daisuke Togawa	Medtronic Sofamore Danek
Michael Y. Wang	Aesculap Spine, Biomet, DePuy
William A. Wilson IV	Computational BioDynamics
Hansen A. Yuan	BreakAway Imaging, DePuy Spine, Medtronics, Pioneer Surgical

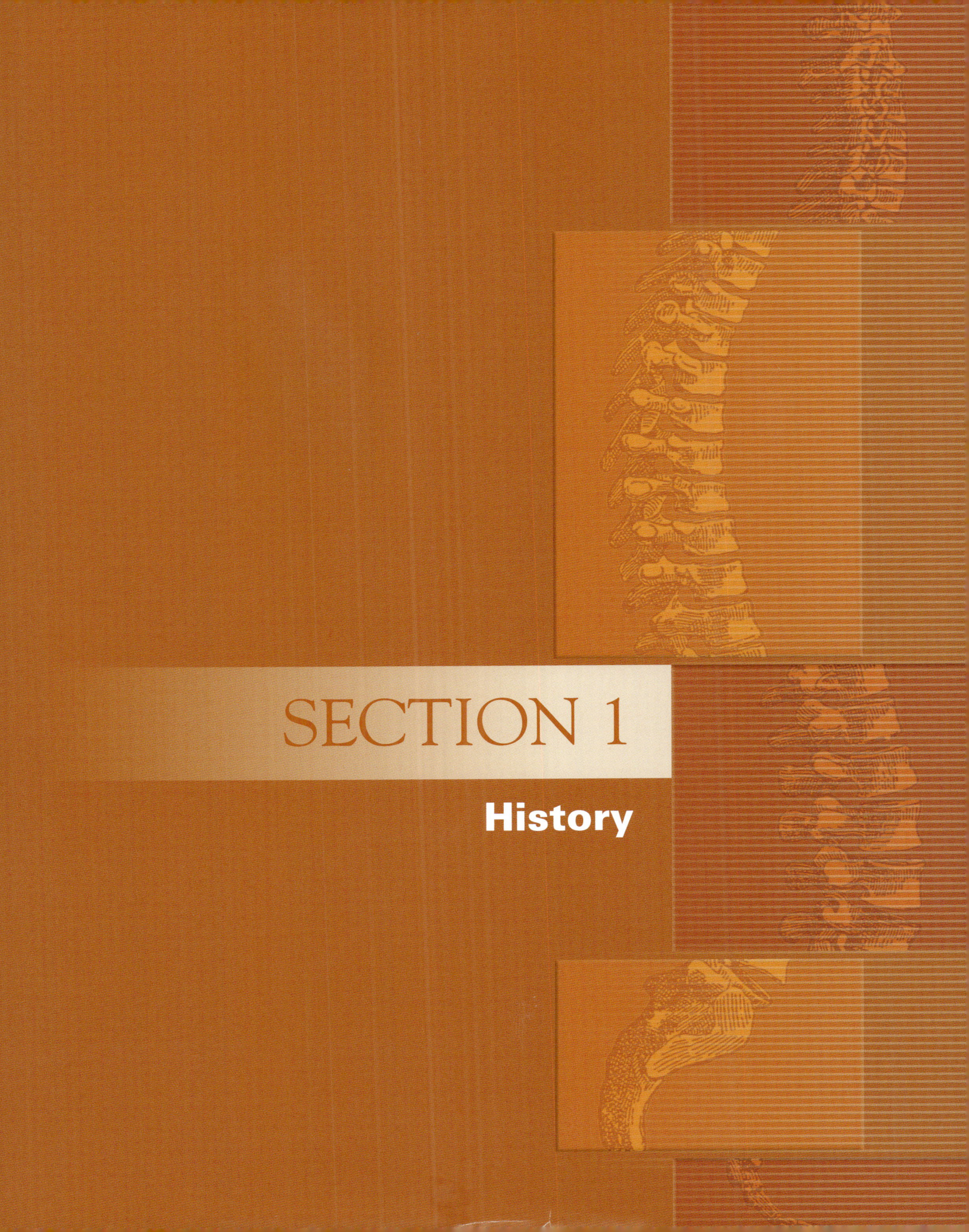

SECTION 1

History

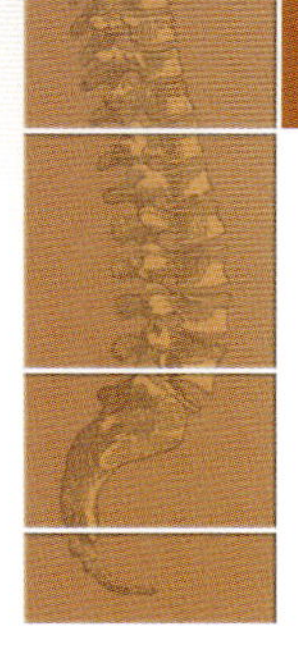

CHAPTER 1

History of Spine Surgery

Sait Naderi | Edward C. Benzel

The evolution of spinal surgery has revolved around three basic surgical goals: decompression, surgical stabilization, and deformity correction. To emphasize their importance, these surgical goals form the framework for this chapter. However, other related fundamental arenas, such as anatomy, biomechanics, nonsurgical treatment modalities, contributed to the development of surgical concepts as well.

Although the main advances in spine surgery occurred in the 19th and 20th centuries, their roots date back several thousand years. Without understanding and appreciating the past, it is not possible to understand and appreciate the advancements of the last two centuries. Therefore, before touching upon the last two centuries' history of the spine, a short examination of spine medicine from the antique period, medieval period, and Renaissance is presented.

Antique Period and Spine Surgery

There is no evidence of surgical decompression and stabilization, or the surgical correction of deformity, during the antique period except for laminectomy in a trauma case reported by Paulus of Aegina. However, it is known that physicians of the antique period were, to some extent, able to evaluate patients with spinal disorders. They in fact used frames for reduction of dislocation and gibbus and applied some of the knowledge gained from human and animal dissections.

Srimad Bhagwat Mahapuranam, an ancient Indian epic (3500–1800 BCE), depicts the oldest documentation of spinal traction. In a passage from this document, it is described that Lord Krishna applied axial traction to correct a hunchback in one of his devotees.[1]

The Edwin Smith Papyrus (2600–2200 BCE) is the most well-known document on Egyptian medicine. This document reports 48 cases. Imhotep (2686–2613 BCE), a late second-dynasty surgeon, authored this papyrus, which reported six cases of spinal trauma. Hence, nearly 4600 years ago, vertebral subluxation and dislocation and traumatic quadriplegia and paraplegia were described.[2] Recently, it was reported that Egyptian physicians described the "spinal djet column concept."[3]

Antique medicine was also influenced by the Greco-Roman period physicians.[4] *Hippocrates* (460–375 BCE) addressed the anatomy and pathology of the spine, describing the normal curvatures of the spine, its structure, and the tendons attached to it. He defined tuberculous spondylitis, posttraumatic kyphosis, scoliosis, spinal dislocation, and spinous process fracture. He addressed the relationship between spinal tuberculosis and gibbus. According to Hippocrates, spinous process fracture was not dangerous. However, fractures of the vertebral body were more important. He described two frames for reduction of the dislocated spine, including the Hippocratic ladder and the Hippocratic board.[5] The details of Hippocratic treatment were recorded by Aulus Cornelius Celsus (25 BCE–50 CE).

Aristotle (384–322 BCE) focused on kinesiology. His treatises—"parts of animals, movement of animals, and progression of animals—described the actions of the muscles." He analyzed and described walking, in which rotatory motion is transformed into translational motion. Although his studies were not directly related to the spine, they were the first to address human kinesiology and, in fact, biomechanics.[6]

Galen of Pergamon (130–200 CE), another physician of the antique era, worked as a surgeon and anatomist. He studied the anatomy of animals and extrapolated his findings to human anatomy. His anatomic doctrines became the basis for medical education for more than 1200 years. He used the terms *kyphosis*, *scoliosis*, and *lordosis*, and he attempted to correct these deformities. He also worked as the official surgeon of gladiators in amphitheaters. Because of this position, he was accepted as "the father of sports medicine." He confirmed the observations of Imhotep and Hippocrates regarding the neurologic sequences of cervical spine trauma. Nevertheless, to the best of our knowledge, he did not operate for spinal trauma.[6,7]

Oribasius (325–400 CE), another physician of the antique period, added a bar to the Hippocratic reduction device and used it to treat both spinal trauma and spinal deformity.[8]

One of the most important figures dealing with spinal disorders during the end of this period was *Paulus of Aegina* (625–690 CE). He collected what was known from the previous 1000 years in a seven-volume encyclopedia. Paulus of Aegina not only used the Hippocratic bed, but also worked with a red-hot iron. He is credited with performing the first known laminectomy. This was performed for a case of spinal fracture resulting in spinal cord compression. He emphasized the use of orthoses in spinal trauma cases.[6,9]

Medieval Period and Spine Surgery

The studies and reports of Paulus of Aegina are the most important source of information regarding this period of medicine. This age was followed by the Dark Ages (ca. 500–1000 CE) in Europe. Although Western medicine showed no progress

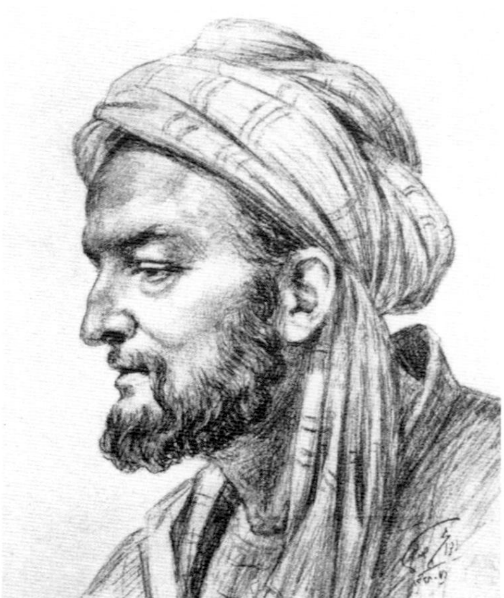

FIGURE 1-1. Avicenna.

during the Dark Ages, the Eastern world developed the science. The early Islamic civilizations realized the importance of science and scientific investigation. The most important books of the antique age were translated into Syrian, Arabic, and Persian. Therefore, using the Western doctrines, the Islamic civilizations discovered new information and were able to contribute further. In terms of spine medicine, several important contributors, including Avicenna and Abulcasis, added to this movement.

Avicenna (981–1037 CE), a famous physician from present-day Uzbekistan, worked in all areas of medicine (Fig. 1-1). His famous book, the *Canon of Medicine*, was a seminal textbook until the 17th century in Europe. He described the biomechanics-related anatomy of the spine, as well as flexion, extension, lateral bending, and axial rotation of the spine.[10] Avicenna also used a traction system similar to the system described by Hippocrates.

Abulcasis (936–1013 CE), a famous Arabian surgeon of the 11th century, wrote a surgery treatise, "At-Tasnif." He described several surgical disorders, including low back pain, sciatica, scoliosis, and spinal trauma. He recommended the use of chemical or thermal cauterization for several spinal disorders. He also developed a device to reduce the dislocated spine.[11]

Serefeddin Sabuncuoglu (1385–1468 CE), a Turkish physician of the 15th century, wrote an illustrated atlas of surgery,[12] in which he described scoliosis, sciatica, low back pain, and spinal dislocations. He delineated a technique for reduction of spinal dislocations, using a frame similar to that designed by Abulcasis.

Renaissance and Spine Surgery

Gradually, the intellectual doldrums of the Dark Ages in Europe evolved into the Renaissance. Academic centers were established in Europe, as well as centers for the translation of documents, similar to centers established in Islamic regions. Thus, the classics from the antique age were translated into Latin from Arabic, making their scientific information available to the scholars and physicians of the Renaissance. During this time, the Western world spawned disciplines, including art, medicine, physics, and mathematics.

The works of *Leonardo Da Vinci* (1452–1519 CE) are of importance in this regard. Da Vinci worked on the philosophy of mechanics and on anatomy in *De Figura Humana*. He described spine anatomy, the number of vertebrae, and the joints in detail. By studying anatomy in the context of mechanics, da Vinci gained some insight into biomechanics. He considered the importance of the muscles for stability in the cervical spine. However, his work was unpublished for centuries, and his brilliant daydreaming had a limited scientific influence on biomechanics.[13,14]

Andreas Vesalius (1514–1564 CE), an anatomist and physician, wrote his famous anatomy book, *De Humani Corporis Fabrica Liberi Septum*, which changed several doctrines described by Galen. Actually, it took several centuries for the world to accept that Galen had made errors that were corrected by Vesalius. Because he described and defined modern anatomy, he is commonly accepted as the father of anatomy. He described the spine, intervertebral disc, and intervertebral foramina. His biomechanical point of view regarding the flexion extension of the head was similar to that of Avicenna.[15]

The early anatomic studies and observations were followed by biomechanical advancements. Prominent among the contributors to those advancements was *Giovanni Alfonso Borelli* (1608–1679 CE), who described the biomechanical aspects of living tissue. He is the founder of the "iatrophysics" concept—a term that subsequently became known as biomechanics. He is accepted as the "father of spinal biomechanics." His book, *De Motu Animalium*, describes the movements of animals. He wrote that the intervertebral disc is a viscoelastic material that carries loads. This is so because he observed that muscles could not bear the loads alone. He concluded that the intervertebral discs should have function during load bearing. He was the first scientist to describe the human weight center (center of gravity).[16,17]

The studies and accomplishments of the Renaissance period were not limited to the aforementioned. Many scientists contributed to the body of the literature in this period. The advancements from this period resulted in the formation of early modern surgery, beginning in the 19th century.

Early Modern Period and Spine Surgery

Spinal Decompression and the Early Modern Period

Although an open decompression of the spinal canal for spinal cord compression was recommended by some surgeons as early as the 16th and 18th centuries (e.g., Pare, Hildanus), there is no evidence of successful intervention except for a case reported by Paulus of Aegina prior to the 19th century.

Spinal decompression in the early modern period was primarily via laminectomy. Throughout most of the 19th century, laminectomy was developed and its utility debated as the only surgical approach to all spinal pathologies, including tumor, trauma, and infection. At the dawn of the 20th century, the indications for laminectomy were extended to the decompression of spinal degenerative disease, an understanding of which had eluded 19th-century surgeons because they failed to appreciate the connection between its clinical and pathologic manifestations.

During the 19th century, spinal surgery was performed almost exclusively for neural element decompression. Numerous nonoperative approaches to deformity correction were attempted over the centuries, but the surgical approach to deformity correction was a 20th-century development. The techniques of spinal stabilization were also a product of the 20th century—both spinal fusion and internal fixation appearing around the turn of the 20th century. Moreover, a failure to recognize the implications for treatment of degenerative spinal disease, including spondylosis and degenerative disc disease, meant that the solution to these problems had to wait for the new century.

Thus, during the 19th century, the indications for spinal surgery were limited to the treatment of tumor, trauma, and infection.[18] Although each of these conditions posed unique clinical and surgical problems, they shared the need for surgical decompression. Throughout the early modern period, surgical decompression of the spine was the single most common reason to undertake the risks of spinal surgery, and laminectomy was the most commonly used technique to achieve it.

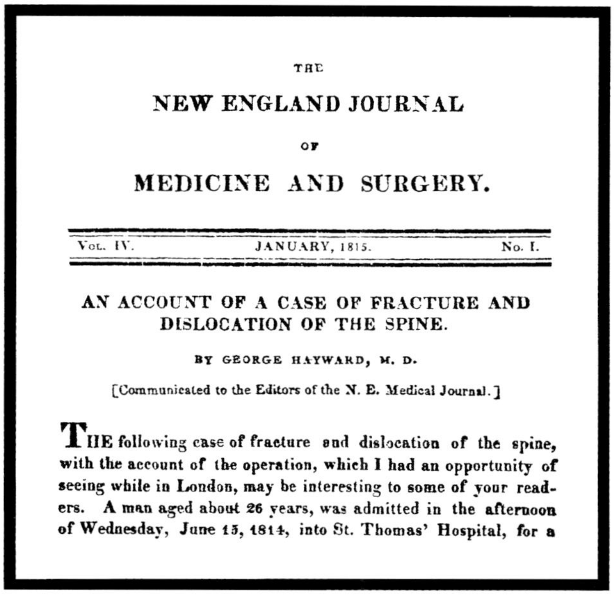

THE

NEW ENGLAND JOURNAL

OF

MEDICINE AND SURGERY.

VOL. IV. JANUARY, 1815. No. I.

AN ACCOUNT OF A CASE OF FRACTURE AND DISLOCATION OF THE SPINE.

BY GEORGE HAYWARD, M. D.

[Communicated to the Editors of the N. E. Medical Journal.]

THE following case of fracture and dislocation of the spine, with the account of the operation, which I had an opportunity of seeing while in London, may be interesting to some of your readers. A man aged about 26 years, was admitted in the afternoon of Wednesday, June 15, 1814, into St. Thomas' Hospital, for a

FIGURE 1-2. First page of H. J. Cline Jr.'s historic laminectomy, as reported by G. Hayward. (From Cline HJ Jr [cited by Hayward G]: An account of a case of fracture and dislocation of the spine. *N Engl J Med Surg* 4:13, 1815.)

Birth and Development of the Laminectomy

H. J. Cline, Jr., and the Argument against Spinal Surgery

At the beginning of the 19th century, the prospects for spinal surgery appeared grim. The dismal results of a well-publicized operation for a traumatic spinal injury stimulated a heated debate over the "possibility" of spinal surgery that persisted for nearly a century. At the center of this debate was H. J. Cline, Jr., a little-known British surgeon.

In 1814, Cline performed a multilevel laminectomy for a thoracic fracture-dislocation associated with signs of a complete paraplegia (Fig. 1-2).[19] The patient was a 26-year-old man who fell from the top of a house. "He was bled previous to his admission" to the St. Thomas's Hospital in London, "and some imprudent attempts were made to relieve him by pressing the knees against the injured part, which only increased the pain and inflammation."[19] Upon admission to the hospital the patient was examined by Cline, who "ascertained that some of the spinous processes . . . were broken off and were pressing upon the spinal marrow . . . [and] who resolved to cut down and remove the pressure from the spinal marrow."[19]

The patient was observed overnight in the hospital, and on the day following admission, Cline performed his proposed operation. Although the operation was performed within 24 hours of injury, Cline was unable to reduce the dislocation or to achieve a complete decompression of the neural elements. The patient survived for 3 days after surgery, with increasing pain and a steadily increasing pulse. On postoperative day 4, however, the patient died, "and on an examination of the body by Mr. Cline, it was found that the spinal marrow was entirely divided."[19] Despite the severity of the neural injury, and the complexity of the fracture-dislocation, the untoward outcome of this unfortunate case would remain a topic of conversation for almost a century, providing ample ammunition for the opponents of spinal surgery.

Of course, the case of Cline was not an isolated mortality. In 1827, for example, Tyrell[20] reported a 100% mortality for a small series of patients with surgically treated spinal dislocation and neurologic injury. Other reports (e.g., Rogers[21] in 1835) were often equally discouraging. Looking back on these early years of the debate about spinal surgery, the early 20th century British surgeon Donald Armour[22] described the controversy this way:

> *This [Cline's operation] precipitated and gave rise to widespread and vehement discussion as to its justification. This discussion, often degenerating into bitter and virulent personalities, went on many years. Astley Cooper, Benjamin Bell, Tyrell, South, and others favored it, while Charles Bell, John Bell, Benjamin Brodie, and others opposed it. The effect of so eminent a neurologist as Sir Charles Bell against the procedure retarded spinal surgery many years—the operation was described with such extravagant terms as "formidable," "well-nigh impossible," "appalling." "desparate [sic] and blind," "unjustifiable," and "bloody and dangerous."*

Of course, surgical fatalities in this period were due as much to septic complications and anesthetic inadequacies as they were to surgical technique. The lack of an effective means of pain control during surgery intensified the problem of intraoperative shock and made speed essential. Furthermore, the problems of wound infection and septicemia were both predictable and frequently fatal. These hindrances to surgery were not ameliorated until the introduction of general anesthetic agents (i.e., nitrous oxide, ether, and chloroform) in the mid-1840s and the adoption of Listerian techniques (using carbolic acid) in the 1870s.[23]

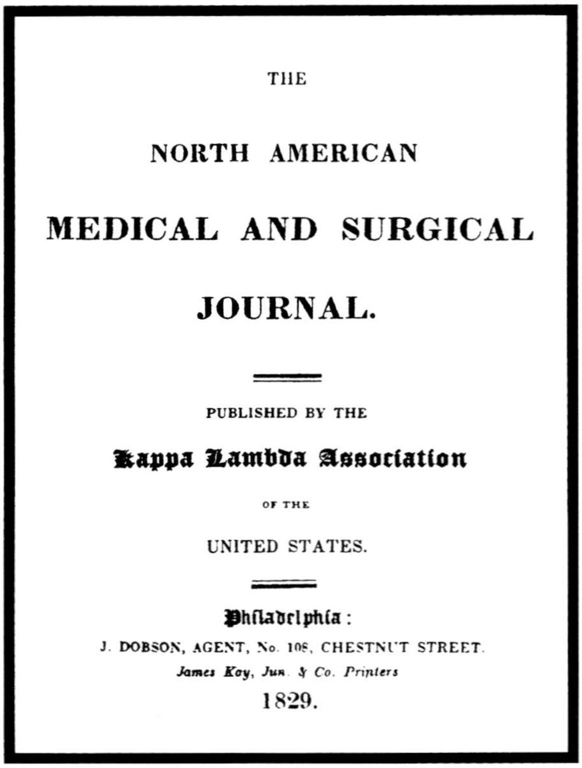

THE

NORTH AMERICAN

MEDICAL AND SURGICAL

JOURNAL.

PUBLISHED BY THE

Kappa Lambda Association

OF THE

UNITED STATES.

Philadelphia:

J. DOBSON, AGENT, No. 108, CHESTNUT STREET.

James Kay, Jun. & Co. Printers

1829.

FIGURE 1-3. Title page of journal that contains the first successful report of a laminectomy. The surgeon, and the author of the report, was Alban G. Smith of Danville, Kentucky. (From Smith AG: Account of a case in which portions of three dorsal vertebrae were removed for the relief of paralysis from fracture, with partial success. *North Am Med Surg J* 8:94–97, 1829.)

A. G. Smith and the First Successful Laminectomy

Despite these risks, a little-known surgeon named Alban G. Smith from Danville, Kentucky, performed a laminectomy in 1828 on a patient who had fallen from a horse and sustained a traumatic paraplegia. To Smith's credit, his patient not only survived the operation but achieved a partial neurologic recovery. The operative technique and surgical results were reported in the *North American Journal of Medicine and Surgery* in 1829 (Fig. 1-3).[24] Smith's procedure comprised a multilevel laminectomy through a midline incision, involving removal of the depressed laminae and spinous processes, exploration of the dura mater, and closure of the soft tissue incision. Although the report of this landmark case appears to have attracted little attention at the time, it is a significant technical achievement and places Smith among the pioneers of the early modern period in spinal surgery.

Laminectomy for Extramedullary Spinal Tumor

During the half century after Smith's historic operation, the primary indication for laminectomy was spinal trauma. In the latter part of the 19th century, the indications for laminectomy were extended to tumor and infection.[25] The first and most celebrated surgical case for spinal tumor in the 19th century, that of Captain Gilbey, was also the first successful one, and it played an important role in the rehabilitation of the laminectomy as a safe and effective procedure.

Captain Gilbey was an English army officer who suffered the misfortune of losing his wife in a carriage accident in which he also was involved. Although Gilbey himself escaped serious injury, he soon began to experience progressive dull back pain, which he attributed to the accident. As the pain became relentless, Gilbey sought the advice of a series of physicians, all of whom were unable to identify the source of his pain. Eventually, Gilbey was referred to the eminent London neurologist, William Gowers, who elicited from the patient a history of back pain, urinary retention, paraplegia, and loss of sensation below the thoracic level (Fig. 1-4).[26]

The neurologist's diagnosis was immediate and unequivocal: the cause of Gilbey's symptoms was located in his spine, where a tumor was causing compression of the thoracic spinal cord. Although no intraspinal tumor had ever been resected successfully, Gowers referred the patient to his London surgical colleague, Victor Horsley (Fig. 1-5). After all, Gowers had himself asserted, in his authoritative textbook, *Manual of Diseases of the Nervous System*, that removal of an intradural spinal cord tumor was "not only practicable, but actually a less formidable operation than the removal of intracranial tumors."[27]

Horsley acted quickly. Within 2 hours of the initial consultation, a skin incision was made at 1 PM, June 9, 1887, at the National Hospital, Queens Square, London. Despite his precipitous decision to undertake this dangerous operation, Horsley did not approach the operation unprepared. Although the Act of 1876 made it a criminal offense to experiment on a vertebrate animal for the purpose of attaining manual skill,

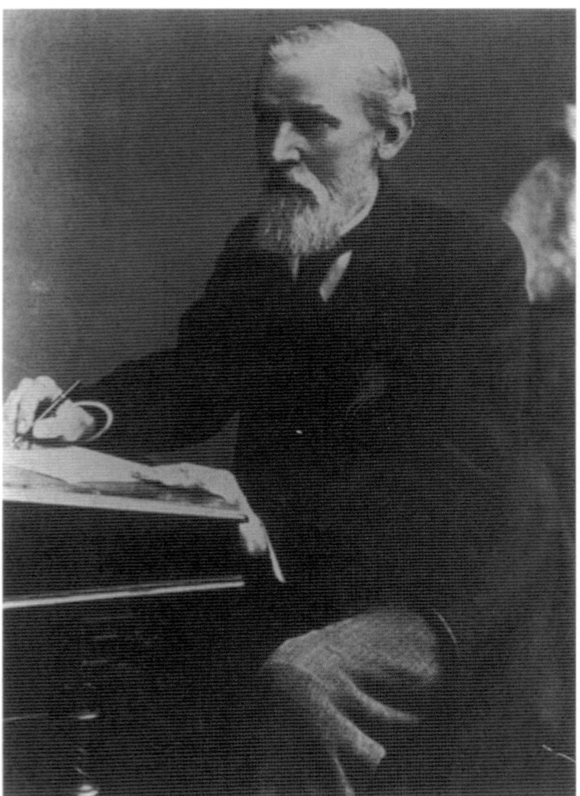

FIGURE 1-4. William R. Gowers.

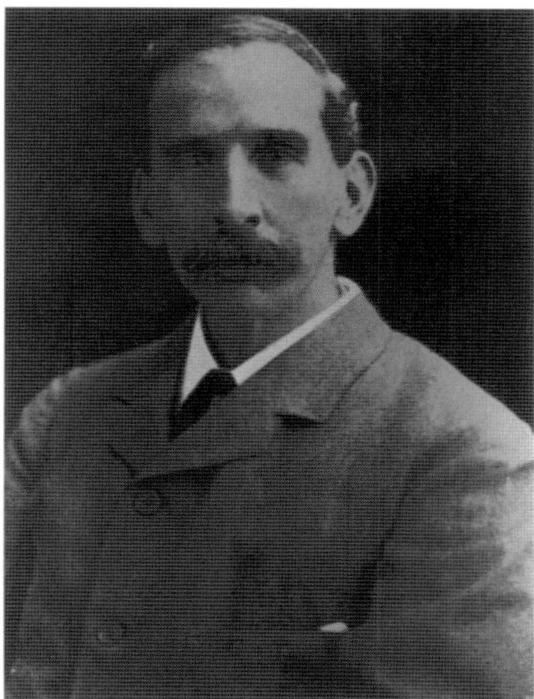

FIGURE 1-5. Sir Victor Horsley.

Horsley had repeatedly practiced the proposed procedure in the course of his surgical experimentation. Despite some initial difficulty in locating the tumor, an intradural neoplasm in the upper thoracic spine causing compression of the spinal cord was identified and safely resected. The pathologic diagnosis was "fibromyxoma of the theca."

Follow-up 1 year later revealed almost complete neurologic recovery. The patient was walking without assistance and had returned to his premorbid work schedule. He remained well, with no evidence of tumor recurrence, up to the time of his death from an unrelated cause 20 years later.

Laminectomy for Intramedullary Spinal Tumor

In 1890, Fenger attempted to remove an intramedullary spinal tumor in an operation that resulted in the patient's death.[28] In 1905, Cushing[29,30] also attempted to remove an intramedullary spinal cord tumor but decided to abort the procedure after performing a myelotomy in the dorsal column. To Cushing's surprise, the patient improved after surgery. In 1907, von Eiselsberg[31] successfully resected an intramedullary tumor.

The unexpected improvement that was observed in the patient reported by Cushing attracted the attention of the New York surgeon Charles Elsberg. Elsberg[32] described Cushing's technique, which he aptly named the "method of extrusion." The technique was intended to remove an intramedullary tumor by spontaneous extrusion of the tumor through a myelotomy made in the dorsal column. The rationale for this method was predicated on the theory that an intramedullary tumor was associated with an increase in intramedullary pressure. Release of this pressure by a myelotomy that extended from the surface of the spinal cord to the substance of the tumor was expected to provide sufficient force to spontaneously extrude the tumor. According to Elsberg, the advantage of this procedure over a standard tumor resection was that it required minimal manipulation of the spinal cord and therefore minimal spinal cord tissue injury.

Because the spontaneous extrusion of an intramedullary tumor occurred slowly, Elsberg performed these procedures in two stages. In the first stage, a myelotomy was fashioned in the dorsal column, extending from the surface of the spinal cord to the tumor (Fig. 1-6A).

When the tumor was identified and observed to begin to bulge through the myelotomy incision, the operation was concluded, the dura mater was left opened, and the wound closed. In the second stage of the procedure, which was performed approximately 1 week after the first stage, Elsberg reopened the wound and inspected the tumor (Fig. 1-6B). Typically, the tumor was found outside the spinal cord, and the few adhesions that remained between the spinal cord and the tumor were sharply divided. After the tumor was removed, the wound, including the dura mater, was closed.

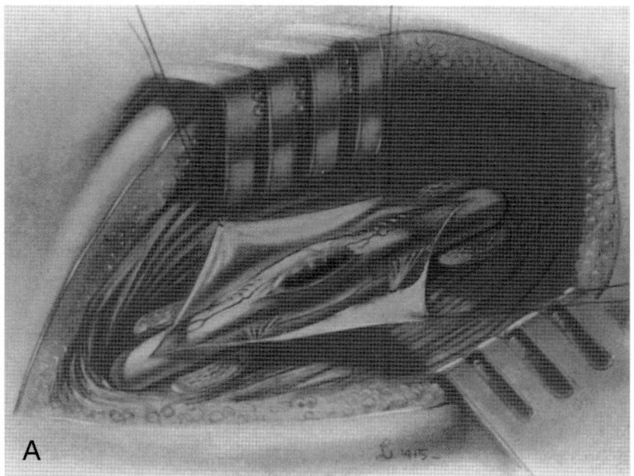

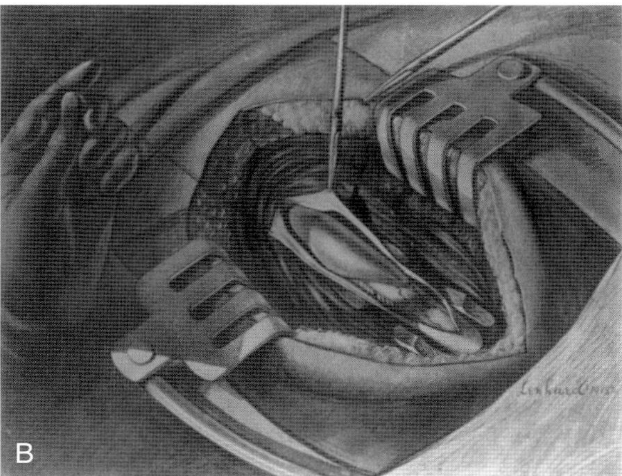

FIGURE 1-6. A, The first stage in an intramedullary spinal cord tumor resection by the extrusion method. Note that the tumor is bulging through the myelotomy incision. The wound was subsequently closed. **B,** The second stage in an intramedullary spinal cord tumor resection by the extrusion method, 1 week after the first stage. Note that the tumor has spontaneously extruded since the first operation, and now may be removed easily. (From Elsberg CA, Beer E: The operability of intramedullary tumors of the spinal cord. A report of two operations with remarks upon the extrusion of intraspinal tumors. *Am J Med Sci* 142:636–647, 1911.)

Variations in Laminectomy Technique

By the last decade of the 19th century, after the case of Captain Gilbey, the possibility of safely performing a spinal operation was established in the collective surgical consciousness. Furthermore, new anesthetic techniques and aseptic methods had become available to most practicing surgeons.[33] All of these factors served to increase the appeal of the laminectomy to surgeons and to widen its range of application. For example, after Horsley's widely publicized success for resecting a spinal tumor, many similar operations were soon described in the literature,[34-39] and in 1896, Makins and Abbott[40] reported 24 cases of laminectomy for vertebral osteomyelitis.

Although the safety and efficacy of the laminectomy had convinced many proponents of the utility of the procedure, toward the end of the century surgeons began to worry about postoperative instability. Advances in operative technique and perioperative management meant that more and more patients survived the operation and ultimately became ambulatory, which further heightened concern about stability.

In 1889, Dawbarn[41] described an osteoplastic method of laminectomy that addressed this concern. Instead of a midline incision, Dawbarn described two lateral incisions that were carried down to the transverse processes. The lateral incisions were connected in an H-like fashion, and a superior and inferior flap—including skin, muscle, fascia, and bone—was then turned. In closing the wound, the intact flaps were reflected back and reapproximated in their normal anatomic positions.

Although not all surgeons subscribed to the osteoplastic method, many turn-of-the-century surgeons were largely preoccupied with modifications of this procedure.[42] At the same time, however, a more important innovation in laminectomy technique, the hemilaminectomy, was developed independently in both Italy[43,44] and the United States.[44]

In 1910, A. S. Taylor of New York described the hemilaminectomy: a midline incision, a subperiosteal paravertebral muscle takedown, and the removal of a hemilamina with a Doyen saw. The advantages of the hemilaminectomy over the cumbersome osteoplastic method were obvious, and Taylor argued that compared with the laminectomy, the hemilaminectomy interfered less with the mechanics of the spine. Despite such detractors as Charles Elsberg, who responded that the field of view was narrow and the effect of laminectomy on spinal mechanics negligible, Taylor successfully championed its use.

Charles A. Elsberg: The Laminectomy in Stride

Charles A. Elsberg was one of the most influential writers on spinal decompression (Fig. 1-7). Working at the Neurological Institute of New York, which he had helped to found, Elsberg[45] published his first series of laminectomies in 1913. In 1916, he published his classic text, *Diagnosis and Treatment of Surgical Diseases of the Spinal Cord and Its Membranes*.[46] Although these publications represent landmarks in the history of spinal surgery, they constitute more of a culmination than an innovation in spinal surgery. Elsberg's work on spinal surgery, coming as it did at the end of a century of evolution of the decompressive laminectomy, effectively codified 19th and early 20th century developments.

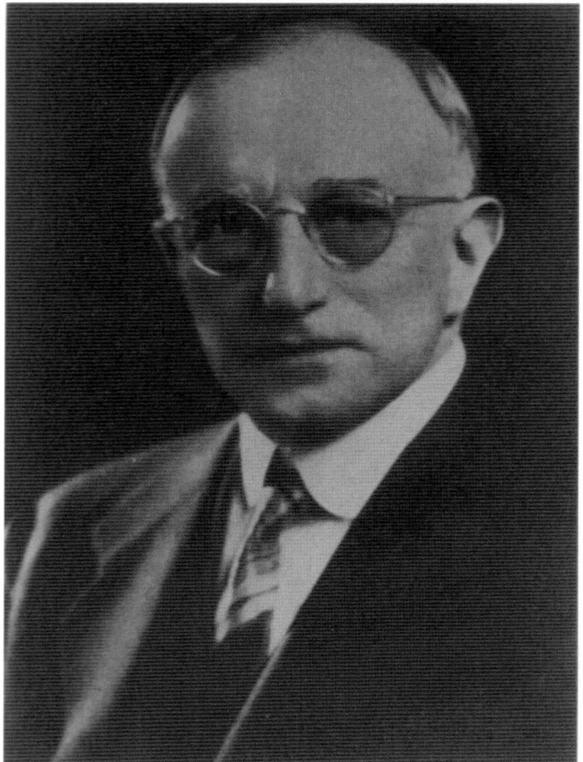

FIGURE 1-7. Charles A. Elsberg.

In his textbook, Elsberg outlined the surgical indications and contraindications for laminectomy. He noted the beneficial effects in his own large series of laminectomies and puzzled over the benefits that may occur in the absence of evident increased intradural pressure, such as in patients with multiple sclerosis. He argued that the primary indications for operation were cases of tumor, trauma, and infection that were associated with symptoms localized to a spinal level. Patients with progressive symptoms should be operated on quickly, in the absence of contraindications such as metastatic cancer or advanced Pott's disease.

Given the exhaustive scope of these early Elsberg publications—which, in addition to tumor, trauma, and infection, also review the management of congenital spine disease—conspicuously little is said about the most common late 20th-century indication for laminectomy: degenerative spine disease. The tardy development of a treatment for degenerative spine disease should be understood in the larger context of 19th and early 20th century knowledge of spinal pathology.

Unlike degenerative disease, tumor, trauma, and infection were already well-known in antiquity. Although the concept of localization of function in the nervous system was undeveloped during the 19th century, the diagnosis and localization of tumor, trauma, and infection, particularly in their late stages, was not especially difficult. Degenerative disease, on the other hand, possessed a more subtle pathophysiology that was not as easily characterized, especially without the help of radiography. Thus, recognition of degenerative spine disease eluded the 19th-century surgeon. This tardy appreciation for the clinical, surgical, and pathologic importance of degenerative spine disease deserves further mention.

Laminectomy for Intervertebral Disc Herniation

Intervertebral disc pathology was first described by Rudolph Virchow[47] in 1857 (Fig. 1-8). Virchow's description of a fractured disc was made at autopsy on a patient who had suffered a traumatic injury.

In 1896, the Swiss surgeon T. Kocher[48,49] identified and described a traumatic disc rupture at autopsy of a patient who had fallen 100 feet and landed on her feet. Although Kocher recognized that the L1-2 disc was displaced dorsally, no clinical correlation was suggested.

The first transdural intervertebral discectomy was reported by Oppenheim and Krause[50] in 1908. However, they reported the disc as "enchondroma."

In 1911, George Middleton,[51] a practicing physician, and John Teacher, a Glasgow University pathologist, described two cases of ruptured intervertebral disc observed at autopsy. Like Virchow and Kocher before them, however, Middleton and Teacher, although they described the pathology, failed to postulate its connection with radiculopathy or back pain.

In 1911, Joel Goldthwaite[52] made this connection. In an article on the lumbosacral articulation, Goldthwaite described and illustrated how weakening of the annulus fibrosus could result in dorsal displacement of the nucleus pulposus. The nucleus pulposus, he argued, could in turn result in low back pain and paraparesis. What eluded Goldthwaite and the surgeons before him, however, was the connection between a herniated disc and radiculopathy.

In a 1929 issue of the *Archives of Surgery*, Walter E. Dandy[53] published a description of two cases of herniated lumbar discs causing a cauda equina syndrome (Fig. 1-9). Dandy correctly described how "loose cartilage from the intervertebral disc" produced the symptoms of cauda equina compression that were relieved alter surgical decompression. He considered that in the second decade of the 20th century, more than 20 years after the first spinal fusion operations, intervertebral disc disease could be added to the list of indications for decompressive laminectomy.

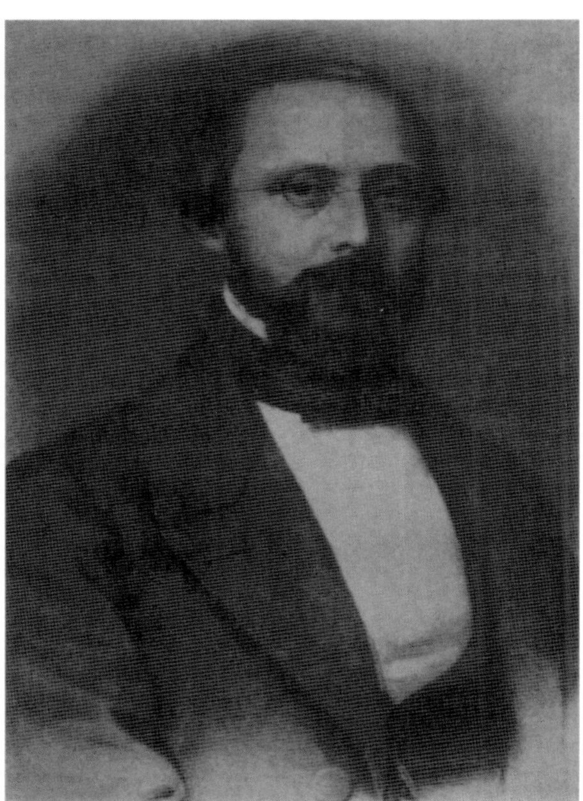

FIGURE 1-8. Rudolph Virchow.

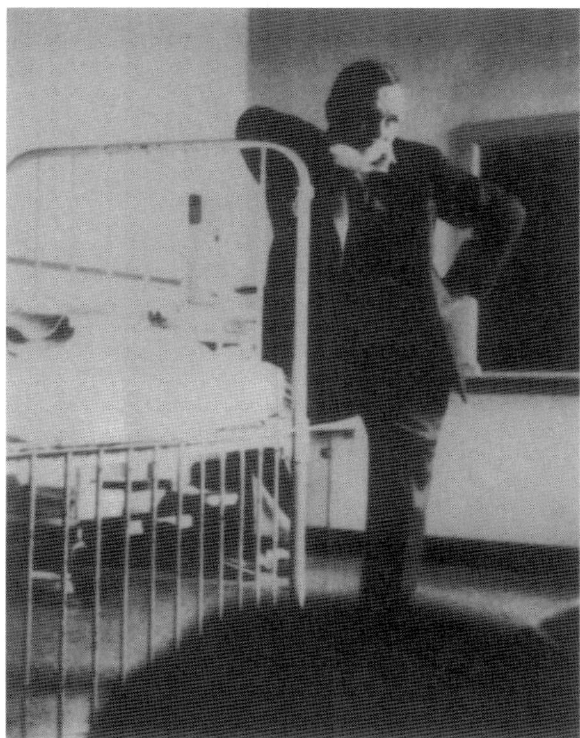

FIGURE 1-9. Walter E. Dandy.

Despite the several aforementioned publications on intervertebral disc herniation, the concept of disc herniation and its relationship to radiculopathy was defined by Mixter and Barr.

Several studies were performed in North America, but an anatomic, radiologic, and microscopic study was performed on 5000 human spines in the Dresden Pathology Institute by *Schmorl* and *Junghanns*. The results of this study were published in a book entitled *The Human Spine in Health and Disease*. In 1932, Barr, an orthopedic surgeon from Massachusetts General Hospital, was assigned to write a critique of this study.

In June of 1932, Barr attempted to treat a patient with an extruded disc herniation. Following a 2-week unsuccessful course of nonoperational treatment, Barr consulted with Mixter. Mixter recommended a myelogram. The myelogram revealed a filling defect. Mixter subsequently operated on the patient and removed the "tumor." Barr studied the "tumor" specimens. Because he contributed to Schmorl's study published in German, Barr remembered the microscopic appearances in Schmorl's study and realized that the specimen from this index patient was the nucleus pulposus. After this finding, Mixter, Barr, and Mallory (pathologist) reevaluated all the cases that were diagnosed (or misdiagnosed) as chondroma in recent years at Massachusetts General Hospital. They retrospectively diagnosed most of these cases as ruptured intervertebral discs. Mixter and Wilson operated on the first ruptured disc herniation diagnosed preoperatively on December 31, 1932.

Mixter and Barr reported the case in *New England Surgical Society* in September 30, 1933.[8,54,55]

In the late 1930s Love[56] from the Mayo Clinic reported on an extradural laminectomy technique. In 1967, Yasargil[57] used the microscope for discectomy. The first results of the lumbar microdiscectomy were reported by Yasargil[57] and Caspar.[58]

Laminectomy for Cervical Disc Herniation

In 1905 Watson and Paul[59] performed a negative exploration for cervical spinal cord tumor. They found an anterior extradural mass in the intervertebral disc at autopsy. This may be the first reported case of cervical disc herniation. The first dorsal approach was performed by Elsberg[60] in 1925. He found a "chondroma" in a quadriparetic patient.

Laminectomy for Spinal Stenosis

Unlike the herniated intervertebral disc, the stenotic spinal canal was described comparatively early in the 19th century. Portal,[61] in 1803, observed that a small spinal canal may be causally related to spinal cord compression, leading to paraplegia. No clinical reports of this entity were published, however, until 1893 when William A. Lane[62] described the case of a woman aged 35 years with a progressive paraplegia and a degenerative spondylolisthesis. The patient improved after a decompressive laminectomy.

Further demonstration of the efficacy of decompressive laminectomy for spinal stenosis came from Sachs and Frankel[63] in 1900. They published an account of a man aged 48 years with neurogenic claudication and spinal stenosis whose symptoms improved after a two-level laminectomy. Recognition of the degenerative nature of the clinical entity of spinal stenosis was established by Bailey and Casamajor[64,65] in 1911 in a report on a patient who was successfully decompressed by Charles Elsberg. In his 1916 textbook, Elsberg[46] later wrote, "a spinal operation may finally be required in some cases of arthritis or spondylitis on account of compression of the nerve roots or the cord by new-formed bone. . . ."

In 1945, Dr. Sarpyener, a Turkish orthopedic surgeon, described congenital lumbar spinal stenosis.[66] This report was followed by a report on adult spinal stenosis from Dr. Verbiest.[67] In 1973 Hattori[68] described the technique of laminoplasty.

Approaches to the Spine

Dorsolateral Approaches to the Spine

In 1779, Percival Pott described a condition involving spinal kyphosis and progressive paraplegia in a now-classic monograph titled "*Remarks on that kind of palsy of the lower limbs which is frequently found to accompany a curvature of the spine and is supposed to be caused by it; together with its method of cure; etc.*" (Fig. 1-10). For the management of this condition, which now bears his name, Pott recommended the use of a paraspinal incision to drain pus from the invariably present paraspinal abscess. For almost a century, this simple surgical procedure became a standard part of the treatment of Pott's paraplegia.

By the late 19th century, however, the laminectomy had received widespread acceptance as a safe and effective method of spinal decompression.[69] This was in part related to the decrease in surgical mortality associated with the adoption of the Listerian methods beginning in the 1870s, and it was only natural then that the laminectomy would play a role in the management of Pott's disease. As in many of its applications, however, disenchantment arose with the results of laminectomy, and alternative approaches were therefore sought.[70] The most promising of these approaches was the so-called "costotransversectomy" of Ménard.

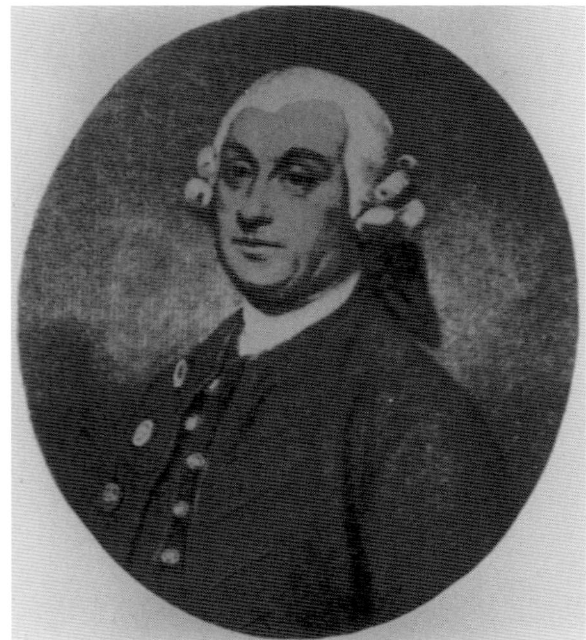

FIGURE 1-10. Percival Pott.

Ménard's Costotransversectomy

Like many surgeons at the beginning of the 20th century, Ménard[71] was disappointed by the surgical results from the laminectomy. In 1894, he described the costotransversectomy as an alternative method for achieving the goal of Pott, namely, drainage of the paraspinal abscess. The advantage of the costotransversectomy over the laminectomy lay in the improved exposure it provided of the lateral aspect of the vertebral column. The procedure was also known as the "drainage latéral," emphasizing that the goal of the procedure was to drain the lateral, paravertebral tubercular abscess.

As described by Ménard, the costotransversectomy involved an incision overlying the rib that was located at the apex of the kyphos. The rib was then skeletonized and divided about 4 cm distal to the articulation with its corresponding vertebra, from which it was disarticulated and removed. These maneuvers provided access to the tuberculous focus, which was exposed and then decompressed directly (Fig. 1-11). Ménard did not intend to totally remove the lesion, but rather to simply decompress the abscess.

The surgical results of Ménard's costotransversectomy far surpassed the results obtained with the laminectomy. Ménard experienced several successes among his first few 23 cases, including significant motor improvement.[72] Regrettably, these promising initial surgical results began to sour with time, as it became increasingly clear that two major complications were occurring with increasing frequency: postoperative development of secondary infection and the postoperative

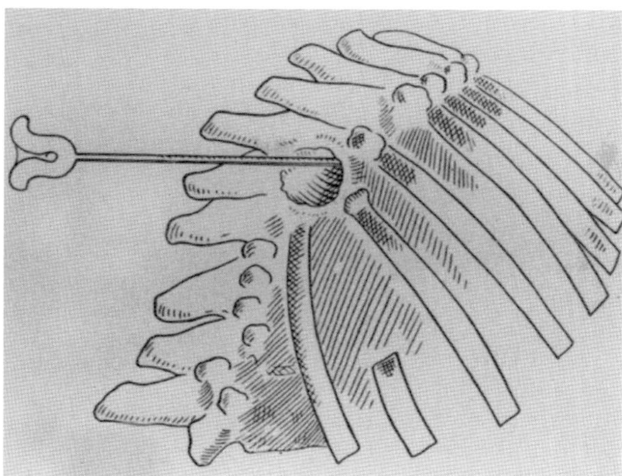

FIGURE 1-11. Drainage of a tubercular abscess via the costotransversectomy of Ménard. (From Ménard V: Causes de la paraplegia dans le mal de Pott. Son traitement chirurgical par l'ouverture direct du foyer tuberculeux des vertebras. *Rev Orthop* 5:47–64, 1894.)

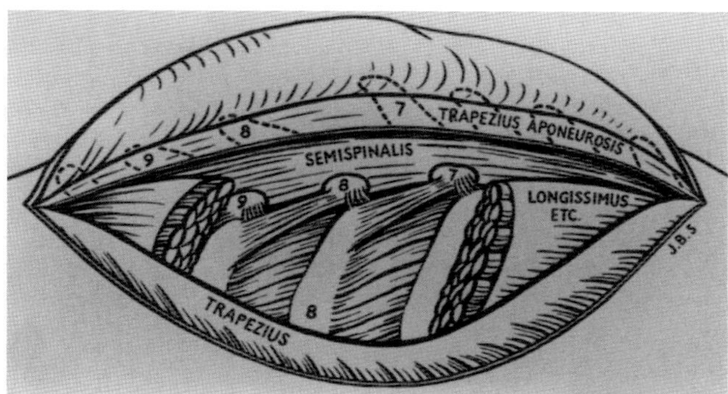

FIGURE 1-12. Dorsolateral exposure via Capener's lateral rhachotomy. Note that the exposure requires a transverse division of the paraspinal muscles. (From Capener N: The evolution of lateral rhachotomy. *J Bone Joint Surg [Br]* 36:173–179, 1954.)

formation of draining sinus tracts. Both problems resulted from the opening up of the abscess. Because no antitubercular chemotherapeutic agents were available at the time, the consequences of the infections that ensued after surgery were frequently disastrous, resulting in significant surgical mortality. As Calot[73] grimly put it in 1930, "The surgeon who, so far as tuberculosis is concerned, swears to remove the evil from the very root, will only find one result waiting him: the death of his patient." The operation of Ménard thus fell into disrepute, and in time even Ménard abandoned it.

Capener's Lateral Rhachotomy

Like Ménard, the English surgeon Norman Capener attempted to find a surgical solution to the problem of Pott's paraplegia. Capener modified Ménard's costotransversectomy in a procedure that he developed and began using in 1933, which was first reported by H. J. Seddon[74] in 1935. Departing from the emphasis of Pott and Ménard, who simply decompressed the tubercular abscess, Capener attempted to directly remove the lesion, which typically consisted of a ventral mass of hardened material. To achieve his more radical goal of spinal decompression, Capener required a more lateral or ventral view of the vertebrae than was afforded by Ménard's approach.

Capener's solution was to adopt Ménard's costotransversectomy but with this difference: whereas Ménard approached the spine via a trajectory that was medial to the erector spinae muscles, Capener[75] transversely divided the muscles and retracted them rostrally and caudally (Fig. 1-12). He named his new approach the *lateral rhachotomy* to distinguish it from Ménard's *costotransversectomy*. The simple change in dissection planes distinguishes these two techniques by producing a significantly different trajectory and surgical exposure. Although the operation was designed for the surgical treatment of Pott's paraplegia, Capener later drew attention to the versatility of the approach and its appropriateness for a variety of pathologic processes, including "the exploration of spinal tumors, the relief of certain types of traumatic paraplegia, and the drainage of suppurative osteitis of the vertebral bodies."[75]

It was perhaps unfortunate that for 19 years the only description of Capener's lateral rhachotomy was in a single case report published by another surgeon.[74] Not until 1954 did Capener himself describe the procedure, and even then he still chose not to publish the results of his 23 cases.[75]

In the interval between Seddon's 1935 description of the lateral rhachotomy and Capener's 1954 report of the same operation, the emergence of a new treatment, antitubercular chemotherapy, was to transform the history of the treatment of Pott's paraplegia. In 1947, streptomycin first became available for clinical use. This was followed by the introduction of *para*-aminosalicylic acid (PAS) in 1949 and isoniazid (INH) in 1952. The effect of the introduction of these new chemotherapeutic agents on the treatment of tuberculosis was spectacular. With the addition of streptomycin alone, the average relapse rate of tuberculosis was decreased by 30% to 35%. Although the effect of antitubercular chemotherapy was not as substantial for the treatment of spinal tuberculosis as for the pulmonary form, its mere availability raised new questions about the optimal management of Pott's paraplegia and, in particular, about the indications for surgical intervention.

Larson's Lateral Extracavitary Approach

In 1976, Sanford J. Larson et al.[76] at the Medical College of Wisconsin published an influential article that helped to popularize Capener's lateral rhachotomy, which they modified and renamed the *lateral extracavitary approach* (Fig. 1-13). This approach has been used more for trauma and tumor than for tuberculosis. The technical difference that distinguishes the lateral rhachotomy from the lateral extracavitary approach lies primarily in the treatment of the paraspinous muscles.

Whereas the procedure of Capener involves transversely dividing these muscles and reflecting them rostrally and caudally, Larson's procedure uses a surgical exposure with a trajectory ventral to the paraspinous muscles, which are then reflected medially to expose the ventrolateral aspect of the spine. Later in the procedure these muscles are redirected laterally to provide access for instrumentation of the dorsal aspect of the spine using the same surgical exposure as that for the ventrolateral approach. Although neurosurgeons, as spine surgeons, had traditionally emphasized spinal decompression over spinal stabilization, an essential aspect of the significance of Larson's overall contribution to the discipline

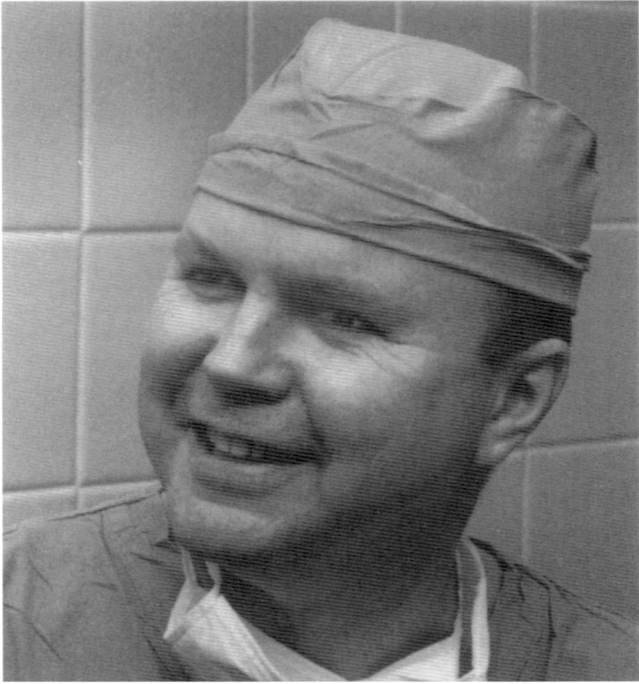

FIGURE 1-13. Sanford J. Larson.

of spinal surgery lies in the fact that, as a neurosurgeon, he dedicated his career to the advancement of reconstructive spinal surgery.

Spinal Stabilization and Deformity Correction

The history of surgical stabilization and deformity correction must include a description of the birth and evolution of spinal fusion and spinal instrumentation. Special emphasis must be given to the role of spinal biomechanics and its influence on the development of internal fixation. Many factors hindered the development of surgical approaches to the decompression, stabilization, and deformity correction of the ventral spine. The development and mastery of the special techniques that were required to safely manage ventral spinal pathologies did not appear until after the beginning of the 20th century, in part because they depended on advances in anesthetic techniques and a more sophisticated approach to perioperative management.

Except for degenerative disease, the technique and indications for the decompressive laminectomy were well established by the turn of the 20th century. The idea of spinal decompression, previously the exclusive province of surgical pioneers, had demonstrated its clinical utility with results that fully justified its acceptance into standard surgical practice. However, the idea of decompression, which had dominated spinal surgery during the 19th century, did not exist alone. Indeed, before the dawn of the 20th century, attention had already turned to another surgical idea: spinal stabilization. Of course, many attempts at surgical stabilization of the unstable spine had been made during the 19th century and before. However, the ancient admonition that vertebral fractures constituted an "ailment not to be treated" was reinforced by the surgeon's singular lack of success. And, thus, despite early attempts at spinal stabilization in the latter part of the 19th century, spinal decompression remained the primary indication for surgery of the spine, until World War II.

Recognition of the idea that compression of the neural elements, in cases of tumor, trauma, and infection, could be responsible for neurologic compromise was the crucial first step needed to develop the idea that spinal decompression could improve neurologic outcome. The invention of a technical means to achieve decompression, namely by laminectomy, represented the next necessary step in bringing this concept into clinical practice. Similarly, the idea of spinal stabilization arose from the observation that the unstable spine was at risk for the development of progressive deformity and that surgical intervention might prevent such deformities. Of course, bringing this concept into practice depended on achieving an adequate technical means. And, indeed, two technical advances were developed around the beginning of the 20th century that provided a means for spinal stabilization that would revolutionize the practice of modern spinal surgery.[77]

Birth and Development of Spinal Fusion and Spinal Instrumentation

Both spinal fusion and spinal instrumentation were born around the turn of the 20th century as methods of stabilizing the unstable spine. For many years, these two technical advances were developed and applied essentially independently, with results that were often complicated by pseudarthrosis. Early attempts at spinal instrumentation in particular failed to gain popularity because of their inability to maintain more than immediate spinal alignment. Spinal fusions were often used to achieve stabilization, but these also frequently suffered a similar fate: pseudarthrosis.[78]

By the 1960s, however, a half century of experience with spinal fusion and instrumentation suggested the concept of the "race between bony fusion and instrumentation failure." The improved surgical results that arose from the application of this important surgical concept provided support for the successful strategy of combining spinal instrumentation with meticulous fusion.

Spinal Fusion

The idea of using spinal fusion for stabilization is attributed to Albee[79] and Hibbs,[80] who, in 1911, independently reported its use (Fig. 1-14). Although these early operations were performed to prevent progressive spinal deformation in patients with Pott's disease, the procedure was later adopted in the management of scoliosis and traumatic fracture. The method of Hibbs, which was most frequently used, comprised harvesting an autologous bone graft from the laminae and overlaying the bone dorsally. Despite later improvements in this technique, however, such as the use of autologous iliac crest graft, the rate of pseudarthrosis, particularly in scoliosis, remained unacceptably high.[81]

In the 1920s Campbell[82] described trisacral fusion and iliac crest grafting. In 1922, Kleinberg[83] used xenograft for

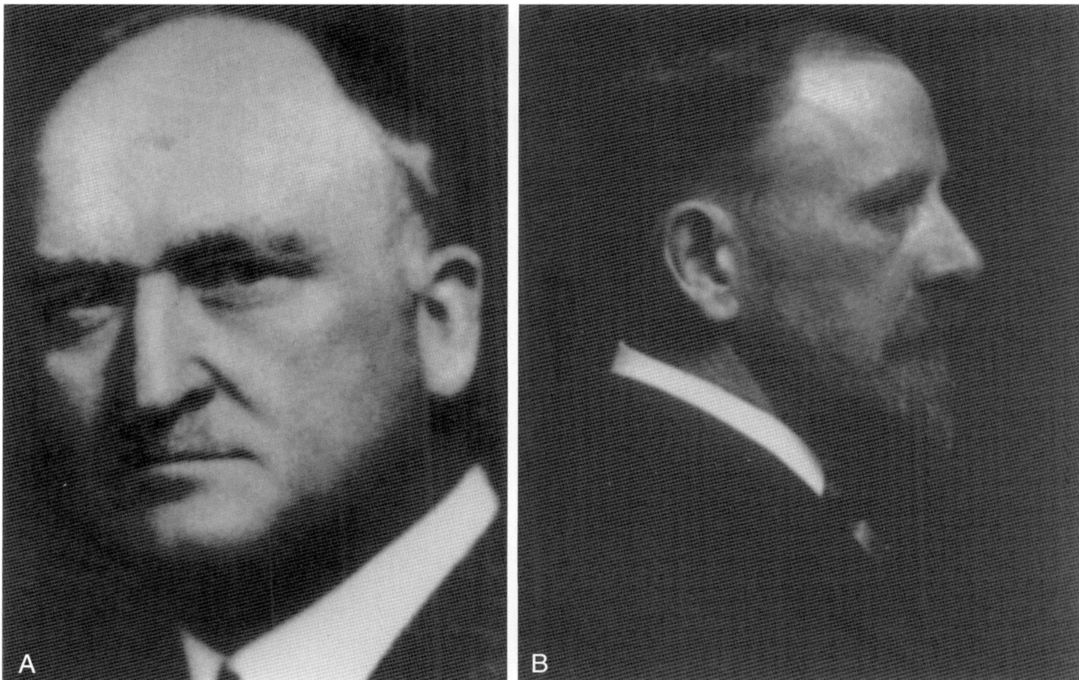

FIGURE 1-14. **A,** Fred Albee. **B,** Russell Hibbs.

spinal fusion. Anterior lumbar interbody fusion (ALIF) was described by Burns[84] in 1933, and posterior lumbar interbody fusion (PLIF) was performed by Cloward[85] in 1940. In the late 1990s transforaminal lumbar interbody fusion (TLIF) was described. In 1959 Boucher described a different spine fusion method.[86] In 1977 Callahan et al.[87] used bone for lateral cervical facet fusion.

Several ventral cervical fusion techniques were described in the 1950s. Robinson and Smith[88] described their technique in 1955, and Cloward[89] described his cervical fusion technique in 1958.

Spinal Instrumentation and Clinical Biomechanics

Like spinal fusion, internal fixation was first applied around 1900. These early constructs used tension-band fixators that were applied dorsally, primarily in cases of trauma. The limitation of the constructs, however, soon became apparent because the metals they contained were subject to the corrosive effects of electrolysis.

With the introduction of vitallium by Venable and Stuck[90] in the 1930s, a metal was found that was previously used successfully as a dental filling material and that had proven resistant to electrolysis (Fig. 1-15).[91] Further attempts at internal fixation during the 1930s and 1940s included fixed-moment arm cantilever constructs. These also failed to maintain alignment.[42,92,93]

F. W. Holdsworth

In the 1950s, the British orthopedic surgeon Sir Frank W. Holdsworth[94] performed perhaps the first large systematic study of the problem of internal fixation for the treatment of posttraumatic fracture. Although the constructs he used, which employed cantilever beams attached to the spinous processes, were traditional, Holdsworth's emphasis on patient selection brought the process of surgical spinal stabilization to a new, more sophisticated, level. His rationale for patient selection was based on a biomechanical definition of instability that he had derived from a study of a large number of spinal-injured patients.

In 1963, Holdsworth[95] published his results and proposed a classification scheme of subaxial spinal fractures based on a two-column model of spinal stability. Four categories of fractures were identified on the basis of the mechanism of injury and on the presence or absence of spinal stability. The latter determination rested significantly on the integrity of

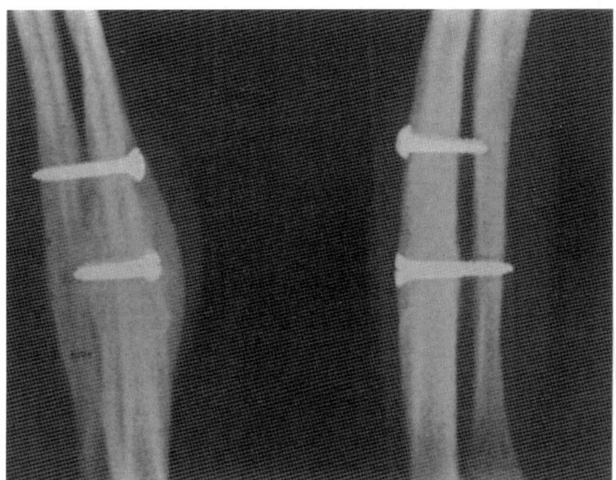

FIGURE 1-15. Radiograph showing no bone changes in dog limb around vitallium screws *(right)*, but erosion of bone around steel screws *(left)*. (From Venable CS, Stack WG, Beach A: The effects on bone of metals; based upon electrolysis. *Ann Surg* 105:917–938, 1937.)

the dorsal ligaments. Holdsworth categorized the fractures as follows:

1. Pure flexion: A pure flexion mechanism is usually associated with an intact dorsal ligamentous complex and no evidence of spinal instability. The vertebral body absorbs the greater part of the impact, and the result is a wedge compression fracture (Fig. 1-16A).
2. Flexion-rotation: A rotation or flexion-rotation mechanism causes disruption of the dorsal ligamentous complex and results in an unstable fracture-dislocation. It is usually associated with paraplegia (Fig. 1-16B).
3. Extension: An extension mechanism, which is usually stable, most frequently occurs in the cervical spine. It may be associated with a fracture of the dorsal elements, with an intact dorsal ligamentous complex (Fig. 1-16C).
4. Compression: A compression, or "burst," fracture is caused by forces transmitted directly along the line of the vertebral bodies. All of the ligaments are usually intact, and the fracture tends to be stable (Fig. 1-16D).

Holdsworth's classification was important, as he himself observed, not as a biomechanical theory (although it was this too), but because it had implications for treatment. At around the same time that Holdsworth's article appeared, several other classifications of spinal fractures were proposed. With the introduction of modern spinal biomechanics, a new era in spinal surgery had begun.[96,97]

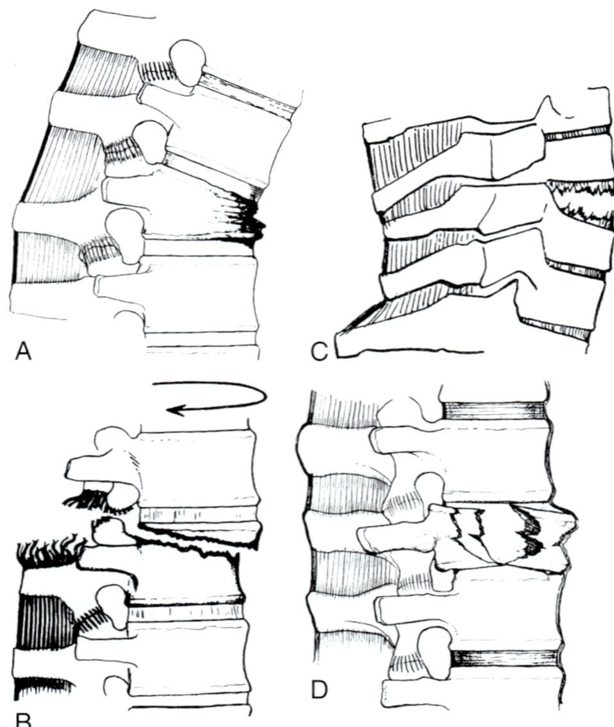

FIGURE 1-16. A, Wedge compression fracture of the vertebral body. Pure flexion mechanism. Note that the posterior ligamentous complex is intact. **B,** Rotational fracture-dislocation of the lumbar spine. The posterior ligamentous complex is disrupted. This is a very unstable injury. **C,** Extension injury. The anterior longitudinal ligament is ruptured. The posterior ligamentous complex is intact. **D,** Burst fracture. All ligaments are intact. (From Holdsworth FW: Fractures, dislocations, and fracture-dislocation of the spine. *J Bone Joint Surg [Br]* 45:6–20, 1963.)

Paul Harrington and the Birth of Modern Surgical Stabilization

In his 1891 report of a case of interspinous wiring for cervical fracture, Berthold Hadra[98] considered in what circumstances his newly described procedure would be indicated (Fig. 1-17). Hadra concluded that his procedure might be indicated for "any deviation of a vertebra."[98] Despite the prescience of his innovation, the substance of Hadra's comment is remarkable, not so much for what it contains, as for what is missing from it; namely, any hint of consideration of biomechanical principles. When one considers the importance of biomechanical principles in Holdsworth's 1963 classification of spinal fractures, Hadra's early 20th-century approach to spinal stabilization serves to underline how much progress was made in the interval. The significance of this new (biomechanical) approach to spinal stabilization, which was heralded by Holdsworth, was brought home in the 1960s with the work of the father of modern spinal stabilization, Paul Harrington (Fig. 1-18).

In 1945, after military service in World War II, Paul Harrington[99] entered into orthopedic practice in Houston, Texas. Within 2 years, Harrington was faced with the orthopedic problems of a large population of poliomyelitis patients, which at that time had reached epidemic proportions. The involvement of the trunk, which afflicted many of these patients, often resulted in scoliotic spinal deformity in association with cardiopulmonary compromise. The presence of cardiopulmonary compromise in a patient with scoliosis often meant that the standard cast corrective measures could not be applied safely. Furthermore, in 1941, the American Orthopaedic Association[100] published a report on the results of treatment in 425 cases of idiopathic scoliosis. The report

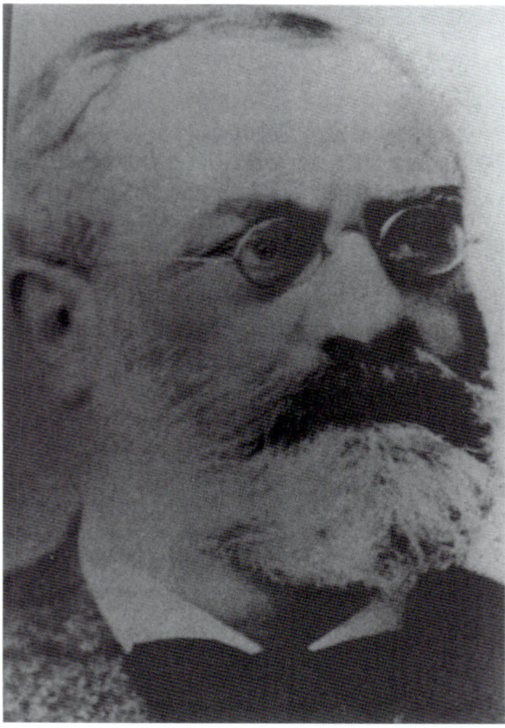

FIGURE 1-17. Berthold Hadra.

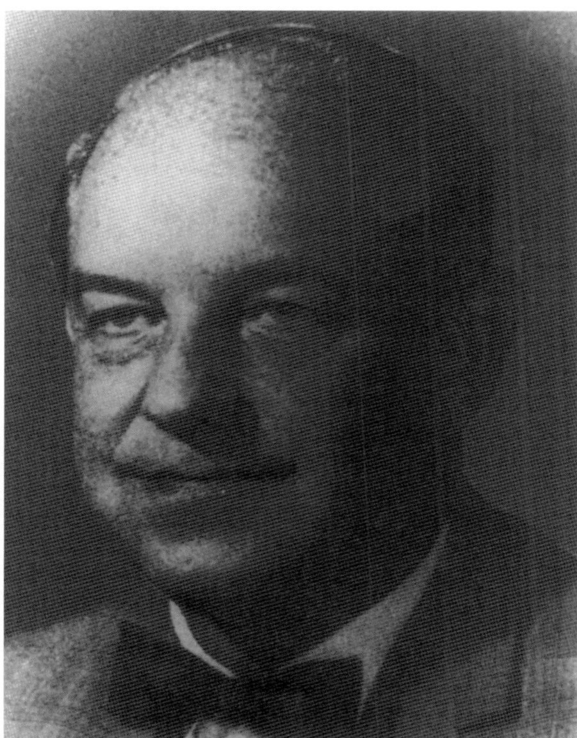

FIGURE 1-18. Paul Harrington.

was quite discouraging. Among those patients treated by exercises and braces, but without spinal fusion, 60% progressed in their deformity and 40% remained unchanged. In another group of patients who underwent surgical correction and fusion, 25% (54 of 214) developed pseudarthrosis and 29% had lost all correction. Among the entire group, the end result for 69% was considered fair or poor, and only 31% were rated good to excellent. It was against this backdrop of dismal results from nonoperative treatment and dorsal spinal fusion that Harrington began his seminal work.

After an initial (unsuccessful) trial of internal fixation with facet screw instrumentation,[101] the method was abandoned in favor of a combination of compression and distraction hooks and rods made of stainless steel. The advantages of these instruments in the establishment of deformity correction became obvious: for the first time in the history of spinal stabilization, spinal instruments provided compression, distraction, and three-point bending forces, which proved equally useful in deformity correction as they did in the maintenance of posttraumatic stability. Nineteen patients were observed during the early phase of Harrington's investigation of dorsal instrumentation. The results of this investigation were published in 1962.[99] The longevity of Harrington's spinal instrumentation system, which remains in use today, is a testimony to both its safety and its efficacy.

Nevertheless, despite a frequent and gratifying correction of the poliomyelitis curvature, the loss of that correction was commonly discovered within 6 to 12 months after surgery. In part, the failure to maintain the alignment achieved at surgery was the result of frequent instrument failure, most commonly instrument fracture and disengagement of the hooks. However, more fundamentally, Harrington recognized that the concept of a dynamic correction system was inherently flawed: the complication of instrument failure would be far less significant if a spinal fusion could maintain the deformity correction achieved by the placement of the implant.[102]

The underlying principles that emerged from Harrington's early failures, then, became clear: (1) because spinal instruments fail over time, they should be applied as a strictly temporary measure; and (2) after instrumentation failure, a successful spinal fusion will maintain stabilization. As a corollary to these principles, Harrington acknowledged that there is a "race between instrumentation failure and the acquisition of spinal fusion." It stands to reason that if fusion is attained before instrumentation failure, the maintenance of deformity correction and stabilization will have been achieved. An understanding of the importance of a successful fusion in an instrumented spine is one of Harrington's most significant contributions to spinal surgery and marks the birth of the modern era of spinal stabilization and deformity correction.

Ventral Approaches to the Spine

Dorsal decompression via the laminectomy had become well established by the turn of the 20th century and was codified by Charles Elsberg in his 1916 textbook, *Diagnosis and Treatment of Surgical Diseases of the Spinal Cord and Its Membranes*. Interestingly, whereas this period marked the culmination of dorsal decompression in spinal surgery, it also signified the beginning of procedures for dorsal stabilization and deformity correction, as pioneered by Hadra (1891), Albee (1911), and Hibbs (1911). The groundwork for further development in this area was laid with the classification scheme of spinal fractures by mechanism and stability, as initially proposed by Holdsworth in 1963. This introduction into clinical practice of the principles of spinal biomechanics is also found in the work of Harrington in the 1950s and 1960s in his development of a novel system of dorsal thoracolumbar instrumentation. Although Harrington later recognized the need to supplement his instrumentation with meticulous spinal fusion, and many modifications and innovations have since been made in dorsal instrumentation, successful outcomes in dorsal decompression, stabilization, and deformity correction had been achieved by the 1960s.

Nothing, however, has been said so far about the achievement of these goals in the ventral spine, where a significant portion of spinal pathology is located. As it happens, the first successful interventions for stabilization of the ventral spine were achieved in the same time frame as the dorsal ones (i.e., in the first half of the 20th century). What is peculiar about surgery of the ventral spine is that a decompressive procedure must be accompanied almost invariably by simultaneous stabilization, which often includes measures taken to obtain deformity correction. Therefore, the history of the major goals of ventral spine surgery—that is, decompression, stabilization, and deformity correction—has been one of parallel developments, not serial ones, as was the case for the dorsal spine. In other words, the history of stabilization and deformity correction of the dorsal spine developed in the half century following the establishment of dorsal decompression. All three goals, in the ventral spine, were achieved during the same 50 years.

Ventral Decompression and Stabilization

The primary difficulty in applying ventral techniques to the spine was in the surgical approach. The relative technical ease and low morbidity associated with a dorsal approach to the dorsal spine provided ample opportunity for the early development of dorsal spinal techniques. By contrast, ventral approaches to the ventral spine required transgression of the abdomen or chest, which (similar to the head) up until the 1880s remained sanctuaries not to be opened, except by accident.[18]

In part, the late development of abdominal and thoracic surgery was a product of the problem of infection: cognizant of the morbidity and mortality related to hospital-acquired gangrene, few of those who entered a surgical ward in the 19th century did so with the hope of leaving alive. The reluctance to adopt the principles of antisepsis as first enunciated by Lister[103] in 1867 and a slowness to accept its theoretical foundation—the germ theory of disease—meant delays for the development of abdominal and thoracic surgery. However, even after the practice of antiseptic surgery became generally accepted, early 20th-century surgeons still approached abdominal surgery with trepidation.

Anyone who would contemplate surgically violating the thoracic cavity had to grapple with the technical problem of the pressure relationships in the chest.[104] Beginning in 1903, Ferdinand Sauerbruch of Breslau conducted a series of experiments that led to the development of an apparatus in which negative pressure for the open thorax could be maintained, and around 1910, endotracheal or insufflation anesthesia became available (Fig. 1-19). This alleviated one of the major technical difficulties confronted by would-be thoracic surgeons, but even then, good control of respiration by a reliable apparatus was not widely available until the late 1930s.

W. Müller

The first report of a successful attempt to approach the ventral thoracic or lumbar spine is attributed to Müller.[105] In 1906, Müller performed a transperitoneal approach to the lumbosacral spine in a patient with a suspected sarcoma.

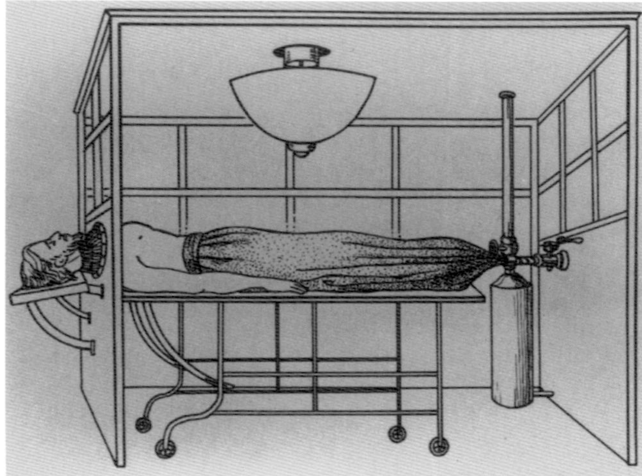

FIGURE 1-19. An early version of Sauerbruch's negative-pressure chamber.

At operation, Müller found tuberculosis. Alter curetting the infected bone, Müller applied iodoform powder and closed. The surgical result was excellent. Notwithstanding the success of this initial operation, however, later attempts at the same procedure failed miserably. After several misadventures that ended in disaster, Müller was forced to abandon further attempts at a ventral exposure.

B. H. Burns

Perhaps the next published report of a successful ventral exposure did not appear until 1933, when the British surgeon B. H. Burns[84] performed a ventral interbody fusion of the lumbosacral spine for an L5-S1 spondylolisthesis (Fig. 1-20). Before the Burns procedure, the only method available to stabilize an unstable spondylolisthesis was a dorsal fusion. However, the results of dorsal fusion for ventral instability, as Burns himself learned firsthand, proved unsound both in theory and in practice. Faced with a high incidence of failed dorsal fusions, Burns chose to take a transabdominal, transperitoneal approach to the lumbosacral spine, which he first investigated on three cadavers before operation. The first operation involved a 14-year-old boy who presented with low back pain and neurogenic claudication after jumping from a height. A radiograph of the lumbosacral spine showed an L5 spondylolysis and a grade II, L5-S1 spondylolisthesis. A tibial autograft was taken and was tamped into a hole drilled obliquely from L5 to S1. Convalescence was uneventful, and pain relief was achieved, even on ambulation at 2 months postoperatively.

Ito and Others

Like the landmark operations of Albee and Hibbs, the first reported series of ventral spinal operations comprised a group of surgical treatments for spinal tuberculosis. In their 1934 article, "A New Radical Operation for Pott's Disease," Ito et al.[106] observed that the surgical stabilization procedure described by Albee and Hibbs did not differ significantly from nonoperative immobilization; the goal in both instances was to rest and unload the diseased spine. Ito, on the other hand, a professor of orthopedic surgery from Kyoto, Japan, proposed a decompressive procedure, which he believed provided a definitive surgical treatment.

Of course, the obstacles that Ito confronted in devising a ventral approach to the spine were considerable. In addition to the obvious anatomic obstacles, all early 20th-century spine surgeons faced the seemingly intractable problem of infection. Although postoperative infections posed major difficulties for the development of (clean) abdominal and thoracic surgical procedures, these difficulties were compounded when the surgical indication *was* infection, as in the case of Pott's disease. Indeed, previous attempts to surgically decompress tuberculosis of the ventral spine via a lateral approach (i.e., a costotransversectomy) met with a high incidence of complications from postoperative secondary infection, permanent fistulas, or persistent spinal tuberculosis resulting from incomplete removal of infected bone.[49,71,107,108]

In part, these operations failed because they were performed prior to 1910, in the age of antiseptic, rather than aseptic, surgery. Perhaps they also failed in part because they predated the introduction of antimicrobial chemotherapy.

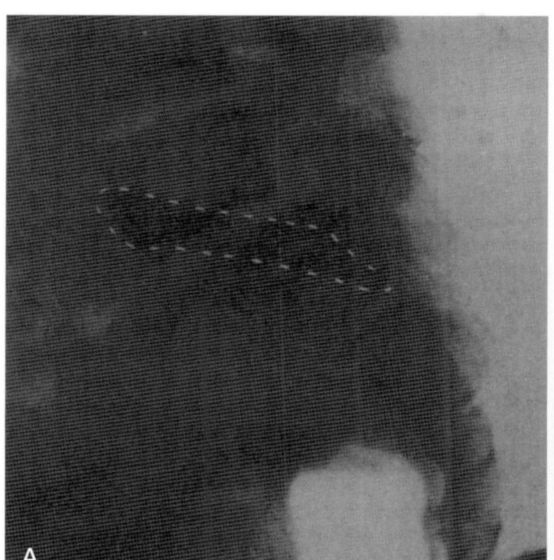

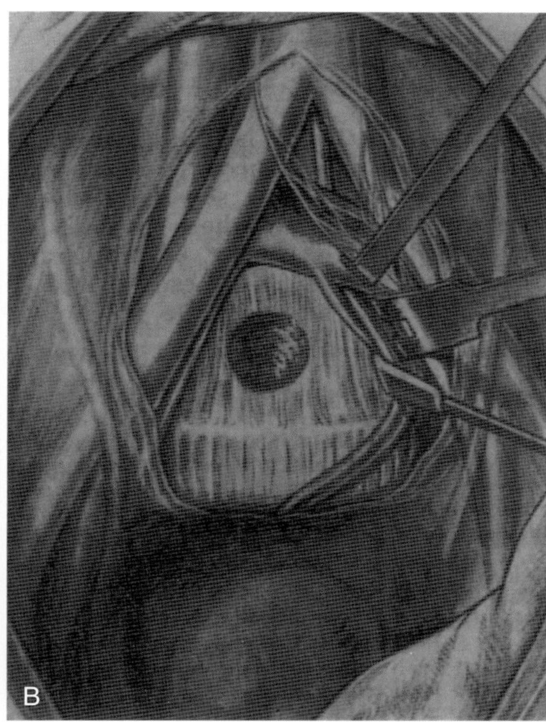

FIGURE 1-20. **A,** Lateral radiograph of lumbar spine showing the graft placement in B. H. Burns's operation for spondylolisthesis. **B,** Illustration of Burns's operation. Ventral view. (**A,** From Burns BH: An operation for spondylolisthesis. *Lancet* 1:1233, 1933, with permission.)

However, the unsatisfactory results that these operations yielded was also importantly attributed to the poor surgical exposure of the vertebral bodies that the lateral approach provided. Recognizing this, Ito proposed a decompression operation that would adequately resect infected vertebrae in order to fully eradicate the presence of tuberculosis in the spine. Drawing on experience with the transabdominal approach, which he had previously used for another purpose, Ito reported his operative technique and surgical results on 10 patients with moderately advanced Pott's disease. The possibility of approaching the ventral spine occurred to Ito et al. after repeated operations using their original technique for lumbosacral sympathetic ganglionectomy. In 1923, Ito and Asaini[109] originated this technique for the purpose of improving lower extremity circulation and reported their results to the Japanese Surgical Society in 1925. The technique was subsequently modified to provide an extraperitoneal approach to the lumbar spine and was adopted for their radical operation for Pott's disease (Fig. 1-21).

Ito et al.'s work was beneficial for several reasons. First, they recognized the need to address the pathology directly, despite the technical difficulties that such an approach presented. Second, at a time when the major surgical treatment for Pott's disease was dorsal fusion, Ito proposed a radical new surgical therapy: decompression. An attempt to eradicate spinal infection by surgical decompression represented an alternative approach to the standard stabilization procedure originated by Albee and Hibbs. In another sense, the idea of decompression harkened back to the 19th-century laminectomy for Pott's disease, which was largely abandoned because of disappointing results, after the introduction of dorsal spinal fusion.[110] Finally, Ito recognized the need, and established the technique, for stabilizing the spine, which, if not already unstable, was certainly rendered unstable by resection of the major load-bearing element. He accomplished this goal by fashioning a ventral interbody fusion, which both provided significant stability and facilitated spinal fusion (Fig. 1-22). However, despite Ito's successes—all except 2 of his

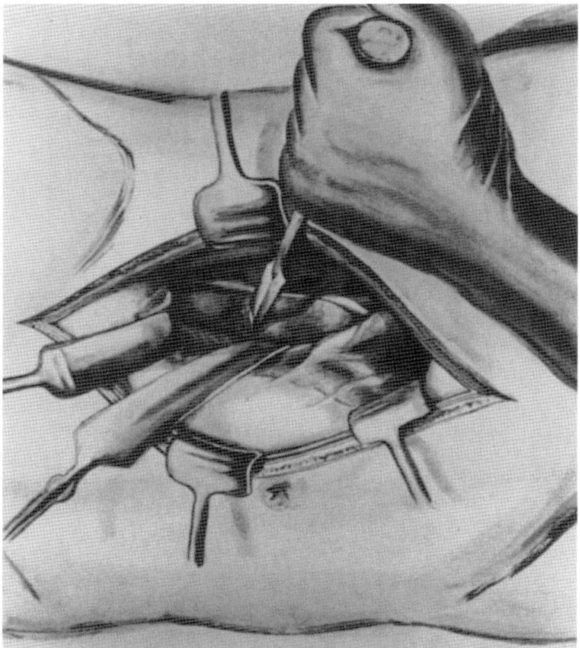

FIGURE 1-21. Extraperitoneal exposure of the body of the lumbar vertebra and resection of the body with a chisel. (From Ito H, Tsuchiya J, Asaini G: A new radical operation for Pott's disease. *J Bone Joint Surg* 16:499–515, 1934.)

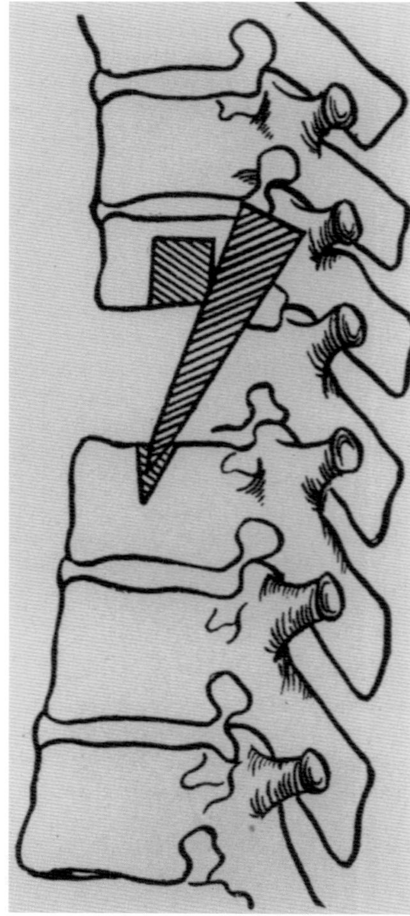

FIGURE 1-22. Schematic illustration of the insertion of ventral bone graft. (From Ito H, Tsuchiya J, Asaini G: A new radical operation for Pott's disease. *J Bone Joint Surg* 16:499–515, 1934.)

10 cases showed a healing by primary intention and despite his acknowledgment of the inadequacies of the dorsolateral approach—Ito himself used the costotransversectomy approach in the 2 cases of thoracic Pott's disease included in his series.

Hodgson and Stock

Thus, it fell to another group of surgeons treating Pott's disease to develop a true ventral approach to the thoracic spine. In 1956, Hodgson and Stock[111] published their first report on ventral spinal fusion for Pott's disease. These authors acknowledged the contributions of Ito et al., and they repeated Ito's assessment of the restricted field of view afforded by the costotransversectomy. They noted that this field of view provided insufficient exposure to determine the extent of the lesion or to confidently undertake its complete resection. What is more, the limited exposure of the costotransversectomy left no room to accurately insert a ventral bone graft, which they considered offered the best chance for fusion because the bone graft would be placed in a compression mode.

Hodgson and Stock also joined Ito et al. in emphasizing decompression, rather than simple stabilization, as a method to arrest further vertebral destruction (which may be responsible for neural element compression and progressive kyphotic deformity), and as a means to eradicate the spinal focus of disease. Their approach to the thoracic spine via a thoracotomy, the first significant series of such an approach described, was facilitated by developments in the medical management of tuberculosis, including the introduction of chemotherapeutic agents (not available to Ito et al.), and safer, more effective anesthetic techniques. The benefits of this approach, then, despite its technical difficulties, were incontrovertible; it facilitated decompression, stabilization, and deformity correction through a single incision and surgical exposure, providing excellent neurologic and anatomic results. The authors took account of the unique anatomic features of the cervicothoracic and thoracolumbar junctions, where the approach was appropriately modified.

Ventral Deformity Reduction and the Development of Ventral Instrumentation

The contributions of Burns, Ito and associates, and Hodgson and Stock were seminal in the history of spinal surgery. They opened new vistas in the management of spinal pathologies, and their techniques were later applied to an increasingly wide range of pathologic conditions, including tumor, trauma, disc disease, and spinal deformity. The methods of Ito and associates were particularly prescient. They accomplished, with a single incision, the goals of both decompression and spinal stabilization, and they achieved both of these goals in the most effective possible manner. The establishment of deformity correction was addressed in the report by Hodgson, who confronted the problem of severe kyphotic deformity causing cardiopulmonary compromise.

On a larger scale, however, the problem of progressive spinal deformity did not receive the attention of these early authors, and no method of ventral internal fixation was yet available to spinal surgeons who wished to establish and maintain a deformity correction via a ventral approach. As mentioned, Paul Harrington addressed the problem of scoliotic deformity by the development of dorsal thoracolumbar distraction rods in the 1960s, and in doing so he initiated the modern instrumentation revolution.

Harrington's method of scoliosis reduction was based on the principle of lengthening the short (concave) side of the curve. After the introduction of a meticulous fusion technique to supplement the immediate rigid internal fixation achieved by the implant, the Harrington instrumentation system proved both a safe and effective corrective measure, an assessment that is corroborated by its long and successful history of clinical application. Nevertheless, the principle of simple dorsal distraction had its drawbacks. First, the Harrington method requires that the fusion be extended at least two levels above and below the extent of the spinal curvature, thus decreasing mobility in otherwise normal spinal motion segments. Second, in most instances, the distribution of force application with the Harrington instrumentation system is uneven, such that the total force applied is borne only by the two vertebrae attached to the upper and lower hooks. Finally, for patients who require a simultaneous ventral decompression and dorsal stabilization procedure, this could be accomplished only through a two-stage operation involving two separate incisions and surgical exposures. Thus, the arrival of a ventral instrumentation system, introduced by Dwyer et al.[112] in 1969, proved an important addition to the spinal surgeon's surgical armamentarium.

A. F. Dwyer

A. F. Dwyer was an orthopedic surgeon from Australia who appears to have originated his method in an effort to provide an alternative to the Harrington technique for treating scoliotic deformity reduction. In his initial report of 1969, Dwyer described a method of ventral instrumentation in which compressive forces are applied to the convex side of the curve at each segmental level. The technique comprises excision of the discs at the motion segments involved and the insertion of vertebral body screws into the convex aspect of the curve. A titanium cable is then threaded through the heads of the inserted screws and tension is applied, providing corrective bending moments at the intervertebral spaces. The tension is maintained by swaging the threaded cable on the screw heads (Fig. 1-23).

In a follow-up article published in 1974, Dwyer and Schafer[113] reported their results of treatment in 51 cases, which demonstrated a generally favorable record of deformity correction and only a 4% rate of pseudarthrosis.[79] Furthermore, some of the disadvantages of the Harrington dorsal instrumentation system were overcome—fusion could be restricted to the motion segments of the curve only; the load borne by the instrumentation device was evenly distributed over the curve; and the exposure necessary for ventral decompression, stabilization, and deformity correction was achieved using a single incision. Although the initial enthusiasm for the Dwyer device was later diminished by the recognition that it encouraged the tendency of the spine toward progressive kyphosis and that it provided no resistance to axial loading, the generally successful application of this ventral instrumentation system stimulated the development of additional ventral implants, such as the instrumentation systems of Zielke and Pellin[114] and Kaneda and associates.[115]

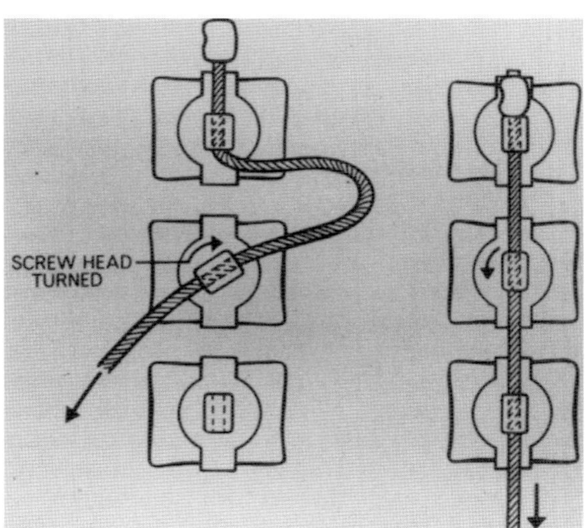

FIGURE 1-23. Dwyer's ventral short segment fixation device. (From Dwyer AF, Schafer MF: Anterior approach to scoliosis. Results of treatment in fifty-one cases. *J Bone Joint Surg [Br]* 56:218–224, 1974.).

Spine Imaging

The diagnosis of the spinal processes could be performed via different diagnostic methods, including plain file radiography, myelography, discography, computed tomography, and magnetic resonance imaging.

X-rays were discovered by Conrad Roentgen (1845–1923).[116] Roentgen, working in Würzburg University, invented the x-ray tube on 8 November 1895. This introduced a new era in the field of medicine. Radiographic imaging using x-rays is now a routine part of diagnostic techniques worldwide. Roentgen was awarded the first Nobel Prize in Physics for his discovery.

The invention of plain film radiography quickly changed diagnostic algorithms. Sicard and Forestier were injecting the radiopaque contrast medium Lipiodol into facet joints during the first World War.[117] In 1920, an incidental injection of contrast medium into the dural sac (instead of the facet joint) provided the first myelogram. In 1942, Steinhausen recommended the use of iodophenylundecylic acid (Pantopaque). Hence, Pantopaque myelography was used routinely for the diagnosis of spinal tumors and disc disorders for decades.[118] Since the 1970s, new contrast media such as Thorotrast, Conray, Dimeray, and Metrizamid have been used for myelography.

Discography has been used since its introduction by Lindblom.[119] It was widely used for both lumbar and cervical imaging throughout 1950s and 1960s. The invention of CT decreased its popularity. After the introduction of spine MRI, however, discography had a resurgence with an increased interest in the black disc, high-intensity zones, and discogenic pain.

In 1972, Oldendorf, Hounsfield, and Ambrose reported the successful use of CT for diagnosing spinal disorders.[120,121] With this invention, Hounsfield was awarded the Nobel Prize for Physiology or Medicine in 1979. Soon thereafter, Damadian invented the MRI scanner.[122]

Summary

The technical accomplishment of performing surgery on the ventral spine provides perhaps a useful marker for the endpoint of the history of "early modern" spinal surgery. By 1970, it may be argued, the basic groundwork had been laid for the subsequent advances, particularly in spinal instrumentation, that have been made over the last 25 years. These advances include an emphasis on location-appropriate decompression; the development of segmental spinal instrumentation by E. R. Luque in the early 1970s,[123-126] the refinement and proliferation of pedicular instrumentation techniques, first described by Harrington in 1969,[127,128] the introduction of universal spinal instrumentation by Cotrel and associates,[129] the further development of ventral thoracolumbar instrumentation by Zielke, Kostuik,[130] and Kaneda; the introduction of ventral cervical instrumentation by Caspar and associates in 1989;[131] and, most recently, the application of endoscopic techniques.[132]

In conclusion, this essay has sought to organize and present the history of spinal surgery as a series of attempts to improve the surgeon's ability to more safely and effectively achieve spinal decompression, stabilization, and deformity correction—the three major goals of spinal surgery. The occasionally formidable obstacles encountered by those surgeons who have participated in this century-long odyssey were frequently managed, if not overcome, by concentrated and indefatigable effort. Alas, many of the same obstacles that faced the early spinal surgeons—including blood loss, pseudarthrosis, instrumentation failure, and neurologic injury—continue to challenge and vex even the best-equipped contemporary spinal surgeons.

KEY REFERENCES

Gruber P, Boeni T: History of spinal disorders. In Boos N, Aebi M, editors: *Spinal disorders: fundamentals of diagnosis and treatment*, Berlin, 2008, Springer, pp 1–35.

Markham JW: Surgery of the spinal cord and vertebral column. In Walker AE, editor: *A history of neurological surgery*, New York, 1967, Hafner Publishing Company, pp 370–371.

Naderi S, Andalkar N, Benzel EC: History of spine biomechanics. Part I. The pre-Greco-Roman, Greco-Roman, and Medieval roots of spine biomechanics. *Neurosurgery* 60:382–391, 2007.

Naderi S, Andalkar N, Benzel EC: History of spine biomechanics. Part II. From the renaissance to the 20th century. *Neurosurgery* 60:392–404, 2007.

Wiltse LL: The history of spinal disorders. In Frymoyer JW, editor: *The adult spine: principles and practice*, Philadelphia, 1997, Lippincott-Raven, pp 3–40.

REFERENCES

The complete reference list is available online at expertconsult.com.

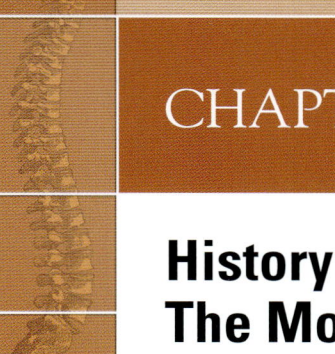

CHAPTER 2

History of Spinal Instrumentation: The Modern Era

Kushagra Verma | John K. Houten | Thomas J. Errico

The use of internal fixation as a tool for both stabilization and correction of deformity was a major advance in modern spinal surgery. A wide experience in the use of internal fixation in the treatment of the appendicular skeleton was extrapolated to the axial skeleton. This experience has culminated in the wide range of surgical implants currently available to the modern spinal surgeon. A thorough knowledge of the evolution of spinal instrumentation should yield a better understanding of both present and future developments.

Dorsal Thoracolumbar Instrumentation

In 1975, the Harrington rod represented the state of the art in spinal instrumentation. The rod system, originally developed by Paul Harrington for the correction of spinal deformities, was soon used in the treatment of traumatic injuries[1,2] (Fig. 2-1), degenerative disease,[3] and metastatic disease.[4,5] The system provided distraction rods as well as compression rods and hooks. Over the years, however, their widespread use led to recognition of their limitations. The use of a distraction system provided excellent correction of coronal plane deformities (scoliosis). Unfortunately, the use of distraction as the sole correction tool resulted in the loss of normal sagittal plane alignment. The loss of normal lumbar lordosis was associated with "flat back syndrome."[6,7] Hook dislodgement and rod breakage also proved to be troublesome complications.[8,9] In addition, casting or bracing was generally required in the postoperative period, which proved to be difficult or impractical in some patients.[10]

In response to the difficulties encountered with Harrington rods, Eduardo Luque advanced a major concept in the mid-1970s that quietly pushed forward the future direction of spinal instrumentation: segmental spinal fixation. The issue of bracing was of particular importance to Luque. Practicing in the warm climate of Mexico City, it was difficult for Luque, from a practical standpoint, to use the postoperative casting required in Harrington rod instrumentation. In addition, a large number of his patients, who were from homes of low socioeconomic status, would travel a great distance to seek treatment and would not comply with bracing or became lost to follow-up.

Luque popularized the use of a 3⁄16-inch steel rod secured at each spinal level with sublaminar wires (Fig. 2-2). Luque reasoned that increasing the number of fixation points along a construct would reduce the force placed upon each individual point and obviate the need for a postoperative cast or brace. Additional beneficial effects of segmental fixation were that it increased the potential corrective power of instrumentation, reduced the potential for construct failure, and resulted in improved fusion rates.

The concept of segmental fixation to a contoured rod was widely embraced because it produced greater construct rigidity and allowed for improved control of the sagittal plane. Sublaminar wires were adopted by some users of Harrington rod instrumentation. A hybrid form of Paul Harrington's technique (from Texas) and Eduardo Luque's technique (from Mexico) was sometimes referred to as the "Tex-Mex" operation.

Although the corrective power of sublaminar wires was well-appreciated, many surgeons had reservations in using them because of reports of neurologic injury resulting either from direct trauma or from epidural hematoma.[11,12] In addition, revision surgery to alter sublaminar wiring is problematic because scarring may preclude the passage of new wires at the same laminae. In response to these concerns, Drummond et al.[13] developed a method for segmental fixation using a button-wire implant passed through the base of the spinous process. This technique does not provide as strong fixation as do sublaminar wires. It avoids, however, passing anything into the spinal canal and thus reduces the risk of direct neurologic injury. This compromise of fixation for less risk of neurologic injury was seen as a prudent choice by many surgeons operating on healthy, neurologically normal adolescents with idiopathic scoliosis. Nevertheless, some pundits referred to the procedure as the "chicken-Luque" procedure.

Increasingly sophisticated multiple hook-rod systems appeared in the 1980s that provided much of the strength of wire fixation but with greater flexibility to address deformities in both the sagittal and the coronal dimensions. The Cotrel Dubousset (CD) system was introduced into the United States in 1986 using a ¼-inch rough-surfaced rod.[14] Multiple hooks allowed spinal surgeons to apply compression and distraction over different areas within the same rod. The multiple-hook design applied the principles of segmental fixation without the need for sublaminar wires. Significantly, the system provided for a unique mechanism for deformity correction: rod rotation. This proved a powerful force in the correction of

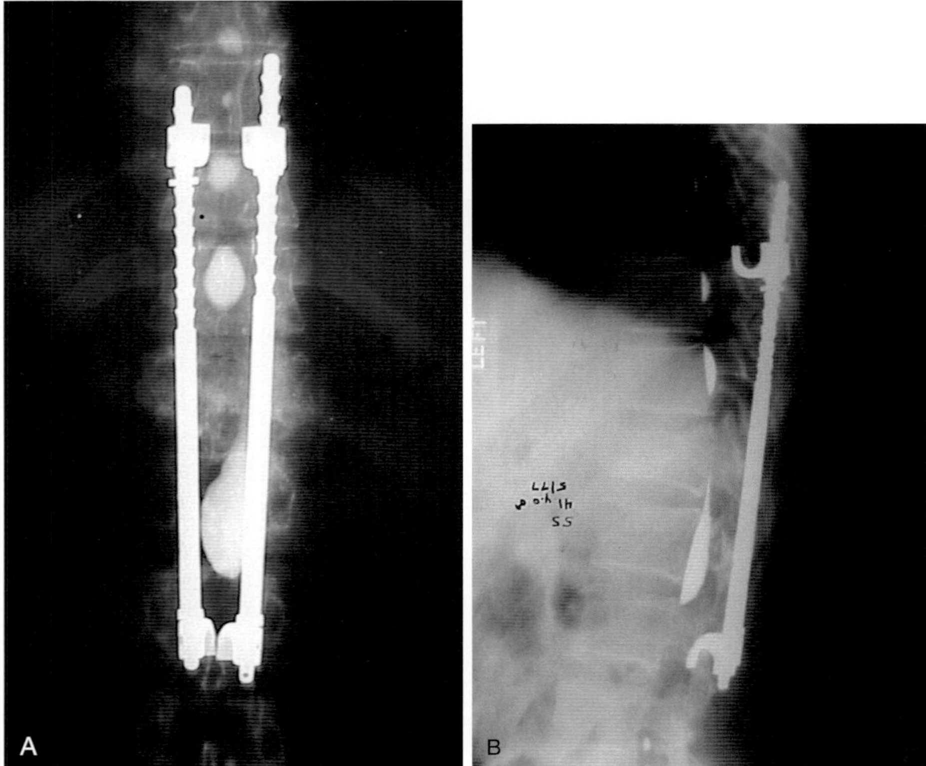

FIGURE 2-1. Anteroposterior (**A**) and lateral (**B**) radiographs after surgical stabilization of a burst fracture of L3 with Harrington rod internal fixation.

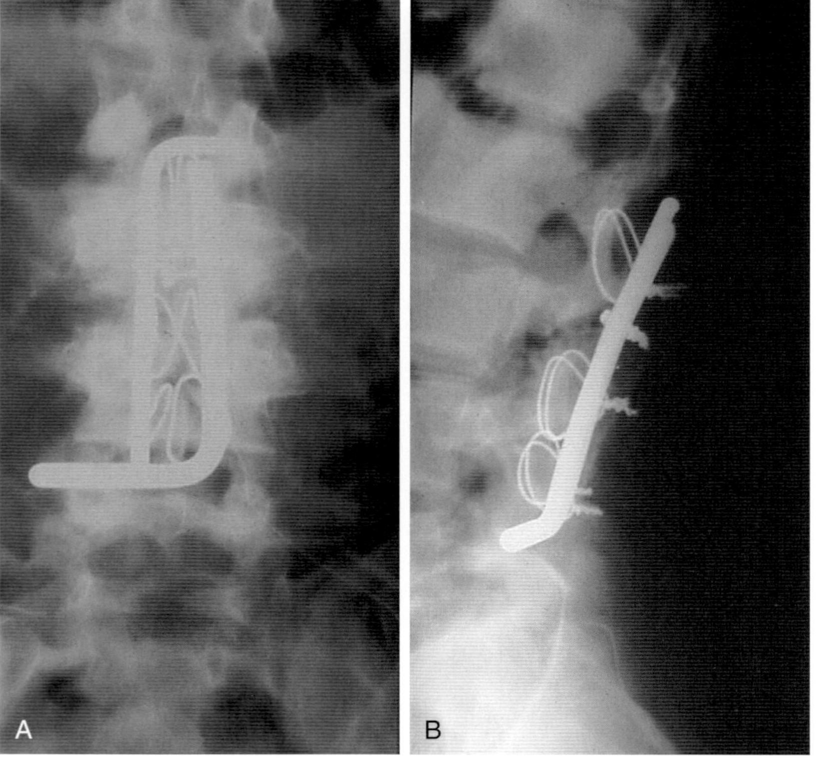

FIGURE 2-2. Anteroposterior (**A**) and lateral (**B**) radiographs after surgical stabilization of a burst fracture of L3 with segmental sublaminar wire fixation to an angled rod using the technique described by Eduardo Luque.

scoliosis. Further stability was provided by cross-linking the two parallel rods together.

The advantages of the CD system were partially offset, however, by the difficulty of removing it. The locking mechanism of the hooks was irreversible without destroying the hook or cutting the rod. The Texas Scottish Rite Hospital (TSRH) system was a design advance that addressed the issue of revision surgery. It was similar to the CD system in its use of multiple hooks and cross links but was designed to allow for the removal of the system's individual components if necessary. Although the features of the TSRH system simplified revision surgery, the top-loading side-tightened system was not universally appreciated. After maturation of the fusion mass, the side-tightened bolts were not always accessible. The following decade saw the introduction of numerous, similar dual-rod systems like Moss-Miami and Isola.[6,15] The major variations revolved around the leading and locking mechanisms: side loading, top loading, side tightening, or top tightening. The last decade has seen the introduction of numerous systems that operate with the same design principles, with a shift toward the use of polyaxial screws that make coupling of the fixation points to the rods easier. Today's systems often have a wide range of screw choices, including monoaxial, polyaxial, uniaxial (screws that are mobile in only one plane to allow for better derotation), as well as monaxial, polyaxial, and uniaxial reduction screws (screws with extended tabs, which allow gradual reduction of the rod into the body of the screw).

A major advance provided by these spinal systems was the exploitation of the pedicle as a site for segmental fixation. This innovation is generally credited to Roy-Camille of Paris. Roy-Camille performed his first operation in 1963 but did not publish the results until 1970.[16] Pedicle screws presented many advantages when compared with other tools for spinal fixation. Pedicle screws are biomechanically superior as a point of fixation[17] compared with hook- or wire-rod constructs and can be placed into the sacrum, an area to which fixation is otherwise difficult. In addition, they can be placed even after a laminectomy has been performed and can be positioned without entering the spinal canal.[18] This advantage allowed for the massive proliferation of spinal instrumentation into the area of degenerative spinal disorders. Prior to the advent of pedicle-screw instrumentation systems, there had been only sporadic reports of the use of instrumentation for degenerative spinal disorders. The Knodt rod (a small distraction rod system) had been used previously in degenerative disease but was associated with localized loss of lordosis and device dislodgement. In addition, the system needed some lamina for device fixation. Pedicle-screw systems, however, can be used after a total laminectomy.

Arthur Steffee popularized the use of pedicle screws in the United States in 1984 using a contourable plate. At about the same time, a screw-rod system, developed by Yves Cotrel of France, was in use in Europe that became incorporated into the "Universal" CD system. Controversy soon followed, with both the screw-plate and screw-rod constructs developing a group of proponents.[19] Proponents of plates noted that plates were stronger. Most surgeons were ultimately attracted, however, to rods because their use provides greater flexibility, reduces encroachment upon the adjacent facet joints, and leaves more surface area for fusion. The marriage of the long dual-rod constructs to lumbar pedicle screws was an important development that enhanced the surgeon's ability to accomplish increasingly difficult and complex spinal reconstructions. The use of the polyaxial pedicle screw has further advanced the ease of spinal reconstructions.

In recent years, there has been an interest in developing dynamic stabilization systems for degenerative diseases. The impetus for these systems arises from clinical evidence suggesting that 100% spinal fusion does not correlate with good clinical outcomes, which may range from 60% to 80%.[20] Spinal fusion may also have kinematic and kinetic consequences at adjacent segments that may increase the rate of adjacent level degeneration.[21] Dynamic stabilization systems aim to restore functional stability while maintaining intersegmental motion.

The most notable advancements in pedicle screw-rod based systems are the Graf ligmentoplasty system, the Isobar TTL Semi-rigid spinal system (Scient'X, West Chester, PA), and the Dynesys system (Zimmer Spine, Minneapolis, MN). The Isobar TTL and the Dynesys have Food and Drug Administration (FDA) approval as an adjunct to fusion, but to date none of these systems have been approved as a dynamic stabilizer (i.e., without fusion).[20-24] The Dynesys system was the only device to undergo an FDA Investigational Device Exemptions (IDE) study as a dynamic stabilizer. The system is composed of titanium pedicle screws connected via a terephthalate cord and polycarbonate spacer. Several authors have recently reported mostly favorable results with a variable incidence of complications.[25-31] At the time of this writing, no system has demonstrated enough evidence to justify widespread use or to be the gold standard.

Interspinous devices that increase the intervertebral space have also been developed to treat a myriad of degenerative conditions. These devices can be categorized as static or dynamic.[32] The most noteworthy static devices include the X STOP (Saint Francis Medical Technologies Inc., Alameda, CA), ExtenSure (NuVasive Inc., San Diego, CA), and Wallis implants (Abbott Spine, Austin, TX). Of these, the X STOP and the ExtenSure implants have been FDA approved for general use.[33] The X STOP has an oblong central core that is stabilized by two lateral wings (Fig. 2-3). The primary indication is mild or moderate neurogenic claudication from spinal stenosis. For dynamic interspinous devices, the Diam (Medtronic Sofamor Danek, Memphis, TN), Coflex (Paradigm Spine, New York, NY), and CoRoent (Nuvasive Inc., San Diego, CA) have been investigationally studied for use in the United States.[34] Of these, only the Diam device has been FDA approved. It attaches at the spinous processes and behind the supraspinous ligament. At the time of writing, numerous dorsal thoracolumbar dynamic systems have been approved by the FDA for investigational use. Outcome data for these systems, however, has been extremely limited.

Ventral Thoracolumbar Instrumentation

Successful use of the Harrington instrumentation kindled interest in developing a ventral system to address neuromuscular scoliosis. Dwyer developed a ventral system for internal fixation using screws connected by a cable.[35] Winter attempted a combined ventral and dorsal approach with Harrington and Dwyer instrumentation to treat painful adult

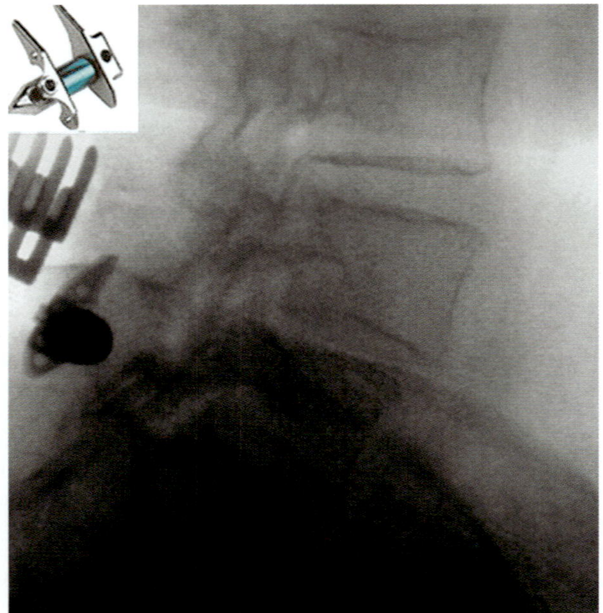

FIGURE 2-3. Intraoperative (lateral) x-ray showing the X STOP spacer placed between the spinous processes. Device shown at top left. (Neurosurg Focus ©2007 American Association of Neurological Surgeons.)

idiopathic scoliosis.[36] This concept was of particular interest in that these patients were at high risk for pseudarthrosis and tended to tolerate bracing less well than adolescents.[36]

The Zielke system, developed in 1975, was the next step in the development of ventral instrumentation. The Zielke device connected transvertebral screws with a threaded rod and nuts and was more rigid than the Dwyer cables. This added both strength and the capacity for incremental correction and derotation, permitting a more powerful correction. The Zielke system produced a lower pseudarthrosis rate and somewhat lower recurrence of the flat back syndrome. In spite of these benefits, the system had many shortcomings. The pseudarthrosis rate remained high when the system was used as a stand-alone device but was lowered with supplementation of dorsal fixation. This system also suffered from the tendency to shorten the ventral columns and to produce kyphosis.

The Dunn device was a ventral implant that consisted of two rods that spanned the distance between two vertebral body bridges: one placed ventrolaterally with a vertebral body staple and the other placed more dorsolaterally with an intervertebral body screw.[37] This system was not widely accepted because it was bulky and was associated with vascular complications.[38]

The ventral Kostuik-Harrington instrumentation was an adaptation of short Harrington rods used in conjunction with a pedicle screw developed by Paul Harrington for use in treating myelomeningocele. Introduced by John Kostuik in the early 1980s, it was an innovative short-segment ventral fixation device. The screw, when placed ventrolaterally in the vertebral bodies, allows for short-segment ventral correction of the kyphotic deformity associated with burst fractures. A second neutralization rod was placed parallel to the first rod to enhance stability (Fig. 2-4). Over time, cross-fixators were added in an attempt to further enhance stability. Two parallel rods rigidly cross-linked are the biomechanical equivalent of a plate. Most ventral short-segment constructs subsequently used plates with vertebral body screws.

Several other plate designs soon followed that had a lower profile. Ryan introduced a plate secured by a rostral and caudal bolt inserted through the vertebral body. The single-bolt design, however, offered less resistance to rotation than the designs that used two screws or bolts above and below.[39] The Yuan I-Plate was an alternative design that consisted of a 3.5-mm stainless steel plate secured with transvertebral screws.[40] Black et al.[41] published their experience with a low-profile, rectangular, stainless steel plate with multiple holes that allowed for the placement of three screws at each vertebral level. The Kaneda device represented another stage in the development of ventral thoracolumbar instrumentation because it allowed reduction of kyphotic deformities after ventral decompression while providing good strength without incidence of vascular injury.[38]

The next generation of ventral plates, including the Z-Plate (Medtronic/Sofamor Danek, Memphis, TN) and the Anterior Thoracolumbar Locking Plate System (Synthes, Paoli, PA), further improved implant design by providing a lower profile and changing the composition to titanium alloys. In addition, the newer systems allow for both the distraction of kyphotic deformities and the compression of the graft.

Dorsal Cervical Instrumentation

The earliest methods to provide internal fixation for dorsal cervical fusions involved the use of spinous process wiring. These techniques, however, are limited in that they often do not provide adequate stiffness or sufficient resistance to rotational movement and extension and cannot be used when the spinous processes have been removed.

For internal fixation of C1-2, the Brooks and Gallie techniques use sublaminar wires to compress an autologous bone graft. Although these techniques are reported to be associated with high fusion rates, they have the disadvantages of potentially producing neurologic injury from the placement of sublaminar wires and the problem that wires may pull through osteoporotic bone. In addition, a small but persistent failure rate is associated with the Gallie fusion that may be caused by inadequate immobilization allowing for "grinding down" of the graft.

Several instrumentation systems were devised as adjuncts or alternatives to wiring. The Daab plate was a stainless-steel implant shaped like an elongated H that could be compressed at either end to fixate it to a spinous process.[42,43] This instrumentation represented no significant advantage over the available wiring techniques, and it was probably inferior, considering that it typically needed the resection of an intervening spinous process and the associated interspinous ligaments.

Halifax clamps are a pair of upgoing and downgoing sublaminar hooks tightened together with a screw that is then secured in position with a locking mechanism (Fig. 2-5).[43,44] Halifax clamps have the advantage of relatively simple and rapid application. In addition, the area of bone contact is broader than that with wiring and is less likely to pull out of soft bone. They offer C1-2 fixation comparable to that

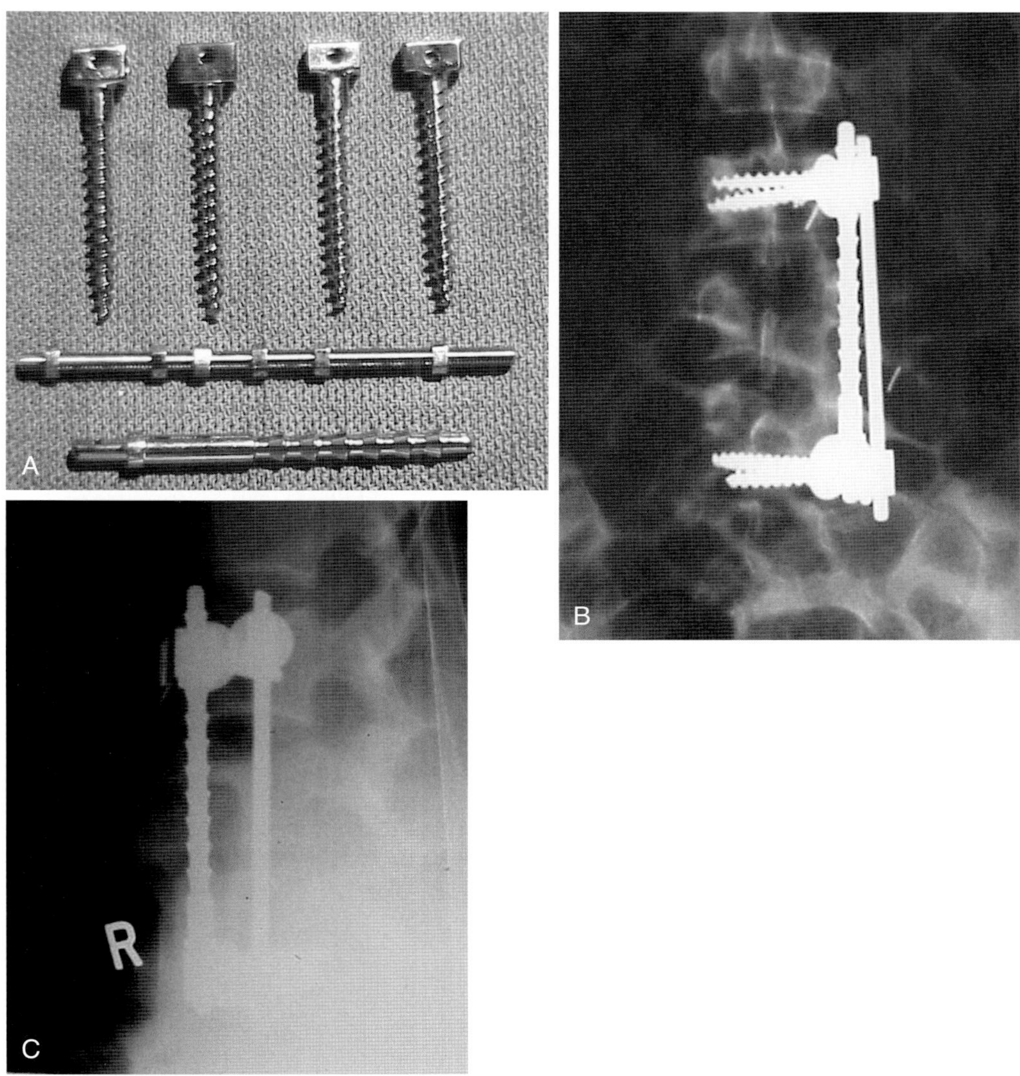

FIGURE 2-4. A, Kostuik-Harrington screws and rods. Anteroposterior (**B**) and lateral (**C**) radiographs after surgical stabilization of a burst fracture of L4 with Kostuik-Harrington instrumentation.

achieved with the Brooks technique.[45] Relative disadvantages of the system are that hooks are introduced into the spinal canal and the implant is relatively "high profile" and has limited application when stabilization is needed over multiple segments.

In the mid-1980s, Magerl introduced transarticular screw placement for internal fixation of C1-2. This is a technically demanding procedure compared with wiring, which achieves better C1-2 stability to flexion-extension and rotation[46] than wiring procedures and is associated with the highest published C1-2 fusion rates.[47] This technique is not always feasible if there is anatomic variation in the course of the vertebral artery, although there is still benefit in unilateral placement.[38] Many practitioners supplement transarticular screws with dorsal instrumentation because broken screws have been seen when used as a stand-alone procedure.

Lateral mass plate fixation with screws was introduced by Roy-Camille et al.[48] This technique of internal fixation is ideal in instances in which the laminae and spinous processes have been removed or fractured. The first technique for screw placement was modified by Magerl and Seeman,[49] Heller et al.,[50] and An et al.[51] The original lateral mass plates were an application of preexisting bone plates with a distance of 13 mm between plate holes. The Haid Plate and Synthes reconstruction plates were soon marketed, each offering a choice of two interhole distances. These systems all suffered from insufficient versatility in accommodating the wide variety of interhole differences often needed.[52] The AXIS system (Medtronic/Sofamor Danek, Memphis, TN) offers plate holes at intervals of 11, 13, and 15 mm and a slotted hole design to allow for limitless interhole variations as well as improved ability to contour the plates.

In recent years, numerous manufacturers have introduced lateral mass plate fixation systems. The most commonly used systems include the Cervifix system (Synthes Spine, Paoli, PA), Starlock instrumentation (Synthes Spine, Paoli, PA), Summit system (Depuy Acromed, Rayham, MA), and others. Advancements and design variations in lateral mass plate fixation have allowed the surgeon flexibility to address variations in anatomy beyond that offered by the AXIS system.

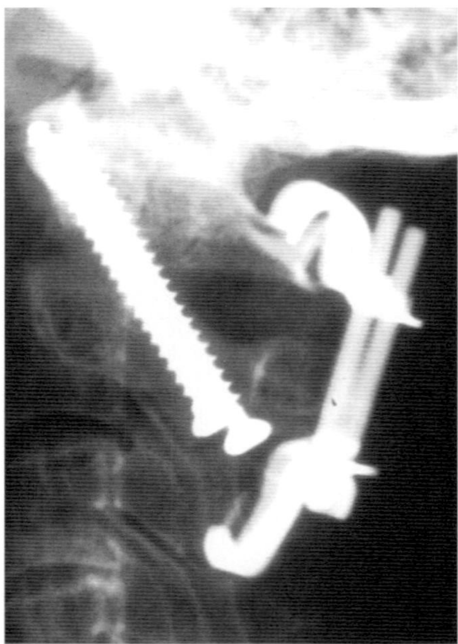

FIGURE 2-5. Postoperative lateral cervical radiograph demonstrating C1-2 internal fixation with Halifax clamps. In this patient, the dorsal clamps were placed to supplement fixation with C1-2 transarticular screws.

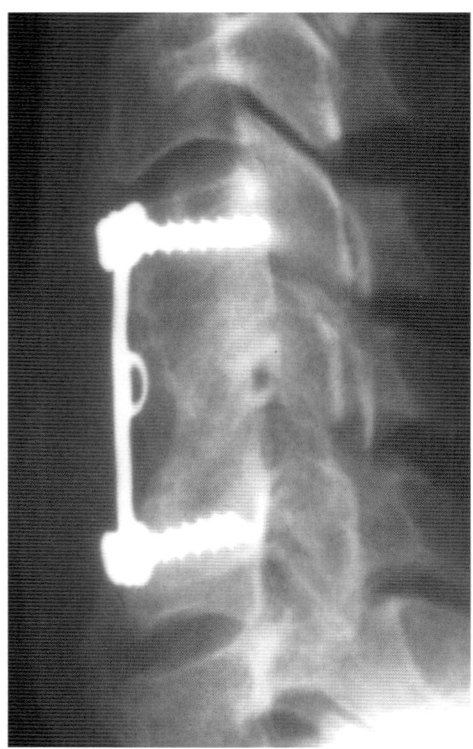

FIGURE 2-6. Postoperative lateral cervical radiograph demonstrating ventral internal fixation with the Orozco plate.

Hybrid plate-rod implants are also available for occipital screw placement in occipito-cervical fusions.

Ventral Cervical Instrumentation

Since the first system was developed by Bohler in the mid-1960s, ventral cervical plating has become a popular means of supplementing a ventral cervical fusion.[53] Early in the development of this instrumentation, the potential for screw backout was recognized as a possible cause of serious complications, including tracheal or esophageal erosion. The first systems widely available were the Caspar (Aesculap, San Francisco, CA) and the Orozco (Fig. 2-6) (Synthes, Paoli, PA). Both of these systems consisted of simple plates with slots or holes but without any locking devices. Constraint of the screws depended on obtaining bicortical purchase and "blocking" backout by screw angulation.

The rate of screw backout or breakage and graft subsidence was high with the first generation of ventral cervical plates. This led to the development of the Cervical Spine Locking Plate (CSLP) (Synthes, Paoli, PA),[54] first introduced in North America in 1991. The CSLP used a titanium expansion screw that secured the screwhead to the plate and, thus, allowed for unicortical purchase without the risk of screw backout. The substitution of titanium for stainless steel allowed for postoperative magnetic resonance imaging. The CSLP reduced the incidence of screw backout[55]; however, its limitations were a rigid screw trajectory and the fact that the plate was wide and difficult to contour.

The Orion ventral cervical plate (Medtronic/Sofamor Danek, Memphis, TN) represented the next major product introduction for ventral cervical plating. The plate was manufactured "prelordosed" with a wide variety of screw lengths to allow for unicortical or bicortical purchase. The drill guide was fixed to the plate, providing 15 degrees of rostral and caudal angulation and 6 degrees of medial angulation. Locking screws were added to fix the screws to the plate by overlapping the screw heads. Although the Orion plate was widely used and had good reported surgical results,[56,57] some surgeons felt that the system was too rigid and shielded the graft from stress, thereby promoting a significant rate of pseudarthrosis.[58]

In response to the perceived deficiencies of rigid ventral plates, dynamic cervical plates have evolved to lower the incidence of graft subsidence and plate failure, while still limiting movement across the diseased segment.[59] There are three main types of dynamic plates: longitudinal, translational, and telescoping. The longitudinal plate allows for toggling of the screw at the plate screw interface, but has the potential for screw loosening and pull-out. Longitudinal plates include the ACCS (Synthes Spine, Paoli, PA), Acufix (Abbott Spine, Austin, TX), Atlantic (Medtronic Sofamor Danek, Memphis, TN), Reflex (Stryker, Allendale, NJ), Slim-LOC (DePuy Spine, Raynham, MA), and Zephir (Medtronic Sofamor Danek, Memphis, TN).[60] In contrast, translational plates have slotted screw holes that allow each screw and vertebra to slide in the axial plane. If improperly placed or with settling over time, translational plates may overlap adjacent disc spaces, leading to ossification and degeneration. Examples include the ABC (Aesculap, Tuttlingen, Germany), C-Tek (Biomet, Warsaw, IN), and Premier (Medtronic Sofamor Danek, Memphis, TN).[60] Telescoping plates are designed to allow axial movement internally (Fig. 2-7). The most notable devices of this type are the DOC and the Swift (Depuy Spine, Raynham, MA). Although thicker in profile, these

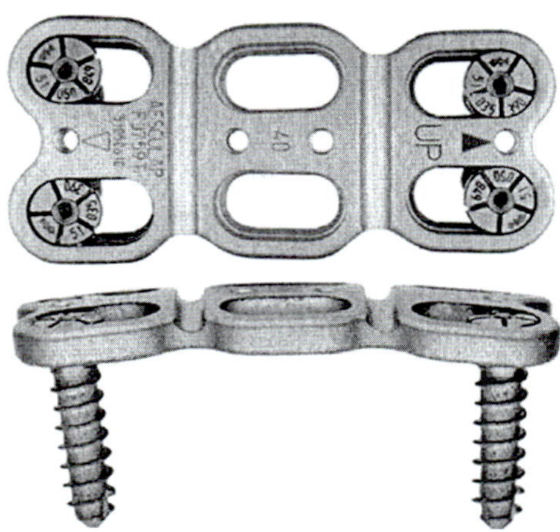

FIGURE 2-7. Anteroposterior (*top*) and lateral (*bottom*) views of the ABC Dynamic ventral cervical plate. The translational design allows for movement of the plate over the screw heads. (Neurosurg Focus ©2004 American Association of Neurological Surgeons.)

devices remain rigidly fixed to bone and therefore do not overlap with adjacent disc spaces. Lastly, hybrid constructs can be created in several ways by utilizing variable or rigidly fixed screws in combination with slotted or nonslotted plate holes.

Ventral fixation of odontoid fractures can be achieved with the placement of one or multiple screws. Although the technique was published in 1971 by Barbour,[61] it did not achieve popularity until the late 1980s.[62] Controversy developed over whether one or two screw placements is optimal for fixation.[63] Several recent papers, however, have not shown improved results with multiple screw placement.[64,65] Some surgeons have advocated the application of cannulated screws placed over Kirschner wires (K-wires) in this procedure, citing improved accuracy and the ability to redirect the screw trajectory as technical advantages. Other surgeons, however, prefer the original noncannulated screws, noting the potential risks of K-wire breakage as well as unintended K-wire advancement during screw placement.[66]

Total Disc Arthroplasty: Cervical and Lumbar

Cervical arthrodesis has been one of the most successful operations in orthopaedic surgery, with 95% of patients reporting significant improvement of symptoms following surgery.[67] However, the rate of adjacent segment disease—as reported by Hilibrand et al.—is 2.9%/year, leading to a significant reoperation rate over the long term.[68] Especially for younger patients with single- or two-level disc disease, motion preservation technology has emerged with hopes to improve outcomes and reduce the incidence of adjacent segment disease.

The Ulf Fernstrom ball bearing device was the first disc replacement method introduced in 1966, which was implanted in the cervical and lumbar spine with disappointing results. To date, the Bryan cervical disc, Prestige disc, and Pro-disc-C are the only cervical disc replacements that have received FDA approval in the United States. The Bryan cervical disc (Medtronic Sofamor Danek, Memphis, TN) consists of a two titanium shells separated by a polyurethane nucleus. Prospective randomized trials demonstrated some benefit of the Bryan disc over one- or two-level fusion in terms of reduced reoperation rate, improved outcome scores, and improved motion at the diseased segment. Complications were related to surgical technique, increased segmental kyphosis, or device failure.[69-73] The newest Prestige ST implant (Medtronic Sofamor Danek, Memphis, TN) underwent a prospective randomized study comparing it with one-level spinal fusion. For patients implanted with the Prestige ST, the study reported improved resolution of neurologic symptoms, less revision procedures, and less revision surgery for adjacent segment disease.[74] The Pro-disc-C (Synthes Spine, Paoli, PA) consists of two end plates of cobalt-chromium-molybdenum alloy with a central keel projecting into each end plate for stability (Fig. 2-8). A prospective randomized trial found no complications, fewer revision procedures, and improved clinical outcomes with the Pro-disc-C compared with spinal fusion for single-level disease.[74] The newest cervical disc replacements with ongoing FDA IDE trials include the Porous Coated Motion (PCM) device (NuVasive, San Diego, CA) and the CerviCore device (Stryker, Allendale, NJ).[74] The PCM is a two-piece device consisting of a cobalt-chrominium-molybdenum end plate with a polyethylene inner core. The CerviCore device, however, is a semiconstrained metal on metal prosthesis. The articulating surface is saddle-shaped, with two keels containing spikes on each end plate.

Total disc replacements for the lumbar spine have also been developed for the same purpose. These devices may be constrained, semiconstrained, or unconstrained. Currently, two lumbar total disc prostheses—the ProDisc-L (Synthes Spine, Paoli, PA) and the SB Charite (DePuy Spine, Raynham, MA)—have FDA approval.[75] The ProDisc-L, designed by Thierry Marnay, a French orthopaedic surgeon, is a semiconstrained device with a fixed center of rotation. The SB Charité disc was designed by Shellnac and ButtnerJans to have a sliding polyethylene core that moved with flexion and extension. At the time of writing, the Maverick (Medtronic Sofamor Danek, Memphis, TN) and the Flexicore (Stryker, Allendale, NJ) devices are awaiting FDA approval. The Maverick was designed by Le Huec et al. as a metal-on-metal ball-and-socket configuration.[76] The Flexicore is also a

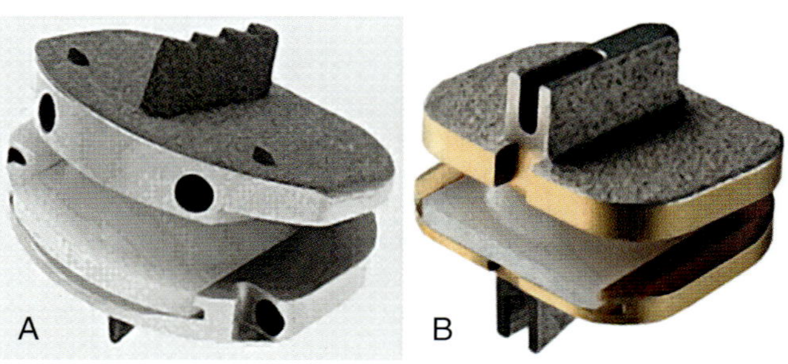

FIGURE 2-8. ProDisc disc replacements: cervical (**A**) and lumbar (**B**). The central keel is utilized for stable fixation to the vertebral body.

metal-on-metal ball-and-socket joint with a semiconstrained designed and fixed center of rotation.

Cage Technology: Horizontal and Vertical

The development of cages to promote interbody fusion traces back to the veterinary work of Bagby in which stainless-steel baskets filled with bone were used to treat wobbler-neck syndrome in race horses.[76] Bagby subsequently pioneered the development of a cage for use in human lumbar interbody fusions.[77,78] The implantation of cages as an interbody device through either a ventral or dorsal approach has become a widely performed procedure. Horizontal titanium-threaded cages include the BAK cage (Sulzer Spine-Tech, Minneapolis, MN) and the Ray Threaded Fusion Cage (Surgical Dynamics, Norwalk, CT), both of which were designed to be stand-alone devices for the ventral column. Brantigan et al.[79] Introduced cages composed of a radiolucent carbon fiber that allowed for improved postoperative imaging. It is also argued that the carbon fiber material has a modulus closer to that of native bone and, thus, should theoretically be a better fusion substrate than metal.[79]

Although the initial cage development was done for the cervical spine, the technology was first widely implemented in the lumbar spine. In April 2002, the FDA approved the use of the BAK-C device (Sulzer Spine-Tech, Minneapolis, MN) for cervical fusion.[80] Recent experience with these implants has indicated that fusion rates are comparable to those seen after procedures using uninstrumented allograft.[46]

To facilitate ventral vertebral reconstruction after ventral and middle column resection, Harms developed a vertical titanium mesh cage that can be packed with bone and is seated into the end plates.[50] This implant has found application in cases of vertebral body destruction resulting from metastatic disease, degenerative conditions, and trauma. The Harms cage was considered a valuable innovation even to those surgeons who preferred using struts made of allograft or autograft because a suitable bone graft is sometimes unavailable. At the time of writing, numerous manufacturers have now developed vertical cage implants of various sizes and materials. These vertical cage implants are most commonly used as ventral column support in combination with dorsal pedicle fixation either inserted ventrally or through a dorsal based interbody approach.

Minimally Invasive Approaches Utilizing Instrumentation

Recently, surgeons have employed minimally invasive approaches to the spine to minimize soft tissue disruption, recovery time, and scar appearance. Transforaminal lumbar interbody fusion (TLIF) has been used most commonly for grade 1 or grade 2 spondylolisthesis with radiculopathy, but also for discogenic back pain.[75,81] Using tubular retractors, METRx (Medtronic Sofamor Danek, Memphis, TN), the technique allows for decompression of the ispilateral exiting and traversing nerve roots. Another emerging technique, extreme lateral interbody fusion (XLIF), has been employed for treating axial back pain but also spondylolisthesis and degenerative scoliosis. From the lateral approach, the spine is accessed through the retroperitoneal fat and psoas muscle using MaXcess tubular retractors (NuVasive Inc, San Diego, CA). For both procedures, preliminary results are promising, but longer-term results have yet to be reported. As with many novel techniques, these approaches have been limited by a steep learning curve.[82] Numerous less invasive spinal instrumentation systems have also been developed for thoracic and lumbar dorsal spinal fusion. Rather than disrupting the paraspinal musculature, pedicle screws have been successfully placed percutaneously with a variety of systems. Under fluoroscopic visualization, tubular retractors are used to spread the paraspinal musculature over the pedicle. Placement of pedicle screws is generally accomplished with cannulated screws over a small guide wire. Placement of the rod or longitudinal connector may vary with the system. Many surgeons may also choose to use stimulated electromyographic neuromonitoring for additional safety.[83]

Kyphoplasty and vertebroplasty are minimally invasive percutaneous procedures that stabilize vertebral compression fractures. These have been indicated for chronic pain secondary to osteoporosis or osteolytic changes within a vertebral body. Vertebroplasty stabilizes a vertebral body fracture with injection of polymethylmethacrylate (PMMA) into the vertebral body, while kyphoplasty may also restore vertebral height by injecting the material within an inflatable device (KyphX, Medtronics Kyphon, Sunnyvale, CA) (Fig. 2-9).[84] Kyphoplasty may afford a smaller risk for cement leakage and associated complications, but advocates of vertebroplasty have claimed that high-viscosity cement may also alleviate these risks at a much lower cost. Both options have been debated in terms of clinical efficacy and complication rate, which has been reported as 1% to 2% for osteoporotic fractures and 5% to 10% for metastatic lesions with either procedure. Complications related to cement extravasation include new fractures of adjacent levels, cord/root compression, subdural hematoma, and embolization.[85]

Instrumentation through video-assisted thoracoscopic surgery (IVATS) has been used recently for thoracic scoliosis. The procedure allows for less disruption of the thoracic rib cage for removal of the disc spaces, release of ligamentous structures, and instrumentation with vertebral body screws and rods. Endoscopic hardware includes variable-angled thoracoscopes and specialized thoracospinal instruments

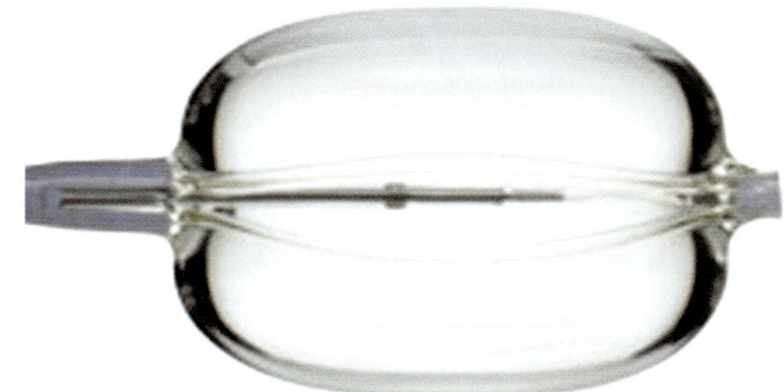

FIGURE 2-9. KyphX inflatable device used to perform a kyphoplasty. The inflatable device is placed within the vertebral body and filled with cement.

(Medtronic Sofamor Danek, Memphis, TN). Although reducing blood loss and improving scar appearance, IVATS has been limited by increased operative times, ICU stays, and complication rates compared with dorsal spinal fusion.[86,87] However, ventral release procedures without instrumentation remain a useful adjunct for scoliosis surgery.

Summary

The development of instrumentation for internal fixation of the spine has dramatically improved the surgeon's ability to successfully provide surgical intervention for a wide variety of spinal disorders. Internal fixation leads to higher fusion rates and provides more powerful means of correcting spinal deformities. In addition, spinal instrumentation allows for reduction or elimination of the need for postoperative external bracing.

Over the past 35 years, there has been an amazing increase in the variety of instrumentation available to provide internal spinal fixation. Surgeons are now able to select a specific type of implant that is best suited to address an individual patient's problem. In the last 10 years, there has been a greater interest in dynamic stabilization technologies and tools for minimally invasive surgery. An improved understanding of biomechanics and clinical experience with today's instrumentation should promote further advancement in internal fixation and even better patient outcomes in the future.

KEY REFERENCES

Bono CM, Lee CK: Critical analysis of trends in fusion for degenerative disc disease over the past 20 years: influence of technique on fusion rate and clinical outcome. *Spine* 29:455–463, 2004.

Cotrel Y, Dnbousset J: [A new technique for segmental spinal osteosynthesis using the posterior approach]. *Rev Chir Orthop Reparatrice Appar Mot* 70:489–494, 1984.

Denaro V, Papalia R, Denaro L, et al: Cervical spinal disc replacement. *J Bone Joint Surg (Br)* 91:713–719, 2009.

Esses ST, Bednar DA: The spinal pedicle screw: techniques and systems. *Orthop Rev* 18:676–682, 1989.

Hilibrand AS, Carlson GD, Palumbo MA, et al: Radiculopathy and myelopathy at segments adjacent to the site of a previous cervical arthrodesis. *J Bone Joint Surg (Am)* 81:519–528, 1999.

Lagrone MO, Bradford DS, Moe JH, et al: Treatment of symptomatic flatback after spinal fusion. *J Bone Joint Surg (Am)* 70:569–580, 1988.

Zucherman JF, Hsu KY, Hartjen CA, et al: A multicenter, prospective, randomized trial evaluating the X STOP interspinous process decompression system for the treatment of neurogenic intermittent claudication: two-year follow-up results. *Spine* 30:1351–1358, 2005.

REFERENCES

The complete reference list is available online at expertconsult.com

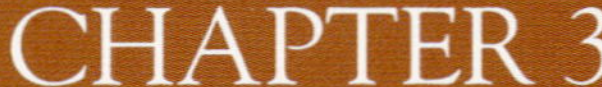

CHAPTER 3

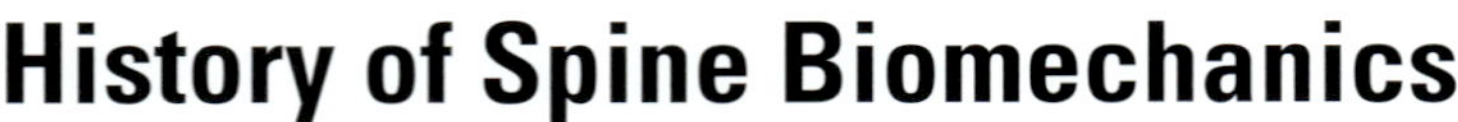

History of Spine Biomechanics

Sait Naderi | Varun R. Kshettry | İlker Gulec | Edward C. Benzel

Biomechanics is the subdiscipline of spine surgery that employs the laws of physics to describe the motion of body segments and the internal and external forces that act upon them. Although the majority of advancements have occurred within the last two centuries, the field of spine biomechanics has evolved over thousands of years. Full appreciation of this field is predicated on a knowledge of the initial discoveries that established the fundamentals of the discipline. In this chapter, the history of spine biomechanics is presented by reviewing major figures in the history of spine surgery, anatomy, and physiology and focuses attention on contributions in biomechanics. Spinal biomechanics presupposes the existence of physics. Therefore, landmark discoveries in physics that later proved to be instrumental for theoretical concepts in spinal biomechanics are discussed as well.

The chapter goes through history in chronological order. Major movements can be conveniently divided into five major time periods with estimated time ranges: Preclassical antiquity (10000 BCE–800 BCE), classical antiquity (800 BCE–500 CE), Middle Ages (500 CE–1500 CE), Renaissance/premodern era (1500–1900 CE), and modern age (1900 CE–present).

Preclassical Antiquity

The oldest known documents related to spine biomechanics were found in ancient Egypt and India. The Edwin Smith Papyrus—named after the American archeologist who purchased the scroll in 1862—is the only surviving copy of a portion of an Ancient Egyptian surgical text.[1] The author is unknown, but postulated to be Imhotep, the well-known physician to the pharaoh. The surviving copy was scribed in 1700 BCE, but the ideas represented date further back to at least the Egyptian Old Kingdom (2600–2200 BCE).[2,3] It contains the first reference to the concept of the spine as a bony column, termed the "djet" column.[4] Among the 48 case presentations of trauma, 6 were cases of spine trauma. Not only does the papyrus contain descriptions of the devastating neurologic consequences of high cervical traumatic injury to the spinal cord, but it also details the first classification of spine trauma. *Sehem* represents vertebral axial failure (likely including both compression and burst fracture), whereas *wenekh* represents dislocation.[3,5,6] Although there is evidence that the Egyptians understood the principle of reduction and immobilization for long bone fractures, they did not advocate treating spinal fractures due to the poor prognosis associated with them.

The oldest Indian reference available for spinal biomechanics is an ancient Hindu mythologic epic, *Srimad Bhagwat Mahapuranam*, written between 3500 BCE and 1800 BCE.[7] The epic includes a description of Lord Krishna correcting the hunchback of one of his devotees by manually applying opposing axial forces on the lady's chin and feet.[8]

Classical Antiquity

Mythologic Period

The early Greco-Roman period, from the Trojan War until the time of Hippocrates, continued the tradition of defining disease in terms of supernatural causes: if you were sick, it was because you displeased the gods. During this period, medicine was not clearly distinguishable from religion or mysticism. Asclepions were formal health care facilities established to honor Aesculapius, the god of health. Ailing visitors would come and while entering a meditation-like state (*enkoimesis*), would hope to be cured by the gods or by priest-physicians, who provided drug therapies and performed minor surgical procedures. Asclepions were opened in many cities, including Titan, Trika, Rhodes, Kos, Epidaurus, Athens, Alexandria, Tiber, and Pergamon.

Homer's *Iliad* contains several references to spinal trauma: "Hector with his sharp spear struck Eioneus on the neck below the well-made helmet of bronze, and loosed his limbs."[9] The Greek word translated into "loosed" or "lysed," probably forms the basis for the development of the term *paralysis*.[10] Empedocles reported data from his studies of the spine in the fifth century BCE. He suggested that the vertebrae were initially unified, forming a rigid spine, and that this solid osseous column subsequently segmented into pieces as a result of movements of the body.[11,12]

Scientific Period

During the scientific period, people gradually became skeptical of the notion of supernatural influence upon diseases and treatments. Hippocrates, the most important figure of this period, is the first physician to reject prevailing superstitions and beliefs and define disease in terms of natural causes; according to him, disease was due to an imbalance of four main bodily fluids, or humors: yellow bile, black bile, blood, and phlegm.

Hippocrates (460–377 BCE)

Hippocrates was a priest-physician born on the island of Cos in 460 BCE. He established an open-air school after he became prominent in the field of medicine. Hippocrates' approach to medicine represented a watershed event for the development of medicine as a scientific discipline. His contributions span all subdisciplines of medicine. The *Corpus Hippocraticum* is a collection of 12 books authored by Hippocrates with contributions from his contemporaries.

Hippocrates made a careful study of the anatomy and pathology of the spine,[12-14] (Fig. 3-1) separating the spinal vertebrae into three parts. The first part included the vertebrae lying above the level of the clavicle (including C7). The second part included the 12 vertebrae at the chest that articulated with ribs, the third part the 5 vertebrae between the chest and pelvis.[13] The sacrum and coccyx were not included as components of the spine by Hippocrates. Hippocrates also described the natural curvature of the cervical and lumbar portions of the spine (although the terms *lordosis* and *kyphosis* were not introduced until Galen in second century CE).[15] He used the term *ithioscoliosis* to describe the natural curves of the spine in the sagittal plane.[13]

Hippocrates classified spinal disorders as follows: (1) kyphosis, including both traumatic and nontraumatic etiologies; (2) scoliosis; (3) burst fractures; (4) vertebral dislocations; and (5) fractures of the spinous processes.[13] He cited spinal tuberculosis as the most common cause for kyphosis, noting that the severity of deformity was greater when it occurred before puberty. Hippocrates was the first to relate traumatic spinal deformities to causative force mechanisms. He found that traumatic kyphosis could result from forceful falls on the shoulder or buttock.[5] He correlated burst fractures with axial loading of the spine. Ventral vertebral dislocation was often secondary to a large force applied to the back such as a fall from a height or a blow from a heavy object.[5] Dorsal dislocations were rare, frequently fatal, and associated with severe abdominal injury.[5] Given the spinal architecture, Hippocrates noted the extreme force needed to create a dislocation: "a great thrusting-out and rupture of the articulation of one or more of them does not very often occur, but is rare. Such injuries, indeed, are hard to produce."[13,16] He also noted that dislocations (which he termed inward curvatures vs. outward curvatures in kyphosis) were associated with a poor prognosis: "In such cases, then, retention of urine and faeces is more frequent than in outward curvatures; the feet and lower limbs as a whole more usually lose heat, and these injuries are more generally fatal. Even if they survive, they are more liable to incontinence of urine, and have more weakness and torpor of the legs; while if the incurvation occurs higher up, they have loss of power and complete torpor of the whole body."[13,16] He noted that isolated spinous process fractures did not result in deformity, healed well, and did not result in clinical impairment.

Beyond his keen observations, Hippocrates also devised several innovative therapeutic interventions for spinal disorders, including the Hippocratic board and the Hippocratic ladder. As a first line of intervention, he recommended manual traction of the spine with application of focal pressure using one's hand or foot over a kyphotic deformity. If this did not work, he recommended use of the Hippocratic board, by which spinal traction could be better obtained using two opposing axial force vectors in combination with manual perpendicular force over the kyphotic deformity (Fig. 3-2). He liked this technique, as he states: "in accordance with nature; for the pressure forces the protruding parts into place, and the extensions according to nature draw asunder the parts that have come together."[13,16]

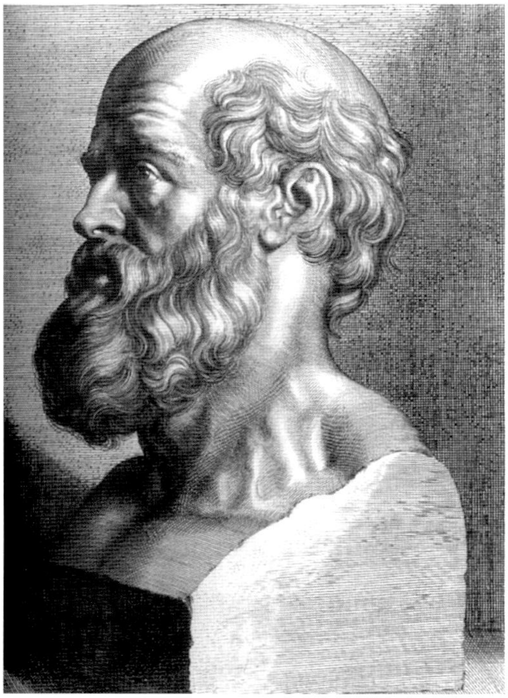

FIGURE 3-1. Hippocrates described anatomy and diseases of the spine.

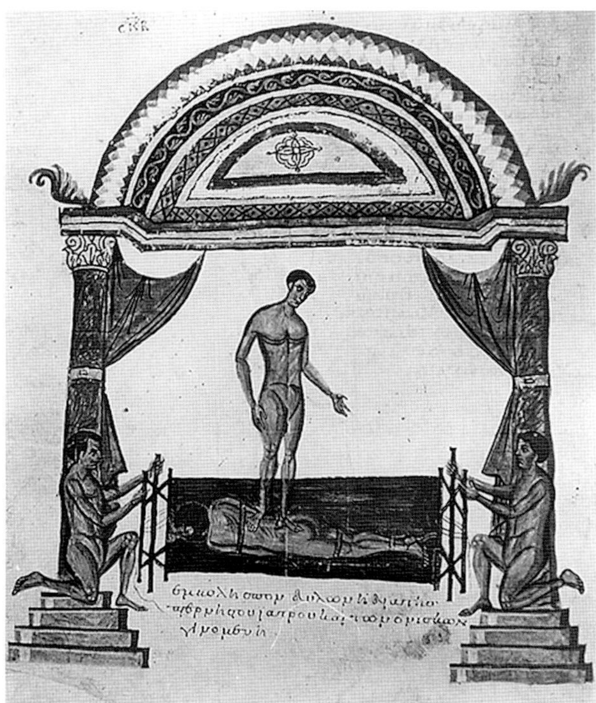

FIGURE 3-2. The Hippocratic board is a device used to manage spinal dislocation and deformities.

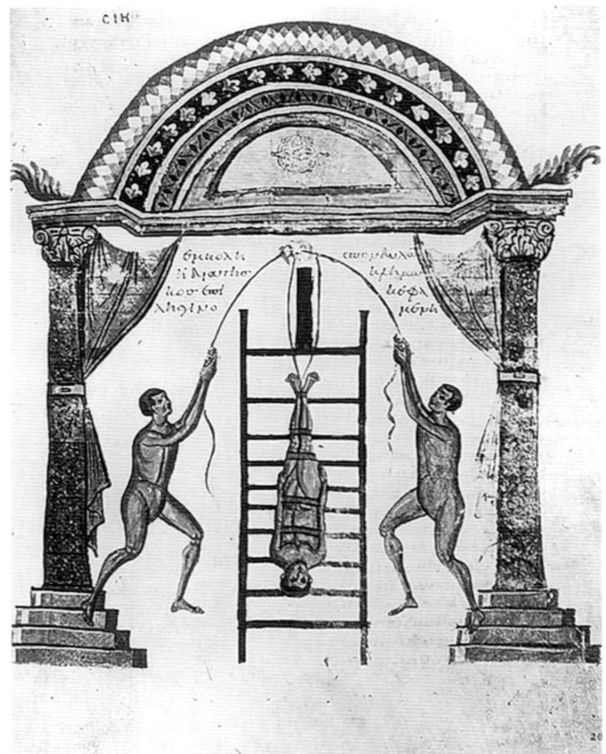

FIGURE 3-3. The Hippocratic ladder was developed to reduce the dislocated spine and its associated deformities.

Although he is credited with developing the Hippocratic ladder, his writings reflect less favorably upon this intervention. By this technique, a patient was fixed upside down on a ladder that was connected to a pulley system from which the ladder was raised, suddenly released, and allowed to fall to the ground, and repeated several times (Fig. 3-3). Hippocrates felt it was more difficult to control the direction and magnitude of force with this technique. Perhaps this is why he warned that this technique, which he called "succussion" (shaking), was better at pleasing the mob then correcting a deformity.[17]

Plato (427–347 BCE)

The great philosopher and mathematician, Plato, was founder of the Academy in Athens, the first institution of higher learning in the Western world. He suggested that mathematics, a system of pure ideas, was the best tool for the pursuit of knowledge. Plato's contributions to mathematics are considered to be the origins and stimulus for the development of the science of mechanics and, consequently, spine biomechanics.[18]

Aristotle (384–322 BCE)

Aristotle provided treatises on many subjects, including physics, metaphysics, poetry, theater, music, politics, ethics, biology, and zoology.[16] He should perhaps be considered the first biomechanist. As such, he recorded detailed information regarding the mechanical system of animals in his first book, *De Motu Animalium* (On the Movement of Animals).[18-23] This work provides the first geometric analyses of isolated muscular movements such as flexion and extension.[5] He commented on the rotational axes surrounding joints and how one type of motion, such as rotation, could be used to create another type, such as translation.

Aristotle discussed the problems of pushing a boat under various conditions from the standpoint of mechanics, describing, in a primitive form, Newton's three laws of motion. Aristotle depicted a qualified understanding of the role of the center of gravity in his analyses of gait.[23,24] Of note, Aristotle's findings were purely observational, he did not perform scientific experiments. Even though his work was not directly related to the spine, Aristotle's work led to the birth of kinesiology and laid further groundwork for spinal biomechanics.[19,22]

Herophilus of Chalcedon (335–280 BCE)

Medical science reached a high point in Greek civilization, but in the third century BCE, the greatest medical minds were to be found in the Egyptian city of Alexandria. The effect of religion and mysticism in the city of Alexandria on medicine was prominent. Archimedes, Euclid, Praxagoras, Herophilus of Chalcedon, and Erasistratus are among the most prominent figures of this period.

Herophilus of Chalcedon, the world's first anatomist, dominated the discussions of anatomic studies during this period. Although Herophilus carried out anatomic dissections on human cadavers, he did not comment on spine anatomy and biomechanics in his works. He did, however, make significant contributions to cerebral neuroanatomy and noted the consequences of spinal cord injuries, suggesting that direct surgical intervention on the spinal column should be avoided.[11,25]

Archimedes (287–212 BCE)

Archimedes was a prominent mathematician, physicist, engineer, inventor, and astronomer of this age. He had the greatest influence on the future of spinal biomechanics through his contributions to theoretical mechanics in his work *On the Equilibrium of Planes*.[19] He is known for his formulation of the hydrostatic principle (known as Archimedes' principle) and the development of the Archimedes screw, a cylinder with an internal revolving screw that was built to pump water against gravity. Archimedes described fundamental theorems concerning the center of gravity and laws of leverage.[5]

Galen of Pergamon (130–200 CE)

In the second century CE, as the Roman Empire rose to prominence, mysticism subsided and scientific thought regained credibility and popularity, albeit under the strict oversight of the Church. Galen (Fig. 3-4) was a physician to the Roman gladiators. More importantly, he made many important discoveries in anatomy and physiology by performing anatomic dissections on animals and extrapolating his findings to humans. Galen's anatomic studies and interpretations affected medicine for more than a thousand years, until the time of Vesalius. His own work corroborated the findings of Imhotep and Hippocrates on the neurologic sequences of cervical trauma.[14,24,26]

Galen was the first to determine the reliance of muscular movements on supplying connections from nerves.[27] He also demonstrated the neurologic implications following transection of the spinal cord at several levels in live animals. He dealt with spinal tuberculosis as well as an abundance of traumatic injuries to the spine and the spinal cord. He appreciated the structure of

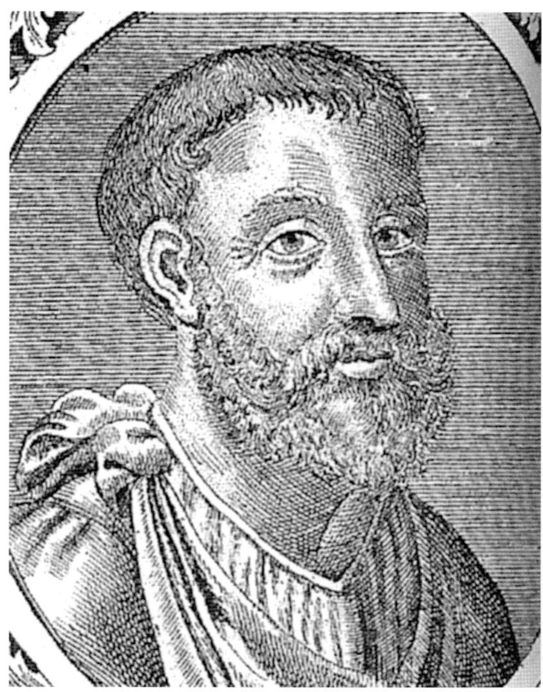

FIGURE 3-4. Galen is referred to as the father of sports medicine.

the spine in allowing an intersecting balance of neural protection and flexibility for mobility.[27] Galen was able to detail the structure of the spine in that the vertebrae were joined ventrally and had articulating components dorsally. He felt that the former allowed for motion and the latter provided greater stability.[5] In addition, he was the first to describe the spinal canal which contained the spinal cord—previously termed the "spinal marrow" in the Greek era. He noted that the spinal cord was an extension of the brain, "like a river having its springs in the brain."[27] He also used the Hippocratic board to treat kyphotic deformities, but unlike Hippocrates, advocated surgery in some cases to remove bony fragments impinging on the spine.[5,25]

Middle Ages (330–1453 CE)

Paulus of Aegina was the last prominent scientist working in the tradition of the Greco-Roman period.[5] As the Dark Ages of Europe settled in, religion governed all aspects of life, particularly science. Yet during this same period, Islamic civilization flourished. Major Greco-Roman scientific texts were translated into Persian and Arabic, and many Islamic scientist physicians led the frontier of medical advancement.

Paulus of Aegina (625–690 CE)

The *Medical Compendium in Seven Books* or *Epitomês Iatrikê Biblio Hepta* was a medical treatise of seven books written by Paulus of Aegina in the seventh century (Fig. 3-5). He used traction tables to treat spinal deformity and employed a new technique of cauterization with a red hot iron to treat various painful illnesses. Paulus of Aegina was the first physician to perform a successful laminectomy for a spinal fracture with symptomatic neural compression. He recommended the use of orthoses for spinal fractures.[25]

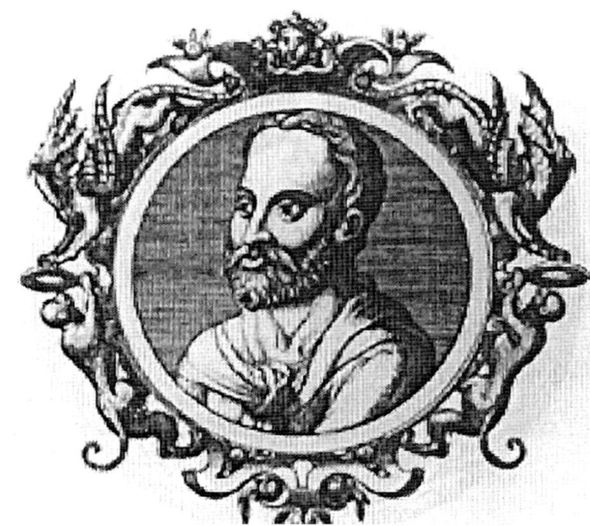

FIGURE 3-5. Paul of Aegina wrote the *Medical Compendium in Seven Books* that is chiefly a compilation from earlier writers.

Avicenna (981–1037 CE)

Avicenna, an Islamic physician, was very interested in the mechanical function of the spine. He studied regional anatomic variations of vertebrae and correlated the different features to their mechanical functions. He described quite accurately the mechanical movements involved in flexion, extension, and lateral bending of the spine. Avicenna studied in detail the mechanics of the craniovertebral junction. He believed that movement at the occiput-C1 joint provides lateral bending, and movement at the occiput-C2 segments provides flexion-extension. Also, during head flexion-extension and lateral bending, C1-2 vertebrae move simultaneously. According to Avicenna, the dens was uniquely developed to protect the high cervical spinal cord and limit motion of C1-2.[28]

Albucasis (936–1013 CE)

Albucasis, also known as Al-Zahrawi, was a prominent Islamic physician and surgeon. He designed instruments and surgical techniques for treating spinal disorders, including lumbar radiculopathy, low back pain, scoliosis, and spinal dislocations. He developed a procedure for cauterization and described a device for reduction of dislocated vertebrae.[29] He classified spinal trauma as complete and incomplete. He observed that a complete dislocation presents itself with abolition of sphincter tone and motor function and that an incomplete trauma causes partial neurologic injury. *Cerrahiyetul Haniye*, a Turkish treatise written by Serafeddin Sabuncuoglu in the 15th century, describes and illustrates the technical details of Albucasis's surgery and treatments for spinal diseases.[30]

Renaissance and Premodern Era

The Renaissance began a new period of scientific exploration unfettered by the restraints of religion. Scientists of this era were able to build on the ideas of the Greco-Roman period thanks to the preservation of texts through Arabic translations. However, seeking to break free from classical traditions, two new trends developed. First, skillful anatomists such as Leonardo Da Vinci (1452–1519) and Andreas Vesalius (1514–1564) rejected the archaic galenic anatomic descriptions of animals and dissected human cadavers in painstaking detail. As Vesalius is known to have stated, it became time to learn from dead bodies rather than dead languages. Second, classical theories were tested under scientific rigor for the first time. Instead of applying traditional treatments without question, doctors developed new practices based on experimentation.[31] Simultaneously, during this time, the fields of mathematics, physics, and mechanics gained significant theoretical developments through the work of René Descartes, Robert Hooke, Isaac Newton, and Thomas Young. As a precursor to more detailed spinal biomechanical research in the 20th century, earlier work was conducted in kinesiology and the biomechanics of gait by Giovanni Alfonso Borelli, the Weber brothers, Christian Wilhelm Braune, and Otto Fischer.

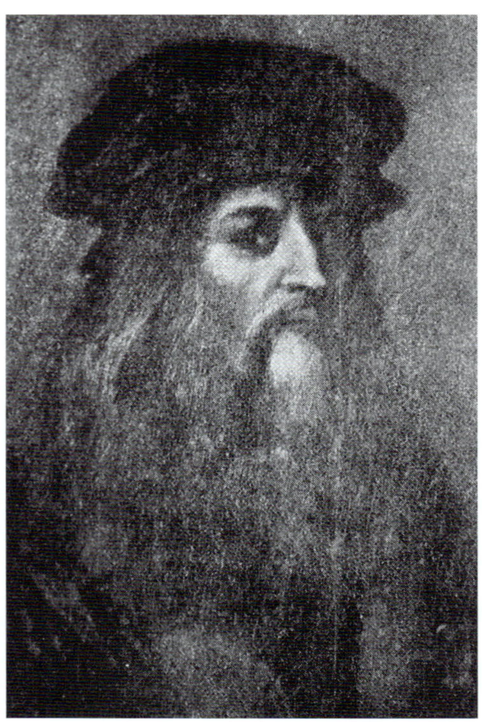

FIGURE 3-6. Da Vinci gave an important contribution to understanding mechanical principles.

Leonardo Da Vinci (1452–1519)

Leonardo Da Vinci (Fig. 3-6) was an intelligent engineer with the skill of a master artist. Da Vinci studied detailed anatomy (Figs. 3-7 to 3-9) using dissections in 10 cadavers, from which he produced over 750 illustrations later published in *De Figura Humana*. He illustrated spinal anatomy with unprecedented accuracy and detail from the variation of regional vertebrae to the natural curvature of the spine, and he included the correct number of vertebrae. He was particularly interested in the mechanics of human movement and therefore focused on the anatomy of motion—muscles, tendons, bones, ligaments, and joints.

He demonstrated an understanding of the components of force vectors, friction coefficients, and the acceleration of falling objects. He clearly demonstrated an understanding of what was to become Newton s third law.[2,32]

He described the mechanical stability of the cervical spine in a methodology around its neutral posture with an emphasis on the cervical musculature in providing stability. He emphasized the importance of leverage systems in animals and their similarity to those in human motion. He examined basic mechanics related to human walking in different positions.

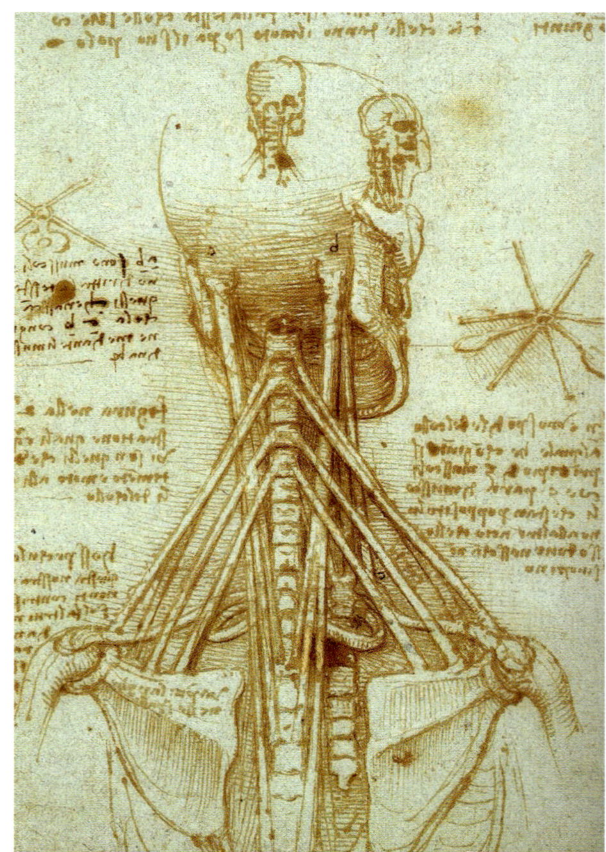

FIGURE 3-7. The musculature of the cervical spine was richly illustrated by Da Vinci.

Andreas Vesalius (1514–1564)

Vesalius rid the study of human anatomy of mythic speculations, which had engulfed it for two millennia. He published *De Humani Corporis Fabrica* (On the Fabric of the Human Body), an encyclopedic work containing more than 200 anatomic drawings.[18,33] Vesalius is credited with being the revolutionary figure of anatomy because the work of Da Vinci remained unpublished and unknown to the medical community for many years.

He termed the spine the "dorsum" (backbone) and confirmed Da Vinci's descriptions of the spinal column, joints, and foramina. Vesalius only disagreed on the number of sacral vertebrae (six) as opposed to Da Vinci, who believed there was five.[34] He was the first to correctly describe the intervertebral disc. He also expounded his view on the mechanics of head movement: "the neck has seven bones...by means of the first of these bones, we move the head directly forward

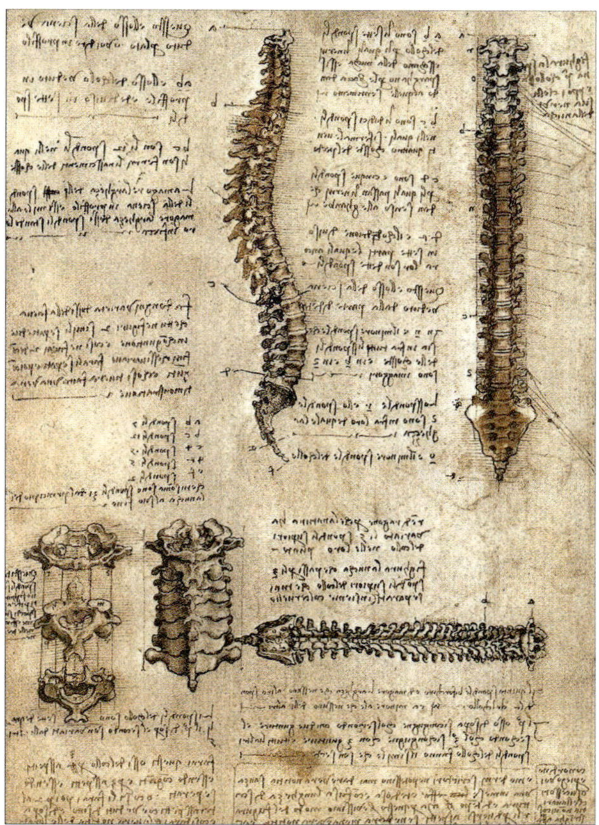

FIGURE 3-8. Da Vinci illustrated bone anatomy of the spine.

and backward. By the use of the second vertebra (to which a prominent process resembling a canine tooth is attached) we turn the head...."[5,34,35] The greatest contribution Vesalius made was to solidify anatomic dissection as a necessary prerequisite to medicine and surgery.

Galileo Galilei (1564–1642)

Galileo is often considered the "first real scientist" because he advocated and practiced the scientific method of hypothesis testing for his experiments.[32] Using the mathematical terminology, he founded the basic principles for kinesiology as a science. In *Discourses on Two New Sciences* (1638), Galileo stated "The mass of animals increase disproportionately to their size, and their bones must consequently also disproportionately increase in girth, adapting to load-bearing rather than mere size," and later added, "the bending strength of a tubular structure, such as bone, is increased relative to its weight by making it hollow and increasing its diameter."[17,31] Although not directly related to the spine, his work laid early groundwork for mathematical analyses of biomechanical properties of load-bearing bone structures.

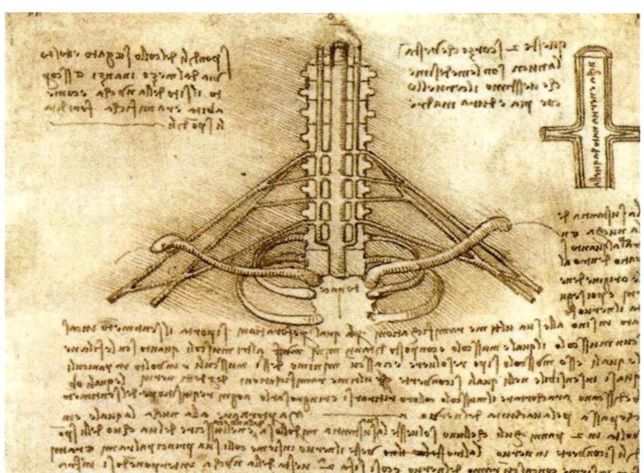

FIGURE 3-9. Cervical nerve roots of the spine were depicted by Da Vinci.

René Descartes (1596–1650)

Descartes, a French philosopher, scientist, and mathematician, is often called the founder of modern philosophy. He was not a major contributor in the field of biomechanics, but his thoughts had an indirect influence on the field. In 1675, Descartes wrote *Tractatus de Homine et de Formatione Foetus* (Treatise on Humans and the Formation of the Fetus). In this treatise, he developed his mechanical view of the universe; movement was the reorganization of matter in a cartesian coordinate system of space. He also equated organisms to God's machines.[32] Aside from inventing the cartesian coordinate system, he is also said to be the founder of analytical geometry. *L'Homme* was Descartes' first systematic presentation of physiology.

Giovanni Alfonso Borelli (1608–1679)

Borelli (Fig. 3-10) was a Renaissance physiologist, physicist, and mathematician.[36] The Accademia del Cimento (Academy of Experiment), an early scientific society, was founded by Borelli and Marcello Malpighi, a mathematician and naturalist. In this academy, he began his first investigations into the science of animal movement. The collaboration between two authors yielded an abundance of scientific work.[18,37]

In *De Motu Animalium* (On the Movements of Animals), one of his most complicated treatises, he investigated in detail the movement of animals. Movement of the musculoskeletal system and internal motions, such as muscle physiology and blood circulation, were also studied.[38] Borelli was the first to determine that muscles acted upon joints with short lever arms, debunking Galen's assumption that muscles acted via long lever arms in order to achieve a biomechanical advantage.[2,31]

Borelli analyzed the biomechanics of individual components of the spine (Fig. 3-11).[39] He described anatomic characteristics that prevent listhesis[39] and demonstrated, with modern experimental calculations, the concept of spinal load sharing (Fig. 3-12): "If the spine of a stevedore is bent and supports a load of 120 pounds carried on the neck, the force exerted by nature in the intervertebral discs and in the extensor muscles of the spine is equal to 25,585 pounds. The force exerted by the muscle alone is not less than 6404 pounds. Therefore, the sum of muscular forces which control the fifth lumbar vertebra and a third of the resistance of the intervertebral disc is equal to 826 pounds. The muscular forces are equal to 413 pounds and the forces exerted by the disc are equal to 1239 pounds."[31,38] He explained that strong fibers of the intervertebral disc are much stronger than those in

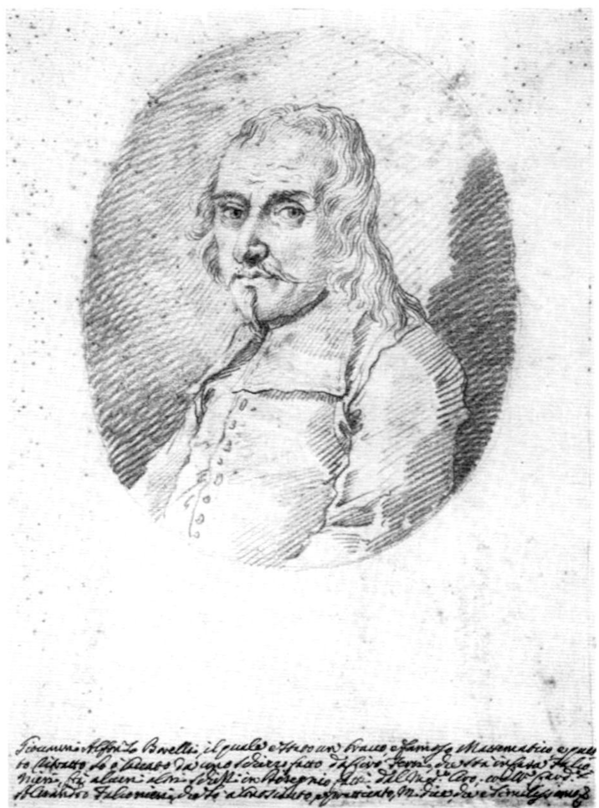

FIGURE 3-10. Giovanni Alfonso Borelli wrote the first modern textbook on spinal biomechanics.

muscle. He suggested that most of the weight of axial loading is carried by the intervertebral discs, with a much smaller portion carried by the spinal musculature.[38]

Borelli was also the first to experimentally demonstrate the human center of gravity as a point between the pelvis and buttocks. He devised a wooden plank resting on a pyramidal fulcrum to conduct his experimental measurements (Fig. 3-13).[26,31] Several centuries later, Braune and Fisher[40] verified that his assessment was correct. After Borelli, biomechanical studies were sparse until the 19th century.

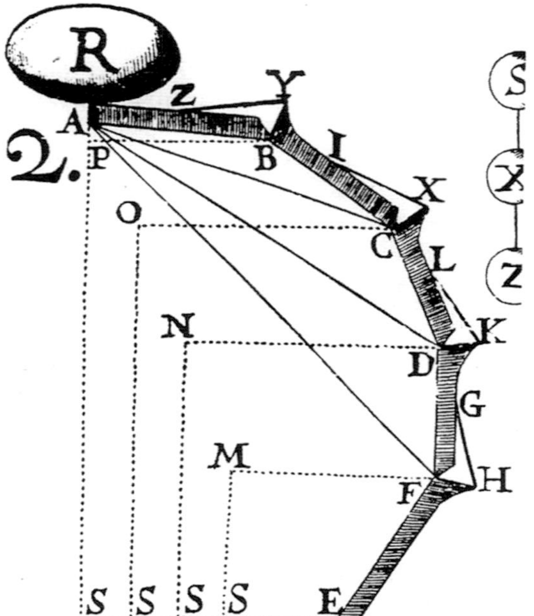

FIGURE 3-11. The spine, muscles, and intervertebral discs were depicted by Borelli, from *De Motu Animalium*.

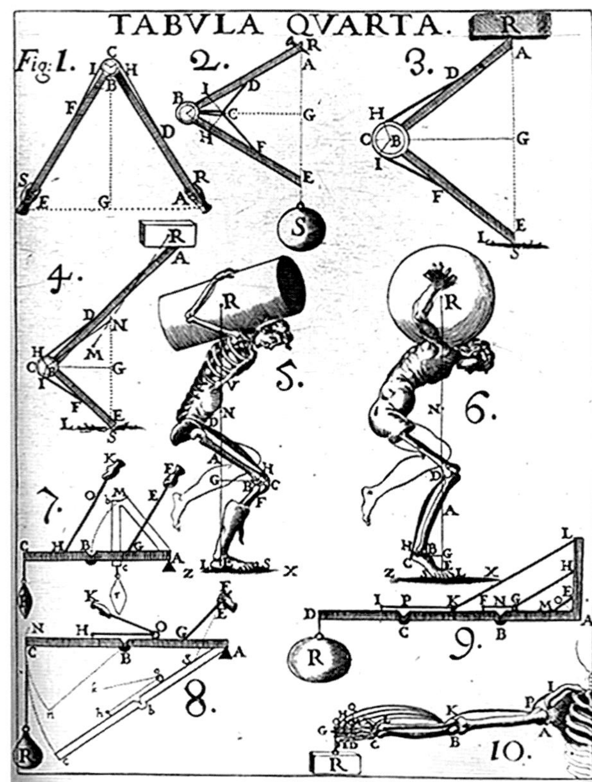

FIGURE 3-12. Illustration by Giovanni Alfonso Borelli analyzing the load-sharing capabilities of the spine.

Robert Hooke (1635–1703)

Robert Hooke, an English philosopher and mathematician, contributed to spinal biomechanics through his theories of the response of solids to deforming forces. Hooke's law states that for small deforming forces, elastic materials will deform to an extent in proportion to the deforming force and the material's elasticity. This physical law is important when designing spinal instrumentation constructs and analyzing in vivo deforming forces.

Hooke went further to describe how solids react under a full range of deforming forces, from zero net sum forces to deforming forces that alter the mechanical properties of the solid. He essentially described the neutral zone, the elastic zone, the plastic zone, and the point of failure.[32]

Isaac Newton (1642–1727)

The English mathematician and founder of classical mechanics, Isaac Newton, invented complex mathematical and engineering principles. Newton described three laws of motion, now known as Newton's laws of motion (laws of inertia, momentum, and interaction).[32,41] With the introduction of these physical laws, biomechanical mechanisms and

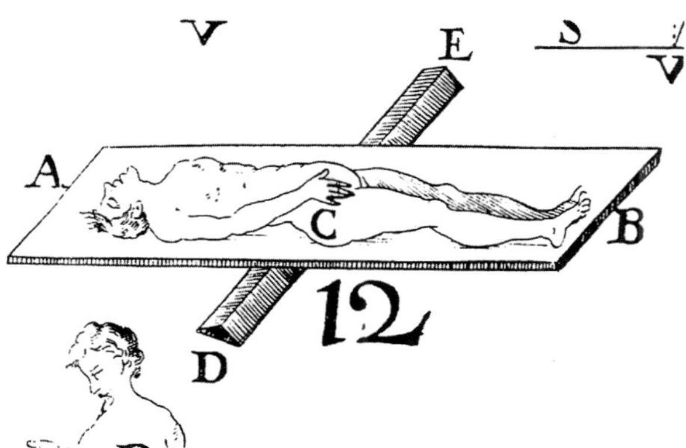

FIGURE 3-13. Center of gravity was more understandable after Borelli's method.

structures could be simulated and studied. He was also credited with calculating resultant force vectors from individual component vectors.

Leonard Euler (1707–1783)

The Swiss mathematician Leonard Euler is known for his work in mathematics, astronomy, and physics. He studied columns under compressive loads and found that columns had a point at which they would deform.[32,41] This point was related to the height and stiffness of the column. At later points in history, the spine was studied as a Euler column.[39]

Thomas Young (1773–1829)

Thomas Young studied the human voice and vibration. He developed Young's modulus, a coefficient that can be calculated to define the relation of stress and strain for a given body. This important concept is employed in contemporary spinal biomechanics to measure the elasticity of both the spine and the spinal constructs.[32]

Weber Brothers

Three brothers, Ernst Heinrich Weber (1795–1878), Wilhelm Eduard Weber (1804–1891), and Eduard Friedrich Wilhelm Weber (1806–1871), in their publication *Die Mechanik der Menschlichen Gehwerkzeuge* (Mechanics of the Human Gait), developed the modern concept of locomotion.[42] It was assumed that the human torso was kept in erect posture primarily via tension of the ligaments, with little or no muscular exertion. The Weber brothers demonstrated that muscle contraction contributed substantially to posture.[43] They also studied the movement of the center of gravity in locomotion.

Christian Wilhelm Braune (1831–1892) and Otto Fischer (1861–1917)

The development of a new three-dimensional mathematical analysis of human gait was published by Christian Wilhelm Braune and Otto Fischer. They described the first plausible theory related to the mechanics of walking and running in *Mechanik der Menschlichen Gehwerkzeuge* (Mechanics of the Human Walking Apparatus).[44] They determined the human center of gravity by suspending frozen human cadavers on thin rods in three perpendicular axes. They observed the center of gravity during locomotion and investigated the forces supplied by the musculature to maintain the center of gravity during locomotion.[40]

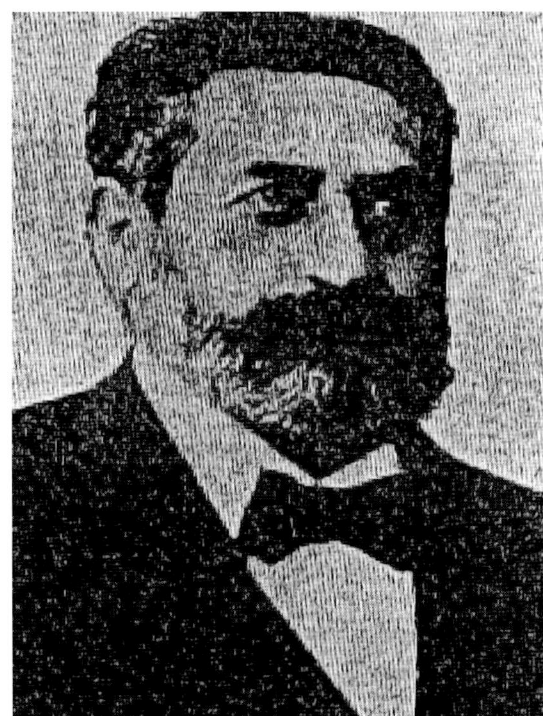

FIGURE 3-14. Trajectoral hypothesis, which forms the basis of one of the most important elements of spine biomechanics, was proposed by Julius Wolff.

Julius Wolff (1836–1902)

Wolff's law embodies the fundamental relationships between applied loads and the body's adaption to such loads. Julius Wolff (Fig. 3-14), a German orthopedic surgeon, studied bony architecture and found that it paralleled mathematically calculated stress trajectories.[45] His law states: "Every change in the form and function of a bone, or of function alone, is followed by specific definite change in its internal architecture and equally definite secondary changes in its external configuration, in accordance with mathematical laws."[31,45] In modern spine biomechanics, this law influences spinal construct design in order to maximize fusion rates.

Emergence of Modern Biomechanics in the 20th Century

An increasing interest in athletics, gymnastics education, and World Wars I and II were major contributors to the development of the field of biomechanics in the 20th century. The technologic advances that emerged during this century led to new and greater force applications to the human body via trauma, such as from motor vehicle and plane accidents and civilian injuries from explosions. These new problems rejuvenated interest in spine biomechanics.[22]

The Human Motor by Jules Amar (1879–1935) was an analysis of the physical and physiologic components of gait and task performance in thousands of disabled veterans in France.[46,47] This was the first biomechanical evaluation derived from human force and motion data.

In World War II, high-speed aircraft with emergency ejection seats provided another inspiration for biomechanical research. Multiple biomechanical studies were conducted to test the safe range of compressive loads tolerable at different levels of the spine. The appropriate spinal posture at the time of ejection was determined by Olof Perey in 1945, and the Martin-Baker aircraft company in England in 1944.[48] Similar studies were performed by the U.S. Air Force in 1945.[48]

Detailed research on the intervertebral disc was performed at Massachusetts General Hospital and Massachusetts Institute of Technology.[48] Parallel to these studies, at Wayne State University, H. R. Lissner and E. S. Gurdjian investigated the effect of applying axial compression and transverse bending on lumbar disc herniation.[48-52]

Friedrich Pauwels (Fig. 3-15) (1885–1980) and Nikolai A. Bernshtein (1896–1966) conducted seminal work in musculoskeletal biomechanics.[13,53] Russell Plato Schwartz established his myodynamics laboratory in the Department of Surgery of the University of Rochester School of Medicine and Dentistry in 1926. The laboratory focused on gait analysis for shoe design and other biomechanical applications. He developed the recording instrumentation and surgical tools necessary to measure normal and abnormal gait.

The mechanical properties of the cervical vertebra in vitro were studied for the first time by Erland Lysell in Sweden. He inserted small steel balls at each cervical vertebra in the cervical spines of 28 fresh cadavers, and using quantitative stereoradiography, he measured intervertebral motion.[31] As an aside, he observed no effect of age on extent of degeneration.[54]

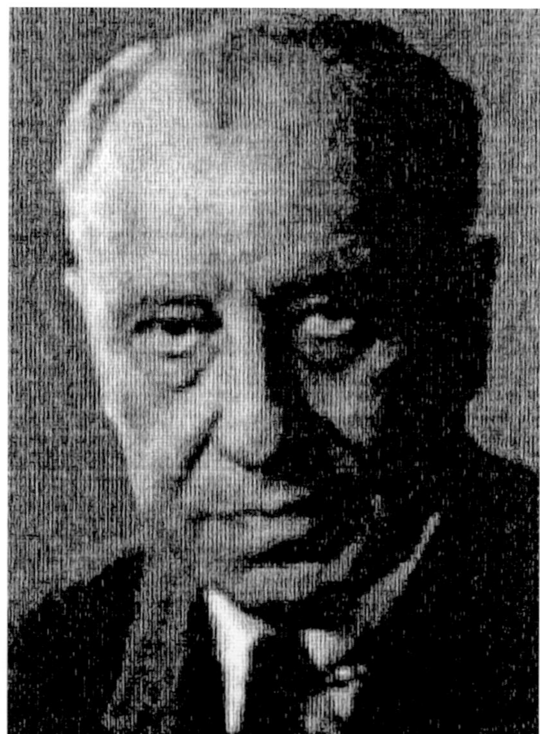

FIGURE 3-15. Friedrich Pauwels focused on musculoskeletal biomechanics research.

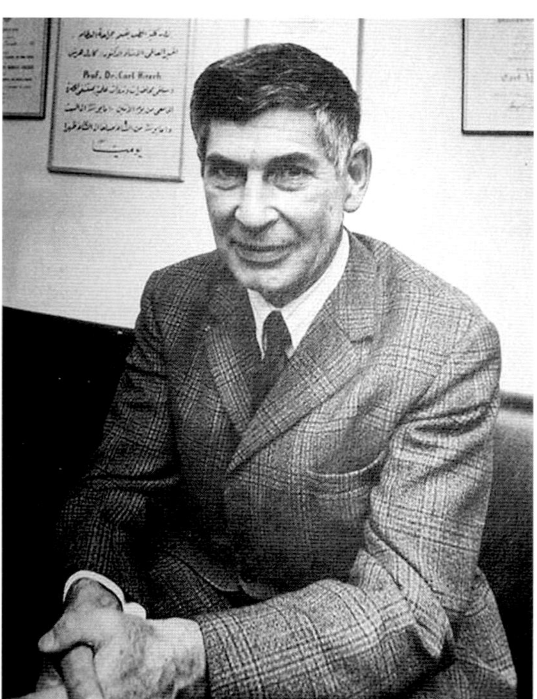

FIGURE 3-16. Carl Hirsch is known as the founder of modern biomechanics.

Advanced studies were performed on the effect of bending moments on the spine. Load-deflection, energy-absorption, and other analyses were performed by Virgin,[55] Hirsch,[56] Hirsch and Nachemson,[57] Hirsch and Schajowicz,[58] Hirsch,[59] Evans,[60,61] Evans and Lissner,[49] Higgins,[62] Friberg and Hirsch,[63] Sylven et al.,[64] and Werne.[65] Carl Hirsch (Fig. 3-16) (1913–1973), a Swedish orthopaedic surgeon, had substantial influence on the development of biomechanics. His interest centered on the knee, hip, and spine in the 1940s.[56] He applied his knowledge and findings to orthopaedic problems. He attracted many visitors and fellows to his laboratory, including Victor Frankel, George Galante, Augustus White, Wilson C. Hayes, and Albert B. Scultz, and many of his fellows went on to establish their own biomechanics laboratories.[31]

Finite Element Analysis

Finite element analysis (FEA), developed by R. Courant and Hilbert[66] in 1943, is a technique originally developed for numerical analysis of complex structural mechanics problems. FEA is based on the idea of building complicated objects from small manageable pieces and is used by engineers in the aerospace industry. Applied to spinal biomechanics, it takes the whole spine and breaks it down into smaller geometric forms at any given level, which can individually be tested and analyzed more easily. Computer programs can then derive composite analyses of discrete finite elements. Using this method, the risk of spinal injury in emergency pilot ejection was investigated for the first time in the second half of 1950s.[67] This technique has become popular for biomechanical testing of the spine in recent years due to its cost-effectiveness.

Clinical Studies

High-quality evidence from clinical trials provided a new valuable source of data. New definitions of "stability" and associated scoring systems were developed and utilized.[68] The column system for spinal stability assessment was first introduced as a two-column system, defined in 1962 by Sir Frank Holdsworth.[69] A three-column system, proposed by Francis Denis,[70] provided further refinement. For tumor-related instability, a six-column system[71] and a cube system for ventral column stability were described.[39] These studies exemplify the transition of evidence obtained from the biomechanical laboratory to clinically applicable knowledge.

Summary

The field of spine biomechanics has evolved from the time of antiquity to the present. The first 2000 years provided the rich seeds with requisite advancements in spinal anatomy, neurophysiology, mathematics, and physics. In the last century, we have seen the field of spinal biomechanics blossom and grow exponentially along with modern technology. Though the technology of today dwarfs historical feats of the past, the essence of the journey remains the same: the pains-staking battle involved in problem-solving and the search for new answers. An appreciation of the previous trodden path can enlighten the footsteps in search of knowledge and innovation.

KEY REFERENCES

Goodrich JT: History of spine surgery in the ancient and medieval worlds. *Neurosurg Focus* 16:E2, 2004.

Hirt S: What is kinesiology? A historical review. *Phys Ther Rev* 35:419–426, 1955.

Marketos SG, Skiadas P: Hippocrates. The father of spine surgery. *Spine* 24:1381–1387, 1999.

Marketos SG, Skiadas PK: Galen. A pioneer of spine research. *Spine* 24:2358–2362, 1999.

Naderi S, Andalkar N, Benzel EC: History of spine biomechanics. Part I. The pre-Greco-Roman, Greco-Roman, and medieval roots of spine biomechanics. *Neurosurgery* 60(2):382–390, 2007; discussion 390–391.

Naderi S, Andalkar N, Benzel EC: History of spine biomechanics. Part II. From the Renaissance to the 20th century. *Neurosurgery* 60(2): 392–403, 2007; discussion 403–404.

REFERENCES

The complete reference list is available online at expertconsult.com.

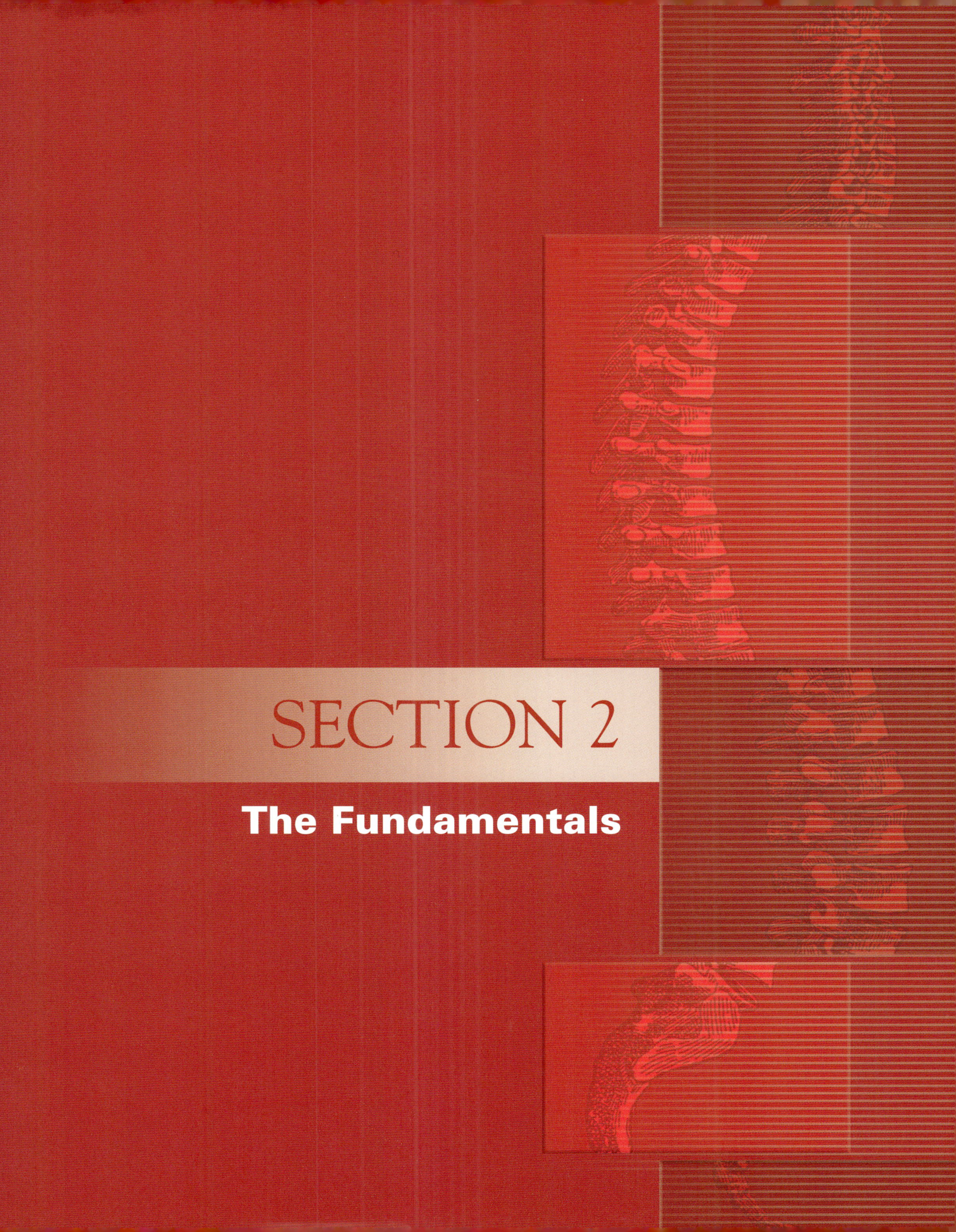

SECTION 2

The Fundamentals

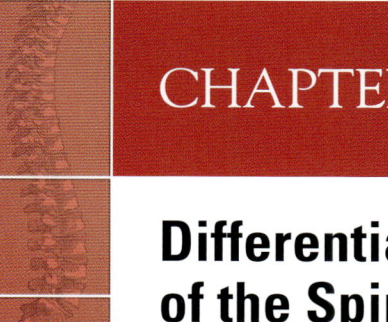

CHAPTER 4

Differential Diagnosis of Surgical Disorders of the Spine

Robert M. Starke | Kai-Ming G. Fu | Justin S. Smith | Christopher I. Shaffrey

Establishing a differential diagnosis of spine pathology starts with the characterization of pain, associated signs and symptoms, and evaluation of any presenting neurologic deficit. Special attention must be paid to the warning signs and symptoms of back pain (Box 4-1), which helps to identify more serious pathology.[1] Assessment of pain in conjunction with fever and weight loss, recumbent position, morning stiffness, acute onset, or visceral component allows for initial categorization. With this information, further laboratory and radiologic evaluation can proceed, and ultimately, a diagnosis with appropriate surgical or medical management can usually be achieved.

This chapter presents a systematic approach to evaluating a patient with a suspected spine disorder (Box 4-2). The first portion of this chapter addresses disorders that usually present with spinal pain, and the second half deals with conditions that present with pain and neurologic deficit.

Spinal Pain

Pain Associated with Fever and Weight Loss

Infectious or neoplastic processes are potential etiologies in patients who present with fever, weight loss, and spinal pain. The most common infectious conditions affecting the spine include vertebral osteomyelitis, discitis, epidural abscess, and granulomatous processes. Neoplastic processes may have similar presentations. Failure to uncover the etiology may lead to neurologic deficits but usually not until pain and systemic symptoms have been present for some time.

Vertebral Osteomyelitis

Vertebral osteomyelitis, the most common pyogenic infection of the axial skeleton, occurs in 2% to 19% of cases of osteomyelitis.[2-4] Adults can present with an indolent or chronic course; the pediatric and immunocompromised groups can present more acutely. Diffuse back pain and fever are the most common symptoms, occurring in approximately 90% and 45% of patients, respectively.[2-4] Weight loss, radicular symptoms, myelopathy, spine deformity, and meningeal irritation also occur. In some cases, neurologic deficits can be the presenting complaint.

A definitive source of infection is found in approximately 40% of cases. The most common organisms that are isolated are the gram-positive cocci, *Staphylococcus aureus* being the most common organism.[2-4] Other organisms such as *Escherichia coli*, *Pseudomonas aeruginosa*, and *Proteus* are potential sources in parenteral drug abusers or immunocompromised patients.

Diagnosis is based on pertinent laboratory findings, including an elevated erythrocyte sedimentation rate, blood and bone cultures, and elevated white blood cell count. MRI is the gold standard for detection of osteomyelitis.[2-5] Bone scans are useful for diagnosis, but care in interpretation is required, as other processes can have similar imaging qualities.

Epidural Abscess

Spinal epidural abscess occurs more frequently in adults. Pain is the most common presentation, but fever, leukocytosis, and neurologic compromise occur more frequently in epidural abscess than in osteomyelitis.[4,6] Epidural abscesses most commonly affect the thoracic spine, followed by lumbar and cervical locations. Common etiologies include a direct extension of a preexisting osteomyelitis, hematogenous spread from a distant focus, or, less likely, trauma.[4,6]

As with vertebral osteomyelitis, the most prevalent species is *S. aureus*, followed by other staphylococcal and streptococcal species or gram-negative rods.[4,6] Laboratory studies, including erythrocyte sedimentation rate and white blood cell count, are elevated in the majority of patients, and MRI is the diagnostic imaging of choice.[4,6]

BOX 4-1. Warning Signs and Symptoms of Lower Back Pain

- New onset of pain in patients >50 years or <20 years
- Pain worse at night
- Pain worse in supine position
- Bowel or bladder incontinence
- Saddle anesthesia
- Motor weakness
- Weight loss
- Fever
- History of cancer or immunosuppression

BOX 4-2. Differential Diagnosis of Surgical Disorders of the Spine

Spinal Pain

Pain with fever and weight loss
- Vertebral osteomyelitis
- Epidural abscess
- Discitis
- Tuberculous spondylitis
- Actinomycosis
- Nocardiosis
- Brucellosis
- Fungal infections
- Coccidioidomycosis
- Blastomycosis
- Cryptococcosis
- Candidiasis
- Aspergillosis
- Wegener granulomatosis
- Syphilis
- Parasitic infections (e.g., echinococcosis)

Pain with recumbency and night pain
- Extradural lesions
  - Metastatic disease
  - Multiple myeloma
  - Chondrosarcoma
  - Chordoma
  - Lymphoma
  - Osteogenic sarcoma and Ewing sarcoma
  - Osteochondroma
  - Giant cell tumor
  - Osteoid osteoma and osteoblastoma
  - Aneurysmal bone cyst
  - Hemangioma and eosinophilic granuloma
  - Synovial cyst
- Intradural-extramedullary lesions
  - Meningiomas
  - Schwannomas
  - Neurofibromas
  - Sarcomas
  - Dermoids
  - Epidermoids
  - Arachnoid cysts
  - Teratomas
  - Ganglion cyst
  - Spinal metastasis
  - Arachnoiditis
- Intradural-intramedullary lesions
  - Ependymomas astrocytomas
  - Metastases
  - Hemangioblastomas
  - Arteriovenous malformation
  - Syringomyelia

Pain associated with morning stiffness
- Ankylosing spondylitis
- Rheumatoid arthritis
- Spinal stenosis
- Spondylolisthesis and spondylolysis
- Herniated nucleus pulposus
- Scoliosis

Acute spinal pain and visceral pain
- Metabolic disorders
- Endocrinologic disorders
- Vascular disorders
- Gastrointestinal disorders

Neurologic Deficits
- Congenital lesions and spinal dysraphism
  - Diastematomyelia, diplomyelia, tether cord, filum lipoma, congenital scoliosis
- Trauma
- Ischemia
- Vascular malformations
  - Arteriovenous fistulas, cavernous malformations, Foix-Alajouanine syndrome
- Intracranial lesions
- Central montine myelinolysis
- Multiple sclerosis
- Transverse myelitis
- Inflammatory disorders
- Infectious disorders
  - Viral myelitis, encephalitis, poliomyelitis, ganglionitis, herpes zoster, cytomegalovirus, herpes simplex, HIV disorders
- Upper motor neuron syndromes
  - Hereditary spastic paraplegia, lathyrism, adrenoleukodystrophy
- Lower motor neuron syndromes
  - Spinal muscular atrophy, muscular dystrophy
- Combined upper and lower motor neuron syndromes
  - Amyotrophic lateral sclerosis
- Miscellaneous
  - Subacute combined degeneration, Guillain-Barré syndrome, diphtheria, acute intermittent porphyria, toxic peripheral neuropathies, paraneoplastic syndromes, postirradiation myelopathy, Kesson disease, familial periodic paralysis

Discitis

Spontaneous discitis is rare in the adult but occurs in 1% to 3% of surgical discectomy patients.[7,8] Clinical presentation reveals back pain at the operated level, usually from 1 to 3 weeks postoperatively. The most common presentation is back pain and painful ambulation, as the lumbar spine is the most common location. Staphylococcal and streptococcal species are the most common organisms. Again, diagnosis is aided by laboratory studies, MRI, and bone scans.

Granulomatous Infections

Granulomatous infections include all processes that produce the classic histologic granuloma. These processes include fungal, spirochetal, and uncommon bacterial organisms (such as *Actinomyces*, *Nocardia*, and *Brucella*) and the most common organism, *Mycobacterium tuberculosis*.

Tuberculous Spondylitis

Although uncommon in developed countries, tuberculous spondylitis is the most common of the granulomatous infections that affect the axial skeleton.[9-11] Recently, there has been a resurgence in developed countries due to the rise of HIV.[12,13] Clinical presentation involves pain over the affected site, fever, malaise, and weight loss.[9-11] In the progressive stages of disease, kyphosis results from erosive bone destruction. Epidural abscesses and paraparesis are possible late sequelae.[9-11] Tuberculous spondylitis is usually caused by M. *tuberculosis*; however, other species of mycobacteria may be encountered. A positive purified protein derivative can be helpful, although false negatives can occur in the anergic patient due to advanced age, malnutrition, or immunocompromise. Diagnosis requires evaluation of urine, sputum, or a sample from a gastric specimen, subcutaneous nodule, or bone biopsy. A chest radiograph reveals no evidence of pulmonary disease in 40% to 50% of cases. MRI is superior to evaluate soft tissue involvement and the presence of abscess formation, and CT provides better bone detail.

Fungal Infections

Fungal infections of the axial skeleton are uncommon. Infections of the spine occur most commonly as the result of pulmonic spread following spore inhalation. Spine osseous involvement with disseminated fungal infection occurs in 10% to 50% of patients with coccidioidomycosis and blastomycosis infections. There is a much lower incidence of *Cryptococcus* infection, candidiasis, or aspergillosis, which may occur in immunocompromised individuals.

Coccidioidomycosis

Coccidioidomycosis, endemic in the southwestern United States, has a high rate of spine involvement and occurs in 20% to 40% of cases of disseminated disease. Vertebral collapse and neurologic compromise are uncommon.[14] Radiographs reveal multiple simultaneous lytic lesions. Diagnosis is made with plain radiographs, immunodiffusion titers, and biopsy.

Blastomycosis

This species is endemic to the Mississippi River Valley and is spread after inhalation and pulmonic infection. Blastomycosis is hematogenously spread with a predilection for ventral vertebral body involvement, resulting in vertebral collapse, joint erosion, and disc invasion. Clinical presentation resembles that of tuberculous spondylitis; however, blastomycosis more commonly is associated with draining sinuses and has a greater predisposition to include the dorsal elements.[15,16]

Cryptococcus

Cryptococcus neoformans is a fungal organism that may cause infection in immunocompromised patients, mostly commonly those afflicted with AIDS. It is usually inhaled and then spreads hematogenously from a pulmonary location, with osseous involvement occurring in only 10% of cases with disseminated disease.[17,18] The usual clinical presentation is swelling, pain, and decreased mobility of the affected vertebral site. Radiographs reveal dorsal vertebral body involvement and disc space sparing. Diagnosis is made via a latex agglutination test, cerebrospinal fluid (CSF) analysis, and blood cultures.

Pain Associated with Recumbency and Night Pain

Nocturnal pain and pain associated with recumbency are hallmarks of destructive lesions of the vertebral column, caused by either a skeletal metastasis or a primary bone tumor. Unfortunately, the majority of spinal column tumors are malignant. Pain is the most frequent clinical presentation, occurring in up to 85% of patients. There are correlations among age, location, incidence, and presentation. Younger patients tend to have a greater incidence of benign bone tumors, whereas those older than age 30 are more likely to have malignancy.

Benign Bone Tumors

Benign bone tumors occur more frequently in patients between ages 20 and 30, in a dorsal location and in the lumbar spine. Oosteochondroma, osteoid osteoma, and osteoblastoma are the most common benign lesions of the axial skeleton and have a lower incidence of recurrence overall compared with malignant bone tumors.

Osteochondroma

These lesions are the most common benign bone tumors, encompassing approximately 35% of all nonmalignant osseous tumors. These tumors arise from the cartilaginous end plates and are slow-growing tumors.[19,20] The majority are asymptomatic lumbar spine lesions found on incidental radiographs. Symptomatic patients commonly present with dull backache, decreased motion, or, rarely, deformity. Plain radiographs demonstrate a protruding lesion with well-demarcated borders in the dorsal elements. On rare occasions, pain, neurologic deficit, or an accelerated growth pattern may be related to malignant transformation.

Osteoid Osteoma and Osteoblastoma

These two tumor types share a common pathologic origin but differ in size and incidence of spine involvement. Both tumors most commonly present in patients less than 30 years of age. Osteoid osteomas are smaller than osteoblastomas (≤2 cm vs. >2 cm). Osteoid osteomas are most commonly located in the lumbar spine and account for 2.6% of all excised primary bone tumors and up to 18% of axial lesions. Osteoblastomas are less common and represent fewer than 3% of benign bone tumors.

Patients with osteoid osteomas commonly present with a dull ache that is exacerbated at night. This condition is believed to be the result of prostaglandin production by the tumor; thus, the classic pain relief with aspirin. Neurologic deficits are rare. Osteoblastomas are more likely to result in spinal deformity and neurologic sequelae, including torticollis in 13% of cervical lesions. Plain films are pathognomonic, revealing a small radiolucent nidus with surrounding sclerosis usually located in the dorsal elements.[21,22]

Giant Cell Tumor

Unlike the majority of primary bone tumors, giant cell tumors occur more commonly in patients in their 30s. The most common presentation is that of pain. However, disease advancement may result in bowel or bladder dysfunction. These aggressive tumors carry some malignant potential and a high incidence of local recurrence. They are responsible for approximately 10% of all primary benign bone tumors and affect the spinal axis in approximately 10% of all cases. These lesions may occur in conjunction with aneurysmal bone cysts (3% to 6%).[23,24] They most commonly occur in the sacral region when the spinal column is involved. Plain radiographs demonstrate cortical expansion with little reactive sclerosis or periosteal reaction.[23,24] Both T1- and T2-weighted MRI scans reveal homogeneous signals, whereas presurgical CT studies can better delineate the degree of vertebral bone involvement. Because of the nondistinct characteristics of giant cell tumors, radiographic investigation, coupled with intraoperative histology, is important to separate this condition from other primary bone tumors.

Aneurysmal Bone Cyst

Although responsible for only approximately 1% to 2% of all primary bone tumors, aneurysmal bone cysts affect the axial skeleton in 12% to 25% of reported cases of aneurysmal bone cysts.[24] They occur more frequently in the thoracolumbar region and dorsal elements in females and patients younger than 20 years of age. Multiple vertebral involvement occurs in 40% of cases. Radiographs demonstrate a single osteolytic lesion with a thin, well-demarcated cortical rim.

Hemangioma

Hemangiomas are found in 11% of general autopsies,[25,26] but symptomatic spinal hemangiomas are exceedingly rare. The most common initial symptom in the case of a solitary lesion is back pain, with or without radiation into the lower extremities.[25,26] These lesions are characterized by slow growth and a female predominance.

Eosinophilic Granuloma

Eosinophilic granuloma is the solitary osseous lesion version of a group of disorders characterized by an abnormal proliferation of Langerhans cells. In its disseminated forms, it is designated Letterer-Siwe disease and Hand-Schüller-Christian disease. The overall incidence for any variety of the histiocytosis X spectrum is one per million people, and it most commonly occurs in patients younger than 20 years of age. Clinical presentation most commonly involves pain in the thoracolumbar region. MRI is the investigative procedure of choice, with definitive diagnosis through biopsy.[27]

Malignant Bone Tumors

Chondrosarcoma

This malignant cartilage-forming primary bone tumor is an uncommon spinal neoplasm. It is more common in adults, in whom it less commonly involves the spine.[28] There is an even distribution of tumor involvement among cervical, thoracic, and lumbar locations.[25] Chondrosarcomas may arise as a primary lesion or secondary to irradiation of lesions, including Paget disease or osteochondroma.[29] The most common presentation is pain (50%) and localized swelling (30%). There is a linear relationship between degree of pain on presentation; a larger, more aggressive tumor; and decreased time of survival.[30,31] Diagnosis is usually based on radiographic studies that reveal bone destruction, a soft tissue mass, and "fluffy" calcifications and pathology from resection.[30,31]

Osteogenic Sarcoma and Ewing Sarcoma

Both osteogenic sarcoma and Ewing sarcoma represent uncommon malignant lesions of the spinal column, with a combined incidence of less than 4% of spinal column tumors.[32-34] Most cases of Ewing sarcoma and primary osteogenic sarcoma (50%) present in the first 20 years of life. Secondary sarcomas arise in the fifth to sixth decades as a result of irradiated bone or a preexisting pagetoid lesion. Almost 70% of clinical presentations are accompanied by a neurologic deficit secondary to epidural compression.[32-34] The most common presentation of Ewing sarcoma is pain.

Chordoma

Chordomas are tumors of the axial skeleton and the skull base arising from the primitive notochord. They encompass approximately 1.4% of all skeletal sarcomas. Although chordomas are histologically low-grade lesions, they are locally invasive tumors, and metastases may occur in 5% to 43% of cases.[35-37] More than 50% of these lesions are located in the lumbosacral region, 35% are located in the clival and cervical area, and the remainder are spread throughout the rest of the vertebral column.[37] Neurologic deficit is usually found in the form of bowel/bladder dysfunction or, less frequently, cauda equina symptoms (20%).[37] Combined imaging, using MRI and CT, provides an evaluation of the tumor and its soft tissue and bony involvement.

Multiple Myeloma

Multiple myeloma and solitary plasmacytoma account for 45% of all malignant bone tumors.[38] These disorders are the result of abnormal proliferation of plasma cells, which are responsible for immunoglobulin and antibody production and affect the spine in 30% to 50% of reported cases. Multiple myeloma is primarily a disease of the sixth and seventh decades of life and has a predilection for the thoracic spine (50% to 60%).

Patients present with back pain in approximately 75% of cases.[38] Unlike the classic metastatic disease presentation of pain with recumbency, multiple myeloma is sometimes relieved by rest and aggravated by mechanical agitation that mimics other sciatic or neurogenic sources. Systemic complications include hyperalbuminemia, renal insufficiency, nephrolithiasis, and characteristic serum protein abnormalities. Plain radiographs and CT can be diagnostic because of the characteristic osteolytic picture without sclerotic edges that involve the ventral portion of the vertebral body and usually spare the dorsal elements.

Lymphoma

Hodgkin disease is a malignant disease of the reticuloendothelial system. Spine involvement occurs in approximately 10% of all extranodal lymphomas.[39,40] Spine osseous involvement occurs at a decreasing frequency as one ascends the spine from the lumbar, thoracic, and, uncommonly, cervical regions. Age at presentation is bimodal, with those ages 15 to 35 and those older than age 50 most frequently affected. Clinical presentation involves concurrent constitutional signs and symptoms of fever and night sweats, and acute cord compression and epidural compression are not uncommon.[39,40]

Metastatic Disease

Metastatic disease in the form of distant foci is evident at autopsy in 40% to 85% of cases of malignancy.[41] The spine is the most common site of skeletal metastasis, and at least 5% of patients with malignancies suffer from this condition.[41,42] The axial skeleton is the leading site of bone metastases that are caused by hematogenous spread through the rich venous network that drains the lungs, pelvis, and thorax. Breast, lung, prostate, and thyroid malignancies account for 50% to 60% of metastatic lesions.[41] Overall, epidural metastases are equally spread throughout the thoracic and lumbosacral spine, but symptomatic metastases occur most commonly in the thoracic spine. Nearly all patients initially complain of back pain, followed by weakness and ataxia. At the time of diagnosis, more than 50% of patients will have a paraparesis or bladder/bowel disturbance.[41,43]

Diagnostic regimens include laboratory studies demonstrating an elevated calcium level, prostate-specific antigen, or alkaline phosphatase. The ultimate diagnosis relies on radiographic studies, including plain radiographs. Bone scans are warranted for suspected occult lesions because approximately 30% to 50% of the trabeculated bone in a vertebral body must be destroyed before the lesions can be detected on plain radiography. Other radiographic modalities, including MRI and CT/myelography and positron emission tomography (PET) scans, are helpful in determining the extent of bone destruction, epidural compression, and disease spread. A metastatic workup, including both a plain chest radiograph and an enhanced abdominal/chest CT, determines the primary focus in the majority of cases. Pathologic confirmation may be made via biopsy of a primary malignant focus or via biopsy or resection of the spinal lesion.

Spinal Cord Tumors

The majority of lesions that involve the spinal cord and meninges occur in the epidural space in the form of metastatic disease. The largest group of neoplastic spinal lesions that involve the spinal cord and meninges occurs in the intradural-extramedullary space (40–50%), followed by the extradural space (30%) and the intramedullary space (20–25%).[43,44]

Back pain is the most common initial complaint in the adult population that harbors spinal neoplasms; the pediatric population with spinal tumors tends to present with neurologic deficit in the form of motor or gait disturbances. The back pain in the adult population is usually diffuse and unrelated to activity, thus prolonging diagnosis until the pain becomes radicular or symptoms that are caused by cord or root compression ensue.

Extradural Lesions

Symptoms may be caused by compression, invasion, or irritation of the involved anatomy. The majority of epidural lesions discussed earlier in the chapter are metastatic in origin. Other epidural pathologies include lipomatous masses, hematomas, and vascular malformations.

Intradural-Extramedullary Lesions

Meningiomas, schwannomas, and neurofibromas constitute more than 50% of all neoplastic processes in the intradural-extramedullary space. Nittner's review of 4885 adults with spinal cord tumors found schwannomas (23%) and meningiomas (22%) to be the most common lesions of the intradural-extramedullary space.[45,46] Symptoms may be nocturnal and most commonly involve pain caused by root irritation. Early neurologic compromise is uncommon because of the adaptive compressibility of surrounding fat, CSF, and adjacent vascular structures. Neurologic compromise occurs when the compliance of surrounding structures is at its nadir and extradural compression is directly transmitted to the spinal cord.

More than 80% of meningiomas are located in the thoracic region, and they occur at a 4:1 ratio in women compared to men. Meningiomas can present with pain from a compressed nerve root as it exits the neural foramina. Although less common in the cervical and lumbar spine, large, slow-growing meningiomas may produce myelopathic symptoms from spinal cord compression, especially at the craniocervical junction.[47] Meningiomas are the most common benign tumor at the foramen magnum.[48,49] CT myelogram and MRI are the best investigative modalities.

Although both meningiomas and nerve sheath tumors are benign lesions that are usually found in thoracic dorsal sites, neurofibromas are a common finding in phakomatoses. Because neurofibromas are almost always lesions of the dorsal roots, patients commonly present with radicular symptoms.[50-52] Although their malignancy potential is low, nerve sheath tumors may be locally destructive if allowed to progress. Caudally located neurofibromas may displace adjacent nerve roots with possible bone erosion of nearby foramina as the neoplasm grows.

Schwannomas, which are commonly found with von Recklinghausen neurofibromatosis, are usually solitary lesions found in thoracic sites in adults between 40 and 50 years of age. These tumors are most commonly found in the intradural-extramedullary space; however, approximately 20% will be found crossing the dura or will be solely extradural. On clinical presentation, patients with these tumors exhibit radicular symptoms, and the tumor is typically easily diagnosed with MRI.

The remaining 30% of intradural-extramedullary tumors include sarcomas, dermoids, epidermoids, arachnoid cysts, teratomas, ganglion cysts, and, rarely, spinal metastases.[53,54] These lesions have characteristic features on MRI that help to delineate them. Arachnoiditis that presents with diffuse constant pain and associated paresthesias is the result of multiple operations on the back or clumping of nerve roots after the administration of the myelographic dye. The diagnosis is made via MRI or myelogram with visualization of characteristic nerve root clumping.

Intradural-Intramedullary Tumors

Intramedullary spinal cord tumors account for 2% to 4% of CNS neoplasms and are of neuroglial origin in 80% of cases, regardless of age.[55-58] More than 90% of these tumors are rostral to the conus in patients under age 15.[55-59] Children are predisposed to astrocytic tumors, whereas adult pathology is more evenly spread over the neuroglial spectrum.[55-59] There is a shift in pathology with increasing age, with ependymomas becoming more common than astrocytomas. The incidence of intramedullary spinal cord tumors increases from rostral to caudal and may present with insidious pain, the most common finding in the adult population, or associated spinal cord dysfunction in the form of band paresthesias or motor deficit. Typically, the pain associated with these lesions is unrelated to mechanical activity. Pediatric patients tend to present with gait or motor disturbances.[55-59]

Other intramedullary disorders such as arteriovenous malformation (AVM), syringomyelia, and metastases are potential but extremely rare causes of spinal pain. AVMs and hemangioblastomas of the spinal cord are potential causes of acute pain with subsequent neurologic sequelae secondary to rupture, resulting in hematoma formation or ischemic effects.

Diagnostic studies include plain radiographs that can reveal widened pedicles or a myelogram that shows a diffuse enlargement of a cord segment. MRI is the gold standard to evaluate spinal cord dysfunction as a result of the aforementioned causes, with the exception of angiography to evaluate AVMs.

Pain Associated with Morning Stiffness

Axial pain, with a prolonged tapering course after the initiation of increasing mechanical activity, heralds the possibility of an inflammatory disorder affecting the spine. The two most common chronic inflammatory processes that involve the axial skeleton are rheumatoid arthritis (RA) and ankylosing spondylitis (AS).

Ankylosing Spondylitis

AS is the most prevalent of the seronegative spondyloarthropathies, with an incidence of up to 2% in the Caucasian population. It is a common cause of axial pain in young adults.[60-62] Unlike RA, it has a male predominance, and it is most commonly found in the axial skeleton with a mild degree of peripheral involvement. The pathogenesis is unclear, but there is a strong immunologic association with HLA-B27 positivity in approximately 95% of patients. The disease progresses in an ascending fashion from caudal to rostral, which can result in severe flexion deformity if allowed to continue.[60,62] The prototypical lesion is enthesopathic, affecting insertion sites of tendons and ligaments to bone. The typical presentation is that of a young white male between ages 15 and 30, with insidious low back pain (LBP) (80–90%), peripheral joint pain in the hip or shoulder (20–40%), and sciatic pain (5%).[60,62] Diagnosis is based on a history of back pain and grades 3 to 4 bilateral sacroiliitis observed on plain radiographs. There have been several revisions of the original criteria for AS, but all accept the radiologic changes with a history of insidious onset of back pain, age younger than 40, persistence for more than 3 months, morning stiffness, improvement with exercise, and limitation of chest expansion.[60-63] Because it takes from 3 to 7 years for the radiographic evidence of bilateral symmetrical sacroiliitis to become evident, a loss of axial mobility, back pain, and morning stiffness are important early signs and symptoms.[60-63] Associated fractures, spinal stenosis, and rotary instability are the end result of a fused vertebral column.[62,64-66]

Rheumatoid Arthritis

RA, a chronic inflammatory process that affects the synovium of peripheral joints, has a quoted prevalence of 1% for both genders by age 65, but is an uncommon cause of back pain. Unlike AS, this disease affects an older patient population, has a female predominance, is found most often in the cervical spine, and often results in spinal instability.[67-71] RA affects the cervical spine most commonly in one of three ways: atlantoaxial subluxation, basilar invagination, and subaxial subluxation.[67-71] Diagnosis of RA is based on the history, the distribution of joint involvement, and a positive rheumatoid factor. Neck pain should warrant a thorough radiographic evaluation, including flexion/extension radiographs and MRI for ligamentous visualization. Radiographic sequelae include soft tissue swelling, narrowing of joint spaces, and, ultimately, bone erosion.

Other rheumatologic disorders of the spine include the remainder of the seronegative spondyloarthropathies such as Reiter disease, Behçet syndrome, Whipple disease, and enteropathic arthritis, as well as osteoarthritis. These conditions represent other possible causes of back pain, with or without deformity.

Mechanical Pain

Anywhere from 40% to 80% of the adult population has LBP sometime before age 50.[1] Ninety percent of cases are a result of mechanical causes. Pain without constitutional signs and symptoms that is initiated and exacerbated by activity is a large category that includes lumbar strain, disc protrusion and extrusion, spinal stenosis, spondylolisthesis, spondylolysis, and soft tissue irritation disorders, such as those in the piriform syndrome. Other entities such as sacroiliac joint dysfunction, facet syndrome, dural ectasia, perineural or ganglion cysts, and collagen disorders (Ehlers-Danlos syndrome) are less well-differentiated causes of LBP and are usually clinically diagnosed. To evaluate degenerative spine disorders, it is necessary to determine the character of pain, whether it be LBP alone or associated with radicular symptoms, symptomatic neurogenic claudication, or, rarely, myelopathy. Clinical history of onset and duration of symptoms, age, presence of a congenital disorder, and spinal deformity help to differentiate among the more common degenerative lesions. MRI and CT/myelogram are most commonly used to evaluate degenerative spine disorders.

Spinal Stenosis

Whether acquired, as in the elderly, or congenital (e.g., in the achondroplastic dwarf), spinal stenosis has a common clinical presentation.[72] The classic bilateral low back, buttock, and thigh pain, consistent with neurogenic claudication associated with activity, can be present whether the patient is standing (94%) or has walked a short distance.[72] Neurogenic claudication must be differentiated from vascular claudication. The clinical picture of vascular claudication reveals progressive calf pain after ambulation, with associated decreased peripheral pulses and chronic tissue changes seen in cool distal extremities. Spinal stenosis is a clinical entity with radiologic confirmation of a decreased spinal canal observed on axial MRI or CT/myelogram views.

Spondylolisthesis and Spondylolysis

Spondylolisthesis and spondylolysis are common causes of back pain in both the pediatric and adult population, with L5 the most common site of involvement.[72-74] The adult population tends to have a more vague and insidious presentation, with back pain as the most common complaint, followed by claudication and hamstring tightness, probably caused by concurrent spinal stenosis. Approximately 20% have spine deformity that can be detected on physical examination.

Herniated Nucleus Pulposus

Herniated nucleus pulposus is a common cause of radicular pain in adults ages 30 to 40. Only 35% of those who present with a herniated nucleus pulposus experience sciatica. The pain is usually sharp and follows a dermatomal pattern. Diagnosis includes clinical findings consistent with the affected nerve root in the form of sensory, reflex, or motor deficits.[7,8]

Other causes of back pain that may present in either a radicular pattern or with diffuse symptoms are a conjoined nerve root or perineural cyst; both may be detected by MRI.

Scoliosis

Scoliosis represents another potential cause of back pain in adults who suffer from LBP. Lumbar degenerative scoliosis with a Cobb angle greater than 10 degrees is reportedly present in approximately 7.5% of the adult back pain population, with an increasing prevalence with age.[75-80] As age increases, the proportion of women who have scoliosis as a cause of both back pain and radicular symptoms increases.[75-80]

Neurologic Deficits

Spinal cord and column dysfunction can be manifested by a variety of pain, motor, sensory, muscle tone, and bladder disturbances. Pain can be of local, radicular, or diffuse (dull ache) origin. Motor weakness can range from complete and acute to chronically progressive, taking the form of clumsiness. Sensory disturbances include dysesthesias, paresthesias, or complete anesthesia. Muscle tone abnormalities range from atonia to spasticity. A spinal lesion results in either a spastic or an atonic bladder, depending on the level of the lesion. Pathologic processes of the spinal cord and column caused by congenital, traumatic, vascular, neoplastic, infectious or inflammatory, degenerative, or environmental causes generally reflect a spinal cord syndrome in the form of neurologic deficit with one or a combination of the aforementioned symptoms.

The time course of a neurologic deficit, in conjunction with a spinal cord syndrome, helps to formulate a differential diagnosis. This diagnosis of spinal cord dysfunction can then be grouped broadly into a compressive or noncompressive neurologic lesion that is further classified by the time course of deficit progression.

Congenital Lesions

In the majority of significant neural tube developmental disorders, a physical examination at birth reveals a spine defect, with or without neurologic dysfunction. Other disorders such as tethered cord or congenital scoliosis may remain occult until symptoms present, secondary to spinal column growth. These lesions will be discussed further in Chapter 7.

Trauma

Patients who present with a history of trauma provide an obvious clue to the differential diagnosis of their acute spinal cord dysfunction. Traumatic injury of the spinal cord and column can be either direct or indirect. In direct trauma, often a knife or gunshot assault, there is violation of the dura mater. In indirect trauma caused by fracture-dislocation, pure fracture, or pure dislocation, the dura mater is often intact. Mechanisms of indirect trauma include flexion, extension, rotation, and compression. Other causes of spinal cord malfunction after trauma include spinal cord contusion, compression of adjacent vessels with resultant ischemia, and epidural compression caused by hemorrhage.

Posttraumatic syringomyelia should be included in the differential diagnosis of any patient who develops deterioration of motor function with an ascending sensory level after traumatic quadriparesis or paraparesis. Approximately 11% of all cases of syringomyelia are reported to be caused by trauma, whereas 3% of cases with severe cervical trauma with paraplegia/quadriplegia are said to result in posttraumatic syringomyelia.[81,82] Its course of symptom development ranges from 2 months to 36 years. It is found most often in the thoracolumbar region. Clinical presentation involves pain, ascending sensory level, motor deficits, and loss of reflexes above the previous lesion. MRI is the imaging procedure of choice to evaluate for a posttraumatic syrinx.

Vascular Lesions

Acute or rapid subacute onset of paraplegia or quadriplegia without evidence of trauma suggests a vascular event involving the spinal cord. A slowly progressive myelopathy or radiculopathy can also be caused by vascular etiologies. These causes include occlusion, inflammatory disorders, hemorrhage, and vascular malformations.

Ischemia

Individuals with circulatory insufficiency in the legs may harbor disease of the abdominal aorta with resultant spinal cord ischemia. Thromboembolic occlusion of spinal segmental arteries (e.g., the artery of Adamkiewicz) and dissection, clamping, or severe atheroma of the aorta are the most common causes of spinal cord infarction.[83] The anterior cord syndrome is a typical clinical presentation of ischemic spinal cord insult. The midthoracic level is the most common site of ischemia because it lies in a vascular watershed zone.

In the less common cases of painless infarction of the spinal cord caused by systemic hypotension, low thoracic and lumbosacral spinal cord central gray matter involvement is observed. Vasculitis and systemic embolism are rare causes of spinal cord ischemia. Polyarteritis nodosa and primary granulomatous angiitis, a neural vasculature disorder without systemic involvement often found with lymphoma, are rare causes of a sometimes painful acute or chronic myelopathy.[84,85] Among the vascular causes of paraplegia and quadriplegia, anterior spinal artery thrombosis is the most common. Although occlusion of the anterior spinal artery is uncommon, ischemia, in its region of supply, occurs relatively often. This is usually caused by disease of the aorta or segmental branches that supply the anterior spinal artery. The anterior spinal artery syndrome, also known as anterior cord syndrome, consists of motor paralysis (upper and lower motor neuron), dissociated sensory loss (pain and temperature), and sphincter paralysis. It results from an infarction in the region of the anterior spinal artery that supplies the vertical two thirds of the spinal cord and is usually the consequence of thrombotic atherosclerotic disease, aortic dissection, embolization, or vasculitis (particularly polyarteritis nodosa). The posterior columns are usually spared, which aids in the diagnosis. This syndrome may result as a complication of aortic angiography, cross-clamping of the aorta for more than 30 minutes, or spine trauma with resulting direct compression of the ventral spinal cord and adjacent vessels.[86,87] Spinal hemorrhages are usually apoplectic in nature, with rapidly developing paralysis and sensory loss. They may occur within the epidural or subdural spaces or within the spinal cord. Trauma, anticoagulant therapy, and vascular malformation are the primary causes.

Vascular Malformations

Spinal vascular malformations are an uncommon cause of neurologic deficit, representing only 10% of spinal epidural hemorrhages.[88,89] More commonly, spinal intradural and extradural malformations present with chronic progressive myelopathy or radiculopathy. Spinal vascular malformations are usually divided into three groups: dural arteriovenous fistulas, intradural vascular malformations, and cavernous angiomas. A vascular malformation infrequently (<3% of cases) may produce an audible bruit over the spinal cord. Dural arteriovenous fistulas occur most often in patients over age 40 and may be exacerbated by changes in posture or activity. These lesions almost always affect the lower half of the spinal cord and produce symptoms in the legs, bladder, and bowel. In contrast, patients with intradural vascular malformations become symptomatic before the age of 40 and often present with an acute onset of symptoms caused by hemorrhage.[89-92]

MRI has replaced myelography as the initial diagnostic study to evaluate these patients; intradural spinal AVMs present as serpentine areas of low signal intensity in the subarachnoid space as a result of signal voids produced by blood flowing in the dilated tortuous vessels. T1-weighted MRI images of intramedullary AVMs usually reveal a low-intensity signal that may be associated with focal widening of the cord. In contrast to MRI, myelography findings are universally abnormal in these fistulas and demonstrate the presence of the lesion, with the exception of cavernous angiomas. In the search for a spinal AVM with a negative MRI and myelogram, arteriography would rarely be indicated. Spine arteriography, however, should be performed in all patients with spinal AVMs that have been diagnosed by means of other studies.[93-95]

Histologically similar to their intracranial counterpart, cavernous angiomas are intramedullary lesions that are characterized clinically by sensorimotor disturbances over an acute or subacute period. These rare lesions of the spinal cord are characterized by acute neurologic dysfunction with intervening episodes of varying recovery.[96-98] They are found most often in thoracic and cervical locations. Cavernous angiomas may not be apparent on findings from myelography, CT imaging, or spine arteriography. MRI remains the investigative procedure of choice, usually revealing residual blood of subacute and chronic hemorrhage, characterized by mixed high- and low-signal components.[97]

Foix-Alajouanine syndrome is a rare form of necrotic myelopathy that results in slowly evolving myotrophic paraplegia in adult males. It has been attributed to spinal venous thrombosis, although its exact nature remains controversial.[99,100]

Trauma to the cervical column can also be a cause of vascular lesions of the spinal cord. These lesions include compression of adjacent vessels, dislocations with dissection or occlusion of the vertebral arteries, or spontaneous epidural hematomas caused by tearing of bridging veins. The time course until the lesion appears ranges from acute to subacute, depending on the type of traumatic vascular injury.

Demyelinating Lesions

Although demyelination might not be the exact pathologic process encountered in the following diseases, this discussion includes disorders, whether inflammatory or destructive, that involve myelin. These disorders include multiple sclerosis (MS) and transverse myelitis (TM).

Multiple Sclerosis

The clinically definite diagnosis of MS requires the presence of six items:

1. Objective CNS dysfunction
2. Two or more sites of CNS involvement
3. Predominant white matter involvement
4. Relapsing-remitting or chronic (>6 months) progressive course
5. Age of onset between 10 and 50 years
6. No better explanation of symptoms

Poser et al.[101] modified these criteria by enhancing the clinical diagnosis with laboratory studies that include analysis of the spinal fluid, evoked potentials, and imaging studies.

The clinical picture of transverse myelitis related to MS accounts for only 0.6% of initial symptoms in these patients. In the majority of these cases, symptoms other than impairment of spinal cord function precede the myelopathy. The most common initial symptoms are limb weakness, paresthesia, optic neuritis, diplopia, vertigo, and urinary difficulty. These are followed by upper and lower motor neuron weakness, spasticity, increased or depressed muscle stretch reflexes, pain, Lhermitte sign, intranuclear ophthalmoplegia and nystagmus, ataxia, impotence, hearing loss, affective disorder, and dementia. Bladder spasticity as an initial presenting symptom is also common. The symptoms and signs may be worsened by exercise or increased temperature (Uhthoff phenomenon). In cases of progressive myelopathy, MS should be differentiated from compressive lesions, leukodystrophies (specifically adrenomyeloneuropathy), and familial spinal cerebellar degeneration. There are a number of MS variants, including neuromyelitis optica or Devic disease, which is a rare form of a rapidly progressive demyelination that is restricted to the optic nerves and the spinal cord.

Among neuroimaging studies, MRI is the modality of choice to confirm the diagnosis. In general, the MRI scan is positive in 85% to 95% of clinically definite MS patients.[102] The clinical diagnosis is supported by laboratory studies, including CSF examination, which may reveal a lymphocytic pleocytosis (usually fewer than 25 cells/mm^3), and normal or increased protein. Oligoclonal bands, lymphocytic reactivity to myelin basic protein, and an elevated IgG/Alb ratio are other laboratory findings that can support a diagnosis of MS.

Transverse Myelitis

Transverse myelitis is a nonhomogeneous group of idiopathic inflammatory processes defined as isolated spinal cord dysfunction over hours or days in patients who demonstrate no evidence of a compressive lesion.[103,104] Transverse myelitis can occur in acute, subacute, or chronic forms. Only the acute forms are discussed here. Transverse myelitis caused by other etiologies usually follows a longer time course and is discussed in later text.

Acute transverse myelitis can be subdivided into the autoimmune and necrotizing types. They are differentiated by an acute versus a subacute time course and associated illness. Autoimmune acute transverse myelitis usually occurs after a viral illness or in association with other autoimmune disorders, such as MS or lupus erythematosus. In several reviews of this process, 37% of patients reported a preceding febrile illness. The initial symptoms were paresthesias, back pain, or leg weakness. The maximal neurologic deficit develops within 10 days in the majority of cases.[104-106] Patients with partial myelitis may have a higher frequency of subsequently developing MS.[106] Acute transverse myelitis has been associated with systemic vasculitis, as in systemic lupus erythematosus, as well as with heroin abuse. Symptoms occur over days to weeks, most commonly in the thoracic spinal cord. Symptoms include ascending paresthesias, weakness, and urinary retention.

Necrotizing acute transverse myelitis (Foix-Alajouanine syndrome) is an acutely progressive necrotizing myelitis that occurs over hours to days.[99,100,107] Clinical manifestations in the typical patient of adult years consist of severe paralysis preceded by tingling or loss of sphincter control. During the acute phase, MRI is normal in approximately half of the cases and is nonspecific in the remainder. Focal spinal cord enlargement on T1-weighted and poorly delineated hyperintensities on T2-weighted scans are the most commonly identified abnormalities. Occasionally, contrast enhancement is observed. Diagnosis is based on the clinical picture and absence of other potential causes of acute myelopathy on MRI, such as acute disc herniation hematoma, epidural abscess, or compression myelopathy.

Degenerative Disorders

Degenerative disorders encompass a broad spectrum of diseases that affect the spinal cord and column. Diseases of the spinal column often present with a combination of pain and neurologic deficits; these were discussed in the section dealing with pain as a primary presenting symptom. Degenerative diseases of the neural tissue are generally referred to as motor neuron diseases and include upper motor neuron syndromes, lower motor neuron syndromes, and disorders that combine upper and lower motor neuron syndromes.

Upper Motor Neuron Syndromes

These rare diseases, which are both inherited and acquired, exhibit degeneration of the descending corticospinal or corticobulbar tracts, with variable involvement of the large pyramidal neurons in the motor cortex. The archetypical disorders in this group are hereditary spastic paraplegia (Strümpell syndrome) and lathyrism, respectively. Hereditary spastic paraplegia is a clinically and genetically heterogeneous disorder that presents with progressive spasticity and mild weakness in the lower extremities. It is inherited more commonly through the autosomal dominant trait. However, in some families, autosomal recessive and rare forms of X-linked inheritance have been reported. Almost 75% of those affected demonstrate difficulty in walking at presentation. Lower extremity spasticity, hyperreflexia, and extensor plantar responses are usually encountered in established cases.

Diagnosis is based on the family history and physical findings and is supported by selected laboratory studies. Peripheral sensory and motor conduction studies, as well as myelography, are usually normal. The peroneal H-reflex, which is normally absent without reinforcement, is obtained in clinically definite cases and in most of those who may be affected. Low-amplitude or absent somatosensory-evoked potentials from the upper- and lower-extremity nerves and slowed spinal cord conduction are usually found. CSF is usually normal; however, elevated levels of protein (≤100 mg/dL) have been reported.

Adrenoleukodystrophy should also be considered in cases of progressive paraplegia. This X-linked recessive disorder of males, manifested most commonly in children, may also be present in adults as adrenomyeloneuropathy, which is a related form. This condition is usually detected in patients older than age 20 who often present with a progressive paraparesis. Unlike hereditary spastic paraplegia, the onset of symptoms is usually abrupt. The motor findings are commonly accompanied by permanent sensory loss in the legs and sphincter dysfunction.

Lower Motor Neuron Syndromes

This group of diseases is dominated by inherited disorders. Spinal muscular atrophy (SMA) is the second most common childhood neuromuscular disease after Duchenne muscular dystrophy, with an estimated 1 in 40 Caucasians harboring a gene for this condition. Degeneration of the anterior horn cells in this group of disorders leads to progressive weakness, characteristic muscle atrophy, and hyporeflexia. Fasciculations are occasionally observed, but sensory involvement, corticospinal tract involvement, and sphincter involvement are absent. In severe childhood cases, contractures and skeletal abnormalities develop. Nerve conduction studies and electromyography are diagnostic and allow differentiation from clinically similar disorders. Nerve conduction studies are usually normal in sensory and motor nerves. Electromyography reveals evidence of denervation in the form of fibrillations, fasciculations, and positive sharp waves. These findings are more prevalent in chronic cases. Neurogenic voluntary motor unit potentials and, in advanced atrophy, myopathic potentials, may be observed. Muscle histology shows group atrophy of type I and type II fibers, pyknotic nuclear clumps, and variable fiber hypotrophy.

Proximal SMAs account for nearly 80% of all SMA cases. Type I, acute infantile SMA (Werdnig-Hoffmann disease) is a progressive disease of infancy that accounts for about 25% of all SMA cases. Usually transmitted by an autosomal recessive gene, this condition presents in a third of the cases that demonstrate decreased fetal movements in the last trimester of pregnancy. The majority of affected infants are floppy at birth. The disease is almost uniformly fatal, usually in the sixth or seventh month of life. About 95% of affected children die by the age of 18 months.[108]

Type II (late infantile and juvenile-onset SMA) constitutes the largest group of these muscular atrophies. This group of childhood diseases includes cases of arrested Werdnig-Hoffmann disease, SMA type II and III, and Kugelberg-Welander disease. In the majority of cases, clinical onset occurs by 5 years of age and is often preceded by infection or immunization. Pelvic and pectoral girdle muscles are weak and atrophied almost universally; tongue and limb muscle fasciculations are common. There may be associated cranial nerve involvement, muscle pseudohypertrophy, mental retardation, hand tremor, and occasionally an eversion deformity of the feet. Electromyography is the study of choice to differentiate this disease from muscular dystrophies. The median survival time is more than 12 years.

Type III (adult-onset) SMA usually develops between the ages of 20 and 50 years with proximal symmetrical muscle weakness, especially in the lower extremities. As in children with the disease, limb girdle weakness and muscle atrophy are typical. The involvement of the face and tongue is more common in adults than in children and occurs in up to half of adult-onset cases, especially in those with a dominant genetic pattern for this disease.

Distal SMA (progressive) (Charcot-Marie-Tooth disease) is a genetically heterogeneous disorder, accounting for about 10% of all cases of SMA, and is mentioned here because it also accounts for 3% to 6% of all cases of the peroneal muscular atrophy syndrome. The scapular-peroneal form is an even less common disorder that belongs to this group, accounting for about 7% of all SMA cases.

Included among the acquired disorders in this group is the poliomyelitis (postpolio) syndrome (postpolio myelitis muscular atrophy, late effects of poliomyelitis, and late progression of old polio myelitis). The postpolio syndrome is defined as a new onset of muscle weakness, pain, and fatigue many years after recovery from acute paralytic poliomyelitis. The new symptoms usually occur 30 to 40 years after acute polio. The age at presentation is between 40 and 50 years. Patients present with fatigue, joint pain, muscle pain, progressive weakness, and atrophy, particularly in previously affected muscles. The following criteria for the diagnosis of postpolio muscular atrophy have been proposed: (1) documented past history of acute paralytic poliomyelitis, (2) incomplete to fairly complete neurologic and functional recovery, (3) a period of neurologic and functional stability of at least 15 years, (4) documented new-onset muscle weakness and/or atrophy in an asymmetrical distribution in previously involved and/or uninvolved muscles, usually with unaccustomed fatigue, (5) electrophysiologic evidence of acute denervation superimposed on chronic denervation-reinnervation, and (6) no other cause demonstrated.

Combined Upper and Lower Motor Neuron Syndromes

Amyotrophic lateral sclerosis (also known as Charcot disease or motor neuron disease) is found in adults and results from degeneration of the upper motor neuron and lower motor neuron.[109,110] The prevalence of amyotrophic lateral sclerosis is four to six individuals per 100,000, and it is familial in 8% to 10% of cases. Familial cases usually follow autosomal dominant inheritance but occasionally demonstrate a recessive pattern.[109-111]

The clinical picture of Charcot disease usually consists of weakness and atrophy of the hands (lower motor neuron), with spasticity and hyperreflexia of the lower extremities (upper motor neuron). Voluntary eye muscles and urinary sphincter muscles are usually spared. If the involvement of lower motor neuron to lower extremities predominates, the hyperreflexia may be replaced by hyporeflexia. As the disease progresses, dysarthria and dysphagia ensue as a combination of upper and lower neuron pathology; tongue atrophy and fasciculations may be seen. Emotional lability is encountered, but only 1% to 2% of cases are associated with dementia. Approximately 20% of patients with corticospinal tract involvement show a Babinski sign. In the familial form, lower motor neuron involvement at presentation is more common (58%), particularly in the legs. Dementia is more often present (15%). Clinical diagnosis is confirmed by electrophysiologic studies.

Miscellaneous Disorders

Subacute Combined Degeneration

Subacute combined degeneration of the spinal cord, caused by a deficiency of vitamin B_{12}, is uncommon today because of the relative ease of diagnosis and treatment. However, when B_{12} levels are reduced for a prolonged period, neurologic sequelae ensue shortly after the anemia. Clinically, this condition presents with both sensory and motor symptoms consistent with thoracic dorsal column involvement, including paresthesias in the feet and loss of vibratory and positional sense. Diagnosis is made through laboratory studies that demonstrate a decreased B_{12} level and a neurologic examination that is consistent with a posterolateral syndrome. Treatment is with vitamin B_{12}.[112,113] Incomplete paraplegia or quadriplegia may accompany myasthenia gravis, an autoimmune disease caused by a defect in neuromuscular transmission with an incidence of 3 per 100,000. Ocular, motor, and bulbar involvement, as well as preserved sensation, often point to the correct diagnosis. A rather stable, nonprogressive myelopathy is observed in degenerative spinal cord diseases, such as hereditary spastic paraplegia or spastic diplegia of cerebral palsy.

Guillain-Barré syndrome, diphtheria, acute intermittent porphyria, toxic peripheral neuropathies (thallium poisoning), or the poorly understood immune response to malignant neoplasms (so-called paraneoplastic syndromes) may present in the form of a subacute myelopathy and evolve over weeks. The symptoms include an ascending or a descending pattern and may produce a combination of upper and lower motor neuron signs. The prognosis for paraneoplastic syndromes is invariably poor.

Guillain-Barré Syndrome

This syndrome is the most common acquired demyelinating neuropathy, characterized by an acute onset of peripheral nerve dysfunction, usually after a viral illness. It presents clinically with symmetrical limb weakness and/or paresthesias.[114] This disease is distinguished from the aforementioned causes of peripheral neuropathies by a history of toxin exposure or ingestion and its tendency to affect proximal muscles initially.

Familial Periodic Paralysis

Diseases that affect primary muscles are rarely acute in their onset. However, in so-called periodic paralysis, attacks of generalized muscle weakness may evolve over minutes to hours. The patient with familial periodic paralysis usually has a medical history of similar attacks or a positive family history. This condition, which is associated with disturbances of serum potassium, is a disease of the young, with initial attacks occurring around puberty.[115] It is extremely rare, with only a few cases being reported each year. Clinically, patients present with weakness or paralysis of either the legs or all muscle groups, usually after a period of rest.

Paraneoplastic Syndromes

These conditions are also common causes of neurologic deficit. Between 7% and 15% of patients with systemic cancer display remote effects of the malignancy known as paraneoplastic syndrome. In more than 50% of these patients, the paraneoplastic symptoms precede diagnosis of the primary cancer. Underlying pathology includes inflammatory, vascular, and autoimmunologic changes. Vascular states are characterized by hypercoagulability, venous thrombosis, nonbacterial or marantic endocarditis, and intravascular coagulopathies. Autoimmune syndromes include myasthenia gravis, the myasthenic syndrome of Eaton-Lambert, and the polymyositis-dermatomyositis complex. The cerebellar syndromes with cortical cerebellar degeneration and myoclonic encephalopathies are thought to have underlying immunologic causes.

Conclusion

The differential diagnosis of pathology of the spine is vast. Therefore, an attempt has been made to delineate the most common causes by age, location, character, site of pain, rapidity of onset, and severity of neurologic deficit and associated systemic illness. The following observations are used to classify spine pathology: (1) the presence or absence of spinal region pain, (2) the characteristics of the pain, (3) the presence or absence of neurologic deficit, (4) the characteristics of the deficit, and (5) the presence of systemic signs and symptoms. Each patient is entered into an algorithm created from these five classifications after a thorough history and physical examination. With this information, further laboratory and radiologic evaluation can proceed, and ultimately, a diagnosis with appropriate surgical or medical management usually can be achieved.

KEY REFERENCES

Harrop JS, Schmidt MH, Boriani S, Shaffrey CI: Aggressive "benign" primary spine neoplasms: osteoblastoma, aneurysmal bone cyst, and giant cell tumor. *Spine (Phila Pa 1976)* 34:S39–S47, 2009.

Oldfield EH: Introduction: Spinal vascular malformations. *Neurosurg Focus* 26:E1, 2009.

Shen FH, Samartzis D, Jenis LG, An HS: Rheumatoid arthritis: evaluation and surgical management of the cervical spine. *Spine J* 4:689–700, 2004.

Smith JS, Fu KM, Urban P, Shaffrey CI: Neurological symptoms and deficits in adults with scoliosis who present to a surgical clinic: incidence and association with the choice of operative versus nonoperative management. *J Neurosurg Spine* 9:326–331, 2008.

Weinstein JN, Tosteson TD, Lurie JD, et al: Surgical vs nonoperative treatment for lumbar disk herniation: the Spine Patient Outcomes Research Trial (SPORT): a randomized trial. *JAMA* 296:2441–2450, 2006.

Yang S, Yang X, Hong G: Surgical treatment of one hundred seventy-four intramedullary spinal cord tumors. *Spine (Phila Pa* 1976) 34:2705–2710, 2009.

Zimmerli W: Clinical practice. Vertebral osteomyelitis. *N Engl J Med* 362:1022–1029, 2010.

REFERENCES

The complete reference list is available online at expertconsult.com.

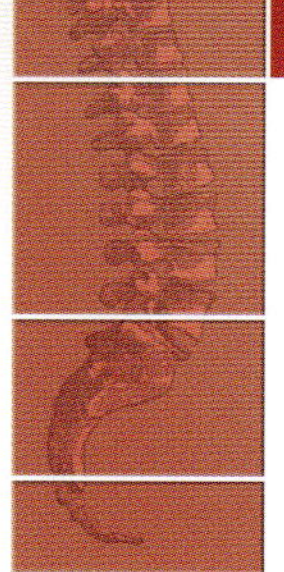

CHAPTER 5

Functional Anatomy of the Spine

Zabi Wardak | Elizabeth Demers Lavelle | Brian J. Kistler | William F. Lavelle

The spine is a complex structure with bony, ligamentous, muscular, and neurologic components. Knowledge of the anatomy and associated pathology of the spine is essential for treating patients with spinal disorders. The focus of this chapter is to develop an understanding of the anatomic and more specifically the functional relationships between these components.

Overview of the Vertebral Column and Spinal Cord

The human spinal column consists of 33 vertebrae separated into five anatomic regions. These regions include 7 cervical (C1-7), 12 thoracic (T1-12), 5 lumbar (L1-5), 5 sacral (S1-5), and 4 coccygeal bones (Fig. 5-1). In utero development plays a large part in the formation of the adult spine, contributing to the primary curvatures: kyphosis in the thoracic and sacral regions. Late in utero, after the development of the primary curvatures and continuing through early childhood, the secondary curvatures of the spine develop (Fig. 5-2). The cervical and lumbar lordosis becomes significant because of the gravitational forces created by the weight of the head and upright posture.[1] The positions taken by the cervical and lumbar spine allow for horizontal gaze while standing in an upright posture.

The development and maintenance of spinal anatomy and posture are not static and vary individually. Variations with intervertebral discs and vertebral bodies can be potentiated by congenital anomalies, age-dependent vertebral changes and osteophyte formation, traumatic injuries, neurologic disorders, and paraspinal muscle imbalances. Commonly occurring variations include sacralization of the fifth lumbar vertebra or lumbarization of the first sacral vertebra, Klippel-Feil anomaly in the cervical spine, and anomalous nerve root anatomy. A myriad of reactive changes may be seen as a response to spinal deformity. The flexibility of the spine may allow a patient to compensate for a deformity in one region with a change in curvature in another. However, a deformity may become so profound that an individual may be severely disabled.

The flexibility of the spine varies from region to region and is based on anatomic constraints. The cervical spine offers the greatest flexibility because of the requisite mobility of the head. This is in contrast to the rigidity of the thoracic spine due to its association with the chest wall.[2] Unique articulations in the cervical region afford flexibility such as those found between the skull-atlas and atlas-axis (C1-2). Flexibility at other regions of the spine is influenced by cartilaginous discs between vertebral bodies and apophyseal joints found dorsal to the vertebral arches, all developed in a manner to provide optimum stability, flexibility, and mobility. The center of gravity of the spinal column and that of the body do not pass through the same points. The former begins cranially at the odontoid process of the axis and passes caudally through the sacral promontory.[3] The latter passes ventral to the sacral promontory caudally. Disability may occur if the center of gravity deviates from the normal position. Studies have found that when the center of gravity passes too far ventral to the sacrum so the work required to maintain erect posture is significantly increased, lumbar muscle fatigue and pain result.

Normal physiologic function is supported by the ligaments and joint capsules of the spine. The ligaments of the spinal column are composed of elastin and collagen[3,4] and may span several segments. The anterior longitudinal ligament (ALL) spans the entire length of the spinal column, extending from the ventral border of the foramen magnum (basion), where it is known as the anterior atlanto-occipital membrane, to the sacrum. The ALL spans 25% to 33% of the ventral surface of the vertebral bodies and intervertebral discs, supporting the annulus fibrosus and preventing hyperextension. The ALL is arranged in three layers: the outermost spanning four to five levels, the middle layer spanning three levels and connecting vertebral bodies and intervertebral discs, and the innermost layer binding adjacent vertebral discs. The posterior longitudinal ligament (PLL) begins as the tectorial membrane at C2 and extends to the sacrum. The PLL runs within the vertebral canal and flares at the level of the intervertebral disc where it is interwoven with the annulus fibrosus and narrows at the vertebral bodies, where it is loosely attached. The layers of the PLL are similar to the ALL but function to prevent hyperflexion.

Interspinous and supraspinous ligaments provide stability to the dorsal elements of the spinal column. Ligamenta flava connect spinal laminae in a discontinuous fashion and are intertwined with the facet joint capsule. The proximal insertion of the ligamentum flavum is the ventral part of the cranial lamina extending to the dorsal part of the caudal lamina. Laterally, the ligamentum flavum is in contact with the ventral

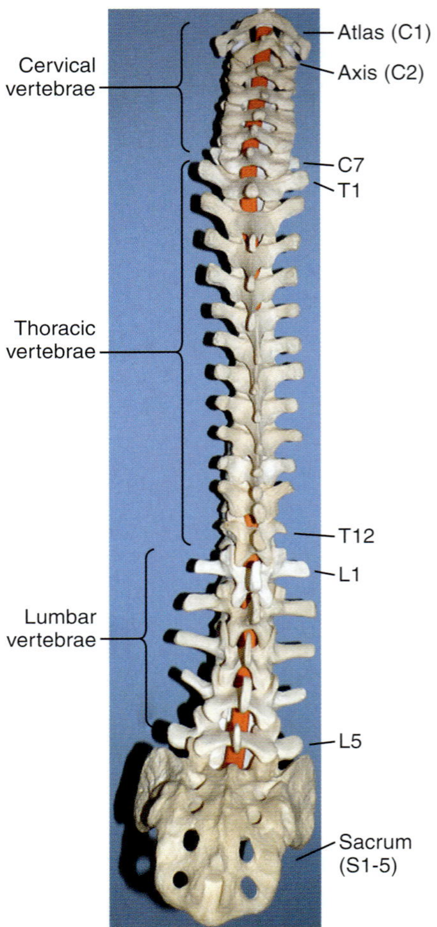

FIGURE 5-1. A dorsal view of the spine demonstrating the cervical, thoracic, and lumbar regions.

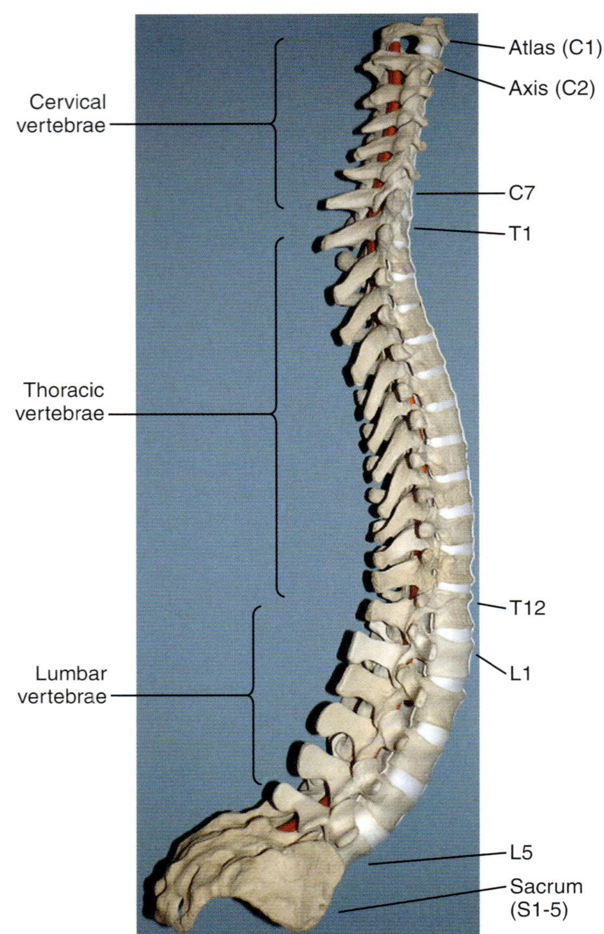

FIGURE 5-2. A lateral view of the spine demonstrating the cervical, thoracic, and lumbar regions. The primary thoracic kyphosis and secondary cervical and lumbar lordosis are illustrated.

capsule of the facet joint. These attachments are significant when excision of the ligamentum flavum is necessary to alleviate spinal stenosis. The microscopic anatomy of the ligamentum flavum is unique due to its approximately 80% elastin content. This is the source of the yellow appearance and the nickname "yellow ligament." The elasticity of the ligamentum flavum allows it to stretch during flexion without limiting motion and allows it to become taut when returning to neutral and during extension. As a person ages, the elastin is replaced with a higher percentage of collagen, causing it to become less elastic, which may lead to buckling into the spinal canal.

The spinal cord is a 40- to 45-cm long structure extending from the foramen magnum to the L1-2 spinal level. The cord transitions at this point into a collection of nerve roots known as the cauda equina. Spinal nerve roots exit neural foramina and consist of a dorsal sensory and ventral motor root, with the exception being C1 and C2 contributions to the spinal accessory nerve. The outermost membranes, or meninges, which cover the spinal cord, are the dura, arachnoid, and pia—the innermost layer of the meninges. Suspension of the spinal cord is accomplished by the dentate ligaments, which interconnect the innermost pia with the outermost dura matter. The spinal cord is divided into regions much like the spine: 8 cervical, 12 thoracic, 5 lumbar, and 5 sacral regions and 1 coccygeal region. The nomenclature of the nerve roots is as follows: the first seven cervical nerves exit above their named vertebrae, with the eighth cervical nerve and all spinal nerves below exiting below their named vertebrae.

The spinal cord is part of the central nervous system and like the brain it is mapped in a somatotopic arrangement. The corticospinal tracts are responsible for motor function. Within these tracts control of the hands is found medially and control of the feet is found laterally. The spinothalamic tracts transmit sensory information, with hand sensation found ventromedially and sacral sensation dorsolaterally. Lumbar regions of the posterior columns of the spinal cord have sacral segments located medially and upper lumbar regions laterally.

Spinal canal dimensions provide adequate space for the spinal cord in all segments except for the midthoracic region. Here, the risk of neural tissue impingement during surgical instrumentation is increased. The lumbar region has a consistent spinal canal size and, along with the cauda equina, the anatomy functions to limit nervous tissue damage due to trauma or degenerative changes.[5]

Decreases in canal dimensions may result in radiographic and clinical spinal stenosis. These decreases in canal size may be either congenital, generally presenting at a younger age, or acquired, presenting at a later age due to degenerative changes. Stenosis is a self-perpetuating loop often beginning with disc degeneration leading to alterations in mechanical stress that cause facet joint degeneration and ligamentous changes, with an end result of a decrease in the canal space. Spinal stenosis may lead to changes in intradural pressure that diminish the blood flow to nerve roots and alter axonoplasmic flow. Acute nerve root constrictions have substantial edema, which can slow electrical conduction and nutrient transport and which are more substantial than chronic conditions. There is also an inflammatory component to stenosis that alters neuropeptide concentrations.

Vertebrae

The intricate design of the vertebrae provides stability to the spinal column along with support and protection for the spinal cord and associated nerve roots. The compressive forces are significant in a stacked column, and the cortical lamellae are arranged vertically to aid in resisting these forces. The cancellous bone found in the inner trabeculae allows for a compromise between strong mechanical support and limiting vertebral weight. All of the structures coincident with the vertebral bodies act to bear weight in compression. The anterior column functions to transfer body weight to the pelvis while standing in an erect posture. Dorsal elements of the spinal column serve to protect the spinal cord. The dorsal elements also function as a tension band and a lever, transferring muscular contractions of the paraspinal musculature through the anterior and middle columns of the spine.

The dorsal bony elements include the pedicles, which arise from the superior aspect of the vertebral body and form the lateral walls of the spinal canal. The laminae extend from the pars interarticularis and fuse to form the dorsal wall of the spinal column. The junction of the laminae, where the spinous processes arise, support functional stability of the spine with their ligamentous and muscular attachments. The relationship between the transverse processes and the dorsal elements is unique to the specific spinal region where they are found. Cervical transverse processes arise from the junction of the vertebral body and pedicle. The shape of cervical spinous processes are bifid, resulting in the great flexibility of the cervical region. Thoracic and lumbar transverse processes have a different anatomic relationship with the dorsal elements, arising from the junction of the pars interarticularis and pedicle. Stability and motion to the spine are also provided by transverse processes with their unique ligamentous and muscular attachments.

Flexion, extension, and rotation of the spine are supported, facilitated, and restricted by the facet joints. A facet joint consists of a superior articular process with an articulating surface projecting dorsally, which is met by the adjacent vertebra's inferior articular process that projects its articulating surface ventrally. The synovial joint formed by the two processes consists of a thin layer of hyaline cartilage between matching articulating surfaces, lined with synovium and surrounded by a joint capsule. Although limited in size, the facet joints provide constraints to extremes of spinal motion.

Atlas (C1) and Axis (C2)

The first cervical vertebra is unique in its articulation with the occipital condyle of the cranium. This articulation is the basis for significant flexion and extension of the head. Another unique aspect of the atlas is that although it lacks a true ventral body it still supports the cranium by the superior facet surfaces of the lateral masses (Fig. 5-3A). The caudal facet surfaces of the lateral mass articulate with the superior facets of the axis (Fig. 5-3B). The transverse process of the atlas houses the vertebral artery within the transverse foramina. Superior and inferior oblique muscles attach to the transverse process. The atlas is hydrostatically held between the cranium and axis. The anterior and posterior occipital membranes attach to the atlas and also contribute to stability. They are continuations of the anterior longitudinal ligament and ligamentum flavum, respectively.

The axis is the second cervical vertebra. The articulation between the atlas and axis, known as the atlantoaxial joint, contributes to the majority of cervical rotation and stability to the upper cervical region. Unlike the atlas, the axis does have a true vertebral body and a unique structure known as the odontoid process projecting cranially from its dorsal aspect (Figs. 5-4A–C). The alar, cruciform, and transverse ligaments are anchored to the odontoid process. Further stability of the cervical region is contributed to by the muscular attachments at the spinous process of the axis, which include the rectus major and inferior oblique muscles. Like the atlas, a transverse foramen encases the vertebral artery.

Ligamentous anatomy of the cervical spine is unique, providing support for the head and maintaining stability despite the tremendous flexibility of this region. Ligaments exist both

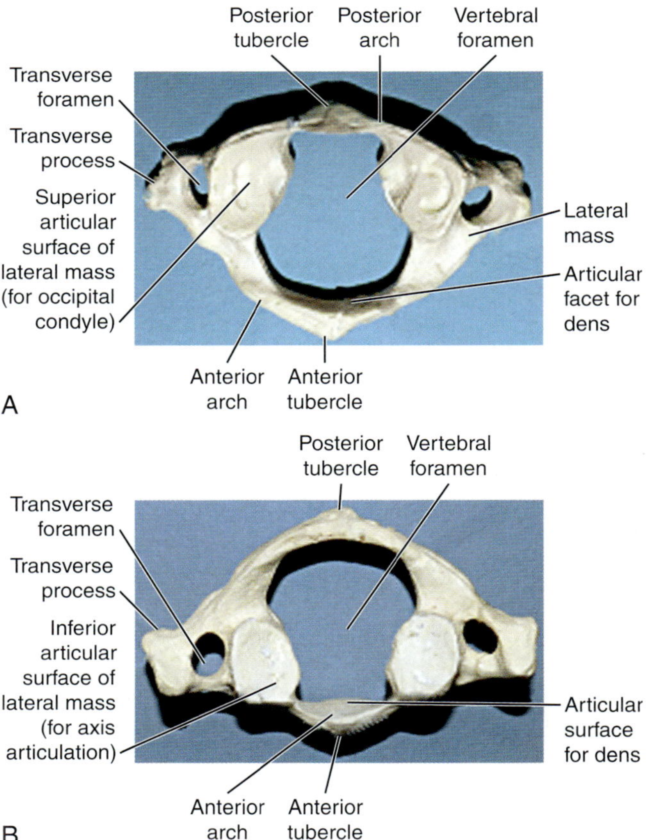

FIGURE 5-3. The anatomy of the atlas (C1) demonstrating its unique osseous anatomy with noted lack of an anterior body and large lateral masses. Superior (**A**) and inferior (**B**) views.

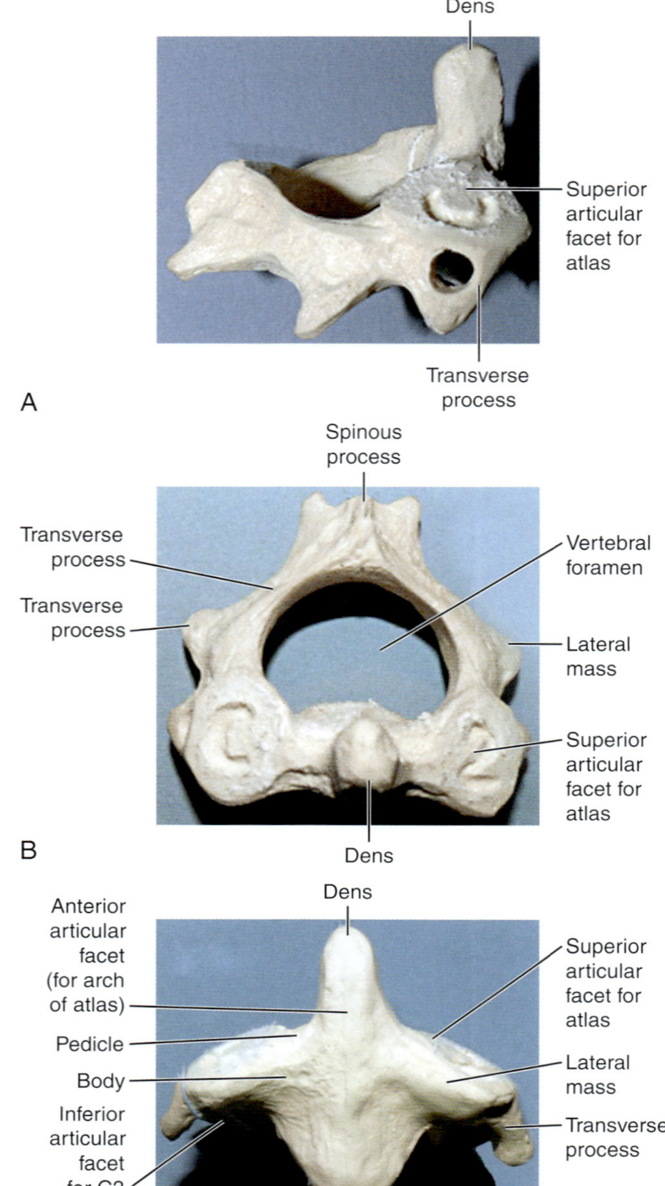

FIGURE 5-4. The anatomy of the atlas (C2) demonstrating its unique osseous anatomy with its large anterior dens that allows for 50% of the cervical spine's rotation through its articulation with the atlas. Lateral (**A**), superior (**B**), and anterior (**C**) views.

within and outside of the spinal canal. Much of the stability of the craniocervical region is provided by the ligaments within the spinal canal, which are ventral to the spinal cord. These are arranged in three layers. The tectorial membrane is the most dorsal of these ligaments and is a continuation of the PLL, attaching dorsally to the cruciate ligament at the basiocciput. The cruciate ligament is the middle layer and functions to constrain ventral translation between C1 and C2. It is a complex ligament with both horizontal and vertical bands. The odontoid ligament, or apical ligament, is the most ventral of the inner ligaments and extends from the lateral aspect of the odontoid to the medial aspect of the occipital condyles. Outside of the spinal canal are fibroelastic bands extending from the foramen magnum to C1. From the ventral portion of the foramen magnum extends the anterior atlanto-occipital membrane. From the dorsal foramen magnum arises the posterior atlanto-occipital membrane. Because these are thin bands, their contribution to the strength of the cervical spine is limited.

Subaxial Cervical Vertebrae (C3-7)

The remaining cervical vertebrae share anatomic features and may be considered separately from the atlas and axis. They are the smallest in size compared with all other regions of the spine and begin the trend of gradually increasing in size with each successively lower level. Descending down the spine, more body weight is supported, which is why the vertebrae increase in size. The end plates of the vertebrae in this region are concave superiorly and convex inferiorly, and they articulate to form the uncovertebral joints (joints of Luschka) (Fig. 5-5). These joints are often the site of arthritic changes, which can cause nerve root impingement. The position of the subaxial cervical spine affects the relative size of the neural foramen (Figs. 5-6A–C). Clinically, this is demonstrated by the Spurling maneuver. If the volume of the neural foramen is compromised by an osteophyte or disc fragment, pain can be elicited by tilting the head toward the affected side, which further reduces the foramen volume.

Pedicles are short and arise from the midpoint of the vertebral bodies. The laminae are fairly narrow. The spinous processes are bifid, with C7 being the largest (Fig. 5-7). The transverse processes, like the atlas and axis, have vertebral foramen that transmit the vertebral artery. The majority of individuals have vertebral arteries passing through the transverse foramen of C1-6, but in 5% of cases these arteries pass through the foramen at C7.[6] The facet joints are horizontal, and the facet capsule is weak, which allows for the mobility of the cervical spine.

The ligamentum nuchae is the primary ligamentous structure in the dorsal cervical spine outside of the spinal canal with attachments to the spinous processes. Descending past C7, the ligamentum nuchae transitions into the supraspinous ligament, which extends to the lumbosacral region, ending between L3 and L5.

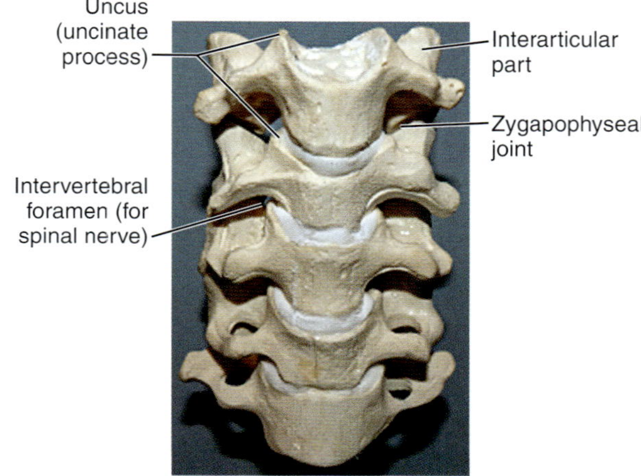

FIGURE 5-5. Dorsal view of the anatomy of the atlas subaxial cervical spine.

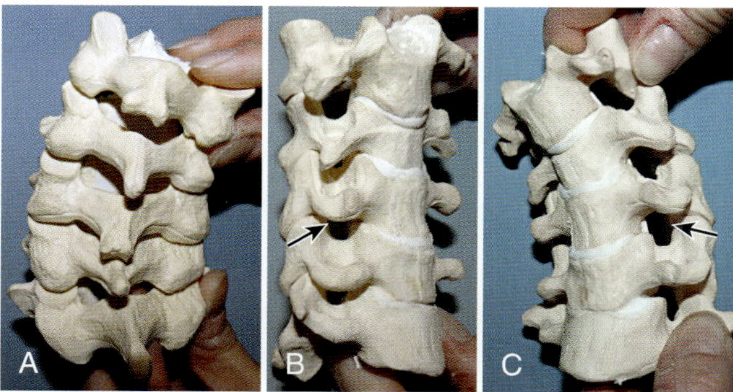

FIGURE 5-6. The alignment of the cervical spine greatly affects the volume of the neuroforamen. **A,** The subaxial cervical spine positioned in lateral bending. **B,** The relative volumes of the neuroforamina (*arrows*) change with the concave side significantly decreasing in volume. **C,** The convex side increases relatively in volume. This becomes important in patients with a cervical disc herniation and an already compromised neuroforamen.

The range of motion measure at the cervical spine can vary due to age, gender, and method of measurement. Visual estimation and radiography are the primary methods used to measure cervical range of motion. Studies of these measurement techniques on active cervical range of motion have found that, on average, the cervical spine has a total of 151 degrees of rotation, a total of 86 degrees of lateral bending, and a total of 126 degrees of flexion-extension. When considering motion in only one direction, leftward and rightward rotation and lateral bending are, on average, half the total values, whereas the cervical spine has, on average, a greater range of extension than flexion.[7]

Thoracic Vertebrae

The thoracic region of the spine contains the largest number of vertebrae, which continue to increase in size from T1 to T12. The first four thoracic vertebrae maintain some cervical features, and the last four possess some lumbar features, maintaining a smooth transition between the adjacent regions. The superior vertebral notch is the cervical feature of T1, and the lumbar features of T12 include lateral direction and inferior articular processes. Laminae in the thoracic region are broader than in the cervical spine and overlap, whereas the transverse processes increase in size as they progress down the thoracic spine[8] (Fig. 5-8). The spinous processes of the thoracic vertebrae are variably arranged in horizontal, oblique, or overlapping vertical arrangements. Horizontal spinous processes are found at T1-2 and T11-12 and oblique spinous processes at T3-4 and T9-10, with the rest of the thoracic vertebrae possessing overlapping, vertical spinous processes (Fig. 5-9). Thoracic facets are primarily arranged in a coronal plane but develop a sagittal orientation near the junction of the lumbar vertebrae. There is less free space in the spinal canal in the thoracic region compared with both cervical and lumbar regions.

A characteristic feature of the thoracic vertebrae is the relationship with the ribs.[9] The ribs articulate with unique costal facets—found where the vertebral body and pedicle meet—as well as on transverse processes, with T10-12 being exceptions to facets on transverse processes. The thoracic spine has maximum stiffness relative to all regions of the spine, which is a function of the relationship between the rib and vertebrae combined with support from accessory

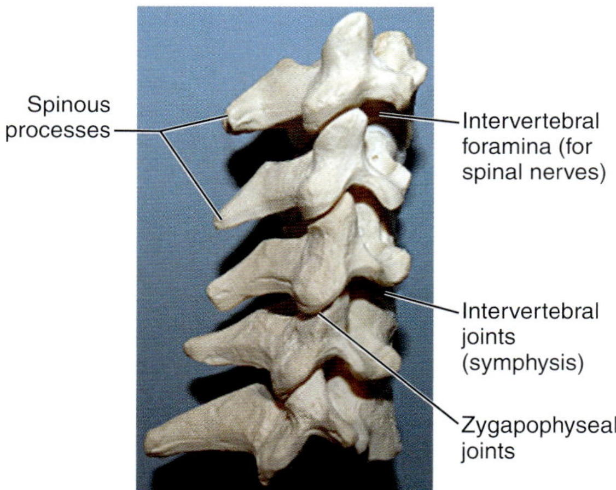

FIGURE 5-7. A lateral view of the subaxial cervical spine. Most striking are the orientation of the cervical facet joints and the bifid nature of the spinous processes, which allow for the extremes of cervical motion.

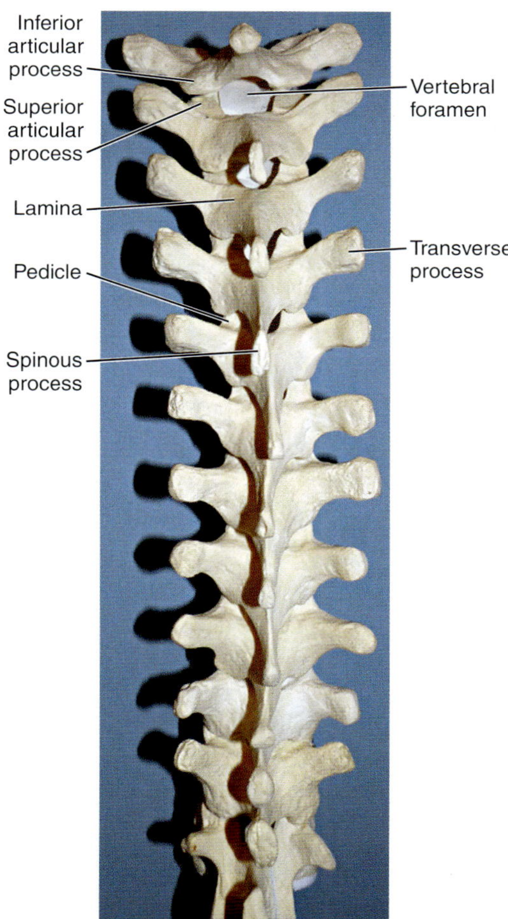

FIGURE 5-8. The dorsal osseous anatomy of the thoracic spine. The large transverse processes are distinctive. Due to the presence of the rib cage (not shown), the thoracic spine is the least mobile spinal segment.

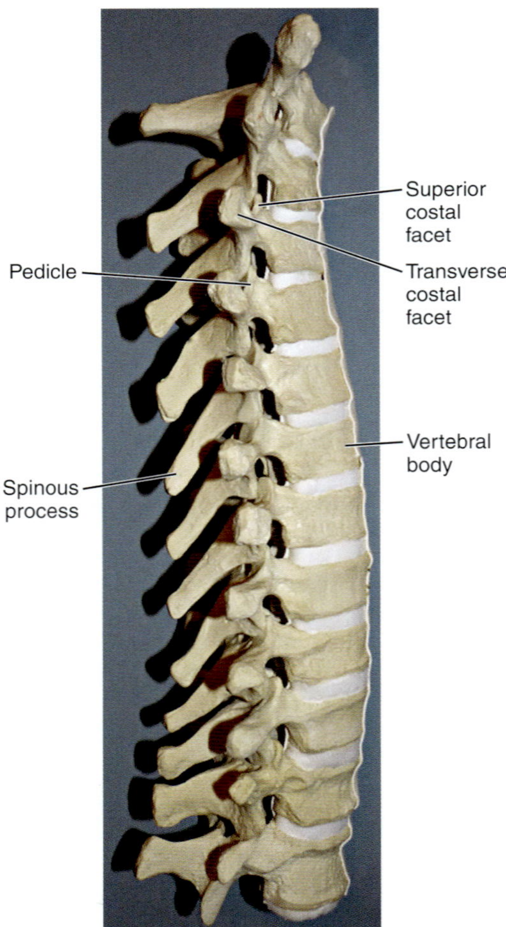

FIGURE 5-9. A lateral view of the thoracic spine. The vertebral bodies increase in size from cranial to caudal as the body imparts greater weight and forces on the spinal column.

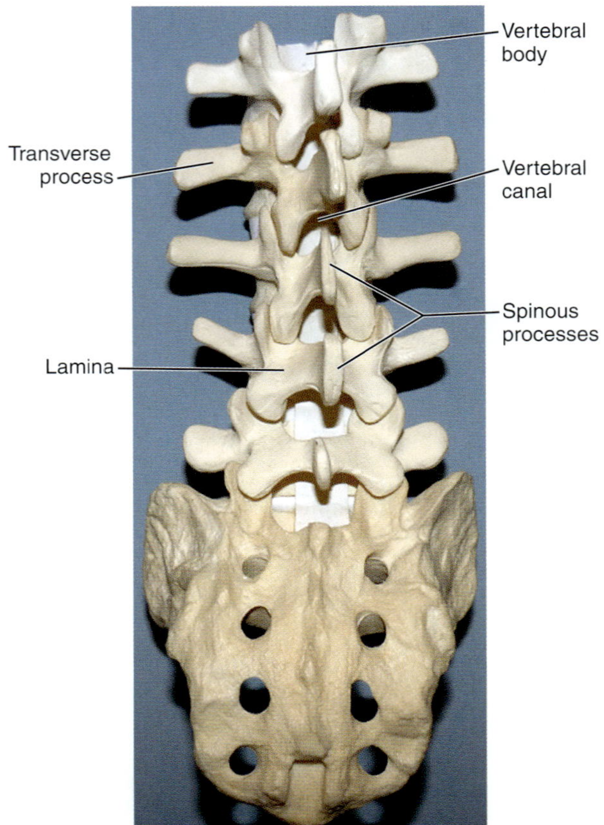

FIGURE 5-10. A dorsal view of the osseous anatomy of the lumbar spine.

ligaments.[9] The "junctional" regions of the spine, such as C7-T1 and T12-L1, are sites of transition from a rigid spinal region to one with maximal spinal motion. These junctional sites are often the sites of natural and iatrogenic pathology.

Lumbar Vertebrae

Descending down the spinal column, we come to the largest vertebral bodies—the lumbar vertebrae (Fig. 5-10). These vertebrae progressively increase in diameter when approaching the sacrum and are greater in transverse width relative to anteroposterior diameter. Within the lumbar region are subregional variations in the anatomy of the vertebrae. These are attributed to the greater weight and forces that these vertebrae must distribute as the spinal column transitions into the pelvis. The L1-2 vertebral bodies have greater depth dorsally, whereas L4-5 vertebral bodies have greater depth ventrally (Fig. 5-11). The two subregions are balanced by the L3 vertebral body, which provides a transitional point between the two. Vertebral body angulation and translation are affected by these locoregional differences in anatomy during flexion and extension. These variations produce changes in intervertebral disc height and foramen cross-sectional area, which are functionally linked to motion during flexion and extension.

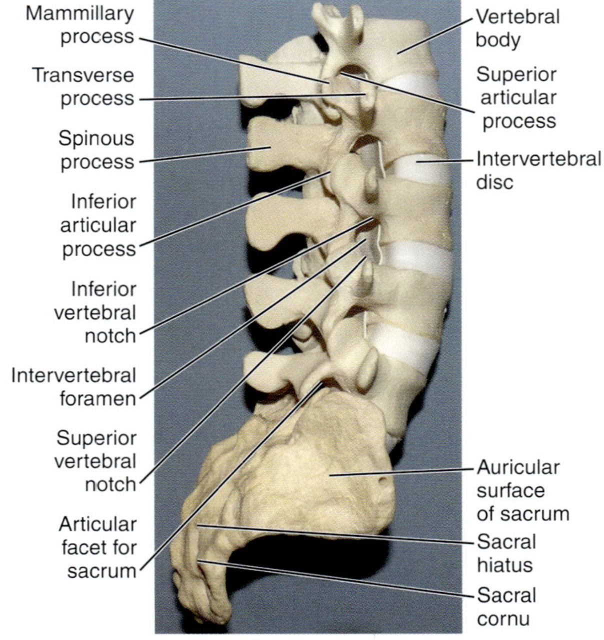

FIGURE 5-11. A lateral view of the osseous anatomy of the lumbar spine.

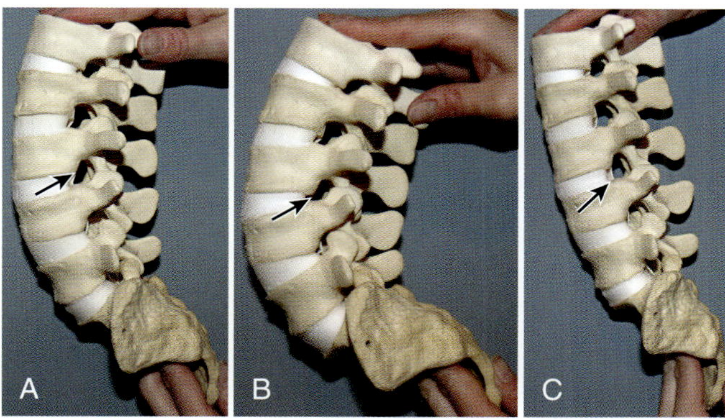

FIGURE 5-12. The positioning of the lumbar spine can greatly affect spinal canal volume. **A,** The neuroforamen volume (*arrows*) in the neutral position. With lumbar extension (**B**), the neural foramen decrease in size, and with lumbar flexion (**C**), the foramen increase in size.

The variations may be associated with susceptibility at lumbar regions for disc herniation, spinal canal stenosis, and other pathology. Cadaveric studies have shown that in the L4-5 region, flexion results in a greater dorsal disc bulge than in the L1-2 region. The cross-sectional area of the foramen in the lumbar region shows that compared with a neutral position, flexion increases the area by 12% (15 mm^2) and extension decreases the area by 15% (19 mm^2). The vertebral bodies move closer ventrally and further apart dorsally during flexion, which increases the dimensions of the spinal canal; the opposite occurs during extension.[10]

The cross-sectional area of the nerve root is linked to flexion and extension as well. The nerve roots traverse beneath the lateral recess of the pedicles and articular facets through the intervertebral foramina. Ventral borders of the nerve root are the vertebral body and intervertebral disc, dorsal borders are lamina and facets, and both superior and inferior borders are adjacent pedicles. Because of the locoregional differences in anatomy of the lumbar region, flexion and extension movements alter these borders and result in changes in nerve root cross-sectional area (Figs. 5-12A–C). These changes can be associated with susceptibility to nerve root impingement. Cadaveric studies have found that the neutral cross-sectional area of the L1-2 nerve root is 28.31 ± 10.48 mm; in flexion it increases to 32.37 ± 9.92 mm, and in extension it decreases to 22.97 ± 7.52 mm.[10]

Pedicles in the lumbar region arise from the rostral aspect of the vertebral body. They can be visualized behind the facet of the named vertebra and supra-adjacent vertebra. The diameter of the L1 pedicle is approximately 9 mm with a medial angle of 12 degrees,[11] which requires consideration with screw placement. Lumbar facets have a sagittal orientation, which limits axial rotation. The L5-S1 facet is unique, with a coronal orientation that resists anteroposterior translation.[2]

Sacrum and Coccyx

Five vertebrae, costal ligaments, and transverse processes are fused to create the sacrum. The sacral bodies are separated by transverse lines. Nerves emerge from rounded dorsal and ventral foramina that are lateral to the vertebral bodies. The unique fusion of vertebrae in the sacrum provides strength and stability to the pelvis, and through articulation with the ilea at the sacroiliac joints the weight of the body is distributed to the pelvic girdle. The coccyx is the terminal portion of the spinal column and commonly referred to as the "tail bone." It can be found as a single fused bone, or the first coccygeal element may be separated from the others. There are no dorsal elements to the vertebrae in the coccyx. The primary function of the coccyx is to serve as a site of attachment for pelvic muscles.

Vertebral End Plates

The vertebral end plates are composed of cortical bone of the vertebral body and cartilage of the intervertebral disc. Approximately 1.3 mm of cortical bone of the vertebral body forms a concave surface that is fused to the thin cartilaginous surface of the intervertebral disc by a layer of calcium known as the lamina cribrosa. Because the intervertebral discs lack a blood supply, nutrients are acquired via passive diffusion from the vertebral end plates. The largest avascular space in the human body is the L4-5 disc space. With aging, the diffusion capacity of the end plate decreases and the disc's nutrition is compromised, narrowing the disc space and increasing susceptibility to pathology.

Intervertebral Discs

The intervertebral discs are a vital component of the spine, contributing to stability, resisting loads in all directions, and restricting intervertebral motion. Twenty-three intervertebral discs are found, starting between C2 and C3 and extending distally to L5-S1. The discs account for roughly 20% to 33% of the vertebral column height and show regional variations much like the osseous structures, such as increasing in cross-sectional size when descending down the spine. The shape of the discs varies based on region of the spine, ellipsoid in the cervical and lumbar regions and resembling a rounded triangle in the thoracic region. In addition to the cartilaginous end plates, the disc components include an annulus fibrosus and the nucleus pulposus. Each component is linked to the other such that pathology of one affects the ability of the others to carry out their physiologic functions.

The cartilaginous end plate is a thin layer of hyaline cartilage that allows nutrient passage via diffusion to the minimally oxygenated disc center. The annulus fibrosus is composed of an outer layer of alternating type I collagen fibers and an inner fibrocartilage component. With torsion, the alternating collagenous fibers become taut while others are lax, which contributes to limitations in motion. This unique structure forms an attachment along the periphery of the vertebral body that maintains spinal stability in combination with the dorsal structures and the soft tissues.

The nucleus pulposus is bounded peripherally by the annulus fibrosus and both superiorly and inferiorly by the end plates. It is made up of negatively charged proteoglycan molecules and collagen. The negative charge makes the nucleus hydrophilic, which contributes to the extensive water component of the disc. Height and resistance to axial loads is maintained by the hydraulic properties of the fluid surrounded by end plates and the annulus fibrosus. Maintenance of disc height keeps the ligaments and capsules of the spine at optimal length and allows them to function physiologically. With aging, the distinct regions of the intervertebral disc are no longer present, and the proteoglycan content and hydration decreases. As disc height diminishes, increased demands are placed on the annulus fibrosus, thus increasing susceptibility to tears and subsequent herniation. Dorsal structures are also affected by the loss of disc height, including facet subluxation and hypertrophy, which may predispose an individual to nerve root compression.

Muscles

With the majority of body weight ventral to the vertebral body, the musculature of the back is crucial to balancing the forces placed on the vertebral column. The muscles can be divided into extrinsic and intrinsic back muscles. The extrinsic back muscles include the latissimus dorsi, trapezius, rhomboid, and serratus posterior muscles. The latissimus dorsi muscle, innervated by the thoracodorsal nerve, is the most prominent and arises from the spinous processes of the inferior six thoracic vertebrae and fans out to the axilla, functioning to raise the trunk when the arms are fixed. The trapezius muscle, innervated by the accessory nerve, is attached to the spinous processes of C7-T12 and functions in scapular movement. The rhomboids, innervated by the dorsal scapular nerve, are attached to the spinous processes of C7-T1 (minor rhomboid muscle) and T2-5 (major rhomboid muscle) and insert on the scapula. They too function in scapular movement. The serratus posterior muscle has two parts: a superior part innervated by intercostal nerves and attached to the spinous processes of C7-T3, and a caudal part innervated by thoracic spinal nerves and attached to the spinous processes of T11-L2. The two parts function to elevate and depress the ribs, respectively.

The intrinsic muscles of the back are superficially the splenius capitis and cervicis muscles, innervated by the dorsal rami of the cervical nerves. The splenius capitis muscle is attached to the ligamentum nuchae and spinous processes of C7-T4 and inserts on the occiput. The splenius cervicis muscle is attached to the spinous processes of T3-6 and inserts on the transverse processes of C1-4. The two muscles function to laterally flex the neck. The intermediate layer of intrinsic back muscles are the erector spinae muscles, which are a trio of columns. From lateral to medial, they are the iliocostalis, longissimus, and spinalis muscles. The columns overlap and have a common broad tendon attached to the iliac crest, sacrum, sacroiliac ligaments, and lumbosacral spinous processes. The erector spinae muscles are the chief extensors of the spinal column and are innervated by the dorsal rami of spinal nerves. The deep layer of intrinsic muscles are the semispinalis, multifidus, and rotatores muscles. All are innervated by the dorsal rami of the spinal nerves. There are three semispinalis muscles: capitis, cervicis, and thoracis. The semispinalis capitis muscle attaches to cervical and thoracic transverse processes and inserts on the occiput. It functions to extend the head. The semispinalis cervicis and thoracis muscles attach to transverse processes and insert on the spinous processes of the more superior vertebrae, respectively. They function to extend their respective region of the spine. The multifidus and rotatores muscles stabilize and rotate the vertebrae.

Anomalous Anatomy

Variants of normal spinal anatomy are not uncommon and can have dramatic effects on the regular function of the spine. Cervical spine anomalies can result in progression of degenerative changes, an example being the Klippel-Feil anomaly. The classic triad of Klippel-Feil is a short neck, low dorsal hairline, and limited neck motion. It is due to the fusion of adjacent cervical vertebrae, which alters the physiologic forces the spine is constructed to handle. Lumbar vertebrae anomalies can lead to functional changes in a region that is already susceptible to pathology. The presence of abnormal numbers of lumbar vertebrae can accelerate degenerative changes or increase susceptibility to herniation. This is commonly found with the presence of only four lumbar segments or the presence of a sixth lumbar vertebra. Nerve root anomalies such as conjoined nerve roots increase the risk of injury from disc herniation, trauma, or iatrogenic injury during surgical procedures.

KEY REFERENCES

Benzel E: Stability and instability of the spine. In Benzel E, editor: *Biomechanics of spine stabilization: principles and clinical practice*, New York, 1995, McGraw Hill, Inc, pp 25–40.

Panjabi MM, Duranceau J, Goel V, et al: Cervical human vertebrae. Quantitative three-dimensional anatomy of the middle and lower regions. *Spine (Phila Pa 1976)* 16:861–869, 1991.

Panjabi MM, Takata K, Goel V, et al: Thoracic human vertebrae. Quantitative three-dimensional anatomy. *Spine (Phila Pa 1976)* 16:888–901, 1991.

Vollmer DG, Banister WM. Thoracolumbar spinal anatomy. *Neurosurg Clin North Am* 8(4):443–453, 1997.

White AA, Panjabi MM: The basic kinematics of the human spine. A review of past and current knowledge. *Spine (Phila Pa 1976)* 3:12–20, 1978.

Woodburne RT: *Essentials of human anatomy*, ed 7, Oxford, England, 1982, Oxford University Press.

REFERENCES

The complete reference list is available online at expertconsult.com.

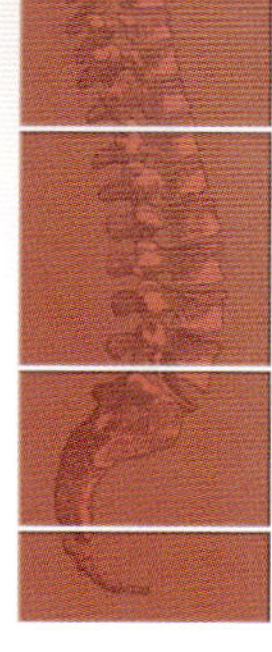

CHAPTER 6

Muscular Support of the Spine

Eric A.K. Mayer | Michael P. Steinmetz

Spinal muscles have long been ignored contributors to spine stability. Paraspinal muscles have been inadequately appreciated and regarded ("lift with your legs, not with your back"), incised with impunity, suffered injury from retraction, neglected through rest/traction, and denervated capriciously. Even in the early 21st century, when bone and collagenous tissue structures (ligaments, tendons, intervertebral discs) are targets of intense basic scientific study, information on spinal muscles often remains empirical, subjective, nonreproducible—and, at worst, harmful. Intended as a compendium of available information and inferences of function, this chapter should challenge the reader to preserve, restore, train, and study the spine.

Muscle, in general, is a highly plastic, adaptable organ. Muscles are classified into three broad categories—striated, smooth, and cardiac muscle—categories that have as much to do with their neurologic control as with their histologic appearance. For the most part, our understanding of muscle form and function is derived from an extensive study of muscles of the *extremities*. Spine muscles, on the other hand, have changed with each phylogenetic selection that produced vertebrates, mammals, and eventually *Homo sapiens*. Histologically, muscle form and function are preserved from other species, but spine muscles have importance in the human beyond that seen in other animals.

The muscles that act as the dynamic control mechanism of the spine constitute the largest collective, coordinated group of muscles in the human body. Human spinal muscle makes us unique among species, allowing us to walk upright exclusively—hence the further ability to carry items to a safe place and thus "accumulate excess." The ability to acquire surplus allows for specialization within a societal structure, impelling the dominance of our species. Without fear of overstatement, our evolutionary success as a species owes everything to the unique structure and function of spinal muscle.

Anatomy

Muscle serves a defined (and seemingly paradoxical) purpose to simultaneously *vitalize with movement* and *protect with strength* the central neural communication link between the brain and periphery. In the past, mischaracterizations of the spine as an overrated "electrical conduit" protecting vital message transduction to the limbs have predominated. This disingenuous oversimplification ignores the fact that interactions with the environment, including force generation, dynamic control, proprioception, and balance, benefit from and often require the intricate coordination of spine function.

The dynamic structure of the spine relies upon muscle to animate with motion its series of paired joints and hydraulically pressurized discs. This dynamic control protects the neural elements while maximizing freedom of mobility. A muscle's function is enhanced by the stability, afferent feedback, and proprioceptive information provided by its associated ligaments, tendons, and joint capsules.[1] This unique combination of motion and stability is demonstrated by the human skill of manipulating objects near the ground from a bipedal stance to lift and carry them to another location. Arguably, the ability to accomplish this "everyday task" has been a key to our success as a species, because the ability to bend efficiently from the waist in combination with squatting and hunkering allows accrual of excess to ensure against environmental pressures like famine and drought. A stable "biomechanical chain" that transfers force efficiently from hands to arms, shoulder girdle, spine, pelvis, and legs and to a stable foot base is essential. In this functional example, the spine musculature acts as a dynamic stabilizer of the biomechanical chain in several ways. It is here that one should recall Panjabi's description of the interplay of the three subsystems of spinal control: muscle control, passive-restraint control, and neural control.[2-4] The cotensioning of abdominal muscles at a distance (force multiplied by a lever arm to generate moment or torque) combined with the collective dorsal force of the erector spinae muscles during flexion-extension allows maintenance of a "balance point."[5-7] At each individual motion segment, the interspinalis, multifidus, and, possibly, intertransverse muscles also provide stability through compressive force spanning only one motion segment.[5,6,8,9] Coupled ventral and dorsal forces have a net compressive force that, in turn, balances motion at the instantaneous axis of rotation for each motion segment, thereby maintaining compression at the disc and minimizing angular change. This net muscle force serves to offset other forces, thereby maintaining the force vector perpendicular to the disc's plane like the guy wires supporting a tent or flagpole or radio tower.[10,11]

In sum, muscles supply dynamic, as well as static, axial compression force to allow for maximal load bearing (for bipedal carrying/lifting) capacity while maintaining function with economy of energy output. Energy is economized via the following mechanical adaptations unique to human musculature: maintaining a balanced plumb line (not working against gravity to maintain posture) with three offsetting curves, sharing tension bands to distribute loads, coupling forces when motion is required, and distributing load/work among the other osteoligamentous static structures.[12]

Form Follows Function

As the father of American architecture, Louis Sullivan stated in 1896, "form ever follows function," and this is true for the human form as for the American skyline. With this in mind, understanding spinal muscle cannot be complete without acknowledging the role of spine muscles in evolutionary change. Evolutionarily, it appears that the common ancestors of land-dwelling vertebrates (including mammals) were ocean-dwelling animals similar to today's fish. Living in water, these animals had to contend with very different forces from creatures that live on land. Large paravertebral muscles provide lateral flexion-extension (crossing the sagittal plane) to propel their bodies through water—demonstrated by the lateral tail motion of the fish. This form of locomotion is evolutionarily conserved in amphibians and land reptiles (even with addition of limbs) as demonstrated by the lateral locomotion of species in the order Crocodylia, including the modern alligator or crocodile. Currently extant reptiles propel themselves forward using lateral spinal motion (side-winding). Propulsion is achieved by alternating contraction of spine muscles that in turn creates alternating sagittal convexities of the spine. This repetitive spine motion allows the ipsilateral foreleg to move forward while the contralateral hindfoot (on the concave side) is brought closer to the contralateral foreleg in preparation for the next reciprocal lateral movement that repeats the motion-event contralaterally.

Adaptation (the results of which are not observed in any reptiles alive today) resulted in a 90-degree transformation of spine muscle motion. This characteristic, seen almost universally in mammals (the platypus and echidna being exceptions), presumably provides an advantage during land locomotion, allowing for explosive growth of the class Mammalia. The transformation allows for flexion-extension (crossing the coronal plane) that enables a greater distance per stride (as seen with the horse or cheetah at full run). Interestingly, land mammals that subsequently repopulated the oceans (whales, seals, manatees) maintained their motion orientation through the coronal plane. This form of spinal locomotion resulted in the vertical orientation of the mammalian tail fluke (a 90-degree transformation compared with fish), even though adaptive pressure has resulted in changes to the other extremities that appear similar to fish.

From an evolutionary standpoint, motion is a balancing act. First, form is intended to maximize the functions of swiftly arriving at a food source or a potential mate while evading a predator. On the other hand, the demand for speed must be balanced with metabolic efficiency that allows the species to survive perturbations in the environment. As stated previously, controlling spine motion (like flexion) with muscles alone is inefficient. Moreover, the space required for the abdominal/thoracic contents further limits the potential size of spine muscles.[13] The evolutionary solution is twofold: (1) strong, elastic dorsal spinal structures (midline ligaments, joint capsules, and lumbodorsal fascia) produce (a) passive restraint, particularly to lumbar spine flexion/extension, and allow (b) static "hanging on the ligaments" subject only to slight, plastic "creep," but without muscular effort; and (2) a lever arm advantage from quadrupeds to use the dorsal pelvic muscles as simultaneous motors and stabilizers of lumbar extension and lower extremity abduction.[14] Specifically, the gluteus and psoas muscles drive the legs more efficiently when the lumbar spine laterally flexes to provide a passive return of energy expended via reciprocal motion.[15] This is of special importance with respect to lumbar and cervical lordosis during surgical procedures as well as in considering the length of construct: excessive fusion length and/or other violations of biomechanical principles lead to decreased efficiency and a painful, less functional patient. Finally, the interplay of the muscles with static structures for metabolic efficiency may have important though insufficiently studied implications for research into so-called motion-preserving technologies.

In summary, the combination of a dorsal ligamentous complex and powerful muscles of the buttocks and dorsal thighs (along with the psoas muscle contributing to controlling the degree of lordosis—discussed later) permits the spine to function like a crane. The boom is the ligament-stabilized flexed spine, the fulcrum is the hips, and the counterweight is the buttocks (maintaining pelvic position with respect to the femurs). Finally, the structure is vitalized by the pelvic extensor musculature that is analogous to the crane's engine.[16,17] This combination of passive and active restraint allows for metabolic parsimony. An important, experimentally observable economy of effort is the tendency of the spine to "hang off its ligaments." This action is a position of comfort and a metabolic conservation frequently observed in stooped laborers and observable in most normal subjects tested. In other words, normal subjects monitored with surface electromyography preferentially flex forward to end range with the lumbar spine (to the point of myoelectrical silence) before adding the component of hip flexion during the initial act of lifting.[18-20] Another efficiency created by muscle is the curvilinear structure of the spine. The combination of cervical lordosis, thoracic kyphosis, and lumbar lordosis creates a balance (and though not myolectrically "silent") requiring minimal muscle output by utilizing the static structure of the thoracolumbar fascia during standing.[12]

The curvilinear structure of the spine that optimizes efficiency is also a prerequisite for human bipedal ambulation and stance. The lumbar lordotic curve converts lateral flexion to torque through the pelvis to the femurs. As noted earlier, this action economizes effort, with upright propulsion leading to a balanced human gait that would be difficult without lumbar lordosis. Conversely, ambulation without lumbar lordosis leads to the shuffling strides of the upright apes whose gait is clearly dissimilar to that of healthy humans (but similar to that of flat back surgical failures). Moreover, the curvilinear structure of the spine permits a greater load to be lifted and carried (so important in human evolution). Spine biomechanical research suggests that cocontraction of spinal and abdominal muscles is the primary generator of the curvilinear structure of the spine that enables greater load bearing than straight-spine models (1200 N vs. 100 N). Furthermore, instantaneous, axial-rotational forces between segments in straight-spine models may lead to rapid failure when the spine is progressively loaded.[21]

This model corroborates observational data of the dynamic contribution of spine muscles to the creation of a compressive-stabilizing force. The cumulative compressive forces applied by the action of muscle, tendon, ligament, and fascia to bony and disc structures enable the spine to withstand greater physiologic forces in sagittal motion as well. This model is analogous to taut guy wires allowing flimsy tent material to withstand 100-mph winds. Tension provided by intrinsic muscle tone and ligamentous passive tension is hypothesized (by the "follower-load" theory) to provide a stabilizing force (in at least the sagittal and coronal planes of motion when standing). This tension directs the force vector to achieve pure compression of the motion segment (which withstands this force largely via the hydraulic force resistance of the disc). The compressive force vector minimizes shear forces implicated as a leading cause of disc degeneration.[10]

Finally, the individual contributions of spine muscles can, alternatively, be seen in the context of function dictating form. Instead of viewing spinal musculature in isolation, one may develop an appreciation of the spinal musculature as an efficiently evolved functional unit, improved upon from earlier iterations, and linking all skeletal muscles to act as one functional unit. The cervicothoracic, shoulder girdle, and upper extremity units are linked by paravertebral, abdominal, buttock, pelvic floor, and hamstring muscles to exert specific force vectors that combine with gravity and the constraint of the passive structures to allow carrying and manipulation while simultaneously maintaining bipedal stance or ambulating. The spinal musculature is the crucial link in a complete biomechanical chain that allows lifting and carrying (of greater than one's own body weight) by the upper extremities while maintaining stable ground contact to haul items out of harm's way or to a safe location. This ability to carry and hoard excess in turn provides maximal evolutionary advantage in an environmental context. The fine balancing act of performance and metabolic economy can tip over into dysfunction when subtle extrinsic (trauma) and/or intrinsic (fear-avoidance) disruptions evolve into a feed-forward system of dysfunction. This concept is ably demonstrated by Panjabi's hypothesis of chronic back pain:[22]

> *Sub-failure injuries of the ligaments and embedded mechanoreceptors . . . generate corrupted transducer signals, which lead to corrupted muscle response patterns produced by the neuromuscular control unit. Muscle coordination and individual muscle force characteristics, i.e., onset, magnitude, and shut-off, are disrupted. This results [sic] in abnormal stresses and strains in the ligaments, mechanoreceptors and muscles, and excessive loading of the facet joints . . . inherently poor healing of spinal ligaments, accelerate degeneration of disc and facet . . . over time, may lead to chronic back pain.*

Physiology and Microanatomy

The relative resistance of muscles due to redundancy and overengineering belies a complex microstructure. Because muscle functions as the dynamic control mechanism of the skeletal system, its structural complexity allows the tissue to respond to environmental cues to be faster, stronger, or more metabolically parsimonious. This very adaptability has very likely made muscle an overlooked and underappreciated structure.

Muscle incorporates many long, overlapping cells specifically adapted for shortening. Voluntary, or skeletal, muscle is by far the most abundant (by volume) muscle type in humans. Muscles controlling spinal movement, in turn, constitute the largest assemblage of skeletal muscles in the body. Of the various muscle-specific organelles and matrix proteins, the most common constituents are actin and myosin isoforms, which represent approximately 25% to 30% of the total body protein synthesis.[15,23] This net metabolic consumption underscores muscles' complexity and versatility, which originates not in its chemistry but in its structure. Sarcomeres, the basic structural units (individual cells) of muscles, are attached end to end to form a muscle filament. Muscle filaments are grouped together in tight formation, with their respective nuclei and organelles pushed to the periphery to form myofibrils.[24] Bathing the myofibrils, nuclei, and organelles is a fluid called sacroplasm whose fluctuating electrolyte concentration is controlled by the external, semipermiable lipid bilayer known as the sarcolemma. The myofibril architecture is highly organized, aligning longitudinally within the sarcolemma, which is indented by a motor axon at its myoneural junction. Myofibrils are bundled to form muscle fibers that are, in turn, covered and connected to other muscle fibers by an endomysium. The axial muscle fibers may be only a few millimeters in diameter but can be 5 cm or more in length. Many fibers are bound together by perimesium collagen to form organized fascicles that are bundled together to form what we call muscle.[24,25] Muscle attaches to bone via a collagenous tissue called tendon. The function of this superstructure depends upon the two-way communication (between the alpha motor neuron and muscle and the Golgi-tendon complex and spinal reflex arc) and the variable neural innervation by one motor neuron that may coordinate contraction for anywhere from 15 to 5000 muscle fibers.

The rigidly organized substructure of the myofilament appears as light and dark striations under a light microscope—hence the designation striated muscle for skeletal muscle. Under normal circumstances, contraction of striated muscle does not occur without neural stimulus, whereas contraction of cardiac and most smooth muscle fibers autopropagates, triggering adjacent fibers to contract without neural stimulation. The cellular mechanics of contractions are relatively simple: actin filaments (occupying the light-colored I band at rest) slide over the myosin filaments (found in the A band and interdigitating with the I band at rest) until, with complete contraction, they completely overlap and eliminate the light H band under microscopic visualization. The biochemical reactions are more complex. Contraction initiates with the release of acetylcholine at the myoneural junction, depolarizing the sarcolemma by changing its permeability to sodium and potassium ions. The sarcolemma-induced ion cascade stimulates release of calcium ions, sequestered in the sarcoplasmic reticulum. These calcium ions bind the troponin complex (C, T, and I), inducing a conformational change that uncovers a "sticky" portion of the actin filament. Myosin, fueled by adenosine phosphate molecules (ATP and ADP), binds and unbinds actin to induce the ratcheting of the myosin along the length of the actin filament. The acetylcholine is rapidly hydrolyzed by acetylcholine esterase, and the calcium is rapidly sequestered back into the sarcoplasmic reticulum so that each nerve firing in skeletal muscle is a discrete, pulsed event rather than a sustained spasm. In this way, multiple stimulations of billions of sarcomeres induce the movements we see that form the basis of dynamic control.

When broken down to its constituent biomechanical parts, it appears that the rate-limiting steps to muscle function are myoneural junction integrity, ionic stability, filament cohesion, and energy. On a more holistic scale, series elasticity, motivation, training, endurance, and energy supply become the rate-determining steps of muscle function. Discrete, independent control of muscle fibers (e.g., only a few motor units contracting or muscle control by multiple motor neurons) permits a gradation of contraction that enables—depending on circumstance—voluntary vacillation between refined control or rapid, maximal contraction. The strength of a single contraction, or "twitch," depends on the number of fibers that contract. The ability to sustain the contraction (endurance) depends on the ability to recruit more muscle fibers with increasingly repeated firing frequency so that *just enough* fibers are recruited to do the minimum necessary to complete a task (muscle efficiency). Other factors, muscle fiber type or fuel source, may independently affect endurance (ability to sustain a contraction), but recruitment adapts through training and neurocognitive, motivational factors.

The fuel for muscle contraction (as well as for most bodily functions) is phosphate from the disassociation of adenosine triphosphate (ATP) to adenosine diphosphate (ADP). How the ATP is derived and the cost associated with fuel manufacture pays the salary of many professionals (and continues to propel an illicit subculture of pseudoscientists in medicine and nutrition). For the scope of this chapter, the major consideration is whether ATP is produced via hydrolysis of glucose into water and carbon dioxide or via the citric acid cycle (Krebs cycle). The implication of emerging research is that exercise may stimulate a more favorable milieu for local and distant cells through a paracrine effect. Lactic acid, when it accrues in "anaerobic" metabolism, is one of the implicated protein-signaling molecules.

As we go to press, the implications of new basic scientific research in muscle metabolism have not seen wide application in clinical care. Research based on the experimental work of George Brooks, termed *lactate shuttle theory*, suggests that higher concentrations of lactic acid produced in the skeletal muscles have beneficial local and possibly distant paracrine effects.[26-28] This growing body of research implies that instead of being a "dead-end metabolite" or mediator of muscle fatigue (as was widely published in the 1960s through the 1980s), lactate may be the mediator of beneficial effects seen empirically in training and exercise. Some research even refutes the implication of lactic acid in fatigue and notes that pH effects of hydrogen ion excess are the primary agents of diminished contractile power.[27] In total, the lactate ion may serve multiple beneficial roles in stimulating change in body milieu in the presence of muscle exertion to maintain constant energy (via conversion of lactate to glycogen); to recruit new energy sources (gluconeogenesis); to stimulate new vascularity (angiogenesis); and to promote a local cascade of healing, plasticity, and hyperplasia.[26,29] Although it is beyond the scope of this chapter, there is an urgent need for research into this area because the raison d'être of spine physicians is based on activity, strength, and maintaining function after the patient leaves our office.

There are several ways to infer how the microstructure we have described influences the function of a healthy spine. Some analysis has focused on structural composition, enumerating the relative contribution of fiber length, fiber size, and fiber directional orientation to classify muscle. This modeling of physiologic cross-sectional area is combined with geometric calculations from the fulcrum (moment arm) to model idealized function and classify muscle type. Alternatively, the ATPase work of Engel in 1962 initiated a body of research demonstrating distinctly different motor units within skeletal muscle.[30] Myotype classification schemes have proliferated based on histology, morphology, or function. Briefly stated, the interaction between the type of myosin heavy chain (ATP-binding site) and actin within individual sarcomeres determines functional differences based on this classification. Furthermore, the rate at which the myosin heavy chains can repetitively bind ATP and release ADP under conditions of physiologic stress defines the function of the sarcomere into one of three broad functional categories.[31] Type I fibers have a slower twitch response (rate or frequency of a single contraction), with good fatigue resistance and lower tension development (power). Type II muscle displays a fast twitch, with broader recruitment for more forceful tension development, but relatively poor endurance as compared with type I muscle fibers. Type II fibers are often subdivided into type IIA (that still show a fast twitch response, but have a fatigue threshold between type I and type IIB) and type IIB, showing the fastest speed, the greatest recruitment force (power), and the most precipitous onset of fatigue.[32,33] Though researchers continue to further subclassify fiber types, type I, type IIA, and type IIB muscles remain the basis of the broadest functional class of voluntary skeletal muscles. Structurally, type I fibers have rich capillary beds with high concentrations of mitochondrial enzymes and relatively low concentrations of glycogen and myosin adenosine triphosphatase—making them appear ideally suited for resisting fatigue associated with aerobic activity. The milieu of type II muscles is very different, with high concentrations of glycogen and a ready supply of ATP for fast, strong contractions in a fixed time period. It should be remembered that in gross structure, each muscle is a heterogeneous, woven tapestry consisting of *all* of the above fiber subtypes. Relative predominance of one particular fiber type is largely based on genetics and anatomic location of a particular muscle. However, one cannot forget the plasticity inherent in muscle and the mutability based on environmental factors of muscle, age of the individual, nutrition, training, demand, and type of exercise.[34,35]

In addition to muscle substructural form, there is also the distance from the joint's axis of rotation. In a simple model, this distance is termed the lever arm or, more correctly, the moment arm. In the case of only one muscle acting on a joint, the moment arm can be represented by the distance of a muscle's action in relation to the joint's axis of rotation. In other words, the amount of muscle shortening causes joint excursion through an arc. From this basic knowledge, it is easy to appreciate that even if a muscle is predominantly type II muscle and built for speed and power, it might not translate to rapid joint angular velocity if there is a large moment arm. Instead, in this scenario, the muscle's activity would be generating high torque at lower angular velocity. The architectural superstructure adds another layer of complexity with multiple intrinsic and extrinsic muscles exerting force to maximize strength and minimize shear, while economizing metabolic expenditure.

Musculature of the Spine Functional Unit

This section offers a brief overview of a compendium of work by McIntosh, Bogduk, Delp, Kamibayshi and Richmond. We refer the reader to these and other sources for more detailed description of the morphometry of individual muscle groups.

Intrinsic Muscles

Erector Spinae Muscles

This large group of interconnected muscles has robust functionality for movement and restraint. It spans the entire spine from the sacrum to the skull. Although the biomechanics of this muscle are still the subject of study, the intricate redundancy of its neural control manifests the importance of this muscle group.[36] The innervation arises from the dorsal rami division of the adjacent nerve root that spreads out to coinnervate up to two levels rostral and caudal (four levels total). The intricately redundant neuromuscular control (as opposed to the single-root control seen in limbs) allows one to infer the importance of this structure. The muscle mass can be divided up into four main divisions whose prefix or suffix (lumborum, thoracis, cervicis, or capitis) denote location—but not necessarily division from the whole. These muscles arise from a robust aponeurosis attaching to the sacrum and pelvis. Medially, the *spinalis* group attaches to the spinous processes. It may be absent in the cervical spine, where it is replaced by semispinalis capitis and cervicis that attach the transverse processes of cervical and upper thoracic vertebrae to the nuchal lines and cervical spinous processes, respectively.[37] Lateral to the spinalis are the longissimus muscles: long, robust sarcomeres probably well adapted to generate great force even when stretched beyond their optimal length.[38] The most lateral group is the intercostalis, connecting the lumbar anoneurosis to the ribs and the rib fulcrum to the neck and head.

Multifidus Muscles

This group of muscles is deep, short, and powerful, acting with short moment arms to generate significant force. Multifidus muscles span the entire length of the spine in the form of bridging, short, overlapping segments. An individual multifidus has several bands that illustrate its multidirectional function to alternatively control and resist rotation, abduction (lateral flexion), and extension. The fascicle length of a single muscle varies from two to four segments, connecting the mammillary process to the rostral spinous process over two to four segments proximally. In the upper cervical spine, these important muscles connect to the facet capsules, and in the lower cervical spine, they attach to the transverse processes of the upper thoracic spine.[38] Like the *erector spinae*, these muscles have a redundant, multilevel innervation, allowing function to be maintained even if a proximate dorsal ramus is injured.

Deep Muscles

The *interspinalis*, *rotator*, and *intertransversarii* muscles are the deep muscles of the spine whose function is only elementarily understood. These muscles are paired, deep muscles on either side of the spine, spanning one segment to contribute dynamic force to the strong, elastic interspinous ligaments. In the lumbar spine, the intertransversarii consist of a pair of muscles bilaterally, spanning the transverse processes of adjacent vertebrae. The *splenius cervicis*, *semispinalis cervicis*, and *capitis* are deep muscles unique to the cervical spine, connecting the spinous process to transverse processes in criss-crossing, overlapping patterns from the thoracic spine to the cervical vertebrae. Their contribution controls lateral flexion, extension, and, to a lesser extent, rotation. These deep muscles are often cavalierly excised during surgical approaches, to the untold detriment of the patient (especially in longer dorsal fusions that often have adjacent segment kyphosis or failure later). Finally, the *rectus capitis* group and *obliquus capitis* group (major/minor, superior/inferior) span C1-2 to control rotation and restraint of this biomechanically tenuous area of fine engineering.

Lateral Control Arms

This group comprises several muscles lateral to the spine with large moment arms. The *quadratus lumborum* originates on the iliac crest and iliolumbar ligament and obliquely inserts on the lowest rib, connecting to transverse processes of the upper four lumbar vertebrae. The innervation is from the ventral rami of T12-L1-L2-L3 roots. The *psoas major* muscle attaches to the transverse processes and vertebral bodies of all the lumbar segments and combines with the *iliacus* (arising from ilium) to form the *iliopsoas* muscle.[36] Though generally thought of as a primary hip extensor (and therefore extrinsic to the spine), the iliopsoas is a primary generator of force ventral to the coronal balance point. Paradoxically, iliopsoas is an intersegmental extensor in the midlumbar spine, even as it produces flexion at the lumbosacral junction in the process of increasing the lumbar lordosis. This action increases lordosis and, like the tent guy-wire model, creates spinal stability during sitting and standing through compressive force.[39] Additionally, the iliopsoas muscle doubles the flexion strength and triples flexion dynamic power compared with that of the abdominals alone.[40] Finally, the contribution of the iliopsoas to lateral flexion is likely responsible for a reciprocal economy of motion in normal gait and restraining shear while sitting.[41] In the authors' (possibly controversial) opinion, these contributions to spinal stability and control make the iliopsoas an intrinsic spine muscle. The psoas major and iliacus muscles are innervated by the femoral nerve (L2 and L3 root segments innervation with minor contribution of L4) and lie in close proximity to the lumbosacral plexus. Proximal weakness resulting in hip and/or back pain is a consequence of poorly conceived surgical approaches that denervate or devascularize via aggressive retraction. The analogue lateral control muscles in the cervical spine are the *sternocleidomastoid* and the *trapezius* muscles. Both of these may be myometrically (categorization of muscles by movement and orientation) divided into three sections, each of which provides flexion, lateral motion, contralateral rotation, and extension based on the direction and length of the fascicles. Like the lumbar lateral intrinsics (iliopsoas and quadratus lumborum), sternocleidomastoid, and trapezius have long moment arms and allow motion while providing a high magnitude of downward force to resist motion. The innervation and control of these two muscles remain debated, with a large motor contribution from the cranial nerve XI (spinal accessory) but proprioceptive, sensory, and possibly motor contributions from the upper cervical root segments. Analogous to lumbar spine motion, the intrinsic control of these lateral control muscles (exerting force through longer moment arms) in the cervical spine is vital for both efficient motion and resistance to shear. More focused investigations of individual muscles and their respective roles are available in other sources.

Extrinsic Spine Muscles

As we have demonstrated, the majority of voluntary muscle in the human skeleton exerts some influence over spine function. Extrinsic to the muscles already discussed are the four layers of abdominal muscles (*transversus abdominis*, *internal obliques*, *external obliques*, and *rectus abdominis*). These muscles have been the subject of much discussion and popular press—mostly centered on the laudable, but poorly defined notion of *core strength*. Despite the popularity of core exercises, there is surprisingly scant research to support the focus on abdominal strength for improving spine function or resistance to injury. To be fair, no information credibly demonstrates harm resulting from exercises focused on abdominal core strength either. Additionally, the large muscles of the buttocks that act as hip extensors or abductors (*gluteus maximus*, *medius*, *minimus*) also have intricate contributions to the spine. In a rudimentary analogy, they act as the "engine" and "counterweight" when the spine approximates a "crane" during lifting/bending activity as well as providing the reciprocal coupled motion across the lumbar spine during ambulation. Thigh muscles (*biceps femoris*, *semimembranosus*, *semitendinosus*) dorsally and (*rectus femoris*) ventrally restrain pelvic translation—thus preventing wasted energy during ambulation as well as providing resistance force when the pelvis serves as a fulcrum during stooping/bending labor. Similarly, the *rhomboid major* and *minor* and *levator scapulae* connect the scapula to the thoracic spine and provide vital scapular stability for lifting or ballistic arm motion. Ventrally, the cervical vertebrae are connected to the ribs by the poorly studied and poorly understood *scalenus* muscles. This muscle group may serve a purpose similar to one of the iliopsoas' functions, but its role remains a subject of folklore rather than hard data. In the thoracic spine, the *latissimus dorsi* and *serratus anterior* are generally associated with arm movement, but with arms or ribs fixed and stabilized, they may actively contribute to trunk mobility. Structurally speaking, there have been good studies of isolated spine muscle contributions, but in terms of integrated motion, adequate data of either normal motion or the sequence of failure that leads to dysfunction, pain, deconditioning, and, occasionally, disability are lacking.

Motion and Strength—Putting It All Together

George Bernard Shaw once said, "The only man I know who behaves sensibly is my tailor; he takes my measurements anew each time he sees me. The rest go on with their old measurements and expect me to fit them." By this definition, those of us involved in spine care in general—and in our regard for muscle in particular—behave NON-sensibly. Even preceding Cady et al.'s work, an empirical understanding of the importance of strength and flexibility to overall health existed.[42] Unfortunately, our rigor in measuring or tracking these fundamental components of function has bordered on lackadaisical. The tendency for nihilism has overcome our best instincts as scientists to rigorously measure what we do and what we advise.[43] Moreover, numerous studies have shown that pain is self-serving, and that following the maxim, "if it hurts . . . don't do it" further reinforces stiffness, atrophy, and psychological fear—exacerbating the "corrupted response patterns" described by Panjabi.[22] This leaves physicians in a conundrum, as they do not wish to advocate activity that leads to injury or to lose patient confidence.[44-47] Only functional measurement to quantify physical deficits will overcome physician nescience when tailoring rehabilitation to meet patient-specific goals. The current expectation of a "one-size-fits-all" evaluate and treat approach lacks sufficient specificity for the physician to help the patient achieve the desirable gains. In 60 years since DeLorme's groundbreaking work in 1945, we have learned much about the secondary physical changes accompanying immobilization and disuse in the spine and extremities.[48,49] Physician intervention combines with spontaneous healing to produce maximum recovery of disrupted collagenous tissues (soft or osseous) in a relatively short period of time—6 to 12 weeks. Exercise science elucidates the effect of training to increasing strength of contraction by enhancing muscular factors, such as muscle size, fiber type, and fiber number, but also (and perhaps to a greater extent) to neural factors.[15] Muscle plasticity is at its apex under the influence of training, and at its nadir with senescence. Between these extremes, certain anabolic hormones (either endogenous or exogenous) may combine with force production to create the characteristic rapid increase in strength and muscle diameter exemplified during hormonal drive of pubescence. Specific exercises, sequences, and frequency of training in healthy normals remain under study. Lost is the understanding of how bulk appearance of muscle translates to function of muscle. The paradox of healthy individual training is demonstrated by data showing that isometric contraction (in which the contracting muscle is not permitted to shorten) is far more effective in increasing muscle bulk. However, exaggerated isometric muscle bulk elevates injury risk and decreases dynamic function with concomitant poor correlation to strength gains. In fact, most research agrees that isotonic and isokinetic training correlate far better with dynamic strength than any isometric regime.

The simplicity of muscle strength gains in healthy individuals (where production of force to failure increases tolerance through training) does not necessarily result in the recovery of coordination, mobility, and force after injury. Injury, pain, and cognitive factors may create a feed-forward system of deconditioning—thereby establishing a pattern of further degenerative change.[50] Functional testing, though in its infancy and poorly remunerated, provides the opportunity for longitudinal measurement coinciding with functional improvement. Specifically, several longitudinal studies correlate spinal strength performance to imaging (e.g., CT and MRI) findings as well as occupational gains.[16,51-53] Based on DeLorme's work, the obvious relationship between extremity joints and strength of their contiguous musculature in normal, athletic (supernormal), and pathologic (subnormal: traumatic, arthritic, or deconditioned) situations has led investigators to study similar relationships in the spine.[54,55] The study of spine muscle strength has suffered from a lack of a gold standard (contralateral limb) against which to test; as well as disagreement over the functional implications of isometric, isotonic, or isokinetic force approximations to real world kinematics. In the end, development of a normative database to assess not just pathologic states, but to verify that rehabilitation has achieved anything meaningful (other than comfort care) is still only sporadically available.

Though "rehab" may be at the outer edge of interest to surgeon readers of this book, a basic familiarity with such seems prudent. Isometric test models employing strain gauges have been in use for over 60 years; however, like the false appearance of strength in a body-builder, isometrics has a wide gaussian distribution when used to predict function versus appearance. Twenty years of data seem to favor isokinetic measures. Multiple papers demonstrate that measurable deficits in strength, endurance, and neuromuscular coordination correlate with dysfunction and disability. Moreover, patients who decrease isokinetic deficits show ability to return to work.[56,57] In short, the crux of assessment requires visual analysis of the area below the curve, plotting force in relation to range of motion. The integral of that curve represents work, and its shape has a relation to effort, injury, and deconditioning. Controversy exists regarding the clinical utility of trunk strength testing, in part because of normal human variability and in part because of unrecognized sources of error related to testing procedures.[58,59] Despite some controversy, clear decrements in the pathologic states are seen with selective loss of extensor strength compared with flexors and an inability to maintain strength at high speeds.[16,51-53,60] By contrast, supernormal individuals or athletes (e.g., female gymnasts, male soccer players, tennis players, and wrestlers) appear to exceed mean torque/body weight strength ratios for the normal population by 15% to 40%. Furthermore, they show no decrease in torque output at high speeds (termed "high-speed drop-off"), which often is the hallmark of pathology, but may be seen in normals, as well. Additionally, supernormals maintain a very stable ratio of extensor to flexor strength (balanced, efficient use of coupled force).[60,61] The precise cause of reduced strength in the face of some pain-producing pathology remains a mystery. This mystery is heightened with advances in computerization making curve analysis possible to show precise measurements of work performed, power consumed, and torque exerted that may give insight to assessment of "effort." Because only maximal muscular effort is truly reproducible, variability of curve shape on test-retest may inform an effort factor. Whereas muscle atrophy undoubtedly occurs with prolonged disuse and deconditioning, pain may inhibit neuromuscular function through a nociceptive reflex feedback mechanism. Similarly, psychosocially induced phenomena (e.g., anxiety, fear of reinjury, or depression changing psychomotor responses) may unconsciously attenuate effort, producing submaximal, variable measurements.[62,63] This unrecognized pathologic feedback loop, in turn, hinders optimal outcomes of spine care, which affects the reputation of our field.

Muscle-Sparing Surgery

In the last decade, improvements in technology, visualization, technique, material innovation, imaging, and device performance have led to greater use of lumbar surgical approaches that are defined as "muscle sparing." These techniques are covered in greater detail in the following chapters, but it is worth examining the claims of muscle sparing. As noted, the lumbar spine is a finely balanced biomechanical wonder that relies on the integration of intervertebral height, joint mobility, proprioception, muscle balance, and osseoligamentous constraint to allow us to function without pain. Though ample redundancy is undoubtedly built into the system, minimizing the disruption of biomechanical integrity hopefully will lead to better functional outcomes for all spine patients.

Lumbar surgery has classically involved extensive dissection of the dorsal muscle, fascia, ligamentous structures, and occasionally joints. The dissection is even more extensive when arthrodesis (with or without instrumentation) is performed. Unintended consequences of denervation, compression, retraction, or vascular injury have led to other biomechanical sequelae.[16,64] Iatrogenic muscle injury related to the aforementioned has been documented histologically, histochemically, and electrophysiologically.[65] Preventive measures of back muscle injury after dorsolumbar spine surgery have been conducted in rats.[16,64-66] It has been hypothesized that this iatrogenic injury may result in instability of the spinal motion segment, loss of the previously described biomechanical balance, and straightening of the lumbar lordosis. All of this may result in a dysfunctional motion segment and pain. Decreased morbidity by sparing vulnerable structures may serve to maintain mobility and function, thereby improving outcomes.

The dorsolateral approach first described by Cloward has been controversial through the years.[67,68] The extensive morbidity of the traditional muscle stripping approaches led to the development of muscle-sparing approaches to the spine. Most such surgery descriptions are based on the approach originally characterized by Wiltse et al.[69] When performed judiciously, the paramedian, or Wiltse, approach allows the erector spinae to be split along the aponeurosis, thus "sparing" the muscle, fascia, and some of the ligamentous structures. Until recently, much larger incisions were still required to perform multilevel decompression or arthrodesis.

Foley and Smith receive credit for describing a percutaneous/minimal access endoscopic approach to the lumbar intervertebral disc.[70] Subsequently, the field exploded, and similar MIS techniques may be applied to virtually every region of the spine. The distinguishing feature of this procedure utilizes the a technique of muscle dilation through a small paramedian incision with multiple dilators until a final tubular retractor is "docked" on the area of surgical interest (e.g., lumbar lamina). The marketing of these methods cite decreased trauma, dissection, blood loss, and pain. However, with increased pressure from tubular retraction denervation/devascularization of the deep muscles is still possible. Additionally, compared with a standard microdiscectomy, only the approach differs. Unfortunately, minimally invasive tubular approaches have not shown improved long-term outcomes over traditional microdiscectomy. Moreover, at least one randomized controlled study shows worse outcome scores for leg or back pain following endoscopic, tubular discectomy compared with standard microdiscectomy.[71] For the most part, the beneficial data associated with the tubular approach are measured in decreased hospitalization time and medication usage.[72,73]

Muscle-sparing technology and approaches have been applied to lumbar arthrodesis. Minimally invasive fusion techniques through tubular retractors were popularized with transforaminal lumbar interbody fusion and now are widely applied to multiple approaches for interbody fusion.[74] Although long-term outcomes with minimally invasive arthrodesis are indistinguishable (and more expensive) than standard fusion, there are data that short-term outcomes with muscle sparing are superior for pain, time to ambulation, hospital length of stay, and medication usage.[75] The implication, awaiting literature confirmation, is that earlier mobilization because patients hurt less may in fact lead to better outcomes. We still await associations of outcomes with studies of muscle bulk, isokinetic strength, biomechanical integrity, and histologic appearance.

The ventral transperitoneal approach has been described since the 1930s in various iterations.[76] A spine surgeon can achieve (indirect) decompression, stabilization, fusion (at a variable rate), and now motion preservation though this approach. Often these surgeries lose the benefit of dorsal muscle preservation when surgeons later elect for additional dorsal stabilization. With newer instrumentation and biomechanical wisdom (outlined later in this book) these surgeries are often performed as a stand-alone ventral procedure. Additionally, retraction can damage abdominal and ventral lumbar muscles that play a key role in maintenance of proper spine balance. The ventral approach has been modified to go retroperitoneally with laparoscopic devices that allow the perceived (unconfirmed) benefit of splitting of the abdominal musculature to provide for more rapid postoperative healing and less perturbation of the abdominal viscera, but often at the cost of crossing and possibly injuring the psoas muscle, which may have a very important role in lumbopelvic coordination of functional tasks. As of the writing of this chapter in 2010, the laparoscopic anterior lumbar interbody fusion has largely been abandoned in the United States because of lack of improved outcomes and increased complications. Keeping in mind the advantages of protecting lumbar musculature and maintaining mobility, there is hope that the functional outcomes of surgical spine procedures will continue to improve.

Summary

Spine muscle has the preeminent role in what we are as a species and what we do as a profession. To the point, everything that we do as physicians (outlined throughout this book) from drug prescription, to injections, to surgery, and beyond are to reestablish a beachhead of stability from which the patient can proceed to maximize strength and flexibility to allow function. Anything we do that does not serve the purpose of function (e.g., harming muscle by excision or excessive retraction during surgery) is a disservice to the patient. Unfortunately, our inability to measure and classify normal spine muscle function hinders our ability to reapproximate normal function. As the specialist whose skill and insight helped to rebuild a traumatized postwar Japan, W. E. Deming can provide surprising insight into what we do as spine surgeons. In applying lessons to restore both Japan and later the Ford Motor Company (in the 1980s) to health, he often used a quote that should serve us well: "If you can't describe what you are doing as a process, you don't know what you are doing" (W. E. Deming).

KEY REFERENCES

Antonio JA, Gonyea WJ: Skeletal muscle fiber hyperplasia. *Med Sci Sports Exerc* 25(12):1333–1345, 1993.

Brooks GA: Intra- and extra-cellular lactate shuttles. *Med Sci Sports Exerc* 32:790–799, 2000.

Mayer T, Vanharanta H, Gatchel R, et al: Comparison of CT scan muscle measurements and isokinetic trunk strength in postoperative patients. *Spine* 14:33–36, 1989.

Neblett R, Mayer T, Gatchel R, et al: Quantifying the lumbar flexion-relaxation phenomenon: theory, normative data and clinical applications. *Spine* 28:1435–1446, 2003.

Newton M, Waddell G: Trunk strength testing with iso-machines: I. Review of a decade of scientific evidence. *Spine* 7:801–811, 1993.

Patwardhan AG, Havey RM, Carandang G, et al: Effect of compressive follower preload on the flexion-extension response of the human lumbar spine. *J Orthop Res* 21:540–546, 2003.

REFERENCES

The complete reference list is available online at expertconsult.com.

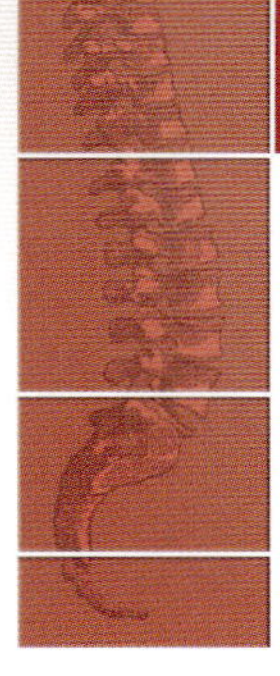

CHAPTER 7

Anatomy and Physiology of Congenital Spinal Lesions

Kai-Ming G. Fu | Justin S. Smith | Christopher I. Shaffrey

The term *congenital spinal anomaly* or *lesion* encompasses a variety of different pathologies affecting the spine, including defects in neural tissue and the vertebral column. This chapter is intended to provide a summary of the possible pathology a spine surgeon may encounter. Discussion of management and operative techniques is generally deferred to other chapters. This chapter discusses abnormalities of the cervical, thoracic, lumbar, and sacral regions, progressing from rostral to caudal.

Preoperative Considerations

In general, congenital spinal anomalies are sporadic, isolated cases.[1,2] A wide variety of associated anomalies often accompany the spinal deformity and often need to be addressed prior to treatment of spinal lesions.[3,4] In fact, the incidence of associated renal abnormalities is roughly 25% and that for cardiac abnormalities is 10%.[5] Intraspinal anomalies, such as stenosis, diastematomyelia, and tethering of the spinal cord, may also occur (5–35%) in association with congenital spinal deformities.[6-9] Therefore, before making treatment decisions, the entire bony vertebral column and spinal cord must be thoroughly analyzed using radiographs, CT, and MRI. Pulmonary function testing and/or arterial blood gases should be obtained when a thoracotomy is planned or when severe thoracic lordosis is present.

Craniovertebral Junction Abnormalities

The craniovertebral junction includes the skull base, atlas, and axis, as well as the neural and vascular structures contained within them. Craniovertebral junction abnormalities encompass a group of conditions that result from abnormal fetal development. Often, these disorders remain undetected during childhood and manifest themselves during adulthood or after minor trauma, as the close association between neural and vascular structures can result in functional compromise during the course of aging or after a traumatic insult.

Basilar Invagination

Basilar invagination results from a defect in the chondrocranium and is often associated with both skeletal and neural axis abnormalities.[10-12] It results from deformation in all three parts of the occipital bone (basiocciput, exocciput, and squamous occipital bone).[11] Two types of basilar invagination have been identified: ventral and paramedian.[10-12] In ventral basilar invagination, the basiocciput is shortened and the associated platybasia raises the plane of the foramen magnum. In paramedian basilar invagination, the exoccipital bone is hypoplastic and the medial portion of the occipital bone is elevated. Clinically, the distinction is not important, and there is admixture between types. One should evaluate patients for an associated elevation of the floor of the posterior fossa that is most pronounced in the region of the foramen magnum. This anomaly may compromise the space available within the foramen magnum.[13] Associated skeletal developmental anomalies found with basilar invagination include occipitalization of the atlas and Klippel-Feil syndrome in addition to neural axis abnormalities such as Chiari malformation, syringobulbia, syringomyelia, and hydrocephalus.[11,12] Although the term *basilar impression* is often used synonymously with *basilar invagination*, this condition refers to an acquired form of basilar invagination caused by softening of the occipital bone, which occurs in conditions such as rheumatoid arthritis, Paget disease, hyperparathyroidism, achondroplasia, and osteogenesis imperfecta.[14]

Patients who are symptomatic from pure basilar invagination most commonly present with weakness and paresthesias in the limbs, whereas those patients with symptomatic Chiari malformations typically have cerebellar and vestibular complaints. Both groups may have evidence of lower cranial nerve dysfunction. Many patients do not develop symptoms until the second or third decade of life.[15] This may be related to increasing instability from ligamentous laxity caused by aging, similar to that from delayed myelopathies reported after atlantoaxial dislocations.[16] If chronic instability is present, granulation tissue may develop and act as a space-occupying mass in the ventral portion of the foramen magnum. Fibrous bands and dural adhesions are common in the dorsal cervicomedullary junction and around the cerebellar tonsils in basilar invagination.[11] A high incidence of vertebral artery anomalies in basilar invagination has been reported (important for surgical planning), and symptoms of vertebral artery insufficiency can occur.[12,17] Diagnosis of basilar impression (or invagination) is based on radiographic evaluation that demonstrates the altered relationship between the occipital bone and the upper cervical spine. Classically, this diagnosis is made by radiographic evaluation of the craniovertebral junction. A series of reference lines have been described to assist with this evaluation.[12] MRI assists in delineating the relationship between the neural structures and the bony abnormalities; however, bony pathology should be evaluated with a thin-section CT.

Assimilation of the Atlas

Assimilation of the atlas represents a failure of segmentation between the atlas and the base of the skull. Embryologically, this entity represents a failure of segmentation between the fourth occipital and first spinal sclerotomes. This condition occurs in 0.25% of the population.[10] The assimilation may be partial or complete and can involve the ventral arch of the atlas, the lateral masses, or the entire atlas. In many instances, assimilation of the atlas occurs with other spinal abnormalities, such as basilar invagination; Klippel-Feil syndrome; or Chiari malformation; as well as systemic congenital abnormalities such as cleft palate or urinary tract abnormalities.[18] Patients with atlanto-occipital fusion often present with symptoms much like those for patients with classic Klippel-Feil syndrome, that is, restricted motion, short neck, low hairline, and torticollis.[10] An increased incidence of atlantoaxial instability occurs with assimilation of the atlas, especially if there is failure of segmentation between the second and third vertebrae.[11]

The onset of symptoms in assimilation of the atlas generally occurs in the third and fourth decades of life. Dull headache and scalp tenderness in the distribution of the greater occipital nerve occurs frequently. Ventral compression of the brainstem from the odontoid processes is also a common finding. Weakness, spasticity, gait disturbances, or cranial nerve dysfunction can be associated problems.[10] Neurologic symptoms have been related to the position of the odontoid process as an indication of the degree of actual or relative basilar impression. Vertical and horizontal nystagmus is related to cerebellum and tonsillar abnormalities. Decreased posterior column function from dorsal compression by the foramen magnum or a dural band is a less common finding. Symptoms may develop precipitously, but in the majority of cases the onset is gradual.

Atlantoaxial Instability

Atlantoaxial instability may result from aplasia or hypoplasia of the odontoid process, from laxity of the transverse ligament, or with assimilation of the atlas. Atlantoaxial instability is associated with Down syndrome, Klippel-Feil syndrome, numerous skeletal dysplasias, osteogenesis imperfecta, neurofibromatosis, and congenital scoliosis.[19] The clinical significance of this condition is the potential for neurologic compromise, which can range from pain and dysesthesias in the distribution of the greater occipital nerve to tetraplegia or death.[10,11] The articulation between the first and second cervical vertebrae is the most mobile segment in the vertebral column and is the least inherently stable. The odontoid process acts as a bony buttress that prevents hyperextension. However, the remainder of the normal range of motion is maintained and depends on the integrity of the ligamentous and capsular structures. Neurologic compromise can occur despite a normal odontoid process. With an attenuated or ruptured transverse atlantal ligament, a relative ventral shift of the atlas over the axis can result in spinal cord injury by impingement against the intact odontoid process such as occurs with atlantal assimilation.[11,20] The risk is less if the odontoid process is absent, fractured, or moves with the axis during flexion, as occurs with most cases of os odontoideum.[21] The stability of the atlantoaxial complex can often be determined using lateral radiographs. The atlantodental interval (ADI) is the distance between the dorsal edge of the ventral ring of the atlas and the ventral edge of the odontoid process. The normal ADI is less than 3 mm in adults and less than 4 mm in children.[22,23] It has been suggested that an ADI greater than 3 mm in adults indicates a disruption of the transverse ligament. An ADI of 5 to 10 mm represents additional ligamentous damage, with total ligamentous disruption occurring in patients with an ADI greater than 10 mm.[22] In congenital anomalies, such as hypoplasia of the odontoid process or os odontoideum, the space available for the cord (SAC) is often a better predictor of potential for neurologic compromise. The SAC is the distance from the ventral edge of the dorsal ring of the atlas or foramen magnum to the dorsal aspect of the odontoid process or the dorsal aspect of the axis. Greenberg suggested that in the adult, spinal cord compression always occurred when the SAC was 14 mm or less and never occurred if the SAC was 18 mm or more.[24] In cases of os odontoideum, a SAC of 13 mm or less is associated with neurologic sequelae.[25] In cases with persistent concerns about atlantoaxial stability, flexion-extension lateral radiographs can be performed. An awake patient should voluntarily perform the flexion-extension movements. MRI should be considered for any patient with a neurologic deficit before obtaining flexion-extension radiographs. MRI with flexion and extension views provides an excellent method of determining the potential for neural impingement with movement.

Anomalies of the Odontoid Process

Aplasia-Hypoplasia of the Dens

Aplasia-hypoplasia of the dens is a rare condition with a spectrum of presentations ranging from a hypoplastic rudimentary dens to complete absence of the dens. Usually, the rudimentary dens does not reach the upper edge of the ventral arch of the atlas, and an associated incompetence of the cruciate ligaments and alar ligaments results in atlantoaxial instability. Distinguishing aplasia or hypoplasia is of limited clinical importance because both conditions can lead to atlantoaxial instability and the treatment is identical. Vascular compromise from stretching and torsion of the vertebral arteries has been reported. Chronic atlantoaxial dislocation may provoke the formation of granulation tissue that can cause neurologic deficit because of constriction of the cervicomedullary junction.[11] The presentation in children with atlantoaxial dislocation and congenital anomalies varies and includes syncope, torticollis, dysesthesia, and tetraplegia.

Os Odontoideum

Os odontoideum is an independent ossicle located rostral to the axis bone in the position of the odontoid process that is separated from a hypoplastic dens by a variable distance.[26] The space between the os odontoideum and the remnant of the odontoid process is above the level of the superior facet of the axis. This leads to potential incompetence of the transverse ligament, which can lead to atlantoaxial instability.[2] In children younger than 5 years, the normal epiphyseal line may be confused with the presence of an os odontoideum or a fracture. In os odontoideum, the free ossicle is rounded or oval, with a smooth cortical border. In the case of an odontoid fracture, the gap is usually narrow and irregular and often extends into the body of the axis at the level of the superior facet of the axis vertebra.[2] The incidence of os odontoideum is increased in Down syndrome, spondyloepiphyseal dysplasia, Morquio syndrome, and after upper respiratory tract infections.[26,27]

There are two types of os odontoideum: orthotopic and dystopic. In the orthotopic variety, the ossicle lies in the location of the normal dens and moves with the axis body and the ventral arch of the atlas. This type is often associated with an intact cruciate ligament. In the dystopic variety, the os is located near the basion and is often fused to the clivus. The ventral arch of the atlas is hypertrophied, and the dorsal arch is hypoplastic. Dystopic os odontoideum has a greater likelihood of causing neurologic compromise than the orthotopic variety. This may occur because of dorsal compromise of the spinal cord by the ventrally located dorsal arch of the atlas during flexion and ventral compromise by the odontoid ossicle.[26] Evaluation of atlantoaxial instability should be performed with flexion-extension films. In cases of chronic subluxation, dense granulation tissue may form, leading to an irreducible state. Os odontoideum has been ascribed to congenital, vascular, and traumatic causes.[26] Trauma or infection during childhood is the most likely cause for the vast majority of cases of os odontoideum. Several cases have been reported in children with a normal odontoid process before trauma who subsequently developed os odontoideum. Many patients have a significant episode of trauma before the diagnosis of os odontoideum. After fracture or vascular compromise, a separation of the bone fragments occurs, probably because of contracture of the apical ligaments. The ossicle continues to receive a blood supply via the apical arcade, but the blood supply in the region of the fracture is disrupted, resulting in poor healing. It is probable that congenital forms of os odontoideum also exist. The congenital form results from failure of fusion of the portions of the dens derived from the proatlas and first cervical sclerotome. Dystopic os odontoideum is thought to be congenital in origin.

Disorders of the Subaxial Cervical Spine

Klippel-Feil Syndrome

Klippel-Feil syndrome was first described as a case report with the clinical triad of a short neck, low dorsal hairline, and marked limitation of cervical range of motion resulting from a single unsegmented vertebral mass extending from the craniocervical junction through the fourth thoracic vertebra.[28] Fewer than half of patients have all three signs. The most consistent finding is limitation of cervical motion.[10] Currently, the term *Klippel-Feil syndrome* is used to describe any congenital fusion of the cervical spine with or without the clinical features of the original description (Fig. 7-1).

Often patients with Klippel-Feil syndrome have associated congenital abnormalities, which are often the conditions that prompt evaluation. The Klippel-Feil syndrome occurs in 25% of patients with congenital scoliosis.[29] Therefore, all patients with congenital scoliosis should have radiographs of the entire spine to exclude the coexistence of the Klippel-Feil syndrome, and, conversely, all patients with a diagnosis of Klippel-Feil syndrome should have radiographs of the thoracic and lumbar spine. Approximately 50% of patients with congenital cervical or cervicothoracic scoliosis have

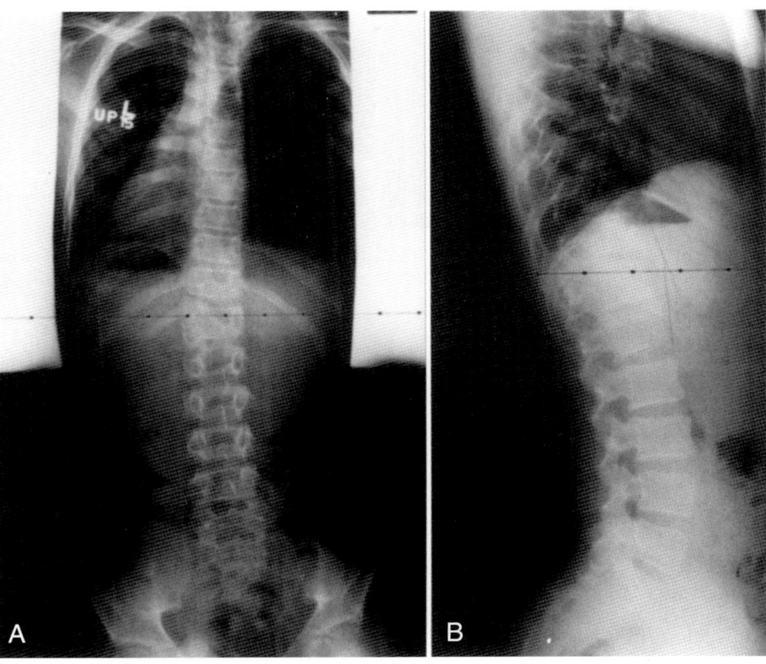

FIGURE 7-1. Frontal (**A**) and lateral (**B**) radiographs of a boy aged 12 years with a shortened neck and congenital hemivertebra at the thoracolumbar junction. Cervical films revealed a Klippel-Feil anomaly with fusion from C3-6.

Figure continues on following page

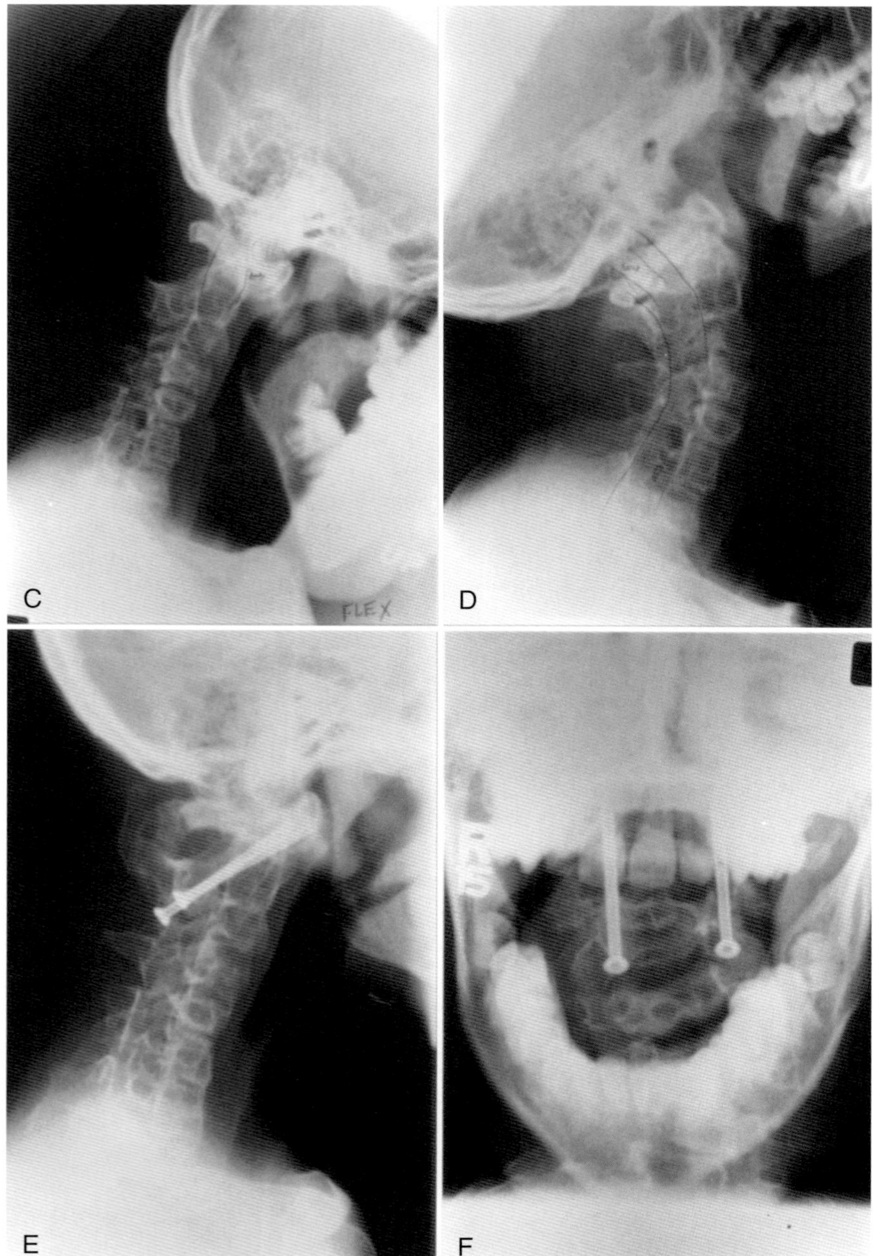

FIGURE 7-1, cont. Flexion (**C**) and extension (**D**) radiographs demonstrated 10-mm instability of C1-2; treatment consisted of a dorsal C1-2 fusion (**E** and **F**). Lateral mass screws were used instead of sublaminar wires because the C1 lamina (**F**) was dysplastic.

associated Klippel-Feil anomalies. Renal anomalies occur in more than one third of patients. It has been suggested that routine screening ultrasonography be performed in all patients with Klippel-Feil syndrome.[30]

Sprengel deformity (an abnormal elevation of the scapula) occurs in 25% to 35% of cases of Klippel-Feil syndrome. It may be unilateral or bilateral.[10] Other less commonly associated anomalies include deafness, synkinesis (involuntary paired movements of the hands and occasionally the arms), congenital heart disease, cervical ribs, ptosis, Duane syndrome (an abducens nerve palsy in which the adducted eye becomes retracted), lateral rectus palsy, facial nerve palsy, syndactyly, hypoplastic thumb, and upper extremity hypoplasia.

Symptoms related to the Klippel-Feil syndrome can be classified as mechanical or secondary to neural compression. Cervical instability and stenosis are potential problems in Klippel-Feil patients. The spinal cord area adjacent to the vertebral fusion may be compressed because of cervical instability, particularly at the occiput-C1 and C1-2 levels. All of these patients should have flexion-extension cervical spine radiographs. Neurologic deficits can range from radiculopathy to sudden death from minor trauma. Overall, 20% of patients who develop neurologic symptoms do so during the first 5 years of life and 65% by the age of 30 years.[10] Neurologic symptoms detected during infancy are usually related to craniovertebral junction abnormalities. Children often have pain with atlantoaxial fusions. Subaxial cervical fusions often do not become problematic until the third decade or later, when degenerative changes begin to develop. Patients with short-segment fusions are less likely to develop symptoms, because of compensatory movement at uninvolved segments.

Iniencephaly

Iniencephaly is a disorder of the cervical spine consisting of congenital cervical synostoses, fixed retroflexion of the head, severe cervical lordosis, and varying degrees of deficits of the dorsal occiput and cervical vertebrae. This condition probably belongs to the spectrum of neural tube defects. The majority of fetuses with this condition are not viable.[10] Parents of a child with iniencephaly have a 5% risk of having another child with a neural tube defect. Ultrasonography and serum or amniotic α-fetoprotein levels can be used to detect this condition in utero.[31] Surviving patients are often handicapped by the cervical lordosis and hyperextension of the head. This posture makes it impossible to see straight without flexing the low back and hips.

Disorders of the Thoracolumbar Spine

Congenital Scoliosis

Congenital scoliosis is an abnormal curvature of the spine in the coronal plane that develops when anomalous vertebrae are present at birth. Congenital scoliosis is distinct from infantile idiopathic scoliosis, although both present with deformity during childhood. Infantile idiopathic scoliosis has no structural vertebral abnormality. Although vertebral abnormalities are present at birth in congenital scoliosis, the spinal deformity is rarely noticeable during infancy and usually presents during childhood or adolescence. Patients with mild or compensated deformities often receive diagnosis as adults when vertebral anomalies are discovered incidentally during routine radiographs. Congenital scoliosis can be associated with a variety of cardiac, genitourinary, and skeletal abnormalities.[1,32] The spectrum of clinical presentations ranges widely based on number, location, and type of vertebral abnormalities. Certain vertebral anomalies result in rapidly progressive scoliosis during early childhood, resulting in severe morbidity, whereas other anomalies cause little or no deformity at any time.[33] In general, 25% of congenital scolioses do not progress, 50% progress slowly, and 25% progress rapidly.[33] Major advancements in the treatment of congenital scoliosis are improved imaging of the spine by CT and MRI, classification by type of vertebral anomaly, improved understanding of the natural history, and clarification of the indications and timing of surgery.

Advances in imaging have aided the diagnosis of associated neural axis abnormalities, such as occult spinal dysraphism and tethering of the spinal cord. Between 10% to 20% of all congenital scoliosis patients have some anomaly of the neural axis.[8] Dorsal midline skin lesions (e.g., hairy patches or deep dimples), asymmetrical foot deformities (cavus or flat feet), muscle weakness, or spasticity all suggest underlying nervous system abnormalities. A thorough imaging evaluation is therefore indicated.

Congenital vertebral anomalies can cause absence, or functional deficiency, of the growth plates on one or both sides of the spine. Asymmetrical spine growth results from a difference in growth between the greater and lesser affected sides of the spine. In some cases, normal growth occurs on one side and no growth on the other, producing a large deformity. The rate of deterioration and the final severity of the congenital scoliosis are proportional to the degree of growth imbalance produced by the vertebral anomalies. The location of the deficient growth plates determines whether a pure scoliosis exists or if some component of sagittal plane deformity is present, resulting in kyphoscoliosis or lordoscoliosis.

Usually, the vertebral abnormalities can be classified by the anomaly in the mesenchymal precursor that results in either a failure of formation or a failure of segmentation. Failure of formation results from a defect in the developmental process that produces an absence of part or all of the vertebrae. The defects range from mild wedging to total absence of the vertebra. A hemivertebra occurs with the complete absence of half of a vertebra and is one of the most common causes of congenital scoliosis. The hemivertebra consists of a wedged vertebral body with a single pedicle and hemilamina (Fig. 7-2).

Segmentation failure causes unilateral or bilateral bony fusion between vertebrae. The defect can involve ventral elements, dorsal elements, or both. The most common segmentation failure is the unilateral unsegmented bar, which results in a bony block that involves the disc spaces and facet joints (Fig. 7-3). A combination of defects of formation and defects of segmentation can coexist in the same patient. An unsegmented bar with contralateral hemivertebrae can cause severe progressive scoliosis.[1]

Three major types of hemivertebrae are classified by the positioning of the hemivertebra and whether the disc spaces above and below the hemivertebra are morphologically normal (Fig. 7-4). A *fully segmented hemivertebra* has a normal disc space above and below the vertebral body that allows near-normal longitudinal growth. A portion of the vertebral body and growth plates are absent on the side of the unformed vertebra, resulting in limited growth potential. Because of full growth potential on one side of the spine and none on the other at the level of the hemivertebra, the potential for a hemivertebra located at the apex of the scoliosis is significant in these cases. The rate of progression and the need for treatment of the scoliosis caused by a fully segmented hemivertebra depends on its location in the spine, with the thoracolumbar and the lumbosacral junction being the most problematic. In general, these scoliotic curves progress at 1 to 2 degrees per year.[34]

The *incarcerated hemivertebra* is a variant of the fully segmented hemivertebra. This type of hemivertebra is set into defects in the vertebrae above and below it. The incarcerated hemivertebra is small, oval, and has poorly formed disc spaces. The defects in the adjacent vertebrae tend to compensate for the hemivertebra, and the poor potential growth of the malformed growth plates results in less scoliotic deformity than with the standard fully segmented vertebrae.[34]

A *semisegmented hemivertebra* is connected to either the vertebra above or below it and causes the absence of one disc space on the side of the hemivertebra with obliteration of two growth plates. Theoretically, this would result in similar growth on both sides of the spine because two active growth plates coexist on each side. However, the wedge shape of the hemivertebra and differences in growth (between sides) can result in some scoliosis.

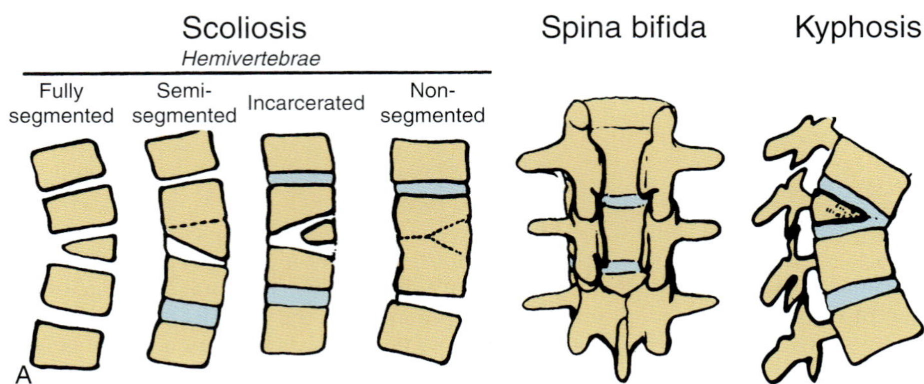

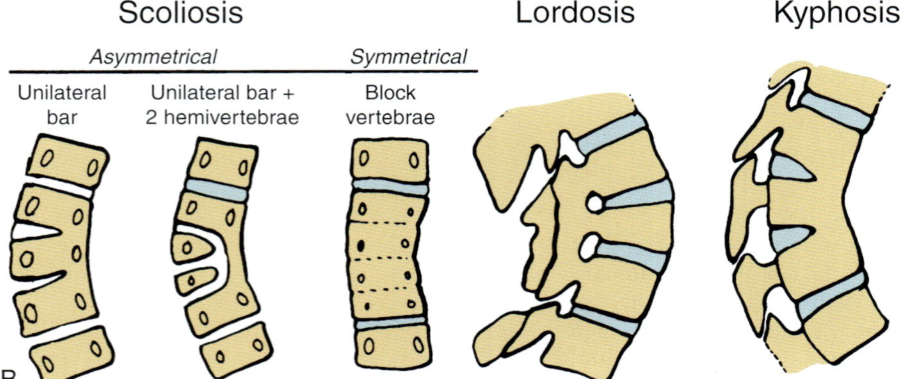

FIGURE 7-2. Structural abnormalities in congenital spine deformity. **A**, Defects in formation resulting in congenital scoliosis, spina bifida, and congenital (type I) kyphosis. **B**, Defects of segmentation that result in congenital scoliosis, congenital lordosis, and congenital (type II) kyphosis.

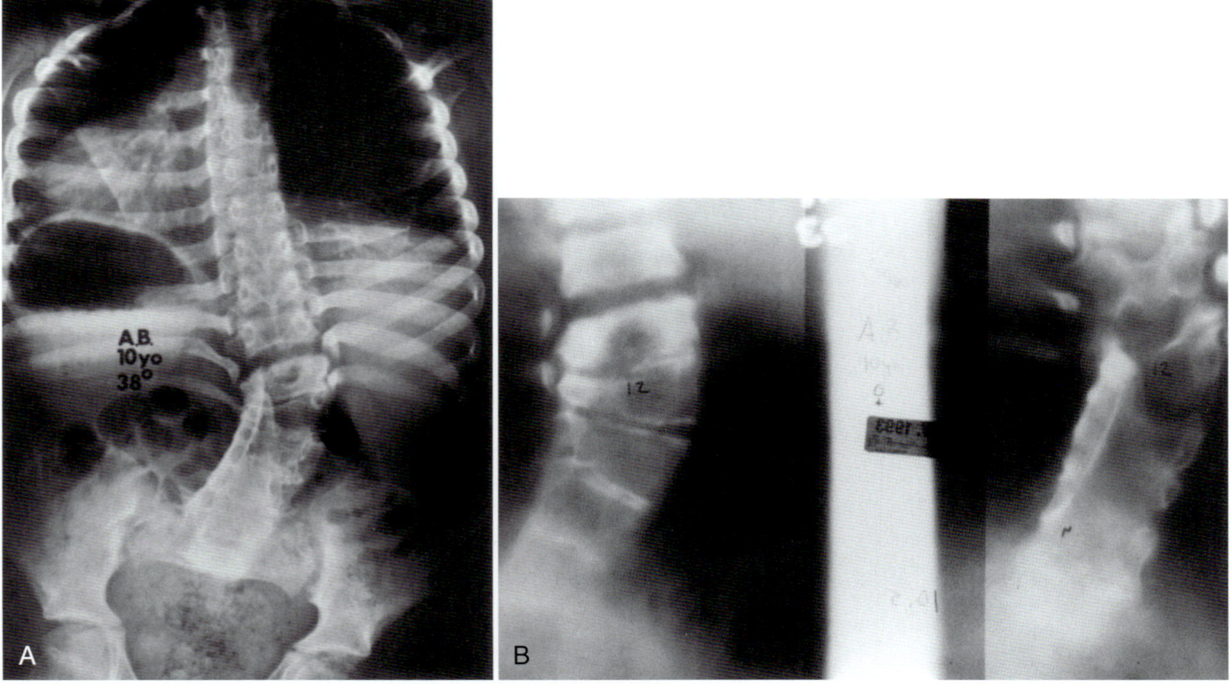

FIGURE 7-3. A, A 4-year-old girl with congenital lumbar scoliosis (measuring 38 degrees) secondary to unilateral bar from T11 to the sacrum. **B,** Anteroposterior tomography showing the laminar synostosis.

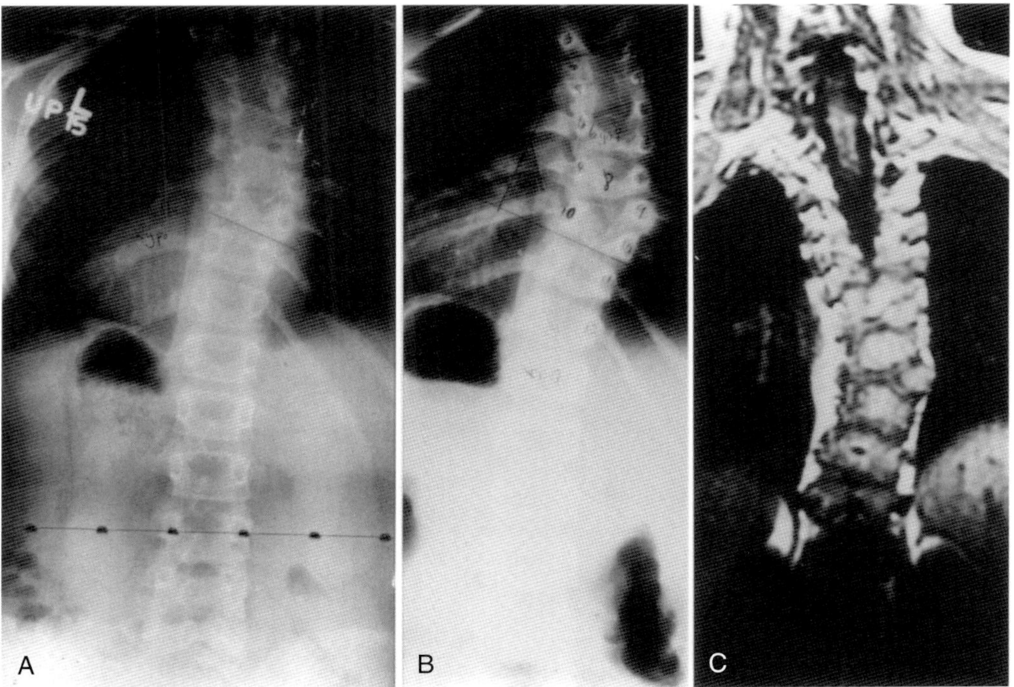

FIGURE 7-4. **A** and **B,** A 6-year-old girl presented with 40 degrees of thoracic congenital scoliosis secondary to a right hemivertebra at T6 and T9, opposite the left rib, and pedicle fusion from T4 to T6. **C,** MRI revealed the fully segmented hemivertebra at T9 and semisegmented hemivertebra at T6.

A nonsegmented hemivertebra is connected to the vertebrae above and below, with no disc spaces and no growth potential. Although the wedge shape of the hemivertebra may cause some deformity, it is not progressive.

Another common cause of congenital scoliosis is a unilateral unsegmented bar.[1] This condition results from a failure of segmentation of two or more vertebrae. The unsegmented bar contains no growth plates, but the unaffected side of the spine continues to grow. The imbalance in growth results in the scoliosis with the unsegmented bar in the concavity. On average, these curves deteriorate at a rate of 5 degrees or greater per year and often result in a significant deformity.[33]

Congenital Kyphosis

Congenital kyphosis is an uncommon sagittal plane deformity, which, if left untreated, is often associated with a neurologic deficit.[35] As with congenital scoliosis, congenital kyphosis is caused by segmentation failure. Winter et al.[36] classified congenital kyphosis into three types: type I is the failure of formation of the vertebral body; type II is the failure of segmentation of the vertebral body, resulting in a ventral unsegmented bar; and type III is the mixed failure of formation and segmentation. The type I kyphosis is the most common and the most likely to lead to both severe deformity and neurologic compromise.[36] The severity of type I kyphosis is directly proportional to the amount of vertebral body or bodies that fail to form. The type II kyphosis is less common, produces less severe deformity, and is much less frequently associated with neurologic compromise than type I. The amount of kyphosis produced is proportional to the discrepancy between the ventral vertebral growth and the growth of the dorsal elements. Type III kyphosis is very rare and probably behaves like type I kyphosis.

Congenital Lordosis

Congenital lordosis is rarer than either congenital scoliosis or congenital kyphosis. This condition results from dorsal defects in segmentation, with normal ventral growth.[37] Often, it has some component of coronal plane deformity, leading to lordoscoliosis because of a dorsolateral location of the unsegmented bar. The most severe consequence of congenital lordosis is an impairment of pulmonary function.[37]

Lumbar Spine Abnormalities

Congenital Spinal Stenosis

Congenital spinal stenosis occurs in a very small number of patients who present with spinal stenosis.[1] It results from a malformation present at birth that predisposes the patient to the development of stenosis, which often manifests itself later in life.

Congenital spinal stenosis can occur as a part of spinal dysraphism.[1] The signs and symptoms are usually not the consequence of stenosis alone, but also of myelodysplasia. Serious radicular pain or dysfunction occurs frequently in this condition.

Congenital stenosis can also result from an area of failure of vertebral segmentation (block vertebrae). Stenosis in the area of the block vertebrae results from a reduction of the midsagittal diameters of the vertebral canal. The signs and symptoms do not differ from those observed with idiopathic developmental stenosis.

A third type is an intermittent stenosis (Morbus de Anquin syndrome) in which the spinous process of S1 is absent and the lamina of S1 has a large medial cleft. There may be a residual island of bone in the area of the cleft. This malformation is associated with a downward hooklike elongation of the spinous process of L5. The patient assumes an increased lordotic posture during standing or walking. The tip of the hooklike spinous process of L5 presses directly on the ligamentum, bridging the spina bifida occulta of S1 or on the rudimentary bony island in its central portion, thus reducing the midsagittal diameter of the upper sacral canal. This condition results in radicular pain during standing or walking and is relieved by sitting.

Developmental Spinal Stenosis

Developmental spinal stenosis usually occurs as the result of an inborn chromosomal error or mutation that alters the fetal and postnatal spinal canal formation. Developmental spinal stenosis commonly occurs in conditions such as achondroplasia, hypochondroplasia, diastrophic dwarfism, Morquio syndrome, and hereditary multiple exostoses. This condition may involve only the lumbar spine or can be associated with developmental stenosis of the cervical spine.[1]

Segmented Spinal Dysgenesis

Segmental spinal dysgenesis is a localized congenital defect in which severe stenosis occurs with malalignment and focal agenesis or dysgenesis in the thoracolumbar or lumbar spine.[1] It was initially described as a form of congenital spinal stenosis with focal narrowing of the spinal canal in the area of the thoracolumbar junction. Neurologic deficits are often present at birth and may range from mild paresis to complete paraplegia. Patients may have congenital absence of nerve root or spinal cord segments. The spinal canal above and below the involved segment is usually normal, and the sacrum is well formed, differentiating this condition from sacral agenesis.[38]

Spondylolisthesis

Spondylolisthesis is the slippage of all or part of one vertebra in relationship with another. The most widely accepted classification of spondylolisthesis is by Wiltse et al.[39] They divided spondylolisthesis into five types: I—dysplastic, II—isthmic, III—degenerative, IV—traumatic, and V—pathologic.

Dysplastic spondylolisthesis accounts for 14% to 21% of cases, with a 2:1 female to male ratio.[40] This type is characterized by structural anomalies of the lumbosacral junction, including dysplasia of the lamina and facet joints. The lack of the normal facet buttress provided by normal facet joints predisposes toward a slippage of the rostral vertebra on its caudal counterpart. The dysplastic articular processes may be oriented in the axial or sagittal planes. In axial dysplasia, the articular processes have a horizontal orientation. This condition is often associated with spina bifida. In sagittal dysplasia the facet joints are often asymmetrical, but the neural arch is usually intact. Therefore, high-grade slippage seldom occurs. Both types can present with hamstring spasm, back or leg pain, or neurologic deficit, including paresthesia, weakness, or, rarely, incontinence of the bowel or bladder. Neurologic deficits are usually associated with high-grade slips.

Axially oriented facet joints associated with spina bifida have an increased risk for high-grade spondylolisthesis. The pars interarticularis is often poorly developed and may elongate, develop a defect, or remain intact. If the pars interarticularis remains intact, neurologic symptoms usually occur only when the spondylolisthesis exceeds 35%. Progression of spondylolisthesis is more likely in younger or skeletally immature patients and in patients with wide spina bifida. Initial treatment should be nonoperative unless progression is documented in younger patients or slippage greater than 50% is observed at the time of the initial evaluation. Fusion in situ is a frequently performed surgical procedure, although some surgeons use reduction and fixation, especially with high-grade abnormalities.[1]

Disorders of the Sacral Spine

Sacral Agenesis

Sacral agenesis is a group of disorders characterized by an absence of variable portions of the caudal spine. Williams and Nixon[41] coined the term *sacral agenesis* in 1957. Sacral agenesis belongs within the spectrum of aplastic vertebral malformations that are loosely grouped under the entity of caudal regression syndrome. It can range from agenesis of the coccyx to absence of sacral, lumbar, and lower thoracic vertebrae.

The clinical severity parallels the number of spinal segments involved with the aplasia or dysplasia. Associated anomalies of the genitourinary, GI, and urinary systems often occur.[42] Patients with sacral agenesis usually lack motor function below the level of the last normal vertebra. It is interesting that in sacral agenesis, compared with other dysplastic syndromes of the lower spine (e.g., myelomeningocele), sensation is relatively spared below the level of the lesion. In the development of the human embryo, the notochord induces the formation of the ventral spinal elements and cells derived from neural crest independently from the dorsal root ganglia. Thus, an insult specific to the notochord/ventral spine could lead to the observed clinical picture in sacral agenesis.[43]

The exact incidence of sacral agenesis is difficult to determine because mild caudal agenesis is often not clinically apparent, and severe cases can result in stillbirth or neonatal death. Sacral agenesis is a relatively rare lesion. An incidence of 1 in 60,000 live births has been reported.[44] Sacral agenesis is considered to have a sporadic, nonfamilial inheritance pattern, although cases of siblings with the disorder have been reported. Maternal diabetes appears to increase the risk of sacral agenesis.[45] Embryonal trauma producing longitudinal kinking of the long embryonic axis, dietary deficiencies, and teratogenic chemicals have caused caudal agenesis in experimental models.[45] Caudal agenesis, as well as other associated congenital anomalies such as imperforate anus and cloacal exstrophy, result from alterations in the normal formation and development of the caudal eminence. The caudal eminence is a mass of undifferentiated cells at the caudal end of the embryo that gives rise to the distal spinal cord, nerve roots, and the vertebral column of the sacral and coccygeal regions.

Pang[42] devised a new classification scheme that combined salient features from other classification schemes (Fig. 7-5). By this method, lumbosacral agenesis is divided into five types, with some of these divided into subtypes. Type I is total sacral agenesis with some lumbar vertebrae also missing. Type II is total sacral agenesis with the lumbar vertebrae not involved.

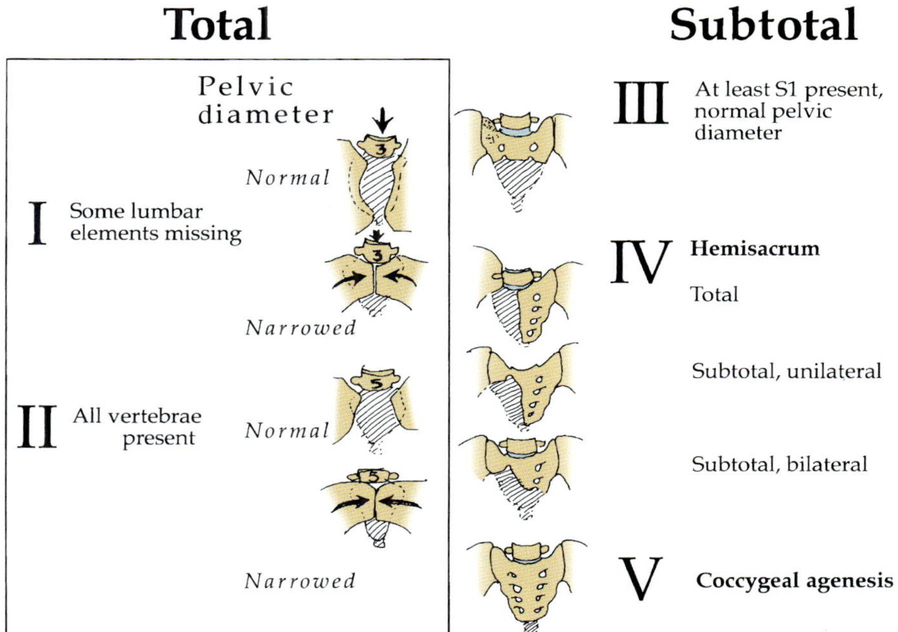

FIGURE 7-5. Classification of sacral agenesis. Types I and II have subtypes with normal and narrowed pelvic diameter. Type III is subtotal and S1 is at least present. Type IV consists of the varieties of hemisacrum possible, and type V splits into total and subtotal subtypes. (Modified from Pang D: Sacral agenesis and caudal spinal cord malformations. *Neurosurgery* 32[5]:755–779, 1993.)

Type III is subtotal sacral agenesis with at least S1 present and the ilia articulate with the side of the rudimentary sacrum. Type IV is a hemisacrum, and type V is coccygeal agenesis.

The clinical features of sacral agenesis can be quite severe. Because of the lack of motor innervation of the lower limbs, intrauterine contractures develop. In severe forms of sacral agenesis, the malformation in the spine-pelvis articulation causes a severe kyphosis to develop. Affected children sit in the "Buddha" position with legs flexed and crossed and lean forward because of the kyphosis. Other spinal deformities develop in children with sacral agenesis. Congenital and developmental scoliosis is common. Klippel-Feil syndrome has also been reported.[1]

Multiple musculoskeletal deformities can present in patients with sacral agenesis. Hip dysplasia, clubfoot, and knee flexion contractures are common.[44] The etiologic factor responsible for sacral agenesis, such as an insult to the caudal eminence, seems to occur during the time of organogenesis. Therefore, children with sacral agenesis can present with multiple abnormalities of the GI, cardiac, and renal systems. Abnormalities of the terminal spinal cord can be associated with sacral agenesis. These include elongated conus medullaris with hydromyelia, tethering of the spinal cord by a thickened filum terminale, lipomas, split-cord malformations, and terminal myelocystoceles. Neurogenic bladder almost always results in cases of sacral agenesis above S2.

Teratomas

Teratomas in the spine almost exclusively occur in the sacrococcygeal region due to their origin from pluripotent tissue derived from the area around Hensen node.[46] This tissue migrates rostrally to lie in the coccyx. These usually benign tumors can undergo malignant transformation if diagnosis and treatment are delayed.

Sacrococcygeal teratoma (SCT) is a common neoplasm in the newborn, with a reported incidence of 1 in 35,000 live births, with a 3:1 female preponderance.[1] The majority of tumors are large, external, and cystic. The tumor mass usually protrudes from between the anus and the coccyx, although some tumors are located predominantly in the presacral space of the pelvis. Although the diagnosis is often possible prenatally by ultrasound, small presacral tumors can be missed in the newborn. The tumors range in size but can average approximately 8.5 cm. The cystic component is usually cerebrospinal fluid (CSF), but is not generally connected with circulating spinal fluid within the thecal sac, instead arising from the choroid plexus contained within the tumor mass. SCTs have been classified into four types: I—totally external, II —almost totally external, III—almost completely internal, and IV—completely internal.[47] Symptoms are largely related to the degree of displacement or obstruction of the bladder, urethra, or rectum.

Surgical therapy by midline or chevron incision is the mainstay for benign SCT. After removal of the tumor with coccygectomy, survival is high.[1] Presacral tumors may require an abdominal approach combined with the usual sacral approach. Multiagent adjuvant chemotherapy is added to surgical therapy for malignant tumors.

Spinal Dysraphism

Dysraphism is an abnormal development of the spinal cord and column, resulting from malformations that arise from the failure of normal embryologic structures to fuse in the midline. These malformations are broadly divided into two groups: spina bifida aperta and spina bifida occulta. The first group involves midline lesions that are (or potentially can) *open* at birth. These lesions include spina bifida cystica (myelomeningocele, meningocele) and myelodysplasia. The second group encompasses malformations that are hidden by complete layers of dermis and epidermis. These lesions include lipomyelomeningocele, neurenteric cyst, and diastematomyelia.[1] In the United States, the incidence of neural tube defects is roughly 1 per 1000. Folic acid supplementation has been credited with decreased rates worldwide.[48]

The degree of the spinal dysplasia depends on the embryologic age at which the malformation is initiated. Malformations that begin before 28 days of gestation induce major defects in neurulation and cause a higher level of defects than malformations occurring after 28 days of gestation, when neurulation is complete. The higher the level of dysplasia, the less survivable the malformation.

Characteristically in spinal dysraphism, the spinal column widens at the level of the defect. If the neural tube does not develop normally, it causes a deficiency of dorsal element formation and the lateral and ventral displacement of the pedicles and lateral elements of the spine. In addition, other abnormalities of the vertebrae, such as wedge vertebrae and hemivertebrae, can be associated with spinal dysraphism. Occasionally, patients who have symptoms of what is thought to be idiopathic scoliosis in fact have some form of occult spinal dysraphism.

Abnormal neural tube development prevents dermis and epidermis closure over the dorsal defect. Dura mater arises ventral to the deformed spinal cord, but then stretches laterally over the expanded pedicles and facets to join the lateral margins of the epidermis. A thin layer of pia-arachnoid and the zona epithelioma, an extremely thin layer of epithelium, covers the dorsal defect.

Usually, spina bifida aperta occurs in the craniocervical and lumbar areas of the spinal column. The morphogenesis of the dysraphism depends on the embryologic period in which the malformation occurs. If the insult occurs before the 28th day, myeloschisis (exposure of the malformed spinal cord) results from failure of neural tube closure. Myeloschisis is common at the thoracolumbar junction. If the insult occurs after 28 days of gestation, however, various forms of meningocele and myelomeningocele may develop.

Occult spinal dysraphism includes a variety of spinal malformations not immediately visible on the skin surface. Spina bifida occulta occurs from a maldevelopment of the dorsal neural arch structures. Some believe that this occurs when an already closed neural tube ruptures. Increased pressure inside the central canal of the neural tube can cause a rupture that spills highly proteinaceous fluid from the canal into the surrounding tissue. With the decrease in pressure, the defect in the neural tube reanneals, but the proteinaceous fluid inhibits normal development of the dorsal elements. Because the neural tube has closed, closure of the dermis and epidermis over the dorsal aspect of the spinal cord is not impeded.

Diastematomyelia

Diastematomyelia is a disorder in which the spinal cord develops into two hemicords, separated by a cartilaginous or bony septum (Fig. 7-6).[49] Diastematomyelia usually occurs from the third thoracic to the fourth lumbar vertebrae. Diastematomyelia is among a spectrum of split-cord malformations. These can occur with two hemicords (each within its own dural tube and split with a rigid osseocartilaginous septum), or they can occur with both hemicords in the same dural covering, with only a fibrous band for separation.

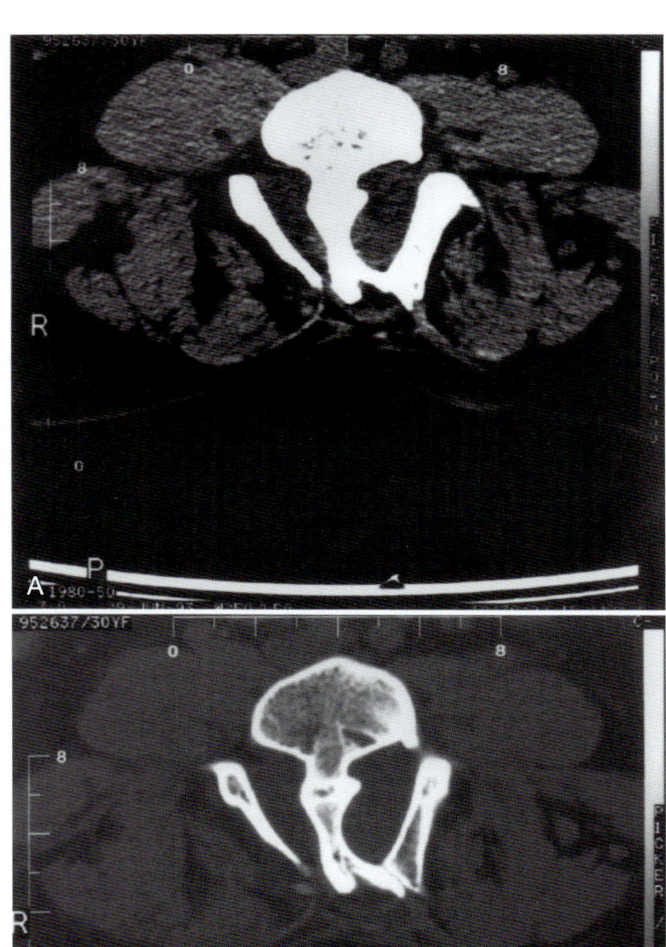

FIGURE 7-6. Diastematomyelia presenting in a 30-year-old woman with spasticity and long tract signs. **A,** Soft tissue window. **B,** Bone window.

Neurenteric Cysts

If endoderm is retained in the tract between hemicords, a neurenteric cyst can result.[50] These rare lesions are retained cystic structures, ventrally located in the spinal canal, derived from embryonic foregut. These cysts occur most commonly in the thoracic and cervical spine. The epithelium of these cysts varies from ciliated columnar lining that suggests a respiratory origin to linings that can resemble gut mucosa. Because of embryonic gut rotation, neurenteric cysts tend to lie to the right of the vertebral column. Neurenteric cysts can cause spinal cord compression usually appearing in childhood.

Lipomas

Lipomas of the spine are a commonly encountered developmental spinal abnormality, often seen with occult spinal dysraphism. They occur in the lumbosacral area 90% of the time. In contrast, intraspinal lipomas not associated with spina bifida occulta account for about 5% of intraspinal tumors in children and show a predilection for the thoracic spine. These lesions most likely result from inclusion of adipose cells from the overlying mesodermal tissue into the developing spinal canal or the folding neural tube. A tethered spinal cord occurs when these lesions traverse both the bony and neural elements of the spine.[51]

Lipomas associated with spinal dysraphism take three principal forms: dorsal, terminal, or transitional. In the dorsal form, the lipoma extends from the subcutaneous space through incomplete neural arches and attaches to the dorsal spinal cord. It is rare for nerve roots to be contained within the substance of a dorsal lipoma. Terminal lipomas insert into the distal conus and may be entirely intraspinal, many times containing nerve roots. Features of both dorsal and terminal lipomas appear in transitional lipomas. The embryology of caudal lipomas most likely arises during secondary neurulation. During secondary neurulation the caudal end of the neural tube blends with a large collection of undifferentiated cells, the caudal cell mass. The last phase of secondary neurulation involves regression of the previously formed tail structures, leaving the filum terminale, coccygeal ligament, and terminal ventricle of the conus as its only remnants. Cell rests with the potential for differentiation may be left in these elements and account for the development of lipomas, hamartomas, teratomas, and the rare malignancy.[51]

Dermoids and Dermal Sinus Tracts

Dermal sinus tracts are lined by squamous epithelium and may penetrate the spinal cord at any level in the midline from the lumbosacral spine to the occiput. Dermoid and epidermoid nodules can frequently accompany dermal sinus tracts. Dermoid and epidermoid tumors may arise within the tract in approximately half of all dermal sinuses.[52] These tumors are also encountered within the subarachnoid space, arising from isolated congenital rests of cells derived from the multipotential caudal cell mass. The embryology of dermal sinus tracts and dermoids of the spine is probably a result of incomplete dysjunction of ectoderm from endoderm during the fourth week of embryologic development. The dermal tract becomes elongated during ascent of the spinal cord within the spinal canal and may traverse several layers of dermis and epidermal space before entering the subarachnoid space. Dermal sinus tracts may frequently be missed on initial examination of the infant and only become apparent when the child has symptoms of recurrent meningitis.

Tethered Cord

Traditionally, the tethered cord syndrome has been defined as a low-lying conus medullaris secondary to a short and thickened filum terminale. Recently, the term has been expanded to include a spinal cord that is tethered by fibrous bands or adhesions or an intradural lipoma. The embryologic origin of the short and thickened filum terminale is unknown. By producing traction on the spinal cord, these lesions can cause profound neurologic deficits.

The degree of spinal cord traction, rather than the type or distribution of the tethering lesions, most likely determines the age of symptom onset. Severe traction on the spinal cord results in presentation in childhood, whereas less severe traction is asymptomatic in childhood but appears later in life (because of repeated tugging of the conus during head and neck flexion), or when abnormal tension is aggravated by trauma or spondylotic spinal canal stenosis.[53]

Syringomyelia

Syringomyelia is a fluid-filled cavity of the spinal cord (Fig. 7-7). Syringomyelia occurs frequently in the cervical and thoracic spine. Although not directly a congenital malformation, it may be considered a developmental abnormality because of its frequent association with Chiari malformations. There is up to a 50% to 75% incidence of cavitation (syrinx) of the spinal cord in the setting of Chiari malformation. The posterior fossa is small because of flattening of the squamous occipital bone. The foramen magnum is enlarged to accommodate the descended cerebellar tonsils.

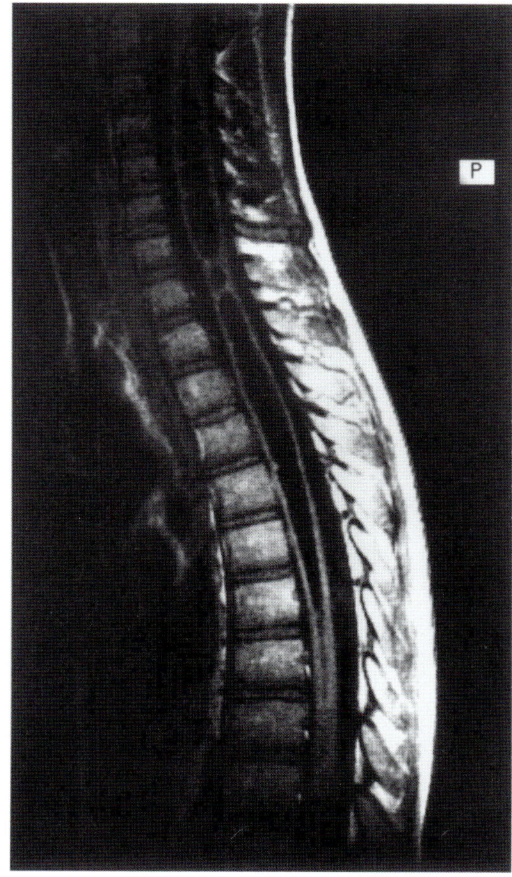

FIGURE 7-7. Congenital syrinx.

Syringomyelia may present with pain in the spine, limb, and trunk. Radiographic features may be widening of the spinal canal and erosion of the vertebrae.[54] In support of the theories of misguided CSF flow around the herniated cerebellar tonsils, posterior fossa decompression without cyst drainage can improve symptoms.

Summary

Congenital spinal abnormalities may result in significant orthopedic and neurologic symptoms. An understanding of the etiology and natural history of these abnormalities will afford improved management decisions.

KEY REFERENCES

Basu PS, Elsebaie H, Noordeen MH: Congenital spinal deformity: a comprehensive assessment at presentation. *Spine (Phila Pa 1976)* 27:2255–2259, 2002.

Belmont PJ Jr, Kuklo TR, Taylor KF, et al: Intraspinal anomalies associated with isolated congenital hemivertebra: the role of routine magnetic resonance imaging. *J Bone Joint Surg [Am]* 86:1704–1710, 2004.

Cavalier R, Herman MJ, Cheung EV, Pizzutillo PD: Spondylolysis and spondylolisthesis in children and adolescents: I. Diagnosis, natural history, and nonsurgical management. *J Am Acad Orthop Surg* 14:417–424, 2006.

Lonstein JE: Congenital spine deformities: scoliosis, kyphosis, and lordosis, *Orthop Clin North Am* 30:387–405, viii, 1999.

McMaster MJ, Singh H: Natural history of congenital kyphosis and kyphoscoliosis. A study of one hundred and twelve patients. *J Bone Joint Surg [Am]* 81:1367–1383, 1999.

Pang D: Sacral agenesis and caudal spinal cord malformations. *Neurosurgery* 32:755–778, 1993; discussion 778–779.

Smith JS, Shaffrey CI, Abel MF, et al: Basilar invagination. *Neurosurgery* 66:39–47, 2010.

REFERENCES

The complete reference list is available online at expertconsult.com.

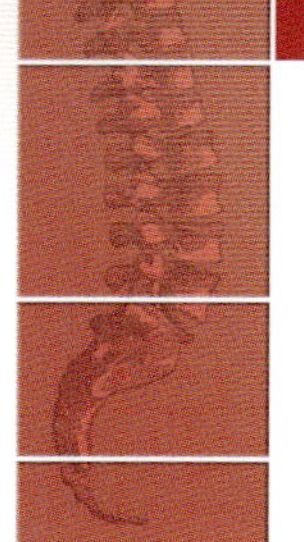

CHAPTER 8

Anatomy and Pathophysiology of Acquired Spinal Disorders

Paul Porensky | Nicholas W.M. Thomas | Gary L. Rea | Philip R. Weinstein

One must understand the anatomy of the affected spinal region and the effects of a particular syndrome on that anatomy as well as the neurology of lesions that impair its function to understand the clinical presentation of a given spinal disorder, predict its natural history, and design treatment algorithms. Such disorders as degenerative disc disease, rheumatoid arthritis, Scheuermann disease, Paget disease, ankylosing spondylitis, ossification of the posterior longitudinal ligament (OPLL), and spondylolisthesis lead to characteristic changes in spinal anatomy, and each results in characteristic radiographic findings, symptoms, and neurologic deficits that dictate indications and planning of surgical therapy. Nonspecific symptoms common to these conditions are due to joint inflammation and nerve root entrapment.

Degenerative Disc Disease and Spondylosis

Degenerative disc disease (with its characteristic clinical syndromes of disc herniation, spondylosis, and radiculopathy) is associated with vascular, biochemical, and anatomic changes in the disc. There is a consistent anatomic pattern of disc degeneration in the spine, with most changes occurring in the midcervical, thoracolumbar, and lower lumbar regions. This pattern is thought to reflect the distribution of the mechanical stresses caused by spine movement and loading, as well as those due to erect posture.[1]

The intervertebral disc consists of three components: (1) the nucleus pulposus; (2) the annulus fibrosus, which surrounds the nucleus pulposus; and (3) the cartilaginous end plates, which attach these structures to the rostral and caudal vertebrae of the motion segment. The annulus is formed by a series of lamellae that have high collagen content and thereby provide significant resistance to tensile forces. The ventral annulus is usually wider and more organized than the dorsal annulus, with which discontinuous lamellae may be present.[2] The nucleus pulposus, derived embyologically from the primitive notochord,[3] has a much higher proteoglycan and water content than the annulus fibrosus. The hyaline cartilage end plates are similar in collagen type to the inner annulus fibrosus and the nucleus pulposus.[4]

Proteoglycans contribute to osmotic pressure elevation, which results in the nucleus pulposus becoming turgid. This turgidity generates an internal pressure that exerts radial stress during axial loading, pushing the surrounding annular fibers outward and the end plates apart, which in turn results in the development of circumferential tensile stress in the annular lamellae, particularly the inner lamellae. Stress also develops in the end plates and is greatest over the nucleus pulposus, diminishing toward the outer annulus.

The disc acts as a deformable, fluid-like material, whose tendency to bulge is resisted by the tensile stress in the annular lamellae and the end plates. Therefore, a substantial intradiscal surface strength is required to resist a high circumferential annular stress and thus prevent excessive disc deformation (bulging). When disruption of the nucleus pulposus and annulus fibrosus reduces intradiscal pressure, bulging occurs.[5]

The disc receives its nutrients through small vessels in the cartilage end plates and from the periphery of the annulus.[6] With aging, however, the end plates calcify, and vessel loss occurs, until nearly the entire disc becomes avascular.[7] The loss of vasculature promotes increased anaerobic metabolism, increasing lactic acid production and cellular necrosis. The water content of the annulus fibrosus decreases from 78% at birth to 70% by the fourth decade, and the nucleus pulposus water content decreases from 90% to less than 70% with maturation.[8,9] With this change in vascularity, and with water loss in the region of the inner annulus and nucleus pulposus, there is a relative increase in fibrocytes and chondrocytes, which are more tolerant of a low-pH environment.[3]

Before the age of 2 years, the nucleus pulposus is translucent and anatomically different from the annulus fibrosus.[10] By the second decade, the inner annulus and nucleus grow increasingly fibrous and lose both height and proteoglycans.[9] In the third decade, nuclear fragmentation and fibrosis appear. Progressive myxomatous degeneration, swelling, and fissure formation occur in the annulus by the fourth decade.[11,12] Eventually the nucleus pulposus may become disorganized, dehydrated, and fragmented with circumferential and radial tears.[10,11,13] Grading systems for these patterns of disc degeneration, using plain radiographs or MRI studies, have been published.[10,14]

On plain radiographs, the degenerative disc changes range from grade I to grade IV. Grade I represents a normal disc.

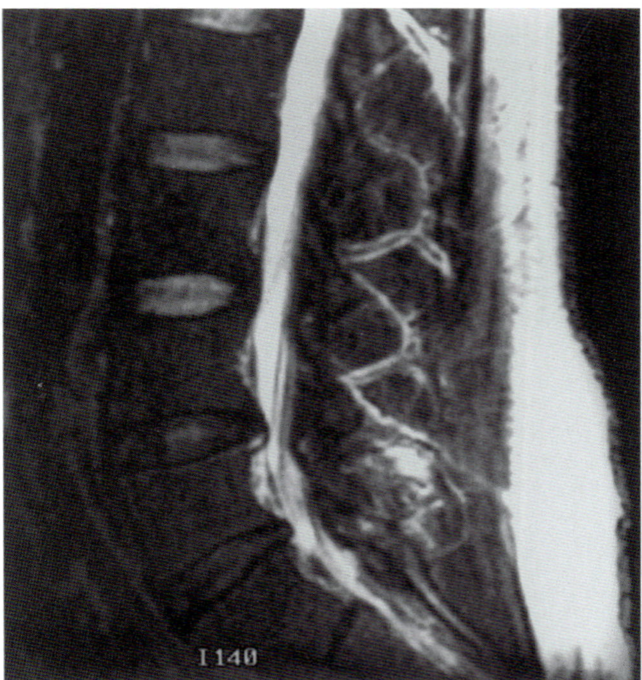

FIGURE 8-1. T2-weighted MRI of lumbar spine demonstrating disc desiccation and herniation at the lower levels.

Grade II demonstrates sclerosis along with disc space narrowing or osteophyte formation. Grade III shows moderate sclerosis, and grade IV is associated with severe sclerosis with disc space narrowing or osteophyte formation.[14] Yu et al.[10] classified changes in the disc, with reference to the age of the subject and to the stage of degeneration, by comparing the anatomic characteristics with the appropriate MRI findings in cadaveric dissections (Fig. 8-1 and Table 8-1). The primitive notochord is present up to age 10. In the second decade of life, a distinct fibrous band forms in the nucleus and disc height diminishes. In the third decade fragmentation and fibrosis of the nucleus occurs. By the fourth decade there is swelling, separation, and myxomatous degeneration of the annular lamellae with fissure formation.[12]

One of the most common disc-related clinical syndromes is a herniated disc with sciatica. With degeneration, fissure formation occurs in a radial distribution. It is likely that the biomechanical cause of disc herniation is related to a combination of complex movements involving compression, lateral flexion, and/or rotation.[15-18] With flexion, the nucleus pulposus moves dorsally. The dorsal annulus has fewer and more disorganized lamellae and may be inherently weaker than the thicker ventral annulus. Degeneration of the annulus results in the development of peripheral, circumferential, and, subsequently, radial tears. With complex stresses applied to the dorsally migrating nucleus, herniation may occur along a radial tear.

Disc herniation can cause associated nerve-root impingement. The typical dorsolateral herniated disc affects the nerve root passing to the next lower foramen, but a more laterally herniated disc can affect the nerve root above. Masaryk et al.[19] used MRI findings to classify the stages of disc herniation. A bulging disc has an MRI signal similar to the rest of the disc, but the bulge is beyond the adjacent vertebral margins. A prolapsed or protruding disc has nearly breached the outer annular fibers and is barely contained. The disc remains contiguous with the rest of the nucleus pulposus by a pedicle that has a high signal on T2-weighted MRI. The disc is extruded when it completely breaches the outer annular fibers and the posterior longitudinal ligament, but remains in continuity with the disc proper. If the fragment is no longer in continuity with the main part of the disc, it is termed a sequestered, or "free," disc fragment. The International Society for the Study of the Lumbar Spine[20] classified the disc as either contained or noncontained, with the latter group including extruded and sequestered discs. Free fragments may migrate in a rostral or caudal direction. It appears that far-lateral herniated discs are more likely to migrate in a rostral direction, thus affecting the nerve root above the disc space.[21]

Disc degeneration without herniation may also lead to changes affecting the biomechanical function and stability of both the intervertebral and articular facet joints. Although opinions differ regarding whether facet or disc degeneration is the initial event that causes spondylosis, the three-joint intervertebral-motion–segment concept emphasizes that disease in each component affects the others. This is to say that unilateral or bilateral facet disease or disc degeneration may lead

TABLE 8-1

Classification of Lumbar Discs

Type of Disc	Anatomic Characteristics	MRI Features
Immature	Nucleus pulposus and annulus fibrosus differentiated, primitive notochord may be present	High-signal intensity from nucleus and annulus
Transitional	Fibrous tissue in equator of annulus	High-signal intensity from nucleus and annulus, low-signal intensity in ventral and/or dorsal region of nucleus pulposus, corresponding to dense fibrous tissue
Adult	Annulus and nucleus not differentiated, annulus intact or marked by small concentric or transverse tears	Moderately high-signal intensity from nucleus and annulus, low-signal intensity from Sharpey fibers and fibrous tissue in midportion of disc
Early degenerated	Radial tear of annulus, diminishing amount and discoloration of fibrocartilage in nucleus	Diminishing signal intensity from nucleus pulposus, low signal from Sharpey fibers disrupted by region of higher-signal intensity at location of annular tear, slightly diminished disc height
Severely degenerated	Replacement of nuclear and annular fibrocartilage with amorphous fiber and cysts	Severely reduced disc height, low (fibrous tissue) or high (fluid) signal intensity from intervertebral disc

From Yu S, Haughton VM, Sether LA, et al: Criteria for classifying normal and degenerated lumbar intervertebral disks. *Radiology* 170:523–526, 1989, with permission.

to progressive changes in the other segmental units. Adjacent bone changes are associated with cartilaginous degeneration in these three joints. Spurs and osteophytes form at the site of peripheral annular attachment to the end plates. These osteophytes are thought to be formed in regions of excessive motion. Kirkaldy-Willis[22] incorporated this concept into a theory regarding the natural history of spinal degeneration. He believed that facet and disc disease occurred with progressive reciprocal dysfunction. This resulted in ligamentous laxity around the facet joint and increased stresses that lead to internal disc disruption. This condition causes subluxation, disc resorption, and, finally, paradiscal osteophyte formation. Enlargement of the facets also occurs as a result of osteophyte formation. These changes may contribute to lumbar stenosis (Fig. 8-2) or a lateral recess syndrome.[23-25]

Patients with significant lumbar spinal canal narrowing resulting in stenosis complain primarily of pain, weakness, and leg numbness while walking. This pain can be relieved when the patient flexes the spine by sitting, by leaning forward while walking (shopping cart sign), or by leaning against counters. The symptomatic improvement associated with these maneuvers is related to an increase in lateral recess and spinal canal dimensions. Flexion results in stretching of the protruding ligamentum flavum and posterior longitudinal ligament, as well as reduction of overriding laminae and facets.[26] This small amount of change in the circumferential spinal canal, lateral recess, and foraminal region alleviates the pressure on the nerve roots and subsequently relieves the symptoms. Returning to the erect posture leads to repeated compression and a further exacerbation of symptoms. During ambulation, some patients experience the onset of symptoms because of an increased metabolic demand in nerve roots that have become ischemic as a result of stenotic compression.

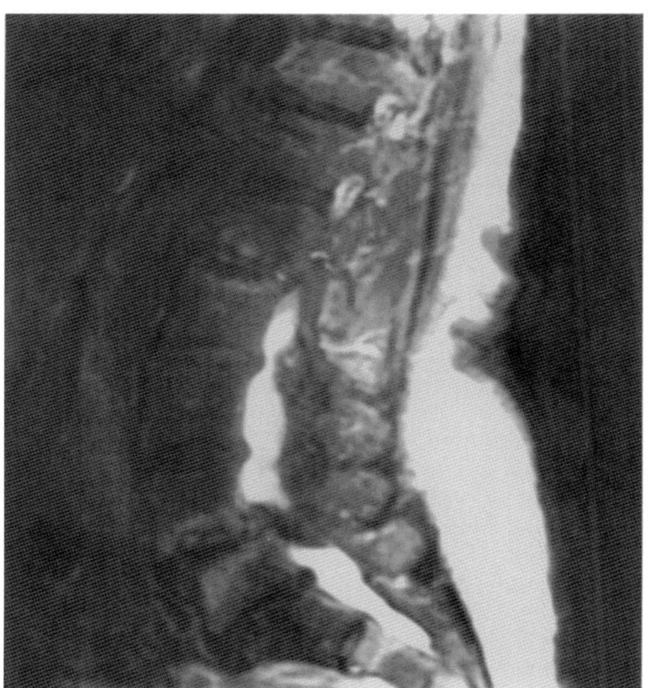

FIGURE 8-2. T2-weighted MRI of lumbar spine demonstrating lumbar spinal canal stenosis, particularly at L4-5. Osteophytic spurs are evident ventrally and hypertrophied ligamentum flavum dorsally.

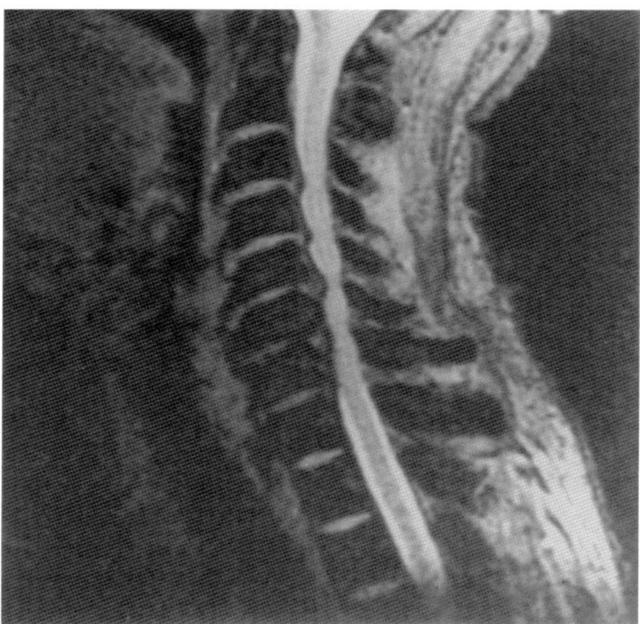

FIGURE 8-3. T2-weighted MRI of cervical spine in a 72-year-old patient. Disc spaces are reduced in height, particularly at the C5-6 and C6-7 levels.

Such "neurogenic claudication" is relieved when the subject sits. Often, bicycling (which is associated with flexion of the lumbar spine) is well tolerated.

Aging discs in the cervical spine cause characteristic spine alterations that may lead to cervical myelopathy or radicular pain and deficit. In young subjects, the cervical spine assumes a lordotic posture. This results in a greater ventral height of the annulus, compared with the dorsal annular height. With aging, however, intradiscal water loss and disc narrowing occur, thus leading to progressive spine straightening. In young patients, the range of intervertebral motion is greatest at C5-6 and C6-7. Narrowing and degeneration with osteophyte formation is most marked at these levels (Fig. 8-3). With these changes there is progressively less movement. In patients older than age 60, motion at C3-4 and C4-5 increases. Increased degenerative instability in older patients, therefore, is associated with translational subluxation, especially retrolisthesis at C3-4 and C4-5.[27] In this scenario the spinal cord of the patient with cervical spondylotic myelopathy may not only be compressed by osteophytes, but may also suffer repeated injuries secondary to intervertebral hypermobility or instability. Dynamic flexion-extension radiographs are necessary to diagnose degenerative spondylolisthesis since static films in neutral position do not demonstrate subluxation, if present. A treatment protocol that does not take these factors into account may be associated with less than optimal success.

Rheumatoid Arthritis of the Spine

Rheumatoid arthritis (RA) affects both the spine and the peripheral joints. It has a prevalence of approximately 1%, with the greatest incidence in the fourth through sixth decades.[28] RA is a disease of the synovial joints. The earliest change in the joints is synovitis, followed by an acute inflammatory response as a result of antibody-antigen complex formation. These processes activate the complement cascade and generate biologically active substances, ultimately resulting in complete destruction of the joint. This acute process is followed by a chronic granulomatous process, or pannus formation, which produces collagenase and other enzymes that destroy surrounding cartilage and bone.[29] This may lead to instability because of ligamentous incompetence.[28,30,31]

Considerable controversy regarding the pathogenesis of cervical spine rheumatoid joint disease revolves around whether the initial site of involvement is (1) the apophyseal joint, with resultant facet destruction and progressive secondary instability of the intervertebral disc, or (2) inflammation in the uncovertebral joint, which leads to primary disc destruction with secondary degenerative involvement of the apophyseal joints. Martel[32] examined 20 RA patients and found instability associated with apophyseal joint involvement. This leads to vertebral end plate destruction, disc space narrowing, and erosion. At autopsy, the discs showed evidence of necrosis and degeneration, with minimal inflammation. Martel proposed that apophyseal changes caused the instability with secondary disc destruction and end plate microfractures. The relative infrequency of cervical spine disease in juvenile-onset RA was explained by the early bony ankylosis of the apophyseal joints observed in these subjects.

Ball[33] reviewed the pathology of 14 RA patients with no radiologic evidence of cervical disease and found that the earliest histologic lesions were in the uncovertebral joints. He suggested that the disc and adjacent bone are then secondarily involved with resultant inflammatory destruction and progressive instability. The fact that uncovertebral joints are not completely developed in the first two decades of life[34] might also explain the infrequency with which cervical rheumatoid disease is seen in juvenile-onset RA.[35]

Cervical spine disease is observed in as many as 88% of patients with RA.[36] The manifestations include C1-2 instability, occipitocervical (OC) instability (with or without vertical displacement of the dens), and subaxial cervical RA. C1-2 instability is the most common form of cervical rheumatoid involvement and may occur in up to 74% of the patients.[37] The dens is surrounded by two synovial joints, one ventrally, between the atlas and dens, and another between the transverse ligament and the dens. With involvement of the synovial joints there is progressive inflammation, destruction, and subsequent transverse ligament laxity, with destruction of the osseous attachments of the ligamentous complex. This loss of ligamentous integrity allows C1 to move ventrally on C2. If there is further significant disruption and osteomalacia of the dens itself, then dorsal C1-2 subluxation can also occur.[38] If the synovial apophyseal joints between C1-2 are involved as well, lateral rotation may also be evident in addition to subluxation at C1-2. OC instability results from involvement of the atlanto-occipital articulations. With significant articular facet destruction, there is progressive collapse of the occiput at C1 and vertical displacement of the residual dens (Figs. 8-4 and 8-5). This has also been termed *atlantoaxial impaction*, *vertical subluxation*, *cranial settling*, and *basilar invagination*.[38] Vertical displacement of the dens occurs in 5% to 32% of RA patients.[29,39,40] It is believed that vertical displacement of the dens represents a more advanced stage of systemic disease burden; indeed, one 10-year retrospective review of patients with RA cervical instability treated with OC fusion noted significantly worse long-term outcomes in the subset of patients with vertical displacement of the dens.[41]

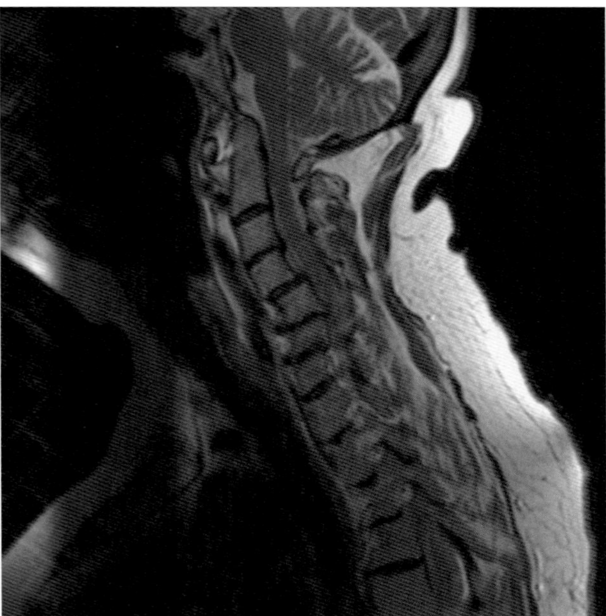

FIGURE 8-4. T2-weighted MRI of cervical spine demonstrating vertical displacement of the dens.

In the subaxial region, the levels most commonly involved with rheumatoid synovitis are C2-3 and C3-4. Subluxation (Fig. 8-6) may occur in approximately 7% to 29% of the patients with RA.[38] Subaxial region subluxation rates as high as 31% have been noted after rostral surgical fusion; however, there was no increased incidence of myelopathy or pain with fusion-adjacent subluxations.[41] These "staircase" subluxations are thought to be caused by significant ligamentous laxity and facet degeneration.[36,42] At any of the various sites of rheumatoid involvement, osseous erosion of adjacent bone, caused by osteoclastic resorption, occurs frequently.[43]

With the significant bony destruction, ligamentous laxity, and the potential for neural compression observed in the rheumatoid cervical spine, the primary emphasis of treatment is reduction of subluxation and fusion/fixation to prevent spinal cord injury. The optimal time to proceed with operative intervention is yet to be determined. Omura et al. stratified their RA population and found that the subset of

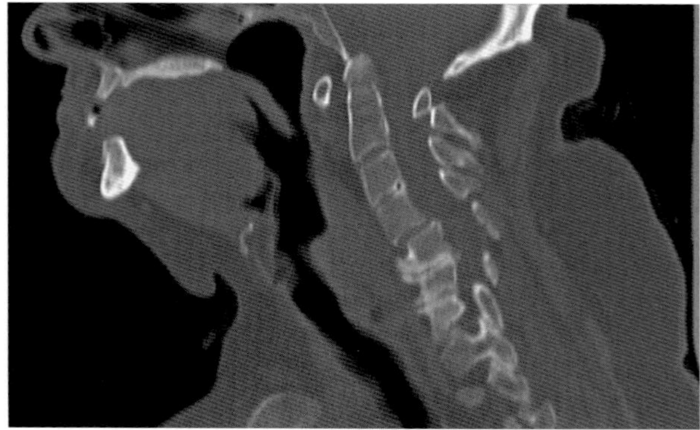

FIGURE 8-5. CT of cervical spine demonstrating vertical displacement of the dens.

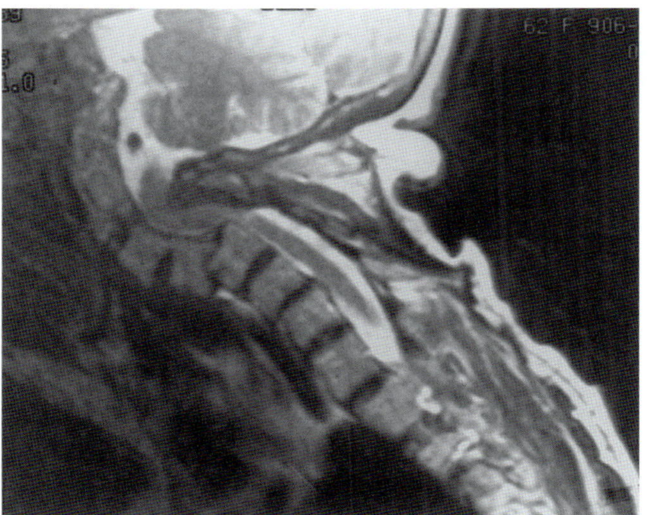

FIGURE 8-6. T2-weighted MRI of cervical spine demonstrating C5-6 subluxation and spinal cord compression in a patient with rheumatoid arthritis. Marked vertical displacement of the dens is also evident.

patients with seropositive disease and systemic evidence of mutilating-type joint involvement are at the highest risk of deterioration of their known cervical lesion.[44] Furthermore, retrospective review of RA patients with cervical disease found that best-medical management faired significantly worse when compared with surgical fusion with respect to both morbidity and mortality.[44] When substratifying the patient population undergoing surgical fusion, patients operated on earlier in their course and with a better functional preoperative score had a more pronounced overall improvement than those undergoing late surgical management. There is strong evidence for early operative intervention for the stabilization of RA-associated cervical disease.[44,45]

Surgical fusion yields multiple benefits, including reduction of both pain and neurologic sequelae; retrospective analysis of long-construct dorsal fusion demonstrates significant recovery of these two characteristics, compared with best-medical management, with improvement of an average of one to two grades on the Ranawat scales for pain and neurologic symptoms (Boxes 8-1 and 8-2).[41,44,45] These improvements were persistent, even in the setting of failed permanent postoperative reduction of deformity and imbalance.[41] The chronic granulomatous pannus decreases in size with the elimination of abnormal movement after successful arthrodesis.[46,47] There is no consensus regarding the optimal type of intervention, but one must keep in mind the inherent poor quality of RA bone, the laxity of ligaments, the insidious inflammatory nature of RA itself, and the destructive effects of the myriad pharmacologic interventions, especially with respect to treatment with corticosteroids.[45]

BOX 8-1. **Ranawat's Scale for Pain**

Stage 0
No pain
Stage I
Intermittent pain responsive to standard analgesics
Stage II
Intermittent pain partially responsive to standard analgesics—need for immobilization by a cervical collar
Stage III
Incapacitating

BOX 8-2. **Ranawat's Scale for Neurologic Involvement**

Class I
No neurologic abnormalities
Class II
Subjective impression of muscle weakness with brisk deep tendon reflexes and dysesthesia
Class IIIA
Moderate objective motor loss leaving some degree of self-sufficiency
Class IIIB
Severe neurologic impairment with complete loss of self-sufficiency

Scheurmann Disease (Juvenile Kyphosis)

Scheuermann[48] first described the progressive dorsal kyphosis of adolescent children in 1920. The deformity is usually evident as a fixed thoracic kyphosis that does not correct with hyperextension, thereby differentiating it from a postural kyphosis. Compensatory hyperlordosis of the lumbar and cervical spine may also be present. A mild scoliosis is noted in 20% to 30% of patients.[49] Sorenson[50] described the characteristic feature of ventral wedging of 5 degrees or more in at least three adjacent vertebrae. Other characteristics include kyphosis of greater than 40 degrees, vertebral end plate irregularity, and disc space narrowing.[51] The prevalence of the disease ranges from 0.4% to 8%.[50] It occurs predominantly in males (91% in one series).[52] Hereditary patterns of transmission have been identified, though genetic loci have yet to be determined.[53]

Basic biomechanical factors and forces may play a role in this disorder. The thoracic spine has a natural kyphosis determined primarily by the shape of the vertebrae; in the adolescent thoracic spine 20 to 40 degrees of kyphosis is normal. The dorsal elements, including the ligamentum flavum and the laminae, resist forward flexion of the spine in tension, whereas the ventral bony elements (vertebral bodies) and disc resist compression.[54] However, the facet joint capsules in the thoracic region are mechanically "weaker" than those in the lumbar region, so that any factor that increases the torque of the spine can result in greater deformity. The more marked the initial angulation of the spine, the larger the load (subject's weight), and the longer the duration of load application, the greater the likelihood of the progression of the deformity.

Scheuermann disease must be differentiated from juvenile postural kyphosis, which, as the name attests, is a kyphosis seen during flexion that will correct with improved posture and extension. The apex of the curve is smooth. The condition will improve with therapy that targets improved posture and core strengthening.[53]

The pathogenesis of the disease remains unclear. Scheuermann believed that aseptic necrosis of the ring apophyses caused interruption of growth, which resulted in ventral vertebral body wedging.[55] Subsequent work has refuted this theory by demonstrating that the apophyses do not contribute to longitudinal growth. Such growth is now known to result from endochondral ossification of the end plates.[55] Schmorl[56] felt that damage to the end plate by herniated disc material was of importance. Schmorl nodes are, however, not limited to the kyphotic region of the spine and are common in otherwise normal patients. It has been postulated that osteoporosis is involved,[57,58] but recent investigations have found no differences in the trabecular bone density between patients with Scheuermann disease and controls matched for age, gender, and race.[52,59] Other factors such as inflammation,[60] hormonal influences,[61] genetic factors,[62] altered calcium metabolism,[63] hypovitaminosis,[64] neuromuscular disorders,[65] extradural cyst formation,[66,67] defective collagen formation of the end plate,[68] and a decrease in the collagen-proteoglycan ratio of the end plate[61] have been implicated, but their roles in the development of the disease have not been substantiated.

There is a high association (>90%) between ventral osseous extensions from the anterior margin of the vertebral body and the diseased vertebrae, a feature that is absent in normal specimens.[52] Histologic examination reveals disorganized endochondral ossification, which may be a result of abnormal stress. Traumatic features of vascular and fibrocartilage proliferation are evident in the ventral end plates in Scheuermann disease.[52,68,69] The dorsal vertebral height in cases of Scheuermann disease is not significantly different from that of controls, implying that either the ventral and dorsal stresses are different or that the kyphotic changes occur after dorsal growth is completed (the normal pattern of ring apophysis closure starts dorsolaterally, then works ventrally).[52] Possibly, the natural thoracic kyphosis, being exacerbated by a rounded back, results in the development of the abnormal kyphosis.

Back pain is uncommon in the growing child with Scheuermann disease. Low back pain has been reported to be common (up to 50%)[51] in adults with progressive, untreated dorsal kyphotic deformities. In other studies pain was not a significant problem.[51] Progression of deformity is documented in 80% of patients older than 25 years of age, but the extent of deformity and pain is generally not severe.[70] The kyphosis most commonly progresses before skeletal maturity, but can occur in adulthood.[71] Disc degeneration is also associated with the deformity. Development of neurologic complications is rare, but is due to thoracic disc hernation, dural tenting, extradural cysts, and vascular compromise.[72]

Examination of the patient with Scheuermann disease can reveal a hyperpigmented lesion at the apex of the thoracic curve—a result of friction injury from the abnormally protruded spinous process. Patients often have a forward-protruding head, flexion contractures of the shoulders and hips, as well as tight hamstrings.[53]

Treatment is often indicated to correct the deformity, prevent its progression, and alleviate pain. The extent of the kyphosis and the age of the patient are important criteria for intervention. The nonoperative forms of treatment, such as bracing (Milwaukee brace) or casting, are the first line of treatment for most cases in which the kyphotic deformity is less than 65 degrees. These cases have a high success rate in correcting the deformity, especially if treatment begins before closure of the iliac apophyses (i.e., skeletal maturation).[73] Operative treatment with fusion is reserved for cases of progressive deformity, pain not responsive to an adequate trial of casting or bracing, degenerative changes in adults associated with the kyphosis, cardiopulmonary compromise, and for a deformity greater than 65 degrees.[71]

Dorsal long-construct instrumentation that extends rostrally and caudally well above the thoracic apex is often adequate for stabilization and correction of the deformity. In the event of extreme kyphotic deformity, both a ventral and dorsal surgical approach is necessary for a more definitive correction,[53] as well as the maintenance of correction until fusion in the setting of greater tension forces opposing the correction. A large retrospective review comparing 78 patients treated with either dorsal instrumentation alone or combined anterior-posterior instrumentation showed a comparable degree of deformity correction. The rates of proximal junctional kyphosis and surgical complications were clinically and statistically significantly increased in the combined procedure. A decreased rate of postoperative loss of correction was observed with the combined procedure. A higher rate of proximal junctional kyphosis was correlated with a greater degree of postoperative kyphosis, greater pelvic incidence, and less imbalance correction. The authors conclude that dorsal arthrodesis and fixation alone should be the favored procedure whenever possible due to the lower complication rate.[74] On the other hand, anterior ligamentous and disc release with video-assisted thoracoscopic surgery (VATS) combined with dorsal spinal fusion may yield lower complication rates and increased sagittal deformity correction, due to the anterior tension band release.[75]

Paget Disease

Paget disease is a metabolic bone disorder thought to be of possible viral origin. Prevalence of the disease has marked geographic variation. In the United States, Paget disease is found radiographically in 3% to 4% of patients older than age 40.[76] Histologically, the disease is characterized by areas of bone resorption and new bone deposition resulting from focal increases in the population of osteoclasts. The individual cells are larger than normal and contain inclusion bodies similar to paramyxovirus capsids. This suggests viral induction of the osteoclastic activity and results in a greater surface bone resorption. There is no disturbance of reactive bone formation; therefore, increased osteoblastic activity compensates for the bone resorption and, in fact, produces a net-positive balance of bone. The bone is usually lamellar, and it is normally mineralized.[76] However, woven bone and occasionally osteoid bone are also present and result in reduced bone quality with disruption of the lamellar structure of both cortical and trabecular bone.

The pelvic bones are the most commonly affected, followed by the spine. Approximately 70% of patients have lumbar spine involvement, 45% have thoracic spine lesions, and the cervical spine is involved in 15% of cases.[77] The frequent involvement of the lumbar spine is thought to be caused by increased loading.[78] The lesions are primarily in cancellous bone. Approximately two thirds of the radiographically evident lesions are asymptomatic.[77] Back pain in Paget disease is related to the combination of the bone deformity and subchondral bone enlargement that alters the contours of the joint surfaces and leads to joint degeneration. The subchondral changes include increased bone deposition and subchondral infarcts from abnormal pressure on expanded bone, each of which causes the bone to lose its normal flexibility and usual biomechanical properties.[76] The involved vertebral body can interfere with nutrition of the intervertebral disc, thus leading to early degenerative sclerotic changes.

Radiographically, the majority of patients with Paget disease have involvement of both the vertebral body and dorsal osseus elements—involvement of only ventral or dorsal structures is rare. Consistent with histologic analysis supporting periosteal bone formation and endosteal absorption, early radiographs show increased density in the osseous periphery contrasted with a central lucency.[79,80] Commonly, sclerotic areas are present as well as localized osteolytic lesions, which may coalesce with time. As a result of the disorganized pattern of bone deposition, biomechanical efficiency is reduced and the risk of fracturing is increased. Healing of fractures is usually efficient. The histologic features of Paget disease are observed in the fracture line.[76] The incidence of neurologic sequelae with thoracic and cervical spine involvement is increased, perhaps caused by the narrower diameter of the spinal canal due to stenosis in these regions.[81,82] Some advocate that a component of epidural fat ossification is a factor, though this may be simply a component of advancing periosteal bone formation that projects into the canal.[79]

Back pain is the most frequent presenting symptom, resulting from multiple possible etiologies, including periosteal stretching, deranged vascularity with resulting zones of ischemia, stenosis, nerve root compression, facet arthropathy, and osseous microfracture.[79] Neurologic sequelae have been reported in 25% to 30% of cases of Paget disease.[81,83] The neurologic deficits are most often caused by bony compression of the spinal canal or the foramina, with the neural arch and the facet joints most commonly affected by the proliferative bone deposition.[81] Fractures and subluxations can also compromise the spinal canal, and progressive platybasia can result in compression of the medulla. Vascular "steal," resulting from the increased vascularity of the pathologic bone, has also been implicated in the development of neurologic deficits.[84]

Treatment centers on reducing the burden of hypertrophied and abnormal bone. Despite the prevalence of stenosis with resultant neural element compression, the first intervention is medical treatment with bisphosphonates and calcitonin, among other agents. Surgical decompression is rarely indicated, owing to the success of medical intervention.[79] If surgery is to be considered, an aggressive preoperative course of treatment should be considered to reduce the volume of abnormal and highly vascularized tissue, which can lead to voluminous blood loss.[80] Pagetic lesions rarely degenerate to benign and malignant neoplasms that require more aggressive surgical management, with osteosarcomas predominating in the latter category.[79]

Ankylosing Spondylitis

Ankylosing spondylitis is an inflammatory disorder affecting synovial and cartilaginous joints, primarily in the axial skeleton. The most noticeable pathologic findings are inflammation of the ligamentous attachments (enthesiopathy), discovertebral erosions, and new bone formation that results in the ankylosis or autofusion of intervertebral joints.

The cause of the disease remains unknown, but it appears to be multifactorial with both genetic and acquired factors playing a role. There is a male predominance, varying from 3:1 to 8:1.[85] Peak age of onset is between 15 and 29 years, with less than 5% beginning after age 50.[86] Prevalence in the United States population is about 0.1%.[87]

The earliest signs of ankylosing spondylitis occur in the region of ligamentous attachment to bone (the enthesis).[88,89] In ankylosing spondylitis the enthesis shows multiple, focal, microscopic inflammatory lesions that eventually destroy the ligament and erode the adjacent cortical bone. This process leads to an osteitis, primarily at the ventral and ventrolateral aspects of the attachment of the annulus fibrosus to the vertebral bone. This is the "anterior spondylitis," or Romanus lesion, that is observed radiographically.[90,91] As the reparative process occurs, woven bone replaces the cortical erosion (ossification in fibrous tissue without preceding cartilage formation). Ultimately, this is replaced by lamellar bone.[33] Syndesmophytes are formed, most conspicuously on the ventrolateral aspects of the vertebrae adjacent to each disc. This results in new enthesis formation above the original level of cortical bone. Further thickening and growth of the syndesmophyte may be caused by inflammatory lesions in this new bone[33] or chondroid metaplasia with ossification.[92]

In the apophyseal joint, osteitis and enthesiopathy occur at the junction of capsule and bone and result in reactive bone formation and ossification of the capsule,[93,94] usually in the presence of well-preserved articular cartilage, implying that the capsule-ligamentous attachment is of primary importance in the apophyseal joint pathology.[33,93] Ultimately the joint may become ankylosed by endochondral ossification. This may be the result of capsular ossification or the general immobility of the spine as a result of discovertebral syndesmophyte formation as described previously.[33,95] However, the observation that apophyseal joint ankylosis may occur in the absence of vertebral ankylosis at the same level makes the former more likely.[94]

Concomitant ossification of the supraspinous and interspinous ligaments also occurs where there is a nonspecific inflammatory process at the attachment of the ligaments.[91] The anterior longitudinal ligament, however, does not usually become ossified, except at its deep fibers adjacent to the annulus fibrosus.[92]

Bone resorption (resulting in squaring of the vertebrae), syndesmophyte formation, bony ankylosis of the intervertebral discs, and apophyseal joint and ligament ossification complete the classic radiographic "bamboo-spine" appearance. Although bone formation at the attachments of the ligaments and at the apophyseal joints is increased, the vertebrae in ankylosing spondylitis are generally osteoporotic. This may be a result of the systemic effects of the disease, immobilization of the vertebrae, the inflammatory process, or drug treatment.[96]

As the bony ankylosis in the discovertebral region and the apophyseal joints progresses, the normal flexibility of the spine is lost. The spine is much stiffer than normal and is unable to absorb and dissipate loading energy in an efficient manner. Indeed, the ankylosing process itself may introduce a "lever-arm" quality to regions of affected neuroaxis,

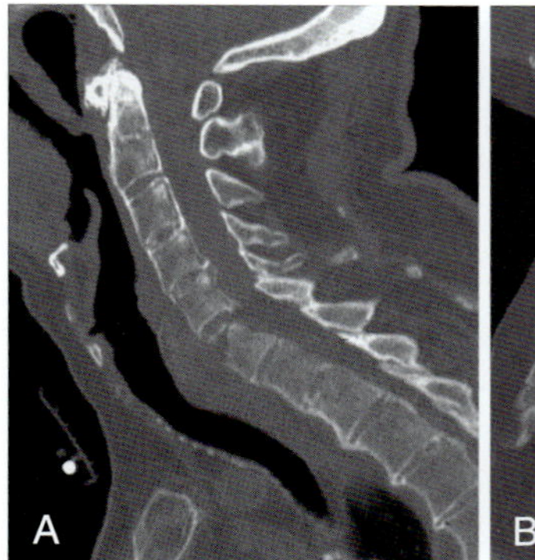

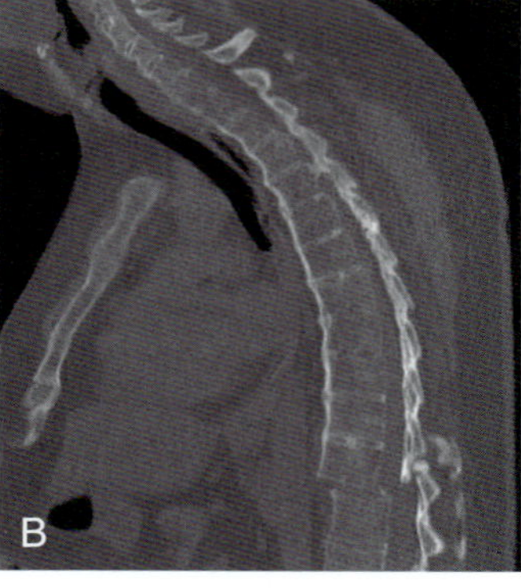

FIGURE 8-7. CT of two patients with ankylosing spondylitis and fracture caused by minor acceleration/deceleration injuries. **A,** C5-6 fracture through the disc space and superior end plate producing sagittal deformity. **B,** Low thoracic fracture dislocation through the disc space and posterior elements resulting in severe canal stenosis. Both fractures are highly unstable.

increasing the magnitude of injury that may be focused at specific spinal levels.[97] Because of these factors and osteoporosis, the bone is much more prone to fracture and subluxation after trivial trauma (Fig. 8-7).[98] Due to the long lever-arm effect of inflexible segments adjacent to the fracture, the spinal cord is significantly vulnerable when dislocation occurs in these fractures. The cervical spine appears to be particularly susceptible; approximately 75% of the spinal fractures occur in this region, primarily in the lower cervical spine.[99] These fractures tend to pass through the ventrodorsal width of the vertebra and may involve the calcified ligaments in the spinous processes. This process may occur either at the level of the disc space or through the vertebral body.[98] A cervical kyphosis is often present, and the neck is especially vulnerable to hyperextension injuries.[99-101] Some authors have attempted to match the mechanism of injury to the fracture location, considering extension to cause transdiscal fractures and flexion to cause transvertebral fractures.[101] Others have not found this relationship.[100]

Injuries to the thoracolumbar spine, though less frequent than cervical traumatic injury, are themselves significantly more frequent in the ankylosing spondylitis patient, occurring at a rate four times that in the general trauma population.[102] The majority of these fractures represent three-column injuries, again an indication of the imbalance, poor osseous quality, and associated disease in adjacent soft tissue structures that is seen with ankylosing spondylitis.

In spondylitic patients with cervical spine fractures, the mortality rate is 35%, as compared with 20% for patients with a normal spine. Also, the risk of severe neurologic sequelae in ankylosing spondylitis is 57% compared with 18% in the normal spine.[98] One review documented an American Spinal Injury Association (ASIA) A posttraumatic grade in 41% of ankylosing spondylitis patients; the mechanism for the majority of these patients was a fall from a standing position.[103] Without ligamentous support, and with multiple ankylosed vertebrae, any spinal movement is concentrated at the fracture site. Therefore, fractures are usually very unstable. The increased risk of bleeding with fracture in ankylosing spondylitis is thought to be related to the enlarged diploic spaces of the pathologic cancellous bone, the extensive nature of the fracture, and damage to adjacent epidural veins.[100,104] Epidural hematomas have been reported to occur in 20% of cases.[30] For these reasons, there is greater potential for neurologic deficit. This is especially problematic because fractures often occur after minor trauma, and often in the lower cervical region. These may be difficult to visualize radiographically, especially in osteoporotic bone. Further complicating the radiographic evaluation of neuraxis trauma is the diffuse and active inflammation that forms the basis of the disease, which is seen as increased signal on the short-tau inversion-recovery (STIR) MRI sequence. Acute injury may be masked during radiographic examination due to these chronic MRI changes.

Operative interventions in the acute setting should focus on restoring preoperative sagittal balance, rather than on attempting to improve the kyphotic deformity that is typically present before injury. Further strain to neural elements by excessive traction, or during patient transfers unprotected by external immobilization, may introduce a devastating additional injury. Correction may proceed at a later time when in a more controlled setting. Additionally, halo vest or other cervicothoracic vest fixation should be used judiciously in cases of ankylosing spondylitis, as these patients often have multiple medical morbidities, including decreased vital capacity and pulmonary insufficiency due to ankylosis of the costovertebral joints, which would be further strained by such intervention.[97,103]

When fractures occur, a normal callus forms at the site, and although inadequate immobilization may lead to pseudarthrosis, healing is typically rapid.[99] Pseudarthrosis of transdiscal fractures in undiagnosed ankylosing spondylitis is often confused with disc space infection or tuberculous spondylitis.

Although atlantoaxial instability is far less common in ankylosing spondylitis than in RA, it may occur.[105,106] Inflammation of the entheses, the apophyseal joints, and the synovial joint between the dens and the transverse ligament results in both bony and ligamentous damage, with subsequent instability similar to that observed in RA. The atlantoaxial joint may be the only remaining mobile segment and the fulcrum of all craniocervical mobility of the cervical spine in patients with advanced ankylosing spondylitis.

Ossification of the Posterior Longitudinal Ligament

Although OPLL was first reported in 1838 in England,[107] it has received increased attention because of the high incidence in Japanese and other Asian populations.[61,108] OPLL appears in approximately 2% of the cervical spine radiographs in the Japanese population, and autopsy studies show an incidence of 20% in subjects older than age 60.[109] More recently it has been recognized in the non-Asian population, but the prevalence is lower in other countries: 0.1% in West Germany,[110] 0.12% to 0.7% in the United States,[110-112] and 1.7% in Italy.[113] The incidence appears to be higher in males, and it increases with age.[109] The pathogenesis of OPLL remains unclear, though recent investigation has narrowed the genetic loci of interest to a site near the human leukocyte antigen (HLA) on chromosome 6p.[114] Routine tests to determine levels of C-reactive protein, rheumatoid factor, and HLA-B27, as well as the erythrocyte sedimentation rate are all normal.[108,109] HLA-BW40 and SA5 alterations are more common in OPLL patients, but there is no clear evidence of an inheritance pattern.[109,115] Metabolic abnormalities such as hypoparathyroidism, acromegaly, vitamin D–resistant rickets, and spondyloepiphyseal dysplasia may occur concurrently with OPLL,[109,114] implying a disturbance of calcium metabolism. However, the significance of these abnormalities in the pathogenesis of OPLL is unclear. The number of growth hormone receptors are often elevated, and bone morphogenic protein (BMP) levels are elevated even in nonossified tissue compared with controls.[114] In one series 28.4% of the OPLL patients were diabetic, and 17.7% had an impaired glucose tolerance test. Patients with diabetes mellitus have an increased incidence of OPLL.[109] Myotonic muscular dystrophy has also been reported in association with OPLL.

Other hyperostotic conditions associated with OPLL are diffuse idiopathic skeletal hyperostosis (with a concomitance rate of 50%),[116] ankylosing spondylitis (with a 2% concomitance rate), and ossification of the yellow ligament (with a concomitance rate of 6.8%).[108,109]

Radiographically, this acquired spine abnormality is characterized by abnormal ossification involving the posterior longitudinal ligament along the dorsal border of the vertebral body. Greater than 70% of disease is located within the cervical spine, and thoracic or lumbar involvement without concomitant cervical involvement is unusual.[114] OPLL is grouped according to its localization along the vertebrae. It has been classified into segmental, mixed, continuous, and localized forms.[109] The segmental type is characterized by calcification or ossification behind each body, with each osteophytic segment separated by the uninvolved disc (Fig. 8-8). The continuous type extends over the bodies and discs of several vertebrae. The mixed type is a combination of these two types. The localized type demonstrates ossification limited to the ligament over the disc space. Early OPLL first presents with small ossification patterns posterior to the disc space, making delineation from more ubiquitous degenerative disc disease difficult. Contrast-enhanced MRI may help with the diagnosis, as the posterior longitudinal ligament (PLL) uniformly enhances in the setting of OPLL, but disc pathology does not.[114] The vertebrae at C4, C5, and C6 are most affected, and the average number of vertebrae involved is 3.1.[109] Ligamentous ossification substantially reduces the size of the spinal canal, particularly in the mixed and continuous types, especially when underlying developmental stenosis is present.

Histologically, the normal PLL contains both type I and type II collagen. In OPLL only type I collagen is identified, suggesting that the process of ossification involves replacement of the original collagen matrix.[117] The heterotopic bone formation observed with OPLL occurs in the superficial layer of the PLL, leaving an unossified gap between the dorsal aspect of the vertebral body and the ligament. The ossified ligament has a typical lamellar bone structure with haversian canals and a few bone marrow canals.[117] Calcification or ossification may also involve the dura mater.

The average radiographic narrowing of the anteroposterior diameter of the cervical spinal cord has been noted to be more than 40% for the mixed and continuous types.[109] Progression of the disease in a single, small series has been documented as a mean annual increase of 4.07 mm rostrocaudally and 0.67 mm in the ventrodorsal direction.[118] Myelopathy is the most common neurologic abnormality. It is likely that a large proportion of cases are asymptomatic when developmental stenosis does not aggravate cord compression.[119] The relative paucity of symptoms has been attributed to the slow rate of progression observed in most cases, as well as the lack of underlying developmental stenosis. However, a critical spinal canal diameter can be reached, where even minimal trauma can result in severe neurologic deficit.

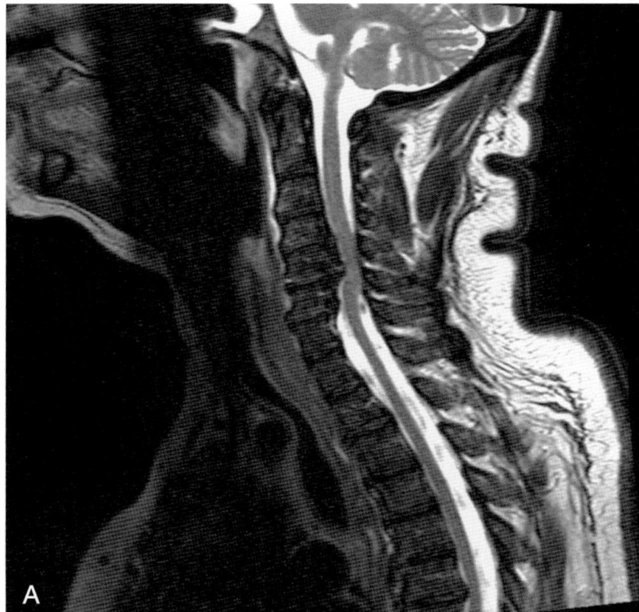

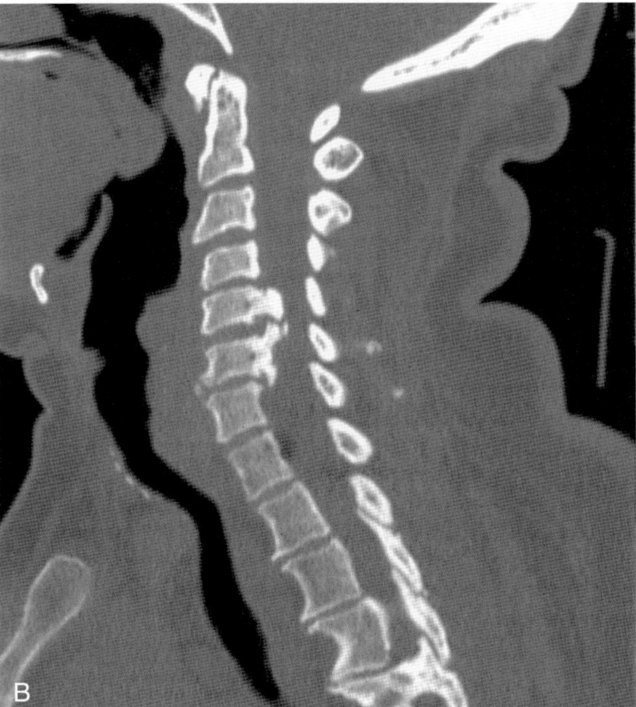

FIGURE 8-8. CT and T2-weighted MRI of cervical spine showing the segmental form of ossification of the posterior longitudinal ligament at C5-6. **A,** MRI demonstrates cord compression. **B,** Ligamentous ossification, however, is best shown by CT.

Management of OPLL must first include a determination of whether a neurologic deficit due to severe stenosis is present or impending, as well as a characterization of other medical morbidity due to OPLL's association with a myriad of metabolic derangements. Conservative treatment of pain and minor neurologic deficits can include NSAIDs, steroids, and external brace immobilization. Studies have shown that early surgical intervention before the onset of neurologic deficit correlates with significantly improved outcomes. Much like patients with other degenerative/inflammatory pathology of the cervical spine, even very minor trauma can lead to devastating neurologic injury due to the derangement of normal cervical dynamics.[114]

The surgical treatment of OPLL has been aimed at enlarging the spinal canal by removing the vertebral bodies and ossified ligament by ventral corpectomy and fusion. Internal fixation may obviate the need for postoperative halo or Minerva immobilization. It is important to note that the dorsal approach for laminoplasty or multilevel laminectomy and posterior spinal fusion with instrumentation does not remove the primary pathologic lesion. With rapid disease progression, ventral surgery may still be required as a secondary procedure. In advanced cases with severe developmental and acquired stenosis over multiple levels, combined or staged dorsal and ventral decompression and fusion may be required. Nevertheless, the anterior approach can be fraught with approach-related complications such as dysphagia and dysphonia. Most notably and unique to this pathology is the complication of iatrogenic durotomy and formation of cerebrospinal fluid (CSF) fistula. Investigation into the predictive value of preoperative radiographic findings has helped to stratify patient risk for CSF leak. Hida et al. first described these CT findings: the single-layer sign, defined as a large focal mass of dense OPLL, and the double-layer sign, with ventral and dorsal hyperdense rims of OPLL surrounding a central hypodense (nonossified) ligament.[75] Evaluation of these two groups allows for further risks stratification; Min et al. described an incidence of dural penetration in 52.6% of patients with the double-layer sign, 13.6% of patients with the single-layer sign, and 1.5% of patients without either sign.[120] Patients with extension of continuous OPLL and cord compression up to the C2 level or caudally to the upper thoracic segments may be best treated with posterior decompression and fusion alone. Whether progression of the OPLL mass effect on the spinal cord in the rostrocaudal or anteroposterior directions is arrested by laminoplasty or laminectomy with fusion remains controversial.

Spondylothesis and Spondylolysis

Spondylolisthesis is the translational movement of one vertebra on another. Spondylolysis refers to a defect in the pars interarticularis and may or may not be observed in spondylolisthesis. Instability of the affected motion segment may cause back pain. Sciatica and radiculopathy are more likely caused by foramen stenosis than by spinal canal constriction. To understand the classification, implications, and radiographic findings of these conditions, the anatomy and biomechanics of the area of the lamina, known as the pars interarticularis, must be considered.

The pars interarticularis, or isthmus, is the bone between the lamina, pedicle, articular facet, and transverse process. This region is able to resist significant forces in excess of 1251 N.[121] It has a cross-sectional area of about 0.75 cm^2, with two layers of cortical bone and intervening trabecular bone.[122] Developmental or traumatic incompetence or disruption of the pars is associated with anterolisthesis due to instability of the motion segment.

Flexion, extension, and rotation all have effects on the disc and, subsequently, on the facet joints and pars interarticularis. With normal lumbar lordosis, with the discs inclined in a ventrocaudal direction, the load is transmitted by the discs.[123] Axial loading therefore places both the disc and the caudal facets under ventral shear stress.[124,125] This stress is parallel to the intervertebral disc and is resisted by the caudal facets of the apophyseal joints, the disc, and the muscles attached to the neural arch.[122,124,125] In the intact specimen under shear stress, approximately 60% of the stiffness is provided by the disc and 15% by the facet joints.[123] The lower lumbar level apophyseal joints lie directly across the plane of the disc and therefore may contribute more to resisting shear than the apophyseal joints in the upper lumbar region, which are at the level of the pedicles.[124] In addition, the upper lumbar disc spaces are more dorsocaudally inclined in the upright position, thus making the apophyseal joints less susceptible.

Exactly which movements cause the mechanical deformation and, ultimately, the failure of the pars interarticularis remains unclear. The contribution of flexion, extension, and rotatory movements has been reviewed.[121,124,125]

It can be demonstrated that as flexion occurs, compression and ventral shear stresses in the lower lumbar region increase.[124] Muscular, and then ligamentous, tension resists the shear stress. The simultaneous application of the shear stress and the resisting forces causes stress concentration at the caudal margin of the pedicle, which progresses across the pars.[124] The pars, which is not as strong as the pedicle, fails as the stress increases with greater flexion. Debate remains about whether a single episode of overload[124] or fatigue[126] causes microfractures that lead to a gross fracture with continuing overload. It is likely that a combination of both processes occurs.[125] The same mechanism that causes the fracture prevents complete healing, and fibrous nonunion results. This may allow progressive listhesis with elongation of the pars.[127]

Research and clinical information also implicate extension movement in generating stresses across the pars interarticularis that may lead to fracture.[125] It has been suggested that the frequency of spondylolisthesis in gymnasts is a result of hyperextension injuries occurring on landing in the upright position with accentuated lumbar lordosis. If the extended spine is accelerating and then is subjected to sudden deceleration, increased shear stress is generated along the disc space, which in the lower lumbar spine is at an angle to the line of deceleration. This results in further extension, increasing shear, and greater stress across the pars.[125] Also, the disc is less stiff in extension, making ventral translation even more probable.[121] Microfractures develop, and once the bone is defective, the forces acting on it result in further microfractures and progression of the lytic lesion. Further support for the importance of lordosis in causing the pars defects is observed in patients with Scheuermann disease, in which a compensatory lumbar lordosis occurs. Asymptomatic lumbar spondylolysis often without spondylolisthesis has been reported in as many as 50% of these patients.[128]

Torque may also play a role in the development of spondylolisthesis, especially in the degenerative type. With degeneration the disc loses its ability to resist shear and torsional stresses.[18,124] Torsional stress, conveyed to the caudal facet, distorts the lamina-pedicle angle and results in the facet being less able to resist shear. The contralateral facet then has to resist more shear stress and may also become damaged.[124] Stress concentration with injury to the pars may occur when torsional forces are applied to the neural arch, and ultimately, ventral subluxation may occur.[124]

The most widely used classification of spondylolisthesis is that of Wiltse et al.[127] Wiltse et al. divide the listhesis types into dysplastic, isthmic, degenerative, traumatic, and pathologic. Degenerative listhesis has a prevalence of 4% to 10%[129,130]; isthmic, 4%; and dysplastic, 1%.[131] Traumatic and pathologic listhesis implies a history of localized trauma or generalized bony disease, which allows forward subluxation to occur.

Dysplastic Spondylolisthesis

Dysplastic spondylolisthesis, which is caused by a congenital defect of the upper sacrum, or the vertebral arch of L5, presents in young children and adolescents.[132] It has two subtypes: type A, with the dysplastic articular facets oriented axially, and type B, with dysplastic articular facets oriented sagittally. When the facets are dysplastic, the ability to resist the ventral shear stress is reduced and can result in listhesis. The pars may be initially intact or even remain intact, but in other cases the ventral shear stress results in microfractures of the pars, with subsequent pars elongation. Thus the pars is not the initiator of the listhesis.[133] In dysplastic cases with a subluxation of greater than 35%, neurologic and muscular symptoms are likely,[132] usually manifested as symptoms of cauda equina or nerve root compression. Paralysis and bowel dysfunction are uncommon. Hamstring tightness and abnormal gait, however, are common.[132]

Isthmic Spondylolisthesis

In isthmic spondylolisthesis a defect occurs in the pars interarticularis (spondylolysis). Facet orientation is normal. The three subtypes depend on the integrity of the pars and the nature of the injury. In subtype A there is distinct separation of the pars interarticularis, as a result of fatigue fracture, a single traumatic episode, or a combination of both (Fig. 8-9). In subtype B the pars is elongated, actually appearing intact, which is thought to be a result of the healing of stress fractures of the pars. Fibrous nonunion is observed in these defects. This can appear similar to a dysplastic lesion with pars elongation. Subtype C is characterized by an acute fracture of the pars, in addition to fractures elsewhere in the vertebra, which are usually a result of severe trauma.

The severity of spondylolisthesis is described by the Meyerding classification of superior vertebral body subluxation over the adjacent inferior vertebral body. The five grades of subluxation are grade 1 (0–25%), grade 2 (25–50%), grade 3 (50–75%), grade 4 (75–100%), and grade 5 (spondyloptysis, >100%).[134,135]

Isthmic spondylolisthesis occurs at L5-S1 in approximately 82%, L4-5 in 11%, L3-4 in 0.5%, L2-3 in 0.3%, and in other levels, in approximately 6% of the cases.[136] The lesion does not appear in other primates, indicating that upright posture is important. Also, true lumbar lordosis, seen only in the human primate, may be a factor.[127]

Infant cadaveric dissections have demonstrated that lytic pars defects are not present at birth.[137] However, bilateral pars interarticularis defects have been documented in a 4-month-old.[138] The most common age for development and diagnosis of isthmic spondylolysis is between the ages of 5 and 7 years.[127] In a study of 500 children,[139] 4.4% of the 6-year-olds and 5.2% of the 12-year-olds had unilateral or bilateral pars defects, whereas the incidence is 6% in adults. It is postulated that with assumption of the upright sitting posture and lordosis of the lumbar spine, subluxation is most likely to develop.[127,140] In adolescent cases participation in contact sports may be a significant factor.[127]

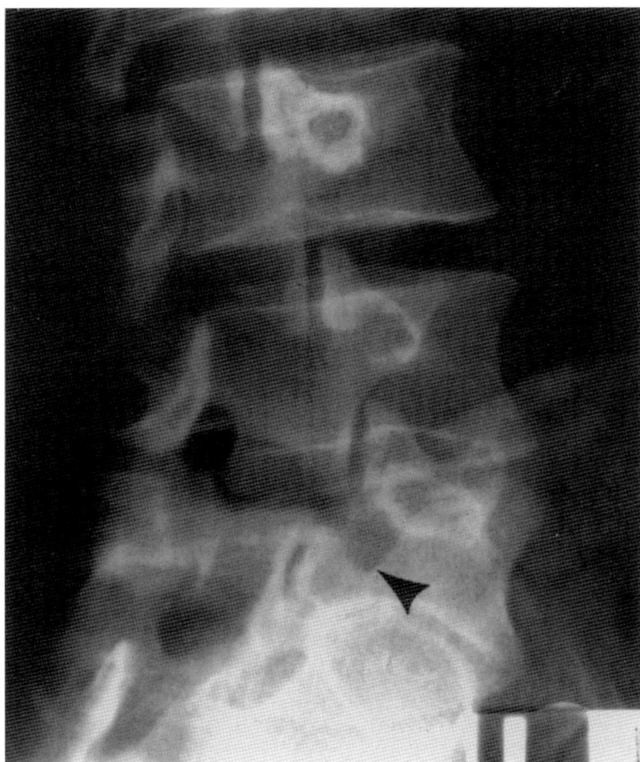

FIGURE 8-9. Oblique plain radiographs of the lower lumbar spine. Arrow indicates subtype A spondylolysis (absence of the neck of the Scotty dog).

There is also evidence that genetics may play a role in isthmic spondylolisthesis.[126,141] White males have an incidence of 6.4%, compared with black women, who have an incidence of 1.1%.[136] There is an association between the dysplastic and isthmic lesions and spina bifida occulta and hypoplasia of the sacrum.[142] The prevalence of spina bifida occulta of L5 or S1 and lumbosacral defects in one series was found to be 94% for the dysplastic type and 32% for the isthmic type.[131] The incidence of the two types of spondylolisthesis has been reported to be increased in first-degree relatives. Thirty-three percent and 15%, respectively, of first-degree relatives of patients with dysplastic and isthmic spondylolisthesis have radiographic evidence of subluxation.[131]

Although the initial degree of slip in isthmic spondylolisthesis can be marked, progression in adulthood is unusual. Slip is more prone to progress at L4-5 than L5-S1, and may be up to 28% in the teenage years.[139] Whether subluxation will progress, however, is difficult to predict. Due to the high prevalence of spondylolysis, spondylolithesis, and low back pain in the general population, it is difficult to attribute low back pain in the individual patient to these anatomic lesions. A subgroup analysis from the Framingham Heart Study found not only a higher prevalence of spondylolysis than previously reported (11.5% vs. 6%), but also found no association of spondylolysis or spondylolithesis with low back pain, which suggests that these lesions are not a major cause of back pain in the general population.[143]

Treatment of each type of spondylolysis depends on the extent of neural compression and motion segment instability. Decompressive laminectomy, foraminotomies, and internal fixation may be required.

Degenerative Spondylolisthesis

Degenerative spondylolisthesis is more common in women than men,[23] with a ratio of 5:1. It is associated with spondylotic changes of the apophyseal joints and disc narrowing. Degeneration of the disc reduces its stiffness and places greater stress on the facets. When subjected to shear forces, subluxation may result without fracture of the pars. Subluxation does not usually exceed 30%.[144] Because of the greater inherent stability of L5 and the prevalence of L5 sacralization,[136] the L4-5 or L3-4 levels are more frequently affected.[145] Stabilization as a result of osteophyte formation usually occurs, and significant progression is rare without destabilizing surgical procedures. Degenerative spondylolisthesis is commonly associated with spinal stenosis and neurogenic claudication caused by lumbosacral radiculopathy. Decompression often relieves symptoms. Fusion with internal fixation may be required in cases with radiographic evidence of instability or severe back pain.

KEY REFERENCES

Bouchard-Chabot A, Liote F: Cervical spine involvement in rheumatoid arthritis: a review. *Joint Bone Spine* 69:141–154, 2002.

Dell'Atti C: The spine in Paget's disease. *Skeletal Radiol* 36:609–626, 2007.

Farfan HF, Osteria V, Lamy C: The mechanical etiology of spondylolysis and spondylolisthesis. *Clin Orthop Relat Res* 8:40–55, 1976.

Katz JN, Liang MH: Differential diagnosis and conservative treatment of rheumatoid disorders. In Frymoyer JW, editor: *The adult spine: principles and practice*, Philadelphia, 1991, Lippincott-Raven, pp 699–718.

Omura K, Hukuda S, Katsuura A, et al: Evaluation of posterior long fusion versus conservative treatment for the progressive rheumatoid cervical spine. *Spine (Phila Pa 1976)* 27(12):1336–1345, 2002.

Scheuermann H: Kyphosis dorsalis juvenilis. *Ugeskr Laeger* 82:385–393, 1920.

Tsuyama N: Ossification of the posterior longitudinal ligament of the spine. *Clin Orthop Relat Res* 184:71–84, 1984.

Wiltse LL, Widell EH Jr, Jackson DW: Fatigue fracture: the basic lesion is isthmic spondylolisthesis. *J Bone Joint Surg [Am]* 57:17–22, 1975.

REFERENCES

The complete reference list is available online at expertconsult.com.

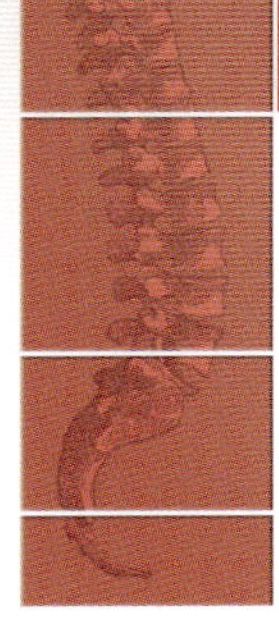

CHAPTER 9

Neural Injury at the Molecular Level

Kevin M. Walsh | Jeffrey P. Mullin | David H. Kim | Alexander R. Vaccaro | Fraser C. Henderson | Edward C. Benzel

The histopathologic appearance of chronic cervical spondylotic myelopathy has been well described and includes the characteristic features of regional demyelination extending axially from the site of compression, preferential lateral column axonal loss, and anterior horn neuron dropout.[1-5] Ongoing research projects are creating a better understanding of myelopathy on a molecular level, and recent studies indicate that a significant portion of cell loss appears to be caused by the process of programmed cell death, also known as *apoptosis*. Although the molecular pathways regulating apoptosis are extremely complex, programmed cell death affects restricted populations of spinal cord cells—including oligodendrocytes and some neuronal and astrocytic subpopulations—suggesting the possibility that targeted antiapoptotic therapy may be a reasonable goal for the treatment or prevention of myelopathy.

Microbiology of the Oligodendrocyte

The oligodendrocyte has been shown to play a pivotal role in several complex biologic processes, including development, injury repair, disease process modulation, and the formation and maintenance of myelin.[6,7] During the early stages of human development, a large oligodendroglial population is generated, and an estimated 50% of these cells eventually disappear by the process of apoptosis.[8] As the central nervous system matures, the oligodendroglia become responsible for the creation and maintenance of myelin sheaths. These sheaths, although formed directly from oligodendroglial cell membrane, demonstrate key biochemical differences from the parent cell membrane in terms of both chemical and protein composition.[9] The biochemical and physiologic characteristics of the relatively small protein constituent are especially important, and absence or alteration of the major protein components (i.e., proteolipid protein or myelin basic protein) can lead to the advent of severe demyelinating disease.[10] Another unique feature of the oligodendrocyte is the high concentration of microtubules, which contribute to formation of an elaborate cytoskeletal framework, allowing myelin sheath formation at remote distances from the cell karyon.[6]

Considerable progress has been made in understanding the response of oligodendroglial cells to injury, and a more complete understanding of this complex process may lead to a greater appreciation of the mechanism of injury in such processes as cervical spondylotic myelopathy. Studies suggest that the oligodendrocyte is particularly sensitive to a wide range of oxidative, chemical, radiation-induced, and mechanical injuries. High iron content and relatively inefficient antioxidant defense mechanisms appear to render the oligodendrocyte vulnerable to oxidative stress.[11-14] Injury-related release of intracellular iron may contribute to the generation of damaging hydroxyl radicals through the Fenton reaction.[15] In addition, in vitro exposure of mature oligodendrocytes to hydrogen peroxide has been shown to induce apoptotic cell death, but preincubation of these cells with an iron chelator, such as deferoxamine, appears to confer some protection from oxidative cytotoxicity and apoptosis.[16,17]

Toxins that impair mitochondrial respiration, such as cuprizone and ethidium bromide, have also been shown to trigger apoptosis in oligodendroglial cells. Subsequently, these chemicals have been used to develop experimental models of demyelinating disease and injury. It has been established that radiation exposure directly damages DNA and has been shown to lead to apoptotic cell death in many cell types. However, several studies of delayed neurologic injury after radiation therapy have revealed that oligodendrocytes are the most radiation-sensitive cell population in spinal cord tissue.[18,19]

In addition to the previously mentioned sources of oligodendrocyte injury, mechanical stress has been repeatedly shown to trigger oligodendrocyte apoptosis. Mechanical injury appears capable of triggering a specific immune response with formation of antibodies and subsequent cytotoxicity directed against oligodendrocyte antigens.[20] This immune-mediated injury may be caused by macrophage activity and appears to involve several different cytokines, such as tumor necrosis factor, lymphotoxin, and gamma-interferon.[21-24] These activated macrophages also generate free radicals and nitric oxide, which have been shown to lead to apoptosis.[25,26] Formation of the membrane attack complex through activation of the complement cascade is another consequence of macrophage activation and has been implicated in oligodendrocyte injury.

In addition to the macrophage, at least two specific subpopulations of T cells may also be involved in oligodendroglial apoptosis. $CD4^+$ T cells adhere to target cells through the Fas receptor identified on oligodendrocyte cells, thereby triggering apoptosis. Gamma-delta T cells have been found to co-localize with oligodendrocytes (expressing heat-shock protein 65), and may trigger cell death through production of gamma-interferon.[27]

Apoptosis

Apoptosis, also known as "programmed cell death," may be the primary cellular process underlying the disappearance of oligodendrocytes in the earliest histologic stages of traumatic spinal cord injury (SCI) and other processes such as cervical spondylotic myelopathy. The process of apoptosis is distinct from necrosis and involves a sequence of intracellular events that includes chromatin aggregation and internucleosomal DNA fragmentation, nuclear pyknosis, and subsequent cell shrinkage.[28,29] Apoptosis ultimately results in phagocytic engulfment of cells without extracellular discharge of cytosolic contents, and without generation of a local inflammatory response.[30]

In contrast to necrotic cell death, apoptosis is a much more abbreviated process that has made its study relatively difficult. Apoptotic cells initially shrink and lose contact with adjacent cells, forming membrane blebs and expressing prophagocytic cell surface signals. The cell chromatin then condenses and fragments, and the process ends in compartmentalization of the entire cell into small, membrane-bound vesicles that are quickly phagocytized. By comparison, cell necrosis is a relatively prolonged affair that is characterized by cell membrane disruption, mitochondrial swelling, random DNA cleavage, and the generation of a local inflammatory reaction.[31]

Several molecular biology assays have been developed for identification of apoptosis in various settings. A marker of DNA cleavage, such as the terminal deoxynucleotidyltransferase (TdT)-mediated nick-end labeling (TUNEL) technique, is a popular assay. Interpretation of studies relying solely on TUNEL staining has been criticized as possibly being limited by the observation that this method has been found to label cells undergoing necrosis as well and may not be as specific for apoptosis as once thought.[31] Internucleosomal DNA cleavage, a hallmark of apoptosis, is demonstrated by a characteristic "laddering" pattern on gel electrophoresis, and this finding can reinforce the results of TUNEL staining. The most specific method for identifying apoptotic cells, however, remains direct histologic examination and the identification of chromatin condensation along the nuclear periphery, condensation of the cytoplasm with intact organelles, and membrane blebbing.[32] A newly developed commercial assay is also available that uses monoclonal antibody to single-stranded DNA (Apostain; eBioscience, San Diego, CA). This method is purported to detect the earliest stages of apoptosis occurring before DNA fragmentation and supposedly has no cross-reactivity for necrotic cells.[33]

Molecular Mechanisms of Apoptosis

The molecular pathways involved in apoptosis have been extensively examined, but were initially studied in the roundworm, *Caenorhabditis elegans*. These studies led to the discovery of one of the first genes associated with apoptosis, which was appropriately named *CED 3* in honor of this worm.[34] Subsequently, a homologous family of apoptosis-related protein products has been identified in mammals and termed the *CED 3/ICE* (interleukin-1β-converting enzyme) family.[35-37] These proteins, also known as *caspases*, serve as functional cysteine proteases.[38] At least 10 distinct members of this gene family have been identified thus far, and at least 2 of these proteins, caspase-3 and caspase-9, have been strongly associated with apoptosis in human cells.[39,40] The intracellular cascade involving caspase-3 ends in activation of specific endonucleases that cleave DNA strands into the characteristic internucleosomal fragments.[41] Production of these 185 base-pair fragments results in the DNA laddering that is one of the histologic hallmarks of apoptosis. Activation of caspase-9 appears specifically to induce mitochondrial release of cytochrome c, which is one of the earliest intracellular events in apoptosis.[42] Targeted inhibition of caspase-1 (ICE) and caspase-3 (CPP-32) in oligodendrocytes has been shown to prevent apoptotic death of these cells.[40]

As previously described, numerous chemical and biologic triggers for apoptosis have been identified. Mature oligodendrocytes are particularly sensitive to oxidative stress.[11] Experimental exposure of oligodendroglial cells to hydrogen peroxide leads to increased expression and nuclear translocation of transcription factors nuclear factor-κB (NF-κB) and activator protein-1 (AP-1), both implicated as critical elements in the apoptotic pathway.[17]

One of the most important biologic triggers of oligodendrocyte apoptosis in SCI may be tumor necrosis factor-α (TNF-α). TNF-α has been shown to induce apoptosis in oligodendrocytes, both in vitro and in vivo.[43-45] Designated death domains located on the intracellular side of the type I receptor for TNF-α (TNFR1) and related receptors have been associated with activation of caspase-3 and caspase-8, which subsequently leads to apoptosis.[40] Gamma-interferon may further enhance susceptibility of oligodendrocytes to TNF-α-triggered apoptosis through up-regulation of the so-called death receptor, Fas.[46] It has also been reported that the p38 and Jun N-terminal kinase (JNK) pathways play a role in the transmission of apoptosis signals following SCI. Further findings indicate that activation of JNK by TNF-α promotes expression of apoptosis signal-regulating kinase 1 (ASK1).[47]

The oligodendrocyte apoptotic signal transduction pathway appears to begin with ligand binding to either Fas (CD95 or Apo1) or p75 (low-affinity neurotrophin receptors) cell surface receptors. These proteins are members of the TNFR family and have been shown to co-localize with cells undergoing apoptosis in a rat model of cervical SCI.[32] Binding of Fas ligand (FasL) to the extracellular cysteine-rich domain of Fas results in formation of oligomers, which allows interaction of the intracellular death domain with Fas-associated death domain protein (FADD).[48] Once the association is made, the death domain of FADD then interacts with procaspases 8 and 10 and triggers a caspase activation cascade that ultimately ends in activation of at least three different effector enzymes, caspases 3, 6, and 7.[32] These effector molecules presumably interact with additional downstream targets, ultimately leading to cell apoptosis.[49] FLICE (FADD-like interleukin-1β-converting enzyme) proteins are proteins demonstrating sequence homology with the caspases, but acting as inhibitors of the apoptosis-triggering pathway.[50]

Another important apoptosis pathway involves the p53 tumor suppressor protein, as well as the proteins p21, Bcl-2, and Bax.[51] In a rat model of SCI, p53 protein appeared within 30 minutes of injury, co-localizing with apoptotic glial cells and spreading in distribution over the course of 2 days.[51] Cellular studies have further demonstrated that exposure of oligodendroglial cells to hydrogen peroxide leads to rapid translocation of p53 from the cytosol to the nucleus and cell death by apoptosis.[52]

Apoptosis in Traumatic Spinal Cord Injury

It has been well established that cell loss in traumatic SCI occurs both at the time of injury and secondarily over a period of days to weeks after the event. At the epicenter of injury, the majority of cell death occurs through necrosis, with macrophages and microglia becoming actively engaged in phagocytosis of necrotic cell debris.[53] However, cell loss in spinal cord white matter continues throughout a much more extensive axial section of the cord for up to several weeks in a process referred to as *secondary injury*. Although it has become apparent that this continued cell loss significantly worsens neurologic outcome in SCI, the underlying biologic mechanisms remain poorly understood. Several studies have suggested, however, that the primary process involves oligodendrocyte apoptosis.[54-59]

Initial evidence that apoptosis contributes to ongoing cell death after acute SCI came from animal studies involving the rat.[60] It was demonstrated that acute compressive cord injury leads to preferential apoptosis of oligodendrocytes along degenerating longitudinal white matter tracts.[55] These initial findings were subsequently supported by similar results in other animal models, including primates.[56] In most of these animal studies, visible signs of oligodendrocyte apoptosis appear within 24 hours and continue for at least 3 weeks after injury.[54-57,60-63]

A histopathologic study of human SCI indicates that oligodendrocyte cell death by apoptosis can continue from 3 hours to at least 8 weeks after injury.[64] In this study, oligodendrocyte apoptosis appeared to correlate with specific patterns of wallerian degeneration and was associated with intracellular activation of caspase-3. Apoptosis was more pronounced in ascending white matter tracts, and the authors speculated that this finding may reflect the histopathologic observation that wallerian degeneration affects ascending tracts before descending ones.[65] The extent of oligodendrocyte apoptosis was shown to correlate with the severity of neurologic injury, being significantly less extensive in patients with incomplete neurologic deficits. This correlation of apoptosis and neurologic impairment is in agreement with previous findings from animal studies.[57] Of note, neuronal apoptosis was not seen, suggesting that neuronal loss occurs through the process of necrosis.

The biochemical trigger for oligodendrocyte apoptosis related to traumatic SCI is currently unknown but is likely to be multifactorial. It has been observed that SCI is characterized by significant intracellular Ca^{2+} shifts, and several apoptotic processes are Ca^{2+} dependent, including DNA fragmentation and proteolysis.[66,67] Similarly, acute SCI has been associated with hypoxia and free radical formation, which are also established triggers of apoptosis.[68,69] Glutamate excitotoxicity has also been implicated in secondary SCI and appears to lead to apoptotic cell death.[70]

Animal models have provided most of the information regarding biochemical responses to SCI. A rat model of SCI has demonstrated increased local TNF-α expression within 1 hour of injury, followed by increased nitric oxide levels at 4 hours.[71] This model used a neutralizing antibody against TNF-α, and significantly reduced nitric oxide levels as well as the extent of apoptosis. Similarly, addition of a nitric oxide synthase inhibitor, N-monomethyl-L-arginine acetate (L-NMMA) also reduced the number of apoptotic cells. These findings suggest that TNF-α signaling triggers apoptotic cell death after SCI, and that this effect is at least partly mediated by nitric oxide. Of note, the amount of decrease in apoptosis after administration of L-NMMA (42%) was less than half that observed after TNF-α antibody administration (89%), implying the existence of multiple parallel apoptotic pathways. A recent study by Genovese et al. demonstrated the neuroprotective effects of selective adenosine A_{2A} receptor agonists, which act by decreasing the overall expression of myeloperoxidase, NF-κB, and inducible nitric oxide synthase (iNOS), and decreasing the activation of JNK mitogen-activated protein kinase (MAPK) in oligodendrocytes.[72] In addition, another recent study found that mice with SCI, when treated with ethyl pyruvate, showed no increase of TNF-α expression and a decrease in oligodendrocyte apoptosis.[73]

Several studies of development suggest that specific trophic factors are produced by axons and that absence of these factors results in oligodendrocyte apoptosis.[74-76] Members of the neuregulin ligand family, in particular the glial growth factor (GGF), bind to the HER4 receptor on the surface of oligodendrocytes and appear to play an important role in cell differentiation and survival.[77] Alternatively, the traumatic event may result in direct release of proapoptotic factors into spinal cord tissue. It is well established that activated microglia release several factors that may cause apoptosis, including TNF-α, reactive oxygen intermediates, and nitric oxide.[78,79] Administration of exogenous thyroid hormone (triiodothyronine [T_3]) during the early period after acute SCI has also been found to increase the population of apoptotic cells.[80]

Apoptosis in Chronic Spinal Cord Compression

Several studies have suggested an important role for ischemic tissue injury in the pathogenesis of myelopathy in the setting of cervical spondylosis. On the cellular level, the sensitivity of oligodendrocytes to hypoxic injury is well established and appears to support the possibility of an ischemic cause.[81] However, neurons are relatively more vulnerable to ischemic injury, and their sparing in early myelopathy makes a purely ischemic cause for cervical spondylotic myelopathy somewhat unlikely.

Although necrosis and apoptosis often occur simultaneously, distinguishing the two processes provides important information regarding the causes of specific disease processes. Although ischemia has been associated with apoptotic cell death, severe ischemia is characteristically thought to result in cell necrosis. Because oligodendrocyte disappearance in both trauma and chronic spondylotic myelopathy is apoptotic in nature, it is thought that mechanisms other than pure ischemia are involved.[55]

Animal models strongly support a role for apoptotic cell death in the tissue degeneration seen in chronic, compression-related cervical myelopathy. The tiptoe-walking Yoshimura (twy) mouse is a specific strain of inbred mouse that has been useful as a model for chronic spinal cord compression.[82] Twy mice become quadriparetic 4 to 8 months after birth because of the development of local hyperostosis along the dorsolateral margins of the C1 and C2 vertebrae, which results in severe cord compression at this level.[83] Histologic examination of spinal cord tissue from these mice has revealed a characteristic pattern of descending degeneration affecting the anterior and lateral columns and ascending degeneration along the posterior columns. These findings are in addition to severe tissue damage at the level of compression.[84] Cavity formation and myelin ovoids (myelin debris) were observed extending from the zone of compression into adjacent levels without gross deformation of the spinal cord. Detection of apoptotic cells using the TUNEL assay revealed a distribution of glial apoptosis that appeared to mirror the pattern of degeneration, whereas cell-specific staining confirmed that apoptotic cells were oligodendrocytes. The investigators included an autopsy study of a human patient dying with cervical myelopathy resulting from ossification of the posterior longitudinal ligament, in which a pattern of neuronal loss, demyelination, and apoptosis was observed that was similar to the findings in the twy mouse. Further studies of the twy mouse showed increased expression of TNFR1 and TNFR2 in chronically compressed spinal cord tissue, which further elucidates the effect of chronic compression on apoptosis and demyelination.[85]

Oligodendrocyte survival depends on the presence of specific so-called survival factors produced by neighboring axons, leading to the possibility that oligodendroglial cell loss merely reflects prior neuronal injury. However, oligodendrocyte apoptosis likely precedes axonal degeneration in chronic myelopathy, as evidenced by both human and animal studies of spinal cord compression demonstrating apoptotic oligodendrocytes in the setting of intact demyelinated axons.[65,86,87]

Prevention of Apoptosis

Oxidative stress has been shown to be a potent trigger for apoptotic death of oligodendrocytes.[16] Conversely, antioxidant therapy with pyrrolidine dithiocarbamate (PDTC) and vitamin E appears to moderate this effect considerably.[17] The asymmetric distribution of phospholipid polar-head groups across the plasma membrane bilayer may play a role in determining vulnerability to oxidative stress.[88] Normally, there is an over-representation of choline phosphoglyceride and sphingomyelin in the outer leaflet, whereas the aminophospholipids, ethanolamine phosphoglyceride (EPG) and serine phosphoglyceride (SPG), are over-represented in the inner leaflet. Apoptosis has been associated with redistribution of SPG and EPG and loss of aminophospholipid asymmetry.[89] The large, polyunsaturated, fatty acid content of both SPG and EPG makes them targets for propagating free radical reactions, leading to generation of lipid peroxides and apoptosis.[15,90] It therefore makes sense that increasing polyunsaturated fatty acid content through addition of docosahexaenoic acid enhances the sensitivity of oligodendrocytes to oxidative stress and thereby results in increased rates of apoptosis.[88] Conversely, reducing EPG synthesis using *N*-monomethylethanolamine and *N*,*N*-dimethylethanolamine (DMEA) supplements appears to rescue cells from apoptotic death.

Methylprednisolone treatment has been shown to protect the spinal cord from injury and has become a standard component of SCI protocols. The protective effect of steroid therapy may be mediated in part by an inhibitory effect on oligodendrocyte apoptosis. Intraperitoneal injection of rats with dexamethasone after SCI significantly decreases the extent of apoptosis in both neurons and glial cells.[91] At least part of this effect may be mediated through inhibition of TNF-α and NF-κB.[92] A more recent study has also shown some additional benefit to the intraperitoneal administration of pregabalin in a post-SCI rat model.[93] Treatment with pregabalin showed a significant decrease in expression of caspase-3, Bcl-2, and p38 MAPK compared with control and methylprednisolone treatment groups. All three of these factors have been shown to be key components of the inflammatory and apoptotic cascades.[94-97]

The role of TNF-α in oligodendrocyte apoptosis appears complex and at times contradictory. Most studies have demonstrated primarily toxic effects, leading to apoptosis in several different models. This form of TNF-α-induced oligodendrocyte apoptosis can be inhibited in vitro by insulin-like growth factor 1 (IGF-1).[45] However, a few studies have suggested that TNF-α may, in certain instances, protect oligodendrocytes from apoptosis.[43,98,99]

The effects of TNF-α can be better understood through a description of its molecular mechanisms. TNF-α exerts its biologic effects through binding of two different cell surface receptors, the type 1 receptor (TNFR1) and the type 2 receptor (TNFR2).[100] TNFR binding has been shown to prevent neuronal apoptosis in several studies.[101-103] TNFR binding leads to increased NF-κB expression, and this TNFR-NF-κB signal transduction pathway has been identified as possibly a key endogenous, antiapoptotic cellular mechanism.[104-107] NF-κB is a transcription factor that increases expression of several genes, resulting in increased production of cellular inhibitor of apoptosis protein 2 (c-IAP2).[108,109] c-IAP2, in turn, inhibits apoptosis through binding TNFR-associated factor 2.

Protein inhibitors of apoptosis have been studied in baculovirus, and homologues to these proteins, referred to as inhibitors of apoptosis proteins (IAPs), have been identified in mammalian cells. IAPs appear to exert antiapoptotic effects through inhibition of the caspase cascade.[110-113]

Recent evidence suggests that activation of the TNFR-NF-κB pathway is important in protecting spinal cord cells from apoptosis after SCI. In an animal model of SCI, rats lacking TNFR1 demonstrated decreased spinal cord tissue levels of NF-κB activity, lower levels of c-IAP2, and increased caspase-3 activity. Apoptosis was significantly increased, the overall lesion size was larger with more extensive demyelination and axonal disruption, and functional recovery was significantly worsened.[114]

These studies suggested that pharmacologic modulation of TNF-α levels may yield benefits in patients with myelopathy or SCI. For example, interleukin-10 reduces TNF-α levels in the spinal cord and has been shown to improve functional recovery from SCI in rats.[115]

Although inflammatory demyelinating disease represents a pathologic process distinct from traumatic injury, the generation of high levels of TNF-α leading to oligodendrocyte apoptosis in both demyelinating disease and SCI implies potentially useful biochemical similarities.[116,117] Bcl-2 is a protein with antiapoptotic properties that is produced by certain types of cells, including oligodendrocytes. The activity of Bcl-2 has been studied in a rat model of human T-lymphocyte virus type I (HTLV-I)-associated myeloneuropathy. In this model, rats develop chronic progressive hind-limb weakness because of apoptotic oligodendrocyte death in the spinal cord.[118] A recent study using this rat model has associated oligodendrocyte apoptosis with enhanced sensitivity to exogenous TNF-α and an associated down-regulation of Bcl-2 in affected cells.[119] It is therefore conceivable that endogenous production of antiapoptotic proteins such as Bcl-2 can be up-regulated therapeutically as a treatment strategy for SCI and cervical myelopathy.[55-57,64,79,120-123]

In the developing central nervous system, oligodendrocytes appear to be protected from apoptosis by molecular, and possibly electrical, signals provided through axonal contact.[124-126] Several studies have demonstrated that exposure to specific cytokines protects oligodendrocytes from apoptosis. IGF-1 prevents TNF-α-triggered apoptosis in cell culture.[45] A study of transgenic mice expressing high levels of IGF-1 demonstrated decreased oligodendrocyte death after exposure to the demyelinating toxin cuprizone.[127] In addition, fibroblast growth factor triggers oligodendrocyte dedifferentiation and confers protection from apoptosis.[128-130]

Serum growth factor deprivation has also been shown to lead to apoptosis in cultured oligodendrocytes. This model of apoptosis has been used to study the role of the complement system in apoptosis. Although assembly of the membrane attack complex, C5b-9, on cell membranes typically leads to formation of transmembrane channels and resultant cell death, sublytic levels of C5b-9 complement components activate the cell cycle and enhance cell survival by preventing apoptosis.[131,132] This antiapoptotic effect appears to involve down-regulation of the proapoptotic cytosolic protein Bcl-2 antagonist of cell death (BAD).[133] Studies suggest that a delicate balance exists between the protective antiapoptotic effects of the membrane-bound Bcl-2 and Bcl-X_L proteins and the proapoptotic cytosolic proteins Bcl-2-associated X protein (BAX) and BAD.[134] This balance appears to determine functional mitochondrial integrity and, consequently, whether a cell will undergo apoptosis.

Glutamate excitotoxicity represents yet another potential trigger for oligodendrocyte apoptosis.[135] Oligodendrocytes express α-amino-3-hydroxy-5-methyl-4-isoxazolpropionic acid (AMPA)/kainite-type glutamate receptors and have been shown to be exquisitely sensitive to glutamate toxicity.[136] The specific receptor antagonist 2,3-dihydroxy-6-nitro-7-sulfamyl-benzo(f)quinoxaline (NBQX) has been shown to protect oligodendrocytes from glutamate both in vitro and in vivo.[136,137]

Finally, the process of apoptosis requires active protein synthesis. Inhibition of protein synthesis in animal models using the chemotherapeutic agent cycloheximide leads to a reduction in apoptotic cell death, less severe histopathologic changes, and improved clinical recovery.[57]

Biomechanical Deformation as an Epigenetic Factor in Neuronal and Oligodendrocytic Apoptosis

Although the environmental sensitivity of oligodendrocytes has been stressed, it should be remembered that specific stresses will trigger apoptosis in neurons. In particular, biomechanical factors have been shown to be an important epigenetic factor in driving neuronal apoptosis. Stretch-related myelopathy and brainstem injury are substantiated in the literature.[138-147] Neuronal strain (stretch) acts on the Na^+ channel mechanoreceptors to increase Na^+ influx, reverse cation exchange pumps, and depolarize voltage-gated Ca^{2+} channels, resulting in pathologic calcium influx.[148] Sublethally damaged neurons also undergo up-regulation of *N*-methyl-D-aspartate receptors, resulting in heightened vulnerability to subsequent challenges of reactive oxygen species and peroxynitrites, concomitant mitochondrial dysfunction, and DNA fragmentation.[149] Stretching neurons induces early calpain activation and contributes to progressive intra-axonal structural damage and apoptosis of neurons and oligodendrocytes.[57,149,150] Stretch injury has been shown to induce phosphorylation of p38 MAPK and apoptosis in vascular, heart, and lung cells.[151] The molecular events in neurons and oligodendrocytes should therefore be viewed within the matrix of environmental biomechanical stresses to which the organism is exposed.

Discussion

Identification of apoptosis per se does not provide much insight into the potential causes of specific disorders, including cervical myelopathy. Many sources of injury can result in histologically identical apoptotic cell death, including both mechanical trauma and ischemia.[55,152,153] Various studies have identified oligodendrocyte apoptosis in response to axonal injury and after exposure to specific cytokines, as well as due to apparent genetic susceptibility.[75,98,154] Adding to the complexity, apoptotic pathways appear to interact with one another in reinforcing relationships. Products of lipid peroxidation-induced cell damage, such as 4-hydroxynonenal (4-HNE), have been shown to enhance extracellular concentrations of glutamate by reducing their uptake, and they also appear capable of inducing apoptosis.[58,155]

Moreover, devising specific treatment strategies based on an incomplete understanding of the complex molecular mechanisms underlying apoptosis can be potentially hazardous. As previously discussed, several studies have pointed out the opposing effects of TNF-α on oligodendrocyte apoptosis.[156,157]

Another example of a molecule with potentially activating and inhibiting effects on apoptosis is nitric oxide. The observation that nitric oxide exposure can trigger both apoptotic and necrotic cell death in oligodendrocytes has led to efforts to protect the spinal cord from secondary injury through modulation of nitric oxide levels.[26,158,159] However, a neurotoxicant-induced model of demyelination in genetically engineered mice lacking inducible nitric oxide synthase (iNOS) revealed significantly more extensive oligodendrocyte apoptosis after cuprizone exposure, compared with control animals.[160] This result suggests a potentially protective effect of nitric oxide in some cases of acute demyelination.

Finally, some investigators warn that attempts to inhibit the wrong molecular events in a cell already committed to apoptosis may merely convert the process to one of necrosis.

Apoptosis is an important determinant of morbidity in cervical spondylotic myelopathy, as well as secondary SCI. Understanding the apoptotic mechanisms involved in these conditions will help to provide insight into potential targets for therapeutic intervention. Recognition that apoptosis plays a principal role in this process has introduced the possibility that the rational design of protease inhibitors active against specific proteins, such as caspase-3, may favorably modulate the response of spinal cord tissue to multiple forms of injury. Nevertheless, the molecular pathways governing apoptosis are extensive and interdependent, and a thorough understanding is absolutely necessary if any attempt at improving myelopathic outcome through modulation of this process is to succeed.

KEY REFERENCES

Casha S, Yu WR, Fehlings MG: Oligodendroglial apoptosis occurs along degenerating axons and is associated with FAS and p75 expression following spinal cord injury in the rat. *Neuroscience* 103:203–218, 2001.

Emery E, Aldana P, Bunge MB, et al: Apoptosis after traumatic human spinal cord injury. *J Neurosurg* 89:911–920, 1998.

Hisahara S, Shoji S, Okano H, et al: ICE/CED-3 family executes oligodendrocyte apoptosis by tumor necrosis factor. *J Neurochem* 69:10–20, 1997.

Inukai T, Uchida K, Nakajima H, et al: Tumor necrosis factor-alpha and its receptors contribute to apoptosis of oligodendrocytes in the spinal cord of spinal hyperostotic mouse (*twyy/twy*) sustaining chronic mechanical compression. *Spine (Phila Pa 1976)* 34:2848–2857, 2009.

Lee YB, Yune TY, Baik SY, et al: Role of tumor necrosis factor-alpha in neuronal and glial apoptosis after spinal cord injury. *Exp Neurol* 166: 190–195, 2000.

Rowland JW, Hawryluk GW, Kwon B, et al: Current status of acute spinal cord injury pathophysiology and emerging therapies: promise on the horizon. *Neurosurg Focus* 25:E2, 2008.

REFERENCES

The complete reference list is available online at expertconsult.com.

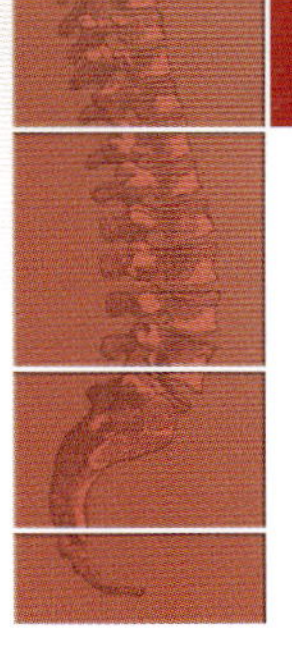

CHAPTER 10

Pathophysiology of Cervical Myelopathy: Biomechanics and Deformative Stress

Fraser C. Henderson | William A. Wilson IV | Edward C. Benzel | Alexander R. Vaccaro

Cervical spondylotic myelopathy (CSM) is a well-described clinical syndrome that evolves from a combination of etiologic mechanisms. The strong association between a narrowed, spondylotic cervical spinal canal and the development of CSM has previously led to the formulation of a relatively simple pathoanatomic concept: a narrowed spinal canal causes compression of the enclosed cord, leading to local tissue ischemia, injury, and neurologic impairment. However, this simple mechanism fails to explain the spectrum of clinical findings observed in CSM, particularly the development of significant neurologic signs in patients without evidence of static cord compression.

Current support for a biomechanical etiology of CSM comes from three areas: clinical studies of cervical mobility in patients with CSM, histopathologic studies of spinal cord tissue from patients with CSM, and biomechanical studies that have led to an improved understanding of the material properties and biomechanical behavior of spinal cord tissue under various physiologic and pathologic conditions. A growing body of evidence indicates that spondylotic narrowing of the spinal canal results in increased strain and shear forces, and that these pathologic deformative forces cause both diffuse and focal axonal injuries in the spinal cord. This biomechanical theory appears to more fully address the clinical and pathologic findings in various studies of spinal cord injury, and better explains the occurrence of clinical myelopathy in patients without static cord compression.

Clinical Patterns of Cervical Spondylotic Myelopathy

Clinical myelopathy typically appears in late adulthood in the setting of progressive degenerative changes, including cervical disc degeneration, osteophytic spur and transverse bar formation, posterior longitudinal ligament calcification, ligamentum flavum thickening, and osteoarthritic facet hypertrophy.[1-3] Progressive encroachment on the spinal canal by ventral and dorsal anatomic structures may first lead to spinal cord compression—compression that occurs only transiently during physiologic cervical range of motion. The appearance of clinical signs and symptoms arising from this condition has been described as "dynamic stenosis." With progressive narrowing of the spinal canal, dynamic compression may eventually evolve into static compression of the enclosed spinal cord and the appearance of classic CSM.

Retrospective observational studies indicate that development of CSM is more common in patients with underlying congenital stenosis of the spinal canal. A sagittal spinal canal diameter of less than 12 mm is strongly associated with signs and symptoms of myelopathy, whereas a diameter greater than 16 mm confers a low risk.[4-8]

Histopathology of Cervical Spondylotic Myelopathy

The theory that ischemic injury is the pathophysiologic basis of CSM originates in early histologic studies of cervical myelopathy, which revealed several changes consistent with ischemic tissue damage. These include cystic cavitation, gliosis, anterior horn cell dropout, and prominent involvement of the central gray matter, as well as wallerian degeneration of the posterior columns and corticospinal tracts.[2,9-11] In these studies, the most severe histologic changes were observed at the level of ventral spondylotic bars, with the most visible histologic changes occurring in the lateral funiculi of the spinal cord, particularly the corticospinal tracts. The anterior columns and dorsal region of the dorsal columns appeared to demonstrate the least extent of injury-related change.

Attempts have been made to correlate the severity of histopathologic findings with the range of clinical findings in patients with CSM. In general, less severe myelopathy has been associated with changes confined largely to the lateral funiculi, whereas more severe cases appear to be associated with involvement of the medial gray area and ventral aspect of the dorsal columns, as well as gliosis and anterior horn cell dropout. In cases of severe CSM there is extensive wallerian degeneration, proceeding proximally and distally from the site of spinal cord compression.

Spinal Cord Ischemia and Cervical Spondylotic Myelopathy

The anatomic basis for the ischemic insult proposed in CSM has been attributed to various mechanisms, including compression of radicular feeders in the neuroforamina, compromise of venous drainage by ventral spondylotic bars, and compression of the anterior spinal artery, as well as its ventral branches.[12,13] Several animal studies support the concept of a potential role for compressive ischemia in the pathogenesis of CSM.[14-16]

Cadaver studies have demonstrated that flattening of the cervical spinal cord is associated with elongation of the laterally directed terminal branches of the central arteries arising from the anterior spinal artery, as well as elongation of the penetrating branches of the lateral pial plexus (corona radiata). It is hypothesized that attenuation of these transversely directed arteries results in decreased arterial blood flow to the corticospinal tracts. Shortening of the ventral-dorsal dimension of the spinal cord, however, results in widening of the arteries directed in the ventral-dorsal direction and relative preservation of blood flow to the anterior columns. These findings might explain the relative vulnerability to injury of the laterally positioned corticospinal tracts, compared with the anterior columns.[17]

Recent clinical studies strongly suggest that compression and ischemia alone do not fully explain the pathogenesis of CSM. Despite observational studies associating CSM with various anatomic factors, such as the presence of decreased ventral-dorsal spinal canal diameter, subluxation, and dorsal osteophytes, at least one study has demonstrated that these factors hold no significant predictive value in terms of identifying which patients are at risk for clinical progression of their myelopathy.[18] Several other studies have also failed to identify an association between the degree of spinal stenosis and spinal cord compression and clinical prognosis.[7,12,19]

Moreover, surgical decompression that results in expansion of the spinal canal and relief of compressive pressures does not consistently alter the natural history of CSM.[20] Ebersold et al.[21] performed a retrospective review of 100 patients with CSM undergoing surgical decompression, with an average 7-year follow-up, and concluded that decompression alone resulted in no clear, long-term improvement. Two thirds of patients experienced initial clinical improvement, but half of these demonstrated subsequent clinical deterioration. At final follow-up, only a third of the original group were improved, leading the authors to conclude that long-term outcome was not predicated on the presence or severity of spinal cord compression and ischemia, but on other, "nonvascular" factors.

Biomechanical Factors and Cervical Spondylotic Myelopathy

There is a growing body of evidence indicating that abnormal or excessive motion of the cervical spine is strongly associated with clinical progression of CSM. In a retrospective clinical review, Adams and Logue[12] demonstrated a cervical flexion-extension arc in excess of 40 degrees was the most significant variable in predicting poor clinical outcome in patients with CSM. Similar retrospective studies have been performed by Barnes and Saunders,[18] as well as by Yonenobu et al.,[19] in which patients with a flexion-extension arc of greater than 60 degrees after laminectomy were at increased risk for development of progressive myelopathy.

In contrast to the relatively poor results after simple decompression for CSM, several studies demonstrate excellent clinical results associated with the elimination of abnormal cervical motion. Using a simple neck brace to restrict cervical motion often leads to improvement in patients with cervical myelopathy from disc protrusions.[22] The largest series of patients undergoing ventral decompression and fusion for CSM demonstrated an 86% improvement rate, with no significant deterioration.[23] Most recently, Uchida et al.[24] discovered that among patients with CSM who had kyphotic deformity in excess of 10 degrees, correction of sagittal alignment of the vertebrae significantly improved neurologic outcomes. Uchida et al. state that " kyphotic alignment may contribute to cervical myelopathy," that longitudinal distraction is a factor in progressive spinal cord dysfunction, and that the pathophysiologic mechanism is similar to that of tethered cord syndrome.[24] Overall, surgical fusion through a variety of approaches has been associated with favorable clinical results, including ventral decompression and fusion without instrumentation[21] or with ventral plating, [25-29] and dorsal decompression with instrumented fusion.[30-33]

The significant clinical recovery experienced by most myelopathic patients after decompression and fusion indicates that neurologic deficits resulting from cervical myelopathy are recoverable.[23,25,26,29-31] Moreover, the rapid improvement experienced by many patients after surgery suggests that these patients do not have irreversible, ischemic histologic changes demonstrated in many early pathologic studies. In contrast, failure of some patients to improve clinically after decompression and fusion may be a result of irreversible spinal cord injury. Histologic examination of spinal cord tissue from these patients may reveal severe ischemic injury.[2]

Pathophysiology of Deformative Stress Injury of the Cervical Spinal Cord

The significance of spinal stenosis and spinal cord compression in early CSM may not be the generation of local ischemia, but rather the creation of a tethering effect, which results in production of local, potentially injurious, tissue strain and shear forces. The concept that increased cervical mobility, coupled with kyphotic deformity, results in spinal cord elongation and increased axial strain forces is well documented.[12,13,17,18,24,34-41] Several studies have demonstrated the adverse effects of even low-grade mechanical stretching on neural tissues. During normal motion, large axial strains occur in the cervical spinal cord.[42] The white matter of the spinal cord can be viewed as an axial array of parallel fibers, with individual fibers demonstrating variable levels of crimping. As a whole the cord is initially compliant to stretch, but it becomes progressively stiffer as the fibers straighten and begin to bear tensile load.[35] Rapid occurrence of these strains can exceed the material properties of the tissue, leading to tissue disruption and transient or permanent neurologic injury. The degree of injury appears to be related to the peak strain of the tissue and the loading rate.[43]

Cadaver studies suggest that even physiologic flexion of the cervical spine leads to stretching and the production of strain forces in the neuraxis.[17] Flexion of the spinal column has been found to result in significant elongation of the spinal canal, with concomitant stretching of the spinal cord. During physiologic flexion of the head and trunk in rhesus monkeys, net movement of the spinal cord occurs from the upper spine downward to the level of C4-5, whereas net movement of the spinal cord occurs upward below this level.[34] Net movement occurs to a greater extent below C4-5, with 1.6 mm of movement at C1 and 6 mm of movement at T3. The amount of spinal cord stretch occurring at each level is proportional to the degree of flexion at the adjacent intervertebral disc space. Thus, forces that are generated in the spinal cord upon flexion can be visualized with neutral and flexion MRIs of the cervical spine. Flexion of the neck results in significant elongation of the enclosed spinal cord (Fig. 10-1). The increase in length (l) over the original length of the same section of the spinal cord (l_o) provides the strain (ε), thus:

$$E = l / l_o$$

At the lower cervical and upper thoracic spine, where the amount of flexion tends to be greatest, local spinal cord strain can reach 24%. Thus, the strain produced at the cervicothoracic junction can exceed 0.2, the strain level at which the giant squid axon ceases to function.[43] This phenomenon might explain the clinical observation that signs are often localized to levels apparently remote from the level of stenosis (e.g., hand intrinsic muscle wasting with high cervical stenosis).

In the absence of a compressive pathologic process, the natural elongation of the spinal cord that occurs with neck flexion and hyperextension is distributed over the entire length of the spinal cord. However, with tethering of the spinal cord, as a result of local compression, the axial strain cannot be distributed throughout the cord and is instead limited to the segment of cord between the distracting force and the tethering point. Local spinal cord degenerative changes are frequently identified adjacent to thickened dentate ligaments, which suggests that localization of injurious mechanical forces at these levels may be associated with the tethering effect of the ligaments.[36,44] A biomechanical study of the material properties of the dura mater indicates that elastic behavior is uniform throughout the length of the spinal canal; however, strain forces are significantly greater in the cervical region than in either the thoracic or lumbar region.[45]

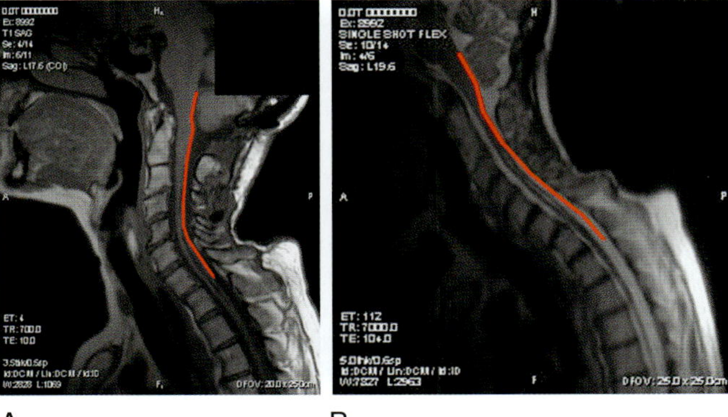

A B

FIGURE 10-1 Strain within the cord on regular flexion. **A,** The red line represents a hypothetical white matter tract measured from the base of the C7 level to the pontomedullary line. **B,** The same tract is shown in flexion. The indicated portion of the tract increases in length from 94 mm to 116 mm, representing a strain ε of approximately 0.24.

The tethering action of the dentate ligaments may be responsible for accentuating the effect of tensile spinal cord stress and exacerbating local tissue injury. Moreover, it has been suggested that dorsal displacement of the spinal cord, as a result of the presence of ventral spondylotic bars, may lead to stretching of the dentate ligaments and tethering of the cervical cord through the ventrolaterally positioned nerve root sleeves. Repetitive and persistent microtrauma to these nerve root sleeves may lead to the progressive thickening that has been observed with age.[44] Therefore, axial tension generated in the spinal cord during physiologic motion may be amplified at certain levels, as a result of two separate factors—overall spinal canal lengthening and the local tethering effects of the dentate ligaments.

Several investigators have attributed delayed, progressive cervical myelopathy to a combination of underlying structural kyphosis and abnormal or excessive cervical motion.[12,13,24,38] Dynamic lengthening of the cervical spinal cord that occurs during neck flexion is magnified in patients with cervical kyphosis. Conversely, kinematic MRI studies have demonstrated that lengthening of the spinal cord also occurs during neck extension in some patients with fixed kyphotic deformity of the cervical spine. In the setting of static spinal cord compression and superimposed instability, cervical extension can also lead to aggravation of the cord impingement and significant upper cervical spinal cord elongation.[46]

Mathematical Models of Spinal Cord Stretch Injury

Numerous mathematical models for spinal cord stretch injury have been developed. Levine[36] represented the spinal cord as a simplified solid material with uniform elastic properties to predict the three-dimensional stresses experienced during physiologic motion and in spondylosis. According to this model, flattening of the cord is not a result of ventral-dorsal compression, but rather the consequence of laterally directed tension arising from the dentate ligaments, which tighten in flexion. This model, with a ventral spondylotic bar and tethering dentate ligaments, predicts maximal stresses in the lateral funiculi. The model provides a possible explanation for the characteristic histologic findings in CSM, in which there is relative sparing of the anterior and posterior funiculi. It also explains why histopathologic changes are found over a relatively extended segment of spinal cord tissue, as opposed to being limited to the point of compression. However, the importance of the dentate ligaments in the etiology of CSM is brought into question by the inconsistent results of sectioning these ligaments at the time of surgery.[47]

Breig[38] also developed a mechanical model to explain some of the apparent inconsistencies found in histologic studies of CSM. For instance, in addressing the question of why some chronic, ventral compression injuries result in predominantly dorsal cord injury, cadaver models demonstrated that a compression force applied ventrally to the spinal cord in the presence of stenosis creates a pincer mechanism, resulting in increased axial tension in the cord and fissuring opposite the side of compression. In this model the spinal cord is represented as a viscoelastic cylinder that, when compressed from the sides, exhibits net tissue creep to the free ends of the cylinder. As a result, tension forces are created perpendicular to the plane of compression. With mild compressive deformation of the spinal cord, elastic stretch of the axis cylinders occurs. However, when the ventral-dorsal diameter of the spinal cord is reduced by 20% to 30%, axial tension forces exceed the material properties of the tissue and result in tearing of axial fibers. The stress field produced by this pincer mechanism is multidirectional, and secondary shearing forces are also created. This model explains how ventral compression of the spinal cord in the presence of stenosis might result in stretch and shear injury to myelin and neural elements.

Finite Element Models of Spinal Cord Stretch Injury

More recently, researchers have produced mathematical models of the cord using finite element analysis, a method adapted from materials science and fluid mechanics. Finite element analysis reduces a continuous structure into discrete, finite "brick" elements. This allows the approximation of partial differential equations by a linear system of ordinary differential equations, which can then be solved by numerical methods with the appropriate boundary conditions.[48] In this particular case, the equations concern mechanical strain (stretch), "out of plane" loading (shear due to transverse compression, such as from a retroflexed odontoid process), and material properties such as Young's modulus of elasticity or Poisson's ratio. Ichihara et al.[40] used finite element analysis to simulate the cervical spinal cord under compression and showed different amounts of stress at a given strain rate were to be expected owing to the differing material properties of gray and white matter. Kato et al.[41] showed that the addition of a small amount of flexion to a model with static compression significantly increased predicted stresses, with the majority of stresses in the anterior and posterior horns. Henderson et al.[49] demonstrated that increased deformative stresses in the corticospinal tracts, as predicted by the finite element analysis, were strongly correlated with neurologic deficits in a cohort of children with cervical and medullary symptoms. Elevated stress levels due to strain occurred during normal neck flexion in the spinal cord at the C1 level of one patient (MRIs from this patient are shown in Fig. 10-1); the addition of compression (shear) from a retroflexed odontoid process generates much higher stress levels with the same degree of flexion (Fig. 10-2).

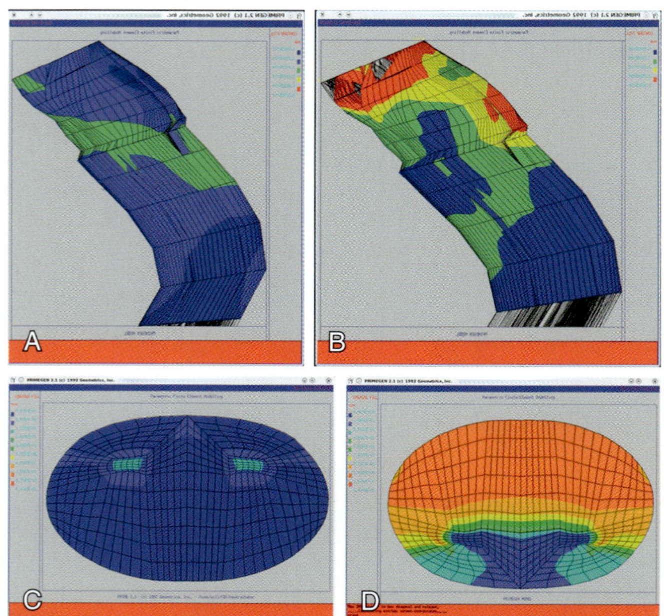

FIGURE 10-2 Finite element analysis of a portion of the cervical spine of the patient whose MRIs are shown in Figure 10-1. **A,** Sagittal view demonstrating the stresses on flexion. **B,** Sagittal view demonstrating more severe stresses on addition of local compression due to retroflexed odontoid with same degree of flexion as in **A**. **C,** Axial view at C1 of **A**. **D,** Axial view at C1 of **B**.

Spinal Cord Tethering and Shear Injury

Studies involving the tethered spinal cord syndrome may also contribute to a better understanding of the pathogenesis of CSM. Stretch injury is now widely accepted as the principal cause of myelopathy in tethered cord syndrome. The symptoms and clinical findings of pain, numbness, weakness, pes cavus, scoliosis, and bowel and bladder dysfunction have all been attributed to stretching injury of the spinal cord.[50-56] The degree or amount of traction on the conus medullaris determines the age of onset of symptoms. Extensive tethering and severe stretching of the conus medullaris results in neurologic disturbances in infancy, whereas a lesser degree of tethering often remains subclinical until adulthood, when symptoms may become manifest in the setting of an acute event (i.e., hyperflexion injury) or chronic process (e.g., development of ventral disc or bone protrusions).[57] Although clinical manifestations of tethered cord syndrome are more commonly referable to the lumbosacral spinal cord, many neurologic findings are referable to the cervical cord. For example, long tract involvement in tethered cord syndrome may lead to hand numbness and poor coordination, as well as upper extremity hyper-reflexia and even speech difficulties. Quadriparesis has also been reported.[58] The phenomenon of increased strain supports the hypothesis that tension in the spinal cord might be transmitted to the brainstem and remote segments of the cord. Injury to the large-diameter fibers of the corticospinal tracts may occur some distance from actual tethering, and result in mixed upper and lower motor neuron deficits.[57]

Experimental studies involving the lumbar and sacral spinal cord of cats have demonstrated that acute tethering is very traumatic to spinal cord tissue, particularly when stretching occurs repeatedly.[59] Spinal cord elongation is most pronounced immediately adjacent to the point of application of the tethering force. Under low levels of tension the spinal cord demonstrates purely elastic behavior and returns to normal resting length. At greater tension, plastic deformation occurs. Portions of the spinal cord near the point of application of stretch remain elongated by 7% over the original length, even after release of tension.

Tissue dysfunction in tethered cord syndrome has been associated with impairment of oxidative metabolism. The relationship of tissue ischemia to spinal cord stretching in this syndrome is unclear. Although a tethered cord may result in permanent neurologic deficit, the fact that surgical untethering usually results in significant improvement of sensorimotor and bladder function indicates a degree of reversibility that militates against a purely ischemic etiology.

A guinea pig model of spinal cord stretch injury has been developed in which the filum terminale was tethered and attached to a 5-g weight. Tethering resulted in significant delay and decreased amplitude of somatosensory evoked potentials. Lipid peroxidation and hypoxanthine levels were significantly increased. Electron microscopic examination of tissue revealed potentially reversible histologic changes, such as edema, destruction of the gray-white junction, axonal injury with loss of neurofilaments, and evidence of myelin sheath damage.[60]

Demyelinization of corticospinal tracts in trauma is similar to the demyelinization and edema seen in the posterolateral funiculi of patients with CSM.[11,13,61-64] Autopsy studies of patients with rheumatoid arthritis and myelopathy have revealed edema localized to the posterolateral funiculi, as well as axonal retraction balls, suggestive of stretch-related injury without evidence of significant ischemia.[37]

The finding that tethering of the spinal cord in one region leads to generation of stretch and shear forces remote from the site of tethering or compression is directly applicable to numerous pathologic processes throughout the spine. The spinal cord can be tethered at any level by scarring, external compression, or spinal deformity. Spinal cord deformation over a large disc herniation at the apex of a thoracic kyphosis can contribute to stretch and shear injury remote from the locus of deformation.[38] Similarly, deformation of the medullospinal junction over the odontoid process in basilar invagination results in both local and remote neurologic dysfunction (e.g., diplopia, dysphagia, dysarthria, vertigo), as well as sensorimotor deficits.[65] Although these effects may also be explained by ischemic injury, local ischemia has not been found.[37] Again, correction of medullospinal deformity through surgical removal of the odontoid process or traction/reduction and occipitocervical stabilization typically results in significant clinical recovery.[66-68] Disturbances of sleep and alterations in central respiratory function have been attributed to ventral deformity of the upper spinal cord and lower brainstem in basilar invagination, and these disturbances have been reversed by correction of the ventral cervicomedullary deformity.[39]

The neurologic dysfunction observed in association with an abnormally acute clivo-axial angle (CAA) is the result of deformation and deformative stress injury of the neuraxis. Kim et al.[69] determined that an abnormal CAA caused subtle deformity of the upper spinal cord and medulla, resulting in headache, weakness, and sensory changes, as well as brainstem-related symptoms. Kubota et al.[70] found that syringomyelia was more likely to resolve after treatment of a Chiari malformation if the CAA was more obtuse and the brainstem therefore straighter. Henderson et al.[49] found that normalizing the CAA (increasing the angle to the normal 160 degrees) significantly improved neurologic function in a cohort of children with cervicomedullary syndrome due to an abnormal CAA. There is significant evidence that an abnormally acute CAA is indicative of a specialized form of brainstem tethering, which may produce the pattern of elevated stresses observed throughout the cord in cervical flexion myelopathy and CSM (Fig. 10-3).

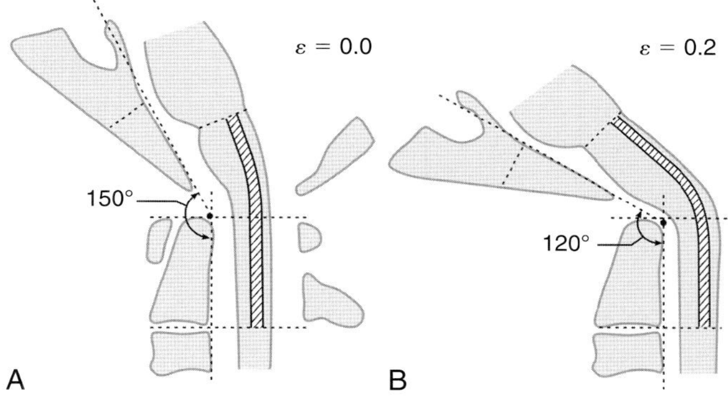

FIGURE 10-3 A, The brainstem and upper spinal cord in the normal individual, with a normal clivo-axial angle (CAA) greater than 150 degrees, shows no strain ($\varepsilon = 0.0$) in a nerve column *(shaded)* in the dorsal neuraxis. **B,** The brainstem and upper spinal cord in a patient with an abnormal acute CAA (in this case CAA = 120°) results in lengthening of the brainstem and spinal cord. The nerve column in the posterior neuraxis becomes stretched ($\varepsilon = 0.2$), resulting in neurologic deficits.

Histopathology of Spinal Cord Shear Injury

If neuraxial deformation, abnormal motion, and stretch injury are the primary causes of CSM and similar neurologic syndromes, then the histopathologic manifestations appear to be myelin edema and reactive axonal changes. A form of spinal axonal injury has been observed that is similar to the diffuse axonal injury (DAI) seen in the brain after deceleration injuries.

DAI is the most common brain injury resulting from blunt head trauma, and patient morbidity has been directly associated with the extent of DAI.[71,72] Experimental primate models have demonstrated that the location and quantity of axonal changes directly correlate with observed morbidity.[73,74] Clinical and pathologic studies have revealed that axonal injury is a component of traumatic brain injury throughout the spectrum of severity, from concussion to severe forms of prolonged coma.[75] Despite these histopathologic observations, the pathogenesis of DAI remains unclear. An early hypothesis speculated that tearing of the axon at the time of injury resulted in expulsion of a ball of axoplasm into the brain parenchyma.[76,77] However, recent DAI studies have demonstrated that axons undergoing shear strain do not undergo immediate disruption, but rather a nondestructive injury manifests as axonal swelling in internodal regions.[78] Axonal stretch at the time of injury results in axolemmal damage, disruption of axon transport and metabolism, and the delayed formation of a retraction ball or reactive axonal swelling.[78,79] This focal swelling is thought to be a prestage secondary axotomy.[80-83]

Studies have demonstrated that traumatic axonal injury results in impairment of anterograde axonal transport. In a guinea pig optic nerve model, 17% of axons demonstrated injury within 15 minutes of an applied stretch injury. The cell body of injured axons retained the ability to incorporate and transport horseradish peroxidase, but local interruption of axonal transport was demonstrated.[84] In a separate study, axonal injury was localized to the nodes of Ranvier and manifested as axolemmal blebs, loss of subaxolemmal density, loss of nodal gap substance, and neurofilament disarray.[82] Although distended, the axolemma remained intact. These findings suggest the possibility that stretch injury disrupts unidentified structural elements located at the node (i.e., membrane-associated proteins) that associate with the cytoskeleton and maintain nodal architecture. Furthermore, the study investigators speculated that nodal disruption leads to local cytoskeletal collapse and impairment of anterograde transport in a grossly intact axon.[82]

The cell ultrastructural events proceeding from axonal injury have been well characterized.[80] Continued anterograde transport to the site of focal impairment appears to result in localized ballooning of the axon and formation of a reactive axon bulb, or "Strich ball." Over the ensuing 1 to 3 days, the proximal axon segment containing the axon bulb continues to expand because of persistent anterograde transport and deposition of smooth endoplasmic reticulum and other intracellular organelles. These deposits become dispersed peripherally around an enlarged neurofilamentous core within the axon bulb. With further enlargement of the bulb, thinning of the overlying axolemma and myelin sheath occurs. Eventually, anatomic disconnection occurs between axonal segments proximal and distal to the original site of injury. The overlying myelin sheath is disrupted and then reforms to enclose the axon bulb, while the distal axonal segment undergoes wallerian degeneration. Meanwhile, the proximal axon bulb continues to expand as a result of continued anterograde transport of intracellular contents from the neuronal soma. In rodent studies, by 14 days, most reactive axons degenerate, become electron dense, and are eventually phagocytized by microglia. By contrast, in studies of mild to moderate head trauma in cats, some reactive axons have been observed to undergo a regenerative process, with outgrowth of regenerative sprouts and growth cones.[85,86]

Axon cytoskeletal collapse and rapid loss of the microtubular network appear to underlie the observed impairment of axoplasmic transport after injury.[87] A quantitative analysis of injury-associated changes in the axoskeleton identified evidence of injury throughout the length of the axon: small axons demonstrated compaction of neurofilaments, larger axons demonstrated enlargement of the para-axonal space, compaction of neurofilaments, loss of microtubules, and reduction in axonal caliber. Neurofilaments have been implicated in maintenance of axon caliber, whereas microtubules are thought to provide the mechanism for fast axonal transport. Neurofilament compaction is thought to precede the cytoskeletal disappearance accompanying wallerian degeneration. Collapse of neurofilaments into tightly packed bundles in the center of the axon may precede secondary axotomy in nondisruptive stretch injury of central nerves.[88]

Injury-associated changes in the axonal cytoskeleton are preceded by alterations in axolemmal permeability. Intra-axonal accumulation of calcium has been demonstrated in focal spinal cord injury.[89-92] Recently, increased calcium influx has been demonstrated in axons suffering stretch injury.[93] Using a guinea pig optic nerve model, a characteristic sequence of cellular events has been observed to occur over 24 hours. Initially, tensile strain leads to mechanical disruption of the myelin lamellae surrounding the nerve. Presumed loss of activity of the ecto-Ca-ATPase pump at sites of myelin disruption is then thought to allow increased calcium influx into the myelin, possibly mediating myelin dissociation, and increased periaxonal space over several hours. Increased calcium influx into the injured axon results in proteolysis of neurofilaments and dephosphorylation of neurofilament side arms.[94] In severe spinal cord injury, calcium-induced neurofilamentous degradation can be detected within 30 minutes.[95]

Abnormal strains in the spinal cord and brainstem from medullary kinking and basilar invagination result in predictable biomolecular changes: altered conformation of the Na^+ mechanoreceptors causes increased intra-axonal Na^+, which can be blocked with tetrodotoxin. The increased Na^+ results in depolarization of the voltage-gated Ca^{2+} channels and reversal of the Na^+/Ca^{2+} exchange pumps, with the consequence of abnormal influx of Ca^{2+} and activation of a deleterious cascade of reactions[93,96-98] (Fig. 10-4).

Although increased calcium influx has been strongly implicated in neurofilamentous degradation by calcium-activated neutral proteases, some investigators question the relationship between calcium influx and the reactive axonal changes seen in stretch-related injury.[80] Povlishock[80] contends that neurofilamentous disarray is either a direct mechanical effect of trauma on the cytoskeleton or the result of increased neurofilament subunit exchange between stable neurofilaments and a pool of soluble kinetically active subunits.

Although changes in axolemmal permeability and cytoskeletal disruption appear to trigger a cascade of intra-axonal changes in moderate to severe injury, in mild injury reactive axonal changes and retraction balls have been demonstrated in the absence of any change in axolemmal permeability and without evidence of neurofilament or microtubule loss. In these instances it has been speculated that a "focal misalignment" occurs at the time of injury, resulting in impaired axoplasmic flow and delayed axotomy.[99] It is conceivable that two different injury patterns exist and that the specific mechanism depends on the severity of tensile strain. In vitro studies have shown that axons under low tensile load undergo disruption of axoplasmic flow without evidence of axolemmal permeability change. High-tensile loading leads to immediate changes in axolemmal permeability and rapid disruption of axoplasmic flow.[100]

Anatomically, axons appear to be disrupted at sites of maximal tension. Large-caliber axons with a long intra-axial course appear to be more susceptible to tensile injury.[57] Reactive changes have been observed in which axons change course, cross blood vessels, and decussate.[101]

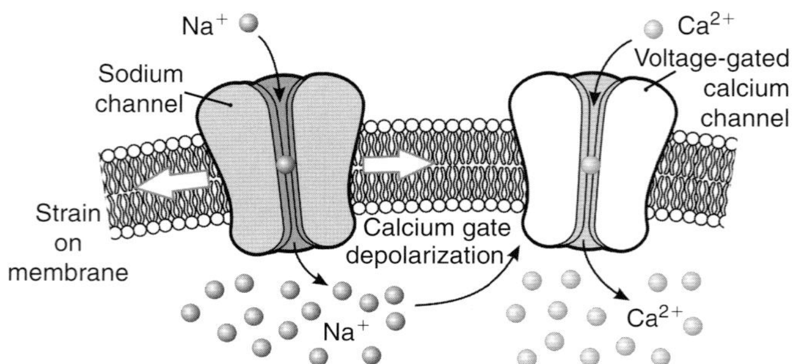

FIGURE 10-4 Mechanisms of calcium entry into stretch-injured axons. Strain on the axonal membrane opens mechanosensitive sodium channels, leading to an abnormal influx of Na^+. Influx of Na^+ and resulting depolarization opens voltage-gated calcium channels, leading to a pathologic influx of Ca^{2+} into the axons.

Relationship between Ischemia and Shear Injury

Stretch injury renders axons more susceptible to secondary injury from other processes, including ischemia.[101] However, the role of ischemia in stretch-related injury is unclear. Reactive axonal swelling occurs against a histologic background that lacks strong evidence of ischemic change. Microscopic studies have failed to identify correlative changes in microvasculature or ischemia-related changes in the neuronal soma, axonal processes, or dendritic processes.[78] Iodoantipyrine studies have revealed no significant changes in regional blood flow.[102,103] Moreover, axons undergoing reactive change are frequently found surrounded by intact neurons, without any evidence of ischemia or injury. When axonal injury is observed near the soma, central chromatolysis has been observed but may be secondary to pathologic processes within the axon. The rapid onset of axonal changes weighs heavily against a process originating in the neuronal soma.

The fact that some axons undergo reactive change while immediately adjacent axons appear uninjured is difficult to explain. It is conceivable, as Povlishock[80] speculates, that specific differences in axonal anatomy, such as location of intra-axial turns, crossing points, and decussations, may make certain axons uniquely susceptible to injury at specific levels.

In the peripheral nervous system, axonal swelling can be seen in response to various insults (e.g., ischemia, severance, and crushing).[80] Caution must be used before assigning a given etiology to the morphologic finding of axonal swelling.

Apoptosis

The pathogenesis of myelopathy is beginning to be investigated on a molecular level. Recent studies suggest that a significant portion of cell loss in chronic compression-related myelopathy is caused by apoptosis.[104] The process of apoptosis is biologically distinct from necrosis and refers to a well-defined sequence of intracellular events that are characterized by internucleosomal chromosome fragmentation, membrane blebbing, and phagocytosis, without generation of an inflammatory response.[105] In contrast, cell necrosis typically involves random DNA cleavage, membrane disruption, mitochondrial swelling, and local inflammation.[106]

Although necrosis and apoptosis often occur concurrently, identifying the dominant biologic process can provide important insight into the causes of specific disorders. In the case of CSM, the identification of primarily apoptotic cell death is significant. Although ischemia is one of numerous triggers associated with apoptotic cell death, severe ischemia such as that implied in the pathogenesis of CSM is more characteristically thought to cause cell death through necrosis. Therefore, the fact that oligodendrocyte disappearance in CSM appears to be apoptotic in nature suggests that a mechanism other than pure ischemia is involved.[107] A prominent role for apoptosis has already been implicated in the secondary cell loss that occurs after traumatic spinal cord injury.[107-111]

Cell loss occurs in spinal cord injury, both at the time of injury and secondarily over a period of days to weeks. At the injury epicenter, most cell death occurs through necrosis and leads to active clearance of necrotic cell debris through macrophage and microglial phagocytosis.[112] However, white matter cell loss continues through a longer segment of the spinal cord for several weeks in a process called *secondary injury*. Animal studies have demonstrated that compressive cord injury leads to apoptosis of oligodendrocytes along degenerating white matter tracts.[107,109] These studies indicate that apoptosis begins within 24 hours of injury and continues for at least 3 weeks.

Strong evidence for the occurrence of apoptotic cell death in chronic compression-related cervical myelopathy comes from studies of an animal model of chronic compression-related cervical myelopathy, the tiptoe-walking Yoshimura mouse.[113] The Yoshimura mouse is an inbred strain that characteristically develops quadriparesis 4 to 8 months after birth because of severe spinal cord compression, a result of hyperostosis along the posterolateral margins of the C1 and C2 vertebrae.[114] Histopathologic examination of cord tissue from Yoshimura mice has demonstrated descending degeneration affecting the anterior and lateral columns, ascending degeneration along the posterior columns, as well as severe injury at the level of compression.[104] Glial cell apoptosis mirrored the pattern of white column degeneration. Histologic staining using cell type-specific markers confirmed that the apoptotic cells were oligodendrocytes. The study investigators also performed an autopsy of a patient with cervical myelopathy from ossification of the posterior longitudinal ligament, and reported discovering a similar pattern of neuronal loss, demyelination, and apoptosis.

Stretch and strain are major epigenetic factors in trauma. For example, stretch results in the up-regulation of *N*-methyl-D-aspartate receptors. This renders the neuron more susceptible to ischemic insults and the effects of nitrous oxide and free radical species.[115]

Summary

The presence of cervical spine mobility, instability, and kyphosis is strongly predictive of clinical progression in patients with CSM. The cervical spinal cord may be subject to abnormal deformative stresses by spondylotic transverse bars, abnormal cervical kyphosis, deformity at the level of the craniocervical junction due to basilar invagination or abnormal CAA, or by remote tethering of the cord. Both proximate and remote tensile and shear forces generate deformative stresses that alter the biomolecular milieu through the Na and Ca channels and disrupt axoplasmic transport through alteration of the intra-axonal architecture, serving to modulate genetic expression to effect, in aggregate, pain and decreased neurologic function.

Strong support for the shear and strain injury theory of CSM pathogenesis comes from several recent developments, including the clinical concept of "dynamic stenosis," an increased neurobiologic understanding of the pathophysiology of stretch-related myelin and axonal injury, insight into the pathogenesis of spinal cord tethering, histologic studies revealing reactive axonal injury in the spinal cord of patients with CSM, and mathematical and finite element analysis modeling of the neuraxis under conditions of deformative stress.

Axonal injury reproducibly occurs at sites of maximal tensile loading. Mechanical injury to the neuronal axon triggers a well-defined sequence of intracellular and paracellular events. Myelin stretch injury leads to changes in axolemmal permeability. Histologically, cytoskeletal collapse is observed in neural cells in association with alterations in anterograde and retrograde axonal transport. Eventually, delayed axotomy occurs. The stretch and shear model may account for the clinical presentation and recovery potential of milder forms of CSM. Of more importance, a greater understanding of the deleterious effects of stretch and shear on the cervical spinal cord may improve treatment strategies for CSM and other spinal cord injuries.

KEY REFERENCES

Agrawal S, Fehlings M: Mechanisms of secondary injury to spinal cord axons in vitro: role of Na+, Na(+)-K(+)-ATPase, the Na(+)-H+ exchanger, and the Na(+)-Ca2+ exchanger. *J Neurosci* 16(2):545–552, 1996.

Arundine M, Aarts M, Lau A, et al: Vulnerability of central neurons to secondary insults after in vitro mechanical stretch. *J Neurosci* 24(37): 8106–8123, 2004.

Breig A: Overstretching of the spinal cord: a basic cause of symptoms in cord disorders. *J Biomech* 3:7–9, 1970.

Chung RS, Staal JA, McCormack GH, et al: Mild axonal stretch injury in vitro induces a progressive series of neurofilament alterations ultimately leading to delayed axotomy. *J Neurotrauma* 22(10):1081–1091, 2005.

Henderson FC, Wilson WA, Mott S, et al: Deformative stress associated with an abnormal clivo-axial angle: a finite element analysis. *Surg Neurol Int* 1:30, 2010.

Ichihara K, Taguchi T, Sakuramoto I, et al: Mechanism of the spinal cord injury and the cervical spondylotic myelopathy: new approach based on the mechanical features of the spinal cord white and gray matter. *J Neurosurg* 99(Suppl 3):278–285, 2003.

Jafari S, Maxwell WL, Neilson M, et al: Axonal cytoskeletal changes after non-disruptive axonal injury. *J Neurocytol* 26:207–221, 1997.

Wolf JA, Stys PK, Lusardi T, et al: Traumatic axonal injury induces calcium influx modulated by tetrodotoxin-sensitive sodium channels. *J Neurosci* 21(6):1923–1930, 2001.

REFERENCES

The complete reference list is available online at expertconsult.com.

CHAPTER 11

Anatomy of Nerve Root Compression, Nerve Root Tethering, and Spinal Instability

William F. Lavelle | Aaron J. Bianco | Sameer A. Kitab | Edward C. Benzel

The majority of the population will experience spine-related pain at some time in their lives. The greatest component of this pain is low back pain, typically occurring in patients 35 to 55 years of age. Fortunately, the majority of acute back pain is self-limited, with over 90% of patients recovering within 6 weeks. Unfortunately, back pain has a high recurrence rate, with symptoms returning within the year in two thirds of patients. Sciatica-type pain is also common. The majority of sciatic pain is also self-limiting. Certain aspects of lifestyle, such as a lack of physical activity, obesity, and smoking, predispose patients to recurrent episodes of back pain and sciatica.[1] Determining the precise causes of these types of pain presents a challenge to spine care physicians. Understanding the pathology of normal spinal degeneration will aid in the diagnosis and treatment of spine-related pain.

Understanding Motion Segments

The spine is composed of three anatomic sections, the cervical, lumbar, and thoracic spine. The majority of spine-related pain involves the lumbar spine because the lumbar spine bears the weight of the entire body. The lumbar spine is the primary focus of this chapter; however, the concepts described may be generalized to a great extent to the cervical and thoracic spine. As discussed in Chapter 5, vertebrae are linked through facet joints on the posterior spinal column. The facet joints are formed between the superior articular processes of one vertebra and the inferior articular processes of the vertebra directly above.

Between each of the vertebrae is a thick, spongy disc made up of various types of cartilage. The anulus fibrosus is the outer ring that forms the border of the disc. It is composed of sheets of collagen fibers that contain the compressible core. The nucleus pulposus forms the center of the disc and resists compressive loads. The nucleus pulposus consists of proteoglycans, hyaluronic acid, and water. Each disc is approximately ¼ to ¾ of an inch thick. Together, these layers form a strong disc, capable of absorbing the shock produced by spinal movement. When weight is put on the spine, the discs compress, and when the weight is lifted the discs return to their original shape and size. When functioning properly, the spine provides eloquent motion as well as structural support and protection for neural elements.

Causes of Back Pain

Subaxial spine pain is often caused by either muscular spasm or a failure of the joints and discs that comprise the complex anatomy of the spine. When examining the causes of isolated back pain in patients who present to a primary care physician, one study found that 4% had a compression fracture, 3% spondylolisthesis, 0.7% a tumor or metastasis of another tumor, 0.3% ankylosing spondylitis, and 0.01% an infection. Therefore, most patients who present with the complaint of low back pain will leave their primary care physician's office without a definitive diagnosis.[2,3] For most of these patients, some form of spinal degenerative change is the likely cause.

Spinal Degeneration

In spinal degeneration, also termed *spondylosis*, disc degeneration seems to occur first. Changes to the biologic structure of the disc lead to the mechanical failure of that disc. Normally, anulus cells synthesize mostly collagen type I in response to deformation, whereas nucleus cells respond to hydrostatic pressure by synthesizing proteoglycans and fine collagen type II fibrils. Cell density declines during growth and is extremely low in the adult, especially in the nucleus. In adult discs, blood vessels are normally restricted to the outermost layers of the anulus. Metabolite transport is by diffusion, which is important for small molecules, and by bulk fluid flow, which is important for large molecules. Low oxygen tension in the center of a disc leads to anaerobic metabolism, resulting in a high concentration of lactic acid and low pH.[4] Chronic lack of oxygen causes nucleus cells to become quiescent, whereas a chronic lack of glucose can kill them. Deficiencies in metabolite transport appear to limit both the density and metabolic activity of disc cells. As a result, discs have only a limited ability to recover from any metabolic or mechanical injury.[5] Disc cells synthesize their matrix and break down existing matrix by producing and activating degradative enzymes, including matrix metalloproteinases and "a disintegrin and metalloproteinase" (ADAMs). The proteoglycan content of the disc is primarily responsible for the disc's ability to act as a compressive buffer. It is maximal in the young adult and declines later in life,[6] presumably because of proteolysis. Disc cells appear to adapt the properties of their matrix to suit their environment. With increasing age, the overall proteoglycan and water content of the disc decreases, especially in the nucleus.[6] There is a corresponding increase in collagen content, a tendency for fine type II collagen fibrils in the inner anulus to be replaced by type I fibers as the anulus encroaches on the nucleus, and a tendency for type I fibers throughout the disc to become coarser. Loss of proteoglycan fragments from the disc is a slow process owing to the entrapment of the nucleus by the fibrous anulus and the cartilage end plates of the vertebrae.[7] Reduced matrix turnover in older discs enables collagen molecules and fibrils to become increasingly cross-linked with each other, and existing cross-links become more stable.[5] In addition, reactions between collagen and glucose lead to so-called nonenzymatic glycation, causing even more cross-linking and imparting a yellow color to the aging disc. With increasing age, the hydrostatic nucleus becomes smaller and the proteoglycan content of the nucleus decreases. As such, its ability to hold water and withstand compressive loads declines. The anulus becomes stiffer and ultimately weaker.

Ultimately, aged discs fail to function properly and place additional strains on the facet joints and adjacent spinal motion segments. In the disc itself, the accumulated products of degeneration affect the metabolism of the remaining viable cells. This further hastens disc failure, resulting in changes that may be seen on MRI. These MRI changes include decreased water content, which is visible on T2-weighted images and is termed *dark disc disease* (Fig. 11-1). The end result of this cascade of failure is disc collapse.[5]

Isolated back pain may be due to a variety of forms of disc dysfunction. Pain may occur at any point of degeneration. Crock studied pain related to disc failure and coined the term *internal disc derangement* in 1970.[8] The term was used to describe a large group of patients whose disabling back and leg pain worsened after an operation for suspected disc prolapse. Internal disc derangement was intended to describe a condition marked by alterations in the internal structure and metabolic functions of the disc thought to be attributable to injury or a series of injuries that may even have been subclinical.[8] Despite Crock's attempts to categorize disc failure, no direct and reliable relationship between measurable disc failure and pain has been developed.

As the disc fails, additional degenerative changes to the surrounding spinal structures may also occur. Disc failure is often the first of a series of failures in the spine. It has been hypothesized that disc failure causes the spinal ligaments to buckle and hypertrophy because of exposure to excessive forces, including new torsion forces.[1,4] These abnormal forces may cause instability. Facet joint degenerative changes are believed to follow. When pain arises from the facet joints, patients often complain of greater discomfort with spine extension or hyperextension. Once muscles weaken, as is often seen with any form of spinal degeneration, any position can cause discomfort. As the degeneration progresses, further instability and joint hypertrophy may result. Similar to the degenerative changes seen in large appendicular joints such as the knee, significant radiographic degeneration may be seen in patients who have little or no back pain. These degenerative changes may, however, impinge on or stretch the neural elements, causing neuropathic pain.

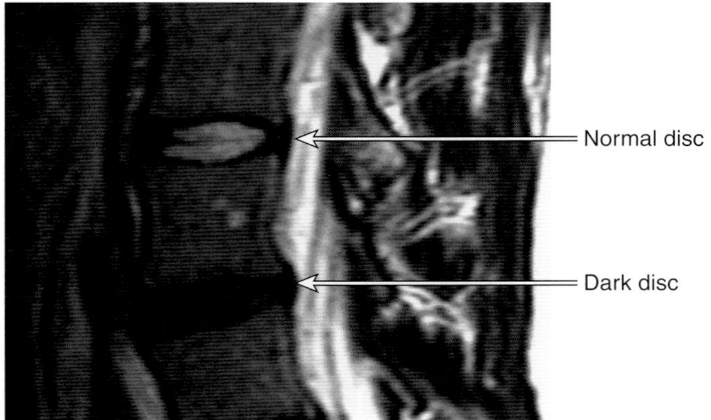

FIGURE 11-1. Sagittal MRI showing dark disc disease. (From Lavelle WF, Carl AL, Lavelle ED, et al: Back pain. In Smith H, editor: *Current therapy in pain*, Philadelphia, 2009, Saunders Elsevier, pp 167–181.)

In the most common scenario, more than one type of degenerative change is responsible for nerve compression. As the nerve roots traverse the spinal canal, they pass through regions adjacent to the facet joints termed the *lateral recesses*. In this region they may be encroached on by any combination of hypertrophic facet joints, infolded ligamentum flavum, and perhaps bulging disc material. All of these changes result in nerve compression within the spinal canal.

Degenerative changes can also cause nerve root impingement in the neural foramen. The anteroposterior diameter of the foramen may be reduced by bulging disc material anteriorly and hypertrophic facets posteriorly. Foraminal height is reduced merely by the loss of intervertebral disc height. Facet subluxation can further decrease foraminal volume, making the exiting nerve roots in these patients even more susceptible to the compression caused be small amounts of disc bulging or facet hypertrophy.[9]

The areas of the degenerating spine may fail at different rates, leading to different clinical pictures of back pain, leg pain, or instability. If the anterior disc and ligaments fail at the same rate as the posterior structures, such as the facet joints, anterior subluxation of one vertebra is a possible result. This is termed *spondylolisthesis*. If failure occurs asymmetrically and there is a rotational or lateral translation, the deformity is termed *olisthesis*. Degenerative spondylolisthesis is most common at the L4-5 level[5] and occurs 6 to 10 times more often here than at any other level. It is more common in women than men and in African Americans than whites.[10] The increased motion caused by disc degeneration, combined with decreased shear resistance, allows for the anterior slip. Degenerative spondylolisthesis at the L4-5 level may result in a combination of central stenosis with lateral recess stenosis that compresses the traversing L5 nerve roots. Degenerative spondylolisthesis rarely exceeds 35% translation of the vertebrae.[11]

The posterior elements of the vertebra may also be disrupted by a stress fracture of an area of the spine called the *pars interarticularis*. The pars interarticularis is the lateral part of the posterior element that connects the superior and inferior facets (the term literally means "part between the articulations"). Repetitive flexion-extension and rotation lead to microtrauma at this junction and thereby fracture. Studies show that most patients with a spondylolysis or isthmic spondylolisthesis are unlikely to be at risk for increased back pain symptoms.[12]

Neuropathic Pain in Spinal Degeneration

There are primarily two types of pain that result from degenerative spinal disease: radicular pain and claudicant pain. Radicular pain, or radiculitis, is pain that radiates along a dermatome of a nerve. This may be due to inflammation, pressure, or stretch of the nerve root. Claudicant pain is more difficult for patients to describe. When forced to describe this type of pain, patients may describe it as leg cramping, "aching," or heaviness that reliably occurs with walking. Claudication is often associated with spinal stenosis. Spinal stenosis is the narrowing of the spinal canal due to any of the causes described previously, including hypertrophy of the ligaments, facets, or discs. This topic is reviewed in detail in a later chapter.

The exact pathophysiology of the mechanisms of radicular and claudicant pain remains elusive. The sequences of neuropathologic changes that result from neurologic compression in the lumbar spinal canal have been investigated in animal studies. Delamarter et al.[13] used a dog model in which they created varying degrees of stenosis and demonstrated deleterious effects on the neural elements by increasing the degree of the stenosis. They found that cortical evoked potentials were highly sensitive to this compression and were affected long before any clinical signs occurred. These authors also demonstrated venous congestion and arterial constriction around compressed nerve roots and dorsal root ganglia. The result was blockage of axoplasmic flow, with resulting edema, demyelination, and wallerian degeneration of motor and sensory fibers. Other authors have shown that sensory fibers are more susceptible to pressure and slower to recover than motor fibers,[14] which may explain the presence of subjective sensory changes in the absence of objective physical findings. Arnoldi et al.[15] suggested that increased venous pressure may explain the symptoms of neurogenic claudication. Others have suggested that narrowing of the spinal canal may lead to a reduction in blood supply to the cauda equina, resulting in ischemic changes from the diffusion of metabolites.[16] These changes may stimulate the sinuvertebral nerve or lead to secretion of pain mediators, such as substance P, from the dorsal root ganglion. Perineural inflammation of unknown origin may also result in pain generation.

Most of the literature examining the causes of neurologic pain resulting from spinal pathology attributes compression as the principal cause.[17-27] There are, however, instances where patients have persistent neuropathic pain, particularly radicular symptoms, in the absence of imaging studies displaying compressive pathology.

Motion of Neural Elements in the Spine: How Nerve Roots Can Be Stretched

Breig and Marions[28] and Breig and Troup[29] initially described movements of the nerve root sleeve in relation to a change in posture. They hypothesized that these patterns of movement might be related to changes in the length of the spinal canal during postural changes and motion.

To understand fully the impact of motion on neural elements, a basic understanding of the anatomic relationships of the nerve roots within the functional spinal unit (FSU) or motion segment is required. In the FSU, nerve roots are enclosed in a mobile osteoligamentous space and are exposed to dynamic stretch and compressive strains. This is most often observed in the situation in which nerve roots traverse a particularly long course through the central and lateral recess. Although compression is the mechanism most commonly associated with pain, inflammation as well as nerve root tethering are also possible causes.[17,30] Tethering of the nerve root has been shown to be deleterious to nerves in clinical scenarios other than pathologic spinal degeneration, such as scoliosis, spina bifida occulta, and intrathecal spinal tumors.[31] Stretch-induced nerve injury is also a well-known complication of lumbosacral spondylolisthesis reduction.[32]

As described earlier, lumbar nerve roots are enclosed in the lateral recess, a hollow, hemicylindrical recess that traverses mobile FSUs. The lateral recess is bordered laterally by the pedicle, posteriorly by the superior articular facet, and anteriorly by the dorsolateral surface of the vertebral body and the adjacent intervertebral disc (Fig. 11-2).

The unique and often underappreciated characteristic of this anatomic region is that lumbar nerve roots are dynamic neural structures with the ability to move alongside the deforming intervertebral disc and articulating adjacent facet joints. The lateral recess has been defined using a three-zone model,[33,34] comprising the entrance zone, midzone, and exit zone. The entrance zone is located medial to and below the superior articular process, with the disc and facet joint forming the anterior and posterior walls, respectively. The midzone is the region through which the nerve root passes beneath the pars level of the lamina. Finally, the exit zone consists of the intervertebral foramen.

The lumbar nerve root may be compressed by or tethered to the surrounding structures primarily in two locations. The first is at the neck of the nerve root sheath as it exits the dural sac and the second is the lateral aspect of the foramen, where the nerve root is attached to both pedicles both rostrally and caudally by the foraminal ligaments (Fig. 11-3).

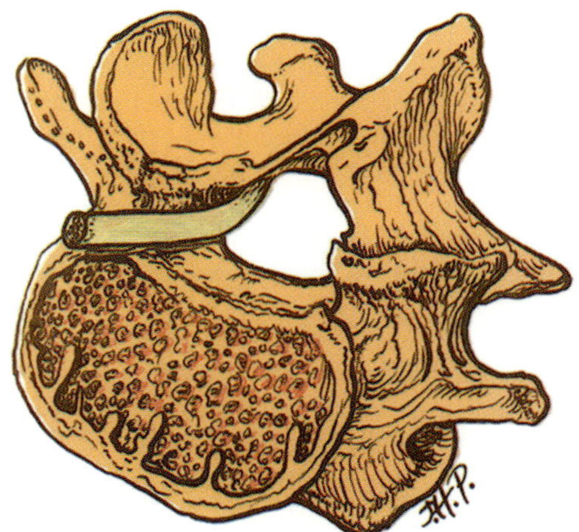

FIGURE 11-2. Drawing of the lateral recess, normal anatomy, at the L5 vertebral level. Note that the height of the lateral recess increases in a rostrocaudal direction. (From Ciric I, Mikhael MA, Tarkington JA, et al: The lateral recess syndrome: a variant of spinal stenosis. *J Neurosurg* 53:433–443, 1980.)

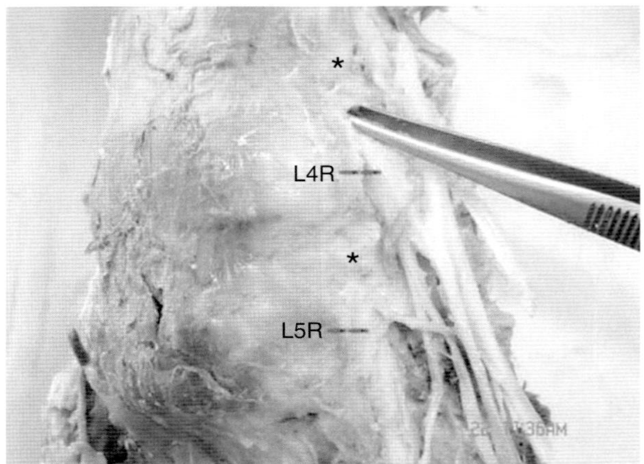

FIGURE 11-3. Cadaveric photograph depicting the extraforaminal vertebral transverse ligaments *(asterisks)* from a ventral-lateral approach. The L4 and L5 nerve roots (L4R, L5R) are tethered by the effect of the ligaments. The angles vary between the exiting nerves and the ligament at each vertebral level. These ligaments are important with regard to the stretch effect at the spinal nerve level. (From Kitab SA, Miele VJ, Lavelle WF, et al: Pathoanatomic basis for stretch-induced lumbar nerve root injury with a review of the literature. *Neurosurgery* 65:161–168, 2009.)

These ligaments limit nerve root excursion and increase in size and strength distally in the lumbar spine.[35] The foraminal ligaments have been shown to play an organizational and protective function by equalizing stresses on neural structures during movements of the spine and extremities.[35-38]

Static lateral recess syndrome can be defined anatomically by the fixed, permanent entrapment of neural structures within the lateral recess.[19,33,34] When a motion segment has erratic or excessive motion, such as that seen with instability associated with a spondylolisthesis, a dynamic lateral recess syndrome may occur. In the foramen, the exit zone of the lateral recess, the nerve root occupies 30% to 50% of the cross-sectional area. As such, there is ample room for the exiting nerve root. The dorsal root ganglion (DRG) is located just proximal to the origin of the spinal nerve. Its position relative to the foramen can vary considerably. The most common location of the DRG is directly beneath the foramen, except for the S1 DRG, which is usually located in the spinal canal.[39] Therefore, if tethering occurs at two points close to the pedicle, nerve root stretch at the area of the DRG may occur. Also, because the DRG cells are the primary sensory neurons that send projections to peripheral and central targets, stretch deformation of the DRG may cause a variety of clinical responses, including pain.

It has also been shown that the more caudal lumbosacral nerve roots traverse a longer path to their extraspinal destination. Thus, the L4, L5, and S1 nerve roots traverse two or more mobile segments. Theoretically, this exposes them to a greater risk of either compression or stretch injury. This may partially explain the higher incidence of pain related to these nerve roots.[19,33,34,37]

Ventral Olisthesis and Loss of Disc Height

In a ventral olisthesis (translational/rotational deformity) of L4 on L5, the lateral recess of L4 moves forward, along with its neural contents. The L5 nerve root is subject to strain (change in length). The tethering effect of the foraminal ligaments combined with the anterior motion of the lateral recess causes the aforementioned strain. Further, the trefoil shape of the spinal canal is associated with reduced height of the lateral recess, which may increase the strain as well as compression seen at the L5 nerve root (Fig. 11-4).

Stretch of the lumbar nerve root can be thought of as occurring through either a dynamic or quasistatic process. The nerve root may be subject to out-of-plane loading and shear by the dorsal-rostral L5 vertebral margin consequent to the dynamics of spine flexion. The presence of an osteophyte or disc bulge may add to the stretch effect by tethering the nerve root. In addition, with lateral recess stenosis and reduced disc height, the exiting nerve root may experience compression at the foraminal level by over-riding facets.

Sagittal plane deformity such as focal kyphosis may also play a role in stretch of the lumbar nerve root. In a simulated ventral olisthesis of L4 on L5, a significant and deleterious differential strain is seen on the nerve root (Fig. 11-5). The maximum strain appears to occur at the L5 nerve root. Sagittal plane deformities are also known causes of axial back pain, requiring greater efforts by the paraspinal muscles to maintain an erect posture.

Lateral Olisthesis

Lateral olisthesis of L4 on L5 exerts a strain on the extraforaminal portion of the L4 root. This occurs because the entire lateral recess and its neural contents move with the olisthetic segment. Lateral olisthesis also stretches the subjacent L5 root on the side opposite to the olisthesis direction.[27] The L5 pedicle on the ipsilateral side of the olisthesis acts as a fulcrum on the intraspinal portion of the subjacent part of the L5 nerve root. An investigation of degenerative scoliotic curves, in which lateral translation is associated with rotation, did not show that neural canal dimension was reduced with this particular deformity.[39]

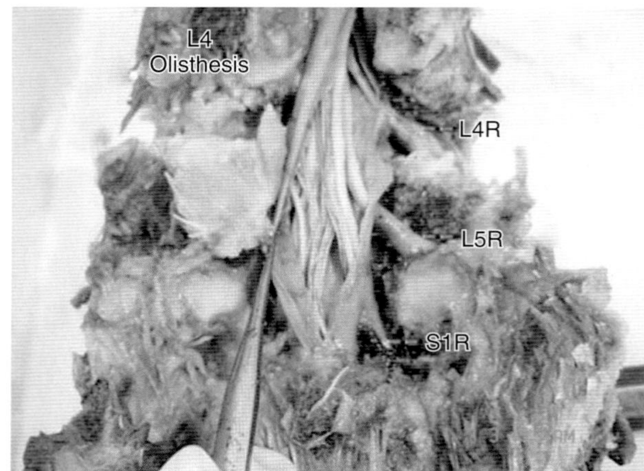

FIGURE 11-4. Cadaveric photograph showing compression of the L4 nerve root (L4R), stretch of the L5 nerve root (L5R), and a normal relationship of the S1 nerve root (S1R) to its surrounding structures during ventral olisthesis of the L4 to L5 motion segment. (From Kitab SA, Miele VJ, Lavelle WF, et al: Pathoanatomic basis for stretch-induced lumbar nerve root injury with a review of the literature. *Neurosurgery* 65:161–168, 2009.)

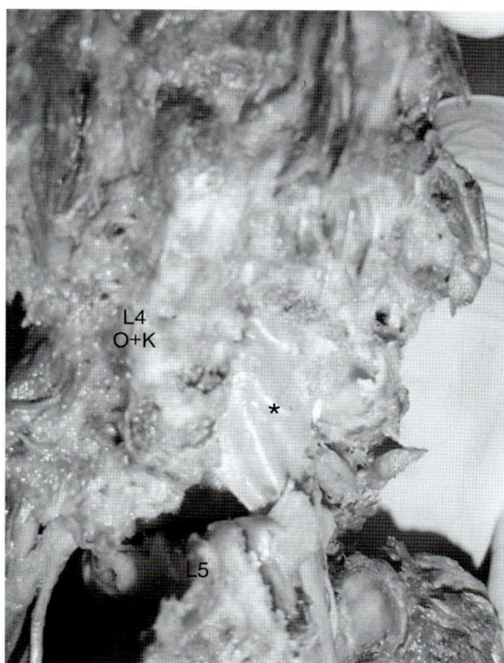

FIGURE 11-5. Ventral olisthesis with rotation and kyphosis (O+K) of L4 on L5 results in varying strains on intraspinal nerve roots, particularly the L5 nerve root at the site of olisthesis *(asterisk)*. (From Kitab SA, Miele VJ, Lavelle WF, et al: Pathoanatomic basis for stretch-induced lumbar nerve root injury with a review of the literature. *Neurosurgery* 65:161–168, 2009.)

Neural, Biomechanical, and Physiologic Considerations of Nerve Stretch

In the previous section we described the pathophysiology of nerve stretch and compression. To understand the development of axonal pathology in response to stretch, the relationship between the applied mechanical forces and the structural and functional response of the axon must be understood.[27,40-46] The literature shows that strain rate is a time-dependent viscoelastic behavior that differs with variation in the histologic composition and diameter of the nerve root.[46-49] The material properties of nerve roots are influenced by their relative proportions of protein and collagen. Spinal nerve roots contain approximately 20% of the amount of collagen in peripheral nerves and six times more collagen than the spinal cord.[43,50,51] Conversely, the DRG is a mechanically and physiologically delicate structure. It has been shown that nerve roots are much less resilient than peripheral nerves, with a strength of only 10% and a stiffness of 20% of those of peripheral nerves.[43] This may suggest that stretch through nerve roots in part occurs through dural or epineural tissues. It is thus apparent that the relative "mechanical friability" of nerve roots can be explained by these variations in histology and collagen composition.

Although stretch-induced neural injury of both the central and peripheral nervous system is well described in the literature, little is known regarding the biomechanical-physiologic responses to stretch at the nerve root level in humans.[17,25,52-54] Animal models have provided some indirect evidence for the mechanisms of clinically observed pain syndromes. Such studies, however, should be interpreted with caution because the majority of animal models do not precisely reproduce the extent of damage, the biologic milieu, and the time course of axonal injury seen in humans.[20,25,36,43-49,55,56]

The magnitude of stretch required to cause a nerve root injury that results in pain or electrophysiologic dysfunction remains unknown. Furthermore, there is a paucity of information regarding the specific response of human nerve roots to varying rates of stretch.

The amount of quantitative data available on the mechanical properties of human spinal nerve roots exposed to the low strain rates that occur at unstable FSUs is limited. Kwan et al. reported that human spinal nerve roots had a tensile strength of 0.17 ± 0.59 MPa and an ultimate strain of 15.0% ± 3.5%, at a strain rate 0.17 mm/sec.[36] Sunderland and Bradley reported the ranges of maximum tensile stress and load to be 3.9 to 29.4 MPa and 0.2 to 3.3 kg, respectively, in human S3 nerve roots stretched at a rate of 1.27 mm/sec.[57]

Nerve roots have characteristic viscoelastic material properties that are strain rate dependent and exhibit higher tensile stress at higher strain rates.[47-49] In vivo studies of rat L5 dorsal nerve roots subjected to a predetermined strain range (<10%, 10% to 20%, >20%) at a specified displacement rate (0.01 mm/sec and 15 mm/sec) demonstrated a threshold rate of complete nerve conduction loss at strain increases of 16% and 9% for the quasistatic 0.01 mm/sec and dynamic 15 mm/sec strain rates, respectively.[47-49] These studies suggest that the modulating effects of excessive loading events (magnitude, rate of application, and duration) on electrophysiologic and possible pain responses may determine the extent of injury.

Basic Science of Chronic Spinal Pain and Stretch-Induced Nerve Root Injury

The actual mechanism by which neural tissue injury causes or contributes to chronic pain syndromes remains speculative. It has previously been suggested that injuries adjacent to the DRG produce pathologic reactions that manifest in differing severities of symptoms and animal behavioral responses.[18,20,26,30,32,34,44,55,58-63]

Stretch injury to peripheral nerves has been shown to induce local and central changes at the DRG and dorsal horn levels.[17,32,54-56] Nerve root injury, on the other hand, may produce more robust, centrally mediated responses than a peripheral nerve injury. It has been suggested that a partial dorsal rhizotomy may activate injury signals in the dorsal root that are primarily transmitted to the central terminals of the spinal cord.[18,21,27,39,44,55,58,59] These injury signals are manifested by sensitization of specific nociceptors or a variety of dorsal horn neurons with a short duration of pain persistence.[18,47-49]

The DRG itself, with its central and peripheral components, may represent the primary focus of stretch deformation during the pathomechanical behavior of a failing FSU. The mechanical deformation of DRG cells is well known to induce alterations in membrane properties that manifest as ectopic discharges and increased excitability. These, in turn, trigger chronic changes in excitability or synaptic plasticity of dorsal horn neurons.[20,30,34,40,58,60,61]

Although biomechanical and electrophysiologic data suggest a possible role of stretch deformation in painful neural element injury, the precise physiologic mechanism of this remains unclear. Nerve root injury, however, is hypothesized to induce central nervous system sensitization through a mechanism that is modulated by synaptic, neuroimmune, and neuroinflammatory events.[24,26,46,58,62] These events mimic synaptic plasticity and remodeling similar to that observed in learning and memory.[26]

Role of Nerve Root Vascularization and Perfusion

Vascular hypoperfusion is another proposed mechanism for the physiologic and structural changes of neural tissues in response to stretch. Ischemic changes occur in response to an elongation of 15%.[49] Histologic changes are also observed between 4% and 50%. Conduction disturbances have been reported at degrees of elongation ranging from 6% to 100%.[49]

The DRG has an abundant intrinsic vascular supply. The volume of blood flow in the DRG is approximately twice that of the nerve root and is similar to that of the gray matter of the spinal cord. Although the effect of compression on the DRG and nerve root blood flow is well documented in the literature, little is known about the effects of quasistatic or dynamic stretch on the nerve root or DRG venous pressure dynamics, blood flow, or blood-neural barrier function.[24]

Conclusion

Spinal degeneration is a common cause of axial back pain, radiating extremity pain, and claudicant pain. There are complex anatomic relationships between spinal nerve roots and their surrounding environment of osteoligamentous structures. In a typical scenario, disc degeneration occurs first through disc desiccation and collapse. Disc regeneration is often followed by failure of the dorsal spinal structures. All of these degenerative changes may be responsible for back pain or neuropathic spinal pain. Nerve roots also have a limited ability for excursion secondary to the dural and foraminal ligamentous structures that provide a tethering force during lower limb function and spinal range of motion. The stretch effect, however, is more dynamically driven and thus may not be easily delineated by current neuroradiologic studies in patients with neuralgic pain. Little is known of the immediate events during and after dynamic nerve root deformation and the differential responses of the various root components (i.e., the DRG itself or its central and peripheral radiations).

Spine care physicians must "think three-dimensionally" and consider all possible sources of nerve compression, nerve irritation, and stretch when planning treatment for pain attributable to the nerve root level. Spinal and paraspinal tissues, such as the intervertebral disc, the facet capsules, ligaments, and muscles, are all potential contributors to mechanical stretch deformation. Such a model will provide new insight into the prevention and management of spinal pain syndromes.

KEY REFERENCES

Arnoldi CC, Brodsky AE, Cauchoix J, et al: Lumbar spinal stenosis and nerve root entrapment syndromes: definition and classification. *Clin Orthop Relat Res* 115:4–5, 1976.

Bain AC, Raghupathi R, Meaney DF: Dynamic stretch correlates to both morphological abnormalities and electrophysiological impairment in a model of traumatic axonal injury. *J Neurotrauma* 18:499–511, 2001.

Chung RS, Staal JA, McCormack GH, et al: Mild axonal stretch injury in vitro induces a progressive series of neurofilament alterations ultimately leading to delayed axotomy. *J Neurotrauma* 22:1081–1091, 2005.

Delamarter RB, Bohlman HH, Dodge LD, et al: Experimental lumbar spinal stenosis: analysis of the cortical evoked potentials, microvasculature, and histopathology. *J Bone Joint Surg [Am]* 72:110–120, 1990.

Kawakami M, Weinstein JN, Chatani K, et al: Experimental lumbar radiculopathy: behavioral and histologic changes in a model of radicular pain after spinal nerve root irritation with chromic gut ligatures in the rat. *Spine (Phila Pa 1976)* 19:1795–1802, 1994.

Kitab SA, Miele VJ, Lavelle WF, et al: Pathoanatomic basis for stretch-induced lumbar nerve root injury with a review of the literature. *Neurosurgery* 65:161–168, 2009.

Wall EJ, Massie JB, Kwan MK, et al: Experimental stretch neuropathy: changes in nerve conduction under tension. *J Bone Joint Surg [Br]* 74:126–129, 1992.

REFERENCES

The complete reference list is available online at expertconsult.com.

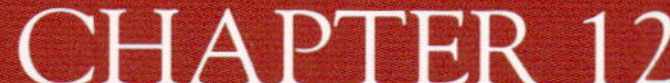
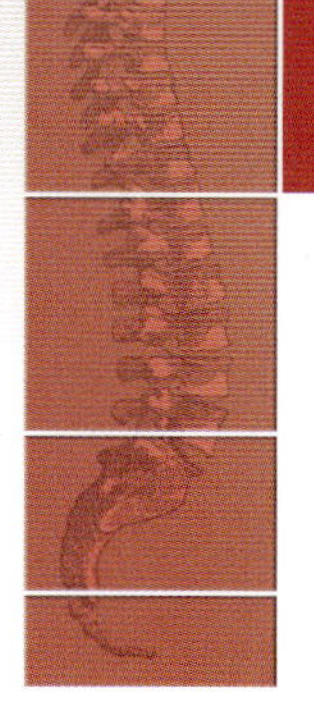

CHAPTER 12

Physical and Neurologic Examination

Chandan Krishna | Andrew D. Livingston | Paul J. Holman | Edward C. Benzel

Recent advances in medical technologies and changes in health care systems have dramatically altered the practice of medicine and the physician-patient relationship. One consequence of these changes, unfortunately, is that the physical examination is no longer the focus of many physician-patient encounters and is often overlooked when important clinical decisions are made. In the field of spinal surgery, the widespread availability of neuroimaging of the spinal column and modern health care policies regulating coverage of elective surgery are two factors that have contributed to this change. Patients who are often referred for their initial consultation with their MRI "in hand" worry more about the radiologist's interpretation of the scan than their symptoms. In many instances, patients are required to consult with multiple surgeons and receive conflicting recommendations regarding the appropriateness of surgical treatment. In this environment, it is essential for the surgeon to place a priority on the fundamentals of history taking and the neurologic examination to establish good rapport with patients and guide them in choosing the best therapy.

History Taking

A surgeon's ability to efficiently obtain a thorough history is the cornerstone of treating patients with spinal disorders. The foundation of good history taking lies in being a good listener. Communicating a genuine interest in the patient and a willingness to offer both surgical and nonsurgical treatment are of paramount importance. This is true in both straightforward and complicated patients (such as those suffering from chronic pain syndromes). Using simple, open-ended questions early in the interview allows patients to articulate their perception of the problem and helps the physician identify treatment goals. The physician can then ask a patient more focused questions to obtain the necessary information to formulate a preliminary differential diagnosis. For example, asking the patient to point to the area of maximum pain and to trace the pattern of their pain or paresthesia often yields valuable diagnostic information.

Careful review of the patient's past medical history is important to uncover conditions with symptoms commonly seen in patients with spinal pathology. Diabetes, peripheral vascular disease, inflammatory arthropathies, and neoplastic disorders are common examples. Any history of trauma involving the spine and related surgical procedures should be noted, in addition to injuries involving the shoulder, hip, and long bones. Unrecognized compression neuropathies secondary to casting, for example, can subsequently be confused with radiculopathy. Retroperitoneal hematoma may present as a femoral or an upper lumbar radiculopathy.[1] It is also important to inquire about a history of any psychiatric disorders and pain syndromes associated with joints, muscles, or connective tissues. Fibromyalgia and reflex sympathetic dystrophy can alter perioperative pain management and may require additional attention. Inquiry about smoking history is also important because smoking has been demonstrated to increase the incidence of pseudarthrosis compared with nonsmoking.[2]

Taking a good history regarding pain associated with spinal disorders deserves special attention. Radicular pain tends to be constant but may be exacerbated by movement or Valsalva maneuvers. The pain occurs in the distribution of the affected nerve root and may have dysesthetic qualities. Mechanical back pain resulting from degenerative disc disease, spondylotic changes of the facets, or gross instability from trauma or cancer tends to be worse with movement and relieved with rest. The pain associated with neurogenic pseudoclaudication is typically an aching or cramping pain in the buttocks, thighs, or legs that becomes worse with standing and walking short distances and is relieved with bending, sitting, or reclining. Pain or paresthesia in the hands that awakens the patient at night and is relieved by shaking the hand is a red flag for nerve entrapment. Pain or paresthesia radiating to the upper extremities that is associated with medial scapular pain is more likely to be radicular in origin.

It is noteworthy that not all patients in neurosurgical consultation have neurologic disease processes. Other etiologies mimicking neurologic syndromes must be considered.

General Physical Examination

Although a comprehensive general physical examination may not be feasible in every patient, details gathered from the patient's medical history serve as a guide to performing an examination of other organ systems. Basic vital signs should be recorded in most patients. Hypertension and atrial fibrillation are two examples of disorders easily identified by physical examination that could significantly affect diagnosis and operative risk in a patient with transient cerebral ischemia.

Auscultation of the lungs and palpation of the abdomen are essential in the setting of metastatic spine disease. Emphysema, chronic obstructive pulmonary disease, pleural effusion, extensive atelectasis, and ascites have an impact on anesthetic risk and may influence patient positioning and surgical approach. Gallbladder disease may refer pain to the back or scapula and may be mistaken for cervical radiculopathy. Nephrolithiasis or ureterolithiasis is often mistaken for a lumbar radiculopathy and may be screened for by gentle percussion over the lumbar paraspinal musculature. Examination of peripheral pulses and distal skin integrity is important in patients with diabetes and possible vascular claudication.

Components of the Neurologic Examination

After completing the relevant portions of the general examination, the neurologic examination is performed. The surgeon may choose to focus the examination on a particular spinal region, but patients often complain of symptoms referable to both the cervical and thoracolumbar spine, particularly those with extensive spondylosis. A comprehensive examination may also be beneficial, for example, by uncovering signs of cervical myelopathy in a patient who needs lumbar decompression and may be at risk for neurologic deterioration during positioning or intubation. Evaluation of cranial nerve function should be included in patients with bulbar symptoms or with coexisting head and spinal trauma. A comprehensive examination should include (1) generalized inspection of the patient, emphasizing cutaneous features, posture, and gait analysis; (2) inspection and palpation of the entire spinal column, with range of motion (ROM) testing of both the spine and joints of affected extremities; (3) sensory and motor evaluation; (4) an assessment of normal and pathologic reflexes; and (5) provocative nerve root testing if previous examination has raised the suspicion of radiculopathy. The order in which these modalities are tested is dictated by surgeon preference, but minimizing patient movement and reserving maneuvers that may cause pain for the end of the examination are important considerations.

Inspection

A generalized inspection of the patient with emphasis on cutaneous features, posture, and gait is carried out as the patient first appears for evaluation and the history is reviewed.

Cutaneous Abnormalities

The skin should be inspected for café au lait spots and other sequelae of neurofibromatosis, in addition to scars from old trauma or prior surgery. The dorsal midline skin should be carefully inspected for a sinus tract, dimpling, abnormal pigmentation, fatty masses, and tufts of hair, all of which could signal an underlying congenital spinal anomaly. In patients with symptoms of claudication, the peripheral pulses are palpated and the skin of the distal extremities is inspected for edema, skin ulceration, loss of hair, and other signs of peripheral vascular disease.

Posture

Inspection of the spinal column as a single unit should be performed from both a lateral and posterior viewpoint in standing and forward bending positions. Abnormalities in spinal balance in both the sagittal and coronal planes can be pathologic and have important implications when considering surgical deformity correction. Asymmetry of paravertebral muscles, spinous processes, skin creases, shoulders, scapulae, and hips may be appreciated in patients with scoliosis.[3] Coronal imbalance can be assessed clinically by examining the standing patient from behind and measuring the distance between a plumb line dropped from C7 and the gluteal cleft. Sagittal imbalance may be implied when a patient stoops forward when walking or sitting. It is best determined by a plumb line from C7 to the sacrum on lateral radiographs.[4] A compensatory forward rocking of the pelvis and flexion of the knees while standing may be seen in severe cases. The recognition of sagittal imbalance is paramount to precise surgical planning, especially when planning for deformity correction.

Gait Analysis

Examination of a patient's gait is an invaluable component of the neurologic examination. Watching patients walk as they appear for consultation, even before formal testing begins, can be of diagnostic value.

Alterations of Gait Associated with Cord Compression

A wide-based, unsteady gait is frequently seen in myelopathic patients and can be accentuated by evaluating tandem walk. Unfortunately, a wide-based gait is not specific for myelopathy and is common in patients with cerebellar pathology, decreased proprioception resulting from peripheral neuropathy, and conditions affecting posterior column function, such as tabes dorsalis, vitamin B_{12} deficiency, and spinocerebellar ataxias. A spastic gait can be seen in patients with stroke or in those with an old cord injury and is manifested by circumduction of a hemiplegic leg or "scissoring" of the legs in a paraparetic patient. The diagnosis of Parkinson's disease should always be kept in mind when patients referred for possible myelopathy display a shuffling gait (festination) with either forward (propulsion) or backward (retropulsion) walking.

Other Characteristic Gaits

Patients suffering from compression of neural elements of the lumbosacral spine often show characteristics of "antalgic gait." This term is somewhat nonspecific but involves alteration of the movement of the affected extremity in an attempt to silence the pain generator. Lumbar radiculopathy associated with weakness of several different muscles can alter gait. Weakness of ankle dorsiflexors and foot drop may cause a patient to walk with a "steppage gait." To clear the ground while the patient pushes off, the hip is flexed excessively and the foot may slap the ground. Weakness of gluteus medius (L5) hip abduction or gluteus maximus (S1) hip extension may cause the patient to rock the thorax, or "waddle," to compensate for poor hip fixation. Patients with advanced lumbar stenosis and neurogenic claudication tend to walk in a flexed-forward position, commonly referred to as the "anthropoid posture." The spinal surgeon should keep psychiatric disorders on his or her list of differential diagnoses when assessing gait. Gait and posture disturbances are the presenting symptom in up to 10% of patients with psychogenic disorders such as anxiety and depression.[5]

Palpation and Range of Motion Testing of the Spine and Related Areas

Formal palpation and ROM testing of the spinal column, shoulders, hips, and pelvis are also included in a comprehensive examination. The spinous processes of the entire vertebral column are palpated and assessed for tenderness and associated paravertebral muscle spasm. Splaying of adjacent spinous processes or a palpable stepoff may indicate spondylolisthesis. Patients with fibromyalgia and related disorders frequently complain of pain exacerbated by stimulation of multiple trigger points. Axial rotation, flexion, extension, and lateral bending are assessed for each region of the spine.

Cervical Spine

In the cervical spine, the resting head position is noted before evaluation of ROM. A patient with a fixed rotation or tilt to one side may have an underlying unilateral facet dislocation. Although precise quantitative evaluation of ROM is not typically performed, the clinician should note obvious limitations and which maneuvers generate pain. Pain or restricted rotation of the head, 50% of which occurs at C1-2,[6] may indicate a pathologic process at this level. Head rotation associated with vertigo, tinnitus, visual alterations, or facial pain may be nonspecific, but occlusion of the vertebral artery should be included in the differential. Selecki[7] showed that rotation of the head more than 45 degrees could significantly kink the contralateral vertebral artery. Extension and rotation of the head can exacerbate pre-existing nerve root compression, and flexion in the setting of cord compression often causes paresthesia in both the arms and legs (*Lhermitte sign*).

Thoracic Spine

Examination of the thoracic spine should focus on the detection of scoliosis or a kyphotic deformity. The patient is observed from behind for symmetry in the level of the shoulders, scapulae, and hips. If a scoliotic deformity is noticed on inspection, flexion and lateral bending are assessed to further characterize the curve and determine its flexibility. Asymmetry in the paravertebral musculature with forward flexion can generate an angle in the horizontal plane that can be followed for progression. In the upper thoracic spine, there are 4 degrees of sagittal plane rotation, 6 degrees of lateral bending, and 8 to 9 degrees of axial rotation at each segment. In the lower two to three segments, these median figures are 12 degrees, 8 to 9 degrees, and 2 degrees, respectively.[6]

Lumbar Spine and Related Areas

Palpation should include not only the spinous processes and paravertebral muscles but the greater trochanter, the ischial tuberosity, and the sciatic nerve itself. The greater trochanter is palpated for focal tenderness when the patient's chief complaint includes thigh discomfort. The bursa is usually not palpable unless it is boggy and inflamed. Acute trochanteric bursitis is included in the primary differential diagnosis of lumbar radiculopathy and can also be a chronic secondary pain generator. The sciatic nerve can be palpated at the midpoint between the greater trochanter and ischial tuberosity, when the patient's hip is maximally flexed. Tenderness can occur with peripheral nerve compression by a tumor or an enlarged piriformis muscle or when the contributing roots are compressed in the spine.

The most important aspect of ROM testing in the lumbar spine is flexion-extension. A simple clinical test is to ask the patient to bend forward with the knees fully extended, and measure the distance from the patient's fingertips to the floor. Patients with facet arthropathy or spondylolisthesis often have back pain that is exacerbated by extension. Lateral bending and axial rotation are strongly coupled in the lumbar spine and more restricted because of sagittal facet orientation. It is critical to exclude the hip as a potential pain generator in the evaluation of possible lumbar spine disease. The *Patrick* or *FABERE test* is used to detect pathology in the hip or sacroiliac (SI) joint. The patient is tested in the supine position and the extremity in question is flexed, abducted, and externally rotated at the hip. This can be accomplished by asking the patient to place the lateral aspect of the foot on the involved side on the opposite shin. Pain with this maneuver is likely from the hip joint. Pain from the SI joint itself is suspected when simultaneous downward pressure on the flexed knee and the opposite anterior superior iliac spine increases symptoms. The SI joint can also be tested as a pain generator by performing the *pelvic rock test*. The examiner places both hands around the iliac crest with the thumbs on the anterior superior iliac spine and compresses medially.

Motor Examination

Muscle weakness is frequently seen in patients suffering from compression of specific nerve roots or the spinal cord itself. Weakness may be the patient's primary symptom or discovered only after physical examination. Motor deficits may be acute and rapidly progressive (i.e., after traumatic disc herniation) or more insidious in onset, similar to the setting of cervical myelopathy. A detailed motor examination and muscle grading (Table 12-1) of the key muscles innervated by the cervical and lumbar nerve roots should be performed in every patient. Evaluating strength systematically allows the clinician to identify common patterns of muscle weakness seen in cord compression and brachial plexus syndromes and reduces the likelihood of missing nonsurgical pathology.

TABLE 12-1
Grading of Motor Function

Grade	Description
0	No palpable/visible contraction
1	Muscle flicker
2	Movement with gravity eliminated
3	Movement against gravity with full range of motion
4	Movement against gravity and some resistance
5	Movement against full resistance

Cervical Spine

Figure 12-1 and Table 12-2 summarize the motor tests used to grade muscle strength for the cervical nerve roots that contribute to motor function of the upper extremity. It is important to remember that the configuration of the brachial plexus (prefixed or postfixed) can alter the typical pattern of innervation by one level. The anatomic relationship of the cervical vertebrae and motor roots must be kept in mind when attempting to correlate motor deficits to nerve root compression seen on an MRI or myelogram. A C5-6 disc herniation, for example, typically compresses the origin of the C6 root before it exits the neural foramen above the C6 pedicle. It has recently been demonstrated that forearm pronation weakness is the most frequent motor abnormality in C6 radiculopathy.[8] Such evidence illustrates the necessity of a detailed motor examination.

Lumbar Spine

Figure 12-2 and Table 12-3 summarize the motor tests used to grade muscle strength for the lumbar nerve roots commonly affected in clinical practice. Again, correlating clinical findings with radiographic abnormalities is imperative. With a typical paracentral L4-5 disc herniation, for example, the root of origin (L5) is compressed as it courses toward the undersurface of the L5 pedicle. A far lateral disc herniation at the same level may compress the root of exit (L4). Detecting motor deficits in the lower extremity, particularly in a large, muscular patient, can occasionally be difficult. Testing the patient's ability to heel (tibialis anterior) and toe (gastrocnemius) walk, maneuvers that require a patient to overcome body weight, can uncover a subtle weakness.

Sensory Examination

The key sensory dermatomes of the upper and lower extremities are depicted in Figures 12-1 and 12-2. The nipple line (T4) and umbilicus (T10) are useful thoracic landmarks. It is emphasized, however, that these landmarks are variable. Of particular note is that the T2 dermatome may be as low as the nipple line, and that it demarcates the C4 to T2 dermatome junction. The clinician should always compare dermatomes from one side with the other and ask the patient to quantify differences. Both light touch and pain perception should be tested, and proprioception and vibratory sense should be included in patients suspected of having cord compression, peripheral nerve entrapment, or sensory neuropathy. The sensory examination is particularly critical in the evaluation of the spinal cord-injured patient to determine the level of injury and to monitor for a progressing deficit. A rectal examination should usually be performed to assess for sphincter tone and perianal dermatomes. Preservation of perianal sensation in the presence of a discrete sensory level defines an incomplete lesion and may dramatically affect management and prognosis for recovery. Special mention should be made here of provocative sensory tests for nerve entrapment syndromes that can occasionally be confused with cervical radiculopathy. Median nerve compression (C6) in the carpal tunnel, ulnar nerve entrapment (C8) in the cubital tunnel or Guyon canal, and radial nerve compression (C7) in the forearm

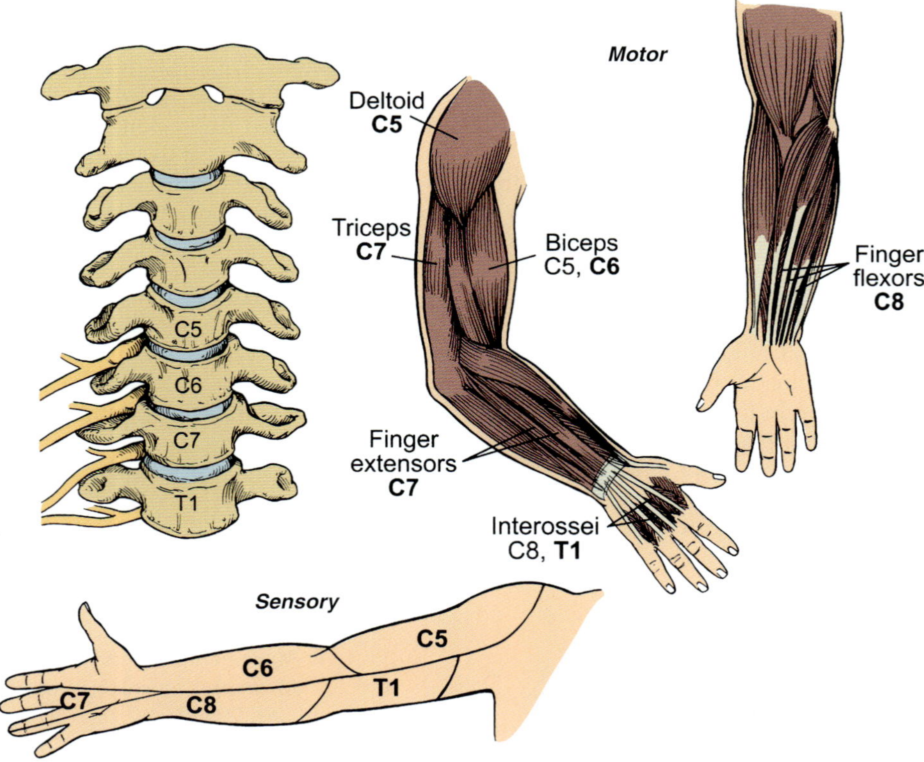

FIGURE 12-1. Examination of the cervical spine.

TABLE 12-2

Clinical Examination for Cervical Radiculopathy

Disc Herniation	Affected Root (Root of Origin)	Motor Test/Muscle	Sensory Test	Reflex
C4-5	C5	Shoulder abduction/deltoid	Lateral deltoid	Biceps
C5-6	C6	a. Elbow flexion/biceps b. Radial wrist extension/extensor, carpi radialis longus and brevis c. Forearm pronation/pronator teres	Thumb and lateral forearm	Brachioradialis and biceps (<C5)
C6-7	C7	a. Elbow extension/triceps b. Finger extension/extensor digitorum communis c. Wrist flexion/flexor carpi radialis	Middle finger	Triceps
C7-T1	C8	a. Finger flexion/flexor digitorum superficialis and profundus b. Hand intrinsics/interossei (<T1)	Little finger	Finger jerk (finger-thumb)
T1-2	T1	Hand intrinsics/interossei	Medial arm	—

are important differential diagnoses and occasionally coexist with root compression in the neck, the "double crush phenomenon."[9] Tapping on the nerve proximal to the site of compression can reproduce symptoms (*Tinel sign*) in the middle course of nerve root compression while the nerve is attempting to regenerate. Sustained wrist flexion over 60 seconds can produce signs of median nerve compression (*Phalen sign*), and similar testing can be done by flexing the elbow (ulnar nerve compression) or pronating the forearm (radial nerve compression).

Reflex Examination

The neurologic examination also includes an evaluation of the deep tendon (stretch) and superficial reflexes.

Deep Tendon Reflexes

The deep tendon reflexes are used to assess the integrity of a monosynaptic reflex arc at various levels of the cord. Table 12-4 depicts the common system for grading deep tendon reflexes. Hyperactive reflexes generally indicate an upper motor neuron lesion, and diminished or absent reflexes can be seen in lower motor neuron lesions. Metabolic abnormalities, such as hypothyroidism or hyperthyroidism, should always be excluded as an etiology for abnormal reflexes. Neuromuscular disorders and neuropathies may also present with abnormal reflexes. Reflexes are compared from one side to another, and reinforcement maneuvers that require isometric contraction of other muscle groups can be used to eliminate cortical modulation of the reflex arc. The Jendrassik maneuver can

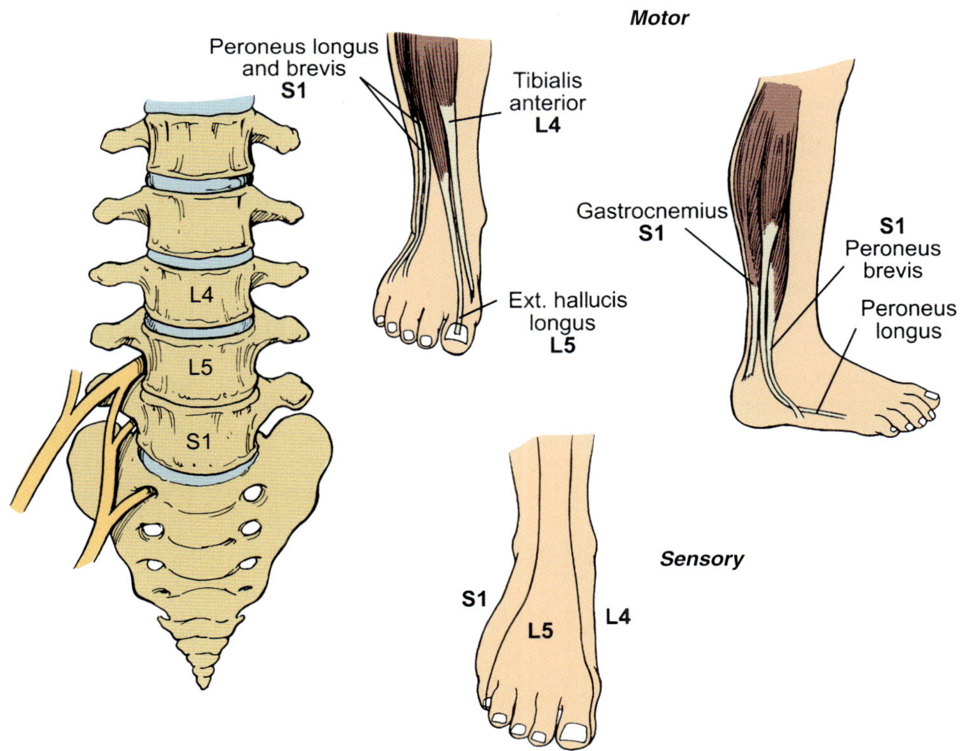

FIGURE 12-2. Examination of the lumbar spine.

TABLE 12-3
Clinical Examination for Lumbar Radiculopathy

Disc Herniated	Affected Root (Root of Origin)	Motor Test/Muscle	Sensory Test	Reflex
L3-4	L4	a. Knee extension/quadriceps b. Ankle dorsiflexion (>L5)/tibialis anterior	Posteromedial leg	Patellar
L4-5	L5	a. Great toe extension/extensor hallucis longus b. Ankle dorsiflexion (<L4) ankle plantar flexion/gastrocnemius, soleus	Anterolateral leg and dorsum of foot	—
L5-S1	S1	—	Lateral malleolus and lateral and plantar foot	Achilles

accentuate lower extremity reflexes and requires the patient to pull interlocked fingers apart while the reflex is tested. Asking the patient to clench the teeth or push down on the examination table with the thighs can accentuate upper extremity reflexes.

One uncommonly practiced reflex is the finger jerk or finger-thumb reflex. Mediated by mainly the C8 nerve root, it is elicited with patient's palm upturned and the fingers half-flexed. The surgeon then holds the tops of the fingers with his or her own half-flexed fingers, which are then tapped. The patient's fingers will be felt to flex and, most strikingly, the free thumb will be seen to flex.[10] Although the commonly tested reflexes are truly mediated by multiple nerve roots, Tables 12-2 and 12-3 outline the dominant nerve roots involved.

Superficial Reflexes

The superficial reflexes are mediated by the cerebral cortex with the afferent limb being supplied by cutaneous stimulation. The absence of a normal cutaneous reflex may signal an underlying upper motor neuron lesion. In the thoracic spine, the *upper abdominal* (T8-9), *mid-abdominal* (T9-10), and *lower abdominal* (T11-12) superficial reflexes can be used to assess the integrity of motor efferents from these levels.[10] As the appropriate dermatome is stroked from lateral to medial, the ipsilateral abdominal muscles will contract. In a thin, muscular patient the examiner will occasionally observe movement of the umbilicus toward the stimulated side. In the lumbar spine, the *superficial cremasteric reflex* is mediated by L1 and L2. Stimulating the upper medial thigh in a male patient will cause elevation of the testicle on the ipsilateral side. The anocutaneous reflex, or "anal wink," is used to assess S2 through S4 and involves contraction of the external anal sphincter in response to stimulation of the perianal skin. The importance of testing this reflex in the setting of spinal cord injury has been previously mentioned.

TABLE 12-4
Grading of Deep Tendon Reflexes

Grade	Description
0	No response
1	Diminished
2	Normal
3	Increased
4	Hyperactive (with clonus)

Pathologic Reflexes

Upper motor neuron (corticospinal tract) lesions should be suspected in patients harboring the classic pathologic reflexes. These include the plantar response in the lower extremity and a positive *Hoffmann sign* in the hand. The plantar reflex is typically assessed by using a sharp instrument to stroke the plantar surface of the foot from the heel dorsally, then lateral to medial across the metatarsal pads. A normal plantar reflex results in flexion of all the toes. A positive test (*Babinski sign*) involves dorsiflexion of the great toe alone or in combination with ankle dorsiflexion and hip flexion ("triple response"). The same reflex can be elicited by stroking the lateral side of the foot (*Chaddock test*) or the crest of the tibia (*Oppenheim test*).

The upper extremity analogue of the plantar response is the *Hoffmann sign*. The palmar surface of the hand is lightly supported as the patient's middle finger is flicked into extension or flexion at the distal interphalangeal joint. A positive response involves reflex flexion of the thumb and fingers and is commonly observed in myelopathic patients with cervical spinal cord compression. A recent study[11] of 536 patients with spine-related problems found 16 patients with a positive Hoffmann sign and no pain or neurologic symptoms referable to the cervical spine. Interestingly, 15 (94%) of these patients had some degree of cord compression on cervical MRI. The clinical significance of this study is unclear, however, because prior studies[12] have documented cervical cord impingement in up to 20% of asymptomatic adults older than 40 years of age.

Provocative Nerve Root Testing

If the history and basic physical examination raise the clinical suspicion of a radiculopathy, performing a series of provocative nerve root tests can further improve diagnostic accuracy. These tests were designed to reproduce clinical symptoms by accentuating nerve root irritation due to compressive pathology.

Cervical Spine

Patients with cervical radiculopathy often complain of worsening pain with Valsalva activities or when rotating the head toward the symptomatic extremity. A foraminal closing test (Fig. 12-3) is performed by hyperextending the patient's head and rotating it toward the affected side, thus decreasing the size of the intervertebral foramen. An axial load is then

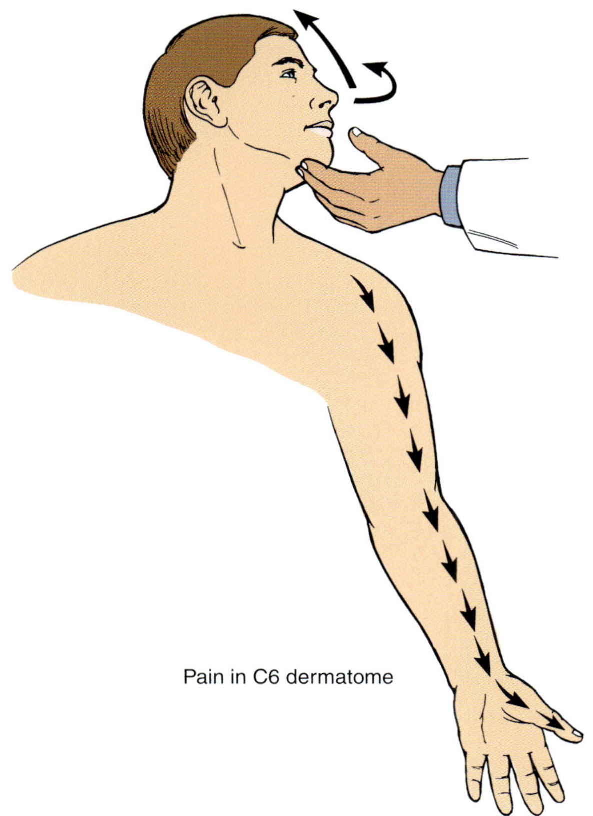

FIGURE 12-3. Foraminal closing maneuver positive for a C6 radiculopathy.

often applied by pressing down on the patient's head. A positive test reproduces the patient's radicular symptoms and is often referred to as the *Spurling sign*. A recent review of the Spurling test,[13] which was administered before electromyelographic testing of 255 patients referred for possible cervical radiculopathy, found poor sensitivity (30%) but excellent specificity (93%). Similar maneuvers can be used to reproduce radicular symptoms, including pure axial compression followed by traction, but these tend to be poorly tolerated by patients. Patients with cervical radiculopathy may also get relief by placing the affected extremity behind the head (the shoulder abduction relief sign).[14]

Lumbar Spine

There are several well-described nerve root tension signs that are useful when testing for lumbar radiculopathy.[15]

Straight Leg Raising Test (Lasègue Sign)

The most widely used test to differentiate leg pain resulting from hip pathology versus nerve root irritation is the straight leg raising test (SLR). The test was discovered by the French pathologist Ernest Charles Lasègue[16] and described in 1881 by one of his pupils, J. J. Forst. In the supine position, the patient's fully extended leg is slowly raised and the patient reports any pain that is elicited. The SLR is considered positive if pain or paresthesia occurs in a radicular distribution at less than 60 degrees of elevation (Fig. 12-4). Lowering the affected leg and dorsiflexing the ankle will exacerbate the

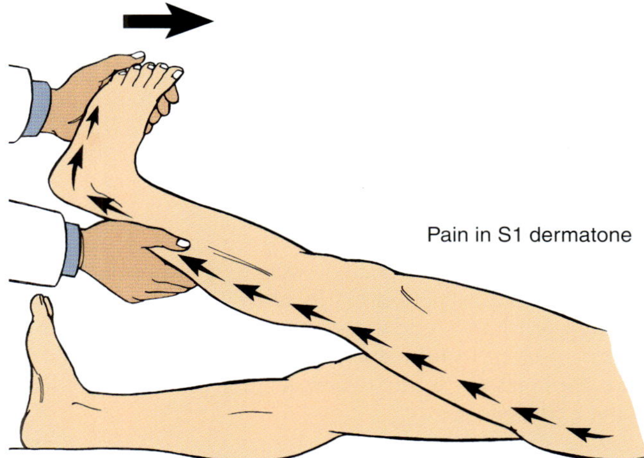

FIGURE 12-4. Positive straight leg raising test for an S1 radiculopathy.

pain. Allowing the foot to rest on the examining table by flexing the knee will typically ease the pain (*bowstring sign*). Pain limited to the low back, hip, or posterior thigh is not indicative of a radiculopathy. SLR is most specific for L5 or S1 radiculopathy.

Reverse Straight Leg Raising Test (Femoral Stretch Test)

This test is more sensitive for pain caused by radiculopathy involving L2, L3, and L4. In the prone or lateral decubitus position, the patient's knee is maximally flexed as the hip is extended (Fig. 12-5). A positive test involves pain in the distribution of the affected nerve root.

Crossed Straight Leg Raising Test (Well Leg/Straight Leg Raising Test)

The crossed straight leg raising test (CSLR) is performed by raising the unaffected leg with the patient in the supine position and is positive when radicular pain occurs in the clinically affected extremity. This phenomenon is also referred to as the *Fajersztajn sign*, in honor of the Polish neurologist

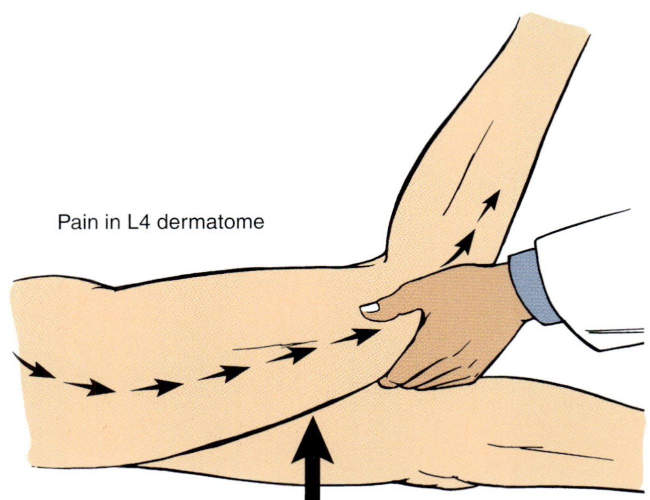

FIGURE 12-5. Positive reverse straight leg raising test for an L4 radiculopathy.

who first described it[17] and, interestingly, also suggested that foot dorsiflexion would aggravate sciatica. The test is typically positive when the patient has a large central disc herniation. It is more specific but less sensitive than SLR.[18] A meta-analysis done by Devillé et al. demonstrated that SLR is 91% sensitive and 26% specific, whereas CSLR is 29% sensitive and 88% specific.[19]

Hoover Test

This test is included to exclude weakness of nonorganic origin and should be performed in series with the SLR. After placing both hands under the patient's heels, the examiner asks the patient to raise one leg. If the examiner cannot feel downward pressure in the resting leg, the patient is not likely giving a true effort.

Differentiating Spinal Cord and Peripheral Nerve Pathology from Bony or Soft Tissue Pathology

Abnormalities of the joints of the upper and lower extremities may occasionally mimic or present simultaneously with neurologic signs and symptoms. The spinal surgeon should be aware of some common maneuvers used to diagnose joint and soft tissue pathology.

Cervical Radiculopathy versus Upper Extremity Pathology

Shoulder

Patients often present with cervical radiculopathy complaints that also include pain or tenderness of the shoulder joint. Possible causes of shoulder pain include bicipital tendon subluxation, frozen shoulder syndrome, and shoulder dislocation. The Yergason test consists of externally rotating the humerus against resistance with the patient's elbow flexed. Resulting pain suggests an unstable biceps tendon. The drop arm test is a quick test for a rotator cuff tear. The patient's arm is abducted to 90 degrees by the examiner and is dropped. If the patient can hold the arm steady, the rotator cuff is likely normal. A rotator cuff injury is possible if the arm falls and the patient is unable to slowly lower it to his or her side. The apprehension test aids in the diagnosis of chronic shoulder dislocation. The arm is abducted and externally rotated. If the shoulder joint is about to dislocate, the patient may exhibit a look of apprehension or fear.[20]

Elbow

Lateral epicondylitis or tennis elbow is a common condition that may be confused with cervical radiculopathy owing to weakness of the forearm extensors. Patients with lateral epicondylitis experience exquisite pain at the insertion of the wrist extensor's origin when asked to dorsiflex the involved wrist against resistance.[20]

Summary

Meticulous history taking and physical examination skills are critical to the surgeon caring for patients with spinal disorders. The value of the neurologic history and physical examination must not be overlooked despite today's advances in imaging technology.

KEY REFERENCES

Boden DS, McGowin PR, Davis DO, et al: Abnormal magnetic-resonance scans of the cervical spine in asymptomatic subjects. *J Bone Joint Surg [Am]* 72:1178–1183, 1990.

Chabrol H, Corraze J: Charles Lasègue, 1809-1863. *Am J Psychiatry* 158:28, 2001.

Devillé WL, van der Windt DA, Dzaferagić A, et al: The test of Lasègue: systematic review of the accuracy in diagnosing herniated discs. *Spine (Phila Pa 1976)* 25:1140–1147, 2000.

Glassman SD, Bridwell K, Dimar JR, et al: The impact of positive sagittal balance in adult spinal deformity. *Spine (Phila Pa 1976)* 30:2204–2029, 2005.

Rainville J, Noto DJ, Jouve C, et al: Assessment of forearm pronation strength in C6 and C7 radiculopathies. *Spine* 32(1):72–75, 2007.

Sung RD, Wang JC: Correlation between a positive Hoffmann's reflex and cervical pathology in asymptomatic individuals. *Spine (Phila Pa 1976)* 26:67–70, 2001.

White AA III, Panjabi MM: Basic biomechanics of the spine. *Neurosurgery* 7:76–93, 1980.

REFERENCES

The complete reference list is available online at expertconsult.com.

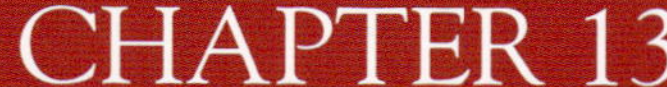

CHAPTER 13

Intervertebral Disc Process of Degeneration: Physiology and Pathophysiology

Scott Tintle | David Gwinn

In the United States alone, nearly 5.7 million people are diagnosed with intervertebral disc disorders each year.[1,2] These disorders are responsible for widespread disability and account for tremendous costs associated with their treatment and loss of productivity. The intervertebral disc is a unique multifunctional structure. It provides a major stabilizing effect for the spine and allows for the dissipation of axial load, and yet is still flexible enough to confer significant mobility. Despite these essential roles in spinal mechanics, the disc also begins to show signs of biochemical and structural change almost immediately after birth, and signs of degeneration are present at an extremely young age.[3-5] Unfortunately, these degenerative changes are often progressive, rendering the disc biochemically and biomechanically incapable of absorbing the forces necessary for normal physiologic spinal function and potentially leading to rapid degeneration of the spine.

Understanding the anatomy and function of the normal disc serves as the framework for comprehension of the complex processes of aging and the pathologic degeneration that afflict the disc. One of the most significant challenges to a complete understanding of disc disease is the lack of consistency with which radiographically detectable signs of disc degeneration translate to clinical symptomatology.[6] As such, there is abundant evidence to suggest that aberrant disc morphology does not necessarily equate with back pain.[6,7] This poses a significant challenge to researchers in this field because individual variation in disc degeneration makes it difficult to distinguish between age-related alterations and pathologic premature degenerative changes.[5,8] In the future, the ability to make this distinction will lead to improved clarity regarding the complex process of disc degeneration.

Normal Intervertebral Disc

The intervertebral disc is composed of water, proteoglycan, collagen, and a small amount of noncollagenous proteins. There are three major regions to the intervertebral disc with differing structural compositions: the nucleus pulposus, anulus fibrosus, and cartilaginous end plates. Each has different functions. Of significant note, the intervertebral disc is one of the most hypocellular structures in the body[9] (Fig. 13-1).

Anulus Fibrosus

The anulus fibrosus is the outer circumferential portion of the disc and is often subdivided into the inner and outer anulus. The outer anulus is a collection of highly organized, densely packed collagen fibrils, creating a lamellar structure of up to 25 lamellae in the mature disc.[9,10] These collagen fibrils insert into the adjacent vertebral end plates and join them together to stabilize the spine. In addition to its predominantly collagenous structure, a small amount of elastin is present in the anulus, which helps it to restore and recoil after stretching in response to compression and tensile forces.[9,11] The strong anulus provides the ability to absorb significant hoop stresses and maintain stiffness in the presence of the tensile forces induced by bending and twisting of the spine.[12,13] The importance of this ability to resist hoop stress has been shown in large animal studies, which demonstrated that even a partial-thickness laceration into the anulus rapidly produced advanced disc degeneration.[12,14] The outer anulus is populated with a low density of fibroblast-like cells.[15] It is the only tissue in the mature disc that remains innervated and is capable of producing pain when exposed to noxious stimuli.[16-19]

The inner anulus appears to serve as a transition zone to the vastly different biochemical composition of the nucleus. It is less dense and lacks the organized lamellar structure of the outer anulus. It is populated with rounder, chondrocyte-like cells, and the concentration of proteoglycans and water content is increased.[20]

Nucleus Pulposus

The nucleus pulposus, the inner, less-organized region of the disc, occupies the middle and posterior thirds of the intervertebral disc.[21] It consists of a rich proteoglycan matrix with a lesser amount of disorganized collagen than in the anulus.[20,22] There is a significantly higher content of water in the nucleus. The large amount of proteoglycan and water present in the nucleus make it ideal for developing the "swelling pressures" necessary to resist the compressive forces of the spine. At birth, the nucleus is populated almost exclusively with notochordal cells. These cells rapidly begin to necrose shortly after birth and by the age of 4 to 10 years they are completely replaced by rounder, chondrocyte-like cells of mesenchymal origin[9] (Table 13-1).

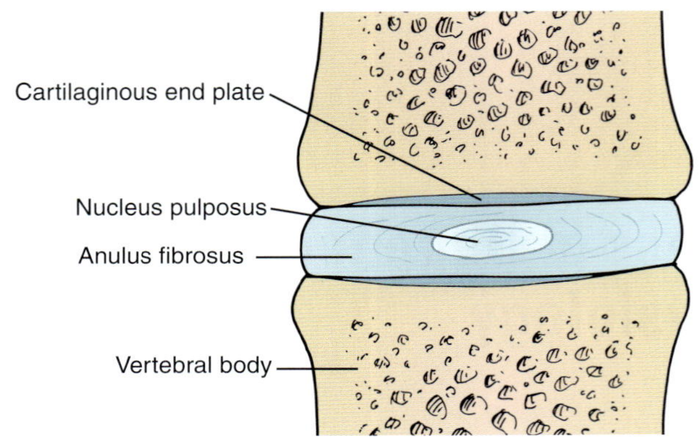

FIGURE 13-1. The three major structural portions of the normal intervertebral disc: the nucleus pulposus, anulus fibrosus, and cartilaginous end plates. (Redrawn and modified from Raj PP: Intervertebral disc: anatomy-physiology-pathophysiology-treatment. *Pain Pract* 8:18, 2008.)

TABLE 13-1

Composition of the Intervertebral Disc

Component	Anulus Fibrosus	Nucleus Pulposus
Collagen (mainly types I and II; others present include types III, V, VI, IX, XI, XII, and XIV)	70% of dry weight 80% type I collagen	20% of dry weight 80% type II collagen
Proteoglycan	25% of dry weight	50%–70% of dry weight
Water	Lowest content	Highest content

Cartilaginous End Plate

The cartilaginous end plate is a hyaline cartilage layer separating the disc from the adjacent bony vertebral end plate. It is usually less than 1 mm thick in the mature disc and lies immediately adjacent to the perforated bony end plate. It is loosely cemented to the underlying bony end plate by a thin layer of calcium that is absent near the perforated areas of the bony plate, which allows for nutrient diffusion from the vertebra to the disc.[21]

Matrix of the Intervertebral Disc

The matrix content of the intervertebral disc is critical to disc function. The uniquely hydrophilic nature of proteoglycans provides the swelling pressure required to increase the intradiscal water content necessary to resist compressive strains on the spine.[9,23,24] The matrix composition changes with age, and the quantitative loss and qualitative deterioration of the proteoglycans is thought to represent the single largest biochemical contribution to disc degeneration.[20,25]

Proteoglycans are highly negatively charged molecules consisting of a core protein and chains of glycosaminoglycans radiating from the core. The chains are composed mainly of keratin and chondroitin sulfate. Multiple proteoglycans then are linked to hyaluronic acid to form large proteoglycan aggregates capable of producing even larger swelling pressures. The aggregates are held together by type II collagen and are cross-linked by type IX collagen.[23,26]

Aggrecan is the most abundant proteoglycan in the disc.[20] It is responsible for 70% of the dry weight of the nucleus pulposus and 25% of the anulus fibrosus. Other proteoglycans present at lower levels include decorin, biglycan, fibromodulin, lumican, versican, and perlican.[20,27]

Nutrition of the Intervertebral Disc

The intervertebral disc is the largest avascular tissue in the human body. Nutritional support for cell survival, matrix production, and disc homeostasis occurs through diffusion of nutrients through the vertebral end plates.[28-30] In the newborn and young child, small blood vessels penetrate the cartilaginous end plates and enter the disc anulus and nucleus.[21] These vessels rapidly become less efficient, yet remain partially functional until about 8 years of age. They then become completely nonfunctional over the next two decades of life.[5,21,28,31,32]

The vertebral body is supplied by an arterial network that drains into a subchondral venous plexus within the bone.[28,33] Capillaries from this region penetrate into the subchondral plate and terminate in loops at the bony end plate–cartilaginous end plate junction.[28,34,35] Through these capillaries, the nutrients necessary for disc metabolism are delivered and diffuse through the cartilaginous end plates to reach the center of the disc.[28] The end plate acts as a semipermeable membrane, letting smaller neutral charges (water, amino acids, oxygen) through more easily than larger, positively charged molecules[28,36-38] (Fig. 13-2).

Modulation and Regulation of Disc Matrix

Anabolic Influences

The intervertebral disc matrix is in a constant state of dynamic flux. Anabolic and catabolic influences on the disc matrix continuously interact with the disc to alter the physical

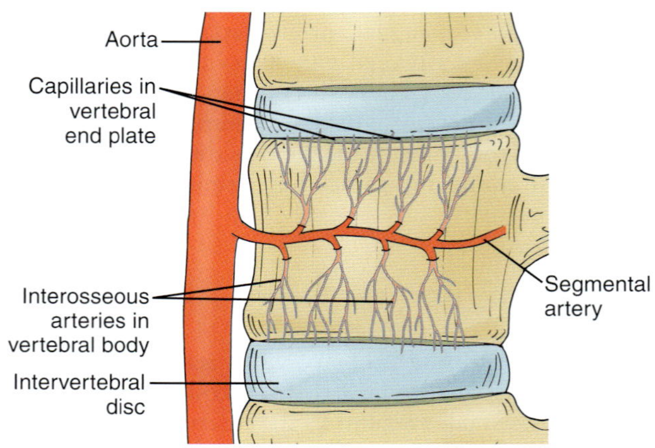

FIGURE 13-2. The normal circulation to the vertebral body and vertebral end plates. (Redrawn and modified from Raj PP: Intervertebral disc: anatomy-physiology-pathophysiology-treatment. *Pain Pract* 8:18, 2008.)

TABLE 13-2

Key Anabolic Modulators (Growth Factors) of the Intervertebral Disc

Growth Factor	Role
Insulin-like growth factor-1 (IGF-1)	Stimulates proteoglycan synthesis Reduces cellular apoptosis
Epidermal growth factor (EGF)	Stimulates matrix synthesis Cellular proliferation
Basic fibroblast growth factor (bFGF)	Stimulates proteoglycan synthesis Cellular proliferation
Platelet-derived growth factor (PDGF)	Decreases cellular apoptosis
Transforming growth factor beta (TGF-β)	Greatly increased proteoglycan synthesis Cellular proliferation
Bone morphogenetic protein-2 (BMP-2)	Increased proteoglycan synthesis Cellular proliferation Increased mRNA for type II collagen, aggrecan, sox9, and osteocalcin Up-regulates gene expression of BMP-6, BMP-7, and TGF-β
Bone morphogenetic protein-7 (BMP-7; osteogenic protein-1 [OP-1])	Increased proteoglycan synthesis Increased collagen synthesis Cellular proliferation
Link protein N-terminal peptide	In concentrations of 10–100 μg/mL stimulates matrix assembly

From Masuda K, Oegema TJ, An H: Growth factors and treatment of intervertebral disc degeneration. *Spine (Phila Pa 1976)* 29:2757, 2004.

composition of the matrix.[23] Metalloproteinases (MMPs) modulate the matrix composition by breaking down aged proteoglycans under catabolic influences while newly synthesized matrix takes the place of the degraded proteoglycans.[23,39] A very complex, multifactorial, poorly understood interaction of mechanical and biochemical factors defines whether a disc is capable of remodeling in response to loading conditions in order to maintain disc homeostasis.[1] If the disc is unable to remodel and maintain a balance of anabolic and catabolic influences, then damage accumulates in a process that may eventually self-perpetuate into a state of continued degeneration.

The key anabolic modulating growth factors work by stimulating the chondrocyte-like cells to produce matrix while inhibiting the MMPs present in the disc.[1] In addition to various growth factors, tissue inhibitors of MMPs (TIMPs) are present to suppress the activation of the MMPs[23,40] (Table 13-2).

Catabolic Influences

Catabolic modulation in the disc occurs mainly through cytokine-induced and metalloproteinase degradation of matrix components.[23] MMPs 1, 2, 3, 8, 9, and 13 are all present in the disc and serve to degrade collagen, aggrecan, versican, link protein, and the other proteoglycans.[9,41-45] The aggrecanases ADAM-TS-4 and ADAM-TS-5, from the ADAM (*a d*isintegrin *a*nd *m*etalloproteinase) protein family, are also present in the disc and mainly function to degrade aggrecan and versican.[9,46] These MMPs and aggrecanases allow for the large proteoglycans to be degraded into smaller components that may be more easily leached from the intervertebral disc by diffusion.[20] In a pathologic catabolic state when the MMPs are working with little opposing matrix production, a significant net loss of proteoglycan and water content occurs, rendering the disc incapable of producing the swelling pressure necessary to resist compressive forces on the disc.[20] Overproduction of MMPs can thus lead to increased forces on other spinal structures and contribute to disc and overall spinal degeneration.

In addition to the catabolic effect of MMPs, growing evidence suggests that inflammatory cytokines may have a significant catabolic influence on the disc.[23,47,48] Animal studies have indicated that in the presence of injury to the intervertebral disc there are increased levels of interleukin (IL)-1, tumor necrosis factor alpha (TNF-α), and IL-8 near the injured regions of the disc.[49] These cytokines have negative catabolic effects on the disc and also stimulate the disc cells to produce chemokines, which are responsible for macrophage attraction and stimulation, especially in the presence of disc herniation.[48,50] Macrophages in the disc usually reflect an attempt to break up or remove herniated disc fragments, but their presence also leads to further inflammation and cytokine release, which may prove damaging to the disc.[23,51] These inflammatory substances are also responsible for the activation of multiple cascades within the disc cell nuclei that lead to the production of metalloproteinases, which in turn contribute to matrix breakdown.[48,52] In addition, these inflammatory cytokines are thought to contribute to the pain-producing effects of disc degeneration[48,49,53,54] (Table 13-3).

TABLE 13-3

Key Catabolic Modulators of the Intervertebral Disc

Catabolic Modulators	Actions
Interleukin-1 (IL-1)	Inhibits synthesis of matrix Promotes metalloproteinase production Stimulates nitric oxide synthetase to produce nitric oxide Enhances caseinase activity Triggers the translocation of transcription factors to cell nuclei that target genes that include collagenases and COX-2
Tumor necrosis factor alpha (TNF-α)	Inhibits synthesis of matrix Promotes metalloproteinase production Stimulates nitric oxide synthetase to produce nitric oxide Triggers the translocation of transcription factors to cell nuclei that target genes that include collagenases and COX-2
Nitric oxide	Produces free radicals that damage cell membranes and induce degenerative pathways Inhibits tissue inhibitors of metalloproteinases (TIMPs)
Interleukin-6 and interleukin-9 (IL-6, IL-9) fibronectin superoxide	Proinflammatory and pro-nociceptive effect stimulates proteoglycan degradation Degrades hyaluronic acid, causing aggregate breakdown

COX-2, cyclooxygenase-2.

Data from references 1, 9, 48; and Anderson DG, Tannoury C: Molecular pathogenic factors in symptomatic disc degeneration. *Spine J* 5(6 Suppl):260S, 2005.

Degeneration

It is very difficult to differentiate the normal degenerative changes of an aging disc from those of pathologic disc degeneration.[5,8] It is also crucial to understand that even pathologic disc degeneration is not always accompanied by back pain, and therefore degeneration as discussed here does not necessarily translate to clinical symptomatology. The biochemical and cellular structure of the intervertebral disc begins changing almost immediately after birth, and the process progresses through life.[3-5] It is useful to divide disc changes into the following two categories:

1. Gross and histologic changes
2. Biochemical changes

The gross structural/histologic and biochemical changes affect the disc's overall ability to function effectively and ultimately both contribute to progressive disc failure in pathologic states.

Gross and Histologic Changes

The hallmark histologic finding in intervertebral disc degeneration is the progressively diminishing vascular supply, which begins shortly after birth and leads to tissue breakdown as early as the second decade of life.[5] Changes in the nucleus pulposus also begin immediately after birth. Within the first two decades of life the nucleus begins to undergo mucoid degeneration, increasing cleft formation, and granular changes consistent with granulation tissue formation at sites of disc injury. These clefts and granular changes eventually lead to frank tears that communicate with anular rim lesions.[5,21]

In the anulus, peripheral rim lesions appear late in the second decade of life and eventually progress to frank tears that communicate with the nuclear clefts. The end plate also shows degenerative changes that begin with the loss of the end plate vessels early in childhood. After the loss of these vessels, cartilage disorganization increases and cracks in the cartilaginous end plate begin to appear. Microfractures in the adjacent subchondral bone follow and new subchondral bone formation and eventual sclerosis of the plate occur. All of these changes eventually lead to a "burned-out" state,[5] apparent in the seventh and later decades of life. At this time, all components of the disc begin to resemble scar tissue and there is no longer a distinction between the different regions of the disc[5,21] (Table 13-4 and Figs. 13-3 to 13-6).

The cellular content of the disc also changes over time. The earliest changes occur shortly after birth and include replacement of the rapidly decaying notochordal cells with mesenchymal chondrocyte-like cells.[9] Cell density in both the nucleus and the anulus also rapidly declines after birth. This occurs as the matrix grows along with the expanding volume of the intervertebral disc. The cell density in the nucleus pulposus shortly after birth is approximately 4×10^6 cells/cm^3 and in the anulus fibrosus, 9×10^6 cells/cm^3. This is significantly lower then the cellular density of even relatively acellular hyaline cartilage,[9] which has about 1.4×10^7 cells/cm^3. As the disc continues to age, cell death accelerates and large numbers of decaying cells can be found in clusters. By adulthood, more than 50% of the disc's cells are necrotic[55] (Fig. 13-7 and Table 13-5).

Biochemical Changes

The most significant biochemical change in the degenerating disc is the net loss of proteoglycan.[20,25] In addition to this quantitative loss of proteoglycan, the quality of the remaining

TABLE 13-4

Gross Degenerative Disc Changes by Age

Age (Years)	Cellularity	Nucleus Pulposus	Anulus Fibrosus	End Plate
0–1 months	Increase in chondrocyte density Increase in decayed cells	Slight mucoid degeneration present	No significant changes	Increased cell density and cartilage disorganization
2–10	Substantial increase in chondrocyte density Substantial increase in decayed cells Complete loss of all notochordal cells	Mild cleft formation present Increasing granular changes	No significant changes	Complete loss of end plate blood vessels Cell density and cartilage disorganization continue to increase Cartilage cracks first appear
11–20	Substantial increase in chondrocyte cell death and proliferation	Increasing clefts and tears present Increasing granular changes	A few rim lesions first appear	Cartilage cracks frequent Microfractures in the adjacent subchondral bone and new bone formation present
21–50	Cell density continues to increase	Increasing clefts and tears present Increasing granular changes Mucoid degeneration	A few rim lesions with edge neovascularity present	Previous changes occur with increasing frequency: cartilage cracks, microfractures, and new subchondral bone formation
51–70	Huge clones of hypertrophic chondrocytes near damaged areas	Huge clefts and tears filled with granular material	Large tears and edge neovascularity predominate	Microfractures and subchondral bone sclerosis present Scar formation present
>70	"Burned-out" appearance: all tissue resembles scar tissue	"Burned-out" appearance: all tissue resembles scar tissue	"Burned-out" appearance: all tissue resembles scar tissue	New bone and cartilage disorganization predominate

From Boos N, Weissbach S, Rohrbach H, et al: Classification of age-related changes in lumbar intervertebral discs. 2002 Volvo Award in basic science. *Spine (Phila Pa 1976)* 27:2631, 2002.

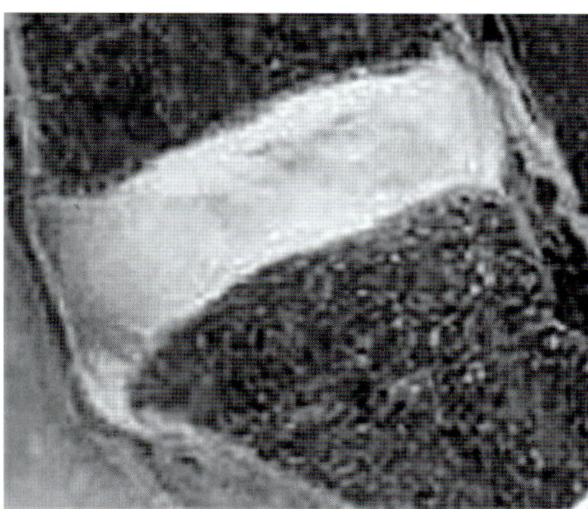

FIGURE 13-3. Sagittal section through a normal intervertebral disc. (From Thalgott J, Albert T, Vaccaro A, et al: A new classification system for degenerative disc disease of the lumbar spine based on magnetic resonance imaging, provocative discography, plain radiographs and anatomic considerations. *Spine J* 4[6 Suppl]:167S, 2004.)

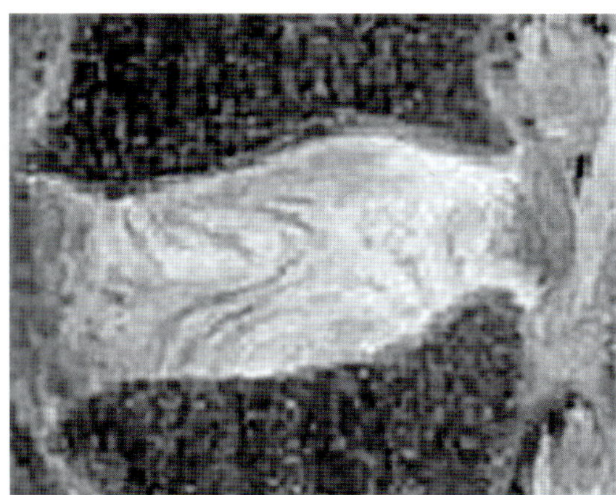

FIGURE 13-4. Sagittal section through a disc with mild degeneration. (From Thalgott J, Albert T, Vaccaro A, et al: A new classification system for degenerative disc disease of the lumbar spine based on magnetic resonance imaging, provocative discography, plain radiographs and anatomic considerations. *Spine J* 4[6 Suppl]:167S, 2004.)

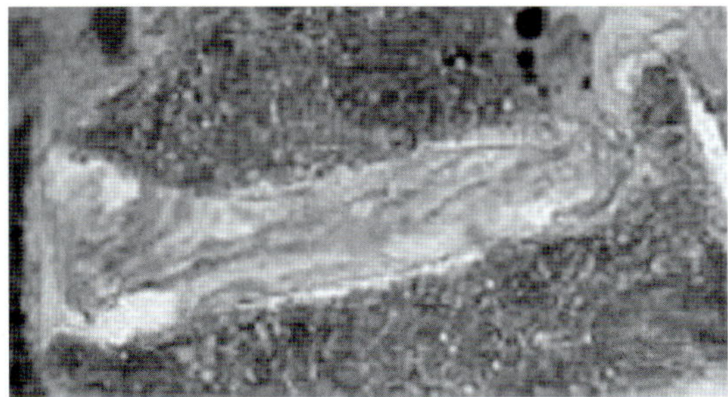

FIGURE 13-5. Sagittal section through a disc with moderate degeneration. Note loss of disc height and irregular end plates. (From Thalgott J, Albert T, Vaccaro A, et al: A new classification system for degenerative disc disease of the lumbar spine based on magnetic resonance imaging, provocative discography, plain radiographs and anatomic considerations. *Spine J* 4[6 Suppl]:167S, 2004.)

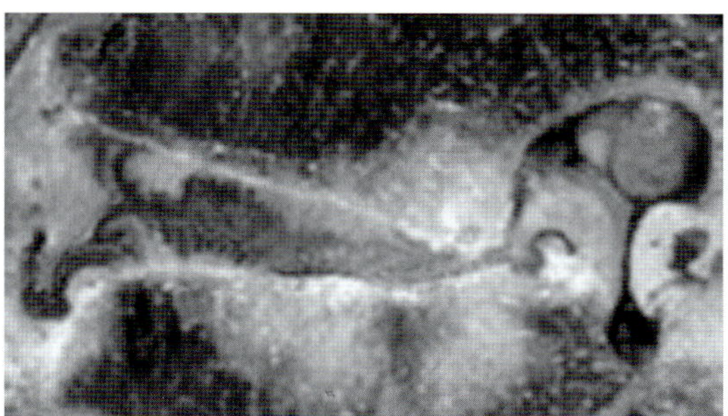

FIGURE 13-6. Sagittal section through a disc with severe degeneration. Note end plate sclerosis, osteophytosis, and severe loss of disc height. (From Thalgott J, Albert T, Vaccaro A, et al: A new classification system for degenerative disc disease of the lumbar spine based on magnetic resonance imaging, provocative discography, plain radiographs and anatomic considerations. *Spine J* 4[6 Suppl]:167S, 2004.)

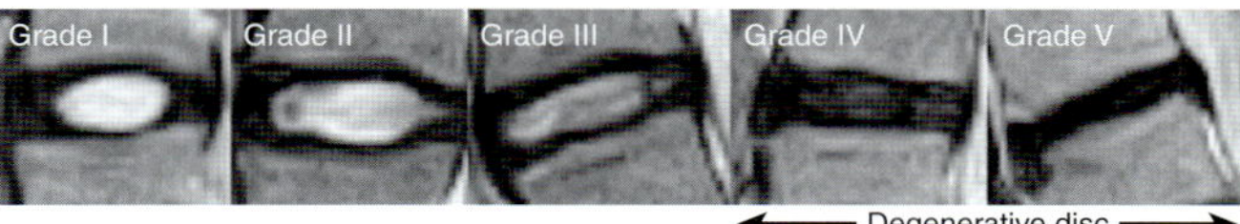

FIGURE 13-7. Midsagittal view on T2 density-weighted MRI of discs graded according to a modified Pfirrmann classification (see Table 13-5). (From Hangai M, Kaneoka K, Kuno S, et al: Factors associated with lumbar intervertebral disc degeneration in the elderly. *Spine J* 8:732, 2008.)

TABLE 13-5

Modified Pfirrmann Classification as Evaluated on Midsagittal T2-Density-Weighted MRI

Grade	Signal Intensity of Nucleus Pulposus	Distinction between Nucleus and Anulus
I	Hyperintense or isointense to CSF (bright white) and homogeneous	Clear
II	Hyperintense of isointense to CSF (white) and inhomogeneous	Clear
III	Intermediate to CSF (light gray) and inhomogeneous	
IV	Hypointense to CSF (dark gray) and inhomogeneous	
V	Low intense to CSF (black) and inhomogeneous	

CSF, cerebrospinal fluid.

Adapted from Hanagai M, Kaneoka K, Kuno S, et al: Factors associated with lumbar intervertebral disc degeneration in the elderly. *Spine J* 8:732, 2008.

proteoglycan is compromised.[9,27,56] With the loss of large quantities of aggregated proteoglycan, the disc's ability to create the swelling pressure necessary to absorb the forces imposed on it decreases. These changes also begin shortly after birth, when the rich proteoglycan matrix composition is altered. At birth, chondroitin sulfate is the predominant glycosaminoglycan in the disc, but as the blood supply is progressively lost and the disc volume increases, the disc contents become increasingly anaerobic. Because of the lack of oxygen, chondroitin sulfate is progressively replaced by keratan sulfate chains, which are created in the absence of oxygen.[9,57-59]

In addition to the changing glycosaminoglycan composition in the disc, the overall structure of the large proteoglycans changes. In the young disc, aggrecan is the predominant proteoglycan. Multiple aggrecan molecules bind to hyaluronan to form an even larger structure called an *aggregate*. In the fetal and newborn disc, aggregating proteoglycans predominate and are extremely effective in creating large swelling pressures.[9,60,61] The amount of aggregating proteoglycan is rapidly diminished with age by proteolytic degradation of the large aggregates. By 6 months of age, only 50% of the anular and 30% of the nuclear proteoglycan content is in aggregated form. In the mature adult disc, only 10% of the proteoglycan is aggregated and these aggregates are smaller and have a higher keratan sulfate composition compared with their younger equivalents.[27,62] These degenerative features of disc proteoglycans may make them less effective in creating the swelling pressure necessary to resist compressive forces[9] (Fig. 13-8).

The collagen content of the disc is not immune to change, also exhibiting signs of degeneration. The disc collagen demonstrates evidence of proteolytic collagenase action, which accumulates and eventually contributes to the weakening mechanical properties of the disc.[9,57,63] It is significant that the triple helix structure of disc collagen is more denatured and damaged than that of the collagen in articular cartilage, which may indicate less effective repair mechanisms in the disc.[57] In addition, the collagen present in the disc appears to be nonenzymatically cross-linked by advanced glycation end products (AGEs).[9,64-66]

AGEs are protein modifiers formed through the Maillard reaction when an amino acid and a reducing sugar react.[66] With age, AGEs accumulate in various tissues in the body such as the skin, myocardial cells, renal cells, chondrocytes, and intervertebral discs.[66-70] AGEs originally were given substantial attention because of their increased presence in diabetes.[71] After research elucidated the presence and negative effect of AGEs on articular cartilage, their presence and potential role in intervertebral disc degeneration were sought.[66,72,73] in vitro and animal studies suggest that AGEs play a role in disc degeneration. Their increased concentration in diabetes may contribute to the increased relative risk for disc herniation seen in at least one study of patients with diabetes.[74]

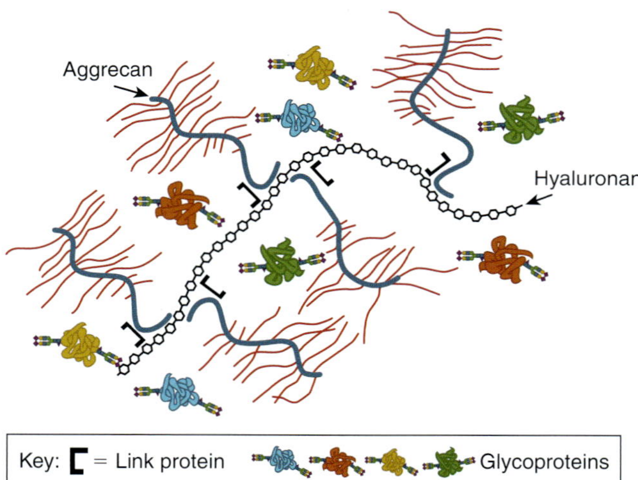

FIGURE 13-8. **The large aggrecan molecule forms an aggregate with hyaluronan and link protein.** (From Esko JD, Kimata K, Lindahl U: Proteoglycans and sulfated glycosaminoglycans. In Varki A, Cummings RD, Esko JD, et al., editors: *Essentials of glycobiology*, ed 2, Cold Spring Harbor, NY, 2009, Cold Spring Harbor Laboratory Press. Online text version available at www.ncbi.nlm.nih.gov/books/NBK1900/.)

AGEs likely influence disc degeneration through negative biologic and biomechanical contributions. Biomechanical studies have demonstrated that the accumulation of AGEs leads to alterations in the disc's physical properties, the most significant of which is increased mechanical stiffness.[75] This increased stiffness of the disc also likely leads to a decreased ability to produce the swelling pressure necessary for normal disc function.[9,69] Biologic in vitro studies have also demonstrated that the accumulation of AGEs in intervertebral disc cells leads to a down-regulation in the production of aggrecan.[66] In addition, a recent bovine study documented the increased expression of the receptor for AGEs (RAGE) in intervertebral discs in the presence of an inflammatory state with increased IL-1β. All of these studies noted a decrease in aggrecan production, which may at least partially explain the increased disc degeneration seen in the presence of chronic inflammation.[48,76]

Disc Material Properties and Disc Degeneration

The gross structural and biochemical changes associated with early degeneration lead to changes in the intervertebral disc's mechanical properties, which make it less capable of performing its necessary functions.[77] Cadaveric studies conducted on discs of various ages and degrees of degeneration have demonstrated an increased shear modulus in aged and degenerated discs, indicating a decreased ability of the disc to absorb energy.[77-79] In essence, the discs become increasingly stiff and appear to undergo a transition from "fluid-like" behavior to "solid-like" behavior with increasing degeneration.[80] Alterations in disc viscoelasticity have also been seen, including both increased creep and creep rate. In addition to these changes, which more drastically affect the nucleus, alterations in the anulus result in a decreased Poisson's ratio as well as decreased radial permeability, which transforms the anisotropic hydraulic permeability of the normal disc to a more isotropic permeability in degenerated discs[81] (Box 13-1).

With the compromised material properties demonstrated in degenerative models, abnormal motion segments are to be

BOX 13-1. Physical Properties of the Degenerated Disc

Nucleus Pulposus

Shear modulus: eightfold increase

Swelling pressure: significantly decreased

Anulus Fibrosus

Poisson's ratio: decreased

Hydraulic permeability: increasingly isotropic

From Iatridis J, Maclean J, Roughley P, et al: Effects of mechanical loading on intervertebral disc metabolism in vivo. *J Bone Joint Surg [Am]* 88(Suppl 2):41, 2006.

expected and have been demonstrated in cadaveric models.[82] These studies suggest that early human disc degeneration and the changing physical properties of the disc may affect the overall mechanical function of the spine, leading to altered dynamics and increased intradiscal pressure as well as increased internal stress and strain patterns on the disc, which ultimately may contribute to further disc degeneration.[82-84]

Etiology of Disc Degeneration

We have discussed the basic components of the disc and the structural and biochemical changes that occur with disc degeneration; in the following sections, we examine the etiology of disc degeneration. As recently as the 1990s, the general belief was that age, sex, occupation, cigarette smoking, and vibration were the leading contributory factors to disc degeneration.[85] Ironically, the contributions of height, weight, and genetics were less certain. Monozygotic twin studies performed over the past two decades have, however, provided tremendous insight into the etiology of disc degeneration and have strongly suggested that environmental and constitutional risk factors are only minor contributors to disc degeneration. Variations in disc degeneration can instead largely be explained by genetic factors.[85-87]

Even with the insight monozygotic twin studies have provided into the importance of the genetic contribution to disc degeneration, there is still a large amount of variation in the process that remains to be explained. This variation is probably the result of a complex, multifactorial set of gene-gene and gene-environment interactions that will not be amenable to linear regression modeling.[85,88,89] The following sections discuss the proposed genetic and environmental influences on disc degeneration.

Genetic Influences

In 1995, Battié et al.[86] published a study on the determinants of lumbar disc degeneration in which they looked at risk factors for disc degeneration in monozygotic male twins discordant for suspected environmental risk factors. Their findings provided strong support for the hypothesis that disc degeneration could largely be explained by a combination of genetic influences and still unidentified factors, which may represent complex, unpredictable genetic or other interactions. When looking at the upper lumbar region, they found that physical loading could explain only 7% of the variability in degeneration summary scores. Age could explain an additional 9%, but genetics could explain 61% of the variability. In the lower lumbar region, physical loading could explain 2%, age 7%, and genetics 34% of the variability.

With twin studies suggesting a strong genetic component to disc degeneration, further investigation to characterize the genetic influence on disc disease followed. At present, uncertainty remains as to whether a single gene has a predominant effect on disc degeneration or if degeneration is due to the smaller influence of many genes. Osteoarthritis, a similar degenerative condition of the musculoskeletal system, is considered to be an oligogenic, multifactorial genetic disease; disc degeneration is likely to be as well.[85,90]

To date, several gene loci have been identified as associated with disc degeneration or related pathology.[91] These associations have been identified predominantly with small sample sizes and there has been significant variation in phenotypic definition. Despite small sample sizes and the challenges of phenotypic definition, there currently exists reasonable reproducible evidence among different ethnic populations to suggest the association of disc degeneration with the vitamin D receptor gene (*VDR*), the collagen IX genes (*COL9A2*, *COL9A3*), and the metalloproteinase-3 gene (*MMP3*).[91] Despite their well-documented associations with disc degeneration, each of these genes has demonstrated only modest effects, suggesting that the most significant genetic susceptibilities have yet to be identified.[91]

The genetic contributions studied most frequently thus far relate to the biologic processes associated with matrix morphology, synthesis, and degradation, and the collagenous structures of the disc.[85,91] Despite these probable genetic contributions to disc degeneration, other mechanisms and risk factors for disc degeneration likely exist. In recent studies by Videman et al.,[92,93] some of the physical characteristics with genetic correlations were evaluated, including body height, weight, fat content, axial disc area, isokinetic lifting performance, and lifetime routine physical activities at work and leisure. Body weight, lifting strength, and axial disc area were more highly associated with disc degeneration than occupational and leisure physical activities, although all of them had minor influences on disc degeneration. In addition, higher body mass, greater lifting strength, and heavier work were all associated with increased disc height narrowing but less disc desiccation, confusing the matter. Smaller discs also appeared to have beneficial effects in these studies.

Videman et al.[92,93] demonstrated the complexity of the genetic contribution to disc degeneration. As genetic research continues, gene-gene and gene-environment interactions will continue to be discovered, and a complete understanding of this complex process will be difficult to attain. For this reason, linear regression models will probably fail to capture the complexity of genetic influence on disc degeneration, and more advanced analytic techniques will be required.[85,89] A summary of the major gene loci that have been associated with intervertebral disc degeneration is given in Table 13-6.

TABLE 13-6

Verified Gene Associated with Disc Degeneration

Gene	Effect
Taq1 tt genotype of vitamin D receptor	Increased disc desiccation Increased anular tears
Taq1 TT genotype of vitamin D receptor	Increased disc bulging Increased osteophytes
Taq1 and *Fok1* genotypes of vitamin D receptor	Increased bulging and disc height
Taq polymorphisms	Increased severity of osteophytosis Disc narrowing
5A5A and *5A6A* gentoypes of *MMP3* gene	More degenerative findings than with the *6A6A* genotype
COL9A2 and *COL9A3*	Collagen IX genes associated with disc pathology and symptoms

From Battié M, Videman T, Parent E: Lumbar disc degeneration: epidemiology and genetic influences. *Spine (Phila Pa 1976)* 29:2679, 2004.

Nutritional Influences

Significant evidence exists to suggest a nutritional contribution to disc degeneration.[5,30,94-96] In the young disc, as previously discussed, a vascular supply penetrates the vertebral end plate and is in close contact with the disc's cartilaginous end plate. By maturity, only small blood vessels that reach the outer 1 to 2 mm of the disc periphery are present. This decreased vascular supply is likely a large contributor to disc degeneration.[5,21]

The inevitable decreased oxygen content that follows the loss of these blood vessels may explain the loss of the notochordal cells early in life, which require higher oxygen concentrations for survival.[9] Decreasing oxygenation may also explain the increased substitution of keratan sulfate for chondroitin sulfate on aggrecan molecules, as well as leading to the increasingly glycolytic metabolism of the disc cells. In addition to the loss of the vascular supply, sclerosis of the subchondral plate negatively affects its porosity, leading to poor diffusion to the relatively avascular disc.[28,30,94,97-99]

Because of the low oxygen concentration within the disc, disc cell metabolism is anaerobic and thus consumes glucose and produces lactic acid. In low glucose states, the disc cells will eventually die. In addition, when cell pH drops below 6.4, cellular viability is compromised.[28] In low pH states, cellular homeostasis is altered and a catabolic state is favored.[28] Cell matrix production is inhibited while production of MMPs continues.[100] These conditions, coupled with the decreased capability to diffuse lactic acid and other waste products, are thought to contribute to disc degeneration. Decreased diffusion also leads to difficulty with removal of degraded proteoglycans from the disc, both stiffening the disc structure and negatively affecting its ability to produce the swelling pressures necessary to function properly.[9]

Further support is garnered for the nutritional contribution to disc degeneration in specific pathologic states such as atherosclerotic disease, avascular necrosis due to decompression sickness, Gaucher disease, and nicotine exposure, which are all detrimental to the local blood supply to the vertebral body. The capillaries of the vertebral end plate in these disease states are narrowed and eventually blocked. This inhibits the transport of oxygen and other nutrients to the disc as well as limits the escape of lactic acid and proteolytic degradation products from the disc.[28,101,102]

Mechanical Influences

The mechanical influence on the metabolic state of the disc has long been debated. Occupational medicine literature has favored the catabolic effects of occupational loading on the intervertebral disc, whereas the sports and exercise physiology literature has often viewed mechanical loading of the disc as beneficial and anabolic.[86,103-109] Monozygotic twin studies have also revealed that variations in mechanical loading of the spine play a relatively small role in explaining variations in disc degeneration.[86] Over the past decade, the concept of the "threshold of stimuli" has developed, which may partially explain the possible anabolic and catabolic effects seen with disc loading at various magnitudes and frequencies.[77,110,111]

With this concept in mind, multiple small rodent studies have been conducted that have shown anabolic effects when tail discs have been loaded within a certain threshold, including increased messenger RNA expression, increased up-regulation of disc proteins, increased matrix production, and down-regulation of proteolytic enzymes. Outside the threshold of loading ranges (i.e., too little or too great a stimulus), negative effects are seen.[78,110,111]

The intervertebral disc experiences substantial forces and frequent loading on a daily basis, including fluid and osmotic pressures, interstitial fluid flow, and compressive, tensile, and shear stresses. These almost constant forces place a significant mechanical demand on the disc and have been thought to contribute to the tissue failure—anular and nuclear tears, as well as end plate damage—associated with disc aging and degeneration.[109]

Significant injury to the intervertebral disc has been associated with catastrophic disc overload.[78,112-114] In cadaver models, when the motion-restricting effect of the facet joints is removed by facetectomy, torsional stress on the anulus results in posterolateral anular tears that radiate centrally. Changes such as disc narrowing, anular fissuring, and nuclear migration have all been seen in this setting. Although disc overload has been shown to lead to significant damage to the disc, it remains uncertain whether the daily wear and tear associated with normal physiologic loads leads to increased degneneration.[23,115,116]

In an effort to evaluate the daily stresses experienced by the intervertebral disc and to assess the cumulative injury model, a recent monozygotic twin study was conducted by Videman et al. on twins with an 8-kg or greater weight discordance.[92] They discovered that higher body mass was not harmful to the intervertebral disc. In fact, the higher body mass actually resulted in a slight delay in lumbar disc desiccation. These findings significantly challenge the common belief that increased weight and the resulting increased loading of the intervertebral disc lead to increased disc degeneration. The findings of this study support the notion that "physical activity strengthens both the vertebrae and the discs,"[117] and are also supportive of the threshold of stimuli model.[93]

Whole-body vibration has been incriminated in the pathogenesis of disc degeneration in the past. Both animal and in vitro studies have suggested a negative impact of vibration on the disc.[23] Epidemiologic studies have also provided evidence to suggest that vibration plays a negative role in disc health.[23,118-120] Data also suggest that helicopter pilots, truck drivers, and tractor operators have a high rate of back pain.[23,121-124] Despite these findings, a monozygotic twin spine study has called into question the effect of whole-body vibration on disc degeneration. The study, performed by Battié et al.,[85,125] arguably the best-controlled study to date evaluating this variable, found no evidence to suggest that whole-body vibration led to accelerated disc degeneration.

Toxic Exposure

The most common toxic exposure suggested to contribute to early disc degeneration is smoking. Nicotine has both direct and indirect negative effects on the disc. Indirectly, nicotine has been shown in a rabbit model to reduce the density of the vascular buds as well as narrow the vascular lumina to the vertebrae, resulting in decreased nutrient diffusion and necrosis and hyalinization of the nucleus pulposus.[126] Nicotine has also been shown in in vitro and animal studies directly to affect the cellular and matrix components of the disc by decreasing the production of collagen and proteoglycans and inhibiting cell proliferation.[127,128] In addition, an increased level of IL-1 and other inflammatory cytokines has been shown in animal discs.[129] Despite the convincing in vitro evidence to suggest the negative role that nicotine plays in the degenerating disc, monozygotic twin studies have demonstrated only a small effect of long-term cigarette smoking in disc degeneration. The total variance explained by long-term smoking in the lumbar spine was less than 2%.[86]

Disc Degeneration and Back Pain

It is well accepted that the degenerated disc can lead to secondarily painful states such as disc herniation, nerve root impingement, deformity, and spinal stenosis.[49,130] What has been more controversial has been the notion of the disc itself as the primary source of pain. Multiple imaging studies support the concept that disc degeneration is asymptomatic in many individuals yet painful in others.[7,49,131,132] This evidence suggests that the painful degenerative disc process differs from asymptomatic degeneration and may be more related to unique biochemical changes than the morphologic changes evident on imaging (Box 13-2; see Fig. 13-5).

The concept that a disc is capable of producing painful stimuli assumes that the disc is innervated. The healthy adult disc is only peripherally innervated by mechanoreceptors, which are thought to take part in proprioception. Innervation is limited to the outer anulus, where substance P-producing nociceptors have been found that are potentially involved with inflammatory pain.[18,133,134] The bony vertebral end plate is also innervated and is likely also involved in primary disc pain.[135] Evidence to support end plate pain perception has been provided by pain resolution after vertebroplasty as well as by pain provocation tests in humans.[19,136] In degenerated discs in which anular tears attempt to heal by formation of granulation tissue, neovascularization as well as neoinnervation spread into the planes of tissue damage, thus providing the degenerated disc with additional innervation.[14,137-141] Nerve growth factor is also up-regulated at this time and may actually lower the disc's threshold to noxious stimuli.[142-144] This increased density of nerve fibers along with a lower threshold to noxious stimuli may contribute to painful disc degeneration.

Growing evidence also suggests that the presence of inflammatory cytokines may be the distinguishing factor between nonpainful and painful disc degeneration. IL-1, IL-6, IL-9, and TNF-α have all been measured in degenerating human discs and have been associated with pain.[48,49] The mechanism and reason for their elevation in the pathologic state are unknown. Animal models have shown, however, that after acute loading or injury a short-term inflammatory cascade is initiated as a part of the healing process. This proinflammatory status usually lasts approximately 1 to 3 weeks, depending on the severity of the injury. When chronic aberrant loading or a pathologic stimulus is present, however, a more persistent inflammatory state arises.[48,52] This prolonged inflammation has been seen in animal tail stab models and has been shown to produce Modic changes in the adjacent vertebrae in the presence of a prolonged inflammatory cascade.[48] In addition to its destructive modulation, the proinflammatory response may be responsible for pain sensitization through production of cytokines and mediators such as prostaglandin E2, IL-6, and IL-8.[53,54,145]

BOX 13-2. Potential Protein Therapies for Intervertebral Disc Degeneration

Growth Factors
Transforming growth factor beta (TGF-β)
Bone morphogenetic proteins (BMPs)
Insulin-like growth factor-1 (IGF-1)
Fibroblast growth factor (FGF)
Growth and differentiation factor-5 (GDF-5)
Epidermal growth factor (EGF)

Cytokine Antagonists
Interleukin-1 receptor antagonist (IL-1Ra)
Tumor necrosis factor alpha (TNF-α) antagonists

Proteinase Inhibitors
Tissue inhibitor of matrix metalloproteinase (TIMP)

Intracellular Regulators
Sox9
Link protein N-terminal peptide
SMADs
LIM mineralization protein (LMP-1)

From Fassett DR, Kurd MF, Vaccaro AR: Biologic solutions for degenerative disk disease. *J Spinal Disord Tech* 22:297, 2009.

Future Treatment for Intervertebral Disc Degeneration

Current treatment strategies in spine surgery are mainly reactive and their goal is to alleviate the pain associated with the pathologic changes resulting from disc degeneration. Advanced clinical therapies, however, are undergoing intensive research. These therapies aim to treat intervertebral disc degeneration at the genetic, cellular, and molecular levels. The goal of these therapies is to stop the progression of disc degeneration, restore the disc to a normal biochemical composition, recreate the normal biomechanical properties of a healthy disc, and maintain disc homeostasis.

The potential advantages of these treatments are numerous, including the preservation of normal anatomy, maintenance of normal biomechanics, and conservation of normal motion segments.[146] One of the key concerns with these therapies, however, remains the lack of vascularity and nutrition to an already degenerating disc.[28,147] Molecular, genetic, and cellular therapies all require the presence of healthy nuclear cells or the ability to sustain these cells after implantation in order to produce matrix and prevent further degeneration.

The majority of the current molecular, genetic, and cellular studies do not seem to consider the avascular and austere physiologic status of the disc, which may lead to unfavorable results in vivo. One possible way of dealing with the lack of nutrition and low metabolic rate of disc cells would be to focus on decreasing the catabolic influences within the disc. This would require less energy and less cellular activity, yet still decrease disc degeneration.[148]

Molecular Therapies

In an effort to promote an anabolic state in the disc, various growth factors have been tested in animal studies and have shown the capability to increase cellular proliferation, up-regulate proteoglycan and collagen production, and increase disc height.[146,149-153] The potential for a number of select growth factors to reverse degenerative disc changes has been reproducibly demonstrated in animal studies.[146,154-156] The catabolic influences on the degenerating disc have also been addressed by the use cytokine inhibitors in an effort to down-regulate the proinflammatory cytokines TNF-α and IL-1 and shift the disc to a more anabolic state.[146,157] Proteinase antagonists such as TIMPs also inhibit the breakdown of proteoglycans and may serve a role in future molecular therapy.[146]

Although early in vivo and in vitro studies have suggested a tremendous potential for these molecular therapies, the half-life of most of these molecules is relatively short.[146] For these therapies to be clinically effective, repeated infusions or a long-term delivery device will likely be needed. For this reason, genetic therapy, with its ability to increase the translation of desired molecules, may prove more promising in the future (see Box 13-2).

Genetic Therapies

Genetic therapy transfers an exogenous gene into a cell along with a promoter in order to induce the translation of a desired target protein. Genetic therapy has the potential to overcome the major problem with molecular-based growth factor treatments by using existing disc cells to create a continuous, prolonged production of a desired protein.[146] Genetic transfer has been performed most frequently using a viral vector, which for safety reasons has been the key limiting step in genetic therapy. Genes encoding for key anabolic growth factors and catabolic antagonists have been successfully transferred to disc cells using viral vectors, resulting in an improved anabolic state.[146,158-161] Despite these promising results, the key challenge remains the safety of genetic transfer. Adenoviral vector transfer has been associated with death and life-threatening immune reactions.[146,162-164] Alternative, nonviral methods of genetic transfer are under investigation and may play a key role in the future.[148,165-168]

Cellular Therapies

Cellular therapies attempt to address the primary disadvantage of molecular and genetic therapies, which is the common lack of viable cells in the disc because of its degenerative state. In the absence of viable, healthy disc cells, molecular and genetic therapies will not work. Although the transplantation of new cells into the disc may solve this dilemma, the continued nutrition and survival of these cells remains a significant challenge.[28,147] Cell-based therapies have used both allograft and autograft nucleus pulposus cells, as well as a variety of stem cells, to regenerate discs. All three cell types have been successfully used in in vivo animal studies, resulting in improved disc biochemical profiles.[146,169]

In addition to these animal studies, one human clinical trial is underway in Europe investigating the role of autologous disc cell reimplantation 12 weeks after microdiscectomy and culture. Interim results were recently reported, indicating that 29 patients with 2 years of follow-up had improved clinical outcomes and visual analogue scores and less disc desiccation, but no difference in disc height. Although these results are encouraging, there is concern regarding the study because it is not blinded and a significant placebo effect may be detrimental to the study conclusions.[146,170,171]

Stem cell transplantation has also seen a surge in research interest. Multiple stem cell lineages have been studied, but mesenchymal stem cells have become the most popular owing to ethical concerns with fetal/embryonic stem cells, and their ready availability. Although good outcomes with in vivo animal studies using stem cells have been demonstrated, only one nonrandomized, uncontrolled study using autologous hematopoietic stem cells has been performed, which revealed no significant improvement in low back pain after treatment.[146,172] One of the most significant challenges facing this technology is that the exact phenotype of the chondrocyte-like cells of the disc is not fully understood and, as such, it is currently impossible to reproduce these cells exactly.[146,169]

Summary

The enormous scale of the disability and cost associated with the loss of productivity and the treatment of pathology resulting from degenerating discs underscores the importance of understanding disc physiology and pathology. The structure and function of the intervertebral disc have been intensively studied and are relatively well understood. The key cellular and biochemical components of the disc and their rapid change with aging and degeneration have been documented and routinely accepted. The nutritional deterioration due to the loss of the disc's direct vascular supply and resulting in a cascade of changes and likely degeneration has been well demonstrated with gross and histologic studies. The complex interplay of growth factors and catabolic mediators, as well as the key histologic, cellular, and biomechanical changes that accompany the degenerative process, continue to be elucidated. In the past decade, the paramount role of genetics and the lesser importance of environmental risk factors in disc degeneration have been discovered.

The internal processes and mechanics of disc degeneration may be partially understood, but the key initiating factors and the interactions of the various processes, including nutritional, molecular, cellular, genetic, inflammatory, and environmental influences, as well as why the disc begins degenerating almost immediately after birth, are poorly understood. Despite our relatively poor understanding of these interactions and the key factors promoting degeneration, research in molecular, genetic, and cellular therapies has rapidly advanced and provides a promising outlook for combating these degenerative changes in the future. Despite the significant challenges facing investigators in translating research into successful clinical treatments, the increasing amount of research in these fields as well as our improved understanding of disc physiology and pathology suggest that significant laboratory and clinical progress may be seen in the very near future.

KEY REFERENCES

Battié MC, Videman T, Gibbons LE, et al: 1995 Volvo Award in clinical sciences. Determinants of lumbar disc degeneration: a study relating lifetime exposures and magnetic resonance imaging findings in identical twins. *Spine (Phila Pa 1976)* 20:2601, 1995.

Battié MC, Videman T, Kaprio J, et al: The Twin Spine Study: contributions to a changing view of disc degeneration. *Spine J* 9:47, 2009.

Boos N, Weissbach S, Rohrbach H, et al: Classification of age-related changes in lumbar intervertebral discs: 2002 Volvo Award in basic science. *Spine (Phila Pa 1976)* 27:2631, 2002.

Roughley P: Biology of intervertebral disc aging and degeneration: involvement of the extracellular matrix. *Spine (Phila Pa 1976)* 29:2691, 2004.

Thompson J, Oegema TJ, Bradford D: Stimulation of mature canine intervertebral disc by growth factors. *Spine (Phila Pa 1976)* 16:253, 1991.

Ulrich J, Liebenberg E, Thuillier D, et al: ISSLS prize winner: repeated disc injury causes persistent inflammation. *Spine (Phila Pa 1976)* 32:2812, 2007.

REFERENCES

The complete reference list is available online at expertconsult.com.

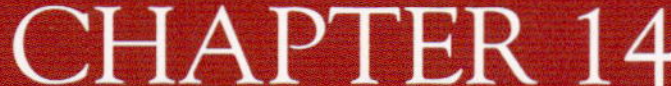

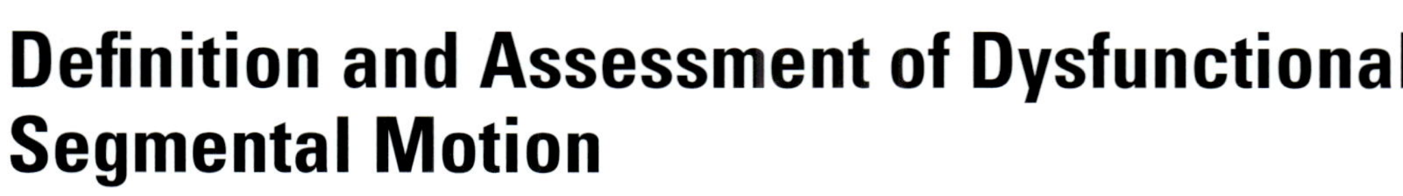

CHAPTER 14

Definition and Assessment of Dysfunctional Segmental Motion

Serkan İnceoğlu | Edward C. Benzel

Biomechanics of Stable Motion Segment

The spine is responsible for providing a smooth motion of the trunk in all planes of motion, while protecting the neural structures. The smallest unit of the spine that exhibits the biomechanical characteristics of the spinal column is termed a *motion segment* or *functional spinal unit* (FSU), and is composed of two vertebral bodies and a disc.

Normal motion of vertebral bodies relative to each other is provided by the soft connective tissue, such as the intervertebral discs and ligaments. Ligaments can only resist tensile loading owing to their fibrous hierarchical structures. Normal motion of the healthy spine is realized through the harmonic interaction of the ligaments with the unique design of gross spinal anatomy. During sagittal motion, for instance, dorsal ligaments (posterior longitudinal, capsule, interspinous, and supraspinous ligaments) are activated in flexion while the others are at rest. In extension, the anterior longitudinal ligament and, to varying degrees, the capsular ligaments, are stretched while the others are at rest.

This functional order of the ligaments is orchestrated by the center of rotation of the FSU, which is located toward the dorsal one third of the disc space in the healthy spine. The line connecting the centers of rotation for all vertebral levels is termed the *neutral axis* of the spine. A load passing through this line would theoretically cause pure compression of the spine, with no rotation and bending moment. Moreover, in flexion, ligaments dorsal to this axis would be stretched and those ventral would be lax. Similarly, in extension, ligaments ventral to this axis would be stretched and those dorsal would be lax. Any change in the location of the neutral axis would influence the function of the ligaments, and vice versa.

The contribution of the disc to spinal motion is more complex than that of the ligaments. In a healthy disc, the gel-like nucleus is filled with water, thanks to the water-trapping proteoglycans. It is nearly incompressible and is pressurized in the unloaded state. When loaded, the nucleus resists compression by pushing against the end plates and the surrounding anulus fibrosus. The anular lamellae, which are compacted and pressurized by the transverse loads exerted by the nucleus, become stiffer and capable of resisting compressive loading exerted by the vertebral bodies. With the aforementioned in mind, it is noted that the water content of the disc plays a key role in maintenance of disc height and FSU biomechanics.

Biomechanics of a Dysfunctional Motion Segment

Dysfunction of a motion segment refers to the functional state of the disc associated with pathologic or abnormal motion segment biomechanics. The most common cause of such dysfunction is disc interspace degenerative changes. With dysfunctional segmental motion, "mechanical pain" may arise. Mechanical back pain is characterized as a deep and agonizing pain that is worsened with loading and relieved with unloading. This triad (deep and agonizing, worsened by loading the spine, and improved by unloading the spine) clinically characterizes mechanical pain and represents the clinical correlate of dysfunctional segmental motion.

Degenerative changes initially influence the structural elements of the spine, particularly the disc. These changes, in turn, result in pathologic motion of the FSU. The most striking biomechanical reflection of degenerative changes is observed in the stiffness characteristics of FSU motion. The loss of water content in the nucleus pulposus results in a decreased central disc interspace pressure. This results in a less taut anulus fibrosus and a decrease in the ability of anular layers to withstand applied compressive and tensile forces. In advanced stages of the degenerative cascade, the anulus fibrosus loses its mechanical strength because of fissures and clefts in the lamellae. The overall effect of these changes is a diminution of stiffness and a resultant laxity of the FSU.

Biomechanical evaluation of the FSU is achieved mainly through cadaveric specimen studies. Much of the body of knowledge regarding spinal biomechanics is based on in vitro assessment of specimens obtained from fresh-frozen cadavers. Specimens, stripped of musculature, are loaded to predetermined bending load levels to quantify the biomechanical response of the FSU. Although limited, the in vitro analysis of FSU motion can be highly controlled and detailed. Numerous researchers studying in vitro FSU biomechanics have shown that the response of the FSU to external loading is associated with two characteristic flexibility zones: the neutral zone (NZ) and the elastic zone (EZ). The NZ is a segment of the flexibility curve within which small loads can generate large displacements. The EZ is a segment within which lesser displacements result from greater load application—without causing mechanical injury to the spine. The sum of the two zones (neutral plus elastic zones) comprises the total range of motion (ROM) of the spine under physiologic loading conditions.

It has been suggested that the width of the NZ is the best indicator of spinal instability (due either to injury or degeneration).[1-5] Panjabi et al. studied the influence of traumatic ligamentous injury on the stability of the thoracolumbar spine.[6] They demonstrated that both ROM and the NZ increased after destabilizing trauma. However, the NZ was observed to be a more sensitive indicator of instability.

Mimura et al. studied multidirectional flexibility of FSUs with a variety of degeneration grades.[7] They observed that the ROM decreased in the sagittal and lateral planes and increased in axial rotation. In addition, they noted an increase in the laxity at the joint, which was associated with the instability index (the ratio of the NZ to the ROM; i.e., the NZ ratio).

Tanaka et al. investigated the effect of degeneration on the flexibility of 114 FSUs obtained from 47 cadaveric lumbar spines.[8] They categorized specimens in five degeneration grades based on radiographic (MRI) and cryomicrotome section analyses. All specimens were tested biomechanically for flexion, extension, lateral bending, and axial rotation. Rotations and translations were recorded. Both techniques seemed to be in an agreement regarding the advanced stages of degeneration, more so than for early stages. The investigators did not report any data regarding the NZ, but did demonstrate that the upper lumbar FSUs were associated with a significantly increased ROM (in rotations and translations) during sagittal bending and axial rotation as the degeneration progressed toward grade IV. ROM decreased at the grade V level. For the lower lumbar FSUs, ROM increased up to the grade III level of degeneration, followed by a decrease at grades IV and V. This observation was statistically significant only during axial rotation and lateral bending.

Schmidt et al. investigated the stiffness of cadaveric lumbar motion segments with radial tears in discs detected by MRI and cryomicrotome sections under sagittal, lateral, and axial rotations.[9] They used normal control specimens ($n = 4$) and degenerated specimens ($n = 16$) with radial tears in the anulus. Specimens with radial tears exhibited loss of stiffness at varying degrees in all planes of motion.

Zhao et al. studied the effect of the depressurized nucleus fibrosus with end plate disruption on FSU motion characteristics.[10] Twenty-one thoracolumbar motion segments, of which four were normal, were studied. Sixteen specimens had pre-existing moderate degeneration, and one had pre-existing severe degeneration. All specimens were tested for bending motion using an *eccentric* (i.e., off-axis) axial loading mechanism. The investigators loaded the specimen in creep (i.e., prolonged exposure to a constant load) to remove the water content from the nucleus and then loaded the specimen in compression-to-failure to generate end plate disruption, which simulated advanced degeneration. They monitored their procedures by pressure measurements within the disc. The comparison of the flexibility tests before and after the degeneration-inducing maneuvers demonstrated that there were substantial increases in NZ and ROM as well as the instability index (NZ/ROM) in flexion and lateral bending.

Fujiwara et al. studied the effects of disc degeneration and facet joint osteoarthritis on the segmental flexibility of the lumbar spine.[11] They graded the degeneration (grades I to V) of 110 lumbar motion segments obtained from 19 female and 25 male cadavers using MRI films and biomechanical tests. They observed an increase in ROM in axial rotation, flexion, and extension as the degeneration advanced (grades II to IV), followed by a decrease at degeneration grade V. In lateral bending, ROM increased at grade III and decreased in more advanced levels. This observation was true for both sexes.

Gay et al. studied the effect of degeneration on spinal flexibility during stepwise loading and continuous loading conditions in an in vitro evaluation.[12] The NZ and ROM have been observed to be larger with stepwise loading compared with continuous loading.[13] The effect of degeneration on spinal flexibility had not previously been studied for both assessment techniques in the same experimental model. Gay et al. demonstrated that the NZ and ROM, assessed using both stepwise and continuous loading techniques, showed a trend similar to that observed with macroscopic evaluation of disc degeneration. In other words, spinal flexibility increased with degeneration up to grade III and decreased at grade IV.

Oxland et al. investigated the relationship between bone density, disc degeneration, and flexibility in cadaveric spinal specimens.[14] They demonstrated a significant increase in ROM in axial rotation, as well as a significant decrease in the NZ in lateral bending, as the degeneration grade increased. There were no significant changes observed in ROM and NZ associated with degeneration level during sagittal motion. In this study, the investigators used axial loading during bending testing to simulate muscle forces, which may have influenced the alterations of the NZ.

There are ample data supporting the destructive effect of degeneration on spinal stability (at least at the early stages of the degeneration cascade). Evidence, however, is lacking regarding characterization of NZ and ROM behavior changes that occur with degeneration, despite strong theoretical foundations. The causes of this deficiency may lie in the variation in biomechanical testing protocols from laboratory to laboratory, the subjectivity associated with grading degeneration, and the adaptive changes in the FSU in response to disc degeneration.

In Vivo Assessment of Three-Dimensional Functional Spinal Unit Kinematics

In addition to the aforementioned limitations associated with the assessment and characterization of the NZ and ROM, an intrinsic deficiency of in vitro biomechanical testing is the fact that muscle forces cannot be accurately reproduced. Therefore, the natural motion of the spine is not properly reproduced in the laboratory setting. Thanks to developments in technology, the detailed in vivo assessment of three-dimensional (3D) spinal kinematics has become feasible and popular.

External markers that are percutaneously attached to the pedicles or spinous processes have been used to assess spinal motion in vivo. Rozumalski et al. analyzed the motion of the lumbar spine during walking with markers attached to the spinous processes of 10 healthy subjects.[15] They reported intervertebral rotations in all planes during walking. Dickey et al.

investigated the correlation of pain and vertebral motion in patients with chronic low back pain using external fixators attached to the pedicles.[16] Although these techniques have produced invaluable data, they have not gained wide acceptance because of patient-associated risks and pain.

MRI provides a noninvasive technology for researchers to analyze in vivo spinal kinematics. Fujii et al. measured intervertebral motion in the lumbar spine in 10 healthy subjects. They applied passive trunk rotations using a rotation device tightly strapped to the pelvis, while the shoulders were fixed.[17] They measured lumbar 3D kinematics from neutral to maximum position with 15-degree passive pelvic axial rotation increments. Each step required a 5-minute imaging time. The researchers successfully measured the intervertebral rotations and translations in all planes. The main shortcoming of the study was the fact that the fixed axis of rotation of the device was not designed to be coaxial with that of the subject's spine. This could result in non-natural rotation.

A dual-fluoroscopy approach has also been used to quantify the 3D kinematics of the human spine. Although this technique is associated with radiation exposure to the subject, it is otherwise noninvasive and allows unrestricted normal motion of the trunk. Li et al. studied the intervertebral motion of the lumbar spine in all planes in 11 asymptomatic subjects.[18] 3D reconstructed images of subjects in neutral posture were registered with images obtained with using dual fluoroscopy during sagittal, axial, and lateral motions. They reported rotations and translations in all planes.

Ahmadi et al. analyzed the kinematics of lumbar motion in patients with lumbar segmental instability using video-assisted fluoroscopy.[19] They compared 15 matched healthy subjects with patients with chronic low back pain who were diagnosed with lumbar instability according to the clinical test of Hicks et al.[20] The authors reported significant differences in intersegmental sagittal translations at the L5-S1 level. They also showed that the instant axis of rotation moved in a larger area for patients with low back pain compared with healthy control subjects at both the L1-2 and L5-S1 levels.

Passias et al. recently compared in vivo lumbar segmental motion between patients with low back pain and healthy control subjects.[21] All patients with low back pain had pathology at the L4-5 and L5-S1 discs, which was confirmed clinically and radiographically. Significant differences were observed between the degenerative and control group ROMs at the L3-4 disc in lateral bending and axial rotation, and at the L4-5 disc in flexion.

Although assessment of the effect of degeneration on FSU motion would be best accomplished by in vivo studies, the quality and extent of the data that can be obtained in vivo are not as great as in in vitro analyses. Moreover, assessment of the extent of disc degeneration is an important factor inhibiting a fair comparison of the data in the literature.

Nevertheless, it is apparent that changes in spinal flexibility (i.e., ROM) increase at degenerated levels, as shown in both in vitro and in vivo studies. With future advances in technology, researchers will most certainly be able to categorize the quality and quantity of these changes in relation to degeneration and pain. Such advances will greatly assist surgeons in the surgical decision-making process.

KEY REFERENCES

Fujiwara A, Lim TH, An HS, et al: The effect of disc degeneration and facet joint osteoarthritis on the segmental flexibility of the lumbar spine. *Spine (Phila Pa 1976)* 25:3036–3044, 2000.

Mimura M, Panjabi MM, Oxland TR, et al: Disc degeneration affects the multidirectional flexibility of the lumbar spine. *Spine (Phila Pa 1976)* 19:1371–1380, 1994.

Oxland TR, Lund T, Jost B, et al: The relative importance of vertebral bone density and disc degeneration in spinal flexibility and interbody implant performance: an in vitro study. *Spine (Phila Pa 1976)* 21:2558–2569, 1996.

Panjabi MM: The stabilizing system of the spine: Part II. Neutral zone and instability hypothesis. *J Spinal Disord* 5:390–396, 1992.

Tanaka N, An HS, Lim TH, et al: The relationship between disc degeneration and flexibility of the lumbar spine. *Spine J* 1:47–56, 2001.

Yue JJ, Timm JP, Panjabi MM, et al: Clinical application of the Panjabi neutral zone hypothesis: the Stabilimax NZ posterior lumbar dynamic stabilization system. *Neurosurg Focus* 22:E12, 2007.

REFERENCES

The complete reference list is available online at expertconsult.com.

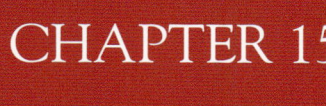

CHAPTER 15

Bone Modeling and Remodeling

Fernando Techy

The structure and composition of bone provide it with excellent failure resistance while retaining relatively low mass. These are close to ideal properties for its function within the musculoskeletal system. Even though frequently perceived as an inert material, bone is an extremely live tissue with extensive remodeling activity in response to injuries or simple wear due to everyday stresses. Its high metabolic activity plays a fundamental role in the body's mineral homeostasis, and yet it gives bone a unique characteristic among tissues: the ability to heal without scar formation.

This chapter discusses bone structure, cells, and extracellular matrix, the mechanical and chemical stimulants and inhibitors of bone activity, and the interaction among these components that leads to bone formation and remodeling both in physiologic situations and in response to injury.

Types of Bone

Based on general shape, bones can be classified into three groups: short, flat, and long or tubular. The femur, tibia, and phalanges are examples of long bones. Tubular or long bones have an expanded metaphysis and an epiphysis at either end of a thick cortical wall diaphysis.[1] The shaft (diaphysis) is responsible for withstanding primarily torsional and bending stresses, whereas the metaphyseal portion, with its greater deformation under the same load, has become specialized in absorbing impact to protect the articular cartilage.[1-3]

Short bones, such as the vertebral bodies and tarsal and carpal bones, measure approximately the same length in all dimensions and are roughly cuboid in shape, with slight variations. They are all mainly composed of loose trabecular bone, like the metaphysis of the long bones. The main function of this bone aggregate is, again, absorbing the body's weight. The carpals and tarsals have very thin cortices,[1] whereas the vertebral bodies have a thin shell of compact trabecular bone with no true cortical structure.[3]

The iliac crests, the skull vault, and the vertebral laminae are examples of flat bones.

Long and short bones ossify using a previously formed cartilage model (endochondral ossification), whereas flat bones form from the condensation and mineralization of loose mesenchymal tissue (intramembranous ossification).[3,4] A third type of ossification that occurs when osteoblasts line the periosteum of an existing bone surface and start secreting osteoid in layers, hence making the bone thicker, is termed *appositional*.[3-6]

Immature bone is woven.[1,3,4,7,8] It is found in the embryonic skeleton, fracture callus, and bone neoplasms. It is less organized, weaker, and more flexible, and has increased turnover compared with mature bone. Woven bone does not have the ability to remodel following the stress pattern.[1,3,4]

Mature bone is lamellar.[1,3,4,7,8] Lamellar bone is stress oriented, stronger, and less flexible, and has slower turnover compared with woven bone.[1,3,4] There are two different types of lamellar bone: cortical (compact) and cancellous (spongy or trabecular).[1,3,4,8-12] Even though cortical and cancellous bone have the same structure and composition, their mechanical properties are very different because of their differences in density and distribution.[9,13] Cancellous bone is 50% to 90% porous, whereas cortical bone has a porosity of approximately 10%. This difference in density makes cortical bone 10 times stronger in compression than the trabecular variant.[8,14-16]

Cortical bone, composed of tightly packed osteons, makes up 80% of the skeleton.[1,4,10] Trabecular bone has a surface area per unit volume approximately 20 times that of cortical bone. Almost all of its cells lie between lamellae or on the surface of trabeculae, in close contact with the bone marrow, which makes them much more metabolically active than the cortical bone cells surrounded by bone matrix.[9,17]

Bone Formation

The formation and maintenance of the skeleton require that bone be produced constantly. Osteoblasts fabricate bone in response to many stimuli and under different conditions, including growth, physiologic remodeling, fracture healing, and heterotopic ossification.[18-20] Several studies have also shown that new bone is formed in response to tumors and infections.[21-24] It has been shown that osteoblasts have the ability to form bone during distraction osteogenesis,[25-31] depositing new bone in the void initially filled by autologous or allogenic bone graft, demineralized bone matrix, or synthetic bone substitutes. In anterior cervical discectomy and fusion (ACDF) and plating, a 97.5% rate of fusion with new bone formation has been achieved with either autograft or allograft.[32] In a recent study, Jensen et al. showed an 86% union rate after single- and multiple-level ACDF using patellar allograft and plating.[33] In a study from Japan, Momma et al. reported complete bone remodeling on CT scan 6 to 12 months after the use of β-tricalcium phosphate to fill a partial vertebrectomy defect created for cervical decompression surgery.[34]

Vertebral Bone Formation

Because the vertebrae are short bones, they ossify through endochondral ossification.[3-5] The process begins with the concentration of undifferentiated cells that transform into chondrocytes and secrete a hyaline or hyaline-like cartilaginous matrix.[5,6,10,35,36] The chondrocytes enlarge and vascular buds invade the cartilage, bringing other progenitor cells that differentiate into osteoblasts that in turn start forming bone on the cartilaginous frame. Osteoclasts then reabsorb the ossified cartilage and immature bone. Osteoblasts finally fill this space with mature lamellar bone.[3-5]

Ossification Centers of the Vertebrae

By the sixth gestational week, centers of cartilage formation (chondrification) develop in each vertebra. Two chondrification centers develop in each half of the central vertebral body. A hemivertebra occurs when these centers fail to form in one side of the vertebral body. Centers of cartilage formation also develop in each half of the vertebral arches. Next, cartilaginous transverse and spinous processes develop from the primitive arches.[37] It has been shown that bone morphogenetic protein 4 is required for the development of the cartilaginous spinous process.[38]

The primary ossification centers develop in utero. In the vertebra, three primary centers form around the eighth week of gestation. One is located in the center of the body and one in each vertebral arch. Bone forms on the pre-existing vertebral cartilage template.[3-5,37] Primary ossification begins in the lower thoracic spine, then progresses in the cranial and caudal directions.[39] The five secondary centers of ossification develop after birth: one at the tip of the spinous process, one at the tip of each transverse process, and one anular center at the ventral portion of the superior and inferior end plates. They start to ossify at approximately 15 to 16 years of age and fuse with the remaining osseous vertebra by the middle of the third decade of life.[37,40]

Bone Modeling and Remodeling

In general, *modeling* alludes to bone turnover that alters the shape of the bone, whereas *remodeling* is the turnover that recycles bone without changing its shape. Bone turnover approaches 100% during the first year of life.[41] Most of the bone turnover during skeletal growth derives from modeling. After the completion of skeletal growth, bone turnover results primarily from remodeling. Bone modeling and remodeling are the end results of the activity of a vast array of cells that work in harmony to create bone while maintaining the body's mineral homeostasis.[3-5,10]

Bone Modeling during Growth

During growth, coordinated osteal resorption and formation change the size and shape of bone.[17] The physes grow and make the bone longer and narrower. The metaphysis also changes its shape, becoming narrower to match the rest of the bone. Appositional periosteal ossification increases the diaphysial diameter.[5] At the same time, the cortices becomes thinner and the medullary canal larger owing to intensified bone resorption on the endosteal side.[42,43]

Physiologic Bone Remodeling after Growth

Throughout life, in situ removal and replacement of bone take place without changing bone form or density. Remodeling occurs on both the surface and the interior of the bone (internal remodeling). Both processes basically start with osteoclast activation. Internal remodeling commences with osteoclasts reabsorbing bone by cutting conical spaces through old osteonal systems.[3-5,17,44] Spindle cells, osteoblasts, and blood vessels fill the conical spaces cut by the osteoclasts. Osteoblasts deposit successive lamellae of new osteoid matrix, which will later mineralize. It takes about 50 osteoblasts to fill the cone cut by 1 osteoclast. Internal remodeling is seen in cortical bone.

Surface remodeling occurs on trabecular (which comprises most of the vertebral body), endosteal, and periosteal bone and is very similar to internal remodeling, except that instead of cutting cones, osteoclasts run on the surface of the lamellae excavating a cavity, the so-called Howship lacuna. The rest of the process resembles internal remodeling. Physiologic remodeling serves to repair damaged bone matrix as well as to maintain mineral homeostasis.[3-5]

Bone Modeling and Remodeling and the Basic Multicellular Unit

Bone modeling and remodeling are performed by the basic multicellular unit (BMU), a temporary anatomic structure comprising osteoclasts and osteoblasts that replace older packets of bone with new bone tissue.[44,45]

Osteoclasts are derived from hematopoietic stem cells. They exit the circulation close to the site to be remodeled.[45] The mononuclear hematopoietic cell's fusion into a polykaryon (immature osteoclast) requires the presence of macrophage colony-stimulating factor (M-CSF), a growth factor, and the receptor activator of nuclear factor κB ligand (RANKL), a tumor necrosis factor produced by osteoblasts.[46,47] Further differentiation of the immature osteoclast occurs under the influence of RANKL and many other genes, including the activator protein-1 (AP-1) family member c-*fos*,[48,49] microphthalmia-associated transcription factor (MITF),[50,51] and nuclear factor of activated T cells, calcineurin dependent-1 (NFAT-c1).[51,52]

The receptor on the osteoclast for RANKL is called RANK.[53] Concomitantly, another factor, also produced by stromal cells and osteoblasts, was found that inhibits the activity of RANKL; it was named osteoprotegerin (OPG).[54] OPG is a soluble decoy receptor for RANKL, and its function is to reduce osteoclastogenesis by competitively occupying the stromal RANKL binding sites on osteoclast RANK receptors.[55-57] The RANKL/OPG signaling axis provides a mechanism through which stromal cells control osteoblastic activity. Factors that exhibit a strong effect on resorption (e.g., parathyroid hormone, prostaglandins, interleukins, vitamin D, and corticosteroids) all signal to the osteoblast/stromal cell, which then appears to translate the message to

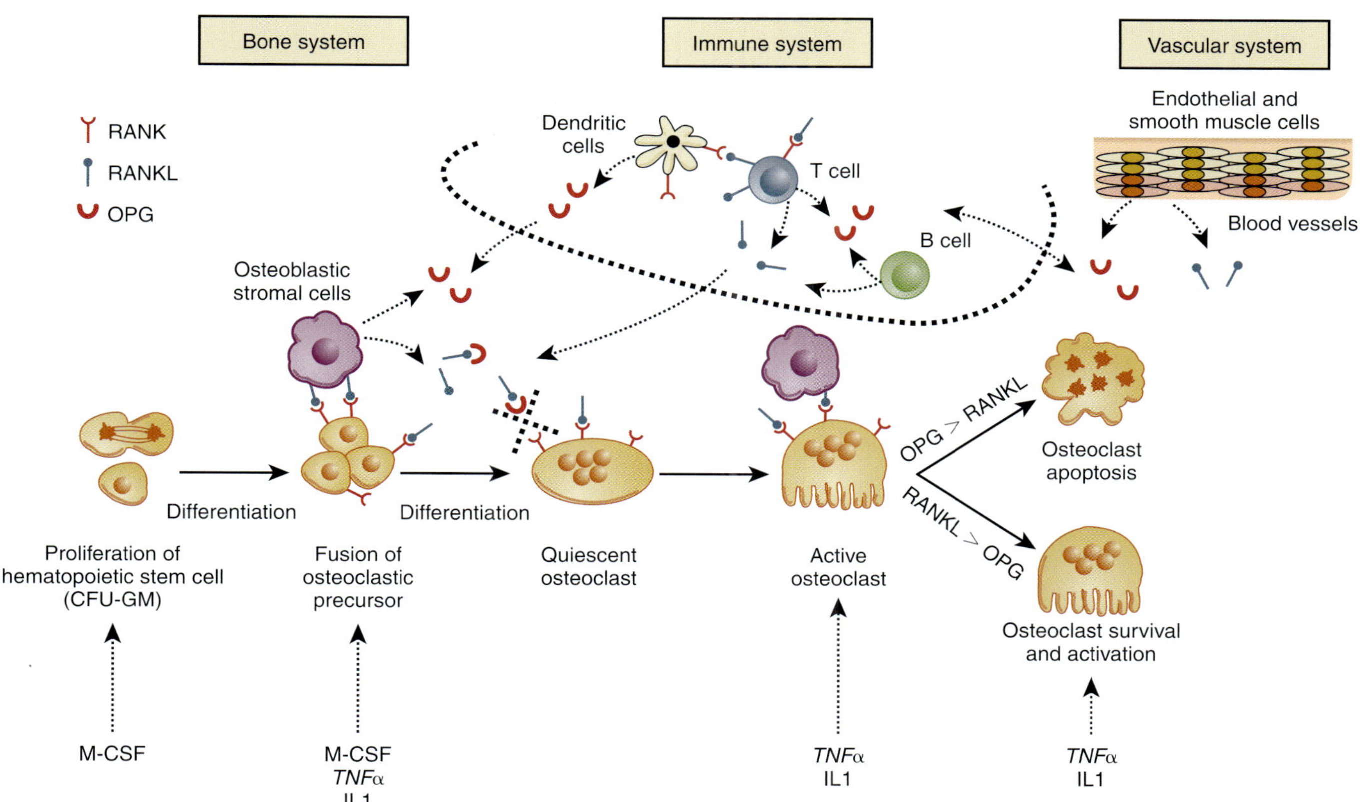

FIGURE 15-1. Osteoprotegerin (OPG), receptor activator of nuclear factor κB (RANK), and RANK ligand (RANKL) are produced selectively by numerous cell types and a variety of tissues, such as lymphocytes, osteoblasts, and endothelial cells. There are three main biologic systems where this molecular triad is particularly important, the osteoarticular, immune, and vascular systems. RANKL is not only a dendritic cell survival factor, but strongly induces osteoclastogenesis and then bone resorption through its binding to RANK. OPG inhibits osteolysis and blocks RANKL-RANK interaction. Although the OPG/RANK/RANKL triad is the main modulator of bone apposition-resorption coupling, other controls of osteoclastic differentiation also exist, such as tumor necrosis factor-α (TNF-α) and interleukin-1 (IL-1), which can modulate the biologic activities of the triad. OPG/RANKL/RANK should be considered as an osteoimmunomodulator complex. (From Theoleyre S, Wittrant Y, Kwan Tat S, et al: The molecular triad OPG/RANK/RANKL: involvement in the orchestration of pathophysiological bone remodeling. *Cytokine Growth Factor Rev* 15:457–475, 2004.)

the osteoclast through the RANKL/OPG axis.[58] The only exception to this is the hormone calcitonin, which does not use the RANKL/OPG axis, instead acting directly on the osteoclast receptors.[3,4] The mature osteoclast then engages in bone resorption by peripheral attachment to the bone matrix using the β3 integrin,[59] which creates a microcompartment between the osteoclast's ruffled basal border and the bone surface. Hydrogen ions are pumped into the compartment by the osteoclast to digest the mineral component. Next, protease is released to degrade the organic matrix[60] (Fig. 15-1).

Osteoblasts are derived from mesenchymal stem cells from the bone marrow and periosteum.[3-5,45] Expression of the transcription factors runt-related transcription factor-2 (Runx2), distal-less homeobox-5 (Dlx5), msh homeobox homologue-2 (Msx2),[61-65] and osterix (Osx), as well as activation of several components of the Wnt signaling pathway,[62,66-69] are required for osteoblastic differentiation (Fig. 15-2).

The mature osteoblast produces proteins like type I collagen, osteocalcin, and alkaline phosphatase, the latter a key enzyme in bone mineralization. Osteoblasts become entrapped in their own osteoid matrix and extrude long cytoplasmic processes to remain in contact with surrounding cells.[70] They then start expressing a whole new set of genes to continue bone turnover and maintain mineral homeostasis. These cells are now considered osteocytes, the mature bone cell[45] (Fig. 15-3).

Age-Related Bone Remodeling (Bone Loss)

Bone density changes drastically with age.[3-5,41,45,71] Peak bone mass is reached approximately 10 years after cessation of skeletal growth. Subsequently, bone mass begins to decline and reaches approximately 50% of its peak value by the eighth or ninth decade of life.[5] Men lose an average of 30% less bone mass than women in a lifetime. In women, extensive loss of bone density starts immediately after menopause and lasts for about 10 years. It is believed to be closely related to the decline in estrogen levels.[41,72-74] Trabeculae decrease more in number than in thickness and the rate of endosteal resorption begins to exceed the amount of periosteal apposition. The bone, with fewer trabeculae and thinner cortices, becomes more fragile. Interestingly, Jaworski and Uhthoff have demonstrated that loss of bone mass due to disuse is caused by increased endosteal resorption in older dogs but mainly by slowing of periosteal apposition in younger dogs with growing skeletons.[75,76]

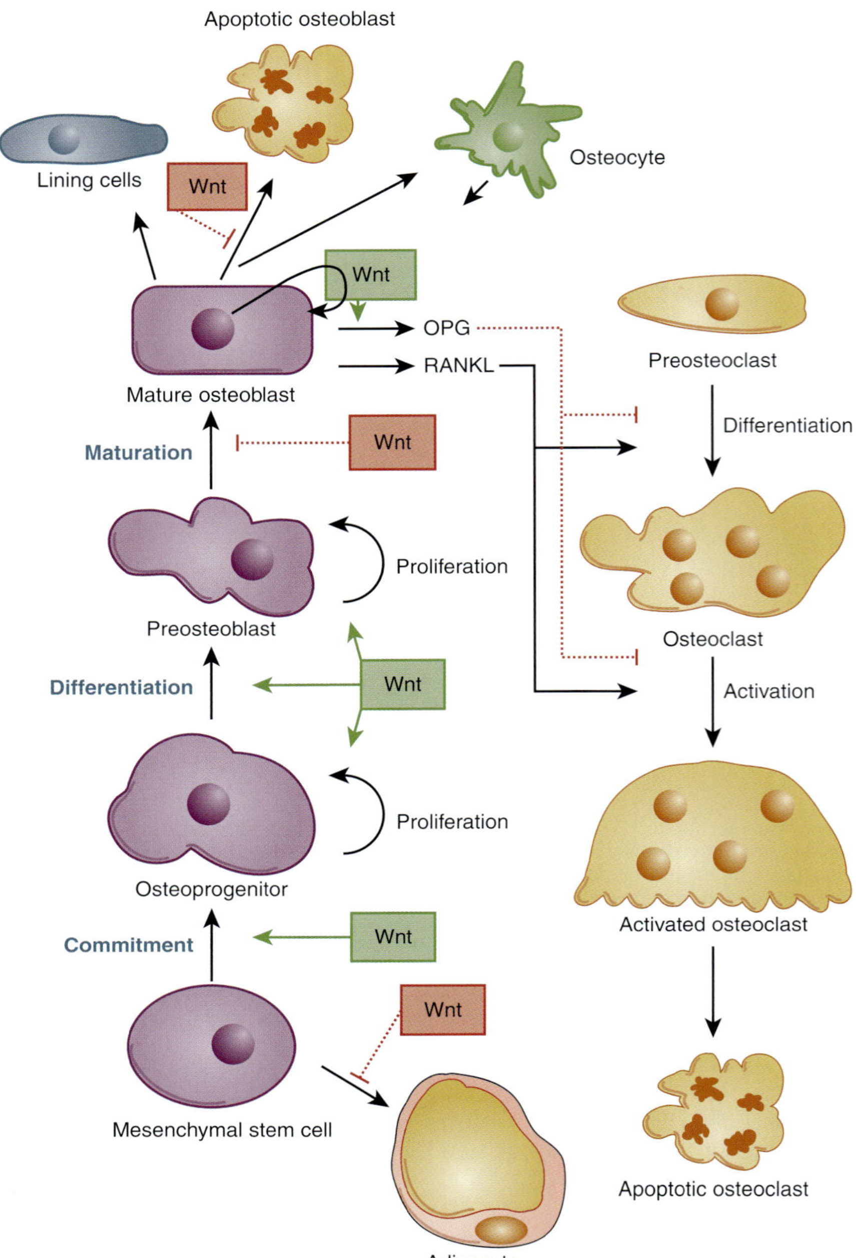

FIGURE 15-2. Schematic representation of the role of Wnt signaling in osteoblast differentiation and function and, indirectly, in osteoclast differentiation and activation. OPG, osteoprotegerin; RANKL, receptor activator of nuclear factor κB ligand. (From Baron R, Rawadi G, Roman-Roman S: Wnt signaling: a key regulator of bone mass. *Curr Top Dev Biol* 76:103–127, 2006.)

Modeling and Remodeling in Response to Mechanical Forces

For many years, the effect of mechanical forces on bone remodeling has intrigued investigators. In the 17th century, Galileo had already noted the correlation of bone size and body weight and activity.[77] In the 19th century, Wolff made the landmark observation that bone structure and remodeling have a clear relationship with loading, and that this association can be expressed mathematically.[3-5] The adaptive changes of bone in response to loading are therefore frequently referred to as following Wolff's law. Several studies have shown that bone adapts to loading and that maintenance of adequate bone density requires cyclic loading.[78-83] Goodship et al. have experimentally proved with animal studies that after resection of the ulna, the radius increases in size and compensates or nearly compensates for the loss.[78] Excessive repetitive loading and vigorous exercise are also known to stimulate bone formation.[79,80] Increased shaft circumference and bone density have been noted on the dominant humerus of tennis players.[81,82] Although not precisely quantified, the absence of loading has a negative effect on bone mass. Uhthoff et al. have reported on loss of bone mass after immobilization/bed rest due to skeletal traction, and adjacent to rigid implants.[76,83]

Regaining bone mass after prolonged disuse may take several months, even in children. In some individuals, especially the elderly, it may never return to its previous level.[5] Disuse results in suppressed periosteal apposition in growing bone and enhanced endocortical resorption in mature bone.[75,76]

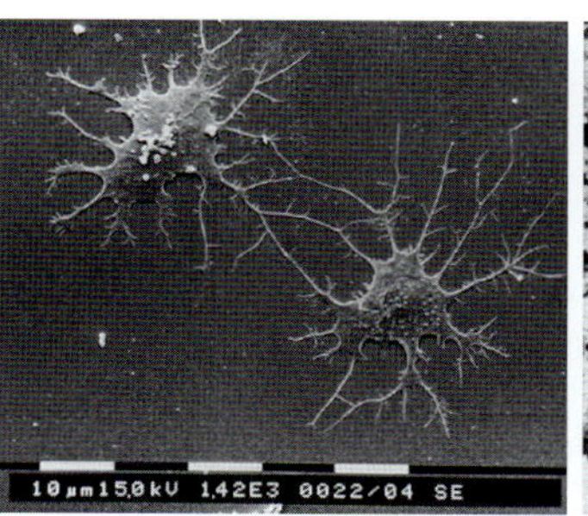

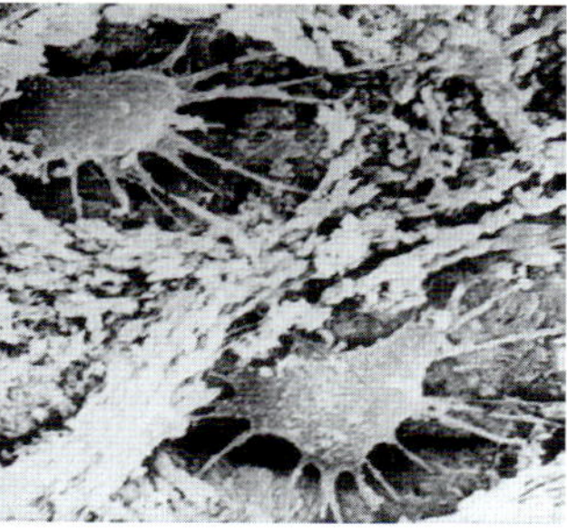

FIGURE 15-3. Osteocyte morphology. *Left,* Scanning electron micrograph of isolated osteocytes in culture. After attachment, osteocytes form cytoplasmic extrusions in all directions. *Right,* Scanning electron micrograph of osteocytes embedded in calcified bone matrix. Note the many cell processes radiating from the osteocyte cell bodies. Magnification ×1000. (From Klein-Nulend J, Bacabac RG, Mullender MG: Mechanobiology of bone tissue. *Pathol Biol [Paris]* 53:576–580, 2005.)

Mechanotransduction

It is currently believed that the mechanical adaptation of bone is governed by the osteocytes, which respond to a loading-induced flow of interstitial fluid through the lacunocanalicular network by producing signaling molecules[70] (Fig. 15-4).

It has been shown that mechanical load induces fluid flow in the canalicular network.[84] Weinbaum et al. suggested that this fluid flow is a physical mediator of mechanosensing by osteocytes in vivo.[85] The osteocytes respond to mechanical stimuli with the production of signaling molecules that modulate the activities of osteoblasts and osteoclasts, thus converting mechanical stimuli into cellular signals that affect bone modeling and remodeling.[86]

Loading results in adaptive changes in bone, making it stronger. This adaptive response is regulated by the ability of resident bone cells to perceive and translate mechanical energy into a cascade of structural and biochemical changes within the cells, a process known as *mechanotransduction*.[44]

Osteocytes probably do not respond directly to mechanical strain (deformation) of bone tissue, but respond indirectly to extracellular fluid flow caused by loading. When osteocytes

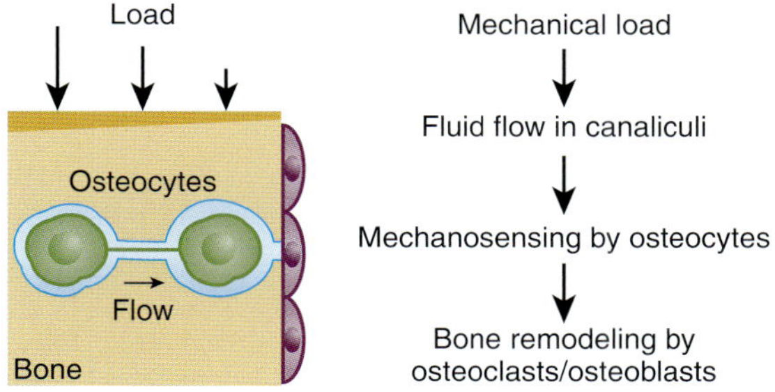

FIGURE 15-4. Model for the transduction of mechanical strain to osteocytes in bone. The diagram at left depicts the network of osteocytes and lining cells of a piece of bone tissue under stress *(vertical arrows)*. Loading results in flow of interstitial fluid in the canalicular nonmineralized matrix *(horizontal arrow)*. (From Klein-Nulend J, Bacabac RG, Mullender MG: Mechanobiology of bone tissue. *Pathol Biol [Paris]* 53:576–580, 2005.)

and osteoblasts are subjected to these changes in fluid pressure, they release several bone-forming growth factors, including nitric oxide and prostaglandins.[86] Certain prostaglandins, particularly PGE2, are anabolic with a demonstrated capacity to stimulate osteoblast activity and new bone formation.[87] Nitric oxide, a strong inhibitor of bone resorption, works in part by suppressing the expression of RANKL and increasing the expression of OPG.[88]

Fluid flow along cell bodies produces drag force, fluid shear stress, and an electric potential. Each of these signals might activate bone cells, although cell culture experiments by Hung et al. and Reich et al. suggest that cells are less sensitive to electrical potentials than they are to fluid forces.[89,90]

There are several hormones that might amplify or transduce the effects of mechanical loading, including parathyroid hormone,[91] estrogen,[92] and insulin-like growth factors.[93] Sawakami et al. suggest that an important event linking mechanical loading to bone formation is Wnt signaling through the LRP5 receptor pathway.[94]

Genetic Factors

Bone modeling and remodeling can be deeply affected by genetic imprint. Diseases like osteogenesis imperfecta, fibrodysplasia ossificans progressiva, and pycnodysostosis result from well-established genetic abnormalities.[95-97] The same holds true for some types and grades of osteoporosis.[98]

Systemic Hormones

The hormones that most directly affect bone turnover and mineral hemostasis are parathyroid hormone (PTH) and calcitonin. Vitamin D also plays an important role. Modeling and remodeling of bone and mineral hemostasis are secondarily influenced by thyroxine (thyroid hormone), glucocorticoids, and estrogen.[3-5]

PTH is a single-chain polypeptide secreted by the chief cells of the parathyroid gland. It increases extracellular calcium levels by raising the renal tubular reabsorption of calcium and also by intensifying calcium release from bone due to increased bone resorption. PTH also stimulates the production of 1,25-dihydroxyvitamin D, which increases renal and gastrointestinal absorption of calcium, as well as its release from bone.[3-5]

Calcitonin is a polypeptide synthesized by the C cells of the thyroid gland. It lowers serum calcium levels by inhibiting osteoclastic bone resorption.[3-5,99,100] Contrary to PTH, which acts on the osteoblasts to activate osteoclasts, calcitonin has a direct effect on osteoclast inhibition.[3,4]

The active form of vitamin D (1,25-dihydroxyvitamin D) is formed in the kidneys. Although its primary function is to increase the blood level of calcium by increasing calcium absorption in the gut and kidneys, it is also a powerful stimulator of bone resorption by osteoclasts.[4,5,101,102]

Thyroid hormone can stimulate resorption of bone by osteoclasts that can lead to loss of bone mass.[103-106] Recent studies suggest that the bone loss seen in hyperthyroidism may be caused by the catabolic action of the elevated thyroid hormone itself or by the decreased anabolic action of thyroid-stimulating hormone.[105,106]

Glucocorticoids decrease bone mass not only by decreasing osteoid formation through osteoblast inhibition, they increase bone resorption by stimulating osteoclast activity.[107] Studies have found that glucocorticoids cause an early and profound reduction in formation of bone through direct inhibition of osteoblasts.[108,109] Glucocorticoids also increase bone resorption by stimulating production of OPG-L and inhibiting the production of OPG by osteoblasts, hence stimulating bone resorption by osteoclasts.[110] Glucocorticoids have also been shown to stimulate the apoptosis of osteoblasts.[111]

Finally, estrogens exert a series of complex effects on bone, either directly by inhibiting bone resorption and total turnover or indirectly by acting on calcitonin, vitamin D, or parathyroid hormone.[5] A recent study suggests that estrogen partially controls osteoblast and osteoclast function, is possibly involved in regulating mechanotransduction, and also interacts with the Wnt/β-catenin pathway.[112]

Exercise

Various authors have demonstrated that repetitive bone loading increases bone mass and decreased loading reduces it.[75-83] Brighton et al. demonstrated that cyclical strain can stimulate bone cell function in culture.[113,114] It is currently accepted that loading results in adaptive changes in bone, making it stronger. Bone's adaptive response is regulated by the ability of resident bone cells to perceive and translate mechanical energy into a cascade of structural and biochemical changes within the cells, a process known as *mechanotransduction*.[44,45]

Strain is defined as the deformation or change in dimension or shape caused by a load in any structure or structural material. Strain is expressed in microstrain units (millionths of a 100% strain), where 1000 microstrain units in compression would shorten a bone by 0.1% of its length.[115] The amount of strain suffered by the bone during load application also influences the organization and density of newly formed bone. Minimal strain will cause the formation of a dense, well-organized bone. Moderate strain will result in formation of less dense, woven bone.[116] A large amount of strain will lead to the formation of fibrous tissue. All of these strain effects are probably mediated through the mechanotransduction pathway.

Prostaglandins and Growth Factors

Cytokines play an important role in local control of normal bone turnover, as well as in neoplastic and inflammatory conditions. Cytokines can be divided into those that primarily form bone, those that primarily cause bone resorption, and those that do both. Interleukin (IL)-1 stimulates the resorption of bone by increasing the proliferation of osteoclast precursors and enhancing their activity.[117-120] IL-1 stimulates osteoclasts through up-regulating activity of the RANK system.[119,120] IL-1 has been also associated with the bone resorption of chronic inflammation and malignancy.[5,120] Platelet-derived growth factor, IL-1, and IL-6 have been shown to be present at the implant-bone interface, contributing to the osteolysis that loosens joint implants.[121-123] Debris from total-joint arthroplasties is associated with the secretion of proinflammatory cytokines such as IL-1β, tumor necrosis factor-α, IL-6, and IL-8. Activation of local (and systemic) inflammation results not only in decreased osteoblast function but in increased osteoclast activity.[123] There is evidence that transforming growth factor beta (a member of the bone morphogenetic protein family) is released during bone resorption and that its presence further inhibits osteoclasts and stimulates osteoblastic activity.[124,125]

Certain prostaglandins, particularly PGE2, are anabolic and have a demonstrated capacity to stimulate osteoblast activity and new bone formation.[87] As mentioned previously, nitric oxide is a strong inhibitor of bone resorption and works in part by suppressing the expression of RANKL and increasing the expression of OPG, which in turn leads to decreased recruitment of osteoclasts.[88]

Bone morphogenetic proteins (BMPs) are a group of growth factors originally defined by their ability to induce the formation of bone and cartilage. Seven proteins from this group were initially discovered. Of these, six (BMP2 through BMP7) belong to the transforming growth factor beta superfamily of proteins, whereas BMP1 is a metalloprotease involved in cartilage development. Since then, more BMPs have been discovered, making a total of approximately 20 today.[126] Induction of bone formation by BMP is a sequential cascade. The key steps in this process are chemotaxis, mitosis, and differentiation, as shown in early studies by Reddi and Huggins.[127] BMPs are known to stimulate osteoblasts and inhibit osteoclasts.[124,125] Currently, only BMP2 is approved by the U.S. Food and Drug Administration for use in humans as a bone growth inducer.

In summary, *modeling* refers to bone turnover that alters its shape, whereas *remodeling* is the recycling of bone without changing its form. Modeling and remodeling occur as physiologic responses to everyday stresses and microtrauma to bone, or to repair a greater insult such as a fracture, infection, or neoplasm. This complex mechanism is also fundamental to maintaining mineral homeostasis. Bone modeling/remodeling is performed by a vast array of cells and is regulated by a variety of mechanisms that range from cyclic loading of bone and mechanotransduction to hormones, local growth factors, and specific genes and proteins. Although it has been a subject of inquiry for hundreds of years, we are only now starting to understand the biomolecular interactions that underlie the coexistence of bone modeling, remodeling, and mineral homeostasis.

KEY REFERENCES

Bono C, Parke W, Garfin S: Development of the spine. In Herkowitz HN, Garfin SR, Eismont FJ, et al, editors: *Rothman-Simeone the spine*, ed 5, Philadelphia, 2006, Elsevier, pp 3–15.

Buckwalter JA, Glimcher MJ, Cooper RR, et al: Bone biology. Part II: Formation, form, modeling, remodeling, and regulation of cell function. *J Bone Joint Surg [Am]* 77:1276–1289, 1995.

Klein-Nulend J, Bacabac RG, Mullender MG: Mechanobiology of bone tissue. *Pathol Biol* 53:576–580, 2005.

Miller JD, McCreadie BR, Alford AI: Form and function of bone. In Einhorn TA, O'Keefe RJ, Buckwalter JA, editors: *Orthopaedic basic science*, ed 3, Rosemont, IL, 2007, American Academy of Orthopaedic Surgeons, pp 129–159.

Robling AG, Castillo AB, Turner CH: Biomechanical and molecular regulation of bone remodeling. *Annu Rev Biomed Eng* 8:455–498, 2006.

Theoleyre S, Wittrant Y, Kwan Tat S, et al: The molecular triad OPG/RANK/RANKL: involvement in the orchestration of pathophysiological bone remodeling. *Cytokine Growth Factor Rev* 15:457–475, 2004.

REFERENCES

The complete reference list is available online at expertconsult.com.

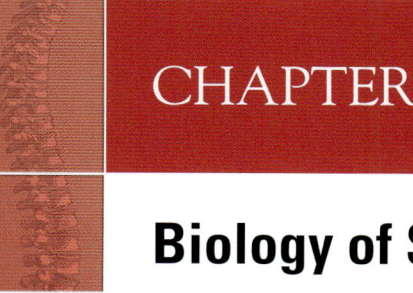

CHAPTER 16

Biology of Spine Fusion

David M. Benglis, Jr. | Scott D. Boden | Michael Y. Wang

In 2001, more than 185,000 spinal arthrodeses were performed in the United States, the majority of which were posterolateral lumbar intertransverse process fusions. From 1997 to 2003, spine fusions climbed from the 41st most common inpatient procedure to the 19th, with resultant increases in spending on lumbar fusion procedures (from 75 to 482 million dollars).[1,2] The number of fusion procedures continues to increase, as does the complexity of devices available for treatment of various spine disorders. Nonunion rates, however, for single-level fusions have been reported to be as great as 35% and even higher in multilevel procedures.[3] Pseudarthroses often result in outcomes that are less than optimal, and often necessitate further surgery.

Changes in the field of spine surgery since the previous edition of this book include specific technical advancements in segmental instrumentation applicable to both open and minimal access surgical approaches, and the widespread implementation of bone morphogenetic protein (BMP) as an alternative to autograft iliac crest harvest in spine fusion. Along with these advancements on the clinical side, the physiologic, molecular, and mechanical requirements for successful fusion also continue to be elucidated.

Local Factors

To achieve a successful fusion, multiple factors must work in concert. These include the local environment of the fusion and systemic factors, with or without the use of fusion enhancers (Box 16-1). Mechanical and biologic factors are closely linked, and any cogent discussion of the biology of spine fusion must be limited to a particular mechanical situation (e.g., compressive forces–anterior column, tensile forces–intertransverse process). This chapter focuses primarily on the biology involved with fusion in the submuscular lumbar intertransverse process environment. To cover the differences and details of all potential fusion environments in the spine is beyond the scope of this chapter. Moreover, one must be cautious in extrapolating results of healing and fusion properties for bone graft substitutes in one region of the spine for another.[4] Nevertheless, some of the principles are applicable and important for anyone who has dedicated a career to the advancement of spine surgery.

Graft Properties: Osteoinduction, Osteogenicity, Osteoconduction, and Connectivity

The choice of graft material has profound implications for the success or failure of arthrodesis. The ideal graft is osteogenic, osteoinductive, and osteoconductive. A balance of these entities, with or without instrumentation, ensures a favorable environment for fusion. Osteoinduction is the stimulation of multipotential stem cells to differentiate into functioning osteogenic cells. This is mediated by growth factors in the bone matrix itself (i.e., BMPs). Urist et al. introduced this concept in their studies of the osteoinductive properties of demineralized bone matrix (DBM).[5,6]

Osteogenicity refers to the presence of viable osteogenic cells, either predetermined or inducible within the graft. These cells are important in the early stages of the fusion process, uniting graft and host bone into a functional unit. Only fresh autologous bone and bone marrow are osteogenic.

Osteoconductivity refers to a material's capacity to foster neovascularization and infiltration by osteogenic precursor cells via creeping substitution. A material may lack inductive stimuli and viable bone precursor cells, but still be osteoconductive. Such grafts act only as scaffolding for bone healing. Calcium phosphate ceramics, coral, and collagen are such materials, whereas allograft bone is osteoconductive and osteoinductive, and autograft bone is osteoconductive, osteoinductive, and osteogenic. Connectivity is the ability of an osteconductive graft material to be "connected" to local bone. This is determined by the surface area available for incorporation into the fusion mass.

Graft Material

Autograft

Autogenous iliac crest bone in the past has been considered the "gold standard" of graft material. Historically, it has been the most successful graft source in spine fusion. Cancellous autograft has the requisite matrix proteins, mineral, and collagen for the ideals of osteoinductivity, osteogenicity, and osteoconductivity. Its large trabecular surface makes it highly connective as well. Donor site complication rates as high as

BOX 16-1. Factors Affecting the Success of Spine Fusion

Local Factors
Bone graft: source and quantity
Mechanical stability and loading
Graft site preparation
Soft tissue bed
Systemic Factors
Nicotine
Drugs
Osteoporosis
Hormones
Fusion Enhancers
Electrical stimulation
Growth factors

25% to 30% have been reported, although a rate of 8% seems more realistic and is more commonly cited.[7,8] Morbidity may be associated with an increased incidence of blood loss, chronic donor site pain, increased operative time, infection, and nerve injury. Furthermore, the quantity of bone available is limited, and may be insufficient for long-segment fusions, or in patients who have had previous graft harvests.

Autogenous cortical bone is useful when structural support is needed at the graft site. Otherwise, it is less desirable than cancellous bone because of the absence of robust bone marrow and, as a result, fewer osteoprogenitor cells. Additionally, these cells are less likely to survive, because they are embedded in a compact matrix where the diffusion of nutrients essential for cell proliferation is impeded compared with the cancellous environment. Cortical bone also has less surface area per unit weight with matrix proteins exposed, and, therefore, connectivity is marginal. Vascular ingrowth into cortical bone is slow. Mechanical strength lags because incorporation takes longer. Although cancellous bone is incorporated fairly rapidly and remodeled, portions of cortical graft may remain necrotic for extended periods. When the likelihood of avascular graft healing is low, as in previously irradiated tissue beds, vascularized grafts may be more desirable due to the presence of greater numbers of osteogenic cells.

Demineralized Bone Matrix

Demineralized bone matrix (DBM) is present in a variety of forms, each of which has a variable degree of osteoinductivity.[4] Current data support its use as a bone graft extender but not as a pure substitute or enhancer.[9] Autogenous and allograft DBMs are osteoinductive due to the presence of low doses of BMPs (~0.1% by weight).[10] Collagenous and noncollagenous proteins serve as osteoconductive material that is left after the demineralization process. Preliminary animal studies have shown efficacy of DBM as a carrier molecule for recombinant human bone morphogenetic protein (rhBMP-2) in ectopic bone formation or as a graft alternative in experimental posterolateral arthrodesis.[11,12] A study by Louis-Ugbo et al. used a non-human primate posterolateral fusion model to test a specific formulation of DBM, which was more porous than its predecessor. With this new formulation they found robust fusions and suggested that it exhibited properties of both a graft enhancer and extender.[13] A recent prospective randomized study by Cammisa et al. looked at 2-year fusion rates in the posterolateral environment in 120 human patients. They concluded that DBM could function as an adequate graft extender and promote adequate fusions when mixed with a small amount of autogenous bone graft.[14]

Allograft

The desire to avoid donor site morbidity led to increased use of allograft bone in spine surgery. This was made practical by advances in procurement, sterilization, preparation, and storage.[15] Although allograft bone is widely used in spine surgery, concerns regarding fusion rates and disease transmission remain. Allograft is not osteogenic, because there are no surviving cells in the graft. Because of the processing and storage requirements of allograft, some of the osteoinductive potential is lost. It also carries a small but real risk of disease transmission and may elicit an immune response from the recipient.[16-21]

Sterilization, donor screening, and sterile harvesting of donor bone help to keep the risks just cited to a minimum. Bone must be harvested in a sterile fashion within 24 hours of death, cultured, and processed for storage. Large tissue banks are available at most academic institutions.

Immunogenicity and maintenance of osteoinductive and osteoconductive properties are affected by these processing and preservation techniques. Bone usually is frozen or freeze-dried as soon as possible after harvest. Both methods decrease immunogenicity and allow for extended storage. Freezing does not diminish the mechanical properties of the bone, and it may be stored at −70°C for 5 years. Freeze-drying further reduces immunogenicity and inactivates viral agents, but it reduces the mechanical strength of the graft.[22-24] Freeze-dried bone may be stored under vacuum, at room temperature, for an indefinite period.

The most common sterilization methods are high-dose gamma irradiation and ethylene oxide gas sterilization.[18] Both alter the structure of matrix proteins, decreasing the osteoinductive capacity and mechanical strength of the bone.[23] Other sterilization methods such as autoclaving are even more destructive, and generally are not used.

Although allograft usually has performed well in both cervical and lumbar interbody fusions, in which the graft is subject to compression, the results in the posterolateral lumbar environment, in which primary tensile forces exist, have not been as favorable.[25-33] This result has led many surgeons to use allograft as an autograft expander rather than a pure substitute for posterolateral arthrodeses.

Xenograft

The use of bone graft taken from other species has been reported in the orthopaedic literature, but these alternatives to autograft never were incorporated into widespread use. Despite processing, xenografts remain immunogenic and provoke a host response. The graft may become encapsulated from the host's response, with resultant blockade to revascularization. Ivory and cow horn resist incorporation into host bone and are no longer used. Bovine bone, both freeze-dried and deproteinized, remains weakly antigenic. Both of these types of xenografts have been used in spine surgery with limited success, and therefore they are not recommended as a graft material.[34-37]

Ceramics

Calcium phosphate ($CaPO_4$) ceramics, including hydroxyapatite (HA) and tricalcium phosphate (TCP), have been widely used in orthopaedic and spine surgery.[38] These osteoconductive, biodegradable materials are compatible with the remodeling of bone necessary to achieve optimal strength of a construct. Other, nonresorbable materials remain in the fusion mass, leaving permanent stress risers and prolonging strength deficiencies.

To be useful as a graft material, synthetic materials must have several properties. They must be compatible with local tissues, remain chemically stable in body fluids, and be able to withstand sterilization. Furthermore, they must be available in useful shapes and sizes, be cost-effective, and have reliable quality control. $CaPO_4$ ceramics qualify, and have been widely used in dentistry and maxillofacial surgery, as well as in animal models for experimental spinal research.[21,39-47] A wide body of literature exists discussing the use of these materials in human spine surgery.[38,46,48-51]

Both HA and TCP ceramics are inherently brittle. They may be prepared as either a compact or a porous material. The greater crystallinity and density of the compact form results in greater strength and resistance to dissolution in vivo, whereas porous versions more closely approximate cancellous bone and enhance bony ingrowth (at the expense of more rapid degradation). Under physiologic conditions, HA is resorbed very slowly, whereas TCP generally is resorbed within 6 weeks of implantation.[25]

Natural coral has been used to augment or even replace autograft, with some success.[52-55] The calcium carbonate ($CaCO_3$) in coral is hydrothermally converted to $CaPO_4$. The structural geometry of coral is similar to that of cancellous bone, making it highly osteoconductive and connective.

Animal Studies

The use of $CaPO_4$ ceramic as a spine fusion bone graft substitute has been studied extensively in animal models. Flatley et al. used porous blocks of a 1:1 ratio of calcium HA and TCP ceramic in a rabbit posterolateral fusion model.[21] At 12 weeks, histologic sections demonstrated bone ingrowth reaching the central portion of the block with no fibrous barrier between the new bone and the ceramic. Holmes et al. used coralline HA in a canine posterior facet model.[46] Although the distribution of bone ingrowth was similar to that seen in autograft controls, they reported no solid fusions, even at 6 months. Using coral porites (calcium carbonate) and a 65:35 HA:TCP biphasic ceramic, Guigui et al. found a 100% rate of fusion in a sheep model, comparable to the fusion rate of autograft in another study by this same group.[56,57]

The use of composites of ceramic and an osteoinductive agent such as DBM, autograft, or recombinant BMP also has been investigated (see Growth Factors, later in this chapter).[58-60] Ragni and Lindholm, in a rabbit interbody fusion model, found that the addition of DBM enhanced the incorporation of an HA block. Animals treated with an HA/DBM composite showed significantly earlier fusion consolidation than those treated with autograft or either HA or DBM alone. By 6 months, however, results of the autograft were comparable to those with the composite.[61] Zerwekh et al. compared a collagen/HA-TCP ceramic/autograft composite with autograft alone in a canine posterior fusion model.[62] Histologic comparisons of bone ingrowth were similar in both groups at 12 months, as were the results of biomechanical testing. Working in a canine segmental posterior spine fusion model, Muschler et al. compared fusions with autograft, collagen/HA-TCP ceramic composite, collagen/HA-TCP ceramic/autograft composite, and collagen/HA-TCP ceramic/bone matrix protein composite, and with no graft.[63] Autograft had a significantly superior union score. Ceramic composite alone performed no better than the no-graft control. The addition of bone matrix protein, however, improved the union score, making it comparable with the composite/autograft treatment.

Human Studies

The clinical efficacy of ceramics, either alone or as part of a composite, has yet to be fully elucidated. Studies suggest that these entities do have beneficial effects. Passuti et al., in a study of 12 severely scoliotic patients, used internal fixation and blocks of 3:2 HA-TCP ceramic alone or mixed with autogenous cancellous bone.[49] After 15 months average follow-up, radiographs demonstrated fusion in all patients. Histologic examination of biopsy material from two of the subjects revealed new bone formed directly on the ceramic surface and ingrowth into the macropores. Similarly, Pouliquen et al. successfully used natural coral as a graft substitute in 49 patients with idiopathic scoliosis.[54] Although the results were favorable, their small patient populations, single diagnosis, and average patient age of 14 years limited these studies. Acharya et al. designed a prospective matched case study examining the effect of a hydroxyapatite–bioactive glass ceramic composite as a stand-alone graft versus autogenous bone in posterolateral spine fusion.[64] The study was halted early, because at 1 year fusion was found to be inferior with the bone substitute as a stand-alone graft compared with autograft.

The use of ceramics and composites as a graft replacement or extender of autograft holds promise in spine fusion. Later discussion in this chapter covers the relevance of ceramics in combination with BMPs.

Mechanical Stability

Fusion rate is affected by the mechanical stability of the involved segments.[65-70] As a result, internal segmental instrumented fixation has commonly been used to achieve higher rates of fusion, an approach that is supported by various studies in the literature.[65-67,70-72] Even in the presence of a rigid construct, nonunion still occurs in up to 10% to 15% of patients, especially when hardware loosening or failure occurs.[71-75] Fusion level, number of segments involved, patient weight and activity level, and postoperative bracing all influence the rate of fusion.[76]

Animal Studies: Spinal Instrumentation

The effects of spinal instrumentation and stability have been investigated in various animal models.[77-81] Although this approach can tell us much about short-term effects of instrumentation failure, caution must be exercised in extrapolating this information to the long-term effects in the human body at the bone/instrumentation interface. McAfee et al. created a canine instability model to study both the effect of spinal instrumentation on fusion success and the radiographic incidence of fusion with respect to spinal stability.[66-68] At 6 months, radiographs revealed a greater probability of fusion in the instrumented animals than in the noninstrumented animals. The instrumented fusions also were more rigid. Likewise, Zdeblick et al. demonstrated both an increased rate of fusion and a more rigid fusion when anterior instrumentation was used in a canine model of an unstable burst fracture at L5.[70] These results also were replicated by Shirado.[82] Kotani et al. showed that after solid posterolateral arthrodesis was achieved in a sheep model, transpedicular fixation continued to provide mechanical support.[83]

The biologic activity of the graft material may partly determine the need for internal fixation. Fuller et al. showed that rigid fixation improved bone ingrowth into a calcium carbonate block in a canine anterior thoracic interbody fusion model.[84,85] Because ceramics are not osteoinductive, a mechanically stable environment is crucial for ingrowth. Osteoinductive graft substitutes, on the other hand, may not be as reliant on construct rigidity.

Nagel et al. developed a sheep model of delayed union and nonunion.[69] Posterior lumbar laminar and facet fusions with iliac crest graft were performed on seven sheep. Six of the seven sheep developed nonunions at the L6-S1 interspace; all cephalad interspaces fused (21 of 21). Eight normal sheep underwent in vivo flexion-extension radiographs. Five normal sheep spines were studied ex vivo, using displacement transducers to test stiffness, displacement, and strain in flexion-extension. The lumbosacral level demonstrated significantly more motion than the other levels, suggesting that motion was a major factor in determining the success of fusion in this sheep model. Similar observations have been made in dogs.[86] The increased stability and decreased motion that instrumentation provides would seem valuable in such instances.

Human Studies: Spinal Instrumentation

Contradictory human studies of the effects of spinal instrumentation have been widely reported. Zdeblick discussed 124 patients undergoing fusion for different conditions.[72] Patients were randomized into three groups, all having dorsolateral autograft fusions. Patients in group 1 were not instrumented, those in group 2 were instrumented with a semirigid pedicle screw system, and individuals in group 3 had rigid pedicle screw instrumentation implanted. The rigid group had a significantly higher fusion rate (95%) than the noninstrumented group (65%). The instrumented groups together had 95% excellent or good results, whereas the noninstrumented patients had only 71% good or excellent outcomes (a statistically significant result).

Bridwell et al. described 44 patients with degenerative spondylolisthesis.[71] Patients were individualized into three groups: no fusion; noninstrumented posterolateral fusion; and pedicle screw instrumented posterolateral fusion. Patients with more than 10 degrees or 3 mm of motion were automatically assigned to the instrumentation group. There was an 87% fusion rate in the instrumented group versus a 30% rate in noninstrumented patients, yet there was no significant clinical difference in successful outcomes between the noninstrumented and unfused groups (30% vs. 33%). Successful outcomes in the instrumented group (83%) were significantly greater than in the nonfusion group. Fischgrund et al. also demonstrated a markedly increased rate of fusion in their patients with instrumentation (83% vs. 45%), yet found no difference in clinical outcome.

In their meta-analysis, Mardjetko et al. reviewed 25 papers describing 889 patients with degenerative spondylolisthesis.[87] Five of the included studies described patients undergoing decompression and posterolateral arthrodesis with pedicle screw instrumentation. Although there was a trend toward an increased rate of fusion in the instrumented versus noninstrumented patients (93% vs. 86%), it did not reach significance ($P = .08$). The clinical outcome was better in the uninstrumented group: 90% versus 86%. However, the authors acknowledged several limitations of their review: data from different treatments over 20 years; variable study designs and quality; and possible dilution of data from the stronger, better-designed studies that suggested an advantage to instrumentation.

Fusion success is also affected by the physical stresses placed on the graft.[88] In human beings, 80% of the load at a motion segment is transmitted through the intervertebral disc. Graft placed ventrally, in the interbody region, is thus primarily subjected to compression. This compressive force promotes fusion, presumably by stimulating vascular ingrowth and the proliferation of mesenchymal cells. Dorsally placed graft experiences tensile forces, as does graft placed in the intertransverse process region. Under these less favorable mechanical conditions, fusion is more dependent on biologic factors.

Facet preparation for fusion has been shown to increase motion of the involved segment. Although many surgeons routinely include facet fusion in posterolateral intertransverse process arthrodeses, biomechanical studies have demonstrated a resultant decrease in stability.[89,90] The developing fusion preparation decreases the surface area incorporated into the fusion mass, and may result in a less rigid fusion. Rigid instrumentation allows the facets to be prepared and incorporated without sacrificing stability. However, in the osteoporotic patient, the screw-bone interface often is weak. Even with instrumentation, facet preparation may not be appropriate in these individuals.

Overall, it is generally agreed that spinal instrumentation decreases the rate of pseudarthrosis. However, in some situations, especially with single-level fusions, no significant clinical benefit may be obtained. Additionally, although a positive relation exists between radiographic fusion and clinical outcome, no absolute convincing correlation has been demonstrated.[91] Currently, prospective randomized blinded clinical trials examining the effects of instrumentation have not yet been completed.

Graft Site Preparation

Preparation of the bony anatomy into which the graft is placed is of paramount importance in achieving a successful fusion. The exposed area of viable, vascular bone should be maximized. This is done by decortication, which may be accomplished with curettes, rongeurs, osteotomes, or a power bur precision drill. Use of a high-speed bur may result in thermal necrosis, which may be minimized with continuous irrigation, use of a drill with deep flutes, and minimizing contact time between bur and bone. As the surface area of decorticated bone increases, so does the connectivity and the availability of osteogenic cells and exposed matrix proteins. Furthermore, a large surface is helpful in forming a bony bridge strong enough to carry the mechanical load.

Soft Tissue Bed

Spine fusion depends on the influx of osteoprogenitor cells, inflammatory cells, nutrients, and endocrine stimuli from the local soft tissues to support bone graft healing. An adequate blood supply in this environment is a critical requirement for success, and nonviable, traumatized tissues should be removed from the graft site.

Hurley et al. evaluated the role of these factors in a canine dorsal spine fusion model.[86] Thirty-seven animals underwent a modified Hibbs fusion (control), a Hibbs fusion with a fluid-permeable/cell-impermeable membrane interposed between fusion site and muscle mass, or with a membrane impermeable to both cells and fluids. Fusion was achieved in all 12 animals with the semipermeable membrane, whereas no animals with the impermeable membrane had a successful fusion.

Radiation has a detrimental effect on a healing spine fusion that is especially pronounced in the first few postoperative weeks. This effect may be caused by cytotoxicity, but is probably a product of the resultant vasculitis and inhibition of angiogenesis that follows radiation treatment. In the long term, radiation also can induce osteonecrosis and dense hypovascular scars, creating a poor fusion environment. Studies suggest that a 3- to 6-week delay in radiation would be beneficial to the fusion process.[92,93] Use of vascularized grafts anastomosed to nonirradiated vessels also may increase the chance of successful fusion.

Systemic Factors

Nicotine

Smokers have a higher rate of pseudarthrosis than do nonsmokers.[27,28,73,94,95] Cigarette smoke retards osteogenesis and inhibits graft revascularization. Tobacco smoke extracts calcitonin resistance, increases fracture end resorption, and interferes with osteoblastic function.[8,96,97]

A direct relation between systemic nicotine and spinal pseudarthrosis has been demonstrated in a rabbit model. Silcox et al. performed L5-6 posterolateral intertransverse process arthrodeses with autologous iliac crest graft in 28 rabbits.[98] The animals were implanted with osmotic mini-pumps, delivering either saline (control) or nicotine equivalent to a human who smokes 1 to 1.5 packs per day. At 5 weeks, 56% of control animals had a solid fusion by manual palpation; no solid fusions were seen in the nicotine-exposed animals ($P = .02$).

Drugs

Drugs taken during the perioperative period can have a detrimental effect on the process of fusion. Chemotherapeutic agents administered in the early postoperative period inhibit bone formation and arthrodesis.[99-101] Nonsteroidal anti-inflammatory drugs (NSAIDs) suppress the inflammatory response, and may inhibit spine fusion.[102]

Dimar et al. performed three-level dorsal fusions in 39 rats. Half the animals received indomethacin, 3 mg/kg/day, on 6 of 7 days, and the other animals received saline.[103] Treatment was started 1 week preoperatively, and continued for 12 weeks after surgery. In the control rats, 27 of 60 levels achieved solid or moderate fusions, whereas only 4 of 42 levels were similarly fused in the indomethacin group ($P < .001$). Weaknesses of this study included the following: the experimental model used had not been well characterized, fusion assessment was not rigidly defined, and the indomethacin dose was significantly greater on a milligram-per-kilogram basis than that used in human beings.

Glassman et al. performed a retrospective review of 288 patients who had undergone L4-S1 instrumented, autologous iliac crest graft spine fusions.[104] Ketorolac had been administered to 167 of them; the remaining 121 did not receive NSAIDs. Using surgical exploration, hardware failure, and tomograms to determine fusion, they found 4% pseudarthroses in the control group, versus 17% in the ketorolac group ($P < .001$). The odds ratio indicated that nonunion was approximately five times more likely in those individuals who received ketorolac. There are several problems with this retrospective study: the number of surgeons involved in the cases varied, and the patients received varying numbers of ketorolac doses, beginning at different postoperative times. Their results, however, are supported in a more controlled animal study by Martin et al., who, working in a rabbit model, compared fusion in animals receiving ketorolac or saline.[105] They found 35% fusions in the ketorolac-treated animals versus 75% in the controls ($P = .037$).

Cyclo-oxygenase 2 (COX-2) inhibitors are specific for the isoform of the enzyme targeted by NSAIDs. Long et al. investigated the effect of orally administered celecoxib on spine fusion in the rabbit model.[106] They compared rabbits receiving celecoxib, 10 mg/kg daily, with groups receiving either indomethacin, 10 mg/kg, or saline. They found a significant difference between the rate of fusion in controls versus that of the indomethacin group, while animals that received celecoxib fused at an intermediate rate. The study was limited by its small size and the use of a relatively high dose of indomethacin compared with that used in humans.

Osteoporosis

The most common metabolic bone disease in the United States, osteoporosis commonly is assumed to be a negative factor in bone healing. The decreased bone density that is the hallmark of osteoporosis makes stabilization with instrumentation difficult in this population. Additionally, there may be changes in marrow quality and bone turnover rate. Older animals have a decreased capacity for osteoinduction.[107] In terms of fusion potential, a decrease in the number of osteogenic stem cells in elderly patients may be more important than absolute bone mass.

Hormones

Hormones affect bone formation both directly and indirectly and probably influence spine fusion as well. These chemical messengers have complex interactions, both positive and negative, with bone-forming and bone-absorbing cells.

Growth hormone, via somatomedins, exerts a stimulatory effect on cartilage and bone formation.[108,109] In vivo experimental research has revealed that growth hormone stimulates bone healing by increasing gastrointestinal absorption of calcium, as well as by increasing bone formation and mineralization.[110,111] Thyroid hormone, which acts synergistically with growth hormone, is required for somatomedin synthesis by the liver. Furthermore, thyroid hormone has a direct stimulatory effect on cartilage growth and maturation, thereby positively influencing bone healing.

Corticosteroids have been shown both experimentally and clinically to be detrimental to bone healing, increasing bone resorption and decreasing bone formation. They inhibit and promote osteoblastic differentiation and also decrease the synthesis of viable bone matrix.[112-114]

Estrogens and androgens play important roles in skeletal maturation, as well as in the prevention of age-associated bone loss. Their effects on bone healing, however, remain controversial. Some studies indicate they may stimulate bone formation, whereas others do not support this positive effect.[115-117] Neither affects bone collagen synthesis, but estrogens may increase bone mineralization by increasing serum levels of parathyroid hormone and vitamin D3.[118]

Fusion Enhancers

Electrical Stimulation

Since 1974, when Dwyer et al. first demonstrated improved spine fusion rates,[119] electrical stimulation has been increasingly accepted as an aid to spine fusion. Electrical stimulation theoretically alters the naturally occurring strain-generated charges present in healing bone toward those that are ideal for bone fusion.[120] Since that time, various devices have gained approval from the U.S. Food and Drug Administration (FDA) for use as adjuncts to fusion: (1) direct current electrical stimulation (DCES), (2) inductive coupling devices such as pulsed electromagnetic fields (PEMFs) and combined magnetic fields (CMFs), and (3) capacitive coupling devices. These devices have been shown to have varying effectiveness.[119]

Electrical Devices

DCES uses an implanted generator that delivers a constant 20- to 40-microampere (μA) current to the fusion bed, for 6 to 9 months. The effective stimulation area is 5 to 8 mm from the cathode. Although the exact mechanism of action is not fully understood, several physiologic effects have been demonstrated. The current attracts charged proteins by electrophoresis, bone, cartilage, and endothelial cells by galvanotaxis, and depolarizes cell membranes. Faradaic reactions at the bone-electrode interface reduce oxygen tension and increase pH, similar to what is seen at the growth plate in healing fractures. Increased pH has been shown to increase osteoblastic bone formation and to inhibit resorption by osteoclasts.[121,122]

PEMFs utilize inductive coupling to generate an electromagnetic field across the fusion area via external coils that are worn from 3 to 8 hours per day for 3 to 6 months. A varying magnetic field induces an electric current, which is hypothesized to stimulate bone healing, possibly by depolarizing cell membranes and increasing calcium influx into bone cells.[123-125] Regardless of the exact mechanism, PEMFs have been shown to increase the levels of BMP-2 and BMP-4 in rat calvarial cells.[126,127]

A less commonly usedtilized inductive coupling device is the CMF. Like the PEMF, it also is worn externally, usually for 30 minutes per day, and combines a static magnetic field with a time-variable field. Although animal data showed increased bone stiffness at the 30-minute dose, the effect was far greater with treatment given 24 hours per day.[128]

Capacitive coupling devices also are noninvasive and employ alternating currents, conductive gels, and electrodes. Fredricks et al.[129] in a rat fusion model (previously described by Boden et al.[130]) showed up-regulation of various factors required for bone fusion with the use of this form of electrical stimulation.

Human Studies

Kane published the first large multicenter study of the use of DCES in dorsolateral spine fusion.[131] Eighty-two patients treated with DCES were compared to a historical control population of 150 patients fused without electrical stimulation. The DCES group had a 91% fusion rate, significantly higher than the 81% in the control subjects. Of note, the DCES group had a significantly higher rate of revision surgery for pseudarthroses. The report also described a prospective, randomized control study in a "difficult to fuse" population of patients who had failed one or more previous attempts at fusion, were undergoing multilevel arthrodeses, had grade II spondylolisthesis, or had other risk factors. The 31 patients in the stimulation group had a significantly higher fusion rate of 81%, compared with 54% of the 28 patients in the control population.

Recent work has lent further support to the use of DCES in dorsolateral spine fusion. Reports indicate that DCES increases the percentage rate of fusion in dorsolateral pedicle screw–instrumented fusions.[132,133] Furthermore, DCES has been shown to increase the fusion rate in smokers from 66% to 83%.[133]

Simmons was the first to report on the use of PEMF in spine fusion. He described treatment of pseudarthroses after posterior lumbar interbody fusion in 13 patients, 77% of whom progressed to fusion without further surgery.[134] In the more demanding environment of posterior pseudarthroses, Lee reported a 67% success rate with PEMF.[135] Bose followed 48 patients who received posterolateral fusion in addition to instrumentation.[136] He reported fusion success of 98%; however, there was no control population in this study. Marks demonstrated twice the percentage of successful lumbar fusions in females when compared with control populations without the device.[137]

Linovitz et al. reported on a double-blind, randomized, placebo-controlled population of patients on the use of CMF in noninstrumented fusions.[138] The study found that 64% of patients with active devices had fused by 9 months, compared with 43% of patients with placebo devices. Stratification by gender showed that the difference was significant only for the female patients in the study. The reasons for this remain unclear.

Although there seems to be support for the use of electrical stimulation in spine fusion, not all modalities are equally effective. Currently, DCES appears to have the greatest effect. Furthermore, all of these devices are expensive. Guidelines for determining which patients would best be served by their use has yet to be fully elucidated.

Growth Factors

BMPs are a group of proteins belonging to the transforming growth factor (TGF)-β family. During the more than 35 years since they were first described by Urist,[5] they have been found to play important roles in both endochondral and intramembranous bone formation, as well as in fracture healing. Recently, a great deal of attention has been paid to a possible role for these proteins in spine fusion, and also to concerns over adverse events and increased costs associated with these molecules.

BMPs bind to receptors on multiple cell types, including osteoblasts, osteoclasts, and mesenchymal stem cells. Their effects are exerted through a second messenger system. At low concentrations, this leads to cartilage formation; at higher levels, direct bone formation is fostered. This bone is histologically and mechanically normal.

Several BMP preparations are in or are nearly in clinical evaluation. Recombinant human BMP-2 (rhBMP-2) and BMP-7 (rhBMP-7), which is more commonly termed *osteogenic protein-1 (OP-1)*, are manufactured by recombinant DNA techniques, and are pure preparations. Two BMPs currently are FDA approved for use in human surgery. rhOP-1 (rhBMP-7) is approved for long bone defects (Stryker Corp., Kalamazoo, MI), and rhBMP-2 has been approved for use in anterior lumbar interbody fusions (ALIF; Medtronic Sofamor Danek, Memphis, TN). A third preparation, bovine BMP extract (bBMPx), is derived from bovine bone and, thus, contains several different BMPs, along with other proteins.

Animal Studies

Preclinical work on the use of BMP in posterolateral spine fusions has been reported by many researchers.[139-145] Many of these early experimental studies demonstrated faster fusion rates when compared to controls. Cook et al., using osteogenic protein 1 (OP-1) in a canine facet and interlaminar fusion model, obtained solid fusions in 12 weeks, as compared with 26 weeks for autogenous graft.[146] In a similar model, Muschler et al. found no difference between autograft and rhBMP-2 at 3 months, though the model was criticized for its intrinsically high fusion rate of the control arm.[147]

A canine intertransverse-process fusion model demonstrated solid fusion with rhBMP-2 within 3 months, whereas autologous iliac crest graft animals had not fused at that point.[143] This same model was used to demonstrate that rhBMP-2 could produce solid fusions without decoration.[144] Using a rabbit intertransverse process fusion model they developed, Schimandle et al. achieved 100% fusion with rhBMP-2, compared with 42% fusion in the autograft group.[148] Martin et al. demonstrated that rhBMP-2 was further able to overcome the inhibitory effect of ketorolac in the model used by Schimandle and Boden.[105] Grauer et al. and Patel et al. then established that OP-1 had the same effects in reference to fusion, but required higher dosages of the BMP compound.[149,150]

Sandhu et al. and Fishgrund et al. reported improved fusion rates with an rhBMP-2 soaked collagen sponge in a canine model for spine fusion compared to controls.[140,142] Martin et al., on the other hand, failed to show improvement in posterolateral fusions in nonhuman primates when using the same concentration of rhBMP-2 as in the canine studies. They listed one potential cause of this discrepancy originating from compression of the BMP out of the sponge by the surrounding tissues. A protective shield was then placed over the absorbable collagen sponge (ACS), and they were then able to achieve successful fusions at lower concentrations.[151]

Several other studies also have examined the effectiveness of these agents in nonhuman primates. Boden et al. tested bBMPx in the lumbar spine of adult rhesus monkeys.[152] Four of the four animals implanted with 3 mg or more of the bovine protein achieved a posterolateral intertransverse process fusion, whereas none of the six animals implanted with a lower dose fused. However, a second study demonstrated only 40% fusion with this same dose, and 54% with a 5-mg dose, although the autograft animals showed only 21% fusion.[153]

A more robust carrier than the collagen sponge alone may be needed to promote fusion in the posterolateral environment. Boden et al. developed a more rigid porous biphasic calcium phosphate (BCP) ceramic carrier that provided a scaffold for new bone and then resorbed over time. They were able to achieve fusion at three different concentrations of rhBMP-2/ACS.[139] Additional carriers have been developed that are based on the original BCP ceramic concept with the same excellent results in the rabbit and primate models.[154,155]

Akamura et al. and Barnes et al. used compression resistant matrix (CRM) carriers (15% hydroxyapatite, 85% β-tricalcium phosphate ceramic collagen matrix) and noted that the carrier, collagen sponge, and concentration of rhBMP-2 are all important in promoting a solid fusion in nonhuman primates.[156,157] Barnes et al. failed to achieve a solid posterolateral arthrodesis when the CRM was not used with rhBMP-2 and the collagen sponge. Like the BCP ceramic carrier in the study by Boden discussed earlier, one explanation for this observation by Barnes et al. could be that the CRM provides a better scaffold for bone growth than the ACS alone.

Human Studies

Human trials using rhBMP-7 and rhBMP-2 in posterolateral fusion have been reported, both with and without instrumentation.[158-165] A safety and efficacy study of OP-1 for posterolateral spinal arthrodesis had been completed by 2001.[166] Sixteen patients with degenerative spondylolisthesis, undergoing noninstrumented posterolateral fusion, were randomized to receive either autograft and OP-1 or autograft alone. At 6 months, 9 of the 12 autograft/OP-1 patients had fused, versus only 2 of 4 autograft-alone patients, although the difference was not statistically significant. Clinically, 83% of the OP-1 patients had 20% or better improvement in their Oswestry score, whereas only 50% of the autograft-alone patients had this level of success. Again, the difference was not statistically significant. Of note, OP-1 had no adverse effects.

This initial pilot study has since turned into a larger prospective series with long-term follow-up. The rhOP-1 (rhBMP-7) data for posterolateral spine fusion support increased rates of fusion in the rhBMP-7 group versus control (55% vs. 40%).[162] At 4 years of follow-up, Vaccaro et al. have achieved similar fusion results with rhOP-1 when compared with iliac crest autograft in posterolateral fusions.[167]

Luque[168] and Boden et al.[159] pioneered early clinical studies of rhBMP-2 in the posterolateral fusion environment. Luque examined two patient cohorts in a prospective, randomized, open-label trial of rhBMP-2, with a biphasic calcium phosphate (BCP) carrier in patients undergoing single-level lumbar fusions for degenerative instability. The first group (seven patients) received rhBMP-2/BCP unilaterally, with autograft on the contralateral side. Eighty-six percent of the rhBMP-2 sides fused by 12 months, whereas only 57% of the autograft-treated sides fused. The second group received a higher rhBMP-2/BCP dose bilaterally, without autograft; at 12 months, 100% had fused. Oswestry scores improved by 15 or more points in 85.7% of cohort 1 patients and in 100% of cohort 2 individuals. Boden et al. performed a prospective randomized clinical pilot trial of rhBMP-2 with BCP carrier versus autograft. All 20 patients with BMP-2 and the BCP carrier had solid fusions judged by CT scans, as evaluated independently. Nine of these patients had no internal fixation. The BMP-2 patients did better than autograft patients at an average of 17 months of follow-up in terms of fusion success and clinical outcome.

Dimar et al. also demonstrated that the rhBMP-2 group had better fusion rates compared with iliac crest bone graft (83% vs. 73%, respectively) for patients receiving posterolateral instrumented fusions in a large prospective randomized study comparing rhBMP-2 with iliac crest (98 patients). Outcome measures such as the Oswestry Low Back Pain Disability Index, and leg and back pain scores, however, were similar over time.[160] These trends toward improved posterolateral fusion rates and outcome scores also were reported by Dawson et al. using rhBMP-2, ACS, and a ceramic bulking agent in a multicenter prospective randomized pilot study without instrumentation.[158]

Bone Morphogenetic Proteins: Adverse Events

Benglis et al. have listed a number of adverse events linked to the use of BMPs, including ectopic bone formation, swelling/hematoma/dsyphagia with anterior cervical discectomy and fusion (ACDF), bony resorption/graft subsidence with lumbar interbody fusions, and painful seroma/mass effect in minimally invasive lumbar surgery.[169]

Ectopic Bone Formation: Animal Studies

Ectopic bone formation and its association with the use of BMP has been documented in both animal and clinical studies. The proposed mechanism is leakage of the molecule into unwanted sites from the carrier causing new both growth over the canal, inside the foramen, or the fusion of unwanted levels. This theory, however, is controversial, and many authors have failed to show any ectopic bone formation in both experimental and human studies, even in the presence of a laminectomy defect.[142,151,170-172] Two studies in lower mammals (rabbits[173] and mice[174]) examined the effects of high doses of BMPs on the exposed thecal sac. In both models, analysis revealed new bone growth and some compression on the neural elements; however, both studies failed to demonstrate any changes in behavior (e.g., motor) in the experimental animals versus the controls. Hsu et al. failed to induce ectopic bone formation in rodents when rhBMP-2 was used in high concentrations without an ACS. They raise the question of the significance of BMP elution without association of a carrier.[175]

Ectopic Bone Formation: Human Studies

Posterior and Transforaminal Lumbar Interbody Fusions

In the FDA-approved investigational device exemption (IDE) study examining rhBMP-2/ACS in posterior lumbar interbody fusions (PLIF), the study was stopped due to evidence on postoperative CT scans of bone encroachment into the spinal canal when compared with the control patients with autograft.[176] There were, however, no clinical symptoms due to this nerve root compression. A later publication by Villavicencio et al. describes the use of rhBMP-2/ACS in transforaminal lumbar interbody fusion (TLIF) without bone encroachment into the vertebral canal.[177] These authors recommend that the sponge be placed ventrally in front of the graft and away from the thecal sac to potentially avoid this complication.

Swelling, Hematoma, and Dysphagia in Anterior Cervical Discectomy and Fusion

Neck swelling, hematoma, dysphagia, and respiratory failure have been reported with the use of rhBMP-2/ACS in ACDF surgery. Five clinical reports totaling 264 patients were analyzed by Benglis et al. in their review on adverse events of BMPs.[169] The studies were by no means standardized, varying in the concentrations of rhBMP-2/ACS used, types of interbody, location of the rhBMP-2, levels fused, and type of anterior construct (discectomy vs. corpectomy).[178-182] The reported complication rates associated with these studies ranged from 5% to 27%, which were higher than historical controls examining complications following ACDF without the use of BMPs. These adverse events, in general, appear to be related to the use of increased dosages and the potential initiation of inflammatory cascades in the soft tissues of anterior cervical procedures. As noted in a study by Baskin et al., only very small doses of rhBMP-2 are needed per level to induce postoperative fusion (one-seventh of a small Infuse kit, Medtronic Sofamor Danek, Memphis, TN).[183]A large, prospective IDE study currently is underway to investigate the clinical outcomes, fusion rates, and adverse events for single-level ACDFs with rhBMP-2.

Bony Resorption and Graft Subsidence

Some in vitro studies have shown that BMPs also may exhibit some osteoclastic activity.[184] This phenomenon could be a function of its interaction with certain interleukins.[185] Various groups are beginning to note robust bone loss during the resorption phase of bone growth associated with the use of BMPs in interbody fusions of the lumbar spine, ranging from resultant instrumentation failure, graft loosening, and subsidence, to migration.[186-190]

Painful Seroma and Mass Effect in Minimally Invasive Lumbar Spine Surgery

Levi and Wang conducted an informal survey with several minimal access surgeons who revealed that a painful seroma from rhBMP-2 is another potential complication (Levi AD, Wang MY, unpublished data, 2010). On reexploration or aspiration of the collection, clear fluid is found, and, following its release, the patient's symptoms disappear. Origins may be due to inflammatory cascades induced by the BMP within a relatively small contained space.

Bone Morphogenetic Proteins and the Rising Costs of Health Care

With the rising cost of health care and current legislation targeted at reducing these costs, the pressures on surgeons to perform more "economical" surgery becomes increasingly relevant.[169] Hospitals traditionally receive a particular payment for a procedure referred to as a *diagnosis related group* or *DRG*. They often do not receive additional funding to cover the cost of devices used in the spinal procedure (e.g., interbody fusion cages, BMP). Despite these upfront increases in initial costs, some groups have published literature supporting a long-term reduction in expenses when using rhBMP-2 versus iliac crest autograft in spine fusions.[191-194] Nevertheless, rhBMP-2 is an expensive molecule, averaging $3600 to $5200 in 2010 for a small and large kit, respectively (personal correspondence with Medtronic/Sofamor Danek), with the hospital carrying most of the cost burden.[192]

A recent article published by Cahill et al. examined the increasing trends in the usage of BMPs in spine fusion surgery. They reviewed a retrospective cohort of 328,468 patients undergoing spine fusion procedures from 2002 to 2006, focusing on certain aspects such as complications, length of stay, and hospital charges. Usage within the United States has increased from 0.69% of all fusions in 2002 to 24.6% of all fusions in 2006. The main point of the article was that increases in hospital charges were noted to be between 11% and 41% (greatest increase seen for anterior cervical fusion).[195]

Future Directions and Emerging Technologies

Mesenchymal stem cells (MSCs) are the precursor cells to the bone-producing osteoblast. The osteoblast cell produces an extracellular matrix that ultimately becomes calcified. Research in bone marrow aspirate (BMA) fusion models has not shown clear evidence supporting its use as a stand-alone bone substitute, but it is potentially effective as a graft extender.[196] Decortication is one traditional means of "recruiting" these osteoprogenitor cells to the site of a fusion. Work is ongoing in the development of techniques to increase the concentration of MSCs by either cellular retention (e.g., membranes that facilitate attachment of MSCs) or cellular expansion (e.g., in vitro culture of an aspirate) methods.[197] The next step in the evolution of therapies to promote bone fusion may lie in the field of tissue engineering, where genes inserted into in vitro cultures of MSCs could be placed into a site of fusion and provide a continuous extracellular supply of proteins such as BMPs.[196, 198, 199] Current work in gene therapy modulation exists only in preclinical animal experiments and has not yet been extended to human clinical studies.[200]

KEY REFERENCES

Benglis D, Wang MY, Levi AD: A comprehensive review of the safety profile of bone morphogenetic protein in spine surgery. *Neurosurgery* 62(5 Suppl. 2):ONS423–ONS431, May 2008; discussion ONS431.

Boden SD: Overview of the biology of lumbar spine fusion and principles for selecting a bone graft substitute. *Spine (Phila Pa 1976)* 27(16 Suppl. 1):S26–S31, 2002.

Boden SD, Kang J, Sandhu H, Heller JG: Use of recombinant human bone morphogenetic protein-2 to achieve posterolateral lumbar spine fusion in humans: a prospective, randomized clinical pilot trial: 2002 Volvo Award in clinical studies. *Spine (Phila Pa 1976)* 27(23):2662–2673, 2002.

Gan J, Glazer P: Electrical stimulation therapies for spinal fusions: current concepts. *Eur Spine J* 15:1301–1311, 2006.

Resnick DK, Choudhri TF, Dailey AT, et al: Guidelines for the performance of fusion procedures for degenerative disease of the lumbar spine. Part 12: pedicle screw fixation as an adjunct to posterolateral fusion for low-back pain. *J Neurosurg Spine* 2(6):700–706, 2005.

Vaccaro AR, Lawrence JP, Patel T, et al: The safety and efficacy of OP-1 (rhBMP-7) as a replacement for iliac crest autograft in posterolateral lumbar arthrodesis: a long-term (>4 years) pivotal study. *Spine (Phila Pa 1976)* 33(26):2850–2862, 2008.

REFERENCES

The complete reference list is available online at expertconsult.com.

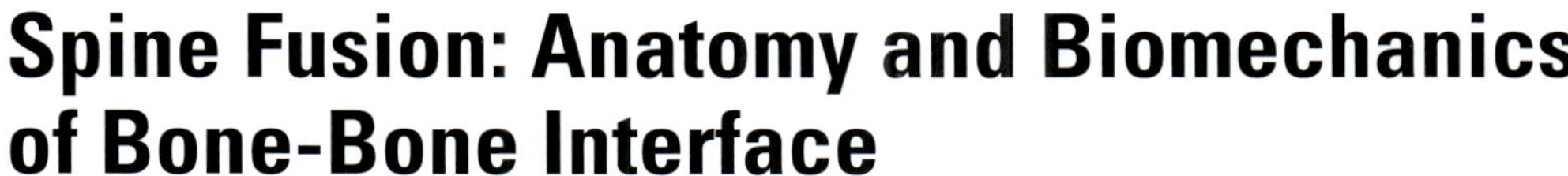

CHAPTER 17

Spine Fusion: Anatomy and Biomechanics of Bone-Bone Interface

Fanor Manuel Saavedra | Rodolfo E. Alcedo-Guardia

In the late 19th century, Sir William Macewen firmly established bone grafting as a treatment option for replacing missing bone and enhancing bone formation. His interest in bone grafting led him to perform allografts and autografts in his patients.[1] In the United States, spine fusion was first reported in the early 1900s by Albee[2] for the treatment of Pott disease and by Hibbs,[3] who used fusion surgery to halt the progression of scoliotic deformity. Since that time the indications for and number of spine fusions have increased. In fact, the numbers doubled between 1980 to 1990,[4] with an increase of 77% between 1996 and 2001.[5] Spine arthrodesis is now one of the most common surgical procedures performed in the United States.

Unfortunately, a number of complications have been associated with spine fusion. Pseudarthrosis can occur in as many as 35% to 40% of multilevel lumbar fusions.[6] Donor site morbidity can also be considerable.[7] To achieve successful bony fusion, minimize complications, and achieve a good functional outcome, it is important to understand the various structural, biologic, and biomechanical aspects of bone fusion.

Bone grafts involve transplanting bone tissue from one site to another in order to obtain bone fusion. The terms used for describing them are usually derived from the bone's origin, anatomic placement, or composition. *Autograft* is a transplanted tissue within the same individual; *allografts* are tissues coming from a genetically different individual of the same species; *xenografts* are tissues transplanted from one species to a member of a different species; *isograft* is tissue obtained from a monozygotic twin. A graft transplanted to an anatomically appropriate site is defined as *orthotopic*, whereas if it is transplanted to an anatomically dissimilar site, it is termed *heterotopic*. Grafts are also categorized by composition as *cortical, cancellous, corticocancellous*, or *osteochondral*.[8]

Anatomy of the Bone-Bone Interface

Histologic Components

On a gross level, all bones are composed of two basic components: cortical (compact) bone and cancellous (trabecular) bone. Cortical bone is a dense, solid mass, except for its microscopic channels, and contains parallel stacks of curved sheets called *lamellae*, which are separated by bands of interlamellar cement. Regularly spaced throughout the lamellae are small cavities, or *lacunae*. Lacunae are interconnected by thin, tubular channels called *canaliculi*. Entrapped bone cells (osteocytes) are located in the lacunae, and their long, cytoplasmic processes occupy canaliculi. The cell processes within canaliculi communicate by gap junctions, with processes of osteocytes lying in adjacent lacunae. Canaliculi open to extracellular fluid at bone surfaces, thus forming an anastomosing network for the nutrition and metabolic activity of the osteocytes. Cortical bone possesses a volume fraction of pores less than 30% and has an apparent density of up to about 2 g/mL. Its compressive strength is approximately 10-fold that for a similar volume of cancellous bone.

Cancellous bone is porous and appears as a lattice of rods, plates, and arches individually known as *trabeculae*. It has a greater surface area and can be readily influenced by adjacent bone marrow cells. Because of this structural difference, cancellous bone has a higher metabolic activity and responds more readily to changes in mechanical loads.[9]

Cortical and cancellous bone may consist of woven (primary) or lamellar (secondary) bone. Woven bone forms the embryonic skeleton and is then resorbed and replaced by mature bone as the skeleton develops.[10] In the adult, woven bone is found only in pathologic conditions, such as fracture healing and in tumors. Woven and lamellar bones differ in formation, composition, organization, and mechanical properties. Woven bone has an irregular pattern of collagen fibers, contains approximately four times as many osteocytes per unit volume, and has a rapid rate of deposition and turnover. The osteocytes of woven bone vary in orientation, and the mineralization of woven bone follows an irregular pattern in which mineral deposits vary in size and in their relationship to collagen fibrils. In contrast, the osteocytes of lamellar bone are relatively uniform, with their principle axis oriented parallel to that of other cells and to the collagen fibrils of the matrix. The collagen fibrils of lamellar bone lie in tightly organized, parallel sheets, with uniform distribution of mineral within the matrix.[11,12]

The irregular structure of woven bone makes it more flexible, more easily deformed, and weaker than lamellar bone.[9] For these reasons the restoration of normal mechanical properties to bone tissue at the site of a healing fracture requires eventual replacement of the woven bone of the fracture callus with mature lamellar bone.[11]

Biomechanical Properties of Graft Material

In vivo, the mechanical performance of a bone graft is a function of the intrinsic property of the graft and the properties of the graft-host interface.[13] Intrinsic properties of a graft are related to its geometry and composition and include its fracture toughness, yield strength, and elastic modulus.[8]

In a clinical setting, where the graft has geometric and mechanical properties similar to the host bone, it may function almost immediately.[14] Nevertheless, in the case of inferior bone graft mechanical properties, the construct should be designed with additional graft material or incorporate internal fixation until remodeling occurs and the graft can provide adequate load-bearing function.[14] A graft's load-bearing capacity is achieved after complete biologic incorporation by the host, which is related to the mechanical and biologic properties of the graft-host interface.

Iliac crest wedges are the most commonly used graft material. The percentages of cortical and cancellous bone remain constant at 41% and 59%, respectively, regardless of the total cross-sectional area of the wedge. Donor age also does not affect this physical parameter.[15]

To reduce the immune response and also as methods of preservation and sterilization, allografts undergo certain modifications. These modifications have a profound effect on the biomechanical properties of the graft. Freezing has minimal effects compared with freeze-drying, which significantly reduces both the yield strength and stiffness of the bone graft.[16] Autoclaving produces a dose-dependent decrease in strength and stiffness.[17] The relationship between gamma radiation and mechanical properties has yet to be established at doses between 0 and 25 kGy (standard dose). But it becomes dose-dependent at 25 kGy for cortical bone or 60 kGy for cancellous bone.[18] Complete demineralization of the bone graft results in loss of almost all of its mechanical properties. Comparison testing of various graft materials shows allograft or fresh-frozen cancellous bone to be the weakest, failing at 863 N of compression. Air-dried, ethylene oxide-sterilized, tricortical bone failed at an average load of 2308 N, and fresh-frozen, tricortical allograft bone failed at an average load of 2257 N. Rehydrated iliac crest wedges are more deformable than freeze-dried wedges.[19] During loading, freeze-dried wedges fail dramatically, fracturing into many small pieces; this occurrence is secondary to its brittle nature. Rehydrated wedges fail with a circumferential fracture along the side of the wedge where the cortical bone is thinnest. It has been recommended that freeze-dried wedges be rehydrated in a vacuum before clinical use.[19] When water or saline is added to the vacuum-sealed container holding the wedge, the wedges gain 100% of their wet weight within 5 minutes of addition of the fluid. Graft collapse occurred more frequently with freeze-dried allografts (30%) than with autografts in anterior cervical fusions.

The loads at the lumbar spine have been well documented in various positions and levels of activity.[20] Either autograft or allograft iliac crest wedges are biomechanically sound in an interbody fusion of the lumbar spine, since such fusions would provide load-bearing capacities approximately four-fold greater than would be applied in vivo. Specimens from the anterosuperior iliac spine could bear substantially greater axial loads (average 3230 N) compared with specimens from the posterosuperior iliac spine (average 1458 N).[21] Fibular strut grafts are the strongest and have been shown to have a compressive strength of 5070 N.[22] However, their cross-sectional area, which is important in preventing telescoping of the graft, is much smaller. In interbody fusion, the cross-sectional area of the graft should be substantially greater than 30% of the end plate to provide a margin of safety.[23]

Incorporation of Bone Graft

Bone graft incorporation is a prolonged process with a sequence of complicated steps involving the interrelationship of the graft and host. This ultimately leads to the envelopment of a complex of necrotic old bone with viable new bone.[24] The complex develops through resorption of the necrotic old bone with viable new bone being laid down. The incorporation of the bone graft is a dynamic process involving the following processes: osteoinduction, osteoconduction along with the availability of osteogenic cells, and the *structural integrity*, which provides mechanical support.[14,19,25,26] This ultimately leads to the replacement of the graft by host bone in a predictable pattern under the influences of load bearing.[14,27]

At the beginning, the inflammatory response at the host-graft interface results in migration of inflammatory cells and fibroblasts into the bone graft. In addition, the developing hematoma enhances the release of both cytokines and growth factors. *Osteoinduction* is the process whereby a tissue is influenced to form osteogenic elements through chemotaxis, mitosis, and differentiation of the host osteoprogenitor cells. Induction requires an inducing stimulus, such as a piece of bone or an osteogenic cell, and an environment favorable for osteogenesis. *Osteoconduction* is the process by which capillaries, perivascular tissue, and osteoprogenitor cells from the recipient bed grow into the graft. It can occur within a framework of nonbiologic materials or nonviable biologic materials. In viable bone grafts, osteoconduction is facilitated by osteoinductive processes and therefore occurs more rapidly than in nonviable or nonbiologic materials.[28] Ultimately, this process results in the resorption of the original graft tissue and replacement with new host bone. Remodeling is a response to weight bearing.

Differences in Cancellous and Cortical Bone Graft Incorporation

Cancellous grafts are revascularized more rapidly and completely than cortical grafts. The open trabecular pattern of cancellous bone facilitates vessel ingrowth. Revascularization has been reported to begin within a few hours after grafting[29] and may be complete by 2 weeks. In contrast, the dense structure of cortical bone prevents neovascular penetration during the first several weeks after grafting, and hence revascularization of cortical bone may take several months. Because of the dense architectural structure of cortical bone, new vessel incorporation follows preexisting haversian and Volkmann canals.[30]

Several differences exist between the cellular process of repair in cancellous and cortical grafts. With cancellous grafts, primitive mesenchymal cells that originate in the trabeculae may differentiate directly into osteoblasts, thereby resulting in relatively early new bone formation. The new bone forms on the dead trabeculae of the graft. This is followed by a resorptive phase. Cancellous bone initially undergoes an appositional new bone formation phase called *creeping substitution*, which is the process of new tissue invading along channels made by invasive blood vessels or along preexisting channels in the transplanted bone.[31] The necrotic areas within the cancellous bone graft eventually are entirely resorbed by osteoblastic activity and totally replaced with new viable bone. As the revascularization of cancellous bone graft proceeds, primitive mesenchymal cells differentiate into osteogenic cells. These osteogenic cells form osteoblasts that line the edges of dead trabeculae and deposit a seam of osteoid that is annealed to, and eventually surrounds, a central core of dead bone. This process of alignment of osteoblasts on existing bone surfaces, with the synthesis of osteoid in successive layers to form lamellae, is termed *appositional bone formation*. Thus initially, there is an increase in the size of the graft. Cancellous grafts tend to repair completely with time. The areas of entrapped necrotic bone are resorbed by osteoclasts. In time the cancellous bone graft is completely replaced by viable new bone.

Cortical grafts must undergo osteoclastic resorption before osteoblastic new bone formation occurs. In cortical grafts the repair process is initiated by osteoclasts with preferential early resorption of the external cortical surface. Osteoblasts appear only after bone resorption has begun, and the initial deposition of osteoid usually occurs in resorbed areas. Cortical grafts remain as admixtures of necrotic and viable bone. In cortical grafts, revascularization is primarily the result of vascular infiltration through Volkmann and haversian canals.[19] Osteoclasts initiate resorption of bone approximately 2 weeks after vascularization. Resorption is maximal at 6 weeks, and then gradually the graft recovers normal strength by 1 year. New bone is formed and seals off the remaining necrotic bone from further encroachment beginning at around 12 weeks. Thus if a biopsy specimen is obtained from a cortical graft years after placement, it demonstrates an admixture of necrotic and viable bone.

Biomechanics of Graft Incorporation

Porosity is a dominant factor in determining the material properties of bone. It is directly related to the stiffness of the tissue and yield of strength.[13,14,32] Therefore, any change in porosity result in important effects on the bone graft material properties. Cortical bone grafts initially may have as little as 5% to 10% porosity, whereas cancellous grafts may be as high as 70% to 80%. This explains the material strength of cancellous graft, which is roughly equivalent to 4% of that of cortical bone.[13]

Cancellous grafts are incorporated by an early appositional phase. New bone formation onto the necrotic trabeculae of the graft tissue leads to an early increase in graft strength. It has been shown that necrotic bone maintains its mechanical strength.[30] Cancellous grafts therefore initially strengthen with the addition of new bone. As the necrotic cores are resorbed, the mechanical strength of the graft area normalizes.

Cortical bone grafts first undergo osteoclastic bone resorption, which significantly increases graft porosity and thus decreases the graft strength. In the canine model of autogenous cortical transplant, the greatest compromise in mechanical strength occurs at 12 weeks[30] (Fig. 17-1). The strength returns to normal between 1 and 2 years after transplantation. Human data suggest that cortical grafts lose approximately half their biomechanical strength during the first 6 months—a decline that persists for another 6 months.[33] This process is related to osteoclastic graft resorption and is slowly reversed during the second year after implantation. These observations correlate with the highest incidence of mechanical graft failure between 6 and 8 months after transplantation. If the graft is allogenic, this process is further prolonged. Hence it is important to protect segmental grafts during the critical phase when the resorptive phase outstrips the appositional phase. This is usually accomplished by load sharing with spinal instrumentation or a spinal orthosis.

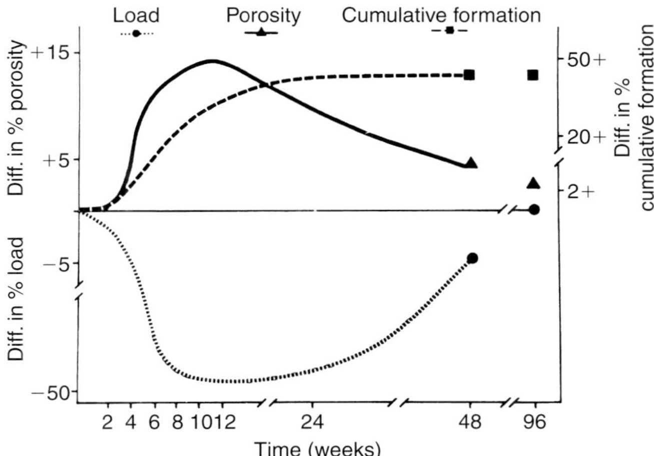

FIGURE 17-1. Graph illustrating the quantitative temporal interrelationships between the physical integrity and the biologic processes of repair within a segmental autogenous cortical bone transplant. The initial persistence of strength (0–4 weeks after transplantation) indicates the subsequent loss was caused by reparative processes rather than any intrinsic weakness in the material. The sudden loss in strength at 6 weeks is caused by the increased internal porosity. From 6 to 12 weeks, the decrease in mechanical strength is reduced by 50%. The level of porosity continues to increase until week 12 because of the temporal lag in the apposition of new bone formation. At 24 weeks, there is no significant improvement in strength, despite the beginning reduction in the porosity of the transplant and maturation of the callus. At 48 weeks, however, the physical integrity of the transplant has returned toward normal, primarily as the result of decreased material porosity, since the amount of callus has not increased. By 2 years, the physical integrity of the transplant has returned toward normal, primarily as a result of decreased material porosity, since the amount of callus has not increased. By 2 years, the physical integrity of the transplant and the internal porosity of the remaining transplanted material are normal. The biologic completeness of repair (i.e., approximately 50% of the graft is viable) is not significant, because mechanical strength has been retained. The admixture of necrotic and viable bone remains for the life of the individual's skeletal metabolic activity. (From Burchardt H: Biology of cortical bone graft incorporation. In Friedlaender GE, Mankin HJ, Sell KW, editors: *Osteochondral allografts: biology, banking, and clinical applications,* Boston, 1983, Little, Brown, p 55.)

Temporal Profile of Graft Incorporation

During the first week after grafting, both cancellous and cortical grafts have similar histologic features. Both are surrounded by coagulated blood, and the graft is the focus of a tissue response characterized by vascular buds infiltrating the grafted bed. By the second week, fibrous granulation tissue becomes increasingly dominant in the graft bed, the number of inflammatory cells decrease, and osteoclastic activity increases. Within the confines of the graft, osteocytic autolysis proceeds, resulting from anoxia and injury by surgery, with necrosis delineated by vacant lacunae. Some cells, however, survive by diffusion of nutrients from surrounding host tissues. Creeping substitution of cortical bone grafts progresses transversely and parallel to the long axis of the transplanted segment. Thus the repair is found to be greater at the graft-host junctions.[34]

A study done in rabbits[35] showed the sequence of events during the process of dorsolateral intertransverse fusion. Three phases were identified. Phase 1 represents the early reparative phase (1–3 weeks). It consists of hematoma formation and granulation tissue. There is minimal ossification. Phase 2 represents the middle reparative phase (4–5 weeks), when the fusion solidifies. Finally, phase 3 represents the late remodeling phase (6–10 weeks).[35]

Both membranous and enchondral ossification play a role in the fusion process. Membranous ossification is the predominant mechanism that begins at the termini of the fusion mass and emanates from the decorticated transverse process. The central portion of the fusion mass, where the vascular supply is poorer and movement is greater, heals by cartilage formation and enchondral ossification.

Host Response and Incorporation of Autograft and Allograft

Autograft remains the gold standard in most fusion applications. In certain situations in which available autologous bone is insufficient or when large structural grafts are needed, allograft fusion rates can approach or equal those of autograft rates, without donor site morbidity. A successful spine fusion requires a sufficient area of decorticated host bone, ample graft material, minimal motion at the fusion site, and a rich vascular supply.[36]

Histocompatibility matching has an important influence on the process of incorporation. Allograft that is mismatched for major histocompatibility complex antigens functions poorly compared with autogenous grafts.[37,38] Bone cells display class I and class II histocompatibility antigens, and there are both cellular and humoral responses to bone allografts.[39] Syngeneic grafts are the most successful. Grafts with major histocompatibility mismatch have delayed and incomplete revascularization, compared with syngeneic grafts. In addition, marked resorption of bone often occurs, resulting in almost complete loss of graft.[38] Freezing the graft, followed by thawing, disrupts and kills the cells. It mutes the antigenicity in major mismatches and thus enhances incorporation of such grafts. However, the killing of cells also diminishes the biologic activity of the graft. It is the osteoinductive component that is mainly affected. The function of an allograft as an osteoconductive system seems virtually unimpaired.

In fresh cancellous allografts, the initial phase consisting of hemorrhage and necrosis is identical to that of the autograft. The fibrin clot and the same inflammatory response develop. However, in the allograft the fibrin clot breaks down, and the granulation tissue, which provides nutrition to the repair site, is invaded by chronic inflammatory cells rather than fibroblasts and blood vessel elements. The major portion of the delay appears to occur in osteoclastic resorption and new bone formation. Final graft incorporation remains incomplete.

In cortical allografts the length of time of creeping substitution is greatly prolonged. The invasion by host vessels and recruitment and differentiation of cellular elements to become osteoblastic and osteoclastic cells are greatly diminished. The proportion of necrotic graft bone to viable host bone is much greater in allogeneic grafts. In fact, the active process of graft substitution may last several years.

Modeling and Remodeling Associated with Spine Fusion

The bone modeling associated with spine fusion is extremely complex. Variables that may affect bone remodeling after graft insertion include (1) the design of implant, materials used, and methods of fixation; (2) the local bone, including its density and shape; and (3) the patient characteristics, including age, gender, hormonal balance, and activity.[40] Osteoblasts and osteoclasts are influenced by the magnitude and state of strain imposed on them by load applied to the bone. Stresses or strains within a given range seem to be required to maintain a steady state remodeling of bone in which the rate of bone formation equals the rate of resorption. Stresses below the optimum are often associated with stress shielding, leading to bone resorption. Stresses and strains exceeding upper limits can also produce resorption of bone as a result of pressure necrosis. Cyclic stresses are required to maintain osseous homeostasis. Constant loads, even when within the desired range, can result in insufficient stimulus to maintain bone mass. Observations of strain-related electric potentials in bone, biopotentials, and electrical stimulation of osteogenesis suggest that bioelectric phenomena function as the regulators of adaptive remodeling of bone.

Growth Factors and Cytokines in Regulating Bone Remodeling

Bone cells carry out diverse functions and are mainly derived from two cell lines: mesenchymal and hematopoietic. The mesenchymal stem cell line consists of undifferentiated cells, or preosteoblasts, that differentiate into osteoblasts, bone-lining cells, and osteocytes. The hematopoietic stem cell line consists of circulating marrow monocytes that differentiate into preosteoclasts and osteoclasts. These cells are regulated by various cytokines.

Bone formation in spine fusion is a complex and regulated process. The cellular events involved in bone formation include chemotaxis of osteoblast precursors, proliferation of committed osteoblast precursors, and differentiation and expression of regulatory factors and structural proteins of bone and mineralization.[41] These processes require tight regulatory control. They may be modulated by systemic hormones, such as parathyroid hormone, but predominant control is by local factors or cytokines. Cytokines are small proteins that serve as signaling agents for cells. Cytokines are classified based on their cellular origin and principal biologic activities.[42] The main families include interleukins, tumor necrosis factors, growth factors, colony-stimulating factors, interferons, and chemokines.

Bone morphogenetic protein (BMP) is a member of the transforming growth factor beta (TGF-β) superfamily. The BMP constitutes a growth family of more than 12 proteins, 9 of which have been shown individually to induce ectopic bone formation.[43] They are water soluble, noncollagenous substances found in the bone matrix with osteoinductive activity. BMPs 2, 4, and 7 are specially increased in the primitive mesenchymal and osteoprogenitor cells, fibroblasts, and proliferating chondrocytes present at the fracture site.[18,44,45] During the phases of healing, the expression of BMPs 2, 4, and 7 is strongly present in undifferentiated mesenchymal cells during the inflammatory phase. During intramembranous ossification, these BMPs are strongly present in the proliferating osteoblasts. During chondrogenesis and endochondral ossification, BMPs 2 and 4 are found in proliferating chondrocytes and strongly in osteoblasts near the endochondral ossification front. BMP 7 is found in later stages of healing in proliferating chondrocytes and weakly in mature chondrocytes.[18,45] BMPs also affect the expression of other growth factors that may function to mediate the effects of BMPs on bone formation.

They are the most widely investigated osteoinductive growth factor in spine fusion.[43,46] Several animal studies have shown that recombinant human (rh) BMPs 2, 4, and 7 induce bone formation at an orthotopic site at which the integration with the preexisting bone is structurally sound. It has also been shown that BMP plus marrow yields the highest union rates (100%) and is three times better than autogenous cancellous graft.[46-54]

However, other factors may play a role in the biologic response to rhBMP in vivo, including the time course activity of rhBMP on the bone formation process, its interaction with other growth factors, and the influence of delivery vehicles.

Biomechanics of Fusion

There is a wealth of literature on the biomechanics of fusion, but the vast majority involves in vitro models. In vivo, a variety of biologic factors influence the mechanical properties of fusion mass. The type of surgical construct and choice of bone graft should be individualized, based on the biologic and mechanical considerations. The main indications for a spine fusion are listed in Box 17-1.

Biomechanics of the Fusion Mass

In dorsal and dorsolateral fusion, healing occurs through callus formation. As ossification proceeds, the callus is converted from a low-stiffness, rubbery quality to a hard tissue type of resiliency. The mineralization of the callus progressively increases its tensile strength. The fusion site during all stages of the reparative process is highly susceptible to mechanical forces directly related to the amount of motion between the graft fragment and host surface. The amount of relative motion determines the morphologic patterns of fracture repair. As healing proceeds, the amount of motion decreases. When mechanical stability is compromised, more cartilage always forms and, occasionally, an exuberant callus. Frequently, with excessive motion the fusion mass is incomplete and a pseudarthrosis develops. Rigid internal fixation has been demonstrated to reduce pseudarthrosis rates in most clinical applications.

BOX 17-1. Primary Indications for Spine Fusion

Deformity: To correct and prevent progression of deformity
Eradication of disease: Examples include metastatic disease and osteomyelitis in which diseased bone is removed and stability restoration is required
Instability: To restore the structural integrity
Painful motion segment: Includes low back pain caused by segmental instability

Positioning of Bone Graft

As White and Panjabi[20] describe, "The placement of a fusion mass at the maximum distance from the instantaneous axes of rotation will be more effective in preventing the movement around those axes" (Fig. 17-2). The instantaneous axis of rotation (IAR) is defined as the point in the body, or some hypothetical extension of it, that does not move when a rigid body moves in a plane. An axis perpendicular to the plane of motion and passing through the point is the IAR for that motion at that instant (Fig. 17-3). It can be defined more simply as the axis around which the vertebral body rotates. It is like a fulcrum. Usually, but not always, the IAR passes through the confines of the vertebral body. With isolated destruction of columns of the spine, the IAR migrates to the remaining intact structures, as shown in Figure 17-4.

The greater the distance of the fusion mass from the IAR, the greater the leverage in preventing motion around those axes of rotation. Examples include dorsal, dorsolateral, and intertransverse lumbar fusion, in which the fusion mass is located at a distance from the IAR (which is located in the region of the vertebral body). A ventrally placed graft is closer to the IAR and applies less leverage, but can still be extremely effective, especially in cases of anterior column deficiency.

The concept of rigidity is also important. A fusion mass that involves all the dorsal elements and transverse processes provides more rigidity than a fusion that only involves the spinous process. In some situations it can be disadvantageous to place the graft at a distance from the IAR. For example, after a dorsal fusion to treat discogenic pain, motion may still occur at the disc interspace, even when all dorsal elements except the pedicle are fixed.[55,56] In such situations an interbody fusion may be considered (Fig. 17-5).[57]

The production of biomechanical changes as a function of different types of lumbar fusion has been studied.[58,59] The three types of fusion evaluated included dorsal, bilateral lateral, and ventral. All types of fusion increased bending and axial stiffness. There is increased stress on the adjoining segments that were not fused, especially the facet joints. Overall, bilateral intertransverse fusion is a superior method because it provides good stabilization to the fused segments and has less effect on adjacent, unfused segments, especially the facet joints. Dorsal (intraosseous) fusion is the least beneficial, producing the highest amount of stress in adjoining segments and allowing superficial motion in the disc space.

The spine experiences compressive forces on the concave side and tensile forces on the convex side of a curve. In the lumbar spine, if the graft material is placed in the intervertebral disc space, it is subjected to compressive loading. It is believed that compressive forces acting on the graft will promote fusion by stimulating the osteoconductive healing process. In contrast, a graft placed in a dorsal location experiences only tensile forces and will not be stimulated in a similar manner (Fig. 17-6).

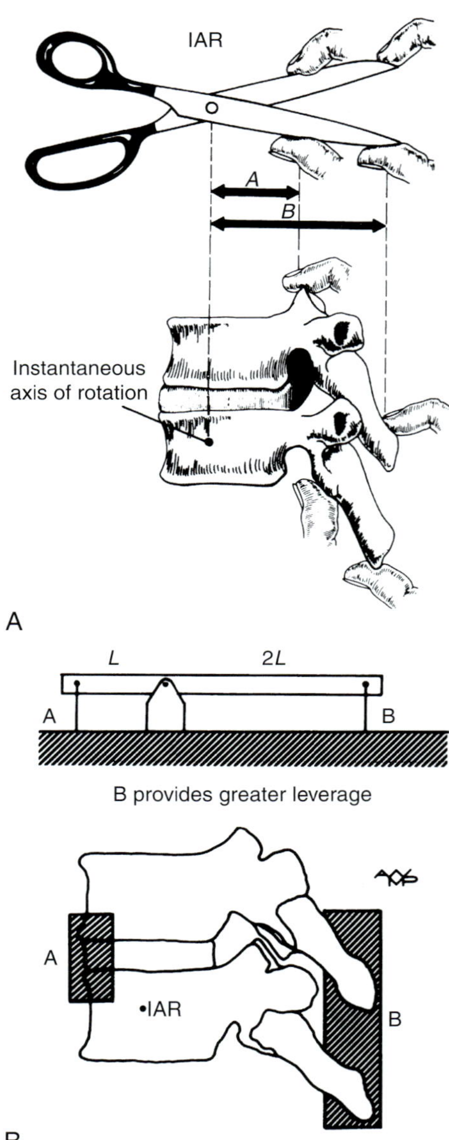

FIGURE 17-2. **A,** To prevent the opening of the blades of the scissors by holding them together, it is distinctly easier to pinch the blades together at the tips (distance *B*) rather than at the midpoint of the blade (distance *A*). Because distance *B* is farther from the instantaneous axis of the rotation (IAR), there is greater leverage. The same concepts apply to the vertebral functional spinal unit. Flexion, separation, or opening of the spinous processes is more readily prevented by placing the fingers at the tips of the spinous processes (distance *B*) rather than at the facet joints (distance *A*). Thus, with regard to a flexion movement, a healed bone graft at distance *B,* at the tips of the spinous processes, is more effective than one closer to the IAR, other factors being constant. These concepts partially explain the efficacy of the rather delicate interspinous and supraspinous ligaments. **B,** The concept of leverage is shown again here. The anterior bone graft A is a short distance (analogous to *L*) from the IAR and therefore provides less leverage than bone graft B, which is a greater distance (analogous to 2*L*) from the instantaneous axis of rotation. (From White AA, Panjabi MM: *Clinical biomechanics of the spine,* Philadelphia, 1990, JB Lippincott, p 533.)

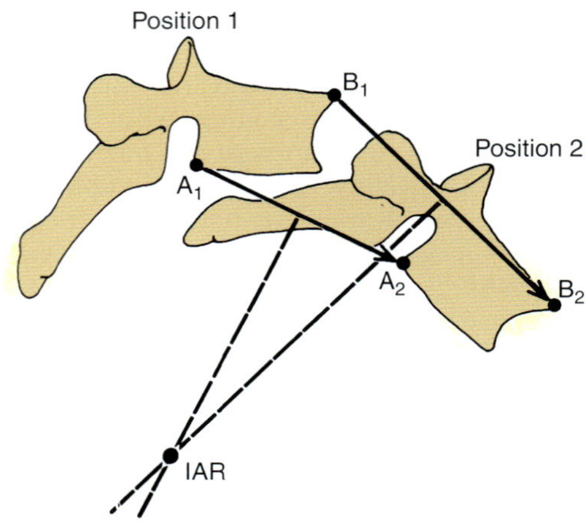

FIGURE 17-3. Instantaneous axis of rotation (IAR). A construction for determining the IAR is shown. A_1–A_2 and B_1–B_2 are translation vectors of points *A* and *B.* (From White AA, Panjabi MM: *Clinical biomechanics of the spine,* Philadelphia, 1990, JB Lippincott, p 660. Reprinted with permission.)

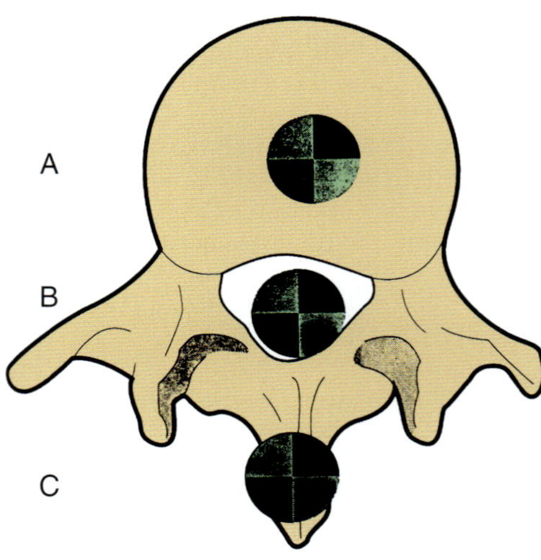

FIGURE 17-4. Location of the axis. The location of the IAR for the intact and compromised specimens. **A,** Facet joints compromised. **B,** Intact spine. **C,** Facet joints and anulus compromised. (From Haher TR, O'Brien M, Felmly WT, et al: Instantaneous axis of rotation as a function of the three columns of the spine. *Spine [Phila Pa 1976]* 1992:17[6S]:S153. Reprinted with permission.)

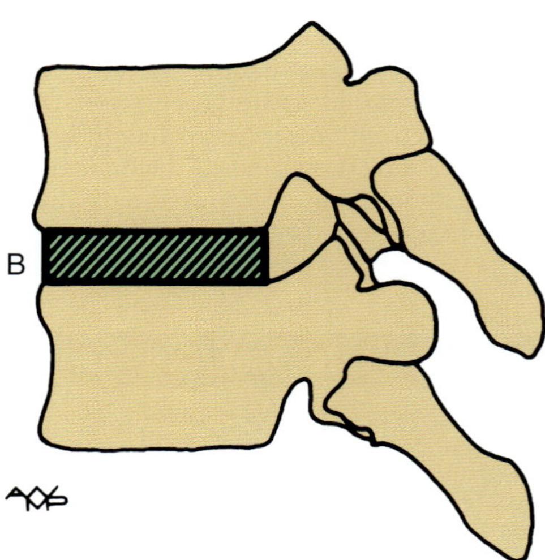

FIGURE 17-5. Illustration of the position of a bone graft (B), which can provide maximum rigidity by eliminating interbody motion. (From White AA, Panjabi MM: *Clinical biomechanics of the spine,* Philadelphia, 1990, JB Lippincott, p 535. Reprinted with permission.)

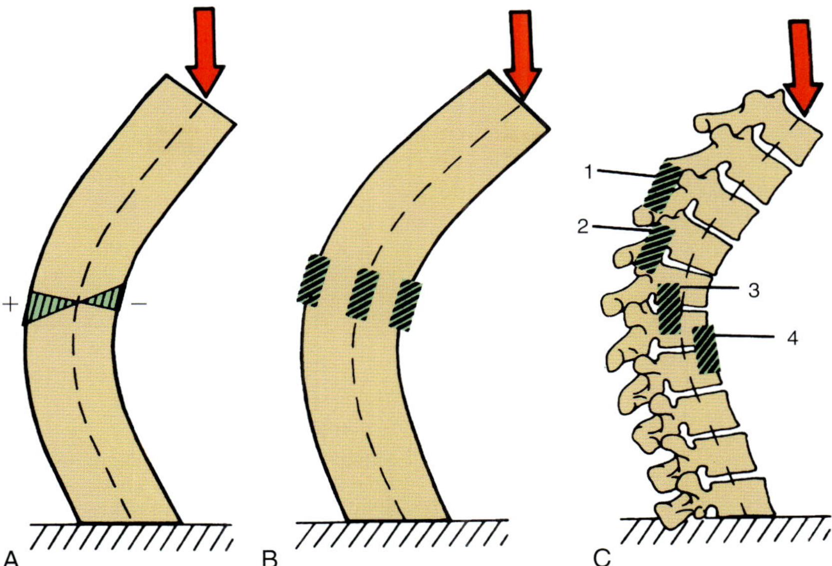

FIGURE 17-6. **A,** The spinal column may be analyzed by regarding it as similar to a beam. There is tension on the convex side of the curve and compression on the concave side. The dashed line is the neutral axis, and there is neither tension nor compression along this line. **B,** Bone grafts inserted at the various points tend to behave as follows. The graft on the convex side of the curve is mainly under tension and cannot resist deforming forces until fully attached at both interfaces. The graft at the dashed line (neutral axis) provides little or no resistance to bending in the plane of the page. **C,** In the spine, the graft at position 1 is well away from the neutral axis and when biologically fused at both interfaces can offer effective tensile resistance against progressive kyphosis. The graft at position 2 can do the same, but is less effective because it is closer to the neutral axis. The graft at position 3 is not likely to be as effective as those at position 1 or 2 in preventing progression of deformity because it is even closer to the neutral axis. The graft at position 4 is effective because it immediately begins to resist compressive forces and therefore tends to prevent additional deformity and angulation at that point. The graft is also some distance away from the neutral axis, giving it a mechanical advantage. (From White AA, Panjabi MM, Thomas CL: The clinical biomechanics of kyphotic deformities. *Clin Orthop Relat Res* 8:128, 1977.)

Kyphotic Deformity and Bone Graft Positioning

At the IAR, there is neither compression nor tension. The farther instrumentation or bone graft is placed from the IAR, the greater the stress. For instance, in a kyphotic deformity, dorsal instrumentation is subjected to severe tensile stress. To reduce stress on a dorsal implant, some structural graft should be placed as ventrally as possible, away from the IAR. This counteracts the tensile stress dorsally. At times, with severe kyphotic deformity, multiple ventral grafts may be required (Fig. 17-7). It has been demonstrated that ventral and dorsal fusions are associated with a better correction and maintenance of correction than the dorsal group, but only with congenital kyphosis.[60]

Load Sharing

Denis[61] introduced the three-column theory of the spine to classify and assist with the management of thoracolumbar spine injuries. Of these three columns, the anterior and posterior columns are the principle support structures.[62] The anterior column resists compression and axial loading, and the posterior column maintains the tension. To maintain an erect posture, all forces and movements must be balanced about the IAR. The IAR is located dorsal to the anulus fibrosus in the intact spine.[63]

Deficiencies in the anterior or posterior column in the thoracolumbar spine usually lead to kyphosis.[64] Kyphosis is

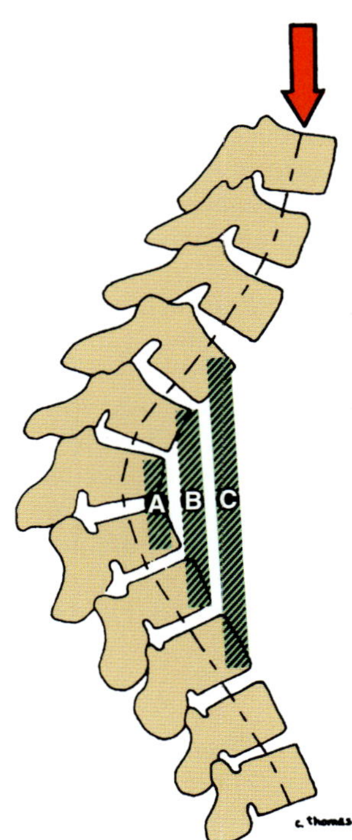

FIGURE 17-7. Illustration of the various locations of ventral bone grafts for kyphotic deformity. The biomechanical considerations involved in choosing graft A, B, or C are discussed in the text. (From White AA, Panjabi MM, Thomas CL: The clinical biomechanics of kyphotic deformities. *Clin Orthop Relat Res* 8:128, 1977.)

corrected by lengthening the anterior column or shortening the posterior column. If the anterior or middle column is destroyed, alignment can be restored by a ventral structural graft and the resulting fusion. In this situation the axial load is shared by both anterior and posterior columns. When deciding on whether to perform a ventral or dorsal fusion, or a combination of both, the principles of load sharing should be considered. If both the ventral and dorsal elements are involved, both columns usually must be instrumented and fused. For example, a burst fracture will be compromised if the dorsal elements frequently require both ventral and dorsal spine reconstruction. With persistent posttraumatic kyphosis after a dorsal instrumentation procedure to treat a cervical or thoracolumbar fracture, anterior column load sharing is eliminated. Instrumentation such as a pedicle screw implant is exposed to high cantilever bending loads and may therefore fail.[65] With correction of a kyphotic deformity, ventral surgery may not be necessary if the weight-bearing line is shifted behind the axis of rotation.[66] By shifting the center of gravity dorsally, the anterior column does not have to support as much axial load. The prerequisites for such a strategy include (1) correction or overcorrection, if surgically feasible; (2) intact dorsal elements; and (3) good osteogenic potential. If sagittal correction is not accomplished, the load on the anterior column is high, and anterior column reconstruction is needed to prevent dorsal instrumentation failure.

Ventral instrumentation, without structural bone grafting, usually fails. A strong structural graft is required to resist axial loading and flexion.[67] Tricortical ilium, fibula, humerus, or titanium cages packed with autogenous graft provide excellent anterior column support. However, single-rib grafts do not provide adequate structural support. Load sharing, in this case, implies a balance between ventral structural bone grafts and ventral or dorsal instrumentation. As the fixation length of ventral and dorsal constructs is reduced, load sharing with the anterior column has become increasingly important in reducing the incidence of failure of the shorter devices. The conditions frequently requiring both ventral and dorsal reconstruction include tumors involving both anterior and posterior columns, fractures involving all three columns, and postlaminectomy kyphosis.[64]

In dorsolateral spine fusion, instrumentation adds to the stability of the fusion by significant load sharing. In a human spine model where bilateral facetectomies were performed and transpedicular screws were used to restore stability, the spinal instrumentation provided 68% of the load sharing, along with the anterior and middle columns.[68] As the fusion mass develops in vivo the load-sharing component of the instrumentation decreases. If an adequate fusion mass does not develop, the cyclical stresses placed on the instrumentation will lead to hardware failure (Fig. 17-8).

Stress Shielding

In a canine model, dorsolateral fusion without instrumentation resulted in fusion in only 57%, compared with a 100% fusion rate with pedicle screw fixation and a 71% fusion rate with Luque rods. Histologic evaluation of the vertebral body at the level of the fusion demonstrated osteoporosis in animals that had received instrumentation. This has been corroborated in humans.[69] Patients who had undergone instrumented dorsolateral lumbar fusion were found to have decreased vertebral body mineral density at the level of fusion, compared with matched controls. This phenomenon has been termed *stress shielding*. However, in animal models the spine fusions that had been instrumented demonstrated increased areas of bone incorporation and biomechanical stability,[70-72] and for any preexisting osteoporosis, compensation was more than adequate. In general, rigid fixation results in better union. Ventral interbody fusions are more prone than dorsal-only fusions to the negative effects of stress shielding.

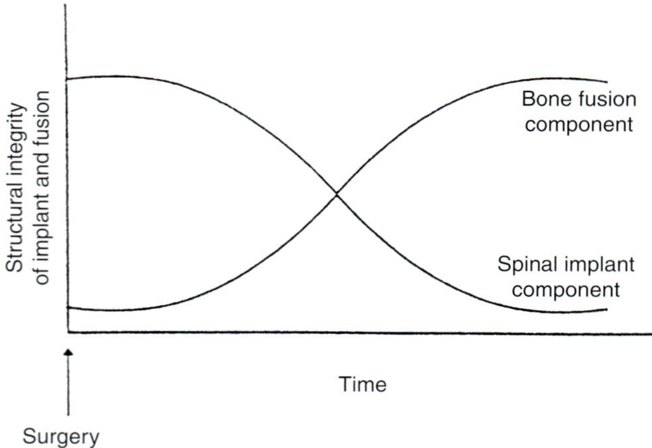

FIGURE 17-8. The relationship between bone fusion acquisition and spinal implant integrity changes with time after surgery. (From Benzel EC: *Biomechanics of spine stabilization,* New York, 1994, McGraw-Hill, p 104.)

Biomechanical Consideration at Specific Sites

Ventral cervical spine fusions are commonly performed using the Smith-Robinson technique. It achieves a wide decompression and provides an optimal load-bearing capacity (Fig. 17-9). The end plates are left intact. The cancellous portion of the graft is in contact with the vertebral end plates and readily permits revascularization. It is important to remember that transplanted bone weakens as resorption proceeds and, consequently, the graft is weaker at 6 months than at the time of implantation.

In the thoracic spine, segments of ribs may be used to provide structural support. However, they have a low compressive strength, which is related to their unfavorable length-to-width ratio, curvature, and small area of contact with the end plate. Fibular strut grafts or iliac crest grafts can be used, if structural support is important. Figure 17-10 demonstrates the relative strengths of various grafts used in ventral thoracic/lumbar fusion.

In the lumbar spine, despite the potential for surgical complications, interbody fusions are being increasingly performed. The lumbar spine experiences static loads in the range of 759 to 1600 pounds and up to 2000 pounds for high loading. The compressive strength of iliac allografts ranges from 396 to 1475 pounds, whereas femoral cortical rings have a strength in excess of 15,000 pounds. Some surgeons thus prefer femoral cortical allografts.[73] Interbody cages are another option because they eliminate the associated iliac crest harvest complications.

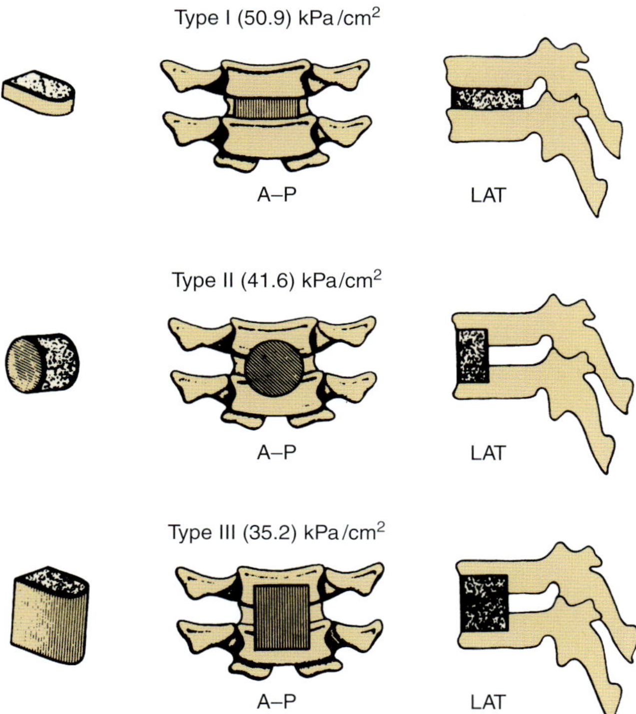

FIGURE 17-9. Graft configuration: How the graft fits into vertebrae, and how the vertebrae are altered to receive it. Type I: Smith-Robinson. Type II: Cloward. Type III: Bailey-Badgeley (modified). The numbers are mean values for load-bearing capacity of each of the three surgical constructions. LAT, lateral. (From White AA, Jupiter J, Southwick WO, et al: An experimental study of the immediate load-bearing capacity of three surgical constructions for anterior spine fusions. *Clin Orthop Relat Res* 91:21, 1973.)

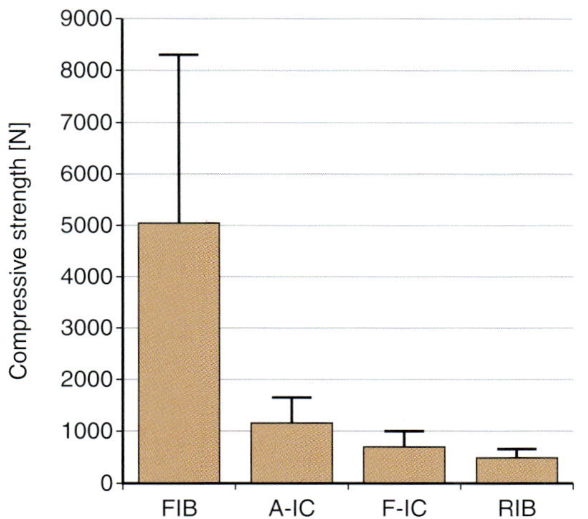

FIGURE 17-10. Compressive strength of anterior thoracic/lumbar grafts. The fibular graft (FIB) was significantly stronger in compression ($P = .05$) than the anterior (A-IC) and posterior (P-IC) grafts and the rib (RIB) graft. (From Wittenberg RH, Moeller J, Shea M, et al: Compressive strength of autologous and allogenous bone grafts for thoracolumbar and cervical spine fusion. *Spine [Phila Pa 1976]* 15:1076, 1990.)

The dorsolateral intertransverse fusion is the most commonly performed fusion procedure. It involves the facet joints, the pedicles, the transverse process, and the gutter between them. This fusion provides greater stability with axial rotation and lateral bending. Motion can persist, even after solid fusion, and can cause discogenic pain, particularly when the facet joints are not included in the arthrodesis. This motion occurs through the pedicles and can be minimized by augmenting the fusion with spinal instrumentation.[74,75]

Summary

Bone is a complex and constantly changing structure. The dynamic nature of bone and its remarkable healing potential determines the final outcome of spine fusion. The surgeon's technical skill and implant design only facilitate this healing process. An augmented understanding of the basic structure and biomechanics of bone interfaces is advantageous to the surgeon in choosing appropriate grafts for specific situations and in minimizing the risk of late complications such as pseudarthrosis. There is currently an explosion of knowledge regarding the mechanisms of bone formation and the control of bone cell function. In the near future we will have the opportunity to exploit this to significantly enhance the outcomes of fusion procedures.

Acknowledgment. Our thanks to Drs. Ajith J. Thomas, Russ P. Nockels, and Christopher I. Shaffrey, who authored prior editions of this chapter. Their work laid the foundation for this third rendition.

KEY REFERENCES

Boden SD, Schimandle JH, Hutton WC, et al: The use of an osteoinductive growth factor for lumbar spinal fusion. Part 1: The biology of spinal fusion. *Spine (Phila Pa 1976)* 20:2626–2632, 1995.

Bostrom MP, Lane JM, Berberian WS, et al: Immunolocalization and expression of bone morphogenetic proteins 2 and 4 in fracture healing. *J Orthop Res* 13(3):357–367, 1995.

Davy D: Biomechanical issues in bone transplantation. *Orthop Clin North Am* 30(4):553–563, 1999.

Lieberman JR, Friedlaender GE: *Bone regeneration and repair: biology and clinical applications*, Totowa, NJ, 2005, Humana Press, pp 57–65.

McCormack T, Karikovic E, Gaines RW: The load sharing classification of spine fractures. *Spine (Phila Pa 1976)* 19:1741–1744, 1994.

Pelker R, Friedlaender G, Markham T: Biomechanical properties of bone allograft. *Clin Orthop Relat Res* 174:54, 1983.

Urist M: Bone transplants and implants. In Urist M, editor: *Fundamental and clinical bone physiology*, Philadelphia, 1980, Lippincott, pp 331–368.

REFERENCES

The complete reference list is available online at expertconsult.com.

CHAPTER 18

Bone Void Fillers: Bone and Bone Substitutes

Hikaru Morisue | Isador H. Lieberman | Lisa A. Ferrara | Edward C. Benzel

One of the most common types of graft (second only to blood) is bone, with over 450,000 procedures using bone performed annually in the United States, and 2.2 million worldwide.[1] Spine arthrodesis is the most common reason for autogenous bone harvest, with approximately 250,000 spinal fusions performed in the United States each year.[2] Autogenous cancellous bone is the gold standard against which all other bone graft materials are compared. The osteogenic, osteoinductive, and osteoconductive properties of autograft are unequaled in stimulating bone repair. The procurement site of choice is the iliac crest because of the quantity and quality of available bone. Nevertheless, there are significant drawbacks to autograft, including procurement morbidity, limited availability, and increased operative time. In fact, iatrogenic complications originating from the graft procurement site represent a significant source of patient and physician concern. The primary operation may be successful, but the secondary procedure can result in increased patient recovery time and disability.[3-6]

Allograft is a commonly chosen alternative to autograft, especially when autografting is either impractical or impossible. However, this convenience comes at a price. Just like any organ allograft transplant, the allograft has the potential to transfer disease and trigger a host immune response. The allograft is heavily processed to mitigate these risks at the expense of impaired osteoinductivity and diminished mechanical properties. This renders allograft inferior to autograft as a bone graft material. In addition, processing adds to the already significant procurement costs.

By virtue of these drawbacks to both auto- and allograft, synthetic alternatives have been a very active area of research over the past 30 years. Nevertheless, only about 10% of the 2.2 million bone graft procedures annually performed worldwide involve synthetics, because of their perceived inferiority to native autograft and allograft.[1] Drawbacks of many synthetics include poor resorbability, inclusion of animal or marine-derived components, variable handling characteristics, limited availability, and added cost. Until recently, synthetic grafts provided only osteoconductive properties, lacking osteoinductive and osteogenic potential. However, composite grafts that combine a synthetic osteoconductive matrix with osteoinductive growth factors and osteogenic cells have the potential to provide the advantages of autogenous bone graft—without its disadvantages. Numerous preclinical and clinical trials are under way to determine whether this potential can be realized.

Use of Cancellous Bone Grafts versus Substitutes

Role of Cancellous Bone

Cancellous bone can be considered a scaffold within which a variety of cell types interact to perform a wide array of essential functions, in addition to its importance as the nurturing microenvironment for hematopoiesis, myelogenesis, and platelet formation. Cancellous bone serves as an incubator that protects and grows the sources of its own maintenance and the renewal of pluripotent osteoprogenitor stem cells. The growth, migration, and differentiation of these bone-forming cells are regulated by local growth factors that are elaborated by the cells and platelets within the cancellous bone.[7] In line with its role as a cell incubator, cancellous bone is highly porous and vascular. It demonstrates a limited weight-bearing function and is susceptible to collapse under compressive forces. Cortical bone surrounds and protects the cancellous bone. This dense structural material makes up the bulk of the skeleton and provides for its axial load-bearing capabilities.

General Characteristics of a Successful Bone Graft

A bone graft functions similarly to cancellous bone, supporting new tissue growth by providing the bone and blood cells with a matrix substrate. For a bone graft to be successful, three processes—osteogenesis, osteoconductivity, and osteoinductivity—that mimic natural events in cancellous bone must take place.

Osteogenesis

Osteogenesis is the process of bone formation through cellular osteoblastic activity, which depends, in turn, on the presence of osteoprogenitor stem cells. Osteogenic grafts provide cells with the direct ability to form new bone.

Osteoinduction

Osteoinduction is the biologically mediated recruitment and differentiation of cell types essential for bone formation. Osteoinductive grafts supply factors that induce undifferentiated tissue to differentiate into bone.

Osteoconduction

Osteoconduction involves the apposition of growing bone to the three-dimensional surface of a suitable scaffold provided by the graft.[8] Osteoconduction requires the structural and chemical environments that simulate those found in cancellous bone.[9] The ideal scaffold provides dimensional stability and degrades at a rate commensurate with the speed of new bone formation.[1]

In addition, material for a successful bone graft must have good handling characteristics, be nontoxic (e.g., not leach chemicals into the circulation), and exhibit biomechanical characteristics (e.g., tension, compression, modules of elasticity) similar to those of cancellous bone. Spine surgeons currently are using a variety of materials, both stand-alone and in combination. Table 18-1 summarizes the biologic properties that constitute a graft's osteointegrative capabilities (i.e., the formation of bony tissue around the implant without growth of fibrous tissue at the bone-implant interface).[10,11]

Potential Uses of Natural and Synthetic Bone Grafts

Surgeons introduce bone graft, natural or synthetic, for many types of repair procedures: in fusion (e.g., cervical fusion after discectomy, as an onlay lumbar graft, an interbody lumbar graft, and in fractures) and as a bone void filler (e.g., collapsed vertebral body, autograft donor site repair, bony defects as a result of trauma or tumor resection, osteonecrosis). Synthetic graft material also can be used in conjunction with either autograft or allograft as a bone graft extender.

TABLE 18-1

Osteointegrative Properties of Bone Graft Materials

Graft Material	Osteo-genesis	Osteoin-duction	Osteocon-duction
Autograft	2*	2	2
Allograft	0	1	2
Xenograft	0	0	2
α-TCP	0	0	1
β-TCP (porous)	0	0	2
Hydroxyapatite	0	0	1
Injectable calcium phosphate cement (e.g., Norian SRS†)	0	0	1
BMA	3	2	0
β-TCP plus BMA	3	2	2
DBM	0	2	1
Collagen	0	0	2
BMP	0	3	0
Hyaluronic acid	0	0	0
Bioactive glasses	0	0	1
Degradable polymers	0	0	1
Porous metals	0	0	1

α-TCP, α-tricalcium phosphate; β-TCP, β-tricalcium phosphate; *BMA*, bone marrow aspirate; *BMP*, bone morphogenetic protein; *DBM*, demineralized bone matrix; SRS, skeletal repair system.
*Score range 0 (none) to 3 (excellent).
†Synthes-Stratec, Oberdorf, Switzerland.
Data from references 24, 45, 59, 63, 70.

Graft Materials

Autograft

Pro

Autograft includes osteogenic bone and marrow cells as well as an osteoconductive matrix of cartilage, minerals, matrix proteins, and osteoinductive proteins associated with the matrix.[12] Neither host rejection nor disease transmission is an issue with an autograft. The combination of these properties can result in high graft success rates. Many spinal fusion procedures (e.g., dorsal cervical. thoracic, and intervertebral) that use autogenous graft produce fusion rates higher than 90%.[2]

Con

Because the separation of body tissue from its blood supply results in cell death,[2] the viability of autogenous bone as a living graft and host is severely compromised when it is harvested. Furthermore, the quality of the donor stock is not constant; it depends on many factors, such as the patient's age, gender, health, and genetic disposition. Thus, the use of autograft does not always effect repair. This opens the door for alternatives. Although some spinal fusion procedures result in high fusion rates, the results are not uniform. Many common procedures, such as dorsolateral lumbar fusion, produce fusion rates as low as 56%.[2,13] Although autogenous bone is regarded as the gold standard, its biologic performance is less than ideal.[14]

However, probably the greatest drawback to autograft use is the need for a second fascial incision and surgical dissection, with the attendant potential for complications.[15] In fact, minor complications such as superficial infection, seroma/hematoma, temporary sensory loss, and mild or transient pain are common. Major complications occur at the donor site range in 0.7% to 39% of patients.[2,16] These include infection, prolonged wound drainage, herniation of muscle and abdominal contents through the donor defect, deep hematomas, need for reoperation, pain lasting longer than 6 months, profound sensory loss, vascular and neurologic injury, unsightly scars, subluxation, gait disturbances, sacroiliac joint destabilization, enterocutaneous fistula, pelvic or iliac fracture, and heterotopic bone formation.[17-19] Life-threatening complications include major vessel or visceral injury.

Neurologic injury may occur from dissection close to several nerves in the area (e.g., sciatic, lateral femoral cutaneous, and cluneal).[6] Vascular injury to the superior gluteal vessels may occur from dissection too close to the sciatic notch. Chronic pain at the donor site, present in up to 25% of cases,[20] may be attributable to excessive removal of bone from the sacroiliac region with violation of the sacroiliac joint.[6]

Hu and Bohlman[6] reported a series of 14 patients who suffered a fracture at the iliac bone graft procurement site after spine fusion. Most of these patients were elderly women with chronic medical diseases. The authors, therefore, recommend iliac bone graft procurement with caution in this group to minimize the potential for these iatrogenic fractures. Based on subsequent cadaver studies, the authors recommend leaving at least 3 cm between the anterosuperior iliac crest and the graft procurement site[21] and a maximum distance of 3 cm from the dorsal ilium.[22]

Although the risk of surgical complications theoretically can be minimized, certain procurement issues remain. These include increased operative time and blood loss, temporary disruption of donor-site bone structure, pain, vascular injuries, and cosmetic defects.[12,20]

Bone also can be obtained from the local decompression site or from a remote site such as the rib or tibia. These sites have their own problems, however, and typically are a choice of last resort.

Osteoconductive Matrices

Most other bone grafts serve primarily as an osteoconductive matrix, with minimal to no self-supplied osteogenic or osteoinductive properties. The trade-off is greater source availability and elimination of the need for a second operative site. The structural properties of the three-dimensional scaffold matrix (especially the degree of porosity) are the primary determinants of the speed and completeness of incorporation and remodeling. The osteoconductive scaffold provides an appropriate environment into which bone cells and bone morphogenetic proteins (BMPs) can migrate, adhere, and proliferate.

Allograft

Allografts initially were used only for massive grafting where autograft use was impossible. However, by 1996 allografts constituted 34% of all bone grafts performed in the United States, an increase in use of more than 14-fold compared with just a decade earlier.[14] Allograft has become the most common autograft substitute or extender for autograft.

Pro

Three factors have led to the surge in popularity of allograft.[14] First, the National Organ Transplant Act increased overall availability. Second, donor screening and tissue processing have improved safety and quality of donated tissue. Third, the manufacture of new allograft forms (e.g., dowels) has greatly improved overall allograft utility and versatility. Perhaps the greatest advantage of allograft is its wide availability in a variety of physical forms that can be customized to specific applications. Machine tooling to shape structural allograft into forms such as wedges or threaded bone dowels can allow allograft to function as both bone graft and fixation device.[2] Other advantages include the reduction of procurement morbidity, the potential for immediate structural support, and a reasonable success rate (>60%) reported for specific procedures (e.g., hip revision surgery, management of tumors in bone).[23] Success rates for ventral-spinal lumbar fusions with allograft are comparable to those with autograft.[24]

Con

Allografts do not generate results equivalent to those of autografts.[24] Allografts can vary greatly in initial bone quality, be of higher initial expense, transmit disease, and evoke immunogenic reactions.[25] Processing constraints, required for patient safety, do not guarantee the absence of disease transmission or immunogenic reaction, but they do minimize risks posed by these adverse responses. One study of 1146 femoral heads considered suitable for bone-bank donation found unexpected disease in 8%, including three undiagnosed malignant bone tumors.[26] Minimal processing of allograft (i.e., freezing freshly obtained bone) is not sufficient to inactivate the AIDS virus, as HIV transmission has been reported by this means.[24]

Processing renders the graft nonviable and mitigates osteoinduction potential by destroying proteins useful in recruiting bone cells and inducing new bone formation. Because the processed allografts are less representative of human tissue compared with autografts, allografts are not as readily received and incorporated by the host. Allografts are slower to be resorbed and not as completely replaced by new bone compared with autografts.[24] The structural integrity of the processed bone complex also is compromised, and stability at the defect site, critical for rapid healing and return to function, is more difficult to achieve.[2,27] Results are especially poor for dorsal lumbar fusion,[24] and lower reported fusion rates for allograft implants compared with autograft-only implants were found in two studies.[2]

The quantity of allograft material is constrained by limited supply; tissue banks report difficulty with procurement because of fear of gross disfigurement at the donor site.[28] Donor-to-donor variation results in uncertain, nonuniform quality.[29] Bone quality varies with donor age and gender; even same-size bones from different anatomic sites in a single donor can vary in strength by as much as 20%.[27]

A low-grade inflammatory reaction typically is associated with allograft.[25] This immune response may contribute to allograft failure (i.e., fracture and nonunion).[24,30,31] Because of an initial intense inflammatory reaction, new capillaries are easily thrombosed, resulting in a delay in vascularization and osteoinduction.[24] Even at maturation, necrotic bone can account for as much as 50% or more of the graft.[24]

A literature review of animal studies suggests a correlation between histocompatibility difference and allograft failure, both biologically and biomechanically.[30] In a mouse model, the immunologic reaction appears to be specific to donor antigen and consists of killer/suppressor T cells, which are associated with soft tissue rejection.[30] In humans, alloreactivity appears similar to the animal findings, resulting in an overall sensitization rate of 67%, higher than that seen after blood transfusion (12–50%).[23,32] The immune response system may share common bone marrow-derived precursors and cytokines with the bone remodeling system, explaining the potential interaction of the immune response with bone remodeling.[30] The most convincing evidence of a causal relationship between immunogenicity and poorer outcome is that among 29 patients studied who received allograft, those lacking sensitization to class II antigens achieved better clinical results than did sensitized patients.[23]

The two types of allograft in common use, fresh-frozen and freeze-dried, differ in their processing, which gives each different advantages and disadvantages. Fresh-frozen allografts retain BMP, are stronger and more completely incorporated in host bone than freeze-dried grafts,[24] but also are the most immunogenic and have produced documented HIV transfer. Freeze-dried allograft is the least immunogenic and has caused no documented HIV or viral disease transmission. However, its BMP is destroyed, and it has the most compromised mechanical integrity, with decreased graft strength of up to 50% relative to freshly frozen allograft.[2,27]

In summary, although allograft tissue processing is necessary, it adds expense, reduces graft function both biologically and mechanically, and does not eliminate allograft risks entirely. Despite processing, histologic evidence of a low-grade inflammatory reaction is typical. These factors indicate that allograft is an inferior graft compared with autograft.

Demineralized Bone Matrix

Demineralized bone matrix (DBM) is thought to possess more osteoinductive properties than regular allograft because of enhanced bioavailability of growth factors following the demineralization process.[2,25] DBM gels and putties have become widely used in spinal fusion surgery since 1990, with about 500,000 mL used for implants each year in the United States.[2] The first widely available DBM preparation was a gel consisting of DBM combined with a glycerol carrier. One retrospective study assessed the augmentation of local bone autograft with a DBM/glycerol composite for dorsolateral lumbar spine fusion as a means to avoid second-site autologous bone harvest. The control group used iliac crest autograft alone. The percentage of patients undergoing fusion was similar in both groups (60% and 56% for DBM and controls, respectively; $P = .83$).[33] Although prospective clinical studies are under way, available data suggest a role for DBM as a bone-graft extender, rather than as a bone-graft substitute, in spinal surgery.[2] Now there are several commercially available DBM substances for clinical use. Wang et al. studied the osteoinductibility of each DBM by comparing the usefulness of the different types of DBM as a bone graft substitute in an athymic rat spine fusion model. He reported that there are significant differences between some of the tested products, although all products claim to have significant osteoinductive capabilities. He noted that several factors such as differences in preprocess handling, varying demineralization times, final particle size, terminal sterilization, the differences in the carrier, and donor viability are expected to influence the properties of a DBM product. He also emphasized that a specific, sensitive, and reliable screening assay of the osteoinductive properties of DBM and objective information about each product's osteoinductivity are much needed.[34]

Xenograft

Xenograft bone tissue is harvested from animals. Because of their immunogenicity, xenograft preparations generally have proven impractical for clinical use. Removal of proteinaceous and fatty materials during processing, as is done in the preparation of Kiel bone, Bio-Oss (Osteohealth, New York), or Oswestry bone, reduces immunogenicity to a degree.[35] However, the processing required to produce this type of graft removes the osteoinductive matrix proteins. To guarantee viral inactivation, all such proteins must be removed. Processing strategies, such as freezing and freeze-drying, are less common than in the past because of unacceptable disease-transmission risk. Chemical washes have become more prevalent, but these tend to reduce or eliminate osteoinductivity.

Ceramics

Noninjectable Ceramics

Synthetic ceramics are osteoconductive but do not intrinsically possess any osteoinductive potential. The most common ceramics in current use are hydroxyapatite [$Ca_{10}(PO_4)_6(OH)_2$], tricalcium phosphate [$Ca_3(PO_4)_2$], calcium sulfate dihydrate [$CaSO_4\ 2(H_2O)$], and combinations thereof.

Although they exhibit different chemical properties from tissue grafts, ceramics provide off-the-shelf availability of consistently high-quality synthetic materials that have no biologic hazards. After incorporation, the strength of the repaired defect site is comparable to that of cancellous bone.[36] Therefore, ceramics can be used as an alternative or as an addition to either cancellous autograft or allograft[37] or as a cancellous bone void filler or bone graft extender or in sites where compression is the dominant mode of mechanical loading.

In a randomized, prospective study of 341 patients undergoing dorsal spinal fusion for idiopathic scoliosis, patients received autograft or synthetic porous ceramic blocks (macroporous biphasic calcium phosphate [MBCP], Triosite, Zimmer, Inc., Warsaw, IN; a mixture of hydroxyapatite and tricalcium phosphate).[38] Curve correction, curve maintenance, pain, and function were comparable between the two groups 18 months postoperatively. However, wound complications were more common in the autograft group—14 patients experienced delayed healing, infection, or hematoma compared with only 3 wound complications in the MBCP group. In addition, 15 autograft patients had pain at the donor site at 3 months. Other donor-site complications at 3 months included seven infections, two hematomas, and four cases of delayed healing. Histologic findings showed new bone incorporating into the MBCP—evidence of good osteoconduction. These results suggest that synthetic porous ceramic is a safe and effective substitute for iliac graft autograft in this patient population.

Another prospective study of 106 cases of lumbar spinal fusion used MBCP granules mixed with autogenous bone chips and bone marrow obtained from the local spine.[39] Dorsal deformity correction using semi-rigid instrumentation was performed in all patients. Only six nonunions were observed (three resulting from primary spondylolisthesis), suggesting a high success rate for MBCP in spinal fusion involving a semi-rigid instrumentation. The authors conclude that because the degenerative spine is not favorable to fusion, this technique offers an alternative to autograft to reduce patient morbidity from iliac bone harvest.[39]

Cost may become prohibitive in selected cases. This and unproven clinical efficacy make assumptions regarding widespread clinical applications tenuous.

Rapidly Resorbing Ceramics

Scaffolds of tricalcium phosphate (the α and β forms have different crystalline structures but the same elemental and stoichiometric characteristics; the α form is formulated at 1200°C and the β form is formulated at 800°C) and calcium sulfate have been used as synthetic bone void fillers for more than 20 years.[40,41] Calcium phosphate contains stoichiometric amounts of calcium and phosphorus, 39% and 20% by weight, respectively, similar to those found in natural bone.[42] It produces calcium-phosphate–rich microenvironments that

TABLE 18-2

Resorption Characteristics of Ceramics

Ceramic	Speed of Resorption
Hydroxyapatite	Slow
β-Tricalcium phosphate	Intermediate
α-Tricalcium phosphate	Rapid
Calcium sulfate	Very rapid

TABLE 18-3

Porosity and Osteoconductivity of Ceramics

Ceramic	Porosity/Osteoconductivity
Calcium phosphate	Very little
Hydroxyapatite	Little
α-Tricalcium phosphate	Intermediate
β-Tricalcium phosphate	Very high

stimulate osteoclastic resorption and then osteoblastic new bone formation, resulting in new bone formation within the resorbed implant.[43] Less porous formulations resorb before complete bone ingrowth is achieved.[25] The rate of resorption and the porosity of several bone substitutes are presented in Tables 18-2 and 18-3.

Calcium sulfate (plaster of Paris) is available in pellet form. Although calcium sulfate is considered an osteoconductive bone graft substitute, its rapid resorption rate creates doubt about its ability to maintain a three-dimensional framework to support osteogenesis.[44]

Intermediate Resorbing Ceramics

β-Tricalcium phosphate (β-TCP) is one of the most commonly used bone graft alternatives. In the process of being resorbed, it can enrich the local environment with osteogenic substrates that, in turn, can be used by activated osteoblasts. Many highly porous β- TCP ceramics are commercially available. Currently they differ from previous β-TCP formulations in that they have a broad range of pore sizes (<1 μm to 1000 μm), and sponge-like interconnected microporosity endowed with excellent wicking and hydrophilic properties. These attributes facilitate the migration of bone-forming cells, growth factors, and phagocytic cells into it, enhancing the process of new bone development and its resorption.[45]

Slowly Resorbing Ceramics

Hydroxyapatite, another ceramic-based synthetic bone graft, can be formed into a three-dimensional structure that is rigid and stable. Controlling its pore diameter and the degree of pore interconnection can allow for rapid incorporation of new bone into it, which leads to a rigid mechanical bond between the implanted material and the host tissue. Although hydroxyapatite itself has some drawbacks, such as slow resorption and brittleness,[46] a mixture of hydroxyapatite, β-TCP, and calcium carbonate can provide better osteoconduction for bone production, as well as long-term stability, leading to successful incorporation into a bone fusion mass.[47]

Thalgott et al. reported a 100% fusion rate using a hydroxyapatite with a pore diameter of 200 μm in combination with rigid plating for ventral cervical decompression and fusion.[48]

Injectable Ceramics: Calcium Phosphate Cement

Injectable calcium phosphate cement (CaP cement) is a paste of inorganic calcium and phosphate that hardens in situ with a low exothermic temperature, and cures by a crystallization reaction.[44] It then slowly transforms into bone over 3 to 4 years. The resulting bone filler has a biologic response and compressive strength similar to that of cancellous bone, and has shown promise for some clinical applications such as use as an adjunct to fixation in both femoral neck and intertrochanteric hip fractures.[44,49]

The primary drawbacks to injectable calcium phosphate are slow resorption, low porosity, and high commercialization costs. Extravasation into surrounding soft tissues, or intra-articular extrusion also may occur, although these adverse events have been rarely reported.[49]

Many attempts recently have been made to apply CaP cements instead of polymethylmethacrylate (PMMA) in vertebral augmentation procedures. One clinical study using calcium phosphate cement reported resorption and fragmentation of the cement mantle. The authors noted two problems specific to calcium phosphate: an increased washout tendency and a lower flexural and shear resistance. They concluded that routine use of CaP cement is not currently recommended for vertebral augmentation.[50]

Collagen

Animal-derived collagen has been used with synthetic calcium phosphate bone fillers to modulate physical properties of bone-filling agents and to deliver factors that stimulate bone formation. The admixture of collagen imparts a putty-like consistency to the bone graft that facilitates handling and placement at the time of surgery. Various configurations are now available for clinical use.[51] These products are designed to be hydrated and implanted with autogenous bone marrow or bone graft, and have been used as bone graft extenders to increase the volume of bone graft into a defect when a sufficient volume of autograft is not readily available.[44]

One formation of a type I collagen/hydroxyapatite matrix, prepared in 50- × 20- × 5-mm sheets, was studied in 50 cases of lumbar posterolateral spine fusion combined with bone marrow aspirate (BMA) as the graft material and achieved a 92% radiographic fusion rate.[51] In contrast, an animal study reported that solid spinal fusion was not detected by manual palpation or on radiographs in any of the rabbits treated with the same collagen matrix combined with heparinized bone marrow.[52]

Nonbiologic Osteoconductive Substrates

The advantages of nonbiologic osteoconductive substrates include absolute control of the final structure, no immunogenicity, and excellent biocompatibility.[43] Examples include degradable polymers,[53] bioactive glasses, and porous metals such as tantalum.

Qualitative Assessment of Ceramics

A summary of the overall advantages and disadvantages of various bone graft materials is presented in Table 18-4. The table provides an overview of the clinical and economic aspects of the ceramics available today. These ceramics can perhaps be best judged by their resorption and porosity characteristics (see Tables 18-2 and 18-3). Of particular note in this regard is the importance of using a bone substitute that resorbs (and remodels) at a rate similar to that of cancellous bone (intermediate; see Table 18-2) and that is highly porous (see Table 18-3).

A canine study was undertaken to determine the rate of new bone ingrowth into defect sites repaired with either porous β-TCP synthetic cancellous bone void filler or hydroxyapatite-coated calcium carbonate.[54] Cylindrical canine metaphyseal defects measured 10 × 25 mm in canine humeri. Bone ingrowth and scaffold resorption were quantified using standard histomorphometric techniques for specimens examined up to 1 year postimplantation.

Approximately 80% of the implanted β-TCP resorbed at 12 weeks, compared with only 34% of hydroxyapatite-coated calcium carbonate ($P < .05$). By 24 and 52 weeks, the remaining β-TCP implant volume was 3% and 1% of original implant size, respectively.

As early as 3 weeks, β-TCP showed resorption (clearing) from the center outward and some immature bone formation (Fig. 18-1). At 6 weeks, the volume of new bone formed throughout the implants exceeded, by approximately 20%, the volume of original bone in areas adjacent to the defects (Fig. 18-2). Remodeling was essentially complete in 6 to 12 weeks, with bone density in the normal range and the scaffold almost completely resorbed by the end of the period. By 24 weeks, the trabecular orientation of the implant approximated the normal stress patterns of adjacent bone. Serial histologic and radiographic assessments made at 12, 24, and 52 weeks demonstrated comparable architecture and density between new bone within the defect sites and the adjacent original bone. The stress-strain curve of β-TCP was nearly identical to bone at 24 weeks and at 52 weeks (Fig. 18-3). In contrast, the calcium carbonate stress-strain curve differed markedly from bone at 24 weeks. Radiographic diffraction data of the β-TCP implants confirmed a 95% match to normal bone at 1 year.[55]

The study suggested that normal bone remodeling occurred with the β-TCP scaffold within 6 to 12 weeks after implantation. In contrast, about one third of the hydroxyapatite-coated calcium carbonate–implanted defect showed new bone formation (mainly at the periphery). No foreign-body response to either ultraporous β-TCP or hydroxyapatite-coated calcium carbonate was observed. The ultraporous β-TCP was manipulated easily at surgery, despite its very high porosity.

These results were superior in several respects to those of earlier, similar studies using other ceramics. Bruder et al.[56] had found that a ceramic composed of hydroxyapatite and β-TCP produced no callus around the defect site or the host bone in the first 16 weeks after implantation, indicating inadequate bone healing. Both Bruder et al.[56] and Kon et al.[57] found that, using traditional synthetics, bone formation was most prevalent at the periphery of the defect. Bruder et al.[56] noted that the only new bone that formed as a result of the osteoconductivity of the porous ceramic was an extension of the outgrowth from the cut ends of the host bone. In contrast, one of the striking observations about β-TCP is the initiation of resorption and osteogenesis at the center of the repaired defect site. In summary, Bruder et al.[56] found that hydroxyapatite bone substitute was not ideal for the treatment of segmental defects because of its brittle nature, susceptibility to fracture, and lack of completely interconnected pores.

TABLE 18-4

Summary of the Defining Advantages and Disadvantages of Bone Graft Materials

Graft Material	Advantages	Disadvantages	Clinical Results*
Autograft	Osteogenic, osteoinductive, osteoconductive	Procurement morbidity, limited availability	56–100%[64]
Allograft	Osteoconductive, weakly osteoinductive	Immunogenic, disease transfer risk	60–90%*[28]
DBM	Osteoconductive, osteoinductive	Lacks structural strength[70]	60%[65]
Ceramics	Osteoconductive, limitless supply, biocompatible	Not osteogenic or osteoinductive, expensive	Equivalent to autograft in scoliosis, but decreased complications[58,61]
β-TCP/BMA composite	Osteogenic, osteoinductive, osteoconductive, limitless supply, biocompatible	R&D, commercialization costs	Not available
Collagen	Good delivery vehicle for other synthetic graft materials	By itself, a poor graft material	Preclinical only
Nonbiologic substrates	Osteoconductive	Foreign body reaction with degradable polymers	Preclinical only
BMP/synthetic composite	Osteogenic, osteoinductive, osteoconductive, limitless supply, biocompatible	R&D, commercialization costs	Ongoing clinical studies using rhBMP-2 combined with either ceramic or collagen sponge show results comparable to autograft[2]

β-TCP, β-tricalcium phosphate; *BMA*, bone marrow aspirate; *BMP*, bone morphogenetic protein; *DBM*, demineralized bone matrix; R+D, research and development.

*Numeric clinical results are the overall incidence of vertebral body fusion in spine surgery, except for the entry for allograft, which represents the clinical, radiographic, and biologic assessments of massive osseous and osteochondral allografts as quoted in the cited reference.

Data from references 14, 25, 45, 60, 64, 71.

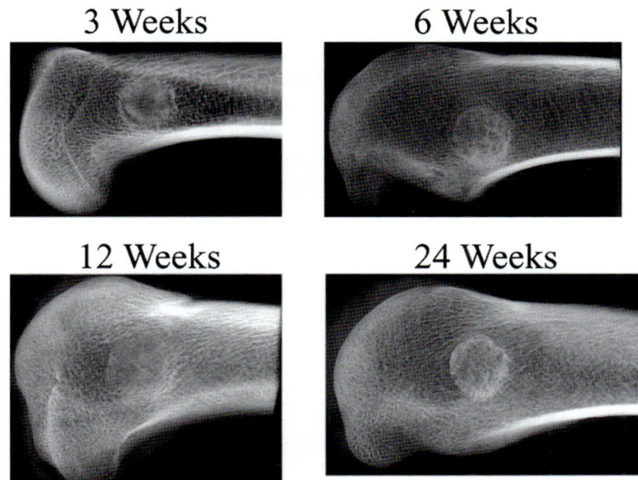

FIGURE 18-1. Radiographs of β-tricalcium phosphate (β-TCP) implant from 3 to 24 weeks.

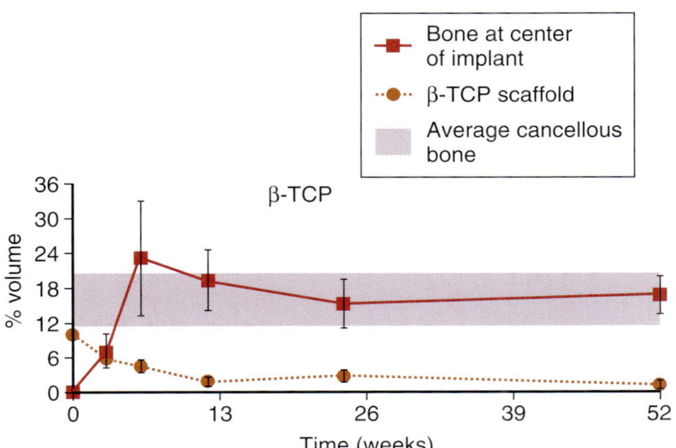

FIGURE 18-2. Rates of new bone ingrowth and resorption. β-TCP, β-tricalcium phosphate. (Redrawn and modified from Erbe E, Clineff T, Lavagnino M, et al: Comparison of Vitoss™ and ProOsteone 500R in a critical-sized defect at 1 year [abstract]. Presented at Annual Meeting of the Orthopaedic Research Society, February 25–28, 2001, San Francisco. Abstract 975.)

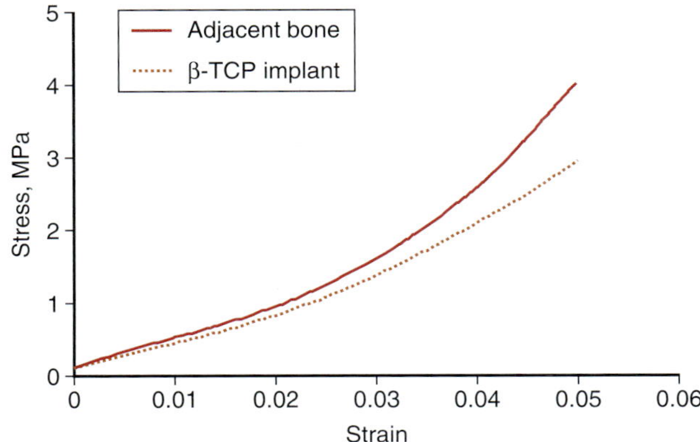

FIGURE 18-3. Results of compression testing of the β-tricalcium phosphate (β-TCP) implant compared with adjacent bone at 52 weeks. MPa, megapascal.

Biologic and Synthetic Composite Grafts

A composite graft can be defined as any combination of materials that includes both an osteoconductive matrix and an osteogenic or osteoinductive material. The carrier matrix could be any of the osteoconductive materials listed in Table 18-1. When the osteoconductive scaffold is mixed with bone marrow aspirate (BMA), the newly formed composite graft may acquire osteogenic and osteoinductive potential, thus providing a competitive alternative to autograft. Other biologic agents that may impart this potential include osteoblastic progenitor stem cells, blood, platelet-rich plasma, and osteoinductive growth factors such as BMP, transforming growth factor, and fibroblast growth factor.[58]

Osteogenic and Osteoinductive Bone Marrow Aspirate

Background

In theory, osteoblast progenitor cells could be obtained from the periosteum of long bones, the peritrabecular connective tissue, or the bone marrow, and combined with a synthetic scaffold.[59] This strategy is designed to minimize the need for chemotaxis and massive proliferation of osteoblast progenitor cells into the defect. Logically, the direct implantation of progenitor cells should lead to more rapid, uniform, and reliable healing of bone defects. A major challenge to this approach is the need to identify more fully the proper type and source of cells for autologous cell therapy.[56] However, for now, extensive clinical experience with bone marrow transplantation makes bone marrow a practical choice as a source of progenitor and osteoinductive cells.[60]

A number of studies have looked at BMA and its positive effects on bone formation both in vitro[61] and in vivo.[15,61,62] All of the critical cellular components that contribute to bone growth are present in BMA. Identifiable cell types include both fibroblasts and undifferentiated stromal cells. Osteoprogenitor stem cells are estimated to constitute 1 in 50,000 bone marrow cells in young patients and 1 in 2,000,000 cells in elderly patients. They are the most useful of bone tissue cells because they can differentiate into four other cell types (osteoblasts, adipose cells, chondroblasts, and fibroblasts) and modify their morphologic/functional attributes as needed.[63] The mesenchymal stem cells have the potential to differentiate into a variety of tissues, including bone, cartilage, tendon, ligament, and adipose aggregations. Consequently, BMA is an abundant source of osteogenic cells for immediate transplantation. Animal research suggests that precursor cells in bone marrow proliferate and differentiate after transplantation. Among the cells derived from such proliferation are active osteoblasts that drive the process of new bone formation.[60,64]

Many investigators are engaged in characterizing the progenitor populations present in bone marrow, and in vitro studies of bone marrow–derived osteoblastic progenitors have helped define the potential role of the many growth factors involved in regulating osteoblast differentiation.[7] Uncontrolled clinical trials suggest that mixtures of aspirated bone marrow and autograft may be effective in treating nonunions,[5,65] but prospective trials using bone marrow alone have not been performed.[66]

Another advantage of BMA is its availability and the relative safety of its harvest. It is the only source that requires neither an open surgical procedure nor the added time and cost of in vitro cell growth.[25] Cell progenitors derived from bone marrow can be harvested by aspiration from patients, with limited dilution by peripheral blood, as long as the volume of aspirate from a single site is held to 2 mL or less.[60] Furthermore, the number of progenitors available in a graft site can be increased by concentration, if necessary, to further enhance the biologic result of bone grafting.[67,68] For subsequent use in transplantation, stem cells also can be cultured and expanded to many times their original number.

Bone Marrow Aspirate and Bone Composites

Bone marrow has been used successfully to stimulate healing in tibial fractures, suggesting a promptly renewable and reliable source of osteogenic cells without the disadvantages of standard open-grafting techniques.[17] In a study using human BMA taken from the femoral head and the iliac crest, the recovered cells demonstrated osteogenic potential in vivo in nude mice. The osteogenic potential was maintained as the cells were expanded in culture and enriched for grafting purposes.[69] Autologous bone marrow aspirated from the iliac crest had a beneficial effect on osteogenesis in 25 of 28 patients when implanted with xenograft bone graft material (Kiel bone).[70] The addition of bone marrow to autograft iliac crest bone graft facilitated greater bone formation and fusion success rates than did autograft alone ($P < .05$) in a rabbit dorsolateral spine fusion model.[62] Furthermore, a study of 23 pediatric patients found that xenograft bone and other bone substitutes could be rendered osteogenic by combining these materials with fresh autologous bone marrow.[71]

Bone Marrow Aspirate and Synthetic Composites

A number of studies have assessed composites of bone marrow and synthetics for bone grafting.[36,57,72] Ceramics of tricalcium phosphate, hydroxyapatite, and collagen hydroxyapatite were evaluated alone and with added BMA to assess their ability to heal defects created surgically in the canine radius. These implants also were compared with a graft of autogenous cancellous bone. The addition of BMA was essential for tricalcium phosphate and hydroxyapatite to achieve results comparable to those obtained with cancellous bone at 24 weeks.[72]

Studies on healing of canine femoral defects with implanted calcium phosphate cylinders loaded with cultured autologous mesenchymal stem cells showed that the addition of the cells augmented the development of new periosteal bone around the implants.[56] Similarly, although porous hydroxyapatite bioceramic (HAC) alone was effective for repair of tibial defects (at 6 months), the introduction of bone marrow stromal cell populations into the composite resulted in far more extensive bone defect repair over a 2-month period.[57] However, in both studies, even in the cell-loaded scaffold, a higher concentration of new bone began in the periphery. The authors speculate that this is the result of better survival of loaded cells within the outermost portions of the HAC cylinder, which probably are vascularized faster and more efficiently than more internal regions. They note that this may be related to the design of the implant device. The β-TCP animal study, which showed bone formation initiating within the center of the β-TCP carrier, supports this explanation. As early as 3 weeks after implantation, β-TCP showed resorption beginning from the center of the implant, perhaps because of the concentration of nutrients in the center.

The new generation of β-TCP implants brings unique biomechanical properties that make them particularly well suited for use with BMA in a composite graft. The broad range of interconnected porosity (1 μm to 1 mm) allows nutrient fluids to percolate throughout the structure and to support the migration of parenchyma into the scaffold, enhancing the processes of new bone development and scaffold resorption. The unique structure of ultraporous β-TCP is conducive, therefore, to rapid vascularization that is necessary for nourishing the seeded bone marrow, including bone-forming cells. In this respect, a β-TCP/BMA composite may be superior even to autograft, which suffers from anoxic cell death in the center of the graft because of the absence of vascularization (Fig. 18-4). One of the striking features of grafting with β-TCP compared with other synthetic constructs is the central pattern of bone formation, suggesting penetration of cells and nutrients.[73]

Thus, a composite made up of ultraporous β-TCP seeded with aspirated autologous bone marrow could deliver many of the positive qualities of an autograft and avoid most of the negative ones. The β-TCP scaffold supplies an osteoconductive surface for bone and tissue ingrowth. Ultraporosity facilitates infusion of bone matrix proteins and growth factors, making the β-TCP osteoinductive.[74] Local and recruited osteogenic cells penetrate the composite and interact with the seeded bone-forming cells to impart osteogenic properties to β-TCP (Fig. 18-5). β-TCP seeded with BMA therefore can provide all three properties necessary for a successful bone graft that was previously satisfied by autografts, namely, osteogenesis, osteoinduction, and osteoconduction.

Bone Morphogenetic Protein and Synthetic Composites

Human recombinant bone morphogenetic proteins, including recombinant human BMP-2 (rhBMP-2) and recombinant human osteogenic protein 1 (rhOP-1 or rhBMP-7), are being investigated in human clinical trials and show promise as autologous bone graft substitutes.[47,75-77] A carrier that can maintain optimal regional concentrations of BMP over a prolonged period is essential for the efficient utilization of BMPs. To date, several biomaterials have been used as carriers for BMP.[46] Of these, hydroxyapatite (HAp) is considered particularly useful, because of its high affinity with BMP. To further enhance their osteogenic potential, HAp and other ceramics are now routinely combined with various active biologic substances.[47]

In Boden's clinical trial, 25 patients underwent posterolateral lumbar spine fusion using 20 mg of rhBMP-2 with a carrier consisting of 60% hydroxyapatite and 40% tricalcium phosphate granules, resulting in a 100% fusion rate, although some patients did smoke during the postoperative period.[66] Dawson performed a clinical study to investigate the use of rhBMP-2 on an absorbable collagen sponge combined with a ceramic-granule bulking agent as a bone graft substitute in single-level posterolateral lumbar spinal fusion, and achieved

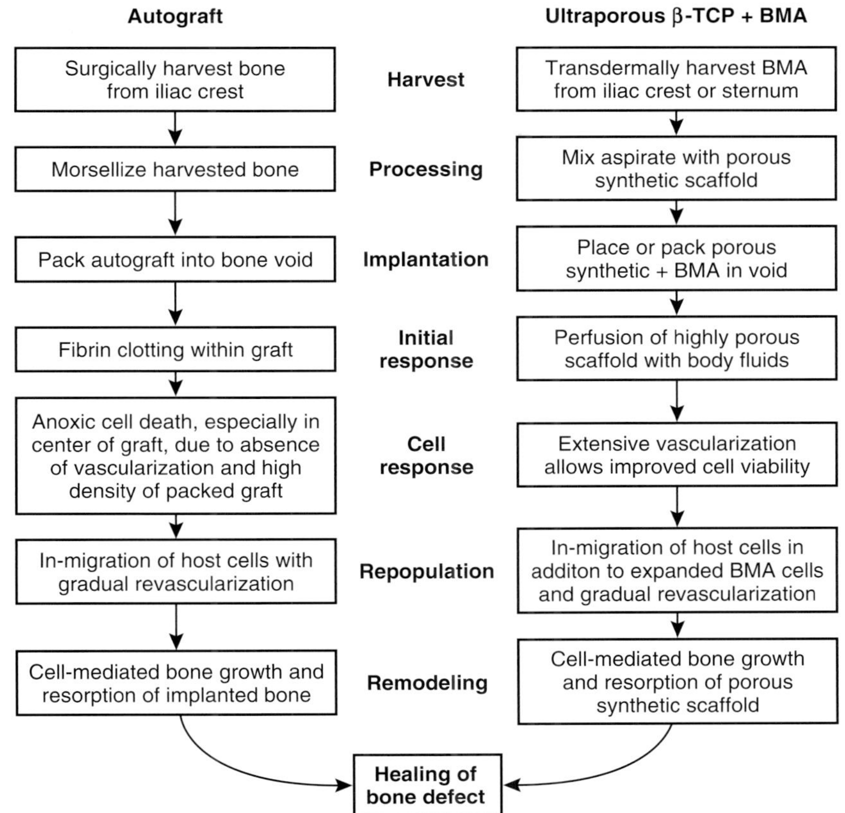

FIGURE 18-4. Processes in filling bone voids with either autograft or porous synthetic (e.g., β-TCP) seeded with BMA. Both are expected to support the osteogenesis, osteoconduction, and osteoinduction needed for healing. β-TCP, beta-tricalcium phosphate; BMA, bone marrow aspirate.

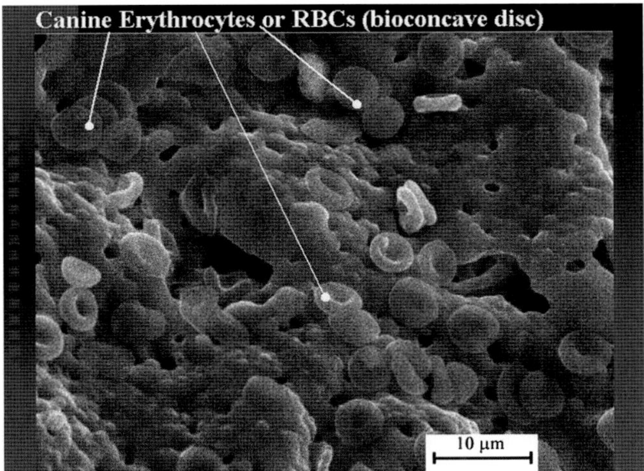

FIGURE 18-5. Scanning electron microscopy image at magnification × 2000, showing a large number of canine erythrocytes (~4–5 μm diameter) in the center of the β-TCP scaffold. Cells can be transported via β-TCP; this includes mesenchymal stem cells, which are approximately 15 μm in diameter. β-TCP, beta-tricalcium phosphate.

an 88% fusion rate.[78] Human clinical trials also have shown the efficacy of OP-1 as both an alternative and an enhancer to autologous bone graft or spinal fusion. OP-1 putty (3.5 mg rhOP-1 to 1 g bovine bone collagen to 230 mg carboxy methyl cellulose) is now approved for use as a carrier.[79]

The delivery systems currently available for recombinant BMPs include DBM, synthetic polymers, type 1 collagen hyaluronic acid gels, and a variety of bone graft substitutes. However, Crawford et al. reported the higher incidence of dorsal cervical wound complications with rhBMP-2 on an absorbable collagen sponge, and emphasized the importance of determining optimal dosing and carrier to achieve the desired results of fusion.[80] An alternate approach that may allow BMPs to produce even greater therapeutic effects may be attained in the future with gene therapy, which provides for the transfer of genetic information to a host cell that would express and produce endogenous BMP protein.[75]

Summary

After blood, bone is the most commonly transplanted tissue. Autogenous bone grafting is one of the most common orthopaedic procedures, performed in about 200,000 cases annually in the United States.[81] Although materials of biologic origin are now generally used, their preference may diminish as well-characterized inorganic materials with off-the-shelf availability offer potential to eliminate procurement morbidity associated with autograft and to eliminate risk of disease transmission associated with allograft.

However, the development of a usable osteoconductive carrier has lagged behind the isolation and synthesis of osteoinductive growth factors. Preclinical data indicate that the enhanced capillarity of ceramics such as β-TCP may bring these bone-healing elements together in better balance. Advances in tissue engineering of synthetic composite grafts should demonstrate a synergy between components with results superior even to autogenous bone grafts.[82] The improved understanding of osteoprogenitor cell function, and advances in procurement and cell separation, will provide for increased osteogenic capabilities with negligible harvest morbidity. Finally, BMPs and synthetic composites show significant promise in the arenas of bone healing and bone fusion. Further clinical information verifying the utility of BMA/bone composites, BMPs, and synthetic composites will be available in the near future.

KEY REFERENCES

Boden SD, Kang J, Sandhu H, Heller JG: Use of recombinant human bone morphogenetic protein-2 to achieve posterolateral lumbar spine fusion in humans: a prospective, randomized clinical pilot trial: 2002 Volvo Award in clinical studies. *Spine* 27:2662–2673, 2002.

Connolly J, Guse R, Lippiello L, Dehne R: Development of an osteogenic bone-marrow preparation. *J Bone Joint Surg [Am]* 71:684–691, 1989.

Fernyhough JC, Schimandle JJ, Weigel MC, et al: Chronic donor site pain complicating bone graft harvesting from the posterior iliac crest for spinal fusion. *Spine* 17(12):1474–1480, 1992.

Fleming JE Jr, Cornell CN, Muschler GF: Bone cells and matrices in orthopedic tissue engineering. *Orthop Clin North Am* 31:357–374, 2000.

Heary RF, Schlenk RP, Sacchieri TA, et al: Persistent iliac crest donor site plan: independent outcome assessment. *Neurosurgery* 50(3):510–516, 2002.

Ludwig SC, Boden SD: Osteoinductive bone graft substitutes for spinal fusion: a basic science summary. *Orthop Clin North Am* 30:635–645, 1999.

Muschler GF, Boehm C, Easley K: Aspiration to obtain osteoblast progenitor cells from human bone marrow: the influence of aspiration volume. *J Bone Joint Surg [Am]* 79:1699–1709, 1997.

Wang JC, Alanay A, Mark D, et al: A comparison of commercially available demineralized bone matrix for spinal fusion. *Eur Spine J* 16:1233–1240, 2007.

REFERENCES

The complete reference list is available online at expertconsult.com

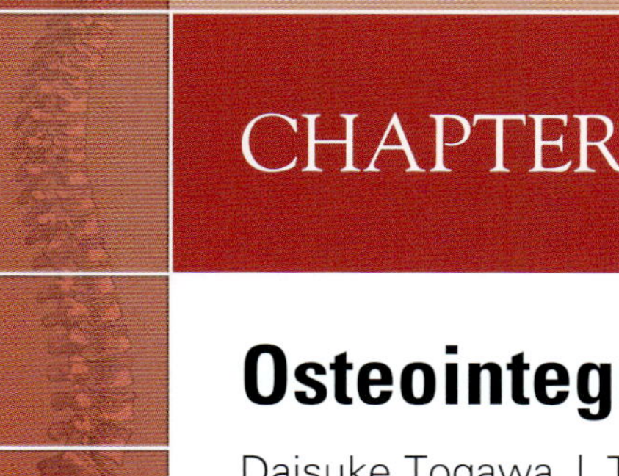

CHAPTER 19

Osteointegration (Osseointegration)

Daisuke Togawa | Thomas W. Bauer | Edward C. Benzel

Recent advances in spine surgery have led to expanded use of synthetic biomaterials. The interface between host bone and a synthetic device has an important influence on the clinical efficacy of that device. These interfaces have been described as abutting (e.g., interbody bone graft, interbody cement), penetrating (e.g., nail, staple, screw), gripping (e.g., hook, wire), conforming (e.g., polymethylmethacrylate), and osteointegrating (e.g., some types of metal and ceramics).[1] The word *osteointegration* is derived from the Latin word *integratus* and the Greek *osteon*, meaning renewing or making new bone. However, because the prefix *osseo-* is also derived from the Latin for bone,[2] the term *osseointegration* is often (or preferably) used instead of *osteointegration*.

Since Brånemark, a Swedish dentist, introduced the term *osseointegration* to describe the process by which some oral implants interface with bone,[3] this term has been widely used in the dental and orthopaedic arenas. Brånemark originally defined osseointegration as "direct structural and functional connection between ordered, living bone and the surface of a load carrying implant."[3] During the past 30 years, however, the term *osseointegration* has been used in a number of scientific publications regarding both structural (morphologic) and functional (physiologic) senses. Various factors influence this process at the implant-bone interface, including preparation of the surrounding bone, the surface preparation and sterilization procedures to remove organic residues from the implant, surface topography, overall implant design and composition, and load transmission.

Direct bone apposition to an implant suggests attachment of the implant to the bone over the entire contact surface, allowing load transfer from the implant to bone over a large surface area. Most surgeons expect direct bone apposition for interbody fusion devices, artificial discs, pedicle screws, and various spacers. However, it remains unclear how often, and to what extent, this is achieved.

Osteoconductivity

An osteoconductive material promotes bone apposition along its surface. The term *osteoconduction* is not absolute and is best understood in the context of a comparison in which variables of the substrate material, porosity, surface geometry, and surface chemistry are highly controlled and defined.[4] For example, when matched by size, shape, and surface texture, hydroxyapatite is more osteoconductive than titanium, but titanium is more osteoconductive than a similar segment of cobalt-chromium alloy, or stainless steel; and rough stainless steel is more osteoconductive than polished stainless steel. Thus, several different factors influence the extent to which osteoblasts bind to a surface and produce bone matrix.

Biomaterials

Metals

Metals have been used in various forms as implants, including stainless steels, cobalt-based alloys, pure titanium, and titanium-based alloys. Each metal has different characteristics and behaves differently in vivo. For example, titanium alloys differ from stainless steel by having less resistance to abrasive wear, but provide better corrosion resistance, biocompatibility, less MRI distortion, and increased modulus of elasticity. Because of these advantages, titanium alloy is often used for orthopaedic and spine implants. As described by Wolff's law, bone grows in response to applied stress and often is resorbed if a mechanical stimulus is lacking.[5] Note, however, that the stiffness of many metals may shield the underlying bone from stress. Alloys with elastic moduli less than that of stainless steel, such as Ti6Al4V, have been successfully used in fracture fixation, but stress shielding is still observed.[6,7] At the implant-bone interface, most of these metals demonstrate variable osteoconductivity. Titanium implants generally have a better biocompatibility and osteoconductivity than many other metals, and their surface chemistry and texture are more influential during bone ingrowth.

Surface Texture

Early investigations were undertaken by Smith in the 1960s, using a porous surface ceramic.[8] Currently, a wide variety of surface textures have been utilized to help achieve bone ingrowth into prosthetic devices in both dental and orthopaedic implant applications. Three dimensionally porous surfaces of sintered beads or wire, roughened surfaces created by etching the implant surface, and rough surfaces created by the application of metal by plasma spray or other methods have been tested in a number of animal and clinical studies[9-12] (Figs. 19-1 and 19-2). For example, Friedman et al. tested various biomaterials with different surfaces in the rabbit

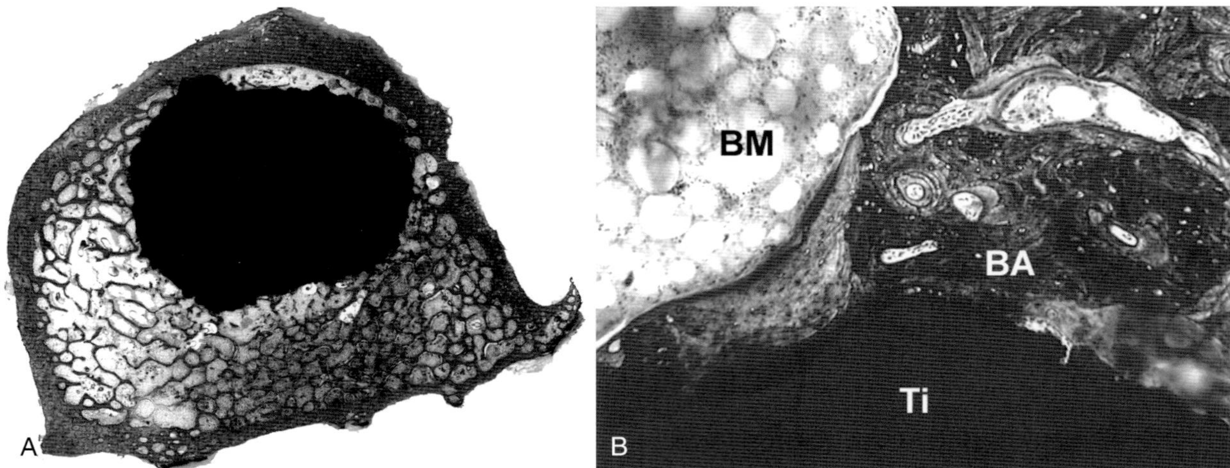

FIGURE 19-1. A, Gross view. **B,** Direct bone apposition to metal hip implant. Direct bone apposition (BA) and healthy bone marrow (BM) are observed without an intervening layer of fibrous tissue on this experimental canine femoral titanium implant (Ti; surface: arc apatitic titanium). (From Togawa D Bauer TW, Mochida Y, et al: Bone apposition to three femoral stem surfaces in canine total hip arthroplasty. *Transactions of the 27th Annual Meeting of the Society for Biomaterials,* 251, 2001.)

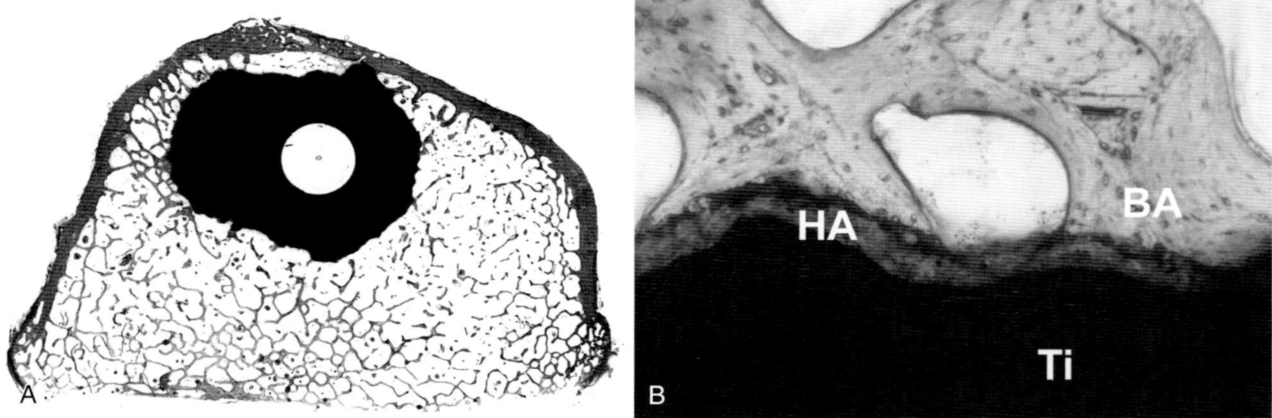

FIGURE 19-2. A, Gross view. **B,** Direct bone apposition to hydroxyapatite (HA)-coated titanium implant. HA-coated titanium femoral stems (Ti) show extensive bone apposition (BA) compared with non–HA-coated stems (canine total hip arthroplasty model). (From Togawa D, Bauer TW, Mochida Y, et al: Bone apposition to three femoral stem surfaces in canine total hip arthroplasty. *Transactions of the 27th Annual Meeting of the Society for Biomaterials,* 251, 2001.)

femur and showed that the shear strength and bone apposition of implants with arc-deposited titanium coating and with one and three layers of cobalt-chromium beads were significantly greater than those of implants with plasma-sprayed cobalt-chromium texture and grid-blasted titanium alloy.[13] Moreover, previous studies have suggested that the metal surface texture of a biomaterial can influence cell attachment and bone apposition. Martin et al. showed that surface texture affects cell attachment as well as cell morphology, proliferation, and differentiation.[14] Thomas and Cook showed that roughened implants yielded more direct bone apposition in vivo than smooth implants of the same materials.[15] Similarly, Turner et al. demonstrated greater bone apposition to titanium canine hip implants with an average texture of 45 μm than implants with texture of 8, 4, and 1 μm.[16]

Excellent clinical results for joint arthroplasty have been reported with several surface treatments.[10,11] However, the optimal surface texture for each implant remains controversial. A number of manufacturers continue to investigate new surfaces in an attempt to improve fixation and lower cost. Thus, a surface topography that incorporates such surface modifications can alter the tissue and/or cell interactions with bone and appears to affect biomechanical interactions as well.[17]

Other Materials

Various other biomaterials have been used at the bone-implant interface for spine surgery, including polymethylmethacrylate (PMMA), calcium phosphate cement, ceramics (hydroxyapatite, bioactive glasses), and polymers (polylactic acid [PLA], polyglycolic acid [PGA], hydrogels, carbon fiber-reinforced polymer, and polyetheretherketone [PEEK]). All foreign materials induce some response when implanted in a host; so strictly speaking, all materials are bioactive. This response is often inflammatory, but some materials induce relatively little inflammation and instead promote bone formation by osteogenic, osteoconductive, or osteoinductive processes. Although PMMA and carbon have excellent biocompatibility, both are less osteoconductive than calcium phosphates or some metals. PMMA has been used for years to help stabilize pathologic fractures, but its exothermic curing and poor osteoconductivity are disadvantages for some clinical applications. Carbon fiber-reinforced polymer and PEEK can yield wear debris,[18-21] but in the spine, carbon fiber-reinforced polymer has been used as an interbody stabilization device and has been associated with clinically successful outcomes without significant particle-induced osteolysis.[22,23] Nevertheless, there is no evidence that these cages have direct bone apposition around them.

Hydroxyapatite (HA) is an osteoconductive calcium phosphate that can be prepared as granules, blocks, or a coating on implants.[24] When placed in a suitable host site, HA is osteoconductive and has some compressive strength, but in general blocks of sintered HA are difficult to machine. In addition, they are brittle and very slow to resorb. Injectable cements are composed of either calcium phosphates or bioglass derivatives. The calcium phosphate cements are highly osteoconductive, develop about 55 MPa compressive strength, cure isothermically, are very slow to resorb, and very weak in tension and shear. The bioglass cements are not as osteoconductive, but offer greater shear strength.[25] Bioabsorbable materials like PLA and PGA, are less osteoconductive in general, but since Kulkarni et al. introduced resorbable polymers for use in surgical implants, these materials have been used successfully in selected applications.[26-30] The use of resorbable polymers in spine surgery has only been advocated recently. The main theoretical advantage of a resorbable material is that it confers initial and intermediate stability without having any of such long-term complications as stress shielding or migration of the implant, but this requires degradation of the implant at a rate that coincides with new bone formation. The gradual degradation of bioabsorbable spinal implants can theoretically allow axial loads that were initially borne by the implant to be progressively transferred to the bone.[31] Another advantage of such materials is that they do not interfere with radiographic studies. Resorbable polymers have been used as plates and interbody fusion devices,[32-34] but again there is little histologic evidence of direct bone apposition to the implant, and the rate of degradation has not always been coupled with new bone formation.

Surgical Applications

Osseointegration of spinal implants is desirable for many clinical applications, and a variety of biomaterials have been used in spine surgery to achieve that result.

Interbody Fusion

Interbody fusion devices are widely used for spinal arthrodesis and have demonstrated their clinical effectiveness for various degenerative disorders of the spine. Numerous types of spinal fusion cages have been developed from titanium and carbon fiber-reinforced or bioabsorbable polymer composites.[35-39] They also have been created in many shapes: horizontal cylinders; vertical rings; or mesh, rectangular, and open boxes. All can be packed with bone graft or graft materials to promote interbody fusion. Variations in cage design in the extent of the end plate, material stiffness, and other characteristics may be factors affecting success. Successful spinal fusion with interbody cage devices has been radiographically confirmed in a number of clinical studies.[22,38,40,41] The results of some animal studies have shown histologic evidence of bone graft incorporation and good connectivity between the bone inside the cages and adjacent vertebral bodies.[36,42-44] The extent of direct bone apposition to clinically satisfactory cages is unknown, but clinically failed cages show no direct bone apposition, even when viable bone is present in the center of the cages[21,45] (Figs. 19-3 and 19-4).

Pedicle Screws

Pedicle screw, rod, or plate systems utilized in conjunction with a dorsal intertransverse bone graft maintain spinal alignment and provide immediate structural stability, thereby allowing early mobilization of the patient while promoting arthrodesis. However, pedicle integrity can be poor in osteoporotic vertebrae, in part due to low screw-bone interface strength. Different methods of improving the purchase of these screws have been investigated, including modifications of the design of the thread, its shape, and surface properties.[46-51] Sandén et al. investigated the effects

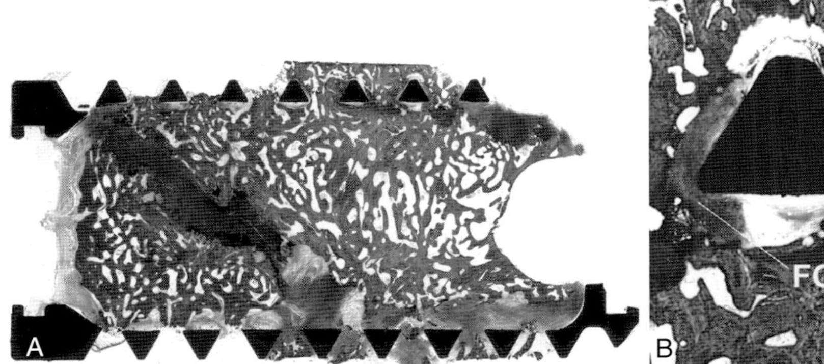

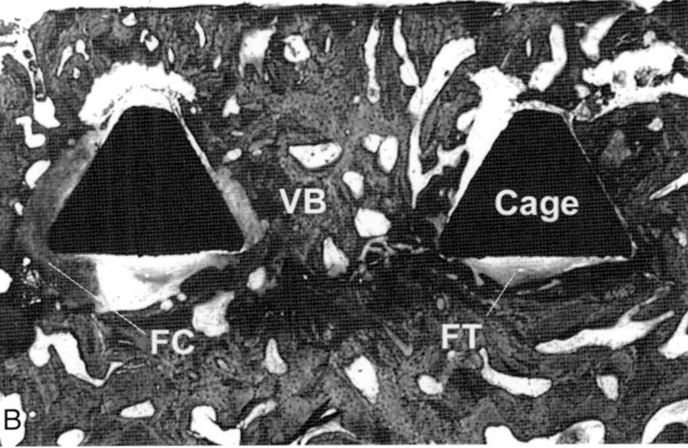

FIGURE 19-3. No direct bone apposition to metal cage. This clinically failed metal cage (**A**) contained viable bone (VB) extending through the openings along one side (**B**). The bone must have connected to bone outside the cage, but there is no direct bone apposition to the metal of the cage. Instead, fibrous tissue (FT) and fibrocartilage (FC) surround each strut of metal. (From Togawa D, Bauer TW, Lieberman IH, et al: Lumbar intervertebral body fusion cages—histological evaluation of clinically failed cages retrieved from humans. *J Bone Joint Surg [Am]* 86:70–79, 2004.)

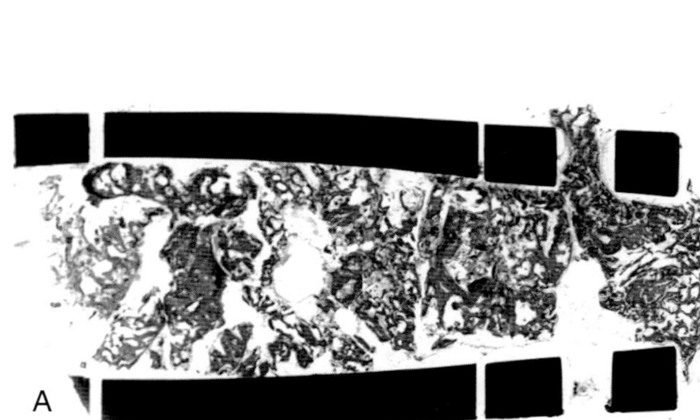

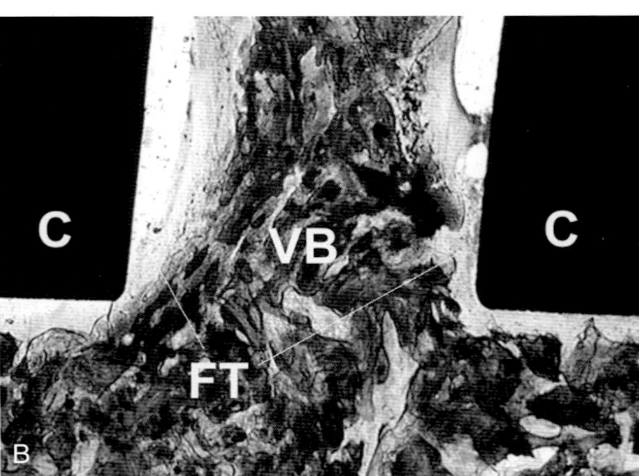

FIGURE 19-4. No direct bone apposition to carbon fiber-reinforced polymer. This clinically failed carbon fiber-reinforced polymer cage (**A**) retrieved from the cervical spine showed no direct bone apposition to the carbon fiber polymer (C) (**B**), even if most of the bone inside the cage was viable bone (VB). The viable bone extends through the lateral hole, but fibrous tissue (FT) separates bone from the cage. (From Togawa D, Bauer TW: The histology of human retrieved body fusion cages: good bone graft incorporation and few particles. *Transactions of the 47th Annual Meeting of the Orthopaedic Research Society,* San Francisco, 950, 2001.)

on purchase of both partial and total HA coating of pedicle screws in a series of the patients with lumbar and lumbosacral degenerative disorders.[52] Approximately 1 year after the surgery, the instruments were removed in some patients, and the authors measured both insertion and extraction torques. The results demonstrated that both insertion and extraction torques for fully coated screws were significantly higher than for uncoated or partly coated screws. Of particular note, the extraction torques exceeded the upper limit of the torque wrench (600 Ncm) for many HA-coated screws, suggesting that HA-coated pedicle screws improved fixation with reduced risk of loosening of the screw.

Augmenting cancellous bone with cement to increase its stiffness and strength represents another modification to improve the chances of successful fixation with pedicle screws.[1,53,54] For example, Turner et al. tested an HA composite resin cement (Kuraray Co., Krashiki, Japan) to determine whether it could stiffen the screw-bone interface in a human cadaveric study.[53] Cement augmentation significantly improved the initial load-carrying capacity (116%), the load-carrying capacity after mechanical testing (165%), and the initial rate of decrease of the implant-bone interface (159%). These results suggested that cement augmentation of pedicle screws increased the stiffness and stability of the screw-bone interface. Furthermore, the pressurized injection of cement into the screw hole causes the cement to penetrate into the trabecular bone, effectively increasing the diameter of the screw.[1]

Spacers, Scaffold, Carrier

Sintered blocks and granules of HA have been occasionally used as a spacer, especially for ventral cervical spine fusions and laminoplasty procedures.[55-61] Radiographic evaluation in these studies have suggested excellent osteoconductivity of these HA spacers. Reported clinical results appear to be good, and there seem to be few complications. Histologic evaluation of three spinous processes of the cervical spine removed from a patient with a recurrent intramedullary tumor 1 year after laminoplasty confirmed direct bone apposition of bone to an HA spacer at three of the six bone-hydroxyapatite interfaces.[61]

Clinically, HA and tricalcium phosphate (TCP) have been shown to be effective as bone graft expanders in dorsal spinal fusion surgery,[62,63] but it may be difficult to distinguish bone from residual synthetic calcium phosphates when radiographs are used as outcome measures in fusion studies. Human biopsies obtained from fusion mass 1 year after dorsolateral fusion using HA/TCP granules show extensive bone apposition[64] (Fig. 19-5).

HA, TCP, and collagen can also be used as carriers of bone morphogenetic proteins (BMPs).[65-68] The combination matrices mixed with HA could have some compression resistance and act as a carrier for BMPs.[69] Akamaru et al. used granules (15% HA, 85% TCP) combined with human recombinant BMP-2 in an adult monkey dorsolateral spine fusion model.[69] Histologic results showed that most of the ceramic had resorbed by 24 weeks after surgery, but some was still present and encased in normal bone, suggesting that the ceramic served as a scaffold and became incorporated with new bone before it could be resorbed.

Artificial Discs

A functional disc interspace prosthesis has been sought at least since the 1950s, and several devices are currently available in Europe and in the United States.[70,71] The Charité artificial disc prosthesis (DePuy Spine, Inc., Raynham, MA) was developed in Germany in the early 1980s,[72] and the third generation of the Charité lumbar total disc replacement prosthesis has been used in more than 5000 patients worldwide since 1987. Originally available as just a grit-blasted titanium ongrowth surface, recent models include calcium phosphate coating. Theoretically, if adequate initial stability is achieved, then the unconstrained design of the prosthesis should reduce the stress at the bone-metal interface and lead to more favorable porous ingrowth characteristics than a constrained prosthesis. In their baboon study, McAfee et al. reported that 14 of 14 hydroxyapatite-coated SB Charité prosthetic vertebral end

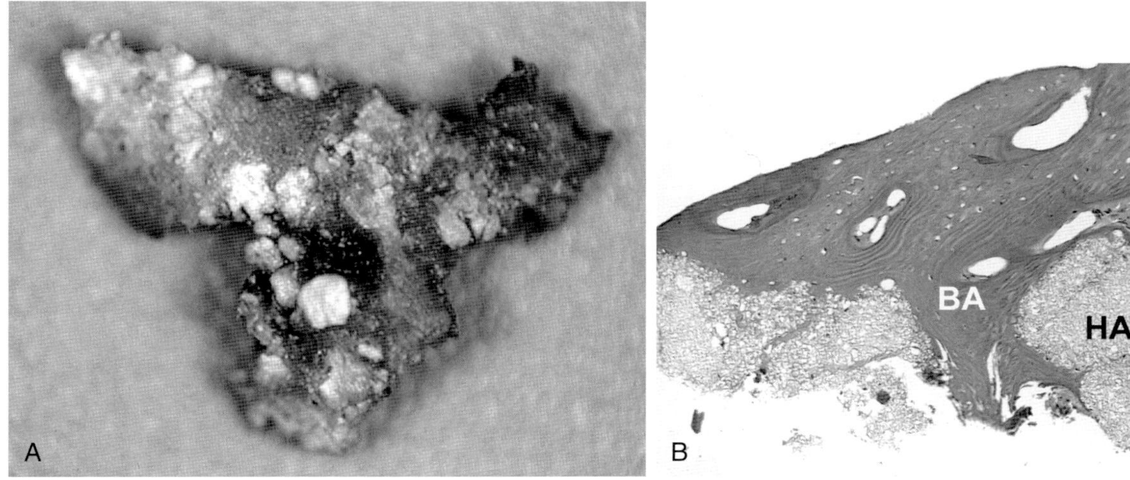

FIGURE 19-5. Direct bone apposition to hydroxyapatite/tricalcium phosphate (HA/TCP) granules. A, Gross view. B, Biopsy specimens obtained from human posterolateral fusion with HA/TCP mixed with autograft showed partial direct bone apposition (BA) to the residual HA/TCP granules approximately 1 year after the surgery. (From Togawa D, Bauer TW, Kanayama M, et al: Histological evaluation of human posterolateral lumbar fusion mass induced by osteogenic protein-1. *Transactions of the 71st Annual Meeting of the American Academy of Orthopaedic Surgeons,* San Francisco, Poster, P396, 2004.)

plates were well-fixed with no evidence of loosening.[73] And a coronal histologic section illustrated in that study shows excellent bone apposition to the HA-coated end plates without evidence of fibrous tissue or synovium 6 months after surgery. Early clinical results, however, have demonstrated migration of some SB Charité implants, suggesting that achieving consistent fixation in humans may still be a problem in some cases.

The few published studies with long duration of follow-up have provided conflicting information, with some reporting success[74] and others describing multiple complications and unfavorable outcome.[75,76] For example, Devin et al. reported a patient who developed osteolysis and failure of a lumbar total disc replacement (AcroFlex, DePuy Spine, Inc.) after 19-year follow-up.[77] Long-term implant fixation depends on bone ingrowth (osseointegration) into the surface of the prosthesis. This case report suggested that although the short-term results were rated as good due to good osteointegration, in long-term follow-up the clinical course can be poor due to associated osteolysis (wear and particles).

Vertebral Augmentation

Vertebral augmentation has been extensively used to treat vertebral bodies involved with osteolytic metastases, myeloma, and osteoporotic compression fractures. PMMA is the most commonly used material for such procedures. Since PMMA is not as osteoconductive as HA, it cannot be expected to promote bone apposition. Technically, under fluoroscopic guidance, PMMA is injected into the weakened vertebrae until the cement is interdigitated into trabecular bone within the vertebrae. A recent report describing the histology of excised human specimens shows absent or only very limited direct bone apposition to the cement. Instead, a thin membrane of fibrous tissue separated bone from the PMMA[78] (Fig. 19-6). To bypass perceived limitations of PMMA, alternative cements that have variable osteoconductive properties have been tested. For example, several animal studies with injectable calcium phosphate cements confirm their feasibility, mechanical effectiveness, biocompatibility, and osteoconductivity[79,80] (Fig. 19-7). Grafe et al. reported a prospective trial comparing 3-year clinical and morphologic outcomes after kyphoplasty to treat painful osteoporotic vertebral fractures with a calcium phosphate cement (CaP, Calcibon, Biomet Merck, Darmstadt, Germany) or with PMMA cement.[81] Their results showed no significant differences between the CaP and the PMMA cement regarding visual analogue scale scores, mobility scores, or height restoration at any time point. Furthermore, there was no significant difference in the occurrence of subsequent compression fractures during the 3-year follow-up period. On the other hand, Blattert et al. reported unfavorable results in kyphoplasty using CaP cement (Norian SRS, Norian Corp., Cupertino, CA) in a prospective randomized controlled clinical study.[82] They reported subtotal cement washout and radiographic loss of correction due to cement failure in the CaP cement group, while there was no case of cement failure in PMMA group.

Composite cements (acrylic cements in conjunction with ceramics) are bioactive, highly radiopaque, and feature excellent mechanical properties. One such cement, Cortoss (Orthovita, Malvern, PA), could be a potentially valuable alternative to PMMA. Palussiere et al. reported that vertebral augmentation with Cortoss rapidly reduced pain, decreased disability, and improved physical functioning in patients with painful vertebral compression fractures.[83] The degree, timing, and maintenance of pain relief seen following Cortoss augmentation in this investigation is similar to that previously reported with PMMA treatment of vertebral fractures.

Summary

In this chapter, the terminology of osseointegration and osteoconductive materials and their clinical applications were discussed. The term *osteointegration* (*osseointegration*) has been used in both structural and functional applications. In order to satisfy both conditions, the material must achieve direct bone apposition and be clinically effective. Many types of spine implants have achieved osseointegration in the broadest

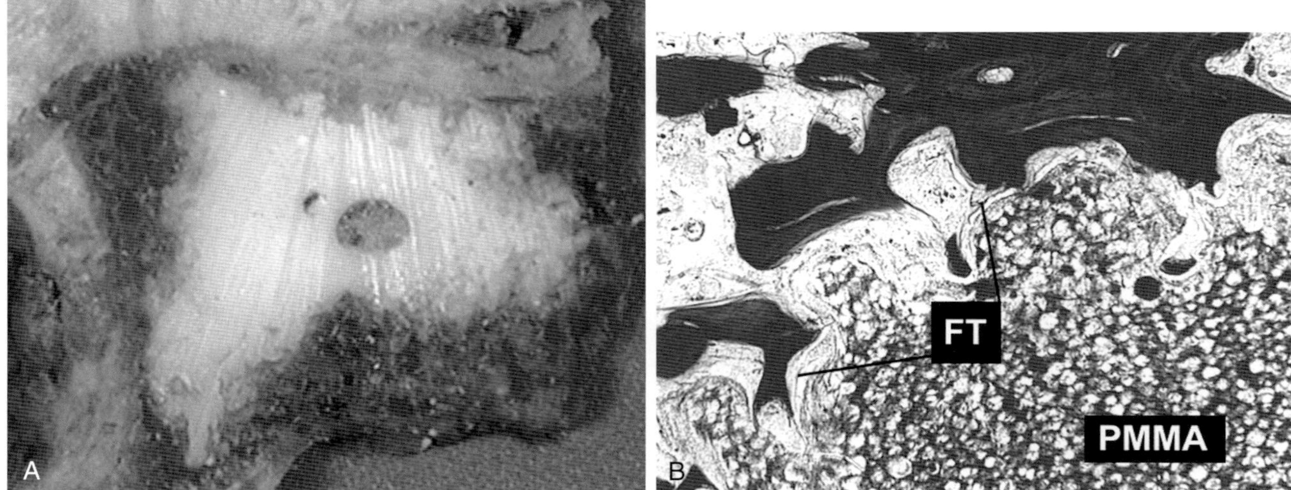

FIGURE 19-6. Interface between polymethylmethacrylate (PMMA) and bone. **A,** Gross view. **B,** Although PMMA interdigitated into trabecular bone of this vertebral body obtained after kyphoplasty, there is no direct bone apposition to the PMMA. Instead, a thin fibrous tissue (FT) separates bone from the PMMA. (From Togawa D, Bauer TW, Lieberman IH, et al: Histologic evaluation of human vertebral bodies after vertebral augmentation with polymethyl methacrylate. *Spine [Phila Pa 1976]* 28:1521–1527, 2003.)

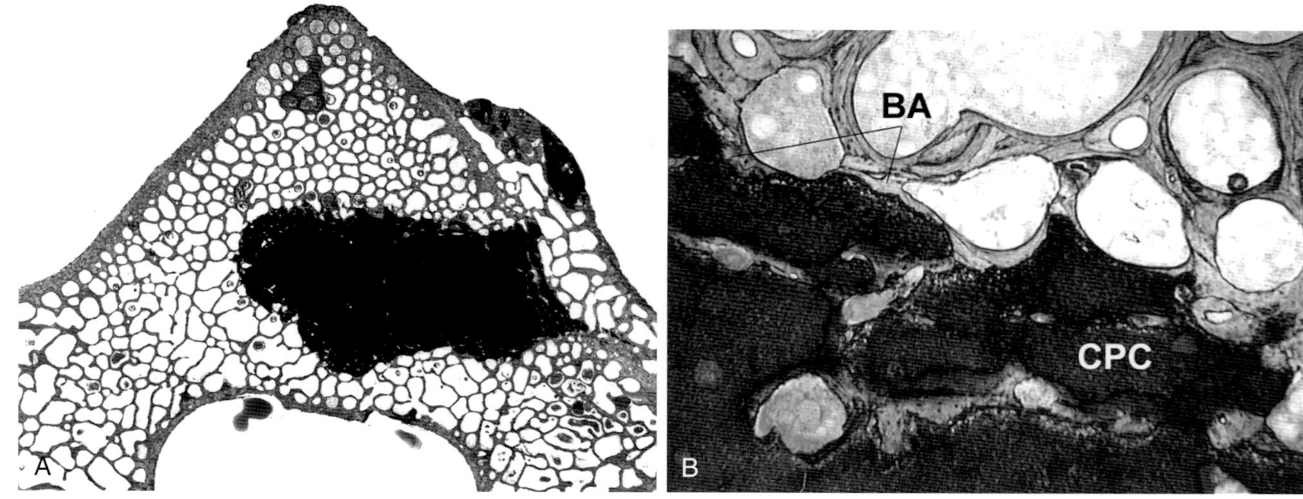

FIGURE 19-7. Interface between calcium phosphate cement and bone. **A,** Gross view. **B,** Calcium phosphate cement (CPC; BoneSource, Stryker Orthopaedics, Mahwah, NJ) injected into a defect in a vertebral body showed extensive bone apposition (BA) 24 months after the surgery. (From Takikawa S, Bauer TW, Turner AS, et al: Comparison of injectable calcium phosphate cement and polymethylmethacrylate for use in vertebroplasty: in-vivo evaluation using an osteopenic sheep model. *Transactions of the Society for Biomaterials* 231, 2002.)

functional sense, but it is often unknown whether direct bone apposition to the implant has been achieved; or for that matter, if it is even necessary. Thus, osseointegration is desirable, but it may not always be necessary. It is necessary for surgeons to understand the importance of material properties, implant characteristics, implant design, and the properties of the local environment (blood flow, load transmission) to achieve clinically successful osseointegration in spine surgery.

KEY REFERENCES

Brånemark PI, Zarb G, Albrektsson T: *Tissue integrated prosthesis: osseointegration in clinical dentistry*, Chicago, 1985, Quintessence.

McAfee PC, Cunningham BW, Orbegoso CM, et al: Analysis of porous ingrowth in intervertebral disc prostheses: a nonhuman primate model. *Spine (Phila Pa 1976)* 28:332–340, 2003.

Phillips FM, Garfin SR: Cervical disc replacement. *Spine (Phila Pa 1976)* 30:S27–S33, 2005.

Sanden B, Olerud C, Petren-Mallmin M, et al: Hydroxyapatite coating improves fixation of pedicle screws. A clinical study. *J Bone Joint Surg [Br]* 84:387–391, 2002.

Thomas KA, Cook SD: An evaluation of variables influencing implant fixation by direct bone apposition. *J Biomed Mater Res* 19:875–901, 1985.

Togawa D, Bauer TW, Lieberman IH, et al: Histologic evaluation of human vertebral bodies after vertebral augmentation with polymethylmethacrylate. *Spine (Phila Pa 1976)* 28:1521–1527, 2003.

Watts TL: Osseointegration is Latin. *Oral Surg Oral Med Oral Pathol Oral Radiol Endod* 89:532, 2000.

REFERENCES

The complete reference list is available online at expertconsult.com.

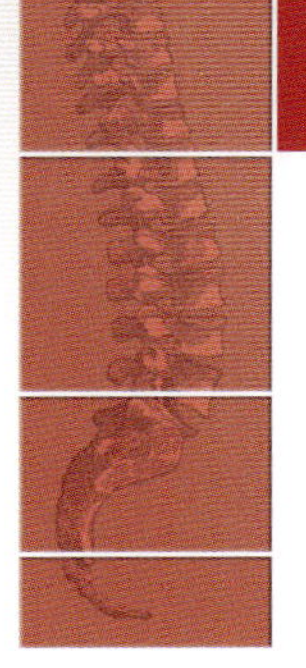

CHAPTER 20

Materials and Material Properties

Steven M. Falowski | Edward H. Scheid, Jr. | Ashwini D. Sharan | Gregory Bennett | Vijay K. Goel | James S. Harrop

The goals of most spine surgeries are to decompress the neural elements and restore spinal alignment and stability. Previously, spinal reconstructive or stabilizing materials consisted only of autograft, allograft, or, in limited circumstances, polymethylmethacrylate (PMMA). Through a better understanding of spinal alignment, bone healing, and fusion principles, and an improvement in implant technology, there has been significant advancement in the field of biomaterials for bone fusion. Traditionally, stabilizing implants have been made of surgical grade stainless steel. The favorable properties of stainless steel include strength, corrosion resistance, and toughness, but, regrettably, its use impairs imaging quality, because stainless steel causes extensive artifacts on MRI.

The next generation of spinal implants consisted of titanium alloys. These implants provided better corrosion resistance, less distortion on MRI, and a decrease in ductility and scratch sensitivity, but with less strength.

Spine surgeons must be aware of these general differences in implants in order to maximize outcomes. A decreased risk of implant failure can be achieved by making an educated decision as to what material would best suit an individual patient. A practical knowledge of the principles of materials also is helpful to evaluate the design of new implants, to anticipate design limitations, and to further lessen the risk of implant failure. For example, allograft bone is a composite material with widely varying properties, depending on its composition and configuration. In the future, ceramic and composite materials may be increasingly available for use as bone substitutes. Another modality that has come into favor is the use of bone morphogenetic protein (BMP) products. The properties of these materials are very different from metals and require different considerations in design as well as surgical application.

The first recorded use of a metallic implant device was in 1804, when a steel implant was used in a fracture repair.[1,2] Later, in 1924, stainless steel, which contains 18% chromium and 8% nickel, was first applied for medical purposes. The next major advance in metallurgy was the aircraft industry's development of light-weight but resilient metals known as titanium alloys.[1,2] In the 1950s, the biomedical field began to make use of titanium. Currently, titanium is one of the most advantageous metals for implant use because of its high strength, low modulus, and high corrosion resistance.[1]

Most of the spinal implants used today include either a stainless steel (iron-based) or titanium-based alloy. This chapter reviews the forces and physical properties of implants, the terminology for material properties, the nature of atomic bonds and various strengthening mechanisms of alloys, the nature of biologic materials, and biocompatibility. In addition, properties of specific spinal implant alloys are explored.

Forces

The International System (SI units), which is based on the metric system, is the nomenclature used by the biomedical engineering profession. The newton (N) is a direct measure of force and is recorded as intrinsic units: kg(m)/sec^2. As defined by Newton's second law, force is equivalent to the product of mass and acceleration. Forces, when applied to the spine, not only consist of a magnitude but also have a directional component. The combination of a force with direction is a vector. Vectors can be displayed graphically or by trigonometric relationships. Vectors can be used to analyze biomechanical forces acting simultaneously on a biologic structure or implant material by making a free body diagram that assumes a state of equilibrium, thereby defining the forces inside the structure or implant material as dependent and proportional to those outside the structure (Fig. 20-1).

A very important principle for the spine surgeon to understand is the force-deformation relationship (Fig. 20-2). When force and deformation are graphically displayed, the result is a characteristic curve. The force-deformation curve has a straight or elastic region in which materials can deform and recover to their original shape (see Fig. 20-2, first portion of curve). As the load increases beyond the elastic region, the deformation increases into the curved or plastic region (see Fig. 20-2, second portion of curve); when the specimen is unloaded, it will be permanently deformed. If deformation is continued, the specimen will eventually fail (e.g., fracture; see Fig. 20-2, third portion of curve).

The integrity of the spine is multifactorial. The vertebral body ossifies from three primary centers, one for the centrum, which will form the major portion of the body, and the other two for neural arches. The cartilaginous growth plate is mainly responsible for longitudinal vertebral growth. The vertebral body design, therefore, provides the requirement for optimal load transfer by maximal strength with minimal weight. Bone mineral density (BMD), bone quality, microarchitecture, and material properties are the important factors that contribute to bone strength.[3] In addition, force and displacement have

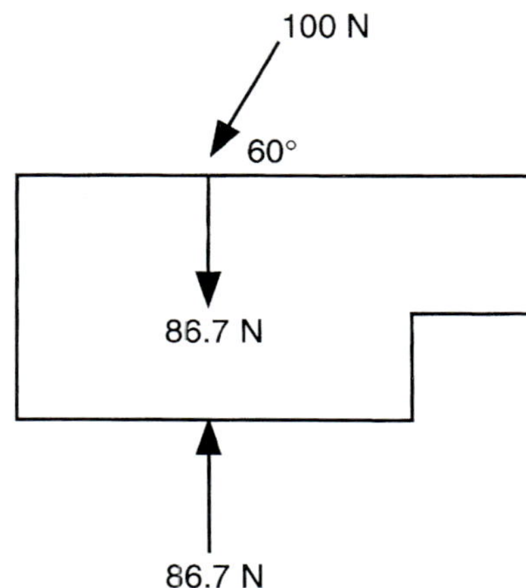

FIGURE 20-1. Free body diagram of a lumbar vertebra with an externally applied load of 100 N at an incident angle of 60 degrees. The vertebra will have to resist the shear component as well (horizontal component—not shown in the figure—of the incident force). The resultant downward force on the vertebral body is sin (60) × 100 N = 86.7 N. The vertebra is in equilibrium with its surroundings and not moving. Therefore, a force of the same magnitude is acting on the caudal end plate.

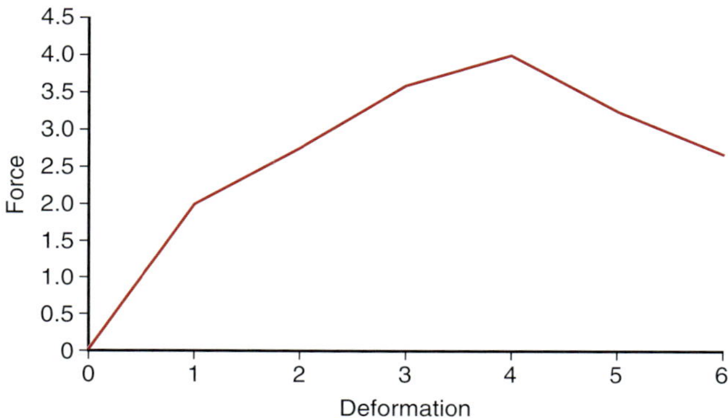

FIGURE 20-2. Force versus deformation curve. The force has a straight or elastic region in which materials can deform and recover to their original shape. As load increases beyond the elastic region, the deformation increases into the plastic region; when the specimen is unloaded, it will be permanently deformed. If the deformation is limited, the specimen eventually will fail (i.e., fracture).

been demonstrated in animal spine models. It has been demonstrated in a biomechanical cadaver study that after dorsal laminectomy and partial discectomy, the neutral zone and range of motion were not different from those in the native spine specimen. However, after pedicle screw-rod fixation, the neutral zone and range of motion of the instrumented specimen decreased significantly compared with the native specimen and the specimen after dorsal laminectomy.[4]

Atomic Bonds, Structures, and Property Relationships

All materials are composed of molecules that interact via intermolecular forces. These bonds determine the properties of the material as a whole. If materials were composed of only one type of molecule and these molecules were perfectly consistent in their orientation, then chemistry alone would be sufficient for deriving all of the elements' properties. However, materials typically are composed of numerous molecules of considerable diversity. Nevertheless, despite the variety of molecules in metals, certain observations can be made from their chemical composition.

Metals are created through the interaction of crystals. These crystals are formed when the electrons that surround the atoms in clouds are given up and conducted as electricity. Metal structures are polycrystalline (i.e., they are formed by a multitude of crystals). Atoms within a crystal can form one of several relationships, which define the crystal structure. They include body-centered cubic, face-centered cubic, and hexagonal close-packed arrangements (Figs. 20-3 to 20-5).

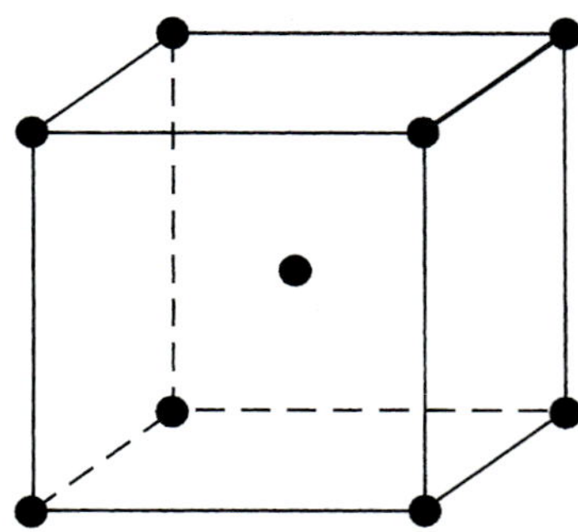

FIGURE 20-3. The unit cell is the smallest group of atoms showing a characteristic structure. The body-centered cube is the most ductile.

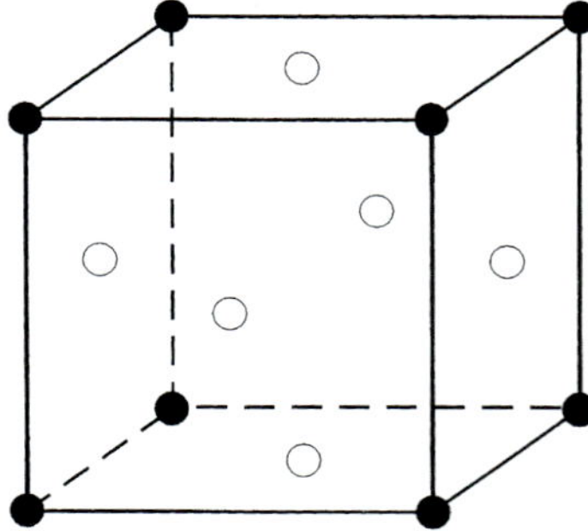

FIGURE 20-4. The face-centered cube is moderately ductile.

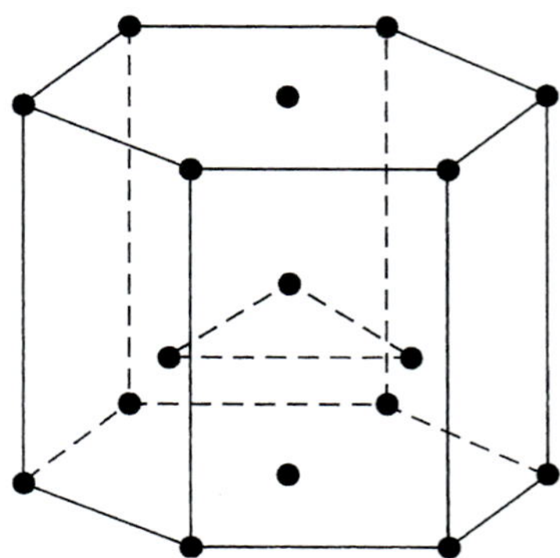

FIGURE 20-5. The hexagonal close-packed cube is the least ductile.

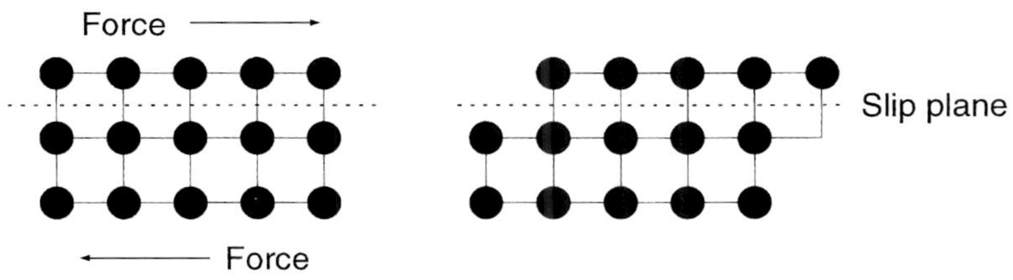

Force
Slip plane
Force

FIGURE 20-6. During stress, individual atomic bonds are disrupted and the atoms slip along a plane.

In addition to variations in the unit cell of the crystal, metals have many imperfections in the crystals, consisting of line defects, point defects, missing atoms, additional atoms, and impurities with foreign atoms. Metals can be further contaminated with larger impurities from nonmetallic elements such as oxides and sulfides.

Point defects occur when a lattice site within a crystal is empty and not occupied by an atom.[1,5] Point defects are present in all metals and provide a mechanism for diffusion, which is the movement of solute through a solvent.

Line defects are microscopic dislocations and are the major defect affecting a given metals mechanical properties. Line defects occur when there is an incomplete chain of atoms inside a crystal. This results in a local distortion of the structure of the crystal because of the resultant dislocation. There is considerable internal strain in the immediate vicinity of the dislocation. When a force is applied, the line defect can propagate through the crystal structure, resulting in a permanent structural change (Figs. 20-6 and 20-7). This is termed *plastic deformation*. When a metal is plastically deformed, a permanent structural change persists after the force is removed from the metal.[1]

An example of an area defect is a grain boundary.[1] When metal begins the solidification process, crystals form independently of one another. Each crystal grows into a crystalline structure, or grain. The size and number of grains developed by a certain amount of metal depend on the rate of nucleation, which is the initial stage of formation of a crystal. Rapid cooling usually produces smaller grains, whereas slower cooling produces larger grains. The orientation of crystal boundaries (grain boundaries) is very influential in the spread of dislocations that become cracks.

A high nucleation rate yields a high number of grains for a given amount of metal. Therefore, the grain size will be small. If the rate of growth of the crystals is high relative to their nucleation rate, however, fewer grains will develop, and they will be of larger size.

As a grain grows, it eventually comes in contact with another grain. The surfaces that separate grains are termed *grain boundaries*. Grain boundaries are the junction areas of the many metal crystals that compose an implant. The grain size has a significant effect on the mechanical properties of a metal. A higher number of grain boundaries increases strength. Grain boundaries prevent line defects from propagating from one grain to another. A higher number of grain boundaries necessitates a higher force required to induce a plastic deformation. Since a higher number of grain boundaries occurs in alloys with smaller grains, smaller grains yield an increase in strength, whereas larger grains are generally associated with low strength and ductility.

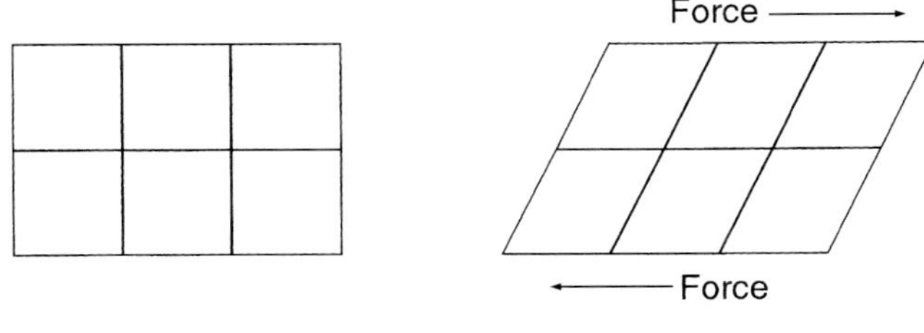

FIGURE 20-7. Deformation occurs when parallel and opposite forces are applied to a structure with one side immobilized.

The many ways in which a metal can acquire defects affecting its strength has led to the development of various strengthening mechanisms to improve the performance of a metal or alloy. All strengthening mechanisms act on the theory that impeding line defects results in increased strength.

Solid solution strengthening occurs when one or more elements are added to a metal. Atoms of the solute will take places within the crystalline lattice by substituting for a solvent (metal) atom. Alternatively, the solute atom may occupy a site not previously occupied by a solvent atom by lying in an interstitial site. Interstitial atoms usually are much smaller than the solvent, whereas substituting elements often are similar in size to the solvent. Interstitial solid solution strengthening often is more effective. The effect of solid solution strengthening is to stop line defects from spreading a dislocation by developing solute-rich regions in the area surrounding the line defect. As a result, increased force is needed to induce a plastic deformation.

Cold working deforms the metal and results in an increase in strength. Deformation of a metal increases the amount of line defects within the metal. These dislocations then entangle with one another. The result is an increasing amount of energy that continues to move these line defects within the grain. The increase in strength from cold working comes at the expense of a decrease in ductility.

Hot working involves the use of high temperature to deform the metal. This often is used to allow a metal to form a shape while altering the microstructure of the alloy. It is possible to obtain a reduction in grain size by hot working. By increasing the temperature to a level that causes a deformation, the dislocations become disentangled. The metal then undergoes recrystallization, and new dislocation-free grains are formed.

Mechanical Properties

Knowing the dimensions of a material, when a force is applied, permits the stress or load per unit area to be determined. Stress is recorded as N/m^2 (Pascal) and is a small quantity. Therefore, most materials are tested with thousands of N/m^2, or megapascals. Strain is a dimensionless unit that is the percentage of elongation (or shortening) during application of force. When both the load and the deformation are divided by the original area or length of the specimen, respectively, the result is stress and strain, which can be displayed graphically (see Fig. 20-7).

Spine surgeons should have a basic understanding of the typical stress-strain curve (see Fig. 20-2). The stress-strain curve defines the mechanical behavior of a metal under various degrees of stress and strain. The ratio of stress to strain is the modulus, or elastic modulus. The relationship is as follows:

$$E = \text{stress/strain}$$

The modulus (E) reflects the stiffness of the material. Stiffness, in turn, depends on the relative difficulty of stretching atoms from their resting position in a crystal lattice. It is important to note that the modulus is not affected to a significant degree by line defects.

At a certain amount of stress, plastic deformation occurs. At this point, line deformations begin to cause structurally relevant deformations, which propagate through the grain. The linear relationship between stress and strain breaks down, and the slope of the modulus decreases. The point at which this occurs is the proportional limit. *Yield stress* is arbitrarily defined as the point at which permanent deformation reaches 0.2% of the metal. *Ultimate stress* is defined as the highest stress reached during testing of the metal. *Percent elongation*, a measure of ductility, is the degree of plastic deformation acquired prior to failure.

Fatigue strength is another property of metal that is important when considering bioimplantation. Fatigue is a process whereby repetitive stress or strain is applied to a metal, eventually leading to breakdown, crack formation, and eventual failure of the metal. By definition, the *fatigue strength* is the cyclic stress required to cause failure of the metal at a given number of cycles. When a metal fails from fatigue, it usually takes much longer and a greater number of cycles to form the initial crack than to achieve complete failure. Consequently, any material that acts to prevent crack formation will improve the metal's resistance to fatigue.

Fatigue failures have become less common in implants because of improved materials and strengthening processes. When they do occur, crack formation usually is the inciting factor. Most of these cracks form at the alloy surface. Therefore, surface conditions become very important in preventing fatigue failure.

Spinal Implants: Rigid versus Dynamic

Spinal implants can be described as rigid, dynamic, or hybrid. Dynamic implants allow some subsidence between segments. The advantage of a dynamic implant is that it is capable of offsetting stress at the implant-bone interface and therefore does not provide stress shielding of the bone graft.

The purpose of a rigid construct is to completely immobilize the spine. Because of the properties of bone, this is rarely achieved. Movement in a rigid system often increases with the passage of time, through weakening of the implant-bone interface. Repetitive movement under sufficient stress eventually will lead to failure at the interface, unless bony fusion occurs first.

Rigid fixation does not completely optimize bony fusion acquisition because of stress shielding. The goal of rigid fixation is only to hold long enough for bony fusion to take place.

The widespread use of instrumentation in the lumbar spine has led to high rates of fusion. This has been accompanied by a marked rise in adjacent-segment disease, which is considered to be an increasingly common and significant consequence of lumbar or lumbosacral fusion. Numerous biomechanical studies have demonstrated that segments fused with rigid metallic fixation lead to significant amounts of supraphysiologic stress on adjacent discs and facets. Although this form of arthrodesis does not completely prevent adjacent-segment disease, the dynamic component of this stabilization technique may minimize its occurrence.[6] Posterior dynamic stabilization (PDS) devices have shown a substantial reduction in stress-shielding characteristics. Higher axial load was noted with the PDS devices, which could slow the degeneration process of bony structures and lower the possibility of implant failure.[7]

The purpose of a dynamic construct is to provide for intersegmental subsidence. Although excessive movement can inhibit fusion, the minimal intersegmental movement (which facilitates compression) increases the rate of bone fusion. Also, the minimal intersegmental movement absorbs some of the strain that is encountered at the implant-bone interface.

Biologic Materials

Bone is the "gold standard" of implant materials as a biologic material. It consists of a framework of type I collagen fibers, a matrix of calcium hydroxyapatite, and small amounts of protein polysaccharides and mucopolysaccharides (ground substance or cement). The organic content of bone is relatively constant at 0.6 g/mL, whereas the mineral content varies (up to 2 g/mL). Bone is slightly viscoelastic, in that rapid deformations result in 95% of the eventual displacement caused by slow deformations. Because of this difference, the *energy* required for fracture is higher under rapid loading conditions. Under very rapid (ballistic) conditions, bone shatters into comminuted fragments. The total energy required to create a fracture is thus reduced. Bone is anisotropic, with a fiber pattern that is parallel to the predominant axis of loading. It displays both elastic and plastic behavior.

The stiffness of bone is approximately 10% that of stainless steel and 20% that of titanium alloy (Ti-6Al4V, or simply 116-4). This means that the stiffness of bone is closer to that of titanium than steel implants. This fact has been used to suggest that there is a better "match" between titanium and bone than between stainless steel and bone. In certain circumstances this might be important, such as when a permanently implanted device will be subjected to repeated deformations while the bone-implant juncture could loosen. Alternatively, the use of steel implants creates a construct of higher stiffness. Surgical constructs of higher stiffness have been associated with higher fusion rates, both clinically and experimentally. Because the optimal stiffness of a surgical construct for bone healing is unknown, the selection of implant material should not be influenced by minor variations in the stiffness of materials.

Stainless Steel

Stainless steel implants are iron- and carbon-based alloys. Medical grade stainless steel alloys typically contain chromium (18–22%), nickel (18–22%), molybdenum (2.5%), manganese (2.5%), and carbon (0.03–0.08%) by weight.

Initial trials of stainless steel as an implant showed that resisting corrosion by improving resistance to chloride degradation was insufficient. The addition of molybdenum and chromium reduced the incidence of corrosion and pitting by aiding the defense against chloride degradation.[1,5]

The 316 stainless steels, which have a face-centered cubic structure, are the steels that are used most commonly for spinal implants. There are two grades, grade 1 (316) and grade 2 (316L), of which grade 2 has the lower carbon content. The lower carbon content aids in reducing the formation of metal carbides, which leads to a decrease in the corrosion resistance of the alloy.[1,8] These 316 alloys are commonly used in fracture fixation devices. They are commonly hot- or cold-worked and solid solution–strengthened.

Titanium-Based Alloys

Titanium-based alloys currently are the alloys most commonly used for bioimplantation. Pure titanium (cP-Ti) and an alloy with aluminum and vanadium (Ti-6Al-4V) are the most common compositions for titanium in the United States.[1,5]

Titanium-based alloys are advantageous for several reasons. They have both high strength and fatigue resistance. Commercially pure titanium has a hexagonal, close-packed structure; various grades differ in their oxygen concentration. In small quantities, oxygen serves to solid-solution strengthen the alloy by interstitial placement of the atom. However, in excessive amounts, oxygen can weaker the material by decreasing the number of grain boundaries. This results in a much lower fatigue strength and surface ductility.[1,5,8] Titanium-based alloys also have decreased stiffness when compared to stainless steel. The reduction in stiffness facilitates transfer of the stress at the bone-implant interface to the alloy; this minimizes bone resorption at the interface. Titanium-based alloys have higher fatigue strength when compared with stainless steel. However, titanium alloys are vulnerable to any surface flaws. Any scratch or notch can rapidly accelerate the fatigue failure process. Titanium, in its pure form, is generally weaker than stainless steel, but it can be cold-worked to increase its strength.[1,2] Titanium alloys also lack any known immunogenicity, an important advantage for any foreign body implant.

Surface Structure and Modifications of Alloys

As discussed previously, any surface component that prevents crack formation will decrease an alloy's sensitivity to fatigue. Implant alloys typically use an oxide film for their surfaces. These oxide films are considered passive films because they are the result of oxidation of the outermost metal atoms on the surface of the alloy.[1]

Corrosion is an oxidative process that is a threat to alloys. Corrosion would ensue rapidly without passive films. Stainless steels have oxide films composed of Cr_2O_3, FeO, and Fe_2O_3. This thin film separates the metal from its surrounding, corrosive environment and is the major factor in resistance to decay. Titanium alloys form TiO_2, which plays a similar role to that of chromium oxide with stainless steel. Oxide films also serve as a protective barrier on articulating surfaces of the alloy.

Immersion of steel alloy surfaces in nitric acid baths also delays corrosion. Nitric baths dissolve impurities anywhere they exist on the surface of the metal implants, thereby ensuring an intact oxide film.

Surface modification is used to increase local strength and hardening of implants. Two types of surface modification include ion implantation and vapor deposition.[1,5] Ion implantation, the direct implantation of gas phase ions into the alloy, involves the acceleration of ions toward the surface of the alloy. The ions penetrate and increase the number and type of subsurface defects and dislocations, which leads to an increase in the durability of the metal surface and a reduction in its susceptibility to corrosion.[1,9]

Another method of surface modification is either chemical or physical vapor deposition. This technique adds a new hardened coating to the alloy surface, usually composed of chromium nitride (CrN) or titanium nitride (TiN). One shortcoming of hardened coatings is that they have variable adhesion with the alloy.

Finally, *nitriding* is a process that modifies the surface of a material by a chemical reaction with nitrogen, which places nitrides on the surface. A portion of the surface of stainless steel or titanium can undergo nitriding by causing the surface to react with either gaseous ammonia or molten potassium cyanate.[1,5] The result is a great increase in surface hardness of the alloy.

Ceramics

In contrast to metals, ceramics have chemical bonds that are predominantly ionic, with a densely packed array of oppositely charged atoms (Fig. 20-8). These atoms have limited mobility because of the interaction of charges of nearby atoms. This charge interaction results in a stiff material with low ductility and no plasticity. Ceramics are composed of crystals oriented randomly in a dense framework that consists of metallic oxides. They may have inorganic chain molecules, such as silicon dioxide in a glass phase. Traditional ceramic materials often have impurities and internal microporous inclusions that limit their strength to less than the theoretical maximum. Newer ceramics are synthesized with chemically pure materials with high densities or as composites with greatly increased strength.[10-12]

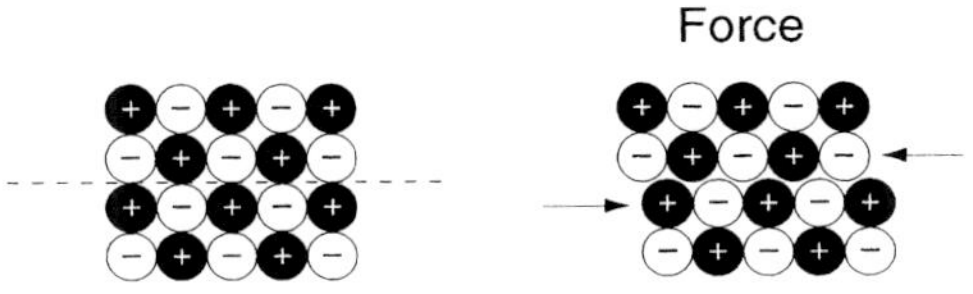

FIGURE 20-8. Ceramics have strong ionic bonds and these charge interactions result in a stiff material with low ductility and no plasticity.

An advantage of oxide ceramics is their wear reduction compared to that of alloys.[1,10] Metals and alloys have a protective oxide film that can be peeled off by adherence to opposing surface polymers.[1,10] This causes local ion release from the alloy. This loss and reformation of the oxide film is a repetitive process that can accelerate degradation of the surface of the alloy implant. Oxide ceramics do not have a passive oxide film and may, as a result, have less long-term breakdown.

Synthetic Polymers

Synthetic polymer production is a rapidly expanding field of implant technology. Polymers, commonly known as plastics, typically are very large molecules made from a large number of individual subunits called *monomers*. Polymers are chemical compounds that are formed by combining these smaller, repeating structural units. The subunits repeat in various patterns, following principles similar to those of molecular biology. The covalent bonds in polymers have a fixed length. The complex folding of polymers is created by weak hydrogen bond cross-links that permit unfolding and elongation. The two most commonly used polymers are polymethylmethacrylate (PMMA) and ultra-high molecular weight polyethylene (UHMWPE).[1]

Stiffening the "backbone" molecular chain and increasing the cross-links, the polymer can be made less flexible. Numerous other properties can be influenced by chemical changes, including density, crystallization, solubility, thermal stability, and strength. UHMWPE has been extensively used for artificial joints because of its favorable surface wear and creep properties. In spine surgery, PMMA has been used extensively because of the additional polymerization that occurs when the powder and liquid are mixed.

The intermediate phase of polymerization yields a doughy material that can be worked and shaped into complex defects before it hardens. PMMA has many molecular and macroscopic defects that contribute to its characteristically weak tensile strength. These defects originate in the powder phase, which consists of microspheres. The microspheres are bound together as the methylmethacrylate monomer (liquid phase) polymerizes into a matrix that incorporates the microspheres. Even after hardening, the juncture between the powder phase microspheres and the liquid phase remains relatively weak. Additionally, the polymer chains have very few cross-links. For all these reasons, the polymerized PMMA has a low tensile strength.

Composite materials are a combination of a filler and matrix. Traditionally, the filler is glass or carbon fibers, whereas the matrix is epoxy, carbon, UHMWPE, PMMA, or a variety of other materials. The fibers can be particulate or relatively large and stiff, in which case they are termed *whiskers*. Composites with whiskers have high tensile strength but can be brittle. Fiber orientation in relation to the direction of loading is important. A complex variety of stress responses can be obtained in polymer matrix composites, making these materials anisotropic. Biologic materials such as bone, ligament, and tendon also are composites with anisotropy. An example of a composite used in spine surgery is the carbon fiber cage for interbody fusion, which is composed of long-fiber carbon and Ultrapek (polyether ketone; BASF Aktiengesellschaft, Germany).[13]

Bone Morphogenetic Protein

Bone morphogenetic protein (BMP) is a group of proteins of the transforming growth factor beta (TGF-β) family that can induce bone growth. Currently, they are synthesized using recombinant DNA and work via signal transduction through BMP receptors. Of the several BMPs, the most commonly used is BMP-2, a disulfide-linked homodimer that induces bone and cartilage formation, playing a key role in osteoblast differentiation and making it a useful adjunct in spinal fusion.

The use of growth factors such as BMPs is showing great promise in spinal surgery and has been used successfully in spine fusion and fracture healing.[14] Several animal models have demonstrated that BMP-containing allograft or synthetic carrier medium is as effective as or superior to autograft bone in promoting spinal fusion.[15] Burkus et al. have illustrated that in ventral lumbar fusions, allograft cortical bone with rhBMP had equivalent fusion rates as autogenous bone graft without the associated graft site morbidity.[16]

Recombinant human bone morphogenetic protein type 2 (rhBMP-2) has been demonstrated to be safe and effective in posterior lumbar interbody fusion procedures when used as an absorbable collagen sponge carrier as an alternative to iliac crest bone graft.[17] The efficacy of rhBMP-2 in augmenting fusion also has been shown when used in non-instrumented posterior lumbar decompressive surgery and leads to satisfactory outcomes, specifically improved pain relief, function, and bone formation, in elderly patients without the use of instrumentation.[18] In addition to lumbar surgery, a prospective nonrandomized study in patients undergoing anterior cervical discectomy and fusion has demonstrated that those performed with BMP allograft are as effective as iliac bone graft in terms of patient outcomes and fusion rates.[19]

Biocompatibility

All surgical procedures are associated with a disruption of normal anatomic tissue planes. This results in an accumulation of exudative fluid, fibrin, platelets, and polymorphonuclear leukocytes. From days 3 to 5 after surgery, macrophages accumulate and remove the surgical debris. By 10 days, the macrophages are no longer present, and lymphocytes predominate. This stage is followed by fibroblasts, which complete the cellular phase of healing. Ceramic implants are very biocompatible, because the cellular response to wound healing is not significantly altered.

However, in the presence of a metal implant, the immune system is activated, with the production of protein-metal hapten complexes, complement activation, and the resultant cellular and humoral immune responses. A chronic inflammatory state with sustained populations of macrophages, lymphocytes, and occasional plasma cells persists for several weeks or months. Eventually, as the inflammatory response subsides, these foreign bodies are sequestered by dense fibrous tissue. Direct apposition of bone to an implant, without an interposed fibrous layer, is very rare, with the exception of titanium and bioactive ceramics such as calcium hydroxyapatite.

In total joint replacement, wear debris accumulates as a function of the force across the joint, the relative displacement of the articular surfaces, and a variety of wear mechanisms, including abrasion, corrosion, fretting (micromotion), and third-body wear resulting from wear debris between the articular surfaces. Wear debris also can cause adverse local responses to the implant, such as osteolysis and regional lymphadenopathy. These phenomena are of increasing interest to neurosurgeons, because articulating artificial discs have become more widely used as an alternative to spinal fusion.[20-22]

For most surgical constructs, stainless steel implants are sufficiently nonreactive to permit bone fusion before the deleterious consequences of the normal inflammatory response, such as severe pain or loosening. The presence of a metal implant may lead to an increased risk of infection. In vitro testing of stainless steel and cobalt alloy materials has shown inhibition of macrophage chemotaxis and phagocytosis, which may contribute to the increased risk of infection. The avascular fibrous layer that accumulates around metal implants in bone also may contribute to this risk. Sites associated with PMMA are especially vulnerable, most likely due to the 0.1- to 0.5-mm layer of necrotic bone that is created by the direct toxicity of the methacrylate monomer and the heat released during hardening.

The fibrous layer around implants may be associated with painful late loosening of the device. For example, after an intertransverse lumbar fusion has occurred, micromotions may persist between the vertebral bodies, resulting in painful movements of vertebral bone in relation to pedicle screws. In theory, bone in-growth and direct adhesion to an implant (such as what occurs with titanium) may lessen the risk of infection and painful late loosening.

Metal allergy is widely prevalent and well recognized, but is poorly understood. Metal ions alone will not stimulate the immune system. When linked with proteins, metals such as cobalt, chromium, and especially nickel are immunogenic. The characteristic immune response to metals is delayed hypersensitivity. This has been proposed as the cause of premature loosening in total hip arthroplasties. Delayed development of sensitivity after prolonged exposure to a metal implant has been well documented, using the leukocyte migration inhibition test.[23] The clinical significance of metal allergy in spinal surgery is unknown, but these data suggest that patients reporting skin sensitivity to metal should be considered for titanium implants rather than stainless steel before elective spinal surgery.

The mechanical strength immediately after instrumentation is determined by the worst case of device-graft subsidence; after instrumentation, bone will adapt itself to the changed loading conditions and therefore reduce the risk of subsidence.[24] Knoller et al. demonstrated a relationship between the stability of a spinal instrumentation and bone mineral density and a significant influence of bone mineral density on range of motion.[25]

Osteolysis, or periprosthetic bone loss, may occur at the site of an implant. Structural remodeling of surrounding bone occurs in response to stress shielding. This bone destruction can lead to loosening and possible failure of the implant. Factors that are thought to play a role in osteolysis include the formation of particulate debris and loosening, or motion, of the implant.[6] Once the particles are generated, macrophages proliferate and attack the periprosthetic space. This leads to activation of an inflammatory cascade and the induction of osteoclastic pathways.

Summary

Contemporary spinal surgeons are faced with the task of making informed decisions regarding the choice of implant for stabilization. The spinal surgeon must have an understanding of the physical and chemical properties of any material that he or she is contemplating implanting into the patient. Various advantageous properties of alloys, and biomaterials in general, include strength, ductility, modulus, hardness, and biocompatibility. Each material possesses different advantages and disadvantages. It is up to the surgeon to understand this increasingly complex aspect of the field and to make decisions accordingly.

KEY REFERENCES

Highsmith JM, Tumialan LM, Rodts GE Jr: Flexible rods and the case for dynamic stabilization. *Neurosurg Focus* 22(1):E11, 2007.

Merritt K, Brown SA: Biological effects of corrosion products from metals (195-206). In Fraker AG, Griffin CD, editors: *Corrosion and degradation of implant materials*. ASTM STP 859, Philadelphia, 1985, American Society for Testing and Materials.

Wang X, Dumas GA: Evaluation of effects of selected factors on intervertebral fusion-a simulation study. *Med Eng Phys* 27(3):197–207, 2005.

White A, Panjabi M: *Clinical biomechanics of the spine*, Philadelphia, 1990, Lippincott-Raven, pp 86–87.

REFERENCES

The complete reference list is available online at expertconsult.com.

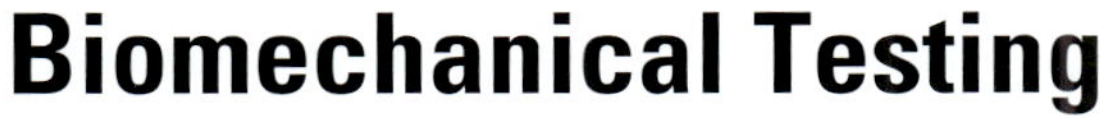

CHAPTER 21

Biomechanical Testing

Vikas Kaul | Ali Kiapour | Vijay K. Goel

Background

In the second half of the 20th century, the research area of biomechanics encompassed a problem that, at one time, was of interest to Leonardo daVinci–the human spine.[1] In the 1970s and 1980s, in particular, there was a rapid increase in the biomechanical analysis and quantitative understanding of the anatomy of the spine and clinical issues related to its treatment.[2-8] This new insight enabled researchers to design and develop devices that aimed to restore normal physiologic movement.[9,10] However, one of the unforeseen consequences of this flurry of scientific activity was a lack of standards.[9,11-13] Depending on the laboratory and the application, devices were being evaluated under different conditions, making comparison difficult. Limitations related to the peculiar nature of the spinal anatomy and testing made standardization difficult. Eventually, however, consensus was achieved and standards evolved.[9,13] From the economic point of view, spine biomechanics seems to have delivered on its promise. According to Epsicom, a global market research company, the spinal implant market saw a growth of about 8 billion dollars in 2008. It is estimated that by 2012, the worldwide spinal market will realize revenues of 10 billion dollars.

Another avenue of inquiry has been aiming at resolving clinical issues without the use of any "mechanical" devices. This field, tissue engineering, has started to show great promise in the field of spine biomechanics. With U.S. federal funding available for stem cell research, a global market of 4.8 billion dollars, and about 200 companies working on designing newer and better orthopaedic biomaterials, the future is bound to see a growing influence of tissue engineering in spine deformity correction. Although challenges exist,[14,15] our understanding of issues related to the regeneration of the nucleus pulposus[16,17] and anulus fibrosus[18] has increased manifold. As a case in point, much interest is being paid to scaffolding.[19,20] Interested readers are advised to review a classic publication by Lanza et al.[21]

Back- and neck-related issues led to 86 billion dollars in health care expenses in the United States from 1997 to 2006.[22] In the same decade, an increase of nearly 50% was found in the number of patients seeking spine-related healthcare expenditure.[22,23] In parallel, a 65% increase in health care expenditure in general was measured. Numerous types of surgical procedures are performed on the spine to prevent further deterioration of spinal components or escalation of pain, and various devices are being conceived, designed, tested, and implanted to aid in these treatments. Most of this instrumentation—for example, interlaminar hooks, transpedicular screws, interbody spacers, and cages—is relevant to spinal fusion.[24] The goal of such instrumentation is to fuse two or more vertebrae together to eliminate pain and allow the patient to return to normal activities. Alternatives to fusion include the hydrogel-based prosthetic nucleus, the liquid polymer-based nucleus, motion preservation devices, and artificial discs.[24]

As shown in Figure 21-1, almost everything that is done in biomechanical testing flows from an existing spinal disorder and the perspective of the individual researcher. We do not claim that this algorithm is comprehensive, a case in point being the regulatory part of the process. Other variables include the types of perspectives (e.g., material science), concepts, and tests. Based on his or her perspective and the clinical objective, a researcher may come up with a concept of a solution, for example, a tissue-engineered nucleus for a damaged intervertebral disc. This concept is tested, proving or disproving a predefined hypothesis. The nature of the specific test may be purely mechanical, biomechanical, or based on biocompatibility. In the case of an engineered nucleus, for example, a test could be any of these (except in vivo, which is rare).[20] For the nucleus, such a test could involve measurement of motion after surgical implantation in a cadaveric spine model or, perhaps, a purely mechanical study assessing its compressive modulus (i.e., a bench-type test). On the other hand, if the clinical objective is being met from a mechanical perspective, resulting in a mechanical device, the range of tests would include pure mechanical tests such as fatigue and wear tests. Determination of the chemical composition following corrosion and wear testing complements these mechanical tests. At some stage, testing using animal spine models, cadaveric spines, analogue spines, or computer simulations (i.e., in silico), and, eventually, clinical trials on human subjects, will follow.

Although all types of testing modalities are important in the process of concept evaluation and assessment as shown in the algorithm, this chapter focuses on three: bench type; in vitro, or, more appropriately cadaveric; and in silico testing of devices and engineered tissues under the overarching term of *biomechanical testing*. Moreover, we differentiate between construct testing and implant testing. The terminology, testing procedures, apparatuses, and protocols that have evolved over the years in testing of spinal implants also are reviewed. We also speculate regarding future prospects for

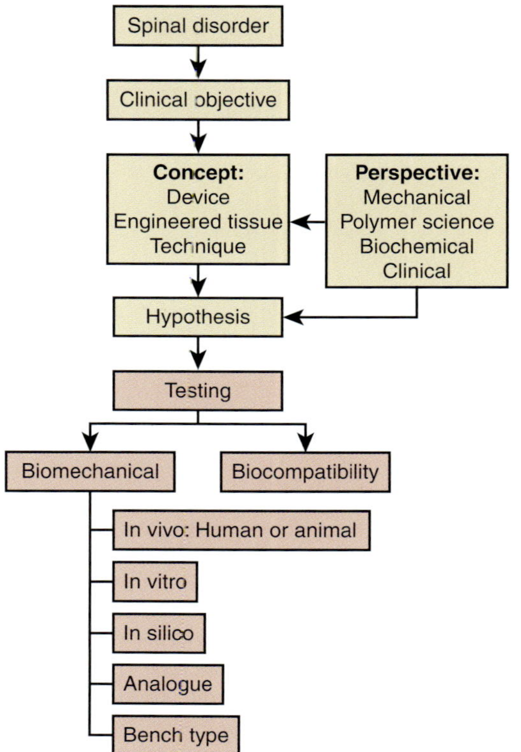

FIGURE 21-1. A testing algorithm for spinal implants.

biomechanical devices and note the areas that may need more attention from the spine biomechanics community.

Bench-Type Tests for Approval by the U.S. Food and Drug Administration

To evaluate the endurance and strength of orthopaedic implants, various mechanical and materials testing protocols have been proposed by ASTM International (formerly known as the American Society for Testing and Materials) as standards for testing of such devices under different dynamic and static loading profiles (Table 21-1). These protocols allow researchers to estimate the static strength and fatigue limits of an implant assembly and its individual components in a consistent way, thereby enabling a fair comparison of results. Guidelines also are proposed by ASTM and the International Organization for Standardization (ISO) for evaluation of fixation of the parts and loosening effect at the interface of implant components.

Data from these standardized tests are used by the medical device industry to seek approval for commercial distribution of devices from the U.S. Food and Drug Administration (FDA). Medical devices are categorized by the FDA in classes—class I, class II, and class III—based on the degree of regulatory control. Most class II devices, such as the pedicle screw–based instrumentation systems, require submission of a Premarket Notification 510(k), whereas class III devices—devices that pose a significant risk of illness or injury—require premarket approval (PMA; Fig. 21-2). Motion preservation systems, for instance, are categorized as class III devices. The test protocols listed in Table 21-1 pertain to class II devices. Class III devices also may be assessed using these protocols, but approval for commercial distribution of such devices requires submission of clinical data in support of the manufacturers' claims.

Similar tests sometimes are carried out on ligamentous motion segments. These tests include subsidence tests, pull-out[25] or push-out testing of pedicle screw systems[26] and cages, respectively, and fatigue tests. Subsidence is a phenomenon in which one or both vertebral end plates adjacent to the implant collapse and allow the implant to move in, increasing the probability of deformity progression and worsening of the fusion.[27] Static, quasi-static, or dynamic tests such as pull-out tests also are performed on pedicle screws to measure bone-implant interfascial strength under such forces. New ASTM guidelines are available for the assessment of facet replacement technologies, wear characterization, and motion preservation systems such as artificial discs.

Wear testing is carried out on a wear simulator (Fig. 21-3). One such simulator (MTS Bionix, MTS Systems Corp., Eden Prairie, MN) consists of six active stations (test stations) and one control station.[28]

Polymeric components in a disc replacement device are soaked in a bath for a week before the test. These are then cleaned and dried in accordance with ASTM F2423-05 (see Table 21-1). Flexion-extension, lateral bending, and rotations are simulated under a constant preload as per ASTM standards. Mass measurements are performed both before and after testing to assess the wear rate. Particulate characterization and element contributions are evaluated using computer-controlled scanning electron microscopy.

Analysis

Conversion of three-dimensional (3D) marker placement data is carried out to evaluate the Cardan or the Euler angles. To determine the motion of the specimen, the data are entered onto the global coordinate system. Relative motion of a component of the construct also may be determined with respect to a static fixture, for example, the mounting platform. Appropriate statistical analysis is performed to assess the impact of a surgical procedure. In most cases, a two-tailed *t* test, a Tukey test, or a one-way analysis of variance (ANOVA) turns out to be sufficient.

Some of the terminology and parameters associated with the analysis of load-displacement data from a typical in vitro test are as follows:

Elastic zone: The amount of total deformation that offers resistance to the applied load. It is measured by evaluating the tangent to the curve at the load that causes maximum deformation (Fig. 21-4; points 5 and 6).

Elastic zone stiffness: This is the stiffness that characterizes the amount of elastic (or recoverable) deformation of the specimen.

Energy dissipation: To characterize the viscoelasticity or plasticity of the specimen being loaded, the area enclosed by the load-displacement curve is evaluated. This quantity provides a measure of the dissipated energy.

Neutral zone: The amount of unrecovered deformation once the specimen is under no load. In cycle 3 shown in Figure 21-4, NZ is the neutral zone. It also may be defined as the part of the range of motion wherein the specimen offers the least resistance to the applied deformation.

TABLE 21-1

ASTM and ISO Standards for Device Evaluation*

Standard or Guide	Status	Focus	Use
ASTM F1798–08: Standard Guide for Evaluating the Static and Fatigue Properties of Interconnection Mechanisms and Subassemblies Used in Spinal Arthrodesis Implants	Reapproved 2008	Fusion devices	Procedures for measuring the uniaxial static and fatigue strength, and resistance to loosening of components used as interconnecting mechanisms of spinal fusion implants
ASTM F2706–08: Standard Test Methods for Occipital-Cervical and Occipital-Cervical-Thoracic Spinal Implant Constructs in a Vertebrectomy Model	Approved 2008	Fusion devices	Methods for static and fatigue testing of occipital-cervical and occipital-cervical-thoracic spinal implants and assemblies in a vertebrectomy model
ASTM F2193–07: Standard Specifications and Test Methods for Components Used in the Surgical Fixation of the Spinal Skeletal System	Reapproved 2007	Fusion devices	Methods for static and fatigue testing of components of devices used in fixation
ASTM F1717–11: Standard Test Methods for Spinal Implant Constructs in a Vertebrectomy Model	Reapproved 2011	Fusion devices	Methods for static and fatigue testing of constructs with focus on the assessment of short-term stability while fusion takes place
ASTM F2077–11: Test Methods for Intervertebral Body Fusion Devices	Approved 2011	Fusion devices	Guidelines for static strength and fatigue testing of interbody devices under axial compression, compressive shear, and torsion
ASTM F2267–04: Standard Test Method for Measuring Load-Induced Subsidence of an Intervertebral Body Fusion Device under Static Axial Compression	Approved 2004	Fusion devices	Testing methods for axial compressive subsidence of nonbiologic fusion devices and implants designed to promote arthrodesis at a given spinal level in a motion segment
ASTM F2790–10: Standard Practice for Static and Dynamic Characterization of Motion-Preserving Lumbar Total Facet Prostheses	Approved 2010	Total facet prostheses	Guidelines for the static and dynamic testing of lumbar total facet prostheses
ASTM F2694–07: Standard Practice for Functional and Wear Evaluation of Motion-Preserving Lumbar Total Facet Prostheses	Approved 2007	Motion-preserving implants	Guidelines for the functional, kinematic, and wear testing of motion-preserving total facet prostheses for the lumbar spine
ASTM F2624–07: Standard Test Method for Static, Dynamic, and Wear Assessment of Extra-Discal Spinal Motion-Preserving Implants	Approved 2007	Motion-preserving implants	Testing guidelines for the static, dynamic, and wear testing of extra-discal motion-preserving implants
ASTM F2423–11: Standard Guide for Functional, Kinematic, and Wear Assessment of Total Disc Prostheses	Approved 2011	Artificial discs	Testing methods for the assessment of wear or functional characteristics, or both, for total disc prostheses (lumbar and cervical)
ASTM F2346–05: Standard Test Methods for Static and Dynamic Characterization of Spinal Artificial Discs	Approved 2005	Artificial discs	Testing methods for static and dynamic testing of artificial discs under compression, compressive shear, and torsion
ISO 12189:2008: Implants for surgery—Mechanical testing of implantable spinal devices—Fatigue test method for spinal implant assemblies using an anterior support	Approved 2008	Artificial discs	Methods for fatigue testing of spinal implant assemblies (for fusion or motion preservation devices) using an anterior support; provides a framework for evaluating the intrinsic static and dynamic strength of spinal implants
ISO 18192–1:2011: Implants for surgery—Wear of total intervertebral spinal disc prostheses—Part 1: Loading and displacement parameters for wear testing and corresponding environmental conditions for test	Approved 2011	Artificial discs	Test guidelines for relative angular movement between articulating components; specifies the pattern of the applied force, speed, and duration of testing, sample configuration, and testing environment to be used for the wear testing of disc prostheses
ASTM WK33006: New Guide for Impingement Testing of Lumbar Total Disc Prosthesis	Draft	Artificial discs	Procedures for static and dynamic behavior of total disc replacements under worst case loading scenarios that can result in impingement damage
ASTM F2789–10: Standard Guide for Mechanical and Functional Characterization of Nucleus Devices	Approved 2010	Nucleus replacements	Guidelines on the methodology for testing of various forms of nucleus replacement and nucleus augmentation devices
ASTM F1582–03: Standard Terminology Relating to Spinal Implants	Reapproved 2003	General spinal device testing	Basic terms and considerations for spinal implant devices and their mechanical analyses

ASTM, American Society for Testing and Materials; ISO, International Organization for Standardization.
*Some of these are currently approved and others are under revision.
More data available at ASTM at www.astm.org/Standards.

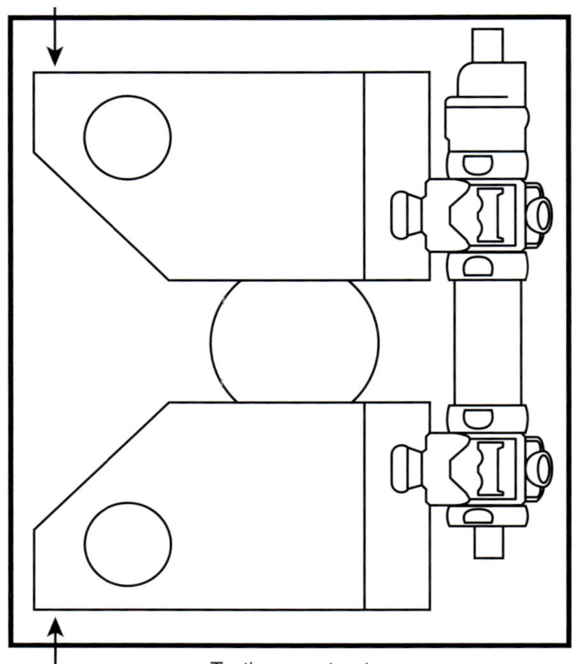

FIGURE 21-2. A schematic view of a typical motion preservation system undergoing hybrid testing for premarket approval (PMA). To the right of the figure, a motion preservation system can be seen. The arrows show the direction of applied force.

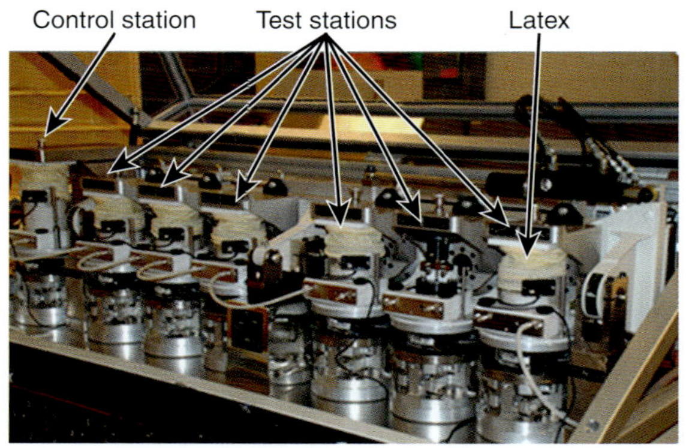

FIGURE 21-3. MTS spine wear simulator (MTS, Eden Prairie, MN). Test stations have 6 degrees of freedom, whereas the control station is under compressive load only. (Adapted from Bhattacharya S, Nayak A, Goel VK, et al: Gravimetric wear analysis and particulate characterization of a dynamic posterior system, PercuDyn™. Presented at the 55th Annual Meeting of the Orthopaedic Research Society, February 22–24, 2009, Las Vegas, NV, Orthopaedic Research Society, Rosemont, IL.)

Neutral zone stiffness: The stiffness of the specimen in the neutral zone, determined by the slope of the load-displacement curve at the point of no deformation

Preconditioning: Cycles of load applied to the specimen—intact or otherwise—to mitigate the impact of the viscoelastic nature of the tissues. From Figure 21-4, cycles 1 and 2 are the preconditioning cycles.

Range of motion (ROM): The linear or the angular distance that a specimen (intact or injured or construct) travels in a plane with the application of load in that plane. From the load-displacement curve of Figure 21-4 the ROM can be calculated as (+ROM) − (−ROM).

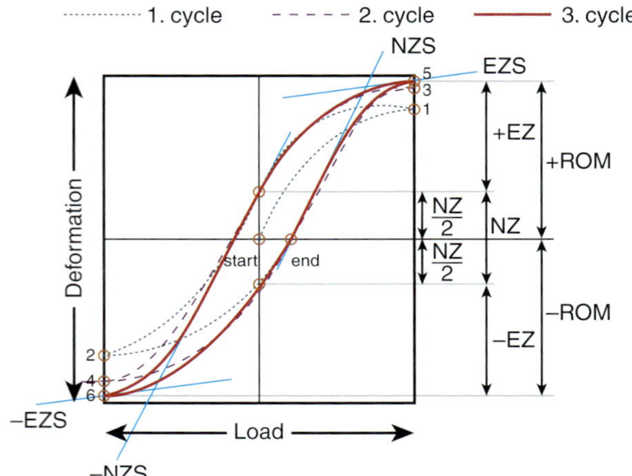

FIGURE 21-4. As the load is applied, deformation of a specimen follows a typical curve that reveals hysteresis. The unloading part of the curve does not retrace the loading part of the curve. EZ, elastic zone; EZS, EZ stiffness; NZ, neutral zone; NZS, NZ stiffness; ROM, range of motion. (Adapted from Wilke HJ, Wenger K, Claes L: Testing criteria for spinal implants: recommendations for the standardization of in vitro stability testing of spinal implants. *Eur Spine J* 7:148–154, 1998.)

Relative range of motion (RROM): The relative motion for the entire spine or a segment or even a vertebral body with respect to the static mounting platform

Sigmoidity: A measure of the non-linearity present in the mechanical behavior of the specimen,[29] calculated as the ratio of the neutral zone stiffness and elastic zone stiffness.

Stiffness: The mechanical resistance of a specimen to an applied load, measured by the slope of the load-deformation or load-displacement curve along a linear region or regions in a nonlinear curve.

In Vitro Testing

The human spine is a complex structure composed of hard and soft, active and passive tissue. This structure has multiple degrees of freedom at each one of several joints formed by intervertebral discs. Ideally, from a biomechanical and biochemical point of view, the most physiologically relevant model for testing the efficacy of a device, surgical technique, or engineered tissue is the human spine of a live subject. However, this is not a practical option. In vitro testing offers significant advantages, even though factors such as intra-abdominal pressure and muscular forces are hard to replicate.[13] In vitro studies have the advantages of the possibility of standardization, ease of estimation of the impact of a surgical procedure, or a simulated injury or stabilization using an implant, because the loads can be varied with relative ease. Such protocols enable researchers to compare different devices designed and developed for the same clinical requirement. Once the device components have been tested using protocols cited in Table 21-1, in vitro testing brings their performance evaluation closer to in vivo use in patients.

Terminology

Some of the terms most commonly used in in vitro studies are defined in this section.

Anatomic planes: To make it possible to specify the locations and angular configurations of the vertebrae, a coordinate system is defined that has three mutually orthogonal planes: the sagittal plane (side view), the frontal or coronal plane (front view), and the transverse plane (top view). Figure 21-5 shows the three anatomic planes along with the terminology for forward/backward, left/right, and up/down directions.[30]

Center of rotation (COR) or instantaneous axis of rotation (IAR): In a general planar motion, the axis of rotation may move. If this movement is broken down into steps, the *instantaneous* axis of rotation can be identified at every step of the motion. Such an axis may pass through the rigid body (in the case of a spinning top) or lie outside it (in the case of the flexion or extension of a spinal segment). To specify the IAR completely, one must provide three numbers: two for translations and one for rotation or any combination of these parameters. The IAR is specified only for plane motion, not for 3D motion—that is, there is no IAR for lateral bending or axial rotation because these involve 3D motion, whereas flexion and extension are considered planar motions for all practical purposes.[31] However, there is evidence that relatively small coupled motions are present even in flexion and extension.[32]

Coordinate system: An orthogonal, right-handed, 3D reference system that makes it possible to define the position and motion of vertebral bodies. In Figure 21-6, the *x*, *y*, and *z* axes represent the three orthogonal directions with the origin of the coordinate system located at the base.[29] The positive *x*-axis represents the left lateral direction, whereas the positive *y*-axis represents the rostral direction and the positive *z*-axis represents the ventral (anterior) direction. Such a system is known as a *global coordinate system*.

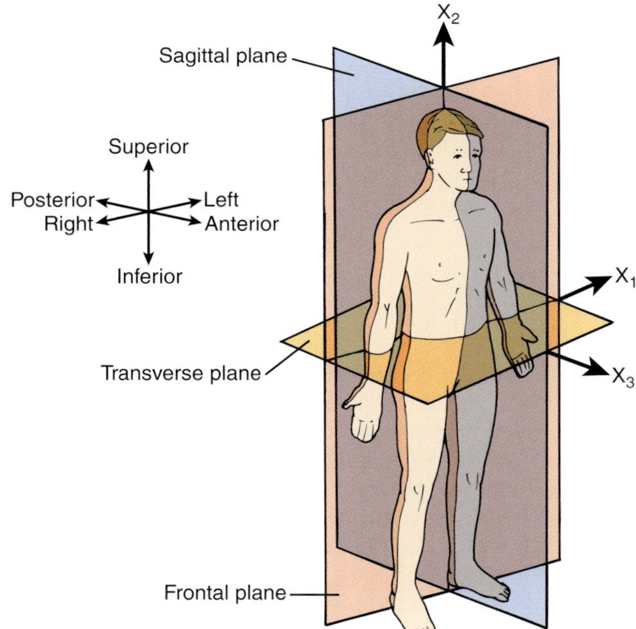

FIGURE 21-5. Primary anatomic planes for the human body. The sagittal plane is the side view, the frontal plane is the view from the front, and the transverse plane is the view from the top. The frontal plane is also known as the coronal plane. x_1, x_2, and x_3 are also referred to as x, y, and z coordinates. (Adapted from Tozeren A: *Human body dynamics: classical mechanics and human movement.* New York, 2000, Springer-Verlag.)

A reference system can be local, however, in the sense that it allows for the position and motion of rigid bodies to be defined with respect to each other. Wilke et al.[29] suggest, for most cases, "the mid-point in the frontal plane of the dorsal (posterior) margins of the two adjacent" vertebral endplates as the origin of the local coordinate system.

Degrees of freedom: The number of independent coordinates necessary for complete specification of the position of a particle or a rigid body in space. Under an applied load, a rigid body may move, in total, in six directions: that is, it has 6 degrees of freedom: three translational and three rotational. In comparison, a particle can have only 3 translational degrees of freedom. A general motion by the vertebra may be broken down into six components of these pure motions.

Envelope of the helical axis of motion: The surface generated by various helical axes of motion of a moving rigid body.

Follower load: A compressive load applied to the spinal segment (through strategic points on each vertebral body) that aims at minimizing the coupled flexion-extension changes in motion and shear force in the disc by following the COR of each functional spinal unit of a specimen.[33] In cadaveric experiments, a compressive follower load is applied to the specimen to mimic the upper body weight and muscle force application on the lumbar spine. The application of follower load works well only in flexion and extension.[31] Bilateral cables are used to apply this load.

Functional spinal unit (FSU) or motion segment: The macrostructural unit of the spine, representing the broad mechanical behavior of two adjacent vertebrae, ligaments, the intervening intervertebral disc, and zygapophyseal (or facet) joints. Studying the biomechanics of an FSU is convenient and relatively straightforward. Figure 21-7 shows with an FSU with an intact intervertebral disc.

Helical axis of motion (HAM) or screw axis motion: As an alternative to *x*, *y*, and *z* coordinates and Euler angles, motion of a rigid body can be decomposed into a translation and rotation about the axis of translation. This axis is known as the *screw axis* or *helical axis* of motion. It can be visualized by observing the motion of a screw being driven into a pedicle of a vertebra. As the screw is being tightened,

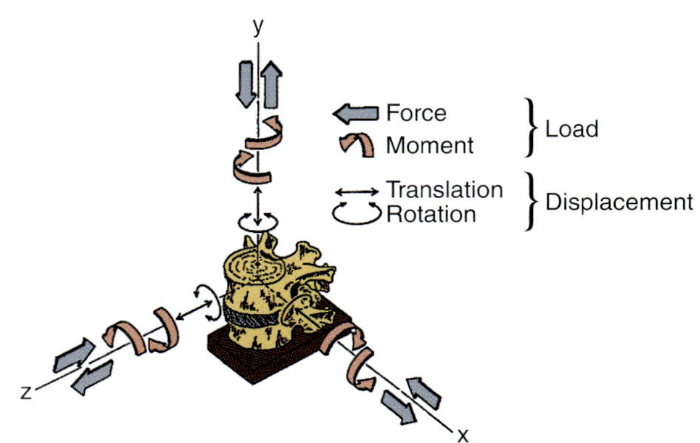

FIGURE 21-6. A functional spinal unit in a three-dimensional coordinate system. Forces and moments are shown by straight and curved arrows, respectively. (Adapted from Goel VK, Panjabi MM, editors: *Roundtables in spine surgery. Spine biomechanics: evaluation of motion preservation devices and relevant terminology,* Vol 1, St. Louis, MO, 2005, Quality Medical Publishing.)

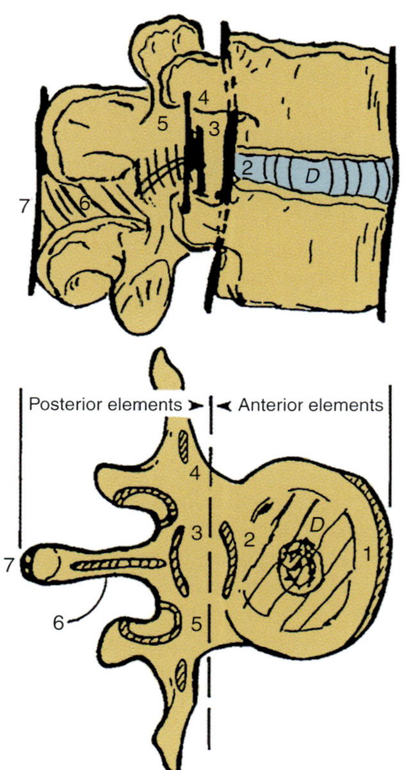

FIGURE 21-7. A functional spinal unit shown with ligaments: (1) anterior longitudinal; (2) posterior longitudinal; (3) ligamentum flavum; (4) transverse; (5) capsular; (6) interspinous; and (7) intraspinous. *D* represents the intervertebral disc. The center line separates the anterior ligaments from the posterior ligaments. (Adapted from Goel VK, Weinstein JN, editors: *Biomechanics of the spine: clinical and surgical perspective.* Boca Raton, FL, 1990, CRC Press.)

it not only rotates but also translates into the pedicle along an axis running through the screw. Consistent with the 6 degrees of freedom for a freely moving rigid body in the 3D coordinate system, six scalar quantities are required to define 3D motion using HAM: two for the orientation of the axis, two for its position, one for the amount of rotation about the axis, and one for the amount of translation along the axis. The helical axis of motion, although difficult to visualize, particularly for clinicians, may provide quality of motion when compared with an end-point parameter such as range of motion (ROM), which determines simply the quantity of motion. For example, it recently was found that axial rotation causes the helical axes to migrate dorsally, correlating well with high facet joint forces.[34]

Injured specimen: A spine specimen with existing or simulated clinical pathoanatomy in terms of injury of ligaments, disc(s), and/or bony tissue

Instability: From a purely mechanical perspective, instability of a specimen undergoing in vitro testing may be characterized by a significant change in the range of motion relative to the intact specimen, for example, 3.5 mm of translation will make a specimen unstable.[35] Instability may be related to spinal degeneration and pain.

Intact spine specimen: A portion of the fresh-frozen cadaveric spine consisting of one or more contiguous functional spinal units with intact ligaments and disc(s). Fascia, muscles, and fatty tissues are dissected.

Muscle force simulator (MFS) or replicator (MFR): A system that simulates muscle forces on a spinal motion segment. Unfortunately, this experimental setup was found to be so arduous that repeating similar experiments became unrealistic.[36,37]

Plane motion: Motion characterized by translation(s) and/or rotation(s) in a single plane. For instance, flexing the vertebra (or, in other words, forward bending) is a plane motion occurring in the sagittal plane. In Figure 21-6, flexion will be fully specified in the y-z plane. Flexion of the vertebral body at the top will involve not only rotation but also translation. Furthermore, there may be some varying degree of out-of-plane motion as well.[38]

Primary and coupled motion: In terms of plane motion, the motion occurring in the same direction as the one in which the load is applied is known as *primary motion*. The out-of-plane motion is known as *coupled motion*.

Primary loading directions: In most cases, spinal motion segments are tested in the following directions: flexion-extension, left-right bending, and left-right axial rotation. Pure moments are applied in one of these directions, and motion is measured. In a complex system such as a spine, application of a pure moment results in six motions. So, in an experiment that involves applying 6 pure moments on a segment, 36 load-displacement curves exist. A specimen may be loaded in a number of ways, which may be understood in terms of their orthogonal constituents or components in a global coordinate system. Reaction loads, for example, can be understood as being composed of three forces and three moments acting at a point of interest, such as the base of the specimen shown in Figure 21-6.

Relative motion: The motion of a rigid body with respect to another rigid body, for example, the motion of a vertebral body with respect to an adjacent vertebral body. However, the motion of a vertebral body *relative* to the static floor is absolute (or global) motion.

Rigid body: A system of particles in which the distance between any two particles remains unchanged regardless of external loads (forces or moments) applied. In other words, a rigid body does not deform. A rigid body is an idealization of a solid body of finite dimensions for the purpose of analysis. In construct testing, vertebrae are considered as rigid bodies.

Rotation: The vertebra in Figure 21-6 can rotate about three orthogonal axes in a clockwise (positive) or counter-clockwise (negative) direction. Curved arrows in Figure 21-6 show these degrees of freedom. In a 3D global coordinate system, Euler or Cardan angles specify the rotation of a rigid body.

Spinal construct: A portion of the spine instrumented with an implant or several implants of interest. Its characteristic motion is different from that of the intact spine. Figure 21-8 shows a spinal construct prepared for testing. The vertebra at the bottom is embedded in a polyester resin or low-melting-point alloy of choice for attachment to the test fixture, and a loading frame is rigidly secured to the superior-most vertebra for the application of loads.

Spine loading simulator: An apparatus to hold spine specimens and test them under different loading scenarios. Several research groups have come up with various designs of a loading simulator, ranging from fully automated to a system of pulleys and dead weights, for manual application of loads.

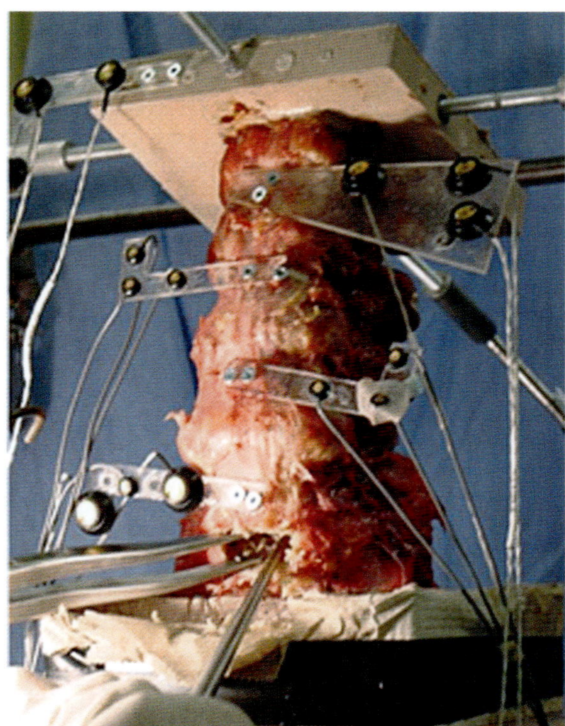

FIGURE 21-8. A spinal construct mounted on a base ready for testing.

Three-dimensional motion: The type of motion seen in a rigid body in a global coordinate system that is free to translate or rotate in one or more of its six degrees of freedom

Translation: As shown in Figure 21-6, a vertebra can translate along three axes, that is, positive or negative x, y, and z axes. These are shown by straight arrows.

Specimen Selection

Species

Several functional animal models have been evaluated for testing the efficacy of spinal implants.[29,39] Calf, sheep, and baboon spines have been used previously. It has been found that larger primates such as baboons are needed for simulating the load, although calf and sheep spines may be valid for range of motion studies. Animal models have several limitations, including appropriate shaping and sizing of implants for the animal tissue, comparable human surgical technique, and differences in the functional anatomy and motions between the human and the animal spine.

Human cadaveric spine models have their own set of limitations. The spine specimens tend to be from elderly individuals who may have suffered some sort of degeneration of the bone (e.g., osteoporosis) or disc (e.g., stenosis) or the spine itself (e.g., spondylolisthesis). Specimens in which such degeneration is apparent are excluded.[29]

Classification

Documentation of the species, age, race, height, weight, gender, cause of death and any pathoanatomy is beneficial in making reasonable conclusions from the data. Bone mineral density is obtained using a dual-energy x-ray absorptiometry (DEXA) scan. Moreover, radiographs and CT scans help with the assessment of spinal degeneration and other anomalies.

Sample Size

Goel and Weinstein[40] suggest using 6 to 10 specimens, whereas Wilke et al.[29] suggest using at least 6 specimens. It is not clear whether they performed a priori or post hoc power analyses.

Number of Segments

At least two FSUs must be included in any given in vitro study.[40]

Sequence

Due to the inherent variability among specimens, the same specimen sometimes is used for comparison among different devices.[41] Usually, the intact state of the FSU is tested first, followed by the injured state and then by the stabilized state.

Testing Environment

Two key factors that may influence the mechanical performance of the construct are temperature and humidity, which is maintained by constant spraying of an appropriate solution, either manually at regular intervals or in an automated fashion using a peristaltic pump. Most experiments are carried out at room temperature. It is known that body temperature causes a slight expansion in ligaments, whereas discs and tendons creep at a higher rate.[42] Evidence for changes in the extensibility and fatigue life of bone also exists.[42] Wilke et al. showed that moisture plays a significant role[43] and recommended intermittent spraying of specimens with 0.9% saline.[29]

Specimen Handling and Preparation

Safety

Proper biohazard safety precautions must be taken before handling biologic tissues. It is common practice for individuals who prepare spinal specimens for testing to wear full protective surgical gear, consisting of a surgical gown, gloves (double), head scarf, face mask, goggles, and shoe covers. Proper procedures are kept in place as for medical emergencies. Furthermore, for ethical reasons, no noticeably identifiable major tissues are discarded in the biohazard bins; such tissues are cremated.

Storage

Musculature is removed from fresh cadaveric specimens as quickly as possible using typical surgical tools. Care is taken to prevent any damage to ligaments and bony structures. Next, the specimens are sealed in double or triple plastic bags and then frozen at −20°C to −30°C. Specimens may be frozen after being wrapped with saline-soaked gauze.

Preparation

Before testing a spinal segment, a specimen is thawed at room temperature for several hours. Preparation may involve casting in resin, attachment of light-emitting diode (LED) marker plates for motion measurement, surgical insertion of implants, guides for follower load cables, and insertion of transducers for facet joint load or disc pressure measurement.[44] A surgical procedure is simulated to represent a clinical scenario as closely as possible. Such procedures may be necessary to imitate a pathologic state. For instance, a vertebral compression fracture may be simulated as a wedge-shaped excision.[45,46]

Testing Apparatus

Two main components of in vitro spinal construct testing are the spinal loading simulator, which allows the application of loads on the spinal segment, and a motion measurement system, which allows evaluation of the 3D motion of the various rigid bodies that are part of the construct.

Spinal Loading Simulator

The spinal loading simulator allows 6 degrees of motion for a spine segment. Different types of simulators have been designed: pulley- and cable-based,[47-49] orthogonal stepper motor–based,[50,51] robotic arm–based,[52-56] Stewart platforms,[57] and others.[58,59] These systems use different control paradigms: constrained load control, unconstrained load control, and displacement control.[60] More recently, newer simulators have been designed[60-62] to minimize apparatus-related errors. These systems aim at applying pure moments on the spine,[9] because applying forces on the spine results in nonuniform loading of the construct, rendering a direct comparison of results challenging. The literature, however, is not clear regarding the accuracy and precision of each of these systems. There is evidence that the apparatus may induce significant artifacts.[63] Although most researchers acknowledge the lack of standardized protocols, a gold standard still remains elusive.

Motion Measurement System

The motion measurement system allows the measurement of 3D motion of a set of markers. A plate carrying at least three non-collinear markers is screwed into a vertebra to assess the rigid body motion of that vertebra. All six motions—three translations and three rotations—are evaluated, first in a local coordinate system and then in a global coordinate system. This motion measurement system, like the load simulator, may have inherent errors associated with the camera system or the marker configuration.[61] Publishing the accuracies inherent to the various setups (including marker configuration) would be beneficial to the scientific community in general.

Other transducers also provide relevant information.[13] For instance, film force sensors, pressure sensors, accelerometers,[13] buckle transducers, and strain gauges[64] have been used to measure facet joint loads, disc pressure, and vibration in the spine and strain in the instrumentation,[65] respectively.

Testing Methods

Static Strength Testing

Until the early 1980s, spinal constructs were tested destructively. These strength tests involved loading an intact spine until some type of failure occurred (either plastic deformation or fracture).[66] High ultimate strength was considered to correlate with higher stability.[11] Parameters like load-to-failure, work-to-failure (or energy-absorbed-to-failure), and stiffness are determined in this type of test, but these are relevant only to catastrophic failures, which are rare. Fatigue failure of implants (e.g., pedicle screw instrumentation) is more common,[67] leading to the evolution of nondestructive testing of spinal segments under subfailure loads. However, cyclic testing rarely produced any failures of implants in the laboratory[11] because tissue properties change in the time required to carry out such tests.[11] Wilke et al. recommend that the total duration of the test be no more than 20 hours.[29,43]

Stability Testing

Stability (or rigidity) testing involves loading the construct to levels that do not result in an apparent failure of any of the components of the construct. Stiffness of the construct may be measured in terms of Newton per millimeter (N/mm) in force-displacement tests or Newton-meter/degree (N-m/deg)[9] in cases of pure moment application and angular motion. Although instability has been used to define the inverse of stability, we recommend flexibility to determine a motion for an applied load. Flexibility is measured in mm/N or deg/N-m as the case may be. The stiffness protocol and flexibility protocol[68] come under the umbrella term of stability testing, but the stiffness protocol entails application of one component of motion at a time to assess loads applied on the vertebra and other components of the FSU. The flexibility protocol involves applying one component of load at a time to determine intervertebral motions.

Hybrid Testing

A hybrid protocol was propounded by Panjabi[31,69,70] as a part of stability testing in order to measure changes on the adjacent levels due to a surgical procedure. The protocol is a four-step procedure.

Presurgery

An intact segment is prepared for the measurement of parameters of interest, such as ligament strains, facet joint loads, or ROM, in response to applied pure unconstrained moments to the segment.

Postsurgery

Uninhibited pure moments are applied to the construct until the total ROM of the construct is equal to the ROM of the intact spine segment. This protocol allows testing for the assessment of adjacent level effects commonly observed in fusion surgical procedures.[69] The argument used in support of this protocol is that, postsurgery, patients undertake the same day-to-day activities that they would carry out presurgery, thus actualizing the same range of motion.[55]

Load versus Displacement Control

Most cadaveric testing has been performed using load as the control variable, pure moments, in particular, because the magnitude of the bending moment does not vary as a function of the spinal level or even the state of the spine—be it intact, injured, or stabilized.[9,71] However, Edwards et al.[72] favor displacement-controlled testing of spinal segments under combined displacements because in vivo motion can be simulated accurately in the laboratory environment, whereas in vivo loads are unknown. The disadvantage of complex loading patterns in displacement-controlled testing, however, makes this method less straightforward. Also, comparison with simulated injuries and stabilizations is not possible. However, it may be beneficial to perform displacement-controlled testing after collection of basic load-displacement data from load-controlled testing.[71]

Additional Applications of Construct Testing

Although the overall methodology of testing remains the same as described earlier for animal specimens, the magnitude of parameters selected will change. Pre- and postsurgical biomechanical and histomorphometric analyses also have been performed on animal spine specimens ex vivo as a function of time in addition to characterization of biomechanical parameters.[73] Spine specimens also are used to delineate the cyclic[74] and viscoelastic behavior of young and old spines.[75] Individual spinal components also may be tested to determine their characteristics, such as the load-displacement behavior of spinal ligaments or vertebral body strength (intact spine vs. one that has a fractured vertebra vs. one that has undergone surgery like kyphoplasty or vertebroplasty).[40]

Analogue Tissue Testing

Three main areas in which tissue engineering has gained some ground are the repair of nucleus pulposus (tissue-engineered or hydrogel-based), the repair of anulus fibrosus, and optimal scaffolding. Like the previous section on in vitro testing, this section also is discussed from the perspective of mechanical testing.

The three main categories of nucleus replacement devices are hydrogel-based, polymer-based, and mechanical. Several types of mechanical tests usually are carried out on these devices. Pure compression tests are performed to determine the compressive modulus for the device or the "apparent" modulus at a given load. Some studies report stress relaxation data.[16,76] Displacement-controlled fatigue testing also is carried out for several million cycles.[77-79] Disc height changes[80] and typical viscoelastic parameters such as loss tangent, viscous modulus, and elastic modulus also are estimated in these studies.[81] Testing is conducted while keeping the device either radially unconfined or confined in a constant-temperature bath filled with Hanks' balanced salt solution or a phosphate-buffered solution.[16,78] Cadaveric axial compression, extrusion tests, and regular loading in all three anatomic planes also are performed to test the integrity of the device. Failure load and strains are assessed from such tests.[77,79] Although similar tests are carried out on anulus replacement devices, destructive tensile testing also is carried out to judge the tensile strength and elongation of the device.[82]

Scaffolds provide a stable structure for tissue growth. A scaffold is a 3D collagen matrix that allows cells (usually multi- or pluripotent stem cells) to attach, divide, proliferate, migrate, and differentiate into a specific phenotype.[83] Certain growth factors may be necessary for these functions to take place while nutrient supply is maintained.[81] Certain cell types have been found to be capable of detecting the stiffness of the surrounding substrate, and such sensitivity (*mechanosensitivity*) has been shown to affect mesenchymal stem cell differentiation.[20] Chan and Leong[20] stress the importance of understanding the impact of interfascial shear stress. Most tissue engineering work specific to the spine has been directed toward the goal of engineering an intervertebral disc in a laboratory setup. However, the challenge lies in fine-tuning the stiffness of the scaffolding for both the nucleus and the anulus replacement. Some of the key issues that still must be resolved include matching the complex in vivo tissue loading, porosity, nutrient supply, cell supply, viscosity and stiffness, and the state of disc degeneration of the native disc.[14]

In Silico Testing

Background

Computational and numeric methods have long been employed to assess the biomechanical behavior of biologic systems. Continuous development of powerful computing systems, in addition to improvement in the emerging computational packages in computer-aided engineering with enhanced modeling features, has enabled scientists to develop more rigorous models of biologic systems. These models are able to predict the behavior of these systems under different biologic conditions. The latest advances in medical imaging technologies have helped obtain better resolution of geometric and anthropometric specifications of individual organs in the human body. These images have helped to develop high-resolution and microscale computational models of the knee, hip, and spine.

One of the most applicable computational approaches used in biomechanical studies is finite element (FE) modeling. In this analytical technique, the object or system of interest is represented by a geometric model consisting of multiple, linked representations of discrete regions called *elements*. The material properties and governing relationships are assigned to these elements, and appropriate loads and boundary conditions are applied to the model to represent in vitro or in vivo conditions. The FE model is validated against available cadaveric or clinical data (such as those described earlier), and this validated model is used to measure important biomechanical parameters such as load and stress distribution across the various components under different static or dynamic loading patterns. It usually is not practical to determine these parameters experimentally; these experimentally validated models, therefore, complement the cadaver studies. Finite element models of individual spinal components such as the vertebra and disc also can be developed to study their behavior. Bench-type tests also can be simulated using the FE technique to help the designer with the development of the device.

Over the last few decades, FE analysis (FEA) has served well in studying the biomechanics of the spine in different physiologic circumstances such as growth, injuries, trauma, and surgical procedures. In these studies, the FE models of spine segments have predicted changes in biomechanical parameters such as load sharing, stress distribution, and segmental kinematics at sections of interest.

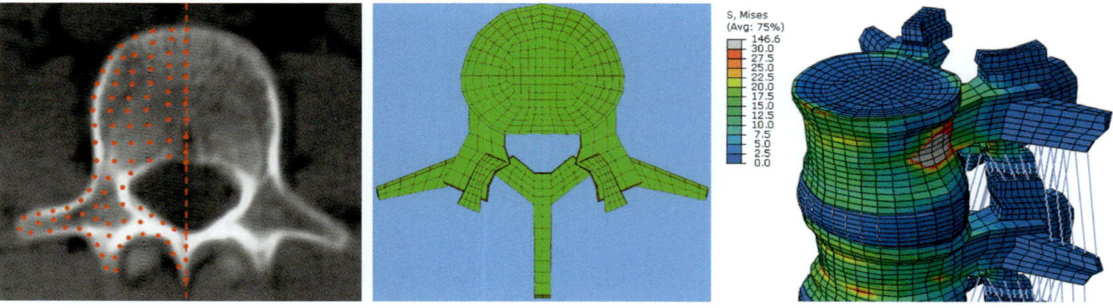

FIGURE 21-9. Steps in the development of a finite element model of a lumbar spine segment using CT scans.

Model Development

FE models can be created in several ways. If a tissue or pathoanatomy is of significance, the current approach is to develop the model based on existing CT or MRI scans of the area. Figure 21-9 shows the steps that were taken to develop an FE model of the L3-S1 lumbar spine segment.[84] First the CT and/or MRI scans of the subject's lumbar spine were acquired. Transverse scans, usually taken at 1-mm intervals, were used to develop the geometry. A node grid was superimposed over each transverse image with appropriate node density to represent a precise geometry of the cross-section, specifically at the outer boundaries and interfaces. The grids were assembled to create a cloud of nodes that represented the 3D geometry of the entire section. Next, the nodes of each of the two adjacent sections were interconnected using 3D hexagonal (brick) elements to develop a solid structure. Facet joints were simulated using GAPUNI contact elements available in ABAQUS (Simulia, Providence, RI). Rebar elements were used to mimic the anulus fibrosus component of intervertebral discs. Finally, the ligaments were simulated by 3D truss elements. After development of the geometry, an appropriate material property was assigned to each group of elements, representing associated structures in the spine such as vertebral bodies, capsular joints, intervertebral discs, and ligaments.[84,85]

The kinematics of this FE model was validated by comparing its segmental rotations with data obtained from an in vitro experiment under similar loading and boundary conditions. Other parameters such as center of rotation and intradiscal pressure (IDP) also were compared for further validation of the model.[86] This validated FE model was used in several biomechanical studies for investigation of biomechanical changes in the spine (e.g., load distribution, kinematics, stresses, and strains) after simulation of surgical and implanted cases.[84,87,88] Figure 21-10 shows FE models of C3-7 and L3-S1 spine segments that were developed using this technique.

To make the predictions of a spine FE model relevant, the following considerations must be taken into account while developing the model:

- It is not practical to obtain a model with geometry that thoroughly matches that of the real spine, but the geometric model must be as close to the actual geometry as possible, specifically at the locations where the geometry may have a significant impact on biomechanical outputs. Contact definition, intervertebral discs, and angle of the articular facet joints are examples.
- Cancellous and cortical regions of the bone should be designated with appropriate thickness and material properties across the vertebrae.
- Each aspect of the model must be assigned a proper element type. For example, bony regions and discs usually are assigned hexagonal or tetragonal elements, whereas for ligaments, 3D truss or beam elements connecting two aspects of the model are suggested. Ligaments can be modeled as a bundle with appropriate cross-sections for each fiber. A no-compression behavior should be assigned to each such fiber to ensure that only tensile loads are allowed.
- The intervertebral disc should be modeled as a nonhomogenous composite structure including an amorphous matrix reinforced by collagenous fibers. Proper element types should be used for each area of the disc.

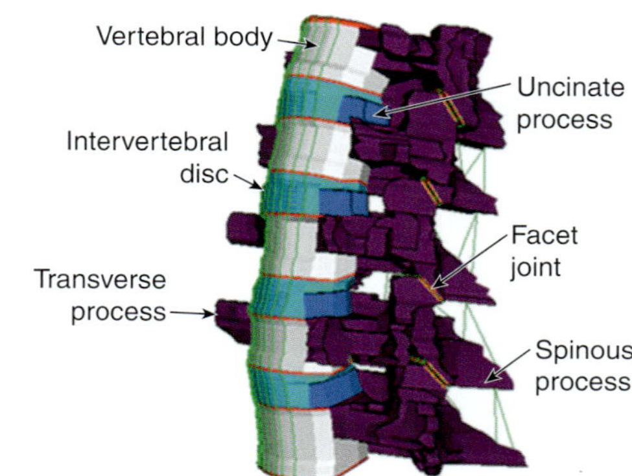

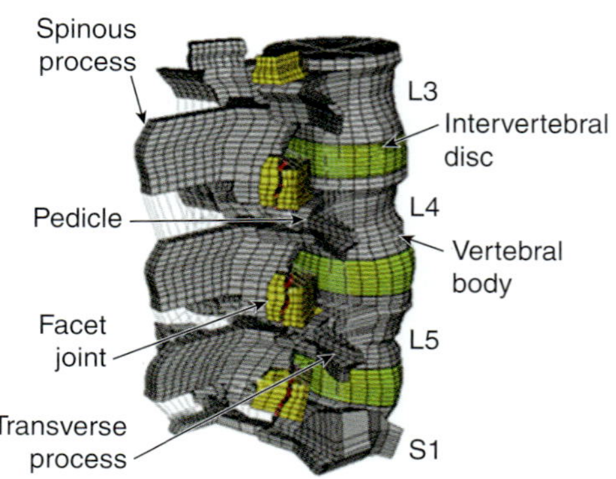

FIGURE 21-10. Finite element model of C3-7 (*top*) and L3-S1 (*bottom*) spine segments. The models have the main physiologic features of the real spine, including bony structure, capsular joints, discs, and ligaments. (Adapted from Sasa T, Yoshizumi Y, Imada K, et al: Cervical spondylolysis in a judo player: a case report and biomechanical analysis. *Arch Orthop Trauma Surg* 129[4]:559–567, 2009; and Pearcy MJ, Bogduk N: Instantaneous axes of rotation of the lumbar intervertebral joints. *Spine [Phila Pa 1976]* 13[9]:1033–1041, 1998.)

For example, the nucleus can be modeled with noncompressible fluid elements. On the other hand, the anulus may be modeled with solid, elastic elements that are assigned mechanical properties and volume fraction. These elements, at appropriate angles, represent the radial variation of the collagenous fibers. It may be necessary to change element types to model a degenerated disc.

- A proper contact profile assignment is required at the articulating surfaces of the facet joints.
- In case a nonstatic simulation, such as dynamic loading, impact, long-term creep, or wear, is of interest, the time-dependent behavior of elements, materials, contact profile, and boundary conditions must be input into the model prior to any simulation run.
- The loads and boundary conditions also must be defined correctly. For example, to simulate physiologic loading such as flexion-extension, left-right bending, and left-right axial rotation, the most caudal section of the model (e.g., S1) should be fixed in all degrees of freedom, and pure bending moments should be applied to the most cephalad vertebra (e.g., L3). To simulate the upper body weight, a follower load may be applied to the spine using actuator-type connector elements. These elements can be activated through each loading step to apply any compressive force across segments.[49,86]

In Silico Study

Figure 21-11 shows the FE spine that was modified to simulate the implantation of a novel 360-degree motion preservation system at the L4-5 segment.[88,89] FEA was performed to investigate whether this motion preservation system would be able to regenerate the kinematics of the intact spine. The 360-degree system included a pair of posterior dynamic stabilizers (PDS) matched with dorsal discs. The surgical procedure for placement of the implants required removal of the entire nucleus and partial anulus, total bilateral facetectomy, and removal of dorsal longitudinal ligaments. Surgery was simulated by removal of associated elements at each section. After placement of the implants, sliding contacts were

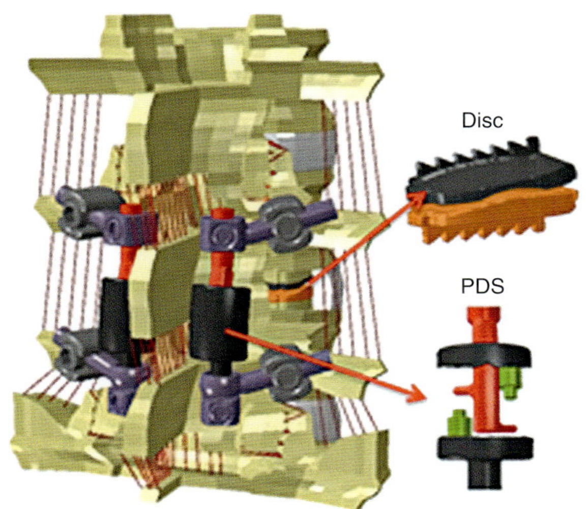

FIGURE 21-11. Finite element model of L3-S1 spine implanted with a posterior dynamic stabilization (PDS) and disc system at L4-5.

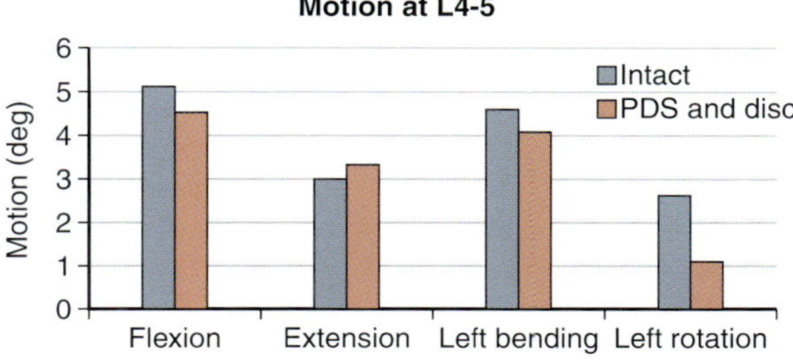

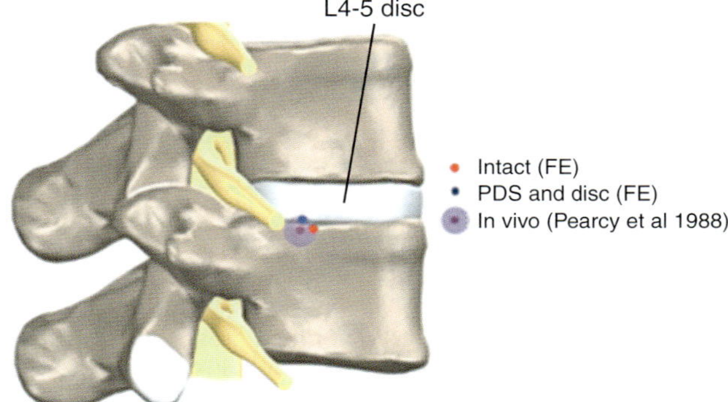

FIGURE 21-12. **Segmental motion and extension-to-flexion center of rotation at index level of finite element (FE) model of the lumbar spine before and after replacement of posterior dynamic stabilization (PDS) and disc system.** (Adapted and modified from Kiapour A, Goel VK: Biomechanics of a novel lumbar total motion segment preservation system: a computational and in vitro study. *BONEZONE* Fall 2009, pp 86–90.)

defined between implant components while rigid fixations were simulated at the interface of bone with pedicle screws and discs. Both intact and implanted models were subjected to the same boundary conditions and loading profiles, including a 10-Nm bending moment plus a 400-N follower load. The kinematic results predicted by the model showed that in most loading conditions (except in axial rotation), the implanted segment had motion close to that of an intact segment (see Fig. 21-11).

The extension-to-flexion center of rotation (COR) remained close to intact after replacement of the 360-degree system, which indicates that the quality of motion also was preserved after implantation (Fig. 21-12). Both CORs were found to be within the in vivo range.

The stress distribution contour and maximum von Mises stress at PDS and disc are shown in Figure 21-13. The maximum stress ranged from 69 MPa to approximately 146 MPa in PDS and 166 to 244 MPa in discs.

Clinical Objective

Decisions on the type and length of specimen, types of tests and protocols, types of statistical analysis, and finite element analysis, among other variables, are made keeping in mind the clinical objective. Some of these decisions may have to be made within the existing standards and requirements of the FDA.[39] In vitro tests may have different clinical objectives. For example, they may be done to (1) perform a comparative study with an existing standard or to evaluate the

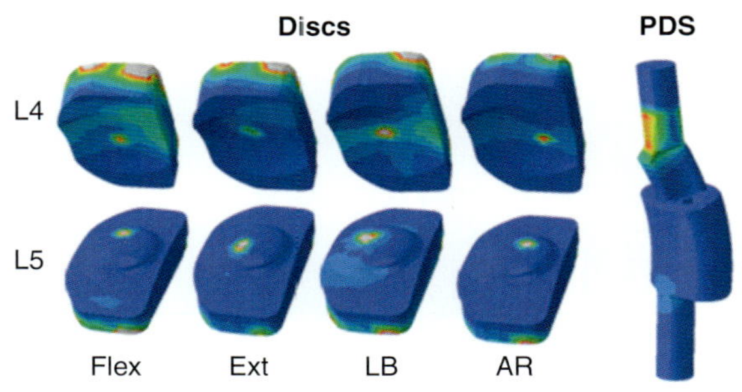

Load: 400 N compression + 10 Nm bending	Maximum von Mises (MPa)	
	PDS	Disc
Flexion	69	166
Extension	78	244
Lateral bending	94.2	260
Axial rotation	145.2	173

FIGURE 21-13. Stress distribution and maximum von Mises stress values at components of posterior motion preservation (disc and PDS) during different loadings. MPa, megapascal; PDS, posterior dynamic stabilization.

performance of a device by measuring relevant parameters, (2) quantify a clinical or surgical procedure using existing or novel parameters using existing or novel protocols relevant to its eventual application, or (3) quantify physiologic data, for example, biocompatibility of a new device, disc height postmortem,[42] and spinal curvature in a given pathology, among several other parameters.[13]

Summary

With emerging standards, rapid progress in the device market, an aging population, and continued growth in the areas of tissue engineering and computational efficiency, testing of spinal implants not only will remain an important step in the path[90] along which a device makes its way to the clinic but also will have a larger role to play. A strong relationship among tissue engineers, clinicians, the finite element analysis community, and mechanical testing experts will be crucial in meeting the challenges of the future. We believe that the spine biomechanics community will benefit greatly by agreeing upon a standard phantom spine made from nondecomposable materials.[61,91-93] Using such a specimen, research groups may document accuracies of their loading methods and measurement systems, making a reasonable comparison of results possible. This approach may also be suitable for the training of students, residents, and fellows.

This chapter has provided an overview of the test protocol–related practices in the area of spine biomechanics. Interested readers may find other reviews of interest, particularly those by Goel et al.,[24,31,39] Wilke et al.,[29] and Panjabi et al.[9,10,32,94] Literature reviews of protocols in the context of specific devices [24,95] also have been published.

Acknowledgment. Thank you to Lars Gilbertson, PhD, for his input regarding the production of this chapter.

KEY REFERENCES

Ashman RB, Birch JG, Bone LB, et al: Mechanical testing of spinal instrumentation. *Clin Orthop Relat Res* 227:113–125, 1988.

Goel VK, Kiapour A, Faizan A, et al: Finite element study of matched paired posterior disc implant and dynamic stabilizer (360° motion preservation system). *SAS J* 1(1):55–62, 2007.

Goel VK, Panjabi MM, editors: *Roundtables in spine surgery. Spine biomechanics: evaluation of motion preservation devices and relevant terminology*, Vol 1, St. Louis, MO, 2005, Quality.

Goel VK, Weinstein JN, editors: *Biomechanics of the spine: clinical and surgical perspective*, Boca Raton, FL, 1990, CRC Press.

Panjabi MM, Oxland TR, Yamamoto I, Crisco JJ: Mechanical behavior of the human lumbar and lumbosacral spine as shown by three-dimensional load-displacement curves, *J Bone Joint Surg [Am]* 76(3):413–424, 1994.

Puttlitz CM, Goel VK, Pope MH: Biomechanical testing sequelae relevant to spinal fusion and instrumentation, *Orthop Clin North Am* 29(4):571–589, 1998.

Wilke HJ, Wenger K, Claes L: Testing criteria for spinal implants: recommendations for the standardization of in vitro stability testing of spinal implants, *Eur Spine J* 7(2):148–154, 1998.

REFERENCES

The complete reference list is available online at expertconsult.com.

CHAPTER 22

Computational Modeling of the Spine

Yunus Alapan | Serkan İnceoğlu | Vijay K. Goel

An anatomic experimental approach has been the gold standard for the biomechanical evaluation of spinal structures. In vitro biomechanical investigations commonly use cadavers, animal carcasses, or synthetic models. Among these options, cadaveric investigations produce the most reliable and realistic results. However, despite its high clinical relevance, fresh-frozen cadaveric spinal specimens may be very expensive (>$1000 in the United States) or difficult to acquire. Animal models such as calves, sheep, and pigs, on the other hand, are relatively inexpensive (~$100). Animal models offer two main advantages. First, bovine, ovine, and porcine spine models exhibit gross anatomic structures (e.g., facets, processes, ligaments) similar to those of the human spine, which permits the convenient application of the instrumentation used in surgery. Secondly, between-subject variability is minimal with animal models, which reduces the statistical sample size demand. Synthetic models usually involve polyurethane foam surrogates, which are available in any density and geometry, ranging from blocks to any anatomic shape. They are quite inexpensive (<$100). In addition, synthetic models can be produced homogeneously, presenting little or no interspecimen or intraspecimen variation. Although synthetic models can represent the human anatomy better than animal models, and have less specimen-related variability, they are considered the least clinically relevant models because they cannot match the material properties of the natural bone.

Some investigators, facing the shortcomings of all of these approaches, turn to computational techniques. With the recent advances in computer and imaging technologies, finite element models of spinal segments or vertebrae can be developed and validated rapidly and inexpensively. Finite element analysis, a mathematical method performed by fictively dividing structures into simpler substructures such as triangles or cubes, can determine the stress or strain response of complex structures under imposed conditions by performing calculations on the simpler substructures. Once the anatomic model is introduced into the finite element analysis software, kinetic and kinematic analyses, as well as thermal, flow, and time-related problems, can be solved.

Computational techniques, especially finite element analysis, have provided substantial help for researchers in the area of musculoskeletal biomechanics for decades. The reduced costs and time (in most cases) and the ability to simulate sophisticated loading conditions and vary certain parameters (such as treatment strategies) in a perfectly controlled analysis environment are the major advantages of finite element analysis. Finite element modeling will become much more pervasive with developments in the hardware and software technology that provide the ability to build complex and comprehensive models that truly reconstruct real-life structures and conditions of the spine.

In this chapter, common finite element modeling procedures (i.e., obtaining three-dimensional [3D] models of spinal segments, determining structural and material properties, and assigning contact, loads, and boundary conditions) and some biomechanical applications are discussed.

Finite Element Models

Even though the finite element method has been applied to structural engineering problems since the 1950s, it was first applied to the biomechanics of the spine in the 1970s.[1,2] With improvements in numerical techniques and computer technology, its use in the field has gained momentum and it has become an integral part of spine biomechanics that is viewed as a complementary and insightful analysis (Fig. 22-1).

Modeling of Spinal Elements

Finite element modeling of spine segments or vertebrae, similar to other engineering solutions, involves the transfer of the physical sample into the 3D reconstructed form in the computer environment, assignment of structural and material properties, definition of contact properties, and application of loads and boundary conditions. Although the finite element modeling procedure is essentially the same in most of the studies, many different techniques and properties are used in these steps.

Three-Dimensional Reconstruction and Structural Modeling

In the finite element method, geometric accuracy of the model has a significant effect on problem solving and can cause marked differences in the results.

Several methods have been commonly used to model spinal units, including touch probe digitizer,[3] laser scanner,[4] CT,[5] and MRI.[6] Even though precise, highly accurate geometric models can be obtained using the touch probe digitizer and laser scanner

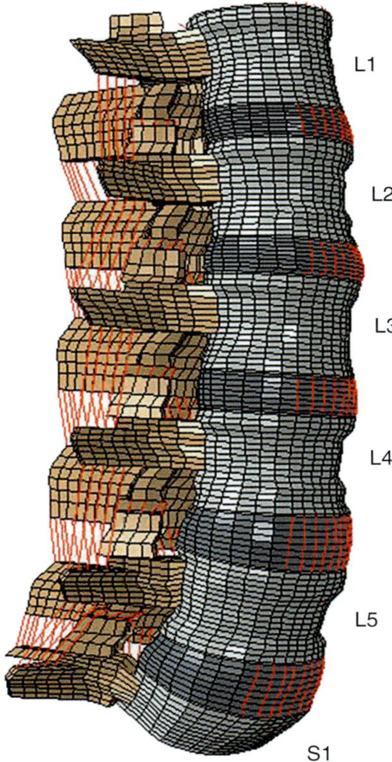

FIGURE 22-1. A typical finite element model of the lumbosacral spine. Material property differences among the spinal elements are depicted by various colors. Ligaments are demonstrated with links (*red*). For the flexibility test simulation, loads typically are applied at the L1 superior end plate while the S1 inferior surface is held steady.

methods, noninvasive techniques such as CT and MRI often are preferred because of their ability to retrieve data on internal features of the specimens—and even from live subjects—with ease. Some techniques also combine some of the methods mentioned earlier for the reconstruction of spinal units.[7]

In thorough finite element models, vertebral bodies usually are modeled in several sections, as cortical shell, cancellous core, dorsal bony elements, bony end plates, and cartilage layers, due to their unique material properties.[5,7,8]

In almost all studies, intervertebral discs are formed by three significant parts: the nucleus pulposus, the anulus fibrosus, and the cartilaginous end plates. The anulus is further divided into subcomponents such as ground substance and anulus fibers. Anulus ground substance is modeled as several layers surrounding the nucleus. The anulus fibers are angled 30 degrees and 150 degrees with respect to the transverse plane in adjacent layers.[9,10] Some studies have used more realistic approaches in the design of these fibers by considering the increase in fiber angle from ventral to dorsal, and also fiber angle variation between anulus layers[5,11] motivated by the histologic findings.[12,13]

After a solid model of the spine is built, each of its components is carefully divided into simpler substructures called "elements" for mathematical calculation purposes. Generally, hard tissues such as cortical shell, trabecular core, and dorsal elements are composed of tetrahedral (pyramid) and pentahedron (wedge) elements.[14,15] With soft tissues, such as the anulus ground substance or cartilage layers, it is necessary to use hexahedral (rectangular prism) elements due to low-elasticity modulus and high Poisson ratio properties. In most studies, bilinear link or spring elements (cables), which are only capable of sustaining tension, are employed for ligaments and anulus fibers.[5, 9-11]

Material Definition

Material definition is one of the most sensitive and intrinsic parts of finite element modeling of the spine. Due to variability within and among test specimens, different researchers have defined many material properties for the different components the spine.

Vertebral Bodies, End Plates, and Facet Cartilages

Even though bone is a poroelastic, anisotropic, and viscoelastic structure, in reality,[16] vertebral cortical shell and cancellous bone usually are considered as linear elastic isotropic or transversely isotropic. Dorsal bony elements most commonly are modeled as linear elastic and isotropic (Tables 22-1 to 22-3). Researchers have either neglected the end plate due to its low elasticity module or modeled it as a composite structure (i.e., bony and cartilaginous layers). End plates most commonly were modeled as linear elastic and isotropic bone with a cartilaginous layer (Table 22-4). Cartilage layers also are added to the facets in most modeling paradigms (Table 22-5).

TABLE 22-1
Material Properties Considered for the Cortical Shell

Model	E [MPa]	v	References
Linear elastic, isotropic	5000–15,000	0.2–0.3	8–10, 13, 20, 22–25, 38, 45, 49–61

E [MPa], Young's modulus; v, Poisson ratio.

TABLE 22-2
Material Properties Considered for the Trabecular Core

Model	E [MPa]	v	G [MPa]	References
Linear elastic, isotropic	100–500	0.2–0.3	41.7	7, 10, 17, 18, 22, 23, 32, 37, 38, 44, 45, 49, 52, 53, 56, 59, 62–64

E [MPa], Young's modulus; G [MPa], shear modulus; v, Poisson ratio.

TABLE 22-3
Material Properties Considered for the Posterior Elements

Model	E [MPa]	v	G [MPa]	References
Linear elastic, isotropic	3000–6000	0.25–0.3	1400	5, 7–10, 14, 17, 18, 20, 22–25, 28, 29, 37, 44, 51, 53, 56, 59, 60, 63, 65–69

E [MPa], Young's modulus; G [MPa], shear modulus; v, Poisson ratio.

TABLE 22-4

Material Properties Considered for the End Plates

Model	E [MPa]	v	References
Bony, linear elastic, isotropic	500–12,000	0.3–0.4	5, 8, 20, 28, 29, 33, 39, 50, 59, 63, 65, 66, 70–72
Cartilaginous, linear elastic, isotropic	23.8–25	0.3–0.4	5, 8, 20, 28, 29, 33, 39, 50, 59, 63, 65, 66, 70–72

E [MPa], Young's modulus; v, Poisson ratio.

TABLE 22-5

Material Properties Considered for the Facet Cartilage Layers

Model	E [MPa]	v	References
Linear elastic, isotropic	0.7–35	0.1–0.4	8, 14, 15, 20, 30, 34, 39, 40, 41, 45, 52, 57, 65, 74

E [MPa], Young's modulus; v, Poisson ratio.

Intervertebral Disc: Anulus Fibrosus and Nucleus Pulposus

The intervertebral disc plays a crucial role in the movement and load-bearing functions of the spinal segments. It probably is the most intricate part of the functional spinal unit (i.e., vertebra-disc-vertebra complex) in finite element modeling, due to the composite structure of the anulus fibrosus and fluid-like behavior of the nucleus pulposus. The anulus fibrosus is formed by a matrix, anulus ground substance, and direction-dependent fibers. Even though there are a few homogeneous models for the anulus fibrosus, more realistic composite models that include matrix and angled fibers have been widely accepted and used (Tables 22-6 to 22-8). Anulus fibers are most commonly modeled with bilinear link, truss, or spring elements, and, in a few cases, with reinforced membrane elements. The material modeling of fibers is almost independent of the modeling technique.

Ligaments

Ligaments are uniaxial structures that do not bear compressive loads. Like the anulus fibers, ligaments are modeled with link, truss, spring, or membrane elements. In general, it is assumed that linear, multilinear, or nonlinear elastic constitutive laws apply for these tissues (Table 22-9).

TABLE 22-6

Material Properties Considered for the Nucleus Pulposus

Model	E [MPa]	v	Other	References
Incompressible fluid	—	—	—	9, 14, 17, 18, 20, 24, 25, 35, 45, 49, 51, 61, 64, 73
Poroelastic	1.5	0.49	Poroelasticity $k_x = k_y = 1.82e\text{-}16$ $k_z = 1.56$ 1e-04 mm^4/Ns	40–42, 74
Fluid-like solid, linear elastic, isotropic	0.2–3.4	0.499	—	7, 8, 10, 17, 22, 23, 32–34, 37, 38, 56, 58, 59, 62, 63, 65, 66
Incompressible, hyperelastic, Mooney-Rivlin	—	0.499	Mooney-Rivlin $c_1 = 0.12$ $c_2 = 0.03–0.09$	5, 28, 29, 50, 70–72

E [MPa], Young's modulus; v, Poisson ratio.

TABLE 22-7

Material Properties Considered for the Anulus Ground Substance

Model	E [MPa]	v	Other		References
Linear elastic, isotropic	3.15–4.2	0.4–0.45	G [MPa] 1.6		8, 10, 17, 18, 23, 32–35, 37, 44, 49, 51, 53, 56, 61, 62, 73, 75
Hyperelastic, neo-Hookean	—	—	Neo-Hookean $c_{10} = 0.3448$ $D_1 = 0.3$		5, 9, 24, 25, 71, 72
Hyperelastic, Mooney-Rivlin	≈=4.2	0.45	Mooney-Rivlin $c_1 = 0.18–0.56$ $c_2 = 0.045–0.14$		5, 28, 29, 38, 70
Poroelastic	Neo-Hookean	—	Neo-Hookean	Poroelasticity	11, 68, 76, 77
Poroelastic	Hyperfoam, nonlinear	—	$c_{10} = 0.25$ MPa	$k_0 = 7.5e\text{-}16\ m^4/Ns$	
Poroelastic	2.56–12.29	0.35	K = 0.67 MPa	$e_0 = 2.3$	
Poroelastic	2.5	0.17		M = 8.5	

E [MPa], Young's modulus; G [MPa], shear modulus; v, Poisson ratio.

TABLE 22-8

Material Properties Considered for the Anulus Fibers

Model	E [MPa]	v	Specifications	References
Nonlinear elastic	Nonlinear curve	—	Ratio of E through layers 1.0–0.9–0.75–0.65	11, 14, 17, 18, 24, 29, 37, 56, 60, 67, 68, 70, 78
Nonlinear elastic	Nonlinear	—	Ratio of stiffness through layers 1.0–0.9–0.75–0.65	9, 25, 48, 49
Linear, elastic	60–500	0.3–0.35	—	8, 10, 33–35, 50, 53, 56, 64, 73, 75, 77, 79, 80

E [MPa], Young's modulus; v, Poisson ratio.

TABLE 22-9

Material Properties Considered for Ligaments in the Literature

Model	ALL	PLL	LF	ITL	CL	ISL	SSL	References
Nonlinear			Nonlinear Stress–Strain Curve					
CS area (mm²)	24–49.1	14.4–22.2	71.7–75	4–12	36–130.9	40–49.2	30–70.3	17, 18, 37, 60
Linear								
E [MPa]	20	70	50	50	20	28	28	
v	0.3	0.3	0.3	0.3	0.3	0.3	0.3	8, 34, 35, 53, 64
CS area (mm²)	38	20	60	10	40	35.5	25.5	

ALL, anterior longitudinal ligament; CL, capsular ligament; CS, cross section; E [MPa], Young's modulus; ISL, interspinous ligament; ITL, intertransverse ligament; LF, ligamentum flavum; PLL, posterior longitudinal ligament; SSL, supraspinous ligament; v, Poisson ratio.

Articular Facet Joints

The facet joint plays an important role in load bearing and restriction of motion in segmental movements. It functions in tandem with the intervertebral disc in load transfer between adjacent vertebral bodies.[17,18] The articulating structure must be modeled with realistic attributes and proper procedures in computational modeling of spinal segments because it has a significant effect on the quality and quantity of the motion. The articulation characteristics and relative motion depend on many factors, including cartilage layers, gap distance, the condition of the intervertebral disc, loading type, and geometric features of the articulating surface.

Kumaresan et al.[19] compared different techniques for modeling of cervical facet joints. They reconstructed the joint capsule using four different methods: slide-line, contact plane, hyperelastic, and fluid models. The slide-line and contact plane models lacked the synovial fluid and synovial membrane. In the slide-line model, interaction was defined by using slide-line elements (gap elements), whereas in the contact plane model it was achieved by defining a contact plane between the cartilage surfaces. A friction coefficient of 0.01 was assigned for both models. The other models, hyperelastic and fluid, did not have elements for contact modeling; instead, they included synovial fluid between the cartilage layers modeled using noncompressible hyperelastic solid elements and hydrostatic noncompressible fluid elements, respectively. They concluded that fluid modeling of the facet joint matched both actual facet joint anatomy and its function better than the other three models. Similarly, Wheeldon et al.[20] used full anatomic parts, such as facet joint cartilage, facet joint synovial fluid, and facet joint membrane, for modeling of the articular facet joints.

Shirazi-Adl et al.[17,18] viewed the articulation process as a general moving contact problem and assigned 1 mm for the initial gap between the articulating surfaces. Guan et al.[7,21] used 3D surface-to-surface contact to simulate the articulation phenomenon and assigned the initial gap between the surfaces according to CT images. Three-dimensional eight-noded compression-only gap elements were used to simulate the articulation between the facets in a study by Goel et al.[22] Based on the CT images, they assigned the value of 0.45 mm for the initial gap between the surfaces.

The facet joints also are modeled with 3D gap contact elements with cartilage layers modeled using a parameter of "softened contact," which exponentially adjusts force transfer between facet surfaces, according to the size of the gap.[9,23-27] An initial gap of 0.5 mm was assigned, and at full closure, the joint was assumed to have the same stiffness as the surrounding bone material.

Schmidt et al.[28,29] modeled the facet joints as nonlinear, with frictionless contact. They assigned the value of 0.6 mm for the initial gap between the cartilage layers. In other studies,[30,31] the facet joints were simulated using frictionless surface-to-surface contact elements in combination with the penalty algorithm with a normal contact stiffness of 200 N/mm, and the initial gap between the cartilage layers assumed to be 0.4 mm.

Some researchers viewed the facet joints as a 3D contact problem with friction.[8,32-34] To allow random motion of the surfaces, such as separation, sliding, and rotation, they defined a finite sliding interaction. For the friction characteristic, they chose a classic isotropic Coulomb friction model and assigned a relatively high friction coefficient of 0.1 as a worst-case scenario.

Lu et al.[35] modeled the facet joints using sliding contact elements and assumed the contact pressure to be between 0 and 5000 megapascals (MPa), depending on the gap size. Pressure has been considered to be 0 MPa at a gap size of 0.5 mm and 5000 MPa when the gap is closed completely.

Loads and Boundary Conditions

Application of loads and boundary conditions varies according to the aim of the study. Generally, loading types used in the computational analysis of the spine are simple static or incrementally altering quasistatic loads. In general, the inferior end plate of the lowest vertebra is fixed rigidly, and loads (or displacements) are applied to the superior end plate of the uppermost vertebral body.

In most cases it is easy to simulate tension or compression loads. It is more complicated to apply moments, add muscle forces and upper body weight effects, or realize coupled motions.

Shirazi-adl et al.[17,18] and Polikeit et al.[8,34] applied a linearly varying distribution of axial loads to the top of the upper vertebra to simulate pure bending moments, with no net axial force. Kumaresan et al.[36] and Wheeldon et al.[20] succeeded in producing pure moments by using a force couple acting on the rigid plate attached to the superior vertebra.

Sharma et al.[37] simulated pure flexion-extension moments using a pair of concentrated axial loads on top of the upper vertebra. They also studied the effect of anteroposterior shear during sagittal motion by a horizontal force applied at the center of the upper vertebral body. Two equal and opposite forces at the nodes at the edge of the sagittal or medial periphery of the upper vertebral body were applied to produce a force couple yielding a pure moment.[38-42]

Researchers have used the follower load technique, suggested by Patwardhan et al.,[43] extensively for the last decade to simulate upper-body weight and the stabilizing effects of muscle forces seen in vivo without inducing any intervertebral rotations.[9,25-28,30,44,45]

Biomechanical Applications

Perhaps the greatest advantage of the finite element method for researchers in the area of musculoskeletal biomechanics is its ability to predict the consequences of surgical applications; age-related changes such as disc degeneration, osteophytes, and osteoporosis; or effects of daily activities on a spinal segment. It also is a great tool for the development and analysis of fusion instrumentation or motion preservation devices.

Disc Degeneration and Vertebral Osteoporosis Simulation

Disc degeneration is one of the most widely studied questions using finite element analysis of the spine because of the complex natural history of the disease and its high impact on clinical practice. Since the 1980s, a large body of literature on the modeling of the normal and degenerated disc has been published. The difficulty in proper simulation of the disc and disc degeneration arises from the hierarchical structural organization of the disc, the coexistence of multiple physical states (i.e., void, solid, fluid) presenting a nonhomogeneous material property distribution, and the influence of the degeneration cascade on these variables at various levels. The "weakest link" in modeling of the healthy disc and disc degeneration is validation of the model, because a significant challenge is presented by experimental evaluation of the material properties of the disc components.

In one of the earliest studies, Shirazi-Adl et al.[45] modeled the degenerated disc by simply omitting a nucleus section. In another study, Shirazi-Adl et al.[18] modeled the healthy disc as noncompressible fluid and suggested the loss of noncompressibility as a means to simulate the degenerated disc.

Goel et al.[10] modeled the aging disc with a great deal of complexity by realistically simulating the radial and circumferential fissures in the anulus fibrosus that appear with age and discectomy. They simulated the radial crack in two ways: "out-in" injury started from the outermost layer and went through the innermost anulus layer with step-wise removal of the anulus elements, whereas "in-out" injury started from the innermost layer and went through the last layer of anulus simulated by replacing material of the anulus's elements with nucleus material. They simulated the circumferential injury by removing the fourth anulus layer along the circumference, starting from posterior and extending through lateral.

Rohlmann et al.[24] investigated the mechanical effects of three different grades of intervertebral disc degeneration—mild, moderate, and severe—compared with the healthy disc. They modeled the degeneration by reducing the disc height to 20%, 40%, and 60% of the healthy disc for mildly, moderately, and severely degenerated discs, respectively. In the finite element model, the laxity in all disc fibers and surrounding ligaments, seen on in vivo conditions after reduction of the disc height, was simulated by offsetting their nonlinear stiffness curves. They assigned the compressibility values for the nucleus pulposus of 0.0005, 0.0503, 0.0995, and 0.15, respectively, for healthy disc and mildly, moderately, and severely degenerated intervertebral discs. They assumed no effect on the material properties of the anulus fibrosus from degeneration of the disc.

Hussain et al.[41,42] modeled two different degenerated discs, moderately and severely degenerated, to study the effects of disc degeneration on the facet loads. They simulated the degeneration according to the signs of Thompson disc grades 2 and 3 (moderate) and 4 and 5 (severe). They decreased the disc height, increased the disc area, and reduced the nucleus portion to simulate the degenerated disc. They also reduced the Poisson's ratio in severely degenerated discs and increased the Young's modulus of anulus and nucleus in both moderately and severely degenerated discs.

Galbusera et al.[11] meticulously modeled the degeneration of the disc based on five different degenerative characteristics: (1) loss of water content in nucleus and anulus, (2) calcification and thickness reduction in end plates, (3) loss of disc height, (4) formation of osteophytes, and (5) diffuse sclerosis. They obtained ten different spinal segments by scaling the size of the finite element model to represent different stages of each degeneration level (mild, moderate, and severe). They changed the initial void ratio to model the degeneration in the nucleus and anulus, and they formed three different types of anular lesions: a rim lesion, a radial tear, and a circumferential tear. They modeled end plate cartilage degeneration by reducing its height and changing its material properties. Degeneration of the disc also was modeled with reduction of its height. When simulating the osteophytes, they used solid elements with the same material attributes of bone and anulus between them. They simulated sclerosis by interchanging the material properties of cancellous bone with the cortical bone in certain areas. They divided the lower half of L4 and the upper half of L5 into four regions and randomly assigned the sclerosis deficiency to these sections.

Polikeit et al.[46] investigated the effects of osteoporosis and disc generation on the load transfer characteristics of an L2-3 segment. Initially, they modeled an osteoporotic vertebra by decreasing the elasticity modulus of trabecular bone by 66% and other bony parts by 33% compared with healthy model. Next, they simulated the progress of osteoporosis by modeling the cancellous bone transversely isotropic (i.e., the elastic modulus in the horizontal direction was one third of that in the vertical direction, using the same material properties as for the isotropic case) and increasing the anisotropy gradually. They postulated five steps of degeneration based on the isotropic osteoporotic vertebra model. At the first step, they changed the material definition of the nucleus pulposus from noncompressible to deformable. In the second step, the nucleus pulposus was hardened by assigning the same material properties as the ground substance of the anulus, and subsequently the Young modulus of the whole disc was doubled. In the fourth step, the innermost anulus layer was removed, other layers were thickened, and increased space between the fibers resulted. In the last step, they further reduced the elasticity modulus of the last remaining fiber layers. They also modeled a worst-case scenario by using transversely isotropic osteoporotic vertebral bodies in conjunction with the degenerated intervertebral disc.

Modeling and Analysis of the Instrumented Spine

A strong statistical power can be obtained in experimental approaches to spinal biomechanics by using a paired design analysis in which the same specimen is used in all experimental and treatment groups. This makes it possible to limit the variables and provide controlled analysis conditions. However, paired analysis design may not always be an option, especially in destructive studies, and the measurement of some parameters may not be possible without introducing confounding factors. Finite element analysis is an effective tool for observing changes in outcome parameters in response to varying input while controlling all other factors.

Analysis of Fusion

Guan et al.[21] studied the range of motion, disc pressure, and facet joint loading following ventral fusion at L4-5 or L5-S1 under flexion-extension loading. They simulated fusion by replacing the whole disc with either a bone graft or a porous tantalum. They assumed an elasticity modulus of 100 MPa and 3.3 gigapascals (GPa), respectively, and a Poisson's ratio of 0.2 and 0.1, respectively, for bone graft and porous tantalum. They found that caudal fusion, compared to rostral, and tantalum, compared to bone graft, caused less range of motion, and that rostral fusion induced more facet joint loads and less adjacent disc stress than caudal fusion.

Park et al.[33] investigated the biomechanical effects of the number of ventral fixation rods, with or without dorsal fixation, on the spinal stability of thoracolumbar burst fracture constructs. They prepared ten separate models, composed of combinations of the following parameters: ventral rod number (0 to 2), with or without midcolumn compression and with or without dorsal fixation. They used different corpectomy procedures for the compression. They placed a cage in the center of L1. To simulate the surgical effects of the posterior fixation, the supraspinal ligament, interspinal ligament, and ligamentum flavum were removed. Pedicle screws and a ventral screw also were placed to simulate dorsal and ventral fixation. They concluded that two-rod ventral fixation ensured enough spinal stability and one-rod ventral fixation with posterior fixation hindered excessive motion.

Kim et al.[47] focused on the biomechanical alterations after removal of the dorsal stabilization device in a fused lumbar segment. They modeled the fusion mass between the transverse processes of L3 and L4 as bilateral rectangular columns. To model the decompressed condition, the supraspinous ligament, the interspinous ligament, a portion of the spinous process, the distal region of the L3 lamina, and the ligamentum flavum were removed. Fixation was achieved with posterior pedicle screws. They inserted the screws into the pedicles at an inward angle of 10 degrees with respect to the horizontal plane and used a rod 5.5 mm in diameter. After intact testing, the fusion state with or without posterior support was studied. They concluded that removal of pedicle screws could lower the stiffness value of the fused segment, which would, however, decrease the stress levels at the adjacent discs.

Polikeit et al.[8] investigated the effects of intervertebral cage applications on the load transfer and stress levels of adjacent tissues. They used a box-shaped cage model with titanium and carbon fiber for the material properties. They simulated the surgical effects by removing the anterior longitudinal ligament, nucleus pulposus, and ventral portion of the anulus. The gap elements with a high friction coefficient of 0.8 were used to define contact between cage surfaces and end plates. They found that intervertebral cage application increased the stress and changed the load transfer at the adjacent segments.

In an optimization study, Zhong et al.[32] sought to devise a new intervertebral cage design that would allow more bone graft volume. They used a dorsal approach to implant the titanium cages and then carried out laminectomy and partial discectomy procedures on the model. They removed the dorsal elements, supraspinous ligament, interspinous ligament, ligamentum flavum, and part of the disc to simulate the procedure. The posterior support was modeled with pedicle screws and rods. The cages were placed between the vertebral bodies within two-thirds of the area of the disc. Cages could bear only compression loads. In the optimization step, they prioritized the gain of volume for bone ingrowth without sacrificing the biomechanical characteristics. They obtained a new cage with a volume of 1603 mm^3 in comparison with the initial cage model with a volume of 2058 mm^3. The new design was satisfying in terms of range of motion and stress levels at the adjacent disc, but had higher stress levels than the original cages.

Analysis of Arthroplasty

Goel et al.[23] used a hybrid approach, a combination of finite element method and biomechanical testing, to investigate the mechanical effects of the Charité artificial disc (DePuy Spine, Inc., Raynham, MA) on the adjacent segments. They assumed that the surfaces of the artificial disc were smooth and flat. Furthermore, they also simulated the surgical procedure by resecting the anterior longitudinal ligament and ventral anulus and excising the nucleus pulposus. They concluded that arthroplasty increases mobility in flexion and extension by 19% and 44%, respectively, with minimal adjacent disc pressure changes. They also found that shear stress levels were higher at the superior bone interface with the artificial disc than at the inferior interface.

Rohlmann et al.[48] investigated the biomechanical effects of artificial disc implant position and height, as well as gradual removal of the disc and contribution of the anterior longitudinal ligament to the biomechanical behavior of the lumbar spine. They used three different disc heights—10, 12, and 14 mm—placed in various locations in the anterior-posterior plane. Removal of the disc was modeled in steps: the ventral anulus, the nucleus, and, finally, excision of the whole disc. To study the contribution of the anterior longitudinal ligament, two models were used, with and without the ligament, simulating a ligament repair after implantation. They concluded that implant position had a great effect on intersegmental rotation for standing and flexion. The increase in disc height increased intersegmental rotation, and when lateral portions of anulus were preserved, intersegmental rotations were found similar to the intact model.

Schmidt et al.[30] studied two hypotheses: (1) that increasing the artificial disc implanted segment number increased the mobility of the spine and facet joint loads, and (2) that incorrect positioning of the implanted disc caused instability. They used the SB Charité 3 Disc in the finite element model. They used chrome-cobalt alloy for the metallic end plates, with an elasticity modulus of 300 GPa and a Poisson's ratio of 0.27. They chose ultra-high-molecular-weight polyethylene for the core with a Young's modulus of 2 GPa and a Poisson ratio of 0.3. The anterior longitudinal ligament, ventral anulus, and nucleus were removed. They obtained a perfect osteointegration between the metallic end plates and the vertebral bodies by using a perfect bond contact. Eleven cases were studied, involving combinations of two, three, or four levels of implantation. The effect of misalignment of the discs also was studied. The results showed that the increase in motion ranged from 51% for two implants up to 91% for four implants. The increase in facet joint loads was 24% for two implants and up to 38% for four implants for the centrally positioned, extension situation. They found that misalignments in the position of the artificial disc induced high facet joint loads, unfavorable kinematics, and lift-off phenomena.

Analysis of Dynamic Systems

Zander et al.[49] studied a hybrid construct with a dynamic implant placed adjacent to a fused segment with a spinal fixator. A pedicle screw–based dynamic implant was placed at the L3-4 segment. An L2-3 fusion initially was modeled with a bone graft and a rigid dorsal fixator. The location of the fusion was tested by moving the fusion and fixators to the L4-5 level. They concluded that the dynamic implant decreased intersegmental rotation of the implanted level in walking, flexion, and extension, and reduced facet joint loads in axial rotation.

Rohlman et al.[9] compared the mechanical performance of dorsal dynamic implants and dorsal rigid fixators. They inserted a pair of dorsal dynamic implants with fictional material attributes to the L3-4 segment. To compare the dynamic and rigid devices, the dynamic system was substituted with the rigid system. They also divided the dynamic implant investigation by studying the construct both with and without distraction to the height of a healthy disc. Furthermore, they studied the effect of implant stiffness on intersegmental rotation by changing the longitudinal rod stiffness in several steps. They found that a dynamic implant decreased the intersegmental rotation and facet joint loads at the implanted level, and that it reduced intradiscal pressure in a healthy disc in extension and standing. They also found that intradiscal pressures were reduced only for the rigid fixator after distraction.

In a recent probabilistic study, Rohlmann et al.[27] investigated the effects of ten variables inherent in a pedicle screw–based motion preservation system on the intradiscal pressure, facet loads, and intervertebral rotations. They used different lengths of implants in the study with titanium screws and polycarbonate-urethane rods. The parameters that varied were elastic modulus, diameter of the rods, angular rigidity of the screw head, interval between the rod and the pedicle screw entry point, orientation of the screws, whether cranial or caudal levels were bridged, and several kinds of defects. They observed that motion preservation systems reduced levels of intersegmental rotation, intradiscal pressure, and facet joint loads in most cases. They concluded that the loading conditions, Young's modulus and the diameter of the rod, the distraction of the segment, and the torsional stiffness of the connection between the screws and rod had a greater effect on the output parameters.

In a parametric study, Schmidt et al.[29] sought the optimal axial and bending stiffness values for a dorsal dynamic implant while validating their findings with an in vitro study. They used a simplified model of the stabilization system, including rod and screws, to investigate the range of axial and bending stiffness of the rod, which represented the nonfixed and fixed situations. They found that lower stiffness values of the rod provided acceptable stiffening to the segment and higher stiffness values of the rod had negligible effects.

Analysis of Cement Augmentation

Polikeit et al.[34] investigated the influence of cement augmentation on load transfer by using an L2-3 finite element model. After adapting the material properties of the osteoporotic vertebral body, they considered polymethylmethacrylate (PMMA) as the bone cement material. In the first case, they simulated the effects of cement augmentation of the whole trabecular bone by changing the cancellous bone material properties to that of PMMA in L2 and L3, subsequently. They modeled unipedicular and bipedicular cement augmentations with one or two vertically placed cement barrels filling up one sixth of the vertebral body volume according to observations on radiographs of treated patients. The results of the study showed that augmentation increased the intradiscal pressure and deflection of the end plate into the adjacent vertebra. They found that augmentation changed the stress levels and distribution in the adjacent vertebrae.

Baroud et al.[50] investigated the effects of vertebroplasty on load transfer in the segment. They modeled the material properties of bone cement composition after vertebroplasty as linear isotropic elastic, 46 times stronger and 12 times stiffer than the osteoporotic bone. To simulate the cement-infiltrated vertebra, they modeled the whole volume of L5 as augmented cement. They found that augmentation reduced bulging of the end plate of the augmented vertebra, which caused stiffening of the intervertebral joint.

Rohmann et al.[51] studied vertebroplasty and kyphoplasty for compression fractures and to investigate the importance of the center of gravity shift compensation of the upper torso on muscle forces and intradiscal pressure. They prepared an intact model, a vertebroplasty model, and a kyphoplasty model. They simulated the vertebroplasty model by reducing the ventral height of L3 by 35% compared with an intact disc, forming a wedge fracture. They simulated the kyphoplasty model by reducing the ventral height of L3 by 90% of the intact disc, assuming a nearly full fracture. In addition, they simulated the upper torso center of gravity shift compensation with three different scenarios. They concluded that the shift of the upper body center of gravity played a greater role in vertebral body fractures at the adjacent segments compared with kyphoplasty or vertebroplasty.

Summary

Although experimental techniques traditionally have commanded a higher position in the hierarchical order of scientific approaches to investigating real-life questions in spine biomechanics, it is not always possible to use them, due to limitations of technology or specimen morphology. Finite element analysis has become an invaluable and relatively inexpensive tool for researchers to investigate questions that are either costly to answer using an experimental model or require measurements that cannot be performed without destroying the specimens. Computational studies, therefore, have contributed significantly to the literature to help in the understanding of complicated biomechanical principles such as facet loads, the relationship between osteoporosis and disc degeneration, as well as the effects on intervertebral load transfer, and implant design.

Despite the advantages of finite element analysis, one must be aware that information obtained using this approach does have limitations. Finite element analysis is founded on four major pillars: modeling, materials, interactions, and boundary conditions. Thanks to the progress in imaging technology, the modeling capabilities have been improved significantly, which has made possible the modeling of the details of bone, even at microscopic levels. The greatest limiting factor in finite element analysis is the material property definitions. Material properties of the elements of the spine (e.g., bone, ligaments, cartilage) are approximated from the previously existing information in the literature. This is associated with a totally separate set of limitations. Interactions between the facet surfaces or the implant-bone interface are based on assumptions such as gaps, friction, or fused surfaces. Loading usually is defined as pure moment, with or without the presence of axial compression. Therefore, the quality of the information obtained in finite element analysis depends on how realistic these assumptions were. The results of the finite element analysis should be treated as predictions rather than absolute facts. If the hypotheses were reasonably appropriate to the question studied, one can gain the most from the results of the computational analyses by observing such characteristics as relative changes in study groups, characteristics of the parameter behaviors during the course of loading, or qualitative analysis of stress or strain distributions.

Nevertheless, computational approaches will continue to complement the experimental science of spine biomechanics and become an increasingly useful tool for the study of complex problems, including the design of implants. Educational environments that provide surgeons with, at minimum, the foundations of finite element analysis are critical. There is no doubt that patient-specific finite element studies can help surgeons better prepare for surgical procedures. The field will most certainly advance by the development of faster modeling capabilities and techniques that can determine patient-specific material definitions.

KEY REFERENCES

Galbusera F, Schmidt H, Neidlinger-Wilke C, et al: The mechanical response of the lumbar spine to different combinations of disc degenerative changes investigated using randomized poroelastic finite element models. *Eur Spine J* 20(4):563–571, 2011.

Goel VK, Monroe BT, Gilbertson LG, Brinckmann P: Interlaminar shear stresses and laminae separation in a disc. Finite element analysis of the L3-L4 motion segment subjected to axial compressive loads. *Spine (Phila Pa 1976)* 20(6):689–698, 1995.

Kumaresan S, Yoganandan N, Pintar FA: Finite element modeling approaches of human cervical spine facet joint capsule. *J Biomech* 31(4):371–376, 1998.

Polikeit A, Ferguson SJ, Nolte LP, Orr TE: Factors influencing stresses in the lumbar spine after the insertion of intervertebral cages: finite element analysis. *Eur Spine J* 12(4):413–420, 2003.

Polikeit A, Nolte LP, Ferguson SJ: Simulated influence of osteoporosis and disc degeneration on the load transfer in a lumbar functional spinal unit. *J Biomech* 37(7):1061–1069, 2004.

Rohlmann A, Zander T, Bergmann G: Spinal loads after osteoporotic vertebral fractures treated by vertebroplasty or kyphoplasty. *Eur Spine J* 15(8):1255–1264, 2006.

Schmidt H, Heuer F, Drumm J, et al: Application of a calibration method provides more realistic results for a finite element model of a lumbar spinal segment. *Clin Biomech (Bristol, Avon)* 22(4):377–384, 2007.

REFERENCES

The complete reference list is available online at expertconsult.com.

CHAPTER 23

Intervertebral Disc: Anatomy, Physiology, and Aging

James K.C. Liu | Edward C. Benzel

The intervertebral disc (IVD) is an integral component of the vertebral column. The disc serves a dual purpose, one as part of a joint complex that allows for the various movements of the spine, including bending, flexion, and torsion. The IVD also plays a vital role in the proper absorption and distribution of stress during compressive load bearing. The individual components of the disc are each unique in their molecular composition and work in conjunction to be able to resist the forces that are subject to it. Understanding the mechanism in which the disc performs its task mandates an understanding of the anatomy of each of the components of the IVD. An understanding of the molecular environment of the disc interspace is also critical, as proper maintenance of this environment is essential to maintaining the proper balance between synthesis and degradation of the products that constitute the extracellular matrix. Finally, changes that occur on a microscopic and macroscopic level are relevant to the functioning of the disc interspace. Each of these components is discussed in this chapter.

Anatomy

Intervertebral Disc

The spinal column has 23 IVDs, starting from the C2-3 interspace to the L5-S1 interspace. These discs constitute approximately 25% of the total height of the spinal column. The discs vary in thickness from the thinnest disc in the thoracic region to the thickest in the lumbar region.[1] The IVD is a vital component of the joint system present at each spinal level. This system allows for the range of motion permitted at each segment.[2] Each IVD works in conjunction with the paired dorsal zygapophyseal joints to form a "three-joint complex." The function of the individual components of this complex are intimately related, as are their effects on one another during the degenerative process.

The IVD is constructed of three distinct components. The bulk of the disc is made up of a central nucleus pulposus (NP) and the surrounding anulus fibrosus (AF) (Fig. 23-1). The disc is flanked rostrally and caudally by cartilaginous end plates that serve as a transitional zone between the disc and the adjacent vertebral bodies.[3]

Nucleus Pulposus

The central core of the IVD is composed of the NP. It is formed from remnants of the notochord, a derivation of the endoderm—unlike the remaining components of the IVD, which are derived from the mesoderm.[4] The NP is composed of a soft gelatinous material consisting of proteoglycans, surrounded circumferentially by the AF. The NP is 80% water, with proteoglycans contributing to 50% of its dry weight. Aggrecans, a type of proteoglycan known as leucine-rich repeat proteins, are the predominant type of proteoglycans in the NP.[5] The high-proteoglycan content allows for the NP's ability to maintain an increased hydration state, which creates the viscoelastic properties of the NP, which are essential to its load-bearing properties in the spine. The NP is rich in type II collagens, which constitute 80% of the collagen content in the NP.[6] There is a clear distinction between the NP and the surrounding AF; however, this distinction becomes less obvious during the course of aging.[1] Elastin fibers can also

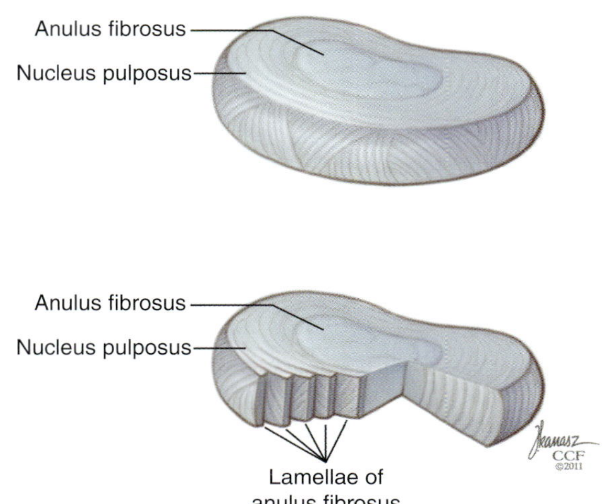

FIGURE 23-1. Axial and lateral views of the intervertebral disc (IVD). **A,** The IVD is composed of a central nucleus pulposus surrounded circumferentially by the anulus fibrosus. **B,** The anulus fibrosus is composed of multiple concentric lamellae made up of fibers oriented in alternating directions to create maximal tension resistance. (Copyright Cleveland Clinic Foundation.)

be found in the NP. These fibers are observed to be situated in both a radial distribution from the center to the periphery in the NP, as well as in a vertical orientation, anchoring the NP to the end plates.[7] This orientation likely contributes to maintaining the structure of the NP within the AF, restoring the NP to its original form following load bearing, as well as playing a role in load transmission to surrounding AF.

Anulus Fibrosus

The AF is a concentrically organized structure that surrounds the NP, occupying the majority of the disc space. It is composed of bundles of collagen fibers that are arranged in concentric lamellae. Approximately 15 to 25 lamellae compose each anulus.[8] The collagen fiber bundles within the lamellae are generally oriented at 30 degrees from the horizontal axis, although closer examination shows that throughout the course of the lamellae, the fiber angle can vary from 20 to 55 degrees.[9] Collagen fibrils in adjacent lamellae run in the opposite direction, allowing for greater tensile strength during stretching.

The AF can be further separated into an outer and inner anulus. The outer AF is a tougher, less flexible component, composed primarily of densely packed type I collagen fibers. The cells in the outer AF are more ellipsoidally shaped cells and are fibroblast-like in nature. At the periphery of the outer anulus, fibrillar bundles known as Sharpey fibers extend superiorly and inferiorly to anchor the disc into the periosteal fibrils of the adjacent vertebral bodies.[10] The inner AF is a softer, less dense, and more fibrocartilagenous component, composed primarily of type II collagen fibers. It possesses a less structured cellular morphology with more widely spaced cells than that of type I collagen. Type II collagen has been shown to be able to maintain 50% to 100% greater water content than type I collagen.[11] The outer lamellae are composed of up to approximately 70% type I collagen and only 20% type II collagen, whereas in the inner AF the percentage of type II collagen increases to 70%. There is also a progressive increase in the concentration of proteoglycans from 10% to 30% when moving from the outer to inner AF.[12] Other types of collagen are also present in the anulus, with type VI collagen making up as much as 10% of the collagen in the AF.[5]

Cartilage End Plates

On the superior and inferior surfaces of the IVD lies the cartilage end plates. They are composed of a thin layer of hyaline cartilage, which serves as the interface between the bony vertebral body and the disc itself. Their composition is similar to the disc; that is, made up of proteoglycans, type II collagen, and water.[13] The end plates range from 0.5 to 1.5 mm in thickness. They are thinnest at the center where they interface with the NP.[14] Each end plate is attached to the adjacent vertebral body by a thin layer of calcium. The calcium is absent in areas where numerous perforations exist throughout the end plates. These perforations in the end plates allow for the passage of vascular channels that traverse from the adjacent vertebral body into the disc.[1] These channels become progressively rare and eventually nonexistent, as the disc ages past the second decade of life.[15] The end plate serve as a stiff but porous barrier between the vertebral body and the IVD. They allow for the diffusion of nutrients and fluid movement into and out of the disc and prevent protrusion of the soft malleable disc material into the vertebral body (Schmorl nodes). Weaknesses in the end plates resulting in Schmorl nodes may be due to a dysregulation of the end-plate composition since those areas have been found to have significantly less proteoglycan concentration.[16]

Vascular Supply

The IVD is generally considered to be an avascular tissue structure, but this is only partially accurate. In infancy, the native disc has a direct vascular supply. This, however, nearly completely regresses by the third decade of life. Vascular "buds" extend from the vertebral bodies through the porous channels in the cartilage end plates and traverse into the disc to supply nutrients.[16] These channels are overtaken by scarring or collapse, likely as a result of weight bearing, past the second decade of life and become occluded and eventually nonexistent.[15,17] Without a direct vascular supply, nutrient exchange occurs through diffusion from blood vessels that surround the periphery of the anulus. The surrounding blood supply comes from segmental branches of the spinal artery.[18]

Innervation

The IVD receives innervations primarily from two sources: the sinuvertebral nerve and the sympathetic trunk via the multiple gray rami communicantes (Fig. 23-2). The sinuvertebral nerve is formed from a branch of the ventral primary ramus and the gray ramus communicans, which branches from the sympathetic trunk. The sinuvertebral nerve enters the spinal canal caudal to the pedicle through the intervertebral foramen and branches into a larger superior division and a lesser inferior division. The superior division travels lateral to the posterior longitudinal ligament in the ventral aspect of the spinal canal, supplying sensation to the dorsal and

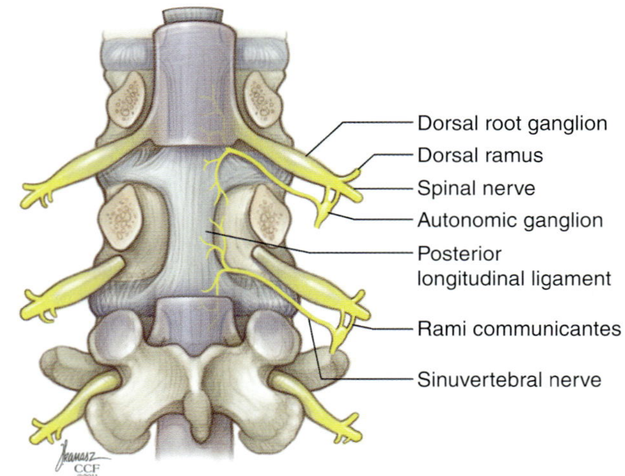

FIGURE 23-2. Innervation of the intervertebral disc. The sinuvertebral nerve is formed from branches off the ventral primary ramus and the gray ramus communicans. The nerve enters the spinal canal caudal to the pedicle through the intervertebral foramen and branches into a larger superior division and a lesser inferior division. This nerve provides sensation to the dorsal and dorsolateral anulus, as well as the posterior longitudinal ligament. (Copyright Cleveland Clinic Foundation.)

dorsolateral anulus, as well as the posterior longitudinal ligament. The inferior trunk passes medially and caudally. The lateral and ventral portions of the AF are supplied by multiple gray rami communicantes from the nearby sympathetic trunk.[19,20] The sympathetic trunk runs in parallel, ventral and lateral to the vertebral column, composed of nerve root contributions from the thoracic and upper two segments of the lumbar spinal cord. The sympathetic trunk provides a number of gray rami comminicantes that help supply the anulus. At least one, but often more, rami communicantes travel around the vertebral body deep to the psoas muscle to join with each ventral primary ramus. Rami communicantes also traverse the psoas to join with the ventral primary ramus. In addition, "paradiscal" rami run along the surface of the IVD in the perianular connective tissue.[19] Innervation of the end plate extends from intraosseous nerves that branch from the ventral primary rami and the basivertebral nerve, a branch of the sinuvertebral nerve, which enters the end plate dorsally.[6]

Innervation of the disc interspace is restricted to the outer anulus. A quantitative analysis of nerve density in multiple IVDs showed innervation to extend to a depth of four to seven lamellae ventrally and no more than three lamellae dorsally. This is indeed very shallow, given that a usual AF contains an average of 15 to 25 lamellae.[8] Unlike the anulus, innervation of the end plate is densest near the center, adjacent to the NP. Innervation of the end plates originates from the intraosseous nerves that penetrate the caudal portion of the vertebral body ventrally and dorsally and travel to the center of the end plate.[21]

Physiology

Extracellular Matrix

The main purpose of the IVD is to serve as a load-bearing structure. The disc performs this task by absorbing axial loads and redistributing them across the entire disc. The capacity for load redistribution is determined, in part, by the molecular structure of the disc. The extracellular matrix is primarily composed of collagen and proteoglycan. These molecules allow the different components of the disc to complete the aforementioned tasks. As previously noted, the AF is a mix of type I and type II collagen, which gives it its necessary tensile strength. In addition to type I and II collagen, multiple other collagen types, including types V and XI, are present in smaller amounts. These collagens play a role in interlinking the collagen fibrils, thus contributing to the overall strong fibrillar collagen network.[5,22] The differences in the composition in different areas of the disc create a dynamic structure that is able to bear and distribute loads across the entire structure. When axial loading takes place, the NP and inner AF absorb the weight and conform to generate hydrostatic pressure that is distributed evenly to the adjacent outer anulus. The alternating lamellar structure of the type I collagen network in the outer AF creates the tensile strength to absorb the redistributed loading force.

Proteoglycans are the other main molecular component of the disc. They constitute 50% of the cells in the NP. Numerous types of proteoglycans are present in the extracellular matrix, including aggregan, versican, decorin, biglycan, fibromodulin, lumican, and perlecan. Aggregan is the most important proteoglycan found in the NP. Proteoglycans comprise a central core protein with attached side chains of keratin sulfate and chondroiton sulfate. Early in life, aggrecans are rich in chondroitin sulfate chains, but these side chains are gradually replaced by keratin sulfate as the disc matures. At their N-terminus, aggrecans attach to hyaluronic acid,[12] and at their C-terminus, they can attach to various molecules in the extracellular matrix, including collagen.[23] The proteogylycans are attached to hyaluronic acid molecules through link proteins, which allow them to form aggregates.[5] Proteoglycans have negative charges on their surface and are therefore hydrophilic molecules able to bind water—thus allowing the NP to retain its hydrated state. The percentages of proteoglycan aggregates are highest in infancy and decrease with age. Breakdown of aggregans that occurs with aging causes them to be replaced by nonaggregated proteoglycans, which are less able to absorb water than their aggregated counterparts.

Metabolic Balance

The extracellular matrix of a healthy intervertebral disc is a dynamic environment, which is maintained at equilibrium due to a fine balance between anabolism and catabolism. The mature NP is essentially void of any vascular supply, and therefore diffusion and glycolysis are the primary sources of nutrient metabolism. Several growth factors, including insulin-like growth factor (IGF), bone morphogenetic protein (BMP), and transforming growth factor-β (TGF-β), contribute to the anabolism within the IVD. IGF and TGF-β have been shown to play a role in stimulating prostaglandin synthesis. BMP-2 also has been shown to stimulate prostaglandin synthesis, as well increase cell proliferation and expression of type II collagen and aggregans.[24] These growth factors work against catabolic factors that lead to breakdown of matrix products. Multiple forms of a zinc-dependent family of enzymes called matrix metalloproteinases (MMPs) are responsible for the degradation of several types of collagen and noncollagenous matrix proteins, including proteoglycans and glycoproteins.[25] MMPs are a vital component of the disc's natural biologic balance between synthesis and breakdown of the extracellular matrix, but have been shown to be up-regulated in diseased discs.[26] The activity of MMPs is tempered by the expression of countering enzymes known as tissue inhibitors of metalloproteinases (TIMPs). TIMPs act to inhibit the activity of MMPs so a proper balance between tissue construction and degradation is achieved.[27] Dysregulation of this system can be seen in degenerative disc disease.

Disc Nutrition

Several factors must be considered to fully understand the nature of the nutrient supply to the IVD. To make things more complex, this landscape changes with age. Only a direct vascular supply exists in the immature disc, which travels from the adjacent vertebral bodies and passes through porous channels in the cartilage end plate. These channels decrease with age and are nearly nonexistent past the second decade as a result of calcification. In addition to the reduction in direct vascular supply, in the early stages of disc maturation, the disc height increases, thus making it more difficult for a direct blood supply to exist in the deeper areas of the disc. Therefore, the nutritional supply and removal of metabolic waste products for the majority of the life of the disc is restricted to diffusion or convection transport. Smaller molecules such as glucose and oxygen are able to effectively diffuse through the disc aided by brownian movements as a result of concentration gradients.[28] This occurs either through the AF circumferentially or through the end plates from the vertebral bodies. The end plates act as a selectively permeable barrier to certain solutes. Calcification of the end plates that occurs with aging can hinder nutrient supply through this pathway.[29] Convection transport, as a result of bulk fluid flow, is the alternative method of solute transport and is likely the preferential method for the transport of larger molecules that are not effectively transported via diffusion. Cycling of mechanical loading between activity and rest can mobilize almost 22% of the total disc volume.[30] Therefore, the diurnal loading cycle can account for a substantial amount of metabolite transfer and is a necessary element of IVD metabolism.[31]

Despite these mechanisms of nutrient supply, the disc lives in a relatively hypoxic environment. The periphery of the disc receives the greatest nutrient supply. This is evident in the increased cell density at the periphery of the AF.[32] In the center of the disc, the levels of glucose and oxygen are lower, due to restrictions in solute diffusion, resulting in increased lactic acid concentration and a more acidic environment, which can hinder proper maintenance of the cell matrix.[28,33] As a result of the natural course of aging and degeneration, further inhibition of nutrient supply pathways can occur, which results in an even more accelerated degeneration within the disc matrix. External factors such as smoking, which can hinder vascular supply, or accelerated calcification of the end plates, as seen in scoliosis, can compound this effect.[34]

Biomechanics

The three components of the IVD work in conjunction to enable its load absorption function. The disc is able to perform this task secondary to its viscoelastic properties, which in turn are secondary to the high concentrations of proteoglycans in the NP. Proteoglycan aggregates facilitate the retention of water, thus allowing it to function essentially as a fluid under static conditions. The NP absorbs weight-bearing compressive loads by conforming its shape to redistribute the load radially to the adjacent AF through hydrostatic forces. Bulk fluid flow from the disc also contributes to its viscoelastic properties. In addition to its utilization for nutrient transport, fluid flow out of the disc allows compressive forces to be absorbed. When the spine is at rest, the axial-loading forces are removed and the hydrostatic pressure decreases. This therefore allows the disc's reabsorption of water to return to its natural conformation. These mechanisms allow the NP to be the first to absorb the compressive load, followed by redistribution of load equally in all directions to the anulus, capitalizing on the structure of the AF to contain tensile stresses. The alternating lamellar structure of the outer AF, which is composed of dense type I collagen fibrils, is optimally designed to resist these tensile strains. This mechanism allows the AF to share in compressive load bearing without being exposed to direct compressive forces. This is not to say that there is no direct compressive force applied to the anulus, but rather that different regions of the AF exhibit varying degrees of load sharing, depending on the posture of the spine when the load is borne.

Load sharing is also performed by the dorsal zygapophyseal joints of the three-joint complex.[6] Aging of the IVD, leading to loss of disc height, can transfer additional load-bearing responsibilities to the joints, and vice versa. The interplay between the IVD and the zygapophyseal joints constitutes the interaction of the three-joint complex, which is a key part of the degenerative process. Despite the interaction between the individual components, studies have shown that degeneration of the disc occurs before that of the joints, indicating the importance of the role of the disc in this sytem.[35]

Aging

Extracellular Matrix Changes

Maturation of the IVD is characterized by a general shift from a thick, well-hydrated, elastic material capable of absorption of compressive loads to a thin, stiff, fibrous material that has lost its ability to properly distribute loads. This is related to the fact that several changes take place at the microscopic level. One of the main changes is the degradation of type II collagen and an increased percentage of type I collagen. This is evident in the elderly in whom less than 30% of the collagen is type II. This is due to selective collagen degradation by various types of MMPs. The collagen fibers also change in composition, as they develop cross-links to adjacent collagen fibers. In addition to enzymatic cross-linking, uncontrolled nonenzymatic cross-linking also occurs, which results in an excessively cross-linked collagen network that increases the stiffness of the entire matrix.[36] Nonenzymatic glycation of this type is a result of a lack of turnover of the collagen supplies in the matrix, which is a consequence of the avascular nature of the disc precluding optimal material turnover. This type of cross-linking results in a yellow-brown pigmentation that is commonly seen in aging discs.

In the NP, significant changes occur to proteoglycans during the course of aging. Early in the disc's life, proteoglycans are rich in chondroiton sulfate side chains, with few surrounding collagen fibers. The proteoglycans interact with nearby hyaluronic acid to form proteoglycan aggregates.[37] As the disc ages, the percentage of proteoglycans in aggregate form significantly decreases, probably secondary to proteolytic degradation. Also, as the number of chondroiton sulfate chains decreases, the number of keratin sulfate chains increases. Further aging is associated with the degradation of the proteoglycan aggregates as well as the link proteins. These effects reduce the NP's ability to create a hydrophilic environment, which in turn leads to decreased water retention in the disc.

Although the exact mechanism is unclear, there appears to be an imbalance between the anabolic and catabolic mechanisms within the disc. An up-regulation of MMPs in herniated and diseased discs has been observed.[38] Proinflammatory cytokines, such as interleukin-1 (IL-1) and tumor necrosis factor alpha (TNF-α), are stimulated from collagen degradation products and lead to further activation of MMPs. TNF-α has been shown to decrease aggregan and type II collagen synthesis and induce the expression of multiple MMPs and aggrecanases.[39] Interestingly, an up-regulation of tissue inhibitors of metalloproteinases (TIMPs),[26] is also noted, suggesting that a repair mechanism is attempting to compensate for the increase in catabolic activity. Nitric oxide has also been shown to play a role in the evolution of the extracellular matrix during aging and degeneration. Although the mechanism by which this is performed is unclear, studies have shown the nitric oxide can inhibit proteoglycan synthesis in response to hydrostatic pressure.[40] This course of events indicates that during the course of disc aging and into degeneration, an imbalance toward catabolism develops, which disrupts the normal equilibrium of the extracellular matrix. The disc's natural ability to compensate for these mechanisms is overtaken, leading to continued activation of these mechanisms and eventually resulting in disc degeneration.

Structural and Functional Changes

The molecular changes that occur during the course of aging result in significant structural and functional changes in the IVD. The NP, which was once a thick viscoelastic substance, becomes thinner and more fibrous, and consequently unable to conform to the compressive loads placed upon it (Fig. 23-3). The distinction between the AF and the NP becomes less clear as the collagen composition becomes stiffer and more fibrous. Anular degeneration results in a reduced number of layers of lamellae, although the thickness of the AF remains the same due to thickening of the remaining lamellae.[8] The proteoglycan concentration decreases, resulting in decreased water content in the NP and a loss of its hydrostatically related ability to dissipate the compressive loads. This, along with thinning of the NP, forces the AF to become directly exposed to the axial-loading pressures of the spine, which in turn results in further injury to the anulus. During the course of aging, reduction in the functional diameter of the NP results in an increase of stress forces applied to the outer AF of up to 160%.[41] In essence, the central NP load-bearing characteristics of youth are transformed directly into a peripheral or perimeter AF load bearing as we age.

Degenerative Cascade

The IVD at each level is a vital component of the three-joint complex, which provides both motion and stability in the spine. The healthy, juvenile disc participates in this joint complex by absorbing the compressive loads and dissipating them to the AF lamellae. The extracellular matrix of the NP and AF allows the disc to function in conjunction with the paired zygapophyseal joints so that no one joint is overly stressed. During the aging process, the IVD loses hydration and becomes thinner and stiffer and consequently less able to properly absorb the load and translate such to the anulus.

Yong-Hing and Kirkaldy-Willis categorized the aging and degeneration of the spine into three stages to further define how the natural history of the IVD and zygapophyseal joint relate to each other.[2] The first state is the dysfunction stage, which is characterized by synovial reaction in the dorsal joints and small tears in the IVDs. These injuries occur as a result of natural load bearing and the inevitable aging process of the disc. This progresses to the destabilization stage, which may be better described as the stage of instability. This stage is defined as a progression of the disc past the normal aging process into a degenerative process that involves all components of the three-joint complex. Disc degeneration in this stage results in a loss of disc height and load-bearing capacity of the disc, thus increasing the loading pressure delivered to the zygapophyseal joints. Excess load bearing on the joints in turn can lead to joint capsule laxity and subluxation of the joints. Instability in the joints can lead to anterior translation of the rostral vertebral body with respect to the caudal vertebral body. Such translation of the vertebral segments, in combination with loss of disc interspace height, can result in further narrowing of the neural foramina (Fig. 23-4). Weakness of the joints and movement of the vertebral bodies result in an even greater load applied to the already damaged discs, continuing a cycling cascade of injury within the joint complex.

The final stage is the restabilization stage. As a result of the joint instability and bony movement, osteophyte formation occurs between the vertebral segments. Further disc degeneration and calcification combined with extensive osteophyte formation results in fusion of the intervertebral level and loss of joint motion, thus restabilizing the given motion segment. At this stage, the IVD essentially becomes obsolete since its original role in maintaining joint mobility and load bearing has been eliminated. Once this fusion has occurred, the degenerative process is complete.

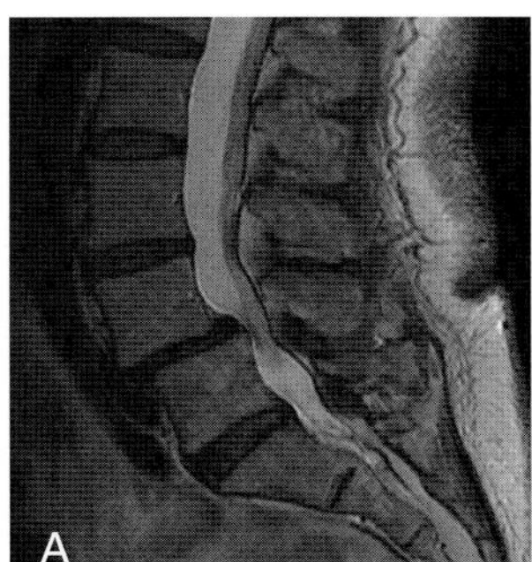

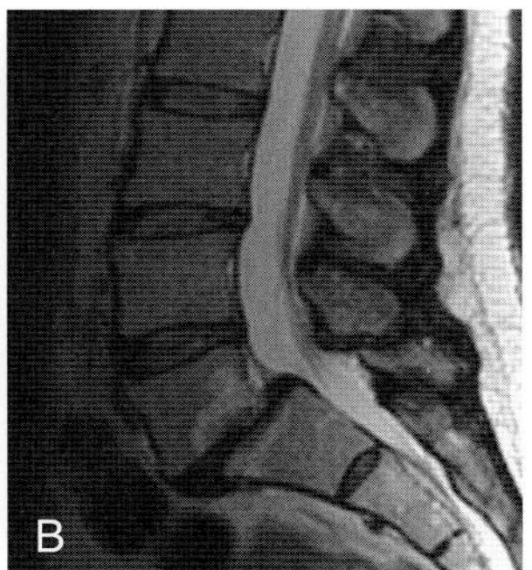

FIGURE 23-3. Spondylolisthesis. **A,** Disc degeneration can be seen at the L4-5 intervertebral disc. As a result of loss of disc height, excess stress is placed on the zygapophyseal joints at that level, which can fail and result in the L4 vertebral body being displaced ventral to the L5 vertebral body (spondylolisthesis). This results in abnormal segment motion, which can result in pain from that level as well as foraminal narrowing and radiculopathy. **B,** Disc degeneration and spondylolisthesis at the L5-S1 level.

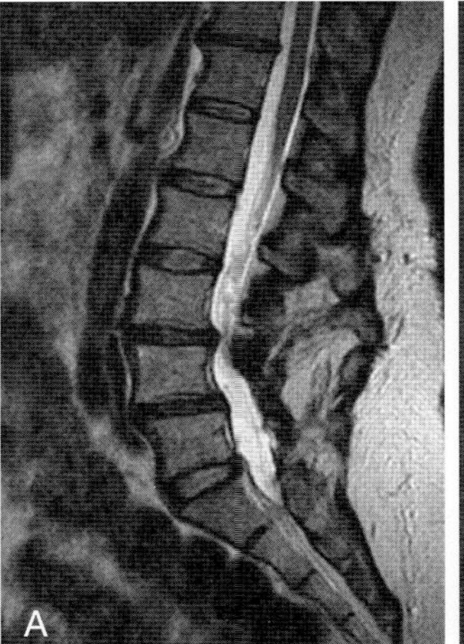

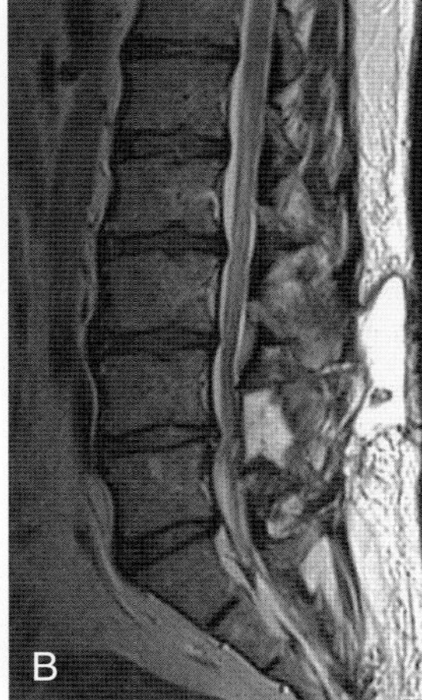

FIGURE 23-4. Intervertebral disc degeneration. **A,** Sagittal MRI showing disc degeneration at the L4-5 disc interspace with a decrease in disc height and signal intensity, representing a decrease in fluid hydration, compared to the other disc level. **B,** Sagittal MRI with multiple levels of disc degeneration at the L1-2, L2-3, and L3-4 levels. Disc herniation into the rostral and caudal veretebral bodies penetrating through the cartilage end plate (Schmorl nodes) can be seen at each of those levels.

Summary

The IVD not only physically occupies a large proportion of the spine, it plays a vital role in the function of the spine in weight bearing and motion preservation. It is a multicompartment structure in which the unique makeup of each component contributes to the overall dynamic functioning of the disc. Despite existing in a relatively nutrient-deprived environment, the disc maintains its complicated extracellular matrix by sustaining a fine balance between catabolism and anabolism. The disruption of this balance is inevitable during the course of aging and is sometimes accelerated to evolve into a degenerative process. As each component of the spine is intimately related to the adjacent structures, the evolution of the IVD initiates a cascade of events that results in the overall remodeling of the spine.

KEY REFERENCES

Adams MA, McNally DS, Dolan P: "Stress" distributions inside intervertebral discs. The effects of age and degeneration. *J Bone Joint Surg [Br]* 78:965, 1996.

Antoniou J, Steffen T, Nelson F, et al: The human lumbar intervertebral disc: evidence for changes in the biosynthesis and denaturation of the extracellular matrix with growth, maturation, ageing, and degeneration. *J Clin Invest* 98:996, 1996.

Buckwalter JA, Einhorn TA, Simon SR: *Orthopaedic basic science: biology and biomechanics of the musculoskeletal system*, Rosemont, IL, 2000, American Academy of Orthopaedic Surgeons.

Philips FM: *Lauryssen: the lumbar intervertebral disc*, NewYork, 2010, Thieme Medical.

Roberts S, Caterson B, Menage J: Matrix metalloproteinases and aggrecanase: their role in disorders of the human intervertebral disc. *Spine (Phila Pa 1976)* 25:3005, 2000.

Yong-Hing K, Kirkaldy-Willis WH: The pathophysiology of degenerative disease of the lumbar spine. *Orthop Clin North Am* 14:491, 1983.

REFERENCES

The complete reference list is available online at expertconsult.com.

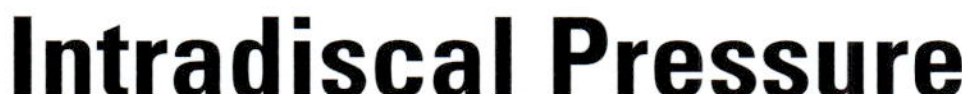

Intradiscal Pressure

Serkan İnceoğlu | Edward C. Benzel

The intervertebral disc is composed of a central gel-like nucleus pulposus (NP) and surrounding anulus fibrosus (AF) with a unique lamellar structure. Each layer of the AF is composed of mainly type I collagen,[1] in which the collagen fibers are organized in an oblique direction that alters at sequential layers. In contrast, the NP has a gel-like structure mainly made by proteoglycans embedded in a type II collagen matrix.

The NP is capable of attracting water molecules and expands its volume through swelling. In a healthy normal state, the NP is, thus, pressurized because the expansion of the volume is restricted by the surrounding AF lamellae and end plates. It has been shown that the disc is a highly viscoelastic fluid-like material with limited compressibility.[2] The water content and, therefore, the intradiscal pressure, are critical for maintenance of normal motion of the spinal segments and for avoiding neurologic complications. The pressurized disc provides the normal intervertebral spacing and smooth motion of the spine and allows balanced load transfer among the adjacent vertebral bodies.

Intradiscal Pressure in the Normal and Degenerated Discs

Early efforts of measurement of disc pressure began in the 1960s. Nachemson and Morris were the first to assess intradiscal pressure.[3] In 1965, Nachemson observed that the pressure in the AF and NP were different and that disc degeneration could alter the pressure.[4] They measured in vivo loading of the spine during different postures via assessing disc pressure. Similar to their subsequent studies, they used the disc as a "load transducer" and did not characterize the pressure properties of the disc itself. A similar study was again performed on a volunteer by Wilke et al. in 1999. They demonstrated similar pressure levels to those shown by Nachemson.[5]

The first comprehensive characterization of disc pressure was accomplished by McNally and Adams.[6] They used a small needle with a pressure transducer mounted at the tip to measure pressure changes within a cadaveric lumbar disc loaded under a variety of conditions. They also collected pressure measurements in both axial and transverse directions by simply rotating the needle during placement in the disc. They demonstrated that a healthy normal disc had a uniform pressure distribution due to hydrostatic pressure that was confirmed in both vertical and horizontal measurements. In contrast, degenerated discs demonstrated an irregular stress distribution across the disc. In the degenerated disc, they observed slight differences in horizontal and vertical directional measurements. They also demonstrated that the pressure (stress) characteristics of the disc depended on the loading conditions.

Sato et al. also performed in vivo experiments using a similar technology.[7] Confirming the findings of McNally and Adams, they reported that normal healthy discs yielded an isotropic pressure profile evidenced by similar pressures in axial and transverse directions. This was in contrast to degenerated discs, in which axial and transverse pressures were found to differ. They also showed that disc with loss of water content, detected by MRI, was associated with less pressure under physiologic loading. McNally et al. noted an association between pain and pressure.[8] They showed that painful discs (after provocation) determined by provocative discography were associated with less pressure in the NP in both vertical and horizontal directions.

The loss of water content in the disc due to degeneration translates into the loss of disc height of the intervertebral space, because the NP becomes more compressible and the anular layers lose their ability to withstand axial compressive loading. The loss of disc height results in the decrease of the gap in the facet joint and subsequent changes in the facet loads. This gradually changes the load transfer patterns in the dorsal and ventral spine and end plates.

Pollintine et al. measured the intradiscal pressure profiles in normal and degenerated cadaveric spines loaded axially or in flexion.[9,10] They demonstrated that the percentage of load transferred via the dorsal spine increased with disc degeneration. Similarly, the loading profile of the end plates lost its homogeneity in healthy normal specimens and shifted toward the perimeter. They also confirmed that the degeneration of the disc was associated with anisotropy of pressure within the disc.

As shown in the aforementioned stress profilometry experiments, the AF in the degenerated discs is associated with increased stress levels and localized stress concentrations. When the anular layers are compressed under axial loading, they bulge inward and outward. This stress profile and deformation pattern, in contrast to healthy normal disc where anular layers are compacted and able to withstand axial loading, sets the stage for anular tear and clefts. These, in turn, may be a cause of pain.

The effect of the disc degeneration on the segmented spinal motion, especially the neutral zone, was discussed in an earlier chapter. Cannella et al. investigated the relationship of intradiscal pressure coupled with the degeneration and motion.[11] They looked at the pressure changes in the intervertebral disc under axial compression as they gradually removed the nucleus via a vacuum tissue removal system. They showed that denucleation of the ventral spinal column unit caused increased instability, confirmed by an increased range of motion and a larger neutral zone. Parallel to this phenomenon, they also measured decreasing intradiscal pressure by means of a pressure transducer placed on a needle. The researchers studied various increasing levels of compression. They did not, however, assess pressure changes in the other planes of motion (e.g., sagittal, lateral).

Disc pressure is also a mechanism by which a painful disc is delineated from other normal discs. Discography, a procedure in which a contrast agent is delivered into the disc through a needle to increase the pressure within the disc, is a widely used method to manually provoke pain in suspect discs. Recently, a group of investigators tested the hypothesis that discography-related pressure could be an indication of disc degeneration and a quantitative marker for the painful disc.[12] Unlike previous studies seeking the minimum discography pressure that provokes pain, they collected the opening pressure, the pressure required to inject contrast agent into the disc, and compared it with the MRI signal—which is an indicator of degeneration. They showed that the opening pressure decreased with increasing levels of disc degeneration and that painful discs had a lower opening pressure than those with no pain. The disc pressure was also shown, in another study, to be transferred to the adjacent levels to some extent during provocative pressurization of a lumbar disc.[13]

As a biomechanical indicator, the disc pressure also has a diagnostic value. Gradual changes in the pressure might provide biomechanical evidence of biochemical changes in the disc during degeneration or regeneration. As the technology develops and measurement of the intradiscal pressure becomes easier, safer, and more reliable, it might be an adjunct evaluation technique to MRI in delineating symptomatic degenerated discs. Similarly, Buser et al. used the disc pressure as an evaluation method for the regeneration of pig intervertebral discs.[14] They studied the effect of fibrin injection in the regeneration of the nucleus in pigs who had undergone complete nucleotomy. In their study, they showed that fibrin inhibited the encroachment of the anulus and facilitated proteoglycan redevelopment. They confirmed histologic findings of new nucleus formation with recovery in the disc pressure.

Limitations and New Technologies in Intradiscal Pressure Measurement

In vivo and in vitro disc pressure measurements have gained popularity since they were first tried by Nachemson. Many researchers have used intradiscal pressure assessment as a tool for understanding load transfer and load sharing in the spine, evaluating disc degeneration, or assessing the spinal kinetics after interventions performed on the spine. Although the intradiscal pressure can be a source of various types of information, all of these studies have a common limitation—the methodology by which the pressure measurements are acquired.

The majority of the studies in the literature used a miniature pressure transducer that is attached at the tip of a needle or rigid substrate vehicle, which is designed to deliver the transducer to the NP or AF. The introduction of the needle to the disc causes the destruction of the anular layers to a degree depending on the size of the needle used. The effect of this disruption may be minimal in terms of the overall kinetics and kinematics of the spine in cadaveric human lumbar spine studies. However, it increases the risk of NP herniation under axial loading.[15-17] As in cadaveric cervical studies,[18] this technique becomes more unreliable due to the decreased ratio of disc height to needle diameter and the orientation of the end plates in animal studies, especially small animal models. In addition, because of the dramatic difference between the stiffness of the needle and the surrounding anulus, the natural stress distribution within the disc may be altered during the experimental procedure.

In vivo animal studies have shown that with a sufficiently thick needle, the normal physiology of the disc can be interrupted by a single anular puncture, which in turn causes a rapid and complete degeneration of the disc.[19] Therefore, traditional methods of intradiscal pressure measurements have an intrinsic risk of influencing the results of an experiment.

Moreover, the measurement of disc pressure is difficult and not of high fidelity because the majority of the pressure transducers are contact based and directional. Therefore, the form of the anular layers and consistency of the nucleus and their interaction with the transducer influence the measurements. Due to the lack of visibility while the transducer is within the disc, control of these variables is usually not possible and their effect on the results remains unknown. Similarly, calibration of the transducer for the unique material properties of an individual disc is another limitation in contact-based transducers.

Researchers have vigorously sought improved devices and techniques for disc pressure measurement because of these limitations. Nesson et al. have developed a fiberoptic pressure sensor for intradiscal pressure measurement in rat spines.[20] The device has an outer diameter of 366 μm and can measure up to 70 kPa with the resolution of 0.17 kPa. Dennison et al. used a custom-made pressure sensor using a new fibre-Bragg gratings.[21] Their device was 0.5 mm in diameter and able to measure up to 50 MPa. They placed the device, through a 25-G hypodermic needle, in human cadaveric lumbar discs and measured the pressure under 2000-N axial compression incrementally with a sensitivity of −0.7 to 1.07 kPa/N. Glos et al. utilized microelectromechanical systems (MEMS) technology to miniaturize the pressure sensor.[22] The device, with an overall size of 3.2 × 15 × 1 mm, was composed of a stainless steel carrier and a silicon-based piezoresistive sensor (2 × 2 × 0.9 mm) mounted at the tip.

In conclusion, disc pressure is an indicator of the state of disc composition and a tool for assessing the kinetics and kinematics of the segmented spinal motion. With improving technology, the limitations intrinsic to the technique may be overcome and intradiscal pressure data may be used for improving surgical outcomes. Benzel et al., for instance, have studied wireless technology that can be implanted into a patient and used to monitor disc pressure telemetrically.[23] However, it appears that more in vitro studies need to be performed in order to establish the theoretical foundations for such technologies.

KEY REFERENCES

Cannella M, Arthur A, Allen S, et al: The role of the nucleus pulposus in neutral zone human lumbar intervertebral disc mechanics. *J Biomech* 41(10):2104–2111, 2008.

McNally DS, Adams MA: Internal intervertebral disc mechanics as revealed by stress profilometry. *Spine (Phila Pa 1976)* 17(1):66–73, 1992.

McNally DS, Shackleford IM, Goodship AE, Mulholland RC: In vivo stress measurement can predict pain on discography. *Spine (Phila Pa 1976)* 21(22):2580–2587, 1996.

Nachemson A: In vivo discometry in lumbar discs with irregular nucleograms. Some differences in stress distribution between normal and moderately degenerated discs. *Acta Orthop Scand* 36(4):418–434, 1965.

Nachemson A, Morris JM: In vivo measurements of intradiscal pressure. Discometry, a method for the determination of pressure in the lower lumbar discs. *J Bone Joint Surg [Am]* 46:1077–1092, 1964.

Sato K, Kikuchi S, Yonezawa T: In vivo intradiscal pressure measurement in healthy individuals and in patients with ongoing back problems. *Spine (Phila Pa 1976)* 24(23):2468–2474, 1999.

Wilke HJ, Neef P, Caimi M, et al: New in vivo measurements of pressures in the intervertebral disc in daily life. *Spine (Phila Pa 1976)* 24(8):755–762, 1999.

REFERENCES

The complete reference list is available online at expertconsult.com.

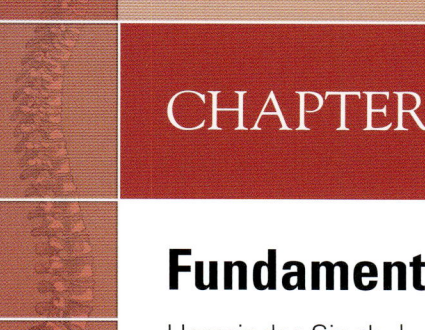

CHAPTER 25

Fundamentals of Spine Surgery

Harminder Singh | James S. Harrop

Decision-Making Process

Clinical decision making is one of the most challenging tasks for any physician, particularly for spine surgeons. Multiple factors influence the surgical and medical decision-making process. Although the patient is the surgeon's first priority, other factors such as financial and social pressures also must be taken into consideration. This chapter addresses some of the fundamentals of this process, including patient selection, informed consent, surgical planning, biomechanics, technology, and medical economics.

Patient Selection

Patient selection is the most important and difficult task in the surgical treatment of spine disorders. A technically perfect operation in the wrong patient might fulfill the surgical goals of the procedure but is unlikely to resolve the patient's initial complaints and deficits. Unfortunately, a proper study investigating the indications for spine surgery is not only difficult to design but also equally difficult to execute.

The Spine Patient Outcome Research Trial (SPORT) highlights some of the difficulties in executing a randomized, multicentric trial.[1-3] SPORT was the first comprehensive study to look at different ways of treating low back and leg pain and the effectiveness of those treatments. Even though this was a prospective, randomized trial, the amount of crossover between the surgical and nonsurgical arms ultimately rendered the analyses nonrandomized. Additionally, blinding was not possible in a surgical trial, which could have also introduced several confounders into the analyses.

Consequently, there is little evidence to guide the spine surgeon concerning operative indications, techniques, and timing of surgery. This lack has impeded the ability of physicians to collect and analyze clinically relevant data. Without such data to guide clinical decision making, the problem of patient selection and management strategy determination will remain difficult.

Previous attempts at analyzing the natural history and postsurgical outcome of spine disorders have yielded equivocal results, primarily because most studies were done retrospectively, and the data generated were, at best, level 2 or 3 evidence. Currently, there is a drive in the spine community to provide more prospective analyses, comparing treatment strategies along with outcome analyses using recognized scales, such as the Oswestry Low Back Pain Disability Questionnaire and the 36-Item Short Form Health Survey (SF-36). These analyses report patient satisfaction and quality of life after procedures, rather than fusion rate and neurologic recovery. The former are the ultimate goals and the true determinants of treatment efficacy.

In addition to increasing patient satisfaction and quality of life, other factors such as personal or financial considerations, defensive practice strategies, and third-party payers have motivated surgeons to address the challenges and difficulties of patient selection. In particular, third-party payers are reluctant to reimburse physicians, hospitals, and patients for procedures that lack clear indications or documented evidence of efficacy. In the current environment of cost-containment, surgeons are increasingly pressured by outside influences to demonstrate that they practice safe and appropriate surgery, by documenting their surgical outcomes. Although the motivations that underlie these powerful forces often are not altruistic, it should be evident that the results of so-called outcome research will benefit both the patient and the surgeon.

The excellent design and timely execution of carotid endarterectomy studies such as the North American Symptomatic Carotid Endarterectomy Trial (NASCET) and the Asymptomatic Carotid Atherosclerosis Study (ACAS) provide a paradigm for the potential benefits of outcomes research.[4,5] These studies clearly defined objective criteria for surgical treatment, based on risk and benefit ratios. Although outcome assessment is obviously more straightforward for carotid endarterectomy than spine surgery, the carotid endarterectomy trials nevertheless serve as a reminder of the powerful influence such trials can exert on surgical practice. These trials not only have established the safety and efficacy of the procedure itself, but also have provided unambiguous guidelines for patient selection. However, the suboptimal prospective study of extracranial-to-intracranial bypass for ischemic stroke, which concluded that surgical treatment was less effective than medical therapy, does illustrate some weaknesses of this type of study.[6]

Newer studies such as the Carotid Revascularization Endarterectomy versus Stenting Trial (CREST) and the Carotid Occlusion Surgery Study (COSS) are using the prospective, randomized study design in an attempt to generate level 1 data to guide evidence-based medicine practices.

Consent for Surgery

When the surgeon's clinical judgment supports surgical treatment for a disorder, the traditional relationship between the patient and the surgeon has been such that the surgeon recommends surgery and the patient, if willing, agrees. The modern "legal" contract that attempts to formalize this interaction is the consent for surgery form. This form is used to document that the patient has agreed to allow the surgeon to perform an operation, with an understanding of the risks, benefits, and alternative treatment options. This form is what most patients and surgeons conceptualize as *consent for surgery*.

However, this consent for surgery form is not just a piece of paper. It manifests the patient's right to determine how he or she will be treated. Physicians' recognition of this distinction has led to a more thoughtful and meaningful agreement or consent that satisfies stringent ethical and legal requirements. This is what is referred to as *informed consent*.

Informed Consent

Patient autonomy, the most fundamental of all patients' rights, is portrayed through the informed consent. It is the permission a patient grants to a physician to administer a treatment. The patient should understand the rationale for the treatment, the alternatives to the treatment, the nature of the treatment, the intended result of the treatment and its chances for success, and the nature and risks of adverse consequences of the treatment. During the interval of informed consent, the physician is able to define the problem facing the patient, based on limited prospective studies, suspected natural history course, alternative treatments, and risks and benefits, along with the goals of surgical treatment. This conference also allows the physician to address any fears and expectations the patient might have about his or her disease process and possible treatment schemes.

In the context of clinical decision making, several objections have been raised regarding the logic, and even the possibility, of informed consent. The defense of the doctrine of informed consent is beyond the scope of this chapter. However, a few points in response to objections about informed consent are worthy of consideration. Some argue that because the physician possesses a superior knowledge of the medical situation and proposed procedures, the patient cannot properly decide about informed consent. This argument is based on a misconception that gives undue primacy to patient understanding. In fact, one's right not to be assaulted is not conditional on one's understanding of the motivation for the assault. In the context of clinical decision making, then, it seems reasonable to argue that a patient's limited understanding of the consequences of the choice does not abrogate the right to decide what is to be done.

Several studies have shown that patients often are unable to recall the content of the information that the physician conveyed during the session at which informed consent was supposedly obtained.[7-9] Sometimes these scenarios are the basis for legal claims against unsuspecting physicians, who are accused of not informing the patient adequately of potential complications. Physicians can avoid these confrontations by carefully documenting their conversations with patients and their families in the medical record, indicating both the time and the date of the conversation as evidence that it occurred before any intervention. Note that this documentation should be in addition to written patient consent. However, legal repercussions aside, the demonstration that patients often do not remember information provided by physicians is certainly not a logical argument against the virtue of informed consent. There are many instances in life when one is unable to recall the reasons or motivations for making even the most important decisions.

Finally, the patient should be afforded the right to make a decision that is *not* consistent with the best medical prognosis. Many factors must be considered in every medical decision. This is especially true of such an important decision as the one to undergo surgery, which is influenced by a wide array of circumstances and beliefs, such as occupation, lifestyle, state of health, family, and the patient's idea of what constitutes a life that is worth living.

Beyond Informed Consent

What informed consent implies, but does not explicitly state, is that medical decisions should be a cooperative effort involving the patient, his or her family, and the physician. This combined effort has the goal of effectively managing the patient's pathologic process in a timely and efficient manner. The fragile interaction between patient and physician in this decision process can be interrupted if the physician dominates the relationship. Physicians are, as would be expected, more knowledgeable than patients about medical matters. Therefore, the physician can influence the patient's decision by creating a sense of urgency or necessity to accept their preferred course of action. This manipulation of the decision usually is unconscious. The result is that a course of treatment is initiated that the patient may be hesitant or reluctant to pursue.

The responsibility of the physician is to help the patient make a decision that is truly in the patient's best interest, not simply the one that matches the physician's preference. Patients have a natural tendency to experience fear and intimidation if they choose to defy the physician's implied or stated wishes. This is not to say that the physician is obligated to refrain from stating or implying his or her preference, but, rather, that the patient should be made to feel comfortable to ask questions and participate actively in the decision-making process.

This process by which a decision is reached, and the decision itself, should be documented in the medical record, and the time and date should be recorded. This serves to protect the physician in case of future litigation, and to solidify in the physician's mind the rationale for the course of action that is taken. The importance of engaging the patient in the process of clinical decision making cannot be overemphasized.

Surgical Considerations

Spinal Anatomy and Biomechanics

Once the physician and the patient have decided to pursue surgical treatment of the spine disorder, the surgeon must define the goal of the procedures and a course to obtain that goal. A surgical approach and objectives are defined during this interval. Because of the lack of prospective data on surgical treatments, the spine surgeon often must rely on personal experiences, along with common sense, in the treatment of spine disorders.

Spine surgeons have a fund of knowledge that is based on common teachings and practice. Included in this knowledge base is a basic understanding of what may be termed the fundamentals of spinal surgery, which includes spinal anatomy and biomechanics. It is efficient for the surgeon to think in terms of principles. To illustrate how spinal anatomy and biomechanics can be applied to the process of clinical decision making, 10 principles of spinal biomechanics, and their implications for clinical practice, are listed here:

- **Principle 1.** *The ventral surgical approach is generally the preferred approach in patients with a loss of cervical lordosis.* The ventral approach decompresses ventral mass and tends to preserve the dorsal tension band. This minimizes the risk of further kyphotic deformation. Conversely, the dorsal approach is relatively contraindicated in patients with a loss of cervical lordosis, because it weakens the dorsal tension band, which tends to exacerbate progressive spinal deformity.
- **Principle 2.** *Dorsal distraction of the lumbar spine is an undesirable force application because it tends to produce a flattened back.* The loss of lordosis is not uncommon as a complication of lumbar spine surgery. The flattened back is a common cause of chronic low back pain, because it alters the normal spinal sagittal balance. Fortunately, this problem can nearly always be avoided if the surgeon obeys this principle.
- **Principle 3.** *With a dorsal fusion operation, a more dorsally placed fusion mass more effectively resists kyphotic deformation.* The dorsal fusion mass resists kyphotic deformity in direct proportion to the length of the moment arm through which it acts. The moment arm is defined as the distance between the fusion mass and the more ventrally located instantaneous axis of rotation (IAR). Therefore, the greater the distance from the fusion mass to the IAR, the longer the moment arm available for the resistance of kyphotic deformation.
- **Principle 4.** *The effectiveness of a spinal brace is inversely proportional to the axial distance between the spine and the inner shell of the brace, and is directly proportional to the length of the brace.* These relationships are explained by the theoretical principle that the efficacy of bracing is related to the cosine of the angle defined by the edge of the brace, the IAR at the unstable segment, and the long axis of the spine. The implication is that a long, tight-fitting spinal brace will result in more effective spinal stabilization than a short, loose-fitting brace.
- **Principle 5.** *In general, a ventrally placed short-segment fixation device should be applied in a compression mode.* This mode of force application allows the fixation device to share the axial load with its associated interbody strut. Conversely, when such an implant is placed in the distraction mode, there is an undesirable allocation of forces. In this case the spinal implant bears the entire load, which greatly increases the chance of implant failure. The principle of load sharing versus load bearing is a key principle in the practice of spinal stabilization.
- **Principle 6.** *Three-column spinal injury (circumferential injury) indicates overt spinal instability, which usually requires spinal stabilization.* This principle is based on the three-column theory of spinal stability. The three columns are divided into: (1) an anterior column, which consists of the ventral half of the vertebral body; (2) a middle column, which consists of the dorsal half of the vertebral body; and (3) a posterior column, which consists of all of those elements that are dorsal to the vertebral body. Interruption of any one, or even two, of these columns does not necessarily lead to spinal instability. However, significant interruption of all three columns almost invariably destabilizes the spine. In these cases, surgical spinal stabilization helps protect the neural elements from initial or progressive injury, and facilitates early mobilization of the patient.
- **Principle 7.** *With time, spinal instrumentation will almost certainly fail without the acquisition of a concomitant bony fusion.* This principle emphasizes the limited role of spinal instrumentation in maintaining spinal alignment. As a corollary to this principle, it is often said that there is a race between spinal implant failure and the acquisition of a bony fusion. The implication is that the surgeon must be cognizant that the goal of spinal instrumentation is to maintain spinal alignment only as long as it takes to acquire an adequate fusion. It follows from this that the execution of a meticulous arthrodesis procedure is imperative.
- **Principle 8.** *Spinal decompression procedures that decompress the neural elements are performed at the expense of spinal stability.* This principle does not imply that neural element decompression (such as is accomplished by lumbar discectomy) invariably results in spinal instability. It should, however, serve as a reminder to the surgeon that the question of spinal stability must always be included in the process of surgical decision making and surgical planning. Appropriate measures must always be taken to avoid or to compensate for this problem. For example, a medial facetectomy greater than one-third the size of the facet tends to destabilize the joint, and may require an instrumented fusion.
- **Principle 9.** *Herniated midline thoracic discs usually should be approached ventrally though a thoracotomy.* Lateral extracavitary and transpedicular approaches to the thoracic spine allow for paramedian decompression of ventral elements. However, for midline ventral pathology (such as a herniated disc), a ventral approach though a thoracotomy is advisable because of the high rate of neurologic injury associated with dorsal decompression of ventral elements in the thoracic spine. The significant rate of postoperative neurologic deficits after laminectomy for thoracic disc herniation is thought to be due to a combination of vascular insufficiency and microcontusions secondary to spinal cord manipulation.[10]
- **Principle 10.** *Closed reduction of cervical spine dislocations entails "recreating" the mechanism of injury while applying traction.* This helps to unlock the facets and allows them to fall back into realignment. For example, in the case of bilateral jumped facets secondary to hyperflexion, the neck must be maintained in flexion while traction forces are applied to achieve successful reduction. Similarly, for a unilateral jump, the rotational forces of the mechanism of injury must be recreated for the facets to unlock.

And, finally, the golden rule: The surgeon should violate any of the aforementioned principles if they conflict with more reasonable or more general principles, or if they conflict with what is obvious (common sense).

Technology and the Spine

There is concern regarding the increasing application of spinal instrumentation, for which few supporting clinical data are available. The increasingly rapid development of expensive implants, with little documented efficacy, should cause surgeons to pause and reflect on basic surgical goals and principles. Typically, goals include neural decompression, the acquisition of surgical spinal stability, and the correction of spinal deformity. These goals should be formulated with no emphasis on using newer technology or techniques. Therefore, the surgeon should not formulate the surgical goals based on how he or she can use technology to benefit the patient. Rather, the directive of the treatment should be what is best for the patient, and only secondarily on the technology that best achieves this goal.

Economics

Managed care and third-party payers have directed physicians to analyze costs and benefits not only for the individual patient, but also for society as a whole, while still achieving the highest quality of care for the individual. Society aims to achieve a health care system with the highest value to the individual, in which value is equated to quality, divided by cost:

$$\text{Value} = \text{quality/cost}$$

In spine surgery, the quality of patient care has improved drastically over the last several decades, because of a better understanding of biomechanical principles and the use of sophisticated spinal implants for stability augmentation during fusion. However, surgeons must be cognizant of the cost of spinal implants and the true quality (of life) these devices afford the patient. Does the use of a device that raises the cost of the implant 200% improve the quality twice as much? In most instances, the answer is: most likely not. Therefore, the overall value, based on the aforementioned equation, is decreased. This is not to say new technology should not be used, but, rather the surgeon should evaluate its indications and goals individually for each surgical procedure. Once again this emphasizes the importance of prospective outcome assessments to evaluate these devices in an unbiased manner.

Economic assessments in the spine surgery arena are difficult, because so many treatment options and strategies are available. The managed-care environment is based on the objective of cost-containment, which emphasizes economic efficiency at the expense of clinical outcome. Therefore, surgery may be underused because of its high cost. Unfortunately, this fails to recognize the overall goal of achieving high quality and of the value of health care for the patient. A dangerous situation may be created in this manner (i.e., clinical decisions may be predominantly motivated by cost, rather than by value). Ultimately, physicians and payers must assess both cost and quality to establish an appropriate approach to patient management.

The importance of clinical outcome studies can never be overemphasized; however, as with any research material, their results should not be taken for granted. This unquestioning acceptance could happen in a health care system that is driven solely by cost and not value or quality of health care. Conversely, the quality of a health care service cannot be assumed just because the service is expensive. Physicians should strive to be cost-effective, and simultaneously to produce high-quality outcomes, which results in higher quality of care for the patient and society. If cost and quality of information were available for large populations of patients with well-defined medical problems, who received care via similar medical management algorithms, both quality and cost-efficiency could be assessed and, therefore, optimized.

The use of actuarial-derived data as the sole determinant influencing clinical decision making is ill-advised and perhaps dangerous, because it is based only on cost and resource use. The following example illustrates this point:

> *A surgical procedure is chosen on the basis of actuarial-derived data, to be "optimally performed" at an annual rate of 50 procedures per 100,000 cared lives. In the managed care environment "optimally performed" is defined as the lowest achievable utilization rates. However, the annual community surgical rate for this procedure is 100 procedures per 100,000 cared lives. The implication of this discrepancy is that the community surgery rate is twice what it should be (100 procedures versus 50).*

This analysis fails to take into account two very important factors: (1) the quality of clinical outcome, and (2) financial savings associated with surgery via indirect costs. (Indirect costs are defined as costs that cannot be specifically traced to an individual service or product.)

The maximization of net revenue and the minimization of the cost of operative management are important to the spine surgeon. An analysis of the overall cost of a procedure must consider not only the cost of performing the procedure (direct costs), but also the cost of *not* performing the procedure (hidden cost or indirect costs). The determination of the savings associated with not performing a procedure is not as simple as computing the cost of the procedure. The surgical procedure may obviate the need for additional nonsurgical care, which may be more costly than the operation alone. The actuarial-derived data (on which many attempts at cost-containment are based) merely provide information about the number of procedures performed (and secondarily, their direct costs). What is not readily obvious is that if surgery were not performed, nonsurgical management would be provided instead, at an additional cost (indirect). The economic relationship between surgical and nonsurgical care may be depicted as follows:

Cost of surgical management = surgical management costs + *routine* nonsurgical management costs

Cost of nonsurgical management = *routine* nonsurgical management costs + *additional* nonsurgical management costs*

Savings associated with surgical management = additional nonsurgical management costs (i.e., performed in lieu of surgery when surgery was not performed) − surgical management costs

*Hidden cost is associated with not performing an operative procedure.

The withholding of surgical treatment eliminates the cost of surgical management. However, the indirect and hidden cost must be calculated, along with social costs (e.g., loss of work and function), before the actuarial data–derived treatment can be declared a strategy success, from both a financial and a social perspective. The hidden costs and indirect costs associated with additional nonsurgical management also must be considered in the overall financial benefit. The aforementioned example can be extended further to emphasize this point:

> *Assume that 50 of the 100 patients who normally would have undergone surgery did not undergo the procedure. Of the 50 patients denied surgery, assume 25 received nonsurgical care that was more expensive than the surgical care (e.g., physical therapy, pain management schemes, and chiropractic treatments for the management of a cervical disc herniation). In this scenario we may conclude that the so-called optimal rate of surgery was not cost-effective. If we assume that the cost of additional nonsurgical management for the remaining patients was less expensive than surgical care would have been, the surgical rate that results in the minimum overall cost is about 75 cases per 100,000 cared lives per year, not 50.*

The analysis previously described considers neither quality of patient care, nor outcome or value. It is merely a cost analysis that considers the effects of savings. However, if surgeons can demonstrate cost-effective and favorable outcomes, then patients, third-party payers, and surgeons all stand to benefit.

Summary

Clinical decision making in spine surgery is affected by myriad influences. This chapter has attempted to describe only a few of these influences. The surgeon should be aware of the complexities that affect such important decisions as informed consent, the use of technology, patient selection, surgical planning, and cost. In the presence of an ever-increasing number of threatening influences, surgeons must remain focused on their principal goal of optimizing patient care.

KEY REFERENCES

Byrne DJ, Napier A, Cuschieri A: How informed is signed consent? *Br Med J* 296:839–840, 1988.

Executive Committee for the Asymptomatic Carotid Atherosclerosis Study: endarterectomy for asymptomatic carotid artery stenosis. *JAMA* 273:1421–1428, 1995.

Herz DA, Looman JE, Lewis LK: Informed consent: is it a myth? *Neurosurgery* 30:453–458, 1992.

North American Symptomatic Carotid Endarterectomy Trial Collaborators: Beneficial effect of carotid endarterectomy in symptomatic patients with high-grade carotid stenosis. *N Engl J Med* 325:445–453, 1991.

Surgery vs non-operative treatment for lumbar disk herniation: the Spine Patient Outcomes Research Trial: a randomized trial. *JAMA* 296(20):2441–2450, 2006.

REFERENCES

The complete reference list is available online at expertconsult.com.

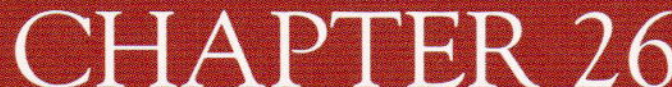

CHAPTER 26

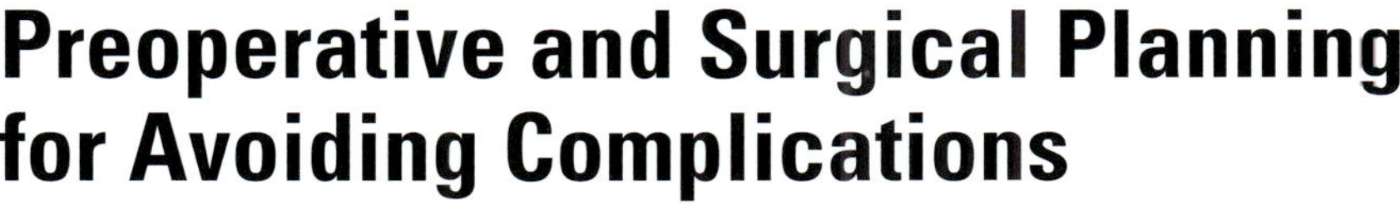

Preoperative and Surgical Planning for Avoiding Complications

Mehmet Zileli | Sait Naderi | Edward C. Benzel

Technical complications in spine surgery usually arise from the overaggressive handling of soft tissue or from hardware "failure" (when hardware "fails," the cause of the "failure" usually rests squarely on the shoulders of the surgeon). Other reasons for complications include poor patient selection, incorrect diagnosis, ill-chosen approach, inadequate operation (e.g., incomplete decompression of a compressive lesion), and injury to normal anatomic structures.

The surgeon should have clearly established a diagnosis and a clear, three-dimensional understanding of the pathologic anatomy, as demonstrated by imaging studies. Finally, an astute surgeon should use common sense by measuring twice, cutting once, and paying meticulous attention to detail.

General Precautions

Antibiotics

The role of preoperative and perioperative antibiotics in spine surgery remains controversial. The average infection rate for spine operations is relatively low. Evidence suggests that the incidence of infections may be decreased further if antibiotics are administered before the operation.[1-4] Indeed, a review of the literature provides support for the use of perioperative antibiotics.[2] Because the most frequently detected organism is a *Staphylococcus* species, a first-generation cephalosporin is usually satisfactory, unless an allergic propensity is recognized.[5]

Steroids

The role of perioperative steroids in spine surgery is also controversial. The administration of steroids before spinal cord injury confers greater benefit than administration after injury.[5,6] Although the literature is inconclusive, some surgeons choose to administer 4 to 8 mg of dexamethasone (or an equivalent dosage of methylprednisolone) preoperatively and to continue steroid administration for 24 hours postoperatively in high-risk cases. Because the short-term use of steroids is effective in experimental studies[6,7] and long-term administration is associated with an increased risk of complications, its use for more than 24 hours seems unnecessary (and possibly harmful).

Intubation

Neck positioning during intubation is important in patients with cervical spinal cord compression. C1-2 extension is most commonly associated with intubation and is usually well tolerated by the patient. In patients with severe stenosis at or above the level of C3-4, intubation with fiberoptic guidance, while the patient is awake and under local anesthesia, is usually preferred. Preoperative skull or halter traction may facilitate intubation and surgery by providing gentle traction and extension. Some surgeons suggest that patients with severe cervical myelopathy should be positioned before the induction of general anesthesia.[1]

Positioning

Numerous complications are associated with improper positioning, including air embolism, quadriplegia, peripheral nerve palsies, pyriformis syndrome, posterior compartment syndrome, and excessive bleeding.

Elastic bandages or sequential compression devices should be placed on the lower extremities before the induction of anesthesia. The legs must not be lower than the hips in the sitting position. Great care should be taken in moving the patient to the prone position. Three-point skull fixation in the prone position may be used, although it can be associated with a variety of complications (generally minor).

Extreme rotation, extension, or flexion of the head may cause cervical spinal cord damage. Older patients with cervical spondylotic bars are more prone to this complication. Awake positioning, awake intubation, and evoked-potential monitoring may be helpful. Loss of somatosensory evoked potentials, with neck flexion and recovery with repositioning, has been reported.[8] In patients with severe spinal canal narrowing, the neutral or near-neutral position is preferred.

A stretch injury of the brachial plexus may occur in both the prone and supine positions by abducting the arm greater than 90 degrees. An axillary roll should be used to prevent injury, with the lateral decubitus position when the dependent arm is compressed. The ulnar nerve could be injured because of its superficial position at the elbow. A pad under an extended elbow helps prevent this injury. Elbow extension minimizes exposure of the ulnar nerve to compression. The radial nerve may be injured if the arm hangs over the operating table edge. Padding under the arm may prevent compression injury. Common peroneal nerve injury with resulting footdrop may occur in the supine, the sitting, and the lateral decubitus positions. The superficial location of the nerve at the head of the fibula may increase the risk of compression. The superficial femoral nerve may be compressed in the prone position and cause a postoperative transient meralgia paresthetica.

Compression and stretch injury of any nerve is possible during positioning. A general rule of thumb is to use a position without excessive compression of the extremities and to place appropriate pads beneath potentially exposed nerves. If the patient appears comfortable, nerve injury is less likely. Injury to the lateral femoral cutaneous nerve has been reported to be as high as 20%.[9] External pressure at the anterior superior iliac spine during prone position is the main reason for the injury of the nerve. The nerve can also be injured at the retroperitoneum by hematoma or traction, as well as during bone graft harvesting at the ventral iliac crest.

Compression of the eyes, with resulting blindness, has been reported with the use of the horseshoe headrest.[10-12] The head should be positioned to prevent it from slipping on the horseshoe headrest. Three-point skull fixation is a viable alternative to the horseshoe and should significantly reduce the incidence of this complication.

Air Embolism

Air embolism is one of the most serious complications encountered. It is predominantly related to operations performed above the level of the heart.[13] Two precautions to avoid air embolism are suggested: (1) if possible, avoid the sitting position; and (2) monitor the patient at risk meticulously with Doppler ultrasound and end-tidal P_{CO_2}. In such patients a central venous catheter should be used so that if an air embolism is detected, air can be emergently evacuated from the right atrium. The central venous pressure should be maintained at greater than 10 cm, so that the pressure in epidural veins does not decline.

One should not administer nitrous oxide when using the sitting position. The incidence and clinical importance of air embolism is greater in the sitting position than in other positions.[14] Its incidence has been reported to be as high as 50%.[13] If air embolism occurs, a central venous catheter may be used to withdraw air from the left atrium. At the same time, the surgeon should flood the wound with Ringer solution and inspect and control any open veins with bipolar coagulation. Bleeding bone surfaces should be treated with wax, and the wound should be precisely packed with wet gauze. If signs of air embolism persist, the patient should quickly be placed in a side-lying position, with the right side facing up, to aid the removal of air via the central venous catheter from the right atrium.

Paradoxic Air Embolism

A patent foramen ovale, or another right-to-left shunting, causes paradoxic air embolism. It is optimally prevented by an accurate preoperative diagnosis with an echocardiogram. Saline injection during echocardiography (if performed) is suggested for the patients in whom a sitting-position operation is considered. If shunting from the right atrium to the left atrium is encountered, the sitting position should not be used.[15] If the patient is placed in the sitting position, positive end-expiratory pressure should not be used, because it increases the right atrial pressure, which increases the risk of paradoxic air embolism. In this case, air may enter the cerebral arteries, resulting in coma, quadriplegia, or death.

Doppler and End-Tidal CO_2 Monitoring

Both Doppler and end-tidal CO_2 monitoring are useful in all sitting-position operations. Although the Doppler is not necessarily a vital monitoring technique (i.e., it may show very small volumes of air that do not change P_{CO_2} and vital signs), the surgeon should immediately search for a source of air entrance into the venous system. If a vessel is identified, it should be coagulated. If not, the wound should temporarily be packed with wet sponges. If the end-tidal CO_2 drops, the wound must be packed. If hemodynamic stability is diminished, the wound must be closed.

Intravascular Volume Control

Central and arterial lines should be placed preoperatively if there is a risk of excessive bleeding. If the sitting position is used, adequate hydration of the patient is imperative. If sympathetic tone is diminished or lost as a result of severe spinal cord compression, a central catheter should be placed. The sitting position in such patients is particularly troublesome.

Intraoperative Radiographs

Intraoperative imaging can ensure the correct level of the operation and may provide information about the degree of decompression, realignment, or stabilization.

Incidental Durotomy, Cerebrospinal Fluid Fistula, and Pseudomeningocele

Unintended tear of the dura mater is a common complication of spine surgery. Its incidence has been reported between 3.1% and 14% in different series.[16-18] Immediately after surgery, a tear causes headaches, wound infection, and cerebrospinal fluid (CSF) fistulae. In the long-term, persistent CSF leakage, pseudomeningocele, neurologic deficit, and arachnoiditis are common problems associated with durotomy.[16] The tear should be better recognized and treated appropriately.

CSF leakage may cause wound dehiscence and subsequent infection. If the fistula is substantial, fluctuations in conscious state may be observed.[19] In fact, an intracranial hemorrhage may develop.[20] After ventral cervical spine surgery, the fistula may even cause airway obstruction,[21] and after ventral or dorsolateral surgery of the thoracic spine, it may even cause a subarachnoid-pleural fistula.[22,23]

Fibrin sealants may be used to prevent leakage. They are biologically derived substances consisting of fibrinogen solution and thrombin, with a calcium cofactor.[24] They are used as adhesives to augment other layers of closure. A retrospective review of fibrin sealants noted that the incidence of postoperative CSF leaks and tension pneumocranium was reduced, while also reducing overall management costs.[24] Nakamura et al.[25] have found that autologous fibrin tissue adhesive was superior to that of commercial fibrin tissue adhesive in terms of cost.

CSF cutaneous fistula and pseudomeningocele are end-stage complications of an improperly treated dural tear. Because these complications may lead to increased morbidity, increased cost, increased pain, and increased neurologic deficit, they must be treated properly and aggressively.[26] The first priority is to implement CSF diversion (i.e., external lumbar drainage). A percutaneous blood patch may also be used. A revision surgery to repair the dural defect may also be indicated. If a pseudomeningocele is noted and the leakage of CSF persists, it may become necessary to perform dural and myofascial closure via an open reoperation surgical procedure. In difficult cases, a shunt (possibly lumboperitoneal shunt) may also be necessary.

Graft Donor Site Complications

If a graft has been taken from dorsal iliac crest, possible complications are superior gluteal artery injury, sciatic nerve injury, or deep wound infection, among others. If the donor site is the ventral iliac crest, donor site herniation, meralgia paresthetica, and pelvic fracture may result.[27]

Thromboembolism

Venous thromboembolic disease, including deep vein thrombosis and pulmonary embolism, is a serious and potentially life-threatening complication in spine surgery. In a recent meta-analysis, the prevalence of deep vein thrombosis was 1.09%, and the prevalence of pulmonary embolism was 0.06% following elective spine surgery.[28] The use of pharmacologic prophylaxis significantly reduced the prevalence of deep vein thrombosis relative to no prophylaxis ($P < 0.01$).

In a recent retrospective study conducted by the Scoliosis Research Society,[29] the complication rate in 9692 lumbar microdiscectomies was 3.6%. In anterior cervical discectomy and fusion, the complication rate was 2.4%, and with 10,329 lumbar stenosis decompressions, it was 7%. Overall rates of pulmonary embolism were 1.38%, death due to pulmonary embolism 0.34%, and deep vein thrombosis 1.18%.[29]

Operative Technique

General techniques for complication avoidance include (1) adequate visualization, (2) use of a high-speed drill, (3) use of microcurettes with varying angles and sizes, and (4) adequate positioning. The decision to operate, the approach, the operative technique, and the use of internal fixation and fusion are all important considerations.

Upper Cervical Spine: Complication Avoidance

The reducibility of a subluxation is a critically important consideration for upper cervical spine pathologic processes. If the lesion is reducible, only a dorsal fixation and fusion procedure may be indicated. If the lesion is not reducible, the optimal operation depends on the localization of the compression. For an extradural lesion located between the midclivus and the C3 vertebral body, a transoral approach may provide the trajectory and exposure of choice. If the lesion is intradural, a dorsal or lateral transcondylar approach may be more appropriate. Complex pathologic lesions with lateral extension that are located between the C1 and midcervical levels may involve a transmandibular, transglossal approach. For more limited pathologic lesions located between the lower clivus and the C2 vertebral body, a ventrolateral or ventromedial retropharyngeal approach may be appropriate. In general, if stabilization is required, a dorsal or lateral transcondylar approach with instrumentation should be considered.

Transoral Approach

Cerebrospinal Fluid Fistula

For intradural pathology, a lateral, transcondylar, or dorsal approach is associated with a significantly lower risk of a CSF fistula, compared with the transoral approach. If the latter approach is used and a CSF leak occurs, the dural leaves may be covered with fascia and fibrin glue. A lumbar drain is usually placed postoperatively to treat a CSF fistula.

Severe Tongue Swelling

Intermittent release of the tongue retractor can be used to minimize tongue swelling. Other methods to avoid tongue swelling include the intravenous administration of dexamethasone and postoperative massaging of the tongue to reconstitute venous and lymphatic flow.[30] Patients who are prone to tongue swelling should not be extubated prior to the complete resolution of the tongue swelling itself.

Hemorrhage

Because bleeding may accumulate in a deep and narrow wound, meticulous hemostasis is imperative. The careful control of bleeding should be maintained throughout the operation. Injury to the vertebral artery may require clipping or compression occlusion of the artery.

Meningitis

Meningitis is commonly associated with intradural operations. Mouth irrigation with an antibiotic solution may be used preoperatively for 2 to 3 days, after preoperative cultures of the oropharynx are obtained. Intraoperatively, the mouth is swabbed with povidone-iodine (Betadine) solution. The presence of a retropharyngeal abscess is a contraindication to surgery. In patients with meningitis, postoperative antimicrobial therapy is administered.

Retropharyngeal Abscess and Palatal and Pharyngeal Wound Dehiscence

In the presence of late wound dehiscence, a retropharyngeal abscess should be sought. Palatal and pharyngeal wound dehiscence is often related to inadequate wound closure. If complications develop, they commonly occur 1 week after the operation.

Neurologic Worsening and Instability

Neurologic worsening is often related to inadequate decompression. It may also be caused by loss of alignment or an iatrogenic injury. Injury during surgical positioning or intubation may be avoided by the use of fluoroscopy during positioning and an awake fiberoptic intubation. Instability can be investigated with postoperative dynamic (flexion/extension) radiographs. If instability is present, an occipitocervical fusion may be necessary.[30]

Median Labiomandibular Glossotomy

Median labiomandibular glossotomy is a very morbid operation that requires a preoperative tracheotomy or the maintenance of tracheal intubation, until the edema of the tongue, palate, and pharynx resolves. If the dura mater is opened, meticulous closure with the application of fibrin glue is useful to avoid CSF fistulae and resulting meningitis. To obtain optimal cosmetic results, the assistance of a plastic surgeon may be appropriate.

Transcervical Retropharyngeal Approach

Hypoglossal nerve injury and carotid artery injury are commonly observed with a transcervical retropharyngeal approach. To avoid intraoperative stroke via embolization, some surgeons use preoperative angiography or Doppler examination of the carotid artery.[30]

Lateral Transcondylar Approach

The most feared complications of the lateral transcondylar approach are vertebral artery injury, air embolism, CSF leakage, and hypoglossal nerve injury. Appropriate decompression and protection of the vertebral artery minimizes the risk of injury. Air embolism may be prevented by the previously mentioned neuroanesthetic techniques. To prevent CSF leakage, an inverted J-shaped incision may provide a more precise closure of the muscle flaps than that achieved with a paramedian vertical incision. A CSF fistula is a less common and less serious complication of this procedure, compared with the transoral approach. The hypoglossal nerve injury is another complication of the transcondylar approach. The hypoglossal nerve may be injured during a condylectomy procedure. A preoperative bone window and CT images of the occipital condyle may help localize the hypoglossal canal and its inner and outer orifices.

Subaxial Cervical Spine: Complication Avoidance

Surgical intervention in a patient with a complete traumatic spinal cord lesion and overt instability may be necessary to reestablish spinal stability. Systemic complications of trauma such as hypotension, respiratory difficulties, and metabolic derangements should be well controlled before embarking on a stabilization procedure.

For cervical spondylotic pathologies, the shape of the cervical curvature should be considered in deciding on the operative approach. In general, cervical kyphosis is a specific indication for a ventral approach, to avoid postoperative instability[31] and to provide adequate ventral decompression.[32]

Often, intradural tumors are optimally approached dorsally, whereas vertebral body tumors are best approached ventrally. A burst or wedge fracture with spinal canal compromise is best approached ventrally. However, severe three-column instability may require both a ventral and a dorsal approach. The indications for the ventrolateral approach are laterally situated tumors, nerve root decompression,[33,34] and the rarely observed symptomatic vertebral artery compression.

Potential Injuries Associated with Ventral Approaches

Spinal Cord Damage

To avoid spinal cord damage, attention should be paid to (1) patient positioning, (2) illumination and visualization, (3) anesthetic and surgical techniques, (4) position of the surgeon, and (5) evoked-potential monitoring. It is perhaps best to place the patient in a neutral position, although mild extension may aid exposure. Care must be taken to avoid hyperextension, which may cause or exacerbate already existing spinal cord compression. Neurologic examination of the awake patient in a test-extension posture before surgery may help avoid neurologic injury related to positioning.

For optimum illumination and visualization, an operating microscope may help avoid injury to neural and vascular structures, especially in narrow surgical fields, such as those associated with the transoral approach.[35-38]

An anesthetic technique without paralytic agents may be useful to monitor motor responses from unwanted irritation of the spinal cord or nerve roots. Only bipolar coagulation should be used. It may help to avoid using Kerrison rongeurs for bone removal and instead to use a Leksell rongeur or a high-speed drill—to minimize the incidence of neural injury. Curettes may be used for the last pieces of bone. To avoid injury to the spinal cord and nerve roots, the graft should not be pushed into the recess with great force, and its depth should not be greater than 13 mm.

Frequently, the surgeon inadvertently obtains a more extensive decompression on the side opposite the side of the approach.[39] This complication may be prevented either by working alternately from both sides of the patient or by using the correct angle of view of the operating microscope.

Although evoked-potential monitoring is controversial, its use is considered helpful by some surgeons.[40,41]

Cervical Nerve Root Injury

A cervical nerve root may be injured during far-lateral dissection as a part of the ventrolateral approaches. Therefore, lateral dissection should not be performed dorsal to the anterior tubercle of transverse process.

C5 Radiculopathy

The C5 motor nerve root is most frequently adversely affected by surgery. This may occur in association with both ventral and dorsal operations. Because its mechanism of injury is not well understood, its prevention is also controversial. It has been suggested that excessively wide exposures result in tethering of the nerve roots. Saunders[42] recommends that the ventral cervical decompression should not exceed 15 to 16 mm in diameter, because an excessive degree of spinal cord displacement may cause traction on a relatively fixed cervical nerve root. The natural history of this complication is spontaneous resolution in most cases.[42]

Dural Tears

Dural tears, CSF fistulae, and pseudomeningoceles may occur, especially in cases of ossification of the posterior longitudinal ligament (OPLL) or severe trauma. Using good illumination, the operating microscope, and diamond-tip burrs in the vicinity of the dura mater may decrease the frequency of these complications. Of note, the posterior longitudinal ligament thins out laterally, and therefore the spinal cord is relatively less protected in this region.

If a violation of the dura mater occurs, repair from a ventral approach is not always possible. A tear is best managed with a piece of fascia with hemostatic gelatin (Gelfoam) and fibrin glue application, with a lumbar drain placed postoperatively (for 48 to 72 hours). If the dura mater has been excised, a Gelfoam and fascia application under the bone graft, without suturing, together with lumbar drainage, may be used. Prophylactic insertion of a lumbar drain before surgery should be considered in high-risk patients.

Major Vessel Injury

Brachiocephalic Vein Injury

The brachiocephalic vein may bleed during dissection for low cervical and upper thoracic inlet exposures.

Vertebral Artery Injury

Vertebral artery injury occurs in approximately 1% of cases and is usually caused by lateral use of the cutting burrs. The surgeon should respect the midline. Longus colli muscles and uncovertebral joints are the key structures for the identification of the midline. Because the uncinate processes are the lateral borders of the spinal canal, bony removal or dissection lateral to the uncinate processes may cause damage to the vertebral artery and nerve roots. Therefore, the uncinate processes should be clearly defined, and careful high-speed drilling of the uncinate processes should be just medial to the vertebral artery.

Ventral cervical bone resection should not be carried out wider than 18 to 20 mm. The medial border of the foramen transversarium from one side to the opposite side is 30 mm. An anomalous position of the vertebral artery should be carefully sought on the preoperative CT and MRI scans. During the ventrolateral approach, the vertebral artery may be displaced laterally with a narrow-tipped retractor, but not more than 1 to 2 mm.[38]

If an injury develops, it may be controlled by application of Gelfoam or bone wax. However, to see if a pseudoaneurysm has developed, a postoperative angiography should be performed.[43] It may be treated using an endovascular approach.

Carotid Artery Injury

The risk of carotid artery injury is greater with a ventrolateral approach than with the more common ventromedial approach. To avoid an injury to the carotid artery and internal jugular vein, it is necessary to identify the artery before retraction, to retract the artery laterally without opening its sheath, and to place the blades of the self-retaining retractors under the longus colli muscles. Inspection of the carotid sheath and the jugular vein should be conducted before closure to detect inadvertent injury of these structures.

Dysphagia

Dysphagia after ventral cervical surgery is a known entity. The reported incidence and prevalence of postoperative dysphagia and risk factors associated with its development vary widely in the literature. In a systematic review of a total of 126 articles,[44] the rates of dysphagia were too high just after surgery and it declined at 1 year to a range of 13% to 21%. Risk factors were multilevel surgery and female sex.

Esophagus and Trachea Injury

Injury to the esophagus is a rare but life-threatening complication that may result in disastrous consequences, including septicemia, mediastinitis, pneumonia, and meningitis. Some authorities suggest the use of finger dissection, rather than a sharp dissection, below the superficial cervical fascia. The surgeon should be aware of any preoperative problems with esophageal dysmotility (observed in 10% of patients, mostly in the elderly). In addition, he or she should avoid injury to the pharyngeal muscles during dissection in the upper cervical region. During lengthy operations, it may be necessary to release the medial blades regularly to avoid esophageal necrosis. The surgeon should conduct inspection of the esophagus and the trachea before closure, to detect inadvertent injury to these structures. Graft dislocations or implant failure with loosened screws may also cause perforation of the esophagus.[45,46]

Fiberoptic endoscopy is the procedure of choice to detect injury to the esophagus or trachea. Esophageal motility films may also help in the diagnosis. If leakage from the wound arouses suspicion a few days after surgery, one can simply have the patient drink methylene blue and look for that color in drainage fluid.

Broad-spectrum antibiotics and primary repair form the basis of management in early cases. In delayed cases, however, it may not be possible to place primary sutures to the esophagus. In case of a perforation with abscess formation, incision and drainage, broad-spectrum antibiotics, and opening a gastrostomy should be instituted. If the infection has subsided, suturing and covering the defect with a myofascial flap may be applied.

Recurrent Laryngeal Nerve Injury

Hoarseness after surgery is usually related to traction of the recurrent laryngeal nerve. It occurs in 3% to 11% of patients. It is usually transient. The recurrent laryngeal nerve passes under the subclavian artery on the right side and under the aorta on the left side. Although the right recurrent laryngeal nerve was thought to be more susceptible to stretch as midline structures are retracted, a recent study comparing the incidences of recurrent laryngeal nerve injury in right- and left-sided surgeries showed that there is no difference in incidence of recurrent laryngeal nerve injury with the side of surgical approach.[47] The same study also showed that reoperative surgery causes significantly more injuries than primary surgery.

Although recurrent laryngeal nerve palsy after ventral cervical spine surgery was thought to be the result of direct injury to the nerve, no data support this hypothesis. Apfelbaum et al.[32,35] have proven that the most common cause of vocal cord paralysis after ventral cervical spine surgery is compression of the recurrent laryngeal nerve within the endolarynx. We recommend monitoring the endotracheal cuff pressure and release after retractor placement. In the series of Apfelbaum et al.[35] about instituting this maneuver, the rate of temporary paralysis has decreased from 6.4% to 1.69%.[16]

Excessive retraction of the medial structures may result in postoperative stridor, hoarseness, and dysphagia. A rare complication is an esophageal fistula. To prevent excessive medial retraction, the following suggestions are made: (1) rostral and caudal dissection should be greater than is needed, (2) retraction should be relaxed on an hourly basis, and (3) the medial retractor should be inserted under the longus colli muscles, if possible.

Hypoglossal Nerve Injury

Twelfth cranial nerve injury is rare, but possible, during high cervical dissections. Knowledge of its anatomy and course should minimize its injury. The hypoglossal nerve runs downward, lateral to the internal and external carotid arteries. Lateral to the occipital artery, the nerve usually turns forward a little above the level of the hyoid bone to disappear deep to the suprahyoid muscles. As it turns around the occipital artery, it gives off the superior root of the ansa cervicalis.

Thoracic Duct Injury

The thoracic duct is on the left side. Because this structure is located laterally, it is uncommon to injure the thoracic duct, at least in exposures medial to the sternocleidomastoid muscle.

Sympathetic Chain Injury

Injury to the sympathetic chain is associated with an ipsilateral Horner syndrome. It is usually attributed to dissection of the longus colli muscles too far from the midline. They are easily injured during the ventrolateral approach. The sympathetic chain is located between the carotid sheath and the longus colli muscles in the midcervical region. Lateral retraction of the longus colli muscle during transverse foramen or uncovertebral joint exposition at the lower cervical levels may injure the sympathetic chain.[48] Horner syndrome, visual symptoms, and an odd sense over the face may result. To avoid this complication, it is necessary to mobilize the sympathetic chain and longus colli muscle over the length of the exposure and insert the medial retraction blade after the lateral blades.

Excessive Bleeding

Excessive bleeding may arise from bone, epidural space, and posterior longitudinal ligament bleeding.

Because extensive bone waxing may prevent fusion, it is often better to use Gelfoam, even for bone bleeding. Bipolar coagulation and Gelfoam may be useful to control bothersome epidural bleeding. Venous bleeding from the plexus around the vertebral artery is a common nuisance. Care must be taken to avoid injury to the vertebral artery during control of venous bleeding.

Postoperative Hematoma

To prevent postoperative hematomas, suction drains may be kept in place for 24 hours postoperatively. The use of drains for this purpose, however, is controversial.

Graft Bed Preparation

If a fibular graft is to be used, the ventral width of the decompression should be no more than the greatest diameter of the graft to ensure a good lateral bony approximation.[38] This width is not usually necessary for the iliac crest graft, which may be fashioned to fit the decompression site.

Graft Dislocation

Allografts have a higher incidence of pseudarthrosis and an associated small risk of transmitting viral infections. Although autografts may also be complicated by pseudarthrosis, they are preferred in most instances. The graft should not be placed deeper than 13 mm. It should distract the intervertebral space approximately 2 mm and be recessed approximately 3 mm. Excessive end plate removal may increase the incidence of graft subsidence.

Graft dislocation may occur ventrally or dorsally. Dorsal dislocation is rare but more serious, because it may cause significant compression of the spinal cord. Partial graft extrusion is of little consequence and usually does not require treatment. Three technical considerations may help prevent graft dislocation:

1. Contour the graft into a shape that fits snugly into the mortise of the graft bed. The graft should be recessed so that the ventral cortical bone is a few millimeters dorsal to the ventral vertebral body. This border, however, should not be confused with the ventral vertebral osteophytes. An obsessive tailoring of grafts is appropriate.
2. Placement of a ventral cervical plate may help avoid graft dislocation.
3. Postoperative bracing may decrease the risk of graft dislocation.

Graft Pseudarthrosis

The pseudarthrosis rate, using different graft techniques, varies from 0% to 26%.[8,37,49,50] The risk of pseudarthrosis increases if more than one level is fused. If one long piece of cortical-cancellous graft or cortical bone is used, however, the risk is lower.[37,51] It should be emphasized that the presence of pseudarthrosis does not necessarily compromise the clinical results of surgery.[52]

Vertebral Avascular Necrosis

Avascular necrosis of the vertebrae is encountered with the use of grafts at individual interspaces.[11] The Cloward technique for a ventral cervical fusion at two adjacent levels may cause avascular necrosis. If a multilevel fusion is needed,

Cloward[52] suggests that a Smith-Robinson graft may be inserted at one disc level, and a bone dowel may be inserted at an adjacent level.[52]

Ventral Plating Complications

Screw breakage, plate breakage, esophageal erosion, pain, and difficulty swallowing may complicate the results of ventral plating. Many surgeons do not advocate placing a screw into a graft, for fear that such a screw may dislodge or weaken the graft.

Most patients should improve neurologically after surgery. If no improvement occurs but is expected, the use of CT or MRI is prudent. The most likely reason for lack of improvement is an inadequate decompression. It is common for a right-handed surgeon operating from the right side to leave residual compression on the right side. Another cause of failure to achieve neurologic improvement may be OPLL, which may easily be overlooked on the preoperative MRI scan. Obtaining a preoperative CT scan is helpful in ruling out the possibility of OPLL.

Dorsal Approaches

Neurologic Deterioration

Patients with cervical kyphosis are poor candidates for cervical laminectomy. A lordotic or neutral position is preferred. Instrumentation under the lamina in the cervical region can cause neurologic damage. The predominant risk during the keyhole foraminotomy is direct nerve root trauma. To avoid this, dissection should only be performed from the axilla of the root.

Lateral mass plating may also cause nerve root injury, and occasionally, vertebral artery injury. With transarticular screw fixation, if a vertebral artery injury is detected after a screw is placed, a second one should be placed. The screw causing the vertebral artery injury may be left in place. It may effectively serve to tamponade vertebral artery bleeding. Residual bleeding may be effectively managed with oxidized cellulose (Surgicel).

Postoperative Instability and Kyphosis

Respect for the facet joints and joint capsules is necessary to prevent postlaminectomy instability.[53] Two additional precautions may be taken to prevent this complication: (1) the use of laminoplasty instead of laminectomy may decrease the risk of instability (although this is not proven); and (2) lateral mass fixation and fusion may be carried out to prevent deformity, minimize instability, and decrease the movement associated with the degenerative process.

Cervicothoracic Junction (C7-T3): Complication Avoidance

Because degenerative diseases in this region are rare, and surgical indications most commonly consist of tumor, trauma, and infection, decision making is usually not difficult. Dorsal pathology located at the cervicothoracic junction is usually exposed with the standard dorsal midline approach.

Ventral approaches to the cervicothoracic junction are technically demanding. Because the kyphotic angle of the upper thoracic spine may compromise the surgical view, the need to access lesions at and below T1 and T2 necessitates a more caudal exposure than is afforded by the ventromedial cervical approach in most patients. Although surgery to the T3 vertebral body is feasible with the ventromedial approach, the surgical view is so limited that only a biopsy of a tumor or partial decompression may be possible. With adequate extension of the neck, it is possible to perform a T1-2 discectomy in nonobese patients with long necks. If only a partial decompression or biopsy without instrumentation is anticipated in a nonobese patient, the standard ventromedial cervical approach with mild neck extension is appropriate for ventral pathologies in the cervicothoracic region.

If, however, extensive resection, with or without instrumentation is required, an upper sternal osteotomy, with or without a medial claviculotomy, may be performed. Another option is transpleural thoracotomy through the fourth rib. Because the latter approach is associated with high morbidity, sternotomy is a last resort.

Ventral Surgery Complications

Recurrent Laryngeal Nerve Injury

When using a right-sided approach, the surgeon can identify the recurrent laryngeal nerve between the trachea and the esophagus. The right recurrent laryngeal nerve exits the carotid sheath at a variable level, coursing medially and entering the tracheoesophageal groove behind the upper pole of the thyroid gland. Because the highly variable course on this side increases the risk of injury, a left-sided approach for a cervicothoracic lesion is warranted.[54]

Thoracic Duct Injury

With left-sided incisions, the thoracic duct may be identified as it enters the dorsal aspect of the subclavian vein. Injury to thoracic duct results in chylothorax. If this occurs, the duct should be ligated.[54,55]

Major Vessel, Lung Apex, and Gland Injuries

Major vessel injury may occur via coarse tissue manipulation or excessive traction.[56,57] Lung apex injury may be detected by filling the wound with saline solution and applying positive-pressure ventilation. If a ventromedial exposure is used, the esophagus, trachea, and thyroid gland are susceptible to injury and should be carefully inspected before wound closure.

Brachial Plexus Injury

The brachial plexus may be injured during the transaxillary and supraclavicular approaches. Stretch injuries of the plexus may be sustained by improper surgical positioning. Meticulous attention paid to surgical positioning helps prevent the occurrence of these injuries. Any change in patient positioning during the course of surgery, whether inadvertent or intentional, should prompt a reevaluation of the patient's position.

Intercostal Neuralgia

Intercostal neuralgia may occur as a complication of the transaxillary injury. Incision of the nerve proximal to the dorsal root ganglion (disrupting the nerve by destroying the cell body) should eliminate this complication.

Chest Wall Deformity and Scar

Chest wall deformities and scars are particularly associated with transsternal and transmanubrial approaches. This must be considered during preoperative planning and when obtaining the patient's consent.

Thoracic, Lumbar, and Sacral Spine: Complication Avoidance

If thoracic, lumbar, and sacral lesions are completely dorsal, a dorsal approach with laminectomy is appropriate. A vertebral body lesion between L1 and L4 may be exposed via a retroperitoneal ventrolateral approach. If the lesion is located between the L5 and S1 levels, and a limited operation such as a biopsy or simple discectomy and interbody fusion is required, a pelvic brim extraperitoneal approach may be suitable. If the lesion is located between the L5 and S1 levels and requires extensive exposure (e.g., a high-grade spondylolisthesis or an L5 tumor), a direct ventral approach such as the transperitoneal approach may be suitable.

Dorsal Surgery Complications

Some of the complications frequently encountered during dorsal spine surgery were discussed previously in the section on dorsal cervical spine surgery. Neurologic deterioration, incidental durotomy, and postoperative instability can also be seen during dorsal, thoracic, and lumbar spine surgery.

The lateral extracavitary approach has been reported to have a high incidence rate (55%) of complications. Pulmonary complications are predominant.[58]

Instability and Deformity

Instability and deformity after surgery depend on the level and amount of decompression and preoperative instability. Disruption of the dorsal ligaments and facet capsules and extensive laminectomy are the main reasons for instability. Avoiding excessive facetectomy and laminectomy in children, as well as using alternative methods such as microdiscectomy and costotransversectomy may prevent postoperative instability.

Neurologic Deterioration

Many factors may cause neurologic deterioration during dorsal approaches to the thoracolumbar spine. In this regard, the insertion of hooks[31] or wires may injure and compress the spinal cord. In a study by Davne et al. examining the complication rates of pedicle screw fixation,[59] the neural injury rate was 1.1% and the technical problem rate was 8.1%.

Ventral Surgery Complications

To avoid complications during the thoracotomy or retroperitoneal approach, the surgeon should have a firm grasp of the retroperitoneal anatomy. The incidence of intraoperative soft tissue injuries is increased by the use of high-speed drills.

Pulmonary Injury

Atelectasis, pneumothorax, pneumonia, and pleural effusions may occur after thoracotomy. A tube thoracostomy may be necessary to treat these complications. It should be removed only after drainage diminishes significantly. A pneumothorax usually clears in 2 to 3 days.

Lumbar Sympathetic Plexus Injury

The lumbar sympathetic plexus, located on the lateral aspects of the lumbar vertebrae, consists of "line structures," which may be stretched and injured during ventral spine dissection. This injury often causes a "warm leg" on the ipsilateral site and reportedly occurs in 10% of ventral lumbar surgeries.[12] It usually resolves spontaneously.

Superior Hypogastric Plexus Injury

Superior hypogastric plexus injury may result in bladder dysfunction in females and either retrograde ejaculation or sterility, or both, in males. The superior hypogastric plexus is situated in the bifurcation of the aorta on the fifth lumbar vertebral body and the sacrum. This sympathetic plexus innervates the smooth muscles of the seminal vesicle, which contracts as the bladder neck closes during ejaculation. It also activates the transport of spermatozoa from the testes to the seminal vesicles. Thus, injury can cause a retrograde ejaculation and sterility. Although it is rare (0.42%),[60,61] careful dissection of the fascia ventral to the promontory and avoidance of electrocautery in this region may help prevent this complication.

Great Vessel Injury

Iliac vessel mobilization is usually difficult with retroperitoneal dissections at lower lumbar levels. Care should be taken to protect the iliolumbar veins that emerge from the iliac veins laterally. An experienced surgeon with an excellent knowledge of vascular anatomy is a prerequisite for ventral lumbar surgery. At the L5-S1 level, working between two iliac arteries and veins may be easier for disc surgery and cage insertion. However, L4-5 and upper levels sometimes need excessive retraction of great vessels. Fine retractors and meticulous use of high-speed drills are necessary for protection of the vessels.

Major vascular injury may also occur during a dorsal approach (lumbar disc surgery). The mortality of such complications may be as high as 50%.[56,62] Most frequently, vascular injury is caused by pituitary forceps during overaggressive disc resection. Up-angled pituitary forceps and marked instruments may help avoid penetration beyond the anterior longitudinal ligament. Decompression of the abdomen by proper positioning facilitates displacement of the great vessels away from the spine.[57]

Visceral Injury

Injury to the liver, spleen, or kidney is a severe complication. This occurs most commonly with transdiaphragmatic approaches to the thoracolumbar spine. Because handheld retractors are responsible for some of these injuries, meticulous care must be taken during their use.

The ureter may be difficult to identify, particularly in obese patients. The anatomy may also be obscured in patients with metastatic cancer. In these circumstances, the preoperative placement of a ureteral catheter or stent may help the surgeon identify the ureter intraoperatively.

Artery of Adamkiewicz

The artery of Adamkiewicz plays an important role in the vascular supply of the thoracic spinal cord. It is usually found on the left side at the level of T9. Some surgeons routinely obtain a preoperative angiogram to identify its anatomy and location. Based on this information, the surgeon may prefer to approach the spine from the side opposite the artery.[32]

Deep Vein Thrombosis

Deep vein thrombosis is a common problem related to retraction of the venous structures. Careful vessel retraction, avoidance of vessel injury, and use of a compressive stocking intraoperatively may prevent this complication. Perioperative prophylactic anticoagulants or intermittent compression boots, if used routinely, may help avoid this complication.

Abdominal Incisional Hernia, Prolonged Ileus, and Hemorrhage

Abdominal wall hernias can be avoided by meticulous reapproximation of the muscle layers at closing. After the retroperitoneal approach, a postoperative ileus may last 24 to 48 hours. After the transperitoneal approach, an ileus may last even longer. Blood loss may be reduced during dorsal exposures by anticipating the presence of the dorsal branch of the interarticular artery, which emerges just lateral to the facet joints in the thoracic and lumbar regions.

Shoulder-Girdle Dysfunction

Dorsal surgery in the cervicothoracic region involves the division of strong scapular and latissimus dorsi muscles. They should be closed in a thorough manner to prevent postoperative shoulder-girdle dysfunction.

KEY REFERENCES

Apfelbaum RI, Kriskovich MD, Haller JR: On the incidence, cause, and prevention of recurrent laryngeal nerve palsies during anterior cervical spine surgery. *Spine (Phila Pa 1976)* 25:2906–2912, 2000.

Banwart JC, Asher MA, Hassanein RS: Iliac crest bone graft harvest donor site morbidity: a statistical evaluation. *Spine (Phila Pa 1976)* 20(9):1055–1060, 1995.

McCormack BM, Zide BM, Kalfas IH: Cerebrospinal fluid fistulae and pseudomeningocele after spine surgery. In Benzel EC, editor: *Spine surgery: techniques, complication avoidance, and management*, Philadelphia, 2005, Elsevier.

Riley LH, Vaccaro AR, Dettori JR, Hashimoto R: Postoperative dysphagia in anterior cervical spine surgery. *Spine (Phila Pa 1976)* 35(Suppl 9):S76–S85, 2010.

Roberts MP: Complications of positioning for neurosurgical operations on the spine. In Tarlov EC, editor: *Complications of spinal surgery*, Park Ridge, IL, 1991, AANS Publishing, pp 1–13.

Smith JS, Fu KM, Polly DW Jr, et al: Complication rates of three common spine procedures and rates of thromboembolism following spine surgery based on 108,419 procedures: a report from the Scoliosis Research Society Morbidity and Mortality Committee. *Spine (Phila Pa 1976)* 35(24):2140–2149, 2010.

Zdeblick TA: The treatment of degenerative lumbar disorders. A critical review of the literature. *Spine (Phila Pa 1976)* 20:1265–1269, 1995.

REFERENCES

The complete reference list is available online at expertconsult.com.

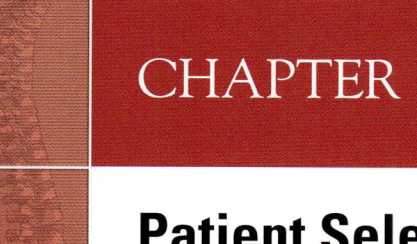

CHAPTER 27

Patient Selection for Spine Surgery

Sharon Walton | Fernando Techy

Between 70% and 85% of all people will have back pain at some time in their lives.[1] Lumbar spine disorders are the most common cause of disability in persons younger than 45 years of age.[2] More than 500,000 lumbar procedures are performed each year for the treatment of lumbar spine disorders.[3] Of those with low back pain (LBP), approximately 151,000 undergo a lumbar fusion each year.[4] Given the large number of individuals that experience back pain, one can only surmise that the number of surgeries performed on the lumbar spine will continue to increase. The vast majority of patients with lumbar spine problems do not require surgery. Nonoperative treatment, however, is very expensive, and the data regarding its efficacy demonstrate equivocal results, at best. It is important for the physician to truly appreciate the indications for lumbar spine surgery, and also to become adept at determining the optimal surgical procedure when surgery is indeed indicated. Based on the best evidence available, this chapter addresses patient selection, clinical management results, and surgical outcomes of surgery for LBP.

Patient Evaluation

Most commonly, the preoperative evaluation should include the history, physical examination, and any warranted imaging tests, such as radiographs, MRI, and CT. Occasionally, blood work, electromyographs (EMGs), and bone scans are used in the evaluation as well. The bone quality should be evaluated with a dual-energy x-ray absorptiometry (DEXA) scan whenever osteoporosis is of concern, especially when major reconstructive surgery is contemplated.

The history is certainly the most important component of the diagnostic process. It also is used to guide treatment. It should include the duration of symptoms, location of pain, any exacerbating and relieving maneuvers, a very detailed description of the radiation of pain, and any constitutional symptoms. The past medical history also is very important, particularly smoking habits. The history of, and response to, conservative management strategies employed for the current complaint (e.g., physical therapy, acupuncture, chiropractic treatments, injections, weight management) must be documented. The quality, intensity, and quantity of the conservative management should also be determined. The type of, number of, and response to injections also should be documented. Selective nerve root blocks, even if the relief given the patient is for only a few days or even hours, provide the surgeon with a great deal of information. Finally, the assessment of the patient's level of energy, mood, affect, and pain pattern is paramount to diagnose problems such as depression, fibromyalgia, and anxiety that may very well manifest as back pain. It is much easier to recommend surgical treatment for the lumbar spine when clear symptoms of radiculopathy and/or claudicant central stenosis are present, especially with associated loss of sensation and/or motor strength. Imaging evidence of instability makes the surgeon's decision a bit easier, especially when coupled with "hard" neurologic findings. Greater difficulty arises when no deficits are present. In such cases, conservative nonoperative treatment should be considered most strongly.

The differential diagnosis of identifiable causes for back pain overlaps with psychosocial diseases and conditions, which can be the source of significant frustration for both surgeon and patient. Medications also should be recorded. Every attempt should be made not to place the patient with chronic back pain on narcotic medication. The detoxification process is a difficult and long one, but is paramount for the success of the treatment. The help of a pain management specialist and psychosocial support usually is quite beneficial.

The intensity and duration, as well as the disability caused by the pain, also play a major role in the decision-making process. A patient who rates the pain as a 1 or 2 on a scale from 1 to 10 and is still working and able to perform daily activities will be managed differently from a person who cannot work, is on disability, and rates the pain 8 out of 10.

Use of the visual analogue scale (VAS) to assess the extent and distribution of pain should also be considered. With the VAS, the patient specifies the level of pain by indicating a position along a continuous line between two end points (0 and 10). The VAS obtained preoperatively and postoperatively can be compared to examine efficacy of treatment.

Individual factors such as work-related injuries and psychosocial support also should be assessed. Low job satisfaction, litigation, and workers' compensation can be predictive of a poor outcome.[5] Trief et al. looked at 160 patients who underwent lumbar spinal fusion. The patients completed preoperative questionnaires regarding their mental health, functional status, workers' compensation, and job satisfaction. Patients with higher mental component scores reported less back and leg pain.[5] In randomized controlled trials (RCTs) from Fairbank et al.[6] and Fritzel et al.,[7] patients in litigation did worse after spinal fusion than their counterparts who were not in litigation. With these studies, however, both subgroups that underwent surgery (with and without litigation) did better than the matched patients who underwent conservative management. The group of patients with the worst response overall were the patients in litigation who received conservative treatment. This, however, was not statistically significant. In another RCT by Haag et al.,[8] several sociologic factors were analyzed 2 years after fusion (workers' compensation, disability pension, unemployment, sick leave due to back pain, cohabitant/married). Overall, the operative group did better than the conservative treatment group. However, the groups that realized the greatest improvement were patients with a lighter job, not cohabiting/married, and not on sick leave. In a recent literature review, Mroz et al.[9] demonstrated that people in litigation usually fare poorly. Nevertheless, they do even worse with conservative treatment. They concluded that socioeconomic factors should not be the sole factor to contraindicate surgical treatment for back pain. Health-related factors such as obesity and smoking also play a role. Recent studies have demonstrated an increase in surgical site infections in morbidly obese patients.[10] Elderly obese patients undergoing lumbar surgery report a high rate of dissatisfaction with the surgery outcome compared with nonobese patients.[10] Smoking is known to be a predictor of poor surgical outcome in lumbar fusion surgery. Habitual nicotine use is thought to decrease the revascularization of the graft, slowing healing rates and increasing the risk of infection and of pseudarthrosis.[11] There are no clear guidelines on preoperative lumbar fusion and cessation of smoking. However, patients should be encouraged to stop smoking as early as possible before undergoing surgery to increase the chance of long-term success.

Chronic LBP may trigger anxiety, depression, and fear, thereby changing the way people perceive pain. The Minnesota Multiphasic Personality Inventory (MMPI) is one of the most widely used personality tests. Patients are asked to answer questions regarding their anxiety and depressive symptoms. The scale attempts to identify patients who are preoccupied with their symptoms, are depressed, or feel a high level of anxiety, because these individuals tend to fare worse.[12] These factors are more predictive of a good outcome than physical findings or radiographic measures. Studies have suggested that fear-avoidance beliefs about physical activity and work might form specific cognitions intervening between LBP and disability.[13] A Fear-Avoidance Beliefs Questionnaire (FABQ) was developed, based on theories of fear and avoidance behavior and focused specifically on patients' beliefs about how physical activity and work affected their LBP. FABQ screening could be useful in patient evaluation for lumbar surgery because it could accurately identify subjects with elevated levels of fear.[13]

After the history is collected, the physical examination should focus on deficits in sensation, muscular weakness, deep tendon reflexes, and any abnormal reflexes such as a Hoffman or Babinski reflex.[14] The clinician also should be aware of any suspicious symptoms or signs that are consistent with malingering. These physical examination findings include pain at the top of the tailbone, entire leg pain or numbness, giveaway weakness, persistent pain, intolerance to treatment, and multiple emergency admissions to hospitals with simple backache (Waddell signs). Clinicians should also be wary of patients who present with a gross limp, use of physical supports (e.g., corset, crutches, transcutaneous electrical nerve stimulation [TENS] unit), or any continuous or repetitive movement.[15] A well-performed hip examination that includes palpation of the greater trochanter to rule out bursitis as well as rotational maneuvers to rule out primary hip joint pathology is imperative when examining the lumbar spine, as are the shoulder and upper extremity peripheral nerves examination when examining the neck. It is very important to be aware of and not miss the "red flag" signs in a patient with pain of spinal origin. The clinician should consider ordering imaging studies after the first encounter in patients with a history of trauma, night pain, weight loss, cancer, persistent weakness, urinary or fecal incontinence, saddle anesthesia, or constitutional symptoms.[16]

In summary, it is very difficult to determine whether a surgical intervention will be beneficial to a patient who presents with LBP. Radiographic evidence of instability may support the argument for surgery. A thorough understanding of the psychosocial situation is imperative. The optimal surgical candidate is a patient who is highly motivated to improve, preferably is not involved in litigation, is not on disability, is not depressed, is physically fit, and does not smoke. This patient has undergone extensive medical management and still is not happy with the result, has significant pain or disability, has a concordant physical examination and imaging tests, is familiar with the results of surgery for LBP, trusts his or her surgeon, and is willing to proceed with surgery. Such patients with back pain represent a significant minority of all back pain patients.

Case Presentation 1: The Importance of Standing Films

The patient presented with a chief complaint of L3, L4, and L5 radiculopathy in the right lower extremity. The MRI examination (Fig. 27-1A) shows stenosis, predominantly foraminal (not shown in this cut). No deformity or instability is observed. On standing radiographs (Figs. 27-1B and C), 12-cm coronal and 17-cm sagittal imbalances are discovered. The imbalances significantly affect the clinical decision-making process.

Low Back Pain: Evidence for Treatment

Certain criteria have been historically accepted in discussing the indications for lumbar fusion. Trauma-related injuries such as unstable fractures, fracture-dislocations, or traumatic spondylolisthesis are all acceptable reasons to perform a lumbar fusion. Scoliosis, infection, and tumor with instability or neurologic deficit also may be indications for surgery. With other pathologies, the indications are not nearly as clear.

Low Back Surgery for Adult Low-Grade Spondylolisthesis

Conservative versus Surgical Treatment

Two RCTs[,18] (same population, different follow-up) comparing low-grade spondylolisthesis patients with those who presented with either chronic LBP or radiculopathy, or both, treated either with fusion or conservative treatment, found that the surgical group did statistically and clinically better, as assessed by pain scores and the Disability Rating Index (DRI). Even

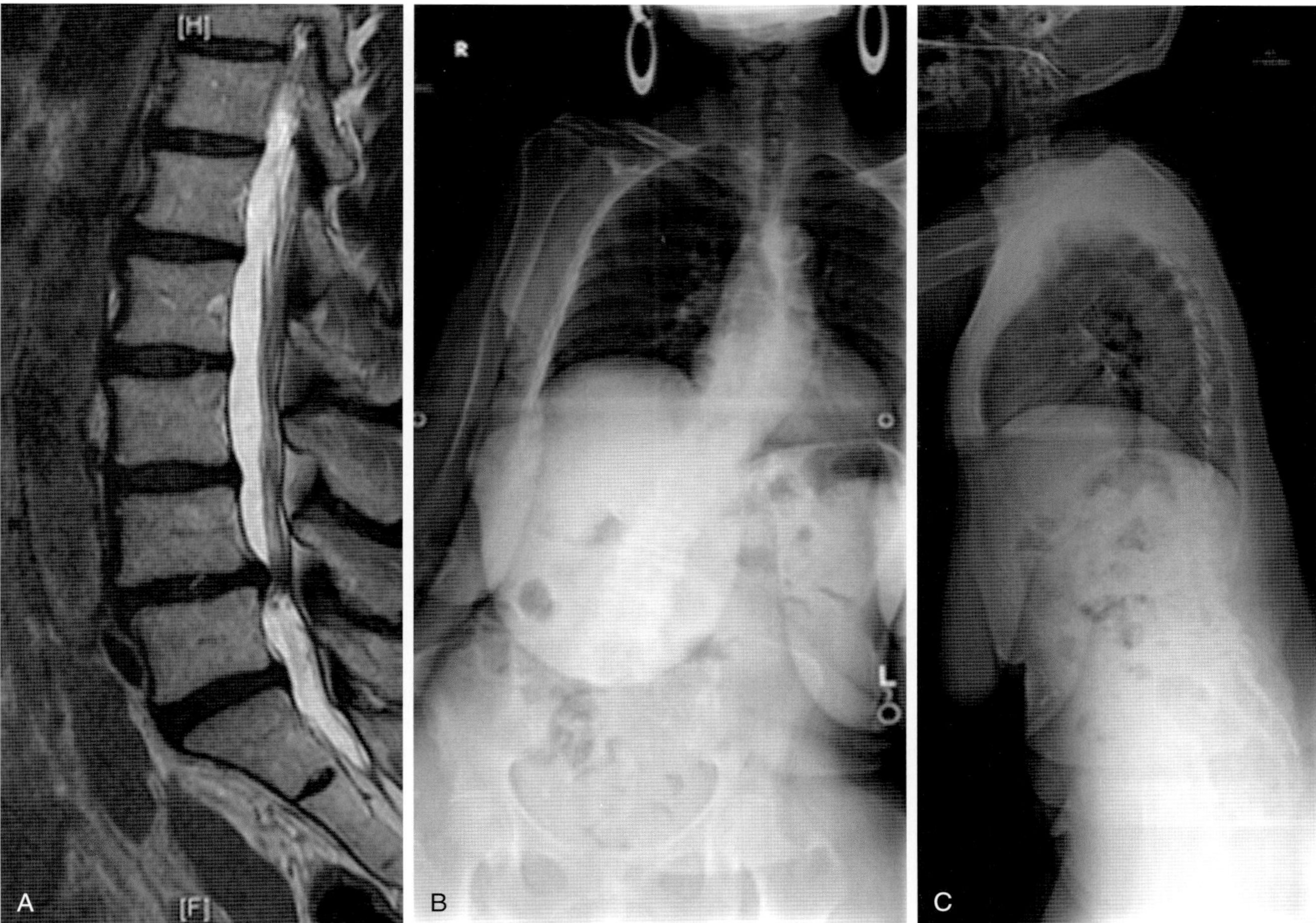

FIGURE 27-1. Case presentation 1:The importance of standing radiographs in the preoperative evaluation. See text for details.

though the long-term follow-up (5 years) showed that some of the initial improvement (1–2 years) had been lost, 76% of the patients in the surgical group still considered their overall outcome as "much better" compared with only 50% in the conservative group. Another prospective RCT found significant difference when treating patients with low-grade spondylolisthesis with an advanced core strengthening program performed by a specialist physical therapist and a control group that performed simple exercises prescribed by their primary physician at 3, 6, and 30 months. The advanced exercise group had better outcomes.[19] Sinaki et al. have shown, in a retrospective analysis, significant benefit of flexion exercises in comparison with extension exercises to control the symptoms of low-grade spondylolisthesis.[20] Daniel et al. reported very poor results with conservative treatment for spondylosis, including the use of a full-time thoracolumbar orthosis. Twenty-nine of 31 patients failed treatment and progressed to surgery.[21]

Low-Grade Spondylolisthesis: To Fuse or Not to Fuse? Role of Instrumentation? Best Approach?

When assessing the role of fusion in the management of adult low-grade spondylolisthesis, Herkowitz and Kurz[22] performed an RCT comparing decompression alone with decompression and uninstrumented PLF (posterolateral fusion). A mean 3-year follow-up demonstrated better outcomes for leg and back pain for the fusion group (P = .0001). Other authors in prospective nonrandomized[23] and retrospective[24-26] series also support decompression and fusion over decompression alone when spondylolisthesis is present.

The role of instrumentation in achieving fusion and improving clinical outcomes in low-grade spondylolisthesis was studied by Fischgrund et al.[27] in an RCT. Patients were divided into two groups: (1) decompression and noninstrumented PLF and (2) decompression with instrumented PLF (pedicle screws). The fusion rate was 83% versus 45%, respectively, for the instrumented versus noninstrumented groups. Clinical outcomes, however, were similar for both groups (78% vs. 85%, instrumented vs. noninstrumented). Kornblum et al. [28] combined the noninstrumented patients from both the Fischgrund[27] and the Herkowitz[22] studies to compare 47 patients with either a solid fusion or a nonunion. The solid fusion group had a satisfactory result in 86% of patients, whereas patients in the nonunion group had 56% satisfactory results at 5 to 14 years of follow-up.

Two additional RCTs were performed. In these studies, instrumentation was associated with higher fusion rates and better clinical outcomes for low-grade spondylolisthesis. Zdeblick[29] reported a 65% fusion rate and 71% satisfactory clinical outcome in the noninstrumented group, versus a 95% fusion rate and 95% satisfactory clinical outcome in the rigid instrumentation group. Bridwell et al.[30] randomized 43 patients into three groups: (1) decompression only, (2) decompression with uninstrumented posterolateral fusion, and (3) decompression with rigid pedicle screw instrumentation posterolateral fusion. The fusion rates were 33% and 87.5% for groups 2 and 3. Clinical improvement was 30%, 33%, and 83.3% for groups 1, 2, and 3, respectively.

Kwon et al.[31] reviewed the literature regarding surgical approaches to low-grade spondylolisthesis (ventral/dorsal/360 degrees). In a total of 1100 patients from 34 studies (4 of which were RCTs), the clinical results and fusion rates were better when the combined ventral/dorsal approach was used. When comparing anterior lumbar interbody fusion (ALIF) plus PLF with instrumentation versus ALIF plus instrumentation without PLF, Shofferman et al.[32] found that both groups had improvement in function, but no difference in results could be detected.

In 2005, the Scoliosis Research Society released a consensus statement on the treatment of low-grade acquired/isthmic spondylolisthesis,[33] making the following points:

- The achievement of a solid fusion is associated with better clinical outcomes.
- The adjunctive use of pedicle screw instrumentation improves fusion rates.
- While instrumentation does not show significant improvement on patient-scored outcome measures, the positive effect on fusion alone warrants its use.
- There is no consensus regarding the approach for fusion—interbody, dorsolateral, or combined.

Lumbar Fusion for Back Pain without Signs of Instability

Lumbar fusion or surgery to treat low back pain–related symptoms, presumably from intervertebral disc disease (IDD), black disc syndrome, or "discogenic" LBP, is arguably the most controversial surgical indication in spine surgery. One reason is that the natural history of IDD is poorly defined, and the condition often is self-limiting and benign. Questions that must be asked include: What specifically causes the pain in IDD? Does selective fusion of a segment lead to pain relief? Is the disc the only source of pain? How important is facet arthritis, inflammation of adjacent tendons, or muscle fatigue in LBP generation? Are other levels involved?

Pain in the anular region may be triggered by chemical and mechanical sensitization of dorsal anular nociceptors.[34] In the 1940s and 1950s, the disc itself was thought to have no nerve supply and, therefore, to have no possibility of generating pain. Subsequent studies have proved this theory wrong. In the normal human disc, sensory nerves extend into the outer third of the anulus. In the degenerated disc, the innervation is deeper and more extensive, with some nerve fibers penetrating into the nucleus pulposus.[35] Pain also may be produced by the sensitization and irritation of nerve endings in the end plate.[34-38] This model of chemical nociception is supported by numerous studies showing disc immunoreactivity to inflammatory mediators such as substance P and calcitonin as well as elevated levels of prostaglandin E2, interleukin (IL)-2, IL-6, IL-8, phospholipase A2, leukotrienes, thromboxane B2, and tumor necrosis in the degenerated intervertebral disc.[39-41] It is now generally accepted that intervertebral discs can be a significant source of back pain. Normal discs resist pain with stimulation because they lack both the chemical sensitization and the mechanical overloading seen in diseased discs.

Since its advent more than 50 years ago, the use of discography has been mired in controversy. Discograms are pain-provoking tests that show radiographic abnormalities of the disc. The procedure is performed with the patient awake in order to assess the level of pain he or she experiences upon injection of normal saline or a water-soluble dye into the intervertebral disc at different segments of the lumbar spine suspected of being abnormal.[42] A positive discogram is associated with the elicitation of a concordant pain response coupled with pain-related behavior (e.g., grimacing, guarding, withdrawing, and verbalizing). Provocative discography is no longer used for the routine evaluation of radiculopathy, having been largely replaced by the advent of noninvasive, more sensitive tests such as CT and MRI. The evidence that these modalities are not only safer but also more accurate than plain discography in detecting herniated nuclear material is irrefutable.[42]

Several authors have attempted to determine the prevalence of discogenic pain in patients suffering from LBP. In one of the most cited studies, Schwarzer et al. found the incidence of IDD (defined in his study by positive discography) to be 39% in 92 patients with chronic LBP.[43]

The first study to question the validity of discography was published in 1968 by Holt, who found false-positive results in 37% of 30 asymptomatic subjects. All participants were prisoners.[44]

Some studies have attempted to correlate discography results with surgical findings and outcomes. Colhoun et al. evaluated surgical outcomes in 162 patients who underwent preoperative discography for axial LBP. In the 137 patients whose discography provoked pain, 89% had a favorable outcome at a mean follow-up of 3.6 years. In the 25 patients whose discs showed morphologic abnormalities but no provocation of symptoms, only 52% reported significant benefit.[45]

Although Colhoun reported successful data, some other studies have not had such positive conclusions. The predictive value of provocative discography on surgical outcome also was assessed in a study by Madan et al. involving 73 patients with chronic LBP. Thirty-two patients underwent spinal fusion based on pain provocation during discography; the remaining 41 patients had surgery without discography. In the discography group, 75.6% of patients had satisfactory outcomes at a minimum 2-year follow-up versus 81.2% in the group who did not have preoperative discography.[46] In summary, the lack of strong evidence for the use of discography in fusion surgery to treat degenerative disc disease (DDD) and the methodologic flaws in the existing studies make interpretation of the data exceedingly difficult. Based on the data that are available, the results are mixed as to whether or not preoperative discography improves surgical outcomes in patients with discogenic LBP.[47,48]

Extensive studies have been performed regarding the use of temporary external fixation before lumbar fusion surgery to help distinguish the area of disease. The aim of externally fixing a lumbar spinal motion segment is to prevent movement, therefore alleviating pain. This may be predictive of subsequent surgical success.[49,50] Although some authors have observed improvement in pain[51] and found good prediction for satisfactory fusion surgery outcomes with this technique, others found a high rate of complications such as pin site infection, neurologic compromise, and cerebrospinal leakage,[52] and found that the technique is a poor predictor of successful fusion surgery.[52,53] Currently, this practice has fallen out of favor.

Clinical Results for the Conservative and Surgical Treatment of Mechanical Low Back Pain

The fact that many patients with DDD suffer from other concomitant causes of back pain that may not respond to operative intervention continues to bring significant controversy to the clinical decision-making debate. Although outcome studies for spinal arthrodesis vary widely, it is generally acknowledged to be less beneficial than surgery for radicular pain, with success rates ranging from less than 50% to almost 90%.[54] Fritzell et al., in a multicenter RCT, compared conservative treatment to spinal fusion for the treatment of chronic LBP. Forty-six percent of the surgical group reported good to excellent results, while only 18% of patients in the conservative group achieved similar results.[7] In another RCT comparing conservative treatment with PLF to treat chronic LBP, Brox et al. report no difference between the two groups.[55]

In the Pro-Disc total disc replacement IDE RCT (2-year follow-up), Zigler et al. report successful outcomes in 54.9% of patients undergoing ALIF plus PLF, compared with a 69% success rate in patients receiving the disc replacement (P = .03).[56] Guyer et al.[57] recently published the results of the 5-year follow-up of the U.S. Food and Drug Administration's IDE trial of the Charité disc. Success results were 57.8% for total disc replacement and 51.2% for the fusion group (ALIF; P = .03). There was no difference between groups in the Oswestry Disability Index (ODI), visual analogue scale, or 36-Item Short Form Health Survey (SF-36) scores. The authors concluded that there was no clinical difference between groups, and that these results were consistent with the 2-year Charité outcomes previously published.[58] Greater clinical success (i.e., good results between 70% and 90%) in lumbar fusion surgery for back pain (using different techniques, e.g., uninstrumented and instrumented PLF, ALIF, posterior lumbar interbody fusion, transforaminal lumbar interbody fusion) are found in smaller, less strictly controlled studies. Most of them were case series.[59-63]

Case Presentation 2: Each Case Is Unique

A 21-year-old female college student presented with a history of LBP for 6 years despite multiple trials of physical therapy and oral medication. Pain was worsened in extension and better in flexion. There was no radiculopathy. Sagittal MRI (Fig. 27-2A) showed degeneration of the L4-5 and L5-S1 discs. Coronal MRI showsed L4-5 bilateral facet joint incompetence with an increased amount of synovial fluid and early degenerative changes (Fig. 27-2B). Fig 27-2C showed normal L3-4 facets for comparison. The patient enjoyed 100% pain relief (at 1 and 4 months) with bilateral L4-5 facet injections with steroids and bupivacaine.

Case Presentation 3: Patient Selection Is Paramount

A 42-year-old female physical therapist and runner (Fig. 27-3) had given up running due to a 2-year history of mechanical LBP. She exhibited no radicular symptoms. Pain had become incapacitating and was interfering not only with running but with daily activities. Preoperative radiographs were obtained (see Figs. 27-3A and B). On MRI (see Fig. 27-3C), the only abnormality was degeneration of the L5-S1 disc. After several months of aggressive medical management and after thorough psychosocial evaluation, the patient underwent an L5-S1 ALIF with percutaneous pedicle screw fixation (Figs. 27-3D and E). She is pain free following surgery. She won a 10K race 6 months postoperatively.

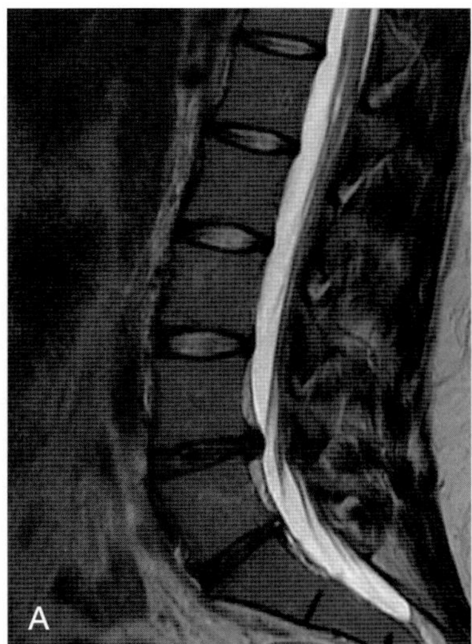

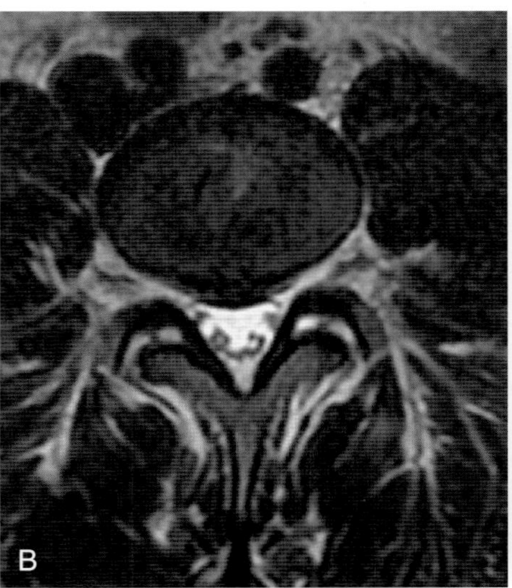

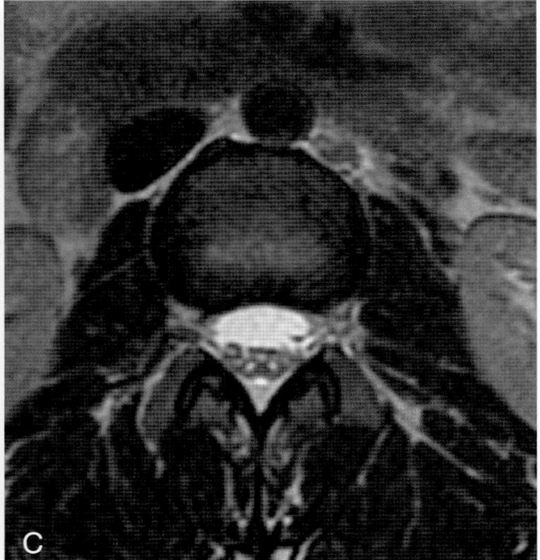

FIGURE 27-2. Case presentation 2: It is extremely difficult to determine the location of the pain generators in low back pain. Attention to detail in the history, physical examination, and imaging components of the evaluation may be helpful. Each case is unique. See text for details.

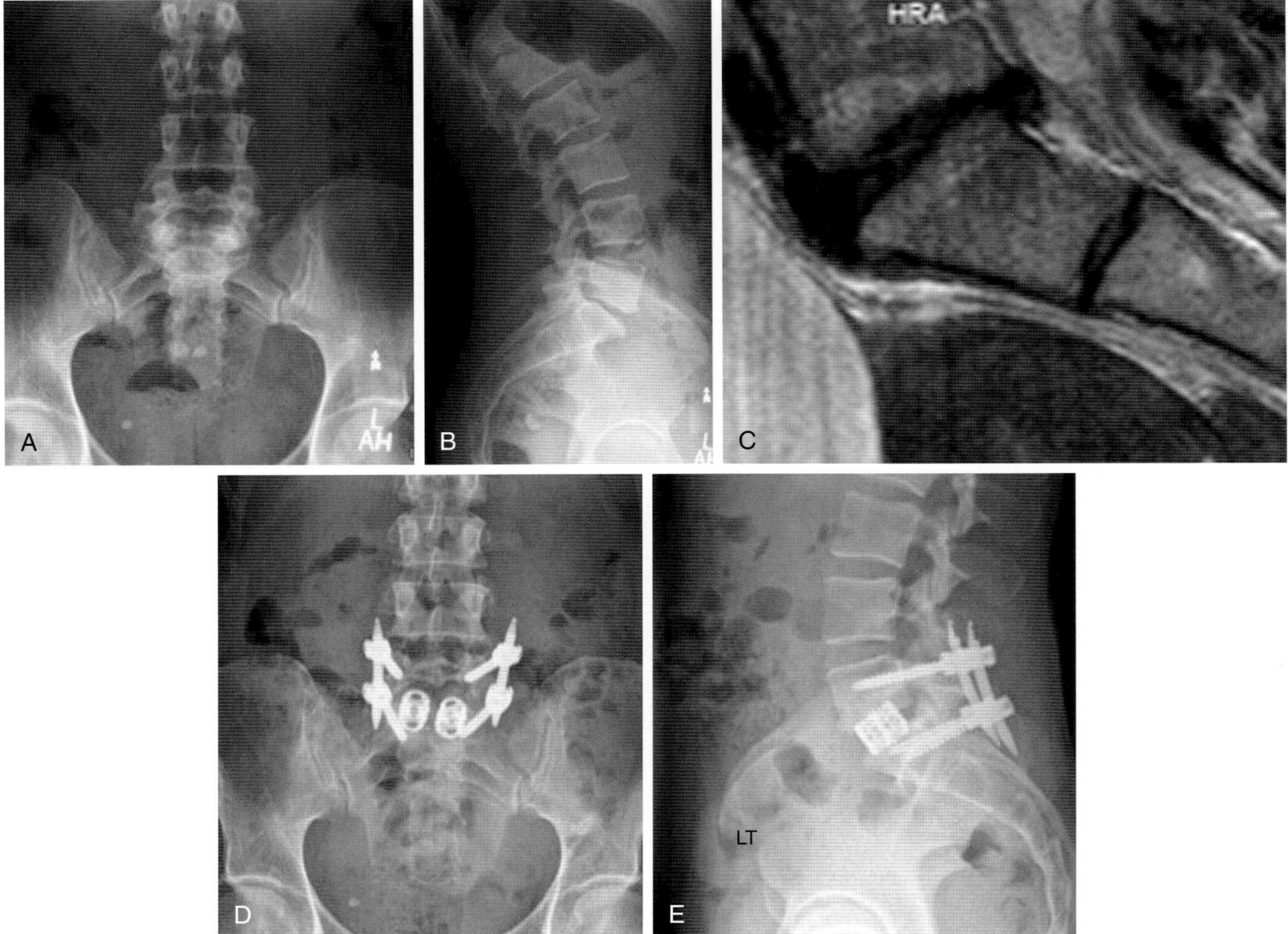

FIGURE 27-3. Case presentation 3: Preoperative radiographs (**A** and **B**) and MRI scan (**C**) show degeneration of the L5-S1 disc. **D** and **E**, The patient underwent an L5-S1 anterior lumbar interbody fusion (ALIF) with percutaneous pedicle screw fixation. (Case courtesy of Robert McLain, MD, Cleveland Clinic, Cleveland, Ohio.)

Conclusions

Many indications for surgery in the lumbar spine have been well established. The most controversial of these is for the treatment of back pain with no neurologic deficit, no radicular pain, no instability, and no deformity present, and that does not respond to an extensive medical management regimen. LBP often is an illness, not a disease. An abnormal illness behavior cannot be treated by a spine operation, not even by a perfectly executed fusion using the ultimate spine fixation device, or by replacing the disc. A multidisciplinary approach with spine medical specialists, physical therapists, psychiatrists, psychologists, pain medicine specialists, bariatric physicians, and the spine surgeon often is needed. Many patients eventually develop a lifestyle based on suffering and despondency. Spine surgeons must be aware of the psychosocial issues that surround the diagnosis of LBP. Only a very demanding and precise selective process, understanding all anatomic and emotional aspects of the history, physical examination, and auxiliary tests, will be able to pinpoint the patients who will benefit from LBP surgery.

KEY REFERENCES

Esses SI, Botsford DJ, Kostuilk JP: The role of external skeletal fixation in the assessment of low-back disorders. *Spine (Phila Pa 1976)* 14:594–601, 1989.

Ghogawala Z, Benzel EC, Amin-Hanjani S, et al: Prospective outcomes evaluation after decompression with and without instrumented fusion for lumbar stenosis and degenerative grade I spondylolisthesis. *J Neurosurg Spine* 1:267–272, 2004.

Holt EP: The question of lumbar discography. *J Bone Joint Surg [Am]* 50: 720–726, 1968.

Katz JN: Lumbar disc disorders and low-back pain: socioeconomic factors and consequences. *J Bone Joint Surg [AM]* 88(Suppl 2):21–24, 2006.

LaCaile R, DeBerard M, Masters K: Presurgical biopsychosocial factors predict multidimensional outcomes of interbody lumbar fusion. *Spine (Phila Pa 1976)* 5:71–78, 2005.

Olerud S, Sjostrom L, Karlstrom G, Hamberg M: Spontaneous effect of increased stability of the lower lumbar spine in cases of severe chronic low back pain. The answer of an external transpeduncular fixation test. *Clin Orthop Relat Res* 203:67–74, 1986.

Waddell G, McCulloch JA, Kummel E, Venner RM: Nonorganic physical signs in low-back pain. *Spine (Phila Pa 1976)* 5:117–125, 1980.

REFERENCES

The complete reference list is available online at expertconsult.com.

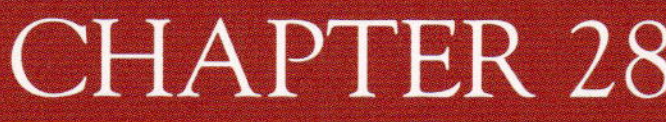

Masqueraders of Spinal Pathology

Rick Placide | Michael DePalma | Daniel J. Mazanec

It is not rare for spinal pathology to refer various symptoms to other parts of the body. In fact, conditions of the spine can present with a multitude of signs and symptoms masquerading as any number of pathologic conditions. A classic example is a C5 radiculopathy from a disc herniation that presents as shoulder pain. Conversely, nonspinal disorders may present with pain thought to be of spinal origin. For example, trochanteric bursitis commonly presents with symptoms that may appear to be originating from the lumbar spine. This chapter will review a number of nonspinal conditions that produce symptoms seemingly of spinal origin despite actually originating from a structure or process outside of the spine. These conditions mimicking spine pathology range from the relatively benign to the serious and life threatening, and they may mimic axial spine pain, radiculopathy, or myelopathy.

Musculoskeletal System

A variety of conditions involving the musculoskeletal system are known to mimic spine pathology.[1-6] Typically, degenerative conditions in the upper and lower extremities such as arthritis, tendonitis, and bursitis are the primary culprits that bring the patient to the spine specialist, suspecting that their complaints are of spinal origin (Box 28-1). Many musculoskeletal structures in the extremities can present with signs and symptoms that seem to be originating from the spine; however, the most common extraspinal musculoskeletal masqueraders of spine disease are the shoulder, hip, and sacroiliac joint.

Shoulder

The term *shoulder* describes a region of the body and not a specific joint. In fact, the shoulder complex includes four separate articulations: the glenohumeral, scapulothoracic, sternoclavicular, and acromioclavicular joints. Any of these joints are subject to trauma and degenerative changes and can therefore cause pain and dysfunction that can be confused with cervical spine pathology. Two of the more common conditions involving the shoulder are impingement syndrome and osteoarthritis. The presenting signs and symptoms often overlap with those of cervical radiculopathy and neck pain. A thorough history and physical examination are often required to differentiate between cervical spine and shoulder pathology. It is necessary to recall that pain coming from shoulder pathology typically does not radiate distal to the elbow and that shoulder and cervical spine disease may coexist.

Impingement Syndrome

Impingement syndrome is a condition caused by repeated mechanical insult to the rotator cuff, with the tendons forced against the overlying coracoacromial arch as the arm is elevated overhead. A variety of anatomic, biomechanical, and neurologic factors either narrow the space available for the rotator cuff or cause abnormal arthrokinematics, leading to

BOX 28-1. Selected Conditions of the Musculoskeletal System with Potential to Mimic Cervical or Lumbar Radiculopathy

Upper Extremity
- Impingement syndrome
- Rotator cuff tear/tendonitis
- Osteoarthritis (glenohumeral, acromioclavicular)
- Glenoid labral tear, glenoid cyst
- Lateral/medial epicondylitis
- DeQuervain tenosynovitis
- Flexor/extensor tendonitis

Lower Extremity
- Osteoarthritis, avascular necrosis (hip)
- Greater trochanteric bursitis
- Abductor/adductor/iliopsoas tendonitis
- Acetabular labral tear
- Femoral neck fracture
- Pes anserine bursitis
- Iliotibial band friction syndrome
- Exertional compartment syndrome
- Plantar fasciitis

General
- Polymyalgia rheumatica
- Myofascial pain syndrome
- Fibromyalgia

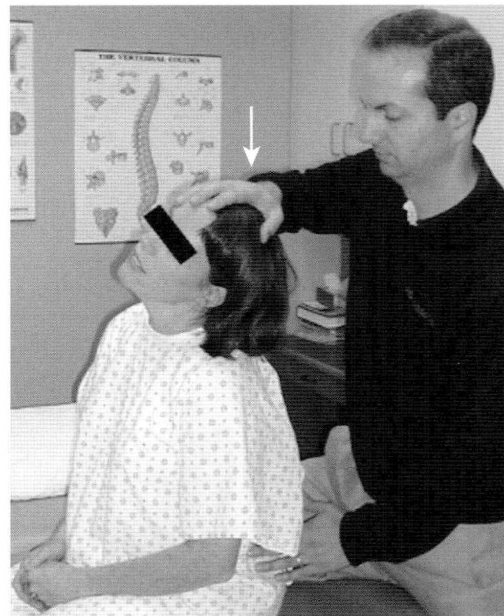

FIGURE 28-1. Spurling examination. Rotation and lateral flexion to the involved side with mild extension and axial load reproduces upper extremity radicular symptoms.

impingement of the tendons. Classically, there are three stages of impingement (described by Neer). Stage 1 is characterized by subacromial edema and hemorrhage; stage 2 progresses to tendonitis and fibrosis; and, ultimately, stage 3 results in tearing of the rotator cuff, either partially or completely.[7]

The patient with impingement syndrome generally complains of activity-related shoulder pain that extends from the top of the shoulder into the arm laterally—to the level of the deltoid tuberosity. This is especially true with overhead activities. Night pain and the inability to lie on the affected side may be additional complaints, particularly if a rotator cuff tear is present. Ultimately, the patient develops movement compensation patterns that place abnormal stresses on associated structures, leading to symptoms such as scapular and cervical muscle strain. Although cervical spine provocative maneuvers such as the Spurling test are negative[8] (Fig. 28-1), a variety of physical examination maneuvers have been developed to diagnose shoulder impingement and are designed to reproduce the patient's symptoms by compressing the rotator cuff under the subacromial arch.[7] The Neer impingement sign and the Hawkins sign are two such tests (Figs. 28-2 and 28-3). The Neer impingement sign can be particularly useful; this overhead position is not well tolerated in the patient with impingement syndrome but may bring relief to the patient with cervical radiculopathy, because it decreases neural tension (shoulder abduction relief sign).[9] Palpation may elicit tenderness over the rotator cuff tendons or the acromioclavicular joint. This joint can be a source of impingement due to degenerative changes, such as spurring and synovitis. In the presence of a rotator cuff tear, weakness of abduction (supraspinatus) and external rotation (infraspinatus) may be noted. However, other structures innervated by C5 and C6, such as the deltoid and bicep muscles, remain intact. In addition, impingement syndrome is not typically associated with sensory loss or reflex changes that may be found with cervical radiculopathy.

A subacromial injection of local anesthetic can implicate or rule out impingement as the cause of the patient's symptoms. Plain radiographs, including anterior-posterior, lateral, axillary, and scapular outlet views, as well as advanced imaging techniques such as MRI, can be helpful. Care must be taken in interpreting the MRI scans in the absence of a quality physical examination because the prevalence of abnormal studies in asymptomatic subjects ranges from 15% to 60% for the cervical spine and from 4% to 54% for rotator cuff tears, depending on the age of the patient.[10,11]

Glenohumeral Osteoarthritis

Osteoarthritis (OA), also known as degenerative joint disease of the glenohumeral joint, is not as common as knee or hip OA but is by no means rare. Causes of glenohumeral OA may be primary (idiopathic) or secondary. Examples of secondary causes are posttraumatic, infectious, metabolic, and inflammatory. The patient with early glenohumeral OA presents with activity-related pain that is relieved by rest. The pain is generally located about the shoulder, and there may be mild range of motion (ROM) restrictions. The distribution of pain is similar to that which a patient with a C5 or C6 radiculopathy might present.[12] As the disease progresses, pain may persist at rest, and night pain may become a complaint. ROM becomes more restricted, particularly external rotation, due to anterior capsular and subscapularis contracture. Motion restrictions are similar for active and passive ROM. Rotator cuff strength is usually maintained but may seem limited secondary to pain. Palpation may demonstrate tenderness, especially about the posterior glenohumeral joint line, and crepitus may be noted with ROM activities. Plain radiographs (anteroposterior [AP], lateral, and axillary views) of the shoulder are usually conclusive in the case of glenohumeral OA. Diagnostic intra-articular injections can help differentiate shoulder OA from cervical spine disease.

Hip

The hip joint is the articulation between the head of the femur and the acetabulum. However, when patients refer to the *hip,* they may be referring to any number of associated and neighboring structures. Due to the proximity of the hip to the lumbar spine, conditions about the hip are often confused with lumbar spine pathology, particularly radiculopathy. When discussing pathology around the hip, it is sometimes useful to separate the conditions into intra-articular and extra-articular processes. Examples of intra-articular pathology include OA and a torn acetabular labrum, whereas extra-articular examples are greater trochanteric bursitis, hamstring muscle strain, and piriformis syndrome.

Hip Osteoarthritis

OA of the hip, as in the shoulder, can be primary or secondary. It can be unilateral or bilateral. When systemic or inflammatory disease processes are responsible for the condition, involvement is more likely to be bilateral. Primary OA is by far the most common form of hip OA. It increases in frequency with increasing age, although the precise interrelationship between aging and arthritis is not clear. Patients with

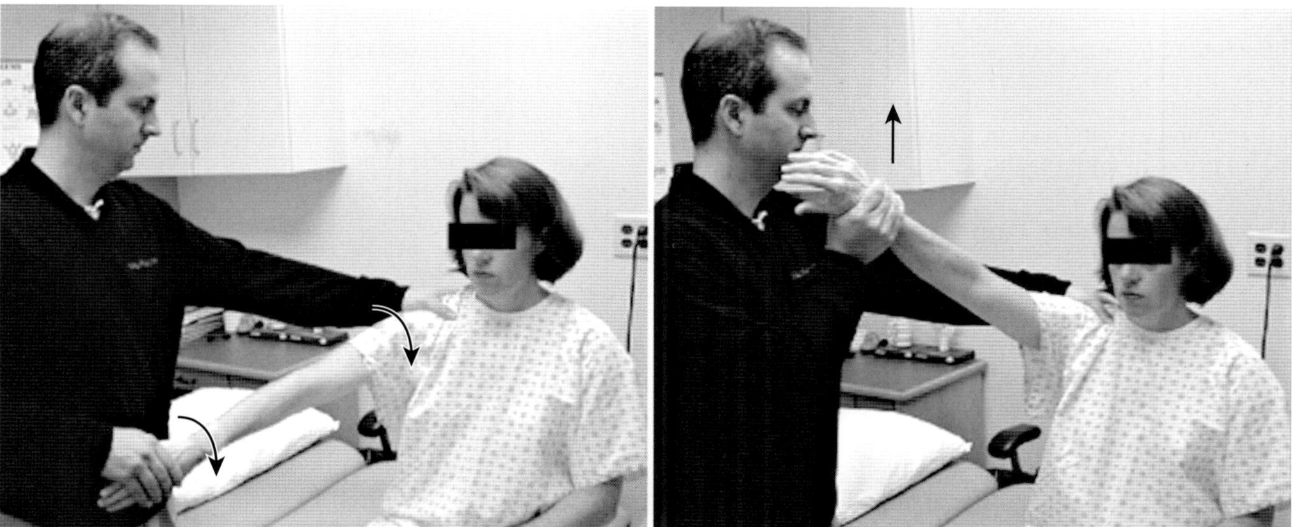

FIGURE 28-2. The Neer impingement test causes rotator cuff impingement against the anterior edge of the acromion with shoulder flexion.

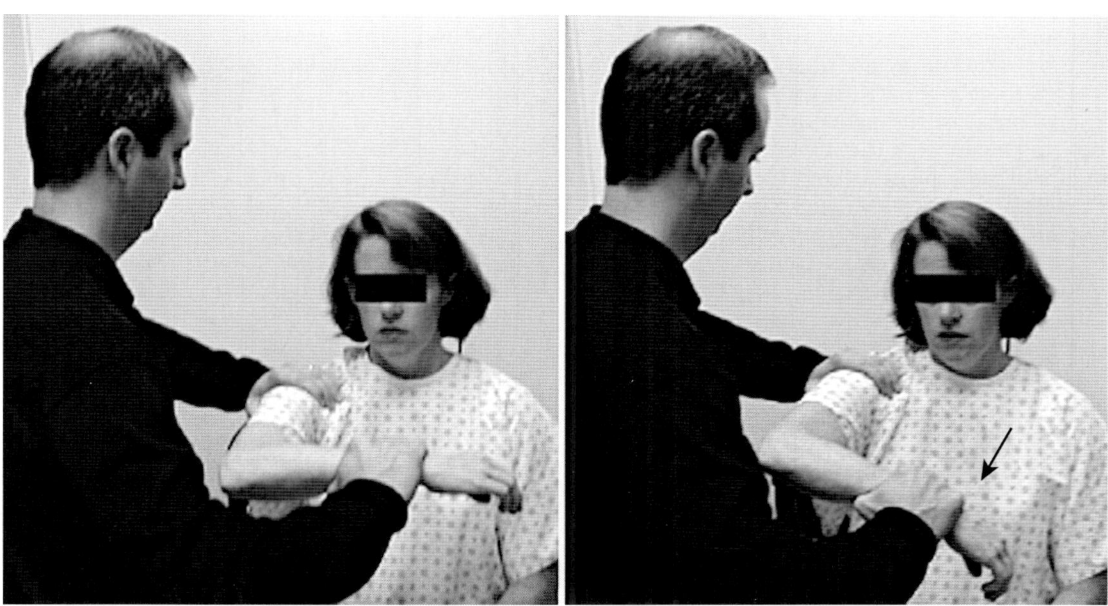

FIGURE 28-3. The Hawkins impingement test causes rotator cuff impingement against the coracoacromial ligament in this position.

primary hip arthritis complain of activity-related pain that is relieved by rest. Those with severe degenerative changes may even have pain at rest. Their ambulation distance is decreased due to pain, and they may develop an antalgic gait pattern. As the disease progresses, patients may complain of difficulty with tasks such as donning shoes and socks due to limitation in hip ROM. As with any intra-articular hip pathology, OA causes groin pain that typically radiates down the ventromedial thigh to the knee. However, hip arthritis may refer pain distal to the knee in more than 40% of patients.[13] In addition to mimicking lumbar radiculopathy, hip arthritis can mimic somatically referred pain from the intervertebral disc, lower lumbar facet joints, and sacroiliac joints. Secondary involvement of the gluteus musculature and trochanteric bursa due to an altered gait pattern may cause lateral hip and thigh pain as well.

Physical examination may demonstrate gait abnormalities such as a trunk lean over the affected hip during weightbearing (to decrease the abductor moment about the hip, thus reducing compressive load across the joint). Patients may display apparent and/or true leg length discrepancy due to hip flexor/adductor contractures and/or hip joint cartilage loss, respectively. There may be weakness of the hip abductors, and they may be tender to palpation. ROM tends to be limited, primarily in hip internal rotation. The most provocative maneuver with hip OA is to flex the hip of the supine patient to at least 90 degrees and then apply adduction and internal rotation. In the case of unilateral disease, this motion is restricted and painful on the involved side. Patients with OA of the hip do not typically have sensory or reflex changes as part of their clinical picture unless there is coexisting neuropathy or spinal pathology. Occasionally, a diagnostic, intra-articular hip injection with local anesthetic is required to differentiate hip and spine symptomatology with a calculated sensitivity of 88% and specificity of 100%.[14] The standard radiographic workup for primary hip OA is an AP pelvis radiograph and AP and lateral radiographs of the involved hip. This is usually confirmatory (Fig. 28-4).

Greater Trochanteric Pain Syndrome

Greater trochanteric pain syndrome (GTPS) is a term that has been used to describe lateral hip pain of soft tissue origin in the region of the greater trochanter. Trochanteric bursitis is the most common etiology of this syndrome. However, other conditions have been described such as tendonitis or tears of the gluteus medius and iliotibial band irritation.[2,15] These conditions are likely related to overuse, abnormal biomechanics, or local trauma. Patients with GTPS complain of pain about the hip laterally that may radiate proximally to the buttock and distally along the lateral aspect of the thigh to the lateral knee. Several lumbar dermatomes share this distribution, allowing GTPS to mimic lumbar radiculopathy. It has been reported that up to 20% to 25% of patients being evaluated for lumbar spine pathology have GTPS as the source of their complaints. In addition, greater trochanteric bursitis has been found in 25% to 35% of patients with low back pain.[2,5]

Physical examination of the patient with GTPS reveals local tenderness to palpation of the involved structure (tendon or bursa). Tenderness may be ventral, dorsal, rostral, or directly over the greater trochanter, depending on the structure involved. Similarly, patients complain of increased symptoms when sleeping on the involved side due to direct pressure on the inflamed structures. Resisted hip abduction or external rotation also compresses or stresses the tissues in GTPS, reproducing the symptoms. Once the physical examination has implicated a particular structure but lumbar radiculopathy has not been ruled out, an injection of a local anesthetic can help in the differentiation between local pathology and referred pain. Some authors suggest the use of fluoroscopy for the injection to ensure that the anesthetic reaches the site of pathology.[15] Plain radiographs are useful to help to rule out hip arthritis and other local pathology such as a fracture of the greater trochanter. Often, patients complain of tenderness on palpation in this region, even when this is not the presenting complaint. Recognizing the existence of the various conditions under the umbrella of GTPS, coupled with a careful history and physical examination, is usually sufficient to differentiate between hip and lumbar spine disease. One must realize, however, that these conditions can coexist.

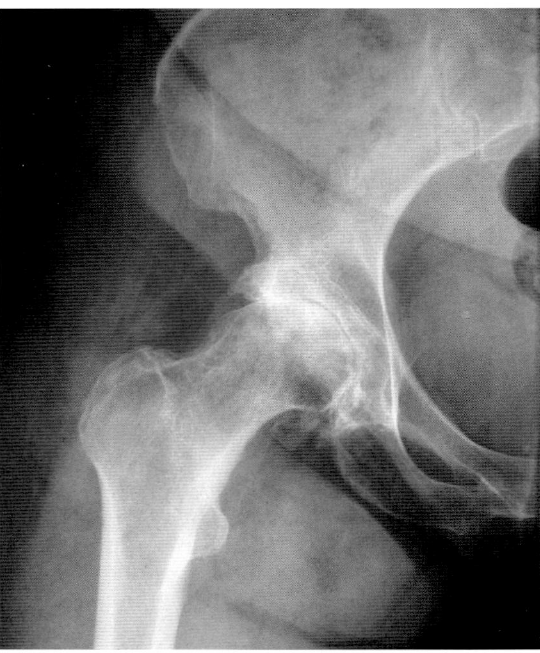

FIGURE 28-4. Radiograph demonstrating hip osteoarthritis. Note the joint space narrowing, osteophytes, subchondral sclerosis, and subchondral cysts, which are the hallmark radiographic signs of osteoarthritis.

Sacroiliac Joint

The sacroiliac joint (SIJ) is certainly capable of producing pain locally. SIJ pain is also in the differential diagnosis as an extraspinal cause of low back and lower extremity pain. A variety of pathologic processes can affect the SIJ, including SIJ pain syndrome, OA, sacroiliitis (as in ankylosing spondylitis and Reiter syndrome), septic arthritis, and traumatic SIJ instability or dislocation. Many of these conditions have an obvious history as well as objective radiographic findings, implicating the SIJ as a pain generator. However, in the absence of "hard" findings on examination or radiographs, attributing a patient's pain to the SIJ has in recent decades been met with skepticism due to the controversy over the joint's ability to be a source of pain and the thought that the SIJ does not move in most individuals. Recent injection studies have demonstrated the SIJ to be a potential source of pain in the low back, buttock, and lower extremity, and studies involving radiostereometric analyses have shown small but definite motion at the SIJ.[4,16]

Sacroiliac Joint Dysfunction

The clinical presentation of the patient with SIJ dysfunction can be highly variable. In patients with a diagnosis of low back pain, the prevalence of this condition has been reported to range from 13% to 30%. Injection studies of the SIJs of asymptomatic volunteers produced pain in the low back, posterior superior iliac spine (PSIS) area, buttock, and thigh. Further studies on symptomatic subjects demonstrated that SIJ injection with a local anesthetic relieved a variety of pain patterns, including pain in the low back, PSIS region, abdomen, buttock, groin, thigh, leg, and foot.[4] Clearly, SIJ dysfunction can mimic lumbar spine pathology, including discogenic pain, lumbosacral facet joint arthropathy, and radiculopathy.

Patients with SIJ dysfunction typically present with pain in the lateral low back, in the parasacral region with radiation to the buttock and posterolateral proximal thigh. They may complain of tenderness in the area of the sacral sulcus. Some authors have suggested that a painful SIJ can refer pain into the calf and foot, although much less commonly. There are many tests described in the literature to test for SIJ dysfunction; to review all of these is not within the scope of this chapter. Two categories of SIJ testing include tests designed to stress the SIJ and reproduce the patient's symptoms and those designed to detect abnormal or asymmetrical motion by palpation of certain anatomic landmarks about the pelvis.[17]

Some tests used to stress the SIJ include the Gaenslen and Faber tests and SIJ compression/distraction maneuvers. Motion palpation tests include the standing flexion test and Gillet test. However, using physical examination tests to provoke SIJ pain through manually stressing the joint, detecting motion abnormalities by palpation, or relying on features of the patient history have traditionally all correlated poorly with the response of fluoroscopically guided intra-articular SIJ injections.[4] However, more recent data suggest that by using a composite of manual tests, a practitioner can reliably implicate or rule out the SIJ as a source of low back pain.[18] Even with these new data, the diagnostic test of choice for SIJ dysfunction seems to be a fluoroscopically guided intra-articular SIJ injection of a local anesthetic.

Nervous System

Conditions of both the central and peripheral nervous systems can mimic spine disease. Pathology of the peripheral nervous system is more likely than that of the central nervous system to mimic spine pathology, but occasionally, an intracranial condition will do so. Intracranial conditions known to have signs and symptoms overlapping those of spine pathology include intracranial neoplasms, Chiari malformation, cerebrovascular accidents, normal pressure hydrocephalus, and spontaneous intracranial hypotension.[19-21]

As previously stated, peripheral neuropathy is one of the more common masqueraders of spinal pathology, particularly radiculopathy and myelopathy. There are many etiologies of peripheral neuropathy, including compression or entrapment; metabolic, nutritional, toxic, hereditary, autoimmune, neoplastic disorders; and disorders associated with neuromuscular disease[22-27] (Box 28-2). Even in the face of an extensive workup, the etiology of peripheral neuropathy is frequently not identified. When this is the case, the initial serologic studies should include vitamin B_{12}, folate, hemoglobin A_{1C}, erythrocyte sedimentation rate, and thyroid-stimulating hormone. The following section will concentrate on the more common peripheral nervous system conditions mimicking spine disease. There are certainly many more causes of peripheral neuropathy than are discussed in this section. The list is too exhaustive to review in this chapter, and the authors suggest a neurology text for further detail.

Compression Neuropathy

Compression or entrapment neuropathy is a type of mononeuropathy resulting from local compression on a peripheral nerve. One well-known example is carpal tunnel syndrome. Compression neuropathies can present with varying degrees of motor, sensory, and autonomic disturbances and can be confused with myelopathy and radiculopathy. However, a careful history, physical examination, and special studies such as electromyography and nerve conduction velocity (EMG/NCV) help localize the site of compression. Injections of local anesthetics at the suspected site of compression can be performed easily in the office and can often help differentiate between several diagnoses. There are numerous peripheral nerve compression syndromes of the upper and lower extremities. Therefore, only a select few are discussed in detail, with others represented in table format (Tables 28-1 and 28-2).

BOX 28-2. Selected Conditions Associated with Peripheral Neuropathy

Metabolic
- Diabetes
- Hypothyroidism
- Uremia
- Combined subacute system degeneration

Nutritional
- Pyridoxine (vitamin B_6), cobalamin (vitamin B_{12}), and vitamin E deficiency
- Alcoholism
- Generalized malnutrition

Toxicity
- Lead
- Mercury
- Isoniazid
- Cisplatin

Infection
- Diphtheria
- Lyme disease
- Herpes zoster

Autoimmune Disease
- Rheumatoid arthritis
- Systemic lupus erythematosus
- Polyarteritis nodosa
- Sjögren disease

Neoplastic
- Paraneoplastic syndromes
- Pancoast tumor
- Peripheral nerve tumors

Hereditary
- Hereditary sensory-motor neuropathy (Charcot-Marie-Tooth)
- Amyloidosis

Idiopathic
- Brachial neuritis (Parsonage-Turner syndrome)

Upper Extremity Compression Neuropathies

Thoracic Outlet Syndrome

Thoracic outlet syndrome (TOS) is a controversial diagnosis. Some authors even question the existence of this condition. The terminology describing this entity is confusing, as well. In fact, more than 10 different terms are used to describe this syndrome in the literature.[28] In any event, TOS has persisted as the most widely recognized term for this condition and will therefore be used in the following discussion.

TOS has been divided into two major categories based on clinical presentation: vascular and neurogenic. The vascular syndrome can be further divided into arterial and venous. The neurovascular structures primarily involved in TOS include the subclavian artery and vein as well as the brachial plexus. The neurogenic form is caused by brachial plexus entrapment. It is the most common type encountered clinically.

Coursing from proximal to distal, the neurovascular bundle first passes between the anterior and middle scalene

TABLE 28-1

Compression Syndromes of the Upper Extremity

Compressive Syndrome	Anatomy	Masquerading As
Thoracic outlet syndrome	Brachial plexus compression at the level of the scalenes, clavicle, first rib, or coracoid process	Cervical radiculopathy, primarily C8, T1
Suprascapular nerve compression	Suprascapular nerve compression at the transverse scapular ligament or at the spinoglenoid notch	C5, (C6) radiculopathy
Carpal tunnel syndrome	Median nerve compression at the wrist	C6 radiculopathy
Pronator syndrome	Median nerve compression about the anteromedial elbow	C6 radiculopathy
Anterior interosseous nerve (AIN) syndrome	AIN compression in the proximal volar forearm	Not commonly confused with cervical radiculopathy because there are no sensory disturbances, only motor abnormalities (weakness of the flexor digitorum profundus to the index finger, flexor pollicis longus, and pronator quadratus)
Cubital tunnel syndrome	Ulnar nerve compression about the medial elbow	C8, T1 radiculopathy
Ulnar tunnel syndrome	Ulnar nerve compression in the canal of Guyon at the wrist	C8, T1 radiculopathy
Wartenberg syndrome	Superficial radial nerve compression between the brachioradialis and extensor carpi radialis longus in forearm	C6 radiculopathy
Posterior interosseous nerve (PIN) syndrome	PIN compression in the proximal forearm	C6, C7 radiculopathy
Radial tunnel syndrome	Radial nerve compression at or distal to the elbow	C6 radiculopathy

TABLE 28-2

Compression Syndromes of Lower Extremity

Compressive Syndrome	Anatomy	Masquerading As
Lumbosacral plexopathy	Compression of the lumbosacral plexus, (e.g., tumor, hematoma)	L1 through S4 radiculopathy
Piriformis syndrome	Sciatic nerve compression at the level of the piriformis muscle	S1 radiculopathy
Meralgia paresthetica (LFCN)	LFCN compression at the level of the inguinal ligament	L2, L3 radiculopathy
Obturator neuropathy	Compression due to many intrapelvic and hip pathologies	L1, L2, L3 radiculopathy
Saphenous neuropathy	Saphenous nerve compression at Hunter's canal or from direct trauma	L4 (L3, L5) radiculopathy
Peroneal neuropathy	Common peroneal nerve compression at the level of the fibular head	L4, L5 radiculopathy
Tarsal tunnel syndrome (tibial nerve)	Tibial nerve compression at the posteromedial ankle	L5, S1 radiculopathy

LFCN, lateral femoral cutaneous nerve.

muscles. This is referred to as the scalene triangle, with the first rib forming the base of the triangle. The subclavian vein is the exception, because it usually passes ventral to the anterior scalene muscle. Next, the neurovascular structures pass through the costoclavicular space, bordered by the clavicle rostrally and the first rib caudally. Finally, the neurovascular bundle passes beneath the coracoid process of the scapula through the subcoracoid space. This space is bordered by the coracoid process rostrally, the scapula dorsally, and the tendon of the pectoralis minor and costocoracoid ligament ventrally.

Etiologies of TOS can be divided into congenital, traumatic, and acquired categories.[28] An example of a congenital anomaly causing TOS is the presence of a cervical rib or fibrous cervical band. The presence of this anomaly causes the neurovascular structures to be stretched and kinked as they are draped over the extra rib or cervical band on their way to the upper extremity. Cervical ribs can be noted on careful inspection of plain radiographs of the cervical spine (Fig. 28-5). An unusually large C7 transverse process seen on AP cervical spine radiographs suggests the presence of a cervical band[29] (Fig. 28-6). Traumatic factors can also play a role in developing TOS. One example is a clavicle fracture that heals in a malreduced position or one that develops a significantly large callus. This can decrease the size of the costoclavicular space, leading to compression of the neurovascular structures. The most common cause of TOS, which falls into the acquired category, is posture related. Upper thoracic and cervical spine posture influences the flexibility and tone of the scalene muscles. Forward shoulder posture with scapular depression narrows the costoclavicular space and causes adaptive shortening of the pectoralis minor muscle and the costocoracoid ligament.

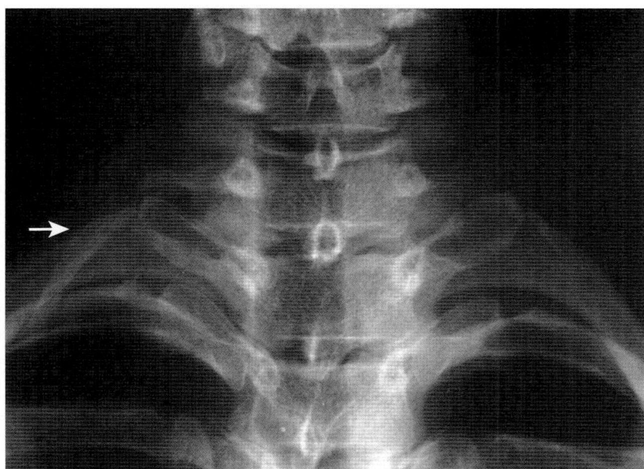

FIGURE 28-5. Anteroposterior cervical spine radiograph demonstrating a unilateral cervical rib *(arrow)*.

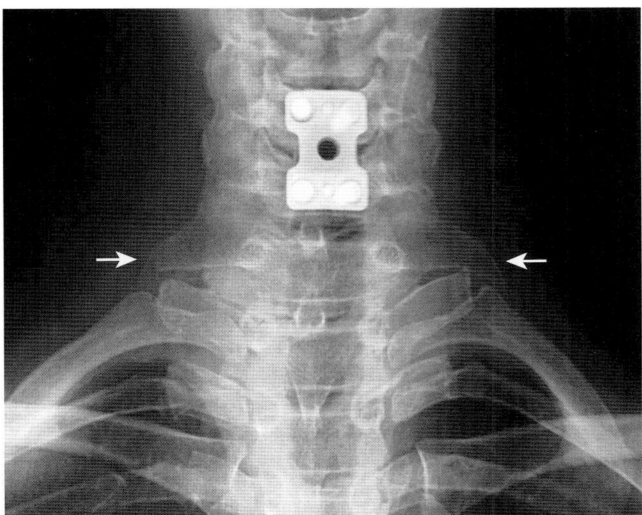

FIGURE 28-6. Anteroposterior cervical spine radiograph demonstrating large C7 transverse processes *(arrows)*. In the proper clinical setting, this may suggest the presence of cervical fibrous bands. This patient underwent C5-6 anterior cervical discectomy and fusion and bilateral carpal tunnel releases without resolution of her bilateral upper extremity paresthesias. Her symptoms finally resolved after surgical release of left and right fibrous cervical bands.

Signs and symptoms in the patient with TOS include pain, paresthesias, motor weakness, and autonomic disturbances in the involved upper extremity. Pain can be reported from the supraclavicular and periscapular regions down the arm to the fingers, not necessarily in a dermatomal pattern. Paresthesias, including tingling or numbness, may be more often described in the C8-T1 distribution. Motor deficits may be noted in the hand, particularly the intrinsic muscles. Even without objective weakness or visible atrophy, patients may complain of hand weakness and poor dexterity. Chronic cases of TOS have been known to cause trophic changes in the hand. Vasomotor signs and symptoms, including periodic pallor or cyanosis, may indicate involvement of the sympathetic fibers or vascular compression.[28]

Many cases of TOS are diagnoses of exclusion. However, once other diagnoses have been ruled out and TOS is being considered, several physical examination maneuvers assist in establishing the diagnosis. Unfortunately, none of these tests are specific or sensitive. They, however, are used together along with clinical judgment and other tests (radiographs, EMG/NCV) to rule out related pathology. The physical examination maneuvers are designed to reproduce the patient's symptoms by compressing the brachial plexus at various points. The Adson maneuver is probably the most recognized physical examination method of testing for TOS. With the patient standing or seated, the examiner locates the radial pulse and then extends, externally rotates, and slightly abducts the shoulder while keeping the elbow straight. The patient is then instructed to rotate the cervical spine toward (or away from) the test extremity, then take a deep breath and hold it. Disappearance of the pulse indicates a positive test, as does the reproduction of paresthesias. Unfortunately, some individuals with no symptoms lose their pulse with this maneuver, so interpretation of this test must be made in the context of the entire clinical picture. Additional tests for TOS include the Roos test, Wright test, and costoclavicular syndrome test. Finally, tapping or gently applying pressure to the supraclavicular fossa may reproduce the patient's upper extremity paresthesias. Eliciting a positive Tinel sign in this manner is consistent with TOS.

Median Neuropathy

The most common peripheral neuropathy of the upper extremity is compression of the median nerve at the level of the wrist, known as carpal tunnel syndrome. The median nerve is formed by the lateral and medial cords of the brachial plexus and therefore carries fibers from C5, C6, C7, C8, and T1. The carpal tunnel is a fibro-osseous channel containing nine flexor tendons and the median nerve. The causes of carpal tunnel syndrome are too numerous to mention but can be divided into two major categories: (1) those conditions that decrease the size of the carpal tunnel such as distal radius fracture; and (2) those that take up space in the tunnel such as flexor tenosynovitis and ganglion cysts. (Additional median nerve compression neuropathies that occur about the elbow and proximal forearm include the pronator syndrome and the anterior interosseous syndrome [see Table 28-1].)

Carpal Tunnel Syndrome. The clinical picture of carpal tunnel syndrome includes pain and paresthesias in the palmar-radial aspect of the hand, which are often worse at night and aggravated by repetitive use of the hand. Occupational and recreational risk factors should be elicited in the history, including vibration exposure and repetitive use of the hands and wrists. The most common pattern of median nerve sensory distribution in the hand is shown in Figure 28-7A, and comparison with the typical C6 and C7 dermatomes is shown in Figure 28-7B. EMG/NCV testing can help delineate anomalies such as Martin-Gruber anastomosis. The physical examination may demonstrate decreased sensation in the median nerve distribution, particularly with threshold testing using Semmes-Weinstein monofilament. A late finding may be thenar muscle atrophy and weakness, particularly of the abductor pollicis brevis. Additional physical examination maneuvers are directed at reproducing the patient's hand paresthesias. The Tinel

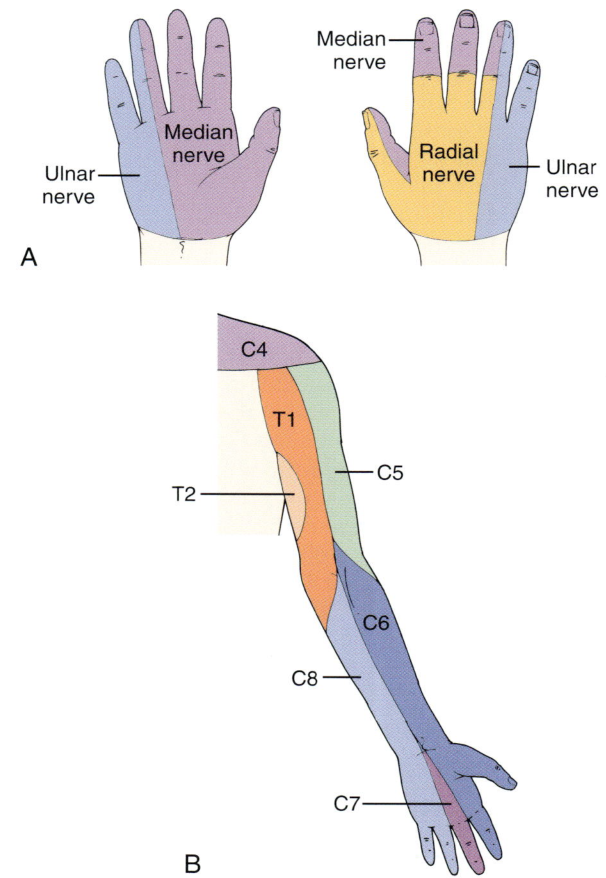

FIGURE 28-7. A representation of peripheral nerve sensory distribution (**A**) versus dermatomal distribution (**B**) for the upper extremity.

percussion test is probably the most commonly performed test. The examiner uses a finger to lightly tap over the carpal tunnel in an effort to reproduce paresthesias in the median nerve distribution; the occurrence of paresthesias indicates a positive test (sensitivity 0.60, specificity 0.67). The tapping should be performed from the wrist to the proximal forearm to rule out more proximal sites of median nerve compression. The Phalen test requires maintaining the wrist flexed to 90 degrees. Numbness and tingling in the median nerve distribution within 60 seconds is considered a positive test (sensitivity 0.75, specificity 0.47). The carpal compression test is performed when the examiner applies direct pressure over the median nerve at the wrist. The occurrence of paresthesias within 30 seconds is considered a positive response (sensitivity 0.87, specificity 0.90).[30]

When the diagnosis of carpal tunnel syndrome is suspected, cervical radiculopathy and proximal median nerve compression should be ruled out. Cervical radiculopathy can be placed higher or lower on the differential diagnosis list by a careful examination of hand and forearm sensation, wrist extensor strength, deep tendon reflexes (brachioradialis), the Spurling test, and cervical spine ROM. Signs and symptoms have been shown to be very useful in differentiating carpal tunnel syndrome from cervical spondylosis.[31] Certainly cervical radiculopathy and carpal tunnel syndrome can coexist, making EMG/NCV testing an invaluable part of the workup. When a patient presents with signs and symptoms of bilateral carpal tunnel syndrome, systemic and metabolic etiologies such as hypothyroidism, diabetes, and amyloidosis (to mention a few) should be considered.

Ulnar Neuropathy

The ulnar nerve is prone to compression at several sites in the upper extremity and can mimic lower cervical spine radiculopathy. The ulnar nerve is a terminal branch of the medial cord of the brachial plexus and usually carries spinal levels C8 and T1. The most common site of ulnar nerve compression in the upper extremity is at the dorsomedial elbow, referred to as cubital tunnel syndrome. Cubital tunnel syndrome can be caused by fascial and anomalous muscle tissue, various soft tissues such as tumors and ganglion cysts, subluxating ulnar nerve, bone spurs, and cubitus valgus deformity. The ulnar nerve can also be compressed in the canal of Guyon at the wrist, a condition called ulnar tunnel syndrome. The canal of Guyon is a fibro-osseous tunnel where the ulnar nerve and artery pass from the forearm into the hand. Several of the more common pathologies implicated are ganglion cysts, ulnar artery aneurysm (or thrombosis), and fractures of the hook of the hamate.[30]

Cubital Tunnel Syndrome. Patients with cubital tunnel syndrome complain of numbness and/or paresthesias in the ulnar side of the hand. There is also numbness in the distribution of the dorsal sensory branch of the ulnar nerve but a lack of sensory disturbance in the medial forearm, which is supplied by the C8 dermatome (see Fig. 28-7B). This helps differentiate cubital tunnel syndrome from cervical radiculopathy. Patients may also complain of worsening symptoms when the elbow is in a flexed position for a prolonged period, such as when driving or sleeping. This is due to increased intraneural pressure and decreased cubital tunnel space with elbow flexion or from subluxation of the ulnar nerve over the medial epicondyle as the elbow is flexed. Tapping over the cubital tunnel (Tinel sign) can often reproduce the patient's paresthesias. In addition to sensory changes, there may also be interosseous wasting and related weakness, which is usually a late finding. The more common sites of ulnar nerve compression about the elbow, from proximal to distal, are arcade of Struthers, medial intermuscular septum, medial epicondyle, cubital tunnel, and proximal edge of the pronator aponeurosis. A careful physical examination can usually differentiate cervical radiculopathy from cubital tunnel syndrome. EMG/NCV can confirm the level of compression, and plain radiographs of the elbow can rule out bony pathology as a source of compression.[30]

Radial Neuropathy

The radial nerve has several regions of potential compression in the upper extremity, rarely proximal to the elbow and more commonly in the forearm. The radial nerve carries fibers from C5, C6, C7, C8, and inconsistently T1, and it is one of the terminal branches of the posterior cord. Syndromes involving compression of the radial nerve include radial tunnel syndrome, Wartenberg syndrome, and posterior interosseous nerve compression syndrome. These are compression neuropathies of the forearm, which can usually, but not always, be differentiated based on patient complaints and careful physical examination. Radial neuropathy is most likely to be confused with a C6 or C7 radiculopathy (see Fig. 28-7).

Lower Extremity Compression Neuropathies

Piriformis Syndrome

Piriformis syndrome refers to entrapment of the sciatic nerve as it passes beneath or through the piriformis muscle, causing pain along the distribution of the sciatic nerve (buttock, dorsal thigh, and dorsal leg). This distribution is also a common source of pain in a patient with an L5 or S1 intervertebral disc herniation, thereby causing a diagnostic dilemma. The piriformis syndrome is a controversial diagnosis; some authors deny its existence, others believe that it should be a diagnosis of exclusion, and yet others consider it a primary diagnostic entity.[32] The sciatic nerve is the largest nerve in the body and is actually composed of two nerves: the common peroneal nerve and the tibial nerve. The peroneal portion arises from the ventral rami of spinal levels L4-S2, and the tibial portion arises from the ventral rami of L4-S3. The sciatic nerve exits the pelvis, coursing through the greater sciatic foramen, usually caudal to the piriformis muscle; however, great variability exists in the relationship between the piriformis muscle and the sciatic nerve.

Many reported etiologic factors are associated with sciatic nerve compression at the level of the piriformis muscle. As mentioned, anatomic anomalies altering the relationship between the piriformis muscle and the sciatic nerve may increase the potential for nerve entrapment.[33] Abnormal mechanics about the lumbar spine, pelvis, hips, and lower extremities have also been implicated in piriformis syndrome due to chronic stretching of the piriformis muscle or chronic overuse of the muscle, both of which can increase compression of the nerve. Patients' symptoms can be intermittent and dynamic, precipitated by particular activities and positions.[34]

Patients with piriformis syndrome usually complain of unilateral buttock, posterior thigh, and trochanteric pain. The pain occasionally refers distal to the knee. Physical examination may demonstrate an antalgic gait, and the affected side may be held in an elevated and externally rotated position, a so-called positive piriformis sign. Palpation of the piriformis region/greater sciatic notch may elicit tenderness and may precipitate pain in the distribution of the sciatic nerve. Patients may also have a positive straight-leg raising test or worsening of their symptoms as the piriformis muscle is stretched with hip adduction and internal rotation. In fact, the Freiburg sign is manifested by reproduction of pain on forced internal rotation of the hip. Resisting hip abduction and external rotation while the patient is in the seated position, known as the Pace sign, may also reproduce symptoms in the patient with piriformis syndrome. Most patients with piriformis syndrome are diagnosed on physical examination, with or without the use of a diagnostic injection. The role of imaging studies in the workup of piriformis syndrome seems to be most important for ruling out other causes of sciatica-type pain. Special testing such as EMG/NCV may demonstrate abnormalities in the patient with piriformis syndrome, but negative electrical studies do not rule out the condition.

Meralgia Paresthetica

Meralgia paresthetica is a term used to describe pain, paresthesias, and/or numbness in the ventrolateral thigh due to neuropathy of the lateral femoral cutaneous nerve (LFCN) and is also referred to as Bernhardt disease. The term *meralgia* comes from two Greek words, *meros* (thigh) and *algos* (pain).[35] The LFCN typically originates from the dorsal branches of the ventral rami of L2, L3, and occasionally L1 and therefore has the ability to mimic upper lumbar radiculopathy. The most common site of entrapment is thought to be the site at which the nerve passes above, below, or through the inguinal ligament just medial to the anterior superior iliac spine. There is considerable anatomic variation as the nerve courses past the inguinal ligament from the pelvis to the thigh.[16]

Some authors have divided the etiology of meralgia paresthetica into spontaneous and iatrogenic forms, but this section will discuss only the spontaneous etiologies. Most noniatrogenic causes of LFCN neuropathies are either mechanical compression or metabolic neuropathy. Mechanical compression can result from external causes such as obesity and pregnancy due to increased intra-abdominal pressure and direct compression at the level of the inguinal ligament, as well as from wearing tight, low-lying pants or belts. Compression can also come from within by way of intra-abdominal and intrapelvic tumors, for example (Fig. 28-8). The LFCN bypasses many potentially entrapping structures prior to reaching the level of the inguinal ligament. Several metabolic conditions, including diabetes mellitus and alcoholism, can be causative or at least associated with neuropathy of the LFCN.

Patients with meralgia paresthetica complain of pain, burning, paresthesias, numbness, or hypersensitivity in the distribution of the LFCN, which overlaps the dermatomal distribution supplied by L2 and L3 (Fig. 28-9). The LFCN carries only sensory fibers. Therefore, weakness on examination should raise suspicion of conditions other than meralgia paresthetica to explain the patient's symptoms.[36] Physical examination may demonstrate decreased sensation in the LFCN distribution, which is different than the true L2 or L3 dermatome distribution. Extending the hip, which places the nerve under tension, increases intraneural pressure and exacerbates the compressive pathology; this maneuver may

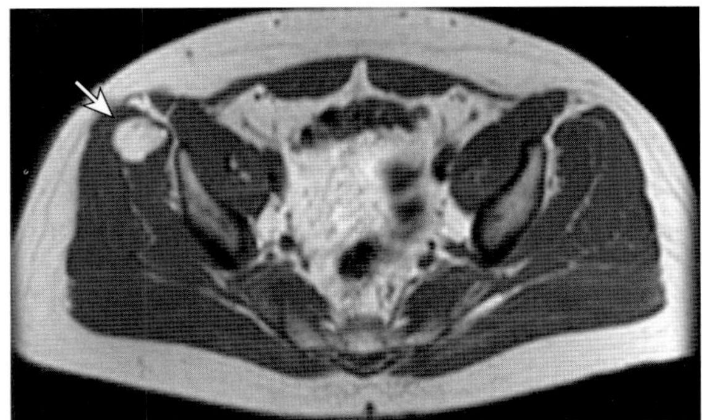

FIGURE 28-8. Axial cut from an MRI scan of the pelvis. This patient had pain and paresthesias in the right anterolateral thigh, thought to be a lumbar radiculopathy. Note the lipomatous lesion *(arrow)* that was compressing the lateral femoral cutaneous nerve.

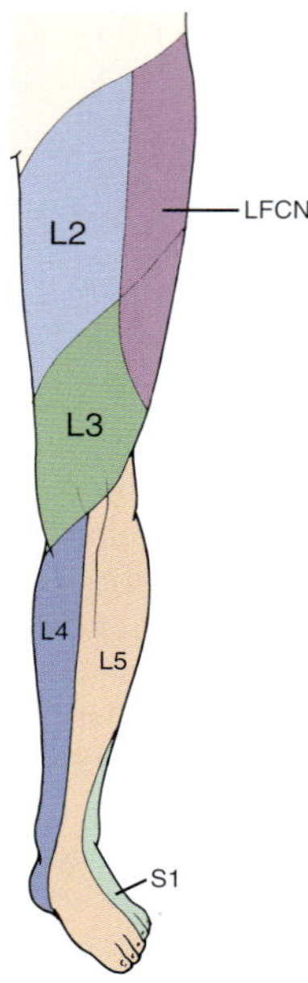

FIGURE 28-9. A representation of lower extremity dermatomal sensory patterns of innervation versus that of the lateral femoral cutaneous nerve (LFCN; *shaded region*).

reproduce patients' paresthesias and pain. Additionally, palpation or Tinel percussion about the site of compression may also reproduce their symptoms. If the history and physical examination are equivocal, electrodiagnostic testing can be helpful. As with most peripheral compression neuropathies, injection of a local anesthetic at the site of compression can be used as a diagnostic test.

Metabolic Neuropathy: Diabetic Neuropathy

Patients with diabetes mellitus may present with a wide variety of signs and symptoms with respect to peripheral neuropathy because their disease process can affect sensory, motor, and autonomic fibers. Although the causative factors for neuropathy in patients with diabetes are multiple and complex, several studies support hyperglycemia as playing an important role in the development of neuropathy.[37] Classifying neuropathy in diabetes is difficult. However, one simple classification distinguishes between mononeuropathy (isolated or multiple) and polyneuropathy. This section will discuss the three most common presentations: sensory mononeuropathy, proximal motor neuropathy, and distal sensory neuropathy.

Diabetic mononeuropathy includes several common peripheral compression neuropathies that patients with diabetes are at greater risk for developing more frequently than patients without the disease. Some examples are carpal tunnel syndrome, cubital tunnel syndrome, meralgia paresthetica, and peroneal neuropathy near the head of the fibula. Additionally, patients with diabetes (and other endocrinopathies) may present more commonly with bilateral symptoms due to the systemic nature of the neuropathy. These mononeuropathies are not limited to the periphery, because patients with diabetes can suffer from truncal neuropathy. Patients describe pain and paresthesias in a bandlike distribution about the chest and abdomen. As far as the spine specialist is concerned, these neuropathies can certainly mimic extremity and truncal radiculopathy.

Proximal motor neuropathy (also known as diabetic amyotrophy or diabetic polyradiculopathy) is another clinical presentation in patients with diabetes, typically in older patients with type 2 diabetes. Presenting signs and symptoms include pain, weakness, and atrophy of the proximal lower extremity musculature.[28] It can present unilaterally or bilaterally, with bilateral findings being asymmetrical. These clinical findings can be similar to those found in patients with lumbar spinal stenosis, and coexisting pathology makes diagnosis and treatment more difficult.

Distal sensory neuropathy is the most common neuropathy found in the diabetic population. These patients can present with a wide variety of symptoms ranging from significant burning pain, paresthesias, and numbness to an insensate foot with Charcot arthropathy. Distal sensory neuropathy usually develops gradually. However, an acute form may develop during a period of poor glycemic control. The legs and feet are commonly involved in a stocking-like distribution, and less commonly the hands are affected in a glovelike distribution. Proprioception may also be impaired; patients may complain of progressively worsening balance with increasing falls as well as demonstrating increased sway with Romberg testing.[37] Many of these signs and symptoms overlap with those of spinal stenosis.

Visceral Organs and Related Systems

The visceral organs of the thoracic, abdominal, and pelvic cavities are associated with pathologic conditions that may present with signs and symptoms that can be confused with spine pathology (Box 28-3). The mechanism responsible for this is generally thought to involve a referred pain mechanism. Although the majority of patients with these conditions have signs and symptoms related to the organ system involved, back pain or radiculopathy could be the sole presenting complaint. This section will discuss spinal masqueraders as they relate to the cardiovascular, pulmonary, gastrointestinal, genitourinary, and gynecologic systems.

Cardiovascular System

Myocardial Ischemia

Cardiac ischemia can result in multiple signs and symptoms, occurring either together or in isolation. Patients with ischemic heart disease can present with any combination of the following signs and symptoms: retrosternal pain; pressure, tightness, or burning; nausea; diaphoresis; epigastric discomfort; pain and numbness in the shoulder, arm, or hand; and interscapular, neck, jaw, or face pain. Many of these signs and symptoms are referred to as angina "equivalents."[38] In fact, there are several case reports of patients presenting to their dentist with complaints of jaw or tooth pain, which is ultimately discovered to be of cardiac origin.

Of particular interest to the spine surgeon is the upper extremity and interscapular back pain that can be of cardiac origin. In patients with myocardial ischemia, the prevalence of arm pain or numbness has been reported as high as 46% to 67% and that of back pain approximately 6%.[39,40] When arm

BOX 28-3. Visceral Organ Conditions Known to Mimic Spine Pathology

Cardiovascular
- Myocardial ischemia
- Aortic aneurysm
- Vascular claudication
- Infectious endocarditis

Pulmonary
- Pancoast tumor
- Lung carcinoma with paraneoplastic syndromes (peripheral neuropathy)

Gastrointestinal
- Peptic ulcer disease
- Cholecystitis
- Pancreatic disease (pancreatitis, carcinoma)
- Colon disease, carcinoma (lumbosacral radiculopathy)

Genitourinary
- Urolithiasis
- Pyelonephritis, polycystic kidney disease, renal infarct
- Prostate disease
- Malignancy

Gynecologic
- Ovarian cyst
- Endometriosis
- Uterine malpositioning
- Carcinoma

pain does occur due to cardiac ischemia, it is more common on the left side and typically refers to the shoulder, medial arm, and forearm. An additional useful aspect of the patient's history is that the symptoms are exertional. Fortunately, the majority of patients with ischemic heart disease have more than just arm pain, and an appropriate history and review of systems help lead to the correct diagnosis.

Aortic Aneurysm

Patients with an aortic aneurysm may be asymptomatic or may have variable pain from mild to significant. For example, aortic arch aneurysms can refer pain to the neck, whereas aneurysm or dissection of the thoracic aorta causes pain in the midback region. Patients with abdominal aortic aneurysms (AAAs) can present with mid and lower back pain.

Patients with AAAs may have no symptoms. Studies have indicated the prevalence of asymptomatic AAAs (>3 cm) is 3% to 10% in patients older than 50 years of age in the Western world, with an increasing incidence partly related to an aging population and improved detection methods.[41] When patients do have symptoms, this is likely related to leakage, rupture, or acute expansion of the aneurysm. Most AAAs rupture dorsally, and the retroperitoneal space provides a tamponade effect to slow or contain the hemorrhage, which can produce chronic low back pain. When they rupture ventrally, the peritoneal cavity provides little tamponade, resulting in significant hemorrhage and acute patient deterioration. The classic triad of abdominal or back pain, pulsatile abdominal mass, and hypotension is present in only about 25% of cases with confirmed AAA rupture.[42] AAAs increase in diameter approximately 0.2 to 0.5 cm per year on average.[43]

The most common complaint is an acute onset of abdominal or back pain, which may radiate to the groin or flank. Other symptoms include those related to compression of neighboring structures by the aneurysm. Duodenal compression can lead to nausea and vomiting, and compression of the ureter(s) may cause hydronephrosis and urinary tract symptoms. Dorsal aneurysm expansion can erode adjacent vertebral bodies, causing back pain. Additionally, aortic aneurysms may compromise blood flow to the spinal cord by aneurysm location and/or thrombus formation. Affected patients can present with back pain, radicular complaints, and varying degrees of myelopathy or paralysis from spinal cord ischemia.[44] Even in the absence of bony erosion and spinal cord ischemia, AAA can cause chronic back pain that is quite vague.

Diagnosing an asymptomatic AAA on physical examination is difficult. Variables that make this problematic include the skill and experience of the examiner, size of the patient, size of the aneurysm, and whether or not the examination is focused. Diagnosing a symptomatic AAA can also be difficult. In a study looking specifically at misdiagnoses of ruptured AAAs, 30% were initially misdiagnosed. Misdiagnoses included renal colic, diverticulitis, gastrointestinal hemorrhage, myocardial infarction, and idiopathic back pain. Fifty-four percent of patients complained of back pain, and it was the second most common complaint after abdominal pain.[42]

Because physical examination for diagnosing AAA is not reliable, imaging becomes crucial. Ultrasound, CT, and MRI are all useful in certain situations, but CT is the most used because of its rapidity, availability, cost, and ability to provide detail for surgical planning. Plain radiographs occasionally demonstrate an AAA (Fig. 28-10). The calcified aneurysmal vessel wall may be seen, as well as softer signs such as loss of the psoas or kidney shadow. If an AAA is discovered

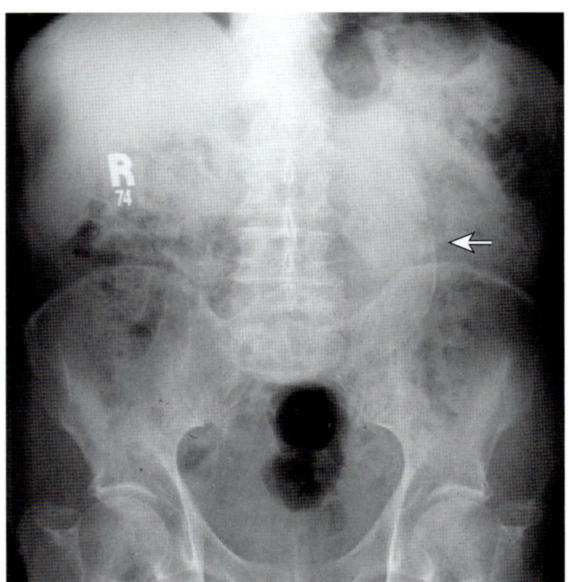

FIGURE 28-10. Anteroposterior lumbar spine radiograph demonstrating lumbar spondylosis as well as an abdominal aortic aneurysm. Note the enlarged calcified aortic wall *(arrow)*. This patient had a 3-month history of low back pain prior to presentation. Vascular surgery consultation resulted in an aortic grafting procedure.

or suspected, a prompt vascular surgery consult is in order. Aneurysms less than 5 cm in diameter can be followed with ultrasound every 4 to 6 months, with a risk of rupture ranging from 0% in 5 years to 6% per year. In aneurysms greater than 5 cm, the risk of rupture is approximately 25% at 5 years.[43]

Vascular Claudication

Intermittent vascular claudication is a disease of the cardiovascular system that must be distinguished from neurogenic claudication due to spinal stenosis. It is a symptom of chronic arterial insufficiency. Chronic arterial insufficiency can be categorized into two major groups: (1) aortoiliac disease affecting the distal aorta and iliac arteries and (2) femoral-popliteal-tibial disease affecting the arteries of the leg. Chronic arterial insufficiency of the lower extremities may have two distinct presentations: intermittent claudication and ischemic rest pain. Ischemic rest pain is typically nocturnal, diffusely involving the forefoot. In this case, the patient soon learns that the pain is relieved through dependency (effect of gravity on perfusion pressure) of the involved limb and sleeps with the involved foot in a dependent position.

The more common condition mimicking spine pathology is intermittent vascular claudication. These patients can present with buttock, thigh, calf, and/or foot claudication, depending on the site of the occlusion. Calf claudication is the most common presentation. Like any of the lower extremity vascular claudication symptoms, they are reliably reproduced after a certain amount of exercise or ambulation distance and are relieved after a few minutes of rest. This is also seen in spinal stenosis with neurogenic claudication symptoms. However, there are signs and symptoms that are useful in differentiating these two conditions.

Generally, either disease can present with a variety of lower extremity complaints, including numbness, weakness, cramping sensation, pain, and a feeling of tiredness in the legs. In the case of foraminal stenosis, the findings may include a dermatomal distribution of sensory changes and a myotomal pattern of weakness. Numbness is a common complaint in either condition. A complaint of weakness in arterial insufficiency is typically a sense of hip and thigh weakness, especially with proximal occlusion. Cramping in the calves is a classic complaint of vascular insufficiency but occurs in either disease, as does the vague complaint of lower extremity fatigability and tiredness with ambulation. The lower extremity symptoms caused by arterial insufficiency are relieved with rest (stopping ambulation), whether standing or sitting. That is to say, a change in patients' spine posture does not affect their symptoms. In patients with spinal stenosis, standing itself may produce symptoms and sitting (lumbar spine flexion) relieves the symptoms.[45] Some patients with neurogenic claudication volunteer that they can walk further when shopping and leaning on a cart. This position allows the lumbar spine to flex, which increases the dimensions of the spinal canal and intervertebral foramen, thereby relieving neural element compression. When impotence is a complaint, it is commonly associated with buttock and thigh claudication as a result of aortoiliac insufficiency.

In addition to presenting symptoms, some physical examination findings are unique to each condition. In neurogenic claudication, the involved spinal levels may correspond to diminished deep tendon reflexes and positive nerve root tension tests. Physical examination maneuvers associated with lumbar spinal stenosis include a wide-based gait, abnormal Romberg test, thigh pain after 30 seconds of lumbar extension, and neuromuscular deficits.[45] Intermittent vascular claudication may present with diminished pulses (femoral, popliteal, dorsalis pedis, and posterior tibial) and bruits. Ankle-brachial indices (ABI) will also be diminished. Normal ABI is 1, whereas vascular "claudicators" have an ABI between 0.6 and 0.9. An ABI less than 0.5 may be associated with rest pain and ulceration. It is necessary to realize that the calcified vessels in patients with diabetes yield a falsely elevated ABI. In those patients with vascular claudication, there may also be trophic changes in the feet and distal legs (thin, shiny, atrophic skin, thickened and ridged nails, and loss of hair) and they may feel cool. One may also find that elevating the limb produces pallor (cadaveric) of the foot and a dusky rubor when placing the foot in the dependent position (Buerger sign). Finally, the van Gelderen bicycle test can help differentiate vascular and neurogenic claudication.[46] Exercising on a stationary bike should reproduce the symptoms of vascular disease more rapidly and reliably because the disease is one of ischemia, so the type of exercise (walking or cycling) should not matter. However, in spinal stenosis, sitting or positions of lumbar spine flexion (as on a stationary bike) often relieve the lower extremity symptoms, and therefore patients with spinal stenosis are able to ride a stationary bike without necessarily reproducing their symptoms. Certainly, patients can have both spinal stenosis and arterial occlusive disease; therefore, consultation with a vascular surgeon may be warranted in this situation.

Infective (Bacterial) Endocarditis

The term *infective endocarditis* (IE) is used to describe an infection of the endocardial surface of a heart valve. The clinical picture of IE can be extremely varied, and of all the potential presenting symptoms, musculoskeletal complaints are frequent and often the initial complaints.[47-49] Several series have reported that more than 40% of patients with IE manifest musculoskeletal signs and symptoms, and as many as 25% of patients have musculoskeletal complaints as the initial symptoms.[47] Of particular interest to the spine specialist are the complaints of neck and back pain and lower extremity myalgias in the thighs and calves. As many as 5% to 20% of patients with IE have back pain as their presenting symptom, and this may be the only complaint for several months, delaying the correct diagnosis. Lower extremity myalgias, although not radicular in distribution, may be severe enough to make the clinician consider radiculopathy in the differential diagnosis, particularly when accompanied by back pain.[48]

The low back pain associated with IE can be quite severe and can present with paraspinal tenderness, muscle spasm, and decreased ROM. The pain may be accentuated by straight-leg raising and Valsalva maneuvers and may be accompanied by lower extremity myalgias, all suggesting a herniated lumbar intervertebral disc.[47] Generally, in patients with complaints of back pain, they are unable to obtain positional relief. Some patients with low back pain and IE have a disc space infection or vertebral osteomyelitis; however, the majority of musculoskeletal manifestations are thought to be related to arterial emboli containing bacteria and immune complexes causing a vasculitic reaction. It has also been suggested that the low back pain in some patients may be a nonspecific manifestation of the infection. Other common symptoms of IE include fever, chills, weakness, anorexia, and headache. Additional signs include heart murmur (changing or new) and dermatologic manifestations such as splinter hemorrhages and petechiae.

Pulmonary System: Pancoast Tumor

The most significant pulmonary condition to present with signs and symptoms, seemingly of spinal origin, is a tumor at the superior pulmonary sulcus (Pancoast tumor). This region lies in close proximity to the C8 and T1 nerve roots and the lower trunk of the brachial plexus, making cervical radiculopathy as well as peripheral neuropathy high on the differential diagnosis in the patient with a Pancoast tumor. Several signs and symptoms can help raise suspicion of a superior sulcus tumor. The majority of patients with a Pancoast tumor are smokers. Unfortunately, respiratory symptoms rarely dominate the initial clinical picture. One of the first and most significant symptoms is shoulder pain, and this is the presenting symptom in more than 90% of patients.[50] The lower trunk of the brachial plexus, the subclavian artery and vein, and the sympathetic chain and stellate ganglia are a few of the important structures in close proximity to the superior pulmonary sulcus that help explain some of the signs and symptoms in these patients. In addition to shoulder pain and lower plexus neuropathy, other findings include Horner syndrome, supraclavicular fullness, upper extremity swelling or discoloration, and hand intrinsic muscle wasting. Many authors state that Pancoast tumor should be in the differential diagnosis whenever lower brachial plexopathy exists, and some include this in their differential diagnosis even with C8 and T1 radiculopathy. If the diagnosis of Pancoast tumor is entertained, chest imaging beginning with routine chest radiographs, including an apical lordotic view, remains a crucial step in the workup (Figs. 28-11 and 28-12). Unfortunately, the average lag time between the onset of symptoms and definitive diagnosis is 7 to 7.5 months.[50]

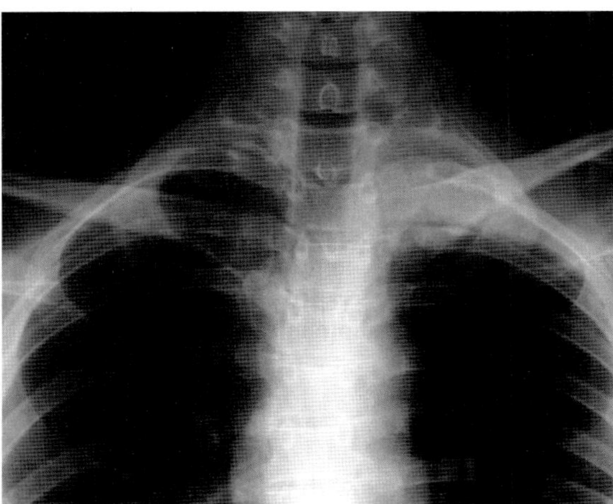

FIGURE 28-11. Anteroposterior chest radiograph demonstrating left upper lobe opacity, an expected appearance with a Pancoast tumor.

Gastrointestinal System

Although not common, patients with gastrointestinal pathology present with pain referred to the spine. Pathology of the stomach/small intestine (ulcer disease), gallbladder, pancreas, and large intestine can all mimic spine pathology.[51] Peptic ulcer disease, cholecystitis, and pancreatic conditions can all refer pain to the thoracic region and thoracolumbar junction, whereas pathology of the colon can refer pain to the lumbar region or can cause compression on the lumbosacral plexus, mimicking lumbar radiculopathy.[51-57] Although signs or symptoms related to the primary structure involved are usually present, there are occasions when back pain or radiculopathy is the presenting symptom.

The patient with peptic ulcer disease and biliary colic due to cholelithiasis may present with back pain, from the interscapular to the thoracolumbar region. In fact, a German gastroenterologist named Ismar Boas (1858–1938) described a tender spot (Boas point) to the left of the T12 vertebra dorsally in patients with gastric ulcer disease. The literature reflects this with cases of patients being treated for musculoskeletal thoracic spine problems only to have resolution of their pain after diagnosis and treatment for peptic ulcer disease. In patients with cholelithiasis and biliary colic, 50% complain of periscapular back pain. Often, these patients complain of intermittent abdominal pain and nausea and may have a positive Murphy sign.[5]

Genitourinary System

The kidneys, ureters, and bladder can be a source of referred pain to the abdomen, flank, back, and groin and can therefore mimic spine disease.[51,58] Several conditions known to cause either flank, back, or groin pain include urolithiasis, pyelonephritis, urinary tract infection, renal artery occlusion, and neoplasm.[59] Disease of the prostate such as prostatitis has also been associated with low back pain, often radiating to the rectum. As with most organ systems, these conditions usually have presenting complaints other than referred pain such as abdominal pain, abdominal mass, dysuria, hematuria, nausea, and/or fever, depending on the underlying process.

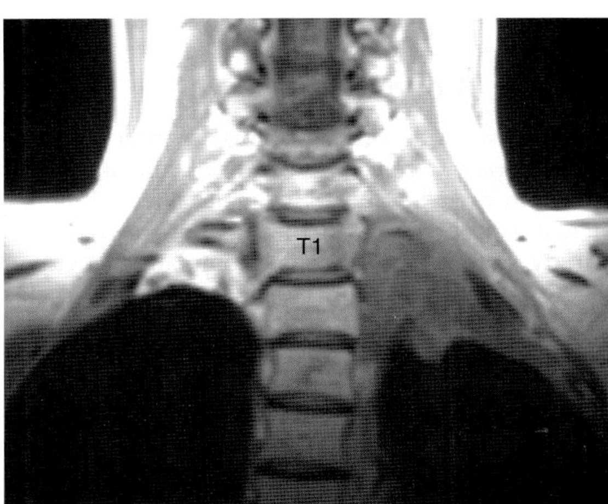

FIGURE 28-12. Coronal MRI scan of the patient in Figure 28-11. Note the left upper lobe tumor encroaching on the lower portion of the brachial plexus. When upper extremity paresthesias continued after cervical spine surgery, additional workup revealed the Pancoast tumor.

CHAPTER 29

Data Management

Micheal J. Speck | Irene Katzan | Ajit A. Krishnaney

The incorporation of true evidence-based models into the care for spinal disorders necessitates the collection of outcomes metrics throughout the continuum of patient care. Until this is realized, the clinical decision process will continue to rely on subjective, anecdotal evidence, with a risk that ineffective treatments will continue to be performed at both high financial and patient expense. Although this is not a problem among skilled practitioners, this subjective model does nothing to promote improved outcomes at a macro level and does not translate well across health systems.

Ultimately, significant barriers pose a challenge to create a system to capture and evaluate outcome measures consistently. At a very fundamental level, the data collection process has a negative effect on the bottom line. Any system designed to capture outcomes data requires human resources, hardware, and software. At its outset, even the most basic system adds to the cost per visit or admission. Worse yet, the data collection process has the potential to disrupt clinical work flows, and the information collected may not always be immediately useful (some data elements will be clinically relevant, but many will not prove their significance until much later).

All of these factors serve as disincentives to implement a system for collecting information about outcomes of care. However, external forces, such as public reporting of outcomes data and value-based purchasing, are starting to drive demand and will eventually overcome the barriers. In the long term, ignoring the call for objective clinical outcomes will prove to be incredibly costly. Appropriately designed systems will allow practitioners to measure the effectiveness of available treatments against the relative cost. Once this type of analysis is available at the point of clinical decision, physicians can finally apply their clinical expertise for the exceptions and depend on evidence for the "regular" cases. This outcome will allow the provider and the health care delivery system to contain cost while maintaining high standards of care.

Most importantly, a patient-centric approach to spine surgery means that specific clinical characteristics, interventions, and outcomes should be considered in context. Data management for such a varied and distributed dataset is extremely complex. It will require a thoughtful and intentional plan that is executed by a strong team with a wide array of skills, from the clinical through the technologic.

Building a Successful Outcomes Information System

The database itself is but one component of an efficient scheme for data collection, storage, and retrieval. At this point it is necessary to highlight a crucial aspect of understanding outcomes information systems (outcomes systems). The word *system* is used here to accent the simple distinction between the data "store," or database (i.e., the electronic data storage mechanism), and its functional environment. Although each system typically has a database at its core that is responsible for data storage, the overall system is much broader, including database management software, data processing software, presentation applications (i.e., browsers), user interfaces (i.e., input and output screens), and the hardware on which it operates (Fig. 29-1). The term *database* simply refers to the data storage mechanism. Within the context of an overall information system, the database can perform properly, but the database is entirely useless outside of the system. Ideally, a well-designed database drives the development of its interrelated technical components (i.e., hardware and software), resulting in an efficient and elegant solution for outcomes research.

Too often, the term *database* is used to describe not only the database but also the database management software used to create and administer it. Although the difference is subtle, it is important. Database management software has drastically simplified the database administration process (maintenance and data management) in recent years, and this has fostered the idea that the underlying databases are simple as well. This is a common and costly misconception. A poorly designed database that is at the heart of an outcomes system invariably leads to faulty data processing and an unsuccessful project. Unfortunately, poor database design is not always immediately evident, and a substantial amount of time, effort, and resources can be wasted before the inherent problems manifest themselves.

This discussion is intended to help bridge the divide between individuals who desire a medical outcomes information system and those who possess the knowledge and skills to build and maintain it. There is often a significant gap between the perceived resource requirements, in terms of time, technology, and human resources, the creation of such

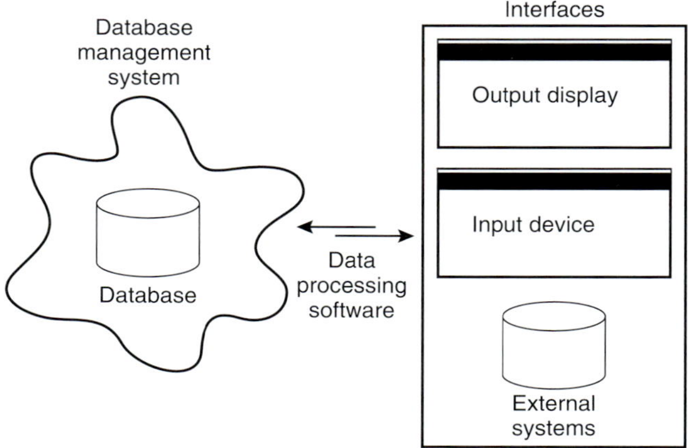

FIGURE 29-1. Schematic of database management.

a system, and the actual requirements. This is especially true with respect to the time necessary for design and development. However, effective communication between the users and the technical staff (i.e., the individuals commissioned to build and maintain a system) can drastically shorten the development cycle. Therefore, here this relationship is analyzed throughout all of the system development stages, beginning with the initial conceptual development and finishing with implementation. The system development process is deconstructed into three key stages: definition, design, and deployment.

System (Project) Definition

Defining the Research Focus

Defining the research focus of the outcomes information system must be a thoughtful, deliberate exercise by the principal investigator, coinvestigators, and clinical project leadership. Carefully defining the question(s) to be answered by the data collected, stored, and ultimately retrieved from the outcomes system is both necessary and critical. A clear vision of the questions at hand, the statistical analysis, and hence the system purpose establishes a solid platform on which the entire system can be built. The result of the definitional phase is the determination of the system/project size and scope from a clinical, technologic, and operational standpoint. Once defined, the ability to obtain answers to the proposed questions serves as the benchmark against which the final system will be evaluated.

A common mistake with system development is to postpone the process of defining the goals, consciously or unconsciously. Individuals who adopt this approach view the definitional phase of the outcomes information system as an evolutionary process in which the defining elements theoretically become evident as the project takes shape, rather than take specific steps to determine them. This inevitably leads to a poorly designed database at the heart of the outcomes system, which functions neither efficiently nor appropriately. Conversely, thorough investigation and due diligence during the definitional phase of the project foster the establishment of a blueprint from which the entire system can be built, thus maximizing the system's efficiency and its ability to achieve the stated objectives.

Understanding the Clinical and Operational Environment

It is impossible to design an appropriate model for data management without a clear understanding of a physician's working environment. This includes cataloging the types of disorders that are treated, the available treatment options, and the factors that influence treatment decisions (i.e., patient age, comorbidities, and medical history), the myriad of possible outcome patterns, the nature and impetus of patient-physician interactions, and measures by which treatments are validated. Clearly, it is the clinician who can best describe this environment, and the transfer of this information to the information technology personnel on the project team is critical. Any disconnect between the clinician and the analyst is most damaging during this phase. However, if this divide can be overcome in the early stages of the process, subsequent tasks become increasingly more manageable.

The establishment of clear project objectives primarily provides a blueprint for the information system and also delivers a number of secondary benefits. It is during this phase that the original concept is validated. Participants (e.g., clinicians, nurses, administrators, analysts) have the opportunity to consider every aspect of the project, and most importantly, the outcomes information system has a distinct model for comparison. Without this objective model, there is no clear way to determine whether the overall project goals have been satisfied.

Describing the Patient Population

The first definitional requirement relates to the description of the patient population. A method by which individual patients and their associated treatments can be compared as a subset of a heterogeneous patient population needs to be established. Some of the critical metrics such as age and gender are universal and relatively straightforward, whereas others such as education level and workers compensation status are more directed and often relate to specific research questions. Core elements that indicate the patient's medical profile include diagnoses, symptoms, and physical signs.

Determining Data Elements

Pursuant to the definition of the outcomes model, difficult decisions surrounding the inclusion of data elements need to be made. The natural tendency is to attempt to collect enough data to potentially answer any question that may surface. This, however, becomes very onerous for both clinician and patient. In this arena, considering patient and provider burden, parsimony is essential.

Input from multiple participants is important during this phase of the process so that critical data elements are not overlooked. However, it is equally important to exclude data elements that do not contribute significantly to the overall goals of the project. Great attention to detail is a requirement in the definitional phase to achieve a proper balance in the data model; the inclusion of too many data elements adds unnecessary strain on the systems resources (both human and technologic), and the exclusion of critical data elements renders the system ineffective.

Beyond the selection process, all of the data elements must be presented in a standardized and concise manner that can be readily adopted by all of the system participants (patients and health care providers). For provider-entered data elements, standardizing the terms used to describe spinal disorders and their manifestations is necessary to allow accurate categorization of patients within each specific disorder. This standardization process is essentially the process of establishing the common language that is subsequently used by all participants. Health care providers will use it to describe their patients, patient symptoms, pathologies, treatment options, and the course of therapy. For patient-reported data, using validated scales and questions that are at the appropriate education level is good practice and optimizes the accuracy of the information.

System Design

Data Mapping and Modeling

Once the nature of the data to be gathered has been defined, the source of the data must be determined. Primary data collection (i.e., patients and clinicians) and electronic sources (i.e., cost and procedure-related data from the operating room and financial systems) must both be considered. The availability and accessibility of these resources varies among institutions. Hence, data acquisition must be tailored to fit. Efficient data acquisitions can be realized through the automation of the data collection process, and automated processes should be introduced to the model wherever and whenever possible. This, of course, is dependent on the availability of data "feeds" from alternate information systems (i.e., patient demographic data retrieved from a patient scheduling system). However, some information will need to be collected directly from clinicians, patients, or both. Outcomes systems must merge all of the data sources gracefully to succeed.

Data sources are not nearly as important, however, as the data destinations. The most critical aspect of system design is found in the modeling of data. Because the components of a clinician's environment have been clearly outlined during the initial (definitional) phase of the project, the definitions are now readily available for use while designing the outcomes information system. Most effective information systems are merely reflections of real-world models. The outcomes information system is no exception. The entire process shifts from a definitional into a translational role as the descriptions of real-world entities become definitions used in the construction of a virtual model. This process is not academic, but accurate descriptions of the data, the environment, and the relationships among them can markedly simplify the process.

In the initial phase, definitions of the patients and their diagnoses, symptoms, and treatments directly describe the observable aspects of the clinician's environment. In the design phase, these definitions are abstracted, assuming a role of data description within the database. Hence, the definitional phase determines *what* data should be stored, and the design phase determines *how* it should be stored. The design phase is also the stage at which the primary responsibility shifts from the clinician to the system analyst. The system analyst, working from the model constructed by the medical and administrative staff, must develop a database model suitable for accurate, meaningful data processing. The data elements selected and defined earlier must now be organized logically into an overall data design that facilitates consistent data storage and retrieval. New questions will be considered for the same data elements determined in the definitional phase. These are directed at defining the nature of the data.

For instance, if a patient's medical record number is to be used as the main form of identification, a series of questions about the data element itself need to be addressed. First and foremost, is the medical record number an appropriate identifier? Is it truly unique, or are there circumstances in which multiple patients can share a medical record number? Will the medical record number be readily available at the time the information is collected? Are there any legal or business constraints on the use of a medical record number as a tracking measure within the information system? In this example, although medical record numbers are generally suitable for identifying specific patients, a number of privacy issues concern their use. Current law requires the use of a separate, unique identifier for each patient that is independent of the medical record number. As a result, sensitive information cannot be directly linked back to a given patient outside of the outcomes system itself. Consequently, even though the medical record number is an *effective* identification technique for patients (and patient records), it may not be an *appropriate* identifier in the overall data model.

Additional questions regarding the information pertain to the type of the data to be acquired. Drawing from the previous example, is the medical record number numeric, or can alphabetic characters be included? If character data can be used, the medical record number must be stored in a character format. Otherwise, it could make sense to store the data numerically (character formats can include numeric data, but numeric formats cannot accommodate alphabetic characters; for example, "123456" can be stored numerically, whereas "4B3R589" cannot). Once this distinction has been made, it is still necessary to decide which character or numeric format should be implemented. For instance, if a data element is to be used in any mathematical calculations, a numeric data type is necessary. However, numeric data types can be further subdivided into integer, long, float, and double, each with its own range of values, storage space requirements, and functionality (i.e., the float data type typically requires more storage space than an integer data type but permits the use of decimal places, whereas integers do not).

Columns are assigned specific data types during the database design process. Data type assignment is based on the data storage requirements of each column, and valid data entries must conform to their data type designations. The data type selection effectively restricts the allowable values in a given column (i.e., a column storing "date of service" allows only date values). In relational databases (defined later in this chapter), data types provide an excellent example of how the data are controlled implicitly through the actual structure of the data. As a result, it is important to consider current and future data needs while selecting the data type for any column. If used effectively, data typing protects the quality of the data and reduces data entry vulnerabilities.

On a grander scale, the system analyst must also consider established protocols for patient care to design a system that can be incorporated into the clinical workflow with the least amount of resistance. This includes assessing the physical layout of clinical areas, clinical and support staff availability for outcomes system functions, and patient flow throughout the clinical areas, and so on. If workstations are available in a waiting area, perhaps a patient can complete an electronic survey while he or she is waiting to see a physician. Otherwise, paper surveys can be used, but it must be determined whether the surveys, once collected, will then be scanned into the data store or whether data entry will be the responsibility of a staff person.

The most fundamental questions in the design phase address the type of database appropriate for the outcomes research project. If the study includes one clinician and a small patient population, a simple desktop database is more than adequate. In this case, the data store might even take the form of a series of files saved on the investigator's computer in lieu of a traditional database. However, if the data store must be accessed from numerous physical locations, or if there are many users sending and consuming data, the desktop approach quickly becomes unmanageable. Clearly, quantitative information, including the number of unique patients and patient visits anticipated in a given time, has significant implications concerning the type of database that is to be used. As the demands on the data collection and storage system (i.e., number of data elements, users, and simultaneous research queries) increase, the viable options are narrowed to the realm of database servers, in which the data are centrally stored and managed. Access can be offered over a network (whether local or global). Regardless of the type of database implemented in the outcomes information system, the core principles of database design are applicable. Because the relational database model is the de facto standard in this arena, it is the focus of this discussion.

Relational Database

The relational model takes its name from the mathematical term *relation*, which can roughly be translated to mean *table*, the building block for relational databases. Regardless of the method by which the relational system stores the data, presentation to the user for viewing and modification takes a tabular form, constructed of tuples (pronounced like *couples*) and attributes, commonly referred to as rows and columns, respectively. Although the mathematical terms (i.e., relation, tuple, and attribute) provide the greatest precision in database description, this discussion uses the more familiar terms (i.e., table, row, and column) for greater clarity and comprehension. The relational model presents information stored in each table in such a way that every column contains "like" data. More formally, the data contained in each column are of the same domain, or data type. The data type selection actually restricts the possible values of a column. For instance, the selection of an integer data type prohibits the entry of alphabetic characters in that column. The use of a character format permits both numeric and alphabetic values to be entered, but the values are stored in such a manner that calculations are not possible without first converting them to a numeric data type. For this reason, character formats should not be selected for any columns that store data that may be used in any type of calculations (i.e., scores, ages). However, they are appropriate for identification numbers or text fields.

Each row groups attributes of a specific entity. In a table that stores patient information, every row stores attributes of a specific patient. This contrasts the columnar view, which provides a longitudinal perspective of one specific attribute across the entire population (i.e., all of the ages of patients are stored in the same column). Consequently, the intersection of a row and column is a special occurrence within each table. The intersection represents a specific characteristic of the entity being defined by the row. For example, the patient table in Figure 29-2 contains the columns "PatientKey," "LastName," "FirstName," "Birthdate," "Physician," "AppointmentDate," and "Diagnosis." The intersection of the first row and the column called "FirstName" indicates that the entity being described (in this case, a patient) has the first name "Jane."

The reliability of these intersections is inextricably bound to the ability to distinguish each row from every[1] other row. This requires the assignment of a unique identifier, or primary key, to every row within the table. A common instinct for the row identification in a table that houses patient information is to use the patient's name as the primary key. This solution, however, breaks down as soon as two different patients with the same name are entered. The medical record number is usually a better alternative, providing a completely unique value for identifying each patient. However, for reasons discussed previously (patient privacy law), the medical record number is not generally a viable option. A more appropriate method is to assign an independent, arbitrary value as a primary key for the row. One column within the table is dedicated to the primary keys (see Fig. 29-2), and will be structured to require that each value is unique.

By assigning a distinct value as primary key for each row, two different patients with the same name can now be identified unambiguously. The uniqueness of the primary key is important because it serves as a device to connect different tables within the database. Establishment of these connections, or relationships, across tables becomes essential as the database is normalized (a process of "tuning" the data storage system, discussed later in this chapter). If each row cannot be identified and referenced individually, relationships between

Patient Table

PatientKey	LastName	FirstName	Birthdate	Physician	AppointmentDate	Diagnosis
1	Smith	Jane	01/01/1950	Jones	02/01/2003	Spondylolisthesis
2	Smith	Jane	02/01/1960	White	03/01/2003	Scoliosis
3	West	Robert	03/01/1970	Jones	04/01/2003	Rheumatoid arthritis
4	Smith	Jane	02/01/1960	White	03/01/2003	Kyphosis

Two different patients with the same name can be distinguished by using a unique key value.

FIGURE 29-2. The relational model-patient table.

Patient Table

PatientKey	LastName	FirstName	Birthdate	PhysicianForeignKey	AppointmentDate	Diagnosis
1	Smith	Jane	01/01/1950	1	02/01/2003	Spondylolisthesis
2	Smith	Jane	02/01/1960	2	03/01/2003	Scoliosis
3	West	Robert	03/01/1970	1	04/01/2003	Rheumatoid arthritis
4	Smith	Jane	02/01/1960	2	03/01/2003	Kyphosis

The Key/Foreign Key relationship allows data from separate tables to be "joined" in the creation of derived tables.

Physician Table

PhysicianKey	Physician
1	Jones
2	White

Derived Table (Join of Patient and Physician Tables)

LastName	FirstName	Birthdate	AppointmentDate	Diagnosis	Physician
Smith	Jane	01/01/1950	02/01/2003	Spondylolisthesis	Jones
Smith	Jane	02/01/1960	03/01/2003	Scoliosis	White
West	Robert	03/01/1970	04/01/2003	Rheumatoid Arthritis	Jones
Smith	Jane	02/01/1960	03/01/2003	Kyphosis	White

Data from patient table — Data from physician table

FIGURE 29-3. Derived tables.

separate tables become confused and unreliable. In the relational model, a table's primary key provides a means for other tables to reference its information. When the primary key of one table is stored in another as a link between them, it is called a foreign key, and it establishes the relationship between the two tables. As a result, data elements that are stored in separate tables in a database can be combined to form new tables (called derived tables), as Figure 29-3 demonstrates. By linking records from the patient and physician tables through the "PhysicianForeignKey" column, a derived table is created that contains the relevant data from both tables.

Although this example is somewhat trivial, the ability of the primary/foreign key model to connect otherwise disjointed tables is clear. As the discussion develops, the importance of this concept will become more evident. The application of the primary/foreign key model is one of the building blocks for normalizing the relational system.

Normalization

The rules of normalization, originally defined by Dr. E F. Codd, deal primarily with the elimination of data redundancies that lead directly to flawed data and impractical, inefficient data management in relational systems.[2] The rules of normalization provide solid guidelines for building effective relational database systems. Normalization leverages the actual structure of the database to improve the integrity of the data. In practice, normalization is manifested as a "spreading" of the data, as information is stored throughout the database in many separate tables that are interrelated. Entities should be grouped and related in the same manner that they would be observed in their real-world roles. In the same way, the differences should be maintained by using separate tables (i.e., a patient table should not contain information concerning the physician). Although this idea is fairly simple, it is the foundation of normalizing the database.

Originally, there were only three rules of normalization, but subsequent rules have been added. The rules of normalization are ordered by their degree of specificity, and each higher-order rule is contingent on compliance with each of the previous rules. A database that is in second normal form (term used to describe a database that complies with the second rule of normalization) must also be in first normal form. Each rule is more rigid than its predecessor and more difficult to use. The highest-order rules, in fact, are so strict that they can actually cause a decline in the performance of a relational system. It is uncommon for a production database to achieve anything higher than third normal form.

First Rule of Normalization

The first rule of normalization is somewhat academic: each column in a given row contains one—and only one—value. Violation of this principle is relatively easy to recognize and correct. It would seem unnatural, for instance, to include a column with the head "Physician/Diagnosis" that contains both the name of the physician and the patient's diagnosis. This problem is easily resolved by separating the two independent values into two distinct columns, "Physician" and "Diagnosis." A subtler example is demonstrated in the storage of a patient's name in a single column, rather than creating one column for the first name and another for the last name. Arguments can be made that this is not truly a violation of first normal form, but the two-attribute approach is more suitable because of the common use of last name as an identifier and sort item for groups of patients.

The higher-order rules of normalization deal more specifically with the reduction of data in the relational system. The storage of duplicate information in multiple locations causes the process of modification to become unruly. For example, in the database depicted in Figure 29-2, if Dr. Jones gets married, triggering a name change, two rows are affected (those with values of 1 and 3 in the "PatientKey" column). As a result, the physician values stored in the "Physician" column of each record must be updated, signaling a data storage redundancy. In Figure 29-3, this redundancy is corrected by isolating the physician information into its own table ("Physician"). The data have been effectively reduced, so that the same change requires the update of only one row. This type of data reduction demonstrates the importance of the primary key in the relational model. Separate, related tables are "bridged" by storing the primary key from one table (i.e., "PatientKey") as a foreign key in another (i.e., "PatientForeignKey").

Second Rule of Normalization

Although this design strengthens the overall structure of the database, Figure 29-3 has yet to satisfy the standard set by the second rule of normalization: every nonkey attribute must be irreducibly dependent on the primary key.[3] The second rule deals with the logical grouping of data elements. Tables should be designed to mirror their real-world counterparts. A table commissioned to store patient data should contain attributes of the patient only, completely separate from other entities, such as diagnosis or physician.

To achieve second normal form, the tables must be restructured. Duplication can be easily identified while reviewing the content of the database, as shown in Figure 29-3. The patient named Jane Smith, who was born February 20, 1960, has two rows in the "Patient" table. As a result, her name and date of birth are repeated unnecessarily. This repetition is caused by the inclusion of the attribute "Diagnosis" as part of the "Patient" table, even though it is functionally independent. To rectify this situation, the "Patient" table must be separated again into a set of smaller tables. This process, known as decomposition, must be "lossless" to maintain the integrity of the data. Just as the term implies, lossless decomposition is a process that retains all essential data and removes redundant values while preserving the ability to reproduce the content of the original table, as needed. This process is demonstrated in Figure 29-3, in which the "Patient" and "Physician" tables are stored separately but can be joined to form a derived table that contains the data from both. It should be noted that derived tables are temporary and should not be included in the long-term data storage design. Derived tables simply provide a convenient, short-term view of related data from separate tables.

In the current example (see Fig. 29-3), the "Diagnosis" column is the source of the redundancy and must be sequestered to its own table. However, this separation must be done without any data loss. To accomplish this, an "Appointment" table should be added to serve as a bridge between each patient and his or her associated diagnoses. The "Appointment" table also connects patients and physicians.

The relationship between patients and appointments is established by storing the "PatientKey" for each patient in the "PatientForeignKey" column. The relationship between the "Patient" and "Appointment" tables in the database mirrors the relationship between patients and appointments in reality. The relationship can be best described as "one-to-many," in which one patient can have many appointments. If this relationship is built into the database design, a patient can have multiple appointments (requiring multiple entries in the "Appointment" table) but only one entry is required in the "Patient" table. As a result, the data redundancy visible in Figure 29-3 (in columns "LastName," "FirstName," and "Birthdate") is eliminated.

The process of decomposition continues as the diagnosis and physician information are also separated. The relationships between the patient and the associated physician and diagnoses must be maintained. The "Appointment" table is used to connect the "Patient," "Physician," and "Diagnosis" tables. Once again, the database design draws from a real-world example. An appointment is the point in the treatment process at which the patient meets with the physician and the physician determines the diagnosis. The database model is a natural extension of this relationship. The restructured database is shown in Figure 29-4.

Two tables worth mentioning have been introduced into the model "PhysicianAppointment" and "DiagnosisAppointment." Up to this point, all of the tables included in the database have been based in the real world, but the new tables are more abstract. Their sole function is to establish a link between tables in such a way that the principles of normalization are not compromised. As a result, they do not have real-world counterparts.

The new tables are necessary because of the nature of the relationships between both appointments and diagnoses and appointments and physicians. These relationships are best described as "many-to-many." For example, every appointment can be associated with multiple diagnoses, and every diagnosis can be associated with multiple appointments. "Junction" tables must be included in the database model to account for this interaction and eliminate data redundancy. In the absence of these tables, multiple diagnoses in any given appointment would cause the unnecessary repetition of appointment data.

Third Rule of Normalization

Third normal form addresses redundancies that stem from transitive data elements (information from one table is implied by information stored in another table). The specific details of third normal form reach beyond the scope of this discussion, but the possibility of higher forms of normalization is noteworthy. The underlying and driving force in normalization is the minimization of redundancies in the relational model. A glaring exception to this rule is the primary/foreign key relationship, in which the redundancy itself is the mechanism by which relationships among tables are established. This anomaly is a necessary byproduct of normalization and is the only desirable form of redundancy in the relational model. However, if the effectiveness of the database would be compromised through compliance with any of the rules of normalization, that rule must be breeched. The effectiveness of the database should outweigh all other considerations.

Technologic Vulnerabilities

The most important factor when considering system vulnerabilities is the protection of data. Access to the database should be restricted to legitimate users, and the nature of access

In the normalized model, data elements are logically separated (i.e., Patient, Appointment, Physician). Relationships are built into the database structure in order to maintain the connections while reducing data redundancy.

Patient Table

PatientKey	LastName	FirstName	Birthdate
1	Smith	Jane	01/01/1950
2	Smith	Jane	02/01/1960
3	West	Robert	03/01/1970

Patient Jane Smith (born 02/01/1960) has an appointment on 03/01/2003.

Appointment Table

AppointmentKey	AppointmentDate	PatientForeignKey
1	02/01/2003	1
2	03/01/2003	2
3	04/01/2003	3

There is one physician for the 03/01/2003 appointment.

PhysicianAppointment Table

PhysicianAppointmentKey	AppointmentForeignKey	PhysicianForeignKey
1	1	1
2	2	2
3	3	1

PhysicianTable

PhysicianKey	Physician
1	Jones
2	White

There two diagnoses for the 03/01/2003 appointment.

DiagnosisAppointment Table

DiagnosisAppointmentKey	AppointmentForeignKey	DiagnosisForeignKey
1	1	1
2	2	2
3	3	3
4	2	4

DiagnosisTable

DiagnosisKey	Diagnosis
1	Spondylolisthesis
2	Scoliosis
3	Rheumatoid arthritis
4	Kyphosis

FIGURE 29-4. Appointment tables.

should be structured to fit the use patterns of each specific user. Full access to every component of the database should be limited to the database administrator. Read-only access for all other users is preferred, reserving write access (update) for situations that require it. For example, a physician will need to update the tables used for any direct data entry (i.e., symptoms, diagnosis), implying write access. However, the same physician will not need permission to update a patient survey table, in which read-only access will suffice. Provision of full access to the database for all users can easily result in the corruption of data.

Control of permissions to the database can be managed with the database management systems built into most commercial database packages. Access can be restricted on a table-by-table basis (by the administrator), allowing for access customizations to fit the use patterns, as previously discussed. Additional layers of software can also be built on top of the database to further control access. Customized software applications can be written to limit user interaction with the database and provide data verification functions. These added tiers act as a buffer for the outcomes system and can effectively monitor the quality of the information before it reaches the database.

A subtler vulnerability relates to the timeliness of the data. The timing and availability of information stored in the database vary significantly, depending on the method of data collection. This becomes critical when some data elements are dependent on others. For example, an outcomes system that tracks patients by appointment creates such a scenario. At each appointment, the patient completes a survey and the physician completes an assessment of the patient's health. In the database model for such a system, the appointment provides the bond between the patient survey and the physician assessment. Relationships have been established in the database design that link the table of appointments with the tables for surveys and assessments. If a particular appointment is not present in the appointment table, it cannot be referenced by either of the other tables, and any attempt to do so will result in an error, preventing the database from being updated.

Participation provides another interesting challenge in the pursuit of an outcomes system. Data collection systems that are too costly in terms of time, effort, or resources will not succeed. A successful model is one that leaves the smallest possible footprint, a prospect that is best realized through collaboration. In the health care industry, the availability of information has increased exponentially in recent years.

Pursuant to this, outcomes systems are afforded the opportunity to draw from many sources within the organization. Data are collected and retained for every patient throughout the scheduling, registration, treatment, and billing processes as the trend of paperless patient care continues. Consequently, information is typically stored in many different systems throughout the organization, and effective outcomes systems draw from these disparate data sources whenever possible. Not only does the sharing of data reduce the possibility of errors stemming from data entry, but it also minimizes the level of effort necessary from the participants (both patients and physicians). For example, if a patient's demographic information is gathered for the registration process, it should not be necessary to collect it again when the patient completes a survey. As multiple systems are leveraged within the outcomes system, the resulting automation can significantly reduce the risk of unverified data. Moreover, participation levels improve as the required effort decreases.

Building the System

As mentioned previously, the three major components of any electronic information system are technology, people, and processes in which the human and technologic components interact. When analyzing the requirements for building a system and diagnosing any shortfalls or failures of a system once it is built, it is useful to categorize the required inputs and/or desired outputs (i.e., expectations) of these three component parts. The preceding sections of this chapter have been devoted primarily to technology and processes; this section focuses on understanding the people involved and their roles in creating the system.

As a prerequisite for success, human resources from the clinical, information technology, and administrative areas of the organization must be dedicated to the project. Participating individuals must be highly skilled in their respective disciplines, and ideally (to help champion the project), they should command a high degree of respect among their peers before joining the project team. Furthermore, they should be able to sustain a high degree of personal commitment to the success of the project over the long range (typically a period of 3–5 years) and possess excellent interpersonal and team-building skills (i.e., listening, speaking, demonstrating a collaborative work style, showing sensitivity to individual differences). Each member of the project team must fully understand and agree to accept a defined role in the process of system development and implementation.

First and foremost, a project leader, director, or manager must be identified. The project leader is responsible for the overall success of the system via effective management of all aspects of the project. It is recommended that a clinician fill this role in any health care information system project, because clinicians are the key stakeholders in these projects. Clinical support, guidance, and direction are vital to the development of a system that will actually meet the needs of physicians and nurses. This is true from both an input (i.e., the data elements to be collected and collection process requirements in the clinical setting) and output (i.e., the data and information produced and provided to clinicians by the system) perspective. If the end result of all of the time, money, and effort invested in the system does not satisfy the clinical participants and stakeholders, the project surely has failed. If the perceived benefits do not outweigh the actual and perceived costs of participating in the system, it has failed as well.

All project team members are expected to take responsibility for ensuring the success of the system as it relates to their respective disciplines. For example, the physicians and nurses are responsible for the clinical success of the system. As such, they must ascertain that the data elements to be collected and information outputs are meaningful and relevant to clinicians, that the collection process is user-friendly to their colleagues and patients, and that the data collected will produce appropriate, clinically valid, and meaningful output for clinical outcomes measurement and research. The entire team relies exclusively on the clinical contingent to assess and decide all clinical parameters.

A system analyst is required to assume responsibility for the technical success of the system. Regardless of his or her actual title or position within the organization, this person must be highly skilled and knowledgeable, with respect to efficient and effective data management strategies, project management strategies, and the fundamental principles of information systems. Most importantly, relationships must be fostered between the technical and clinical personnel, so that each has a keen understanding of the other's working environment. The system analyst will not be able to build a system tracking clinical activity and patient outcomes without a clear description of the physicians' working environment. Inefficiencies in the project will develop if clinicians cannot describe this setting in a manner that the system analyst can comprehend.

Finally, an administrative representative is relied on to manage the operational and financial aspects of the project. For the project to be successful, the system must ultimately "fit" into the constraints of a busy and demanding clinical setting, especially because it requires collecting data from both physicians and patients at the time of an outpatient visit. This is typically the greatest challenge in developing such systems and has been noted as a major obstacle to outcomes measurement systems development. Data collection methods must be evaluated from a cost-benefit perspective and for user-friendliness. Securing "buy in" from affected operational and clinical personnel is essential, and this task is typically shared by the entire team, although the administrative representative carries the main responsibility for this function throughout the project. The administrator also handles tasks such as securing copyright permission for patient surveys or Institutional Review Board (IRB) approval of clinical studies when applicable, preparing a budget and securing approvals, informing clinical and operational personnel as to project milestones, implementation schedules, and so on. It is recommended that at least one management representative join the team for the entire duration of the project, whereas other operational or financial personnel may be called on to participate in or consult with the project team for defined project tasks.

Deployment

Successful deployment of the system is predicated on clear communication about the implementation schedule, tasks, and implications for all involved. This includes communication among the team members, and perhaps most importantly, between the team and all affected parties. Advanced notification and discussion of timeframes, expectations, and the roles of all operational and clinical personnel in assisting patients and physicians in data collection are needed. The establishment of feedback loops for communicating implementation problems and issues is essential to the deployment process. People need to know, on a real-time basis, how to report technical malfunctions or process issues. In turn, responsive troubleshooting by members of the project team is equally essential. It is suggested that the project leader or his or her designee give timely project updates and process statistics to key stakeholders, including clinical departments, medical staff, and management, to keep people informed of the implementation schedule and milestones.

Measuring Success

Both objective and subjective indicators can gauge the success of an outcomes information system. Establishing the metrics by which the system's success will be measured is ideally done early in the project development phase. This ensures that the system created is, in fact, that which is desired by the stakeholders. A simple report that presents the results of objective and subjective evaluations is useful and recommended. Ideally, monthly reports are generated during the first year or two of implementation.

In the final evaluation of any outcomes system, both objective and subjective measures must be considered. Both measures combine to form a critical component of an ongoing monitoring and evaluation of the system. Feedback will not only help to determine the effectiveness and relevance of the outcomes project but will also be used as the primary tool to develop enhancements and refinements as the system evolves.

Objective Metrics

- The number/percentage of all patients seen, in the target population, from whom patient-reported data are collected. Example: 89 of 100 (89%) patients seen in March 2002 completed the required data collection survey.
- The number/percentage of all patients seen, in the target population, for whom physician-reported data were collected. Example: Physicians submitted data on 90 of 100 (90%) patients seen in March 2002.
- The number/percentage of survey "matches" between physician and patient-collected data. Example: For the 200 surveys collected from patients during March 2002, 190 (95%) surveys were collected on the same patients by physicians.
- The number/percentage of surveys (either physician or patient) completed entirely (no questions or sections left blank or illegibly marked). Example: 95 of 100 (95%) surveys completed by physicians (or patients) were complete.
- The average and range of time required for patients to complete a survey. Example: Patients spent between 10 and 35 minutes to complete a survey (average, 15 minutes).
- The average and range of time required for physicians to complete a survey. Example: Physicians spent between 5 and 15 minutes to complete a survey (average, 7 minutes).
- Based on a random cross-check of selected fields from 20 completed physician-reported surveys with the corresponding patient medical record, the number and percentage of surveys in which the survey data were in agreement with the medical record. Example: In 16 of 20 (80%) physician surveys, the selected data fields were in complete agreement with the medical record.
- Quantification of individual physician participation relative to other physicians within the department (e.g., physician A provided data on 62% of patients compared with a department-wide percentage of 84%).

Subjective Metrics

- Patient-reported perceptions of the time required and user-friendliness of the surveys
- Perceptions of the operational and clinical personnel with respect to the ease of administration of the patient surveys, user-friendliness, and so on
- Patient expectations about treatment
- Patient satisfaction with the clinical encounter and health care providers
- Measures of pain and functional limitation
- Usefulness and appropriateness of output reports that are produced and provided to the clinicians, as well as the clinicians' impressions about the data
- Clinicians' impressions and those of the entire project team, as to the cost-benefit ratio of system inputs versus outputs

KEY REFERENCES

Codd EF: A relational model of data for large shared data banks. *Communications of the ACM* (Association for Computing Machinery) 13(6):377–387, 1970.

Date CJ: *Introduction to database systems*, Reading, MA, 2000, Addison Wesley Longman.

Frymoyer JW, Cats-Baril WL: An overview of the incidences and costs of low-back pain. *Orthop Clin North Am* 22:263–271, 1991.

REFERENCES

The complete reference list is available online at expertconsult.com.

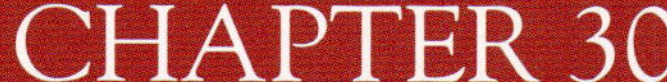

CHAPTER 30

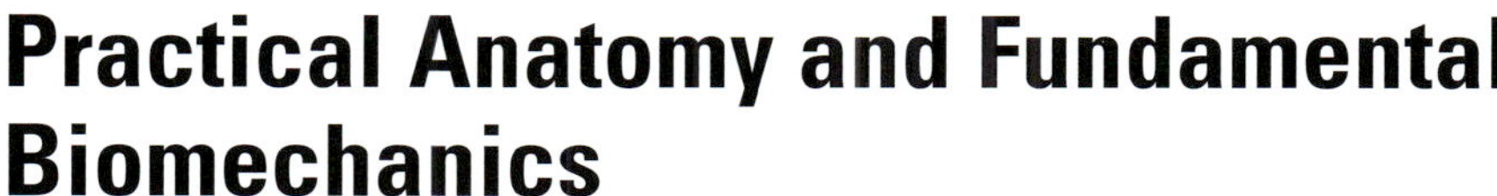

Practical Anatomy and Fundamental Biomechanics

Narayan Yoganandan | Curtis A. Dickman | Edward C. Benzel

Vertebral Column

The human spinal column consists of 33 vertebrae interconnected by intervertebral discs, facet capsules, and ligaments. Normally, there are 7 cervical (C1-7), 12 thoracic (T1-12), 5 lumbar (L1-5), 5 fused sacral (S1-5), and 4 separate coccygeal bones. The first three regions are flexible. The most common variations include sacralization of the fifth lumbar vertebra or lumbarization of the first sacral vertebra. Ventral and dorsal views of the spinal column with the skull are shown in Figure 30-1. The normal adult vertebral column has four curvatures. The cervical and lumbar regions are lordotic and the thoracic and lumbosacral regions are kyphotic. The lordotic curvature is convex ventrally, and the kyphotic curvature is concave ventrally. The thoracic and lumbosacral kyphotic curvatures exist in utero and are called the primary curvatures. The cervical and lumbar lordotic curvatures develop with the raising of the head postnatally and the assumption of the erect posture. The cervical curvature is shallow; it begins at the dens of the axis and terminates at T2. The lumbar lordosis develops due to the upright position of the trunk. The sacral curvature is relatively smooth and concave. Variations in the disc and vertebral body dimensions form and maintain these curvatures; they are often modified by age-related changes of the vertebrae, osteophyte development, trauma, congenital malformations, neurologic disorders, and imbalances of the paraspinal muscles. The center of gravity of the spinal column generally passes from the dens of the axis through the vertebra to the promontory of the sacrum.[1] The center of gravity of the body is located just ventral to the sacral promontory (Fig. 30-2). The vertebral column has different types of articulations: cartilaginous joints between the vertebral bodies, apophyseal joints between vertebral arches, unique articulations between the axis (C2) and atlas (C1), and skull-C1 articulation.

Vertebrae

Each vertebra consists of a cylindrically shaped body ventrally and an arch dorsally, and all encase the spinal cord and nerve roots. The outer shell of the vertebral body consists of a thin layer of relatively rigid compact cortical bone. This outer shell houses an inner core of soft and porous cancellous bone containing bone marrow. The structure of the cortical bone is aligned in vertical lamellae to resist compressive forces. The trabeculae of the cancellous bone are ordered like columns, and they resist a variety of loads. The rostral and caudal surfaces of the vertebral body are generally concave and are separated and bound together by the fibrocartilaginous discs. The dorsal arch is composed of the laminae, pedicles, spinous processes, and facet joints. Pedicles are stout bars of bone extending dorsolaterally from the rostral aspect of the vertebral body. The laminae extend dorsally, immediately from the pars interarticularis. They fuse in the midline to form the dorsal wall of the spinal canal. The laminae are oblong plates with a sloping surface. The spinous process arises from the junction of the laminae. The orientation of the spinous process depends on the region of the spine (cervical, thoracic, and lumbar). The cervical transverse processes arise from each side of the vertebral body near the junction of the pedicle and body. The thoracic and lumbar transverse processes arise from the junction of the pars interarticularis and pedicle. The transverse and spinous processes serve as attachments for muscles and ligaments. The articular processes arise from the pars interarticularis, interposed between the pedicles, laminae, and facet joints. Generally, superior articular processes project cranially with the articulating surface of facet on the dorsal surface. Typically, the inferior articular processes project caudally with the articular surface facing ventrally. A thin layer of hyaline cartilage lines the surface of each facet, which is a synovial joint, lined with synovium, and surrounded by a capsule. Characteristic features of cervical, thoracic, and lumbar vertebrae are described in what follows.

Cervical Vertebrae

These vertebrae are smaller in size compared with those in the thoracic and lumbar regions. They are cylindrically shaped and are wider in the transverse than anteroposterior (AP) diameters. The size gradually increases from C3 to C7. The pedicles are short and project dorsolaterally. They arise from the vertebral body midway between the rostral and caudal surfaces. The arch is composed of paired pedicles and articular facets, as well as the lamina and spinous processes. The laminae are narrow and overlap. The spinous processes are short and are usually bifid from C3 to C6. The transverse processes are unique. They contain the transverse foramen from C1 to C6, which transmits the vertebral artery. The anatomy of a typical cervical vertebra (C3-7) is shown in Figure 30-3. The pars interarticularis in the cervical spine is termed the *lateral masses*. The superior

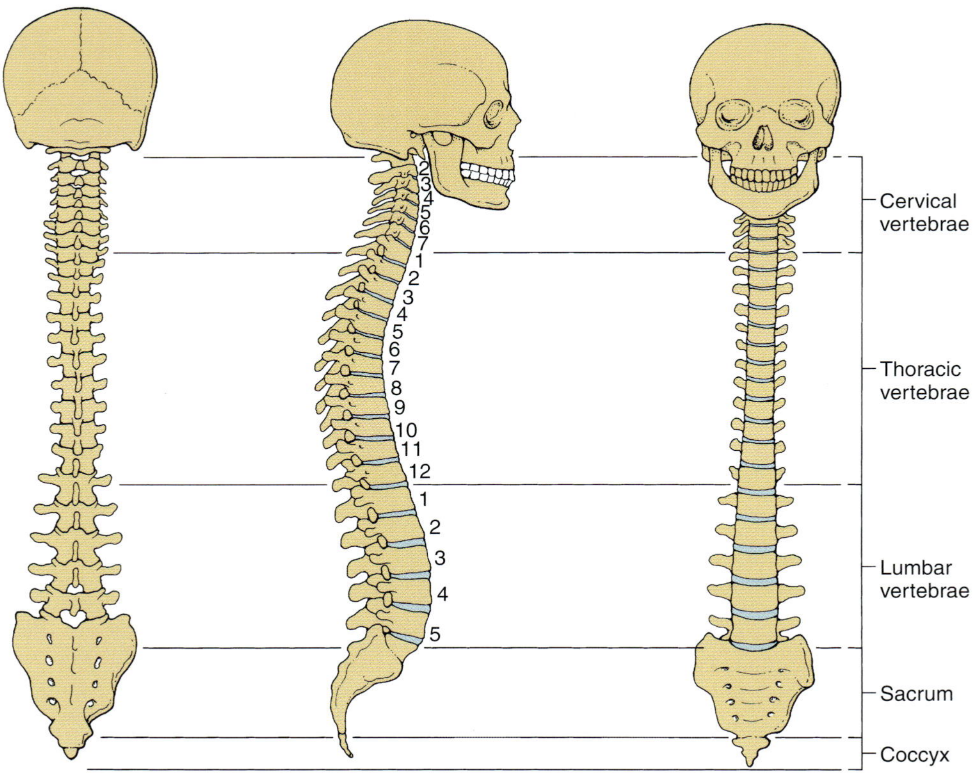

FIGURE 30-1. Human spinal column and skull: dorsal view (*left*); right lateral view (*center*); anterior view (*right*), all illustrating the cervical, thoracic, and lumbar vertebrae, sacrum, and coccyx. (From Sances A Jr, Weber RC, Larson SJ, et al: Bioengineering analysis of head and spine injuries. *Crit Rev Bioeng* 5:79–122, 1981.)

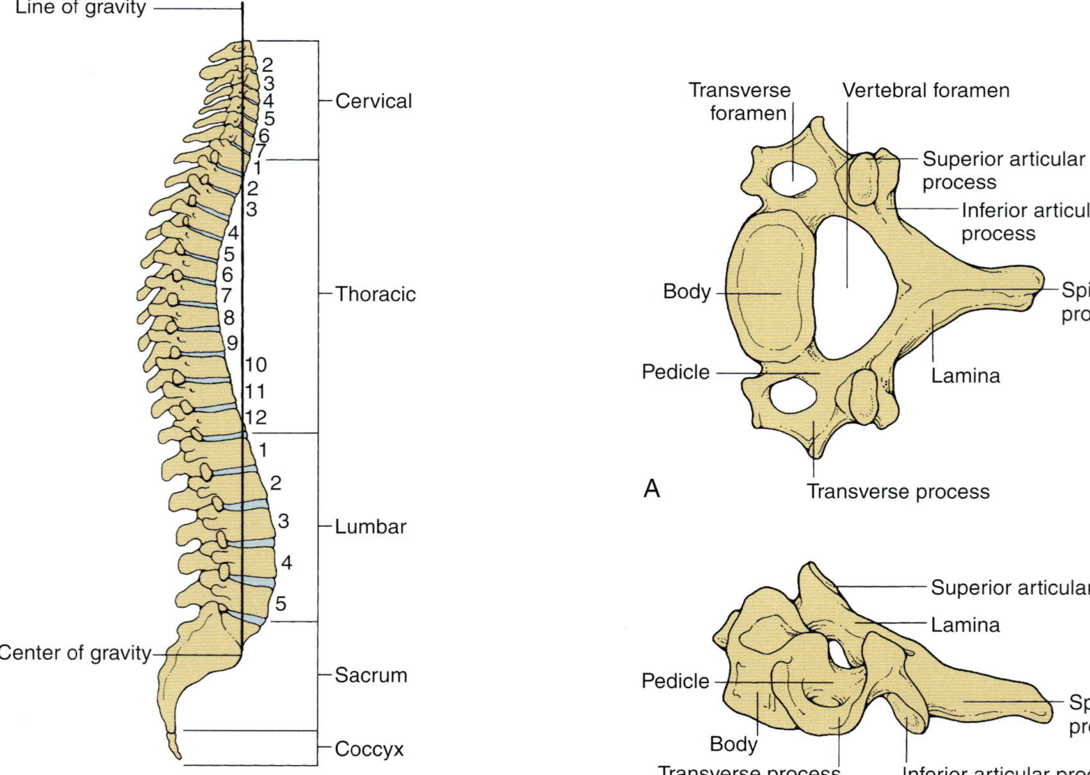

FIGURE 30-2. Human vertebral column showing the line of gravity. (From Woodburne RT: *Essentials of human anatomy,* 7th ed, Oxford, England, 1982, Oxford University Press.)

FIGURE 30-3. **A** and **B,** Anatomy of a typical cervical vertebra.

and inferior facets extend from the lateral masses. The facets from C2-3 to C6-7 are oriented approximately 45 degrees with respect to the horizontal and are aligned with a coronal orientation to their surfaces. The first cervical vertebra (C1), or atlas, is ring shaped and supports the cranium. The atlas consists of a bony ring with stout lateral masses and anterior and posterior arches. It has large lateral masses containing the horizontally oriented facet surfaces. Rostral facets articulate with the occipital condyles of the skull, and the inferior facets articulate with the rostral facets of C2. The axis (C2) has a unique shape with a transitional morphology; it has a well-developed vertebral body with the odontoid process projecting rostrally. Its broad sloping superior facets extend laterally from the body.

Thoracic Vertebrae

These vertebrae are somewhat heart shaped and are intermediate in size between the lumbar and cervical vertebrae. The anatomy of a typical thoracic vertebra is shown in Figure 30-4A. It exhibits costal facets on each side at the junction of the body and pedicle and on transverse processes. These facets are unique (Fig. 30-4B). The costal facets are also seen on the transverse processes (except for T10-12). Vertebrae at the rostral and caudal regions have some transitional morphologic features; that is, T1 to T4 vertebrae have some cervical features, and T9 to T12 have some lumbar features. The surface area gradually increases from T1 to T12. The middle four vertebrae have almost equal lateral and AP dimensions. Lateral dimensions increase toward the cervical and lumbar extremes of the thoracic region. The spinous processes of the first, second, eleventh, and twelfth vertebrae are horizontal; the third, fourth, ninth, and tenth are oblique; and the fifth to eighth spinous processes overlap and are long and vertical. The size of transverse processes increases progressively from T1 to T12. The cervical features of T1 include the superior vertebral notch, and the lumbar features of T12 include the lateral direction of the inferior articular processes. The laminae are broad and sloping, and they overlap one another like shingles on a roof. The thoracic facets are oriented along the coronal plane. At the thoracolumbar junction, they assume a more oblique sagittal orientation.

Lumbar Vertebrae

Vertebral bodies in this region are the largest and typically increase in the diameter caudally. They are larger in the transverse width than their AP diameter; a concavity of the vertebral body gives rise to an hourglass profile and a kidney-shaped cross section. The bodies of L1-2 vertebrae are deeper dorsally. The L4-5 vertebrae are deeper ventrally, whereas the L3 vertebra is transitional. The laminae are relatively broad, wide, and minimally overlap. The interlaminar spaces are covered by the ligaments and by large oblong and horizontal spinous processes. Long, thin, slender horizontal transverse processes incline slightly rostrally in the lower two lumbar segments. The transverse process of L3 projects the farthest and that of L5 spreads ventrally. The fifth lumbar vertebra represents the transition from the lumbar to the sacral spine. It is substantially taller ventrally. This contributes to the lumbosacral angle. The thick and conical transverse process arises from the junction of the pars and the pedicle of L5. The anatomy of a typical lumbar vertebra is shown in Figure 30-5.

Sacrum and Coccyx

The sacrum is formed by the fusion of the costal ligaments and the transverse processes. It is triangular in form, concave, and relatively smooth on its pelvic surface. It is convex and highly irregular dorsally. Five sacral bodies are demarcated by four transverse lines that end laterally in four pairs of ventral sacral

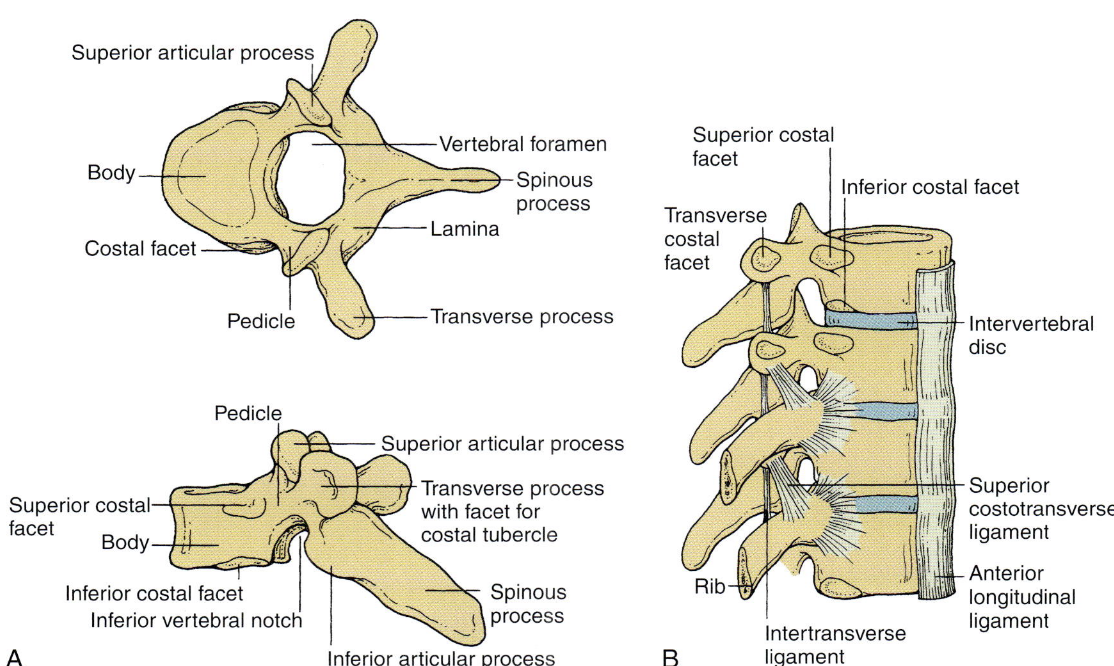

FIGURE 30-4. Typical thoracic vertebra. **A,** In addition to the rib articulations, note the orientation of the articulating facets. **B,** Drawing of thoracic spine showing nature of rib articulation to two vertebrae each.

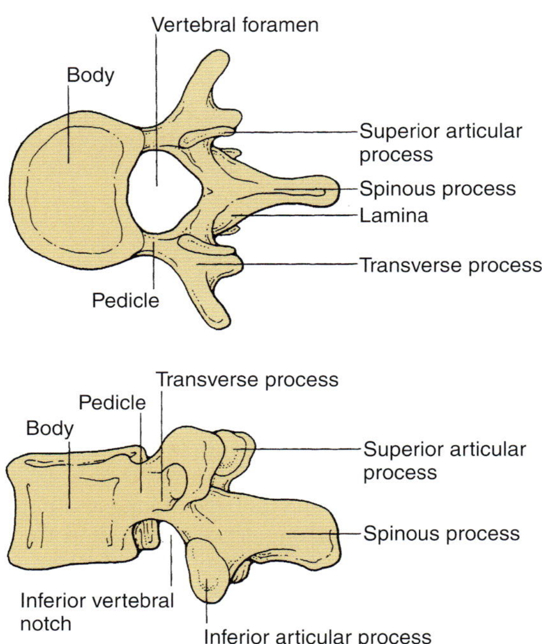

FIGURE 30-5. Anatomy of a lumbar vertebra.

foramina. The bilateral foramina are rounded laterally to indicate the courses of the emerging nerves. The coccyx may be a single bone fused from coccygeal elements, or the first segment may be separate from the other. These vertebrae are reduced in size, and they have no laminae, pedicles, or spinous processes.

Vertebral End Plates

These are formed by the rostral and caudal surfaces of the vertebral body. They are composed of concave surfaces of approximately 1.3-mm-thick cortical bone. The cartilaginous end plates are the superior and inferior thin planar surfaces of the intervertebral disc. They are the transition components between the fibrocartilaginous disc and the vertebral end plates. Each cartilaginous end plate is fused to the vertebral end plate by a calcium layer termed the *lamina cribrosa*, a sievelike surface that permits osmotic diffusion. Nutrients for the disc penetrate through the small pores at the lamina cribs.

Intervertebral Discs

The most rostral intervertebral disc space is located between the second and third cervical vertebrae and the most caudal disc is between the L5 and S1 vertebrae. Twenty-three discs span the vertebral column between C2 and S1. Discs demonstrate regional geometric variations that parallel morphologic differences in the vertebral bodies. The discs account for approximately one third to one fifth of the total height of the vertebral column. Four concentrically arranged components are often identified in the intervertebral discs: an outer alternating layer of collagen fibers that form the peripheral rim of the anulus fibrosus, a fibrocartilage component that forms a major portion of the anulus fibrosus, a transitional region between the central nucleus pulposus where the anulus and nucleus merge, and the nucleus pulposus. The core of the disc, termed the *nucleus pulposus*, is made of a soft, pulpy, highly elastic mucoprotein gel. The nucleus contains various mucopolysaccharides with relatively few collagen fibers and a high water content. The anulus fibers pass obliquely from the vertebral body above and below and are arranged in a helicoid manner. The anulus is composed of concentric layers of fibrous tissue. The orientation of the fibers within each layer is the same. The orientation of the fibers in adjacent layers differs by 30 degrees (Fig. 30-6). The disc undergoes age-related changes. At birth, the disc has four distinct anatomic regions. However, the distinguishing features disappear as age transforms the disc into fibrocartilage and the number and size of the collagen fibers increases. With age, the macromolecular framework consists of collagen, proteoglycans, a noncollagenous matrix of proteins, glycol proteins, and small amounts of elastin. The elastic fibers are made of a central amorphous zone and a peripheral rim of dense microfibers. The arrangement of the fibers in the nucleus is irregular. The disc is approximately cylindrical with different ventral and dorsal heights. Typical cross sections of the disc resemble an ellipse in the cervical region, a rounded triangle in the thoracic region, and an ellipse in the lumbar region. Generally, midthoracic discs are mostly circular in cross section. In contrast, midcervical intervertebral discs are less circular. Like the vertebral body, cross-sectional areas of the disc increase from C2 to T1.

Ligaments

Ligaments are multilayered and are composed primarily of elastin and collagen. Ligaments connect adjacent vertebrae and may extend over several segments along the spinal column. Ligaments and joint capsules, while permitting normal spinal motion, restrict excessive motion.

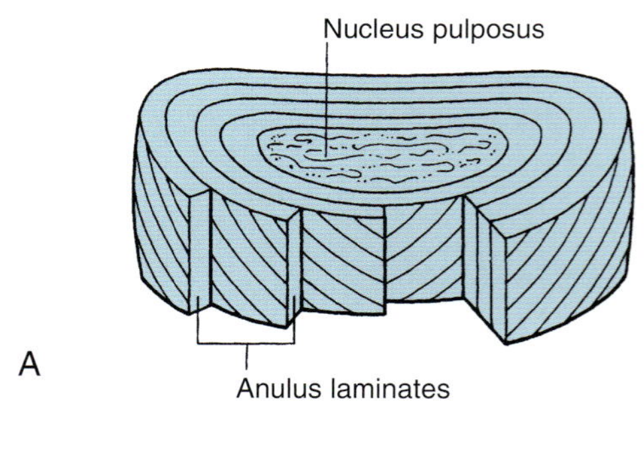

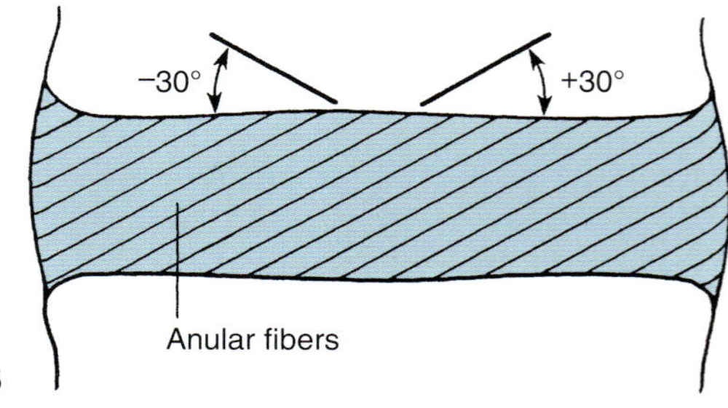

FIGURE 30-6. Intervertebral disc. **A,** The nucleus and anulus fibrosus. The anulus is made of laminated bands of fibers arranged concentrically. **B,** The anulus fibers and their orientation. (From White AA, Panjabi MM: *Clinical biomechanics of the spine*, ed 2, Philadelphia, 1990, JB Lippincott.)

Anterior Longitudinal Ligament

This ligament is continuous and spans the entire length of the vertebral column. It begins at the occiput as the anterior occipitoatlantal membrane and continues down to the sacrum covering one fourth to one third of the ventral circumference of the vertebral bodies and discs. It consists primarily of long-ranged collagen fibers aligned in interdigitizing layers. The deepest layer extends between the adjacent vertebrae, binding to the edges of the intervertebral discs. The middle layer binds the vertebral bodies and the discs over three levels, and the superficial fibers extend approximately four to five levels. The ligament is thickest over the concavity of the vertebral body blending into the periosteum.

Posterior Longitudinal Ligament

This ligament also traverses the entire length of the spinal column. It begins at C2 as the tectorial membrane and continues to the sacrum with fibers spreading out at the disc level and narrowing at the middle of the vertebral body. This ligament consists of several layers with the deep fibers extending only to adjacent vertebrae and the stronger superficial fibers spanning several levels. Whereas the ligament closely adheres to the disc anulus, it attaches only marginally to the vertebral body. This ligament is much thinner over the vertebral body and over the disc (by a factor of approximately one half) and is thickest in the thoracic region. Both the posterior and anterior longitudinal ligaments have a longitudinal (rostral to caudal) fiber orientation.

Ligamenta Flava

These are broad paired ligaments that connect spinal laminae. They arise from the ventral surface of the caudal lamina and attach to the dorsal border of the adjacent rostral lamina. They are discontinuous at midvertebral levels and in the midline. They extend laterally to the joint capsules and become confluent. These ligaments extend from C1-2 to L5-S1 levels. They have a high elastin content and are yellow. The ligamenta flava are the most elastic tissues in the human body. The capsular ligaments attach the adjacent vertebra to articular joints. The fibers are longer and slacker in the cervical region than in the thoracic and lumbar regions. The fibers are perpendicular to the plane of the articular surfaces.

Interspinous and Supraspinous Ligaments

These ligaments connect the adjacent spinous processes. They are composed predominantly of elastin. The interspinous ligaments attach from the base to the tip of each spinous process. They start at C2-3 and terminate at L5-S1. Both spinous ligaments are most prominent in the lumbar region. In contrast, the supraspinous ligament begins at the most dorsal aspect of the spinous process of C7 and continues into the lumbosacral region. The supraspinous ligament is primarily associated with the ligamentum nuchae of the neck contacting the spinous processes at their tips. It is the continuation of the ligamentum nuchae in the cervical spine. The ligament fibers end between the L3 and L5 levels. Figure 30-7A illustrates the ligamentous structures in the sagittal and axial planes.

Upper Cervical Spine Ligaments

Upper cervical ligaments span from the occiput to C2 (see Fig. 30-7B). Beginning ventrally, the anterior longitudinal ligament is renamed as the anterior atlanto-occipital membrane from C1 to the occiput. The apical ligament attaches from the tip of the odontoid process of C2 to the basion of the occiput. The alar ligaments connect the rostrolateral aspect of the odontoid process and run obliquely to the occipital condyles. The cruciate ligament has ascending and descending bands and a strong transverse portion that courses dorsal to the odontoid process and attaches to tubercles on the medial aspects of the lateral masses of the atlas. The vertical cruciate ligament attaches from the occiput, just dorsal to the apical ligament, and intertwines with its transverse portion. The descending band attaches to the dorsocaudal aspect of the body of C2. The tectorial membrane attaches to the ventral one third of the basiocciput just dorsal to the vertical cruciate ligament. This ligament tapers caudally to become continuous with the posterior longitudinal ligament. Finally, the posterior atlanto-occipital membrane connects the rostral aspect of the dorsal arch of C1 to the occiput.

Muscles

The superficial muscles of the rostral thoracic region and dorsal neck originate from thoracic spinous processes and insert laterally on the scapula. The muscles are attached medially to the ligamentum nuchae, which is a fibrous intermuscular septum. The sternocleidomastoid muscles arise from the sternum and the clavicle, and they insert into the mastoid process of the occipital bone. In the lower thoracic and lumbar regions, several muscles make up the superficial layer. The most prominent muscle is the latissimus dorsi, which arises from the spinous processes of the lower thoracic vertebrae and extends as a sheet across to the ventral axilla. Both the intercostal muscles and serratus posterior muscles arise from the ribs in different directions. Muscles encircling the abdominal region include the external and internal obliques and the transversus abdominis. The rectus abdominis muscle is located in the ventral abdominal wall. Deeper muscles ventral to the vertebral column are less prominent than the dorsal muscles. In the cervical region, the longus coli muscle passes from the atlas to the transverse processes of C3 to C6. Deep lateral muscles include the anterior scalenus, the longus capitis, and the intertransverse muscles. They also attach to the transverse processes.

In the thoracic region, the longus coli muscle extends only a few segments. In the lower thoracic and upper lumbar region, however, the lateral muscle groups are prominent, especially the psoas, intertransverse, and quadratus lumborum muscles. The iliopsoas muscles originate from the lateral aspects of the vertebral bodies and extend to the femur. As in the rest of the spine, the intertransverse muscles extend between the transverse processes. The quadratus lumborum also originates from the transverse processes and runs obliquely to the lateral ileum. Beneath the trapezius muscle, the splenius capitis muscle arises from the lower ligamentum nuchae and the cervical and upper six thoracic transverse processes, to attach to the occiput. The narrowest muscle, the splenius cervicis, originates only from the upper six thoracic

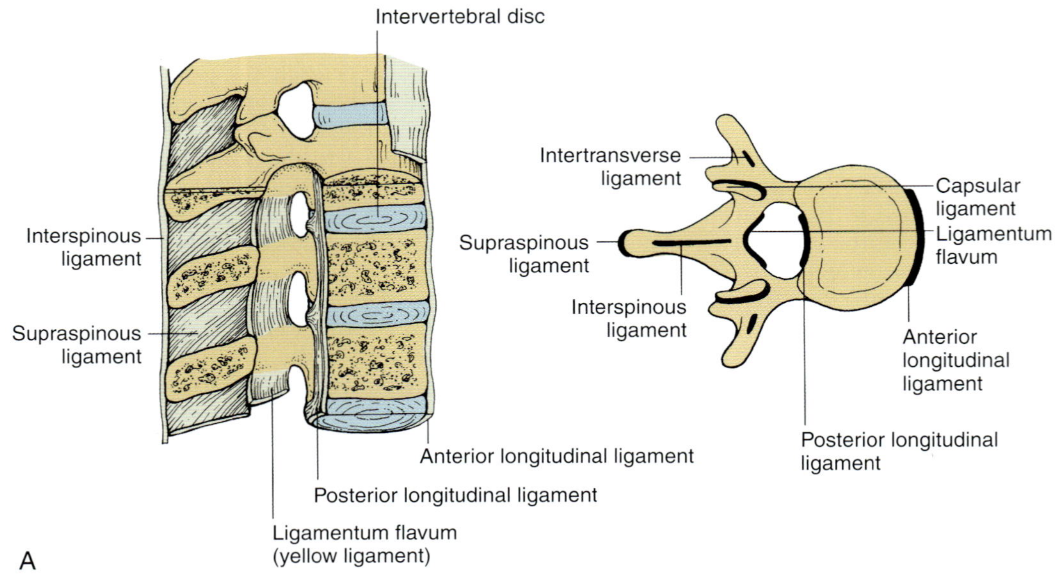

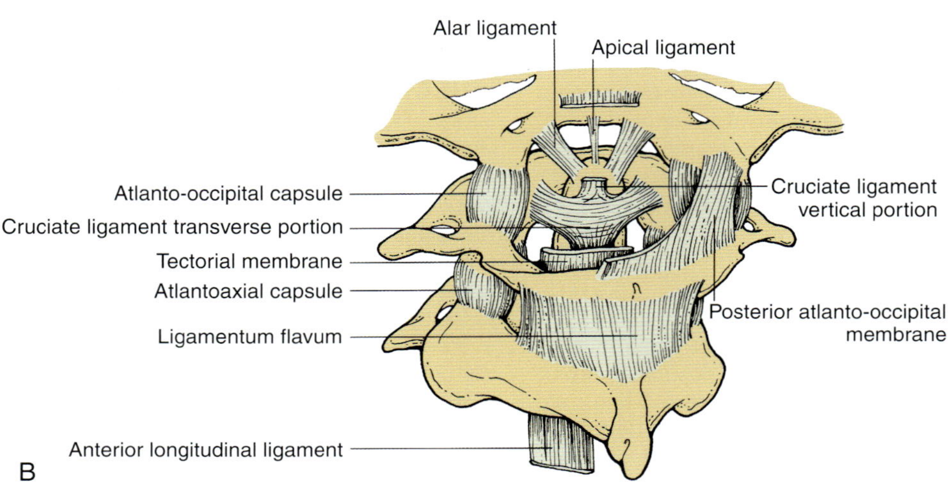

FIGURE 30-7. A, Sagittal and axial section through the lumbar spine demonstrating the associated ligaments. **B,** Schematic diagram of the upper cervical (occiput-C1-2) spinal region emphasizing the ligaments. Cut-away posterolateral view showing the relative location of the major ligaments. (**A,** From Sances A Jr, Myklebust JB, Maiman DJ, et al: The biomechanics of spinal injuries. *Crit Rev Biomed Eng* 11:1–76, 1984, with permission.)

spinous processes to insert on the posterior tubercles of C1 to C3. The adjacent deeper layer includes the semispinalis capitis and semispinalis cervicis muscles. The more medial semispinalis cervicis arises from the transverse and articular processes of the upper thoracic vertebrae inserting into the spinous process of the cervical spine. The lateral muscle originates from the transverse processes of C3 to C6 and inserts on the occipital bone. The deepest muscles of this group include the iliocostalis and longissimus cervicis, which arise from the upper thoracic ribs and transverse processes, respectively, to end on the transverse processes and facets of C4 to C7. Other deep muscles include the rectus capitis and capitis obliques, which serve as head extensors.

In the thoracic and lumbar regions, the erector spinae muscle group lies in the vertebrocostal groove directly under the thoracolumbar fascia. This muscle group begins as a tendon attached broadly to the dorsocaudal sacrum and iliac crest and extends the entire length of the spine. Its columns are composed of shorter fascicles. The lateral column represents the iliocostalis muscles, the intermediate column represents the longissimus muscles, and the middle column represents the semispinalis muscles.

The iliocostalis muscles arise from the iliac crest and insert on the angles of each of the ribs (iliocostalis lumborum and thoracis) as well as the cervical transverse processes. The longissimus represents the largest column. It arises from the transverse process at the lowest spinal levels and inserts into the transverse processes rostrally with the most rostral fibers inserting onto the mastoid process of the skull. The narrow spinalis muscle arises from the spinous processes of the sacrum and inserts into the higher spinous processes.

Deep to the erector spinae muscle lie the paravertebral or transverse spinal muscles. These muscles, including the semispinalis discussed previously, have their origins primarily from the vertebral transverse process and insert into the spinous process. The semispinalis group is continuous in the cervical and thoracic regions. The multifidus muscle is different in the cervical and lumbar areas, where the attachments are to the articular joint, but in the thoracic region the attachments are to the transverse processes. This muscle is thickest in the lumbar region.

Spinal Cord

The spinal cord and nerve roots traverse the spinal canal. The spinal cord is approximately 40 to 45 cm long in the adult and usually terminates at L1-2. The rostral cord at the level of the foramen magnum is continuous with the medulla oblongata. The dura mater, the pia mater, and the arachnoid are the three membranes that cover the spinal cord. The spinal cord is suspended in the spinal canal by dentate ligaments. These arise from the pia and are attached to the dura. Usually, the spinal cord terminates approximately at the caudal aspect of the L1 vertebral body. The cauda equina consists of the nerve roots, which have not exited through their neural foramina. Spinal nerves are composed of a dorsal sensory root and a ventral motor root. With the exception of the C1 and C2 contributions to the spinal accessory nerve, nerve roots leave the spinal canal via the neural foramina. Anatomically, the spinal cord is divided into five sections: 8 cervical, 12 thoracic, 5 lumbar and 5 sacral, and 1 coccygeal. Figure 30-8A shows a schematic of the spinal cord, indicating the relationship among spinal segments, nerves, and vertebral bodies.

The tracts within the spinal cord in the cervical and thoracic regions and nerve roots in the lumbar region are somatotopically oriented. The cortical spinal tracts are somatotopically arranged so that hand function is located more medially, whereas the foot function is located laterally. The spinothalamic tract is arranged so that hand sensation is located most medially and ventrally, and the sacral sensation is located most dorsally and laterally. The posterior columns are similarly arranged in a somatotopic manner. In the lumbar region, the nerve roots are arranged so that the lower sacral segments are located most medially and the exiting upper lumbar regions most laterally (Fig. 30-8B).

In a normal spine, spinal canal dimensions and hence the subarachnoid space are generous except in the midthoracic region (Fig. 30-8C). In the case of preexisting spinal stenosis, the factor of safety is reduced. This is important during a spinal instrumentation procedure that might impinge on the neural elements (e.g., sublaminar wire or hook placement). The lumbar spinal canal depth does not change significantly as one descends from the upper to the lower lumbar regions; however, its width increases (see Fig. 30-8C). The lumbar and sacral spinal canal cross-sectional areas are also more generous than in other areas of the spine. It contains the cauda equina, which consists of peripheral nerves and is relatively resistant to traumatic insults. For both reasons, posttraumatic neural element injury in the lumbar region is less severe than that associated with comparable deformation in the other regions of the spinal column, particularly the midthoracic area. The respective shapes of the typical spinal canal in the cervical, thoracic, and lumbar regions are depicted in Figure 30-8D.

Fundamental Biomechanics

Biomechanics is defined as the application of the principles of engineering and computers to solve biologic problems. Clinical biomechanics of the spine refers to the understanding of the normal and the pathologic functions of the human vertebral column due to the application of mechanical insult. The insult could be in the form of traumatic dynamic forces, deformations, and/or slowly applied loads to the spine.[2] Several terms are explained to facilitate a better understanding of clinical spinal biomechanics.

Scalar and Vector

A scalar is a quantity defined by its magnitude. It is directionally independent. Energy absorbed by the cervical spine due to the application of a load is an example of a scalar. In contrast, a vector possesses both magnitude and direction. Forces applied to the spine can be broken down into the components of vectors. To accomplish this, a reference system must be chosen. Force can be defined as an action that tends to change the state of the rest of the body to which it is applied. Force is a scalar. Force applied in a particular direction is often termed as the *force vector* or *load vector*. In biomechanics, force and load are used synonymously. Because the spine is not rigid, the application of force results in deformations.

Cartesian Coordinate System

The right-handed Cartesian system of reference is commonly adopted in spine biomechanics. The system consists of three axes: x, y, and z. Rotational and translational movements can occur along and about these axes. Translational movements are considered positive if the movements occur along the positive direction of the axis; it is considered negative if the moments are in the negative direction. Similarly, a clockwise rotation around an axis looking from the origin of the coordinate system toward the positive direction of the axis is termed *positive* rotation, whereas the counterclockwise rotation is termed *negative*. Figure 30-9 illustrates the right-handed Cartesian coordinate system of reference with the z-axis oriented along the caudal to rostral direction, the x-axis along the dorsal to ventral direction, and the y-axis along the right-to-left direction. For the right-handed system, this results in a positive flexion moment (extension being negative), positive moment left-to-right lateral bending (right-to-left lateral bending is a negative moment), and positive twisting right axial rotation moment (left axial rotation is a negative moment). This reference system has been adopted by the American Standard for Testing Materials. Once the coordinate system of reference is chosen, the force vector can be divided into its components.

Deformation

Deformation can be translational and/or rotational. Translational deformation results in a change in the length of the body. Rotational deformation results in a change in the angle of the body to which the force is applied. Deformations result in strains.

Strain is defined as the change in unit length (linear) or change in unit angle (shear) in the body subjected to a force (vector). There are two types of strain: normal and shear. Normal strain is defined as the change in the length divided

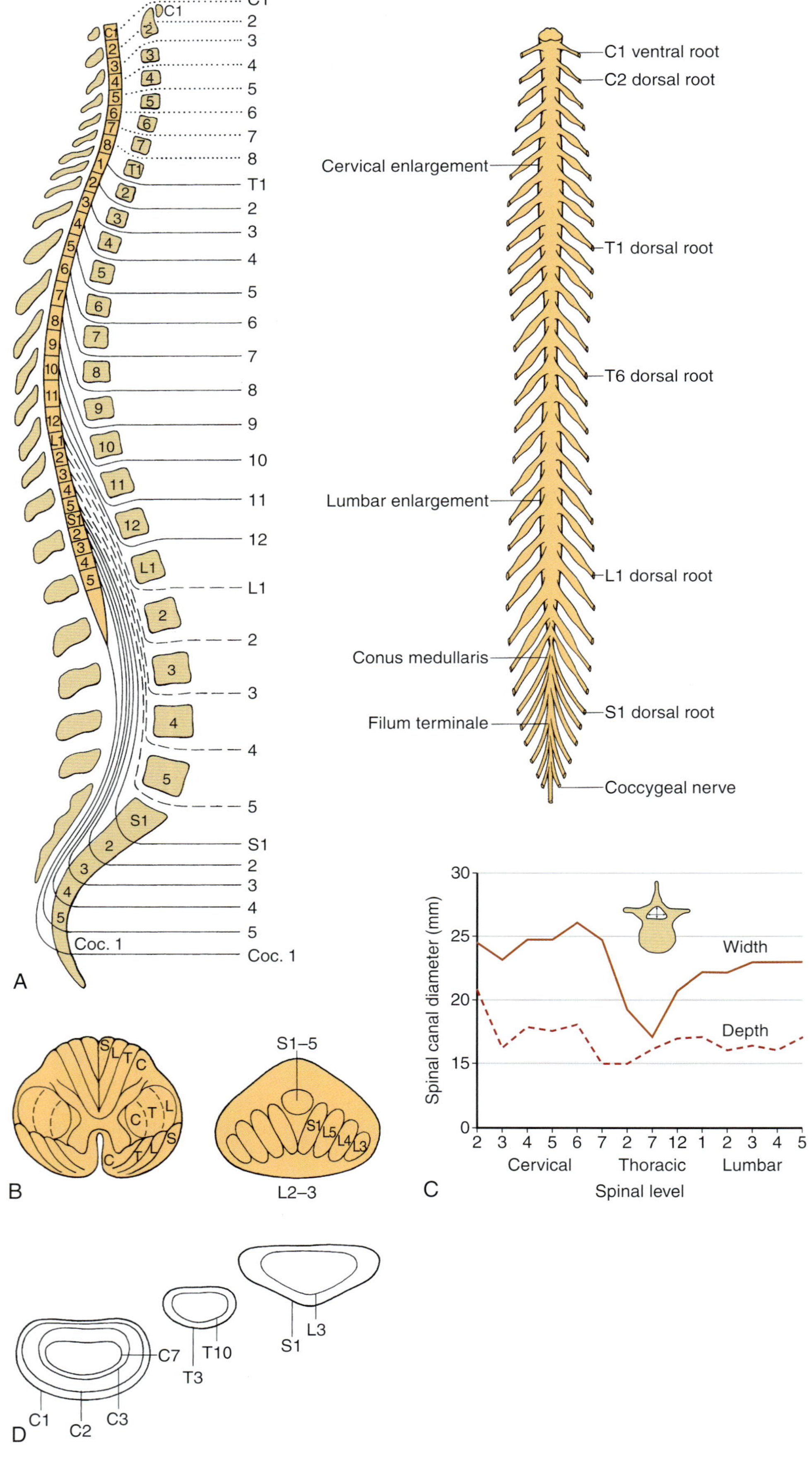

C1
2
3
4
5
6
7
8
T1
2
3
4
5
6
7
8
9
10
11
12
L1
2
3
4
5
S1
2
3
4
5
Coc. 1
A
C1 ventral root
C2 dorsal root
Cervical enlargement
T1 dorsal root
T6 dorsal root
Lumbar enlargement
L1 dorsal root
Conus medullaris
S1 dorsal root
Filum terminale
Coccygeal nerve
B
S1–5
L2–3
C
Spinal canal diameter (mm)
Width
Depth
Cervical
Thoracic
Lumbar
Spinal level
D
C1
C2
C3
C7
T3
T10
S1
L3

FIGURE 30-8. Diagrams of the human spinal cord. **A,** Sagittal view showing relationships among spinal segments, spinal nerves, and vertebral bodies (*left*); dorsal view illustrating various spinal land masses (*right*). **B,** Diagrammatic axial section of the spinal cord demonstrating the somatotopic orientation of spinal tracts (*left*); diagrammatic axial section of the spinal canal at the level of the midlumbar spine (*right*). Note the orientation of the neural elements (*clusters*); the lower elements are situated most medially and those preparing to exit the spinal canal most laterally. **C,** Spinal canal diameter versus spinal level. The width (*solid line*) and depth (*dashed line*) of the canal are depicted separately. **D,** A diagrammatic representation of the respective shapes and sizes of a typical spinal canal in the cervical (*left*), thoracic (*middle*), and lumbar (*right*) regions. (**A,** Modified from Carpenter MB: *Human neuroanatomy,* 7th ed, Baltimore, 1976, Williams & Wilkins. **B,** From Benzel EC: Stability and instability of the spine. In Benzel EC, editor: *Biomechanics of spine stabilization, principles and clinical practice,* New York, 1995, McGraw-Hill, pp 25–40. **C,** Data from references 67–70. **D,** From Sances A Jr, Weber RC, Larson SJ, et al: Bioengineering analysis of head and spine injuries. *Crit Rev Bioeng* 5:79–122, 1981.)

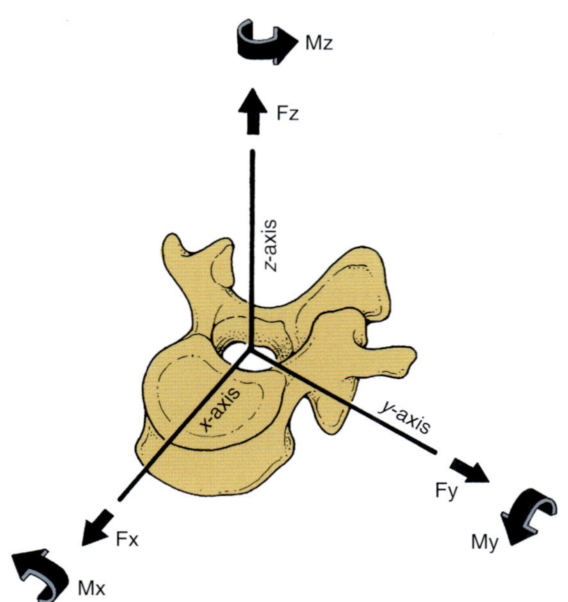

FIGURE 30-9. Schematic representation of the spine and three-dimensional coordinate axes. Linear forces are designated Fx, Fy, and Fz, and moments are designated Mx, My, and Mz. A positive *x*-force is dorsal to ventral, a positive *y*-force is from right to left, and a positive *z*-force is from caudal to rostral. A positive *x*-moment is right-lateral bending, a positive *y*-moment is flexion, and a positive *z*-moment is left axial rotation.

by the original length. Shear strain is defined as the change in the right angle (90 degrees). When a deformable body is subjected to a load vector, deformations occur, resulting in strains. The deformation along the direction of the force application is termed *axial strain,* whereas the deformation transverse to the direction of application of the force is often termed the *transverse strain.* The ratio of the lateral (transverse) to the longitudinal (axial) strain is termed *Poisson's ratio.*

Kinetics and Kinematics

The study of the mechanics of the body in relation to the forces and the deformations is *kinetics.* In contrast, *kinematics* deals with the motion of the body (deformations) independent of the forces responsible for the deformations. Both the terms are applicable to the biomechanics of the spine.

Force Deformation Response

Because of the deformability characteristics of the spine, the application of an external force or a load vector results in deformations. Energy is frequently used to relate the force and the deformation; it represents the amount of work done by a force on a body. It is defined as the area under the force deformation curve. In contrast, stiffness is defined as the ratio of force to deformation. Because the force deformation characteristics of a spinal structure are not always linear (Fig. 30-10), the most linear portion of the curve is often selected for obtaining the maximum stiffness of the structure. Analysis of the typical force deflection characteristics of the spinal structure (example of a functional unit) is given subsequently. Response is nonlinear; that is, force does not increase linearly with the deformation or vice versa. Within the principles of structural mechanics, this biomechanical load deflection response has been classified into the physiologic loading phase; the traumatic loading phase; and the failure, or the posttraumatic, loading phase. The stiffness response of the structure has been used to derive these biomechanical classifications. This system has been used to design a schema to evaluate the onset of spinal injury due to external load. This may help define the mechanism of spinal disorders.

In the physiologic loading phase, the spinal structure acts as an integral unit, and the stiffness increases gradually to a maximum value. During this phase, the structure obtains its highest stiffness; consequently, its resistance increases

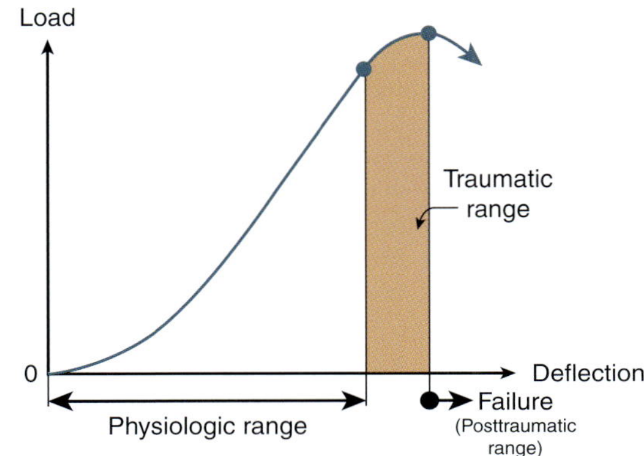

FIGURE 30-10. Typical nonlinear response of the lumbar spine, indicating the different stages in the biomechanical characteristics of the structure. (From Yoganandan N, Larson SJ, Gallagher M, et al: Correlation of microtrauma in the lumbar spine with intraosseous pressures. *Spine* 19:435–440, 1994.)

with the externally applied loads. This region represents the highest mechanical efficiency domain in the structural response. Trauma does not occur during this region of loading. With the increase in the application of load, yielding of the structures occurs. This is identified biomechanically by the onset of decreased stiffness for the first time during the loading process. Previous studies have demonstrated microfailures during this phase of loading.[3] The end of this traumatic range is characterized by changes in the stiffness that correspond to the ultimate load-carrying capacity of the structure. After reaching its peak during the physiologic loading phase, the stiffness gradually decreases to zero at the end of the traumatic loading phase, indicating that the structure has reached its ultimate load-carrying capacity. In the subsequent phase (i.e., the posttraumatic loading phase), the structure responds with negative resistance; that is, an increase in the deformation results in a decrease of the load. Trauma has been identified on radiographs when the structure has been loaded to this level. Based on the simple fundamental force deformation response and using the stiffness as a mechanics-based criterion, studies have indicated that microtrauma may initiate the loss of a local component before the structure has reached its ultimate load-carrying capacity.[4,5] In other words, even under subfailure loading, the structure may exhibit signs of weakness or microfailure.

Flexibility, Stiffness, and Range of Motion

Flexibility is defined as the inverse of stiffness (i.e., ratio of the deformation to an applied load). Flexibility and stiffness are inversely interchangeable in spinal biomechanics. Another quantity, the range of motion, is frequently used in spinal biomechanics. This refers to the deformation from one extreme to the other extreme under the physiologic range of translation or rotation of an intervertebral joint.

Coupling

Because of the three-dimensional nature of the spinal structure, motions are coupled. Coupling is defined as the capacity of the spine to move in translations and/or rotations independent of the principal motion. In other words, it represents obligatory movements of the spine (translations or rotations) that always accompany a primary motion. Both principal and coupled motions exist in the spine.[6] Principal motion can be defined as the motion associated with the direction or the plane of application of the external force. Any out-of-phase motion is the coupled motion. For example, axial rotation of the upper cervical spine is usually coupled with lateral bending.[7] Similarly, in the lower cervical spine, axial rotation and lateral bending of the vertebra in the opposite direction are usually coupled (Fig. 30-11).

Bending Moment

The force vector may act on a lever arm to cause a bending moment. A diagram indicating the amount of bending moment at various sections of the structure is termed the *bending moment diagram*. Frequently, in spinal biomechanics, three-point bending (Fig. 30-12A) and four-point bending (Fig. 30-12B) are often used. In three-point bending, the force is applied at the middle of the length of a structure with the structure being supported at its two ends.[2] This results in a triangular-shaped bending moment with the maximum moment under the point of load application. In four-point bending, the spinal structure is subjected to two equal loads placed at equal distances from the center, and the structure rests on two simple supports. This results in a trapezoidal-shaped bending moment diagram, in which the bending moment is constant between the points of load application. In this region, the sheer force is zero. A pure moment is sustained by the structure between the points of loading, and consequently the results obtained using a four-point bending technique can be applied for a pure bending moment situation.

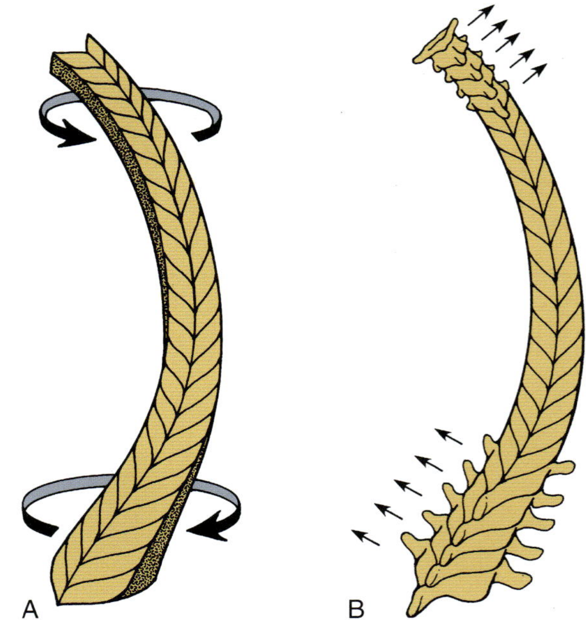

FIGURE 30-11. **The coupling phenomenon is the relationship between lateral bending and rotation in the cervical and lumbar regions. This is depicted (A) diagrammatically and (B) anatomically. The coupling phenomenon results in rotation in opposite directions of these two regions. The thoracic spine does not exhibit significant coupling.** (From Benzel EC: Stability and instability of the spine. In Benzel EC, editor: *Biomechanics of spine stabilization, principles and clinical practice*, New York, 1995, McGraw-Hill, pp 25–40.)

Instantaneous Axis of Rotation

If the load is applied along the spinal long axis, it is called an *axial* or a *longitudinal load*. This load may result in structural buckling. The buckling load represents the highest load that the column can sustain before failure when the load is applied in the longitudinal manner. The instantaneous axis of rotation (IAR) defines characteristic movements during rotation of a vertebra. It is the point about which the vertebra rotates. The IAR is defined as the axis perpendicular to the plane of the motion of the body and passing through a point within the confines of the body or outside the body that does not move is the IAR for that motion at that point in time. Table 30-1 includes additional details.

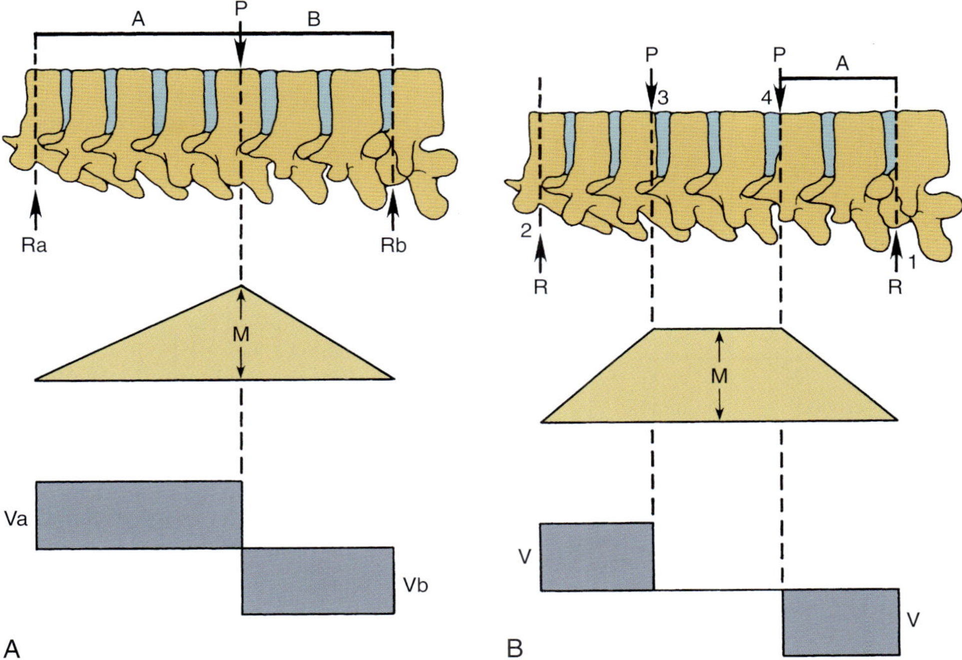

FIGURE 30-12. **A,** Three-point loading diagram in response to lateral bending (*upper*). A bending moment diagram verifying that maximum moment is under the loading point (*middle*). A shear diagram, depicting opposite but equal values (*lower*). **B,** Four-point bending diagram (*upper*); bending moment (*middle*) is maximal between loading points. There is no shear force medial to loading points (*lower*).

TABLE 30-1

Units of Some Commonly Used Parameters

Description	Units
Displacement	mm
Elastic modules	N/cm^2
Energy	N-m, J
Force	N
Moment	N-m
Rotation	Degrees, rad
Strain	Nondimensional
Stress	N/cm^2, MPa
Torque	N-m
Stiffness	N/mm
Flexibility	mm/N

TABLE 30-2

Terminologies Used Synonymously

Clinical	Bioengineering
Extension	Rearward bending
Flexion	Forward bending
Lateral flexion	Lateral bending
Angulation	Rotation
Rotation	Torque/twist
Stretch/distraction	Tension
Subluxation	Shear

Clinical Biomechanics

Internal Deformation

The human spinal column resists external mechanical forces by undergoing internal deformations. The mechanical and structural changes depend on the type of force vector applied to the spine. The following terms are used routinely: flexion, extension, subluxation, rotation, and distraction (Table 30-2). Flexion refers to a forward bending moment. Extension refers to a backward bending moment. Subluxation refers to an AP or posteroanterior shear. Rotation refers to an axial twist or torsion. Distraction refers to stretch or tension. Due to the anatomic characteristics of the vertebral column, the human spine is under the action of compressive force applied in an eccentric manner. Depending on the location of the center of gravity (see Fig. 30-2), this force generally induces a flexion moment. One of the principal actions of the vertebral body is to resist compressive forces. The compressive force resisted by the body gradually increases from the cervical to the lumbar levels. As described earlier, the width, depth, and height of the vertebral bodies increase from the rostral to caudal direction. This geometric phenomenon permits an efficient load-carrying capacity of the structure of the lumbar region compared with the cervical region. The exception is the height of the C6 vertebral body, which is less than C5 and C7; the height of the lower lumbar vertebral body is usually less than that of L2. Although the general shape of the vertebral body is cylindrical, the concave geometry of the dorsal aspect of the vertebral body (the surface facing the spinal canal) is significant in ventral spinal operations where screw purchase of the dorsal vertebral body cortex is critical. Misinterpretation of the lateral radiograph may lead to neural impingement by the screw. Figure 30-13 presents properties of the vertebrae from the cervical to the lumbar region. The compression strength of the vertebral body shown in Figure 30-13C

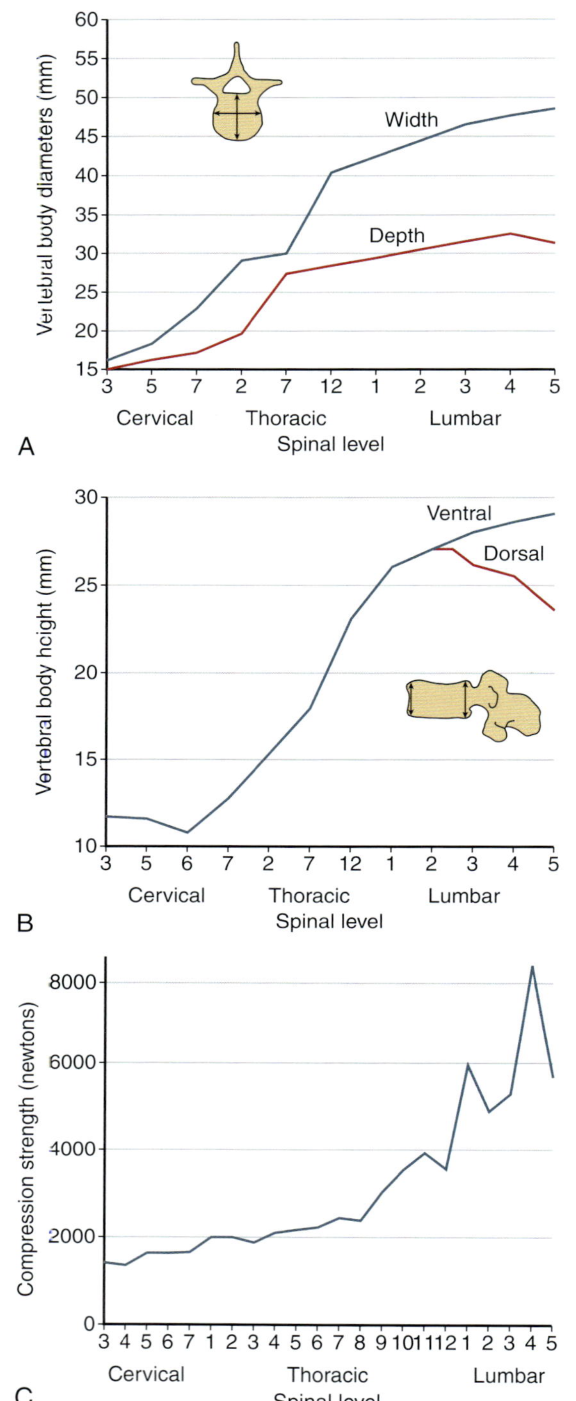

FIGURE 30-13. **A,** Vertebral body diameters versus spinal level. The width (*blue line*) and depth (*red line*) of the vertebral bodies are depicted separately. **B,** Vertebral body height versus spinal level. The dorsal height (*red line*) and ventral height (*blue line*), where significantly different, are depicted separately. **C,** Vertebral compression strength versus spinal level. (**C**, Data from references 11 and 70–72.)

indicates the general trend. Variations are due principally to the sample size, population, and age-dependent characteristics of specimens tested in the literature. An understanding of the tolerance levels under compression for the vertebral bodies is important in fracture fixation techniques.

Facet Joints

The facet joints do not substantially support axial compressive loads unless the spine is in extension. Change in the orientation of the facet joints alters the mobility—and hence the load-carrying capacity—of the spinal column under different force vectors. For example, the primarily coronal orientation of the facet joints in the cervical spine, compared with an intermediate orientation in the thoracic region and a sagittal orientation in the lumbar region, account for the alterations in the magnitudes of the rotations of these regions. In particular, the facet joint orientation changes substantially from L1 (approximately 25 degrees) to L5-S1 (approximately 50 degrees). Figure 30-14 depicts the orientation of the facet joints in the cervical, thoracic, and lumbar regions. The general sagittal plane orientation of the facet joints in the lumbar region renders the lumbar spine unable to resist flexion or translational movements, whereas the ability to resist rotation is substantial (Fig. 30-15). Relatively decreased incidents of subluxation found clinically can be attributed to a nearly coronal facet orientation at the L5-S1 level. It is well known that the subluxation is more common at L4-5 than at L5-S1 despite the relatively oblique orientation of the L5-S1 disc interspace. The ability of the cervical spine facet joints to resist flexion and extension, lateral bending, and rotation is relatively reduced because of the coronal plane orientation. Consequently, such movements are substantial in the cervical spinal region.

Spinal Cord

The spinal cord participates with the vertebral column in configuration changes due to alterations in body positioning. The susceptibility to injury varies with the specific abnormalities of the column. The physical properties of the spinal cord and related nerve roots, dentate ligaments, and pia and dura mater have been reported.[8,9] The spinal cord is part of a continuous tract originating in the mesencephalon and extending to the point where the nerve roots exit. This structure participates in the physical alterations, with the predominant effects occurring at the local level of distraction. Similar to the biomechanical response of a functional spinal unit, distraction in the cadaver cord demonstrates a load displacement curve with two phases. Large initial displacements occur with small force levels, demonstrating the elastic flexibility of the cord. However, this initial flexibility is followed by stiffening in which additional stretch or distraction requires higher load levels.[10]

In flexion, the spinal cord elongates within the spinal canal and decreases in the AP diameter. This induces increased axial tension in the axon cylinders of the white matter tracts and lesions of the vertebral canal that compromise the cross-sectional area; especially those processes ventral to the spinal cord call for the local and generalized increases in axial tension within the spinal cord. In extension, the spinal cord shortens and increases in the AP diameter with relative relaxation of the axon cylinders. The corresponding decreased cross-sectional area of the canal occurring from the dorsal bulging of the anulus, as well as the infolding of the ligamentum flavum and scaffolding of the lamina, may result in a "pincerlike" action on the cord. Studies indicate that irreversible spinal cord damage occurs when the compression exceeds approximately 30% of the initial cord diameter. Tensile forces applied to the spinal cord in the neutral position produce a relatively even load distribution

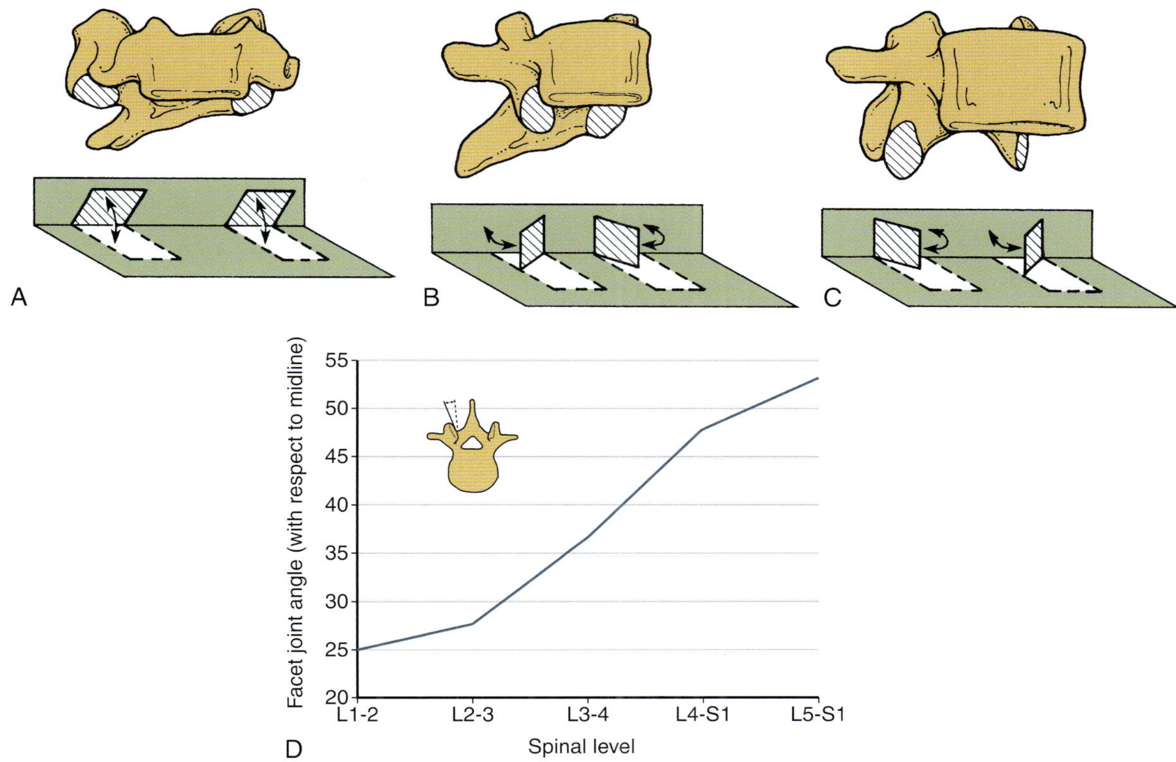

FIGURE 30-14. Facet joint orientation. **A,** The relative coronal plane orientation in the cervical region. **B,** The intermediate orientation in the thoracic region. **C,** The relative sagittal orientation in the lumbar region. **D,** The facet joint orientation changes substantially in the lumbar region; here the facet joint angle (with respect to midline) is depicted versus spinal level. (Data from references 11 and 71–73.)

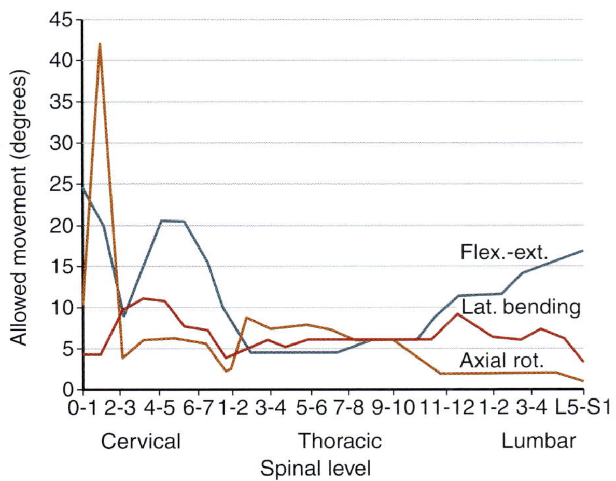

FIGURE 30-15. Segmental motions allowed at the various spinal levels. Combined flexion and extension (*blue line*), unilateral lateral bending (*red line*), and unilateral axial rotation (*orange line*). (Data from references 11, 74, and 75.)

across the structure, but if the cord undergoes bending, compressive forces increase on the concave side, causing increasing distractive forces on the convex side (Fig. 30-16). Shear forces, in contrast to tensile forces, are maximal toward the center of the cord. By definition, shear forces act in a perpendicular plane to the tensile forces. Interaction of these force vectors applied to the various regions of the spinal cord during flexion indicates the potential for a complex pattern of injury. Increases in the shear stresses in the central region of the cord occur due to the "pincerlike" action, during a sudden forceful hyperextension.

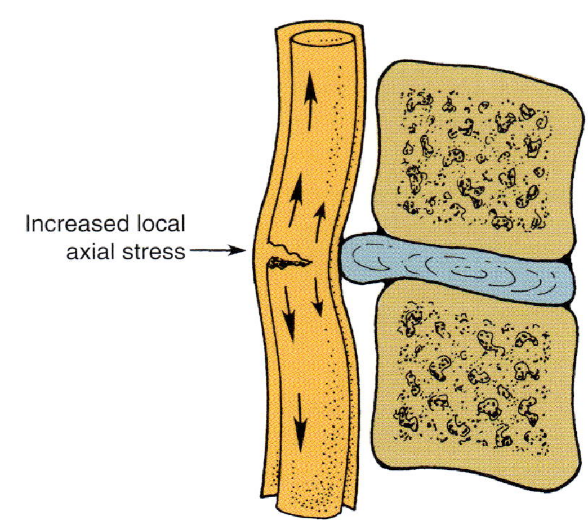

FIGURE 30-16. Illustration of the increased tensile stresses in the dorsal half of the spinal cord during flexion, with an increasing compressive stress imposed by a ventrally placed osteophyte. (From Cusick JF: Pathophysiology and treatment of cervical spondylotic myelopathy. *Clin Neurosurg* 37:661–681, 1991.)

Pedicle

The sagittal pedicle height increases gradually from the cervical to thoracolumbar region and decreases caudally in the lumbar spine. The transverse pedicle width decreases from the cervical to the midthoracic area and then increases caudally in the lumbar spine, favoring the placement of pedicle screws in the lumbar spine (Fig. 30-17). Because of the

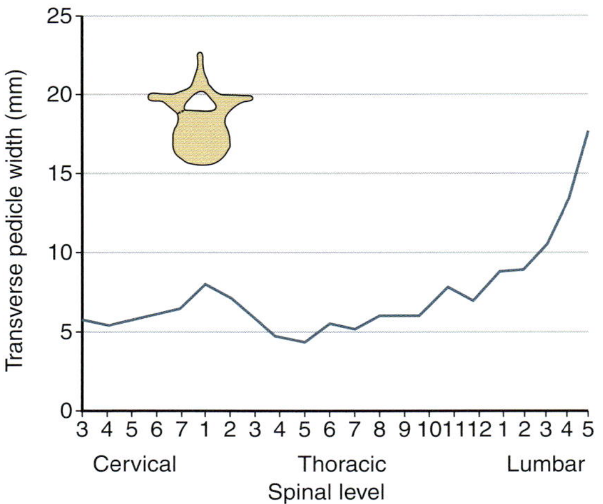

FIGURE 30-17. Transverse pedicle width versus spinal level. (Data from references 68, 76, and 77.)

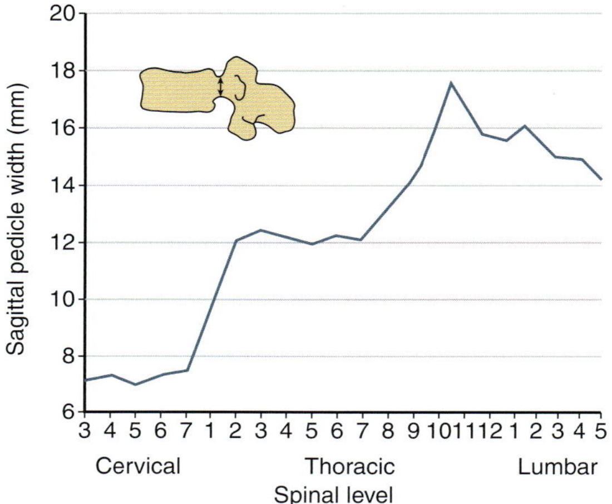

FIGURE 30-18. Sagittal pedicle width versus spinal level. (Data from references 68, 76, and 77.)

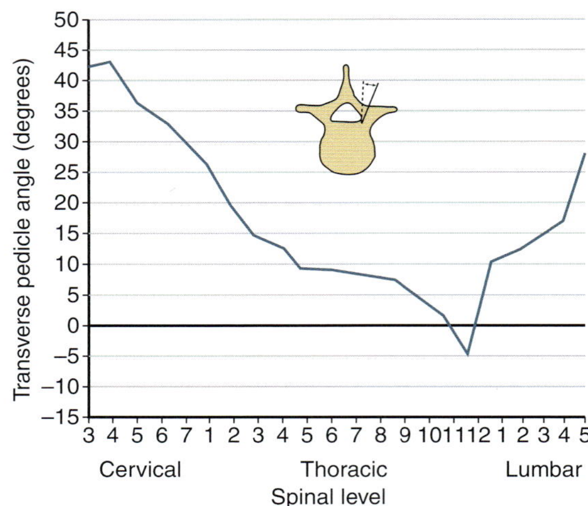

FIGURE 30-19. Transverse pedicle angle versus spinal level. (Data from references 68, 76, and 77.)

generous dimension, a small variation in the pedicle height in the lumbar region is clinically insignificant (Fig. 30-18). The decrease of the transverse pedicle angle from the cervical to the thoracolumbar region, and then a caudal increase in the lumbar spine, necessitates a wider angle of approach for the placement of pedicle screws in the lower lumbar spine (Fig. 30-19). An appreciation of vertebral anatomy is important for pedicle screw placement in the sacral region. There is, however, usually a great margin of safety for screw placement in this region of the vertebral column.

Intervertebral Disc

Any load resisted by the vertebral body is transferred to the adjacent one (generally caudal) through the disc. Because of the inhomogeneity and anisotropy of the material properties of the body and disc, the mechanism of load transfer is complex. Differences in the age-related changes between the disc and vertebral body add to the complexity. Because of the relative flexibility of the disc compared with a very rigid cortical shell enclosing a relatively soft cancellous core, the intervertebral disc resists compression, tension, shear, bending, and torsion forces. Depending on the age and magnitude of the external load vector, any combination of these forces resulting in complex three-dimensional deformations is possible. Consequently, this component of the spine has received great attention by researchers. Similar to the vertebral body geometry, changes in the disc geometric properties account for the increases in the load to be resisted by the lumbar disc in contrast with the cervical intervertebral discs.

Unlike the vertebral body, discs cannot be tested in isolation, that is, the adjacent supports of the vertebra are necessary to determine its gross biomechanical properties. Routinely, functional segments (vertebra-disc-vertebra structure with or without the posterior complex) are used to determine the strength.[11] Biomechanical testing has indicated that the first component to fail in a functional spinal unit is the end plate.[3,12] In the lumbar spine, normal discs respond with higher load-carrying capacity and higher stiffness compared with degenerated discs.[4] Studies have also demonstrated the movement of the nucleus material into the cancellous core of the vertebral body under discographic techniques.[13] Initiation of trauma identified biomechanically by the first decrease of stiffness within the specimen still able to resist further increases of load, occurs with the movement of the nucleus pulposus into the vertebral end plate, causing its rupture.[14] Under symmetrical axial compressive loading, the disc bulges in the transverse plane.[15] The compressive structural property of the disc does not contribute to the commonly observed disc herniation in the dorsal lateral direction; it depends primarily on the specific loading situations, which include compression, combined with other loading modes.[16] Although the disc is never subjected to a direct uniform tension along its entire cross section, certain modes of loading induce tensile forces in different regions of the disc. For example, under physiologic conditions, the anulus of the disc is subjected to tensile forces. Under flexion, the dorsal aspect of the disc is subjected to tension; in extension the ventral part of the disc experiences tension. In right lateral bending, tensile forces are resisted by the disc on the left side; in left lateral bending, tensile forces are resisted on the right side of the disc. From this point of view, the disc resists tensile forces locally, although the applied load vector may be in a different loading mode.

Depending on the spinal level, the disc resists a considerable amount of rotation or torsional forces. The average failure torque for a nondegenerated disc is 25% higher than a degenerated disc. Similar to the case of an axial compressive load-deflection curve on a spinal unit, the torque versus angle curves are nonlinear. With increasing rotation, the torsional stiffness increases. Whereas the end-plate integrity alters in compression, under torsion the end plates generally remain intact. In experimental in vitro human cadaver studies, cracking sounds emanate secondary to injury to the anulus. This may have a clinical correlation in the fact that patients with low back pain often report that they have experienced a "pop" in the back.

Ligaments

Although ligaments possess three-dimensional geometry in terms of attachment and insertion, from a biomechanical perspective they are uniaxial structures; that is, they respond to direct tensile forces. Figure 30-20 illustrates the tensile load-carrying capacity of spinal ligaments. The effectiveness of a ligament depends on the morphology and the moment arm through which it acts. To appreciate the contribution of a ligament to the load-carrying capacity of the spine, one must consider the anatomic location as well as the strength of the ligament under tensile forces. A very strong ligament that functions through a relatively short lever arm may contribute less to the stability than a weaker ligament working through a longer lever arm (Fig. 30-21). For example, although the posterior longitudinal ligament is relatively strong, it offers little resistance to flexion because of its ventral attachment. In other words, because the ligament is closer to the IAR than the interspinous ligament, it is less effective (Fig. 30-22). This is similarly true for the ligamentum flavum. This ligament is deficient in the midline; that is, a longitudinal midline cleavage plane exists. This property facilitates surgical entrance to the epidural space. The ligamentum flavum is not lax except under hyperextension. This factor, along with its high elastin content, minimizes the likelihood of buckling during extension, which might result in dural sac compression. The dorsal location of the posterior longitudinal ligament relative to the IAR, combined with a shorter moment arm, renders it a weak resistor of flexion. Although the capsular ligaments have a shorter lever arm, particularly in the cervical spine, they play a large role in the maintenance of spinal stability. This stems from their increase of strength compared to their counterparts in the thoracic and lumbar regions.

Biomechanical studies have shown that the ligaments farthest from the IAR, in general, demonstrate the highest amount of strength.[17,18] Variations in strength and stability can be related to anatomy and loading characteristics.[19] The

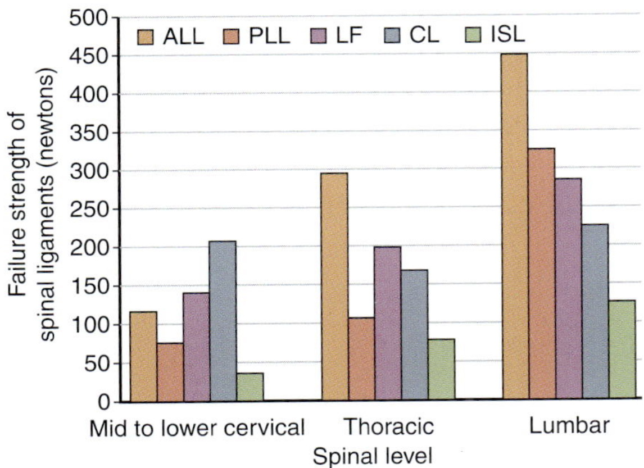

FIGURE 30-20. Failure strength of spinal ligaments versus spinal region. ALL, anterior longitudinal ligament; CL, capsular ligament; ISL, interspinous ligament; LF, ligamentum flavum; PLL, posterior longitudinal ligament. (Data from references 11, 20, 26, 68, and 78–83.)

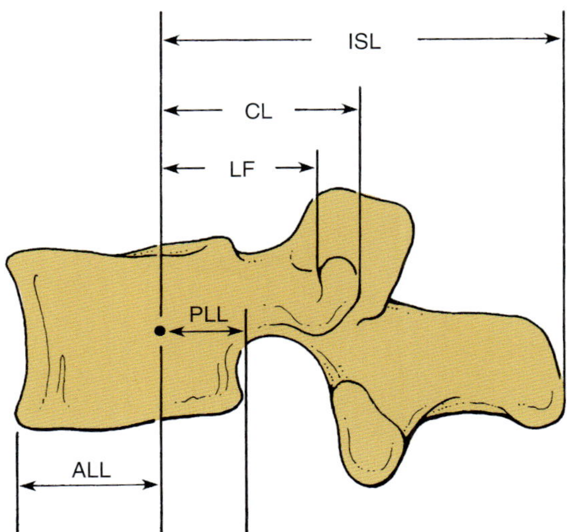

FIGURE 30-21. The relative lever arm (moment arm) length of ligaments causing flexion (or resisting extension). This length depends on the location of the instantaneous axis of rotation (IAR; *dot*). An "average" location is used in this illustration. ALL, anterior longitudinal ligament; CL, capsular ligament; ISL, interspinous ligament; LF, ligamentum flavum; PLL, posterior longitudinal ligament.

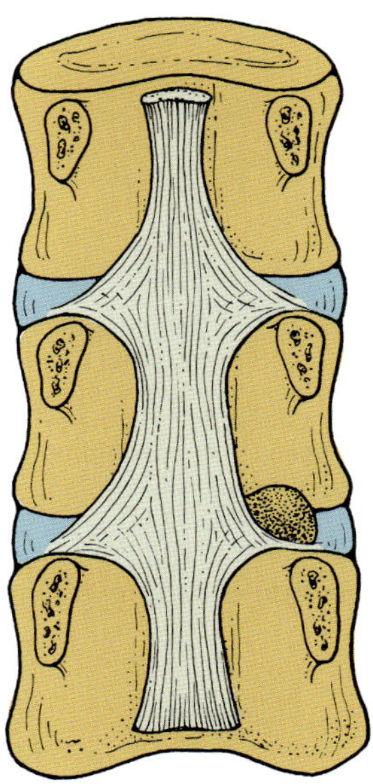

FIGURE 30-22. The posterior longitudinal ligament is narrow in the region of the vertebral body and attached laterally (at the level of its widest point) in the region of the disc interspace. The most common site of disc herniation is the dorsal paramedian region of the intervertebral disc. This injury has been reproduced by flexion, lateral bending (away from the side of the prolapse), and the application of an axial load. (From Adams MA, Hutton WC: Prolapsed intervertebral disc. A hyperflexion injury. 1981 Volvo Award in Basic Science. *Spine [Phila Pa 1976]* 7:184–191, 1982.)

failure deflection generally increases with the distance from the vertebral center of rotation with a general increase in strength moving from cervical to lumbar levels. Ligaments in the convex side of the spinal curvature are generally stronger. Additional increases in the strength are observed at the thoracolumbar and cervicothoracic junctions. Based on an exhaustive study of 132 samples, Pintar et al. determined the biomechanical parameters for the six major ligaments of the lumbar spine.[20] Responses based on mechanical characteristics and anatomic considerations were grouped into T12 to L2, L2 to L4, and L4 to S1 levels maintaining individuality and nonlinearities. Using nondimensional analyses and accounting for interspecimen variability, biomechanical parameters in terms of the stiffness, energy, stress, and strain to failure, along with cross-sectional area and original length have been computed for the longitudinal ligaments, joint capsules, ligamentum flava, and interspinous and supraspinous ligaments (Fig. 30-23 and Tables 30-3 to 30-5). Upper cervical ligament data are available in the literature (Table 30-6).[20]

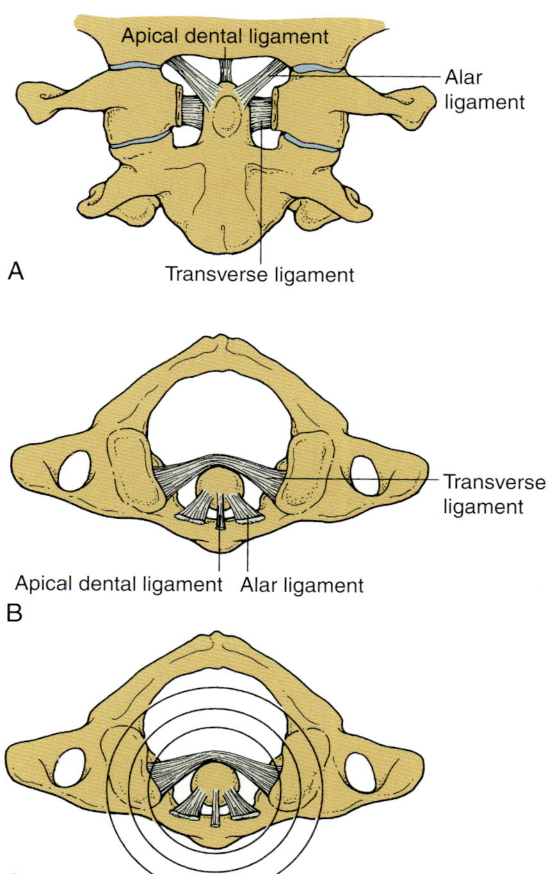

FIGURE 30-23. **A,** The occiput-C1-2 ligaments as viewed from a ventral orientation with the anterior arch of C1 removed. **B,** The same ligaments viewed from a rostral orientation. **C,** The predominance of rotation of the cervical spine is allowed between C1 and C2 about the odontoid process peg (instantaneous axis of rotation).

Yoganandan et al. conducted an analysis of mid- to lower cervical spine ligaments.[21] Using in situ testing and cryomicrotomy, properties of the C2-5 and C5-T1 ligaments were determined. Data were reported in the form of stiffness, energy, stress, strain, and modulus of elasticity (Table 30-7) and area and length (Table 30-8). In the original article, Yoganandan et al. provided force-deflection curves as a function of ligament type and vertebral level.

Muscles

The force resisted by the muscle depends on factors such as its length at the initiation of contraction. The maximum force develops at approximately 125% of the resting length of the muscle; in contrast, at approximately 50% of its resting length, the muscle develops very low force. The muscle stress (the maximum force per unit area) ranges from 30 to 90 newtons/cm^2.[22] Electromyographic (EMG) studies are used to determine muscle action. Generally, the relationship between an EMG and a muscle's distractive force is monotonic. Whereas muscles contribute significantly to maintain the stability of the spinal column under physiologic conditions, the action of the muscles is not clearly understood under dynamic forces. During flexion, most of the back muscles are active; at full flexion, however, they often become inactive except for the iliocostalis dorsi. EMG activity in the back muscles occurs at the beginning and at the completion of the full extension from the neutral position, with only slight activity between these two extremes. The abdominal muscles, in contrast, respond with increasing activity during bending, and in this mode, the activity of the muscle increases primarily on the ipsilateral side. During axial rotation, the erector spinae muscles on the ipsilateral side and musculi rotators on the contralateral side are active. Abdominal muscles show slight activity during rotation.

TABLE 30-3

Values of Cross-Sectional Area and Original Length for Ligaments of the Lumbar Spine (T12-S1)

		CROSS-SECTIONAL AREA (mm²)		ORIGINAL LENGTH (mm)	
Ligament	**N**	**Range**	**Mean ± SD**	**Range**	**Mean ± SD**
ALL	25	10.6 – 52.5	32.4 ± 10.9	30.0 – 48.5	37.1 ± 5.0
PLL	21	1.6 – 8.0	5.2 ± 2.4	27.8 – 36.7	33.3 ± 2.3
JC	24	19.0 – 93.6	43.8 ± 28.3	12.8 – 21.5	16.4 ± 2.9
LF	22	57.2 – 114.0	84.2 ± 17.9	13.0 – 18.0	15.2 ± 1.3
ISL	18	13.8 – 60.0	35.1 ± 15.0	6.7 – 20.0	16.0 ± 3.2
SSL	22	6.0 – 59.8	25.2 ± 14.0	17.0 – 33.5	25.2 ± 5.6

ALL, anterior longitudinal ligament; ISL, interspinous ligament; JC, joint capsules; LF, ligamentum flavum; PLL, posterior longitudinal ligament; SD, standard deviation; SSL, supraspinous ligament.

From Pintar FA, Yoganandan N, Myers T, et al: Biomechanical properties of human lumbar spine ligaments. *J Biomech* 25:1351–1356, 1992.

TABLE 30-4
Biomechanical Parameters of Human Lumbar Spine Ligaments

		SPINAL LEVEL					
Parameter	**Type**	**T12-1**	**L1-2**	**L2-3**	**L3-4**	**L4-5**	**L5-S1**
Stiffness (N/mm)	ALL	32.9 ± 20.9	32.4 ± 13.0	20.8 ± 14.0	39.5 ± 20.3	40.5 ± 14.3	13.2 ± 10.2
	PLL	10.0 ± 5.5	17.1 ± 9.6	36.6 ± 15.2	10.6 ± 8.5	25.8 ± 15.8	21.8 ± 16.0
	JC	31.7 ± 7.9	42.5 ± 0.8	33.9 ± 19.2	32.3 ± 3.3	30.6 ± 1.5	29.9 ± 22.0
	LF	24.2 ± 3.6	23.0 ± 7.8	25.1 ± 10.9	34.5 ± 6.2	27.2 ± 12.2	20.2 ± 8.4
	ISL	12.1 ± 2.6	10.0 ± 5.0	9.6 ± 4.8	18.1 ± 15.9	8.7 ± 6.5	16.3 ± 15.0
	SSL	15.1 ± 6.9	23.0 ± 17.3	24.8 ± 14.5	34.8 ± 11.7	18.0 ± 6.9	17.8 ± 3.8
Energy (J)	ALL	3.30 ± 2.01	3.88 ± 2.34	5.31 ± 1.98	5.35 ± 4.54	8.68 ± 7.99	0.82 ± 0.54
	PLL	0.22 ± 0.15	0.22 ± 0.21	0.33 ± 0.11	0.11 ± 0.04	0.07 ± 0.05	0.29 ± 0.27
	JC	1.55 ± 0.55	4.18 ± 2.15	3.50 ± 1.61	2.35 ± 1.88	2.05 ± 0.99	2.54 ± 1.31
	LF	2.18 ± 1.89	1.58 ± 0.93	0.56 ± 0.46	2.63 ± 2.09	3.31 ± 1.20	2.47 ± 0.60
	ISL	0.72 ± 0.47	2.65 ± 0.25	1.06 ± 0.73	0.59 ± 0.29	1.13 ± 0.91	0.78 ± 0.56
	SSL	3.75 ± 2.78	4.09 ± 2.00	4.72 ± 5.77	11.64 ± 5.39	3.40 ± 2.59	3.18 ± 1.94
Stress (MPa)	ALL	9.1 ± 0.6	13.4 ± 3.9	16.1 ± 6.2	12.8 ± 7.0	15.8 ± 1.9	8.2 ± 2.5
	PLL	7.2 ± 4.1	11.5 ± 10.0	28.4 ± 11.3	12.2 ± 1.9	20.6 ± 7.3	19.7 ± 7.1
	JC	13.2 ± 1.1	10.3 ± 2.9	14.4 ± 1.4	7.7 ± 1.6	3.5 ± 1.2	5.6 ± 2.5
	LF	4.0 ± 1.2	2.5 ± 0.8	1.3 ± 0.4	2.9 ± 1.7	2.9 ± 1.4	4.1 ± 0.5
	ISL	4.2 ± 0.2	5.9 ± 1.8	1.8 ± 0.1	1.8 ± 0.3	2.9 ± 1.9	5.5 ± 0.1
	SSL	8.9 ± 3.2	15.5 ± 5.1	9.9 ± 5.8	12.6 ± 2.7	12.7 ± 7.1	14.0 ± 1.7
Strain (%)	ALL	31.9 ± 24.5	44.0 ± 23.7	49.0 ± 31.7	32.8 ± 23.5	44.7 ± 27.4	28.1 ± 18.3
	PLL	16.2 ± 9.3	15.7 ± 7.4	11.3 ± 0.2	15.8 ± 3.7	12.7 ± 6.3	15.0 ± 8.4
	JC	78.2 ± 24.3	90.4 ± 17.7	70.0 ± 27.5	52.7 ± 7.2	47.9 ± 5.4	53.8 ± 28.8
	LF	61.5 ± 11.9	78.6 ± 6.7	28.8 ± 8.2	70.6 ± 13.6	102.0 ± 12.9	83.1 ± 19.3
	ISL	59.4 ± 36.1	119.7 ± 14.7	51.5 ± 2.9	96.5 ± 35.8	87.4 ± 6.7	52.9 ± 23.2
	SSL	75.0 ± 7.1	83.4 ± 21.4	70.6 ± 45.0	109.4 ± 2.5	106.3 ± 9.7	115.1 ± 49.1

ALL, anterior longitudinal ligament; ISL, interspinous ligament; JC, joint capsules; LF, ligamentum flavum; PLL, posterior longitudinal ligament; SD, standard deviation; SSL, supraspinous ligament.
From Pintar FA, Yoganandan N, Myers T, et al: Biomechanical properties of human lumbar spine ligaments. *J Biomech* 25:1351–1356, 1992.

TABLE 30-5
Overall Mean Values of Stiffness (N/mm^{-1}) for Ligaments of the Lumbar Spine (T12-S1)

Ligament	Mean ± SD
ALL	33.0 ± 15.7
PLL	20.4 ± 11.9
JC	33.9 ± 10.7
LF	27.2 ± 9.2
ISL	11.5 ± 6.6
SSL	23.7 ± 10.9

ALL, anterior longitudinal ligament; ISL, interspinous ligament; JC, joint capsules; LF, ligamentum flavum; PLL, posterior longitudinal ligament; SD, standard deviation; SSL, supraspinous ligament.
From Pintar FA, Yoganandan N, Myers T, et al: Biomechanical properties of human lumbar spine ligaments. *J Biomech* 25:1351–1356, 1992.

TABLE 30-6
Mean and Standard Deviation Values of Force and Deflection at Failure for Human Upper Cervical Spinal Ligaments

Ligament Type	Levels	Load (N)	Deflection (mm)
Anterior atlanto-occipital membrane	OC-C1	233 (± 23)	18.9 (± 2.7)
Posterior atlanto-occipital membrane	OC-C1	83 (± 17)	18.1 (± 2.7)
Anterior longitudinal	C1-2	281 (± 136)	12.3 (± 6.7)
Apical	OC-C2	214 (± 115)	11.5 (± 10.5)
Alar	OC-C2	357 (± 220)	14.1 (± 7.2)
Joint capsules	OC-C2	315 (± 134)	11.4 (± 7.2)
Ligamentum flavum	C1-2	113 (± 85)	8.7 (± 5.2)
Vertical cruciate	OC-C2	436 (± 69)	25.2 (± 14.6)
Tectorial membrane	OC-C2	76 (± 44)	11.9 (± 2.5)

OC, occiput.
From Myklebust JB, Pintar F, Yoganandan N, et al: Tensile strength of spinal ligaments. *Spine (Phila Pa 1976)* 13:526–531, 1988.

TABLE 30-7

Properties of the C2-5 and C5-T1 Ligaments

Biomechanical Data of C2-C5 Ligaments (n = 25)

		PARAMETER			
Type	**Sample Size**	**Stiffness (N/mm)**	**Energy (N-m)**	**Stress (MPa)**	**Strain (%)**
ALL	10	16.0 ± 2.7	0.61 ± 0.25	8.36 ± 1.76	30.8 ± 5.0
PLL	7	25.4 ± 7.2	0.21 ± 0.1	6.29 ± 2.28	18.2 ± 3.21
JC	8	33.6 ± 5.53	1.49 ± 0.54	5.67 ± 1.47	148 ± 28.5
LF	12	25.0 ± 7.04	0.49 ± 0.17	2.64 ± 0.79	77.0 ± 12.9
ISL	8	7.74 ± 1.61	0.13 ± 0.03	2.97 ± 0.76	60.9 ± 11.2

Biomechanical Data of C5-T1 Ligaments (n = 25)

		PARAMETER			
Type	**Sample Size**	**Stiffness (N/mm)**	**Energy (N-m)**	**Stress (MPa)**	**Strain (%)**
ALL	7	17.9 ± 3.44	0.54 ± 0.13	12.0 ± 1.41	35.4 ± 5.86
PLL	10	23.0 ± 2.39	0.4 ± 0.11	12.8 ± 3.38	34.1 ± 8.77
JC	11	36.9 ± 6.06	1.5 ± 0.37	7.36 ± 1.27	116 ± 19.6
LF	11	21.6 ± 3.65	0.91 ± 0.22	2.64 ± 0.34	88.4 ± 13.1
ISL	8	6.36 ± 0.69	0.18 ± 0.06	2.88 ± 0.74	68.1 ± 13.8

Bilinear Young's Modulus (MPa) of Cervical Ligaments (n = 25)

	C2-5			C5-T1		
Type	E_1	E_2	ε_{12}	E_1	E_2	ε_{12}
ALL	43.8	26.3	12.9	28.2	28.4	14.8
PLL	40.9	22.2	11.1	23.0	24.6	11.2
JC	5.0	3.3	56.8	4.8	3.4	57.0
LF	3.1	2.1	40.7	3.5	3.4	35.3
ISL	4.9	3.1	26.1	5.0	3.3	27.0

Note: ε_{12} denotes the strain transition between the two bilinear moduli (E_1 and E_2).
ALL, anterior longitudinal ligament; ISL, interspinous ligament; JC, joint capsules; LF, ligamentum flavum; PLL, posterior longitudinal ligament.
From Yoganandan N, Kumaresan S, Pintar FA: Geometric and mechanical properties of human cervical spine ligaments. *J Biomech Eng* 122: 623–629, 2000.

TABLE 30-8

Area (n = 4) and Length (n = 4) of Cervical Spine Ligaments

	C2-5		C5-T1	
Type	**Area (mm²)**	**Length (mm)**	**Area (mm²)**	**Length (mm)**
ALL	11.1 ± 1.93	18.8 ± 1.04	12.1 ± 2.68	18.3 ± 0.5
PLL	11.3 ± 1.99	19.0 ± 1.04	14.7 ± 6.77	17.9 ± 0.54
JC	42.2 ± 6.39	6.92 ± 0.68	49.5 ± 12.28	6.72 ± 0.45
LF	46.0 ± 5.78	8.45 ± 0.85	48.9 ± 7.9	10.6 ± 0.64
ISL	13.0 ± 3.27	10.4 ± 0.77	13.4 ± 1.03	9.87 ± 0.69

ALL, anterior longitudinal ligament; ISL, interspinous ligament; JC, joint capsules; LF, ligamentum flavum; PLL, posterior longitudinal ligament.
From Yoganandan N, Kumaresan S, Pintar FA: Geometric and mechanical properties of human cervical spine ligaments. *J Biomech Eng* 122: 623–629, 2000.

Regional Characteristics

Cervical Spine

Upper Cervical Spine and Craniocervical Junction

Atlanto-occipital joints allow flexion-extension. A minimal degree of lateral bending coupled with minimal rotation is allowed. Most cervical rotation occurs about the occiput-C2 complex. The movements allowed in the craniocervical region are shown in Table 30-9. Although movement in the upper cervical region does not occur in all planes and in rotation at each spinal level, its sum from occiput to C2 exceeds that observed in any other region of the spine (see Fig. 30-23). Anatomic features of the upper cervical spine offer several fixation points for instrumentation constructs and sites for bony fusion attachment. Upper cervical spine surgery is complicated by difficulties associated with calvarial fixation, unique anatomy of the upper cervical vertebrae, and substantial spinal movements in this region.[23]

TABLE 30-9

Movements Allowed in the Craniocervical Region

Joint	Motion	Range of Motion (degrees)
Occiput-C1	Combined flexion/extension	25
	Lateral bending (unilateral)	5
	Axial rotation (unilateral)	5
C1-2	Combined flexion/extension	20
	Lateral bending (unilateral)	5
	Axial rotation (unilateral)	40

From Maiman DJ, Yoganandan N: Biomechanics of cervical spine trauma. *Clin Neurosurg* 37:543–570, 1991.

The atlantoaxial region represents a unique integration of anatomy and function, allowing three-dimensional movement of the head through both individual and coupled motions. At the atlanto-occipital joint, 13 to 16 degrees of flexion-extension occurs. In addition, more than 8 degrees of lateral bending occurs without rotation. At the atlantoaxial junction, flexion-extension is significant (10–13 degrees). The most significant motion at C1-2 is 40 degrees of unilateral axial rotation, which represents 40% of the total rotation seen in the cervical spine. In any forced rotation of the entire cervical column, maximum rotation occurs at C1-2 before use of potential rotation in the lower cervical spine.[24]

Translation also occurs in the upper cervical spine, although it is normally limited to approximately 2 mm, primarily because of the anatomic relation between the odontoid process, arch of C1, and transverse atlantal ligament. Other motion limiters include those that inhibit hyperflexion: the relationship between the anterior lip of the foramen magnum and the odontoid process at the occiput-C1 and low elasticity of the tectorial membrane at C1-2. Extension limiters include the tectorial membrane and anterior longitudinal ligament. Rotation is contained by the contralateral C1-2 alar ligament.[24]

Mid- and Lower Cervical Spine

Orientation of the facet joints in the coronal plane does not excessively limit spinal movement in any direction or in rotation. An exception is extension. This orientation facilitates spinal instrumentation in certain situations. With the integrity of the facet joints and pedicles maintained, the vertebral bodies are able to equally resist axial loading, and translation instability may be effectively managed by the application of a tension band fixation construct (Fig. 30-24). Facets and the joint capsules are injured under internal tension secondary to spinal hyperflexion. Normally, they absorb approximately one fifth of the total compressive loads applied to the lumbar spine segment.[25] They have an important role in resisting pathologic forces. In facetectomy studies, the shear and combined compression-flexion strength and kinematics of the spine are significantly compromised.[25-29]

In the lower cervical spine, primary spinal motions are related to disc integrity. Flexion-extension is distributed throughout the cervical spine a total of 60 to 75 degrees. Sagittal translation is limited to 2 to 3 mm at all cervical levels. This is a function of facets, ligaments, and discs. Thus, even small increases in translations may be harmful. Lateral bending, on the other hand, is a prominent motion, particularly

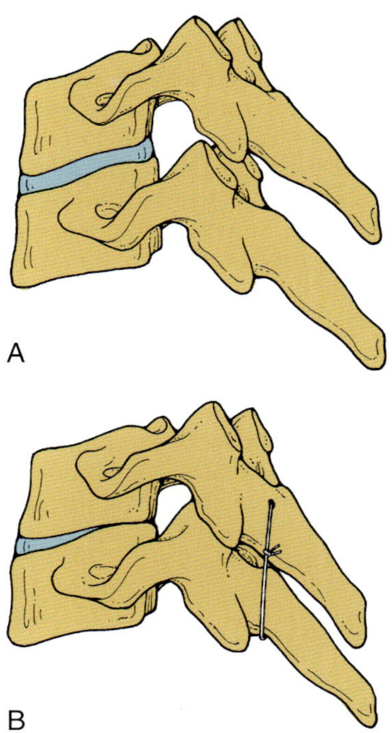

FIGURE 30-24. In the cervical spine, the orientation of the facet joints can be used to advantage via cerclage wiring techniques. **A,** The compression of two spinous processes together in a tension-band manner prevents subluxation by bringing the rostral and caudal facets together. **B,** Because the facet joints are oriented coronally, the close approximation of the superior and inferior facets causes them to abut each other and thus prevent translational deformation. (From Benzel EC: Stability and instability of the spine. In Benzel EC, editor: *Biomechanics of spine stabilization, principles and clinical practice*, New York, 1995, McGraw-Hill, pp 25–40.)

TABLE 30-10

Normal Motion of the Cervical Spine

	Maiman et al.*	Johnson et al.†
Lateral bending	64.2 (± 6.8)	
Rotation	134.2 (± 17.1)	
Flexion-extension		
OC-C1	16.7 (± 10.0)	13.6 (± 6.0)
C1-2	11.6 (± 4.7)	15.2 (± 3.8)
C2-3	17.1 (± 4.5)	17.1 (± 3.9)
C3-4	18.1 (± 6.1)	18.8 (± 2.2)
C4-5	13.7 (± 1.7)	12.0 (± 1.2)
C5-6	17.6 (± 1.5)	20.1 (± 1.6)
C6-7	21.8 (± 1.6)	20.7 (± 1.6)

*Maiman DJ, Yoganandan N: Biomechanics of cervical spine trauma. *Clin Neurosurg* 37:543–570, 1991.
†Johnson RM, Hart DL, Simmons EF, et al: Cervical orthoses. A study comparing their effectiveness in restricting cervical motion in normal subjects. *J Bone Joint Surg [Am]* 59:332–339, 1977.

above C6. Between C2 and C5 there is 10 to 12 degrees of lateral bending per spinal level, and at C7-T1 there is 4 to 8 degrees. Typically, lateral bending is coupled with axial rotation.[6] This coupling in which the spinous processes are rotated in the opposite direction of the lateral bending may be a consequence of muscle contraction or the three-dimensional spatial orientation of the spinous processes (Table 30-10).[2]

Thoracic Spine

The thoracic spinal cord is shielded from injury by the massive regional paraspinal muscle masses and by the thoracic cage. The narrow spinal canal diameter in the upper thoracic region, however, complicates the issue. The former protects the neural elements; the latter contributes to neural injury. This may explain the increased incidence of catastrophic neurologic injuries associated with thoracic fractures. The significant paraspinal muscle mass protects the spine from injury. However, the narrow spinal canal leaves little room to spare for the spinal cord, which is easily compromised by malalignment of the spine or retropulsion of bone due to a fracture[30] (Fig. 30-25). The normal kyphotic posture of the thoracic spine, with its associated predisposition to spinal fracture, amplifies all of these factors. Biomechanical effects of laminectomy on thoracic spine stability are reported.[31]

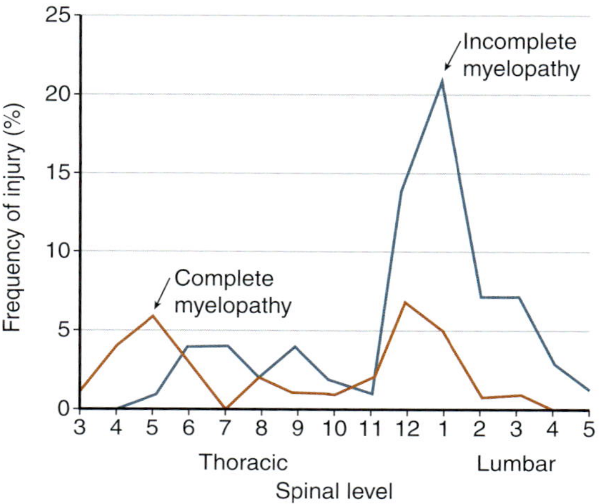

FIGURE 30-25. A representation of the frequency of the level of vertebral injury in patients with traumatic spinal cord injury, contrasting complete myelopathies (no function preserved below the level of injury; *red line*), and incomplete myelopathies (some function preserved below the level of injury; *blue line*). Note that in patients with complete myelopathies, the curve is shifted to the left. (From Benzel EC, Larson SJ: Functional recovery after decompressive operation for thoracic and lumbar spine fractures. *Neurosurgery* 19:772–778, 1986.)

Lumbar Spine

Its relatively large proportions and the resumption of lordosis make this region relatively resistant to failure. Furthermore, the transition of the spinal cord into the cauda equina makes catastrophic spinal injury from trauma less likely. The caudal end of the column is associated with significant logistical therapeutic dilemmas. Frequently, an inability to obtain a solid point of sacral fixation creates surgical problems. Similarly, an appropriate bending moment is not often resisted by the instrumentation construct because of an inadequate length of the lever arm below the injury.[30,32-34] Furthermore, the relatively steep orientation of the lumbosacral joint exposes the lumbosacral spine to increased translational deformations.

Spinal Stability

The original two-column stability concept presented by Holdsworth was based on the clinical experiences of Holdsworth and Nicoll, and the experimental work of Roaf.[35-37] In the two-column definition, the dorsal column consists of the posterior ligamentous complex (i.e., the interspinous and the supraspinous ligaments, ligamentum flavum, and apophyseal joints). The anterior column consists of the vertebral body, intervertebral disc, and anterior and posterior longitudinal ligaments. Holdsworth contended that the stability depends principally on the integrity of the dorsal ligament complex.[35] Consequently, a simple burst fracture with no dorsal involvement was deemed stable. A compression burst fracture with an intact dorsal complex also is stable. Unstable fractures consist of the loss of integrity of the posterior ligament complex and at least one of the components of the anterior column.

The consideration of "columns" in defining the extent of stability helps the physician conceptualize and categorize case-specific phenomena. The theory of Louis is that the spine bears weight principally by sustaining axial loads along the vertebral body, the disc, and the two facet joint complexes (Fig. 30-26) at each spinal level.[38] This concept assists in the instability assessment process when predominantly axial loads are involved. Because of its obvious

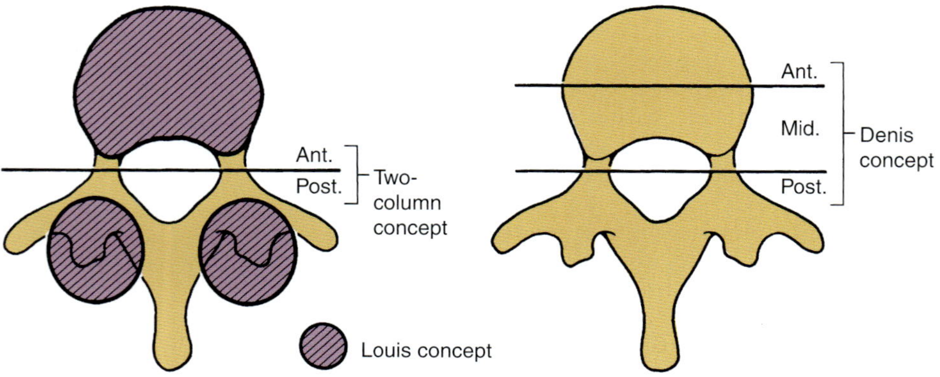

FIGURE 30-26. The "column" concepts of spinal instability. The concept described by Louis (*left*) assigns significance to the vertebral body and the facet joint complexes (lateral masses) on either side of the dorsal spine. Denis's three-column concept (*right*) assigns significance to the region of the neutral axis and the integrity of the posterior vertebral body wall (middle column). The two-column construct (*right*) relies on anatomically defined structures, the vertebral body (anterior column), and the posterior elements (posterior column). Louis's three-column concept (*left*) similarly relies on anatomically defined structures. (From White AA, Panjabi MM: *Clinical biomechanics of the spine*, ed 2, Philadelphia, 1990, JB Lippincott, with permission.)

association with the bony columns of the spine (vertebral body and facet joints), this three-column concept of Louis assesses the bony component failure more effectively than soft tissue damage.[38] Conventional radiographs and CT scans are tools to assess this type of instability. However, except for the case of a significant vertebral body failure, a correlation between the external bony injury and chronic instability may be tenuous.[33] In addition, this theory does not facilitate the assessment of the distraction, flexion, and extension components of injury. The three-column concept of Denis is more applicable to this situation.[39,40] This theory assists in assessing bony collapse associated with axial load bearing; it also provides insight into the assessment of the distraction, flexion, and extension components of injury (injury to the dorsal elements) of the spinal column. The three-column theory adds the concept of a middle column to the two-column theory and allows specific assessment of that component to the spinal column in the region of the neutral axis.[39,40]

The neutral axis is that longitudinal region of the spinal column that bears a significant portion of the axial load and about which spinal distraction or compression does not necessarily occur with flexion or extension (Fig. 30-27). Usually, the neutral axis is located in the region of the midposterior aspect of the vertebral body (i.e., the middle column of Denis).[39] This also encompasses the IAR in the sagittal plane.

The middle-column definition of Denis was based on experimental studies demonstrating that transection of the entire dorsal ligament complex alone was insufficient to produce instability. However, when the posterior longitudinal ligament and the dorsal portion of the disc were also transected, instability ensued. Therefore, in the three-column spine of Denis, the middle column consists of the posterior longitudinal ligament, the dorsal anulus fibrosus, and the dorsal wall of the vertebral body; the anterior column consists of the anterior longitudinal ligament, the ventral anulus fibrosus, and the ventral wall of the vertebral body. The posterior column is the same as in the two-column approach of Holdsworth. Of the major spinal injuries defined by Denis, only minimal and moderate compression fractures with an intact posterior column should be considered stable. The two- and three-column theories differ in classifying burst fractures in terms of stability. Denis classifies the burst fracture as unstable because both anterior and middle columns are affected. All fractures and fracture/dislocations categorized as unstable by Denis demonstrated trauma in at least two of three columns. Many other definitions of clinical instability also exist. Clinical instability is also defined as the loss of the ability of the spine under physiologic loads to maintain its pattern of displacement so that there is no initial or additional neurologic deficit, no major deformity, and no incapacitating pain.[11]

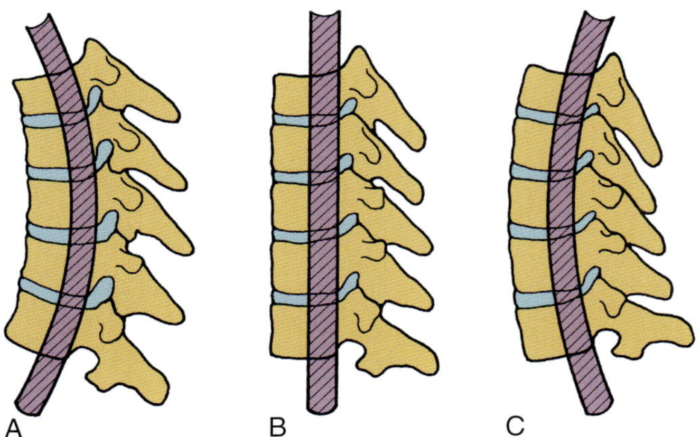

FIGURE 30-27. The depiction of the neutral axis (*shaded areas*). The neutral axis is the longitudinal region of the spinal column that bears much of the axial load and about which spinal element distraction or compression does not significantly occur with the assumption of flexed (**A**), neutral (**B**), or extension (**C**) postures. (From Benzel EC: Stability and instability of the spine. In Benzel EC, editor: *Biomechanics of spine stabilization, principles and clinical practice*, New York, 1995, McGraw-Hill, pp 25–40.)

In biomechanical literature, stability and instability are used interchangeably. Instability is the inverse of stability. Benzel defined instability as the inability to limit excess or abnormal spinal displacement. The use of the word *excessive* reflects the difficulty of quantifying instability in clinical situations.[33] Stability has also been classified as acute and chronic. Acute instability may be categorized as vertical and limited. Chronic instability can similarly be classified into two subgroups: glacial instability and the instability associated with dysfunctional segmental motions.

Quantification of Acute Instability

Numerous authors have attempted to quantify the degree or extent of acute instability by a point system approach. White and Panjabi described a region-specific point system in which an accumulation of five or more points indicates an unstable spine.[11] The system emphasizes the differences between the cervical, thoracic, and thoracolumbar and lumbar regions. These are the essential assessments of overt and limited instability as defined subsequently. The primary purpose of a stability determination is to delineate the most appropriate management scheme for patient care. Recently, Benzel presented the quantification of acute instability in subaxial cervical, thoracic, and lumbar regions based on the point system suggested earlier by White and Panjabi.[33] In principle, the earlier classification was combined in such a way that regional differences were eliminated so that the point system was independent of spinal region.

The stretch test for the assessment of acute cervical spine instability by White and Panjabi involves a progressive addition of cervical traction up to 33% of the patient's weight with serial radiographic and clinical assessments. A positive test indicating the presence of instability is the one that shows a disc interspace separation of more than 1.7 mm or a change in the angle between the vertebrae of more than 7.5 degrees between the prestretch and poststretch conditions. The merits of this test are debatable. First, it is clearly not without risk, whether those risks be immediately obvious or occult. A risk of tethering the spinal cord over a ventral mass may also exist. The most significant and least immediately recognized risk of this procedure is that of a false-negative test (i.e., the presence of stability in a real unstable circumstance). This test has been used as a determinant of eligibility for participation in contact sports.[33] It should be noted that the resistance of stretching by muscle action (voluntary or involuntary) may conceal ligament deficiencies, particularly in an athlete.

Flexion-extension radiographs may also not be helpful, and in certain cases, could be misleading, particularly following trauma. If pathology is observed and iatrogenic injury via the act of flexion and extension is not incurred, they are useful.[33] They are, however, not without risk if spinal instability is present. A "normal" flexion-extension radiograph may not always indicate stability (i.e., the test may be a false negative). Incomplete patient cooperation and "guarding" against excessive spinal movement due to underlying acute pathology can also disguise an injury process that, if not treated properly, may lead to catastrophe.

The definition of stability in clinical practice must address the integrity of each component. Whether the two-column or the three-column approach is used initially, each component must be subsequently analyzed to reach a clinical decision. The problem of simple definitions of stability is that clinical cases are not always simple. Examination of a burst fracture should lend itself to additional questions, such as the nature and extent of vertebral body compression, as well as the number of ligament(s) in the posterior column stretched beyond their elastic limits or even torn. These questions deal with component-related problems. Understanding of the biomechanical characteristics and an interrelationship among spinal components is limited. Additional research that relates component attributes to acute and chronic instability must be undertaken. The clinician should have a detailed understanding of the biomechanical properties of the individual components (discs, ligaments, facet joints, and vertebra) and the relationship of their integrity to the overall stability and load-carrying capacity of the spine.

Anomalous Anatomy

This feature is occasionally associated with structural, biomechanical, or neurologic sequelae. For example, the Klippel-Feil anomaly in the cervical spine can place excessive stress on adjacent motion segments via the application of an abnormally lengthy moment arm. This, in turn, could result in the acceleration of degenerative changes at adjacent motion segments. Similarly, the lumbarization of the L5 vertebral body (i.e., the presence of 4, instead of 5, lumbar segments) could place excessive stress at the L4-5 disc interspace. Conversely, the presence of six lumbar vertebrae could result in excessive lordosis and abnormal loading patterns that expose the lower lumber motion segments to significant stress that may lead to increased rates of disc herniation and degenerative changes. Anomalous nerve root anatomy, such as conjoined nerve roots (Fig. 30-28), can expose the patient to injury from disc herniation or trauma, due to the restriction of normal nerve root motion and mobility. In addition, the unaware surgeon may cause intraoperative iatrogenic injury if the presence of this anomaly is not evident to the surgeon prior to surgery.

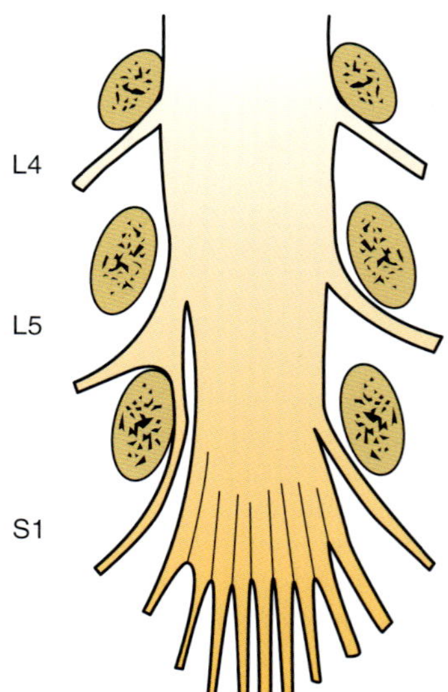

FIGURE 30-28. Anomalous nerve root.

Soft Tissue Biomechanics

As discussed, integrity of soft tissues is vital to maintain spinal stability and physiologic function. Physiologic dysfunction in the form of pain to the neck or headache occurs due to motor vehicle rear impacts, and these injuries do not often result in osseous damage. These injuries, often termed whiplash trauma, are soft tissue related.[41] Studies conducted by Yoganandan et al. have explained the mechanisms of headache and neck pain, the two most common complaints of whiplash patients. Using biomechanical tests, Yoganandan et al. documented soft tissue injuries in the form of ligament and facet joint compromise secondary to single rear impact acceleration using intact whole-body postmortem human subjects.[42] Cusick et al. discussed the formation of a reverse curve during the earlier stages of the rear impact acceleration wherein the spine attains a nonphysiologic curvature (i.e., upper cervical spine flexion associated with lower cervical spine extension).[42-48] Using kinematic analysis as a biomechanical basis, these studies indicated that flexion at the upper segment may stretch the posterior suboccipital structures, creating tensile forces, which may affect the related neural structures and be responsible for suboccipital headaches. The local lower cervical spinal extension indicated that the facet joint slides from the anterior to the posterior direction and the joint stretches ventrally while compressing dorsally, indicating a pinching mechanism. The sliding and the pinching mechanism result in a stretch of the joint itself. This local stretch of the lower cervical spine facet joint may be responsible for neck pain in whiplash patients. A diagrammatic representation of the facet joint pinching mechanism resulting in a stretch of the facet joint is shown in Figure 30-29. Differences

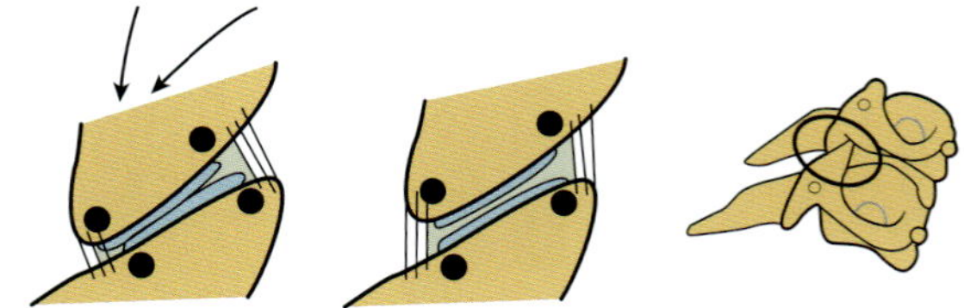

FIGURE 30-29. Diagrammatic representation of the facet joint pinching mechanism occurring in the lower cervical spine under whiplash loading because the compression is more pronounced in the posterior facet joint and the sliding is approximately the same. This mechanism causes the posterior aspect of the facet to be pinched. (From Cusick JF, Pintar FA, Yoganandan N: Whiplash syndrome: kinematic factors influencing pain patterns. *Spine [Phila Pa 1976]* 26:1252–1258, 2001.)

have been reported between men and women with regard to cervical spine motions during rear impact, in particular, during the time of formation of the nonphysiologic S curve.[48,49] Specifically, female intervertebral joints have shown a higher degree of motion than male joints at the lower cervical spine levels. These studies appear to support the clinical and epidemiologic finding that females are more susceptible to soft tissue–related injuries than males.[50,51] The role of gender on the anatomic variations is discussed in the next section.

Gender Effects

The human spine exhibits anatomic and biomechanical differences between genders. It is well known that the rate of maturation process is earlier in women than men. Men have larger vertebral dimensions than women.[52-54] Lumbar vertebral body heights and cross-sectional areas are greater in men than women.[55] In addition, lumbar body sizes in adult and pediatric women are smaller than men, after accounting for age, stature, and total body mass.[56-58] Widths of lumbar vertebrae are also smaller in women. In the adult cervical spine, sizes of vertebrae are also greater in men than women, and in particular, vertebral bodies are longer in the midsagittal plane, and the canal-to-body ratio is greater.[52,53,56] Lumbar ligaments in women have decreased collagen and increased elastin.[59] In a quantitated CT study of 98 adult healthy human volunteers from the North American population between the ages of 18 to 40 years, Yoganandan et al. showed that the trabecular bone densities of cervical vertebrae are greater than those of lumbar vertebrae, and furthermore, the density increases caudally in the cervical region.[60,61] Also, lumbar spine density was the best predictor of cervical vertebral density. Using the same group of 98 volunteers and size-matching based on sitting height and circumference, the following parameters were extracted: vertebral width, disc-to-facet depth, and segmental support area, combining interfaced width and disc-to-facet depth.[62] Vertebral width was defined as the distance between the most lateral extents of the right and left articular masses. Disc-to-facet depth was defined as the distance between the most anterior vertebral body extent and the most posterior articular mass extent. Interfacet width was defined as the distance between the posterior extents of the right and left articular masses. Segmental support area was defined as the triangular area formed by the interfacet width and disc-to-facet depth. These parameters (i.e., vertebral width, disc-to-facet depth, and segmental support area) were significantly greater in men than in women.

Regions of cervical vertebrae with specific relevance to posterior surgical procedures were evaluated for gender dependence using the quantitated CT study on 98 human volunteers.[62] Pedicle width, height, length, axis length, and medial and sagittal offsets, as well as transverse and sagittal angulations, significantly depended on gender and vertebral level.[63] All six linear parameters showed gender and level bias; they were larger in men than in women. In addition, the angular parameters were also gender dependent. The mean pedicle width and height data were 19% and 18% greater in men than in women. These findings are consistent with the results of a study involving the Japanese population; pedicle width and height data are 5% and 19% greater in men.[64] Variations in pedicle lineal dimensions and angulations may be important in presurgical planning. Further evaluations of the mean lateral mass width and bicortical screw lengths for the Roy-Camille and Magerl techniques also indicated greater dimensions in men than women in the subaxial cervical column, although these parameters showed level dependence.[65] Additionally, using unembalmed human cadaver cervical spinal columns coupled with cryomicrotomy, facet joint width, cartilage thickness, and cartilage gap (defined as the distance from the most ventral or most dorsal region of the facet joint to the location where the cartilage began to appear) were extracted from occiput to T1 levels.[66] The cartilage gap in the dorsal region was greater in women than in men, and the overall mean facet cartilage thickness was lower in men than in women. The lack of adequate cartilage in females may expose the underlying adjacent subchondral bone to direct stresses during normal physiologic and traumatic loads.

Acknowledgment. This research was supported in part by DOT NHTSA DTNH22-07-H-00173, the Office of Naval Research through Naval Air Warfare Center Division contract N00421-06-C-0046, and the Department of Veterans Affairs Medical Research.

KEY REFERENCES

Cusick JF, Yoganandan N, Pintar FA, et al: Biomechanics of sequential posterior lumbar surgical alterations. *J Neurosurg* 76:805–811, 1992.

Yoganandan N, Knowles SA, Maiman DJ, et al: Anatomic study of the morphology of human cervical facet joint. *Spine* 28:2317–2323, 2003.

Yoganandan N, Kumaresan S, Pintar FA: Geometric and mechanical properties of human cervical spine ligaments. *J Biomech Eng* 122:623–629, 2000.

Yoganandan N, Larson SJ, Gallagher M, et al: Correlation of microtrauma in the lumbar spine with intraosseous pressures. *Spine* 19:435–440, 1994.

Yoganandan N, Maiman DJ, Pintar F, et al: Microtrauma in the lumbar spine: a cause of low back pain. *Neurosurgery* 23:162–168, 1988.

Yoganandan N, Maiman DJ, Pintar FA, et al: Biomechanical effects of laminectomy on thoracic spine stability. *Neurosurgery* 32:604–610, 1993.

Yoganandan N, Pintar FA, Larson SJ, et al: *Frontiers in head and neck trauma: clinical and biomechanical.* Amsterdam, 1998, IOS Press.

Yoganandan N, Pintar FA, Stemper BD, et al: Level-dependent coronal and axial moment-rotation corridors of degeneration-free cervical spines in lateral flexion. *J Bone Joint Surg [Am]* 89:1066–1074, 2007.

Yoganandan N, Ray G, Pintar FA, et al: Stiffness and strain energy criteria to evaluate the threshold of injury to an intervertebral joint. *J Biomech* 22:135–412, 1989.

Yoganandan N, Stemper BD, Pintar FA, et al: Normative segment-specific axial and coronal angulation corridors of subaxial cervical column in axial rotation. *Spine* 33:490–496, 2008.

REFERENCES

The complete reference list is available online at expertconsult.com.

CHAPTER 31

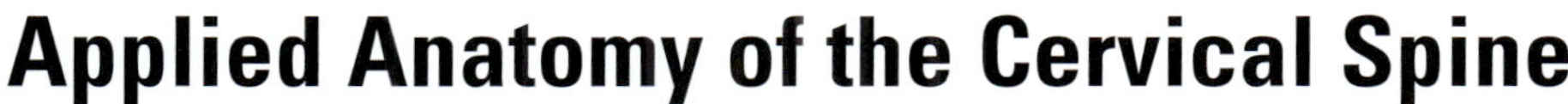

Applied Anatomy of the Cervical Spine

Srinivas Prasad | Wolfgang Rausching

The cervical spine is composed of seven vertebral bodies, spanning the interval between the occiput, rostrally, and the thoracic spine, caudally. Individual segments are connected by an extensive complex of viscoelastic structures to form a single flexible but constrained column serving both neuroprotective and structural functions. A thorough understanding of the normal relationships between these osseous, discoligamentous, and neural elements is essential for safe and effective surgical intervention. These relationships, moreover, have important implications for the biomechanical and clinical presentation of spinal pathology.

Spinal Column

The cervical spine may be divided into two morphologically distinct zones: the occipitocervical junction and the subaxial cervical spine. These zones are discussed separately to facilitate more detailed examination of their unique osseous and discoligamentous structures.

Occipitocervical Junction

Osseous Elements

The first and second vertebral segments attach to the occiput to form the craniocervical junction, which is a complex articular system permitting rotational and nutational movement. The first cervical segment, also known as C1 or the *atlas*, is composed of a ventral and dorsal arch, joined laterally by symmetrical lateral masses (Figs. 31-1 to 31-3). The superior and inferior articulating surfaces of the lateral mass are concave to enable articulation with the occipital condyles, superiorly, and the shoulders of the axis, inferiorly (Figs. 31-4 and 31-5). The ventral arch forms a short bridge between the lateral masses, with a dorsal articular surface forming a synovial joint with the odontoid process of C2 and an anterior tubercle ventrally to which the longus colli muscle attaches. The dorsomedial walls of the C1 lateral masses form a small tubercle that serves as the attachment for the transverse atlantoaxial ligament. The dorsal arch of the atlas typically forms a posterior tubercle in the midline that is a rudimentary equivalent to subaxial spinous processes. Caution should be exercised in dissection of this structure because the dorsal arch may be incomplete. The dorsal arch is round in cross-section in the midline and attenuates laterally to form a flatter surface where it attaches to the dorsal lateral masses. The superior surface of the lateral dorsal arch forms a groove known as the *sulcus arteriosus* on which the vertebral arteries run bilaterally; it is often thin or even dehiscent and great care must be taken when exposing the inferior surface of the C1 lateral mass. The lateral masses are bounded laterally by short transverse processes that are fenestrated by the transverse foramen, or foramen transversarium. As in the subaxial spine, the vertebral artery traverses the transverse foramen of C1 before turning 90 degrees medially to run along the superior surface of the dorsal arch, as described previously. This genu lies 1.5 to 2 cm lateral to midline[1] and dorsal dissection should seldom require exposure of this precarious region.

The second vertebral segment, or *axis* (see Figs. 31-1 to 31-4), is a distinctive osseous structure. The odontoid process, a peglike rostral projection, forms a synovial joint with the atlas along its ventral border and allows the atlas to rotate on C2, with translational restriction created by a complex of ligamentous

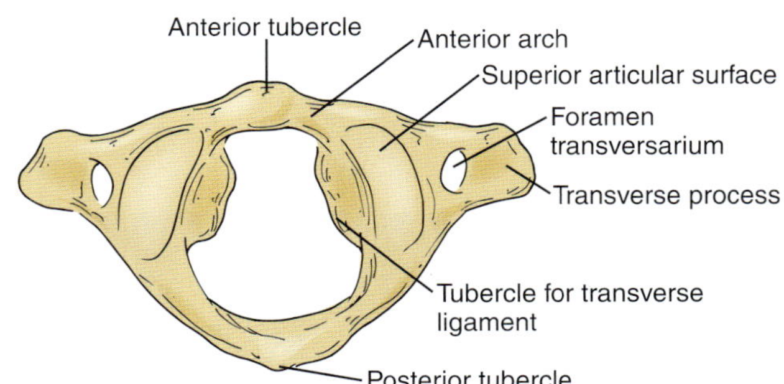

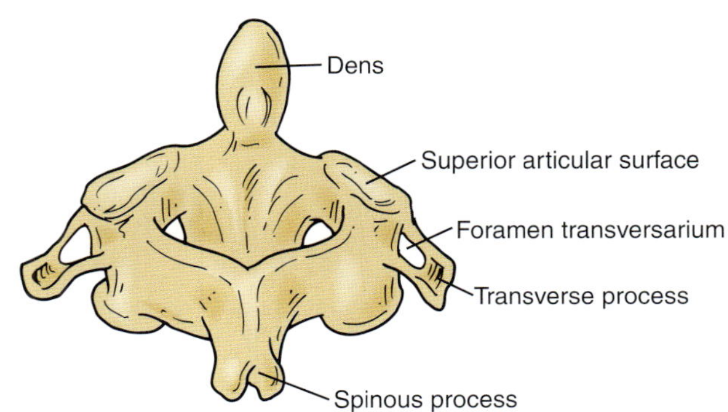

FIGURE 31-1. Atlas and axis osseous anatomy and landmarks.

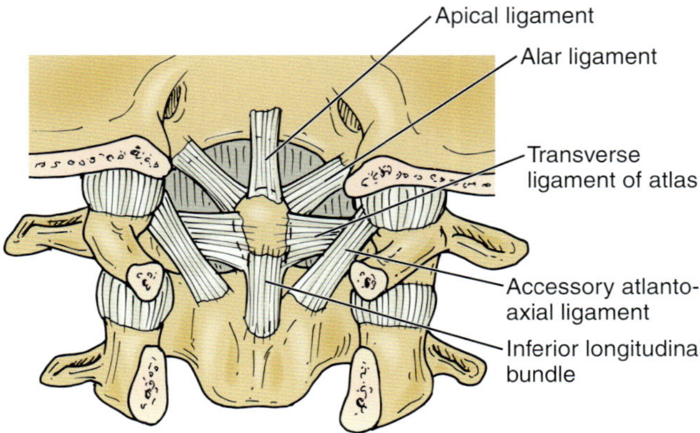

FIGURE 31-2. Occipitocervical junction ligaments. The cruciate ligament, accessory atlanto-axial ligaments, and alar ligaments are shown.

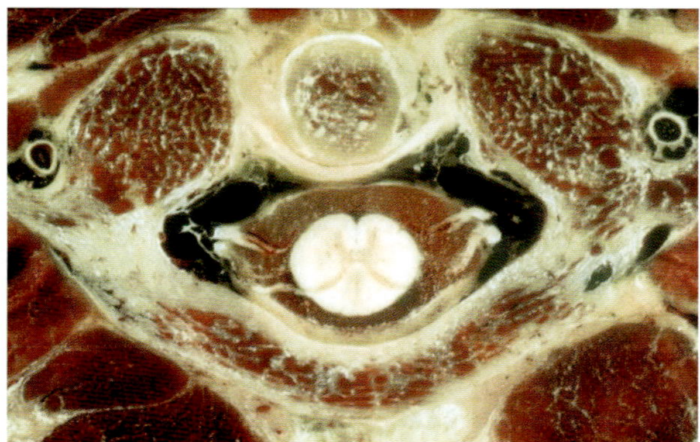

FIGURE 31-3. Cross-section of atlantoaxial complex. The transverse atlantoaxial ligament inserts on tubercles along the posteromedial wall of the lateral masses. The synovial joint between C1 and C2 is visualized. Note foramen transversarium with traversing vertebral artery.

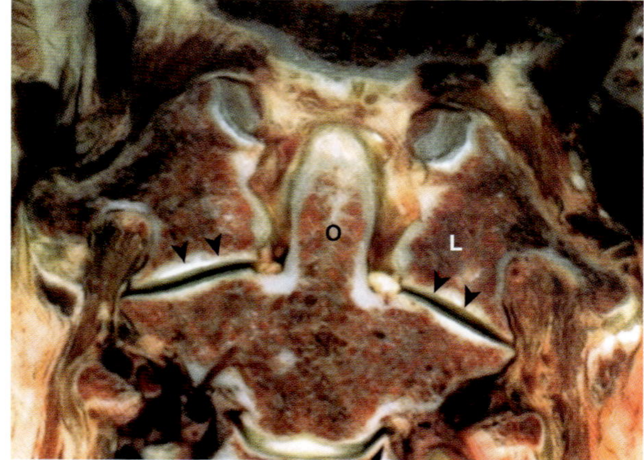

FIGURE 31-4. Coronal section through occipitocervical junction. *Double arrowheads* show inferior articular surface of C1 lateral mass on shoulders of C2 superior articular process. The odontoid process (O) and C1 lateral mass (L) are shown. Note section of transverse atlantoaxial ligament flanking the odontoid process; alar ligaments are also visible.

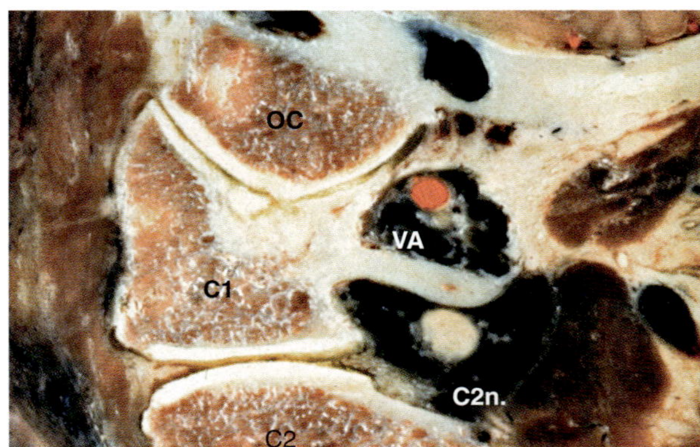

FIGURE 31-5. Parasagittal section showing articulations of occipital condyle (OC), C1, and C2. Note location of the vertebral artery (VA) above the posterior arch of C1 and the C2 nerve root (C2n) below.

structures. The tip of the odontoid process serves as the attachment for the apical ligament, which connects C2 to the basion (the ventral lip of the foramen magnum). The tip is flanked by two bony prominences that serve as the attachments for the paired alar ligaments that span the divide between C2 and the occipital condyles. The transverse atlantoaxial ligament traverses the dorsal border of the odontoid process, which often carries a groove for this strong ligament. The neck of the odontoid process narrows to meet the vertebral body of C2 and is a common site for C2 fracture. The vertebral body culminates rostrally to form two bilaterally symmetrical "shoulders" that flank the odontoid process and articulate with the lateral masses of C1. A relatively long pars interarticularis spans the interval between superior and inferior articulating processes and is laterally bounded by the transverse process of C2. The disproportionate length of the C2 pars interarticularis has important clinical implications. Because the superior and inferior articulating processes of C2 are coronally offset, extension applies significant strain on the C2 pars interarticularis. Under forceful hyperextension, the pars interarticularis may fracture, giving rise to the mechanism and morphology of the so-called hangman's fracture. As at other levels, this process is fenestrated by the transverse foramen, which lies immediately lateral to the C2 pedicle and serves as the conduit for the vertebral artery. Unlike at other levels, the C2 foramen is angulated 45 degrees laterally so that the vertebral artery is partially roofed by the superior articular process.[2] The inferior articular process forms an articulation with the C3 superior articular process and assumes the more typical orientation of subaxial lateral masses.

Ligamentous Structures

Although the articular surfaces of the occipitocervical junction are oriented to permit constrained flexibility, a complex of intervening ligamentous structures acts in concert to restrict excessive translation and rotation (see Figs. 31-2 to 31-4). Three ligaments span the divide between the odontoid process and the occiput. In the midline, the apical ligament spans the interval between the basion and the tip of the odontoid process. This ligament, also known as the *middle odontoid ligament* or *suspensory ligament*, is of unclear biomechanical significance because it has been described as absent in 20% of specimens.[3] The alar ligaments are bilaterally symmetrical structures approximately 1 cm in length spanning from the dorsolateral odontoid tip to the medial occipital condyles. Each alar ligament restricts excessive rotation to the contralateral side and excessive lateral bending to the contralateral side.[4]

The cruciate, or cruciform, ligament is the most important ligamentous structure of the craniovertebral junction. It is composed of four limbs that unite over the dorsal odontoid process. The superior limb, or ascending band, inserts on the occiput, whereas the inferior limb, or descending band, inserts on the dorsal body of C2. The transverse atlantoaxial ligament forms the transverse limbs of this complex and attaches to bony tubercles on the medial borders of the C1 lateral masses. The transverse ligament is a strong, inelastic structure composed of primarily dense collagen with a ventrolateral transition to fibrocartilaginous tissue near its insertion on the C1 lateral masses. As a consequence, this lateral transition portion is the zone most susceptible to traumatic rupture, and the transverse atlantoaxial ligament has been demonstrated to rupture under loads of 400 to 1100 N.[5] Rupture of this ligament may be identified on MRI, particularly on gradient-echo sequences,[6] and is associated with atlantoaxial instability. On occasion, the insertion of this ligament will fracture off the medial wall of one or both lateral masses while the ligament itself remains intact. CT and MRI characterization of these disruption patterns has important implications for the management of traumatic atlantoaxial instability.

The anterior atlanto-occipital membrane is the rostral continuation of the anterior longitudinal ligament (ALL), extending from the atlantoaxial complex to the basion. The posterior atlanto-occipital membrane is the occipitocervical homologue to the ligamentum flavum. It extends from the posterior arch of C1 to the posterior rim of the foramen magnum, or opisthion.

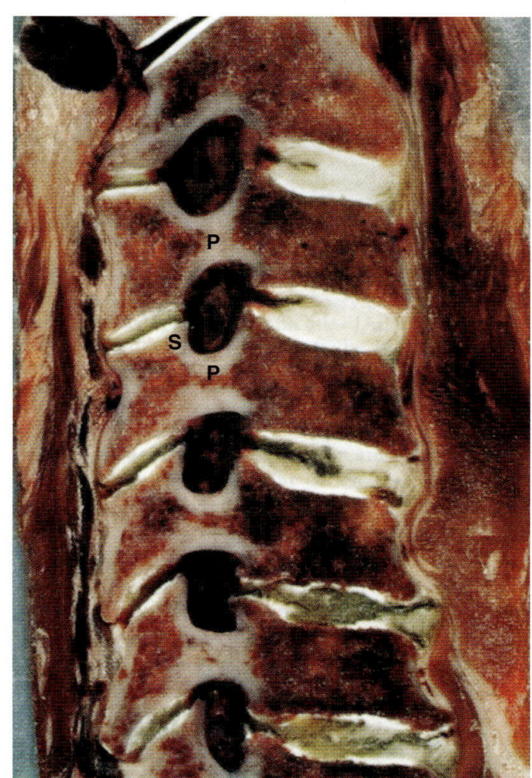

FIGURE 31-6. Oblique sagittal section along axis of pedicles (P). Note superior articular process (S) and its relationship to the neuroforamen. Progressive caudal degenerative changes include disc desiccation, uncovertebral hypertrophy, and ventral osteophyte formation.

Subaxial Cervical Spine

The third through seventh cervical vertebral segments share a similar morphology by virtue of their homologous embryologic origin. Because of this uniformity, the osseous and discoligamentous features of a single canonical vertebral segment and level are described.

Osseous Structures

Each vertebral segment can be divided into a ventral portion, the vertebral body, and a dorsal portion, the dorsal or vertebral arch. The cervical vertebral body is roughly cylindrical in geometry, although the anteroposterior diameter is typically smaller than the transverse diameter. Relative to the vertebral arch, the cervical vertebral bodies are smaller than the vertebral bodies of the thoracolumbar spine, likely because they bear significantly less load. The superior and inferior surfaces of the vertebral body serve as the superior and inferior end plates, respectively. The lateral edges of the superior end plate curve sharply upward to form the uncinate processes bilaterally, a unique feature of the cervical spine. These processes articulate with complementary bevels on the lateral surfaces of the adjacent inferior end plate. Although this articulation is referred to as the "uncovertebral joint," it contains no synovial fluid and as a consequence is not a true joint[7] (Figs. 31-6 and 31-7).

The most distinctive feature of the cervical spine is the fenestration of the transverse processes that flank each vertebral body. The transverse process projects ventrolaterally with a deep groove along its superior surface; this serves to carry the cervical

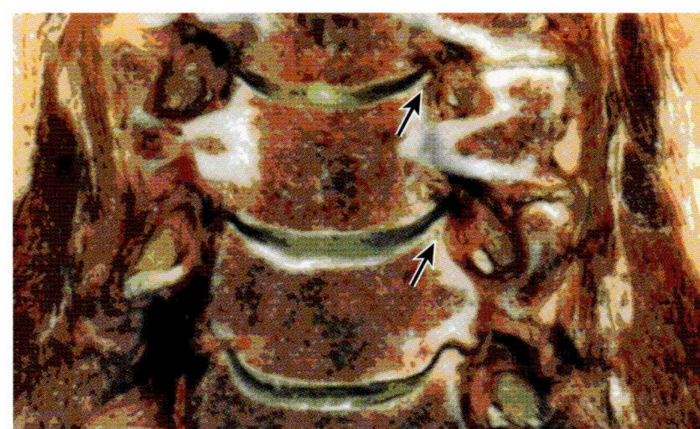

FIGURE 31-7. Coronal section through midcervical spine. Note prominent uncinate process and uncovertebral joints (*arrows*).

spinal nerves. The transverse process terminates laterally with two prominences—the anterior and posterior tubercles. The anterior tubercle serves as an attachment for the ventral cervical musculature and the posterior tubercle serves as an attachment for the dorsal cervical musculature. The transverse foramen, or foramen transversarium, fenestrates the transverse process and carries the vertebral arteries bilaterally (Figs. 31-8 to 31-10).

Importantly, the cervical pedicle serves as the dorsomedial wall of the foramen transversarium, exposing the vertebral artery to hazard when pedicle screws breach laterally. The cervical pedicles connect the dorsal arch with the vertebral body and are angled medially between 38 and 48 degrees from the midsagittal plane.[8] The pedicles of C3 through C7 range in outer diameter from 6.0 to 6.5 mm[9] and in inner diameter

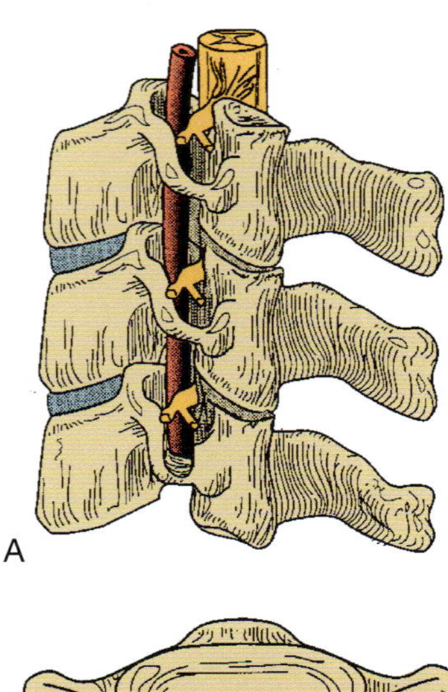

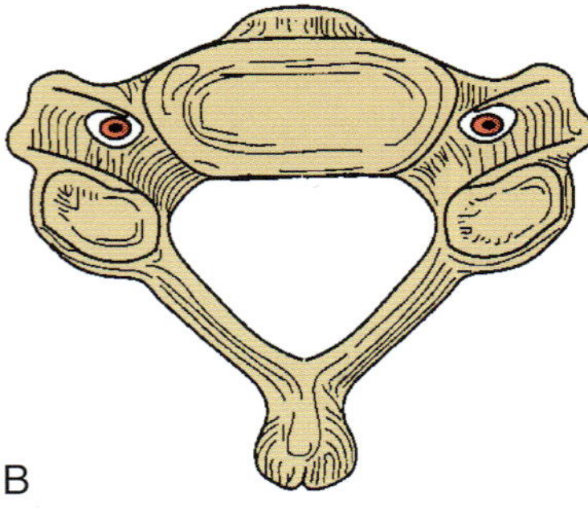

FIGURE 31-8. Subaxial cervical spine, sagittal (**A**) and axial (**B**) views. Note relative positions of transverse processes, which are fenestrated by the foramina transversaria, and adjacency to lateral masses and cervical nerve roots.

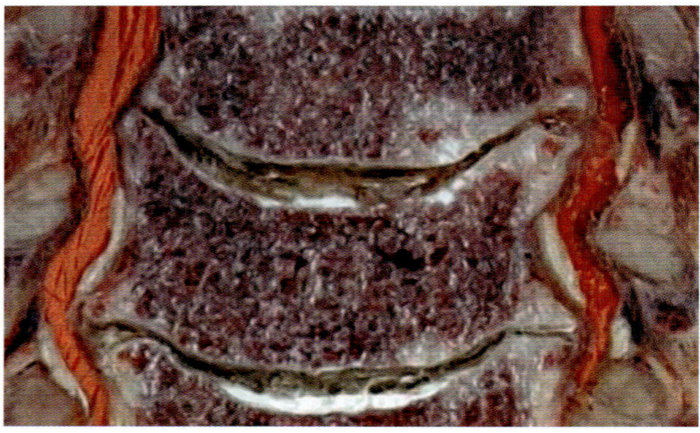

FIGURE 31-9. Coronal section through foramina transversaria showing vertebral arteries traversing adjacent foramina. Note proximity to uncovertebral joints and tortuosity caused by uncovertebral hypertrophy.

from 2.7 to 3.1 mm.[8] The pedicle is thinnest along its lateral wall. In aggregate, these features make safe placement of cervical pedicle screws a challenge. The medial wall is close to the thecal sac, the lateral wall is close to the vertebral artery, and the superior wall is close to the superjacent nerve root.

The superior and inferior articular processes of the cervical spine are oriented obliquely on sagittal projection, with complementary surfaces on adjacent segments. Together with the intervening bone, these articular processes combine to form lateral masses at each level that are parallelogram-shaped in sagittal cross-section. Adjacent lateral masses in the subaxial cervical spine are in close apposition so that in aggregate they form a flexible, cylindrical column of bone dorsolateral to the vertebral bodies. This pillar-like architecture affords axial load-bearing capacity to the dorsal vertebral arches. The oblique configuration of articular surfaces imparts a shingle effect to the lateral masses and allows for flexion and extension while restricting translation, affording osseous neuroprotection for the enveloped cervical spinal cord and nerve roots (see Fig. 31-6). The lateral mass serves as a common anchor point for instrumentation, but an awareness of adjacent neurovascular structures is essential for safe placement of lateral mass screws that avoid the vertebral artery and cervical nerve roots. A rostral screw trajectory is protective of the exiting nerve root, whereas a lateral trajectory protects the vertebral artery (Figs. 31-11 to 31-13).

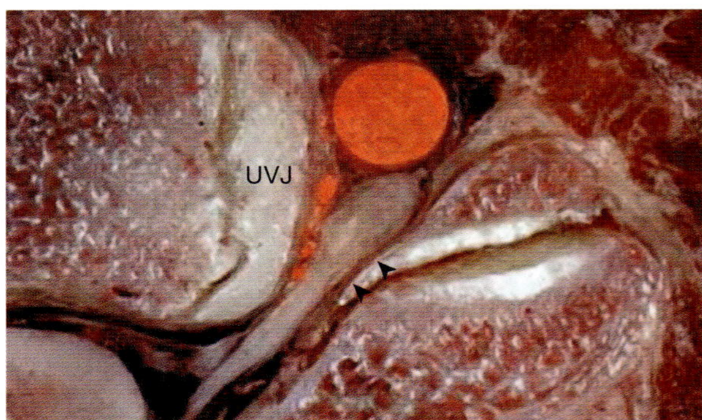

FIGURE 31-10. Axial section showing vertebral artery. Note proximity to exiting nerve root (*double arrowheads*) and uncovertebral joint (UVJ) in section.

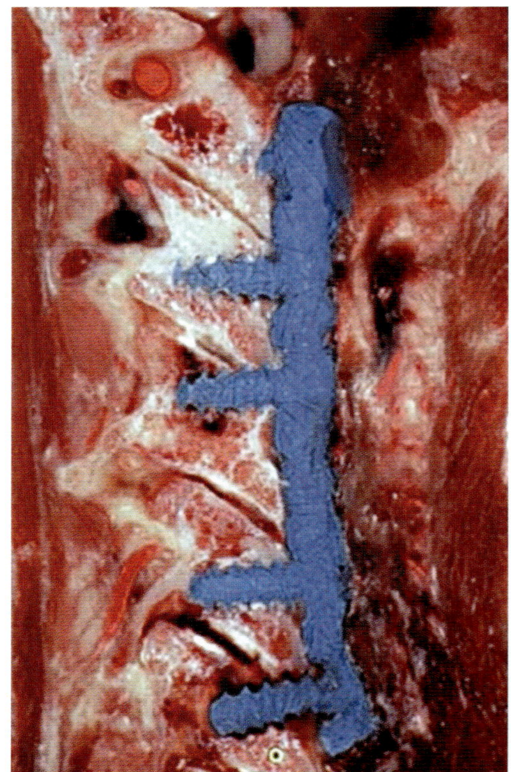

FIGURE 31-11. Parasagittal section showing satisfactory lateral mass screw trajectories.

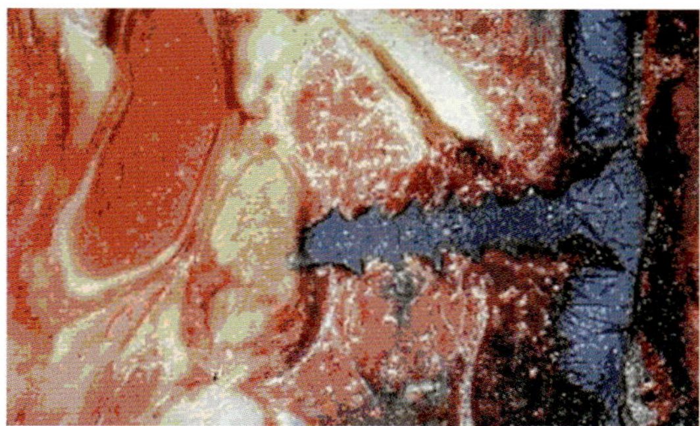

FIGURE 31-12. Parasagittal section showing unsatisfactory screw trajectory with violation of neural foramen, causing nerve root distortion. Failure to maintain a rostral trajectory jeopardizes the nerve root.

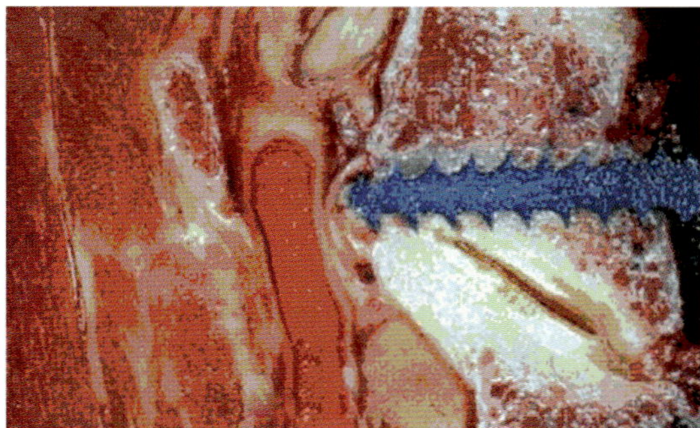

FIGURE 31-13. Sagittal section showing unsatisfactory screw trajectory with vertebral artery distortion. Failure to maintain a lateral trajectory jeopardizes the vertebral artery.

The dorsal arch is completed by bilateral laminae that unite in the midline to form a bifid spinous process rostrally (typically from C3 to C5) and a monofid spinous process caudally (typically from C6 and below). The laminae are narrow, with a thinner superior than inferior edge. The height of the lamina is 10 to 11 mm at C4, whereas the thickness of the lamina is about 2 mm at C5.[10] The spinous processes act as insertions for the semispinalis cervicis muscle. In aggregate, the pedicles, lateral masses, laminae, and spinous processes form the dorsal vertebral arch, which circumscribes the spinal cord and affords neuroprotective function (see Fig. 31-8).

Discoligamentous Structures

The cervical disc space is created by the interval between adjacent superior and inferior vertebral end plates. The inferior end plate is typically concave, creating a ventral lip on the superjacent vertebral body and taller disc space at midbody. Together, the cervical discs constitute 20% of the total cervical height.[11] In a normal cervical spine the disc space height increases with consecutive levels from C3-4 to C7-T1 and the disc space depth increases from approximately 16 mm at C3 to 20 mm at C7.[12] These progressive dimensional changes must be factored into instrumentation selection for ventral cervical procedures.

The intervertebral disc is composed of two components: a central nucleus pulposus that is circumscribed in axial cross-section by the anulus fibrosus. The nucleus pulposus is an

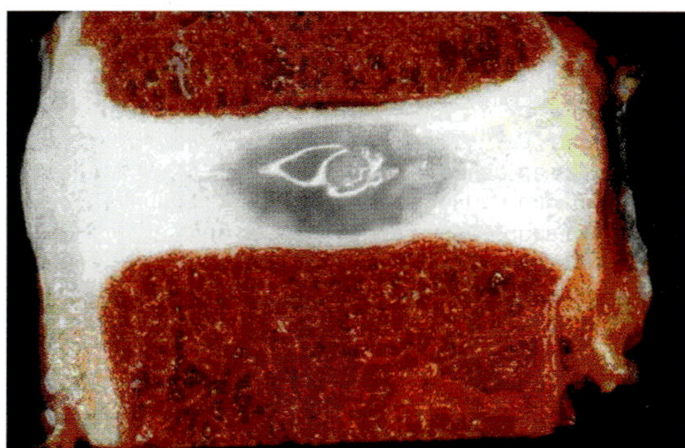

FIGURE 31-14. Sagittal section through intervertebral disc showing central nucleus pulposus and peripheral anulus fibrosus merging with adjacent anterior and posterior longitudinal ligaments.

avascular structure composed of loose fibrous strands suspended in a proteoglycan gel. It has a high water content that can be readily evaluated on MRI and its hydration declines with normal aging, with 88% water content at birth declining to 64% by the seventh decade[13] (see Fig. 31-6). The intervertebral disc receives nutrition by diffusion[14] and creates an immune-isolated avascular space susceptible to infection. The anulus fibrosus is composed of concentric rings of obliquely oriented fibers spanning the disc space from one vertebral body to the other. These fibers insert on the epiphyseal ring of the end plate, where the anchoring fibers are called *Sharpey fibers*. These concentric fibrous rings confer multiaxial shear resistance, like the steel belt of an automobile tire (Fig. 31-14).

The ALL is composed of interdigitating collagen fibers running longitudinally from the anterior tubercle of C1 along the ventral vertebral bodies to the sacrum. It is a broad-based, flat structure without clear lateral boundaries that attenuates laterally where it merges with paramedian, prevertebral connective tissue. The fibers of the ALL are lamellated, with the deepest fibers spanning only adjacent levels, its more superficial layers spanning two to three levels, and its most superficial layers spanning many levels. It serves to restrict hyperextension and excessive axial traction and is adherent to the underlying vertebral bodies and intervertebral discs. Along with the anulus fibrosus, the ALL is the predominant restricter to hyperextension. The posterior longitudinal ligament runs along the dorsal vertebral bodies from C2 to the sacrum. Its rostral extension, called the *tectorial membrane*, inserts at the basion, along the clivus of the occiput. Like the ALL, it is a flat band of fibrous collagen tissue, although it is composed of two layers. The ventral layer is adherent to the dorsal vertebral bodies and intervertebral discs and the dorsal layer is adjacent to the thecal sac. The epidural venous plexus is sandwiched between these two layers. The posterior longitudinal ligament is three to four times thicker in the cervical spine than in the thoracolumbar spine and serves to restrict hyperflexion and axial traction.[15] It is believed to provide further resistance to disc herniation and neural compression (Fig. 31-15).

The dorsal elements are spanned by numerous ligamentous structures that permit constrained flexibility in the cervical spine. The ligamentum flavum is a two-layered structure that spans the interlaminar space between adjacent segments, originating on the ventral surface of the superjacent lamina approximately halfway up the lamina and inserting on the

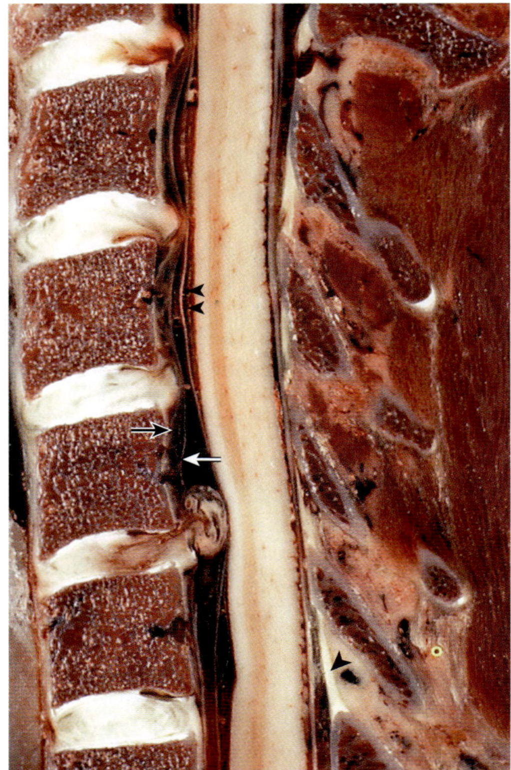

FIGURE 31-15. Midsagittal section showing varying degrees of disc disruption. Note three visible membranes oriented longitudinally dorsal to the vertebral bodies. From ventral to dorsal, these membranes are the two layers of the posterior longitudinal ligament (PLL; *black arrow* and *white arrow*) with intervening epidural venous plexus visible, and the ventral dura (*double arrowheads*). The caudalmost disc extrusion appears to have herniated through both layers of the PLL, whereas the rostral extrusions have not. The anterior longitudinal ligament is similarly visible in close apposition to the anterior vertebral bodies. The ligamentum flavum is seen spanning adjacent laminae (*single arrowhead*), and the interspinous and supraspinous ligaments are seen spanning adjacent spinous processes.

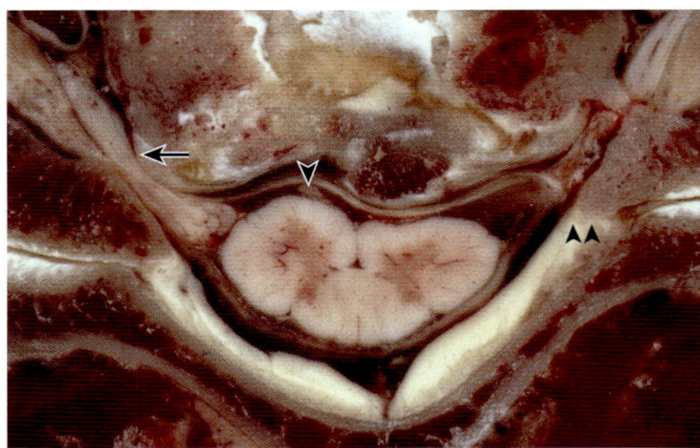

FIGURE 31-16. Axial section through a herniated intervertebral disc, seen distorting the left side of the cervical spinal cord. Note one right-sided ventral rootlet (*single arrowhead*) and its proximity to midline. Central and paracentral disc herniations may cause ventral rootlet symptoms. Right-sided foraminal stenosis is seen as a consequence of uncovertebral hypertrophy (*arrow*). Note ligamentum flavum attachment to superior articular process of subjacent level (*double arrowhead*). Circumferential spinal cord demarcations include ventral median fissure, anterolateral and posterolateral sulci, and posterior median sulcus. Note gross distinction between central gray matter and peripheral white matter.

superior edge of the subjacent lamina.[16] Importantly, it also inserts laterally on the medial edge of the superior articular process. The ligamentum flavum derives its name from its high elastin content, which confers a yellow appearance to it.[13] The ligamentum flavum restricts hyperflexion; with aging, the contractile elasticity of the ligamentum flavum diminishes and hyperextension creates redundancy in this structure, which may narrow the anteroposterior diameter of the spinal canal, potentially contributing to spinal cord compression.

Intertransverse ligaments are short bands of fibrous tissue that bridge adjoining transverse processes. These ligaments serve to restrict lateral cervical bending. The interspinous ligaments are paired midline structures that bridge adjoining spinous processes. In the cervical spine the nuchal ligament represents the rostral extension of the supraspinous ligament. It spans the interval from the occipital protuberance rostrally to the spinous process of C7 caudally. It is a thick, elastic fibrous band that serves to resist hyperflexion. These ligaments are predominant elements of the so-called posterior tension band (Fig. 31-16; see also Fig. 31-15).

Neural Elements

Although a detailed review of cervical neural anatomy is outside the scope of this chapter, a general discussion is provided with an emphasis on relational anatomy as it applies to clinically and pathologically relevant adjacent structures.

Cervical Spinal Cord

The spinal cord is a roughly cylindrical neural continuation of the caudal medulla. In cross-section, the spinal cord is bilaterally symmetrical and can be separated into the central, butterfly-shaped gray matter and the circumferential white matter, which is mostly composed of longitudinally oriented spinal tracts. The perimeter of the spinal cord is demarcated by longitudinally oriented sulci and fissures that serve to divide the spinal cord longitudinally into white matter columns. The ventral median fissure is a true, pia-lined space in which the anterior spinal artery runs. The other circumferential demarcations are less defined. The posterior median sulcus separates the left and right hemicords, the anterolateral sulcus is marked by the emergence of the ventral/motor roots, and the dorsolateral sulcus is marked by the entry of the dorsal/sensory roots. These sulci divide each half of the spinal cord into three principal columns: the anterior column (in the interval between the ventral median fissure and the anterolateral sulcus), the lateral column (between the anterolateral and posterolateral sulci), and the posterior column (between the posterolateral sulcus and the posterior median sulcus). In the cervical spinal cord, the posterior column is further subdivided by the intermediate sulcus into a lateral fasciculus cuneatus and a medial fasciculus gracilis. In the cervical spine, the spinal cord segment is at approximately the same level as the same-numbered spinal column segment (see Fig. 31-16).

Cervical Spinal Nerves

The cervical spinal nerves represent the union of ventral and dorsal roots that arise independently from the cervical spinal cord, as outlined previously. Each root, in turn, represents the union of numerous rootlets that arise from the anterolateral sulcus (for the ventral root) and posterolateral sulcus (for the dorsal root). The anterolateral sulcus is only 1 to 3 mm lateral to midline, and, as a consequence, midline ventral compressive lesions may exert pressure on these exiting ventral rootlets[17] (see Fig. 31-16). Moreover, this branching architecture allows for intradural anastomoses between nerve roots, which may cause atypical dermatomal or myotomal distribution of radiculopathy.[18-20] Within the dorsal root, before splitting into numerous dorsal rootlets, large fibers for proprioception run medially and ventrally and small pain fibers are located laterally and dorsally. The ventral and dorsal roots both traverse the intervertebral neural foramen above their same-numbered pedicle (i.e., the C5 nerve roots exit in the C4-5 neural foramen, above the C5 pedicle). The C8 pedicle exits the C7-T1 intervertebral foramen. The first cervical root does not have a dorsal root ganglion and consequently does not have a corresponding sensory dermatome.

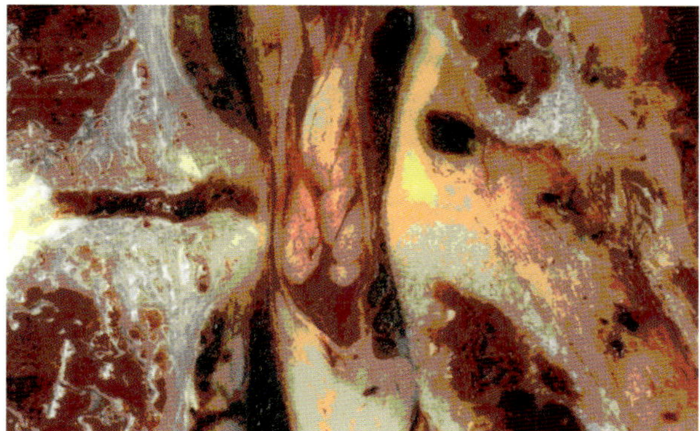

FIGURE 31-17. Disc-osteophyte complex exerting pressure on obliquely oriented ventral and dorsal rootlets.

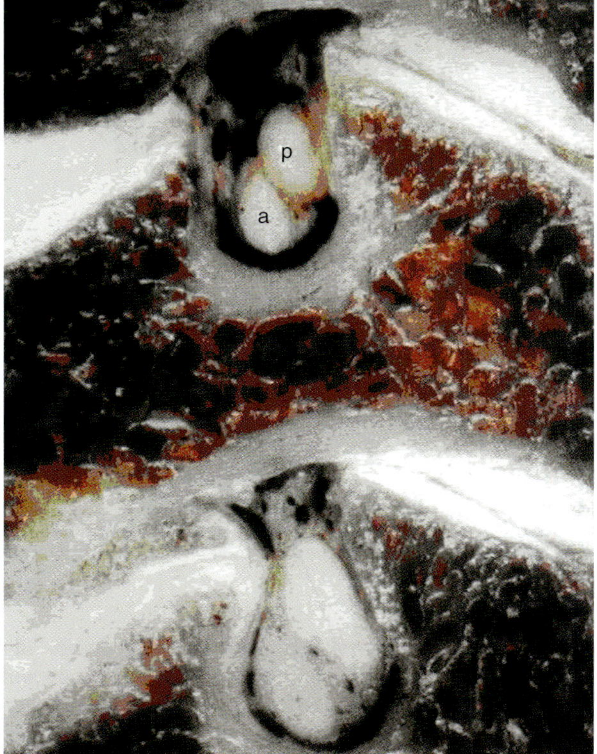

FIGURE 31-18. Topographic organization of exiting nerve roots. The ventral root (*a*, anterior) is inferior and anterior to the dorsal root (*p*, posterior). Even a small disc bulge may cause notable foraminal stenosis, as shown at the caudal level. The boundaries of the foramen include the cranial and caudal pedicles as well as the disc-uncovertebral complex and facet joint.

The cervical spinal nerve roots traverse the intervertebral foramen close to numerous adjacent osseous, discoligamentous, and vascular structures. A thorough understanding of these relationships facilitates safe and effective decompression when clinically indicated. The nerve root exits the neural foramen immediately above the like-numbered pedicle, as described previously. Within the intervertebral foramen, the dorsal root is located more rostrally than the ventral root; hence, compressive pathologies may disproportionately affect the ventral or dorsal root, causing dissociation of radicular symptoms. The course of the exiting nerve root is oblique with a ventrolateral trajectory that varies across levels. At its origin, the foramen is bounded ventromedially by the uncovertebral joint; more laterally, the nerve root and dorsal root ganglion abut the vertebral artery. Uncovertebral hypertrophy and lateral disc extrusions may cause compression or distortion of the nerve root, triggering radiculopathy (Fig. 31-17). The vertebral artery, which lies immediately lateral to the uncovertebral joint, may also become distorted by this uncovertebral hypertrophy, causing a secondary compressive effect on the exiting nerve root or, more typically, the dorsal root ganglion[21] (see Fig. 31-9). The dorsolateral wall of the foramen is defined by the superior and inferior articular processes of the adjacent vertebral bodies, and facet hypertrophy may similarly precipitate radiculopathy. This topography gives rational basis to the Spurling maneuver on physical examination, in which an irritable nerve root may be triggered by hyperextension and lateral bending toward the affected nerve root. Although the cranial and caudal bounds of the foramen are defined by the superjacent and subjacent pedicles, the cervical nerve roots lie more caudally within this interval, often directly abutting the roof of the subjacent pedicle (Fig. 31-18).

Vascular Anatomy

Although the anatomy of both the arterial and venous systems is described here, a more detailed examination of the former is provided. A comprehensive description of spinal vasculature is outside the scope of this chapter; however, spinal cord perfusion and large-vessel anatomy are described, with an emphasis on surgically relevant relationships.

Arterial Anatomy

Spinal Cord Perfusion

The spinal cord is perfused by three principal arteries: the anterior spinal artery (ASA) and the paired posterior spinal arteries (PSAs; Fig. 31-19). None of these vessels represent

arteries or posterior inferior cerebellar arteries.[11] The paired PSAs run in the dorsolateral sulci and form a peripheral anastomotic plexus perfusing the dorsal one third of the spinal cord.

The cervical segmental vessels are paired and arise from the vertebral artery and branches of the subclavian arteries. They provide perfusion to the spinal roots and dorsal root ganglia before entering the intervertebral foramen and giving rise to three branches: the dural, radicular, and medullary branches. The dural branch perfuses the spinal dura and nerve root sleeve, the radicular branch penetrates the dura and perfuses the ventral and dorsal nerve roots, and the medullary branch anastomoses with the ASA within one or two levels of its origin.

Vertebral Artery Anatomy

The vertebral arteries are paired vessels that lie close to the cervical spine. The vertebral artery arises from the subclavian artery, from the innominate artery, or directly from the aorta. The course of the vertebral artery is divided into four segments. The V1 segment represents the segment from origin until the artery enters its first foramen transversarium. In 87.5% of cases, this is at the C6 level; in 5.4% it is at C7; in 6.6% it is at C5, and in 0.4% it is at C4.[26] The V2 segment is the portion that traverses the foramina transversaria and terminates after the C2 foramen transversarium. This is the most vulnerable segment of the vertebral artery in most common cervical spine surgeries. The V2 segment may have a tortuous course, and awareness of these anomalies must be achieved radiographically before performing cervical surgery (Fig. 31-20). Moreover, the foramen transversarium is closer to the uncovertebral joint at more rostral levels, warranting more cautious uncovertebral drilling. The V3 segment continues until the vertebral artery penetrates the dura. The V4 segment is the intradural portion of the vessel, ending at the vertebrobasilar junction (Fig. 31-21).

Numerous muscular and osseous branches arise from the vertebral artery at each level. At each level in the subaxial spine, anterior and posterior central arteries contribute to an epidural plexus that provides perfusion to the vertebral bodies. Anterior and posterior ascending arteries arise from the vertebral arteries at the C2 level and anastomose to perfuse the atlantoaxial complex. Collateral arterial supply is recruited from the thyrocervical and costocervical trunks in the lower cervical spine and the ascending pharyngeal and occipital arteries in the upper cervical spine. The odontoid process is perfused by an arcade of arteries, with the base of the odontoid supplied by the ascending branches of the vertebral artery and the tip supplied by the apical artery of the odontoid process, a branch of the hypoglossal artery.[27]

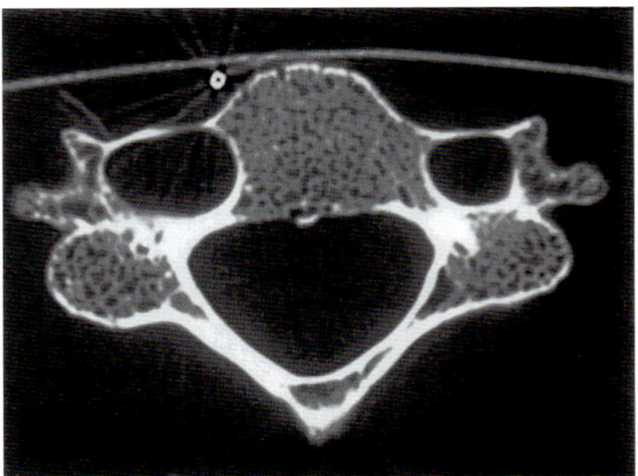

FIGURE 31-20. Axial CT image showing anomalous foramina transversaria. The right-sided vertebral artery is especially vulnerable to iatrogenic injury if this anomaly is not appreciated preoperatively. (Reprinted with permission from Felton DL, Shetty AN, editors: *Netter's atlas of neuroscience*, ed 2, Philadelphia, 2009, Saunders. All rights reserved.)

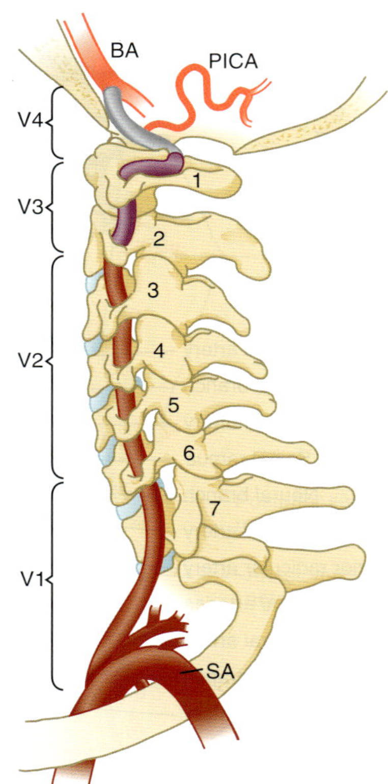

FIGURE 31-21. Vertebral artery anatomy. BA, basilar artery; PICA, posterior inferior cerebellar artery; SA, subclavian artery. (Used with permission from Dickman CA, Fehlings MG, Gokaslan ZL, editors: *Spinal cord and spinal column tumors*, New York, 2006, Thieme.)

Venous Anatomy

The intrinsic spinal cord is drained centrifugally by radially oriented veins that empty into a circumferential venous plexus called the *vasa corona*. The dorsal half of the spinal cord venous drainage empties into this plexus, eventually converging on the median dorsal longitudinal vein, whereas the ventral half of the spinal cord drainage empties into a comparable plexus, eventually draining into the median ventral longitudinal vein. These two principal longitudinal veins collateralize through the venous vasa corona and empty into the epidural venous plexus by way of medullary veins. The epidural venous plexus is a complex but organized system of valveless vessels that allow bidirectional flow, eventually draining into the vena cava and azygos veins. Just as the Batson venous plexus is implicated in the migration of neoplastic and infectious processes in the caudal spine, the pharyngovertebral veins have been implicated in the migration of parapharyngeal infections to the cervical intradural and epidural compartments.[28]

Surgically Relevant Adjacent Structures

Surgical approaches to the ventral cervical spine are common and a thorough understanding of adjacent structures is imperative to minimize morbidity and iatrogenic injury. A comprehensive treatment of this topic is outside the scope of this chapter, but a number of significant surgically relevant structures are reviewed.

Several structures are readily visible or palpable along the ventral neck and serve as landmarks for underlying structures. The hyoid bone is the most rostral palpable landmark in the midline and roughly correlates with the C3 vertebral body. The thyroid cartilage, immediately inferior to this, corresponds to the C4 vertebral body. The cricoid cartilage is a general landmark for the C6 vertebral body. On occasion, the anterior tubercle of the C6 transverse process, also known as the Chassaignac tubercle, may be palpable. Palpation of these structures facilitates optimal placement of ventral neck incisions (Fig. 31-22).

The platysma muscle lies immediately deep to the skin and subcutaneous tissue. It can be divided to expose the medial border of the sternocleidomastoid and strap muscles. As its name implies, the sternocleidomastoid runs from the mastoid rostrally to the sternum and clavicle caudally. Deep to this muscle is the carotid sheath, containing the carotid artery, internal jugular vein, and vagus nerve. In the midline, the trachea and esophagus are critical adjacent structures that lie immediately ventral to the ventral cervical spine. A dissection plane may be developed medial to the sternocleidomastoid and carotid sheath, lateral to the trachea and esophagus, dividing the pretracheal fascia and bluntly extending the plane down to the prevertebral fascia. This plane may be traversed by the omohyoid muscle, which runs from the scapula to the hyoid bone obliquely approximately over the C5 level. It may be retracted rostrally or caudally to facilitate exposure; however, if needed, it may be divided without significant clinical consequence (Fig. 31-23; see also Fig. 31-22).

The recurrent laryngeal nerve, a branch of the vagus nerve, descends into the chest and on the left side loops around the aortic arch before coursing into the tracheoesophageal groove. This relatively consistent course makes surgical approaches to the cervical spine from the left less hazardous to the recurrent laryngeal nerve. On the right, the recurrent laryngeal nerve generally loops around the subclavian artery before coursing into the tracheoesophageal groove, although there is more variability in this course. The superior laryngeal nerve also originates from the vagus nerve and travels with the superior thyroid artery below the hyoid bone at or above the C4 level. It branches into the external and internal laryngeal nerves. Caution must be exercised in ventral cervical exposure to avoid disruption of this innervation; most iatrogenic injuries to these nerves result from excessive traction causing neurapraxia rather than unintentional division of these nerves.

The longus colli muscles flank the ventral cervical vertebral bodies, originating on the anterior tubercle of C1 and extending down to the T3 level, where they insert on the ventral T3 vertebral body. The sympathetic chain runs on the ventral surface of the longus colli muscles and injury must be avoided to prevent an iatrogenic Horner syndrome.[29] Although the longus colli may be safely elevated to facilitate placement of ventral cervical retractor blades, awareness of vertebral artery tortuosity is necessary to avoid iatrogenic arterial injury (Fig. 31-24).

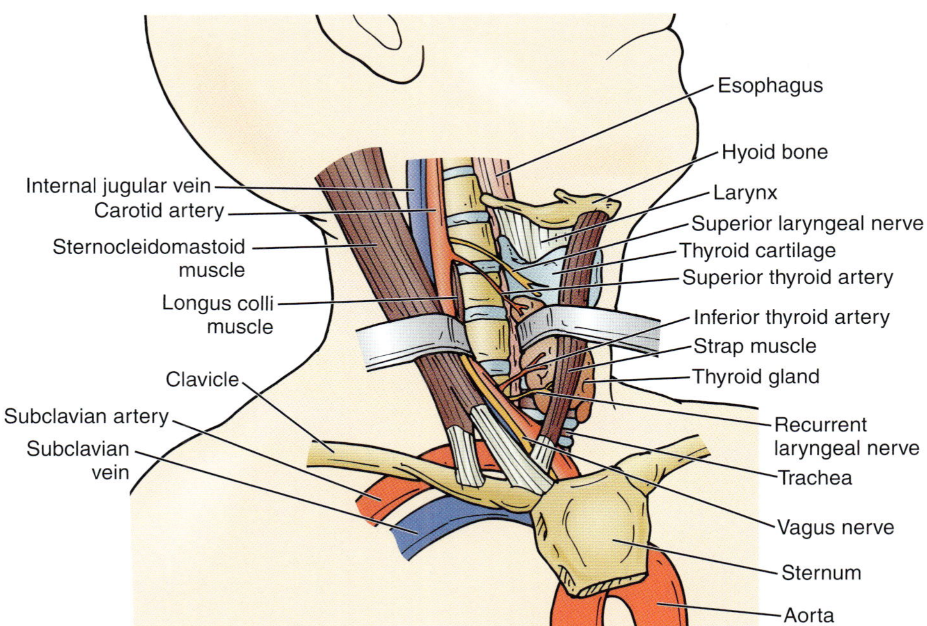

FIGURE 31-22. Anterior landmarks and their vertebral level correlates. Note important adjacent structures encountered during ventral approaches to the cervical spine.

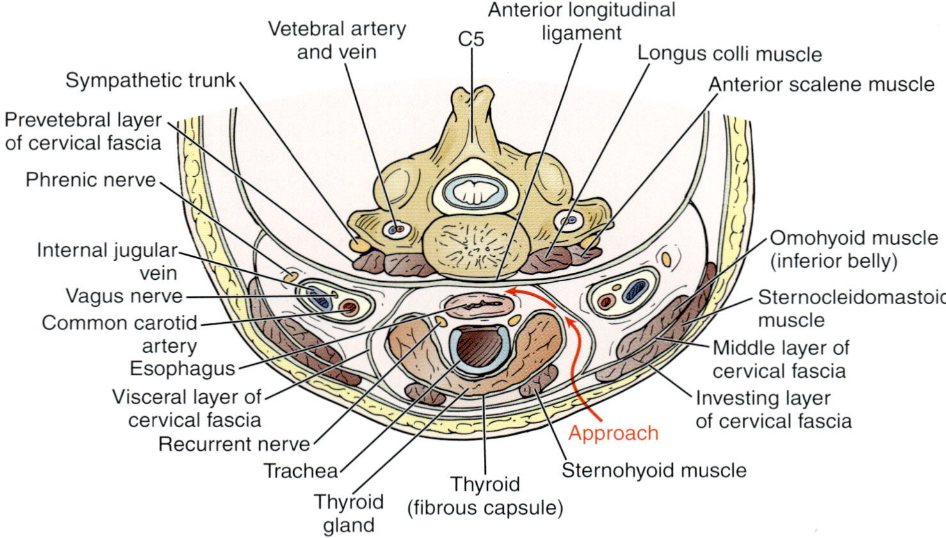

FIGURE 31-23. Ventral cervical dissection plane.

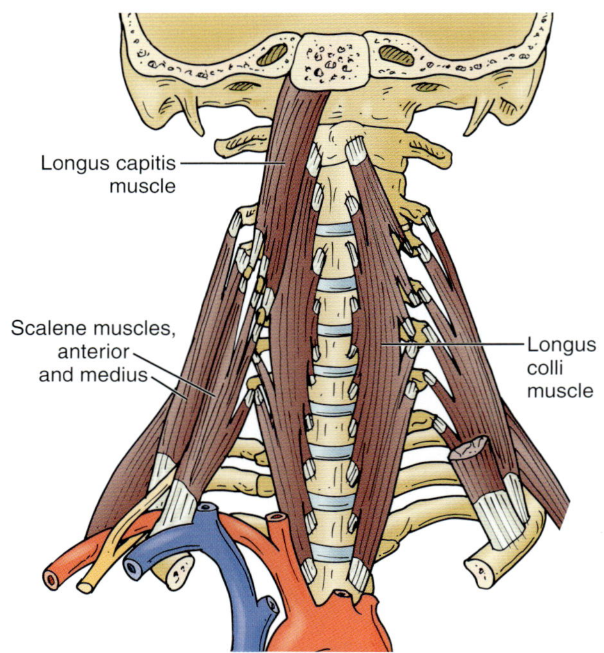

FIGURE 31-24. Longus colli muscle flanking cervical spine. The sympathetic chain overlies the longus muscles bilaterally.

KEY REFERENCES

Hassler O: Blood supply to human spinal cord: a microangiographic study. *Arch Neurol* 15:302–307, 1966.

Lu J, Ebraheim NA, Nadim Y, et al: Anterior approach to the cervical spine: surgical anatomy. *Orthopedics* 23:841–845, 2000.

Maiman DJ, Pintar FA: Anatomy and clinical biomechanics of the thoracic spine. *Clin Neurosurg* 38:296–324, 1992.

McCormick PC, Stein BM: Functional anatomy of the spinal cord and related structures. *Neurosurg Clin N Am* 1:469–489, 1990.

Pait TG, Killefer JA, Arnautovic KI: Surgical anatomy of the anterior cervical spine: the disc space, vertebral artery, and associated bony structures. *Neurosurgery* 39:769–776, 1996.

Rhoton A, de Oliveira E: Anatomical basis of surgical approaches to the region of the foramen magnum. In Dickman CA, Spetzler RE, Sonntag VKH, editors: *Surgery of the craniovertebral junction*, New York, 1998, Thieme, pp 13–57.

REFERENCES

The complete reference list is available online at expertconsult.com.

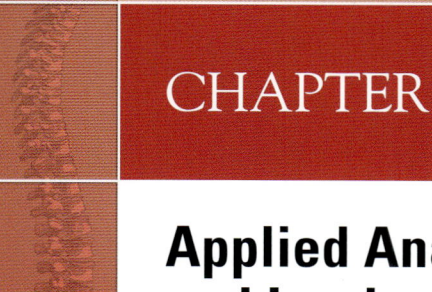

CHAPTER 32

Applied Anatomy of the Thoracic and Lumbar Spine

S. Scott Lollis

The normal human spine consists of 33 vertebrae: 7 cervical, 12 thoracic, 5 lumbar, and 5 fused sacral vertebrae. At the caudal portion of the sacrum, four or five ossicles comprise the coccyx. Thoracic vertebrae are defined by their articulations with ribs, though variation in rib number is commonplace.

The complexity of the thoracic and lumbar spine is rooted in the gradual transformation of anatomic structures as one descends along the rostral-caudal axis. The safe application of anatomic knowledge to surgical procedures requires that the surgeon be at least as familiar with the differences within regional groupings as with the commonalities that typically characterize those groupings.

Spine Alignment

The acquisition of upright posture and bipedal locomotion during human evolution imposed specific demands on the thoracic and lumbar spine. These demands are reflected in its overall structure (Fig. 32-1). Upright posture requires added load-bearing capacity; along the rostral-caudal axis, there is a substantial increase in the robustness not only of the vertebral bodies, but also of other stabilizing structures, such as the articular processes and spinous processes. Bipedalism requires spinal balance; this is reflected in normal spinal curvature. Unlike our quadruped ancestors, who possessed a single, broad spinal curvature, humans exhibit a combination of thoracic kyphosis and lumbar lordosis. These curves are formed by relatively small variations in intervertebral disc and vertebral body morphology. In the absence of spine deformity, the thoracic and lumbar curvatures are balanced, and the midportion of the C7 vertebral body sits atop the L5-S1 pivot point, located at the dorsal aspect of the L5-S1 intervertebral disc. With normal spinal balance, the degree of thoracic and lumbar curvature may vary considerably without adverse effect. However, deviations from normal sagittal alignment are mechanically unfavorable, imposing stress on axial musculature and resulting in pain and acceleration of the degenerative process.

Vertebrae and Ligaments

Vertebral Body

Because of graded variation in morphology between the upper thoracic spine and the lumbar spine, it is difficult to make accurate, dichotomous generalizations about the structure of thoracic and lumbar vertebrae. The 11th and 12th vertebral bodies, in particular, possess a mixture of thoracic and lumbar morphology. Generally, when viewed in cross section, thoracic vertebrae possess a heart shape, while lumbar vertebrae are more kidney shaped; a concavity along the dorsal aspect of each marks the ventral portion of the spinal canal. On the left side of thoracic vertebrae, a shallow depression marking the course of the aorta may be visible.

Sagittal vertebral morphology also changes along the rostral-caudal axis (Fig. 32-2). Thoracic vertebral bodies are wedge shaped, ventral height being shorter than dorsal height. This results in the normal thoracic kyphosis. In the lumbar spine, ventral and dorsal heights are generally comparable, and it is the disc shape, rather than vertebral body shape, that is the principal contributor to lumbar lordosis. At L4 and L5, some reverse wedging of the vertebral body may occur, with increased ventral height further contributing to the lower lumbar lordosis. The vertebral body gradually increases in cross-sectional area and height from the thoracic spine to the midlumbar spine (Figs. 32-3 and 32-4). From L2 to L5, vertebral height is usually stable and may decrease slightly. Changes in cross-sectional area are reflected in compression strength (Fig. 32-5).

Intervertebral Disc and Vertebral End Plate

The general function of the intervertebral disc is twofold: (1) It deforms to accommodate compressive loads, a role assumed by the nucleus pulposus, and (2) it resists tensile and torsional stresses, a role assumed by the anulus fibrosus (Fig. 32-6). At a microscopic level, the nucleus pulposus consists of a semifluid, gel-like substance embedded in a fine meshwork of fibrous strands. This structure results in a viscoelastic property that allows the disc to withstand and absorb axial stress. The anulus fibrosus has a lamellated boundary of intersecting fibrous strands. Anular fibers known as Sharpey fibers penetrate the dense cortical bone that makes up the outer ring of the vertebral end plate. The outermost fibers blend with overlying periosteum and longitudinal ligaments. Viewed in histologic cross section, the transition from nucleus pulposus to anulus fibrosus is a gradual one.

The bony vertebral end plate is a concave depression. At its central portion, the cancellous bone of the vertebral body is directly apposed to a cartilaginous plate, which fills the depression up to the level of the apophyseal ring, or marginal ring. The apophyseal ring is composed of cortical bone and is

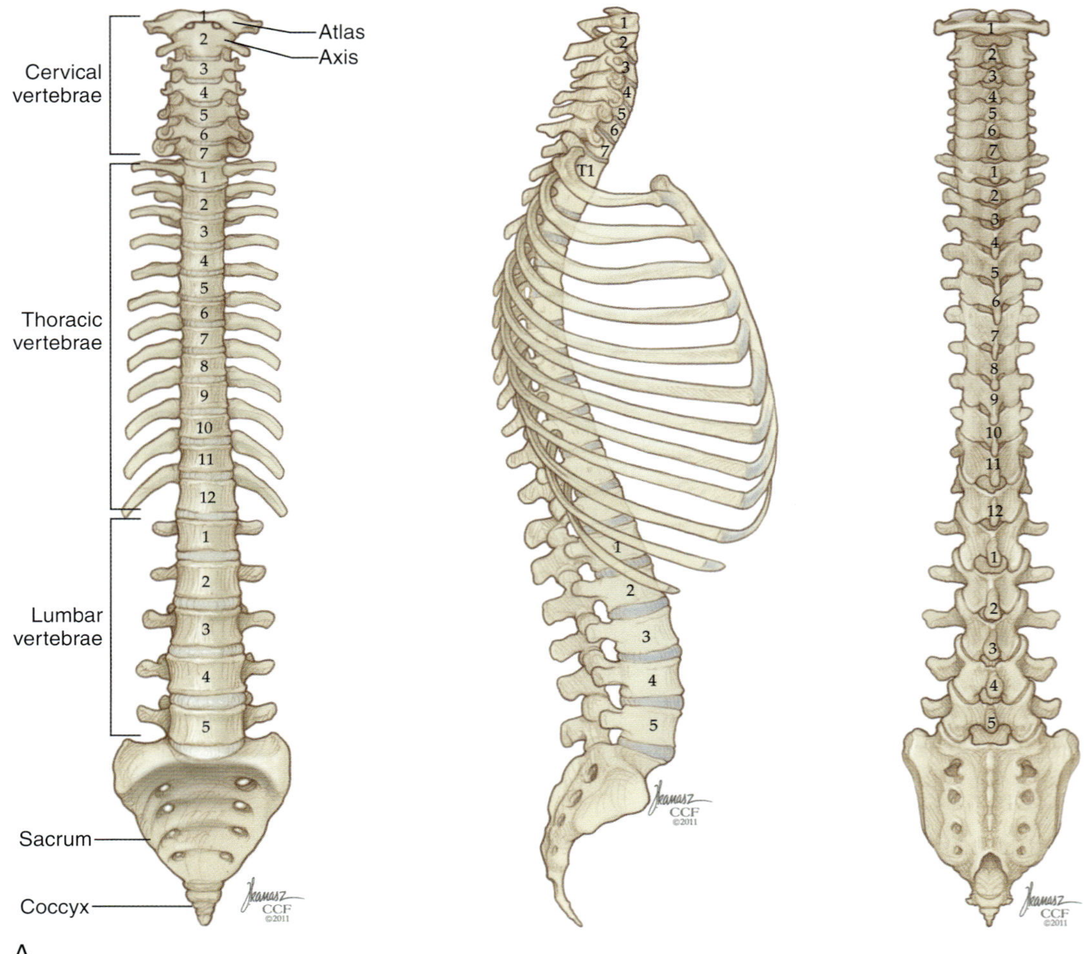

FIGURE 32-1. Ventral (**A**), lateral (**B**), and dorsal (**C**) views of the thoracic, lumbar, and sacral spinal column. (Copyright Cleveland Clinic Foundation.)

more resistant to compression failure than is the central end plate. Biomechanical studies have shown the strongest region of the lumbar end plate to be the dorsal, lateral aspect of the marginal ring, adjacent to the pedicle.[1]

As part of the normal degenerative process, disc bulging and the resultant traction on Sharpey fibers result in bony osteophyte growth along this outer ring. Thus, the degree of concavity of the vertebral body, when viewed in profile, increases with age. Because the stress on Sharpey fibers is greatest along the concavity of a curve, these changes will be most evident along the ventral surface of the thoracic vertebral bodies and the dorsal surface of the lumbar vertebral bodies.

The cross-sectional profile of the intervertebral disc changes along the rostral-caudal axis in accordance with the changing profile of the end plate. In the thoracic spine, the nucleus pulposus is centrally located. In the lumbar spine, it is closer to the dorsal aspect of the disc.

Anterior Longitudinal Ligament

The anterior longitudinal ligament (ALL) is a strong, broad ligament that spans the ventral surface of all the vertebral bodies. Its width increases along the rostral-caudal axis; at the lower lumbar levels, it encompasses almost half of the total circumference of the vertebral body. The ALL has multiple layers. The innermost layer inserts on each vertebral body and is only loosely adherent to the anulus fibrosus of the intervertebral disc. The middle layer bridges two or three vertebral bodies. The outer layer bridges up to five levels at a time.

Because of relative strength, the ALL is an important contributor to spine stability, particularly in the lumbar spine. It resists hyperextension and, to a lesser degree, translational motion.

Posterior Longitudinal Ligament

The posterior longitudinal ligament (PLL) also spans the full rostral-caudal axis of the spine but is less substantial than the ALL. It is located along the dorsal surface of the vertebral bodies, within the spinal canal (Fig. 32-7). At the midbody level, it is relatively narrow, but it widens considerably at the level of the disc before narrowing again as it transitions to the level below. It is adherent at the level of the end plate and anulus but elevated from the concave dorsal surface of the midvertebral body. Along the lateral margins of the PLL, there are often areas of adhesion with the underlying dura. Although the PLL's contribution to spine stability is modest, it serves to direct disc herniations dorsolaterally, away from the central portion of the spinal canal.

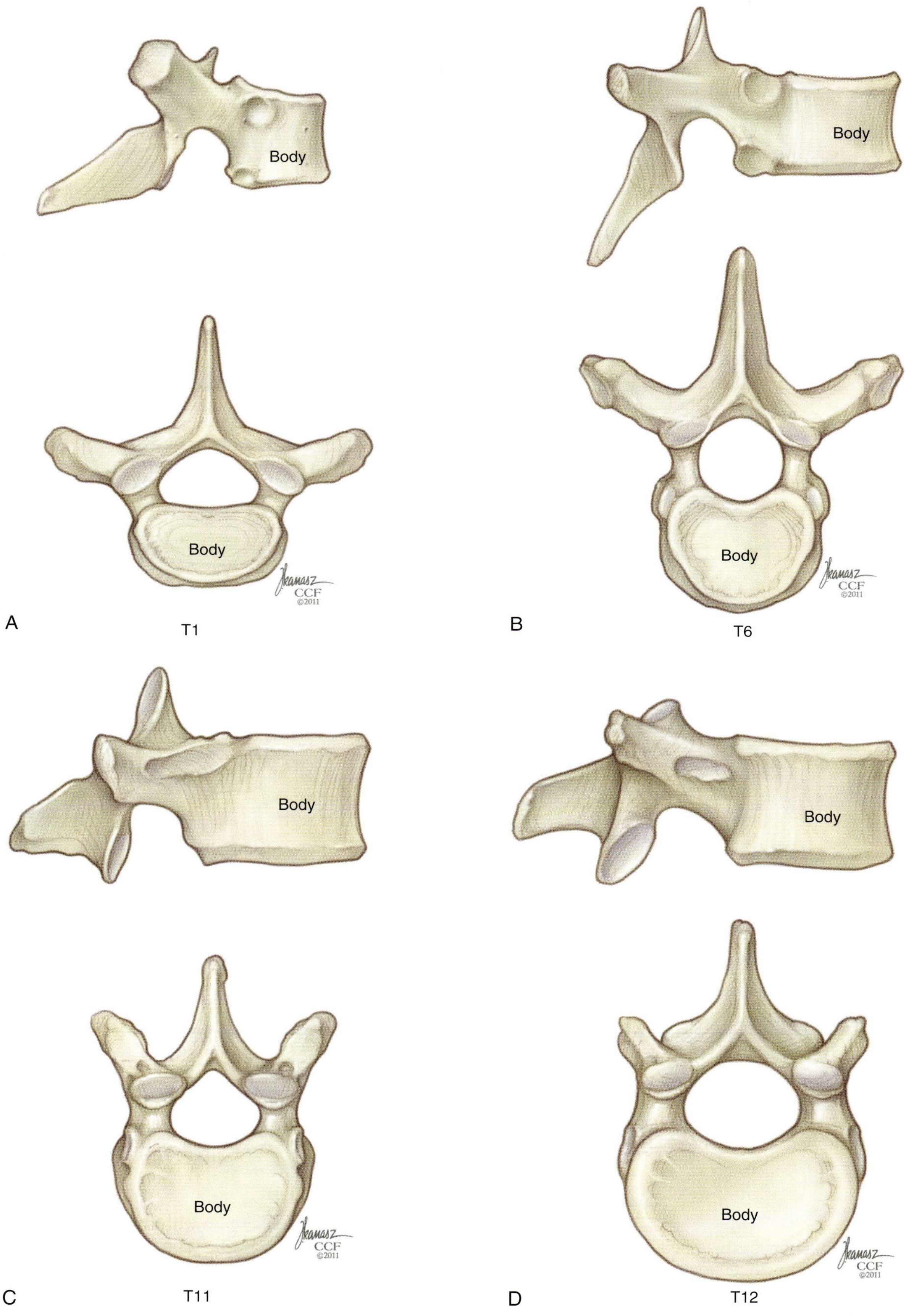

FIGURE 32-2. Lateral and superior views of T1 (**A**), T6 (**B**), T11 (**C**), T12 (**D**).

Figure continues on following page.

the vertebral body. The intervertebral foramen at these levels is formed almost exclusively by the inferior vertebral notch; the superior vertebral notch is small or nonexistent. By the lower thoracic spine, a relative increase in pedicle height has resulted in the caudal pedicle surface inserting somewhat lower, in plane with the lower one third of the vertebral body. In the lumbar spine, the pedicle is positioned progressively lower on the vertebral body and the superior vertebral notch is more pronounced.

Sagittal angulation of the pedicle with respect to the vertebral body also differs between the thoracic and lumbar spine. In the thoracic spine, the pedicle angles downward to meet the vertebral body, while in the lumbar spine, the pedicle is approximately coplanar with the vertebral body in a sagittal view. In thoracic pedicle screw placement, the so-called anatomic trajectory follows this pedicular axis; however, many surgeons employ a "straight-on trajectory," in which the sagittal angulation of the screw is coplanar with the vertebral end plate rather than the pedicle itself. This oblique passage is possible because of the excess of pedicle height relative to pedicle width.

Transverse pedicle width, rather than pedicle height, is the dimension that limits the size of a pedicle screw that can be placed at a given level. In the thoracic spine, pedicle height is commonly double that of pedicle width. Pedicle width is smallest in the region of T4-6, but increases only minimally until one arrives at the thoracolumbar junction. A graphical depiction of changes in these two dimensions across the neuraxis is shown in Figures 32-8 and 32-9.

For the same reason that pedicle width constrains screw placement more than pedicle height does, transverse pedicle angle is a more relevant anatomic variable than is sagittal angle in the placement of thoracic pedicle screws. If a screw's medial-lateral trajectory differs from that of the pedicle by even a relatively small amount, medial or lateral breach may result. Transverse pedicle angle declines fairly steadily as one proceeds down the thoracic spine until a nearly "straight-ahead" trajectory is encountered in the lower thoracic vertebrae; it then increases steeply across the lumbar levels, such that the L5 pedicle has a transverse angle of 25 to 30 degrees (Fig. 32-10).

Transpedicular instrumentation in the thoracic spine is more challenging than that in the lumbar spine because of the presence of the adjacent spinal cord, the smaller pedicle diameter, and the relative proximity to neural structures (see Figs. 32-8, 32-9, and 32-14). In the lumbar spine, there is approximately 1.5 mm of epidural space between the medial pedicle wall and the thecal sac.[2] In the thoracic spine, the medial pedicle border is contiguous with the edge of the thecal sac.[3] In the lumbar spine, the distance from the upper edge of the pedicle to the nerve root above is approximately

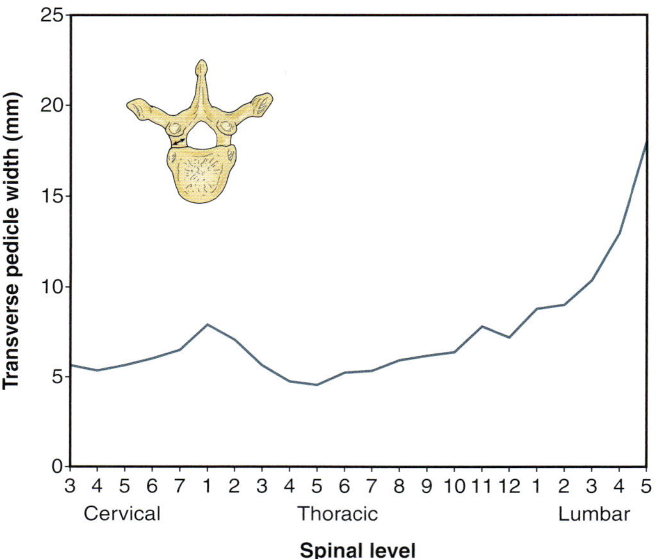

FIGURE 32-8. Transverse pedicle width by level. (Benzel EC: *Biomechanics of spine stabilization*, New York, 2001, Thieme, p 6, reprinted with permission.)

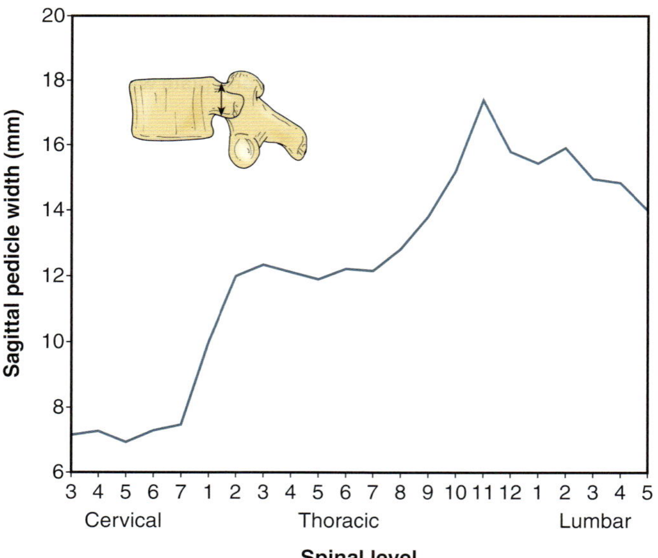

FIGURE 32-9. Sagittal pedicle width by level. (Benzel EC: *Biomechanics of spine stabilization*, New York, 2001, Thieme, p 6, reprinted with permission.)

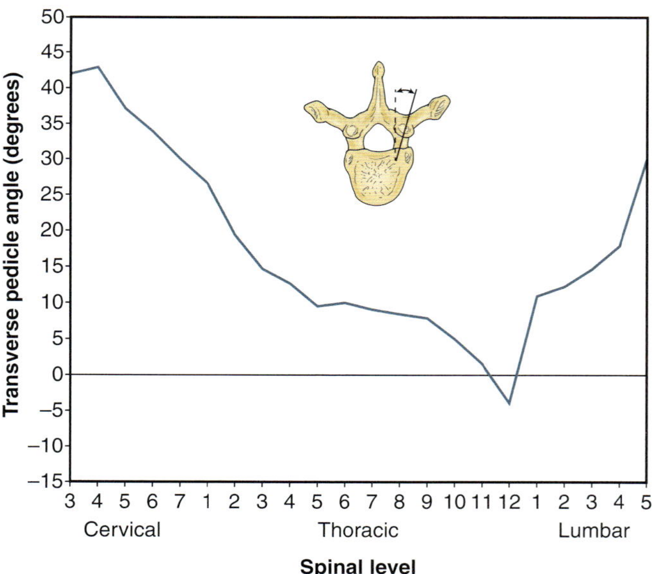

FIGURE 32-10. Transverse pedicle angle by level. (Benzel EC: *Biomechanics of spine stabilization*, New York, 2001, Thieme, p 6, reprinted with permission.)

5 mm, and the distance from the lower edge of the pedicle to the nerve root below, approximately 1.5 mm.[2] In the thoracic spine, the distance from the upper edge of the pedicle to the nerve root above is approximately 2 to 4 mm and the distance from the lower edge of the thoracic pedicle to the nerve root below is approximately 2 to 3 mm.[3]

Facet and Pars Interarticularis

The facet joint, or zygapophyseal joint, is formed by an inferior articulating process emanating from the level above and a superior articulating process emanating from the level below. The facet joint is a synovial joint, possessing a true joint capsule. This capsule has two layers: an outer layer, composed of parallel bundles of collagenous fibers, and an inner elastic layer, similar in composition to the ligamentum flavum.[4] Gliding articulation at the facet joint is limited by the capsular fibers, which are relatively lax in the cervical region but increase in tautness along the rostral caudal axis.

The facet joint functions primarily as a motion-limiting structure; only in extension does it function in an axial load-bearing capacity. The way in which a facet joint constrains motion depends on the alignment of its articulating surfaces (see Fig. 32-2). Lumbar facets occupy a plane that is intermediate between the sagittal and coronal planes. In the lumbar spine, there is a progression from relatively sagittal (25 degrees from sagittal) at L1-2 to relatively coronal (50 degrees from sagittal) at L5-S1. To the surgeon approaching the dorsal lumbar spine, the entry into the facet joint will be found progressively more laterally as one descends toward the lumbosacral junction. This more coronal orientation at the lumbosacral junction is an important element in preventing spondylolisthesis. Thoracic facets have an alignment that is oblique to all three cardinal planes; the articulating surface faces dorsally and slightly superolaterally. Thus, the superior articulating process is positioned relatively medial to the inferior articulating process; this is in contrast to the lumbar spine, where the superior articulating process occupies a lateral position. The transition from thoracic facet orientation to upper lumbar orientation occurs abruptly at the thoracolumbar junction.

Coincident with this transition in facet angulation in the lower thoracic spine is a change in overall facet morphology. Viewed from the back, thoracic facets have a flat, monotonous, shingle-style arrangement; the facet complex resides in a trough between the dorsally directed lamina and the dorsally directed transverse process. Lumbar facets are more protuberant, pedunculated structures that occupy an elevated position relative to the lamina and transverse processes. The transition between the two occurs in the lower thoracic spine. In the lumbar spine, the mammillary process is visible as a slight bony prominence at the junction of the superior articulating process and transverse process; it serves as a site of attachment for deep paraspinous musculature and is an important landmark for pedicle screw insertion.

Transverse Process

The transverse processes of the thoracic spine and the lumbar spine are relatively thin, consisting of both cortical and cancellous bone. In the thoracic spine, the transverse process projects dorsolaterally and articulates at its tip with the like-numbered rib. In the lumbar spine, the transverse processes project straight laterally and are easily fractured during wide dorsal exposure for dorsolateral fusion. The transverse processes of T11 and T12 are hypoplastic relative to their neighbors and do not articulate with their corresponding ribs. Commonly, the T11 transverse process is a dorsolaterally directed bony stump. In lieu of a T12 transverse process, there are only three small tubercles: a superior tubercle, which is equivalent to the lumbar mammillary process; an inferior tubercle, which is equivalent to the lumbar accessory process; and a lateral tubercle, which represents a very small equivalent of a transverse process. Variation in transverse process morphology can be seen in Figure 32-2.

Rib Articulations of the Thoracic Spine

The relationship of each rib to its corresponding vertebral body changes along the rostral-caudal axis of the thoracic spine (see Fig. 32-1). The 1st rib articulates exclusively with T1 via a single, complete facet located at the lateral aspect of the vertebral body. The 2nd through 9th ribs articulate with their like-numbered vertebrae, as well as the vertebra below, via paired demifacets. These demifacets are also located on the lateral aspect of the vertebral body but in a progressively dorsal position. By the lower thoracic spine (T10-12), two important changes have occurred, First, the pattern of articulation has returned to that of a single, complete, unpaired facet; second, the gradual dorsal movement of the articulation has resulted in the joint being located on the lateral surface of the pedicle, not the vertebral body. However, the size of the rib head and its joint capsule are such that ventrolateral access to the disc space or neural foramen inevitably requires removal of some or all of the adjacent rib head, regardless of level (Fig. 32-11). Because the parietal pleura obscures much of the relevant anatomy, palpation of the rib head is an important orienting maneuver during transthoracic approaches to the spine; often the only recognizable structure that is visible through the pleura is the sympathetic chain, coursing over the rib heads (Fig. 32-12).

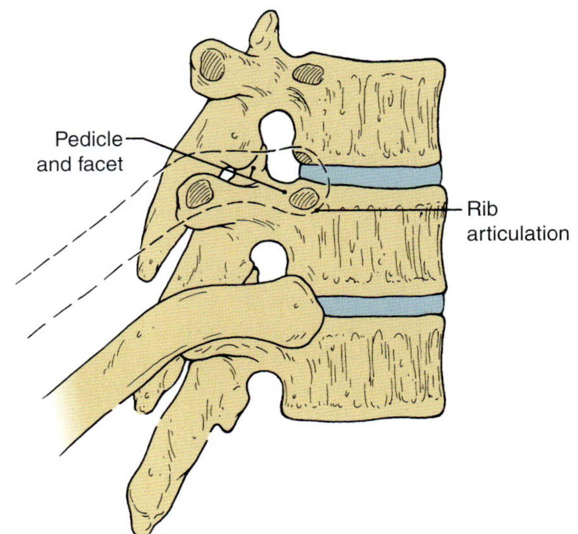

FIGURE 32-11. Rib removal is required for access to the thoracic neural foramen and intervertebral disc.

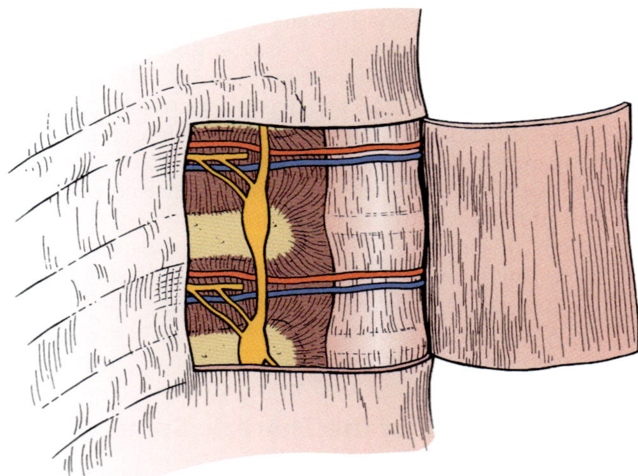

FIGURE 32-12. Lateral view of thoracic spine with segmental vessels and sympathetic chain located deep to the parietal pleura.

A second site of rib articulation, the costotransverse joint, is located at the ventral aspect of the tip of the transverse processes of T1-10. Ribs 11 and 12 fail to make contact with their respective transverse processes, a fact that can be appreciated during dorsolateral approaches at the thoracolumbar junction.

Lamina and Spinous Process

In general, the laminae are arranged in a shingle-like array, in which the lamina above overlaps the one below (see Fig. 32-1). During laminectomy, the deeper position of the more rostral portion of the lamina is readily appreciated. In the thoracic spine and the lumbar spine, the pars interarticularis consists of the lateralmost portion of the lamina. This is the portion of lamina that resides between, and functionally connects, the superior articulating process and the inferior articulating process. The pars interarticularis is important for spine stability; without it, the stabilizing effect of the facet joint below is lost.

When viewed from a dorsal approach, laminae of the upper thoracic region are horizontally oriented and relatively narrow in the rostral-caudal axis. Though the spinous process has a caudal angulation, this angulation is relatively minor (approximately 40 degrees from horizontal); hence, the relative prominence of the upper thoracic spine to dorsal palpation. As one moves into the middle thoracic region, the laminae become more V-shaped, giving rise to a more caudally directed spinous process. The laminae also become broader along their rostral-caudal axis. In both the upper and middle thoracic spine, the interlaminar space is small, if not nonexistent, when the patient is in a nonflexed, prone position. In the lowest two thoracic vertebrae, this V-shaped configuration is diminished; the laminae again become relatively horizontal, and the caudally directed angulation of the spinous process is less. Concomitant with this is an elongation of the superior and inferior articulating processes in the rostral-caudal axis. The result of these changes is the development of an interlaminar space between the paired facet complexes.

In the lumbar spine, the elongation of the articulating processes, combined with the nature of their confluence with the laminae, gives the dorsal elements the appearance of an H. The interlaminar space becomes more prominent with further caudal descent. At the same time, the spinous processes transition from a slight caudal angulation to completely horizontal at L5. As a result of these changes, the interlaminar space at L5-S1 is sufficiently large to permit inadvertent passage of tissue dilator during minimally invasive procedures.

Laminar anatomy is commonly appreciated during dorsal exposure for decompression or fusion procedures. Particularly for dorsal fusion procedures, understanding the relationships between the lamina, the pars interarticularis, the facet joints, and the transverse process is essential to obtaining good exposure without unnecessary destabilization of the facet complexes. The surgeon dissecting the paraspinous muscles off the spinous process arrives at the midportion of the lamina, the cross-bar of the H. As the surgeon proceeds laterally, the lateral edge of the lamina is encountered; this is the lateral boundary of the pars interarticularis. Just above and below this bony edge, the humps of the facet articulations with the levels above and below can be palpated. By following this edge of the pars interarticularis rostrally and slightly laterally, taking care to remain lateral to the facet joint capsule, the surgeon can expose the outer edge of the superior articulating process and the transverse process, without destabilizing the supra-adjacent facet articulation. The pars interarticularis tends to be thinner at its rostral-medial portion and thicker in its caudal-lateral portion.

Ligamentum Flavum

The ligamentum flavum is a thick, yellow ligament that goes from the sacrum to C2. Its characteristic appearance and consistency result from a relatively increased ratio of elastic to collagen fibers. The ligamentum flavum is discontinuous, emanating from the rostral surface of the lamina below, spanning the interlaminar space, and inserting on the ventral surface of the lamina above (Fig. 32-13). It is absent along the rostral half of the ventral laminar surface. This has practical significance for the surgeon who is relying on the ligamentum flavum to help prevent incidental durotomy during laminectomy for lumbar stenosis. The ligamentum flavum has two layers, between which exists a virtual, "gliding" space; the outer layer is discontinuous in the midline.[5] Even in cases of spondylosis, in which the ligamentum flavum has assumed an exuberant or redundant posture, careful inspection will reveal a midline cleavage plane. This can be a useful point of entry in attempting the safe division of this structure without violation of the dura below.

Interspinous and Supraspinous Ligaments

The interspinous and supraspinous ligaments form a single sheet of soft tissue support in the midline (see Fig. 32-13). The interspinous ligaments span one motion segment; they originate along the superior ridge of the spinous process below and insert at the base of the spinous process above. The supraspinous ligament occupies a position superficial to the tips of the spinous processes. It has two fiber layers: a deep layer that spans one or two motion segments and a superficial layer that may span several segments. Because of their distance from the instantaneous axis of rotation, the interspinous and supraspinous ligaments serve a valuable role as a tension band. In

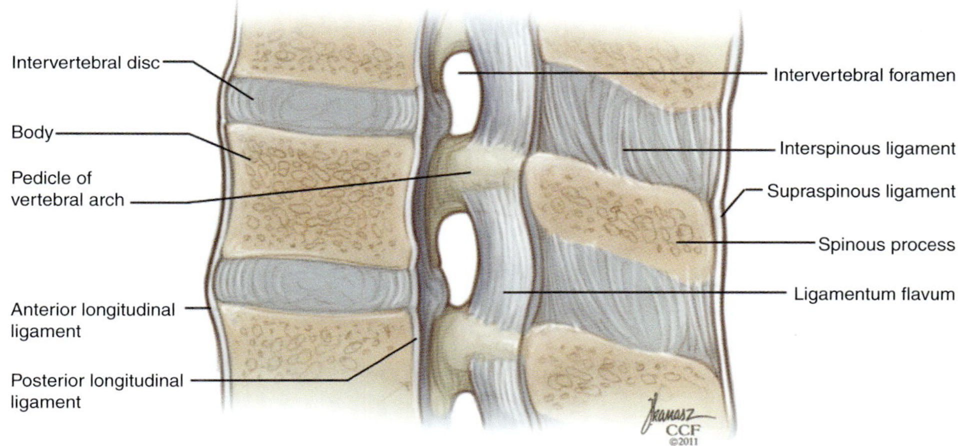

FIGURE 32-13. Lateral view of lumbar spine with associated ligaments. (Copyright Cleveland Clinic Foundation.)

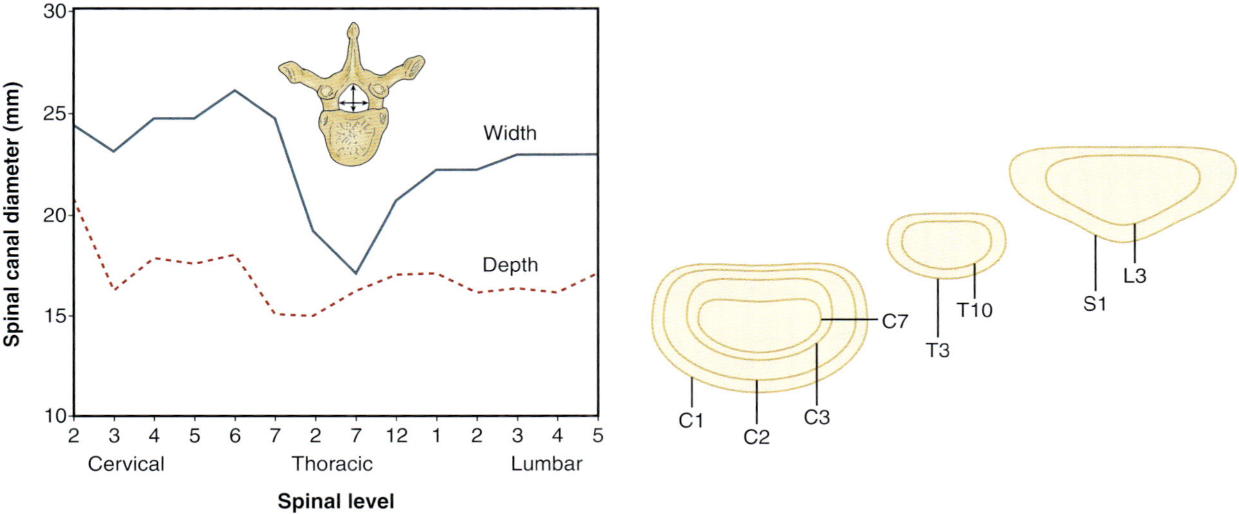

FIGURE 32-14. Spinal canal diameter by level.

surgeries in which complete laminectomy is not performed, preservation of these ligaments can reduce the likelihood of iatrogenic postoperative kyphotic deformity.

Spinal Canal

Spinal canal dimensions vary along the rostral-caudal axis, being greatest in the cervical region and smallest in the midthoracic region. This variation is principally due to changes in the ventral-dorsal diameter (Fig. 32-14).

Neural Anatomy

Spinal Segmentation

During fetal development and childhood, the vertebral column grows faster than the spinal cord, resulting in ascension of the conus medullaris within the spinal canal. In the normal adult, the conus typically terminates at L1, though it may occupy positions ranging from T11-12 to the upper vertebral body of L3.[6] Fig. 32-15 depicts the normal discordance between spinal level (the level defined by spinal rootlets' origin) and vertebral level (the level of the neural foramen). A fracture-dislocation in the upper and midthoracic spine will typically cause cord injury at the level of injury or one level below. A fracture-dislocation in the lower thoracic spine would be expected to cause cord injury two or more levels caudal to the bony injury. In both cases, concomitant injury to descending nerve roots may result in a relative concordance between bony injury and its associated neurologic syndrome.

Spinal Cord

The gray matter of the spinal cord is divided into a ventral motor portion and a dorsal sensory portion. The ventral horns contain the cell bodies of lower motor neurons, while the dorsal horns contain the cell bodies of second-order sensory neurons; interneurons can be found in both. Major white matter tracts are depicted in Figure 32-16. Somatotopy of white matter tracts is usually such that fibers to rostral segments are positioned medial to fibers to more caudal segments; an

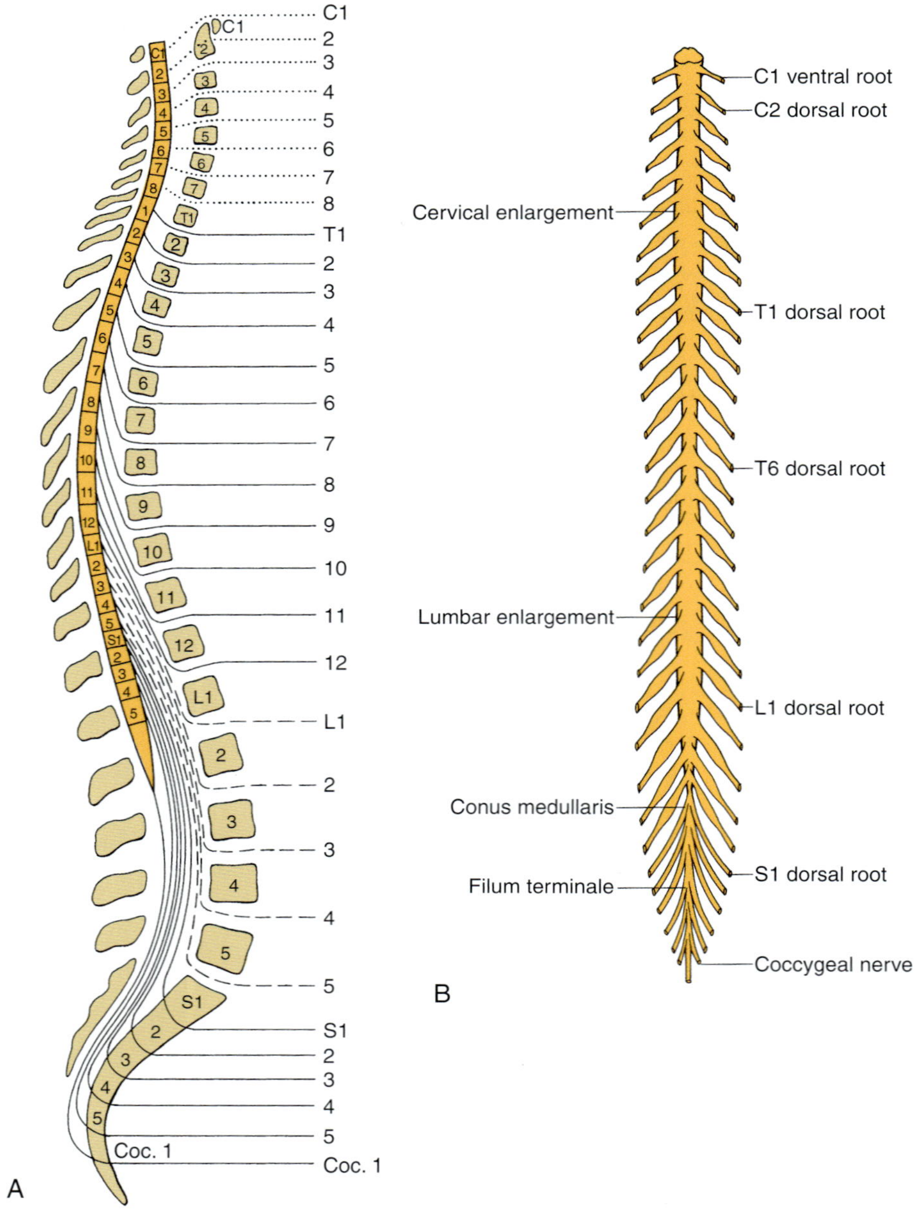

FIGURE 32-15. **A,** Relationship of spinal cord segmentation and vertebral segmentation. **B,** Anatomy of the cervical and lumbar enlargements.

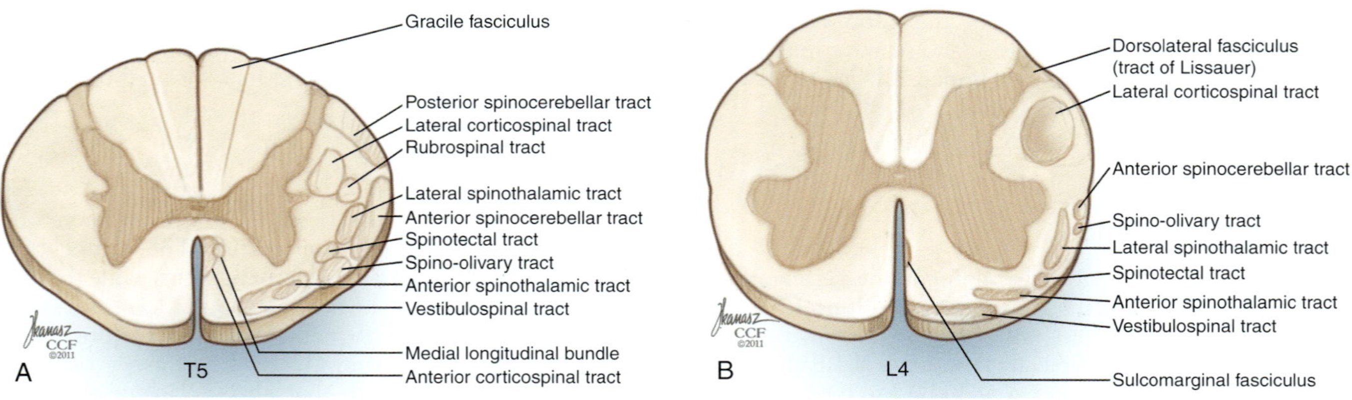

FIGURE 32-16. Spinal cord tracts. **A,** Thoracic cross section; **B,** lumbar cross section. (Copyright Cleveland Clinic Foundation.)

important exception is the dorsal columns, in which fibers to more caudal segments are positioned medially.

The diameter of the spinal cord increases in two regions, known as the cervical enlargement and the lumbosacral enlargement (see Fig. 32-15). The cervical enlargement results from the increased number of cell bodies present in gray matter innervating the upper extremities; it is found at vertebral levels C4-T1. The lumbosacral enlargement results from the expansion of gray matter at levels innervating the lower extremities and is found at vertebral levels T9-12.

Intradural Roots and the Cauda Equina

The descending intradural roots of the cauda equina possess a rough somatotopy that may be of practical use during intradural procedures. Sacral roots tend to occupy a more central position within the canal (having emanated from the tip of the conus), while lower lumbar roots are located in a paramedian position and upper lumbar roots are located most laterally.

Lateral Recess, Neural Foramen, and Intraforaminal Root

At the lateral border of the thecal sac, each root becomes ensheathed in dura. In the lumbar spine, this shoulder angles obliquely downward to pass below the like-numbered pedicle; in so doing, it crosses the plane of the intervertebral disc. In the cervical spine, by contrast, the nerve takes a relatively horizontal course to its corresponding foramen (above the like-numbered pedicle). This has significance during dorsal operations for dorsolateral disc herniation. During cervical foraminotomy/discectomy, the disc fragment is typically located within the root axilla and can be found with gentle elevation of the nerve root, while during lumbar laminotomy/discectomy, the disc fragment is usually located at the shoulder and is uncovered with medially directed traction on the shoulder. In the upper and midthoracic spine, the course of the ensheathed nerve root is more complicated; anatomic studies have shown downward angulation of the intradural root, followed by upward angulation after the root enters the dural sleeve, followed again by downward angulation once the root has left the neural foramen.[7]

Before entering the neural foramen, a nerve root traverses the lateral recess. Though it is been variously defined by different authors,[8-10] the most intuitive explanation of the lateral recess is a space defined medially by the edge of the thecal sac and laterally by the medial pedicular plane at the level of the midvertebral and lower vertebral body (Fig. 32-17). In the lumbar spine, it is located ventral to the ligamentum flavum and facet complex, dorsal to the vertebral body, and just rostral and medial to the neural foramen. Lateral recess stenosis results from spondylotic redundancy of the ligamentum flavum and facet hypertrophy.

The neural foramen is a space defined rostrally by the pedicle, caudally by the pedicle, ventrally by the inferior portion of the vertebral body and the intervertebral disc, and dorsally by the superior articular process of the level below, with its capsular covering (Fig. 32-18; see also Fig. 32-17). The dimensions of the neural foramen are greater on the rostral-caudal axis than on the ventral-dorsal axis. In the lumbar spine, the neural foramen is approximately 12 to 19 mm high but only 6 to 8 mm wide in the sagittal plane. Thus, the nerve is particularly susceptible to compression from in front (the intervertebral disc) and behind (the superior articular process of the level below). Symptomatic foraminal stenosis commonly results from loss of disc height with secondary impaction of the superior articular process into the neural foramen. Since the height of the neural foramen is commonly two or three times its width, neural compression is usually the result of narrowing in the dorsal-ventral axis rather than the rostral-caudal axis. Restoration of disc height may alleviate symptoms, but this is

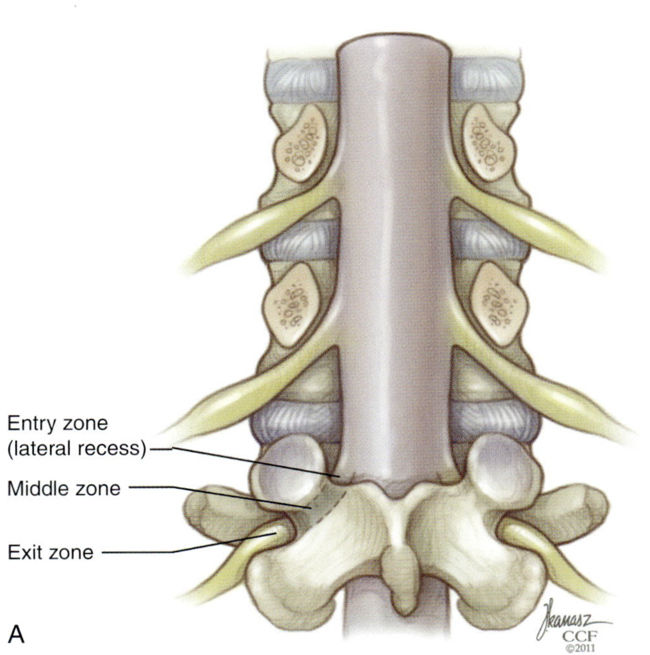

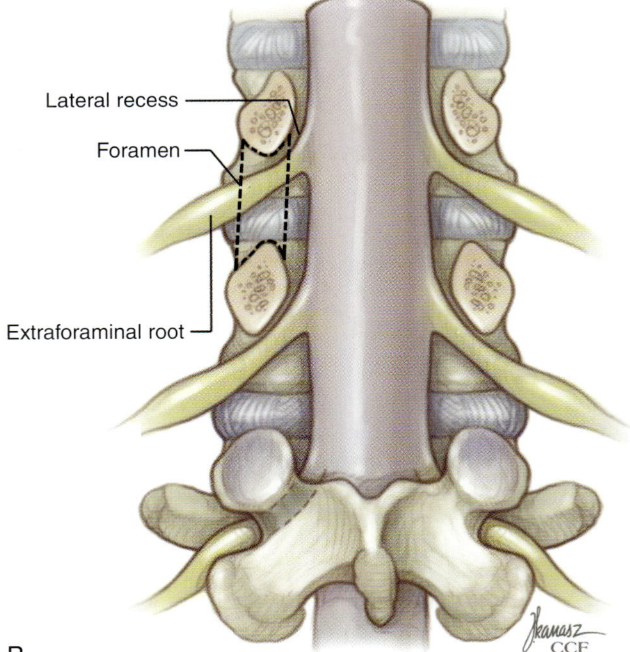

FIGURE 32-17. Dorsal view of the lumbar neural foramen demonstrating the boundaries of the lateral recess and neural foramen, as well as two common nomenclatures for nerve root anatomy (**A** and **B**). (Copyright Cleveland Clinic Foundation.)

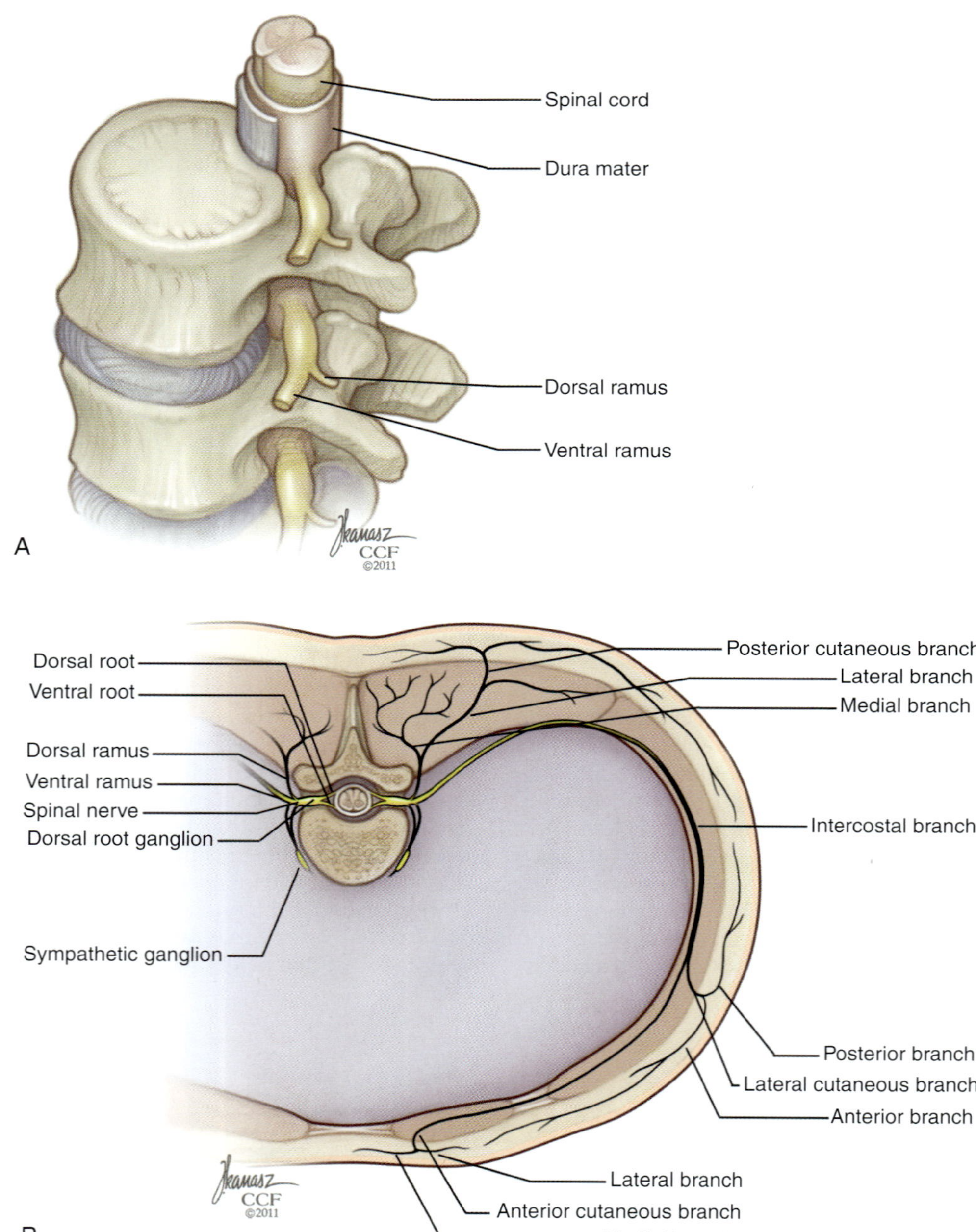

FIGURE 32-18. A, Lateral view of lumbar neural foramen. **B,** Thoracic cross section showing distal nerve branches. (Copyright Cleveland Clinic Foundation.)

more commonly the result of an associated increase in foraminal sagittal width than foraminal height per se.

The relationship between exiting nerve roots and associated bony structures is a common source of confusion. In the thoracic spine and the lumbar spine, unlike the cervical spine, nerve roots exit *below* their like-named pedicle. Because the dura of the exiting root is closely apposed to the medial and inferior aspects of the pedicle, the exiting root leaves the spinal canal at some distance above the intervertebral disc. Indeed, it is only when the root has exited the bony foramen that it crosses the plane of the disc. Understanding the different manifestations of a lumbar dorsolateral disc herniation and a far lateral disc herniation requires that one understand this fundamental anatomic concept. A dorsolateral L4-5 disc herniation occurs just lateral to the PLL and compresses the shoulder of the L5 root as that root begins to descend along the medial border of the L5 pedicle. A far lateral L4-5 disc herniation occurs 1 to 2 cm more laterally, beyond the neural foramen, and causes compression of the L4 root.

The origin of the spinal nerve is defined by the union of the dorsal and ventral roots. This usually occurs within the neural foramen, after the roots have entered a common dural root sleeve. The dorsal root ganglion is located distally on the dorsal root and usually occupies a foraminal position. Variation is common, however, and a significant percentage of ganglia are located proximal or distal to the neural foramen.

Extraforaminal Spinal Nerve

After leaving the neural foramen, the spinal nerve bifurcates into ventral and dorsal primary rami (Fig. 32-19). In the thoracic spine, the ventral primary ramus is called the posterior intercostal nerve. This nerve travels laterally and joins the intercostal neurovascular bundle of the like-named rib. Thus, the ninth thoracic spinal nerve exits through the T9-10 foramen and gives rise to the ninth posterior intercostal nerve, which joins the intercostal bundle beneath the 9th rib. In the lumbar spine, the spinal nerve travels obliquely caudally and laterally between the transverse processes, ventral to the intertransverse muscles and ligaments. Bifurcation into ventral and dorsal primary rami occurs at the level of the intervertebral disc. The lumbar ventral primary rami continue along the oblique course of the spinal nerve and make up the lumbar and lumbosacral plexi.

The dorsal primary ramus innervates the dorsal elements of the spinal column and the dorsal paraspinous musculature. In the lumbar spine particularly, its medial branch is often a target for injections and ablative procedures to alleviate axial back pain. At its origin, each lumbar dorsal primary ramus turns dorsally and pierces the intertransverse ligaments. At 5 mm from its origin, it bifurcates into a lateral and a medial branch. The lateral branch passes into the longissimus and iliocostalis muscles. The medial branch turns dorsally and caudally, wrapping around the junction of the superior articulating process and transverse process at the next caudal level and then passing along the surface of that lamina.

Innervation of the Spine

The innervation of the spine is complex, varied, and incompletely understood. The medial branch of the dorsal primary ramus is believed to be important because it is a major source of innervation to the facet joint. The sinuvertebral nerve is believed to be important because it contributes to the innervation of the intervertebral disc and ventral spinal dura.

As the medial branch of the dorsal primary ramus travels along the dorsal elements of the next caudal level, it gives off branches to the facet capsule, periosteum of the neural arch, and dorsal ligaments. Each medial branch gives off twigs to the adjacent and subadjacent facet joints. Thus, the medial branch of the L2 dorsal primary ramus supplies the L2-3 facet joint via proximal zygapophyseal nerves and the L3-4 facet joints via the distal proximal zygapophyseal nerves.[11]

The sinuvertebral nerve (nerve of Luschka or ramus meningeus) is a recurrent nerve that may originate from the distal margin of the dorsal root ganglion, the spinal nerve, or the rami communicantes (Fig. 32-20). It then passes, either singly or in multiple fibers, back through the rostral portion of the neural foramen to innervate the intervertebral discs above and below, as well as the ventral dura (see Fig. 32-16).[12] Encapsulated as well as nonencapsulated nerve endings have been demonstrated in these terminal branches, suggesting possibly a proprioceptive function as well as a nociceptive function.

Anomalous Root Anatomy

Anomalies of nerve roots are relatively common, occurring in over 10% of nerve roots studied.[13] Intradural connections, or conjoined roots, are more common than extradural anastomoses, which often have no demonstrable neural connection when viewed histologically. Additionally, roots may have anomalous relationships with their respective foramen, exiting low in the foramen or through a different foramen altogether. Figure 32-21 depicts a variety of anomalies demonstrated in one oft-cited cadaveric study.[13] The possibility of anomalous

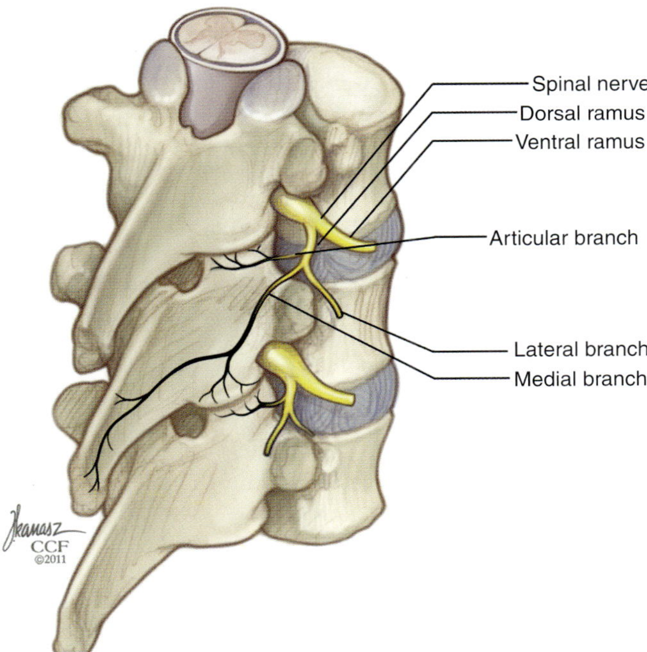

FIGURE 32-19. Extraforaminal nerve root with ventral primary ramus and dorsal primary ramus and its associated medial and lateral branches. (Copyright Cleveland Clinic Foundation.)

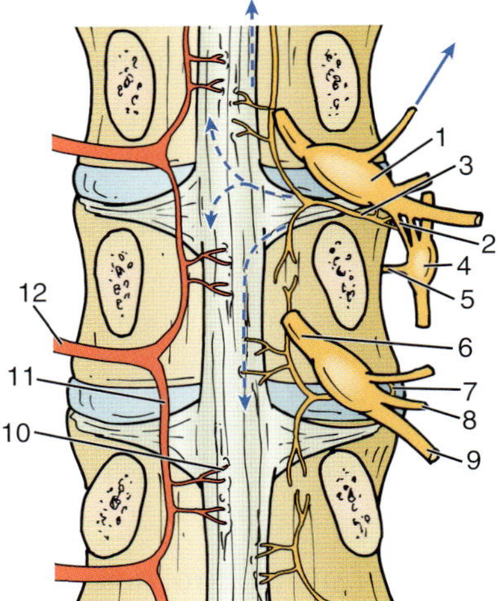

FIGURE 32-20. Sinuvertebral nerve. 1, dorsal root ganglion; 2, rami communicantes; 3, sinuvertebral nerve and its origin; 4, autonomic ganglion; 5, nerve to anterior longitudinal ligament; 6, spinal nerve roots; 7, sinuvertebral nerve arising from distal pole of ganglion; 8, dorsal primary ramus of spinal nerve; 9, ventral primary ramus of spinal nerve; 10, arteries entering basivertebral sinus to supply cancellous bone; 11, descending dorsal central branch of vertebromedullary (spinal) artery; 12, ventral branch of vertebromedullary artery. (From Herkowitz H, editor: *Rothman-Simeone the spine,* Philadelphia, 2011, Saunders, p 31.)

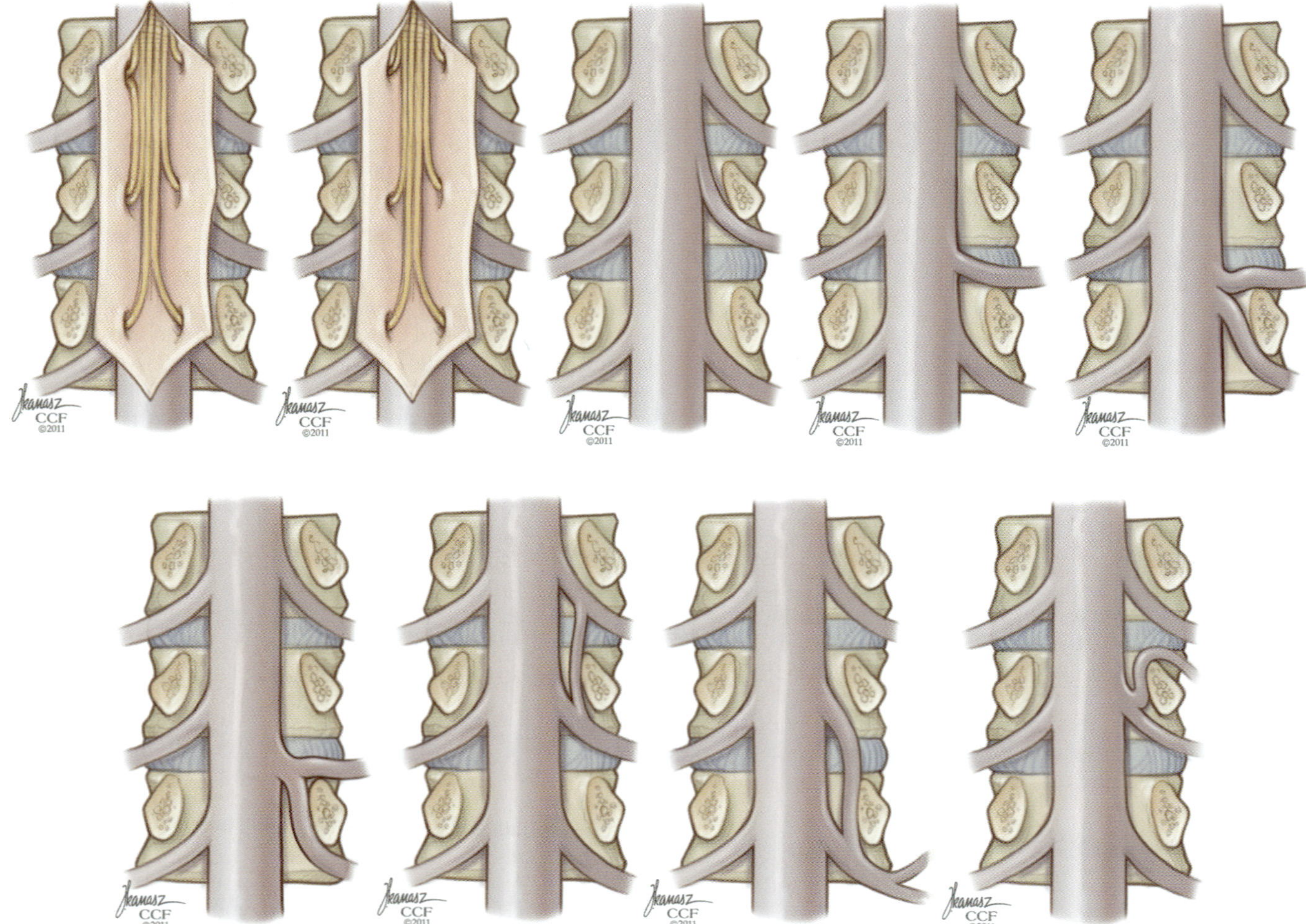

FIGURE 32-21. Common nerve root anomalies. (Copyright Cleveland Clinic Foundation.)

anatomy should be considered when there is discordance between radiographic and clinical findings.

Vascular Anatomy

Upper Thoracic Spine Arterial Supply

The lower cervical (C6, C7) and upper thoracic (T1, T2) spine receives its principal arterial supply from costocervical branches of the subclavian artery. These branches have a variable pattern between individuals. Anastomotic connections also exist with the more rostral cervical arterial supply, which consists of branches from the vertebral arteries and deep cervical arteries.

Middle Thoracic, Lower Thoracic, and Lumbar Arterial Supply: The Segmental System

The descending aorta begins on the left side of the fourth thoracic vertebra and descends ventromedially to reside on the ventral surface of the fourth lumbar vertebra. Just below the fourth lumbar vertebra, the aorta bifurcates into the common iliac arteries. The orifices of the segmental vessels are positioned on the right side of the aorta in the upper thoracic spine, but as the aorta assumes a more ventral, midline position with its caudal descent, the orifices move dorsomedially, so in the lumbar spine, they occupy a midline position on the dorsal wall (Fig. 32-22).

There is variation in the rostral-caudal course of the segmental arteries from level to level (Fig. 32-23).[14] Arteries that originate in the middle thoracic spine have a steeper upward trajectory, crossing as many as two vertebral bodies before reaching their final segmental position. This angle is reduced as the aorta descends. In the lower thoracic and upper lumbar spine, segmental arteries usually ascend one level. At the third and fourth lumbar levels, they course horizontally. Each segmental vessel ultimately courses laterally over the midportion of the destined vertebral body.

Segmental vessels are named differently depending on their location and destination. In the thoracic spine, segmental arteries destined for the intercostal bundles of the 3rd through 11th ribs are termed posterior intercostal arteries; the segmental artery destined for the intercostal bundle of the 12th rib is termed the subcostal artery. Lumbar segmental arteries are termed lumbar arteries. These names are also used to describe the lateral branch of each segmental artery, which may lead to confusion.

The segmental arteries have three major branches (Fig. 32-24). Ventral to the neural foramen, each segmental artery

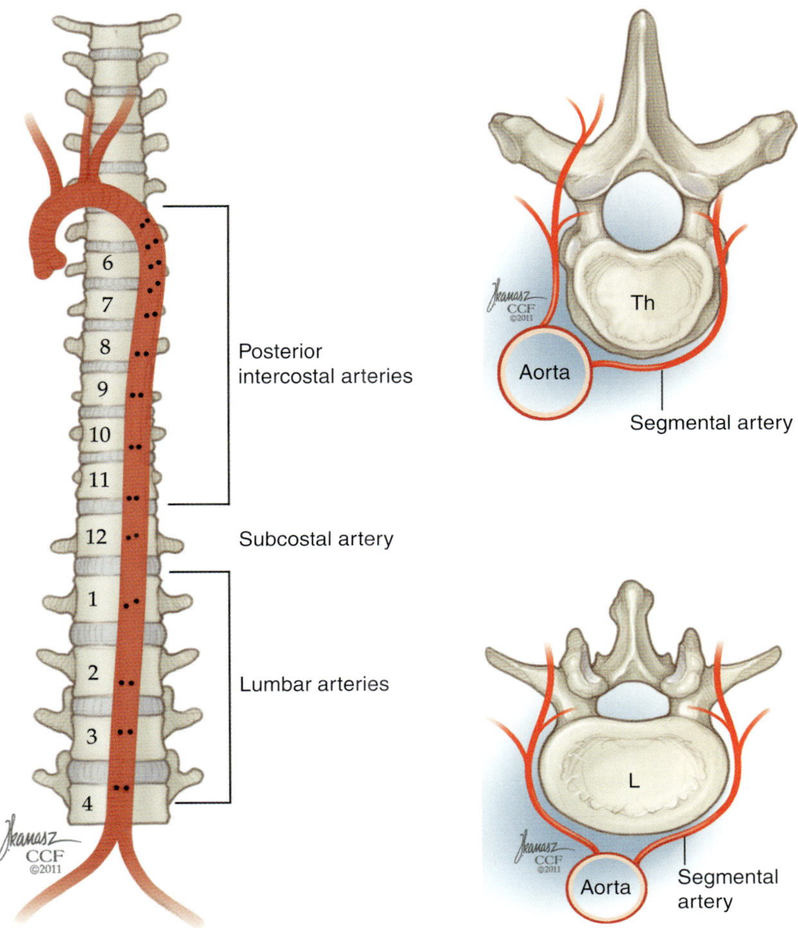

FIGURE 32-22. Medialization of segmental artery origins. (Copyright Cleveland Clinic Foundation.)

branches into a dorsal (or middle) and a lateral branch. One or more spinal (or medial) branches will arise from either the parent segmental artery or the dorsal or lateral branches. The spinal branch courses into the neural foramen and gives rise to four types of vessels: (1) posterior central branches, which remain in the epidural space, supplying the dorsal vertebral body and PLL; (2) prelaminar branches, also epidural, which supply the inner surface of the lamina and ligamentum flavum; (3) dural branches, which supply the dura of the root sleeve and adjacent spinal dura; and (4) neural branches, which supply the roots and spinal cord. The foraminal spinal branch should not be confused with the anterior and posterior spinal arteries, which are major intradural arteries supplying the spinal cord.

Neural branches travel in apposition to the spinal nerve, perforating the dura at approximately the level of the dorsal root ganglion–ventral root complex, within the neural foramen. A neural branch is termed a radicular artery if it terminates in small branches along the root, a radiculopial artery if it traverses the length of the root and anastomoses with the pial arterial plexus on the surface of the spinal cord, and a radiculomedullary artery (or segmental medullary artery) if it anastomoses with the anterior spinal artery. The posterior spinal arteries are functionally part of the periaxial network, so neural branches anastomosing with them are properly termed radiculopial arteries. Neural branches may be further classified as ventral or dorsal, depending on whether they are apposed to the ventral or dorsal roots.

After giving off the spinal branch, the dorsal branch continues dorsally, passing between the transverse processes and supplying branches to the dorsal elements and dorsal musculature. In the thoracic spine, the lateral branch, or posterior intercostal artery, ascends obliquely upward across the intercostal space toward the angle of the rib. It travels first between the parietal pleura and the posterior intercostal membrane and then pierces the membrane and lies between it and the external oblique muscle. Upon arriving at the angle of the rib, the posterior intercostal artery enters the costal groove with its associated vein and nerve.

Spinal Cord Arterial Supply

The arterial system of the spinal cord consists of a single anterior spinal artery and two paired posterior spinal arteries, all of which are variable in diameter along the length of the spinal cord. The anterior and posterior spinal arteries are supplied by radiculomedullary arteries that are variable in number and location. Branches of this arterial network may be broadly divided into two systems (Fig. 32-25). On the surface of the spinal cord, the pial arterial plexus (or corona radiata or vasa

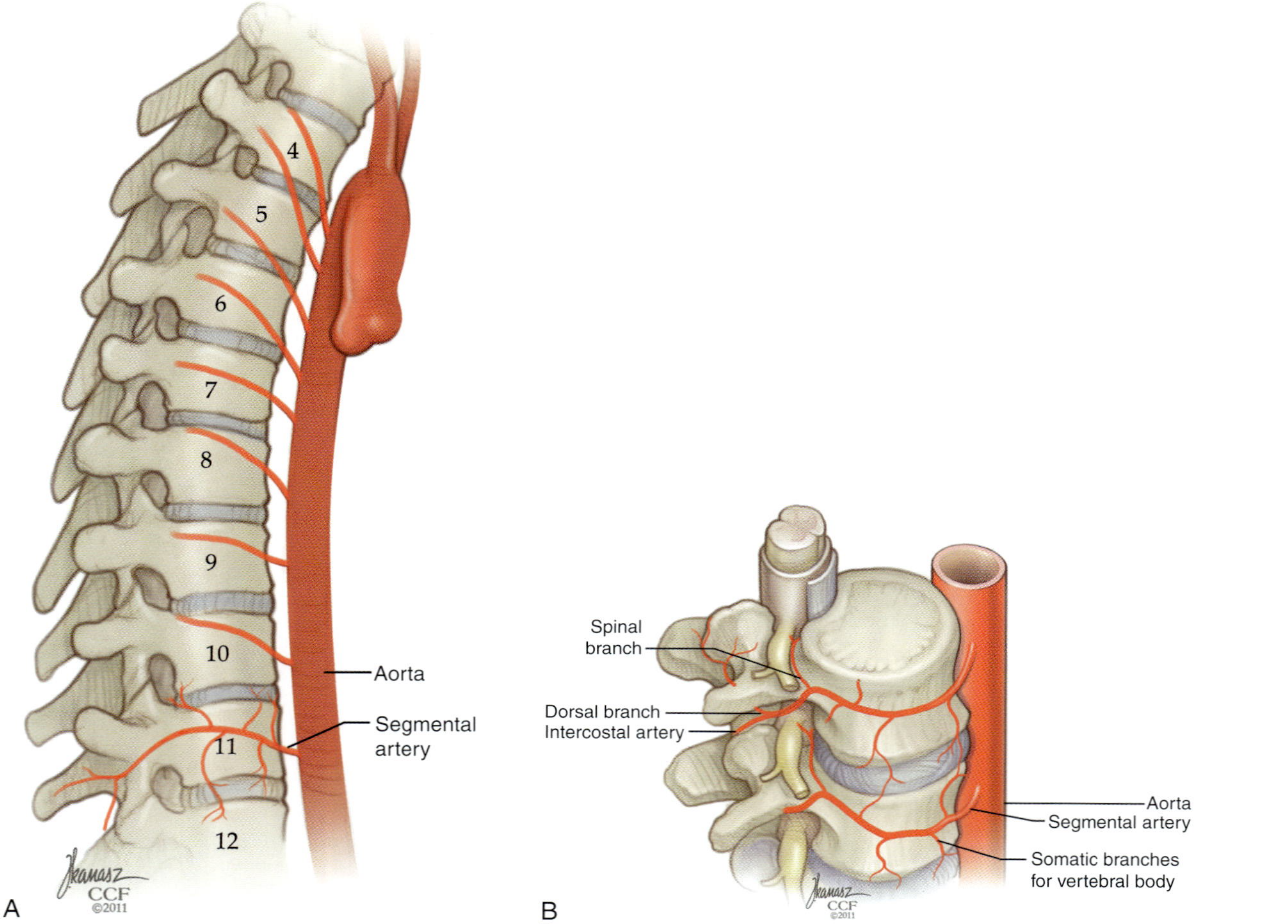

FIGURE 32-23. **A,** Decreasing ascension of segmental arteries along the rostral-caudal axis. **B,** Segmental artery and its major branches. (Copyright Cleveland Clinic Foundation.)

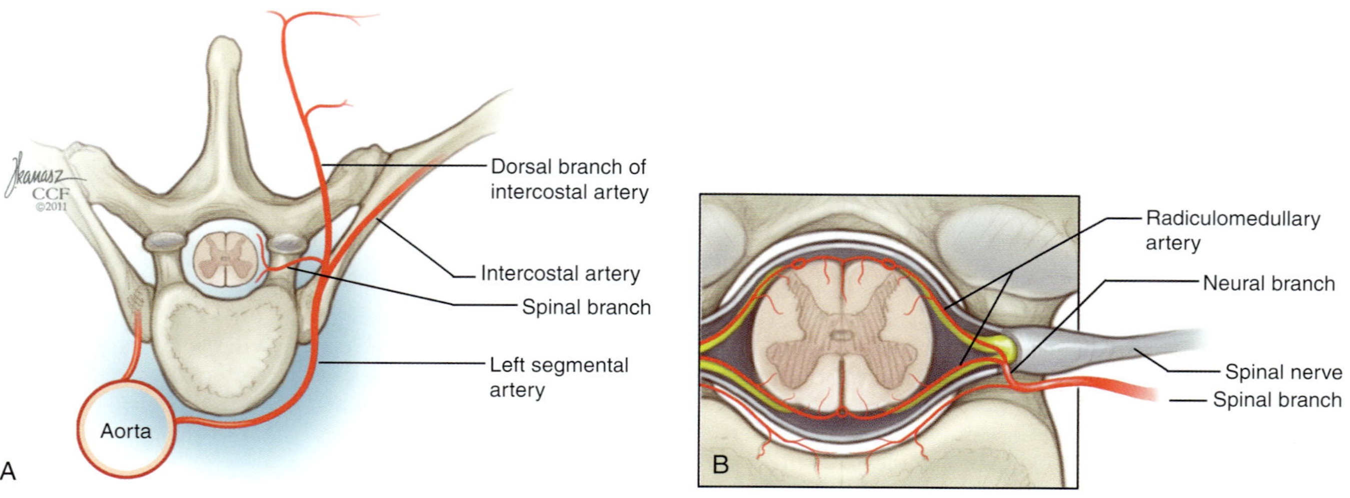

FIGURE 32-24. **A,** Major branches of a thoracic segmental artery. **B,** Major intradural and extradural branches of the spinal branch of a segmental artery. (**A,** Copyright Cleveland Clinic Foundation.)

corona) participates in a pial, or periaxial, anastomotic network that connects the anterior and posterior spinal arteries, supplying peripheral white matter tracts. The gray matter of the spinal cord, including both dorsal and ventral horns, is principally supplied by central arteries (sulcal branches, or arteriae sulcocommissurales) emanating from the anterior spinal artery. Though intra-axial anastomoses do exist in the form of vertical connections between adjacent central arteries, these are small in caliber and of limited functional significance.

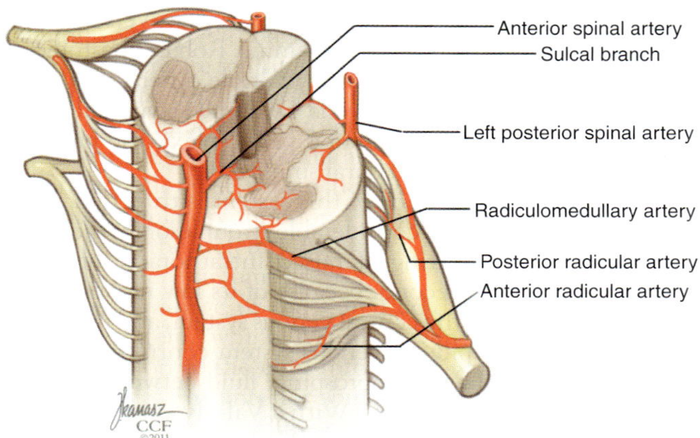

FIGURE 32-25. Arterial supply of the spinal cord and proximal nerve roots. (Copyright Cleveland Clinic Foundation.)

Three regions of the spine may be distinguished on the basis of the richness of arterial supply and anastomosis. The superior or cervicothoracic area encompasses the cervical and upper thoracic spinal cord and thus includes the cervical enlargement. It is supplied by multiple branches of the vertebral arteries, the deep cervical artery, and the ascending cervical artery. The anterior spinal artery is usually fairly robust in size. The intermediate, or midthoracic, zone (T4-8) has a sparser arterial supply. It is supplied by radiculomedullary vessels from the segmental system, which are inconsistent in number and size; often only one major radiculomedullary vessel supplies this zone. The anterior spinal artery is usually of a smaller diameter and may be absent. The lower, or thoracolumbar, zone (T9 to conus) includes the lumbar enlargement and benefits from a more robust segmental supply compared to the midthoracic zone. The principal radiculomedullary artery to this zone is known as the artery of Adamkiewicz; its inadvertent occlusion may result in paraplegia. The anterior spinal artery is relatively large in the lower zone, and it participates in a constant circumferential arterial anastomosis with the posterior spinal arteries at the level of the conus medullaris.[15]

The richness of anastomotic connections within each of the three zones is also variable. Compared with the upper and lower zones, the midthoracic region has a dearth of periaxial and intra-axial anastomoses. The central arteries emanating from the anterior spinal artery are fewer in number and smaller in diameter.[15] Thus, the midthoracic region is vulnerable as a watershed zone during prolonged periods of global ischemia.

Artery of Adamkiewicz

The artery of Adamkiewicz (AA) is the largest radiculomedullary artery, possessing a diameter of 0.5 to 0.8 mm, which is comparable to that of the anterior spinal artery. It anastomoses with the anterior spinal artery, following a characteristic hairpin loop that is visible on an anteroposterior projection during spine angiography. Ligation or occlusion of the AA will commonly result in spinal cord infarction. The artery typically arises at a variable level between the ninth intercostal artery and the second lumbar artery (in 85% of cases), most commonly on the left side (in approximately 75% of cases)[16,17]; however, its origin is sufficiently variable that individual radiologic investigation is necessary when its course must be determined preoperatively. Within the foramen, the AA is found in the rostral or middle portion, ventral to the dorsal root ganglion–ventral root complex, where it pierces the dura before joining the ventral root.[16]

Nerve Root and Cauda Equina Arterial Supply

The arterial supply of nerve roots follows a common scheme. Proximal radicular arteries emanate from the spinal cord's arterial system and supply the portion of the root closest to the cord; dorsal proximal radicular arteries course along the dorsal roots and are usually direct branches of the posterior spinal artery, and ventral proximal radicular arteries are derived from the pial plexus and course along the ventral roots. The root's distal portion is perfused by distal radicular arteries emanating from the segmental arterial system. The intervening middle portion of each root relies on a series of progressively smaller anastomotic vessels between these two systems. Radiculomedullary vessels, such as the AA, that traverse the entire length of the root and anastomose directly with the anterior or posterior spinal arteries are usually not significant contributors to root perfusion and often travel in a separate pial investment from the radicular arteries.[18]

Roots that make up the cauda equina are considerably longer than their rostral counterparts. As a result, there is a longer region in the midportion of each root with a less robust vascular supply. This may have relevance in the clinical entities of neurogenic claudication and cauda equina syndrome. In both, the time dependency of symptoms suggests reversible, or potentially reversible, ischemia of nerve roots. Some authors have suggested that the smaller vessels that predominate in the roots' middle portions may be more vulnerable to traction or compression.[18,19]

Venous Drainage of the Spinal Cord and Cauda Equina

The vertebral column is drained by a single large venous plexus. The veins are valveless, permitting bidirectional flow within the system; the assignation of different names to different "plexi" within the system belies its true nature as a single functional unit. The term Batson plexus, which alludes only to the epidural component, is somewhat misleading. Nonetheless, the use of a terminology based on anatomic location is useful. The venous drainage of the spine can be subdivided into an anterior external venous plexus, located along the ventral surface of the vertebral body; the anterior interior venous plexus, located in the epidural space ventral to the thecal sac; the posterior internal venous plexus, located in the epidural space dorsal to the thecal sac; and the posterior external venous plexus, located along the dorsal surfaces of the laminae, facets, and spinous processes. Basivertebral veins radiate through the vertebral body, connecting the anterior internal and anterior external plexi. Dorsally, venous channels traverse the laminae as well. The anterior and posterior internal vertebral venous plexi both resemble ladders, with laterally positioned longitudinal veins connected by transverse anastomoses (Fig. 32-26). In the anterior internal vertebral venous plexus, these anastomoses occur at the level of the midbody and include a connection with the corresponding basivertebral vein. In the

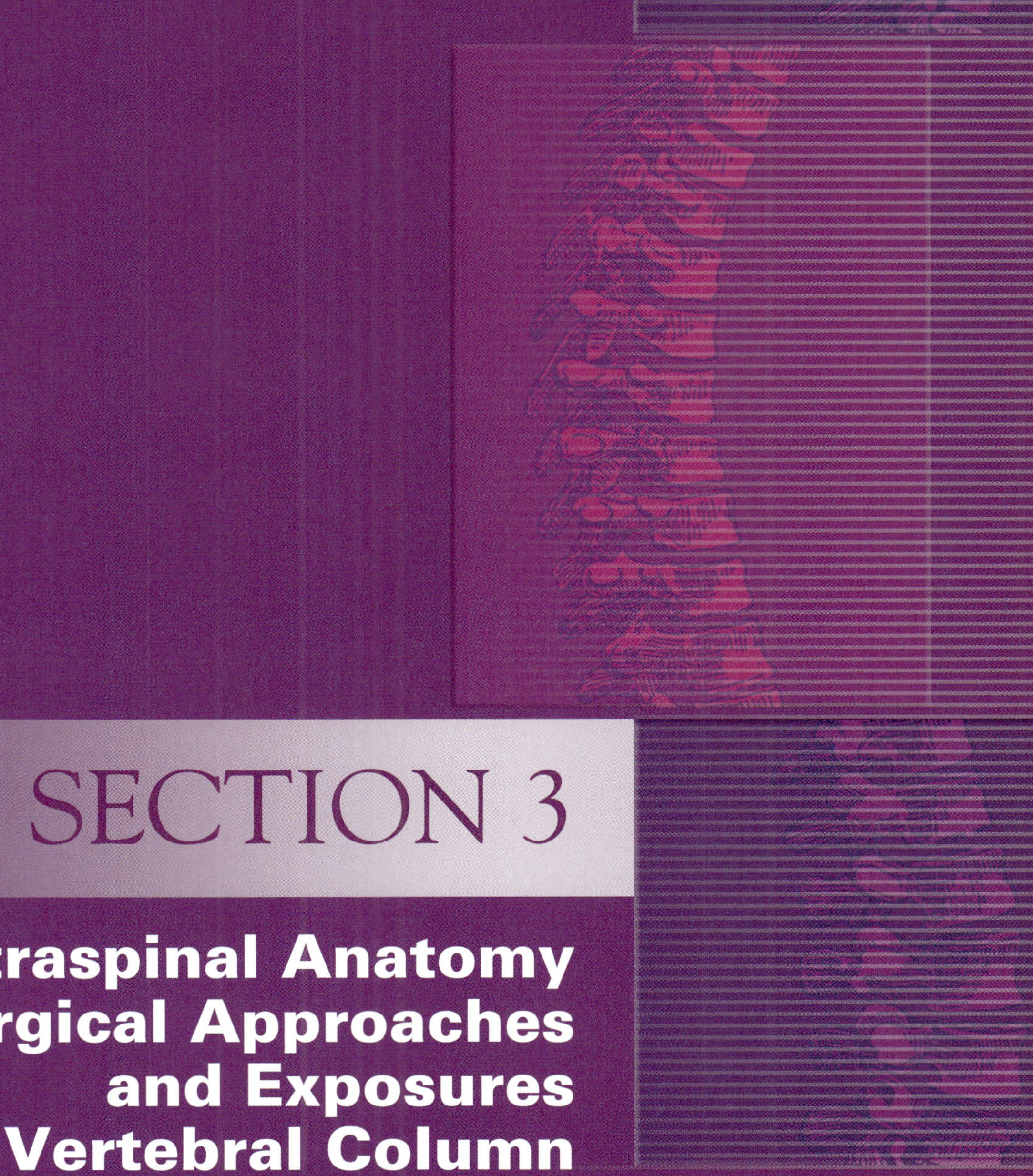

SECTION 3

Extraspinal Anatomy and Surgical Approaches and Exposures of the Vertebral Column

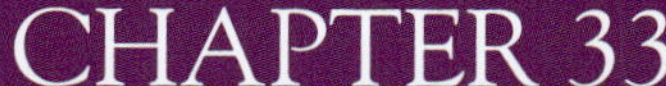

CHAPTER 33

Occipitocervical Region

Robert A. McGuire, Jr. | Ashraf A. Ragab

Although fewer procedures are performed at the occipitocervical (OC) junction when compared with subaxial cervical procedures, there are specific indications where the exposure of the OC region is necessary for surgical intervention. Indications include trauma, which may lead to instability or compressive lesions arising from tumors or infection. Vague symptoms such as pain, headaches, or limitations of motion may develop as a result of these lesions. Once the origin of these symptoms is correctly identified and the indications for surgery arise, the remaining challenge is the surgical approach. In order to approach these lesions safely, a thorough understanding of the regional anatomy of the OC junction, the surgical approaches available, and complications that may occur is mandatory. This chapter discusses the surgical anatomy and the ventral and dorsal approaches to the OC region.

Surgical Anatomy

Dorsal Surgical Anatomy of the Occipitocervical Region

Dorsal approaches to the OC area are most commonly used for OC fusions. During the approach, dissection through several muscular layers is required. The trapezius muscle constitutes the first superficial layer. The trapezius arises from the external occipital protuberans, the ligamentum nuchae, and the spines of the seventh cervical and all thoracic vertebrae.[1] The upper fibers insert into the lateral third of the clavicle and form the curve of the shoulder. The middle fibers insert into the medial edge of the acromion and the superior margin of the spine of the scapula, and the lower fibers ascend also onto the scapular spine (Fig. 33-1). The nerve supply of the trapezius muscle is the accessory nerve.

The second muscle layer consists of the levator scapulae. This muscle originates as slips from each of the transverse processes of the upper four cervical vertebrae. The muscle inserts onto the medial border of the scapula and is supplied by the ventral rami to the third and fourth cervical nerves and the fifth through the dorsal scapular nerve. The splenius muscle originates from the lower aspect of the ligamentum nuchae and the spines of the seventh cervical and upper six thoracic vertebrae. Its fibers pass rostrally, and it is divided into cervical and cranial components. The splenius cervicis is the lateral component, which inserts into the transverse processes of the upper three cervical vertebrae, deep to the levator scapulae muscle. Meanwhile, the splenius capitis muscle inserts on the lower aspect of the mastoid process of the temporal bone. Its nerve supply is the dorsal rami of the cervical nerves. Beneath the splenius lies the cervical component of the erector spinae muscle. The erector spinae muscle is composed of three main columns (from lateral to medial): the iliocostalis, longissimus, and spinalis muscles. The longissimus capitis muscle is a long muscle that lies under the splenius muscle immediately dorsal to the transverse processes. It arises from the transverse processes of the upper four thoracic vertebrae and passes upward to be inserted into the back of the mastoid process. The ligamentum nuchae is a strong fibrous substance, which is median between the muscles of the two sides. It is considered a continuation of the superior spinous and interspinous ligaments from the spine of the seventh cervical vertebra through the external occipital protuberans.

The main vessels in the dorsal OC area are the occipital artery and the vertebral artery. The occipital artery arises from the external carotid artery in the front of the neck and runs dorsally and rostrally deep to the mastoid process and then courses dorsally immediately deep to the muscles attached to the superior nuchal line. It then pierces the trapezius muscle 2.5 cm from the midline to ramify on the back of the head (see Fig. 33-1). As for the vertebral artery, only the third part of this artery is significant during the approach. It emerges from the foramen and the transverse process of the atlas and hooks dorsomedially around the dorsal surface of the lateral mass of the atlas (see Fig. 33-1). It is partly separated from the arch of the atlas by the first cervical nerve (Fig. 33-2; see also Fig. 33-1). It then passes ventromedially in front of the thickened lateral edge of the dorsal atlanto-occipital membrane, which forms an arch over the artery. Occasionally, this arch may be ossified and is referred to as the *ponticulus posticus*.[2] This condition must be recognized preoperatively because failure to do so can lead to catastrophic results if the lateral mass C1 screws are placed through the vertebral arteries. The artery then pierces the dura mater and enters the vertebral canal. The suboccipital plexus of veins is a network of veins that drains into the deep cervical vein and into the vertebral venous plexus around the vertebral artery. The greater occipital nerve is the medial branch of the dorsal ramus of the second cervical nerve, which is the thickest cutaneous nerve in the body. It appears at the middle of the lower border of the

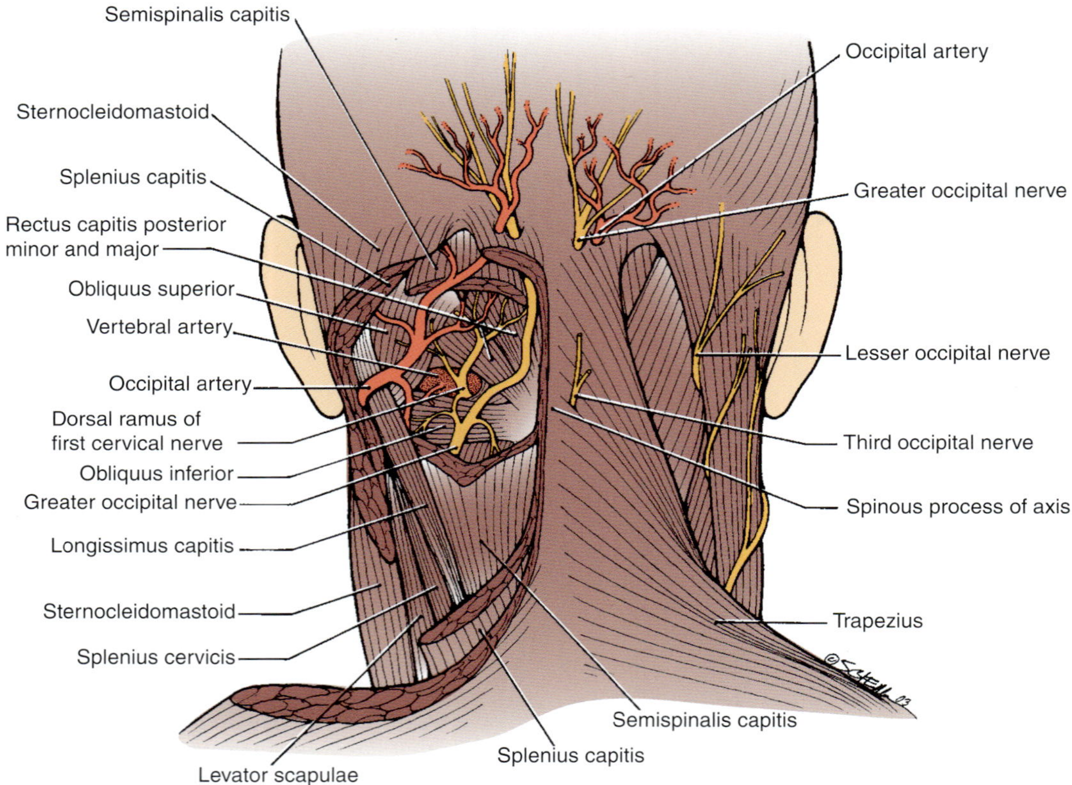

FIGURE 33-1. Dorsal surgical anatomy of the occipitocervical region. Superficial *(right)* and deep *(left)*.

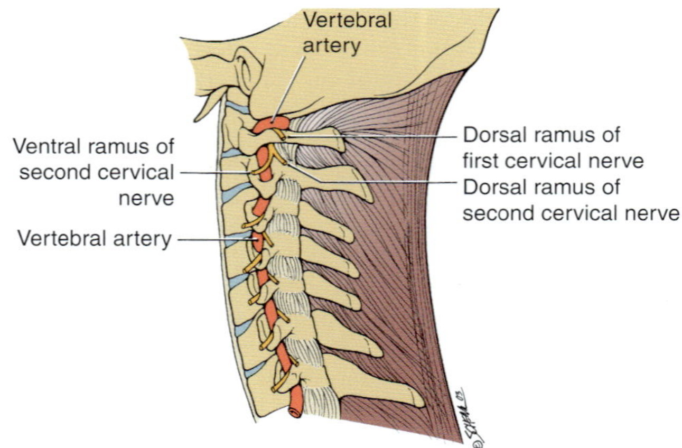

FIGURE 33-2. Course of the vertebral artery. The dorsal ramus of the first cervical nerve runs between the arch and the vertebral artery.

inferior oblique muscle and curves superior medially across the suboccipital triangle. It runs rostrally on that muscle and then pierces the trapezius muscle about 2 cm lateral to the occipital protuberans (see Fig. 33-1).

Ventral Anatomy of the Occipitocervical Junction

Three muscles originate from the ventral aspect of the atlas: longus colli, rectus capitis anterior, and rectus capitis lateralis (Fig. 33-3).

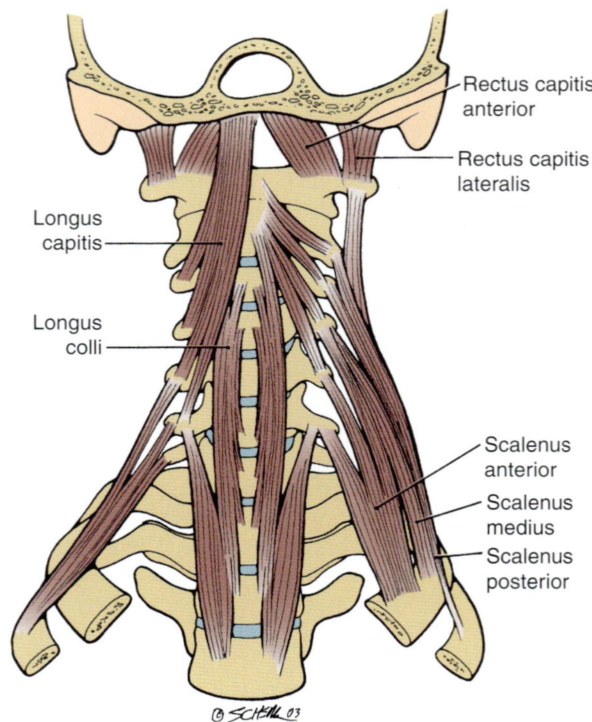

FIGURE 33-3. Ventral muscles of the occipitocervical region.

1. The longus colli muscle is the longest and most medial of the muscles. It extends from the anterior tubercle of the atlas to the lower part of the body of the upper thoracic vertebrae. Between these points it is attached to all the vertebral bodies and into the third to sixth cervical transverse processes.
2. The rectus capitis anterior is a short, wide muscle that originates from the ventral surface of the lateral mass of the atlas and is inserted into the base of the skull ventral to the occipital condyle.
3. The rectus capitis lateralis is a short muscle that runs vertically between the rostral surface of the transverse process of the atlas and jugular process of the occipital bone. It lies dorsal to the jugular foramen and is separated from the rectus capitis anterior by the ventral ramus of the first cervical nerve, which supplies both muscles. The function of these muscles is to stabilize the skull on the vertebral column (see Fig. 33-3).

Ventral to the prevertebral muscles is the retropharyngeal space. The anterior tubercle of the atlas may be palpated through the dorsal pharynx during a transoral approach.

Vertebral Artery

The anatomy of the vertebral artery must be understood because injury to this artery may have dire consequences. The artery starts as a branch of the subclavian artery and passes to the transverse process of the sixth cervical vertebra.[1] The artery then ascends vertically through the foramina transversaria accompanied by the vertebral veins and plexus of sympathetic nerve fibers derived from the cervicothoracic ganglion of the sympathetic trunk. Between the transverse processes, it lies medial to the intertransverse muscles and ventral to the ventral rami of the cervical nerves. Upon entering the axis it turns laterally under the superior articular facet in the foramen transversarium and enters the foramen transversarium of the atlas, which is placed farther laterally than the others. Therefore at this level, the artery takes a lateral course (see Fig. 33-2). The artery then emerges on the rostral surface of the atlas between the rectus capitis lateralis muscle and the superior articular process of the atlas. Here it lies with the ventral ramus of the first cervical nerve and curves with it horizontally around the lateral and dorsal aspect of the superior articularis process. It then traverses the articular process and the dorsal arch of the atlas, where it lies rostrally to the dorsal ramus of the first cervical nerve. The artery then turns rostrally and pierces the dura and arachnoid mater. It enters the cranial cavity through the foramen magnum. It then runs ventrally and rostrally over the ventral surface of the medulla oblongata to meet and join the opposite vertebral artery at the inferior border of the pons to form the basilar artery. Through the branches of these vessels, blood is supplied to the hindbrain, midbrain, and dorsal aspect of the cerebrum and the rostral aspect of the spinal medulla. The vertebral vein originates from a plexus of veins that is formed by the union of veins from the internal venous plexus and suboccipital triangle. It accompanies the vertebral artery through the foramina transversaria and exits the sixth cervical transverse process. It passes ventral to the subclavian artery and ends by entering the dorsal surface of the brachiocephalic vein near its origin.

Atlanto-Occipital Joint

The atlas is a ring of bone with a lateral mass on each side (Fig. 33-4, *top*).[1] The lateral masses are articulated rostrally with the occipital condyles and caudally with the superior articular facets of the axis. Each has a transverse process projecting laterally from it. The atlas is attached to the occiput by strong ligaments, which hold these bones together. However, the articular surfaces, which the atlas has with the skull and axis, are of two different configurations. The kidney-shaped occipital condyles lie on the ventrolateral aspect of the foramen. They fit into the superior articular facets of the atlas, which are also kidney shaped (see Fig. 33-4). The joint allows flexion and extension and slight side-to-side rocking of head motion, but no rotation. The stability of these joints depends on the aid of ligaments, the tectorial membrane, and the longitudinal bands of the cruciate ligament, which all bind the skull to the axis. The ligaments of the joints of the atlas include the anterior longitudinal ligament, which tapers rostrally to be attached to the tubercle of the axis and continues as a narrow band to the base of the skull. The dorsal atlanto-occipital membrane is a rostral continuation of the ligamentum flavum. This membrane passes from the dorsal arch of the atlas to the margin of the foramen magnum dorsal to the atlanto-occipital joint. The lateral margins of the membrane arch over the corresponding vertebral artery and the first cervical nerve. In some cases, these margins may be ossified. The tectorial membrane is a broad ligamentous sheet, which is the rostral continuation of the posterior longitudinal ligament. It passes from the dorsal surface of the body of the axis to the cranial surface of the occipital bone, and it holds the axis to the skull and covers the dorsal surfaces of the dens with its ligaments and the ventral margin of the foramen magnum.

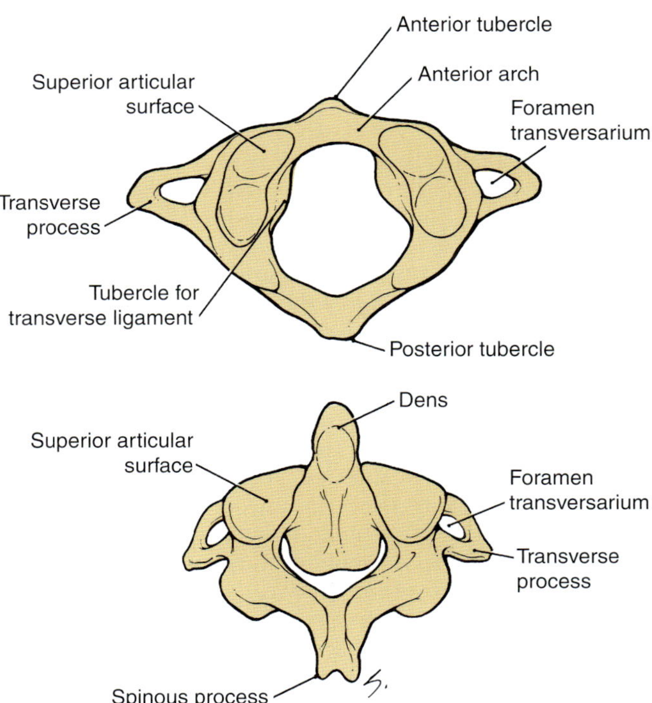

FIGURE 33-4. Bony anatomy of the atlas *(top)* and the axis *(bottom)*.

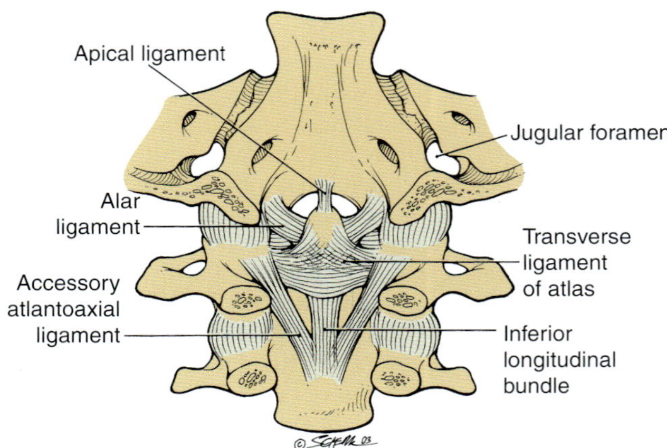

FIGURE 33-5. Ligamentous anatomy of the occipitocervical region.

The cruciate ligament is formed by rostral and ventral longitudinal bands, which pass from the transverse ligament to the cranial surface of the occipital bone and the body of the axis, respectively. The apical ligament of the dens is a cordlike ligament, which stretches from the apex of the dens to the cranial surface of the occipital bone, immediately above the foramen magnum. The alar ligaments are strong ligaments that arise from the sloping sides of the dens (Fig. 33-5). They pass laterally and upward to the medial sides of the occipital condyle and tighten when the atlas, carrying the skull, rotates around the dens. They are the main factor in limiting rotation of the atlantoaxial joint. The first and second cervical spinal nerves pass dorsally to the OC and C1-2 joint capsules, respectively, and not ventral to the articular facets, as is the case with the remaining subaxial cervical vertebrae.

Approaches to the Occipitocervical Region

Dorsal Approach to the Occipitocervical Region

The dorsal approach is most commonly used when fusion of the OC region is indicated. This approach has been described by different authors, including Grantham et al.[3] and Wertheim and Bohlman.[4] Key in the approach is positioning of the patient to allow safe intubation and protect the neural elements. Longitudinal traction should be applied preoperatively to provide stability during the intubation process. The patient is then logrolled into the prone position. Support for the head may also be provided using a Mayfield three-point headrest. Radiography or intraoperative fluoroscopy is used to confirm the alignment of the occiput to the atlas and the remainder of the cervical spine. The skin is then prepared, and the subcutaneous tissues are injected with a solution of epinephrine 1:500,000. A midline incision is made, extending from the external occipital protuberance to the spinous process of the fourth or fifth cervical vertebra. The spinous process of the C2 is the most prominent of the spinous processes encountered during the approach. The spinous process of C2 is bifid, allowing the short external rotators of the head to be attached to the cervical spine. Once the skin is incised, the incision is extended into the deep fascia and then into the ligamentum nuchae. It is very important to remain in the midline to avoid excessive bleeding. This placement can be confirmed by palpating the alignment of the spinous processes and by visualizing the avascular midline plane of the ligamentum nuchae. By staying in the midline, the paramedian venous plexuses are avoided. The paravertebral muscles are stripped off the spinous processes and the lamina subperiosteally to avoid excessive bleeding.

Although some may believe that it is safe to use Cobb elevators in dissecting the muscles subperiosteally off the lamina, the authors do not recommend this technique. The fact that the laminae are weaker in this region than in the lumbar spine may lead to fracture of the lamina because of excessive force, as well as increased blood loss caused by uncontrolled stripping of the musculature. However, a Cobb elevator may be used to gently retract the muscles, placing them under tension, while the muscles are stripped off of the lamina using a freer elevator or cautery in a controlled manner. At the base of the skull, full-thickness scalp flaps are reflected along the occipital ridge about 2 to 3 cm laterally. The extensive lateral dissection along the lamina of the cervical spine should be to the groove, which indicates the junction of the lamina along with the articular facet. Once the occipital exposure is completed, special care must be taken during the dissection of the arches of C1. The vertebral artery runs on the rostral surface of the arch and the lateral third of the arch (see Figs. 34-1 and 34-2). To expose this area safely, only 1 cm on each side of the dorsal arch of C1 is dissected. In this area, it is important to elevate the muscles subperiosteally. Cauterizing in this area is not recommended because of the thin membrane that attaches the base of the skull to the arch of atlas. Once exposure of the bony occipital protuberance, the dorsal arch of the atlas, and the remainder of the laminae of the cervical spine is accomplished, arthrodesis may be completed. This may be performed using the technique described previously by Grantham or modifications that were introduced by other authors.[3] With this technique, 24-gauge stainless-steel wires are used along with an iliac crest bone graft that is contoured to span the distance from the occiput and the upper cervical laminae after the laminae and occiput are decorticated with a burr. Occipital plates or rods that are inserted into the lateral mass of C1 and C2 using screws may also be used to provide more rigid fixation.

Ventral Approaches

Indications for ventral approaches include ventral bony tumors with neural compression, extradural tumors, intradural midline lesions, and irreducible subluxations.[5-9] The ventral approach may also be used for repair of nonunion of C2 odontoid fractures and for odontoid resection.[10] The ventral aspect of the OC junction may be approached via an extension of the ventral retropharyngeal/extrapharyngeal approach to the upper cervical spine or via a transoral approach.

Ventral Retropharyngeal Approach

The ventral retropharyngeal approach to the upper cervical spine has been described by Whitesides[11] and McAfee et al.[12] This approach allows exposure of the ventral aspect of the axis and atlas and also may allow exposure of the clivus and ventral aspect of the foramen magnum. Decompression and OC fusion may be performed through this approach.

Cortical somatosensory-evoked potentials may be measured. The patient is positioned on the operative wedge frame, and the neck is extended as far as allowed while the patient is awake without signs of neurologic compromise. A modified transverse submandibular incision is used (Fig. 33-6). The incision is made on the patient's right side, if the surgeon is right handed. This exposure is the rostral extension of the ventral lateral exposure to the midpart of the cervical spine. The fascial planes that are dissected through are the same as those described in the ventral approach to the cervical spine, consisting of the superficial fascia and the deep fascia layers. The submandibular incision is made through the platysmal muscle and the superficial fascia and skin are immobilized in the platysmal plane of the superficial fascia. The marginal mandibular branch of the facial nerve is found with the aid of the nerve stimulator by ligating and dissecting the retromandibular veins superiorly. The common facial vein is continuous with the retromandibular vein, and the branches of the mandibular nerve usually cross the latter vein superficially and superiorly. The superficial branches of the fascial nerve are protected. The ventral border of the sternocleidomastoid muscle is mobilized by longitudinally transecting the superficial layer of deep cervical fascia. The submandibular salivary gland is resected, and the duct is sutured adequately to prevent the formation of a salivary fistula. The jugular-digastric lymph node from the submandibular and carotid angles can be resected and sent for frozen section if a neoplasm is in question. The dorsal belly of the digastric muscle and the stylohyoid muscle are identified, and the digastric tendon is divided and tagged for later repair. As described by Whitesides,[11] rostral traction at the base of the origin of the stylohyoid muscle can cause injury to the facial nerve as it exits from the skull. After the digastric and stylohyoid muscles are divided, the hyoid bone and the hypopharynx are mobilized medially. The hypoglossal nerve, which is identified with a nerve stimulator, is then completely mobilized from the base of the skull to the ventral border of the hypoglossal muscle (see Fig. 33-6). It is retracted rostrally through the remainder of the procedure. The dissection then proceeds to the retropharyngeal space between the carotid sheath laterally and the pharynx medially. Rostral exposure to the atlas and the base of the skull is facilitated by ligating the branches of the carotid artery and internal jugular vein (see Fig. 33-6). The vessels to be ligated (from caudally and progressing rostrally) include the superior thyroid artery and vein, lingual artery and vein, ascending pharyngeal artery and vein, and facial artery and vein. After ligation, the carotid sheath is easily mobilized laterally. The superior pharyngeal nerve, which is also identified with the help of the nerve stimulator, is mobilized from its origin near the nodose ganglion to the entrance into the larynx. The alar and prevertebral fasciae are transected longitudinally to expose the longus colli muscle, which runs longitudinally. It is

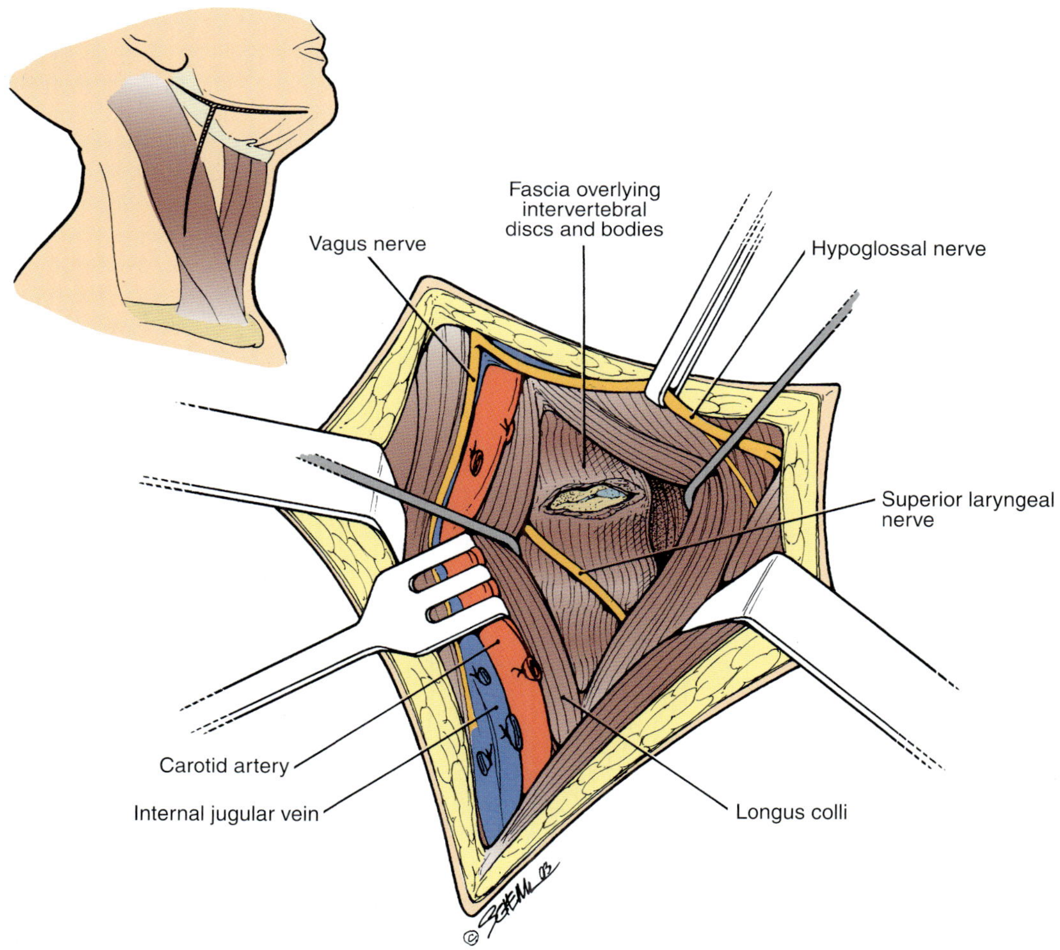

FIGURE 33-6. Surgical exposure of the occipitocervical region through a ventral retropharyngeal approach.

important at this point to maintain the orientation of the anterior tubercle of the atlas because rotation and lateral dissection may endanger the vertebral artery. The dissection along the prevertebral fascia may be extended cranially to reach the base of the skull and the clivus through this approach. Once this exposure is achieved, ventral decompression and, if necessary, fusion of the OC junction may be initiated.

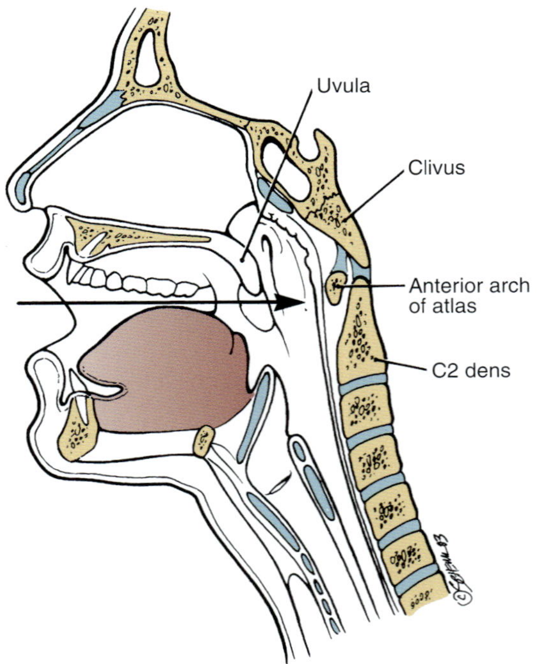

FIGURE 33-7. The clivus, ventral arch of C1, and dens are accessible through the transoral approach.

Transoral Approach

The transoral procedure allows exposure of the clivus, the arches of the atlas, and the ventral aspect of C2 (Fig. 33-7). Adequate interdental distance (at least 25 mm) is necessary for this exposure. If this is not achievable or there is a disease involving the temporomandibular joint, a transmandibular splitting approach or other more extensive approaches may be necessary.[13]

Preoperative management includes assessment of the interdental space. After this is found to be adequate, the dorsal pharynx should be cultured to allow adequate preoperative antibiotic coverage. Palpation of the dorsal pharynx is then performed to identify the landmarks. This is performed after the dorsal pharynx is anesthetized with topical anesthetic to prevent the gag reflex. The anterior tubercle of C1 and the ventral body of C2 are palpable because they are directly dorsal to the mucous membrane. A tracheotomy is performed, although some authors avoid tracheotomy by using a nasal tracheal fiberoptic intubation while the patient is awake. The nasal tracheal tube does not impinge on the surgical field for lesions below the foramen magnum. They reserve tracheotomy for patients for whom long-term ventilatory problems are expected.[7,14] A nasogastric tube may be used to retract the uvula and soft palate to allow adequate exposure (Fig. 33-8). The nasogastric tube is passed through the nose and out of the mouth to elevate the soft palate. Intraoral retractors are used to depress the tongue to allow better exposure. The uvula of the palate may also be sutured to the roof of the mouth, and the tongue is retracted interiorly (see Fig. 33-8). Before the midline incision of the

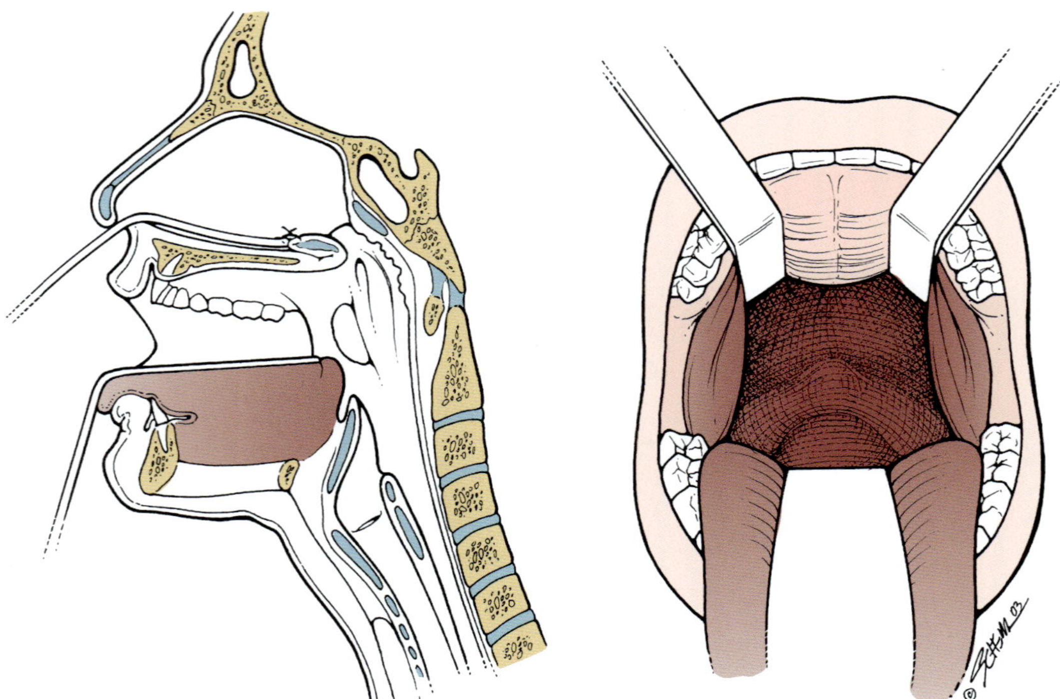

FIGURE 33-8. Placement of retractors for exposure during the transoral approach. The ventral arch of C1 and the dens may be palpated through the pharynx *(right)*.

mucosa is made, the area is infiltrated with a 1:600,000 solution of epinephrine. The midline incision is then made, extending about 2 cm above the ventral arches of the atlas and 2 cm below the prominence of the arch. The desired structures can be accessed by retracting the mucosa laterally. This retraction assists exposure of the clivus of the occiput, C1, and C2. The rotation of the atlas may be deceiving, and the ventral aspect of the lateral mass may be mistakenly perceived as the anterior tubercle of C1.[14] This wall places the vertebral artery at risk of being injured; it will also come closer to the midline because the atlas is rotated. If access to the clivus more superiorly is necessary, the hard palate may be split with a reciprocating saw to allow more access. When access to the retropharyngeal space using the transoral approach is limited either due to a transdental distance of less than 25 mm or to severe macroglossia, other approaches may be used. These include extended maxillotomy or mandibular osteotomy approaches.[13,15,16]

Extended Approaches to the Craniocervical Junction

Extended Maxillotomy

James and Crockard[16] described surgical access to the base of the skull and upper cervical spine by extended maxillotomy, which provides a much wider surgical access to the base of the skull. With this technique, a tracheotomy and placement of the gastric tube are performed first. Next, the patient is positioned in the supine or three-quarter supine position with some degree of neck extension to assist access to the palate. Surgical exposure of the cranial base is performed through an incision made above the mucogingival reflection from the first molar tooth on either side, and the soft tissues are reflected subperiosteally to expose the ventral and lateral walls in the maxilla (Fig. 33-9). The osteotomy sites include (1) a transverse standard LeFort osteotomy cut that is made using an air-powered reciprocating saw, and (2) a sagittal cut that separates the two parts of the maxilla by sawing to the side of the midline suture (see Fig. 33-9). The bone between the central and incisor teeth is divided using a fine osteotome to avoid damage to the adjacent dental roots. This median section is completed with division of the soft palate in the midline. This exposure allows larger access to the clivus, through which a clivectomy can be performed. Excision of tumors and approaches to aneurysms can also be performed through this exposure. Complete details of the procedure may be found in the technique described by James and Crockard.[16]

Bilateral Sagittal Split Mandibular Osteotomy

Another approach that may be of use in gaining access to the retropharyngeal space when there is limited exposure is the bilateral sagittal split mandibular osteotomy (as described by Vishteh et al.[13]). In their technique, the sagittal split mandibular osteotomy is performed on both sides of the mandible, as an adjunct to the transoral approach to the ventral craniovertebral junction. They described the osteotomy as a stair-step split mandibulotomy (Fig. 33-10). Before the osteotomy is performed, a plate is placed in the appropriate position across the lateral osteotomy site on which the procedure is to be performed. A drill hole is made on each side, and screws are placed. The remaining drill holes are drilled, and the plate is removed and set aside. The osteotomy site courses through the lateral cortex medially above the lingula along the ventral border of the ramus lateral to the second and third molars and through the lateral cortex.

Transcondylar Approach to Craniovertebral Junction (Extreme Radial Craniocervical Approach)

Access to the craniovertebral junction through a ventral approach sometimes has it limitations, including inadequate exposure or inability to perform craniocervical fusion; difficulty in reaching lateral located lesions; narrowing of the interdental distance less than 25 mm, and thereby limiting the exposure; and the risk of infection from a contaminated

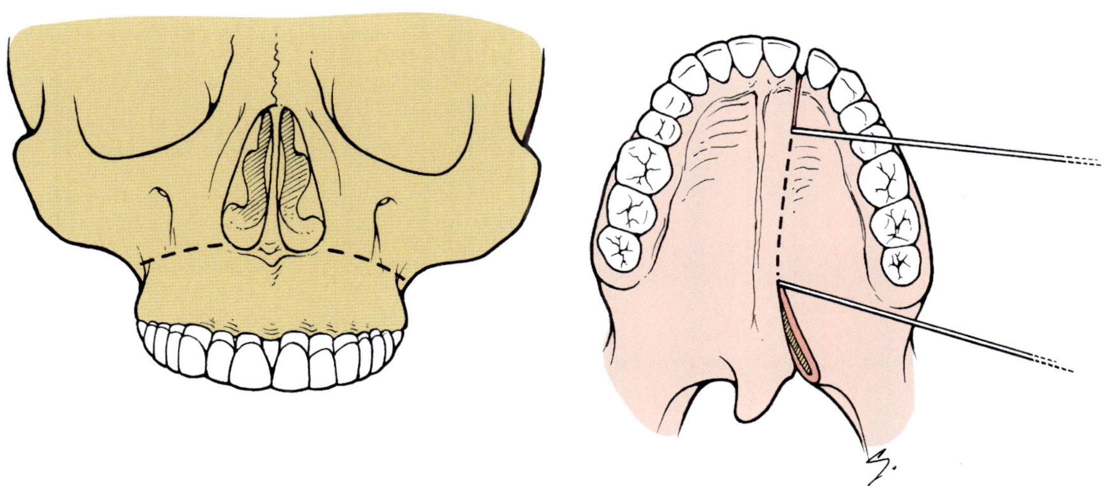

FIGURE 33-9. Access to the occipitocervical junction by extended maxillotomy. Transverse standard LeFort osteotomy *(left)* and sagittal cut to maxilla *(right)*.

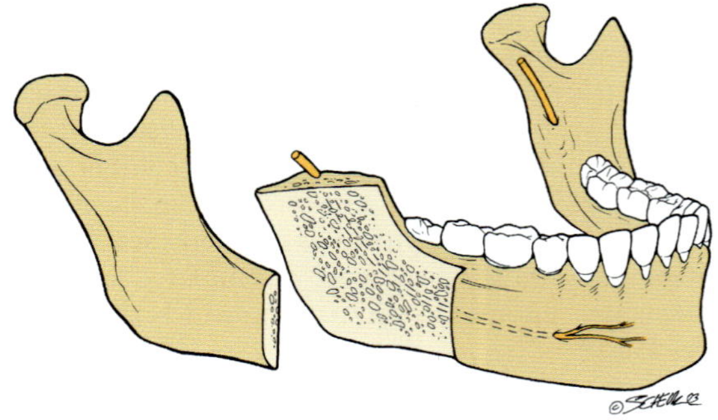

FIGURE 33-10. Bilateral sagittal split mandibular osteotomy.

field. The extreme lateral/transcondylar approach has been described by al-Mefty et al.[17] and Bejjani et al.[18] to access extradural non-neoplastic lesions of the ventral craniovertebral junction, where decompression and stabilization are necessary. The advantages of this approach include a more direct access to the lesion and direct visualization of the dural sac, eliminating manipulation of the brainstem or upper spinal cord. Identification and control of the ipsilateral vertebral artery are also assisted, along with direct visualization and protection of the lower cranial nerves. This approach also provides a more sterile field than the transoral approach. OC fusion and instrumentation can be performed during the same procedure, as opposed to the transcondylar approach.

The patient is placed in a halo brace with the neck and head in the neutral position. The positioning of the patient is in the supine position with the entire body being rotated 45 degrees to the opposite side. Intubation is performed while the patient is awake. Intraoperative monitoring is also recommended, including bilateral somatosensory-evoked potentials, bilateral brainstem auditory-evoked response, and the cranial nerves 10, 11, and 12.[17] The skin incision begins behind the ear at the level of external auditory canal and extends medially to the midline and inferiorly to level of C4, where it curves ventrally to reach the ventral border of the sternomastoid muscle. The skin flap is elevated ventrally. This elevation exposes the greater auricular nerve and the sternomastoid muscle. Blunt dissection is performed along the ventral border of the sternomastoid muscle and falls superiorly to the mastoid process, where it is attached. The sternomastoid, splenius capitis, longissimus, and semispinalis muscles are detached from the mastoid in one layer and retracted. The eleventh cranial nerve must be identified and preserved where it enters the middle third of sternomastoid muscle. The dorsal belly of the digastric muscle is kept in place to protect the facial nerve as it exits the stylomastoid foramen. The deep muscular layer forms the suboccipital triangle, which is delineated by the major and minor rectus capitis muscles medially, the superior oblique muscle superiorly, and the inferior oblique muscle inferiorly. The apex of the triangle is the transverse process of C1. The horizontal segment of the vertebral artery and C1 root can be seen in this triangle. The C2 nerve root can be followed laterally where it crosses over the vertebral artery and its vertical segment between C1 and C2. The nerve root is protected. The vertebral artery is then identified from the transverse foramen of C2 to its entry to the dura mater. The vertebral artery is moved out of the foramen of C1 after this foramen is opened with a diamond drill, and the artery is then held inferomedially. The C1 nerve root may be sacrificed. After exposure is complete, the mastoid tip is drilled to expose the occipital condyle and the jugular bulb. The occipital condyle and the condylar surface of C1 are exposed widely and drilled out. The hypoglossal canal is then identified and the 12th nerve is preserved. After the lateral bone structures are resected, the odontoid process and the surrounding ligaments are clearly seen. The odontoid process is drilled until the contralateral condyle is identified. In patients with severe odontoid invagination, the jugular bulb must be skeletonized to permit a more superior extension. Complete details of the procedure may be found in the technique described by al-Mefty et al.[17]

Salas et al.[19] described variations of the extreme lateral cranial cervical approach in an anatomic study and clinical analysis of 69 patients. The variations include the transfacet oral approach, the retrocondylar approach, the partial transcondylar approach, the complete transcondylar approach, the extreme lateral transjugular approach, and the transtubercular approach.[19,20] These are all variations to allow improved access and exposure to the pathology, depending on the location of the pathology.

Summary

Approaches to the craniocervical junction are not as frequently used as those used in gaining access to the subaxial cervical spine. However, when the indication for surgery at the craniocervical junction arises, a thorough understanding of the anatomy and techniques of exposure is mandatory to avoid injury of vital neurovascular structures encountered during the approach. The specific approach chosen will vary according to the pathologic process encountered, the location of the lesion, and the need for adjuvant stabilization.

KEY REFERENCES

Al-Mefty O, Borba LA, Aoki N, et al: The transcondylar approach to extradural nonneoplastic lesions of the craniovertebral junction. *J Neurosurg* 84(1):1–6, 1996.

Crockard HA: Anterior approaches to lesion of the upper cervical spine. *Clin Neurosurg* 34:389–416, 1988.

Grantham SA, Dick HM, Thompson RC Jr, Stinchfield FE: Occipitocervical arthrodesis. Indications, technic and results. *Clin Orthop* 65:118–129, 1969.

McAfee PC, Bohlman HH, Riley LH Jr, et al: The anterior retropharyngeal approach to the upper part of the cervical spine. *J Bone Joint Surg [Am]* 69:1371–1383, 1987.

REFERENCES

The complete reference list is available online at expertconsult.com.

CHAPTER 34

Cervical Spine and Cervicothoracic Junction

John W. German | Tyler J. Kenning | Alexander J. Ghanayem | Edward C. Benzel | Joseph T. Alexander

Cervical and Nuchal Anatomy

An understanding of anatomy is the most basic tenet of surgery. Because both ventral and dorsal approaches are commonly used when operating on the cervical spine, it is essential that the spine surgeon be familiar with the anatomy of both the cervical and nuchal regions.[1]

Anatomic Overview of the Neck

Frick et al. have presented an overview of the anatomy of the neck with the cervical spine as the centerpiece.[2] Dorsal to the cervical spine lies the nuchal musculature, which is covered superficially by two large muscles: the trapezius and the levator scapulae. Just ventral to the vertebral bodies lies the visceral space, which contains elements of the alimentary, respiratory, and endocrine systems. The visceral space is surrounded by the cervical musculature and portions of the cervical fascia. Dorsolateral to the visceral space but separated from the visceral space, as well as the cervical musculature, lie the paired neurovascular conduction pathways. Thus, in this scheme, the neck may be divided into five distinct regions: cervical spine, nuchal musculature, visceral space, cervical musculature, and neurovascular conduction pathways.

Surface Anatomy of the Neck

Knowledge of the surface anatomy of the neck is essential when planning cervical spine surgery. These relationships help establish the site of the skin incision and dictate which vertebral level(s) may be approached. Classically, several superficial anterior neck structures have been used to identify the approximate cervical spinal levels for the purposes of the skin incision. These include the hyoid bone (C3), thyroid cartilage (C4-5), cricoid cartilage (C6), and carotid tubercle (C6). These landmarks, however, may not be universally reliable because, depending on a patient's body habitus, they may be difficult to palpate reliably. Therefore an understanding of the overall relationships of the surface anatomy is essential for operative planning.

The most prominent structure of the upper dorsal surface of the nuchal region is the inion, or occipital protuberance. This may be palpated in the midline and is a part of the occipital bone. The spinous processes of the cervical vertebrae may then be followed caudally to the vertebral prominence, variably corresponding to the spinous process of C6, C7 (most common), or T1.

The prominent surface structure of the ventral neck is the laryngeal prominence, which is produced by the underlying thyroid cartilage. The thyroid cartilage is composed of two broad plates that are readily palpable. This cartilage protects the vocal cords, which lie at the midpoint of the ventral surface. Rostral to the thyroid cartilage lies the horseshoe-shaped hyoid bone, which is easy to palpate with the neck extended. The hyoid bone lies in the mouth-cervical angle[3] and mediates the muscular attachments of the muscles of the floor of the mouth (middle pharyngeal, hyoglossus, and genioglossus muscles), as well as those of the six hyoid muscles (stylohyoid, thyrohyoid, geniohyoid, omohyoid, mylohyoid, and sternohyoid). The hyoid bone provides some movement during swallowing. This movement is limited caudally to the fourth cervical vertebral body by the stylohyoid ligament.[2] The transverse process of the atlas may be palpated at a point marked by a line between the angle of the mandible and a point 1 cm ventrocaudal to the tip of the mastoid process.[3]

Caudal to the thyroid cartilage lies the signet-ring–shaped cricoid cartilage. The cricoid cartilage marks the laryngotracheal transition of the respiratory system and the pharyngoesophageal transition of the gastrointestinal system. Caudal to the cricoid cartilage lies the trachea. The isthmus of the thyroid gland overlies the first few rings of the trachea, which may make palpation of these rings difficult. The trachea may be followed caudally to the jugular notch, which is the rostral depression of the manubrium. The trachea may be palpated dorsally and the sternal heads of the sternocleidomastoid muscle may be palpated laterally. The sternocleidomastoid muscle is the key landmark of the ventral neck, with respect to the traditional division of the neck into triangles.

Triangles of the Neck

The sternocleidomastoid muscle divides the neck into two large triangles, posterior and anterior, which are then subdivided into two and four triangles, respectively. Knowledge of these triangles includes a definition of the borders and the contents of each triangle (Fig. 34-1).

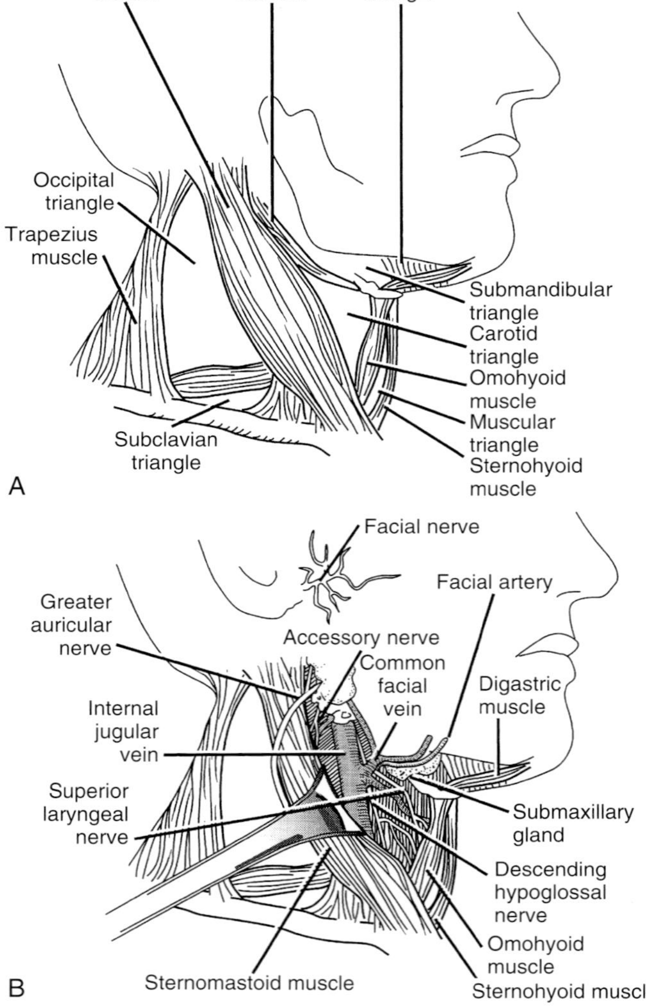

FIGURE 34-1. A, Cervical triangles. **B,** Carotid triangle and its contents. (Copyright University of New Mexico, Division of Neurosurgery, with permission.)

Posterior (Dorsal) Triangle

The borders of the posterior (dorsal) triangle are the dorsal edge of the sternocleidomastoid muscle, the ventral edge of the trapezius muscle, and the middle third of the clavicle. The deep cervical fascia covers the dorsal cervical triangle, thus forming its roof. The floor of the dorsal cervical triangle is formed by the scalenus posterior, scalenus medius, levator scapulae, and splenius capitis muscles, as well as the lateral extension of the prevertebral fascia that overlies these muscles. The dorsal belly of the omohyoid muscle partitions the dorsal cervical triangle into a large rostral occipital triangle named for the occipital artery exiting at its apex and a small caudal subclavian triangle named for the subclavian artery, which lies deep to it.

The spinal accessory nerve leaves the deep surface of the sternocleidomastoid muscle to enter the dorsal triangle of the neck, which it crosses to innervate the trapezius muscle. The two important structures found in the dorsal cervical triangle, which arise above the spinal accessory nerve, are the occipital artery and the lesser occipital nerve. The occipital artery leaves the dorsal cervical triangle at its apex where the sternocleidomastoid and trapezius muscles approach one another on the superior nuchal line. This artery then ascends to supply the dorsal scalp. The lesser occipital nerve ascends along the dorsal surface of the sternocleidomastoid muscle before dividing into several superficial branches that supply the scalp dorsal to the ear.

Caudal to the spinal accessory nerve are many important anatomic structures. The external jugular vein, which is formed by the confluence of the posterior auricular and the posterior division of the retromandibular vein at the angle of the mandible, courses over the sternocleidomastoid muscle obliquely to enter the dorsal cervical triangle caudally, en route to joining the subclavian vein approximately 2 cm above the clavicle.[3] Two branches of the thyrocervical trunk cross the dorsal cervical triangle. The suprascapular artery runs rostral to the clavicle before passing deep to the clavicle to supply the periscapular muscles. The transverse cervical artery lies 2 to 3 cm rostral to the clavicle and also runs laterally across the dorsal cervical triangle to supply the periscapular muscles.

Three superficial nerves also exit the dorsal triangle below the spinal accessory nerve. In all cases, these nerves arise from the cervical plexus, which is formed by the ventral rami of the rostral four cervical spinal nerves. The plexus lies within the lateral neurovascular conduction pathways located between the internal jugular vein and the sternocleidomastoid muscle. The superficial nerves then arise along the middle portion of the dorsal border of the sternocleidomastoid muscle to supply the skin of the neck and scalp between the mastoid process and the inion. The great auricular nerve crosses the sternocleidomastoid muscle and ascends toward the parotid gland, branching into dorsal and ventral rami that supply the skin in an area stretching from the angle of the mandible to the mastoid process and the skin of the neck. The transverse cervical nerve also crosses the sternocleidomastoid muscle to supply the skin overlying the ventral cervical triangle. The supraclavicular nerves arise from a single trunk that trifurcates into lateral, intermediate, and medial branches that innervate the skin of the neck, ventral chest, ventral shoulder, sternoclavicular joint, and acromioclavicular joint. The phrenic nerve arises, in part, from the cervical plexus and, in part, from the brachial plexus. The brachial nerve arises near the scalenus anterior muscle, where it crosses ventromedially and deep to the transverse cervical and suprascapular arteries and the prevertebral fascia, to descend through the superior thoracic aperture near the origin of the internal mammary artery. The upper, middle, and lower trunks of the brachial plexus lie deep to the floor of the posterior cervical triangle. They emerge between the scalenus medius and scalenus anterior muscles and cross deep to the transverse cervical and suprascapular arteries to descend under the clavicle to enter the axilla.

Anterior (Ventral) Triangle

The borders of the anterior (ventral) cervical triangle are the ventral edge of the sternocleidomastoid muscle, the inferior border of the mandible, and the midline of the neck. The ventral cervical triangle may be subdivided into four smaller triangles: submental, submandibular, carotid, and muscular.

The submental triangle is bounded by the hyoid body and laterally by the ventral bellies of the right and left digastric muscles. This triangle has, as its floor, the two mylohyoid muscles that connect to each other in the midline by forming a median raphe. Within this triangle lie the submental lymph nodes that drain the ventral tongue, the floor of the oral cavity, the middle portion of the lower lip and the skin of the chin, and several small veins that ultimately converge to form the anterior jugular vein.

The boundaries of the submandibular triangle are the anterior and posterior bellies of the digastric muscle and the inferior border of the mandible. The floor of the submandibular triangle is formed by the mylohyoid, hyoglossus, and middle constrictor muscles. The submandibular gland fills a significant portion of this triangle, and its duct passes parallel to the tongue to open into the mouth. The hypoglossal nerve also passes into this triangle along with the nerve to the mylohyoid muscle, a branch of the inferior alveolar nerve, and portions of the facial artery and vein.

The carotid triangle is bounded by the ventral border of the sternocleidomastoid muscle, the rostral edge of the rostral belly of the omohyoid muscle, and the caudal edge of the dorsal belly of the digastric muscle. Within the carotid triangle lie the bifurcation of the common carotid artery, the internal jugular vein laterally, the vagus nerve dorsally, and the ansa cervicalis (see Fig. 34-1B).

The muscular triangle is bounded by the median plane of the neck, the caudal edge of the rostral belly of the omohyoid muscle, and the medial border of the sternocleidomastoid muscle. Within this triangle lie the infrahyoid muscles and neck viscera.

Cervical Fascia

An understanding of the cervical fascia aids the surgeon approaching a targeted cervical spine level by providing an avascular plane of dissection. There are three layers of the cervical fascia: investing, visceral, and prevertebral (Fig. 34-2). The investing fascia surrounds the entire neck, splitting to enclose the sternocleidomastoid and trapezius muscles and the submandibular and parotid glands. Rostrally, the investing fascia is connected to the hyoid bone, caudal border of the mandible, zygomatic arch, mastoid process, and superior nuchal line. Caudally, the investing fascia splits to attach to the ventral and dorsal surfaces of the sternum, thus forming the suprasternal space.[3] The investing fascia forms the roof of both the ventral and dorsal cervical triangles.

The visceral, or pretracheal, fascia courses deep to the infrahyoid muscles and surrounds the visceral space, including the thyroid gland, trachea, and esophagus. The visceral fascia is attached to the hyoid bone and the thyroid cartilage rostrally and extends caudally to the dorsal surface of the clavicles and sternum and into the mediastinum. Laterally, this layer blends into the carotid sheath. The thyroid vessels are located deep to this layer.

The prevertebral layer of cervical fascia surrounds the vertebral column and its musculature, including the scalene and longus groups of muscles. Ventral to the vertebral bodies, the prevertebral fascia splits into a ventral alar layer and a dorsal prevertebral layer, forming a potential space. This space is referred to as the "danger zone" because it extends from the skull base rostrally to the level of T12 caudally and communicates with the mediastinum. Within the prevertebral fascia, and in front of the longus colli muscle, lies the cervical portion of the sympathetic chain.

Cervical Sympathetic Chain

The cervical sympathetic chain (CSC) usually consists of three cervical ganglia that lie at the levels of the first rib, the transverse process of C6, and the atlantoaxial complex, respectively. The CSC lies directly over the longus colli muscles and beneath the prevertebral fascia.[4] The chain runs in a superior and lateral direction with an average angle of 10.4 ± 3.8 degrees relative to the midline.[4] The superior ganglion is typically located at C2-3[4] or C4[5] and lies more laterally on the splenius capitis. The average distance between the CSC and the medial border of the longus colli muscles at C6, however, is 10.6 ± 2.6 mm.[4] Therefore the CSC is considerally more vulnerable to damage at lower levels due to its

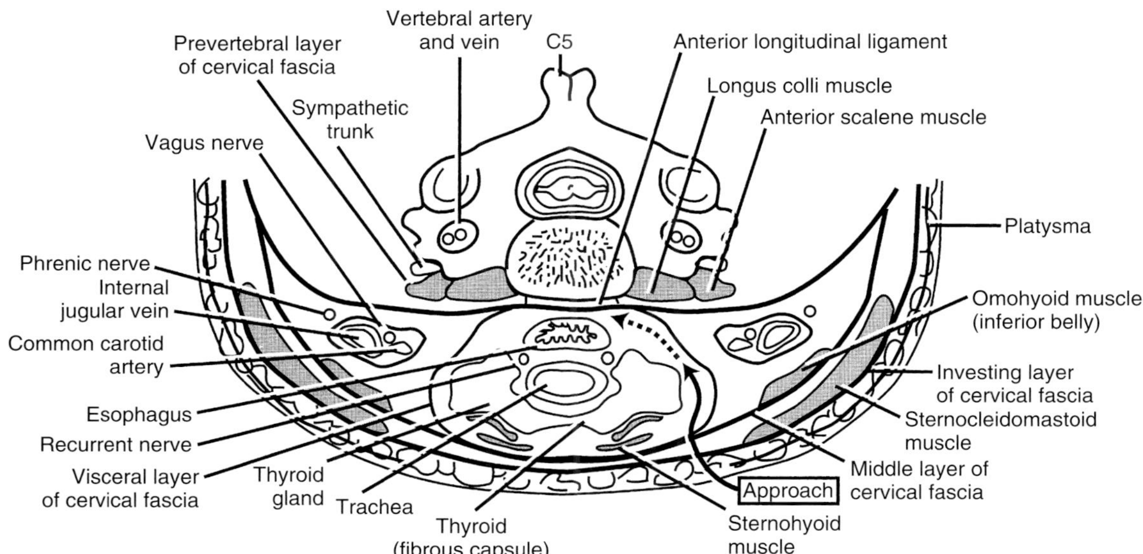

FIGURE 34-2. Cervical fascia. (Copyright University of New Mexico, Division of Neurosurgery, with permission.)

more medial location. While the longus colli diverge laterally when descending down the cervical spine, the CSCs converge medially at C6.[4] The average diameter of the CSC at C6 is 2.7 ± 0.6 mm.[4] Potential damage to the CSC may result during longus colli dissection off the anterior vertebral bodies or during lateral rectraction of the carotid sheath and/or longus colli.[4] Fibers from the superior cervical ganglia pass to the internal carotid artery to innervate the pupil. Interruption of the sympathetic trunk in the neck results in an ipsilateral Horner syndrome.

Cervical Musculature

The cervical musculature is divided into two layers: superficial and deep. The muscles of the superficial layer include the platysma, the sternocleidomastoid, and the infrahyoid group. The platysma lies just under the surface of the skin and is one of the muscles of facial expression, innervated by the cervical ramus of the seventh cranial nerve. It is draped like an apron from the mandible to the level of the second rib and laterally as far as the acromion processes. The sternocleidomastoid muscle arises from the region of the jugular notch and courses rostrolaterally to the mastoid process. It is dually innervated by the 11th cranial nerve and ventral branches of the C2-4 spinal nerves. The spinal accessory nerve enters the deep surface of the muscle at the border of the middle and rostral thirds. The two main actions of the sternocleidomastoid muscle are to turn the head to the contralateral side and to flex the head ipsilaterally. The infrahyoid group represents the rostral continuation of the rectus muscular system of the trunk.[2] This group contains four muscles: sternohyoid, sternothyroid, omohyoid, and thyrohyoid. The first three members of this group are innervated by the ansa cervicalis, and the thyrohyoid receives its innervation from the C1 spinal nerve via the hypoglossal nerve. The main actions of the infrahyoid group are to assist in swallowing and mastication. This group, together with the suprahyoid group, determines the rostrocaudal location of the larynx between the hyoid bone and the rostral thoracic aperture and can help flex the cervical spine and lower the head.

The deep layer of cervical musculature includes two groups: scalene and longus groups. The scalene group includes three muscles: anterior, medius, and posterior. These muscles form a roof over the cupula of the lung. As a group, these muscles arise from the transverse processes of the subaxial cervical spine and project to the first and second ribs. The scalene muscles are innervated by the ventral rami of C4-8. They help to elevate the rib cage during respiration. The longus group also includes three muscles: rectus capitis anterior, longus capitis, and longus colli (Fig. 34-3). As a group, these muscles arise from the ventral vertebral body, transverse processes, and basilar portion of the occiput. They project caudally along the ventrolateral aspects of the cervical and upper thoracic vertebral bodies. These muscles are innervated by the ventral rami of C1-6, and their main action is to flex the head and the cervical spine.

Longus Colli

The longus colli attach to the anterior atlas, the vertebral bodies of C3-T3, and the transverse processes of C3-6.[6] The distance between the medial borders of the longus colli muscles increases in a rostral to caudal direction, measuring 7.9 ± 2.2 mm at C3, 10.1 ± 3.1 mm at C4, 12.3 ± 3.1 mm at C5, and 13.8 ± 2.2 mm at C6.[6] A great deal of variation exists in this musculature, so care should be taken in using it as a landmark for lateral dissection.

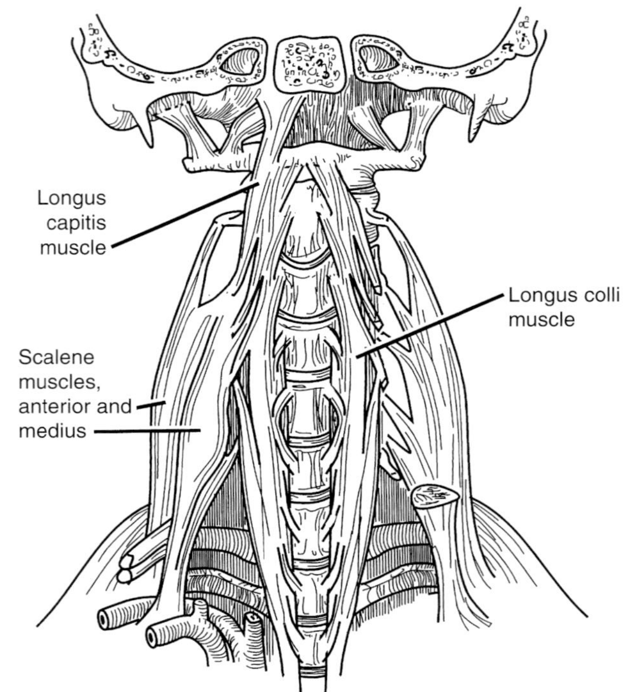

FIGURE 34-3. The scalene and longus muscles. (Copyright University of New Mexico, Division of Neurosurgery, with permission.)

Cervical Viscera

The cervical viscera are arranged in three layers: a deep gastrointestinal layer, containing the pharynx and esophagus; a middle respiratory layer, containing the larynx and trachea; and a superficial endocrine layer, containing the thyroid and parathyroid glands. These structures are not covered in detail here, and much of the anatomy of the larynx and trachea has already been described in other sections of this chapter. As previously noted, these structures are contained within the visceral or pretracheal fascia.

The pharynx is a fibromuscular tube that projects from the pharyngeal tubercle of the clivus to its transition into the esophagus near the level of C6. The dorsal surface of the pharynx lies on the prevertebral fascia and must be mobilized during ventral approaches to the cervical spine. The muscles of the pharynx may be divided into two groups: constrictors and internal muscles of the pharynx. The constrictor group includes three muscles whose main action is to sequentially constrict the pharynx during swallowing, propelling food caudally. All of the constrictors are innervated by the pharyngeal plexus, which receives its branches from both the glossopharyngeal and vagus nerves. The constrictors do not form a continuous tube but are open at four points, allowing certain structures to pass into the pharynx. Rostral to the superior constrictor, the ascending palatine artery, the eustachian tube, and the levator veli palatini muscles pass to enter the pharynx. Between the superior and inferior constrictors pass the glossopharyngeal nerve, the stylohyoid ligament, and the stylopharyngeus muscle. In the gap between the middle and inferior constrictors pass the internal laryngeal nerve and the superior laryngeal artery and vein. Caudal to the inferior constrictor pass the recurrent laryngeal nerve and the inferior laryngeal artery. The internal muscle groups of the pharynx have a common function of elevating the larynx and pharynx during swallowing and a common innervation by the glossopharyngeal nerve. At the level of C6, the pharynx blends into the esophagus, which passes through the superior thoracic aperture to the stomach. In the root of the neck, the esophagus is in close approximation to the thoracic duct as it empties into the left subclavian vein.

Thoracic Duct

The thoracic duct is located on the left side within a triangle bounded medially by the longus colli muscles and the esophagus, laterally by the anterior scalene muscle, and inferiorly by the first rib.[7,8] Although it may ascend as high as C6, it is most often found between C7 and T1, before it descends to empty into a variable termination at the jugulosubclavian junction.[7,8] The rostral extension of the thoracic duct appears to vary by gender, as in patients who have a narrow thoracic inlet, as most women do, the duct may ascend as high as the level of the C6 vertebral body. Conversely, in patients who have a wide thoracic inlet, as most men do, the duct may ascend to the level of the C7-T1 disc, never truly leaving the mediastinum. Many have cited the increased possibility of injuring this structure in the left upper thorax as a reason for preferring a right-sided approach, especially to the upper thoracic vertebrae.[7]

The isthmus of the thyroid gland usually overlies the first two or three tracheal rings. The isthmus is the center bridge of glandular tissue that connects the right and left lobes. The entire gland is surrounded by a fibrous capsule, which should be differentiated from the pretracheal fascia. The thyroid gland is heavily vascularized and receives its blood supply from the superior and inferior thyroid arteries, which are branches of the external carotid and thyrocervical arteries, respectively. The recurrent laryngeal nerve is in close approximation to the inferior thyroid artery, and if this artery must be ligated, it is best ligated at a distance from the thyroid gland to avoid the nerve. A similar relationship exists between the superior thyroid artery and the external laryngeal nerve, again dictating arterial ligation distal from the substance of the gland. The thyroid gland is drained by the superior, middle, and inferior thyroid veins. The inferior thyroid veins may cover the ventral surface of the trachea and represent a potential source of bleeding during tracheotomy.

Laryngeal Nerves

The vagus nerve, or cranial nerve X, emerges from the brainstem, exits the intracranial space via the jugular foramen, and passes through the neck, chest, and abdomen, where it contributes to the innervation of the viscera. In the cervical region, both the right and left vagus nerves lie within the carotid sheath, lateral to the carotid artery. Near its passage through the thoracic inlet, the vagus nerve branches, giving rise to the recurrent laryngeal nerves (RLNs), which subsequently ascend toward the larynx. Before doing so, however, each RLN assumes a different course. The right RLN leaves the main trunk of the vagus and passes anterior to and then under the subclavian artery. This loop occurs at the T1-3 level. Meanwhile, the left RLN passes under and posterior to the aorta at the site of origin of the ligamentum arteriosum, a loop that is found at the T3-6 level.[9] The right RLN also courses rostrally in a more oblique fashion (in a superior and medial direction at an angle of 25 ± 4.7 degrees relative to the sagittal plane) than the left RLN (4.7 ± 3.7 degrees).[9] In the neck, the left RLN lies in the tracheoesophageal groove, entering at the midpoint of its course. The right RLN, however, lies 6.5 ± 1.2 mm anterior and 7.3 ± 0.8 mm lateral to the tracheoesophageal groove at C7, with high variability at this site and throughout its course.[9] The left RLN, therefore, is better protected from iatrogenic injury. Anatomic variations of the RLN such as nonrecurrence on either side or the nerves' entering the larynx directly after their takeoff from the vagus are overall extremely rare.[9]

Nearing their entrance into the laryngeal structures at C5-7, the RLNs lie in close association with the inferior thyroid arteries (ITAs). The RLN length between the superior margin of the clavicle and the ITA is 23 ± 4.4 mm on the left and 22.8 ± 4.3 mm on the right.[9] The RLNs' relation to the ITA branches, however, is highly variable; on the right, the RLN is more commonly found anterior (26–33% of the time) or between the arterial branches, whereas on the left, the RLN is more commonly posterior (50–55%).[9]

Although unilateral RLN palsy is reported to be the most common nerve-related injury after anterior cervical surgery, the overall incidence of the resultant hoarseness is relatively low at 2% to 4%. This may be avoided by recognizing the sites at which the RLN is most vulnerable. The nerve is susceptible to injury if the dissection plane is not maintained entirely medial to the carotid sheath, if the longus colli dissection is not limited to the area between the muscle and the vertebrae, or if the dissection is carried superficial to the esophagus.[7] As mentioned earlier, the right RLN is vulnerable to injury if ligation of the inferior thyroid vessels is not performed as laterally as possible or with prolonged retraction without intermittent interruption.[9] The superior laryngeal nerve (SLN) originates from the inferior vagal ganglion at the C2 level and then descends medially toward the thyrohyoid membrane.[10] At the C3 level, the SLN branches into external and internal branches deep to the internal carotid artery.[10,11] The external branch of the SLN (EBSLN) travels with the cricothyroid artery and descends deep to the superior thyroid artery (STA) toward the cricothyroid muscle.[10] The internal branch travels with the superior laryngeal artery and passes deep to a loop of the STA before piercing the thyrohyoid membrane.[10,12] Both the external and internal branches of the SLN are within the fascia overlying the longus colli muscles.[11]

Conduction Pathways

The neck has two major neurovascular conduction pathways: cervicocranial and cervicobrachial (Fig. 34-4). The cervicocranial neurovascular bundle is outlined by the carotid sheath, which contains the common carotid artery medially, the internal jugular vein laterally, the vagus nerve dorsally, and the lymphatic plexus. As a whole, the cervicocranial neurovascular bundle lies laterally to the visceral space and ventrally to the prevertebral fascia. The bundle passes rostrally from the

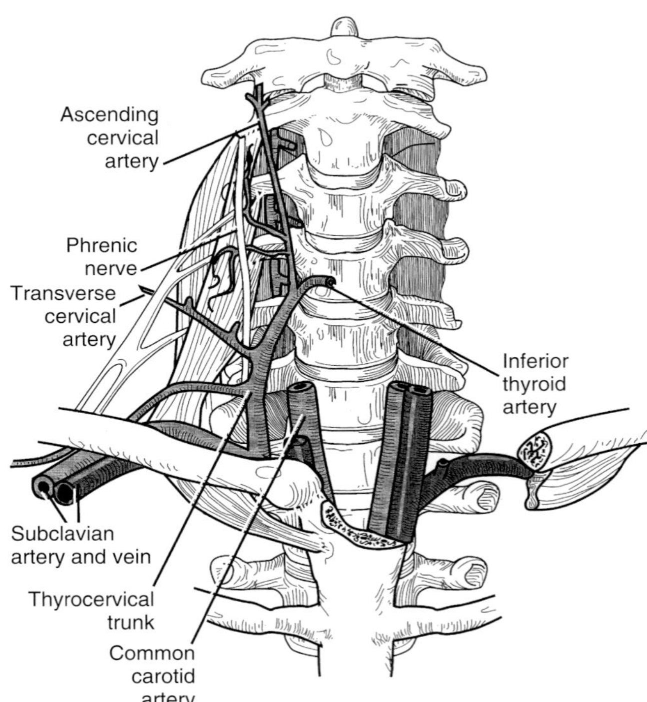

FIGURE 34-4. The conduction pathways. (Copyright University of New Mexico, Division of Neurosurgery, with permission.)

thorax and enters the carotid triangle, where the common carotid artery bifurcates into the internal carotid artery dorsolaterally and the external carotid artery ventromedially.

Within the carotid triangle, the external carotid artery provides a total of eight branches: three ventral, one medial, two dorsal, and two terminal. The ventral branches include the superior thyroid, lingual, and facial arteries. The superior thyroid artery descends from its origin caudal to the greater cornu of the hyoid to supply the thyroid gland. The lingual artery also arises at the level of the greater cornu of the hyoid bone and crosses under the hyoglossus muscle to supply the tongue. The facial artery is the final ventral branch of the external carotid artery. It runs under the submandibular gland before crossing the mandible and arriving to supply the face at the ventral surface of the masseter muscle. The sole medial branch is the ascending pharyngeal artery, which arises from the medial external carotid artery to supply the pharyngeal wall. The two dorsal branches are the posterior auricular and occipital arteries. The posterior auricular artery runs from underneath the parotid gland to the mastoid process. The occipital artery also reaches the mastoid but on its medial aspect in the groove named for the artery. The two terminal branches are the superficial temporal and maxillary arteries. The internal jugular vein originates in the jugular foramen as the superior bulb turns dorsolaterally to enter the carotid sheath lateral to the common carotid artery. It eventually drains into the subclavian vein.

Five of the cranial nerves—facial, glossopharyngeal, vagus, spinal accessory, and hypoglossal—traverse the neck. The facial nerve exits the skull at the stylomastoid foramen and ramifies into five branches within the parotid gland. The most caudal branch, the marginal mandibular, courses under the mandible and may be encountered in retropharyngeal approaches. Damage to this ramus results in drooping of the ipsilateral lip. Arising from the jugular foramen are the vagus, glossopharyngeal, and spinal accessory nerves. The vagus travels dorsally in the carotid sheath and gives off two important branches that run in the neck to supply the larynx.

The superior laryngeal nerve exits just below the inferior vagal ganglion and bifurcates into a small external laryngeal nerve that supplies the motor innervation to the inferior pharyngeal constrictor and cricothyroid muscles. This nerve also bifurcates into a large internal laryngeal branch that receives the sensory input of the laryngeal mucosa above the glottis. Damage to the superior laryngeal nerve results in early fatigue of voice, difficulty in producing high notes, and decreased gag reflex, resulting in a risk of aspiration. Both inferior laryngeal nerves ascend from the thorax in the tracheoesophageal groove, enter the inferior pharyngeal constrictor to supply motor innervation to the intrinsic laryngeal muscles, and receive all sensory innervation below the glottis. Damage to the inferior laryngeal nerve results in hoarseness.

The glossopharyngeal nerve exits the skull from the jugular foramen in close approximation to the vagus nerve and courses between the internal carotid artery and the internal jugular vein before passing between the stylopharyngeus and styloglossus muscles to enter the base of the tongue. The caudal ganglion of the glossopharyngeal nerve has two branches. The tympanic nerve, which supplies sensory innervation to the tympanic mucosa, divides into the tympanic plexus, from which the lesser petrosal parasympathetic fibers form to supply the otic ganglion. The communicating rami join the auricular ramus of the vagus. Below the inferior ganglion, the glossopharyngeal nerve divides into the following branches: stylopharyngeal ramus, carotid sinus ramus, tonsillar ramus, lingual ramus, and pharyngeal ramus. Both the vagus nerve and the glossopharyngeal nerve contribute to the pharyngeal plexus, which mediates motor and sensory innervation of the pharynx.

The spinal accessory nerve traverses the rostrodorsal corner of the carotid triangle to reach the deep surface of the sternocleidomastoid muscle one third of the distance from the mastoid to the clavicle and then continues through the occipital triangle to supply the trapezius muscle. The hypoglossal nerve exits the skull from the hypoglossal canal, enters the carotid triangle deep to the dorsal belly of the digastric, and courses between the carotid artery and the internal jugular vein before turning medially to enter the substance of the tongue. The hypoglossal nerve gives off the superior branch to the ansa cervicalis, which innervates the strap muscles and may be divided at the time of surgery.

The other major neurovascular conduction pathway is the cervicobrachial pathway, which supplies the upper extremities. The subclavian artery and the components of the brachial plexus exit the neck over the first rib and between the anterior and middle scalene muscles and then proceed through the posterior triangle of the neck to enter the axilla. The subclavian artery gives off the following arteries: vertebral, thyrocervical, internal thoracic, costocervical, and dorsal scapular. The vertebral artery is the vessel of most interest to the spine surgeon (Fig. 34-5). It arises from the dorsal aspect of the subclavian artery and courses medial to the anterior scalenus to enter the foramen transversarium of the sixth cervical vertebra. It then ascends in the foramen transversarium until the level of the axis, where it courses medially in a groove bearing its name and through the atlanto-occipital membrane to enter the cranial

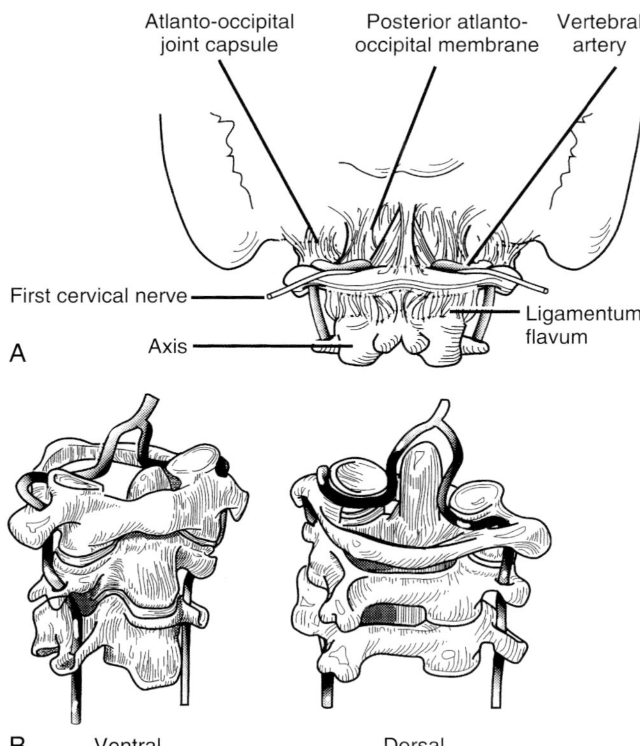

FIGURE 34-5. The cervicocranium and the vertebral artery relationships. **A,** Dorsal soft tissue and bony relationships of the vertebral artery; **B,** ventral *(left),* dorsal *(right),* and bony relationships of the vertebral artery. (Copyright University of New Mexico, Division of Neurosurgery, with permission.)

cavity. The subclavian vein runs ventral to the artery and to the scalenus anterior muscle just under the clavicle.

Vertebral Artery

The vertebral artery (VA) usually originates from the subclavian, or innominate, artery on the right and the aortic arch on the left. The artery is typically divided into four anatomic segments: the first segment, V1, consists of the artery's origin to the C6 transverse foramen; the second segment, V2, passes cranially from the C6 to the C2 transverse foramen; the third segment, V3, exits C2 and extends to the level of the foramen magnum; and the final portion, V4, passes through the foramen magnum and reaches to the vertebrobasilar junction.[13]

Due to the frequency of operative procedures in the subaxial spine, the anatomy of the V2 segment has been thoroughly reviewed. After ascending cranially, V1 passes by the transverse process of C7 anteriorly and laterally before entering the transverse foramen of C6.[14] V2 then extends from the artery's entry into the C6 foramen to the transverse foramen of C2.[15] In 94.9% of specimens, C6 is the first transverse foramen entered, but variations do exist (C4 in 1.6%, C5 in 3.3%, and C7 in 0.3%).[13] Within the intertransverse space, the vertebral artery and nerve root are encased in a fibroligamentous band. This band is attached to the lateral aspect of the uncinate process and the uncovertebral (UV) joint, combining the artery, nerve root, and uncinate process as a unit.[16] Before resection of the uncinate process or UV joint (i.e., uncoforaminotomy), it is necessary to dissect this fibroligamentous tissue off of the uncinate process.[16] In addition, it must be noted that the posterior and medial portion of the VA gives rise to numerous spinal and muscular branches in the intertransverse space.[15,17]

For a number of reasons, the V2 segment of the vertebral artery is more at risk during decompression of more cephalad vertebrae.[14,16,17] First, the diameter of the artery decreases from C2-3 to C6-7 (4.88 ± 0.63 mm at C2-3 to 4.27 ± 0.63 mm at C6-7),[17] and the anteroposterior diameters of the transverse foramina decrease from C6 to C3 (5.4 ± 1.1 mm at C6 to 4.7 ± 0.7 mm at C3).[14] The amount of the intertransverse space occupied by the artery, therefore, increases at more rostral levels.[17] Second, the artery ascends medially from C6-3 at an angle of approximately 4 degrees relative to midline, making it more likely to be encountered in the surgical field at higher cervical levels.[18] Finally, a series of other relationships places the VA at greater risk of iatrogenic injury at more cephalad levels. These include decreased interforaminal distance (27.4 mm ± 2.3 mm at C6 to 22.6 ± 1.8 mm at C3), width of the vertebrae (25.6 ± 2 mm at C7 to 19.2 ± 1.8 mm at C3), interuncinate distance (24.6 ± 2.1 mm at C7 to 19.2 ± 1.5 mm at C3), and distance from the lateral tip of the uncinate process to the medial border of the transverse foramen (3.3 ± 1 mm at C6 to 1.7 ± 0.8 mm at C4) at higher levels.[14] In addition, it should also be noted that because the vertebral artery is more anterior at C6 and becomes more posterior as it travels toward C3, there is greater risk with anterolateral uncinate resection in more caudad levels and with posterolateral decompression in more cephalad levels.[19]

Three possible risk factors have been identified for vertebral artery injury: motorized dissection with a high-speed diamond burr used off midline, excessive lateral dissection of bone and disc, and the bone of the lateral part of the spinal canal being pathologically softened by infection or tumor.[20] Intraoperative VA injury can be largely avoided by following a number of guidelines. If far lateral decompression is necessary, the anterior wall of the transverse foramina should be removed, the vertebral artery retracted laterally, and small rongeurs and curettes used, rather than a high-speed drill.[14,16] In performing foraminotomies, lateral dissection can generally be carried safely to the medial margin of the UV joint in most patients. Care should be taken, however, when extending farther laterally and should likely not exceed 5 to 6 mm beyond the nerve root's emergence from the thecal sac.[19] This is because the posterior surface of V2 rests on the anteromedial aspect of the cervical nerve roots at each level of the intertransverse space, and the mean length of the nerve root between the dural sac and the VA is 6.3 ± 1.06 mm.[15]

In posterior approaches, injury to the vertebral artery is more common than in ventral surgery. Whereas in anterior cervical procedures, the artery is most at risk during osseous decompression, the placement of posterior instrumentation is the portion of that procedure during which there is greatest risk for VA injury. It is, therefore, important to recognize the artery's relationship to the osseous structures of the posterior column. The shortest distance from the artery to the cervical pedicle increases from C3 to C5 (0.5 ± 0.2 mm at C3, 1.1 ± 0.4 mm at C4, 1.4 ± 0.8 mm at C5), decreases at C6 (0.9 ± 0.5 mm), and then dramatically increases at C7 (7.3 ± 2.7 mm).[21] As the VA emerges from the C2 transverse foramen, it travels in a groove extending horizontally from the medial border of the transverse foramen to the medial edge of the posterior ring.[19] To avoid injury, exposure of the posterior ring of the atlas should remain medial to that groove.[19] In about 80% of patients, the VA makes an acute lateral bend in the C2 lateral mass just under the superior articular facet.[19] If the trajectory of a C1-2 transarticular screw is aimed too low, the VA may be injured here.[19] In C2 pedicle screws, lateral perforation of the pedicle puts the VA at risk, and in C1 lateral mass screws, the VA is vulnerable near its exit from the C2 transverse foramen where it lies in close proximity to the C1 lateral mass.[19]

Nuchal Musculature

The intrinsic musculature of the dorsal neck may be divided into three layers: superficial, intermediate, and deep (Fig. 34-6). All of these muscles are innervated by the dorsal rami of several consecutive spinal nerves. The superficial layer contains the splenius capitis and the splenius cervicalis, which take their origin from the ligamentum nuchae and the spinous processes of C6-T1. The splenius capitis inserts along the lateral third of the superior nuchal line and on the mastoid process. The splenius cervicalis muscle inserts into the posterior tubercles of the transverse processes of C1-4. These muscles produce extension, lateral bending, and rotation of the head or neck.

The intermediate layer is composed of the massive erector spinae group, of which there are three columns: spinalis medially, iliocostalis laterally, and longissimus muscle between. All three columns share a common origin from the iliac crest, sacrum, and caudal lumbar spinous processes. The spinalis group inserts along the spinous processes of the cervical spine. The longissimus group inserts onto the mastoid process, and the iliocostalis group inserts into the posterior tubercles of the transverse processes of C4-6. As a group, the erector spinae muscles act to extend or laterally bend the head or neck.

The deep layer of the spinal musculature is also termed the *transversospinalis group* because it lies in the angle of the spinous and transverse processes. This layer is divided into three groups. The semispinalis group lies most superficially and has both capitis and cervicalis divisions. The semispinalis capitis muscle arises from the transverse processes of T1-6 and inserts medially between the superior and inferior nuchal lines. The semispinalis cervicalis muscle originates from the transverse processes of the lower cervical and upper thoracic spine and inserts on the cervical spinous processes. Beneath the semispinalis division lies the multifidus division, which comprises short muscles that span only one to three spinal segments. These muscles pass from the lamina caudally to the spinous process of the adjacent level. The deepest divisions of the transversospinalis group are the rotators that arise from the transverse process of one vertebral level and insert on the base of the spinous process at the adjacent rostral level. As a group, the transversospinalis muscles produce rotation and extension of the head or neck.

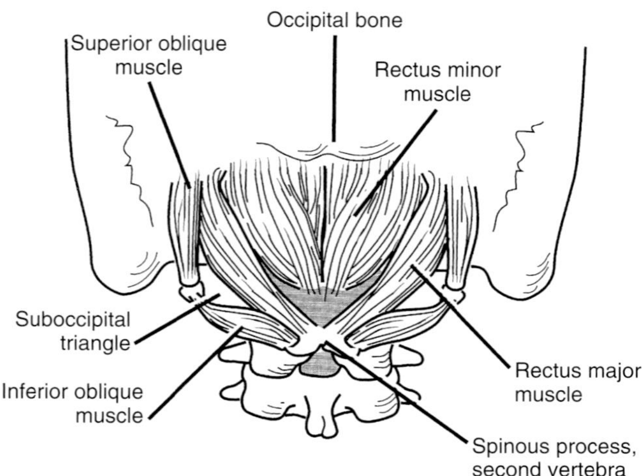

FIGURE 34-6. The suboccipital region. (Copyright University of New Mexico, Division of Neurosurgery, with permission.)

Spinal Anatomy

The upper cervical spine is characterized by the axis and its "anatomic neighbors" (Fig. 34-7). The subaxial cervical spine varies minimally from level to level and is discussed as a single unit (Fig. 34-8). The components of the subaxial vertebrae include the body, upper and lower articular processes, pedicles, lamina, and spinous process. The vertebral bodies are the axial load-bearing elements of the spine. In the subaxial cervical spine the vertebral body height increases as the spine is descended with a slight reversal of this relationship at C6, which is usually shorter than either C5 or C7. Each body has a dorsally directed concavity that forms the ventral spinal canal. From each body arise three body projections: rostrally the uncus, laterally the ventral ramus of the transverse process, and dorsolaterally the pedicle.

The rostral aspect of each of the lower cervical vertebral bodies contains the uncus, a dorsolateral bony projection. The uncus gives the body a rostrally concave shape in the coronal plane and enables the vertebral body to receive the rounded caudal aspect of the immediately adjacent vertebral body, sometimes overlapping the next level by a third of the vertebral body height. The uncovertebral joints limit lateral translation and contribute to the coupling of lateral bending and rotation of the cervical spine.

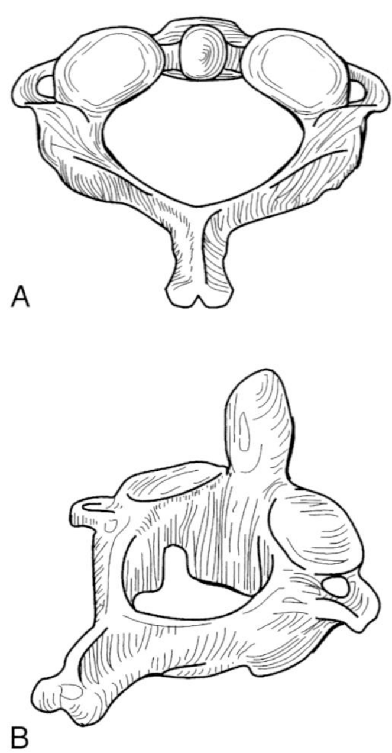

FIGURE 34-7. The axis. **A,** Axial view from above. Note that the articular facets and odontoid are anterior to the spinal canal. **B,** Posterior view. (Copyright University of New Mexico, Division of Neurosurgery, with permission.)

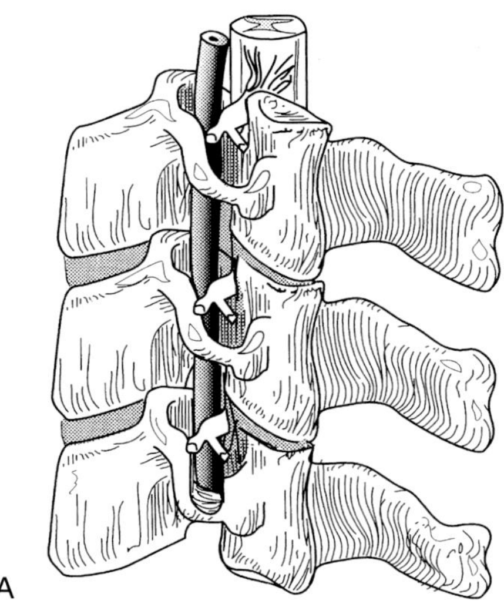

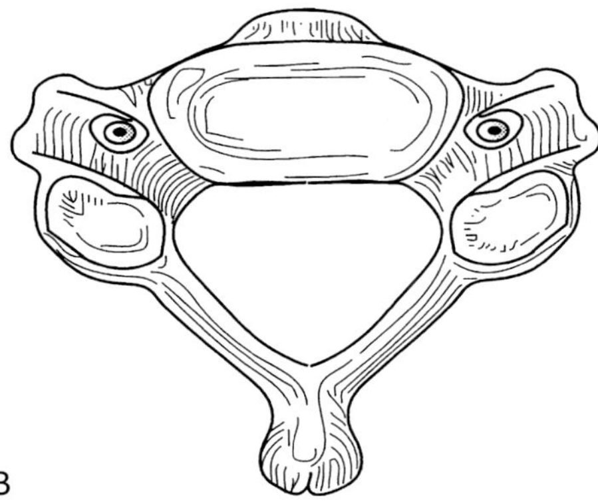

FIGURE 34-8. The subaxial spine. **A,** Lateral view; **B,** axial view. (Copyright University of New Mexico, Division of Neurosurgery, with permission.)

The anterior tubercle arises from the rostral vertebral body and projects laterally while the posterior tubercle arises from the midportion of the lateral mass and projects ventromedially to join the anterior tubercle. The lateral surface of the pedicle, the dorsal surface of the anterior tubercle, and the ventral surface of the posterior tubercle form the foramen transversarium, which transmits the vertebral artery from C6 to the atlas. The anterior scalene, longus colli capitis, longus colli cervicalis, and ventral intertransversus muscles take their origin from the anterior tubercles. The splenius cervicalis, longissimus, levator scapulae, middle scalene, posterior scalene, and iliocostalis take their origin from the posterior tubercle. On the rostral surface of each transverse process there is a prominent groove carrying the exiting nerve root.

The pedicles of the subaxial cervical spine connect the vertebral bodies with the lateral masses and are small and medially oriented. The lateral masses of the subaxial cervical spine consist of superior and inferior articulating surfaces that form the facet joint. The facet joint is a coronally oriented synovial joint that is protected by a thin capsule. The vascular supply to the joint capsule arises from the vertebral, ascending pharyngeal, deep transverse cervical, supreme intercostal, and occipital arteries. The facet joints are innervated by the dorsal branches of the spinal nerves, which enter the joint at the center of the dorsal capsule. The laminae are thin, and the spinous processes of the midcervical spine are small and often bifid.

Discs

The intervertebral discs adjoin each of the subaxial vertebral bodies and contribute significantly to the flexibility of the spine. The cartilaginous end plates of the bordering vertebral bodies are the rostral and caudal boundaries of the disc space, and the anterior and posterior longitudinal ligaments overlie, respectively, the ventral and dorsal surfaces of the intervertebral disc space. Laterally, the disc space is limited by the uncal process. The end plate is more substantial on its periphery than centrally and is composed of hyaline cartilage. The disc itself is composed of the gelatinous nucleus pulposus surrounded by a fibrous ring. The fibrous ring contains intersecting layers of predominantly collagen and, to a lesser extent, elastin fibers.

Ligaments

The ligaments of the cervical spine are essential for the maintenance of alignment and stability. The ligaments of the subaxial spine include the anterior longitudinal ligament, the posterior longitudinal ligament, the interspinous ligament, the supraspinous ligament, the capsular ligaments, the ligamentum flavum, and the intertransverse ligaments (Figs. 34-9 and 34-10). The anterior longitudinal ligament is attached to the ventral surfaces of the vertebral bodies and the intervening discs. It spans the entire length of the spine from the skull base to the sacrum. The main biomechanical feature of the anterior longitudinal ligament is resistance of hyperextension. The superficial fibers extend for four or five vertebral bodies, and the deep fibers span two vertebral bodies.

The posterior longitudinal ligament is attached to the discs on the dorsal surface of the vertebral bodies and rostrally fans out to become continuous with the tectorial membrane. The main biomechanical effect of the posterior longitudinal ligament is resistance of hyperflexion. The interspinous and supraspinous ligaments attach adjacent spinous processes and are represented in the cervical region as the ligamentum nuchae, which runs from the inion to the spinous process of C7. This fibromuscular septum divides the paraspinal muscles and serves as an attachment site for the nuchal musculature. This represents the midline avascular plane, which may be transversed when exposing the dorsal cervical spine. These ligaments can limit flexion to a significant degree because of their long lever arm, with respect to the instantaneous axis of rotation. The capsular ligaments are loose under normal cervical spine movement and become taut with movement, thus limiting excessive flexion and rotation. The ligamentum flavum is an elastic ligament that traverses adjacent laminae in a shingle-like fashion, arising from a ridge on the inner surface of the lamina and projecting to the inner surface of the next rostral lamina. The intertransverse ligaments connect adjacent transverse processes, which have little biomechanical effect in the cervical spine.

Ligamentum Nuchae

The ligamentum nuchae (LN) is a triangle-shaped intervertebral syndesmosis, a bilateral fibroelastic intermuscular septum interposed between paired groups of paravertebral muscles of the cerviconuchal region.[22] It is formed by the aponeurotic

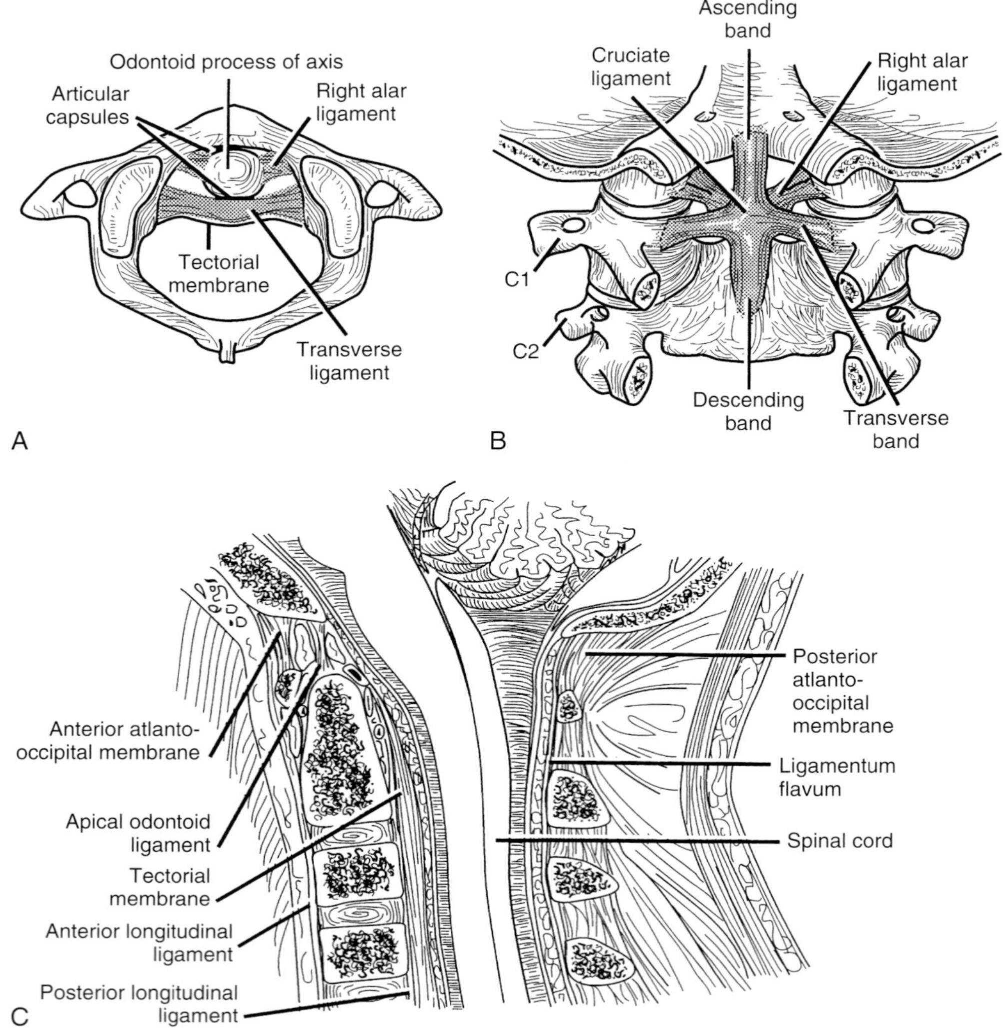

FIGURE 34-9. Ligaments of the cervical spine: **A,** axial, **B,** dorsal (after laminectomy), and **C,** midsagittal views. (Copyright University of New Mexico, Division of Neurosurgery, with permission.)

fibers of the trapezius, splenius capitis, rhomboideus minor, and serratus posterior superior muscles.[23] Functionally, the LN serves to maintain lordotic alignment and stabilize the head during rotation of the cervical region.[22] Extending from the external occipital protuberance, or inion, to the spinous process of C7, it is covered by layers of cervical fascia and the aponeurosis of the trapezius muscle.[22] During posterior exposure of the cervical spine and suboccipital region, it is important to identify and maintain the dissection plane within the LN in order to minimize tissue damage, blood loss, and the possibility of injury to lateral structures such as the vertebral arteries.

The LN consists of two components: the lamellar portion ventrally and the funicular portion dorsally. The latter is a fibrous raphe that corresponds to the fusion of the underlying layers of the lamellar portion. The dorsal component is attached to the inion and the C7 spinous process and is freely mobile between these two structures.[24] The lamellar portion is a double-layered midine septum with fatty areolar tissue interposed between its layers. It inserts into the medial side of the cervical vertebra's bifid spinous processes.[22] Attached rostrally at the inion and external occipital crest, the lamellar portion is superficial at C6-7 and deepest at C1.[22,24] Anteriorly, it seems to be continuous with the interspinous ligament, suboccipitally with the atlanto-occipital and the atlantoaxial membranes, as well as the posterior spinal dura, and rostrally with the periosteum of the occipital bone.[22,25] Although it is laterally continuous with the deep fascia of the semispinalis capitis and the splenius capitis, a cleavage plane separates the adjacent semispinalis capitis, allowing for a relatively easy intraoperative division.[24]

To ensure that the midline plane is respected with a posterior dissection, three strategies should be used: (1) Dissection should be maintained within the fatty areolar tissue of the LN's lamellar portion; (2) isolation and incision of the funicular portion should be carried from inside to outside; and (3) retrograde dissection of the cerviconuchal muscles attached to the occipital bone should be performed in a subperiosteal plane.[22]

Intervertebral Foramen

The cervical spinal nerves exit from the spinal canal through the intervertebral foramen. True foramina, with four distinct walls, are found in the subaxial cervical spine, and partial

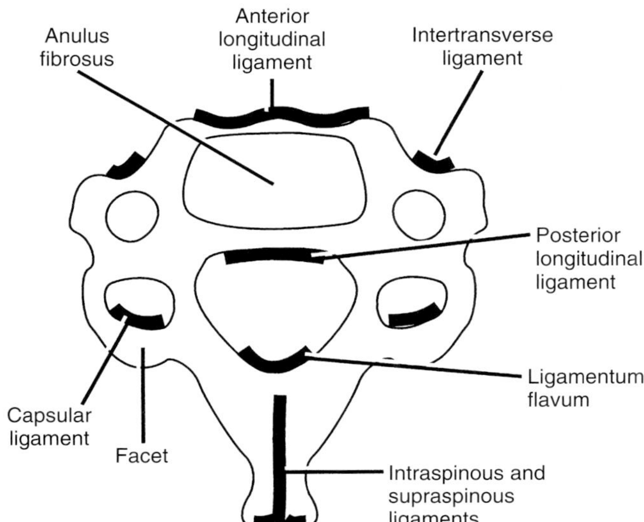

FIGURE 34-10. Ligaments of the subaxial cervical spine (axial view). (Copyright University of New Mexico, Division of Neurosurgery, with permission.)

foramina are present at the atlanto-occipital and atlantoaxial levels.

The pedicles form the rostral and caudal boundaries of each foramen. The cervical spinal nerves exit above the like-numbered pedicle in close proximity to both the cervical disc and the uncovertebral joint at that level. The ventral wall of the intervertebral foramen is formed rostrally by the vertebral body and caudally by the uncovertebral joint that overlies the disc space. The dorsal wall is formed by the capsule of the facet joint, which covers the underlying superior articular process. The superior articular process often projects above the uncal process of the same intervertebral foramen. Degeneration of either the uncovertebral joint or the facet joint can cause stenosis of the intervertebral foramen, resulting in radiculopathy. The spinal nerve crosses dorsally to the vertebral artery as it ascends in the foramen transversarium.

Blood Supply

The blood supply of the subaxial cervical spine is derived mainly from the vertebral artery with additional and variable contributions from the ascending pharyngeal, occipital, and deep cervical arteries.

The vertebral artery branches segmentally to supply the cervical spine through two main branches: ventral branch and dorsal branch. The ventral branch is transmitted across the midportion of the lateral surface of the vertebral bodies below the transverse process and below the longus colli muscles. It contributes to the blood supply of the ventral vertebral body through the accompanying ventral vertebral body arterial plexus.

The dorsal branch enters the intervertebral foramen and, in turn, gives off three branches. The first is transmitted along the nerve roots and supplies the spinal cord itself, anastomosing with the anterior and posterior spinal arteries. The second branch supplies the inner surface of the lamina and the ligamentum flavum. The third branch contributes to the blood supply of the dorsal vertebral body through the accompanying dorsal vertebral body arterial plexus, which passes underneath the posterior longitudinal ligament.

The venous drainage of the cervical spine includes an internal and external system. The internal vertebral venous plexus (Batson plexus) extends from the coccyx to the occiput. It consists of numerous small valveless veins that run ventral and dorsal to the thecal sac and merge at the intervertebral foramen. The internal system then exits the spinal canal along the nerve roots and flows into the external vertebral plexus, which is represented in the cervical region by the vertebral veins. The vertebral veins form a peripheral veil around the vertebral artery and, subsequently, anastomose with the condylar, mastoid, occipital, and posterior jugular veins.

KEY REFERENCES

Ebraheim NA, Lu J, Haman SP, Yeasting RA: Anatomic basis of the anterior surgery on the cervical spine: relationships between uncus-artery-root complex and vertebral artery injury. *Surg Radiol* 20:289–292, 1998.

Ebraheim NA, Lu J, Heck BE, Yeasting RA: Vulnerability of the sympathetic trunk during the anterior approach to the lower cervical spine. *Spine (Phila Pa 1976)* 25:1603–1606, 2000.

Ebraheim NA, Lu J, Martin S, et al: Vulnerability of the recurrent laryngeal nerve in the anterior approach to the lower cervical spine. *Spine (Phila Pa 1976)* 22:2664–2667, 1997.

Hart AK, Greinwald JH, Shaffrey CI, Postma GN: Thoracic duct injury during anterior cervical discectomy: a rare complication. Case report. *J Neurosurg* 88:151–154, 1998.

Lu J, Ebraheim NA, Georgiadis GM, et al: Anatomic considerations of the vertebral artery: implications for anterior decompression of the cervical spine. *J Spinal Disord* 11:233–236, 1998.

Mercer SR, Bobgduk N: Clinical anatomy of ligamentum nuchae. *Clin Anat* 16:484–493, 2003.

REFERENCES

The complete reference list is available online at expertconsult.com.

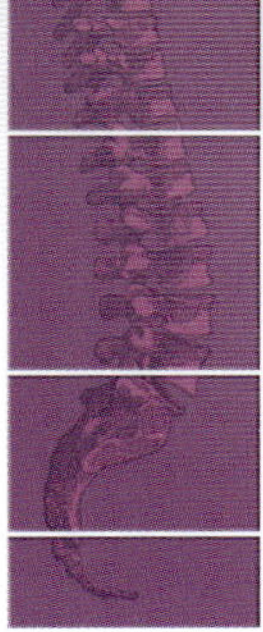

CHAPTER 35

Extraspinal Anatomy and Surgical Approaches to the Thoracic Spine

Brendan Killory | M. Yashar S. Kalani | Timothy Uschold | Nicholas Theodore

The thoracic spine contains more vertebrae than any other segment of the spinal column. With its 12 vertebrae, the thoracic spine is responsible for the load bearing and flexibility that has allowed *Homo sapiens* to stand erect. Given its critical role in the biomechanics of movement and its large contribution to the spinal column (almost a third of the total vertebrae), it is not surprising that the thoracic segment is also a frequent site of pathology (Table 35-1). Trauma, primary and metastatic tumors of the column, infections, vascular malformations, congenital disorders, and deformity all affect the thoracic column, making the ability to operate in this region an essential skill set for the competent neurosurgeon.

Anatomy

The thoracic vertebrae arise from a mesodermal origin. There are three primary centers of ossification in the cartilaginous template of the vertebra, the centrum and the two neural arches.[1,2] These initial three centers of primary ossification mature into five secondary centers at the tips of the transverse processes, the spinous processes, and the annular epiphysial discs.[1,2] Development of the spinal column proceeds postnatally and continues into adolescence, whereby the lordotic and kyphotic curves necessary for weight-bearing are established and completed.

During early development, the intricate connection between the ribs and the thoracic spine begins to contour the posture of humans. The ribs articulate with the vertebral bodies via the costovertebral joints, the transverse processes via the costotransverse joints, and the pedicle of the vertebrae. As is the rule in the spinal column, the size of a vertebra increases from the cervical to the lumbar regions. Therefore the size of the thoracic vertebrae is intermediate compared with their adjacent vertebrae (Fig. 35-1).[3] From T1 to T12, the length of the transverse processes decreases. The spinous processes of the thoracic vertebrae are not uniform. At the midthoracic levels, the spinous processes are long and oriented inferiorly compared with their more horizontal orientation at the lower thoracic levels. From T1 to T4, the spinal canal is heart shaped and gradually transitions to a more circular shape from T4 to T8. An imaging study of the thoracic spine frequently shows a vascular groove caused by the impression of the descending aorta. Relative to their cervical counterparts, the thoracic laminae are thicker and deeper, albeit their width is considerably decreased.[4] The thoracic pedicles are short, and their height and radius increase from T1 to T12.[3,5]

Throughout the thoracic spine, the angle between the pedicle and midsagittal plane changes dramatically depending on the level.[5] This observation has important clinical implications, such as for the placement of pedicle screws for fixation.[6] At T1 the angle between the pedicle and the midsagittal plane is wide, but by T12 the pedicles are parallel to

TABLE 35-1

Indications for Surgery

Indication	Type
Trauma	Vertebral body fracture causing spinal cord compression
Infection	Tuberculosis of the vertebral body
Deformity	Scoliosis, kyphosis
Degeneration	Any type
Tumor	Primary and metastatic

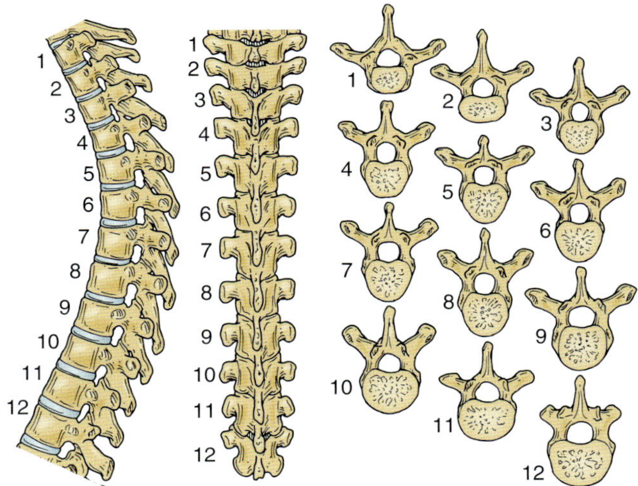

FIGURE 35-1. Schematic representation of the thoracic vertebrae.

the midsagittal plane. The thoracic pedicles are shorter and thinner than their lumbar counterparts, making them more susceptible to perforation during screw placement.

The relationship between the transverse process and the pedicle is variable in the thoracic spine; this variability makes the use of intraoperative fluoroscopy a necessity for thoracic cases.[7] At the upper thoracic levels, the transverse process is located rostral to the pedicle; at the lower levels, the transverse process is caudal to the pedicle with the crossover occurring at T6-7.[7]

From T1 to T10 the facets are oriented coronally. The orientation becomes oblique between T10 and T12.[8] The coronal orientation is important for flexion-extension movements in the lower thoracic spine. The thickness and width of the laminae overlying the facets increase as they progress from rostral to caudal in the thoracic spine. Throughout the thoracic levels, the short and broad laminae in the upper and middle thoracic spine prevent hyperextension.[3] The multitude of ligamentous connections, most notably the anterior longitudinal ligament, provides additional stability by increasing the tensile strength of the column. The articular surface of the superior facets is on the ventral aspect, whereas the articular surface of the inferior facets is dorsal. The articular surfaces of the facet joints are flat and slope in an oblique coronal plane, in the same plane as the lamina.

TABLE 35-2

Approaches to the Thoracic Spine as a Function of Level of Pathology

Approach	Vertebral Level
Standard ventral cervical	T1-4
Transsternal	T1-4
Transthoracic	T3-11
Transthoracic, transdiaphragmatic, retroperitoneal	T11-L1

TABLE 35-3

Surgical Approaches to the Thoracic Spine

Approach	Incision/Position	Indication	Contraindications	Advantages	Disadvantages
Ventral					
Ventral	Supine position	Ventral	Dorsal or dorsolateral neural compression	Ventral exposure of dura	Limited to T1-3
Cervicothoracic	Ventrolateral cervical/median sternotomy			May use instrumentation	Recurrent laryngeal nerve and esophageal injury
Transthoracic	Lateral decubitus position, thoracotomy incision	Ventral compression of spinal cord or roots	Dorsal neural compression	Ventral exposure of dura	Morbidity of thoracotomy
		Ventral release to treat thoracic scoliosis		Excellent for correction of thoracic scoliosis	Staged instrumentation may be necessary
				Control of radicular vessels	Requires mobilization of diaphragm for T10-L1 access
				May use instrumentation	
Dorsolateral					
Costotransversectomy	Prone position	Accessible lateral neural compression without significant ventral component	Polytrauma and medical complications	Lateral and dorsal neural exposure	Extensive muscle dissection
Lateral extracavitary	Hockey stick incision			Dorsal instrumentation can be done simultaneously	Difficult to visualize ventral dura and contralateral pedicle
				Minimal risk of injury to lung and great vessels	
Dorsal					
Laminectomy	Prone position, midline thoracolumbar incision	Dorsal laminar fractures with neural entrapment incision	Ventral neural compression or dorsal epidural hemorrhage with incomplete spinal cord or cauda equina injury	Less surgery Dural tears easy to repair Dorsal instrumentation may be performed	Cord compression May be destabilizing with ventral pathology

Approaches

The choice of the approach to the thoracic spine largely depends on the location of the pathology that the surgeon is treating (Tables 35-2 and 35-3; Fig. 35-2). Traditionally, the operative technique of choice for treatment of pathology involving the thoracic spine has been laminectomy. Although this approach is useful for reaching dorsal pathology, it can cause great damage if used to treat ventral lesions.[9,10] With the recent advent of novel microsurgical techniques and hardware for ventral stabilization, ventral approaches have become commonplace for the treatment of ventral pathology.

The dorsal approaches include laminectomy, the lateral gutter approach, and the transpedicular approach. These approaches usually involve the removal of facet and pedicles with a high-speed drill.

Approaches to ventral lesions of the thoracic spine include dorsal, dorsolateral, lateral, and ventrolateral approaches. Each approach provides a unique visualization of the ventral thoracic spine, and the utility of each approach depends on the location of the pathology. The simplest ventral approach for lesions from T4 to T11 is via a thoracotomy incision with the patient in the lateral decubitus position. Dorsolateral approaches including costotransversectomy, lateral extracavitary, and parascapular approaches are performed via an incision in the back and require mobilization of the rib and transverse process to gain access to the vertebral body.

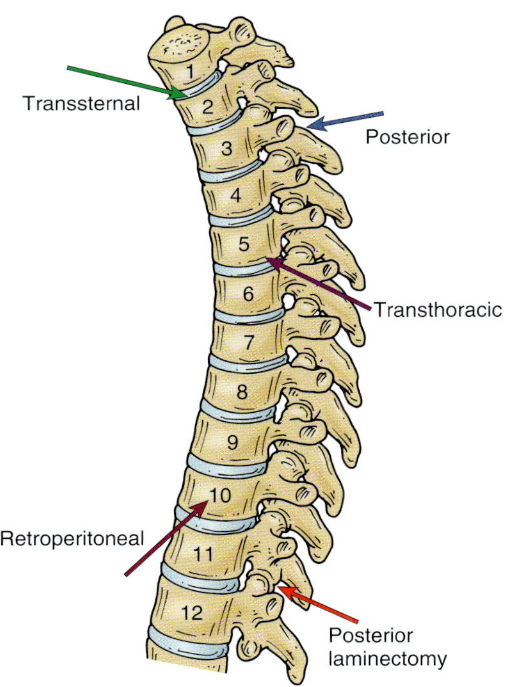

FIGURE 35-2. The choice of approach to the thoracic region depends on the location of the lesion that the surgeon hopes to treat. For posteriorly located lesions, the approach is posterior. Ventral lesions can be approached via a thoracostomy or by using one of the dorsolateral approaches. The approach to each thoracic level is complicated by the intricate anatomy of the mediastinum and abdomen, and the surgeon must be cautious to avoid complications.

Dorsal Approaches

Dorsal approaches can be used to gain access to the entire spinal column. Although the approach is relatively straightforward, the adjacent muscles are likely to be damaged. With the advent of minimally invasive spinal approaches, many surgeons now use muscle-splitting approaches to minimize such damage to the paraspinal muscles. The indications for the use of this approach include correction of spinal stenosis, correction of disc herniation, correction of deformity and thoracolumbar factures caused by trauma, resection of thoracic level tumors, and the treatment of infections.

The patient is positioned on the operating table in the prone position. A padded headrest should be used to minimize pressure on the patient's face. The patient's abdomen must be free and hanging to avoid compression and congestion of the venous networks, which can be a significant cause of bleeding during this approach. Fluoroscopy should be used to identify the spinal level requiring treatment, thus minimizing the occurrence of surgery performed at the wrong level. The landmarks for dorsal approaches are the spinous processes, iliac crest, and posterior superior iliac spine.

The skin is incised in the midline above the spinous process, and the subcutaneous tissue is dissected (Fig. 35-3A). The thoracolumbar fascia is incised with electrocautery. The paraspinal muscles are detached subperiosteally from the spinous process and lamina (Fig. 35-3B). A sponge may be used to perform the blunt dissection of the paraspinal muscles laterally. The sponge may also be used to control bleeding. During the blunt dissection it is important to ensure that the joint capsule of the facet is not damaged.

If this approach is used for spinal fusion, the dorsolateral bed must be prepared for a bone graft. The multifidus muscles must be detached from the lamina, facet joint, and transverse process. While the transverse process is dissected, the periarticular vessels that cross around the facet joint tend to bleed. Closure must involve layer-by-layer correction of the fascia. If necessary, a drain should be inserted and the tissue layers closed using interrupted or running suture.

Ventral Surgical Approaches

Historically, the impetus for the development of spinal approaches and stabilization was the treatment of trauma, tumors, and Pott disease caused by the tuberculosis pandemics of the late 1800s and early 1900s. Hodgson and Stock described the first ventral approach with an acceptable morbidity rate of 2.9% for the debridement of a tuberculosis abscess.[11]

The ventral approaches can be divided on the basis of the level on the thoracic column that they reach (see Table 35-2). Generally, the higher thoracic levels (T1-3) are readily accessible using a standard ventral cervical approach, occasionally extended with a median sternotomy or sternal window. This approach is excellent for ventrally located disease with minimal paraspinal involvement. The T2-11 vertebrae can be approached through a dorsolateral

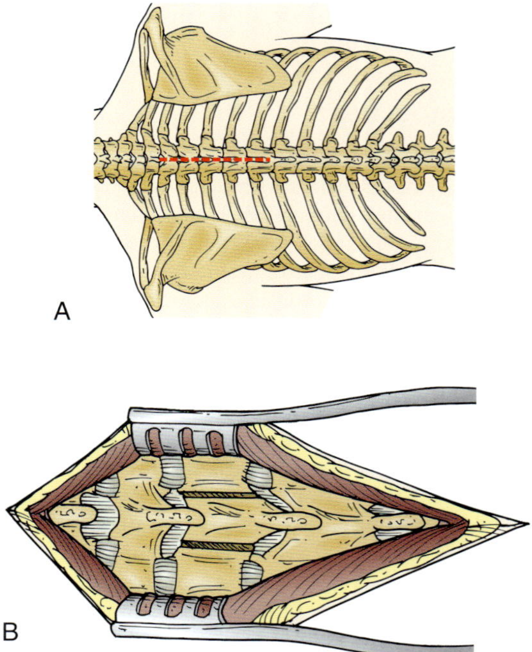

FIGURE 35-3. **A,** The posterior thoracic approach. **B,** The dissection shows the spinous process and paraspinal muscles. Dissection of the paraspinal muscles exposes key bony portions of the vertebra, which can be removed during decompression or used as a platform for instrumentation.

thoracotomy, usually from the left side to avoid the liver and azygos vein. However, some surgeons prefer the right-sided approach to avoid the aorta. When the approach is used to correct a deformity, the rule is to use the side of the apex or convexity of the curve to allow application of interbody devices. The lower thoracic region and the thoracolumbar junction can be approached via a left thoracotomy combined with dorsal detachment of the diaphragm via a retroperitoneal approach. Again, the preference of the side depends on the surgeon's comfort and the location of the pathology.

Regardless of the approach used, the patients at the authors' institution are intubated with a double-lumen endotracheal tube and arterial and venous lines are placed. Baseline somatosensory and motor-evoked potentials are recorded in all major spinal cases.

Cervical Exposure with a Median Sternotomy/Transmanubrial Approach

The high thoracic levels can be accessed via a standard cervical approach (Fig. 35-4A). A cervical approach paralleling the medial border of the sternocleidomastoid muscle is usually appropriate for T1 and T2 lesions. A medial sternotomy or sternal osteotomy is occasionally necessary to extend the surgical field to the level of T3 or T4. Most surgeons prefer a left-sided approach, which lowers the risk of injury to the recurrent laryngeal nerve on this side.[12] A preoperative CT scan can be helpful in determining the relationship of the clavicle and sternum to the spine and for planning purposes.

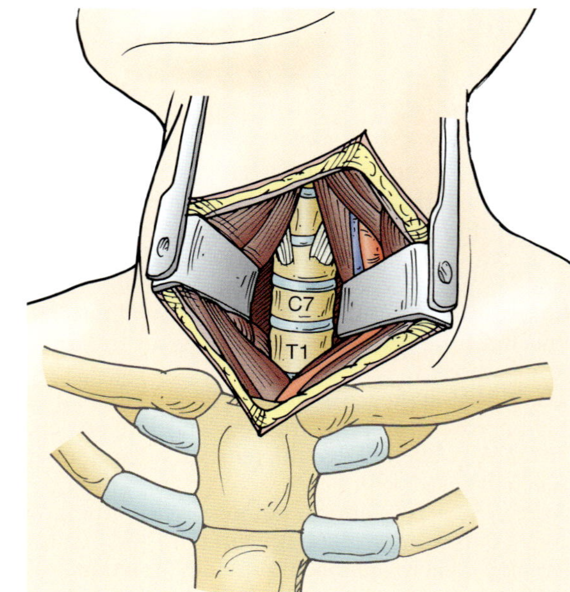

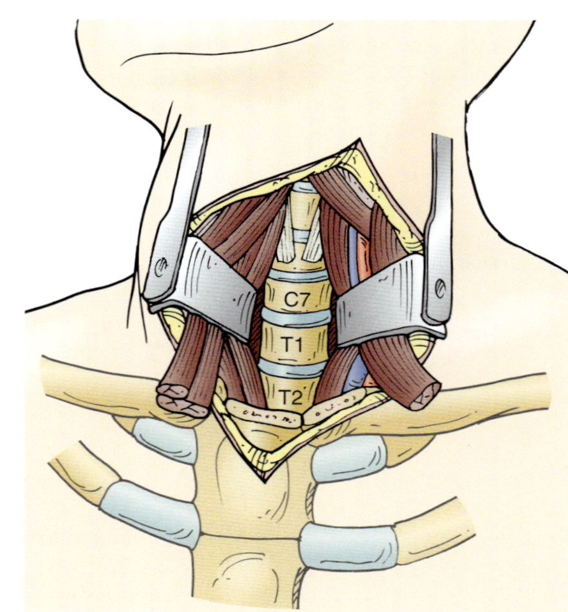

FIGURE 35-4. **A,** Cervical exposure via a median sternotomy/transmanubrial approach. The critical anatomy exposed during this approach involves the carotid artery, esophagus, and trachea. **B,** During this approach, the muscles, clavicle, and sternum can all be mobilized to improve the exposure for reaching the vertebra.

The patient is positioned supine with the midline of the head placed on a donut and the neck extended. A roll can be used between the scapulae to augment the manubrium. The incision is made in a T-shaped or cervicosternal fashion parallel to the border of the sternocleidomastoid muscle. During the dissection it may be necessary to sacrifice veins in the surgical path. The sternocleidomastoid muscle can be detached from its origin to increase the field of view. The sternohyoid and sternothyroid muscles are sectioned above the clavicles and sternal notch. The platysma is divided along its fibers in the direction of the incision. If necessary, the medial third of the clavicles can be sectioned and disarticulated from the manubrium. The inferior thyroid vein is ligated and sectioned. The carotid sheath is identified and retracted laterally. Similarly the trachea and esophagus are mobilized medially to create a plane for dissection. Next, the sternohyoid muscle is mobilized from the medial clavicle and sternum (Fig. 35-4B). Finger dissection is used to create a plane beneath the sternum and into the upper mediastinum. The superior thyroid artery should be identified and ligated.

A median sternotomy is performed down to the manubrium, and the mediastinum is opened with a retractor.[13] The pleura is opened, and the left innominate vein is divided with ligatures for adequate caudal exposure. A plane is developed beneath the esophagus and above the prevertebral fascia. The longus colli muscles are elevated, and self-retaining retractors are placed. Care must be taken to avoid damage to the recurrent laryngeal nerve. The area of interest is identified using fluoroscopy. At the end of the case, the manubrium is fixed with stainless steel wires and the clavicle with plates and screws.

The remainder of the wound is closed in layers with nonabsorbable sutures and with either suture or clips to the skin. If necessary, a drain should be placed and attention should be paid to pneumothoraces.

Transaxillary Approach

The patient is positioned in the lateral position and tilted 15 degrees dorsally, with the arm abducted and the elbow flexed. An axillary roll is placed under the armpit. A skin incision is made at the third intercostal space between the ventral and dorsal axillary skinfolds. The intercostobrachial nerve is identified and sectioned. The pleural cavity is entered through the second or third intercostal space. The third rib may be removed. Small rib retractors are used to split the ribs aside. The ipsilateral lung is then deflated and retracted. One must use care not to damage the sympathetic chain. The parietal pleura is incised between T1 and T3 to expose the corresponding ventral vertebral bodies.

During closure, a single chest tube is inserted before the pleura is closed with a 3-0 absorbable suture. Three to six interrupted nonabsorbable no. 1 pericostal sutures are used to ensure that the intercostal nerve is not damaged. The remainder of the wound is closed in layers.

Thoracotomy

This approach traverses the thorax to gain access to the spinal column, most notably the vertebrae from T3 to T10.[14,15] A thoracotomy can be performed from either the right or left side, and the approach largely depends on the location of the pathology. The indications for thoracotomy are correction of deformity, degenerative disease, repair of fractures, resection of tumors, stabilization after trauma, and treatment of infection involving the thoracic column. When the approach is used to correct a deformity, the approach is always from the side of the apex of the curve of the spine. This approach provides excellent visualization of the thoracic vertebrae but is also associated with complications. Among the most avoidable of such complications are procedures performed on the wrong side or the exposure being too high or too low relative to the pathology. These problems can be largely avoided by using fluoroscopy and image-guided systems in the operating room (OR) and the use of standard OR time-outs. Preoperative marking by a radiologist can also be helpful.

Patients are placed in the lateral decubitus position with the arms placed orthogonally, elevated, and flexed at the elbows. The legs are positioned with knees bent and padding placed to prevent the formation of pressure sores. Both the sacrum and symphysis should be well padded and supported.

The incision should be placed as close over the pathology as possible. During this approach, the rib resected usually dictates the highest vertebral level that can be accessed and the best exposure for the vertebra two levels below it. The skin incision starts at the lateral border of the paraspinous muscles and extends to the sternocostal junction of the ribs. After the incision is made through the subcutaneous tissue, the latissimus dorsi and serratus anterior muscles are divided. In the authors' experience it is best to incise the latissimus dorsi only partially and to lift it with a retractor to minimize the risk of damage to underlying tissues (Fig. 35-5). The serratus anterior muscle should be dissected as far distally as possible, especially in the higher thoracic levels, to minimize damage to the long thoracic nerve.

Once the ribs are exposed, the periosteum is dissected in the midline and the rib is liberated with blunt dissection and the aid of a rib stripper. The liberated rib is cut with a rib cutter as far ventrally and dorsally as possible to obtain a good exposure. When a rib-preserving thoracotomy is performed, the intercostal muscle is cut in the lower half to preserve the neurovascular bundle lying in the inferior edge of the rib. Immediately deep to the rib lies the parietal pleura, which is mobilized and removed. At this point the anesthesiologist deflates the lung to increase the surgeon's exposure. The intercostal space can be increased with a retractor, and the lung can be wrapped with a moistened sponge and retracted to further augment the exposure of the vertebral column.

The vertebral pleura, which is frequently covered by the parietal pleura, is lifted from the column and opened to expose the segmental vessels. The segmental vessels may be mobilized and ligated 3 to 4 cm ventral to the head of the rib. At this juncture, it is important to note the contribution of the segmental vessels to the blood supply of the spinal cord. To ensure the safety of the spinal cord and to prevent unwanted ischemic damage, the vessels can be temporarily occluded with an aneurysm clip to test whether ligation affects the blood supply of the spinal cord as indicated by evoked potential monitoring (motor and somatosensory evoked potentials). Once the surgeon is certain that sacrifice of the vessel will not lead to vascular compromise of the spinal cord, he or she can safely ligate the vessel.

Once the segmental vessels are released, the aorta can be mobilized to the right side and the prevertebral area exposed for surgery (Fig. 35-6). A sponge stick can be used to further expose the vertebral bodies. For approaches to T11-L1, monopolar cauterization is used to divide the diaphragm about 1 cm from the costal margin. The retroperitoneal space is then entered.

The technique for closure is important because several critical structures, including the lung, azygos vein, and aorta, are in the surgeon's path. One or two chest tubes are placed,

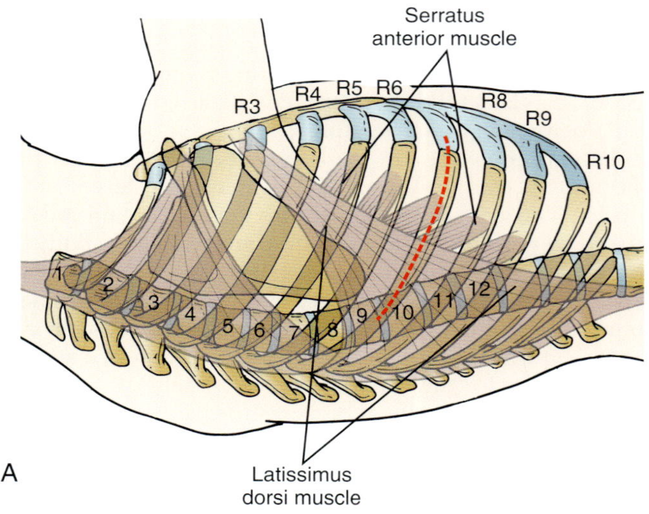

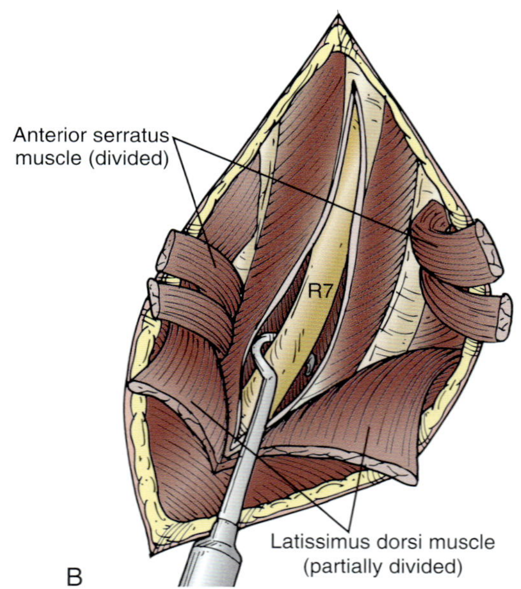

FIGURE 35-5. **A,** The approach for a thoracotomy. **B,** Partial dissection of the latissimus dorsi muscles exposes the underlying tissues during dissection.

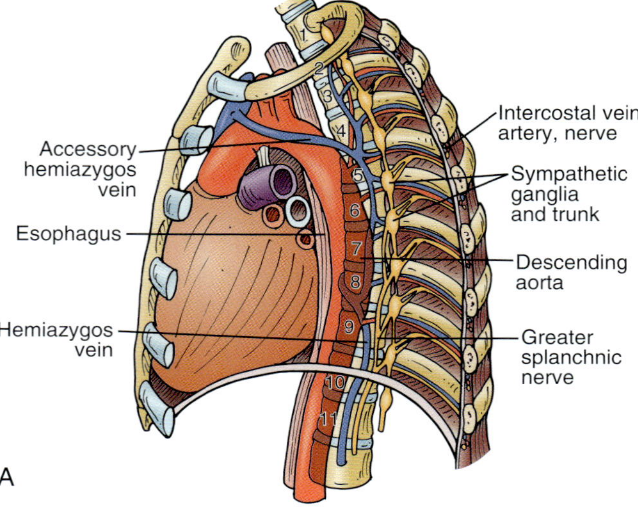

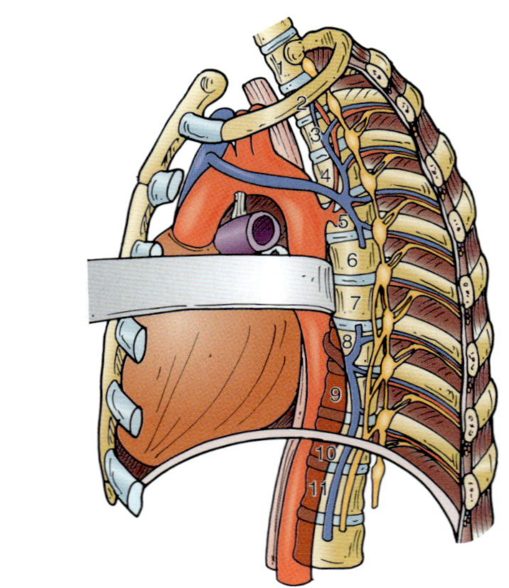

FIGURE 35-6. **A,** Anatomy of the mediastinum. **B,** The release of segmental vessels allows the aorta to shift to the right, exposing the paravertebral area for surgery.

and the operative site is irrigated with antibiotic solution. The chest tubes are set to suction and remain in place until drainage decreases to less than 100 mL/day. Chest tubes are placed to water seal in cases where the dura has opened or cerebrospinal fluid has been encountered. The parietal pleura should be closed whenever possible. At our institution we use thoracic drains. The skin incision for the thoracic drains should be placed one level below the targeted intercostal level. A rib approximator may be used to narrow the cavity between the ribs created by the retractor. The ribs may be reapproximated with a suture. The surgeon must ensure that the neurovascular bundle is excluded. At this point the anesthesiologist can test the patency of the lung by reinflating it. Reinflation of the lung is critical to avoid unwanted atelectasis. The soft tissues are closed sequentially. Other potential sources of complication include the risk of injury to the lung, segmental vessels, azygos vein, and aorta or entry into the intervertebral foramen.

Postoperatively, the patients who require prolonged bedrest or immobilization receive either 5000 U of subcutaneous heparin or 30 mg of subcutaneous enoxaparin sodium twice daily. A thoracolumbosacral orthosis is used in some cases. Serial postoperative radiographs are obtained to assess stability and healing.

Thoracoabdominal Approach

This approach is excellent for the thoracolumbar junction, most notably from T9 to L5.[16,17] Although this approach is feasible from both the right and left sides, a left-sided approach is preferred because the liver and vena cava are not in the trajectory of the surgeon's approach. For a left-sided approach, the patient is placed on the right side. The table can be bent above the pelvis to increase the distance between the pelvis and ribcage, adding exposure to this region. Depending on the target level, it is recommended to resect the ninth or tenth rib. After the skin and subcutaneous tissues are incised at the thoracolumbar junction, the muscle is split in the direction of its fibers to open the superficial muscular layer of the rectus anterior, latissimus dorsi, and external oblique muscles.

Starting with a retroperitoneal approach, the external oblique, internal oblique, and transversus muscles are split. The peritoneum is mobilized to the midline and freed with a sponge stick from the diaphragm. The ninth or tenth rib is resected as in a thoracotomy. This rib can be used later as a structural bone graft or morcellized and placed in a cage. The ventral resection is performed as near the cartilage-bone junction of the rib as possible. The costal cartilage is split, and the diaphragm is transected about 2 cm medial to its insertion into the thoracic wall. The transected diaphragm should be mobilized by using holding sutures, which are used during closure to approximate the tissues. The mobilized diaphragm is transected about 2 cm above the medial and lateral arcuate ligaments. The parietal pleura is incised at the thoracic level of the pathology. The psoas muscle should be mobilized dorsally to augment the field of view. The segmental vessels may be ligated at the level of the pathology to minimize bleeding during the approach and operation (Fig. 35-7).

Closure begins with suturing the parietal pleura. The bilateral stay sutures placed in the diaphragm make its repair simpler. The ribs are reapproximated, and the abdominal wall is closed in three layers.

Complications associated with this procedure include entry into the peritoneal space and damage to the greater splanchnic nerve, ascending lumbar vein, sympathetic trunk, thoracic duct, or the great vessels.

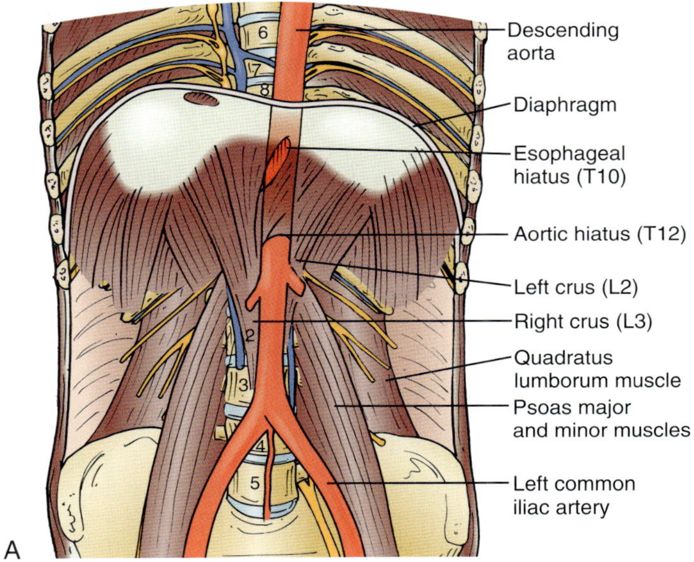

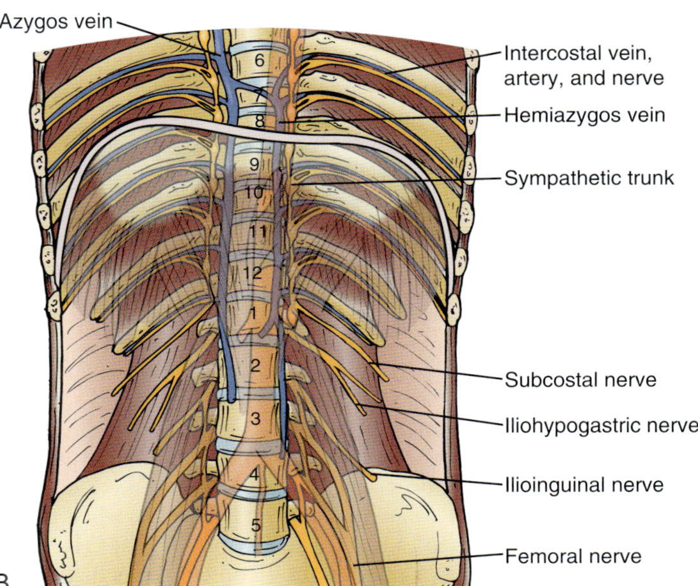

FIGURE 35-7. The critical anatomy observed during a thoracoabdominal approach to the thoracic spine. **A,** The descending aorta passes through the diaphragm at the level of T12. The left crus and right crus attach to vertebral bodies of L2 and L3, respectively. **B,** The diaphragm and aorta are ghosted to demonstrate the locations of the sympathetic chain, azygos and hemiazygos veins, and segmental arteries.

Dorsolateral Surgical Approaches

Costotransversectomy

The patient is typically placed in the prone position; some surgeons also use the lateral decubitus position.[18,19] A roll may be placed under the scapula to augment the exposure of the chest. The choice of incision depends on the location and extent of the pathology and may include either a longitudinal paraspinal incision or a midline or transverse paraspinal incision. The paraspinal incision is made in a curvilinear fashion almost 2 inches from the midline of the vertebra of choice. Cautery is used to cut the paraspinal muscle and thoracolumbar fascia, and a Cobb elevator is used to separate the muscles at the level of interest (Figs. 35-8A and B).

The pleura lies immediately deep to the ribs; therefore the surgeon must use caution during the resection. Using sharp periosteal dissection, the surgeon separates the periosteum from the rib (Fig. 35-8C). The costotransverse joint is incised, and the periosteum of the rib is elevated circumferentially. During the dissection, the neurovascular bundle should be identified and care exerted to preserve it. The rib is cut at its angle and disarticulated from the costovertebral joint to enable dissection of the parietal pleura and endothoracic fascia. A self-retaining retractor or a rib spreader can be used to augment the exposure.

At this juncture, the transverse process is brought into the field of view. Further dissection leads to the pedicle and vertebral body. The exiting nerve root can be identified by tracing it to its foramen. After the nerve root is identified and secured, decompression or manipulation can be performed. In dissections ventral to the vertebral body, vital soft tissues are avoided by elevating the prevertebral fascia from the vertebral body and using it to protect structures. A multiple-layer closure is used.

Lateral Extracavitary Approach

This approach is an extension of the costotransversectomy, as described earlier.[20] As in a costotransversectomy, the patient is placed in the prone position. This approach can be from the right or left; the most important determinant is the location of the lesion.

Given the nature of the thoracic cord and its location in a vascular watershed zone, it is important to identify the location of the artery of Adamkiewicz via preoperative angiography. Although not always feasible, temporary clip occlusion of a suspected radicular artery with concurrent motor evoked potential monitoring can be attempted. Once this artery is identified, the surgeon should modify the approach to enter from the side that does not place the artery in the entry trajectory. A midline, semilunar, hockey stick, or paramedian skin incision can be used. As explained earlier, a muscle-splitting technique must be used to minimize trauma to the bountiful spinal muscles.

The dissection proceeds deep to the thoracodorsal fascia. The fascia is opened in a paramedian or T-shaped fashion and retracted, revealing the erector spinae muscles, which are detached and retracted medially. Rib dissection proceeds as described earlier; the ribs can be removed and used as bone grafts as needed. The neurovascular bundle is preserved and followed to the neural foramina. The radicular vessels are identified and cauterized. Using a subperiosteal dissection along the lateral aspect of the vertebral bodies, the pedicles are exposed and removed using rongeurs, a Kerrison punch, or

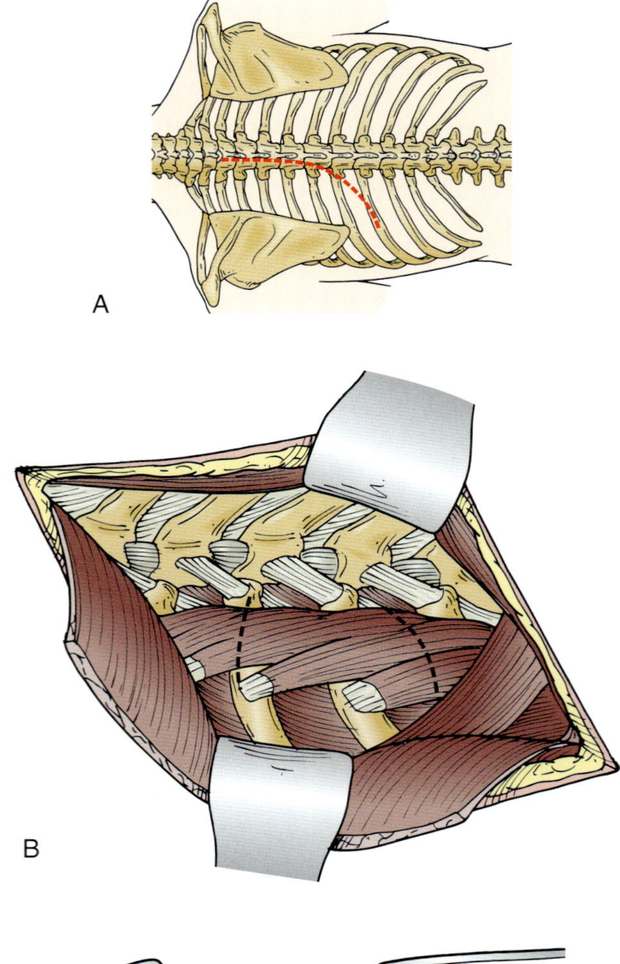

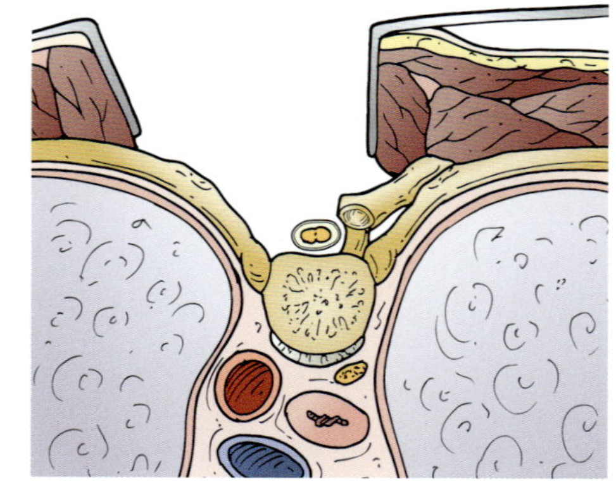

FIGURE 35-8. **A,** The approach for a costotransversectomy. **B,** The skin incision and blunt dissection of the paraspinal muscles show the thoracic vertebrae. **C,** Using sharp periosteal dissection, the surgeon separates the periosteum from the rib.

a high-speed drill. The wound is closed, as described earlier, in multiple layers.

Summary

The thoracic spine may be approached from the front or back and from either side. The complex anatomy of the mediastinum and the abdomen means that a multidisciplinary team of thoracic surgeons, general surgeons, and neurosurgeons is required to approach, treat, and stabilize the spinal column. Given the diversity of pathology that involves the thoracic spine, comfort with approaching the thoracic levels is requisite for a spinal surgeon.

KEY REFERENCES

Chaynes P, Sol JC, Vaysse P, et al: Vertebral pedicle anatomy in relation to pedicle screw fixation: a cadaver study. *Surg Radiol Anat* 23(2):85–90, 2001.

Dias MS: Normal and abnormal development of the spine. *Neurosurg Clin North Am* 18(3):415–429, 2007.

Ebraheim NA, Xu R, Ahmad M, Yeasting RA: The quantitative anatomy of the thoracic facet and the posterior projection of its inferior facet. *Spine (Phila Pa 1976)* 22(16):1811–1817, 1997.

Lesoin F, Thomas CE III, Autricque A, et al: A transsternal biclavicular approach to the upper anterior thoracic spine. *Surg Neurol* 26(3):253–256, 1986.

Maiman DJ, Pintar FA: Anatomy and clinical biomechanics of the thoracic spine. *Clin Neurosurg* 38:296–324, 1992.

McCormack BM, Benzel EC, Adams MS, et al: Anatomy of the thoracic pedicle. *Neurosurgery* 37(2):303–308, 1995.

Overby MC, Rothman AS: Anterolateral decompression for metastatic epidural spinal cord tumors. Results of a modified costotransversectomy approach. *J Neurosurg* 62(3):344–348, 1985.

REFERENCES

The complete reference list is available online at expertconsult.com.

CHAPTER 36

Lumbar and Sacral Spine

Robert E. Isaacs | Richard G. Fessler

Surgical approaches to the lumbar and sacral spine should be dictated by the location and extent of the pathology to be addressed. Knowledge of the pertinent adjacent structures, whether neural, visceral, muscular, or vascular, aids in limiting potential complications while facilitating the procedure. Complex spine reconstruction and minimally invasive techniques require the surgeon to use this knowledge, given limited information. For these reasons, surgical decision making begins with an appropriate overview of anatomy.

Anatomy

Osseous Anatomy

In the lumbar spine, the large osseous ring that surrounds the spinal canal is bordered ventrally by a cancellous cylindric mass (the vertebral body), dorsally by the vertebral arch, and dorsolaterally by the pedicles. Three other key vertebral elements are located near the pedicle and laminae: transverse process and superior and inferior articular processes. With its neural and bony relationships, the pedicle is key to conceptualizing the lumbar spine. The pedicles are wide and thick and are widely spaced on the rostral dorsolateral aspect of the body. In the rostral/caudal dimension, their height is one-half that of the vertebral body. The angles in the transverse and sagittal planes increase and decrease, respectively, as the lumbar spine is descended[1] (Fig. 36-1).

The transverse processes are flat and long in the first four lumbar vertebrae; they are small stubs at the fifth lumbar vertebra. The mamillary processes are large in the lumbar area, providing attachment sites for the origins of the thick lumbar muscles.

The articular processes bear complementary relationships rostrally and caudally. The rostral facet is concave and faces dorsomedially to meet the caudal facet from above. The caudal facet, an extension of the lumina, faces ventrolaterally and complements the superior articulating facet of the vertebral body below. The junction of the two facets forms the roof of the neural foramina (Fig. 36-2).

The sacrum consists of five fused vertebrae. It has a triangular shape and forms the dorsal aspect of the pelvis. It joins with the fifth lumbar vertebra via the L5-S1 disc and facets. The five

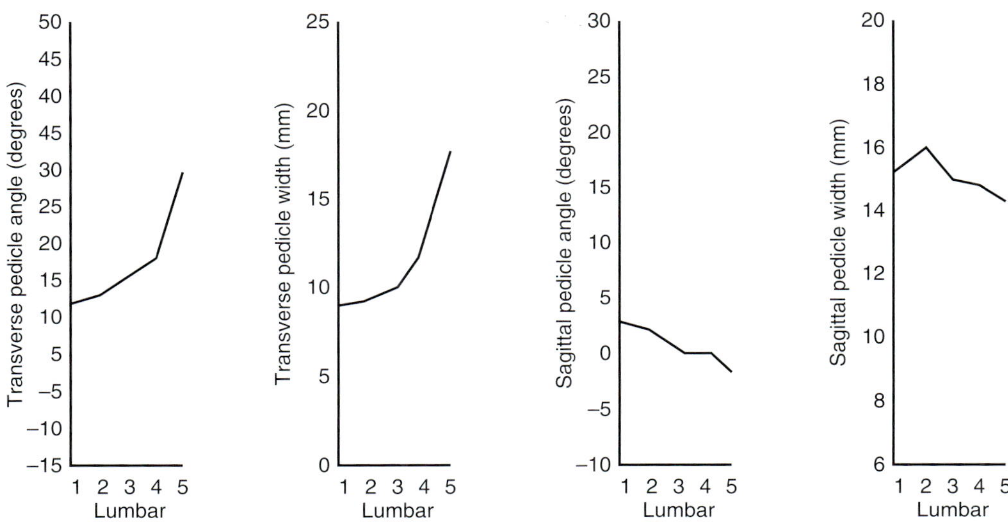

FIGURE 36-1. Lumbar pedicle angles and dimensions: transverse pedicle angle, transverse pedicle width, sagittal pedicle angle, and sagittal pedicle width. (Data from Watkins R: Anterior lumbar interbody fusion surgical complications. *Clin Orthop* 284:47, 1992; Newman MH, Grinstead GL: Anterior lumbar interbody fusion for internal disc disruption. *Spine [Phila Pa 1976]* 17:831, 1992; Eisenstein S, O'Brien JP: Chylothorax: a complication of Dwyer's anterior instrumentation. *Br J Surg* 64:339, 1977.)

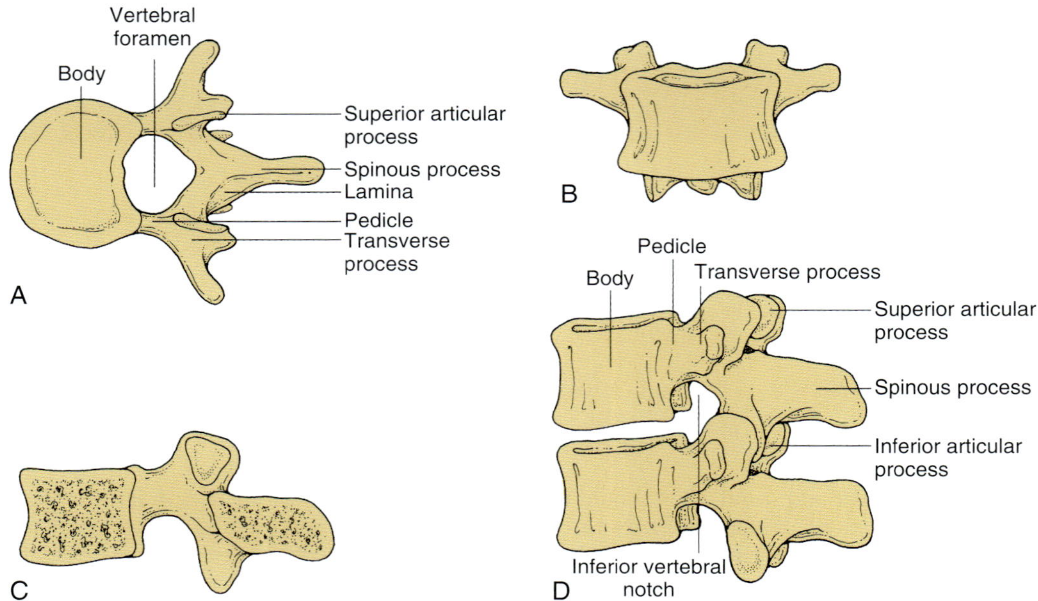

FIGURE 36-2. **A,** Lumbar vertebra viewed from above; **B,** ventral; **C,** median sagittal; **D,** in articulation.

fused vertebrae have homologous structures referable to the lumbar spine. The transverse processes are the laterally projecting alae that articulate with the pelvis. A prominent midline dorsal ridge represents the fused spinous processes. More laterally, another ridge forms the sacral articular crest with a functional superior articular process at S1. This facet faces caudally and dorsally. Because of the sacrovertebral angle created by the tilt of the sacrum as it joins the fifth lumbar vertebra, this joint functions to prevent ventral displacement of the lumbar spine on the sacrum. Ventrally, transverse ridges represent fused vertebrae and enclose remnants of intervertebral discs. Foramina dorsally and ventrally provide sites of exit for the ventral and dorsal divisions of the sacral nerves. The sacrum is the most variable portion of the spine. Lengthening or shortening of the lumbar spine by deletion or addition of segments to and from the sacrum is not uncommon[2] (Fig. 36-3).

Thoracic vertebrae T2-9 have points of articulations for each rib: one on the vertebral body and the other on the corresponding transverse process. T11 and T12 have a single costal facet on their pedicles (Fig. 36-4). The typical rib has a head, a neck, a tubercle, and a shaft or body. The crest of the head is joined to the intervertebral disc by an intra-articular ligament with two surface articulations: one on the numerically corresponding vertebra and one on the vertebra above it. The neck is the nonarticulating portion of rib between the head and tubercle. The tubercle is on the dorsal portion of the rib at the junction of the neck and shaft. The tubercle of most ribs has a smooth convex facet that articulates with the transverse process of the corresponding vertebra and a rough nonarticular surface to which the lateral costotransverse ligament attaches. The body of the rib is thin and flat, with its greatest diameter in the rostral to caudal orientation. The point of greatest curvature is called the *angle of the rib*. The costal groove and the flange formed by the caudal border of the rib accommodate and protect the intercostal vessels and nerve that accompany the rib. The 11th and 12th ribs are short and capped with cartilage. They have a single facet on their heads and no neck or tubercle. The 11th rib has a slight angle and a shallow costal groove. The 12th rib has neither of these features. Minet[3] classifies the 12th rib as long, medium, or short. The long type is parallel to the 11th rib, and the short type is horizontal and less oblique than the long type. For thoracolumbar surgery, it is important to understand the relationship of the pleural sac to the 12th rib. The pleural sac passes caudally over the inferior border to the 12th rib and continues in this direction for 1 to 2 cm. From there it passes horizontally, crossing caudally, and 3 to 4 cm lateral to the 12th rib head, it continues to pass along the 12th rib for another 7 to 8 cm[3] (Fig. 36-5).

Soft Tissue Anatomy

Around the bony cylindric canal of the lumbar spine and triangular sacrum, soft tissue structures have intimate and crucial anatomic relationships. These include (1) synovial and nonsynovial tissue, (2) muscles and ligaments that attach directly or indirectly to the spine, (3) exiting nerve roots that form a plexus of nerves in and around muscle structures or important autonomic plexuses, and (4) soft tissue structures such as vasculature and viscera that are adjacent to bony structures.

Lumbar Spine

Muscles and Ligaments

The ligaments important to the lumbar spine include the ligamentum flavum (which bridges the space between adjacent laminae, attaching to the ventral surface of the upper lamina and rostral lip of the lower one), the intertransverse ligaments, the interspinous ligaments, and the unpaired supraspinous ligament.

The intrinsic and extrinsic musculature adjacent to the spine is commonly dissected in approaches to the spine and provides important landmarks in specific approaches. Intrinsic muscles consist of the erector spinae, multifidus, quadratus lumborum, and deep muscles. The large erector spinae muscle

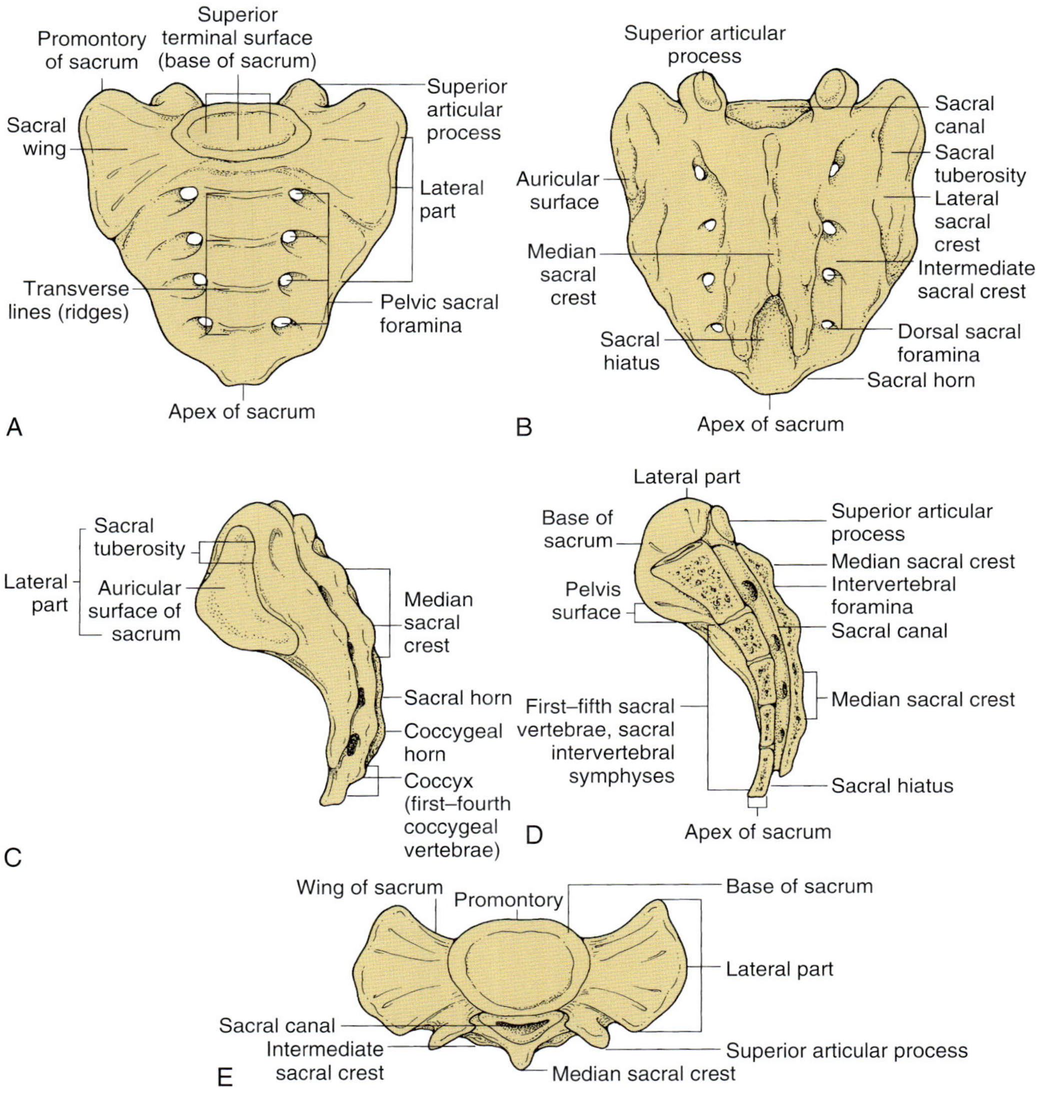

FIGURE 36-3. The sacrum: **A,** ventral, **B,** dorsal, **C,** sagittal, **D,** medial sagittal, and **E,** rostral views.

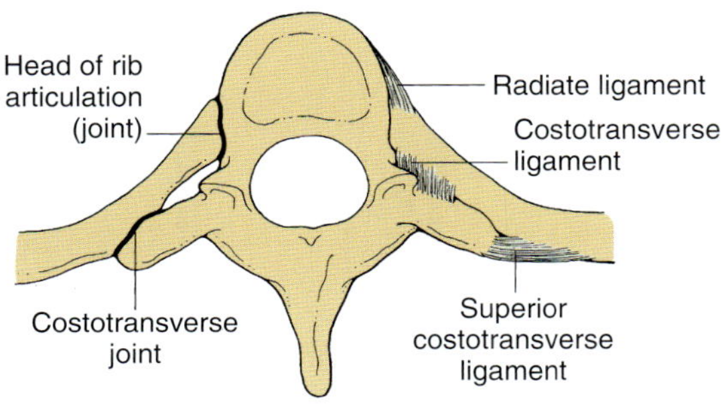

FIGURE 36-4. Cross section through thoracic vertebra and costovertebral joints.

is divided into three columns: iliocostalis, longissimus, and spinalis muscles. The iliocostalis muscle, as its name indicates, is the most lateral of the group and arises from the iliac crest and inserts into the ribs. The longissimus muscle, intermediate in the column, runs between the transverse processes of the vertebrae. The spinalis muscle, the most medial, inserts and attaches to spinous processes in the lumbar and thoracic region. All three columns of the erector spinae muscle extend the vertebral column and bend the vertebral column laterally.

Central to the erector spinae muscles are several short muscles that interconnect adjacent and nearby vertebral bodies. This group of small muscles, called the *multifidus muscles*, originates on the mamillary processes of the rostral facets and runs rostrally and medially to insert on the spinous processes of vertebrae two to four segments above. The quadratus lumborum muscle is located ventral and lateral to the erector spinae muscles. This muscle originates on the iliac crest and iliolumbar ligament and runs obliquely to insert ventrally on the lowest rib and transverse processes of the upper four lumbar vertebrae. Ventral and medial to this muscle are the small intertransversarius muscles that span the transverse processes. Ventrolateral and adjacent to the lumbar vertebral bodies are the psoas muscles, which originate from the lateral aspects of the vertebral bodies and transverse processes of L1-5 and pass through the pelvis and into the thigh dorsal to the posterior inguinal ligament (Figs. 36-6 and 36-7).

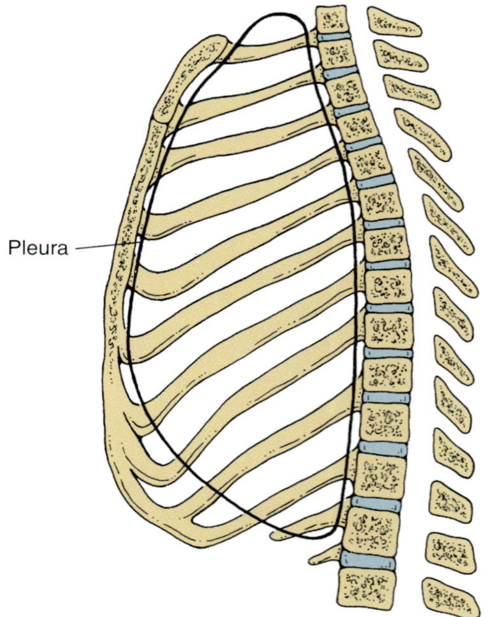

FIGURE 36-5. Relationship of pleura to costal margin.

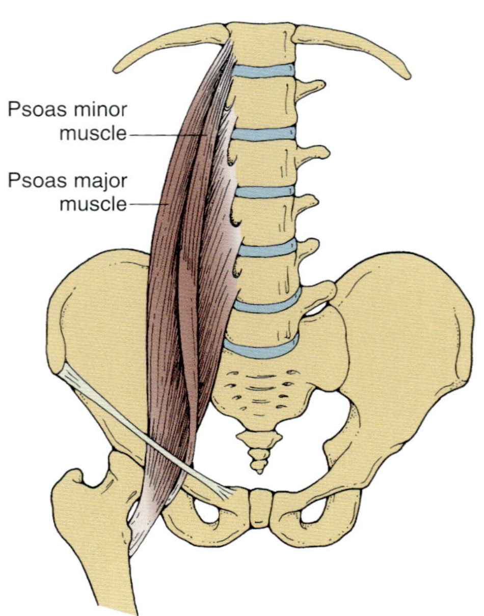

FIGURE 36-6. Psoas muscle relationships to lumbar and sacral vertebrae and pelvis.

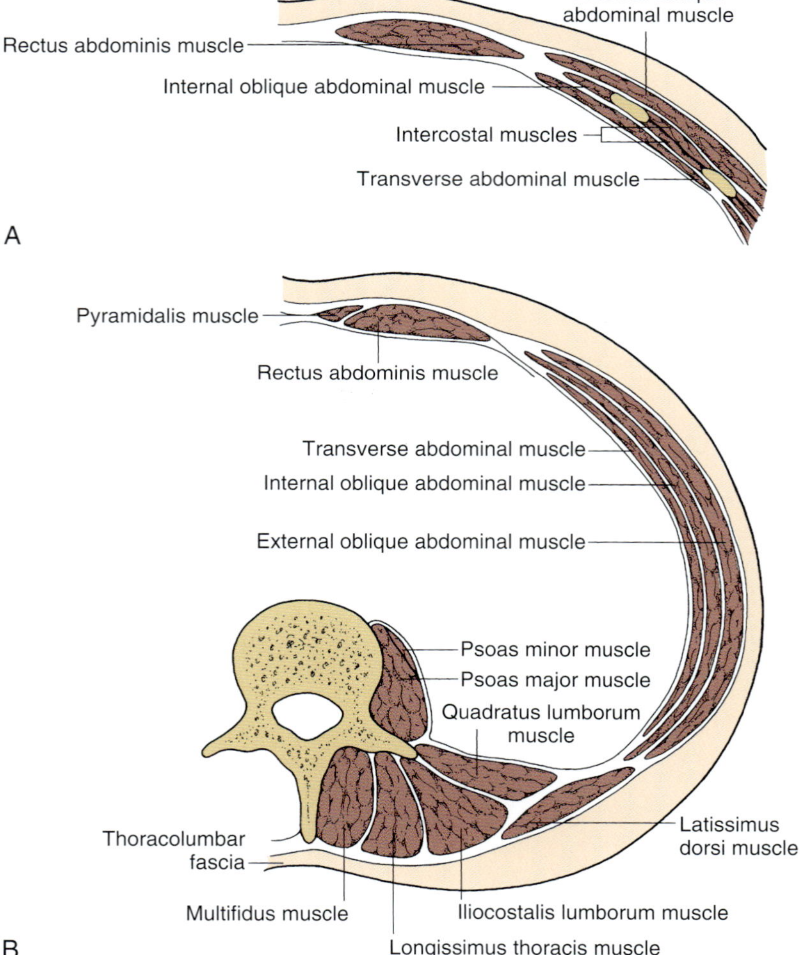

FIGURE 36-7. Coronal sections through the thoracoabdominal musculature above (**A**) and below (**B**) the umbilicus.

The extrinsic musculature consists of the rectus abdominis, external oblique, internal oblique, transversalis, latissimus dorsi, and serratus dorsalis caudalis muscles (see Fig. 36-7). The rectus muscles run bilaterally on the ventral abdominal wall from the pubis to the middle ribs. The internal and external oblique muscles and the transversalis muscles are layered superficial to deep as described. They arise from the ribs and thoracodorsal fascia dorsally and insert on the iliac crest caudally and the linea alba medially. The latissimus muscle is a large and diffuse muscle that originates on the sacrum, dorsal iliac crest, and 10th, 11th, and 12th ribs. The fibers in the costoiliac interval run rostrally and laterally. The serratus dorsalis caudalis muscle originates from the lower four ribs, runs caudally and medially, and inserts on the thoracolumbar fascia ventral to the latissimus dorsi muscle.

Exiting Nerve Roots

The lumbar plexus is formed within the psoas major muscle. The largest and most important branches of the lumbar plexus are the obturator and femoral nerves (L2, L3, and L4). The ilioinguinal and iliohypogastric nerves are derived from L1, enter the abdomen dorsal to the medial arcuate ligament, and pass inferolaterally, ventral to the quadratus lumborum muscle, piercing it near the anterior superior iliac spine. The genitofemoral nerve (L1 and L2) pierces the fascia iliaca and the ventral surface of the psoas major muscle and divides lateral to the common and external iliac arteries into two femoral and genital branches. The lumbosacral trunk (L4 and L5) is a large, flat nerve, from which the L4 component descends through the psoas major muscle on the medial part of the transverse process of the L5 vertebra and passes closely over the ala of the sacrum to join the first sacral nerve (Fig. 36-8).

The sympathetic and parasympathetic nerves are distributed to the abdominal viscera via a tangle of plexuses and ganglia located on the ventral surface of the aorta. The principal components of this system are the celiac plexus ganglia, which are located on each side of the celiac trunk at the level of the rostral aspect of the first lumbar vertebra. The greater, lesser, and lowest splanchnic nerves are branches of thoracic sympathetic ganglia 5 to 12. The hypogastric plexus runs on the ventral surface of the aorta. It receives contributions from the lateral rami of the right and left lumbar sympathetic trunks and from median rami of the celiac plexus and the superior and inferior mesenteric plexuses. It spans the distance from the fourth lumbar to the first sacral vertebra. Its shape and bifurcations can be variable.[4] In males the plexus innervates the bladder, vas deferens, and seminal vesicles and is important in the neurophysiology of ejaculation (Fig. 36-9).

Soft Tissue Structures

The thoracolumbar junction is one of the more complicated areas of the vertebral column and has important soft tissue anatomic structures that require special attention. The thoracolumbar fascia is made up of dorsal, intermediate, and ventral

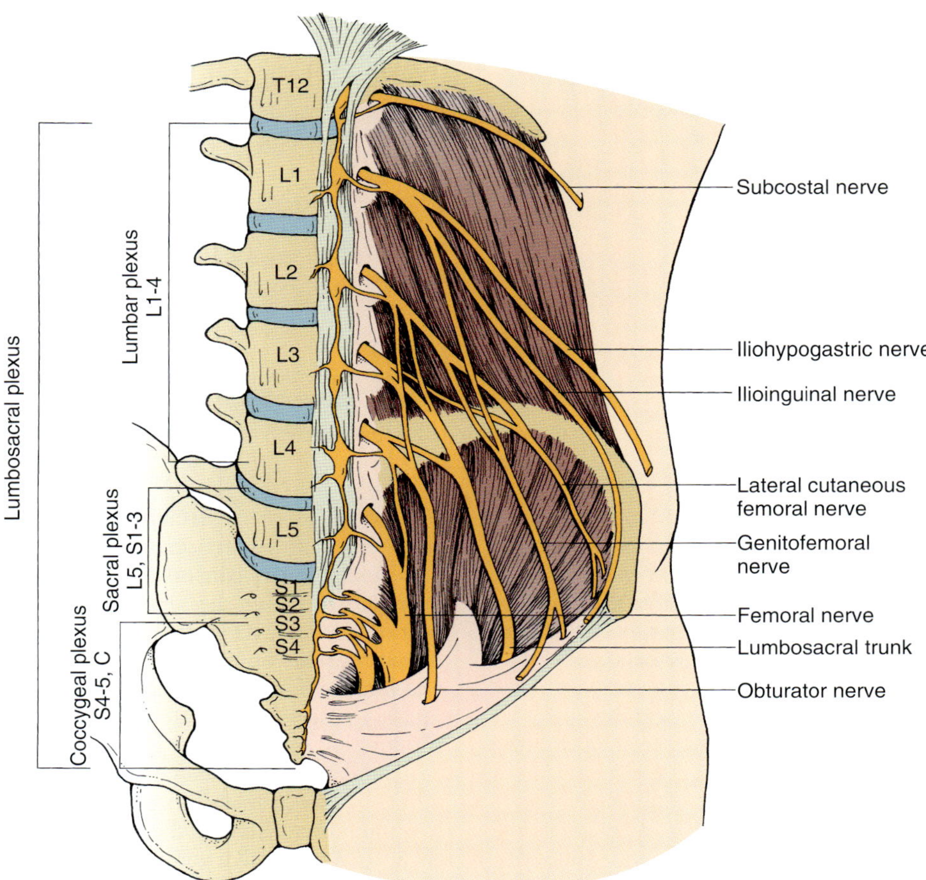

FIGURE 36-8. Anatomic representation of the lumbosacral plexus with the psoas muscle removed on one side.

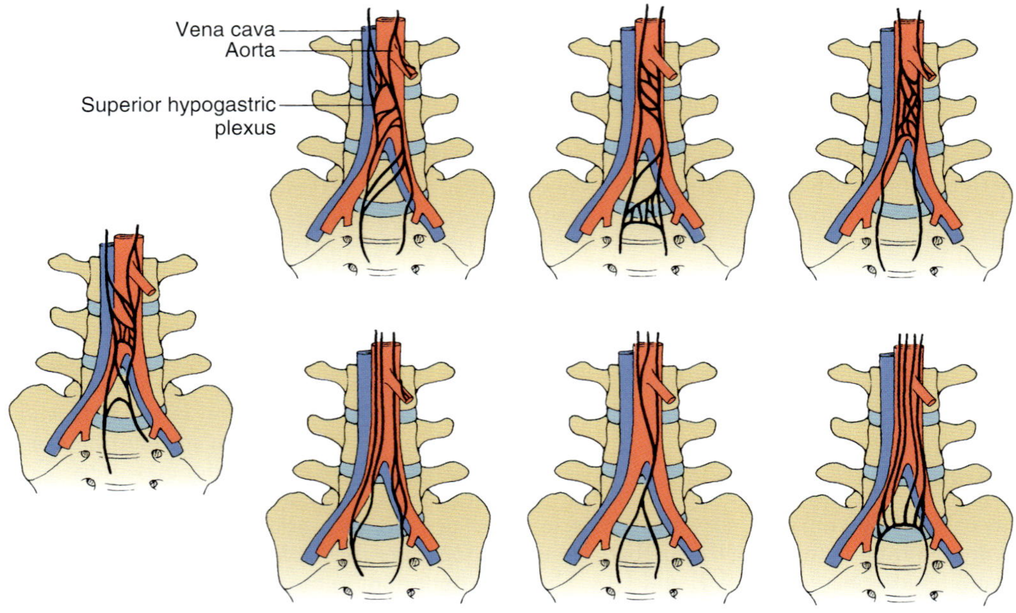

FIGURE 36-9. Variations of the superior hypogastric plexus.

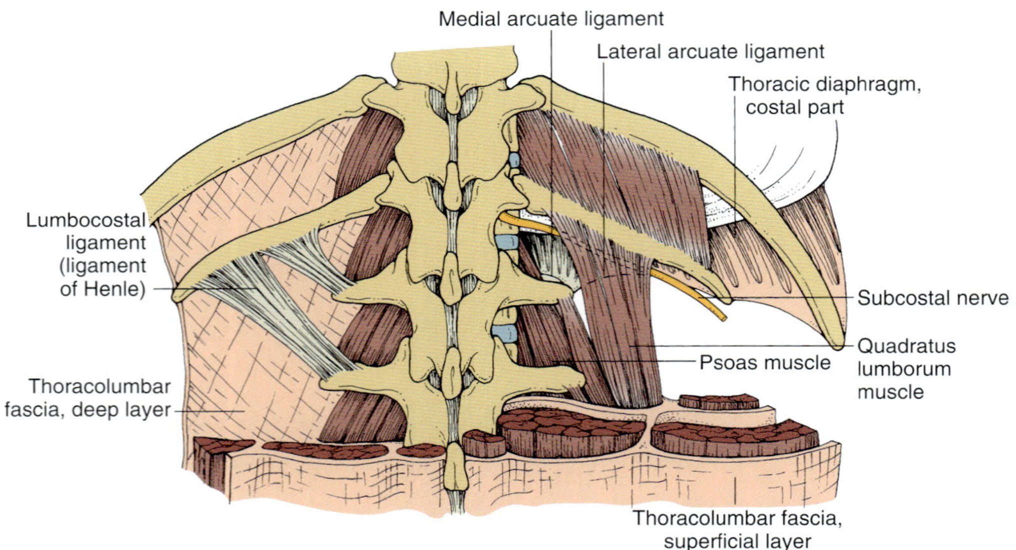

FIGURE 36-10. Fascial planes of thoracolumbar junction: dorsal view.

layers. The dorsal layer surrounds the erector spinae muscles dorsally. It arises with the tendon of the latissimus dorsi on the sacrum and iliac crest and attaches on the spinous processes of the lumbar vertebrae. The intermediate layer of the thoracolumbar fascia attaches to all of the transverse processes of the lumber vertebrae and to the caudal border of the 12 rib. The lumbocostal ligament of Henle arises from the transverse process of L1 and runs rostrolaterally, inserting to the caudal border of the 12th rib close to its medial end. The ventral layer of the thoracolumbar fascia is attached to the lateral arcuate ligament rostrally, to the iliac crest caudally, to the transversalis fascias laterally, and to the psoas fascia medially. This layer covers the quadratus lumborum muscle and is in contact with the retroperitoneal contents[5] (Fig. 36-10; see also Figs. 36-6 to 36-9).

The lateral arcuate ligament arises from the L1 transverse process and crosses the proximal portion of the quadratus lumborum muscle to attach to the lower border of the 12th rib lateral to the insertion of the quadratus lumborum muscle.

The diaphragm consists of a muscular portion and a central aponeurosis termed the *central tendon*, on which the muscular portion converges (Fig. 36-11). The muscular portion is divided into three parts on the basis of its fibers' origins: sternal, costal, and lumbar. The sternal part of the diaphragm arises from the xiphoid process. The costal part of the diaphragm arises from the internal surface of the caudal six ribs at the costal margin. The lumbar part of the diaphragm arises from the lumbar vertebrae by two crura and three arcuate ligaments. The musculotendinous crura envelop the aorta and attach ventrolaterally to the rostral two lumbar vertebral bodies on the left and the upper three on the right. The crura blend with the anterior longitudinal ligament of the lumbar spine. Three arcuate ligaments give rise to fibers of the diaphragm. The median arcuate ligament

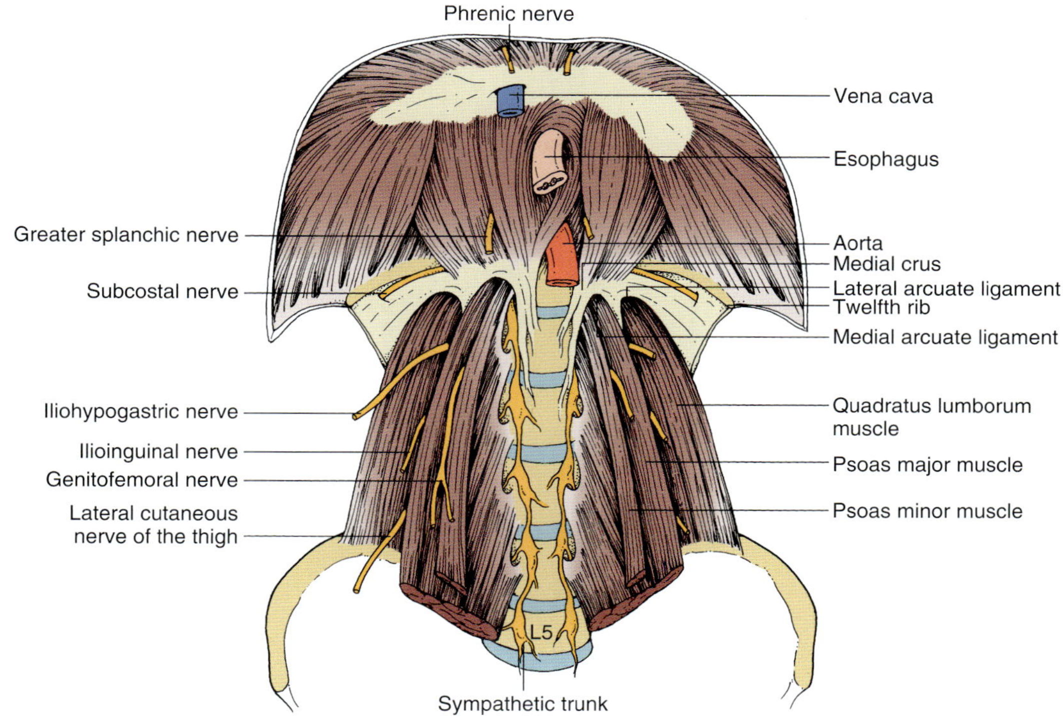

FIGURE 36-11. Anatomic representation of the diaphragm in relationship to lumbar spine and intimate structures.

unites the medial sides of the two crura. The medial arcuate ligament on each side is a thickening of the ventral thoracolumbar fascia over the rostral part of the psoas muscle. From the medial insertion on the vertebral body, it runs over the psoas and has an attachment to the transverse process of the first lumbar vertebra. The lateral arcuate ligament is a thickening of the anterior thoracolumbar fascia running over the rostral aspect of the quadratus lumborum muscle forming attachments to the 12th rib and transverse process of the first lumbar vertebra.[6]

The abdominal aorta begins at the aortic hiatus in the diaphragm at the level of the T12-L1 intervertebral disc and ends at about the level of L4 by dividing into the two common iliac arteries. The inferior vena cava begins ventral to the fifth lumbar vertebra by the union of the common iliac veins and ascends to the right of the median plane. It pierces the central tendon of the diaphragm at the level of the eighth thoracic vertebra. Five anatomic variants of the aortocaval axis are outlined according to the level of bifurcation and origin of the aorta and vena cava, respectively[7] (Fig. 36-12). The aorta is ventral to the vena cava and lumbar vertebral bodies and sits slightly to the left, and the vena cava is located slightly to the right.

The branches of the abdominal aorta may be grouped into four types: (1) those arising rostrally to the celiac (T12), superior mesenteric (L1), and inferior mesenteric (L3) arteries; (2) those arising laterally—the renal (L1), the middle suprarenal (L1), and the testicular or ovarian (L2) arteries; (3) those arising dorsolaterally—the parietal branches of the inferior phrenic arteries, which give rise to the superior suprarenal arteries and the four pairs of lumbar arteries; and (4) an unpaired parietal artery, the sacral artery, which arises from the dorsal surface of the aorta just proximal to its bifurcation (Fig. 36-13). The lumbar arteries pass dorsomedially. On the right they run dorsal to the inferior vena cava, dividing between the transverse processes into the ventral and dorsal branches. The ventral branch passes deep to the quadratus lumborum muscle to anastomose with the inferior epigastric arteries. Each dorsal branch passes dorsally lateral to the articular processes and supplies the spinal cord, cauda equina, meninges, erector spinae muscles, and overlying skin.[8] The radicular arteries, which supply blood to the posterior and anterior spinal arteries, arise from these dorsal branches. The largest of these, the arteria radicularis magna (spinal artery of Adamkiewicz), supplies most of the blood to the caudal spinal cord including the lumbosacral enlargement (Figs. 36-14 and 36-15).

Tributaries of the inferior vena cava are the common iliac veins (L5), the lumbar veins, the right testicular or ovarian vein (the left drains into the left renal vein), the renal veins, the azygos vein, the right suprarenal vein (the left also drains into the renal vein), the inferior phrenic veins, and the hepatic veins. The lumbar veins consist of four or five segmental pairs. They may drain separately into the inferior vena cava or the common iliac vein, but they are usually united on each side by a vertical connecting vein, the ascending lumbar vein that lies dorsal to the psoas major muscle. Each ascending lumbar vein passes dorsal to the medial arcuate ligament of the diaphragm to enter the thorax. The right ascending lumbar vein joins the right subcostal vein to form the azygos vein, and the left subcostal vein forms the hemiazygos vein.[6]

The cisterna chyli is saclike and is located between the origin of the abdominal aorta and the azygos vein. It lies on the right sides of the bodies of the first two lumbar vertebrae and is located dorsal to the right crus of the diaphragm. The thoracic duct begins in the cisterna chyli.

Each kidney lies dorsal to the peritoneum on the dorsal abdominal wall. The kidneys lie along the vertebral column against the psoas muscle. The ureter is retroperitoneal throughout its length. It adheres to the peritoneum and is usually retracted with it during retroperitoneal approaches to the spine. The ureter descends nearly vertically along the psoas major muscle. On the right, it is next to the vena cava, and on

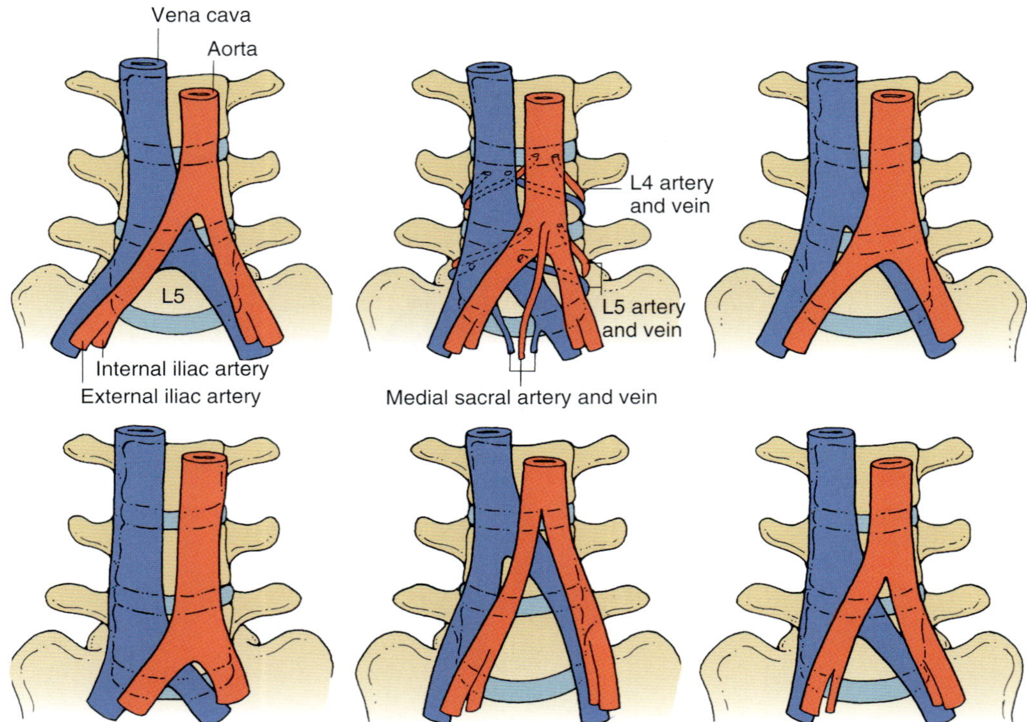

FIGURE 36-12. Variations of the aortocaval junction and tributary vessels.

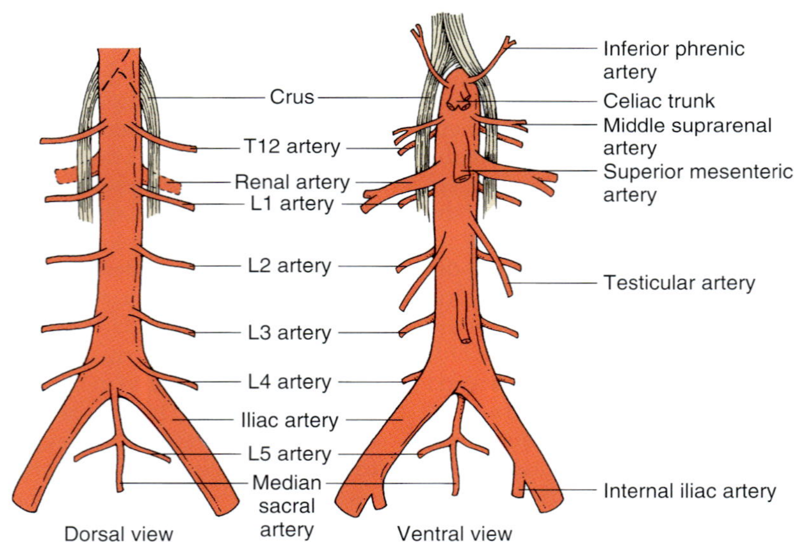

FIGURE 36-13. Abdominal aorta and its branches.

both sides, it crosses the brim of the pelvis and the external iliac artery, just beyond the bifurcation of the common iliac artery.

Sacral Spine

Synovial and Nonsynovial Tissue

The joints of the sacrum consist of the superior bilateral facet joints with the fifth lumbar vertebrae, the sacrococcygeal joint, caudally with the coccyx via the cornua, and the sacroiliac joints laterally with the innominate bone. The anterior longitudinal ligament passes over the sacral promontory. The posterior longitudinal ligament runs across the dorsal surface of the lumbosacral disc, forming the ventral margin of the sacral canal. The sacrococcygeal joint contains a disc and is secured by four ligaments (ventral, dorsal, and two lateral ligaments). The sacroiliac joint is strengthened ventrally by ventral and lumbosacral ligaments. Other accessory ligaments are the sacrospinous, sacrotuberous, and iliolumbar ligaments.

Nerve Roots

The sacral canal contains sacral and coccygeal nerve roots. The filum terminale consists of two parts: interna and

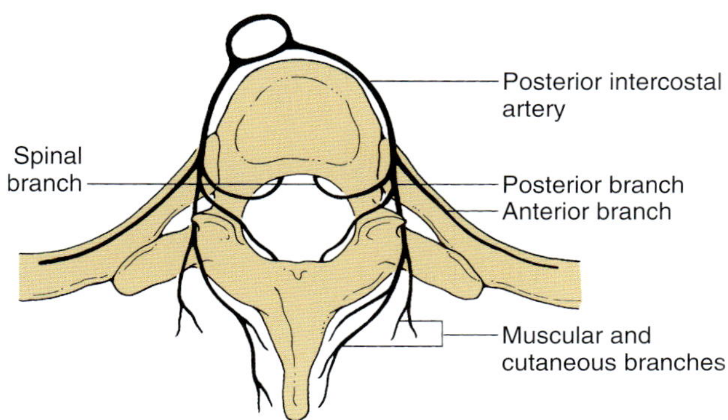

FIGURE 36-14. Blood supply to the spinal cord and vertebral canal in transverse section.

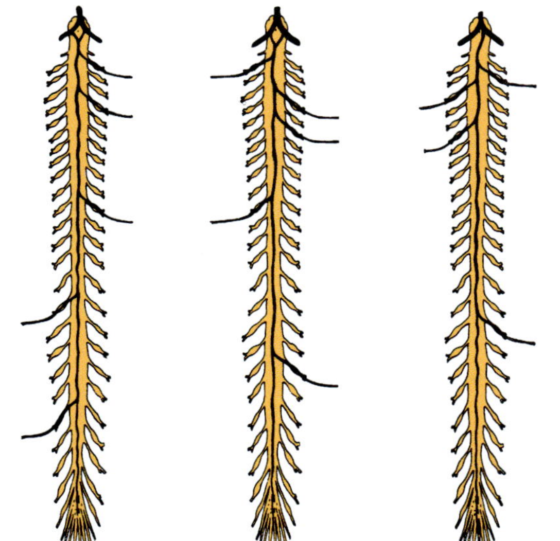

FIGURE 36-15. Segmental arterial supply of the spinal cord.

externa. The interna extends from the tip of the conus to the level of the second sacral neuroforamen. The externa begins at the level of the second sacral neuroforamen and attaches to the first coccygeal vertebra. The dorsal root ganglia is in the sacral canal, central and rostral to the foramina, from which their respective rami emerge. The sacral plexus is complex[9] (Fig. 36-16). The predominant nerves of the plexus are the superior and inferior gluteal, sciatic, posterior, femoral, and pudendal nerves. The sympathetic trunk passes deep to the common iliac artery to run on the ventral surface of the sacrum. Each trunk continues caudally to the coccyx to form a single ganglion, the ganglion impar. The pelvic plexus lies embedded in the subperitoneal serosa lateral to the sacrum on the rostral surface of the obturator internus (Fig. 36-17).

Soft Tissue Structures

Important muscles in the sacral region include the gluteal, piriformis, and levator ani muscles. The floor of the pelvic cavity is made up mainly of the levator ani muscle. This muscle originates on the body of the pubis and the ischial spine and inserts on the central perineal tendon, the wall of the anal canal, the anococcygeal ligament, and the coccyx. It forms a sheet extending from the pubis ventrally, ischium laterally, and coccyx dorsally and encircles the urethra and anus in the middle. It is divided into three parts: pubococcygeus, puborectalis, and iliococcygeus muscles. The anococcygeal raphe of the ligament is the median fibrous intersection of the pubococcygeus muscle from each side and extends between the anal canal and the coccyx. Muscles in the gluteal region that become important are the gluteus maximus and the piriformis. The gluteus maximus originates on the external surface of the ileum (including the iliac crest), dorsal surface of the sacrum and coccyx, and sacrotuberous ligament. The piriformis muscle originates on the ventral surface of the sacrum and the sacrotuberous ligament.

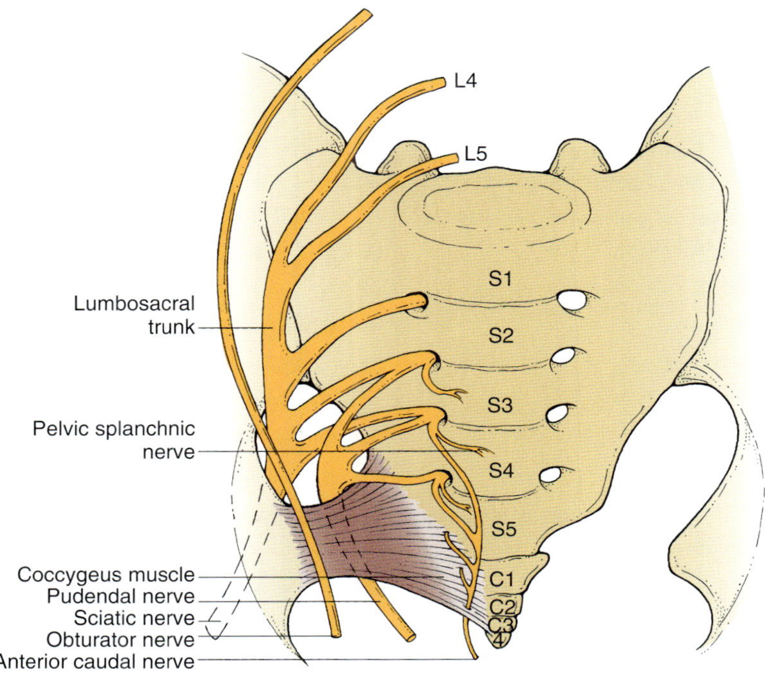

FIGURE 36-16. Sacral plexus.

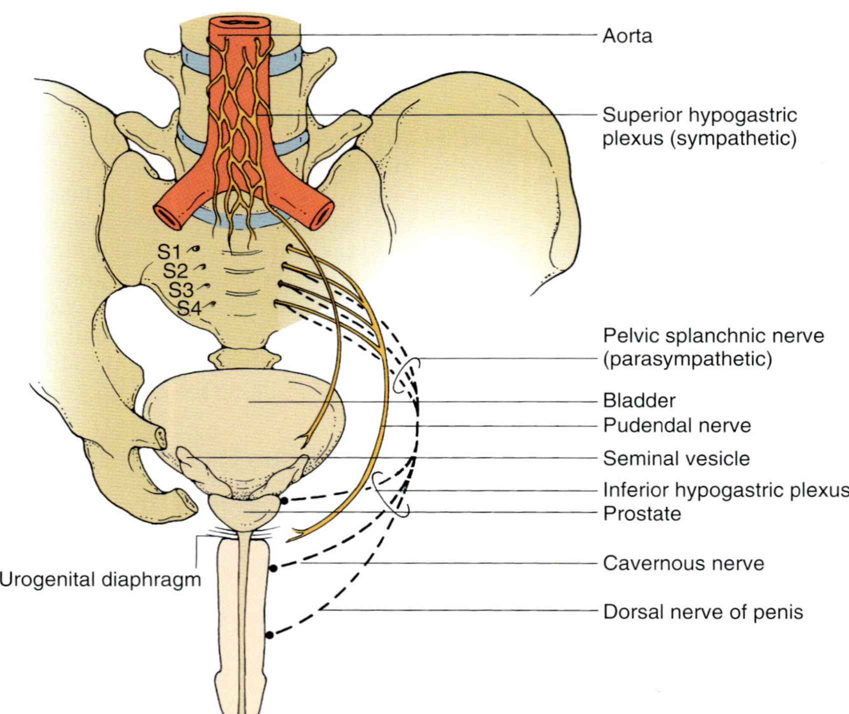

FIGURE 36-17. Superior hypogastric and sympathetic innervation of the bladder.

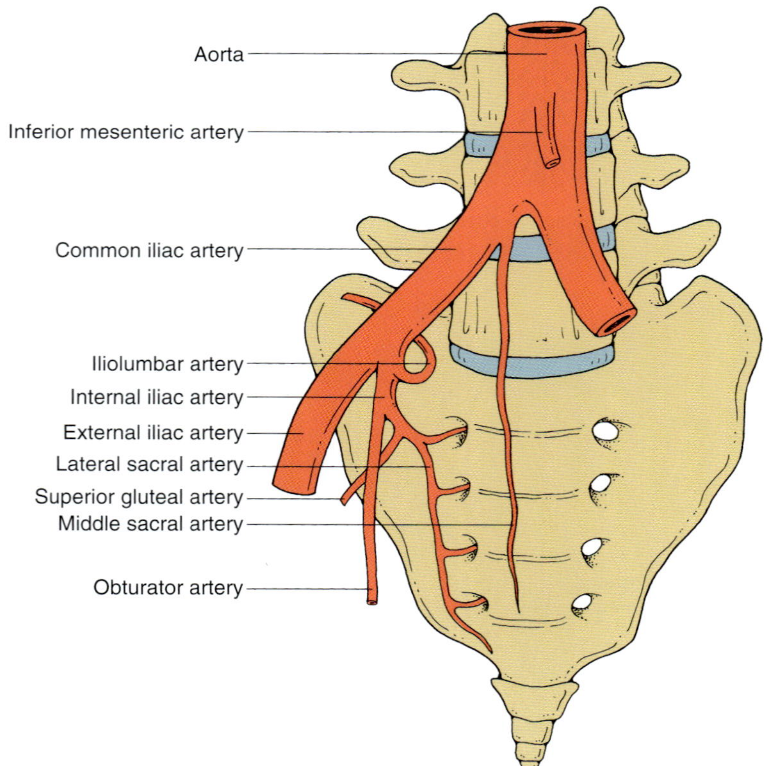

FIGURE 36-18. Vascular supply of the sacrum.

The common iliac arteries pass caudally and laterally to bifurcate into the external and internal iliac arteries at the level of the lumbosacral disc. The right common iliac artery crosses over the right common iliac vein to lie lateral and ventral to it at the point of bifurcation of the artery. The left iliac artery runs parallel and lateral to the left iliac vein. Branches of the common and internal iliac arteries are the iliolumbar, lateral sacral, and superior and inferior gluteal arteries (Fig. 36-18). The venous anatomy is also variable, but on the whole it mirrors the arterial anatomy.

In adults, the bladder lies in the pelvis minor, dorsal to the pubic bone. The pelvic part of the ureter courses dorsocaudally, external to the parietal peritoneum on the lateral wall of the pelvis and ventral to the internal iliac artery. In males, the ureter enters the bladder dorsorostrally, just above the seminal vesicle. In females, its entrance to the bladder is the same, but it is in close proximity to the uterine artery and fornix.

Surgical Approaches

Dorsal Approach

After endotracheal intubation, the patient is carefully log rolled onto a spinal table. Pressure points (i.e., eyes, elbows, genitalia, and abdomen) should be routinely checked and padded as needed. The abdomen should hang freely in order to decrease intra-abdominal pressure. This will decrease venous bleeding intraoperatively. Fluoroscopy or plain radiography may be used to mark the surgical level and to plan the appropriate incision length.

After a thorough preparation, the usual incision is in the midline over the previously palpated spinous processes. Fatty tissue is dissected with a sharp scalpel or Bovie. Achieving hemostasis early prevents "rundown" later in the case. Once the thoracoabdominal fascia is reached, it is precisely incised over the spinous processes to allow optimal closure at the end of surgery. The muscle attachments to the spinous processes, laminae, and facet joints are then dissected subperiosteally. This can be achieved with a Cobb elevator or a Bovie. In this manner, the lamina can be exposed for laminectomy or laminotomy to gain access to the conus medullaris, cauda equina, and disc interspace. With further lateral muscle dissection over the facet joint, the erector spinae muscles can be fully removed from their attachments and the facets, pedicle, and transverse processes can be fully exposed. Care must be taken to avoid disrupting the facet joint capsule.

The ligamentum flavum is found between the laminae originating in the middle of the undersurface of the rostral laminae and inserting under the rostral edge of the caudal laminae. It is thinnest in the midline and is made up of two layers that extend laterally to the facet joint to form the ventral portion of the facet capsule.

Depending on the goals of surgery, partial or complete removal of laminae, facet joints, and pedicles can be performed. An ability to mentally visualize the location of the pedicle from dorsal bony structures is crucial to successful bony dissection and preservation of neural structures.

The disc space at L5-S1 is located at the level of the interlaminar space. As one proceeds rostrally, each disc space becomes more rostral in relation to the interlaminar space. As a rule, one half of the laminae must be removed to approach the L3-4 or L4-5 discs (Fig. 36-19).

The lumbar epidural plexus can be a source of profuse bleeding. Proper visualization using appropriate lighting, bone removal, and retraction will generally enable adequate hemostasis with bipolar electrocautery or direct compression.

The dorsal exposure of the sacrum is the same as that described earlier, except that as one dissects laterally over the sacrum, the dorsal foramina can be inadvertently entered, causing damage to the dorsal nerve roots. En bloc and combined procedures for approaching tumors of the sacrum are discussed later.

The closure is performed in multiple layers, with special attention being paid to tight closure of the fascia.

Ventral Approach

Although most approaches are dorsal, in selected cases a ventral approach is indicated. This approach has been used for lumbar sympathectomy, osteomyelitis, and ventral interbody fusion for many years.[8,10-14]

The location of the lesion dictates the exposure. For T12-L1, a thoracoabdominal or lateral extracavitary approach is preferred. For L2 to L5, a retroperitoneal approach through the flank is optimal, if the pathology can be addressed from one side. If bilateral L2-5 exposure is required, a transperitoneal approach can be used. The best exposure of the L5-sacrum complex can be achieved through a transperitoneal ventral midline approach. Occasionally, this can be combined with a perineal approach for greater sacral exposure. Combined approaches are dictated by the surgical goals and the need for stabilization. A complete sacrectomy may require ventral, dorsal, and perineal exposures, and a ventral T12-L1 decompression may require a simultaneous dorsal exposure for placement of instruments.

Approach to T12-L1

The patient is placed in the right lateral decubitus position. Pressure points are checked including elbows and knees. A right-sided approach can also be used if dictated by the pathology, but the left side is preferred to avoid retraction of the liver and the fragile vena cava.

The length of the incision is dictated by the number of vertebrae to be exposed, and the thoracic ribs guide the rostral aspect of the incision. If the T11 body is to be adequately visualized, the T10 rib should be removed. If the body of T12 is to be exposed, the T11 rib should be removed, and for L1, the T12 rib should be removed. The incision is begun dorsally, near the midline, and it follows the appropriate rib ventrally and obliquely downward on the upper middle abdomen. Its end point is determined by the number of lumbar vertebrae to be exposed (Fig. 36-20).

The abdominal muscle layers are transected in line with the skin incision. Beginning superficially they are transected in the following order: (1) latissimus dorsi and external oblique, (2) serratus posterior inferior and internal oblique, (3) transversus abdominis, and (4) sacrospinal and multifidus. The latter muscles are transected at the spinous process level of T12, perpendicular to the muscle fiber direction, and are elevated subperiosteally 2.5 cm rostrally and caudally for assisting medial exposure. At times, the sacrospinalis muscle can be retracted medially without transecting it. The transversalis fascia is opened, and the peritoneum identified. Usually, there is a certain amount of fat in the preperitoneal space. A history of abdominal surgeries dictates that great care be taken to not open adherent peritoneum or bowel. Once a plane is established, and the peritoneum is bluntly dissected from the transversalis fascia, the rest of the transversalis muscle is opened. Retractors are placed, and the peritoneum is sharply separated from the abdominal wall with finger or sponge dissection. For difficult adherent areas, sharp dissection may be carefully performed.

With retraction of the sacrospinalis muscle, the intermediate layer of the thoracolumbar fascia is identified and

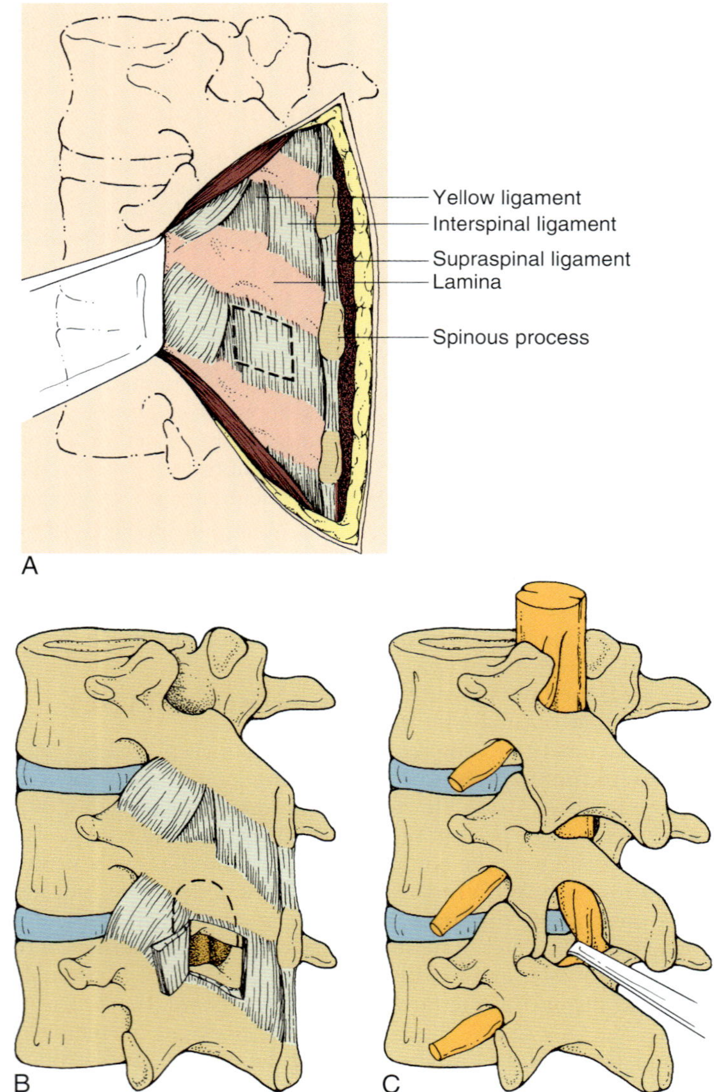

FIGURE 36-19. **A,** Dorsal subperiosteal exposure of the lumbar spine. **B,** Removal of the ligamentum flavum. **C,** Exposure of the lumbar disc.

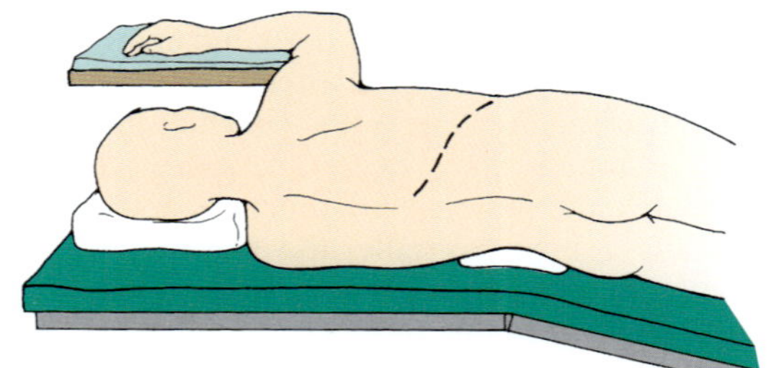

FIGURE 36-20. Skin incision for extrapleural retroperitoneal approach.

followed to the ligament of Henle. This ligament is detached from the L1 transverse process at its lower border that is contiguous with the rostral insertion of the quadratus lumborum muscle. The parietal pleura is gently separated from the ventral surface of the quadratus lumborum muscle and retracted above the 12th rib. The medial half of the rib is resected after detaching the quadratus lumborum muscle from the 12th rib. The pleura is retracted upward with the periosteum of the 12th rib, and the quadratus lumborum muscle is retracted downward with the lower half of the periosteum of the 12th rib. The insertion of the lateral arcuate ligament is also detached from the transverse process of L1, leaving enough for reattachment. After verification that the pleura and peritoneum have been freed, the diaphragm is transected above the arcus lumbocostalis (medial arcuate ligament). The right medial crus of the diaphragm is also divided, following application of stay sutures. Phrenic and subcostal vessels may require ligation and incision. The subcostal nerve should be preserved (Fig. 36-21).

To expose the vertebrae, the retroperitoneal tissue and the parietal pleura are split at the thoracolumbar junction. The psoas muscle is retracted medially. A plane is established between the vertebral body and the psoas attachment to the bodies. If a body is collapsed or filled with tumor, it is important to locate normal landmarks above and below this body because tissue planes may be disrupted at the site of

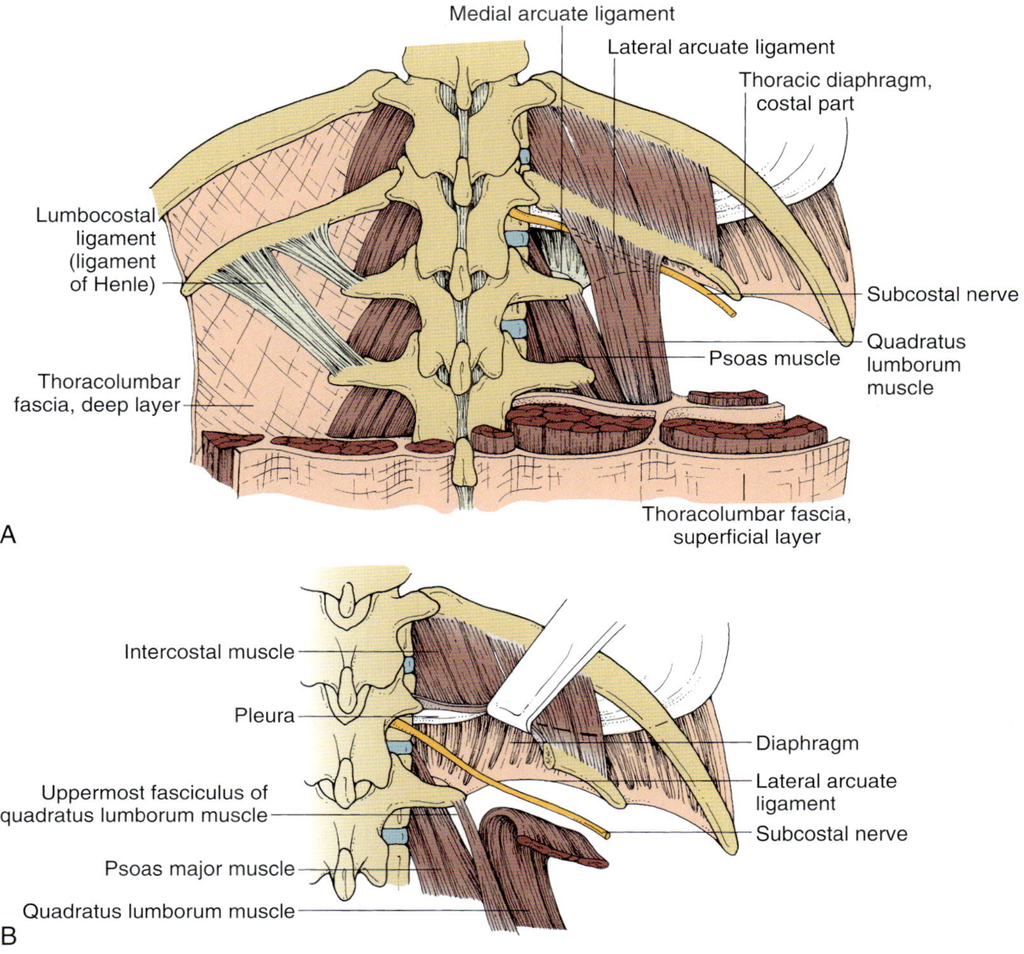

FIGURE 36-21. Thoracoabdominal exposure. **A,** Important relationships of thoracolumbar fascia and lumbocostal ligament of Henle, quadratus lumborum, and diaphragm. **B,** Sectioning of quadratus lumborum, medial 12th rib, and diaphragm.

pathology. The psoas muscle is dissected medially until the base of the pedicle is palpated, and the ventral neural foramen is exposed. Transecting the parietal pleura in line with the vertebral bodies exposes the segmental vessels that run transversely over the vertebral bodies. They are mobilized, ligated, and transected as needed. The anterior longitudinal ligament can then be loosened with a periosteal elevator to establish the ventral plane in front of the pathologic site. When exposing the vertebral bodies, dissection should begin over the intervertebral discs, using the hinged anterior longitudinal ligament and the medially placed psoas muscle to protect the sympathetic chain and great vessels. If a more rostral exposure is required, the parietal pleura can be further retracted and the medial half of the 11th rib can be resected. During this dissection, it is important to recall the location of the ascending lumbar vein, azygos vein, thoracic duct, splanchnic nerves, and sympathetic plexus.

Closure is performed in multiple layers with careful reapproximation of the diaphragmatic crus. The diaphragm above the medial arcuate ligament is closed using the stay sutures. The quadratus lumborum muscle is resutured to the rostral half of the periosteum of the 12th rib. The abdominal musculature is closed in multiple layers, and the iliocostal, serratus posterior, serratus inferior, and latissimus dorsi muscles are sutured.

Retroperitoneal Approach to L2-5

The patient is placed in the lateral decubitus position, with the side of surgery dictated by the pathology. If one has a choice of sides, the left side is preferred to avoid liver retraction and manipulation of the vena cava. The spleen is smaller and can be easily retracted, although injury has been reported.[15] The table is angled so that the middle of the patient's body is concave and arched downward. This opens the space between the ribs and the iliac crest and allows the viscera to fall away. The upper hip should be flexed to relax the psoas muscle. The incision is dictated by the level to be exposed (Fig. 36-22). The umbilicus can be used as a guide. To expose L5-S1, an incision is made between the symphysis pubis and umbilicus, with a slightly higher incision used for L4-5. The incision for L3-4 is made at the umbilicus; for L2-3, the incision is above the umbilicus. If L2 exposure is desired, the skin incision begins near the midline at the level of the spinous process of T11 and continues along the 12th rib before running obliquely and vertically toward the rectus sheath. The caudal distance of the incision is dictated by the number of vertebral bodies to be exposed.

The latissimus dorsi, external oblique, internal oblique, and transversus muscles should be cut in line with the skin incision. The transversalis fascia is opened, and the retroperitoneal space is entered. The peritoneum is thin and blue and needs to be dissected thoroughly from the abdominal wall in all directions. The peritoneum is thickest laterally and is easier to separate from the transversalis in this location; toward the midline, it is thinner and more attached. A sponge or sharp dissection for adhesions can be used as needed. The correct plane of dissection may not be clearly obvious. The dissection follows dorsal to the kidney in the potential space between the renal fascia and quadratus lumborum and psoas muscles. The retroperitoneal fat and contents, along with the ureter (identified by its cylindric shape and peristaltic movements), are gently retracted medially. The quadratus lumborum muscle is identified. When palpating through this muscle, the transverse processes can be mistaken for the vertebral bodies. If in the correct plane, the psoas muscle will come into view. A common mistake is to enter the retropsoas space, which is a blind pouch between the psoas and the quadratus lumborum muscles (Fig. 36-23). On the surface of the psoas muscle, the genitofemoral nerve is noted as a small white structure lying on the belly of the psoas muscle. This nerve should be protected. The lumbar spine is immediately medial to the psoas muscle and can be obscured by this muscle. If access to L2 is required, it is helpful to resect the 12th rib. The periosteum is incised over the 12th rib, and the peripheral portion of the rib is resected, with care taken to not open the pleural cavity.

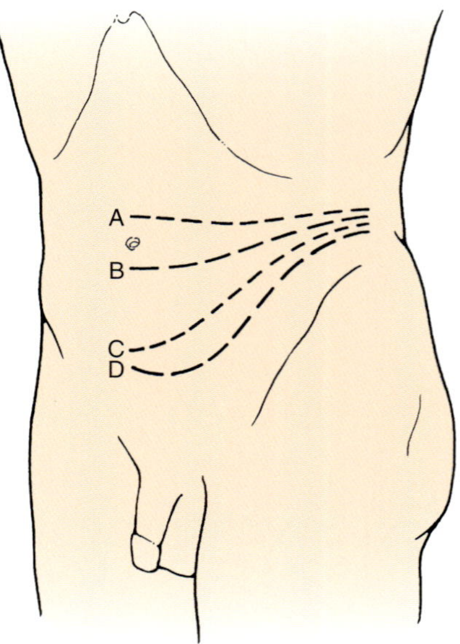

FIGURE 36-22. Retroperitoneal incisions: L2-3 (A), L3-4 (B), L4-5 (C), and L5-S1 (D).

A Finochietto rib retractor or Bookwalter retractor is used to open the wound longitudinally, and a padded Deaver retractor is used to retract the kidney and peritoneal contents medially. To expose the ventrolateral borders of L2-5, the psoas muscle can be mobilized dorsally with a Cobb elevator or Bovie. The sympathetic trunk, which lies just medial to the psoas muscle, should be preserved as much as possible. It should be remembered that the ascending iliolumbar vein crosses the L4-5 disc space and needs to be ligated and separated to expose the disc space and the L5 vertebral body. The segmental vessels located at the midportion of each vertebral body should be isolated, ligated, and cut outside the neuroforamina without retraction of the vessels. Once the segmental vessels have been incised, the aorta can be mobilized medially to expose the ventral aspect of the vertebral bodies. Next, the Cobb elevator can be used to separate the anterior longitudinal ligament from the ventral vertebral bodies. This provides

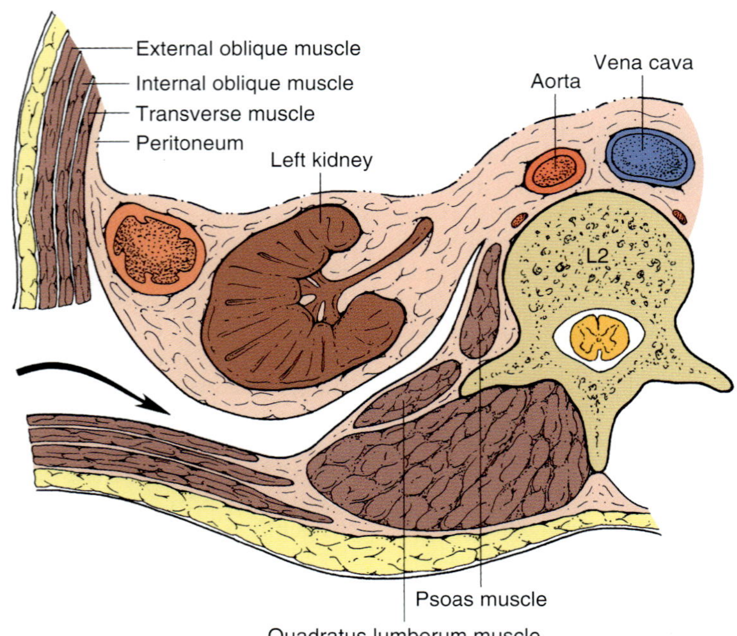

FIGURE 36-23. Retroperitoneal approach in the coronal plane and anatomic relationships to muscle and retroperitoneal contents.

a barrier of protection as the surgeon works on the selected vertebral body. If the pathology is not obvious or the sacral promontory is not evident, a radiograph should be obtained to determine the appropriate level.

The closure begins with the rib bed, which is reapproximated. The muscle closure is undertaken in multiple layers.

Transperitoneal or Retroperitoneal Paramedian Rectus Approach

Although L4-5 can be approached retroperitoneally, exposure of L5 and the sacrum can be achieved more readily through a direct ventral approach. Before surgery, the patient should be prepared with a bowel cathartic. The supine position is augmented with a sacral bolster to elevate the sacrum and provide better exposure. The Trendelenburg position allows the peritoneal contents to rest upward. The level of incision should be subumbilical, several centimeters above the pubis. If exposure of more rostral vertebral bodies is desired, the length of the incision can be extended to the umbilicus. The abdominal wall is opened para midline at the border of the left rectus muscle. If the midline is used and the linea alba opened, the preperitoneal fat will be identified immediately.

One can decide at this point whether to use a transperitoneal or a retroperitoneal approach. A retroperitoneal approach on the left side is safe, with the viscera and hypogastric plexus being protected, but it has the disadvantage of a less direct route and less than maximal exposure of the spine.[16] The parietal peritoneum can be retracted from the lateral abdominal wall with a swab stick or blunt hand dissection. Once the retroperitoneal contents are packed and retracted upward and lateral, the psoas muscle and genitofemoral nerves are visualized. The common iliac artery ventral to the vein can be seen through a layer of retroperitoneal fatty tissue. At the caudal margin of L4, the ureter and testicular vessels cross the common iliac artery laterally to medially. Midway above the aortic bifurcation runs the superior hypogastric plexus, which fans out ventrally to the promontory. For exposures above L5, the plexus is retracted medially; for exposures below L5, it is retracted laterally (Fig. 36-24). The psoas muscle is detached laterally, and the iliolumbar and segmental vessels are ligated and separated as needed. For lower lumbar access, the iliac vessels are freed from the anterior longitudinal ligament and mobilized contralaterally.

Transperitoneally, the peritoneum is a thin, blue membrane that is freed from the abdominal wall and opened in a linear fashion. The greater omentum, small bowel, and the mesenteric root are retracted rostrally. The mesocolon is retracted laterally, and the sigmoid colon retracted caudally. After the bowel is mobilized, the aortic bifurcation and sacral promontory are identified through the dorsal peritoneum. The dorsal peritoneum is opened in a linear fashion along the right common iliac artery from the aortic bifurcation to the bifurcation of the internal and external iliac arteries. Care should be taken to identify the ureter, which should cross the right external iliac artery and the hypogastric plexus, which is directly ventral to the fifth lumbar vertebra and the L5-S1 disc space. To aid in dissection, saline solution is infiltrated into the dorsal peritoneal tissue before incision. This elevates the peritoneal tissue while leaving the superior hypogastric plexus adherent to the aorta.[5] The plexus is best

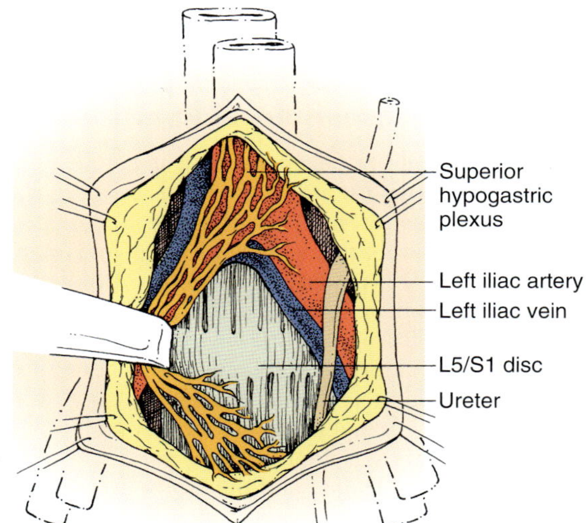

FIGURE 36-24. Superior hypogastric plexus laterally retracted.

preserved by finding the plane between the anterior longitudinal ligament and the prevertebral tissue and mobilizing the structures en bloc. The sacral vein and artery may be adherent to the sacrum. Ligation and incision may be necessary to mobilize the large vessels laterally. L3 and L4 may also be exposed in this dissection by ligating and transecting appropriate segmental vessels to allow lateral retraction of the aorta and common iliac arteries (Fig. 36-25). If the aortic bifurcation is located more rostral than usual, an interiliac approach may be used.

The parietal peritoneum is closed with running absorbable suture. Before the omentum is pulled down, one must ensure that no torsion is present on the mesenteric root. The ventral

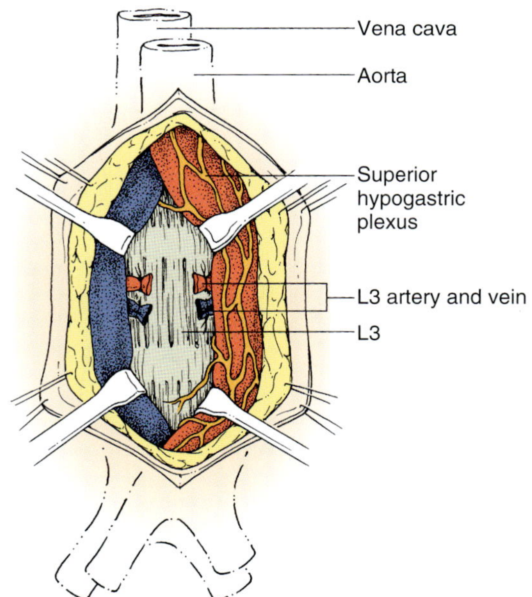

FIGURE 36-25. Transperitoneal L3-4 exposure with the segmental vessels ligated and aorta and common iliac arteries retracted laterally.

peritoneum is also closed, as was the dorsal peritoneum. The rectus and skin are closed in multiple layers.

Laparoscopic Transperitoneal Approach

Especially for the case of disc pathology at L5-S1, a laparoscopic approach allows for a direct ventral exposure without the need for open laparotomy. As with the standard open procedure, a routine bowel prep, a Foley catheter, and an orogastric tube are used. The patient is positioned supine in steep Trendelenburg to aid in retracting the peritoneal contents toward the upper abdomen. Portals are placed in a diamond shape, with the superior/periumbilical portal being used for the camera, the middle or lateral portals for dissection and retraction, and the suprapubic portal for the spinal instrumentation (Fig. 36-26). The spinal working portal is not placed until the disc space is defined and the dorsal peritoneum and vasculature have been dissected free from it.

Dissection of the peritoneum is performed through a right-sided vertical incision as described earlier, with care taken to avoid coagulating on or near the hypogastric plexus. For exposure to the L5-S1 disc space, the middle sacral artery and several small veins may need to be clipped and then ligated. Once the disc space has been exposed, a long needle may be used to determine the angle of the L5-S1 disc space. This technique allows for optimal positioning for the spinal working portal, and it greatly assists the procedure (Fig. 36-27). Once completed, each portal is removed and each incision is closed in layers.

Approaches to the Sacrum

Surgical approaches to the sacrum vary according to the location of the pathologic lesion and according to whether debulking or en bloc resection is the surgical goal. This area is surgically challenging because of (1) its relationship to the pelvis, (2) dorsal tilt, (3) concavity, (4) long intraosseous course of the vertically positioned sacral nerve roots, and

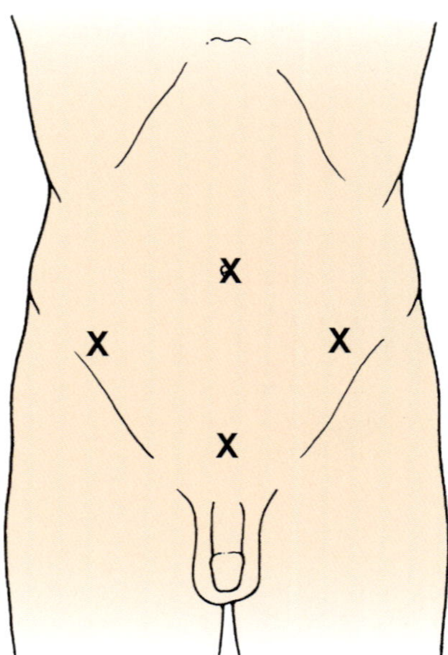

FIGURE 36-26. Ventral abdominal wall showing the configuration of the laparoscopic portals.

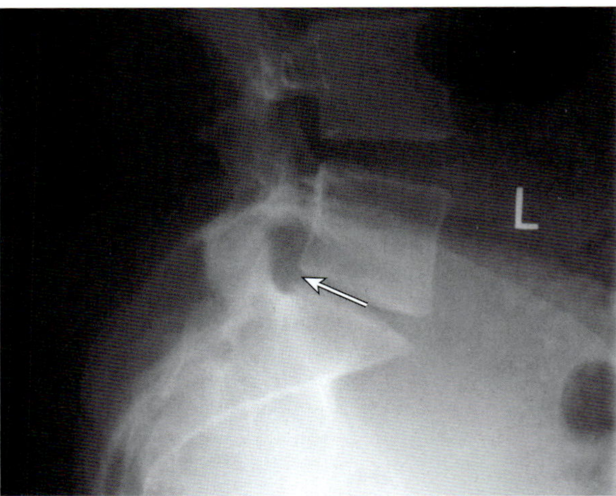

FIGURE 36-27. Lateral radiograph showing the correct working angle *(arrow)* for the suprapubic portal to allow entry into the L5-S1 disc space.

(5) approximation to the iliac wings and overhang of the superior iliac crests.[17] Often, combined approaches are necessary because of these anatomic constraints. Ventral and dorsal approaches that have been described for the low lumbar spine are often applicable to the sacrum. Other approaches that are useful are the lateral sacroiliac approach and the perineal approach (if the pathology is caudal or extending laterally outside of the sacrum into the iliac wings). A combined ventral/dorsal abdominosacral approach or a radical sacrectomy is useful if en bloc resection is desired.[17,18]

The dorsal transsacral approach is indicated for lesions contained within the sacral canal (no presacral extension). Incisional biopsy or intralesional debulking is easily performed via the dorsal approach. Routine subperiosteal dissection and sacral laminectomy, followed by intraspinal or intrasacral tumor removal using standard microsurgical technique, is the method of choice. For marginal resection of tumors with presacral extension, a combined dorsal/ventral approach is indicated.

The ventral approach is preferred for complete visualization of the presacral space and can be achieved with either transabdominal or retroperitoneal exposure.[19] The former is preferred if bilateral visualization of the sacrum is desired, as in the case of large tumors. Ventral access allows exposure of the iliac and sacral vessels and other viscera for early control of the vascular supply of the tumor and for dissection of the tumor-viscera junction. These approaches provide good exposure of the mid sacrum and upper sacrum. Intradural or intraspinal tumors cannot be adequately exposed from a ventral approach.[20] The main advantage of the retroperitoneal approach is the option for a combined retroperitoneal/dorsal exposure for intraspinal en bloc tumor resection.

For lesions below the mid sacrum or upper sacrum (Fig. 36-28), the perineal approach is indicated.[7] The patient is positioned in the flexed prone (i.e., Kraske) position. A single longitudinal incision is made, extending below the coccyx. Separating the anococcygeal raphe and releasing the gluteal and levator ani muscles exposes the presacral space. The anal canal and rectum are bluntly dissected from the tumor surface. After the tumor margins are identified, the lateral sacral attachments of the piriformis muscle and the

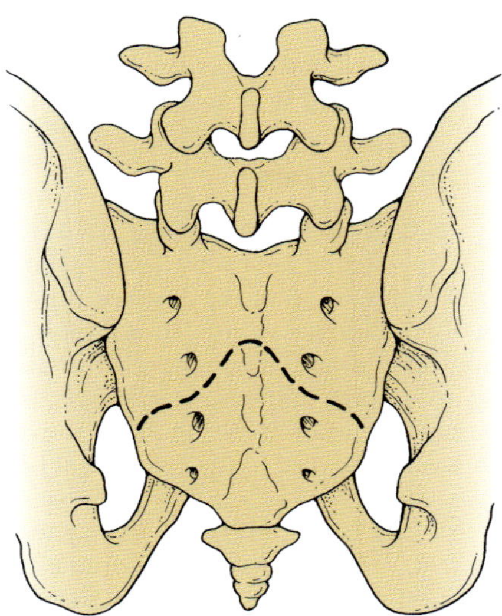

FIGURE 36-28. Dorsal representation of the lower third of sacrum that can be removed through a perineal approach.

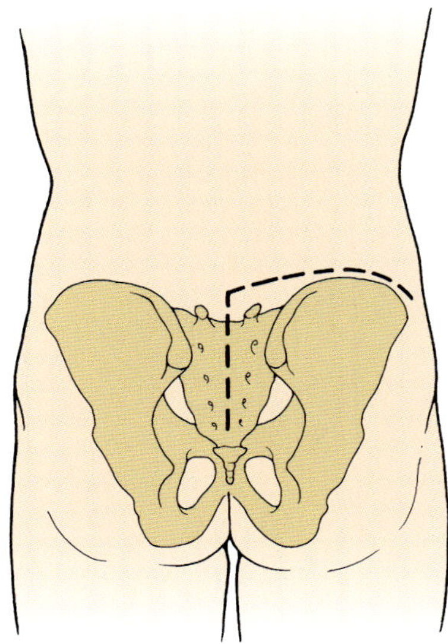

FIGURE 36-29. Hockey-stick incision for the lateral approach to the sacroiliac joint.

sacrospinous and sacrotuberous ligaments are incised bilaterally. A laminectomy is performed dorsally at the foramina, one space above the lesion. The filum externa and nerve roots caudal to the determined level are divided and sectioned. An osteotome is used to section the sacrum ventrally through the perineal opening at the appropriate level, usually below S3. The tumor can then be removed en bloc or with wide margins. The wound is closed in layers over a suction drain.

The lateral approach to the sacroiliac joint allows simultaneous exposure of the dorsal and ventral surface of the sacroiliac joint for resection of tumors that involve the sacroiliac joint, lateral ala, and medial iliac wing. The incision is shaped like a hockey stick, starting over the sacrum and curving laterally over the iliac crest (Fig. 36-29). The muscular attachments of the abdominal, erector spinae, and gluteus muscles and the lumbodorsal fascia are detached and reflected. The gluteus muscles are elevated using a subperiosteal technique down to the sciatic notch. The gluteal vessels and nerves should be preserved. Ventrally subperiosteal elevation of the iliac and psoas muscles exposes the sacroiliac joint. Care must be taken to not injure the lumbosacral nerve trunk as it passes ventral to the surface of the sacroiliac joint. The osteotomy is performed in a dorsoventral direction. The sacral osteotomy is begun lateral to the upper three dorsal neuroforamina and directed ventrally. Laterally, the iliac osteotomy is carried down to the sciatic notch. The entire specimen is removed en bloc. The bony margins are covered with bone wax and Gelfoam, as desired, and closed in layers over drains.[17]

The abdominosacral approach is a combination of a low ventral sacral approach and a dorsal sacral approach.[8] It is also used for the sacrectomy, if en bloc resection is indicated.[18] The incision for the ventral approach varies, depending on whether rectum resection is required. If it can be preserved, the peritoneum need not be opened. A generous, semicircular incision provides adequate exposure of the sacrum after retracting the peritoneal contents rostrally. The patient is positioned supine with legs bent and flexed. The semicircular incision is made just above the pubis bone, cutting through the tendon of the rectus muscle, 1 cm above its attachments bilaterally (see Fig. 36-28). The peritoneum is swept upward to expose the common and external and internal iliac vessels. Vessel loops are applied for vascular control. This dissection is performed medially under the dorsal parietal peritoneum, preserving the superior hypogastric plexus and ureter, and meets in the midline behind the rectum.

If the rectum is resected, the peritoneal cavity is opened through a caudal midline incision. It will be necessary to ligate the superior rectal vessels, cut the bowel through the ureterosigmoid junction, and invaginate the tissue of incised bowel. The peritoneum is incised through the bottom of the rectovesical pouch, and the rectum is released ventrally. With the patient in the lithotomy position, an inverted U incision is made around the anus and the anal canal and rectum are dissected free.

The internal iliac arteries and veins are separated and controlled with vessel loops. The lateral and medial sacral veins and arteries are incised and ligated. If a sacrectomy above S1 is to be performed, iliolumbar vessels must also be taken. The periosteum is stripped, and the sympathetic nerve trunk is incised ventral to S1. Lateral to the sympathetic trunk, the lumbosacral nerves L4 and L5 pass ventral to the sacral wing and the sacroiliac joint. These must be released and protected. Finally, the sacrum is removed via osteotomy. It is advised that the osteotomy line be carried past the sacroiliac joint so that it can be palpated during the dorsal approach (Fig. 36-30). Also, if an en bloc resection is desired, the osteotomy should be performed one level above the tumor. The wound is closed in multiple layers or is closed temporarily, if the rectum is to be resected.

For a combined procedure, the patient is turned and a dorsal midline incision is made from L5 to the coccyx. The iliac attachments of the gluteus muscles are transected, leaving a cuff for reattachment. The sacral attachments of the gluteus maximus and underlying piriformis muscles and the anococcygeal, sacrospinous, and sacrotuberous ligaments are transected, also leaving a cuff. The gluteal nerves and vessels are preserved, if possible. The sciatic nerves are dissected through the sciatic notch and preserved. A partial lower L5 and upper sacral laminectomy is performed to expose the dural sac, which is ligated just below

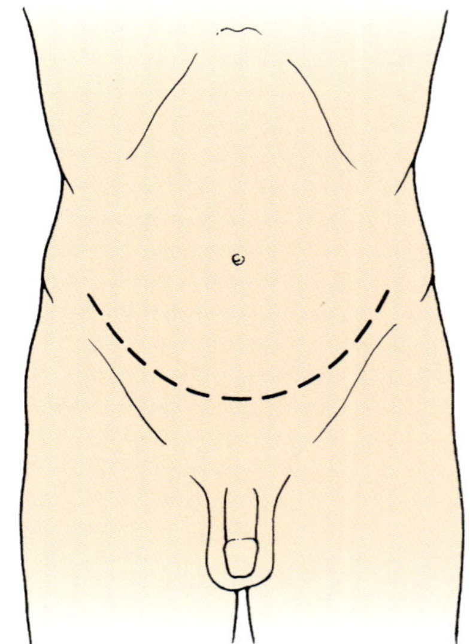

FIGURE 36-30. U incision for ventral sacrectomy.

the last nerve root to be preserved. The ventral osteotomy line is then palpated, and the dorsal osteotomy is performed. This should extend from the midline through the sacroiliac joint. Stabilization of the lumbar spine to the ileum may be required, if the L5-S1 joints are taken. However, if the S1 vertebral body is left intact, stabilization is usually not necessary. Once the osteotomy is complete, the distal ends of the sacrificed sacral nerve roots are divided just proximal to their entry into the sciatic nerve. Bleeding is usually profuse. Hemostasis should be quickly achieved with bone wax and electrocautery. If the rectum can be preserved, the anal region is released from the dissecting bands that attach it to the coccyx. However, if it is to be included, the levator ani is transected on each side. In an en bloc procedure, the sacrospinal muscles are taken with the specimen to avoid violating the tumor wall. The wound is closed in multiple layers over a drain. If the rectum has been included in the specimen, the patient is placed in the supine position and the abdomen is opened again. The sigmoid colon is removed from its mesentery, a colostomy is performed, and the pelvic peritoneum is closed. The wound is again closed in a standard fashion.

Complications

Visceral Complications

Perforation of the peritoneum is common, especially if there has been previous surgery, scarring, or infection. If this should happen, immediate repair is indicated. With the retroperitoneal approach, the abdominal wall is well developed laterally and, therefore, the transverse abdominis muscle and peritoneum can be readily identified and separated. For a pararectus retroperitoneal approach, the peritoneum can be identified just lateral to the rectus sheath.

With the retroperitoneal approach, the ureter is usually identified on the undersurface of the peritoneal sac. It should be swept medially and ventrally. With the transperitoneal approach, the ureter is lateral and is usually not a problem. If the ureter was incised, primary repair is indicated.

Injury to bowel, bladder, kidneys, spleen, or any other visceral organ during direct or retroperitoneal approaches should be dealt with by the appropriate surgical specialist.

Vascular Complications

To prevent vascular complications, one should be aware of the variations in vascular anatomy (e.g., a large left iliac vein, an unusual bifurcation of the aorta or vena cava, atypical positions of the lumbar veins). In addition, osteophytic spurs associated with reactive changes in the disc can cause the vena cava to become adherent to the disc. Because most vascular structures are injured during disc removal, a layer of tissue is left between the disc (or disc/vertebral body) and the great vessels.

Lumbar veins can be variable in location, especially the fifth, or iliolumbar, vein. This vein drains into either the vena cava or left iliac vein and can become a tether, if it becomes necessary to move the vena cava from left to right. The risk of avulsion of the vein directly off the vena cava exists and can cause rapid blood loss. As the left iliac vein courses over the disc space at L5-S1, it can be stretched and flat. It must be identified and controlled to avoid injury when opening the L5-S1 disc space.[21] This vein can also be large, bulbous, and difficult to retract. If it is lacerated, proximal and distal control must be obtained before repair.

Arterial injury can occur in the form of clot formation or laceration. The most common injury reported is to the left iliac artery during an approach to the L4-5 disc space. This vessel must be partially mobilized to approach the disc space. Once it is mobilized, retractors must be carefully positioned and checked periodically to avoid kinking or compressing the large vessels.

Pulmonary Complications

Pleural tears should be treated with a tube thoracostomy. Chylothorax has been reported because of damage to the thoracic duct during ventral surgery while mobilizing the right crus of the diaphragm.[22]

Neural Complications

Neural injury can occur to the superior hypogastric plexus, sympathetic chain, cauda equina, or lumbosacral plexus. The superior hypogastric plexus is responsible for closure of the bladder neck during ejaculation. If the plexus is damaged, the result may be retrograde ejaculation.[20] This damage may be avoided by careful dissection of structures within the bifurcation of the aorta. By entering this area to the right of the left iliac artery and vein and sweeping the tissue from left to right, one can retract this tissue en bloc to preserve the plexus (see Fig. 36-24). Blunt dissection with gentle retraction of the prevertebral tissue must be used and excessive electrocautery avoided.

The paraspinous sympathetic lumbar chain must usually be stretched or cut in the normal course of the ventral approach. Usually, the patient complains of a cold foot on the opposite side of the dissection. In fact, the ipsilateral foot is abnormally warm because of the lack of vasoconstrictive ability on the side of the surgery.

Cauda equina damage results from direct penetration into the spinal canal. Correct graft measurement, controlled impaction technique, and good visualization of pathologic anatomy should minimize the risk of cauda equina injury.

The lumbosacral plexus is located in the psoas muscle. Penetration or aggressive retraction must be avoided to prevent significant plexus damage. Often the psoas muscle is markedly enlarged and bulging over the spine. Psoas muscle dissection should begin at the midline (at the disc space). A pin retractor can be used to hold the muscle away from the surgical site after dissection is completed.

Summary

Adequate exposure of ventral lumbosacral anatomy is limited by the physical impediments imposed on this region by the thoracic cage and pelvis, thoracic and abdominal viscera, and great vessels. Because of these constraints, a number of specific surgical approaches have been designed to maximize exposure of specific regions. To perform these operations safely and effectively, the surgeon must have a thorough understanding of the three-dimensional anatomy of the lumbosacral region and the potential anatomic variants, and a detailed plan for achieving the surgical goal within existing constraints. In addition, by understanding where the majority of complications arise and how to avoid them, the safety of these procedures can be improved significantly.

KEY REFERENCES

Benzel EC: Biomechanically relevant anatomy and material properties of the spine and associated elements. In Benzel EC, editor: *Biomechanics of spine stabilization: principles and clinical practice*, ed 1, New York, 1995, McGraw-Hill, p 3.

Found EM, Weinstein JN: Surgical approaches to the lumbar spine. In Frymoyer JW, editor: *The adult spine: principles and practice*, ed 1, Philadelphia, 1991, Lippincott-Raven, p 1522.

McCormick PC, Post KD: Surgical approaches to the sacrum. In Doty JR, Rengachry SS, editors: *Surgical disorders of the sacrum*, ed 1, New York, 1994, Thieme, p 257.

Sacks S: Anterior interbody fusion of the lumbar spine. *J Bone Joint Surg [Br]* 47:211, 1965.

Watkins R: Anterior lumbar interbody fusion surgical complications. *Clin Orthop* 284:47, 1992.

REFERENCES

The complete reference list is available online at expertconsult.com.

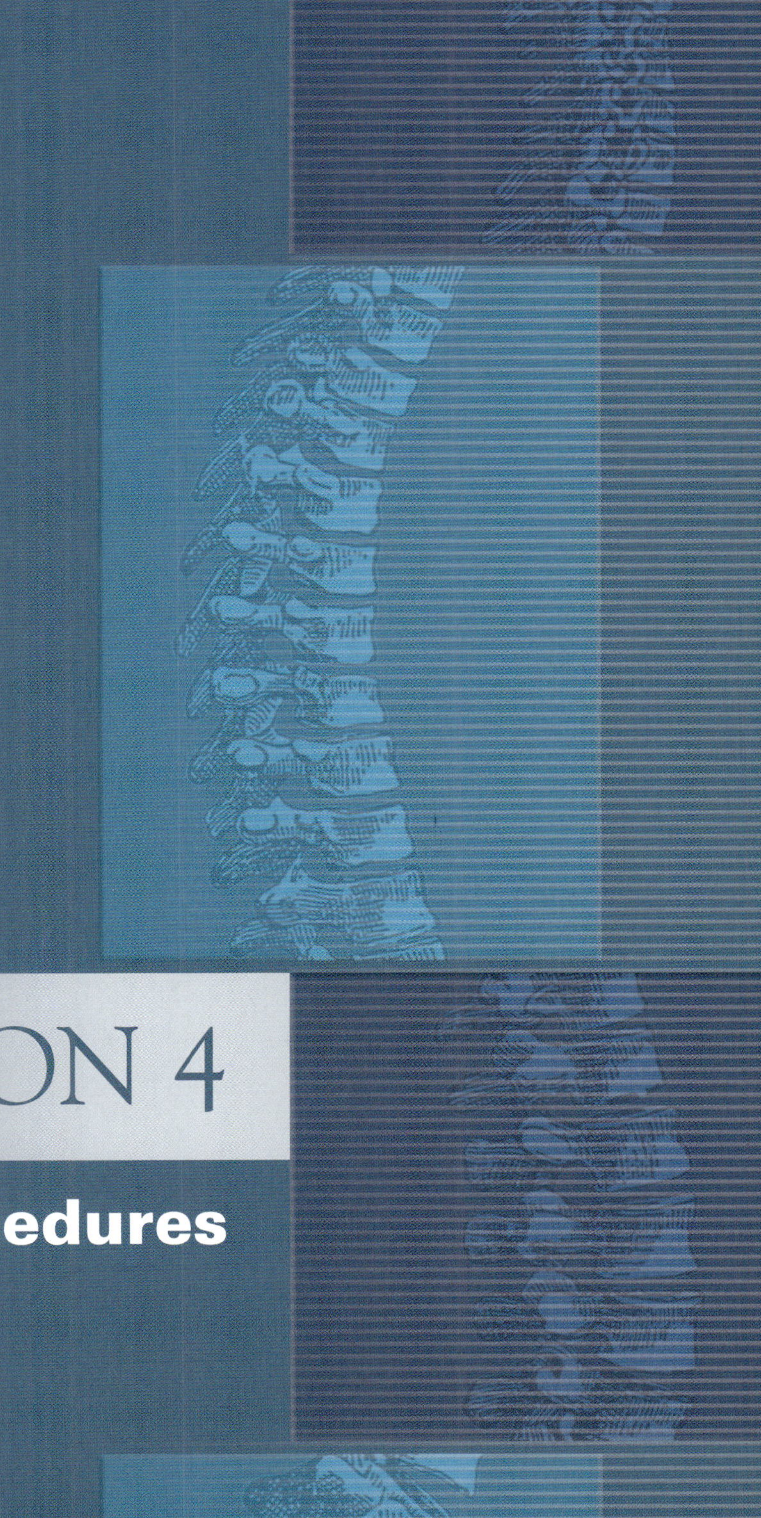

SECTION 4

Surgical Procedures

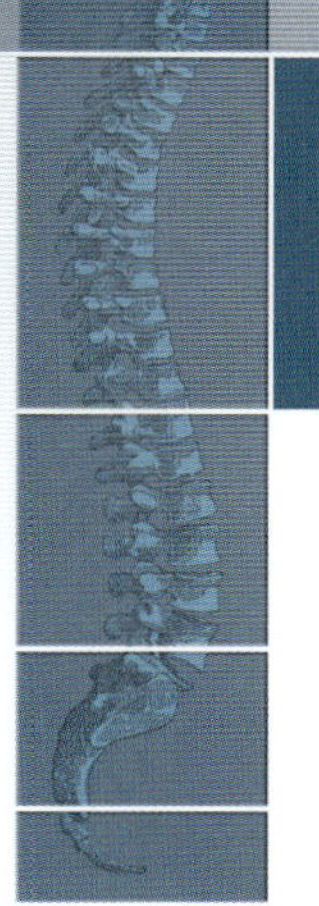

4.1 Decompression and Arthrodesis of the Cervical Spine

CHAPTER 37

Upper Cervical and Craniocervical Decompression

Brian R. Gantwerker | Volker K.H. Sonntag | Robert F. Spetzler

The posterior fossa and craniocervical junction house the structures vital for basic human functions. Deformities and pathology in this region place these structures at risk. Compression in this region may cause neurologic deficits related to the cerebellum, brainstem, and spinal cord. Operative decompression of endangered structures helps alleviate neurologic dysfunction. On radiography the presence of an obvious pathology in this region that correlates with a neurologic deficit makes the decision to operate straightforward. A more difficult question arises when there is discordance among a patient's films, history, and neurologic examination. The operative approach is dictated by the location of the pathology and the anatomy of local structures. Complication avoidance and management are paramount to good surgical outcomes. This chapter focuses on the choice of operation (ventral, lateral, dorsal, or combined) and on potential pitfalls associated with operating on complex pathologies in the posterior fossa, craniocervical junction, and upper cervical spine.

Pathology Overview

The pathologies possible at the craniocervical junction are varied.[1] Most lesions requiring surgery are approached dorsally through a posterior fossa craniectomy and C1 laminectomy. Table 37-1 lists the pathologies encountered by category. In a more basic organization, the abnormalities can be divided into congenital abnormalities and developmental/acquired pathologies. In Box 37-1 the material is reorganized in an empirical fashion.

Ventral Approaches

Several routes to the ventral clivus and upper cervical spine are accepted. Standard approaches to the ventral cervical spine are limited by the mandible and oropharynx.[2-4] Transoral routes to the lower clivus and upper cervical spine are acceptable and safe for addressing pathologies that cause craniocervical instability and that compress neurovascular structures. In 1917 Kanavel[5] described the first transoral procedure, which he performed to remove a bullet lodged between the clivus and ventral atlas. In 1962 Fang and Ong[6] reported the first series of six patients who underwent transoral decompression for atlantoaxial instability or congenital anomalies. Their high complication rate contributed to the slow acceptance of this approach.

A resurgent interest in the transoral approach led to the development of better techniques and instrumentation.[7] Current techniques and practices have lowered complication rates considerably.[8] Modern antibiotics and instruments have revolutionized and revitalized this operation. An extrapharyngeal approach for exposing the high cervical region is technically difficult but a reasonable alternative when the transoral approach cannot be used.[9] The transoral approach remains an excellent tool in the surgeon's armamentarium for ventral decompression. It is also versatile in that the upper clivus rostrally and C3 vertebral body caudally can be accessed. The authors prefer this route for extradural pathology. Dural closure is difficult in the transoral setting, and a lateral approach is preferable for intradural lesions. The far-lateral approach is quite robust for this purpose.

As minimally invasive surgery becomes more prevalent and patient demand for it increases, approaches to the upper cervical spine and clivus have become the target of efforts to minimize incisions and complications. In 2008 an endoscopic endonasal approach to odontoid resection was reported.[10]

Surgical Technique

General anesthesia is used for all ventral cases. A reinforced endotracheal tube is used to preserve the airway. Cervical stability is maintained by using fiberoptic endoscopy or awake-intubation techniques. At the authors' institution they routinely monitor somatosensory evoked potentials (SSEPs), and often motor evoked potentials (MEPs), intraoperatively. Baseline recordings are obtained before final positioning of the patient.

The patient is placed in the supine position on a standard operating room table with the head fixated in a Mayfield three-pin head holder (Codman, Inc., Randolph, Mass.) or a halo-ring adapter. A Spetzler-Sonntag transoral retractor (Aesculap, San Francisco) is positioned over the mouth. Retractors are used to form a rectangle of exposure. The palate is elevated cephalad, and the tongue and endotracheal tube are retracted caudally. The tonsils and lateral oropharyngeal

TABLE 37-1

Pathology of the Craniocervical Junction

Location	Congenital	Acquired	Primary Neoplastic	Secondary Neoplastic	Intra/Extradural	Neural "Tumors"
Clivus and foramen magnum	Segmentation failure	Basilar invagination Basilar impression (Paget disease, rickets, osteogenesis imperfecta, acro-osteolysis, rheumatoid arthritis) Paramesial invagination (achondroplasia)	Eosinophilic granuloma Fibrous dysplasia Chordoma Chondroma Chondrosarcoma Plasmacytoma	Prostate Breast Nasopharyngeal cancer Ectopic pituitary	Neurofibroma Meningioma Chordoma Glomus tumor Rhabdomyosarcoma	Tumors of brainstem, cerebellum Aneurysms Arachnoid and ependymal cysts Chiari II malformation
Atlas	Assimilation with segmentation failures	Stenosis (e.g., achondroplasia) Chronic dislocation (Morquio syndrome, Down syndrome, rheumatoid arthritis, other arthropathies)	Chordoma Chondroma Giant cell tumor Osteoid osteoma Osteoblastoma	Metastasis Plasmacytoma Local extensions of primary malignancy	Neurofibroma Meningioma Chordoma	Spinal cord glioma Syringohydromyelia Chiari malformation
Axis	Segmentation failure Os odontoideum Neurenteric cysts	Basilar invagination Basilar impression (Paget disease, rickets + hyperparathyroid arthropathies, osteogenesis imperfecta, rheumatoid arthritis, skeletal dysplasias) Chronic dislocations Osteomyelitis	Aneurysmal bone cyst Plasmacytoma Chordoma Giant cell tumor Osteoblastoma Chondroma	Metastasis Local extensions of primary malignancy	Meningioma Neurofibroma	Spinal cord glioma Syringohydromyelia

Modified from Menenzes AH: Pathology encountered at the craniocervical junction. *Oper Tech Neurosurg* 8(3):116–124, 2005. Used with permission from Elsevier.

BOX 37-1. Origin of Pathology at Craniocervical Junction

Congenital

Occipital bone malformations

- Occipital vertebrae
- Clivus segmentation
- Remnants around foramen magnum
- C1 variants
- Dens segmentation
- Basilar invagination
- Condylar hypoplasia
- Assimilation of atlas

Atlas malformations

- Atlas assimilation
- Atlantoaxial fusion
- Incomplete arch

Axis malformations

- Segmentation abnormalities
- Dens dysplasias
- Os odontoideum
- Ossiculum terminale persistens
- Hypoplasia-aplasia
- C2-3 segmentation failure

Developmental/Acquired

Foramen magnum abnormalities

- Secondary basilar invagination
- Rheumatoid arthritis
- Rickets
- Paget disease
- Osteomalacia
- Foraminal stenosis (e.g., achondroplasia)

Atlantoaxial instability

- Metabolic errors (e.g., Morquio syndrome)
- Down syndrome
- Infectious
- Inflammatory (e.g., rheumatoid arthritis)
- Trauma
- Os odontoideum
- Tumors (e.g., neurofibromatosis, syringomyelia)
- Miscellaneous

Modified from Menenzes AH: Pathology encountered at the craniocervical junction. *Oper Tech Neurosurg* 8:116–124, 2005. Used with permission from Elsevier.

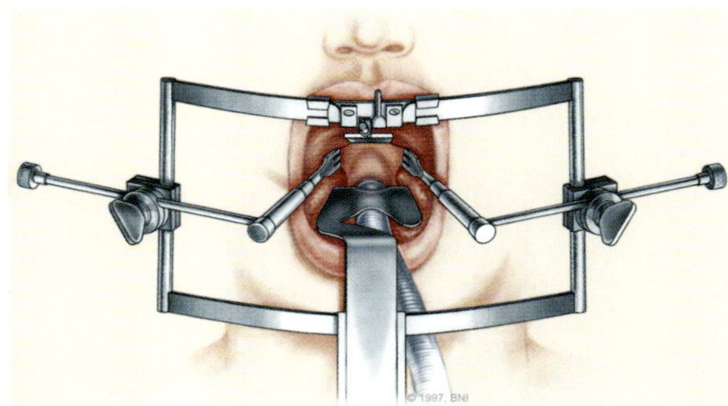

FIGURE 37-1. Placement of the Spetzler-Sonntag retractor system. The reinforced endotracheal tube and tongue are held by the lower blade. The upper blade retracts the soft palate away from the oropharynx. The depth of the lateral "fork" retractors can be adjusted to retract the tonsils first and then the soft tissue of the back wall of the oropharynx as the operation progresses. (Used with permission from Barrow Neurological Institute.)

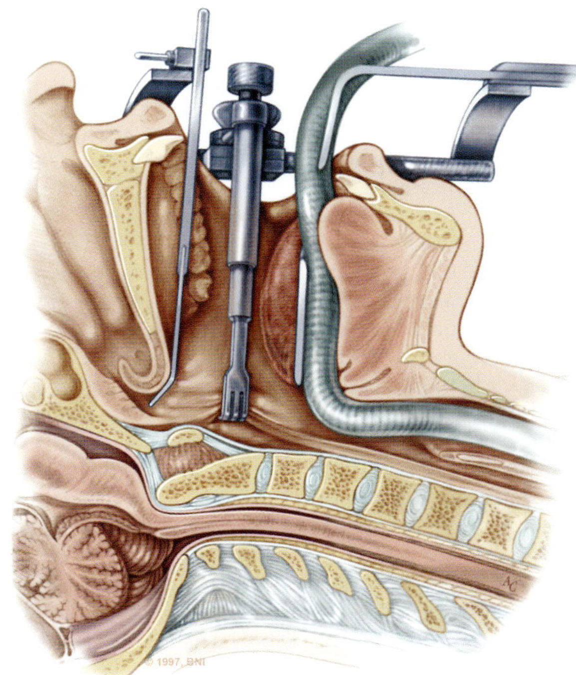

FIGURE 37-2. Lateral view of the retractor system in place. The lateral retractors lift the soft tissue up and away from the resection bed. Retraction of the palate and tongue provides excellent exposure. (Used with permission from Barrow Neurological Institute.)

walls are covered with moist gauze and retracted outward (Figs. 37-1 and 37-2). Transnasal catheters and palatal retraction sutures can be used in lieu of the Spetzler-Sonntag retractor. If the mouth cannot be opened sufficiently, a mandible-splitting approach can be used[11] and a tracheostomy performed before the surgical approach begins.

After the retractor is placed in its final position, the oral cavity is cleansed with povidone-iodine (Betadine). A preoperative dose of antibiotics that includes coverage for oral flora should be administered. The authors prefer cefepime and metronidazole. The surgeon sits at the patient's head, necessitating an adjustment in orientation for the duration of the case. An operating microscope is brought into the field. Stereotactic guidance may be used to guide the angle of approach and to confirm the location before the palatal incision is made.[12] Alternatively, fluoroscopy can be used for confirmation. Electrocauterization is used, and the incision proceeds down to bone. Subperiosteal dissection is used to expose the lower clivus, atlas, and axis. The authors seldom find it necessary to divide the soft palate unless the upper clivus is the target. Self-retaining retractors are placed to maintain exposure.

A high-speed air drill is used to remove the ventral arch of C1. The ventral arch of the atlas is the load-bearing portion of the bone.[13] An effort should be made to preserve a portion

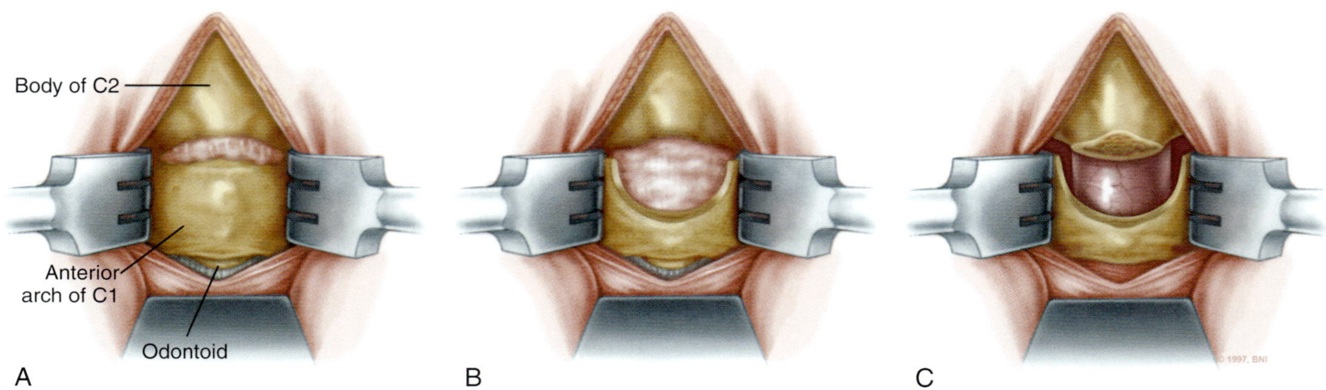

FIGURE 37-3. Stepwise resection of the odontoid. **A,** The back wall of the oropharynx is incised from the top of C1 to the bottom of C2. Subperiosteal dissection is extended laterally. The anterior arch of C1 is identified, and the midline is maintained by preserving part of the anterior arch. Frameless stereotactic guidance is also helpful. **B,** The anterior arch of C1 is partially drilled away, and the lesion encompassing the odontoid is clearly in view. **C,** The posterior portion of the odontoid is removed, and the dura is visible. The superior part of the anterior arch of C1 is intact. (Used with permission from Barrow Neurological Institute.)

of the arch to prevent spread of the lateral mass and to maintain orientation relative to midline. Approximately 70% of patients undergoing ventral decompression require supplemental internal fixation. This number increases to 90% in patients with rheumatoid arthritis.[14] The remaining anterior tubercle of C1 is left as a landmark for posterior screw fixation (Fig. 37-3A–C). Stereotactic navigation may be useful in cases requiring hardware fixation, especially if a large ventral portion of C1 and surrounding bone must be removed. Various instruments can be used to remove bone and tissue carefully. Long-handled curettes and rongeurs, as well as bipolar cautery, are useful adjuncts (Figs. 37-4 to 37-6). The average distance between the vertebral arteries is approximately 3 cm. The anatomic "safe zone" is 1.5 cm lateral to midline in both directions (Fig. 37-7). Preoperative radiographs must be evaluated carefully. In many cases, CT angiography can delineate aberrant or asymmetrical vasculature. Further lateral dissection places the hypoglossal nerve, vertebral artery, and cervical neurovascular bundle at risk.[15]

During a transoral odontoidectomy, cautious dissection and a methodical approach are essential to minimize the risk of cerebrospinal fluid (CSF) fistula. The superior ligamentous complex (consisting of the apical and paired alar ligaments) must be sectioned to remove the dens. This step should be performed first with curved curettes. This region is often adherent to the dura, and great care must be taken to avoid durotomy.[16,17] A thin shell of bone can be left to avoid a dural tear. Once the last of the odontoid is removed, the frameless guidance or a lateral radiograph can be checked with a radiopaque instrument in the field.[18]

Hemostasis is achieved using bipolar cautery and a thrombin hemostatic matrix (Floseal, Baxter Healthcare, Fremont, Calif.). Dural integrity is checked with a Valsalva maneuver held for 10 seconds. The pharynx is closed in a single layer with an absorbable suture. An enteric feeding tube is placed before anesthesia is reversed. Patients are left intubated 24 to 48 hours to avoid the trauma of reintubation if the upper airway or tongue swells. A feeding tube is placed under microscopic vision to avoid violating the mucosal suture line. After 1 week, the patient is allowed fluids. A swallow evaluation and modified barium swallow study may be undertaken before oral feedings are resumed. Dorsal stabilization may be performed during the same sitting or delayed several days to allow reassessment.

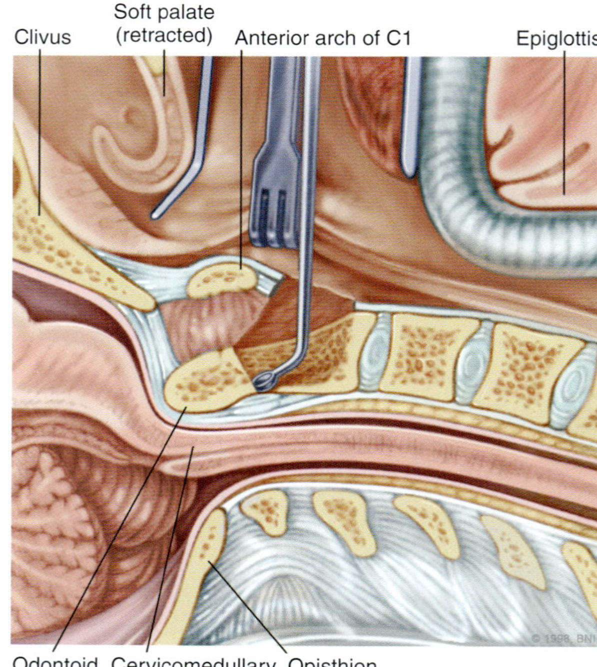

FIGURE 37-4. Decompression of the cervicomedullary junction by resection of the odontoid. A midline incision is made in the oropharynx, and a long, curved curette is used to resect the bone or mass. Orientation to midline is crucial during the compressive stage. A portion of C1 should be left to maintain the appropriate trajectory. (Used with permission from Barrow Neurological Institute.)

Pitfalls and Complication Avoidance

Preoperatively, many patients requiring ventral decompression may be severely debilitated. Postoperatively, they may need a course of parenteral nutrition, long-term rehabilitation

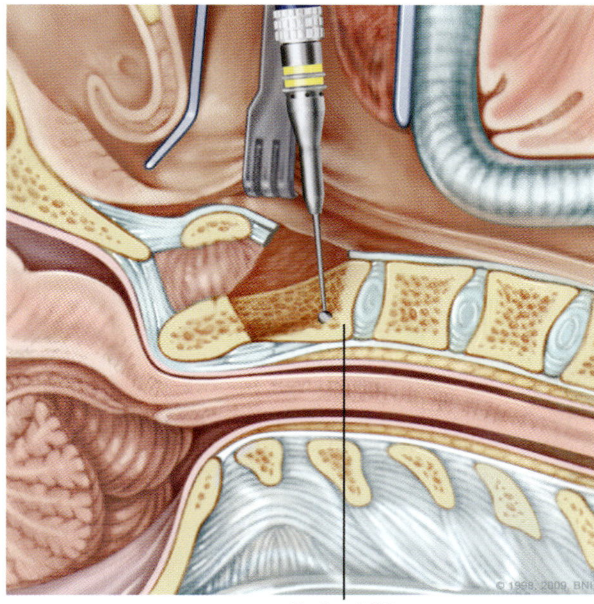

FIGURE 37-5. Further decompression is achieved with a high-speed drill. A handpiece with an angled bur works well in the depths of the resection bed. (Used with permission from Barrow Neurological Institute.)

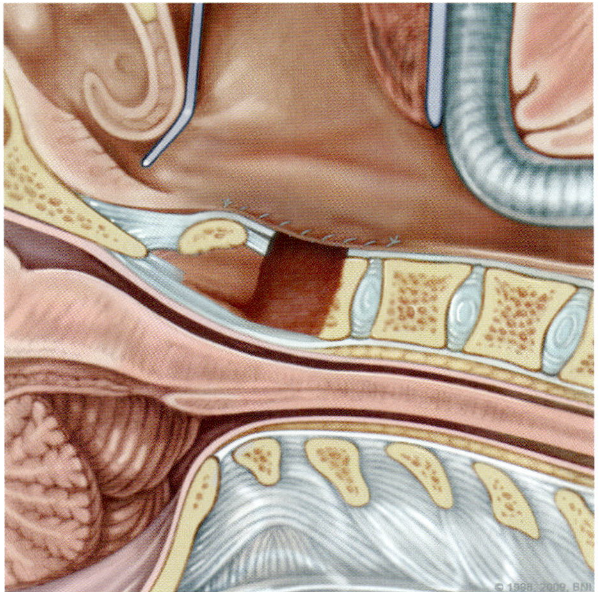

FIGURE 37-6. A watertight closure of the oropharyngeal incision is important to prevent postoperative cerebrospinal fluid leakage. The brainstem is well decompressed and in anatomic position. (Used with permission from Barrow Neurological Institute.)

or skilled-nursing care placement, and a long convalescent period. The surgeon should make it a priority to ensure that patients and their loved ones have appropriate and realistic expectations about outcomes and that they understand the possible risks and complications associated with the procedure.

Checking and rechecking midline orientation and depth of resection are key to safety. Dissection planes may be obscured by local pathology and may never emerge during the course

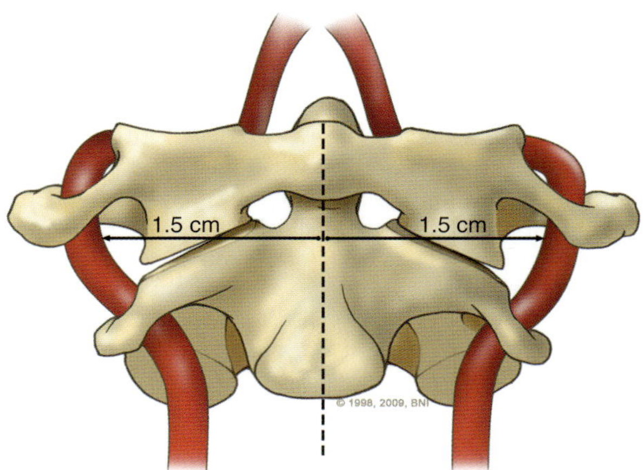

FIGURE 37-7. Illustration showing the lateral "safe zone" for resection of the odontoid, the average distance of which is 1.5 cm from midline. (Used with permission from Barrow Neurological Institute.)

of a case. As the resection proceeds deeper, meticulous dissection is crucial. A clean and bloodfree field must be maintained. Should the dura become lacerated, the surgeon should make every effort to repair it primarily. Fibrin glue or a fascial graft should be considered for adjuncts. Postoperatively, a lumbar subarachnoid drain should be placed and left for several days. The patient should be under constant surveillance, and fluid cultures should be followed to observe for signs of meningitis. Preoperative antibiotics should be maintained postoperatively if contamination is suspected. Before extubation, upper airway and tongue swelling should have abated enough to avoid obstruction and the precipitous decline of a patient with a difficult, swollen airway. Should this situation develop, an emergent tracheostomy or cricothyrotomy is option for reestablishing the airway.

Lateral Approaches

The lateral craniocervical region is rarely involved with bony compressive lesions. Most of these lesions are strongly associated with assimilation of the atlas into the occiput when segmentation fails between the last (fourth) occipital and first cervical sclerotomes. The sclerotomes fail to separate and remain fused, resulting in an incompletely separated atlas and sometimes a bifid lamina. This defect is associated with various syndromes (e.g., achondroplasia, Morquio syndrome) and usually occurs in conjunction with other occipitocervical bony anomalies. Astute clinicians should be wary of such entities, which may be common, such as Chiari I malformations and Klippel-Feil syndrome. Rarer but no less significant entities such as basilar invagination and congenital fusion of C2 and C3 also occur.[19,20] Thus lateral approaches may need to be part of a larger operative plan and used in conjunction with other techniques to completely address the pathologies present.

Lateral compression can be unilateral or bilateral. Stenosis of the foramen magnum leads to pain (usually occipital or high cervical) and possibly myelopathy. Instability may be present, and a fusion procedure may be necessary in addition to decompression. Other lesions located ventrally in the foramen magnum such as vertebrobasilar aneurysms and meningiomas can be approached laterally. A lateral approach allows adequate exposure while protecting delicate neural structures.

Lateral approaches to the upper cervical spine have been in development for decades. These surgeries eventually resulted in the techniques commonly used today. Henry described a technique for gaining access to the V2 and V3 segments of the vertebral artery through a similar incision.[21] Whitesides and Kelly further developed lateral approaches for spinal fusion using a similar incision.[22] Their technique was based on dividing the sternocleidomastoid muscle at its origin in the mastoid and reflecting it dorsally. Since then, numerous authors have modified, refined, and expanded this approach to the lateral upper cervical spine and foramen magnum for both extradural and intradural lesions.[23-26] Some authors have reported more aggressive approaches involving mobilization of the vertebral artery and sectioning of the sigmoid sinus when exposure needs to be increased.[27] Approaches have been modified to allow resection of lesions traversing the foramen magnum and into the upper cervical spine—the so-called "extreme lateral" approaches.[28] Either a laterally or medially based incision can be used with the muscle flap directed medially or laterally, respectively. The authors' preferred method is based on a dorsal midline approach.

Surgical Technique for Far-Lateral Approach

Intraoperative stereotactic navigation can be helpful with the far-lateral approach. During resection of tumors it can be useful to monitor the lower cranial nerves in addition to SSEPs. The patient is placed in the three-pin head holder with one pin on the forehead in the supraorbital area of the ipsilateral forehead. The two-pin portion is placed low on the contralateral occipital bone, above the level of the inion, leaving the retroauricular area to the midline open (Fig. 37-8A).

The patient is placed in a modified park-bench position.[29] The lower arm is slung off the table and cradled with the arm padded and the sling taped to the Mayfield adapter. The head is flexed and rotated contralaterally to bring the lesion to the highest point in the field. The surgeon should guard against the tendency for the patient's head to translate forward during positioning. Bending the head away from the ipsilateral shoulder opens the angle between the upper cervical spine and occiput. The upper shoulder is pulled caudally and taped to the bed. Care is taken not to tape over the clavicle, as doing so puts tension on the upper brachial plexus and can cause Erb palsy. The axilla is well padded. A beanbag may be used. Foam padding should be used generously. The body, especially the upper hip, should be well taped to the bed, permitting full vertical and lateral rotation of the operating table. While the patient is positioned, the evoked potentials should be monitored closely for changes (Fig. 37-8B).

A satisfactory stereotactic film and registration are critical. Either a curvilinear "hockey stick" or paramedian incision can be used. A paramedian incision is simpler, but stereotactic guidance should be used to avoid injury to the vertebral artery (Fig. 37-9). If used, a curvilinear incision is curved rostromedially below the superior nuchal line. The inferior part of the incision extends caudally to about C4. In heavier patients C4 may be difficult to identify. A cuff of muscle and fascia can be left near the superior nuchal line to aid in closure. Using subperiosteal dissection, the surgeon elevates the remaining muscle and fascia in one flap and retracts it laterally. This maneuver exposes the occiput down to the spinous process of C2. Fish hooks or heavy "0" sutures can be used to hold the flap away with a Leyla bar or other retractor system. The C2 ganglion is preserved throughout its course.

The ring of C1 can usually be palpated deeper to and above the spinous process of C2. Subperiosteal dissection

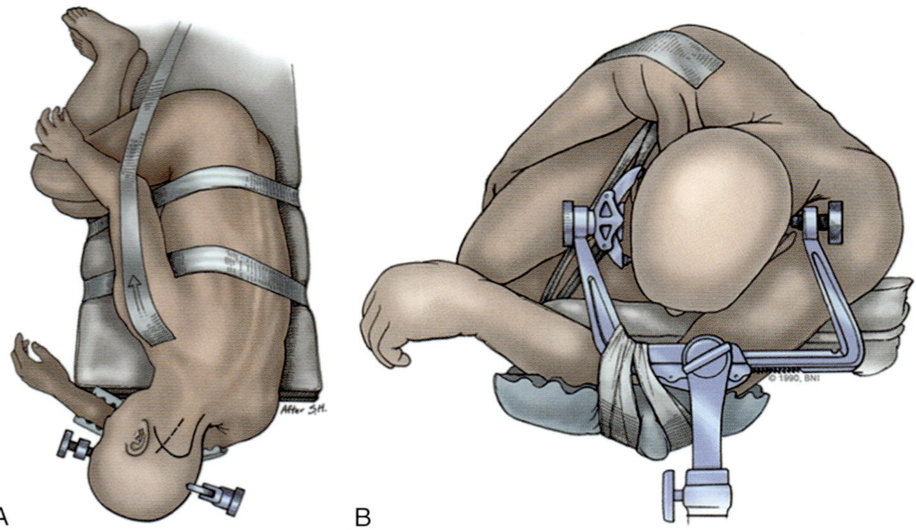

FIGURE 37-8. A, Patient position for a far-lateral craniotomy. Both the standard and paramedian linear *(dashed line)* incisions are shown. Note the position of the lower arm, which is slung in egg crate from the Mayfield head holder. The upper shoulder is taped on the lateral side to open the working space and to avoid injury to the brachial plexus. **B,** Another view of patient position. The Mayfield pins are placed to maximize exposure. Two pins are placed anteriorly. The third is placed far on the side opposite the operative side. The neck is flexed slightly. Care should be taken to avoid too much traction on the shoulder. The lower arm is slung from the head holder. (**A,** From Baldwin HZ, Miller CG, van Loveren HR, et al: The far lateral/combined supra- and infratentorial approach: a human cadaveric prosection model for routes of access to the petroclival region and ventral brain stem. *J Neurosurg* 81:60–68, 1994. **B,** Courtesy of Barrow Neurological Institute.)

proceeds laterally onto the lateral mass of C1. The suboccipital triangle is composed of the superior oblique, inferior oblique, and splenius capitis muscle. Deep to the triangle is the vertebral artery. The lateral point of the triangle is the C1 tubercle. The vertebral artery usually courses along the upper border of the C1 lamina (Fig. 37-10). Familiarity with the particular patient's anatomy, especially the vertebral artery and its segments (Fig. 37-11), is important. The V1 (ostial) segment arises from the subclavian artery and courses superiorly to the transverse foramen of C6. The V2 (transverse) segment extends from C6 to the C2 foramen. The V3 (suboccipital) segment courses from the C2 foramen until it penetrates the dura and enters the subarachnoid space. When the artery penetrates the dura, it becomes the V4 (intracranial) segment. V4 courses anteromedially along the medulla and joins its twin segment at the vertebrobasilar junction to form the basilar artery.

During operative exposure, the surrounding venous plexus can cause troublesome bleeding. Bipolar cautery, surgical

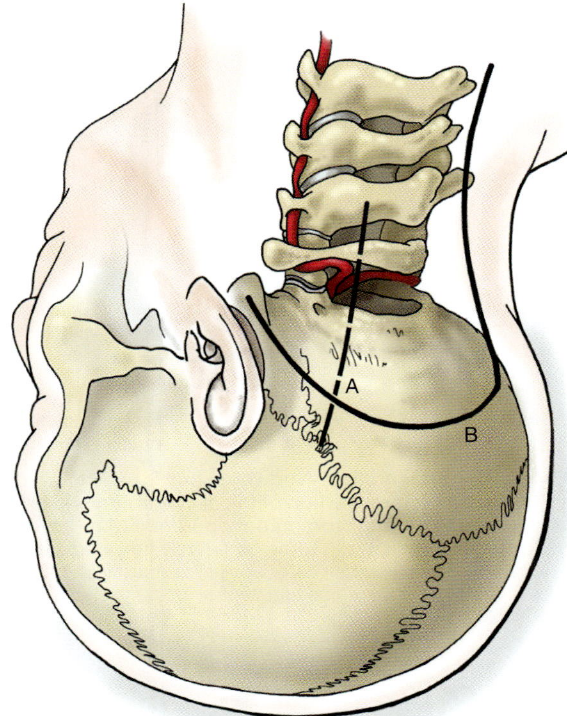

FIGURE 37-9. Linear incision for a far-lateral craniotomy, which is the simplest method for exposure *(A)*. Great care should be taken to avoid the vertebral artery, which is near the deep portion of the incision, just inferior to the foramen magnum. The classic "hockey-stick" or "inverted J" incision *(B)*. The lateral portion begins at the mastoid tip and is directed medially to the midline. The long arm of the incision is at midline, ideally in the avascular midline (the nuchal line). (From Baldwin HZ, Miller CG, van Loveren HR, et al: The far lateral/combined supra- and infratentorial approach: a human cadaveric prosection model for routes of access to the petroclival region and ventral brain stem. *J Neurosurg* 81:60–68, 1994.)

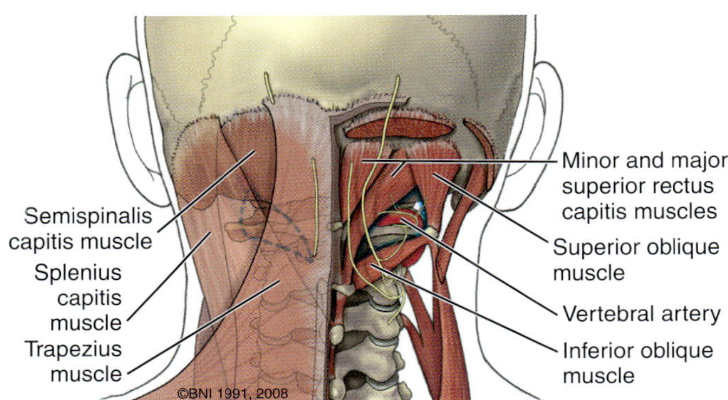

FIGURE 37-10. Regional anatomy of the suboccipital triangle. The vertebral artery lies in the deep portion of the triangle formed by the superior oblique, inferior oblique, and rectus capitis muscles. (Used with permission from Barrow Neurological Institute.)

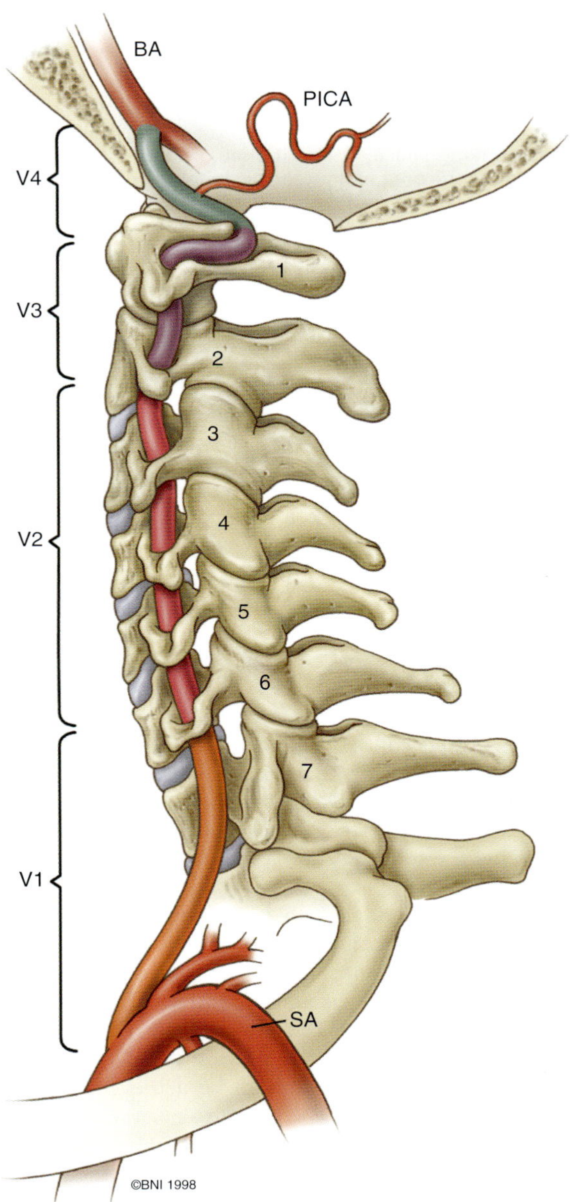

FIGURE 37-11. Segmental anatomy of the vertebral artery. The four segments are V1, ostial; V2, transverse; V3, suboccipital; and V4, intracranial. See text for details. BA, basilar artery; PICA, posterior inferior cerebellar artery. (Used with permission from Barrow Neurological Institute.)

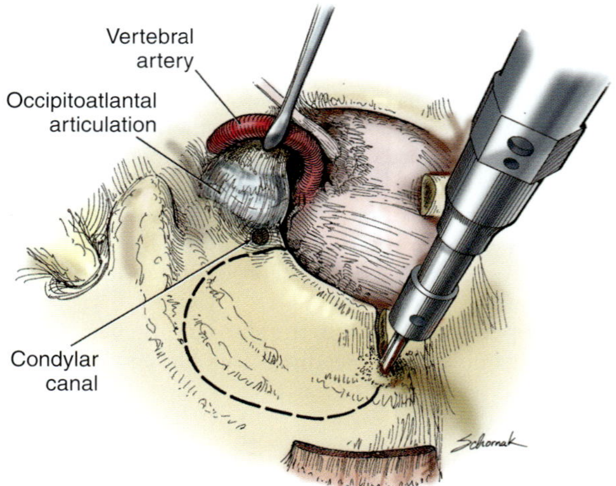

FIGURE 37-12. Craniotomy for a far-lateral approach. The C1 hemilaminectomy is completed first and provides decompression and a useful working space. The foot plate of the drill is guided from the midline to the area behind the occipital condyle. The vertebral artery is gently retracted. Its normal position is directly behind the occiput-C1 facet. (From Baldwin HZ, Miller CG, van Loveren HR, et al: The far lateral/combined supra- and infratentorial approach: a human cadaveric prosection model for routes of access to the petroclival region and ventral brain stem. *J Neurosurg* 81:60–68, 1994.)

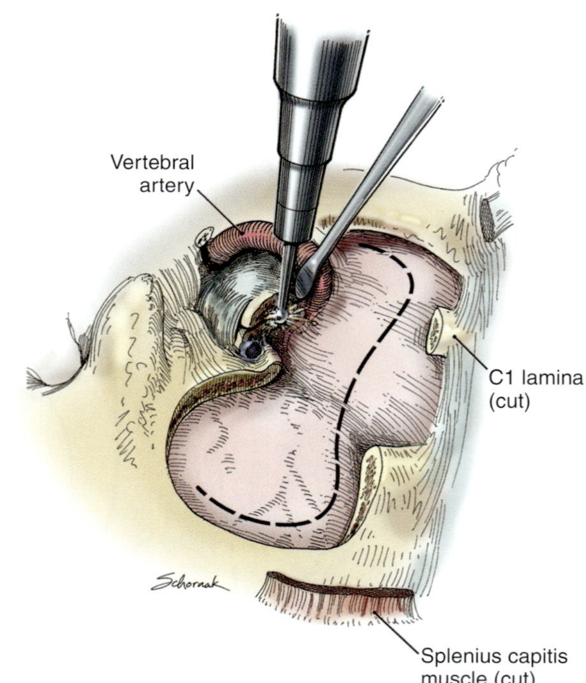

FIGURE 37-13. Condylar drilling. A powered drill is used to gradually remove the posterolateral portion of the occipital condyle to maximize access to the anterior foramen magnum. (From Baldwin HZ, Miller CG, van Loveren HR, et al: The far lateral/combined supra- and infratentorial approach: a human cadaveric prosection model for routes of access to the petroclival region and ventral brain stem. *J Neurosurg* 81:60–68, 1994.)

cellulose (SURGICEL NU-KNIT, Ethicon, Somerville, N.J.), and liquid hemostatic agents (Floseal) usually control any bleeding encountered.

A C1 hemilaminectomy is performed from just beyond midline to the ipsilateral sulcus arteriosus. The artery can be unroofed from the foramen to mobilize it. A lateral suboccipital craniotomy is performed with a foot-plate drill (Fig. 37-12). The craniotomy is enlarged using rongeurs until the lateral mass of C1 and the occipital condyle are exposed. The bony lesion is exposed extradurally. The vertebral artery is kept moist and protected. A high-speed air drill is used to remove the lesion extradurally. A diamond bur is useful, but care should be taken to avoid heating the bit near the artery. Upbiting curettes can be used for lesions that are difficult to reach. If a dural breach is seen, primary closure or a patch graft should be used with fibrin glue. If deemed necessary, a stabilization procedure may be performed. The wound is closed in anatomic layers, and a lumbar drain is placed if the dura is violated.

The occipital condyle can be removed to assist further decompression of the foramen magnum (Fig. 37-13). The hypoglossal foramen runs in a posteromedial to anterolateral direction with the occipital condyle (Fig. 37-14). The posterolateral portion of the condyle can be removed to increase access to the anterior portion of the foramen magnum. A wide surgical corridor can be achieved, with access to the anterior portion of the foramen magnum (Figs. 37-15 and 37-16). The relation of the occipital condyles can vary greatly from patient to patient. Some patients have anteriorly or posteriorly displaced configurations (Figs. 37-17A–C). Drilling carefully and gradually can achieve the desired access to the anterior foramen magnum. If brisk bleeding from the dorsal condylar emissary vein is encountered, it can be controlled with NU-KNIT or bone. The anatomy of the hypoglossal canal must be understood to avoid injuring the

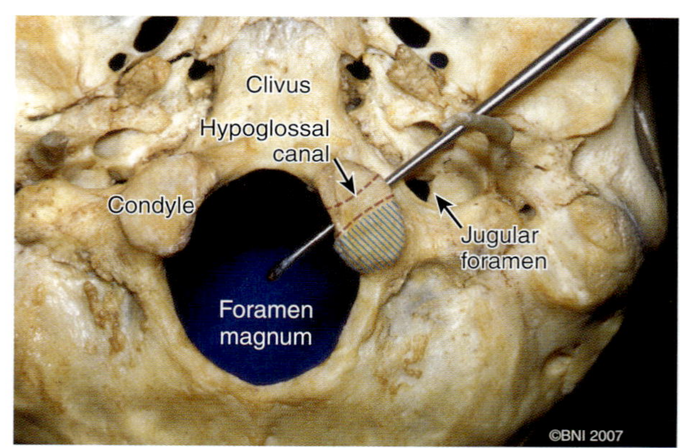

FIGURE 37-14. The hypoglossal canal and occipital condyle. The posterolateral portion of the condyle can be drilled to increase anterior exposure. The metal probe indicates the location of the hypoglossal canal within the condyle. (Used with permission from Barrow Neurological Institute.)

12th cranial nerve. The canal runs anterolaterally to posteromedially. The dorsal portion of the condyle can be removed with a high-speed drill. Using navigation at this depth is difficult. In select cases, occipitocervical stabilization should be considered. Biomechanical stability is altered when more than 50% of the condyle is resected.[30] Stability is also reduced significantly if the ventral portion of the condyle is removed. Options for fusion include occipitocervical plating with lateral mass screws, Steinmann pin fixation, or sublaminar wires.[31,32]

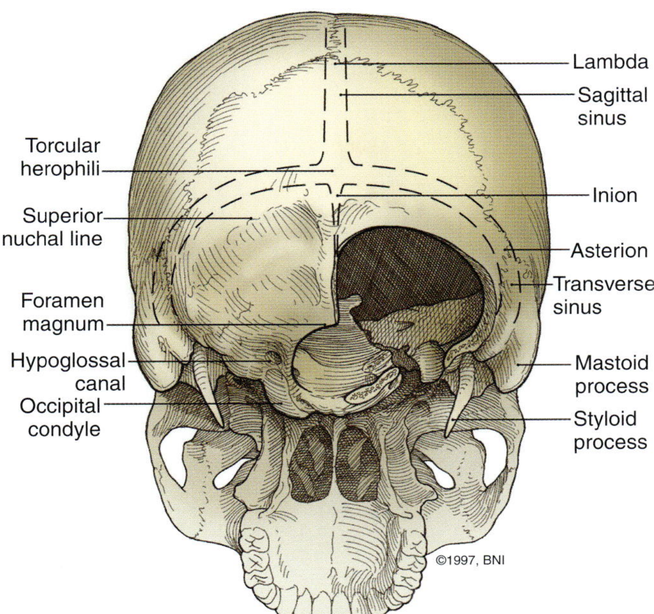

FIGURE 37-15. Detailed bony anatomy of the access provided by a far-lateral craniotomy. Much of the anterior foramen magnum can be accessed through this corridor. (Used with permission from Barrow Neurological Institute.)

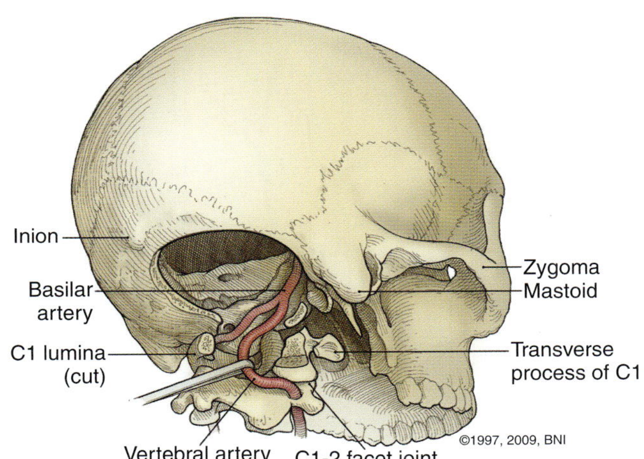

FIGURE 37-16. Oblique view of anterolateral access provided by a far-lateral craniotomy. The vertebrobasilar system is included to show the relevant regional arterial anatomy. (Used with permission from Barrow Neurological Institute.)

Pitfalls and Complication Avoidance

Patients usually present with cervical pain and various degrees of neurologic compromise. Potential complications are closely associated with the surgical angle of approach. The vertebral artery is at risk from surgical manipulation. Arterial lacerations should be repaired primarily. If a rent is too large, an end-to-end anastomosis should be performed with nonabsorbable monofilament suture of the surgeon's choice (usually 6-0 to 10-0). Although most patients may tolerate occlusion of the vertebral artery, the procedure should be avoided. Other possible vascular complications include thromboembolic stroke or ischemia from an arterial dissection. If available, endovascular therapies may be considered. Postoperatively, CT angiography or vessel-specific angiography should be completed expeditiously if vascular injury occurs.

Other complications reported with this technique and its variants[25,27,28] include venous air embolism, lower cranial nerve palsies, CSF leakage, hydrocephalus, brainstem edema, and death. Complications are most common with ventral and lateral tumors that require some brain retraction and cranial nerve dissection. If hydrocephalus is present preoperatively, it may be prudent to place an external ventricular or lumbar drain before surgery. Theoretically, doing so may reduce the need for retraction and lessen the likelihood of a CSF fistula.

Dorsal Approaches

In the early years of neurosurgery most, if not all, decompressions for the craniocervical junction were performed dorsally. Posterior fossa craniectomy with upper cervical laminectomy for the treatment of ventral pathology was soon found to be inadequate. In fact, in some instances, the patient's neurologic status worsened. With the advent of more direct approaches, the surgical strategy is now based on the location of the pathology and local anatomy. Dorsal decompression still holds a prominent place in the surgical methods of contemporary neurosurgeons.

Described by Hans Chiari in 1891,[33] Chiari I malformations result from descent of the cerebellar tonsillar below the level of the foramen magnum. Others have also been involved in the elucidation of this neurologic abnormality.[34,35] Patients usually suffer from headaches. Cervical myelopathy and hydrocephalus can be a part of the constellation of findings. Myelopathy may result from direct compression from tonsillar herniation or syringomyelia. Hydrocephalus reflects alterations in CSF flow patterns. Both conditions usually resolve after posterior fossa decompression and duraplasty.[36] Syringomyelia most often resolves 3 to 6 months after surgery.[37] Type II Chiari malformations are often associated with spina bifida and may necessitate decompression if symptoms occur (Fig. 37-18C).

The most common form of dwarfism, achondroplasia, is often associated with craniocervical deformities.[38] Most cases are sporadic. The foramen magnum becomes narrowed due to craniovertebral abnormalities related to thickening of the occipital bone. A thick epidural band can accompany the bony changes.[39] Spinal stenosis leads to spinal cord compression and hydrocephalus.[39] The major threat is respiratory compromise and the risk of sudden death.[40] Newborns with achondroplasia may benefit from early neurologic and respiratory screening, MRI of the craniocervical junction, and early decompression for severe cases.[41,42] Rheumatologic and degenerative diseases can also cause chronic subluxation and basilar settling. Irreducible cervicomedullary compression often results. Dorsal decompression and C1 laminectomy with dorsal stabilization are often used to correct the deformity, decompress neurologic structures, and halt progression.

Surgical Technique for Chiari Decompression

Monitoring SSEPs is a useful adjunct. Baseline readings should be obtained before the patient is positioned. Lower cranial nerve monitoring is not used routinely at our institution.

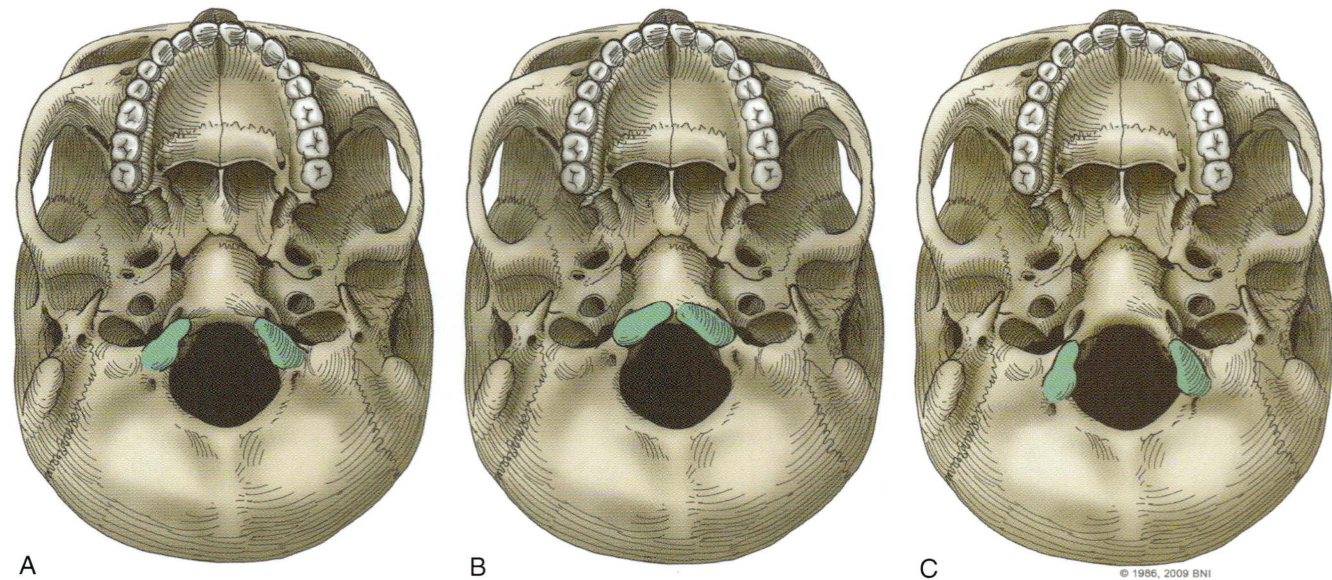

FIGURE 37-17. **A,** Normal configuration of the occipital condyles (*green*) at the "10" and "2" o'clock positions. Anterior (**B**) and posterior (**C**) variants of the occipital condyles (*green*). (Used with permission from Barrow Neurological Institute.)

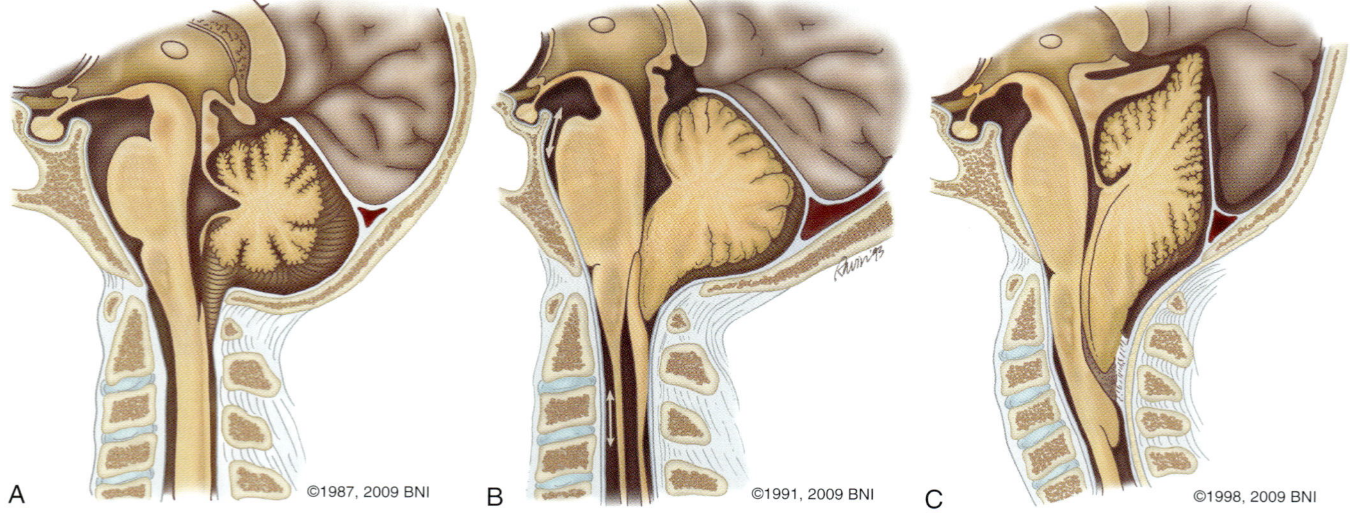

FIGURE 37-18. **A,** Type I Chiari malformation with cerebellar tonsillar herniation only. **B,** Type I Chiari with an associated syrinx. The bidirectional arrow indicates an altered pattern of cerebrospinal fluid flow. **C,** Type II Chiari malformation associated with various types of spina bifida. (Used with permission from Barrow Neurological Institute.)

Preoperative halo traction or Gardner-Wells tongs may be placed to assist reduction of the deformity or maintain stability. Often patients undergo further reduction when under general anesthesia. Before the incision is made in patients in traction, a lateral radiograph should be obtained to ensure their optimal alignment.

Patients are turned prone onto chest rolls, and the arms are tucked at the sides. The chin is tucked forward, against the neck in a military tuck position (Fig. 37-19). The planned craniectomy borders the venous sinuses on all borders. Care should be taken to avoid an overaggressive lateral decompression to prevent cerebellar sagging (Fig. 37-20). A midline incision is planned from the inion to C4. The nuchal line is an anatomic bloodless plane in the midline. Dissection proceeds in this plane to the occiput and spinous process of C2. The muscle attachments of C2 are left intact, but the top of C2 should be exposed (Fig. 37-21). The region around C1 and the foramen magnum is often the deepest part of the exposure. The occiput is exposed laterally and inferiorly in a subperiosteal fashion. Near the foramen magnum, curettes can be used to expose the foramen magnum carefully. A sharp ventral curve of the occipital bone indicates the margin of the foramen magnum. The C1 lamina is identified. A bifid C1 is often associated with a Chiari I malformation, and the surgeon should be cautious while finding the lamina. On both sides of midline, the exposure is continued laterally onto the

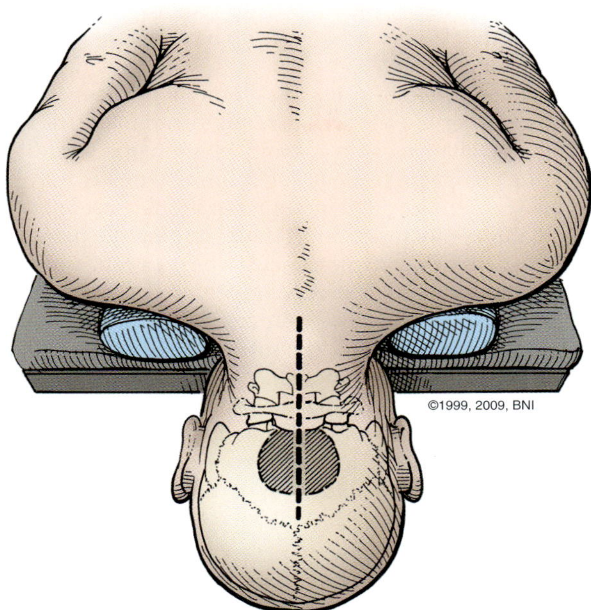

FIGURE 37-19. Patient position for suboccipital craniectomy. The patient is placed prone on soft gel rolls with the chin in a "military tuck." The incision is made from just above the inion to the spinous process of C2 in the midline. The proposed craniectomy (*cross-hatched area*) incorporates the posterior foramen magnum. Cervical laminectomies of C1 and C2 may be necessary to achieve adequate decompression. (Used with permission from Barrow Neurological Institute.)

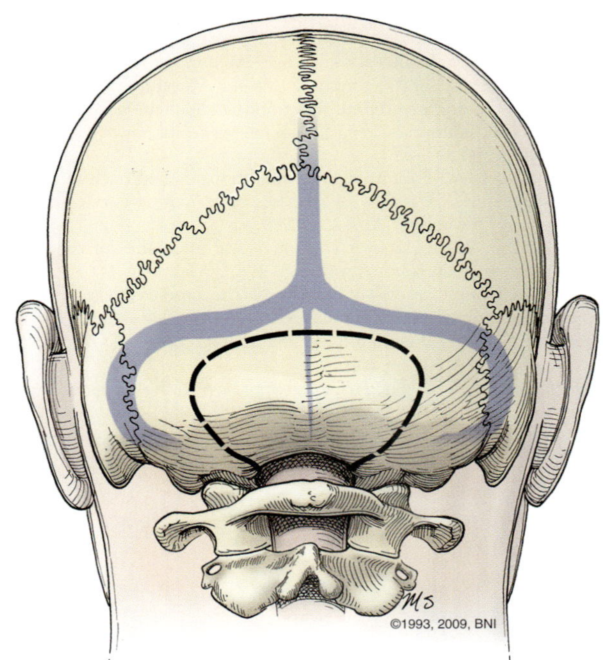

FIGURE 37-20. Suboccipital craniectomy. The venous sinuses border the proposed craniectomy. Care should be taken to avoid overzealous bone removal. (Used with permission from Barrow Neurological Institute.)

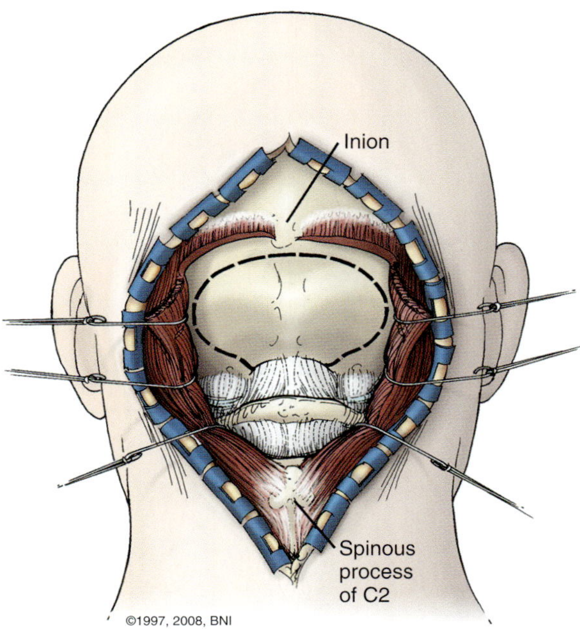

FIGURE 37-21. Midline incision for decompression. The avascular midline plane is followed, and exposure extends to C2. Bone is removed with a drill, Kerrison punches, or both. (Used with permission from Barrow Neurological Institute.)

ring of C1 using periosteal elevators and curettes. Laterally, the paravertebral venous complex can cause brisk bleeding. Such bleeding can be avoided by the use of bipolar forceps as a periosteal dissector on the lateral portion of the atlas and by use of Metzenbaum scissors to cut the coagulated muscle. SURGICEL and Floseal are helpful hemostatic adjuncts. Small, curved curettes are used to palpate under the ring of C1 and foramen magnum.

The bone of the occiput is removed with a high-speed drill. Two bur holes can be placed on either side of the midline "keel." The holes can be used both as depth gauges for drilling the bone and as access to strip the dura from a particularly deep keel with Penfield dissectors. The amount of bone removed depends on the anatomy of the pathology. In some cases, the foramen magnum only needs to be opened minimally. In the case of a Chiari malformation, a generous dorsolateral decompression allows adequate room for the cerebellum. At this time, a C1 laminectomy should be performed before the dura is opened. If instrumentation is anticipated, it can be placed before duraplasty.

A thick fibrous band, which can be quite vascular, is often present at the foramen magnum, especially in achondroplastic patients. If a duraplasty is planned, the dura is opened in a Y-shaped fashion. This configuration allows hemostatic clipping of the occipital sinus in the posterior fossa midline. Clips are placed sequentially along the dural incision. Arachnoid adhesions obstructing the foramen of Magendie should be lysed. The authors do not use bipolar cautery near the cerebellar tonsils. The practice of plugging the obex has also fallen from favor. A chevron-shaped patch is used for grafting. Historically, autologous fascia lata or skull periosteum is the graft best tolerated. Bovine pericardium, cadaveric dura, or paravertebral fascia are all reasonably reliable substitutes.

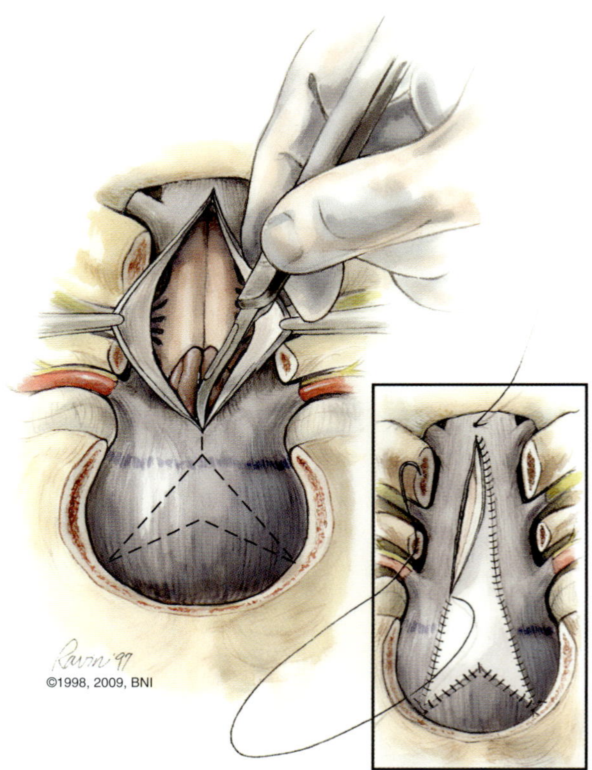

FIGURE 37-22. A midline dural incision is used, and a patch graft of autologous fascia lata or other suitable substitute is sewn in place. Watertight closure is critical to prevent postoperative complications. (Used with permission from Barrow Neurological Institute.)

A watertight closure is critical, and special attention should be paid to the inferior corner when the graft is sewn in place (Fig. 37-22). At this stage, CSF leaks can occur from a small dural defect in closure. More critical is the cervical fascial closure. The junction of the cervical fascia and galea at the inion should be closed meticulously. Here, most CSF leaks occur due to inadequate closure, especially in the corners of the durotomy. If allograft is used, some surgeons prefer a short course of low-dose steroids to reduce the rate of postoperative chemical meningitis.

Pitfalls and Complication Avoidance

The most commonly reported complications associated with dorsal approaches are CSF leaks, hydrocephalus, and pseudomeningoceles. Dural closure is therefore paramount to prevent complications. There have been no prospective, randomized studies on preoperative placement of a ventriculostomy, and only class III data are available. Many have reported their experiences with achondroplasia. Aryanpur et al.[43] reported four documented CSF leaks in 15 cases; 1 patient developed meningitis. Three of their patients required postoperative shunting. Other studies on this entity have reported low rates of CSF leakage.[36,39,41,44]

Neurologic outcomes are also limited to class III data. Lower cranial nerve dysfunction, respiratory difficulties, weakness, sensory changes, and chemical meningitis are all possible. Poor preoperative neurologic status tempers hopes for a good outcome. The diligent clinician should ensure respiratory and alimentary function in the postoperative period and during the patient's convalescence. Often, a swallowing evaluation is necessary both preoperatively and postoperatively to assess the patient's recovery. Increased weakness and sensory changes should prompt the surgeon to obtain postoperative imaging or, if severe enough, should warrant immediate reoperation. Patients with delayed signs should be screened for iatrogenic instability with dynamic films. Chemical meningitis, which is usually a diagnosis of exclusion, should be entertained if a spinal fluid assay is negative for infection. Usually, low-dose dexamethasone taken orally brings relief to the patient.

Summary

Advances in instrumentation, imaging, and intraoperative monitoring have opened new horizons and afforded increasingly effective and safe methods of decompression and stabilization of this vital region. A clinical presentation well correlated with a neurologic examination and radiographic findings is the basis for surgical evaluation. Choosing the appropriate approach, effective execution of the surgery, and an astute knowledge of the regional anatomy and pathology are all critical factors to obtaining satisfactory patient outcomes.

KEY REFERENCES

Batzdorf U: Chiari I malformation with syringomyelia. Evaluation of surgical therapy by magnetic resonance imaging. *J Neurosurg* 68:726–730, 1988.

Dickman CA, Spetzler RF, Sonntag VKH, Apostolides PJ: Transoral approach to the craniovertebral junction. In Dickman CA, Spetzler RF, Sonntag VKH, editors: *Surgery of the craniovertebral junction*, New York, 1998, Thieme, pp 355–370.

Hadley MN, Spetzler RF, Sonntag VK: The transoral approach to the superior cervical spine. A review of 53 cases of extradural cervicomedullary compression. *J Neurosurg* 71:16–23, 1989.

Klimo P Jr, Rao G, Brockmeyer D: Congenital anomalies of the cervical spine. *Neurosurg Clin North Am* 18:463–478, 2007.

Menezes AH: Complications of surgery at the craniovertebral junction: avoidance and management. *Pediatr Neurosurg* 17:254–266, 1991.

Menezes AH: Pathology encountered at the craniocervical junction. *Oper Tech Neurosurg* 8:116–123, 2005.

Spetzler RF, Grahm TW: The far-lateral approach to the inferior clivus and the upper cervical region. *BNI Q* 6:35–38, 1990.

REFERENCES

The complete reference list is available online at expertconsult.com.

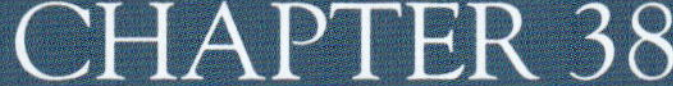
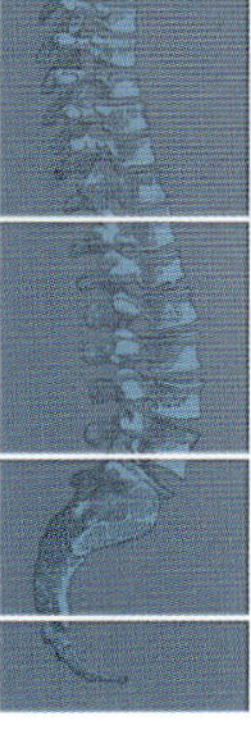

CHAPTER 38

Upper Cervical and Occipitocervical Arthrodesis

M. Yashar S. Kalani | Udaya K. Kakarla | Volker K.H. Sonntag | Nicholas Theodore

The cervicomedullary junction (CMJ) is a challenging region in which to perform surgical maneuvers. Although most pathologic changes affecting the CMJ are traumatic in origin, large skull-base tumors requiring extensive manipulation of the high cervical vertebrae also contribute to instability in this region. With the majority of the flexibility and motion of the neck centered on the high cervical vertebrae, a competent spine surgeon must be able to manipulate and stabilize the CMJ while minimizing morbidity to the patient.

Advances in imaging, spinal surgical technique, and instrumentation have provided novel means of approaching, stabilizing, and treating pathology at the CMJ. Key advances in instrumentation, including novel occipital fixation devices, C1 lateral mass screws, and C2 pedicle screws, [1-3] have promoted the development of numerous methods for fixation of the upper cervical spine. This chapter emphasizes the technical aspects of the different types of fixation and fusion of the upper cervical spine and CMJ. Methods for fixation of odontoid fractures, atlantoaxial instabilities, and occipitocervical instabilities—with special emphasis on the latest developments and instrumentation methods—are discussed.

Although a variety of techniques are emphasized in this text, several key points are common to all of the fixation methods. Given the importance of postoperative imaging, implants compatible with MRI, such as titanium, should be used whenever possible.

Ventral Approaches

Odontoid Fixation

Odontoid fractures, a common injury of the cervical spine, are found in conjunction with almost 60% of atlas fractures and with 10% to 20% of all cervical fractures.[4,5] Based on the Anderson and D'Alonzo nomenclature for odontoid fractures, almost 40% are type II fractures[6] (Fig. 38- 1). Although conservative management should be considered, given the high rate of nonunion associated with these lesions, surgery is the gold standard of treatment. Historically, dorsal wiring techniques, such as C1-2 arthrodesis with halo-vest immobilization for 3 months, offered an excellent fusion rate (as high as 97%).[7] The main shortcoming of wiring methods is the long-term loss of patient mobility from sacrifice of the atlantoaxial joint and prolonged halo-vest immobilization immediately after surgery.[7] Odontoid screw fixation, introduced by Bohler[8] and Nakanishi's group,[9] has eliminated the need for halo-vest immobilization, while preserving motion at C1-2: the fusion rate can be as high as 100% (92–100%),[10] and it is one of the only motion-preservation stabilization procedures available in spine surgery.

Patient selection is the key to obtaining good outcomes. Odontoid screw fixation is indicated for patients with an acute (more recent than 4–6 weeks) type II fracture. The high rate of sclerosis associated with fracture margins causes a high rate of nonunion in patients with chronic fractures.

Other key contraindications to this procedure include exclusion of patients with disruption of the transverse atlantal ligament as seen on MRI,[11] osteopenia with poor bone quality, inability to reduce a displaced fracture, and the presence of a type II fracture that extends across the base of the odontoid in an oblique plane. A disrupted transverse atlantal ligament results in dorsal migration of the fusion fragment during screw insertion; it does not address rupture of the transverse ligament even if the fracture heals. The inability to reduce a fracture appropriately to restore alignment and an oblique fracture line make capture of the fractured dens challenging. Osteopenia is a key contraindication that can result in "windshield wiping" of the screw with the potential to cause neurologic injury.

In the case of a ventral dislocation, the patient is placed supine with the neck extended or hyperextended and in a three-pin holder or halo tongs if preoperative traction is necessary. In the case of a dorsal dislocation, the patient is placed in a military chin-tuck position under fluoroscopic guidance. At our institution, we use intraoperative stealth image guidance to visualize bony anatomy in the coronal plane, eliminating the need for two image intensifiers. In a patient with a large barrel chest, it is difficult to obtain the necessary sagittal trajectory for screw placement. This problem can be corrected by translating the head and neck ventrally by hyperextending the neck with direct visualization using lateral fluoroscopy (Fig. 38-2). A very large chest can make the procedures technically impossible.

A transverse skin incision is made at the level of the cricothyroid junction, and the platysma is divided longitudinally to the ventral border of the sternocleidomastoid muscle. The dissection is performed using natural planes to the level of C4-5 (Fig. 38- 3). Blunt dissection proceeds rostrally to the level of the C2-3 disc space, and the retropharyngeal space is opened at C2. The medial borders of the longus colli muscles

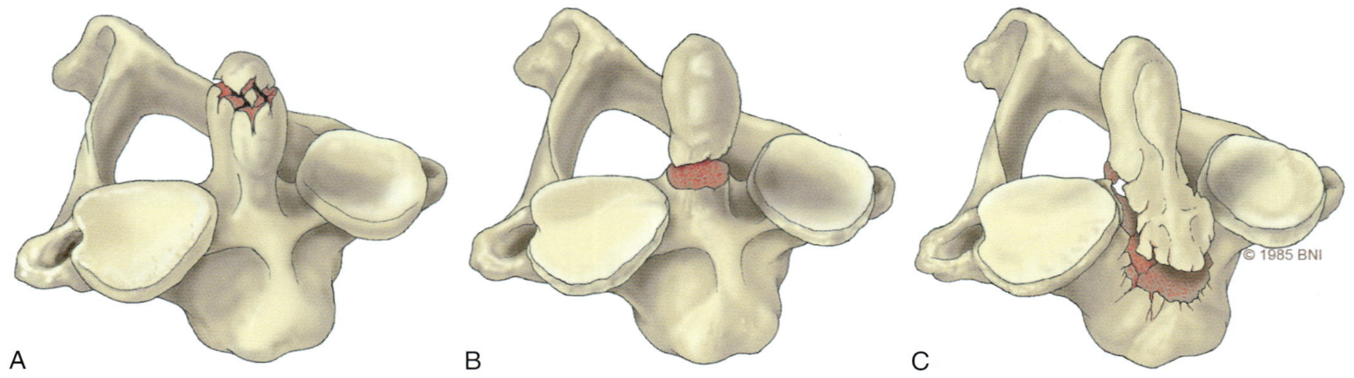

FIGURE 38-1. Anderson and D'Alonzo nomenclature for odontoid fractures. **A,** Type I fracture involving the odontoid tip. **B,** Type II fracture at the base of the odontoid. **C,** Type III fracture involving the body of C2. (Used with permission from the Barrow Neurological Institute.)

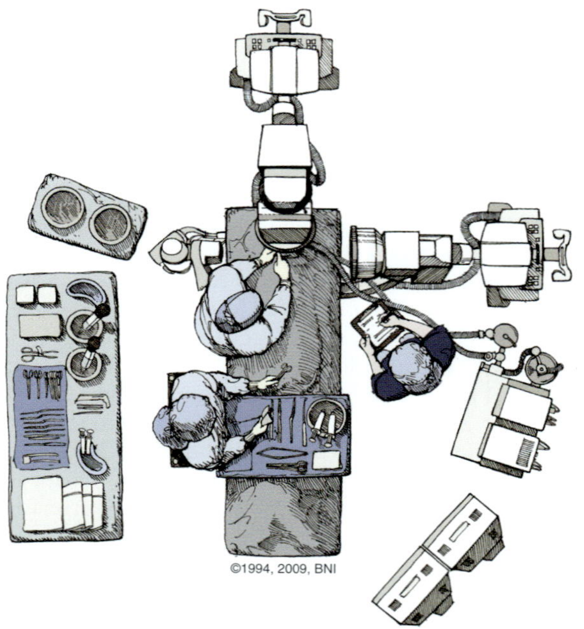

FIGURE 38-2. Positioning of two C-arm fluoroscopes for odontoid screw fixation. (Used with permission from Barrow Neurological Institute.)

are coagulated and elevated laterally to maintain exposure. Next, it is important to expose the midline of the body of C2 because the midline keel of C2 is the landmark for screw placement. Doing so requires creating a midline trough through the anulus and disc at the C2-3 interspace. The placement of this entry site is critical because rostral placement of a screw can cause the shaft of the screw to lie too close to the overlying ventral cortex of C2. In this scenario the screw can cut out, or windshield-wipe out, of the C2 body, and pseudarthrosis can then develop.

More recently, image-guided navigation for placing odontoid screws has been employed. When this technique is used, the patient's head is placed in a three-point fixation device and secured to the operating table. Using isocentric C-arm fluoroscopy, intraoperative images are obtained and 3D reconstruction is performed using the StealthStation (Medtronic, Minneapolis, MN). Using the coronal trajectory on the StealthStation, the midline of the C2 body is identified and a K-wire is advanced through the odontoid fracture. Real-time lateral fluoroscopy is used to monitor progress in the lateral plane until the K-wire approaches the cortex of the odontoid tip. Although the sagittal trajectory on the StealthStation may be used, it is not reliable. As force is applied on the C2 body during K-wire insertion, the body is pushed down and an error in sagittal trajectory is introduced, which can result

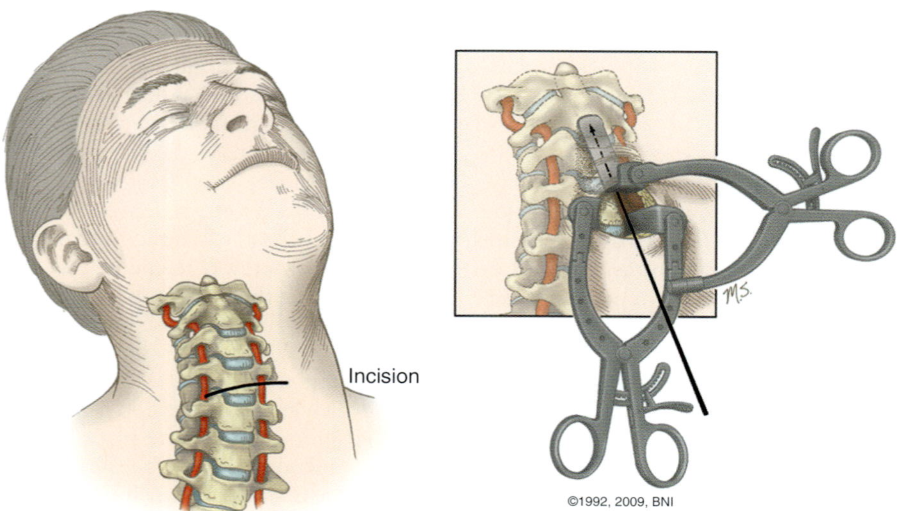

FIGURE 38-3. The incision used for exposure of the ventral cervical spine and pertinent anatomy of the vertebrae and vasculature. (Used with permission from Barrow Neurological Institute.)

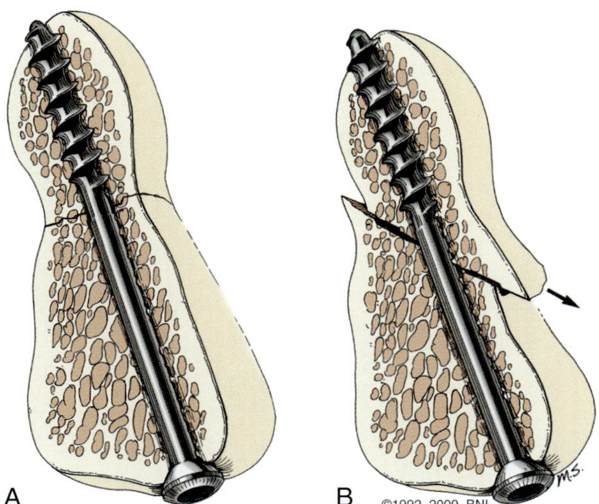

FIGURE 38-4. Ventral screw fixation of the odontoid with ideal (**A**) and suboptimal (**B**) screw placement. (Used with permission from Barrow Neurological Institute.)

in misplacement of the screw. As a result, we use image guidance for the coronal trajectory of the screw and lateral fluoroscopy for the sagittal trajectory and to monitor real-time progress of the K-wire and screw. Once the K-wire is placed, the bone can be drilled if it is very dense. The path is then tapped and a 4-mm screw is advanced under fluoroscopic guidance until it approaches the distal cortex of the dens. At this point, a cannulated titanium screw is selected (lag or fully threaded 4 mm). The screw is advanced and tightened until the screw head is just countersunk with respect to the body of C2 (Fig. 38-4). The screw length can be customized by measuring the K-wire depth on the fluoroscopic image.

A screw protruding into the C2-3 interspace can cause a lever effect that results in screw loosening and failure. Although a two-screw technique can be used, one screw is sufficient to achieve a stable union in most cases. Closure involves copious irrigation and hemostasis followed by layer-by-layer closure. Placement of the screw does not ensure complete restoration of the strength of the dens, and the patient must wear a cervical orthosis for at least 6 to 8 weeks. In the presence of contraindications to odontoid screw fixation, standard dorsal atlantoaxial fixation is performed.

Ventral Atlantoaxial Facet Screw Fixation

Ventral atlantoaxial facet screw fixation is similar to its odontoid counterpart, but the screw trajectory differs. This technique should only be performed when the appropriate alignment of C1-2 can be restored before screw insertion. It can also be performed in cases of transverse atlantal ligament disruption or in the presence of dorsal arch fractures. It is primarily a salvage procedure when a dorsal C1-2 fusion has failed.

With the patient positioned supine and the neck extended, the surgeon makes a small incision at the level of C4-5. Dissection is carried out to expose the inferior lateral mass of C2. The trajectory used is parallel to the ventral surface of the cervical spine. Screws shorter (about 20–25 mm) than those used in odontoid fusion are inserted to enter the C2 vertebral body in the recess between the vertebral body and the inferior C2 facet. The screw is then directed rostrally and about 35 to 40 degrees laterally into the lateral mass of C1. Although not performed as frequently as dorsal C1-2 fixation methods, this technique rigidly stabilizes C1-2 and sacrifices all motion at C1-2. One disadvantage of ventral C1-2 fixation compared to the dorsal alternative is the inability to place a bone graft to promote fusion except to curettage the C1-2 facet. This procedure is not commonly performed.

Hangman's Fracture

Traumatic spondylolysis of the C2 isthmus, also known as *hangman's fracture*, can be treated surgically or with an external orthosis, depending on the extent of dislocation and angulation. There are three types of hangman's fractures, according to the classification devised by Effendi and modified by Levine and Edwards.[12] In type 1 injuries there is a normal C2-3 intervertebral disc and less than 3-mm displacement without angulation. The mechanism of injury is hyperextension with axial loading, and the fracture can be treated in an external orthosis. Type 2 injuries consist of disruption of the C2-3 disc space and ventrally angulated or displaced fractures. The mechanism is combined hyperextension and axial loading followed by hyperflexion. This injury can be treated surgically or by placing the patient in an external orthosis. Type 3 injuries involve ventral displacement with hyperflexion of the axis associated with unilateral or bilateral facet dislocations. The mechanism of the dislocation is flexion and distraction, with hyperextension responsible for the spondylolisthesis. This injury is treated surgically.

A type 2 hangman's fracture can be treated via ventral C2-3 discectomy and fusion using a plate-screw type fixation. Fluoroscopy is used to place a small incision over the C2-3 interspace, and a discectomy is performed. Appropriate alignment under gentle traction is performed, and an appropriately shaped bone graft is placed in the interspace before placing a correctly sized plate. The fusion is completed by placing two screws in C2 and two screws in C3. Postoperatively, the patient wears a hard collar for 6 to 8 weeks.

Direct reduction and fusion of a type 2 hangman's fracture is possible by placing a screw through the pars and into the vertebral body. This cannot be performed in most cases given the size of the pars and the morphology of the fracture. If dorsal fusion of a hangman's fracture is preferred, then screws are placed into the C1 and C3 lateral masses with the connecting rods as described in the section on dorsal upper cervical fixation. With a rib graft placed over the C1-3 dorsal arches, a multistranded titanium cable is passed under the rods and over the rib graft. With appropriate tensioning of the cable, the fractured C2 pars can be reduced, which enhances the fusion (Fig. 38-5).

Dorsal Upper Cervical Fixation

Occipitocervical Fixation

Occipitocervical fixation is used to correct deformities or instability at the occipitocervical junction. This fixation technique also can be used to treat atlantoaxial instability in patients who are not candidates for atlantoaxial fixation or who have failed previous attempts at C1-2 fusion.

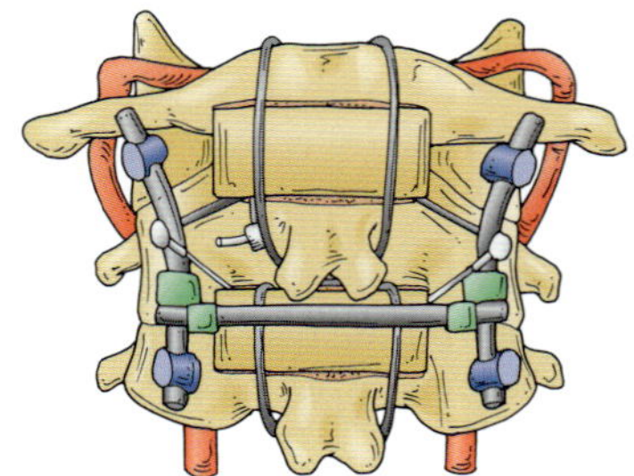

FIGURE 38-5. With a rib graft placed over the C1-3 dorsal arches, a multistranded titanium cable is passed under the rods and over the rib graft. With appropriate tensioning of the cable, the fractured C2 pars interarticularis is reduced and fusion is achieved.

Determining which cervical levels to include in an occipitocervical fusion depends on the patient's diagnosis, presentation, and radiographic findings. In cases of isolated occipitocervical instability associated with intact dorsal elements but no evidence of basilar invagination, an occipital-to-C1 or occipital-to-C2 fusion is sufficient for fixation. Isolated occipitoatlantal dislocation without atlantoaxial injury may be treated with occiput-to-C1 fixation alone. Similarly, unstable Jefferson fractures with disruption of the transverse ligament often require occiput-to-C2 fixation. When basilar invagination or ventral compressive deformities complicate a case, the fusion can be extended lower, possibly to C4, to provide sufficient fixation, depending on the degree of deformity or basilar invagination. If the dorsal arches are deficient, the fusion should extend at least two levels below the absent lamina. Alternatively, rigid external fixation can be used postoperatively.

Various methods can be used, but the general approach is as follows. After the patient is placed in a prone position in a three-point fixation device, it is critical to ensure appropriate neutral alignment of the head and the neck using lateral fluoroscopy and direct observation. Eyes must be looking forward and without a lateral tilt. Extensive flexion or extension should be avoided. A military chin-tuck position may be used to aid in exposure of the craniocervical junction and for placement of the C1 lateral mass screws (Fig. 38-6). Alternatively, the patient's head and neck should be realigned appropriately before the final securing of the construct.

A midline incision is made from the inion to the inferior aspect of the proposed construct. The length of the incision can be increased or decreased depending on the number of segments to be fused. Dissection proceeds within the midline avascular plane, ensuring adequate exposure of the foramen magnum and dorsal arches of the facet joints of the vertebrae to be fused. The authors favor the use of the operating microscope to expose the C1 lateral masses. During dissection of the lateral mass of C1, frequent venous bleeding is encountered. FloSeal Hemostatic Matrix (Baxter International Inc., Deerfield, IL) and a 1 × 1 cottonoid are essential and often achieve hemostasis without difficulty. Injury to the vertebral artery as it emerges from the transverse foramen of the atlas and courses medially on the ventral portion of the rostral surface of the dorsal ring must be avoided. An angled curette is used to detach the dorsal occipitoatlantal membrane from the rim of the foramen magnum and C1. Subperiosteal resection of the muscle attachments using a Cobb elevator strips

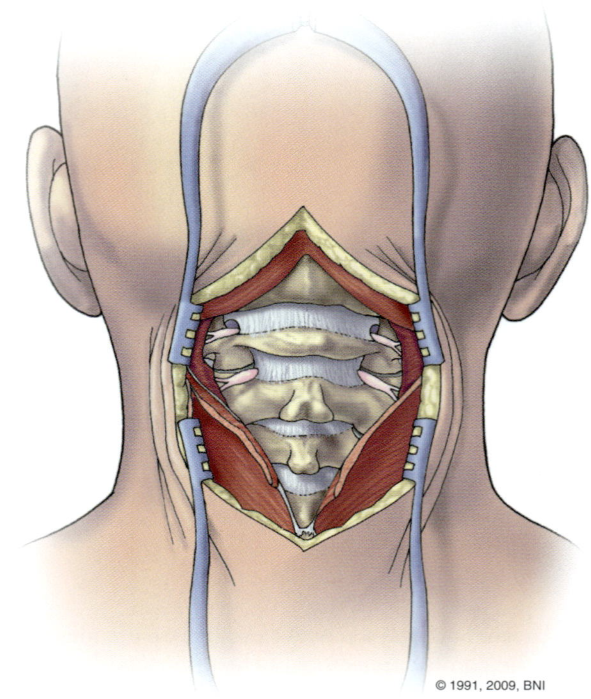

FIGURE 38-6. The incision used to expose the dorsal cervical spine. (Used with permission from Barrow Neurological Institute.)

the muscle and veins with minimal bleeding. The facet joints are the lateral extent of the exposure. Preservation of the spinous process at the lowest level included in the fusion is recommended to preserve the interspinous ligaments and to prevent the subsequent development of kyphosis below the fusion.

Adjunct Tools for Occipitocervical Fixation

Occipital Plate

An occipital plate system may be used as an adjunct for occipitocervical fixation. This technique depends on using the thick surface of the occipital keel to insert fixating bone screws and the use of a plate to provide stabilization between the upper cervical vertebra and occiput. Because the occipital bone is usually very thick, the screw holes must be drilled and tapped to the full depth before screw insertion. Although a bicortical screw is desirable, it is not necessary and it also increases the risk of spinal fluid leak.

Occiput-to-C1 Screw Fixation

In cases of isolated occipitoatlantal dislocation, an occiput-to-C1 fusion may be performed via an occipital keel plate and the insertion of lateral mass screws into C1 or via a transarticular screw placed into the O-C1 joint[13] (Fig. 38-7). The technical difficulty with insertion of a C1 lateral mass screw rests in the approach and placement of an entry point into C1.

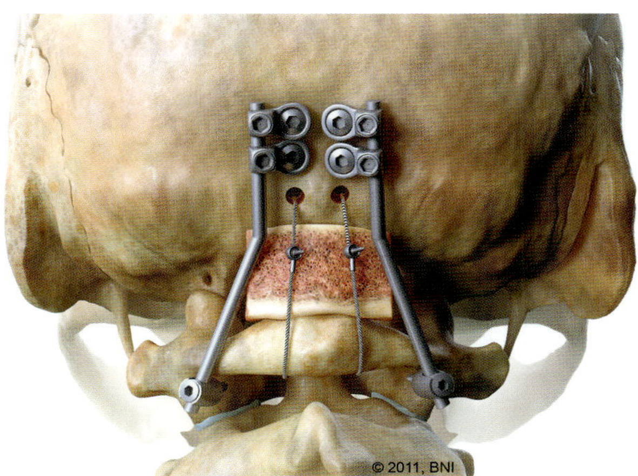

FIGURE 38-7. Representation of occiput-C1 fusion with occipital keel screws, posterior lateral mass screws, and rib graft, augmented with intralaminar wiring. (Used with permission from Barrow Neurological Institute.)

The C2 nerve root and its associated venous plexus are intimately associated with C1, and identification of the medial border of C1 as well as preparation for insertion of the lateral mass screw may result in injury or significant blood loss, especially in a small child.[14] The depth of the anterior tubercle of C1 varies considerably and should be studied carefully on preoperative computed tomography scans before using lateral fluoroscopy of this structure to guide depth of C1 lateral mass screw placement.[15] The entry point for placement of the pilot hole for a C1 lateral mass screw is in the middle of the lateral mass. The entry point for an O-C1 transarticular screw is similar to placement of a C1 lateral mass screw but is aimed more rostrally (usually 1 cm above the tip of the odontoid) to avoid the hypoglossal canal. The screw is placed via a K-wire similar to the technique described in the section on dorsal C1-2 transarticular screws. The judicious use of fluoroscopic or isocentric C-arm guidance minimizes damage to underlying tissues.

C1-2 Lateral Mass Fixation

The bilateral insertion of polyaxial-head screws in the lateral mass of C1 and the pars interarticularis or the pedicle of C2, followed by a fluoroscopically controlled reduction maneuver and rod fixation, also known as the Goel or Harms technique, is a newer method for fixation of the C1-2 joint.[1] Dorsal exposure of the C1-2 complex is performed and 3.5-mm polyaxial screws are inserted into the lateral masses of C1. Next, using fluoroscopy, two polyaxial screws are inserted into the pars interarticularis or pedicle of C2.

The pars interarticularis of C2 is the portion of the vertebra between the superior and inferior articular surfaces. A C2 pars screw is placed in a trajectory similar to that of a C1-2 transarticular screw, except that it is much shorter. The entry point for the C2 pars screw is generally 3 mm rostral and 3 mm lateral to the medial aspect of the C2-3 facet joint. The screw follows a steep trajectory paralleling the C2 joint. There is a medial angulation of approximately 10 degrees. To avoid injury to the vertebral artery, the tip of the screw should end before the dorsal cortex of the C2 vertebral body. Although longer screws can be placed, stopping at the dorsal aspect of the C2 vertebral body as confirmed on fluoroscopy ensures avoidance of the vertebral artery in almost all cases. If necessary, reduction of C1 onto C2 can be accomplished after placement of two 3-mm rods. This step is routinely followed by C1-2 interspinous fusion.

In cases of traumatic occipitoatlantal or atlantoaxial dislocation, the C1 ring is often free floating and unstable, which can preclude placement of C1 lateral mass screws. A free-floating C1 ring is easily susceptible to torsion during screw insertion and can result in vertebral artery injury, neurologic injury, or both. Therefore, during dissection and insertion of the lateral mass screw, it is imperative to stabilize the ring manually with a clamp to avoid complications. If this is not possible, C1 should not be instrumented. It can later be wired into the construct if desired.

Dorsal C1-2 Transarticular Screws

Initially described by Grob and Magerl,[12] this technique is used to fuse C1 to C2 by passing screws from the dorsal aspect of the C2 facet through the C1-2 joint so that it engages the middle of the ventral bone surface of the C1 lateral mass. When used in conjunction with an interspinous wired graft, this method of fixation is biomechanically a very stable construct.[16]

After the patient is placed prone and C1 and C2 are aligned anatomically, the laminae and lateral masses of the first two vertebrae are exposed. Deep to the C2 nerve lies the C1-2 joint and its medial limit in the spinal canal. With gentle C1-2 interlaminar distraction and the C2 nerve retracted, it is possible to curettage and decorticate the C1-2 facet capsule to promote fusion. In cases of significant instability or deformity, we pass the cable around C1 so that the atlas can be reduced and held firmly in that position during drilling. An entry pilot hole is drilled on the lateral mass of C2, which is located 3 mm lateral from the medial border and 3 mm rostral to the C2-3 facet. Using lateral fluoroscopy and aiming 5 to 10 degrees medially and toward the middle of the C1 tubercle, a K-wire is advanced through the C2 pars interarticularis into the C1-2 facet joint, capturing the C1 lateral mass. This is done under continuous fluoroscopic image guidance. The wire is advanced until the tip reaches the dorsal aspect of the C1 ventral arch. After lateral fluoroscopy, an appropriate screw tap is done for placement of a 4-mm titanium screw over the K-wire, and a cannulated titanium screw is placed. This step is routinely followed by performance of C1-to-C2 interspinous wiring and bone grafting.

This technically challenging method of fixation is associated with significant hazards and potentials for complication. The technique is unsuitable for cases with a long-standing irreducible deformity, lateral mass destruction, torticollis, or rotatory subluxation of the joint. Vertebral artery injury is the most feared complication; therefore, an aberrant course of the vertebral artery in the C2 lateral mass is a strong contraindication.[17] When the course or status of the vertebral artery is unclear, preoperative CT angiography is needed to study the vertebral artery to determine whether this technique is feasible. If the vertebral artery is damaged during placement of the first screw, it is important not to proceed with placement of the second screw. Unilateral transarticular C1-2 fixation, when combined with interspinous wire graft, provides sufficient immobilization and promotes fusion similar to bilateral fixation.[18]

C2 Intralaminal Fixation

Bilateral crossing C2 laminar screws have become popular as an alternative technique for C2 fixation.[19] The authors reserve this technique when other types of C2 fixation are not possible or as a bail-out maneuver.

After the exposure, a high-speed drill is used to place a pilot hole pointed opposite the lamina to be fixated. The hole is drilled to a depth of 20 to 28 mm, and a 3.5- or 4.0-mm polyaxial screw is advanced into the lamina. To ensure that any possible cortical breakthrough is pointed dorsally through the laminar surface as opposed to ventrally into the spinal canal, the trajectory for screw insertion is kept less than the downslope of the lamina. A dental instrument is placed under the lamina during screw insertion to help detect any breakouts. In its correct final position, the head of the screw is at the base of the spinous process while lying flush within the lamina. A second screw is placed from the opposite base of the spinous process into the lamina similar to the first screw. Reported disadvantages of this technique include early hardware failure, breach of the dorsal lamina or ventral canal, and difficulty in bone graft or rod placements due to the position of the screw heads.[20]

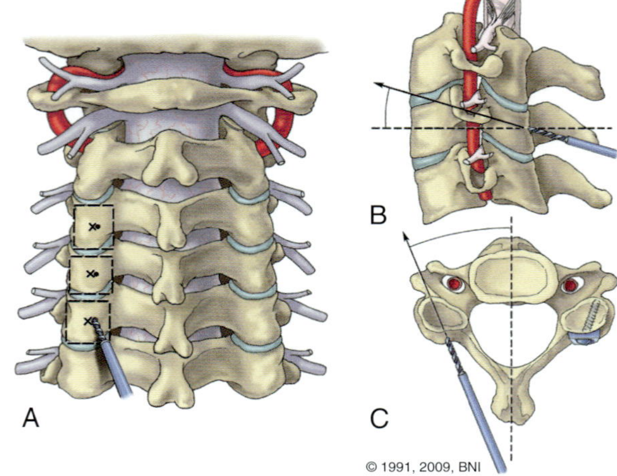

FIGURE 38-8. Target area for placement of lateral mass screws. Screws are inserted into the bone 1 mm medial to the center of the lateral masses (**A**) and directed 20 to 30 degrees cephalad (**B**) and 20 to 30 degrees laterally (**C**). (Used with permission from Barrow Neurological Institutue.)

Gallie-Brooks-Sonntag Fusion

The Gallie-Brooks fusion, as modified by Sonntag, allows fixation of atlantoaxial instability via preparation of the dorsal lamina of the atlas and axis and preservation of the C2-3 interspinous ligament.[21] Initially, the inferior aspect of C1 and superior aspects of C2 are roughened with a drill to create a suitable interface for fusion. A Kerrison punch is used to notch the inferior C2 hemilamina, and a loop of cable is passed under the dorsal arch of C1 in a caudal to rostral direction. A rectangular graft, approximately 1.5 cm × 3.5 cm, is then harvested (dorsal rib is now used instead of iliac crest) and trimmed to fit snugly between the dorsal arch of C1 and the lamina of C2. The loop cable is drawn over the spinous process of C2, and its ends are tightened. This one-point fixation construct does not counter rotatory or translatory movements. Therefore, it is recommended that this technique be used in combination with another form of fixation, such as placement of C1-2 transarticular screws or C1-2 lateral mass screws. Postoperatively, a hard collar is worn for approximately 6 weeks.

Lateral Mass Fixation (C3-6)

Lateral mass fixation does not depend on the spinous process or lamina for fixation. It can be used to treat laminar or spinous process fractures and overcomes the shortcomings inherent to wiring techniques. Lateral mass fixation can be achieved with a screw-plate or a screw-rod construct.

Screws are placed in the center of the lateral mass, which is defined by the groove between the lamina and the beginning of the lateral mass medially and the curving lateral edge laterally (Fig. 38-8). The trajectory is 30 degrees lateral and 30 degrees rostral (see Fig. 38-8). Screw lengths may be measured on a preoperative CT or intraoperatively by stopping the drill before it reaches the dorsal aspect of the lateral mass on lateral fluoroscopy. Placing the screws from the contralateral side of the table helps achieve correct angles. Good bone quality is key, and poor screw fixation invariably results in early screw pullout. Lateral mass screws are relatively contraindicated in patients with poor bone quality. The technique is associated with a risk of damage to a nerve root or vertebral artery. With appropriate rostral and lateral trajectories, both risks are minimized. Bicortical screw purchase is unnecessary and offers no biomechanical advantage compared to unicortical screws.[18]

Bone-Grafting Techniques

The techniques described in this discussion all rely on the support of a bone graft. The type of bone graft used depends on the surgical procedure and the surgeon's preference. The options for bone graft include autografts and natural and synthetic allografts. Grafts may be cortical, cancellous, or mixed. Cortical bone is the strongest form of graft and is typically used when strong structural support is required. Pure cancellous bone is quite weak and should only be used in cases that do not require the graft to withstand compressive forces. Autografts are the gold standard and are associated with the highest rates of fusion. Obtaining autograft, however, is associated with complications such as pain and infection. At times the quality of autografts can be inadequate, and the risks of complications can be too high. In such cases cadaveric allografts can be used. Compared to autografts, allografts tend to revascularize more slowly; the rate of bone fusion is slower; and the risk of bone resorption, infection, or rejection is higher. When neither autographs nor cadaveric allograft can be used, methyl methacrylate is an option. Methyl methacrylate is used as an immediate stabilizing method and should be reserved for patients with a short life expectancy because its usage does not lead to bony fusion.

Possible sites for harvesting autologous grafts include the ribs, iliac crest, skull, and fibula. Grafts from the rib and iliac crest, which are good sources of tricortical, bicortical, or cancellous chips, are preferred. The rate of arthrodesis for grafts from ribs or the iliac crest is the same, but the rate of complications associated with harvesting a rib is lower.[22]

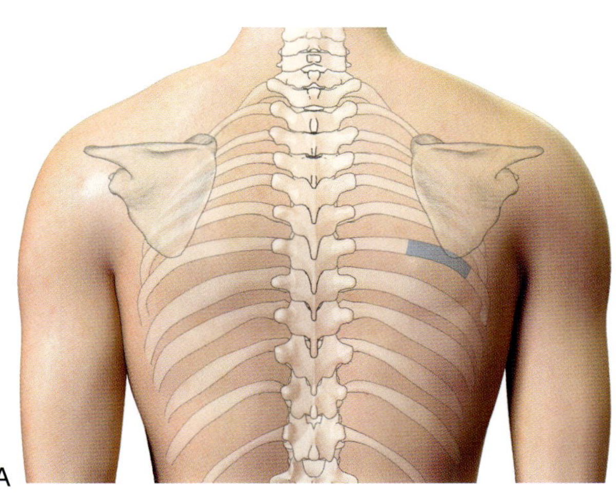

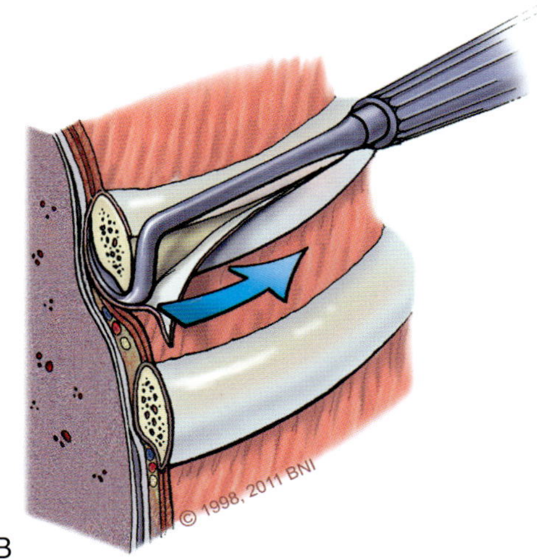

FIGURE 38-9. Technique for harvesting rib graft. **A,** Extent of rib needed for harvest. **B,** Technique of graft harvest. (Used with permission from Barrow Neurological Institute.)

To harvest rib grafts, a linear incision is made in the skin over the rib surface (Fig. 38-9A). Blunt dissection with a Doyen rib dissector is used to detach the intercostal muscles and parietal pleura from the undersurface (Fig. 38-9B). The ends of the rib graft are cut sharply using a rib cutter or oscillating saw and smoothed to avoid a pneumothorax.

In the young child, the iliac crest is largely cartilaginous and ribs are small. In such cases, bone from the parietal skull can be harvested through a bicoronal flap. If identical free flaps are taken and split carefully, half-thickness skull bone replacements at both sites facilitate solid and cosmetically acceptable reconstruction within 3 months.

Bone grafts also can be harvested from the fibula. As a graft source, the fibula offers a high cortical-to-cancellous bone ratio; long segments up to 25 cm can be harvested safely. To obtain a fibula graft, the leg is prepared and a tourniquet is applied to the thigh. After a straight lateral incision over the fibula is made, the peroneal muscle is separated from the ventral aspect of the fibula. The muscles of the dorsal compartment of the leg are also dissected free, and a Gigli saw is used to divide the fibula, paying due attention to the peroneal artery and nerve. The fibula is elevated in a distal-to-proximal fashion, and the fibular diaphyseal segment and peroneal vessels are ligated and dissected. The site is closed with suction in place.

The dorsal iliac crest can serve as another source to obtain tricortical grafts, cortical-cancellous plates, cancellous bone strips, or cortical matchstick grafts. Using a curved skin incision beginning at the posterior iliac spine and extending superolaterally, dissection is carried out through the fascia and opened over the iliac crest. Dissection is continued subperiosteally to minimize damage to the gluteal artery, sciatic nerve, ureter, and ilioinguinal nerve. The graft is obtained using bone curettes, and the incision is closed in layers. It is important not to remove graft more than 8 cm from the iliac spine to avoid damaging the superior cluneal nerves. It is also important not to harvest the graft too medially because this can place the sciatic notch and the sacroiliac joint in danger.

After harvesting a structural autograft, careful carpentry comes into play. The graft must be fashioned to maximize the bony contact between the surfaces needing to be fused. At C1-2, for example, a notch in the bone is often fashioned to allow the graft to "sit" on the spinous process of C2. At the occipitocervical junction, the graft should be fashioned so that there is solid contact with the skull, C1, and C2. This can be done by cutting an oblique angle into the graft and drilling a trough into the suboccipital bone into which the graft is wedged. All structural grafts should be augmented by wiring to ensure that the bone is under compression.

KEY REFERENCES

Brockmeyer DL: Lateral mass screw fixation of C-1. *J Neurosurg* 107(Suppl 2): 173–177, 2007.

Dickman CA, Mamourian A, Sonntag VK, Drayer BP: Magnetic resonance imaging of the transverse atlantal ligament for the evaluation of atlantoaxial instability. *J Neurosurg* 75(2):221–227, 1991.

Galler RM, Dogan S, Fifield MS, et al: Biomechanical comparison of instrumented and uninstrumented multilevel cervical discectomy versus corpectomy. *Spine* 32(11):1220–1226, 2007.

Gonzalez LF, Klopfenstein JD, Crawford NR, et al: Use of dual transarticular screws to fixate simultaneous occipitoatlantal and atlantoaxial dislocations. *J Neurosurg Spine* 3(4):318–323, 2005.

Grob D, Magerl F: Surgical stabilization of C1 and C2 fractures. *Orthopade* 16(1):46–54, 1987.

Hadley MN, Browner C, Sonntag VK: Axis fractures: a comprehensive review of management and treatment in 107 cases. *Neurosurgery* 17(2):281–290, 1985.

Maughan PH, Horn EM, Theodore N, et al: Avulsion fracture of the foramen magnum treated with occiput-to-C1 fusion: technical case report. *Neurosurgery* 57(3):E600, 2005.

Song GS, Theodore N, Dickman CA, Sonntag VK: Unilateral posterior atlantoaxial transarticular screw fixation. *J Neurosurg* 87(6):851–855, 1997.

Wait SD, Ponce FA, Colle KO, et al: Importance of the C1 anterior tubercle depth and lateral mass geometry when placing C1 lateral mass screws. *Neurosurgery* 65(5):952–956, 2009.

REFERENCES

The complete reference list is available online at expertconsult.com.

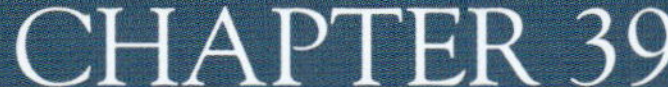

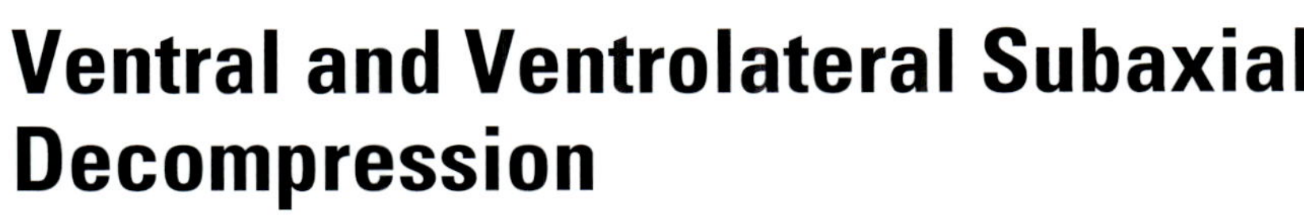

CHAPTER 39

Ventral and Ventrolateral Subaxial Decompression

Fadi Hanbali | Ziya Gokaslan | Paul R. Cooper

Ventral compression of the spinal cord or the nerve roots is the most common indication for ventral decompression. Clinical conditions such as cervical trauma with ventral disc herniation or bone fragments, acute cervical disc herniation, cervical spondylosis, ossification of the posterior longitudinal ligament, neoplastic processes, and infection can all be successfully managed by a ventral decompressive technique. Ventrolateral decompression may be required for vertebral artery stenosis secondary to tumor, spondylosis, or compression of the cervical nerve roots. Although these decompressive measures are quite effective and generally safe, they nevertheless may be associated with a number of complications that can be quite serious and even devastating. Ventral cervical discectomy, although considered relatively safe and simple, is one of the most common procedures involved in malpractice litigation.

General Considerations

The first step for avoiding complications associated with any surgical procedure is to perform the appropriate operation on the appropriate patient. Although a detailed discussion of various indications for surgery and criteria for patient selection is beyond the scope of this chapter, the importance of correlating the clinical picture with the imaging abnormalities cannot be overemphasized. The majority of middle-aged patients will have at least some degree of degenerative changes of the cervical spine, but only a few will have symptomatic spinal cord or nerve root compression. Therefore, a careful analysis of patient history and meticulous neurologic examination are essential to accurately correlate the imaging abnormalities with the patient's clinical picture.

The ventral approach to the cervical spine is performed through a plane between the sternocleidomastoid muscle and the carotid sheath laterally and the strap muscles and tracheoesophageal viscera medially. This approach is appropriate for ventral cervical discectomy, vertebrectomy, fusion, and instrumentation (Fig. 39-1).

The ventrolateral approach, however, is more suitable for decompression of the vertebral artery in the transverse foramen or between the foramina or spinal nerve roots outside the spinal canal. Two different techniques are described in the literature. Verbiest's[1] technique is performed through the same plane as the ventral approach. However, further exposure is performed lateral to the longus colli muscle on the ipsilateral side. This exposure allows visualization of the costotransverse lamella, which forms the roof of the foramen transversarium covering the vertebral artery. Hodgson,[2] on the other hand, approached the cervical spine lateral to the sternocleidomastoid muscle and the carotid sheath. These structures, along with the musculovisceral column, are retracted medially (Fig. 39-2). The remainder of the exposure is similar to that described by Verbiest, with the exception that the longus colli muscles are retracted medially to laterally to gain access to the vertebral artery.

Essentially, the structures at risk of injury are the same with either the ventral or the ventrolateral approach. In Hodgson's approach, the tracheoesophageal viscera and recurrent laryngeal nerve (RLN) are protected, whereas the nerve roots, sympathetic chain, and vertebral artery are at greater risk.

Specific Complications, Avoidance, and Management

Preoperative Period

In patients with a significant neurologic deficit, the preoperative use of corticosteroids may be considered. However, there are no convincing data in the literature to support the efficacy of the routine use of corticosteroids in patients undergoing decompressive operation.

Although hyperextension of the neck usually facilitates exposure during the operation and restores normal lordotic curvature of the cervical spine, excessive hyperextension during intubation or during the operative procedure may further narrow the spinal canal and exacerbate a preexisting neurologic deficit, especially in patients with spinal canal compromise. The amount of hyperextension that can be tolerated by the patient can be assessed in the preoperative period by placing the neck in the amount of extension anticipated during the operation or intubation. If the patient can maintain this position for 30 minutes without motor or sensory symptoms, the operation can be performed safely in that position. If, however, any symptoms are induced during the testing, the neck must be kept neutral throughout surgery and the patient should be intubated fiberoptically.

Intraoperative evoked potential monitoring can be used to identify and avoid dangerous manipulation of the neural

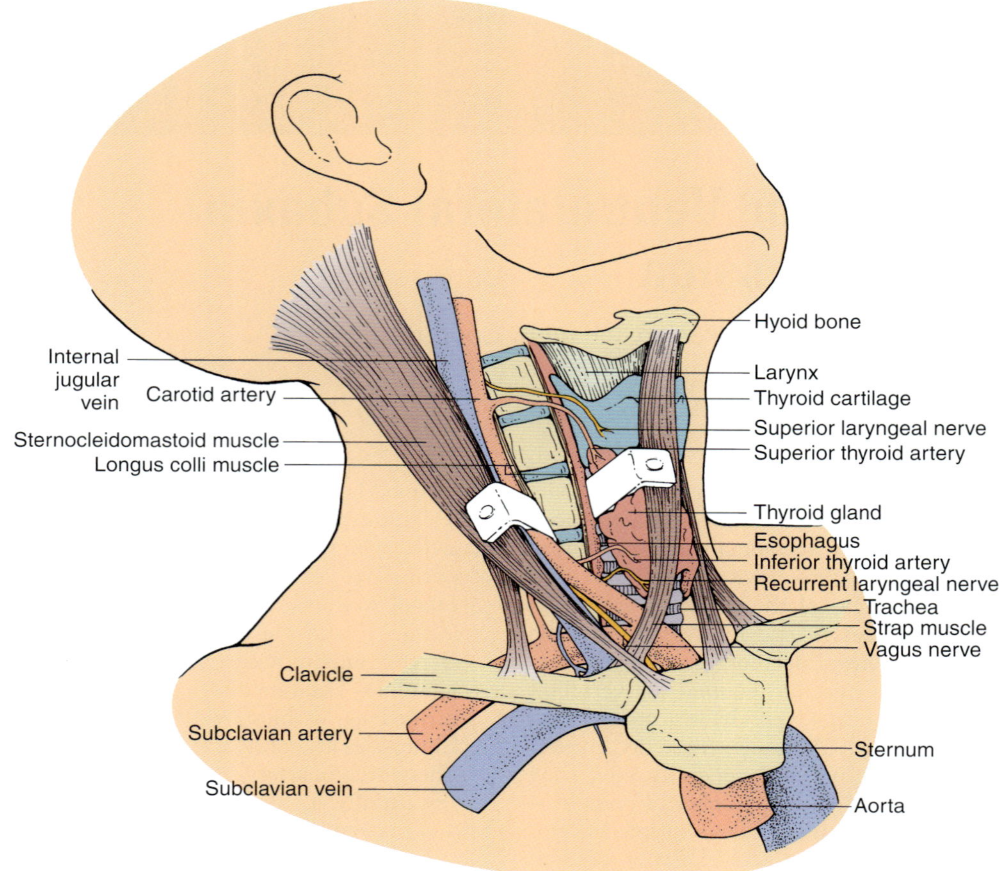

FIGURE 39-1. Ventral exposure of the cervical spine and anatomic structures of surgical importance.

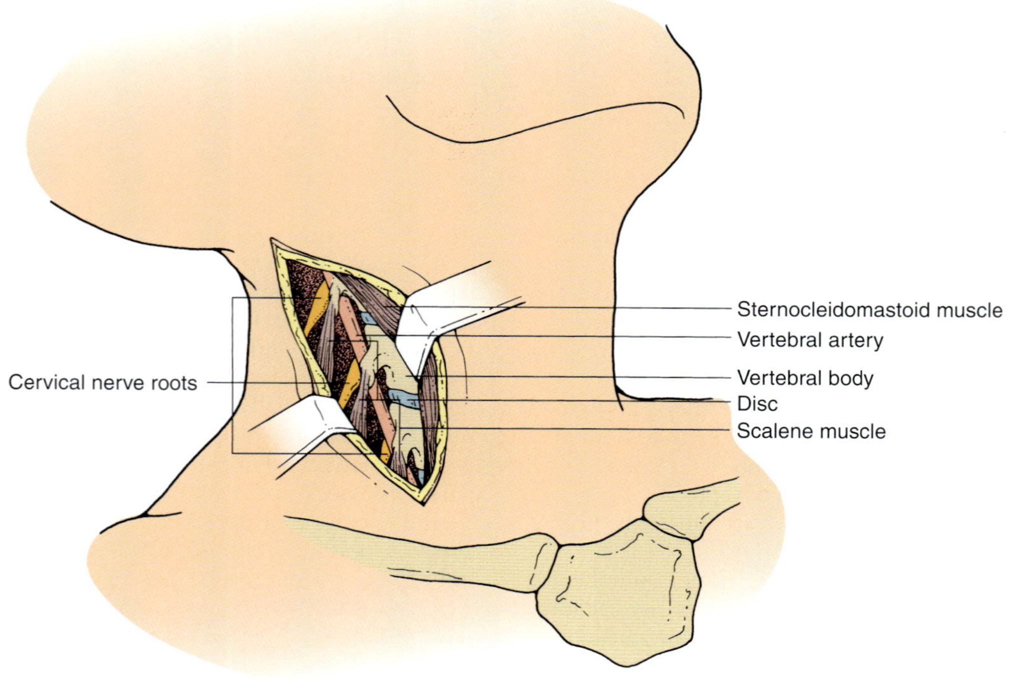

FIGURE 39-2. Ventrolateral exposure of the cervical spine as described by Hodgson.

tissue during surgery.[3] However, there is currently no convincing evidence that the use of this modality improves outcome after decompressive surgery. Somatosensory evoked potentials (SSEP) are most commonly used for this purpose. However, this type of monitoring may be associated with false-positive intraoperative SSEP changes, thus creating significant anxiety for the surgeon and possibly unnecessary anesthetic and surgical maneuvers. Motor evoked potential monitoring reflects the function of the ventral spinal cord tracts more reliably than does SSEP monitoring and may avoid some of the false-positive intraoperative changes observed with SSEP.

To facilitate identification of the lower cervical segments on the localizing radiograph, caudal traction is applied to the shoulders or arms. In this case, excessive traction should be avoided because there is potential risk for traction injury of the upper brachial plexus.

Intraoperative Period

A right-sided approach is generally recommended because it is easier for the right-handed surgeon. Some authors, however, believe that a right-sided approach is associated with higher risk of injury to the RLN, especially in the lower cervical spine. The risk, however, is low.

The risk is probably balanced by the convenience of the position for right-handed surgeons. A left-sided approach, on the other hand, carries the risk of injury to the thoracic duct during exposure of the lower cervical spine. A recent review of 328 patients who underwent ventral cervical spine fusion procedures showed no association between the side of the approach and the incidence of RLN symptoms.[4]

The skin incision is usually transverse and localized in a skin crease. Alternatively, a diagonal skin incision along the medial border of the sternocleidomastoid muscle may be used for multilevel disease. After the skin incision is made, the platysma muscle is dissected both rostrally and caudally. One should look for branches of the external jugular vein because these may be inadvertently transected with sharp scissors during the dissection. If identified, the blood vessels can be coagulated and sharply divided. The platysma is then incised vertically parallel to its fibers throughout the limits of the exposure to prevent undue traction.

For a ventrolateral approach, more complete exposure of the sternocleidomastoid muscle is required. During the opening of the ventral cervical fascia, the greater auricular nerve and other ventral cutaneous nerves are at risk of injury. Injury to the greater auricular nerve results in decreased sensation of the skin of the face in the area of the parotid gland. This nerve penetrates the deep fascia on the dorsal surface of the sternocleidomastoid muscle at approximately midbelly and travels rostrally on the surface of the sternocleidomastoid muscle toward the ear. The anterior cutaneous nerve, on the other hand, takes a more horizontal course across the sternocleidomastoid muscle before dividing into ascending and descending branches. The ascending branch provides cutaneous innervation of the skin overlying the mandible. Damage to this nerve can result in decreased sensation over the mandible. The key to avoiding injuries to these structures is to identify them and to be aware of their anatomic location.

During lateral retraction of the sternocleidomastoid muscle for a ventrolateral approach, the eleventh cranial nerve is also at risk of injury and must be identified. This nerve enters the sternocleidomastoid muscle two to three fingerwidths below the mastoid tip and exits the muscle obliquely, caudally passing across the posterior triangle of the neck to the ventral border of the trapezius muscle.

After the superficial cervical fascia is incised and the plane is developed between the sternocleidomastoid muscle laterally and the strap muscles medially, certain structures are at risk of injury. These include the larynx and trachea, esophagus and pharynx, laryngeal nerves, carotid artery, internal jugular vein, vagus nerve, sympathetic chain, and pleura. The complications related to these structures are discussed separately.

Injury to the Larynx and Trachea

Perforation of the trachea, though a rare and unusual complication of this procedure, can occur during medial dissection. If it does occur, direct repair is usually possible. Severe laryngeal retraction can result in significant laryngeal edema that may appear as an immediate postoperative emergency. Many measures can be undertaken to reduce the severity of the postoperative glottic edema, including systemic corticosteroids, cold mist, and inhalation of racemic epinephrine. If these measures are not successful, reintubation may be attempted. If these maneuvers fail, a tracheotomy should be performed.

Injury to the Esophagus and Pharynx

Dysphagia is a common problem after ventral cervical surgery and is usually secondary to edema from retraction. This symptom usually resolves within a few days without any treatment. In certain cases, however, it may persist as long as several weeks; rarely, it may be permanent. It is more common in elderly patients and in those who had extensive mobilization of the upper esophagus or hypopharynx. In a questionnaire mailed to 497 patients who had undergone ventral cervical fusion procedures, 60% reported some dysphagia after the surgical procedure compared to 23% in the control group.[5]

Esophageal or pharyngeal lacerations can occur, especially in the upper cervical region where the hypopharynx is thinner, either from sharp dissection or from the teeth of self-retaining retractors. If esophageal perforation is recognized intraoperatively, it should be repaired primarily. The wound should be drained and the patient placed on nasogastric drainage for at least 7 to 10 days. Fusion in these circumstances is contraindicated. Subsequently, a swallow study with a water-soluble contrast agent should be obtained to confirm that the perforation has sealed. In the majority of cases, the injury to the esophagus is not recognized during surgery and shows symptoms later as a local infection, fistula, sepsis, or mediastinitis.[6,7] The presence of crepitus or an enlarging mass in the neck or mediastinal air on a chest radiograph usually suggests the strong possibility of an esophageal perforation. Diagnosis can be confirmed with an esophagogram. However, this test may not always be positive when esophageal injury is present. Esophagoscopy or a postesophagogram CT scan may also demonstrate a perforation. Treatment of a delayed perforation consists of nasogastric drainage, antibiotics, and reexploration of the incision. If a defect is found, it should be repaired and a wound drain placed.[6] To avoid this complication, the longus colli muscles should be freed enough rostrally, caudally, and laterally so that the sharp teeth of the self-retaining retractors can be placed safely under them

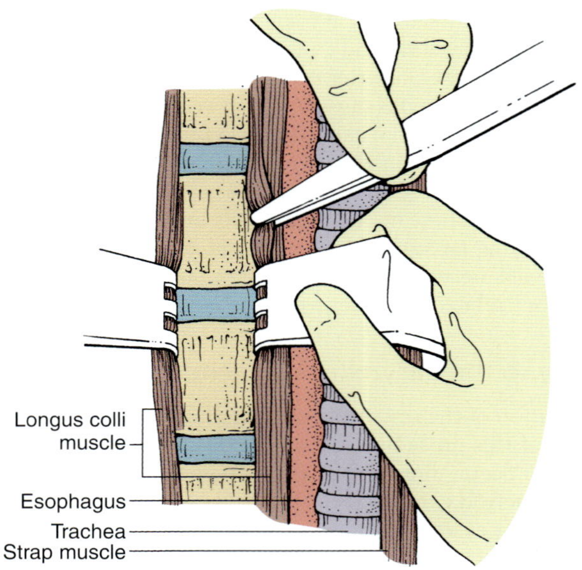

FIGURE 39-3. Placement of self-retaining retractors under the longus colli muscle to prevent dislodgement during surgery.

without risk of dislodgement during the procedure (Fig. 39-3). In addition, the esophagus and other soft tissue structures should be hidden by the retractors to avoid injury by the high-speed drill during bone removal.

Occasionally, perforation of the esophagus can result from a displaced graft.[8] To avoid this problem, some surgeons recommend reapproximation of the longus colli muscles over the graft. When a displaced graft perforates the esophagus, reexploration is required. Either replacement or removal of the graft may be indicated, depending on the need for the graft to maintain stability. The esophageal perforation should be repaired, if possible, and the patient treated with antibiotics and nasogastric drainage.

Injury to the Laryngeal Nerves

Minor hoarseness or sore throat after a ventral cervical operation is common; it has been reported in approximately 50% of patients. It resolves without further intervention in weeks or months in the majority of patients. The cause is usually edema from tracheal intubation. However, injury to the laryngeal nerves can also occur and may result in permanent laryngeal dysfunction.

Both the superior and inferior (recurrent) laryngeal nerves are at risk during exposure of the ventral cervical spine. Some proposed mechanisms of this complication include direct surgical trauma, nerve division or ligature, pressure or stretch-induced neurapraxia, and postoperative edema.

The superior laryngeal nerve is a branch of the inferior ganglion of the vagus nerve and innervates the cricothyroid muscle. The superior thyroid artery, encountered above C4, is an important anatomic landmark for the superior laryngeal nerve. Damage to this nerve may result in hoarseness, but it often produces symptoms such as easy voice fatigue.[9] To avoid injury to this nerve, one should be aware of its anatomic location.

On the left side, the inferior (recurrent) laryngeal nerve loops under the arch of the aorta and is protected in the left tracheoesophageal groove. On the right side, however, the RLN travels around the subclavian artery, passing dorsomedially to the side of the trachea and esophagus. It is vulnerable as it passes from the subclavian artery to the right tracheoesophageal groove. The inferior thyroid artery on the right side is an anatomic marker for the RLN. The nerve usually enters the tracheoesophageal groove, the point at which the inferior thyroid artery enters the lower pole of the thyroid. Damage to the RLN may result in hoarseness, vocal breathiness or fatigue, weak cough, dysphagia, or aspiration.[10]

Preoperative insertion of a nasogastric tube not only allows easier identification of the esophagus for protection against an esophageal injury, but also allows localization of the tracheoesophageal groove and the avoidance of the plane. Endotracheal tube-related RLN injury has also been cited. Monitoring of the endotracheal cuff pressure and its release after retractor placement decreased the rate of RLN temporary paralysis from 6.4% to 1.7% in one series.[11]

One should also be aware of the anatomic variations, especially on the right side, where the RLN may be nonrecurrent. However, the frequency of this aberration is well below 1%.[12] In this situation, the RLN travels directly from the vagus nerve and the carotid sheath to the larynx. If a suspected nonrecurrent nerve is encountered, it may be identified with a nerve stimulator and laryngoscopic examination of the vocal cords. If it cannot be retracted safely, it is best to abandon the procedure and use a left-sided approach.

The RLN is better protected during Hodgson's approach than it is during a standard ventral cervical approach. However, it should be kept in mind that this nerve is still vulnerable at the position at which it enters the right tracheoesophageal groove. It is important to remember that during Hodgson's procedure, the midline is first identified after the prevertebral fascia is incised and the longus colli muscle retracted from medial to lateral position. The key to avoiding injury to the important anatomic structures during Hodgson's approach is to recognize that the approach is lateral to the sternocleidomastoid muscle, as well as to the carotid sheath. However, during the opening of the prevertebral fascia, the midline is identified, and the longus colli muscles are retracted medially to laterally.

The true incidence of RLN injury is difficult to determine but is probably about 1% to 2%.[4,13] Beutler et al.[4] reported that the incidence of RLN symptoms was 2.1% with anterior cervical discectomy, 3.5% with corpectomy, 3% with instrumentation, and 9.5% with reoperative anterior surgery.

Because many patients have some degree of voice change after ventral cervical operations, a thorough investigation is not required in most cases. However, a laryngoscopic examination should be performed in persistent cases. If RLN palsy is present, the vocal cord will be faced in the paramedian position. Immediate treatment is not usually required for a paralyzed vocal cord because, in most instances, the nerve has not been severed, and the condition will resolve with time.[13] In some patients, hoarseness or voice dysfunction may be minimal, not requiring treatment. However, patients with persistent hoarseness after several months can be treated with injections of hemostatic gelatin (Gelfoam) or Teflon into the vocal cord. Gelfoam produces a temporary improvement and may be used as an interim measure pending spontaneous return of function. Teflon injection is a permanent treatment modality that is used in patients in whom no recovery is expected.

Injury to the Structures in the Carotid Sheath

To avoid injury to the carotid artery, internal jugular vein, or vagus nerve, care must be taken not to enter the carotid sheath. Laceration of the carotid artery may result from the sharp teeth of retractor blades or during dissection with sharp instruments. In most cases, carotid artery lacerations can be repaired primarily. However, one may consider abandoning the procedure if such an injury occurs early in the course of the operation.

It is important to recognize that manipulation of the carotid artery may result in a stroke secondary to either mechanical compression of the artery or dislodgement of debris from a preexisting carotid plaque.[14] In some cases, it may be useful to monitor the temporal artery pulse after placement of the self-retaining retractors to avoid the risk of stroke as a result of carotid occlusion from retraction.

Injury to the internal jugular vein results from either sharp dissection or the sharp teeth of a dislodged self-retaining retractor, usually causing a significant amount of bleeding, and it can also compromise the exposure of the other important anatomic structures. Bleeding should be controlled, and either the laceration should be repaired or the jugular vein should be ligated.

Injury to the vagus nerve can result from entry into the carotid sheath. This is an unusual complication, but if transection is observed intraoperatively, primary anastomosis should be attempted.

Injury to the Vertebral Artery

Injury to the vertebral artery may result from asymmetrical and far lateral bone removal and is most likely to occur on the left side during a standard right-sided approach (Fig. 39-4). In a cadaveric study, the course of the vertebral artery was analyzed in 222 cervical spines. A 2.7% incidence of tortuous vertebral artery was identified.[15] Injury to the vertebral artery can also result from aggressive dissection of the longus colli muscles, which injures the vascular structures between the transverse processes.[16] Although primary repair of the vertebral arteries has been recommended, this is usually very difficult. Commonly, bleeding can be controlled with gentle compression using a muscle pledget, Gelfoam, or oxidized cellulose (Surgicel), after which an angiogram should be obtained to rule out the development of an arteriovenous fistula or pseudoaneurysm.[17] To avoid this injury, one should identify the midline carefully and proceed with drilling accordingly.

Occasionally, transection of the vertebral artery can occur inadvertently during decompression of the vertebral artery via a ventrolateral approach. When this occurs, it requires control of the bleeding by a ligature at the level above and below the lesion. The risk of neurologic deficit after a unilateral vertebral artery occlusion is low.[16] Thorough mobilization of the vertebral artery invariably causes bleeding from the surrounding venous plexus; consequently, vigorous retraction and aggressive mobilization of the vertebral artery should be avoided to minimize hemorrhage.

Injury to the Sympathetic Chain

The sympathetic chain may be more vulnerable to damage during ventral lower cervical spine procedures because it is situated closer to the medial border of the longus colli muscles at C6 than at C3. The longus colli muscles diverge laterally and the sympathetic chain converges medially at C6.[18] Injury to the cervical sympathetic chain, which results in Horner

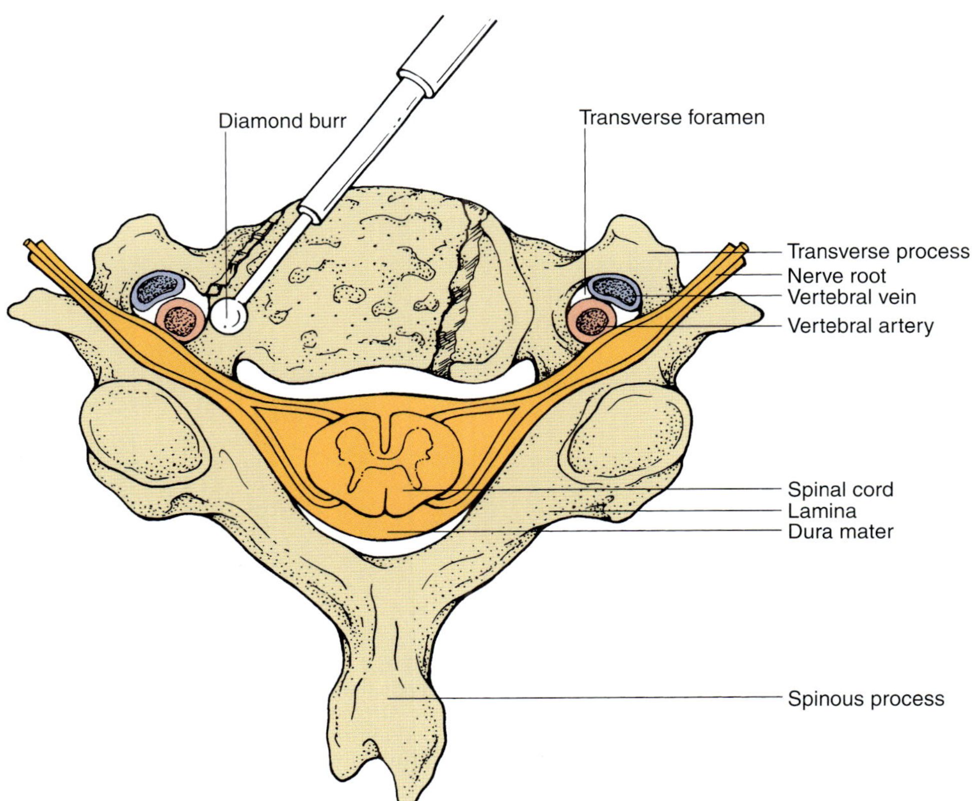

FIGURE 39-4. Mechanism of injury at the vertebral artery as a result of misassessment of the midline or asymmetrical drilling.

syndrome, is unusual but can result from either retraction or transection of the sympathetic chain. The incidence of permanent injury is less than 1%.[19] To avoid this injury during a ventral approach, the soft tissue dissection should be limited to the medial aspect of the longus colli muscles.

During a ventrolateral approach, the sympathetic chain is particularly at risk of injury. The sympathetic chain is located ventral to the transverse processes. It is either embedded in the dorsal carotid sheath or lies on the connective tissue between the sheath and the longus colli muscle. To avoid injury, the superior cervical ganglion at C1 and the middle cervical ganglion at C6 should be included with the sympathetic chain as it is retracted laterally to medially together with the longus colli muscle.

Increased Neurologic Deficit

Increased neurologic deficit after a ventral cervical operation is unusual. Most spinal cord or nerve root injuries are associated with technical mishaps (excepting most C5 deficits). Although the exact figure is difficult to determine, Flynn[19] reported a 1.3% incidence of additional radicular dysfunction and a 3.3% incidence of worsening myelopathy.

To avoid neurologic injury, certain measures should be undertaken at every step of the procedure. Important precautionary measures regarding positioning, neck hyperextension, intubation, and electrophysiologic monitoring have been described. During intraoperative localization, the localizing needle (18-gauge spinal needle) in the disc space should be bent at the tip, as shown in Figure 39-5, so that inadvertent advancement of the needle into the spinal canal is impossible.

During the removal of spondylotic ridges, it is important that osteophytes not be disconnected from the vertebral bodies until they have been thinned sufficiently to permit removal with fine curettes. Otherwise, further attempts to drill may result in compression of the spinal cord (Fig. 39-6). Achieving a complete decompression before placement of the bone graft is also crucial. As shown in Figure 39-7, in instances of incomplete decompression, tapping of the bone graft may result in compression of the spinal cord. During the final advancement of the bone graft, a bone tamp should be positioned in such a way that one half of the surface of the tamp is placed against the remaining rostral or caudal vertebral body (Fig. 39-8). This placement avoids an inadvertent advancement of the graft into the spinal canal and thereby prevents spinal cord compression. Countersinking of the bone graft can be accomplished by angling the tamp but maintaining the position of the tamp relative to the vertebral body (see Fig. 39-8). Occasionally, misplacement or displacement of a bone graft may cause nerve or cord compression. To avoid this injury, the depth of the graft should be measured

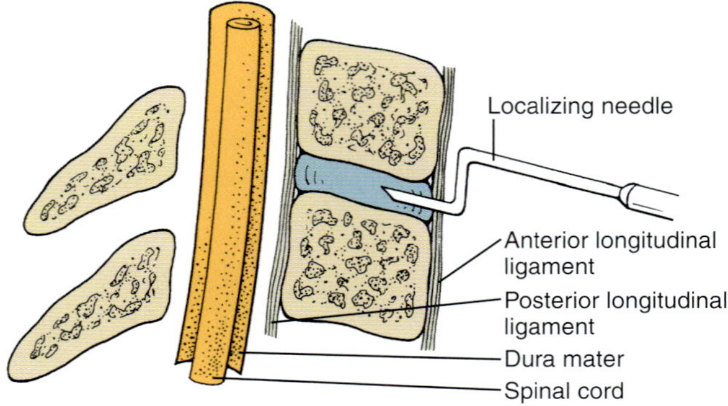

FIGURE 39-5. The localizing needle (18-gauge spinal needle) should be bent at the tip to prevent inadvertent penetration of the spinal cord.

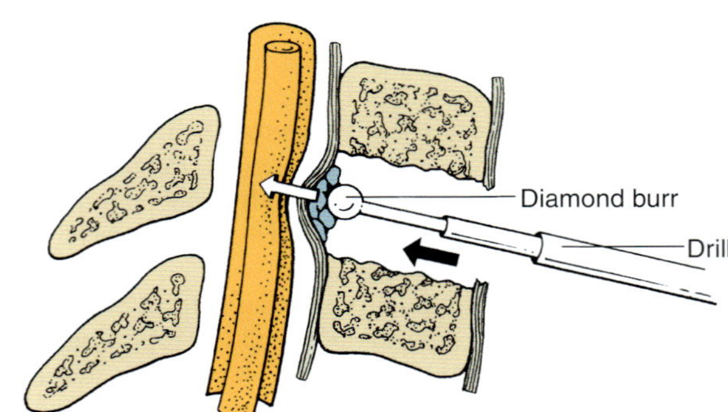

FIGURE 39-6. Possible mechanism of injury if the bone fragments become disconnected from the vertebral bodies before they have been completely thinned out during the removal of spondylotic ridges. In this case, the remaining mobile fragment may cause neural impingement during further drilling.

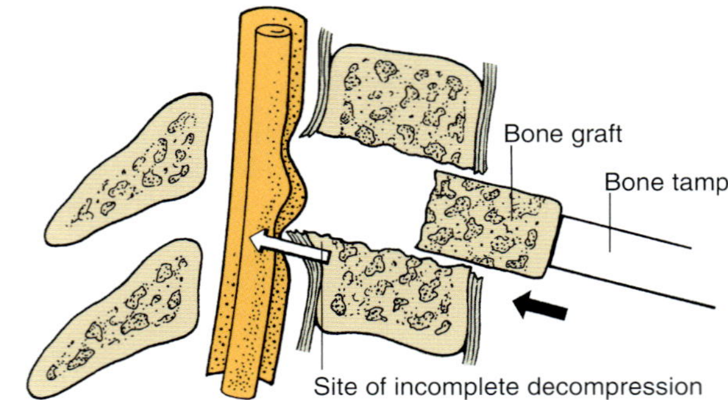

FIGURE 39-7. Possible mechanism of spinal cord injury in cases of incomplete decompression as a result of "water hammer" effect during the placement of bone graft. Impaction of the bone graft may result in transmission of force vectors to the spinal cord via the persistent osteophyte.

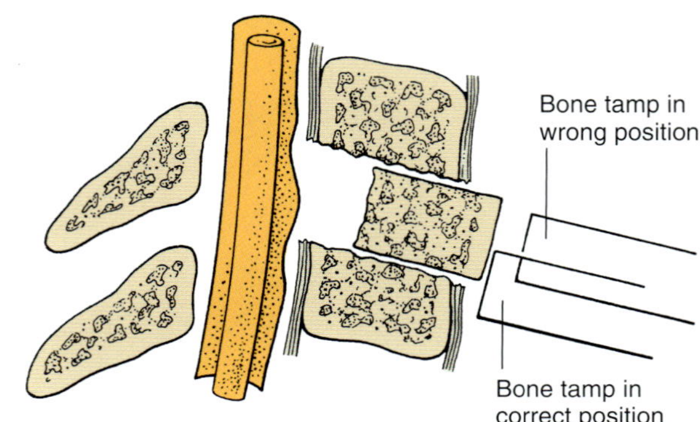

FIGURE 39-8. Recommended position of the bone tamp during the final positioning of the bone graft to prevent inadvertent advancement into the spinal cord. The tamp cannot pass beyond (dorsal) to the ventral margin of the vertebral body. The seating of the bone graft into a recessed position may require the angling of the tamp, while maintaining the obligatory positioning of the tamp partially over the vertebral body.

carefully, and the depth of the vertebral body should be measured on preoperative imaging studies. If the depth of the bone graft in an anteroposterior plane is limited to 13 mm, penetration of the spinal canal is unlikely. Nerve root injuries are less common than spinal cord injuries, but for unclear reasons, the C5 nerve root is very sensitive to trauma.[20]

If a neurologic deficit is not present immediately after the patient awakens but appears within hours, the possibility of an epidural hematoma should be considered. In the case of suspected epidural hematoma with rapidly deteriorating neurologic function, the patient should be returned to the operating room for immediate exploration, without delay for diagnostic studies. In patients who have neurologic deficits immediately after surgery, one should consider administering glucocorticoids and should obtain lateral cervical spine radiographs to determine the position of the bone graft. If the patient's neurologic status is stable, MRI may be valuable to determine the cause of the deterioration. If a hematoma or bone graft misplacement is suspected, expeditious reexploration is required.

If neurologic worsening occurs within days after the operation, an epidural abscess must be considered in the differential diagnosis. Obviously, the abscess should be drained as soon as possible, and the patient should be treated with appropriate antibiotics.

Sleep-induced apnea has been reported as an unusual complication of ventral cervical spine surgery. It is usually a self-limited process. Supportive respiratory therapy is occasionally needed.[21]

Dural Laceration and Cerebrospinal Fluid Fistula

Dura mater laceration and cerebrospinal fluid leak may occur during removal of the posterior longitudinal ligament or during drilling. Direct repair is usually not feasible. A piece of Gelfoam should be placed over the dural defect, and lumbar subarachnoid drainage should be performed for 4 to 5 days. To minimize the chance of dural laceration from the drill bit, one should consider switching to a diamond drill when the dorsal cortex or the slope of the uncovertebral joints is encountered. The surgeon must also be aware that the nerve roots are more ventrally located than the spinal cord. Therefore, if one were to continue drilling laterally at the same ventrodorsal depth as the midline dura mater, violation of the dural sleeves of the nerve roots and, possibly, of the vertebral artery could occur.

Postoperative Period

Soft Tissue Hematomas and Respiratory Problems

Cervical soft tissue hematomas after ventral cervical operation are unusual, and many can be managed nonoperatively. However, a large hematoma may lead to airway obstruction and is a potentially life-threatening complication. To avoid this problem, careful hemostasis before closure is imperative. A Jackson-Pratt drain, inserted in the prevertebral space before closure, should be left in place for 24 hours in case adequate hemostasis was not achieved. The patient should be monitored very carefully in the recovery room after the operative procedure for signs of respiratory insufficiency or cervical swelling. If a palpable hematoma is noted immediately after the cervical procedure but the patient does not have any respiratory compromise, the hematoma may be treated expectantly. However, a large or expanding hematoma should be drained, even if the patient is otherwise asymptomatic. If respiration is compromised, emergency treatment is required. The patient should be reintubated, if possible, and the wound opened. If intubation is not easily accomplished, the wound should be reopened in the recovery room and, if necessary, the airway reestablished via a tracheotomy or cricothyroidotomy.

Postoperative Infection

Infectious processes can occur after a ventral cervical operation and can affect only the superficial layers or can involve the deeper structures. These are reported in 0.4% to 2% of patients with spine complications.[22] Superficial infections external to the platysma muscle can be treated by simple opening of the incision, followed by dressing changes and administration of appropriate antibiotics and secondary closure.

Cellulitis or abscess in the deeper tissues, however, requires a more thorough evaluation. Perforation of the esophagus or pharynx should always be considered a possibility and a potential source of infection. This is especially true when an unusual mixture of organisms is identified. In such instances, the incision should be explored under general anesthesia to drain the abscess and investigate the possibility of an esophageal perforation with intraoperative inspection. Subsequently, a postoperative esophagogram and CT scan should be obtained to assess the status of the perforation.

The issue of bone graft removal in the presence of infection is complex. We choose to leave the graft in place, treat with antibiotics, and follow the status of the graft with cervical spine films. If the graft is collapsing, removal and replacement with autograft would be indicated; in most cases, bone healing will take place.

Epidural abscesses and meningitis have also been reported in association with ventral cervical operations. However, these complications are quite rare.[23] If a patient has progressive postoperative spinal cord dysfunction, with or without evidence of osteomyelitis or systemic signs of sepsis, epidural abscess should always be considered in the differential diagnosis. Either MRI or CT myelography should be used to establish the diagnosis. Meningitis should be considered in a septic patient if a dural laceration was observed or suspected intraoperatively. Lumbar puncture is required to confirm the suspicion.

Graft-Related Complications

The predominant complications related to the bone graft are graft collapse, extrusion and migration, and nonunion. These may occur from suboptimal sizing, vertebral endplate fracture, postoperative trauma, or inadequate immobilization. Graft collapse is most frequently observed in elderly patients with osteoporotic bone. If there is any question regarding the structural integrity of autologous bone, an allograft should be used. However, in younger patients, autologous graft is stronger than allograft in resisting axial compression. The majority of patients with graft collapse are asymptomatic and do not require reoperation.

Graft extrusion and migration are reported in 2.1% to 4.6% of single-level fusions and in 10% to 29% of multilevel fusions with bony or ligamentous instability after ventral cervical discectomy and fusion. Graft displacement may require reoperation if the patient reports dysphagia, respiratory compromise, or neurologic deficits.[24,25] A well-fitting graft and placement under compression may help reduce this complication.

Graft pseudarthrosis has been reported in 5% to 10% of patients who undergo single-level fusion, in 15% to 20% of two-level fusions, and in 30% to 63% of three-level fusions.[24] Despite radiographic nonunion, the majority of these patients are clinically asymptomatic, and reoperation is not indicated. However, persistent neck pain, progressive angulation, and subluxation mandate graft revision.

Failure to Improve

The patient with nerve root compression should have immediate or nearly immediate relief of arm pain after the surgical procedure. There is a group of patients, however, who do not follow this pattern but who ultimately have a good result. Some patients may have arm discomfort persisting for several weeks. Usually immediate imaging studies are not required in such cases. However, if the pain is severe or increases during the period of observation, one should obtain cervical spine radiographs to be certain that the surgical level is correct and the graft has been properly placed. If the symptoms persist for more than 3 months, the patient will require reevaluation using MRI or CT myelography.

The patient with persistent or worsened myelopathy presents a more difficult problem. Although most patients, after a satisfactory decompression, should have immediate improvement of some symptoms, overall improvement of myelopathic symptoms may take longer than recovery from radicular symptoms. If a patient does not have any significant neurologic recovery, imaging studies should be obtained at some point to rule out the possibility of an inadequate decompression. In such instances, reoperation may then be considered.

KEY REFERENCES

Ardon H, Van Calenbergh F, Van Raemdonck D, et al: Oesophageal perforation after anterior cervical surgery: management in four patients. *Acta Neurochir (Wien)* 151:297–302, 2009.

Bose B, Sestokas AK, Schwartz DM: Neurophysiological detection of iatrogenic C-5 nerve deficit during anterior cervical spinal surgery. *J Neurosurg Spine* 6:381–385, 2007.

Ebraheim NA, Lu J, Yang H, et al: Vulnerability of the sympathetic trunk during the anterior approach to the lower cervical spine. *Spine* 25: 1603–1606, 2000.

Eskander MS, Connolly PJ, Eskander JP, Brooks DD: Injury of an aberrant vertebral artery during a routine corpectomy: a case report and literature review. *Spinal Cord* 47:773–775, 2009.

Kahraman S, Sirin S, Erdogan E, et al: Is dysphonia permanent or temporary after anterior cervical approach? *Eur Spine J* 16:2092–2095, 2007.

Miscusi M, Bellitti A, Peschillo S, et al: Does recurrent laryngeal nerve anatomy condition the choice of the side for approaching the anterior cervical spine? *J Neurosurg Sci* 51:61–64, 2007.

REFERENCES

The complete reference list is available online at expertconsult.com.

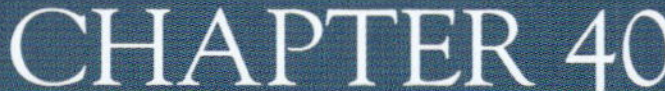

CHAPTER 40

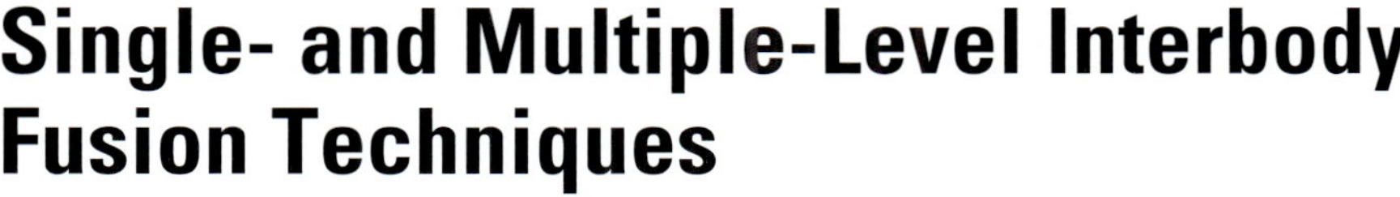

Single- and Multiple-Level Interbody Fusion Techniques

Robert F. Heary | Reza J. Karimi | George L. Sinclair III | Edward C. Benzel

Cervical discectomy via a ventral approach, better known as anterior cervical discectomy (ACD) or anterior cervical discectomy and fusion (ACDF), is one of the most common procedures performed by spine surgeons. Complication rates are low and the clinical results are gratifying. Some surgical complications are treatable at the time of their detection intraoperatively or in the immediate postoperative period, and other complications may have no reasonable treatment once detected. Avoiding irreversible complications is the only logical solution to their management. Overall, complication rates for ACDF operations vary from approximately 5%[1-4] to 15%.[5-9] The operation itself can be divided into stages, including general surgical considerations, discectomy, donor site considerations, and bony fusion.

Surgical complications may be categorized as occurring in the preoperative, intraoperative, or postoperative period. A majority of the complications that occur during an ACDF are avoidable with appropriate patient selection, careful preoperative planning, meticulous surgical technique, and close follow-up and monitoring of the clinical and radiographic conditions of the treated patient.

A brief history of ACD and ACDF is useful. More than 400 years ago, Vesalius described the intervertebral disc.[10] It was not until 1928 that Stookey described a number of clinical syndromes that resulted from disc protrusions. These protrusions were thought to be neoplasms of notochordal origin and were incorrectly identified as chondromas.[11] During this same era, other investigators provided a more precise understanding of the pathophysiology of the intervertebral disc.[12-14]

In the 1950s, the first reports of ventral approaches to cervical disc pathology appeared. The two most common methods for ACDF were described by Robinson and Smith in 1955[15] and by Cloward in 1958.[16] Robinson and Smith described an operation for removal of cervical disc material with replacement of a rectangular bone graft, obtained from the iliac crest, to allow for the development of a cervical fusion.[15] With the Cloward technique, the discectomy was performed by a cylindrical dowel technique.[16] Although numerous modifications have been developed since the 1950s, the great majority of spine surgeons currently use either the Cloward or the Smith-Robinson technique.[9,17-26]

Preoperative Considerations

The best predictor of a good postoperative clinical result is proper preoperative patient selection. ACD and ACDF are indicated for myelopathy, radiculopathy, and degenerative disc disease with mechanical pain. The presence of clinical symptoms, a consistent physical examination, and confirmatory imaging studies lead to the best postoperative result. In addition, a meticulous evaluation of the general overall medical condition of the patient is mandatory. Postoperative mortality may be caused by myocardial infarction,[6,10,27,28] respiratory failure,[29] pulmonary embolism,[30] or laryngeal edema,[28] among many other potential complications.

General considerations that may directly affect ACDF include the presence of diabetes mellitus or immunocompromised states such as AIDS, autoimmune disturbances, or systemic medical conditions that require corticosteroid administration. A history of smoking is clearly associated with diminished postoperative fusion rates.[27,31-37]

The deleterious effects of smoking are manifested by inhibition of the neovascularization necessary for incorporation of a bone graft.[38-40] A current preoperative recommendation is cessation of smoking for a minimum of 8 weeks before surgery and for a minimum of 12 weeks postoperatively. A preoperative dependence on narcotic analgesics has been associated with suboptimal outcome. This is particularly true if the clinical surgical indication is axial neck (mechanical) pain in the absence of radiculopathy or myelopathy. An important concern is preoperative difficulty with swallowing, which is more common in the elderly; it should be investigated, as necessary, before surgical intervention. If possible, the use of estrogen replacements or oral contraceptive pills in female patients should be discontinued preoperatively. These medications are known to increase the development of deep vein thromboses in the postoperative period. In addition, corticosteroids and nonsteroidal anti-inflammatory agents have a known deleterious effect on spine fusions and should be discontinued 10 days before surgery, if possible.

Preoperative radiographic imaging studies are necessary to confirm the history and physical examination findings. Plain radiographs remain a cornerstone of the preoperative radiographic evaluation. Lateral cervical spine radiographs allow for an assessment of the sagittal plane alignment and a rough assessment of bone mineralization. Flexion and extension views are useful to establish the presence of spine instability that may alter the surgical decision-making process. Finally, the dorsal elements should be assessed for splaying of the spinous processes or for facet joint abnormalities.

For many years, the gold standard imaging study for ventral cervical surgery was the myelogram, followed by a postmyelogram CT scan. This study provides excellent anatomic detail of both the spinal cord and the cervical nerve root sleeves. Recently, MRI has become more popular. MRI allows for greater soft tissue detail and is useful for identifying disc degeneration. However, MRI is extremely sensitive and may overestimate the extent of surgical pathology. A recent study has demonstrated a significant incidence of abnormal MRI findings in asymptomatic patients.[41] As a result, it is important to remember that an abnormal MRI is not necessarily an indication for surgery. However, note that MRI allows for the evaluation of pathology in both the axial and sagittal planes. In some cases of previously instrumented cervical spine surgery, CT myelogram may be preferable to MRI because it is less affected by metallic artifacts. Finally, reports of lower cervical spine ventral surgery performed in patients with significant pathology of the foramen magnum and the upper cervical spine should increase the surgeon's index of suspicion for such lesions.[2,5]

Intraoperative Considerations

The majority of intraoperative complications may be avoided by careful preoperative planning and meticulous intraoperative technique. If intraoperative complications occur, they are usually best managed at the time of detection. However, some may not be detected until the postoperative period. Thus, there is considerable overlap between the management of intraoperative and postoperative complications. Intraoperative considerations include positioning, incision, dissection, retraction, distraction, discectomy, donor site considerations, and fusion.

Positioning

The patient is positioned supine on the operating table, and general endotracheal anesthesia is administered. If significant spinal cord compression or myelopathy is present, consideration should be given to a fiberoptic nasotracheal intubation on a patient who is awake. After successful intubation, the patient's neurologic examination results are confirmed to be unchanged before the induction of general anesthesia.

The patient's head should be supported with either a foam donut or a Mayfield horseshoe headrest. The neck should be supported dorsally with a firm support to prevent intraoperative motion. In addition, an attempt at achieving a normal lordotic cervical curvature should be made to optimize the postoperative sagittal plane alignment. Ordinarily, a degree of neck extension is preferable to improve the lordotic curvature, as well as to aid in the dissection process. This is particularly true for upper cervical dissections. It is important to evaluate the patient's ability to extend the neck preoperatively and to not exceed this degree of extension intraoperatively. Hyperextension of the neck in a narcotized patient may lead to spinal cord compression.[4]

The operating table is flexed slightly at its midpoint, and a sandbag or other bolster is placed beneath the iliac crest to facilitate bone graft harvesting. All bony prominences must be padded, with particular attention paid to the protection of the ulnar nerves at the elbow. The knees are flexed and the heels are padded. Antiembolic stockings may be placed, and sequential compression devices are used to prevent the development of an intraoperative deep vein thrombosis.

After patient positioning and before preparation, the endotracheal cuff is deflated for 5 seconds and then reinflated. This maneuver was described by Apfelbaum[42] and has been used to limit compression of the vocal cords at the level of the arytenoid cartilage in the larynx. The recurrent laryngeal nerve (RLN) terminates at the arytenoid cartilage, and if it is compressed by the endotracheal tube, an RLN palsy may result.

A Doppler probe may be used to auscultate a baseline signal for the superficial temporal artery. During intraoperative retraction (of the carotid artery), the Doppler pulse can be reevaluated. If skeletal traction is to be used, the tongs are placed at this stage.

Incision

The selection of the ideal side for approach is controversial, with advocates for both right- and left-sided approaches. As a general rule a right-handed surgeon can approach the operation more easily from the patient's right side, but the more variable anatomic course of the right RLN may render the nerve more vulnerable to injury during a right-sided approach.[43-45] This vulnerability is particularly true with lower cervical dissections (Fig. 40-1). The reported incidence of postoperative RLN palsies presenting as postoperative hoarseness varies between 0.8% and 3.7%.[4-7,9,28,43-51] From a left-sided approach, the RLN has a longer course and may be less likely to be injured, but the thoracic duct is vulnerable with left-sided approaches to the lower cervical spine[9] (Fig. 40-2). In addition, the thoracic duct may be bifid, and injury to one of the limbs of the thoracic duct may not be recognized intraoperatively. If chyle is observed, simple ligation of the thoracic duct is usually all that is necessary. With lower cervical discectomies there is a theoretical risk of pneumothorax or mediastinitis with approaches from either side.[10,16,52,53]

It is essential to make the skin incision at the proper level. The most common error is to place the incision too caudal, thereby obligating the physician to operate at an awkward, upward oblique angle. This can limit visibility during the discectomy. It is much easier to gain access caudally from a rostrally placed incision than the converse.

With one- or two-level discectomies a transverse incision is most commonly used. This is placed in a skin fold that allows for a more cosmetic postoperative result. If discectomies at three or more levels are to be performed, an oblique incision that parallels the medial border of the sternocleidomastoid muscle is preferable. This incision is commonly used for carotid endarterectomies because it allows for a better exposure of multiple spine levels. We prefer to make our transverse incisions for lower cervical approaches at the level of the upper border of the crossing omohyoid muscle. This incision will be at the C5-6 level and provides comfortable access to both the C5-6 and C6-7 intervertebral discs.

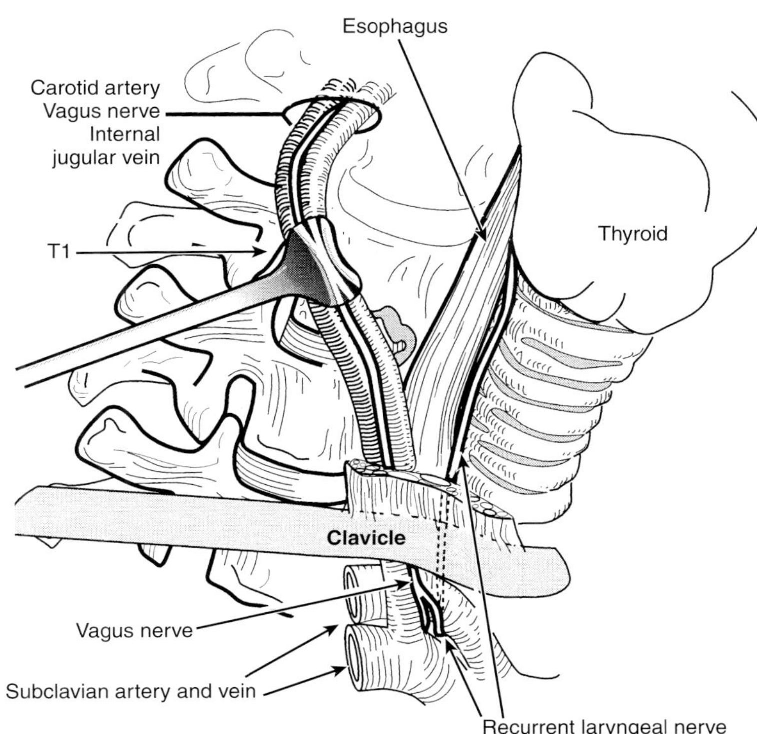

FIGURE 40-1. Right-sided low cervical exposure places the right recurrent laryngeal nerve at risk. The regional anatomy is depicted. (Copyright University of New Mexico, Division of Neurosurgery.)

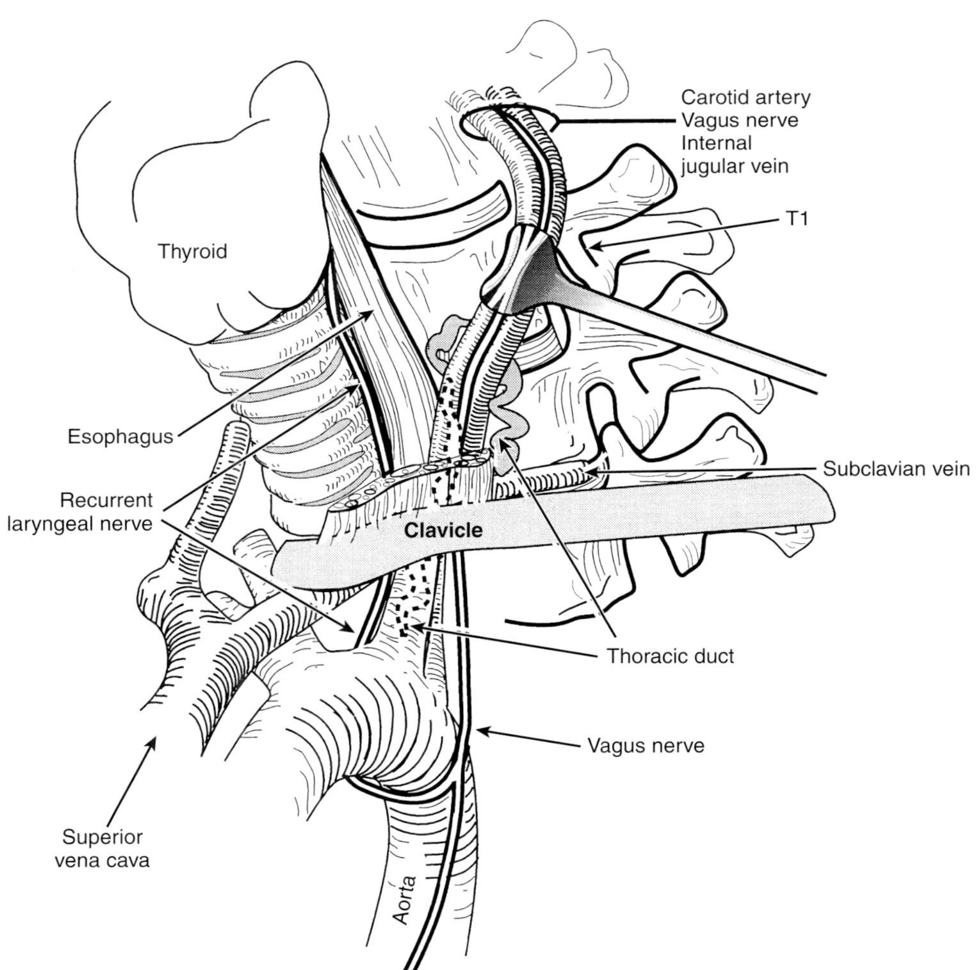

FIGURE 40-2. Left-sided low cervical exposure places the thoracic duct at risk. The regional anatomy is depicted. (Copyright University of New Mexico, Division of Neurosurgery.)

Maintaining the dissection plane rostral to the omohyoid muscle and depressing it inferiorly as necessary has resulted in an extremely low rate of postoperative RLN palsy in our practice.

Dissection

The dissection is carried sharply through the subcutaneous tissue and the platysma muscle. The platysma muscle may be sharply divided in a transverse fashion or split longitudinally for access to the subplatysmal space. As a general rule, transecting the platysmal muscle is preferable for exposures of two or more levels. If access to multiple levels of the upper cervical spine is necessary, a generous subplatysmal dissection is used to limit the extent of soft tissue retraction required to gain adequate exposure. After the subplatysmal dissection is completed the fascia overlying the medial border of the sternocleidomastoid muscle is sharply divided, and the deep dissection is performed, either sharply or bluntly. The plane of the deep dissection is between the sternocleidomastoid muscle and carotid sheath laterally and the trachea, esophagus, and strap muscles of the neck medially. Careful dissection, with identification of the carotid artery by palpation and gentle finger dissection, is required to avoid carotid artery injuries.[6,30,54,55] This trajectory allows for exposure of the prevertebral fascia. In patients who have not undergone previous ventral cervical surgery, blunt dissection is easily and safely accomplished. Excessive soft tissue stretching should be avoided because occasional RLN injury has been hypothesized to be secondary to stretching. In this case, avoiding high endotracheal cuff pressures may reduce the incidence of such injuries.[42]

In patients who undergo reoperation sharp dissection may be necessary. It is important to confirm that the dissection remains dorsal to the hypopharynx and the esophagus. With reoperation, a nasogastric (NG) tube should be placed. This may be palpated to confirm the location of the esophagus and hypopharynx. The incidence of hypopharynx perforation during upper cervical discectomies varies between 1%[8,46,47,56] and 5%.[48,57,58] Esophageal perforation has also been reported in cervical discectomies.[47,59-64] If the hypopharynx or esophagus is penetrated, a drain should be placed, a layered closure performed, and an NG feeding tube inserted. The latter must be maintained for at least 1 week postoperatively to allow for the soft tissue to heal and prevent the development of a fistula.

If there is a question of perforation of the alimentary tract, the NG tube should be withdrawn so that the tip of the tube is in the esophagus. After this maneuver, instillation of a colored inert dye, such as methylene blue or indigo carmine, should assist with demonstration of the violation. Unrecognized esophageal perforations can lead to the development of deep soft tissue infections (including mediastinitis). These manifest as high fevers, severe retrosternal pain, and subcutaneous emphysema. Other severe complications of esophageal perforation include esophagocutaneous fistula[57] and even death.[61]

Retraction

On entering the prevertebral space a radiographic marker must be placed and a lateral cervical spine radiograph obtained. This mandatory step ensures that the operation is performed at the correct level. There have been reports of ACDs being performed at the wrong level.[2,9]

Establishing that the correct level is being operated on is readily accomplished by placing a radiopaque 18-gauge spinal needle into the intervertebral disc space and obtaining a lateral fluoroscopic image. Alternatively, the authors prefer to place the spinal needle into the ventral aspect of the vertebral body cortex rather than the intervertebral disc, which avoids perforation of the anulus. Should the first attempt at localization demonstrate exposure of an intervertebral disc not to be operated upon, perforation of the outer anulus with a spinal needle may lead to accelerated adjacent-segment disc degeneration at this level. Thus, placement of the spinal needle through the ventral vertebral body cortex potentially avoids this complication.

When the appropriate level has been identified, it is useful to mark the true anatomic midline. This is best accomplished by marking a point midway between the most medial borders of the longus colli muscles. After the midline is identified, the longus colli muscles are elevated from the vertebral bodies and discs bilaterally. Longus colli dissection should be limited laterally to 3 mm of muscle. If the longus colli muscles are dissected excessively, a Horner syndrome—the triad of ipsilateral ptosis, myosis, and anhydrosis—may result. The incidence of postoperative Horner syndrome varies from 0.2% to 2%[2,4-6,46,47,65-67] after ventral cervical spine surgeries.

After the longus colli muscles are elevated, a self-retaining retractor system is used. Toothed retractors are placed under the longus colli muscles bilaterally. With single-level discectomies there is rarely a need to place vertical self-retaining retractors. When operating on the lower cervical spine, it is essential to avoid retraction of the RLN, which is particularly problematic when a right-sided cervical approach is used. If necessary, vertical retractors should be smooth at the tips, and care should be taken to avoid excessive retraction.

The self-retaining lateral retractors should be carefully placed to avoid excessive retraction on the esophagus, which may lead to postoperative dysphagia. The exact mechanism responsible for the development of postoperative dysphagia is unknown; however, it is thought that retraction-induced pressure on the esophageal wall leads to local ischemia with subsequent hyperemia and swelling.[68] This in turn may lead to postoperative dysphagia. A mild, transient, postoperative dysphagia is common after ventral cervical surgery. However, in the majority of patients this resolves within 3 months.[69-71] Dysphagia rates have been reported to vary from 1.8% to 9.5%,[1,7,10,17,27,28,48,53,69-72] to between 21.2% and 35%.[5,9,46] Intermittently releasing the retractor pressure during prolonged surgical procedures helps to avoid this complication. Most dysphagia episodes are transient and do not require a gastrostomy tube. In cases of severe postoperative dysphagia, a gastrostomy tube may be needed for enteral feedings.

Excessive lateral retraction may also compress the carotid sheath. In patients with significant preoperative atherosclerosis, prolonged pressure against the carotid artery can lead to thrombosis with cerebral ischemia. To avoid this problem, after the lateral self-retaining retractors have been placed, the pulse of the superficial temporal artery above the level of the zygoma may be auscultated with a Doppler probe or palpated by the anesthesiologist intraoperatively. This measure confirms blood flow in the external carotid artery. Because the common carotid artery bifurcates into its external and internal branches at the C3-4 level, this maneuver indirectly increases the degree of confidence that blood flow in the internal carotid artery has not been significantly compromised. In addition, the retractors may alter the position of the endotracheal tube. Release of the endotracheal tube cuff for 5 seconds, followed by re-inflation to the lowest pressure that eliminates air leak, confirms that the vocal cords are not being excessively compressed.[42]

Distraction

After the retractors have been firmly positioned, the anulus fibrosus is incised and the ventral two thirds of disc material is removed with a combination of rongeurs and curettes. Distraction techniques may improve the visualization of the disc interspace. Commonly, Gardner-Wells tongs are placed before draping, and additional weights may be added to augment distraction. Holter distraction may also be used. Improved visualization may be achieved by the use of intervertebral body disc spreaders. Alternatively, posts may be placed into the vertebral bodies above and below the desired disc exposure, with a distractor placed over the posts.

After the distractor is placed, an operating microscope may be used to improve the magnification and lighting. Alternatively, a head light or high-quality overhead light, with or without loupe magnification, may be used. Adequate visualization is essential for performing the discectomy procedure safely. We routinely utilize the operating microscope in all ventral cervical spine surgeries.

Discectomy

The adequacy of neural decompression is directly related to the completeness with which the discectomy itself is performed. In addition, most neurologic complications occur at this stage of the procedure. The disc is removed, including the entirety of the dorsal anulus fibrosus in the midline. The depth of the dissection necessary to achieve this may be estimated from the preoperative MRI and CT scans. Small, upbiting microcurettes and rongeurs allow for removal of the anulus fibrosus. Hemostasis is achieved with judicious use of bipolar electrocautery, hemostatic gelatin (Gelfoam) soaked in thrombin, and cotton patties. After removal of the anulus fibrosus, the underlying posterior longitudinal ligament (PLL) will be seen.

The need to open the PLL is debated. Numerous authors recommend routine opening of the PLL after removal of the dorsal anulus fibrosus.[42,48,51,73-75] However, others do not agree with the routine sectioning of the PLL after good quality preoperative radiographic imaging studies.[76-78] Although preoperative imaging studies may suggest that the disc material has not protruded dorsally, the PLL may be safely sectioned to allow for entry into the epidural space. On entry a blunt nerve hook may be used to search for disc material. In addition, the PLL itself may be thickened and may be responsible for ongoing neural compression. As a result, if there is any doubt about the adequacy of decompression, the PLL should be opened sharply to allow a direct look at the underlying dura mater. Any disc fragments dorsal to the PLL are removed. Likewise, ridges from dorsal osteophytes may compress the spinal cord or nerve roots. If osteophytes are detected, either by preoperative imaging studies or during the surgical procedure, they should be resected using small Kerrison rongeurs.[1,7,24,50,76,79-82]

Tearing of the underlying dura mater is possible during the opening of the PLL. This is particularly likely in cases of ossification of the PLL and in patients who have undergone previous ventral procedures.[83,84] In a series of 450 patients who underwent ventral cervical surgery, Bertalanffy and Eggert reported 8 patients (1.8%) who sustained damage to the dural sac. Of these 8 patients, 1 developed meningitis.[46] If a dural tear occurs, it is usually impossible to repair the defect primarily. The methods used to prevent egress of cerebrospinal fluid (CSF) include placing free muscle and fascial grafts and using Gelfoam soaked in thrombin or fibrin glue. Additionally, newer dural substitutes made from synthetic materials, bovine grafts, and collagen can also be used.[85-88] With a dural tear, placement of a lumbar subarachnoid drain must be considered to divert CSF in the immediate postoperative period. Once the PLL is opened, instead of electrocautery, thrombostatic agents such as Gelfoam and cotton patties should be used for hemostasis. Our philosophy has been to routinely open the PLL in all cases of radiculopathy and myelopathy. In our practice, only surgery for axial mechanical neck pain, which constitutes less than 5% of our cases, is performed without opening the PLL.

The width of the decompression is determined on a case-by-case basis. Care must be taken to maintain the orientation of the midline, which is essential when determining the width of decompression. Useful techniques include referring to the marking of the true bony midline made before the longus colli muscle dissection, as well as being aware of the anatomic bony structures, such as the uncovertebral joints. As a general rule a 15-mm bony dissection centered over the midline is necessary for an adequate decompression.[89] If nerve root compression is present, the dissection may be extended laterally. The medial border of the uncovertebral joint serves as a bony anatomic marker of the lateral extent of a cervical discectomy. Limiting the dissection to this point will allow for a good decompression of the shoulder of the nerve root. Once again, the majority of intraoperative neurologic injuries that occur are the result of loss of orientation of the bony anatomic midline. A useful intraoperative maneuver to prevent an excessively wide discectomy is frequent placement of a cotton patty in the discectomy defect. A standard cotton patty measures 13 mm and allows for reorientation throughout the procedure.

As mentioned earlier in this chapter, the majority of neurologic injuries occur during the deep portion of the discectomy procedure. The most common complications include dural tears, damage to the neural elements, and vertebral artery injuries. Intraoperative nerve root injuries and spinal cord contusions occur in less than 1% of ACDs.[2,4,7,16,28,46,90,91]

If the discectomy is too wide, the vertebral artery may be injured. The vertebral artery and its accompanying venous plexus are at risk during removal of the lateral disc material.[6,8,54,55,92,93] Profuse arterial bleeding occurs after a vertebral artery injury. If the patient's head was rotated as part of the initial operative positioning, the head should be immediately returned to the midline before attempts are made to control bleeding.[94] Immediate tamponade should be used for the initial management of vertebral artery injuries. If the

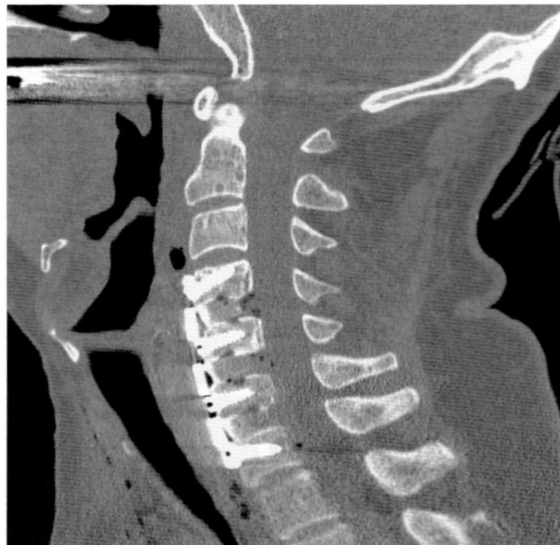

FIGURE 40-4. Early postoperative sagittally reconstructed CT scan following three-level anterior cervical discectomy and fusions from C4 to C7. The open end of the tricortical autograft is directed dorsally, and the ventral aspect is countersunk 1 mm below the ventral vertebral body surface. Screw trajectories are directed superiorly and inferiorly at the rostral and caudal extremes of the construct, respectively. The plate sits flush with the ventral aspect of the vertebral bodies and is lordotically contoured to allow for maintenance of a normal sagittal alignment of the cervical spine.

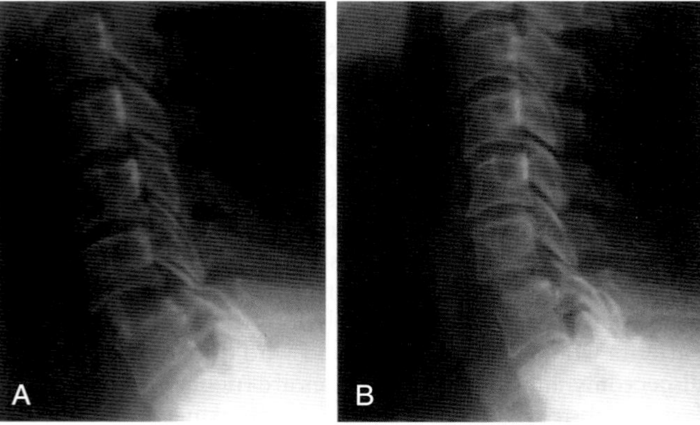

FIGURE 40-5. A noninstrumented anterior cervical discectomy and fusion at C6-7 with a generous, oversized bone graft with the crest portions of the graft oriented ventrally. **A,** Note that the graft is seated 2 mm below the ventral-most surface of the vertebral bodies above and below. **B,** A subsequent radiograph (3 months postoperatively) demonstrates an acceptable degree of subsidence.

replaced or modified to fit the interspace accordingly. After the bone graft is in place, the interbody distraction device is removed. A lateral cervical spine radiograph is obtained, with distraction pins in place, to confirm correct graft placement and spine alignment and to determine the optimal screw length if a screw-plate stabilization construct is to be placed. Proper screw length is determined by examining the radiographic appearance of the known distraction pin screw lengths.

If multiple interbody fusions are to be performed, the interbody distractors are then placed sequentially at each level and the interbody graft is placed. After placement of all interbody grafts, all distraction devices and pins are removed, all traction is discontinued, and a lateral cervical radiograph is obtained. The radiograph should be studied to confirm spine alignment and the depth of the bone graft(s) and to reconfirm that the facet joints are not overdistracted (Fig. 40-5A).

Ventral cervical plating is now often employed when performing ACDF. The potential benefits of plating include higher fusion rates, decreased pseudarthrosis and strut graft dislodgement, resistance to segmental kyphosis, and less need for external immobilization. A recent meta-analysis suggests that ventral plating increases fusion rates regardless of the number of levels involved.[107]

When using ventral cervical plating the basic technique is as follows: proper identification of the midline and the alignment of the plate along its centerline, meticulous preparation of the ventral vertebral bodies to facilitate plate contact, selection of a properly sized plate, selection of a screw size that provides maximal cortical purchase based on preoperative or intraoperative imaging, screw placement within the vertebral body, and engaging the screw-plate locking mechanism (see Fig. 40-3). The exact plating system chosen will determine any variations to screw placement.

It is important for the rostral end of the plate system to sit as flush as possible with the ventral vertebral bodies. This is accomplished through meticulous preparation of the ventral vertebral bodies to accommodate the plating system, in addition to the specific technique used to place the screw-plate system. Once the centerline of the plate is aligned with the midline and the correctly sized plate is chosen, which will allow screws to be placed in the vertical center of the vertebral bodies to be fused, the first screw hole is drilled at the caudalmost level on the surgeon's side. A self-tapping screw is then placed and tightened until approximately 90% of the screw threads are engaged within the vertebral body. The two rostralmost screw holes are then drilled, the screws are placed, and the screws are fully engaged within the vertebral body to allow the plate to sit as flush as possible at its rostral end. The caudal screw is then fully engaged and a screw is placed on the contralateral side of the caudally fixated vertebra. If a multilevel fusion is being performed, screws may then be placed at each intermediate level to achieve additional points of fixation. A final lateral radiograph is obtained to confirm graft position, screw-plate position, spine alignment, and the appearance of the dorsal facet complexes. After this confirmatory radiograph is obtained, the final locking mechanism of the plate is engaged. Once again, it is essential to release the distraction pins or the tongs before placing the spinal instrumentation to prevent inadvertent loading of the instrumentation with stress shielding of the bone graft or cage.

The most common complication of the fusion portion of the operation is the development of a delayed nonunion, or pseudarthrosis. Complications related to improper positioning of the bone graft are less common. Useful intraoperative maneuvers to avoid nonunion include placement of the graft under tension and the use of an adequately sized bone graft. Preservation of the vertebral body end plates above and below minimizes the chance of collapse or pistoning (Fig. 40-5B). Graft collapse has been detected on follow-up imaging studies in 0.8% to 5.8% of cases.[17,27,65,77,100,110] Foreign bodies should be avoided at all times. Bone wax limits bony fusion rates and should be avoided.

After the bone graft is placed, hemostasis must be attained. Generous irrigation is performed. A drain may be placed in the prevertebral space, ventral to the bone graft, and it is brought out through a separate stab wound in the skin. However, as with the iliac donor site, drains are not mandatory.

Complications

Postoperative complications are categorized as problems related to the decompression (neurologic) and those related to the fusion (pain). In the immediate postoperative period, neurologic complications are the most common. Overall, complications include esophageal injury, postoperative airway compromise, vertebral artery injury, dural tear, spinal cord injury, dysphagia, dysphonia, graft dislodgement, infection, and hematoma.[30,38,111]

The most catastrophic immediate postoperative complication is the development of an epidural hematoma, with an accompanying neurologic dysfunction. Symptomatic epidural hematomas occur in 0.2% to 0.9% of cases.[2,46,55,75,92] This complication is managed by immediate surgical evacuation of the hematoma. Any unnecessary delay in the evacuation of an epidural hematoma may lead to an irreversible neurologic deficit. If a postoperative neurologic decline that suggests an epidural hematoma is observed, either a CT scan and a myelogram or an MRI study should be performed immediately. Alternatively, if a high index of suspicion suggests the presence of spinal cord compression, the patient can be brought back to the operating room immediately without advanced neuroimaging studies being obtained.

If an epidural hematoma is identified on postoperative neuroimaging, the patient is immediately returned to the operating room, the bone graft is removed, and the hematoma is evacuated. If there is no evidence of compression of neural tissue on the neuroimaging study, expectant observation is proper. In the absence of imaging evidence of neural compression, the majority of neurologic deficits resolve.

An additional complication during the postoperative period is an unrecognized dural tear. If this occurs, a lumbar drain is placed and maintained for 1 week to divert the flow of CSF and allow the durotomy to spontaneously close. If this is unsuccessful, surgical reexploration and direct operative treatment of the durotomy may be necessary.

Wound infections may occur at variable periods during the postoperative course. These are best identified by persistent pain, as well as by an elevation of the erythrocyte sedimentation rate. Fever or an elevated white blood cell count is not a reliable indicator of postoperative wound infections. Wound infections occur in 0.1% to 2% of cases.* If a cervical wound infection is identified, the treatment is prompt surgical reexploration, culture, irrigation, and closure of the wound, with the placement of a drain. Appropriate antibiotics are used postoperatively. If an iliac crest wound infection occurs, the wound must be reopened, debrided, and drained. Prevention of cervical and iliac crest wound infections is best accomplished by avoiding the use of foreign bodies (e.g., bone wax) and by obtaining meticulous hemostasis. Some surgeons argue that the use of drains may decrease the development of hematomas and subsequently decrease wound infection rates. Others argue that they provide an access route for microorganisms.

*References 2, 5, 7, 17, 28, 35, 46, 67, 78, 80, 81, and 112.

Iliac region pain is ordinarily secondary to the development of a subperiosteal hematoma. The majority of these resolve spontaneously. If the hematoma is excessively large or painful, surgical reexploration and evacuation of the hematoma may be necessary. Persistent occult blood loss during the postoperative period may be secondary to enlargement of a retroperitoneal hematoma. This may dictate the need for reexploration of the iliac crest graft harvest site. A wound infection must also be ruled out. In questionable situations, obtaining a bone scan and a C-reactive protein level may be helpful in establishing the diagnosis. A postoperative hernia secondary to violation of the transversalis fascia may present with chronic donor site pain postoperatively. This may be diagnosed by an intraluminal contrast study such as a barium enema. If a painful hernia is present or if a bowel obstruction occurs, surgical reexploration, with closure of the hernia defect, is usually successful.

Postoperative neck pain in the first few weeks is usually transient and self-limited. Persistent postoperative pain in the neck, arm, and interscapular region has been observed in 4% to 20% of cases.[7,46,48,80,97] Wound infections or the development of a deep hematoma should be ruled out. We have found that surgery at the C6-7 level is most frequently associated with postoperative interscapular pain. Fortunately, this pain is usually transient.

A bony nonunion, or pseudarthrosis, after an ACDF often presents with persistent axial neck pain. This may or may not be associated with radicular symptoms. Bony fusion is typically well under way by 12 weeks postoperatively. This may be delayed in smokers, immunocompromised patients, or patients undergoing multilevel discectomies. A pseudarthrosis is diagnosed by persistent axial neck pain with evidence of a radiographic lucency at the vertebral body–graft junction at 6 or more months after surgery. Bone graft collapse is diagnosed by a 2-mm or greater loss of graft height detected on radiographs taken 12 months postoperatively.[35]

If a pseudarthrosis develops, imaging studies should be performed to confirm whether neural compression is also present. If neural compression is present, a repeat ventral operation is necessary to remove the bone graft, perform a neural element decompression, and re-fuse the cervical spine. If axial neck pain is present and neuroimaging studies do not demonstrate evidence of neural compression, a cervical pseudarthrosis is best treated with either a ventral or dorsal fusion of the involved motion segment. A successful dorsal fusion for the treatment of a pseudarthrosis secondary to an ACDF most often results in a stable circumferential fusion. In exceptional cases it may be necessary to revise a pseudarthrosis ventrally and perform a dorsal fusion at the same time. This leads to a higher fusion rate, but is considered excessive by some.

If the patient develops persistent axial neck pain and plain radiographs cannot demonstrate a lucency suggestive of a pseudarthrosis, further diagnostic studies may be necessary. Tomograms are more sensitive than plain radiographs for detecting pseudarthroses. In addition, flexion and extension views may help confirm the diagnosis. CT scans with sagittal reconstructions are very effective at identifying nonunions.

The issue of postoperative immobilization is controversial. Some authors use no postoperative bracing after a single-level ACDF. Others use a cervical collar for a variable period of 6 to 12 weeks. In rare circumstances, a postoperative Minerva jacket or halo vest may be used for prolonged immobilization.

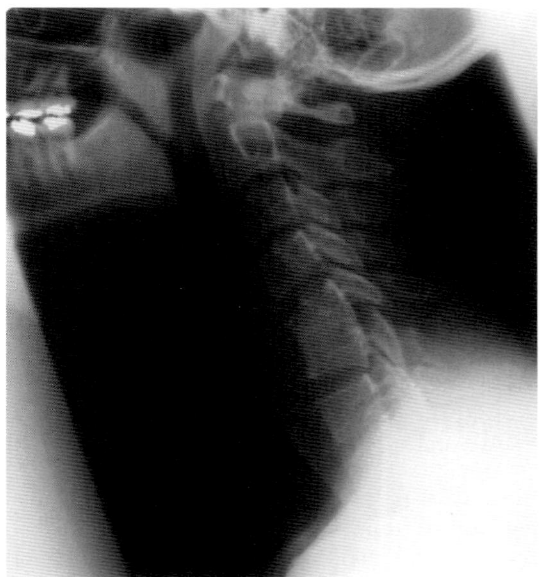

FIGURE 40-6. Graft collapse with kyphotic angulation is seen in this noninstrumented C5-6 anterior cervical discectomy and fusion 3 months after surgery. This collapse is frequently the result of excessive removal of the bony vertebral end plates or an undersized graft.

A spinal implant may be indicated in a patient who is likely to suffer fusion failure. Such patients include smokers, immunocompromised patients, and those undergoing multilevel discectomies.

In the postoperative period, serial radiographs are obtained until a bony fusion is confirmed. Patients should be followed for a minimum of 12 months postoperatively and should only be discharged after evidence of a successful clinical and radiographic fusion. We typically discontinue patient follow-up after 24 months in patients with good outcomes.

Other delayed complications that may occur after an ACDF include a loss of cervical lordosis. This is most commonly observed after the use of undersized grafts, graft material of insufficient integrity, or excessive end plate removal, possibly leading to the development of a kyphotic deformity (Fig. 40-6).[2,57,100,110] In general, no surgical intervention is necessary for this problem, unless it is severe. Graft subsidence without angulation may also occur.

Some neck motion is lost postoperatively. As a general approximation, there is a 10-degree loss of cervical motion for each fused motion segment. For a single-level discectomy this loss of motion is not ordinarily discernible. With multilevel discectomies the patient and physician may notice a loss of neck motion.

Graft protrusions or dislodgements occur in 0.4% to 4.6% of cases.* The treatment of a graft dislodgement involves a surgical reexploration and fusion.

Discitis or osteomyelitis may also occur as a delayed complication.[1,24,46,57,65,66,77] This warrants antibiotic therapy and, usually, surgical debridement.

Some patients (as many as 50%) develop persistent radiographic nonunion without clinical symptoms. Lateral radiographs from these patients have a persistent lucency, but no clinical neck pain or radicular symptoms. Such patients should be followed clinically with serial imaging studies. Delayed radiographic fusion may occur in some of these cases. If radiographic fusion is not demonstrable but no clinical symptoms are present, there is no indication for surgical reexploration.

After an ACDF, there is an increased risk of disc degeneration at the levels adjacent to the fused segments (accelerated degenerative changes or adjacent segment disease). This is most common and is clinically significant at the interspace immediately rostral to the fusion. Adjacent-level disc degenerations may occur after longer cervical fusions, and longer-term follow-up is necessary after a multiple-level ACDF, both to monitor the fusion itself and to monitor for degenerative changes at adjacent levels. Adjacent-segment disease may require treatment if symptomatic.

Accelerated degenerative changes at motion segments adjacent to a spine fusion may occur as a result of increased biomechanical stresses and hypermobility. Some surgeons have advocated the performance of a total disc arthroplasty (TDA) in an off-label fashion, for the treatment of adjacent-segment disease, as a well-intentioned effort to preserve motion at the affected spine level. However, since the pathophysiology of adjacent-segment disease is hypermobility itself, we recommend an ACDF rather than a "mobility-sparing" TDA (Fig. 40-7). In addition, we strongly recommend the use of autograft in this clinical scenario because a more rapid spine fusion is likely to be obtained, and thus there will be a shorter time in which the screw-plate construct is exposed to the increased biomechanical stresses at this excessively mobile spine level.

Hospitalization for ACDF can range from less than 24 hours to 3 to 4 days. Given the low overall complication rate of ACDF, it seems feasible that this surgery could be performed on an outpatient basis. Doing so could significantly lower the cost of performing this procedure. Although class 1 data on this topic are lacking, recent studies have attempted to evaluate the safety of performing outpatient ACDF.[113-115] The results of these studies suggest that this surgery can be safely performed on outpatients with a short observational period. Until further studies are available, the surgeon must continue to evaluate the preoperative, intraoperative, and immediate postoperative considerations when deciding the length of hospitalization for patients.

Multiple-Level Anterior Cervical Discectomy and Fusion

The complications associated with multiple-level discectomies and fusions are similar to those for single-level operations, with respect to each fused segment. However, certain complications are more prevalent with multiple-level operations. The rate of pseudarthrosis increases with the addition of each fused segment.[8,10,27,53,86,100,102,116-118] Thus, the indication for each fused level must remain as strict as the indications for a single fused level. Dysphagia rates are higher because of the longer duration of surgery with prolonged retraction of the esophagus. Similarly, the incidence of hoarseness secondary to RLN dysfunction is higher with multiple-level discectomies. This is particularly true if the C6-7 space is fused. Multiple-level discectomies require a longer operative time, which increases the complications related to anesthesia, as well as general medical problems. In addition, larger iliac crest bone grafts are necessary for multiple-level

*References 2–4, 6, 7, 19, 26, 53, 65, 72, 77, and 97.

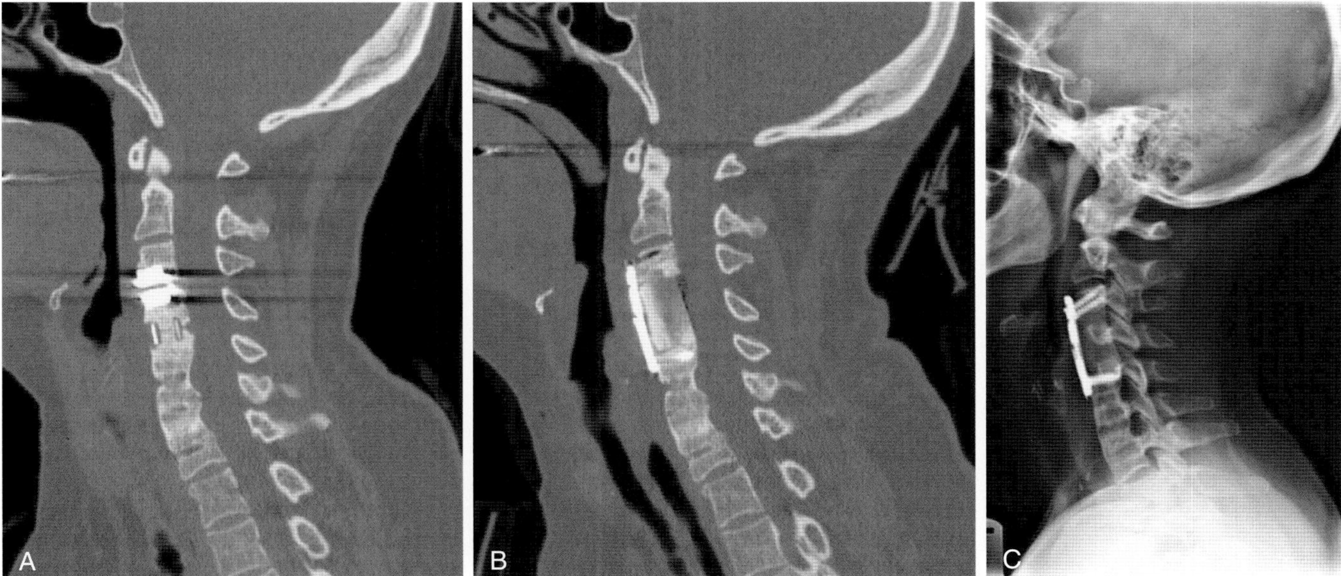

FIGURE 40-7. **A,** Sagittally reconstructed CT scan of a 48-year-old female who previously underwent three-level anterior cervical discectomy and fusions from C4 to C7. After 3 years, a herniated disc at C3-4 was treated by a total disc arthroscopy (TDA) with the Prodisc device for adjacent-segment disease. The goal of this total disc arthroscopy was to preserve motion at that adjacent level; however, immediately after the TDA, the patient developed severe axial neck pain that was unresponsive to conservative treatment. A reoperation was performed to remove the TDA and stabilize and fuse the unstable segment. Due to the keel on the device and rigid incorporation of the TDA at the TDA-C4 surface, a C4 corpectomy was necessary for its removal. **B,** The previously placed polyetheretherketone cage at C4-5 was also removed and structural autograft was placed from C3 to C5. The TDA had not incorporated into the inferior C3 bony end plate, and it was removed from C3 without substantial damage to the C3 end plate. The patient experienced immediate relief of axial neck pain in the early postoperative period. **C,** Lateral cervical spine radiograph at 1-year follow-up, demonstrating full incorporation of the bone graft and fusion from C3 to C7. Improved spinal sagittal alignment was obtained, and graft position remains optimal.

discectomies. The incidence of bleeding, pain, and infections at the iliac crest donor site may thus be increased. The strategies for avoiding and managing each of the individual complications are identical for multiple-level and single-level discectomies.

Summary

Many of the complications associated with ACDF can be avoided by performing properly indicated surgery, employing careful preoperative planning, and using meticulous surgical technique. When intraoperative complications occur, many of them can be managed immediately. However, some complications do not develop until the postoperative period. When postoperative complications are detected, immediate imaging studies and treatment, as necessary, are warranted. As a rule, the postoperative neurologic results depend on the adequacy of the decompression. Pain relief depends on the adequacy of the bony fusion.

Long-term follow-up is essential to confirm both the clinical and radiographic successes of the ACDF. With proper preoperative patient selection, careful preoperative planning, meticulous intraoperative surgical technique, and diligent postoperative follow-up, the incidence of complications after ACDF can be minimized.

KEY REFERENCES

Apfelbaum RI, Kriskovich MD, Haller JR: On the incidence, cause, and prevention of recurrent laryngeal nerve palsies during anterior cervical spine surgery. *Spine* 25:2906–2912, 2000.

Cloward RB: The anterior approach for removal of ruptured discs. *J Neurosurg* 15:602–614, 1958.

Frazier JF, Hartl R: Anterior approaches to fusion of the cervical spine: a meta-analysis of fusion rates. *J Neurosurg Spine* 6:298–303, 2007.

Hilibrand AS, Carlson GD, et al: Radiculopathy and myelopathy at segments adjacent to the site of a previous anterior cervical arthrodesis. *J Bone Joint Surg [Am]* 81:519–528, 1999.

Matz PG, Ryken TC, et al: Techniques for anterior cervical decompression for radiculopathy. *J Neurosurg Spine* 11:183–197, 2009.

Monfared A, Kim D, Jaikumar S, et al: Microsurgical anatomy of the superior and recurrent laryngeal nerves. *Neurosurgery* 49(4):925–932, 2001.

Smith-Hammond CA, New KC, Pietrobon R, et al: Prospective analysis of incidence and risk factors of dysphagia in spine surgery patients: comparison of anterior cervical, posterior cervical, and lumbar procedures. *Spine (Phila Pa 1976)* 29:1441–1446, 2004.

REFERENCES

The complete reference list is available online at expertconsult.com.

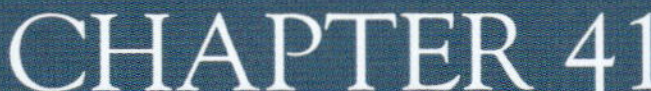
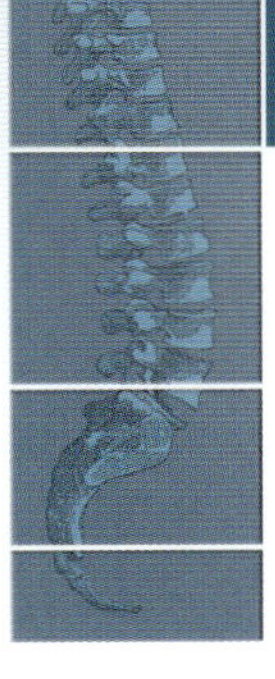

CHAPTER 41

Threaded Cylindrical Interbody Cage Fixation for Cervical Spondylosis and Ossification of the Posterior Longitudinal Ligament

Hiroshi Nakagawa | Yasunobu Itoh | Junichi Mizuno | Hidenori Matsuoka | Yoshitaka Hirano

With advances in neuroimaging using CT and MRI, the diagnosis of cervical disc herniation, spondylosis, and ossification of the posterior longitudinal ligament (OPLL) has become more precise and less invasive in recent years.[1] In addition, routine microsurgery with refined drills and implants such as interbody cages has facilitated less invasive and more efficient ventral cervical spine procedures.[2,3]

Preoperative Workups and Surgical Considerations

In Japan, two factors must be taken into consideration that result in the need for a different approach than that used in North America and Europe. These factors significantly affect the surgical strategies for cervical discogenic diseases.

The first factor is the frequent association of cervical spondylosis and disc herniation with OPLL and hypertrophy of the posterior longitudinal ligaments,[4] causing myelopathy rather than radiculopathy.[5-7] Radiologically, OPLL of the cervical spine has been classified into four types: (1) the local, bridge, or circumscribed type, which is located behind the disc space; (2) the segmental type, which usually is limited to the posterior aspect of one or two vertebral levels; (3) the continuous type, which usually extends continuously over several vertebral bodies; and (4) the mixed type, which is a combination of the continuous and segmental types.[1]

In epidemiologic studies, OPLL of the cervical spine is found in 3.2% of those age 50 years and older in Japan and is relatively common in south Asian countries. It is also found not infrequently in New York, Utah, and Hawaii in the United States and in some European countries. Therefore, understanding of this condition (OPLL) is important in determining surgical strategies to treat patients with cervical discogenic disease.[8]

The second factor resulting in the need for a different surgical approach in Japan is unique: allografts are not available in Japan. Therefore, autografts or other alternatives have to be used for anterior cervical fusion.[9,10]

In preoperative workups, a routine study with dynamic plain radiographs, thin-slice CT with sagittal reformation, and MRI is mandatory, because less advanced OPLL, such as local or segmental types, may be easily missed with plain radiograph and MRI alone. With the advent of multislice CT with sagittal reformation, conventional and CT myelography may not be necessary; hence, it is not used in our practice. With advanced CT and MRI, the precise diagnosis of spurs, disc protrusion, and OPLL, along with the extent of cord and root compression, can be easily made and surgical strategies properly crafted.

Deciding which surgical strategy—ventral versus dorsal approach—to use can be determined based on the number of spinal levels involved, the extent of OPLL, the presence of canal stenosis, and the alignment of the cervical spine, but more often depends on the surgeon's experience and philosophy. Generally speaking, the ventral approach is applied to single-level or two-level lesions and the dorsal approach is usually applied to three-level or four-level lesions.[3,5,11,12] The surgical techniques of expansive laminoplasty have been well described.[13-15]

Evolution of Surgical Techniques

Over the past three decades, our surgical techniques for cervical spondylosis and OPLL have significantly changed and advanced to a less invasive method with more refined implants and technologies.

Corpectomy with Iliac Bone Graft

From 1980 to 1991, multilevel corpectomy with iliac crest interbody graft was carried out for multilevel OPLL and spondylosis, but graft problems, donor site discomfort, and the necessity of postoperative application of a halo brace were drawbacks of this method. Development of ventral plate fixation dramatically reduced the usage of halo brace application.[5,7,11,16]

Corpectomy with Vertebral Graft

From 1992 to 1997, limited or keyhole corpectomy with vertebral graft using a Williams microsurgical saw (Ace Medical Co., Los Angeles) was carried out with reasonable results in 60 patients with cervical spondylosis with segmental OPLL.

One of the pitfalls of this method is that bone grafts taken from the cervical spine are often more fragile than iliac grafts, especially in heavy smokers and elderly women with osteoporosis.[17-19]

Microdiscectomy without Grafting

Microdiscectomy for central and paramedian discs and spurs without grafting has been done with reasonable results, but the small opening is often not adequate to decompress lateral spurs or OPLL.[20-22] Ventral transuncal foraminotomy was also added to lateral or foraminal discs and spurs with satisfactory results.[23,24]

Threaded Cylindrical Interbody Cage Fixation

Threaded cylindrical titanium cages were first introduced for posterior lumbar interbody fusion (PLIF) of lumbar spine instability in the early 1990s.[25] In 1997, the cylindrical Bagby and Kuslich cervical interbody cage (BAK/C; Spine-Tech, Minneapolis, MN) became available in Japan for ventral cervical fusion.[26] However, these instruments were made for macrosurgery and were too large and difficult to use under the operating microscope. Therefore, we developed smaller and more slender instruments, so that the entire procedure of decompression and cage fixation could be done under microsurgical control as a less invasive procedure (M-cage, Ammtec Inc., Tokyo).[2,3,27]

Modified Keyhole Microsurgical Approach

By using the advantages of keyhole discectomy and limited corpectomy and at the same time avoiding the pitfalls of the aforementioned procedures, a modified keyhole microsurgical technique with interbody cage fixation for cervical spondylosis and OPLL was developed.[3,28]

In this chapter, the surgical indications and techniques for both the twin-cage method and single-cage method are presented, as well as a combined method.

Surgical Technique

Under general endotracheal anesthesia, the patient is placed supine with the head slightly extended. The ventral cervical procedure is approached almost always from the right side of the neck, because the right-sided approach is much more comfortable for right-handed surgeons than the left-sided approach. The skin incision is made transversely along the crease for cosmetic reasons even in a two- or three-level approach. The subcutaneous tissue is dissected rostrally and caudally, and the platysma muscle is sectioned obliquely along the ventral border of the sternocleidomastoid muscle.

The ventral aspect of the cervical spine is then approached by dissecting the deeper fascia, usually rostral to the omohyoid muscle, while the right carotid tubercle of C6 is palpated as a landmark with the surgeon's left index finger. The level of the intervertebral disc space is identified with fluoroscopy with a needle inserted into the disc space at one or two levels, and a small amount of dye, usually indigo carmine, is injected through the needle for further confirmation of level location. The blue coloring of the disc is quite useful in contrasting the bony spur with the disc when drilling the spur. After the introduction of the operating microscope, which enables the surgeon and an assistant to see the operative field at almost the same depth, retractors are placed and the discectomy and osteophytectomy are carried out.

Twin-Cage Method for Cervical Spondylosis and Herniated Disc

In cases of cervical spondylosis and herniated discs, with or without instability, two smaller M-cages of 6, 7, or 8 mm in inner diameter are used side by side in a twin-cage fashion after decompression (Fig. 41-1).

First, after complete discectomy, the ventral spur of the upper vertebra is removed with a Kerrison rongeur; while the disc space is opened using a spreader, the dorsal spur is carefully drilled out using a high-speed drill with a 4- to 5-mm diamond bur and the posterior longitudinal ligament (PLL) is incised with a microknife to expose the decompressed and bulging dura. The fragments of the herniated disc, which are often located between the two layers of the PLL but sometimes are found in the epidural space, are completely removed. It is important to drill out the dorsal spur far laterally enough to decompress the medial portion of the foramen containing the nerve root, especially when the far lateral disc or foraminal stenosis is responsible for the radiculopathy.

Originally the disc space was opened with a reamer for cage insertion[3]; however, this reaming was soon abandoned to avoid subsidence of the cages into the vertebrae. Now, by using the spreader efficiently and by drilling the medial portion of the uncinate process after fine adjustment, cylindrical cages, most frequently 7-mm cages, are snugly inserted side by side in a locking fashion. Cages are usually packed with small bone chips of the vertebrae and hydroxyapatite granules (Apaceram, Hoya Corp., Tokyo). The ventral surface of the cages is leveled to the ventral cortex of the vertebral body to avoid subsidence of the cages.

Single-Cage Method for Ossification of the Posterior Longitudinal Ligament

In cases of OPLL, usually of the local or segmental type, some degree of corpectomy is often necessary to remove the ossified ligament that extends behind the vertebrae (Fig. 41-2). For this reason, a larger M-cage of 10, 12, or 14 mm in inner diameter (most frequently 12 mm) is usually used in the single-cage method. After complete discectomy, a Williams microsurgical saw or an ultrasonic bone scalpel (Sonopet, Stryker, Kalamazoo, MI) is used to perform an 8- to 9-mm square corpectomy followed by 10-mm reaming to make a round hole; usually a 12-mm cage packed with bone chips and hydroxyapatite granules is snugly inserted after decompression.[3,29]

If a Williams saw or Sonopet is not available, a round hole can be made stepwise by using progressively larger reamers. Through this keyhole, the remaining vertebra, spur, and ossified ligament are drilled out with great care, making the OPLL paper-thin by using a high-speed drill with a diamond bur and an ultrasonic bone curette (Sonopet, Stryker). The thinned-out OPLL and hypertrophied ligament, as well as associated disc fragments, are then carefully separated from

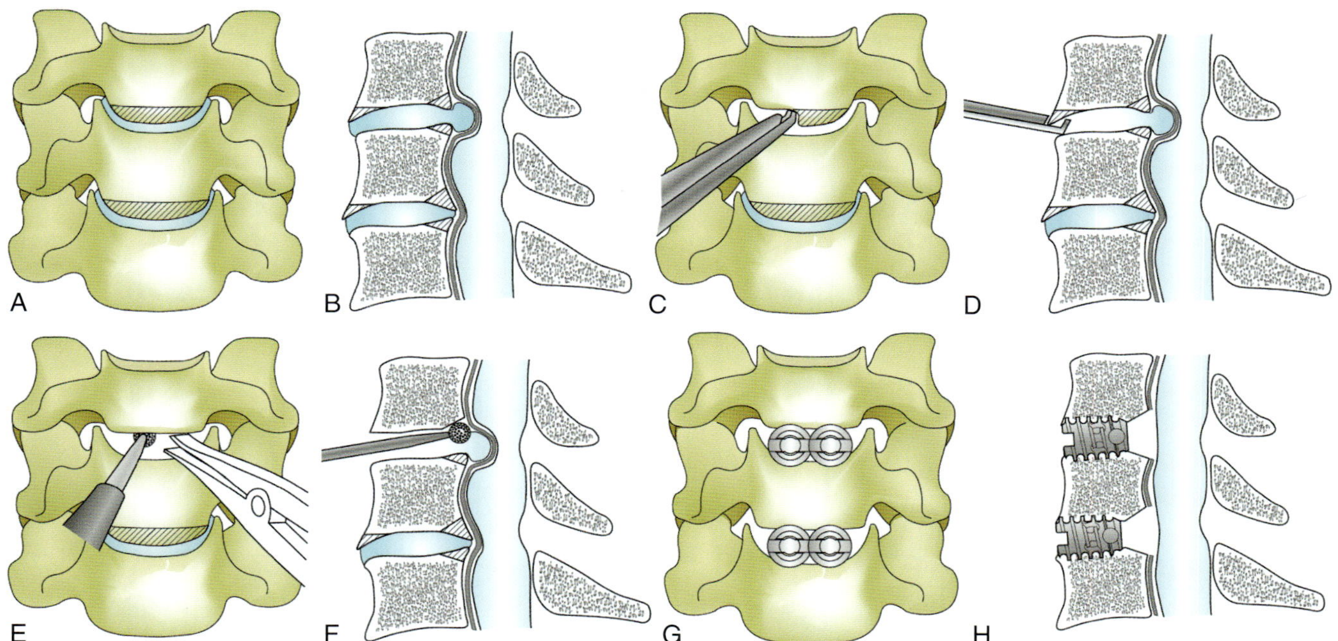

FIGURE 41-1. Twin-cage method of treating cervical spondylosis and herniated discs. **A** and **B,** Cervical spondylosis and disc protrusion with cord compression. *Striped areas* in the vertebrae indicate portions to be removed. **C** and **D,** Anterior spurs are removed with a Kerrison rongeur. **E** and **F,** Dorsal spurs are eliminated with a high-speed drill and protruded discs removed. **G** and **H,** Cages are inserted into the disc spaces in the twin-cage and locking fashion after decompression.

the dura and excised by using a microdissector, microknife, curettes, and Kerrison rongeurs.

Most of the ossified ligament behind the vertebrae can be removed through this keyhole and through the adjacent disc space above or below the keyhole (see Fig. 41-2). After good hemostasis a cage is inserted with its ventral surface leveled to the ventral cortex of the vertebrae to minimize subsidence. For the past decade, dural ossification has not been removed; instead, it is left alone after good decompression of the dura to avoid leakage of cerebrospinal fluid (CSF). Dural ossification is found in 15.3% of all cases of OPLL, in 10.5% of segmental types, and in 41% of nonsegmental types.[30]

Surgical Cases

Between August 1997 and December 2007, a series of 449 cases was operated on with cervical interbody cage fixation. There were 312 (69.5%) males and 137 females, with the average age being 57.2 years. The main symptom was myelopathy in 81% and radiculopathy in 19%. Among these 449 cases, 314 (69.9%) had cervical spondylosis and herniated discs; 135 (30.4%) had OPLL. Seven cases received a second cage fixation at an adjacent level within these years.

In 319 operations of cases with cervical spondylosis and herniated discs, one-level cage fixation was done in 186 (58.3%), two-level in 126 (39.5%), and three-level in 7 (2.2%); in 137 operations of cases with OPLL, one-level cage fixation was performed in 36 (26.3%), two-level in 89 (64.9%), and three-level in 12 (8.8%).

Surgical results were satisfactory (excellent and good) in 88% judging by Odom's criteria and the Neurosurgical Cervical Spine Scale (NCSS)[31]; 56% returned to their previous work and 32% to lighter work. No significant difference in surgical results was observed between patients with cervical spondylosis and those with OPLL. The group aged 70 years and older had less favorable results but showed significant neurologic improvement—as much as 72%. The younger group showed satisfactory results in 91%. The most influential factor for poor prognosis was the severity of preoperative neurologic status. Cases with severe myelopathy disclosed satisfactory results in only 65%, and cases with mild to moderate myelopathy disclosed satisfactory results in 93%.[27,28]

Major complications in cervical cage fixation are relatively rare. CSF leakage resulting from dural tear or defect occurred in several cases with prominent OPLL but was well managed with local repair and lumbar drainage when necessary. By not removing dural ossification, the frequency of CSF leakage was reduced significantly. Subsidence is a problem in ventral cervical fusion with any kind of graft or cage, particularly in heavy smokers and elderly patients with osteoporosis, but it has not been the major problem after reaming of the disc space was abandoned to minimize subsidence of the cages, especially in use of the twin-cage method in cervical spondylosis and disc herniation. Two elderly female patients with two-level cage fixation developed kyphotic deformity with compression fracture of the vertebra after a fall, causing deterioration of myelopathy; both were successfully treated by performing multilevel corpectomy with an elongated cage and plate fixation, one with and the other without additional posterior fixation.

Postoperative wound hematoma and infection were present in less than 1% of patients. Postoperative temporary dysphagia was seen in 2%. No neurologic deterioration was seen, except for one patient with temporary root sign and another with temporary worsening of a long tract sign.

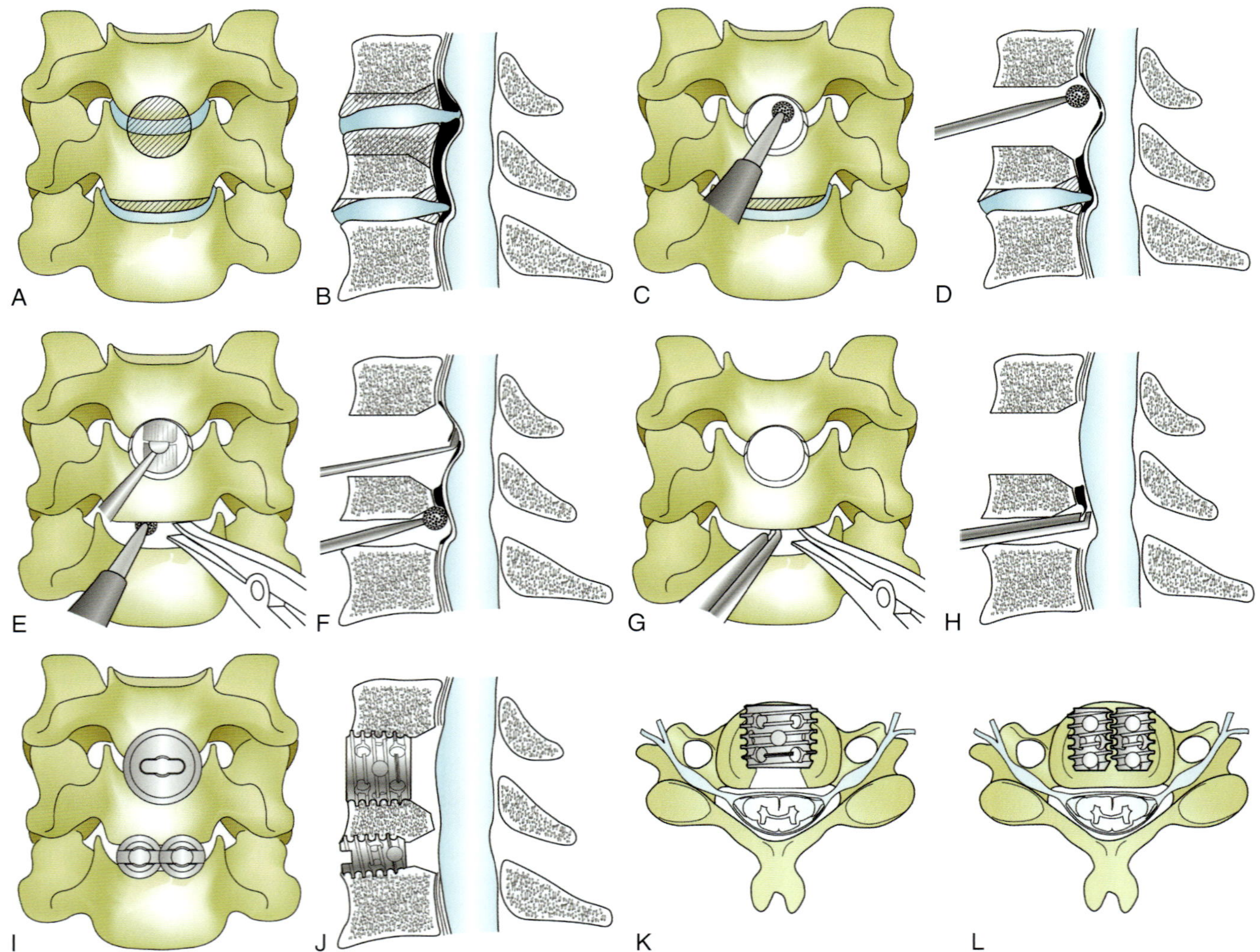

FIGURE 41-2. Single-cage and combined methods in cervical ossification of the posterior longitudinal ligament (OPLL). **A** and **B,** OPLL of segmental type with cord compression. *Striped areas* in the vertebrae indicate portions to be removed. **C** and **D,** Drilling of OPLL through a keyhole with a high-speed drill. **E** and **F,** Separation of paper-thin OPLL from the dura and excision for decompression and drilling of OPLL through the adjacent disc space. **G** and **H,** Removal of residual OPLL behind the vertebra through the keyhole and disc space for decompression. **I–L,** Solid cage fixation in the single-cage and twin-cage methods.

Fusion in cervical cage fixation has been evaluated by dynamic radiographs in flexion and extension and multislice CT in sagittal and coronal reformation. Fusion rate in 1-year follow-ups was 90% and bony formation encasing the cages was easily observed. However, even in cases with some motion at operated sites, it did not affect surgical results.

Discussion

Since the ventral approach with interbody fusion for cervical discs was introduced by Cloward and Smith and Robinson in 1958, ventral discectomy with iliac bone graft, with or without the help of an operating microscope, has been the standard procedure with reasonably satisfactory results.[32-34]

However, postoperative kyphotic deformity, graft collapse, and donor site discomfort cannot be totally disregarded. To avoid these disadvantages, microdiscectomy without bone graft has been advocated by many authors with excellent results.[20-22] This method, however, is often not appropriate for spondylosis with prominent bilateral spurs and OPLL. Allografting is one solution to the problems of the autograft, but is reported to have a lower fusion rate compared with autograft. Therefore, ventral plate fixation seems to be necessary for allografting.[10] Because allografting is not available in some countries, including Japan, hydroxyapatite, coralline, and titanium threaded cages have been introduced as a substitute for autogenous grafts for cervical interbody fusion.[9,26,33,35] Threaded cylindrical cages, which were initially introduced for lumbar interbody fusion,[25] have been used for a cervical ventral approach for cervical spondylosis and local and segmental OPLL for the past decade.[3,26-28]

OPLL of the cervical spine, which was first reported in an autopsy study by Tsukimoto in 1960,[36] has been extensively studied for its pathophysiology and surgical management over the past 30 years, especially in Japan.[6,13,37-39] OPLL is often associated with cervical spondylosis and disc herniation and is one of the major causes of cervical compressive myelopathy in Japan, but it is also found in other countries to a lesser degree.[18] Therefore, it is absolutely vital to establish the precise diagnosis in patients with cervical myelopathy or radiculopathy by using routine radiographs, CT with sagittal reformation, and MRI to make the right and appropriate decision for surgical treatment.

If segmental or local type OPLL is present with cord compression at one or two levels (sometimes at three levels in cases with kyphotic spines), the ventral approach is often selected by surgeons with expertise in microsurgery.[12,28] In extensive OPLL of continuous or mixed type with multilevel cord compression over three to four levels, expansive laminoplasty (open-door or double-door) is commonly used because multilevel decompression is readily obtained and the procedure is less risky compared with the ventral approach.[13-15]

Since 1997, ventral interbody cage fixation with autologous vertebral graft and hydroxyapatite granules became our standard surgical technique for cervical spondylosis and OPLL of local and segmental types, because this method provides immediate stabilization with rare cage-related complications and no donor site problems in addition to sufficient space for microsurgical decompression. However, the surgeon's microsurgical technique must be further refined and adjusted to the relatively smaller keyhole corpectomy, compared with wide corpectomy, to perform safe decompression.

The twin-cage method is more commonly used than the two-levels method to treat single-level cervical spondylosis and herniated discs. In cases associated with OPLL, keyhole corpectomy with the single-cage method with a larger cage is the procedure of choice to access OPLL behind the vertebral body, but more frequently the combined approach, in which the single-cage and twin-cage methods are performed at adjacent levels, is carried out in two-level operations (65%). The three-level cage fixation is relatively rare in cervical spondylosis (2.2%) but is sometimes indicated in cervical OPLL (8.9%). Surgical results are generally satisfactory with rare complications and early ambulation, short hospital stays, and early return to work. Biomechanical testing of cervical interbody cages has indicated better stability with the twin-cage method compared with the single-cage method, and no significant difference in design variations between the cages.[40,41] Good bony fusion was observed in 90% at 1-year follow-up.

Conclusion

Threaded cylindrical interbody cage fixation after microsurgical decompression is a safe, effective, and less invasive method for a ventral approach to treat cervical spondylosis, herniated discs, and OPLL with few complications. The single-cage and combined methods are commonly used for OPLL; the twin-cage method is normally used for cervical spondylosis and herniated discs. The surgical method is tailored to the pathology of each level after precise diagnosis from preoperative neuroimaging. This procedure facilitates early ambulation, short hospital stays, and early return to work.

Acknowledgement. The authors wish to thank Mr. Shunji Ono for preparing the figures and Ms. Emiko Nagase for her editorial assistance.

KEY REFERENCES

Epstein N: The surgical management of ossification of the posterior longitudinal ligament in 51 patients. *J Spinal Disord* 6:432–455, 1993.

Matge G: Anterior interbody fusion with the BAK-Cage in cervical spondylosis. *Acta Neurochir (Wien)* 140:1–8, 1998.

Mizuno J, Nakagawa H: Outcome analysis of anterior decompressive surgery and fusion for cervical ossification of the posterior longitudinal ligament: report of 107 cases and review of the literature. *Neurosurg Focus* 10:E6, 2001.

Mizuno J, Nakagawa H: Ossified posterior longitudinal ligament: management strategies and outcomes. *Spine J* 6:282s–288s, 2006.

Nakagawa H, Mizuno J: Threaded interbody cage fixation for cervical spondylosis and ossification of the posterior longitudinal ligament. In Benzel EC, editor: *Spine*, ed 2, Philadelphia, 2005, Elsevier Churchill Livingstone, pp 363–369.

Nagata K, Sato K: Diagnostic imaging of cervical ossification of the posterior longitudinal ligament. In Yonenobu K, Nakamura K, Toyama Y, editors: *OPLL ossification of the posterior longitudinal ligament*, ed 2, Tokyo, 2006, Springer, pp 127–143.

REFERENCES

The complete reference list is available online at expertconsult.com.

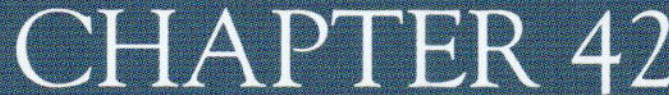

CHAPTER 42

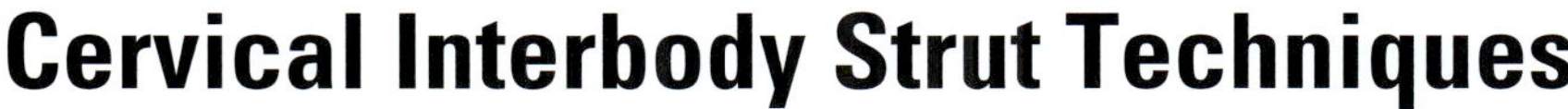

Cervical Interbody Strut Techniques

John O'Toole | Sanford E. Emery | Vincent C. Traynelis

Since the 1980s, extensive ventral decompression via corpectomy for cervical spondylotic myelopathy and spinal deformity has become routine.[1] Although neurologic outcomes remain similar between multilevel anterior discectomy and corpectomy,[2-5] certain clinical scenarios favor corpectomy (e.g., ossification of the posterior longitudinal ligament, trauma, osteomyelitis, neoplasms). Moreover, fusion rates after anterior decompression procedures across more than two disc levels may be higher for corpectomy than discectomy, particularly in uninstrumented cases.[4,6,7] Therefore, spine surgeons must be comfortable with anterior decompression by corpectomy and also with the subsequent intervertebral strut grafting, the focus of this chapter.

Technologic advances now permit a wide variety of materials to be used as interbody devices; these newer products are covered elsewhere in this textbook (see Chapters 41 and 43). Furthermore, in the majority of clinical situations today, anterior corpectomy strut grafting is supplemented with anterior spinal plate instrumentation to reduce graft migration and enhance fusion rates.[4,6-8] However, certain scenarios, for either clinical or logistical reasons, may dictate uninstrumented strut grafting. The techniques of interlocking bone grafting discussed in this chapter are most germane to the latter category of corpectomy cases. Even in instrumented strut grafts, however, some of the principles delineated here remain important for successful integration of the bone graft.

Fundamentals of Grafting

Three fundamental concepts need to be recognized for successful strut grafting. First is a clear understanding of the surgical objectives of the procedure in general. The primary goal for cervical spondylotic myelopathy typically is adequate and durable decompression of the neural elements. Although this generally would seem obvious, concerns over reconstruction can alter the operative plan and possibly subvert the primary goals of the surgery (Fig. 42-1). Ideally, the reconstruction must be fit to the decompression, and not vice versa.

The second essential component of strut grafting is an understanding of the factors affecting spinal stability (Box 42-1).[9] An uninstrumented, unstable spine requires prolonged external bracing (e.g., halo brace or Minerva jacket). This is relatively independent of the surgical fusion technique. The stable spine reconstructed with a short-segment strut graft may be managed with a rigid cervical orthosis.

The third fundamental concept of strut grafting is knowledge of the material characteristics of the intervertebral graft. Appropriate choices for bone are somewhat limited, and in practice surgeons have only iliac crest and fibula, either as allograft or autograft, as options. Autograft calvarium has been used for struts, but it is not surprising that this source has not been embraced widely.

Bone Graft

Both the origin of the graft material and its proper handling are important considerations in bone graft selection. Autogenous iliac crest tends to fuse rapidly, which is a distinct advantage. Its incorporation, however, can be compromised by suboptimal harvesting techniques (see Chapter 123), osteoporosis, and injudicious tailoring. Technical constraints typically limit its use to replacing two or three vertebral segments. In fashioning iliac crest to the bony defect, it is ideal to preserve at least two contiguous cortical surfaces from one end of the graft to the other to optimize axial loading strength. Surgeons must also keep in mind the real complications associated with iliac crest harvest, which fortunately only rarely result in long-term problems.

With a fibular implant, however, there are different characteristics to consider: (1) it is a strong, circumferential cortical strut with a higher modulus of elasticity than mixed cortical–cancellous implants, and as such must be used with caution in the osteoporotic spine; (2) it can be tailored to any needed length; and (3) it provides a central channel for the packing of autograft cancellous bone to enhance fusion. The disadvantage of fibula is the mismatch of the density with that of the vertebral body. As a general rule, the receiving vertebra will fail before the fibula graft does. This generally results in "pistoning," in which the fibula penetrates through the vertebral body and can even enter the next motion segment. Some subsidence may be unavoidable, especially in osteoporosis, but is usually of no significant clinical consequence (Fig. 42-2). Subsidence may theoretically be limited by using minimal distraction during graft placement and by using an orthotic brace postoperatively to limit flexion. Too much graft loading and excessive neck flexion early in recovery predispose to graft pistoning. Minimal disruption of the

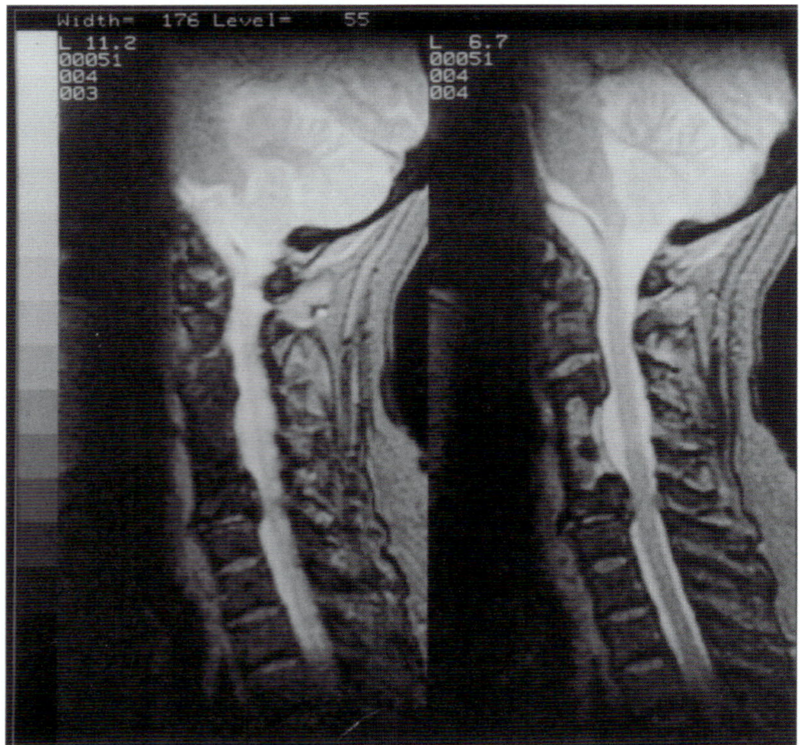

FIGURE 42-1. Postoperative MRI scan of a two-level decompression. Note the persisting spinal canal stenosis at the subjacent level.

vertebral body graft bed site is also important in maintaining the final height of the fusion. A fibula grafted to a partial corpectomy will almost invariably result in substantial subsidence and loss of height. If necessary, an additional vertebral level may need to be resected to preserve the resistance to subsidence at the graft site.

Allograft fibula is slower to incorporate than autologous iliac crest.[8] Autograft fibula is less commonly used owing to the increased operative times and blood loss and significant complications associated with its harvest.[10] One method to enhance fusion but attenuate graft harvest morbidity is to use allograft fibula packed with autograft cancellous bone, taken from the iliac crest or from the resected corpectomy bone itself.[11] Autogenous cancellous bone may be accessed via the superficial surface of the iliac crest through a 3-cm skin incision. The medial and outer surfaces of the iliac crest are not disturbed, as would be needed for the harvest of tricortical grafts. This ideally reduces blood loss and postoperative pain. A 1-cm cortical defect is created in the iliac crest with

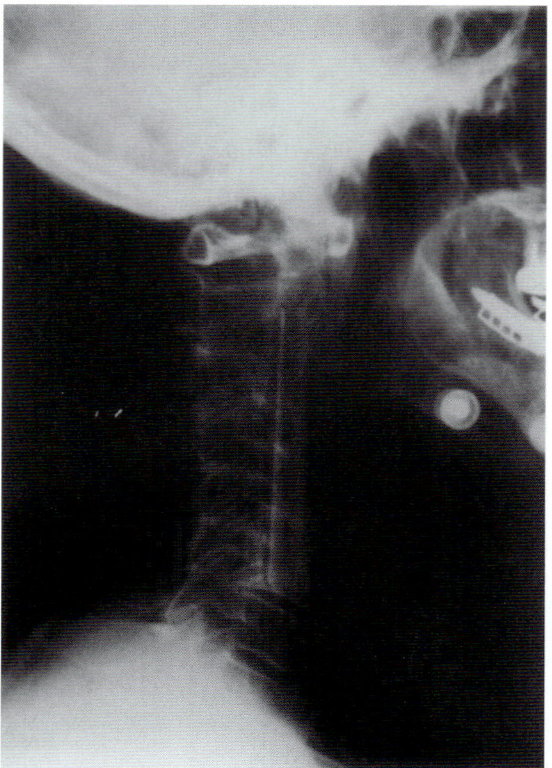

FIGURE 42-2. Lateral radiograph taken 3 years postoperatively after corpectomy and fibula strut grafting. Note the subsidence into both the rostral and caudal mortise (i.e., "pistoning"). No symptoms were present and no further treatment was needed.

BOX 42-1. Factors Influencing Stability

- Ventral element integrity
- Dorsal element integrity
- Dynamic radiographic elements
- Sagittal plane translation >3.5 mm
- Sagittal plane rotation >20 degrees

From White AA, Panjabi MM: *Clinical biomechanics of the spine*, ed 2, Philadelphia, 1990, Lippincott-Raven, p 314.

a high-speed bur, and cancellous bone is taken with a large curette. This, in turn, is packed into the central canal of the allograft fibula with a 3-mm diameter rod. No bone need be placed around the outside of the fibula strut after insertion.

Despite the differences between iliac crest structural autograft and fibular allograft, a significant difference in pseudarthrosis rates has not been consistently demonstrated.[2,5,12,13]

Strut Graft

Preparation of Vertebral Defect for Strut Grafting

The paramount concern in preparing the vertebral end plates for arthrodesis is the prevention of graft displacement. Although plates and screws prevent graft displacement and improve graft incorporation, even instrumented grafts in rare cases can retropulse toward the spinal cord. The bed for the graft must be prepared in such a manner that the avenue toward the spinal canal is shorter or narrower than the graft itself. If graft migration were to occur, the direction should be away from the spinal cord. When anterior plating is used, deep slots or mortises in the vertebral body are limited by the need for adequate remaining vertebral body volume for screw purchase. When hardware insertion is not anticipated, spinal canal protection may be attained by one of four strategies (Figs. 42-3A–C): (1) the keystone mortise and tenon, (2) the dovetail technique, (3) the lateral step method, or (4) the anterior peg method of Niu et al.[11] The primary focus here is on the keystone method.

Keystone Technique

The keystone graft method places the graft close to the middle column of the vertebral body. It is secured by means of mortises or slots in the opposing vertebral end plates (see Fig. 42-3A).

Proper preparation of the mortises in the keystone technique requires consideration of the angling of the cervical disc space (Fig. 42-3D). This disc space angling is the consequence of the ventral vertebral surface being slightly more caudal than the dorsal vertebral surface. The caudal mortise can be fashioned into the face of the vertebral end plate without removal of the anterior cortical corner of the vertebra. Thus, the sloping of this end plate away from the spinal canal provides the opportunity for creating the ideal mortise. The dorsal mortise lip is longer than its ventral counterpart. This ensures that any potential displacement of the graft occurs across the shallower ventral mortise lip. Because the caudal vertebral mortise can be readily fashioned with preservation of the cortical vertebral margins, this is the strongest mortise construct (see Fig. 42-3D).

Creation of the rostral mortise is more complex. Again, the critical consideration is the disc space angle. At the caudal end plate of the rostral mortise, the angle is such that to ensure a shorter ventral mortise lip, a portion of the anterior vertebral body must be resected. To avoid undue anterior

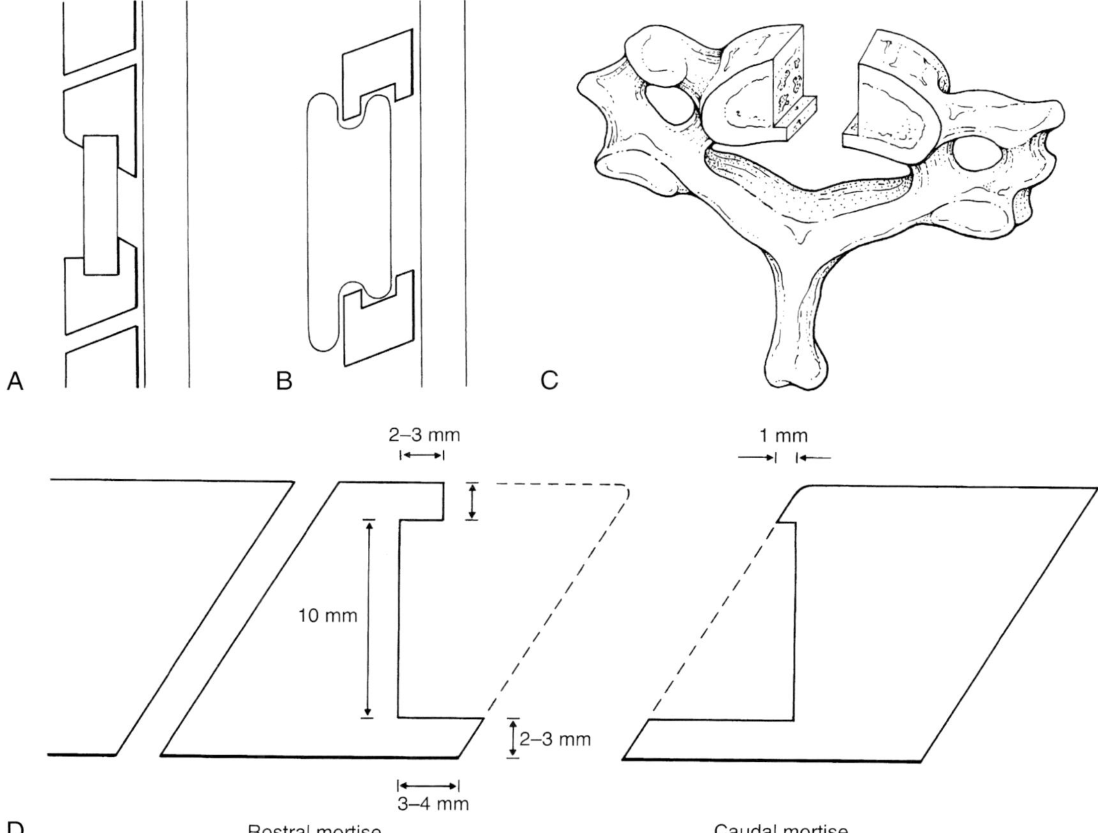

FIGURE 42-3. Schematics of keystone (**A**), dovetail (**B**), and Voorhies lateral bone step (**C**) techniques, and the measurement details of keystone mortises (**D**).

resection while ensuring adequacy of the posterior mortise lip, appreciable resection of the dorsal vertebral margin in the decompression is precluded. Should any dorsal vertebral body decompression be pursued, the remaining vertebral body may be inadequate for proper mortising (see Fig. 42-3D).

Dovetail Technique

The dovetail grafting method refers to fashioning a segment of the graft that is placed ventral to the anterior vertebral surfaces and is longer than the length of the decompression defect. *Dovetail* refers to the bipartite shape of both ends of the graft, one slightly longer than the other. This is not unlike the tail of a dove (see Fig. 42-3B). The shorter of the two "tail feathers" at both ends is placed into matching slots drilled into the opposing end plates of the cephalic and caudal vertebrae. The rostral slot is of a depth such that the respective dovetail can be inserted to a depth that allows the clearance of the distal "tail" into its respective slot with moderate cervical traction. The graft, thus in place, is then shifted distally for a final locking-in position. The advantage of this construct is that it can be prepared in such a way that it is unequivocally too large to be displaced into the spinal canal. The disadvantages are that it can place excessive vertical loads on the ventral vertebral body cortex and may not allow significant impaction of the cancellous components of the graft and vertebra. In theory the graft is located within the anterior column. Therefore, vertebral failure may not be via impaction but via anterior displacement. Obviously, this construct does not lend itself to plating. Finally, the dovetail graft may lead to some increase in postoperative dysphagia given its position anterior to the anterior vertebral body walls.

Lateral Bone Step Technique

As described by Awasthi and Voorhies,[1] lateral bone steps can be fashioned on either side of the anterior spinal canal, after completion of decompression by widening of the trough superficially (see Fig. 42-3C). The graft is then tailored so that it is wider than the width of the decompression and is placed superficial to the lateral steps. Potential disadvantages of this technique include possible inadequate canal decompression to maintain the posterior vertebral body wall steps and possible trapping of epidural bleeding behind the steps and graft with subsequent epidural hematoma (a fortunately rare complication[14]).

Preparation of the Strut Graft

The keystone graft (see Fig. 42-3A) is tailored for intimate lateral surface contact with the sides of the decompression trough. This fit should not require more than firm pressure for positioning. Forcefully hammering a slightly wide graft past a tight lateral contact point risks subsequent displacement by a lateral levering mechanism, which may occur with minimal neck movement. Width tailoring is usually accomplished with a high-speed bur or oscillating saw. A rongeur may cause cortical microfractures, which may lead to subsequent postoperative midshaft graft fracture. The width is repeatedly checked by placing both ends of the graft into the vertebral trough until a fit that allows no lateral play is achieved. By a similar tailoring sequence, the rostral tip of the graft is fashioned to fit its mortise exactly. Because the ventral mortise lip is foreshortened deliberately, the strut can be angled into the mortise, and the fit can be assessed before the final determination of the strut length. After the exact graft width and rostral fit have been determined, the length is ascertained by marking the caudal aspect of the graft with the graft fully positioned rostrally while manual cervical traction is applied. Traction will usually provide at least 1 mm of trough distraction. This, in turn, results in the graft marked 1 mm longer than the defect. The caudal mortise graft fit is then tailored similar to the rostral end. The graft can then be put into place, rostral end first, using firm pressure or very light tapping with a small mallet. It is important to advance the caudal portion of the graft into the trough until it contacts the posterior mortise and lies deep to the anterior mortise lip. Caution should be used to avoid overdistracting the spine, resulting in "too tight" a fit, because this may predispose it to increased axial loading and fracture of the caudal vertebrae.

Once in place, the graft can be stressed, if desired, with a flexion and then an extension movement of the neck by the anesthesiologist. This nestles the graft into the mortises and determines whether levering will cause displacement. It is done under direct vision after removal of the soft tissue retractors.

Similarly, the dovetail graft (see Fig. 42-3B) is fastidiously tailored. However, as already noted, the strategy of locking the graft by caudal engagement requires a greater vertebral slot or mortise depth. Because tailoring of the anterior mortise lips, as in the keystone method, is not necessary with the dovetail technique, the anterior vertebral cortical edges should ensure the utmost vertebral resistance to fracture. A cortical surface of the iliac crest graft should be placed toward the depth of the decompression to ensure a strong graft construct. The positioning of the cortical margin of the bone graft within the confines of the vertebral body (i.e., dorsal to the ventral vertebral body margins) helps minimize the chance of ventral bone graft migration. Because the fibula has a tendency to cut or penetrate into its receiving vertebral bodies, it should be used sparingly for this purpose.

Complications of Strut Grafting

Strut grafts across the cervicothoracic junction are subjected to unique forces due to the long lever arm of the thoracic cage.[15] The potential for fracture (either of the vertebra, strut, or both) with the use of a multisegment intervertebral graft may be significant and merits consideration of anterior plating with or without supplemental posterior instrumentation.

In general, correction of kyphotic deformity is ideal in anterior reconstructions, in particular to prevent the spinal cord from draping over the ventral apex of a kyphotic spine.[16] Nevertheless, forceful correction of such a deformity often loads anterior strut grafts substantially, subsequently risking graft complications. In these situations, segmental posterior instrumentation should be strongly considered.

Complications of anterior cervical approaches in general are discussed elsewhere in this volume (see Chapters 35 and 40). Fortunately, hematoma and infection of the anterior neck are uncommon, but there are no specific management schemes unique to strut grafting for preventing these complications. The use of a suction drain for 24 hours may lessen their incidence. Persistent severe neck pain early in the course of recovery should raise concern for infection. Infection, especially after the first postoperative week, should prompt suspicion of esophageal leakage. Infection alone may not require graft or hardware removal, but typically incision and drainage are necessary.

Specific types of graft complications include displacement, midgraft fracture, mortise fracture, pistoning, and angulation.

Graft Displacement

Displacements and displaced graft fractures almost always occur early after surgery and are usually best handled by repeat surgery. The incidence of graft migration increases with the number of levels involved and the proximity to the cervicothoracic junction.[15] Displacement alone often reflects a technical error and is often accompanied by an associated vertebral fracture (Fig. 42-4). Vertebral fractures are usually caudal and, unless minor, will require extending the fusion across the next motion segment. This does not require further decompression but does require a new strut and the creation of a bed across the fractured vertebra. In such a situation, many surgeons will opt for anterior plating, prolonged bracing, or circumferential fixation after graft revision.

Graft Pistoning

As mentioned above, subsidence, or pistoning, is frequently seen to at least a minor extent, particularly when fibula is used (see Fig. 42-2).[17] It is important to avoid circumferential sharpening of the fibula strut ends. This may in part be averted by not overdistracting at the time of graft insertion. The degree of penetration may appear alarming on a radiograph. An average of 6 to 7 mm of settling of the fibula strut graft is typical after two- or three-level corpectomy; this has been reported to have no impact on postoperative pain, neurologic outcomes, or fusion rates.[16,17] When the graft penetrates into the adjacent disc space (frequently the caudal disc space), the options are to observe clinically ot to revise the graft. Anecdotally, both approaches may result in good outcomes.

Graft Angulation

Graft angulation, usually at the rostral mortise, occurs infrequently. The incidence of this complication is not necessarily proportional to strut graft length (Fig. 42-5). Clearly, plating should minimize the incidence of this problem. The revision of an angulated graft is not typically necessary. Extensive bracing with a halo vest or Minerva jacket may be the most appropriate first line of treatment.

Pseudarthrosis

Late complications of strut grafts include pseudarthrosis (Fig. 42-6) and midshaft graft fracture[18,19] (Fig. 42-7). If these are associated with compressive osteophyte formation or persistent neck pain, a posterior instrumented arthrodesis is a viable revision option. Ventral revision of a pseudarthrosis is also feasible. However, a simultaneous posterior fusion and stabilization procedure may be prudent if stability has been significantly threatened. Anterior revision of a midgraft fracture requires a new strut graft and plating. Late graft fractures may heal with the passage of time alone (see Fig. 42-7).

The clinical significance of pseudarthrosis after strut grafting is as uncertain as it is after an anterior cervical dissection and fusion. The incidence of this complication in uninstrumented cases has been reported as less than 5% (typically single-level

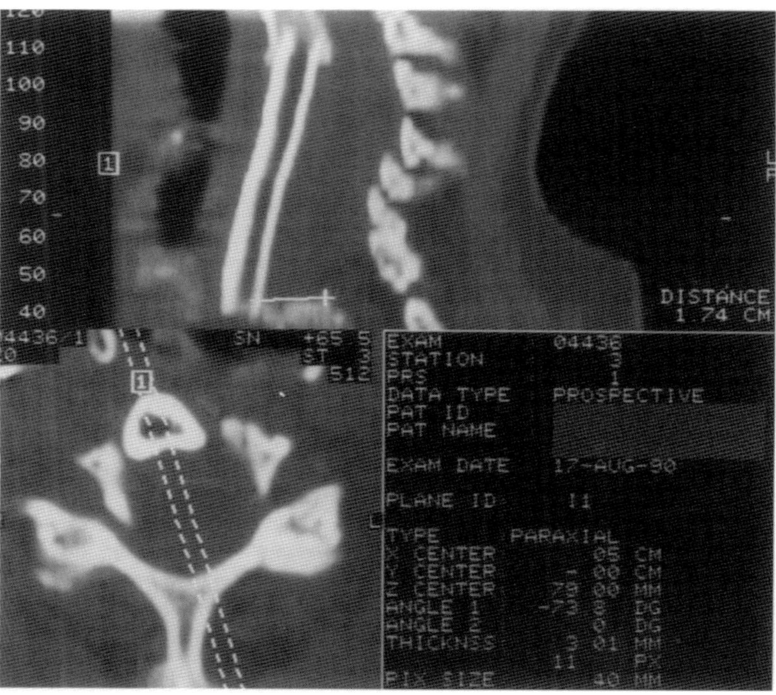

FIGURE 42-4. CT scan of a displaced fibula graft associated with a ventral fracture of the caudal vertebral body.

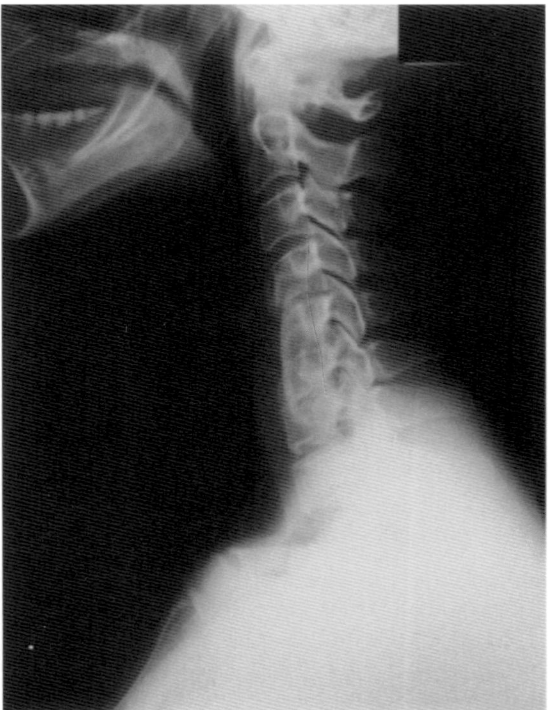

FIGURE 42-5. Lateral radiograph of a graft associated with kyphosis, without clinical consequence. We have observed angulations as great as 20 degrees that have been effectively managed without revision.

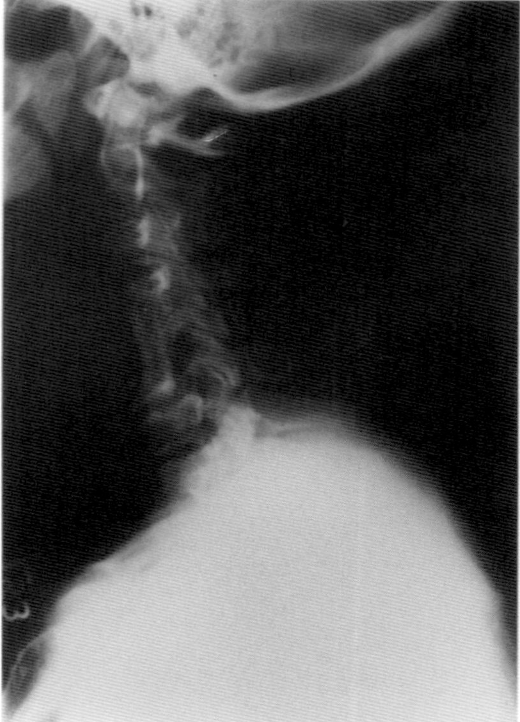

FIGURE 42-6. Lateral radiograph showing hypertrophic changes and lucency at the caudal graft–vertebral body interface. This is consistent with pseudarthrosis. The patient was asymptomatic. Dynamic films demonstrated no motion.

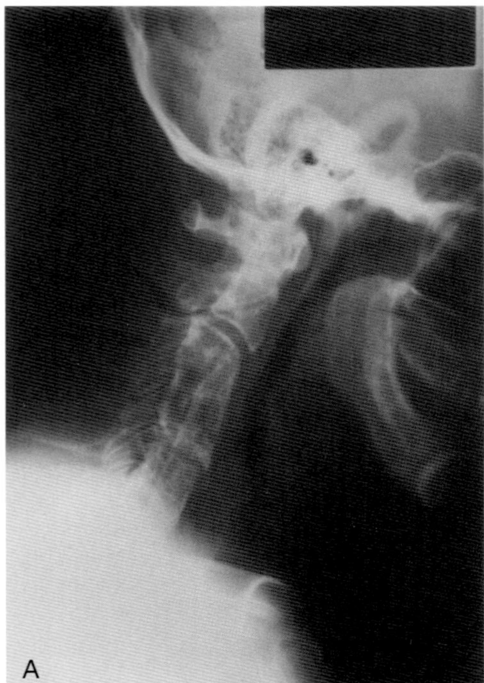

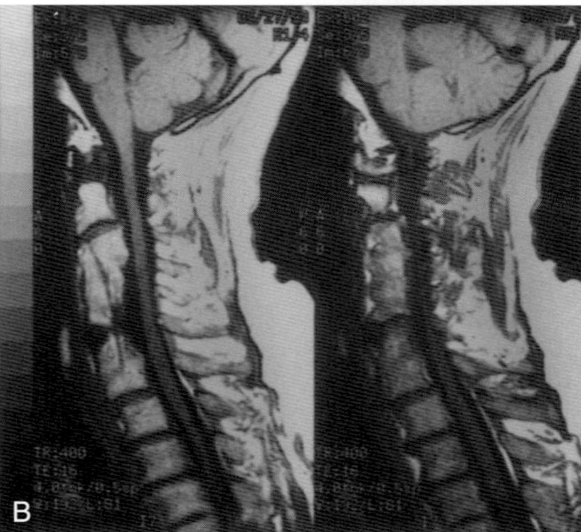

FIGURE 42-7. Lateral radiograph (**A**) and MRI scan (**B**) are consistent with an old, healed midgraft fracture. The patient had no neck symptoms.

cases with autograft) to as high as 30% (higher rates associated with multilevel corpectomies and possibly with allograft).[2,5,12,13] Instrumentation clearly improves fusion rates[4,6] and tends to eliminate differences between autograft and allograft.[8,20] Late recurrent myelopathy may occur in these patients due to a pseudarthrosis with hypertrophic changes or new adjacent-segment disease.[2]

Treatment options after radiographic pseudarthrosis are largely based on clinical symptomatology. If pseudarthrosis is associated with intolerable neck pain, the patient may be offered a posterior arthrodesis. When the etiology of persistent neck pain is unclear, a posterior exploration of segmental motion may be undertaken and instrumented arthrodesis employed if abnormal mobility is found. This latter strategy is plausible during the period of anterior graft immaturity in the first year postoperatively. Radiographic findings after this time on CT and flexion/extension x-rays are such that a determination of nonunion is somewhat more straightforward (Fig. 42-8). Patients with fibrous unions and late graft fractures can potentially be relieved of persistent neck pain by successful posterior fusion.

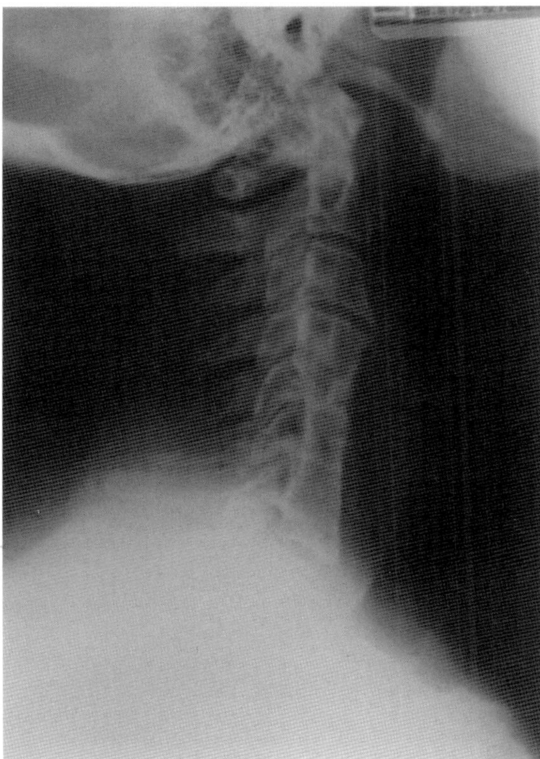

FIGURE 42-8. Lateral radiograph taken 5 years after strut grafting. Note continuity of cortical lines and complete absence of demarcation between vertebra and graft. Such a film excludes pseudarthrosis; dynamic films are unnecessary. This complete bony incorporation may require a year or more to achieve with autograft, and substantially longer with fibular allograft.

Summary

Strut grafting after ventral cervical decompression ordinarily requires fastidious graft fit. With careful technique, ventral fusion is successful and complements the original objective of neural decompression. If the uninstrumented graft cannot be displaced intraoperatively, it should remain in place, even with some minor subsidence over time. Any concern for spinal instability, inadequate graft fit, or undue forces placed on the graft at the time of the initial surgery, however, should prompt the use of instrumentation or prolonged external bracing.

KEY REFERENCES

Emery SE, Bohlman HH, Bolesta MJ, Jones PK: Anterior cervical decompression and arthrodesis for the treatment of cervical spondylotic myelopathy. Two- to 17-year follow-up. *J Bone Joint Surg [Am]* 80:941–951, 1998.

Hankinson TC, O'Toole JE, Kaiser MG: Multilevel ACDF vs. corpectomy for cervical kyphosis. In Mummaneni PV, Lenke LG, Haid RW, editors: *Spinal deformity: a guide to surgical planning and management*, St. Louis, 2008, Quality Medical.

Hughes SS, Pringle T, Phillips F, Emery S: Settling of fibula strut grafts following multilevel anterior cervical corpectomy: a radiographic evaluation. *Spine (Phila Pa 1976)* 31:1911–1915, 2006.

Ikenaga M, Shikata J, Tanaka C: Anterior corpectomy and fusion with fibular strut grafts for multilevel cervical myelopathy. *J Neurosurg Spine* 3:79–85, 2005.

Nirala AP, Husain M, Vatsal DK: A retrospective study of multiple interbody grafting and long segment strut grafting following multilevel anterior cervical decompression. *Br J Neurosurg* 18:227–232, 2004.

Saunders RL: Anterior reconstructive procedures in cervical spondylotic myelopathy. *Clin Neurosurg* 37:682–721, 1991.

Wang JC, Hart RA, Emery SE, Bohlman HH: Graft migration or displacement after multilevel cervical corpectomy and strut grafting. *Spine (Phila Pa 1976)* 28:1016–1021, 2006.

REFERENCES

The complete reference list is available online at expertconsult.com

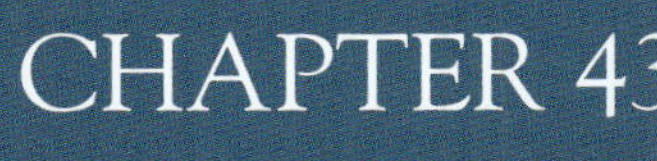

CHAPTER 43

Interbody Cages

Anthony A. Virella | Donald A. Smith | D. Mark Melton | David W. Cahill | Edward C. Benzel

Anterior cervical discectomy and cervical corpectomy for decompression of degenerative disease, trauma, tumor, and infection are commonly performed spinal operations. Options for reconstruction of the ventral column include structural autografts and allografts, as well as an evolving genre of prosthetic devices. The objectives of reconstruction are to restore a stable load-bearing ventral column, to maintain intervertebral height, and to establish an anatomic cervical lordosis when possible. The ultimate goal is for the construct to become biologically integrated into the native spine and to be replaced by living bone over time. For simple discectomy and single-level corpectomy, these end points are usually achievable with tricortical autografts harvested from the iliac crest or commercially available prefabricated cadaveric bone grafts. Complications such as graft collapse or extrusion are occasionally encountered. The primary objection to the use of structural autografts, however, is the relatively high rate of morbidity at the donor site from chronic pain, numbness, infection, hematoma, and cosmetic deformity. Such complications are reported to occur in 10% to 25% of cases.[1-4] A common observation among spine surgeons is that the morbidity associated with the bone graft harvest frequently exceeds the morbidity related to the primary procedure. Pain at the bone graft harvest site has traditionally been reported by patients to be worse than that at the primary surgical site. This high rate of donor site morbidity has spurred the search for alternative reconstructive possibilities. Cadaveric prefabricated allografts have gained popularity over the past several years because of concerns over this donor site morbidity. Recently, several authors have advocated use of donor site alternatives to iliac crest (e.g., manubrium)[5]; however, long-term follow-up after using such an alternative is lacking. Structural allografts eliminate donor site problems but are associated with a slightly increased risk of pseudarthrosis and graft resorption, especially in smokers and diabetics. Although highly processed, lingering patient concerns remain about potential risk for disease transmission from allografts.

Reconstruction of a multilevel corpectomy bed poses yet a greater challenge. In fact, in a recent study by Uribe et al., the rate of early hardware failure and pseudarthrosis was higher after cervical corpectomy than after anterior cervical discectomy, suggesting that in the absence of specific pathology requiring removal of a vertebral body, multilevel anterior cervical discectomy and fusion (ACDF) using interbody cages and autologous bone graft could result in lower morbidity.[6] Iliac crest and fibula are the best options available for autograft, but harvest of suitably long struts contributes significantly to patient morbidity. It can also be very difficult to match the graft to the cross-sectional and longitudinal geometry of the recipient site. These obstacles have prompted many surgeons to substitute fibular allograft as a simpler expedient. Fibular allografts are very straight and have a much smaller diameter than does material from the cervical corpus. These features enable it to fit readily into the recipient bed, but may not indicate optimal load transfer characteristics. Fibular allograft is composed almost exclusively of hard cortical bone. The mismatch in cross-sectional diameters and physical characteristics between the graft and recipient bone contributes to "pistoning" of the fibular strut through the adjacent central end plates, a condition commonly observed as the reconstructed segment foreshortens during graft incorporation, with resultant loss of lordosis.[7] An additional concern is the heightened risk of nonunion that accompanies long-segment allograft constructs.

Interbody Cages

A variety of prosthetic interbody cages are now available for use in the cervical spine, both for disc space arthrodesis and to bridge the larger voids created by single- or multilevel corpectomy. Current devices are fabricated, either from titanium alloy or polymer, and can be classified into four categories: (1) screw-in, (2) box-type, (3) interbody fusion cage with integrated ventral fixation, or (4) a cylindrical design.[8,9] Devices approved by the U.S. Food and Drug Administration (FDA) include hydroxyapatite spacer grafts, bioabsorbable implants, and artificial discs; they are now widely used and are not the primary focus of this chapter.

Interbody cages are intended to confer immediate structural integrity to the ventral spine and to provide instant support through the instantaneous axis of rotation. Although some surgeons have placed these as naked implants,[10] more typically, they are employed as carriers for osteoinductive or osteoconductive materials whose purpose is to secure long-term stability through biologic integration with the recipient spine. In our experience, interbody cages are usually loaded with morselized autograft obtained from the cervical spine itself or from cancellous harvest from the sternum or iliac crest with negligible added morbidity.

Alternatives such as allograft bone, hydroxyapatite, and "biologics," including recombinant human bone morphogenetic protein (rhBMP), may even obviate this need.

Devices designed for disc space arthrodesis come prefabricated in a variety of sizes for direct implantation. Cages used for vertebral body replacement are provided as stock material, which can be rapidly modified to match an individual patient's unique anatomic need. Many of these implants remain in development and have not been released by the FDA for clinical application in the United States at this time. The literature that bears on these devices includes animal-testing data,[11] biomechanical studies,[8,12,13] and clinical reports[2,10,14-29]; it is comparatively sparse and is devoid of any class 1 evidentiary material.

Screw-in Devices

The Bagby and Kuslich cervical cage (BAK/C, Sulzer Spine-Tech, Minneapolis, MN) is the prototypic example of a screw-in design. The BAK/C cage is fundamentally an adaptation of a spinal instrumentation system already validated for disc space arthrodesis in the lumbar spine. After successful completion of a prospective randomized multicenter trial, it received FDA approval for use in the cervical spine.[20] Similar to the larger lumbar devices, a BAK/C implant consists of a hollow, threaded cage with multiple side-wall fenestrations. The cages are manufactured from a titanium alloy and are provided in a 12-mm length, with a choice of 6-, 8-, 10-, and 12-mm diameters. Using a modification of the Cloward technique,[30] it is usually inserted as a single, midline cage after reaming and tapping of the adjacent central end plates (Fig. 43-1). Alternatively, two smaller (6- or 8-mm) cages may be applied in a side-by-side fashion, although this necessarily limits the height of disc space distraction that can be achieved

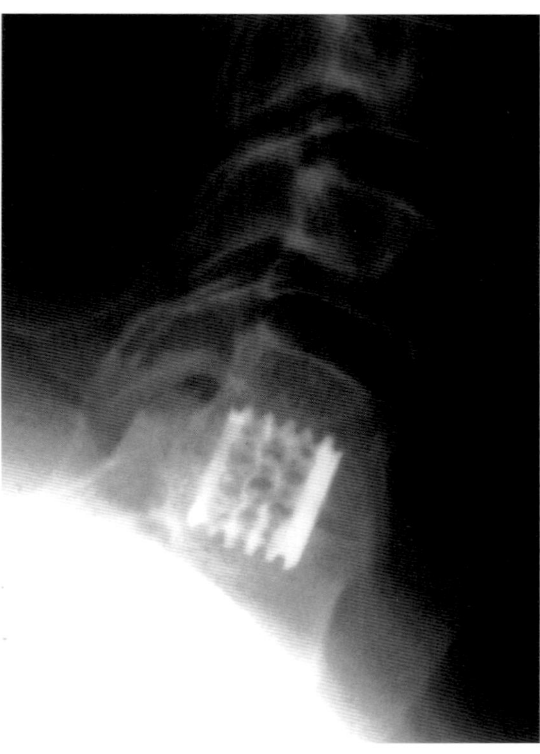

FIGURE 43-1. Bagby and Kuslich cervical cage.

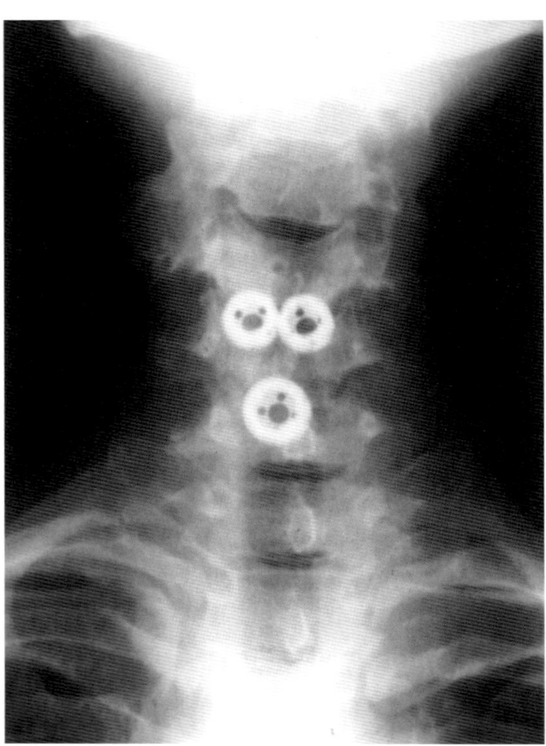

FIGURE 43-2. Side-by-side Bagby and Kuslich cervical cages with adjacent single-level cage.

(Fig. 43-2). The cages are loaded with locally derived bone shavings, sometimes supplemented with allograft, according to volumetric needs. Sofamor Danek (Memphis, TN) has recently released the Affinity cage in North America. This is similar in concept to the BAK/C, but has a conically tapered configuration whose purpose is to help establish cervical lordosis.

In the BAK/C study a single-level "fusion rate" of nearly 100% was reported. No device-related failures or complications occurred, and other measures of clinical outcome appeared comparable to the noninstrumented ACDF "control" patients.[20] Furthermore these outcomes were achieved without the morbidity associated with iliac crest bone graft harvest observed in the control group. However, certain concerns linger about the consequences of violating the central vertebral end plates, as is required for insertion of this device. Hacker observed a 20% incidence of postoperative "sagittal alignment abnormalities" at follow-up.[2] Lordotic reaming and tapping techniques and a tapered expansile cage (Varilift, Advanced Spine, Irvine, CA) have been developed in an effort to address this issue.

Because screw-in cages have a cylindrical cross section, the contact surface available for load transfer (and for fusion) is a comparatively narrow trough whose width is less than half of the cage diameter. This difference is mechanically disadvantageous in resisting lateral flexion, and the potential for subsidence of the implant with concomitant loss of cervical lordosis may be magnified if two or more adjacent segments are instrumented. Disc space restoration to an average height of 6 to 8 mm requires implantation of 8- to 10-mm diameter cages. When this is attempted at two or more adjacent levels, the resultant encroachment into the intervening body can be substantial and may necessitate offset placement of the devices and result in significant subsidence (Fig. 43-3). When Wang et al.[31] studied 64 patients who underwent ventral decompression and interbody fusion with BAK/C, they found that the ventral height of intervertebral space decreased significantly after 1 year, when compared with the ventral height immediately after surgery. BAK/C subsidence was observed in nine patients, including five with single-level fusion, one with two-separated-level fusion, and three with double-adjacent-level fusion, according to the standard of loss of intervertebral height of more than 3 mm. BAK/C fusion was generally effective; however, neck pain tended to reoccur in the patients with cage subsidence and two of them needed revision surgery because of the recurrence of myelopathy with progressive neck pain. Although BAK/C was generally effective, the pitfalls in the design of the device have resulted in the observation of clinical subsidence, which, in some cases, required reoperation for the recurrence of symptoms.

Box Cages

In Smith-Robinson–type interbody fusions, the bony end plates are left intact, and a block-shaped structural graft with large, flat, superior and inferior contact surfaces is countersunk into the disc space.[32] From a biomechanical standpoint this construct is superior because it retains the integrity of the end plates and provides a large surface area for load transfer and arthrodesis. Several box-type implant designs have been explored as alternatives to the more traditional tricortical autograft or structural allografts for Smith-Robinson fusion. These share a more or less rectangular configuration with a hollow core and fenestrations in their superior and inferior surfaces to allow the through growth of bone. Both titanium and polymer cages have been produced. The Rabea cage (Signus Medizintechnik, Alzenau, Germany), the Syncage (Synthes, Davos, Switzerland), and the Tibon cage (Biomet-Merck, Berlin, Germany) are representative of titanium box designs.

With FDA approval, the Rabea cage is currently available as a "cement restrictor." It is made of forged titanium to ensure MRI compatibility and is prefabricated in a 12-mm width, 12- and 14-mm depths, and in heights ranging from 4 to 8 mm (Fig. 43-4). The Rabea is offered as a parallel end-plate design and as a "lordosed" version, with 5 degrees of divergence built in. The rostral and caudal surfaces also bear retentive serrations to engage the end plates and resist implant extrusion during neck flexion. Published experience with the Rabea cage is limited, but preliminary biomechanical studies and clinical reports are both favorable.[10,12,15] As with other metallic devices, it is hard to judge fusion according to criteria of radiographically demonstrable bridging bone across the disc space and end plates. Alternative criteria including less than 2 degrees of angulation in dynamic radiographs and absence of any peri-implant bony lucency are substituted.

Carbon fiber box cages have found favor as intervertebral implants in the lumbar spine.[33] These devices appear to be largely inert biologically; they exhibit good strength in all axes of applied stress, they are impact and fatigue resistant, their elastic modulus is purported to match well with that of the cortical bone of the recipient spine, and because they are radiolucent, they afford an opportunity for direct graft visualization and fusion assessment. Extending these advantages to a cervical interbody application, box-type polymer cages have been under active development abroad and are poised to enter

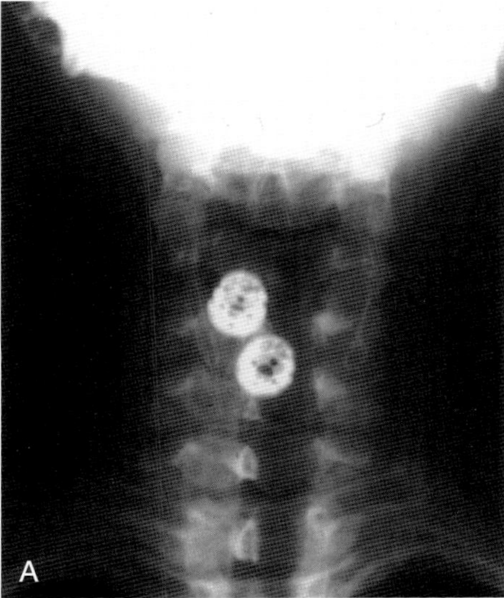

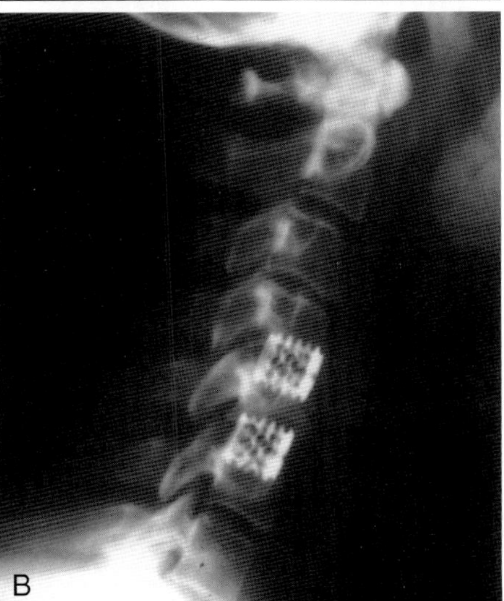

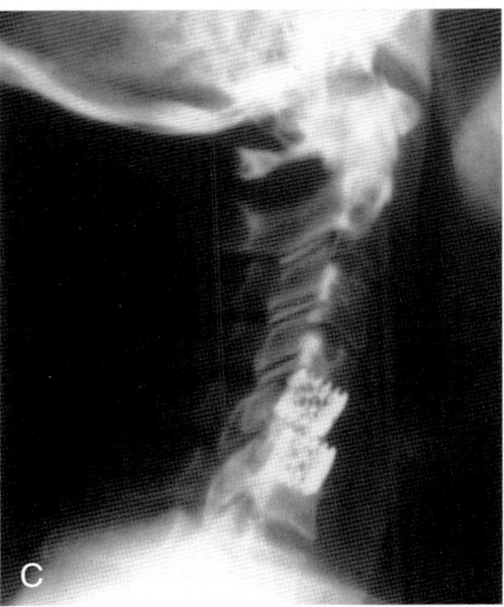

FIGURE 43-3. **A,** Two-level Bagby and Kuslich (BAK) cervical cages, anteroposterior view. **B,** Two-level BAK cages, lateral view. **C,** Same case, two-level BAK cages at 1-year follow-up showing subsidence.

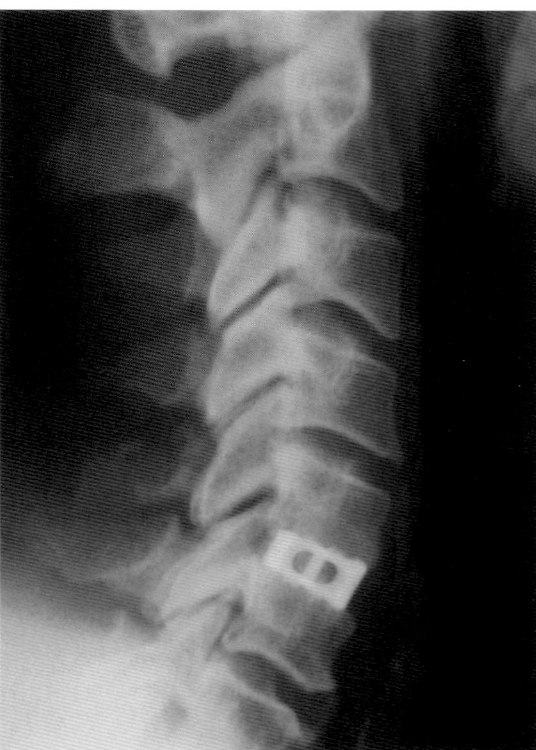

FIGURE 43-4. Single-level Rabea cage.

the U.S. market. Most designs have been fabricated from polyetheretherketone (PEEK), some also including a carbon fiber component (Cervical IF Cage, DePuy AcroMed, Raynham, MA). The Rabea device is now offered as a PEEK cage, again with approval in the United States for use as a cement restrictor. Other major vendors, including Stryker Instruments (Kalamazoo, MI [Solis PEEK cage]), Medtronic Sofamor Danek (CornerStone-SR), and Synthes (CR), have polymer cages already in place in overseas markets (Fig. 43-5). Like the Rabea cage, they are offered in a variety of sizes and configurations, including parallel end-plates, lordotic, and superiorly convex designs to conform to individual disc space anatomic requirements. Shared features include a large central opening to contain graft material, ridged end plates to resist implant extrusion, and imbedded radiopaque markers to allow radiographic visualization of the device.

Cho et al.[18] have recently reported on their preliminary experience with the Solis PEEK cage loaded with cancellous autograft in 40 patients undergoing mostly one- and two-level cervical discectomy and fusion.[18] Although the term of follow-up is unclear, the authors reported good functional outcomes, no device-related complications or failures, increased cervical lordosis, enlargement of neural foraminal cross-sectional area, and a 100% fusion rate. The complication rate was 2.5% in PEEK cage patients compared with a rate of 17.5% in a concurrent control group undergoing conventional discectomy and structural autografting in whom problems with graft collapse, dislodgement, and donor site morbidity were encountered. Other reports[34] have found a high subsidence tendency of box cages into predominantly C7; this illustrates the need for a modified box cage design that improves and extends contact with the inferior surface.

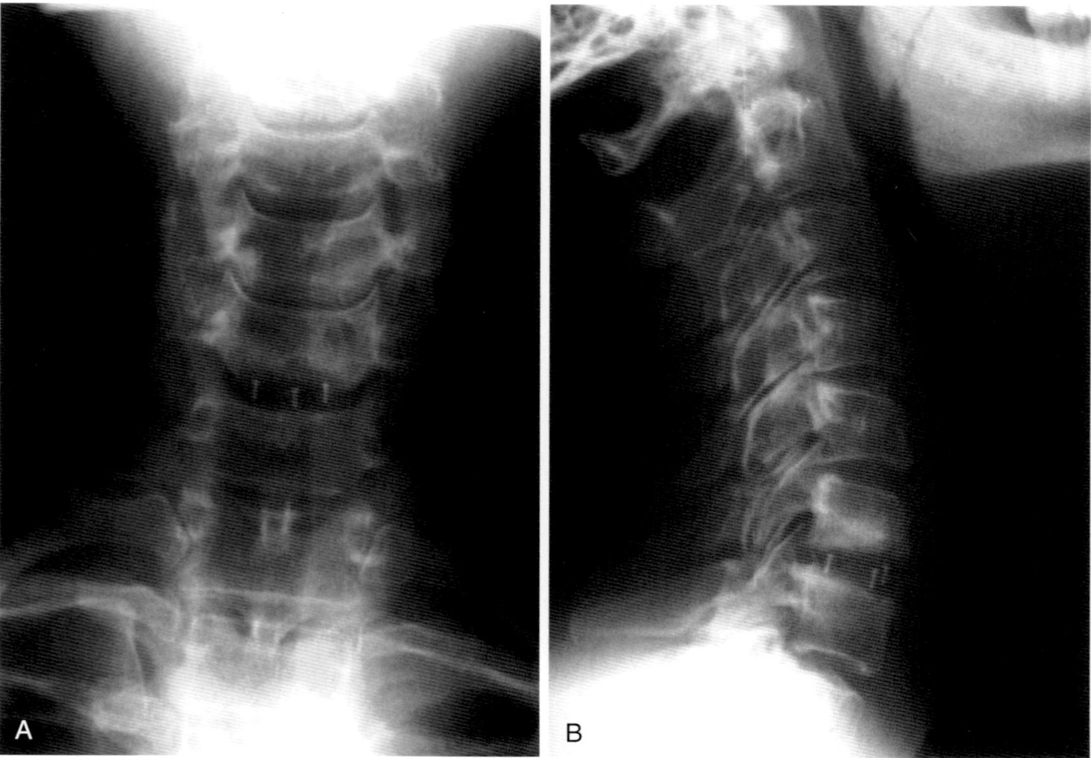

FIGURE 43-5. A, Single-level Synthes CR cage, anteroposterior view. **B,** Single-level Synthes CR cage, lateral view.

Radiolucent polymer cages are easily inserted; they appear to be biomechanically sound, and they hold much promise as interbody prostheses in the cervical spine, pending the outcome of more comprehensive clinical studies.

Interbody Fusion Cages with Intergrated Ventral Fixation

Recently, newly developed interbody spacers with integrated ventral fixation components have been gaining popularity in clinical use.[9] The low profile of these devices allows the surgeon to treat ventral pathology without having to disrupt indwelling hardware. An example of the clinical utility of such a device is an adjacent-level disc herniation after an anterior cervical discectomy. These devices can often be inserted at the adjacent site, after the discetomy is performed, without the need to disrupt the indwelling ventral cervical plate at the previously fused adjacent level. The anchored spacer provides similar biomechanical stability to that of the established ventral fusion technique and has potentially lower associated perioperative and postoperative morbidity, such as dysphagia or swallowing difficulties.[9] Two of these FDA-approved devices are the ROI-C VerteBRIDGE (LDR Inc., Austin, TX) interbody device and the Mosaic cervical implant system (Spinal Elements, Inc., Carlsbad, CA). See Figure 43-6. To date, more than 2500 of these devices have been used in the United States. Studies on the long-term efficacy of these devices are in progress.

Cylindrical Mesh Cages

Vertically oriented cylindrical cages fabricated of titanium mesh are now gaining use in the cervical spine, both for disc-space arthrodesis and for segmental reconstruction after corpectomy. The Harms cage (DePuy AcroMed, Warsaw, IN) is the primary example of this type of device; the SynMesh cage (Synthes) and Pyramesh cage (Sofamor Danek) are fundamentally similar designs. The FDA has approved use of this instrumentation in the thoracic and lumbar spine. Published biomechanical data and clinical studies describing its use in the cervical spine are sparse.

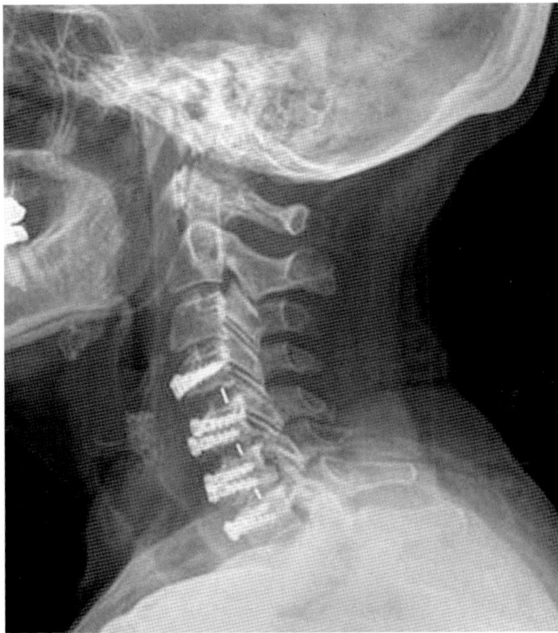

FIGURE 43-6. Three-level anterior cervical discectomy and fusion utilizing Mosaic cervical interbody spacers with integrated ventral fixation screws.

Similar to the box cage designs, mesh cages are intended to interface with intact end plates at the rostral and caudal ends of the construct. This increases the strength of the construct and reduces the risk for subsidence. Manufacturers provide stock material as sleeves with both circular and oval cross section and in a variety of lengths and diameters. Cage diameters between 10 and 16 mm are most suited for use in the cervical spine. In general the largest diameter that can be safely accommodated within the bed of the decompression is used because the cage will then bear on the end-plate perimeter, the apophyseal ring, which is its strongest part. The mesh can be trimmed to any desired length and tailored to the particular reconstructive need if a stock length is not an exact match. All three systems can fit end caps to the top and bottom of the cylinder, thereby enlarging the metal-bone interface and lessening the risk of end-plate perforation. Large central apertures within the end caps permit through growth of bone. The palisading teeth of the cage ends project slightly above the plane of the end caps, or the end caps themselves are serrated to grip the adjoining vertebral end plates and resist ventral cage extrusion. The Harms instrumentation provides a large selection of precut straight and custom-lordosed cages suitable as "off the shelf" implants for cervical disc space arthrodesis. Cylindrical cages are usually loaded with densely packed autograft. As with other metallic devices, the radiographic evaluation of fusion status within mesh implants is indirect.

There is a paucity of literature pertaining to the use of mesh cages for cervical disc space arthrodesis.[19,23] Our own experience with these devices in single- and multilevel discectomy operations suggests a significant potential for subsidence when these devices are used in a stand-alone mode. We attribute this to the relatively small contact area at the bone-implant interface in small-diameter disc space cages, despite the use of end caps.[23] To retard subsidence, we came to augment almost all ventral mesh cage reconstructions for degenerative disc disease with a dynamic ventral cervical plate. Although the addition of a ventral plate contributes only minimally to the duration and risk of operation, it does constitute a significant added expense. It is hoped that some of the newer box cage designs may yield satisfactory clinical results without a need for supplemental ventral fixation.

Mesh Cage Reconstruction of Corpectomy Defects

A more distinct advantage of using cylindrical mesh cage constructs is in the reconstruction of corpectomy defects. Indications for cervical corpectomy can include spondylosis, ossification of posterior longitudinal ligament, trauma, tumor, deformity correction, and occasional cases of infection. We and others have come to favor it in treatment of adjacent segment cervical disc disease as well.[21,24] Removal of a cervical corpus and the adjoining discs, and any associated osteophytes, can frequently be accomplished more expeditiously than two separate microdiscectomies (Fig. 43-7). The quality of the decompression is unsurpassed, and ample bone is acquired from the corpectomy material to satisfy any need for graft.

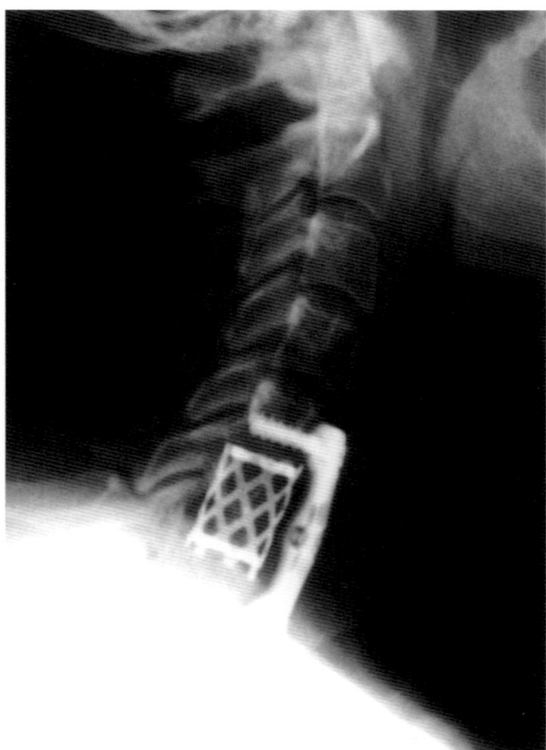

FIGURE 43-7. Harms cage, one-level corpectomy.

Except in cases of total spondylectomy for tumor, the central corpectomy bed is flanked on either side by a shell of lateral cortex and disc material. The method of decompression is addressed elsewhere in this volume. Ventral reconstruction seeks to restore the normal height of the vertebral column, which is frequently foreshortened with loss of cervical lordosis by the underlying conditions dictating the need for decompression. In the course of decompression, axial distraction is routinely applied via halter or cranial tong traction, and a thin interscapular roll is placed to help establish slight neck extension. Screw-in posts are inserted into the ventral midbodies of the rostral and caudal vertebrae adjacent to the decompression. Powerful forces can then be applied using a rack and pinion distraction arm, which has the combined effect of lengthening the ventral column of the spine and restoring lordosis. In significantly kyphotic deformities, divergent distraction techniques may be advantageous. As a consequence of this maneuver, the planes of the recipient rostral and caudal end plates are brought more nearly to a parallel alignment. Some divergence usually persists, however, and this needs to be accounted for in the subsequent fashioning of the construct. Often a small ledge of osteophyte projects caudally from the ventral caudal edge of the rostral vertebral body. This should be removed to create a relatively planar end-plate surface that will allow unimpeded insertion of the construct. The cartilaginous end plates are scraped down with curettes, but every effort is made to leave the bony end plates inviolate.

Once the desired degree of distraction in the corpectomy bed has been obtained, calipers are used to measure the desired construct length at both its ventral and dorsal limits. Because of the divergence of the end plates, the ventral height is often 1 to 2 mm longer than the dorsal measure. We are most experienced with the Harms system, which provides cages suitable for use in the cervical spine as straight cylindrical stock ranging from 12 to 16 mm in diameter and from 30 to 50 mm in length. Oval stock 15 mm × 12 mm is also available, as well as prelordosed tubular stock. We advise selecting the largest cage that can be safely accommodated within the corpectomy bed, without intruding on the ventral spinal canal. The desired ventral and dorsal heights of the cage are marked according to caliper measurements, and the cage is cut accordingly. For straight mesh stock spanning three or more levels, it may be advantageous to cut the lower end of the cage on a slight bias to optimally accommodate the divergence of the end plates to which they will be paired. Other systems offer end-fitted, lordotic end caps as an alternative to direct cage modification. Intraoperative lateral fluoroscopy showing the rostral and caudal recipient end plates, with distraction applied, is helpful in forming an image of the desired cage geometry. Ideally, full cross-sectional contact will be achieved between each end of the cage and the adjoining end plate.

An appropriately sized end cap is fitted to one end of the cage. The bias cut is never so severe as to preclude a snug fit. The cage can then be loaded with morselized autologous bone obtained from the corpectomy bed itself or elsewhere. This bone is repeatedly tamped down to create dense packing within the construct without any internal voids. Good packing of the construct is achieved when graft material is seen extruding centrifugally through the interstices of the mesh. Only in cases of tumor and infection is locally derived graft material quantitatively or qualitatively insufficient. If necessary, it is easily supplemented by cancellous autograft obtained from the iliac crest or combined with allograft. The second end cap is seated, and a final bit of additional graft is packed into the central orifice of each end cap. Just before the cage is to be inserted, the distractor mechanism is opened to lengthen the corpectomy trough an additional 1 to 2 mm. The cage is then seated in the corpectomy bed until a good friction fit is achieved. Small impactors are applied alternately over the rostral and caudal ends of the cage, tapping the cage deeper into the corpectomy trough until its presenting edge is recessed just below the ventralmost cortices of the adjacent vertebrae. At this point, axial traction is removed to allow elastic recoil of the soft tissues to lock the construct in place. A nerve hook can be inserted behind the cage to assess the tightness of the fit and confirm the patency of the ventral spinal canal. Anteroposterior and lateral fluoroscopy are then used to control proper placement in the coronal and sagittal planes, and any indicated adjustments are performed.

Reconstruction of one- and two-level corpectomies is generally straightforward. For degenerative conditions, we secure the construct with a dynamic plate and screw system, which provides additional rigidity during neck extension and helps limit subsidence during healing. If bone quality and screw purchase are good, use of an external orthosis is optional in single-level corpectomy. In weakened osteoporotic bone, bicortical screw fixation of the ventral plate and an orthosis are used. Especially precarious constructs or trauma cases with dorsal ligamentous disruption are supplemented with dorsal instrumentation and fusion. For acute spinal traumas, a rigid plate and screw system is preferred because of the frequently associated soft tissue injury and the heightened risk of instability. A minor degree of subsidence is routinely observed during healing, but graft or plate dislodgement or significant cervical straightening is most unusual.

As an alternative to long-segment corpectomy or multilevel discectomy in patients who need decompression/fusion

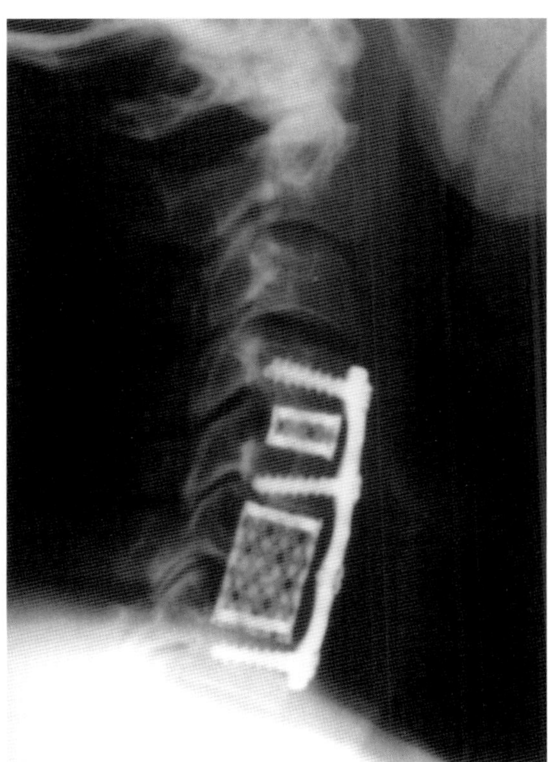

FIGURE 43-8. Harms cages, one-level corpectomy and adjacent disc space arthrodesis.

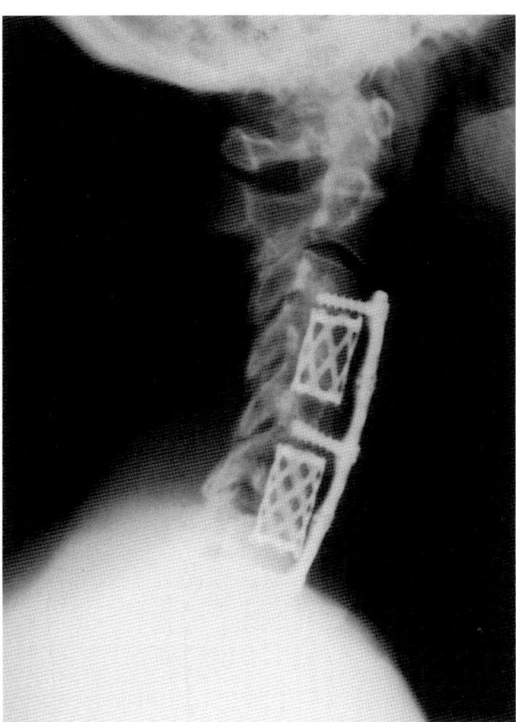

FIGURE 43-9. Harms cages, two-level discontinuous corpectomies.

at three or more motion segments, we have performed corpectomy plus adjacent-level discectomy (three motion segments), or "discontinuous corpectomies" with retention of an intervening body (four motion segments). A ventral plate is thereby afforded at least two extra intermediary points of fixation (Figs. 43-8 and 43-9). The advantage of this technique over multilevel discectomy is the speed and completeness of the decompression and the provision of locally derived autograft. We have experienced no instances of plate loosening or graft migration in this group of patients.

Reconstruction of three- and four-level corpectomies is more problematic. The potential for graft migration, plate loosening, and end-plate fracture is considerably greater. Frequently, such patients are being operated on for correction of a kyphotic deformity, and the bone quality can be suboptimal. Long-segment ventral plates fixated only at their rostral and caudal ends are very prone to failure. Failure typically occurs at the inferior end of the construct where the hardware either fractures or levers off of the caudal body (Fig. 43-10). Simple "kick plates" fitted to the vertebral bodies at the rostral and caudal ends of the construct are worthy of consideration in this circumstance. They do not contribute to the inherent stability of the construct other than to prevent ventral extrusion of the implant. Immediate stability is secured by supplemental, instrumented dorsal spinal fusion and/or halo immobilization (Fig. 43-11).

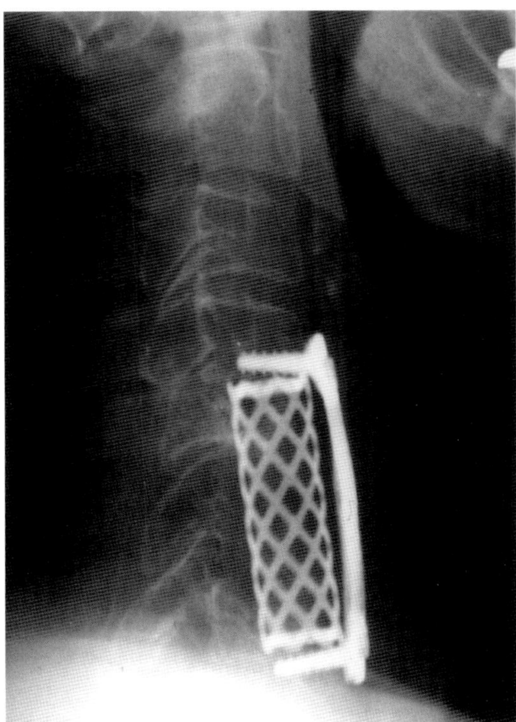

FIGURE 43-10. Long-segment cage failure at caudal end of construct.

Summary

Structural autografts and allografts have proved themselves generally satisfactory in single-level disc space arthrodesis and in the reconstruction of single-level corpectomy defects. The risk of graft fracture, resorption, extrusion, and nonunion increases as fusion is extended over an increasing number of motion segments. A variety of interbody devices has been developed with shared advantages of strength, resistance to

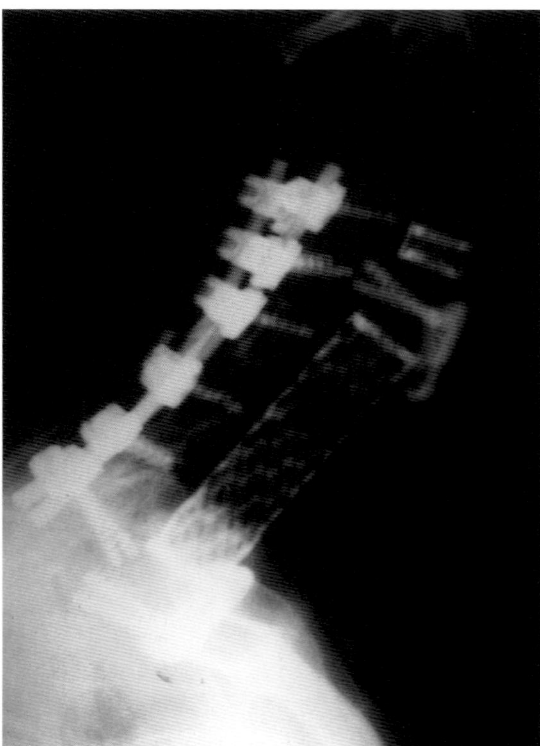

FIGURE 43-11. Long-segment reconstruction with kick plate and dorsal fixation.

collapse and extrusion, and an ability to function as carriers of bone graft "generators" while averting the morbidity associated with structural autograft harvest. Polymer cages have the additional benefits of radiolucency and a more physiologically elastic modulus. Recently, ventral interbody cages with integrated ventral fixation systems have been gaining popularity in clinical use.

Interbody cages have a mechanical function as spacer devices, restoring structural integrity to the load-bearing ventral column of the spine. The development of so-called biologies such as rhBMP will begin to shift the focus from the mechanical properties of these devices to their biologic role as delivery systems for the mediators of bony fusion. Once fusion has been achieved, the function of the prosthesis itself has been supplanted. Bioabsorbable devices, which are "digested" after this function has been fulfilled, are therefore a logical next step in the future evolution of interbody device design. However, the ultimate role for interbody devices may be in the preservation or restoration of the physiologic motion segment rather than in its abolition

Acknowledgment. Dr. Cahill, now deceased, received grant and research support from Medtronic Sofamor Danek and Synthes. Some of the devices described in this chapter have not received approval from the FDA for use as implants in the cervical spine. Please refer to product labeling information for approval status.

KEY REFERENCES

Kandziora F, Pflugmacher R, Schaefer J: Biomechanical comparison of cervical spine interbody fusion cages. *Spine (Phila Pa 1976)* 26:1850–1857, 2001.

Saunders RL, Traynelis VC: Interbody strut techniques. In Benzel EC, editor: *Spine surgery*, New York, 1999, Churchill-Livingstone, pp 241–248.

Uribe JS, Sangala JR, Duckworth EA, Vale FL: Comparison between anterior cervical discectomy fusion and cervical corpectomy fusion using titanium cages for reconstruction: analysis of outcome and long-term follow-up. *Eur Spine J* 18(5):654–662, 2009.

REFERENCES

The complete reference list is available online at expertconsult.com.

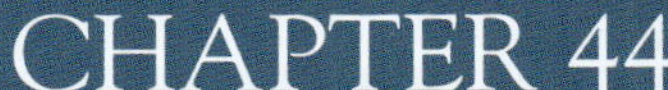
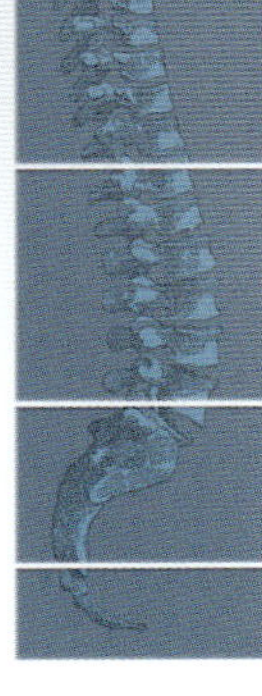

CHAPTER 44

Cervical Laminectomy and Laminoforaminotomy

Paul K. Maurer

General Principles

Cervical spondylosis, disc herniation, and allied pathologies are a common cause of neurologic compression. Cervical spondylotic myelopathy is the most common cause of spinal cord dysfunction in adults.[1]

In spite of more than 40 years of evaluation of various techniques, there is no class I or class II evidence to strongly support one procedure over another, be it anterior or posterior, in the overall group of patients.[2] The natural history of the compressive myelopathies varies, eroding the efficacy of procedural long-term outcomes.[1] The origin of cervical spondylotic myelopathy appears to originate from two principle forces on the spinal cord and associated structures:

1. Reduction in the ventral/dorsal cervical canal volume leading to direct neurologic compression.
2. The dynamic forces (i.e., "stretch") on the spinal cord during head motion in the presence of such compressive forces.[3-5]

In essence, the compressed spinal cord is stretched, or distracted, through a compromised canal, leading to damage in the spinal cord. Interestingly, the damage is often in the lateral cord region in early to moderate cases of myelopathy.[4] It has long been felt that, given the frequent ventral location of the compressive spur, the procedure must be directed to that location. It appears that it is the *combination* of compressive and dynamic motion of the spinal cord that leads to compromised function. In light of the static (compressive) and dynamic forces involved in the genesis of myelopathy, all the ventral and dorsal surgical options that address either one, or both, of the involved factors have a role.[4,5]

Given the preceding two underlying factors (compression and motion) in the genesis of cervical spondylotic myelopathy (CSM), a wide variety of procedures are available to address the problem. As a primary goal, decompression should be achieved (i.e., the spinal canal volume enlarged). This can be accomplished with anterior discectomy-spurectomy and fusion, anterior corpectomy and fusion, cervical laminectomy, cervical laminoplasty, and cervical laminectomy and fusion.[2-6] Each procedure has its attendant downside in the form of various complications. All have been shown to be effective and in the overall population of CSM patients, but no one procedure has clearly outclassed the other options.[2] Cervical laminectomy for decompression of the spinal cord and/or nerve roots has been shown to be effective in the treatment of CSM.[2,7] It addresses the compressive forces in CSM, but does not reduce the dynamic forces. Nevertheless, many patients do well with this option, and in appropriately selected patients the procedure is a safe, relatively simple, and effective option. A number of advantages can be ascribed to cervical laminectomy/decompression:

- A relatively simple technique with a moderate number of technical steps
- An effective means of decompressing an extensive rostral/caudal compression (two to five levels)
- No potential pseudarthrosis, as no fusion is included; similarly, no hardware-related failures or complications
- No hypermotility segmentation stress and delayed adjacent segment concerns because the motion of the spine is preserved (a motion-sparing procedure)
- Usable in elderly patients in whom osteoporotic bone may not favor successful hardware implantation
- Fairly rapid multilevel procedures possible, which may be advantageous in the patient with multiple subsystem issues (e.g., cardiac, renal) that increase perioperative risk

As with all surgical options in the treatment of CSM, there are a number of potential limitations:

- May represent same risk of delayed kyphosis over time secondary to loss of the posterior tension band (lamina and intraspinous ligaments).[8] The exact incidence of postlaminectomy kyphosis is not well established, and the published reviews have generally been limited in patient numbers. Clinically relevant, as opposed to radiographically identified, incidental sagittal balance change is probably in the 5% to 10% range.[8] This problem, to some degree, can be limited by proper technical performance[9] (see section on technique).
- In light of the preceding point, cervical laminectomy should be limited to patients with reasonable lordosis, and not utilized in those with a frank kyphosis. Patients younger than age 20 are at greater risk for delayed cervical kyphosis after laminectomy.[7,8]
- In patients with advanced CSM, reducing the dynamic component of CSM by adding simultaneous dorsal instrumentation (arthrodesis *may* be beneficial, but at the time of this writing, the exact subgroup to benefit from this is uncertain).[2,5]

Patient Selection

Cervical laminectomy addresses the compressive aspects of CSM and associated disorders, but not the dynamic forces.[2,5,7] If concerns arise regarding frank stability, or it is felt that the dynamic aspects must be addressed, simultaneous dorsal instrumentation and fusion can be utilized in addition to simple decompression. The decision to select one posterior option or another, and even the consideration of anterior options, is often a combination of science and surgeon preference and experience.[2,5,7] Over the years, and over the course of 400 cases, I have used the following general guidelines:

A cervical laminectomy is considered in the following circumstances:

- For patients with multilevel (more than two) canal size reduction and reasonable lordosis
- In cases where decompressive laminectomy alone is used if an early to moderate myelopathy is present, but not dramatic signal change within the spinal cord on MRI (myelomalacia). In advanced cases of CSM, I generally favor simultaneous reduction of motion/dynamic forces by adding dorsal instrumentation (lateral mass screws) and fusion to the procedure. This preference is based on outcome trends, and no strong scientific data exist to bolster any dogmatic decision.
- Cervical laminectomy is a reasonable option in patients with a relatively "clean" canal (i.e., without dramatic ventral spurs, such as can be seen in congenital narrowing).
- A good option in the elderly multilevel CSM patients with poor bone stock and severe subsystem diseases that would increase morbidity in more complex procedures.

Technique

Positioning

Two basic positions are available: prone or sitting. A less common approach is lateral decubitus.

1. Prone—The patient is placed on appropriate padding material. The head is fixed in neutral position. Care must be taken to get a solid purchase in bone with the head holder because the weight of the head and neck in the prone position can lead to slippage with attendant lacerations and head shift. It is important to flex the knees to prevent migration of the patient on the table, which can lead to neck extension if the patient slides down the table during the procedure.
2. Sitting—Over the years, the trend had been to avoid the sitting position as inherently hazardous because of the risk of air embolization.[10,11] Recently, a trend back to this option has been noted. Although air ingress can be seen in 5% to 8% of the sitting cases, clinically significant air embolization in sitting cervical cases is unusual.[10,11] The risk of air embolization in cranial cases is higher because of the noncollapsible venous structures of the cranium. Over 1500 sitting cases accumulated in the literature attest to the safety, with proper technique, of the sitting position.[10,11] The sitting position provides a fairly bloodless field due to dependent flow of blood to the bottom of the field and reduced epidural venous tension. Nerve root decompression via dorsolateral foraminotomy can be facilitated for this reason in the sitting position.

Monitoring

Historically, a panoply of monitoring devices is used for dorsal decompression.[12,13] Over the last 10 years, I have gravitated to two peripheral intravenous catheters and a systemic arterial line *if* subsystem diseases suggest such a line may be beneficial. No Foley catheter is generally used since the procedure is brief (80–110 minutes). The literature supports the use of the sitting position *without* the use of a central line.[10,11] I have not used central venous pressure lines in such cases in more than 10 years.

After many years of using electrophysiologic monitoring, I no longer use "routine" physiologic monitoring in standard decompressive laminectomies. There is extensive literature regarding the option of physiologic monitoring, but no clear scientific data or consensus exists.[13] It may have a more credible role in tumor resections, spinal reconstruction, and so on, but even in these cases, there is sufficient variability to consider such monitoring on a case by case basis.

Incision and Dissection

A skin incision adequate for the proposed decompression is utilized. Excessive attempts to limit the incision may jeopardize the ease and safety of deep dissection. A standard subperiosteal dissection is employed to just lateral to the laminar facet groove (Fig. 44-1). There is no need nor benefit to carrying the dissection more laterally into the facet/facet capsule because this only exacerbates the risk of delayed kyphosis. Remember that a small group of patients may have an occult spina bifida, so care must be taken to avoid dissection through such a midline breach.

Laminectomy

Many techniques have been used over the years to complete the dorsal lamina arch resection, thereby affording decompression. I have used the Leksell technique, a high-speed drill, and so forth, but in recent years I have settled on a "trough technique," using a drill and thin foot-plate, 2-mm Kerrison rongeur. The key features of this technique are as follows:

1. The trough is started at the caudal, lateral area of the lamina (Fig. 44-2). Be certain to begin the bone removal *medial* to the laminar facet groove. A more lateral dissection only leads to more facet damage and does not allow an effective trough to be fashioned through the lamina.
2. The Kerrison rongeur is carefully inserted, slowly and carefully fully approximating the inner cortical surface of the lamina. Note: No "bowling" is allowed, that is, no intrusion into the canal and pulling back to the bone. Whether a drill, Kerrison rongeur, or other instrument is used, pushing into the canal and pulling back to the inner bone surface can cause cord or root compression. The thin foot-plate, cervical Kerrison rongeur "walks" in a rostral direction using a 10 o'clock and 2 o'clock bone punch sequence. This alternating direction of each

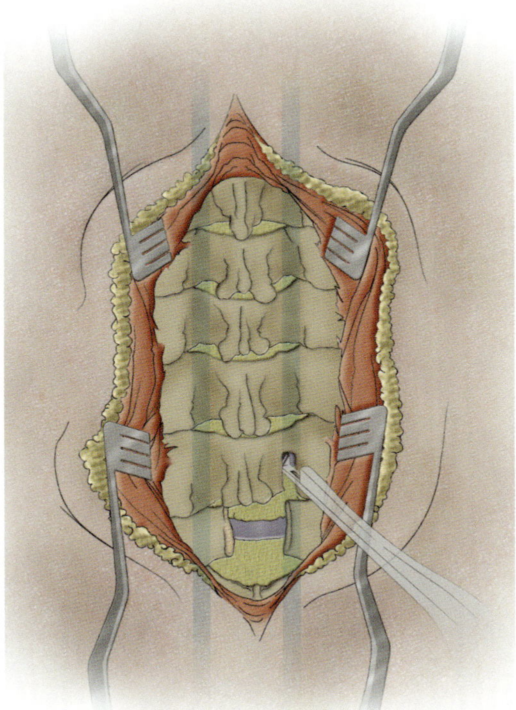

FIGURE 44-1. The soft tissue dissection should not be extended laterally beyond the medial third of the facet. This helps reduce facet capsule damage with potential delayed kyphosis. A 2-mm thin foot-plate Kerrison rongeur is used in a lateral "trough" to remove each laminar segment en bloc. This reduces potential canal compromise over the cord. Each bone bite should be in a 10 o'clock, then 2 o'clock fashion to prevent trapping the instrument in the trough.

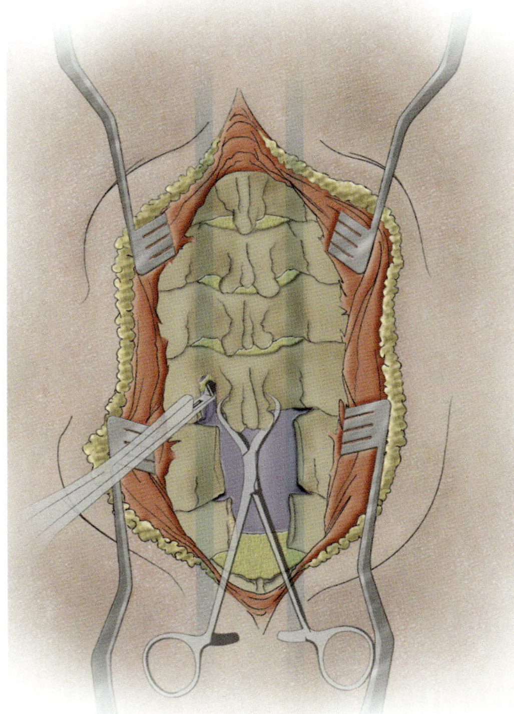

FIGURE 44-2. Each laminar segment is carefully tractioned as it is freed laterally. A medium-sized towel clip (Adair clamp) is used to gently but firmly elevate the lamina off the spinal canal with a caudal and dorsal traction technique. Note that the trough laterally is centered on the laminar facet groove.

successive site of bone prevents the instrument from being trapped in the bone trough, which makes smooth movements more difficult. By staying in the lateral lamina, the likelihood of cord compression is reduced (Fig. 44-3).

3. The contralateral bone trough is fashioned, a medium-sized towel clip is inserted near the base of the spinous process, and gentle traction is applied inferior and dorsal to the wound, that is, "down and out" of the wound, which elevates the laminar segment safely off the spinal cord as the second trough completes the freeing of the lamina from its boney attachments. The *ligamentum flavum* is sectioned with the lamina gently tractioned off the dura. A Kerrison punch (2-mm thin foot plate) can be used to section the lamina and free it from its soft tissue attachments. Each laminar segment, or occasionally two lamina, can be removed en bloc segmentally. If the troughs have been properly placed, an "equator to equator" decompression of the spinal cord results, and the proximal nerve roots are just visualized.

Laminoforaminotomy

A moderate foraminotomy (3–4 mm) is generally completed or progresses until a microspatula easily passes the foramen (Fig. 44-4). If a specific radiculopathy is a concern, a more extensive laminoforaminotomy can be completed. The nerve root almost always arises within 4 to 5 mm rostrally or caudally to the facet articular line. The 2-mm Kerrison rongeur, (or drill and curette, etc.) can now be directed laterally, forming a series of successive "crescent moon" bone removals at the medial facet. As the proximal nerve is identified, simply tightly "hug" the bone with the foot plate (or curette) and remove bone from the rostral to caudal line of the nerve. (Again, the facet articular line is a good guideline as the center of the crescent moon.) A microspatula can be passed over the dorsal nerve surface to ensure adequate decompression of the nerve root. It is *rarely* necessary to remove more than 6 to 7 mm of the medial facet to accomplish this task.

Although I used to pursue the ventral root/bone area for spurs, the literature and experience suggest that a thorough foraminotomy alone (exclusive foraminotomy) is successful and limits the morbidity resulting from attempts at spur removal.[9,10] A large soft disc can be approached via the axilla or the shoulder of the nerve depending on where the fragment predominates. A small group of patients have a conjoint nerve, so care must be taken when "sweeping" the nerve in the axilla to avoid damaging a conjoint nerve. The incision into a disc fragment should be very shallow (just enough to release the fragment). The vertebral artery is deep to the nerve and can be damaged. Hemostasis can be readily established (particularly in the sitting position) with judicious microbipolar use or a *small* piece of hemostatic agent.

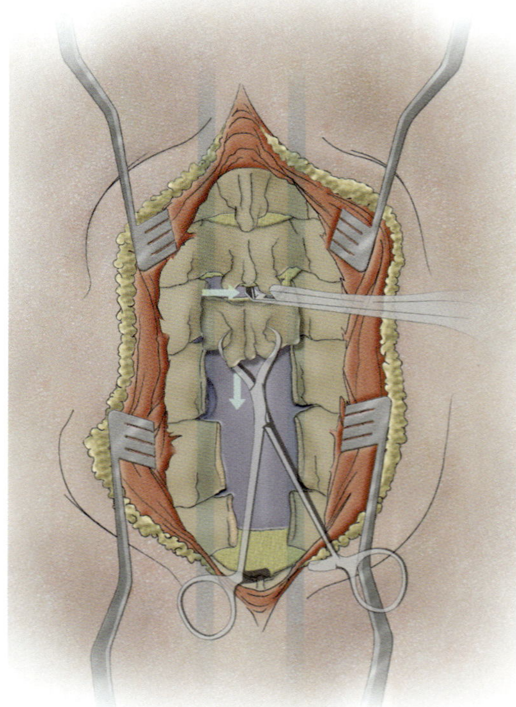

FIGURE 44-3. As the laminar segment is pulled down and away (caudal and dorsal), the ligament moves dorsally off the dura and can be sectioned with the Kerrison 2-mm thin foot-plate instrument of the #11 scalpel.

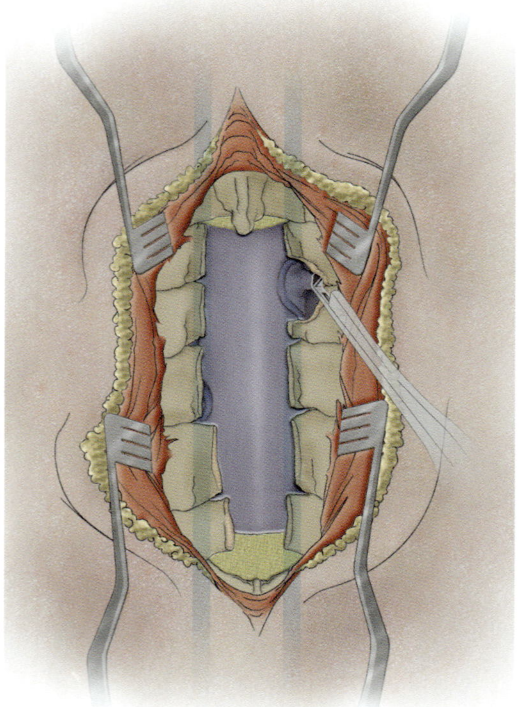

FIGURE 44-4.. On completion of sequential laminectomies, an "equator to equator" decompression is achieved. Laminoforaminotomy can be added as deemed necessary. The foraminotomy is centered on the articular facet groove. Note that an important part of the laminoforaminotomy is the resection of the lateral-rostral lip of the caudal lamina. Much of the nerve compression is located in this region.

The wound is closed using standard layered technique. Polyglactin 910 #0 sutures are used in the fascia and #2-0 in the subcutaneous plane. Adhesive skin closures (Steri-Strips) are then applied. No drain is used unless the conditions favor such placement. As with all surgical events, the drain can be helpful, but it is "the devil's highway" for introducing bacteria. No collar is needed for cervical laminectomy cases.

Summary

Cervical laminectomy is a relatively straightforward and effective procedure for treating a significant number of cervical degenerative conditions. The procedure can be accomplished effectively in multisegmental disease and has no associated hardware or delayed hypermotility issues. It can be used in patients with poor bone quality, the elderly, with coexistant subsystem disease, and in patients with reasonable preservation of lordosis. No definitive scientific data absolutes guide selection in the menu of surgical options in the cervical spine. Each case must be selected on its individual characteristics and the experience of the surgeon.

KEY REFERENCES

Benzel EC: *Biomechanics of spine stabilization*, Rolling Meadows, IL, 2001, American Association of Neurological Surgeons.

Fehlings MG, Arvin B: Surgical management of cervical degenerative disease: the evidence related to indications, impact, and outcome. *J Neurosurg Spine* 11:97–100, 2009.

Henderson FC, Geddes JF, Vaccaro AR, et al: Stretch-associated injury in cervical spondylotic myelopathy: new concept and review. *Neurosurgery* 56:1101–1113, 2005.

Kaptain GJ, Simmons NE, Replogle RE, et al: Incidence and outcome of kyphotic deformity following laminectomy for cervical spondylotic myelopathy. *J Neurosurg* 93:199–204, 2000.

Matz PG, Anderson PA, Holly LT, et al: The natural history of cervical spondylotic myelopathy. *J Neurosurg Spine* 11:104–111, 2009.

Maurer PK, Ellenbogen RG, Ecklund J, et al: Cervical spondylotic myelopathy: treatment with posterior decompression and Luque rectangle bone fusion. *Neurosurgery* 28:680–683, 1991.

Mummaneni PV, Kaiser MG, Matz PG, et al: Cervical surgical techniques for the treatment of cervical spondylotic myelopathy. *J Neurosurg Spine* 11:130–141, 2009.

REFERENCES

The complete reference list is available online at expertconsult.com.

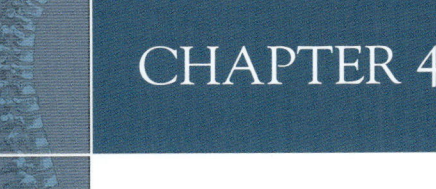

CHAPTER 45

Cervical Skip Corpectomy

Sedat Dalbayrak | Mesut Yilmaz | Sait Naderi

The ventral approach to the cervical spine was first suggested by Dr. Leroy Abbott in 1952. The approach was used and subsequently described by Bailey and Badgley.[1] During the late 1950s and 1960s many approaches and techniques were defined to obtain a successful neural decompression and cervical spine arthrodesis.[2] All these frontier studies focused on anterior cervical discectomy and arthrodesis.

Evolution of new techniques facilitated the complex surgical procedures, leading surgeons to use more aggressive techniques in cases with traumatic, degenerative, infectious, and neoplastic disorders. As a result, the first cervical corpectomy procedures were performed in 1970s. With time cervical ventral and dorsal plating techniques were developed.[3]

Cervical corpectomy is an effective procedure decompressing the ventral spinal cord. The existing literature indicates that the success rate usually is good for single-level or two-level cervical corpectomy, but not for multilevel corpectomy.[4-15] On the other hand, although this surgery is associated with good results in terms of neurologic recovery, many complications, such as strut graft fracture, graft pistoning, graft dislodgement, hardware failure, and pseudoarthrosis, are also part of its history.

Vaccaro et al. demonstrated high rates of early construct failure in multilevel fusions: 9% for two-level corpectomy, and 50% for three-level corpectomy.[15] A similar high rate of construct failure after multilevel corpectomy was reported by others as well.[6,7,10,11,15-19] The reported high rate of failure indicates that reconstruction of a multilevel corpectomy defect in the cervical spine remains a challenge.

Biomechanics of Cervical Corpectomy

The evidence of failure of long constructs has been investigated in biomechanical studies.[20-22] Cadaveric biomechanical studies showed that the longer plate generates greater motions at the fusion sites under physiologic loads because of its longer lever arm,[23] and that the stabilizing potential indices significantly decrease after fatigue for the three-level corpectomy, but not for the one-level corpectomy.[16,17,23-25] This explains the lesser rate of construct failure in one-level cervical corpectomies.

Cervical corpectomy results in a posterior shift of the center of rotation, as the anterior aspect of the spine is cut. Addition of an anterior cervical plate shifts the center of rotation to the anterior, thus changing the loading pattern.[16,17,24] In other words, whereas the stand-alone strut graft is loaded in flexion and unloaded in extension,[16,17] the addition of a plate completely reverses the loading pattern. The outcome is reversal of the loading pattern in anterior-plated long-strut grafts so that loading of the graft does not occur under flexion moments, and excessive compression of the graft occurs under extension loads, resulting in the graft pistoning into the caudal vertebral end plate and, subsequently, in plate kicking.[16,17]

Alternative Solutions

Based on clinical experiences and biomechanical facts, many alternative techniques have been developed to avoid graft plate-related problems in cases of multilevel corpectomy.[4,6,8,13,26-30]

Based on the evidence of the high stress in the lower end of the construct, the use of a buttress (junctional) plate alone was recommended. However, Riew et al.[27] and MacDonald et al.[8] reported high rates of complication after the use of a buttress plate alone in multilevel corpectomy. They recommended that the buttress plate be supplemented with posterior fixation.[8,27,30]

Others focused on the 360-degree fixation using long plates.[4,6,13,26] However, the 360-degree procedure is a lengthy, sometimes staged procedure.

Different combinations of multilevel anterior cervical discectomy and fusion (ACDF) with or without corpectomies are other alternatives. As ventral alternative approaches to three-level corpectomy, Rhee and Riew[31] proposed (1) multilevel ACDF, (2) single corpectomy combined with additional ACDFs, and (3) two single-level corpectomies separated by an intact intervening vertebra. As another alternative, Ozer et al. described an open-window corpectomy technique.[32]

Indications of Skip Corpectomy

The skip corpectomy is indicated and is applicable in compressions extending from C3-4 to C6-7, particularly when the area of compression at the C5 level is confined to the adjacent disc spaces (Fig. 45-1A). This is so because skip corpectomy allows optimal decompression of the C3-4, C4-5, C5-6, and C6-7 intervertebral disc levels and C4 and C6 vertebral body levels (Fig. 45-1B). However, the limited work angle does not

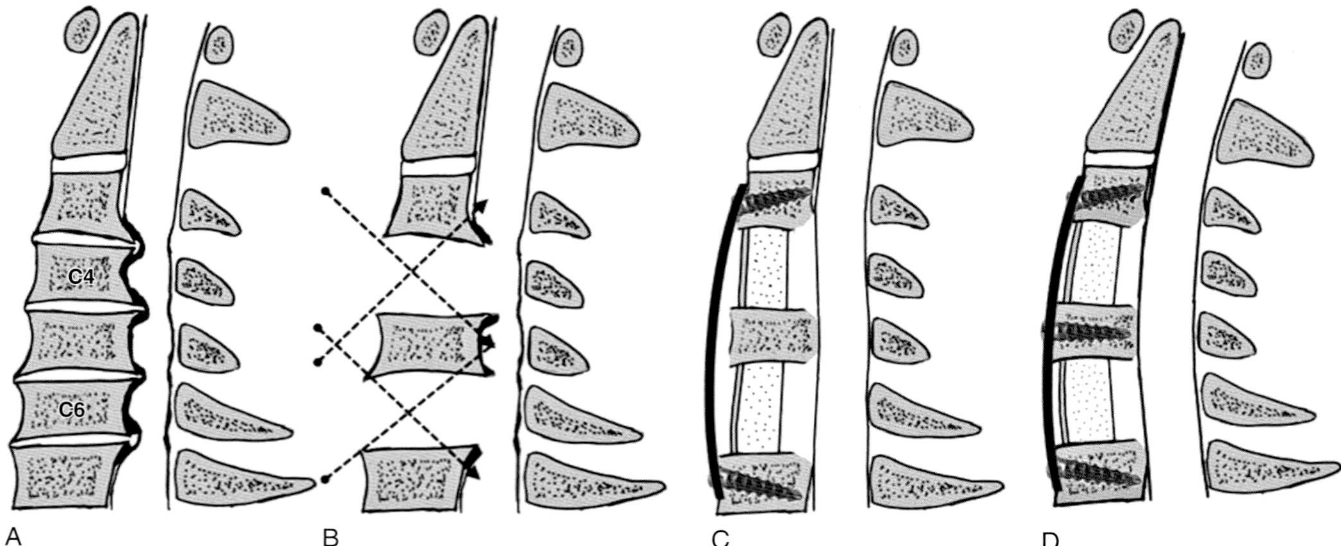

FIGURE 45-1. An illustration of a case indicative for skip corpectomy. **A,** Spondylotic and ossification of the posterior longitudinal ligament; compression is confined to the level of the C3-4, C4-5, C5-6, and C6-7 intervertebral discs and posterior to the dorsal wall of the C4 and C6 vertebral bodies. **B,** The best surgical view for optimum decompression in skip corpectomy. **C,** The illustration shows the placement of grafts and fixation of caudal and rostral vertebrae. **D,** Final fixation of the cervical spine after skip corpectomy. Note that the screw placement into the middle vertebra brings the C5 vertebral body to the plate.

allow for optimum decompression of the posterior aspect of the C5 vertebral body, as seen in continuing ossification of the posterior longitudinal ligament (OPLL) cases. Note, however, that the surgeon may change strategy during the procedure and can add a C5 corpectomy if the decompression behind the C5 vertebral body is not satisfactory. Such an additional C5 corpectomy means a three-level corpectomy and should be combined with a posterior stabilization procedure.

Skip Corpectomy Technique

The skip corpectomy technique is exemplified by a C4 and C6 corpectomy, C5 osteophytectomy, and decompression of dorsal-rostral and dorsal-caudal aspects of the C5 vertebra. Preservation of the C5 vertebral body and the use of this vertebra for screw fixation are the most important aspects of this technique. Reconstruction can be performed using either iliac crest autograft or fibula allograft. After placement of the C3-5 and C5-7 bone grafts, a fixed rigid ventral cervical spine plate is placed (Fig. 45-1C). The plate is contoured in lordosis. The intervening vertebral body that is left after C4 and C6 decompression (i.e., the C5 vertebral body) serves as an intermediate point of construct fixation. The plate is first secured at the rostral and caudal ends (the C3 and C7 vertebral bodies). Next, screws are placed into the intervening vertebral body (the C5 vertebral body). As the C5 vertebral body screws are tightened, the spine is "brought to the cervical plate" (Figs. 45-1D and 45-2). Figure 45-3 shows preoperative and postoperative images of a patient who underwent skip corpectomy.

Advantages of Skip Corpectomy

The skip corpectomy technique achieves four healing surfaces, representing fewer than an equivalent number of multilevel ACDFs (eight surfaces), while avoiding problems with long-strut grafts. The fixation is obtained at the top, bottom, and middle of the constructs. The technique was suggested in recent years.[31,33,34] Ashkenazi et al. reported results after skip corpectomy, what they called hybrid decompression, in 13 cases.[34] They noted fusion in all cases and experienced mechanical failure of the construct in only one case (4%). Using this technique, Agbi and Paquette[33] reported successful outcomes in four cases. The results of the current series are in line with those reported by Ashkenazi et al.[34] Dalbayrak et al. reported a high fusion rate (100%) and a low graft hardware-related complication rate (3.4%) using skip corpectomy.[35] The technique is biomechanically superior to ventral plating alone for three-level corpectomy.

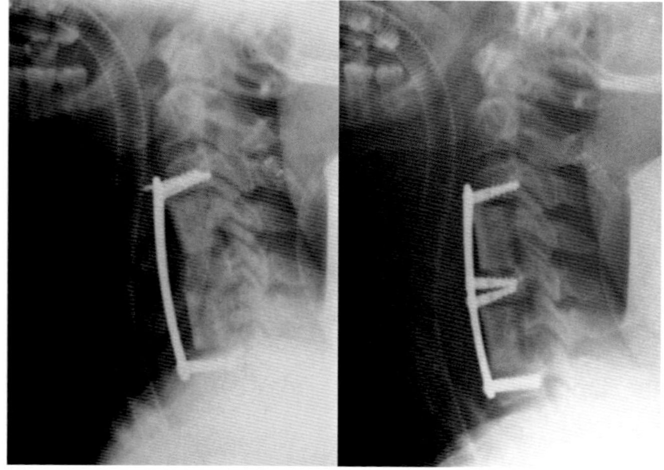

FIGURE 45-2. Radiograph indicating placement of screw into the middle vertebra, bringing the C5 vertebral body to the plate during the surgery.

Singh et al.[36] compared the biomechanical aspects of different hybrid discectomy and corpectomy models and

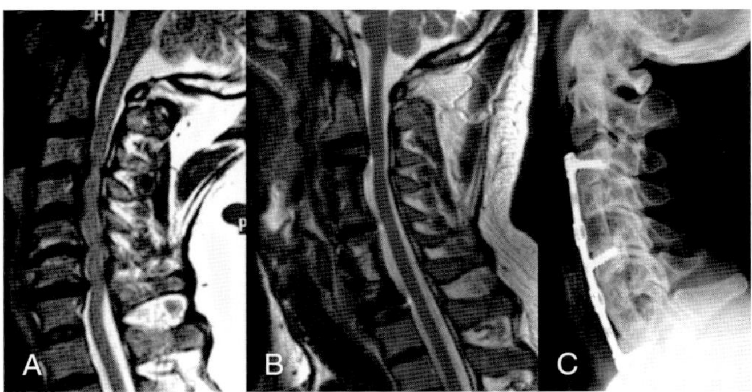

FIGURE 45-3. A, Preoperative T_2-weighted sagittal cervical spine MRI showing the multiple ventral compressions. **B,** Postoperative T_2-weighted sagittal cervical spine MRI showing decompression of the spinal cord. **C,** Postoperative lateral cervical spine plain radiograph showing the position of the grafts and screws.

reported that the increased rigidity afforded by segmental fixation may significantly decrease the likelihood of plate dislodgement in the setting of anterior instrumentation alone. Addition of intermediate points of fixation also provided a better translational stability.

In a recent biomechanical study, Yüksel et al. compared the skip corpectomy with standard three-level corpectomy.[37] They reported that skip corpectomy allowed a slightly smaller range of motion during lateral bending and axial rotation than did standard three-level corpectomy. However, high pull-out forces still occurred at superior and inferior vertebral screws during axial rotation. They concluded that skip corpectomy provided a better stability during lateral bending and axial rotation movements of the neck, and because of the high pull-out forces seen in the superior and caudal screws during the axial rotation, the patient's axial rotation should be restrained.

The size of the grafts is another advantage of the skip corpectomy. Whereas one-level or two-level corpectomy can be reconstructed using iliac crest graft, a three-level corpectomy requires a long fibular graft. Skip corpectomy allows the use of two short iliac crests or fibular grafts.

The technique also has the advantage of adding stability to the construct without requiring an additional surgical approach. Although the addition of a second approach provides the greatest stability for the construct, it comes at the expense of increased operative time and the potential for higher surgical morbidity.

Summary

Skip corpectomy allows for effective decompression and stabilization in most cases with CSM and OPLL extending from C3-4 to C6-7.

KEY REFERENCES

Dalbayrak S, Yilmaz M, Naderi S: Skip corpectomy: an alternative approach to multilevel cervical spondylotic myelopathy and ossified posterior longitudinal ligament. *J Neurosurg Spine* 12:33–38, 2010.

DiAngelo DJ, Foley KT, Vossel KA, et al: Anterior cervical plating reverses load transfer through multilevel strut-grafts. *Spine (Phila Pa 1976)* 25:783–795, 2000.

Naderi S, Alberstone CD, Rupp FW, et al: Cervical spondylotic myelopathy treated with corpectomy: technique and results in 44 patients. *Neurosurg Focus* 1(6):e5, 1996.

Ozer AF, Oktenoğlu BT, Sarioğlu AC: A new surgical technique: open-window corpectomy in the treatment of ossification of the posterior longitudinal ligament and advanced cervical spondylosis: technical note. *Neurosurgery* 45:1481–1485, 1999.

Panjabi MM, Isomi T, Wang JL: Loosening at the screw-vertebra junction in multilevel anterior cervical plate constructs. *Spine* 24:2383–2388, 1999.

Sasso RC, Ruggiero RA Jr, Reilly TM, Hall PV: Early reconstruction failures after multilevel cervical corpectomy. *Spine (Phila Pa 1976)* 28:140–142, 2003.

Vaccaro AR, Falatyn SP, Scuderi GJ, et al: Early failure of long segment anterior cervical plate fixation. *J Spinal Disord* 11:410–415, 1998.

Wang JL, Panjabi MM, Isomi T: The role of bone graft force in stabilizing the multilevel anterior cervical spine plate system. *Spine (Phila Pa 1976)* 25:1649–1654, 2000.

REFERENCES

The complete reference list is available online at expertconsult.com.

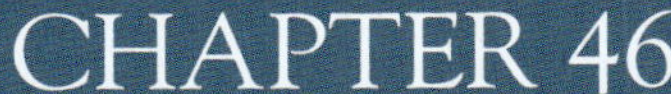

CHAPTER 46

Cervical Laminoplasty

Noboru Hosono | Kazuo Yonenobu

General Principles and History

Laminectomy was first introduced to release the spinal cord compressed at multiple levels, although it fell into relative disfavor due to complications such as laminectomy membrane, segmental instability, kyphosis, and late neurologic deterioration. Ventral decompression and fusion or posterior fusion in addition to laminectomy was a solution in the United States and European countries, whereas laminoplasty was created in Japan, especially for treating ossification of the posterior longitudinal ligament (OPLL). Such ossification is difficult to remove directly via a ventral approach because the extremely hard ossification often tightly adheres to the dura mater. Direct resection of the ossification, therefore, was strongly associated with the potential risk of disastrous cord damage, and postoperative displacement of the grafted bone or pseudarthrosis was not rare, because a long bone graft was needed to span the trough after resection of the long OPLL. All of these complications kept most surgeons away from employing ventral surgery for cervical OPLL. Laminoplasty was developed as a safer and more reliable procedure to treat OPLL in 1971 by Hattori et al.,[1] who expected to enlarge the spinal canal and to relieve neural compression while maintaining a skeletal and ligamentous dorsal arch to prevent epidural scarring and malalignment of the cervical spine. Although this procedure, the so-called Z-shaped laminoplasty, was rather complicated, simpler and more feasible laminoplasty procedures were devised and are now divided into two categories: unilateral (hinge) laminoplasty and bilateral (hinge) laminoplasty. Given that the patients with compressive myelopathy generally have a developmentally narrow spinal canal, decompression over the entire cervical spine with laminoplasty seems more reasonable than ventral decompression surgery, in which operated levels are restricted and adjacent segment disease can take place several years later. Thus, the number of patients with compressive myelopathy who undergo laminoplasty is increasing each year. Several trials to eliminate the disadvantages of laminoplasty are discussed herein.

Indications

The surgical indication for compressive cervical neuropathy is a myelopathy that progresses despite treatment. It is, however, difficult to determine when to apply surgery to cervical myelopathy, because its natural history remains obscure. Apparent ambulatory disturbance is a definite indication, but symptoms no more profound than finger numbness are debatable indicators. Some surgeons prefer the less popular prophylactic laminoplasty to prevent accidental spinal cord injury for patients with a narrow spinal canal even if they have only slight neurologic symptoms. It is, however, difficult to eradicate the risk of spinal cord injury by doing laminoplasty; some patients with OPLL who have residual cord compression after laminoplasty can sustain cord injury due to minor trauma.

Indications for laminoplasty should be discussed in contrast with those for ventral and other dorsal techniques. Generally speaking, a patient with spinal cord compression at one or two levels is a good candidate for anterior decompression and fusion unless the anteroposterior canal diameter is equal to or less than 13 mm. Because most patients with myelopathy who require surgical decompression have a developmentally narrow canal, they are candidates for laminoplasty. Although the spinal cord is assumed to migrate dorsally and escape from anterior lesions by laminoplasty, such a mechanism may not work in two special conditions: kyphosis and the presence of a large anterior lesion. In a kyphotic cervical spine, dorsal cord migration may not be expected after lamina opening, yet some surgeons argue that kyphosis of less than 5 or 10 degrees can benefit from laminoplasty. The extent of kyphosis for which laminoplasty can effectively release the spinal cord remains unknown. The spinal cord does not seem to escape from large and/or steep ventral lesions, even after sufficient dorsal space is provided by laminoplasty. Herniated nucleus pulposus, however, is successfully treated by laminoplasty. Neurologic improvement is excellent after laminoplasty for disc herniation, regardless of whether the herniated nucleus is absorbed after surgery. Beak-type OPLL, in contrast, does not seem to be successfully treated by laminoplasty. Resection or floating of the ossification via the anterior approach should be considered for these patients, although these methods are technically demanding and associated with a high rate of surgical morbidities.

Contraindications

A cervical kyphosis of greater than 5 to 10 degrees is considered a contraindication for laminoplasty, because the spinal cord cannot be released from the anterior lesion if the dorsal space is made by laminoplasty.

Elderly patients who tolerate general anesthesia may be candidates for laminoplasty because the operative impact of laminoplasty is acceptable. There exist, however, arguments regarding the operative outcome for elderly patients. Potential risks for postoperative delirium and cardiovascular accidents should be taken into account.

Subaxial lesions in rheumatoid arthritis (RA) have been treated with arthrodesis, although reduction of neck motion, swallowing disturbance, and adjacent segment disease are not rare after spinal fusion. Laminoplasty is an alternative to diminish the drawbacks associated with arthrodesis. Retrospective investigation in our series revealed that patients with nonmutilating-type RA can benefit from laminoplasty if subaxial subluxation is mild.[2] In contrast, mutilating-type RA and/or RA with vertebral slippage more than 5 mm is a contraindication for laminoplasty. Cervical myelopathy associated with athetoid cerebral palsy may be best treated with laminoplasty combined with fusion. A screw-rod system or a long bone graft spanning all fused levels with a postoperative halo vest is a common technique to attain spinal fusion. Laminoplasty alone has little effect on the myelopathy of athetoid cerebral palsy. Patients undergoing hemodialysis may be candidates for laminoplasty, unless they have destructive spondyloarthropathy, in which spinal instability should be managed by spinal fusion. Pyoderma on the nape skin is a contraindication for laminoplasty, because of the high risk for surgical site infection. Pyoderma is an infectious dermal disease well observed on buttock skin, although head and neck regions may also be affected.

Although laminoplasty was originally developed to treat OPLL, occasional neurologic deterioration is reported immediately after laminoplasty for massive OPLL. The reason for this complication is unclear, but surgeons with expertise have a good reason for choosing ventral surgery for OPLL that has a thickness greater than 50% of the spinal canal.

Techniques

Various types of laminoplasty are in clinical use. They are divided into two major categories: unilateral (hinge) laminoplasty and bilateral (hinge) laminoplasty. In unilateral laminoplasty, or open-door procedure, two bony gutters are drilled on either side of the lamina-facet junction. The gutter on one side is cut out and the lamina is opened by elevating this edge, while the gutter on the other side functions as a hinge by following gentle fracture. The side to be opened does not depend on the laterality of compression. A left-side opening is generally convenient for right-handed surgeons. The opened lamina is kept in situ by sutures placed between holes drilled in the lamina and the facet joint capsule. Postoperative reclosure of the lamina, however, can take place, and the opening space may be spanned by a spacer to maintain the enlarged spinal canal. Resected spinous processes or ceramic spacers are often inserted at every two laminae and fixed by sutures between the lamina edge and the lateral mass. The nonfixed laminae are also kept open by a yellow ligament attached to the adjacent fixed laminae (Fig. 46-1). Small metal plates are alternative implants to maintain the opened lamina, although they are not as popular in Japan as in Western countries. Metal plating adds to the complexity of the operation, is time-consuming, and adds to the expense.

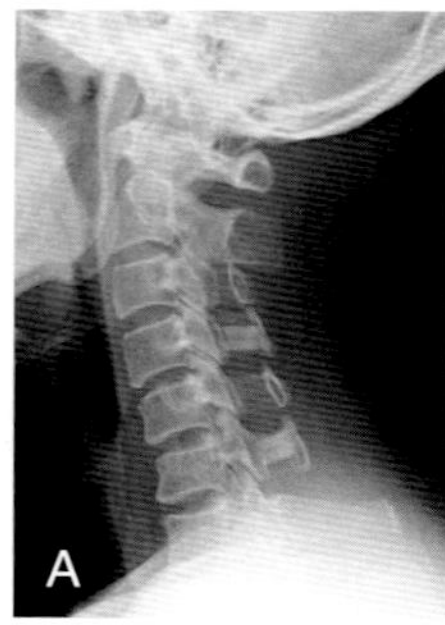

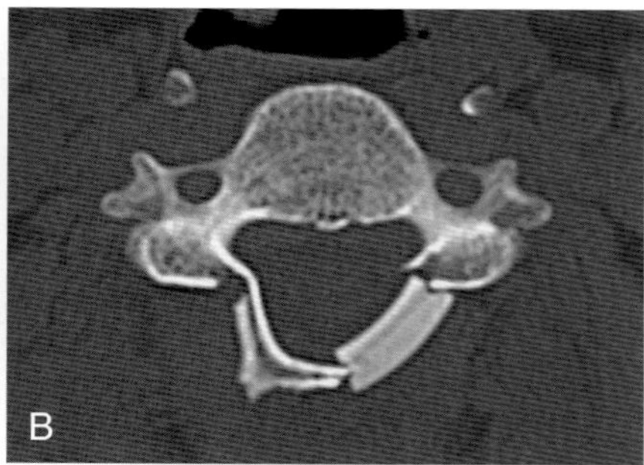

FIGURE 46-1. **A,** Lateral radiograph after unilateral laminoplasty. **B,** CT scan after unilateral laminoplasty. A ceramic spacer is fixed between the opened lamina and the lateral mass with a suture.

With bilateral laminoplasty, or the double-door (French door) procedure, three bony gutters are drilled not only on either side of the lamina-facet junction but also in the midst of the spinous process. After the midline cut is made, each half of the lamina is opened laterally, similar to opening French doors. The lamina was originally kept in situ by inserting a bone graft between each half of the lamina; at present the most popular insertion materials are ceramic spacers. Although ceramic spacers are usually fixed by sutures, they often become displaced in the early postoperative period. The more dorsally the spacers are inserted, the more often the spacers become displaced.

Although the superiority of unilateral or bilateral laminoplasty has been discussed, significant differences between them have not been found so far. Intraoperative blood loss, operating time, outcome, and morbidities are all supposed to be similar between the two kinds of laminoplasties. One more bone gutter to be made in the midst in bilateral laminoplasty seems to be time-consuming for surgeons who prefer unilateral laminoplasty, whereas occasional epidural bleeding from the open side gutter in unilateral laminoplasty seems troublesome for surgeons who advocate bilateral laminoplasty.

When radiculopathy accompanies myelopathy, nerve roots can be released by foraminotomy in addition to laminoplasty. In unilateral laminoplasty, foraminotomy facilitates nerve root exposure on the open side. In bilateral laminoplasty, aggressive foraminotomy might destroy the bony gutter and result in lamina separation. Much care should be taken not to violate the bony gutters. Microsurgical foraminotomy is an alternative method of releasing the nerve roots.

Electrophysiologic monitoring with somatosensory-evoked potentials, motor-evoked potentials, and electromyography is not mandatory for laminoplasty. Inadvertent neural injury cannot be avoided by intraoperative monitoring, and laminoplasty is a relatively safe procedure. Arguments exist over whether electrophysiologic monitoring can detect complications such as C5 palsy. This is doubtful.

During the introduction period of laminoplasty in Japan, a cervical collar was generally applied for a few months after surgery. Surgeons thought that external support was a prerequisite to facilitate bony union of the hinged gutters or grafted bones. However, as unfavorable spine fusion and aggravation of axial neck pain were recognized as the adverse effects of collar application, many surgeons discontinued this practice. In contrast, patients are encouraged to perform isotonic muscle exercises in the early postoperative period to prevent muscle weakness.

Modifications of the Procedure

Reattachment of the Nuchal Muscles to the Spinous Process of the Axis

The rectus major, inferior oblique, and semispinalis cervicis muscles attached to the axis are considered to lend mechanical stability to the cervical spine. These muscles are, therefore, best preserved with laminoplasty, although they often disturb access to the C3 lamina by covering it. Formerly, we cut the tips of the spinous process of the axis along with the origin of these muscles. After opening all laminae, the bony fragments to the axis are replaced, so that these muscles can exert traction force again after laminoplasty.[3] Aggressive retraction, but not cutting, of these muscles is an alternative way, and some surgeons recommend C3 laminectomy to preserve the muscles attached to the axis.

Preservation of the Spinous Process/ Ligament-Muscle Complex

To preserve muscle function, the deep extensor muscles are stripped from the laminae on the side of approach, and the contralateral muscles are preserved by cutting the spinous processes at their bases along with the muscle attachments. The spinous process/ligament-muscle complex is retracted during the process of gutter drilling and lamina opening and reattached to the opened laminae by sutures.

Outcomes

The operating time for laminoplasty is 1 to 3 hours and intraoperative blood loss is 100 to 500 mL. Allogenic transfusion is not usually required. Neurologic gain after laminoplasty is generally excellent. The recovery rate averages from 55% to 60% when the patients are evaluated by the JOA (Japan Orthopedic Association) score, which has subsets for motor and sensory functions of the extremities and bladder function. The operative outcomes, however, vary depending on the outcome measures, including the JOA score, Nurick's scale, and various kinds of performance tests. The grip-and-release test that counts finger motion cycles in maximum effort in 10 or 15 seconds reveals 100% recovery after laminoplasty. It is unclear that laminoplasty produces superior neurologic outcome over laminectomy or anterior surgery, because few studies have conducted a randomized controlled comparison of these surgical procedures. Factors that can predict the outcome of laminoplasty include the patient's age, period of disease, preoperative neurologic status, transverse area of the spinal cord, and preoperative signal changes on MRI. Low-intensity changes on T_1-weighted images and high-intensity changes spanning multiple levels on T_2-weighted images are indicators of poor functional recovery. The outcome of laminoplasty for large OPLL is considered to be especially poor when the anteroposterior occupying ratio to the spinal canal is more than 60%.

Long-term outcomes of laminoplasty are also excellent and maintained for 5 years from surgery, after which neurologic gain is gradually lost in some patients. Approximately 30% of the patients who underwent laminoplasty were reported to encounter neurologic deterioration in the 10-year follow-up.[4] Late deterioration is more frequent in cases of OPLL (27–30%) than in cases of spondylosis (16–30%).[4] Neurologic deterioration after laminoplasty can be attributed to osteoarthritis of the hip or knee joints, degenerative lumbar diseases, cardiovascular and cerebrovascular diseases, minor trauma, age-related dysfunction, progression of cervical OPLL, and thoracic spine ossification, although no causative factors can be identified in some patients. Increase in OPLL thickness is as frequent as 70% of cases in the 10-year follow-up after laminoplasty, although neurologic deterioration results in only 3% to 7%.[5] Thus, the long-term outcome of laminoplasty can be concluded to surpass that of anterior surgery, which definitely has adjacent segment diseases.

Complications

Perioperative Complications

One of the most disastrous complications of laminoplasty is spinal cord injury. In drilling bony gutters with a high-speed drill, it is possible for the bur on the drill to injure the dura mater or even the spinal cord. If the bleeding is such that a clear field cannot be maintained in the drilling area, the bur can go dangerously deep. Because the loss of resistance method is not reliable for preventing inadvertent perforation of the lamina, every effort should be made to minimize bleeding so the drilling area is easy to visualize. Bleeding from the bone marrow of the pedicle, which often makes the irrigation water opaque, may be addressed by applying bone wax. A surgical microscope is not required for the common type of laminoplasty, as long as a clear visual field is maintained by the measures described here. Spinal cord injury with laminoplasty is rare compared with that in the anterior surgery, in which the visual field and working space are smaller than those in laminoplasty.

Another cause of spinal cord injury is the stepwise decompression nature of the procedure. If the laminae are drilled and opened one by one, the decompressed spinal cord migrates dorsally with each opening. The spinal cord can be kinked at the edge of the residual lamina, causing cord injury. Laminae should therefore be opened en bloc over the total decompression area.

Epidural bleeding is a common complication of spinal surgery. The typical blood loss for laminoplasty is about 100 to 500 mL. The epidural venous plexus is rich in the lateral part of the spinal canal, but it is sparse in the midline. In unilateral laminoplasty, bony gutters are made just on the rich epidural vein and bleeding can be massive. Surgeons should take care not to perforate the inner cortex of the lamina, especially when using a steel bur. The best way to cut off the lamina on the opened side is to crack the evenly thinned lamina by rotating the elevator inserted in the gutter (Fig. 46-2). Even after every lamina is cut off in this way, massive bleeding can occur during lamina opening. If a suction tube is effective to allow visualization of the dural surface, lamina opening should be continued to the last lamina prepared because dural expansion by lamina opening often squeezes dilated veins. If bleeding is overwhelming and far beyond suction capacity, the opening process should be transiently interrupted and surgeons may have to wait for a few minutes after placing hemostatic collagen onto the vein until the blood flow decreases. Huge vein networks are difficult to cauterize using a bipolar

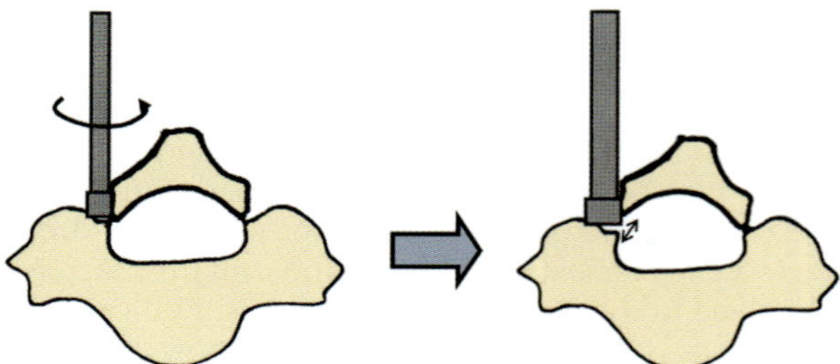

FIGURE 46-2. The best way to cut off the lamina on the opened side is to crack the evenly thinned lamina by rotating the elevator inserted in the gutter.

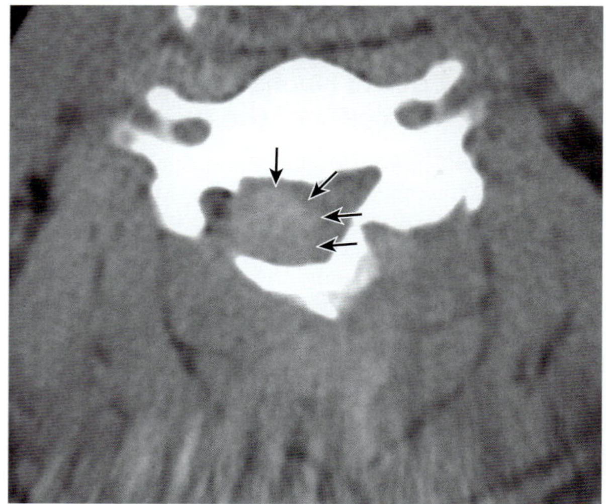

FIGURE 46-3. A 60-year-old man with cervical spondylotic myelopathy. A CT scan just after unilateral laminoplasty indicates that an epidural hematoma (*arrows*) is compressing the spinal cord. Note that the hematoma is limited to the enlarged spinal canal; deep extensor muscles have normal contours without any fluid collection on the lamina.

coagulator. Bleeding, however, is minimal in most cases of unilateral laminoplasty.

Epidural hematoma formation is another common complication of spinal surgery. A subfascial closed wound drain tube should be placed to prevent hematoma formation, although the tube placed on laminae often has no effect in evacuating blood collection under laminae (Fig. 46-3). Laminoplasty has an advantage in that an opened lamina functions as a protector against posterior muscles that may compress the spinal cord, whereas with laminectomy, the exposed spinal cord is susceptible to compression by hematoma or muscles.

Wound dehiscence can occur, especially in patients with athetoid cerebral palsy, in whom dense sutures with nonabsorbable material are recommended to approximate the fascia. Surgical site infection is not frequent after laminoplasty, except in patients with infectious skin diseases such as pyoderma. When the dura mater is injured, most often by a high-speed drill, cerebrospinal fluid leaks postoperatively. The fascia should be sutured densely in a water-tight manner if dural laceration is recognized during surgery. Other treatments for cerebrospinal fluid leak are discussed in another chapter.

Postoperative displacement of an implanted ceramic spacer is more often observed after bilateral laminoplasty than after unilateral laminoplasty (Fig. 46-4). Although ceramic spacers usually migrate dorsally, they can cause not only dural laceration but also cord injury if they displace ventrally.[6] Lamina dropping, or falling forward, on the hinged side is one of the most common complications of laminoplasty. When surgeons realize the complete separation of the hinged side cortex, they should remove the floating lamina to avoid neural injury. Making the bony hinge appropriately flexible is a critical point of laminoplasty, because too loose a hinge makes the lamina drop and too rigid a hinge results in reclosure of the opened lamina (Fig. 46-5).

Palsy of C5 has been the biggest topic of debate in cervical spine surgery. Scoville[7] and Stoops[8] described this complication after laminectomy in 1961, but it was first reported after laminoplasty in 1986. Postoperative C5 palsy is defined as paresis of the deltoid muscle and/or the biceps brachii muscle after cervical decompression surgery without any deterioration of myelopathy symptoms. The vast majority of C5 palsies occur within a week following surgery, and recent studies reveal a shorter latency between surgery and the onset of the C5 palsy than had been previously considered. Some patients present with palsy on the day of surgery. Although the reason why the palsy occurs exclusively in the unilateral C5 nerve root has been extensively discussed, recent papers reveal that the palsy occurs in every root, including C5, C6, C7, and C8, individually or in combination.[9,10] The incidence of palsy is 5% for only the C5 root but 10% for all roots. The incidence of palsy is similar between laminoplasty and anterior cervical surgery. C5 palsy generally recovers spontaneously as long as the palsy is mild. Most mild palsy with a manual muscle testing (MMT) grade of 3 or 4 fully recovers within 6 months, whereas severe palsy with an MMT grade 2 or less recovers only up to a useful level, often taking more than 6 months.

The cause for C5 palsy or upper limb palsy in a broader sense still remains unknown. Inadvertent injury to the nerve root during surgery, nerve root traction caused by consecutive dorsal shifting of the cord following decompression surgery ("tethering phenomenon"), spinal cord ischemia due to decreased blood supply from radicular arteries, segmental spinal cord disorder, and reperfusion injury of the spinal cord have been proposed so far, although none of these alone can effectively account for all of the clinical characteristics of C5 palsy. Tethering phenomenon has been considered the most likely pathogenesis of C5 palsy for a long time. Some authors, however, report that C5 palsy does not necessarily emerge in patients whose dorsal migration of the spinal cord is excessive after laminoplasty.[11,12] Spontaneous recovery of C5 palsy or the palsy after anterior surgery cannot be accounted for by this tethering theory. Reperfusion injury has been advocated recently as a possible cause of C5 palsy. A chronically compressed spinal cord may be injured by free radicals after being exposed to rapid reperfusion of the blood flow. However, the distribution of palsy restricted to a single segment is difficult to explain by reperfusion of the spinal cord. The most recent hypothesis for C5 palsy is thermal damage to the nerve roots. The experimental data suggest that tissues adjacent to drilled bone, especially nerve roots, can be damaged by friction heat from a high-speed drill, which is often beyond 100°C without water irrigation.[13] In experiments simulating hyperthermia therapy, not only the latent period between thermal damage

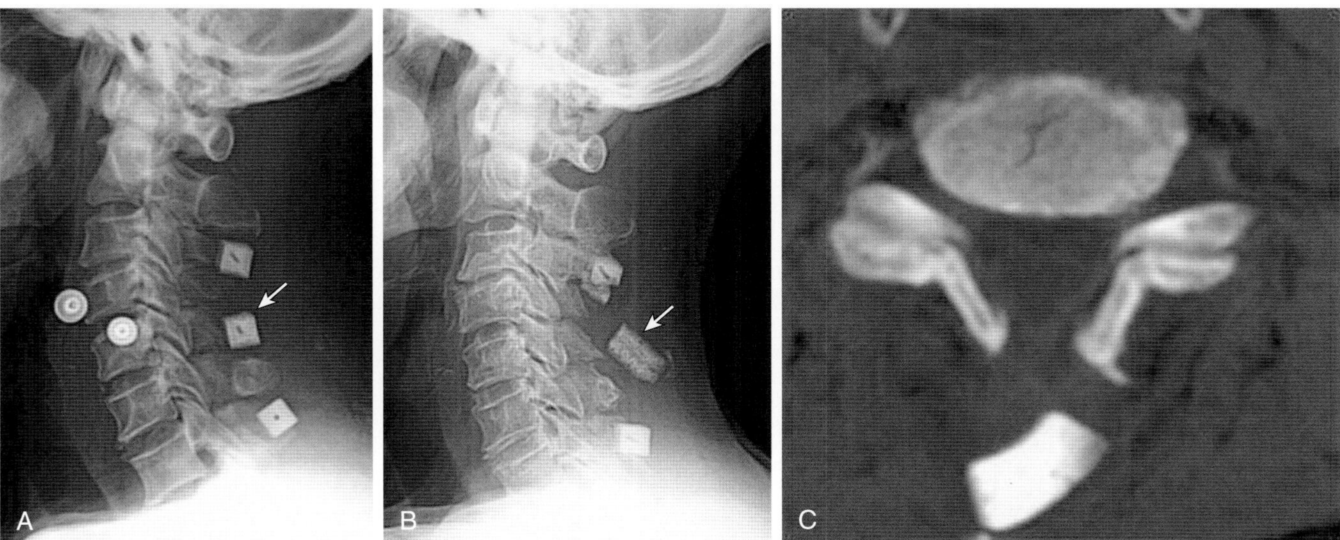

FIGURE 46-4. A 74-year-old woman with cervical spondylotic myelopathy. A ceramic spacer at C5 is displaced dorsally with no concomitant symptoms. **A,** A lateral radiograph just after laminoplasty. **B,** A lateral radiograph 4 years after laminoplasty. **C,** A CT scan 4 years after laminoplasty.

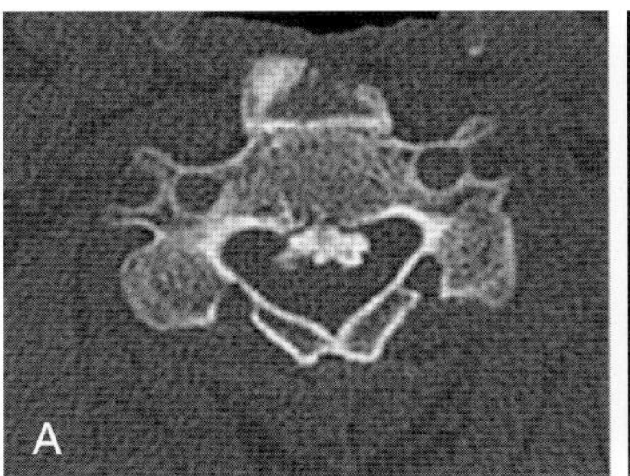

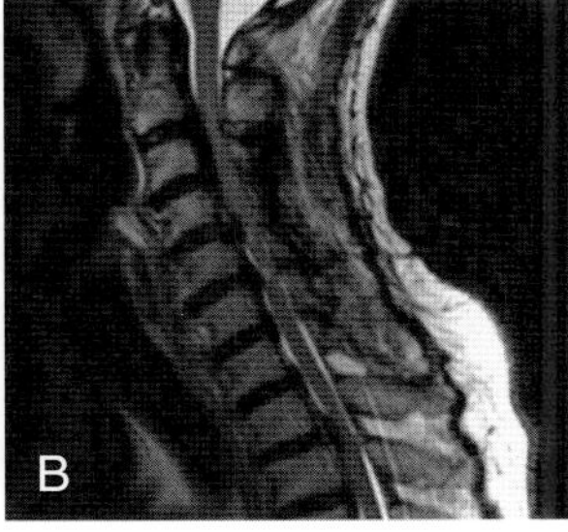

FIGURE 46-5. A 53-year-old man with ossification of the posterior longitudinal ligament. After bilateral laminoplasty, opened laminae returned to their original position, compressing the spinal cord again. When the patient visited our hospital 12 years after the initial laminoplasty, he was experiencing severe tetraparesis. Because the midline gutter had already fused, we chose unilateral laminoplasty as salvage surgery. **A,** CT scan before salvage surgery. **B,** MRI before salvage surgery.

and palsy but also motor recovery after several weeks is indicated. This characteristic coincides with the clinical course of C5 palsy.

Axial neck pain is the most frequent complication of laminoplasty, with an incidence of 10% to 20%. It can be defined as the appearance of neck and shoulder pain after cervical spine surgery. Since its first report in 1992, many attempts were made to reduce this notorious complication. The most effective preventive measure is to discard the cervical collar after surgery. Long-term collar application definitely aggravates axial pain, and no collar application decreases the incidence and intensity of axial pain. A trend of not using a collar after laminoplasty has emerged. The pathogenesis of axial pain, however, is still obscure. Because axial pain is much more frequently observed after laminoplasty than after anterior surgery, the disruption of posterior neck tissues is suspected to be the origin of pain. Intermittent decompression by skip laminectomy[14] or minimally invasive laminoplasty using a tubular retractor seems promising to decrease axial neck pain by preserving posterior neck tissues. Such procedures, however, appear complicated and time-consuming. We realized that postoperative axial pain significantly decreased by limiting the range of laminoplasty from C3-7 to C3-6.[15] The C7 spinous process with various tissue attachments has a critical biomechanical importance and should be spared from the range of laminoplasty. Given the rarity of cord compression at C6-7 in cervical spondylosis, C3-6 laminoplasty seems to be a necessary and sufficient procedure, although another strategy may be needed in treating OPLL.

Late Complications

Long-term outcome of laminoplasty is generally good, and late neurologic complications such as adjacent segment disease are seldom reported so far. Late complications are largely radiologic changes, which are divided into alignment change, range of motion change, and instability development including slippage. Sagittal alignment tends to be kyphotic after laminoplasty, although one of the advantages of laminoplasty is the paucity of postoperative kyphosis compared with conventional laminectomy. Lordotic alignment accounts for 70% of patients before laminoplasty and 50% after laminoplasty in both patients with spondylosis and OPLL. However, severe kyphosis resulting in neurologic deterioration seldom develops. Range of cervical motion significantly decreases to 20% to 35% of the preoperative range 10 years after laminoplasty. The reduction in range of motion is greater after laminoplasty than after anterior corpectomy surgery that fuses 2.5 interspaces on average. Although the unintended fusion of facet joints or of opened laminae is supposed to cause the reduction in range of motion, no application of a cervical collar and early postoperative neck exercise can be expected to minimize the reduction in range of motion. Segmental instability, vertebral slippage, and adjacent segmental degeneration that requires treatment are rare after laminoplasty.

KEY REFERENCES

Chiba K, Ogawa Y, Ishii K, et al: Long-term results of expansive open-door laminoplasty for cervical myelopathy: average 14-year follow-up study. *Spine (Phila Pa 1976)* 31:2998–3005, 2006.

Hosono N, Miwa T, Mukai Y, et al: Potential risk of thermal damage to nerve roots by a high-speed drill: a possible cause of C5 palsy after cervical spine surgery. *J Bone Joint Surg [Br]* 11:1541–1544, 2009.

Hosono N, Sakaura H, Mukai Y, et al: C3-6 laminoplasty takes over C3-7 laminoplasty with significantly lower incidence of axial neck pain. *Eur Spine J* 15:1375–1379, 2006.

Iwasaki M, Kawaguchi Y, Kimura T, Yonenobu K: Long-term results of expansive laminoplasty for ossification of the posterior longitudinal ligament of the cervical spine: more than 10 years follow up. *J Neurosurg* 96(2 Suppl): 180–189, 2002.

Kaito T, Hosono N, Makino T, et al: Postoperative displacement of hydroxyapatite spacers implanted during double-door laminoplasty. *J Neurosurg Spine* 10:551–556, 2009.

Shiraishi T: A new technique for exposure of the cervical spine laminae. Technical note. *J Neurosurg* 96(Suppl 1):122–126, 2002.

Yonenobu K, Wada E, Ono K: Laminoplasty for myelopathy. Indications, results, outcome and complications. In Clark CR, editor: *The cervical spine*, ed 4, Philadelphia, 2004, Lippincott Williams & Wilkins, pp 1057–1071.

REFERENCES

The complete reference list is available online at expertconsult.com.

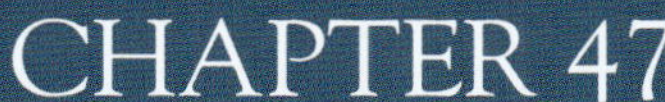

Interspinous, Laminar, and Facet Fusion

Noel I. Perin | Joseph F. Cusick

Basic to the details of therapeutic intervention, either operative or nonoperative, is an understanding of the biomechanical principles of cervical spine function. These considerations permit the most effective planning of a specific treatment, especially the details of surgical intervention. Generally, in the cervical region, the major mechanism of injury is transmission of force through the head. The corresponding changes are usually related to flexion, extension, or rotation, with associated axial compression or distraction. Clarification of these factors assists the surgeon in designing the most appropriate procedure. A surgeon therefore desires to counteract the major force vectors responsible for the principal injury pattern. (One would not accentuate an extension-compression or extension-distraction injury by increasing extension forces with certain posterior fixation procedures.) The selected method of treatment should be based on the biomechanics of the injury and the experience and preference of the surgeon. This chapter covers the factors predisposing to instability in the subaxial (C3-7) cervical spine and the management of instability, using wire and cable techniques. Allen et al.[1] proposed a mechanistic classification based on biomechanical considerations of the injury vectors. Panjabi and White[2] proposed a working classification, especially for acute instability, in which more than 3.5 mm of anterolisthesis or more than 11 degrees of angulation constitutes instability in the lower cervical spine; this classification may be helpful in evaluation. In awake patients who fail to demonstrate radiologic evidence of instability with routine cervical spine films, flexion-extension lateral radiographs should be obtained. Dynamic radiographs, however, should be approached with a level of caution. The situation is often best approached initially by CT, with sagittal reconstruction for full definition of the possible injury patterns. If instability is not demonstrated with the aforementioned studies yet is suspected from the increased prevertebral soft tissue swelling and the severe neck pain, these patients should be placed in a firm cervical collar and the flexion-extension films repeated in 2 weeks. The elapsed time allows muscle spasm to abate and allows demonstration of ligamentous instability on the flexion-extension radiographs.

Initial Management

An accident victim with suspected cervical spine injury should have the head and neck immobilized in a firm cervical collar, or with sandbags, before being transported. In the emergency department, after stabilization of the respiratory and hemodynamic status, a rapid neurologic assessment is undertaken. Radiographs of the cervical spine are obtained, paying special attention to visualization of C7-T1 levels. Patients with evidence of instability on the initial evaluation are placed in traction using Gardner-Wells tongs or a halo ring. Traction is initiated at 10 lbs, with appropriate head and neck positioning dependent on the mechanism and radiologic appearance of the injury.

Muscle relaxation with agents such as diazepam (Valium) assists reduction of the subluxation and alignment of the spine. Weights are added in 5-lb increments to a maximum of 35 to 40 lbs. Lateral cervical spine radiographs are obtained after each weight or position change to monitor cervical spine alignment. Patients with injuries that do not reduce on graded cervical traction, as well as those who cannot tolerate traction, are considered for early surgical reduction and stabilization. All patients with spinal cord injury with moderate to severe neurologic deficit are started on the Solu-Medrol protocol.[3]

Imaging Evaluation

After initial evaluation with plain radiographs, patients who are neurologically intact as well as those with residual neurologic function below the level of the injury should have an MRI scan or a myelogram with postmyelographic CT scan. These studies demonstrate the presence of any soft tissue compression (disc herniation) on the neural elements. If an MRI scan is performed, a CT scan with bone windows should be obtained to assess the bony anatomy of the fracture. In patients without neurologic function below the level of the injury, it may be sufficient to obtain CT images only to assess the anatomy of the fracture.

Timing of Surgery

Surgery for cervical spine instability may be performed ultra early (in <6–8 hours), early (in 24–72 hours), or late (several days to weeks later). The temporal course of events may be conditioned by the presence of other associated injuries, but generally most surgeons operate on these patients between 24 and 72 hours, unless during this period there is deterioration of the patient's neurologic status since admission.

Deterioration of the neurologic status may suggest corresponding vertebral artery compromise or other events that may indicate consideration for emergent surgery. In patients with partial neurologic injury and nonreduction of the subluxation, the ongoing bony or soft tissue compression may suggest a theoretical advantage to early surgery in reducing secondary neurologic injury; the full validity of this concept has not been fully defined, however.[4] In neurologically intact patients and patients with a complete neurologic deficit noted from the outset, timing is not as critical. However, early mobilization should minimize pulmonary and other complications.

Operative Techniques

Positioning, Intubation, and Monitoring

Patients in traction are brought to the operating room in their beds. Patients with normal neurologic function and those with residual neurologic function below the level of the injury are potential candidates for somatosensory-evoked potential (SSEP) and motor-evoked potential (MEP) monitoring. Oral endotracheal intubation entails extension of the neck, which may be hazardous in patients with instability. In the presence of significant instability, after awake fiberoptic intubation the patient is turned to the prone position while awake, in a firm cervical collar or in traction. A rapid neurologic examination is carried out before anesthesia is given.

The patient is turned to the prone position, in a firm cervical collar with manual traction applied to the head ring by the surgeon. The head is supported in a cerebellar head rest, and traction is reestablished (Fig. 47-1). Mayfield skull clamps can be used if alignment can be maintained without traction. The latter mode of fixation minimizes problems with pressure necrosis of the face and potentially disastrous ocular injury. A lateral cervical spine radiograph is obtained to check alignment after turning and positioning the patient.

Exposure

The neck (up to the occiput) and the area around the iliac crest and posterior superior iliac spine are routinely prepared and draped. A midline incision is made in the neck; the length of the incision depends on the number of segments to be addressed. It is critical to stay in the midline to avoid excessive bleeding. The paracervical muscles are stripped subperiosteally from the spine and laminae and retracted laterally. The possibility of preexisting bony or ligamentous incompetence with associated instability or dural exposure cautions the surgeon to exercise care in the exposure of the dorsal elements. Supported by preoperative imaging information, dissection is accomplished sharply. Blunt dissection and monopolar cautery are avoided. The dissection is carried to the lateral edge of the facet joints. When possible, the supraspinous and interspinous ligaments are preserved. Once the spine is exposed, a lateral radiograph is obtained with a marker on the spinous process to identify the levels to be fused.

Reduction of preoperatively unreduced, unilateral, or bilateral locked ("jumped") facets should be attempted at this time. The tip of the superior facet is drilled. Using two straight curettes between the adjacent laminae in the "tire-lever" B-type maneuver and working from medially to laterally toward the facet joint, the surgeon removes the superior facet ventral to the inferior facet (Fig. 47-2). In cases in which there is a facet fracture with encroachment into the neural foramen, this fragment of bone should be removed to relieve pressure on the exiting nerve root. The surgeon should always be aware of the potential for a lateral mass fracture that mimics a unilateral facet displacement.

Wire and Cable Fixation

The dorsal anatomic configuration of the subaxial cervical spine favors the use of adjunctive wire and cable fixation techniques. Wire and cable can be passed through and around spinous processes, through facet joints, and underneath the

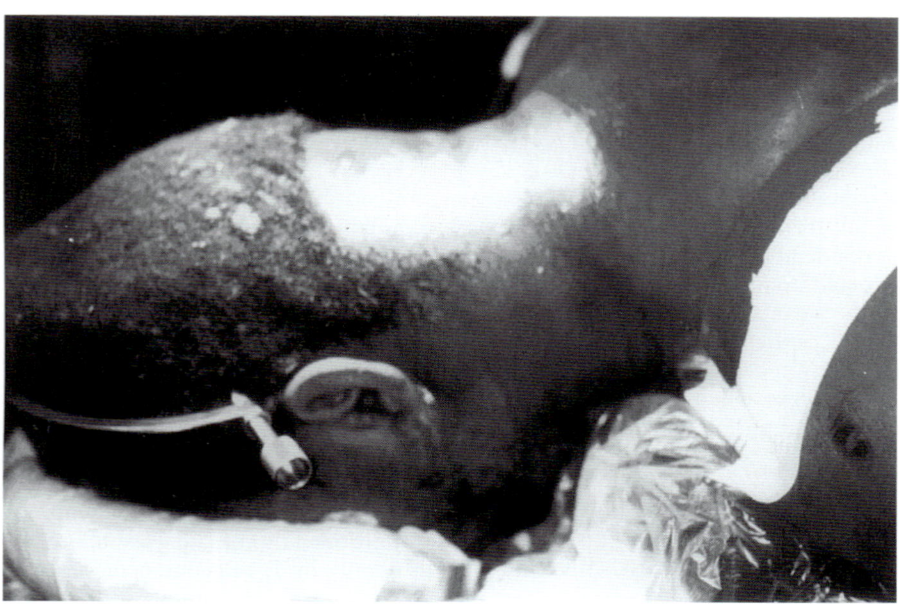

FIGURE 47-1. Patient prone in cervical traction.

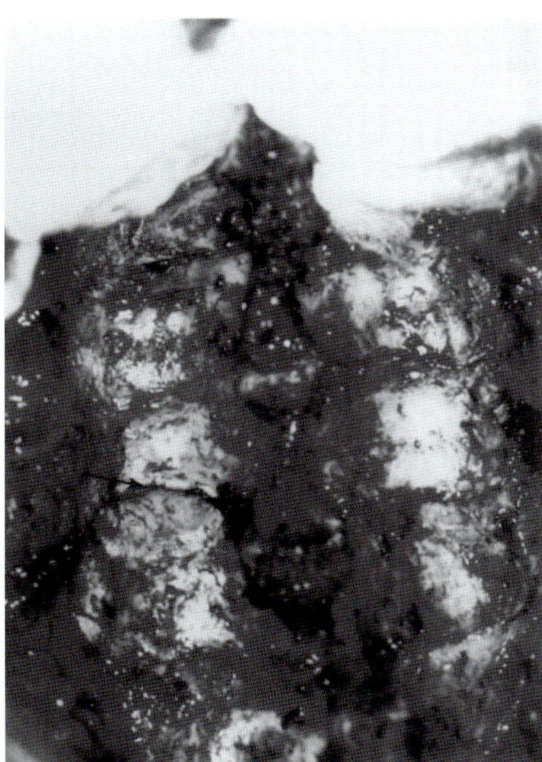

FIGURE 47-2. Reduction of jumped facet.

laminae. Sublaminar passage of wire in the subaxial spine may injure the spinal cord. Thus most surgeons restrict the use of sublaminar cables and wires to the more capacious upper cervical spine only, avoiding the regions of cervical spinal cord enlargement. These wires and cables can also be used to hold the bone graft to the spine, laminae, and facets.

For maximum efficiency, the wire and cable should be strong, malleable, and MRI compatible. The cable systems on the market, in addition to fulfilling these criteria, are coupled with high-quality instrumentation and have generated a renewed interest in the use of wiring in the cervical spine.

Interspinous Wiring

The majority of patients with cervical spine instability can be treated with wiring. Since Rogers first reported a high success rate for cervical fusion with a single, interspinous wiring, numerous techniques of dorsal wiring have been defined. As previously noted, the availability of commercially prepared, braided-wire (cable) systems has improved the technical ease of applying some of these wiring methods. Basically the systems are 18 gauge (Songer) and 20 gauge (Codman), with varying characteristics that may offer improved usage in different constructs. Each system is available in stainless steel or titanium, with specific force application limits that are dependent on the specific type of metal. The braided character of the cables markedly improves strength and malleability. These characteristics are not meant to imply a universal acceptance of the cable systems in creating dorsal constructs; some surgeons prefer the less malleable Luque wire, especially when applying compression techniques with spinous process wiring.[5]

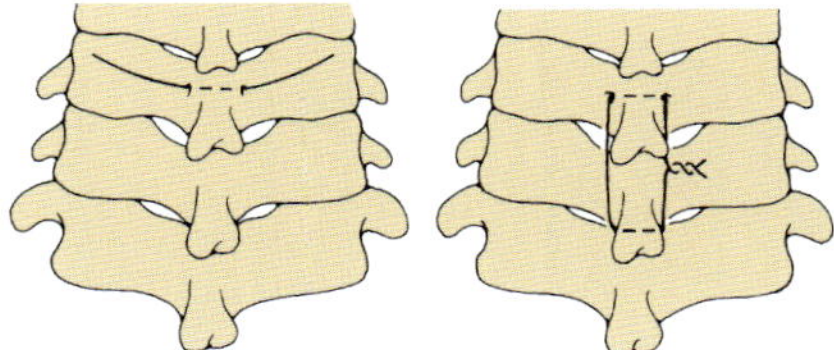

FIGURE 47-3. Interspinous wiring technique (single-level fusion).

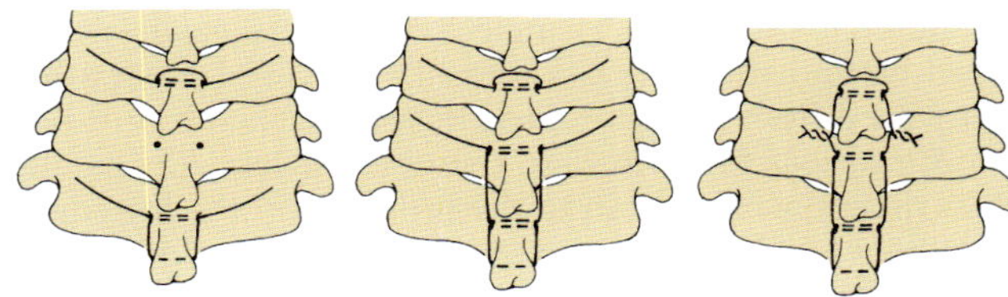

FIGURE 47-4. Interspinous wiring in multilevel fusion with equalization twists.

After exposure of the appropriate levels in the cervical spine and confirmation by radiography, the process of wiring can begin. For spinous process wiring, a transverse hole is made at the junction of the spinous process and lamina of the most rostral level to be fused. This can be made using a power drill and can be completed with a large towel clip. Care should be taken not to angle the drill ventrally and enter the spinal canal. The use of a right-angled dental drill appliance permits a straight lateral drill path. The leader wire of the cable system is passed through the drill hole at the spinolaminar junction and then carried distally, parallel across the interspace, down to the next most rostral spinous process. The cable ends are then passed in opposite directions around the caudal aspect of that spinous process (Fig. 47-3A and B). The cable is tightened with the Tensioner-Crimper, as defined by the recommendations of the system's manufacturer. The wire can also be looped around the rostral border of the spinolaminar junction of the upper level and then threaded in opposite directions through the drill hole at the spinolaminar junction, before being carried caudally.[6] Alternatively, the cable can be passed in the form of a loop through two drill holes at the base of the two spinous processes to be fused. In multilevel fusion each level is wired individually, beginning at the rostral end (Fig. 47-4). This latter construct places the majority of the stress between the donor bone and wire, rather than between the spinous process and wire.

With dorsal cervical interspinous compression wiring in the subaxial spine,[7] the base of the most rostral spinous process to be fused is cannulated. Double-stranded, 22-gauge, stainless-steel wire is passed through the hole in the upper spinous process and around the base of the lower spinous process. A single-stranded, 22-gauge wire (compression wire) is placed between the two spinous processes and underneath the twisted wire. Then it is used to secure the bone graft to the spinous processes. The two ends of the double-stranded cerclage wire are twisted together to achieve the required alignment of the cervical spine (Fig. 47-5).

Triple-Wire Technique

Three wires are used in the triple-wire technique.[8] A drill hole is made at the spinolaminar junction, as described previously. Both levels to be fused have drill holes made at the

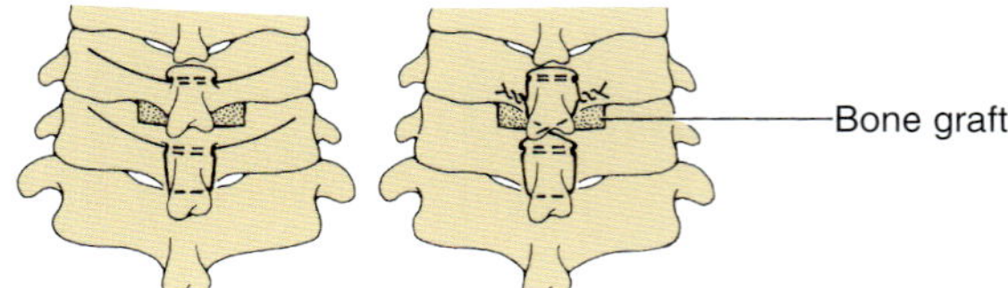

FIGURE 47-5. Compression wiring: two-wire crossover technique.

spinolaminar junction. A single-stranded, 20-gauge wire is looped around the rostral border of the rostral process and then passed from opposite directions through the drill hole in that process. The wires are then passed caudally, parallel across the interspace down to the drill hole in the lower process. One end of the wire is passed through the drill hole at the caudal process and then looped around the base of the spinous process at that level, before coming back through the same drill hole. It is torqued to the opposite end of the wire that is emerging from the rostral drill hole (Fig. 47-6). This wiring arrangement is described as the tethering wire. Two separate 22-gauge wires are passed from either side through the same holes to secure the bone graft. After decortication, the two corticocancellous strips of bone are wired down snugly. Biomechanical studies have verified the strength of this construct, and case reviews have described excellent union with this technique.[8]

Oblique Wiring

Most wiring techniques are effective in restricting flexion, but are less effective in limiting extension and especially rotation. Modification of wire fixation has been developed to aid in the treatment of rotational instability, especially as encountered with facet dislocation.[9] A standard dorsal midline incision is made in the neck, with the patient in the prone position. The segments to be fused are exposed, with care taken not to take down the supraspinous, interspinous, and capsular ligaments. After the segmental level is confirmed with lateral cervical radiographs, the facet joint capsule at the level to be fused is taken down. If the facet dislocation is not reduced, this can be achieved manually, as described in the previous section. A small, angled curette is used to remove articular cartilage from within the facet joint to be fused. The facet joint is opened using a Penfield, or periosteal, elevator, which is also used to protect the superior facet below during drilling. To open the facet joint and ease the wire passage, it is advisable to bur down the superior facet. Often the frustration of passing a facet wire is caused by the lack of a widely opened facet joint. A 3⁄32-inch drill, or bur, is used to make the hole in the inferior facet (Fig. 47-7). The drill hole is made at the center of the inferior facet, angled slightly medially and caudally. A 22-gauge braided wire or cable is passed through the drill hole, with the facet joint kept open by the Penfield dissector. The end of the wire, or "leader," of the cable is picked up within the joint with a curved hemostat. By a combination of pushing and feeding the wire from above, together with pulling from below, the wire is threaded. Vigorous pulling and pushing will produce a "Gigli saw" effect and cut through the inferior facet. The upper limb of the wire is passed through the interspinous ligament above the spinous process to be wired, and the lower limb of the wire is passed through the interspinous ligament below the spinous process to be wired (Fig. 47-8). The wire is twisted, or the cable is torqued and crimped on the opposite side of the lower spinous process. The application, in a bilateral fashion, establishes both flexion and rotational stability.

If the inferior facet is fractured and cannot take a wire or cable, the wiring must skip to the next intact rostral inferior facet. The upper limb of the wire or cable, in this instance, instead of passing between the middle and caudal spinous processes, passes above the middle spinous process and then joins the caudal limb and passes below the caudal spinous process, as described previously.

Other variations on the technique depend on the injury and fracture pattern and include unilateral and bilateral oblique wiring with interspinous wiring and bone grafting.

Facet Wiring

The facet joints are major determinants of cervical motion. Numerous studies have demonstrated that facet joint instability occurs with both dorsal ligamentous and dorsal bony injuries.[10-12] Functional unit studies have shown approximately a 30% decrease in stiffness to flexion-compression load with unilateral facetectomy and approximately a 50% decrease in stiffness with bilateral facetectomies. Facet-to-facet or facet-to-spinous process fixation resulted in significant restoration to intact levels but demonstrated persistent interspinous motion.[10] This latter finding suggests that facet wiring techniques should be associated with spinous process wiring, if available. Other in vitro studies have verified the relative contribution of the facet joint to stability and the merits of fixation.[11,12]

The technique of wire placement is similar to oblique wiring. Again, the wide opening formed in the facet joint by drilling down the upper portion of the superior facet assists wire or cable passage. A bicortical, biconcave bone graft is laid over the decorticated facets to be fused, and the two limbs of the facet wires are brought around the bone graft and twisted (Fig. 47-9).[13] This construct, however, may not provide adequate stiffening and is best considered primarily a method to secure the graft to the facets. A similar technique may also be used to wire down contoured rods and Luque rectangles, especially in postlaminectomy patients. This latter form of

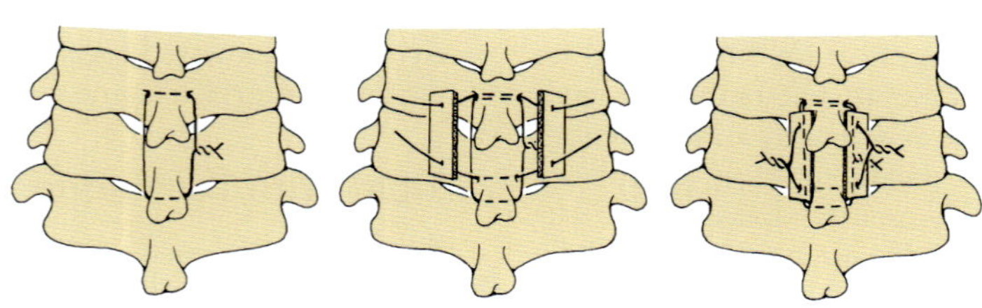

FIGURE 47-6. Triple-wire technique.

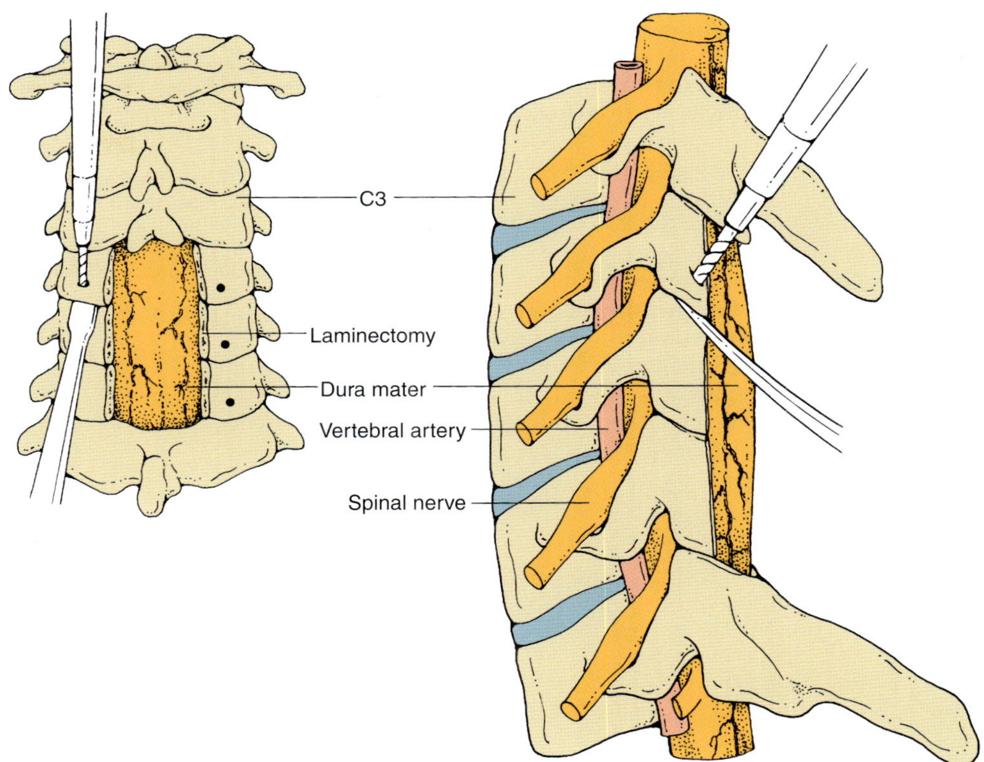

FIGURE 47-7. Drilling for facet fusion. The hole is being drilled through the inferior facet into the joint.

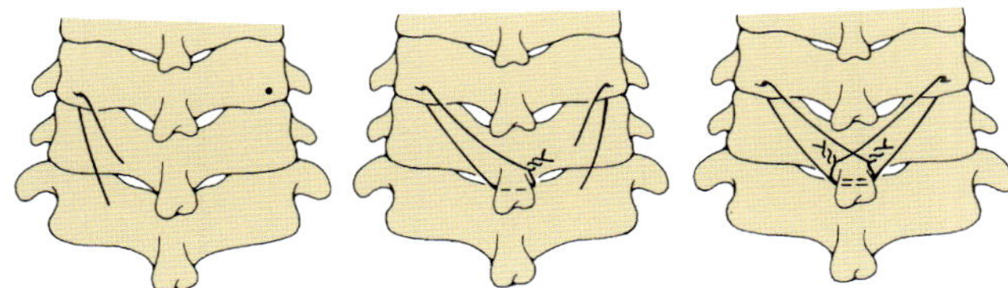

FIGURE 47-8. Oblique wiring technique: bilateral facet to spinous process wiring.

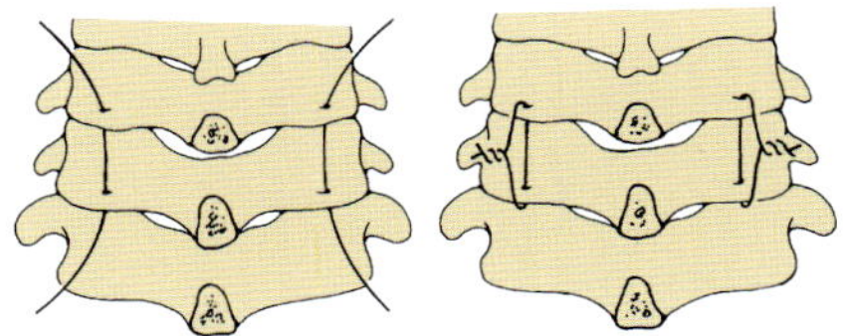

FIGURE 47-9. Interfacet wiring with ipsilateral wires.

stabilization will significantly decrease flexibility, offering a firmer construct with improved expectations for resistance to flexion, extension, and rotation.[14]

Often, securing the Luque rectangle, or similar metal construct, requires sublaminar and facet wiring, in conjunction with autologous bone grafting of the facets and facet joints. In the passage of sublaminar wires, the operator must again consider the potential of compromising underlying neural structures, especially at the level of the cervical spinal cord enlargement. In this aspect, preoperative MRI will assist in clarifying the epidural and subarachnoid space at the C2 and T1 levels. Some surgeons prefer Songer cables at the proximal and distal sublaminar points and soft-wire cables (Codman) for facet passage.

Fusion

Bone fusion should be performed in all patients who undergo dorsal subaxial wire or cable fixation. Autograft should be used in all cases for best results. The iliac crest is the best source of bone for grafting. An incision is made over the posterior superior iliac spine and extended laterally over the dorsal iliac crest. The incision should not extend more than 6 to 7 cm lateral to the posterior superior iliac spine. The cluneal nerves may be injured beyond this point, which can lead to postoperative gluteal numbness and painful neuralgias. The iliac crest is exposed subperiosteally, and the greater sciatic notch is palpated. The superior gluteal artery emerges from the greater sciatic notch and traverses between the gluteus medius and minimus muscles. Injury to the artery may be difficult to control because the injured proximal stump of the vessel can retract into the pelvis, necessitating a pelvic exploration to control bleeding. Subperiosteal stripping of the gluteal muscles and avoiding the greater sciatic notch will prevent this complication. Strips of corticocancellous and cancellous bone are obtained for onlay grafting.

The dorsal elements of the subaxial spine to be fused are decorticated with a cutting bur. Roughening of the bone is usually sufficient in the cervical spine to assist onlay bone fusion. The facet joint to be fused is denuded of capsule, and a small, curved curette is used to remove the joint cartilage and roughen the opposing surfaces of the facet joint. Cancellous bone graft is interposed into the facet joint before the wire or cable is tightened. Further bone graft is laid around the wires over the decorticated spines and laminae. In the technique of facet wiring, bicortical bone graft, contoured in two planes, is laid over the decorticated lateral masses and facets to be fused and wired.

Summary

Injuries to the dorsal osseoligamentous complex are most suited for dorsal wire or cable techniques. The introduction of cable systems into the market has renewed an interest in wire fixation of the cervical spine. The particular technique chosen to stabilize an unstable cervical spine will depend on the injury pattern, the experience, and the preference of the surgeon.

KEY REFERENCES

Benzel EC, Kesterson L: Posterior cervical interspinous compression wiring and fusion for mid to low cervical spinal injuries. *J Neurosurg* 70:893–899, 1989.

Cooper PR, Cohen A, Rosiello A, Koslow M: Posterior stabilization of cervical spine fractures and subluxations using plates and screws. *Neurosurgery* 23:300–306, 1988.

Cusick JF, Yoganandan N, Pintar FA, Hussain H: Biomechanics of cervical spine facetectomy and fixation techniques. *Spine (Phila Pa 1976)* 13: 808–812, 1988.

McAfee PC, Bohlman HH, Wilson WL: Triple wire technique for stabilization of acute cervical fracture dislocations. *Orthop Trans* 10:455–456, 1986.

Zdeblick TA, Zau DD, Warden KE, et al: Cervical stability after foraminotomy. *J Bone Joint Surg [Am]* 74:22–29, 1992.

REFERENCES

The complete reference list is available online at expertconsult.com.

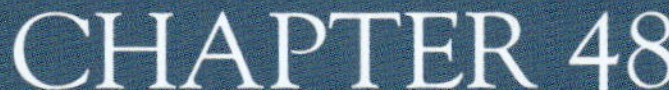

CHAPTER 48

Combined Ventral-Dorsal Surgery

Amrendra S. Miranpuri | Gregory R. Trost

Disorders of the cervical spine can be considered for combined ventral and dorsal surgery in one setting. The indications for these cases may be small in number but when necessary can be technically demanding with associated significant morbidity.[1,2] Traditionally, such operations were most appropriate for trauma patients having three-column instability, much like that seen in the thoracolumbar model described by Denis.[3] With anterior and posterior ligamentous and osseous disruption, combined ventral and dorsal surgery may provide short- and long-term stability and prevent late kyphotic deformity.[4,5]

Acute trauma of the cervical spine, kyphotic deformity, symptomatic pseudarthosis, rheumatoid arthritis, ankylosing spondylitis, neoplasms, and cervical spondylotic myelopathy have benefitted from combined ventral and dorsal operations from a biomechanical and symptomatic relief standpoint. Consideration of patients for a combined ventral and dorsal operation includes several factors. Patient age, comorbidities, bone quality (e.g., osteoporosis), degree of ligamentous and bony disruption, and surgeon's level of expertise can all influence the results of a combined versus single side approach.

It is clear that a combined operation under a single anesthetic offers savings in blood loss, incidence of wound infections, hospital stay, and total cost.[1,2] This chapter summarizes some indications for performing combined surgery, as well as the technical and complicating factors associated with such procedures.

Acute Cervical Spine Injury

Patients who suffer traumatic cervical spine injury will have plain radiographs taken or CT imaging performed. Although these methods can demonstrate osseous injury, ligamentous injury is not accurately depicted. Advanced imaging such as MRI should be considered in the patient who is stable and is being considered for a ventral, dorsal, or combined procedure.[6]

The three-column framework for managing spinal instability in the thoracolumbar spine can likewise be incorporated in acute cervical spine injury patients.[3] Before the use of MRI, Cybulski et al. reviewed the factors that make three-column disruption more likely: (1) disruption of anterior and posterior longitudinal ligaments; (2) dislocation of facets; and (3) disruption of the posterior interspinous ligaments with sufficient force to cause shear dislocation of one vertebra on another.[6]

Although posterior tension band stabilization procedures can be performed on most reduced cervical fracture-dislocations, Cybulski et al. recommend consideration of circumferential surgery in cases of significant three-column instability. Distractive-flexion or compressive-flexion injuries corrected with posterior fusion were the most likely to need a ventral fusion. These injuries apply horizontal shearing forces that destabilize all three columns.[6]

In defining the most optimal procedure, most shortcomings arise from a lack of standardized nomenclature or a scoring system.[7] Vaccaro et al. proposed a scoring system (subaxial injury classification, SLIC) based on three key features: (1) injury morphology as determined by mechanism of injury from existing imaging studies; (2) integrity of the discoligamentous soft tissue complex (DLC) based on anterior and posterior longitudinal ligamentous structures and the intervertebral disc, and (3) patient neurology (Table 48-1).[8] An ideal classification system would be based on fracture pattern,

TABLE 48-1

Subaxial Injury Classification

	Points
Morphology	
No abnormality	0
Compression	1
Burst	+1–2
Distraction (e.g., facet perch, hyperextension)	3
Rotation/translation (e.g., facet dislocation, unstable teardrop, advanced-stage flexion-compression injury	4
Discoligamentous complex	
Intact	0
Indeterminate (e.g., isolated interspinous widening, MRI signal change only)	1
Disrupted (e.g., widening of disc space, facet perch, dislocation)	2
Neurologic Status	
Intact	0
Root injury	1
Complete cord injury	2
Incomplete cord injury	3
Continuous cord compression in setting of neurologic deficit (neuromodifier)	+1

Data from Vaccaro AR, Hurlbert RJ, Fisher CG, et al: The sub-axial cervical spine injury classification system (SLIC): a novel approach to recognize the importance of morphology, neurology and integrity of the discoligamentous complex. *Spine (Phila Pa 1976)* 32(23):2365–2374, 2007.

suspected mechanism of injury, spinal alignment, neurologic injury, and prognosis of long-term stability.[8] The Vaccaro classification was derived from literature review and surveys done with the Spine Trauma Study Group (STSG, founded in 2004, consisting of 50 surgeons from 12 countries dedicated to improving interpretation and management of traumatic spine conditions). The results demonstrated that DLC is the most difficult to objectify on the basis of low interrater and intrarater intraclass correlation coefficient (ICC). There was a high degree of validity, with 93.3% of raters agreeing on a treatment plan based on the SLIC algorithm.[8]

Dvorak et al.[7] described an algorithm for deciding the choice of surgical approach on the basis of a systematic review of the literature, as well as opinions of 48 spine surgeons comprising the STSG. On the basis of the scoring system from the SLIC scale, algorithms were created by the STSG. Although many approaches described are for either ventral or dorsal approaches, some algorithms conclude with a combined approach. In distraction injuries with hyperextension injury with or without avulsion fractures, the fusion construct can be addressed ventrally. However, in cases of severe spondylosis, diffuse idiopathic skeletal hyperostosis, or ankylosing spondylitis, the adjacent level stiffness is best neutralized with an additional dorsal approach. For bilateral facet subluxations (perches facets without fracture) there is a higher incidence of kyphosis after posterior fusion alone speculating progressive disc space collapse as a cause for failure. End-plate compression fracture with facet fracture/dislocation almost always requires a combined approach. In those who have a ventral surgery alone, there may be early mechanical failure of the fusion. Severe ventral vertebral body fractures including teardrop fractures and burst-fracture dislocations have posterior element failure as a common feature (Fig. 48-1). These patients are candidates for a combined approach. In unilateral or bilateral facet fracture dislocations (no vertebral body fracture) a posterior approach is often used. However, if prereduction MRI demonstrates a disc fragment displaced into the spinal canal or the patient declines neurologically after closed reduction, a concomitant anterior discectomy, reduction, and fusion approach is recommended.[7]

Kyphotic Deformity

Cervical kyphosis can occur because of several conditions, including trauma, malignancy, inflammatory disease, infection, spondylosis, and iatrogenic processes. Postlaminectomy kyphosis, or "swan neck" deformity, occurs in approximately 20% of adult patients after multiple cervical laminectomy.[9] Risk factors associated with postoperative kyphosis include preoperative loss of cervical lordosis, extent of laminectomy, facet capsule destruction, tumor, and radiation.[9] In postlaminectomy kyphosis, a ventral decompression and fusion are associated with significant graft complications and instability. Graft complications can include dislodgement, pseudarthrosis, and acceleration of adjacent level degeneration.[10] In advanced disease, further degeneration resulting in foraminal stenosis and subsequent radiculopathy; progressive spinal cord shift to the anterior portion of the spinal canal, resulting in myelopathy; as well as swallowing, breathing, and forward gaze difficulties can be present and are reasons for surgical intervention.[11]

A combined approach has the potential for correction of severe postlaminectomy kyphotic deformity. Various methods of reduction exist. Beginning in a supine position, the patient is intubated, placed in prongs and traction, and positioned in an extended position. A lateral cervical radiograph confirms kyphotic correction. An anterior approach is begun with an anterior cervical discectomy and fusion. The patient is then turned to the prone position. Lateral cervical radiograph confirms stable alignment, and a dorsal fusion with placement of lateral mass screws and rods is performed (Fig. 48-2). Alternatively, Sin et al. describe a ventral-dorsal-ventral, or 540-degree fusion, for correction of nearly 90-degree cervical kyphosis secondary to C5-6 *Pseudomonas* discitis. In this case, the anterior approach was suboptimal due to scar and inability to reduce the deformity after partial C5-6 corpectomies because of dorsal element fusion from the remote infection. The wound was closed, and a dorsal approach with radical removal of the C5 lamina, posterior facets, and lateral masses was performed. This approach allowed for significant enough reduction posteriorly to proceed with fusion. Sin et al. then

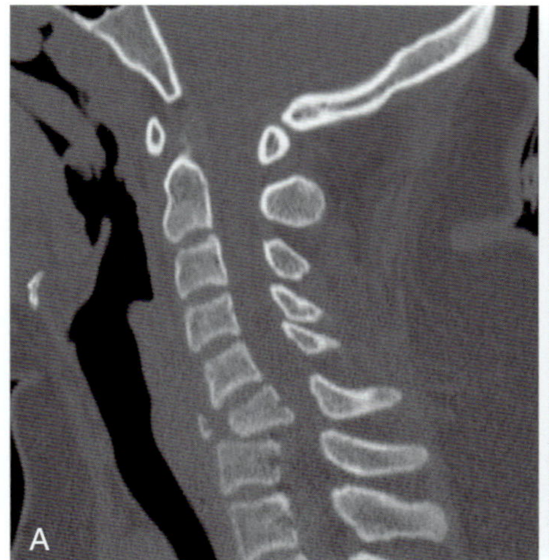

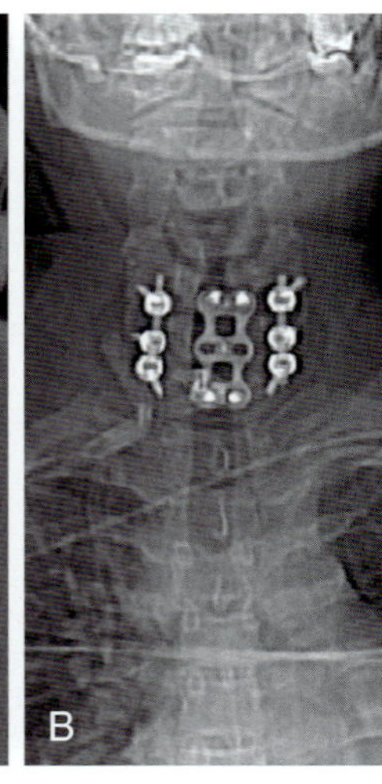

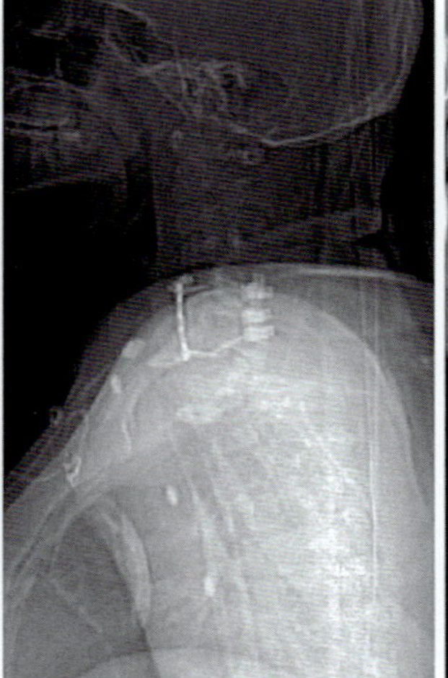

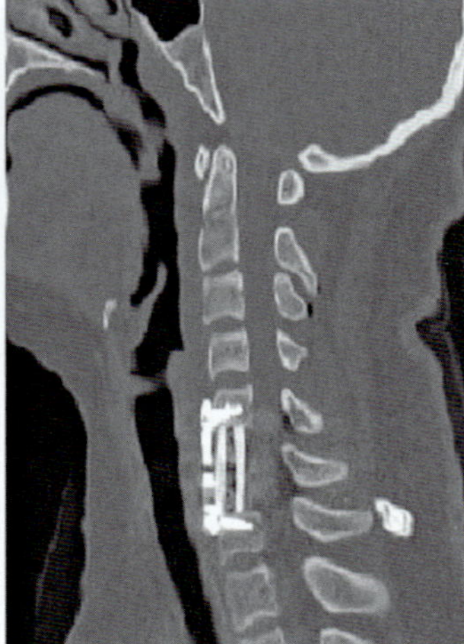

FIGURE 48-1. This 12-year-old patient fell into shallow pool and incurred a C6 burst fracture and C7 ASIA A spinal cord injury. **A,** Preoperative sagittal CT demonstrating C6 burst fracture. **B,** Postoperative anteroposterior and lateral cervical radiographs demonstrating C6 corpectomy, anterior C5-7 arthrodesis, posterior cervical instrumented fusion with lateral mass screws bilaterally at C5 and C6 with pedicle screw fixation at C7, and improved alignment.

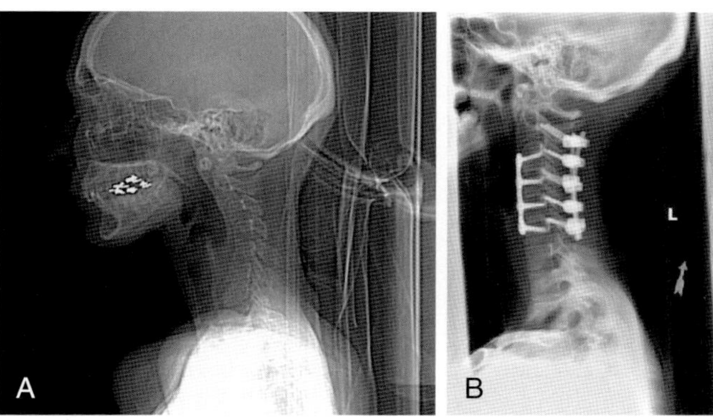

FIGURE 48-2. **A,** Preoperative lateral cervical radiograph demonstrating postlaminectomy kyphotic deformity. **B,** Postoperative lateral cervical radiograph demonstrating relatively straight spine without instrumentation failure.

returned ventrally and completed the C5-6 corpectomies followed by graft placement and ventral plating.[12]

Combined ventral and dorsal approaches to correct cervical kyphosis have several advantages. The dorsal osteotomy works synergistically with the return to lordosis offered by ventral osteotomy and reconstruction by shortening the posterior column and lengthening the anterior column. There is also a reduction in stress forces, which reduces the risk of graft migration and pseudarthosis.[13]

Numerous studies exist on ventral or dorsal approaches for managing kyphotic deformity. However, few reports exist in the literature about combined cervical reconstruction of kyphotic sagittal plane deformity. Few studies demonstrate the amount of preoperative kyphosis, amount of deformity correction, and maintenance of correction. Nottmeier et al. reviewed the charts of patients who underwent 360-degree reconstruction over a 6-year period. Forty-one patients with average follow-up of 19 months had a mean sagittal angle correction of 22 degrees and a mean fusion rate of 97.5%. However, three patients had adjacent segment kyphosis, one of whom required extension of the fusion.[11] Mummaneni et al. had a mean follow-up of 2.6 years in 27 patients. Mean Ishihara index values improved from −17.7 to +11.4, demonstrating a significant return to cervical lordosis. They had a 95% fusion rate. The complication rate was 33.3%, none of which were neurologic deficits after surgery. All patients had neuromonitoring (motor evoked potentials, somatosensory evoked potentials, and electromyogram).[13] These studies suggest a role of combined approach for cervical kyphotic deformity with a potentially superior fusion rate. The adjacent segment kyphosis and complication rates will need further scrutiny.

Neoplasms

The differential diagnosis for intramedullary spinal tumors includes metastasis, astrocytoma, ependymoma, hemangioblastoma, ganglioglioma, and vascular malformations. Extremely rare cases of schwannoma, lymphoma, lipoma, primitive neuroectodermal tumors, and meningioma have been described.[14]

The goals of surgery include pain control, neurology preservation, and stable fusion construct, all while maximizing a safe tumor resection. Tumors that invade ventral and dorsal neural elements and cause kyphotic deformity are considered for a combined approach. Patients with a life expectancy greater than 2 years, including those with breast carcinoma and myeloma, should be carefully evaluated for a combined approach that provides multiple areas of stabilization when circumferential tumor destruction has occurred.[2]

Large cervical neurofibromas extending around the spinal cord can be challenging and should be considered for a combined approach.[15] Neurofibromas with extensive paraspinal involvement have a particularly high recurrence rate. In addition, tumor revision cases have longer operation times and higher complication rates.[15] Chordomas and giant cell tumors are rare occurrences in the cervical spine. However, both have a high local recurrence rate with subtotal resection. Total spondylectomy (combined ventral and dorsal approach) has been described for both tumors in this region. Furthermore, total spondylectomy with wide surgical margins followed by adjuvant radiation therapy can lead to oncologic cure.[16,17]

Ankylosing Spondylitis

Minor trauma in patients with ankylosing spondylitis can cause cervical fractures extending through all three columns and resulting in significant instability and neurologic deficits. Although some advocate more conservative measures with halo immobilization, others see the benefits of surgical fusion. In certain patients a combined ventral and dorsal fusion construct is necessary.

Ankylosing spondylitis commonly results in kyphotic deformity. Patients have difficulty looking straight ahead and difficulty chewing. Chronic inflammation, inactivity atrophy, and steroid use are all responsible for osteoporosis of the spine in these patients.[18] Ankylosing of the facet joints and ossification of the anulus fibrosus and ligaments render the spine stiff.[19] The lower cervical spine is most commonly affected during trauma.[19]

Most cervical fractures in ankylosing spondylitis can be surgically managed with a posterior approach alone. Taggard and Traynelis described their results of posterior instrumentation in a group of seven ankylosing spondylitis patients with cervical fractures. All five patients available at follow-up had 100% fusion. All patients underwent MRI, which evaluated ligamentous injury and epidural hematoma. Epidural hematoma occurs with increased incidence in the ankylosing spondylitis population and can contribute significantly to neurologic deficit. Each patient underwent lateral mass plating at least two segments above and below the level of injury. Due to the extensive fusion that occurs in ankylosing spondylitis, facets may be indistinguishable and can make screw placement difficult. The authors recommend screws of less than 14 mm to avoid nerve root injury. In addition, at C7 and below the authors use a medial trajectory for pedicle incorporation and neural avoidance. None of these cases had significant enough anterior column fracture to warrant an additional ventral approach.[20] However, when there is concern about inadequate anterior column support or kyphotic deformity at the fracture site, a combined approach should be considered (Fig. 48-3).

Payer presented his results of four patients managed with a combined ventral and dorsal approach. All patients

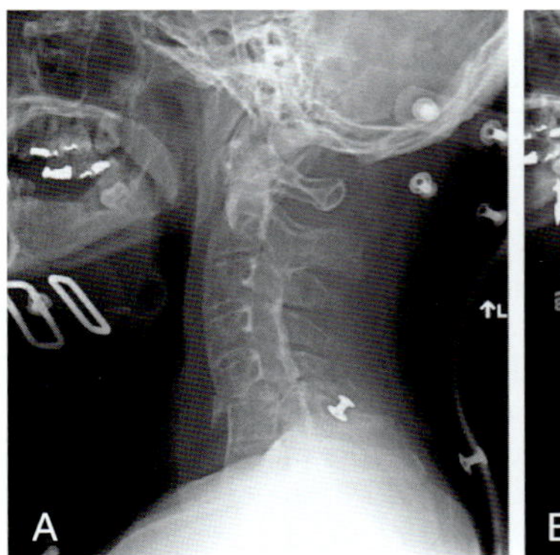

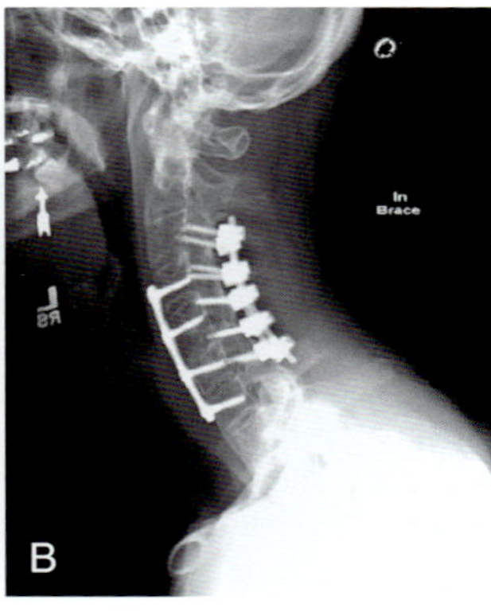

FIGURE 48-3. A 53-year-old man with ankylosing spondylitis suffered C5-6 fracture dislocation after a fall. **A,** Preoperative lateral cervical radiograph showing slight subluxation and significant angulation in Minerva brace standing upright. **B,** Postoperative lateral cervical radiograph demonstrating reestablishment of normal alignment and no instrumentation failure.

had transverse fractures at the C6-7 disc level with varying degrees of lordotic opening (8 to 35 degrees). Except for a single case, all patients were managed with posterior fixation three levels above and below followed by anterior single-segment corpectomy and fixation. This patient had a C6-7 level disc transverse fracture with a 38-degree lordotic opening and an 11-mm anterior sagittal gap, ventral epidural hematoma, and cord compression. A ventral approach reduced the lordosis to 26 degrees. Six days later there was back-out of the plate, suggesting inadequate biomechanical construct from a ventral approach alone. Dorsal fixation followed by ventral refixation was performed. All patients had stable fusion constructs during the postoperative observation periods of 6 to 18 months.[19]

Cervical Spondylotic Myelopathy

Cervical spondylotic myelopathy is a progressive degeneration of the cervical spine associated with disc height loss and facet and uncovertebral joint motion abnormalities. Uncovertebral joint disease leads to disc herniation and osteophyte formation leading to ventral stenosis. Facet disease and dorsal ligamentous hypertrophy lead to dorsal and lateral recess stenosis. The natural history is one of progressive circumferential spinal stenosis resulting in neurologic decline. Ventral and dorsal approaches alone have been performed for cervical spondylotic myelopathy with varying results in fusion, clinical improvement, and adjacent segment motion. In some cases a combined approach may be favorable for adequate decompression of both ventral and dorsal elements causing stenosis.[10]

In patients needing more than two-level corpectomy, the rate of failure has been shown to dramatically increase.[21] Thirty-three patients underwent two-level corpectomy and fusion compared with seven with three-level corpectomy and fusion. The two-level group had two failures (6%) manifesting as pseudarthrosis. The three-level group had five failures (71%) involving graft dislodgement, which were more serious in nature. Three of the patients with three-level and subsequent failure underwent posterior fusion and have all done well. The addition of dorsal instrumentation biomechanically moves the instantaneous axis of rotation dorsally, thus preserving the graft during extension.[21] Vaccaro et al. also noted unacceptably high failure rates for three-level versus two-level anterior cervical corpectomy and fusion (50% vs. 9%, respectively).[22] Thus circumferential surgery should be considered in patients undergoing long-segment corpectomy reconstruction.

Recently, Mummaneni et al. performed a systematic literature review and evidence-based medicine to describe the efficacy of various anterior and posterior cervical approaches for the treatment of cervical spondylotic myelopathy. Anterior cervical discectomy and fusion (ACDF) and cervical corpectomy and fusion (ACCF), laminoplasty, laminectomy, and laminectomy with fusion have improved functional outcomes. ACDF and ACCF have similar results in multilevel spine decompression for the same level lesion. With anterior plating they have equivalent fusion rates. Without anterior fixation, ACCF may have better fusion rates but also higher graft complication rates than multilevel ACDF (class III). There exists class III evidence for late deterioration with laminectomy compared with laminectomy with arthrodesis. Manuscripts reviewed by the authors were deemed class III evidence for several reasons, including absence of a control group, nonblinded allocation of a control group, nonvalidated outcome measures, and unblinded outcome assessors.[23] The importance of a prospective, randomized, controlled clinical trial is validated by the equivalent outcomes with these procedures without good class I or II evidence.

There may be a subgroup of patients who would benefit from a combined ventral and dorsal approach. Acosta et al. studied the biomechanical stability and clinical results of anterior cervical fusion level 3 or higher and circumferential reconstruction using titanium mesh cage (TMC) and dorsolateral fixation. They had 15 patients with cervical spondylotic myelopathy. Each patient had a halo ring secured to a Mayfield frame. Corpectomy and decompression (including posterior longitudinal ligament) was performed. Corpectomy bone was harvested and packed into an appropriate-size TMC. All TMCs had a lordotic curvature. Cervical traction was applied by anesthesia, TMC was inserted, and finally traction was relieved. An anterior plate was inserted in each case. The patient was then turned prone, and posteriolateral screw-rod fixation was performed at least one level above and below the corpectomy. Average follow-up was 33 months. There was a 100% fusion rate, and there was no significant cage subsidence or case of instrument failure.[24]

Summary

Combined ventral and dorsal cervical spine surgery can be technically difficult with high morbidity. Cervical spine trauma, malignancy, ankylosing spondylitis, kyphosis deformity, and cervical spondylitic myelopathy are all pathologies for which a combined approach may be biomechanically advantageous. Predicting which patients will benefit from this combined approach can potentially improve fusion rates, prevent delayed deformities, decrease hospital readmissions, and thereby be more cost-effective.

KEY REFERENCES

Dvorak MF, Fisher CG, Fehlings MG: The surgical approach to subaxial cervical spine injuries: an evidence-based algorithm based on the SLIC classification system. *Spine (Phila Pa 1976)* 32:2620–2629, 2007.

Mummaneni PV, Dhall SS, Rodts GE, Haid RW: Circumferential fusion for cervical kyphotic deformity. *J Neurosurg Spine* 9:515–521, 2008.

Mummaneni PV, Kaiser MG, Matz PG, et al: Cervical surgical techniques for the treatment of cervical spondylotic myelopathy. *J Neurosurg Spine* 11: 130–141, 2009.

Nottmeier EW, Deen HG, Patel N, Birch B: Cervical kyphotic deformity correction using 360-degree reconstruction. *J Spinal Disord* 22:385–391, 2009.

Vaccaro AR, Cook CM, McCullen G, Garfin SR: Cervical trauma: rationale for selecting the appropriate fusion technique. *Orthop Clin North Am* 29:745–754, 1998.

Vaccaro AR, Hurlbert RJ, Fisher CG, et al: The sub-axial cervical spine injury classification system (SLIC): a novel approach to recognize the importance of morphology, neurology and integrity of the disco-ligamentous complex. *Spine (Phila Pa 1976)* 32:2365–2374, 2007.

Witwer BP, Trost GR: Cervical spondylosis: ventral or dorsal surgery. *Neurosurgery* 60(Suppl 1):S130–S136, 2007.

REFERENCES

The complete reference list is available online at expertconsult.com.

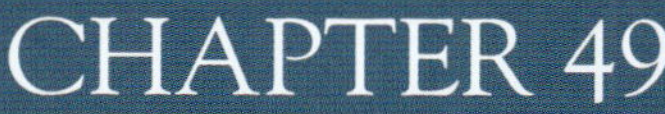

CHAPTER 49

Percutaneous and Minimally Invasive Approaches to Decompression and Arthrodesis of the Cervical Spine

Youssef R. Karam | Richard G. Fessler

Degenerative disease of the cervical spine can cause compression of neural elements through disc herniation, ligament and facet joint hypertrophy, and the formation of vertebral body end-plate osteophytes. The effects of these changes can be exacerbated by a congenitally narrow spinal canal, segmental instability, and deformity. These dynamic processes can contribute to radiculopathy, myelopathy, or both, depending on the degree to which nerve roots and/or the spinal cord are affected. Surgical decompression is indicated for selected patients with neurologic signs and symptoms of radiculopathy and/or myelopathy with corresponding radiographic evidence of neural compression. The cervical spine can be decompressed through an anterior or a posterior approach, each of which has relative advantages and disadvantages. Although the choice of approach is sometimes relatively clear, often the problem can be addressed from either direction, with the ultimate decision balancing the risks and benefits of each method. In the past 2 decades, the minimally invasive and percutaneous techniques have been shown to preserve healthy tissues, shorten hospital stays, cause less postoperative pain, and enable faster patient recovery. This chapter discusses these different techniques (anterior and posterior approaches) with descriptions of the procedures and outcomes.

Dorsal Minimally Invasive Approaches for the Cervical Spine

Dorsal decompressive procedures are fundamental tools in the surgical treatment of symptomatic cervical degenerative spine disease.[1-4] Even as ventral cervical procedures have gained prominence, posterior cervical laminoforaminotomy still provides symptomatic relief in 92% to 97% of patients with radiculopathy from foraminal stenosis or lateral herniated discs.[3,5] Similarly, dorsal cervical decompression for cervical stenosis achieves neurologic improvement in 62.5% to 83% of myelopathic patients undergoing either laminectomy or laminoplasty.[4,6-8] Moreover, these operations avoid the complications attendant to ventral approaches to the cervical spine, namely, esophageal injury, vascular injury, recurrent laryngeal nerve paralysis, dysphagia, and accelerated degeneration of adjacent motion segments after fusion.[9-11]

However, open dorsal approaches to the cervical spine require extensive subperiosteal stripping of the paraspinal musculature that leads to postoperative pain, spasm, and dysfunction and can be persistently disabling in 18% to 60% of patients.[4,9,12,13] Furthermore, preoperative loss of lordosis and long segment decompressions increase the risk for postoperative sagittal plane deformity,[14-17] a complication that frequently prompts instrumented arthrodesis at the time of laminectomy. Employing these extensive posterior fusion techniques increases operative risks, time, and blood loss; exacerbates early postoperative pain; and potentially contributes to adjacent-level degeneration.

The fundamental tenet of minimal access techniques is reduction of approach-related morbidity. To that end, the advent of muscle-splitting tubular retractor systems and the use of endoscopic technology or the microscope have allowed for the application of minimally invasive techniques to dorsal cervical decompressive procedures[13,18-35] and fixation.[36-40]

Spurling, Scoville, and Frykholm were the first to describe the open cervical foraminal decompression between 1944 and 1947.[41-43] In 1983 Williams reported the first microsurgical technique for dorsal cervical foraminotomy.[44] Several minimally invasive dorsal cervical techniques were described after that.[18-40] To avoid confusion, and to simplify the description of all these techniques, we divided them into two main approaches: (1) the minimally invasive midline cervical approach, and (2) the minimally invasive paramedian (transtubular or transmuscular) cervical approach. An endoscope or microscope could be used in either approach. These approaches are used to perform laminotomy/foraminotomy/discectomy, laminectomy, laminoplasty,[34,35] and lateral mass fixation.[36-40]

Indications

The operative indications for minimally invasive laminotomy/foraminotomy/discectomy are (1) unilateral single-root (Fig. 49-1) or multiple-root cervical radiculopathy from lateral disc herniations or foraminal stenosis (single-level or multilevel), without instability, significant kyphosis, or severe axial neck pain; (2) persistent or recurrent root symptoms following anterior cervical discectomy and fusion; (3) cervical disc disease in patients for whom anterior approaches are relatively contraindicated (e.g., ventral neck infection, tracheostomy, prior irradiation); and (4) cervicothoracic disc herniation and radiculopathy, to avoid ventral approach potential complications and when the ventral approach is not feasible (short neck or others). A ventral approach should be considered in case

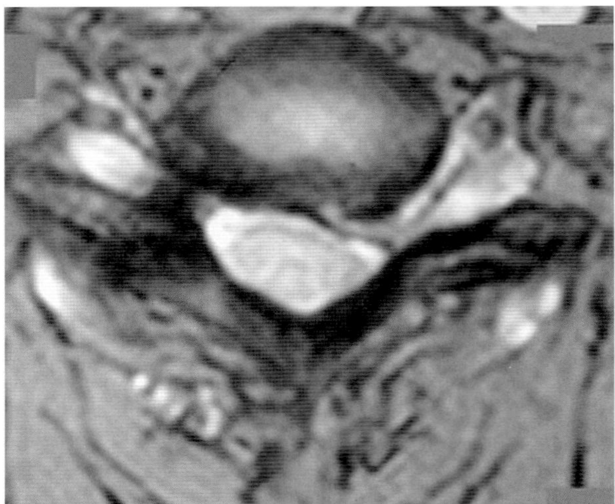

FIGURE 49-1. Axial T2-weighted cervical spine MRI demonstrates laterally herniated disc to the left with resultant effacement of the lateral thecal sac and compression of the exiting nerve root.

of same-level bilateral radiculopathy, central disc herniation, significant kyphosis, and severe axial neck pain.

Most patients who are candidates for a noninstrumented, dorsal cervical decompression are also candidates for a minimally invasive cervical decompression. These are selected patients with clinical myelopathy or myeloradiculopathy, radiographic evidence of spinal cord compression from one to three adjacent cervical levels, and a lordotic cervical spine (Fig. 49-2). Contraindications include loss of the normal cervical lordosis, severe ventral disease (disease that extends for more than three levels), and segmental instability.

Minimally invasive dorsal cervical fixation could be applied in case of facet dislocation or segmental instability or to support ventral instrumentation. Few clinical reports are available in the literature.[36,37,39] Minimally invasive cervical laminoplasty is still undergoing investigation.

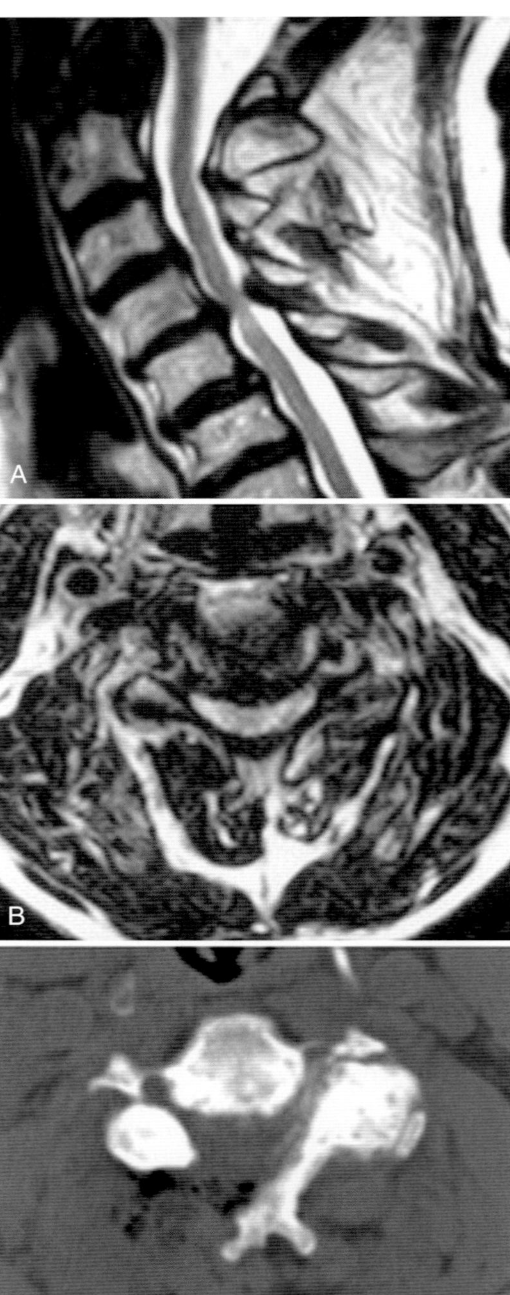

FIGURE 49-2. An 80-year-old male presented with chronic myelopathy from cervical stenosis and underwent right-sided approach for C4-5 microendoscopic decompression for stenosis. **A,** Sagittal T2-weighted MRI demonstrates focal C4-5 spondylotic stenosis with signal change in the spinal cord. **B,** Axial T2-weighted MRI reveals severe focal compression at C4-5. **C,** Postoperative axial CT image shows typical extent of bony resection required to achieve adequate decompression of the spinal cord. Note the preservation of the dorsal spinous process and contralateral lamina and facet. Also note the minimal impact on paraspinal soft tissues on the approach side (postoperative air is seen on the approach side and at the site of the laminotomy).

Preoperative Evaluation

The preoperative radiographic evaluation follows a detailed history and physical examination and should include MRI or postmyelographic CT, in addition to anteroposterior (AP), lateral, and dynamic cervical radiographs. Electromyography (EMG) and nerve conduction studies (NCS) may also assist to confirm the localization of radicular compression. Selective nerve root blocks can also be a useful additional therapeutic and diagnostic tool. All patients with pure radiculopathy who go on to surgery have failed conservative therapy, including oral medications, physical therapy, and/or steroid injections. Cervical spondylotic myelopathy patients undergo a careful analysis of their disease progression, physical examination, radiographic studies, and comorbidities. All patients are carefully counseled regarding the risks, benefits, and alternatives to surgery.

Operative Setup

General endotracheal anesthesia is induced on a standard electric operating table. A neurophysiologic monitoring array with capabilities for somatosensory evoked potentials

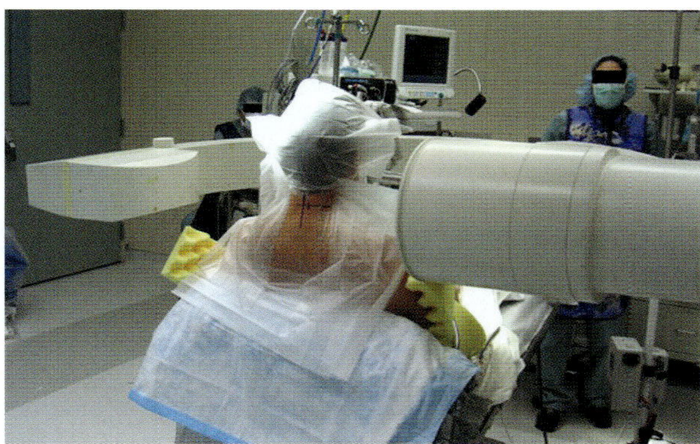

FIGURE 49-3. Sitting position with C-arm in place.

(SSEPs), motor evoked potentials (MEPs), and free running electromyography (EMG) is put in place. In cases of myelopathy, a fiberoptic intubation may be elected and evoked potentials are compared before and after positioning to identify positioning-related cord ischemia. Maintenance of normotension to avoid spinal cord hypoperfusion is best directed with continuous blood pressure measurements afforded by an arterial line. Measures to detect and treat air embolism, such as a precordial Doppler and a central line, are options but have not yet proven necessary. Given the small exposure, the risk of air embolism is low. A urinary catheter is generally not necessary for one- or two-level procedures. Routine perioperative antibiotics are administered. Relaxants are minimized after induction to allow for effective neurophysiologic monitoring.

Posterior cervical approaches might be performed with the patient in the prone or sitting position. With the prone position, the head is held with a Mayfield pin-holder or a well-padded horseshoe-shaped headrest, with slight flexion. The operating table is tilted in a reverse Trendelenburg position to ensure that the cervical spine is parallel to the floor. The senior author (RGF) prefers the sitting position (Fig. 49-3) because it confers advantages of decreased epidural bleeding, decreased pooling of blood in the operative field, decreased anesthesia time, and gravity-dependent positioning of the shoulders for better lateral fluoroscopic images. The table is turned 180 degrees relative to the anesthesiologist. The patient's head is fixed in a Mayfield head holder. The table is manipulated to place the patient in a semisitting position with the head flexed and the neck straight and perpendicular to the floor.

Midline Approach

A 3-cm skin incision is made in the dorsal midline with the disc space centered on the incision. Larger incisions extending over several segments may be necessary for multilevel disease. The operative level(s) and entry point are confirmed on lateral fluoroscopy. The superficial fascia is incised in the midline to the level of the ligamentum nuchae. The ligamentum nuchae is incised just off the midline ipsilateral to the site of interest. Care should be taken to avoid penetration into the erector spinae muscles, by staying along the margin of the bloodless deep fascia. After reaching the spinous processes of the site of interest, paraspinous muscles are dissected from the spinous processes, laminae, and facet joint, using a monopolar cautery or subperiostal dissection with a Cobb. A self-retaining retractor is placed to reflect the paraspinous muscles from the interlaminar space of interest. The remaining steps are performed under microscopic magnification or using loops and an endoscope.

Paramedian Approach

The operative level(s) and entry point are confirmed on lateral fluoroscopy with a K-wire. A 1.8-cm longitudinal incision is marked out approximately 1.5 cm off the midline on the operative side and injected with local anesthetic. For two-level procedures the incision should be placed midway between the targeted levels. After an initial stab incision, the K-wire is advanced slowly though the subcutaneous tissue and docked on the cervicodorsal fascia. Once an optimal trajectory is established, the fascia is incised with a scalpel to accommodate dilators. The fascia is retracted, and the smallest dilator is placed through the posterior cervical musculature under fluoroscopic guidance and docked at the lamina-facet junction of the level of interest. A slightly lateral trajectory is advised to avoid the spinal canal and ensure contact with the lateral mass. Successive tubular muscle dilators are carefully and gently inserted, remembering that the axial forces that are routinely applied during muscle dilation in the lumbar spine are hazardous in the cervical spine. After dilation, the final tubular retractor is placed and secured over the junction of the lamina and the facet with a table-mounted flexible retractor arm and the dilators are removed. The following steps are performed under microscopic magnification or using loupes or an endoscope. The endoscope is inserted and attached to the tubular retractor (Fig. 49-4). Monopolar cautery and pituitary rongeurs are used to clear the remaining soft tissue off of the lateral mass and lamina of interest, taking care to start the dissection over solid bone laterally.

Laminotomy/Foraminotomy/Discectomy

The medial facet/interlaminar space junction is identified. Using a high-speed drill, a partial laminotomy-facetectomy is performed beginning at the medial facet/interlaminar space and going laterally, without exceeding 50% facet removal, to maintain biomechanical integrity. The dorsolateral portion of the superior lamina and the medial part of the inferior articular facet are removed first. This will permit the removal of the lateral corner of the inferior lamina and the medial part of the superior articular facet, exposing the medial border of the caudal pedicle. The nerve root is located directly above the caudal pedicle and anterior to the superior articular facet. The ligamentum flavum can be removed medially after the foraminotomy to expose the lateral edge of the dura and proximal portion of the nerve root. Progressive lateral dissection can then proceed along the root as it enters the foramen. The venous plexus overlying the nerve root should be carefully coagulated with bipolar cautery and incised. With the root well visualized, a fine-angled dissector can be used to palpate ventrally to the nerve root for osteophytes or disc fragments. Should an osteophyte be present, a down-angled curette may be used to tamp the material further ventrally into the disc space or fragment it for subsequent removal. In the case of a soft disc herniation, a nerve hook may be passed ventrally and inferiorly to the root to gently tease the fragment away from the nerve for ultimate removal with a pituitary rongeur.

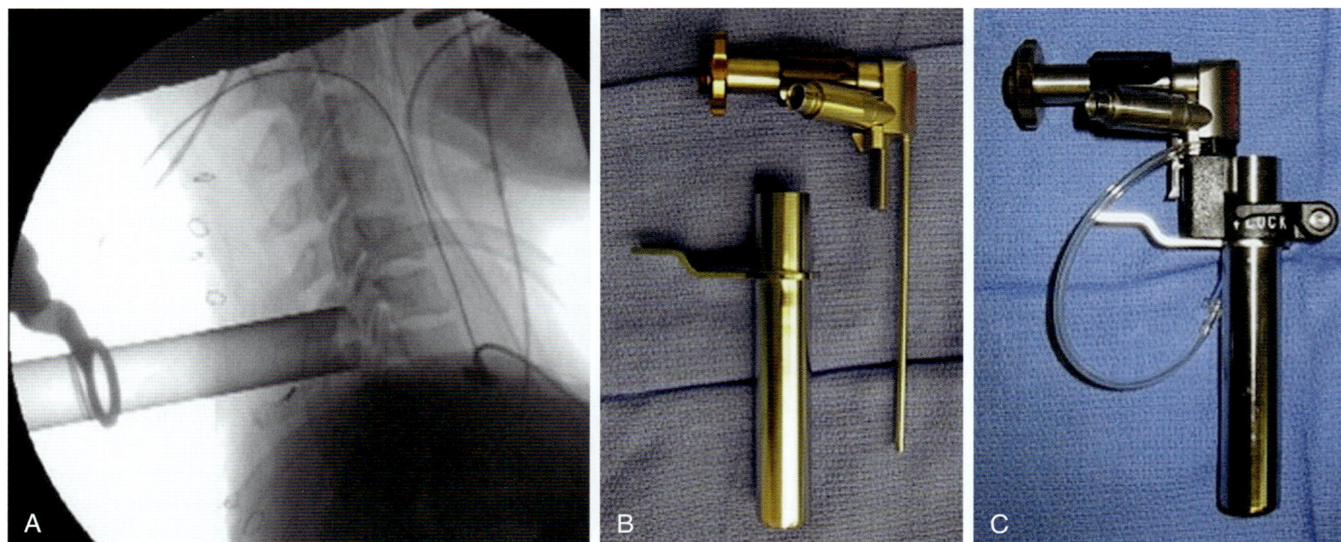

FIGURE 49-4. **A,** Fluoroscopic control verifying the right placement of the table-mounted retractor after removal of the dilators. **B,** The endoscope and the retractor separately. **C,** The endoscope mounted on the tubular retractor.

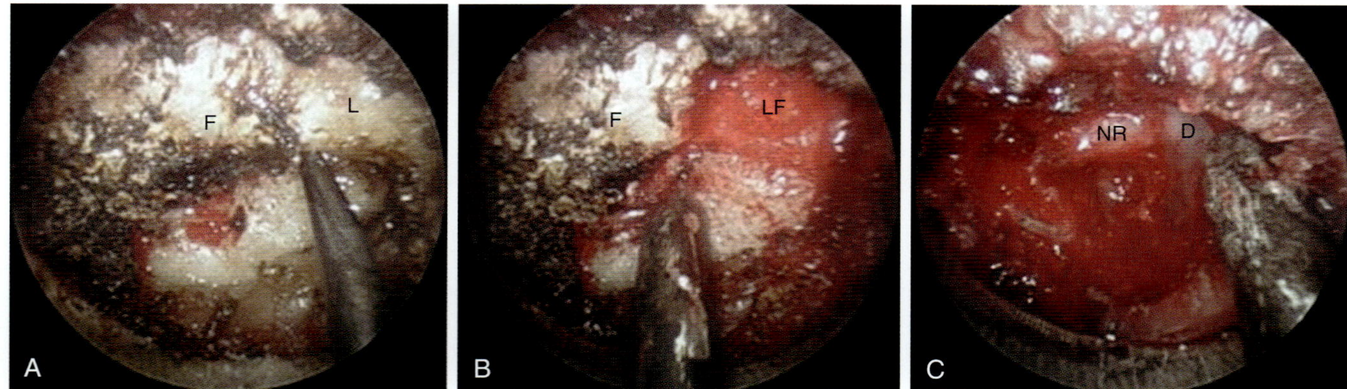

FIGURE 49-5. Intraoperative endoscopic photographs during left-sided cervical microendoscopic foraminotomy. In all photos, rostral is to the top and medial is to the right. **A,** Initial exposure reveals lateral edge of lamina (L) joining the medial facet (F) with fine up-going curette inserted under caudal edge of laminofacet junction. **B,** After initial laminotomy, the ligamentum flavum (LF) is seen with adjacent facet (F). **C,** After foraminotomy, the lateral edge of dura (D) and decompressed nerve root (NR) in the proximal foramen are revealed.

In either case, additional drilling of the superomedial quadrant of the caudal pedicle allows greater access to the ventral pathology and obviates the need for excessive nerve root retraction superiorly (Fig. 49-5).

Decompression for Stenosis

In this case, ipsilateral laminotomy of the levels of interest is performed and the ligamentum flavum is left in place to protect the dura. The tube is then angled about 45 degrees off the midline such that the tube is oriented to visualize the contralateral side. A plane between the ligament and undersurface of the spinous process is gently dissected with a fine curette. The drill with guard sleeve extended is then used to progressively drill the undersurface of the spinous process and contralateral lamina all the way to the contralateral facet. This initial decompression allows greater working space within which to remove hypertrophied ligament while avoiding downward pressure on the dura and spinal cord. Dissection and removal of the ligament with curettes and Kerrison rongeurs may now proceed safely. Any compressive elements of the contralateral facet or the superior edge of the caudal lamina may also be drilled off or removed with Kerrison rongeurs at this time because their impact on the dura is more apparent with the ligament removed. After gently confirming decompression over to the contralateral foramen with a fine probe, the tube is returned to its original position to complete the ipsilateral removal of ligament and bone. This should then reveal completely decompressed and pulsatile dura (Fig. 49-6). If indicated, ipsilateral foraminotomy, as described earlier, also may be performed at this time.

Lateral Mass Fixation

After exposure of the facet joint, a hand drill is used to create a pilot hole. The starting point is 1 mm medial to the midpoint of the lateral mass, and the trajectory will be 25 degrees lateral and parallel to the facet joint. Appropriate dimension

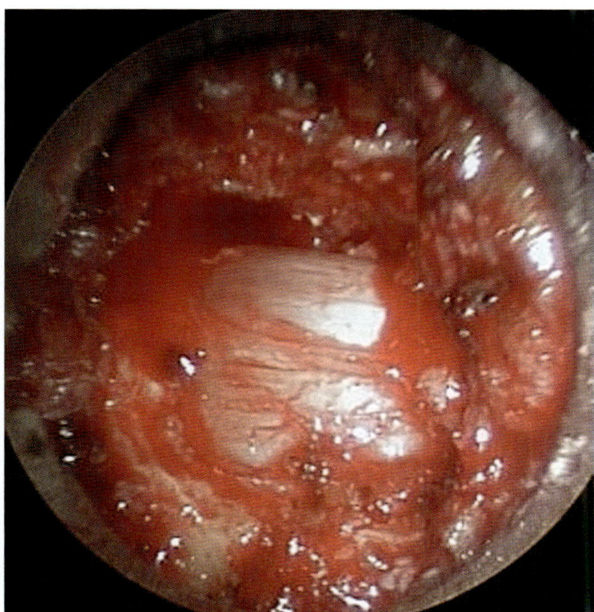

FIGURE 49-6. Intraoperative endoscopic photograph during right-sided approach. The dura is seen to be completely decompressed in this image, following removal of offending bone and ligament. Rostral is to the right and lateral is to the bottom.

screws are inserted after taping, and a rod is fixed with set screws. A midline incision is preferred in this case for the transmuscular approach. The same incision could be used for both sides. Also, fluoroscopic guidance is preferred.

Closure and Postoperative Care

Local anesthetic is injected into the fascia and muscles surrounding the incision. The wound is closed using one or two absorbable stitches for the fascia, two or three inverted stitches for the subcutaneous layer, and a running subcuticular stitch and Dermabond for the skin. After awaking from general anesthesia, the patient is brought to the postanesthesia care unit and mobilized as early as possible. No collar is necessary. The patient is discharged the same or next day, if medically stable.

Outcomes and Results

Favorable outcomes were reported in the literature for posterior cervical foraminotomy with a range between 75% and 100%.[1,3,9,44-48] Krupp et al. separated the outcomes by soft, hard, and mixed pathology, with favorable outcomes of 98%, 84%, and 91%, respectively.[45] Jodicke et al. reported a significantly better outcome for soft discs compared to hard discs in early follow-up, but no difference was found at long-term follow-up.[47]

The reports of minimally invasive, microscopic, and microendoscopic posterior cervical formainotomy have demonstrated equivalent efficacy to the open technique, but the blood loss, length of stay, and postoperative pain medication usage were reduced with the minimally invasive techniques.[9,13,20,21,25,26,48] The senior author and Khoo prospectively used cervical microendoscopic posterior foraminotomy in 25 patients and compared the results with another 26 patients treated via open cervical laminoforaminotomy.[9] The microendoscopic group had a lower overall operative time (115 vs. 171 minutes), less blood loss (138 vs. 246 mL), shorter postoperative hospital stay (20 vs. 68 hours), and fewer postoperative narcotic medications (11 vs. 40 equivalents) when compared with the open technique group.

Ruetten et al. conducted a prospective, randomized, controlled study with lateral cervical herniations, operated either in a full endoscopic posterior foraminotomy (89 patients) or conventional microsurgical anterior technique with fusion/plating (86 patients), with 2 years of follow-up.[20] There was no significant difference between the groups in the clinical outcome, revision, or complication rates. Preservation of motion was conserved in the full endoscopic posterior group.

Perez-Cruet and the senior author have reported on five patients undergoing cervical microendoscopic decompression for stenosis at one, two, or three levels.[16] All patients demonstrated improvement in their myelopathy and returned to work with the only complication being one unintended durotomy that sealed spontaneously. Yabuki et al. performed endoscopic partial laminectomy in 10 patients with degenerative cervical compressive myelopathy.[28] All patients experienced symptomatic improvement with slight postoperative wound pain. The mean operative duration was 164 ± 35 minutes and the intraoperative blood loss was 45.5 ± 27 mL. Boehm et al. reported the results of 13 patients who were operated on under the microscope through a transmuscular tubular approach.[30] Nine of these patients suffered from cervical myelopathy. The average follow-up was 17 months. The neck disability index score and visual analogue scale score were significantly improved. Thirty-three percent showed complete recovery of the preoperative neurologic deficit, while 67% had improvement.

Wang et al. reviewed retrospectively 18 patients treated with lateral mass screws placed in a minimally invasive fashion.[37] In two cases, the minimally invasive technique was converted to the standard open technique because of inability to visualize anatomic landmarks on fluoroscopy (bulky shoulders). Successful fusion was documented in all cases, and there were no hardware failures during the minimum 2 years of follow-up. Two patients were lost to follow-up after 6 months.

Complications

The posterior cervical foraminotomy is a safe procedure associated with a low rate of complications (1–15%),[1,3,9,13,20,21,25,26,44-48] with wound infection and dural tear contributing to the majority of them. The senior author has no infection to date in his microendoscopic series, and the unintended durotomy rate has dropped from 8% in the initial series of patients[9] to around 1% more recently. Direct suture repair of durotomy is difficult through the narrow-diameter tubes or small incisions. Therefore one technique for handling small defects is to simply cover the durotomy with muscle, fat, hemostatic gelatin (Gelfoam, Baxter Healthcare, Glendale, CA), or dural susbstitute followed by fibrin glue or synthetic sealant such as Coseal (Baxter Healthcare, Glendale, CA). Using this approach, overnight bedrest is usually sufficient to seal the defect. For larger dural tears that cannot be primarily closed, 2 to 3 days of lumbar cerebrospinal fluid (CSF) drainage may prevent a leak. Ultimately, the small opening and relative lack of dead space after minimally invasive procedures have made the incidence of postoperative pseudomeningoceles and CSF49-cutaneous fistulae negligible.

Potential neurologic complications include radicular injury from manipulation within the tight foramen or direct mechanical spinal cord injury during dilation or decompression. Vertebral artery injury can be avoided by early detection of dark venous bleeding from the venous plexus surrounding the artery that may arise from accidental dilation lateral to the facet or during overly aggressive dissection laterally in the foramen. This type of bleeding can typically be controlled by packing with Gelfoam or another hemostatic product.

Postoperative muscular pain and spasm from subperiosteal dissection are minimized with the transmuscular miscroscopic and microendoscopic techniques.

Ventral Minimally Invasive Approaches for the Cervical Spine

Anterior cervical discectomy and fusion (ACDF) was first described by Smith and Robinson and then by Cloward in the 1950s.[49-51] Orozco introduced anterior plating in 1970 as adjunctive treatment in cervical fractures.[52] Since then, several types of plates and grafts were developed. ACDF has now developed as a standard procedure in the treatment of cervical radiculomyelopathy. It is described as a safe and efficacious procedure with good fusion rates. However, several problems can occur, mainly because of access complications and adjacent segment degeneration as a disadvantage of fusion. Hilibrand et al. postulated that up to 25% of the patients who undergo a ventral cervical fusion could require treatment for degenerative changes of the adjacent segments within 10 years.[53] With the fascination of minimally invasive techniques and the intent to preserve motion and prevent adjacent segment disease, several anterior alternative approaches have been reported: (1) ventral cervical foraminotomy (microsurgical and endoscopic); (2) percutaneous ventral cervical procedures for discectomy, anuloplasty, and stabilization; and (3) cervical arthroplasty. The final approach is not discussed in this chapter.

Ventral Cervical Foraminotomy (Microsurgical and Endoscopic)

In 1968, Verbiest described a ventrolateral approach to the cervical neuroforamen, which involved sectioning of the longus colli muscle, exposure of the transverse process, mobilization of the vertebral artery, and performing discectomy with and without fusion.[54] In 1976, Hakuba described the transuncodiscal approach. In his approach the vertebral artery was not displaced, and a complete discectomy was performed with and without fusion.[55] In 1989, Snyder and Bernhardt published a new anterior cervical fractional interspace decompression technique, which consisted of a 6-mm-wide cylindric bur hole in the lateral third of the intervertebral disc, and fragmentectomy. They reported minimal disc space collapse and a 4% rate of spontaneous fusion.[56] In 1996, Jho described the anterior cervical foraminotomy with resection of the uncus process, lateral portion of the rostral end plate, and lateral portion of the intervertebral disc. This technique required cutting of the longus colli muscle and exposure of the vertebral artery along its medial surface.[57] In 2002, Saringer proposed a modification of Jho's technique by preserving a thin piece of cortical bone of the lateral wall of the uncinate process, avoiding exposure of the vertebral artery,[58] and he added the endoscope to his procedure in 2003.[59] Again in 2002, Jho reported an upper vertebral transcorporeal foraminotomy technique. The hole in this technique was drilled at the most lateral and inferior 4 to 5 mm of the upper vertebral body.[60] The cartilage end plate was exposed and entered in its posterior third. In 2007, Choi et al. described a modification of the upper vertebral transcorporeal Jho's approach, made by drilling the hole more medially, to avoid cutting the longus colli muscle and exposing the vertebral artery.[61] The evolution of this technique has led to (1) having less disc disruption, (2) avoiding exposure of the vertebral artery, and (3) avoiding cutting the longus colli muscle, which could result in the injury of the sympathetic chain.

Indications and Contraindications

This procedure is indicated in patients with unilateral radicular symptoms, at single or multiple levels, due to a dorsolateral soft-herniated disc or uncovertebral osteophytes. Contraindications include bilateral radiculopathy, instability, central herniated disc, severe spinal canal stenosis, instability, and severe axial pain.

Preoperative Evaluation

History taking and the physical examination should confirm the unilateral radicular pain, with absence of significant neck pain. Standard anteroposterior, lateral, oblique, and flexion/extension radiographs help to visualize the bony anatomy, especially the uncovertebral joints and the foramens, and rule out instability. MRI evaluation is sufficient most of the time to visualize the herniated disc or osteophytic compression in the foramen. Vertebral artery anatomy and possible variations or anomalies should be reviewed to avoid access injury and possible catastrophic complications. Sometimes, a thin-slice CT scan is requested if better bony anatomy details are necessary.

Surgical Technique

The initial steps for this technique are similar to the open ventral cervical approach. It is performed under general anesthesia and on a standard operating room table. The patient is positioned supine with the head in neutral position and slight extension. A roll is placed between the shoulders. The shoulders are taped with down longitudinal traction, to allow visualization of the lower cervical levels if necessary. Fluoroscopy is used to mark the transverse 3- to 4-cm skin incision at the side of the radiculopathy, with one third of it lateral and two thirds medial to the medial border of the sternocleidomastoid muscle. Preparation and draping are done as usual.

After the skin incision, the platysma muscle is sectioned along the same line. The superficial cervical fascia is opened medial to the sternocleidomastoid muscle and blunt dissection is directed deeply to the spinal column, with the vascular structures retracted laterally and the trachea and esophagus medially. The prevertebral fascia is opened, and the anterior part of the vertebral bodies with intervertebral discs and longus colli muscles are exposed. The level of concern is again checked with fluoroscopy. As mentioned earlier, several techniques and modifications have been reported. These can be divided into two main approaches: (1) the transuncal approach and (2) the transcorporeal approach.

Transuncal Approach

The medial border of the longus colli muscle is cut perpendicularly and retracted or excised to expose the medial aspect of the transverse process and the uncinate process of the lower vertebrae. Care should be taken when exposing the C6-7 level because the vertebral artery lies between the transverse process of C7 and the longus colli muscle. The next steps are performed under microscopic magnification or using the endoscope as described by Saringer in his 2003 technique modification.[59] According to Jho, in his first description,[57] the uncinate process is undertaken with a 2-mm high-speed drill, leaving a thin dorsolateral rim of cortical bone that limits the vertebral artery laterally and the nerve root dorsally. The thin cortical bone is removed with a curette and a Kerrison rongeur. The posterior longitudinal ligament is exposed, which covers the nerve root posteriorly. At this point, the foraminotomy is completed and the uncovertebral osteophyte is removed. In case of a herniated disc, the posterior longitudinal ligament should be excised with a curette and Kerrison rongeur and the disc fragment removed. Epidural bleeding could be troublesome and should be controlled with bipolar cauterization or by application of Gelfoam and cottonoid. Saringer, in his microscopic[58] and endoscopic[59] techniques (Figs. 49-7 and 49-8), described two essential modifications to Jho's transuncal approach: (1) leaving the lateral cortical rim of the uncinate process to protect the vertebral artery, and (2) extending the foraminotomy by removing more bone from the caudal dorsolateral aspect of the rostral vertebrae.

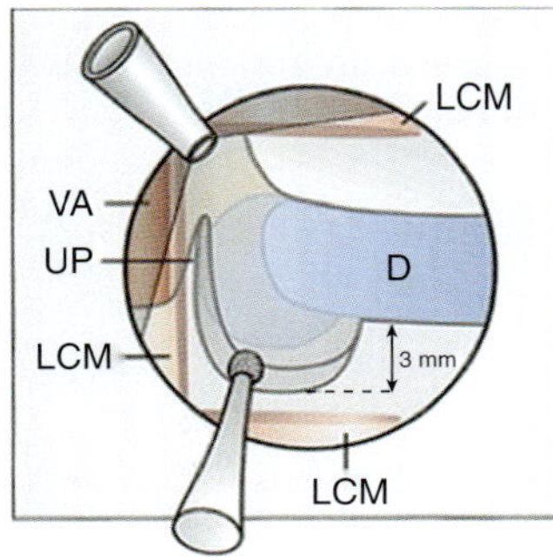

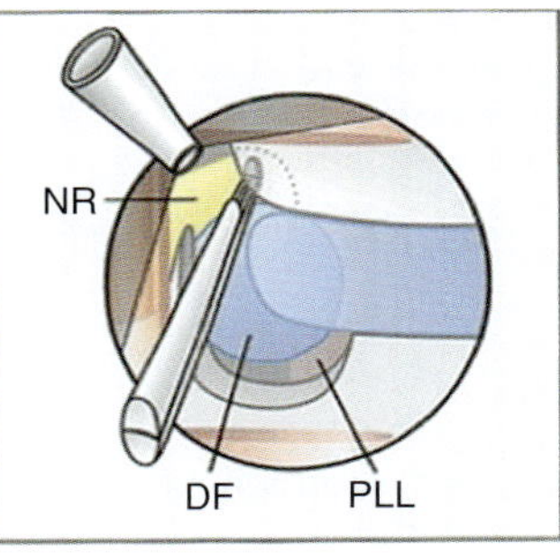

FIGURE 49-7. *Left,* Under the endoscope, the medial portion of the longus colli muscle (LCM) is excised and the lateral portion of the disc (D) and the uncus process (UP) are exposed. The UP is drilled up. A thin piece of the lateral wall of the UP is left, serving as a landmark and protective layer for the underlying vertebral artery (VA). Periosteum covers the nerve root, disc fragments, and lateral portion of the posterior longitudinal ligament (PLL). The intervertebral disc is maintained in its form. The VA is intentionally not exposed. *Right,* The periosteum and cartilaginous and degenerative fibrous tissue between the tip of the UP and the rostral end plate and osteophytes at the dorsolateral cephalad end plate are removed using a 1- or 2-mm thin-foot Kerrison rongeur. Disc fragments (DF), parts of the nerve root (NR), and lateral parts of the PLL are exposed. (Modified from Saringer WF, Reddy B, Nöbauer-Huhmann I, et al: Endoscopic anterior cervical foraminotomy for unilateral radiculopathy: anatomical morphometric analysis and preliminary clinical experience. *J Neurosurg* 98[2 Suppl]:171–180, 2003.)

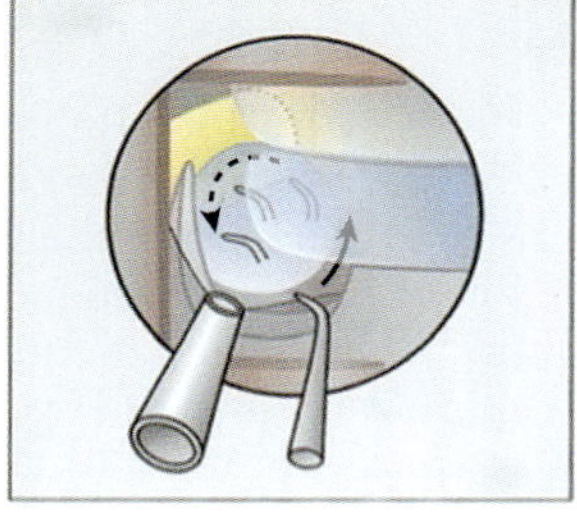

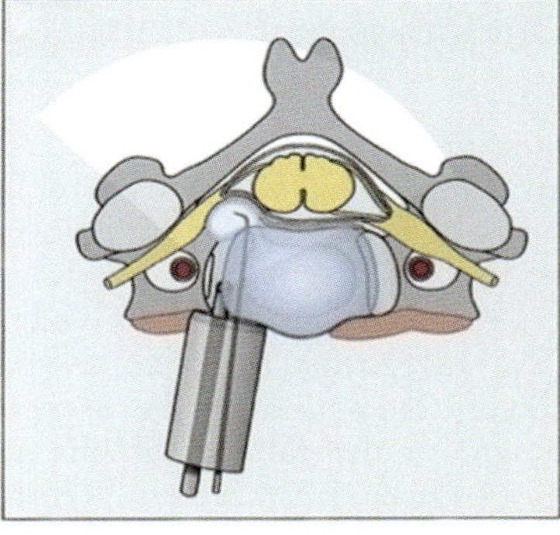

FIGURE 49-8. *Left* and *right,* Transtubular and axial depiction of the last step of the operation shown in Figure 49-7. To improve visualization, the endoscope is positioned with its tip inside the drilled canal. Herniated disc fragments are mobilized with a microhook. (Modified from Saringer WF, Reddy B, Nöbauer-Huhmann I, et al: Endoscopic anterior cervical foraminotomy for unilateral radiculopathy: anatomical morphometric analysis and preliminary clinical experience. *J Neurosurg* 98(2 Suppl):171–180, 2003.)

Transcorporeal Approach

In his technique modification of the transcorporeal approach, Jho describes drilling a hole through the ventral caudolateral portion of the rostral vertebrae[60] that extends dorsally to reach the dorsal portion of the uncinate process. Only this dorsal portion is removed. The uncovertebral osteophyte is removed, and as described earlier, the posterior longitudinal ligament should be opened if a disc fragment has to be removed. This approach reduced the disc disruption comparatively with the transuncal approach. Choi et al. more recently described a modification of this technique made by starting the hole more medially on the upper vertebrae, to avoid cutting the longus colli muscle and its related possible complications.[61] They also stated that a transcorporeal approach through the inferior vertebrae could be feasible, especially for the upper cervical levels (Fig. 49-9).

Once the decompression is completed, the platysma is closed as usual with 3-0 absorbable sutures. The skin is closed with a subcuticular suture. No cervical collar is necessary postoperatively, and activity is advanced as tolerated.

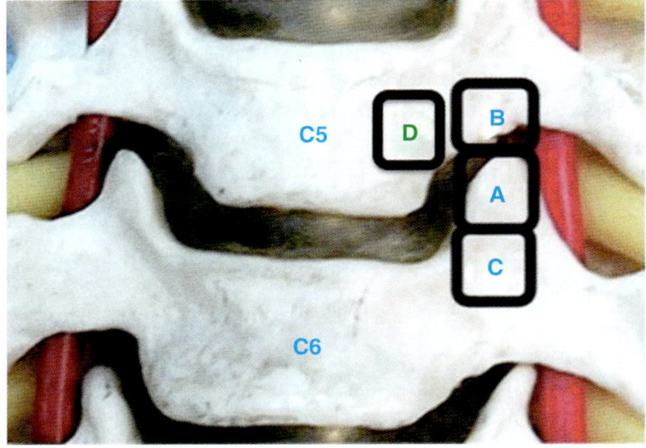

FIGURE 49-9. Photograph of a cervical spine model demonstrating bone entry sites: Transuncal approach as originally discribed by Jho (A); upper transcorporeal approach as described by Jho (B); lower transcorporeal approach (C); and upper transcorporeal approach as described by Choi et al. (D).

Outcomes and Results

The microscopic or endoscopic ventral cervical foraminotomy for unilateral cervical radiculopathy has been shown to be an effective and safe procedure. Johnson et al. reported their series of 21 patients operated on by Jho's original technique and followed between 6 and 36 months.[62] Nineteen patients (91%) had improved or resolved radicular symptoms, and two (9%) had persistent radicular symptoms necessitating further surgery. No patients had evidence of instability or loss of disc height on lateral radiographs at 3 months postoperation. Tascioglu et al. reported their result of the same technique for three patients with long-term follow-up.[63] The three patients were symptom free in the immediate postoperative period, and their follow-up examinations demonstrated findings within normal limits at 37, 36, and 36 months, respectively, after surgery. Saringer et al. reported in 2002 his results of 34 patients operated with microscopic uncoforaminotomy.[58] The follow-up period varied from 2 to 17 months with a mean of 8.2 months. The large majority (97%) of patients were pleased with the results of their operation. The relief of neck pain and redicular pain in the affected dermatome was immediate in all patients. Motor weakness and sensory deficit improved dramatically immediately postoperatively, and improved to normal in the majority of patients within 3 to 6 months. One of the patients had a repeat herniation on the second postoperative day but recovered completely after reoperation and continued to do well at the 6-month follow-up. In 2003, Saringer et al. reported their results from 16 patients operated on with endoscopic uncoforaminotomy.[59] During a mean follow-up period of 13.8 months, an average absolute improvement of 44% ($P > .05$) in the neck disability index score and of 96% ($P > .05$) in the visual analogue scale score for radicular pain (compared with the preoperative score) was observed. Jho et al. reported their results for 104 patients.[60] Ninety-nine percent experienced excellent or good results. One patient developed discitis, which resulted in bony fusion. All other patients maintained their motion segments. Lee et al. reported their results for 13 patients operated on with the transuncal approach[64]; the mean follow-up was 19 months. All patients experienced complete relief of their radiating pain. The mobility was conserved, and no instability was detected on neuroimaging follow-up. Choi et al. also reported their results from 20 patients operated on by their technique.[61] The maximum follow-up was 1 year. All patients experienced immediate postoperative relief of their radicular symptoms and recovery of their neurologic symptoms. The percentage change in disc height was only 6% from the baseline value, but the difference was statistically significant ($P = .005$). They noted that the loss in disc height seemed to stabilize after 3 months postoperation. Balasubramanian et al. also reported 94% good to excellent results in 34 patients.[65]

Hacker and Miller are the only researchers to report a significant number of poor outcomes (poor 35% and fair 13%) and a high reoperation rate (30%).[66]

Hong et al. compared the results of the transuncal approach (40 patients) and the transcorporeal approach (20 patients).[67] The mean follow-up period was 9.5 months. They analyzed postoperative changes of disc height, the spinal instability, the average length of hospital stay, the degree of patients' satisfaction, and complications from each approach. They stated that the transcorporeal approach is a better surgical technique than the transuncal approach, considering the preservation of disc height, spinal stability, length of hospital stay, degree of satisfaction, and complications.

Complications

Possible complications are mostly the same as for a standard anterior cervical approach. As in some of these techniques when the longus colli muscle is cut, risk of injury of the sympathetic chain could be higher. This outcome is true especially at the lower cervical levels, where the sympathetic chain becomes more medial on the longus colli muscle. Jho reported 2 transient Horner syndromes in his 104-patient series.[60] With Choi's technique, this complication could be avoided. Injury of the vertebral artery is another concern of these techniques. Meticulous review of the anatomy of the vertebral artery on the imaging studies and good knowledge of the anatomy of this region should help to avoid this complication.

Percutaneous Ventral Cervical Procedures for Discectomy, Nucleoplasty, and Stabilization

In 1963 to 1964, Smith introduced the chemonucleolysis with chymopapain to treat herniated discs.[68,69] In 1975, Hijikata developed the percutaneous lumbar discectomy and reported his series of 136 cases 12 years later.[70] In 1986, Ascher reported the laser discectomy.[71]

The percutaneous ventral cervical approach was first described by Smith and Nicole in 1957, as the cervical discographic technique for the diagnosis of discogenic pain.[72] Despite its low complication rates (0.16–2.48%),[73-75] its use was limited due to the catastrophic consequences that can occur if a complication developed. Although controversies still exist, several reports of related percutaneous cervical discectomy (PCD) procedures have been reported: (1) PCD with chemonucleolysis,[76] (2) automated/coblation PCD,[77-82] (3) PCD with laser,[83-90] (4) PCD with endoscopic manual and laser,[83,91-95] and (5) PCD with stabilization.[83]

Indications and Contraindications

Patients who present with new onset of cervicobrachial neuralgia, due mainly to recent soft disc herniation (contained), and who are nonresponsive to conservative treatment and without severe neurologic deficit could be considered for PCD with laser, coblation, or chemonucleolysis. In case of the same scenario, but with noncontained herniated disc, PCD with endoscopic manual and laser is recommended. Percutaneous stabilization is indicated when axial symptoms predominate, in case of angular instability (kyphosis), and when cervicoencephalic pain is reproduced by discography.[83]

These procedures are contraindicated in patients with migrated or calcified discs, advanced spondylosis, significant anterior bony spurs that could block the entry into the disc, cervical canal stenosis, myelopathy, or evidence of instability, and in those who had previous neck surgery.[83,92,94]

Surgical Technique

The procedures could be performed under local or general anesthesia. The patent is placed in the supine position, as for a conventional ventral cervical approach. A roll is placed under the shoulders, and the shoulders are taped down for better visualization of the lower cervical levels as needed. Preparation and draping are completed as usual. The choice of the side of approach depends on the surgeon's preference, but an approach contralateral to the side of the lateral herniated disc is preferable. Fluoroscopic guidance is used through the procedure for anatomic orientation and avoidance of complications. The level of work is identified with fluoroscopy, using a K-wire. The point of skin entry will be at the medial border of the sternocleidomastoid muscle. Firm pressure is applied digitally at this level between the sternocleidomastoid muscle and the trachea, and pointed toward the cervical spine. The larynx and esophagus are displaced medially, and the carotid artery is displaced laterally (Fig. 49-10). The esophagus could be made more prominent with the insertion of a nasogastric tube, and the carotid pulse is augmented with sympathomimetics. After palpation of the anterior cervical spine, an 18-gauge spinal needle is placed in the disc space of concern under fluoroscopic guidance. A guidewire is passed through the spine needle and then removed. A 3- to 5-mm skin incision is made, depending on the procedure and instruments to be used. To assist the placement of the endoscope or the working cannula, 3- to 5-mm dilators are passed through the K-wire. Specific instruments are then used to perform the discectomy, with papain (chemonucleolysis), loop-shaped electrode (automated PCD), laser, microcurette, and microforceps, as well as graft for fixation (Figs. 49-11 to 49-14).

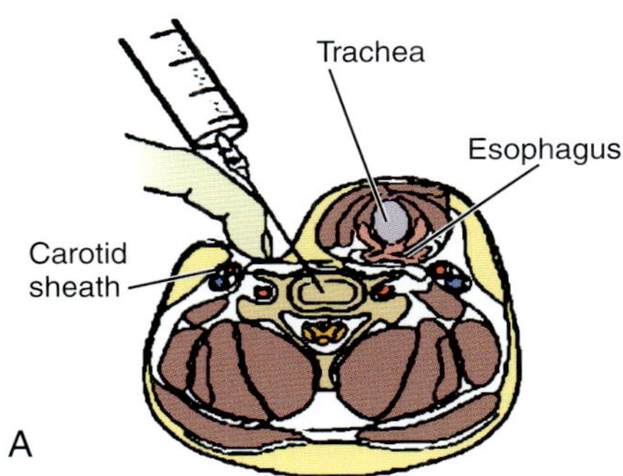

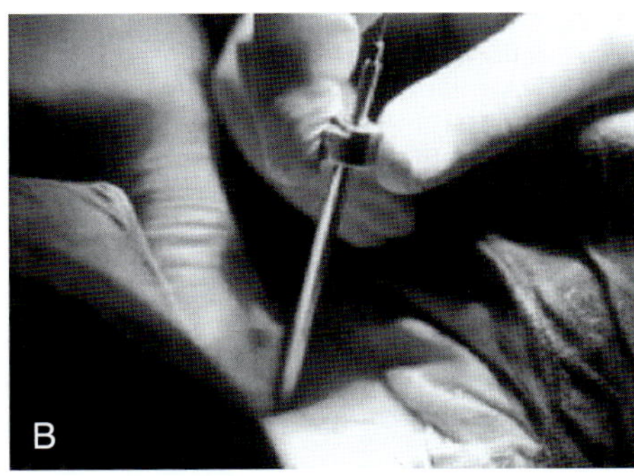

FIGURE 49-10. Illustration of needle insertion (**A**) and intraoperative view of serial dilation (**B**). The tracheoesophagus is displaced medially, and the carotid artery is displaced laterally with the surgeon's finger. An 18-gauge spinal needle is then inserted into the disc space under fluoroscopic monitoring and percutaneous approach using sequential dilation is performed. (Modified from Lee SH, Ahn Y, Choi WC, et al: Immediate pain improvement is a useful predictor of long-term favorable outcome after percutaneous laser disc. *Photomed Laser Surg* 24:508–513, 2006.)

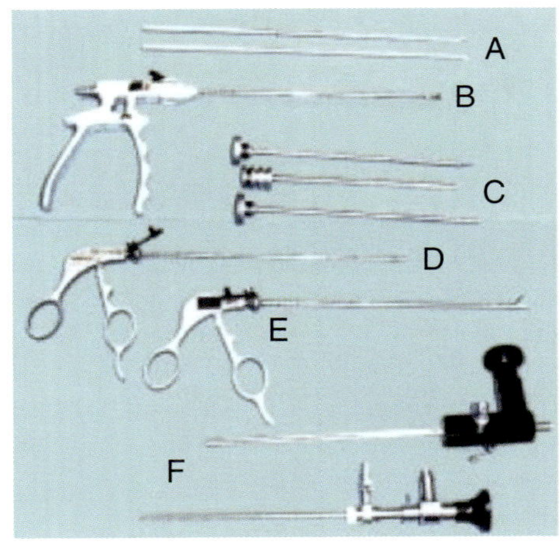

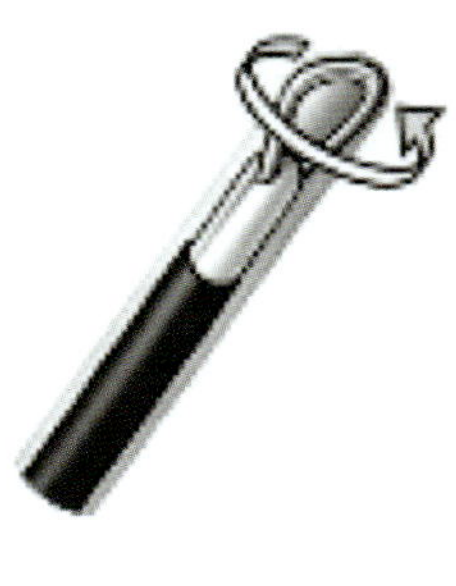

FIGURE 49-11. Minimally invasive spine surgery instruments. *Left:* minicurettes (A), discectome (B), discectomy dilator/cannula/trephine (C), cutter forceps (D), grasper forceps (E), and endoscopes (F). *Right:* Loop-shaped electrode. (*Left,* Modified from Chiu JC, Clifford TJ, Greenspan M, et al: Percutaneous microdecompressive endoscopic cervical discectomy with laser thermodiskoplasty. *Mt Sinai J Med* 67:278–282, 2000. *Right,* Modified from Bonaldi G, Baruzzi F, Facchinetti A, et al: Plasma radio-frequency-based diskectomy for treatment of cervical herniated nucleus pulposus: feasibility, safety, and preliminary clinical results. *AJNR Am J Neuroradiol* 27:2104–2111, 2006.)

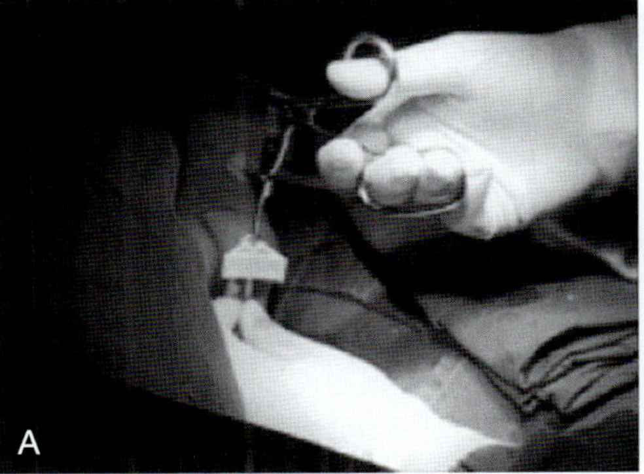

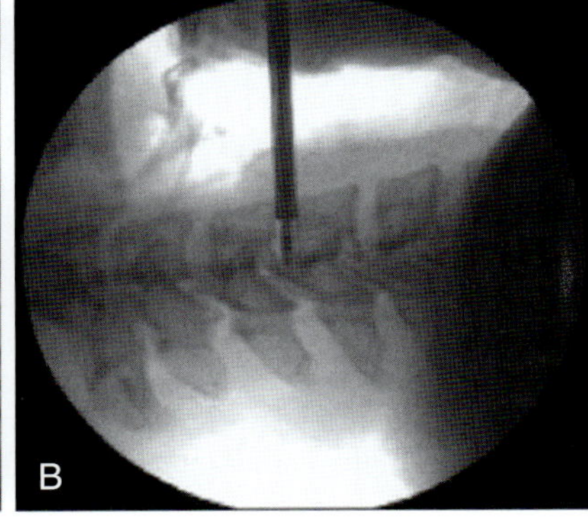

FIGURE 49-12. Intraoperative view (**A**) and C-arm view (**B**) of manual discectomy using microforceps. (Modified from Lee SH, Ahn Y, Choi WC, et al: Immediate pain improvement is a useful predictor of long-term favorable outcome after percutaneous laser disc decompression for cervical disc herniation. *Photomed Laser Surg* 24:508–513, 2006.)

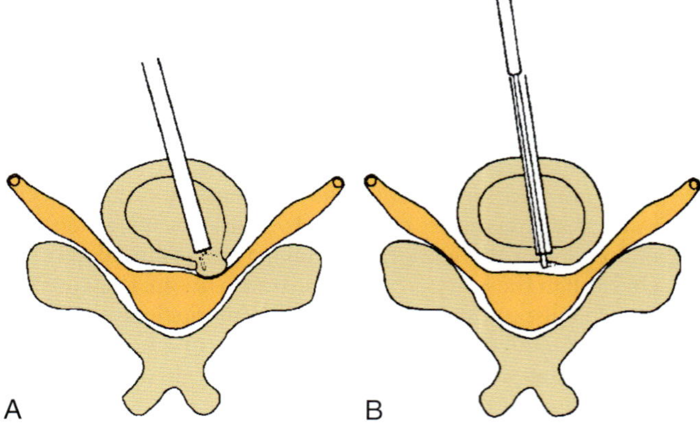

FIGURE 49-13. Schematic diagram of percutaneous endoscopic cervical discectomy. **A,** Cross-sectional view through the disc level. The disc fragment is removed by microforceps under high-resolution endoscopic visualization. **B,** Cross-sectional view through the uncovertebral joint level. The side-firing Ho:YAG laser can safely ablate the osteophytes. (Modified from Ahn Y, Lee SH, Shin SW: Percutaneous endoscopic cervical discectomy: clinical outcome and radiographic changes. *Photomed Laser Surg* 23:362–368, 2005.)

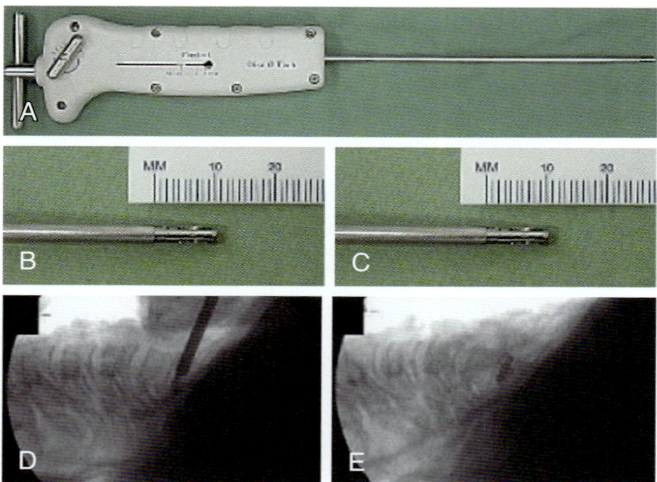

FIGURE 49-14. The cervical B-Twin with its delivery system (**A**), in its reduced form (**B**) and its expanded form (**C**). After its proper positioning in the cervical disc space (**D**), manual rotating leads to expansion of the implant and then the implant is released from the delivery system (**E**). (Modified from Lee SH, Lee JH, Choi WC, et al: Anterior minimally invasive approaches for the cervical spine. *Orthop Clin North Am* 38:327–337, 2007.)

Outcomes, Results, and Complications

Good-to-excellent clinical outcomes were reported in the literature, ranging from 80% to 85% for automated PCD,[78-81] 75% to 94.5% for laser PCD,[86,87,89,90] 80.2% to 94.5% for PCD with manual resection and laser,[91-94] and 86.36% for chemonucleolysis.[76] Predictors of good outcome were found to be related to radiating arm pain, lateral disc location herniation, and immediate postoperative pain relief.[91,93] Radiographically, Ahn et al. showed a significant decrease in the disc height by 11.2%, with maintenance of overall and focal sagittal alignments.[92] There was no segmental instability or spontaneous fusion noted. Interestingly, complication rates were less than 1%, without any catastrophic ones.[76,80,81,86,87,89-91,94] Most serious complications were infection[81] and postoperative hematoma due to rupture of the inferior thyroid artery,[80] not of major vessels. Good knowledge of the cervical anatomy, understanding the safety zone of work for each level,[96] and frequent fluoroscopic checking will help to avoid complications in these procedures.

Li et al. compared retrospectively the percutaneous cervical disc nucleoplasty (42 patients) with the percutaneous cervical discectomy (38 patients).[97] The average follow-up was 12 ± 4 to 5 months. There was no significant difference of the clinical outcomes for the two groups, but operative time was significantly lower for the nucleoplasty group.

Ruetten et al. conducted a prospective, randomized, controlled study to compare the results of full-endoscopic anterior cervical discectomy (FACD) (60 patients) with those of ACDF (60 patients) in mediolateral soft disc herniations.[98] Patients were followed for a period of 2 years. Operative time and blood loss were less in the FACD group. There was no significant difference in the clinical outcomes, the progression of preexisting adjacent disc degeneration, or the increase of the postoperative kyphotic angle at the operated segment between the two groups. Revision rates were 6.1% for the ACDF group and 7.4% for the FACD group.

The clinical outcomes of these techniques seem promising, but they are not widely accepted because of the doubt that the clinical success could be due to the natural history of the disease, rather than the therapeutic effect.

Summary

Minimally invasive techniques have gained popularity in recent decades. Benefits from these approaches include less surgical trauma, preservation of the anatomic structures, early recovery, better cosmesis, and good clinical outcomes. Ventral and dorsal cervical applications seem promising. Careful patient selection, good knowledge of the anatomy, and technical skills are required for achieving good results. More clinical comparative studies with open techniques will be the basis of evidence in using these techniques.

KEY REFERENCES

Jho HD: Microsurgical anterior cervical foraminotomy for radiculopathy: a new approach to cervical disc herniation. *J Neurosurg* 84:55–56, 1996.

Khoo LT, Perez-Cruet MJ, Laich DT, Fessler RG: Posterior cervical microendoscopic foraminotomy. In Perez-Cruet MJ, Fessler RG, editors: *Outpatient spinal surgery*, St Louis, 2006, Quality Medical Publishing, pp 71–93.

Lee SH, Lee JH, Choi WC, et al: Anterior minimally invasive approaches for the cervical spine. *Orthop Clin North Am* 38:327–337, 2007.

Perez-Cruet MJ, Samartzis D, Fessler RG: Microendoscopic cervical laminectomy. In Perez-Cruet MJ, Khoo LT, Fessler RG, editors: *An anatomic approach to minimally invasive spine surgery*, St Louis, 2006, Quality Medical Publishing, pp 349–366.

Santiago P, Fessler RG: Minimally invasive surgery for the management of cervical spondylosis. *Neurosurgery* 60(Suppl 1):S160–S165, 2007.

Saringer W, Nöbauer I, Reddy M, et al: Microsurgical anterior cervical foraminotomy (uncoforaminotomy) for unilateral radiculopathy: clinical results of a new technique. *Acta Neurochir (Wien)* 144:685–694, 2002.

REFERENCES

The complete reference list is available online at expertconsult.com.

CHAPTER 50

Ventral and Ventrolateral Spine Decompression and Fusion

Eric M. Massicotte | Michael G. Fehlings | Alexander R. Vaccaro

Ventral spinal decompression was described by Royle[1] as early as 1928. This approach remained unused until 1956, when Hodgson and Stock[2] reported the use of ventral spinal decompression in the treatment of tuberculous lesions. A progressive increase in the use of ventral and ventrolateral approaches for spinal decompression in treating various spinal lesions such as tuberculosis, pyogenic osteomyelitis, kyphotic deformities, neoplasms (primary and metastatic), and burst fractures[3-6] has been observed. The types of ventral approaches used for different spinal levels are summarized in Table 50-1. Ventral and ventrolateral decompression principles for spinal tumors are discussed in depth. This discussion is followed by the management of other types of spinal pathology that may be treated through a ventral decompression.

Spinal Tumors

The surgical management of patients with spinal tumors and associated spinal cord compression has shifted from a laminectomy approach to ventral approaches with ventral decompression.[3,7-9] Because most spinal tumors are located ventrally, a laminectomy can limit the degree of ventral resection and can exacerbate, or worsen, existing spinal instability associated with tumors that have destroyed spinal body segments. Several authors[10,11] have reported that the results of ventral decompression of spinal tumors with spinal cord compression are significantly better in most cases when compared with radiation therapy (RT) alone or in conjunction with laminectomy. Patchell et al. demonstrated the superiority of combined surgery and radiation in their randomized study.[12] Ambulation as their primary end point was significantly better in the combined surgery and radiation cohort. Dorsolateral approaches can also provide some degree of ventral spinal decompression, with the advantage that they allow for both ventral and dorsal decompression and dorsal stabilization with a single exposure. Because of the limited access of the contralateral ventral dural sac, however, this exposure is more suitable in cases with unilateral spinal canal and vertebral involvement. The results of ventral decompression suggest that this is an effective method to preserve and improve neurologic function in patients with neural compromise from primary and metastatic tumors of the thoracic and lumbar spine.[3,4,13,14]

TABLE 50-1
Classification of Ventral Surgical Approaches

Spinal Segment	Surgical Approach
Cervicothoracic C7-T2 (see Fig. 50-11)	Extended ventral cervical (division of strap muscles)
	Transsternal
	Cervicosternotomy ("trapdoor" approach)
Upper thoracic T2-5 (see Fig. 50-10)	High dorsolateral thoracotomy (third-rib approach with mobilization of scapula)
T6-12	Dorsolateral thoracotomy
Thoracolumbar T12-L2 (see Figs. 50-2 to 50-7)	Transthoracic/retroperitoneal with 10th to 12th rib resection; division of diaphragm
Lumbar	Retroperitoneal/flank
L2-5	Transabdominal
Lumbosacral L5-sacrum	Ventral retroperitoneal ("pelvic brim" approach)

The principal indications for ventral decompressive surgery in patients with ventrally located spinal tumors are (1) progressive neurologic deficits, (2) pathologic fracture or impending spinal instability, and (3) mechanical or compressive pain. In rare circumstances, resection of a lesion to make the diagnosis is required. A CT-guided needle biopsy can and should be undertaken if the lesion has characteristics of a primary tumor. The issue of pain can be controversial; if the etiology of the pain is from compression of the neural tissues or mechanical instability, justification for decompression and fixation can be made. The authors have intervened surgically on terminal patients with a life expectancy of 3 to 4 months for whom conservative measures have failed to provide sufficient pain relief. Life expectancy is therefore an important factor to consider, but one must appreciate the collective limitations in arriving at an exact figure.

The radiosensitivity of the tumor plays an important role in overall management. Radiosensitive tumors (e.g., lymphoma, myeloma, Ewing sarcoma, neuroblastoma) can be treated with radiation therapy initially, if the cord compression is the result of epidural tumor alone. Surgical decompression should be the initial treatment when a significant degree of compression can be attributed to bony or ligamentous fragments or spinal deformity, as a result of destruction by tumor. In cases of failed radiation therapy with persistent or recurrent spinal cord compression, surgical intervention is also recommended. The increased complications associated with operating on a previously radiated site also favor surgery before radiation. Surgical decompression can be considered for radiation-resistant tumors such as melanoma or renal cell carcinoma and intermediate radiosensitive tumors such as those of the lung, breast, or prostate. The rate of clinical progression provides the surgeon with valuable information when deciding the optimal timing of intervention. Rapid progression of symptoms is best managed with surgery because the effects of radiation can initially be associated with swelling. The medical status of the patient and ability to tolerate the surgery are also taken into consideration. The issue of radiation sensitivity of tumors is changing. The field of radiation treatment, much like the surgical field, has seen significant advances. Stereotactic delivery of radiation and image modulation are just two examples.

Preoperative Assessment

Initially, plain spine radiographs (anteroposterior and lateral) are used to determine the level and extent of tumor involvement. The spinal alignment can also be observed from these films. A CT scan without intravenous contrast at the appropriate spinal levels allows better definition of the degree of bony destruction of the spinal column. Although MRI is less precise than CT in outlining bony destruction, it provides the most precise means for illustrating the site and degree of spinal cord compression by tumor or soft tissues (Fig. 50-1). Myelography and postmyelography CT scan can be used

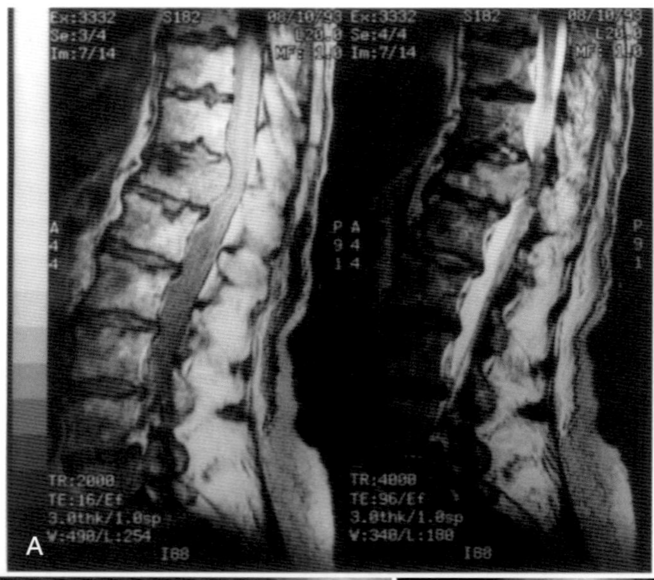

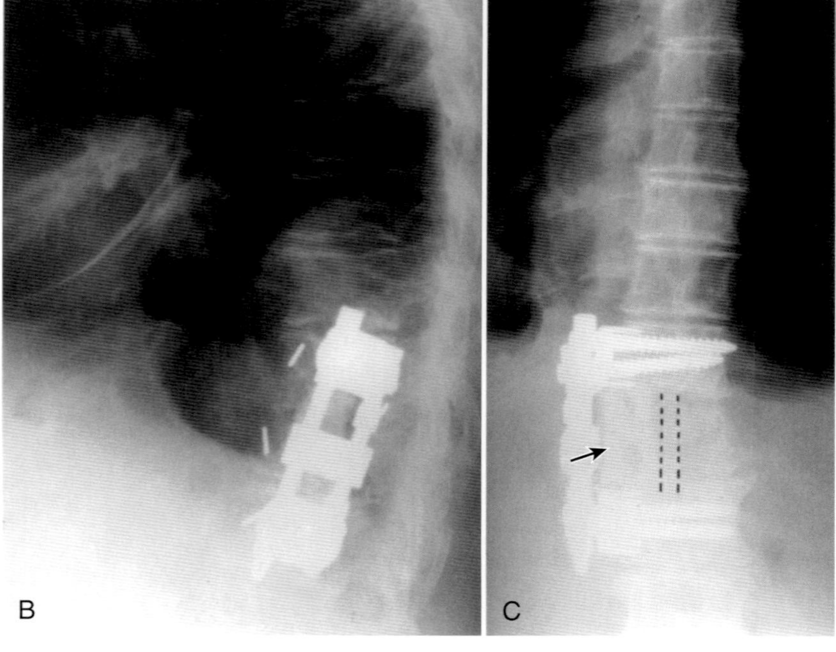

FIGURE 50-1. **A,** Proton density and T2-weighted sagittal MRI of metastatic carcinoma of the breast to the T12 vertebral body with angulation and severe spinal cord compression. **B** and **C,** Postoperative lateral and anteroposterior radiographs after T12 vertebral body resection showing the placement of a rib bone graft, methylmethacrylate, and Kaneda instrumentation. (*Arrow* in **C** indicates spinal canal.) Postoperatively, the patient recovered full neurologic function and was pain free. In view of the isolated vertebral body involvement, it was believed that good long-term survival was possible (thus the use of additional bone graft in the reconstruction). The patient, however, died of systemic metastatic cancer 8 months postoperatively.

when MRI is contraindicated or unavailable. The use of contrast for determining the degree of vascularity of the tumor with either CT scan or MRI is still at the research level. CT angiographies are becoming more useful in the spine as their resolution is increasing.

To avoid complications from intraoperative and postoperative instability of the spinal column, it is important to assess the spinal stability before performing a vertebral decompression. Stability can be considered in terms of the three-column theory, after the extent of bony destruction produced by tumor has been determined from imaging.[15,16] Single-column involvement can be considered relatively stable. The additive destabilizing effects of decompression, however, must factor into the decision-making process.

Anterior column and middle column involvement is the most common finding in symptomatic patients with spinal

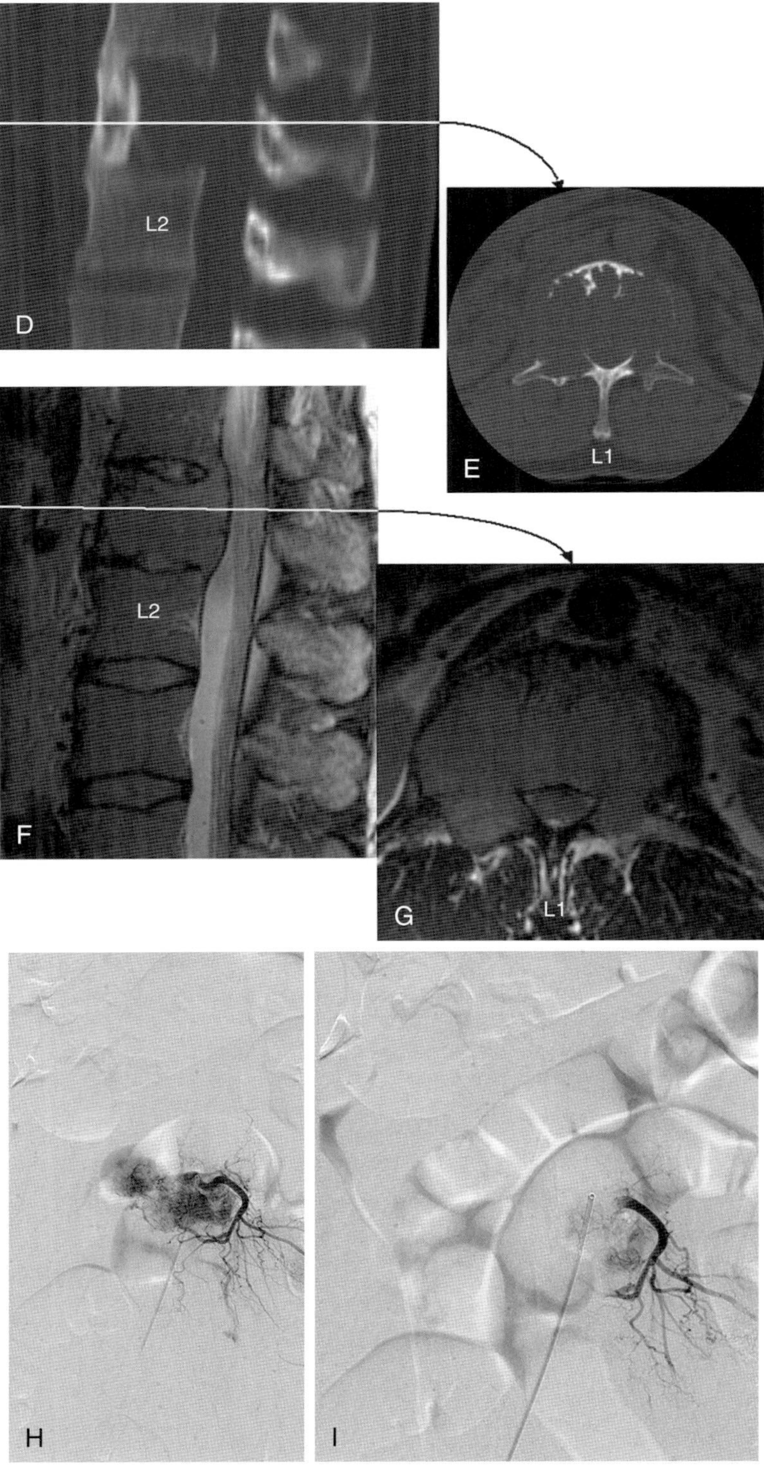

FIGURE 50-1, cont. D, Sagittal reconstruction CT scan and corresponding axial image of (**E**) a patient with plasmacytoma involving the L1 vertebral body. T2-weighted sagittal (**F**) and axial (**G**) MRIs of the same case. Images of the CT scan illustrate the bony destruction, whereas the MRIs show the spinal cord compression more accurately. **H,** Preembolization angiogram showing the vascular supply of the L1 lesion with a tumor blush. **I,** Postembolization angiogram with a significant reduction in tumor blush in the same case.

tumors and is frequently associated with some degree of vertebral body collapse and bony retropulsion into the spinal canal (see Fig. 50-1A). If these conditions are treated by corpectomy, with a strut graft used for fusion (see Figs. 50-1B and C), stability of the spinal column can be achieved.

Careful review of the degree of involvement of the dorsal elements is required. The need for augmentation of ventral fixation with dorsal instrumentation will be based on the integrity of the laminae, lateral masses, pars interarticularis, and facets. Corpectomy and vertebral replacement techniques can result in persistent dorsal element instability if overdistraction and opening of the facets are achieved. This instability can prevent subsequent fusion and result in failure of the ventral fixation. The ease with which distraction can be obtained following decompression can also provide the surgeon with information regarding the degree of dorsal instability. Intraoperative radiographs can be taken to ensure the proper amount of distraction. In cases when the dorsal instability is deemed significant, dorsal stabilization should be undertaken. Discretion of the surgeon will be used to decide if and when the dorsal stabilization procedure is required.

When planning surgery for spinal tumors, an assessment of stability must also take into account angulation and alignment.[16] Higher failure rates will be observed with a poorly aligned construct. It is also important to consider the nature of the tumor in terms of its capacity to infiltrate and destroy bony tissue and its response to RT or chemotherapy.

Preoperative Angiography and Embolization

Angiography, with a view to embolization, is recommended for patients with known vascular tumors (e.g., melanoma, renal cell carcinoma, metastatic thyroid tumor, primary giant cell tumor) or in patients in whom imaging suggests a relatively vascular tumor. If these tumors are amenable to embolization, it should be performed no more than 48 hours before surgery. Waiting too long after embolization may result in recanalization. The expertise of the interventional neuroradiologist will influence greatly the impact of presurgical embolization by reducing intraoperative blood loss. Additional information concerning the vascular supply of the spinal cord can also be obtained. Performing a spinal angiogram, however, for the sole purpose of defining the anatomy is unwarranted.

Surgical Management

Intraoperative Monitoring and Anesthetic Management

The authors recommend electrophysiologic monitoring, if available, including somatosensory and motor evoked potentials, at all vertebral levels involving the spinal cord. Electromyography (EMG) monitoring is also useful in the lumbar region, if segmental pedicular fixation is contemplated. Monitoring setup time and cost are definite drawbacks to this type of technology, although its use is generally supported in the literature.[12,17-19] In approaches of the upper and middle thoracic spine, a double-lumen endotracheal tube allows the lung in the operative field to be deflated, improving the surgical exposure. In lesions of the lower thoracic and thoracolumbar regions, the lung can be retracted easily. Invasive arterial pressure monitoring and central venous pressure (CVP) monitoring and access are recommended in order to address any blood loss during the surgery.

Positioning

Patients are positioned in the full lateral decubitus position (Fig. 50-2) with an axillary roll placed under the dependent axilla to prevent neurovascular compromise. A mild flexion in the hip will assist mobilization of the psoas muscle should the exposure require it.

Incision and Exposure

The side of approach and the level of the spine that is involved are important factors in determining where to make the incision. To maximize resection, the decision to perform a right-sided or left-sided skin incision and approach should be determined by the side of the spine with greater tumor involvement. If neither side is predominantly involved by tumor, the spine is generally approached from the right side, at or above the T5 vertebral segment, to avoid the arch of the aorta. Below T5, the spine is generally approached from the left side to minimize retraction on the liver. Careful review of the axial images in order to appreciate the corridor of access between the great vessels and the lateral aspect of the spine is essential. This information may, in fact, push a surgeon to the other side and to tolerate the liver retraction.

Lesions involving the cervicothoracic (C7-T1), upper thoracic (T1-5), lower thoracic (T6-11), thoracolumbar (T12 and L1), and lumbar and sacral (L2 to sacrum) segments require specific approaches (see Table 50-1) and considerations that have been described in other chapters of this text.

Spinal Decompression

Spinal decompression requires a sequential approach that can be divided into four stages, which are discussed in the next four sections.

Exposure

The pleura is sharply incised and reflected. A rib that overlies the level of the pathology in the midaxillary level is resected. The appropriate rib is identified using intraoperative imaging. The segmental vessels at the level of the pathology and of the

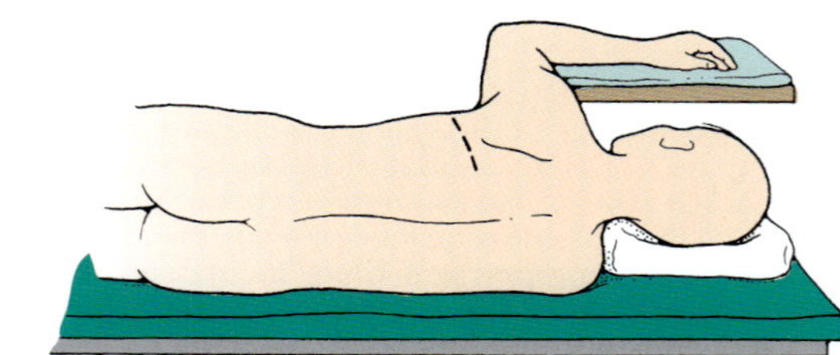

FIGURE 50-2. Patient is in the lateral position, and a dorsolateral thoracotomy skin incision is placed below the scapula.

vertebral bodies above and below the lesion (Fig. 50-3) are ligated and divided. Division of segmental vessels over the vertebral body in the middle of the body reduces the risk of vascular compromise of the spinal cord by taking advantage of collateral vessels from adjacent levels. The periosteum is reflected medially, and the anterior longitudinal ligament is identified.

Vertebral Body Decompression

The intervertebral discs above and below the involved vertebral body are identified and resected initially by sharp dissection (Fig. 50-4). Disc material is cleared with curettes and pituitary rongeurs. Removing the rib head will allow identification of the ipsilateral pedicle and its continuation into the vertebral body. The pedicle is an important marker for the orientation and position of the spinal canal. Using sharp curettes, rongeurs, and a high-speed drill, the vertebral body is resected ventrally to dorsally, except for a rim of the ventral portion of the vertebral body. This rim protects the aorta and inferior vena cava from accidental trauma. Resection of the vertebral body can progress as far as the opposite pedicle (Figs. 50-5 and 50-6), and the entire dorsal aspect of the vertebral body can be removed. Sufficient bone needs to be removed to clear the posterior longitudinal ligament of any compression of the dura. The dissection can also be continued dorsolaterally to allow decompression of the spinal nerve roots. The tumor involvement and the quality of the residual bone for instrumentation will determine the extent of bony removal. Techniques to augment the strength of the purchase into the bone are discussed in subsequent paragraphs.

Rostrocaudal Dissection

Special care is afforded to the cartilaginous end plates and the central regions of cancellous bone of vertebral bodies adjacent to the corpectomy site. Removal is performed using a small high-speed bur or curette (Fig. 50-7) or osteotomes and rongeurs, depending on the bone consistency. This allows troughs to be created in the vertebral bodies above and below the corpectomy site to allow subsequent reconstruction with a bone graft, an implant, or an acrylic graft. Preparing the end plates to accommodate the construct requires special attention. When the construct involves bone, either autograft or allograft, an eventual fusion will be desired. In this circumstance the end plates require adequate vascular supply for achieving fusion. The structural integrity of the graft can also fail if it is suboptimal or radiated. Methylmethacrylate (MMA), on the other hand, will not fuse, and the overall construct strength can be weakened by aggressive removal of the end plates. The risk of telescoping and the graph imploding into the vertebral body can also occur when the end plates are destroyed. MMA, however, will tolerate radiation.

Intraspinal Decompression

After adequate bony resection, decompression, and removal of all devitalized bone and tumor tissue, the posterior

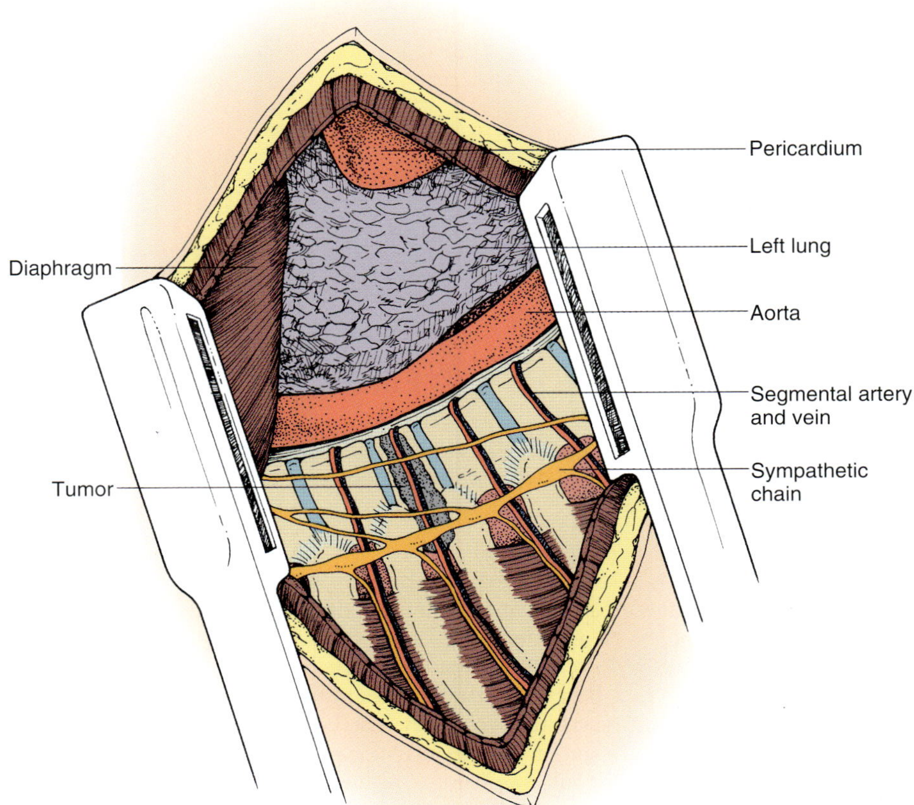

FIGURE 50-3. Exposure of the thoracic spine after entry into the thoracic cavity and placement of a self-retaining chest retractor. The parietal pleura has been separated from the ribs and spinal column with the segmental vessels along the side of the vertebrae identified.

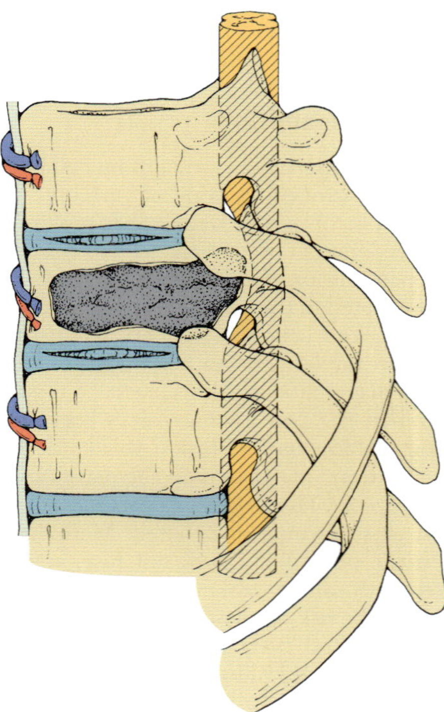

FIGURE 50-4. After a thoracotomy via resection of a rib located one level rostrally, the pleura is reflected off the ventral spine. The segmental vascular bundles are isolated and ligated as shown. Vertebral decompression of the tumor begins by the excision of intervertebral discs above and below the involved vertebra. Following this, 1 to 2 cm of the rib head is drilled down to expose the ipsilateral pedicle.

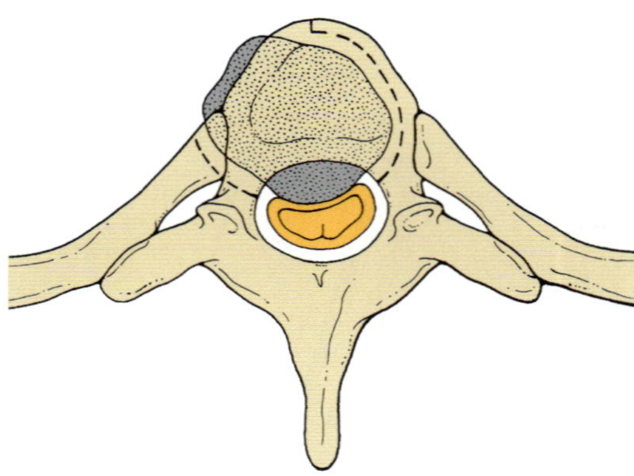

FIGURE 50-5. Axial section through vertebra involved with spinal tumor showing the extent of bony decompression necessary to allow adequate tumor resection.

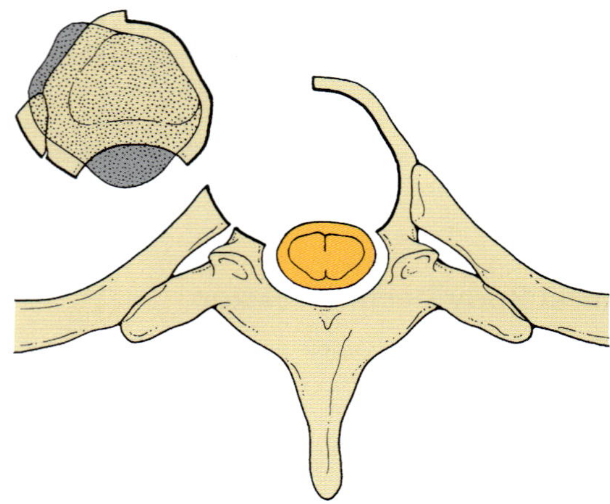

FIGURE 50-6. Remaining vertebra after bony decompression and tumor removal showing that the decompression extends from the ipsilateral pedicle to the contralateral pedicle.

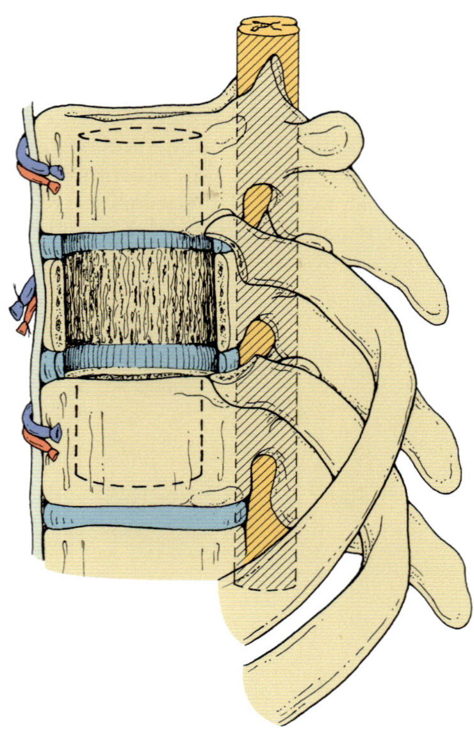

FIGURE 50-7. After tumor resection, the end plates and cancellous bone of adjacent vertebral bodies are removed to the degree shown *(dotted line)* using an angled high-speed drill or angled curettes.

longitudinal ligament is resected to expose the dura mater that encloses the spinal cord and segmental nerve roots. Any tumor or bone impinging on the dural sac or nerve root is carefully removed to allow decompression of these structures. The goal of surgery should be radical tumor resection and decompression. In patients who have previously received RT, the posterior longitudinal ligament is frequently adherent to the dura mater and may be difficult to separate. In these cases, it may be advisable to leave it in situ. In most virgin cases the dissection plane between tumor and dura is easily exploited.

Avoiding Complications during Spinal Decompression

Complications Related to the Approach

A thoracotomy carries pulmonary risks such as atelectasis and pneumonia. The retroperitoneal exposure may injure the spleen, kidney, or ureter, and a prolonged postoperative ileus may occur. Any unrepaired defect in the abdominal wall or diaphragm may be the site of visceral herniation. Using vertebral body screws with manual confirmation of bicortical penetration requires considerable dissection of the contralateral aspect of the vertebral body, placing the aorta, inferior vena cava, and iliac vessels at risk if this is not done meticulously. Injury to the lumbar hypogastric plexus at L5 in males may be complicated by retrograde ejaculation. Chyle leak from damage to the thoracic duct is best managed with immediate repair.

Inadequate Spinal Decompression

Inadequate decompression or incomplete tumor resection reduces the chance of adequate neurologic recovery. It is important that the decompression be performed to the contralateral pedicle. Complete visualization of the dura mater and confirmation with intraoperative radiograph that the appropriate level has been decompressed are required.

Neurologic Injury

A carefully staged approach to spinal decompression with adequate exposure and identification of segmental vessels, nerve roots, and the dural tube markedly reduces the risk of nerve root and spinal cord injury. Nuwer[20] concluded that intraoperative neurophysiologic monitoring is a cost-effective way of reducing the potential for a neurologic deficit. Intraoperative information is valuable not only to the prognosis but also by altering intraoperative and postoperative management. Hardware revision and removal during the operation may be performed on the basis of intraoperative neurophysiologic changes.

Dural Tears

Dural tear from direct surgical trauma may occur while the tumor is being dissected or because of erosion of the dura caused by the tumor. In these cases, the precise site of dural tear should be identified and the tear repaired with a nonabsorbable suture (e.g., 4-0 Nurolon [Ethicon]). In less discrete or poorly visualized dural tears, fibrin glue can be layered over the cerebrospinal fluid leakage site and allowed to adhere to underlying dura mater. A lumbar drain should be placed for 5 days postoperatively to assist dural closure and reduce cerebrospinal fluid leaks.

Excessive Epidural Bleeding or Bleeding from Tumor

Preoperative angiography and embolization of vascular tumors reduce the risk of such intraoperative bleeding. After careful identification and mobilization, segmental vessels above and below the corpectomy site should be ligated and cut to avoid bleeding from these vessels when the vertebral bodies adjacent to the corpectomy site are spread apart. Other sites of epidural bleeding should be identified, and hemostasis should be attained with bipolar coagulation. Epidural bleeding can be particularly troublesome and require the use of various packing agents such as hemostatic gelatin (Gelfoam, Baxter Healthcare, Glendale, CA) and thrombin. Dealing with epidural vessels by coagulation before sharp dissection is the optimal strategy. Tumor bleeding can also be difficult to address. Remember to remove all visible tumor, because the most frequent site of bleeding is from the tumor bed. Preoperative planning and gross total resection of the lesion is the best strategy for tumor bleeding. Tumor bleeding can also be controlled using various packing material as described earlier. Polymethylmethacrylate (PMMA) in the resection cavity can be used. The primary function is to reconstruct, but one of the secondary benefits will be from the thermal reaction of the cement, which can cauterize the remaining tissues.

Spinal Reconstruction

Graft Material

The appropriate type of material to use for spinal column reconstruction depends on the nature of the lesion and the patient's life expectancy. In cases of trauma, for benign lesions, or for patients with malignant tumors who have a relatively long life expectancy (>2 years), reconstruction is best when using autogenous bone from the iliac crest or rib for single vertebral body defects. If two or more vertebral levels are involved with the neoplasm, an allograft (e.g., from the fibula or humerus) can be used. It is often useful to supplement the allograft strut with local autograft bone (Fig. 50-8).

In patients with malignant disease and a short life expectancy, autogenous bone grafts have certain disadvantages: (1) If life expectancy is less than 1 year, solid bony fusion over the long term is unnecessary; (2) the use of adjunctive radiation and chemotherapy will slow or prevent the bony fusion needed for stability; (3) any remaining local tumors may infiltrate the bone graft and weaken the construct; and (4) autogenous donor sites may not be suitable because of tumor involvement.

For patients with an expected survival of 18 months or less, a synthetic construct using PMMA with or without titanium cages can be used. Expandable cages with only titanium construct have also been used to provide ventral support and reconstruction in difficult cases (see Fig. 50-8D and E). Biomechanical studies looking at intervertebral fixation have shown resistance of the implants to cyclical fatigue within typical normal physiologic loading and superior reduction of intervertebral motion and increased spinal stiffness.[11,21-27] The use of expandable vertebral protheses or cages is gaining popularity. An example of such a device can be found with the X-mesh cage (DePuy Spine, Raynham, MA).

Reconstruction Technique

Reconstruction techniques aim to provide solid fixation of adjacent spinal segments. Failure of these constructs is usually the result of reconstruction material dislodging at proximal and/or distal ends where the material fits into adjacent spinal segments. Early spinal changes in the cancellous bone of adjacent vertebral segments, seen on postoperative MRI scans, can be an indication of potential failure of these regions to anchor the construct. Another important situation is one in which adjacent vertebral segments are involved with disease but are not collapsed and are not causing spinal cord compression. PMMA can be used to strengthen the adjacent bone. Alternatively, supplemental dorsal instrumentation may be required. The technique of vertebroplasty has grown significantly in popularity for osteopenic fractures in the elderly.[28-32]

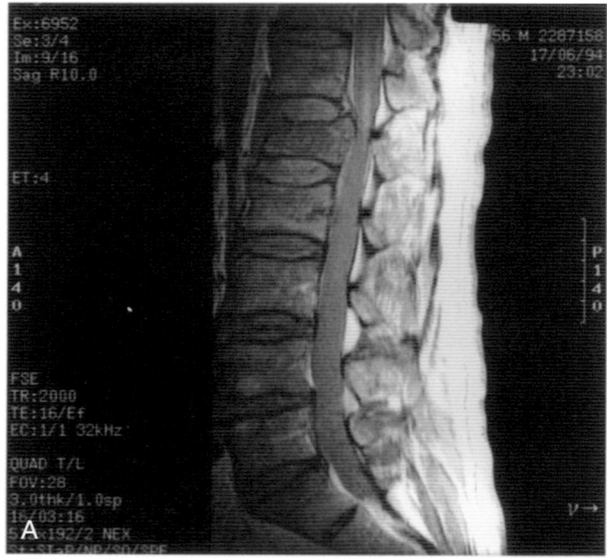

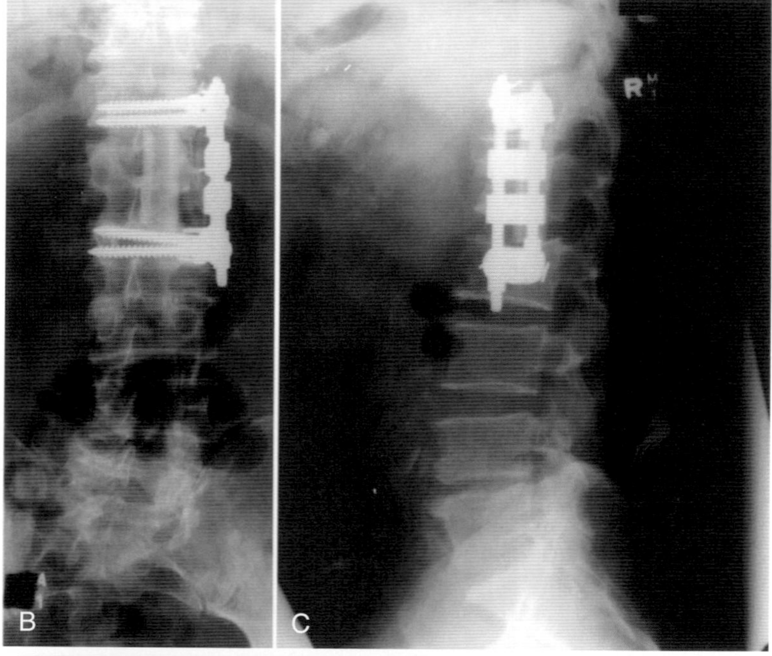

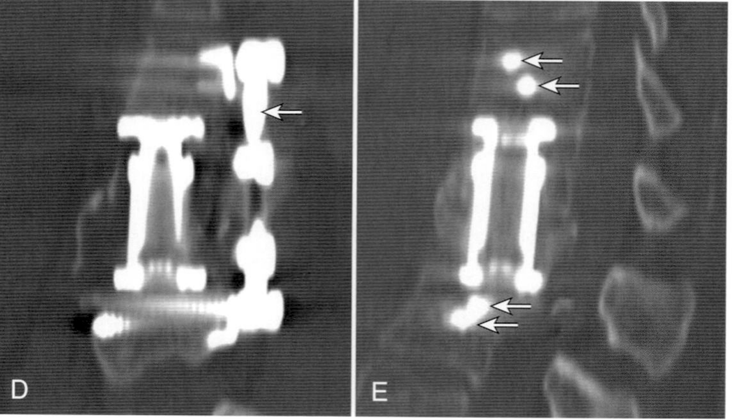

FIGURE 50-8. A, Proton density sagittal MRI scan illustrating an L1 burst fracture with compression of the conus. **B** and **C,** Postoperative anteroposterior and lateral radiographs after anterior decompression and stabilization using bone graft (combination of humeral allograft and rib autograft) and Kaneda instrumentation. Coronal (**D**) and sagittal (**E**) CT scan images showing an expandable cage for the reconstruction of a two-level corpectomy. The Kaneda system is added to the construct for additional support to the anterior and middle column. The *arrows* in (**E**) identify the Kaneda screws into the body above and below the cage, while the *arrow* in (**D**) shows the connecting rods.

This technique can complement and add strength to a ventral or even dorsal construct.

Synthetic Constructs

The technique of Errico and Cooper,[7] in which PMMA is pressure injected into a Silastic tube that is fitted against the vertebral bodies above and below, provides an ideally suited construct for patients with metastatic lesions (Fig. 50-9). Silastic tubing of varying diameters (typically 15–20 mm) is cut to a measured length (from the outer edge of the upper and lower troughs of adjacent vertebral segments to the corpectomy site). One 6-mm-diameter hole is made in the center of the tubing with a rongeur, and three small holes are made laterally, two at the rostral end and one at the caudal end. Small bites are also made at the ends of the tubing to allow extrusion of cement overflow. The three smaller lateral holes allow air bubbles and excess cement to flow out easily. The side of the Silastic tubing facing the spinal cord is free of the central and lateral holes to avoid cement extrusion into the spinal canal. The Silastic tubing is passed into the space between two adjacent vertebral bodies at the corpectomy site and positioned so that there is no bending of the tubing that could obstruct cement flow. Low-viscosity, slow-curing PMMA is prepared and is kept in a large 50-mL syringe. When it has become semiliquid, the PMMA is injected through the center hold of the Silastic tubing, filling the tubing until PMMA can be seen passing out from the ends of the tube (see Fig. 50-9). Certain PMMA mixtures are now available, allowing for more controlled timing of the reaction and more reliable handling characteristics. The tube must be observed carefully to avoid spilling the PMMA into the spinal canal. Curved Penfield dissectors can be used to protect the dural tube. As the PMMA in the Silastic tubing becomes harder, more PMMA is prepared and placed ventral and lateral to the Silastic tube until it is continuous with the borders of the upper and lower vertebrae. During polymerization and hardening of the PMMA, copious saline irrigation is used to help dissipate the heat. Hemostasis is attained with bipolar coagulation.

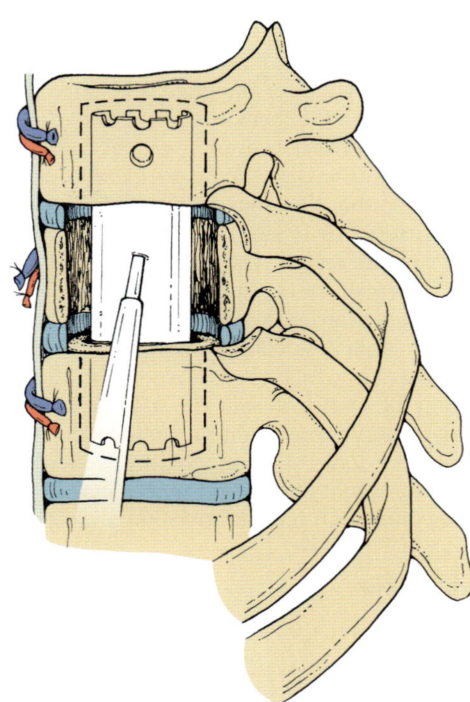

FIGURE 50-9. After the Silastic tubing is inserted into the spinal defect, a syringe is used to fill the tube with slow-curing, low-viscosity polymethylmethacrylate.

Using Silastic tubing instead of K-wires, in conjunction with PMMA, for reconstruction of the vertebral body defect has certain advantages. First, the pliable Silastic tubing can be positioned with its ends sitting against the graft beds of the rostral and caudal adjacent vertebrae. This ensures the tubing is anchored against the adjacent vertebral bodies and does not remain unanchored in an open defect, thus reducing the risk of extrusion of the cement into the spinal canal and enhancing fixation to the adjacent vertebral column. Second, passing PMMA into the cancellous bone of adjacent vertebral segments further reinforces the vertebral bodies above and below the corpectomy site. Third, the pliable plastic filled with hardened PMMA becomes a long rigid construct that encompasses the length of the corpectomy site defect to assist anchorage into adjacent vertebrae, which reduces the risk of the construct dislodging from this position.

Degree of Vertebral Involvement

Most forms of metastatic spinal disease usually involve the vertebral body. When there is significant involvement of the dorsal elements, dorsal resection of the pathology can be performed by laminectomy. The decision to decompress using a ventral or dorsal approach is based on the location of the pathology and the compression. Combined approaches are required when the destruction of the native spinal column is circumferential. Many surgeons prefer to proceed with ventral decompression initially because this approach will more often provide a greater degree of decompression. Dorsal instrumentation will supplement the ventral construct and can be done either in combination with the initial operation or in a delayed fashion. Circumferential stabilization is recommended to prevent subsequent spinal instability, spinal deformity, or excessive spinal movement that may predispose to loosening and dislodgement of the spinal construct at the corpectomy site. The length of the dorsal instrumentation will be based on the quality of the pedicular purchase and the overall alignment of the construct. Instrumentation should not be terminated in the midthoracic curve to minimize the chance of pulling out the screws at the end of the instrumentation. Added consideration is given to the transition zones at the cervicothoracic and thoracolumbar levels. Bridging of these areas is often required to reduce the chance of failure of the spinal segment adjacent to the construct.

Bony Graft Fusion in Malignant and Nonmalignant Disease

In patients with nonmalignant disease, or with malignant disease with a relatively longer survival period (usually >2 years), a bone graft is used to supplement the synthetic construct described earlier (see Fig. 50-1).

Fusion

Distraction

After initial vertebral decompression, vertebral distraction is attained by using a vertebral distracter or by applying distraction after placing vertebral screws.

Graft Site Preparation

The end plates of vertebral bodies adjacent to the decompression site are prepared to accept a graft. The underlying cancellous bone should not be exposed by complete removal of the end plates. Destruction of the end plates will lead to reduction of the mechanical strength of the vertebral body and increase the risk of the strength of the vertebral body. It will also increase the risk of the graft telescoping into or penetrating the weakened vertebral bodies. The rostral and caudal end plates are of different shapes. This difference must be kept in mind, and selective drilling must be used to ensure that the graft site has parallel surfaces with adequate cortical bone remaining to support the graft. One common mistake is the failure to remove sufficient ventral and dorsal end plate lip, resulting in a central gap between the bone graft and vertebral end-plate. Another mistake that has more serious consequences is the "ramp effect," which occurs when excessive bone is removed from the ventral two thirds of the lower vertebral body. This excessive removal results in a graft site that is longer ventrally than dorsally, predisposing to ventral dislocation of the graft.

Grafting

A firm, well-fitted graft is the result of not only a well-prepared graft site but also a well-proportioned, appropriately sized bone graft. A caliper and depth gauge should be used to measure the length and depth of the graft site accurately to determine the dimensions of the bone strut. The depth of the graft site is measured from the dorsal cortex to the ventral cortex along the midline of the vertebral body. The length of the graft site is measured with the vertebral bodies maximally distracted and is the distance between the end plates.

A tricortical iliac crest bone graft can be used up to a two-level corpectomy. More extensive decompression may necessitate a humeral or fibular allograft. Such an allograft strut has greater biomechanical strength than an iliac crest, with an acceptable fusion rate. The high cortical bone content, however, means that it may take up to 1 year for the graft to incorporate.[33] A supplemental local autograft (e.g., from rib or vertebral body) enhances the rate of fusion when using allografts (see Fig. 50-8). If grafts are taken from the iliac crest, the osteotomies should be perpendicular to the surface to the iliac crest and parallel to each other. A double-bladed oscillatory saw is useful in obtaining parallel surfaces. When these grafts are to be used for subtotal or total vertebral body replacement, several extra millimeters should be taken to allow for further reshaping. In the midthoracic and upper thoracic spine, rib strut grafts taken at the time of the thoracotomy are usually adequate if combined with cages.

With the vertebral bodies distracted, the graft is gently placed into position and should fit without excessive force or hammering. Tactile inspection of the final position of the graft should be done using a blunt hook alongside the graft. Small pieces of cancellous bone can be gently impacted into the remaining gaps. However, care should be taken to avoid spinal canal compromise or compression of neural structures by these smaller pieces of bone. It is important to use a drill to remove any irregularities of the ventral surface of the vertebral bodies so that the plate can sit flush against them. A greater plate-to-bone contact allows increased structural stability of this construct.

Avoiding Complications Related to Fusion

To reduce the morbidity that can be associated with this procedure, specific fusion-related complications must be considered.

Hemorrhage

Although hemorrhage cannot be totally avoided, it is important to minimize the amount of blood loss during fusion by giving special consideration to the following three factors:

1. Careful positioning of the patient on the operating table will avoid unnecessary pressure on the abdomen. This is particularly relevant in the lateral and prone positions. Obstruction of the vena cava and collateral flow from the lower extremities into the paravertebral plexus will have an impact on the venous congestion of the epidural venous plexus and contribute to blood loss.
2. Timing of the end-plate preparation and decortication may be associated with additional blood loss; this should only be done after the bony exposure has been completed, soft tissue has been excised, and bone graft has been harvested. Bleeding from decortication sites should not be treated with bone wax, because this reduces the capacity for osteogenesis.[34] Excessive bleeding usually slows after the graft is inserted and may be controlled with Gelfoam.
3. Avoiding inadvertent injury and excessive bleeding, the segmental vessels should be clearly identified and dissected so that they may be suture ligated and divided in a controlled, safe manner. In the lower thoracic and upper lumbar region, the artery of Adamkiewicz and other radicular arteries supplying the anterior and posterior spinal arteries should not be sacrificed. Preoperative angiogram of selected spinal levels is recommended in instances in which there is a concern that these vessels may be at risk during the approach. The authors usually reserve preoperative spinal angiography for cases with a long-standing fixed kyphotic deformity in which the spinal cord blood supply may be tenuous or for cases in which preoperative embolization is desired.

Pseudarthrosis

Pseudarthrosis refers to a lack of bony union and may account for a poor clinical result. It is worth noting, however, that fibrous pseudarthrosis may limit spinal movement and allow a good clinical outcome with symptomatic relief. Moreover, even when bony fusion has occurred, patients can remain symptomatic. Meticulous attention to graft site preparation and use of autograft, where possible, enhances fusion rates. In cases of traumatic lesions, the supplementation of the fusion with a local vertebral body autograft, where possible, enhances fusion rates. In cases of traumatic lesions, the supplementation of the fusion with a local vertebral body autograft that is osteoinductive may be appropriate.

Harvesting Autogenous Iliac Crest Bone

The iliac crest is the most common site from which bone grafts are taken. Consideration of the following complications during this procedure may help reduce the donor site morbidity associated with this procedure.[35-38] Donor site pain is common and can continue to be a problem in one out of five patients, lasting up to 2 years postsurgery.[39]

Cosmetic deformity can be a problem when full-thickness grafts are taken from the iliac crest. When larger grafts are taken and cosmetic deformity becomes a concern, three techniques are useful in preventing crest deformities: (1) The trapdoor method uses the crest as a hinge; (2) the subcrestal window avoids resection of the rostral margin of the crest;[40] and (3) oblique sectioning of the crest allows the crest to be reconstituted.[39,41] Reconstruction of the crest, using different techniques, has been described: rib,[42-44] bioactive apatite and wollastonite-containing glass ceramic,[45] or methylmethacrylate.[46] Although infection is not a major concern, it does occur occasionally. A deep wound infection at the iliac donor site is treated like other wound infections adjacent to bone. It will require drainage, irrigation, and appropriate antibiotic coverage. Hematoma is common at the wound site. Gelfoam or bone wax can be used, but microcrystalline collagen is best for reducing bleeding from cancellous bone.[47] Suction drainage, although not a proven method, may be used to reduce the incidence of wound hematomas. Gait disturbance, with a limp or abductor lurch as a result of considerable stripping of the outer table muscles, can cause hip abductor weakness. With bone graft taken from the dorsal crest, patients may have difficulty with hip extension, which is evident when climbing stairs or rising from a chair.

Stress fractures can occur after full-thickness grafts are taken from the ventral iliac crest.[48] Stress fractures, as a result of the pull from the sartorius and rectus femoris muscles, can be avoided by harvesting the graft well away from the anterior superior iliac spine.[49] Moreover, taking long strips of bone along the iliac crest increases the risk of ilium fracture.

Perforation of the peritoneum can occur with a ventral approach to the inner table of the iliac crest because the peritoneum is closely related to the inner surface of the abdominal wall and iliacus muscles.[50] Herniation of abdominal contents can occur after removal of full-thickness grafts that include the iliac crest.[51]

Placing the skin incision behind the anterior superior iliac spine can minimize injury to the lateral femoral cutaneous nerve. Anatomic variation of the lateral femoral cutaneous nerve places this nerve at risk in less than 10% when dissection is 3 cm dorsal to the anterior iliac spine.[52]

Instrumentation

The need for supplementary instrumentation depends on the spinal level involved and the degree of bony involvement.

T1 to T9

When the corpectomy involves only the thoracic spine, supplementary instrumentation is generally unnecessary because the thoracic spine, unlike the lumbar spine, is supported by the rib cage. However, if there is three-column involvement, additional instrumentation will be necessary (Fig. 50-10).[3] For the upper thoracic spine (T1-3), ventral cervical plates can be used (Fig. 50-11).

T10 to L5

The T12 vertebral body and lumbar spine receive little or no additional support from the rib cage, and in this region there is a greater degree of extension of the spine with spinal motion. Ventral instrumentation is necessary to supplement the reconstruction and to prevent excessive extension that can lead to extrusion of the graft or synthetic construct.[13,53,54]

Supplemental Ventral Instrumentation

The rationale for using ventral instrumentation can be understood best by considering the biomechanics of the ventral fixation device. Shono et al.[55] and Gertzbein[56] have described the biomechanics of thoracolumbar ventral fixation devices when loss of anterior and middle column integrity is present. The Kaneda device,[53] which has two cross-fixed rods linked to four vertebral body screws (see Figs. 50-1 and 50-8), allows rigid stabilization against forces of axial compression, flexion, extension, and rotation. The quadrangular construct created by the two independent rods linked by the two cross-fixed bars provides greater resistance to flexion-extension and rotation than a single-rod system such as the Zielke system. The insertion of the vertebral body screws in nonparallel (triangular) alignment controls ventral and downward displacement. In the ventrally destabilized spine, the Kaneda construct provides superior fixation compared with dorsal instrumentation (such as a laminar hook or pedicle screw system), especially against flexion and axial compression forces. The vertebral body screws should be placed in a triangular fashion to avoid pullout and the need to engage the contralateral cortical bone of the vertebral body (see Fig. 50-11). If disruption of dorsal elements is present, ventral instrumentation alone is insufficient to provide stability (see Fig. 50-10). Most important, regardless of the rigidity of instrumentation, the spinal construct will eventually fail unless solid bony fusion occurs. One of the key concepts of ventral fusion is that the bone graft should be placed under compression to allow greater graft stability and fusion to adjacent vertebral bodies.[41]

Instrumentation Technique

The basic principle of this technique entails inserting screws into the midpoint of the vertebral bodies above and below the corpectomy site and connecting these by a rod or plate. Initially, Kostuik-Harrington instrumentation was used. This has been supplanted by the Kaneda device, CD Horizon Antares Spinal System, and Z-plate system. Multiple instrumentation systems are now available from most spinal implant companies. Above T10, the small size of the vertebral bodies may make screw placement difficult, although screws can

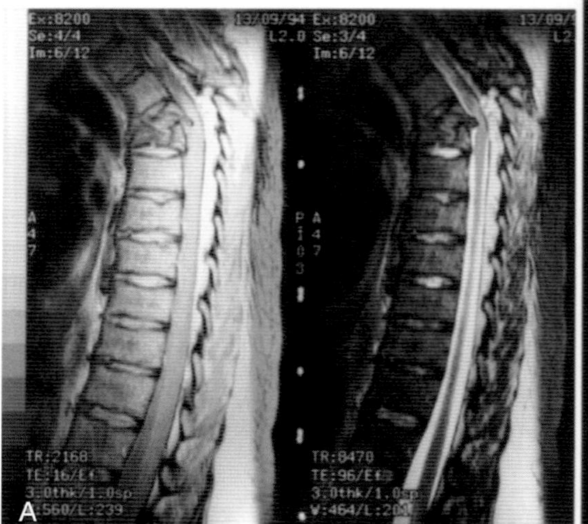

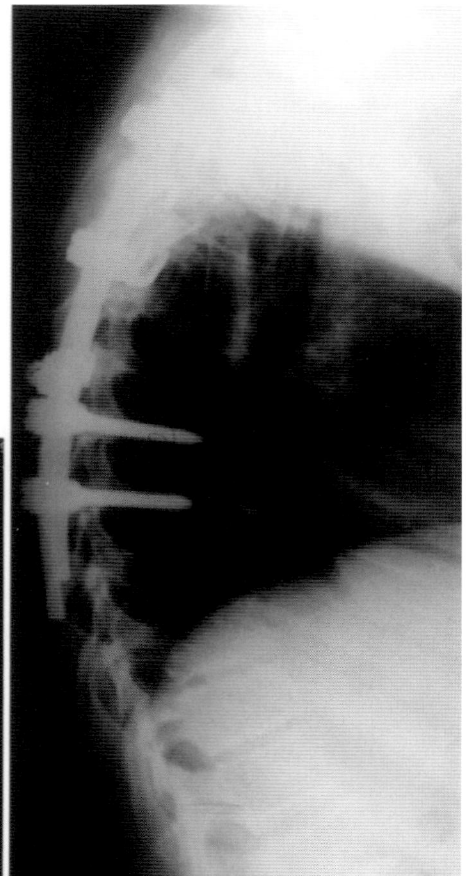

FIGURE 50-10. **A,** Proton density and T2-weighted sagittal MRI scan showing a T4-5 fracture dislocation with angulation and spinal cord compression in a 24-year-old woman with an incomplete spinal cord injury. A left third rib thoracotomy approach was used to perform a ventral decompression and reconstruction with rib autograft. In view of the three-column injury with associated rib fractures, posterior instrumentation (AO Universal Spine System) was performed. **B,** Postoperative lateral radiographs show correction of the kyphotic deformity with posterior segmental stabilization.

usually be placed as high as T6 in select cases. Below L4, the iliac veins and origin of the inferior vena cava tend to impede the safe placement of some of these systems. The Z-plate system, which has a lower profile, has recently been modified to allow ventral instrumentation of the midthoracic and lower thoracic spine. Most systems now use the fixed head screws, which can be placed in the vertebral body through a staple or perforated plate, allowing greater stability of the screw-vertebral body interface. By having screws in place, the surgeon can then distract the corpectomy and resection cavity in order to accommodate the vertebral body reconstruction. Rods are then placed in position, and compression can be applied to the anterior column support, which eventually leads to a solid construct with optimal alignment. The plate systems, by nature, do not allow the flexibility and finer degree of adjustments required for a complex reconstruction.

Avoiding Complications Related to Instrumentation

The role of instrumentation in the context of any spinal pathology is to provide stability either transiently, while fusion occurs, or permanently. Placement of instrumentation, however, carries risks and can cause complications. Direct trauma related to poorly positioned instruments is typically noted immediately. Erosion of screws into soft tissues can present in a delayed fashion. Poorly placed instruments can also fail to achieve the primary goal of providing stability. Patients will often complain of persistent mechanical pain. Assessment of the bone quality is often limited, and bone density studies can only provide limited information preoperatively. The interface between the instrumentation and the bone, also described as the purchase, can be improved by injecting PMMA into the vertebral body. The technique of vertebroplasty can be performed intraoperatively,[57-59] using radiopaque PMMA and injecting it while in liquid form under fluoroscopy to ensure safe distribution in the vertebral body and avoid the spinal canal (see Figs. 50-11D and E).

Other Spinal Pathology

In addition to metastatic spinal disease, several other conditions require ventral spinal decompression and are discussed in the following sections. Because the principles of ventral spinal decompression, fusion, and instrumentation are similar, only factors that are unique to these situations are outlined.

Osteomyelitis of the Spine

The most common infections of the spinal column are (1) infections caused by pyogenic organisms (*Staphylococcus aureus* and coliform bacilli are the most common pyogenic bacteria found), (2) infections caused by fungi (actinomycetes and blastomycetes are the most common organisms found), and (3) tuberculosis (Pott disease) (see Fig. 50-11).

These organisms usually reach the spinal column by hematogenous spread. The seeding of these infections is typically localized to the disc space because this avascular compartment is harder for the patient's own immune system to control. This "disc"-centric pathology is important when reviewing the images and trying to distinguish infectious from neoplastic pathology. Infection becomes symptomatic as a result of neural compromise from an associated extradural abscess or bony deformity from vertebral collapse with adjacent bone overgrowth that compromises the spinal canal (gibbus formation).

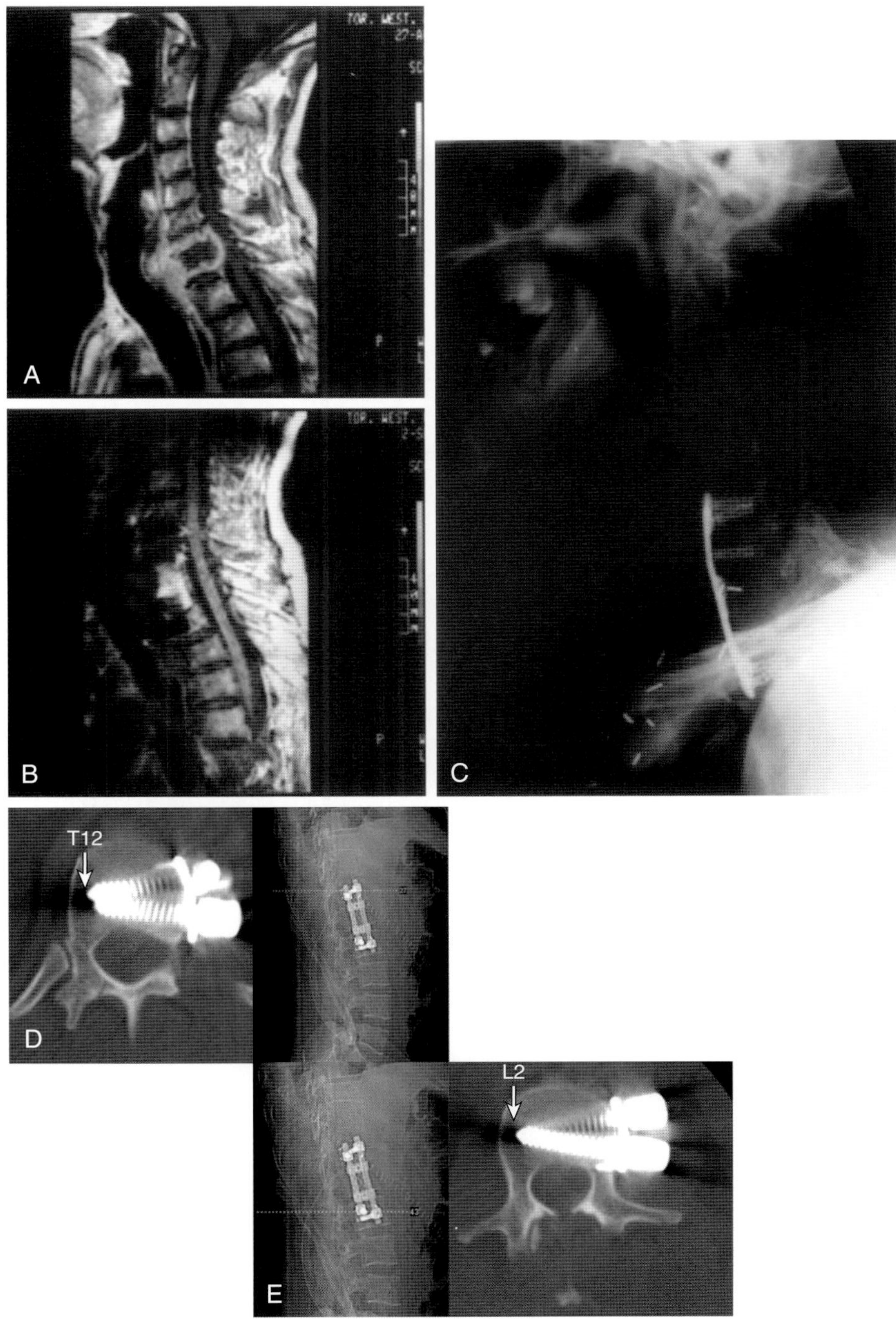

FIGURE 50-11. **A,** Gadolinium-enhanced T1-weighted sagittal MRI scan of a patient with tuberculosis of the cervicothoracic junction showing vertebral body involvement of T1 and extension into the spinal canal with severe spinal cord compression and paraspinal extension. Surgical exposure of this lesion was achieved via a right-sided cervicosternotomy approach. **B** and **C,** Postoperative T1-weighted sagittal MRI scan and lateral cervical spine radiograph after vertebral body resection and stabilization with an iliac crest bone graft and Synthes plate. These axial CT scan images at T12 (**D**) and L2 (**E**) demonstrate the suboptimal screw placement (Kaneda system). The screws are convergent but do not engage the second cortex; the *arrows* show the gap.

Figure continues on following page

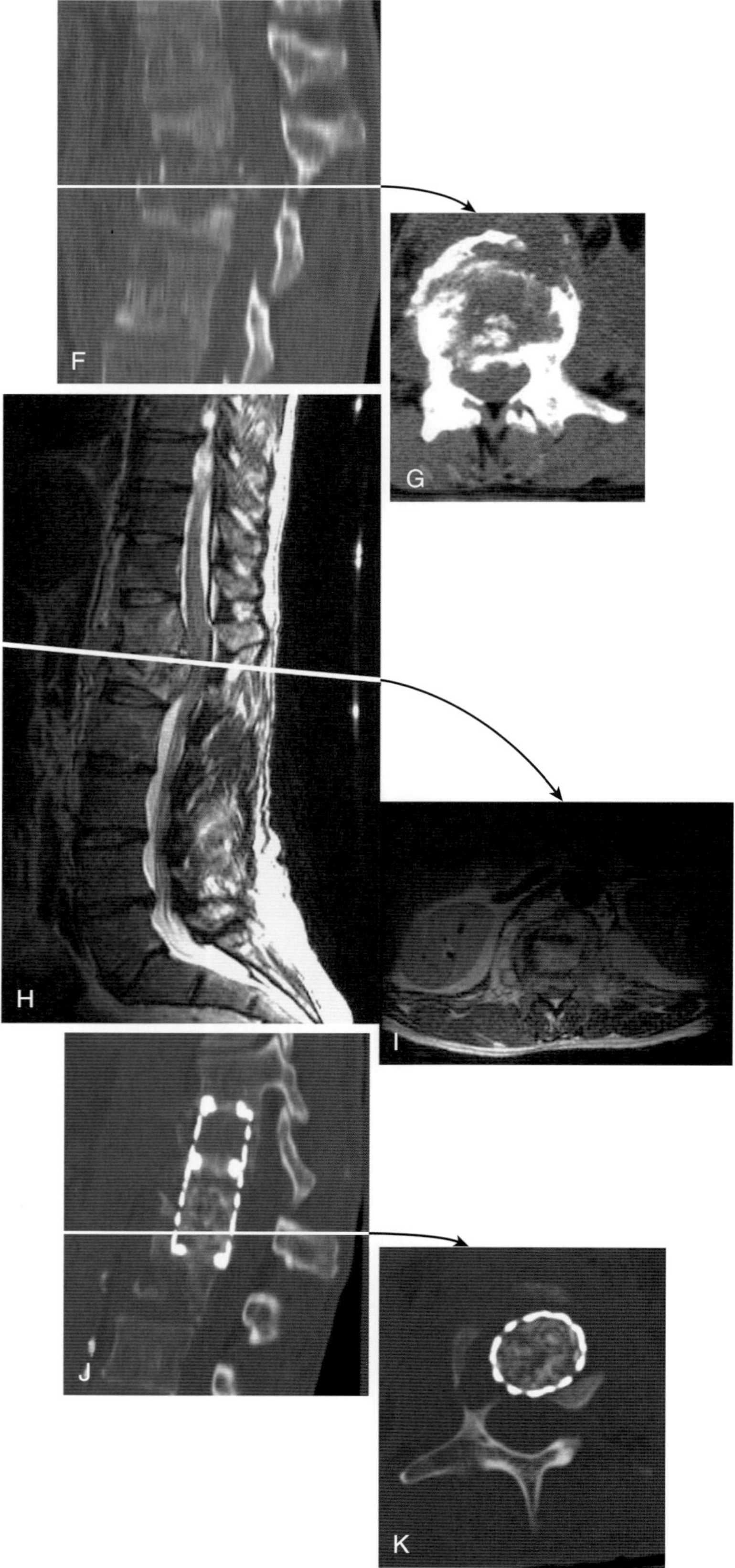

FIGURE 50-11, cont. The CT scan images, sagittal (**F**) and corresponding axial images (**G**), show the bony destruction in this case of Pott disease at the T12 and L1 level. The MRIs, T2-weighted sagittal (**H**) and corresponding axial image (**I**), show the spinal cord compression. **J** and **K,** A postoperative CT scan demonstrates the anterior reconstruction with a titanium cage filled with autologous bone graft. This construct was subsequently complemented with posterior instrumentation using pedicle screws above and below the cage *(not shown here).*

Identification of predisposing factors for infection following spinal surgery has been described by Wimmer et al.[60] Medical conditions such as diabetes, obesity, corticosteroid therapy, chronic infection, and smoking were identified in patients with a higher rate of infection. Surgical variables such as previous spinal surgery, extended preoperative hospitalization ($P < .001$), and high blood loss ($P < .01$) were identified as risk factors. The role of prophylactic antibiotic administration has been demonstrated by Horwitz and Curtin[61] to reduce wound infection with spinal surgery. Some institutions have adopted a prolonged duration of antibiotic doses for patients at higher risk, using the factors mentioned previously.

Patients with osteomyelitis usually have symptoms of back pain, local spinal tenderness, and paraspinal muscle spasm. Associated fever and leukocytosis are common. Erosion of several adjacent vertebral bodies with collapse and involvement of associated intervertebral discs is characteristic and an early radiographic finding on lateral and anteroposterior spine films. Bone scans are often positive at regions of vertebral infection, and the serum alkaline phosphatase level is often elevated.

In these infective cases, it is important to assess, using axial CT images, the degree of spinal canal narrowing from vertebral collapse or gibbus formation (see Fig. 50-11F and G). In the absence of spinal canal narrowing, an extradural abscess or granuloma is the likely cause of spinal symptoms. MRI or myelography to delineate neural (spinal cord or nerve root) compromise is also indicated for these patients before surgical decompression (see Figs. 50-11H to K).

Surgical decompression is indicated in patients with progressive symptoms of spinal cord compression. The thoracic region is the most common site of osteomyelitis, and dorsolateral spinal approaches (e.g., costotransversectomy) usually allow adequate spinal decompression. Occasionally, ventral decompressive procedures are necessary when there is (1) progressive spinal compression; (2) osteomyelitis of the cervical spine; (3) spinal infections with kyphotic angulation in the lower lumbar spine, in which a retroperitoneal approach with corpectomy can be performed; and (4) extensive involvement of the vertebral body that cannot be adequately decompressed by the dorsolateral approach (see Fig. 50-11).

The method of vertebral decompression and reconstruction is similar to that described earlier. The use of autogenous bone is favored in the setting of osteomyelitis. Internal fixation use is controversial. Some surgeons advocate its use in the setting of osteomyelitis provided that a good local debridement is achieved. For pyogenic infections, appropriate intravenous antibiotics are necessary for 4 to 6 weeks, followed by oral antibiotics, until the infection resolves both clinically and radiographically.

Some patients with tuberculosis of the spine and mild neurologic signs of spinal cord compression improve with antituberculous drugs and rest, and without requiring surgical decompression. However, close neurologic follow-up is required to ensure that symptoms are not progressive. It is important to remember that spinal infections can result in spinal cord symptoms without actual spinal cord compression. These symptoms occur as a result of vascular thrombosis secondary to the inflammatory process. It is important, then, to confirm radiologically any evidence of spinal cord compression because these patients do not benefit from surgical decompression.

Kyphotic Deformities

Ventral corpectomy and fusion allow the correction of severe, symptomatic deformities. Surgical exposures are performed as described earlier, depending on the spinal level of the deformity. A ventral release with section of the anterior longitudinal ligament and discectomies is helpful for correcting the deformity. The adjacent discs involved in the kyphosis are identified and excised, and autologous bone (cortical iliac bone, section of rib, or fibula) is used for bone struts. This may be supplemented by ventral instrumentation to allow early ambulation of the patient. Most severe fixed kyphotic deformities require supplemental dorsal instrumentation and fusion.

Resection of Hemivertebra

A hemivertebra may become symptomatic and cause a severe, progressive deformity of the spine with neurologic compromise.[9] This usually occurs when the anomaly lies low in the lumbar spine and results in congenital scoliosis with the hemivertebra as the apical part of the curve. The hemivertebra is resected ventrally to dorsally, back to the level of the epidural space, with the base of the pedicle also resected. An autologous bony strut graft with ventral instrumentation can be used for stability. Either during this procedure or during a second operation, a dorsal approach is used to resect the dorsal elements of the hemivertebra.

Thoracic and Thoracolumbar Fractures

These fractures can be approached by a ventral, ventrolateral (see Figs. 50-8 and 50-10), dorsolateral, or dorsal approach depending on certain features.[20,62-64] When lesions are ventral in the thoracic spine, available options for surgical exposure that allow decompression and stabilization include costotransversectomy, a lateral extracavitary approach, a transthoracic extrapleural approach, or a transthoracic transpleural approach. The authors favor the latter approach when neural decompression is an important goal, as in the patient with incomplete spinal cord injury (see Figs. 50-8 and 50-10). For burst fractures at the thoracolumbar junction, a transthoracic/retroperitoneal (10th rib approach) exposure is used to achieve ventral decompression and reconstruction (see Fig. 50-8). For midlumbar fractures (L2 or L3), a retroperitoneal approach is used. Low lumbar fractures (L4 or L5) are approached via a dorsolateral approach because the nerve roots may be retracted with greater facility, allowing easier decompression.

The transthoracic and retroperitoneal approaches allow a single-stage procedure with decompression and removal of pathologic material ventral to the dura mater over several vertebral segments and reconstruction with bone graft and instrumentation. Three-column injuries necessitating the use of ventral decompression require supplemental dorsal instrumentation (see Fig. 50-10).

Decompression and Stabilization

Surgical exposures to other thoracic and lumbar levels (T1-3 and T3-L2) are described in other chapters in this text. The fractured or retropulsed bone segment is identified under the microscope and removed, using curettes and a high-speed pneumatic drill. The intervertebral discs and end plates of adjacent vertebral bodies are removed to allow adequate fusion of the bony graft inserted between the intact adjacent vertebral bodies above and below the decompression. Important principles of direct visualization of neural elements should be observed in spinal decompression associated with spinal trauma.

The decompression can often be performed without removing the entire vertebral body. The aim is to remove only the bony segment that is compromising the spinal canal. Using a high-speed bur, this can be performed by drilling away the bone ventral to the bony segment that protrudes into the spinal canal, which creates a vacant area ventral to the bony fragment impinging into the spinal canal. Using an angled curette, the retropulsed fragment can then be gently pushed away from the ventral aspect of the dura into the empty ventral space. This technique is similar to that used for the removal of a herniated thoracic disc. For fracture decompressions, however, one third to one half of the vertebral body should be resected to allow adequate spinal decompression.

After a herniated disc or retropulsed bony fragment is removed, the spinal column needs to be stabilized. Rib struts, prepared from the resected rib, can be used for the bony graft in the upper thoracic and midthoracic spine. An iliac crest bone graft is used in the lower thoracic spine, thoracolumbar junction, or lumbar spine. Alternatively, allograft humerus or fibula supplemented with local autograft (rib or resected vertebral body) may be used. Unlike the neoplastic condition, local bone from the vertebrectomy can be used for achieving fusion. Subjacent intervertebral discs and cartilaginous end plates should be removed from vertebral bodies adjacent to the bony graft. Any spinal column deformity that is not fixed should be corrected using an appropriate distraction system. This is particularly useful in cases with significant kyphosis extending over several vertebral levels. Slots are drilled into vertebral bodies immediately above and below the decompression site to allow the bone grafts to be held in position. The decompressed vertebral segment is measured, and a bone graft of appropriate size is prepared. The bone graft is gently tapped into the prepared interval between the two vertebral bodies using the bone set. A number of instrumentation systems are currently available for ventral instrumentation of the thoracolumbar spine.

Transthoracic Discectomy

Symptomatic thoracic intervertebral disc herniations are relatively uncommon, with an incidence of 1 per million,[65] constituting approximately 0.25% to 0.75% of all symptomatic disc lesions. They usually occur between T4 and T12. Patients may appear with radicular symptoms or spinal cord compression, depending on whether the disc has herniated laterally or centrally. MRI is the imaging technique of choice for the diagnosis (Fig. 50-12). Initially, thoracic disc herniations were approached by laminectomy with poor results.[26,27,44,46,59,66-69] Although patients with lateral disc herniation had slightly better outcomes compared with central disc herniation, in both cases a number of patients failed to improve, continued to deteriorate, or had postoperative paraparesis as a complication.[26,27,44,46,59,66-69] In 1960, a lateral approach via a costotransversectomy was used with encouraging results.[70] Recently, a more direct ventral transpleural approach has provided further reduction in neurologic morbidity.[59,68]

Transthoracic (Transpleural) Discectomy

This approach allows direct exposure of the ventral and lateral regions of the intervertebral disc. If the surgeon is inexperienced in this approach, exposure should be performed by a thoracic surgeon. The patient's medical and pulmonary condition should be evaluated before surgery to ascertain the patient's ability to tolerate the procedure. A standard chest radiograph should be included as part of the pulmonary assessment and also to ensure the patient has 12 ribs. This anatomic detail is important when confirming the appropriate level intraoperatively.

The surgical approach to the appropriate vertebral level by thoracotomy is described in other chapters in this text. The vertebral bodies above and below the herniated intervertebral disc are identified using the rib as a guide. The rib will articulate with the vertebral body above; therefore the eighth rib head will point to the seventh and eighth disc spaces. Using a radiograph to confirm the correct level is highly recommended.

An operating microscope may be used once the appropriate vertebral levels are identified. Dissection and proper visualization of the disc space, as previously described, is integral before proceeding with the discectomy. The amount of dissection is typically less extensive and limited to the rostral and caudal levels. The primary objective is to avoid retraction or manipulation of the dural sac at any time during the discectomy. To ensure adequate decompression and to allow smaller remnants of herniated disc to be removed, the floor of the spinal canal is palpated gently with flat instruments such as the Penfield dissector. These are then used to gently remove small, sequestered disc fragments. If the anulus fibrosus or posterior longitudinal ligaments are lax, or free, they can be pushed back into the intervertebral space and removed from this region. The operative site is then irrigated, and hemostasis is ensured once the spinal cord appears adequately decompressed.

Thoracic Endoscopic Surgery

Thoracic endoscopic surgery was first described for treatment of Pott disease in 1951.[71] The expansion of video technology in the early 1990s affected endoscopic capabilities, providing a better-quality image with small equipment.[69,72] Thoracoscopic approaches to the thoracic spine for sympathectomy, discectomy, and paraspinal neurogenic tumor with low morbidity and mortality have been described.[8] Thoracoscopic-assisted treatment of thoracic and lumbar fractures has been carried out on more than 371 patients to date.[73] Expansion of these new minimally invasive techniques seems appealing when reported by a small number of authors.[8,13,74] Caution should be exercised when adopting

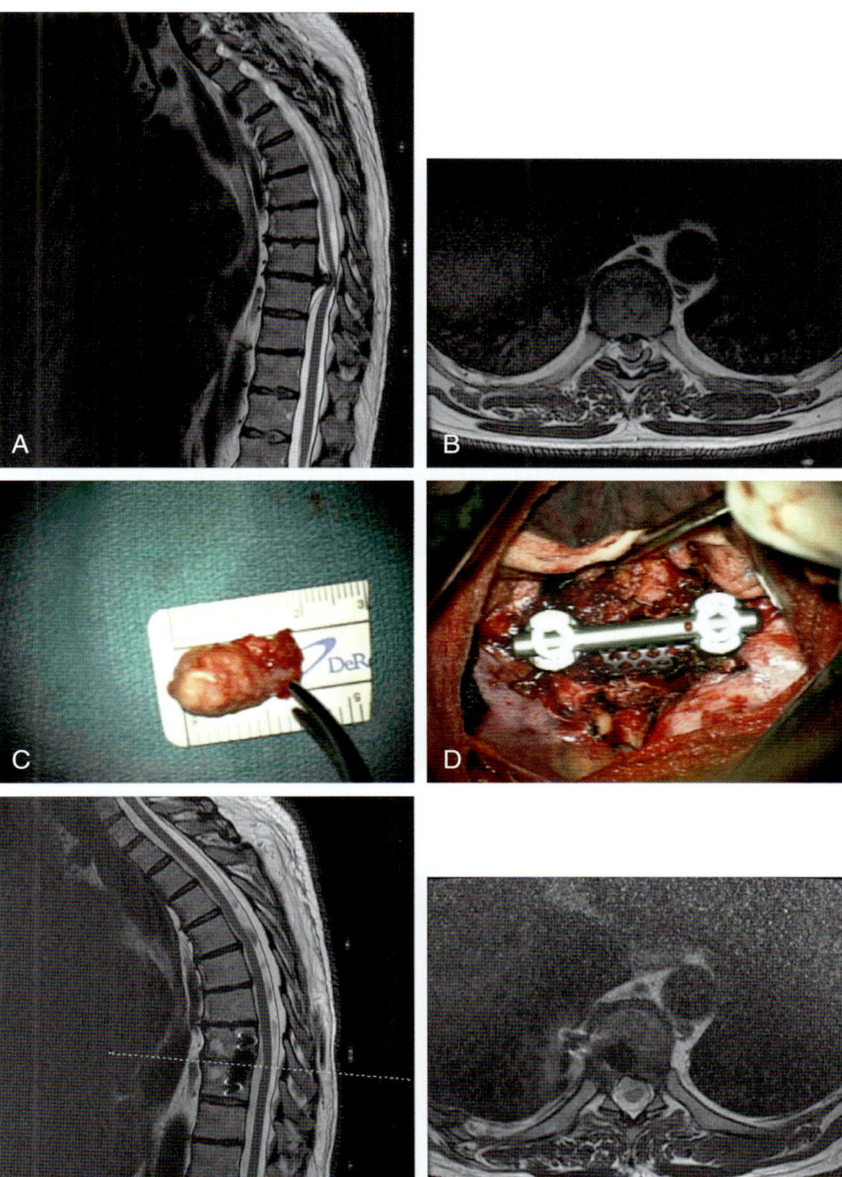

FIGURE 50-12. **A,** T2-weighted sagittal MRI of a patient with thoracic herniated disc. **B,** T2-weighted axial MRI of the same patient. **C,** Removed disc measuring 2 cm. **D,** Intraoperative image of the reconstruction with a titanium cage (SynMesh, Synthes) filled with locally harvested bone graft. The construct consisted of two vertebral screws connected with a single rod (Expedium, DePuy Spine). **E,** Postoperative T2-weighted sagittal MRI of the same patient. **F,** Postoperative T2-weighted axial MRI of the same patient.

these new surgical techniques because there is a significant learning curve. Certain pathologic entities still require open procedures to achieve adequate decompression and control bleeding.

Closure and Postoperative Care

Routine closure with approximation of all muscle layers in surgery involving the thoracic cavity is performed with one or two thoracostomy tubes, one passing to the apex and/or one to the dependent region of the chest cavity, connected to an underwater suction seal allowing drainage of air and blood. The drains are removed once the drainage is less than 100 mL over a 12-hour period, which usually occurs by postoperative day 2 or 3. A major complication of both the transpleural and the ventrolateral approaches to the thoracolumbar spine is blood loss, which occurs during both the decompressive procedure and the fusion. The blood loss occurs from the cancellous surfaces of the bone graft and vertebral body sites. The blood lost should be estimated and replaced intraoperatively, and the hematocrit should be followed closely postoperatively. Pulmonary complications are low if relatively young, healthy patients are selected for these procedures.[75] Daily chest radiographs will help the physician monitor for pneumothorax and pleural effusions.

Patients who have undergone transthoracic surgery begin ambulation soon after removal of throacostomy tubes. Sufficient analgesic must be given at all stages of postoperative care to reduce pain associated with this type of surgery. Intercostal nerve blocks can be used before closure of the thoracostomy. Intrathoracic catheters for administration of narcotic analgesics are also helpful. Depending on neurologic recovery and capability for independence and support at home, the patient may return home or require further rehabilitation at an appropriate facility.

Summary

Ventral and ventrolateral decompression, fusion, and instrumentation assist spinal canal and spinal cord decompression and provide stability in conditions with loss of anterior and middle column integrity, as in trauma (e.g., burst fracture), tumor, infection, degenerative disease, and congenital deformities. The techniques described allow decompression, correction of kyphosis, and stabilization to be performed as one-stage procedures and provide a stable construct with fixation involving the minimal number of segments. Postoperatively, excellent results for degree of decompression and rates of fusion have been obtained with minimal complications related to the surgical procedure.

KEY REFERENCES

Denis F: Spinal instability as defined by the three-column spine concept in acute spinal trauma. *Clin Orthop Relat Res* 189:65–76, 1984.

Errrico TJ, Cooper PR: A new method of thoracic and lumbar body replacement for spinal tumors: technical note. *Neurosurgery* 32:678–680, 1993.

Nuwer MR: Spinal cord monitoring. *Muscle Nerve* 22:1620–1630, 1999.

Patchell RA, Tibbs PA, Regine WF, et al: Direct decompressive surgical resection in the treatment of spinal cord compression caused by metastatic cancer: a randomized trial. *Lancet* 366:643–648, 2005.

White AA III, Panjabi MM: *Clinical biomechanics of the spine*, Philadelphia, 1978, Lippincott-Raven.

REFERENCES

The complete reference list is available online at expertconsult.com.

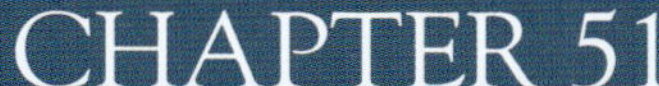

CHAPTER 51

Lateral Extracavitary Approach to the Thoracolumbar Spine

Michael Martin | Kevin Cooper | Dennis J. Maiman

The lateral extracavitary approach (LECA) can be used in the thoracolumbar spine to access both the ventral and dorsal elements of the spinal column. Through this approach, discectomy, spondylectomy, fusion, and deformity reduction may be accomplished. In addition, other approaches, including transpedicular decompression and laminectomy, can be added to allow a 360-degree approach through one incision. LECA was first used as a derivation of lateral costotransversectomy in the treatment of tuberculous spondylitis (Pott disease) by Capener in 1933 and first reported by Seldon in 1935.[1] It was also described in 1960 by Hulme, who advocated it as an alternative to laminectomy for ventral thoracic pathology, including disc herniation, secondary to the high incidence of poor surgical outcome of laminectomy attributed to inadequate exposure of ventral elements and the requirement of direct manipulation of the thoracic spinal cord and its extradural vasculature.[2] The approach was further refined by Larson et al. at the Medical College of Wisconsin, and it has been applied to traumatic lesions, thoracic disc herniations, tumors, and other pathologic conditions[1,3-7] (Figs. 51-1 to 51-5). This approach has recently been modified in a cadaver study to be used via minimally invasive retractor systems for deformity correction.[8] Minimally invasive LECA has also been used successfully in thoracic disc herniation.[9]

This approach can be applied to ventral spinal lesions located between T1 and L5 and, if necessary, can be performed in a bilateral fashion for more extensive pathology.[10] In addition to decompression and the removal of pathology, ventrolateral instrumentation can be accomplished through LECA with additional instrumentation placed dorsally as needed.

Surgical Preparation

Before undertaking any surgical procedure, a careful history and physical examination are essential, along with proper diagnostic imaging. For lesions that can be approached via LECA, imaging should consist of plain radiographs, MRI, and possibly CT. MRI is most useful for disc surgery and tumors, and CT is often obtained to evaluate fractures and the size and orientation of the pedicles if transpedicular instrumentation is planned for augmentation. The importance of plain radiographs in preoperative evaluation cannot be overstated because it is vitally important to understand with certainty the true number of ribs that the patient has before undertaking LECA. Overall spinal alignment is also important and best assessed with plain radiographs. In the case of tumors, consideration must be given to preoperative angiography with embolization (just before surgery, if possible) to prevent excessive blood loss.

Operative Technique

Following the induction of general anesthesia, the patient should have a Foley catheter placed and appropriate preoperative antibiotics administered. The Jackson table provides optimal padding and available positioning for LECA, and all pressure points should be checked after positioning. The patient should be safely secured to the table at all points because the bed will be rotated later in the case. For discectomy or fractures, the use of intraoperative monitoring is not essential; for deformity correction and tumor cases, such monitoring may provide an additional measure of safety. Following induction and proper positioning, the next step is appropriate fluoroscopic localization of the lesion. This is critical because the exposure provides a direct view of specific vertebrae, and extending the exposure more than one level in either direction can be difficult. It is imperative to have a clear understanding of the bony anatomy on radiograph before surgery to aid in localization. The typical anatomy of the rib and thoracic spine interface is also an important fact to keep in mind. In most patients a rib abuts disc space in the thoracic spine, and this rib typically corresponds to the caudal vertebrae at the segment.[11] For example, at T7, the rib typically articulates with the T6-7 disc space. This anatomy holds true down to the T10-11 space. The 11th and 12th ribs typically articulate with the corresponding vertebral bodies below the disc spaces. It is generally advisable to count ribs in the thoracic spine from above and below and to compare this count with preoperative radiographs for confirmation.

Once the location has been confirmed and marked, attention is given to planning the incision. Various shapes have been used (Fig. 51-6), but the hockey stick–type incision is generally performed. The incision should generally extend from at least one segment cranial to the pathology to one segment caudal to it, with the caudal limb angling out toward the pathologic side with attention paid to the need for approaching the dorsal elements or placing instrumentation.

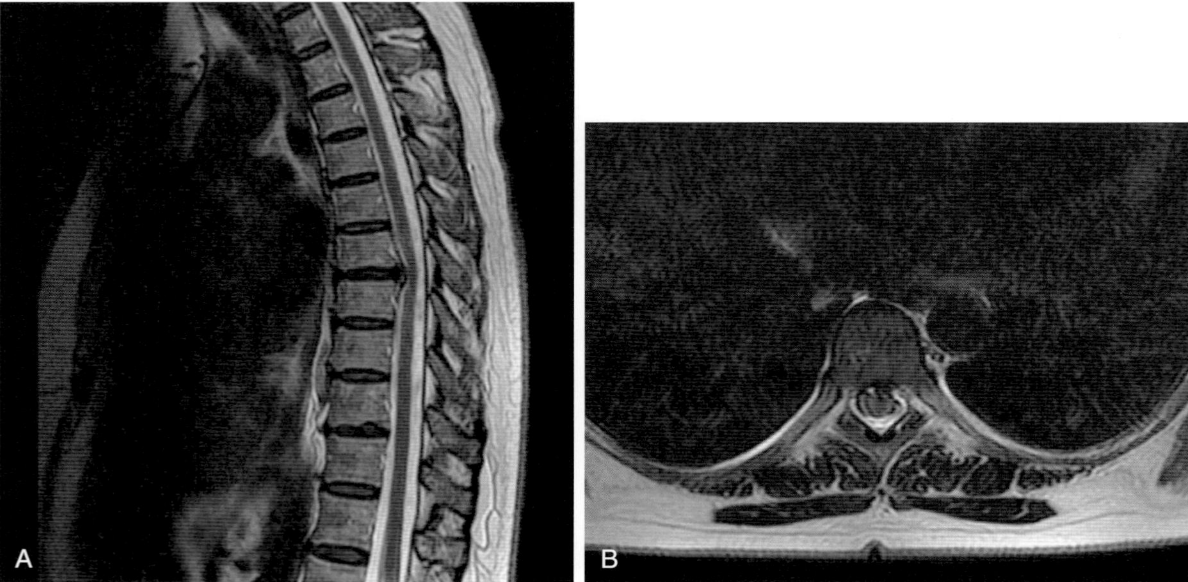

FIGURE 51-1. Sagittal (**A**) and axial (**B**) T2-weighted MRI of a thoracic herniated disc.

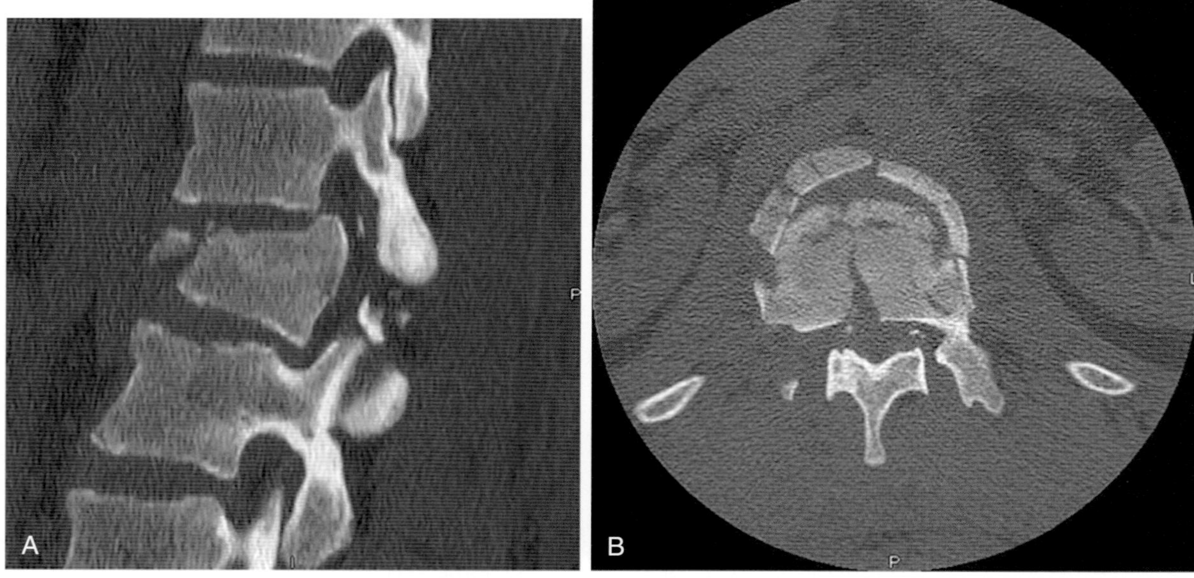

FIGURE 51-2. Sagittal reconstruction (**A**) and axial (**B**) CT images of a traumatic L1 fracture in a 24-year-old male. The patient had an incomplete spinal cord injury with bladder dysfunction.

For procedures involving dorsal fixation and fusion, the straight midline portion of the planned incision should extend to the segments to be included in the construct. In the case of single-level discectomy without a need for dorsal exposure, a paramedian incision may be used and may be as small as 5 cm in length.

The incision is opened down to and just through the thoacodorsal fascia so that a flap consisting of skin, subcutaneous tissue, and fascia can be retracted laterally. At this point, with the erector spinae muscles visible, the rib of interest can be palpated just lateral to the bulk of the muscle. This should be marked and confirmed again with a radiograph. Once this is done, the muscles overlying the rib can be retracted medially to expose the costovertebral junction.

After the incision is made, the approach varies little. Usually one rib should be exposed for discectomy; two ribs must be exposed to widen the field for tumor or fracture where a vertebrectomy is planned. At this point, a Doyen rib-stripping tool is used to free the rib of soft tissue and the intercostal vein, artery, and nerve complex that travels on the caudal surface of the rib. The rib is then cut approximately 10 cm from its insertion and disarticulated at the costovertebral joint (Fig. 51-7). This piece can often be removed intact and should be kept for possible use as graft. For lumbar spine pathology, the same general approach applies, with the transverse processes serving the localizing function for which the ribs are used in the thoracic spine. Careful attention must be paid to the

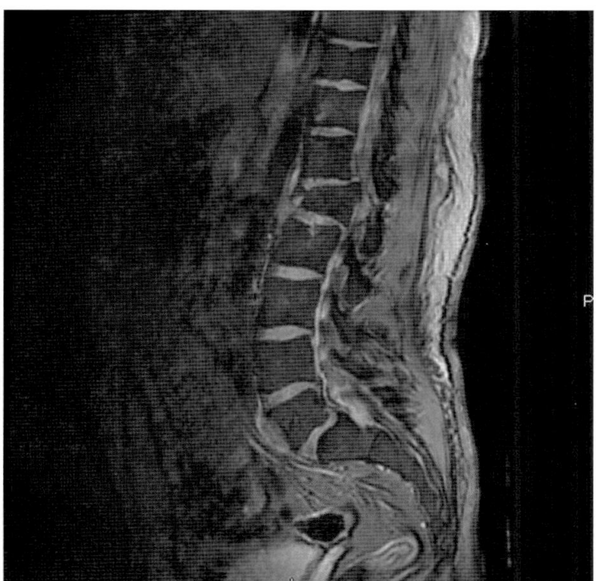

FIGURE 51-3. Sagittal T2-weighted MRI of the patient in Figure 51-2.

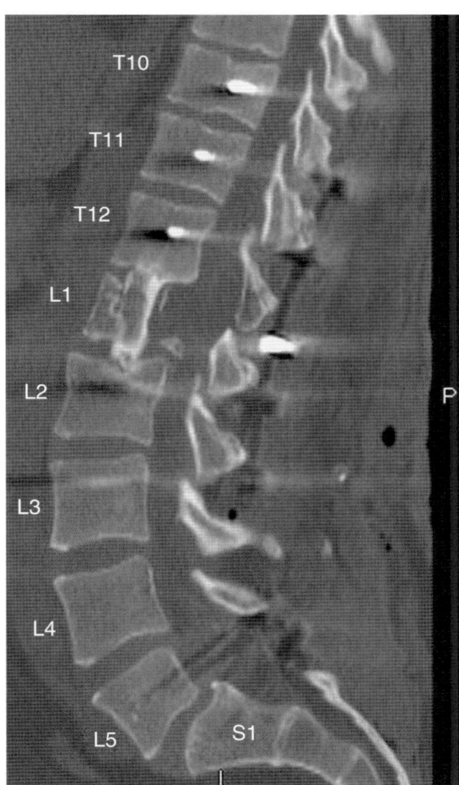

FIGURE 51-4. Postoperative sagittal CT reconstruction of the patient in Figures 51-2 and 51-3. The patient underwent a lateral extracavitary partial corpectomy of L1 with allograft and posterior instrumentation.

location of the nerve roots and possibly prefixed lumbosacral plexus.

At this point, it is helpful to rotate the table 20 to 30 degrees away from the surgeon so that the vertebral body comes into view. The lateral surface of the body can be cleared with blunt dissection and bipolar cautery. With the rib removed, the intercostal nerve is followed proximally to the neural foramen, which should then be enlarged with a Kerrison rongeur. There may be a vascular bundle at the foramen, which can usually be coagulated safely. With the foramen enlarged, attention is turned to the exposed pedicle. It should be thinned with a drill and removed completely, which will allow full visualization of the lateral thecal sac and exposure of the disc space and cranial portion of the vertebral body. For vertebrectomy, the rib and pedicle caudal to the lesion can be removed as well. At this point, it is wise to reconfirm the level of interest with a radiograph.

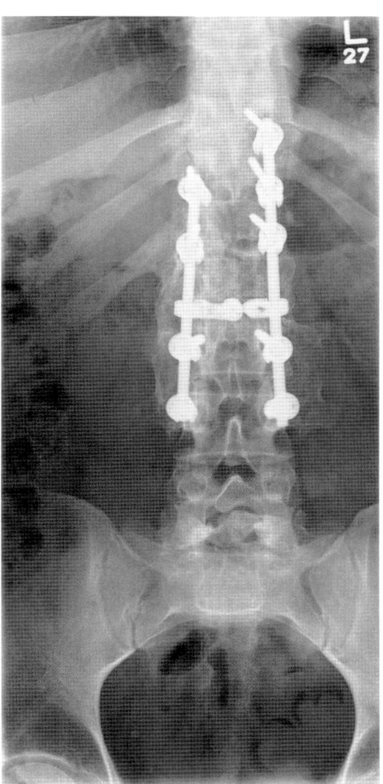

FIGURE 51-5. Anteroposterior radiograph demonstrating T10-L3 instrumentation in the patient from Figures 51-2 to 51-4.

LECA then proceeds in a logical sequence of decompression, stabilization, and fusion. If the surgery is for discectomy, the operation may proceed in a standard fashion at this point, with an anular incision followed by removal of herniated fragments. This incision can be continued through LECA until the opposite side of the thecal sac is visualized. Down-pushing curettes across the disc space may help in accomplishing this. If the goal of the surgery is vertebrectomy, the entire affected body may be removed using a combination of high-speed drill, curettes, and rongeurs. In the case of fractures, it is sometimes safer to leave a few millimeters of bone attached to the dura to prevent injury. To achieve adequate vertebrectomy and proper fusion bed preparation, the disc spaces above and below must also be cleared until the end plates of the rostral and caudal vertebrae are visible (Fig. 51-8). These can then be decorticated using the drill or curettes. After this, the graft material of choice is inserted and lateral plating applied to the upper and lower vertebral bodies. In the case of discectomy, no additional instrumentation is necessary and fusion in the absence of overt instability is unnecessary. If fusion is necessary, the

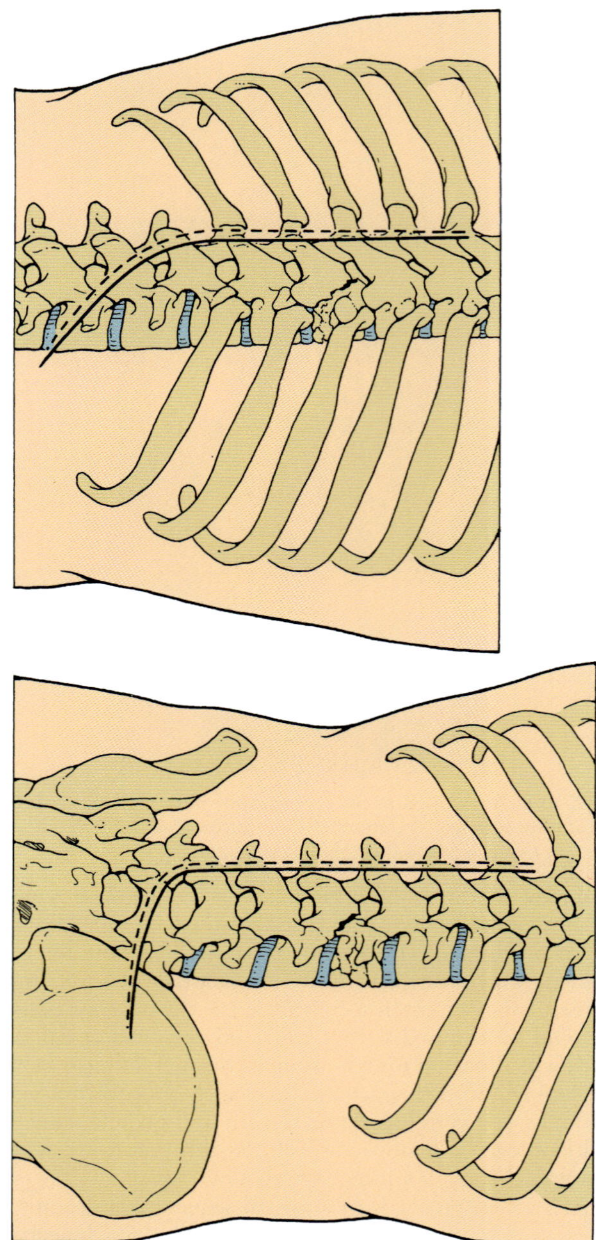

FIGURE 51-6. Two variants of the standard hockey stick–style incision for the lateral extracavitary approach.

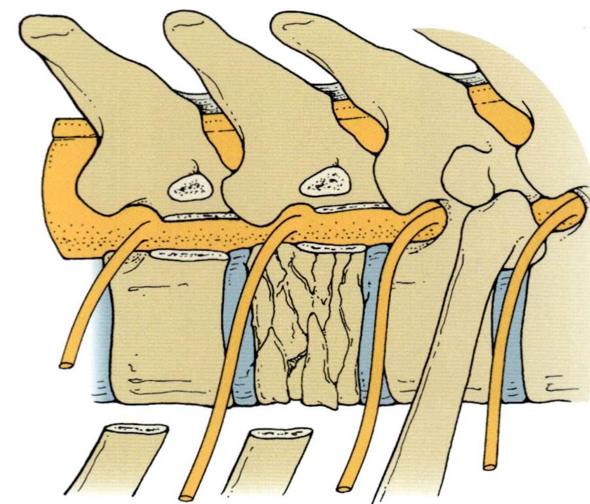

FIGURE 51-7. View provided via lateral extracavitary approach following rib and pedicle removal.

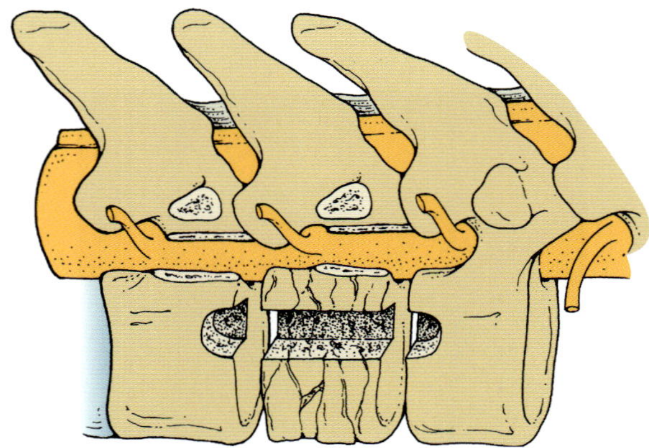

FIGURE 51-8. Lateral extracavitary approach following partial vertebrectomy.

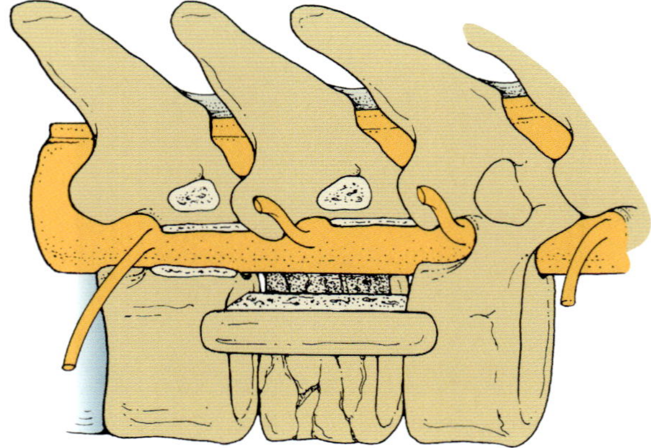

FIGURE 51-9. One possible method of grafting using structural autograft following partial vertebrectomy.

removed rib pieces can be used as structural autograft or alternately taken to the back table and morselized for use with expandable cages (Fig. 51-9). If necessary, dorsal instrumentation can be used as well for further support if overt instability is noted. This instrumentation should be compressed very little to avoid loosening the ventral graft and is best placed before the addition of the interbody or other ventral graft.[12]

The wound is then irrigated with saline, and attention should be paid to the presence of bubbles in the field, which may signal a pneumothorax. If one is suspected, careful observation of the pleural fascia should be undertaken and any visible defects repaired. The retractor holding the spinae muscles can then be removed, and the muscle bundle allowed to lie in its normal anatomic position. The fascia and skin should be closed in the standard fashion.

A chest radiograph should be taken in the recovery room to check for pneumothorax, even in the absence of frank pleural wall breech. Patients can be mobilized after recovery from anesthesia, and the average length of stay following discectomy alone is 1 day.[12] Length of stay for trauma and neoplasm is longer and often depends on the patient's other comorbidities. The incidence of pneumothorax following LECA is about 8% (although some report a higher incidence), and infection rates are less than 2%.[12,13] Vascular and pleural injuries are rare but possible complications; subarachnoid pleural fistula has been reported but is also rare.[14] Postoperative atelectasis and pneumonia are also a concern, as is ileus.[1,13,15] If roots must be sacrificed, care should be taken to divide them proximal to the dorsal root ganglion to avoid excessive pain afterward.[15]

LECA is a technically demanding and sometimes time-consuming procedure, but it offers an unparalleled view of vertebral and disc pathology while avoiding some of the morbidity of transabdominal or transthoracic exposure. Decompression, tumor removal, and fixation can all be accomplished via a well thought out and executed LECA, which make it an invaluable tool in spinal surgery.

KEY REFERENCES

Larson SJ, Holst RA, Hemmy DC, Sances A Jr: Lateral extracavitary approach to traumatic lesions of the thoracic and lumbar spine. *J Neurosurg* 45:628–637, 1976.

Lifshutz J, Lidar Z, Maiman D: Evolution of the lateral extracavitary approach to the spine. *Neurosurg Focus* 16:E12, 2004.

Maiman D: Lateral extracavitary apporach to the thoracolumbar spine. In Wolfla C, Resnick D, editors: *Neurosurgical operative atlas: spine and peripheral nerves*, New York, 2007, Thieme, pp 156–160.

Maiman DJ, Larson SJ, Benzel EC: Neurological improvement associated with late decompression of the thoracolumbar spinal cord. *Neurosurgery* 14:302–307, 1984.

Maiman DJ, Larson SJ, Luck E, El-Ghatit A: Lateral extracavitary approach to the spine for thoracic disc herniation: report of 23 cases. *Neurosurgery* 14:178–182, 1984.

REFERENCES

The complete reference list is available online at expertconsult.com.

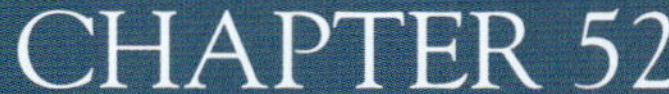

CHAPTER 52

Retropleural Approach to the Ventral Thoracic and Thoracolumbar Spine

Paul C. McCormick

Two of the most widely used approaches to the ventral thoracic and thoracolumbar spine are the transpleural thoracotomy and the lateral extracavitary approach.[1,2] Each approach has its advantages and disadvantages. The major advantage of the ventrolateral transpleural thoracotomy is that it provides unparalleled exposure of the ventral vertebral column over several segments. Nevertheless, this exposure has several disadvantages. First, this approach is characterized by an extensive incision and soft tissue dissection that are necessitated by a deep operative field. Second, because with this approach the chest cavity is entered from the ventrolateral chest quadrant, significant retraction of the unprotected lung is required. Finally, identification and decompression of the ventral spinal canal are also problematic, because the rib head partially obscures the spinal canal and the epidural veins are difficult to control via this trajectory. The aforementioned factors can create a less secure operative environment, increase surgical morbidity, and hinder the attainment of the surgical objective(s).

The lateral extracavitary approach is particularly useful when circumferential spinal exposure is needed, but it is impractical for isolated ventral vertebral column exposure. Ventral vertebral exposure with this technique requires an extensive and often bloody paraspinal muscle and foraminal dissection. Intercostal nerves are sacrificed to optimize exposure, which may result in a painful neuroma or abdominal wall muscle weakness at lower thoracic and thoracolumbar levels. The foraminal dissection may inadvertently occlude a medullary vessel, which may risk spinal cord infarction. Finally, despite the extensive dissection, direct ventral spinal canal visualization extends only to the midline and provides insufficient exposure to place a lateral spinal implant.

A retropleural thoracotomy, ideally, is more suited for a ventral exposure of the thoracic and thoracolumbar spine.[3-7] Similar to the situation in ventrolateral thoracotomy, the line of vision provided with a retropleural thoracotomy is ventral to the ventral aspect of the spinal canal, but because the chest cavity is entered more dorsally, there is a significantly shorter distance to the ventral vertebral column and canal. The extrapleural nature of the dissection allows safer and more secure lung retraction and avoids postoperative tube thoracostomy placement. This approach allows for earlier identification and entry into the lateral spinal canal, via a resected pedicle. It greatly facilitates ventral spinal canal decompression through the disc space and vertebral bodies. Unlike the lateral extracavitary approach, however, mobilization or sacrifice of the foraminal neurovascular structures is avoided. Thus, retropleural thoracotomy represents a hybrid surgical approach, incorporating the advantages of both standard transpleural ventrolateral and dorsolateral extrapleural approaches while avoiding their limitations.

Operative Planning

Retropleural thoracotomy is an appropriate approach for localized ventral thoracic and thoracolumbar vertebral lesions between T3 and L2. The side of the operative approach is determined primarily by the location of the lesion. Eccentric lesions are approached ipsilaterally. The choice of the approach for central lesions is determined by the proximity of the great vessels and viscera. For high thoracic lesions, the aortic loop favors a right-sided approach. Either side is appropriate at midthoracic levels, although an ectatic aorta in older patients may obscure the field with a left-sided approach. At the thoracic and thoracolumbar levels, a left-sided approach is preferred to avoid the vena cava and retraction of the liver.

Consistency must be ensured between the methods of preoperative and intraoperative determination of pathologic level to avoid a discrepancy. This discrepancy is particularly likely to occur when the preoperative levels are determined by MRI. MRI identifies levels according to an end-vertebrae reference point. For a lower thoracic lesion, for example, the pathologic level is numbered by counting up from the sacrum. This creates two areas of uncertainty. First, there may be transitional lumbosacral vertebrae. Second, MRI does not identify the number of ribs, size of the end rib, and number of nonrib lumbar vertebrae. From a surgical perspective, intraoperative localization is usually performed according to a surgically verifiable landmark, such as the end rib. Therefore, these two study methods must be consistent before surgery. If the location of the pathology has been identified with MRI, plain radiographs should be obtained to determine the size of the end rib and the number of nonribbed lumbar vertebrae.

Surgical Technique

After appropriate arterial and venous line access has been established, induction and intubation are performed. A double-lumen tube is used for lesions above the T6 vertebral level.

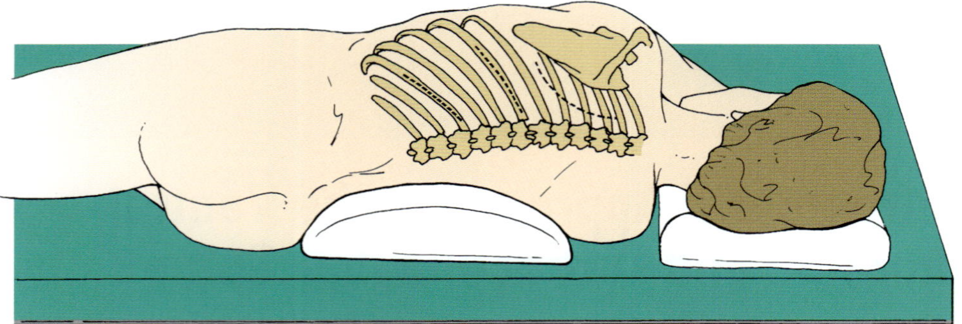

FIGURE 52-1. Patient positioning and skin incisions for retropleural thoracotomy.

An epidural catheter may be placed after intubation or at the conclusion of the procedure for postoperative pain management. A broad-spectrum antibiotic is usually administered 30 minutes before the skin incision, and this may be continued for two postoperative doses. The patient is carefully turned into a lateral position on a beanbag chair, with a small, soft roll under the dependent axilla. The upper arm is supported on a pillow or sling. The lower leg is slightly flexed at the hip and knee to help secure the position. All bony prominences and subcutaneously coursing nerve trunks must be well padded. The ulnar nerve at the elbow and the peroneal nerve at the fibular neck are particularly vulnerable areas. Thoracolumbar lesions should be centered over the kidney break. The skin incision is planned according to the level of exposure. For midthoracic lesions (T5-9), a 14-cm skin incision should extend from a point 4 cm off the dorsal midline to the dorsal axillary line. Extension of the incision toward the midaxillary line expands ventral access and may be required in some cases (Fig. 52-1, *center incision*). A curved incision that parallels the medial and inferior scapular border is used for upper (T3-4) thoracic lesions (see Fig. 52-1, *right incision*). For thoracolumbar exposure (T10-L2), the incision should parallel the rib one spinal segment above the pathologic level because of the more caudal inclination of the proximal portion of the lowest ribs (see Fig. 52-1, *left incision*). Therefore, whereas the approach to a T7-8 disc is exposed through the T8 rib bed, a T12 lesion is approached through the bed of the T11 rib.

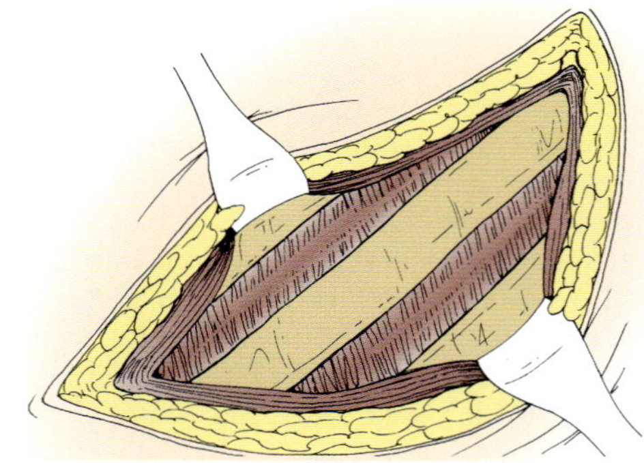

FIGURE 52-2. Skin incision is carried down to expose the rib to be resected.

The skin incision is carried down to the rib (Fig. 52-2). A 10- to 12-cm rib segment, extending from the costotransverse ligament to the dorsal axillary line, is subperiosteally exposed and removed with rib shears (Fig. 52-3). The exposed bone surfaces are waxed. Note that the proximal 4 cm of the rib, extending from the costotransverse articulation to the rib head, has yet to be removed. The bed of the resected rib is now inspected. Muscle fibers of an inconstant subcostal muscle may be seen. At thoracic levels above T10, the endothoracic fascia will be identified in the rib bed. The endothoracic fascia is analogous to the transversalis fascia of the abdominal cavity.[8] Both types of fascia line the walls of their respective visceral cavities and are reflected onto the surface of the diaphragm. The endothoracic fascia is tightly applied to or is continuous with the inner periosteum of the rib and vertebral bodies. The parietal pleura maintains its attachment to the chest wall through a surface tension seal with the inner surface of the endothoracic fascia. The intercostal vessels, nerves, and sympathetic chain are contained within the endothoracic fascia. Although only a potential (subendothoracic) space exists between the endothoracic fascia and the parietal pleura, a small amount of fluid and loose adipose tissue is occasionally identified, particularly dorsally near the rib head and vertebral bodies. Because the endothoracic fascia is continuous with the inner periosteum of the rib, it may be inadvertently torn during rib dissection and removal. This is common in older patients. If the endothoracic fascia is intact, it should be incised in line with the rib bed (Fig. 52-4). The underlying parietal pleura is bluntly and widely separated from the endothoracic fascia, either manually or with a Kittner (peanut) clamp (Fig. 52-5). The endothoracic fascia incision is continued dorsally to the margin of the cut surface of the remaining proximal rib. Blunt dissection

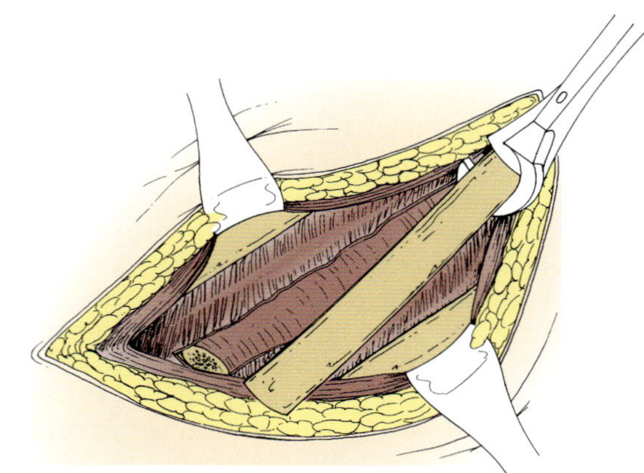

FIGURE 52-3. After a careful subperiosteal dissection, a 10- to 12-cm rib segment is removed.

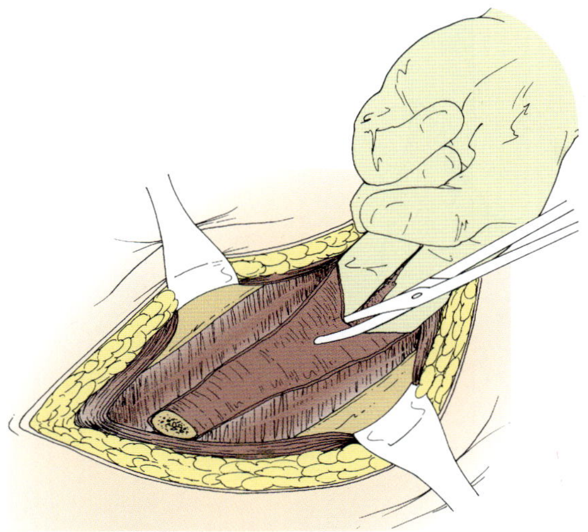

FIGURE 52-4. The endothoracic fascia is incised in line with the bed of the resected rib. Note that the underlying pleurae are bluntly freed from the undersurface of the endothoracic fascia with gloved fingers.

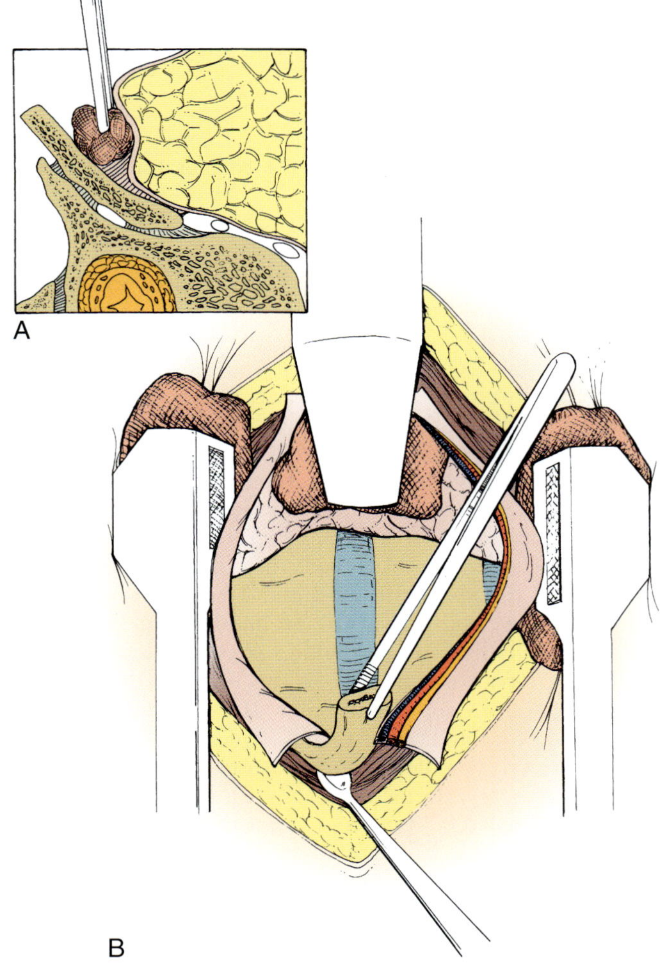

FIGURE 52-5. A, The pleurae are bluntly freed from the inner surface of the endothoracic fascia with a Kittner clamp. **B**, After a wide pleural dissection, the remaining endothoracic fascia overlying the remaining rib head and vertebral bodies is incised, and the rib head is removed.

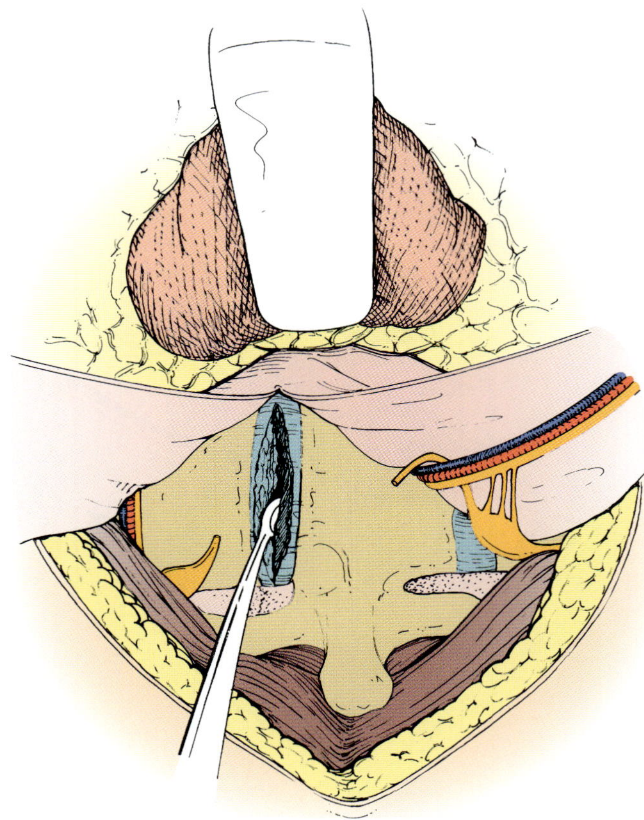

FIGURE 52-6. The endothoracic fascia opening has been continued onto the lateral aspect of the vertebral bodies. It is reflected away from the disc. The intercostal vessels remain within the reflected tissue. The thoracic sympathetic chain has been divided, and the disc has been incised.

of the pleura off the proximal rib head extends dorsally to expose the vertebral bodies and disc space. When the ventral convex border of the vertebral body has been exposed, a self-retaining, table-mounted retractor maintains exposure of the vertebral column (Fig. 52-6).

The endothoracic fascia incision is continued dorsally over the remaining proximal rib segment and onto the vertebral body with electrocautery. This divides the sympathetic chain that descends within the endothoracic fascia, just ventral to the rib head insertion on the surface of the vertebral column. The musculoligamentous attachments, including the costotransverse and stellate ligaments, are detached from the rib head segment, which is then removed. Removal of the rib head is critical because it allows identification of the pedicle (through which the lateral spinal canal entry will subsequently be accessed). For thoracic disc removal, the incised endothoracic fascia and vertebral body periosteum are elevated in either direction from the disc space to the midvertebral body. The intercostal vessels, which run transversely at the midvertebral level, are preserved within the reflected tissue. The margins of the pedicle are defined with angled curettes and nerve hooks. The pedicle is resected with a high-speed drill or Kerrison rongeurs. Removal of the pedicle provides lateral spinal canal identification and entrance. This lateral canal entrance, unlike the lateral extracavitary approach, avoids a bloody foraminal dissection as well as possible nerve root and radiculomedullary artery injury.

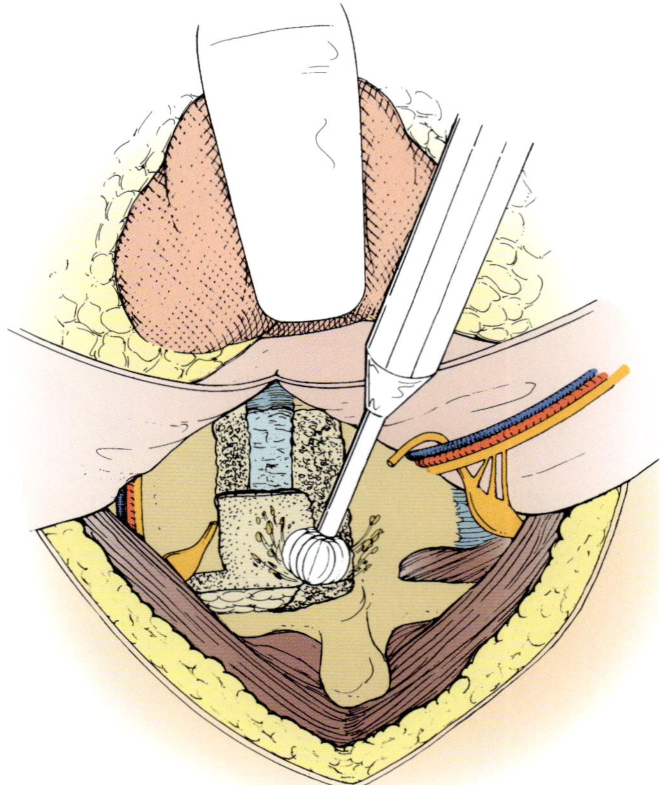

FIGURE 52-7. After disc curettage, the adjacent vertebral end plates and pedicle are removed with a high-speed drill.

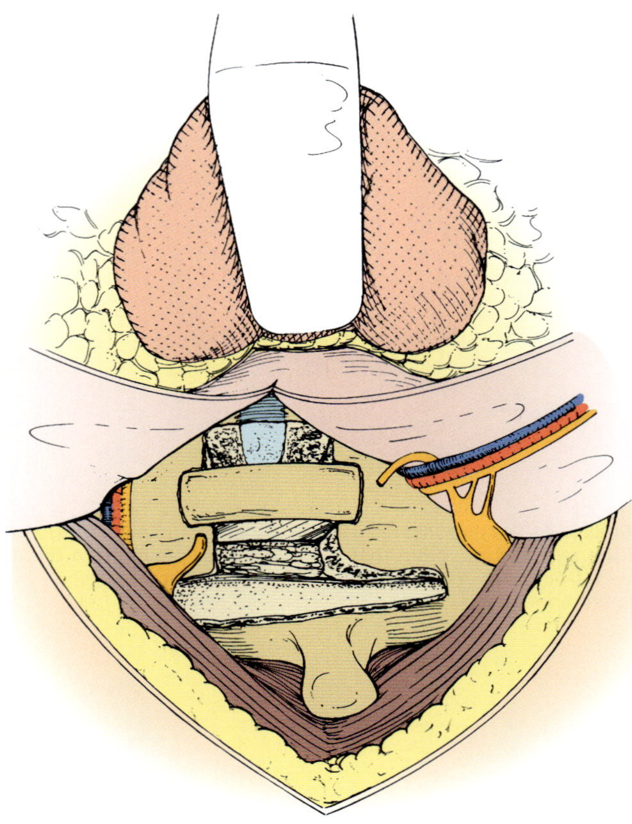

FIGURE 52-8. An interbody rib graft is placed after discectomy and spinal canal decompression.

The lateral disc anulus fibrosus is sharply incised. The disc is evacuated with curettes and rongeurs. The adjacent endplate and vertebral body margins are removed with a high-speed drill. The width and depth of the disc and adjacent vertebral body dissection must be adequate to ensure ventral spinal canal exposure and decompression. The depth should extend 3 to 3.5 cm from the lateral body vertebral margin to reach the contralateral pedicle. The width should extend about 1 cm on either side of the disc into the adjacent vertebral bodies (wider for larger calcified discs that have migrated, usually caudally, behind the vertebral body). The dissection is continued dorsally toward the spinal canal with disc curettage and a high-speed drill (Fig. 52-7). Spinal canal identification through the disc space and adjacent vertebral bodies is readily achieved because of the previously exposed lateral spinal canal entrance through the resected pedicle bed. When the dissection is carried back to the dorsal cortical margin and dorsal anulus fibrosus, a sharp, reverse-angle curette is passed through the lateral spinal canal entrance to displace these structures away from the spinal canal and into the bed of the resected disc and adjacent vertebral bodies. This maneuver may precipitate epidural bleeding that can be effectively managed with bipolar cautery forceps, introduced through the lateral spinal canal margin or with small pieces of Surgicel. As in the ventral cervical region, a thin dorsal layer of posterior longitudinal ligament (PLL) often remains after resection of the thicker ventral portion of the PLL (which is firmly attached to the dorsal disc anulus). Many calcified thoracic disc fragments are suspended within this thin dorsal PLL layer and are not located intradurally as often as the literature suggests. The ventral spinal canal should be probed with a microdissector and nerve hook for identification and delivery of these fragments that are suspended within this layer of ligament. The dura mater should be clearly identified before the decompression is considered complete. After adequate spinal canal decompression has been achieved, an interbody autologous rib graft is placed, although its efficacy after routine discectomy has as yet to be established (Fig. 52-8).

A more extensive dissection is required for vertebral corpectomy, particularly if stabilization with a lateral metallic implant is planned. For a T8 corpectomy, after the initial exposure through the T8 rib bed, the T8 and T9 rib heads are removed to expose the T7-8 and T8-9 disc spaces. The segmental artery and vein at the T8 midvertebral body level are individually ligated and divided as ventrally as possible. After resection of the pedicle of the vertebral body to be resected, the discs above and below the vertebral body are incised and evacuated (Fig. 52-9). Rongeurs and a high-speed drill are used to complete the corpectomy. Appropriate stabilization is then performed (Fig. 52-10). If a lateral implant is planned, the lateral aspects of the instrumented segments must be well exposed. This includes subperiosteal reflection of the endothoracic fascia and suture ligation and division of the segmental vessels at the midvertebral body level. The rostral margin of the rib of the rostral instrumented vertebrae may also have to be removed to achieve adequate exposure for plate placement.

The retropleural approach is modified at the thoracolumbar junction (T10-L2), because of the caudal rib angulation and diaphragm attachments (Fig. 52-11). At these levels,

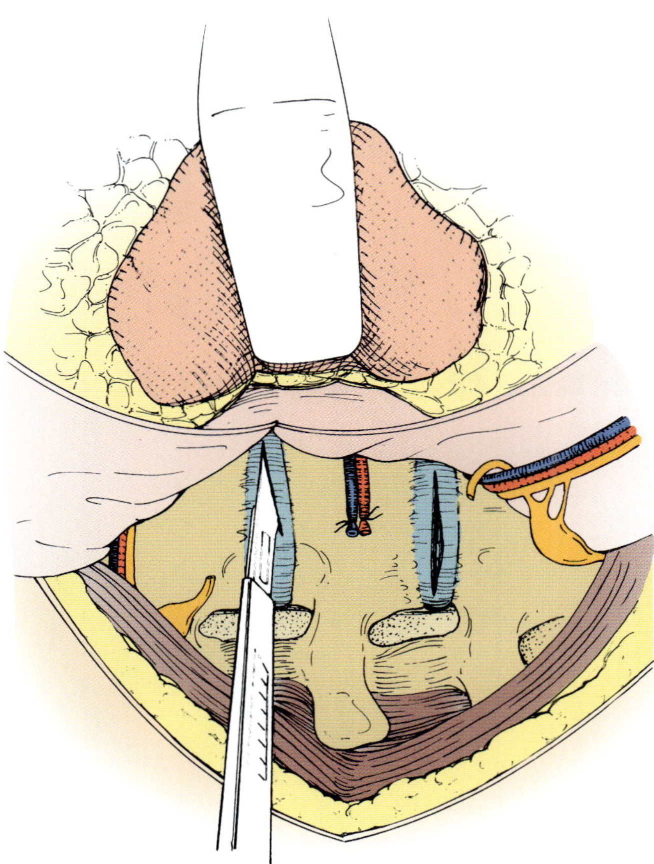

FIGURE 52-9. Adequate exposure for a corpectomy requires the additional removal of just the proximal rib head at the lower margin of the vertebral body to be resected. The segmental vessels are ligated and divided.

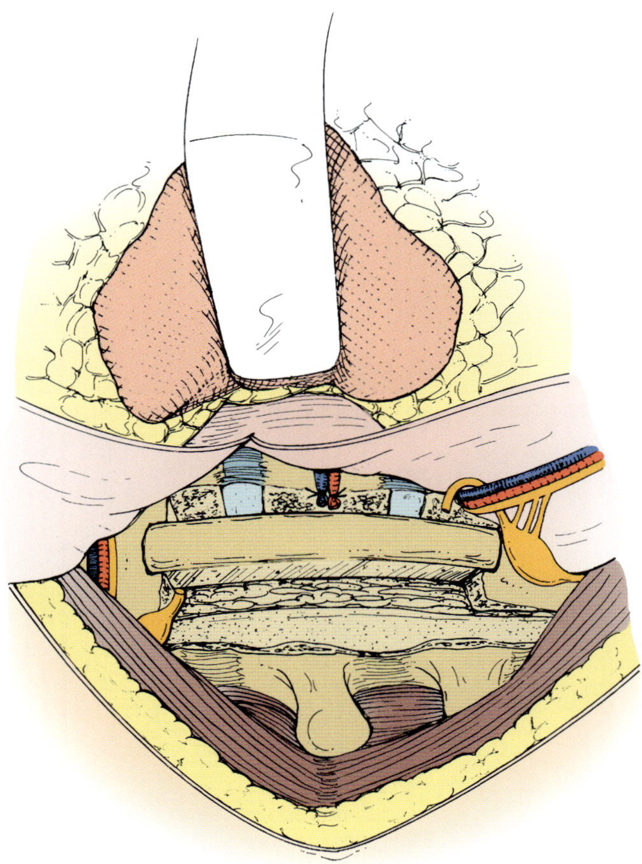

FIGURE 52-10. After corpectomy, reconstruction is accomplished with bone graft.

the approach is through the rib, one level above the pathologic segment. When the initial rib segment is removed, the diaphragm, rather than the endothoracic fascia, remains in the bed of the rib at the lowest three rib levels. A Cobb elevator is used to detach the dorsal diaphragm margins from their attachment to the inner surfaces of the rib origins. This immediately unites the retropleural and retroperitoneal compartments. The dissection continues dorsally to elevate the diaphragm from the dorsal abdominal wall attachments to the quadratus lumborum muscle (lateral arcuate ligament), the psoas muscle (medial arcuate ligament), and the vertebral body (crus). The exposure is maintained with table-mounted retractors. Elevation of the psoas muscle with electrocautery is required at the L1 and L2 levels. Decompression and stabilization are then performed by using the previously described techniques and principles. After decompression and stabilization, the diaphragm is reattached to the psoas and quadratus muscles with suture.

The pleurae are inspected before closure. Ideally, pleural tears should be repaired with sutures as soon as they occur. If the lung remains adherent to the parietal pleura at the conclusion of the procedure, no tube thoracostomy is placed, even if a prior pleural tear has been incurred. If separation between the lung and parietal pleura is present, indicating either an air leak (i.e., lung parenchymal entry) or a non-airtight pleural tear closure, a no. 32 tube thoracostomy is placed and brought out through a separate stab incision. It can usually be removed the next day. The remainder of the wound is closed carefully in layers with suture and skin staples.

Postoperative Care

Postoperative care is fairly standardized. If a tube thoracostomy has been placed, it can be removed on postoperative day 1 unless an air leak or excessive drainage is present. The epidural catheter, through which a long-acting narcotic is instilled for perioperative pain relief, is removed 36 hours postoperatively. Ambulation or mobilization is encouraged on the first postoperative day. Ambulatory patients are usually discharged on postoperative day 3 or 4. Skin staples are removed on postoperative day 10.

Follow-Up

In the author's experience, the morbidity and complications are less than were seen in previous experience with the standard transpleural ventrolateral thoracotomy. Postoperative pain is similar to that encountered with dorsolateral approaches, which suggests that the pleural incision accounts for much

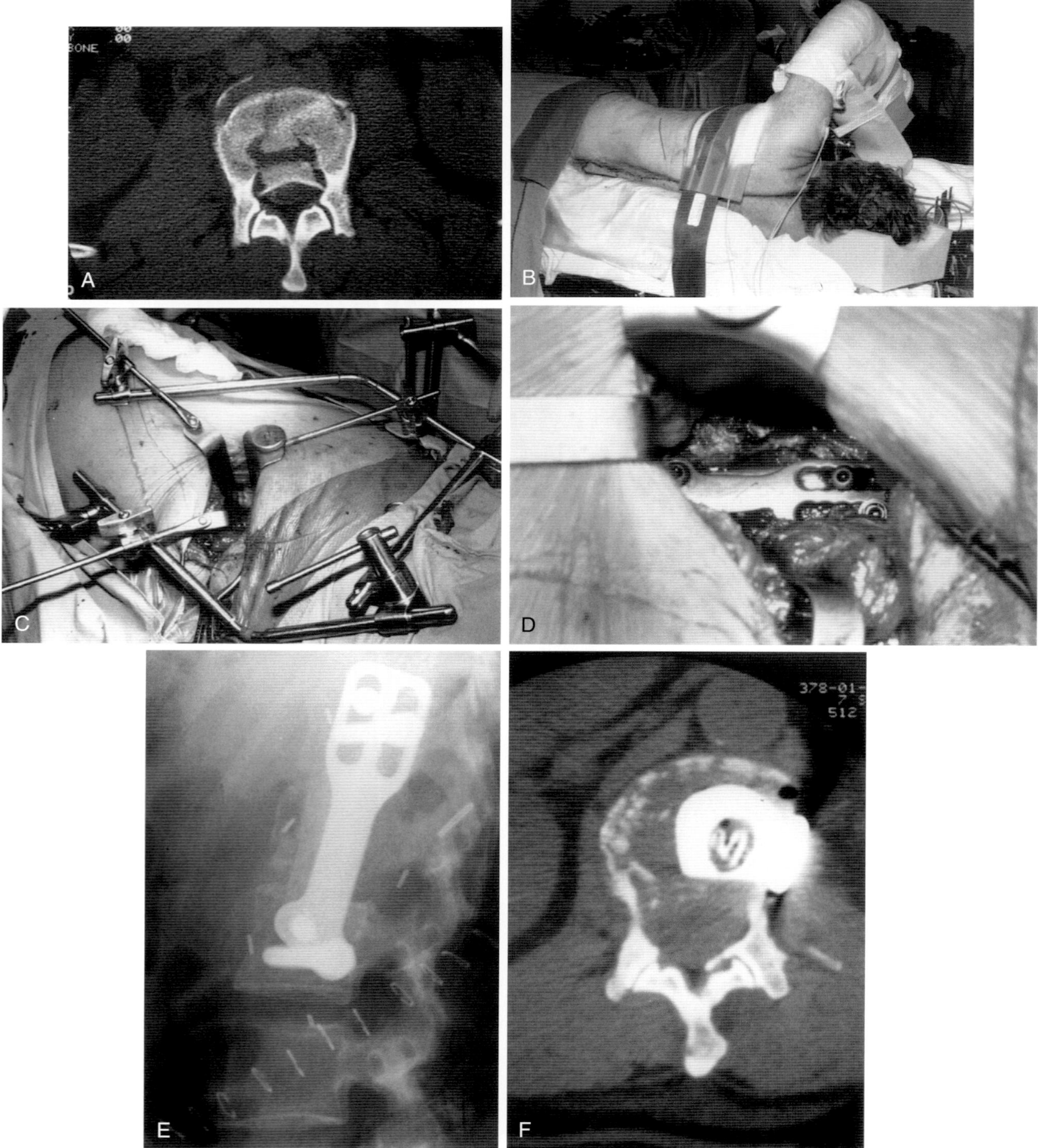

FIGURE 52-11. **A,** CT scan of L1 burst fracture with large retropulsed fragment into the spinal canal. **B,** Operative photograph demonstrating position and skin incision for a thoracolumbar approach for an L1 burst fracture. **C,** After the initial dissection and exposure, an operative photograph demonstrates the table-mounted retractor that maintains retraction. **D,** After corpectomy, a reconstruction with interbody graft and a lateral plate has been accomplished. **E,** Lateral radiograph after decompression and stabilization shows lateral plate and a large structural graft extending from T12 to L2. **F,** Postoperative CT scan demonstrates spinal canal reconstruction and placement of a large, structural femoral shaft allograft that has been filled with rib autograft. The lateral plate is in good position.

of the postoperative intercostal neuralgia that has occurred in fewer than 10% of patients. In some patients, postoperative intercostal pain and dysesthesias eventually lessened and evolved into a mildly annoying numbness or hypersensitivity. For lower thoracic and thoracolumbar approaches (T7-L1), abdominal wall outpouching (i.e., pseudohernia) has also occurred, particularly in middle-aged men.

Summary

Retropleural thoracotomy has proved to be useful for ventral exposure of the thoracic and thoracolumbar spine. It incorporates the advantages of both the ventrolateral transpleural thoracotomy (i.e., direct ventral canal exposure) and the lateral extracavitary approach (extrapleural dissection and initial lateral spinal canal entry via the pedicle or foramen) while avoiding the disadvantages of each approach, such as the extensive incision and soft tissue dissection, deep operative field, and oblique spinal canal exposure of the transpleural thoracotomy and the bloody paraspinal and foraminal dissection, intercostal nerve sacrifice, and incomplete direct ventral spinal canal exposure associated with a lateral extracavitary approach. Retropleural thoracotomy should be considered when ventral exposure of up to three vertebral segments of the ventral thoracic and thoracolumbar spine is required.

KEY REFERENCES

Angevine PD, McCormick PC: Retropleural thoracotomy. *Neurosurg Focus* 10:1–5, 2001.

Angevine PD, Parsa AT, Schwartz TH, McCormick PC: Ventral approach: extrapleural thoracotomy. *Tech Neurosurg* 8(2):122–129, 2003.

Bohlman HH, Zdeblick TA: Anterior excision of herniated thoracic discs. *J Bone Joint Surg [Am]* 20:1038–1047, 1988.

Louis R: *Surgery of the spine*, New York, 1983, Springer-Verlag, pp 228–231.

McCormick PC: The lateral extracavitary approach to the thoracic and lumbar spine. In Holtzman RNN, McCormick PC, Farcy JPC, editors: *Spinal instability*, New York, 1993, Springer-Verlag, pp 335–348.

McCormick PC: Retropleural approach to the thoracic and thoracolumbar spine. *Neurosurgery* 37:908–914, 1995.

REFERENCES

The complete reference list is available online at expertconsult.com.

CHAPTER 53

Laminotomy, Laminectomy, Laminoplasty, and Foraminotomy

Gordon R. Bell | Edward S. Connolly

Thoracic and lumbar laminotomy and laminectomy are two of the more commonly performed spine procedures. They have changed little since the 1930s but have been refined with the advent of magnification and microtechnique, microinstrumentation, and power tools. These advances, along with use of perioperative antibiotics and better neurodiagnostic tests, have reduced the incidence of complications of these procedures.

The surgical management of thoracic and lumbar laminectomy, laminotomy, laminoplasty, and foraminotomy may be divided into four strategies and components: (1) positioning, (2) exposure of the spine, (3) decompression, and (4) wound closure. Important perioperative aspects include prophylactic antibiotics, which should be administered within 1 hour prior to surgery to reduce risk of infection, and mechanical prophylaxis measures, such as pneumatic compressive stockings, which should be utilized to reduce the risk of deep venous thrombosis.

Positioning

Positioning for thoracic and lumbar decompressive surgery is dictated by the level of the spine being operated upon. Exposure of the upper thoracic spine requires that the patient be prone with the neck moderately flexed, the arms at the side, and the shoulders depressed (Fig. 53-1). Middle and lower thoracic spine exposure requires that the patient be prone, with the arms either at the side or abducted at the shoulders and flexed at the elbows (Fig. 53-2). We recommend that head tongs, such as Gardner-Wells tongs, be used to allow the head to hang freely, thereby avoiding external pressure on the eyes and reducing intraocular pressure. In addition, we prefer that the head of the bed be elevated to reduce facial swelling, which can contribute to airway edema (see Fig. 53-2B). Lumbar exposure may be facilitated in either the prone position, kneeling position (Fig. 53-3), knee-chest position, or lateral decubitus position. The important common feature of all of these positions is the absence of abdominal compression, reducing intra-abdominal pressure and epidural bleeding. It is important to limit hip and knee flexion to approximately 90 degrees or slightly greater to avoid hyperflexion of the knees, which can result in calf swelling and possible compartment syndrome (see Fig. 53-3C). The prone and kneeling position, as compared with the lateral decubitus position, allows complete exposure of the dorsal elements from the cranium to the sacrum. It allows the surgical assistant to have an adequate view of the vertebral column and allows at least four hands to be available to help with the procedure. Surgeries are currently rarely done in the lateral decubitus position. There are, however, potential disadvantages of the prone position. These include restriction of thoracic expansion, compression of the abdominal viscera (producing increased venous pressure in the epidural venous plexus), and the potential for ocular and peripheral nerve compression. These disadvantages can be obviated by use of a Jackson operating table with Gardner-Wells skull traction, as was noted earlier in the chapter (see Fig. 53-2B). This setup allows the abdomen to hang freely, thereby eliminating abdominal compression, and suspends the head, thereby eliminating the potential for ocular pressure and facial abrasions.

To position for upper thoracic procedures (T1-5), the head is placed in three-point fixation using Mayfield tongs (see Fig 53-1) to provide stability to the lower cervical and upper thoracic spine. Ophthalmic ointment is applied to the eyes, which are taped shut prior to prone positioning. If head tongs are not employed, plastic goggles may be utilized to minimize the risk of pressure on the eyes. Compression stockings and serial venous compression devices should be placed on the patient's legs to reduce the likelihood of deep venous thrombosis and possible pulmonary embolus. In turning the patient to the prone position, care is taken to prevent twisting the

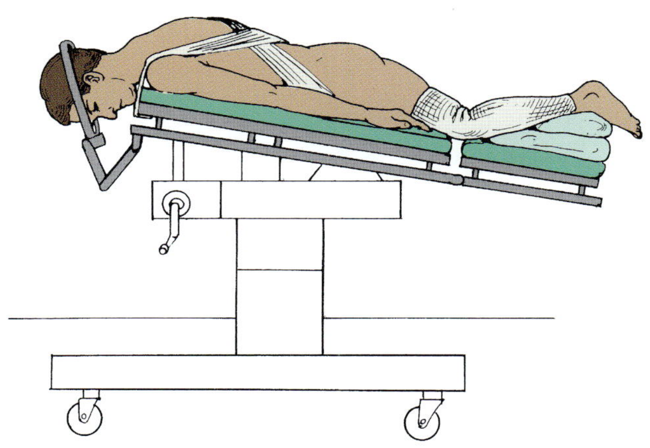

FIGURE 53-1. Prone position for upper thoracic laminectomy.

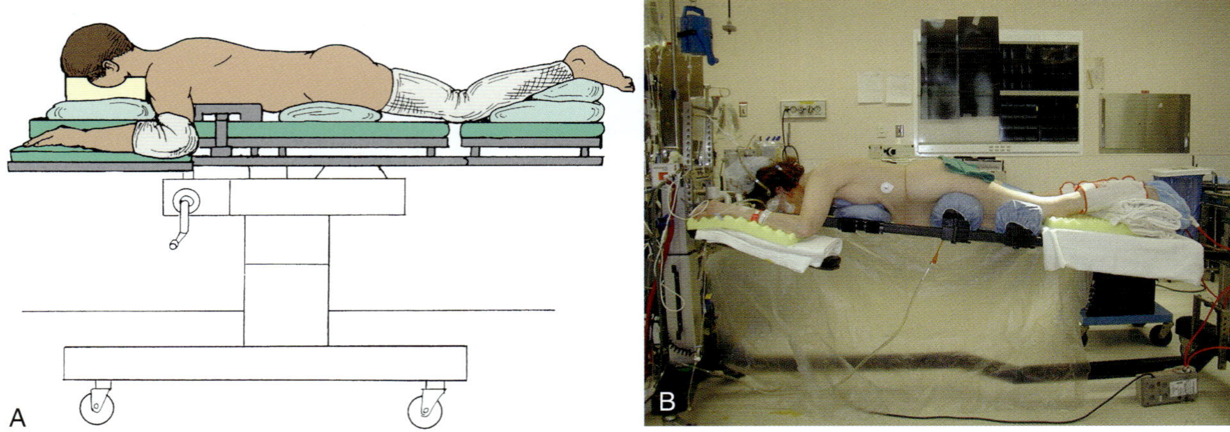

FIGURE 53-2. **A,** Prone position for middle and lower thoracic laminectomy. **B,** Prone position on a Jackson operating table with Gardner-Wells tongs to suspend the head to reduce the risk of ocular injury and facial swelling. Note that the abdomen is hanging freely and that the head of the table is elevated in relation to the feet to further reduce the amount of facial swelling.

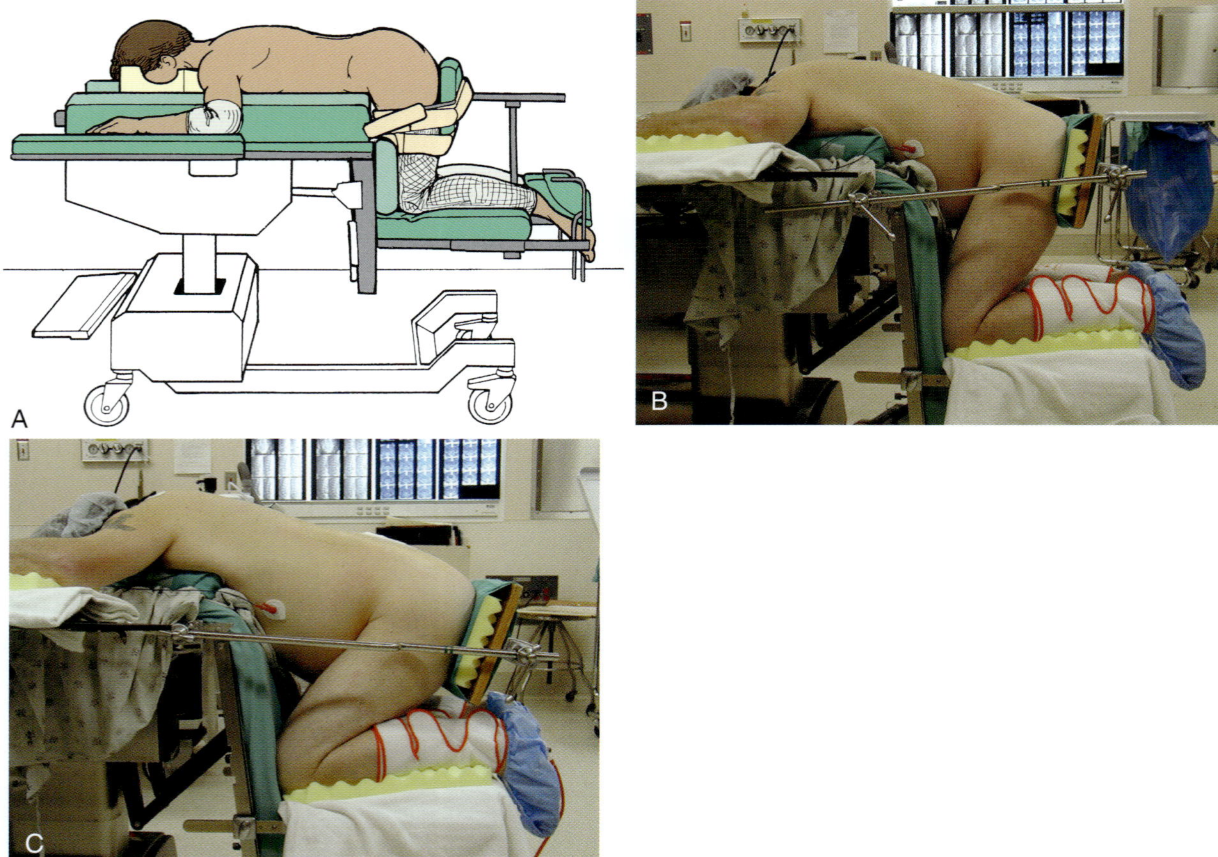

FIGURE 53-3. **A,** Knee-chest position on an Andrews operating table for lumbar laminectomy. **B,** Patient in a kneeling position using a fabricated kneeling frame. This position allows the abdomen to hang freely, thereby reducing intra-abdominal pressure and epidural venous pressure. Note that the hips and knees are flexed to only slightly more than 90 degrees. **C,** Patient positioned with hips and knees hyperflexed. Note that this position promotes excessive flexion at the knees, thereby risking a compartment syndrome in the lower leg.

neck. The patient is log-rolled onto soft bolsters that extend from the shoulders to the pelvis, allowing the weight to be carried at these four points and allowing the chest to expand and the abdomen to be free from compression. The skeletal head holder is positioned so that the cervical spine is mildly flexed ("military position"). All bony prominences, particularly the elbows, are padded, and the arms are tucked to the side. Exposure can be facilitated by using 3-inch-wide adhesive tape to depress the shoulders by extending the tape from the tip of one shoulder to the opposite side of the table in a crisscross fashion, ensuring that the cross occurs at the thoracolumbar region and does not involve the upper thoracic region. Care must be exercised to avoid extreme shoulder depression, which can produce a traction injury to the brachial plexus. The operative table is then tilted in a mild, reverse Trendelenburg position to elevate the head in relation to the feet and to place the upper thoracic vertebrae parallel to the floor (see Figs. 53-1 and 53-2B).

Positioning for exposure of the lower thoracic spine is identical to that for the upper thoracic spine except that the arms may be either left at the side or abducted to 90 degrees at the shoulder with the elbows flexed 90 degrees. It is important to check the patient's shoulder motion preoperatively to be sure that the shoulders are capable of 90 degrees of abduction. In addition, care must be exercised to avoid shoulder abduction beyond 90 degrees, which can result in a painful shoulder postoperatively.

Positioning for lumbar spine exposure may be prone, lateral decubitus position, or knee-chest position. Our preference is either the kneeling position on an Andrews operating table (see Fig. 53-3A) or modified kneeling frame (see Fig. 53-3B) or the knee-chest position. These positions avoid abdominal compression, thereby reducing epidural bleeding. It is important to check preoperatively that the patient is able to flex both hips and knees to 90 degrees. The kneeling types of positioning are generally not appropriate for patients who weigh more than 300 pounds because of the risk of pressure blisters on the knees with prolonged kneeling. For most adults, this is an excellent method of positioning for lumbar exposures. The authors have used this position without difficulty for many patients in the late stages of pregnancy. If the Andrews table is used, it is important to measure the chest-to-knee distance accurately before turning the patient to the prone position. As with all face-down positioning, eye protection is necessary, and venous compression stockings and alternating leg compression devices (pneumatic compression stockings) are important. The patient's feet should be padded before they are placed in the stirrups of the Andrews table. As the patient is being slid into the knee-chest position, it is important to keep sliding until the thighs are flexed 90 to 95 degrees. The buttocks board should be placed high on the buttocks so that it does not compress the sciatic nerves in the upper thigh. The arms are abducted 90 degrees at the shoulders, and the elbows are flexed 90 degrees, with padding of the axilla and the elbow to prevent peripheral nerve compression.

Exposure of the Spine

It is mandatory that the correct operative levels are identified and confirmed radiographically. In comparing intraoperative levels to the preoperative imaging study, it is important that the counting be done in a standardized manner. This is straightforward in the lumbar spine, where both the radiographic level and the intraoperative level are counted upward (cephalad) from the sacrum. It is also straightforward in the cervical spine, where the counting is performed caudally, beginning from the occiput. However, the identification of the precise level can be difficult in the midthoracic spine, where easily identifiable radiographic landmarks are not usually present. Two radiographs spanning both the lumbar and lower thoracic spine to accurately identify a mid-lower thoracic vertebra, or two radiographs spanning the cervical and upper thoracic spine to identify an upper-mid thoracic level may be required. Radiographic confirmation of thoracic levels can also be obtained by intraoperative fluoroscopic imaging.

The skin preparation should be much larger than the area that is to be exposed so that if additional unanticipated exposure is necessary, the incision can be extended without entering an unprepped area. Hemostasis may be improved by injecting 0.5% lidocaine (Xylocaine) with epinephrine 1:200,000 along the incision line. The incision is carried down to the deep fascia. The subcutaneous fat is reflected off the deep fascia with a periosteal elevator. Small perforating vessels are coagulated and divided as they penetrate the thoracolumbar fascia. If unilateral exposure of the vertebral column is performed, as in the case of a unilateral hemilaminotomy or hemilaminectomy, the deep fascia is incised just lateral to the spinous process, leaving a few millimeters of fascia to facilitate closure. Electrocautery can be used to dissect the paraspinous muscle tendinous attachments from the spine and laminae. Alternatively, a periosteal elevator and sponge packing can be used to expose the laminae and obtain hemostasis. Care is taken not to injure the facet capsules as the muscles are retracted laterally. The exposure should be extensive enough that the laminae overlying each pathologic level of neural compression are exposed. A long muscle release also allows less retraction of the muscles. The muscles may be held by a self-retaining retractor. Particular attention should be paid to obtaining meticulous hemostasis before proceeding with the bony decompression.

Decompression

It is important that the surgeon be aware of all the potential sources of nerve compression (stenosis). These include central stenosis, lateral recess stenosis, foraminal stenosis, and extraforaminal compression. When more than one site of neural compression exists, the surgeon may elect to treat all of the sources or limit the decompression to the more severe sources when there is a concern about potential instability from excessive bone removal.

For complete (bilateral) laminectomies, the spinous processes are removed with a Horsley rongeur. The base of the spinous process and superficial lamina can be thinned with a Lexel rongeur. The laminectomy can be completed with either a high-speed drill or a Kerrison rongeur. Once the laminae have been removed and the underlying cauda equina or spinal cord is exposed, it is important that instruments not be passed over the exposed dura, since an inadvertently dropped instrument could produce significant spinal cord or nerve injury. Care must be exercised in using a high-speed power bur, as it can "jump," even in expert hands. Using two hands may provide additional stability and prevent dural or neural injury. Paradoxically, there is more stability and less tendency for the bur to jump in drilling at a higher rate of speed than at a very slow rate.

In decompressing a highly stenotic canal at the spinal cord level, it is always safer to begin the decompression at a normal or minimally stenotic segment rather than at the most stenotic segment. Decompression of a highly stenotic L4-5 segment, for example, is more safely initiated at the L5-S1 level, which is rarely severely narrowed. Thinning the lamina with a high-speed bur will facilitate decompression by permitting use of a smaller Kerrison rongeur having a smaller foot plate. Trying to force a bigger rongeur with a larger foot plate into a stenotic canal can result in inadvertent injury to the spinal cord or cauda equina (Fig. 53-4). An alternative technique is to use a high-speed bur to create bilateral troughs in order to remove the lamina en bloc. This also offers the option to leave the dorsal arch intact so that it may be replaced and secured with miniplate fixation if considering a laminoplasty (Fig. 53-5). Although not commonly performed in the lumbar spine, this has been described as an option in a skeletally immature spine to prevent a delayed spine deformity.

Some surgeons prefer to remove as much bone as possible before removing the ligamentum flavum, since the latter provides additional protection to the underlying nerves or spinal cord. Since the ligamentum flavum attaches approximately halfway up on the ventral surface of the cephalad lamina, removal of the inferior half of the lamina exposes the origin of the ligamentum. A small straight or angled curette can be used to separate the ligamentum from the ventral surface of the lamina to facilitate insertion of a Kerrison punch. A dural separator can then be passed beneath the ligamentum, which can then be incised longitudinally by using a scalpel and then removed piecemeal with a Kerrison rongeur (Fig. 53-6). It is essential that the ligament be completely free of any adhesions to the underlying dura before it is removed. When the dura is tightly adherent to the overlying ligamentum flavum or to a synovial cyst, dural tears are more likely to occur. Great care and gentle dissection are required to free such adhesions before the ligament is removed.

The laminectomy may be widened by undercutting the facet joints by using a high-speed bur, a Kerrison rongeur, or even a sharp chisel. Since large bites with an angled punch could result in excessive bone removal from the facet joint or the pars interarticularis, a high-speed bur may be used to thin the lamina so that a smaller punch can be used to remove residual compressive bone without injuring the facet joint. In using a high-speed bur to undercut the facet joint, a cottonoid should be placed over the dura for protection (Fig. 53-7). Although not commonly used any more, a sharp chisel can also be used to loosen the bone before removing it with a small angled Kerrison punch. Epidural venous bleeders should be controlled with bipolar coagulation, and bone bleeding can be reduced with bone wax. If a lumbar facet is inadvertently fractured, the fractured fragments are generally removed.

Although inadvertent durotomy may occur with either a high-speed power bur or a Kerrison rongeur, it is the latter that is the most common cause of dural injury. When a durotomy is encountered, it is important that it be repaired promptly. In general, it is better to repair a durotomy when it is noted rather than later in the case, as loss of the turgidity of the intact dural sac with its enclosed cerebrospinal fluid will result in excessive bleeding from loss of the tamponade effect of the full dural sac on the epidural vessels. Most durotomies can be repaired by direct suture of the defect. The author prefers a running #6-0 or #5-0 silk suture if possible. The use of end sutures, in which each end of the durotomy is sutured with a separate suture to allow gentle retraction and elevation by a surgical assistant, facilitates closure by elevating and profiling the defect. This technique also separates the edges of the dura from the underlying nerve roots or spinal cord, thereby reducing the likelihood of inadvertent incarceration of the underlying neural structures. The dural repair can then be augmented with a

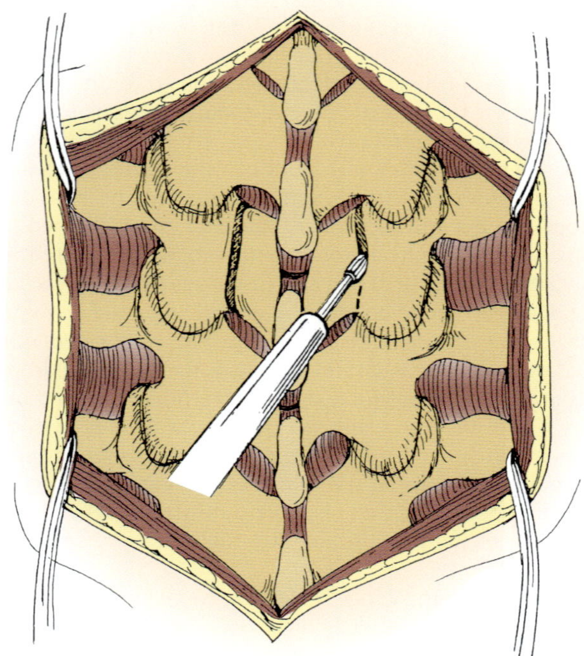

FIGURE 53-4. Laminectomy with high-speed drills reduces the need for placing instruments into the spinal cord and allows replacement of the dorsal arch (laminoplasty).

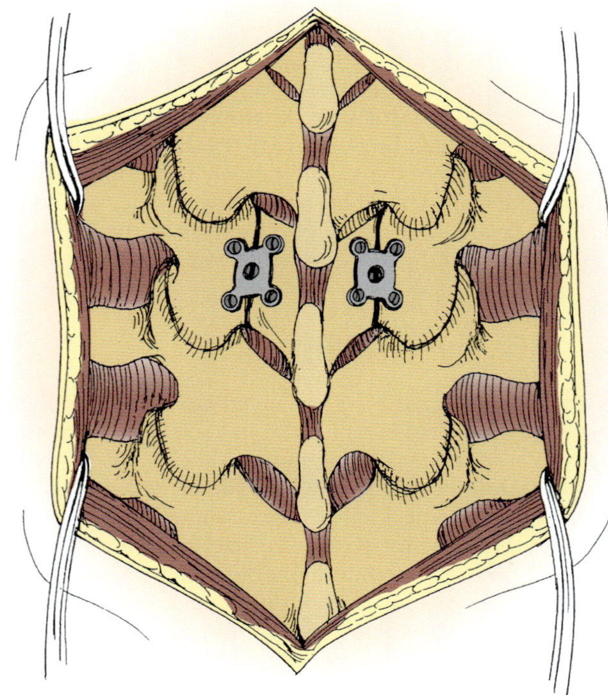

FIGURE 53-5. The use of miniplates and screws to replace the dural laminar arch in a laminoplasty.

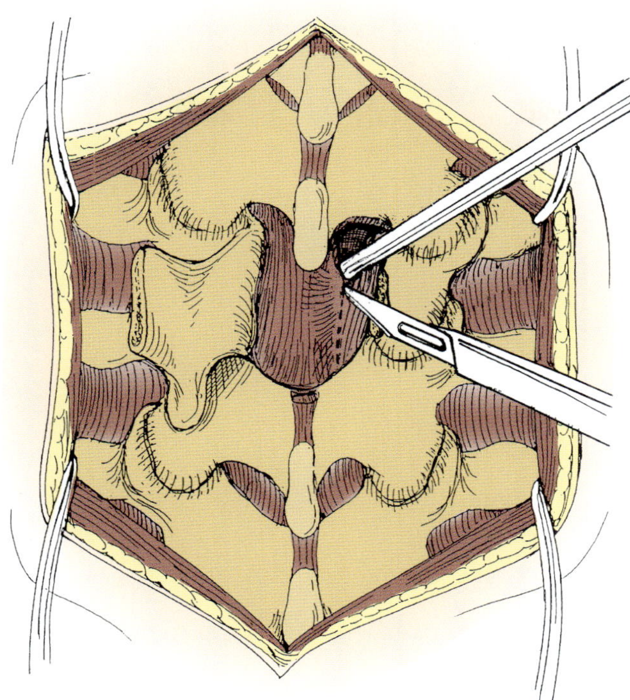

FIGURE 53-6. Ligamentum flavum is opened over a dural separator or other angled instrument to prevent injuring the dura mater.

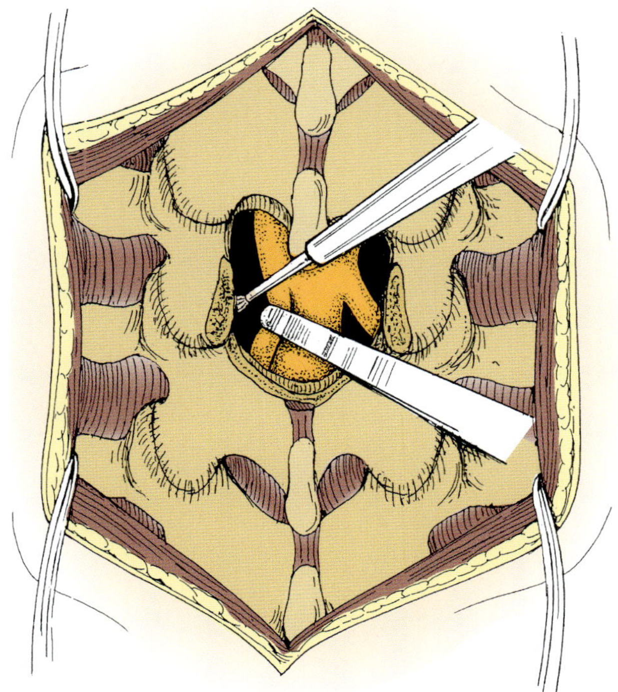

FIGURE 53-7. The dura mater and nerve root should be protected by a malleable retractor when a medial facetectomy is performed with a high-speed drill.

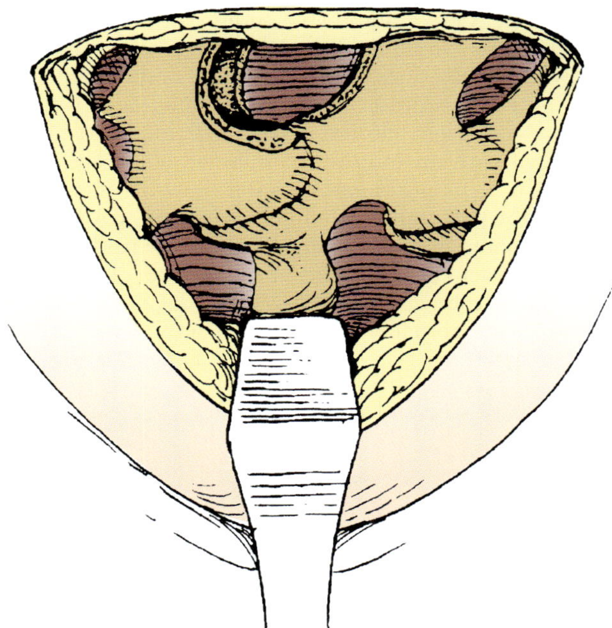

FIGURE 53-8. Left-sided laminotomy (cranial to left, caudal to right, left side down, right side up). Laminar bone removal is frequently not required above the insertion of the ligamentum flavum.

fibrin glue sealant if necessary. If direct suturing is not possible because of the location of the tear, a piece of fascia, a collagen matrix patch, or fibrin sealant may be used.

Distraction laminoplasty is a technique that has been described as an alternative to standard laminectomy. Distraction between two adjacent spinous processes with a laminar spreader allows visualization and access to a stenotic canal and requires only minimal dorsal bone resection. Limited bone is removed from the inferior spinous process and lamina of the cephalad vertebra and the superior aspect of the caudal vertebra. Ligamentum flavum can be removed, and the lateral recess can be decompressed by performing a limited partial medial facetectomy.

Lumbar laminoplasty, in a manner analogous to that performed in the cervical spine, has been described.[1] Although rarely performed, it may have a role in the skeletally immature patient with central stenosis, as described previously.[2] The lamina of the stenotic segment may be hinged and opened on the opposite side, using a small plate to keep the hinged side open, or the lamina can be removed and reapplied by using miniplates and screws bilaterally (see Fig. 53-5).

The amount of bone and ligament removal required for unilateral neural compression from disc herniation or focal, unilateral stenosis is dictated by the extent of concomitant pathology and the ease with which the primary compressing pathology can be accessed. Usually, decompression is required only to the proximal origin (insertion) of the ligamentum flavum (Fig. 53-8).

Wound Closure

It is important to obtain a good closure of the deep thoracolumbar fascia, since this provides the major strength of the closure. The deep thoracolumbar fascia should be closed with a heavy, interrupted, absorbable suture, although a nonabsorbable suture can be used. If a durotomy has occurred, an oversewn, running, locking suture of the deep fascia should be performed in addition to the interrupted deep suture to provide a watertight closure. The subcutaneous tissues are then closed with an interrupted inverted absorbable suture material. In the upper thoracic region in which there is tension from the pectoral girdle muscles, the skin may be closed with interrupted mattress sutures or staples with deep retention sutures over bolsters to prevent separation of the wound. The wound is then covered with a light, dry, sterile dressing. The sutures are normally kept in place in the upper thoracic spine for approximately 2 weeks.

KEY REFERENCES

Kawaguchi Y, Kanamori M, Ishihara H, et al: Clinical and radiographic results of expansive lumbar laminoplasty in patients with spinal stenosis. *J Bone Joint Surg [Am]* 86:1698–1703, 2004.

Tsuji H, Itoh T, Sekido H, et al: Expansive laminoplasty for lumbar spinal stenosis. *Int Orthop* 14:309–314, 1990.

REFERENCES

The complete reference list is available online at expertconsult.com.

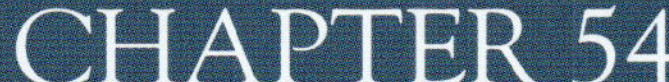
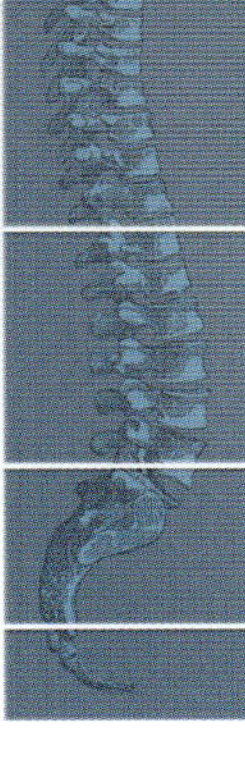

CHAPTER 54

Posterior and Transforaminal Lumbar Interbody Fusion

Davis L. Reames | Justin S. Smith | Christopher I. Shaffrey

History and Description

Dr. Ralph Cloward, who spent the majority of his professional life in Hawaii as one of the only practicing neurosurgeons during the period encompassing World War II, is credited as one of the original proponents of the posterior lumbar interbody fusion (PLIF). Although Mercer had theorized an interbody fusion as the "ideal" operation for spinal stabilization in 1936 and reportedly Jaslow performed the first PLIF in 1946, Cloward popularized the technique the following decade through presentations of his own cases at various meetings of organized neurosurgery.[1-4] In his 1952 description of 321 patients treated with PLIF for ruptured intervertebral discs, Cloward mentions the unacceptably poor durability of symptomatic relief afforded by lumbar discectomy at the time as an impetus for reexamining the more conservative treatment of disc herniations. He implied a general lack of appreciation in the spine community of the primary etiology, namely instability resulting from a broken or damaged vertebral joint as the causative factor in the generation of lumbar disc disease. Cloward argued that effective treatment for the radicular symptoms as well as the mechanical symptoms of low back pain present in many of his patients required not only decompression but immobilization of the damaged joint. He advocated for intervertebral body fusion as opposed to fusion of the dorsal elements alone because this allowed for restoration of the intervertebral space (and thus indirectly the neural foramen and central canal) while incorporating the chief load-bearing elements into the fusion.[1] As Cloward wrote in 1953, "The purpose of this procedure was to maintain the normal width of the intervertebral space and the intervertebra foramen. At the same time all false movement between the vertebra resulting from injury and collapse of the intervertebra disc was arrested."[2]

Approximately 30 years after Cloward's initial presentations regarding PLIF, Lin modified the original concept to include four central principles.[5] Preservation of the posterior elements of the motion segment (by maintaining the supraspinous and interspinous ligaments and limiting bony decompression to a medial facetectomy) and total (80%) discectomy (thought to improve fusion rates) represented the first two principles. Partial decortication, but not complete removal of the bony end plates, and the concept of the "unigraft" represented the remaining two principles. The "unigraft" concept was analogous to the model of the interbody graft used in anterior cervical discectomy and fusion surgery, namely the packing of all remaining interbody space with autologous bone to achieve a single solid fusion mass.[5]

Lin also described the notion of "dynamic decompression," which refers to the combining of two motion segments into one in a state of relative decompression. Widening of the neural foramen is achieved through both direct decompression and indirectly through the use of an interbody graft.[5] This restoration of the normal anatomic relationship between the motion segment and neural structures achieved in part through maintenance of disc height and restriction of motion was thought to protect the nerve roots. Immobilization of the unstable degenerative area arrested further degeneration; some authorities thought that this helped to protect the nerve roots. Investigators have cited reestablishment of weight bearing to ventral structures, prevention of recurrent disc herniations (at that level), and placement of the anulus under tension as advantages of PLIF over more conservative decompressive procedures such as discectomy, laminectomy, and foraminotomy.[6,7]

The PLIF has seen many changes and procedural variations since its first description nearly 80 years ago.[1,2,8] Modifications to the surgical technique have mainly focused on the expansion of available methods for achieving decompression, access to the disc space, and fusion. Unilateral versus bilateral exposures with unique methods of introducing grafts into the disc space and decompression strategies ranging from midline to far lateral, incorporating laminotomy, laminectomy, various extents of facetectomy, or foraminotomy have been devised. Additionally, the application of minimally invasive options for achieving interbody fusion has likely increased its attractiveness. An assortment of interbody grafts has been proposed, including various autologous sources such as morselized or structural elements of the posterior neural arch, bicortical or tricortical grafts, cancellous sources, or iliac crest.[9] Allograft sources ranging from morselized cancellous bone chips to numerous shapes of structural cadaveric bone graft such as bone pegs, trapezoids, crescents, or other configurations designed in part to prevent retropulsion or graft migration have also been described. Titanium mesh cages, threaded cages (BAK cage, Ray cage), polymeric rectangular cages (Brantigan carbon cage, polyetheretherketone [PEEK] cage, bioabsorbable cages (Hydrosorb cage), and ceramic cages (hydroxyapatite blocks) have been developed, all with variable biomechanical and bioabsorptive properties and similar clinical outcome in most reviews.[10-13] Facilitation of bony fusion and sound construction, applying concepts such as load sharing to complement the native spine successfully in its endurance of biomechanical forces, are among the fundamental properties used by these various grafts. Studies characterizing available interbody grafts generally describe variations such as sagittal contour, posterior disc height, fusion rates, clinical outcome, and biomechanical advantages in load sharing and the modulus of elasticity.[9,14-19] One investigation found cylindrical cages to be associated with a higher rate of nerve root damage than wedge-shaped bone allografts.[20] Some class III evidence supports general trends such as improvement in radiographic and functional outcome using artificial cages over bone chips. However, incorporating bilateral pedicle screw fixation may attenuate some of the differences described for the various interbody cages, and no consensus has been reached regarding efficacy among interbody grafts.[21-25]

Although some early pioneers of PLIF believed that a posterior fusion was redundant and perhaps unnecessary given the construction of a good anterior fusion, a description of supplementation with posterolateral bony fusion appeared early in the history of the PLIF.[1,26] More recently, evidence has accumulated for the use of posterior instrumentation, which, among other advantages, provides immediate internal fixation and facilitates fusion, as well as helps prevent loss of disc space height, progressive kyphosis, and graft migration.[13,27-30] The widespread use of transpedicular screw fixation for posterior spinal fusion began in the late 1980s and has generated necessary adaptations to the original concepts of PLIF as described by Mercer, Cloward, Lin, Jaslow, and others.[1-6,31-33] This has spawned a plethora of outcomes studies describing new techniques.[6,34,35]

The use of PLIF was not widespread until the 1990s, when advances in instrumentation and surgical technique revitalized its popularity.[36,37] Although the procedure is biomechanically sound conceptually and most reviews demonstrate significant improvement in various radiographic and functional outcomes when applied to spinal disorders commonly treated with decompression and fusion, comparison studies with other fusion techniques show mixed results.[13,37-46] Spondylolisthesis, which is thought by many surgeons to require rigid internal fixation to better withstand inherent instability from factors such as shear forces, has varying results regarding need for interbody fusion.[42,47-50] A recent international study comparing open pedicle screw instrumented fusion with and without posterior interbody fusion for spondylolisthesis found the PLIF group to have a better fusion rate and the other group to have a higher rate of hardware complications related to biomechanics; however, there were no significant differences in clinical outcome.[7] Studies of degenerative spondylolisthesis suggest evaluation of preoperative segmental instability may be an important factor in determining whether to perform additional interbody fusion.[47]

More recently, the transforaminal approach to the intervertebral disc, known as transforaminal lumbar interbody fusion (TLIF), has gained popularity.[13,19,51,52] Originally described by Harms in the late 1990s, the TLIF has arguably developed into the most commonly performed and efficacious posterior interbody fusion method in modern spine surgery.[51,53,54] Although there are many variations on specific surgical techniques, the underlying concept is access to the intervertebral disc space from a more lateral trajectory; this is generally accomplished through unilateral exposure of the neural foramen and exiting nerve root using a greater degree of facetectomy.[55] It should be noted, however, that although the "traditional" TLIF uses a less invasive unilateral approach to the disc space, whereas the "traditional" PLIF uses a more extensive bilateral exposure, both can be performed in a unilateral or bilateral fashion.[55] The impetus for the development of the TLIF grew out of concern regarding damage to the cauda equina and lumbosacral nerve roots because the more midline exposure performed for the PLIF requires more retraction of the dura to achieve adequate operative exposure for the interbody fusion. Reflective of this concern is the limitation of PLIF to the levels of L3-S1 to avoid damage to the conus medullaris, whereas the TLIF may be performed at higher levels. Therefore, a major advantage to the TLIF is the potential for less damage to the dura or nerves.[36,56] A recent prospective study evaluating TLIF for degenerative and isthmic spondylolisthesis found a median decrease in the Oswestry Disability Index (ODI) score of 10 points (23.5 to 13.5), with a fusion rate of 95%. There was a 7.6% serious postoperative complication rate requiring operative revision.[57]

Although both PLIF and TLIF are regarded as technically demanding, repeated studies have shown them to be safe and effective means of establishing circumferential fusion with similar clinical outcomes.[58] Numerous outcomes studies evaluating the efficacy of PLIF and the plethora of technical modifications are varied, however.[45] With regard to fusion, it is now widely accepted that interbody grafts result in higher fusion rates, often exceeding 90% to 94%.[59] Multilevel PLIF cases appear safe and effective, and although mention is made regarding increased invasiveness, good clinical outcomes and lumbar lordosis have been described.[60] However, although both techniques include positioning of an interbody graft under compression, maintenance of the posterior tension band, and to an extent correction of deformity through restoration of lumbar lordosis, recent reports have found additional benefits of TLIF over PLIF.[13,52,61] These include better improvement in lumbar lordosis given placement of interbody graft within the anterior column, greater enlargement of the neural foramen, and the option for using an effective unilateral approach; all these preserve other aspects of the posterior column integrity such as the contralateral lamina, facet, and pars, which may also provide a greater surface area for bony arthrodesis.*[13,48,57]

Compared with TLIF, it would appear that the larger dural exposure required for PLIF may carry with it added risk of durotomy during dissection of scar tissue in revision surgery. Fusion rates, however, are similar between the two and range between 89% and 95% in most studies.[13,48,57] Humphreys et al. performed a comparison of operative characteristics and complications between TLIF and PLIF.[57] Although for one-level surgeries, there was no significant difference in blood loss, operative time, or length of hospitalization, there was a statistically significant decrease in overall complications as well as blood loss for two-level surgeries in the TLIF group.[56] Preservation of the interspinous ligaments and preservation of the contralateral laminar surface were cited as additional advantages of TLIF in this study.[56] Biomechanical studies

*A report of unilateral PLIF has also been described.

focusing on the destabilizing effects of surgical approach for TLIF suggest no significantly increased spinal flexibility with the exception of axial rotation at L4-5. However, this was corrected with bilateral (but not unilateral) pedicle screws.[62] No consensus can be made on the effect of exposure on destabilization or the ability of pedicle screws to correct this effect between TLIF and PLIF, however, because other studies have demonstrated good results with unilateral PLIF surgery.[63]

Many additional variations to both TLIF and PLIF have been described. TLIFs incorporating more aggressive decompressions through total bilateral facetectomies and resection of the pars (in combination with instrumented fusion), enabling placement of bilateral interbody graft placement as in PLIF, have been reported.[55] Alternatively, less invasive procedures (e.g., LI-PLIF), which advocate the use of percutaneous pedicle screws if needed and "preservation of posterior elements and avoidance of far lateral dissection over the transverse processes," have been described.[35]

Although outcomes studies often cite a steep "learning curve" for the necessary acquisition of new skills and familiarity of equipment as limitations, minimally invasive techniques (described elsewhere) have several unique advantages that make them attractive alternatives to open surgery.[35] Quicker and less painful postoperative recovery and less destruction of adjacent tissue are commonly mentioned advantages.[64-66] Recent studies have also demonstrated reduced hospital charges and lower transfer rates to inpatient rehabilitation facilities.[67] Investigators have described similar clinical results for spondylolisthesis, including similar reductions in listhesis when original slip is less than 50%, between open and minimally invasive PLIF.[66] Researchers recently reported a minimally invasive method of interbody fusion for isthmic spondylolisthesis.[68] This technique, called the extraforaminal lumbar interbody fusion (ELIF), uses a prone position and several small parasagittal incisions and fluoroscopic guidance to achieve decompression and percutaneous pedicle screw fixation. This approach appears to be limited to decompression of the exiting nerve root, however. Another recent series describes minimally invasive TLIFs using unilateral percutaneous pedicle screw fixation and demonstrates results similar to those of previously published open TLIF/PLIF procedures.[64] Reports of other approaches such as minimally invasive presacral approaches for intervertebral discectomy and fusion at L5-S1 exist in the literature.[69] Although exposure to radiation and operative times may be longer for minimally invasive PLIF or TLIF, reported differences in long-term clinical outcomes with open surgery are not consistent.[70,71]

Although new reports refining and validating old techniques and innovative descriptions of novel concepts continue to represent a majority of the available literature, one appreciates some commonly debated concepts. These include trends in the preservation of various posterior elements, trajectories for accessing the disc space, strategies for achieving fusion, less invasive techniques, and advancements in materials research.[72-74]

Indications for Surgery

Controversy regarding the indications for PLIF has existed since its inception.[1,2,26,45,75] Cloward designated broad indications for PLIF that included essentially all symptomatic lumbar disc disease (low back pain with or without radiculopathy resultant from a pathologic disc). Current treatment guidelines consist mainly of class III evidence, because class I and II data are lacking. Outcomes studies have generated a more extensive and specific list of indications; however, in light of the current trend of cost-benefit analysis and increasing costs of health care, controversy remains.

Degenerative disc disease (generally associated with Modic changes), lumbar segmental instability (iatrogenic, degenerative, or other causes), spondylolisthesis, degenerative scoliosis, pseudarthrosis after previous fusion surgery, spinal stenosis, deformity, and recurrent disc herniations are common indications for PLIF or TLIF surgery.[13,59,76-78] Cloward, in his review of 100 patients with 30 to 40 years of follow-up after treatment for spondylolisthesis, has described PLIF in combination with laminectomy of the entire separate neural arch as a "superior operation."[32] Citing poor durability of posterior decompressive surgery for symptomatic spinal stenosis (15–20% short-term failure and 50% long-term failure), Hutter combined the benefits of anterior fusion and posterior decompression afforded by the PLIF and applied them to the treatment of this disorder. In 142 patients with a minimum of 3 years of follow-up, he described good or excellent results in 78% and a fusion rate of 91%.[79] In a relatively large, long-term (12-year), single-surgeon comparison study of PLIF versus standard laminotomy and discectomy for lumbar disc disease, Hackenberg described similar results in clinical outcome; however, he found PLIF to reduce the rate of revision surgery, and overall he thought that it represented an improvement in the management of lumbar disc disease.[49] Although one-level disc disease (at L5-S1) was well treated with either technique, additional instrumentation and stabilization were recommended for spondylolisthesis and severe multilevel lumbar disc disease.[49] Lumbar instability has been debated for some time, and clear evidence of instability is not always found. Some authors state that a difference of 10 degrees of angulation on lumbar flexion and extension films or spondylolisthesis of 4 mm or more may support this diagnosis, whereas other surgeons rely more heavily on intraoperative findings of instability such as "rocking of the vertebral bodies one on another with two Kocher clamps on adjacent spinous processes" (as described by Brown).[80,81] Segmental instability as defined by Frymoyer et al. refers to a "loss of motion stiffness such that force application to that motion segment produces greater displacement than would be seen in a normal structure, resulting in a painful condition and the potential for progressive deformity."[82] In a prospective study comparing discectomy to PLIF for massive disc herniations and/or segmental instability, some superiority of PLIF over discectomy was demonstrated within 5 years of follow-up.[75] PLIF and TLIF have been shown to be more effective at deformity correction than posterolateral fusion and more cost-effective than anterior-posterior lumbar interbody fusion with similar outcomes.[39,41,44] Most proponents of PLIF cite protection from pain resultant from recurrent disc herniations (attributed to the complete discectomy performed in preparation for the interbody fusion) as a primary indication for fusion surgery over more conservative decompressive procedures.[49,75,83] Data regarding the durability of lumbar disc surgery for controlling radiculopathy describe recurrence rates between 10% and 29%, and reduction in the recurrence of radicular symptoms subsequent to disc herniations has been demonstrated with PLIF.[49] Controversy remains regarding how many conservative lumbar discectomies should be performed (if any) prior to PLIF.

Attempts have been made to clarify the more subjective indications for PLIF. Evidence positively correlating preoperative level of disability (in the setting of degenerative disc disease) to functional recovery has been described.[72] Acute disc herniations with significant and protracted pain, chronic mechanical axial low back pain ("discogenic" pain), central disc prolapse at the L4-5 level, high demand activity, the "failed back syndrome," and chronic back pain following chemonucleolysis are all supported to some degree as indications for decompression and/or interbody fusion.[26,36,81] Chemonucleosis, although currently not as commonly performed due to concerns regarding side effects such as allergic reactions and neurologic deficits, is proposed to lead to loss of intervertebral disc height and progression of degenerative disc disease similar to the standard model of degenerative lumbar disc disease.[81]

Contraindications to PLIF may include arachnoiditis, active infections, short life expectancy (<3 months), severe osteoporosis, severe subchondral sclerosis with failure to demonstrate viable bone marrow with MRI, and potentially significant epidural fibrosis.[6,84]

Techniques

The PLIF as proposed by Cloward in 1953 was described as a 2- to 3-hour surgery for an experienced surgeon. Recent studies have demonstrated similar operative times and have associated longer operative times with increased perioperative complications.[85] Cloward described three separate surgical phases: harvest of the iliac crest bone graft, laminectomy and discectomy, and spinal fusion.[1] Modern technical advances have generated some necessary adaptations to the original descriptions.

In contrast to most current positioning techniques, which maintain a more neutral position through slight hip extension and elevation in an attempt to preserve lumbar lordosis (i.e., Jackson spine frame which in addition facilitates use of 360-degree fluoroscopy), some surgeons may prefer the original position described by Cloward, which used a prone flexed position (knee-chest position) favoring an opened posterior lumbar spine. Although flexion of the hip reduces lumbar lordosis, it facilitates access to the spinal canal. Interestingly, however, a recent study failed to find a difference in the maintenance of lumbar lordosis after PLIF whether a Wilson frame or a Jackson table was used.[86] An important aspect of either position is the elimination of pressure on the abdomen. A decrease in intra-abdominal pressure decreases epidural venous bleeding by reducing epidural venous plexus pressure. For the same reason, as well as to prevent damage from an overly distended bladder, most surgeons place a Foley catheter prior to positioning. Attention should also be given to properly supporting the chest to ensure adequate ventilation. Orbital pressure must be avoided to prevent visual loss through mechanical damage to the cornea or globe. A slightly reversed Trendelenburg position is used by many surgeons to help attenuate the increased intraocular pressure generated by the prone position. Although relatively controversial, it is thought to be especially important in possibly preventing visual deficits, including blindness, in patients with preexisting diseases that prevent proper ocular pressure regulation (i.e., glaucoma). Arms are positioned in such a way as to prevent brachial plexus injury, quickly assess an infiltrated intravenous line, eliminate pressure from superficial peripheral nerves, and support and protect all joints. This is accomplished with shoulder abduction and elbow flexion to 90 degrees and zealous use of padding. The feet should be slightly elevated to prevent venous stasis, and care should be given to protecting the lateral femoral cutaneous nerve because the anterior iliac crests often bear a large degree of the patient's body weight and should be appropriately padded.[87] Appropriate deep venous thrombosis prophylaxis is recommended.

Facilitated by external landmarks, palpation of the spinous processes, and/or the use of preoperative fluoroscopy, a midline incision is planned over the levels to be fused. A standard approach to the posterior lumbar spine is performed.[88] Dissection is carried through the subcutaneous tissue to the lumbosacral fascia. This may be done sharply using the scalpel or alternatively with electrocautery. Care is used with dissection through the fascia to maintain the supraspinous and infraspinous ligaments if so desired. This is thought to be especially critical if there are no plans for instrumented internal fixation. Once the correct levels are identified using intraoperative imaging studies, a subperiosteal technique is used to expose the laminae above and below the level to be fused (i.e., for the L4-5 disc, the L4 and L5 laminae are exposed). This is commonly performed by maintaining tension on the paraspinal musculature with the Cobb periosteal elevator while electrocautery or mechanical dissection with gauze sponges cleans the bone of the surrounding soft tissue. The laminectomy described by Cloward involved removal of only the laminae and spinous processes adjacent to the level to be fused (i.e., L4 and L5 laminae and spinous processes for L4-5 fusion). He stated that only a deep notch be made in the laminae and spinous processes rather than a complete laminectomy. Exposure was also facilitated by an instrument designed by Cloward called the *vertebra spreader*, although other methods are commonly used for distracting the adjacent segments (see later discussion). Cloward also advocated maintaining the attachment of the ligamentum flavum medially to the spinous process and preferred to superiorly reflect this ligament bilaterally after sharply dissecting it free from the facet laterally and laminae superiorly and inferiorly. Although a great deal of variation exists regarding the degree of bony resection, commonly it is carried laterally as far as the pedicle, removing at least half of the superior and inferior facets. Great care is taken not to damage the facet joint capsules, especially if a fusion is not to be performed. A greater degree of facetectomy improves visualization; however, controversy exists regarding its effect on the development of adjacent-level disease (ALD).[89-92]

Once the bony removal is performed, the dura is retracted medially with either the use of handheld retractors or a self-retaining retractor as described by Cloward (Fig. 54-1). A standard discectomy using a scalpel to incise the anulus and a series of pituitary rongeurs to remove the majority of the disc is performed. A variety of instruments used to prepare the vertebral end plates, such as end-plate scrapers, shavers, curets, or rasps, have been developed since the use of the chisel in many of the first descriptions of the PLIF.[1] After the

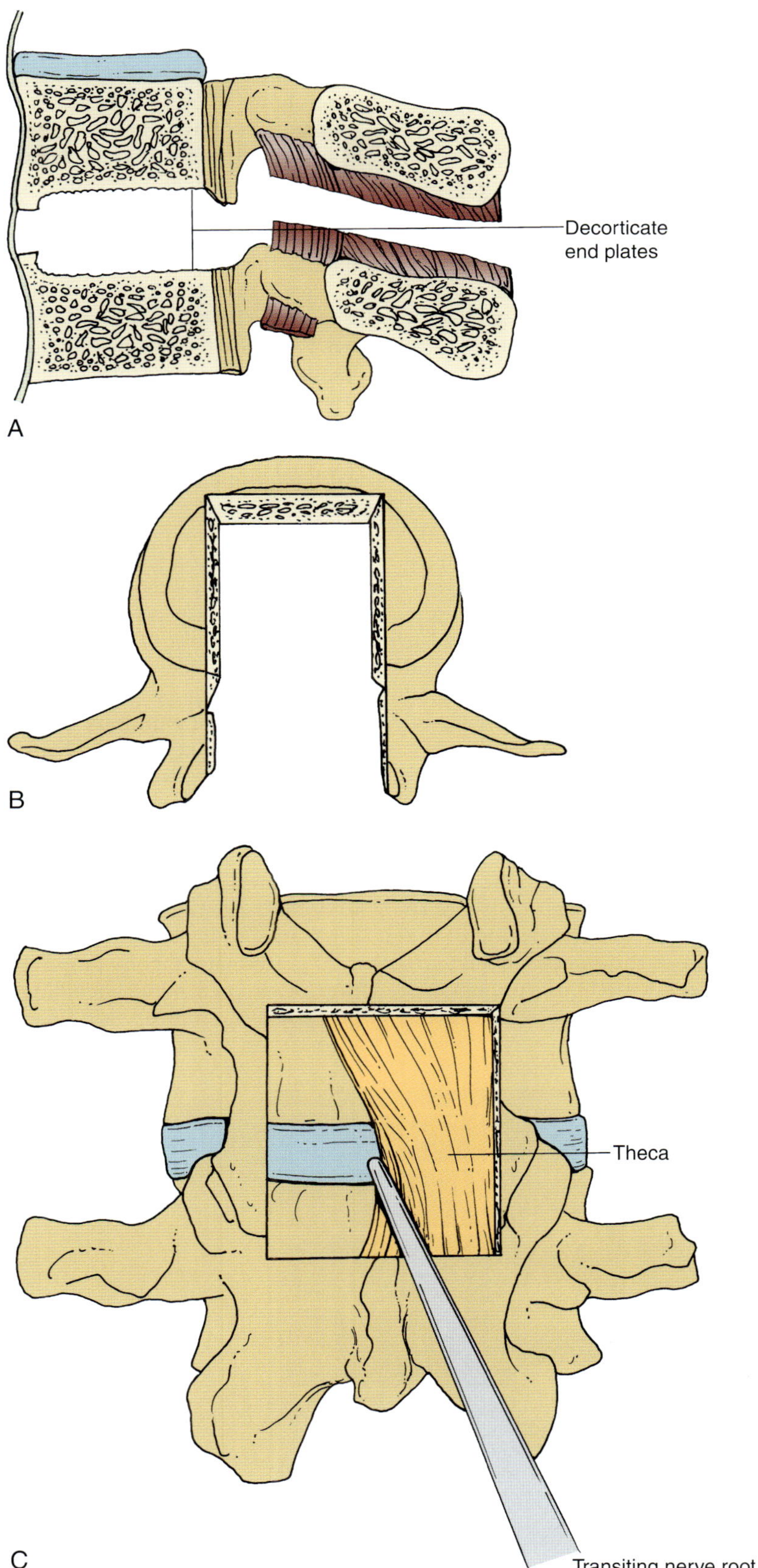

FIGURE 54-1. Sagittal (**A**), axial (**B**), and operative (**C**) views of the exposure.

discectomy is performed and the end plates are adequately prepared using a series of reamers, shavers, rasps, curets, and other available instruments, the grafts are ready to be placed (Fig. 54-2A).[59] Careful attention should be paid to the insertion depth of all instruments while working within the disc space, however, because the average depth of the disc space often ranges from 25 mm under the facet to 35 mm in the center of the interspace.[6] Original descriptions of the PLIF include bilateral exposures with bilateral graft placement, and although this is still commonplace, more recent descriptions of unilateral graft and/or pedicle screw placement exist.[17] Many modern instrumentation sets contain trial grafts that are used to verify correct size of the interbody graft prior to its actual placement (Fig. 54-2B). Studies have demonstrated maximal biomechanical advantage with graft coverage representing greater than 30% of the intervertebral body surface area; a larger surface area of contact between cage and vertebral body has shown lower stress distribution patterns (Fig. 54-2C).[13,93,94] A variety of cage materials and designs have been developed, including carbon fiber implants (Fig. 54-3).

When performing a TLIF (unilateral or bilateral), to gain access to the intervertebral disc, the pars interarticularis is identified and resected. Next, a hemifacetectomy of the superior and inferior facets of the levels to be fused is accomplished, often with an osteotome, high-speed drill, and a series of rongeurs.[51,56] The inferior nerve root is retracted medially along with the thecal sac. In initial operations, the superior nerve root is easily visualized because it courses inferiorly to the pedicle of the superior vertebral body. Revision cases may require extensive dissection for complete exposure of this nerve root as it exits the neural foramen. Although this nerve rarely requires any retraction, exposure is critical for ensuring protection during cage placement. Discectomy is then performed in standard fashion, although with care to preserve the medial portion of the anulus. Distraction of the disc space to facilitate placement of the intervertebral graft may be accomplished with a variety of methods. A temporary rod may be placed in the contralateral pedicle screws under gentle distraction. Care must be taken at this step not to overdistract; this may cause screw pull-out, screw breakage, or pedicle fracture. Overdistraction at the L4-5 level has also been shown to increase rates of ALD.[95] Once discectomy and preparation of the end plates have been accomplished, a trial may be used for verifying correct graft size. Whether structural allograft or an intervertebral cage is used, a combination of morselized autograft or allograft is often placed within the disc space. Positioning of the TLIF graft in the anterior versus middle column has not been shown to affect stability.[27]

Based on biomechanical studies, pedicle screw fixation is suggested for single-level TLIFs and PLIFs and felt to be necessary when two levels are fused.[27] If pedicle screw instrumentation and/or posterolateral bony fusion is planned, additional exposure of the transverse processes of the levels to be fused is generally performed for appropriate localization of the pedicle and drilling of a small pilot hole or defect in the cortical bone using a high-speed drill or rongeurs. Pedicle screws are placed by introducing a pedicle finder through the pedicle into the vertebral body, followed by assessment of the trajectory for breach using a ball-tip probe. A tap is used to generate an appropriately sized trajectory, and a ball-tip probe is used once again to assess for evidence of a cortical breach, prior to final placement of the pedicle screws. Appropriate training in pedicle screw instrumentation is necessary, because misplaced or inappropriately placed screws may significantly increase surgical morbidity. Inadvertent durotomy, neurovascular injury, or compromise in construct biomechanics may result. Proper knowledge of the instrumentation set is critical in selecting instrumentation of appropriate caliber, length, and size in relation to the anatomy. Although the addition of a cross-link has been found through biomechanical studies to have measurable effects on added stability (mainly in axial rotation), general consensus regarding its clinical usefulness is lacking.[96]

If posterolateral bony fusion is to be performed, decortication of exposed bone, including the lamina and transverse processes, is achieved using a cutting bur on a high-speed

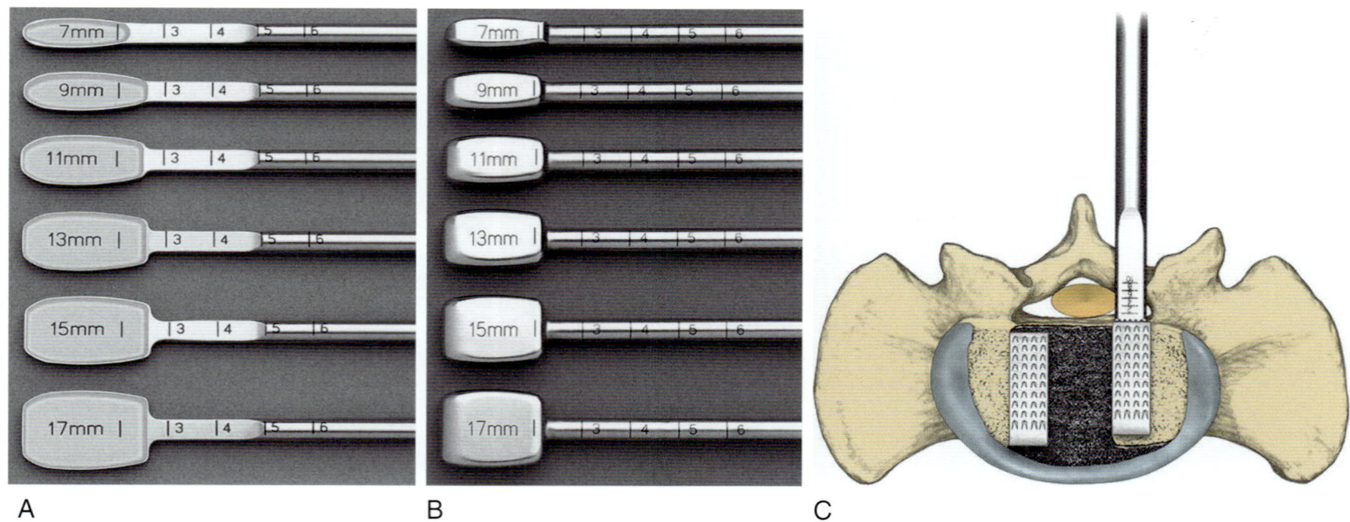

FIGURE 54-2. A, Examples of intervertebral disc shavers. These allow breakdown of the nucleus pulposus to facilitate removal while also removing cartilaginous tissue from the end plate. **B,** Intervertebral disc sizers. These help in the determination of the optimal size of interbody spacer to be implanted. **C,** An example of two posterior lumbar interbody fusion spacers within the disc space. The spacers are contoured, wedge-shaped cortical allograft. (From Synthes, West Chester, PA, with permission.)

drill. Morselized bone chips (autograft and/or allograft) are used to pack the lateral gutters between transverse processes and lateral to rods or plates if pedicle screw fusion is performed. Although bone morphogenetic protein (BMP)-soaked collagen sponges are not currently approved by the Food and Drug Administration (FDA) for posterior lumbar fusion, some surgeons choose to use them as an adjunct for augmenting fusion.[36]

Minimally invasive surgical techniques have been developed for posterior interbody fusion and instrumentation of the lumbar spine. Schwender et al. described a minimally invasive technique for TLIF[97] and subsequently reported favorable outcomes using this technique in patients with spondylolisthesis at a minimum follow-up of 2 years.[71] Although whether the minimally invasive approach for TLIF is superior to the traditional open techniques remains a controversial topic,[98] several reports have documented potential benefits of the minimally invasive approach compared with the open approach. These include decreased infection rates, shorter hospital stays, reduced postoperative narcotic use, and faster return to work.[99-102]

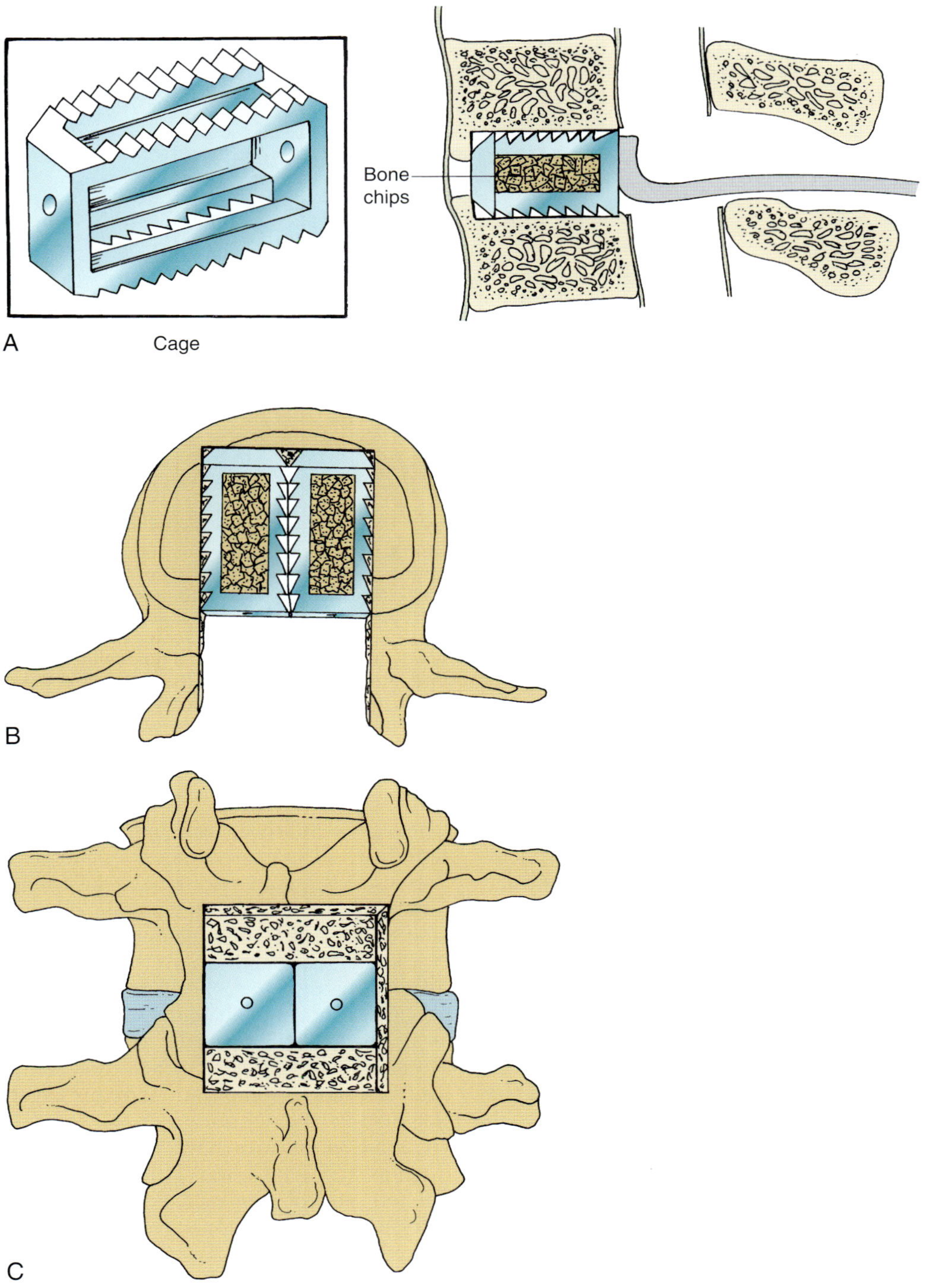

FIGURE 54-3. Sagittal (**A**), axial (**B**), and operative (**C**) views using Brantigan carbon fiber fusion.

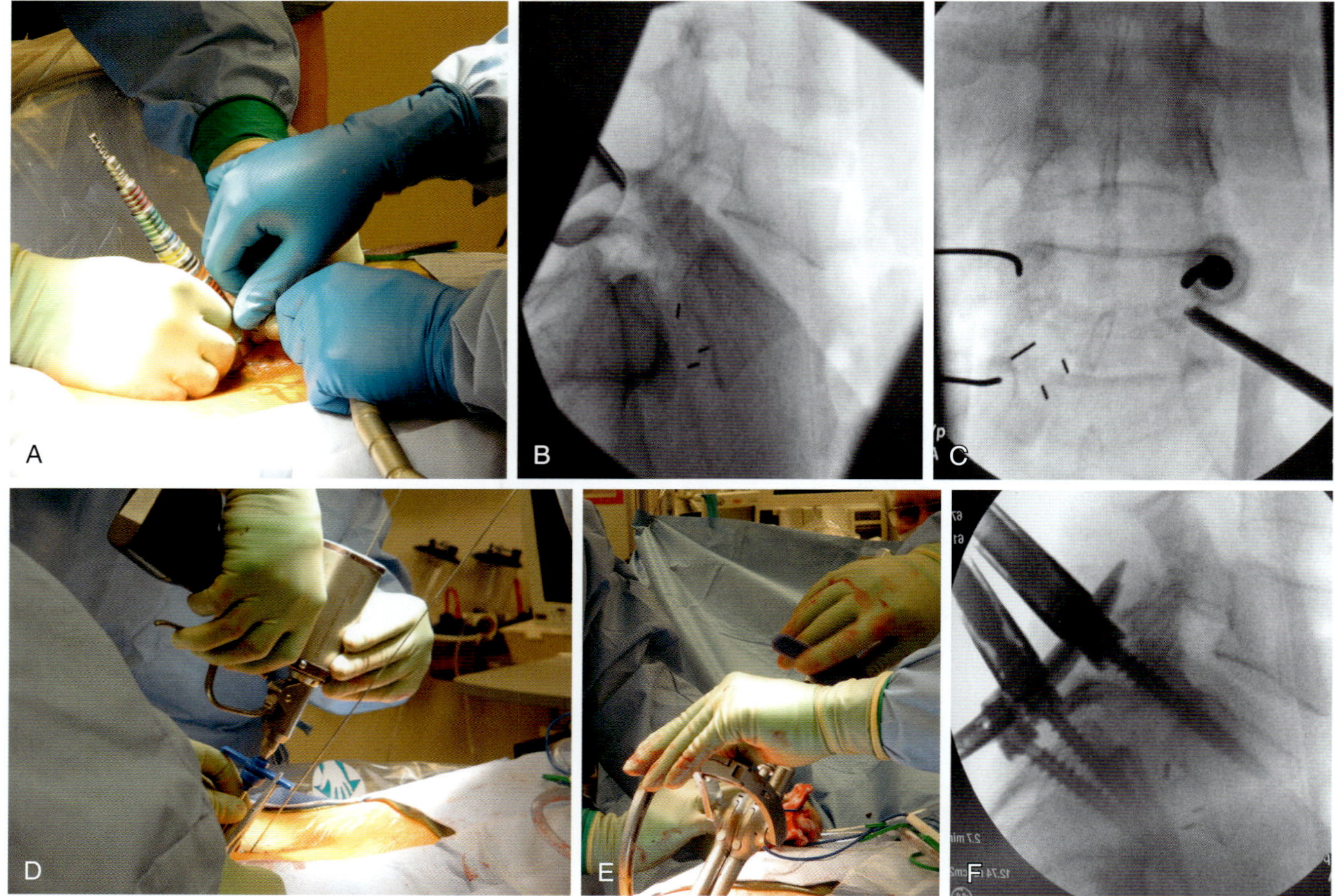

FIGURE 54-4. Minimally invasive transforaminal lumbar interbody fusion. **A,** A minimally invasive tubular retractor system is placed. Image shows dilators still in place with working port is being secured to the operative table with a flexible arm. **B,** Facetectomy, discectomy, and placement of graft and interbody spacer are performed through the tubular retractor. Shown is a fluoroscopy image with the tubular retractor visualized (*left*). Radiopaque markers delineate the interbody spacer in the disc space. **C,** The "bulls-eye" technique is used to align a Jamshidi needle with the pedicle on anteroposterior fluoroscopic imaging (*right*). Shown on the left are two pedicles with guidewires already in place. **D,** A guidewire is placed through the Jamshidi needle with the aid of a guidewire driver. **E,** After tapping of the trajectory with a cannulated tap and placement of cannulated screws into each pedicle over the guidewire, the rod is passed using a minimally invasive approach. Most systems include temporary extenders that attach to the heads of each screw and facilitate passing and securing the rod. **F,** Fluoroscopic image showing passage of a rod through the heads of the screws with screw extenders in place.

In brief, a standard approach for minimally invasive TLIF includes paramedian dilation to the underlying facet (Fig. 54-4A), followed by facetectomy, discectomy, and placement of an interbody spacer and graft material through the tubular retractor (Fig. 54-4B). Percutaneous pedicle screw placement can then be accomplished with alignment of a Jamshidi needle with the pedicle (Fig. 54-4C) and placement of a guidewire through the Jamshidi needle (Fig. 54-4D). Cannulated screws can then be placed over the guidewires, and rods can be passed and secured with minimally invasive techniques (Figs. 54-4E and F). Radiographically, the final appearance of the minimally invasive TLIF is very similar to that of the open approach (Fig. 54-5).

Complications

There are specific concerns and limitations to PLIF.[59] Most surgeons agree about the technically demanding nature of the surgery and have reported difficult intraoperative cases with poor outcomes.[59,103] The necessary acquisition of autologous interbody graft and/or selection of appropriate interbody allograft or composite material are potential limitations. ALD, graft migration or subsidence, collapse of the intervertebral space with resultant neuroforaminal stenosis, and the potential for segmental instability or pseudarthrosis are among the complications that may be associated with this type of surgery.[72,92,103-106] If not supplemented with pedicle screw fixation, immediate instability prior to bony arthrodesis is also of concern, especially with aggressive decompressions. Postoperative neurologic deficit, however, is arguably one of the most serious complications of this surgery, with rates ranging from 9.0% to 24.6%.[13,85,90]

Some authorities have reported complication rates as high as 37.5% for initial PLIF surgery, whereas others have quoted rates of new radiculopathy ranging from 13.0% to 16.4%.[48,59,85,107] Postoperative neuralgia is a known complication after PLIF, and there are reports of rates in the order of 7% (no significant difference in subtotal vs. total facetectomy) in the literature.[108] Nerve damage secondary

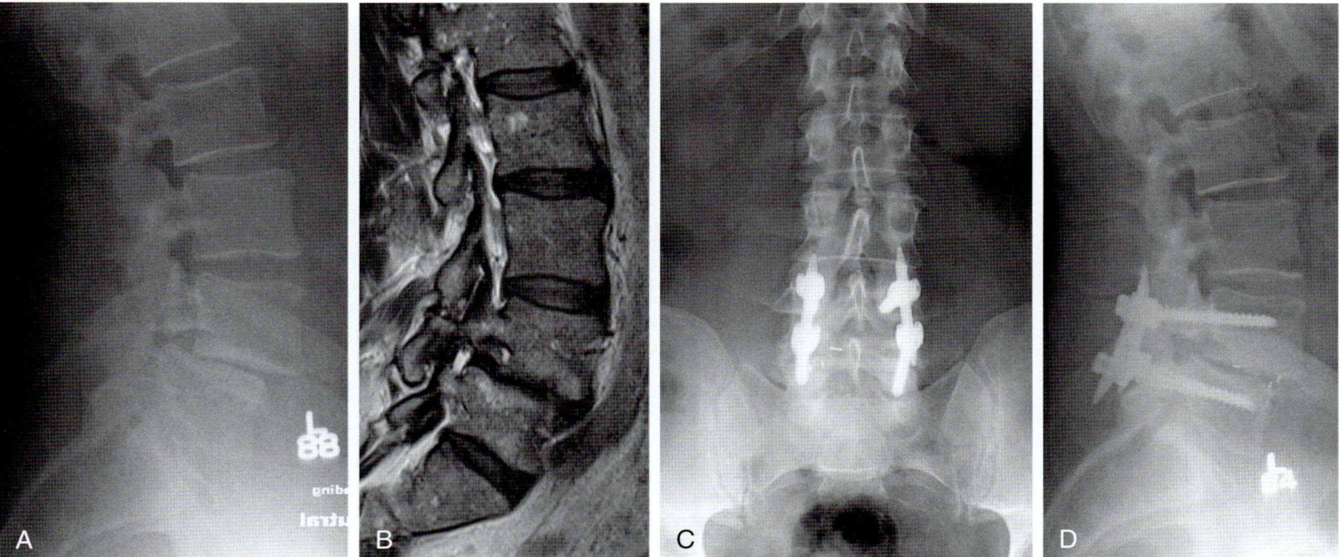

FIGURE 54-5. Case of 67-year-old man with back and leg pain. **A,** Lateral radiograph demonstrates L4-5 spondylolisthesis. **B,** Sagittal T2-weighted paramedian image demonstrates severe foraminal stenosis with nerve root impingment. Anteroposterior (**C**) and lateral (**D**) radiographs following L4-5 minimally invasive lumbar interbody fusion.

to retraction with resultant endoneural fibrosis and chronic radiculopathy is possible, especially if the dorsal root ganglion is damaged. A recent study of 1680 patients with a mean follow-up of 5 years found a 13.2% rate of revision surgery after PLIF. No statistically significant difference occurred in the rate of revision for single-level versus multilevel PLIF, although a trend toward a greater rate of ALD was apparent in the multilevel group.[109] Most authors agree that revision surgery for failed PLIF surgery is technically difficult, with limited surgical options; clinical outcomes are poor.[110] In a recent outcome study of PLIF of elderly patients (≥70 years of age), although no obvious differences in the clinical results were observed, collapsed and delayed unions were more common and postoperative ALD was less frequent in the elderly patients, compared with younger patients (<70 years of age).[111] ALD is a well-described complication after spinal fusion.[92,112] Although preoperative individual anatomic factors (e.g., facet sagittalization or tropism and laminar inclination) have been linked with its development, studies have failed to demonstrate correlation of radiologic degeneration of adjacent levels and clinical outcome.[92] Not all results have been statistically significant. However, in a recent comparison of the development of ALD among groups who have had PLIF, posterolateral fusion, and ligamentoplasty, PLIF appeared to develop ALD earlier and require revision surgery more often than in the other two groups.[113] Attempts have been made to attenuate the development of ALD through innovations in surgical technique with some measurable results.[114] Presumably a result from the more lateral trajectory of the graft placement for TLIF, anecdotal reports exist that suggest cage migration after TLIF may not cause neural compression as often as after PLIF and may not always necessitate revision surgery.[115,116] Cage migration rates as high as 8% have been seen after uninstrumented PLIF surgery (and are also associated with total facetectomy) and in contrast to TLIF, often require revision surgery, which is more technically difficult.[116] Cage type and positioning have also been found to influence rate of migration.[117] Vascular complications may result from graft migration, and care should be taken in compacting graft material ventrally.[106]

Other complications not unique to PLIF/TLIF warrant mentioning. Increased blood loss, higher rates of durotomy (5.4–10.0%), and development of arachnoiditis are disadvantages compared with posterolateral fusion.[36] Wound infection (0.2–7.0%), iliac crest bone harvest site pain, delayed wound healing, hematoma, screw misplacement, intraoperative pedicle fracture, postoperative urinary retention, pulmonary embolism, cerebellar infarction or hemorrhage, mass effect from epidural fat grafts, seroma, and epidural fibrosis/scar are among the reported complications.[5,6,13,34,49,59,103,104] Although surgical debridement and prolonged antibiotics are often required for the treatment of wound infection after PLIF, the removal of the cage itself is not always warranted.[118]

Recombinant BMP has been demonstrated to facilitate bone fusion and is currently FDA-approved for use in "stand alone" anterior lumbar interbody fusion (ALIF) surgery. Off-label use is not uncommon, including in PLIF/TLIF surgery.[119,120] Anecdotal reports of complications of its use exist. Theoretically, increased risk of cage migration and subsidence subsequent to loosening during the early resorptive phase have been postulated during the use of PEEK cages.[121] Although previously thought to represent a benign radiologic finding, limited reports of symptomatic ectopic bone formation with the use of BMP exist.[122,123]

Future Directions

Advancements in surgical techniques will continue to be described. The use of radiofrequency ablation for end-plate preparation has recently been described.[124] As minimally invasive techniques continue to be explored and incorporated by spine surgeons, its use will be expanded. Currently, surgeons are in need of longer follow-up for many early studies comparing minimally invasive and open techniques.[125] Technologic advancements in spine navigation surgery may increase its attractiveness may provide safer instrumentation techniques. Materials development will continue to advance the repertoire of interbody grafts and instrumentation. Biomechanical studies will help guide the application of new technology.

Summary

When performed by experienced surgeons, PLIF and TLIF can provide safe and effective options for a variety of spinal disorders. Most reports demonstrate similar results among the various methods with which to achieve PLIF. The TLIF has emerged as a potentially superior modification to the original surgery described by Cloward almost 70 years ago. Although based mainly in retrospective case series, PLIF remains a biomechanically sound technique that when used by experienced surgeons can provide relief for many patients.

KEY REFERENCES

Cloward RB: Posterior lumbar interbody fusion updated. *Clin Orthop Relat Res* 193:16–19, 1985.

Dickerman RD, Reynolds A, Bennett M, et al: Posterior lumbar interbody fusion. *J Neurosurg Spine* 6:194–195, 2007; author reply 195.

Ekman P, Moller H, Tullberg T, et al: Posterior lumbar interbody fusion versus posterolateral fusion in adult isthmic spondylolisthesis. *Spine (Phila Pa 1976)* 32:2178–2183, 2007.

Harms J, Jeszensky D: The unilateral, transforaminal approach for posterior lumbar interbody fusion. *Orthop Traumatol* 6:88–99, 1998.

Harris BM, Hilibrand AS, Savas PE, et al: Transforaminal lumbar interbody fusion: the effect of various instrumentation techniques on the flexibility of the lumbar spine. *Spine (Phila Pa 1976)* 29:E65–E70, 2004.

Humphreys SC, Hodges SD, Patwardhan AG, et al: Comparison of posterior and transforaminal approaches to lumbar interbody fusion. *Spine (Phila Pa 1976)* 26:567–571, 2001.

Okuda S, Miyauchi A, Oda T, et al: Surgical complications of posterior lumbar interbody fusion with total facetectomy in 251 patients. *J Neurosurg Spine* 4:304–309, 2006.

REFERENCES

The complete reference list is available online at expertconsult.com.

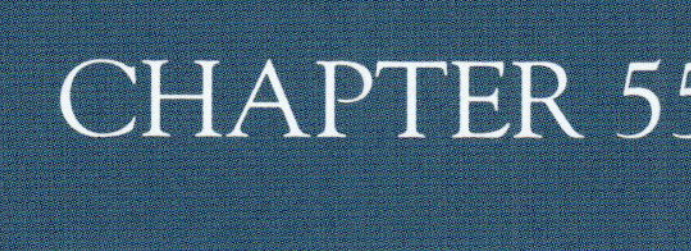

CHAPTER 55

Anterior Lumbar Interbody Fusion

Robert F. Heary | Daniel S. Yanni | Edward C. Benzel

Anterior lumbar interbody fusion (ALIF) reconstructs the anterior column of the lumbar spine. It also facilitates restoration, or at least improvement, of normal lumbar lordosis. In addition, the neural foramina may be enlarged secondary to the increased intervertebral height produced by the cage or graft replacing the degenerative disc. Its popularity has been maintained, mainly because of improved understanding of the biomechanics of the spine and the relatively large size of the graft. In addition, the relative ease of performing the surgical procedure has been a positive factor.

Dorsal decompression without fusion has suffered from difficulties that involve the development of chronic low back pain. Posterior lumbar interbody fusion can be associated with complications, as well as slightly higher rates of fusion failure, compared with ALIF. The biomechanically superior construct that results from ALIF has also enhanced its popularity. More recently, the biomechanical strength afforded by a large ventral graft has improved the attractiveness of other approaches, such as the lateral approach.

Possibly more than any other spinal surgical procedure, a careful consideration of the indications for ALIF is essential for a good surgical outcome. Chronic low back pain is a frequent indication for ALIF.[1-10] ALIFs are not ordinarily used to decompress the neural elements because of less-than-optimal visualization. Therefore, safe ventral decompression is difficult to perform.[1,11,12]

ALIF is associated with a low complication rate. Complications include difficulties with respect to the approach, the discectomy, the donor site, and the fusion, and can be divided into preoperative, intraoperative, and postoperative components.

ALIF may also provide a powerful revision strategy for pseudarthrosis after a dorsal lumbar fusion without interbody fusion. Typically, ALIF can be performed for failed dorsal lumbar fusion at L3-4, L4-5, and L5-S1, lending a significant biomechanical advantage with a large interbody graft.

History

Anterior lumbar interbody fusion has evolved considerably over the past century. Ventral approaches to the lumbar spine were first reported for the treatment of tuberculosis. In 1892, Vincent[13] described a costotransversectomy that was used to treat tuberculosis of the ventral lumbar spine. In 1906, Muller[14] described a transperitoneal decompressive operation for the lumbar spine. Ito et al.,[15] in 1934, described a transperitoneal approach to the lumbar spine that incorporated fusion.

Spondylolisthesis has been treated with ventral lumbar surgery since 1933. At that time, Burns described a transperitoneal approach using a tibial graft for fusion of the L5-S1 interspace.[16] Numerous other investigators have followed with modifications of ventral lumbar surgery for spondylolisthesis.[17-26] The retroperitoneal approach to the lumbar spine was first reported by Iwahara[27] in 1944. In 1948, Lane and Moore[28] described a series of patients with isolated lumbar disc disease who were treated with ALIF.

The ventral approach to interbody lumbar fusion avoids the neural elements. Most early experiences with this surgical procedure were those of orthopaedic surgeons. Over the past two decades, increased experience with this technique has been shared by both orthopaedic and neurologic surgeons. Although modifications to the standard technique have been devised, the basic tenets of the operation continue to be removal of the disc through a ventral approach, followed by placement of a spacer to maintain or improve disc space height, provide anterior column stability, and facilitate bony fusion.

Preoperative Considerations

Proper patient selection is vital to the success of an ALIF procedure[12] and is the best predictor of a good surgical outcome. Operative indications for ALIF include degenerative disc disease with intractable back pain.[2,6,9,10,29,30] Degenerative spondylolisthesis with back pain often accompanies degenerative disc disease.[4,30-36] A failure of prior dorsal surgery may also be an indication for ALIF.[1,2,7-9,11,12,31-33,37,38] Most important, the symptoms should have persisted for a prolonged period. In general, symptoms are present for 6 months or more before a patient undergoes ALIF. Likewise, a prolonged trial of conservative therapy should have been attempted and failed before planning an ALIF procedure.[6,29,38,39] Contraindications to ALIF are absolute or relative. The only true absolute contraindication is advanced osteoporosis that prevents the vertebral bodies from maintaining a bone graft.[1] Relative contraindications occur in varying degrees. Neural compression as a result of either disc disease or stenosis is a relative contraindication. If neural compression is present, it is most safely and thoroughly approached from a dorsal approach. Other relative contraindications to ALIF include prior retroperitoneal surgery, severe peripheral vascular disease,[1,40-42] an active disc space infection, a neoplasm,[42] an infrarenal aortic aneurysm, an anomalous genitourinary system[3] with only a single ureter, and systemic medical illness that precludes the surgery. Also, ALIF may be relatively contraindicated in men who wish to reproduce because a small but present risk of retrograde ejaculation has been described.[43-49] As a general rule, an ALIF procedure is associated with less blood loss and is better tolerated than the majority of dorsal lumbar surgical procedures.[5,8,50]

A trial of nonoperative therapy is mandatory before undergoing ALIF.[6,29,38,39,51] Mainstays of nonoperative treatment include optimizing body weight, which usually consists of weight loss in most patients. Cessation of smoking is also important because smoking is known to decrease fusion rates.[39,52,53] In addition, a core-strengthening exercise program that includes back and abdominal muscle strengthening and stretching exercises should be instituted. Consultations with a pain management specialist,[7] as well as a psychological evaluation,[7,10,13,31,33,35,38,51,54-56] may be useful adjuncts in determining the optimal candidates for this procedure. Chronic pain may cause varying degrees of depression, anxiety, and aggression, and these behavioral changes can be reversed if the cause of pain is discovered and corrected.[54,57] The efficacy of other conservative therapies such as epidural steroid injections, acupuncture, chiropractic, and biofeedback is more debatable. A preoperative trial of bracing is often recommended, and advocates of preoperative bracing believe that surgical results are superior if there is a good response to preoperative use of an external orthosis.[58-60]

It is important to assess the patient's level of function before surgery. It should be determined whether the patient is able to maintain employment and enjoy recreational activities. In addition, simple parameters such as walking distances in a pain-free state, as well as total walking distance, should be assessed. If the preoperative level of function is equivalent to the level that a good surgical result would yield, ALIF should not be performed. Back pain of a magnitude sufficient to consider a fusion procedure should substantially limit a patient's level of function.

It is essential for both the surgeon and the patient to have realistic expectations of the surgical outcome, and this is one of the reasons for a prolonged, conservative trial. Surgical success should be evaluated by a return to normal activities of daily living rather than by the hope for a return to high-level athletic activities. Surgical success cannot be fully evaluated until a minimum of 6 to 12 months after the operation.[6,9,29,31-33,37,38,54] In general, it is not until the fusion process has been completed that surgical success can be fully evaluated.

Well-known negative prognostic indicators include involvement in workers' compensation or litigation cases,[8,9,31,39,50,51,55] because these patients are known to have suboptimal long-term clinical results. This is particularly worrisome because the operative indications for ALIF are often subjective (low back pain) rather than objective (neurologic deficit).

Before considering an ALIF procedure, a detailed radiographic imaging workup is required. The initial workup includes a plain-film radiographic series with flexion and extension lateral views.[50] Flexion and extension radiographs may not reveal segmental instability because many painful motion segments are caused by rotational destabilization.[61] These radiographs are used to evaluate spinal stability as well as to confirm the number of true lumbar vertebrae. In preoperative planning, these images are correlated with advanced radiographic imaging studies, such as MRI, CT scans, and myelography with postmyelography CT scanning. It is important to evaluate lumbar interspaces beyond the zone of the previous spinal surgery to identify additional sources of pain.

In cases of L4-5 fusion, it is important to review the anteroposterior (AP) radiographs to note the position of the L4-5 interspace relative to the pelvic brim. Some surgeons have advocated that patients with a low-seated L4-5 interspace in relation to the pelvic brim have a higher success rate in fusion and clinical outcome than patients with a higher-seated L4-5 interspace. The higher-seated L4-5 interspace may also be complicated by a more difficult exposure.

A myelogram, with a postmyelography CT scan, is considered by some to be the gold standard to rule out neural compression.[7,20,29,37,50] A myelogram and CT scan are particularly useful in cases of lateral recess stenosis. In addition, CT scanning is an excellent tool for evaluating bony pathology and recording measurements of the cross-sectional diameters of the vertebral bodies on axial views.

MRI is extremely useful in defining soft tissue pathology. In particular, T2-weighted sagittal images are valuable in determining disc dehydration as evidenced by decreased signal intensity.[10,62] In addition, MRI can evaluate motion segments adjacent to a previously operated level, neural compression secondary to a herniated lumbar disc, and central stenosis. Furthermore, axial measurements to be used in preoperative planning can be accurately obtained from MRIs. MRI will also reveal the presence of facet disease or other dorsal disease, which may influence the decision to back up the ALIF with a dorsal fusion. An ideal candidate for ALIF would have an isolated degenerative disc at L5-S1 with at least 50% loss of height.

Discography is a more controversial preoperative radiographic imaging technique. Some advocates of discography promote the use of a provocative discogram to evaluate patients who are considering lumbar interbody fusion.[8,12,29,37,39,50,53,56,63] With a provocative discogram, the patient's typical pain pattern must be reproduced at the involved level in an awake, nonsedated state. In addition, injection at other levels of the lumbar spine must not reproduce the patient's typical low back pain pattern. Discography should be used to confirm MRI findings. It can be most effective in determining the number of levels to be fused in cases of multilevel disease. In patients who show discrepancies between the results of discography and MRI, consideration should be given to delaying surgical therapy and pursuing other conservative treatments. In other words, diagnostic imaging techniques should be used to decrease, *not increase*, the percentage of surgical candidates.

The number of levels to be fused is an important yet controversial topic. Many studies have clearly demonstrated that pseudarthrosis rates are increased with each additional level of fusion.[9,33,37,39,41,56] Thus, clinical success rates are lessened with each additional fused level.[33] Furthermore, there is an increased chance of adjacent motion segment degeneration with longer fusions, which is particularly problematic at the level immediately rostral to a lumbar interbody fusion.[29,64]

The number of levels fused is most frequently determined by a review of the radiographic imaging studies. Typically, plain flexion and extension radiographs that demonstrate pathologic motion at the proposed fusion site are helpful in demonstrating segmental instability.[50,65] In addition, MRI scans, especially T2-weighted sagittal images, which demonstrate loss of signal consistent with disc dehydration, may help to define the involved segments.[10,62] Finally, it is the opinion of some authors that a provocative discogram confirming the results of the MRI or the flexion and extension radiographs may be useful in determining the number of levels to be fused.*

Before undergoing ALIF, a detailed general medical evaluation should be completed. Smoking is known to decrease fusion rates in spinal surgical procedures,[39,52,53] and as a general guideline, patients are requested to quit smoking a minimum of 8 weeks before surgery and to continue to not smoke until radiographic fusion has been confirmed. Additional factors known to detrimentally affect both clinical and radiographic fusion rates include diabetes mellitus, an immunocompromised state, and chronic corticosteroid use.

ALIF is performed for chronic low back pain. As such, patients who have experienced prolonged courses of narcotic analgesic use have a poorer clinical outcome with respect to overall pain control than patients who have not used narcotics preoperatively.[38,54] It is unclear whether the worsened clinical outcome in patients requiring narcotic analgesics before surgery is due to more severe disease, changes in the pain receptor mechanisms, or psychological factors.

The use of oral contraceptives or any drugs containing estrogens is known to increase the incidence of deep venous thromboses during the postoperative period.[67] As a result, these drugs should be discontinued for a minimum of 3 months before surgery. If there is any chance that an ongoing spinal infection or neoplastic process is present, it should be thoroughly evaluated before considering ALIF surgery.[10] The presence of peripheral vascular disease should also be investigated preoperatively, with a detailed evaluation by physical examination of the aorta and lower extremities.[1,41,65] Likewise, if there are genitourinary abnormalities, imaging studies should be performed to confirm the presence of two functioning kidneys and two functioning ureters. Abnormalities of the reproductive system, particularly evidence for ejaculatory dysfunction in a male patient, should be evaluated before surgery. The presence of osteoporosis should be evaluated by bone mineral density testing before any consideration of surgery.[42]

The preoperative regimen for ALIF may include a bowel preparation the night before surgery. A bowel preparation makes retraction of the intraperitoneal structures easier and increases safety by decreasing the possibility of an iatrogenic bowel injury.[6,8,40] In addition, routine preoperative antibiotic coverage directed at *Staphylococcus* and *Streptococcus* species should be administered. This is usually accomplished with a first-generation cephalosporin antibiotic.

Intraoperative Considerations

Most complications of ALIF can be avoided by following strict preoperative indications, careful preoperative planning, and meticulous intraoperative technique. When intraoperative complications do occur, most can be managed immediately during the surgical procedure. Some complications are not detectable until the postoperative period. In the following discussion, the operation is broken down into each of its components, which are considered separately.

Positioning

Operative positioning depends on the level to be operated on. Most ALIFs are performed at the two most caudal motion segments of the spine, L4-5 and L5-S1.†

General principles of spine surgery should be followed for operative positioning. As a rule, all bony prominences must be padded, with particular attention paid to protection of the ulnar nerve at the elbow[38] and the peroneal nerve at the fibular head.[53] In addition, antiembolic stockings and sequential compression devices are useful intraoperative adjuncts. Because no neural decompression is performed during an ALIF procedure, there is no need for intraoperative evoked potential monitoring or the use of electromyography. The operating table must allow for both AP and lateral fluoroscopy because this feature is essential for accurate placement of a bone graft or intervertebral cage.

The best operative positioning is obtained by placing the lumbar spine in a position of lordosis. This position is achieved by reversing the flex on the table and placing a roll or bump under the low back region. These maneuvers help open the interspace ventrally, improve the sagittal plane alignment, and facilitate the discectomy. In addition, the left iliac crest should be prepared and draped and included in the operative field if iliac crest autograft is to be used.

When possible, it is best to keep the patient in a true supine position. This is ordinarily achievable without difficulty at the L4-5 and L5-S1 levels. At progressively rostral levels, it may be necessary to position the patient slightly in a right lateral decubitus position. Lateral positioning may be necessary to aid in retraction of the intraperitoneal contents during retroperitoneal exposure. Any lateral positioning leads to increased difficulty in maintaining orientation to the true bony midline, making the placement of the interbody graft more difficult. As a general rule, thin patients can be maintained in a true neutral supine position, whereas more obese patients require some lateral rotation on the operating table to allow gravity to assist with retraction of the intraperitoneal contents.

Incision

In any surgical procedure, a properly placed skin incision is essential for achieving optimal exposure. The usual approach for an ALIF procedure is by retroperitoneal exposure from the patient's left side. The left side is safer than the right because it allows the great vessels to be approached from the side of the aorta. It is easier to retract the infrarenal aorta from left to right than to retract the inferior vena cava from the patient's right side. A left-sided retroperitoneal approach minimizes the need for any retraction of the inferior vena cava and thus decreases the possibility of injuring[5,69] or thrombosing[13] this structure. Some surgeons advocate the use

*See references 1, 4, 6, 8, 12, 29, 33, 37, 39, 50, 53, 56, 62, 63, and 66.

†See references 1, 4, 6, 8, 25, 29, 39, 53, 56, and 68.

of contrast-enhanced CT to identify the arterial and venous anatomy to help with surgical planning.

The nerves, muscles, and ureters that surround the lumbar spine are ordinarily symmetrical. Only vessel asymmetry determines the need for a left-sided incision. Occasionally, prior abdominal or retroperitoneal surgery may determine the need to perform ALIF from the patient's right side.

Incisions vary based on the level of surgery. Single-level ALIF at either the L4-5 or L5-S1 interspace may be performed using a right-angled incision. The standard retroperitoneal incision includes a horizontal limb extending from the midline to the linea semilunaris (lateral border of the rectus abdominis muscle). This horizontal limb is located at a point between the umbilicus and the pubic tubercle. The vertical limb of the incision extends up the linea semilunaris for a variable length, depending on the number of levels to be fused. For a single-level ALIF, the vertical limb is approximately the same length as the horizontal limb (Fig. 55-1). When multiple levels are to be fused, the vertical limb extends a longer distance than the horizontal limb. At progressively higher levels, it is necessary to orient the incision in an oblique fashion, extending toward the tip of the left 12th rib. This oblique incision may be necessary to gain access to the retroperitoneal space of the L1-2 and L2-3 interspaces. At more rostral levels, care must be taken to avoid retraction on the spleen, which is susceptible to minor blunt trauma from the retractors.[70]

Exposure

Anterior lumbar interbody fusion can be approached by a variety of exposures. The most commonly used technique is a left-sided retroperitoneal dissection. Other methods include a transperitoneal open procedure as well as a laparoscopic approach.[52,64,71-78] The difficulties with transperitoneal surgery include prolonged postoperative ileus, as well as problems with fluid management and "third spacing" secondary to fluid shifts from an edematous bowel. As such, the open transperitoneal approach is less frequently used in favor of retroperitoneal exposure. Laparoscopic techniques are discussed elsewhere; however, they do not have long-term follow-up data that support their use because they typically have a steep learning curve and prolonged operative time. Although laparoscopic approaches were popularized in the 1990s, they have recently become less often used owing to prolonged operative times.

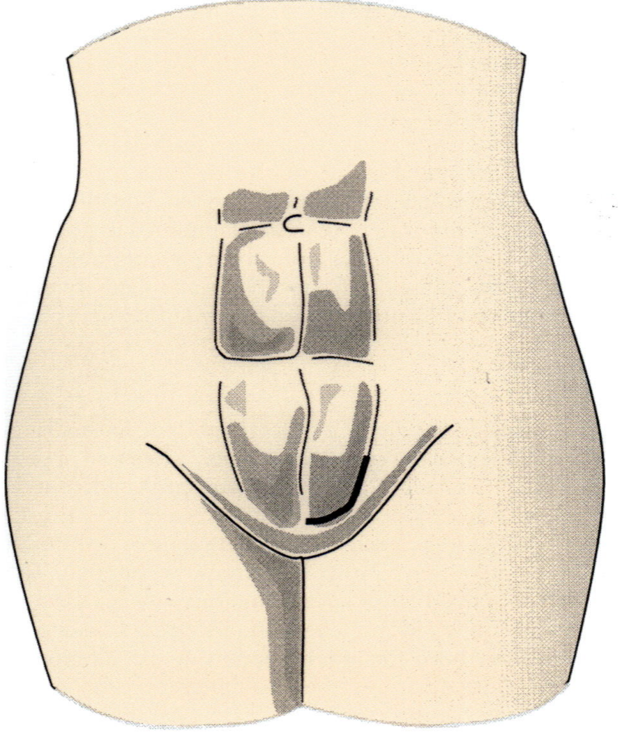

FIGURE 55-1. Incision for an L5-S1 or L4-5 anterior lumbar interbody fusion. (Copyright University of New Mexico, Division of Neurosurgery, with permission.)

It is mandatory that a surgeon who is comfortable with the surgical approach provide the exposure. This procedure can be performed by a general surgeon or a vascular surgeon familiar with the retroperitoneal region, as well as management of the potential complications that may occur during the operation. Proper techniques of vessel ligation are vital to successful exposure of the disc spaces.[2] With a left retroperitoneal approach, the intraperitoneal contents are dissected away from the retroperitoneal space from the left side toward the midline. The ureter must be identified and protected. During the exposure, it is best to avoid cutting longitudinally oriented structures.[10,42] The dissection must be performed ventral to the psoas muscle. In thin patients, it is possible to dissect into the retropsoas space, which can result in excessive postoperative fluid collections, blood loss, and the possibility of injury to the genitofemoral and ilioinguinal nerves.

In patients who have not undergone prior retroperitoneal surgery, gentle blunt dissection is the safest, quickest, and easiest technique. If the peritoneum is violated during the retroperitoneal approach, it should be immediately closed to prevent development of a postoperative hernia.[57] Closure is accomplished by isolating the edges of the peritoneum and using an absorbable suture with a continuous stitch. An unrecognized peritoneal violation can result in a postoperative hernia and subsequent bowel obstruction or incarceration. If the bowel proper is violated during retroperitoneal exposure, it should be treated with immediate irrigation, followed by layered closure, with the mucosal and serosal layers repaired separately, and abortion of the ALIF procedure. In addition, broad-spectrum antibiotics with anaerobic coverage should be instituted immediately. In spite of the excellent bony and vascular anatomic landmarks present in the ventral lumbar spine, radiographic confirmation of the correct level is mandatory before performing ALIF. Intraoperative radiographs should be compared with preoperative plain radiographs to confirm the appropriate level.[65,67,68] Surgery at the incorrect level has been previously reported.[9]

Each level of the lumbar spine has distinct anatomic structures that must be addressed during a retroperitoneal approach. In general, lumbar segmental arteries should be preserved unless specific arterial damage has occurred. There is no need routinely to ligate these vessels, which are involved in supplying blood to the vertebral body proper.[67]

At the L5-S1 interspace, there is no need to mobilize the iliac vessels. This interspace is routinely located between the right and left common iliac vessels and is easily visualized without vessel dissection. Important structures at the L5-S1 level include the autonomic nerves that traverse the prevertebral space at this level. These nerves may be damaged by a monopolar electrocautery, and this can lead to autonomic dysfunction. In men, this is manifested as retrograde ejaculation. To avoid this complication, a monopolar electrocautery should not be used in the prevertebral space. In addition, a vertical opening of the midline prevertebral space should be used with gentle blunt dissection laterally to free all overlying soft tissues and, in the process, to gently dissect the hypogastric plexus away from the ventral disc space at the L5-S1 level[10,65] (Fig. 55-2). Rates of postoperative retrograde ejaculation have been reported as ranging from 0.42% to 22.5%, with the transperitoneal approach carrying an approximately 10-fold greater risk.[43-49]

At the L4-5 interspace, the left common iliac vessels routinely traverse the prevertebral space and thus prevent direct access to the space. These vessels must therefore be mobilized from left to right to expose the bony midline. Before mobilizing the iliac vessels, however, vessel loops should be passed proximally and distally to obtain vascular control of both the left common iliac artery and the left common iliac vein. In addition, the left iliolumbar vein routinely enters the left common iliac vein laterally at a variable distance caudal to the inferior vena cava. It is necessary to locate and ligate the left iliolumbar vein before medially mobilizing the left common iliac vein. This ligation will allow for better exposure of the L4-5 interspace because the vessel typically courses over the L5 vertebral body and tethers the iliac vein.[79,80] If the left common iliac vein is mobilized without ligation of the iliolumbar vein, extensive hemorrhaging can occur secondary to avulsion of this vessel[5,69] (Fig. 55-3A). If an iliac vein is damaged, direct pressure should be applied and proximal and distal vascular control obtained. Fine, nonabsorbable suture is used to close the venous defect primarily with a continuous suturing technique. Common iliac vein injuries have been described in 2% to 4.5% of cases.[35,57,81,82] Although they have been reported, injuries of the common iliac artery[82] and inferior vena cava[5,69] are very rare.

At the L3-4 disc space, the iliac vessels must be mobilized medially. In addition, a minimal amount of mobilization of the distal aorta from left to right is necessary (Fig. 55-3B). There is no need to mobilize the inferior vena cava during a left-sided approach to the lumbar spine at any level. If surgery

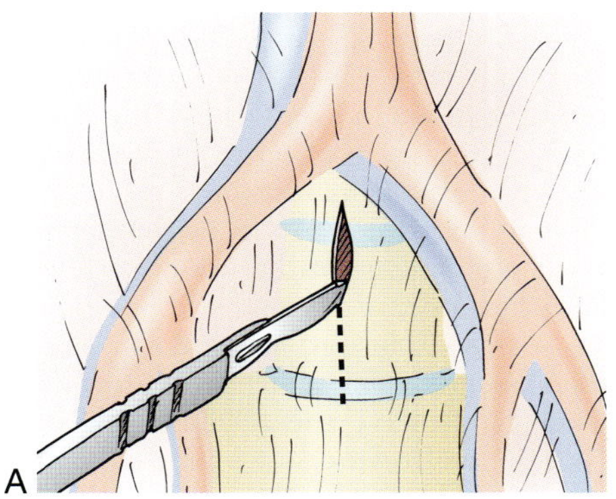

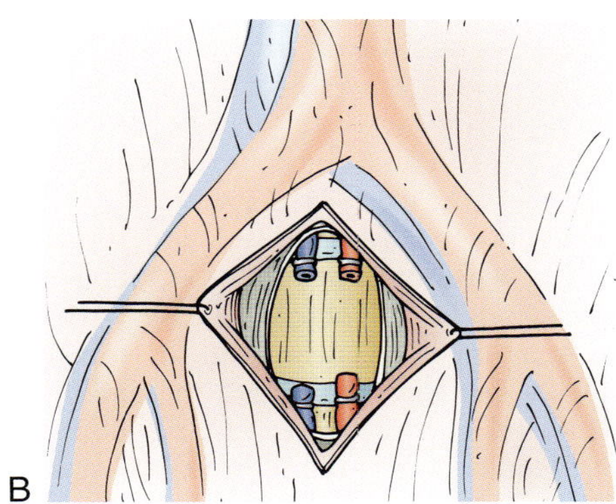

FIGURE 55-2. After retraction of the retroperitoneal and abdominal structures, a vertical incision is made in the prevertebral space. **A,** Gentle retraction laterally gains access to the L5-S1 and, occasionally, the L4-5 disc interspace. **B,** Vessels are ligated and clipped or tied. (Copyright University of New Mexico, Division of Neurosurgery, with permission.)

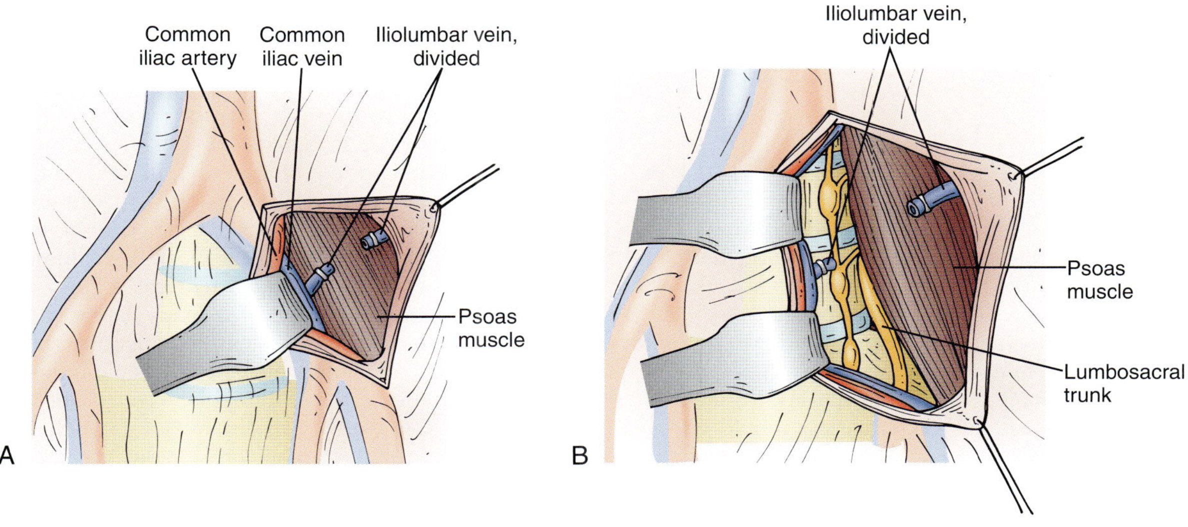

FIGURE 55-3. At the L4-5 interspace, lateral retraction initially exposes the left common iliac vein beneath the left common iliac artery (**A**). The iliolumbar vein is then clipped and ligated or tied. After this, further retraction gains access to the ventral L4-5 and L3-4 disc interspaces (**B**). (Copyright University of New Mexico, Division of Neurosurgery, with permission.)

is necessary at the L1-2 levels, the aorta will need to be mobilized from left to right to gain exposure to the true bony midline. In addition, care must be exerted at the L1-2 level to avoid iatrogenic injury to the left renal artery if overly vigorous medial displacement of the aorta is performed.

Retraction

After exposure of the retroperitoneal space, a table-mounted, self-retaining retraction system is useful. It should have malleable, broad-bladed retractors to disperse pressure evenly. Laparotomy pads are used to cover the retractor blades to protect the sensitive intraperitoneal structures. After the self-retaining retractor system is positioned and the correct level identified, a lateral fluoroscopic image can confirm the appropriate level.[10,65,67,68] An AP fluoroscopic image is necessary to mark the true bony midline with an indelible marking pen or methylene blue dye. Maintaining orientation to the bony anatomic midline is critical to the safe performance of an ALIF procedure.

Excessive retraction can lead to injuries to the peritoneum, the intraperitoneal structures, or the major blood vessels. The intraperitoneal contents are best retracted using the self-retaining retractor system; however, the iliac vessels and the aorta should not be retracted by this method. The use of self-retaining retractors on these vessels can be associated with an increased risk of vascular injury and an increased risk of thrombosis of either the artery or the vein.[1,67,68] The major vessels are best retracted by hand-held instruments manipulated by a surgical assistant under direct vision. Thus, pressure on the vessels can be frequently released, which helps to prevent development of an intramural thrombus. If one of the iliac vessels or the aorta is injured, the umbilical tapes, which provide distal and proximal vascular control, are used to halt the bleeding. This is followed by primary vessel repair using nonabsorbable sutures. This repair is ordinarily performed by either a general or vascular surgeon. Iliac artery thrombosis can be detected by carefully monitoring peripheral pulses and skin color in the lower extremities. If a thrombus is detected or strongly suspected, an intraoperative angiogram should be obtained immediately. Thrombectomy is the treatment for a positive angiogram.[41] In addition, if the ureter is injured during the retraction or exposure, placement of a ureteral stent is ordinarily performed by a general or urologic surgeon.[83]

Discectomy

After the correct level has been confirmed with lateral fluoroscopy and an AP fluoroscopic image has confirmed the midline, the midline is marked on the vertebral bodies above and below the disc space to help maintain orientation. At this stage in the operation, long-handled instruments are useful. Commercially available curets and rongeurs 13 to 15 inches long facilitate performance of the discectomy. To determine the depth of the discectomy, confirmation should be made based on the preoperative MRI study or CT scan. Particularly at the L5-S1 interspace, it is important to confirm that all tissue overlying the disc space has been gently and bluntly swept laterally before incising the ventral anulus fibrosus. Once again, avoidance of monopolar electrocautery diminishes the incidence of postoperative autonomic dysfunction.[2,8,10,33,67,84]

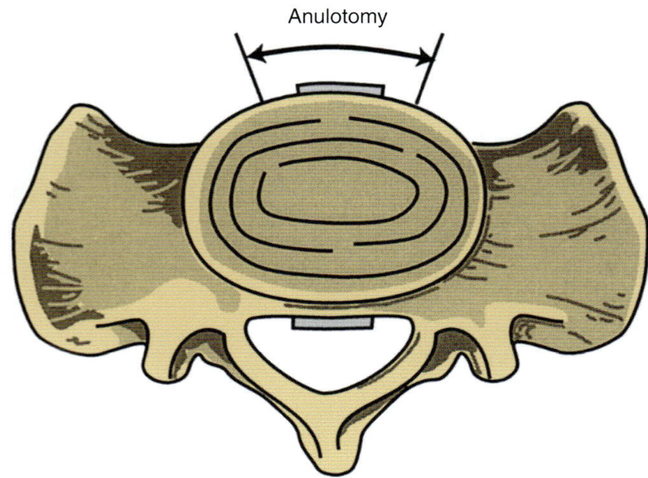

FIGURE 55-4. An anulotomy is performed as depicted, taking great care not to proceed too far laterally. (Copyright University of New Mexico, Division of Neurosurgery, with permission.)

A symmetrical window is cut into the ventral anulus fibrosus, taking care to preserve the lateral aspects of the disc bilaterally (Fig. 55-4). It is essential to maintain orientation to the midline and stay within the anulus fibrosus, with care being taken not to violate the anulus laterally or dorsally. The nucleus pulposus is removed, up to the dorsal anulus fibrosus. Calibrated tips on the instruments are useful at this stage. With use of some of the newer cage techniques, a predetermined cylinder of disc material is removed. In a standard lumbar interbody fusion, all articular cartilage is removed from the bony end plates above and below the disc space, with care taken to preserve the subchondral bone of the end plates. As a general rule, disc material is removed 25 to 30 mm in depth and 30 to 35 mm in width, centered at the bony midline. These measurements are quite consistent for the lower lumbar motion segments. Variations exist in the AP dimensions of the vertebral bodies. The oval shape of the lumbar vertebrae accounts for a larger depth in the midline than in the lateral portions of the vertebrae.[2] It is important to avoid use of bone wax for bleeding cancellous bone because foreign bodies may decrease the postoperative fusion rates.

Excessive depth of the discectomy can be catastrophic. The dorsal anulus fibrosus is not well visualized from an ALIF approach, and if it is violated, epidural bleeding or a dural injury can occur. These are usually not well controlled by a limited exposure and are best avoided. If the dorsal anulus fibrosus is violated, the disc space must be observed for bleeding or a cerebrospinal fluid (CSF) leak. Bleeding is best controlled with copious amounts of irrigation, as well as with the use of thrombin-soaked Gelfoam. Patience is the key because access in this area is extremely poor. It is unrealistic to attempt bipolar cautery on a bleeding epidural vessel unless it is directly visualized. Monopolar electrocautery must be avoided at all times in the epidural space. If a CSF leak occurs, free muscle and fascia grafts, with or without fibrin glue, are used to attempt to control the egress of CSF. Consideration should be given to placement of a lumbar subarachnoid drain to divert CSF during the immediate postoperative period.[85] Safe and reliable decompression of the thecal sac or nerve roots is not realistic from an ALIF approach, and if neural decompression is necessary, it should be performed using a dorsal procedure or as part of a combined procedure.

Distraction

Several commercially available systems have been developed for ALIF. These systems have disc space distractors with calibrated tips to prevent excessively deep disc space distraction (Fig. 55-5). Improved distraction can also be obtained by proper patient positioning. This helps to maintain lumbar lordosis and in the process opens up the ventral aspect of the interspace. Particularly in larger patients, the operating surgeon may choose to wear a headlamp to improve visualization.

The interspace can be distracted with either a system developed specifically for ALIF or with a laminar spreader, a straight osteotome, or a Cobb periosteal elevator. The danger of excessively deep placement of a distractor is violation of the dorsal anulus fibrosus, with subsequent entrance into the epidural space. This can be associated with epidural bleeding, which may be difficult to control, or neurologic injury or durotomy, which cannot be adequately visualized and repaired. In most cases, no distraction is necessary after an aggressive discectomy is completed in a well-positioned patient.

Bone Graft Harvest

Excellent fusion rates are obtained when autograft bone is used as a fusion substrate. This bone can be used alone, in combination with allograft bone, or with a cage. If the iliac crest is within 5 cm of the retroperitoneal skin incision, dissection through the same skin incision allows access to the iliac crest for harvesting autologous bone graft. If more than 6 cm separates the skin incision from the iliac crest, a separate skin incision will be necessary to harvest the bone graft.

When harvesting iliac crest autograft, the most medial aspect of the skin incision should be at least 2 cm lateral to the anterior superior iliac spine. The lateral femoral cutaneous nerve is subcutaneous in this location and typically runs within 2 cm of the anterior superior iliac spine. If this nerve is transected, permanent anesthesia of the ventrolateral skin of the thigh can result.[7,85] If it is compressed, a temporary sensory deficit, caused by neurapraxic injury, results. When ALIF is performed using structural iliac crest autograft as the sole graft source, the medial and lateral aspects of the crest need to be exposed and an oscillating saw used to harvest tricortical strut grafts. Osteotomes can also be used; however, they have been shown to be associated with an increased incidence of microfractures of the tricortical bone graft.[86] If the iliac crest autograft is being used to augment allograft bone or a cage, then a small cortical window can be opened on either the medial or lateral surface of the iliac crest, and curets and gouges can be used to remove cancellous bone from the iliac crest. In extremely thin patients, the medial crest is favored for its cosmetic advantages; in heavier patients, the lateral crest is more easily accessible. Ordinarily, harvesting iliac crest autograft does not result in cosmetic deformity.

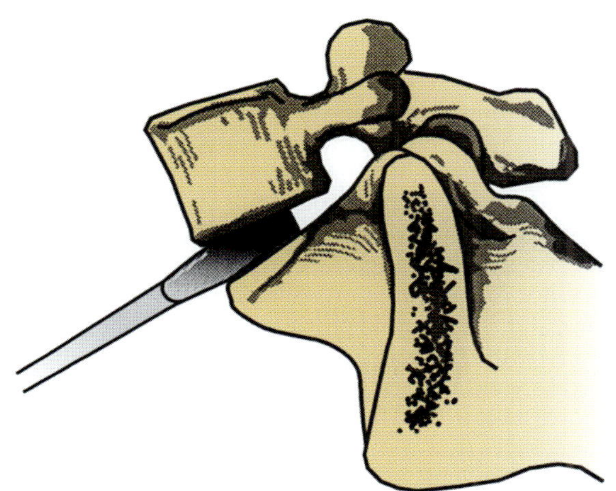

FIGURE 55-5. An interbody strut, several types of which are available, can be used to increase disc interspace height. (Copyright University of New Mexico, Division of Neurosurgery, with permission.)

Excessive exposure of the medial iliac crest can lead to a hernia through the transversalis fascia. If the transversalis fascia is violated, it should be repaired immediately to prevent development of a postoperative hernia. After removal of the iliac autograft, the wound should be copiously irrigated and packed with thrombin-soaked gauze. Bone wax should be avoided because it is associated with an increased incidence of wound infections. After removal of all packing and copious irrigation, hemostasis is obtained. A drain should also be considered, followed by a routine layered closure.

Complications associated with iliac crest autograft harvesting include lateral femoral cutaneous nerve palsies that result from medial placement of the skin incision. A postoperative hematoma may develop in the event of inadequate hemostasis.[8] This complication can be avoided by paying attention to hemostasis, and perhaps with the use of a drain. Postoperative wound infections and subsequent pain may also occur,[29,37,82] and are avoided by use of generous quantities of irrigation, drainage of the wound, use of prophylactic antibiotics, and consideration of pulse lavage after graft harvest.

Bone Morphogenetic Protein

In 2002, the U.S. Food and Drug Administration (FDA) approved the use of recombinant human bone morphogenetic protein-2 (rhBMP-2) for use in the Medtronic (Minneapolis, MN) LT Cage at the L4-5 and L5-S1 interspaces.[87] The study compared the use of rhBMP-2 with iliac crest autograft, citing clinical success with fusion rates of 96.9% versus 92.6% at 12 months and 94.5% versus 88.7% at 24 months. The rhBMP-2 group also did not complain of donor site pain or cosmetic appearance, as opposed to the small percentage (2–10%) of the iliac crest group who did experience these complaints.[87]

To date, rhBMP-2 is the only osteoinductive growth factor that is FDA approved for use in ALIF. Its presumed mechanism is the stimulation of pluripotent stem cells from bleeding cancellous bone to form bone.[87] Other, subsequent studies have used rhBMP-2 in femoral ring allograft, threaded cortical bone dowels, and threaded cylindrical titanium cages, and found similar clinical and radiographic success rates.[88,89] In the initial FDA study group's 6-year follow-up, the clinical and radiographic results remained durable.[90]

Fusion

Anterior lumbar interbody fusion is performed for low back pain, and long-term bony fusion is necessary for the best postoperative results.[9,33,68] Fusion can be judged both clinically, as evidenced by the relief of back pain, and radiographically, as evidenced by radiographic incorporation of the graft. The meticulous performance of ALIF is critical.

After the discectomy is completed, a spacer must be placed in the involved interspace. A variety of materials have been used to function as spacers. Iliac crest autograft can be used as a spacer, in which case two or more tricortical grafts are typically placed side by side. Allograft bone can also be used. The different forms of allografts used in ALIF procedures include femoral ring, tibia, humerus, and iliac crest. Of these, femoral ring is the best choice because it can be sculpted to anatomically fit the defect and then be packed with cancellous autograft bone. The use of iliac crest allograft is a poor choice because this bone does not have the same structural strength as comparable autografts. Threaded dowels of bone derived from femoral allograft have also been used.[91] They are placed in predetermined channels, a method similar to the Cloward technique used for the cervical spine. Recently, the use of cages as spacers in ALIF procedures has gained popularity.[52,92,93] These cages received FDA approval in 1996 and are available in many forms; threaded titanium cages, polyetheretherketone (PEEK), and carbon fiber–reinforced PEEK cages can be obtained. These cages are routinely packed with iliac crest cancellous autograft bone or rhBMP-2 soaked sponges.

Titanium cages are threaded cages that lie flat within the interspace, side by side, and are filled with autograft iliac crest cancellous bone. In addition, a titanium cage is available that stands upright as a single trapezoidal cage within the interspace. Typically, carbon fiber–reinforced PEEK cages are placed as two cages flat within the interspace, side by side. More recently, PEEK cages have been used to allow a more customizable footprint. These PEEK cages have been used in stand-alone fashion and with a ventral plate, an interference plate, or an integrated plate.

Spacers are used to maintain disc height after discectomy and to facilitate bony fusion. Ideally, a spacer is slightly larger than the disc height as measured by preoperative sagittal plane imaging studies. Likewise, an optimal spacer has a slightly trapezoidal configuration, with the larger end placed ventrally to maintain or increase lumbar lordosis. The depth of the spacer is determined by careful examination of the preoperative axial images from CT or MRI. Spacers perform a variety of functions, including restoration of lumbar lordosis and improvement of sagittal plane alignment of the lumbar spine. In addition, a spacer serves to improve disc height, and in so doing, increases the size of the corresponding neural foramina. The PEEK cage implants are available in a variety of lordotic or straight angles and may be customized to improve or preserve a patient's lordosis and coronal and sagittal balance.

Two principles of bony fusion are applicable to ALIF: (1) the need for compression, and (2) the need for immobilization to increase the chances of acquiring stable bony fusion. Unlike dorsal fusion, with ventral fusion the graft can be maintained in a position of compression.[2,6,38,65,67,68] Compression is best achieved by distracting the interspace and placing a slightly oversized spacer in this disc space. Compressive forces felt by a spacer in the intervertebral space are many times greater in magnitude than any compression achieved by an onlay graft dorsally. Immobilization is obtained by firmly fitting a spacer into the intervertebral disc space. In addition, an external orthosis may be used to diminish motion at the lower lumbar spine. There is less need for internal instrumentation with ALIF. Historically, interference plates were placed to prevent cage backout. Newer devices have been used for implantation with ventral plate/screw fixation or with integrated plate/screw fixation in the cage itself.

In sizing the spacer or choosing the number of spacers to place, recent unpublished data recommend 60% vertebral body end-plate coverage.[94] Because approximately 80% of the load on the spine and 90% of the articular surface area is supported ventrally,[95] this larger footprint is biomechanically more advantageous in stability and allows for optimum fusion across the intervertebral space.

The grafting technique itself involves removal of all articular cartilage overlying the surfaces to be fused. The interspace is distracted, and a slightly oversized spacer is selected. A portion of cancellous bone from the vertebral body immediately above and below the interspace is exposed using a drill, curet, or gouge. The exposed cancellous bone of the vertebral body should be aligned with the exposed cancellous portion of the bone graft or the center of the cage, which allows for optimal fusion as well as providing immediate hemostasis. The ventral-most aspect of the spacer should be slightly countersunk beneath the ventral-most surface of the vertebral bodies above and below. Bone wax should be avoided because it decreases fusion rates; hemostatic agents or grafting agents may be used instead. When placing a spacer, meticulous attention to maintenance of the orientation of the bony midline is important. If two spacers are used, they should be symmetrically placed on each side of the midline, and if a single spacer is used, it should be centered on the midline. After placement of the spacer, AP and lateral fluoroscopic confirmation should be obtained immediately.[65,67,68,96] If any modification of the positioning of the spacer is necessary, it should be addressed immediately. A particular concern regarding the placement of two spacers side by side is assurance that when the second spacer is positioned, it does not cause loosening of the first spacer. This must be confirmed after placement of the second spacer, and if the initial spacer has been loosened, modification must be made before wound closure. Strict adherence to symmetrical placement of the spacers with respect to the midline helps avoid this problem.

Plating

Recent biomechanical studies have shown improved stabilization with ventral fixation devices. Stand-alone interbody implants do not confer significant stabilization in extension or rotation compared with flexion and lateral bending.[97] The historic buttress/interference plate has evolved into a ventral plate, similar to a cervical plate, to allow for stabilization. Ventral plates can eliminate the need for a separate dorsal approach for instrumentation. The presumed increase in biomechanical stability would protect against graft migration and allow for better bony healing. Biomechanical studies have shown that ventral plating significantly enhances stability in flexion, extension, and lateral bending.[98-100] Clinical studies have also supported the effectiveness of ventral plating for ALIF, with excellent fusion rates and improvement in visual analogue pain scores and the Oswestry Disability Index.[101]

Newer technologies have incorporated the plate and screw into the interbody graft. These devices have also shown improved biomechanical stability over stand-alone ALIF. The long-term clinical outcome of these devices is still under investigation. The benefit of an integrated plate and screws is that it allows for less dissection of soft tissues and mobilization of blood vessels. Some surgeons have reported blood vessel complications such as erosion when the vessels overlie the ventral plate,[95] lending further advantage to cages with integrated plate and screws.

Ventral plating entails the placement of a plate ventrally or ventrolaterally to the interbody implant overlying the superior and inferior vertebral bodies. Screws are then placed in a convergent manner in the superior vertebral body in a rostrally aimed trajectory and in the inferior vertebral body in a caudally aimed trajectory. Care should be taken to maintain native blood vessel anatomy with respect to the ventral plate when the retractors are removed.

Dorsal Supplementation

In situations in which circumferential instability is present, anterior/posterior circumferential fusion should be considered. This procedure involves a significantly larger operation, more operative time, and greater operative blood loss. If neural compression is present, requiring a dorsal operation, and there is a need for anterior column restoration, then both a ventral and dorsal operation may be preferable. In addition, ventrodorsal fusions may be indicated in conditions with known diminished fusion rates, including smokers, patients with diabetes, immunocompromised patients, and patients with chronic corticosteroid use.

Biomechanical studies have shown that pedicle fixation offers the strongest construct to resist forces in flexion, extension, axial rotation, and lateral bending.[98,100] Novel methods in minimally invasive percutaneous pedicle fixation may be used in patients with facet disease, instability, or dorsal pathology. These patients may have dorsal fixation for enhanced biomechanical stabilization with minimal blood loss and tissue disruption. In experienced hands, surgical times are often short for these percutaneous procedures.

Postoperative Complications

Postoperative complications related to ALIF can be divided into four categories: (1) complications related to the operative approach, (2) neurologic complications, (3) complications related to the bone graft, and (4) complications related to the fusion. Neurologic complications are quite unusual in properly performed ALIF procedures. They tend to appear in the first 2 days after the operation and require prompt diagnosis and intervention. Complications related to the operative approach and those related to the iliac crest donor site both occur between 3 and 14 days after surgery. Complications related to the fusion proper tend to consist of the development of chronic pain syndromes. Fusion problems are usually not detectable until 6 to 12 months after surgery.

Operative Approach Complications

After ALIF, it is possible to develop a postoperative hernia,[30,56,82] which can lead to bowel obstruction[1,20,102] and possible bowel infarction. Violation of the peritoneum during ALIF with the retroperitoneal approach, or violation of the transversalis fascia during iliac bone graft harvest, can lead to the development of both internal hernias and subsequent bowel obstruction. When the peritoneum or the transversalis fascia is violated, postoperative hernias are best prevented by immediate operative repair of the defects during the index surgical procedure.[57] If these structures are violated and are inadequately repaired or not appreciated, a hernia may result.

An injury to the bowel may occur during retroperitoneal exposure, and this extremely rare complication requires immediate detection and treatment. The treatment is aggressive irrigation followed by direct repair of the bowel, with separate, layered closures of the mucosal and serosal layers. Prophylactic antibiotics are administered and the ALIF procedure is aborted at this point. If not already present during the surgery, a general surgeon should be summoned to perform or assist in the bowel repair. Bowel injuries are best avoided by using a preoperative bowel preparation, including an enema to help decompress the loops of bowel, as well as placement of a nasogastric tube before the retroperitoneal procedure is performed.[6,8,41]

Major blood vessel injuries are rare during operative exposure. Injuries to the iliac arteries or veins, the inferior vena cava, and the aorta occur in 2% to 4% of ALIF operations.[5,35,57,69,81,82] To avoid vessel injuries, a self-retaining retractor should not be used on the vessels during the exposure portion of the operation.[1] In addition, before mobilizing the iliac vessels or the aorta, proximal and distal control should be obtained with vessel loops, which are used when a major vessel is injured. Should this type of injury occur, a vascular surgeon should perform or assist in vessel repair. Major vessel injuries are repaired primarily using nonabsorbable sutures. Sometimes smaller vessels are injured. The left iliolumbar vein can be avulsed if it is not ligated before the left common iliac vein is mobilized.[5,69] This vessel is safely ligated at any time and should be ligated before common iliac vein mobilization. Likewise, lumbar segmental arteries can be ligated safely at any level; however, these vessels ordinarily are spared during the surgical procedure.

Retrograde ejaculation is a serious complication that may occur in male patients after ALIF.[8,33,41,84] It occurs when the autonomic nerves are injured, usually at the L5-S1 level. The hypogastric plexus is a continuation of the preaortic sympathetic chain that extends down from the thoracic region ventral to the aorta and lumbar vertebrae in the retroperitoneal space.[10,42,84] As stated, the use of monopolar electrocautery over the L5-S1 interspace has been associated with an increased incidence of retrograde ejaculation and should be avoided.[2,8,10,33,67,84] The rates of retrograde ejaculation have been reported as ranging from 0.42% to 22.5%, with a transperitoneal approach carrying a 10-fold greater risk.[43-49] The mechanism of retrograde ejaculation involves the presence of dry ejaculate secondary to relaxation of the internal bladder sphincter, with retrograde flow of ejaculate into the bladder.[42,84] There is no surgical management for this complication, and it becomes prograde in 25% to 33% of patients by the end of the second year.[45,102]

Thrombosis of either venous or arterial structures may occur after ALIF. Venous thrombosis has been reported in 1% to 11% of all ALIF procedures, but arterial thrombosis is extremely rare.* To avoid thromboses, retraction should not be prolonged, and self-retaining retractors should not be used on major vessels. If thrombosis is suspected, an immediate angiogram or venogram should be obtained. The treatment is open surgical thrombectomy.[41] Likewise, an embolus in the arterial vascular tree in the lower extremities can occur rarely and is particularly likely if the patient is elderly. To avoid arterial embolization, retraction should not be prolonged and care should be taken not to use self-retaining retractors on blood vessels. An arterial embolus is detected in the perioperative period by loss of distal pulses and a cool extremity and is best treated by immediate vascular surgical intervention.

General systemic medical problems may arise during the postoperative period. Urinary retention occurs in 5% to 27% of cases and is usually temporary.[2,4,18,29,33,39,68] It may be related to the use of perioperative narcotic analgesics. If urinary retention occurs, it is important to rule out an injury to the ureter or cauda equina syndrome. If urinary tract dysfunction occurs in the late postoperative period, obstruction of the distal ureter from retroperitoneal scarring must be ruled out.[81] Ileus is also common during the postoperative period and usually resolves less than 1 week after the operation. Prolonged postoperative ileus has been reported in 1% to 8% of all ALIF procedures† and also may be related to the use of perioperative narcotic analgesics. An internal hernia that causes bowel obstruction secondary to violation of the peritoneum or transversalis fascia must be ruled out in cases of prolonged postoperative ileus. Serious general medical problems that have been reported include both fatal[66,105] and nonfatal[4,9] cardiac arrest, fatal[4,38] and nonfatal[4,5,8,9,53] pulmonary embolus, and aortic aneurysm rupture.[82]

Neurologic Complications

Neurologic complications are quite rare after ALIF because the epidural space ordinarily is not entered, and no attempt is usually made to decompress the neural elements during this procedure. Most neurologic complications are related to injuries to the nervous structures during the operative procedure. If neurologic deterioration occurs during the postoperative period, immediate neuroimaging with either MRI or CT myelography should be performed. If an epidural hematoma that causes neurologic dysfunction is detected, the patient should be immediately returned to the operating room. Epidural hematomas are best treated using a dorsal approach, which provides the safest and easiest access to the thecal sac and nerve roots to decompress the hematoma. An incomplete neurologic deficit requires that imaging studies be promptly performed. The surgeon's judgment determines whether repeat surgery or expectant observation is the solution. Cauda equina syndrome must be ruled out and, if detected, treated with laminectomy. The decision to observe or explore a patient for postoperative bowel and bladder dysfunction is based on postoperative neuroradiographic imaging studies.

Specific nerve root syndromes are manifested as radiculopathies and should be worked up immediately with neuroimaging studies. Based on the results of these studies, either expectant observation or dorsal exploration should be undertaken. Injuries to the genitofemoral or ilioinguinal nerves may occur after an ALIF procedure.[6,29,41] These injuries are characterized by postoperative numbness in the groin and/or the medial thigh region. They are most common in patients who undergo ALIF procedures at the upper lumbar levels. Palsies in these nerves frequently resolve spontaneously and are usually treated by observation alone.

Compression of the thecal sac during the postoperative period secondary to hematoma, infection, or retropulsed disc material is best treated with dorsal exploration.[37,106] A dural tear is ordinarily detectable during surgery. However, it usually cannot be adequately treated through an ALIF approach. Placement of a lumbar subarachnoid drain to divert the CSF during the first week after surgery is the usual treatment for an intraoperative dural tear resulting from an ALIF procedure.[85] Injury to the sympathetic nerves on the side ipsilateral to the retroperitoneal approach may occur. Usually, partial sympathectomy occurs and is manifested by vasodilation of vessels in the ipsilateral foot.[29,39,107] The usual patient complaint is a cold sensation in the contralateral foot.[41,42] Sympathectomy symptoms usually resolve spontaneously in the first 3 to 6 months after surgery. Discitis[68,108] and osteomyelitis[63,109] each occur in approximately 1% of all ALIF procedures. Their treatment involves reexploration for a confirmed abscess, using either a ventral or a dorsal approach, and wound culture and drainage of the abscess. If infection is present without an abscess, treatment with prolonged antibiotics and immobilization can be used. Surgical exploration may also be necessary in some cases.

Bone Graft Harvest Complications

Postoperative infections of the iliac crest donor site wound occur in 1% to 9% of all ALIF procedures[29,37,82] and are usually detected secondary to pain, which is followed by eventual purulent discharge from the wound. Iliac wound infections are best prevented by avoiding the use of foreign material in the wound (e.g., bone wax) and using perioperative prophylactic antibiotics, copious irrigation, and meticulous intraoperative hemostasis. The use of large-bore drains in iliac wounds may prevent accumulation of a hematoma and decrease wound infection rates; however, they lead to an egress of organisms through and around the drain. When iliac crest wound infection occurs, treatment requires surgical reexploration of the wound, cultures, and drainage.

Postoperative iliac crest wound hematomas usually are manifested as pain in the iliac crest region, which may radiate toward the groin.[8] These hematomas are best avoided by meticulous hemostasis and generous intraoperative wound irrigation. The use of a postoperative large-bore drain may diminish the incidence of postoperative hematomas. Most of these hematomas resolve spontaneously and can be managed by observation. Based on the surgeon's preference, it may be necessary to drain them if they become large or painful.

Fusion Complications

Problems related to the bony fusion portion of the operation are the most common complications of ALIF. Persistent low back pain is the most frequent complaint and is usually the result of pseudarthrosis, or nonunion, of the fusion. This complication is reported at extremely variable rates, ranging from

*See references 1, 5, 8, 9, 29, 33, 56, 64, 68, and 103.
†See references 4, 8, 9, 29, 33, 37, 41, 56, 57, 68, and 104.

3% to 58%.* It is not possible to diagnose lumbar pseudarthrosis secondary to an ALIF procedure until 6 to 12 months after surgery.[6,9,29,31-33,37,38,67] The workup includes plain radiographs to detect evidence of a persistent lucent line between the graft and the vertebral body. Tomograms and CT scans with sagittal reformations also may be useful for detecting this lucent line.[112] Flexion and extension lateral radiographs can detect persistent motion consistent with pseudarthrosis.[39] MRI is difficult to interpret after ALIF and is not particularly useful in revealing postoperative pseudarthrosis.

The treatment of symptomatic pseudarthrosis secondary to ALIF is prolonged immobilization of the patient, which can be accomplished with a thoracolumbosacral orthosis or with a body cast. Electrical stimulation or a bone growth stimulator may also be helpful. In addition, reoperation using a ventral or dorsal approach may be necessary. Rarely, a ventrodorsal combined procedure is necessary for treatment of pseudarthrosis. Several authors have stated that there is no correlation between radiographic pseudarthrosis rates and clinical outcome results.[4,8,35,55,105,111] No treatment is required for asymptomatic pseudarthrosis and the patient should be observed with serial radiographs and clinical evaluations.

Graft collapse occurs in 1% to 2% of all ALIF procedures,[1,39,96,103] and ordinarily results from excessive removal of subchondral bone from the vertebral body bony end plate.[37] A kyphotic deformity may develop. The treatment is surgical reexploration through a ventral approach. Graft resorption may occur and is particularly likely in patients who are smokers,[39,53,113] have diabetes, or are immunosuppressed. Graft dislodgement occurs in 1% of all ALIF procedures, and the treatment is reoperation using a ventral approach.[9,39,41] Graft displacement may be minimized using a ventral buttress/interference plate, ventral/ventrolateral plate fixation, or dorsal pedicle fixation to enhance stability.

Other revision strategies include midline open dorsal fusion and stabilization with pedicle fixation and dorsolateral fusion. Alternatively, minimally invasive dorsal fusion options, from percutaneous pedicle fixation to paramedian tubular retractor–assisted fusion and stabilization, can be performed, although their long-term outcomes are still under evaluation. The extreme lateral transpsoas approach can also be used as a salvage technique at the L4-5 level if above the pelvic brim, or at more rostral segments. Using this technique, the disc space can be approached laterally through the psoas muscle to allow removal of the failed implant, placement of a new interbody device, and placement of a lateral fixation plate.

After a successful ALIF procedure, the motion segments immediately adjacent to the fusion are exposed to increased stress. Months to years after a successful procedure, adjacent-level disc herniation or degeneration may occur and is particularly likely to take place at the motion segment rostral to the ALIF.[29,64] Detection of adjacent-level disc problems is best accomplished with diligent long-term follow-up.

Multilevel Anterior Lumbar Interbody Fusion

Complication rates increase when multiple motion segments are fused. Several investigators have described a direct correlation between the number of levels fused and postoperative pseudarthrosis rates. With each additional level fused, the overall pseudarthrosis rate increases.[9,29,33,37,39,41,56] Likewise, clinical success rates decrease for each additional level fused.[33] In addition, because of the longer lever arms that result from multilevel ALIF, adjacent-level disc problems increase after multilevel procedures. Complications with the retroperitoneal approach also increase because of the larger surgical exposure. Furthermore, systemic medical problems secondary to the longer duration of surgery with increased blood loss are more common in multilevel procedures. Finally, iliac donor site problems are increased when additional bone harvesting is necessary to fuse multiple levels.

Minimally Invasive Anterior Lumbar Interbody Fusion

Following the lead developed by gynecologic and general surgeons, clinicians have developed laparoscopic approaches to the lumbar spine for ALIF procedures, and they are particularly useful at the L5-S1 level.[71,72,74-77,114] In this region, the iliac vessels are located lateral to the L5-S1 space, providing direct access for an ALIF procedure to be safely performed laparoscopically. Once again, it is essential to avoid using a monopolar electrocautery over the L5-S1 disc because this may result in higher rates of retrograde ejaculation in male patients.[2,8,10,33,42,67,84] The laparoscopic approach provides good visualization but makes hemostasis difficult. Likewise, maintaining orientation to the true bony midline is more difficult laparoscopically. AP and lateral fluoroscopy are essential to the laparoscopic approach. Because of the need to mobilize the large blood vessels (iliac artery and vein, inferior vena cava, aorta) at levels rostral to the L5-S1 interspace, laparoscopic methods are more dangerous at these levels.[78] There are no long-term data available on the success rates of laparoscopic ALIF. Some surgeons have abandoned laparoscopic ALIF because of the steep learning curve, lack of three-dimensional visualization, and associated complications.

Summary

In properly selected patients, the results of ALIF in treating patients with chronic low back pain secondary to degenerative disc disease have been encouraging (Fig. 55-6). ALIF offers the advantages of immediate immobilization of the motion segment, a larger fusion area than is achievable with dorsal or dorsolateral techniques, a fusion construct under compression, improved sagittal plane alignment that can restore lumbar lordosis, restoration of intervertebral disc height, and an increase in the height of the neural foramina. In addition, the spinal canal is avoided, as well as many of the difficulties attributed to scarring that commonly occur with dorsal approaches.[11,29] ALIF is generally well tolerated and is associated with less operative blood loss compared with equivalent dorsal procedures.[8,37,50]

The end result of an ALIF procedure should be a biomechanically strong construct. Long-term follow-up is necessary until both clinical and radiographic fusion are demonstrated. Complication rates are reasonable and many problems can

*See references 1, 5, 9, 20, 29, 31, 33, 37–39, 41, 50, 63, 68, 82, 96, 103, 105, and 110–112.

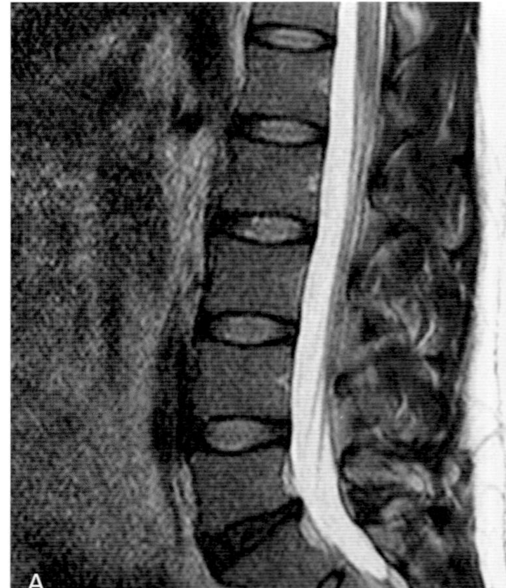

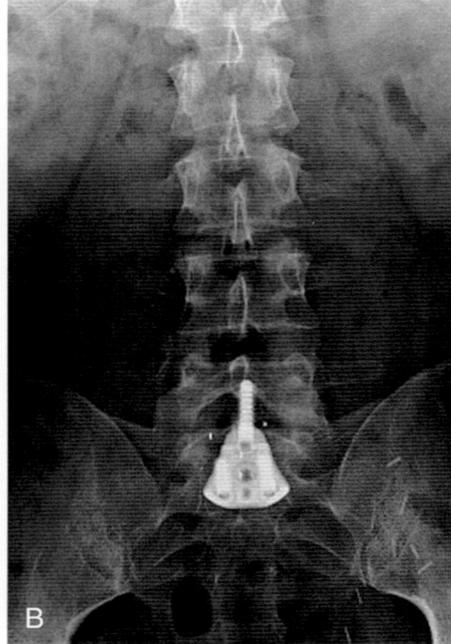

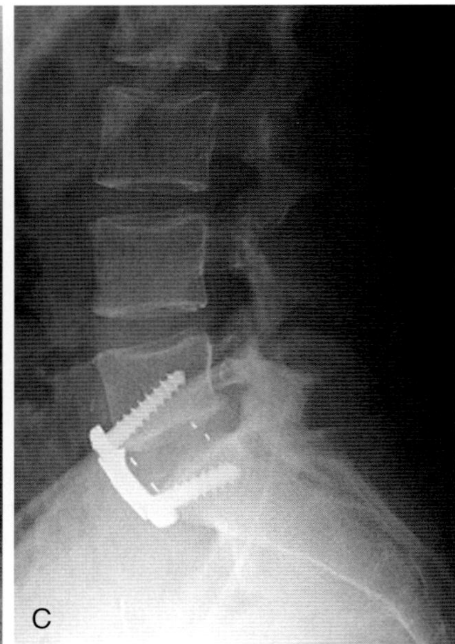

FIGURE 55-6. A 38-year-old man in a motor vehicle accident presented with low back pain 4 years after the accident. His visual analogue score for back pain was 10. Prolonged attempts at conservative treatment were not successful. Neurologic examination was positive only for a left S1 sensory deficit. Preoperative MRI demonstrated a small left-sided herniated L5-S1 disc with degenerative disc changes at this level only (**A**). A provocative discogram was positive at L5-S1 and negative at the L3-4 and L4-5 levels. An anterior lumbar interbody fusion at the L5-S1 level was performed through a left retroperitoneal approach. Postoperative anteroposterior (**B**) and lateral (**C**) plain radiographs demonstrate excellent alignment of the interbody cage and ventral screw/plate fixation construct. The patient was pain free and neurologically intact at late follow-up with evidence of a solid bony arthrodesis. (Copyright University of Medicine and Dentistry of New Jersey, New Jersey Medical School, Department of Neurological Surgery, with permission.)

be treated during the index surgery. Complications are (1) related to the operative approach, (2) neurologic, (3) related to the iliac donor site, and (4) directly related to the fusion proper. Fusion complications are the most common. It is the adequacy of the long-term bony arthrodesis that provides long-term pain relief in patients undergoing ALIF procedures, and the long-term results are promising. Continued modifications, including the use of laparoscopic approaches, minimally invasive approaches, rhBMP-2, and integrated fixation cages, must undergo long-term scrutiny to determine their efficacy.[1,4,6,8,12,29,35,115]

Acknowledgments. The authors thank Abhishek Chaturbedi and Linda Chaman for their time and help, and acknowledge all the sources used in the preparation of this chapter.

KEY REFERENCES

Burkus JK, Gornet MF, Schuler TC, et al: Six-year outcomes of anterior lumbar interbody arthrodesis with use of interbody fusion cages and recombinant human bone morphogenetic protein-2. *J Bone Joint Surg [Am]* 91:1181–1189, 2009.

Crock HV: Lumbar vertebral interbody fusion. In Lin P, Gill K, editors: *Lumbar interbody fusion*, Rockville, MD, 1989, Aspen, pp 115–125.

Faciszewski T, Winter RB, Lonstein JE, et al: The surgical and medical perioperative complications of anterior spinal fusion surgery in the thoracic and lumbar spine in adults: a review of 1223 procedures. *Spine (Phila Pa 1976)* 20:1592–1599, 1995.

Long DM, Filtzer DL, BenDebba M, et al: Clinical features of the failed-back syndrome. *J Neurosurg* 69:61–71, 1988.

Sasso RC, Kenneth Burkus J, LeHuec JC: Retrograde ejaculation after anterior lumbar interbody fusion: transperitoneal versus retroperitoneal exposure. *Spine (Phila Pa 1976)* 28:1023–1026, 2003.

Watkins R: Anterior approaches to the lumbar spine. In Torrens MJ, Dickson RA, editors: *Operative spinal surgery*, New York, 1991, Churchill Livingstone, pp 161–171.

REFERENCES

The complete reference list is available online at expertconsult.com.

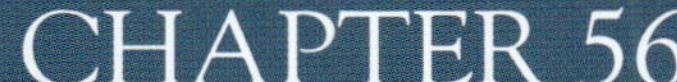

CHAPTER 56

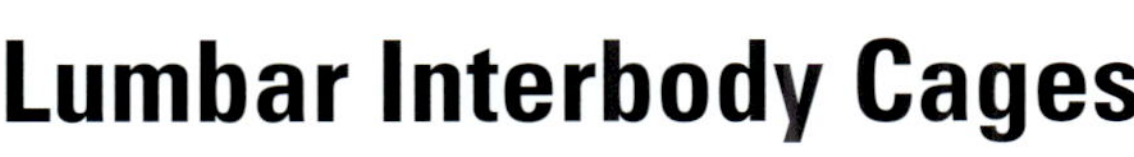

Lumbar Interbody Cages

Steven S. Agabegi | Camille Connelly | Jeffrey S. Fischgrund

Lumbar fusion procedures have become increasingly common in the treatment of degenerative conditions of the lumbar spine. The use of interbody cages to add structural stability and to improve fusion rates has become more common over time. It has been demonstrated biomechanically that the most effective means of eliminating motion between two vertebrae is through the disc space rather than the facet joints, transverse processes, or spinous processes.[1] Traditionally, dorsolateral fusion has been associated with a higher pseudarthrosis rate than has a circumferential fusion. Furthermore, it has been shown that posterolateral fusion does not completely achieve immobilization of the motion segment despite the presence of a solid dorsolateral fusion.[2] This result makes intuitive sense, as 80% of spinal loads are transmitted through the anterior column.

Interbody Fusion

Interbody fusion procedures offer several potential advantages: The interbody grafts are placed in the weight-bearing position with fusion-promoting forces (Wolff's law): There is an increased surface area for fusion, and there is good blood supply after decortication of the vertebral end plates; the neural foramina are increased in height and diameter, thus relieving compression of nerve roots; and the disc, which may be a source of pain, is removed. Furthermore, proponents of interbody fusion argue that disc height and lumbar lordosis are restored, thereby improving overall sagittal balance. Most patients with degenerative conditions of the lumbar spine affecting one or two levels do not have significant sagittal imbalance. However, if segmental lordosis is not restored at each level at the index operation and those segments are fused in a hypolordotic position, future adjacent segment degenerative changes may compound the problem and may ultimately result in a flat back deformity.

Despite the aforementioned theoretical advantages of anterior column fusion, it is not yet clear whether clinical outcomes are improved in comparison with a dorsolateral fusion alone. The disadvantages of including an interbody device include the added cost; increased operative time; the risk of neurologic injury due to nerve root or dural sac retraction; and the long-term, potentially deleterious, effects of complete immobilization of a motion segment on the adjacent lumbar levels. One study found that at long-term follow-up (average 14 years), clinical outcomes were not correlated with disc height after ventral fusion using tricortical iliac bone.[3]

Lumbar interbody fusion can be performed from either a ventral approach (anterior lumbar interbody fusion) or dorsal approach (dorsal or transforaminal lumbar interbody fusion).With a ventral approach, greater access to the disc space allows a more complete discectomy. However, a substantial portion of the disc can also be removed from the dorsal approach, although it is difficult to remove disc material from the side opposite the approach. Approximately 70% of the disc can be removed from a unilateral dorsal approach, which is likely sufficient to obtain an optimal surface area for fusion. Advocates of ventral approaches argue that improved access to the disc, more complete discectomy, and superior end-plate preparation are likely to yield a higher fusion rate and improved lordosis. It is much easier to restore segmental lordosis from a ventral approach because circumferential release of the anulus fibrosus allows more effective restoration of disc space height, and a larger cage can be inserted in terms of both height and width.

Also, cages that are inserted from a ventral approach can have varying degrees of lordosis (Fig. 56-1). The first tapered cage that was developed was the Lumbar Tapered Cage (LT cage; Medtronic, Memphis, TN) (Fig. 56-2). Most implants on the market today are tapered and have built-in lordosis. Although lordotic cages can be inserted from a dorsal approach, this degree of lordosis is limited. Most cages that are inserted from a dorsal approach have a tapered tip to allow initial insertion of the cage into the disc space. Therefore, the degree of lordosis that is achievable with a cage inserted from a dorsal approach is somewhat limited.

One purported advantage of interbody fusion is the ability to obtain indirect decompression by increasing the size of the neural foramina. However, a recent study found that while an anterior lumbar interbody fusion (ALIF) restored foraminal height by 18.5% and lumbar lordosis by 6.2 degrees, transforaminal lumbar interbody fusion (TLIF) decreased foraminal height by 0.4% and decreased lumbar lordosis by 2.1 degrees.[4] This decrease may be due to subsidence of the cage into the end plates. Also, after insertion of the cage from the dorsal approach, many surgeons apply compressive force across the pedicle screws to lock in the cage, and this may lead to a decrease in foraminal height.

In the standing position, 80% of spine loads are transmitted through the anterior column.[5] The implant or graft

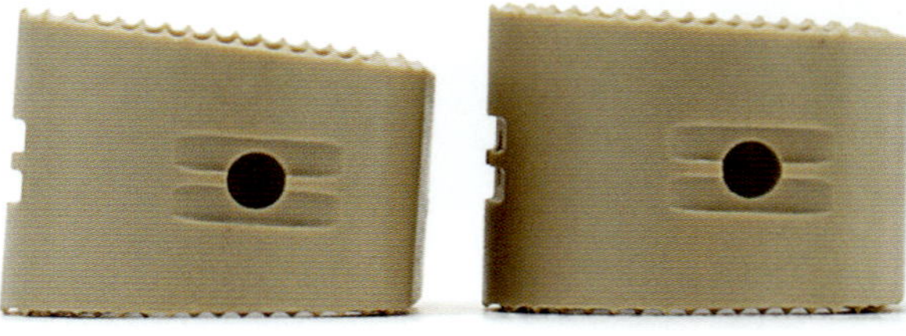

FIGURE 56-1. Anterior lumbar interbody fusion cages in different degrees of lordosis. (Courtesy of Stryker Spine, AVS AL cage.)

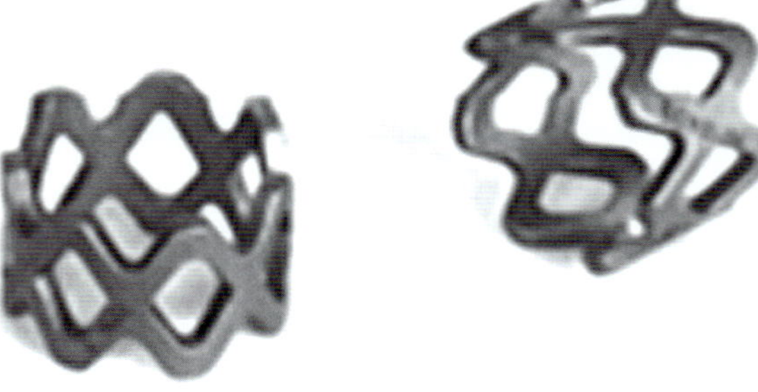

FIGURE 56-3. Harms cage. (Courtesy of DePuy Spine.)

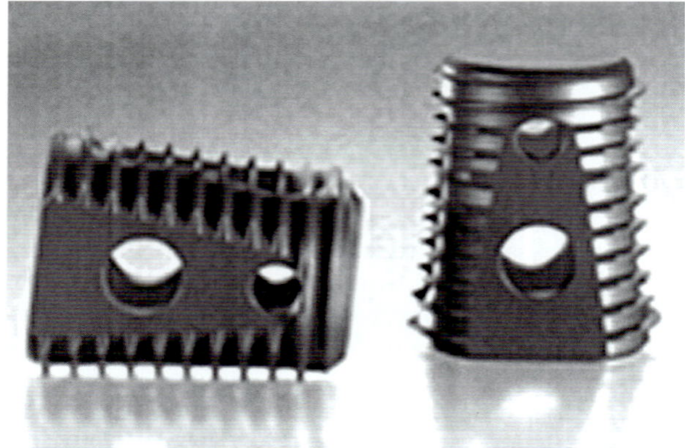

FIGURE 56-2. Lumbar tapered cage. (Courtesy of Medtronic.)

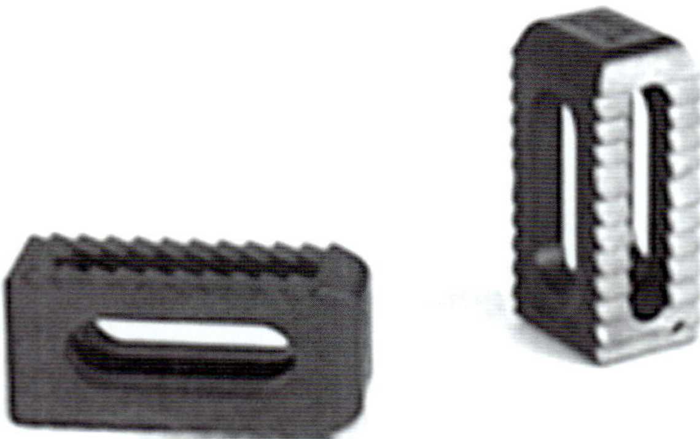

FIGURE 56-4. Brantigan cage. (Courtesy of DePuy Spine.)

must be capable of withstanding these loads to allow fusion to occur. Early on, autologous bicortical iliac crest autograft was the gold standard, supplemented with a screw and washer to keep the graft in place. However, high rates of pseudarthrosis, graft collapse, migration, and loss of correction were observed with the use of autologous iliac crest alone.[6-11] Lumbar interbody cages have become more popular because of the high rate of pseudarthrosis associated with use of interbody bone graft alone.[12,13] A cage provides immediate rigid axial mechanical support and stability postoperatively, allowing the graft material inside the cage as well as surrounding the cage to form a solid biologic fusion. There are a number of options to provide anterior column support, including fibular allograft, vascularized autograft (usually rib or fibula), vertical mesh cages (e.g., Harms cage; Fig. 56-3), carbon fiber cages (Brantigan cage; Fig. 56-4), cylindrical threaded cages (BAK, LT cages), and polyetheretherketone (PEEK) cages.

Anterior lumbar interbody fusion may be achieved with a stand-alone cage or supplemented with dorsal instrumentation. At present, there is no industry consensus for performing one procedure over the other. Proponents of the stand-alone ALIF contend that an exclusively ventral approach allows for superior preparation of the fusion surfaces while preserving the dorsal elements,[14] which avoids perioperative morbidity related to the dissection of the spinal muscles and complications from the dorsal instrumentation.[15] On the other hand, advocates for dorsal instrumentation assert that supplementary dorsal stabilization increases system constraint, creating an environment that is more conducive to fusion.[16]

A number of biomechanical studies have investigated the stabilization provided by stand-alone ALIF cages versus those supplemented with dorsal instrumentation. In general, stand-alone interbody cages significantly reduce flexion and lateral bending compared to intact spines.[14,17,18] Constraint of axial rotation, however, has not been as successful,[14,16,19,20] although studies suggest that ALIF procedures generate better stabilization in torsion than does posterior lumbar interbody fusion (PLIF).[21] Regardless of the surgical approach, interbody cages do not stabilize in extension,[18,21-23] although it is unclear whether the lack of stabilization in extension is clinically relevant and should warrant dorsal instrumentation.[21]

It is widely accepted that supplementary dorsal instrumentation further increases range of motion constraint and stiffness in one or more planes compared to stand-alone ALIF cages.[16,18,19,23] However, the constraint parameters that are ideal for facilitating fusion have not been defined. If supplementary dorsal instrumentation is required to achieve a stable environment for fusion, the advantages of ALIF over dorsal procedures are lost.

Clinical studies comparing stand-alone interbody cages and cages with dorsal stabilization have been equivocal. Fusion rates of between 82% and 98% have been reported for both procedures,[24,25] and patient satisfaction rates have also been similar between stand-alone and circumferential procedures. In a study of 71 patients who underwent stand-alone ALIF with bilateral low-profile interbody fusion cages, the overall fusion rate was 86% with an average time to fusion of 10 months. While the single-level fusion rate was 93%, the rates for two- and three-level procedures were lower, at 55% and 67%, respectively. This is consistent with other published data reporting fusion rates for both ALIF and PLIF procedures of around 90% to 94%, with lower fusion rates for multilevel procedures. This may suggest that stand-alone procedures are most beneficial for single-level fusions.[24]

Additionally, Greenough et al. concluded that ALIF for a single level was associated with significantly less perioperative morbidity than were dorsolateral fusion and instrumentation, although he did not find a significant difference in clinical outcome between the two approaches.[15] Nichols et al. found that the addition of a ventral plate to ALIF provided stability similar to that of supplemental dorsal fixation, with dorsal fixation providing only additional constraint in lateral bending.[26]

Historical Perspective

The concept of interbody fusion was first introduced in the 1940s by Ralph Cloward, who pioneered the posterior lumbar interbody fusion technique. Toward the end of the 1970s, Dr. George Bagby introduced the stainless steel basket as an adjunct to spinal arthrodesis. He implanted a cervical interbody cage made of stainless steel in a racehorse with successful fusion. He called his technique *distraction-compression stabilization*. In the 1980s, Kuslich and others adapted Bagby's basket for human use. Subsequently, threaded PLIF cages were introduced.[27] Threaded PLIF cages were thought to have biomechanical advantages over traditional dorsolateral fusion, including providing anterior column support, placement closer to the vertebral center of rotation, and a reduced bone graft requirement.[28] The FDA approved anterior lumbar interbody fusion cages in 1996. Until the end of the 1990s, most cages were made of titanium. It was not until the late 1990s that the first radiolucent polymer implants (PEEK cages) were introduced. Over the last decade, the field of interbody cage technology has exploded, and a variety of implants have been introduced into the market.

Cage Material and Design

A variety of cages for lumbar interbody fusion surgery are currently available from a number of manufacturers. Cages come in various sizes and shapes and include circular, tapered, and rectangular, with and without curvature. Some devices have design features such as radiolucency that allow assessment of fusion; some have end-plate interdigitation with serrations, screw threads, or spikes; and others are modular. Modular cages are designed to customize the fit of the cage to each patient's intervertebral geometry.

The following features are desirable in the design of an interbody cage:

- A cage should ideally have a hollow region of sufficient size to allow packing of bone graft or bone graft substitute.
- It should be structurally sturdy so that it can withstand the great forces applied to it in the immediate postoperative period.
- It should have a modulus of elasticity that is similar to that of vertebral bone to optimize fusion and avoid subsidence.
- It should have ridges or teeth to resist ventral migration or retropulsion into the canal. Serrations on the top and bottom surfaces of the cage may improve fixation strength.
- It should be radiolucent to allow visualization of fusion on radiographs.
- If inserted from a dorsal approach (TLIF or PLIF) it should be tapered, with a bullet-shaped tip to allow easier initial insertion into the disc space.

The stiffness of a cage has been found to influence fusion rates.[29,30] Ideally, a cage would have a modulus of elasticity that is similar to that of vertebral bone, which would optimize the load transfer between the cage and the adjacent vertebral bodies and reduce the effects of stress shielding on the graft material. Carbon fiber cages have a modulus of elasticity closer to that of cortical bone.[31] In contrast, metal and titanium cages exceed the stiffness of the vertebral bone. The modulus of elasticity of stainless steel and titanium implants is 200 and 110 GPa, respectively,[32] compared with that of vertebral trabecular and cortical bone, which is 2.1 and 2.4 GPa, respectively.[33,34]

Titanium cages have the disadvantage of incomplete radiographic assessment of the fusion mass. Furthermore, owing to the mismatch of modulus of elasticity of titanium and vertebral bone, the stiffness of titanium cages may cause subsidence into the vertebral end plates. PEEK is a semicrystalline aromatic polymer used as a structural spacer that has gained popularity because of its similar modulus of elasticity to that of bone and its radiolucency. It can be used in conjunction with carbon fiber reinforcement or as pure PEEK. Radiomarker dots are used at the ventral and dorsal aspects of the cage so that the surgeon can see the implant on radiographs. PEEK is also MRI and CT compatible and does not create significant implant artifact on these imaging studies. PEEK cages come in a variety of sizes (Fig. 56-5).

There is some biomechanical evidence showing lower primary fixation and initial stability of PEEK cages compared to titanium cages of equal dimensions.[18] Despite this evidence, PEEK implants have been shown to have good to excellent clinical outcomes[35-37] and are widely used. Particularly when augmented with dorsal instrumentation, PEEK cages have been shown to provide stability similar to that of titanium cages, reduce stress at the end plates adjacent to the cage, and increase load transfer through the graft.[38]

In a study of lordosis correction in circumferential arthrodesis using PEEK cages, Rousseau et al.[37] found that immediate postsurgery increases in lumber lordosis were lost at subsequent follow-up. Lordosis loss was statistically related to the initial increase in lordosis, cage size, patient age, and presence of dorsal instrumentation and level of fusion. This tendency to restore preoperative sagittal balance occurred despite a 98% fusion rate and 86% excellent or good clinical outcomes. Similar loss of lordosis correction, despite solid

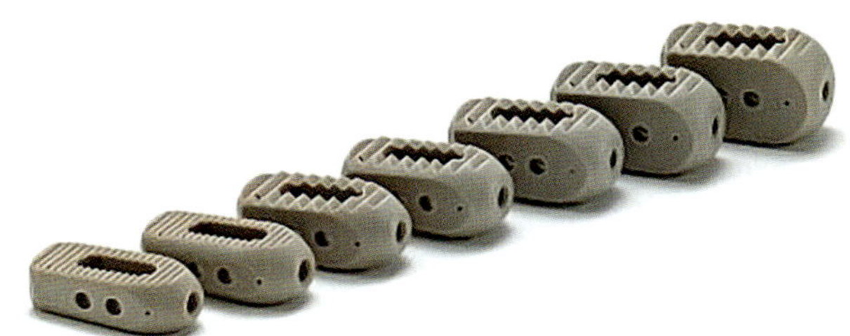

FIGURE 56-5. Tapered PEEK (polyetheretherketone) cages for transforaminal lumbar interbody fusion. (Courtesy of Stryker Spine, AVS PL cages.)

fusion and good clinical outcomes, has been found in other studies regardless of interbody cage material.[3,39]

Bioabsorbable cages have also been designed. These cages are absorbed over time, thus leaving only a bony fusion between vertebrae without any foreign material in the spinal segment. There is limited experience with the clinical application of resorbable implants in lumbar fusion surgery, and studies are contradictory. Jiya et al.[40] randomized 26 patients to undergo instrumented posterior lumbar interbody fusion with either a nonresorbable PEEK cage or a resorbable poly(L-lactide-co-D,L-lactide) (PLDLLA) cage. The fusion rate was significantly higher with the PEEK cage compared with the PLDLLA cage. Furthermore, the PLDLLA cage showed a significantly higher rate of subsidence compared with the PEEK cage. Other studies have evaluated the fusion rate and its relationship to cage stiffness, evaluating a poly-L-latic acid (PLLA) cage versus a titanium cage.[29,30] After 6 months, increased interbody fusion was seen with the PLLA cages. An in vitro study showed that PLLA cages were mechanically sufficient directly after implantation.[41] Other studies have supported the use of resorbable cages, with fusion rates being comparable to those of nonresorbable implants without adverse effects related to the implant.[42-44]

Subsidence

One of the goals of interbody fusion is to increase disc space height and maintain segmental lordosis. Increasing disc space height is relatively easy to accomplish in the prone or supine patient intraoperatively and even on short-term follow-up. However, over time, settling of the cage into the vertebral end plates can occur. If significant subsidence occurs, it can lead to segmental loss of lordosis and loss of anterior column support. These changes may result in an unfavorable biomechanical environment contributing to pseudarthrosis and possibly compression of the neural elements.

Several reasons have been proposed to explain the relatively high incidence of subsidence, including regional strength of the end plate, degree of osteoporosis, size and/or shape of the cage, degree of end-plate removal during end-plate preparation, and the addition of supplemental fixation.

Intraoperatively, during discectomy and end-plate preparation, the surgeon should aim to remove the cartilaginous end plate but preserve the bony end plate. Removing the cartilaginous end plate is important for improving the vascularity to aid the process of fusion. However, removing the bony end plate may compromise the stability of the end plate, weaken the compressive strength of the vertebral body, and lead to subsidence of the interbody device. There is some evidence to support this claim: Oxland et al. reported that strength was mechanically reduced by approximately 33% with resection of the bony end plate compared to the rate without resection.[45] While removal of the end plate to expose bleeding cancellous bone is advantageous from a fusion standpoint, it may weaken the bone and increase the risk of implant subsidence. Although the bony end plate itself is very thin (usually <0.5 mm thick),[46,47] it likely serves to distribute loads evenly over the underlying cancellous bone. Most surgeons leave the bony end plate intact to preserve structural support.

The periphery of the end plate is stronger than the center, and the dorsolateral portions (just ventral to the pedicles) are the strongest regions of the end plate. The dorsolateral sites have more than twice the strength of the central end plate. Given this pattern, if a small portion of the end plate is removed in the central portion of the end plate, the risk of subsidence may not be substantially increased,[45] and the exposed central cancellous bone may improve fusion. Removal of the end plate in the peripheral regions, particularly in regions where the cage is in contact with the end plate (depending on cage design), likely increases the risk of subsidence.

Cage material can affect the degree of subsidence. Previous studies have shown that anterior lumbar interbody fusion using iliac allograft or autograft has a very high rate of subsidence.[48] Hollowell et al.[49] loaded thoracic vertebrae in compression comparing a titanium mesh cage, humerus, tricortical iliac graft, triple-rib strut graft, and single-rib graft on intact vertebrae or on a cancellous trough of vertebrae. The titanium mesh cage construct provided the greatest resistance to axial load. However, there is concern that rigid metal cages have a high incidence of subsidence. Unfortunately, interstudy comparison of subsidence is complicated by inconsistency in defining criteria and the lack of a standard measuring technique. Schiffman et al.[24] studied the radiographs and clinical outcomes from 56 patients at least 12 months following surgery with bilateral low-profile interbody fusion cages (BAK/Proximity; Minneapolis, MN) and found minimal evidence of subsidence (<2 mm) and no significant differences in amount of subsidence between one- and two-level procedures. Additionally, he found no association between the amount of subsidence and disc height, fusion status, change in lordosis, or patient satisfaction. In other studies, Beutler and Peppelman[39] and Eck et al.[50] found subsidence greater than 2 mm in 10% and 14% of patients, respectively, who underwent noninstrumented ALIF with titanium mesh cages. Likewise, subsidence incidence was not associated with loss of lordosis or patient satisfaction. Increased subsidence was associated with greater reaming depth and with larger cage diameters.[39] Furthermore, ideal positioning of interbody cages at the dorsolateral sites was identified as an important factor to limit subsidence. Another study found that the addition of dorsal instrumentation did not change the compressive strength of the cage-vertebra interface, indicating that dorsal fixation was unlikely to contribute to subsidence.[51]

Factors Affecting Construct Rigidity

The rigidity provided by interbody cages is influenced by a number of factors, including cage design and size, anular tension and device preload, end-plate strength, and the location of the cage within the interbody space. In addition, supplemental instrumentation has a substantial effect on the stability of the construct.

Anular tension is influenced primarily by the vertical height of the cage. Axial "oversizing" of the cage leads to increased anular tension, which may improve the rigidity of the construct.[52] Most systems have trials that can be inserted into the disc space to assess ligament tension. One method of assessing the size of the implant is to measure the height of a normal lumbar disc one level above or below the level to be fused on preoperative imaging studies. This height approximates the desired height at the diseased level. However, intraoperative assessment of anular tension with trial implants is the most reliable method of determining cage size. Undersized cages with anular tissue relaxation may lead to device loosening, fusion failure, and possibly migration of the implant.

Vertebral bone quality, or end-plate strength, is critical to cage stability.[45,49,53-55] The dorsolateral region of the end plate, the region near the pedicle base, has the greatest resistance to subsidence, while the central region provides the least resistance.[56] The additional cortical bone at the pedicle base may account for this improved strength.[56] This is of clinical importance in performing a TLIF, in which smaller cages are used. Positioning the cage dorsolaterally in these cases maximizes stability of the construct.[56] The disadvantage of this position is that it may increase the likelihood of cage retropulsion into the canal. For this reason, cages that are inserted through a dorsal approach are typically countersunk relative to the dorsal vertebral body by at least 3 to 4 mm.

Cage size also affects construct stability. In compression, larger cages have greater maximum load to failure of the end plates than smaller cages do.[55] Wider implants that are supported by the periphery of the end plate provide superior stability.[57] For this reason, cages that are inserted through the lateral approach (e.g., extreme lateral interbody fusion or direct lateral interbody fusion approaches) likely provide superior compressive stability in comparison to smaller cages that are inserted through the dorsal approach. Closkey et al. have shown the association between contact area of the cage and compressive strength.[53] A smaller cage applies more load to the central portion of the end plate, which is much weaker than the periphery of the end plate. Many cages, particularly those that are inserted through the dorsal approach, have too small an area of graft bone/host bone contact surface area. The small total contact surface area between the device and the vertebral end plates may also result in subsidence.

Cage features such as serrations or spikes may also affect the overall stability. There is biomechanical evidence for this. Buttermann et al. compared three cage types: a PEEK spacer with small ridges, a modular interbody device with end-plate spikes, and a dual tapered threaded interbody cage. Cages with end-plate spikes provided improved motion segment rigidity in bending modes and particularly in torsion.[14] End-plate engagement with spikes is beneficial in limiting torsion.[14] Like the threaded cage, the spiked cage engages the end plates, but with spikes instead of threads (Fig. 56-6).

The question that remains is how much rigidity is necessary. The degree of micromotion that would not compromise biologic fusion is not known. Pilliar et al.[58] studied the effect of micromotion on bone ingrowth into porous surfaced implants and found that while a small amount of micromotion of up to 28 μm does not affect bone ingrowth, a large amount of micromotion of over 150 μm can produce fibrous tissue development at the implant–end plate interface. If optimal construct rigidity is not obtained, supplemental fixation should be considered, particularly in cases of osteopenia, end-plate disruption, or excessive anular laxity. In osteoporotic spine, supplemental fixation has been recommended.[55]

Complications and Management

The majority of cage complications are related to the approach and technique. When the cage is inserted through a dorsal approach, the neural elements are at risk of injury. Particularly through a TLIF approach, the exiting nerve root is at risk of "crush" injury if it is not adequately visualized and protected. The exiting nerve root is particularly at risk in certain clinical circumstances. If the disc space is severely collapsed, the exiting nerve root may be lying on top of or just above the disc, and this allows for less room for insertion of the cage. Patients with spondylolisthesis are at risk for the same reason. An attempt at inserting an oversized cage may also lead to nerve root injury. It is critical that care be taken to protect the dural sac and exiting nerve root during discectomy, end-plate preparation, and cage insertion. Nothing should be done blindly, and visualization and protection of all neural structures are mandatory to prevent neurologic complications.

Failure to achieve adequate distraction of the anulus fibrosus and undersizing the cage can risk pseudarthrosis and cage migration with potential injury to the neural elements. Vascular injury can occur if the cage migrates ventrally in the lower lumbar spine. Furthermore, ventral migration of the graft can lead to loss of correction and segmental kyphosis. Dorsal fusion and instrumentation, with compression across the pedicle screws, add further stability and enhance the fusion rate. The use of fluoroscopy during end-plate preparation and cage insertion may lower the incidence of complications that are related to suboptimal positioning of the cage. In placing cages from the dorsal approach, countersinking the implant by 3 to 4 mm may lower the risk of neural element impingement if micromigration of the implant occurs (Fig. 56-7).

If dorsal cage migration occurs after a TLIF procedure such that the neural elements are at risk, a ventral approach is the safest method of retrieving the cage without causing nerve root injury. In such a setting, if a repeat dorsal approach is utilized, the surgeon is likely to encounter scarring around the nerve

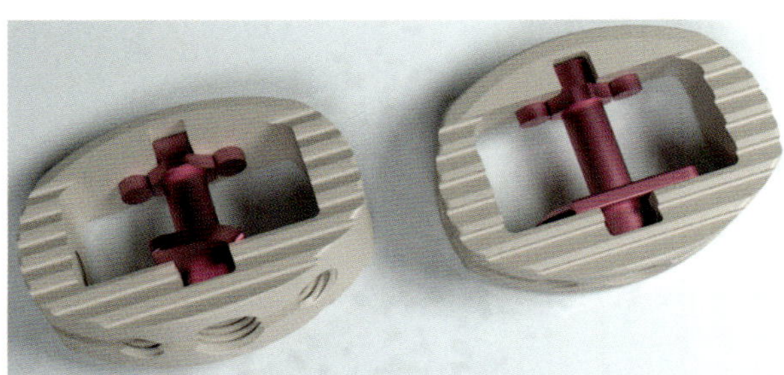

FIGURE 56-6. Anterior lumbar interbody fusion cages with built-in spin plate/locking plate to engage the vertebral end plates for additional stability. (Vu aPOD cage courtesy of Integra/Theken Spine.)

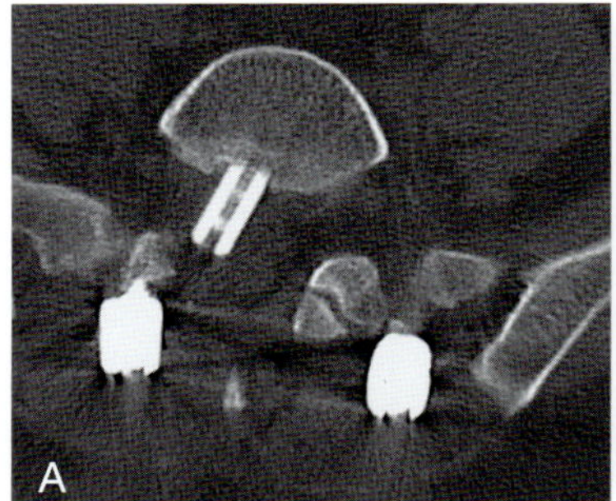

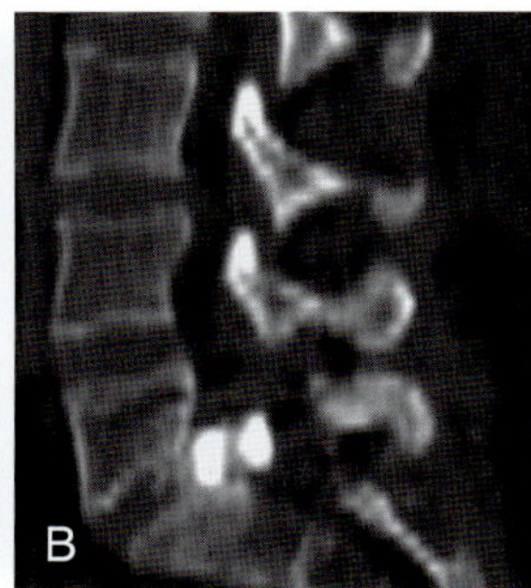

FIGURE 56-7. Axial (**A**) and sagittal (**B**) CT scans of posterior migration of a transforaminal lumbar interbody fusion cage causing severe neural element impingement.

roots, and retrieval of the cage can lead to nerve root injury or a ventral dural tear. For these reasons, a ventral approach may be the safest technique to remove the implant. This approach would also allow an effective anterior interbody fusion, as pseudarthrosis was likely the cause of the implant migration.

KEY REFERENCES

Bagby GW: Arthrodesis by the distraction-compression method using a stainless steel implant. *Orthopedics* 11:931–934, 1988.

Brantigan JW, Steffee AD: A carbon fiber implant to aid interbody lumbar fusion: two-year clinical results in the first 26 patients. *Spine (Phila Pa 1976)* 18:2106–2117, 1993.

Hollowell JP, Vollmer DG, Wilson CR, et al: Biomechanical analysis of thoracolumbar interbody constructs: how important is the endplate? *Spine (Phila Pa 1976)* 21:1032–1036, 1996.

Kuslich SD, Danielson G, Dowdle JD, et al: Four-year follow-up results of lumbar spine arthrodesis using the Bagby and Kuslich lumbar fusion cage. *Spine (Phila Pa 1976)* 25:2656–2662, 2000.

Lowe TG, Hashim S, Wilson LA, et al: A biomechanical study of regional endplate strength and cage morphology as it relates to structural interbody support. *Spine (Phila Pa 1976)* 29:2389–2394, 2004.

Oxland TR, Grant JP, Dvorak MF, et al: Effects of endplate removal on the structural properties of the lower lumbar vertebral bodies. *Spine (Phila Pa 1976)* 28:771–777, 2003.

Rousseau MA, Lazennec JY, Saillant G: Circumferential arthrodesis using PEEK cages at the lumbar spine. *J Spinal Disord Tech* 20:278–281, 2007.

REFERENCES

The complete reference list is available online at expertconsult.com.

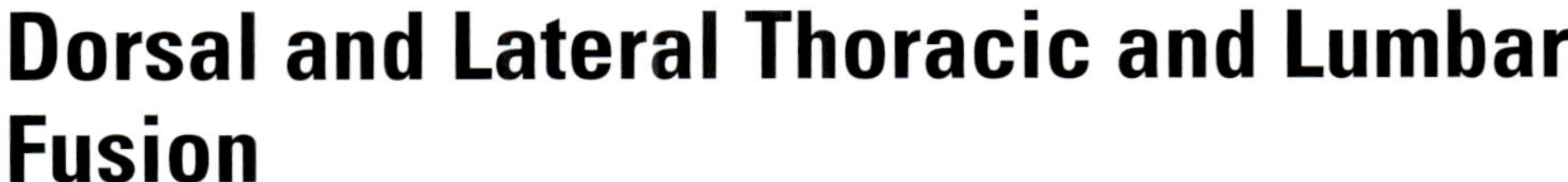

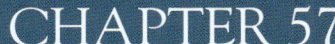

CHAPTER 57

Dorsal and Lateral Thoracic and Lumbar Fusion

Umesh S. Metkar | Andrew P. White | Paul A. Glazer

Thoracic and lumbar spine fusion procedures are typically performed to provide pain relief, to preserve neurologic function, and to maintain or restore spinal stability and alignment. Dorsal and lateral thoracic and lumbar fusion procedures are performed as part of the treatment of many spinal disorders. These include traumatic, neoplastic, infectious, iatrogenic, and certain degenerative conditions associated with deformity or instability.

When surgical treatment of degenerative disorders is required, following neurologic decompression, fusion may be indicated in cases associated with spondylolisthesis or significant scoliosis. One well-known study,[1] for example, demonstrated better clinical and radiographic outcomes following decompression and noninstrumented fusion, compared to decompression alone in the treatment of degenerative spondylolisthesis. Spine fusion may also be useful in cases in which significant iatrogenic instability has been created by wide decompression or by resection of significant lesions. Lumbar spine fusion as a treatment of degenerative disc disease alone, however, is generally not indicated.

The addition of segmental instrumentation has been shown to increase fusion rates and improve clinical outcomes.[2,3] While internal fixation may be associated with complications, particularly in the setting of osteoporosis, it should also be considered for patients who are thought to be candidates for spine fusion.

Historical Background

Albee[4] and Hibbs[5] were the first surgeons to independently describe the technique of arthrodesis. They created greenstick fractures of spinous processes in patients with Pott disease. Albee used tibial autograft to augment the fusion. Mackenzie-Forbes[6] and Hibbs[7] introduced the technique of laminar decortications extending the fusion further laterally. Hibbs also described the concept of facet joint fusion in a series of his scoliosis patients.[7] The technique was further modified by Howorth,[8] McBride,[9] and Moe.[10]

The subsequent introduction of intertransverse process fusion by Mathieu and Demirleau provided an alternative technique to dorsal fusion that proved beneficial for patients in whom laminectomy was contemplated.[11] Adkins[12] implemented this technique in spondylolisthesis patients. Watkins[13] described a paramedian approach to gain access to transverse processes lateral to paraspinous musculature, thus sparing the spinous processes and interspinous ligaments. Wiltse et al.[14] devised a muscle-splitting approach between the longissimus and multifidus muscles to gain access to the intertransverse process region. The introduction of spinal instrumentation further improved the fusion results.

Biology of Bone Grafting and Spine Fusion

Bone healing following fracture involves a regenerative process, usually leading to complete restoration of the structural integrity of the affected bone. The physiology of spine fusion is similar to the physiology involved in fracture healing. The process of fusion begins by hematoma formation at the surgical site. The rich vascular arcade around the dorsal elements delivers oxygen to the fusion site and also leads to an influx of various inflammatory cells. The healing process begins within hours after surgery. The macrophages infiltrating the hematoma remove the necrotic debris at the fusion site. During this process, the macrophages secrete a number of inflammatory cytokines that stimulate migration of other inflammatory cells into the fusion area.[15] Platelets within the hematoma secrete platelet-derived growth factor, which is chemotactic to fibroblasts and other mesenchymal cells in the area.[16] The inflammatory markers secreted by platelets and other inflammatory cells promote proliferation and differentiation of primitive mesenchymal cells into cells of osteoid or chondroid lineage.[17] Bone morphogenetic protein plays an active role in bone synthesis.[18-20]

The second phase of fusion involves a repair process.[21] Inflammatory markers secreted during the repair process promote ingrowth of new blood vessels. Formation of cartilaginous matrix by chondroblasts as well as osteoid formation by osteoblasts leads to new bone formation. Mineralization of the matrix leads to primary or woven bone formation. Compression and distraction forces[22] at the fusion site may provide a stimulus for remodeling[21] and consolidation of the fusion mass. Incomplete ossification may lead to fibrous nonunion or pseudarthrosis.

Graft Selection for Dorsal and Lateral Thoracolumbar Fusions

A host of factors are necessary to achieve a solid arthrodesis. These factors include the preparation of an optimal fusion bed as well as application of appropriate bone graft material. The graft material that is selected for fusion may serve osteogenic, osteoconductive, and/or osteoinductive functions. Osteogenic grafts provide an ample number of osteoprogenitor cells necessary for the fusion process. Osteoinduction is the process whereby undifferentiated mesenchymal cells divide and transform into osteoid and chondroid cells. Osteoconductive grafts provide a biologically appropriate scaffold for ingrowth of vascular and bone progenitor elements from the recipient host bed.

The ideal graft contains an ample number of viable osteoprogenitor cells. Cortical and cancellous autografts and allografts are the most commonly used graft[23-26] materials for thoracic and lumbar fusions. Autogenous cancellous grafts are considered more likely to promote fusion than are cortical bone grafts because they are more rapidly vascularized and are more osteoinductive.[19,20,27,28] However, cortical autografts are used for their structural integrity in ventral fusion procedures of the thoracic and lumbar spine. Autograft is limited in quantity, however, and is associated with significant morbidity from the autologous bone harvest.[27,29-32]

Allografts may provide an osteoconductive matrix necessary for fusion. They have limited osteoinductive properties, however, and are inferior to autogenous grafts. Allografts may evoke significant host immune response.[33,34] Allografts are considered useful in patients with a limited bone supply or when a large quantity of graft material is needed.[35] Adequate fusion rates can be achieved with autograft or allograft when supplemented with segmental instrumentation in young patients with thoracolumbar scoliosis.[23-26] Thoracolumbar spine fusion rates are much higher, however, when autograft is used in comparison to allograft alone. A higher pseudarthrosis rate has been demonstrated with the use of allograft as compared to autograft for intertransverse and interlaminar fusion in the lumbar spine.[36-39]

Surgical Technique

Dorsal thoracic and lumbar fusions are usually performed in the prone position. After intubation, compressive calf devices may be applied to prevent deep venous thrombosis. Urinary catheterization is required in performing surgeries greater than 2 to 3 hours in length. The patient is then gently positioned in the prone position on either chest rolls or a spinal frame. Pressure points are padded to prevent skin breakdown. No pressure should be placed on the eyes in the prone position. The arms should be abducted less than 90 degrees. The elbows are flexed and placed on arm boards. The elbows should be adequately padded to prevent ulnar nerve injury. In patients with restricted shoulder range of motion and in cases of upper thoracic fusions, the arms should be tucked by the patient's side. The hips should be positioned in extension to maximize the lumbar lordosis. If there are significant hip flexion contractures, the lower extremities should be positioned with the hips flexed, however. The pelvis and knees should be adequately padded, and the legs should be supported by pillows.

Approaches to the Thoracolumbar Spine

A midline approach is used for the majority of thoracic and lumbar fusions. The dissection is carried down through superficial fascia to reach the deep thoracolumbar fascia. Self-retaining retractors are placed at each end. The spinous processes are palpated through the deep fascia, and the fascia is divided over the spinous processes. Once the tip of the spinous processes is visible, the dissection is advanced laterally in a subperiosteal plane with the use of a Cobb elevator. With use of a Bovie electrocautery, the paraspinal musculature is cut at its attachment to the spinous processes. The dissection is advanced laterally and subperiosteally along the spinous process and lamina to expose the pars interarticularis and medial portion of the facet joints. The facet capsule should be preserved until the levels of fusion are confirmed radiographically. Dissection is further advanced lateral to the facet joint to expose the dorsal surface of the transverse processes. Bipolar cautery should be used to cauterize the terminal branches of the lumbar segmental artery that are located rostral, caudal, and lateral to the facet joints. The self-retaining retractors are advanced to expose the transverse processes. The lateral surface of the pars and facet joints should be cleared of their muscular attachments. Transverse processes in the thoracic spine can be exposed by lateral and rostral extension of the subperiosteal exposure of the lamina. Exposure of the L5 transverse process and sacral ala requires elevation of the multifidus and sacrospinalis origin from the sacral ala and dorsal sacrum. The L5 transverse process, lateral surface of the facet joint, and sacral ala should be denuded of the soft tissue attachments and decorticated to provide an optimal fusion bed for lumbosacral fusion.

Paraspinal (Wiltse) Approach to the Lumbar Spine

In the paraspinal (Wiltse) approach,[14] two paramedian incisions are made approximately 5 cm from the midline just medial to the posterior superior iliac spine. The incision can be planned from the preoperative MRI images by measuring the distance of the plane of separation between the multifidus and longissimus muscles and the midline (Fig. 57-1). The dissection is advanced to the deep dorsal fascia. The fascial incisions are curved medially at their caudal ends to provide adequate muscular retraction. The dissection is further advanced through muscle fascia. The interval between the longissimus and the multifidus muscles can be separated by blunt finger dissection. The dissection should be directed medially to reach the transverse processes and lateral surface of the facet joints. Self-retaining retractors are placed deep to the fascia, and the transverse processes are exposed subperiosteally.

Preparation of Fusion Bed and Bone Grafting

Preparation of Interlaminar and Intertransverse Region

The dorsal surface of the lamina, lateral surface of the facet joint, mamillary body, and lateral pars should be cleared of soft tissues. The exposed area is decorticated by using either

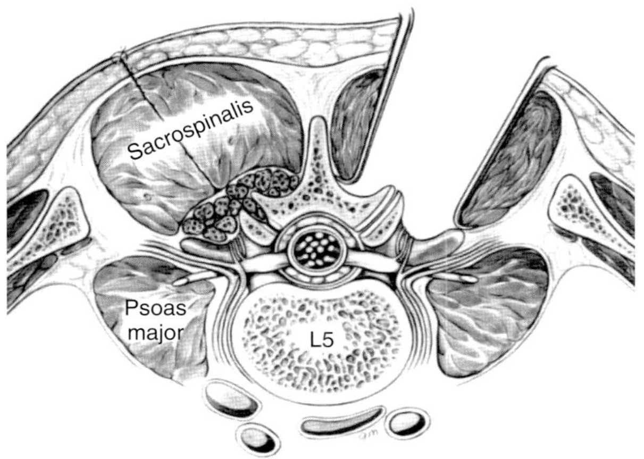

FIGURE 57-1. Paraspinal sacrospinalis muscle-splitting approach (Wiltse approach) for lumbar spine.

a rongeur or a high-speed bur. Graft material is then placed over the decorticated bony elements (Fig. 57-2A).

Facet Joint Fusion

In the thoracic spine, the inferior articular process can be excised by using an osteotome or a Capner gouge to expose the facet joint and cartilaginous surface of the superior articular process.[40] The cartilage is then removed to expose bleeding cancellous surface. The bone graft can then be placed on this exposed surface (Fig. 57-2B).

In the lumbar spine, the facet joints can be exposed by excising the facet capsule. Once exposed, the cartilage from the joint can be excised by using a narrow rongeur or a high-speed bur. The exposed bleeding joint surface can then be packed with cancellous bone chips to facilitate fusion across the joint (see Fig. 57-2A).

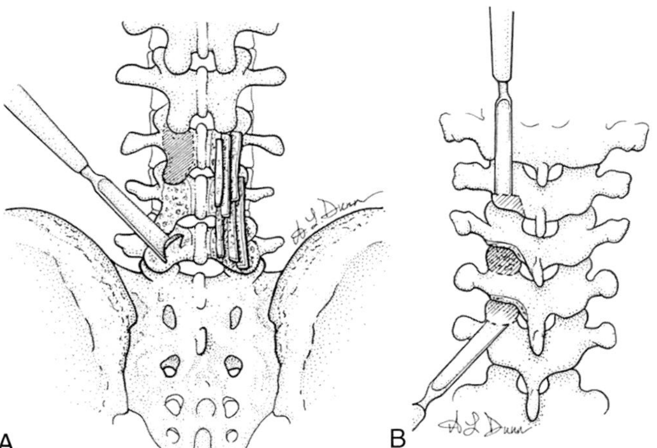

FIGURE 57-2. Technique of preparation for interlaminar and facet joint fusion. **A,** Diagrammatic representation showing interlaminar and facet joint fusion. Cortical surfaces of lamina and facet joint surface are decorticated using a high-speed bur. Corticocancellous graft is then placed over the decorticated surface. **B,** Facet joint preparation in thoracic spine. The inferior articular process is excised to expose the articular surface of the joint. The articular surface is decorticated by using a high-speed bur, and bone graft is onlaid over the decorticated surface.

Complications and Avoidance

Hemorrhage

Perforation of terminal branches of lumbar and thoracic segmental arteries during the exposure of the facet joints, lateral pars interarticularis, and transverse processes can lead to significant blood loss. These arteries are found deep to the paraspinal muscles at the superior and inferior aspects of the facet joints (rostral and caudal articular arteries) and on the dorsal surface of the transverse process (communicating artery) (Fig. 57-3). Bleeding from these vessels can be reduced by identification and cauterization prior to dissection. Venous bleeding in the lumbar spine can be avoided by careful positioning of the patient to avoid increased intra-abdominal pressure. Autologous blood donation and the use of cell savers should be considered in patients in whom excessive intraoperative blood loss is anticipated. Intraoperative venous bleeding can be greatly decreased by reducing pressure on the abdomen. This decreases pressure on the vena cava, thus reducing the pressure in the epidural and paravertebral venous plexus.[41]

Loss of Lumbar Lordosis

Normal lumbar lordosis can be maintained intraoperatively by keeping the lower extremities in an extended position by limiting flexion at the hips.[42]

Pressure and Traction Injuries

Pressure injuries to skin at the bony prominences can be avoided by proper padding of the bony prominences of the upper and lower extremities. Traction injury to the brachial plexus can be avoided by limiting the shoulder abduction to less than 80 degrees. Pressure on the eyes should be avoided to prevent injury to the globe. Elbows should be properly padded to prevent ulnar nerve compression.

Pseudarthrosis

Successful fusion is defined as the presence of continuous bridging trabeculae of bone between spinal segments. A successful fusion inherently requires the absence of motion between the segments and may provide relief of symptoms caused by mechanical instability. Failure of fusion at the surgical site at or after 1 year from index surgery indicates a pseudarthrosis and needs further investigation into etiology and treatment. Pseudarthrosis is one of the leading causes for revision lumbar spine surgery.[43]

A variety of factors are thought to be responsible for pseudarthrosis, including metabolic abnormalities, smoking, infection, and persistent motion at the fusion site. Smoking has been shown to be associated with increase in nonunion rates from 8% in nonsmokers to 40% in smokers.[44] Persistent motion across the fusion segments is thought to be associated with pseudarthrosis. The incidence of pseudarthrosis increases with increase in the number of levels fused owing to the presence of a longer area that needs to be bridged by the fusion process as well as the presence of more motion across the fusion area.[45,46] Spinal instrumentation has been shown to increase the fusion rate by limiting the motion across the fusion segments.[3,46-48] A prospective randomized study by

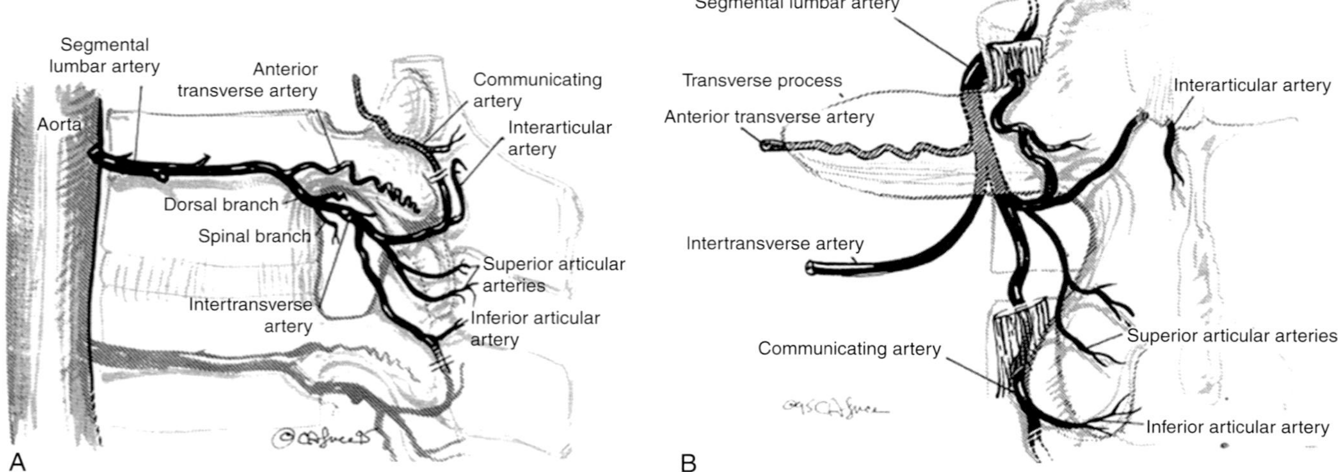

FIGURE 57-3. The arterial arcade formed by terminal branches of lumbar segmental arteries. Cauterization of these terminal branches around the facet joint helps in reducing the total blood loss. Lateral (**A**) and posterior (**B**) views of the transverse process.

Fischgrund et al. showed significantly improved fusion rates at the end of 2 years when lumbar decompression and dorsolateral fusion were combined with instrumentation as compared to noninstrumented decompression and dorsolateral fusion.[49]

Use of flexion/extension radiographs for diagnosis of pseudarthrosis is controversial and is affected by high interobserver variability.[50] Thin-cut CT scans are considered more accurate than are plain radiographs in determining the integrity of the fusion. The presence of metallic artifacts in instrumented fusion, however, decreases the sensitivity of CT scan as the diagnostic modality of choice. Thin-slice CT scan combined with a high index of clinical suspicion may be considered a most reliable diagnostic option. However, exploration of the fusion mass is considered the most specific and sensitive test for diagnosis of pseudarthrosis.

Failure of fusion may present with persistence of back pain, progression of deformity in scoliosis surgery, or recurrence of symptoms in spondylolisthesis. Pseudarthrosis is associated with worse clinical outcomes.[51] The treatment of pseudarthrosis should begin with identification of biologic and mechanical factors that contribute to poor bone healing after spine fusion. Correction of endocrine and nutritional factors may assist in achieving solid fusions. Addition of nonrigid mechanical fixation has also been shown to lead to higher fusion rates. The incidence of pseudarthrosis is higher at the thoracolumbar junction as well as the lumbosacral junction. Surgical treatment includes repair of pseudarthrosis by exposure of the fusion area, removal of instrumentations, thorough decortication, and bone grafting with large quantity of autogenous iliac crest bone graft. Instrumentation is then reapplied with compressive forces across the fusion area. RhBMP-2[52] and osteogenic protein-1 (OP1) have been found to be useful in increasing the fusion rates in lumbar spine fusion surgeries.

Infection

The rate of infections following spine surgery procedures has been shown to correlate with the duration of the procedure, associated patient comorbidities, and the use of instrumentation. The rate of infection is 2% to 4% in noninstrumented spine fusion and 6% to 11% in instrumented spine fusion.[53] *Staphylococcus aureus* is the most common organism responsible for postoperative spinal infections. Postoperative infections may result from direct inoculation or through hematogenous spread of infection from a remote source of infection. Statistically significant preoperative risk factors that are associated with increased risk of infection include age more than 60 years, smoking, diabetes, previous surgical infection, increased body mass index, and alcohol abuse. Intraoperative factors that are associated with increased risk of infection include staged procedure, operative time more than 5 hours, and fusions involving 7 to 13 levels.[54]

Attempts to reduce preoperative and intraoperative risk factors may decrease the risk of infection and improve patient outcomes following spine fusion surgery. Surgeon familiarity with decortication, bone harvesting, and instrumentation techniques may reduce the operative time and decrease the risk of bacterial colonization. Preoperative antibiotics[55] and repeat administration of antibiotics every 4 hours for long-duration surgeries, adequate intraoperative wound irrigation, intermittent repositioning of self-retaining retractors, and limiting the use of monopolar cautery may also decrease the incidence of postoperative infections. The risk of a hematogenous spread of infection can be decreased by recognition and treatment of remote sources of infection. Early patient mobilization and the use of incentive spirometery may help to decrease the risk of pulmonary infections. Careful sterile technique is essential during administration of the Foley catheter.

Surgical treatment of postoperative wound infections should include debridement of infected and necrotic tissues and obtaining sufficient cultures. Exposure of the fusion mass and the hardware with removal of infected unincorporated bone graft material followed by thorough irrigation with a pulsatile lavage system should be carried out. Bone grafting material can then be replaced. Postoperative wound infection can usually be treated without removal of hardware.[56]

Minimally Invasive Transpsoas (Lateral) Interbody Fusion

The lateral transpsoas fusion procedure has been developed as an alternative to the well-established anterior lumbar interbody fusion (ALIF) procedure. Compared to dorsally based interbody procedures, such as posterior lumbar interbody fusion and transforaminal lumbar interbody fusion, ALIF is thought to have superior biomechanical and biologic attributes. Specifically, ALIF is likely to be associated with better restoration of lumbar lordosis, improved indirect decompression by achieving greater height restoration between vertebrae, and higher fusion rates with improved graft-host interface.

The ALIF procedure is typically performed through a transperitoneal or ventral retroperitoneal approach. These open approaches require retraction of the peritoneum and its contents. Postoperative ileus is a common condition following an ALIF procedure. Manipulation of the major retroperitoneal vascular structures may also be required. This can be associated with increased risk of vascular injury.[57] While the open ventral approach provides excellent and reliable exposure of L5-S1, exposure of the L4-5 disc requires control of the recurrent iliolumbar vein and segmental vessels to achieve safe retraction of the iliac vessels. Ventral exposure can also be complicated by injury to the sympathetic chain leading to retrograde ejaculation.[58] The direct ventral approach can also be more challenging in obese patients and as such may be associated with increased risk of complications in this group of patients.

The lateral transpsoas approach to the lumbar spine was developed as an alternative to the traditional ALIF. The goal was to achieve the interbody biomechanical and biologic benefits of the open ALIF procedure but with reduced complications and reduced invasiveness.[59] The transpsoas (lateral) interbody fusion offers certain biomechanical and biologic advantages of the traditional ALIF approach but does not require vascular or visceral retraction.

The lateral transpsoas approach requires a small flank incision and placement of a laterally based retractor. This provides access to the lateral aspect of the disc through the psoas muscle. After bilateral anular release and complete discectomy, interbody grafts or devices can be introduced through this minimally invasive approach. This provides a large fusion surface in the compressive environment of the anterior columns. Since the laterally placed interbody graft or device bears weight bilaterally over the apophyseal ring, it provides excellent interbody mechanical support to maintain restoration of interbody height and resist subsidence[60] (Fig. 57-4).

The lateral transpsoas approach maintains the integrity of the anterior and posterior longitudinal ligaments. Coronal and sagittal plane deformities can be corrected via excellent height restoration in concert with lateral soft tissue releases. Patient obesity creates less risk with a lateral approach, as the abdomen remains out of the way in the lateral decubitus position.

Indications and Clinical Applications[61]

As currently developed, the transpsoas lateral interbody fusion procedure can be applied from the thoracolumbar junction to L5 but is most frequently used in the midlumbar segments. However, thoracic procedures including discectomy and fusion as well as corpectomy have been performed. More typically, this minimally invasive approach is used for interbody lumbar fusion in the setting of adult degenerative disorders, including scoliosis. With coronal plane deformities, the approach is usually performed on the concave side of the curve to provide access to multiple disc spaces through a single flank skin incision (Fig. 57-5). After ipsiplateral and contralateral release of the anulus and Sharpey fibers from the end plates, placement of large interbody spacers can achieve gentle correction of the scoliosis. In patients with degenerative spondylolisthesis, placement of an interbody spacer through a transpsoas technique may help in the restoration of segmental lordosis as well as to increase the foraminal height. Similar results can be obtained in patients with low-grade isthmic spondylolisthesis. The transpsoas technique may be an adjunct to the dorsal treatment of pseudarthrosis and may also be applied to the treatment of patients with adjacent segment disease. We have also used this technique to perform open biopsies and curettage of spinal tumors that were not amenable to CT-guided biopsy (Fig. 57-6). Application of the transpsoas fusion procedure, like any fusion procedure, for the treatment of degenerative disc disease without instability is controversial and is unlikely to be well indicated.

Currently, laterally placed interbody implants should typically not be considered adequate as stand-alone ventral fusion devices. Dorsally and laterally based instrumentation is recommended as an adjunct. Dorsal instrumentation may be placed in a minimally invasive fashion, particularly if a direct neurologic decompression is not required after interbody correction. Dorsal instrumentation may also be placed by traditional open techniques, with or without direct decompression. Laterally based instrumentation can be carried out by using a laterally based plate and screw construct or vertebral body screws passed through the interbody device.

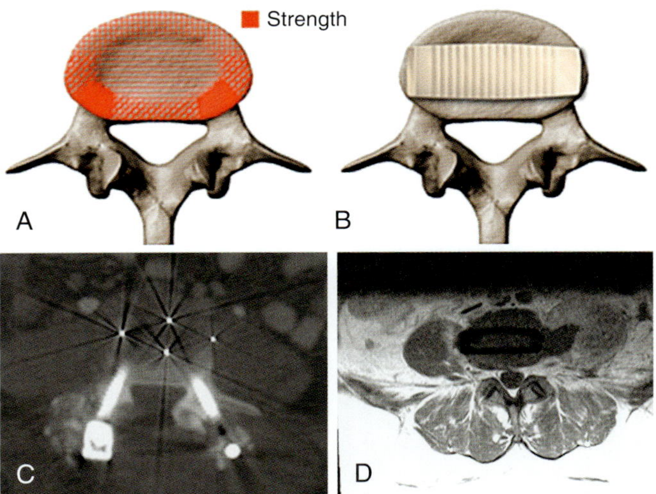

FIGURE 57-4. The weight-bearing portion of a vertebra. **A,** Diagram showing the ring apophysis, the strongest area of a vertebral body. **B,** Positions of a transpsoas lateral lumbar interbody fusion implant resting on the ring apophysis. Postoperative CT scan (**C**) and MRI (**D**) showing position of implants.

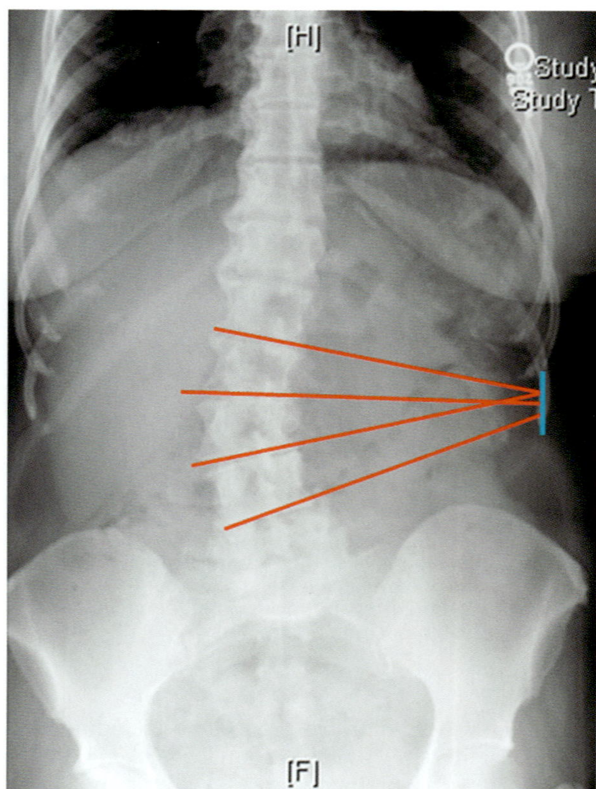

FIGURE 57-5. Transpsoas lumbar interbody fusion for adult degenerative scoliosis. Approach through concave side of the deformity provides access to multiple disc levels through a small incision.

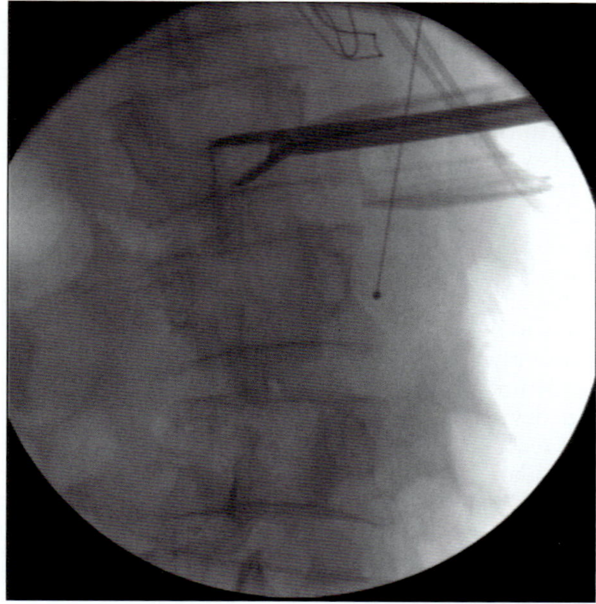

FIGURE 57-6. Use of transpsoas lateral approach for biopsy of a sclerotic lesion in L3 vertebra not accessible for CT-guided biopsy.

We have used this lateral transpsoas interbody fusion technique most frequently in degenerative deformity or adjacent segment degeneration cases that require direct decompression. It should be noted, however, that in many cases, indirect neurologic decompression can be achieved by restoring the normal interbody anatomic relationship. For example, we have treated isthmic spondylolisthesis in this manner (Fig. 57-7).

Surgical Technique of the Lateral Transpsoas Procedure[61]

A familiarity with the anatomy of the psoas muscle is useful to guide surgical technique. The psoas muscle originates from the vertebral body, transverse processes, and intervertebral discs from T12 to L4 and covers the vertebral column laterally. The psoas muscle is larger in the lower lumbar region than in the upper lumbar region. A lateral approach through the psoas provides spinal access dorsal to the great vessels and between the segmental vessels, thus minimizing the blood loss and risk of injury to the great vessels. The lumbar plexus traverses the psoas, however, and there is a potential for injury during the approach. Moro et al.[62] in their cadaveric study analyzed the distribution of the lumbar plexus within the psoas muscle (Fig. 57-8). The ventral half of the psoas was considered to be the safest to traverse, and the risk was found to increase rostral to caudal. Surgeons should use neuromonitoring while traversing the psoas at the L4-5 level. Care also should be taken to avoid injury to the genitofemoral nerve. The genitofemoral nerve is formed from the branches of the L1 and L2 nerve roots. It traverses the psoas muscle from dorsal to ventral, typically surfacing on the psoas between L3 and L4 and coursing along the ventral surface of the psoas thereafter.[62] The nerve ultimately supplies the medial thigh.

Preoperative planning can be very helpful. Posteroanterior and lateral radiographs are assessed to determine whether the lateral approach is applicable to the patient's anatomy. The iliac crest prevents direct lateral access to L5-S1 and can also interfere with direct lateral access to L4-5 in some patients. This pelvic anatomy is more commonly seen in male patients and can be assessed on radiographs. The presence of long 11th and 12th ribs may also interfere with the approach to the upper lumbar levels. Traversing between ribs or resecting a rib can facilitate the approach (Fig. 57-9).

The determination of a left- versus right-sided approach can also be made on the basis of imaging. Radiographs are used to guide the approach in treating scoliosis. An approach from the convex side of the curve provides easier entry to the disc space because the convex side of the interspace provides more space between the lateral aspect of the end plates in comparison to the concave side. For this reason, we will often approach from the convex side of the deformity when treating at a single level. When treating L4-5 in the setting of coronal malalignment, typically only one side can be used because the iliac crest will obscure the opposite side. This frequently dictates the side of the approach when treating scoliosis. In treating multilevel coronal plane deformities, however, an approach from the concave side may provide access to multiple disc spaces through the same small flank incision (see Fig. 57-5).

Cross-sectional imaging such as MR or CT can be helpful in determining a right- or left-sided approach. Axial images are used to examine the psoas muscle as well as other retro-

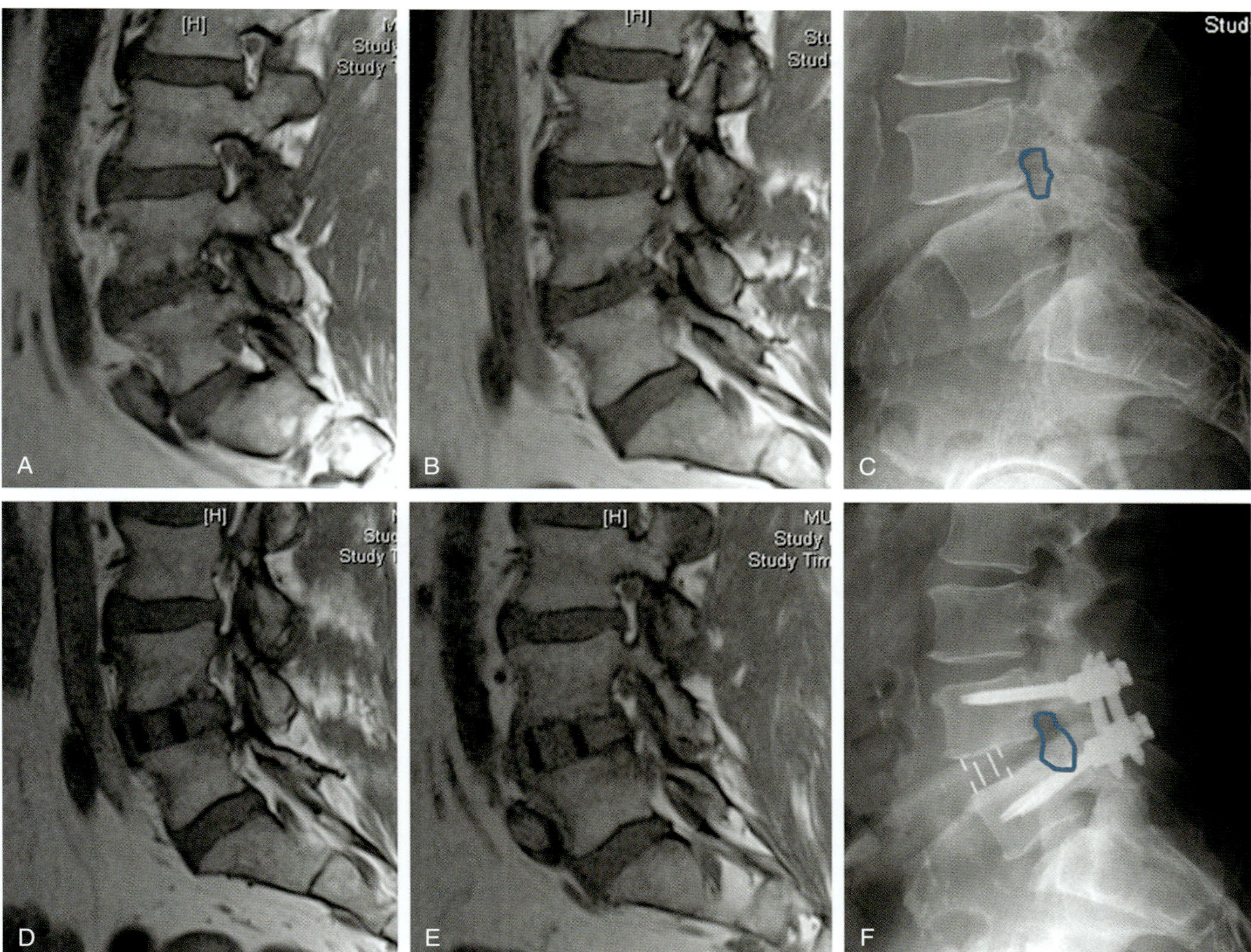

FIGURE 57-7. Preoperative and postoperative images after transpsoas lateral lumbar interbody fusion. Preoperative MRI images (**A** and **B**) and radiograph (**C**) compared with postoperative MRI images (**D** and **E**) and radiograph (**F**) illustrate the restoration of foraminal height after placement of the implant.

peritoneal structures in determining whether there is a left or right preference. For example, a psoas that is relatively large and relatively ventral may be associated with an increased risk of encountering the nerves of the lumbosacral plexus as compared to a psoas that is slender and relatively dorsal. Additionally, we make it routine practice to identify the path of the ureter from kidney to bladder on MRI, if possible, to help prevent injury. In certain deformities, the path of the ureter has guided the approach.

Intraoperative electrophysiologic neuromonitoring should be used to prevent injury to the lumbosacral plexus. We use multimodal monitoring but rely most heavily on free-running and triggered electromyogram (EMG) modes to navigate through the psoas muscle and avoid the neurologic structures within it. While there are monitoring systems that are commercially available through various spinal implant vendors, we have found intraoperative electrophysiologic neuromonitoring provided by experienced neuromonitoring services to be superior. The placement of "redundant" intramuscular leads into the vastus lateralis, vastus medialis, quadriceps femoris, and adductor longus muscles by an experienced neuromonitoring technician has been very useful. For example, we have seen significant responses to triggered EMG in only one or another of the quadriceps leads, such as only the vastus lateralis, while the rectus and medialis leads remain quiet. We also routinely place a cremaster lead in males to monitor the genitofemoral nerve. As well, we routinely use intermittent transcranial electrical motor potential (tcMEP) and find it to be more sensitive in detecting pressure injury to the lumbosacral plexus caused by compression between the retractor blade and transverse processes.

Proper patient positioning speeds the procedure and improves its safety. After intubation and after placement of the neuromonitoring leads, the patient is placed in the lateral decubitus position on an articulating operating table. The pelvis is then secured with 3-inch cloth tape to the operating table just below the table articulation. The hips and knees are flexed to relax the iliopsoas muscle on the operative side. The upper thigh and leg are also secured to the table with 3-inch cloth tape (Fig. 57-10). Bony prominences and upper extremities are well padded, and an axillary role is placed and secured in safe position.

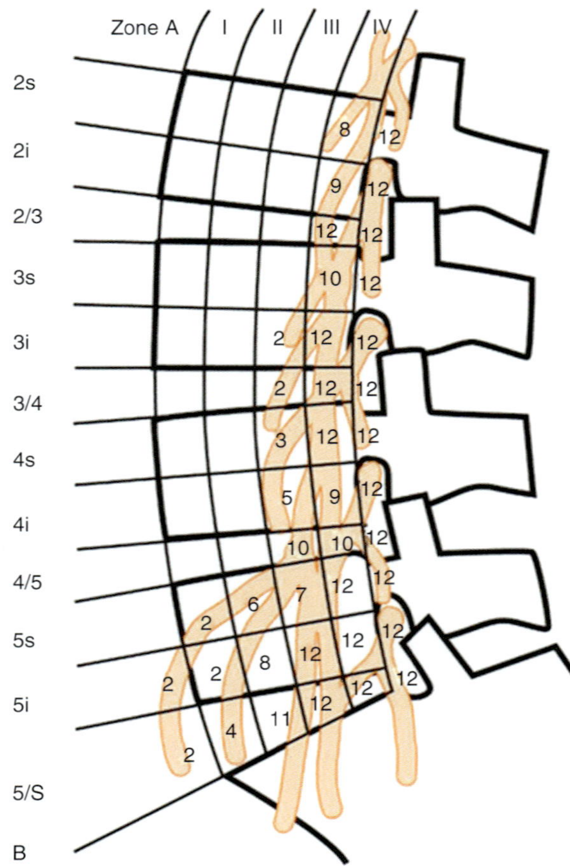

FIGURE 57-8. Position of exiting lumbar plexus and nerve roots in relation to the vertebral body and psoas muscle. The ventral half of the muscle is considered safe for the transpsoas approach. The risk of nerve injury increases from rostral to caudal.

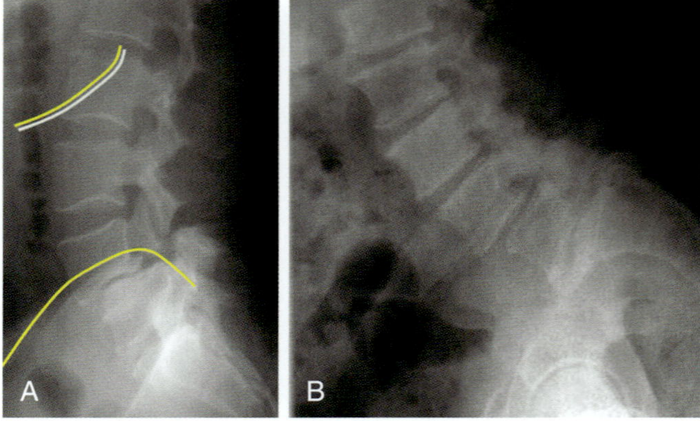

FIGURE 57-9. Unfavorable anatomy for transpsoas lateral approach. **A,** Long 11th and 12th ribs. The intervertebral discs can be approached through the intercostal space or by partial resection of the ribs. **B,** High iliac crests. Found to be more problematic in males. Meticulous positioning helps in approaching the disc space in these patients.

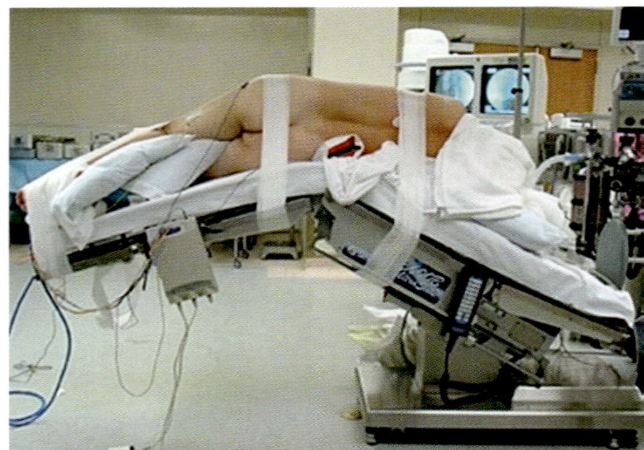

FIGURE 57-10. Positioning of patient for transpsoas lateral lumbar interbody fusion.

The operating table is then maximally flexed to open the space between the 12th rib and the iliac crest. Biplanar fluoroscopy is used to assess the orientation of the operative vertebrae. The operating table is then moved (in rotation and Trendelenburg planes) so that the vertebral end plate is oriented orthogonally to the walls and floor of the operating room (Figs. 57-11A and B). To achieve this, the cross-table C-arm is positioned so that the beam is parallel to the wall and perpendicular to the floor of the room, and the vertebrae are moved to create a true PA view of the vertebrae. Subsequent placement of the C-arm with its beam parallel to the wall will provide lateral images of the vertebrae. Positioning of the vertebrae in this manner allows the surgeon to approach and traverse the disc in a direct lateral trajectory simply by proceeding straight down. This may reduce the risk of traversing the disc obliquely and inadvertently entering the spinal canal or ventral vascular structures. The skin is then marked directly lateral to the operative disc(s). A transverse incision is used for one- or two-level procedures, and a longitudinal incision is used for three or more levels.

After appropriate prepping and draping, the skin is incised at the marked level (Fig. 57-12). The subcutaneous tissue is dissected to expose the lateral fibers of the external oblique muscle. These are gently split in the line of muscle fibers. Gentle manual retraction in this interval under direct visualization reveals internal oblique muscle fibers 90 degrees to the external oblique muscle. Splitting the fibers of internal oblique muscles reveals transverse running fibers that are separated. The separated fibers are retracted by using hand-held McBurney retractors to provide direct visualization of the transversalis fascia, which is opened to reveal retroperitoneal fat. Blunt finger dissection is then performed so that the retroperitoneal fat is moved ventrally. The quadratus lumborum muscle can be felt by dorsal palpation. Further ventral palpation along the quadratus leads to the tip of the transverse processes of lumbar vertebrae as well the (ventrally) overlying psoas muscle. The dorsolateral and ventral aspects of the psoas muscle belly are determined.

Narrow Wylie renal vein retractors are then placed to allow direct visualization of the lateral surface of the psoas muscle. Using direct visualization may reduce the risk of injury to abdominal structures, including peritoneal contents, as compared to approaches relying on radiographic guidance

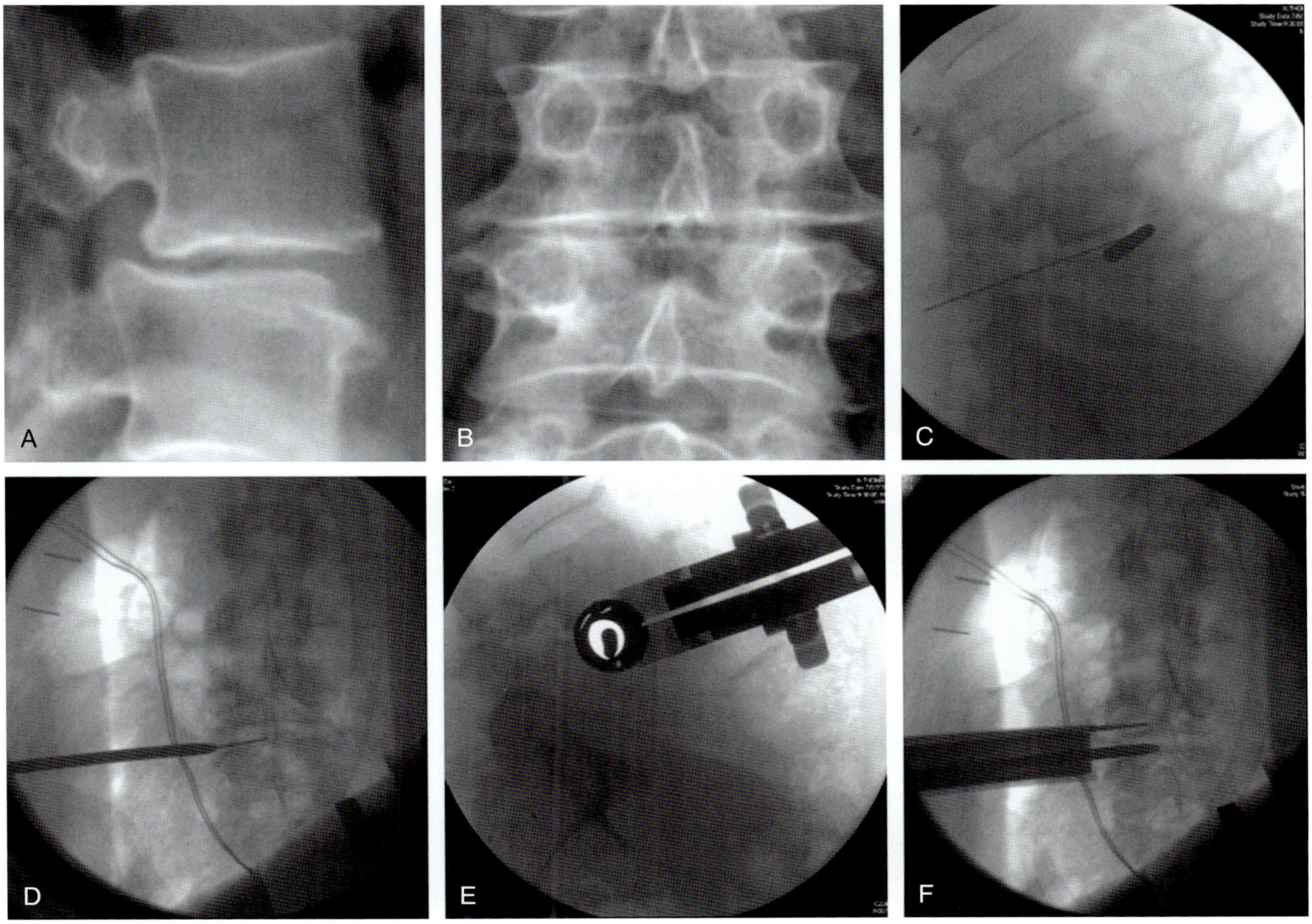

FIGURE 57-11. Series of intraoperative fluoroscopy images during transpsoas lateral lumbar interbody fusion. **A** and **B,** Orthogonal orientation of vertebral end plates. **C–F,** Localization of the disc space and insertion of serial dilators under fluoroscopic guidance.

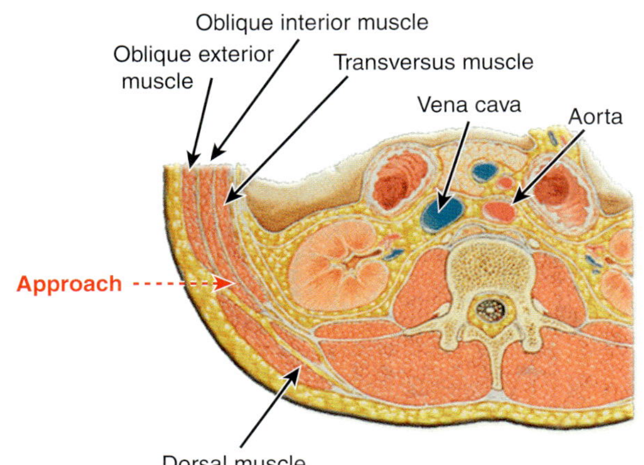

FIGURE 57-12. Diagrammatic representation of the transpsoas approach for lateral interbody fusion.

alone. The surface of the psoas muscle is inspected for identification of the genitofemoral nerve and the ureter. A triggered EMG stimulator probe is then placed upon the lateral aspect of the psoas muscle at the desired surgical level. This is done under direct visualization with confirmation by biplanar fluoroscopy. Stimulation is then applied to assess for potential underlying or adjacent neurologic structures. Biplanar fluoroscopy is used to confirm the optimal position of entry at the lateral surface of the disc and at the junction of the ventral one third and middle one third of the vertebral body (Figs. 57-11C to F).

A guidewire or probe is then placed into the disc. Its position is confirmed by biplanar fluoroscopy. Serial dilation is then performed, and retractor length is determined. The retractor is assembled and passed over the outermost dilator. After removal of the dilators from within the retractor, the lateral aspect of the disc space is inspected. A triggered EMG stimulator is used to stimulate within and around the periphery of the retractor. Subsequently, osseous fixation of the retractor can be performed with certain retractor systems. This is placed adjacent to the end plate, care being taken to not traverse the segmental vessel. The retractor is fixed to the table with a rigid articulating arm (see Fig. 57-11F).

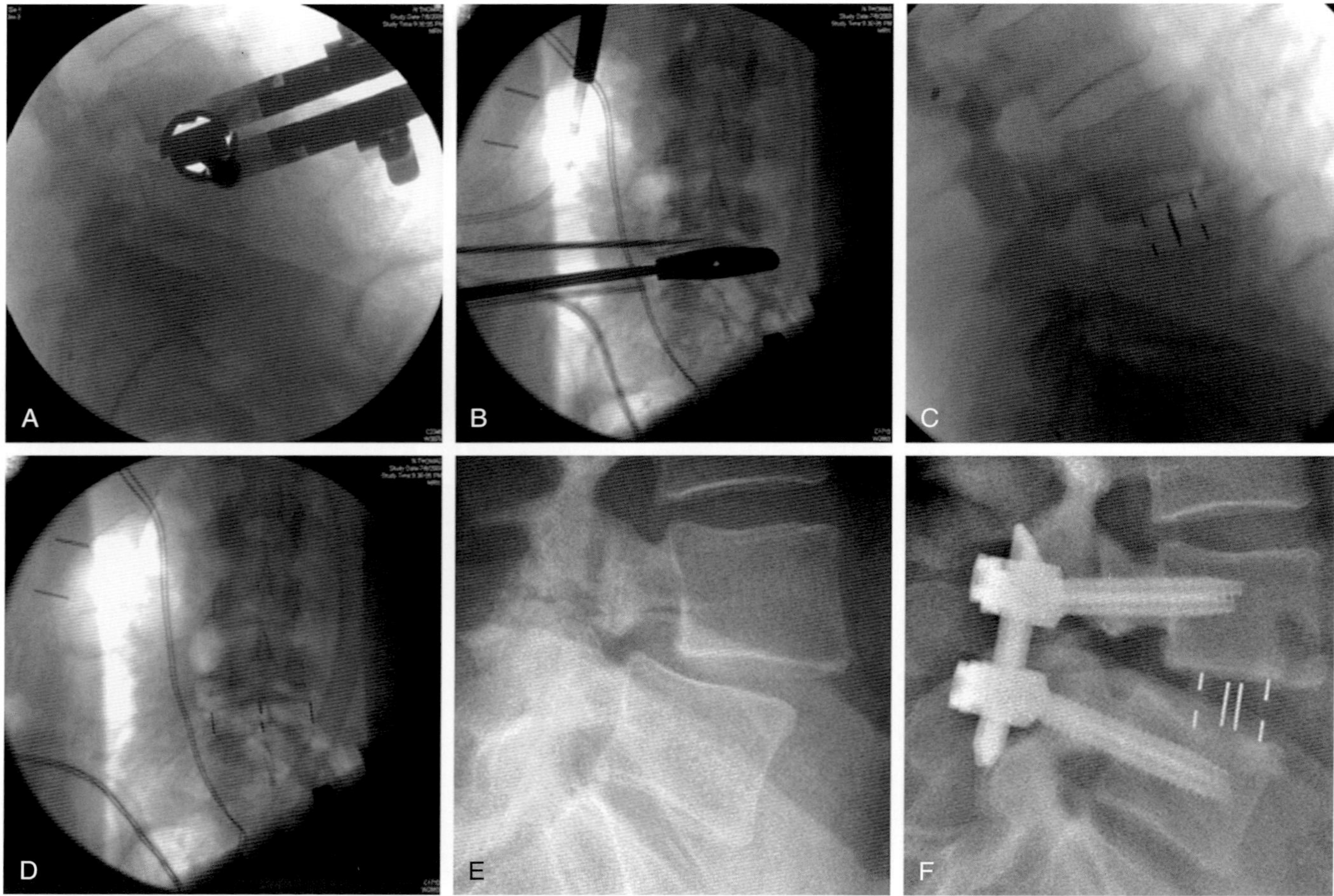

FIGURE 57-13. Intraoperative fluoroscopy images during transpsoas lateral lumbar interbody fusion. **A** and **B,** Insertion of trial implants after preparation of the disc space. **C** and **D,** Final images after insertion of the implant. **E** and **F,** Preoperative and postoperative images of transpsoas lumbar interbody fusion with minimally invasive dorsal instrumented fusion.

After inspection of the lateral aspect of the disc, a bayoneted anulotomy knife is used to perform a box anulotomy. Pituitary forceps are used to remove indwelling nucleus pulposus. Fluoroscopy is used to confirm the direct lateral approach through the disc as shavers, curettes, rasps, and rotary shavers are used to perform a thorough discectomy, taking care not to traverse the end plates. The vertebral end plates are then prepared with rasps and rakes to remove the cartilaginous portion of the end plate but not breach the bony aspect of the end plate. Finally, a Cobb elevator is used to perform a lateral release across the opposite side of the disc space under direct visualization as well as biplanar fluoroscopy.

Trial implants of sequentially increasing size are passed to select the proper implant size (Figs. 57-13A and B). The appropriate size spacer is selected and packed with bone graft or bone graft substitute. The implant is advanced between the vertebral bodies under direct biplanar fluoroscopy to ensure proper placement of the implant (Figs. 57-13C to F). Free-running EMG and the more sensitive intermittent tcMEP provide monitoring of the integrity of the local nerve roots throughout the procedure.

The operative site is inspected under direct visualization to ensure complete hemostasis before and after removal of the retractor blades. The wound is then closed with absorbable suture ligatures in layers approximating each layer of muscle fiber as well as fascia. The patient may then be transferred to the prone position for pedicle screw placement.

Outcomes

The use of the lateral lumbar interbody fusion technique for lumbar interbody fusion is associated with shorter operative times, minimal blood loss, early postoperative patient mobilization, and shorter hospital stays. Diaz et al., in their series of 18 patients, had a mean operative time of 125 minutes, and intraoperative blood loss of 50 mL. The average hospital stay was 2 days.[63] The technique led to significant improvement of visual analogue scale and Oswestry Disability Index scores at the end of 1 year. Bergey et al., in their series of 21 patients, observed an average operative time of 149 minutes, average blood loss of 150 mL, and average postoperative hospital stay of 4.1 days.[64] Immediate clinical improvement was seen in 84% of patients. The average visual analogue scale score decreased by 5.9 at the end of 6 months, and an excellent clinical outcome was seen in 60% of patients at 6 months. No cases of implant migration or pseudarthrosis were observed in any of the patients.

Complications

The most common complications seen with the lateral interbody fusion technique are transient groin and thigh paraesthesias. Recent papers describing the lateral interbody fusion technique have reported the varying rate of such complications to be bewteen 0.7% and 62.7%.[64-67] In a large clinical series by Rogers et al., postoperative neurologic deficit was reported to be 0.7% (4/600 patients).[65] Transient thigh paraesthesia and numbness were seen in 30% (6/21) of patients in a clinical series by Bergey et al.[64] Improvement from the paraesthesia was seen in 4 weeks in four of these six patients. Uncommon complications such as transient psoas hematoma and transient iliopsoas weakness on the side of surgical approach are also possible. In another clinical series, Wang et al. found postoperative thigh numbness, pain, weakness, and dysaesthesia lateralized to the side of the approach in 30.4% (7/23) of patients.[66] The symptoms resolved during the postoperative period in all but one patient, who needed admission to the rehabilitation unit to facilitate recovery. In another clinical series, Cummock et al. reported the incidence of postoperative neurologic deficit to be 62.7%.[67] Fifty percent of these patients had their symptoms resolved in 3 months, and 90% within the first postoperative year. Considering the high incidence of postoperative ipsilateral thigh symptoms, we advise discussing this possibility with patients prior to surgery.

The rate of complications may be reduced in the future with more widespread use of tcMEP, attention to surgical techniques such as hemostasis, minimizing trauma to the psoas by careful dissection and avoiding tension on the muscle, performing gentle dilation to the disc space, use of local medications such as intramuscular dexamethasone (in psoas), and performance of a rapid procedure to reduce retraction time.

Summary

The use of the lateral lumbar interbody fusion approach creates a minimally invasive way to achieve a ventral fusion in the lumbar spine. The approach is now being applied to a multitude of degenerative conditions, including spinal deformities. The use of neuromonitoring and accurate intraoperative fluoroscopy reduces the rate of complications with this novel approach.

KEY REFERENCES

Buttermann GR, Glazer PA, Bradford DS: The use of bone allografts in the spine. *Clin Orthop Relat Res* 324:75–85, 1996.

Cummock MD, Vanni S, Levi AD, et al: An analysis of postoperative thigh symptoms after minimally invasive transpsoas lumbar interbody fusion. *J Neurosurg Spine* 15(1):11–18, 2011.

Fischgrund JS, Mackay M, Herkowitz HN, et al: 1997 Volvo Award winner in clinical studies: degenerative lumbar spondylolisthesis with spinal stenosis: a prospective, randomized study comparing decompressive laminectomy and arthrodesis with and without spinal instrumentation. *Spine (Phila Pa 1976)* 22(24):2807–2812, 1997.

Jorgenson SS, Lowe TG, France J, Sabin J: A prospective analysis of autograft versus allograft in posterolateral lumbar fusion in the same patient: a minimum of 1-year follow-up in 144 patients. *Spine (Phila Pa 1976)* 19(18):2048–2053, 1994.

Kornblum MB, Fischgrund JS, Herkowitz HN, et al: Degenerative lumbar spondylolisthesis with spinal stenosis: a prospective long-term study comparing fusion and pseudarthrosis. *Spine (Phila Pa 1976)* 29(7):726–733, 2004; discussion 733–734.

Moe JH: A critical analysis of methods of fusion for scoliosis: an evaluation in two hundred and sixty-six patients. *J Bone Joint Surg [Am]* 40(3):529–554, 1958.

Ozgur BM, Aryan HE, Pimenta L, Taylor WR: Extreme lateral interbody fusion (XLIF): a novel surgical technique for anterior lumbar interbody fusion. *Spine J* 6(4):435–443, 2006.

Rogers WB, Gerber EJ, Patterson J: Intraoperative and early postoperative complications in extreme lateral interbody fusion: an analysis of 600 cases. *Spine (Phila Pa 1976)* 36(1):26–32, 2011.

Simpson AK, Chambliss H, White AP: Lateral lumbar transpsoas interbody fusion. *Tech Orthop* 26(3):156–165, 2011.

Wang MY, Mummaneni PV: Minimally invasive surgery for thoracolumbar spinal deformity: initial clinical experience with clinical and radiographic outcomes. *Neurosurg Focus* 28(3):E9, 2010.

REFERENCES

The complete reference list is available online at expertconsult.com.

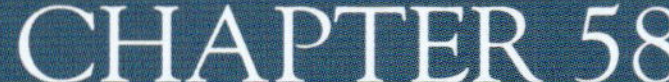

CHAPTER 58

Indications for Spine Fusion for Axial Pain

Daniel J. Hoh | Zoher Ghogawala | Richard Schlenk

Low back pain (LBP) is among the leading reasons for individuals to seek medical attention. One out of 17 patients seen by a family practitioner presents primarily with LBP, with approximately 31 million patient visits for back pain occurring in the United States annually.[1] It is estimated that 70% to 85% of individuals will suffer an acute episode of LBP in their lifetime. Most people experience a benign course with near complete resolution of symptoms within a few months of onset.[2] Unfortunately, a small percentage, approximately 5% to 10%, continue to develop persistent or chronic LBP.[3]

Persistent LBP is often a significant source of personal anxiety, distress, and disability. In addition, chronic LBP weighs heavily on society. It is estimated that 28% of the working population in the United States will be disabled by LBP at some time during their professional lives, with approximately 8% of the entire work force disabled in a given year.[3] Acute LBP occurs across a wide range of ages. Chronic LBP, however, is the primary cause of disability in individuals less than 50 years of age, when most people expect to be at their peak productivity. The total socioeconomic burden of LBP, including both health-care costs and lost wages, is estimated at $100 billion to $200 billion annually, with two thirds of this cost due to work-related disability.[4] Of alarming concern is that while the incidence of diagnosed chronic LBP has been stable for 30 years, the rate of LBP-related disability claims has increased by 14 times that of population growth.[5]

These individual and socioeconomic problems are further compounded by a lack of consensus in the health-care community regarding the appropriate diagnosis and management of chronic LBP. LBP is a generalized somatic complaint that may be the manifestation of one or a combination of various processes. The underlying pathophysiologic mechanisms may be inherent to the spinal column or nerves or may be referred from various supporting musculotendinous structures. Furthermore, which anatomic structures, whether internal or external to the spine, are the actual source of pain for a given individual is often unclear. Potential LBP etiologies include the intervertebral discs, facet joints, bony vertebral column, neural elements, muscles, ligaments, tendons, and fascia. While these various structures are associated with certain LBP syndromes, such as "axial low back pain," "discogenic pain," "facetogenic pain," "mechanical back pain," and "myofascial pain," the true relationship between an anatomic structure, pathophysiologic process, and pain transmission remains difficult to confirm. As a result, definitive diagnosis and appropriate treatment intervention remain challenging at best.

Of these LBP syndromes, axial LBP has undergone the most intense scrutiny by the health-care, scientific, and general communities. Axial LBP is described as a pain disorder of the lumbosacral region that is theorized to be secondary to advanced degeneration of the intervertebral discs. The term *axial LBP* is often used interchangeably with other, more anatomically directed terms such as *discogenic pain*, *degenerative disc disease*, *internal disc disruption*, *black disc disease*, and *disc prolapse*. The presumed pathophysiology of axial back pain is that accelerated disc degeneration results in abnormal alterations in the mechanical and chemical nature of the disc. Pain generation is believed to be due to the ensuing change in segmental biomechanics as it leads to instability, abnormal motion, or loss of stiffness. Alternatively, pain may be transmitted by changes in the biochemical environment through release of inflammatory cytokines or nociceptive neurotransmitters.

Controversy regarding axial LBP is due to a number of factors. First, there is a lack of definitive scientific evidence identifying the disc as the pathoanatomic source of pain. The validity and reliability of current diagnostic modalities for discerning which disc or discs are the primary pain generators are unresolved. Second, general medical journals and popular media have generated controversy by suggesting that surgeons are overtreating axial LBP without any proven basis for diagnosis and intervention. Subsequently, many people have made the claim that current trends for operative management of axial LBP have been propagated by ulterior interests from the surgical community and medical device industry. In fact, survey and national inpatient data sample results have indicated that lumbar fusion surgery for degenerative spinal conditions has been steadily increasing. Approximately 300,000 spine fusions are performed annually in the United States, which is a relative increase of 220% between 1990 and 2001. Of these fusion operations, about 75% are performed for degenerative disc disorders and spinal stenosis. A national inpatient data sample identifies degenerative disc disease as the diagnosis that accounts for the largest increase in the number of lumbar fusions during this period.[6]

Spine fusion for axial LBP is predicated on the theory that pain is related to the degenerated disc's causing abnormal movement across a motion segment. Painful disc degeneration may be analogous to other arthritic joint pathology involving the hips or knees, in which the degenerated joint causes altered local mechanical and chemical processes that generate pain. Arthrodesis across these degenerated joints in the appendicular skeleton is known to eliminate pain successfully. Spine surgeons have adopted fusion across a degenerated disc as a method for stabilizing the abnormal motion segment to similarly relieve pain.

Unfortunately, the spine surgical literature has failed to demonstrate consistent successful clinical outcomes after fusion surgery in patients with axial LBP. Critics of fusion surgery for axial LBP again raise the issue that current imaging and functional diagnostic modalities do not accurately identify the source of LBP in most patients that lack evidence of nerve compression or neurologic deficit.[7] Therefore, difficulties with patient selection and determining which levels to fuse may account for suboptimal rates of clinical success. Furthermore, the relationship between solid arthrodesis and LBP relief remains equivocal. This uncertainty is accentuated by an overall lack of improvement in successful outcomes despite increasing fusion rates with advancing surgical technique, fixation devices, and osteobiologic agents.

Alternatively, proponents of fusion surgery argue that patients with axial LBP who ultimately undergo surgery are unlike other lumbar spine surgery patients. Often, these patients have had debilitating pain for years with failure of multiple nonsurgical therapies. Axial LBP patients often suffer from psychosocial disorders, chronic narcotic use, and prolonged disability, which negatively affect outcome with any intervention. Even a modest rate of improvement in pain, narcotic use, or ability to return to work represents a positive result for an otherwise desperate patient population that has frequently exhausted all other therapeutic resources.

The controversy regarding fusion surgery for axial LBP continues today. In 1989, Nachemson issued an editorial stating that for the majority of patients, basic science has yet to demonstrate the true origin of back pain.[8] He further stated that our present-day treatments are mostly ineffective, as evidenced by the epidemic increase in back pain related disability in all industrialized societies. Twenty years later, these issues remain subjects for debate, and several recent highly contested studies suggest that there is a lack of clinical evidence to support the surgical treatment for a number of degenerative lumbar disorders.[6,9] To gain a better understanding of axial LBP and the indications for spine fusion, this chapter provides an overview of the pathophysiology and current literature with regard to diagnosis, surgical treatment, and outcomes for axial LBP.

Pathophysiology

The normal lumbar intervertebral disc consists of fibrocartilaginous tissue designed to absorb and dissipate load applied to the spinal column. The two components of the disc are the nucleus pulposus and the anulus fibrosus. The nucleus pulposus is composed of proteoglycan aggrecan molecules with 70% to 80% water content. Absorption of water into the nucleus provides disc height and resistance to compression. With loading, water defuses out of the disc, and subsequent reabsorption occurs with unloading. The anulus is an interlacing collagen network that provides tensile strength in axial rotation. With bending or compression of two adjacent vertebrae, the nucleus pulposus changes volumetrically, causing bulging of the disc away from the internal axis of rotation. The anulus also functions to limit and contain expansion or herniation of the nucleus.

With aging, the disc gradually becomes less hydrated, and the concentration of proteoglycans decreases. Normal disc metabolism shifts toward catabolic processes, which further deplete proteoglycans and lead to increasing matrix degeneration. As a result, the disc becomes progressively dysfunctional as the nuclear material is replaced by desiccated fibrocartilaginous material. Loss of fluid results in decreased hydrostatic pressure as a mechanism for effective load transference. Thinning or microfracture of the end plates can occur, and subsequent loss of end-plate vascularity reduces transport of nutrients and waste products out of the disc. Eventually, with cyclic loading of the degenerated disc, radial fissures or cracks propagate through the anulus, with migration of nuclear material peripherally. With complete anular disruption, disc material can herniate into the central canal, lateral recess, or foramen. These degenerative processes are estimated to occur in 90% of normal individuals by 50 years of age.[10]

In 1970, Crock first associated back pain with the pathophysiologic process of disc desiccation and subsequent radial fissure formation of the anulus.[11,12] He termed this entity *internal disc disruption*, which was characterized by the progressive disruption of the internal architecture of the disc while essentially maintaining the external shape such that nerve root compression did not occur. Crock hypothesized that pain is generated when degradation of the disc matrix causes release of inflammatory cytokines, which then migrate through the disrupted inner anular fibers to irritate the high concentration of sensory nerve endings in the outer anulus. His conclusion was supported radiographically by the relative absence of any nerve root compression but the high correlation of concordant pain in discs that exhibited severe radial fissures with intradiscal contrast injection.

Since then, several theories regarding the relationship between degenerative disc disease and pain generation have developed. The mechanical theory suggests that degeneration results in alteration in the biomechanical properties of the disc. As the disc degenerates and the anulus becomes disrupted, increasing instability occurs at the motion segment. Therefore, with normal physiologic loading, the motion segment responds with excessive compression, bending, or rotation, which can trigger pain transmission in surrounding nociceptors. CT and MRI studies have quantified the response of the lumbar spine to rotatory torque and have correlated increased axial rotation in degenerated discs with pain provocation on discography.[13,14] Also as the disc desiccates, it loses hydrostatic pressure, so with normal physiologic loading, more stress is transferred to the anulus and the end plate, where pain-sensitive nerve fibers are in high concentration. Increased stress to the end plate can lead to end-plate fracture and disc herniation into the vertebral body, which may further propagate pain generation.

The chemical theory suggests that catabolism of the disc results in release of proinflammatory chemical mediators. Nitric oxide, phospholipase A_2, prostaglandin E, matrix metalloproteinases, and other cytokines have been implicated as chemical agents that infiltrate through radial fissures to irritate nociceptors that are present in the outer aspect of the anulus and the end plate. Proteoglycan breakdown is known to have a high concentration of the neurotransmitter glutamate, which may in turn stimulate glutamate-specific receptors in the dorsal root ganglion, resulting in back or radicular pain in the absence of nerve root compression. Nociceptors are also known to be present in high concentrations elsewhere within the spinal canal, such as the posterior longitudinal ligament, dura, and blood vessels.

Alternatively, although the disc may demonstrate signs of degeneration, pain may arise from other associated structures. The facet joints, ligaments, fascia, nerve roots, and dura are capable of transmitting pain. While disc degeneration may be the initial inciting pathology, one or more of these structures may in fact be the source of pain. Progressive disc disease results in increased load transference to surrounding structures such as the facet joints, ligaments, and paraspinal muscles, which may eventually exceed their capacity for resistance. Cyclic loading to these structures can lead to increased arthropathy, ligamentous hypertrophy, and muscle fatigue, which may contribute to pain. The medial branch of the dorsal primary rami courses around the facet and innervates the joint capsule and may be a particularly pain-sensitive fiber signaling back pain with increased stress. Diagnostic blockade of various spinal and paraspinal structures with injected anesthetic may be performed to evaluate certain areas as potential pain generators. Studies performed in patients with similar presentations of LBP have demonstrated a wide range of sources of pain, including the disc, facet joints, and sacroiliac joints. Therefore, while the degenerated disc may be implicated in the pathophysiology of LBP, it remains unclear whether the disc itself or other surrounding structures are the actual source of pain.

Diagnosis

Patients with axial LBP generally present with a deep, aching pain localized to the lower back, sacral, or gluteal region. The pain is characteristically worsened with mechanical activities such as bending, twisting, or lifting and is relieved with recumbency. Pain is also increased with lumbar flexion, such as when ascending stairs, and is presumed to be secondary to increased ventral loading on the degenerated discs. Also, patients often describe increased pain with prolonged sitting. Interestingly, patients may also describe buttock or leg pain (generally limited to above the knee) that is not radicular in nature but may be referred sclerotomal pain.

Physical examination rarely provides information in facilitating the diagnosis of axial LBP or the level of disease. Often, the physical and neurologic assessment is normal. The clinical history and the physical and neurologic examination, however, are critical in evaluating other potential etiologies of LBP such as nerve root compression, spinal deformity, fracture, spinal instability, spondylolisthesis, tumor, or infection. Masqueraders that closely mimic axial LBP symptomatology and that can be assessed on physical examination include myofascial pain, sacroiliac joint pain, piriformis syndrome, and hip osteoarthritis.

In light of a normal physical examination and relatively ubiquitous symptomatology, the diagnosis of axial LBP is made clinically using various radiologic studies. Because of the overt dependence on imaging for determining the source of pain, there has been intense scrutiny of radiologic criteria for identifying which discs are painful and which patients may ultimately benefit from fusion surgery.

Plain Radiographs

Plain radiographic findings in patients with axial LBP may demonstrate characteristics consistent with degenerative disc disease. While radiography does not visualize the soft tissue disc, plain films may reveal decreased disc height consistent with a collapsed or dehydrated disc (Fig. 58-1A). Sclerotic end plates or bone-on-bone appearance are commonly seen with severely degenerated discs (Fig. 58-1B). Plain radiographs can be performed with patients in weight bearing, flexion, or extension to demonstrate the alignment of the spine and the nature of the motion segments under normal physiologic loading. The presence of hypermobility or malalignment

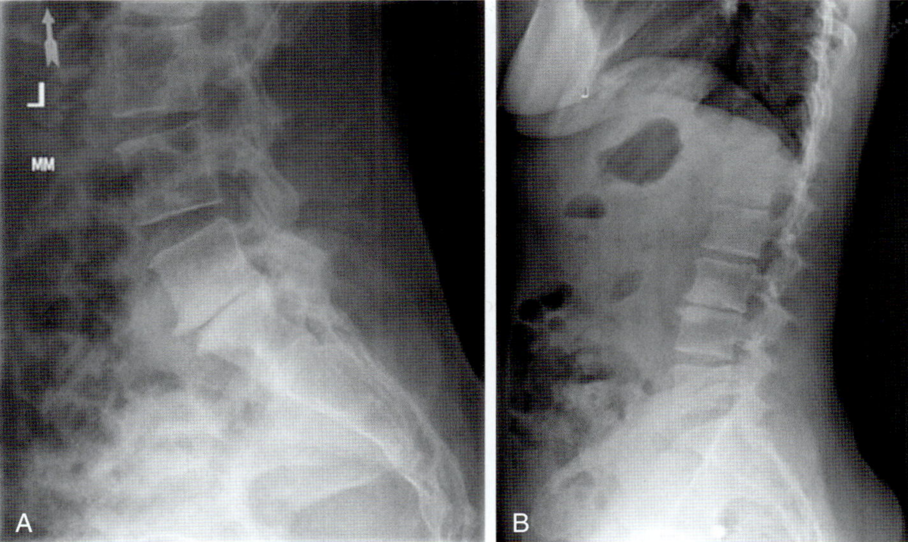

FIGURE 58-1. **A,** Lateral radiograph demonstrating a degenerated, collapsed L5-S1 intervertebral disc space. **B,** Lateral radiograph demonstrating a degenerated L3-4 intervertebral disc space with sclerotic end plates.

under such stresses may help to identify which levels are symptomatic or may suggest other pathologic processes.

In evaluating lumbar plain radiography in symptomatic patients, Scavone et al. observed that radiographs alone were uniquely diagnostic in only 2.4% of patients.[15] Liang and Komaroff found that lumbar radiographs did not provide diagnostic value in differentiating patients with acute versus chronic LBP.[16] Coste et al. reported that there was a high degree of variability in interpretation of plain films performed in LBP patients, underscoring the poor diagnostic value of these studies for this condition.[17] Many clinicians conclude that the degenerative findings that are seen on lumbar plain radiographs may in fact represent normal age-related changes and as such provide little information with regard to differentiating symptomatic degenerated discs from asymptomatic age-appropriate discs. Plain radiographs, however, are useful in the assessment of axial LBP for effectively ruling out other etiologies of back pain. Fractures, osteomyelitis, tumor, spondylolisthesis, and deformity can often be quickly assessed with lumbar weight-bearing or 36-inch standing plain films. Therefore, plain radiographs are indicated in LBP patients who are of pediatric age, are at high risk for osteoporosis, have a history of prior surgery, present with neurologic deficit or gross deformity, or have clinical signs suggestive of trauma, infection, or malignancy.

Discography

The ability of discography to diagnose degenerated disc disease and identify painful symptomatic discs has been the subject of ongoing debate. Discography is an invasive procedure by which a needle is placed percutaneously into the nucleus pulposus under fluoroscopic or CT guidance. Contrast is injected into the nucleus, and images are generated on plain radiographs and/or axial CT images. The flow of contrast within the disc provides information regarding disc morphology and the integrity of the anulus. Contrast filling of a degenerated, desiccated disc may highlight a collapsed narrow disc space. Radial fissures may be revealed by contrast leakage from the nucleus into the periphery and, in the case of anular disruption, spilling of contrast into the canal or foramen. The integrity of the anulus can be inferred from the resistance or volume of injection, normal discs having a high resistance and smaller volume of injection. Low resistance or a high volume of injection suggests disruption or a possible tear in the anulus.

One unique feature of discography, in contrast to other conventional passive imaging modalities, is the behavioral component of the diagnostic procedure. Essential to discography is the evaluation of both the suspected symptomatic disc and control or asymptomatic discs. With injection of contrast into an abnormal disc, the discographer assesses for provocation of concordant pain. Pain with disc injection is likely due to either an increase in intradiscal pressure or the displacement of biochemical agents. With pressurized contrast injection, stretching of pain-sensitive nerve endings in the anulus may be stimulated, or stress may be transmitted to the end plates or vertebral body. Alternatively, contrast injection into the nucleus may cause displacement of inflammatory cytokines, which then diffuse through radial fissures to the periphery, where they may stimulate nociceptors in the outer anulus or the surrounding environment. Ideally, the provoked pain is similar to or an exact reproduction of the patient's presenting back pain. Otherwise, the injection provokes dissimilar pain or does not produce pain, and the discogram is inconclusive or negative for that level. The gold standard for diagnostic discography is exact reproduction of pain at the morphologically abnormal level with no pain provocation at control or normal discs.

Several studies provide evidence to support discography as an effective method for identifying degenerated, symptomatic discs. Cadaveric studies have shown a strong correlation between discographic contrast distribution and the severity of degeneration on gross examination. There is also a good correlation between disc morphology on discography and intraoperative findings of disc protrusions and herniations. Importantly, studies have identified morphologic findings on discography that correlate with concordant pain provocation. As expected, pain provocation is most commonly observed in discs that demonstrate dorsal anular tears (65.3%) as compared to simply degenerated discs (36.6%), internal anular disruption (20%), or intraosseous disc herniations (0%).[18] The use of axial CT imaging provides even further morphologic assessment of the disc. Using the Dallas Discogram Description (DDD) for CT-based discography, severe and moderately graded degenerated discs show a strong correlation with exact reproduction of pain, anular disruption being the best predictor of concordant pain.[19] McCutcheon and Thomas found that contrast tracking to the periphery of the anulus suggesting radial fissures and anular disruption has an 87% correlation with concordant pain.[20]

Subsequent studies, however, have failed to consistently reproduce these positive correlations. Several studies have demonstrated pain production with discography in otherwise normal-appearing discs in asymptomatic individuals. Carragee et al. studied discography in a group of patients who did not have back pain but had chronic pain related to iliac crest bone harvest for non–lumbar spine surgery. Of these patients, 37.5% had similar or exact reproduction of donor site pain with lumbar discography. Some have proposed that high-pressure injection is responsible for false-positive pain production in normal discs. However, even with low-pressure discography, pain was produced in the same number of asymptomatic volunteers as LBP patients.[21] Vanharanta et al. found that morphologically normal discs on DDD grading still provoked some pain response in 24% of individuals.[22] Also, they observed that severely degenerated discs resulted in exact reproduction of pain in only 22% of individuals. In their study, even discs with severe anular disruption had exact pain reproduction in only 36% of subjects. The reverse association demonstrated slightly better correlation. Patients who had a positive pain response were also more likely to have evidence of disc degeneration. However, discs with exact reproduction of pain were distributed among a range of DDD grades from slight (20%) to moderate (39%) to severe (37%). The best correlation among patients with exact reproduced pain was for severe anular disruption (77%). Overall, the investigators found that painful discs tend to have higher degrees of degeneration and anular disruption compared to painless discs. However, all discs as they deteriorated were more likely to provoke pain, although often the pain was not similar to the presenting back pain and therefore the degenerating disc could not be conclusively diagnosed as the symptomatic disc.

Further adding to diagnostic uncertainty, studies have shown that nonspinal factors such as abnormal psychometric findings, chronic pain states, and disputed compensation claims also strongly correlate with positive discography.[21]

Despite these conflicting studies, many clinicians have adopted discography as an instrument for presurgical screening and patient selection, with the presumption that positive discography can reliably predict which patients and levels will respond favorably to fusion. Specifically, discs that demonstrate abnormal morphology and/or concordant pain provocation are likely the symptomatic levels. Therefore, fusion across the positive discographic motion segment will result in alleviation of pain. Conversely, discs with normal morphology or discs that do not reproduce similar pain can be reasonably excluded from surgery or the fusion construct. As a result, for many surgeons, discography is assigned a critical role in selecting which patients with chronic back pain are surgical candidates and ultimately in determining which levels to fuse.

Certain studies have demonstrated that positive discography reliably predicts good surgical outcomes. Simmons and Segil studied patients who had discography prior to undergoing lumbar discectomy, discectomy and fusion, or fusion alone. They found that preoperative discography demonstrated 82% diagnostic accuracy in identifying the symptomatic level.[23] This study, however, represented a heterogeneous patient population that included not only back pain patients, but also those suffering from herniated discs and nerve root compression. Colhoun et al. found that among patients undergoing lumbar fusion, 89% of those with a positive preoperative discogram had significant improvement postoperatively, including decreased pain, return to work, and cessation of analgesics.[18] Patients with nondiagnostic preoperative discography had a lower rate of success after lumbar fusion, only 52% of patients reporting a similar satisfactory postoperative outcome.

Varying degrees of success with preoperative discography have been observed. Good clinical outcomes have been demonstrated in 64% to 86% of patients with positive discography who undergo anterior lumbar interbody fusion (ALIF).[24-26] Other studies have shown that more than 90% of patients with positive discography improve after posterior lumbar fusion.[27,28] Derby et al. argue that better correlation is observed when chemically sensitive discs are identified on preoperative discography.[29] Chemically sensitive discs provoke concordant pain under particularly low-pressure injection, suggesting that pain is generated by the displacement of biochemical agents that then stimulate sensory nerve endings in the outer anulus. Therefore, Derby et al. hypothesize that patients with chemically sensitive discs require complete discectomy with thorough removal of the offending disc for pain relief. Among patients with chemically sensitive discs, successful clinical outcome was observed in 89% of patients who underwent discectomy and interbody fusion, compared to only 20% of patients who underwent dorsolateral fusion alone and 12% of patients who were treated nonoperatively. Similarly, Weatherly et al. used discography to identify painful, symptomatic discs within a fused segment in patients with persistent LBP after posterior lumbar fusion.[30] Subsequent ventral discectomy and interbody fusion of the positive discographic levels resulted in complete resolution of pain.

The positive predictive value of discography for success after lumbar fusion, however, has not been borne out through multiple repeated studies. Of particular concern is that the potential for a high false-positive rate may lead to an inappropriate rise in fusion surgery and consequently an unacceptable rate of unsatisfactory outcomes. Carragee et al. evaluated patients with positive single-level discography using low-pressure injection who then underwent lumbar fusion of the abnormal disc.[31] They observed that only 27% of patients had a highly effective outcome as defined by a visual analogue score (VAS) of 2 or less, Oswestry Disability Index (ODI) of 15 or less, full return to work, and cessation of narcotics and analgesics. A minimal acceptable outcome of VAS of 4 or less, ODI of 30 or less, no narcotic use, and at least some gainful employment was reached in only 43% of patients. The authors concluded that in the best case calculation, the adjusted positive predictive value for a minimal acceptable outcome was only 55%. Other studies have similarly found less promising results, with successful outcomes in only 35% to 46% of patients who had undergone lumbar fusion with discography as the primary diagnostic tool.[32] It should be noted, however, that in one of these studies, a particularly low arthrodesis rate was observed (47.9%), which may account for the unexpected poor outcomes.

Overall, discography remains an imperfect instrument for diagnosing and localizing discogenic pain. Particularly, discography has come into doubt as a reliable measure for predicting which patients and what levels will respond well to fusion surgery. Much of this lack of accuracy and consistency may be dependent on discography technique and reporting of pertinent positive and negative findings. Furthermore, patient, discographer, and surgeon expectations may bias toward false-positive results, potentially leading to increasing the number of surgeries or creating unrealistic prospects for successful results. Ultimately, the degree to which discography plays a role in surgical decision making largely depends on the surgeon's prior experience in drawing upon this diagnostic modality and also establishing clear communication with the patient with regard to reasonable expectations for outcome. Given the available data, discography is best indicated for correlating concordant pain in discs that are morphologically abnormal, as the finding of pain provocation in otherwise normal-appearing discs appears to be clinically irrelevant. Discography may also facilitate assessing prior to fusion whether levels adjacent to the symptomatic level are also abnormal and may be included in the fusion construct. Last, in certain circumstances, discography may play a role in evaluating patients who have persistent back pain after posterior lumbar fusion to assess for a painful pseudarthrosis or the presence of a symptomatic disc within the fused segments.

Magnetic Resonance Imaging

MRI is the radiologic study of choice for visualizing the soft tissue structures of the spine, including the discs, ligaments, joints, and neural elements. As a result, MRI is the preferred test for nerve root compression from disc herniation or lumbar stenosis. MRI is also well equipped for clearly visualizing the intervertebral disc. Besides the ability to image in multiple planes, MRI, with good-quality spin-echo T2-weighted images, provides excellent characterization of the morphology of the disc and superb differentiation between the nucleus pulposus and anulus. The signal intensity within the nucleus is related to the concentration of water in the proteoglycan

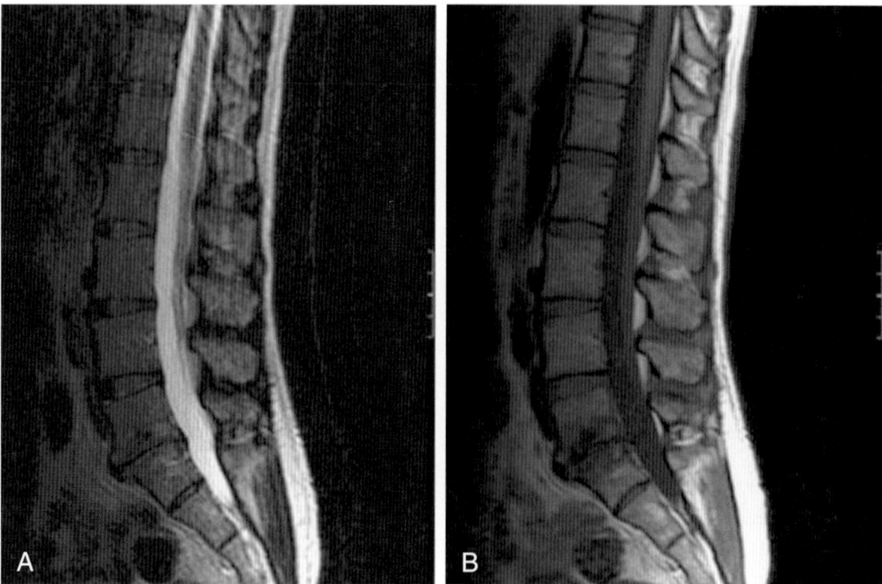

FIGURE 58-2. A, T2-weighted sagittal MRI demonstrating a severely degenerated L5-S1 disc with abnormal signal changes in the adjacent vertebral body bone marrow. **B,** T1-weighted sagittal MRI demonstrating decreased signal in the adjacent vertebral bone marrow consistent with vascularized, fibrous tissue.

matrix. Therefore, a reduction in signal intensity correlates with matrix degradation and disc degeneration (Fig. 58-2A). The ability of MRI to detect loss of water content and disc desiccation has prompted consideration of MRI as a sensitive measure of degenerative disc disease.

MRI also well characterizes the effect of disc degeneration on the adjacent end plates and vertebral bodies. With advanced degeneration of the discs, greater load is transferred to the end plates. In the early phase, the normal vertebral body bone marrow is replaced with vascularized fibrous tissue as a reparative response to injury.[33] This appears on T1-weighted MRI as decreased signal (Fig. 58-2B), and conversely increased signal on T2-weighted images. With chronic degeneration, the normally red bone marrow is converted to yellow marrow as the marrow elements are replaced by fat cells, a situation that appears to represent a chronic, stable state. The prevalence of fat is represented by increased signal on T1-weighted MRI.

Because MRI adeptly characterizes the various stages of disc degeneration and its effects on the discovertebral complex, it is often performed as the initial study in evaluating patients who present with axial LBP. However, it is unclear whether findings of disc degeneration on MRI are in fact age-related changes or abnormal processes that are related to pain generation. Several studies have evaluated MRI in asymptomatic volunteers and found that more than 30% of individuals without back pain have evidence of degenerated lumbar discs.[5,34] These include significant findings of herniated discs (24%) and anular defects (14%) in individuals who are asymptomatic. Boden et al. observed that 28% of asymptomatic individuals had an MRI of the lumbar spine that was characterized as abnormal.[34] The most common finding was bulging discs, which appeared in 79% of individuals older than 60 years of age and in 54% of those younger than 60 years of age. Degenerated discs were seen in all but one subject older than 60 years of age, many having multiple degenerated discs. Boden et al. concluded that given the high incidence of bulging and degenerated discs in asymptomatic subjects, these findings in part represent the normal process of aging.

Several studies, however, have shown that MRI findings correlate well with abnormal discography that is suggestive of symptomatic degenerative disc disease.[35] Horton et al. performed both MRI and lumbar discography in 25 patients presenting with discogenic LBP.[36] They observed that normal-appearing discs on MRI with a high fluid content rarely had concordant pain or abnormal morphology on discography. Alternatively, discs that demonstrated a dark nuclear pattern on MRI, suggesting severe disc dehydration and anular disruption, strongly correlated with pain provocation on discography. The more common finding, however, of a dark or speckled nucleus on MRI, which was interpreted as some degree of disc degeneration, had poor correlation with discographic findings. Subsequent studies observed that painful discs on discography tend to show more evidence of degeneration such as anular fissures, disc prolapse, and decreased disc height on MRI. However, there is no significant difference in pattern or frequency of these degenerative findings between asymptomatic individuals and those with LBP to suggest that MRI can effectively screen for painful, symptomatic discs.[37]

Aprill and Bogduk describe a specific finding on MRI that appears to correlate particularly well with concordant pain on discography.[38] The high-intensity zone (HIZ) is an area in the anulus fibrosus that can appear on T2-weighted MRI and has high signal intensity in an otherwise degenerated dark-appearing disc (Fig. 58-3). The HIZ was found in 28% of 500 patients undergoing lumbar MRI for chronic LBP. All discs with an HIZ on MRI were also noted to have a grade 3 or 4 anular disruption on the DDD scale. The HIZ appears to be related pathologically to injury to the anulus. Importantly, the presence of an HIZ correlated strongly with exact reproduction of pain. The sensitivity and specificity of the HIZ for exact pain reproduction on discography were 82% and 89%, respectively. The positive predictive value of the HIZ for

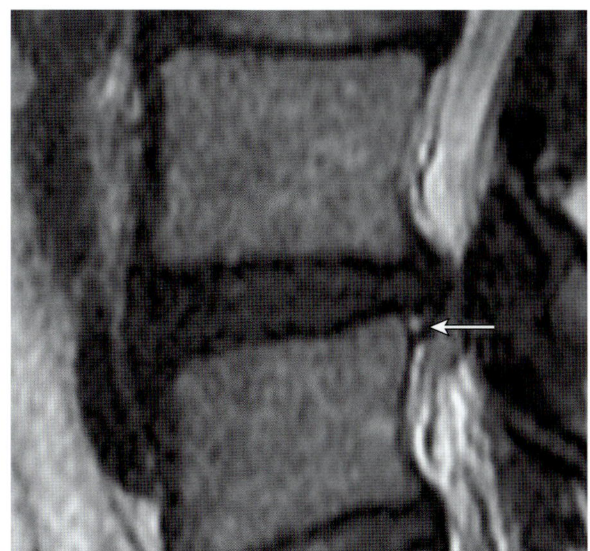

FIGURE 58-3. T2-weighted sagittal MRI of a degenerated disc with a high-intensity zone in the dorsal anulus (*arrow*), suggestive of anular disruption.

concordant pain was determined to be 95%, suggesting that the MRI finding of an HIZ may be a reliable noninvasive measure for anular disruption and pain provocation on discography.

Ultimately, however, there does not appear to be a clear relationship between the mere presence of degenerative changes on MRI and axial LBP. Therefore, one must be careful in interpreting MRI findings and assigning symptomatology to discs that demonstrate radiologic signs of degeneration. Particularly, when evaluating patients for potential surgery, one must consider that the same degenerative changes occur with similar frequency in normal, asymptomatic individuals. Therefore, definitive clinical significance cannot be attributed to abnormal-appearing discs on MRI in the absence of nerve root compression and neurologic symptoms. Modic et al. found that MRI does not appear to have any measurable value in terms of management and outcome of patients with acute LBP.[39] With regard to patient selection for surgery, it does appear that MRI is effective for ruling out normal-appearing discs as the source of pain. The decision whether to treat discs that appear abnormal on MRI, however, warrants either further evaluation with provocative discography and/or the experienced assessment of a spine care provider taking into account the patient's clinical history and symptomatology.

Summary of the Diagnostic Evaluation of Axial Low Back Pain

Diagnosing the source of pain in patients with axial LBP is particularly challenging. Discogenic pain commonly occurs in patients who have a normal physical and neurologic examination. The distribution of pain is somatotopic rather than dermatomal; therefore, identifying the spinal level of pathology is problematic. Imaging findings are also generally nonspecific. Plain radiographs may show decreased disc height and sclerotic end plates. MRI may demonstrate dehydrated, desiccated, or collapsed discs. However, these changes may occur in multiple discs, making it difficult to determine which level is symptomatic. Furthermore, these radiographic and MRI changes commonly occur in asymptomatic individuals, calling into question their clinical relevance.

In 2005, the Joint Section of the American Association of Neurological Surgeons/Congress of Neurological Surgeons published guidelines for the performance of fusion surgery for lumbar degenerative conditions and made recommendations regarding the diagnostic evaluation of axial LBP.[35] MRI allows for the assessment of multiple levels simultaneously and noninvasively. Therefore, one can gain an appreciation of the disease pattern of the discs and determine which discs may have evidence of advanced degeneration, disc prolapse, anular disruption, or disc herniation. Once the degenerated levels have been identified on MRI, discography can be performed to further subselect which discs demonstrate abnormal morphology and concordant pain provocation. In their assessment of MRI and discography, they recommended that MRI be performed initially instead of discography in the evaluation of chronic LBP. They also recommended that normal-appearing discs on MRI should not undergo fusion. Conversely, surgery should not be offered on the basis of discography alone, as patients with positive discography but normal MRI had poor outcomes after fusion surgery.[40] The use of discography to determine which levels to fuse in patients with an abnormal MRI should demonstrate both concordant pain provocation and morphologic abnormalities.

Nonsurgical Treatment

The first line of treatment for axial LBP remains conservative, nonsurgical therapy. While the majority of Americans will suffer an acute episode of LBP at some point in their life, only about 5% to 10% will then continue to develop chronic LBP.[3] Basic symptomatic treatment consists of oral analgesics such as nonsteroidal anti-inflammatory agents, narcotics, and muscle relaxants. Injection therapies with caudal epidural steroid injections, selective nerve blocks, direct injections into the peripheral anulus, facet blocks, and trigger point injections may provide significant long-term benefit for some individuals. Alternatively, they may provide enough short-term relief to allow the patient to engage in a physical therapy program and adaptive lifestyle modification, which may afford better long-term benefits. Spinal injections, in addition to being therapeutic, may also help to diagnose which structure is the primary source of pain. Temporary relief of symptoms after selective nerve root injection may help to predict whether decompression will provide more lasting benefit. Pain relief after facet block has not proven to similarly predict long-term success after fusion, although it can be useful in selecting patients who may benefit from medial dorsal rhizotomy. Ohtori et al. observed that preoperative pain relief after intradiscal injection of bupivicaine correlated well with successful improvement in VAS and ODI after lumbar fusion.[41]

Bracing has a role in the short-term treatment of acute LBP. In general, however, bracing is not recommended for the treatment of chronic LBP, because there is no evidence to suggest that it provides any long-term benefit. Brace therapy has not been shown to decrease the incidence of LBP or lost work days when used as a preventive strategy.[42]

Furthermore, long-term bracing may discourage conditioning and strengthening of low back muscles, leading to atrophy and decreased flexibility. Some clinicians contend that symptomatic relief of axial LBP while wearing a brace is a predictor for successful outcome after fusion surgery, although there is no substantial medical literature to support this strategy.

The most significant advances in nonsurgical intervention have been in the development of specialized physical therapy regimens and the emergence of multidisciplinary treatment strategies consisting of lumbar stabilization exercises, endurance training, cognitive behavioral therapy, education, fear avoidance training, adaptive coping skills, and functional restoration. Therapeutic exercises for treating axial LBP have evolved with a recent focus on improving lumbar spine stability. These exercises aim to increase core muscle control, strength, and endurance to maintain dynamic spinal and truncal stability. Specifically, these exercises improve abdominal, spinal, paraspinal, and pelvic muscle function. The potential benefits of lumbar stabilization exercises are based on limited studies showing that patients with unilateral chronic LBP also demonstrate atrophy of the multifidus muscles on the ipsilateral side of their pain. Multicenter prospective clinical studies have shown that patients with chronic LBP who are treated with lumbar stabilization exercises have meaningful improvements in function, pain, and quality of life; however, clinical outcomes are not significantly better when compared to conventional physical therapy, manual therapy, or spinal manipulative therapy.

The McKenzie method is a physical therapy modality that involves an initial assessment of a "directional preference," in which sustained posture or lumbosacral movement in that direction leads to termination of pain. Proponents of the McKenzie method observe that sequential and eventually lasting abolition of pain can occur in response to repeated movements or sustained postures in this single direction. Once such directional preference has been identified, the patient performs end-range lumbar exercises that match the single direction. In the process, exercises are designed to strengthen muscles, increase soft tissue stability, restore range of movement, improve conditioning, and reduce fear of particular movements.

Multidisciplinary programs have evolved to supplement physical therapy with cognitive behavioral therapy, education, fear avoidance training, adaptive coping skills, and functional restoration. Cognitive behavioral therapy is directed toward replacing maladaptive patient coping skills, emotions, and behaviors with more adaptive ones. Back school is a form of patient education training that teaches patients about lumbar anatomy, physiology, and degenerative disease. Education is directed toward reassurance of safety, fear avoidance, and encouraging activity and self-management. Cognitive behavioral therapy and back school are often provided through group education, training, and exercises. While these interventions do not treat the underlying pathology, they have been demonstrated to reduce pain and anxiety and have become a key component of many multidisciplinary chronic pain management programs.

Functional restoration is a biopsychosocial approach that views chronic pain as an interconnected complex of physiologic, psychological, and social factors, each significantly affecting the patient's clinical presentation. Functional restoration strategies integrate psychosocial and socioeconomic assessment, cognitive behavioral therapy, pharmacologic therapy, and physical therapy combined with an interdisciplinary medical team to provide a comprehensive treatment plan. Ultimately, functional restoration is directed toward rehabilitation to reduce pain, improve function, and, with early intervention, prevent the progression to chronic disability. Certain studies have shown that functional restoration therapy early in the development of chronic pain syndromes results in fewer indices of chronic pain disability, less narcotic use, earlier return to work, and resolution of medicolegal issues when compared to conventional treatment.

Patient Predictors of Treatment Outcome

Several clinical, psychological, and socioeconomic factors have been identified that correlate with outcome after nonsurgical and surgical treatment of axial LBP. Prior to initiating any intervention, particularly treatments that are irreversible or have associated morbidity, proper consideration of individual patient factors may help to predict the likelihood of success. The benefit of assessing for these predictors is fourfold: first, to appropriately select patients for treatment given the inherent risk/benefit profile; second, to increase the likelihood of success by modifying alterable factors prior to treatment; third, to optimize or tailor the treatment strategy on the basis of the patient's positive or negative predictors; and fourth, to align patient and physician expectations for realistic treatment outcomes before initiating any intervention.

Patient age has been identified as a risk factor for the occurrence of LBP; however, it is not an individual risk factor for developing chronic disabling LBP. Studies have revealed conflicting results regarding the influence of patient age on outcome after treatment for chronic LBP. Buchner et al. performed a 6-month follow-up on chronic LBP patients who had undergone a multidisciplinary biopsychosocial therapy approach.[43] The treatment regimen consisted of cognitive behavioral therapy, lumbar exercises, relaxation training, work-related training, medical training, and therapy directed at developing adaptive coping skills. Significant improvement was observed in all age groups compared to pretherapy except that older patients did not demonstrate significant improvement in functional capacity. Overall, younger patients had significantly better results for both functional capacity and pain level compared to older patients.

Elevated body mass index (BMI) has been associated with LBP symptoms, obesity representing an individual risk factor for the development of chronic LBP.[44] The relationship between the BMI and the occurrence of LBP is becoming better clarified. Khoueri et al. evaluated morbidly obese patients with chronic axial LBP who were undergoing elective bariatric surgery.[44] They found a statistically significant improvement in both VAS and ODI in patients who had a decrease in BMI after weight-reduction surgery, despite not undergoing any specific LBP therapy. Obesity is also associated with increased risk for surgical procedures of the spine. A logistic regression analysis demonstrated a positive correlation between risk of significant complication after spine surgery and increasing BMI. While other studies argue that even complex spine surgery can be performed in obese patients with an acceptable morbidity that is comparable to that of nonobese patients, it stands to reason that preoperative weight reduction may improve various aspects of clinical outcome. Overall cardiovascular conditioning, aspects of patient positioning, length of surgery, blood loss, wound healing, and earlier postoperative mobilization and return to activities are potential advantages for patients with an optimal BMI prior to treatment.

Psychological and emotional factors are known to significantly contribute to chronic pain disorders. Anxiety, depression, and maladaptive coping skills that can occur when individuals suffer from longer pain duration result in less improvement in daily activity and work-leisure activity after treatment. Patients with back pain for less than 2 years have significantly better pain relief after treatment than do those with more than 2 years of chronic back pain. The Minnesota Multiphasic Personality Inventory has been well established as a presurgical instrument for predicting outcome after lumbar surgery. Various other measures of psychological and emotional well-being have also been correlated with surgical outcome. Andersen et al. found that the Dallas Pain Questionnaire grading for emotional distress predicted likelihood of significant disability after lumbar fusion surgery.[45] Wasan et al. observed that psychiatric conditions, particularly depression or anxiety, affected the likelihood of positive outcome from medial branch block injections for LBP.[46] Carragee et al. reported that absolute psychometric scores, particularly fear avoidance characteristics, were significant predictors of poor outcome.[31] Derby et al. studied the effect of preoperative psychological and emotional status on patients undergoing single-level lumbar fusion for discogenic LBP.[47] They found that patients with a normal preoperative mental component summary (MCS) score had significantly better surgical outcomes at 1 and 2 years compared to those with abnormal MCS scores. Regression analyses have also shown that tobacco use, depression, and ongoing litigation are the most consistent presurgical predictors for poor patient outcome.

Work status and pending worker's compensation claims prior to treatment appear to be significant predictors of outcome. Beals and Hickman demonstrated that work disability for longer than 6 months was a strong predictor of poor outcome.[48] Only 50% of patients that are disabled from work for more than 6 months eventually return to full work capacity, with only 20% still employed at 1 year and 0% at 2 years after attempting to return to work. Alternatively, patients who are preoperatively employed are more likely to demonstrate good clinical outcomes and return to work function. In a study of patients undergoing dorsolateral fusion for discogenic LBP, all patients who had good or excellent outcomes were employed preoperatively or had been disabled for less than 3 months.[49] Interestingly, they found that preoperative work status was a better predictor of outcome than was positive discography. Anderson et al. observed similar findings in patients undergoing ALIF for discogenic LBP.[50] Patients who were employed preoperatively were 10.5 times more likely to be working at follow-up. Only 43% of patients who were unemployed before surgery were employed at follow-up. Alternatively, 90% of patients who were working before surgery were still working at follow-up. Preoperative work status also predicted posttreatment pain relief. Patients who were employed before surgery demonstrated greater improvement in pain scores, while those with worker's compensation claims had less pain relief. These findings were independent of number of levels treated or other patient demographics. For patients with musculoskeletal injuries in general, it has been shown that continuing even modified work activities prior to surgery had a significant impact on the likelihood of returning to work after treatment.[51,52] Therefore, patients should be encouraged to remain active and continue to work in some capacity, even if work accommodations or restrictions are necessary. Limiting preoperative work disability to less than 3 months may improve outcome and the likelihood of returning to full work capacity postoperatively.

Lumbar lordosis and sagittal balance have recently come to light as independent predictors of LBP and overall health status. An association between LBP and loss of lumbar lordosis has been observed. Jackson et al. characterized lumbar lordosis in asymptomatic individuals and patients with mechanical-type LBP who were matched for age, gender, and size.[53] They observed that two thirds of total lumbar lordosis occurs at L4-5 and L5-S1 and that LBP patients have significantly different segmental lordosis for each motion segment, with particularly less distal segmental lordosis. Significant conclusions regarding the effect of decreased lumbar lordosis on back pain must be considered carefully, as it has also been shown that all people, including asymptomatic individuals, demonstrate progressive positive sagittal balance with normal aging. The absence of back pain in individuals with sagittal imbalance may reflect effective compensatory mechanisms, the development of pain representing eventual failure of compensation.

The relationship between sagittal balance and outcome after surgery may potentially be extrapolated from the spinal deformity literature. Glassman et al. investigated predictors of poor health status in adult scoliosis patients.[54] They found that among both surgical and nonsurgical patients, positive sagittal balance was the most reliable predictor of clinical symptoms. Worse self-assessments in pain, function, and self-image were correlated with positive sagittal balance as compared to other patient factors. They also noted that relative kyphosis of the lumbar spine was correlated with more significant disability than was the case in patients with a normal or lordotic lumbar spine.[55] Takayama et al. reported the incidence of LBP in patients who had previously undergone spinal deformity surgery.[56] They observed that LBP was strongly correlated with sagittal balance, more so than latest Cobb angle or evidence of degenerative changes at the adjacent segments. Therefore, when considering operative intervention, one should carefully assess the overall lumbar alignment, particularly the segmental lordosis at L4-5 and L5-S1, as disc degeneration and collapse at these levels factor significantly in the global sagittal balance. Relative straightening of the distal lumbar segments may help to dictate a surgical plan not only to fuse the abnormal motion segment but also to increase lumbar lordosis and improve sagittal balance.

Surgical Outcome

The surgical treatment of axial LBP due to degenerative disc disease remains controversial. Axial back pain is thought to be due to alterations in the biomechanical and biochemical environment created by the degenerated disc. Pathologic motion or stress transference to pain-generating structures under normal physiologic loads can lead to pain. Disruption of the normal architecture of the disc may result in extravasation of biochemical agents that stimulate surrounding nociceptors. Lumbar fusion surgery, by immobilizing the motion segment, is believed to counteract these pathologic processes to reduce pain generation and decrease disability.

The concern with fusion surgery stems from a lack of consensus regarding the appropriate indications for surgical treatment of axial LBP. Because patients commonly present with generalized complaints, a normal neurologic examination, and imaging studies that are often unreliable in identifying the pain generator, determining which patients are candidates for fusion surgery is challenging at best. Unclear surgical indications likely result in a heterogeneous patient population undergoing spine fusion for symptoms of back pain. Many of these patients may in fact have varying underlying etiologies of back pain. Therefore, it is not surprising that surgeons and institutions demonstrate a broad spectrum of management practices for axial LBP, which consequently is reflected in a wide range of patient outcomes in the surgical literature. To compound the issue, the actual correlation between bony fusion, clinical outcome, and pain relief has yet to be definitively established.[57-59] Studies of lumbar spondylolisthesis–related instability, which is commonly treated with arthrodesis, have failed to demonstrate a clear correlation between successful fusion and outcome. In a randomized, prospective study of patients with lumbar spondylolisthesis and stenosis, dramatically increased fusion rates in patients with pedicle screw fixation did not, however, result in a concomitant improvement in clinical outcomes.[58]

Proponents of fusion surgery for axial LBP contend that a certain percentage of patients do respond well to surgery with improved pain, decreased narcotic use, and return to work compared to the natural history of the disease. While the success rate of lumbar fusion for axial LBP may be less than that of decompression for herniated disc or lumbar stenosis, the axial LBP population is a particularly challenging group that is susceptible to poor outcomes. Often, these patients have failed all other treatment options, are disabled from work, and suffer psychosocial disorders related to long-standing pain and anxiety. There is an arguable need, though, to offer a treatment option for those patients who have exhausted all other resources. Therefore, even in the absence of absolute indications, there may be a role for surgery to provide some measure of pain relief and improve the quality of life for a fraction of patients afflicted with chronic axial LBP.

There are a number of clinical studies that have examined outcomes after fusion surgery for axial LBP and degenerative disc disease. Drawing reasonable conclusions from these studies, however, must be done cautiously. The majority of studies are retrospective case series, with only four prospective, randomized controlled studies comparing fusion to nonsurgical treatment for back pain to date. As previously stated, many of these studies employ wide-ranging practices with regard to diagnostic workup, indications for surgery, procedure performed, and method for assessing outcome. Differences with regard to diagnostic evaluation and patient selection vary in the use of discography, MRI, or relying on clinical judgment for determining which patients and what levels to fuse. A broad spectrum of surgical procedures is also described. Currently, there are a number of ways to arthrodese a motion segment, including anterior interbody fusion (ALIF) (Fig. 58-4), posterior interbody fusion (PLIF), transforaminal interbody fusion (TLIF) (Fig. 58-5), lateral interbody fusion (Fig. 58-6), intertransverse fusion (PLF), and facet fusion. Preferences differ with regard to choice of bone graft material, such as autogenous iliac crest, local autograft, allograft, and synthetic osteobiologic agents. The use of segmental instrumentation and interbody devices is also variable. The specific techniques, nuances, advantages, and disadvantages of these surgical procedures are beyond the scope of this chapter. The literature supporting these general fusion techniques in the treatment of axial LBP will be presented separately; however, ultimately, the common singular objective is to achieve solid arthrodesis of the motion segment, and, therefore, the specific surgical measures to perform the fusion are presumed to be secondary.

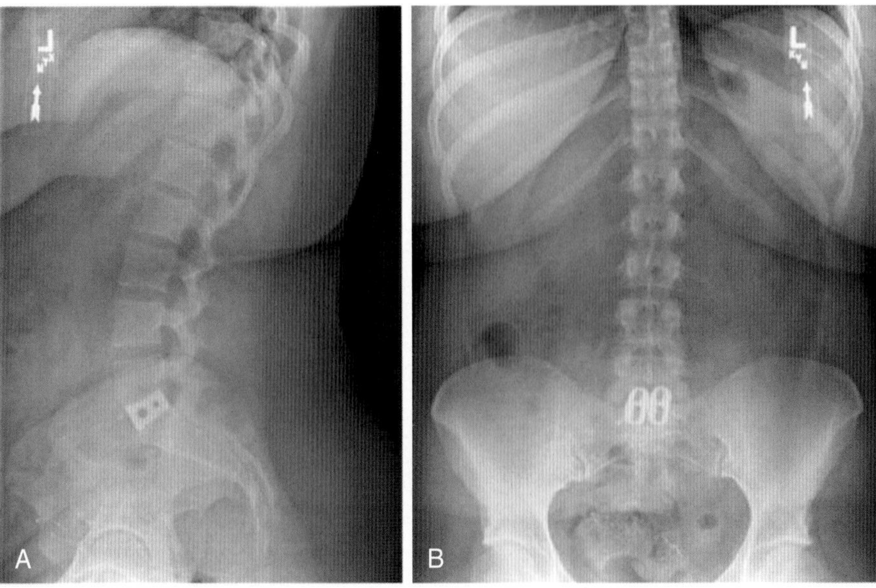

FIGURE 58-4. A, Lateral radiograph demonstrating an L5-S1 anterior lumbar interbody fusion (ALIF) with an interbody cage. **B,** Anteroposterior radiograph demonstrating an L5-S1 ALIF with two interbody cages.

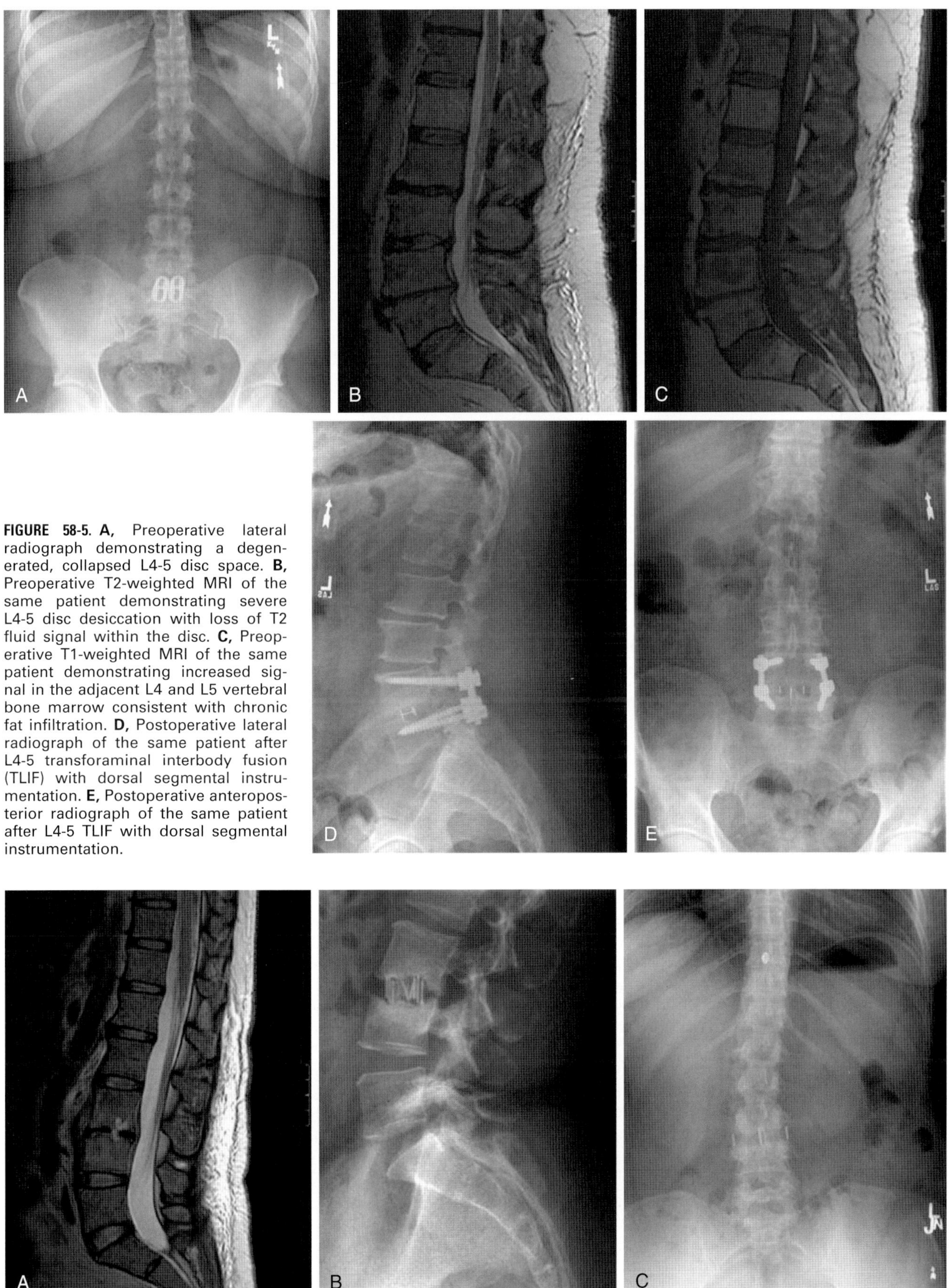

FIGURE 58-5. **A,** Preoperative lateral radiograph demonstrating a degenerated, collapsed L4-5 disc space. **B,** Preoperative T2-weighted MRI of the same patient demonstrating severe L4-5 disc desiccation with loss of T2 fluid signal within the disc. **C,** Preoperative T1-weighted MRI of the same patient demonstrating increased signal in the adjacent L4 and L5 vertebral bone marrow consistent with chronic fat infiltration. **D,** Postoperative lateral radiograph of the same patient after L4-5 transforaminal interbody fusion (TLIF) with dorsal segmental instrumentation. **E,** Postoperative anteroposterior radiograph of the same patient after L4-5 TLIF with dorsal segmental instrumentation.

FIGURE 58-6. **A,** Preoperative T2-weighted MRI demonstrating severe disc degeneration of L3-4 disc. **B,** Postoperative lateral radiograph of the same patient after L3-4 lateral interbody fusion with interbody cage placement. **C,** Postoperative anteroposterior radiograph of the same patient demonstrating L3-4 lateral interbody fusion with interbody cage placement.

Clinical Series: ALIF, PLIF, PLF, 360-Degree Fusion

Studies evaluating outcome after ALIF for axial LBP demonstrate high rates of clinical improvement. Newman et al. evaluated 36 patients who underwent ALIF with autogenous iliac crest bone graft for degenerated discs diagnosed with MRI and provocative discography.[24] Twenty-eight patients underwent single-level fusion, and eight patients had two-level fusions. Overall, 86.1% of patients had a successful clinical outcome, with a fusion rate of 88.9%. Unsuccessful results were observed in 13.9% of patients. Chow et al. similarly reported promising outcomes in 97 patients undergoing ALIF for degenerative disc disease.[60] Complete relief of symptoms occurred in 60%, with an additional 29% having marked improvement in symptoms. Of note, the primary diagnosis of degenerative disc disease and which levels were symptomatic was made by using only the clinical history and plain radiographs in the majority of patients. Only four patients had preoperative provocative discography to facilitate assessment of the symptomatic discs. Blumenthal et al. found a slightly lower rate of successful outcome after ALIF.[26] They observed that 74% of patients with single-level discogenic disease had a good outcome as defined by return to work and cessation of narcotic use.

Lee et al. studied 62 patients undergoing uninstrumented PLIF with autogenous iliac crest bone graft for chronic disabling LBP.[28] Symptomatic levels for fusion were determined on the basis of provocative discography and corresponding morphologic abnormalities on MRI. Overall, 59.2% of patients were free of narcotic use at last follow-up. Eighty-one percent of patients had completely returned to work, with over 92% of patients employed in at least some partial capacity. Seventy-two percent of patients reported that they were completely satisfied with their surgical outcomes, with 80.5% stating that they would undergo the operation again.

Parker et al. assessed 23 patients who underwent instrumented PLF with iliac crest autograft for discogenic LBP.[49] All patients underwent both MRI and discography preoperatively; however, the fusion levels were ultimately determined by which discs demonstrated concordant pain on provocative discography. Overall, only 39% of patients had a good or excellent outcome as defined by a VAS of 4 or less, no analgesic use, and return to at least 75% of premorbid work status. Poor outcomes were observed in 48% of patients, who had a VAS of more than 6, daily narcotic use, and less than 25% of previous work capacity. They noted that pseudarthrosis (22%) and unemployment for more than 3 months preoperatively were associated with poor outcomes. Overall, only 56% of patients reported that they were extremely satisfied with the surgical results.

Combined anterior-posterior or 360-degree fusion for degenerative disc disease has also been reported. Moore et al. studied 58 patients who underwent ALIF with instrumented dorsolateral fusion for discogenic pain.[61] With a minimum of 2 years of follow-up, they observed a 95% arthrodesis rate. At final follow-up, 86% of patients were improved in comparison to their situation preoperatively, with 88% of patients having returned to work. Linson et al. similarly studied patients undergoing anterior-dorsal fusion and reported that 80% of patients had measurable improvement in LBP symptoms.[25]

Leufven and Nordwall studied 29 patients undergoing combined instrumented PLIF and PLF for axial LBP of greater than 2 years' duration.[62] Fusion levels were identified by positive discography. Sixty-nine percent of patients reported either no back pain or improvement of back pain symptoms, with 31% describing complete relief of symptoms, being off all analgesics, and return to full activities. Forty-eight percent of patients had a suboptimal outcome consisting of continued moderate or severe pain, some or total activity restriction, and continued daily use of analgesics. Only 62% of patients were employed at follow-up, and only 76% of patients stated that they would have the surgery again.

Recently, studies have also evaluated surgical outcome for the treatment of disease on three or more levels, challenging the presumption that surgical fusion for degenerative disc disease is best limited to single-level or two-level fusions. Suratwala et al. assessed 360-degree fusion for three or more levels in patients with lumbar degenerative disc disease.[63] Surgical procedures consisted of either ALIF or TLIF with dorsal instrumentation. Diagnostic workup consisted of MRI in all patients, with 60 of 80 patients undergoing discography. Overall, the authors reported a 29.5% improvement in ODI and 30.7% improvement in Roland Morris score at a minimum of 2 years of follow-up.

Lettice et al. compared patients undergoing lumbar fusion for single-level or two-level discogenic disease with those with three or more affected levels.[64] Surgical procedures include PLF plus ALIF or PLIF. Symptomatic discs were identified by using provocative pressure-controlled discography. They found significant improvement in SF-36 physical component scores in both groups at 1-year and 2-year follow-up. The longer-segment group did have a higher pseudarthrosis rate and reoperation rate; however, the number of levels that were treated did not have a significant effect on overall clinical outcome as measured by SF-36.

In 2004, Geisler et al. performed a meta-analysis of the literature to compare various fusion techniques for the treatment of axial LBP.[65] They reviewed 25 papers that had a minimum of 2 years of follow-up for the standardized outcome measures ODI and VAS. They found that patients undergoing ALIF had a mean 45.5% improvement in VAS and a mean 27.9-point reduction in ODI. Similarly, for 360-degree fusion (PLF plus ALIF, TLIF, or PLIF), patients demonstrated a mean 49.1% improvement in VAS and a mean 20.6-point reduction in ODI. In a prospective, randomized controlled trial, Fritzell et al. compared patients who had undergone uninstrumented PLF, instrumented PLF, and instrumented 360-degree fusion.[66] At 2 years of follow-up, there was no significant difference in pain, disability, depressive symptoms, or overall rating between the three surgical groups. While they did observe that the use of instrumentation resulted in increased fusion rates, no correlation between fusion rate and clinical outcome was demonstrated. More complications, lengthier hospitalization, increased blood loss, and new incidence of postoperative leg pain were identified in the patients who had undergone pedicle screw instrumentation.

Prospective, Randomized Studies

The Oxford Centre for Evidence-Based Medicine classifies studies investigating medical treatment effect based on the soundness of their scientific method and the value of their clinical relevance.[67] On the basis of this classification, the majority of existing studies supporting lumbar fusion for the treatment of axial LBP provide only class III or IV evidence (retrospectively collected data; case-control study or case series). To date, there have been only four prospective, randomized controlled trials comparing lumbar fusion to nonsurgical therapy for the treatment of chronic LBP (class I evidence). In 2001, the Swedish Lumbar Spine Study Group published their findings comparing lumbar fusion with nonoperative treatment in patients with chronic LBP.[68] A total of 294 patients were randomized, 222 patients undergoing surgery and 72 patients treated nonoperatively. Inclusion criteria were patients with chronic disabling LBP with disc degeneration. Exclusion criteria were leg pain, spondylolisthesis, spinal stenosis, fracture, infection, or tumor. Surgical patients were then randomized to either uninstrumented dorsolateral fusion, instrumented dorsolateral fusion, or 360-degree instrumented fusion. Nonsurgical therapy was not standardized, with the patient's treating physician deciding from a range of interventions including physical therapy, education, transcutaneous electrical nerve stimulation, epidural steroid injections, cognitive and functional training, and coping strategies.

The surgical group as a whole demonstrated a 33% reduction in back pain and 25% reduction in ODI. Sixty-three percent of surgical patients rated themselves as "much better" postoperatively. Return to work was observed in 36% of surgical patients. Interestingly, there was a 20% reduction in depressive symptoms among the surgical group. Conversely, the nonsurgical group demonstrated only a 7% reduction in back pain and a 6% decrease in ODI. Only 29% of nonsurgical patients rated themselves as "much better" after treatment, with only 13% returning to work. On the basis of these findings, the Swedish Lumbar Spine Study Group concluded that fusion surgery not only decreases chronic LBP and disability but is superior to nonsurgical therapies.

Although this study by Fritzell et al.[68] received the 2001 Volvo Award for clinical studies, it also sparked considerable debate. The primary criticism stems from the nonsurgical group and the lack of a standardized nonsurgical treatment strategy. Because the nonsurgical arm consisted of whichever intervention was offered by the individual treating physician, these patients were subjected to any variety of possible therapies, which are not well detailed in the report. It is certainly possible that the members of the nonsurgical group that had already failed conservative treatment for an average duration of 8 years were potentially being randomized to a treatment arm that consisted of essentially the same continued failed therapy. Therefore, it is not surprising that the nonsurgical group demonstrated modest (if at all) improvement in pain and disability compared to any benefit seen in the surgical group. Additional criticism arises from an unclear algorithm for diagnosing the etiology of back pain and determining the symptomatic levels. Taken a step further, a reasonable concern is that the study could be misconstrued as wholesale advocating of lumbar fusion surgery as a better treatment for chronic LBP than nonsurgical therapy.

In response to these issues, Brox et al. performed a prospective, randomized controlled trial comparing instrumented lumbar fusion and a standardized nonsurgical treatment protocol, which had been shown to be more effective than conventional conservative care.[69] A total of 64 patients with more than 1 year of LBP and evidence of disc degeneration at L4-5 or L5-S1 were enrolled. Nonsurgical treatment consisted of an intensive 3-week program in which patients stayed at a "back hotel" and participated in physical therapy sessions three times per day, with an average total of 25 hours per week of exercises, cognitive intervention, education, and peer counseling.

Both the surgical and nonsurgical groups demonstrated significant improvements compared to baseline at 1 year of follow-up in nearly all outcome measures. The surgical group had an average 15-point reduction in ODI compared to a 12-point decrease in the nonsurgical group. The surgical group had better reduction in leg pain; however, the nonsurgical group had greater improvement in fingertip-to-floor distance and fear avoidance beliefs. No significant differences in back pain, analgesic requirements, emotional distress, life satisfaction, or return to work were observed between the surgical and nonsurgical groups. Overall, both treatment strategies were considered to be effective, with 70% of surgical patients and 76% of nonsurgical patients deemed successful outcomes.

In a subsequent study, the same research group performed a prospective, randomized clinical trial comparing lumbar fusion versus the same nonsurgical treatment protocol in patients with chronic LBP after prior disc herniation surgery.[70] A total of 60 patients were enrolled. The investigators found that the surgical group had a mean ODI reduction of 9 points compared to a 13-point decrease in the nonsurgical group. These differences were not statistically significant, and the overall success rate of the surgical group was 50% compared to 48% of the nonsurgical group. Again, the authors concluded that at 1-year follow-up, lumbar fusion failed to demonstrate any significant benefit over cognitive intervention and exercises in the treatment of chronic LBP.

The primary criticism of these two studies is that the follow-up duration was only 1 year and that both studies were significantly underpowered. Fairbank et al. investigated lumbar fusion versus an intensive rehabilitation program.[71] Three hundred forty-nine patients were randomly assigned, with 176 patients undergoing surgical treatment and 173 undergoing rehabilitation. The surgical procedures varied and were dependent on surgeon and institutional practices. The nonsurgical treatment was a standardized protocol that involved 5 days per week for 3 weeks of outpatient therapy. A total of 75 hours of intervention were performed consisting of cognitive behavioral therapy and various exercises directed toward strengthening, flexibility, endurance, and aerobic conditioning. The surgical group demonstrated an average reduction in ODI of 12.5 points compared to an 8.7-point decrease in the nonsurgical group. This difference was marginal although statistically significant. The authors concluded that the modest advantage of fusion surgery did not provide clear evidence that surgery is more beneficial than intensive rehabilitation for the treatment of chronic LBP. Alternatively, they suggest that their study provides evidence that intensive rehabilitation with cognitive behavioral principles is a viable treatment option and alternative to fusion surgery. Critics of this study point out that 28% of nonsurgical patients crossed over to the surgical arm. Therefore, the patients who were demonstrating the worst outcomes with nonsurgical therapy ultimately had surgery. An intent-to-treat analysis was performed that was inherently biased against surgery, as these patients who were failing nonsurgical therapy may have gained benefit after crossing over, although this was not reflected in the final outcomes assessment.

In 2008, Mirza and Deyo performed a Cochrane summary of these three prospective, randomized controlled studies (Fritzell et al.,[68] Brox et al.,[69] and Fairbank et al.[71]).[72] Mirza and Deyo concluded that in all three studies, surgical treatment demonstrated similar functional improvement with an 8.9 to 15.6 decrease in ODI, which corresponded to a 19% to 37% change from baseline. The nonsurgical group, which ranged from a nonstandardized variety of treatments to standardized protocols for intensive cognitive therapy and exercise, showed an improvement in ODI of 2.8 to 13.3 points and a 5.8% to 30.1% improvement from baseline. Their conclusion was that surgery provided a fairly modest increase in improvement compared to nonsurgical treatment for discogenic back pain. However, none of the observed differences in average back-specific disability outcome were sufficiently large to meet FDA criteria, as defined by a 15-point or more improvement in ODI, for a clinically meaningful difference between treatments.

Analysis of Lumbar Fusion Outcomes in Studies of Total Lumbar Disc Replacement

It is difficult to generate meaningful practice guidelines from the existing literature regarding spine fusion for axial LBP. The majority of the studies are retrospective case series with varying degrees of follow-up and inconsistent outcome assessment measures. A broad spectrum of practices with regard to patient selection, diagnostic workup, procedures performed, and levels fused is presented. Most important, although many of these studies demonstrate an improvement in back disability indices or pain scores compared to preoperatively, it is unclear whether these changes represent a clinically meaningful improvement.

Over the last 20 years, there has been considerable interest in exploring lumbar disc replacement as a surgical treatment for degenerative disc disease. For a full discussion regarding disc arthroplasty, see Chapter 161. However, heightened enthusiasm for this device technology has led to several FDA-approved investigational device exemption (IDE) studies comparing total disc replacement to lumbar fusion for degenerative disc disease. As part of the FDA IDE protocol, study centers maintained meticulous high standards with regard to subject enrollment, preoperative evaluation, standardization of surgical procedure, prospective outcomes assessment, duration of follow-up, and controlling for confounding variables. Although these studies were intended to evaluate the effectiveness of disc replacement compared to fusion, they also provide valuable information about lumbar fusion outcomes in a highly controlled patient population with axial LBP. Therefore, evaluating only the lumbar fusion treatment arm of these FDA IDE studies provides prospective, controlled data regarding lumbar fusion for the treatment of axial LBP. Based on the Oxford Centre for Evidence-Based Medicine, these studies provide class II evidence regarding the use of lumbar fusion to treat axial LBP.

Blumenthal et al. performed a prospective, randomized controlled trial comparing treatment of degenerative disc disease with the Charité total disc replacement versus ALIF with a BAK cage packed with autogenous iliac crest bone graft.[73] Study enrollment included patients suffering from back pain without leg pain, positive discography, single-level disease, failure with conservative therapy, and no prior lumbar fusion surgery. The conclusions of the study were that the Charité total disc replacement demonstrated noninferiority compared to ALIF for the treatment of degenerative disc disease with 2 years of follow-up.

Focusing specifically on only the lumbar fusion group, 99 patients underwent ALIF with outcomes assessment at 24 months. The fusion patients demonstrated a mean 42.4% reduction in ODI and an average 34.1% reduction in VAS at 2 years. However, at 2 years, 80% of patients still required narcotic pain medications. A small increase in employment rate was observed from 57.6% preoperatively to 65% at 2 years. As part of the FDA IDE protocol, a standardized criteria for meaningful clinical success was determined prior to initiating the study. The FDA criteria for overall clinical success were defined as a 25% or greater improvement in ODI, no device failure, no major complications, and no neurologic deterioration. At 2 years, 56.8% of patients undergoing ALIF for degenerative disc disease met FDA criteria for clinical success. A subsequent study that followed a portion of these same patients at 5 years after surgery demonstrated that the employment rate dropped to 46.5% and the overall clinical success rate decreased to 51.2%.[74] Overall, the study by Blumenthal et al. provides class II evidence that slightly more than half of patients undergoing ALIF for single-level degenerative disc disease meet FDA criteria for clinical success at 2 years.

Zigler et al. studied the Prodisc-L total disc replacement compared to 360-degree fusion for patients with back pain due to single-level degenerative disc disease.[75] Patients were prospectively, randomized to either disc replacement or ALIF with femoral ring allograft and dorsolateral fusion with iliac crest autograft and pedicle screw fixation. At 24 months of follow-up, patients who were treated with the Prodisc-L had statistically significant better reduction in ODI than did fusion patients, with an improvement in VAS that trended toward significance. Again focusing specifically only on the fusion group, 75 total patients underwent 360-degree fusion for debilitating back pain due to single-level degenerative disc disease. Of these patients, 84.5% reported some improvement in ODI, with 54.9% demonstrating a 25% or greater improvement in ODI and 64.8% having a minimum 15% or greater improvement in ODI. A mean 32-point reduction in VAS was observed. At 24 months, 70% of fusion patients had improvement in their composite SF-36 physical and mental score compared to baseline. A modest improvement in employment rate was noted, with 78.1% working preoperatively and 85.1% employed at 24 months postoperatively. The FDA criteria for success for this study included a 15-point or higher ODI improvement; improvement in SF-36; device success as defined by absence of reoperation to modify, remove implants, or supplemental fixation; radiographic evidence of fusion without graft subsidence, migration, radiolucency, or loss of disc height; and no evidence of neurologic deterioration. Only 40.8% of patients undergoing 360-degree fusion for single-level degenerative disc disease met FDA criteria for overall clinical success.

Together, these two studies provide class II evidence that lumbar fusion provides meaningful clinical success in 56.8%

and 40.8% of patients undergoing ALIF or 360-degree fusion for axial back pain, respectively. The strength of these studies is that they are prospective, controlled, multicenter studies with rigorous follow-up using validated outcome assessment measures. Strict inclusion and exclusion criteria were maintained with a well-defined medical condition for study enrollment. Importantly, they also evaluated for clinically meaningful success as determined by FDA criteria. On the basis of these findings, one can conclude that lumbar fusion may significantly benefit approximately half of patients with single-level degenerative disc disease who have failed conservative therapy.

These studies must also be interpreted cautiously. Inherently, these studies were not blind; therefore, involved centers may have been biased toward demonstrating benefit of total disc replacement and downplaying the beneficial effects of lumbar fusion. Furthermore, in an attempt to encourage study recruitment and meet study deadlines, investigators may have aggressively enrolled patients whom they normally might not have considered good candidates for lumbar fusion, knowing that a 2:1 disc replacement to fusion randomization scheme was employed. Furthermore, poor outcomes in the fusion group may have been confounded by disappointment from subjects not being randomized to the newer device technology with disc replacement. Last, the strict inclusion criteria might not in fact represent optimal or realistic candidates for lumbar fusion. Several authors found that only about 0% to 6% of patients treated in their practice with a single-level interbody fusion would have met the inclusion criteria of the Charité study.

Conclusion

Axial LBP remains a significant health-care problem, causing pain and disability for many individuals and placing a heavy financial burden on society. The management of axial LBP is challenging. Difficulties stem from our poor understanding of the pathophysiology of axial LBP and inconsistent and unreliable diagnostic modalities for localizing the source of pain. Therefore, the task of treating axial LBP becomes immeasurably more challenging as our confidence in identifying the pain generator falters and consensus for surgical indications remain unresolved. Furthermore, the overall condition of disabling LBP may in fact be multifactorial, as several nonspinal factors such as psychosocial well-being, employment, and duration of pain appear to significantly contribute to the clinical problem and likelihood of treatment success. The existing literature (class I, II, and III evidence) does, however, provide support for the utilization of lumbar fusion as a treatment option for a properly selected group of patients with chronic axial LBP. In fact, both surgical and nonsurgical interventions have demonstrated improvement in pain relief, back disability index measurements, and return to work, with fusion surgery resulting in better outcomes in a limited number of prospective, randomized controlled trials. However, even in highly controlled studies, fusion surgery may be successful in only about one half to three fourths of patients, with a significant percentage of patients gaining no benefit from surgery. This underscores the heterogeneity in the patient population. Further studies are needed to determine which patients have true mechanical back pain that might be reduced by fusion of the lumbar spine.

KEY REFERENCES

Biyani A, Andersson GB: Low back pain: pathophysiology and management. *J Am Acad Orthop Surg* 12(2):106–115, 2004.

Brox JI, Sorensen R, Friis A, et al: Randomized clinical trial of lumbar instrumented fusion and cognitive intervention and exercises in patients with chronic low back pain and disc degeneration. *Spine (Phila Pa 1976)* 28(17):1913–1921, 2003.

Fairbank J, Frost H, Wilson-MacDonald J, et al: Randomised controlled trial to compare surgical stabilisation of the lumbar spine with an intensive rehabilitation programme for patients with chronic low back pain: the MRC spine stabilisation trial. *BMJ* 330(7502):1233, 2005.

Fritzell P, Hagg O, Wessberg P, Nordwall A: Chronic low back pain and fusion: a comparison of three surgical techniques: a prospective multicenter randomized study from the Swedish lumbar spine study group. *Spine (Phila Pa 1976)* 27(11):1131–1141, 2002.

Mirza SK, Deyo RA: Systematic review of randomized trials comparing lumbar fusion surgery to nonoperative care for treatment of chronic back pain. *Spine (Phila Pa 1976)* 32(7):816–823, 2007.

Resnick DK, Choudhri TF, Dailey AT, et al: Guidelines for the performance of fusion procedures for degenerative disease of the lumbar spine. Part 6: magnetic resonance imaging and discography for patient selection for lumbar fusion. *J Neurosurg Spine* 2(6):662–669, 2005.

Zigler J, Delamarter R, Spivak JM, et al: Results of the prospective, randomized, multicenter Food and Drug Administration investigational device exemption study of the ProDisc-L total disc replacement versus circumferential fusion for the treatment of 1-level degenerative disc disease. *Spine (Phila Pa 1976)* 32(11):1155–1162, 2007; discussion 63.

REFERENCES

The complete reference list is available online at expertconsult.com.

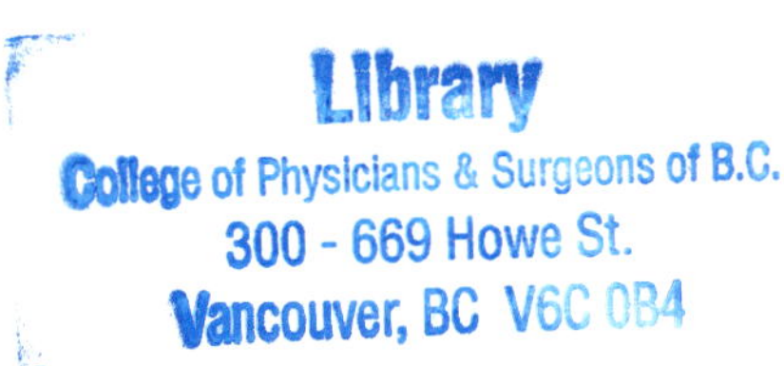

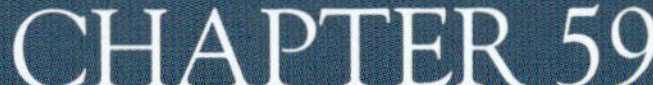
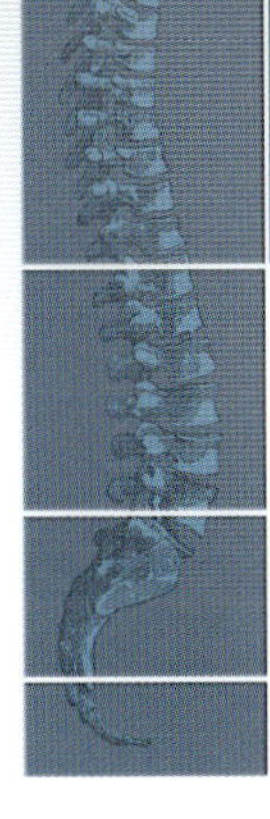

CHAPTER 59

Black Disc: Diagnosis and Treatment of Discogenic Back Pain

Frank S. Bishop | Kenneth S. Yonemura | Hansen A. Yuan

Black disc disease is the common term for the degenerative processes of intervertebral disc dehydration that correlate with imaging changes from a normal white nucleus to a black nucleus on MRI. Despite the intriguing name of its MRI appearance, however, this condition is commonly observed incidentally and does not necessarily indicate the presence of disease that results in clinical symptoms.

Nevertheless, there are likely distinct situations in which disc degeneration alone can cause significant symptoms and, with appropriate screening, may benefit from surgical intervention. The diagnosis and treatment of patients with low back pain from disc degeneration, referred to as *discogenic back pain*, are the focus of this chapter.

The degenerative process of disc dehydration resulting in the "black disc" is common to all disc spaces in the body and is the earliest sign of normal aging and osteoarthritis in the spine. Degenerative disc disease, therefore, must be distinguished as symptomatic or asymptomatic. The symptomatic "black disc" reflects intrinsic changes in the disc itself that can result in primary joint pain without compression of the traversing spinal nerve roots or spinal cord. Discogenic back pain, therefore, is the clinical presentation of lumbosacral pain in the absence of radicular pain or neurogenic claudication.

The fact that intractable axial back pain may be associated with degenerative changes in the lumbar discs has been recognized for over half a century. Discography was introduced by Lindblom in 1948[1] to evaluate the disc anatomy for disc herniations. Four years later, Hirsh and Schazowicz[2] described the provocation and localization of axial back pain with discography despite a normal myelographic study. Since that time, in spite of a general understanding of the condition, a consensus definition of discogenic back pain has not been achieved.

The lack of consistent terminology to describe symptomatic disc degeneration has added to the controversy. In 1970, Crock[3] used the term *internal disc disruption* as an alternative to describe this process. More recently, the term *symptomatic anular tear* has been used because of subtle findings on high-resolution MRI and lumbar discography. For consistency in this chapter, we will use the terms *discogenic back pain*, *anular tear*, and *anular degeneration* in reference to symptomatic disc degeneration. Less specific terms such as *black disc disease*, *dark disc disease*, *postlaminectomy syndrome*, and *failed back syndrome* should be avoided in favor of more specific terminology.

Because of inconsistent terminology and nonstandardized definitions for low back pain, the various causes of back pain have been difficult to differentiate in clinical studies.[4] Furthermore, although axial back pain occurs independently of radicular pain in many cases, clinical studies have not routinely distinguished between the causes and treatments of axial back pain as compared with radicular leg pain. Consequently, accurate or reasonable epidemiologic estimates for the incidence, prevalence, or natural history of discogenic back pain as compared with radiculopathy with or without axial back pain are not available.

Causes of Discogenic Pain

Although the most common source of midline axial back pain remains muscular or ligamentous strain, chronic pain associated with specific postural changes can be attributed to either facet joints or intervertebral discs. More specifically, discogenic pain is classically associated with sitting intolerance and flexion of the spine, as compared with pain with spinal extension in cases of facet syndrome. As the body's largest avascular structure, the intervertebral disc is prone to decreased nutritional uptake and subsequent degeneration. Repetitive motions in the spine from activities of daily life can create shear forces, resulting in microtrauma to the disc. Breakdown of proteoglycans and hydrophilic proteins in the nucleus pulposus leads to disc desiccation, which in turn initiates a cascade of disc height loss, progressive disc collapse, and immobility of the functional spinal unit. This decreased motion may actually lead to mechanical stability through the formation of osteophytes across the affected disc space and gradual resolution of pain, despite continued or progressive degeneration. The natural history and time course of symptoms can vary widely, and a small number of patients remain chronically symptomatic. The dilemma in diagnosis and treatment lies in our lack of understanding of why intervertebral discs with nearly identical morphology can behave differently, some causing patients chronic pain while others remain asymptomatic.[5]

Progress has been made, however, in understanding the pathophysiology of the lumbar disc as a cause of discogenic pain. The lumbar disc is supplied by a network of pain fibers from the sympathetic chain arising from the sinuvertebral nerve,[6] which innervates the outer six layers of the anulus

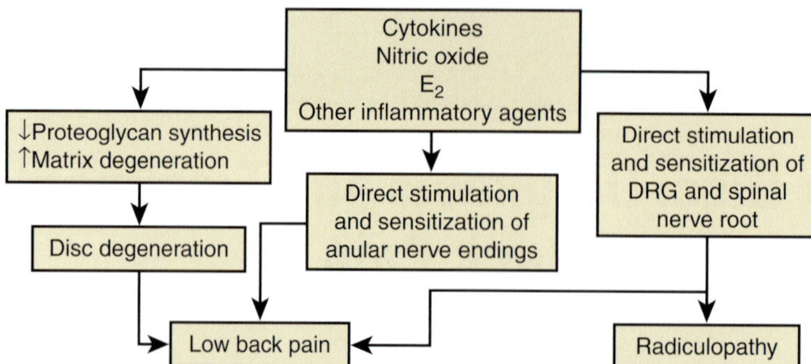

FIGURE 59-1. Diagram showing potential mediators of anular inflammation. DRG, dorsal root ganglion; E_2, prostaglandin.

fibrosus.[7] With progressive disc collapse, the anulus bulges and tears. Activation of anular nociceptive C-fibers then occurs from direct mechanical stimulation from disc material extending into the outer region of the disc. In addition to causing direct pain, anular tears decrease disc integrity and can cause pathologic loading of the facet joints and end plates, with resultant inflammation. Sprouting of pain fibers into the site of anular injury has also been observed and may be a factor in causing symptoms.[8]

Pressure changes within the disc provide yet another mechanical mechanism that causes discogenic pain. Intradiscal pressures have been shown to be greatest in the sitting position[9,10] and correlate with the symptomatic pattern of discogenic pain, which worsens with sitting and resolves with recumbency. Clinically, a lumbar disc herniation can present with an initial history of acute back pain prior to the development of radicular leg pain. Some patients report the resolution of this initial back pain with simultaneous acute new onset of radicular leg pain. Although cause and effect are difficult to prove, it has been postulated that the initial pain from a symptomatic anular tear resolves as internal pressure on the anular pain fibers decreases with herniation of nuclear material into the spinal canal.

In addition to mechanical sources of pain, a wide variety of putative inflammatory agents, such as phospholipase A2, metallomatrix proteinases, and prostaglandins, have been reported to occur in the nucleus pulposus as part of the degenerative process (Fig. 59-1).[11-13] Leakage of these substances into the outer anulus may be another mechanism of pain generation in degenerative disc disease. Exposure of the dorsal root ganglion to these same noxious agents has also been shown to result in histologic damage to the myelin sheaths and ganglion.[14,15] This inflammatory process may be the basis of neuropathic pain, which may accompany discogenic pain.

Clinical Presentation

The hallmark of discogenic back pain is the pattern of activity-related back pain that is characterized by sitting intolerance and significant relief with recumbency. This chronic lumbosacral pain is usually described as a deep midline aching discomfort, not tender to the touch, which frequently extends into the gluteal region and occasionally radiates into the lower extremities. Patients may report an abrupt onset of symptoms with acute anular tears, which typically occur while the person is bent over to lift, and are described as a "pop" in the spine followed by severe pain. Activities that increase intradiscal pressure (e.g., coughing, sneezing, and bending forward) or increase axial loading (e.g., running) can also exacerbate symptoms. Ascending stairs and prolonged periods of driving, which require flexing the spine and load the disc space, are often reported to significantly aggravate the patient's pain.

The leg pain arising from a symptomatic anular tear typically extends into the dorsal thigh but only rarely extends below the knee and may be mistaken for true radiculopathy. Occasionally, pain may present extending distally into the foot but in the absence of nerve root compression on MRI; this pattern would signify referred pain that would be best described as pseudoradiculitis.

Despite the description of significant pain, the physical examination is usually normal; by definition, the diagnosis of discogenic back pain excludes findings associated with nerve compression. On close observation, the patient may exhibit a tendency for frequent position changes, a relative intolerance to sitting, and pain on forward flexion. The absence of physical findings may prompt the diagnosis of malingering or psychogenic pain. Formal psychometric testing should be used liberally to rule out potential psychosocial issues and to quantify the effect of long-standing pain on coping mechanisms.[16,17] Abnormal psychological factors, in addition to the presence of active litigation, tobacco use, and disability, are predictive of a poor outcome with surgical treatment.[18] Close observation of the patient at the time of discography can be helpful in further substantiating the presence or absence of psychological risk factors, and some institutions use video recordings for accurate recording of the patient's response at the time of testing.

In addition to pain of discogenic origin, there are alternative sources of activity-related back pain. Myofascial and ligamentous pain tend to be more superficial, diffuse, and sharp; often have significant local tenderness; and are less associated with sitting intolerance. Facet pain from facet arthropathy typically occurs with extension maneuvers of the spine and improves with flexion. Tumors may present with vague back pain symptoms but are rarely missed with current MRI capabilities. Osteoporotic or pathologic fractures frequently present with isolated back pain but are easily recognized with standard radiographs and CT and with MRI scans in the acute setting. Isthmic spondylolisthesis can result in chronic back pain or be asymptomatic and may present with acute back pain in adolescent patients, while older patients more often present with radiculopathy. An incomplete transitional vertebra syndrome with unilateral or bilateral pseudojoint formation between the enlarged L5 transverse process and sacral ala can also be a potential source of pain and can be easily missed without an angled anteroposterior (Ferguson's) plain radiograph of the lumbosacral junction.

Diagnostic Imaging

Without specialized testing, discogenic back pain secondary to lumbar degenerative disc disease is not adequately assessed by conventional radiography, CT, and MRI scans. Typical radiographic findings include loss of disc space height, end-plate sclerosis, osteophyte formation, and disc bulge, consistent with spondylosis, which may also be found in asymptomatic patients.[19,20] Standard spine radiographs are warranted to rule out spinal instability but are otherwise unhelpful in the diagnosis of symptomatic anular tear. With the advent of MRI, the entire spine can be screened for degenerative processes. While the so-called black disc features nonspecific imaging changes that are consistent with loss of water content (and the disc therefore appears hypointense on T2-weighted imaging), a unique finding referred to as a high-intensity zone (HIZ) in the dorsal anulus has been described on MRI consisting of a discrete hyperintensity within the dorsal anulus.[21] The HIZ lesion has been thought to represent either disc material visualized within an anular tear or edema fluid located within the dorsal anulus (Figs. 59-2 and 59-3). While this finding may be suggestive and helpful in localizing the site of pain, it may also be asymptomatic.[22-24]

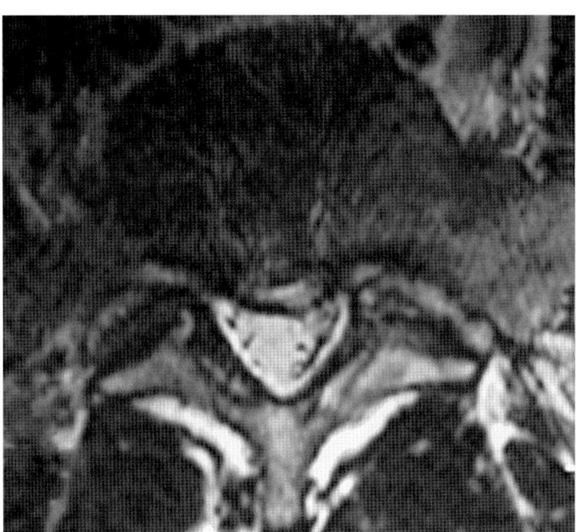

FIGURE 59-3. Axial T2-weighted MRI showing the L5-S1 high-intensity zone lesion without significant central or lateral recess stenosis.

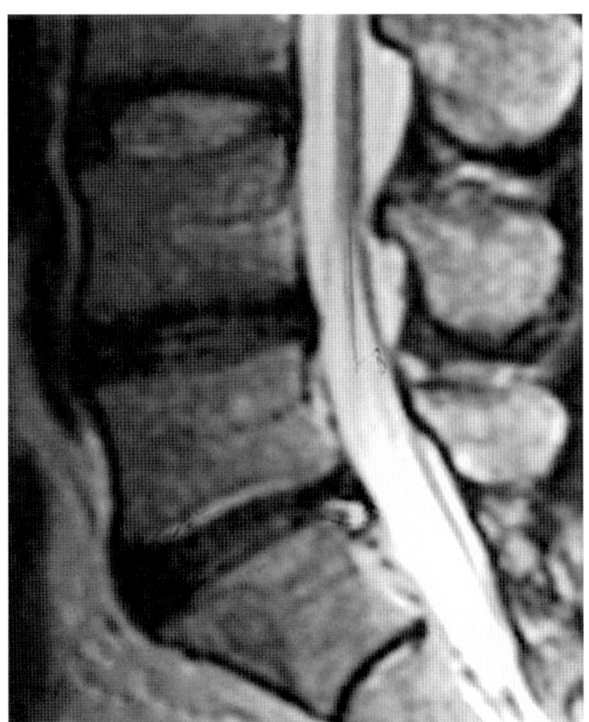

FIGURE 59-2. A 53-year-old man presented with chronic intractable axial back pain and sitting intolerance. Sagittal T2-weighted MRI demonstrating the L5-S1 high-intensity zone lesion.

Additional MRI findings have been characterized by Modic et al.,[25] who described signal changes in the vertebral bodies adjacent to the affected disc space that may have clinical implications correlating with discogenic disease. Modic type I changes are hypointense on T1 and hyperintense on T2 sequences and signify bone marrow edema. These findings are indicative of acute changes in the vertebral body, have a high specificity for discogenic back pain, and may warrant further workup for the possibility of treatment.[26,27] Modic type II changes indicate marrow replacement by fat, are bright on both T1 and T2 sequences, and signify chronic degenerative changes involving the vertebral body and intervertebral disc that are less likely to be associated with discogenic pain.[27] Modic type III changes are dark on both T1 and T2 sequences, indicating sclerotic vertebral end plates that are clinically insignificant.

While these MRI findings may be helpful for localization of a potential pain generator, the diagnosis should be confirmed with provocative testing of the disc space via discography.[28] With the advent of water-soluble contrast agents and MRI, discography has been used primarily for the evaluation of chronic axial discogenic back pain. Patients with a consistent clinical history who have greater than 50% low back pain compared with lower-extremity pain warrant further investigation with discography.

Discography Technique and Interpretation

Discography involves the injection of water-soluble iodine contrast into the disc with observation of the contrast pattern, volume of injection, effect of pressure, and, most important, the patient's pain response (Figs. 59-4 and 59-5). The diagnosis of discogenic pain is made if the patient's pain is identically and consistently reproduced when the contrast is

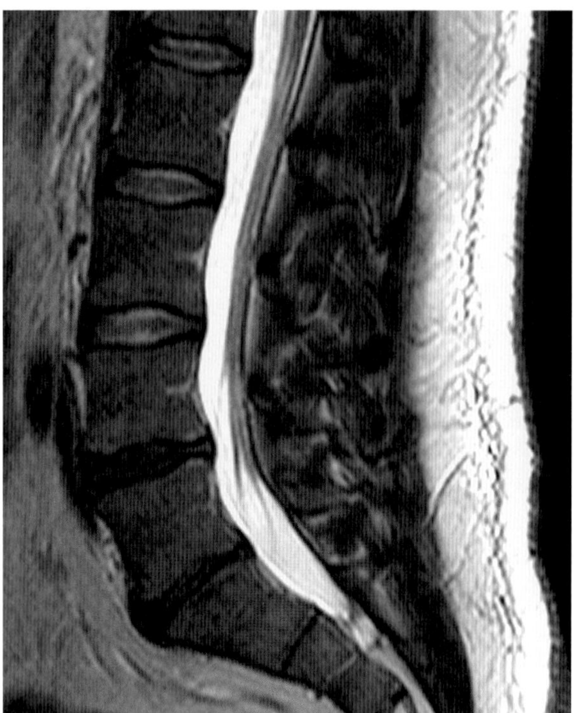

FIGURE 59-4. Imaging from a 37-year-old man presenting with chronic low back pain with sitting intolerance and disc degeneration at L4-5 and L5-S1.

injected into the disc. While the development of concordant pain is key, equally important is the absence of significant pain from a control level. If lateralizing symptoms are described in the history, reproduction of these lateralizing symptoms at the time of discography may be helpful to determine the level of concordance. The patient's typical referred pain should not be confused with radiculopathy.

The technique for discography requires the use of fluoroscopy for localization but does not necessarily require a biplane facility. With an anteroposterior view, a paramedian entry point 8 to 10 cm from the midline aligned with the disc of interest is chosen. A more lateral insertion may be required for obese patients. The needle is directed 45 degrees in the axial plane lateral to the superior articular process, at the midpoint between the two end plates, and medial to the exiting nerve root, which is known as the Kambin triangle. When large facets are encountered, a more lateral entry point may be needed.

We prefer the two-needle technique, which minimizes the potential for iatrogenic discitis.[29] A standard-length 18-gauge spinal needle is first inserted into the interspace of interest. The stylet is then removed, and a 6- to 7-inch 22-gauge spinal needle is placed coaxially through the 18-gauge spinal needle. Placement of the needle tip into the center of the disc space is confirmed with fluoroscopy. Peripheral placement of the needle must be avoided, as an injection into the anular region can result in either a false-positive result or negative pain responses. At L5-S1, entry into the disc space can be difficult because of the limitation of the iliac crests combined with the larger facet joints. Placing a gentle curve in the tip of the 22-gauge needle is usually sufficient for overcoming these anatomic obstacles. Occasionally, a midline transdural approach may be required at L5-S1.

Contrast agent should be injected until a firm pressure resistance is felt, and the volume should be recorded. Typically, 1.5 to 3 mL of contrast can be injected into the lumbar disc spaces. The use of manometry may help to standardize the injection procedure but is not necessary for obtaining accurate useful data. Between 60 and 80 psi, pressure resistance is typically met, and injection of additional contrast agent becomes difficult and potentially painful. Degenerative discs acting as pain generators are often sensitive and may be symptomatic at the time of provocative testing even with lower pressures. These discs that develop concordant pain with relatively small volumes of contrast have been termed *chemically sensitive* discs and may have a higher rate of response to surgical treatment.

Close observation and recording of the pattern and intensity of the pain response must be done during the discography procedure. The reliability of this information is intimately related to the level and clarity of communication between the patient and physician. Sedation during the test should therefore be minimized and even avoided if possible. A discogram should not be considered positive or concordant without exact reproduction of the patient's typical pain, and the

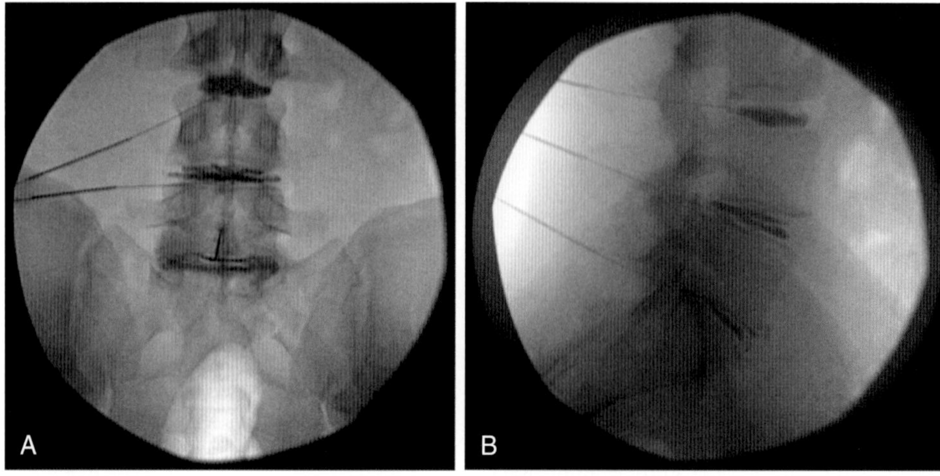

FIGURE 59-5. Anteroposterior (**A**) and lateral (**B**) fluoroscopic images of the discogram demonstrating the needle position and contrast pattern following injection. Only L4-5 had concordant pain.

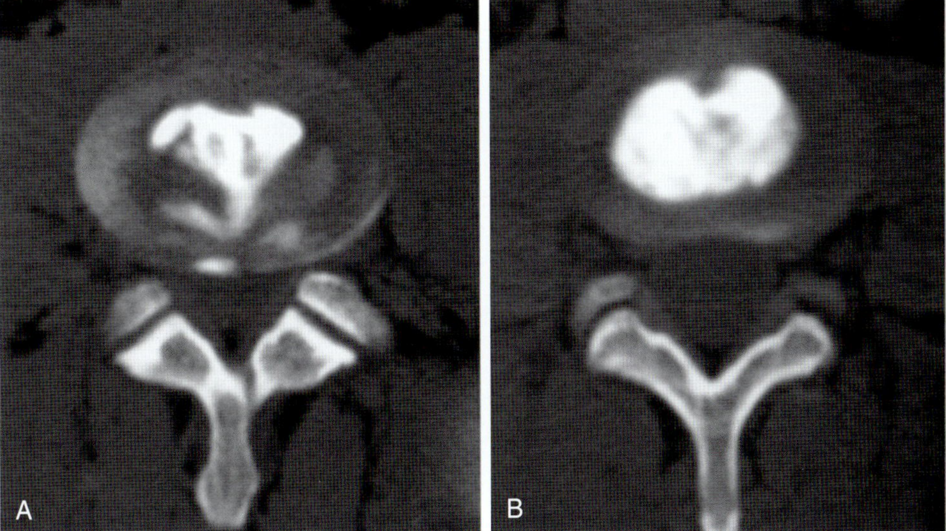

FIGURE 59-6. **A**, Axial CT after a disc injection at L4-5 demonstrating contrast in the disc space extending into the anulus with concordant pain, consistent with a symptomatic anular tear. **B**, Comparison axial CT of a normal discogram with contrast contained within the nucleus pulposus.

patient must remain blind to the disc that is tested during the procedure for accurate assessment of results. Injecting local anesthetic into the disc at the end of the procedure may provide pain relief, further increasing the diagnostic sensitivity. With the addition of intradiscal steroids, there can occasionally be a therapeutic advantage. Because of this need for clinical correlation, the operating surgeon may be in the best position to assess the validity of the test, whether through direct performance of the procedure or by review of a video recording of the procedure.[16]

The various radiographic appearances of the degenerated disc space containing contrast material have been described, and grading systems have been devised.[30,31] The observed contrast patterns have not, however, been shown to consistently result in clinical symptoms.[31] CT is usually obtained within a few hours after the injection and may help with operative planning by providing information regarding the internal architecture of the disc, localizing anular tears, and offering guidance for minimally invasive surgeries (Fig. 59-6). Postprocedure CT images are especially important in cases with planned percutaneous approaches that involve direct treatment of a demonstrated anular tear.

Surgical Treatment of Discogenic Pain

The surgical treatment of discogenic back pain should be reserved for patients with symptoms that are refractory to conservative management, as most patients will note slow resolution of pain over 3 to 6 months with medical and physical therapy.[32,33] Because these patients are neurologically intact, a trial of nonoperative treatment should initially be recommended for all patients.

Various procedural treatment strategies are available for discogenic pain; these have widely differing levels of complexity. Percutaneous treatments are highly desirable from a patient's standpoint but have a limited application, primarily in the early stages of the degenerative cascade. The lack of advanced disc space collapse during early degenerative disease provides an environment that facilitates the manipulation of catheters, electrodes, and endoscopic instruments within the disc space (Figs. 59-7 and 59-8). These treatments are best suited for younger patients with mild disc collapse who are reluctant to undergo total disc replacement or fusion

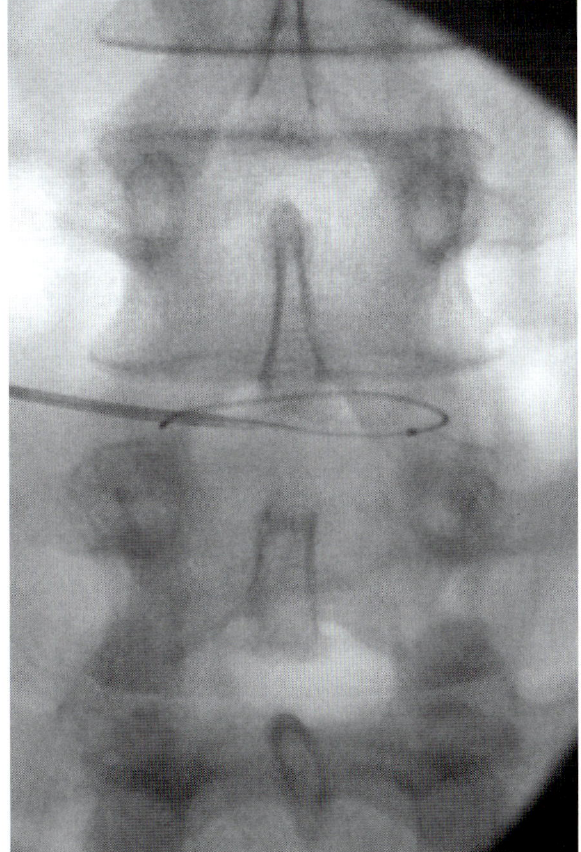

FIGURE 59-7. Anteroposterior fluoroscopic image showing the intradiscal electrothermal therapy catheter positioned within the L3-4 disc space.

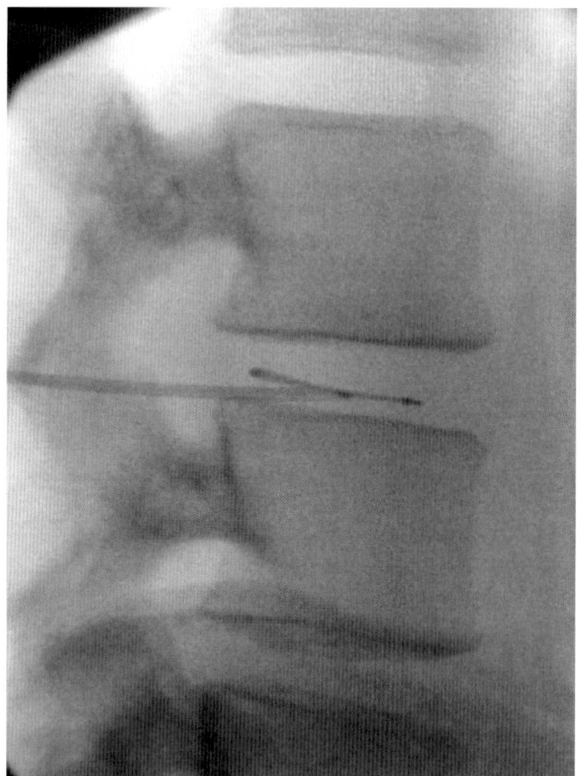

FIGURE 59-8. Lateral fluoroscopic image showing the intradiscal electrothermal therapy catheter located correctly in the dorsal anulus at the site of the high-intensity zone lesion.

procedures. Although patients have the advantage of undergoing a less invasive procedure, they must be informed that the efficacy of the treatment varies widely and that the solution might not be long-term. During the effective time frame of treatment, the hope is that the disease will follow the normal natural history and lead to eventual resolution of symptoms. Percutaneous procedures can also be a treatment bridge until such time as more invasive surgical procedures become available or possible.

The potential for direct percutaneous treatment of an internal anular tear has prompted the development of two forms of treatment. Historically, intradiscal electrothermal therapy (IDET) was performed by placing a resistive heating coil catheter into the dorsal anulus.[34-36] The coils were heated to 90°C, which increased the temperature of the surrounding anular tissue. With temperatures greater than 45°C, denervation of anular pain fibers occurred, and denaturation of collagen fibers occurred at temperatures above 65°C. The denaturation, through cross-link disruption, results in contraction of collagen fibers and may also promote healing of anular tears. Studies comparing the IDET procedure with sham treatment have had mixed results, showing significant improvements in pain, disability, and depression over placebo in some studies[37] and no significant differences between groups in other studies.[38] A second similar form of direct treatment involves the intradiscal treatment of anular tears with percutaneous endoscopy and laser anuloplasty, as well as endoscopically guided radiofrequency probes. Reports have indicated the effectiveness of these treatments, but it remains to be seen whether the technique can be standardized and replicated.[39,40]

For definitive treatment, surgical fusion of the affected disc space can be offered, and multiple studies have substantiated the efficacy of lumbar fusion for the treatment of discogenic pain.[41-44] The patients who can expect to achieve the best outcomes from fusion procedures are those who have failed 6 to 12 months of conservative management, have disc degeneration limited to one to two levels, have a clinical history consistent with discogenic pain, and have concordant pain reproduction on discography. Patients who do not sufficiently meet these criteria or who have questionable symptoms from disc degeneration are less likely to have an optimal outcome from operative treatment. Surgery should be approached with caution and avoided in these cases.[45]

In general, interbody fusion is recommended as the direct treatment for a painful disc, although no significant differences have been reported between fusion techniques.[46,47] In theory, interbody fusion has the advantages of directly addressing the pain with removal of the pain generator and providing maximum biomechanical axial support and compression for fusion. This may be achieved with multiple methods, including anterior lumbar interbody fusion (ALIF), posterior lumbar interbody fusion (PLIF), transforaminal lumbar interbody fusion (TLIF), and extreme lateral interbody fusion (XLIF). Dorsolateral fusion is also an option, especially in cases with advanced disc collapse, but reports of persistent discogenic pain despite development of a solid intertransverse fusion should not be overlooked.[47] The relative indications, merits, and techniques of various lumbar fusion procedures are discussed in other chapters of this text. Fusion procedures may be particularly beneficial for patients with advanced spondylosis and disc space collapse with relatively limited spinal mobility. Minimally invasive procedures, such as percutaneous pedicle screw fixation and arthrodesis, may help to increase the success rates by limiting surgical approach morbidity and pain.

More recently, total disc arthroplasty has emerged as a growing technology and alternative to fusion (Fig. 59-9). For discogenic back pain, total disc replacement has the benefit of removing and replacing the painful intervertebral disc, as with fusion, but with the added advantage of simultaneously preserving spinal mobility. Early results from multiple studies indicate improvements in pain, return to daily activity with the implantation of arthroplasty devices, and low complication rates.[48-50] Furthermore, employment and long-term disability rates have shown to be improved with total disc arthroplasty in comparison to interbody fusion.[51] This procedure may be considered in most patients with discogenic back pain and may become a primary treatment modality as motion preservation devices continue to improve and advance. Surgeon preference, insurance restrictions, and patient reliability for compliance and follow-up will always be significant factors in decisions about surgical treatment.

Conclusions

Studies reported during the past 25 years have substantiated the existence of discogenic back pain associated with discrete anular tears and diffuse anular degeneration. The literature supports the premise that both mechanical and biochemical factors are involved in the genesis of discogenic pain. Standard diagnostic tests alone are insufficient to make the diagnosis; provocative testing with discography is mandatory.

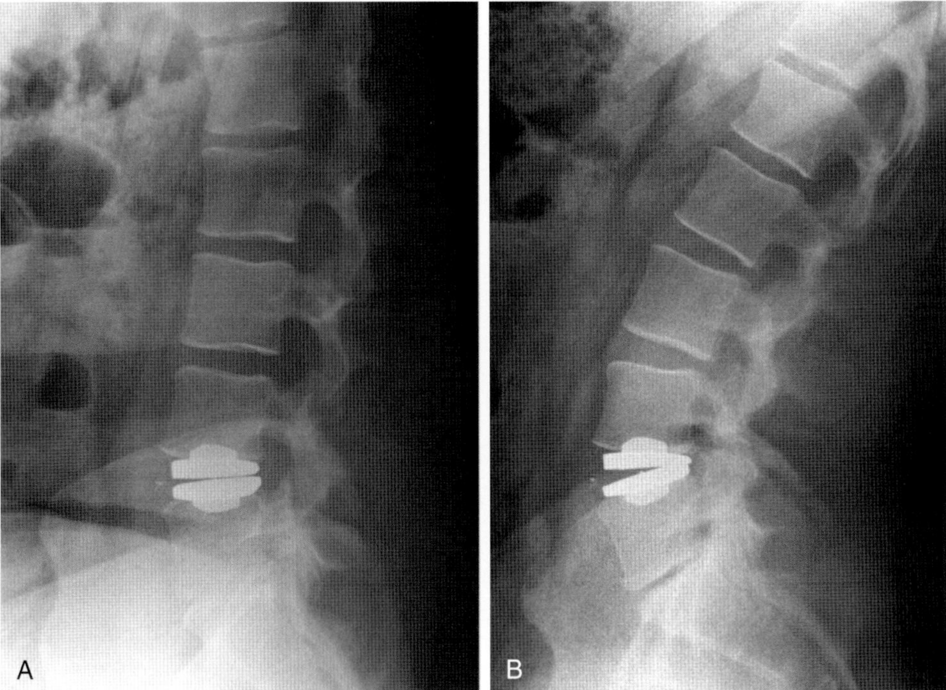

FIGURE 59-9. Lateral radiographs demonstrating placement of the Activ-L arthroplasty device at L4-5 in a patient with L4-5 discogenic pain with flexion (**A**) and extension (**B**) views.

Ultimately, the restoration of biomechanical function, elimination of the painful spinal unit, and avoidance of fusion morbidity should be the goals of future treatment strategies. With the advent of minimally invasive surgical techniques and nonfusion technology, effective treatment for discogenic pain may become a reality.

KEY REFERENCES

Crock HV: The presidential address: ISSLS, internal disc disruption, a challenge to disc prolapse fifty years on. *Spine (Phila Pa 1976)* 11:650–653, 1986.

Dionne CE, Dunn KM, Croft PR, et al: A consensus approach toward the standardization of back pain definitions for use in prevalence studies. *Spine (Phila Pa 1976)* 33(1):95–103, 2008.

Jensen MC, Brant-Zawadzki MN, Obuchowski N, et al: Magnetic resonance imaging of the lumbar spine in people without back pain. *N Engl J Med* 331(2):69–73, 1994.

Nachemson A, Morris JM: In vivo measurements of intradiscal pressure: discometry, a method for the determination of pressure in the lower lumbar discs. *J Bone Joint Surg [Am]* 46:1077–1092, 1964.

Nachemson A, Zdeblick TA, O'Brien JP: Lumbar disc disease with discogenic pain: what surgical treatment is most effective? *Spine (Phila Pa 1976)* 21(15):1835–1838, 1996.

REFERENCES

The complete reference list is available online at expertconsult.com.

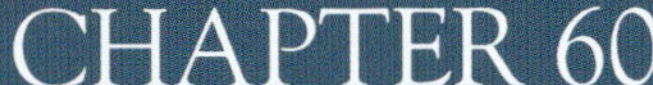

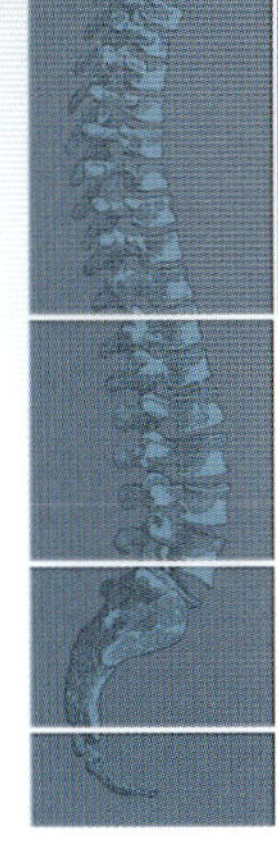

CHAPTER 60

Percutaneous and Minimally Invasive Approaches to Decompression and Arthrodesis of the Thoracolumbar Spine

Kalil G. Abdullah | Michael P. Steinmetz | Thomas E. Mroz

While still considered a burgeoning field, minimally invasive surgery (MIS) of the spine boasts a storied history spanning several decades. Since its inception, many MIS techniques have been developed to treat a wide variety of spinal pathologic conditions. The history of this field, the philosophy and rationale for its use, and an overview of clinical outcomes achieved are thoroughly covered elsewhere in this book. Additionally, Chapter 49 in this book is devoted to MIS of the cervical spine. Herein, we examine surgical approaches limited to the lumbar spine and the thoracic spine, and we analyze their clinical outcomes.

Lumbar Spine

Dorsal Approaches to Arthrodesis

Minimally Invasive Posterior Lumbar Interbody Fusion

The traditional approach for posterior lumbar interbody fusion (PLIF) requires a large dorsal midline exposure with substantial manipulation of overlying ligamentous and muscular processes. When compared to other approaches to the lumbar spine, PLIF results in the highest complication rate, possibly owing to the broad exposure that is traditionally used.[1] This rate makes the possibility of successful minimally invasive approaches particularly attractive. Few studies have examined MIS PLIF, and none have directly compared traditional PLIF to MIS PLIF.

One of the first and most illustrative reports of the use of MIS to limit collateral soft tissue damage during PLIF was presented in 2002 by Khoo et al.[2] Briefly, small incisions were made between 2 and 4 cm from the midline bilaterally at the level of interest (Fig. 60-1). Under fluoroscopic guidance, sequentially larger dilators were then placed over a K-wire to ultimately place a tubular retractor that provided a working corridor 15 to 20 mm in diameter.[3,4] Decompression, hemilaminotomy, and discectomy were then performed endoscopically. During interbody graft placement, the authors used endoscopic visualization to ensure neural element retraction while working within the tubular system.

Percutaneous pedicle screw-rod systems were used in concert to complete the instrumented arthrodesis. Generally (and as reported in all patients in the cited study), cannulation of the pedicles can be performed by using the same incisions that are made for the purpose of decompression after removal of the tubular retractor and endoscope.[2] Fluoroscopy was utilized while a Jamshidi needle was advanced to the pedicle and subsequently swapped for a K-wire using the Seldinger technique. In lieu of traditional fluoroscopy, a fluoroscopic navigation system was used to track the needle in the sagittal, coronal, and axial planes. A tap was passed over the K-wire, and the multiaxial pedicle screws (Sextant, Medtronic Sofamor Danek) were attached to screw extender sleeves and passed over the K-wire into the screw pathway.[2] The remainder of the screw-rod assembly involved mating of the ipsilateral pedicle pairs using Sextant precontoured rods.

Clinical data from this series of three patients undergoing L4-5 MIS PLIF for treatment of bilateral L5 radiculopathies clearly demonstrate the steep learning curve necessary for the MIS procedure. The first operative case took 6 hours and 15 minutes to complete, but time spent in the final case had been whittled down to 4 hours and 30 minutes. Furthermore, blood loss decreased from 208 to 110 mL, as did the length of hospital stay for each patient (from 5.4 to 3 days). The authors cited 100% fusion at 8-month follow-up and an observational decrease in the amount of morphine equivalence units with the MIS approach when compared to previous unpublished open PLIF data.

Another clinical series in 2002 reported positive outcomes in 10 patients who underwent MIS PLIF with pedicle screw fixation.[5] Again, operative time was found to be greatest during the familiarization period and declined with time. Half of the patients were discharged on postoperative day 1 or 2, the remainder being discharged on the third postoperative day. Solid fusions were documented in all patients at 13.8 months of mean follow-up time. In 2007, Park and Ha compared 32 patients who had been treated with traditional one-level PLIF with 29 who had undergone MIS PLIF.[6] Consistent with the aforementioned comparison, there was no statistical difference in fusion rates at 1-year minimum follow-up. The MIS group did show statistically significant differences in postoperative and intraoperative metrics. These included decreased blood loss, postoperative pain, recovery time, and hospital stay.

Interestingly, a recent study has examined the MIS placement of percutaneous pedicle screws using a miniature robotic system.[7] In this procedure, 31 patients received a PLIF with decompression, discectomy, and polyetheretherketone (PEEK) cage implantation along with percutaneous

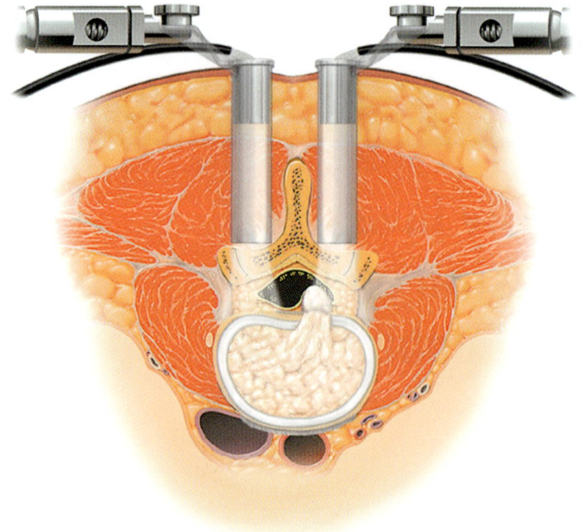

FIGURE 60-1. Posterior lumbar interbody fusion (PLIF) dilation/tubular retraction. METRx Tubular Retraction System for PLIF. (Courtesy of Medtronic, Minneapolis, MN.)

pedicle screw fixation. The SpineAssist (MAZOR Surgical Technologies Ltd., Israel) system was utilized, in which an image-correlated framing system provided an edifice for spinous process clamping and screw guidance. The authors used a modified frame to support pedicle screw fixation and computer-based trajectories. In 29 of 31 cases, seamless percutaneous pedicle screw placement was achieved, with deviations from surgical trajectories of less than 2 mm in the vast majority of cases. While this study was an interesting proof of concept and demonstrated precision in percutaneous screw placement, it utilized a modified MIS approach and did not provide outcomes for the patient population. Further work with this or similar guided systems may be of interest in the future to expand MIS PLIF approaches.

Transforaminal Lumbar Interbody Fusion

As a variation of dorsal lumbar fusion, transforaminal lumbar interbody fusion (TLIF) utilizes a far lateral, or transforaminal, approach that can be applied throughout the lumbar spine. Additionally, complications related to neural element retraction are minimized in comparison to PLIF[1] as TLIF does not necessitate retraction of the traversing nerve root during the discectomy and cage/graft placement. Furthermore, TLIF is not limited to levels L3-4 and below, as is the case with PLIF. When compared to MIS PLIF, MIS TLIF uses a similar but more lateral approach, giving way to an eventual facetectomy, along with complete resection of the inferior and superior articulating facets of the inferior and superior vertebrae, respectively. Discectomy, preparation of end plates, pedicle/facet screw placement, and interbody graft placement are then performed in the usual manner.

Schwender et al.[8] first reported the results of 49 patients who had undergone TLIF with percutaneous pedicle screw placement. Fusion was reported in all patients at a minimum follow-up of 18 months, and narcotic use was discontinued on average between 2 and 4 weeks postoperatively. Other clinical indicators were similarly favorable, with an average blood loss of 140 mL and an average Oswestry Disability Index (ODI) score that dropped from 46 preoperatively to 14 at last follow-up. Jang and Lee also presented a cohort of 23 patients undergoing MIS TLIF with both ipsilateral pedicle screw and contralateral facet screw fixation.[9] In this series, 21 of 24 patients achieved fusion at follow-up (mean of 19 months), with an average blood loss of 310 mL and ODI scores dropping from 33.1 to 7.6 after surgery.

In 2009, Peng et al. presented one of the most comprehensive comparisons of MIS versus open spine surgeries, comparing 29 MIS TLIF procedures to 29 open TLIF procedures.[10] The benefits of MIS TLIF were most pronounced in the immediate postoperative period and included less blood loss, a shorter hospitalization period, diminished postoperative pain, and subsequent lower analgesic use ($P < .05$ for all parameters). However, the MIS procedure also required longer operative and fluoroscopic exposure time. Importantly, follow-up at 6 months and follow-up at 2 years were statistically equivalent when quality-of-life metrics and fusion rates were compared. The authors concluded that MIS TLIF had "retained" positive long-term outcomes associated with TLIF but with fewer immediate postoperative complications (13.8% vs. 6.9%, open vs. MIS). It should be noted that three quarters of complications in the open group likely arose from immobility (two urinary tract infections and one case of atelectasis) and were not directly attributable to the surgical procedure.

Ventral and Lateral Approaches to Arthrodesis

Lateral Interbody Fusion

In 2004, Bergey et al. described an endoscopic lateral transpsoas approach to the lumbar spine in 21 patients undergoing discectomy and fusion.[11] A modification of McAffee's endoscopic approach,[11] the true lateral approach provides a retroperitoneal approach to the lumbar spine without trespassing into the peritoneum or dissecting the great vessels.[12] The exposure typically requires the patient to be in the right lateral decubitus position (Fig. 60-2). An incision is made along the lateral border of the lumbar paraspinal muscle, and a finger dissection is performed through the retroperitoneal space to the psoas.[3] With the use of fluoroscopy to determine the proper starting point along the flank, a counterincision is made directly lateral to the disc space(s) of interest. The dilators are guided to the psoas using the initial incision, and a corridor is developed through the psoas to the disc space of interest. Continuous electromyogram monitoring is utilized to avoid injuring the exiting lumbar nerve roots, which also pass through the psoas muscle. A final expandable retractor is then placed over the final dilator, providing adequate access to the disc space. The discectomy and placement of the interbody graft are then followed by placement of a side plate and/or dorsal fixation of some kind (i.e., pedicle screws, translaminar or facet screws).

While a lateral approach decreases the likelihood of complications arising from anterior lumbar interbody fusion, it presents a unique set of challenges. First, it is essential to note the location of the lumbosacral plexus, as it migrates ventrally from L1 to L5[13] and is at significant risk when approaching the L4-5 interspace.[14] Injury to the genitofemoral nerve is still possible and was noted in 30% of patients

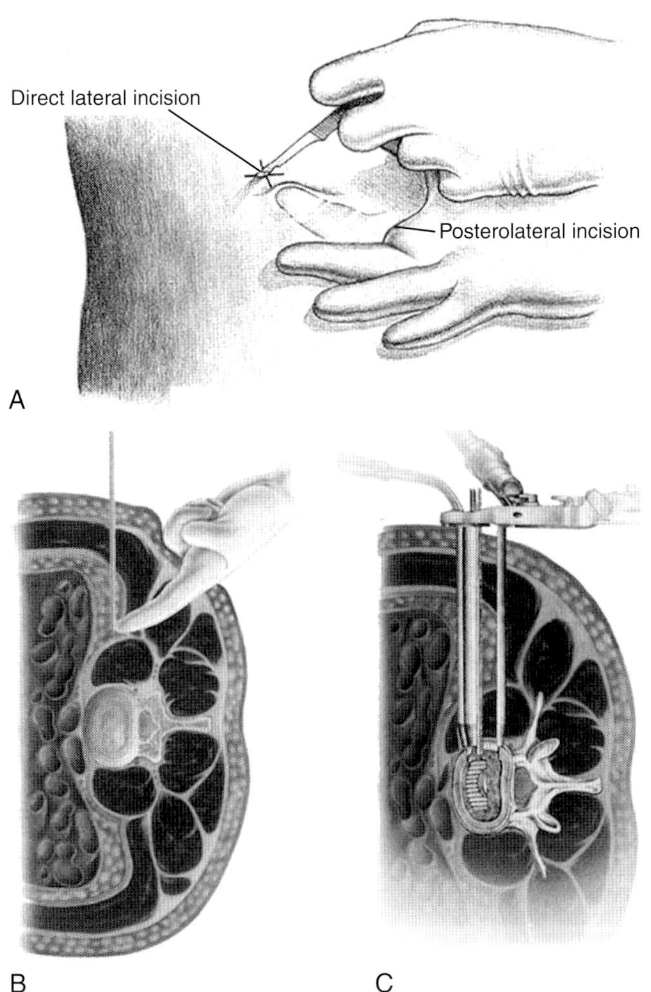

FIGURE 60-2. Extreme lateral interbody fusion procedure. **A,** Incision over the psoas. **B,** Sequential dilation through the retroperitoneal space. **C,** Insertion of the implant. (From NuVasive, San Diego, CA, with permission.)

in Bergey et al.'s 2004 study.[11] This complication was not found in a 2006 study,[15] but staying within the ventral third of the psoas and visualizing the genitofemoral nerve has been recommended.[3] The far lateral approach provides excellent access to the L1-4 levels and ability to restore disc height, but further dissection is necessary to expose any caudal disc spaces and may even require removal of a portion of the iliac crest.[16] Clinical outcomes of extreme lateral interbody fusion are also notable; a recent study shows MIS extreme lateral interbody fusion, unlike traditional open lumbar procedures, to be no more likely to result in complications in the obese patient.[17]

Ventral Limited, Laparoscopic Approaches

Ventral laparoscopic approaches to the lumbar spine have fallen out of favor with the spine surgery community. As late as the mid-1990s, prospective studies demonstrated equivalent rates of complications between laparoscopic and open approaches, encouraging further study.[18] However, the past decade has revealed that complication rates for video-assisted procedures were higher than those in open surgeries.[19] In one series, the laparoscopic approach, utilizing techniques similar to those of abdominal laparoscopy, resulted in higher rates of retrograde ejaculation and new-onset radicular pain. In 11% of cases, the laparoscopic approach required conversion to a more open approach for reasons that included major vessel lacerations and peritoneal tears. The laparoscopic techniques also favored the L4 vertebra and below, as higher approaches were deemed even more technically demanding. Therefore, the authors of that study advocated abandonment of the laparoscopic technique for ventral lumbar fusion.

Nonlaparoscopic, MIS approaches to the lumbar spine have faired far better. In 1997, Mayer introduced a muscle-splitting approach that allowed easy access to the entire lumbar spine.[20] After exposure of the target level, disc removal and graft placement can proceed. In his study, Mayer reported uniform fusion at follow-up, low intraoperative blood loss and postoperative morbidity, and a short recovery period. A 2004 study retrospectively compared 33 patients who had undergone the traditional extraperitoneal approach to 23 who had undergone Mayer's minimally invasive approach.[21] First, unlike the case with most MIS procedures, the authors reported a significantly shorter operative time when compared to the open procedure. Blood loss was significantly less in the MIS group, and complication and fusion rates were similar. In light of these findings and a similar study showing higher complication rates in the open group,[22] it is reasonable to conclude that the MIS approach may be preferred to the traditional extraperitoneal approach. A variety of grafting options can be used for an MIS ALIF approach. The Lumbar Tapered (LT)-Cage (Medtronic Sofamor Danek, Memphis, TN) is a stand-alone tapered titanium cage that is approved by the Food and Drug Administration (FDA)[23] for single-level ALIF with the concomitant use of bone morphogenetic protein-2 (BMP-2) (INFUSE Bone Graft, Medtronic Sofamor Danek, Memphis, TN), with fusion rates reported at 94.5% at 12 months. Other graft options for MIS (analogous to those in open procedures) include the autogenous iliac crest corticocancellous graft, allograft (e.g., femoral ring), and PEEK, carbon fiber, bioabsorbable, and other metallic interbody cages. These materials, when used as stand-alone devices (i.e., no dorsal fixation), result in suboptimal fusion rates and clinical outcomes. Therefore, it is recommended that they be used in conjunction with dorsal fixation. Equally nebulous at the time of this writing is the ideal grafting substrate. The ideal substrate (i.e., iliac crest autograft, allograft, tricalcium phosphate, BMP-2) to be used with the various interbody structural components (non-LT metallic cages, allograft rings, PEEK, and carbon fiber cages) have not been defined clearly in the literature. Appropriately designed and executed studies are necessary to define the ideal cage, graft substrate, quantity, and, in the case of BMP-2, dose for the use of ALIF surgery.

Minimally Invasive Decompression

A thorough treatise on MIS lumbar decompression could fill several volumes. The use of laser dehydration, chemical application, percutaneous extraction, and MIS implants have been evaluated repeatedly and found to be inferior to direct decompression.[24,25] While implants may be an attractive alternative for select patients, it is still not entirely known how patient selection affects outcome, and several studies have shown high failure rates or inconsistent radiographic and clinical factors predicting clinical outcomes.[26,27]

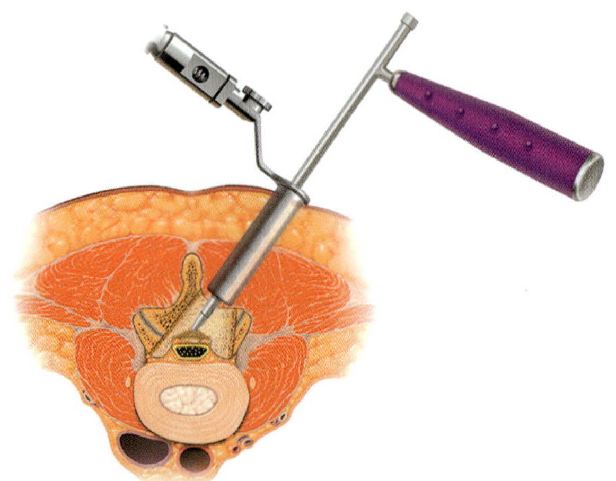

FIGURE 60-3. Contralateral decompression via ipsilateral approach. In the METRx system for lumbar stenosis, after ipsilateral decompression, the retractor can be angled medially toward the spinous process. (Courtesy of Medtronic, Minneapolis, MN.)

Therefore, this chapter focuses on MIS surgical intervention for decompression of the thoracolumbar spine.

The approach to MIS decompression (i.e., laminotomy, laminectomy, foraminotomy) is similar to that of MIS PLIF in that muscle-splitting techniques are used with tubular retractor systems to provide targeted access to the affected vertebra. The placement of the tubular or expandable retractor relative to midline is predicated on the type of decompression being performed (e.g., ipsilateral foraminotomy vs. bilateral decompression via a unilateral approach; Fig. 60-3).[25] A microscope or endoscope can be used for visualization; however, the latter has ergonomic restraints, particularly in working through a narrow retractor. A recent study retrospectively compared 38 patients who had undergone MIS decompression with 126 patients who had been treated with open laminectomy.[28] MIS procedures were associated with shorter operative times, less blood loss, shorter length of hospital stay, and fewer complications. Several other recent studies have also reported excellent clinical results in single-level and multilevel MIS laminotomy or midline decompression.[29-31] A biomechanical study examined lumbar segments with regard to axial compression, flexion, extension, and lateral bending after intervention of isolated fenestration, bilateral decompression via unilateral approach, and medial or total facetectomy.[32] These preliminary results found that bilateral decompression had less effect on stiffness, as did medial facetectomy. This supports the use of a minimally invasive bilateral decompression due to preservation of facet joints.

Thoracic Spine

Minimally Invasive Surgical Approaches to Arthrodesis and Decompression

Application of endoscopic technologies for ventral exposure of the thoracic spine was first reported in the mid-1990s.[33-35] However, both the high complication rate and the steep learning curve, as well as limited access to more cephalad vertebrae, have limited the use of MIS ventral approaches in favor of open approaches that allow greater visibility.[36]

Dorsal MIS approaches were until recently limited to trauma, metastasis, deformity, and infection, entities that are outside the scope of this chapter. In the past few years, however, progress in thoracic MIS approaches has accelerated. In 2006, Ringel et al.[37] assessed the feasibility of MIS percutaneous dorsal pedicle screws in 104 patients with instability in the thoracic and lumbar spine. The authors found "good" screw placement in 87% of cases, and a majority of patients proceeded to ventral MIS fusion; of those patients, all but two reported resolution of radiculopathy. However, this study lacked a control arm or matched comparison to open thoracic screw placement. In 2009, Haufe et al.[38] performed isolated laminoforaminoplasty for the treatment of thoracic radiculopathy in 12 patients. When compared to traditional laminotomy, the authors reported a shorter hospital stay and lower complication rates. Overall, while clinical data for MIS approaches to arthrodesis and decompression are sparse, initial reports dating as far back as 2006 provide positive outcomes and a solid foundation for further study.

Discussion

Minimally invasive surgery has become increasingly popular among both spine surgeons and patients. Over the past decade, MIS technology (i.e., retractors, instrumentation, interbody cages, pedicle and facet screws) has advanced at a rate that has exceeded the literature on the topic. The fundamental premise of MIS surgery is that it is better for the patient because it reduces the amount of tissue trauma associated with open procedures. Certainly, short-term results indicate a benefit for patients following decompression and fusion surgery in regard to narcotic use and hospital stays. However, there is a paucity of articles that define long-term outcomes. There are many studies that have demonstrated that open midline spine approaches are associated with paraspinal muscle damage, and proponents of MIS surgery use this as a springboard to promote MIS techniques.[39-47] However, there is currently a lack of evidence that substantiates less soft tissue damage with MIS techniques. Simple observation may lead one to believe that MIS causes less tissue damage, but this has not been quantified and remains an aspect of MIS surgery that needs to be defined further.

Large-scale, systematic, well-designed and well-executed studies are necessary in order to define the optimal retractor size for each type of MIS procedure, the ideal type of interbody cage (i.e., metal vs. PEEK vs. autograft vs. allograft), the ideal graft substrate, the adverse event profile for the various techniques, the adverse event profile associated with the use of biologics for these techniques, and, most important, long-term clinical outcomes. Last, it is also critical to emphasize that the majority of the MIS techniques require the use of ionizing radiation for intraoperative navigation (i.e., fluoroscopy, intraoperative computed tomography). All surgeons must keep in mind that the adverse effects of radiation are cumulative and that each surgeon must therefore monitor his or her annual exposure. Overall, while percutaneous and MIS approaches to decompression and fusion of the thoracolumbar spine have shown early clinical promise, the outcomes of these procedures must be better characterized and documented for the field to reach its maximum potential.

KEY REFERENCES

Foley KT, Gupta SK: Percutaneous pedicle screw fixation of the lumbar spine: preliminary clinical results. *J Neurosurg* 97:7–12, 2002.

Jang JS, Lee SH: Minimally invasive transforaminal lumbar interbody fusion with ipsilateral pedicle screw and contralateral facet screw fixation. *J Neurosurg Spine* 3:218–223, 2005.

Kawaguchi Y, Matsui H, Tsuji H: Back muscle injury after posterior lumbar spine surgery: a histologic and enzymatic analysis. *Spine (Phila Pa 1976)* 21:941–944, 1996.

Khoo LT, Palmer S, Laich DT, et al: Minimally invasive percutaneous posterior lumbar interbody fusion. *Neurosurgery* 51:S166–S171, 2002.

Mayer HM: A new microsurgical technique for minimally invasive anterior lumbar interbody fusion. *Spine (Phila Pa 1976)* 22:691–699, 1997; discussion 700.

Ozgur BM, Aryan HE, Pimenta L, et al: Extreme lateral interbody fusion (XLIF): a novel surgical technique for anterior lumbar interbody fusion. *Spine J* 6:435–443, 2006.

Schwender JD, Holly LT, Rouben DP, et al: Minimally invasive transforaminal lumbar interbody fusion (TLIF): technical feasibility and initial results. *J Spinal Disord Tech* 18(Suppl):S1–S6, 2005.

REFERENCES

The complete reference list is available online at expertconsult.com.

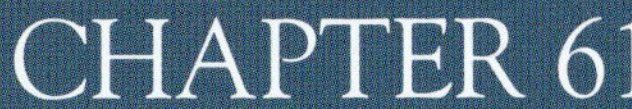

CHAPTER 61

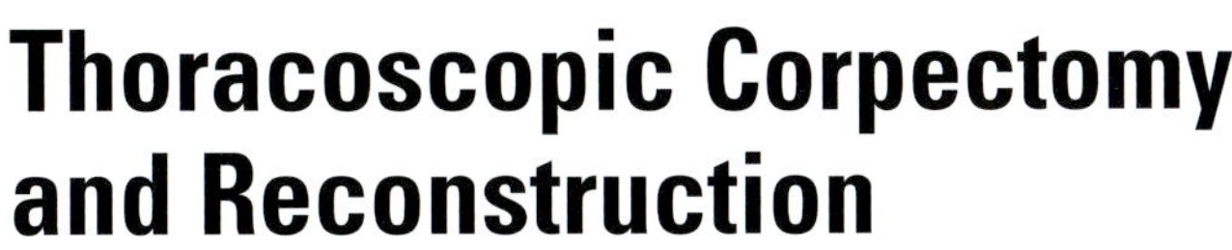

Thoracoscopic Corpectomy and Reconstruction

Frank S. Bishop | Meic H. Schmidt

Thoracoscopic spine surgery, also known as endoscopic-assisted or video-assisted thoracoscopic surgery, is a minimally invasive, closed endoscopic approach to the ventral thoracolumbar spine for decompression and stabilization. It offers an alternative to open thoracotomy for thoracolumbar vertebral body resection from T5 through L2, ventral spinal cord decompression, and spine reconstruction with interbody and ventrolateral plate instrumentation for restoration of biomechanical stability.

Spinal instability caused by trauma or destructive disease has historically been treated through a dorsal approach. Purely dorsal techniques, however, often fail adequately to address ventrally located pathology. Dorsal decompression with thoracic laminectomy of ventral epidural masses has been associated with increased risk of injury to the spinal cord. Ventral spinal canal decompression through dorsal and even posterolateral approaches can be challenging and ineffective.[1-3] Furthermore, dorsal instrumentation may not sufficiently stabilize a significantly disrupted ventral load-bearing spinal column.[4,5]

To more effectively and directly decompress and stabilize the ventral spine, ventral thoracotomy and thoracoabdominal techniques were developed.[6,7] Although these approaches demonstrated improved outcomes and are an acceptable treatment modality for ventral thoracolumbar disease, the high access morbidity of these open procedures often results in post-thoracotomy pain syndromes, postoperative pneumothorax or pleural effusion, shoulder dysfunction, abdominal wall relaxation, and significant scarring of the chest wall.[8]

Spine surgeons have more recently adapted the minimally invasive thoracoscopic techniques that have been applied by thoracic surgeons for many years. Thoracoscopic spine surgery was first used for the treatment of thoracic disc herniations and traumatic fractures. With advances in thoracoscopic video technology, instrumentation, and instrument systems, thoracoscopic spine surgery has improved significantly, and its use has been expanded to include the treatment of most ventral thoracolumbar disorders, including trauma, tumor, and degenerative disease, as well as deformity correction in select cases.[4,9-15]

Specialized tools for endoscopic spine surgery are used to access the thoracic cavity through small chest incisions, and the surgery is performed under two-dimensional video guidance. Minimizing chest wall dissection and retraction through the use of small thoracoscopic incisions has significantly improved outcomes and reduced postoperative morbidity without compromising long-term successful fusion rates.[9-11,16-18] The minimally invasive thoracoscopic approach can now be safely and effectively performed to treat disease that had previously required an open thoracotomy.

Advantages and Disadvantages

Several advantages are offered by the minimally invasive ventrolateral thoracoscopic approach over an open thoracotomy. Multiple vertebral levels and the ventral spinal canal can be visualized and treated without increasing surgical exposure when access ports are properly placed. The surgical field can be imaged with excellent resolution using modern high-definition endoscopic technology. The small intercostal incisions negate the need for rib resection and retraction, unlike open thoracotomy approaches, which necessitate large incisions, extensive dissection of intercostal muscles, rib resection, and retraction of the chest wall. The thoracoscopic approach is associated with reduced blood loss, need for blood transfusion,[19] days of mechanical ventilation, perioperative wound pain, incidence of pulmonary and shoulder dysfunction, length of hospital stay, and days to rehabilitation.[16-18]

For most spine surgeons, the major disadvantage of the thoracoscopic approach is unfamiliarity with the technique and high technical demand. The operation is performed distant from the surgical site in two dimensions based solely on thoracoscopic image guidance, which requires most spine surgeons to acquire a new set of skills. Before operating on a patient, the surgeon must gain familiarity with the new technique in practical and didactic training sessions. The surgeon and operating room staff must overcome a steep learning curve while gaining familiarity with the approach, and this can initially increase operative times by several hours. Anesthesia monitoring and double-lumen ventilation may also increase operative times. Conversion to an open thoracotomy may be required with difficult cases or when intraoperative complications cannot be resolved with the thoracoscopic technique. Finally, extensive intrathoracic disease, whether pulmonary or spinal, may be difficult to address with the thoracoscopic approach.

Indications and Contraindications

The thoracoscopic approach is best suited for patients with thoracolumbar disease limited to one vertebral body and the ventral spinal canal between T3 and L3, although multiple levels may be treated. The most common indication for thoracoscopic spinal surgery is in the setting of trauma. Among patients with traumatic spinal injury, ventral spinal reconstruction for biomechanical instability is the most common surgical indication. Traumatic spinal instability may be secondary to fracture, injury to the intervertebral discs, or significant ligamentous disruption. The mainstay of treatment for thoracolumbar fractures is rigid fixation with transpedicular screw and rod constructs. The decision to add ventral column reconstruction is based on the load-bearing capacity of the injured spinal segment. The load-sharing classification system developed by McCormack et al.[5] established a correlation between failure of dorsal short segment fixation and the characteristics of the most significantly injured vertebrae. Fractures with a high degree of vertebral body comminution, fragment apposition, and postoperative deformity correction were found to be at high risk for dorsal instrumentation failure. Thoracoscopic surgery for reconstruction of the ventral load-bearing elements is indicated in these patients. Although patients with neurologic deficits from fracture intrusion into the ventral spinal canal comprise a minor subgroup of patients with traumatic spine injury, they are also indicated for spinal canal decompression and ventral stabilization.

In cases of spinal tumor, thoracolumbar surgery is indicated for treatment of spinal instability, radiation treatment failures, most cases of spinal stenosis secondary to epidural tumor causing neural compression, and pain intractable to conservative measures or to obtain a histologic diagnosis.[3,20-23] The thoracoscopic approach is indicated for resection of vertebral body tumors with or without ventral spinal canal involvement and for ventral column reconstruction with interbody placement and ventrolateral instrumentation.

The thoracoscopic approach is contraindicated in patients unable to tolerate single-lung ventilation because of severe cardiopulmonary disease such as acute posttraumatic lung failure, significant pulmonary contusions, advanced chronic obstructive pulmonary disease or asthma, or hemodynamic instability. This approach is also contraindicated in patients with significant medical diseases, disturbances in hemostasis, or terminal illnesses precluding surgical treatment. The surgery may be technically challenging in patients with a history of trauma, prior surgery, or infection because of the development of dense pleural adhesions. In cases with substantial dorsal column disruption or involvement, stand-alone ventral surgery may be insufficient to achieve spinal stability, and supplemental dorsal fixation should be considered.

Preoperative Assessment and Planning

Radiographic and Diagnostic Evaluation

As with other spine surgeries, careful preoperative review and understanding of the radiographic studies are essential to identify the most appropriate treatment method and to plan the surgery. The presence or extent of vertebral body disease and bony destruction, instability of the load-bearing spinal column, spinal cord compression and canal stenosis, and anatomic malalignment are noted for surgical planning. Plain radiography can be used as an initial evaluation to localize the levels of involvement; however, CT must be obtained to further assess the anatomy and involvement of the osseous spine, which is important for precise surgical planning of the dimensions of the reconstruction. The spinal cord and neural elements, intervertebral discs, epidural contents, paraspinous anatomy, and soft tissues, including abnormalities such as tumors, are evaluated primarily with MRI. The detail and orthogonal views displayed with CT and MRI allow the best assessment for local anatomy and disease morphology. When necessary, other imaging modalities, such as angiography for vascular spinal tumors, may be used to obtain further information on the disease process.

The preoperative evaluation for thoracoscopic surgery also includes assessing the patient's ability to tolerate surgery under general anesthesia with single-lung ventilation. The patient's overall medical condition, including cardiovascular and hemodynamic stability, is assessed, and laboratory studies, including a complete blood count and coagulation panel, are reviewed. The patient's pulmonary status is also thoroughly assessed before surgery, which may require an evaluation by a pulmonologist, anesthesiologist, or qualified internist. An evaluation by or discussion with a cardiothoracic surgeon may also be warranted in cases of pulmonary disease, previous lung injury, or infection to decide whether the patient is suited for thoracoscopic surgery or open thoracotomy. A cardiothoracic surgeon should be available at the time of surgery, with advance knowledge of the case when possible, in the event that immediate conversion to an open exposure is needed.

Planning of Approach

The patient's imaging studies are examined in detail to develop a thorough understanding of the individual patient anatomy, particularly the relative locations of the chest wall and thorax, thoracolumbar spine and spinal cord, and mediastinal structures. The side of surgery is chosen based on disease lateralization and location with respect to the surrounding anatomy. The locations of the aorta and vena cava are noted in relation to plate placement and the lesion being treated. A left-sided approach is generally preferred at the thoracolumbar junction (T11-L2) and for disease lateralization to the left. For lesions of the upper to midthoracic spine (T3-10), a right-sided approach is typically chosen.

Planning of Resection and Reconstruction

Detailed preoperative examination of the patient's bony anatomy is important for planning the reconstruction. The appropriate lengths of the vertebral body screws are determined by measuring the widths of the vertebrae on the preoperative images. The height of the interbody is approximated by measuring the distance between the inferior end plate of the cranial level and the superior end plate of the caudal level. The plate dimensions can also be approximated preoperatively by measuring the distance between the lower third of the cranial vertebral body and the upper third of the caudal vertebral body. The extent of pathologic canal intrusion is also measured to determine the amount of bony resection needed for sufficient ventral spinal canal decompression.

Operative Technique

Thoracoscopic Instruments and Instrumentation Systems

Minimally invasive thoracoscopic instruments have been specifically developed for this application and are highly specialized. They are designed with adequate length for safe and effective intrathoracic maneuvering, have large handles for improved grip and ease of use, and are made with nonreflective surfaces to decrease glare on the endoscopic view. For illumination and optimal visualization, a high-quality endoscopic camera is essential. A high-definition, 0- to 30-degree angled rigid endoscope with a high-output xenon light source provides the best digital resolution.

The room is set up with the surgeon standing directly behind the patient and operative site. A video monitor with the projected endoscopic image is placed in front of the patient, directly across from the main surgeon, and a monitor displaying the fluoroscopic image is placed beside the endoscopic video monitor. The assistant operating the endoscope stands to the right of the surgeon. The third assistant, when available, stands across from the main surgeon in front of the patient and operates the retractor and suction/irrigation devices.

In addition to specialized instruments, the MACS-TL ventrolateral thoracolumbar spinal implant (Aesculap, Tuttlingen, Germany) was specifically designed for thoracoscopic use (Fig. 61-1). It consists of a rigid plate that is secured to the ventrolateral vertebral body with two pairs of triangulated fixation screws for increased strength: two dorsal polyaxial screws and two ventral stabilizing screws. The screws are implanted into the normal vertebrae adjacent to the diseased vertebra(e). The fixation plate is then rigidly secured to the screws. The biomechanical properties of the MACS-TL plating system have been characterized in monosegmental and bisegmental partial and full corpectomy models both with and without dorsal ligamentous injury. Case series have also demonstrated its clinical efficacy.[10,13,15,24-26]

Anesthesia

The patient is placed under general anesthesia for thoracoscopic spine surgery. For maximum surgical exposure, a double-lumen endotracheal tube is used for single-lung ventilation. The position of the endotracheal tube is confirmed before and after final positioning with a bronchoscope. A Foley catheter, arterial line, and, if necessary, central venous access are placed before patient positioning.

Patient Positioning

The patient is placed on a radiolucent operating table in the lateral decubitus position with the spine parallel to the operating table. Stabilizing supports positioned between the scapulae and against the sternum, sacrum, and coccyx are secured to the operating table for four-point stabilization. An axillary roll is placed and a Krause arm rest is used to support the top-lying arm, which is angled cranially to prevent obstruction of the instrumentation during the operation. The legs are placed in a slightly flexed position. A lateral spine view obtained with the C-arm fluoroscope confirms appropriate alignment of the spine in relation to the operating bed, by aligning the ventral and dorsal vertebral body lines and facet joints.

Localization

The relation of the spine and identified sites of the access portals is determined with intraoperative fluoroscopy. After optimal patient positioning, a lateral image centered over the pathologic area is obtained and projected orthograde onto the chest wall. The level of interest is often evident because of changes in spinal alignment and bony architecture. The skin is marked with a diagram outlining the vertebral bodies of the pathologic and adjacent levels by drawing the ventral and dorsal spinal lines and intervertebral discs. The four portal access sites are then marked (Fig. 61-2). The positioning of these portals determines working distances and is essential for proper retraction and intraoperative thoracoscopic image guidance.

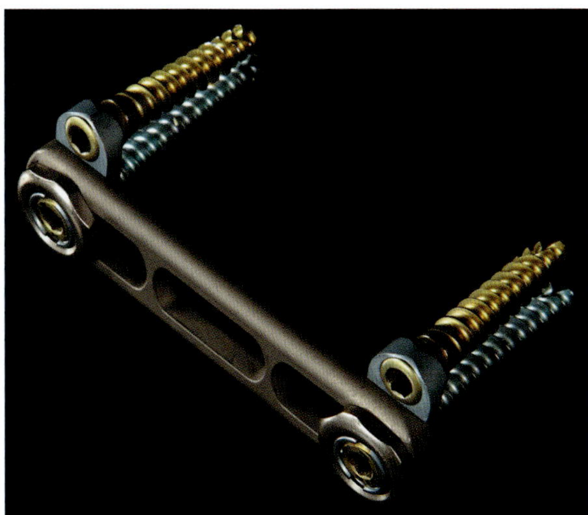

FIGURE 61-1. The MACS-TL ventrolateral thoracolumbar spinal implant (Aesculap, Tuttlingen, Germany) is a minimally invasive rigid fixation plate designed for thoracoscopic spinal stabilization.

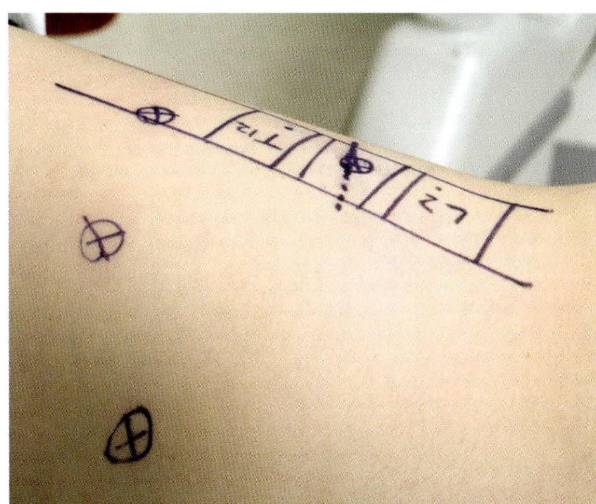

FIGURE 61-2. The skin is marked under fluoroscopic guidance with a diagram outlining the spine and portal sites. The vertebral bodies of the pathologic and adjacent levels are marked first, followed by the four portal access sites.

The operating portal site is centered directly over the pathologic level. Instrumentation and resection can be difficult if this portal site is improperly positioned. Moreover, misdirected instruments may slide along angled surfaces and increase the risk of injury to the spinal cord and vasculature. This access site extends 3 to 4 cm in length and is large enough to insert the fusion instrumentation during the case. The other access sites are approximately half the length of the working portal. The portal site for the thoracoscopic camera is situated along the axis of the spine approximately two to three intercostal spaces from the operating portal. For lesions at the thoracolumbar junction, the access site is marked in the cranial direction. Conversely, the site is marked in the caudal direction for middle to upper thoracic spine lesions. The suction/irrigation portal is located ventral and cranial to the operating portal, close enough to allow for ease in irrigation and suction of the surgical bed. The retractor for the lung and diaphragm is inserted through an access portal slightly caudal to the operating portal and further ventral to the suction/irrigation portal. Maintaining sufficient distance between the retractor and operating portals prevents intraoperative interference of the thoracoscopic instruments.

Access

The entire lateral chest wall is sterilized and draped in case conversion to open thoracotomy is necessary. After the anesthesiologist initiates single-lung ventilation, the surgeon opens the most cranially located portal, which minimizes the risk of injury to the underlying organs and diaphragm. The skin is incised, and a minithoracotomy technique is used to carry the dissection down to the rib. The rib is freed from the subcutaneous tissues and intercostal muscle layers with blunt dissection, without removal of the rib, and the pleural space is entered. The first trocar is inserted through the minithoracotomy between the ribs, and the thoracic cavity is inspected with the 30-degree endoscope to confirm successful single-lung ventilation and the absence of significant pleural adhesions. The retraction and suction/irrigation access ports are placed next using a similar technique under direct thoracoscopic visualization. The operating portal is placed last (because of its proximity to the intra-abdominal organs) and after the diaphragm has been safely retracted away from the access site.

Dissection and Exposure

The spine is oriented horizontally on the video monitor by rotating the endoscope. The aorta is situated ventral to the spine, and its dorsal margin demarcates the ventral border of the vertebral bodies. The dome of the diaphragm is then retracted to expose the diaphragmatic insertion, which is typically located between T12 and L1. The spine is exposed by incising the diaphragm when operating at or below the insertion (Fig. 61-3). The diaphragm is incised with a harmonic scalpel where it is naturally thin, which is parallel to and 1 to 2 cm away from the insertion site. Closure of the diaphragm at the end of the case is also facilitated by this margin of tissue. The layers of the diaphragm are incised in a semicircular line along the spine and ribs. A 2- to 3-cm incision is generally sufficient for lesions at L1. For exposure of L2, the length is increased caudally to approximately 5 cm. For lesions at L3, which may be difficult to approach with the thoracoscopic technique, a more extensive incision is made in the diaphragm, and a thoracoscopic-assisted, mini-open retroperitoneal exposure is used. Once the diaphragm is incised, the retractor is inserted through the opening. The ventral spine is exposed by mobilizing the peritoneal sac and retroperitoneal fat from the psoas muscle fascia with blunt dissection and retracting the tissue ventrally and caudally.

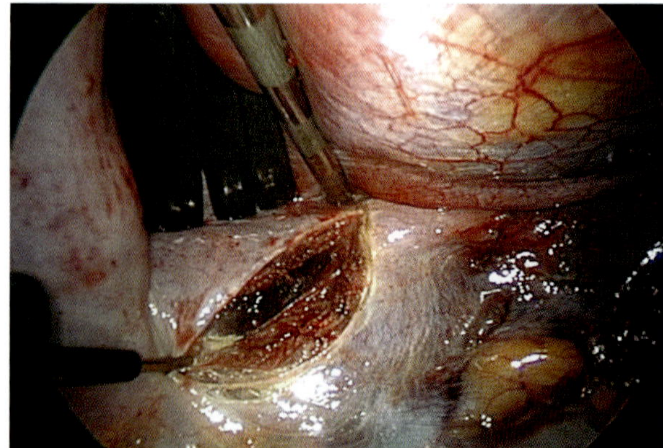

FIGURE 61-3. When operating at or below the insertion of the diaphragm, a harmonic scalpel is used to incise the diaphragm where it is naturally thin, approximately 1 to 2 cm away from and parallel to the insertion site.

The thoracic vertebral bodies and intervertebral discs are exposed by dissecting the prevertebral soft tissue off of the ventrolateral spine. The correct level is identified with intraoperative fluoroscopy and endoscopy, by recognizing local deformity, injury, or masses. The parietal pleura is incised along the spinal axis with the hooked-tip harmonic scalpel and elevated off of the vertebral body surface with blunt dissection. The segmental blood vessels run transverse to the incision and are located at the midportion of the vertebrae. The surgeon must be careful to identify the segmental vessels during the dissection without injuring them. Once identified, they are ligated with endoclips and divided. The pleural incision may be extended along the proximal rib of the pathologic and adjacent levels and elevated. Increasing the mediolateral exposure can increase access to the lateral vertebral body wall, intervertebral discs, and underlying injury or masses. The amount of exposure necessary may be determined by the extent of pathologic involvement of the vertebral body.

Vertebral Body Screw Instrumentation

The ventrolateral polyaxial screws for the MACS-TL plating system are inserted into the uninvolved vertebral bodies adjacent to the pathologic level. The first polyaxial screw is placed into the caudal level, which prevents the surgeon having to "look over" a cranially placed screw and keeps the visual field unobstructed. The screw entry point is positioned approximately 10 mm ventral to the spinal canal and 10 mm away from the end plate in the upper third of the vertebra (Fig. 61-4A), away from the midportion of the vertebral body where the segmental blood vessels lie. A short Kirschner wire (K-wire) is inserted under fluoroscopic guidance perpendicular to the cortical surface with a radiolucent targeting device. When a perpendicular position is attained, the concentric

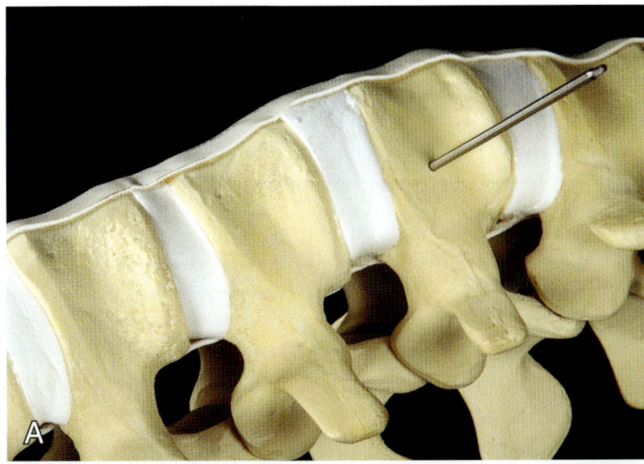

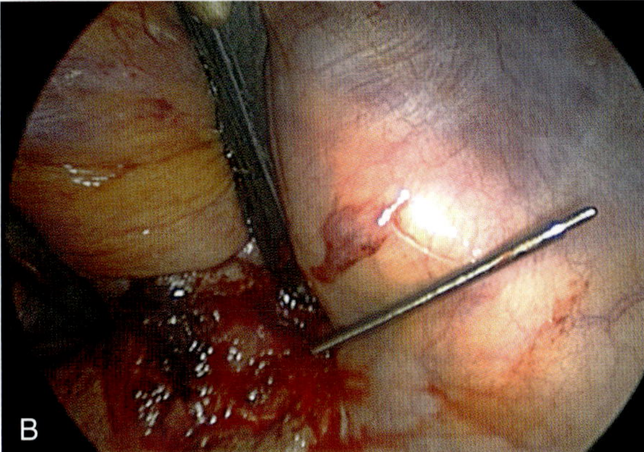

FIGURE 61-4. The entry point for the caudal screw is positioned approximately 10 mm ventral to the spinal canal and 10 mm away from the end plate in the upper third of the vertebra (**A**). A K-wire is driven with a mallet into position away from the midportion of the vertebral body where the segmental blood vessels lie (**B**).

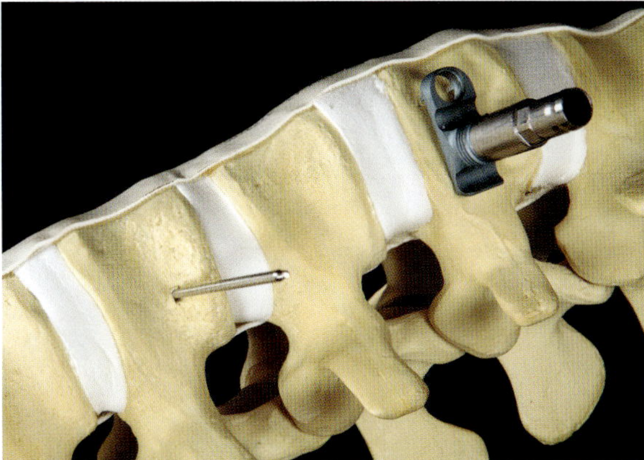

FIGURE 61-5. The screw-clamp assembly is oriented with the holes for the ventral stabilizing screws located ventrally and inserted over the K-wire.

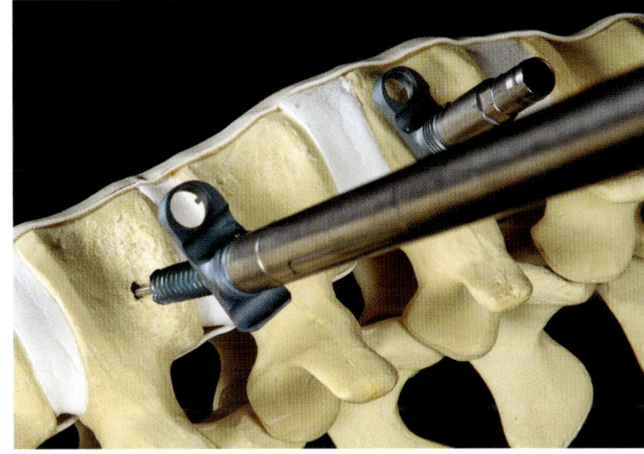

FIGURE 61-6. Inserting the caudal screw first keeps the surgical field clear for screw placement at the cranial level. The screw-clamp assembly at the cranial level is inserted approximately 10 mm ventral to the spinal canal and 10 mm away from the caudal end plate, in the inferior third of the vertebral body.

rings on the targeting device will align and the K-wire will appear on-end. A mallet is used to strike the device attached to the K-wire until a stable depth of approximately 25 mm is reached (Fig. 61-4B). The K-wire is then detached from the targeting instrument. The cortical surface is perforated with a cannulated decorticator, which is inserted over the K-wire, in preparation for screw instrumentation.

The screws for the MACS-TL system are inserted into a specialized polyaxial clamp before placement. The screw-clamp assembly is attached to a centralizer tube and inserted over the K-wire. The clamp is oriented with the ventral stabilizing screw hole located ventrally. The K-wire is removed after the screw is advanced past the cortical surface. Removal of the K-wire prevents its advancement during screw insertion and the possibility of vascular perforation or soft tissue injury. The screw is then safely inserted to its full depth (Fig. 61-5). Screw placement is then performed at the cranial level using a similar technique (Fig. 61-6). The insertion site is approximately 10 mm ventral to the spinal canal and in the inferior third of the vertebral body, approximately 10 mm cranial to the inferior end plate.

Vertebral Body Resection and Spinal Canal Decompression

The corpectomy boundaries are defined cranially and caudally by the intervertebral discs. The polyaxial clamps are oriented parallel to the end plates. The ventral and dorsal edges of the clamps define the ventromedial and posterolateral margins of the corpectomy. These boundaries define an area that includes both the corpectomy region itself and a safety zone that protects critical structures (Fig. 61-7A). The instruments are kept within these safe boundaries during the vertebral body resection.

Thoracoscopic discectomies at the disc spaces above and below the pathologic level are performed using the same technique as in open procedures. A thoracoscopic scalpel is used to perform an anulectomy and thoracoscopic rongeurs are used for disc resection. Cartilage and soft tissue are removed for end-plate preparation. A central corpectomy is performed by removing the vertebral body bone between the resected disc spaces. Osteotomes are used to create a rectangular trough in the vertebrae. Curettes, rongeurs, or a high-speed drill may be used to extend the corpectomy cavity (Fig. 61-7B). The cortical bone of the ventral, dorsal, and contralateral margins is kept intact. The depth of the corpectomy across the midline is confirmed with intraoperative fluoroscopy. In cases of tumor, bone and tissue samples are collected for frozen and permanent pathology sectioning.

Spinal canal decompression is performed for lesions significantly encroaching on the spinal canal beyond the dorsal wall of the vertebral body. The ventral spinal canal is accessed by

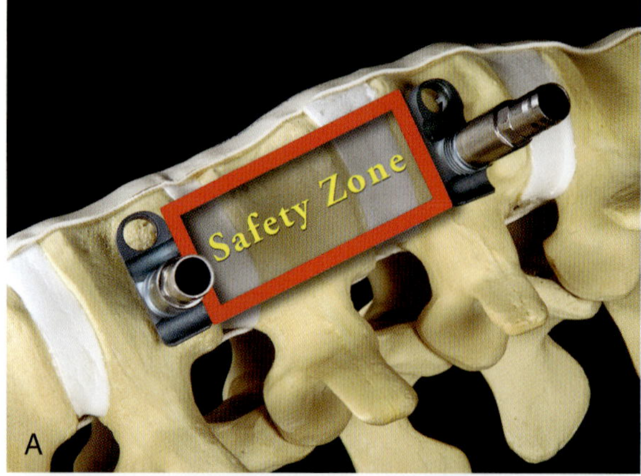

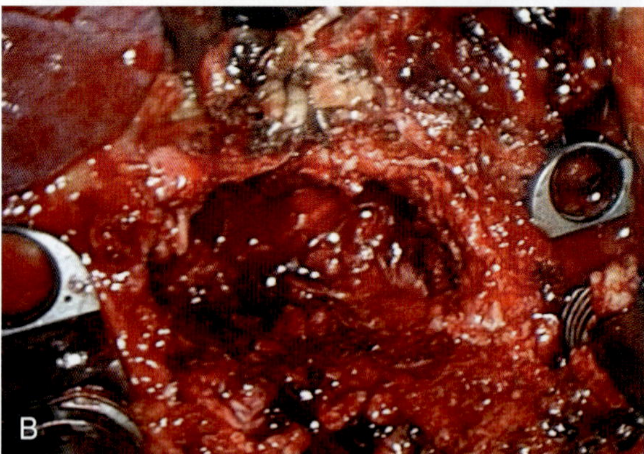

FIGURE 61-7. A safety zone is defined by the borders of the clamps (**A**). Instruments are kept within these safe boundaries, which also define the limits of the corpectomy (**B**). (Copyright Department of Neurosurgery, University of Utah.)

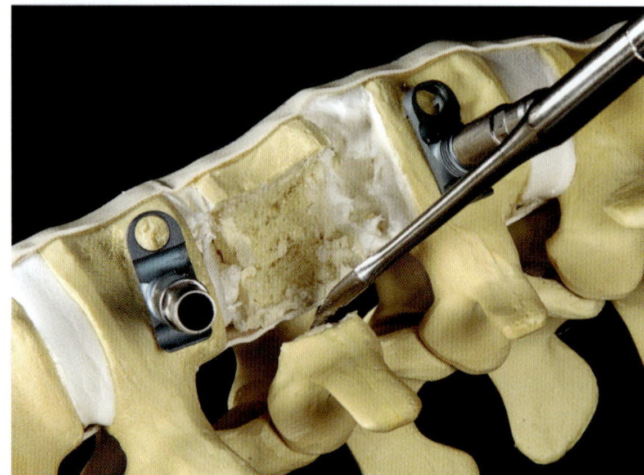

FIGURE 61-8. The ventral spinal canal is accessed and decompressed by removing the proximal rib head and pedicle.

identifying and removing the ipsilateral rib head and pedicle (Fig. 61-8). The rib head is followed to its attachment to the ventrolateral spine and resected with a high-speed drill. Removal of the proximal 2 cm exposes the underlying pedicle, which may be palpated and demarcated with a blunt hook. The pedicle is resected with thoracoscopic rongeurs and a high-speed drill to simultaneously decompress the neuroforamen and provide ventral spinal canal access. The epidural space is carefully cleared of bone and other pathologic tissues, such as blood and tumor, by gentle manipulation into the corpectomy cavity and removal. During this process, direct visualization of the thecal sac prevents injury to the underlying ventral spinal cord. Vertebral body resection is completed after the ventral spinal canal is adequately decompressed and the corpectomy cavity has been enlarged to accommodate the interbody device for reconstruction and stabilization.

Vertebral Body Reconstruction and Completion of Instrumentation

The vertebral body is reconstructed and final stabilization with instrumentation is performed after corpectomy and spinal decompression are completed. For the interbody implant, we commonly use expandable titanium cages, although interbody reconstructions can be performed with iliac crest autograft or with allografts, depending on surgeon preference. Calipers are used to measure the corpectomy cavity dimensions. The operating portal is replaced with a speculum, and the expandable cage is inserted into the corpectomy cavity. Both thoracoscopic and fluoroscopic visualization are used to determine the position of the cage in the coronal and sagittal planes while it is being expanded. To promote fusion, morselized bone autograft or allograft may be placed in and around the cage.

After the vertebral body is stabilized, the ventrolateral MACS-TL plate is fit and secured over the screw-clamp assembly. A suitable plate length is chosen by measuring the distance between the screw heads and adding 30 mm to the measurement. The plate is first mounted over the centralizer and caudal screw-clamp assembly and then positioned onto the cranial assembly (Fig. 61-9). Leaving the screws slightly loose when fitting the plate allows angulation of the polyaxial heads and facilitates plate positioning. Fixation nuts are screwed onto the polyaxial head over the plate and secured with a torque handle and then the centralizers are removed from the polyaxial clamps.

The reconstruction is completed by inserting the ventral stabilizing screws and tightening and locking the polyaxial screws. Final tightening of the polyaxial screws down to the vertebral bodies eliminates the rotational freedom of the screw-clamp assembly and plate. The guide sleeve for the

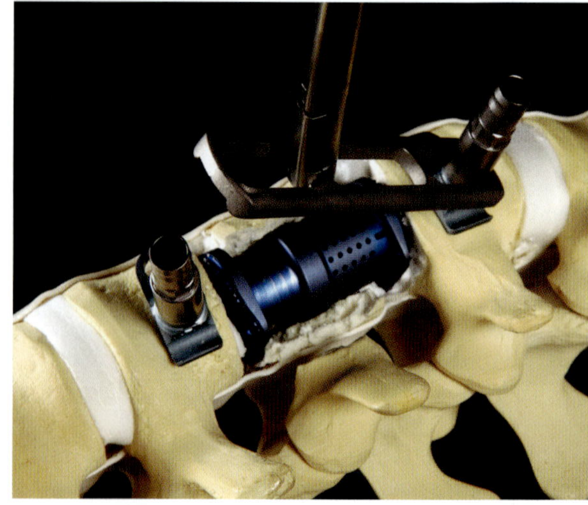

FIGURE 61-9. The ventrolateral plate is fitted over the cranial screw-clamp assembly after secure placement over the caudal assembly. Leaving the screws slightly loose allows angulation and adjustment of the polyaxial heads.

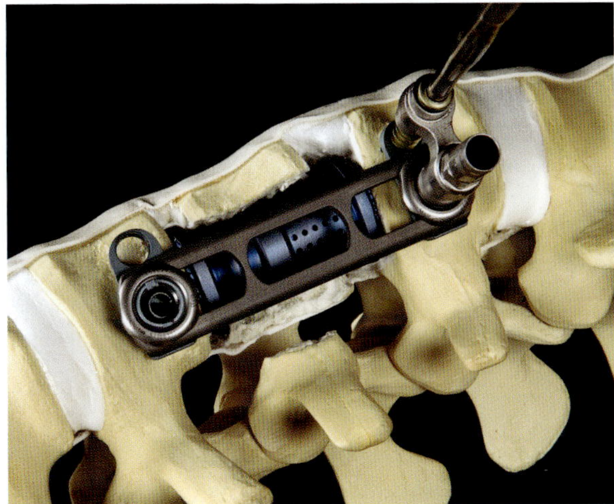

FIGURE 61-10. After fixation nuts are secured and the entire assembly is tightened, ventral stabilizing screws are placed through the screw guide sleeve.

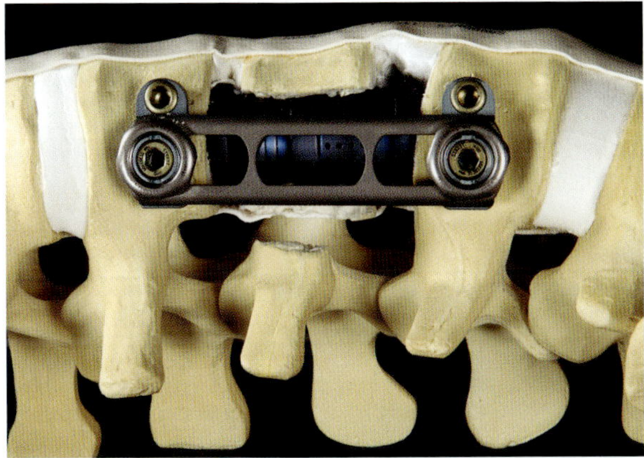

FIGURE 61-11. The construct is completed after securing the locking screws, converting the polyaxial screw-clamp system into a rigid construct.

ventral stabilizing screw is attached to the polyaxial clamp. The decorticator is inserted through the guide sleeve and ventral hole in the clamp. A driver is used to insert the ventral stabilizing screw into the vertebral body (Fig. 61-10), and the guide sleeve is removed. The ventral stabilizing screws for the MACS-TL system are triangulated and should be 5 mm shorter than the posterolateral screw to prevent contact of the two screws. Finally, the gold locking screw is inserted into the polyaxial head and locked with a torque wrench, converting the polyaxial screw-clamp system into a rigid and completed construct (Figs. 61-11 and 61-12). Anteroposterior and lateral fluoroscopic imaging verifies the final construct position.

Chest Tube Placement and Wound Closure

Closure of the surgical site begins by reapproximating the diaphragm. The incision is exposed by rearranging the retractors and closed with interrupted, absorbable sutures or staples. The thoracic cavity is irrigated and inspected for hemostasis, and visible blood clots are removed. A 24-French chest tube is inserted through the suction/irrigation or lung/diaphragm retractor portals under direct thoracoscopic visualization such

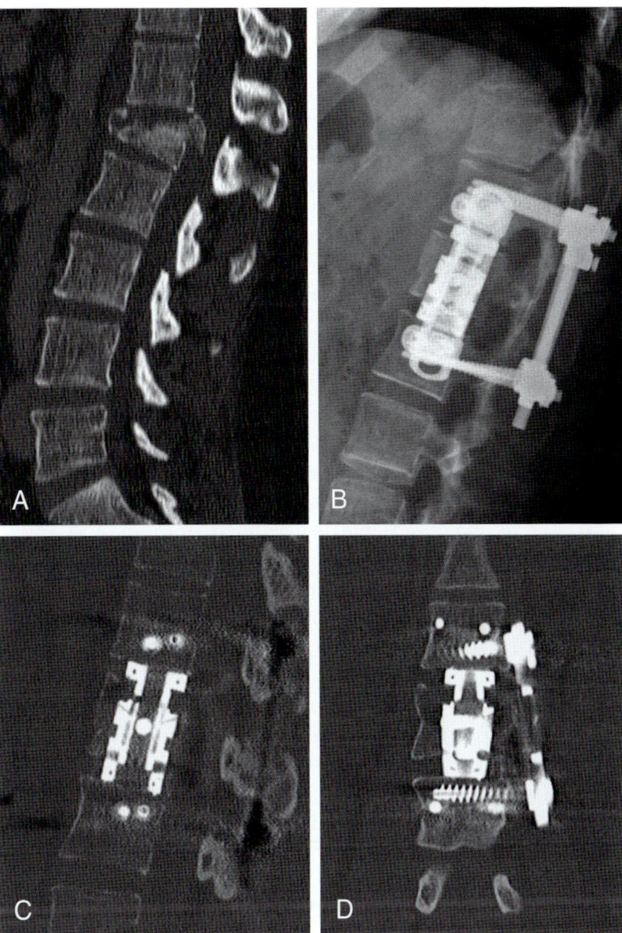

FIGURE 61-12. A 37-year-old woman involved in a high-speed motor vehicle crash suffered an L1 burst fracture without neurologic deficits (**A**). She underwent T12 through L2 dorsal spinal fusion followed by L1 thoracoscopic corpectomy and reconstruction with an expandable titanium cage (**B–D**).

that the end is situated at the chest cavity apex. To ensure that all lobes are properly reinflated, the lung is visualized with endoscopy during reinflation. The trocars are sequentially removed, the incisions are reapproximated in multiple layers, and the chest tube is secured.

The patient may be extubated immediately after surgery. Lung inflation without significant pneumothorax is also verified in the immediate postoperative period with a chest radiograph. Initially, the chest tube is connected to intermittent wall suction. If proper lung inflation is demonstrated on the chest radiograph, the chest tube is advanced to water seal on postoperative day 1. Patient mobilization, incentive spirometry training, and postoperative plain radiographs and CT scans centered on the construct are also obtained on postoperative day 1. Once chest radiographs continue to demonstrate lung inflation without pneumothorax and the chest tube output decreases below 100 mL/day, the chest tube is removed, typically on postoperative day 2. A final chest radiograph is used to verify stable lung inflation after chest tube removal. After discharge, the patient returns to the clinic for follow-up examination and plain radiographs at 1-, 3-, 6-, 12-, and 24-month intervals. Work with light duty is typically allowed after 4 weeks and full activity after 3 months.

Technical Tips

The initial setup largely determines the ease or difficulty of the operation. The operation is more likely to be successfully completed by positioning the patient and access portals correctly. The patient's spine is positioned in a true lateral position by inspecting the edges and end plates of the operative vertebral bodies under fluoroscopy, ensuring that no overlap is present. By correctly positioning the spine, the thoracoscopic instruments and instrumentation are aimed perpendicular to the spine, which increases screw placement accuracy and decreases the potential for injury. Avoiding instrument conflicts and misplacements during surgery also increases the chances of a safe operation, which can be accomplished with proper placement of access ports, with sufficient distance between them.

The complexity of thoracoscopic fusion techniques mandates that technical details are adhered to strictly and that each step is executed in the specified manner and order. Preoperative measurements of the vertebral body dimensions and screw lengths should be communicated to the surgical staff at the beginning of the operation. Optimal preparation of the instrumentation before placement can decrease intraoperative lag time and increase efficiency.

The surgeon must be aware of the surrounding anatomy during the exposure to avoid injury and complication. When operating adjacent to the segmental blood vessels, monopolar electrocautery must be used judiciously to avoid damage to the vasculature. Successfully identifying and ligating the segmental vessels decreases the risk of significant bleeding. The nerve root emerges dorsal to the vertebral body, and electrocautery should not be used in its vicinity. In the event of organ injury or significant hemorrhage, conversion to an open thoracotomy may be necessary. When warranted, the aid of a cardiothoracic surgeon early during the operation or during preoperative coordination may facilitate intervention.

The vertebral body resection is performed within protected margins to avoid complications. The operative safety zone is defined by the edges of the polyaxial clamps attached to the screw heads, and the depth of corpectomy is confirmed with fluoroscopy or by direct measurement by placing a scaled instrument into the resection bed and filling the trough with irrigation fluid. The level of fluid marks the corpectomy depth, which can be compared with the vertebral body width measured preoperatively and the planned dimensions of the corpectomy. The implant can be safely and easily inserted without excessive force, which can damage the surrounding neural and vascular structures.

Patients with poor bone quality may require construct reinforcement to achieve solid instrumented fixation. Cementable MACS-TL screws with increased thread diameter and pitch to prevent pullout are available for this purpose (Figs. 61-13 and 61-14); these have been demonstrated to increase fixation strength and biomechanical stability.[27,28] In challenging cases, these screws can also be used for rescue. Injectable cement is delivered into the hollow screw core and through three longitudinal slits into the surrounding cancellous bone. The posterolateral MACS-TL screws are replaced by the cementable screws in the polyaxial clamps, and screw implantation is performed with the same technique. The construct is tightened flush against the bone into its final position before 1.5 mL of cement is injected because adjusting the position of the construct is extremely difficult once the cement has set. Securing the locking nuts completes the construct.

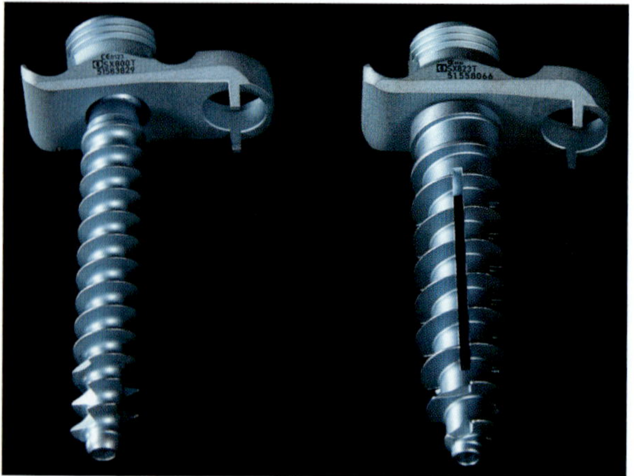

FIGURE 61-13. Cementable MACS-TL screws (*right*) have increased pitch and thread diameter compared with standard screws (*left*) to prevent screw pullout. Injectable cement is delivered into the hollow screw core and through three longitudinal slits into the surrounding cancellous bone.

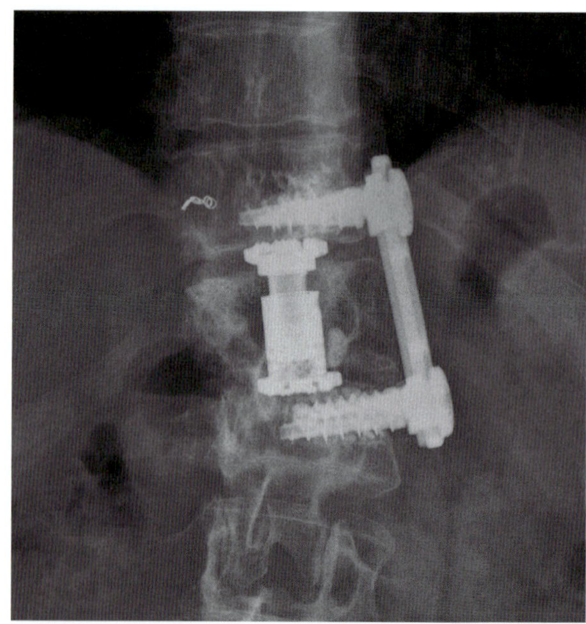

FIGURE 61-14. A 54-year-old man with metastatic lung cancer to T12 undergoing a left thoracoscopic corpectomy and reconstruction with an expandaple cage was found to have significantly osteoporotic bone from his prior treatments. Cementable Polyaxialscrew XL screws (Aesculap, Tuttlingen, Germany) were used in place of the standard MACS-TL screws, and 1.5 mL of polymethylmethacrylate cement was injected into each screw.

Outcomes

Results

Minimally invasive thoracoscopic spine surgery has demonstrated safety and efficacy, with improved outcomes over open surgery. The limited exposure and approach are the primary factors in decreasing overall morbidity. Thoracoscopic procedures have complication rates between 0% and 5.4%,[10,13,16-18] whereas open thoracotomy morbidity rates are between 14% and 29.5%.[8,16-18,29] The complication rate of postoperative pneumothorax, pleural effusion, and intercostal muscle neuralgia for the thoracoscopic approach is reported to be 5.4%, compared with 14% for the open approach.[18] In cases of tumor, the reported mortality rate for open thoracotomy is 8.2%,[8] whereas thoracoscopic surgery has had no reported mortality.[10,16] Both thoracotomy and thoracoscopic surgery are associated with low infection rates of around 0.5%.[16-18]

Postoperative pain after thoracoscopic surgery is significantly reduced.[10] Postoperative analgesic therapy dosages and durations are reported to decrease by 42% and 31%, respectively.[16-18] Although reported rates of chronic pain with open thoracotomy range from 7% to 55%,[18] favorable rates between 4% and 35% are associated thoracoscopic surgery. The median length of stay in the hospital was 7 days (range, 4–10 days) in a series of patients who underwent thoracoscopic tumor surgery,[10] compared with a median of 9 days (range, 4 to 57 days) for patients who underwent open thoracotomy for tumor resection.[8] Fusion rates at 1-year radiographic follow-up have been reported to be up to 90% using the MACS-TL ventrolateral plating system.[17]

While the surgeon and surgical staff learn the new thoracoscopic technique, operative times increase initially to an average of 6 hours or more.[9,10,13,16-18] Once the procedure has been mastered, total surgical time for resection and reconstruction is decreased to 2.5 to 3 hours in cases of trauma[18] and to 4 hours for cases of tumor.[10] The average estimated blood loss for thoracoscopic spine surgery in trauma patients ranges from 250 to 450 mL,[18] which is less than with many dorsal fusion procedures. In cases of tumor, blood loss of 600 mL is reported for thoracoscopic cases,[10] whereas studies of open thoracotomy cases for tumor have reported 1 L of blood loss.[8] Major intraoperative complications such as injury to the viscera or vasculature, uncontrollable hemorrhage, and cerebrospinal fluid or chyle leak can be avoided in most instances with meticulous adherence to surgical technique.[10] In skilled hands, the rate of conversion to an open thoracotomy is 1% or less.[17]

Complications

The incidence of significant intraoperative complications with thoracoscopic surgery is low.[10,11,13,15] Injury to the aorta or vena cava constitutes the most hazardous complication. Direct injury may occur from excessive use of sharp instruments; indirect extension of injury to the segmental vessels may also damage the great vessels. Injury to the segmental vessels themselves can result in considerable blood loss and is typically the result of insufficient exposure and coagulation. The vasculature may also be injured by a breach through the cortex opposite the corpectomy site, where the segmental vessels may be in close proximity to the vertebral body. To prevent a breach through the cortical bone, the integrity of the opposite cortex is verified with direct thoracoscopic visualization and intraoperative fluoroscopy. Overaggressive retraction, suction, or instrument handling can result in local injury to the lung parenchyma, which is usually sufficiently addressed with stapling or suturing as needed. Aggressive diaphragmatic incisions or retraction can cause injury to the kidneys, spleen, and ureters.

Thoracoscopic procedures can also place the neural structures at risk. Spinal cord injury or dural tears can occur with overaggressive maneuvers during decompression of the ventral spinal canal. These same injuries can also occur with insufficient decompression from forced overimpaction of the interbody implant into an inadequately sized corpectomy cavity. Persistent cerebrospinal fluid leaks significantly increase the risk of wound breakdown and infection. If an intraoperative dural defect is discovered, direct repair with suture should be attempted to perform a watertight dural closure; however, if that is not possible, we usually place collagen at the site of the leak, close with fibrin glue, and place a lumbar drain. In the event that a cerebrospinal fluid leak is detected postoperatively, the formation of a cerebrospinal fluid fistula is prevented by keeping the chest tube suction on no more than 20 cm of water suction, which should be changed to water seal as soon as possible. Spinal cord injury from direct manipulation or vascular compromise is most likely to occur during vertebral body resection, ventral canal decompression, or interbody reconstruction. These steps should be performed with careful, precise handling of the instruments and with thoracoscopic or fluoroscopic visual confirmation. Injury to the exiting nerve roots is most likely to occur during the exposure with aggressive electrocautery, which should be avoided along or dorsal to the dorsal vertebral body.

Pulmonary complications are most common during the early postoperative period. Patients may experience atelectasis, persistent pneumothorax or hemothorax, pleural effusions, or pneumonia, and with time may develop intrathoracic adhesions.[17,18] Aggressive pulmonary toilet, early ambulation, avoidance of narcotic overuse, and judicious use of the chest tube can prevent these complications in most cases. Although their incidence is lower than with open thoracotomy, intercostal neuralgia and shoulder pain and dysfunction are still possible. The risk of both superficial and deep wound infections and wound dehiscence exists with all surgeries, and may be decreased with a careful multilevel closure.

Potential late complications include instrumentation and fusion failures. Although minimally invasive technology has undergone major advances and improvements, the potential complications of hardware fracture, pullout, and loosening cannot altogether be prevented. The incidence of hardware complications may be decreased by carefully choosing a suitable construct and by improving surgical technique. Furthermore, patients with significant spinal column disruption, as may be the case in trauma, or with advanced osteoporosis may benefit from dorsal instrumentation for supplementation of ventral thoracoscopic reconstruction and to increase overall spinal stability.[30]

Conclusions

The recent advances in thoracoscopic surgical techniques, instruments, and instrumentation have made this treatment modality one of the standard procedures for thoracolumbar vertebral body resection and ventral spinal canal decompression. The technology continues to be improved and refined. The development of instrumentation specific to thoracoscopic technique has made ventral spinal stabilization and reconstruction achievable after decompression. With current methods, the thoracoscopic technique is safe and effective, and patient outcomes are improved after thoracoscopic surgery compared with open thoracotomy. Given familiarity with the operative technique, an understanding of local and patient-specific anatomy, and appropriate patient selection, a diversity of ventral thoracolumbar disease can be successfully treated with minimally invasive thoracoscopic surgery.

KEY REFERENCES

Beisse R: Endoscopic anterior repair in spinal trauma. In Regan JJ, Lieberman IH, editors: *Atlas of minimal access spine surgery*, 2nd ed, St. Louis, 2004, Quality Medical Publishing, pp 285–320.

Beisse R: Thoracoscopic decompression and fixation (MACS-TL). In Kim D, Fessler RG, Regan JJ, editors: *Endoscopic spine surgery and instrumentation*, New York, 2004, Thieme, pp 180–198.

Beisse R: Thoracoscopically assisted anterior approach to thoracolumbar fractures. In Mayer HM, editor: *Minimally invasive spine surgery: a surgical manual*, New York, 2005, Springer, pp 203–214.

Beisse R, Muckley T, Schmidt MH, et al: Surgical technique and results of endoscopic anterior spinal canal decompression. *J Neurosurg Spine* 2: 128–136, 2005.

Kan P, Schmidt MH: Minimally invasive thoracoscopic approach for anterior decompression and stabilization of metastatic spine disease. *Neurosurg Focus* 25(2):E8, 2008.

Khoo LT, Beisse R, Potulski M: Thoracoscopic-assisted treatment of thoracic and lumbar fractures: a series of 371 consecutive cases. *Neurosurgery* 51(Suppl 5):S104–S117, 2002.

REFERENCES

The complete reference list is available online at expertconsult.com.

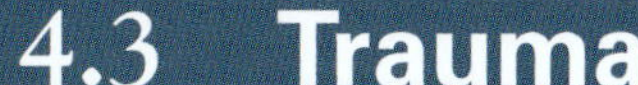
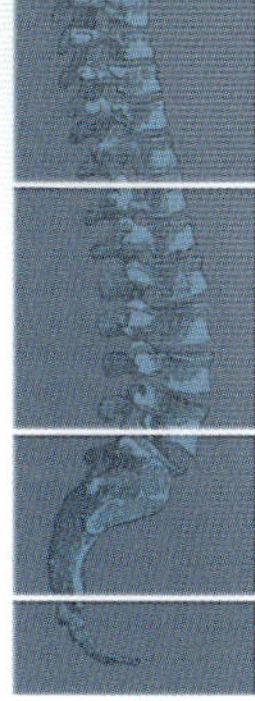

4.3 Trauma

CHAPTER 62

Classification of Thoracolumbar Spine Fractures

Nader S. Dahdaleh | Patrick W. Hitchon

Review of Thoracolumbar Classification Schemes

In this chapter, fractures of the thoracic spine, thoracolumbar junction, and lumbar spine are grouped under the rubric of "thoracolumbar spine fractures."

The biomechanical force vectors acting on the spine can be either rotational or linear. Among the rotational forces are flexion, extension, lateral bending, and torsional forces. Linear forces include compression, translational, and distraction forces. These forces can act alone or in combination, resulting in different and diverse fracture patterns.[1] Although not always possible, categorizing a fracture based on a classification system is crucial to aid the clinician in selecting the appropriate management strategy. An effective classification system should be comprehensive, easy to apply, and directive of appropriate treatment.[2]

Current classification systems base their algorithms on the stability of different fracture patterns. The earliest attempt to classify thoracolumbar spine fractures was reported by Boehler in 1929.[2] He grouped thoracolumbar fractures into five entities: compression, flexion-distraction, extension, shear, and rotational fractures. In 1938, Watson-Jones[3] divided these fractures into simple wedge fractures, comminuted fractures, and fracture-dislocations. He introduced the concept of instability and was the first to associate the integrity of the posterior ligamentous complex (PLC) with spinal stability. In 1949, Nicoll[4] categorized fractures into stable and unstable fractures. He ascribed four structures as contributing to spinal stability: the vertebral body, the disc, the facets, and the interspinous ligaments. In his view, the integrity of the latter was the major determinant of stability. He classified thoracolumbar spine fractures into anterior wedge, lateral wedge, fracture-dislocations, and neural arch fractures.

In his landmark 1963 paper, Holdsworth introduced the two-column theory of spinal stability.[5] He recognized five mechanisms of injury: flexion, flexion-rotation, extension, compression, and shear forces. His classification scheme included anterior compressions; fracture-dislocations; rotational fracture-dislocations; and extension, shear, and burst fractures. He then categorized fractures as stable or unstable. According to his model, the spine was divided into anterior and posterior columns. The anterior column consisted of the vertebral body and the intervertebral disc, and the posterior column consisted of the neural arch, facet joints, and PLC (interspinal and supraspinal ligaments and ligamentum flavum). Fractures that included posterior column injury were unstable. His model thus defined burst-type fractures, which he was the first to describe, as stable.

In a sometimes controversial formulation, White and Panjabi in 1978 defined clinical instability as the inability of the spine under physiologic loads to maintain relationships between vertebrae such that there is neither acute nor subsequent neurologic injury, deformity, or pain.[6] In addition to neurologic deficit, motion, and disruption of the anterior and posterior "elements," their algorithm recognized the significance of pain and the anticipated loading of the spine. The latter, although significant, had not been identified in previous paradigms of fracture severity.

The three-column theory of the spine was introduced by Francis Denis in 1983.[7] He added a third or middle column to Holdsworth's two-column model. According to Denis, the anterior column of the spine comprised the anterior longitudinal ligament and the anterior half of the vertebral body, anulus, and disc. The middle column included the posterior half of the vertebral body, anulus, and disc, in addition to the posterior longitudinal ligament. The posterior column incorporated the neural arch, facets, and PLC, which consisted of the supraspinal and interspinal ligaments, ligamentum flavum, and facet capsules (Fig. 62-1). The middle column was important because for dislocation to occur, it was necessary to disrupt the middle column along with the anterior or posterior column, or both. Denis defined stability based on the integrity of two of the three columns. His classification included four groups: compression fractures resulting from failure of the anterior column under compression, burst fractures resulting from failure of the anterior and middle columns secondary to fractures of the vertebral body under axial loads, flexion-distraction injuries secondary to failure of the posterior and middle columns, and fracture-dislocations resulting from failure of all three columns. Under this scheme, flexion-distraction injuries or seat belt-type injuries were considered unstable in the first degree. Burst fractures with deficit were considered unstable in the second degree, and fracture-dislocations were unstable in the third degree.

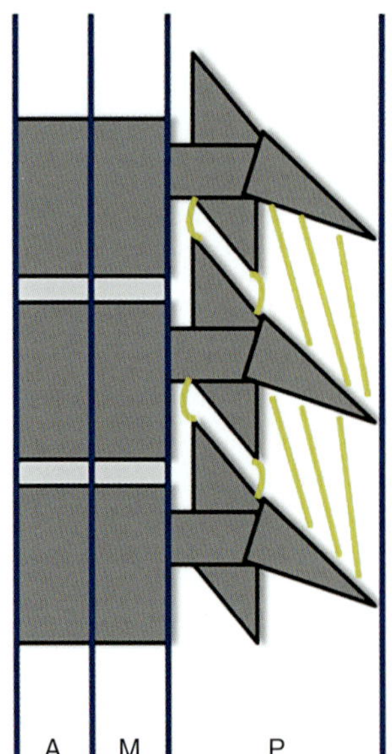

FIGURE 62-1. Denis's three-column model of the spine: anterior column (A), middle column (M), posterior column (P).

This classification system was later supported by in vitro biomechanical studies.[8]

As opposed to Denis, who subdivided basic injury patterns based on review of mostly radiographs of 412 fractures (53 were CT images), McAfee et al. in 1983 based their classification on an examination of CT scans with sagittal reconstruction from 100 patients.[9] They recognized six fracture patterns: wedge compression, stable burst, unstable burst, Chance fracture, flexion-distraction, and translational. They linked the stability of burst fractures with the integrity of the PLC, emphasizing the PLC as the major factor in fracture stability. Shortly afterward, in 1984, Ferguson and Allen[10] introduced the "mechanistic classification." They classified fractures into seven categories: compressive flexion, distractive flexion, lateral flexion, torsional flexion, translation, vertical compression, and distractive flexion injuries.

In 1989, Magerl et al.[11] introduced the AO (*Arbeitsgemeinschaft für Osteosynthesefragen*) classification system, based on a 10-year review of 1445 thoracolumbar fractures. They recognized three main fracture types: type A (compression), type B (distraction), and type C (fracture-dislocation). Subdivisions were created according to the severity of the fracture, resulting in 53 fracture patterns, with A1 being the least severe and C3 the most severe. This schema was generated based on review of radiographs, and as a result of their diligence, the schema was extensive and not always user friendly.

The load-sharing classification, introduced by McCormack et al. in 1994,[12] was derived from analysis of failures of thoracolumbar spine fractures treated with transpedicular short-segment arthrodesis. Fractures were graded according to the degree of comminution of the body, apposition of the fracture fragments, and deformity. A point system from 1 to 3 was applied to each fracture, with a higher number indicating greater severity. Fractures with a score greater than 7 had a high risk of short-segment fixation failure. This algorithm was intended to aid in the surgical decision of whether to use short-segment arthrodesis or anterior column graft support. The classification was validated biomechanically in vitro.[13]

In 2005, the Spine Trauma Study Group introduced the Thoracolumbar Injury Severity Score (TLISS) as a new classification system.[13-15] The system was based on three injury characteristics: mechanism of injury, neurologic status, and integrity of the PLC. Pertaining to the mechanism of injury, compression injuries are assigned one point; compression fractures with coronal plane deformity greater than 15 degrees and burst fractures are assigned two points. Translational or rotational injuries receive three points, and distraction injuries, being the most unstable, receive four points. The severity of neurologic injury is scored based on a five-category system. Patients with a negative neurologic examination receive zero points. In the presence of nerve root injury or complete spinal cord injury, the fracture is assigned two points. Patients with an incomplete spinal cord injury or cauda equina syndrome are assigned three points. The integrity of the PLC can be assessed clinically by the presence of a palpable interspinous gap, by separation of the spinous processes on plain radiographs, or by MRI. Patients with an intact PLC receive zero points. Those in whom the integrity of the PLC is indeterminate receive two points, and those with confirmed injury receive three points.

In the TLISS system, if the injury involves multiple levels, the most severe level is scored. In cases where more than one mechanism involves the same level, the score should represent the summation of mechanisms. The total TLISS reflects the severity of the injury and helps guide treatment. Patients with a score of 3 or less are treated nonoperatively. Those with scores of 5 or above are treated by surgical stabilization. Finally, patients with a score of 4 points fall into the indeterminate category, and treatment is according to the surgeon's preference.

Based on a study that showed fair to moderate inter-rater agreement,[16] the TLISS system, which emphasizes the mechanism of injury, was modified into the Thoracolumbar Injury Classification and Severity Score (TLICS), which emphasizes the morphology of fractures. In cases of multiple mechanisms involving one or more levels, the TLICS, as opposed to the TLISS, would consider only the most severe injury mechanism. Moreover, the one-point addition for coronal plane deformity was eliminated. Subsequent studies showed that both the TLISS and TLICS were comparable.[17,18] Moreover, Lenarz et al.[19] showed that the interobserver reliability of the TLISS system was comparable to that of the Denis and AO systems. The TLICS algorithm encompasses radiographic or mechanistic criteria, clinical criteria, and the integrity of the PLC assessed on MRI. No weight is given to the presence of pain, however.

Iowa Classification System and Algorithm

Recognizing the aforementioned schemes, and based on data collected prospectively on 300 thoracolumbar fractures, a simple classification system and algorithm for thoracolumbar spine fractures were developed (Fig. 62-2). This algorithm is based on three categories of criteria: clinical, biomechanical, and radiographic. The clinical criteria address the presence or absence of pain or neurologic deficit. Biomechanical criteria describe the involvement of one, two, or three columns, referring to Denis's three-column theory. Radiographic criteria address the degree of kyphosis and canal compromise, and the integrity of the PLC.

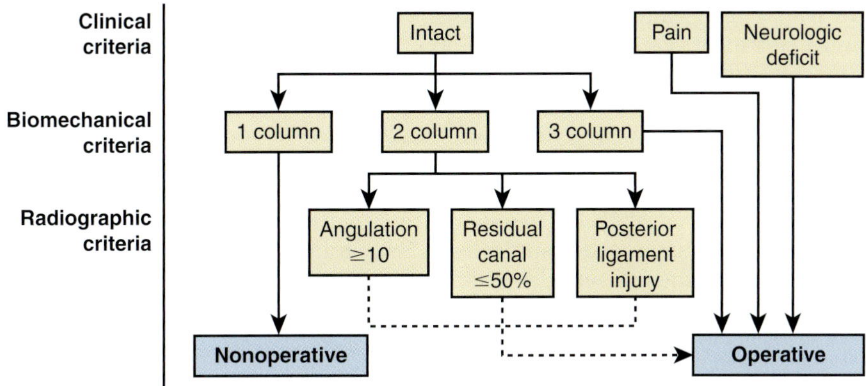

FIGURE 62-2. Iowa algorithm for the classification and treatment of thoracolumbar fractures. Patients who have a neurologic deficit, disabling pain, or a three-column injury undergo stabilization surgery. In patients with burst fractures (two-column injury), the integrity of the posterior ligamentous complex, degree of angulation, and residual canal factor into assessing spinal stability and hence direct management.

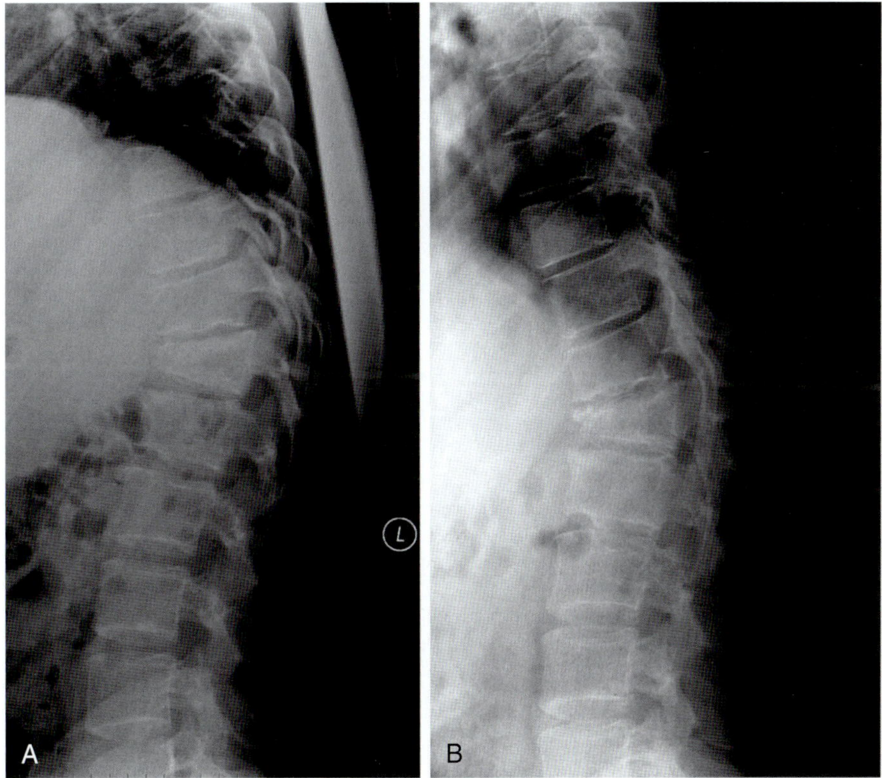

FIGURE 62-3. This patient sustained a thoracic flexion-compression fracture (**A**). He was neurologically intact, and his fracture was treated conservatively with external bracing for 3 months. Eleven months later, the patient was asymptomatic, with minimal progression of angulation at the fracture site (**B**).

Surgical decompression and stabilization is recommended for those patients with neurologic deficit. Surgery is also recommended in those patients who, in spite of a negative neurologic examination, experience persistent pain despite bracing and cannot be mobilized satisfactorily. In patients with a negative neurologic examination, the biomechanical criteria are then used to address three-column involvement using plain radiographs and CT scans. In the presence of three-column injuries (e.g., fracture-dislocations or flexion-distraction injuries), which are inherently unstable, patients are operated on acutely. Patients with a single-column fracture (e.g., wedge compression fracture) are treated nonoperatively with bracing. In a two-column injury (e.g., burst fracture), the integrity of the PLC is assessed with MRI. Disruption of the PLC would render burst fractures unstable and hence qualify these patients for stabilization.

This algorithm recognizes four major types of thoracolumbar spine fractures:

1. *Wedge compression fractures:* These are the most common type of fractures and occur secondary to axial load application in flexion.[1] These fractures involve injury to the anterior Denis column only, sparing the middle and posterior columns (Fig. 62-3). Patients are typically neurologically intact and associated PLC disruption is

rare. Conservative management with bracing and/or analgesia is the usual treatment. Patients with osteoporosis are at risk for these fractures, which can lead to severe kyphosis if multiple levels are involved.

2. *Burst fractures:* These fractures occur as a result of axial load application. They involve injury to both the anterior and middle columns of Denis. Retropulsion of bony fragments into the canal occurs to varying degrees. The occurrence of associated neurologic injury is similarly variable, but when present demands decompression and stabilization. Correlation between the occurrence of neurologic deficit and the extent of canal compromise is controversial.[20-22] Management of these injuries can be challenging, especially in patients who are neurologically intact.[23,24] Disruption of the PLC as ascertained by MRI renders these fractures unstable. An unpublished, prospective review of 70 burst fractures treated at the University of Iowa since 1993 was conducted. Owing to absent or minimal neurologic deficit, this cohort was treated nonoperatively. Ultimately, 20 patients failed nonoperative treatment, mostly because of pain, and underwent surgery. The

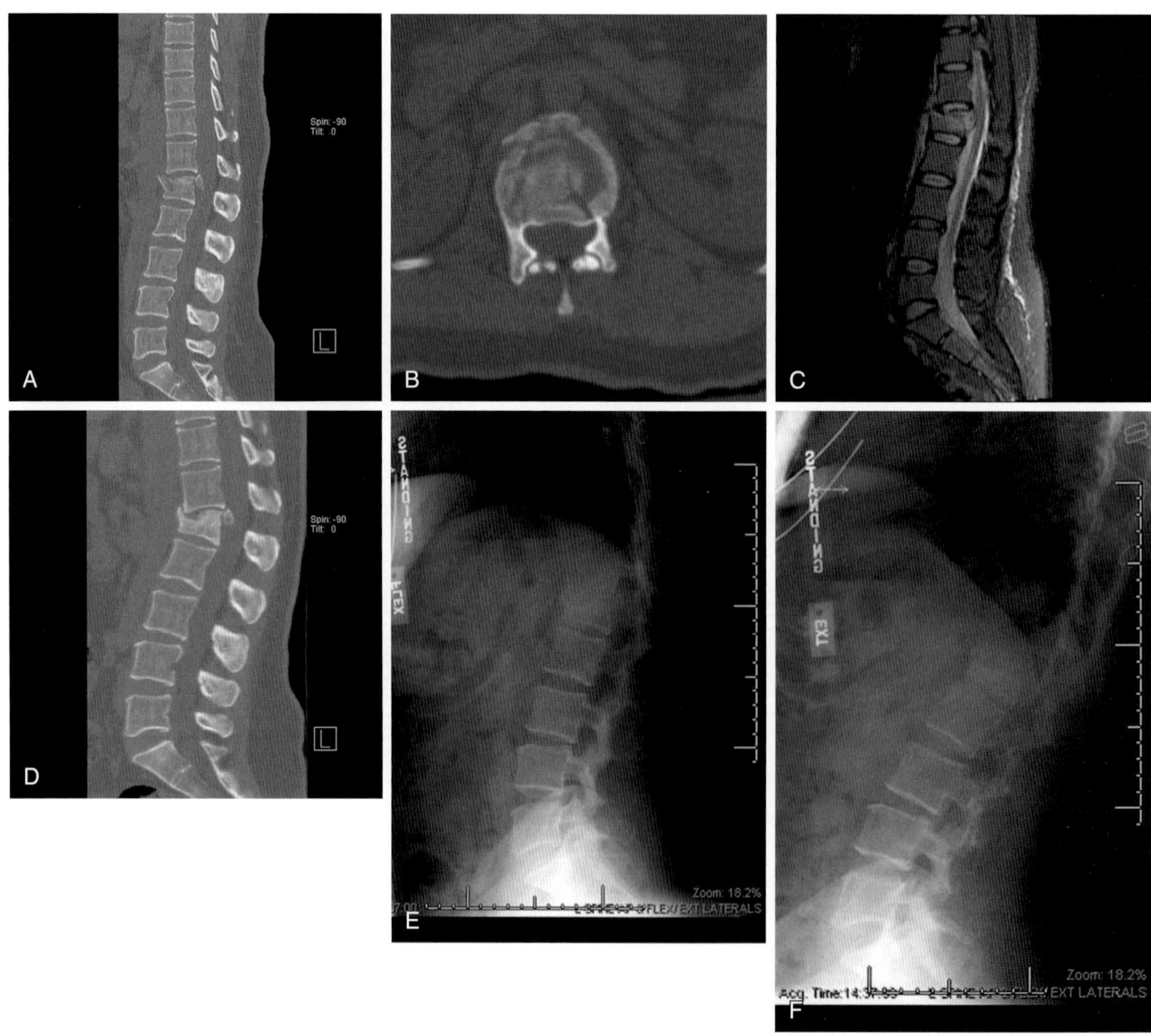

FIGURE 62-4. This patient sustained an L1 burst fracture after falling from a standing position. She was neurologically intact on presentation. CT scan showed a Cobb angle of less than 10 degrees and a residual canal of more than 50% (**A** and **B**). A short tau inversion recovery MRI sequence showed no disruption of the posterior ligamentous complex (**C**). She was treated conservatively with bracing for 3 months. A CT scan obtained after 8 months showed mild progression of her angulation (**D**). The patient was asymptomatic, and dynamic radiographs showed fracture healing and no instability on flexion (**E**) and extension (**F**).

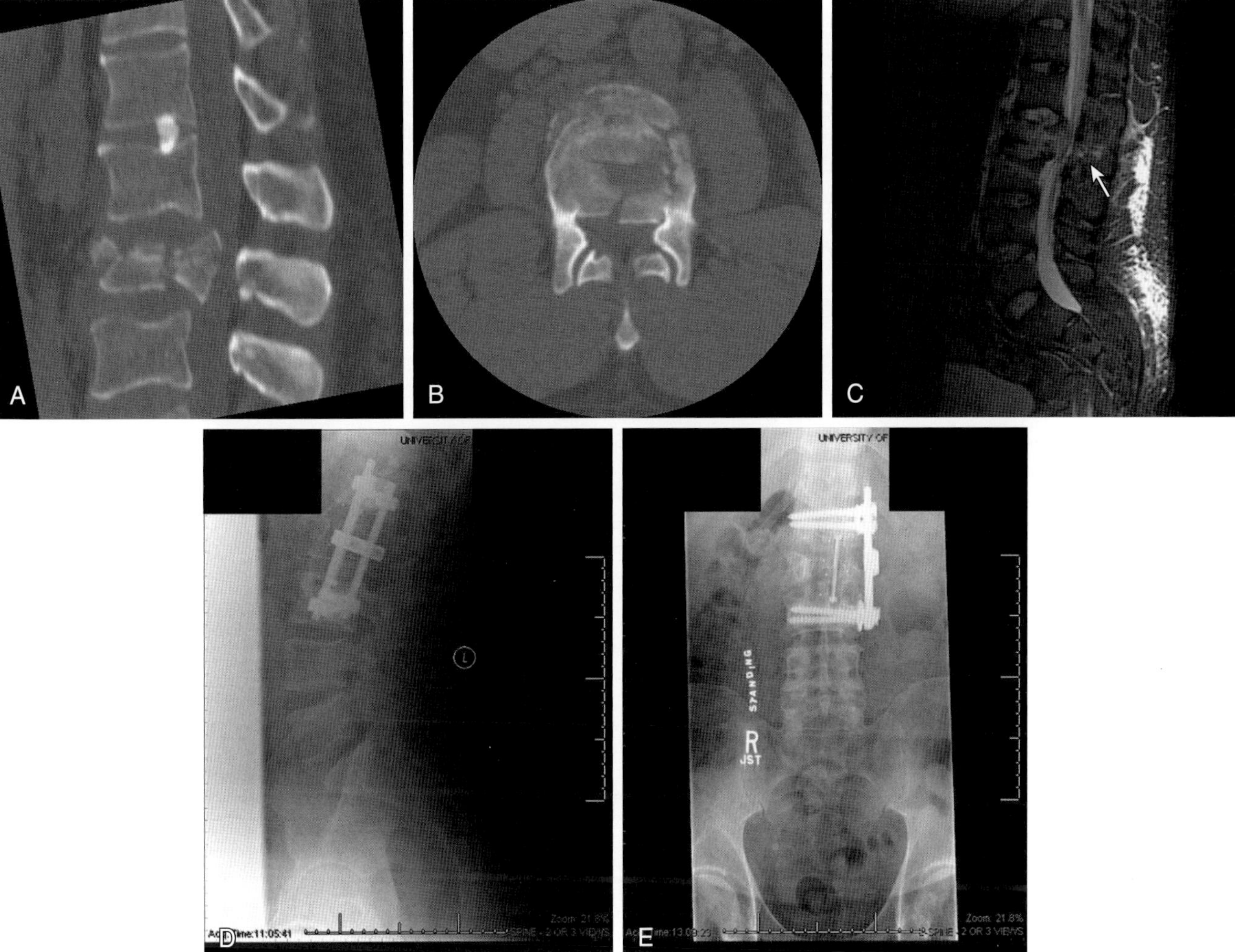

FIGURE 62-5. This patient fell from a horse, sustaining an L2 burst fracture. He was neurologically intact on presentation. A CT scan revealed angulation of less than 10 degrees and a residual canal of at least 50% (**A** and **B**). A short tau inversion recovery MRI sequence showed disruption of the posterior ligamentous complex (**C,** *arrow*). The patient underwent a left anterolateral approach for decompression and stabilization of his fracture (**D** and **E**).

data suggest that in burst fractures, an angulation of more than 10 degrees and a residual canal of less than 50% were associated with failure of nonoperative treatment. On the other hand, patients with burst fractures who are neurologically intact without disruption of the PLC, in whom angulation is less than 10 degrees and the residual canal exceeds 50% of normal, will most likely succeed with nonoperative treatment (Figs. 62-4 and 62-5).

3. *Flexion-distraction injuries:* These fractures occur secondary to failure of Denis's middle and posterior columns, with preservation of the anterior longitudinal ligament. The classic example is the Chance fracture, which involves failure of the middle and posterior bony columns, or can be limited to ligamentous injury traversing the PLC and disc-anulus complex, or a combination of both (Fig. 62-6). Surgical management is the rule because these fractures are inherently unstable.
4. *Fracture-dislocations:* These occur secondary to rotational shear forces, translational forces, or a combination of both. All three Denis columns are involved, rendering these fractures highly unstable (Fig. 62-7). Associated neurologic compromise is common. Surgical management is the rule.

Conclusion

In conclusion, there are many classifications for spinal fractures. The schemas differ in their complexity, completeness, and treatment guidance, but generally overlap to varying degrees. It is up to the spine surgeon to use the system with which he or she feels most comfortable to classify and manage patients with these fractures. In addition to criteria derived from plain radiographs, CT, and MRI, it is important to consider the patient's clinical and neurologic condition before proceeding with management.

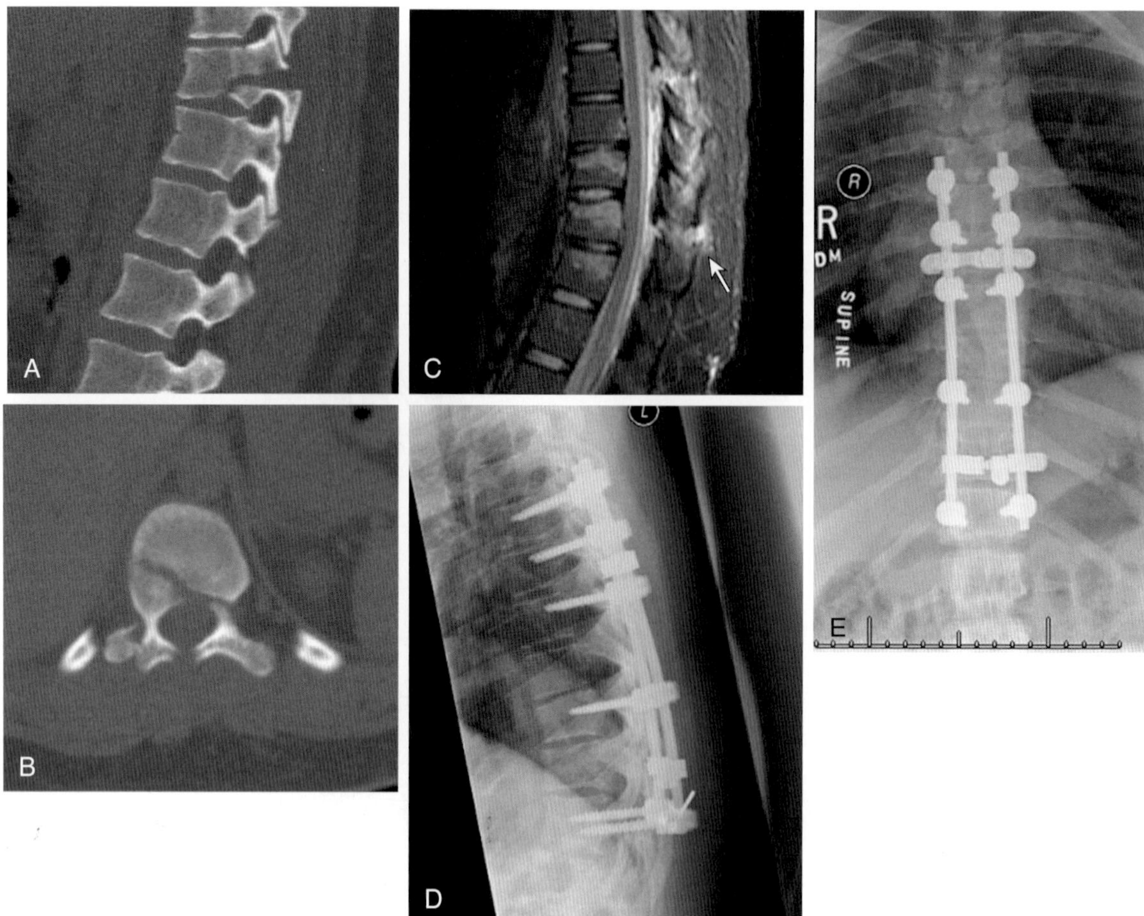

FIGURE 62-6. This patient sustained a flexion-distraction injury after a bicycle fall. She was neurologically intact on presentation. CT scan of the spine showed a flexion-distraction injury with fracture of the left pedicle and both middle and posterior columns (**A** and **B**). Short tau inversion recovery MRI showed disruption of the posterior ligamentous complex (**C**). Lateral (**D**) and anteroposterior plain films (**E**) show pedicle screw fixation.

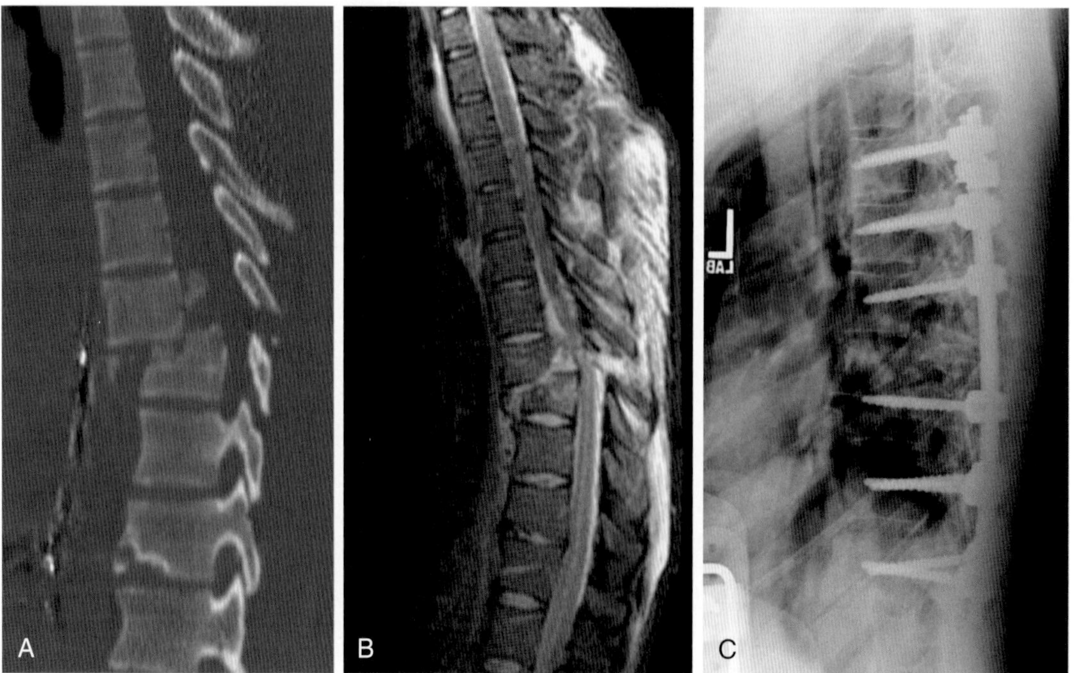

FIGURE 62-7. This patient sustained a T10/T11 fracture-dislocation injury after a car accident while racing. He had a complete spinal cord injury. Sagittal-formatted CT scan shows a fracture-dislocation with anterior displacement of T10 on T11 (**A**). Short tau inversion recovery (STIR) MRI shows spinal cord contusion along with disruption of the posterior ligamentous complex (**B**). The patient underwent dorsal long-segment pedicle screw instrumentation with reduction of the fracture (**C**). There were no change in neurologic status, and the patient is still employed as a mechanic.

KEY REFERENCES

Denis F: The three column spine and its significance in the classification of acute thoracolumbar spinal injuries. *Spine (Phila Pa 1976)* 8:817–831, 1983.

Magerl F, Aebi M, Gertzbein SD, et al: A comprehensive classification of thoracic and lumbar injuries. *Eur Spine J* 3:184–201, 1994.

McCormack T, Karaikovic E, Gaines RW: The load sharing classification of spine fractures. *Spine (Phila Pa 1976)* 19:1741–1744, 1994.

Panjabi MM, Oxland TR, Kifune M, et al: Validity of the three-column theory of thoracolumbar fractures: a biomechanic investigation. *Spine (Phila Pa 1976)* 20:1122–1127, 1995.

Vaccaro AR, Zeiller SC, Hulbert RJ, et al: The thoracolumbar injury severity score: a proposed treatment algorithm. *J Spinal Disord Tech* 18:209–215, 2005.

White AA III, Panjabi MM: *Clinical biomechanics of the spine,* Philadelphia, 1978, JB Lippincott, p 240.

REFERENCES

The complete reference list is available online at expertconsult.com.

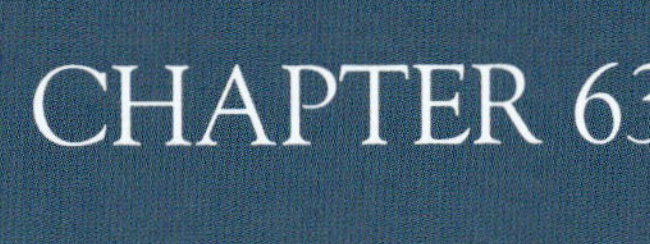

CHAPTER 63

Trauma Surgery: Occipitocervical Junction

Miguel Lopez-Gonzalez | Curtis A. Dickman |
Tanvir Choudhri | Jurgen Harms

The occipitocervical junction includes the skull base at the foramen magnum, C1, C2, and the associated ligamentous, neural, and vascular structures. Because of the important neural and vascular structures in the region, occipitocervical junction injuries have the potential to cause significant neurologic morbidity or mortality. Therefore, careful recognition, diagnosis, and management of these injuries are essential. The association with high-impact trauma and occipitocervical junction injuries is well recognized. However, the potential for injuries even with relatively minor trauma should be remembered, especially with abnormal bone (e.g., osteoporosis) and/or ligaments (e.g., rheumatoid arthritis).

Occipitocervical junction injuries can be classified in several ways (Box 63-1). One useful system describes occipitocervical junction injuries as isolated ligamentous injuries, isolated fractures, or mixed ligamentous and bony injuries. Occipitocervical junction trauma can also be described by the site and/or level(s) of injury. At most sites, classification systems have been developed for specific injury patterns (e.g., C2 odontoid fractures). Finally, occipitocervical junction injuries can be described on the basis of their stability. Stability is generally determined with clinical and radiographic assessment, sometimes using dynamic flexion/extension radiographs. A stable injury does not demonstrate significant radiographic deformity, pain, or neurologic dysfunction with normal physiologic loads and movement. An example of a stable injury would be an isolated C2 spinous process fracture that meets the preceding criteria. Some injuries are clearly unstable, such as occipitocervical dislocations. Other injuries may initially appear stable but have a reasonable chance of developing delayed instability with time, gravity, movement, and/or relaxation of paraspinal muscle spasm. This category reflects the reality that clinical and radiographic assessment of long-term stability may be indeterminate.

The preceding classification systems are helpful in injury assessment and planning management. However, the management of a patient with occipitocervical junction trauma is best determined by considering the nature of the injury (including associated injuries), patient characteristics (e.g., age, medical risk factors, bone quality, desire and ability to tolerate use of a halo orthosis), and the physician's experience. Although much less common, penetrating trauma to the occipitocervical junction presents unique issues that relate to the specific location and trauma modality (e.g., bullet, knife). This class of injuries is not specifically discussed in this chapter but is addressed in Chapter 73. Although most of the principles from blunt trauma are applicable to penetrating trauma, it is important to point out some important differences. Compared with blunt trauma, penetrating trauma typically results in less ligamentous injury and, therefore, for a similar fracture, may be more stable. However, penetrating trauma more commonly results in trauma to vascular or other important regional structures.

General Principles

The initial management of occipitocervical junction injuries is focused on basic trauma management principles, including establishment and maintenance of airway, breathing, and circulation; careful immobilization and transportation; and recognition and management of any associated injuries. These principles have evolved over time and have been published in numerous settings.[1,2]

Occipitocervical junction injuries are frequently recognized on routine cervical spine imaging. However, these injuries may be difficult to detect on initial diagnostic studies. Clinical suspicion based on history and physical examination can aid recognition. Routine radiographs and clinical assessment are often inadequate to fully characterize the injury, and more specialized imaging is usually indicated. Coronal, curved coronal, sagittal, and/or three-dimensional CT reconstruction views can be extremely helpful in characterizing the presence and nature of injury. MRI may be difficult or impossible to obtain acutely but can often provide essential information on spinal canal compromise and may suggest the presence and degree of ligamentous injury. Dynamic imaging with plain radiographs, CT, and/or MRI can be valuable in assessing stability but should be performed carefully. Occasionally, stability is checked with real-time fluoroscopy during careful flexion and extension controlled by a qualified examiner. For example, fluoroscopic flexion/extension imaging may be helpful when there is urgent need to assess the stability of the cervical spine in an unresponsive patient but there is still controversy about its interpretation.[3]

Once occipitocervical junction injuries are diagnosed, management decisions are based on several factors, including the extent and stability of injury, the presence or progression of neurologic deficits, and patient-specific factors that

BOX 63-1. Occipitocervical Junction Injury Classification Systems

A. Location of Bone or Ligamentous Injury

Pure ligamentous injuries

- Occipitoatlantal dislocations
- Transverse ligament injuries
- Rotatory C1-2 dislocations

Isolated fractures

- Occipital condyle fractures
- C1 (lateral mass, ring)
- C2 (odontoid, body, hangman, dorsal element)

Mixed ligamentous and bony injuries

B. Site/Level of Injury

Occipital bone (C0) (e.g., condyle fracture)

C0-1 ligaments (e.g., occipitoatlantal dislocation)

C1 (e.g., lateral mass, ring fractures)

C1-2 ligaments (e.g., transverse ligament injuries)

C2 (odontoid, body, hangman, dorsal element fractures)

C. Degree of Stability

Stable

Low probability of delayed instability

High probability of delayed instability

Unstable

influence the risks with different treatments. Nonoperative management typically includes some type of rigid (halo) or semirigid (collar) orthosis. Operative management is generally indicated for injuries that are unstable, have significant potential for delayed instability, have progressive neurologic deficits, and/or cause significant deficits or symptoms that are not controlled with nonoperative measures. Operative planning may include obtaining additional imaging (e.g., dedicated studies for image guidance), ensuring the availability of appropriate instrumentation, and arranging neurophysiologic monitoring where appropriate.

Diagnosis and Management

Occipitocervical Dislocations

Occipitocervical dislocations are relatively uncommon ligamentous injuries that usually result from hyperflexion and distraction during high-impact blunt trauma.[4,5] These injuries are highly unstable, frequently fatal, and usually result in significant neurologic injury from stretching, compression, and/or distortion of the spinal cord, brainstem, and cranial nerves.[6] In addition, significant morbidity and mortality can result from associated cerebrovascular injury, which varies among trauma series, diagnosis test used (CT, conventional angiogram), and severity of injuries.[7,8] Recognition and rapid management of these injuries may limit further injury, but even with appropriate care, neurologic deficits can progress. Although these were initially felt to be rare, several series of trauma fatalities have revealed an incidence between 8% and 19%.[4]

Lateral cervical spine radiographs may recognize occipitocervical dislocations (sensitivity, 0.57), especially in severe injuries. However, these injuries can be difficult to diagnose with plain radiographs alone, especially with less-severe dislocations. In addition, the frequent presence of coexisting significant head trauma can delay recognition of spinal injury. Diagnostic clues include prevertebral soft tissue swelling, an increase in the dens-basion distance, and separation of the occipital condyles and C1 lateral masses (Fig. 63-1). CT imaging with reconstruction views (sensitivity 0.84) usually provides a better assessment of fractures and alignment than plain radiographs do. The presence of subarachnoid hemorrhage supports but does not confirm the diagnosis. MRI imaging can be helpful for diagnosis (sensitivity 0.86), to assess the extent of spinal cord compression and injury, and to demonstrate compressive hematoma lesions.[2]

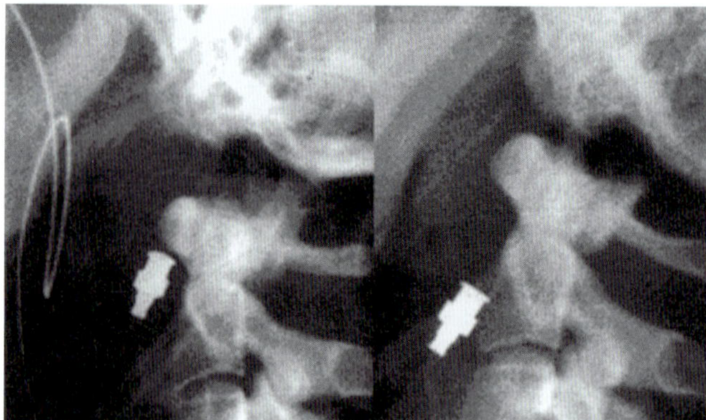

FIGURE 63-1. Lateral cervical radiographs demonstrating occipitocervical dislocation. The craniovertebral instability is apparent in the two images. (From Dickman CA, Spetzler RA, Sonntag VKH, editors: *Surgery of the craniovertebral junction*, New York, 1998, Thieme.)

On the basis of the injury pattern, occipitoatlantal dislocations have been classified by Traynelis et al.[9] into four types: type I (anterior), type II (longitudinal), type III (posterior), and "other" (complex). A number of diagnostic radiographic criteria have been described that assess the relationship between the skull base and cervical spine (Fig. 63-2). Although developed for lateral plain radiographs, these criteria can also be used on sagittal reconstruction CT views, provided that there are no significant artifactual distortions. The Wackenheim clival line extends along the dorsal surface of the clivus and should be tangential to the tip of the dens.[10] Ventral or dorsal translation of the skull in relation to the dens will shift the clival line to either intersect or run dorsal to the dens, respectively. The Powers ratio is based on the relationship of the B–C line (from the basion to the C1 dorsal arch) and the O–A line (between the opisthion and the C1 ventral arch).[11] Normal B–C/O–A ratios average 0.77, while pathologic ratios (>1) typically represent occipitocervical dislocations. However, false negatives can occur with longitudinal or dorsal dislocations.[12] The Wholey dens-basion technique assesses the distance from the basion to the dens tip.[13] Although variability is common, the average distance in adults is about 9 mm, and pathologic distances are greater than 15 mm.[14] The Dublin method, the least reliable method, measures the distance from the mandible (posterior ramus) to the ventral part of C1 (normally 2–5 mm) and C2 (normally 9–12 mm).[15]

Initial management of these injuries focuses on immobilization, almost always with a halo orthosis. Cervical collars

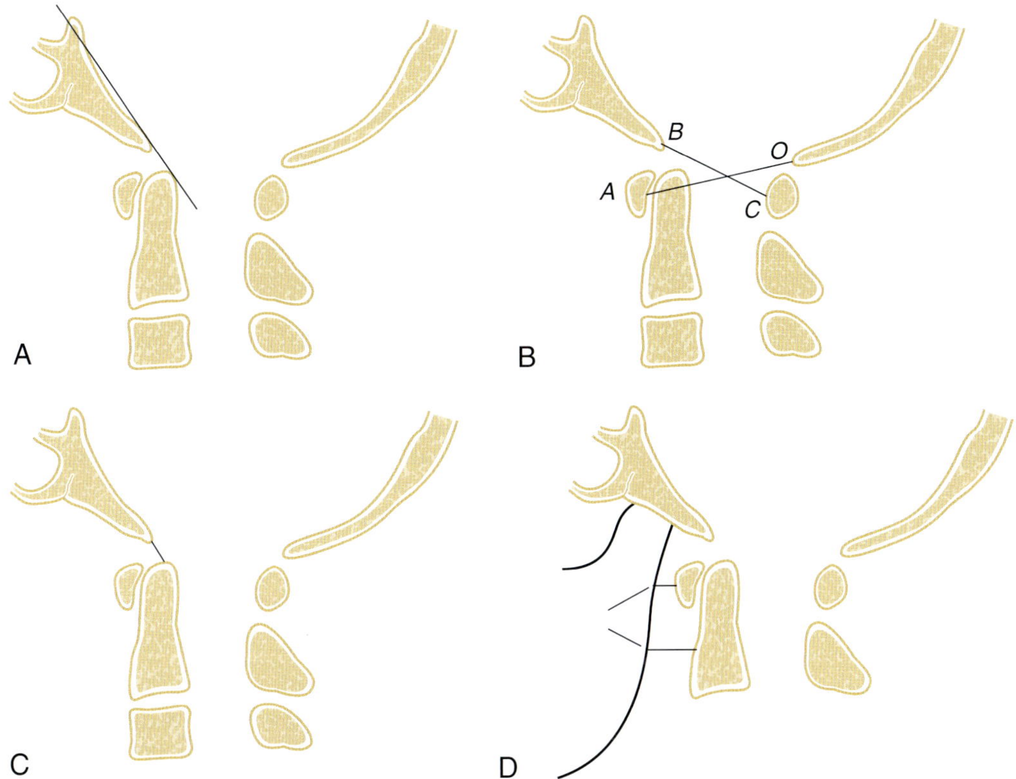

FIGURE 63-2. Four radiographic methods for assessing occipitocervical dislocation. **A,** Wackenheim clival line. **B,** Power ratio (*B–C/O–A*). **C,** Wholey dens-basion technique. **D,** Dublin method. See text for details. (From Barrow Neurological Institute, with permission.)

are potentially dangerous because they may produce distraction and thereby promote further injury. Similarly, traction can cause neurologic worsening (2 of 21 patients) and should be avoided or used with extreme caution.[1,2] Nonoperative management does not provide definitive treatment of these injuries because of the significant ligamentous disruption that cannot be expected to heal even with prolonged rigid (halo) external immobilization (11 of 40 patients had a nonunion and/or neurologic deterioration).[2] Operative stabilization consists of an occipitocervical arthrodesis with rigid internal fixation (discussed later and in Chapter 143). Decompression and restoration of alignment may also be necessary to maximize neurologic recovery.

Transverse Ligament Injuries

Isolated traumatic transverse ligament injuries are unstable injuries that can result in significant upper cervical spinal cord injury either during the initial trauma or afterwards. These injuries are more common in hyperflexion injuries. Because transverse ligament injuries may be difficult to recognize on initial (neutral) plain radiographs, an elevated index of suspicion is required in some settings—for example, high-impact trauma.

Transverse ligament injuries are suggested or diagnosed with radiographic imaging. A widened atlantodental interval on flexion lateral cervical radiographs (>3 mm in adults, >5 mm in children) suggests transverse ligament insufficiency. Thin-cut CT imaging with reconstruction views may suggest the diagnosis by demonstrating a C1 lateral mass avulsion fracture at the ligamentous insertion. Thin-cut MRI with attention to the transverse ligament when using gradient echo sequences can directly demonstrate a transverse ligament injury.[16] If the diagnosis is uncertain, dynamic (flexion/extension) imaging is appropriate for cooperative patients. On the basis of CT and MRI, traumatic transverse ligament injuries can be classified into two categories (Fig. 63-3). Type I injuries involve disruptions of the midportion (IA) or periosteal insertion laterally (IB). Type II injuries involve fractures that disconnect the C1 lateral mass tubercle for insertion of the transverse ligament via a comminuted fracture (IIA) or an avulsion fracture (IIB).[17]

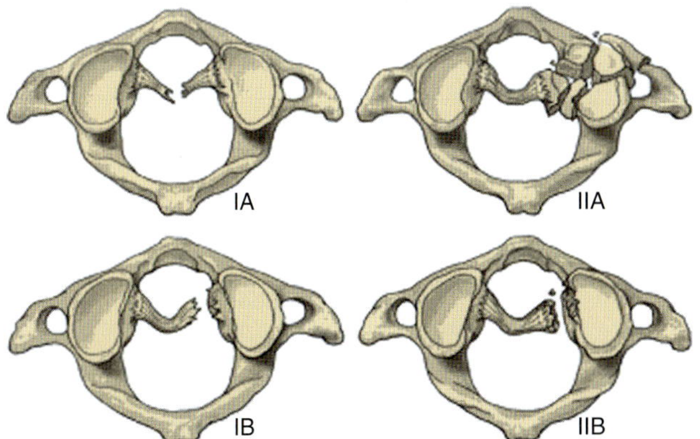

FIGURE 63-3. Classification of transverse ligament injuries. Type I injuries are disruptions of the transverse ligament in its midportion (IA) or periosteal insertion laterally (IB). Type II injuries lead to transverse ligament insufficiency through fractures that disconnect the C1 lateral mass tubercle (insertion of the transverse ligament) via a comminuted fracture (IIA) or an avulsion fracture (IIB). (From Barrow Neurological Institute, with permission.)

The management of transverse ligament injuries is based on the type of injury. Type I injuries are pure ligamentous injuries that cannot be expected to heal with nonoperative external fixation. Therefore, operative stabilization with a dorsal C1-2 arthrodesis and fixation is indicated. The surgical options include C1-2 dorsal wiring, C1-2 Halifax clamps, C1-2 transarticular screws, and/or C1-2 segmental screw fixation (see later section and Chapter 143). Type II injuries have a much higher chance of healing with halo immobilization (up to 74%).[17] If a nonunion is still present after a prolonged period of immobilization (>3 months), then operative stabilization is generally appropriate.

Rotatory C1-2 Subluxations

Rotatory C1-2 subluxations are ligamentous injuries that are more common in children and adolescents. These injuries typically present with neck pain and a fixed, rotated "cock-robin" head position. Open-mouth radiographs may demonstrate an asymmetry of the C1 and C2 lateral masses. CT imaging can confirm the rotatory subluxation diagnosis and demonstrate coexisting fractures. C1-2 axial rotation greater than 47 degrees confirms the diagnosis. Three-view CT imaging (15 degrees to the left, neutral, and 15 degrees to the right) can also be helpful in establishing the diagnosis.[18,19] MRI may detect a coexistent transverse ligament injury.

The treatment of C1-2 rotatory subluxations is generally nonoperative. Axial traction with a halter device or Gardner-Wells tongs can usually achieve reduction of the injury. Prolonged traction and/or the use of muscle relaxants may be needed. Periodic imaging may help to assess progress, but clinical improvement in the alignment and symptoms often provides confirmation of a successful reduction. Operative reduction and fixation are reserved for irreducible injuries, recurrent subluxations, and transverse ligament injuries.

Occipital Condyle Fractures

Occipital condyle fractures generally occur with axial trauma and are almost always unilateral (>90%). These injuries are classified into three types according to Anderson and Montesano.[20] Type I injuries are comminuted fractures that result from axial trauma. Type II fractures are extensions of linear basilar skull fractures. Type III injuries, the most common, are avulsion fractures of the condyle that can result from a variety of mechanisms. The incidence of occipital condyle fractures has been estimated to be between 1% and 3% of blunt craniocervical trauma cases.[21] Although plain radiographs (usually open-mouth radiographs) may occasionally identify the injury, they have an unacceptably low sensitivity (estimated at 3.2%) and should not be relied on when the diagnosis is suspected. CT imaging with reconstruction views provides the best assessment of fracture pattern and alignment.[21,22]

Occipital condyle fractures are generally stable and therefore are typically managed with an external nonrigid orthosis (collar) until the fracture heals (often 12 weeks). Type III fractures are felt to be more prone to instability, and when significant displacement or clinical concern exists, halo immobilization may be appropriate.[23] Operative stabilization with an occipitocervical fusion is generally reserved for situations in which there are associated cervical fractures or significant ligamentous injuries.

C1 Fractures

Isolated C1 fractures account for approximately 5% of cervical spine fractures. These injuries occur with axial trauma with or without lateral bending.[24] Open-mouth radiographs may suggest the injury, but CT imaging with reconstruction views provides the best assessment of fracture pattern and alignment. Fractures can include almost any part of the ring or lateral masses of C1. Aside from unilateral lateral mass fractures, the fractures usually occur at multiple sites (Fig. 63-4). Jefferson fractures are four-part fractures with bilateral ventral and dorsal ring fractures. The assessment of these injuries is focused on evaluating the integrity of the transverse ligament and on recognizing any additional fractures.

The management of C1 fractures is based on the integrity of the transverse ligament that can be assessed indirectly with several radiographic criteria such as a widened atlantodental interval (>3 mm) and increased spread of the lateral masses of C1 over C2 (>6.9 mm, rule of Spence)[25] or directly through high-resolution MRI (Fig. 63-5). If the transverse ligament is intact, isolated C1 fractures are generally stable and can be treated with an external orthosis (e.g., SOMI) primarily for symptom control until the fracture heals. With transverse ligament insufficiency, operative stabilization is indicated by using a C1-2 fusion technique such as dorsal C1-2 wiring techniques, C1-2 transarticular screws, C1 lateral mass-to-C2 pars/pedicle screws, or ventral C1-2 screw fixation (see Chapter 143). The surgical choice is based primarily on patient anatomy and fracture pattern as well as the surgeon's experience and preference. Postoperatively, most operations employing rigid internal fixation can be managed with a nonrigid external orthosis (e.g., a collar, SOMI), but C1-2 dorsal wiring without additional instrumentation generally warrants the use of a halo.[26]

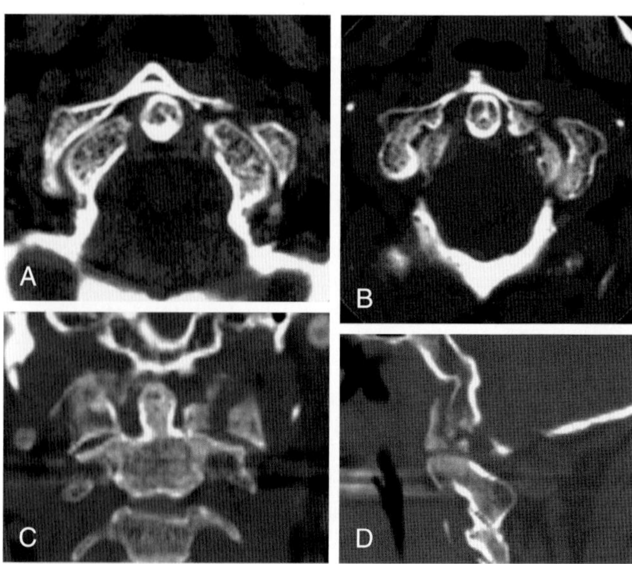

FIGURE 63-4. C1 lateral mass fracture. Axial CT images (**A** and **B**) and coronal (**C**) and sagittal (**D**) CT reconstruction views of right C1 lateral mass fracture from high-speed motor vehicle accident. The fracture healed with 3 months of external immobilization.

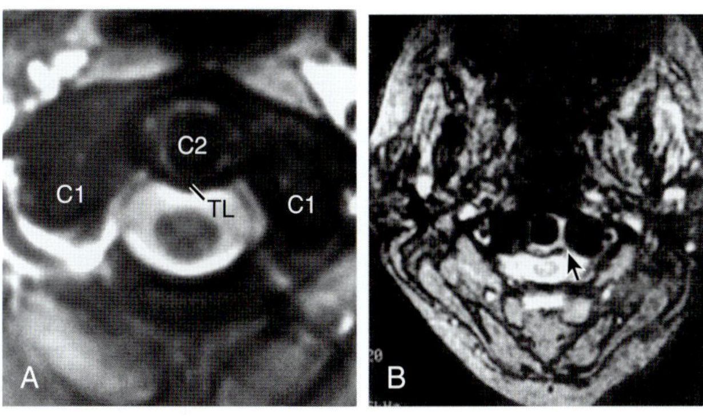

FIGURE 63-5. Axial MRI images demonstrating an intact (**A**) and ruptured (**B,** *arrow*) transverse ligament (TL). (From Dickman CA, Spetzler RA, Sonntag VKH, editors: *Surgery of the craniovertebral junction*, New York, 1998, Thieme.)

C2 Fractures

C2 fractures make up about 20% of all cervical spine fractures and are classified as either odontoid, body, or other fractures (e.g., hangman, laminar, or spinous process).

Odontoid Fractures

C2 odontoid fractures can occur from a number of mechanisms but most often are caused by hyperextension injuries. Although lateral cervical spine radiographs may demonstrate some fractures, especially those with displacement, this technique can easily miss fractures, especially those with degenerative changes or minimal displacement. Open-mouth radiographs are very helpful for diagnosing most odontoid fractures, but these also may be inconclusive. Thin-cut CT images with sagittal and coronal view reconstruction views are the best way to diagnose and characterize odontoid fractures as well as to find associated fractures and plan treatment.[27,28]

Anderson and D'Alonzo classified odontoid fractures into three types based on the location of the fracture line through the odontoid tip (type I), odontoid base (type II), or C2 body (type III)[29] (Fig. 63-6). Type I fractures are essentially avulsion fractures of the odontoid tip and are rare, generally stable, and usually managed with an external semirigid (collar) or rigid (halo) orthosis. Type II fractures are the most common type of odontoid fracture. These fractures are unstable and prone to nonunion because they occur in an area of relatively reduced osseous vascularity. Therefore, rigid halo immobilization or surgical stabilization is often necessary. Hadley et al. described type IIA fractures that are comminuted fractures at the base of the dens with associated free fragments.[30] These fractures are considered particularly unstable, and surgical stabilization is advisable, usually with a dorsal C1-2 fusion. Type III fractures involve the vertebral body and are discussed later.

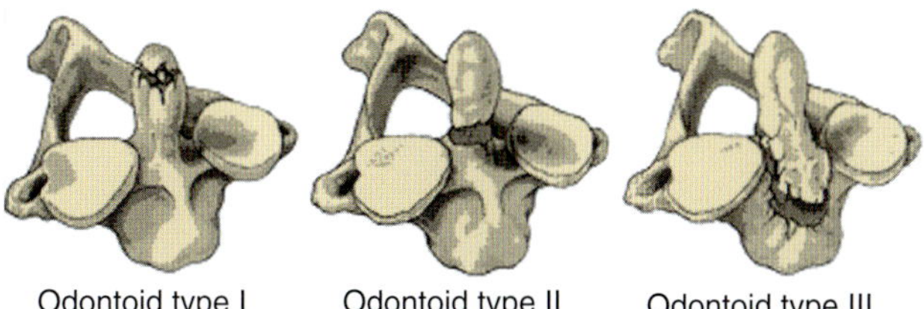

FIGURE 63-6. C2 odontoid fractures as described by Anderson and D'Alonzo. Type II fractures are better described as C2 body fractures, as discussed later in this chapter. (From Barrow Neurological Institute, with permission.)

C2 Body Fractures

The C2 body can be defined as the C2 bone mass caudal to the dens and ventral to the pars interarticularis bilaterally. Benzel et al.[31] have classified C2 body fractures on the basis of the orientation of the fracture line: coronal, sagittal, or transverse (also known as horizontal rostral). The transverse type of C2 body fracture is a more appropriate description of type III odontoid fractures. The coronal and sagittal types represent "vertical" fractures. Of the vertical fractures, the coronal type was much more common (4:1 ratio) and resulted from multiple (four) different mechanisms. Sagittal type C2 body fractures were caused by axial loading trauma. Figure 63-7 shows an example of a C2 body fracture.

Although standard cervical radiographs will often recognize the fracture, the injury is best characterized with high-resolution CT scanning with multiplanar reconstruction views. It is important to look for radiographic evidence of involvement of the foramen transversarium and clinical signs of vertebral artery injury. If there is a significant degree of suspicion, an assessment of the vertebral artery with CT, MRI, or transfemoral catheter angiography should be obtained. The stability of C2 body fractures can be assessed either with fracture characteristics (e.g., displacement) or with careful dynamic (flexion/extension) imaging when stability appears likely.

A majority of C2 body fractures can be managed nonoperatively. Depending on the alignment, degree of displacement,

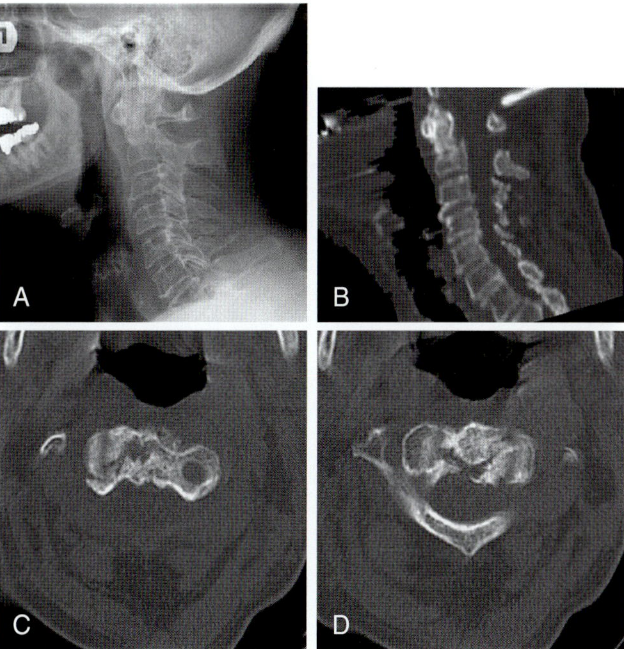

FIGURE 63-7. C2 body fracture. An 80-year-old woman presented with neck pain after a fall. A lateral cervical radiograph (**A**) suggests C1-2 instability from a C2 fracture. A sagittal CT reconstruction image (**B**) suggests a C2 body fracture with a transverse fracture line (also described as type III odontoid fracture) and a vertical (coronal) fracture line in addition. Axial CT images (**C** and **D**) confirm the C2 vertical fracture component.

and fracture location, either a collar or a halo may be advisable. Occasionally, surgical intervention with a dorsal C1-2 fusion is indicated, particularly for highly unstable fractures and in patients who are prone to nonunion.

Other C2 Fractures

Traumatic spondylolisthesis fractures of the axis (also known as hangman fractures) are characterized by bilateral fractures through the C2 pars/pedicle (Fig. 63-8). Although these fractures may be unstable, they do not generally cause significant compromise of the spinal canal or neurologic injury. Effendi et al.[32] have classified these injuries into three groups based on mechanism. Type I fractures are single hairline fractures of the pedicle of axis and occur with axial loading and hyperextension. Type II fractures have displacement of the ventral fragment with an abnormal disc below the axis and are hyperextension injuries with rebound hyperflexion. Type III fractures have displacement of the ventral element with the body of the axis in the flexed position, and the facet joints at C2-3 are dislocated and locked and are primarily flexion injuries with rebound extension. Levine and Edwards[33] modified the system by adding a type IIA, which represents flexion-distraction injuries with mild or no displacement but very severe angulation. Type I and II injuries are generally stable and can usually be managed in a collar. With significant displacement (>4–6 mm), halo immobilization may be advisable. Type IIA injuries are more likely to be unstable, especially with displacement greater than 4 to 6 mm or angulation more than 11 degrees. If one or both of these findings are present, surgical stabilization may be necessary. Type III injuries are unstable and typically require surgical stabilization. Isolated C2 laminar or spinous process fractures are stable and therefore are usually managed with an orthosis (e.g., a collar).

Combination Occipitocervical Junction Injuries

Combination occipitocervical junction fractures involve bony and ligamentous injuries of the foramen magnum (e.g., occipital condyles), C1, and/or C2. These injuries are usually unstable, occur with high-impact trauma, and frequently result in death or major neurologic injury. Management of these injuries is similar to that of occipitocervical dislocations. Initial management involves airway management, craniovertebral immobilization, and medical stabilization. Patients who are medically stable are considered for more prolonged stabilization with rigid external halo immobilization and/or surgical stabilization. For incomplete spinal cord injuries, decompression of any compressive bony or hematoma lesions may also be necessary and is performed when the patient is medically stable. With complete spinal cord injuries, the timing of surgical stabilization and/or decompression is less urgent.

Combined C1-2 fractures occur with axial trauma with or without lateral bending. Although plain radiographs may indicate a combined fracture, a CT with multiplanar reconstruction views is usually necessary to fully characterize the fractures and alignment and to plan treatment. Compared with isolated C1 and C2 fractures, combined C1-2 fractures are typically associated with a higher rate of instability, nonunion, and neurologic injury. Treatment of these injuries is based on the degree and location of bony and ligamentous injuries. Because of the instability, rigid external (halo) and/or

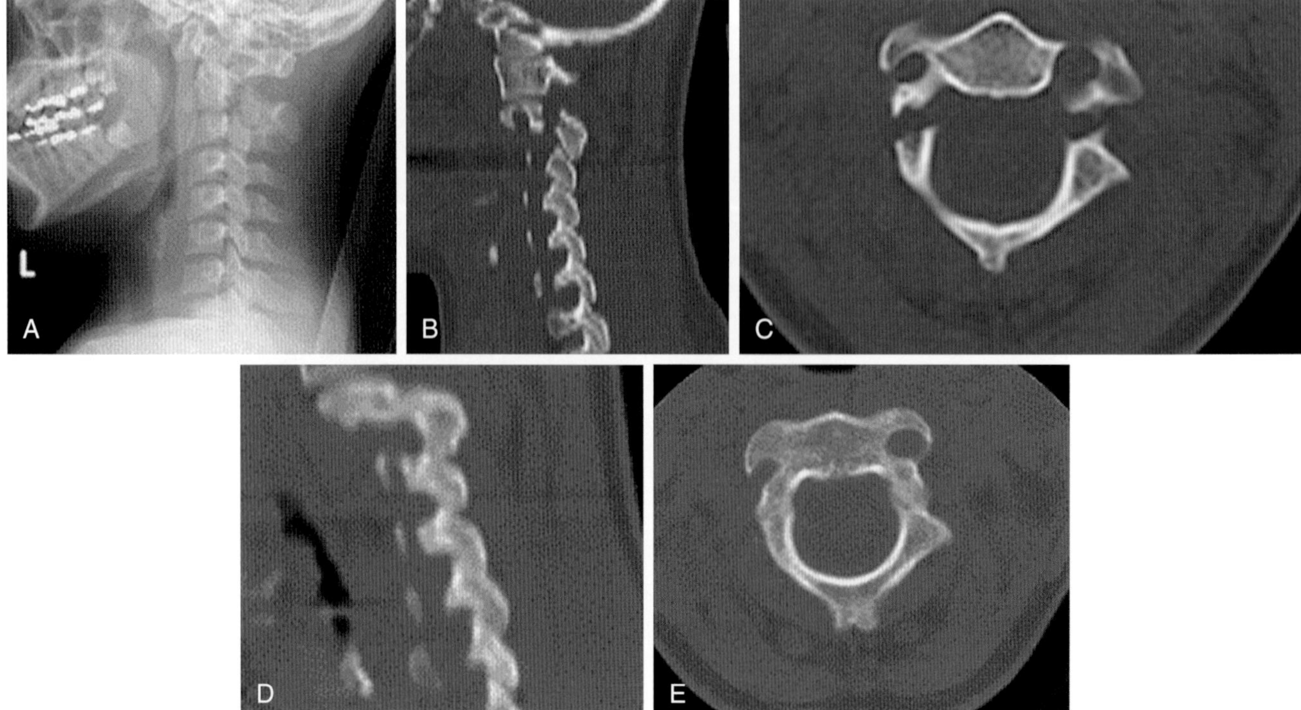

FIGURE 63-8. C2 hangman fracture. A 21-year-old woman presented with neck pain after a motor vehicle accident. Initial studies with a lateral cervical radiograph (**A**), sagittal CT reconstruction image (**B**), and axial CT image (**C**) demonstrate the fracture through the C2 pars/pedicle with moderate displacement. The fracture healed with 3 months of external immobilization, as is evidenced by the delayed sagittal CT reconstruction (**D**) and axial CT (**E**) images.

internal fixation is usually required. Standard surgical procedures (e.g., dorsal C1-2 interspinous fusion) might not be possible because of the extensive fractures. Advances in instrumentation and surgical technique have allowed the development and increased use of newer types of surgical stabilization such as C1-2 transarticular screws or C1-2 segmental fixation.[34,35]

Surgical Procedures

General Principles

Preoperative Care

There are multiple indications for surgical intervention with occipitocervical trauma. Decompression may be necessary to relieve compromise of the spinal canal or neural foramina from bone or soft tissue (e.g., hematoma) lesions. Internal stabilization may be necessary to treat acute or impending instability, to promote fracture healing, and to improve and/or correct alignment.

Preoperative care is focused on optimizing medical stability; obtaining the necessary imaging to assess the injury location, alignment, and stability; and determining the nature and timing of any needed intervention. The timing of surgery is based on the patient's medical stability, the degree of spinal compression, the presence or progression of neurologic deficits, and the availability of optimal operating room equipment and personnel. When appropriate likelihood of benefit exists, incomplete spinal cord injuries with compressive lesions warrant surgical intervention as soon as possible. This is particularly true when there are progressive neurologic deficits. However, it is important to note that neurologic deterioration may be related to the natural history of the neurologic injury and/or medical deterioration (such as hypoxia, hypotension, and/or fever) that would not necessarily be assisted with surgical intervention. Rather, it is possible that the patient would have a better chance of tolerating, and hopefully benefiting from, the procedure by delaying surgery until the medical issues have been optimized. When possible, early surgical intervention is desirable to promote early mobilization and transfer to rehabilitation.

Preoperative planning includes selection of a primary surgical plan as well as backup plans, which may become necessary. When needed, specialized equipment (e.g., image guidance, instrumentation) and/or neurophysiologic monitoring should be reserved or arranged in advance. When possible, preoperative studies should be loaded onto image guidance equipment (if used) in advance to permit preoperative surgical planning.

Intraoperative Care

The intraoperative setup and positioning are directed by the nature of the injury and surgical approach. In general, occipitocervical junction trauma procedures use a midline dorsal approach in the prone position with cranial fixation or a high ventral cervical approach in the supine position. Transoral, transfacial, and far lateral skull base approaches are not commonly used in the trauma setting. When there is sufficient neurologic function and degree of potential new or exacerbated neurologic injury, spinal monitoring (sensory and/or motor evoked potentials) may prove useful for determining whether the final surgical positioning is satisfactory.

Exposure of the occipitocervical junction for trauma may require special considerations. For example, throughout the case, careful attention is advised to maintain appropriate alignment and minimize or avoid pressure on unstable or compressed neurologic structures. Traumatic injuries to the subcutaneous and paraspinal soft tissues can distort and obscure anatomic landmarks. Additional exposure (e.g., length of incision, number of levels) may aid in the recognition and management of the abnormal anatomy because of increased exposure of adjacent normal anatomy.

Decompression and stabilization are two primary objectives of surgery. Decompression of neurologic structures may be accomplished by correcting alignment or removing compressive bone, ligaments, or other space-occupying lesions such as hematomas. The goals of stabilization are to achieve stability and, where appropriate and possible, to maintain or improve alignment, maximize neurologic function, and improve symptoms. Achieving bony fusion is the best way to achieve long-term stability. At surgery, the standard principles of arthrodesis should be followed with careful attention to the exposure and preparation of bone fusion surfaces and the choice of structural or morselized bone graft material. For the majority of cases, internal fixation with instrumentation is utilized to maintain alignment and promote osseous union. Nonrigid external orthoses (e.g., collar, SOMI) do not provide substantial immobilization of the occipitocervical junction. Therefore, instrumentation should be optimized with some (or all) of the following strategies: including all segments involved in the construct, using larger-diameter or longer screws as possible, and achieving bicortical purchase where advisable.

Occipitocervical junction trauma operations may require special closure considerations. For example, these cases may have an increased risk of postoperative infection, as the incision typically extends beyond the suboccipital hairline. Copious irrigation is therefore advised before closure. Leaving one or more Jackson-Pratt or Hemovac drains may reduce the incidence of postoperative hematoma or seroma collections. However, these drains should be used cautiously if the dura was compromised from the trauma or during the procedure. In the event of dural compromise, primary closure and/or augmentation (e.g., patch, fibrin glue product) and extra attention to fascial closure are often used. A running locked suture may be used for the skin closure. For cases with significant dural compromise that is not possible to repair, several days of postoperative spinal drainage via local (through or near incision) or distal (typically lumbar) placement of an intrathecal catheter may reduce chances of a postoperative spinal fluid collection or leak.

Postoperative Care

Postoperatively, a rigid external orthosis (halo) is used if instrumentation is not used or if concern exists regarding the instrumentation or bone quality. Otherwise, some type of nonrigid orthosis is advisable in most cases. Because standard cervical collars do not immobilize the occipitocervical junction well, special orthoses are often used (e.g., SOMI braces). Currently, there is no consistent medical evidence to support or refute the use of bone stimulator devices.[36] Although not officially studied, bone stimulators have been used as a primary adjunct in patients who are prone to nonunion (e.g., smokers) or in an attempt to salvage a nonunion. Patients with spinal cord injury require special attention to nutrition, skin care, pulmonary toilet, deep vein thrombosis prophylaxis, and often psychiatric support. Patients with poor nutrition are prone to wound-healing problems, and sutures may need to be left for a prolonged period (2 to 3 weeks or more).

Postoperative imaging with plain radiographs and/or CT imaging is generally obtained when possible to assess final anatomy and alignment, extent of decompression, and position of instrumentation. Interval imaging is followed as needed to assess bony fusion. When sufficient stability is achieved from the internal fixation and/or bone fusion, the orthosis can be weaned. Dynamic imaging with flexion/extension views can provide an assessment of stability and bony fusion.

Occipitocervical Junction Fusions

Occipitocervical junction fusions are performed through a dorsal midline approach. Ventral occipitocervical junction fusions may be technically possible, but the transoral approach for trauma is prone to infection and may be difficult to expose because of the altered anatomy and difficult to close because of the instrumentation. Finally, the ventral approach is not ideal for placement of instrumentation because the surgeon is limited in the extent of rostrocaudal exposure.

At surgery, careful transfer to the prone position is required. The patient's head is fixed with a Mayfield head clamp unless the patient is already in a halo ring/vest. In this case, it is possible to turn the patient in the halo ring/vest. After the halo ring is locked to the operating table with a Mayfield halo adapter, the dorsal part of the halo vest and connecting bars are disassembled to permit adequate exposure. As much as possible, the head should be positioned in an appropriate alignment such that the patient will naturally look forward (i.e., avoid hyperflexed or hyperextended positioning to maximize patient visualization and comfort). The iliac crest region is prepped to harvest bone graft. The exposure should extend from the inion down to C3 at least, with the ability to continue further caudally as necessary. Decompression of the foramen magnum should be performed if necessary, but the ability to achieve a midline fusion and take advantage of the thicker midline bone is limited by an extensive midline suboccipital decompression.

Structural unicortical strips are harvested from the iliac crest along with cancellous bone. Local autograft from the cranium or dorsal spinal elements is significantly less effective in achieving fusion. Allograft is least likely to achieve fusion and generally should not be relied on. Instrumentation options include inverted U-rods with wiring, inverted-Y-plate/screw constructions, and specialized cranial plate attachments for polyaxial cervical screws.[37,38] The midline bone is thickest and allows placement of longer screws with better purchase. The construct should be extended to at least C2 and sometimes lower to achieve optimal fixation. However, advances in instrumentation have made the longer constructs to the lower cervical spine or cervicothoracic junction uncommon unless additional subaxial cervical spine injuries exist. Dorsal C0-1 transarticular screw fixation has recently been described by Grob[39] and by Gonzales et al.[40] The utility of this procedure is still evolving. The instrumentation options and techniques are discussed further in Chapter 111. Postoperatively, a collar or SOMI brace is used until bony fusion occurs (usually 12 weeks). Halo immobilization is used when the bone quality or fixation is suboptimal.

Dorsal C1-2 Fixation

Dorsal C1-2 fusions are indicated for unstable C1 and/or C2 fractures and are performed through a dorsal midline approach. C1-2 fusion requires sacrifice of the movement at C1-2 (primarily rotation); therefore, for appropriate fractures with an intact transverse ligament, odontoid screw fixation may be preferable.

At surgery, the positioning is similar to that used in occipitocervical junction fusions. However, if transarticular screw placement is planned, the head should be flexed as possible to facilitate screw placement. The exposure should extend from the foramen magnum through C3. If the dorsal elements of C1 and C2 are intact and do not need to be decompressed, then structural autograft from the iliac crest is harvested for placement between or along the dorsal elements of C1 and C2. Careful exposure, preparation, and decortication of the fusion surfaces are important to maximize the chances of achieving fusion. The caudal edge of C1 is a common site for nonunion and deserves special attention.

Instrumentation options include C1-2 wiring alone or with additional screw instrumentation, C1-2 Halifax clamp fixation, C1-2 transarticular screw fixation, and C1-2 segmental screw fixation.[34,35] The wiring options include the Brooks, Gallie, and Sonntag interspinous fusion operations.[41-47] The relative advantages and disadvantages of the various options are listed in Box 63-2. Postoperatively, a collar or SOMI brace is used until bony fusion occurs (usually 12 weeks). Halo immobilization is used when the bone quality or fixation is suboptimal.

Odontoid Screw Fixation

Ventral odontoid screw fixation is appropriate for many unstable C2 odontoid fractures that require operative fixation. The main advantages of odontoid screw fixation are the preservation of C1-2 mobility and the relatively short and well-tolerated

BOX 63-2. Advantages and Disadvantages of Dorsal C1-2 Fusion Operation

C1-2 Wiring (Brooks, Gallie, Sonntag)

Advantages: Familiar technique, avoids screw

Disadvantages: Least rigid, requires more external fixation, higher nonunion rate

C1-2 Transarticular Screw Fixation

Advantages: Most rigid

Disadvantages: Potential for vertebral artery injury

C1-2 Segmental Fixation

Advantages: Familiar technique, avoids screw, very rigid

Disadvantages: Venous plexus bleeding, potential vertebral artery injury

C1-2 Sublaminar Hooks (Halifax Clamps)

Advantages: Avoids screw placement risks

Disadvantages: Less rigid than screws, weak in extension, may narrow canal

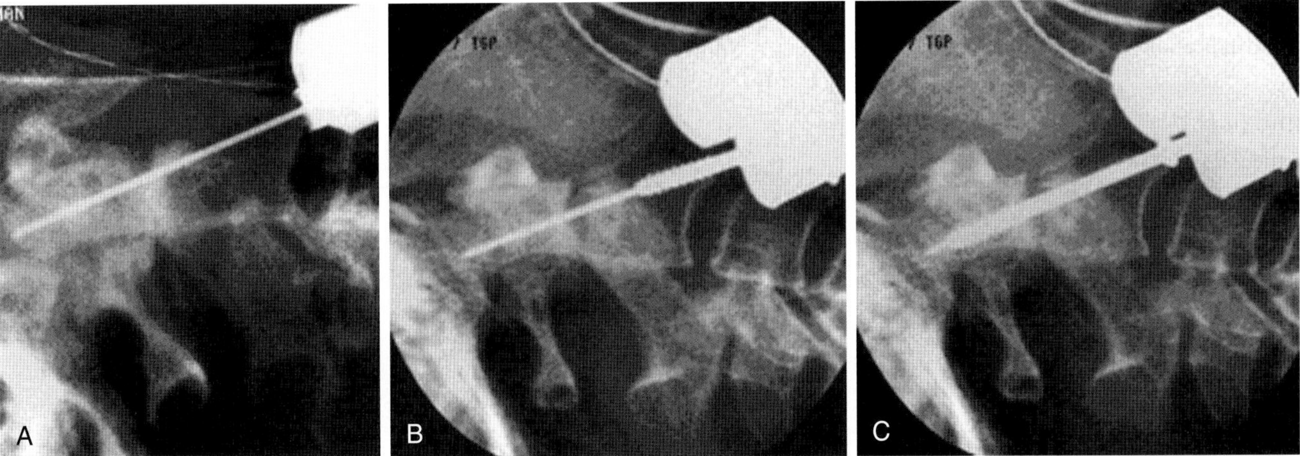

FIGURE 63-9. C2 odontoid screw placement with a cannulated screw system. Initially, a K-wire drill bit is placed (**A**). Next, the screw is carefully threaded over the drill bit under fluoroscopic guidance (**B** and **C**). (From Dickman CA, Spetzler RA, Sonntag VKH, editors: *Surgery of the craniovertebral junction*, New York, 1998, Thieme.)

nature of the procedure. However, the procedure is not possible for many patients and fractures because of anatomic limitations. For example, patients with short necks, barrel chests, inability to tolerate cervical extension, insufficient transverse ligaments, oblique fracture lines, and/or significantly comminuted fractures are poor candidates for this procedure. For these patients, a dorsal C1-2 fusion is typically chosen.

At surgery, the patient is positioned supine with the head extended, usually in a fixed position with a Mayfield head holder. Biplanar fluoroscopy is generally used. Using a lower cervical incision about at C5-6, a standard high ventral cervical approach is followed to the C2-3 region. A variety of standard or specialized retractors can be used to maintain exposure. By using a Kerrison rongeur or high-speed drill, a midline trough is made in the ventral-rostral C3 vertebral body. Next, by using the trough, a power drill with a 2-mm bit is used to drill a pilot hole from the ventral caudal border of C2, across the fracture line, and to the tip of the odontoid process. The appropriate-length screw is determined by preoperative radiograph or CT measurements, intraoperative fluoroscopy, and/or measuring the length of the drill bit. If reduction of the fracture is needed, then a lag screw of an appropriately shorter length should be selected. Even without significant fracture displacement, lag screws can promote fusion by providing a compressive force across the fracture line. The screw is threaded into the pilot hole in the same trajectory. One or two screws may be placed, but one is typically used because the outcomes appear similar.[48,49] Several odontoid screw systems exist with specialized instrumentation and screws.[50] One system includes cannulated screws that can be placed over a threaded drill bit (Fig. 63-9).[51] See Chapter 143 for additional details on the instrumentation.

Patients are managed with a postoperative external orthosis (collar) until the fracture heals (usually 10–12 weeks). Success rates are high, with fusion rates between 81% and 96%.[48,49] In the event of a nonunion, a dorsal C1-2 technique can be used.

Ventral C1-2 Fixation

Ventral C1-2 transarticular fixation can be used if an odontoid screw fixation is not successful during a ventral approach. In addition, the approach may be used if a dorsal approach is not feasible for some reason or a dorsal C1-2 fusion has failed. The technique involves bilateral screws through the lateral vertebral body of C2 into the lateral mass of C1. Careful preoperative assessment of the course of the vertebral artery is essential to determine whether the procedure is feasible.

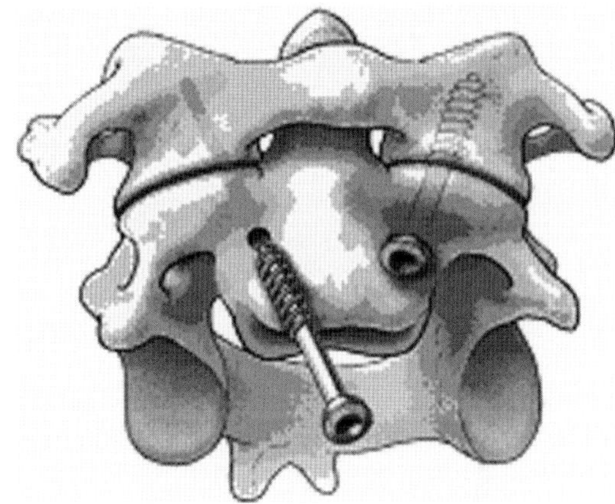

FIGURE 63-10. Anterior C1-2 transarticular instrumentation. (From Barrow Neurological Institute, with permission.)

At surgery, the positioning, approach, and exposure are similar to odontoid screw placement. An entry point is marked with a pilot hole at the groove between the C2 body and superior articular facet. This point is just medial to the vertebral artery. The screw trajectory is about 20 degrees lateral and rostral as needed to engage the C1 lateral mass securely. The screws are placed with fluoroscopic guidance (ideally biplanar) (Fig. 63-10). Although placing an onlay bone graft may be possible, the technique does not allow direct placement of bone between C1 and C2 and aims to have fusion occur at the articulation between the C1 and C2 lateral masses. Therefore, the C1-2 facet should be scraped with a small curette as possible to promote arthrodesis. Postoperatively, a collar or SOMI brace is used until bony fusion occurs (usually 12 weeks). Halo immobilization is used when the bone quality or fixation is suboptimal.

Ventral C2-3 Fixation

Ventral C2-3 discectomy and fusion are used for some traumatic C2 hangman fractures that demonstrate sufficient instability to warrant operative fixation.[52] Using a high cervical incision, a standard high ventral cervical approach and limited C2-3 discectomy are performed. If there is canal compromise from osteophytes or a herniated disc, then a more extensive dorsal osteophytectomy and/or discectomy is performed. The alignment, if abnormal, is optimized as much as possible. After preparation of the end plates, a C2-3 arthrodesis is performed with structural iliac crest autograft or allograft. Then C2-3 ventral cervical plating is performed (see Chapters 143 and 144). Extra attention is required for the C2 screws because of the unique anatomy. A narrow low-profile plate is preferred to facilitate placement. The patient is managed with a postoperative external orthosis (collar) for 6 or more weeks depending on the degree of preoperative instability.

Dorsal C2-3 fixation does not adequately treat these fractures unless direct dorsal C2 screw placement across the fracture is used. C1-3 dorsal segmental instrumentation with intervening screw or sublaminar wiring at C2 is another alternative procedure.

Summary

Occipitocervical junction trauma can result in a variety of injury patterns involving the regional bony, ligamentous, neurologic, and vascular structures. Because of the vital nature of these threatened structures, accurate diagnosis and careful management are required. In particular, careful attention is directed to achieving and maintaining an appropriate alignment from the onset of trauma. After initial airway management and medical stabilization, relevant diagnostic imaging should be obtained. Although many of the injuries can be recognized on plain radiographs, high-resolution CT scanning with multiplanar reconstruction views generally provides the most useful information. MRI may be difficult to obtain but is usually best to assess any spinal canal compromise and the integrity of important ligaments. Flexion/extension imaging is most useful for cooperative patients who do not have significant spinal canal compromise.

The primary focus of the imaging is to identify and characterize injuries and to guide management. If instability is documented or presumed on the basis of imaging, then some combination of external and/or internal stabilization is necessary to protect neurologic function and permit mobilization. If malalignment is present, correction with an orthosis, traction, and/or operation is considered, depending on the degree of deformity and its relationship to current or potential neurologic injury. When needed, traction should be performed cautiously and only with a solid understanding of the injury, as distraction can exacerbate certain injuries (e.g., occipitoatlantal dissociation).

Operative procedures generally require rigid intraoperative fixation via a halo ring/adaptor or Mayfield head clamp. Surgical intervention is focused on decompressing significant compressive lesions (e.g., bone, hematoma), restoring alignment, and achieving stabilization with arthrodesis and usually internal fixation. Advances in instrumentation and surgical technique in the past three decades (e.g., image guidance, surgical innovation) have led to the development of better, stronger internal fixation constructs that can spare motion (e.g., odontoid screw fixation), reduce the number of levels to be fused, and avoid or minimize use of uncomfortable orthoses such as halos, which have inherent risks themselves (e.g., pulmonary compromise, skull pin site complications). These instrumentation techniques are discussed further in Chapter 143. Achieving bony fusion is an important goal of stabilization, and careful attention to technique is required. Although many trauma patients are good fusion candidates (young, healthy patients), liberal use of autograft is advised in most cases, because many patients may be or become critically ill and malnourished because of spinal or systemic injuries. Furthermore, nonunions can be difficult to manage and may require more substantial operative intervention. Overall, the treatment of occipitocervical injuries must be individualized on the basis of patient and injury characteristics, the surgeon's knowledge of the different operative risk factors, complication avoidance and management, instrumentation options, and experience.

KEY REFERENCES

Benzel EC, Hart BL, Ball PA, et al: Fractures of the C-2 vertebral body. *J Neurosurg* 81:206–212, 1994.

Effendi B, Roy D, Cornish B, et al: Fractures of the ring of the axis. A classification based on the analysis of 131 cases. *J Bone Joint Surg [Br]* 63:319–327, 1981.

Garrett M, Consiglieri G, Kakarla UK, et al: Occipitoatlantal dislocation. *Neurosurgery* 66:A48–A55, 2010.

Greene KA, Dickman CA, Marciano FF, et al: Acute axis fractures. Analysis of management and outcome in 340 consecutive cases. *Spine (Phila Pa 1976)* 22: 1843–1852, 1997.

Hadley MN, Browner CM, Liu SS, Sonntag VK: New subtype of acute odontoid fractures (type IIA). *Neurosurgery* 22:67–71, 1988.

Hadley MN, Walters BC, Grabb PA, et al: Management of acute central cervical spinal cord injuries. *Neurosurgery* 50:S166–S172, 2002.

Melcher RP, Puttlitz CM, Kleinstueck FS, et al: Biomechanical testing of posterior atlantoaxial fixation techniques. *Spine (Phila Pa 1976)* 27:2435–2440, 2002.

REFERENCES

The complete reference list is available online at expertconsult.com.

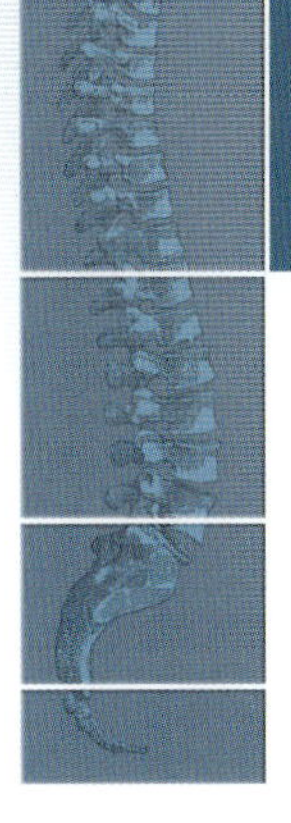

CHAPTER 64

Subaxial Cervical Spine Injuries

Amirali Sayadipour | D. Greg Anderson | Sergey Mlyavykh |
Olga Perlmutter | Alexander R. Vaccaro

Cervical fractures are found in approximately 3% of all trauma patients.[1] The subaxial spine accounts for the majority of cervical injuries, making up approximately 65% of fractures and more than 75% of all dislocations.[2] Approximately 150,000 cervical spine injuries occur annually in North America. In the same region, there are 11,000 new spinal cord injuries (1 per 25,000 people) annually.[3] Trauma in the subaxial cervical spine accounts for almost half of all cervical spine injuries and the largest proportion of new traumatic spinal cord injuries.

Anatomy

The anatomy of the lower cervical spine is unique and contributes to the injury patterns that are observed in this region. The cervical spinal canal houses the delicate spinal cord, which fills much of the canal, leaving relatively little room for displacement of the vertebral osteoligamentous structures without the risk of neurologic injury. The subaxial cervical disc spaces curve upward laterally to form the uncovertebral joints. The uncovertebral joints augment the stability of the segment in rotation but allow a large range of motion in flexion, extension, and lateral bending. The facet joints are oriented at 45 to 60 degrees to the coronal plane and also allow significant flexion, extension, and lateral bending motion. Because the intrinsic bony anatomy of the cervical spine provides relatively limited stability, there is a great dependence on the ligamentous structures to stabilize the subaxial cervical region.

Various authors have modeled the cervical spine as either a two-column[4,5] or three-column system.[6,7] Although both systems have merits, the two-column system probably provides the best understanding of the common injury patterns seen in the lower cervical region. The two-column spine consists of an anterior column and a posterior column. The anterior column contains the anterior longitudinal ligament, intervertebral disc, vertebral body, and posterior longitudinal ligament. The posterior column consists of the posterior bony elements, facet capsules, interspinous and supraspinous ligaments, and ligamentum flavum. The most important stabilizer of the anterior column is the anulus fibrosus, whereas the facet joints are the most important stabilizers of the posterior column.[5]

The ligamentous structures provide a check to hypermobility during normal motion. For example, the anterior longitudinal ligament and ventral anulus become taut during extension, whereas the posterior column ligamentous structures act as a tension band during flexion. Compressive loads are resisted by the vertebral bodies, intervertebral discs, and facet joints. Pure tensile loads are resisted by the anulus, interspinous ligament, ligamentum flavum, and facet capsules. Flexion is resisted by the interspinous ligaments, facet capsules and facet joints, anterior longitudinal ligament, and posterior anulus. Extension is also resisted by the bony block of the facet joints. Maximal sagittal plane translation occurring under physiologic loads is 2 to 2.7 mm.[5] Lower cervical spine injuries can be understood as a failure of the structures designed to resist the forces and moments occurring at the time of the injury. By observing the pattern of bony and ligamentous disruption on imaging studies, the treating physician may generally deduce the force vectors that acted to create the injury pattern and also begin to gain an understanding of the "personality" of the injury, and thus the tendency for displacement under physiologic loads.

Injury Classification

Classification of cervical spine injuries is important for several reasons. First, classification facilitates accurate communication regarding the nature of an injury. Second, a classification system allows the physician to determine the optimal treatment of an injury. Third, classification allows the treating physician to make predictions regarding prognosis of the injury. Fourth, accurate classification is necessary for valid outcomes research to be performed or for data to be compared between centers. Finally, classification may facilitate an improved understanding of the pathomechanics of a particular injury.

Many classification systems have been proposed to describe injuries of the cervical spine. Available classification systems are generally based on specific factors, including mechanisms of injury, radiographic findings, injury severity, and neurologic status.

All classification systems have certain individual strengths and weaknesses. To use a system appropriately, one must understand the rationale of the classification so that an injury can he viewed in the appropriate context.

The simplest method of discussing injuries to the cervical spine is to use radiographic descriptions of the injury. Hence, terms such as *compression fracture*, *burst fracture*, *teardrop fracture*, or *facet dislocation* remain in common usage, although these descriptive terms provide only a broad overview of the injury and do not provide information on injury severity, neurologic status, or treatment options. Mechanistic classifications are useful in promoting an understanding of injury pathomechanics and also assist the surgeon in designing a rational treatment approach, although biomechanical validation of the presumed injury mechanisms is generally lacking. Despite this limitation, these classification schemes are useful in clinical practice and remain the preferred scheme at most trauma centers managing large volumes of cervical trauma.

The "ideal" classification system would allow all injuries to be placed into a specific category. An ideal system would have perfect interobserver and intraobserver reliability. The system should allow the clinician to better understand the injury and would define both treatment and expected outcome. Finally, the optimal scheme would be simple, reliable, and valid across the spectrum of treating physicians. Needless to say, this "ideal" classification system is not yet available.

Although many classification schemes have been proposed, this chapter reviews several schemes that have strong historical significance or practical utility, or are recent additions to the literature, including those proposed by Whitley and Forsyth (1960),[8] Allen et al. (1982),[9] Harris et al. (1986),[10] Anderson et al. (2007),[11] and, finally, Vaccaro et al. (2007).[3]

Whitley and Forsyth[8] described a mechanistic classification of cervical spine injuries in 1960 based on a review of 159 patients with cervical fractures. In their scheme, fractures were divided into flexion injuries, extension injuries, combined flexion-extension injuries, burst-type injuries, and direct trauma. The authors further divided flexion and extension injuries into those occurring with and without compression. This classification system retains historical importance for promoting a mechanistic thinking about cervical spine injuries.

White and Panjabi[5] devised an early checklist for instability after cervical trauma. They hypothesized that a similar injury mechanism might produce different injury patterns because of the complex multidirectional forces, moments, and positions of the affected joints at the time of trauma. They devised a point-based system for assessing stability in lower cervical spine injury, summarized in Table 64-1. To use their system, radiographic criteria, physical examination, and a stretch test are required. A score of 5 or more points in this system is said to predict spinal instability.[12]

The stretch test described by White and Panjabi is performed by securing the patient's head in halter or tong traction with a roller beneath the head to reduce friction. Initial lateral radiographs of the cervical spine with 10 pounds of traction are carefully analyzed to rule out a disruption of the occipitocervical junction. Serial weight is sequentially added in 10-pound increments, performing neurologic testing with each addition of weight. The end point of the test is reached when "instability" is noted on radiographs or when there is a change in neurologic examination, or when the weight limit (65 pounds or one-third body weight) is reached. Instability on the stretch test is defined as distraction of a vertebral interspace by 1.7 mm or greater or a change in segmental alignment of 7.5 degrees or greater compared with the baseline radiographs.[12] Although advocated by several authors, this type of test has not become a standard method for analyzing stability in most trauma centers because of its cumbersome nature and concerns regarding iatrogenic neurologic injury.

TABLE 64-1

Diagnosis of Clinical Instability in the Middle and Lower Cervical Spine

Element	Point
Anterior elements destroyed or unable to function	2
Posterior elements destroyed or unable to function	2
Positive stretch test	2
Radiographic criteria	
Flexion-extension radiographs	
Sagittal plane translation > 3.5 mm	2
Sagittal plane rotation > 20°	2
Resting radiographs	
Sagittal plane displacement > 3.5 mm	2
Relative sagittal plane angulation > 11°	2
Developmentally narrow spinal canal	1
Abnormal disc narrowing	1
Spinal cord damage	2
Nerve root damage	1
Dangerous loading anticipated	1

A total of five or more points indicates clinical instability.

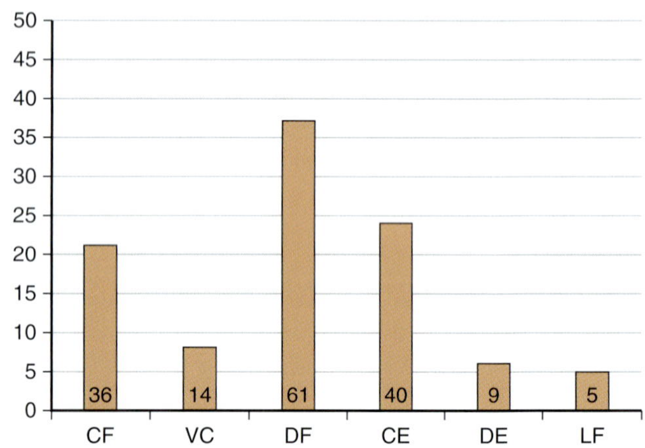

FIGURE 64-1. Distribution of lower cervical spine injuries among 165 patients. CE, compressive extension; CF, compressive flexion; DE, distractive extension; DF, distractive flexion; LF, lateral flexion; VC, vertical compression. (Data from Allen BL, Ferguson RL, Lehmann TR, et al: A mechanistic classification of closed indirect fractures and dislocations of the lower cervical spine. *Spine [Phila Pa 1976]* 7:1–27, 1982.)

In 1982, Allen et al.[9] published a mechanistic classification system that has been widely used in recent years. They based their scheme on the clinical review of 165 patients with indirect lower cervical spine trauma. In this system, subaxial cervical injuries were divided into "phylogenies" based on a common proposed injury mechanism, with an orderly progression of severity ranging from mild to severe. They included six injury phylogenies—compressive flexion, vertical compression, distractive flexion, compressive extension, distractive extension, and lateral flexion (Fig. 64-1). The terms used for each category describe the attitude of the cervical spine at the time of injury and the dominant force vector. The authors acknowledged the presence of minor force vectors that may cause separate or combined injuries. "Rotation" in this system was described as localizing an injury asymmetrically to one side rather than acting as an independent force vector. In general, the risk and severity of neurologic injury were noted to increase with increasing severity stages (Box 64-1).

In 1986, Harris et al.[10] proposed a similar classification system that placed injuries into groups related to a predominant causative force vector or combination of force vectors (Box 64-2). Unlike the Allen scheme, Harris et al. included the rotational vectors combined with flexion or extension but did not emphasize the role of distractive forces.

In 2007, Anderson et al.[11] presented the Cervical Spine Injury Severity Score (CSISS), a scheme allowing the observer to grade the degree of osteoligamentous disruption of the injury based on a four-column concept of the cervical spine modified from the work of Louis. The concept is to correlate increasing amounts of osseous separation or ligamentous disruption with a higher degree of instability using an analogue scale, with the goal of identifying patients who would benefit from surgical stabilization. The authors found excellent intraobserver and interobserver reliability when applying their scheme to a cervical trauma population, perhaps owing to the critical analysis of each of the four columns of the cervical spine. When analyzed, the CSISS was noted to perform well for all fracture types and for a spectrum of injuries from relatively minor to grossly unstable.[11] Patients with scores greater than 7 points were generally subjected to surgical stabilization, suggesting the system produced consensus regarding the need for operative stabilization.

Vaccaro et al.[3] presented a point-based scheme for evaluating subaxial cervical injuries in 2007. The authors reviewed the positive elements of prior classification systems and used the expertise of an experienced group of clinicians in the Spine Trauma Study Group (STSG) to devise a working system known as the Subaxial Injury Classification (SLIC; Table 64-2). The SLIC system applies a severity ranking in three specific areas: (1) a morphologic description of the bony fracture pattern, (2) a rating of the discoligamentous complex, and (3) a rating of the patient's neurologic status.[3] By applying points in each area, the authors were able to produce a severity score that was used to separate treatment into surgical and nonsurgical categories.

To use the SLIC system with a high degree of interobserver and intraobserver consistency, it is important that the clinician adhere to a few simple concepts. First, at a given spinal level, the most severe injury pattern should be graded for morphology. Second, if a cervical spine injury demonstrates elements of both burst and translation, then the injury is classified as a translational injury. Third, if both a nerve root and spinal cord injury coexist, then it is the spinal cord injury that should be used to define the SLIC neurologic score.

Spinal Stability

Spinal stability is one of the most fundamental issues affecting treatment decisions for cervical trauma, yet an absolute method to define stability remains elusive. Many attempts have been made to define instability by various researchers. Spinal stability was defined by White and Panjabi[13] as "the ability of the spine under physiologic loads to limit patterns of displacement so as not to damage or irritate the spinal cord or nerve roots and, in addition, to prevent incapacitating deformity

BOX 64-1. Lower Cervical Spine Trauma Phylogeny Classification System*

1. Compressive Flexion (CF)

CFS1: rounded shape to the anterior superior vertebral body without any posterior ligamentous disruption

CFS2: "beaked" appearance of the anterior vertebral body with loss of anterior height due to compression failure

CFS3: an oblique fracture line traversing from the anterosuperior vertebral body to the inferior end plate

CFS4: up to 3 mm of posterior translation of the posterior vertebral body into the neural canal

CFS5: >3 mm displacement of the posterior aspect of the vertebral body into the neural canal

2. Vertical Compression (VC)

VCS1: failure or "cupping" of either the superior or inferior end plates

VCS2: failure of both end plates with the "cupping" deformity

VCS3: comminution of the vertebral body with a radial displacement of the fragments (± fragments of bone displaced into the spinal canal)

3. Distractive Flexion (DF)

DFS1: forward subluxation of the upper facet in the motion segment with widening of the space between the spinous processes

DFS2: unilateral facet dislocation demonstrating up to 25% forward subluxation of the vertebral body in the motion segment

DFS3: bilateral facet dislocation with approximately 50% anterior subluxation of the upper vertebra in the motion segment

DFS4: gross anterior displacement of the upper vertebra on the lower vertebra in the motion segment, creating the "floating vertebra"

4. Compressive Extension (CE)

CES1: unilateral vertebral arch fracture (pedicle, facet, and/or lamina) with or without rotational displacement of the vertebral body

CES2: bilateral laminar fractures, often at multiple contiguous levels but without evidence of other soft tissue failure

CES3: bilateral disruption of the articular pillars (pedicle, facet, and/or lamina) without displacement

CES4: partial forward subluxation of the fractured vertebra on the vertebra below

5. Distractive Extension (DE)

DES1: failure of the anterior longitudinal ligament and anulus fibrosus with widening of the disc space anteriorly

DES2: posterior displacement of the upper vertebra in the motion segment

6. Lateral Compression (LC)

LCS1: asymmetrical compression failure of the vertebral body with an ipsilateral, undisplaced vertebral arch fracture

LCS2: displacement of the vertebral arch fracture or widening of the contralateral articular processes, demonstrating tension failure opposite the compression injury

*Injuries in 165 patients classified into six categories, or phylogenies, based on a common proposed injury mechanism.

Adapted from Allen BL, Ferguson RL, Lehmann TR, et al: A mechanistic classification of closed indirect fractures and dislocations of the lower cervical spine. *Spine (Phila Pa 1976)* 7:1–27, 1982.

BOX 64-2. Mechanism of Cervical Spine Injuries

I. Flexion
A. Anterior subluxation (hyperflexion sprain)
B. Bilateral interfacetal dislocation
C. Simple wedge (compression) fracture
D. Clay-shoveler's (coal-shoveler's) fracture
E. Flexion teardrop fracture

II. Flexion-Rotation
A. Unilateral interfacetal dislocation

III. Extension-Rotation
A. Pillar fracture

IV. Vertical Compression
A. Jefferson bursting fracture of atlas
B. Burst (bursting, dispersion, axial loading) fracture

V. Hyperextension
A. Hyperextension dislocation
B. Avulsion fracture of anterior arch of atlas
C. Extension teardrop fracture of axis
D. Fracture of posterior arch of atlas
E. Laminar fracture
F. Traumatic spondylolisthesis (hangman's fracture)
G. Hyperextension fracture-dislocation

VI. Lateral Flexion
A. Uncinate process fracture

VII. Diverse or Imprecisely Understood Mechanisms
A. Atlanto-occipital disassociation
B. Odontoid fractures

From Harris J, Edeiken-Monroe B, Kopaniky D: A practical classification of acute cervical spine injuries. *Orthop Clin North Am* 17:15–30, 1986.

TABLE 64-2

Subaxial Cervical Spine Injury Classification System

Characteristic	Points
Morphology	
No abnormality	0
Compression	1
Burst	1–2
Distraction (e.g., facet perch, hyperextension)	3
Rotation/translation (e.g., facet dislocation, unstable teardrop or advanced-stage flexion compression injury)	4
Discoligamentous Complex	
Intact	0
Indeterminate (e.g., isolated interspinous widening, MRI signal change only)	1
Disrupted (e.g., widening of disc space, facet perch or dislocation)	2
Neurologic Status	
Intact	0
Root injury	1
Complete cord injury	2
Incomplete cord injury	3
Continuous cord compression in setting of neurodeficit (neuromodifier)	1

Adapted from Vaccaro A, Hulbert J, Patel P, et al: The subaxial cervical spine injury classification system: a novel approach to recognize the importance of morphology, neurology, and integrity of the discoligamentous complex. *Spine (Phila Pa 1976)* 32:2365–2374, 2007.

or pain due to structural changes." Although this definition is logical, it is notoriously difficult to apply in clinical practice.[13] In contrast, Anderson et al.[11] used a continuous scale for grading stability of the bony and ligamentous structures in the CSISS. This approach seems to have good reliability, but the exact point at which an injury becomes unstable still remains imprecise. Allen et al.[9] defined instability as "greater than normal range of motion within a motion segment" and viewed each injury pattern as a spectrum. However, clinical judgment and experience on the part of the treating physician remain critical in defining stability.[9]

Holdsworth[4] and others[14,15] have emphasized the importance of the posterior ligamentous complex in conferring stability to the spine. In their description, the disruption of the posterior ligamentous complex is the primary determinant of instability. Instability comprises a spectrum, with rare cases of clinically significant instability not being recognizable on initial imaging. Herkowitz and Rothman[16] coined the term *subacute instability* to describe patients with negative initial radiographs and neurologic examinations who were subsequently noted to have unstable cervical injuries on follow-up radiographs. This situation was thought to be due to initial muscle spasm masking the instability. Because of the risk of a missed injury, early removal of cervical immobilization was discouraged. Instead, it was recommended that a patient with a suggestive trauma mechanism and neck pain remain in a secure cervical collar immobilization until the muscle spasm has resolved, at which time clinical and flexion and extension radiographs can be obtained.

Neurologic Classification

Neurologic classification is critical for the spinal cord-injured population. The neurologic examination should be repeated frequently in the early course after a spinal cord injury because the examination can change and affect the management of the patient. Accurate neurologic classification is crucial when performing research in the spinal cord-injured population and should be done in a careful and reproducible manner.[17] Many authors have noted a poor correlation between the severity of the spinal column injury and the severity of the neurologic injury. Total quadriplegia may occur without an apparent spinal column disruption; conversely, a widely displaced cervical dislocation may sometimes occur in a neurologically intact patient.

The first edition of the International Standards for Neurological and Functional Classification of Spinal Cord Injury was published in 1982 by the American Spinal Injury Association (ASIA). Since then there have been three revisions, the most recent in 1996.[18] The ASIA clinical format for recording a neurologic examination is shown in Figure 64-2. Sensory and motor testing are performed separately for each side of the body over 28 standardized dermatomes and 10 standardized myotomes. Sensation is tested for pinprick and

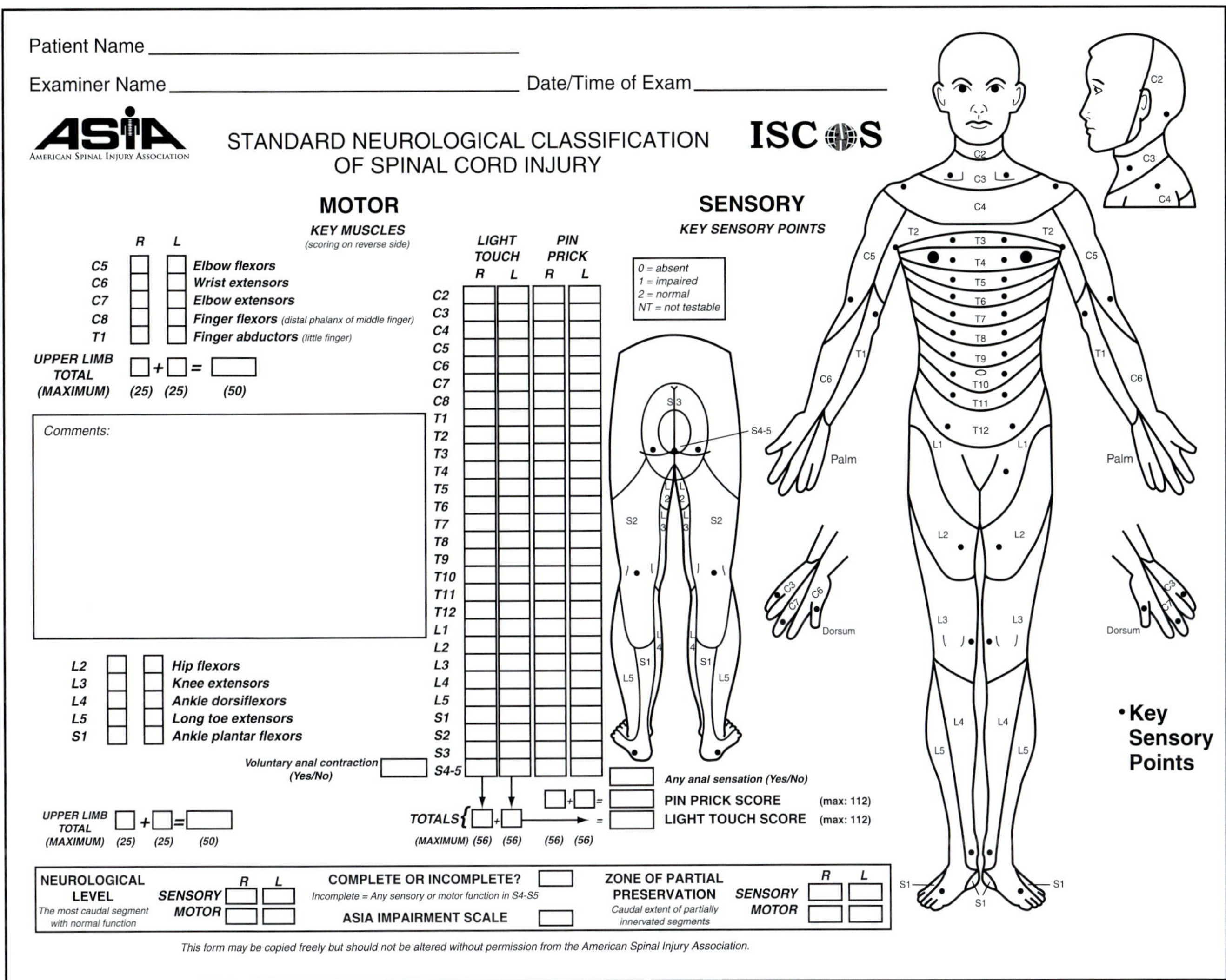

Patient Name ______________________

Examiner Name ______________________ Date/Time of Exam ______________

ASIA AMERICAN SPINAL INJURY ASSOCIATION

STANDARD NEUROLOGICAL CLASSIFICATION OF SPINAL CORD INJURY

ISCoS

MOTOR

KEY MUSCLES (scoring on reverse side)

	R	L	
C5			Elbow flexors
C6			Wrist extensors
C7			Elbow extensors
C8			Finger flexors (distal phalanx of middle finger)
T1			Finger abductors (little finger)

UPPER LIMB TOTAL (MAXIMUM) □+□=□ (25) (25) (50)

Comments:

	R	L	
L2			Hip flexors
L3			Knee extensors
L4			Ankle dorsiflexors
L5			Long toe extensors
S1			Ankle plantar flexors

Voluntary anal contraction (Yes/No) □

UPPER LIMB TOTAL (MAXIMUM) □+□=□ (25) (25) (50)

SENSORY

KEY SENSORY POINTS

LIGHT TOUCH R L — PIN PRICK R L

C2, C3, C4, C5, C6, C7, C8, T1, T2, T3, T4, T5, T6, T7, T8, T9, T10, T11, T12, L1, L2, L3, L4, L5, S1, S2, S3, S4-5

0 = absent
1 = impaired
2 = normal
NT = not testable

TOTALS {□+□ → = □ (MAXIMUM) (56) (56) (56) (56)

Any anal sensation (Yes/No)

PIN PRICK SCORE (max: 112)

LIGHT TOUCH SCORE (max: 112)

NEUROLOGICAL LEVEL — The most caudal segment with normal function — R L SENSORY MOTOR

COMPLETE OR INCOMPLETE? □ Incomplete = Any sensory or motor function in S4-S5

ASIA IMPAIRMENT SCALE □

ZONE OF PARTIAL PRESERVATION — Caudal extent of partially innervated segments — R L SENSORY MOTOR

This form may be copied freely but should not be altered without permission from the American Spinal Injury Association.

FIGURE 64-2. American Spinal Injury Association (ASIA) neurologic classification form used to document the physical examination of a patient after cervical trauma.

light touch modalities. The neurologic level is recorded as the most distal level with normal function. In cases where there is a discrepancy between sides of the body or between sensory and motor testing, each neurologic category should be individually recorded. Because many key muscles have neurologic input from more than one nerve root level, mild weakness may be present when a portion of the normal nerve supply is absent because of a neurologic injury. The motor level is defined as the most distal muscle group with a power score of 3 out of 5 or greater strength given normal motor testing above. It is important to test the most distal sacral levels (S4 and S5) for sensation as well as for anal sphincter motor function to define injury prognosis. Functional impairment can be categorized using the ASIA Impairment Scale (Box 64-3), which is a modification of the original Frankel grading system.

BOX 64-3. American Spinal Injury Association Impairment Scale

A. Complete. No sensory or motor function is preserved in the sacral segments S4-5.

B. Incomplete. Sensory but not motor function is preserved below the neurologic level and extends through the sacral segments S4-5.

C. Incomplete. Motor function is preserved below the neurologic level, and more than half of key muscles below the neurologic level have a muscle grade of less than 3.

D. Incomplete. Motor function is preserved below the neurologic level, and at least half of the key muscles below the neurologic level have a muscle grade of greater than or equal to 3.

E. Normal. Sensory and motor function is normal.

Diagnosis

The spinal literature supports *not* obtaining radiographs in asymptomatic patients who are awake, alert, nonintoxicated, and without distracting injuries who exhibit no neck tenderness or pain with range of motion after trauma.[19] All other patients sustaining significant neck trauma should be evaluated with plain radiographs at a minimum. Although plain radiographs continue to be the most common modality for initial imaging of the cervical spine after trauma, Woodring et al. and others have reported the limitations of plain radiography in detecting certain types of cervical fractures, particularly fractures of the posterior elements.[20-22] In one study, plain radiographs missed 23% of cervical fractures, including some that created the potential for instability. CT scanning has become a common initial imaging modality for patients after high-energy trauma in many trauma centers and is particularly indicated in cases of neurologic deficits or altered mental status.[23] In addition to a high sensitivity for fracture detection, CT with reformatted images provides an excellent assessment of sagittal and rotational alignment of the spine and has proved to be a beneficial tool for preoperative planning of surgical cases.[24]

MRI has been used increasingly in the setting of cervical trauma, particularly in patients with a neurologic deficit. MRI can localize and quantify cord compression, hemorrhage, or signal change within the cord and can detect the presence of nonbony lesions such as epidural hematoma or disc herniation. MRI may also demonstrate disruptions of the cervical ligaments, which are not detectable by plain radiographs or CT.[25] MR angiography can be used to define patency or injury to the vertebral arteries in the setting of high-energy trauma.[26,27]

Lateral flexion-extension radiographs are rarely indicated in the acute trauma setting because pain and muscle spasm may prevent an accurate identification of injuries.[16] Dynamic films, however, are useful when performed in a delayed fashion (10 to 14 days after the injury) to rule out subtle instability before the discontinuation of immobilization. Patients subjected to this technique should have voluntary motion of the neck and an absence of significant muscle spasm for accurate detection of a subtle injury.

Treatment

Simple Compression Fractures

Simple compression fractures (Fig. 64-3) may involve the upper or lower vertebral end plates (or both) and are caused by forceful flexion or axial loading of the neck. This type of injury is common in patients with osteopenia but may also be seen after higher-energy trauma in patients with normal bone. By definition, these injuries have no significant ligament disruption, facet diastasis, or subluxation. Our preferred treatment involves immobilization in a semirigid cervical orthosis for 6 to 8 weeks followed by flexion-extension lateral radiographs to rule out a more serious instability pattern. If no abnormal motion is seen on flexion-extension lateral radiographs, the patient can be weaned from the collar and begin a postinjury rehabilitation program.[28]

Severe Compression/Burst Fractures/Axial Compression Injuries

These injuries are usually seen with high-energy trauma when the cervical spine is subjected to axial loading with various amounts of flexion. The energy of these injuries is sufficient to produce a substantial crush injury to the discoligamentous complex and may, in the case of burst fractures, lead to retropulsion of material into the spinal canal. Unlike the teardrop/compressive flexion injury pattern (see later), the posterior osteoligamentous complex remains competent. Therefore, diastasis of the facets or widening between the spinous processes generally is not present (Fig. 64-4).

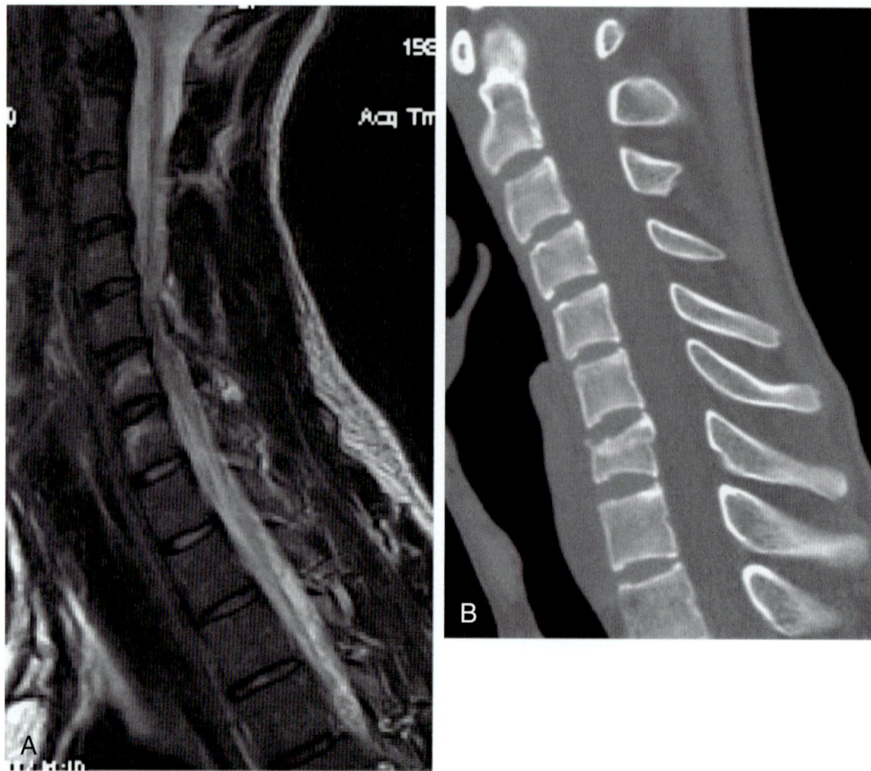

FIGURE 64-3. **A,** Midsagittal MRI of a patient with subtle compression fractures at C6 and C7, showing edema in the vertebral bodies. No ligamentous injuries are evident. **B,** Midsagittal CT reconstruction showing a compression fracture of C7. Note that the dorsal elements show no evidence of diastasis.

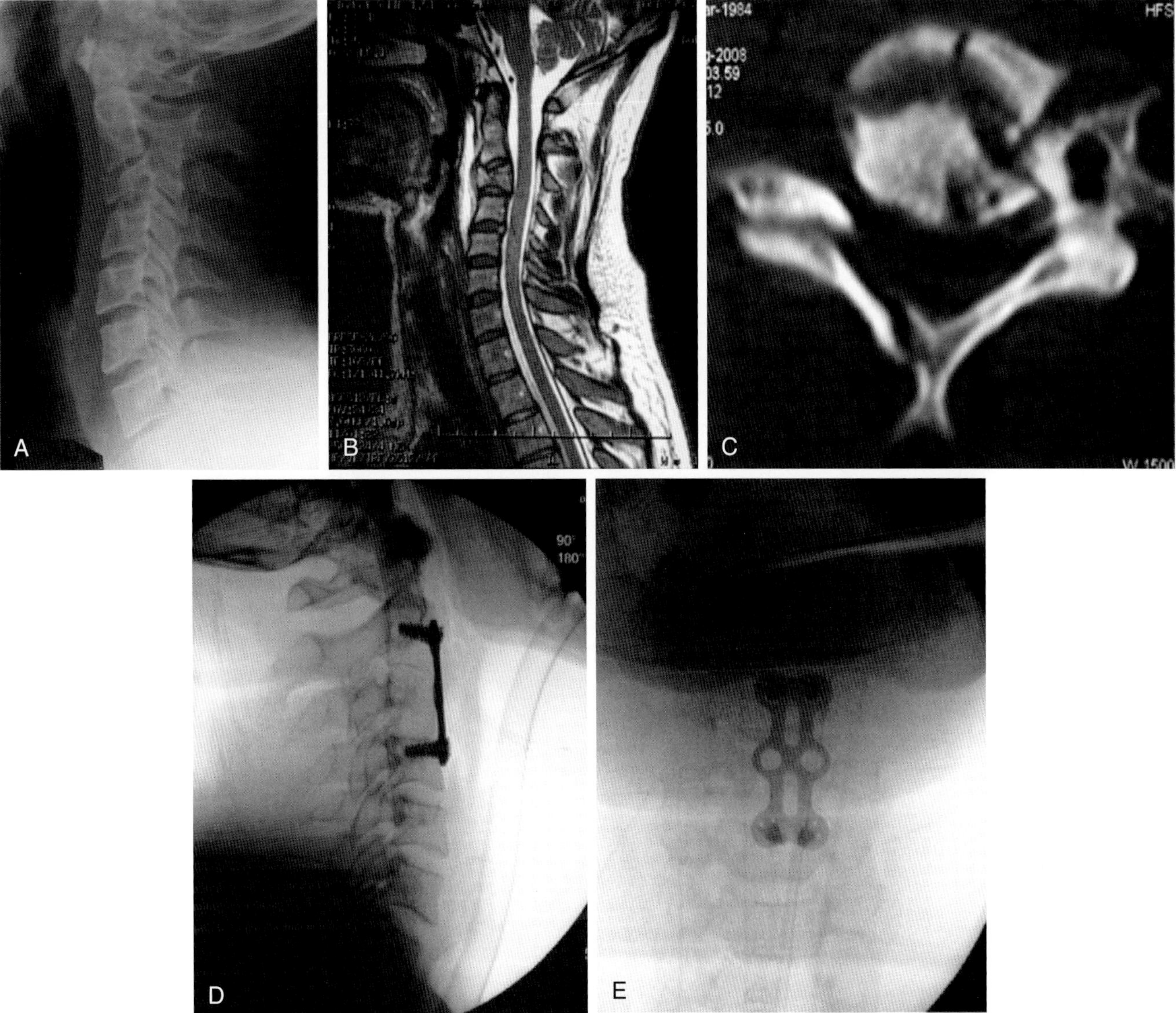

FIGURE 64-4. Plain radiograph (**A**), sagittal MRI (**B**), and CT scan (**C**) of a burst/axial compression injury at C3. Note retropulsion of the vertebral body on the axial CT (**C**). Although a laminar fracture is present, there is no evidence of widening of the dorsal elements on the plain radiograph or MRI. The injury was treated with a corpectomy of C3 followed by strut grafting and ventral cervical plating (**D** and **E**).

Treatment for this injury pattern is dictated primarily by the neurologic status of the patient and secondarily by the presence of significant kyphosis. Patients who are neurologically intact without significant kyphosis are usually amenable to nonoperative treatment. Immobilization in a cervical collar or halo orthosis may be used successfully to treat this injury pattern. Close follow-up radiographs should be taken at frequent intervals, early in the course of nonoperative care, because these injuries may demonstrate progressive collapse.

In cases where there is substantial compression of the spinal cord with an incomplete neurologic deficit, operative intervention is generally recommended. The most common operative approach is anterior, performing a corpectomy of the fractured vertebral body with decompression of the spinal cord and reconstruction using a structural graft and ventral cervical plate.[29] Treatment for patients with complete neurologic deficits or significant kyphosis without a neurologic deficit is more controversial. Many authors have recommended surgery to facilitate early rehabilitation of patients with complete spinal cord injuries or to promote root recovery at levels below the injury. Anderson and Bohlman found an average recovery of one to two root levels below the level of a complete cord injury even with delayed decompression.[30] Substantial posttraumatic cervical kyphosis may lead to problems with chronic neck pain or even delayed neurologic symptoms, and, therefore, such patients are candidates for anatomic reconstruction of the fractured level.

Cervical Facet Dislocations/Distractive Flexion Injuries

Cervical facet dislocations result from hyperflexion and posterior distraction of the cervical spine, with or without rotational forces. These injuries are most commonly seen after high-energy trauma such as motor vehicle collisions, diving accidents, or severe falls.[31] Unilateral facet dislocations generally exhibit up to 25% anterior subluxation of the cranial vertebral body over the caudal level. In contrast, bilateral

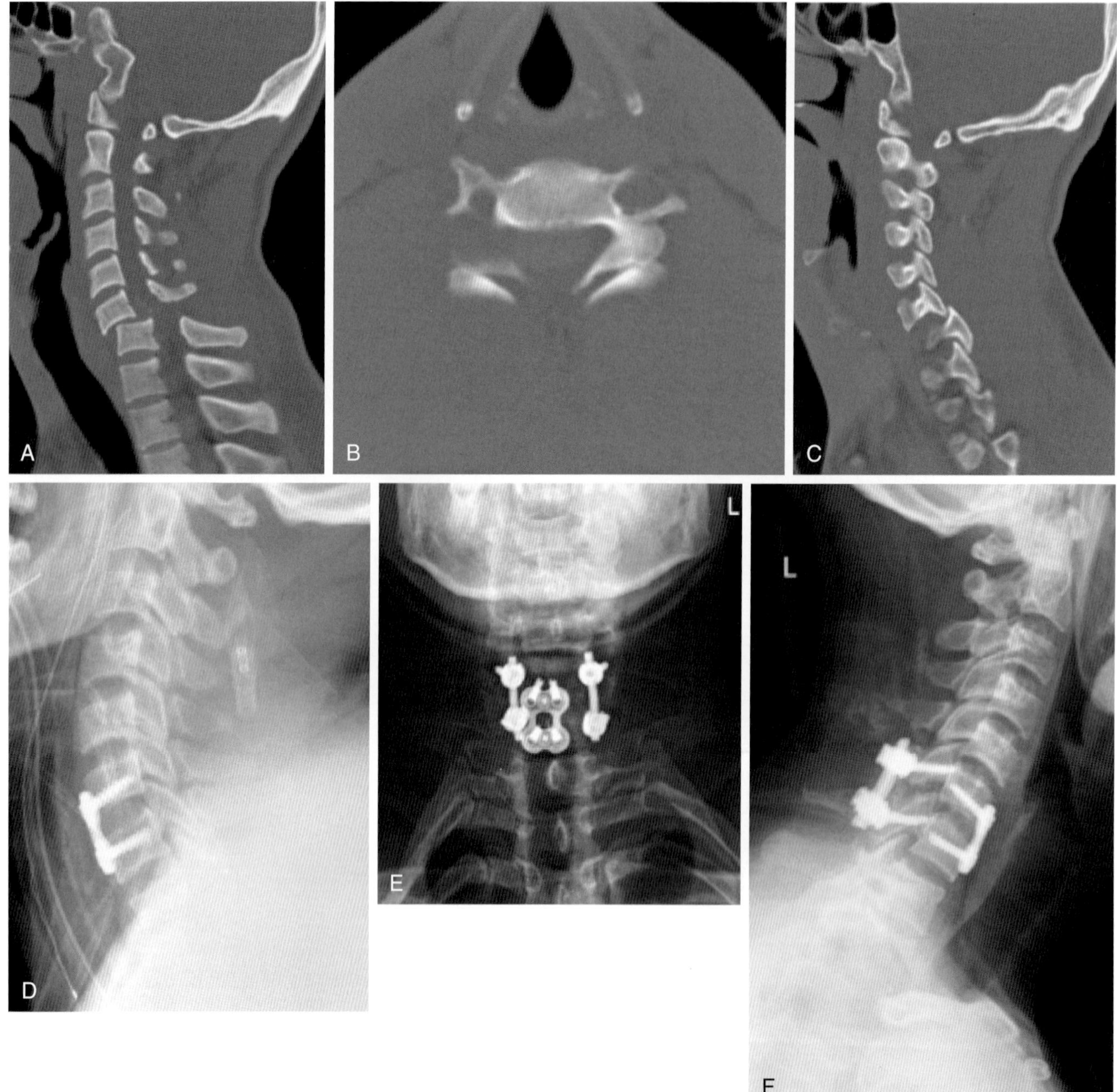

FIGURE 64-5. CT scans of a patient who sustained a bilateral facet dislocation (**A–C**). Note the ventral subluxation of the rostral vertebral body and the caudal articular process, which is ventral to the rostral articular process. MRI (not shown) demonstrated a large traumatic disc herniation dorsal to the C6 vertebral body. Therefore, a ventral approach was performed first to achieve decompression of the spinal cord. Next, a reduction of the facet dislocation was achieved through a ventral approach, followed by interbody grafting and ventral cervical plating (**D**). Finally, the posterior column was stabilized using lateral mass fixation (**E** and **F**).

facet dislocations generally demonstrate 50% or more ventral displacement of the upper vertebral body over the lower (Fig. 64-5). Fracture of the inferior or superior articular processes or comminution of the lateral mass region is commonly seen with facet dislocations, producing a continuum of injury. MRI and surgical exploration commonly reveal massive disruption of the posterior musculature, interspinous ligament, supraspinous ligament, facet capsule, and ligamentum flavum, making this injury pattern intrinsically unstable. Neurologic injuries are commonly seen in patients sustaining bilateral facet dislocations, but are much less common after unilateral facet dislocations. Patients with unilateral facet dislocations may demonstrate evidence of an isolated nerve root injury.

The initial assessment and management of cervical facet dislocations has raised controversy in the literature. Some authors have recommended rapid realignment of the spine through closed traction, followed by surgical stabilization. Proponents of this approach argue that in the awake, alert, and examinable patient, the application of progressive traction to achieve a rapid reduction of the dislocation will achieve the quickest decompression of the cord and thus the highest chance of neurologic recovery.[32] With this approach it is crucial to perform careful serial neurologic examinations and serial radiographs with each application of weight.

An alternative approach for managing a cervical facet dislocation injury has been advocated by Eismont et al.[33] These authors believe that before any significant traction or attempt to reduce a cervical facet dislocation, an MRI should be obtained to rule out the presence of a traumatic disc herniation. Proponents of this approach point to rare case examples of neurologic deterioration that have occurred after closed reduction, particularly if done under general anesthesia where serial neurologic examination is not possible. With the approach of Eismont et al., after obtaining an MRI, the treating surgeon would perform an anterior decompression for those patients with a traumatic disc herniation, followed by reconstruction. Those without a traumatic disc herniation may be reduced either by closed or open reduction, followed by surgical stabilization.[33] The safety and efficacy of each approach for traumatic facet dislocation continue to generate debate.[34]

In comparisons of surgical reconstruction techniques, posterior reconstruction has been shown to be more biomechanically sound than anterior reconstruction.[28] Posterior reconstruction allows the disrupted posterior tension band to be reestablished. Despite this, Elgafy et al. and others (as cited in Jenkins et al.[28]) have reported the development of segmental kyphosis in some cases of bilateral facet dislocation treated with posterior-only instrumentation, particularly if nonrigid forms of instrumentation (i.e., wiring) are used. The most stable reconstruction technique of all is a circumferential approach with both anterior and posterior instrumentation. However, this approach produces increased surgical morbidity and requires additional time under anesthesia.[35]

In the case of a unilateral facet dislocation in the neurologically intact patient, some authors have advocated the use of a halo-vest orthosis or even cervical collar for immobilization without performing a reduction of the displaced joint. However, failure rates with immobilization because of either recurrent instability or chronic pain have ranged as high as 50%, suggesting reconsideration of this strategy.[36] In the cases of an unreduced, unilateral dislocation, there is a significant risk of radiculopathic symptoms from compression of the exiting nerve root.[37] Reduction can be achieved in either a closed fashion (with traction) or in an open surgical procedure, usually from a posterior approach. If the dislocation is reduced with traction, the surgeon has the option of performing either an anterior or posterior approach for stabilization. If open reduction is chosen, a posterior instrumented fusion would normally be performed.[37] Shapiro et al. evaluated reconstructive options (interspinous braided cable/lateral mass plating with spinous process/facet wiring) with a posterior approach in patients with unilateral facet dislocations.[38] Although all of the techniques proved to be effective, the more rigid lateral mass plating techniques were preferred. Henriques et al. reported a small series of patients with unilateral facet dislocations treated with anterior fusion.[39] Successful fusion was achieved in most cases, but reoperation was required in 5.9% of the patients.

There is almost universal agreement regarding the need for surgical stabilization in cases of bilateral facet dislocation. These injuries are highly unstable and may redislocate after reduction, even when immobilized in a halo-vest orthosis.[35] In the absence of an anterior disc herniation, reduction can be achieved by either closed or open means followed by posterior stabilization of the injury, preferably with rigid instrumentation.[35] However, treatment of a bilateral facet dislocation in the presence of a large anterior traumatic disc herniation involves a more complex series of steps. First, a ventral approach is used to remove the disc herniation and decompress the spinal cord. Next, the surgeon can reduce the dislocation using either traction or anterior manipulation, or can proceed to a posterior open reduction. The advantage of achieving the reduction during the ventral portion of the procedure is that it allows the anterior column defect to be grafted. If a posterior approach is required to obtain the reduction, the posterior column of the spine can be stabilized with internal fixation; however, the anterior column must again be approached to graft the defect at the level of the disc space. Great care should be taken to avoid overdistraction of the disc space, which may occur in these grossly unstable injuries.

Although some have described successful treatment of bilateral facet dislocations with ventral stabilization alone, others have found an unacceptable rate of redislocation after this technique.[40] Therefore, many authors recommend dorsal supplemental instrumentation even if the reduction and stabilization are achieved through an anterior approach. If the reduction cannot be achieved from the anterior approach or is not attempted owing to neurologic concerns, the surgeon should close the ventral wound and proceed to the dorsal spine to perform the reduction and stabilization of the segment, followed by a final return to the anterior column to graft the defect. One unique solution to handle a case with bilateral facet dislocation and a ventral disc herniation was described by Allred and Sledge,[41] who placed a small ventral graft after ventral decompression, followed by placement of a ventral cervical plate attached only to the rostral vertebral body to retain the graft. With this technique, they were able to coax the graft back into position (using fluoroscopic guidance) during the dorsal reduction maneuver, thus avoiding the need to return to the ventral spine to graft the defect.[41]

Teardrop Fractures/Severe Compressive Flexion Injuries

The teardrop fracture pattern is thought to result from severe flexion and compression of the cervical spine.[9] This injury pattern demonstrates disruption to both the anterior and posterior columns of the cervical spine and has a high rate of neurologic injury. The injury pattern can be recognized on lateral radiographs by the fracture of the anteroinferior corner of the vertebral body and the commonly associated retrolisthesis of the upper vertebral body on the lower (Fig. 64-6). In addition, the posterior elements usually exhibit diastasis and the segment demonstrates kyphosis. A closely related variant, termed the *quadrangular fracture*, has a larger fracture fragment ventrally, seen on the lateral view, that courses vertically through the vertebral body from end plate to end plate.[28] CT usually demonstrates dorsal fractures of the lamina or lateral mass, diastasis of the facet joints, and a sagittally oriented split through the vertebral body. MRI scanning commonly demonstrates spinal cord compression, cord signal change, and traumatic hemorrhage within the spinal canal, along with disruption of the dorsal ligamentous structures.

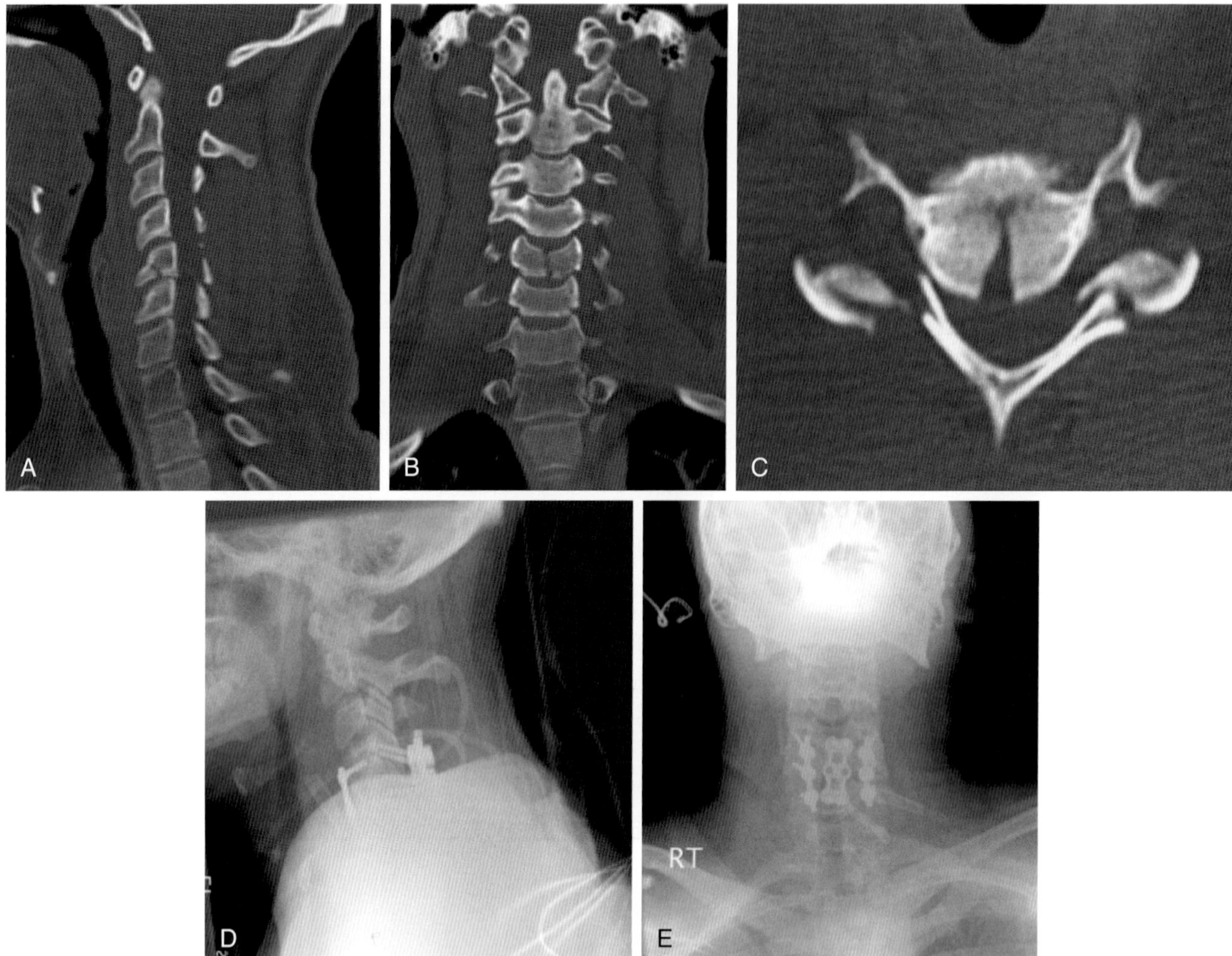

FIGURE 64-6. C5 teardrop fracture. **A,** Note the fracture of the ventral/caudal corner of the vertebral body on the sagittal CT reconstruction, and the widening of the dorsal elements. **B** and **C,** Also note the sagittal plane vertebral body split on the coronal CT reconstruction and axial CT. The dorsal elements show significant comminution and displacement. **D** and **E,** The injury was stabilized by corpectomy of the C5 vertebral body with strut grafting and ventral plating, followed by dorsal stabilization with lateral mass fixation.

Neurologic injuries are exceedingly common in patients with the teardrop fracture pattern. The classic picture is a dense ventral spinal cord injury, although any pattern of injury may be encountered.[28] Treatment for severe teardrop fractures is generally surgical, with the goals of decompressing the spinal canal, correcting the traumatic deformity, and providing stability to allow fusion across the fractured segment.

Some authors, including Toh et al. (as cited in Jenkins et al.[28]), have advocated a ventral approach with corpectomy, strut grafting, and the application of an ventral cervical plate. Although this approach may provide early reconstruction of the spinal injury, concerns regarding the lack of stability of the disrupted posterior column remain. For this reason, many authors have recommended a combined ventral and dorsal fixation strategy to address the more severe versions of this injury pattern. Cybulski et al.[28] identified vertebral body retrolisthesis, facet diastasis, and shearing through the disc as indications for a circumferential fusion. De Iure et al.[28] recommended circumferential surgery for any teardrop fracture in which an anatomic reduction could not be obtained or there was a traumatic listhesis of the segment. With the circumferential approach, the ventral decompression is usually performed first, achieving decompression of the spinal cord and reconstruction of the anterior column by placement of a structural strut graft, followed by posterior stabilization with segmental instrumentation. Dorsal stabilization can be achieved using a variety of techniques, although lateral mass fixation has become popular in recent years.

Hyperextension/Distractive Extension Injuries

Severe extension injuries are most commonly seen in elderly patients or those with a stiff or ankylosed cervical spine, particularly those with diffuse idiopathic skeletal hyperostosis or ankylosing spondylitis. The most common injury mechanism is a ground-level fall or other low-energy trauma causing forced hyperextension of the neck with disruption of the anterior longitudinal ligament and disc. The stiff or ankylosed spinal segments are thought to create a long lever arm that concentrates the traumatic forces to the injury site, which is most commonly the disc space.[28] The more severe forms of this injury pattern also exhibit disruption of the dorsal ligaments, which can be recognized by retrolisthesis of

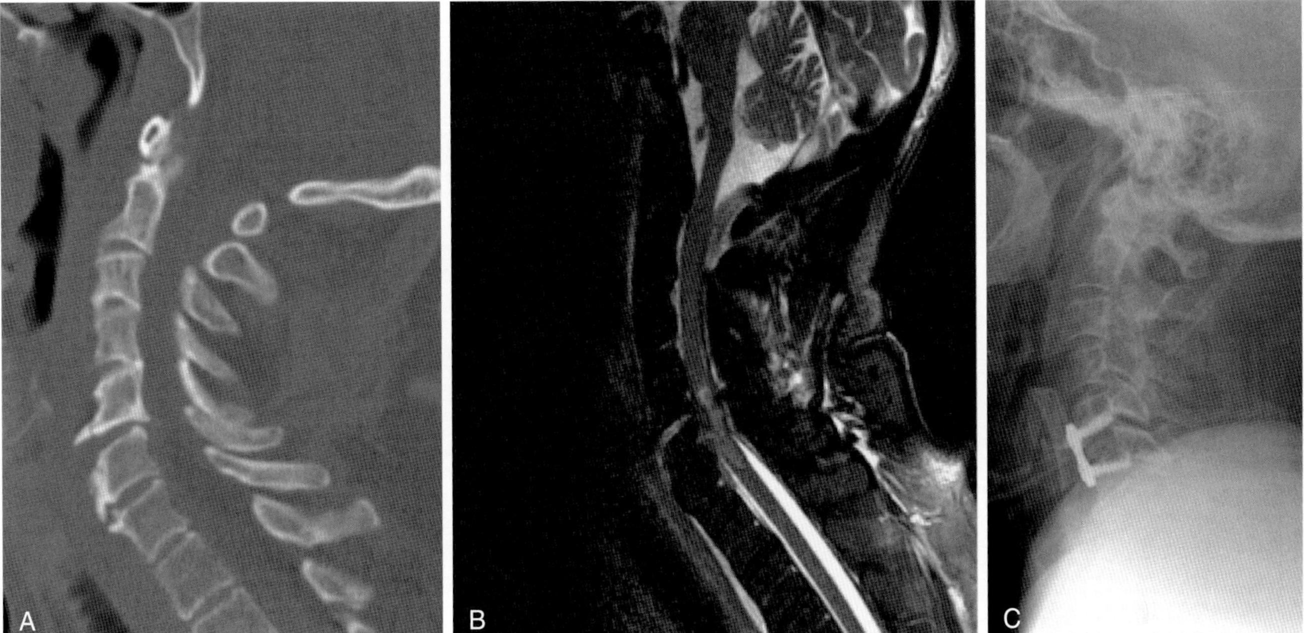

FIGURE 64-7. Extension-distraction injury to the C5-6 interval. Note the underlying spondylosis, creating a stiff cervical spine. Also note that the injury is less evident on the CT scan (**A**) compared with the MRI, where the abnormal signal in the disc space is evident (**B**). The injury pattern was stabilized by ventral fusion and plating of the C5-6 level (**C**).

the rostral vertebral body on the caudal body. The treating physician must have a high index of suspicion when evaluating an elderly patient or a patient with a stiff spine after a suggestive trauma mechanism. Plain radiographs or even CT scans may fail to demonstrate displacement at the site of the disc space disruption, making it difficult to identify the injury. In such cases, an MRI often proves useful because it may demonstrate signal change through the disrupted disc space (Fig. 64-7).

The majority of these injuries benefit from surgical stabilization because the potential for displacement, especially in those with diffuse idiopathic skeletal hyperostosis or ankylosing spondylitis, is substantial. The most common surgical approach for a simple distractive extension injury is anterior, with structural grafting of the disrupted disc and anterior plating to reestablish stability. Supplemental dorsal fixation is indicated when significant retrolisthesis of the rostral vertebral body is observed or when bone quality is insufficient to provide adequate stability with ventral plating alone. In some cases, significant preexisting cervical stenosis may complicate the injury by predisposing to neurologic injury and cord compression. In such a situation, patients with incomplete neurologic deficits may benefit from a more extensive dorsal decompression of the spinal canal, which is best achieved through a dorsal approach with a multilevel laminectomy. In such a situation, rigid segmental fixation at multiple levels can be used to stabilize the injury, with ventral grafting if the anterior column is thought to contain a significant structural defect.

Dorsal Element Fractures

Dorsal element fractures make up a heterogeneous group of injuries, including fractures of the spinous process, lamina, lateral mass, and articular processes or pedicle.

Spinous Process Fractures

Also known as *clay-shoveler's fractures*, these injuries are most commonly seen at the C6, C7, or T1 levels. The injury mechanism can be hyperextension with forceful compression of the spinous processes, hyperflexion with avulsion of the spinous process, or direct blunt-force trauma to the neck. Displaced spinous process fractures due to avulsion or repetitive stress have a high rate of pseudarthrosis.[42] Because spinous process fractures may be a component of a more severe injury pattern, it is important to search for evidence of other injuries when a spinous process fracture is seen. Isolated spinous process fractures are usually stable injuries. After a period of immobilization to allow healing, flexion-extension radiographs are useful to rule out further instability. In the absence of instability, the neck is generally mobilized even if evidence of a nonunion is present.

Lamina, Pedicle, and Lateral Mass Fractures

Lamina, pedicle, and lateral mass fractures are commonly seen in association with other fractures, and thus it is important to search for other injuries that may signify a more severe injury pattern. These injuries are generally thought to be produced by forceful extension and/or rotation of the spine.[42] Like other minimally displaced posterior element fractures, these fractures are easily missed on plain radiographs. Although oblique plain radiographs were previously recommended for diagnosis, these have been largely supplanted by CT, which provides excellent visualization of the posterior element fractures.[42] Most isolated, nondisplaced fractures in this category are stable and are successfully treated with immobilization in a cervical orthosis. After healing, flexion-extension lateral radiographs can be obtained before initiating a structured rehabilitation program.[42]

Fractures of the lateral mass may involve the articular processes and thus could compromise the stability of the

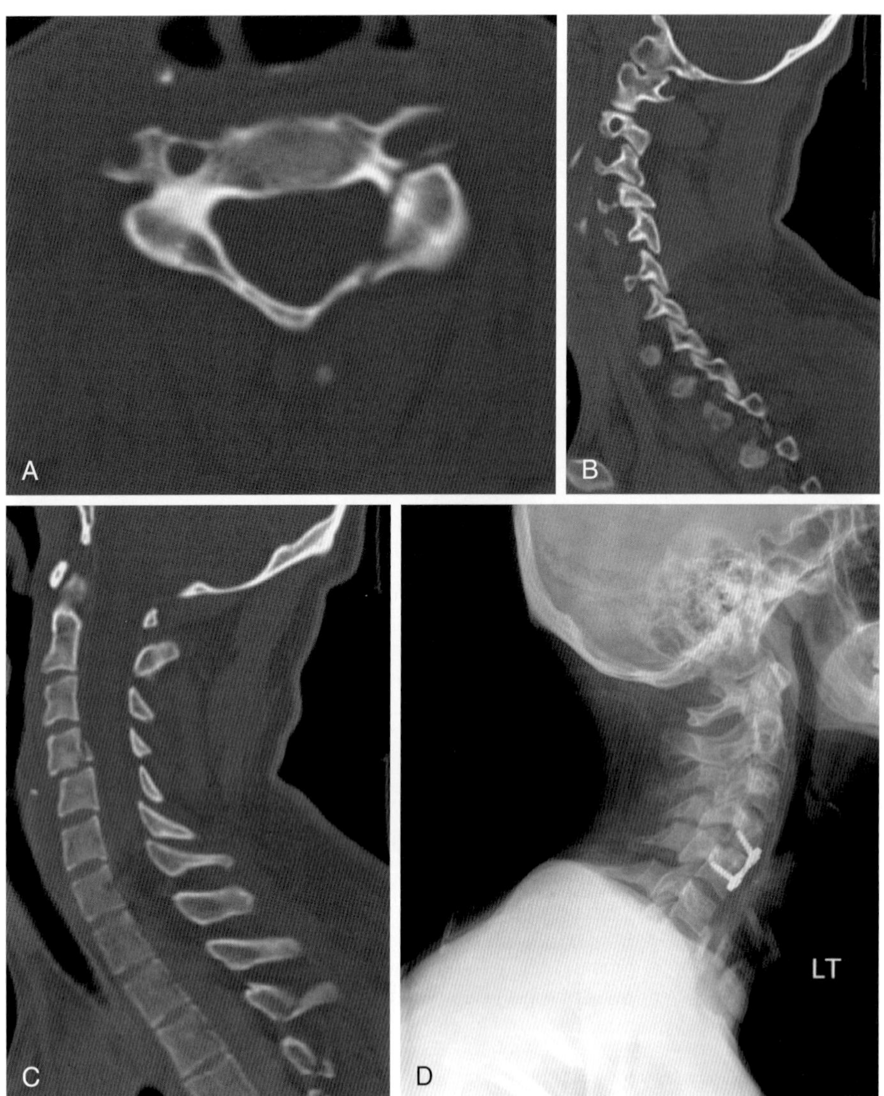

FIGURE 64-8. C4 fracture-subluxation with fracture of the lamina and pedicle creating a floating lateral mass (**A**). Note the disruption of the facet relationship on parasagittal CT reconstruction (**B**) and the slight kyphosis and anterior subluxation on sagittal CT reconstruction (**C**). The injury was stabilized by ventral cervical discectomy and fusion with anterior cervical plating (**D**). Use of the anterior approach allows the fusion to be limited to the C4-5 level.

segment. It is important to examine the imaging studies carefully, looking for evidence of subluxation, which may indicate a more severe instability pattern. According to Allen et al.,[9] subluxation of the spinal segment, substantial comminution of the lateral mass, and/or significant displaced fractures that extend to the articular processes are criteria for surgical stabilization.[43] When surgical stabilization is required, the surgeon can either pursue an anterior approach, which has the advantage of fusing only the compromised segment, or a posterior approach, which generally requires bridging the disrupted segment to obtain stability and thus involves fusion of an additional motion segment.

Kotani et al.,[43] in a retrospective analysis of injuries to the lateral mass and facet joint, described an injury pattern involving an ipsilateral fracture of the lamina and pedicle, thus creating a "floating lateral mass" (Fig. 64-8). This injury is considered to be "unstable" by some because of the loss of both the superior and inferior articular process buttresses on the ipsilateral side of the spine.[43] Others have recommended simple immobilization for the floating lateral mass injury without any evidence of subluxation. Some patients with fractures of the facet joint may experience radicular symptoms that can be managed with a dorsal foraminotomy with or without dorsal stabilization.[42]

Facet Fractures

Facet fractures make up a heterogeneous group of injuries, ranging from small avulsion fractures of the facet to shearing injuries that compromise a large portion of the articular process (Fig. 64-9). These fractures may result from either a hyperflexion or hyperextension mechanism, often combined with rotation. Facet fractures commonly occur in association with other cervical spinal trauma patterns, and thus a careful review of the imaging studies must be undertaken before characterizing a particular injury as an isolated facet fracture. For example, Johnson et al. found that two thirds of patients with an end plate compression fracture associated with a significant facet injury had an instability pattern that failed treatment with a ventral instrumented fusion.[31]

As reviewed by Kalayci et al., several authors have categorized cervical facet injuries.[44] The management of a unilateral facet fracture remains controversial, with the exact indications

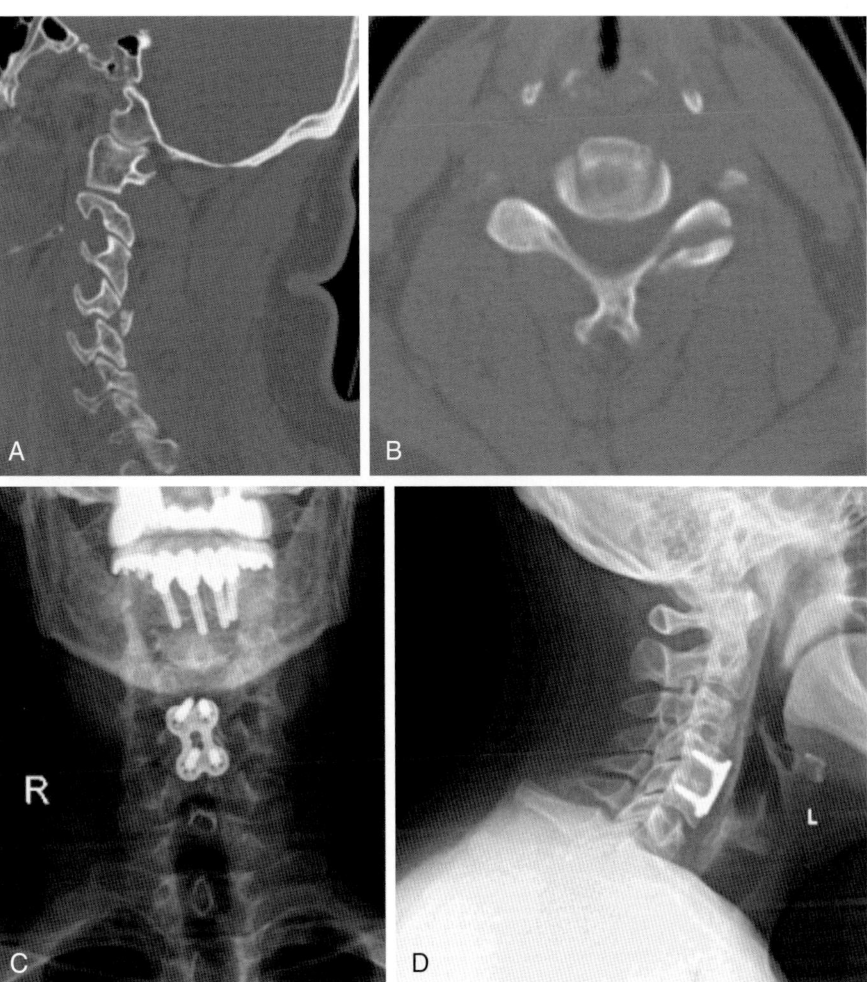

FIGURE 64-9. C4 facet fracture involving a significant percentage of the inferior articular process. **A** and **B,** Note that the fractured facet joint is widened and the fracture is angulated and displaced. **C** and **D,** The injury has been stabilized by ventral fusion with anterior plating.

for surgical stabilization being poorly defined. In part, this is due to the heterogeneous injury pattern and the variable levels of patient compliance with immobilization.

Although simple, minimally displaced fractures of the facet complex can be successfully treated with immobilization, displaced fractures or those involving large portions of the facet joint may be associated with instability and thus may require surgical stabilization. Lifeso et al.[44] reviewed a cohort of patients with unilateral facet fractures and found coexisting spinal cord injury in 18% and root injury in 34%. Rorabeck et al.[44] reported a series of 26 patients with unilateral facet fractures and found healing in only 20%, with a significant rate of chronic cervical pain and even late dislocations. In a series of 36 patients (24 of whom were treated nonoperatively), Beyer and Cabanela[44] found a union rate of only 50%.

Surgical treatment has been suggested by some, using either an anterior or a posterior approach. In cadaver studies performed by Coe et al.,[44] dorsal stabilization techniques (i.e., Rogers wiring, sublaminar wiring, Bohlman wiring, Roy-Camille dorsal plate fixation, oblique dorsal hook plate fixation) were compared without any significant biomechanical differences noted. However, wiring techniques generally are not useful in injuries with associated lamina or spinous process fractures; thus, lateral mass fixation has gained popularity in recent years. Lifeso et al.[44] reported that dorsal stabilization and fusion procedures led to unsuccessful results in 5 of 11 patients using nonrigid stabilization techniques, with late kyphosis and/or poor rotational control of the injury pattern. Ventral discectomy and fusion with anterior cervical plating has also been suggested by some.[44] Although ventral fusion is biomechanically less stable than dorsal fusion for injuries with severe dorsal disruption, it has proven successful for simple facet fractures requiring surgical stabilization.[44] Garvey et al.[44] found a lower rate of complications with a ventral, as opposed to a dorsal, approach. In a prospective study done by Lifeso et al.,[44] patients treated by ventral stabilization with autogenous tricortical iliac crest bone graft demonstrated no nonunions and did not require any additional surgery during a minimum 2-year follow-up period.

Conclusion

Subaxial cervical trauma includes a heterogeneous group of injuries that have been characterized by both morphologic and mechanistic descriptions. It is useful to recognize the common injury patterns but also to note that within each injury pattern, a spectrum of disruption exists that produces advancing degrees of instability. Because the patient's neurologic status is a key factor in determining treatment, a detailed examination according to ASIA standards should be undertaken. Definitions of mechanical stability remain somewhat elusive, although several classification systems provide a useful framework for the surgeon when defining the mechanical stability of the injury. The biomechanics of the injury should be a primary consideration when determining the treatment approach for stabilizing a cervical injury pattern.

KEY REFERENCES

Allen BL, Ferguson RL, Lehmann TR, et al: A mechanistic classification of closed indirect fractures and dislocations of the lower cervical spine. *Spine (Phila Pa 1976)* 7:1–27, 1982.

Anderson PA, Moore TA, Davis KW, et al: Cervical spine injury severity score: assessment of reliability. *J Bone Joint Surg [Am]* 89:1057–1065, 2007.

Harris J, Edeiken-Monroe B, Kopaniky D: A practical classification of acute cervical spine injuries. *Orthop Clin North Am* 17:15–30, 1986.

Moore TA, Vaccaro AR, Anderson PA: Classification of lower cervical spine injuries. *Spine (Phila Pa 1976)* 31(Suppl 11):S37–S43, 2006.

Vaccaro AR, Hulbert RJ, Patel AA, et al: The subaxial cervical spine injury classification system: a novel approach to recognize the importance of morphology, neurology, and integrity of the disco-ligamentous complex. *Spine (Phila Pa 1976)* 32:2365–2374, 2007.

White AA III, Panjabi MM: *Clinical biomechanics of the spine*, Philadelphia, 1978, JB Lippincott, pp 102–107.

Whitley JE, Forsyth HF: The classification of cervical spine injuries. *Am J Roentgenol Radium Ther Nucl Med* 83:633–644, 1960.

REFERENCES

The complete reference list is available online at expertconsult.com.

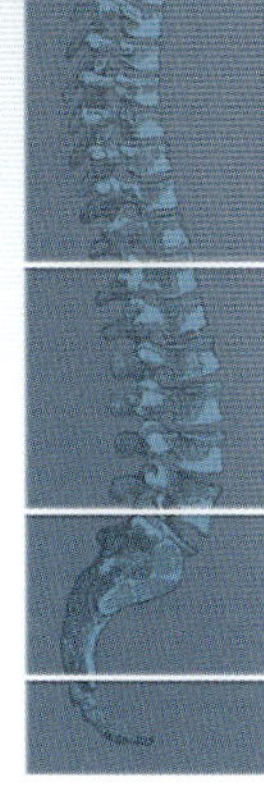

CHAPTER 65

Trauma Surgery: Cervical Spine

Thomas C. Chen | Charles B. Stillerman | Scott D. Daffner | L. Erik Westerlund | Alexander R. Vaccaro

Injury to the cervical spine should be suspected in any patient complaining of neck pain after trauma. Initial management of the multiply injured patient will be dictated by established advanced trauma life support (ATLS) protocols, with priority directed to management of airway, breathing, and circulatory compromise. The "chin lift and jaw thrust" method of securing an airway may decrease the space available for the spinal cord (beyond that seen with nasal or oral intubation) and should be avoided in the patient with a known or suspected cervical spine injury. Spinal precautions (to include cervical spine immobilization) should be maintained throughout the early stages of evaluation and resuscitation of the multitrauma patient.[1] The most common causes of injury to the neck are motor vehicle accidents (MVAs), diving into shallow water, and sport-related activities. A thorough history of a given accident may further influence clinical suspicion for the presence of a cervical spine injury. Did the patient strike his or her head? Was there evidence of cranial impact to the windshield from inside the vehicle? Was the patient ejected? Was there any indication of weakness or paralysis noted at the accident scene? Was the patient neurologically intact at the scene with later deterioration in neurologic function? Information gathered through such questioning will guide clinical suspicion for neck injury and may provide important prognostic information when neurologic compromise is present. Obtaining information regarding prior history of injury, underlying preexisting cervical spine disease, or systemic conditions (e.g., ankylosing spondylitis) is important as well.

The physical examination of the patient with known or suspected cervical spine injury begins at the patient's head and progresses distally. It is complete only after a thorough evaluation of the entire musculoskeletal system has been performed.[1] Abrasions or lacerations about the scalp, face, or neck provide mechanistic clues, alerting the examining physician to the potential for underlying spine trauma. The dorsal cervical spine should be palpated carefully to evaluate for focal tenderness, stepoff, or hematoma. Range of motion should be prohibited until the radiographic evaluation of the neck has been completed. All voluntary motion of the arms, hands, fingers, legs, feet, and toes should be observed, graded, and recorded, along with any noted sensory or deep tendon reflex compromise. Incomplete spinal cord lesions are described by a constellation of characteristic neurologic findings determined by the anatomic location of an injury. Examples include Brown-Séquard syndrome, central cord syndrome,[2] anterior cord syndrome, and posterior cord syndrome (Table 65-1). A rectal examination is essential (particularly in the neurologically injured patient in order to document the degree of sacral sparing, if any) and should be accompanied by bulbocavernosus reflex testing to assess for spinal shock. Spinal shock is the transient loss of all motor, sensory, and reflex function distal to the level of an acute spinal cord injury. The classification of a neurologic deficit as complete or incomplete cannot be determined until spinal shock has resolved.[3]

The radiographic evaluation often begins with the ATLS screening series that includes a cross-table lateral view of the cervical spine from the occiput to C7. Care should be taken that the lower part of the cervical spine is completely visualized; superimposition of the shoulders may be overcome with caudally directed manual traction on the patient's arms. Experience at multiple centers has demonstrated that most missed cervical fractures and subluxations are those present at the lower aspect of the cervical spine.[4,5] A swimmer's view often proves useful for complete visualization of the cervicothoracic junction.[6] An open-mouth odontoid view, an anteroposterior view, and a lateral plain radiograph of the entire spine should be obtained if a fracture is found because of the frequent occurrence of noncontiguous spinal injuries. Radiographic findings suggestive of cervical instability are summarized in Table 65-2.

Segmental injuries are common and the presence of injury at one level should prompt a careful search for subtle injuries elsewhere in the spine. CT should be routinely used to provide a more accurate delineation of osseous injuries. Sagittally reconstructed images are helpful in illustrating the sagittal alignment of the spine as well as injuries at the cervicothoracic junction. Such reconstruction is often helpful in demonstrating those fracture lines passing in the plane of the transaxial CT cuts.[12] MRI is used further to evaluate the nature and extent of neural and connective soft tissue injury. As such, MRI may be used to identify intracanalicular associated disc herniations, spinal cord contusions, ligamentous disruption, and occult fractures.[10,15] Flexion and extension dynamic radiography is frequently used in the awake, neurologically intact patient with isolated neck pain and negative plain radiographs.[11] These films are often repeated in patients with persistent

TABLE 65-1

Incomplete Spinal Cord Injury Syndromes

Syndrome	Characteristics
Central cord syndrome	The central cord syndrome is the most commonly encountered of all incomplete spinal cord injuries. It is characterized by upper extremity motor weakness with relative sparing of the lower extremities. Expected neurologic recovery is fair to poor.
Anterior cord syndrome	Anterior cord syndrome results from damage to the interior two thirds of the spinal cord with sparing of the posterior third. There is loss of motor function and pain and temperature sensation. There is preservation of vibration and position sense. Potential for recovery is variable.
Posterior cord syndrome	Posterior cord syndrome is the least common. Injury to the posterior columns results in loss of vibration and position sense. There may be sparing of crude touch. Potential for functional recovery is fair.
Brown-Séquard syndrome	Brown-Séquard syndrome is an uncommon injury pattern secondary to injury to half of the spinal cord. This is characterized by ipsilateral motor weakness and loss of proprioception, and contralateral loss of light touch, pain, and temperature sensation. Prognosis for ambulation is excellent in this setting.

TABLE 65-2

Radiographic Findings Suggestive of Cervical Instability

Direct Evidence of Instability	Indirect Evidence of Instability
Angulation >11° between adjacent segments[7]	Increased retropharyngeal soft tissue margin[10]
AP translation >3.5 mm[7]	Avulsion fractures at or near spinal ligament insertions
Segmental spinous process widening on lateral view[8]	Minimal compression fractures of the anterior vertebral bodies[11-14]
Facet joint widening[3]	Nondisplaced fracture lines through the posterior elements or vertebral body
Malalignment of spinous processes on AP view	
Rotation of facets on lateral view[9]	
Lateral tilt of vertebral body on AP view[9]	

AP, anteroposterior.

neck pain to rule out masked instability secondary to acute muscle spasm.

Soft Tissue Neck Injuries

Isolated soft tissue injury is a common occurrence that has been variably described as whiplash, cervical sprain, cervical strain, acceleration injury, and hyperextension injury.[4,16,17] Each of these is nearly always the result of an excessive acceleration force acting violently to extend the neck beyond normal restraints. The overwhelming majority of these injuries occur as the result of MVAs.[18,19]

Symptoms may include nonfocal neck pain with or without accompanying radicular symptoms, isolated cervical radiculopathy, cervical myelopathy, and various incomplete spinal cord syndromes. Closed head injuries may be associated with these injuries. Intracranial manifestations include chronic headache, concussion, extra-axial/intracranial bleeding, and sympathetic dysfunction. Psychiatric changes, including sleep disturbance, depression, mood changes, or frank personality changes, also may occur.[16]

The most common radiographic finding is the loss of normal cervical lordosis as seen on a lateral plain radiograph.[8] Delayed flexion and extension radiographs are again obtained approximately 1 week after resolution of acute muscle spasm to evaluate for evidence of potential destabilizing soft tissue disruption if an obvious injury is not present.[3,11] Bone scan has a limited role in screening for occult fractures in selected patients with atypical chronic pain.[8] If the bone scan is positive, a CT may then be performed for further evaluation. Early intervention and treatment are based on the presenting injury subtype, including its pathomechanics and severity, and the overall medical status of the patient. In the setting of a whiplash-type injury, initial use of a soft collar will improve comfort in many patients, although use should be limited to a 2- to 4-week period to minimize dependence, muscle atrophy, and decreased neck range of motion.[20] Isometric exercises and gentle, supervised range of motion should be initiated as soon as symptoms permit (or within 2 weeks of injury). The regimen should be performed several times a day and should include neck flexion and extension, rotation, and lateral flexion. Enlisting the assistance of a physical therapist may be beneficial, particularly in the early phases of recovery.

Transient Quadriplegia

A neurapraxia-type injury to the cervical spinal cord resulting in transient quadriplegia is most commonly seen in athletes participating in contact sports. The incidence among collegiate football players is 7.3 per 10,000 athletes. Plain radiographs are negative in this setting. The mechanism of injury is most often axial compression combined with hyperflexion or hyperextension. Sensory and motor neurologic deficits are bilateral and usually persist from several minutes to 48 hours after trauma. There is an association with developmental cervical stenosis, although effective guidelines for identification of predisposed athletes have been difficult to establish. Efforts to establish sensitive and specific screening methods to reliably identify at-risk athletes are under way.[17,21]

Injuries to the Occipitocervical Articulation

Injuries to the occipitocervical junction are being recognized with increasing frequency while patient mortality rates are declining. Improved outcomes are likely a direct benefit of present trauma protocols that begin at the scene of an injury, supporting those who would not have previously survived. Heightened suspicion and early detection (with current imaging techniques) have further contributed to the aforementioned trends.

The occipital condyles are paired, semilunar-shaped projections from the inferior aspect of the occiput that articulate with the atlantal lateral masses. This articulation bears little intrinsic osseous stability, depending instead on the external and internal craniocervical ligaments for constraint. The internal craniocervical ligaments (tectorial membrane, cruciate ligament, and paired alar and apical ligaments) confer most of the intrinsic occipitoatlantal stability.[22] Injury to the craniocervical junction commonly occurs through three primary forces: distraction, compression, and rotation.[23] Injuries may be mild and stable or life threatening (with complete osteoligamentous disruption).[24]

Occipital Condyle Fractures

Occipital condyle fractures are most often identified incidentally on head CT in the unconscious patient, although awake patients with complaints of deep suboccipital pain or occipital headache should be suspected of having sustained an injury to the occipitocervical junction.[25,26] The incidence is not high, with one trauma center estimating an incidence of 1.7/1000 per year.[27] The neurologic examination in survivors is often negative, although mild cord injury and lower cranial nerve injury have been reported. Classification of occipital condyle fractures is based on CT morphology[25,28] (Fig. 65-1). A type I fracture is a comminuted fracture of the condyle resulting from impaction of the condyle by the lateral mass of C1. The mechanism is often a direct blow to the head. A type II injury is characterized by the presence of a related basilar skull fracture. Type III injuries are avulsion fractures occurring at the attachment site of the alar ligaments. They may be bilateral in up to 50% of cases and, in this circumstance, are associated with an atlanto-occipital dislocation. Treatment of stable type I and II injuries is cervical immobilization in a hard collar, cervicothoracic brace, or halo vest for 8 to 10 weeks. Type II fractures demonstrating separation of the occipital condyle from the occiput may have inadequate lateral column support, thus requiring 8 to 12 weeks of halo-vest immobilization. Instability is commonly noted in type III injuries and is demonstrated by occipitoatlantal anteroposterior displacement, longitudinal diastasis, or joint incongruity. Injuries identified as unstable are best managed with a dorsal occipitocervical arthrodesis.[23,29-32] Recently, Maserati et al. performed a retrospective review of 24,745 consecutive trauma patients over a 6-year period and identified 100 patients with 106 occipital cervical fractures (0.4% incidence). They concluded that immobilization in a rigid cervical collar with delayed radiographic follow-up was adequate as long as there was no evidence of occipitocervical misalignment, which would necessitate the need for occipitocervical fusion or halo fixation.[33]

Occipitocervical Dislocation/Dissociation

Until recently, few cases of patients surviving this entity had been reported.[29-31,34-36] Most reports of survival from occipitocervical dislocation/dissociation have been in children.[37] Occipitocervical dislocation or dissociation often results from high-energy trauma, is highly unstable, and is frequently fatal (Fig. 65-2). High-resolution CT (with or without MRI) is often required to evaluate these injuries because they may be difficult to appreciate on plain radiographs unless significant displacement is present (Fig. 65-3A). MRI is often required to evaluate these injuries. Occipitocervical instability (subluxation and dislocation) is classified according to the direction of displacement of the occiput.[25,33,38] Type I injuries are ventral subluxations of the occipital condyle relative to the atlantal lateral masses. These represent the most commonly observed injury pattern. Type II injuries are vertical displacements of the occipital condyles greater than 2 mm beyond normal. C1-2 distraction injuries are included in this category. Type III injuries are dorsal occipital dislocations and are exceedingly rare. In evaluating these injuries, more than 2 mm of subluxation at the atlanto-occipital articulation indicates a functional loss of integrity of the major occipitocervical stabilizers such as the alar ligaments and the tectorial membrane.[28,39] The treatment of occipitocervical instability is through closed or open reduction and surgical stabilization.[40] Traction is to be avoided in these injuries (Figs. 65-3B and C). There has been a recent trend toward performing occiput-to-C1 fusion (C0-1 fusion) using transarticular screw fixation, instead of occipitocervical fusion, in order to maintain mobility across the C1-2 junction.[35,37]

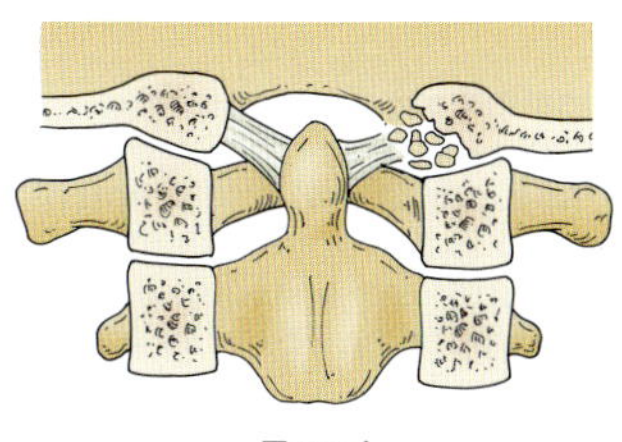

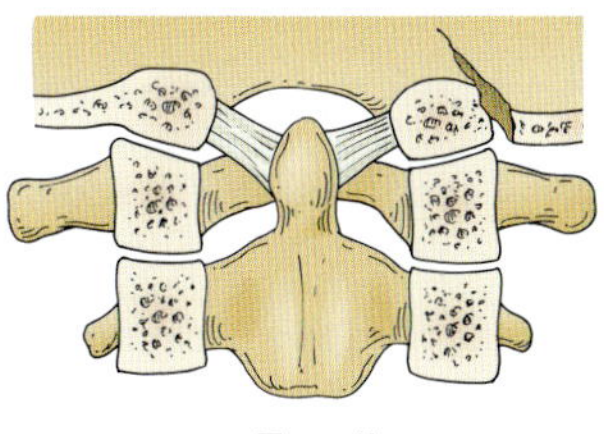

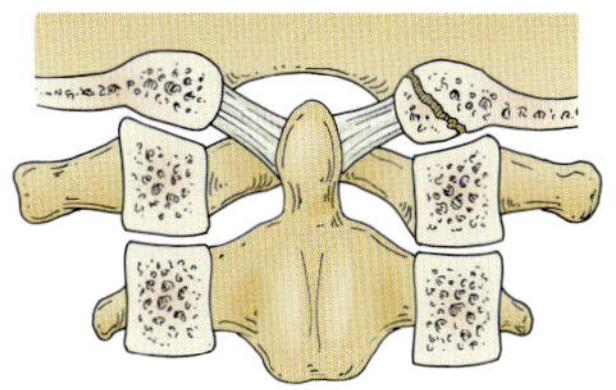

FIGURE 65-1. Occipital condyle fracture classification. A type I fracture is a comminuted fracture of the condyle resulting from impaction of the condyle by the lateral mass of C1. The mechanism is often a direct blow to the head. A type II injury is characterized by the presence of a related basilar skull fracture. A type III injury is an avulsion-type fracture occurring at the attachment site of the alar ligaments.

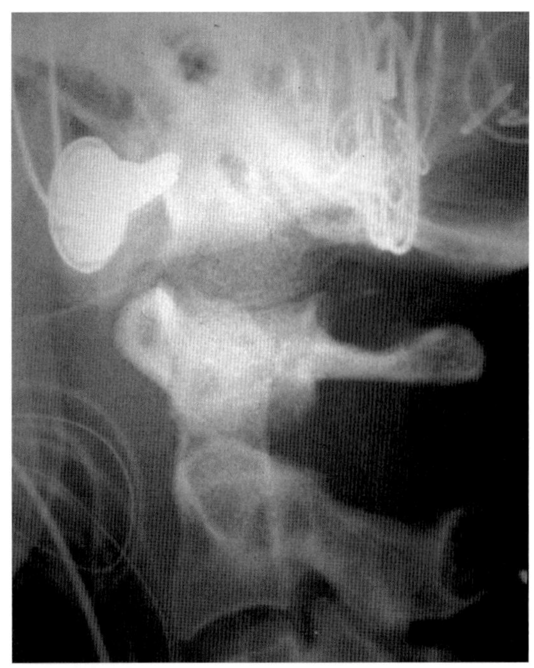

FIGURE 65-2. Lateral plain radiograph revealing longitudinal diastasis of the occipital-C1 articulation.

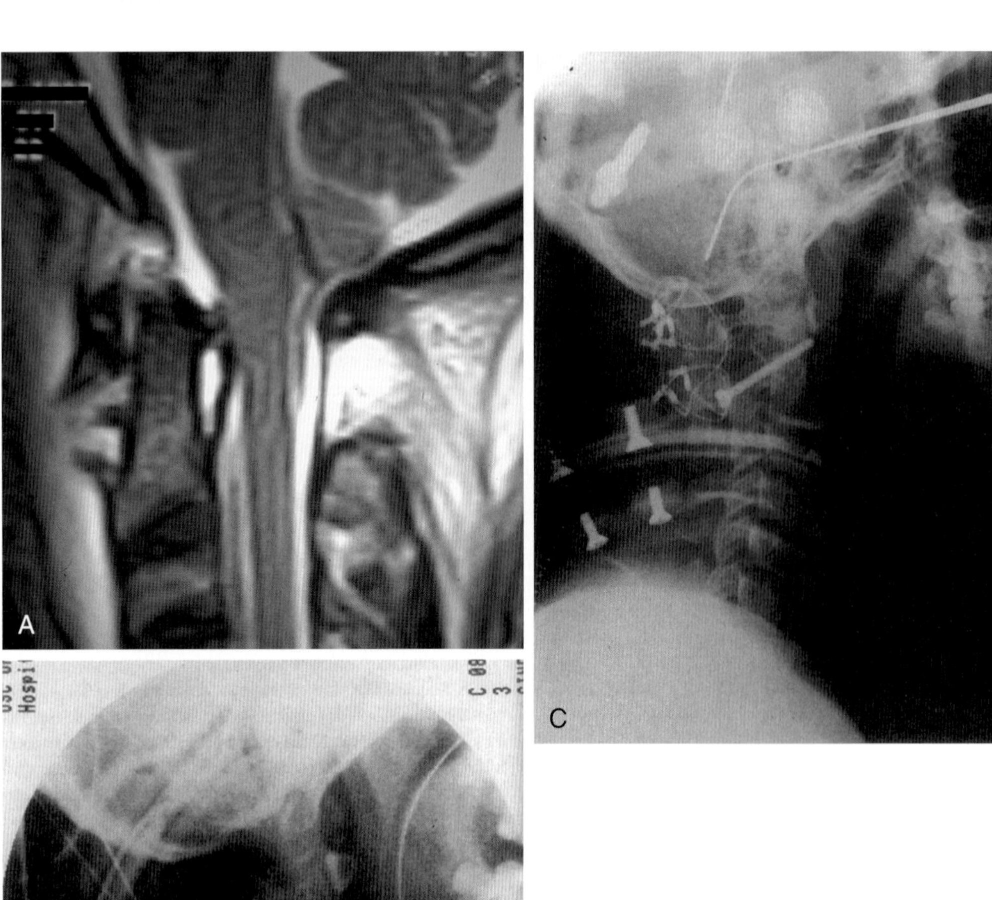

FIGURE 65-3. A, Sagittal MRI revealing longitudinal diastasis of the occipital-C1 and C1-2 articulations. **B,** Lateral plain film of type IIB occipitoatlantoaxial dislocation. Note that in addition to the longitudinal distraction of the occiput relative to the atlas, a distractive injury also exists at the atlantoaxial segment. **C,** Postoperative lateral plain film demonstrates the screw-cable-rib construct used to stabilize this occipitoatlantoaxial instability. Posterior C1-2 transarticular screw fixation was used to provide rigid fixation across the atlantoaxial level, thereby blocking rotational movement at this level. Multiple titanium cables were also placed to achieve occiput-to-C2 fixation. Rib was used because it conforms to the occipitoatlantoaxial contour. (**B** and **C,** From Stillerman CB, Ranjan SR, Weiss MH: Cervical spine injuries: diagnosis and management. In Wilkins RH, Rengachary SS, editors: *Neurosurgery*, vol II, ed 2, New York, 1995, McGraw-Hill, p 2883.)

Injuries to the First Cervical Vertebra

Traumatic Transverse Atlantal Ligament Avulsion

Insufficiency or avulsion of the transverse atlantal ligament (TALA) may occur after a violent flexion force to the upper cervical spine. Associated head injuries are common, and although survival after acute traumatic rupture had previously been thought unusual, it is now being reported with increasing frequency.[41,42] Findings range from normal to transient quadriparesis. Permanent quadriparesis is rare given the fatal sequelae that typically follow complete injury at this leve1.[42-44] Associated clinical signs include cardiac and respiratory changes secondary to brainstem compromise, or dizziness, syncope, and/or blurred vision as a result of vertebral artery disruption. Symptoms may be exacerbated by neck flexion. A lateral plain radiograph often demonstrates abnormal translation (>5 mm) at the atlantodens interval.[45,46] Conservative treatment strategies have generally failed to provide satisfactory results, and the treatment of choice in most patients is a C1-2 arthrodesis. Acute disruption of the transverse ligament may also be noted in association with a Jefferson-type burst fracture of C1.[47-51] Treatment in this circumstance should consist of cervical immobilization for 10 to 12 weeks, awaiting union of the C1 arch. Persistent instability after completion of cervical immobilization may then be addressed with a C1-2 fusion.[48,52] An atlas nonunion has been reported to result in basilar invagination with significant splaying of the C1 lateral masses.[53]

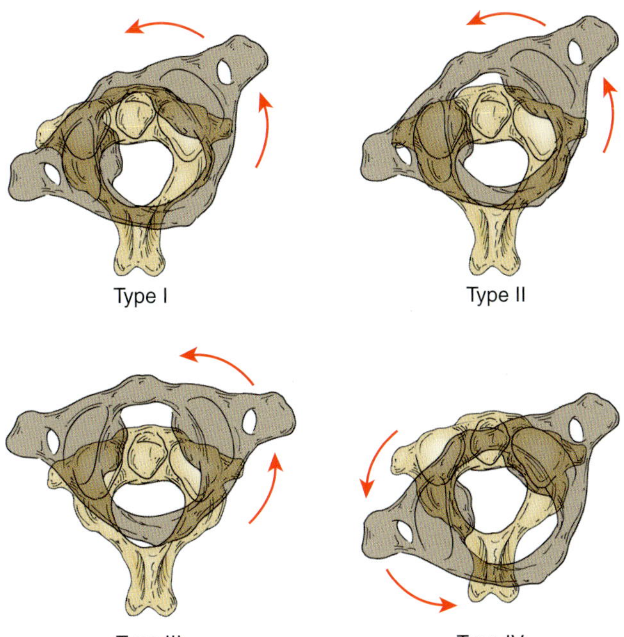

FIGURE 65-4. Classification of rotatory subluxation. Type I, simple rotatory displacement without anterior shift. The odontoid acts as a pivot point. Type II, rotatory displacement with anterior displacement of 3 to 5 mm. The lateral articular process is the pivot point. Type III, rotatory displacement with anterior displacement of more than 5 mm. Type IV, rotatory displacement with posterior translation. (From Fielding JW, Hawkins RJ Jr: Atlanto-axial rotatory fixation [fixed rotatory subluxation of the atlanto-axial joint]. *J Bone Joint Surg [Am]* 59:37–44, 1977.)

Traumatic Rotatory Subluxation

Acute trauma is an unusual cause of acute C1-2 rotatory subluxation. The clinical presentation of C1-2 rotatory subluxation is the complaint of neck pain with findings of torticollis, and it is more commonly seen in children than adults. Four types of fixed C1-2 rotatory injuries have been described[54] (Figs. 65-4 and 65-5). Type I injuries involve fixed rotational changes without associated subluxation. In the type II pattern there is 3 to 5 mm of displacement of C1 on C2 (with one lateral mass acting as a pivot while the other rotates ventrally). Type III injuries have more than 5 mm of forward displacement of both lateral masses. Type II and III injuries are both associated with transverse ligament incompetence, and neurologic involvement is common. Associated C2 fractures (type II and III odontoid fractures) have been reported with severe rotatory atlantoaxial subluxation.[55,56] Conservative treatment consists of halo or Gardner-Wells traction-reduction, followed by external immobilization for 2 to 3 months. Delayed instability is managed with a dorsal stabilization procedure. Severe rotations with associated cervical fractures (i.e., C2) need to be fixed with intraoperative fusion.[55] Fixed or irreducible deformities as well as delayed presentation of this condition are again best managed with surgical stabilization.

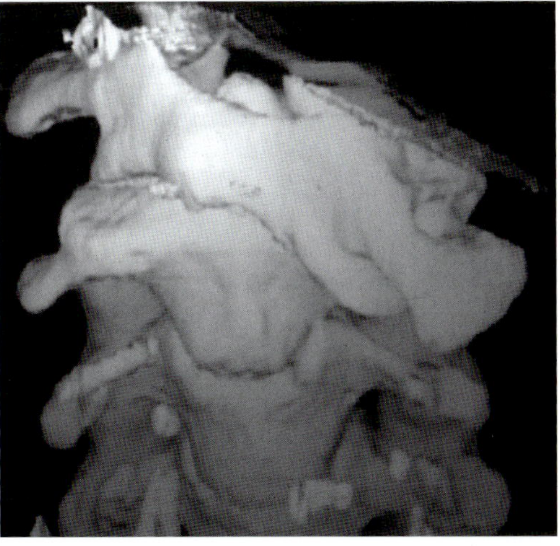

FIGURE 65-5. A three-dimensional CT scan revealing a traumatic rotatory dislocation of C1-2.

Fractures of the First Cervical Vertebra

Fractures of C1 occur either as an isolated injury or often in combination with a fracture to the C2 vertebra. The most common associated cervical spine injuries are a type II odontoid fracture and spondylolisthetic fracture of C2.[48,57,58] Fractures of C1, seen in up to 10% of all spine injuries, are encountered with relative frequency.[59,60] Neurologic injury is unusual.[46]

Fractures of C1 are classified generally into three categories. This classification scheme has proven useful in determining treatment options, expected clinical course, and prognosis[61] (Fig. 65-6). Type I fractures are limited to involvement of the dorsal arch, are often bilateral, and typically occur at the junction of the lateral masses and dorsal arch. This is the most common pattern of C1 fracture and likely occurs secondary to hyperextension in conjunction

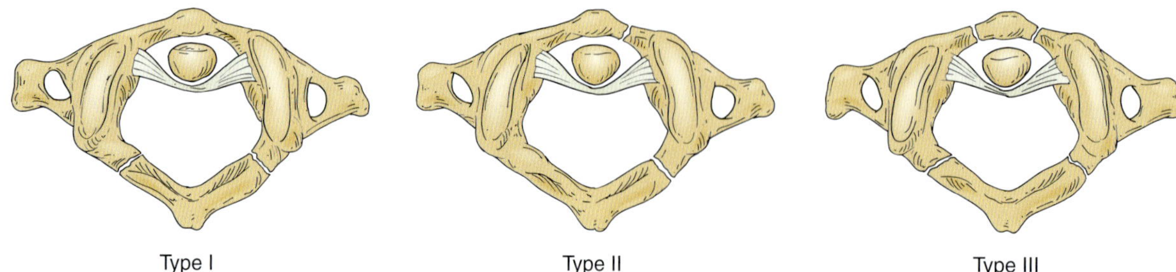

FIGURE 65-6. Classification of fractures of C1. Type I fractures are limited to involvement of the posterior arch, are often bilateral, and typically occur at the junction of the lateral masses and posterior arch. A type II atlas fracture is usually a unilateral injury defined by involvement of the lateral mass (with fracture lines passing both anteriorly and posteriorly) as the result of an asymmetrically applied axial load. A type III (or Jefferson) fracture is a burst-type fracture that involves three or more fractures through the anterior and posterior aspect of the C1 ring.

with an axial load. A type II atlas fracture is a unilateral lateral mass injury that occurs as the result of an asymmetrically applied axial load. Intra-articular extension is not common but is reported.[46,62] A type III (or Jefferson) fracture is a burst-type fracture that involves three or more fractures through the ventral and dorsal aspects of the C1 ring. The mechanism of this second-most-common pattern is that of a pure axially applied load.[63,64]

Plain radiographs are useful in the evaluation of these injuries and often demonstrate widening of the retropharyngeal soft tissue shadow from C1 to C3 (although these changes may take 6 or more hours to develop).[65,66] The open-mouth odontoid view shows lateral displacement of the lateral masses in a Jefferson-type fracture and may appear normal with the more common type I dorsal arch fracture. If total combined lateral displacement of the C1 lateral masses over C2 is greater than 6.9 mm,[65,67] the transverse ligament has been disrupted, resulting in an unstable injury.[48,59,68] Type II fractures appear radiographically as unilateral displacement of the affected lateral mass on an open-mouth odontoid radiograph. Improvements in technique and image quality have made CT in the plane of the C1 ring helpful in fully defining these injuries. The most important factor governing treatment and outcome is the simultaneous occurrence of other injuries.[48,57,69] Treatment of isolated C1 fractures has traditionally been nonoperative, although some European centers have reported the successful surgical reduction and stabilization of markedly displaced Jefferson burst fractures. Results with nonoperative treatment have been good,[49] although mild neck pain is a chronic sequela in up to 80% of these patients.[59] There has been no reported correlation between fracture union/nonunion and functional outcome.[51]

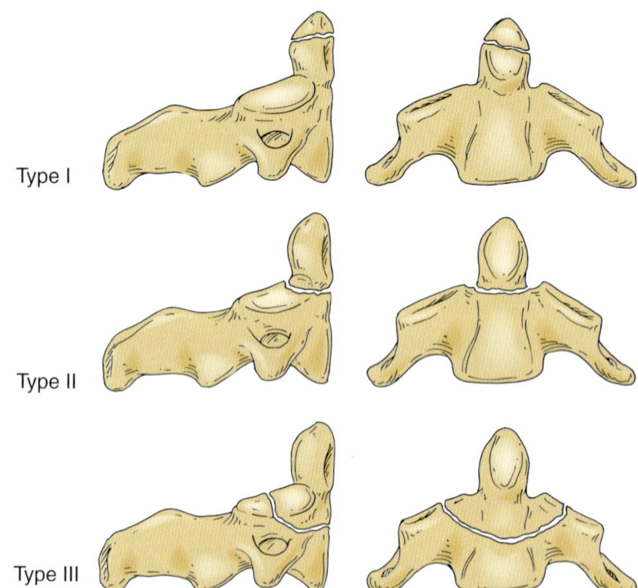

FIGURE 65-7. Classification of odontoid fractures. Type I fractures are the least common and are described as an oblique fracture involving the superior tip of the dens. Type II odontoid fractures, the most common type, occur at the junction of the base of the dens and the body of the axis. Type III odontoid fractures are characterized by the fracture line passing through the cancellous bone of the vertebral body.

Fractures of the Second Cervical Vertebra

Fractures of the Odontoid Process

Fractures of the odontoid process of the axis are relatively common among injuries of the upper cervical spine, although the exact prevalence is not well established. Odontoid fractures in young adults are most often secondary to high-energy trauma, such as MVAs or violent blows to the head.[70-73] Those sustained by the elderly or very young are more commonly due to lower-energy falls.[74-76] As with other upper cervical injuries, clinical suspicion is critical to early recognition because several studies have reported a high incidence of missed injuries, especially in patients with depressed mental status. The degree of neurologic involvement is widely variable; however, the majority of patients have a negative neurologic examination. Odontoid fractures are best visualized on lateral and open-mouth anteroposterior plain radiographs, as well as on reformatted sagittal CT images (because routine axial imaging may miss the fracture).[77]

The most widely adopted classification system is that proposed by Anderson and D'Alonzo[70] based on their experience with 60 patients with odontoid fractures treated over an 8-year period. This classification identifies three fracture types based on the anatomic location of the fracture line[68,70] (Fig. 65-7). Type I fractures are the least common and are described as an oblique fracture involving the superior tip of the dens. Type II odontoid fractures occur at the junction of the base of the dens and the body of the axis. This is the most common of the three types and the most controversial regarding discussing treatment.[70] Type II fractures have the highest rate of nonunion when treated nonoperatively, especially in the

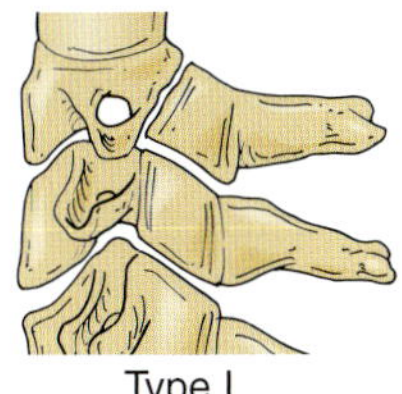

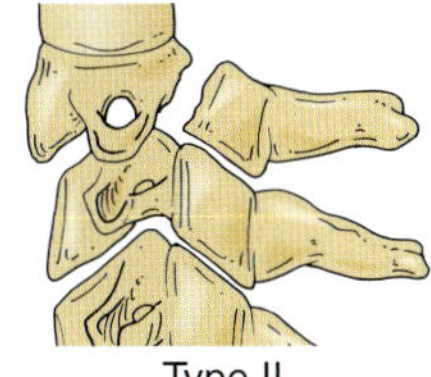

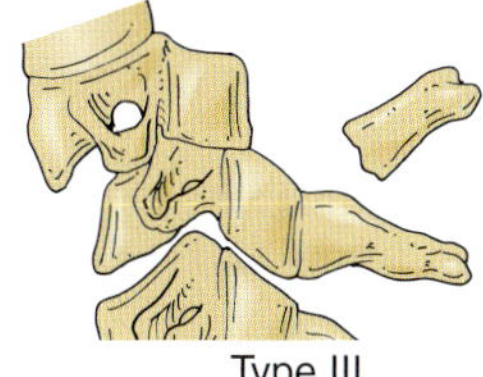

FIGURE 65-8. Classification of traumatic spondylolisthesis of the axis. Type I fractures occur through the neural arch in the region just posterior to the vertebral body. There is less than 3 mm of translation and no angulation at the fracture site. Type II fractures have greater than 3 mm of displacement and significant angulation. Type III fractures describe a type I (pars) fracture with an associated bilateral facet dislocation at C2-3. The critical feature is the classic presence of a free-floating posterior arch of C2.

elderly.[68] In type III fractures, the fracture line occurs in the body of the axis (primarily involving cancellous bone) and exits through the C2 superior articular facet.

Isolated type I odontoid fractures are considered stable (unless they are associated with instability involving the occipitocervical junction) and may be treated with a Philadelphia collar or similar orthosis. Type III fractures are often successfully managed with collar or halo immobilization. Type II fractures, however, lack both periosteum and cancellous bone at the fracture site, increasing the propensity for nonunion.[72,78] Fractures that are significantly displaced may be realigned with traction-reduction and immobilized with a halo vest until definitive treatment measures are selected. Factors considered to be associated with nonhealing of type II fractures include the degree of displacement, angulation, age of patient, loss of fracture reduction, and medical comorbidities. Surgical stabilization, when chosen, may proceed through a ventral or dorsal approach, depending on patient variables and fracture subtype.[69,71,79-81]

Traumatic Spondylolisthesis of the Axis

Traumatic spondylolisthesis of the axis is a pars interarticularis fracture of the second vertebra with disruption of the C2-3 junction; it has been of interest for decades given its unique distinction as the "hangman's fracture."[82-88] The lesion encountered today, frequently a result of an MVA, is similar in terms of location to the originally described hangman's fracture, but from a mechanistic standpoint bears little resemblance to the fracture subtype characteristic of judicial hanging.[78,88-90] The majority of these injuries are the result of MVA trauma and are infrequently associated with injury to the spinal cord (5.5%). The basic mechanism of injury is hyperextension with vertical compression of the posterior column with translation of C2 and C3.[83,87] Each of the three primary fracture types (types I to III; Fig. 65-8) are characterized further by variations of this mechanism. Dynamic radiography may be required to differentiate injury types.

Traumatic spondylolisthesis of the axis can be divided into three types of fractures. Type I fractures occur through the neural arch in the region just dorsal to the vertebral body. There is less than 3 mm of translation and no angulation at the fracture site. This fracture subtype is the result of hyperextension and an axial load. These may be treated with immobilization in a cervical orthosis for 3 months.[75]

Type II fractures are divided further into type II and type IIA injuries. Type II fractures have greater than 3 mm of displacement and significant angulation. The mechanism of injury is a combined force comprising hyperextension and axial loading (extension immediately followed by flexion). Fracture reduction may be achieved with skeletal traction in extension with immediate or delayed conversion to halo-vest immobilization. Vaccaro et al. have recently reported excellent results with early halo immobilization and reduction for type II or IIA hangman's fractures. Decreased fusion rates were found for type II fractures with an angulation of 12 degrees or more, requiring an extended period of traction to ensure proper alignment before long-term fixation with halo immobilization.[91] Surgical stabilization is infrequently necessary, although several surgical options exist for patients in whom a reduction cannot be maintained or those unable to tolerate prolonged halo traction or halo-vest immobilization. In reducible fractures, a primary screw fixation of the pars articularis has been performed with good realignment and fusion.[92] In fractures that are not anatomically reducible, or in cases of displaced nonunion, a ventral C2-3 arthrodesis is a viable treatment option (Fig. 65-9). Recently, Chittiboina et al. performed a cadaveric biomechanical analysis of ventral C2-3 fusion versus dorsal

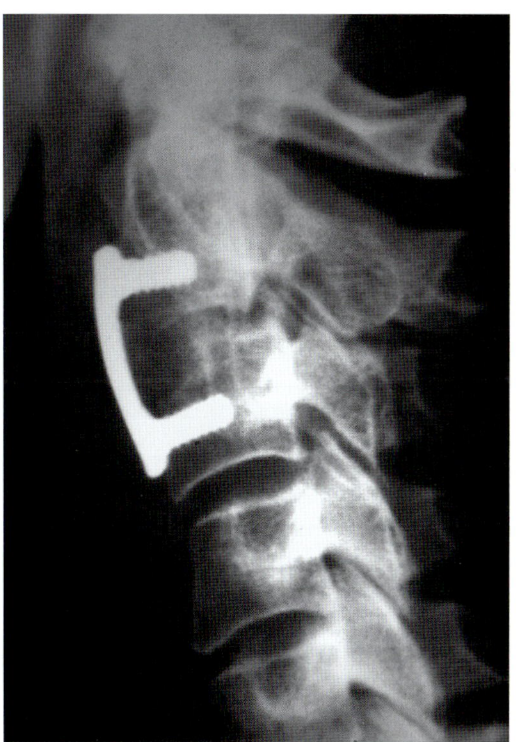

FIGURE 65-9. Lateral plain radiograph after an anterior C2-3 fusion for late instability in a type II hangman's fracture.

fixation with C1 lateral mass screws and C2-3 dorsal fixation. The authors concluded that both methods resulted in a consistent increase in stability.[83]

Type IIA fractures are distinguished by an oblique fracture line often running from dorsal-rostral to ventral-caudal along the length of the pars. The mechanism is a flexion-distraction force. This fracture subtype is seen in less than 10% of hangman's fractures. Reduction is by extension and slight axial loading; axial traction will accentuate the deformity. Reduction should be followed by immobilization in a halo vest for 3 months.

Type III fractures describe a type I (pars) fracture with an associated unilateral or bilateral facet dislocation at C2-3. The critical feature is the classic presence of a free-floating dorsal arch of C2. These are unstable and irreducible by closed means, requiring surgical intervention.[93]

An additional group of injuries may also be described as traumatic spondylolisthesis of C2-3 with either bilateral laminar fractures (type IV) or bilateral facet fractures of the inferior articular processes of C2 (type V). The mechanism of both types is flexion or shear, producing a highly unstable pattern.[82,85]

Injuries to the Lower Cervical Spine

The C3 through C7 vertebrae are similar in anatomy and biomechanics, and generally incur similar fracture patterns. However, the C7 vertebra is exposed to greater axial compression and flexion load because of its location at the junction of the cervical and thoracic spine. Closed indirect injuries to the head and neck therefore often produce patterns of injury that are characteristic to the lower cervical vertebral column. The most severe neurologic sequelae arise as a result of a translational deformity, establishing ligamentous integrity as critically important to stability and treatment.

Both two- and three-column models are used in discussing the traumatic pathoanatomy of the lower cervical spine. The three-column model was originally described in 1984 with specific reference to thoracolumbar injuries[94] but has since been modified to address cervical spine stability. It may be of greater utility to discuss the cervical spine as a two-column entity composed of an anterior and posterior column.[7,95-97] In the two-column model, the ventral spine consists of the posterior longitudinal ligament and all remaining ventral structures, whereas the posterior column consists of all structures dorsal to the posterior longitudinal ligament (Box 65-1). The anterior and posterior columns are then reciprocally affected by flexion and extension moments.

A mechanistic classification of subaxial cervical spine injuries was described by Allen et a1.[95] in 1982. This classification divides middle and lower cervical fractures into six groups based on force vector (initial dominant force) and subsequent incremental tissue failure (based on the attitude of the spine at failure). Abnormal relationships between adjacent vertebrae imply ligamentous failure, suggesting a shear force mechanism (because ligaments do not fail in compression). The three most common injury groups are compressive flexion, compressive extension, and distractive flexion. Vertical compression injuries occur with intermediate frequency, whereas distractive extension and lateral flexion injuries occur the least.[98] The presence of neurologic injury has not been strongly associated with any individual group in the classification, although it is related to progressive osteoligamentous disruption or the severity of injury in a particular subgrouping. Injuries as identified on plain radiographs should undergo further evaluation with CT scanning and possibly MRI. Assessment of plain radiographic, CT, and MRI findings assists in the evaluation of spinal stability.

BOX 65-1. The Two-Column Model of the Lower Cervical Spine

Anterior Column Components
Anterior longitudinal ligament
Intervetebral disc and anulus fibrosus
Vertebral body
Posterior longitudinal ligament

Posterior Column Components
Pedicles and posterior vertebral arch
Posterior interspinous ligament complex

Traumatic Central Cord Syndrome

Traumatic central cord syndrome is the most common incomplete spinal cord injury. It is characterized by a disproportionately greater motor deficit in the upper extremities compared with the lower extremities. It is usually attributed to a hyperextension injury in the presence of osteophytic spurs. Varying degrees of sensory findings may be present. Myelopathic findings may be present. The upper extremities are more involved because the cervical long tract motor fibers for the upper extremities are located more medially than those for the lower extremities. The diagnosis of central cord syndrome is confirmed with an MRI scan, which demonstrates cervical stenosis with degenerative osteophytic spurs. Recovery is usually gradual, with recovery of motor function over a period of 6 to 8 weeks. Timing of surgery is still controversial. The old rule that surgery should be delayed while the patient regains neurologic function has been recently challenged. Subsequently, there has been a movement toward earlier surgery to decompress the spinal cord and prevent further compression due to delayed swelling. The consensus at this time is that early surgery is not harmful.[99] Recently, Chen et al. analyzed 49 patients with traumatic central cord syndrome.[98] They found that there was no correlation in improvement in neurologic recovery if the patients had surgery within 4 days or more than 4 days after their spinal cord injury. There was also no significant correlation in improvement based on the location of the injury or surgical approach used. There was a trend toward better recovery in patients younger than 65 years of age compared with patients older than 65 years.[98] Similar data were reported by Aito et al., who found that subjects younger than 65 years of age had significantly better neurologic and functional recovery than patients older than 65 years.[99]

Spinal Cord Injury without Radiographic Abnormality in Adults

Although spinal cord injury without radiographic abnormality (SCIWORA) is typically attributed to pediatric spinal cord injuries (1.5–16 years of age) in which there is a neurologic deficit but no radiographic abnormality, SCIWORA has also been reported in adults. This section addresses SCIWORA in adults only. The incidence of adult SCIWORA is underreported. Kasimatis et al. recently reported on 166 patients with cervical spine injury treated at a single institution. Seven of these 166 adult patients (4.2%) presented with frank neurologic symptoms but with no acute signs of trauma. On MRI, these patients were found to have intramedullary changes (five of six patients) with varying degrees of compression from a disc or the ligamentum flavum.[100] The mechanism of adult SCIWORA has been explored by Imajo et al.[101] Whereas pediatric SCIWORA has been hypothesized to be secondary to the increased elasticity of the spinous ligaments and paravertebral soft tissue, resulting in a "whiplash" type of effect on the normal cord after impact, adult SCIWORA has been hypothesized to be secondary to degenerative changes and translations.[102] In adult SCIWORA, Imajo et al. performed three-dimensional finite element analysis to analyze biomechanical responses under compression and extension moments. They created facet surfaces from C3 to C5 under varying degrees of angulation, and found that 60 degrees of angulation at C3-4 resulted in the greatest flexibility in extension and the highest total translation. This increased translation, combined with facet and ligamentum flavum hypertrophy in the adult cervical spine, led to increased risk of SCIWORA in the adult patient.[101] Shen et al. reported that diffusion-weighted MRI can detect signal changes that are not depicted on typical T1- or T2-weighted images in patients with thoracic SCIWORA.[103] Tewari et al. have prognosticated recovery for adult patients with SCIWORA on the basis of MRI signal changes, with patients with minimal cord changes on MRI having the best outcome, followed by those with cord edema alone. Patients with parenchymatous hemorrhage and contusions on MRI had the worst prognosis, often with no significant improvement in their Frankel grade.[104]

Compressive Flexion

Compressive flexion injuries are caused by a ventral and axially directed load of increasing intensity. Compressive fractures without facet fracture or subluxation are usually stable injuries. Higher stages of injury involve increased ventral osseous and dorsal ligamentous injury and may be unstable (Figs. 65-10 and 65-11). Treatment is tailored accordingly, although a frequent complication with conservative management is late instability.[13] Surgical intervention often involves a cervical corpectomy and instrumented fusion with a structural graft. Adjunctive dorsal stabilization may be necessary in highly unstable, advanced-stage lesions.[105]

Compressive Extension

Compressive extension injuries result in a spectrum of pathologic processes, ranging from unilateral vertebral arch fractures to bilateral laminar fractures, and finally to vertebral arch fractures with full ventral displacement of the vertebral body (Fig. 65-12). Management is based on injury severity and instability. An initial dorsal reduction and stabilization procedure is often required, followed by adjunctive ventral stabilization if necessary.[106]

Distractive Flexion

Distractive flexion injuries are also known as the flexion-dislocation injuries. There is typically little osseous injury except for minor compression failure of the caudal

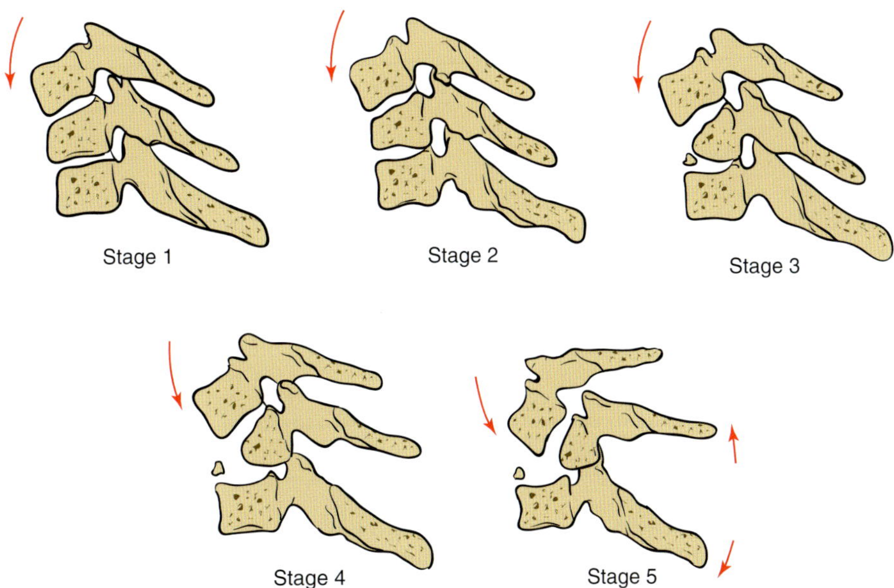

FIGURE 65-10. Compressive flexion injury. Stage 1: blunting and rounding-off of anterosuperior vertebral margin. Stage 2: loss of anterior vertebral height with anteroinferior beaking. Stage 3: fracture line extending from anterior surface of vertebral body extending obliquely through the subchondral plate (fractured beak). Stage 4: less than 3 mm of the posteroinferior vertebral margin into the neural canal. Stage 5: greater than 3 mm of displacement of the posterior aspect of the vertebral body with complete disruption of the posterior ligamentous complex. The vertebral arch is intact. (From Rizzolo SJ, Cotler JM: Unstable cervical spine injuries: specific treatment approaches. *J Am Acad Orthop Surg* 1:57–66, 1993.)

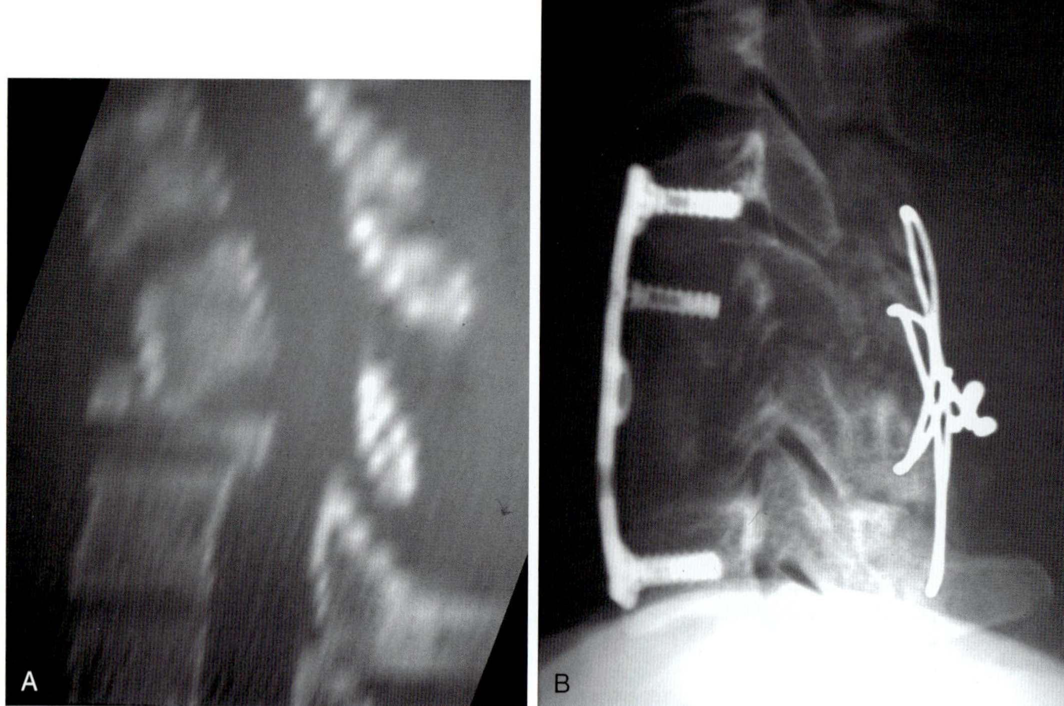

FIGURE 65-11. **A,** Sagittal CT reconstruction revealing an advanced-stage compressive flexion cervical spine injury. **B,** Plain radiograph after an anteroposterior cervical decompression and stabilization procedure.

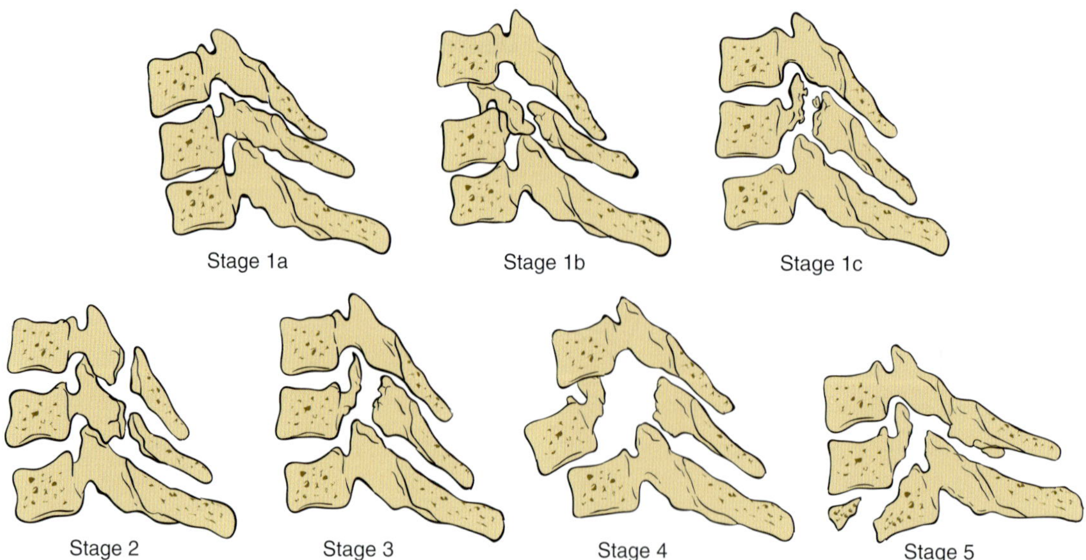

FIGURE 65-12. Compressive extension injury. Stage 1: unilateral vertebral arch fracture through the articular process (stage 1a), the pedicle (stage 1b), or lamina (stage 1c), either with or without a rotary spondylolisthesis of the centrum. Stage 2: bilaminar fracture at one or more levels. Stage 3: bilateral fractures of the vertebral arch with partial-width anterior vertebral body displacement. Stage 4: partial-width anterior vertebral body displacement. Stage 5: complete anterior vertebral body displacement. (From Rizzolo SJ, Cotler JM: Unstable cervical spine injuries: specific treatment approaches. *J Am Acad Orthop Surg* 1:57–66, 1993.)

vertebral segment. However, there is severe ligamentous damage involving the dorsal facet capsule complex, ligamentum flavum, and interspinous ligaments, and (depending on the presence of a unilateral or bilateral dislocation) injury to the posterior longitudinal ligament and intervertebral disc[14] (Figs. 65-13 and 65-14). A significant number of patients with this injury also have an associated closed head injury.[106] Radiographic changes may be minimal in the early stages (flexion sprain) of this injury subtype. MRI is often useful to delineate the full extent of soft tissue disruption (including injury to the disc), although obtaining this study in an awake, alert, and cooperative patient should not delay traction reduction when plain radiographs demonstrate a translational displacement. Some physicians recommend obtaining an MRI before closed or open reduction of this injury subtype.[107] All

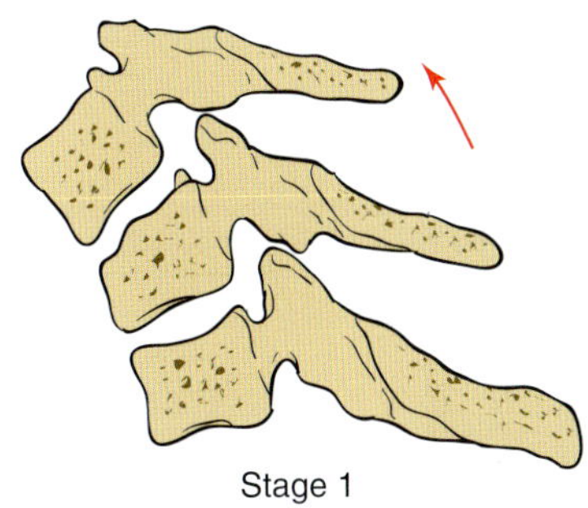

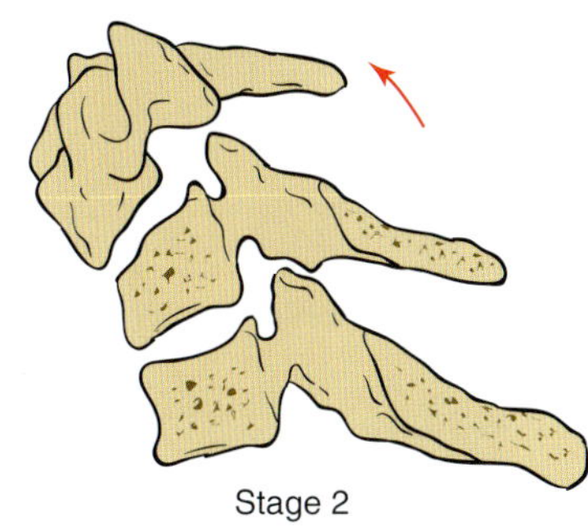

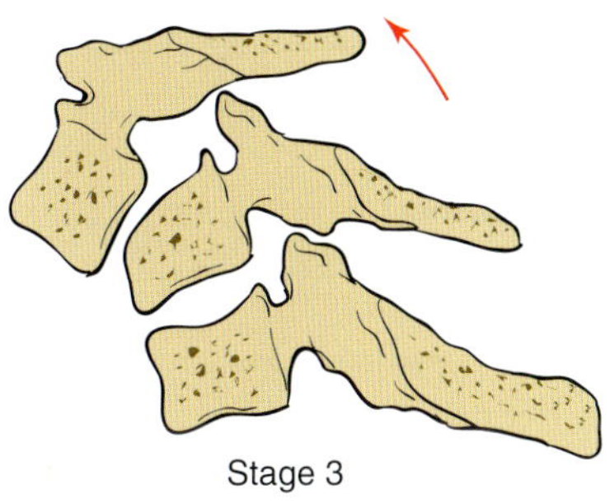

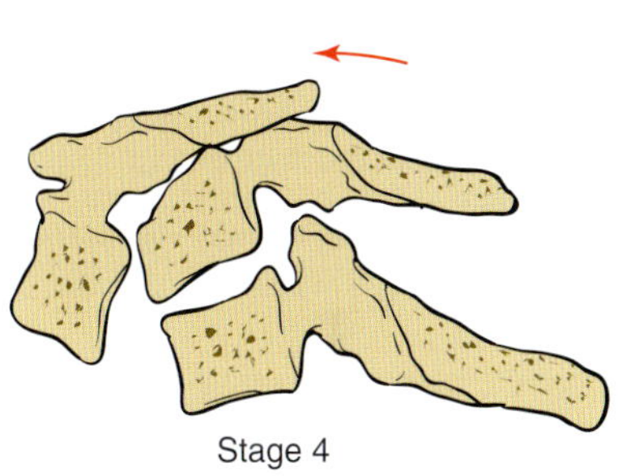

FIGURE 65-13. Distractive flexion injury. Stage 1: flexion sprain injury with facet subluxation in flexion and divergence of spinous processes. There may be some blunting of the anterosuperior vertebral margin (similar to stage 1 compressive flexion injury). Stage 2: unilateral facet dislocation with or without rotary spondylolisthesis. Stage 3: bilateral facet dislocation with up to 50% vertebral body displacement. Stage 4: completely unstable motion segment with full-width vertebral body displacement. (From Rizzolo SJ, Cotler JM: Unstable cervical spine injuries: specific treatment approaches. *J Am Acad Orthop Surg* 1:57–66, 1993.)

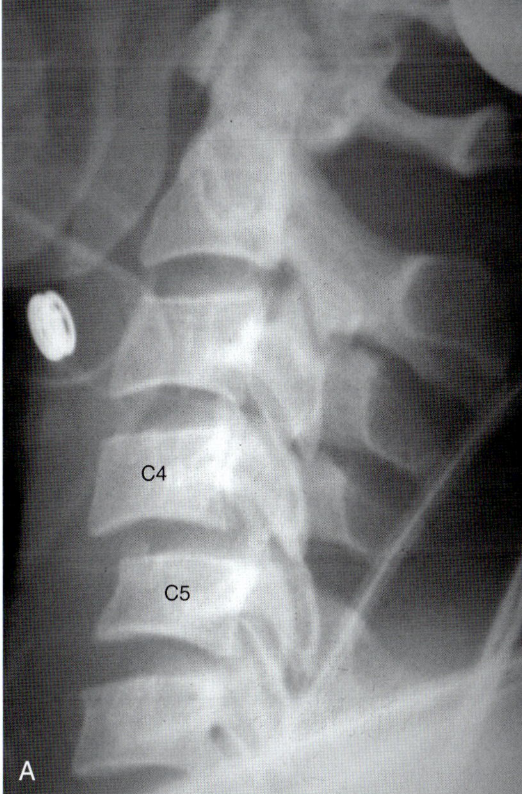

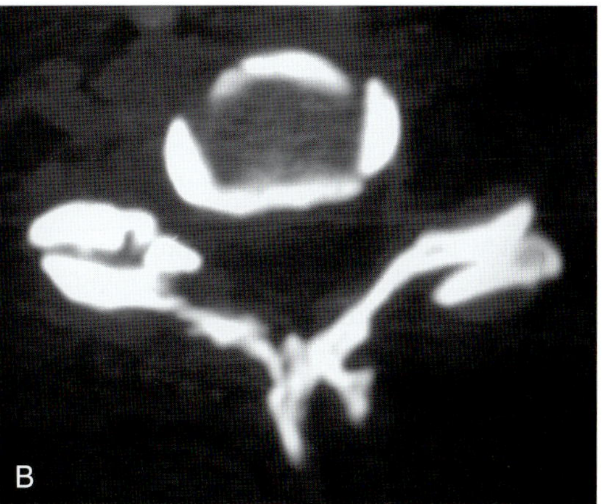

FIGURE 65-14. A, Lateral plain radiograph revealing evidence of a C4-5 unilateral facet dislocation (type II distractive flexion injury). Note the 25% anterior subluxation of C4 on C5. **B,** Transaxial CT scan revealing a left-sided unilateral facet dislocation. Note that the left C4 inferior articular process is anterior to the left C5 superior articular process.

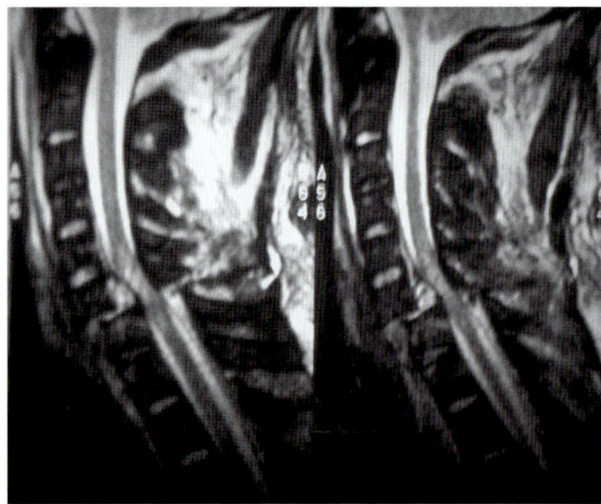

FIGURE 65-15. Sagittal MRI revealing significant cord edema and hemorrhage at the level of a C6-7 bilateral facet dislocation (stage 4 distractive flexion injury). Note the soft tissue density behind the body of C6, which may represent an extruded disc fragment.

injuries in this family should be considered at risk for further displacement, making surgical stabilization the primary mode of treatment.[9,108] After a successful closed reduction, MRI should be obtained to evaluate for the presence of a herniated disc (Fig. 65-15); if present, a ventral decompression and stabilization is the preferred surgical approach. If a closed reduction is not feasible, the surgical approach is predicated on the presence of an extruded disc fragment. If a disc fragment is present, a ventral decompression is required with or without an attempted ventral open reduction followed by a stabilization procedure. Recently, Johnson et al. analyzed the results of 87 patients with either unilateral or bilateral facet dislocations or fracture-dislocations treated with a single-level anterior cervical discectomy and fusion. They, like others, found a 13% incidence of nonunion, and concluded that facet fractures or end-plate fractures were predisposing factors for long-term nonunion.[109,110] Paxinos et al. performed biomechanical studies and concluded that an anterior cervical discectomy and fusion with a locked plate was sufficient to stabilize a flexion-distraction stage 3 injury in the lower cervical spine, provided that osteoporosis was not present.[105] In the absence of an extruded disc fragment, a dorsal open reduction and stabilization procedure may be performed.

Our overall approach has been to treat these injuries as unstable three-column injuries that necessitate a front-to-back fusion. In patients without an extruded disc, dorsal reduction and fixation is first performed; ventral fixation is then performed with an anterior cervical discectomy and fusion. In patients with an extruded disc, the anterior cervical discectomy is performed first. If sufficient reduction is obtained to reduce the facet joint, an anterior cervical fusion is then performed.[105] If that is not possible, dorsal reduction and then anterior fusion are performed.[111]

Vertical Compression

A vertical compression fracture is described as a cervical burst fracture caused by an axial loading mechanism. Osseous

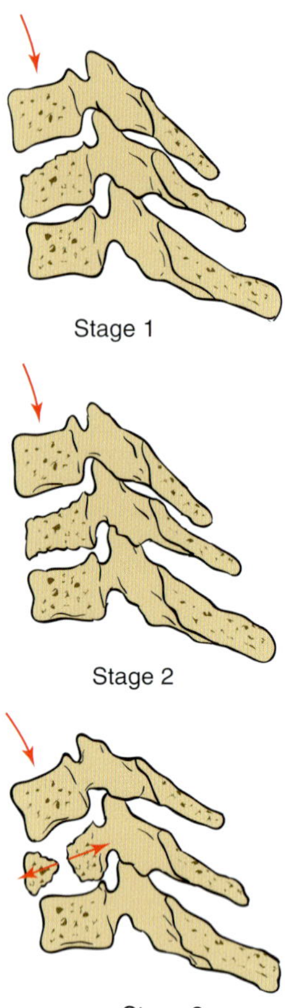

FIGURE 65-16. Vertical compression injury. Stage 1: central "cupping fracture" of the superior or inferior vertebral end plate. Stage 2: fracture of both superior and inferior end plates. Stage 3: displacement and fragmentation of the vertebral body. (From Rizzolo SJ, Cotler JM: Unstable cervical spine injuries: specific treatment approaches. *J Am Acad Orthop Surg* 1:57–66, 1993.)

failure is considered to be much more significant than damage to the ligamentous structures in this type of injury (Fig. 65-16). Treatment with halo immobilization is usually sufficient, although injuries at the cervicothoracic junction (C7) have a tendency to settle into kyphosis, which may require surgical intervention.[96,112-114] Ventral surgical decompression and stabilization is often necessary in patients with an incomplete neurologic deficit.

Distractive Extension

Distractive extension injuries are usually caused by forces that place the ventral elements under tension (Figs. 65-17 to 65-20). Ventral disc space widening is the characteristic radiographic finding, although failure may occur in a ventral-to-dorsal direction through the vertebral body. Less severe injuries may have little displacement, making radiographic detection difficult.[107] The presence of a ventral avulsion fracture resulting from an avulsion of the anterior longitudinal ligament may provide a clue to this injury type, This injury is especially unstable in a patient with ankylosing spondylitis or diffuse idiopathic skeletal hyperostosis,

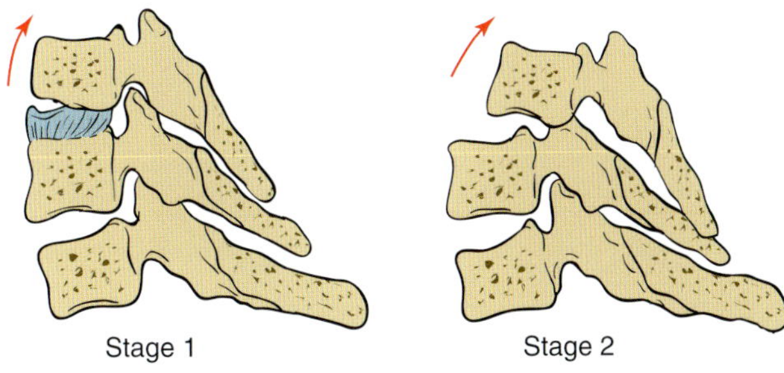

FIGURE 65-17. Distractive extension injury. Stage 1: failure of anterior ligamentous complex, which may present as a widening of the disc space or a nondeforming transverse fracture through the centrum. Stage 2: injury may be identified radiographically by an anterior marginal avulsion fracture of the centrum. Posterior ligamentous disruption may be identified by posterior displacement of the superior vertebra. (From Rizzolo SJ, Cotler JM: Unstable cervical spine injuries: specific treatment approaches. *J Am Acad Orthop Surg* 1:57–66, 1993.)

in which two rigid moment arms are joined at an unstable junction. Distractive extension injuries are commonly associated with neurologic impairment. Patients frequently present with neurologic evidence of a central cord syndrome with significant weakness involving the upper extremities and relative sparing of the lower extremities. Spontaneous recovery is common.[91] Most distractive extension injuries without disc space disruption are stable and may be treated nonoperatively, with late flexion-extension radiographs to confirm stability. Unstable injuries benefit from a ventral reconstructive procedure with ventral plating acting as a ventral tension band.[107]

Lateral Flexion

Lateral flexion injuries are secondary to asymmetrical compressive loading resulting in unilateral vertebral body compression failure and ipsilateral dorsal arch fracture (Fig. 65-21). As noted previously, this is the least common pattern of lower cervical spine disruption and is often stable, requiring cervical immobilization for 6 to 12 weeks.

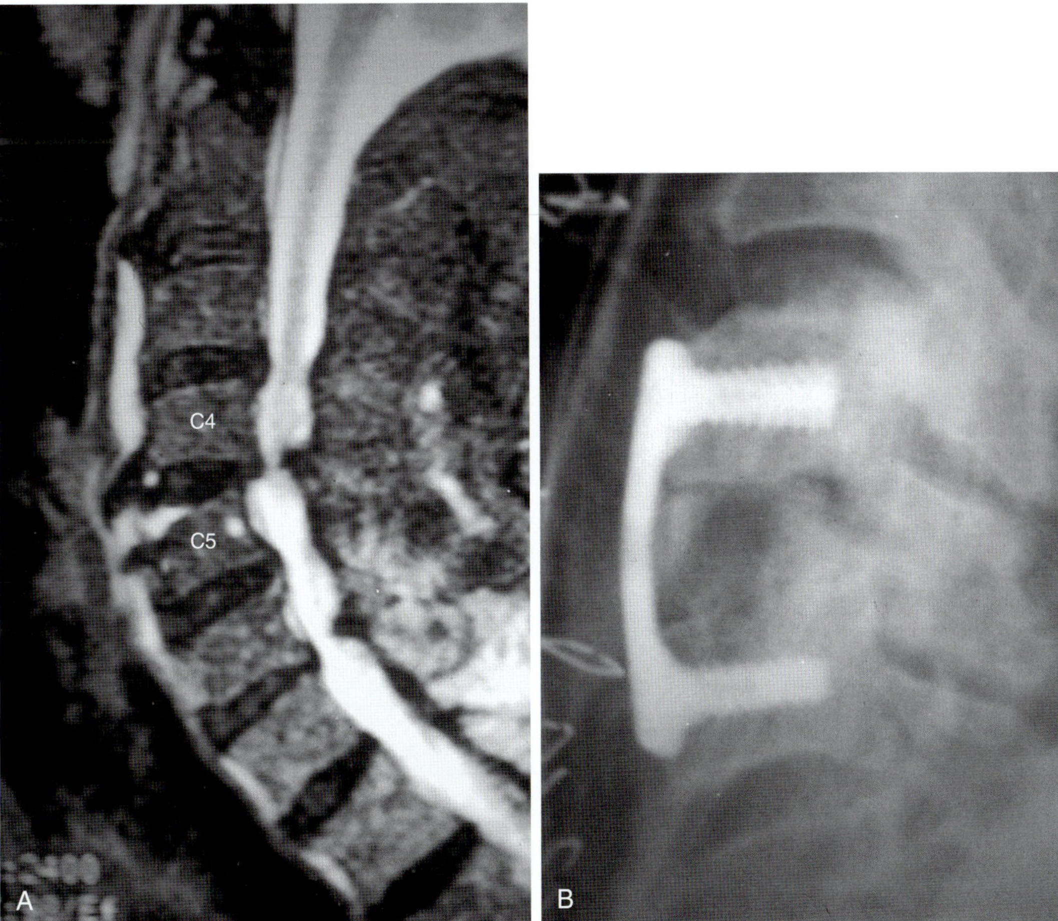

FIGURE 65-18. A, Sagittal MRI revealing a distractive extension injury at the C4-5 level with retrolisthesis of C4 on C5. **B,** Plain lateral radiograph after an anterior tension band (instrumented fusion) reconstruction of the injury.

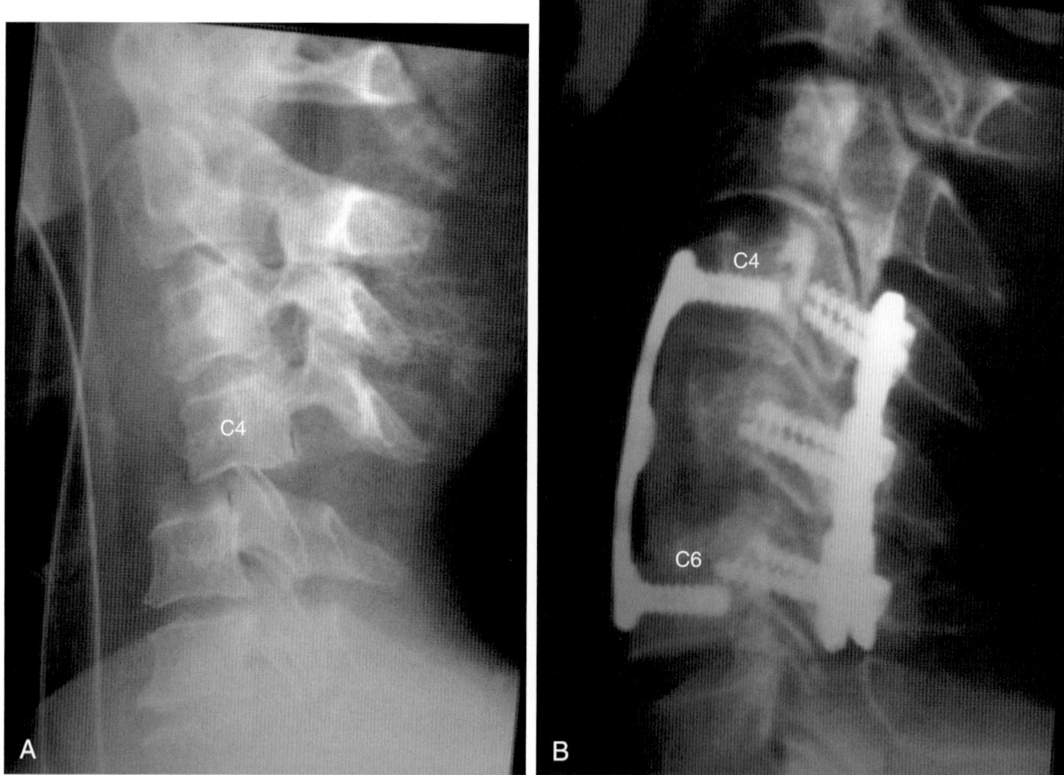

FIGURE 65-19. **A,** Lateral plain film revealing a high-grade distractive extension cervical injury at the C4-5 level. **B,** Lateral plain film after a posterior-to-anterior reconstruction procedure to obtain adequate spinal stability.

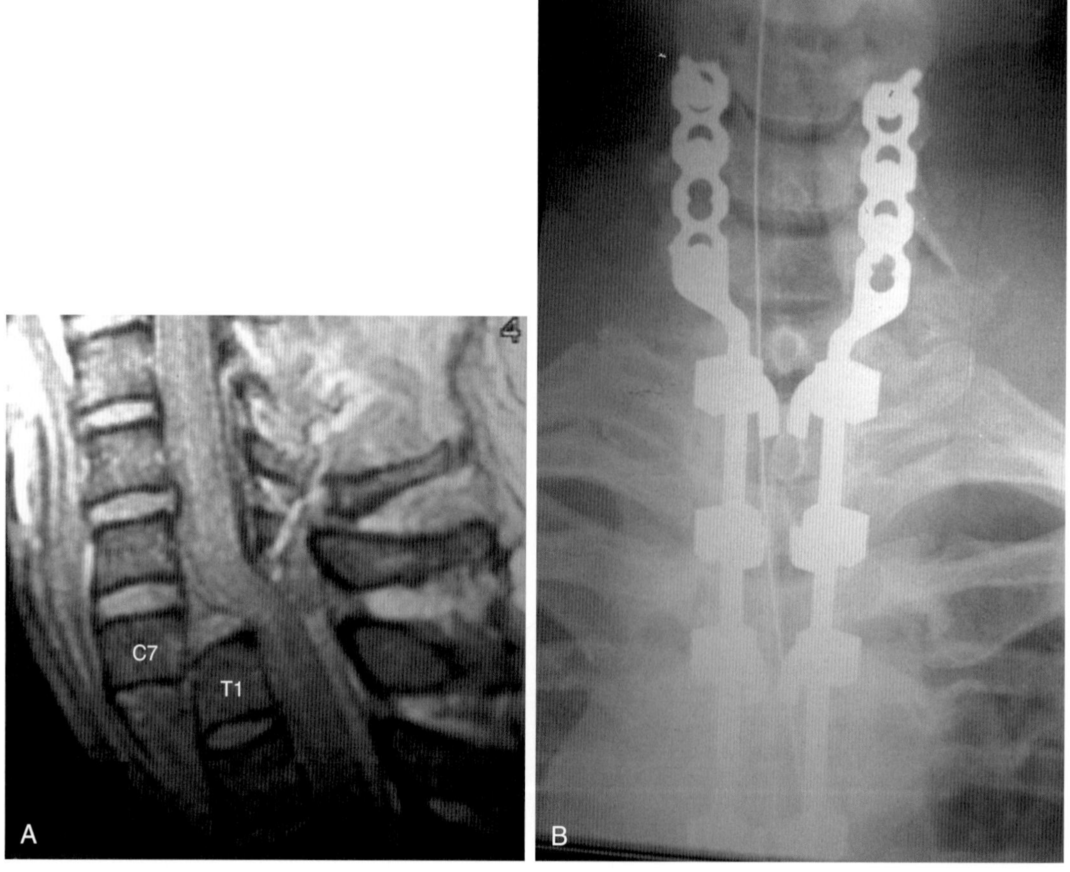

FIGURE 65-20. **A,** Sagittal MRI revealing a high-grade distractive extension injury at the C7-T1 level. **B,** The patient underwent a posterior open reduction and stabilization procedure using a cervicothoracic plate-rod implant to obtain adequate spinal stability.

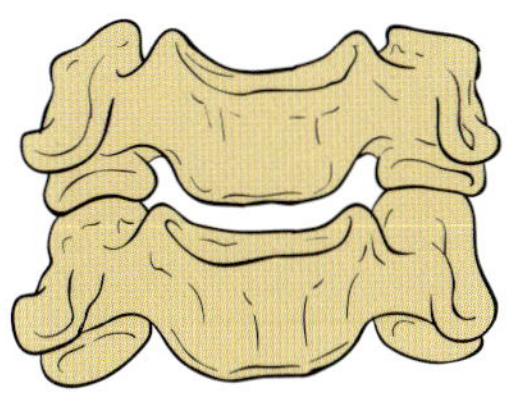

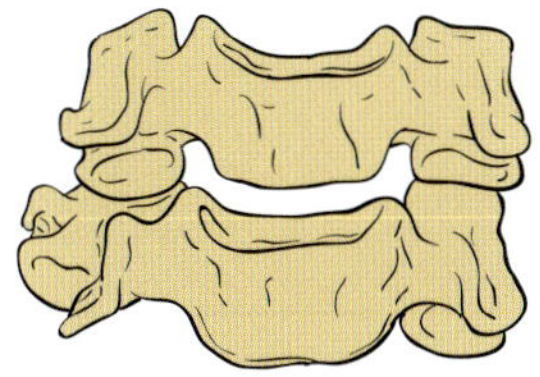

FIGURE 65-21. Lateral flexion injury. Stage 1: asymmetrical compression fracture of the centrum with associated ipsilateral vertebral arch fracture seen on lateral view; no displacement is noted on the anteroposterior (AP) view. Stage 2: displacement is evident on the AP as well as the lateral views. There may also be tension failure of the contralateral ligaments and facet joint. (From Rizzolo SJ, Cotler JM: Unstable cervical spine injuries: specific treatment approaches. *J Am Acad Orthop Surg* 1:57–66, 1993.)

Summary

Over half of the 50,000 new spinal cord injuries reported annually in the United States occur in the cervical spine. Of these, 11,000 have some degree of permanent deficit. Further advancement and implementation of ATLS protocols may be expected to result in an increased number of multitrauma survivors with a proportionately increased incidence of cervical spine trauma presenting in our emergency departments. These trends and statistics underscore the socioeconomic importance of cervical spine trauma, and they add greater emphasis to the critical nature of early injury recognition, evaluation, and proper treatment.

KEY REFERENCES

Anderson LD, D'Alonzo RT: Fractures of the odontoid process of the axis. *J Bone Joint Surg [Am]* 56:1663–1674, 1974.

Daffner RH: Evaluation of cervical cerebral injuries. *Semin Roentgenol* 27:239–253, 1992.

Denis F: Spinal instability as defined by the three column spine concept in acute spinal trauma. *Clin Orthop Relat Res* 189:65–76, 1983.

Jefferson G: Remarks on fractures of the first cervical vertebra. *BMJ* 2:153–157, 1927.

Levine AM, Edward CC: The management of traumatic spondylolisthesis of the axis. *J Bone Joint Surg [Am]* 67:217–226, 1985.

Montane I, Eismont FJ, Green BA: Traumatic occipitoatlantal dislocation. *Spine (Phila Pa 1976)* 16:112–116, 1991.

Pang D, Wilberger JE: Spinal cord injury without radiographic abnormalities in children. *J Neurosurg* 57:114–129, 1982.

White AA III, Panjabi MM: Update on the evaluation of instability of the lower cervical spine. *Instr Course Lect* 36:513–520, 1987.

REFERENCES

The complete reference list is available online at expertconsult.com.

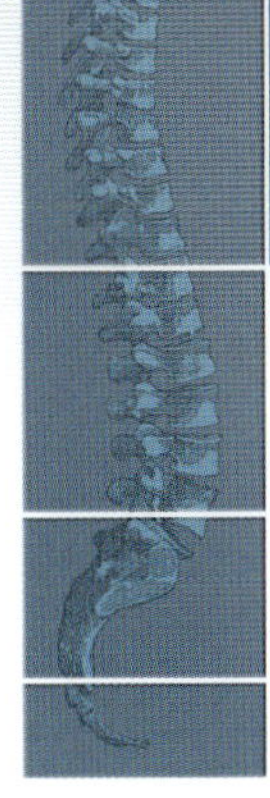

CHAPTER 66

Trauma Surgery: Thoracic and Thoracolumbar Junction

Edward Marchan | Alexander R. Vaccaro | Kevin T. Foley | Iain H. Kalfas | James S. Harrop

Approximately 160,000 patients a year in the United States suffer traumatic spinal column injuries, with 10% to 30% of them having a concurrent spinal cord injury.[1-4] The majority of these injuries consist of cervical and lumbar (L3-5) spine fractures. However, between 15% and 20% of traumatic fractures occur at the thoracolumbar junction (T11-L2), whereas 9% to 16% occur in the thoracic spine (T1-10).[5,6] Forces along the long stiff, kyphotic thoracic spine catalyze an abrupt switch into the mobile lordotic lumbar spine at the thoracolumbar junction. Biomechanically, this transition zone is susceptible to injury and is the most commonly injured portion of the spine. High-energy trauma (i.e., motor vehicle accidents) is the leading cause of injury over this region, followed by falls and sports-related injuries.[7] Men are at four times higher risk than women. Because of the higher-energy mechanisms of injury, involvement of other organ systems is encountered in up to 50% of thoracolumbar trauma patients.[7] These high-energy injuries, such as those causing thoracic-level paraplegia, have a first-year mortality rate of 7%.[3,8]

Thoracic spine and thoracolumbar junction trauma, as a result of regional anatomy and biomechanical characteristics, is categorized according to radiographic presentation, biomechanical deficiencies, and clinical presentation of the patient. Primary goals in thoracolumbar trauma patients are prompt recognition and treatment of associated injuries and expeditious stabilization of the spine and protection of the neural elements.

Anatomy

The vertebral column provides humans with the ability to maintain an upright posture, protects the neural and visceral organs (i.e., heart, lungs, abdominal contents), and helps with motility. It consists of 29 vertebrae arranged in 4 major curves, 2 primary curves (thoracic and sacral), and 2 compensatory or secondary curves (cervical and lumbar).[9] The vertebral column also provides a protective environment for the spinal cord and neural elements. The vertebral body, pedicles, and dorsal elements surround the spinal cord, permitting the spinal nerves to exit through the paired neural foramina. The laminae are formed as dorsomedial extensions of the pedicles and fuse in the midline to create the spinous processes (Fig. 66-1). Nomenclature for the thoracic spine varies; however, in this chapter the thoracic spine is considered to span T1 through T10, and the thoracolumbar junction T11 through L2.

Primary spinal curves are present at birth, are maintained through life, and are relatively rigid or stiff. Secondary curves are more flexible and result from development or adaptation. The first secondary curve is the development of cervical lordosis at approximately 3 to 9 months of age as the infant begins supporting his or her head and sitting upright. The lumbar lordosis develops later (between 12 and 18 months), as the child begins to ambulate and assumes an upright posture.[9] A thorough knowledge of the thoracic spine and thoracolumbar junction anatomy facilitates a greater understanding of the biomechanical, radiographic, and surgical techniques that are used to treat these fractures.

Thoracic Spine

The thoracic spine differs from the cervical and lumbosacral spines as a result of its articulation with the rib cage (T1-12), extensive ligamentous support network, coronal facet joint orientation, and small spinal canal-to-neural element ratio (Fig. 66-2). The thoracic laminae increase in width and thickness from T1 to T12, and this prevents hyperextension.[10] The anterior longitudinal ligament (ALL) provides further stability by increasing the tensile strength from T1 to T12. Moreover, the dorsal, ventral, and lateral diameters of the vertebral bodies increase from T2 to T12.[11-15] The thoracic kyphotic curve results from the greater height of the dorsal vertebral wall as opposed to the ventral vertebral wall. The transverse pedicle diameters decrease from 9 mm at T1 to 5 mm at T5 and then increase in size distally to T12.[14] In the sagittal plane, pedicle width increases from T1 to T11. However, in the transverse or axial plane, the thoracic vertebrae have a triangular configuration and appear heart shaped. There is significant variability in what is considered the "normal" sagittal curvature of the thoracic spine. This value has been reported to be between 20 and 45 degrees,[13,16,17] with each individual vertebral body contributing approximately 3.8 to 3.9 degrees of kyphosis through its wedged-shaped angulation. This variability is further influenced by age (increases with age) and sex; women have a greater degree of kyphosis than men.[16,17] There is also a significant degree of variability on a segmental basis, particularly at the transitional regions with the lordotic cervical and lumbar spines.[12,18,19] The apex of thoracic kyphosis is typically located at the seventh thoracic vertebra, but varies with each individual. The thoracic spine typically has a mild, right-sided lateral curvature.[9,17]

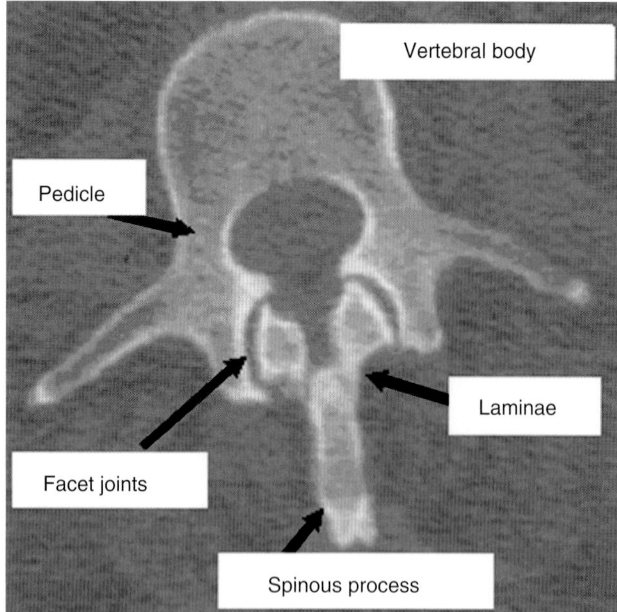

FIGURE 66-1. Axial CT image of L2 vertebral body identifying the dorsal elements.

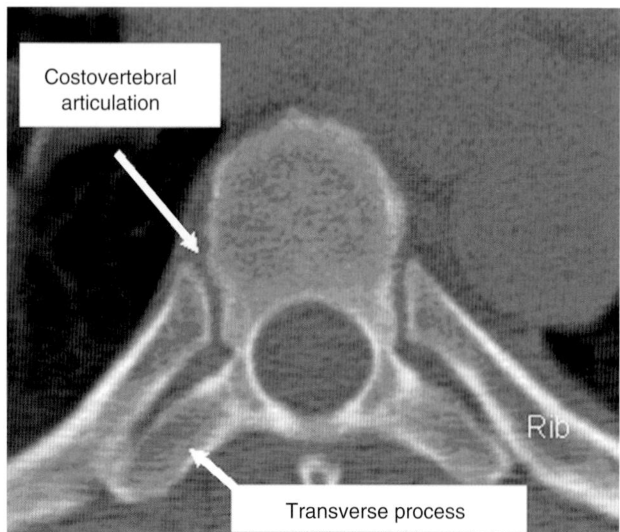

FIGURE 66-2. Axial CT image of T6 vertebral body identifying the relationship between the vertebral body and the rib head's articulations.

The etiology of the right-sided lateral curve is debated but is believed to be either the result of hand dominance (right-hand majority) or created by pulsations of the thoracic aorta.[9]

The thoracic pedicles are situated toward the rostral portion of the vertebral body, close to the superior disc space (Fig. 66-3). The pedicle angle decreases from T1 to T12; it is 251 degrees at T1 and 0 degrees at T12.[11,17,20] The pedicle location on the vertebral body progressively migrates as the spine is descended in a caudal direction. The medial pedicle cortical wall is approximately two to three times thicker than the lateral wall.[21]

The thoracic transverse processes project laterally from the dorsal articular pillars and decrease in length caudally.[5] However, unlike the lumbar spine, the relationship between the transverse process and the midpoint of the pedicle is not as clearly defined. McCormick[22] showed that there is a significant degree of

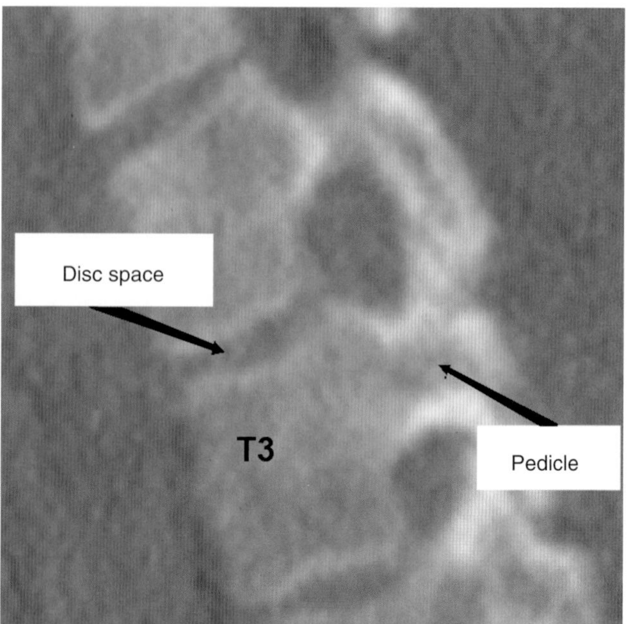

FIGURE 66-3. Sagittal CT reformatted image of T2 and T3 vertebral bodies illustrating the relationship of the pedicle to the intervertebral disc space in the thoracic spine.

variability in the relationship of the transverse processes to the pedicles. The midpoint of the T1 transverse process is approximately 5 mm rostral to the center of the pedicle, whereas at T12 the transverse process-to-pedicle relationship changes to approximately 6 mm caudal.[20] Comparatively, this transverse process to pedicle relationship is greater than 1 cm at both T1 and T2, and is approximately 0 cm when one analyzes T6 and T7.[20]

The thoracic spine facet articulations are considered apophyseal joints and are composed of a ligamentous capsule with a synovial lining. These ligaments in the thoracic spine are thicker than their cervical counterparts. In the thoracic spine, the costovertebral (rib-vertebra) facets are located anterior to the transverse processes. The isthmus of bone between each pair of superior and inferior facets is called the *pars interarticularis*, a site of fracture and bony nonunion for those with a condition known as *spondylolysis*. The joints are located at the rostral and caudal borders of the laminae and situated medial to the transverse processes (Fig. 66-4). The caudal facet's ventral surface articulates with the rostral facet's dorsal surface. Thoracic facet joints are oriented in a coronal plane and therefore limit the degree of flexion and extension of the thoracic spine.[23]

There are several key anatomic features that are essential for understanding the relationship of the ribs and the thoracic vertebrae. First, the ribs articulate with the thoracic vertebrae at two separate locations. The head of the rib articulates with the transverse process of the body at the costotransverse articulation, except at T1, T11, and T12. This articulation is supported with a large superior costotransverse ligament, which connects the rostral rib segment to the caudal transverse process (see Fig. 66-2). It also articulates with the disc space adjacent to the body above by virtue of the rib head of the same-numbered vertebral body articulating with it through the two costal hemifacets (T2-10).

The strong ligamentous structures that compose the costovertebral joint make the thoracic disc the strongest of all the

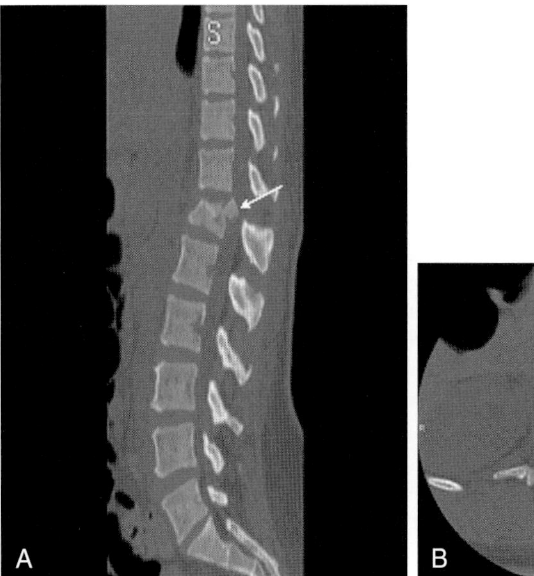

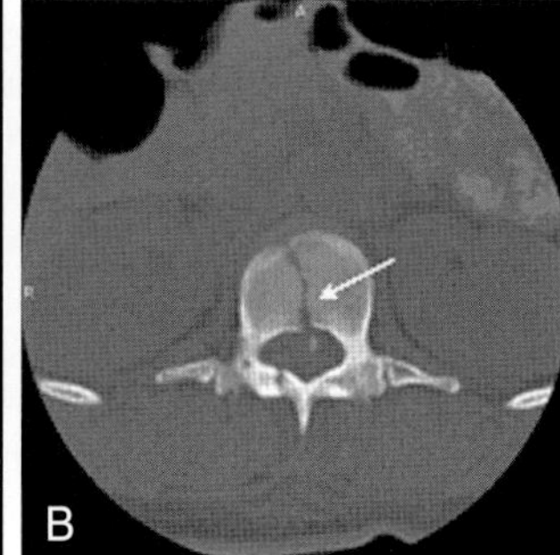

FIGURE 66-4. T12 burst fracture sustained after a motor vehicle accident. Note the high definition of the posterior displaced fragment (**A**, *arrow*), along with the vertebral body sagittal fracture (**B**, *arrow*) and the associated laminae fractures.

vertebral discs.[24] The superior hemifacet (rostral on the vertebral body and caudal to the rib) is located over the pedicle, such that the sixth rib articulates with the fifth and sixth thoracic vertebral bodies and overlies the sixth vertebral pedicle. Because of the rostral location of the thoracic pedicle on the vertebral body, the sixth rib overlies the T5 to T6 disc space. Understanding the anatomic relationship of the rib head with the pedicle allows the surgeon to remove the rib head and identify the neurovascular bundle, along with the neural foramina and thecal sac, at that level.

The spinal canal diameter varies throughout the vertebral column and is the narrowest in the midthoracic region (T3-9).[11,13,25] The transverse spinal canal diameter decreases from T1 to T3 and then increases caudally into the lumbar region. The anteroposterior (AP) diameter, however, is more varied.[13,25] Therefore, in the thoracic region a minor degree of canal encroachment can compromise the narrow canal and may result in neurologic compromise.[26,27] Furthermore, the thoracic spinal cord has the most tenuous blood supply.[13] Thus, small canal size, limited blood supply, and the high degree of energy required to create a thoracic fracture combine to result in a 90% incidence of neurologic deficit in patients who sustain a thoracic fracture.[28]

Thoracolumbar Junction

The transition from a relatively rigid thoracic kyphosis to a mobile lumbar spine occurs at the thoracolumbar junction. This transition generally occurs at T11 to T12, although in elderly female patients the thoracolumbar inflexion point migrates caudally as a result of their increased degree of thoracic kyphosis.[12,17,19]

The caudal thoracic ribs (T11 and T12) afford less stability at the thoracolumbar junction region compared with the rostral thoracic region because there is no connection to the sternum and thus they are "free floating." Only a single rib articulation is present on the T11 and T12 vertebral bodies, and there are no accessory ligamentous attachments, such as the rib's tubercle to the vertebral body by the costotransverse ligament, or the ligamentous attachment to the transverse process.[9] The surrounding thoracolumbar ligaments, such as the interspinous and thoracolumbar fascia, are strongest caudally and provide a significant amount of stability.[14]

The thoracolumbar junction facet joints are again of the apophyseal type and are composed of a ligamentous capsule with a synovial lining. As mentioned previously, the joints of the midthoracic region are oriented in the coronal plane, limiting flexion and extension while providing substantial resistance to AP translation.[5] In the lumbosacral region, the facet joints are oriented in a more sagittal alignment, which increases the degree of potential flexion and extension at the expense of limiting lateral bending and rotation. Depending on the spatial orientation of the spinal column (i.e., flexion or extension), the facet joints may support a third of the axial load. These joints, however, provide substantial support and resistance to approximately 35% to 45% of the torsional and shear forces experienced in this region.[6,29]

At birth, the spinal cord terminates at the end of the vertebral column or lumbosacral junction. However, the end of the spinal cord, or conus medullaris, migrates rostrally as the infant develops.[30] In neonates the spinal cord terminates between the first and third lumbar vertebrae, whereas in adults it is positioned between the twelfth thoracic vertebra and the second lumbar vertebra.[30]

Imaging

It is not uncommon in clinically unstable trauma patients for fractures not to be identified early in the resuscitative period. It has been reported that between 5% and 15% of multisystem trauma patients have occult fractures not diagnosed on their initial evaluation.[31-33] Although thoracic vertebral fractures make up only a minor proportion of traumatic fractures, they are extremely difficult to visualize compared with other vertebral or appendicular fractures. Approximately 20% to 50% of superior thoracic spine fractures are not diagnosed on admission plain radiographs.[5,34,35] Therefore, all suspected spine trauma patients should be immobilized on admission until a thorough and detailed spinal evaluation can be performed. If appropriate stabilization precautions are not taken in this patient population, unforeseen neurologic compromise may result.[6]

Initial radiographic assessment includes AP and lateral spine films. The AP film should be examined for loss of vertical body height, fracture of the oval-shaped pedicles, increased interpedicular distance, transverse process or rib fractures, and malalignment of vertebral bodies or spinous processes without a history of scoliosis. The lateral radiograph should be examined for loss of body height, disruption of the rostral or caudal end plate, dorsal cortical wall fracture with retropulsed bone, fracture of spinous processes, widening of interspinous distance, and subluxation or angulation of vertebral bodies.[36] Malalignment in any plane, but especially in the AP plane, suggests the possibility of a fracture-dislocation.[12] Plain radiographs may not be accurate in determining the involvement of the posterior vertebral wall with a thoracic fracture.[37,38]

Plain radiographs are particularly useful in assessing the patient's overall sagittal and coronal balance. If a deformity exists, a useful radiographic technique to determine the degree of deformity is measurement of the Cobb angle, which is the subtended angle measured between a perpendicular line drawn from the superior end plate of the vertebral body above the injured vertebral body and the inferior end plate one level below the injured body (see Fig. 66-20). This method of measuring spinal sagittal angulation has been shown to have the highest degree of intraobserver and interobserver reliability.[39]

In the presence of a vertebral body injury, the entire spine should be imaged in an orthogonal manner because of the high incidence (5–20%) of noncontiguous spine fractures.[40-42] The rostral thoracic spine can be difficult to visualize on lateral plain radiographs because of the patient's shoulders and body habitus, and a swimmer's view may provide better visualization of the cervicothoracic junction down to the T3 vertebral body.[43] Radiographically, a typical superior end-plate thoracic fracture shows loss of vertebral height, with or without malalignment, a widened paraspinal line, and possibly a widened mediastinum.[35] Because of difficulties in imaging the upper thoracic region (T1-4), a high index of suspicion is required on the physician's part to avoid missing injuries at this level. The physician should have a low threshold for ordering supplemental imaging modalities to assist in the diagnosis, such as CT and MRI.

Computed Tomography

CT is more sensitive in detecting fractures than plain radiographs[44] (see Fig. 66-4). It can also define the three-dimensional anatomy of complex fractures through reformatting in the sagittal and coronal planes. CT better delineates the bony structures once an injury is identified.[45-47] CT reveals the integrity of the middle column and the degree of canal compromise, as well as subluxations or fractures of facets and laminae. The presence of two vertebral bodies on the same axial cut of a CT scan may indicate a fracture-dislocation, but first the radiographer must ensure that the gantry has been angled parallel to the vertebral end plates. Sagittal reconstructions are helpful in visualizing flexion-distraction injuries and fracture-dislocations. Serial CT scans of lumbar fractures have confirmed spontaneous remodeling and the reabsorption of retropulsed bone fragments in the spinal canal at long-term follow-up.[48-50]

CT image reconstruction is also invaluable at the cervicothoracic junction because of the overlap of the scapula, shoulders, and surrounding tissues. In the obtunded patient, this technique has been reported to identify more than 10% of fractures not visualized on plain radiographs.[51] CT, however, has a limited capacity to visualize disc herniations, epidural or subdural hematomas, ligamentous disruption, and spinal cord parenchymal changes.[52]

Magnetic Resonance Imaging

MRI has further improved the ability to visualize and comprehend the pathoanatomy of soft tissues, ligaments, and intervertebral discs, and the neural element disruption that occurs after spine injury. Unfortunately, MRI is not always available because of its expense, because it takes longer to implement, and because it cannot be performed on patients with ferromagnetic implants. Today it has supplanted CT myelography as the imaging tool of choice for the neuraxis because it is faster and noninvasive and allows improved visualization of the spinal cord parenchyma.[53] MRI provides the physician with the ability to identify edema and/or hemorrhage of the spinal cord[53] (Fig. 66-5). These images have been correlated with neurologic outcomes, where the presence of hemorrhage in the spinal cord parenchyma is associated with minimal neurologic recovery.[54]

MRI evaluation is especially useful at the thoracolumbar junction because of the variable location of the cauda equina and conus medullaris in the adult population at this level.[55] A neurologic examination can be difficult to interpret at the conus-cauda equina transition level as a result of the presence of lumbar spinal nerve sparing, the presence of concurrent injuries, sedation, or indwelling catheters, and delayed reflex recovery (Fig. 66-6). Accurate neural visualization may help in clarifying the pathoanatomy in these clinical situations.

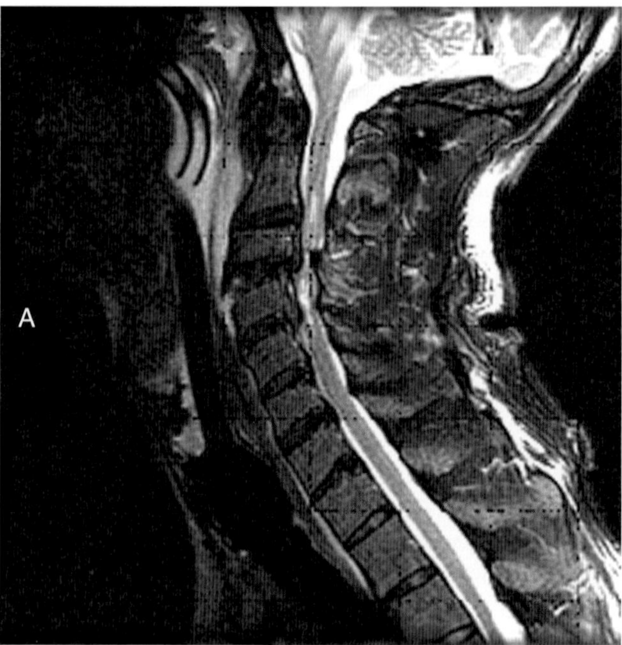

FIGURE 66-5. T2-weighted MRI of cervical spine of C5 ASIA type A spinal cord–injured patient after an automobile crash. Note severe intraparenchymal edema, along with hemorrhage in the spinal cord.

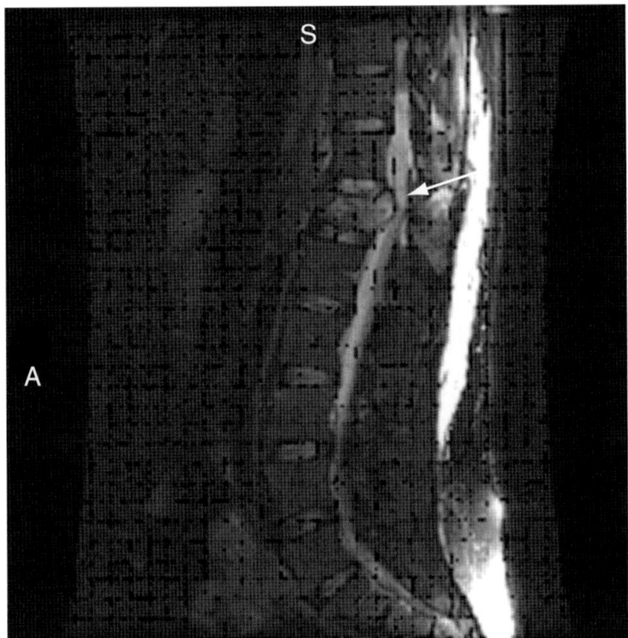

FIGURE 66-6. T12 burst fracture with retropulsion of fragment into canal. Note that the fragment is compressing the conus medullaris (*arrow*) and there is resulting spinal cord edema. Clinically the patient has a severe lower extremity paresis and loss of bowel and bladder function.

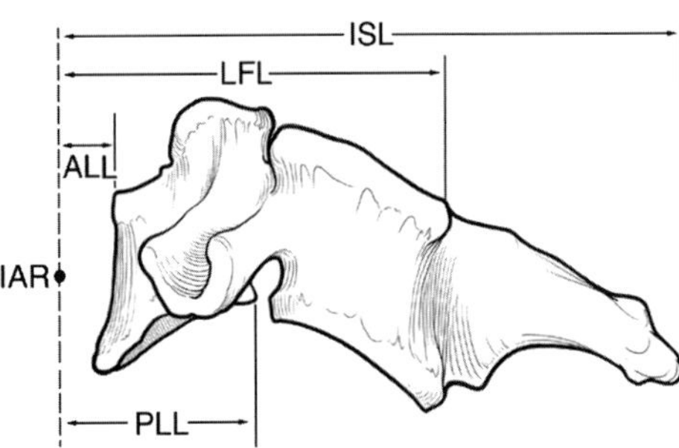

FIGURE 66-7. The lever arm of the ligaments to the instantaneous axis of rotation (IAR) greatly influences the stability of the spine. The weaker interspinous ligaments (ISL) work at the greatest distance from the IAR and therefore provide significant resistance to gravitational influences. ALL, anterior longitudinal ligament; LFL, ligamentum flavum; PLL, posterior longitudinal ligament.

Biomechanics

The vertebral body is the primary load-bearing structure of the spine, with the intervertebral disc transferring all forces applied to the adjacent vertebral bodies.[56,57] The anulus fibrosus of the intervertebral disc supports a significant portion of all applied axial and lateral loads and resists tension and shearing.[58]

The spinal ligamentous structures are essential in maintaining overall sagittal balance. The posterior longitudinal ligament (PLL) is a relatively weak ligament that provides some restriction to hyperflexion, along with the ligamentum flavum. The thicker ALL functions in resisting spinal hyperextension and distraction.[59] This thick ligament has fatigue loading values that are approximately double those of any other spinal ligaments,[57-59] and its strength increases caudally from C3 to the sacrum.[59] The intrinsic strength of the spinal ligaments is only an isolated factor in the overall stability of the spinal column. The lever arm by which these ligaments act on the spine also significantly affects the overall stability of the vertebral column (Fig. 66-7).

Abnormal motion patterns and coupling can be an indication of clinical instability, which ultimately must be treated in some manner. Clinical instability can be quantitatively measured in respect to the moving segment's instantaneous axis of rotation (IAR). The IAR is an axis about which a vertebra rotates at some instant of time.[46] This axis is a geometric concept and does not apply to a specific anatomic location.[60] However, in the normal thoracic and thoracolumbar spine, the IAR is located in the ventral vertebral body. For normal spinal units, the IAR for each of the rotary modes (flexion, extension, lateral bending, and axial torsion) is confined to a relatively small area somewhere within the spinal unit.[14] The facet capsules are very strong ligaments and act with a short lever arm by their relationship to the IAR, whereas the intraspinous ligaments are relatively weak but act with a great lever arm because of their increased distance from the IAR. Based on the ligaments' relative strengths, it would seem that the intraspinous ligaments are not important, but both ligaments significantly affect the strength and structure of the spine.

The thoracic spine differs from the remainder of the spinal column because it is supported by and maintains articulations with the ribs (see Fig. 66-2). The intact rib cage increases the axial load-resisting capacity of the thoracic spine by a magnitude of four. The rib cage and facet articulations limit rotation, and therefore most thoracic spine fractures occur from a flexion or axial compression force vector.[61] The majority of stability in flexion is provided by the costovertebral articulations.[62] A significant factor in the degree and extent of fracture character is the rate of force impact loading.[63]

Gravitational forces exert a significant axial load on the vertebral column in the standing adult human. The center of gravity of the body, located where all forces are counterbalanced such that there is no net movement, is approximately 4 cm anterior to the first sacral vertebra.[14] This results in a ventral bending (angular) vector acting on the spinal column. This bending force draws or attracts the ventral spinal column closer to the center of gravity such that a lower energy state may be achieved by the paraspinous musculature. The dorsal ligamentous complex and dorsal paraspinal musculature, acting as a tension band, counteracts these forces, such that the net sum of the vectors acting on the spine equals zero. Therefore the dorsal ligamentous, osseous, and muscular components are essential for overall support of the spine to prevent a change in the spine's sagittal alignment. Trauma resulting in disruption of the spinal ligaments or osseous structures may change the net vector sum from zero, resulting in the potential for spinal imbalance. These new vectors acting on the spine, if not corrected, may result in a gradual spinal deformity with or without associated pain or neurologic deterioration. Whiteside used the analogy of a construction crane to illustrate this mechanical principle[64] (Fig. 66-8). In this analogy, the weight to be lifted is ventral to the crane, where the boom (anterior vertebral column) is under compression and the guidewires (posterior columns) are under tension. Failure of either supporting structure independent of the other will result in mechanical failure or collapse.

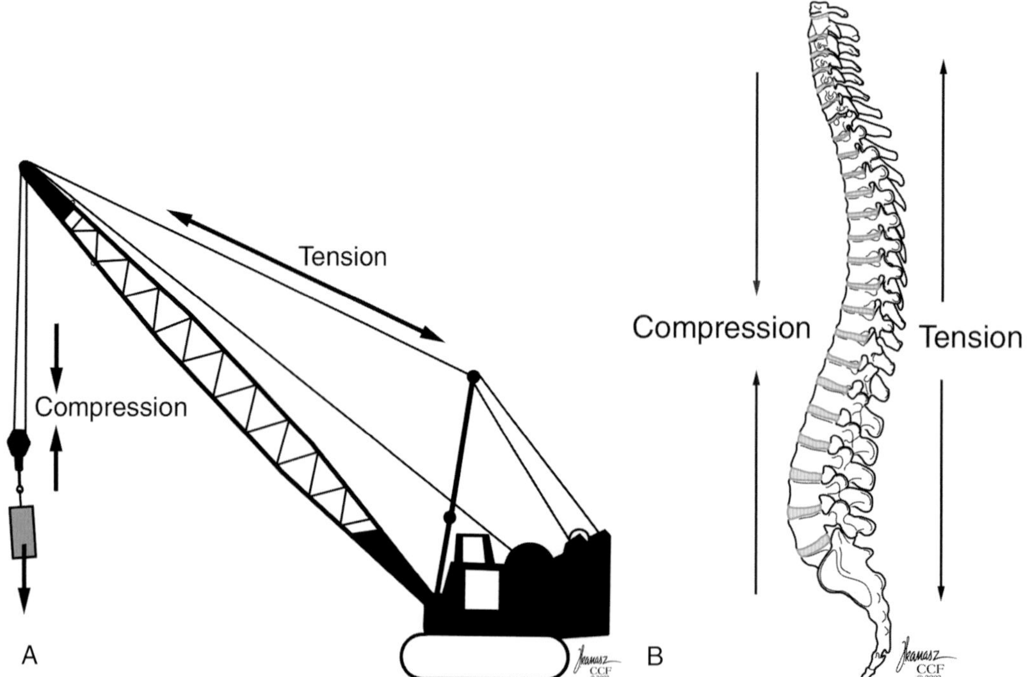

FIGURE 66-8. **A** and **B,** Whiteside's crane analogue of the spine illustrates the delicate equilibrium of the anterior compression vectors against the posterior tension vectors. (Copyright Cleveland Clinic Foundation.)

The thoracic and thoracolumbar vertebrae are at increased risk for development of compression fractures after trauma as a consequence of axial loads resulting from the natural kyphotic curvature of the thoracic spine.[65] The kyphotic posture results in the placement of axial forces on the ventral portion of the vertebral body. An axial load causes all points that are ventral to the IAR of the spine to come closer together while simultaneously all points that are dorsal are spread apart. Therefore, if the strength of the ventral vertebral body is exceeded, a fracture of the vertebral body occurs, resulting in a vertebral compression fracture (VCF). The traumatic forces may also exceed the strength of the dorsal vertebral body and ligamentous elements, resulting in disruption of the dorsal tension band. The destruction of the ventral vertebral stabilizing elements (i.e., vertebral body, disc, ligaments, anulus) causes the IAR to migrate dorsally to the region with intact supporting structures.[65,66] Dorsal migration of the IAR causes the previous mechanical advantage of a longer level arm from which the dorsal ligaments and muscles acted to be shortened. This migration of the IAR also simultaneously increases the distance of the center of gravity to the IAR, thereby placing further distraction on the dorsal spinal column and compression on the ventral spinal column[65,66] (see Fig. 66-7).

Concurrent Injuries

Thoracic Spine Fractures

The thoracic spine's structural integrity—the interaction of its osseous structures and ligaments and the rib cage—provides more protection against potential fracture than the remaining vertebral column. Hence, when a fracture occurs over this region, the physician must be aware that a high degree of energy was required to produce this lesion. These forces on impact are transmitted to the soft tissue and viscous elements contained within and around the thoracic cavity, resulting in a high incidence of concurrent injuries. The incidence of concurrent injuries is reported to be greater than 80%, involving the thorax, appendicular skeleton, and abdominal region.[35,42,67] These high-energy impacts also affect areas remote from the trauma, such as the cranial vault. Petitjean et al.[67] reported a 65% incidence of head injuries after high-velocity impacts that resulted in incomplete thoracic spinal cord injury, with 12% of these injuries classified as severe (Glasgow Coma Scale score <8).

Tearing or rupture of the aorta has been associated with thoracic vertebral fractures.[68] Hemodynamic instability may result from injury to any vascular structure, or even from blood loss secondary to a thoracic vertebral fracture.[67,69,70] Hemothorax has also been reported to occur in 24% to 32% of patients with thoracic fractures.[71,72] Pulmonary injuries have been reported in 85% of patients and typically consist of pulmonary contusions.[28] Infrequently, perforation of the esophagus and tracheal injuries have also been associated with thoracic fractures.[73-75] The mechanism of perforation is believed to be ischemia of the esophageal tissue after becoming devascularized as a result of a deceleration-traction injury.[73,75]

Thoracolumbar Junction Fractures

The thoracolumbar region is more vulnerable to concurrent injuries than the thoracic region because it is not provided the protection of the thoracic rib cage. Petitjean et al.[67] reported a 71% incidence of associated blunt abdominal injuries after thoracolumbar fractures. Typically, these consist of hollow viscus injuries (e.g., intestinal perforation), mesenteric avulsions, or solid organ injuries.[28,67,76]

The most common mechanism of abdominal injury is the distraction or seat belt injury.[28,67,77] Blunt abdominal aortic dissections are associated with distraction-rotation injuries of the thoracolumbar region.[2,77] These aortic injuries can range from an intimal tear to a full-thickness laceration. CT provides accurate imaging of this injury in the stable and asymptomatic patient. A large degree of energy is involved in this distraction-type mechanism, accounting for the large number of associated injuries. Multiple-level thoracic and lumbar fractures are also associated with a high incidence of abdominal injuries.[2]

Axial load injuries, particularly in patients who have jumped or fallen and landed on their feet, may manifest as both thoracolumbar fractures and calcaneal fractures. Isolated transverse process fractures of the lumbar spine should not be overlooked as a minor injury. Miller et al.[78] reported a 48% incidence of concurrent abdominal injuries associated with transverse process fractures. Therefore, a physician treating vertebral column injuries must be aware not only of the presence of spine fractures but also of the possibility of concurrent, nonspinal, soft tissue and bony injuries.

Classification

Injuries to the thoracic and lumbar spine account for more than 50% of all spine fractures and a large portion of acute spinal cord injuries.[17] Given this frequency and the significant impact of these injuries, significant advances have been made in the surgical treatment of thoracolumbar trauma. Nevertheless, although there has been progress in the invention and evolution of spinal instrumentation and surgical techniques, medical decision making in spine trauma remains controversial. To this day, fracture treatment can vary widely, from bracing to invasive 360-degree fusions, based on geographic, institutional, or individual preferences with little scientific basis.

A number of classification systems have been developed in an attempt to better define thoracolumbar trauma and aid treatment decision making. These systems are typically based on either anatomic structures (Denis three-column system) or on proposed mechanisms of injury (Ferguson and Allen).[79,80]

In 1931 Watson-Jones pioneered one of the first spinal fracture grouping systems by type.[81] This schematic categorization was based on diagnostic and treatment of flexion injuries.[82] This was followed by Nicholl,[83] who developed the first detailed thoracic and thoracolumbar spine fracture classification scheme and attempted to define unstable versus stable fractures after trauma in a series of flexion and flexion-rotation injuries. This classification system was originally intended to guide the treatment and work status of injured miners. Nicholl emphasized the importance of the dorsal interspinous ligament in spinal stability.[83] Later, Holdsworth,[84] after clinical failures in immobilizing pure flexion fractures following the recommendations of Watson-Jones, further studied the importance of the spinal ligamentous complexes after thoracolumbar junction injuries. He classified fractures, according to their mechanism of injury, into four main types: flexion, flexion and rotation, extension, and compression. Holdsworth[84] further classified these fractures as unstable if the posterior ligamentous complex, consisting of the intervertebral disc, spinous ligaments, facet capsules, and ligamentum flavum, was disrupted. He noted that in compression, flexion, and extension injuries, the dorsal ligamentous complex is typically not ruptured and these fractures were therefore considered stable. However, he reported that flexion and rotational injuries were at a much greater risk for disruption of the dorsal ligamentous complex and subsequent instability. Subsequently, Rennie and

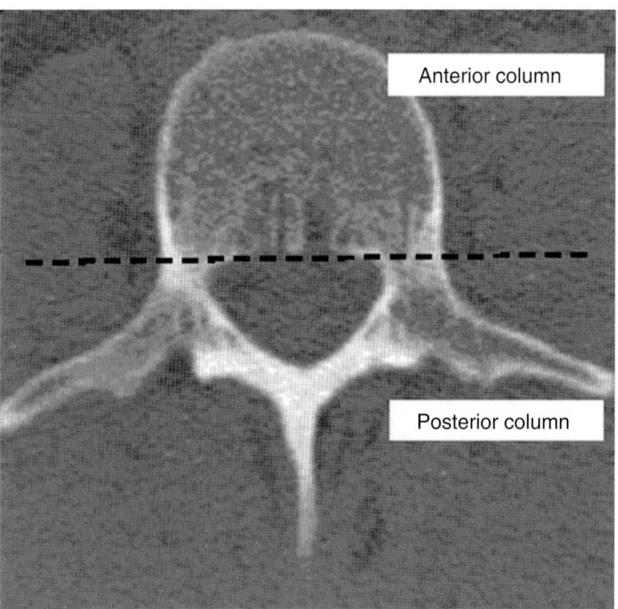

FIGURE 66-9. Axial CT of lumbar vertebral body illustrating Kelly and Whiteside's two-column theory of spine stability, which classifies the spine into equal anterior and posterior columns of support.

Mitchell[85] added a fifth category of thoracolumbar junction fractures consisting of flexion-distraction fractures or seat belt injuries, based on the description and reporting of Chance.[86]

Kelly and Whiteside[87] reported that without dislocation of the dorsal elements of the spinal column, neurologic injuries rarely occur. They classified fractures based on structural criteria and considered the spine to consist of not one, but two separate supportive columns (Fig. 66-9). The primary weight-bearing ventral column is composed of the vertebral bodies, and a second structural column consists of the posterior neural arches and ligaments. The structural classification scheme provided surgeons the ability to predict the degree of instability of the spine based on the degree of resulting structural damage after trauma. Based on this assessment, treatments were devised to enhance neurologic and spinal stability. Later, Louis[88] modified this structural classification scheme by proposing a third column. Louis's three-column concept consisted of one ventral column, the vertebral bodies, and two dorsal columns involving each facet articulation (Fig. 66-10).

Technologic advances in the form of superior imaging studies have allowed a greater understanding of the pathoanatomy of spine trauma. Several biomechanical studies have documented that an isolated rupture of the posterior spinal ligamentous complex is insufficient to create instability.[89-91] Nonetheless, if the PLL, along with the posterior anulus fibrosus, is also disrupted, then the vertebral column will become unstable, particularly in flexion.

Denis[79] used the enhanced CT imaging techniques, along with in vitro biomechanical data, to modify spinal column theories further into a different three-column classification scheme (Fig. 66-11). In this classification, the ventral column consists of the ALL, the anterior anulus fibrosus, and the anterior half of the vertebral bodies. The middle column consists of the PLL, the dorsal anulus fibrosus, and the dorsal half of the vertebral bodies. Last, the posterior column, analogous to what Holdsworth defined as

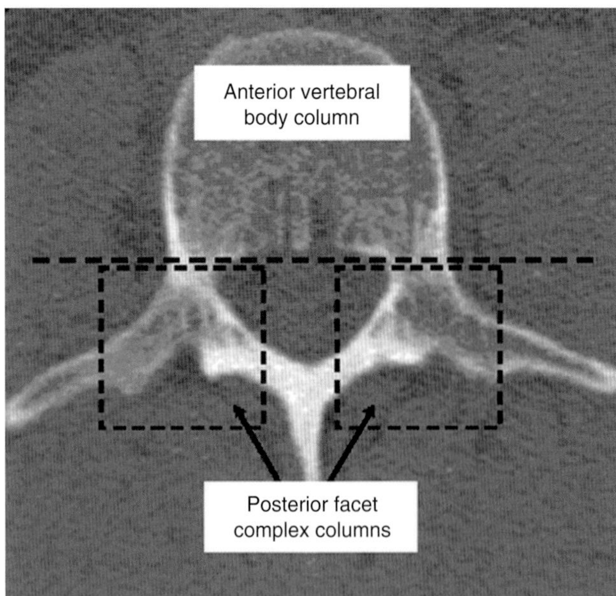

FIGURE 66-10. Axial CT of lumbar vertebral body illustrating Louis's three-column figure theory of spine structure. This classification system divides the spine into an anterior column consisting of the vertebral body and two equal posterior columns consisting of the facet complexes.

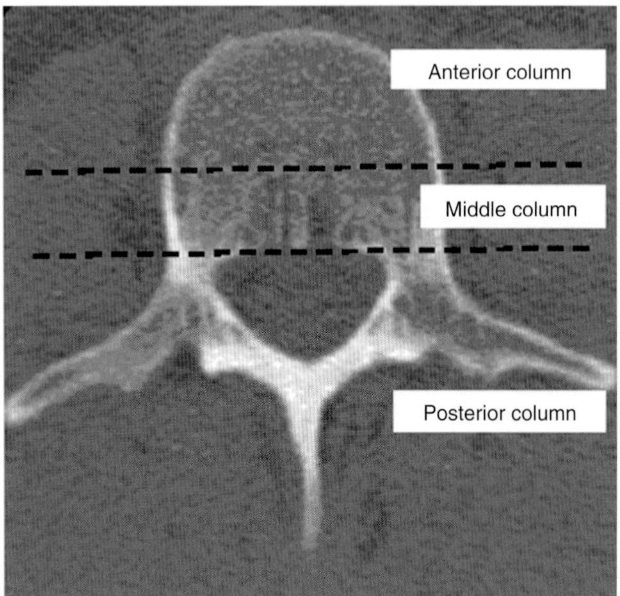

FIGURE 66-11. Axial CT of lumbar vertebral body illustrating Denis's three-column classification scheme of spine stability. This classification system divides the spine into an anterior column consisting not only of the anterior half of the vertebral body but the anterior longitudinal ligament. The middle column consists of the posterior half of the vertebral body and the posterior longitudinal ligament. The posterior column consists of the facets, laminae, and ligamentous complex.

the dorsal ligamentous complex, consists of the bony neural arch, posterior spinous ligaments, and ligamentum flavum, as well as the facet joints. According to the Denis classification scheme, rupture of the dorsal ligamentous complex creates instability only if there is concurrent disruption of at least the PLL and dorsal anulus.

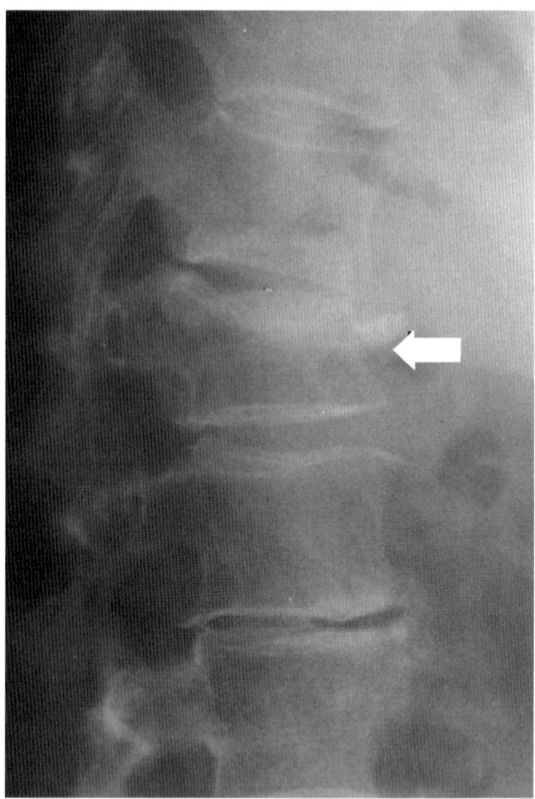

FIGURE 66-12. L1 vertebral compression fracture (*arrow*). Note the posterior vertebral body's height is maintained, and in the Denis classification only the anterior column is disrupted.

Denis[79] defined failure of the anterior column alone under compression (compression fracture) with an intact posterior column as a stable fracture (Fig. 66-12). Burst fractures were defined as being generated through an axial compressive load, and involved failure of the anterior and middle columns (Fig. 66-13). Severe tensile injuries resulted in seat belt fracture or flexion-distraction injuries, which involve a disruption of the posterior and middle columns with an intact anterior column that serves as a fulcrum or hinge (Fig. 66-14). The last category in Denis's scheme is fracture-dislocations, which are defined as a mechanical failure of all three columns, making them extremely unstable injuries (Fig. 66-15).

Denis organized instability into three categories: mechanical, neurologic, or both mechanical and neurologic. Mechanical instability may result in a late kyphotic deformity. For instance, a seat belt or severe compression fracture with compromise to the dorsal ligamentous complex may result in the spinal column falling into kyphosis, rotating around the intact middle column because of the deficient dorsal tension band.

External immobilization and, when appropriate, operative reduction and stabilization, may prevent this progressive deformity. Neurologic instability may occur after a severe burst fracture in which the middle column has ruptured under axial loads. This disruption and retropulsion of bone fragments into the spinal canal predisposes patients to an increased risk for neurologic injury, especially with increased spinal motion. Denis[79] reported that in 20% of patients with severe burst fractures and dorsal ligamentous injuries that were treated nonoperatively with external immobilization, a subsequent neurologic deficit developed. Neurologic and

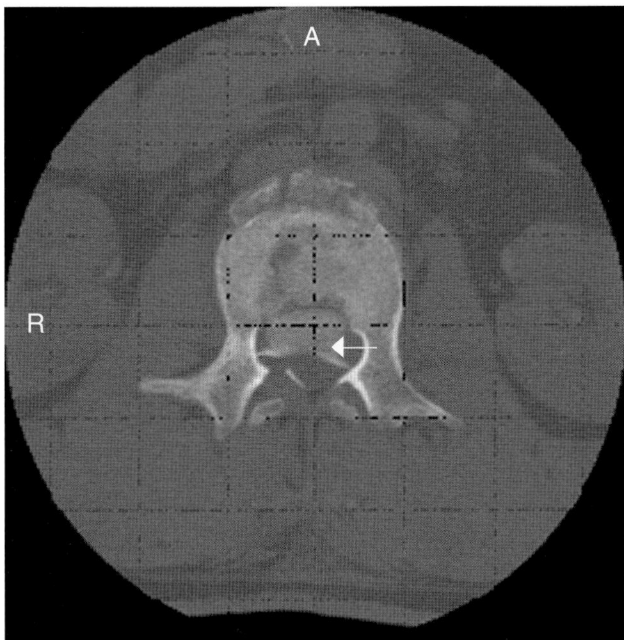

FIGURE 66-13. An 18-year-old man who sustained a 25-foot fall. Axial CT of L2 burst fracture details the canal encroachment of the retropulsed fracture (*arrow*). Note disruption of the posterior vertebral wall and splaying of the pedicles.

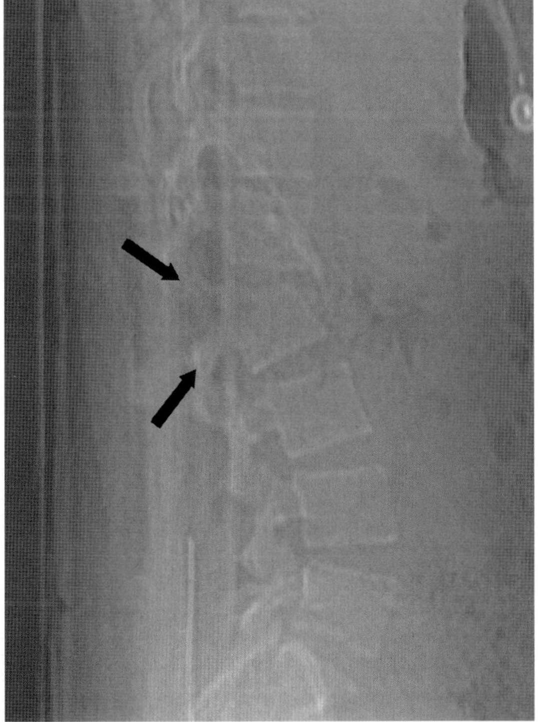

FIGURE 66-14. L2 Chance or seat belt fracture. Note this flexion-distraction injury splits the pedicle and facets (*arrows*), leaving the anterior column intact.

mechanical instability may develop after a burst fracture or fracture-dislocation, with or without an initial neurologic deficit. These are very unstable injuries and according to Denis's analysis require decompression and internal stabilization.

Magerl et al.[92] developed a comprehensive classification scheme based on pathomorphologic criteria. This system is modeled on the AO (*Arbeitsgemeinschaft für Osteosynthesefragen*) long bone fracture classification (developed by Müeller, Schneider, and Willenegger) and consists of a grid with three major fracture types, subdivided into three more groups, which are further subgrouped into three more categories.[92] The main categories are (A) compression injuries of the vertebral bodies, (B) distraction injuries that affect the anterior and posterior elements, and (C) axial torque or multidirectional injuries with translation that also affects the anterior and posterior elements. The severity of the fractures in this scheme increases as they progress from type A through type C. Although this classification system is extremely organized and comprehensive, it is underused clinically because of its complexity.

McCormack et al.[93] created a classification system based on a load-sharing principle that uses a graded point system reflecting the integrity of the vertebral bodies or anterior and middle columns. Points are based on the amount of vertebral body comminution, spread of fragments at the fracture site, and amount of corrected traumatic kyphosis (Fig. 66-16). Trauma associated with the highest degree of energy should result in the greatest dispersion and displacement of bone fragments. This classification can be applied before surgery to quantitatively estimate the extent of disruption of the anterior and middle columns. Patients with high point values (>6) have a large void or gap, resulting in the least supportive anterior and middle columns. Fractures with the greatest dispersion of fragments and least bone-to-bone contact result in the highest degree of cantilever bending loads on the pedicle screw implants, predisposing posterior instrumentation to failure.[15,94] This classification scheme assists the surgeon in deciding if ventral spine support is necessary after dorsal instrumentation, based on the premise that inadequate anterior column support will result in excessive loads being transferred to the dorsal elements (and instrumentation), thus increasing the risk for failure.

In 2009, the Spine Trauma Group created the Thoracolumbar Injury Classification and Severity Score (TLICS) system to address many of its predecessors' limitations.[95-97] The TLICS system defines injuries according to injury morphology, integrity of the posterior ligamentous complex, and neurologic status of the patient. It is the first thoracolumbar injury classification system to use injury morphology combined with the patient's neurologic status and the critically important status of the posterior ligamentous structures in medical decision making.

Consequently, the TLICS system was designed to aid in medical decision making by providing both diagnostic and prognostic information with a weighted injury severity score. Stable injury patterns (TLICS <4) may be treated nonoperatively with brace immobilization and active patient mobilization. Unstable injury patterns (TLICS >4) may be treated operatively with the guiding principles of deformity correction, neurologic decompression if necessary, and spine stabilization followed by active patient mobilization.[95]

So far, the TLICS system has shown good to excellent intraobserver and interobserver reliability in a number of countries, with both orthopedic surgeons and neurosurgeons, and throughout a spectrum of spine treatment providers with varying levels of experience.[95] The TLICS system has been tested in the setting of an academic trauma center, verifying that

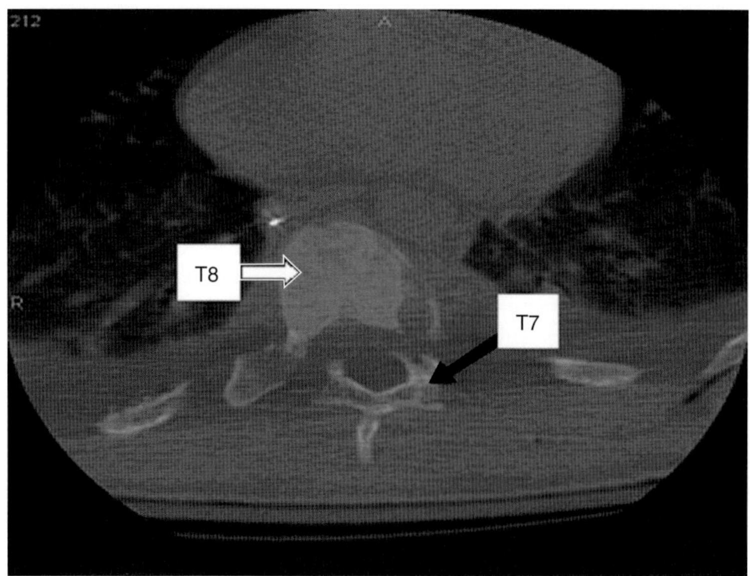

FIGURE 66-15. A 38-year-old man driven over by a truck presented with thoracic T7-8 dislocation and complete loss of motor function and sensation below the injury. The spine was fractured and dislocated, therefore separating all three columns of stability as detailed in the Denis classification.

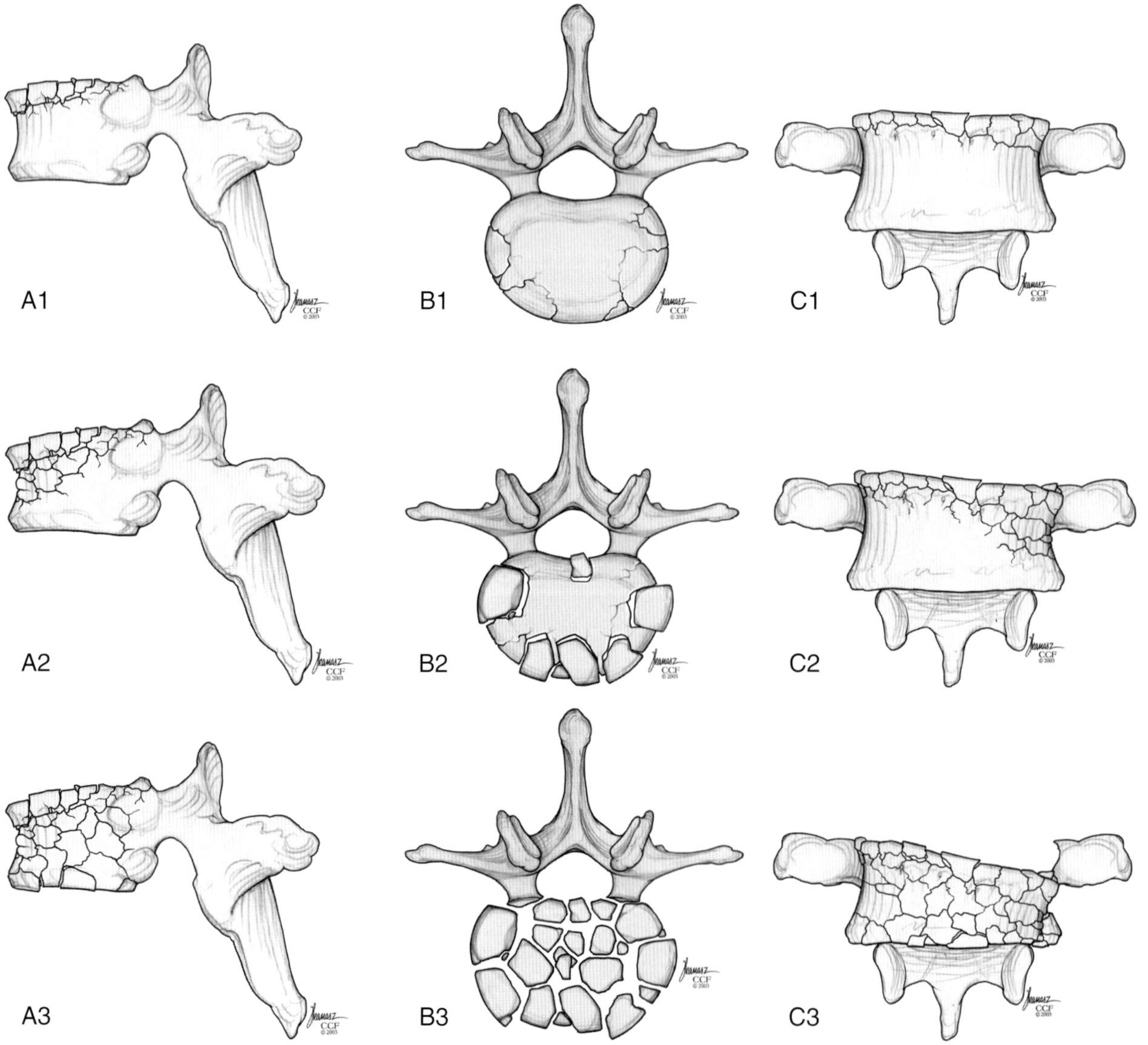

A1 B1 C1

A2 B2 C2

A3 B3 C3

FIGURE 66-16. McCormack grading scheme or load-sharing classification. Comminution of fragments based on a sagittal CT reformat: **A1**, little (<30%), one point; **A2**, moderate (30–60%), two points; **A3**, gross (>60%), three points. Apposition of fragments based on an axial CT scan: **B1**, minimal, one point; **B2**, spread, defined as greater than 2 mm in less than 50% of the body, two points; **B3**, wide, defined as greater than 2 mm in greater than 50% of the body, three points. Kyphosis correction based on plain radiographs: **C1**, less than 3 degrees, one point; **C2**, 4 to 9 degrees, two points; **C3**, greater than 10 degrees, three points. (Copyright Cleveland Clinic Foundation.)

physicians in training (residents and fellows) can readily be taught the TLICS system and incorporate it into patient care.[95] Furthermore, use of the TLICS system has yielded greater than 90% agreement in decision making for the management of thoracolumbar trauma across a number of providers.[98]

Although the TLICS system has demonstrated success, it has inherent limitations. To date, many of the investigations into the TLICS system have been performed by individuals involved with its development.[99] In addition, a prospective application of the TLICS system to the treatment of spine injuries is needed to define any improvements in care and patient outcomes compared with the use of conventional systems.

Treatment Options and Strategies

No definitive treatment algorithm has been universally accepted for thoracic spine injuries, despite the numerous classification systems that exist. Stability of the vertebral column over the thoracic and thoracolumbar region, like the remainder of the spine, depends on the integrity of the osseous and ligamentous components. Once these structures are disrupted, the stability of the vertebral column can become compromised, resulting in an unstable spine. One difficulty in treating these fractures is that spinal instability is difficult to assess, based on clinical and radiographic findings. White and Panjabi give the most detailed description of instability: "the loss of the ability of the spine under physiological loads to maintain relationships between vertebrae in such a way that there is either damage or subsequent irritation to the spinal cord or nerve roots, and in addition, there is development of incapacitating deformity or pain due to structural changes."[14] However, even this definition leaves a large degree of ambiguity because of the large spectrum of spinal disorders.

Nonoperative Strategies

Nonoperative treatment is indicated for stable injuries without the potential for progressive deformity or neurologic injury. One-column injuries such as compression fractures and posterior element fractures are stable by definition and can be treated nonoperatively unless excessive kyphosis is noted, which raises concern for increased pain and deformity in the future.

Treatment of two-column injuries, such as burst fractures, depends to a significant extent on the patient's neurologic status. In neurologically intact patients, nonoperative treatment is generally recommended.[14] A period of bed rest followed by mobilization in a thoracolumbosacral orthosis (TLSO) brace and continued close monitoring for increased kyphosis and neurologic changes are recommended.

Gertzbein demonstrated in a large study that kyphotic deformity greater than 30 degrees correlated with increased back pain.[6,56,82,100] This result has not been duplicated in other studies. There is an array of highly morbid complications that can arise from nonoperative treatment for a kyphosis of greater than 30 degrees. More specifically, acute to subacute neurologic deterioration from avoidance of surgery becomes the most serious untoward event. This has been proven by Denis et al.[45] who witnessed how, in 21% (6/29) of their patients in this series, a concerning and debilitating neurologic deficit developed after nonoperative treatment was undertaken. In a prospective study by Mumford et al. of 41 patients with a nonoperatively treated burst fracture, a neurologic deficit developed in 1 patient.[101]

Notwithstanding the aforementioned surgical experiences for kyphotic deformities, other authors such as Reid et al.[102] and Cantor et al.[40] have not necessarily noted an abrupt, or even progressive, decline in neurologic status by recommending a nonsurgical approach for patients with thoracolumbar burst fractures. It appears that the incidence of neurologic worsening lies between 0% and 20%. The inherent stability of the preserved ligaments and osseous structures usually prevents acute instability; however, a low potential for chronic or glacial instability still remains. Glacial instability usually presents as mechanical pain but could also present as a neurologic deficit.

VCFs, as discussed earlier, consist of a loss of anterior column or ventral vertebral body height as a result of axial compression. Anatomically, these fractures are considered stable if the dorsal ligamentous complex, along with the dorsal vertebral body, is not disrupted. Neurologic function should not be impaired in these fractures because the dorsal cortex of the vertebral body is not violated and there is no encroachment of fracture fragments on or into the spinal canal.

In the elderly, symptomatic compression fractures associated with severe pain and functional morbidity, which have not responded to a minimum of 6 weeks of conservative management, have been treated with polymethylmethacrylate (PMMA) augmentation, either through vertebroplasty or through a cavitation and end-plate elevation procedure (Fig. 66-17). These techniques have been associated with significant improvements in patient function and pain relief.[93,103,104]

Burst fractures, as defined by Denis,[45,79] are vertebral body fractures involving the anterior and middle columns, such that the ALL and vertebral body, including the dorsal vertebral body cortex, are disrupted (see Figs. 66-4, 66-6, 66-11, and 66-13). As stated earlier, a burst fracture in a neurologically intact patient without posterior ligamentous or dorsal element fractures is usually considered a stable injury. James et al.[105] confirmed this clinically in their reported series of patients with burst-type fractures with an intact dorsal bony architecture, all of whom became stable with a bracing regimen. Thoracic burst fractures (T1-10) make up a minor subset of burst injuries, representing approximately 5% to 10% of the total number of burst fractures. Thoracic burst fractures are inherently more stable because of the presence of the costovertebral ligamentous complex, along with the support of the rib cage.[106] Therefore, as with VCFs, conservative therapy using bracing and postural reduction has been the mainstay of treatment.[89,90,107]

The incidence and degree of kyphosis and neurologic deterioration after a thoracic or thoracolumbar burst fracture are not known. In the neurologically intact patient with a mild kyphotic deformity (<15 degrees) and minimal dorsal ligamentous disruption, a bracing strategy may be appropriate[108] (Fig. 66-18). This is corroborated by Rajasekaran,[109] who in 2009 reviewed the major series of burst fracture management in the previous 20 years and found that the results of conservative treatment were equal to those of surgery and also carried fewer complications. He mentions, however, that surgery for

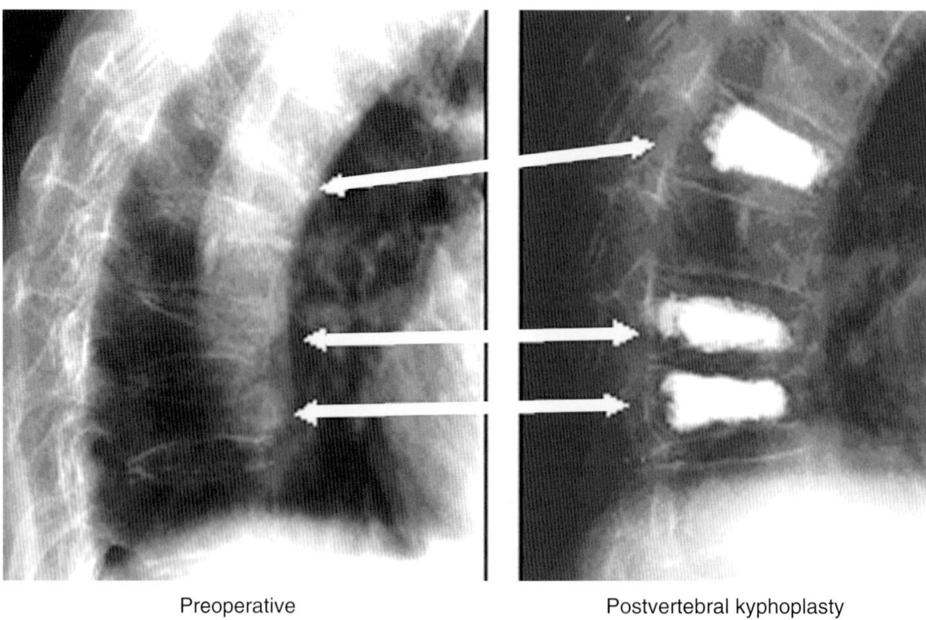

FIGURE 66-17. Three levels of kyphoplasty (vertebral augmentation with polymethylmethacrylate).

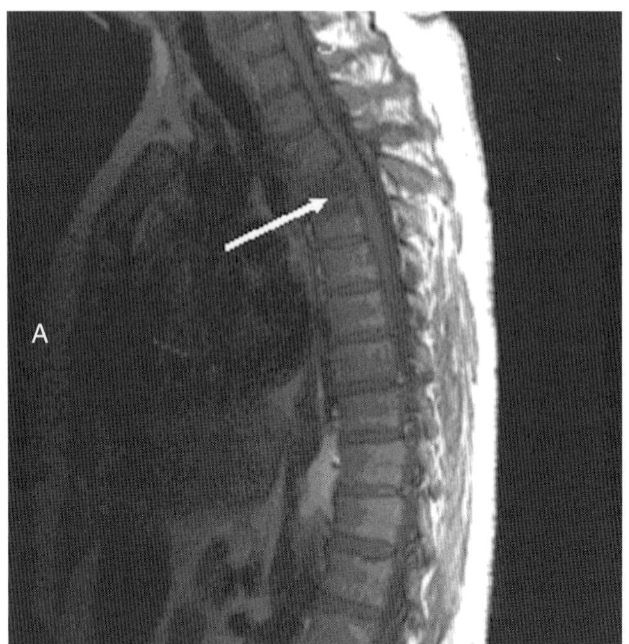

FIGURE 66-18. A 35-year-old man sustained a T4 burst fracture (*arrow*) with minimal retropulsion and normal strength on physical examination. He was treated in a thoracic brace with cervical extension and has had no neurologic decline or progression of kyphosis.

burst fractures may have definite advantages in patients with polytrauma or in the rare event of neurologic deterioration. Thus, nonoperative treatment can be safely adopted in the management of thoracolumbar burst fractures with a normal neurologic status. However, significantly divergent splaying of the spinous processes on lateral plain radiographs, which implies dorsal ligamentous complex disruption, suggests the potential for progressive instability, and in such cases surgical intervention should be considered.

Brown et al.[110] advocated nonoperative treatment of burst fractures with less than 50% of vertebral body collapse, less than 30 degrees of kyphotic deformity, and no more than 3 cm of offset from the standard sagittal vertical angle on lateral scoliosis films. These recommendations are supported by the findings of Cantor et al.,[40] where evidence of dorsal ligamentous complex disruption was present if there was greater than 30 degrees of kyphosis, greater than 50% loss of ventral vertebral body height, splaying of the spinous processes, facet fracture or subluxation, and pars interarticularis fracture. Brown et al.'s management protocol recommended immediate casting of the hemodynamically stable patient in a hyperextension body cast, followed by serial radiographs. Casts were maintained for 6 to 12 weeks, followed by a Jewett orthosis and then serial radiographs every 4 weeks. This management strategy facilitated early mobilization, reduced hospital stays and costs, and, when successful, avoided the risks of surgical therapy.

Nonoperative management therefore may be used in the neurologically intact patient, even with a large degree of spinal canal stenosis from retropulsed bone fragments, as long as there is no significant kyphosis representing significant disruption of the dorsal osteoligamentous complex.[111] CT has confirmed spontaneous remodeling through reabsorption of retropulsed bone fragments in the spinal canal in patients immobilized nonoperatively.[48] However, if there is a decline in the patient's neurologic status during nonoperative treatment, operative intervention is indicated in the presence of documented instability or neural compression.[101]

Operative Strategies

Wood et al.[112] published the first prospective, randomized study comparing operative and nonoperative treatment of a thoracolumbar burst fracture in patients without a neurologic deficit. They found that operative treatment of patients with a stable thoracolumbar burst fracture and normal findings on the neurologic examination provided no major long-term advantage compared with nonoperative treatment.

In general, there are only a handful of strict surgical indications for thoracolumbar burst fractures. Severe burst fractures with a neurologic deficit and canal compromise should be treated surgically. Moreover, in patients who are neurologically intact but have evidence of disruption of the posterior longitudinal ligament, inferred from greater than 25 degrees of kyphosis on radiographs or direct visualization of rupture of the PLL on fat-suppressed sagittal T2-weighted MRI, surgery is warranted.

There has, however, been a trend toward performing short-segment instrumentation at the thoracolumbar junction in an effort to preserve motion at adjacent levels. In this case, the McCormack classification seems useful in determining which patients would require an anterior stabilization in addition to the posterior short-segment instrumentation.[113]

Because of loss of integrity of the posterior column, distraction injuries, seat belt injuries, and Chance fractures require surgical stabilization to restore the posterior tension band. Translation injuries, rotational injuries, and those that shatter through the disc space and ligamentous complexes from ventral to dorsal always require surgical stabilization.

If surgical management is chosen, the next step is determining the most appropriate approach: anterior, posterior, or both.[114,115] Many factors, including fracture morphology and neurologic status, can play a role in this decision. Patients with complete neurologic deficit who are no longer in spinal shock have very little chance of significant neurologic recovery. The primary goal of surgery in this group is realignment and stabilization, typically through a posterior approach.[38]

Another option is anterior decompression and fusion with instrumentation. Surgeon preference often plays a role, as does fracture morphology. Concomitant lamina fractures with posterior canal compromise generally necessitate beginning with a posterior approach because of possible neural entrapment and dural tears.[116]

Flexion-distraction injuries result in disruption of the posterior and middle columns in tension.[117] Very often, the anterior column remains intact, acting as a hinge. Surgical intervention for these fractures typically involves a posterior approach. Anterior approaches are not routinely used in these injuries, to preserve the intact anterior column.

Fracture-dislocation injuries result in disruption of all three columns and hence carry a high incidence of complete spinal cord injury. Therefore, the main objective of surgical intervention is solely to provide posterior stabilization, facilitating early mobilization and rehabilitation. Anterior decompression and stabilization is performed after posterior surgical realignment of the fracture in those rare instances in which a partial neurologic deficit exists in the presence of significant anterior neural compression.

Ventral versus Dorsal Approaches

When a partial neurologic deficit is present, improving residual canal compromise is also a goal of surgery. This situation most typically occurs with burst fractures. If performed early enough (generally within 72 hours), posterior instrumentation allows for distraction and correction of sagittal alignment and successful indirect decompression of the spinal canal. Laminectomy with transpedicular decompression also can improve the canal clearance achieved through a posterior approach. A ventral or dorsolateral approach may effectively decompress the neural elements in the setting of spinal cord compression. The ventral approach is particularly useful for decompressing midline ventral lesions and correcting severe kyphotic deformities.[11,48] Bohlman et al.[26,27] reported superior neurologic outcomes after a ventral, compared with a dorsal, procedure in the setting of an incomplete thoracic spinal cord injury. The major limitation of a ventral exposure is the potential surgical violation of the pleural and/or peritoneal cavities. McCormick[22] reported the effective use of an extrapleural technique for the exposure of the ventral thoracic and thoracolumbar spine, thus avoiding violation of the pleural cavity.

Dorsal decompression by laminectomy after thoracic and thoracolumbar injuries has been shown to be ineffective and should not be performed as an isolated treatment strategy.[11,118] The surgical removal or destruction of the dorsal ligamentous complex, along with the dorsal osseous elements, may permit temporary neurologic recovery. However, the vertebral column may not be able to maintain its alignment with the loss of the dorsal tension band, and instability, along with the potential progression of a kyphotic deformity, may ensue (Fig. 66-19). The immediate result of removing the dorsal osseous components is dorsal migration of the spinal cord if the spine has a lordotic alignment. However, the normal, untraumatized spinal column at the thoracolumbar junction maintains a slightly kyphotic posture. Spine trauma typically results in an increase in the kyphotic deformity or angulation. Therefore, removing the dorsal tension band after trauma in the setting of ventral compression from bone fragments may result in further neurologic compromise, caused by tethering of the neural elements over ventral bony elements (bowstring effect).

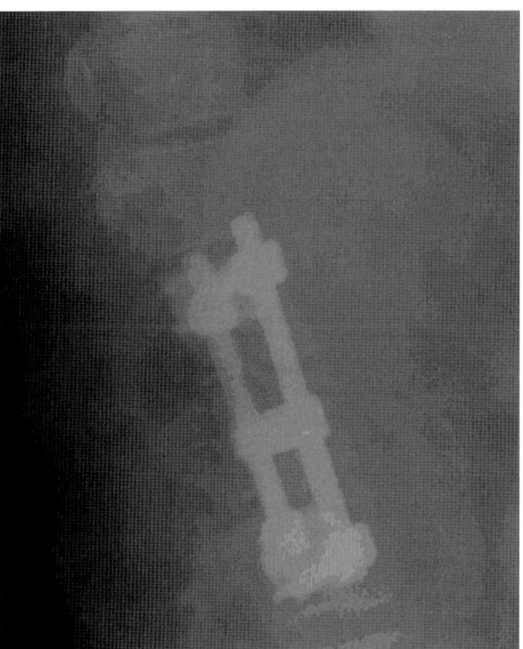

FIGURE 66-19. Anterior corpectomy and decompression after a burst fracture, followed with an anterior iliac crest bone graft fusion with a Kaneda device.

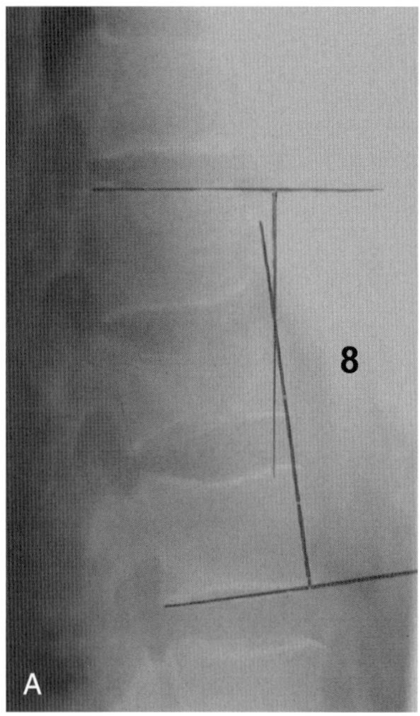

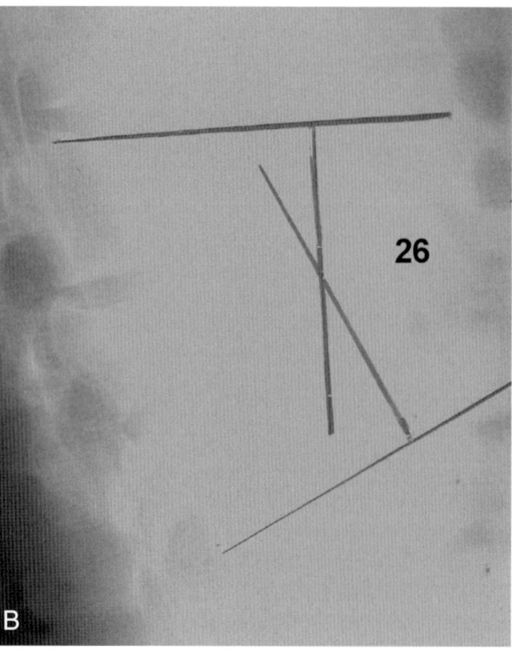

FIGURE 66-20. A 50-year-old man with an L2 burst fracture after a fall. **A,** Plain sagittal radiograph illustrating 8 degrees of kyphosis. **B,** He was treated in a body cast and then braced but had progressive back pain; follow-up radiographs illustrated progression of the kyphosis to 26 degrees.

Biomechanically, ventral as opposed to dorsal reconstruction and instrumentation strategies provide superior mechanical stability over an equal number of spinal segments to compressive loads.[57,119] A patient with midline ventral spinal cord compression, an incomplete neurologic injury, and an unstable thoracic or thoracolumbar junction burst fracture is most effectively treated with a ventral decompression and reconstruction procedure (Fig. 66-20). A variety of ventral instrumentation systems are available that may be applied to the ventral spinal elements after an adequate decompression and fusion procedure. Biomechanically, ventral bicortical screws provide a 25% to 50% increase in screw purchase strength compared with unilateral screws.[120]

An advantage of a dorsal approach is that it provides excellent visualization and access to the dorsal thecal sac. This is useful in certain fracture types because the reported incidence of thecal sac lacerations (with the potential for nerve root incarceration) after traumatic thoracic and thoracolumbar burst fractures is 7% to 16%.[121,122] The lumbar nerve roots are prone to entrapment through these lacerations, and a ventral approach will not provide access to repair this deficiency.[123] The presence of a central split or greenstick fracture of the spinous process on preoperative transaxial CT may be an indicator of a dural laceration, depending on its size and displacement during impact.[124]

Surgical Stabilization Methods

Harrington rods were the first spinal implants widely used for the treatment of vertebral fractures.[125] The dorsal spinal elements are distracted to reduce and realign the vertebral column by ligamentotaxis.[9] Unfortunately, this artificially applied distraction force can result in the loss of the normal spinal curvature (loss of lordosis or exaggeration of kyphosis), resulting in muscles and ligaments working at a biomechanical disadvantage.[126] Harrington rods perform relatively poorly in three-column injuries because of a predisposition to overdistraction and the relatively high incidence of rod breakage and hook cutout (7–10%).

Although Harrington instrumentation can be used, it has mostly been supplanted by newer segmental instrumentation systems initially developed for scoliosis. These systems use multiple fixed anchors along the fixation rod. Application of multiple forces at different points is possible, resulting in a relatively low incidence of fixation failure. Compression, distraction, and translation are all possible using the same construct. Initially, these systems used hooks (sublaminar, pedicle, and transverse process) for fixation, but most now allow for pedicle screw fixation as well.

Pedicle screw fixation allows for instrumentation of vertebrae with fractured or absent laminae. In addition, pedicle screw fixation allows for rigid bony purchase through all three columns. Because of this increased rigidity, it is often possible to use fewer segments for stable fixation, allowing the preservation of more motion segments. Preserving motion segments is of less importance in the thoracic spine because little motion is lost compared with the cervical and lumbar segments. However, limiting instrumentation of distal segments is important in thoracolumbar injuries.[106]

The osseous structures are fused concomitantly with posterior instrumentation. Some surgeons fuse only the injured vertebral segments with subsequent staged removal of hardware. Others fuse the entire length of the instrumentation, which results in loss of motion at additional segments. As mentioned, this is of less importance in the thoracic spine. With modern segmental fixation, fewer segments need to be instrumented to provide stability, and generally, the entire instrumented region is fused.[127]

Individual anatomic factors, such as the presence of lamina fractures, often dictate choice of anchors. In the thoracic spine, it is not uncommon for pedicles to be too small to allow screw placement. Depending on the injury, two to three segments of fixation above and below the level of injury usually are required if hooks alone are used. With pedicle screws, this often can be limited to one or two segments.

The condition of the anterior column also can affect instrumentation choices. If severe comminution or kyphosis is present, extending the length of the dorsal instrumentation should be considered. This will allow for added anterior column support toward the construct as a whole. This is often an issue with burst fractures, with which ventral strut graft fusion may be required.

Neurologic Decompression for Incomplete Injuries

Neurologic injuries are present in 42% of patients with thoracolumbar junction fractures.[56] Approximately 90% of patients with a thoracic fracture, excluding a VCF, have a concurrent neurologic injury, with 63% having a complete neurologic deficit.[128] Compression of the spinal cord after thoracic or thoracolumbar trauma is typically caused by a ventral retropulsed bone fragment from the vertebral body. Complete loss of neurologic function below the level of the injury usually occurs at the moment of trauma, and therefore removing the retropulsed bone in the setting of a complete neurologic injury (American Spinal Injury Association [ASIA] type A) rarely, if ever, enhances neurologic recovery.[48] However, in the presence of an incomplete neurologic deficit with persistent compression of the neural elements, a decompressive procedure may maximize the potential for neurologic recovery.[8]

Hence, timing of surgery becomes an important issue in the treatment of thoracic spine fractures. Progressive neurologic deficit in the presence of continued canal compromise is an accepted indication for immediate decompression and stabilization. Quite often, patients with thoracic spine fractures have concomitant injuries, making the timing of spinal stabilization difficult to plan. Some studies suggest that patients with thoracic spine fractures treated within 72 hours, regardless of concomitant injuries, do much better physiologically after surgery than those in whom stabilization is delayed. Early fixation results in less time in the intensive care unit, less ventilator support, a decreased rate of pulmonary complications, and less overall time in the hospital. Boerger et al.[48] performed a meta-analysis of the world literature to analyze surgical outcome after decompression of the spinal cord after thoracolumbar burst fractures. Patients with an incomplete neurologic deficit who underwent an operative decompression and stabilization procedure in less than 72 hours were shown to have an enhanced neurologic recovery compared with nonoperatively treated patients.[48,129] Operative therapy has also been shown to decrease pain, reduce periods of postural reduction or bed rest, and improve sagittal alignment.[56] At present, surgical decompression in patients with a complete neurologic injury has not demonstrated true benefit in terms of overall neurologic improvement.[27]

Additional Operative Considerations

Fracture-dislocations are the most unstable of traumatic vertebral column injuries. The fractures are created by significant high-energy loads that result in a complete dissociation of the osseous structures and ligamentous complexes. Typically these carry a complete loss of neurologic function[45,130] (see Fig. 66-15). Flexion-distraction-dislocation injuries have a significant distraction component and differ from seat belt–type injuries in that there is a large rotatory or torque component that causes a disruption of all three spinal columns.[79] An injury of this type in the thoracic region almost always results in a complete spinal cord injury. Such injuries are associated with the highest incidence of concurrent neurologic injuries.[79] Denis reported that over 50% of patients with this fracture subtype had a complete paraplegia.[79]

Patients with a complete neurologic injury involving the thoracic spine may frequently benefit from surgical intervention to realign a deformity, provide immediate stability, and prevent further or future neurologic injury. This expedites their transfer to a facility so they can begin rehabilitation and can subsequently be placed erect without further injury to the spinal cord proper.[131] Postural reduction and bed rest mandate at least 6 to 12 weeks of prolonged immobilization before the spine heals enough to attain any degree of intrinsic stability.[130]

Indirect augmentation of the anterior column through a dorsal transpedicular approach, without removal or replacement of the contiguous intervertebral discs, does not appear to provide sufficient anterior column support. Alanay et al.[132] demonstrated that short-segment transpedicular screw fixation through a dorsal approach failed equally (approximately 50%) with and without transpedicular bone graft augmentation. The lateral extracavitary approach provides access to both the ventral and dorsal portion of the vertebral column through a single dorsal incision. However, this approach has limited usefulness in thoracic and lumbar trauma because of its high incidence of associated morbidities. For example, Resnick and Benzel[133] reviewed their series of 33 trauma patients treated with this approach and reported a 55% incidence of morbidity.

Summary

The care of patients with thoracolumbar spine trauma with or without neurologic deficits has evolved dramatically over the past 30 years. The development of more effective spinal instrumentation and anesthesia techniques coupled with the establishment of spine injury care centers where immediate treatment and rehabilitation can be administered successively has definitely improved the care of these patients. Despite these advances, the majority of patients with thoracolumbar injuries are still treated nonoperatively with cast or brace immobilization and early ambulation. More aggressive treatment is guided by the use of classification systems that detail the mechanism of injury, the degree of compromise of spinal structures, and the potential for late mechanical instability or neural injury. Even now, the goal of treatment remains attainment of spinal stability with protection or improvement of the patient's neurologic status, allowing rapid and maximal functional recovery. Guidelines such as the TLICS system are now in place to help the clinician make better-educated decisions as to which patients to treat operatively and which to manage nonoperatively.

Successful management of thoracolumbar spine injuries protects the patient from further spinal deformity and neurologic deficit. As we have seen here, there is no clear consensus as to the absolute indications for surgical intervention in patients with many types of thoracolumbar fractures.

KEY REFERENCES

Denis F: The three column spine and its significance in the classification of acute thoracolumbar spinal injuries. *Spine (Phila Pa 1976)* 8:817–831, 1983.

Haber TR, Filmy WT, O'Brien M: Thoracic and lumbar fractures: diagnosis and management. In Bridwell KH, DeWald PR, editors: *The textbook of spinal surgery*, Philadelphia, 1991, JB Lippincott, pp 857–910.

Magerl F, Aebi M, Gertzbein SD, et al: A comprehensive classification of thoracic and lumbar fractures. *Eur Spine J* 3:184–201, 1994.

McCormack BM, Benzel EC, Adams MS, et al: Anatomy of the thoracic pedicle. *Neurosurgery* 37:303–308, 1995.

Patel AA, Dailey A, Brodke DS, et al: Spine Trauma Study Group: thoracolumbar spine trauma classification: the Thoracolumbar Injury Classification and Severity Score system and case examples. *J Neurosurg Spine* 10: 201–206, 2009.

Rajasekaran S: Thoracolumbar burst fractures without neurological deficit: the role for conservative treatment. *Eur Spine J* 19(Suppl 1):40–47, 2010.

White AA, Panjabi MM: *Clinical biomechanics of the spine*, Philadelphia, 1978, JB Lippincott.

Wood K, Buttermann G, Mehbod A, et al: Operative compared with nonoperative treatment of a thoracolumbar burst fracture without neurological deficit: a prospective, randomized study. *J Bone Joint Surg [Am]* 85:773–781, 2003.

REFERENCES

The complete reference list is available online at expertconsult.com.

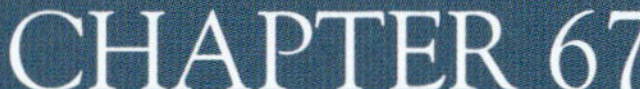

CHAPTER 67

Trauma Surgery: Lumbar and Sacral Fractures

Chris J. Neal | Richard G. Fessler

Fractures of the lumbosacral spine due to trauma involve injury to the portion of the spine that transitions from the relatively immobile thoracic segment to a mobile lumbar segment to the sacrum, which forms the keystone of a relatively immobile pelvic ring. This area also houses the terminus of the spinal cord with its accompanying nerve roots innervating the lower extremities, bowel, bladder, and genitalia. This section of the spine, however, can be divided into four distinct biomechanical segments: the thoracolumbar junction, the midlumbar spine, the lumbosacral junction, and the sacrum. Although the fracture patterns and associated neurologic deficits overlap somewhat in this classification, it is important to understand that similar fractures along the lumbosacral spine require different treatment strategies to optimize patient outcomes.

The upper lumbar spine (L1-2) should be considered as part of the thoracolumbar junction (T11-L2). The thoracolumbar junction is unique in that it transitions from a relatively immobile thoracic spine to the more mobile lumbar spine. Biomechanically, this difference results in a region of high stress at the interface between these two segments. The majority of the thoracic spine is resistant to rotational forces because of the stabilizing effect of the rib cage.[1] However, the thoracolumbar spine lacks attachments to the rib cage and has a transitional facet structure that is unable to resist rotational forces. As a result, 60% of all spinal fractures occur between T12 and L2 and 90% occur between T11 and L4.[2,3]

Fractures of the mid to caudal lumbar spine (L3-5) account for approximately 4% of all spinal fractures. The transition into the lumbar spine results in larger vertebral bodies, designed to sustain greater axial loads, and significantly more muscular attachments, adding to its stability.[4,5] However, the facets in the upper lumbar spine are more oblique in orientation, transitioning to a sagittal orientation at the lumbosacral junction. This results in more translational mobility.[6] The change in facet orientation, the increased mobility, and the lack of a thoracic cage actually make the lumbar spine more susceptible to injury than the thoracic spine.

The lumbosacral junction is a transition zone from a mobile, lordotic segment to a relatively immobile, kyphotic segment. Since the sacrum typically lies at an incline, as measured by the sacral slope and pelvic tilt from horizontal and vertical reference lines, respectively, axial loads result in rotational forces. These rotational forces are resisted by the strength of the sacrotuberous and sacrospinous ligaments, which attach opposite the S4 neural foramina. Fractures of the lumbosacral junction rarely occur in isolation and are typically associated with a sacral fracture.

The sacrum with its intimate attachments to the pelvis is a very stable structure.[7] The relatively immobile sacroiliac joint and strong ventral and dorsal ligamentous attachments between the sacrum and pelvis account for this stability. The sacrum forms a portion of the dorsal pelvic arch and, as a result, most sacral fractures occur in conjunction with pelvic fractures. The sacrum is critical to pelvic ring stability. Removal of the sacrum distal to the S1-2 interspace weakens the pelvic ring by 30%, whereas resection up to S1, which requires removal of half of the sacroiliac joint, weakens the pelvic ring by 50%.[8]

Spine Stability

A discussion of spine fractures necessitates a definition of spine stability since the goal of any clinically applicable characterization of fracture pattern and subsequent treatment paradigm relies on the concept of restoring the spine to its preinjury functional capacity. White and Panjabi define spinal stability as the ability of the spine to maintain physiologic loads without pain, deformity, or neurologic deficit.[9] Conversely, Benzel describes instability as the inability to limit excessive or abnormal spinal displacement.[10] These terms are somewhat nebulous, and we agree with the concept that spinal stability should be considered as part of a dynamic process that takes into account multiple parameters, such as actual segment loading, activity level, and chronicity. A detailed discussion of spinal stability is outside the scope of this chapter, but the spine surgeon must have a general concept of acute and chronic instability. With trauma, the initial decision of whether to operate depends in part on whether the fracture is acutely unstable. As described later in this chapter, multiple classification systems based on radiographic and clinical examination help to determine if the injury is acutely unstable. However, the potential of chronic instability should not be ignored. Recognizing injury patterns that lead to chronic instability and that pose a risk of posttraumatic deformity is essential to the long-term care of trauma patients.

Mechanism of Injuries

In general, the mechanism of injury to the lumbosacral spine is blunt, although penetrating trauma does occur, especially in a military or combat situation. For penetrating injuries, the key component to the extent and pattern of injury is the amount of kinetic energy (KE) released at the time of impact. The formula KE = 1/2 mv^2, where m is mass and v is velocity, explains that the higher the velocity of the projectile, the more kinetic energy it disperses on impact, and, hence, the greater the resulting damage. Most spine injury classifications and subsequent treatment paradigms are based on blunt trauma, with penetrating trauma patterns imposed within that system. Like any injury, the mechanism should be considered when determining a treatment plan, with the understanding that penetrating injuries of the spine are different from their blunt counterparts; this difference is primarily determined by the kinetic energy imparted by the projectile (Fig. 67-1).

Prehospital Management

All patients involved in major trauma should be treated as having a potential spinal injury until proven otherwise. This treatment includes multiperson patient transfers, log rolling, and the use of a cervical orthosis and a backboard. Every attempt should be made to maintain the spinal column in as near neutral alignment as possible. Initial management in the field should follow an advanced life support protocol. A stable airway, adequate ventilation, and hemodynamic stability should be maintained. Preventing hypoxia and hypotension is critical to preserving neural element function after trauma. Once a patient is stabilized, a neurologic examination should be performed, keeping in mind that concomitant head injury, intoxication, or injury to the extremities may make a thorough examination difficult or impossible.[11] A "normal" neurologic examination in the field does not rule out a spinal injury.

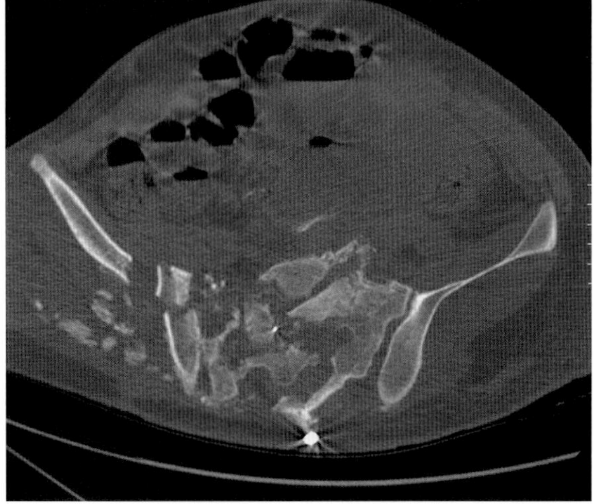

FIGURE 67-1. Fragmentation injury to the abdomen resulting in pelvic and sacral disruption. (Courtesy of Michael Rosner.)

Initial Hospital Management

Because the thoracolumbar spine is relatively resistant to injury, the amount of force required to result in a fracture makes these traumas high risk for associated neurologic and retroperitoneal injury. It has been reported that 4.4% of all patients arriving at a level I trauma center have a fracture in the thoracolumbar spine and approximately 19% to 50% have a neurologic deficit.[12-15] Even with modern spinal immobilization techniques, the concern still exists for an unstable fracture that could result in a new neurologic injury or neurologic deterioration. In a study by Reid et al., fractures of the thoracolumbar spine that were diagnosed in a delayed fashion had a higher incidence of a new neurologic deficit than those diagnosed at the time of admission (10.5% vs. 1.4%).[16] Unfortunately, delay in the diagnosis of thoracolumbar injuries is not uncommon. In a retrospective review, Dai et al. found that 28 of 147 patients with acute thoracolumbar injuries had a thoracolumbar fracture that was not diagnosed at the time of admission. Although some diagnoses were delayed secondary to resuscitation efforts or acute surgical intervention, 37% of these patients (7/19) with fractures did not undergo initial radiographic evaluation because of a lack of clinical suspicion and another 26% (5/19) had radiographs but their fractures were either misclassified or not diagnosed at all.[17] Because of the potential for neurologic injury from a missed injury, some authors have suggested that the thoracolumbar spine should be imaged in all patients with polytrauma.[16,18]

Certain injury mechanisms should raise the suspicion of associated spinal fractures. Patients jumping or falling from heights with significant lower-extremity injury, calcaneal injuries in particular, are at high risk for accompanying lumbar and thoracolumbar spine injuries. Patients involved in motor vehicle accidents and wearing lap belts only are at risk for flexion distraction injuries. Lumbar fractures have been associated with abdominal and urologic trauma, particularly in cases of lap belt injuries.[19] Sacral fractures are often associated with injury to the pelvic ring.

The evaluation of the thoracolumbar spine starts with the primary and secondary surveys to include visual inspection and manual palpation for stepoffs or other bony abnormalities. Bruising of the abdomen may be a sign of an underlying lap belt–type injury. An abnormal posture may be indicative of muscle spasm and associated spinal injury. Using full spinal precautions, the patient should be log-rolled and the skin and contour of the neck and back examined. Bruising, stepoff, deviation from the normal spinal curvature, or pain with dorsal midline palpation may be indicative of an underlying bony and ligamentous injury. In the patient with a head injury, verbal response to questions about pain during palpation may not be entirely reliable.

A neurologic examination should be carried out in a systematic and standardized fashion. Results should be communicated using the American Spinal Injury Association (ASIA) grading system (described elsewhere in this book). This facilitates communication between treating specialties. Progressive neurologic deterioration is a widely accepted indication for acute intervention. It is, therefore, imperative that baseline neurologic function be accurately established. In the confused or obtunded patient, facial grimace or withdrawal to painful stimuli can serve as a gross motor and sensory examination. A rectal examination should be performed to assess perianal sensation, rectal tone, and a bulbocavernosus reflex. Radiographic studies of other areas of injury should be evaluated closely for patterns that may indicate a direction of force through the thoracolumbar spine.

The pattern of neurologic injury observed depends on the location of spinal injury. In the majority of patients, the conus medullaris lies directly opposite the L1 vertebral body. The conus medullaris contains the anterior horn cells of the L5 through S5 nerves. Both upper motor neuron (conus injury) and lower motor neuron (cauda equina) injury can occur. The injury pattern runs the spectrum from a complete injury below L1 to incomplete syndromes resulting in partial motor and sensory preservation with sacral dysfunction. The sacral nerve roots are the most sensitive to injury and the least likely to improve after injury. Injury to the sacral spinal cord and nerve roots can result in loss of bowel and bladder function; sexual function is often less severely affected. Injuries from L2-5 can result in isolated root injuries or cauda equina syndrome. Root injuries can appear as monoradiculopathy or polyradiculopathy. Cauda equina syndrome appears as variable sensory, motor, bowel, and/or bladder dysfunction. Sensory and motor loss tend to be asymmetrical. This tendency is in contradistinction to the conus medullaris syndrome, in which deficits are usually more symmetrical.[20] Sphincteric dysfunction is common and is often permanent.

Radiographic Evaluation

In compliant patients with unaltered metal status, no distracting injuries, and lack of midline spinal tenderness, the spine can be cleared without obtaining screening plain radiographs.[21] However, if the patient does not meet any of the preceding criteria, radiographic evaluation is mandatory. One should bear in mind that between 5% and 20% of all spine fractures are multiple, and 5% occur at noncontiguous levels.[22] Commonly, radiographic evaluation includes anteroposterior (AP) and lateral views of the cervical, thoracic, lumbar, and sacral spine and an open-mouth odontoid view. Flexion-extension studies are generally avoided in the workup of acute fractures. Spinal alignment should be assessed in both planes. The margins of the vertebral bodies and the spinolaminar line, facets, interspinous and interpedicular distances, and position of the transverse process should be studied. Acute kyphotic angulation or loss of lordosis may be indicative of an acute bony or ligamentous injury. Loss of disc height at the level above a vertebral body fracture is often observed in acute flexion injuries, but it may also be seen in cases of degenerative disc disease. Bare, or "naked," facets may be indicative of posterior ligamentous injury as a result of a distraction-type injury. Abnormalities of the soft tissues, such as a paraspinal mass or loss of the psoas stripe, can help identify areas of adjacent bony injury.

Per advanced trauma life support (ATLS) guidelines, all patients sustaining high-energy trauma should have an AP radiograph of the pelvis. However, these images are often inadequate for evaluating the sacrum due to sacral inclination, bowel gas, and, sometimes, the overlying anterior pelvis.[23] Nork et al. identified L5 transverse process fractures and a paradoxic inlet view on AP pelvic radiographs as factors suggestive of sacral fractures.[24] Others have identified the foraminal stepladder sign, caused by a displaced and overriding transverse fracture, and disruption of the anterior sacral foraminal lines or sacral arcuate line as diagnostic clues.[25-27] Sacral fracture should be suspected in any patient with a pelvic ring injury associated with a neurologic deficit.[28-30]

Computed Tomography

In many institutions, AP and lateral radiographs are the standard screening tools for evaluating thoracolumbar fractures. However, plain radiographs have been criticized for their lack of sensitivity, diagnostic inaccuracies, and for the amount of time required for adequate views. Many have advocated the use of CT as the primary means of evaluating the thoracolumbar spine. Multiple studies have shown that CT scans are more sensitive for detecting fractures in the spine than plain radiographs.[31-34] However, CT carries with it concerns about cost and radiation exposure. In 2004, Brandt et al. found that for 50 patients undergoing radiographic evaluation, the average time for a CT of the chest/abdomen/pelvis was 55 minutes ± 32 minutes with a cost of $654. For thoracic, lumbar, and sacral plain radiographs, the average time was 113 minutes ± 43 minutes. The cost of the radiographic evaluation of the spine in addition to dedicated CT scanning of the spine and viscera was $1487.[35] Wintermark et al. found that an average of 4.3 views were needed to adequately evaluate the thoracolumbar spine; 9% of the thoracolumbar films had to be retaken because of insufficient quality. Time needed to perform conventional radiographs was 33 minutes, with 70% (23/33 minutes) devoted to imaging the thoracolumbar spine. This compares with the median time to perform a cervical, thoracic, abdominal, and cranial CT of 40 minutes, including 7 minutes for reformatting and reconstructions of the films.[36] There is no level I evidence regarding the use of CT as a standard for diagnosing spine fractures, but a single series of CT scans that can be reformatted specifically to evaluate the spine has proven to be at least equal to if not superior to, plain radiographs in several studies.[37]

Obtaining appropriate radiographs of sacral injuries is problematic. In one series, 49% of sacral fractures were missed on initial hospital presentation, including 24% with an "unexplained" neurologic deficit that was later explained by the presence of a fracture.[38] The sacrum is poorly visualized on standard AP views of the pelvis, so the treating physician must rely on other cues to prompt a more detailed survey of this region. CT with coronal and axial reformations is the most sensitive modality for defining complex pelvic and sacral fractures. For all radiographic measurement parameters, the Spine Trauma Study Group advocates the use of thin-section (1.0–1.5 mm) axial CT scans with coronal and sagittal reconstruction rather than plain radiographs.[39]

Magnetic Resonance Imaging

MRI can be useful in the study of neurologic deficit to determine the extent of compression on the neural elements. Although current MRI techniques are in many ways more sensitive than CT in detecting areas of acute injury, they do not provide the bony detail provided by conventional CT. Increased signal on T2-weighted imaging may be used to detect fractures that are not well visualized on plain radiographs or CT. Short tau

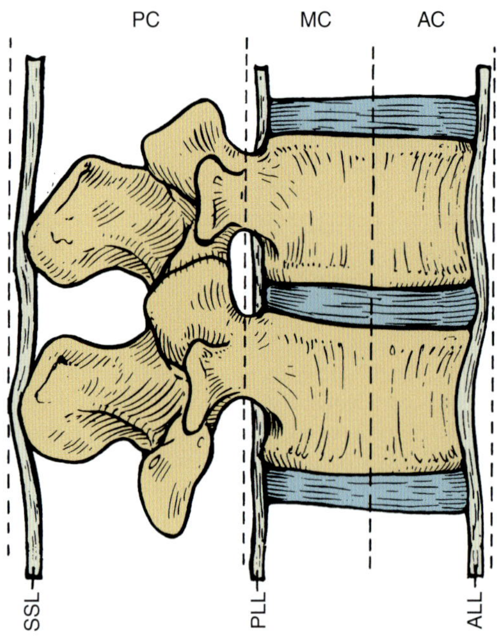

FIGURE 67-2. Three columns of the spine: anterior column (AC), middle column (MC), and posterior column (PC). ALL, anterior longitudinal ligament; PLL, posterior longitudinal ligament; SSL, supraspinous ligament. (From Haber TR, Felmly WT, O'Brien M: Thoracic and lumbar fractures: diagnosis and management. In Bridwell KH, DeWald RL, editors: *Textbook of spinal surgery,* vol 2, Philadelphia, 1991, JB Lippincott, pp 857–910.)

inversion recovery (STIR) sequences are quite sensitive for the detection of ligamentous and intervertebral disc injury not otherwise apparent by plain radiographs or CT.

Classification of Injuries

Several classification systems have been developed to describe fractures of the thoracic and lumbar spine. In 1983, both Denis and McAfee et al. independently published three-column models that have become widely accepted (Fig. 67-2).[2,40] These models are very similar but do have some fundamental differences (Table 67-1).[41] Each model divides the vertebra into three columns: anterior column (anterior longitudinal ligament, ventral half of the vertebral body, and ventral half of the anulus fibrosus), middle column (posterior longitudinal ligament, dorsal half of the vertebral body, and dorsal half of the anulus fibrosus), and posterior column (supraspinous and infraspinous ligaments, ligamentum flavum, articular processes, joint capsules, spinous processes, and laminae). In Denis's model, instability requires injury to at least two columns with an emphasis on preservation of the middle column for the maintenance of stability. Fractures are divided into four groups: wedge compression (Fig. 67-3), burst fracture (Fig. 67-4), lap belt–type injury (Fig. 67-5), and fracture-dislocation (Fig. 67-6). Instability varies in magnitude: first degree (mechanical), second degree (neurologic), and third degree (mechanical and neurologic). McAfee's system places more emphasis on preservation of the posterior column for the maintenance of stability and defines six fracture patterns: wedge compression, Chance fracture, flexion-distraction injury, stable burst, unstable burst, and translational injury.

In 1994, Magerl et al. proposed the *Arbeitsgemeinschaft für Osteosynthesefragen* (AO) system, based on the review of 1445 consecutively treated thoracolumbar injuries. There are three main types of fractures (types A, B, C), with a progression in the severity of injury from type A to type C. Each category contains subclassifications. Type A injuries are compressive forces acting on the vertebral body. Type B injuries are characterized by a distraction mechanism with disruption of the anterior and posterior elements. Type C lesions are rotational injuries involving the anterior and posterior elements.[42] Although more accurately descriptive than the three-column classification, the AO system is often viewed as cumbersome to apply in a clinical setting.

In 2005, the Spine Trauma Study Group devised a thoracolumbar injury classification and severity score scale.[43] This system relies on three characteristics to describe the injury: injury morphology, the integrity of the posterior ligamentous complex, and neurologic status (Table 67-2) Points are

TABLE 67-1

Comparison of Three-Column Classification Schemes

FRACTURE TYPE		SPINAL COLUMN FAILURE			ASSESSMENT OF STABILITY	
Denis	**McAfee**	**Anterior**	**Middle**	**Posterior**	**Denis**	**McAfee**
Wedge compression	Wedge compression	X			Stable*	Generally stable†
Lap belt–type injury	Chance fracture		X	X	Unstable‡	Generally stable§
	Flexion-distraction	X	X	X		Generally unstable
Burst fracture	Stable burst	X	X		Unstable‖	Stable
	Unstable burst	X	X	X		Unstable
Fracture-dislocation	Translational injury	X	X	X	Unstable¶	Unstable

*Severe wedge compression fractures may result in progressive kyphosis over time.
†Multilevel wedge compression fractures may require surgical therapy.
‡Potential mechanical instability.
§Unstable if there is facet dislocation, subluxation, or facet fracture.
‖Burst fractures are either neurologically unstable or both mechanically and neurologically unstable.
¶Fracture-dislocations are both mechanically and neurologically unstable.
Modified from McCormack B, MacMillan M, Fessler RG: Management of thoracic, lumbar and sacral injuries. In Tindall GT, Cooper PR, Barrow D, editors: *The practice of neurosurgery*, vol II, Baltimore, 1996, Williams & Wilkins, pp 1721–1740.

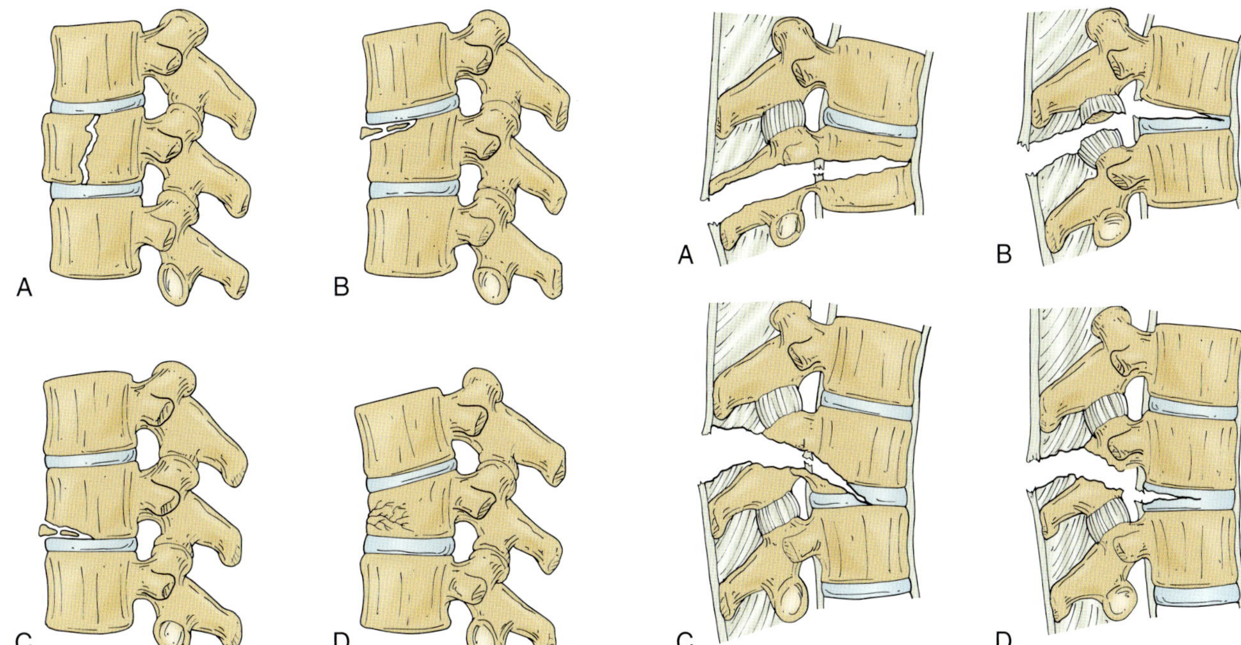

FIGURE 67-3. Four types of compression fractures, as described by Denis: **A,** Compression fracture detaching anterior vertebral body from posterior vertebral body. **B,** Failure of superior end plate. **C,** Failure of inferior end plate. **D,** Failure of superior and inferior end plates. (From Denis F: The three column spine and its significance in the classification of acute thoracolumbar spinal injuries. *Spine [Phila Pa 1976]* 8:817–831, 1983.)

FIGURE 67-5. **A,** One-level lap belt–type injury through the bone (Chance fracture). **B,** One-level lap belt–type injury through the ligament. **C** and **D,** Variants of two-level lap belt–type injuries: two-level lap belt–type injury through the bone (**C**); two-level lap belt–type injury through the ligaments (**D**). (From Denis F: The three column spine and its significance in the classification of acute thoracolumbar spinal injuries. *Spine [Phila Pa 1976]* 8:817–831, 1983.)

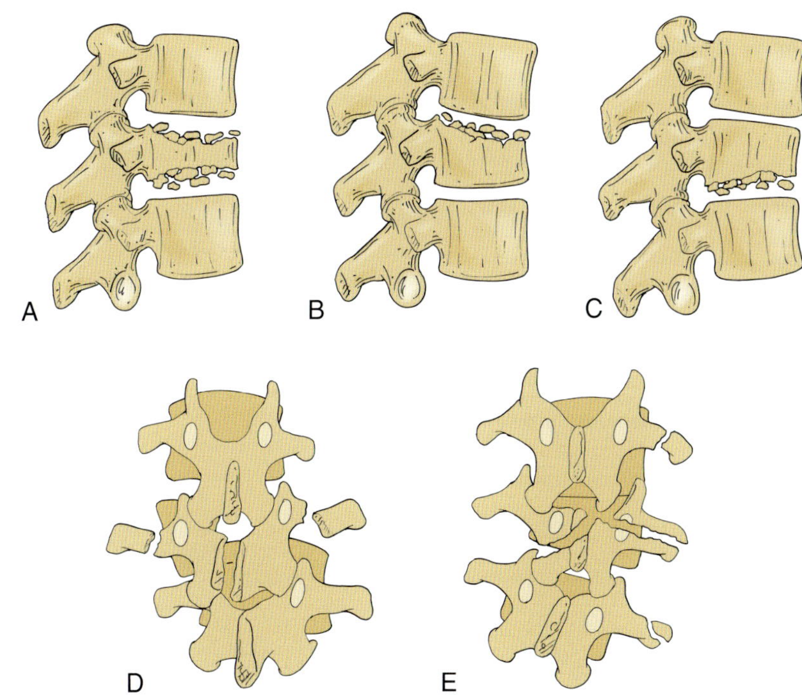

FIGURE 67-4. Classification of burst fractures (by Denis). **A,** Fracture of both end plates. **B,** Fracture of the superior end plate. **C,** Fracture of the inferior end plate. **D,** Burst rotation. **E,** Burst lateral flexion. (From Denis F: The three column spine and its significance in the classification of acute thoracolumbar spinal injuries. *Spine [Phila Pa 1976]* 8:817–831, 1983.)

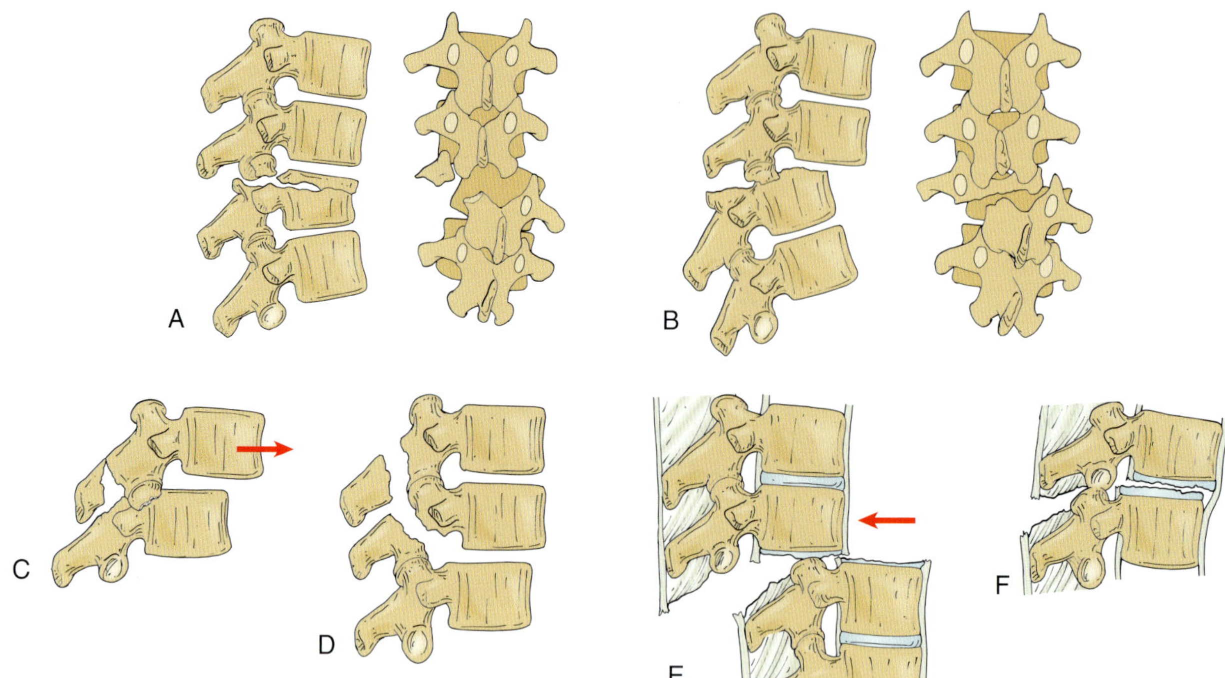

FIGURE 67-6. Fracture-dislocation types (according to Denis). Flexion-rotation type through the bone (**A**) and the disc (**B**). Note the difference in rotation between both spinal segments. **C,** Shear (posteroanterior) subtype; the segment above is sheared off forward on the top of the segment below. **D,** This shearing may leave a floating dorsal arch. A dural tear and complete paraplegia are very common with this type of fracture. **E,** Shear (anteroposterior subtype). **F,** Flexion-distraction type resembles a lap belt–type fracture, but, in addition, there is stripping of the anterior longitudinal ligament during subluxation or dislocation. (From Denis F: The three column spine and its significance in the classification of acute thoracolumbar spinal injuries. *Spine [Phila Pa 1976]* 8:817–831, 1983.)

TABLE 67-2

Thoracolumbar Injury Classification and Severity Score Scale

Category	Points
Injury Morphology	
Compression	1
Burst	1+
Translation/rotational	3
Distraction	4
Neurologic Status	
Intact	0
Nerve root	2
Cord/conus medullaris	
Incomplete	3
Complete	2
Cauda equina	3
Posterior Ligamentous Complex	
Intact	0
Injury suspected/indeterminate	2
Injured	3

A score <3 is generally considered a stable fracture, and a score ≥5 is considered an unstable fracture and typically requires surgical stabilization.

assigned to the various subcategories. The total score among the three categories determines the injury severity score. Scores of 5 or higher suggest the need for operative treatment due to the unstable nature of the injury, and scores of 3 or lower suggest nonoperative management. A score of 4 may be treated either way. If multiple fractures are present, the injury with the greatest score dictates the treatment.

Treatment of Lumbar Spine Fractures

When initiating treatment for lumbosacral fractures, certain objectives should be kept in mind: (1) Decompress neurologic elements in order to maintain or improve neurologic function. (2) Stabilize the spine. (3) Prevent posttraumatic deformity. With these goals in mind, a determination should be made about whether the patient would benefit from surgical intervention or nonsurgical treatment. It is not always appropriate to discuss nonsurgical management as "conservative treatment" since these patients often face a multitude of risk factors during the healing process.

Nonsurgical treatment, usually consisting of a period of bedrest followed by bracing, in patients who are neurologically intact has a long track record, even in the face of a fracture that by the classification schemes is dubbed "unstable."[44] Depending on the type of fracture, the period of bedrest may be as little as 2 weeks or as long as 4 to 6 weeks, depending on the surgeon's comfort with the fracture pattern. In the acute setting, the use of a specialty bed, specifically a rotating bed, has been found to maintain stability of the spine and decrease pressure on the skin to avoid decubitus ulcers. Although this modality inevitably increases the length of hospitalization, it avoids the risk and costs of surgery. This course of treatment must be accompanied by aggressive pulmonary toilet and mechanical prophylaxis and chemoprophylaxis to prevent deep vein thrombosis.

Indications for surgical treatment include, but are not limited to, incomplete or progressive neurologic injury in the setting of neural element compression, an unstable fracture, or a multitrauma situation in which fixation of the fracture would greatly aid in the treatment of other injuries. If surgery is undertaken, it is important to attempt to reconstruct and stabilize the spine in a normal anatomic alignment to promote healing and prevent deformity. Great thought should go into a case in which decompression alone is performed in the setting of an unstable fracture, unless a period of postoperative immobilization is included. When instrumenting the spine, a general practice is to expose and fuse the least number of segments that will accomplish the goals of surgery. Although considerable debate surrounds the need for a long or short construct, each operation should be tailored for the individual pattern of injury.

Although the literature has established very few standards for treating these patients, a few thoughts are worth discussing. In general, stopping a construct at a transition from a mobile to an immobile section of the spine may result in a junctional kyphosis. In the lumbosacral spine, this means that when a multilevel lumbar construct is undertaken, crossing the thoracic junction should be considered if the construct would end at L1. Long thoracolumbar constructs or sacral fractures that result in lumbar-sacral disassociation often require fixation to the pelvis in the form of iliac screws (Fig. 67-7). Whenever the treatment is this extensive, care should be given to restore normal anatomic alignment so that appropriate sagittal balance is maintained.

The next question with surgical intervention becomes a matter of timing: early or delayed. In a retrospective review, Schlegel et al. found that patients treated after 72 hours were at 4.3 times higher risk of being admitted to the ICU, 2.8 times higher risk of being on a ventilator, 12.2 times higher risk for development of pulmonary complications, 4.8 times more likely to develop bed sores, and 3.2 times more likely to develop urinary tract infections than those who had surgery within 48 hours of injury.[45] A concern about performing early surgery is an increased risk of complications. To examine this problem, McLain and Benson reported on 75 patients treated with spinal instrumentation for fractures and found that surgery within 24 hours was as safe as treatment for those provided care between 24 and 72 hours after injury.[46] When specifically looking at the thoracolumbar spine, Chipman et al. found that early surgery (<72 hours) in patients with higher injury severity scores (≥15) was associated with shorter periods in the ICU, shorter hospital stays, fewer ventilator days, and fewer complications.[47] A study by McHenry et al. reviewing 1032 spine fractures echoes these results. They found that surgery performed within 2 days of injury, one of the only variables of the injured patient that the surgeon can control, may decrease the risk of developing respiratory failure.[48] However, not all the studies on early surgery show an improved outcome. Kerwin et al. compared 361 patients that underwent surgical fixation of their spinal fracture within 48 hours with patients who underwent surgery after 48 hours. The only differences found between the two groups was a statistically significant higher mortality rate in the early-surgery group coupled with a shorter length of hospitalization, which the authors suggest may be related to the higher early mortality.[49] In general, each case should be evaluated individually. Although early surgery may be beneficial in a neurologically incomplete injury, the overall status of the patient must be taken into account in order to maximize postoperative function.

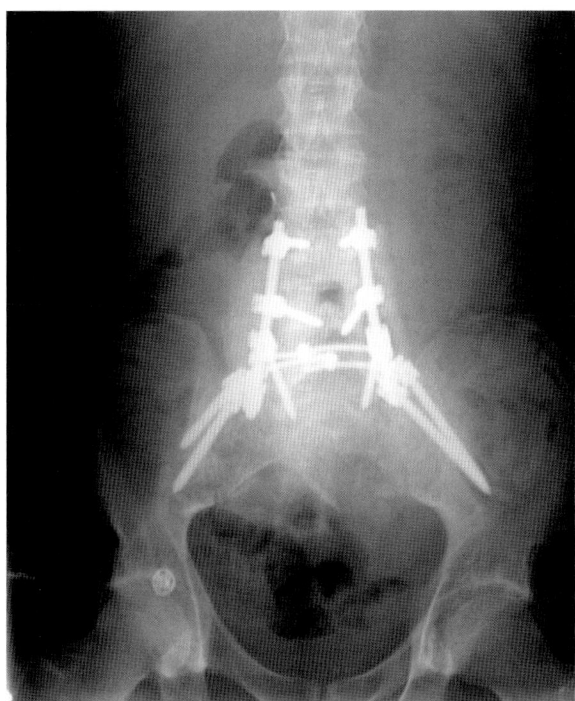

FIGURE 67-7. Lumbosacral dislocation from a gunshot wound to the abdomen treated with an L4 to pelvis posterior construct. (Courtesy of Michael Rosner.)

Outcomes

The ultimate goal of treatment is the restoration of function to a preinjury baseline. To determine the current status of treatment strategies, McLain reported on 70 patients treated with spinal instrumentation for thoracic, lumbar, and thoracolumbar fractures.[50] At 5-year follow-up, he found that 70% of patients were employed at 56% of their previous level of employment. The most significant correlation with return to work status was the degree of neurologic injury. Seventy percent of intact patients returned to full-time employment, whereas only 23% of those with neurologic deficits did. Twelve and one half percent of the intact patients were considered disabled or unemployed, whereas 63% of those with neurologic deficits were considered disabled or unemployed. Although arguments can be made for various treatment modalities and their timing, the preservation and/or recovery of neurologic function should be of the highest priority.

Sacral Fractures

Multiple different classification systems for sacral fractures have been proposed. However, the Spine Trauma Study Group advocates for the use of the Denis system and its modifications.[39,51,52] In 1988, Denis et al. published his classification of sacral fractures based on a retrospective review of 236 patients with sacral fractures.[28] This system divides the sacrum into three anatomic regions: alar region (zone 1), foraminal region (zone II), and region of the central sacral canal (zone III) (Fig. 67-8).

Zone I fractures involve the sacrum lateral to the foraminal line, without injury to the foramina or the sacral canal. These are usually the result of lateral compression of the pelvis with preservation of the sacroiliac ligaments and are composed of two major subtypes: alar fractures and sacrotuberous ligament avulsion. Alar fractures can either be stable if there is minimal displacement or unstable if there is significant displacement. If the vertical shear force on an alar fracture is severe enough for the fracture to become unstable, then the upwardly displaced fragment may stretch the L5 root or entrap it against the L5 transverse process. Displacement of the sacrotuberous ligament represents a severe injury with pelvic instability, typically with some additional anterior pelvic injury. Neurologic deficit was seen in 5.9% of these patients and mainly involved either the L5 root or sciatic nerve. Sacroiliac involvement of zone I fractures should be assessed because this has a deleterious effect on pelvic stability.

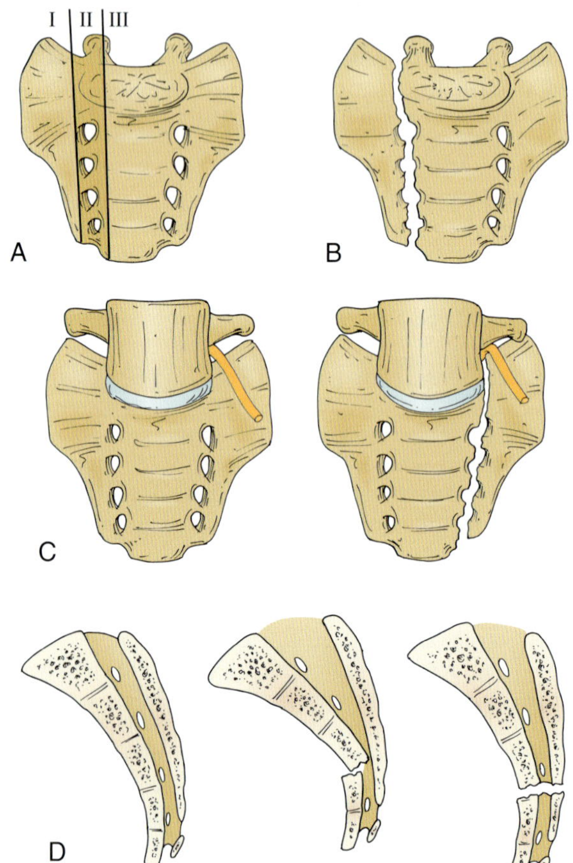

FIGURE 67-8. **A,** Classification of sacral fractures into zone I, region of the ala; zone II, region of the sacral foramina; and zone III, region of the central sacral canal. **B,** Zone II fracture. **C,** Mechanism of L5 nerve root damage or entrapment in the traumatic "far out" syndrome. The L5 root is caught between the sacral ala and the transverse process of L5 as the fragment migrates superiorly and posteriorly. **D,** Sagittal view of zone III fractures: normal sacrum (*left*), sacral burst fracture with a high potential for sacral root compression (*middle*), and sacral fracture-dislocation with a higher potential for sacral root disruption (*right*). (From Denis F, Davis S, Comfort T: Sacral fractures: an important problem: retrospective analysis of 236 cases. *Clin Orthop Relat Res* 227:67–81, 1988.)

Zone II injuries involve one or more of the foramina and may go through the ala but do not violate the central canal. Neurologic injury was seen in 28.4% of these patients, typically involving the L5, S1, or S2 root. Zone II injuries comprise fractures extending through one or more sacral foramina but lateral to the sacral canal. These fractures are often seen in shear-type injuries but may also occur as the result of lateral compression. Vertical shear injuries are the result of significant force transmission to the sacrum and pelvis and usually result in concomitant injury to the sacroiliac joint. As a result, they are unstable. Nerve root injury has been reported in 28% to 54% of zone II injuries.

Zone III fractures include vertical shear injuries, high and low transverse fractures, and traumatic spondylolisthesis of L5 on S1 (highly unstable in flexion). Transverse sacral fractures are commonly seen after falls from great heights. These fractures usually cross the S2-3 level below the level of the sacroiliac joints with ventral and caudal displacement of the spine above the fracture. Zone III fractures primarily involve the central sacral canal, but the fracture line may go through the other two zones. Neurologic deficits were seen in 56.7% of these patients, with 76.1% of the patients with deficits having bowel, bladder, or sexual dysfunction. Zone III fractures have a high incidence of bilateral nerve root injury and cauda equina dysfunction. In addition to the features mentioned, the following are also associated with a risk of instability: high transverse, bilateral sacral, and vertical shear fractures.

Additionally, lumbosacral fracture-dislocations have a high incidence of concomitant transverse sacral fractures and can involve the S1 facet, resulting in instability. The majority of sacral fractures caused by indirect forces are vertical fractures, observed in conjunction with fractures of the pelvis.

Management of Sacral Fractures

The management of sacral fractures remains controversial. Complicating this issue is the fact that 80% of patients with neurologic injury at the time of presentation may recover regardless of whether operative reduction and internal fixation/neural decompression is performed.[29,39,52-54] Cadaveric studies of sacral and pelvic fractures have demonstrated high rates of nerve root avulsion, suggesting that neurologic injuries (other than a cauda equina syndrome) that do not resolve may frequently be root avulsion, for which decompression is not useful.[55]

Stability of sacral fractures is generally defined as greater than 1 cm of displacement.[39,56] However, translation, kyphosis, and comminution can affect treatment decisions, operative approaches, and clinical outcomes. Treatment strategies that involve open reduction and internal fixation appear to produce better results than closed reduction and percutaneous iliosacral screw fixation.[57] Prior to treating a sacral fracture, stability of the pelvic ring should be assessed since these fractures have a high rate of association with pelvic fractures. Typically, these injuries will require treatment separate from or in conjunction with the sacral fracture, usually with an orthopaedic traumatologist.

Most sacral fractures can be treated with bedrest and pelvic immobilization. In the acute setting, application of an external fixator may help to tamponade life-threatening bleeding. However, this may not be enough to stabilize the pelvis in the long term. Treatment for stable, minimally displaced fractures revolves around nonsurgical management with early ambulation and weight bearing as tolerated. Reduction of an alar or zone I fracture may be necessary to decompress an L5 nerve root injury.[58] In some cases, stabilization of the pelvis along with bedrest will suffice, particularly in cases where the dorsal ligamentous complex of the pelvis is intact. Treatment for unstable zone I fractures involves open reduction and stabilization of the pelvis. Zone II injuries causing radiculopathy are best treated by bedrest. Residual symptoms despite conservative therapy can be treated by sacral laminectomy and foraminotomy as needed. Weakness from S1 nerve root entrapment may require early decompression. Transverse zone III fractures are usually not associated with pelvic instability. High transverse fractures are the exception and may require instrumentation and surgical decompression of the neural elements. Transverse fractures may also lead to compression of the cauda equina. Early decompression is advocated in an attempt to restore bowel, bladder, and sexual function.[7] However, early management of sacral fractures is often complicated by significant comorbidity. Damage to the internal iliac vessels and presacral venous plexus can be associated with significant hemorrhage and is a contraindication to anterior approaches to the sacrum.

Conclusions

Trauma to the lumbosacral spine is fairly common, and a high degree of suspicion should be maintained, especially in patients with an appropriate mechanism of injury, another spine fracture, or neurologic deficit. The stability of these fractures, although not always obvious, should be considered in the development and execution of a treatment strategy. Neurologic deterioration in a patient with a known lumbosacral fracture should prompt immediate evaluation for change in the fracture diagnosis and intervention as warranted.

Acknowledgment. The authors wish to thank Dr. Michael Rosner for images used in this chapter.

KEY REFERENCES

Denis F: The three-column spine and its significance in the classification of acute thoracolumbar spinal injuries. *Spine (Phila Pa 1976)* 8:817–831, 1983.

Denis F, Davis S, Comfort T: Sacral fractures: an important problem retrospective analysis of 236 cases. *Clin Orthop Relat Res* 227:67–81, 1988.

Sheridan R, Peralta R, Rhea J, et al: Reformatted visceral protocol helical computed tomographic scanning allows conventional radiographs of the thoracic and lumbar spine to be eliminated in the evaluation of blunt trauma patients. *J Trauma* 55:665–669, 2003.

Vaccaro AR, Kim DH, Brodke DS, et al: Diagnosis and management of sacral spine fractures. *Instr Course Lect* 53:375–385, 2004.

Vaccaro AR, Lehman RA Jr, Hurlbert RJ, et al: A new classification of thoracolumbar injuries: the importance of injury morphology, the integrity of the posterior ligamentous complex, and neurologic status. *Spine (Phila Pa 1976)* 30:2325–2333, 2005.

White AA, Panjabi MM: *Clinical biomechanics of the spine*, ed 3, Philadelphia, 1990, Lippincott.

REFERENCES

The complete reference list is available online at expertconsult.com.

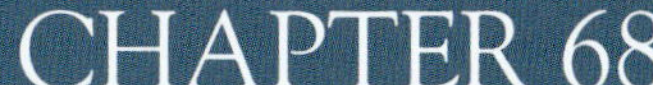
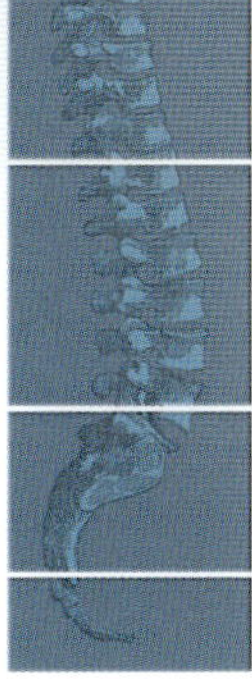

CHAPTER 68

Surgical Indications in Spine Trauma

Eric Roger | Muhammad Zeeshan Memon

Spine surgery should be straightforward. However, complex spinal fracture classification schemes, the mechanism of injury, and the biomechanics of spine trauma and injury itself may, at first, seem intimidating. In this chapter, the surgical indications for intervention for traumatic injuries of the cervical and thoracolumbar spine are identified. Although this topic might be somewhat controversial, a growing body of evidence-based information helps guide strategy determination.

Instability

As defined by White and Panjabi[1] nearly two decades ago, instability is the inability "of the spine under physiological loads to limit patterns of displacement so as not to damage or irritate the spinal cord or nerve roots and, in addition, to prevent incapacitating deformity or pain caused by structural changes." Their description of instability implies concepts of immediate or delayed neural compromise, deformity, and/or pain in conjunction with activities of normal daily living.

Determining spinal instability is not all black or white but, rather, encompasses shades of gray. Many schemes for the classification of instability have been suggested. In general, instability may be acute or chronic. Acute instability may be further defined as overt versus limited (Box 68-1). Acute instability may represent a threat to neural elements, may function as a pain generator, or may lead to progressive deformity if left unattended. Chronic instability may be subdivided as glacial instability, in which deformity occurs slowly over the course of time, similar to the movement of a glacier, or as a dysfunctional segment motion, in which the involved joint shows abnormal motion. As opposed to glacial instability, dysfunctional segment motion does not lead to deformity but rather to a pain syndrome associated with dysfunctional joint movement.

Limited Instability

Limited instability is defined as the loss of either ventral or dorsal spinal element integrity, but not both. Examples include wedge compression fractures with normal dorsal elements; isolated dorsal element fractures, including fracture of the spinous process, lamina, or pedicle; or dorsal ligamentous injuries with normal vertebra and disc integrity. Limited instability may be wrongfully assumed when ligamentous injury is missed. Use of MRI and dynamic imaging (flexion-extension film) is essential in assessing the integrity of the ligamentous structures.

Overt Instability

Overt instability is defined as the inability of the spine to support the weight of the torso. It is generally assumed when circumferential spinal integrity is lost. In effect, both anterior and posterior elements are compromised. Such injuries usually occur with larger force vectors or in patients with poor bone quality or biomechanical disadvantage (see later discussion). Compromise of the ventral elements can easily be demonstrated on plain film, CT, or MRI. Assessment of the dorsal elements, especially ligamentous structures, may be more challenging. Fat suppression or short tau inversion recovery (STIR) sequencing may illustrate ligamentous edema and suggest dorsal instability, but true disruption of the posterior tension band may be difficult to demonstrate.[2] Flexion-extension films may be extremely dangerous in the face of overt instability. Disruption of the posterior ligamentous tension band may be noted on palpation of the affected area (Fig. 68-1).

Surgical Indications

In general, surgical intervention for spinal trauma should be considered in cases of neural compromise, overt instability, or progressive deformity (i.e., glacial instability). Indications for surgery should also include intractable pain.

Neural Compromise

Strong consideration should be given to patients with spinal cord, nerve root, and/or cauda equina compression with resulting neurologic deficits. Although still controversial, a growing body of evidence suggests that early decompression is the single most important predictor of neurologic recovery in spinal cord injury (SCI). Animal studies consistently show that neurologic recovery is enhanced by early spinal cord decompression.[3,4] However, it is difficult to extrapolate the data for the effective application of decompression in the clinical setting from these animal models. To date, the

BOX 68-1. Instability Categorization Scheme

Acute instability
- Overt instability
- Limited instability

Chronic instability
- Glacial instability
- Dysfunctional segment motion

From Benzel EC: *Biomechanics of spine stabilization*, New York, 2001, Thieme.

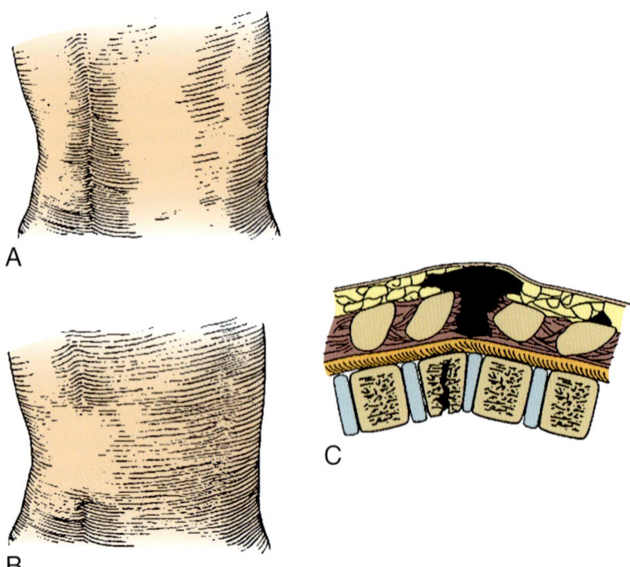

FIGURE 68-1. Dorsal instability in the thoracic and lumbar region can be suggested, particularly in thin patients, by physical examination. The presence of tenderness over the spinous processes or the absence of the normal midline crease (**A**), as a result of swelling or hematoma formation below the skin (**B**), suggests underlying soft tissue injury (**C**). This in turn suggests, but does not prove, the presence of dorsal spinal instability. (From Benzel EC: *Biomechanics of spine surgery*. Copyright © 2001 by the American Association of Neurological Surgeons, Rolling Meadows, IL.)

TABLE 68-1

American Spinal Injury Association Impairment Scale

Class	Description
A	Complete: No motor or sensory function preserved in sacral segments S4-5
B	Incomplete: Sensory but no motor function preserved below the neurologic level (includes sacral segments S4-5)
C	Incomplete: Motor function preserved below the neurologic level (more than half of key muscles below the neurologic level have a muscle grade <3)
D	Incomplete: Motor function preserved below the neurologic level (more than half of key muscles below the neurologic level have a muscle grade ~3)
E	Normal: Sensory and motor function normal

From Frankel HL, Hancock DO, Hyslop G, et al: The value of postural reduction in the initial management of closed injuries of the spine with paraplegia and tetraplegia. I. *Paraplegia* 7:179–192, 1969.

TABLE 68-2

Prognostic Significance of ASIA Grading: Data from the Sygen Study Group

Acute Phase Measurement of ASIA Grade	CHRONIC PHASE MEASUREMENT OF ASIA GRADE (%)*				
	A	B	C	D	E
A	76	15	8	4	0
B		22	22	27	5
C			5	83	15
D				12	82
E					

ASIA, American Spinal Injury Association.
*One year later among patients available for follow-up evaluation.
From Geisler FH, Coleman WP, Grieco G, et al: Measurements and recovery patterns in a multicenter study of acute spinal cord injury. *Spine (Phila Pa 1976)* 26:S68–S86, 2011.

clinical studies that have examined the role of surgical decompression in SCI are limited to class II and III evidence. One randomized controlled trial[5] showed no benefit to early (<72 hours) decompression; however, several recent prospective series suggest that early decompression (<12 hours) can be performed safely and may improve neurologic outcomes.[6,7] La Rosa et al.[8] published a meta-analysis of the literature addressing the issue of early decompression and its role in acute SCI. They reviewed all published clinical studies and extracted data on 1687 patients. Patients were divided into three treatment groups: early decompression (<24 hours), delayed decompression (>24 hours), and conservative management. Statistically, early decompression resulted in better outcomes than either delayed decompression or conservative management. However, on homogeneity analysis, only data for patients with incomplete SCI who underwent early decompression were reliable. These studies concluded that early decompression can only be considered as a practice option. The Surgical Treatment of Acute Spinal Cord Injury Study (STASCIS)[9] is a prospective, randomized controlled, multicenter trial that is currently in progress and seeks to determine the best timing of surgical decompression in SCI. In the authors' opinion, surgery should be attempted in a medically stable patient as early as clinically feasible, often within 24 hours of admission.

The American Spinal Injury Association impairment scale[10] (ASIA), which is a modified Frankel classification,[11] describes the completeness of an SCI. It has two main components: motor and sensory. The ASIA motor score of 0 to 5 is assigned for each muscle group innervated by spinal levels C5 to T1 and L2 to S1. This gives 10 levels on each side of the body, or a maximum possible score of 100. A sensory score of 0 to 2 is assigned for each dermatome from C2 to S4-5, using light touch and pinprick sensation. This gives 28 levels for a possible score of 56 on each side, or a maximum possible score of 112. Table 68-1 describes ASIA grading. The ASIA impairment scale has been shown to have great prognostic value, with chances of marked recovery more frequent in patients with better baseline scores. Table 68-2 shows the prognostic value of the ASIA impairment scale from the Sygen study group data.[12]

Overt Instability

Columns

As previously described, overt instability refers to circumferential loss of spinal integrity. Compromise of only one column (either anterior or posterior) is considered limited instability only. The concept of "columns" is at the center of understanding spinal stability (Fig. 68-2) and dates back to the 1960s. In their seminal article, Kelly and Whitesides[13] describe the concept of two columns as "one of solid bone and one composed of neural arches . . . Working together, these two columns support the body's weight." Later, Denis[14] introduced the concept of a middle column, consisting of the posterior half of the vertebral body and disc and posterior longitudinal ligament. Depending on the pattern of column injury, he suggested four types of spinal fractures: compression, burst, seat belt–type, and fracture-dislocation (Table 68-3). The middle column suggested by Denis is interesting because it allows for specific assessment of the neutral axis. The neutral axis is the longitudinal axial weight-bearing zone about which spinal element distraction or compression does not significantly occur with flexion or extension (Fig. 68-3). As a rule, it is often suggested that compromise of two of the three Denis columns constitutes overt instability.

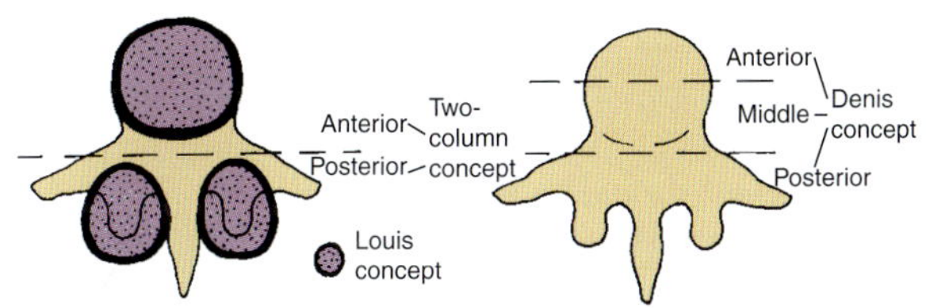

FIGURE 68-2. The "column" concepts of spinal stability. The concept described by Louis[20] (*left*) assigns significance to the vertebral body and the facet joint complexes (lateral masses) on either side of the dorsal spine. Denis's three-column concept (*right*) assigns significance to the region of the neutral axis and the integrity of the posterior vertebral body wall (the middle column). The two-column construct (*left*) relies on anatomically defined structures, the vertebral body (anterior column), and the posterior elements (posterior column). Louis's three-column concept (*left*) similarly relies on anatomically defined structures. (From Benzel EC: *Biomechanics of spine surgery.* Copyright © 2001 by the American Association of Neurological Surgeons, Rolling Meadows, IL.)

TABLE 68-3

Basic Modes of Failure of the Three Columns in the Four Types of Spinal Injuries

	COLUMNS		
Types of Fracture	**Anterior**	**Middle**	**Posterior**
Compression	Compression	None	None or severe distraction
Burst	Compression	Compression	None
Seat belt	None or compression	Distraction	Distraction
Fracture-dislocation	Compression rotation shear		Distraction rotation shear

From Denis F: The three column spine and its significance in the classification of acute thoracolumbar spinal injuires. *Spine (Phila Pa 1976)* 8:817-831, 1983.

Mechanism of Injury Classification

To date, the most commonly used classification scheme for traumatic spinal injuries is the *Arbeitsgemeinschaft für Osteosynthesefragen* system (AO) classification.[15] This scheme categorizes fractures and other spinal injuries by type, groups, subgroups, and specifications. The AO classification is extensive and often difficult to remember in the clinical context if not used regularly. It provides comprehensive coverage of all possible fracture types and therefore is of the utmost importance in research. Nonetheless, knowledge of its basic types and groups is useful in a clinical context, as it provides a helpful template for understanding the mechanism of injury. This classification scheme categorizes fractures in three major mechanisms of injury. Type A fractures are ventral column injuries resulting from axial load, with or without flexion (Box 68-2 and Fig. 68-4). Type B fractures are distraction injuries in flexion or extension, resulting in compromise of ventral and dorsal elements (Box 68-3 and Fig. 68-5). Type C fractures are ventral and dorsal column injuries with translation and/or rotation (Box 68-4 and Fig. 68-6).

Type A fractures are subdivided into simple wedge fractures, split fractures, and burst fractures. Type B fractures are subdivided into ligamentous flexion-distraction injuries (so-called ligamentous Chance fractures), bony flexion-distraction injuries (so-called bony Chance fractures), and hyperextension shear injuries. Type C fractures are subdivided into rotation plus type A, rotation plus type B, and rotational-shear injuries.

Although the classification scheme does not directly address the integrity of the posterior ligamentous complex (PLC), it is indirectly assumed by the mechanism of injury (intact in type A, compromised in types B and C). Corroboration via MRI findings increases the accuracy of the classification.

Type A injuries have compromise of only the anterior column (the posterior column is intact). These injuries are

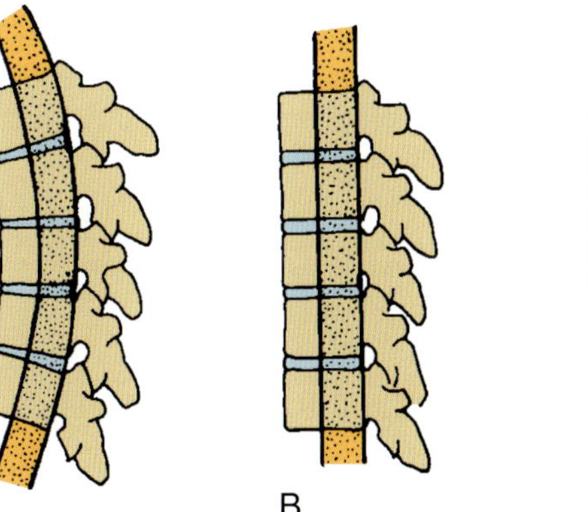

FIGURE 68-3. The depiction of the neutral axis (*shaded areas*). The neutral axis is the longitudinal region of the spinal column that bears much of the axial load and about which spinal element distraction or compression does not significantly occur with the assumption of flexed (**A**), neutral (**B**), or extension (**C**) postures. This is a dynamic and theoretical concept. (From Benzel EC: *Biomechanics of spine surgery.* Copyright © 2001 by the American Association of Neurological Surgeons, Rolling Meadows, IL.)

BOX 68-2. AO Classification: Type A Injuries: Vertebral Body Compression

A1 Impaction fractures
- A1.1 End-plate impaction
- A1.2 Wedge impaction features
- A1.3 Vertebral body collapse

A2 Split fractures
- A2.1 Sagittal split fracture
- A2.2 Coronal split fracture
- A2.3 Pincer fracture

A3 Burst fractures
- A3.1 Incomplete burst fracture
- A3.2 Burst-split fracture
- A3.3 Complete split fracture

AO, *Arbeitsgemeinschaft für Osteosynthesefragen*.
From Magerl F, Aebi M, Gertzbein SD, et al: A comprehensive classification of thoracic and lumbar injuries. *Eur Spine J* 3:184–201, 1994.

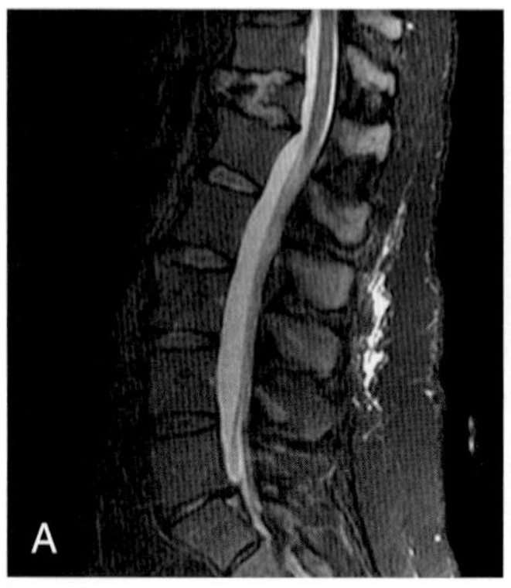

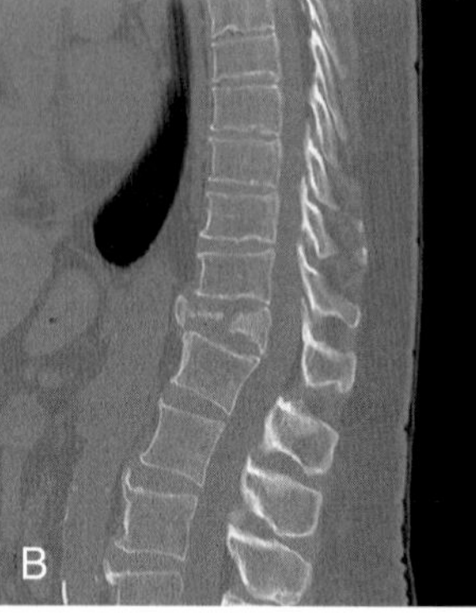

FIGURE 68-4. *Arbeitsgemeinschaft für Osteosynthesefragen* type A fracture. **A,** Short-tau inversion recovery sequence sagittal MRI showing T12 acute fracture with angulation deformity. Note the absence of spinal cord compression and absence of posterior ligamentous edema. **B,** On CT, note the burst (type A3) pattern of fracture, also illustrated on axial imaging (not shown here).

thus considered "stable" and usually do not require surgical stabilization. It is wisest to consider that they may have limited instability and may need to be observed for delayed glacial instability. Furthermore, patients with type A injuries requiring decompression of neural elements may require stabilization due to the "iatrogenic" disruption of the posterior column. In effect, these types of A injuries may "become" B injuries. Types B and C injuries are overtly unstable and should be considered for surgical stabilization.

Resting and Dynamic Radiologic Parameters

Trauma, especially to the ligamentous structures, may result in excessive angulation and/or translation deformity (Table 68-4[1]), which may render the spine grossly unstable (overt instability) or lead to progressive deformity over time (glacial instability from acute limited instability). In the cervical spine, displacement of 3.5 mm and/or angulation of greater than 11 degrees on plain film, or translation of 3.5 mm on flexion-extension film, with rotational motion of greater than 20 degrees should be considered unstable. In the lumbar spine, displacement of 4.5 mm and/or angulation of greater than 22 degrees on plain film, or translation of 4.5 mm on flexion-extension film, with rotational motion of greater than 15 to 25 degrees (depending on the level) should be considered unstable. The thoracic spine is inherently "stabilized" by the rib cage. Therefore, lower values of translation and angulation are considered unstable.

BOX 68-3. AO Classification: Type B Injuries: Anterior and Posterior Element Injury with Distraction

B1 Posterior disruption predominantly ligamentous (flexion-distraction injury)
- B1.1 With transverse disruption of the disc
- B1.2 With type A fracture of the vertebral body

B2 Posterior disruption predominantly osseous (flexion-distraction injury)
- B2.1 Transverse bicolumn fracture
- B2.2 With disruption of the disc
- B2.3 With type A fracture of the vertebral body

B3 Anterior disruption through the disc (hyperextension-shear injury)
- B3.1 Hyperextension-subluxations
- B3.2 Hyperextension-spondylolysis
- B3.3 Posterior dislocation

AO, *Arbeitsgemeinschaft für Osteosynthesefragen*.
From Magerl F, Aebi M, Gertzbein SD, et al: A comprehensive classification of thoracic and lumbar injuries. *Eur Spine J* 3:184–201, 1994.

Progressive Deformity from Limited Instability

As previously discussed, certain fractures with limited instability may be at risk for delayed progression (i.e., glacial instability), leading to deformity. In an attempt to predict the risk of such chronic instability, certain authors have devised point systems, such as the one suggested by White and Panjabi[1] (Table 68-5), which assigns relative scores to the involved columns, the amount of resting and dynamic translation and angulation, the presence of neural injury, and other minor factors. In this system, a score of 5 or more is suggestive of overt instability, and patients with this score should be considered for surgical stabilization. A score of 2 to 4 is suggestive of limited instability, and such patients should be observed for delayed instability.

Acutely, burst fractures result from direct axial loading without ventral or dorsal angulation, as opposed to wedge compression fractures that occur as a result of axial loading with a ventrally or dorsally applied vector force, with a given perpendicular distance for the instantaneous axis of rotation (IAR) of that given vertebra. The force (*F*) at a given distance (*D*) from the IAR results in a given moment arm (M) (Fig. 68-7). The magnitude and speed of the applied moment arm determine the resulting bony and/or ligamentous deformation. The resulting deformity in the sagittal or coronal plane leads to either kyphosis or scoliosis, which increases the distance from the IAR, thus increasing the gravitational moment arm applied to that segment, leading to the progression of the deformity. Hence, "deformity begets deformity."

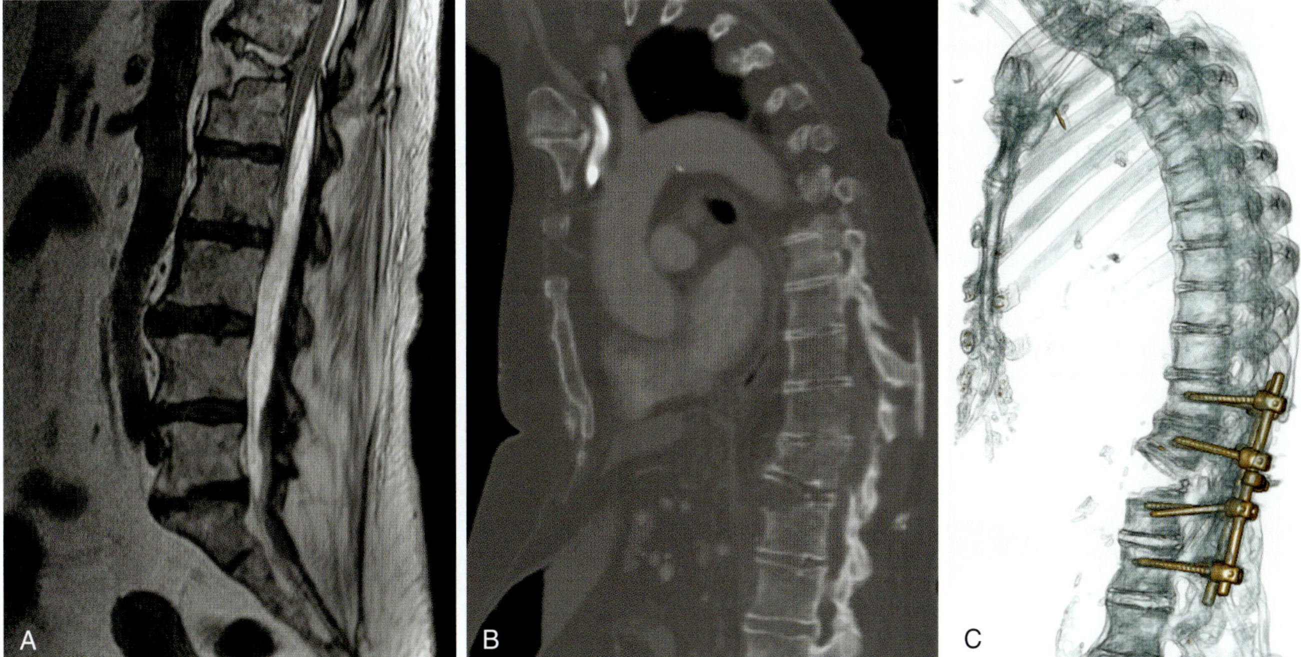

FIGURE 68-5. *Arbeitsgemeinschaft für Osteosynthesefragen* type B fracture. **A,** Sagittal T2-weighted MRI showing T12 avulsion of superior end plate. **B,** Note bony anatomy on CT. Patient had ankylosing spondylosis (not very well illustrated here). This is a hyperextension injury (type B3). **C,** Percutaneous pedicle screw fixation (Longitude, Medtronic, Memphis, TN) and tubular access fusion (Metrx, Medtronic) in this 80-year-old woman with poor overall health. A surgical decision was made to avoid "closing" the fish-mouth to maintain sagittal balance.

BOX 68-4. AO Classification: Type C Injuries: Anterior and Posterior Element Injury with Rotation

C1 Type A injuries with rotation (compression injuries with rotation)
- C1.1 Rotational wedge fracture
- C1.2 Rotational split fracture

C2 Type B injuries with rotation
- C2.1 B1 injuries with rotation (flexion-distraction injuries with rotation)
- C2.2 B2 injuries with rotation (flexion-distraction injuries with rotation)
- C2.3 B3 injuries with rotation (hyperextension-shear injuries with rotation)

C3 Rotational-shear injuries
- C3.1 Slice fracture
- C3.2 Oblique fracture

AO, *Arbeitsgemeinschaft für Osteosynthesefragen*.
From Magerl F, Aebi M, Gertzbein SD, et al: A comprehensive classification of thoracic and lumbar injuries. *Eur Spine J* 3:184–201, 1994.

Intractable Pain

Patients who have spinal fractures with limited or overt instability may have intractable pain despite an aggressive course of conservative management, including narcotics, bedrest, and bracing. Bony pain is often seen in older patients with osteoporotic compression fractures or young patients with type A wedge compression or burst fractures. Vertebroplasty or kyphoplasty may offer excellent pain palliation and increase overall functionality.

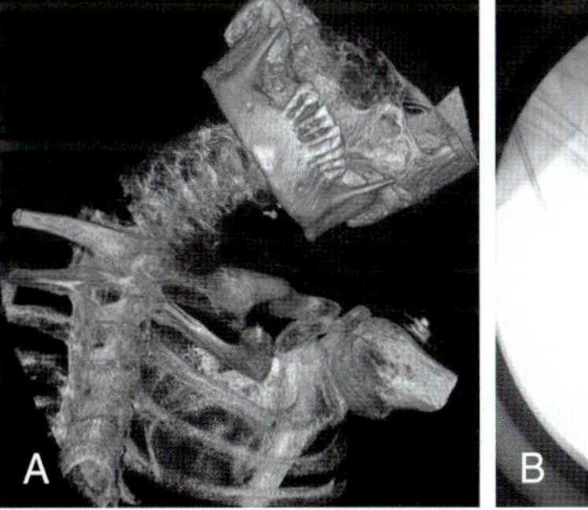

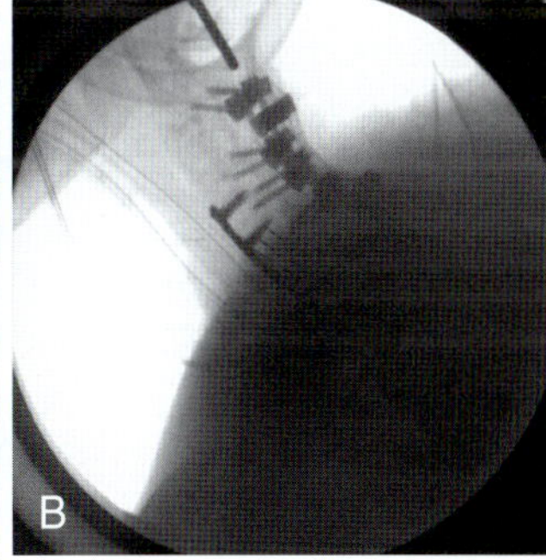

FIGURE 68-6. *Arbeitsgemeinschaft für Osteosynthesefragen* type C fracture-dislocation. **A,** Impressive 3D CT reconstruction showing severe fracture-dislocation at C5-6 in a 58-year-old woman with ankylosing spondylosis who presented with complete tetraplegia below the biceps level. **B,** Postoperative fluoroscopic image showing front/back fusion, corpectomy (Medtronic, Memphis, TN, stackable polyetheretherketone [PEEK] cage), and instrumentation (Medtronic Vertex Max).

Pain may also result from pathologic motion at the level of the injury. Stabilization internally, when external stabilization (brace) fails, may offer excellent pain palliation and may be done in a minimally invasive fashion.

Thoracolumbar Injury Classification and Severity Score

Management of thoracolumbar spinal trauma should be based on comprehensive evaluation of the clinical and radiographic information available at the time of initial assessment. The classification systems mentioned previously (Kelly, Denis, AO, radiologic parameters, and the White and Panjabi point system) have been developed to

TABLE 68-4

Resting and Dynamic Radiologic Guidelines

	Resting	Dynamic
Subaxial cervical spine	>3.5 mm displacement >11° angulation	>3.5 mm translation >20° angulation
Thoracic spine	>2.5 mm displacement >5° angulation	
Lumbar spine	>4.5 mm displacement >22° angulation	>4.5 mm translation >15° L1-4 >20° L4-5 >25° L5-S1

From White AA, Panjabi MM: *Clinical biomechanics of the spine*, ed 2, Philadelphia, 1990, Lippincott.

TABLE 68-5

Quantitation of Acute Instability for Subaxial Cervical, Thoracic, and Lumbar Injuries

Condition	Points Assigned
Loss of integrity of anterior (and middle) column	2
Loss of integrity of posterior column(s)	2
Acute resting translational deformity	2
Acute resting angulation deformity	2
Acute dynamic translational deformity exaggeration	2
Acute dynamic angulation deformity exaggeration	2
Neural element injury	3
Acute disc narrowing at level of suspected pathology	1
Dangerous loading anticipated	1

From White AA, Panjabi MM: *Clinical biomechanics of the spine*, ed 2, Philadelphia, 1990, Lippincott.

help physicians devise a treatment strategy. However, significant interobserver variability has been noted with these mechanistic classifications as injuries are classified by inferring unknown injury patterns rather than by a description of known or presenting injury.[16] To address these limitations, a new classification scheme has been proposed by the Spine Trauma Study Group in 2005 that uses spinal injury morphology combined with the neurologic status of the patient and the critical importance of the posterior ligamentous structures in medical decision making.[17] This new system, the Thoracolumbar Injury Classification and Severity Score (TLICS), assigns numeric values to each injury based on the categories of morphology of injury, integrity of the PLC, and neurologic involvement (Table 68-6).

A numeric value is assigned for each injury subcategory based on the severity of injury. These individual scores are then added to produce an injury severity score, which, in turn, aids in medical decision making by providing both diagnostic and prognostic information with a weighted injury severity score. Stable injury patterns (TLICS <4) may be treated nonoperatively with brace immobilization and active patient mobilization. Unstable injury patterns (TLICS >4) may be treated

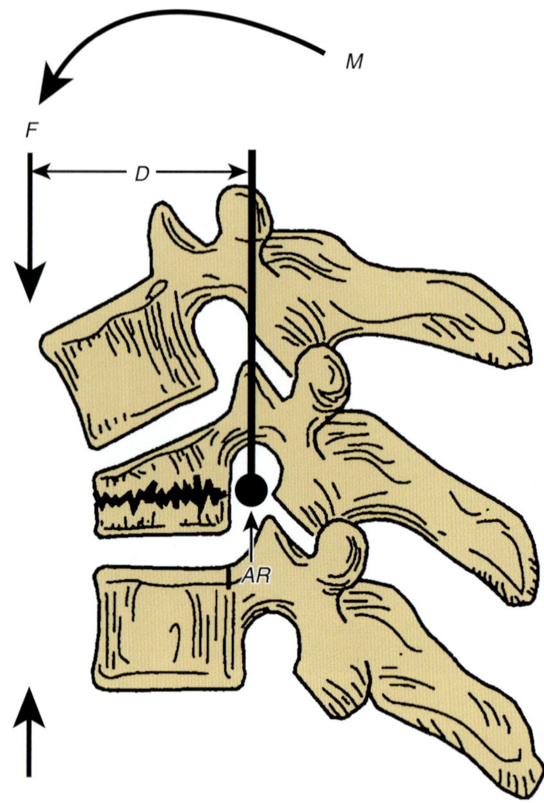

FIGURE 68-7. A depiction of the injury force vector causing a ventral wedge compression fracture. *AR*, axis of rotation; *D*, length of moment arm (from IAR to plane of *F*); *F*, applied force vector; *M*, bending moment. (From Benzel EC: *Biomechanics of spine surgery*. Copyright © 2001 by the American Association of Neurological Surgeons, Rolling Meadows, IL.)

TABLE 68-6

Thoracolumbar Injury Classification and Severity Score Scale

Category	Points
Injury Morphology	
Compression	1
Burst	+1
Translational/rotational	3
Distraction	4
Neurologic Status	
Intact	0
Nerve root	2
Cord, conus medullaris	
Incomplete	3
Complete	2
Cauda equina	3
Posterior Ligamentous Complex Integrity	
Intact	0
Injury suspected/indeterminate	2
Injured	3

From Vaccaro AR, Lehman RA Jr, Hurlbert RJ, et al: A new classification of thoracolumbar injuries: the importance of injury morphology, the integrity of the posterior ligamentous complex, and neurologic status. *Spine (Phila Pa 1976)* 30:2325-2333, 2005.

operatively with deformity correction and neurologic decompression and spinal stabilization, followed by active patient mobilization.

Although the TLICS system has shown good to excellent intra- and interobserver reliability throughout a spectrum of spine treatment providers,[18,19] many of the initial studies were performed by individuals involved with its development. Therefore, a broader application of the system across multiple physicians and trauma centers may further validate or refute this classification system in the future.

KEY REFERENCES

American Spinal Injury Association: *Reference Manual of the International Standards for Neurological Classification of Spinal Cord Injury*, ed 6, Chicago, 2003.

La Rosa G, Conti A, Cardali S, et al: Does early decompression improve neurological outcome of spinal cord injured patients? Appraisal of the literature using a meta-analytical approach. *Spinal Cord* 42:503–512, 2004.

Magerl F, Aebi M, Gertzbein SD, et al: A comprehensive classification of thoracic and lumbar injuries. *Eur Spine J* 3:184–201, 1994.

Vaccaro AR, Lehman RA Jr, Hurlbert RJ, et al: A new classification of thoracolumbar injuries: the importance of injury morphology, the integrity of the posterior ligamentous complex, and neurologic status. *Spine* 30:2325–2333, 2005.

White AA, Panjabi MM: *Clinical biomechanics of the spine*, ed 2, Philadelphia, 1990, Lippincott.

REFERENCES

The complete reference list is available online at expertconsult.com.

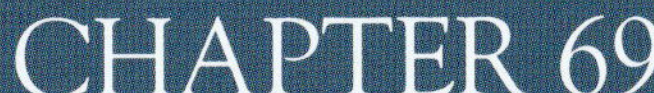
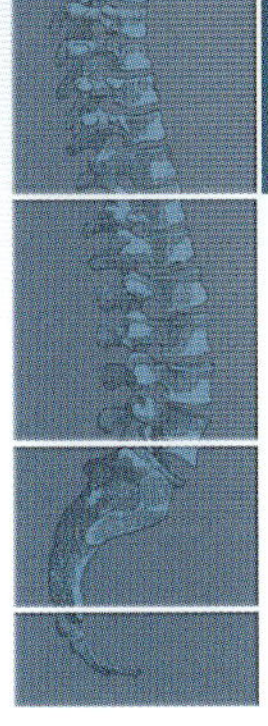

CHAPTER 69

Nonoperative Management and Treatment of Spine Injuries

Mark L. Prasarn | Glenn R. Rechtine II

The morbidity and mortality associated with injuries to the spine have been known since antiquity. Nonoperative methods have been a mainstay of care for such injuries since ancient Egypt. Even with modern-day surgical techniques, the majority of spine injuries should be managed nonoperatively with the goal of healing the spine without any of the inherent risks of surgery. In most spine injuries, a good functional outcome and no long-term disability can be expected with nonoperative care.

Nonsurgical treatment is used in all cases of spine injuries. Nonoperative treatment techniques are employed at the initial evaluation and management at the scene of the accident. In the vast majority of cases, nonsurgical principles are extended as a definitive treatment plan. In addition, during every step of diagnosis and treatment, strict adherence to principles of immobilization must be followed to minimize motion to the injured spine and prevent neurologic injury or deterioration.

The objectives of nonoperative management of spine injuries are the same as those for operative treatment. These include (1) preservation of neurologic function, (2) improvement in neurologic deficit if already present, (3) reduction of spinal deformity and maintenance of acceptable alignment, (4) minimization of loss of spinal mobility, and (5) achievement of a healed and stable spinal column.

At the Scene

According to Advanced Trauma Life Support (ATLS) protocol, life-threatening compromise to airway, breathing, and circulation should be promptly addressed. Although the greatest risk for spinal cord injury occurs at the time of high-energy impact, neurologic deficits can develop thereafter during treatment. In 1983 Podolsky et al. reported that up to 25% of spinal cord injuries had been caused by or aggravated after the patient had come under medical care.[1] Immobilization of the injured spine is the key to preventing such catastrophic decline.

The care of spine trauma patients at the scene has dramatically improved over the past several decades. Extrication and transport of trauma patients with immobilization techniques and adherence to ATLS protocols for resuscitation have been credited for this improvement. ATLS protocol mandates that a spine injury be assumed for all injured patients and rigid immobilization employed. At the scene, the patient should be immobilized with a cervical collar, head immobilization device, and spine backboard.

At the Hospital

The patient should arrive in the emergency department on a backboard with a cervical collar in place. In the face of a global instability, motion can still occur in spite of all attempts at rigid immobilization. The patient should be moved on and off the backboard as few times as possible until the stability of the spine can be adequately assessed. For most injuries the collar provides an increased level of stability. However, it does not provide complete immobilization.[2] With a complete ligamentous disruption, the collar has minimal effect. The person stabilizing the spine is much more significant in restricting motion.[3]

Moving the patient off the backboard for CT should be coordinated so that imaging of the brain, spine, chest, abdomen, pelvis, sinus, or orbits or any other appropriate study is obtained in one trip to the scanner and one movement off and on the backboard.

The risk of decubitus ulceration is directly proportional to the length of time on a backboard—8 hours on a backboard is associated with a 100% likelihood of a decubitus ulcer.[4] The patient should be moved from the board as soon as possible. Appropriate spine immobilization must be continued at all times.

Contrary to all available evidence suggesting that the log roll is an ineffective and potentially dangerous technique for spine immobilization, it is still almost universally used. In fact, studies conducted prior to 2004 showed dramatic and unacceptable motion with a log roll.[5] Recently, many studies have reevaluated this controversial subject. Compared with any other method of transfer, the log roll maneuver has been shown to cause more segmental motion at the level of the unstable, injured segment.[6-13] Lift and slide techniques are far superior since they tend to create less motion at the injured segment.[10]

Imaging Studies

Following review of the initial CT scan, another assessment of spinal stability can be performed. When a closed reduction of a dislocated segment is needed, it should be performed

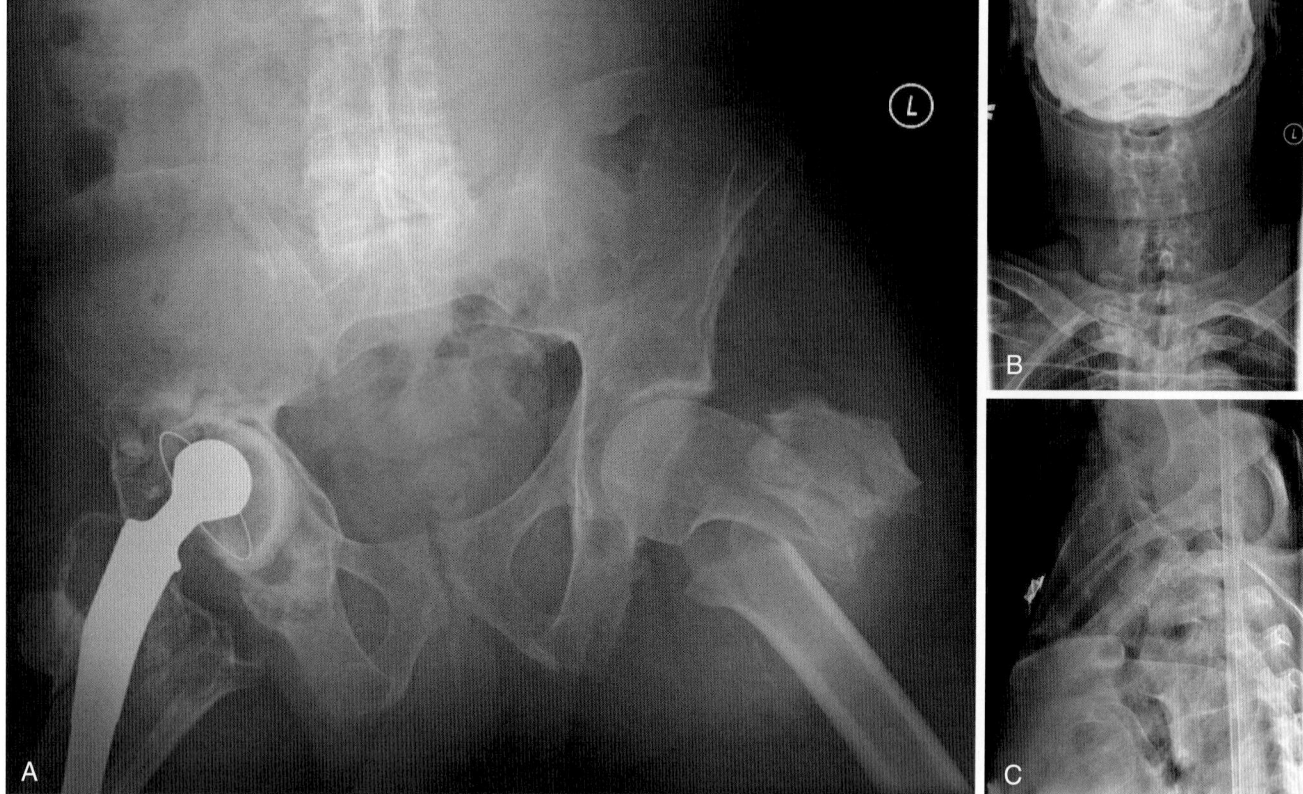

FIGURE 69-1. Initial imaging of a 53-year-old male involved in a motor vehicle accident with bilateral hip pain who was neurologically intact and had no complaints of neck or arm pain. **A,** Anteroposterior (AP) radiograph of the pelvis demonstrating bilateral proximal femur fractures. AP (**B**) and lateral (**C**) radiographs of the cervical spine showing an extension-distraction injury at C6-7 in the same patient.

expediently in the awake and alert patient. Serial neurologic examinations are performed during such a reduction maneuver. If the patient is obtunded or reliable neurologic examinations are impossible, then an emergent MRI should be obtained prior to attempting reduction to rule out significant disc herniation.[14]

In the absence of a facet dislocation and in the presence of significant spine injury, the appropriateness of an MRI scan must be determined. The spinal motion necessary to transfer the patient on and off the MRI table must be kept in mind when deciding the necessity of this imaging modality. The strongest argument for an MRI is a suspected neurologic deficit that is not explained by the injury seen on the CT scan. If the patient has an unstable injury that requires surgery that is identified clinically or by other imaging studies, it is not necessary to obtain an MRI just to assess the dorsal ligamentous complex.

Anteroposterior and lateral radiographs of the cervical, thoracic, lumbar, and sacral spine are standard imaging studies obtained in cases of high-energy impact with suspected spinal injury. Distracting injuries can often mask symptoms secondary to significant spine injury, and meticulous assessment of the spine must always be performed (Figs. 69-1 to 69-3). It is necessary to image the entire spinal column due to a 10% incidence of noncontiguous spinal injuries.[15] Specific injury mechanisms and fracture patterns should prompt the treating team to search for commonly associated nonspinal injuries. Flexion-distraction injuries are highly associated with potentially life-threatening intra-abdominal injuries, so these must be ruled out. Patients with transverse process fractures at L5 have a 61% incidence of a pelvic fracture.[16] Falls from a height with resulting burst fractures are often associated with significant lower-extremity fractures, in particular those of the tibia and calcaneus.

Closed Reduction of the Cervical Spine

Decompression of the spinal cord through closed reduction should be performed as soon as the patient can medically tolerate it. Closed reduction is a means of reducing cervical spine deformity, indirectly decompressing neural elements, and providing stability. It has been shown to be safe and can dramatically improve neurologic status if performed within the first few hours following injury. In animal studies, Carlson et al. showed that decompression within 3 hours showed better and quicker neurologic recovery.[17] A small series of patients with no cord function who received reduction in an emergent manner immediately began to recover.[18] Although this is anecdotal, it is extremely important. The timing question is answered after consideration of the risk-benefit ratio between waiting to obtain a prereduction MRI and proceeding directly with reduction.

Considerable controversy surrounds the order of the reduction and obtainment of an MRI in an acute cervical spine dislocation. Eismont et al. reported on a series of six patients who roentgenographically demonstrated herniation of an intervertebral disc with marked protrusion of disc material into the spinal canal following subluxation or dislocation of a cervical facet. For the first patient in this series, no myelogram or CT scan was performed, and the patient awoke with complete quadriplegia following dorsal open reduction and internal fixation. Following a myelogram and ventral decompression surgery, the cause was identified as an extruded

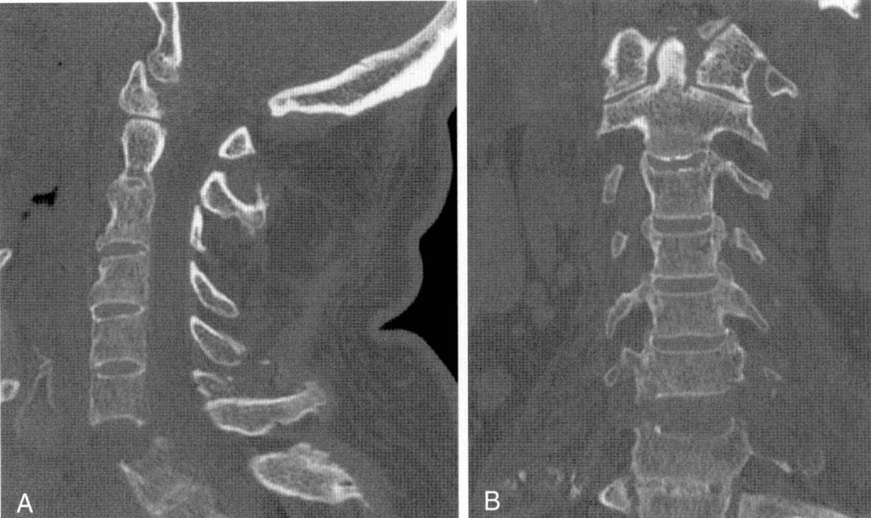

FIGURE 69-2. Further imaging of the cervical spine in the same patient as in Figure 69-1. Sagittal (**A**) and coronal (**B**) CT images demonstrating the ankylosed cervical spine and injury at C6-7.

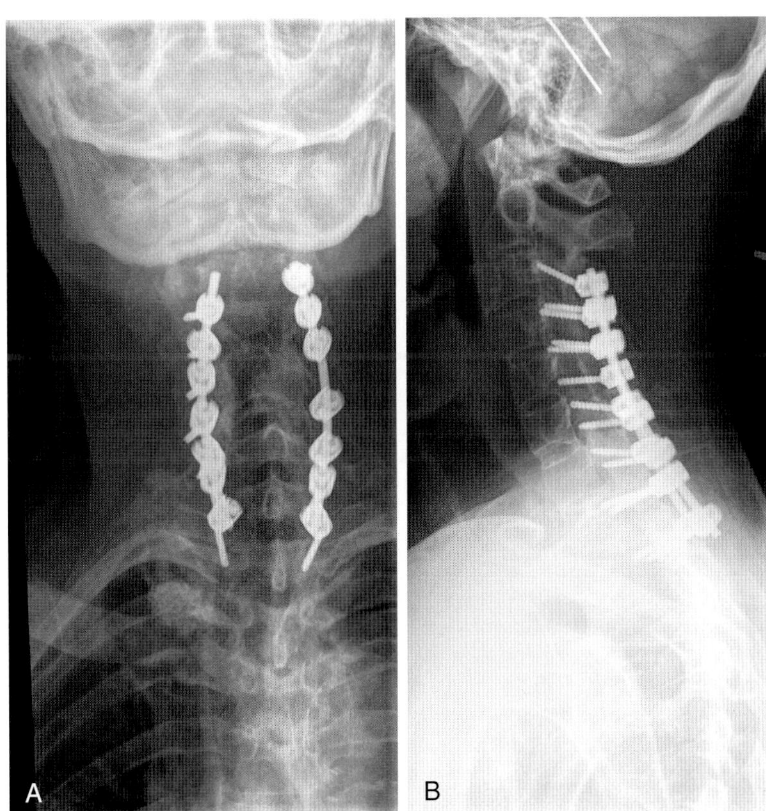

FIGURE 69-3. The same patient as in Figure 69-1 was taken emergently for open reduction and internal fixation of the cervical spine fracture. Anteroposterior (**A**) and lateral (**B**) radiographs at 1 year follow-up after posterior spinal fusion.

intervertebral disc. The authors recommended obtaining an MRI in all patients prior to attempted closed reduction and definitive surgery.[19-21] Several other cases with neurologic deficits after open reduction under general anesthesia have been reported.[20,21] There have also been reports of progression of neurologic deficits during traction while the patient was awake and participating that later resolved.[22]

The group from Thomas Jefferson University advocates performing immediate closed reduction in the patient that is awake and can reliably participate in serial neurologic examinations. Vaccaro et al. published their series of 11 patients who underwent successful awake closed reduction without any neurologic worsening. In their series, two patients had herniated discs prior to reduction, and another five had herniated discs following reduction.[14] Darsaut et al. attempted to determine the effect of disc herniation during closed reduction in a series of 17 patients who had a cervical dislocation that was reduced under MRI monitoring. They demonstrated that at least as a research tool this technique was possible.[23]

A commonly used algorithm is based on the patient's neurologic status. If the patient is unable to participate reliably in the physical examination, then an MRI is obtained as expediently as possible. In cases of mild radicular deficit, MRI has the principal disadvantage of requiring vital time. If the patient has a significant spinal cord injury, the risk is that the cord will remain compressed for a longer time. Therefore, if the patient has minimal or no neurologic dysfunction, an MRI should be obtained. If the patient has an American Spinal Injury Association (ASIA) A, B, or C injury and is able to cooperate with the reduction and serial neurologic examinations, consideration should be given to an immediate, rapid reduction. In this situation, the MRI would be obtained after reduction.

Reduction Techniques

Reduction of a cervical spine dislocation must be performed under image guidance and in a very controlled manner. Gardner-Wells tongs are applied with the pins placed 1 cm above the pinna of the ear just below the equator of the head. Pins are tightened to 3.6 kg of pressure. This is indicated once the precalibrated indicator pins protrude a measured amount. If using weights over 25 kg, titanium pins and MRI-compatible tongs are insufficient. Weights of over 60 kg have been used safely for closed reduction of such injuries.[24] In such instances, stainless steel pins or two sets of tongs must be used. Another option includes the use of a halo that provides four titanium pins to distribute the forces over more pins. The major disadvantage of stainless steel pins is their MRI incompatibility.

It is recommended that the initial applied weight be no more than 4.5 kg. Using more weight can be catastrophic if the patient has an unrecognized instability such as an occipital cervical dislocation. After applying the initial 4.5 kg, a neurologic examination should be performed, followed by a radiograph. Additional weight should be added incrementally until reduction is obtained. Serial examinations, as well as serial roentgenograms, are performed to look for any neurologic deficit following each addition of weight. After reduction, the weight should be decreased to the minimum needed to maintain the reduction. Routine examinations are continued, as are efforts to stabilize the instability when medically appropriate. Pulmonary and skin issues can be addressed with use of a kinetic treatment table until surgery.

Definitive Treatment

Closed treatment remains the standard of care for most spinal injuries. In a few situations surgical intervention is clearly required, including skeletal disruption in the presence of a progressive neurologic deficit and purely ligamentous injuries in a skeletally mature patient. Such ligamentous injuries require spinal fusion to obtain stability. It should also be noted that the presence of a neurologic injury is not an absolute indication for surgery. The remaining gamut of spinal injuries can be treated without surgery. Closed treatment options include bedrest, halo apparatus, external orthosis, or a cast. Many unstable injuries can be treated with an initial period of bedrest in a kinetic treatment bed followed by bracing and mobilization once some early healing has been achieved. The absence of significant pain should be the clinical indicator of the patient's readiness to be cleared from the kinetic treatment bed and mobilized. Upright films in the external orthosis should be obtained to confirm that the spinal column is stable at this point.

Timing of Surgical Intervention

Debate continues over the appropriate timing of traction or surgery in cases of acute spinal cord injury. It is difficult to demonstrate improvement in neurologic function from acute surgical intervention.[25] Complete cord injuries and neurologically intact patients are very likely to remain neurologically unchanged with appropriate surgical or nonoperative care. Incomplete lesions typically improve with either surgical or nonsurgical care. Late surgery with decompression of the spinal canal in incomplete cord injuries has been shown to improve neurologic function even several years following the traumatic event.[26,27] In the acute setting, there is sparse and unconvincing evidence supporting early surgery. Surgery for the purpose of spinal canal decompression in a neurologically intact patient is difficult to defend considering that several series have shown dramatic spinal canal remodeling over time in patients with and without surgery.[28-35]

Upper Cervical Injuries

Occipitocervical injuries are most often fatal and typically found postmortem. When encountering a patient with such an injury, the treating physician must be vigilant about the diagnosis to ensure the patient's survival. Initially, such patients should be meticulously immobilized on a backboard with a collar and the head secured with sandbags and tape. Atlanto-occipital disassociation is then stabilized with a halo vest until definitive surgical stabilization is performed.[36] It should be noted that traction for type II injuries (axial distraction) can be catastrophic and is strictly contraindicated. The injury is treated with dorsal occipital cervical fusion with at least 3 months of halo vest immobilization. Occipital condyle fractures and Jefferson or atlas ring fractures are typically managed with an orthosis or a halo.[37]

Odontoid fractures depend on the injury itself. Many can be treated with a rigid orthosis or halo vest. Type I and type III fractures typically heal uneventfully and have a good prognosis without surgery. Transverse type II fractures through the waist of the odontoid have a high associated nonunion rate and are therefore the ideal fractures for surgical treatment. A dorsally displaced odontoid fracture is more likely to be treated with surgery.[38-43] Polin reported on a series of patients treated with a rigid collar as opposed to a halo. More nonunions were associated with the type II fractures. However, there was no statistically significant difference between the orthoses used.[43] Chronic odontoid nonunions in the elderly can often be followed and may not require surgical intervention. In a series of persistent nonunions, no progression of atlantoaxial instability or neurologic deficit was noted or myelopathic symptoms during the follow-up period.[44]

At later reassessment of stability, transverse ligament ruptures can be managed in an orthosis if a bony avulsion occurs.[45,46] If successful, this avoids the significant loss of motion following an atlantoaxial arthrodesis. Dickman et al. demonstrated a 100% failure to heal in complete ligamentous disruptions. These injuries often result in a significant incidence of neurologic injury, and there is frequent association with other upper cervical injuries. They should be treated with C1-2 arthrodesis.[47]

The vast majority of other axis injuries can be stabilized with an orthosis or a halo vest. Traumatic spondylolisthesis of the axis most commonly occurs secondary to a hyperextension and axial load mechanism. Neurologic deficit rarely occurs, with the exception for the atypical fracture that occurs ventral to the dorsal vertebral body cortex.[48] These atypical fractures may require surgery to prevent neurologic decline. Severe hangman's fractures with instability through the C2-3 disc space require surgery. Most other axis injuries can be managed successfully nonoperatively.[37,40,49-52]

Subaxial Injuries

Isolated minimally displaced subaxial lamina and spinous process fractures can be treated with a cervical collar. Single-level axial compression fractures with intact ligaments can be managed similarly. Minor ventral column injuries due to a flexion-compression mechanism with intact dorsal ligaments should also be stabilized in an orthosis.

The treatment of burst-type fractures is controversial due to how imprecisely mechanical stability is determined. Fractures that are thought to be mechanically stable can be treated nonoperatively but require close follow-up. In the setting of cord compression from retropulsed bone fragments in the neurologically compromised patient, ventral decompression and fusion is clearly indicated. In between is a gray area that certainly requires greater investigation to guide treatment.

In subaxial facet dislocations, the nonoperative management is reduction as soon as medically appropriate. After reduction, surgical stabilization is usually necessary because up to 40% of cases remain unstable even after 3 months of halo immobilization.[53-55]

Hyperextension injuries are common after falls in the elderly and can result in spinal cord injury in the absence of mechanical instability. The resulting central cord syndrome results from neural compression due to narrowing of the canal from long-standing spondylosis and the hyperextended position at impact. Surgery is not performed to address instability but may be utilized to decompress the cord or to prevent further injury. A collar may be placed acutely for patient comfort.

Table 69-1 summarizes the treatment options for cervical fractures.

TABLE 69-1

Treatment Options for Cervical Injuries

Cervical Injuries	Observation	Collar	Halo	Surgery
Atlanto-occipital dissociation				√
Jefferson fracture—stable		√	√	
Jefferson fracture—unstable			√	√
Axis body fracture		√	√	
Type I odontoid fracture	√	√		
Type II odontoid fracture		√	√	√
Type III odontoid fracture		√	√	
Unilateral facet dislocation				√
Bilateral facet dislocation				√
Subaxial compression fracture		√	√	
Unilateral facet fracture		√	√	√
Spinous process fracture	√	√		

TABLE 69-2

Treatment Options for Thoracic and Lumbar Injuries

Thoracic and Lumbar Injuries	Observation	Brace	Cast	Surgery	Bed Rest
Compression fracture	√	√			
Multiple compression fracture		√	√	√	√
Burst fracture—posterior ligaments intact	√	√	√	√	√
Burst fracture—posterior ligaments disrupted			√	√	
Fracture-dislocation				√	√
Flexion-distraction				√	
Osteoporosis	√	√	√		
Transverse process fracture	√				

Thoracic and Thoracolumbar Fractures

Transverse process fractures that are isolated require no treatment and can be mobilized as tolerated. With multiple transverse process fractures, a thorough assessment must be made to determine instability or a fracture-dislocation. An L5 transverse process fracture has a 61% association with a pelvic or sacral fracture.[16] These should be critically evaluated with a pelvic CT scan to rule out an associated pelvic injury.

Compression fractures without injury to the dorsal ligamentous complex can be mobilized as tolerated with an orthosis for comfort. Ohana et al. have even suggested that an orthosis may not be necessary.[56] Multiple-level compression fractures in a young healthy individual suggest a high-energy mechanism. Particular attention must be paid to the dorsal ligamentous complex at all injured levels. If a dorsal ligamentous injury is present, surgical treatment is necessary.

Burst Fractures

Most lumbar and thoracolumbar burst fractures can be managed nonsurgically (Table 69-2). Several excellent studies have shown comparable functional outcome to surgery, with less morbidity from nonsurgical treatment. The key to establishing stability is the intact dorsal ligamentous complex. Wood et al. demonstrated in a prospective, randomized series comparable or better outcomes than in those patients treated surgically.[57] Although Denis et al. in 1984 reported a 17% increase in neurologic deficit with nonoperative treatment, this has not since been reported.[58] There are multiple reports with minimal complications and almost no progression of neurologic deficits. There appears to be little correlation to long-term pain and disability with degree of kyphosis.[28,29,31,32,57-87]

Although the dorsal ligamentous complex is the key to deciding on operative versus nonoperative treatment, a definitive way of defining stability can be elusive in many cases. A palpable interspinous gap or pain that occurs with deep palpation is a good indicator of dorsal ligamentous involvement. Although it has been popularized that kyphosis can be an indicator of dorsal injury, this has not been conclusive. Many utilize MRI to assess the dorsal ligaments, although the findings can often be ambiguous.[83] Lee et al. reported that a fat-suppressed T_2 sagittal MRI was the most reliable way to assess the dorsal ligamentous complex. In their series of 34 burst fractures they identified 30 patients with dorsal ligamentous instability,[88] which seems to be an extremely high number of unstable fractures. Instead, it may be that MRI changes may not necessarily correlate with competency. Oner et al. did a similar study and was unable to correlate the MRI to an *Arbeitsgemeinschaft für Osteosynthesefragen* (AO) classification to determine treatment.[89] The treating physician must therefore exercise a great deal of judgment in deciding which fractures require surgical intervention.

Multiple-Level and Noncontiguous Injuries

In cases of multiple-level injuries, particularly noncontiguous injuries, bear in mind that surgical intervention requires multiple-level fusions at multiple levels of the spine or one long fusion mass. This fact has dramatic effects on the final range of motion, function, and long-term outcome. Avoiding fusion, therefore, greatly benefits this patient population (Figs. 69-4 and 69-5). Another alternative is the Jacobs rod long and fuse short technique (i.e., using long rods to reduce fractures while fusing the minimum number of segments). In this technique, the instrumentation is later removed to restore motion at the unfused segments.[90]

Kinetic Therapy

Whether used as a temporary measure or for definitive treatment, kinetic therapy is a useful adjunct to the management of spinal injury. A specially designed hospital bed achieves kinetic therapy by continually rotating the patient through a minimum of 40 degrees. The Kinetic Concepts, Inc. (KCI, San Antonio, TX) RotoRest bed stabilizes the spine while providing kinetic therapy. The Hill-Rom (Batesville, IN) SPO_2RT and KCI TriaDyne beds provide patient rotation but are not adequate for spinal stabilization. Use of kinetic therapy has demonstrated shorter ICU stays, decreased time on a ventilator, better pulmonary outcomes, and a lower incidence of adult respiratory distress syndrome (ARDS) in trauma patients.[91-103]

Initial Emergency Department Stabilization

A trauma patient who cannot be immediately mobilized can be treated very effectively with kinetic therapy. Until the spine is stabilized surgically or sufficient time passes for bony healing, the KCI RotoRest bed can provide 24-hour-a-day mobilization and pulmonary benefit as well as maintaining spine stabilization.[5,104,105] Even after spine stabilization surgery, kinetic therapy with a SPO_2RT or TriaDyne bed can minimize postoperative pneumonia and ARDS.

Short-Term Treatment

In the setting of multiple-level noncontiguous fractures, the patient can be maintained on a RotoRest bed or in traction to allow for initial osseous healing of some of the fractures.[106] Cancellous vertebral body fractures heal rapidly if the patient is receiving adequate nutrition. A period of 2 to 3 weeks of initial healing may allow for single-level fusion or no surgery at all instead of a multiple-level procedure.

Long-Term Definitive Treatment

For polytrauma patients with multiple fractures and life-threatening associated injuries, surgery is not an attractive solution and in many instances is contraindicated. Four to six weeks of recumbency in a kinetic therapy bed can allow for enough healing to mobilize the patient in a brace.[79]

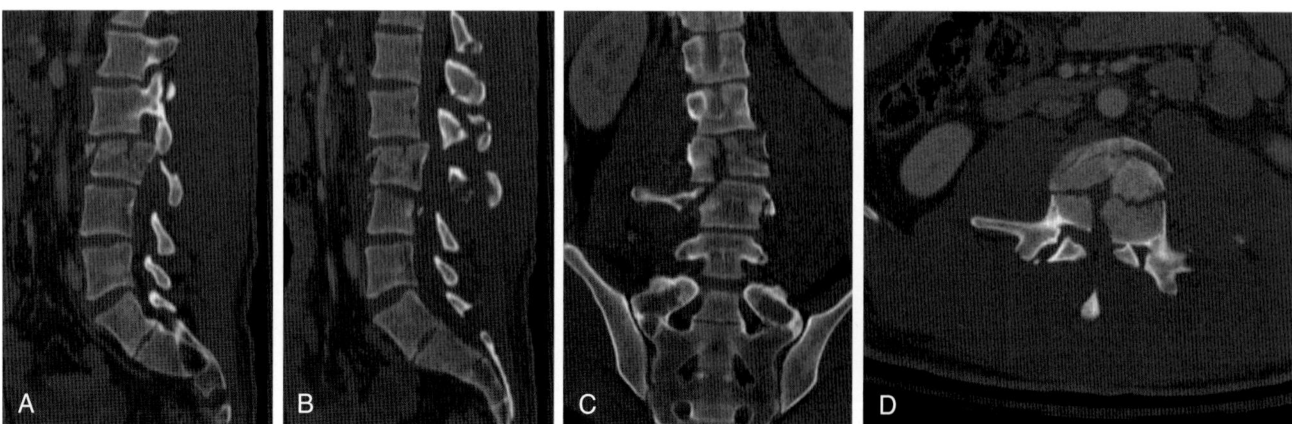

FIGURE 69-4. Thirty-year-old male involved in a motorcycle accident. **A** and **B**, Sagittal CT images demonstrating a burst fracture of L3 and multilevel posterior injury. **C**, Coronal CT image with a sagittal fracture line through L3 and an oblique fracture through the right side of L4. **D**, Axial CT image demonstrating canal compromise.

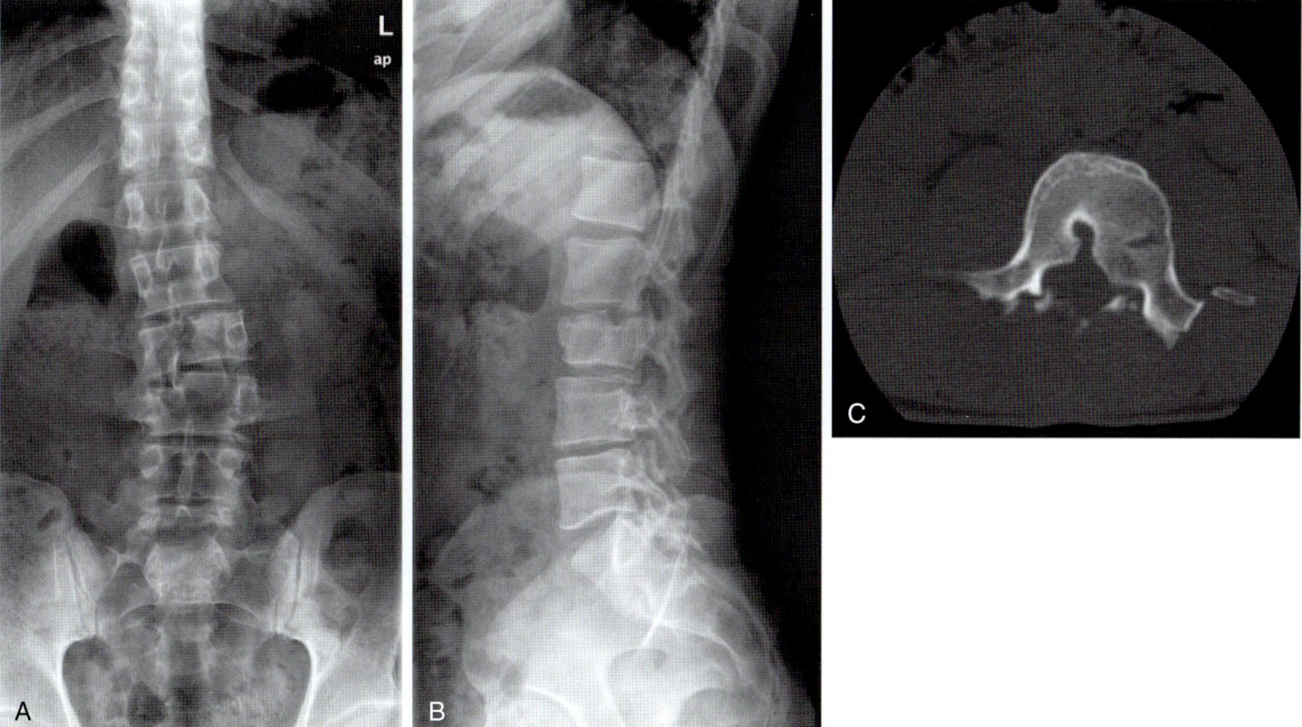

FIGURE 69-5. The same patient as in Figure 69-4 returned to work 3 months following injury, after being treated conservatively in a Roto-Rest bed. Anteroposterior (**A**) and lateral (**B**) radiographs at 2-year follow-up demonstrating adequate alignment and healing of the fractures. **C,** Axial CT image showing canal remodeling at 2 years.

Neurologic Complete Cord Injuries

Although many advocate immediate stabilization for earlier rehabilitation in a patient with a complete cord injury, there is a dramatically increased risk of infection in the long term. In the neurologically complete patient, the incidence of acute wound infection has been reported to be as high as 25% to 40%.[107] Furthermore, these patients experience multiple urinary tract infections over the course of their lifetimes, and these transient episodes of bacteremia or septicemia can lead to late infections.

Penetrating Injuries and Gunshot Wounds

Low-velocity missile wounds to the spine rarely require surgical stabilization. Exploration of missile tracts for vessel or hollow viscous injuries should be determined by the general surgery trauma team. Removal of foreign bodies for spinal canal decompression is not routinely warranted at spinal cord levels. Some investigators report improved neurologic function with canal decompression in the region of the cauda equina. The risk of such acute complications as spinal fluid fistulas, infections, and wound dehiscence is increased with surgical intervention.[108-111] Blood levels can be monitored over time if there is concern of plumbism. In the setting of increased serum lead levels, the bullet fragments can be removed later. This is an uncommon occurrence.[112-114]

High-velocity gunshot injuries (muzzle velocity >1000 fps) require a thorough debridement in the operating suite, a repeat debridement 48 to 72 hours later, and possible spinal stabilization. Fusion may be necessary as the tissue destruction and energy absorbed are orders of magnitude greater than with a nongunshot injury. The energy causing the tissue destruction is directly proportional to the square of the projectile velocity.

Osteoporosis Fractures

All osteoporotic fractures should be treated nonsurgically if possible. Short-term bedrest, bracing, or cement augmentation is usually preferable to surgical stabilization. Constructs that are usually effective in the nonosteoporotic spine may not hold in soft bone. The difference in stiffness between the instrumentation and bone presents a problem at the bone-implant interface, with a high likelihood of implant pullout or failure. Adjacent segment fractures also pose a significant problem due to the stiff instrumented segment producing a stress riser and the presence of osteoporotic bone.[115,116]

Keys to Nonoperative Care

The spine must be accurately assessed and then reassessed to ensure the accurate determination of spinal stability. Stability is reevaluated when the patient is able to be mobilized and examined upright. Upright radiographs in the orthosis or definitive method of treatment provide another chance to determine the level of stability and effectiveness of treatment. Mehta et al. reported that in 25% of their patients, the upright radiographs resulted in a change in treatment.[117]

In cervical injuries, imaging studies must be scrutinized for any subluxation to determine if any ligamentous or facet instability was not previously appreciated. In thoracic or lumbar injuries, the initial upright radiograph is another opportunity to assess dorsal ligamentous instability. Once again, kyphosis alone does not mean dorsal ligamentous disruption. It must be determined whether the kyphosis is a result of ventral column collapse or dorsal column distraction. One of the most effective ways to determine the significance of the dorsal ligamentous injury is to simply palpate the spinous processes.

The original upright radiograph is then used to measure for progressive kyphosis. Keep in mind that increased kyphosis from the original supine film on a backboard may not be meaningful since normal individuals show more kyphosis when standing in the absence of spinal injury.

Summary

Nonoperative management is initiated at the time of injury in all spinal cases, regardless of the method of definitive treatment. In the field, during transport, and while the patient is being evaluated at the hospital, principles of spinal immobilization must be strictly followed. After an appropriate evaluation via history, physical examination, and imaging, an individualized treatment plan is developed. All treatment options should be thoroughly evaluated and considered. The patient should always be involved in the decision-making process. Few spinal injuries actually require surgical intervention.

KEY REFERENCES

Brunette DD, Rockswold GL: Neurologic recovery following rapid spinal realignment for complete cervical spinal cord injury. *J Trauma* 27(4): 445–457, 1987.

Denis F, Armstrong GW, Searls K, Matta L: Acute thoracolumbar burst fractures in the absence of neurologic deficit. A comparison between operative and nonoperative treatment. *Clin Orthop Relat Res* 189:142–149, 1984.

McGuire RA, Neville S, Green BA, et al: Spinal instability and the log-rolling maneuver. *J Trauma* 27(5):525–531, 1987.

Pape HC, Remmers D, Weinberg A, et al: Is early kinetic positioning beneficial for pulmonary function in multiple trauma patients? *Injury* 29(3):219–225, 1998.

Podolsky S, Baraff LJ, Simon RR, et al: Efficacy of cervical spine immobilization methods. *J Trauma* 23(6):461–465, 1983.

Rechtine GR 2nd, Cahill D, Chrin AM: Treatment of thoracolumbar trauma: comparison of complications of operative versus nonoperative treatment. *J Spinal Disord* 12(5):406–409, 1999.

REFERENCES

The complete reference list is available online at expertconsult.com.

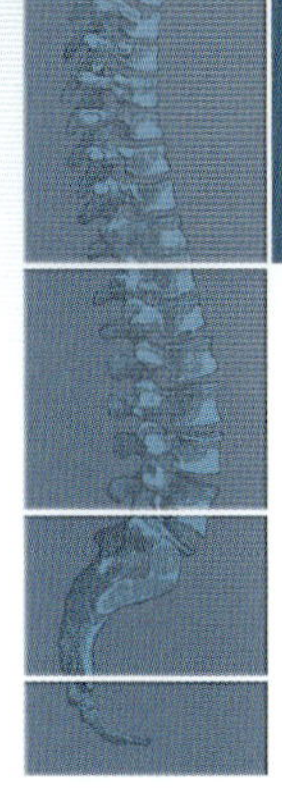

CHAPTER 70

Medical Management of Adult and Pediatric Spinal Cord Injury

James D. Thompson | J. Brad Bellotte | Jack E. Wilberger

The three primary goals of managing both adult and pediatric spinal cord injury (SCI) are to optimize neurologic outcome, provide for early mobilization, and facilitate rehabilitation. These goals are difficult to meet when medical complications supervene. Unfortunately, SCI patients are uniquely vulnerable to a variety of complications that, at a minimum, prolong hospitalization, increase costs, and delay entry into rehabilitation, and at the other extreme may impair neurologic recovery.

Fortunately, mortality after SCI is relatively low and continues to decline. However, morbidity, even in children, remains significant. Thus, attention to the medical management of SCI is essential, and the skills of a multidisciplinary team of spine surgeons, critical care specialists, and physiatrists are often required.

The American Association of Neurological Surgeons published guidelines in 2002 for the management of acute injuries of the cervical spine and spinal cord. This supplement includes medical management strategies for these challenging injuries.[1]

Pharmacologic Intervention

Administration of the steroid methylprednisolone within 8 hours of adult SCI has been shown from the National Acute Spinal Cord Injury Studies (NASCIS II and NASCIS III) to improve American Spinal Injury Association (ASIA) motor and sensory scores in patients.[2-4] In response to SCI, the spinal cord swells, and methylprednisolone is administered to reduce inflammation in hope of preventing further nerve cell death. However, these NASCIS studies are controversial because they failed to address potentially important recovery-influencing details regarding surgical intervention and rehabilitative therapies.[5,6] Furthermore, later analysis revealed that these studies did not demonstrate an improvement in patients' primary outcome measures, which indicates that the improved recovery could be due to random events.[5-8] Because these studies are not entirely credible, evidence is lacking to decisively recommend the use of methylprednisolone following acute SCI.

The studies, however, do demonstrate that it is inadvisable to use methylprednisolone more than 8 hours after SCI because it is associated with a slight decrease in neurologic recovery.[4] Additionally, the NASCIS studies document conclusively that methylprednisolone has serious side effects, such as higher infection rates, respiratory complications, and gastrointestinal hemorrhage. Therefore, methylprednisolone has no benefit in a neurologically intact patient.

Trials with other neuroprotective agents such as the ganglioside GM1, gacyclidine, tirilazad, and naloxone have also failed to demonstrate conclusive effectiveness, and their use cannot be justifiably recommended due to their potential side effects.

Clinical trials involving a new nerve repair drug, BA210 (Cethrin), have been conducted to investigate its safety and effectiveness in restoring neurologic function following traumatic SCI. Cethrin is a recombinant protein that acts as a rho inhibitor to promote neuroregeneration and neuroprotection in the CNS. Rho proteins are involved in a key pathway that promotes apoptosis, and the inhibition of this pathway facilitates axon regeneration at the site of the injury. The clinical trials demonstrated that topical administration of 0.3, 1, 3, or 6 mg of Cethrin following surgical decompression is safe. Recently, a placebo controlled trial has been initiated in order to better assess the drug's clinical efficacy.[9]

Spectrum of Medical Complications

Every organ system can be affected by SCI, irrespective of whether the system is primarily injured in the traumatic event. To reduce the number and severity of overall medical complications, the patient should be transported to a level I or II trauma center with immediate access to a trauma team and imaging capabilities including CT scans and MRI. Once medically stable, and preferably within 24 hours of the injury, movement to a specialized SCI injury center with coordinated state-of-the-art care, if not a component of the level I or II trauma center, is advised. Tator et al. described an almost 50% reduction in hospital length of stay, as well as a significant reduction in mortality and an increase in neurologic recovery when a multidisciplinary team approach was employed in an acute SCI unit.[10] Thus, constant vigilance must be maintained to prevent these complications and to manage them as rapidly and as comprehensively as medically feasible when they do occur.

Because the incidence of pediatric SCI is quite low (<1% of all new spinal cord injury cases per year), the incidence of medical complications in children is not well documented. However, with the exception of pulmonary embolism (PE), it should be anticipated that pediatric medical considerations are not dissimilar to those of adults.

Pulmonary Considerations

The respiratory system is uniquely susceptible to SCI because primary neurologic dysfunction profoundly affects respiratory physiology directly, as well as indirectly. Cervical injury is more commonly associated with pulmonary complications, as 84% of all respiratory complications are the result of C1-4 injuries. However, more than 60% of patients with lower-level injuries develop pulmonary problems, so these may also occur from thoracic-level injuries.[11] Pulmonary complications are the single most common cause of morbidity and mortality after pediatric SCI.

The muscles of respiration include the abdominal, intercostal, diaphragm, and cervical accessory muscles. The abdominal muscles are the primary muscles of active expiration and account for over 50% of expiratory capacity. Thus, thoracic SCI with abdominal muscle paralysis may lead to ineffective expiration, excessive end-tidal volumes, and, subsequently, a diminished lung capacity.[12,13]

To diagnose an abdominal injury in a patient with cervical SCI and hypotension, a Focused Assessment with Sonography for Trauma (FAST) abdominal ultrasound examination is recommended.[14] FAST is a diagnostic tool used to screen for significant hemoperitoneum after blunt trauma.[15] In the absence of or after a positive FAST examination, an abdominal CT scan is advisable to better define the nature of the injury. In a hemodynamically stable patient, a FAST examination is less reliable and the use of a CT scan is necessary to reduce the number of missed injuries.[16]

The intercostal muscles play an important role in stabilizing the chest wall during inspiration. Their paralysis results in a functionally flail chest, in which the chest wall collapses during inspiration and expands during expiration, resulting in an overall loss of tidal volume.

The diaphragm muscles account for approximately 50% to 60% of the inspiratory force generated. When the other muscles of respiration are nonfunctional, however, the diaphragm assumes 100% of the workload and may rapidly fatigue.[17]

Overall, generalized muscle weakness associated with midthoracic injury levels contributes to diminished contraction force for effective coughing and clearing of secretions. These muscle abnormalities, singly or in combination, may ultimately significantly decrease functional residual capacity, tidal volume, and inspiratory and expiratory volumes, while markedly increasing residual lung volumes.[18] Nasotracheal suctioning is often insufficient to mobilize secretion, and consequently, expiratory aids such as mechanical insufflation-exsufflation or quad coughing are necessary.[19,20]

Remember that the vital capacity and the tidal volume of the quadriplegic patient are greater in the supine position than in the upright position. In the supine position, the weight of the abdominal contents helps in forcing the diaphragm rostrally, which leads to a decrease in residual volumes.[21]

Despite attention to these details, some patients may require intubation for respiratory support. The two primary indications are the inability to ventilate effectively (partial pressure of carbon dioxide >50 mm Hg) and the inability to oxygenate adequately (partial arterial oxygen pressure <80 mm Hg). It is critical to monitor these blood oxygen and carbon dioxide levels via pulse oximetry or arterial blood gas measurement early during SCI management.

Endotracheal intubation is often required before the location of an injury can be determined, so it is essential to keep the cervical spine as stationary as possible while securing the airway in case of a cervical-level injury. Succinylcholine is the recommended neuromuscular blocking agent to use during intubation, but only within the first 48 hours after injury due to the risk of hyperkalemia.[22]

Intubation with current endotracheal tubes can be safely maintained for several weeks, although there are some proponents of early tracheotomy. An early tracheotomy should be considered for any patient with high tetraplegia or one who is likely to remain ventilator dependent for an extended period of time, since the tracheotomy simplifies the ventilator weaning process. One review of tracheotomy in critically ill patients illustrated that early tracheotomy reduces the duration of both the stay in the ICU and time needed for mechanical ventilation.[23] Although almost all surgery for acute SCI requires an endotracheal tube, one disadvantage of early tracheotomy is that it may interfere with anterior cervical surgery in those patients who require internal stabilization from such an approach.

Except for quadriplegics with injury at very high levels, most SCI patients can be weaned from ventilatory support during acute hospitalization. A limited number of studies have demonstrated that high tidal volume ventilation of 20 mL/kg or greater (except for patients with adult respiratory distress syndrome or acute lung injury) during rehabilitation reduces the time to ventilator weaning and improves the outcomes for atelectasis.[24] The use of a progressive ventilator-free breathing T-piece protocol also reduces ventilator weaning time.[25] Most patients can be successfully weaned when the vital capacity is greater than 1 L, maximal negative inspiratory force exceeds 30 cm H_2O, and minute ventilation is less than 10 L.[26]

Despite attention to these details, atelectasis and ventilator-associated pneumonia are still common in the SCI population, and thus, constant vigilance is of utmost importance to diagnose and treat pneumonia rapidly. Preventative strategies that reduce the risk of ventilator-associated pneumonia include the maintenance of the patient in a semirecumbent position, the assessment of the patient's readiness for accepted ventilator weaning protocols, and the use of an orotracheal route of intubation.[27-29] The use of prophylactic antibiotics is not encouraged, even in those patients who require prolonged intubation or tracheotomy. Routine use may increase the occurrence of antibiotic-resistant infection.[12,30]

Another potential pulmonary complication of SCI is sleep apnea. Automatic respiration is regulated by spinal cord tracts that lie in the rostral cervical spinal cord. If these pathways are significantly damaged, only voluntary respiration (which is dependent on consciousness) is possible, and breathing may cease during sleep. One should maintain a high index of suspicion of this syndrome in any patient with a high cervical SCI. An apnea monitor or pulse oximeter should be used on a continuous basis for 7 to 10 days after injury in such patients.

Hemodynamic Considerations

The transection of sympathetic pathways after SCI, with concomitant unopposed vagal activity or hyperactivity, accounts for the majority of cardiovascular complications associated with SCI.[31] Monitoring with a Swan-Ganz catheter, however, has documented far-reaching hemodynamic derangements in these patients. The primary immediate concerns are generally bradycardia and neurogenic spinal shock. Although the majority of patients with cervical SCI have bradycardia, only rarely does this become of significant clinical concern to warrant treatment with atropine or use of a temporary transvenous cardiac pacer. Nevertheless, it is important to utilize electrocardiographic monitoring during the early phase after cervical SCI.[32]

In addition to electrocardiographic monitoring, it is necessary to monitor both the temperature and blood glucose level of an SCI patient. Temperature is a factor because the disruption of the autonomic nervous system can cause a loss of vasomotor control, which impairs the patient's thermoregulation. Blood glucose levels are significant because insulin therapy may be needed to maintain normoglycemia in mechanically ventilated patients. A randomized study has shown that regulating blood glucose levels between 80 and 110 mg/dL reduced ICU mortality rates when compared with conventional treatments.[33]

The most important aspect of initial hemodynamic management is to prevent and treat hypotension, particularly in cases of high-level SCI where hypotension is most common. Treatment with early fluid resuscitation, while avoiding fluid overload, is employed to maintain tissue perfusion. Once intravascular volume is restored, vasopressors may be used to constrict the blood vessels to treat hypotension.[34] Fluids and vasopressors are administered to maintain a mean arterial pressure of 85 mm Hg for up to 7 days, and the initial base deficit or lactate level may be useful when determining the need for ongoing fluid resuscitation.[35,36] It is important to raise the blood pressure as soon as possible to improve neurologic recovery, especially in brain-injured patients with reduced cerebral perfusion.[37] A number of experimental models suggest improved outcomes after spinal cord blood flow is maximized by paying careful attention to systemic resuscitation.[38,39]

Neurogenic shock results from inadequate circulating fluid or blood volume due to loss of vascular tone, pooling of blood in the periphery, and third spacing of fluids. Hypotension and systematic vascular resistance, which may be less than 50% of normal, along with an inconsistent heart rate response, are indications of neurogenic shock.[40] However, other injuries should still be investigated as possible causes of hypotension. Neurogenic shock occurs secondary to sympathetic denervation and, when combined with unopposed vagal activity, results in diminished myocardial contractility and bradycardia.

Due to decreased systematic vascular resistance, fluid resuscitation alone may be insufficient to restore normal blood pressure, and pressor agents are frequently required to offset the loss of sympathetic tone and give chronotropic support to the heart. An ideal agent should include both α- and β-adrenergic agonists, such as dopamine, norepinephrine, or epinephrine. On occasion, however, these agents produce a paradoxical effect by decreasing cardiac output and by secondarily decreasing tissue perfusion. Vasopressors should also be chosen as to minimize the exacerbation of bradycardia.

Another manifestation of sympathetic denervation is orthostatic hypotension. Children seem particularly predisposed to this problem. Raising an SCI patient abruptly from the supine to the upright position may result in a significant drop in blood pressure because of an inability to regulate vascular tone. Thus, once the patient has medical and spinal stability, mobilization often requires gradual progressive elevation with elastic stockings, elastic wraps, and abdominal binders.

Deep Venous Thrombosis and Pulmonary Embolism

Deep venous thrombosis (DVT) is another common complication associated with acute SCI. Venous pooling secondary to decreased vascular resistance, combined with a lack of muscle contraction, are the primary factors in its occurrence. Because DVT may not be clinically overt, a high index of clinical suspicion is required, and these patients are best treated with aggressive preventive measures. DVT is dangerous because it can lead to a catastrophic pulmonary embolism (PE), which is fatal in approximately 4% of acutely hospitalized patients. Venous thromboembolism (VTE) has been reported in 6% of more than 16,000 admitted patients with SCI according to California hospital discharge data, and without prophylaxis it is likely to develop in at least 50%.[41] VTE is infrequent in children, and PE has rarely been reported after pediatric SCI.

Early after SCI, it is beneficial to apply a mechanical compression device. Mechanical compression decreases the likelihood of blood clotting by increasing venous outflow and reducing venous stasis.[42] Despite being relatively ineffective in high-risk patients, compression devices are very safe and should therefore be implemented in all patients with acute SCI.[43]

Anticoagulation with low-molecular-weight heparin (30 mg enoxaparin SC every 12 hours) or unfractionated heparin (5000 units every 8 hours) with intermittent pneumatic compression, administered once primary hemostasis is apparent is the mainstay of prophylaxis. Enoxoparin is the preferred low-molecular-weight heparin because the incidence of PE and major bleeding was infrequent in the Spinal Cord Injury Thromboprophylaxis Investigators enoxaparin study.[44] Bleeding should be stabilized before anticoagulants are administered, and potential contraindications include intracranial bleeding, perispinal hematoma, and hemothorax.

The clinical diagnosis of DVT is difficult to establish, and therefore some surgeons advocate the routine use of venous Doppler ultrasonography. Such studies have a 90% accuracy rate in detecting significant venous thrombosis.

An increased vigilance for the possibility of PE should be maintained once DVT is established, because signs and symptoms may be absent or misleading. Fever is often the first manifestation, because SCI patients may not be able to perceive pleuritic pain or mount a tachycardic and tachypneic response to altered pulmonary perfusion. Because of the unreliability of chest radiography and ventilation-perfusion scans in diagnosing PE, pulmonary CT is most often necessary.

If anticoagulation is not possible because active bleeding is expected to continue for 72 hours, a vena cava filter should be considered. However, 26% to 36% of patients with permanent filters eventually developed DVT according to a long-term follow-up study.[45,46] Additionally, a vena cava filter can be a complication for patients with a manually assisted coughing machine because the filter can dislodge when bronchial secretions are cleared.[47,48] To avoid these filter-related complications, a change to pharmacologic prophylaxis is appropriate if the patient's risk of bleeding decreases.

Gastrointestinal Considerations

Gastrointestinal concerns in the SCI patient vary from minimizing gastric and abdominal distension and stress ulcerations to providing nutrition and bowel retraining.

The simplest and most effective means of preventing most acute GI complications is by using nasogastric suction. Gastric atony and paralytic ileus may compromise respiratory function by further decreasing lung capacity or by leading to vomiting and aspiration.

The primary GI concerns for SCI patients are GI bleeding and stress ulceration, which usually occur within the first 4 weeks of injury. The risk of ulceration can be minimized by maintaining a gastric pH above 4. Ranitidine is a histamine H_2-receptor antagonist (H_2RA) that inhibits stomach acid production. It is administered for stress ulcer prophylaxis because it decreases the risk of GI bleeding without increasing the likelihood of ventilator-associated pneumonia or altering the gastric pH.[49] Another option is the use of proton pump inhibitors (PPIs), which block the final common pathway in acid secretion as opposed to H_2RAs, which only block one of three pathways. PPIs are as effective as H_2RAs in preventing upper GI bleeding and more effective for maintaining a pH above 4 for critically ill patients requiring mechanical ventilation.[50] Nevertheless, both options are safe ways to suppress acid levels and prevent stress-related mucosal disease.

More severe and life-threatening acute abdominal complications, such as splenic rupture or liver lacerations, or chronic complications, such as bowel obstruction or perforation or other similar conditions, may be obscured because of a lack of pain perception after SCI. Occasionally, vague pain may be appreciated secondary to autonomic visceral afferent branches that are conducted into the spinal cord via the splanchnic nerves. Also, if the SCI is not above the C5 level, referred pain secondary to diaphragmatic irritation may be felt in the shoulder region. Other signs of ongoing abdominal complications, such as temperature elevation, elevated white blood cell count, or associated ileus are not reliable signs for the identification of abdominal disease in these patients. Similarly, clinical examination may be misleading because localized abdominal tenderness, muscle guarding, and rigidity are likely to be absent, even though peritonitis may be present. Thus, it must be recognized that patients with SCI can develop such abdominal complications. The patient should be observed carefully for any indirect signs that may point to an ongoing acute abdominal problem.[51]

Because SCI patients are hypermetabolic and hypercatabolic acutely, enteral nutrition should be provided for the patient once swallowing is evaluated, resuscitation is complete, and there is no evidence of ongoing shock or hypoperfusion. Enteral feeding is advised because it has a lower incidence of infection and hyperglycemia than parenteral feeding methods.[52,53] The patient's caloric needs during rehabilitation are usually 45% to 90% of the calculated values and are lower for tetraplegics than for paraplegics.[54] The need for caloric support decreases progressively as the SCI patient recovers.

Bowel retraining is a critical component of GI management and should be begun early after injury due to the patient's loss of colonic motility and sacral reflexes. Appropriate procedures for a bowel program can be chosen based on the bulbocavernosus reflex. This reflex is an indicator of upper versus lower motor neuron bowel dysfunction. An effective daily bowel regimen can be implemented using oral medications, suppositories, and digital stimulation.[55]

Urologic Considerations

SCI patients often have the neurologic loss of the ability to void due to the sudden loss of autonomic control. Placement of an indwelling urinary catheter is recommended no later than in the emergency department when IV fluids are initiated in order to monitor urinary output during the early period of hypotension and third fluid spacing. However, the longer the need for an indwelling catheter, the greater the risk of urinary tract infection. Thus, the catheter may be removed once the patient is hemodynamically stable and strict monitoring of fluid status is no longer necessary. If the use of an indwelling urinary catheter is contraindicated, emergent suprapubic drainage will suffice.

Some situations require additional input from a urologist, such as if the patient suffered a urethral injury. For any pelvic fracture or penetrating injury near the urethra, instrumentation such as a urinary catheter should be avoided as it can exacerbate urethral injury. Also, priapism is common during the early period after SCI, but a urethral catheter may still be used, and usually no special treatment is required.

Depending on the level of the SCI, the bladder may be areflexic and flaccid or dyssynergic and spastic. With an areflexic bladder, voiding may be accomplished by using abdominal pressure—the Credé maneuver. However, if residual urine remains high, this maneuver should be supplemented by clean, intermittent catheterization.[56] With a spastic bladder, spontaneous voiding is possible as long as the intravesicular pressure is not too high and there is no overriding sphincter spasticity. In this situation, at least in men, an external condom catheter is acceptable.[57] If the pressure is too high or if the sphincter is spastic, pharmacologic intervention may be helpful. The bladder musculature may be relaxed with anticholinergics such as propantheline or smooth muscle relaxants such as oxybutynin.

Pediatric SCI regimens for bladder management depend on the age, gender, size, and weight of the child and the type of bladder. Fluid intake and output are crucial in establishing programs and schedules. In infants and toddlers, for whom the use of diapers is appropriate, one should ensure adequate emptying of the bladder. With school-aged children, diapers are no longer appropriate, and their continued use may be detrimental to the child's self-esteem and self-image. Clean intermittent catheterization is an alternative and can be instituted at any age.

Skin Care

Development of pressure areas is another complication of SCI. Immobility and the lack of sensation predispose to pressure necrosis of the skin and subsequent skin breakdown. Thus, pressure over the skin should be avoided. Areas that create the greatest pressure points are the bony prominences such as the sacrum, occiput, scapulae, trochanters, ankles, and heels. For patients who must be maintained on a backboard for more than 2 hours, pressure should be relieved every half hour. Those who are immobilized for a prolonged period require a specialized bed that provides pressure reduction and protective surfaces. An appropriate skin care procedure includes repositioning every 2 hours, inspecting the skin regularly, and maintaining a clean, dry area underneath the patient.[58]

Psychological and Rehabilitation Issues

Not only does SCI create a physical disability but it is a severe psychological stress on both the patient and family members. Because this stress may not be readily appreciated initially, it is important to provide appropriate levels of psychiatric support and counseling within a few days of SCI. The patient's mental health status should be regularly assessed, paying attention to depression, posttraumatic stress disorder, life stressors, and any suicidal ideations. It is constructive to foster effective coping strategies, promote healthy behaviors, acknowledge the patient's suffering, and treat for any underlying causes for depression. For some patients who become rapidly depressed because of their physical limitations, the use of antidepressant medications may be appropriate. Any treatment refusal or requests for withdrawal from treatment are serious matters, and the patient's decision-making capabilities should be evaluated under these circumstances.

Additionally, SCI rehabilitation aims to facilitate maximal neurologic recovery while helping the individual develop compensatory strategies for the neurologic loss. The involvement of a rehabilitation specialist, beginning early after injury, is beneficial for the treatment of an SCI patient. Protocols for physical therapy, occupational therapy, and speech and language pathology should be developed and initiated early to ensure the efficiency and effectiveness of the rehabilitation process.

KEY REFERENCES

Consortium for Spinal Cord Medicine: *Respiratory management following spinal cord injury: a clinical practice guideline for health-care professionals*, Washington, DC, 2005, Paralyzed Veterans of America.

Consortium for Spinal Cord Medicine: Clinical practice guidelines: neurogenic bowel management in adults with spinal cord injury. *J Spinal Cord Med* 21(3):248–293, 1998.

Guidelines for the management of acute cervical and spinal cord injuries. *Neurosurgery* 50(3):S1, 2002.

Heyland DK, Dhaliwal R, Drover JW, et al: Canadian Critical Care Clinical Practice Guidelines Committee. Canadian clinical practice guidelines for nutrition support in mechanically ventilated, critically ill adult patients. *JPEN J Parenter Enteral Nutr* 27(5):355–373, 2003.

Kocan MJ: Pulmonary considerations in the critical care phase. *Crit Care Clin North Am* 2:369–374, 1990.

Mansel JK, Norman JR: Respiratory complications in management of spinal cord injuries. *Chest* 97:1440–1452, 1990.

Rogers FB, Cipolle MD, Velmahos G, et al: Practice management guidelines for the prevention of venous thromboembolism in trauma patients: the EAST practice management guidelines work group. *J Trauma* 53:142–164, 2002.

REFERENCES

The complete reference list is available online at expertconsult.com.

CHAPTER 71

Spinal Injuries in Sports

Vincent Miele | Joseph Maroon

Injury to the spine and surrounding structures are common occurrences in athletes with a wide spectrum of consequences ranging from an annoyance to a life-altering event. Although injuries that require minimal intervention are exponentially more common, it is the fear of permanent spinal cord injury (SCI) that causes the trepidation associated with this subject, and the differentiation between minor and serious injuries is the foundation of treatment of the athlete.

This chapter discusses spinal injuries that are unique to the athlete and addresses the spectrum of injury from simple strains/sprains to those resulting in gross instability and permanent neurologic deficits. An optimal response to the athlete with suspected or proven neck injuries has unique facets, which are detailed in this chapter. In addition, the current evidence and expert opinion on return to play following spinal injuries, as well as surgery, is summarized. Section One details the epidemiology of sports-related spinal injuries, broken down by discussion of individual sports with a higher risk of injury. Section Two focuses on the cervical spine, and also covers the on-site management of catastrophic SCI. Section Three deals with the thoracic spine, and Section Four with the lumbosacral complex.

Section One

Sports-Specific Epidemiology

Each year, approximately 10,000 cases of SCI occur in the United States.[1] Participation in sporting activities accounts for nearly 10% of these and is the fourth most common cause of SCI (after motor vehicle accidents, violence, and falls).[2,3] Sports-related SCIs also occur at a younger mean age of 24 and are the second most common cause of SCI in the first three decades of life.[4,5]

Spinal injuries are more common in nonorganized sports such as diving and surfing than in organized sports.[1,6] The challenge in this population is that rules, supervision, and training are limited. These limitations make it difficult to improve injury patterns by enforcing safety guidelines and manufacturer standards. Although less frequent, spinal injury in organized sports have a much higher public profile. Several organized sports, including football, ice hockey, rugby, skiing, snowboarding, and equestrian sports, have been identified as placing the participant at high risk for SCI.[7-10]

Sport-Specific Risks to the Spine

American Football

American football involves approximately 1.4 million athletes at the junior/senior high school level, 75,000 in college, and 1000 in professional play.[11] This total contrasts roughly with 60,000 rugby players in the United States. With the innumerable high-velocity collisions incurred during practice and games, it is the most dangerous sport for SCI in terms of exposure and is responsible for the highest risk of cervical spine trauma among organized sports participants. Although American football has a lower per participant rate of catastrophic cervical spine injuries than ice hockey or gymnastics, the huge number of participants translates into the largest overall number with catastrophic cervical spine injuries.[11]

High school participants are at the highest risk, accounting for over 80% of cervical injuries, largely due to the wide discrepancies in player size, age, maturity, and speed at this level. At the other end of the injury risk spectrum is the preadolescent and early adolescent participant. In this group, disabling spinal injuries are almost nonexistent, a result of the players' small size and the relative lack of high-velocity collisions.

Notably, a significant increase in catastrophic cervical trauma coincided with the development of the modern football helmet. However, rule changes in 1976 prohibiting playing techniques that used the top of the helmet as the initial point of contact for blocking and tackling (spearing) have significantly reduced this trend. From 1976 to 1987, the rate of cervical injuries decreased 70%, from 7.72 per 100,000 to 2.31 per 100,000 at the high school level.[12] Traumatic quadriplegia decreased approximately 82% over the same period.[13] Since most football players are injured during tackling, defensive players (defensive backs, members of the kickoff teams, and linebackers) are at the highest risk of injury. Almost all cervical spine injuries occur when a player strikes an opponent with high velocity using the vertex of the helmet or with the head down. This action results in a significant axial load, often with a degree of flexion. The cervical musculature that is responsible for maintaining extension is much stronger than that used in maintaining flexion. Thus, a player who lowers his head in blocking or tackling increases his vulnerability to cervical injury by placing his cervical spine in a position that is less able to absorb the consequent energy.

Baseball and Softball

Minor spinal injuries are fairly common in baseball and softball, but catastrophic injuries do occur. Participants who slide headfirst into a base have the most risk of catastrophic SCI. If the hands of the runner separate, the top of his head can collide with the leg of the defensive player, creating a great deal of axial load transmission to the vertebral column. Although the use of breakaway bases substantially decreases the risk for occurrence of sliding-related injuries, serious injuries can still occur. The use of even lower profile bases and the outlawing of sliding have also been suggested.[14]

Basketball

Basketball involves rapid changes in direction and explosive movements, causing repeated stresses to the spinal vertebrae. Thus, it is not surprising that the most common neurologic risk in basketball is to the player's spine. A variety of acute back injuries, such as lumbosacral sprains, contusions, and facet joint and pars interarticularis injuries, are common.[15,16] In addition, this sport is a leading cause of sports-related disc disease and has been reported to be the second most common cause of disc herniation among athletes.[17] Herniated discs usually arise dorsally or dorsolaterally and occur as a consequence of numerous microtraumas to the intervertebral disc compounded by chronic overstraining. Cervical cord neurapraxia has also been reported in basketball players.

Cycling

Cycling-related injuries to the spine can be secondary to acute trauma or overuse. The athlete most at risk for serious traumatic injury is the 20- to 30-year-old male considered adept at the sport but not participating in an organized class or team. Over half of the total acute cycling injuries result from contact with motor vehicles. The risk of neck injury increases in cyclists struck by motor vehicles or hospitalized for any injury.

Neck and back pain are common complaints in cyclists, occurring in over half of participants. The odds of female cyclists developing neck and shoulder overuse problems have been reported to be 1.5 and 2.0 times greater, respectively, than for their male counterparts.[18] Neck pain is partially the result of a combination of increased load on the arms and shoulders required to support the cyclist and hyperextension of the neck in the horizontal, bent forward position of riding. These stresses are compounded in bicycles improperly fitted to the cyclist. Lower back pain often results from hyperextension of the angle between the spine and pelvis, which increases stress at the promontorium.

Equestrian Sports

Approximately 20% of the injuries sustained by an equestrian involve the CNS. One study found that 13% of the patients had injury to the spinal cord, with the cervical region most commonly involved.[19] There does not seem to be any correlation between risk of injury and the participant's age, gender, or experience.[20] Equipment failure has been shown to be a common cause of injury. Although jumping events have garnered the majority of attention in the past decade due to catastrophic injuries to celebrities such as Christopher Reeves, the particular type of equestrian activity with the most risk to the spinal cord is unequivocally rodeo rough-stock riding (bull, bareback bronco, and saddle bronco riding).[21] Common spinal injuries include cervical and lumbar sprain, acute torticollis secondary to being thrown, and cervicothoracic strain secondary to missing the animal in the steer wrestling competition.

Gymnastics

Gymnasts are a group of athletes with perhaps the greatest risk of back injury. A National Registry of Gymnastic Catastrophic Injury was established in 1978, and 20 gymnasts injured the cervical spine in its first 4 years. Of these, 17 remained quadriplegic and 3 died secondary to their injury. Notably, most of the injuries occurred in experienced gymnasts during practice.[22] The sport accounts for a significant proportion of all sports-related SCIs, and an 18-month study of elite and subelite female gymnasts reported a back injury rate of 14.9%.[23] Injuries are commonly to the cervical spine, and the sport is by far the leading cause of quadriplegia in women's sports.

The most common cause of nonacute back injury in gymnastics is the repeated hyperextension of the back by the participant, compounded by numerous microtraumas. Spondylolysis, a relatively common injury in the gymnast, can evolve into spondylolisthesis if the condition is not recognized early.

Ice Hockey

The sport of ice hockey has experienced a marked increase in the occurrence of cervical spine injuries through its history.[24] Major vertebral column injury occurred at an increased rate between 1982 and 1993, with a mean of 16.8 fracture-dislocations per year during that period. Checking an opponent from behind, which typically produces a headfirst collision of the checked player with the boards, has been identified as an important causative factor in cervical spine trauma in hockey. Changes in the rules that prohibit checking from behind and checking of an opponent who is no longer controlling the puck seem to be decreasing the incidence of these injuries, and data suggest that fewer cases of complete quadriplegia have been caused by these playing techniques since the rule changes have been instituted.[24]

Mixed Martial Arts

Mixed martial arts (MMA) is a full-contact sport combining elements of boxing, kickboxing, and wrestling. It has evolved since 2001 to become a mainstream sport with improved regulations to minimize injury.[25] Most competitions now forbid head butting; stomping or kneeing on an opponent on the ground; and striking the throat, spine, or back of the head. Also, athletes must fight within a predetermined weight class. Despite the dramatic impacts that a participant receives during competition, the overall injury rate in MMA competitions has been determined to be similar to other combat sports, including boxing.[25,26] While no catastrophic spinal injury has been reported during competition in the past decade, many of the maneuvers seem to be particularly risky.

Maneuvers known as "spinal locks" are often employed in competition. A spinal lock is performed by forcing the spine beyond its normal ranges of motion and is typically accomplished by bending or twisting the opponent's head or upper body into abnormal positions. These maneuvers can be separated into two categories based on their primary area of effect on the spinal column: spinal locks on the neck are called neck cranks, and locks on the lower parts of the spine are called spine cranks. Spine cranks are less commonly performed in competition than neck cranks because they are more difficult to apply. These can commonly strain the spinal soft tissue and musculature and if forcefully and/or suddenly applied could theoretically result in ligament damage, bony fracture or displacement, and SCI.

Four of the most commonly utilized maneuvers in the sport are the O goshi (judo), in which the fighter uses his shoulders to swing the opponent over his hips; the suplex (jujitsu), in which the fighter grabs the opponent around the waist and lifts him up over his shoulder to fall forward onto his face; the souplesse, a variant of the suplex, in which the opponent is rotated and slammed down onto his back; and the guillotine drop (a choke hold). A detailed kinematic and biomechanical analysis of these maneuvers showed that the forces involved are of the same order as those involved in whiplash injuries and of the same magnitude as compression injuries of the cervical spine.[27]

Rugby

Spinal injuries, especially to the cervical region, are common in the traditional tackle games of rugby union, rugby league, and Australian rules football. A retrospective study of SCIs in rugby from 1960 through 1989 identified 117 catastrophic neck injuries. It was also reported that for every serious rugby-associated SCI, 10 severe neck injuries occurred that did not involve the cord.[28]

Three specific activities during the game of rugby—the tackle, tight scrum, and loose play (ruck and maul)—result in the majority of injuries to the cervical spine.[29] Cervical spine injury often results from impact between the tackler's head and the ground or the body of the opponent (usually the thigh). The immediate halt of the head's forward progress results in compression fractures of the vertebral bodies from axial forces transmitted down the spine. These forces are increased significantly if the player's neck is flexed, which eliminates the normal lordosis of the cervical spine. An injury during a high tackle from behind often results from hyperextension secondary to the head being pulled back and down. If the tackle is from the side, hyperflexion injury often results. Rotational forces are also a factor in these injuries, especially if the tackle is performed with only one arm. Double tackles, often referred to as "sandwich" or high-low tackles, are more common near the goal with a concentration of defenders merging on the ball carrier. They can cause injury to both the offensive and defensive player. If the defensive players miss their target, they can collide into each other with considerable force at unexpected angles. If the tackle is successful, the offensive player's body is forced in two directions. This inhibits the player from moving with either force completely, increasing rotational and shearing stresses to the spine.

Water Sports

The water sport with the most risk for spinal injury is by far recreational diving. Mishaps have been reported to account for up to 75% of all recreation-related spinal cord injuries.[30-32] These injuries tend to occur in teenage males involved in unsupervised activities during the summer months. The most common cause of injury is the participant striking his head on the bottom of a pool, lake, or ocean after having miscalculated the depth of the water. Diving injuries occur almost exclusively to the cervical spine and often result in quadriplegia. Forward flexion, often with axial compression, is the usual mechanism of injury. The C5 level is most commonly involved, likely attributable to the wide range of motion and the relatively smaller size of the vertebral canal at this level.[33]

A second water sport with a significant risk of cervical spine injury is surfing. These injuries are usually related to a variety of impact positions, as surfers are propelled by falls or tidal action, striking their heads and necks on the ocean bottom.

Wrestling

The sport of wrestling has been associated with spinal injury, most commonly in the cervical region.[34] Although the intervertebral discs, joints, and ligaments are somewhat resistant to compression stresses, they are very susceptible to injury by rotational and shearing forces. Most injuries result from landing with the body twisted on the head and neck and occur during takedowns and sparring. Various combinations of thoracolumbar spine abnormalities, such as spondylolysis, are also prevalent in this population of athletes.

Section Two

Cervical Spine and Brachial Plexus

A dramatic range of symptomatology may result from trauma to the cervical spine and brachial plexus. Although injuries in this area are almost always transient, the large contribution of this part of the nervous system to normal function predicates that they be taken very seriously.

Cervical Sprains, Strains, and Contusions

One of the most common causes of neck pain in the athlete is the constellation of cervical strain, sprain, and contusion. A *strain* is defined as a stretch injury at the musculotendinous junction or within the muscle itself. If the ligamentous structures of the spine are more involved, it is termed a *sprain*. *Contusions* are blunt-force injuries to soft tissue. Injuries in this group most often occur when a force is applied to a contracting muscle. This creates an eccentric contraction resulting in some degree of tensile failure. The most vulnerable area for this injury is at the myotendinous junction as well as areas of greater type II (fast-twitch muscle fibers) concentration.[35] Most injuries involve an overlap of all three components, with the severity of injury being a consequence of the magnitude and direction of the applied forces.

The natural course of these injuries is a gradual resolution of pain and muscle spasm with conservative treatment. Obviously, an athlete who presents with pain and limited cervical range of motion should undergo a complete clinical and radiographic examination. At a minimum, this imaging should include dynamic (flexion-extension) plain radiographs in at least two orthogonal planes of the entire cervical spine (occiput to C7-T1 junction). If the injury only appears to be a strain, sprain, or contusion, a cervical collar may be continued until any severe muscle spasm has resolved, which usually takes 7 to 10 days. Use of a cervical collar for longer than this length of time has been demonstrated to result in significant deconditioning and weakening of the cervical musculature.[35] Repeat dynamic radiographs can then be taken to ensure that the athlete does not have any delayed instability that could present after the splinting effect of muscle spasm has resolved. If these tests are negative, the collar can be discontinued and physical therapy begun. This should include gentle range-of-motion and isometric strengthening exercises, followed by a more sport-specific regimen.

The athlete may return to play when he or she is asymptomatic, has full range of motion, and has baseline sport-specific neck function. After returning to competition, the athlete should continue stretching and strengthening exercises in an attempt to reduce the incidence and severity of any future injury. The use of a sport-specific protective orthosis (e.g., a "horse collar" in American football) to prevent further injury may be employed, although significant data on their actual benefit are limited. Such orthoses used in American football have been shown to limit hyperextension of the cervical spine while allowing enough extension to prevent axial loading injury.[36]

Facet Injury

Facet joints contain encapsulated mechanicoreceptors that provide proprioceptive information from the cervical spine. They can also play a significant role in protective muscular contraction (spasm) in response to unexpected external forces. Forced flexion-type forces commonly received by the cervical spine of the athlete may lead to damage of the cartilaginous surfaces of these joints, resulting in chronic pain and premature degenerative changes. Chronic pain experienced by some individuals following a cervical whiplash-type injury can usually be managed with rest, physical therapy, and occasionally injection therapy. If the pain becomes intractable, serious consideration should be given to limiting participation in sports.

Brachial Plexus Neurapraxia

Brachial plexus neurapraxia (also known as stinger-burner or transient brachial plexopathy or nerve root neurapraxia) is a transient neurologic event characterized by pain and paresthesia in a single upper extremity following a blow to the head or shoulder. This condition is one of the most common occurrences in collision sport participation and is not the result of an SCI. It was first described in 1965 by Chrisman et al.[37] Because the mechanism was thought to be direct force applied to the shoulder with the neck flexed laterally away from the point of contact, the condition has also been referred to as "cervical pinch syndrome."[38] The symptoms most commonly involve the C5 and C6 spinal roots. The affected athlete can experience burning, tingling, or numbness in a circumferential or dermatomal distribution.[38] The symptoms may radiate to the hand or remain localized in the neck. These athletes often maintain a slightly flexed cervical spine posture to reduce pressure on the affected nerve root at the neural foramen or may hold or elevate the affected limb in an attempt to decrease tension on the upper cervical nerve roots.

Weakness in shoulder abduction, external rotation, and arm flexion is a reliable indicator of the injury.[39] If weakness is a component, it usually involves the C5-6 neurotome. The radiating arm pain tends to resolve first (within minutes), followed by a return of motor function (within 24–48 hours). Although the condition is usually self-limiting and permanent sensorimotor deficits are rare, a variable degree of muscle weakness can last up to 6 weeks in a small percentage of cases.

As mentioned previously, this injury is most commonly the result of downward displacement of the shoulder with concomitant lateral flexion of the neck toward the contralateral shoulder. This is thought to result in a traction injury to the brachial plexus. The condition may also result from ipsilateral head rotation with axial loading resulting in neural foramen narrowing and compression-impaction of the exiting nerve root within the foramen.[40,41] Direct blunt trauma at the Erb point, located superficially in the supraclavicular region, has also been reported to be a cause.[42] This can occur when an opponent's shoulder or helmet drives the affected athlete's shoulder pad directly into this area.

This injury has been graded using the Seddon criteria. A grade 1 injury is essentially a neurapraxia defined as transient motor or sensory deficit without structural axonal disruption. This type of injury usually completely resolves, and full recovery can be expected within 2 weeks. Grade 2 injuries are equivalent to axonotmesis and involve axonal disruption with an intact outer supporting epineurium. This results in a neurologic deficit for at least 2 weeks, and axonal injury may be demonstrated on electromyographic studies 2 to 3 weeks following the injury. Grade 3 injuries are considered neurotmesis, or total destruction of the axon and all supporting tissue. These injuries persist for at least 1 year and show little clinical improvement.

Stingers with prolonged neurologic symptoms are the most common reason for high school and college athlete cervical spine evaluations in an emergency department.[43-45] The athlete commonly demonstrates a full, pain-free arc of neck motion with no midline palpation tenderness on examination. If tenderness is present or unilateral neurologic symptoms persist, a paracentral disc herniation with associated nerve root compression should be considered. This is usually accompanied by the sudden onset of dorsal neck pain and spasm. Monoradiculopathy characterized by radiating pain, paresthesias, and/or weakness in the upper extremity also occurs secondary to compression and inflammation of the cervical root.

Although this injury is usually considered benign, an athlete that suffers an episode of brachial plexus neurapraxia should be immediately removed from competition until symptoms have fully resolved. On-field evaluation should include palpation of the cervical spine to determine any points of tenderness or deformity. Sensation and muscle strength should be evaluated using the unaffected limb as a point of reference. Weakness in the muscles innervated by the upper trunk of the brachial plexus is often observed. These include the deltoid (C5), biceps (C5-6), supraspinatus (C5-6), and infraspinatus (C5-6) muscles.[46,47] The shoulder of the affected limb should also be evaluated, paying particular attention to the clavicle, acromioclavicular joint, and supraclavicular and glenohumeral regions. Percussion of the Erb point can be performed in an attempt to elicit radiating symptoms. Obviously, the athlete should be evaluated for other serious injuries such as cervical spine fractures and dislocations. It is unusual to find lower brachial trunk injury patterns involving the C7 or C8 nerve roots. It is also uncommon to see persistent sensory deficits involving either the lower or upper extremities. This condition is always unilateral and has never been reported to involve the lower extremities. If bilateral upper extremity deficits are present, SCI should be at the top of the differential diagnosis. Localized neck stiffness or tenderness with apprehension to active cervical movement should alert the examiner to a potentially serious injury and the subsequent initiation of full spinal precautions, including spine board immobilization and transport for imaging.

If the player does not complain of neck pain, decreased range of motion, or residual symptoms, he or she can usually return to competition. If symptoms do not resolve or there is persistent pain, prompt imaging of the brachial plexus via MRI is recommended. If the symptoms persist for over 2 weeks, electromyography can be performed to establish the distribution and degree of injury.[48] Residual muscle weakness, cervical anomalies, or abnormal electromyographic studies are exclusion criteria from return to play.[44]

By definition, brachial plexus neurapraxia is a transient phenomenon. It usually does not require formal treatment. The athlete should be followed closely with repeat neurologic examinations since although the condition usually resolves in minutes, motor weakness may develop hours to days following the injury.[39,45] Repeated injury may result in long-term muscle weakness with persistent paresthesias, resulting in permanent removal from competition.[49] Options in participants to decrease the risk of future occurrences are to change their field positions or modify their playing techniques.

Central Cord Syndrome

Injury to the lower cervical cord can result in a spectrum of neurologic dysfunction. Incomplete SCI can occur with partial preservation of sensory or motor function. Central cord syndrome is the most common manifestation of this, followed in frequency by the anterior cord syndrome.

Burning hand syndrome is considered to be a variant of central cord syndrome. It is characterized by burning dysesthesia in both upper extremities and is likely the result of vascular insufficiency affecting the medial aspect of the somatotopically arranged spinothalamic tracts.[50,51] The lower extremities may occasionally be involved and weakness may occasionally be evident. Cervical spine fracture or soft tissue injury is frequently associated with these syndromes, and any athlete exhibiting this condition should be initially treated as having an SCI (see section titled On-Site Evaluation and Management of Spinal Cord Injury).[52]

Cervical Cord Neurapraxia and Transient Quadriplegia

Neurapraxia of the cervical spinal cord (CCN) resulting in transient quadriplegia has been estimated to occur in 7 per 10,000 football players.[53] This alarming injury is characterized by a temporary loss of motor or sensory function and is thought to be the result of a physiologic conduction block without true anatomic disruption of neuronal tissue. The affected athlete may complain of pain, tingling, or loss of sensation bilaterally in the upper and/or lower extremities. A spectrum of muscle weakness is possible, varying from mild quadriparesis to complete quadriplegia. The athlete has a full, pain-free range of cervical motion and does not complain of neck pain. Hemiparesis or hemisensory loss is also possible.

The condition is thought to result from a pincer-type mechanism of compression of the cord between the dorsocaudal portion of one vertebral body and the lamina of the vertebra below.[54] Although this can also occur during hyperflexion, it is more commonly the sequela of extension movements with infolding of the ligamentum flavum, which can result in a 30% or more reduction of the anteroposterior diameter of the spinal canal.[55] The spinal cord axons become unresponsive to stimulation for a variable period of time, essentially creating a "postconcussive" effect.[56]

CCN is described by the neurologic deficit, the duration of symptoms, and the anatomic distribution. A continuum of neurologic deficits that range from sensory only, sensory disturbance with motor weakness, or episodes of complete paralysis may occur. These may be described as paresthesia, paresis, or plegia. An injury is defined as grade 1 if the CCN symptoms do not persist for longer than 15 minutes. Grade 2 injuries are defined as lasting from 15 minutes to 24 hours. Grade 3 injuries persist for 24 to 48 hours. All four extremities may be involved; this is considered a "quad" pattern. Upper- and lower-extremity patterns may also be observed.[57]

By definition, CCN is transient, and complete resolution generally occurs within 15 minutes but may take up to 48 hours. Steroid administration in accordance with the Bracken protocol[58] in this population is controversial. No controlled studies have reported that the administration of steroids has altered the natural history of athletes with CCN.[44] In players who return to football, the rate of recurrence has been reported to be as high as 56%.[57]

A considerable amount of controversy exists regarding whether the presence of cervical stenosis makes an athlete more prone to sustaining CCN and even permanent neurologic injury.[59,60] This controversy is compounded by the imprecise methods of objectifying whether an individual suffers from stenosis. The anteroposterior diameter of the spinal canal (measured from the dorsal aspect of the vertebral body to the most ventral point on the spinal laminar line) determined from lateral cervical spine radiographs is considered normal if there is more than 15 mm between C3 and C7. Cervical stenosis is considered to be present if the canal diameter is less than 13 mm. However, this measurement varies widely secondary to variations in landmarks used for measurement, changes in target distances for making the radiographs, patient positioning, differences in the triangular cross-sectional shape of the canal, and magnification of the canal because of a patient's large body habitus. In an effort to eliminate this variability, Torg and Pavlov designed a ratio method for determining the presence of cervical stenosis, comparing the sagittal diameter of the spinal canal with the sagittal midbody diameter of the vertebral body at the same level.[61] A ratio of 1:1 was considered normal, and less than 0.8 was indicative of significant cervical stenosis. This ratio was found to mislabel many athletes with adequately sized canals but large vertebral bodies as being stenotic. This observation, as well as an unprecedented ability to image the vertebral column, intervertebral discs, spinal canal, cerebrospinal fluid (CSF), and spinal cord directly, have made MRI, and not boney landmarks, the currently preferred method of choice for assessing "functional spinal stenosis." MRI assessment of CSF signal around the spinal cord, termed the *functional reserve*, can be determined, and the visualization of the CSF signal, its attenuation in areas of stenosis, and changes on dynamic sagittal flexion-extension MRI studies are now the standard in diagnosing this condition. An absent CSF pattern on axial and, particularly, sagittal MRI is diagnostic of functional stenosis.

It had been previously accepted that young athletes who suffered an episode of CCN were not predisposed to permanent neurologic injury.[60,62] This assumption has recently been called into question now that a player who experienced a CCN subsequently sustained a quadriplegic injury.[63]

Traumatic Intervertebral Disc Herniation

Acute herniation of an intervertebral disc can occur during participation in sports and in the athletic population. Those involving the cervical spine are less common than lumbar disc injuries and usually involve the older athlete. Compared with the overall incidence of disc herniation in the general public, the incidence is likely increased in the high-performance athlete competing in contact sports such as football and wrestling.[64,65] Conversely, participation in noncontact sports might actually be protective against the development of cervical or lumbar disc herniation. This is likely the result of improved muscular conditioning protecting the disc from stresses transmitted to the spine.[66]

There are two types of disc herniation: hard and soft. Soft disc herniation is a more sudden phenomenon during which the soft nucleus populsus comes through the dorsal anulus. Hard disc herniations, on the other hand, are more of a chronic degenerative issue that likely begins much earlier in life than when the patient becomes symptomatic. This population often demonstrates a diminished disc height, marginal osteophytes, and degenerative disc material bulge and herniation.

Athletes with symptomatic cervical disc herniations most often present with varying degrees of neck or arm pain. Although the types of symptoms are similar in athletes and nonathletes, they may seem to be more severe in the competing athlete due to the demands of the specific sport. A traumatic central disc herniation typically presents with the sudden onset of dorsal neck pain and paraspinous muscle spasm as well as true radicular arm pain or referred pain to the periscapular area.[67] Extrusion of disc material into the central spinal canal can result in acute cord compression and injury. Clinically, the athlete may present with acute paralysis of all four extremities and a loss of pain and temperature sensation.

In almost all cases except for those involving acute neurologic deficit, the initial 6 to 8 weeks of treatment should be nonoperative. This is especially important for an athlete who wishes to return to competition since this will be easier to accomplish without an operative intervention in most circumstances. As in the nonathlete, treatment options include rest, activity modification, anti-inflammatory medication, immobilization, cervical traction, and occasionally therapeutic injections.[35] In most cases, the symptoms slowly resolve with these modalities, and a gradually increasing intensity of exercises can be initiated. These should at first emphasize isometric strengthening and cervical range of motion, followed by more sport-specific exercises. The athlete can return to competition when asymptomatic and after he or she has regained full strength and painless range of motion.

In some cases, radicular symptoms may persist despite conservative interventions or the athlete may develop myelopathy or a progressive neurologic deficit. In these situations, surgical intervention is considered. Although either a traditional ventral or dorsal approach can be performed, minimal disruption of normal anatomy is critical. Anecdotal evidence has suggested that an athlete may achieve a faster recovery following laminoforaminotomy without fusion, but a direct comparison between athletes undergoing the two types of surgery remains to be performed. This nonfusion procedure also has the advantage of preserving the majority of the disc involved, which theoretically decreases the forces that will be received by the adjacent segments when competition is resumed.

Following a dorsal disc procedure, the athlete can generally return to play when he or she is asymptomatic and has regained full strength and mobility. Following anterior discectomy and fusion at up to two levels, return to play can be considered once a successful bone fusion has been documented and the patient is pain free. Obviously, patients with longer fusions are generally considered to be at risk when returning to contact sports, and therefore the participation of these athletes must be individualized. The stability of disc arthroplasty devices in sports has yet to be determined, and, given the risk of extrusion, athletes who undergo an artificial disc placement are generally barred from a return to contact sports.

Minor Cervical Fractures

Compression Fractures

Compression fractures are significantly less common in the cervical spine than in the thoracolumbar spine due to the anatomic shape of the vertebra, decreased axial load, and increased range of motion allowed by the cervical spine. Hyperflexion is the most common mechanism of cervical spine compression fractures. Although they rarely result in any significant angulation or loss of height, the injury mechanism can also cause major dorsal ligamentous disruptions, depending on the magnitude of the applied forces. Because of this, when a fracture is identified, care must be taken to rule out the presence of associated dorsal structure injuries that could lead to instability.

Individuals found to have suffered an isolated cervical compression fracture are usually treated with a semirigid cervical collar for 8 to 10 weeks. At the conclusion of immobilization, dynamic (flexion-extension) radiographs should be obtained to rule out a more severe ligamentous disruption.[35]

Spinous Process Fractures

Fractures of the spinous processes most commonly involve the lower cervical and upper thoracic area, occur as isolated injuries, and are stable. They occur via three mechanisms. The most common involves a strenuous contraction of the trapezius and rhomboid muscles, which avulses the spinous process. The C7 level is the most commonly involved, and this injury was previously termed *clay-shoveler's fracture*. A second mechanism of injury is a hyperflexion or hyperextension injury to the neck, resulting in avulsion of the spinous process by the supraspinous and interspinous ligaments. This mechanism of injury is most commonly associated with a high-energy trauma, such as from a motor vehicle accident, but can also occur during contact sports such as football, gymnastics, and hockey.[68] A less common mechanism described in the literature entails a direct blow to the spinous process.

Although spinous process fractures often occur as isolated stable injuries, vigilance should be maintained for an accompanying unstable injury. As mentioned earlier, isolated injuries are stable and usually heal with no long-term sequelae. The core of management is rest and symptom control. The athlete is usually placed in a semirigid collar to help control pain as well as to guard against delayed instability. Once the fractured area becomes nontender, dynamic radiographs (flexion-extension) can be obtained and, if negative, strengthening and range-of-motion exercises begun. This process can commonly take 1 to 2 months.

Isolated Lamina Fractures

The fracture of a lamina without an accompanying more serious and unstable injury is rare. If the lamina fracture is vertical, the mechanism is usually an axial load, with or without rotation. An injury to the vertebral body is commonly associated with such a fracture. Transverse lamina fractures, on the other hand, are often avulsion injuries and can result from the pull of the ligamentum flavum during extreme hyperflexion. Both of these multiple-column injuries are often unstable.

As would be expected, management strategies for these injuries are dependent on their stability. If the injury is truly isolated and stable, it can be treated with rest and immobilization in a semirigid cervical collar until pain has resolved. Dynamic radiographs can then be performed, and if negative, the athlete can begin rehabilitation.

Catastrophic Cervical Spine Injury

A structural distortion of the cervical spinal column associated with actual or potential damage to the spinal cord is classified as a catastrophic cervical spine injury.[67] Sports-related cervical spine injuries are divided into three groups that provide useful information when deciding when an athlete is ready to return to play.[1,6,69] Type 1 injuries are those in which the athlete sustains permanent SCI. This category includes both immediate, complete paralysis and incomplete SCI syndromes. The incomplete injuries are of basically four types: Brown-Séquard syndrome, anterior spinal syndrome, central cord syndrome, and mixed types. Mixed types include the finding of crossed motor and sensory deficits with more prominent involvement of the upper extremities, which is considered to be a central cord/Brown-Séquard variant. There are, in addition, a few individuals in whom the neurologic deficit is relatively minor but who demonstrate an associated spinal cord pathology on imaging studies. For example, a high-intensity lesion within the spinal cord seen on MRI documents a spinal cord contusion. Type 2 injuries occur in individuals with normal radiographic studies. These deficits completely resolve within minutes to hours, and eventually the athlete has a normal neurologic examination. An example of the type 2 injury is the burning hands syndrome discussed earlier, which is a variant of central cord syndrome characterized by burning dysesthesias of the hands and associated weakness in the upper extremities.[50] Most of these patients have normal radiographic studies, and their symptoms completely resolve within about 24 hours. Although certainly dramatic, these injuries are usually not considered catastrophic. Type 3 injuries comprise those with radiographic abnormality without neurologic deficit. This category includes fractures, fracture-dislocations, ligamentous and soft tissue injuries, and herniated intervertebral discs.

SCIs can also be divided into upper (occiput, atlas, and axis) and lower (C3-T1) cervical spine injuries. A thorough understanding of the normal anatomy and unique motion of the spine at various segments is mandatory when treating these injuries.

Unstable fractures and/or dislocations are the most common cause of catastrophic cervical spine trauma. The most common primary injury vector is axial loading with flexion occurring in football and hockey.[70,71] Eighty percent of injuries to the cervical spine result from the accelerating head and body striking a stationary object or another player.[72,73] The cervical spine is compressed between the instantly decelerated head and the mass of the continuing body when an axial force is applied to the vertex of the helmet. In neutral alignment, the cervical spinal column is slightly extended as a result of its normal lordotic posture, and it is believed that compressive forces can be effectively dissipated by the paravertebral musculature and vertebral ligaments. This buffering cervical lordosis is eliminated when the cervical spinal column is straightened and large amounts of energy are transferred directly along the spine's longitudinal axis.[71] Under high enough loads, the cervical spine can respond to this compressive force by buckling.

Two major patterns of spinal column injury result from the compression injury vector. Compression-flexion injury is the most common variant that results from the combination of axial loading and flexion. It results in shortening of the anterior column because of compressive failure of the vertebral body and lengthening of the posterior column because of tensile failure of the spinal ligaments.[74] If the cervical vertebra is subjected to a relatively pure compression force, both the anterior column and posterior column shorten, resulting in a vertical compression (burst) fracture. The vertebral body essentially explodes, during which disc material extrudes through the fractured end plate, and osseous material retropulses into the spinal canal, resulting in possible cord damage.[75] Alternatively, a significant SCI may occur without major disruption of the spinal column's integrity. This type of injury is the result of transient spinal column distortion with energy transfer to the spinal cord.

Catastrophic cervical trauma caused by the primary disruptive vector flexion generally results from either a direct blow to the occipital region or rapid deceleration of the torso. The flexion-distraction injury most likely to result in spinal cord dysfunction is a bilateral facet dislocation.[76,77] Unilateral facet dislocation, associated with cord injury in up to 25% of cases, can occur with the addition of axial rotation to the distractive force.[78] It should be recognized that unstable cervical fracture-dislocations do not always result in upper motor neuron dysfunction. A unilateral facet dislocation can cause a monoradiculopathy due to foraminal compression of a nerve root on the side of the dislocated articular process. In other cases, major osseous or ligamentous damage produces no neurologic impairment. SCI potential in these scenarios is based on the amount of lost structural integrity of the vertebral column.[67]

Upper Cervical Spine Injury

For the purposes of sports-related injuries, the upper cervical spine is considered to include the occiput, atlas (C1), and axis (C2). The major function of the atlanto-occipital joint is motion in the sagittal plane, which accounts for 40% of normal flexion and extension of the spine and 5 to 10 degrees of lateral bending. The midline atlantodens articulation is stabilized by the transverse atlantal ligament, which prevents forward translation of the atlas. This specialized osseoligamentous anatomy allows the atlas to rotate in a highly unconstrained manner. The atlantoaxial complex is responsible for 40% to 60% of all cervical rotation.[79] This rotation is limited by the alar ligaments extending from the odontoid process to the inner borders of the occipital condyles. The apical ligaments attach the odontoid centrally to the ventral foramen magnum. Atlantoaxial joint strength is provided by the transverse ligament and the lateral joint capsules.[48]

Spinal cord damage due to fractures or dislocations involving the upper cervical spine is rare because proportionately greater space exists within the spinal canal than with the lower cervical segments. Injuries that destabilize the atlantoaxial complex (fracture of the odontoid or rupture of the transverse atlantal ligament) are most likely to result in spinal cord dysfunction. Flexion is the most common cause of injury at the atlantoaxial joint. Odontoid fractures can also result from extension injuries. Unilateral rotary dislocations are usually the result of rotational forces. Cord compression is unusual with a burst fracture of the atlas or traumatic spondylolisthesis of the axis because these osseous injuries further expand the dimensions of the spinal canal. If anteroposterior radiographs demonstrate spreading of the lateral masses of greater than 7 mm, the transverse ligament is likely torn. Bilateral pedicle fractures of the axis may occur from extension of the occiput on the cervical spine. Importantly, although these injuries can result in instability, they usually do not cause neurologic deficits due to the anatomically wide spinal canal that is also present at this level.[48] If an upper cervical cord injury does occur, diaphragmatic paralysis with acute respiratory insufficiency can occur along with quadriplegia since the phrenic nerve arises from three cervical nerve roots (C3-5).

Lower Cervical Spine Injury

The lower cervical spine encompasses the C3 through C7 vertebrae. This area accounts for the remaining arcs of neck flexion, extension, lateral bending, and rotation and has several important anatomic differences with respect to the upper cervical spine. The spinal canal is not as wide at this level, and the facet joints are oriented at a 45-degree angle. Because of this angulation, axial rotation is somewhat limited.

Each motion segment can be separated into an anterior and a posterior column. Stability of a cervical segment is derived mainly from the ventral spinal elements. Compression of the spinal column is primarily resisted by the vertebral bodies and intervertebral disc, whereas shearing forces are opposed primarily by paraspinal musculature and ligamentous support. Instability of the lower cervical spine has been defined radiographically as translational displacement of two adjacent vertebrae greater than 3.5 mm or angulation of greater than 11 degrees between adjacent vertebrae.[80]

The majority of fractures and dislocations occur in the lower cervical region. Lower cervical spine injuries are defined by the forces acting on the area (i.e., flexion, extension, lateral rotation, axial loading). Dislocated joints are usually the result of a flexion mechanism with either distraction or rotation. The ligamentous structures are the primary restraints to distraction of the spine.[79] Compression of the dorsal structures as well as damage to the ventral structures is usually the result of extension or whiplash injuries. This mechanism of injury commonly results in tearing or the anterior longitudinal ligament and fractures of the dorsal elements.[48]

Compressive forces usually result in vertebral body fractures. These are commonly seen in spear tackling, a tackle in football in which a player's entire body is launched head first—spear-like—against an opponent, resulting in significant axial loading on the cervical spine because the top of the head is the "spear point" of contact.[81] This population commonly has a flexed posture to the head and a loss of the protective cervical lordosis.[48] Large axial loads can result in protrusion of disc material or fractured bone into the spinal canal. This is the most common mechanism for sports-related quadriplegia.[82,83] The C3-4 level is most commonly involved in cases of quadriplegia secondary to cervical dislocations.[84,85]

On-Site Evaluation and Management of Spinal Cord Injury

Participation in contact and collision sports carries an inherent risk of injury, for which injuries to the nervous system have the greatest potential for significant morbidity and mortality. Neurologic injuries suffered during athletic competition must be treated promptly and correctly to optimize outcome, and differentiating between minor and serious injuries is crucial to their management. Catastrophic injuries to the head or spinal cord are usually easy to identify, as are those that develop an immediate neurologic deficit. More challenging is the diagnosis of an injury with minimal initial symptomatology. This section is a guide to identifying and managing serious sports-related spinal injuries.

Primum non Nocere

The most important rule in dealing with potentially injured athletes is that an unstable spine injury can be easily converted into an injury with permanent neurologic deficit if mishandled. Because severe athletic-related injuries are relatively rare, the experience of the on-site medical staff is usually limited. Thus, everyone who shares responsibility for treating spine-injured athletes should be adequately trained and receive frequent refresher courses in the care of possible injury situations. The Inter-Association Task Force for Appropriate Care of the Spine-Injured Athlete was formed in 1998 and developed guidelines for the treatment of the catastrophically injured athlete.[86] The five categories of on-field management are (1) preparation for any neurologic injury, (2) suspicion and recognition, (3) stabilization and safety, (4) immediate treatment and possible secondary treatment, and (5) evaluation for return to play.

Prior preparation should ensure that all of the proper equipment (e.g., spine boards, cervical collars or immobilization devices, cardiopulmonary resuscitation equipment, and stretchers) is available on site and easily accessible during a sporting event. Additionally, specific equipment for protective gear removal (e.g., football face mask) should also be readily available. There should be a clear hierarchy among the medical staff, indicating one member as the "captain" who directs the efforts of the team. In addition, arrangements should be made in advance to have ambulance services on site or close at hand. Preparation allays discomfort among providers and fosters efficiency and good decision making in the event of injury.[72] It should also be mentioned that those who would treat injured athletes are legally responsibile for their actions, and precedent exists for legal action against team physicians and trainers who fail to properly care for those players.[80]

On-Site Management

The prevailing goal among the medical team members should be the prevention of secondary neurologic injury as a result of improper handling of the fallen athlete. Cervical spine injury should be suspected, and the athlete treated as if the injury were present whenever the mechanism of injury involves forced movement of the head and neck, even in the absence of neurologic deficit. The head and neck of the player should be immediately immobilized in a neutral position.

The immediate treatment of the player who has suffered an SCI should follow standard trauma protocols that address airway, breathing, and circulation. During this assessment, a rapid evaluation of the athlete's level of consciousness may also be performed. Unless the player is unconscious or airway or breathing considerations exist, he or she should be left in the position in which he or she lies, until safe transfer onto a spine board can occur. If an athlete is wearing protective gear with a face mask, the face mask should be removed. If the player is wearing a helmet, it can usually be left in place until the head and neck can be adequately immobilized.[87] The following situations require removal of the helmet: (1) a loose-fitting helmet that does not hold the head securely, thereby allowing the head to remain mobile; (2) an uncontrolled airway or inadequate ventilation provided even after removal of the face mask; (3) a face mask that cannot be removed after a reasonable period of time; and (4) a helmet that prevents immobilization for transport in an appropriate position.[86] If necessary, the helmet should be removed with concomitant occipital support or simultaneous removal of shoulder pads (in American football). If left in place following helmet removal, the shoulder pads may cause cervical hyperextension. Obviously, if the helmet is removed, cervical immobilization must be maintained during the procedure.

The initial objective in this primary survey is to assess the athlete for immediately life-threatening conditions and to prevent further injury. During this primary survey, appropriate resuscitation procedures are instituted and the emergency medical system is activated immediately on recognizing a life-threatening problem or serious spinal injury.[88]

Following the initial survey, one of three clinical scenarios will become apparent: actual or impending cardiopulmonary collapse, altered mental status but no compromise of the cardiovascular or respiratory system, or normal level of consciousness and normal cardiopulmonary function. In a neurologically intact athlete with a normal mental status, once cervical spine involvement has been excluded, the athlete may be assisted to a sitting position and, if stable in this position, to a standing position. If able to stand, the athlete can then be walked off the field for further evaluation.

Unconscious athletes need to be stabilized before any neurologic appraisal. When sudden unconsciousness without preceding craniospinal trauma occurs, a cardiac etiology should be considered. If the athlete is experiencing cardiopulmonary collapse, the use of advanced cardiac life support principles is essential. If the athlete is lying prone, he or she must be carefully log rolled into a supine position on a rigid backboard if available. Any face mask should be rapidly removed to provide adequate airway access. As mentioned earlier, the removal of the helmet or other equipment is not routinely indicated unless they interfere with resuscitation. If still in place, the mouthpiece should be taken out while manual stabilization of the neck in a neutral position is maintained. Airway evaluation should be performed, understanding that obstruction can be secondary to a foreign body, facial fractures, or direct injury to the trachea or larynx. A depressed level of consciousness can also contribute to the inability to maintain an airway.

If breathing is of insufficient depth or rate, assisted ventilation is required. On the field, this usually is performed by using a bag-valve device and face mask. Hypoxia should be rapidly corrected by providing adequate ventilation with protection of the vertebral column at all times. In a patent airway, respiratory collapse could be the result of an upper cervical SCI due to paralysis of the diaphragm and accessory breathing muscles. Indications for definitive airway control by endotracheal intubation include apnea, inability to maintain oxygenation with face mask supplementation, and protection from aspiration. Circulation must also be addressed during the primary survey. Neurogenic shock due to SCI could result in diminished amplitude of the peripheral pulses in combination with bradycardia. If the femoral or carotid pulses are not palpable, cardiopulmonary resuscitation is required. If this is the case, the front of the shoulder pads can be opened to allow for chest compressions and/or defibrillation.[86]

If the athlete's mental status is altered without cardiopulmonary compromise, a brief neurologic examination can be performed. The prevention of further injury to the cord is of primary importance, and once initial resuscitation and evaluation are performed, focus should be placed on immobilization. The helmet and shoulder pads should remain in place unless removal is required to access the airway. Neutral axial alignment and occipital support must be maintained. If a player is unconscious, he or she should be log rolled into a supine position and any mouthpiece removed.

If, after completion of the primary survey, the athlete is found to have a normal mental status without cardiopulmonary compromise, a neurologic assessment should be performed. If the athlete exhibits symptoms or signs suggestive of cord damage, a catastrophic cervical cord trauma should be assumed. If the neurologic assessment is normal but the athlete exhibits cervicothoracic pain, focal spinal tenderness, or restricted neck motion, an unstable spinal column injury with potential cord compromise is assumed.

The athlete should be taken from the field while maintaining strict immobilization of the spine. A rigid backboard with cervical collar or bolsters on the sides of the head should be used. It is important to remember that the athlete's helmet may cause unintended cervical flexion on a rigid spine board. Once the athlete arrives at the hospital, if they are still in place, the helmet and shoulder pads should be removed before radiographic examination.

Off-the-Field Management

The treatment of the various forms of cervical spine injury has been summarized by numerous authors and follows established guidelines.[1] The initial caregivers of the spine-injured athlete must be aware of the potential for respiratory failure and hemodynamic instability, as well as associated lesions, such as head injuries, which may affect the timing and order of needed treatments. Because of these concerns, patients with acute neurologic deficit from SCIs usually are initially cared for in an intensive care environment. The neurologic deficits from SCI may be improved by the early administration of steroids, but this method is controversial.[78] The early induction of hypothermia has also been anecdotally reported to be beneficial.

After initial resuscitation and radiographic evaluation, informed decisions concerning the management of the injury can be made. Some bony injuries, such as spinous process fractures or unilateral laminar fractures, may require no treatment or only immobilization in a cervical collar. Others, such as the bilateral pars interarticularis fracture of C2 ("hangman's fracture") may require immobilization with a cervical collar or halo vest. Unstable injuries should initially be reduced and temporarily stabilized with cervical traction using Gardner-Wells tongs or a halo ring device. Contrast-enhanced CT scan or MRI of the cervical spine should be obtained before fracture reduction to rule out the presence of retropulsed intervertebral disc material, which has been implicated in the sudden neurologic deterioration of patients undergoing reduction of cervical fractures. Severe comminuted vertebral body fractures, unstable dorsal element fractures, type 2 odontoid fractures, incomplete SCIs with canal or cord compromise, and progression of neurologic deficit to higher levels of spinal cord function may require surgical intervention.

Any permanent neurologic injury should disqualify an athlete from further competition. Likewise, those whose fractures require halo vest or surgical stabilization are usually considered to have insufficient spinal strength to safely return to contact sports, although there may be exceptions. Even after the fracture has healed, the altered biomechanics in surrounding spinal segments and loss of normal motion result in a high risk of future sports-related injury. Athletes without cord injury who have stable fractures as evidenced by flexion-extension radiographs may be allowed to return to their previous level of activity. Athletes with burning hands syndrome or brachial plexus injuries may be considered safe for return to play when their neurologic examination returns to normal and they are symptom free.

Managing traumatic spinal injury in athletes presents a unique challenge for the surgeon. The classification scheme previously described is useful in decision making regarding optimal treatment and ultimate playing status of these athletes. Type 1 athletic injuries (those with permanent neurologic injury) preclude the player from further participation in contact sports. In type 2 injuries (transient neurologic disturbances with normal radiographic studies), if the complete workup reveals no injury, the player may return to competition once he or she is symptom free. Players with type 3 injuries (heterogeneous, including all players with radiographic abnormalities) such as bony or ligamentous spinal instability, or spinal cord contusion, are advised not to return to contact sports. Other radiographic abnormalities, such as spear tackler's spine, dorsal ligamentous injury, congenital fusion or stenosis, herniated discs, or degenerative spondylitic disease, should be evaluated on an individual basis.

Spear tackling puts a group of athletes at high risk for cervical quadriplegic injury and has been considered a relative contraindication for participation in contact sports.[81] Affected athletes have (1) developmental cervical canal stenosis, (2) persistent straightening or reversal of the normal cervical spine lordotic curve, (3) evidence of preexisting, posttraumatic radiographic abnormalities of the cervical spine, and (4) documentation of having previously used spear tackling techniques showing predisposal to injury from cervical spine axial energy forces. When a spine with a congenitally narrowed canal is straightened, impact at the top or crown of the helmet causes buckling of the neck because the movement of the head is momentarily stopped while the trunk continues to accelerate forward. This axial loading impact to the persistently straightened cervical spine, which occurs when athletes deliberately engage in frequent head impact, can result in permanent SCI. Occasionally, if no significant bone or ligamentous instability is present, cervical lordosis may be restored through physiotherapy. If the player can be coached against using head vertex impact, a return to competition may be allowed. Otherwise, these individuals should be withheld from participation in contact sports.

Section Three

Thoracic Spine

Injuries involving the thoracic spine are relatively infrequent in athletes, largely because athletic training provides significant stability gains to the rib cage, sternum, and broad paraspinal musculature. The osseous elements of the rib cage alone have been found to increase the stability of the thoracic spine by 20% to 40%. This has been previously referred to as a "fourth column" of stability in reference to the Denis three-column model of instability for thoracolumbar fractures. Despite the protective advantages to the thoracic region, injuries can occur. Most are minor and can be treated as discussed in the previous section. When an unstable injury does happen, there is a theoretically increased risk of injury to the cord due to a higher ratio of spinal cord to spinal canal diameter.

The thoracic spine can be divided into three separate zones each with varying risks of injury: midthoracic zone, cervicothoracic junctional zone, and thoracolumbar junctional zone. The midthoracic zone is the most structurally stable of the three but does have a higher theoretical risk of minor injuries such as contusions due to the prominence at its apex. The junctional areas have an increased vulnerability for unstable injuries. As mentioned previously, the cervicothoracic junction is a common site for spinous process avulsion fractures.

General return to competition guidelines are similar to those already discussed in the cervical spine section. Athletes requiring surgery in this area can usually return to competition once they are pain free and have regained full range of motion. If a fusion procedure was performed, there should also be radiographic evidence of solid bone fusion. Relative contraindications for return to competition are fusions that cross the cervicothoracic or thoracolumbar junction. Absolute contraindications to return to competition are fusions that terminate at a junctional zone.

Section Four

Lumbosacral Spine

Most population-based surveys of back pain report a point prevalence of 15% to 30%, a 1-year prevalence of 50%, and a lifetime prevalence of 60% to 80%.[89] Given these numbers, it is not surprising that issues with the lumbosacral portion of the spine are fairly frequent in sports. An incidence of 7% has been reported in college athletes, and approximately 30% of college football players miss games due to lumbar spine problems.[90] These injuries become more common as the level of play increases; the majority are simple lumbar strains. Most of these injuries are the result of direct contact causing a significant axial load or repeated hyperextension activities. Fortunately, most are minor and resolve spontaneously or with minimal intervention. This section deals with lumbosacral pathology in athletes, including diagnosis and surgical management. Simple strain, sprain, and contusion management were detailed in the cervical spine discussion.

Disc Herniation

Although lumbar discogenic disease is relatively uncommon in the younger population, its incidence increases with involvement in sporting activity.[22] Pain can be axial mechanical, radicular, or both, and injuries range from anular tears to herniation with nerve root compression. Disc herniation in athletes is a consequence of numerous microtraumas to the intervertebral disc, which are further compounded by chronic overstraining. Although symptoms of other common injuries can resemble disc disease or damage, some mimickers are unusual. For example, a fracture of the lumbar lamina with epidural hematoma simulating herniation of a disc has been reported.[91]

When disc herniations occur in athletes in the teenage years or early twenties, they often present more subtly, with the main symptoms being back pain and muscle spasm. Signs of radiculopathy are less obvious due to the more viscous nature of the younger anulus and the lower likelihood of a free fragment.

Conservative therapies, including limiting participation, activity modification, anti-inflammatory medications, and therapeutic injections, are most commonly the first employed. Although these modalities have an excellent chance of improving symptoms, athletes frequently resist being sidelined and pressure the physician for a "quick fix." This is especially true in the elite athlete.

Intractable symptoms refractory to conservative treatment and signs of progressive neurologic deficit or cauda equina syndrome are often treated operatively. Although true for most surgeries, minimal tissue disruption is particularly important for the athlete with the goal of return to competition. Either standard microsurgical discectomy or percutaneous microendoscopic discectomy is the technique of choice. Since the anulus of the disc is going to be subjected to considerable and frequent tensile forces when the athlete does return to competition, avoiding wide anular disruptions may decrease the incidence of reherniation. Bilateral laminectomies should be avoided to preserve as much bony and ligamentous structural integrity as possible.

Generally, surgical treatment is well tolerated, and the athlete can return to competition without restriction in as little as 3 weeks. Criteria for return to competition following surgery are a completely healed incision and pain-free activity. If more time can be taken off, postoperative physical therapy including core strengthening should be performed.

Facet Syndrome

Damage or inflammation of the facet joints can often result in recurrent axial mechanical pain that worsens during participation. Pain from this source is greatest with hyperextension or twisting of the spine and may be unilateral. It is commonly observed in basketball players and is often associated with disc disease or injury.[92] Management is similar to that discussed in the section on cervical facet injury.

Pars Interarticularis Injury

The majority of sporting activities involve rapid changes in direction and explosive movements. A spectrum of injuries, ranging from stress fractures to complete spondylolysis and pars interarticularis defect, may result from such movements. The younger athlete is more prone to these injuries since this small bony connection is not yet fully developed in early adolescence. Because athletes in this population is also beginning a rapid growth phase, they are also more vulnerable to some of the more significant complications of spondylolysis, such as vertebral slippage and spondylolisthesis.[93,94] Even without the development of deformities or instability, pars defects can result in chronic back pain.[95]

Early detection in the adolescent is critical to arresting and possibly reversing damage. If not corrected, spinal stenosis and narrowing of the foramen can result in chronic lower back pain, radiculopathy, and symptoms of neurogenic claudication. Patients with spondylolysis or spondylolisthesis with less than 50% slippage can be treated with rest, but more severe injuries often require bracing of the lumbosacral spine or surgical fusion.[96-98]

Impending Spondylolysis or Impending Pars Defect

Ideally, stress fractures of the pars interarticularis can be discovered and treated before a frank bony separation occurs. This stage of injury is referred to as an impending spondylolysis, spondylolysis in the developmental stage, pars stress fracture, or impending pars defect. The first sign of such an injury is constant axial mechanical lower lumbar pain in an adolescent athlete that worsens with activity. Point tenderness is often evident at the lumbosacral junction, particularly over the L5 vertebra.[99]

Traditional bone-imaging modalities such as plain radiographs or CT scans are of limited value since no bone displacement has yet occurred, yet several other tests may give objective evidence of this condition.[100,101]

Generally, impending pars defects appear hypointense on T1-weighted MRI sequences and hyperintense on T2-weighted sequences. The extent of the edema can often be appreciated best on fat-presaturated T2-weighted images. MRI has the advantage of not exposing the athlete to radiation.

Nuclear scanning tests such as a bone scan can reveal bone inflammation indicative of an impending pars defect. Single-photon emission computed tomography (SPECT) can also aid in the diagnosis of an impending pars defect. It is similar to conventional nuclear medicine planar imaging but can provide true three-dimensional information typically presented as cross-sectional slices. The disadvantages to these modalities are the radiation exposure required and their fairly nonspecific results. For example, SPECT cannot distinguish between a pars stress fracture and other causes of increased activity in the pars such as arthritis, osteoid osteoma, or infection. Since these conditions are uncommon in the population that would be evaluated for an impending pars defect, this becomes less of a factor.[102,103]

In most cases, athletes, especially in their adolescence, with greater than 3 weeks of axial mechanical back pain and no structural abnormalities evident on normal plain radiographs of the lumbar spine (including oblique views) should be evaluated by MRI. If this testing is negative and a high degree of suspicion remains, nuclear imaging modalities may be employed. Once an impending pars interarticularis defect has been discovered, the treatment goals are the relief of pain, prevention of spondylolysis and spondylolisthesis, and eventual return to unrestricted activity. These goals are met by withholding the athlete from participation and practice involving any strenuous activity and possibly bracing. To our knowledge, there is no evidence that bracing has any benefit in healing versus simply restricting activity. Bracing may play a more important role in the noncompliant athlete who will not adhere to activity restrictions. Bone healing generally occurs after 6 to 12 weeks, and the athlete can gradually be reintroduced to activity when pain free. Numerous studies have demonstrated that the early recognition and treatment of an impending pars interarticularis defect is up to 80% successful in preventing progression.[103-105]

Spondylolysis and Spondylolisthesis

Spondylolysis is a defect of the pars interarticularis, typically resulting from repetitive extension activities. It accounts for a much larger percentage of lumbar spine injuries in adolescent athletes than in adults. Pars defects are more common in athletes involved in activities that involve repetitive hyperextension and axial loading. It is present in more than 10% of college football players and gymnasts, in contrast to an incidence of less than 3% in the general population. In American football, participants playing on the line are the most at risk, again because of the repetitive axial loading and extension involved in the position.[106,107] Because an actual bony defect is present, these injuries are easily identified using plain lumbar radiographs including obliques or CT imaging.

Once a pars defect has occurred, management goals are to alleviate pain and prevent progression and instability. Because the pars consists primarily of cortical bone with a poor blood supply, defects to it do not heal well. The athlete is restricted from activities until the pain subsides and adequate range of motion is achieved. This is followed by a gradual resumption of sporting activity. Typically, all athletic activity is stopped for at least 2 months or until the patient can achieve painless lumbar extension. Should the pain resume, a period of lordotic bracing may be attempted for 3 to 6 months or until pain once again subsides. The use of an external bone growth stimulator has also been suggested.

Surgical management for pars defects with no associated spondylolisthesis is considered when the patient continues to have disabling pain refractory to conservative therapy. Numerous methods of fixation have been described, including dorsal wiring of the transverse process and spinous processes (Scott wiring), translaminar interfragmentary screws (Buck technique), and various pedicle screw to hook constructs within the same vertebra. The prognosis for return to competition is excellent after surgery. In a retrospective case series of four competitive athletes who underwent direct pars repair for symptomatic spondylolysis, all returned to presymptomatic levels of activity.[108] A separate study of 22 similarly treated athletes (13 professional footballers, 4 professional cricketers, 3 hockey players, 1 tennis player, and 1 golfer) also demonstrated the strong likelihood of return to play.[109]

Spondylolysis that progresses to a spondylolisthesis is first managed conservatively. Athletes with low-grade slips can usually return to competition after an aggressive rehabilitation program. Return to play is based on the individual athlete's symptoms and treatment. Patients sufficiently treated conservatively may return to full play after adequate pain control and range of motion are achieved. Typically, all athletic activity is stopped for at least 2 months, or until the patient can achieve painless lumbar extension.

Surgical management is reserved for progressing slips, refractory symptoms, neurologic deficits, or high-grade slips. Although no large series of instrumented or noninstrumented lumbar spine fusions in athletes exists to date, it is believed that the extent of tissue disruption, scarring, and stress placed on adjacent structures greatly increases the likelihood of continued postoperative pain with aggressive activity. Nevertheless, when lumbar fusion surgery is performed, either with lateral fusion alone or with interbody fusion, there is no absolute contraindication to the return to competition after complete recovery from surgery. Criteria for release for return to competition should include resolution of pain, no disabling neurologic deficit, and evidence of bone fusion on imaging. A clear understanding between the physician and the athlete about the possibility and consequences of reinjury is crucial.

Lumbar Fractures

Although fractures of the lumbar spine are rare in sports, when one occurs timely diagnosis and treatment are essential for a good outcome. Compression fracture management was detailed in the discussion on cervical compression fractures. Fractures of the spinous or transverse processes (which more commonly affect the lumbosacral spine) occur secondary to trauma or from strong muscular contraction. These result mainly in axial mechanical low back pain. If a transverse process is significantly displaced, it can also cause radicular symptoms.

Summary

Injuries to the spine and surrounding structures associated with athletic competition are common and have a wide spectrum of consequences, ranging from annoyance to a life-altering event. This chapter gives insight into the complex process of differentiating between minor and serious injuries and the resulting repercussions for management.

KEY REFERENCES

Cantu RC: Cervical spine injuries in the athlete. *Semin Neurol* 20:173–178, 2000.

Torg JS, Corcoran TA, Thibault LE, et al: Cervical cord neurapraxia: classification, pathomechanics, morbidity, and management guidelines. *J Neurosurg* 87:843–850, 1997.

Vaccaro AR, Klein GR, Ciccoti M, et al: Return to play criteria for the athlete with cervical spine injuries resulting in stinger and transient quadriplegia/paresis. *Spine J* 2:351–356, 2002.

Zmurko MG, Tannoury TY, Tannoury CA, Anderson DG: Cervical sprains, disc herniations, minor fractures, and other cervical injuries in the athlete. *Clin Sports Med* 22:513–521, 2003.

REFERENCES

The complete reference list is available online at expertconsult.com.

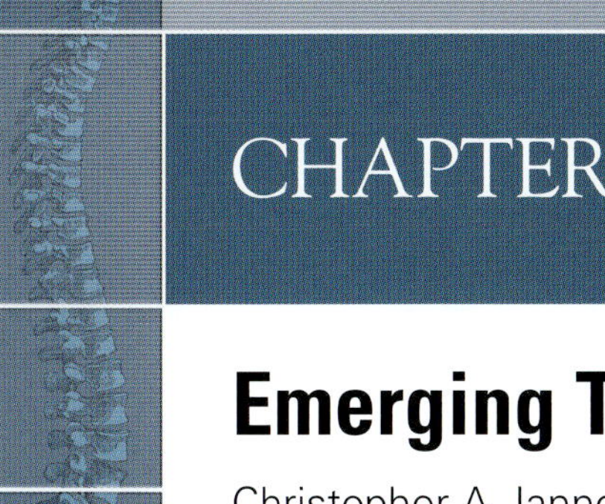

CHAPTER 72

Emerging Therapies for Spinal Cord Injury

Christopher A. Iannotti | Michael P. Steinmetz

The reversal of paralysis following spinal cord injury (SCI) represents one of the greatest challenges in all of neuroscience. Despite significant improvements in the early medical and surgical management of SCI, along with a greatly improved understanding of SCI pathophysiology, there remains no effective treatment to improve neurologic outcomes following SCI. SCI destroys neuronal connectivity by severing descending motor and ascending sensory axonal pathways. Such damage often results in permanent paralysis and loss of sensation below the level of injury. Although SCI causes loss of neurons and glial cells at the lesion site, functional deficits result primarily from loss of white matter axons by direct trauma and from progressive damage to initially intact axons by complex secondary injury mechanisms.[1] To date, numerous potential therapies have been investigated in prospective, randomized, controlled clinical trials, yet all have failed to demonstrate neurologic benefit despite evidence that these agents demonstrated benefit in preclinical animal studies of SCI. This chapter will review previous clinical trials as well as major recent preclinical advances, in pharmacologic and cell-based therapeutic approaches to SCI.

Spinal Cord Injury Epidemiology

SCI is associated with severe physical, psychological, social, and economic burdens on patients and their families. With an annual incidence rate of 15 to 40 persons per million, it has been estimated that at least 10,000 North Americans will suffer an SCI each year.[2] With the average acute-care and rehabilitation charges of approximately $60,000 for each of these phases of care, the societal expense associated with the medical management, as well as lost earnings of this disorder over the course of one's life, is significant.[3] It has been estimated that the lifetime cost of medical care and other injury-related expenses for a 25-year-old patient with SCI who suffers high cervical quadriplegia is approximately $3 million.[4] SCI occurs predominantly in young, otherwise healthy individuals, with injury occurring with the greatest frequency in those between 15 and 25 years of age; the male-to-female ratio for SCI is approximately 4 to 1.[5] Common causes of SCI in the United States are motor vehicle accidents (50%), falls and work-related injuries (30%), violent crime (11%), and sports-related injuries (9%).[6] Injuries most commonly occur in the cervical spine and are associated with the most devastating neurologic impairments (e.g., quadriplegia). A recent report from the U.S. National Spinal Cord Injury Database found that 56% of all SCI cases occur in the cervical spine.

Pathophysiology of Spinal Cord Injury

A detailed understanding of the pathophysiologic processes that occur following SCI is paramount to the development of effective therapies for SCI. The pathophysiology of SCI is best described as biphasic, consisting of a primary and a secondary phase of injury.[7] The primary phase involves the initial, immediate mechanical injury during which failure of the spinal column occurs, and includes compression, contusion, shear, or laceration due to penetrating injury and acute stretching of the spinal cord as a result of vertebral distraction or sudden acceleration-deceleration of the spinal column. The most common underlying primary injury mechanism results from the acute compression and contusion of the spinal cord due to bone or disc displacement within the spinal column during fracture-dislocation or burst fracture of the spine.[2] The primary mechanical trauma to the spinal cord, along with subsequent persistent compression, triggers a complex and delayed pathologic cascade, termed the secondary injury phase, which involves vascular dysfunction, edema, ischemia, excitotoxicity, electrolyte shifts, free radical production, inflammation, and delayed apoptotic cell death. Although neurologic deficits are present immediately following the initial injury, the secondary injury phase results in a protracted period of neuroinflammation and tissue destruction. The spatial extent of secondary injury events spreads both radially and longitudinally along the spinal cord in a rostral-to-caudal manner, resulting in neuronal and glial cell death. The end result is cavitation of central gray matter along with partial or complete loss of adjacent white matter tracts.

The pathophysiology of SCI has been extensively studied in many experimental animal models, including mice, rats, cats, and primates, in order to understand the cellular and molecular mechanisms of tissue damage and the consequent disability.[2] Traumatic SCI initiates a series of destructive cellular inflammatory processes which accentuate tissue damage at and beyond the original site of trauma, and cystic cavitation inevitably occurs due to these secondary injury events. Contusion SCI in animals produces a predictable pattern of progressive injury resulting in neuronal and glial cell death,

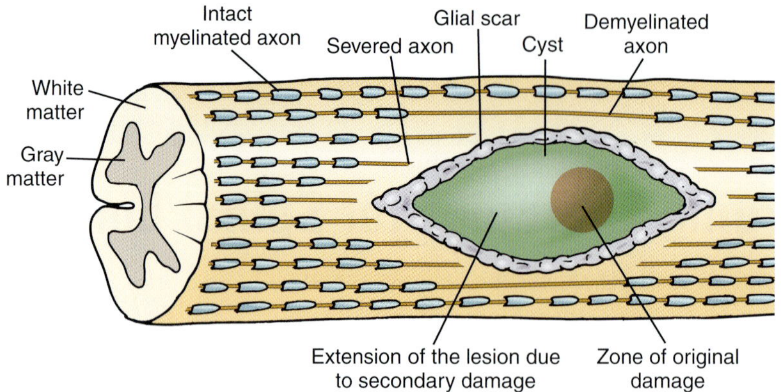

FIGURE 72-1. Schematic diagram depicting the various pathologic events occurring after traumatic spinal cord injury. A zone of primary injury progressively expands because of secondary injury. Acute and chronic inflammatory cascades lead to secondary tissue damage, axonal loss, and demyelination. The result is a cystic cavity surrounded by a rim of preserved white matter. An astroglial scar forms the periphery of the lesion, presenting a physical and chemical barrier to axonal regeneration. (From McDonald JW. Repairing the damaged spinal cord. *Sci Am* 281[3]:64–73, 1999.)

vascular injury, axonal destruction, and demyelination that is analogous to the pattern in human spinal cord contusion injury, the most common type of the human SCI (Fig. 72-1).[7,8] The progressive expansion of the injury from gray to white matter causes secondary damage to initially intact axons within hours to several weeks after injury. The cellular inflammatory response, predominated by macrophages, has been implicated as the primary mediator of progressive secondary injury. The major targets for spinal cord repair include severed and/or demyelinated axons, inflammatory cells and proinflammatory cytokines, and glial scar components.

Past Spinal Cord Injury Clinical Trials: A Synopsis

To date, several therapeutic strategies have been examined in phase I/II clinical trials. Ten randomized controlled trials examining methylprednisolone sodium succinate (MPSS), tirilizad mesylate, GM-1 ganglioside, thyrotropin-releasing hormone (TRH), gacyclidine, naloxone, and nimodipine have been completed. Although the primary outcomes in these trials were negative, a secondary analysis of the North American Spinal Cord Injury Study (NASCIS) II trial demonstrated that MPSS, when administered within 8 hours of injury, produced modest clinical benefits, which need to be weighed against potential complications. TRH (phase II trial) and GM-1 ganglioside (phase II and III trials) also showed some promise. Several clinical trials have explored various surgical interventions, such as early surgical decompression (Surgical Treatment of Acute Spinal Cord Injury Study, STASCIS) and electrical field stimulation.

Emerging Preclinical Spinal Cord Injuries Therapies

The failure of axonal regeneration after CNS injury is the result of two distinct processes: the limited intrinsic regenerative potential of CNS neurons and the inhibitory extrinsic environment of the injured CNS. However, CNS neurons may regenerate when provided with a "permissive" substrate that promotes axonal growth. The ability of CNS neurons to regenerate over long distances after axotomy was first established through pioneering work in which injured CNS axons were found to regenerate into and through growth-permissive peripheral nerve (PN) grafts.[9] The therapeutic potential of PN grafts for use in SCI was then demonstrated by Cheng et al. in 1996,[10] who reported that transplantation of multiple PN grafts stabilized with fibrin glue containing acidic fibroblast growth factor into a rat spinal cord transection model promoted hindlimb functional recovery.

Experimental therapies for SCI can be grouped into several subtypes, based on their general mechanism of action. These general treatment subcategories include therapies that (1) promote neuroprotection, (2) stimulate intrinsic axonal regrowth, (3) enhance remyelination, and (4) remove or block inhibitory molecules within damaged myelin and within the astroglial scar. To date, researchers have identified and characterized a number of molecular signals associated with axonal growth following injury and have developed drug therapies that are capable of stimulating axonal regeneration. Several regeneration-associated genes have been found to be up-regulated after axonal injury, including *L1*, *c-fos*, and *c-jun*, and the 43-kD growth-associated protein (GAP43). Despite these findings, the degree and extent of their up-regulation is apparently insufficient to promote a strong regenerative response in the CNS. Numerous reports have implicated a decrease in the levels of intracellular cAMP after CNS injury as a major cause of intrinsic regenerative failure. The elevation of intracellular cAMP levels by cAMP analogues and/or the phosphodiesterase inhibitor, rolipram, has been shown to increase axonal sprouting and reduce the effects of myelin-associated inhibitors.[11,12]

Multiple inhibitory molecules exist that make the injured CNS a nonpermissive environment for axonal growth. These molecules may be categorically divided into myelin-associated inhibitors and inhibitors associated with the astrocytic glial scar. Recently, major advances in molecular neuroscience have led to the identification of several growth-inhibitory molecules associated with myelin (Nogo, myelin-associated glycoprotein, and oligodendrocyte myelin glycoprotein) and the glial scar (chondroitin sulfate proteoglycans, CSPGs), as well as their receptors and downstream signaling pathways, which make up the inhibitory extrinsic environment of the injured CNS. This chapter will review several recently developed targeted molecular strategies that enable axons to overcome inhibitory influences of myelin-associated proteins and astroglial scar components.

Several clinical trials have been recently initiated or planned using promising potential therapies. These therapeutic strategies, which are both pharmacologic and cell-based (e.g., minocycline, C3 transferase, oligodendrocyte progenitor cell [OPC] transplantation), have been validated by multiple laboratories in experimental and preclinical studies. Unfortunately, some experimental and poorly characterized SCI therapies are being offered without rigorous investigation, which will produce results that are of limited scientific value and risk harm to SCI patients who are understandably desperate for any intervention that might improve their function. However, recent advances have provided a basis for optimism for both patients and clinicians, as safe and effective therapies for SCI may become available over the next decade.

Considering the multifactorial nature of secondary pathologic events attributed to SCI, drug cocktails with multifaceted modes of neuroprotection and axonal growth promotion will likely be useful in preventing or limiting secondary injury progression. Because of the numerous complex pathophysiologic changes that occur after SCI, successful repair may involve strategies that combine the use of neuroprotective drug therapies with those that promote axonal regeneration, such as cell transplantation, genetic engineering to increase neurotrophic factors, neutralization of inhibitory factors, limiting glial scar formation, and neurorehabilitation. Furthermore, neuroprotective drug therapies that function at later time points following SCI will likely have greater clinical relevance than those with small therapeutic windows. There is also a requirement to establish methods for the systematic evaluation of preclinical therapeutic outcomes from the various research SCI centers. In the evaluation of future potential SCI therapies, a clinical basis for the implementation of novel therapies will be required. Refined clinical outcome measures as well as neurophysiologic measures are needed for a precise qualitative and quantitative assessment of spinal cord function in SCI patients, especially at an early stage after injury. This will allow for better detection of improvements in functional recovery and will enable clinicians to precisely monitor the effects of novel therapies.[3,13]

Neuroprotective Strategies

Methylprednisolone

The most extensively investigated pharmacologic intervention for SCI is the glucocorticoid methylprednisolone sodium succinate (MPSS, Solu-Medrol). To date, three major clinical trials evaluating the use of MPSS in acute SCI have been performed. The National Acute Spinal Cord Injury Study (NASCIS I) compared the efficacy of administering an intravenous (IV) loading dose of MPSS (100 or 1000 mg) and a dose of either 25 or 250 mg every 6 hours thereafter for 10 days to SCI patients who had motor or sensory deficits below the level of injury.[14] This study demonstrated that higher-dose MPSS was no more effective than the lower dose in reducing neurologic deficits between the two groups at 6 weeks, 6 months, and 1 year after injury. Although a placebo group was not included in the NASCIS I because of ethical concerns, the use of MPSS became much less prevalent after this trial.

Subsequent animal studies demonstrated that the effective neuroprotective dose of MPSS was much higher than that used in NASCIS I.[15] Therefore, following the NASCIS I study, the NASCIS II trial was conducted to compare the efficacy of high-dose MPSS administered as a 30-mg/kg bolus over the first hour, followed by an infusion of 5.4 mg/kg/hour over the next 23 hours, to that of placebo and that of the opioid receptor antagonist naloxone.[16,17] The trial was also designed to examine the effects of different timing schedules of drug administration following SCI. An analysis of all patients entered into the trial failed to demonstrate a significant difference in motor and sensory function among the treatments. However, upon stratification of the data on the basis of time to loading dose (<8 hours or >8 hours from SCI) and adjustment for the severity of SCI (complete vs. incomplete), analysis of the results from the NASCIS II study at the 6-week and 6-month follow-up revealed that patients who were treated with MPSS within the first 8 hours of injury had significantly improved motor and sensory function, compared to patients who received placebo, naloxone, or MPSS at later times. Furthermore, these differences remained significant 1 year after injury.[18] None of the differences in patients taking naloxone or in patients treated with MPSS more than 8 hours after SCI were statistically significant.

Despite the beneficial therapeutic effects demonstrated with MPSS treatment, the results from the NASCIS II trial have not been universally accepted.[19,20] Concerns about the small sample population size for the groups showing beneficial effects, nonstandardized performance of medical and surgical protocols by participating centers, and lack of defined functional outcome measures to assess whether the improvements seen with MPSS treatments were correlated with clinical significance have reduced enthusiasm for the indication of MPSS for acute SCI. Additional criticisms remained because of concerns about the adverse effects of steroids and the small therapeutic effects that were noted over the short (6-month) follow-up period used as the basis for conclusions about the trial, as well as the differential loss to follow-up between MPSS-treated and untreated patients. The NASCIS III trial resolved some of these issues with the inclusion of a functional independence measure.[21] All patients in this study received an initial MPSS bolus of 30 mg/kg before being randomized to one of three treatment arms: (1) MPSS infusion of 5.4 mg/kg/hour over 24 hours, (2) MPSS infusion of 5.4 mg/kg/hour over 48 hours, or (3) tirilizad mesylate (TM, a lazaroid with inhibitory effects on lipid peroxidation without glucocorticoid side effects) 2.5-mg/kg bolus every 6 hours for 48 hours. The results from this third study concluded that no benefit was associated with extending MPSS treatment beyond 24 hours if MPSS had been administered within the first 3 hours of SCI, while patients who started MPSS therapy at 3 to 8 hours demonstrated improvements in motor capabilities if drug infusion was continued for 48 hours in comparison to 24 hours of infusion.

Research on the neuroprotective mechanism of MPSS in experimental SCI models has demonstrated that in addition to possessing antioxidant properties, MPSS reduces tumor necrosis factor–α (TNF-α) protein synthesis and nuclear factor kappa B (NF-κB) activity, effects that may account for the anti-inflammatory actions exerted by MPSS.[22] However, MPSS treatment is not without adverse effects; high-dose MPSS has been associated with an increased prevalence of wound infections, pneumonia, sepsis, and death due to respiratory complications.[16,21] Furthermore, the anti-inflammatory actions of high-dose MPSS may also have detrimental effects on neuronal regeneration and axonal sprouting while exacerbating postischemic necrosis. These adverse effects may explain the ineffectiveness of MPSS treatment started beyond 8 hours post-SCI observed in the NASCIS II study. The guidelines committee of the American Association of Neurological Surgeons and Congress of Neurological Surgeons Joint Section on Disorders of the Spine and Peripheral Nerves, upon reviewing the evidence regarding the use of MPSS in the treatment of acute SCI in adults, concluded that its use could be supported only at the level of a treatment option (Joint Section on Disorders of the Spine and Peripheral Nerves of the AANS/CNS, 2002). However, criticisms directed toward the NASCIS II and III trials must be balanced by the current lack of alternative neuroprotective strategies for acute SCI. Therefore, MPSS administration may remain justified for acute SCI (within 8 hours) in nondiabetic and nonimmunocompromised patients, given the severity of SCI deficits and current lack of alternatives. Although many neurosurgeons continue to administer steroids, the rationale for this administration appears to have changed over recent years, according to a survey published in 2006, which revealed that the majority of respondents continue to administer methylprednisolone but that this is motivated predominantly by fear of litigation.[23]

21-Aminosteroids

The 21-aminosteroids (lazaroids) are synthetic glucocorticoid analogues that are capable of inhibiting lipid peroxidation without activating glucocorticoid receptors. The 21-aminosteroid TM utilizes three neuroprotective mechanisms: antioxidation, preservation of endogenous vitamin E, and membrane stabilization through the inhibition of lipid peroxidation.[15] TM was administered in comparison to MPSS in the NASCIS III clinical trial and was shown to be as effective as the 24-hour MPSS regimen.[21] However, because TM was not shown to have superior efficacy in comparison to MPSS, and given the absence of proven benefit over placebo controls, 21-aminosteroids have not been adopted for neuroprotection in clinical SCI.

GM-1 Ganglioside

The gangliosides are a group of sialic acid–containing glycosphingolipids located in high concentrations in the outer membranes of nervous tissue. A small randomized, placebo-controlled, double-blind trial, the Maryland monosialotetrahexosylganglioside (GM-1) Ganglioside Study, was conducted to investigate the efficacy of GM-1 in patients with cervical and thoracic SCIs.[24] The test drug protocol consisted of either 100 mg of GM-1 or placebo control administered once daily via IV infusion for a total of 18 to 32 doses, the first dose beginning within 72 hours of the onset of SCI. Results from this study demonstrated that GM-1 improved the motor and sensory recovery of lower extremities only, suggesting that GM-1 had an ability to enhance the function of axons traversing the site of injury but had no effect on the gray matter at the level of trauma. Furthermore, unlike the dosing regimen of MPSS, which appears to be effective when initiated within the first 8 hours of SCI, GM-1 demonstrated neuroprotective effects following initiation of treatment 48 hours post-SCI. The results from this study led to the initiation of a larger clinical trial comparing the effects of low- and high-dose GM-1 to placebo.

The randomized double-blind Sygen Multicenter Acute Spinal Cord Injury Study was completed in the late 1990s and reported in 2001.[25] In this landmark clinical trial, all 797 patients received a 30-mg/kg bolus of MPSS, followed by a 5.4-mg/kg/hour infusion of MPSS for 23 hours initiated within the first 8 hours following SCI, as the standard of care based on the initial report from the NASCIS II. Placebo, low-dose GM-1 (300 mg loading dose followed by 100 mg/day for 56 days), or high-dose GM-1 (600 mg loading dose followed by 200 mg/day for 56 days) was then randomly assigned following the completion of corticosteroid administration to avoid unwanted drug interactions. Recovery patterns were measured by using the American Spinal Injury Association (ASIA) and modified Benzel classification neurologic examination scales.[26] The primary efficacy assessment assigned to this trial was termed *marked recovery*, defined as the proportion of patients who demonstrated a two-grade improvement from baseline examination. Although the primary outcome for this trial was negative, patients who received either low- or high-dose Sygen showed an accelerated motor recovery over the first 3 months postinjury, regardless of their initial severity. There was also a trend toward improved bowel/bladder function, sacral sensation, and anal contraction.[26] Interestingly, the placebo group of this trial failed to confirm the neurologic improvements noted with MPSS for the NASCIS II trial. To our knowledge, no future clinical trials with Sygen are currently planned.

Opioid Antagonists

Following SCI, the release of the endogenous opioid peptide dynorphin A is increased at the injury site along with kappa opioid receptor binding capacity. Although dynorphin A and other related opiates have well-defined roles as inhibitory neurotransmitters in pain reduction, evidence also exists to support the hypothesis that exposure to high concentrations of dynorphins can induce hyperalgesia and allodynia and may contribute to neurodegeneration. Moreover, sustained exposure to dynorphin-derived peptides is neurotoxic, and activation of the kappa-opioid receptor subtype has been associated with reduced spinal cord blood flow, which may contribute to secondary injury after SCI.[27] The use of opioid antagonists for treatment of SCI is controversial. While the nonselective opioid receptor antagonist naloxone has demonstrated an ability to improve spinal cord conduction, reduce edema, and decrease allodynia in animal models of SCI, results from the NASCIS II trial showed that naloxone given as an IV bolus of 5.4 mg/kg followed by an infusion of 4 mg/kg for 23 hours failed to provide benefit.[16] However, further analysis of the effects of timing for initiating naloxone treatment in patients with incomplete SCI showed that naloxone dosing within the first 8 hours of SCI resulted in significant motor recovery below the level of injury.[28] Therefore, further refinement of naloxone-dosing regimens in experimental SCI models may be beneficial.

Thyrotropin-Releasing Hormone

TRH is a tripeptide (Glu-His-Pro) that possesses numerous physiologic actions, in addition to its well-characterized actions on the pituitary gland. TRH and its analogues are capable of antagonizing the effects of endogenous opioids, platelet-activating factor, peptidoleukotrienes, and excitatory amino acids, all of which have been implicated in the biochemical events of secondary SCI.[29] In response to the overwhelming therapeutic benefit demonstrated by TRH in animal models of SCI, a small clinical trial consisting of 20 patients was designed to assess the safety and potential efficacy of TRH in patients with complete and incomplete SCI.[30] The patients were randomized on the basis of the severity of their SCI (complete or incomplete) in a double-blinded fashion to receive either a 0.2-mg/kg bolus of TRH followed by a 0.2-mg/kg/hour infusion of TRH over 6 hours or an equal volume of saline vehicle placebo. The results of the 4-month follow-up revealed statistically significant improvements in neurologic and sensory function. However, this study was hampered by the small patient population that was included in the study and the high variability of neurologic scores obtained within the placebo group. Results for complete SCI patients treated with TRH were negative. Although 1-year data were available, a relatively high number of patients were lost to follow-up, and the data were deemed inconclusive. Considering the amount of evidence in support of neuroprotective effects generated by TRH and TRH analogues from previous preclinical studies and the results obtained from this small clinical trial, larger and more extensive trials with TRH may be beneficial.

Glutamate Receptor Antagonists

The class of glutamate receptor antagonists readily crosses the blood–spinal cord barrier following systemic administration. However, given the fact that glutamate is a key neurotransmitter possessing a variety of physiologic functions, blockade of glutamatergic synaptic transmission results in unwanted psychomimetic effects. Gacyclidine, a potent and specific phencyclidine analogue noncompetitive *N*-methyl *D*-aspartate receptor antagonist, was previously shown to provide neuroprotection through improvement of the functional, histologic, and electrophysiologic status of the injured rat spinal cord following experimental contusion with an absence of dose-related adverse effects.[31] These findings prompted initiation of a randomized double-blind phase II clinical trial with more than 200 patients recruited to test the efficacy of 0.005, 0.01, and 0.2 mg/kg gacyclidine administered via IV infusion within 2 hours of SCI and with a second dose given within the next 4 hours.[32] The subjects of this trial were divided into four strata based on the level of SCI (cervical or thoracic) and the severity of injury (complete or incomplete). The study results, reported for the 1-month follow-up, demonstrated improved overall ASIA scores. However, results for the follow-up at 12 months posttreatment failed to support long-term benefit on neurologic scores. Despite evidence of a trend for improved motor function in the incomplete cervical strata receiving higher gacyclidine dosing, further development of this drug for SCI has been halted.

Calcium Channel Blockade

Calcium influx is believed to be an important mediator of excitotoxic intracellular damage and vasospasm-induced ischemia. Consequently, Ca^{2+}-channel blockers are prescribed in the treatment of systemic hypertension, coronary artery disease, stroke, cardiac arrhythmias, and vasospasm. Vasospasm and the release of endogenous vasoactive amines have been suggested as important contributing factors to the pathobiology of SCI.[2] The dihydropyridine-sensitive (L-type) Ca^{2+}-channel blocke nimodipine represents the most widely investigated therapy for vasospasm. In a rat model of severe spinal cord compression, nimodipine, alone or in combination with dextran, was examined for effects on spinal cord blood flow and spinal cord axonal function.[33] The results of this study demonstrated that the administration of nimodipine alone was associated with systemic hypotension due to vasodilation. However, the combination of nimodipine with dextran resulted in increased cord blood flow within the lesion epicenter and improved axonal function in the motor and somatosensory tracts of the cord.

In 1996, a randomized clinical trial of 100 acute SCI patients was initiated, comparing the safety, efficacy, and neurologic outcome following administration of nimodipine (0.015 mg/kg/hour over 2 hours followed by 0.03 mg/kg/hour for 7 days), MPSS (NASCIS II dosing regimen), both treatments, or placebo control.[34] Results from the 1-year follow-up demonstrated no neurologic benefit beyond the natural course of recovery within the placebo group. The authors also examined the results based on the timing of surgical spinal decompression and stabilization and found no correlation with recovery of neurologic function and the timing of surgery, although the patients were not randomized on the basis of timing of surgery. Although the data from this SCI clinical trial were not suggestive of nimodipine-mediated therapeutic effects, the conclusions made by the authors were susceptible to type II errors owing to the small patient population.

Sodium Channel Blockade

After SCI, there is a deleterious accumulation of intracellular sodium.[35] Injury causes failure of the Na^+/K^+-ATPase and accumulation of axoplasmic sodium through noninactivating Na^+ channels, which, together with membrane depolarization, promotes reverse Na-Ca exchange and axonal calcium overload. Thus, administration of sodium channel blockers may prevent the ensuing calcium-induced cell injury or death. Pharmacologic antagonism of voltage-gated Na^+ channels has been demonstrated to prevent axonal degeneration, preserve the function of injured spinal cord white matter tracts, and reduce damage to myelin.[36] For example, the focal administration of tetrodotoxin directly into the contused rodent spinal cord significantly reduced axonal loss and axoplasmic pathology, as compared to vehicle-treated animals.[36] The benzothiazole anticonvulsant Na^+ channel blocker riluzole is neuroprotective and promotes functional neurologic recovery following SCI in rodents.[37] Riluzole exerts neuroprotective properties in the injured spinal cord following systemic administration by sparing gray and white matter rostral-to-caudal to the injury epicenter,[37] a property that appears to be due to its ability to decrease the levels of intracellular sodium and calcium. The use of riluzole as a therapy for SCI is potentially feasible, as it has already received approval from the Food and Drug Administration (FDA) for treatment of amyotrophic lateral sclerosis. Furthermore, riluzole has been used as an adjunctive therapy in combination with MPSS.[38] However, despite the current in vivo evidence in support of riluzole as a therapeutic drug for SCI, efforts to proceed with clinical testing of this drug are lacking.

Potassium Channel Blockade

Demyelination of intact and injured axons is a prominent feature of SCI. Axonal conduction deficits that arise from demyelination appear to contribute to the neurologic outcome following SCI, although the underlying mechanisms remain unclear.[39,40] It has been suggested that focal demyelination of intact axons, along with altered activity of ion channels, plays an important role in the loss of axonal conduction.[41] The exposure of K^+ channels as a result of demyelination results in a reduced safety factor of action potential propagation (i.e., the ratio of action current generated by an impulse to the minimum amount of action current needed to maintain conduction) across the demyelinated region of the axon. Under normal physiologic conditions, myelinated axons have a high density of voltage-gated Na^+ channels at the nodes of Ranvier, while rapidly inactivating voltage-gated K^+ channels are clustered at the paranodal and internodal regions beneath the myelin sheath. As such, these K^+ channels normally do not play a prominent role in repolarization of the action potential, as their outward current is constrained by myelin. However, when demyelination occurs, there is no myelin to shield the capacitance of the internode, and shunting of the action current occurs due to these fast voltage-gated K^+ channels. Subsequently, the action potential progressively declines, resulting in conduction failure, marked slowing of the conduction velocity, and/or the inability to sustain repetitive discharges.[42]

Experimental studies using K^+ channel blockers on animal nerve preparations have provided the rationale for undertaking clinical trials to assess the safety and efficacy of 4-AP, a blocker of rapidly inactivating voltage-gated K^+ channels, as a therapy in SCI patients. Electrophysiologic studies have shown that 4-AP is capable of restoring conduction in focally demyelinated axons, enhancing synaptic transmission in many types of neurons, and potentiating muscle contraction.[42] Several preclinical trials of intravenously administered 4-AP have demonstrated transient improvements in neurologic function in patients with chronic SCI.[43-45] To date, three multicenter phase II randomized clinical trials of fampridine-SR, a sustained-release oral form of the K^+ channel-blocking compound 4-AP, have been conducted with SCI patients. The first of these studies was a randomized crossover study, which demonstrated that fampridine-SR improved spasticity (modified Ashworth scores), ASIA motor and sensory scores, erectile dysfunction, and bowel function compared to placebo.[46] In another crossover trial involving 60 patients, there was a nonsignificant trend toward reduced erectile dysfunction and decreased spasticity.[47] A double-blind, randomized, placebo-controlled, parallel-group phase II clinical trial was conducted at 11 academic rehabilitation research centers in the United States to assess the safety and efficacy of fampridine-SR in subjects with chronic SCI.[48] The study enrolled 91 patients with motor-incomplete SCI, randomized to three arms: fampridine-SR 25 mg twice daily (group I), fampridine-SR 40 mg twice daily (group II), and placebo (group III) for 8 weeks. Outcome measures included ASIA and Ashworth scores, bladder and bowel management questionnaires, and Subject Global Impression (SGI). A higher discontinuation rate was seen in group II patients, compared to group I and group III patients, due to more frequent adverse side effects such as hypertonia, generalized spasm, insomnia, dizziness, pain, constipation, headache, and seizures. Overall, group I patients showed significant improvement in SGI, and subgroup analysis showed improvement in spasticity in the lower-dose fampridine-SR group compared to the placebo group.[48]

Two large-scale phase III randomized clinical trials of fampridine-SR have been conducted in chronic (>18 months after injury) incomplete SCI patients. Approximately 400 patients were enrolled from 70 clinical centers in the United States and Canada. The primary end points were Modified Ashworth Scale scores and SGI. Both of the trials failed to detect a significant benefit of fampridine-SR over placebo on the primary end points. Although Ashworth scores progressively improved in both groups at a similar rate, there was a nonsignificant but strong positive trend of fampridine-SR toward reducing muscle spasticity in one study. However, Acorda Therapeutics, Inc., has placed the fampridine-SR clinical program for SCI on hold.

Erythropoietin

Erythropoietin (EPO) is a 34-kD hematopoietic glycoprotein that binds to its receptor (EPOR) to induce signals promoting survival, differentiation, and proliferation of erythroid progenitor cells.[49] The expression of EPO and EPOR is widely distributed within the developing and adult human brain and spinal cord, and is up-regulated in the adult brain after injury. Peripherally administered EPO crosses the blood-brain barrier, stimulates neurogenesis and neuronal differentiation, and activates neurotrophic, antiapoptotic, antioxidant, and anti-inflammatory signaling pathways.[50] EPO is the only hematopoietic growth factor whose production is regulated by hypoxia, in which low oxygen tension activates hypoxia-inducing factor-1 to up-regulate EPO gene transcription.

Endogenous and exogenously administered EPO, and EPOR, have been reported to play important roles in SCI.[51] EPO expression is up-regulated after SCI as part of the physiologic response to hypoxia. EPO has been shown to be neuroprotective in vitro and is capable of protecting neuronal cells from hypoxia-induced apoptosis and from excitotoxic cell death.[52] The administration of exogenous recombinant human EPO (rhEPO) has been reported to produce substantial neuroprotection in animal models of SCI, spinal nerve root crush injury, transient spinal cord ischemia, and spinal cord inflammation in experimental autoimmune encephalitis. Although the mechanisms by which EPO exhibits its neuroprotective effects are not fully understood, EPO is capable of preventing apoptosis, reducing inflammation, and restoring vascular integrity. The preventive effects of EPO on neuronal apoptosis have also been demonstrated in a spinal cord compression model in rats, in which EPO administration results in inhibition of caspase-1 and caspase-3 and induction of survival proteins such as Bcl-xL. EPO administration also results in a reduction in neutrophil infiltration after SCI and has been shown to delay the postinjury increase in TNF-α, decrease interleukin-6 (IL-6) levels, and reduce apoptotic cell death.[53-55] EPO has also been shown to prevent endothelial cell apoptosis, stimulate mitogenesis, and promote angiogenesis by restricting vascular endothelial growth factor–induced permeability and strengthening endothelial tight junctions. In addition to the anti-inflammatory properties of rhEPO, the inhibition of lipid peroxidation may contribute to its neuroprotective effects.[56] Results of studies in animal models suggest that treatment with rhEPO may be beneficial after SCI, even when rhEPO was administered up to 24 hours after the initial injury. The delivery of rhEPO appears to protect ventral spinal cord motor neurons in an ischemic injury model in rabbits.[57] Although a study of rat thoracic spinal cord contusion and clip compression injury reported substantial tissue sparing and recovery in locomotor function,[55] an independent SCI research group failed to reproduce similar results, as delivery of rhEPO in the same injury paradigm failed to decrease secondary injury and cystic cavitation or to improve locomotor function.[58]

In a recent phase II clinical trial, intravenously administered rhEPO was shown to be safe and demonstrated a strong trend to reduce infarct size and improve clinical outcome in stroke patients.[59] Although there has been great interest in conducting an SCI clinical trial with rhEPO, given the significance of initial preclinical results following experimental SCI, the use of rhEPO in clinical trials of human SCI deserves caution, and requires further investigation before implementing clinical trials. A major concern of EPO is the inadvertent and unwanted stimulation of hematopoietic activity, increasing the risk for thrombosis. Several EPO analogues have been developed in attempts to address this concern. The administration of the short-lived asialo-erythropoietin, in which sialic acid residues have been removed, has been shown to be neuroprotective in animal models of stroke, SCI, and peripheral neuropathy without causing erythrocytosis.[60] In addition, asialo-erythropoietin was as effective as rhEPO in normalizing motor function after experimental SCI using a clip compression model. Other EPO analogues such as carbamylated EPO do not bind to the EPO receptor, a property that confers a loss of hematopoietic activity.[61] Carbamylated EPO is capable of maintaining its associated neuroprotective properties, resulting in reduced neurologic deficit in comparison to saline or EPO in a chronic rodent model of SCI, and remained effective even when treatment was delayed for 24 hours.[61]

Cyclosporin-A

Agents that suppress the systemic immune response have also demonstrated beneficial effects within the injured spinal cord. Cyclosporin-A (CsA) is a potent immunosuppressive drug that is capable of inhibiting mitochondrial permeability transition, limiting constitutive and inducible nitric oxide synthase activity and expression (thereby diminishing free radical production), and reducing lipid peroxidation.[62] For example, a systemic low dose (2.5 mg/kg) of CsA was shown to reduce lipid peroxidation when administered within the first 6 hours of SCI in rats.[63] The delayed (2, 6, and 12 hours post-SCI) intraperitoneal injection of CsA was shown to inhibit inducible nitric oxide synthase activity, presumably via inhibition of the calcium-dependent calcineurin.[64] Comparison of the efficacy of low-dose CsA alone and in combination with high-dose (30 mg/kg) MPSS demonstrated that CsA alone was superior to MPSS following SCI, as CsA was able to reduce lipid peroxidation to the same extent as that mediated by high-dose MPSS while yielding greater survival.[65] Furthermore, CsA was demonstrated to inhibit autoimmune-mediated demyelination and neuronal cell death and resulted in improved motor outcome following SCI.[66] However, conflicting experimental results have been obtained in various laboratories examining the potential beneficial effects of CsA after SCI. Using a stereologic method to assess lesion volume, Rabchevsky et al.[67] reported that CsA treatment 15 minutes after a moderate experimental contusion SCI failed to alter the amount of spared white matter and did not improve locomotor recovery. However, when CsA was administered 4 days after moderate contusion SCI injury, motor functional recovery was observed in CsA-treated animals 3 weeks postinjury, although no significant difference in lesion volume was observed between CsA-treated and control groups.[68]

A nonimmunosuppressive CsA derivative, termed NIM811, also inhibits the mitochondrial permeability transition pore and is significantly less cytotoxic than CsA is. The effects of NIM811 on apoptosis, lesion size, and tissue sparing have been examined following contusion SCI and oral administration of either 20 mg/kg NIM811 or vehicle 15 minutes postinjury. NIM811 reduced apoptosis during the first 24 hours following SCI and reduced the lesion volume and enhanced the degree of spared gray and white matter at 7 days postinjury.[69] Together, these findings support the need for continued experimental investigation of CsA and its derivatives as potential neuroprotective therapies in animal models of SCI.

Minocycline

Minocycline, a highly lipophilic semisynthetic derivative of tetracycline, is capable of crossing the blood-brain barrier. Minocycline possesses anti-inflammatory properties, which are distinct from its ability to inhibit bacterial protein synthesis. Minocycline can inhibit excitotoxicity, oxidative stress, caspase-dependent and caspase-independent pathways of neuronal death, and proinflammatory mediators released by activated microglia.[70] The anti-inflammatory properties of minocycline include reduction in the expression or activity of inflammatory cytokines, free radicals, and matrix metalloproteinases.[71]

Neuroprotection by minocycline has been demonstrated in animal models of SCI. In these studies, systemically administered minocycline demonstrated convincing neuroprotective ability by decreasing apoptosis of oligodendrocytes, diminishing microglial cell activation, reducing lesion size, and improving neurologic deficit.[70,71] In addition, minocycline was shown to be a superior therapeutic agent to MPSS and maintained neuroprotective efficacy when administered 1 hour following experimental SCI.[71] Minocycline has been shown to improve functional recovery after clip compression SCI in mice and after contusion SCI in rats, in which it inhibits release of cytochrome c from mitochondria.[70-73] After intraperitoneal administration of minocycline in a rat contusion model of SCI, minocycline exerts neuroprotective and anti-inflammatory effects, leading to a reduction in caspase-3 activation, reduced neuronal apoptosis, and improved recovery early after SCI.[74] The proposed mechanisms of minocycline-mediated neuroprotection within the injured spinal cord also include increased mRNA levels of the anti-inflammatory cytokine IL-10 and decreased TNF-α production.[70] Although positive effects with minocycline have been reported in several animal models of injury with different drug administration schemes, an independent replication of the study by Lee et al.[72] using minocycline after experimental contusion SCI did not lead to significant functional or histopathologic improvements.[75] Although minocycline has been demonstrated to have a good safety profile with prolonged use in humans, the use of minocycline following contusive SCI may require further experimental investigation before clinical trials are implemented.

Despite mixed results of minocycline in SCI animal models, a recent double-blind randomized controlled pilot study was initiated in SCI patients presenting within 12 hours after nonpenetrating injury.[76] Patients were randomized to receive IV minocycline 200 mg twice daily, IV minocycline 400 mg twice daily after an 800-mg loading dose, or placebo for 7 days. There were no adverse treatment-related effects. Minocycline treatment improved ASIA motor scores in complete and incomplete cervical SCI patients through 1 year and improved the Functional Independence Measure and SF-36 scores.[76] However, no differences in ASIA motor scores were observed for patients with thoracic complete SCI. On the basis of these results, large-scale clinical trials with minocycline may be anticipated.

Early Surgical Decompression

There is substantial experimental evidence that persistent compression of the spinal cord is a potentially reversible form of secondary injury.[7] The severity of SCI in experimental models appears to vary depending on several factors, including the force of compression, duration of compression, spinal cord displacement, impulse, and kinetic energy. The severity of the pathologic changes and the degree of recovery appear to be directly related to the duration of acute compression, as demonstrated by experimental studies in which longer compression times produced less demonstrable clinical recovery. Furthermore, experimental studies of spinal cord decompression performed after SCI, using both kinetic and static compression models, have demonstrated that neurologic recovery is enhanced by early decompressive surgery.[77] However, it is difficult to determine a time window for the effective application of surgical decompressive intervention in the clinical setting from these animal models. Results of studies on secondary injury mechanisms suggest that early intervention within hours after SCI is critical to attain a neuroprotective effect, but whether the same time window applies to surgical treatment remains unclear.

Clinical studies assessing surgical decompression for SCI have not provided convincing evidence that surgical decompression influences patients' neurologic outcome after SCI or a clear consensus as to the appropriate timing of surgical intervention. Although suggestive evidence is presented in these studies that early decompressive surgery in selected patients may enhance neurologic recovery, most studies were uncontrolled, and any beneficial effects must be considered in the context of spontaneous recovery, which can occur in nonoperatively managed patients with SCI. Several retrospective studies have shown improvement in neurologic function after delayed decompressive surgery in patients with cervical or thoracolumbar SCI whose recovery has plateaued, and there have been reports documenting recovery of neurologic function after performance of delayed decompressive surgery months to years postinjury.[78] Taken together, these studies have suggested that ongoing spinal cord compression is an important contributing factor to neurologic dysfunction.

To better define the role of decompressive surgery in the management of acute SCI, a prospective randomized controlled trial (the Surgical Treatment of Acute Spinal Cord Injury Study, STASCIS) was planned in 2003. This trial was designed to be randomized; however, resistance to randomizing patients to an intentionally delayed decompression led to restructuring as a prospective observational study. This study recruited 170 consecutive patients with subaxial cervical SCI and imaging evidence of spinal cord compression from 10 centers in the United States and Canada. To date, results of this ongoing prospective study suggest that early decompressive surgery significantly improves outcomes and reduces complication rates in patients with SCI. One-year results from the STASCIS trial showed 24% of patients who received decompressive surgery within 24 hours of their injury experienced a two-grade or greater improvement on the ASIA scale, compared with 4% of those in the delayed-treatment group.[3] However, major barriers still exist in achieving early decompression in the SCI population, likely because of delays in hospital transfer and challenges with obtaining appropriate neuroimaging and accessing operating room facilities. Thus, implementation of the STASCIS protocol will require major efforts to influence public policy.

Hypothermia

Hypothermia has long been explored for its putative neuroprotective effects, despite associated risks that include coagulopathy, sepsis, and cardiac dysrhythmia. In addition to reducing the metabolic rate, hypothermia appears to reduce extracellular glutamate, vasogenic edema, apoptosis, neutrophil and macrophage invasion and activation, and oxidative stress. In animal models of traumatic SCI, both regional (epidural) and systemic hypothermia have been studied and have demonstrated inconsistent results. Recent studies have demonstrated the benefits of mild systemic hypothermia (33°C) in promoting tissue sparing and functional recovery in animal models of thoracic and cervical contusive SCI.[79-81]

The effects of modest and severe hypothermia have also been tested in SCI patients.[80] Modest systemic hypothermia was reported to be safe in severely injured SCI patients. In a recently published study, the clinical application of modest hypothermia was evaluated in 14 patients with acute cervical SCI.[82] This safety study included a retrospective analysis on a subset of patients with acute cervical SCI over a 2-year period. An FDA-approved intravascular catheter was utilized according to established guidelines to deliver a rapid and stable hypothermic state in patients. Patients were intubated and sedated by using muscle relaxants and were cooled to the target temperature (33°C) for 48 hours, after which they were rewarmed to 37°C at a controlled rate. Compared with a control group of age- and injury-matched patients, modest systemic hypothermia appears to be relatively safe, with an incidence of potential risk factors, including respiratory complications, pulmonary embolism, and myocardial infarction, comparable to that in the control group. However, because of a lack of sufficient randomized clinical trial data with the use of modest hypothermia, the AANS/CNS Joint Section on Disorders of the Spine and Peripheral Nerves recently decided that not enough evidence is available to recommend for or against the practice of therapeutic hypothermia as a treatment for SCI. Therefore, continued clinical investigations into this experimental therapy will be required.

Cell Transplantation Strategies

Activated Autologous Macrophages

Based on the premise that the relative inability of the CNS to regenerate can be largely attributed to the insufficient recruitment and activation of macrophages within the immune-privileged injured CNS, preclinical studies using transplantation of activated autologous macrophages after experimental SCI were performed.[83,84] Studies from several laboratories have demonstrated the ability for peripheral macrophages to synthesize nerve growth factor following sciatic nerve lesion as well as the capability of these cells to phagocytose myelin,[85,86] providing additional rationale for using hematogenous macrophages to repair the injured spinal cord. In preclinical experiments, local injection of autologous macrophages, activated by incubation with autologous PN or skin, induced partial motor recovery after spinal cord transection in adult rats.[87] In these studies, sciatic nerve- or skin-coincubated macrophages were reported to demonstrate a distinctive profile of cytokine secretion and cell-surface markers indicative of antigen-presenting activity, such as enhanced synthesis of the IL-1α and brain-derived neurotrophic factor, expression of major histocompatibility complex (MHC) class II molecules, and decreased synthesis of the proinflammatory cytokine TNF-α.[88,89] Furthermore, this treatment resulted in a significant recovery of motor function and reduced cystic cavity formation in animal models of contusion SCI.[88]

Based on positive results in preclinical studies, a phase I clinical SCI trial of activated macrophage transplantation was performed in Israel. The treatment, termed ProCord (Proneuron Biotechnologies, Inc., New York, NY), consisted of a single injection of autologous blood-derived macrophages (activated by coincubation with skin) directly into the epicenter of the injured spinal cord. The initial phase I study was a nonrandomized, open-label study that enrolled 16 patients with complete SCI.[89] No adverse treatment-related events were reported. On the basis of these findings, ProNeuron initiated the recruitment of patients into a phase II international multicenter randomized clinical trial to evaluate the safety and efficacy of ProCord for complete SCI. The study enrolled acute complete SCI patients with an injury between C5 and T11 within 14 days of injury. All control and treatment patients underwent SCI rehabilitation and underwent follow-up testing for 1 year. However, the phase II ProCord trial was stopped prior to completion because of several major drawbacks in the design of the clinical trial, including the following: (1) The majority of patients were treated relatively late after injury (day 14 or later), (2) the injection of the macrophages often necessitated a second surgery after an initial surgery for decompression, (3) it was difficult to accurately identify the location of the lesion border at the time of macrophage injection, and (4) the expense was too great.

Human Embryonic Stem Cells and Oligodendrocyte Progenitor Cells

Numerous preclinical studies suggest that embryonic and adult stem cells, along with their lineage-specific progenitors, may improve the outcome after experimental SCI. Transplanted stem cells may potentially act through several proposed mechanisms, which include (1) providing trophic support to promote the survival and regrowth of host tissue, (2) acting as a cellular scaffold to permit axonal elongation through the site of injury, and/or (3) the replacement of lost or damaged cells (e.g., oligodendrocytes). Demyelination of intact axons is a prominent feature of SCI and contributes to loss of function after injury. Therefore, potential therapeutic strategies may involve the replacement of myelin-producing cells through the transplantation of embryonic stem cells, various organ-specific adult stem cells, or lineage-restricted progenitor cells. ES cells provide novel prospects for cellular replacement strategies because of their ability to provide seemingly unlimited numbers of stem cell in vitro, their ability to undergo genetic modification, and their broad developmental capacity.[90] McDonald et al.[91] reported that transplantation of neural differentiated mouse embryonic stem cells into a contusion SCI in rats improved functional recovery and suggested remyelination as a likely mechanism underlying the effect. Despite these findings, the progress of human embryonic stem cells (hESCs) research has been hampered by numerous scientific issues and ethical concerns. One of the many scientific challenges facing hESC research is the production of high-purity cell lineages from pluripotent hESCs, an issue that has become paramount because of the potential of these cells to differentiate into teratomas. As a result, many researchers have turned to pursuing the use of ESC-derived lineage-restricted progenitor cells. Recently, researchers have successfully differentiated hESCs along the oligodendrocyte lineage, obtaining highly purified oligodendrocyte progenitor cells (OPCs). [92] The transplantation of human hESC-derived OPCs into adult rat spinal cord injuries has been shown to enhance remyelination and promote improvement of motor function.[93] In this study, transplantation of OPCs 1 week after SCI resulted in widespread oligodendrocyte remyelination throughout the white matter. The total number of remyelinated axons in the acute transplant group increased by 136% compared to endogenous remyelination in controls, and remyelination in the acute OPC-transplanted group was approximately double the amount of endogenous remyelination observed 1 year after injury in nontransplanted controls. In addition, histologic studies confirmed that substantial remyelination was performed by transplanted OPCs. Transplantation of hESC-derived OPCs 10 months after SCI did not result in increased remyelination compared with control animals that did not receive OPCs, a finding that is paradoxical, considering that a significantly greater density of demyelinated axons is present as compared to the acute injury group. Histopathologic analysis of the chronic transplant group revealed widespread astrogliosis and engulfment of axons by astrocyte processes, suggesting the presence of an inhibitor of remyelination after chronic injury. Several studies have suggested that an established, but not necessarily ongoing, glial scar is largely responsible for the failure of remyelination. Overall, these landmark studies demonstrated the feasibility of predifferentiating hESCs into functional OPCs and demonstrated their therapeutic potential at early time points after experimental SCI. However, it remains unclear whether the improved functional recovery that has been seen in preclinical studies is due to enhanced remyelination, to the secretion of trophic factors by OPCs, or to other neuroprotective effects of OPC transplantation that have yet to be characterized.

On the basis of data from these preclinical studies, Geron Corporation received clearance from the FDA in January 2009 to begin the first clinical trial of hESC-derived OPCs (known as GRNOPC1) for acute SCI. A phase I multicenter trial will assess the safety and tolerability of GRNOPC1 in patients with ASIA A subacute thoracic spinal cord injuries with a neurologic level from T3 to T10. In this trial, the human OPCs will be injected directly into the lesion sites between 7 and 14 days after injury. However, the FDA has placed the Investigational New Drug application on clinical hold pending data from a preclinical animal study being conducted by the company.

Schwann Cells and Peripheral Nerve Grafting

The Schwann cell is one of the most widely studied cell types for repair of the spinal cord.[94-97] These cells play a crucial role in endogenous repair of PNs because of their ability to dedifferentiate, migrate, proliferate, express growth-promoting factors and extracellular matrix molecules, and myelinate regenerating axons.[98] Following SCI, Schwann cells migrate from the periphery into the injury site, where they participate in endogenous repair processes.[8,39] For transplantation into the spinal cord, large numbers of Schwann cells are necessary to fill injury-induced cystic cavities. Several culture systems have been developed that provide large, highly purified populations of Schwann cells, and the development of in vitro systems to harvest human Schwann cells has created the opportunity for autologous transplantation. In experimental SCI models, grafting of Schwann cells or PN into the lesion site has been shown to promote axonal regeneration and myelination.[9,94,95] However, axons do not regenerate beyond the transplant, owing to the inhibitory nature of the glial scar surrounding the injury.[95] Although Schwann cells have great potential for repair of the injured spinal cord, their combination with other interventions is needed to maximize axonal regeneration and functional recovery. To overcome the glial scar inhibition, additional approaches need to be incorporated into therapeutic strategies, such as increasing the intrinsic capacity of axons to regenerate, by using trophic factors or elevating cAMP levels, and removing growth-inhibitory molecules associated with the astroglial scar and damaged myelin.[98]

PN grafting, first described by Richardson et al. in the 1980s,[9] represents a promising treatment strategy for spinal cord repair. In 1996, Cheng et al.[10] performed transplantation of autologous intercostal nerve transplants affixed with fibrin glue containing acidic fibroblast growth factor. These grafts spanned the injury site and joined the rostral white matter to the distal gray matter. Regeneration of the corticospinal tract and recovery of hindlimb function was seen over a 6-month period. However, despite multiple attempts by several independent groups to replicate these results, only one could obtain similar, albeit smaller, effects 6 years later.[99] A second group observed some axonal regeneration in primates, but this did not occur beyond the lesion border and did not result in functional recovery.[100] Despite incomplete preclinical evidence, this strategy has been used to treat patients with SCI. A case report of a single patient with chronic incomplete SCI has shown that autologous sural nerve grafts could improve both motor and sensory function.[101] A similar study was conducted in Brazil over a 5-year period in eight patients in which no motor or sensory recovery was seen.[102] Hence, there is insufficient data to recommend this strategy as a treatment.

To date, the methods used for PN grafting continue to be explored and refined. PN grafting techniques have been developed using segments of sciatic nerve placed either directly between the damaged rostral and caudal ends of the injury site or used to form a bridge across the lesion to restore functional connectivity across the lesion site. This approach has several advantages in comparison to transplantation of other neural tissues:

- The regenerating axons can be directed toward a specific target area.
- The number and source of regenerating axons are easily determined by tracing techniques.
- The graft can be used for electrophysiologic experiments to measure functional recovery associated with axons in the graft.
- Functional recovery due to axonal regeneration within the PN bridge may be confirmed by lesioning experiments.
- Autologous nerve grafts may be used, reducing the possibility of graft rejection.

In this paradigm, regenerated axons that reach the distal end of the PN graft fail to extend back into the spinal cord when PN grafts are used alone. However, regenerated axons have been shown to reenter the distal spinal cord after additional treatment with chondroitinase ABC (ChABC), a bacterial enzyme that degrades inhibitory CSPGs present within the glial scar at the distal graft-host interface. Previous studies have shown that delivery of ChABC, either via an osmotic minipump or by microinjection into the distal lesion site, resulted in extensive CSPG degradation, enhanced axonal regeneration, and functional recovery in the PN grafting-bridging model.[103] Furthermore, the delivery of exogenous growth and neurotrophic factors, through genetic modification of transplanted or host cells or by direct protein delivery, encourages longer-distance axonal regrowth into the spinal cord. The PN grafting approach appears to be effective in promoting axonal regeneration of both acute and chronically injured neurons.

Axonal Regeneration

Phosphodiesterase Inhibitors

The elevation of intracellular cAMP levels represents a promising therapeutic strategy for inducing neurons to overcome myelin inhibitory signals.[11,12] Although there is no spontaneous regeneration of mammalian CNS axons after injury, dorsal root ganglion (DRG) axons have been shown to regenerate if the peripheral branch of these neurons is lesioned prior to CNS injury (termed a *preconditioning lesion*). The axonal regeneration that is seen in preconditioned DRGs is associated with marked elevations in the level of intracellular cAMP. Similarly, the injection of dibutryl cAMP (db-cAMP), a nonhydrolyzable cAMP analogue, into neuronal cell bodies can mimic a preconditioning lesion.[104] Prophylactic administration of cAMP is an impractical clinical therapy for SCI, however, and several strategies have been employed to increase intracellular cAMP levels postinjury. These strategies involve direct injection of db-cAMP or the use of indirect methods such as stimulating adenylate cyclase with forskolin. The transcription factor cAMP response element binding protein (CREB) is activated by elevated cAMP levels in a protein kinase A–dependent fashion and serves as the primary mediator of cAMP-induced transcription.[105] CREB activity has been shown to be essential for overcoming neurite outgrowth inhibition of cerebellar neurons by myelin, as the expression of dominant-negative CREB blocked these effects of cAMP.[106] Several cAMP-regulated gene products have been identified that play a role in overcoming myelin inhibition, including arginase I (Arg I) and IL-6. Arg I expression is increased in cerebellar neurons in response to cAMP, and overexpression of Arg I is sufficient to overcome inhibition by myelin-associated glycoprotein (MAG).[107] Arg I hydrolyzes arginine to ornithine and urea, stimulating the synthesis of polyamines, such as putrescine, spermidine, and spermine. The priming of DRG neurons with polyamines has been shown to enhance neurite outgrowth on MAG, and this effect is lost when pharmacologic inhibitors of polyamine synthesis are administered with cAMP.[107]

As an alternative approach to using cAMP analogues, inhibition of the cAMP-degrading enzyme phosphodiesterase has been extensively studied in animal models of SCI. Rolipram, a specific inhibitor of type IV phosphodiesterase, readily crosses the blood-brain barrier and may be either delivered orally or injected subcutaneously, thereby allowing for simple and clinically relevant means of drug delivery. The therapeutic potential of rolipram has been assessed in several SCI studies.[11,108-110] Rolipram, delivered through a preconditioned subcutaneous priming method, was shown to overcome myelin inhibition in vitro, as DRG neurons from preconditioned animals demonstrated increased neurite outgrowth on inhibitory myelin substrates.[109] The efficacy of rolipram in vivo was assessed after subcutaneous delivery for 10 days via mini-osmotic pumps implanted 2 weeks after spinal cord hemisection lesion, along with acute transplantation of embryonic spinal cord tissue at the injury site. In animals that received rolipram, there was significantly more axonal regrowth into the transplants, particularly that of serotonergic fibers. Rolipram-treated animals also had significantly greater functional recovery, measured by using forelimb paw placement testing. In addition, rolipram treatment resulted in a decrease in astrocytic GFAP expression adjacent to the lesion, indicative of reduced glial scarring.[109] In a contusion SCI model, delivery of rolipram has been shown to prevent a drop in cAMP levels seen in the rostral spinal cord, sensorimotor cortex, and brainstem after injury.[11] Furthermore, the combined treatment of rolipram and Schwann cell transplantation promoted significant supraspinal and propriospinal axonal sparing and myelination.[11] Injection of db-cAMP adjacent to the graft further elevated cAMP levels beyond those in uninjured controls. The combination of rolipram, Schwann cell grafts, and db-cAMP delivered after contusion SCI resulted in enhanced axonal sparing and myelination, promoted axonal regrowth of serotonergic fibers into and beyond the graft site, and improved functional recovery.[11] Rolipram has also been shown to increase phrenic nerve output ipsilateral to an experimental C2 hemisection lesion. Intravenous rolipram restored respiratory-related activity to the phrenic nerve ipsilateral to the injury and significantly enhanced phrenic nerve inspiratory burst activity in both normal and C2 hemisected animals. These results provided evidence that elevating cAMP levels by using a phosphodiesterase inhibitor may enhance phrenic nerve output and restore respiratory-related phrenic nerve function after high cervical SCI.[111]

Although rolipram has been shown to promote axonal regeneration following experimental SCI, recent studies also suggest that the drug promotes robust neuroprotection in experimental models of SCI.[110,112,113] The delivery of rolipram after contusive SCI resulted in significant white matter sparing at the injury epicenter and increased the number of oligodendrocyte-myelinated axons in ventral white matter months after injury.[11,110] Rolipram has been shown to decrease the production of the potent proinflammatory mediators TNF-α and IL-1α, promote myelinated tissue sparing, and improve locomotor function after experimental contusion SCI.[11,110,113] It appears likely that rolipram will enter clinical trials in the future, pending FDA approval based on preclinical studies.

Removal and Blockade of Inhibitory Substrates

Chondroitinase ABC

It is well accepted that significant neuronal regeneration fails to occur following injury to the CNS. The cause is multifactorial, due in part to CSPGs within the forming glial scar and throughout the perineuronal net. The formation of the glial scar after CNS injury presents both a chemical barrier and a physical barrier to axonal regeneration. The up-regulation of axonal growth inhibitors, such as CSPGs, ephrins, and semaphorins, within the glial scar represents a major impediment for axonal regeneration.[114,115] CSPGs function as potent inhibitory extracellular matrix molecules, consisting of a protein core to which many large, sulfated glycosaminoglycan (GAG) chains are covalently attached. These glycosaminoglycans confer most of the inhibitory properties of CSPGs. The CSPGs form a large family of molecules, including aggrecan, brevican, neurocan, NG2, phosphacan, and versican.

The degrading enzyme chondroitinase ABC (ChABC) cleaves the inhibitory glycosaminoglycans from the protein core of CSPGs, thereby removing the axonal growth-inhibitory properties of intact CSPGs.[116] Several studies have demonstrated that axons are able to extend over long distances in vitro following ChABC treatment. Culture of adult sensory DRG neurons on a gradient of inhibitory CSPGs resulted in the formation of dystrophic end-bulbs, which mimics regeneration failure in vivo. Combining inflammation-induced preconditioning of DRG in vivo before harvest with ChABC digestion of proteoglycans in vitro resulted in significant axonal regeneration across a once potently inhibitory substrate.[117]

The degradation of CSPGs using ChABC renders the environment of the damaged CNS more permissive to axon regeneration, and overcoming proteoglycan inhibition using ChABC has been shown to promote axonal growth past the lesion and enhance functional recovery, making it a promising strategy for repair of the injured rat spinal cord.[118-121] The presence of CSPGs within the lesion penumbra appears to be a major factor preventing the regeneration of axons.[122,123] The role of CSPGs in limiting axonal regeneration has been studied in a transgenic mouse model in which the *gfap* promoter was used to express ChABC in astrocytes.[121] In this study, corticospinal axons entered the lesion site but did not extend caudally across a dorsal hemisection lesion in transgenic mice. Accordingly, no significant improvement in motor functional recovery was observed in this model. In contrast, functionally significant sensory axon regeneration was observed, suggesting that ChABC acts on spatially distinct axonal pathways. Intrathecal delivery of ChABC has been shown to degrade CSPGs at the site of injury, up-regulate a regeneration-associated protein (GAP-43), promote regeneration of ascending sensory projections and descending corticospinal axons, and improve functional recovery.[124,125] In addition, microinjection of ChABC induces collateral sprouting in the cuneate nucleus after cervical SCI through digestion of the perineuronal net.[126]

The administration of ChABC has also been used as an adjunctive strategy to promote axonal regeneration in combination with neurotrophic factors and various cell types, such as Schwann cells, PN grafts, olfactory-ensheathing cells, and fetal spinal cord tissue.[103,120,127,128] Recent studies have shown that delivery of ChABC into the rostral and caudal ends of the lesion site enhanced the ability of regenerating axons to enter, as well as exit, PN grafts transplanted into CNS lesions.[103] Despite these findings, recent evidence suggests that axonal sprouting might not be responsible for the functional recovery that is seen after ChABC delivery and that neuroprotective effects of ChABC may exist.[129]

Currently, there are no ongoing clinical trials of ChABC for the treatment of SCI. However, on the basis of an increasing number of preclinical studies supporting a role for ChABC in spinal cord repair, it is likely that ChABC will enter pilot studies and clinical trials for SCI in the near future (Fig. 72-2).

Anti-Nogo-A Antibody (ATI-355)

In the late 1980s, pioneering work by Caroni and Schwab[130,131] demonstrated that oligodendrocyte myelin was a major inhibitor of axonal growth within the CNS. The myelin was then biochemically separated into 35- and 250-kD inhibitory fractions (termed NI-35 and NI-250), and a monoclonal antibody (termed IN-1) was developed that could block their inhibitory properties in vitro.[130] Subsequent in vivo application of IN-1 in rodents resulted in substantial axonal sprouting and long-distance corticospinal axonal regeneration within the adult mammalian CNS and was associated with improved functional recovery. The IN-1 antibody was also used in the characterization and protein sequencing of its target antigen, which has led to the identification of several myelin-associated inhibitors, known as Nogo-A; myelin-associated glycoprotein (MAG); and oligodendrocyte myelin glycoprotein (OMgp). Recent advances in molecular neuroscience have also led to the identification of their receptor complex (consisting of the Nogo receptor (NgR), LINGO-1, and p75^{NTR}/TROY), and a common downstream signaling pathway involving two key proteins, Rho-A GTPase and Rho kinase (ROCK). These landmark findings have prompted the development of targeted strategies aimed at halting the signaling cascade, thereby enabling axons to overcome myelin inhibition and regeneration failure. To date, several experimental and preclinical strategies have been employed, including the development of the following:

- A Nogo-A knockout mouse
- NgR-Fc, a soluble Nogo receptor fusion protein that blocks Nogo-A
- A humanized anti-Nogo-A neutralizing antibody
- NEP1–40, a Nogo-66 receptor antagonist
- Anti-NgR antibodies
- NgR knockdown mice using small interfering RNA (siRNA)
- An anti-LINGO-1 neutralizing antibody (Fig. 72-3B)

The myelin-associated inhibitors (Nogo-A, MAG, and OMgp) utilize a common receptor, the Nogo-66 receptor (NgR), which transduces signals, resulting in the inhibition of axonal regeneration. Recently, a novel vaccine approach has been used to stimulate the production of an anti-NgR antibody to overcome NgR-mediated growth inhibition after SCI.[79] Adult rats immunized with recombinant NgR produced high titers of the anti-NgR antibody, and antisera that was obtained from the immunized rats promoted neurite outgrowth of rat cerebellar neurons on the inhibitory myelin substrate MAG in vitro. In a spinal cord dorsal hemisection model, NgR immunization promoted regeneration of lesioned corticospinal tract axons beyond the lesion site. In a contusive SCI model, NgR immunization markedly reduced the total lesion volume and improved hindlimb locomotor recovery.[79] Thus, the NgR vaccine approach may represent a promising repair strategy to promote recovery following SCI.

The blockade of Nogo-A through the use of a humanized monoclonal neutralizing antibody, termed ATI-355, has been shown to promote axonal sprouting and functional recovery following SCI in numerous animal models, including primates, and represents a clinically relevant and promising strategy to overcome myelin inhibition (see Fig. 72-2). The delivery of anti-Nogo A antibody has been shown to stimulate axonal sprouting caudal to the site of experimental SCI. The axonal sprouting that is seen after treatment with the Nogo-A antibody is accompanied by enhanced functional recovery of manual dexterity in primates, as compared to control antibody.[132] Furthermore, delivery of anti-Nogo-A antibody also reduced retrograde axonal degeneration (axonal dieback) in anti-Nogo-A antibody–treated monkeys. In the cervical cord, anti-Nogo-A treatment enhanced axonal sprouting of corticospinal fibers rostral to the site of injury, and some of these fibers grew around the lesion and into the caudal spinal segments.

Following preclinical studies that demonstrated the safety and effectiveness of humanized anti-Nogo-A antibody, a large-scale phase I clinical trial was initiated by Novartis Pharma in close collaboration with the European and North American Clinical Trial Networks for SCI to assess the safety, feasibility, and pharmacokinetics of this antibody in patients with complete SCI between C5 and T12 at 4 to 14 days postinjury.[13] The agent is being administered via continuous intrathecal infusion, and patients are being enrolled in four increasing dose regimens, the highest dose being delivered over 28 days.

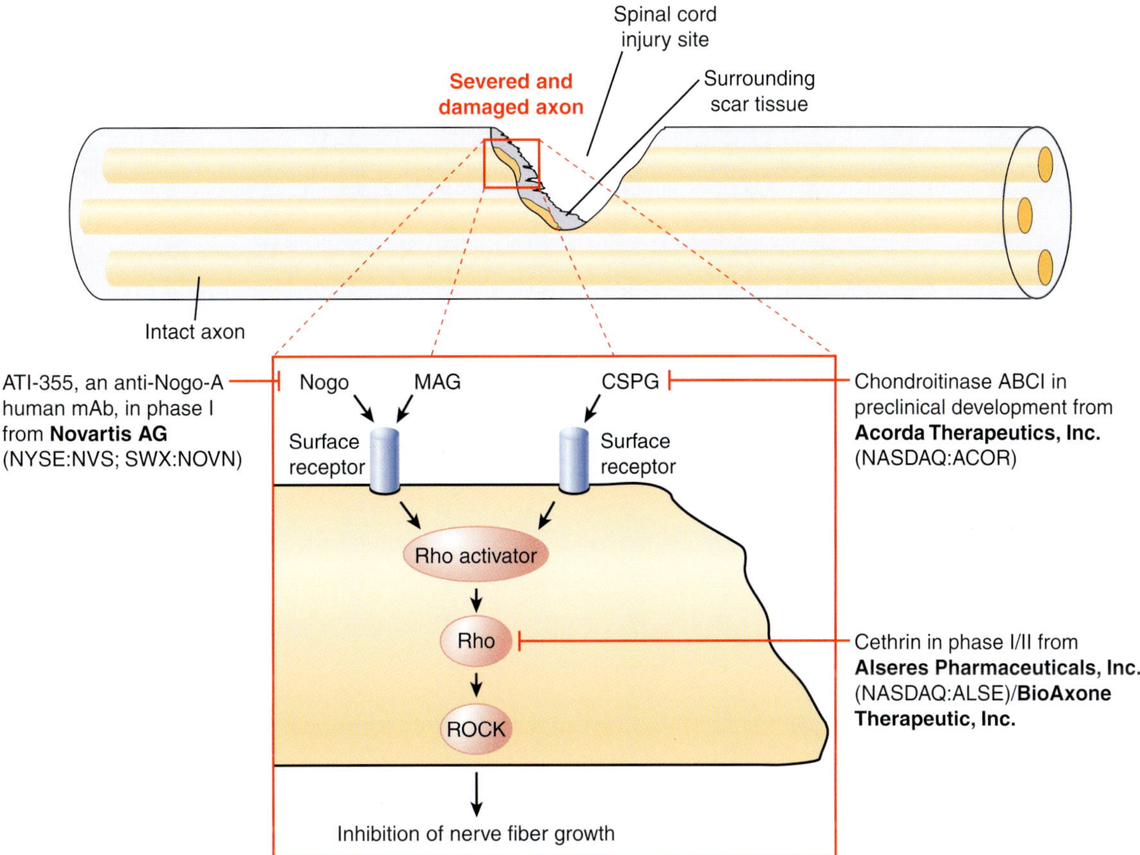

FIGURE 72-2. Schematic diagram depicting key signaling molecules involved in axonal growth inhibition and several experimental preclinical and clinical strategies targeting this pathway. The humanized monoclonal antibody IN-1 (ATI-355) inactivates Nogo-A. The bacterial enzyme chondroitinase ABC (ChABC) degrades inhibitory CSPGs present in the surrounding astroglial scar tissue. Several variations of the *Clostridium botulinum* C3 transferase protein have been designed, including BA-210 (termed Cethrin), which inactivates Rho by ADP ribosylation of its active site. (From scibx.com/scibx_main/20081009.html.)

However, the FDA expressed concerns about the external nature of the infusion pump, and the clinical evaluation has subsequently been limited to Europe and Canada. In addition, neutropenia was recently reported as a severe adverse event associated with this therapy. The results of this trial are currently pending.

Rho Antagonists

The microenvironment of the lesioned spinal cord is not conducive for axonal regeneration, owing in large part to the presence of myelin-associated inhibitory proteins, which include Nogo-A, MAG, and OMgp, and the presence of CSPGs, semaphorins, and ephrins within the glial scar. Many of these inhibitors have been shown to activate a common signaling pathway within neurons, consisting of the RhoA GTPase and its downstream effector, the serine/threonine kinase, Rho-associated coiled kinase (ROCK) (Fig. 72-3A).[133] The Rho/ROCK pathway is an important determinant in the response of axons to growth inhibitory proteins, which exert growth-inhibitory effects through the regulation of the actin-myosin network, leading to stimulation of actin-myosin contractility via myosin light chain phosphorylation, inhibition of myosin phosphatase, and inactivation of the actin-depolymerizing factor cofilin.[133] These molecular events eventually lead to the induction of neurite retraction and subsequently to growth cone collapse.[134]

Rho activity has been shown to increase extensively following transection of the rat spinal cord, and numerous studies have demonstrated that inhibition of the Rho/ROCK pathway results in enhanced axonal regeneration and functional recovery in animal models of SCI.[135,136] Several pharmacologic methods have been used to inhibit the Rho/ROCK pathway, including the delivery of the *Clostridium botulinum*–derived Rho antagonist (C3 ribosyltransferase, dominant negative Rho, or use of the pyridine-derivative Y-27632, a specific inhibitor of ROCK.)[137] In vitro experiments with Rho and ROCK inhibitors have shown that these drugs are capable of preventing the inhibition of neurite outgrowth that is observed on typical inhibitory substrates present within the glial scar and in white matter.[133,138,139] Intravenous and intrathecal delivery of Y-27632 has been shown to enhance sprouting of corticospinal and dorsal column axons and to accelerate locomotor recovery after corticospinal lesions in adult rats.[140,141] The regenerative effects of C3 transferase appear to be greater than those of Y-27632, suggesting the presence of other effectors of the Rho signaling pathway that are inactivated by C3 transferase but not by Y-27632.[138] The administration of Rho pathway antagonists for up to 24 hours following spinal cord transection in mice resulted in a rapid improvement in locomotion, with progressive improvement in forelimb-hindlimb coordination, suggesting that C3 transferase may be a promising option for SCI with a clinically relevant therapeutic

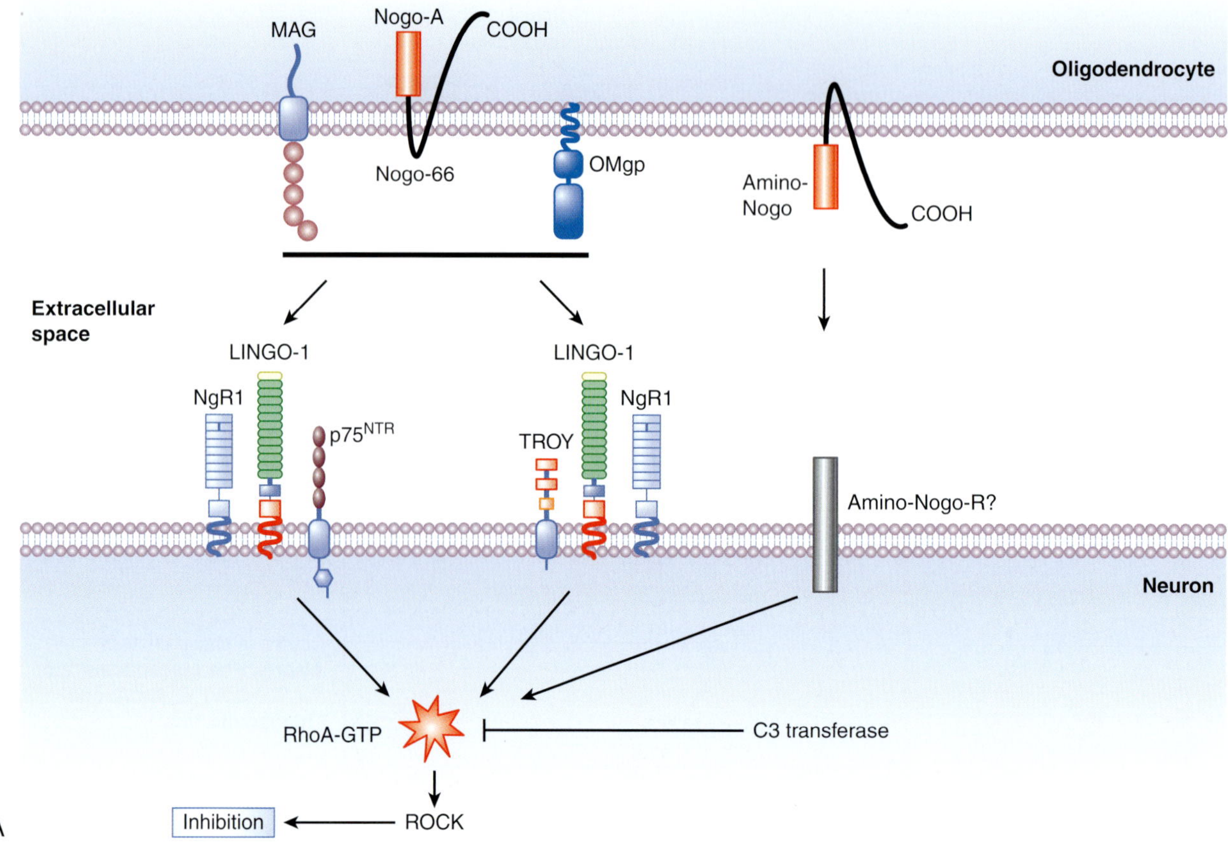

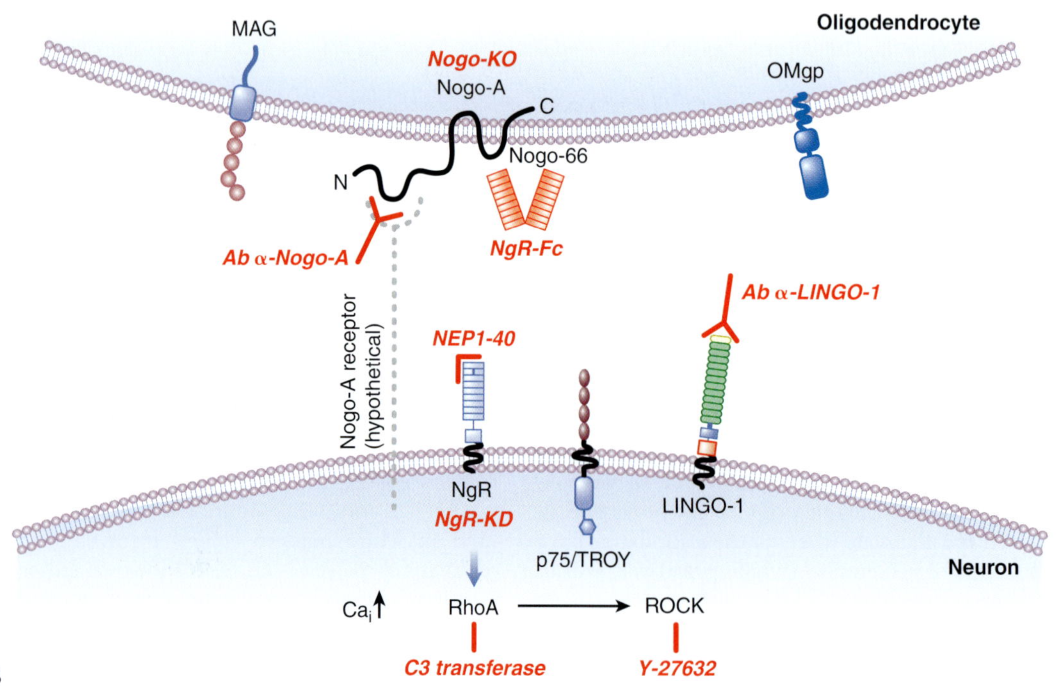

FIGURE 72-3. **A,** Schematic illustration of the molecular mechanisms involved in axonal growth inhibition after SCI. All known myelin inhibitors appear to activate the Rho GTPase, which leads to growth cone collapse. Signaling via NgR has been established for Nogo, MAG, and OMgp. Other known inhibitors, such as CSPGs, also signal using Rho through pathways that have not yet been elucidated. **B,** Diagram illustrating the molecular targeting of specific components involved in transducing myelin inhibition. Several experimental and preclinical strategies have been employed, including the development of a Nogo-A knockout mouse; NgR-Fc, a soluble fusion protein blocking Nogo-A; a humanized anti-Nogo-A neutralizing antibody; NEP1-40, a Nogo-66 receptor antagonist; anti-NgR antibodies (not shown); NgR knockdown mice using siRNA; an anti-LINGO-1 neutralizing antibody; *Clostridium botulinum* C3 ribosyltransferase (C3 transferase); and Y-27632, a selective ROCK inhibitor. (**A,** From Chaudhry N, Filbin MT: Myelin-associated inhibitory signaling and strategies to overcome inhibition. *J Cereb Blood Flow Metab* 27[6]:1096–1107, 2007. **B,** From Rossignol S, Schwab M, Schwartz M, Fehlings MG: Spinal cord injury: time to move? *J Neurosci* 27[44]:11782–11792, 2007.)

window.[138] Neuroprotective actions have also been attributed to the Rho pathway antagonists. For example, C3-mediated neuroprotection appears to involve an ability to enhance the half-life of vascular endothelial nitric oxide synthase mRNA, thereby improving blood flow to ischemic regions.[142]

Following a multitude of preclinical studies in support of axonal regenerative and neuroprotective properties of Rho pathway antagonists, BioAxone Therapeutic, Inc., initiated a phase I/IIa multicenter open-label, dose-escalating clinical trial to assess the pharmacokinetics and evaluate the safety, tolerability, and neurologic status of patients following administration of a single extradural application of the Rho antagonist Cethrin (see Fig. 72-2). Cethrin is a recombinant fusion protein composed of C3 ribosyltransferase in combination with a membrane transport sequence, which allows the protein to cross cellular membranes, where it inhibits RhoA activity by ADP-ribosylation. The patient population in the phase I/IIa Cethrin trial consisted of males and females aged 16 to 70 years of age with an acute thoracic or cervical SCI corresponding to an ASIA grade A who were scheduled to undergo spinal decompression/stabilization within 7 days of injury. Injuries from T2 to T12 and from C4 to T1 were subject to separate analysis, and 6-month and 1-year follow-ups were planned. The study recruited 37 patients and did not include control subjects. The drug was administered an average of 53 hours postinjury, delivered in a single dose with fibrin sealant. Dose levels ranged from 0.3 mg to 9.0 mg. At 6 months follow-up, approximately 28% of the patients had improved by one or more ASIA grades (five subjects improved by two grades, and two subjects improved by three grades). The results of the study show that 19.4% of patients improved by two or more ASIA grades at 6 months, a rate that is 1.5- to 3-fold higher than rates in historical controls. Overall, cervical SCIs appeared to show greater benefit. There were no adverse events related to Cethrin. To date, it appears that local application of the Rho inhibitor Cethrin is both feasible and safe in patients with acute SCI. These results must be interpreted with caution, given the early phase of this trial and its nonrandomized nature. However, this rate of improved neurologic function appears promising, and a subsequent prospective, randomized phase II study is being conducted under the sponsorship of Alseres Pharmaceuticals.

Conclusions

The pathophysiologic events that occur after SCI are formidable challenges to successful neural repair. Despite the best efforts of the scientific and clinical communities, we have yet to meet these challenges. A more comprehensive understanding of the complex biologic processes continues to be essential to our development of highly effective therapies. With the lessons learned from recently completed trials, many new clinical trials for SCI are under way. It is anticipated that several of these promising therapies will be effective. Furthermore, many more potential therapies are in preclinical studies with the promise of entering clinical trials in the near future. To date, efforts to induce regeneration and repair of the injured spinal cord have led to a number of translatable therapies directed at inhibiting myelin-associated inhibitors, targeting intracellular second messenger systems that mediate axonal growth, and degrading inhibitory glial scar components. Additionally, cell transplantation strategies have enormous therapeutic potential, although many scientific and clinical aspects of therapeutic cell transplantation still require resolution. However, the modest functional improvements that have been obtained from the experimental therapies being developed clearly illustrate the need for multifaceted approaches that combine neuroprotective, regenerative, and rehabilitative approaches with the aim of optimizing the recovery of SCI patients. There is a clear basis for researchers, clinicians, and patients to be optimistic. However, it is unfortunate that despite the lessons of the past, many experimental therapies are being tested or used in an unsatisfactory fashion. We hope that the promotion of recently published guidelines will maximize what can be learned from the patients who participate in such trials.

KEY REFERENCES

Bracken MB, Shepard MJ, Collins WF, et al: A randomized, controlled trial of methylprednisolone or naloxone in the treatment of acute spinal-cord injury: results of the Second National Acute Spinal Cord Injury Study. *N Engl J Med* 322(20):1405–1411, 1990.

Houle JD, Tom VJ, Mayes D, et al: Combining an autologous peripheral nervous system "bridge" and matrix modification by chondroitinase allows robust, functional regeneration beyond a hemisection lesion of the adult rat spinal cord. *J Neurosci* 26(28):7405–7415, 2006.

Lehmann M, Fournier A, Selles-Navarro I, Dergham P, et al: Inactivation of Rho signaling pathway promotes CNS axon regeneration. *J Neurosci* 19(17):7537–7547, 1999.

Pearse DD, Pereira FC, Marcillo AE, et al: cAMP and Schwann cells promote axonal growth and functional recovery after spinal cord injury. *Nat Med* 10(6):610–616, 2004.

Richardson PM, McGuinness UM, Aguayo AJ: Axons from CNS neurons regenerate into PNS grafts. *Nature* 284(5753):264–265, 1980.

REFERENCES

The complete reference list is available online at expertconsult.com.

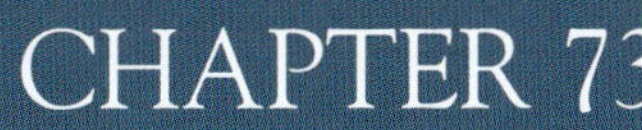

CHAPTER 73

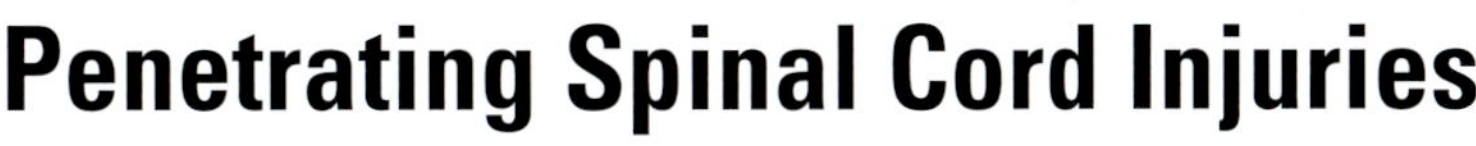

Penetrating Spinal Cord Injuries

Michael P. Steinmetz | William McCormick | Alex Valadka |
Perry A. Ball | Philip A. Yazbak | Edward C. Benzel

Penetrating spine injury is a major cause of spinal cord injury (SCI) in the United States. Gunshot injuries have been reported to be the third leading cause of SCI.[1] Stab wounds and other penetrating injuries tend to occur less in the United States than in some other countries. In South Africa, they account for 25% of all SCIs.[2]

Avoiding complications in the management of patients with penetrating SCIs begins with meticulous attention to evaluation, resuscitation, and operative and surgical techniques.

Military versus Civilian Gunshot Injuries

Most experience with the management of penetrating SCIs has been gained during wartime. During World War I, survival was uncommon after a complete myelopathy (72% mortality). Treatment of these injuries consisted of laminectomy for incomplete myelopathy and debridement of the entry and exit wounds for complete myelopathy.[3] A high operative mortality rate (62%) added to the dismal outcome.

During World War II, advances were made in trauma resuscitation and therapy. These advances dramatically decreased the mortality from penetrating SCIs.[4-6] Some surgeons reported neurologic improvement in patients who were managed surgically.[7] During the Korean War, most patients with penetrating SCIs underwent surgical exploration. There were reports of significant improvement.[8] Further improvements were made in trauma resuscitation, evacuation, and surgical treatment during Operation Iraqi Freedom and Operation Enduring Freedom.[9] The treatment of civilian penetrating SCIs, however, has generated less optimism than previous military reports have.[10-14] Despite these findings, some authors have demonstrated benefit with early surgical intervention following civilian gunshot wounds.[15] This is likely related to the pathophysiology of this type of injury.

Military weapons fire high-velocity missiles, while civilian weapons (typically handguns) fire low-velocity missiles. The pathophysiology of the SCI differs on the basis of velocity. High-velocity missiles may produce SCI by a concussive effect of the bullet passing close to, but not through, the spinal canal.[16] Most SCIs caused by high-velocity missiles fit this pattern. These types of injuries may have a slightly better prognosis. Low-velocity missiles are more likely to injure the spinal cord directly, without a significant concussive effect; therefore, the prognosis for recovery is worse owing to the direct cord injury. This phenomenon may also explain the large percentage of civilian gunshot SCIs that present as complete myelopathies.[10,12,17,18]

Impalement Pathophysiology

A weapon (knife) that penetrates the spinal canal may damage the spinal cord directly or indirectly. The direct injury may range from a dural tear to a total cord transection. Indirectly, there may be spinal cord contusion from the weapon impacting the cord against the bony spinal canal. The anatomy of the spinal canal may protect the spinal cord from a complete transection (Fig. 73-1). The weapon usually enters the spinal canal in the gutter between the spinous process and transverse process, thus leading to an incomplete SCI. Classically, the Brown-Séquard syndrome or a variant results.[19]

Resuscitation

The initial management begins with advanced trauma life support measures. The airway should be evaluated and secured. If necessary, endotracheal intubation should be performed. Oral intubation using manual in-line traction has been shown to be both safe and effective in patients with suspected SCI.[20] Tracheostomy is indicated if the injury involves the trachea or larynx.[21] Chest radiographs and arterial blood gas analysis (if indicated) should be part of the initial evaluation. The incidence of associated visceral injuries may be as high as 25%.[22] These injuries, such as pneumothorax or vascular injury, must be sought early, as their treatment takes priority over spinal cord or spinal column injury.

The patient's early course may be complicated by hypotension, which may be due to blood loss (hypovolemia) or to neurogenic shock from the loss of sympathetic vasomotor tone. Determining the exact cause of the hypotension is often difficult in the acute setting. However, tachycardia and cool extremities are often observed with hypovolemia, while bradycardia is often observed with spinal shock.[19] The treatment for either condition is aggressive volume resuscitation. A central

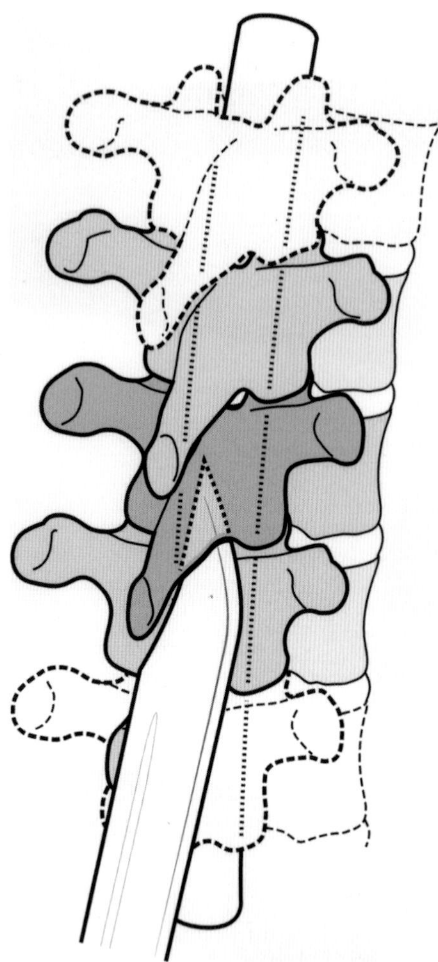

FIGURE 73-1. A depiction of a stab wound to the spine. The weapon enters in the gutter between the spinous process and the transverse process. This anatomy prevents the weapon from crossing midline as it enters the spinal canal. A spinal cord hemisection, rather than a transection, often results.

venous catheter is often helpful for monitoring the volume resuscitation. If the hypotension persists despite adequate intravascular volume replacement, vasopressor agents such as phenylephrine or dopamine should be employed. Vagolytic agents such as atropine may also be used. An indwelling pulmonary artery catheter may be useful if hypotension persists despite the use of vasopressor agents. Enthusiasm for the use of these catheters has waned lately.[23]

A Foley catheter should be placed. This allows bladder decompression and assists with gauging of the effectiveness of volume resuscitation. It also decreases the likelihood of subsequent urologic complications.[19]

Once the patient is stable from a cardiopulmonary standpoint, a more thorough history and physical examination should be performed. Information about the mechanism of injury and the caliber of the weapon should be obtained. The physical examination should note whether the patient has suffered a complete or incomplete myelopathy. If the injury is incomplete, the level of the SCI should be noted. The entry and exit sites should be inspected, and notation of cerebrospinal fluid (CSF) or foreign material should be made.[7]

Treatment of non-neurologic injuries is of primary importance because such treatment is usually lifesaving (rather than function-preserving).[19] Because the course that a penetrating object takes within the torso is unpredictable, there may be an associated visceral injury.[19] A trauma surgeon should assist with the evaluation for such potential injuries. Explorations of the neck, chest, and abdomen take precedence over spine surgeries.[24]

Some clinicians advocate exploration for wounds that penetrate the platysma, whereas others advocate the individualization of surgical planning.[19] The two approaches appear equally effective if injuries to the great vessels, upper airway, and upper gastrointestinal tract can be ruled out via angiography, endoscopy, or swallowing studies.[25-28]

Pharyngeal perforation carries the risk of osteomyelitis.[21,28,29] There are divergent views on the appropriate management of pharyngeal perforation. Some authors advocate broad-spectrum antibiotics, debridement of bone and soft tissue, drainage, and immobilization.[21] Others have reported a lower infection rate with neural decompression and debridement of the wound.[30]

Penetrating thoracic injuries may damage the lungs or mediastinum. Chest radiography, computed tomography, and/or angiography may be used to define the extent of the injury. Tube thoracostomy or surgical exploration may be indicated.

Radiographic Evaluation

Initial evaluation should begin with routine radiographs. Fractures and bullet fragments may be seen (Fig. 73-2). A CT through the area of involvement should be performed next. This modality is generally superior to plain radiographs for the evaluation of the injury and for localizing the fracture or bullet fragments (Fig. 73-3). Compressive lesions may be identified with routine CT imaging. Bone and/or bullet fragments compressing the thecal sac may be identified. The aforementioned will also give the surgeon a sense of spinal stability or instability. CT myelography may be used to assess or confirm neural compression. This modality may also aid in the evaluation of a CSF fistula. If there is a question of spinal instability, passive flexion/extension radiographs may be used, but only in an awake, alert patient in whom there is no neurologic deficit.

MRI may also be used in the evaluation. There will be artifacts from the bullet fragments, but valuable information, such as the presence of extradural hematoma, disc herniation, or spinal cord contusion, may be gained. There is a risk of fragment migration in the magnetic field, so only patients for whom the information gained would have been difficult to obtain with other imaging modalities should undergo MRI.[31]

Steroids and Antibiotics

Experience with large patient populations has shown no improvement in outcome from using steroids in patients with penetrating spine injuries.[19,32-34] This lack of efficacy and the potential adverse effects on wound healing and infection suggest that steroids have no role in patients with penetrating spine injury.

The rate of infection in penetrating SCI during the Vietnam War was lower in comparison to the rates in prior conflicts. The reason for the lower incidence was predominantly the use

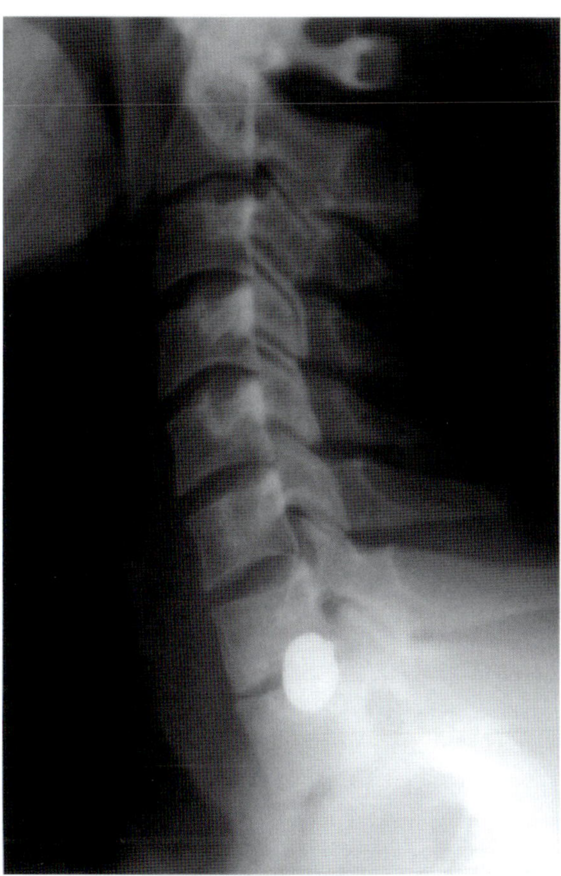

FIGURE 73-2. Lateral radiograph demonstrating a bullet that has entered the spinal canal. It is in the proximity of the neural foramen.

of antibiotics.[35] Therefore, one may reasonably conclude that prophylactic antibiotics are of benefit in penetrating SCI. At least 7 days of antibiotic treatment for penetrating abdominal wounds with accompanying involvement of the spine have been shown to result in fewer infectious complications than do shorter courses of antibiotic treatment.[36] The antibiotic agents should be chosen on the basis of the region of the body injured and local hospital bacterial sensitivities.

There has been some concern regarding infection following associated visceral injury. Roffi et al. reviewed 42 patients with gunshot wounds to the spine involving bullets passing through the alimentary tract.[36] The patients were treated with a 2-week course of broad-spectrum antibiotics, and no evidence of late infection or osteomyelitis was found. Waters and Sie confirmed these findings in over 1000 cases of gunshot wounds to the spine.[37] It may be concluded from these findings that it is not necessary to debride and remove bullet fragments following civilian gunshot wounds, even in the face of viscus perforation. This is not the case with high-velocity missile injuries, which pose a greater risk of contamination. Debriding the wound and removing the bullet fragments plus giving parenteral antibiotics are recommended.[38]

Management

Protection of the integument, support of pulmonary function, and prophylaxis against deep vein thrombosis should be addressed immediately. Specialized nursing care is of the

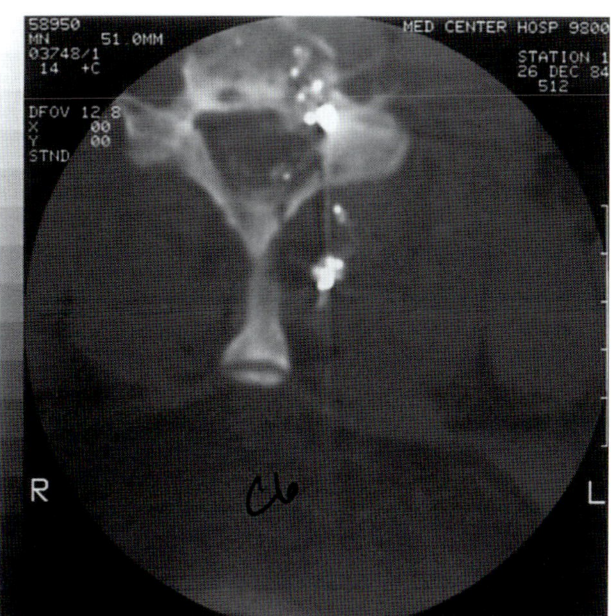

FIGURE 73-3. Axial CT scan of a gunshot wound to the cervical spine demonstrating multiple fragments and a resultant fracture of the vertebral body.

utmost importance. This should begin immediately. The patient should be turned frequently, and an aggressive pulmonary toilet program should be instituted.

Surgical Indications

Missile Injuries

Surgery may be indicated in the following circumstances: (1) cord compression with an incomplete injury, (2) a discrepancy between the clinical examination and the missile trajectory with a complete myelopathy, (3) a migratory missile fragment, (4) spinal instability, (5) associated infection, and (6) persistent CSF leak[17-19] (Fig. 73-4). Consideration should be given to surgical exploration of lesions of the cauda equina regardless of neurologic status. Because such injuries involve nerve roots rather than the spinal cord proper, they have a better prognosis.[7] Surgery to remove a bullet fragment is not warranted unless compression of the cauda equina exists. Removal of the fragment when associated with a spinal cord–level injury remains controversial. As was noted previously, the type of injury may warrant fragment removal. If the injury was caused by a high-velocity weapon, such as during wartime, debridement and fragment removal may be indicated, especially in the face of viscus injury. If incomplete SCI is noted and the fragment is compressive, removal should be strongly considered. The composition of the bullet fragments has not been shown to adversely affect neurologic function.[13,39,40]

Impalement Injuries

Indications for surgery include neural element compression by bone or soft tissue fragments, retained fragments, CSF fistula, and infection. In contrast to gunshot injuries, retained foreign material should be removed after a stab wound. Because stab wounds are rarely delivered with enough force to cause

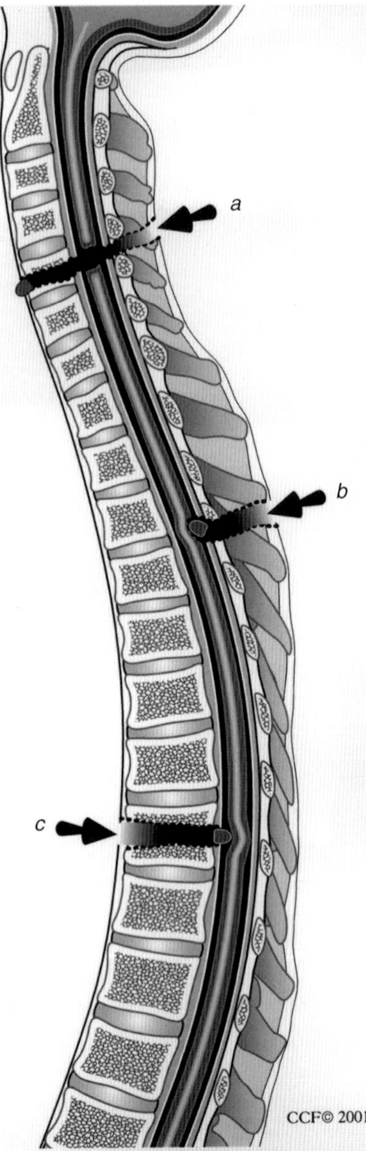

FIGURE 73-4. Depiction of injury types that may be treated surgically. Through-and-through gunshot wound (GSW) that has resulted in a complete myelopathy with spinal instability or a neurologic level of injury that is significantly higher than the level of spine injury (*a*). A dorsal GSW to the spine that has resulted in an incomplete myelopathy with spinal cord compression (*b*). Surgical decompression via laminectomy is indicated. A gunshot wound that has caused a ventral compression and an incomplete myelopathy (*c*). Surgical decompression is warranted. In the thoracic or lumbar spine, a ventral or dorsolateral strategy may be used. (Copyright Cleveland Clinic Foundation.)

spinal instability, this is an uncommon indication for surgery after these types of injuries.

Surgical Technique

Dorsal Approach

The dorsal approach is used most commonly for treatment of penetrating SCIs.[19] A midline incision is made over the area of injury, and a standard subperiosteal dissection is used to gain access to the spine. Laminectomy or laminotomy is performed to expose the area of injury. Care should be taken to remove all compressive elements. Of particular importance is preservation of the facet joints to preserve spinal stability. The dura mater is often opened to expose the injured spinal cord or nerve roots. If an intramedullary mass with associated neurologic deficit is identified, it can be approached via midline myelotomy. Unnecessary injury to the posterior columns can be avoided by strict adherence to the placement of the midline myelotomy, and liquefied clot can be removed from within the spinal cord with gentle irrigation and suction[19] (Fig. 73-5).

Bullet and bone fragments that are compressing neural elements are removed. Not all fragments need be removed, especially if they are intramedullary. Foreign objects associated with an impalement injury should be removed.

Dural closure should be pursued aggressively, care being taken not to compromise intradural contents[19] (Fig. 73-6). Watertight closure should be performed, either primarily or with patching. Every effort should be made to use autologous material, such as local fascia or fascia lata. Ventral dural tears represent a challenge to repair from the dorsal approach. They may be left alone or may be loosely patched with muscle or other tissue. Fibrin-based tissue sealants are often helpful in treating such dural lacerations. CSF diversion is another useful adjunct.

Dorsolateral and Ventral Approaches

If a compressive lesion is lateral or ventral to the spinal cord, a dorsolateral or ventral approach may be indicated. Options include a transpedicular or costotransversectomy approach or a thoracotomy and lateral extracavitary approach for a more ventral exposure. Because these approaches do not provide wide exposure of the dura, they are rarely indicated.[17] If the spine has been judged unstable, appropriate fixation and fusion techniques should be employed.

Closure

All closures should be accomplished in multiple layers. Drains should be avoided if at all possible.

Prognosis

Prognosis is better after an impalement injury than after a missile injury. Overall, 60% of patients with stab wounds are able to ambulate at follow-up, compared to 24% of those with SCI due to gunshot wounds.[41] The prognosis is poor with complete injury in either group.

Complications

CSF fistula may occur at the entrance or exit site. Fistulous connections with the bowel, bladder, and pleural cavity have also been reported.[42-44] The initial management should be with subarachnoid drainage. If this fails, surgical exploration is warranted.

With the institution of prophylactic antibiotics, the incidence of infection after gunshot wounds has dramatically decreased.[36] The antibiotics should be given for 7 to 14 days and should be tailored to the body site violated and to local hospital sensitivities. The combination of removal of retained

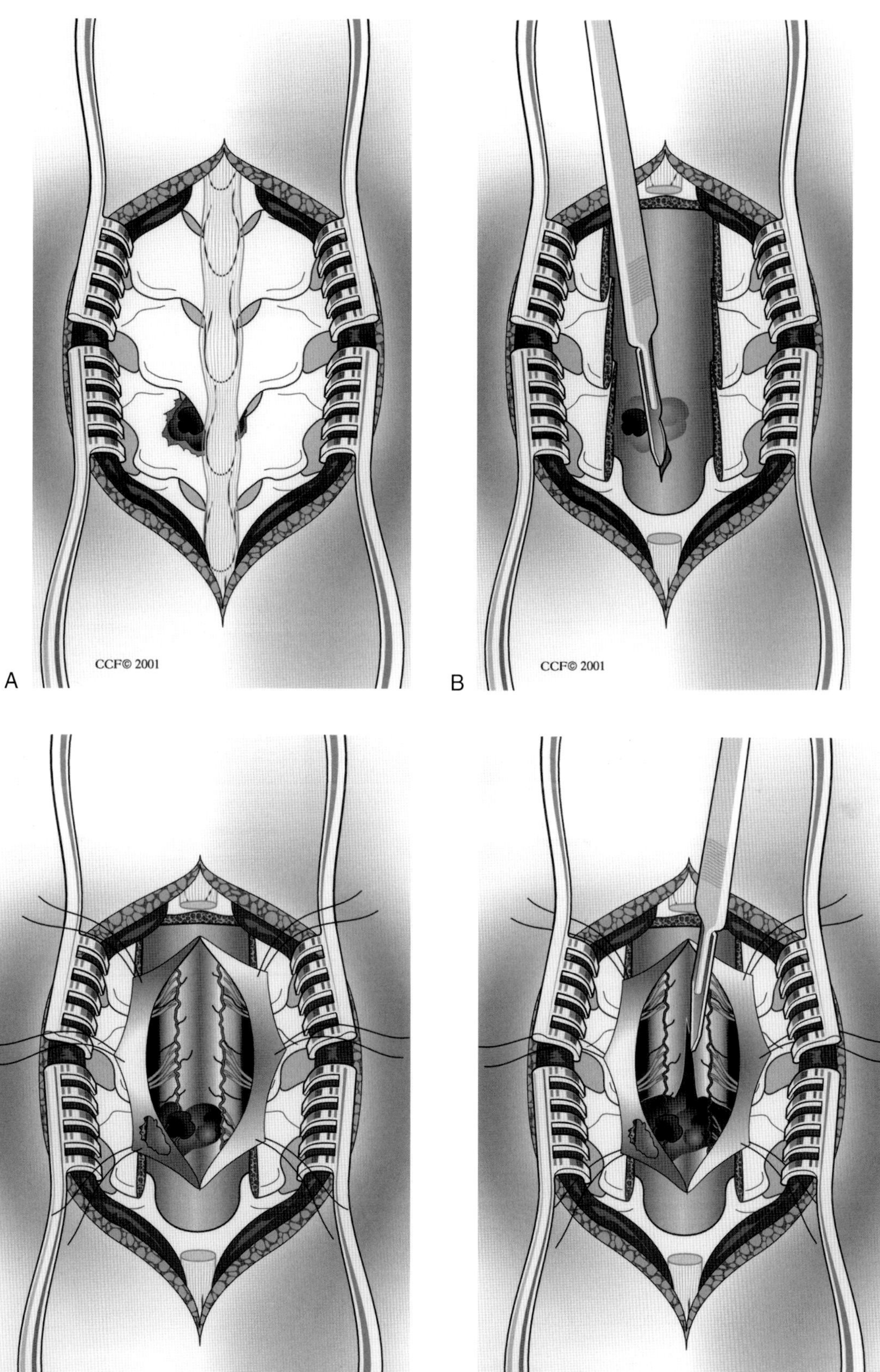

FIGURE 73-5. A, A wide exposure has demonstrated the bullet's entry site. **B,** A generous laminectomy is performed, both above and below the level of entry. **C,** The durotomy should also be generous. **D,** If an intramedullary hematoma has been identified, a midline myelotomy may be performed to evacuate the clot. (Copyright Cleveland Clinic Foundation.)

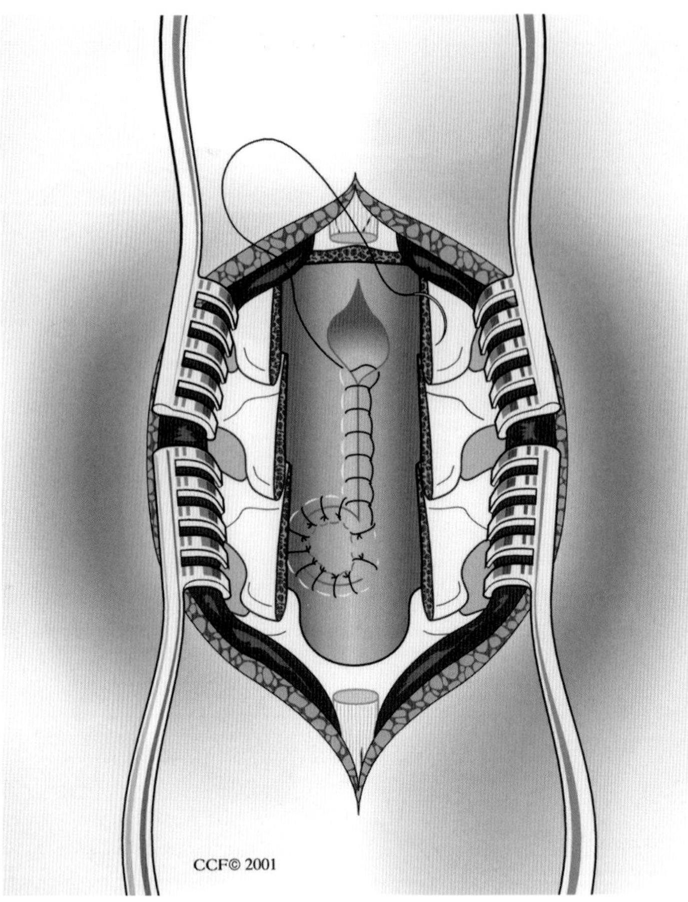

FIGURE 73-6. The dura mater is closed in a watertight fashion. Any dural defect should be patched. (Copyright Cleveland Clinic Foundation.)

foreign material, debridement, and prophylactic antibiotics should achieve a low infection rate after an impalement injury.

Fever should prompt lumbar puncture to rule out meningitis. Late deterioration after penetrating SCI may indicate an infectious source, such as epidural abscess.

Metallic fragments have been reported to migrate in the CNS.[45-48] If there has been migration and the patient is asymptomatic, no treatment may be needed, and the patient may simply be followed. If the patient is or becomes symptomatic (e.g., radiculopathy or paresthesias), the fragment should be retrieved.

Lead intoxication after a gunshot injury is rare. Bullets become encapsulated by poorly vascularized fibrous tissue.[49] In addition, the lead from a bullet is relatively insoluble. Removal of a bullet for the purpose of decreasing lead intoxication is not warranted.

Penetrating spine injuries often lead to deafferentation pain. This pain is problematic in that it is often refractory to treatment.[21] The problem is usually managed medically but often with minimal or no success. Surgery to remove bullet fragments thought to be related to pain has not been shown to provide improvement.[41,50,51] Procedures such as spinal cord stimulation may be an option if medical therapy fails.

Conclusions

Penetrating injuries are significant causes of SCI. Despite a better understanding of the pathophysiology and improved surgical care, the prognosis is still poor. Surgery does not play a significant role in GSWs unless there is an incomplete myelopathy with a surgically correctable cause. Surgery plays a larger role in impalement injuries, which have a better prognosis than gunshot injuries do. Complications such as infection and lead intoxication are rare and do not warrant removal of retained fragments, whereas in stab injuries, retained foreign objects should be removed.

KEY REFERENCES

Bell RS, Neal CJ, Tingo J, et al: Traumatic brain and spinal column injury: a 5-year study of the impact blast and other military grade weaponry on the central nervous system. *J Trauma* 66(4):S104–S111, 2009.

Jacobson SA, Bor E: Spinal cord injury in Vietnamese combat. *Paraplegia* 7:263–281, 1970.

Kitchel SH: Current treatment of gunshot wounds to the spine. *Clin Orthop Relat Res* 408:115–119, 2003.

Turgut M, Ozcan OE, Gurcay O, Saglam S: Civilian penetrating spinal firearm injuries of the spine. *Arch Orthop Trauma Surg* 113:290–293, 1994.

Waters RL, Sie IH: Spinal cord injuries from gunshot wounds to the spine. *Clin Orthop Relat Res* 408:120–125, 2003.

REFERENCES

The complete reference list is available online at expertconsult.com.

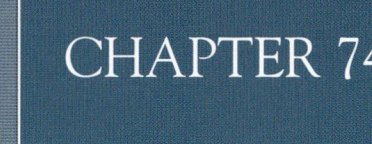

CHAPTER 74

Timing of Surgery Following Spinal Cord Injury

Jamie Baisden | Dennis J. Maiman | Michael G. Fehlings

To date, there have been no level 1 studies to determine the optimal timing of surgery for acute spinal cord injury (SCI). The reasons for this are multifactorial; there are no clear definitions of early or late surgery, every SCI is unique, and designing a randomized prospective clinical trial to determine optimal timing for surgery would be almost impossible. The optimal timing of surgery for SCI remains controversial.[1,2]

Difficulties Associated with Study Design

The difficulties in designing a prospective, randomized, clinical trial are many. Owing to statistical power, the study would need to be multicenter to generate adequate numbers of participants. Some of these patients would be transferred from other institutions to level 1 or appropriate trauma centers. Patients may or may not be given pharmacologic interventions such as the methylprednisolone protocol. They may already be 6 to 8 hours out from their time of injury when they arrive at the designated study institutions. The medical stability of acute SCI patients and their associated injuries, such as head trauma, blunt chest and/or abdominal trauma, and other orthopedic injuries necessitate a multidisciplinary approach. The coordination and orchestration of care of the polytrauma patient may delay the radiographic workup (CT and/or MRI) for SCI. Hypotension, surgery for other life-threatening injuries, and treatment of closed head injuries may further delay surgical intervention.

Basically, every SCI is unique. Controlling for age, sex, level, mechanism of injury, severity of injury, and extent of injury necessitates enrolling patients at different points in their disease.

Confounding the difficulty with study design are the real-life variables of ethics of randomization, potential for litigation, financial impact of both the injury and hospitalization, and the psychological devastation of the SCI itself.

Animal Studies in Timing of Surgery for Spinal Cord Injury

Animal studies have been easier to design and complete than have human studies. Multiple animal studies have shown the benefit of early surgical decompression. Typically, the studies have been performed with extradural balloon, static weight, clip, piston impactor, or circumferential cable models of SCI. The laboratory studies in various animal models have shown that neurologic recovery is improved by early decompression.

Carlson et al. studied 16 dogs undergoing a sustained spinal cord compression for 30 or 180 minutes using a hydraulic piston.[3] Somatosensory-evoked potentials were monitored during a 60-minute recovery period and at 28 days after injury. Functional motor recovery was assessed at 26 days. MRI imaging and histologic analysis were performed to assess the volume of the lesion and tissue damage. Improved motor function and balance were noted in the 30-minute group compared to the 180-minute group. The longer duration of compression produced spinal cord lesions of greater volume, which corresponded to poorer long-term functional outcomes.

Dimar et al. studied the influence of spinal canal narrowing and timing of decompression on neurologic recovery after spinal cord contusion using a spacer model of injury in 40 adult rats.[4] The results of this study concluded that there was strong evidence that the prognosis for neurologic recovery was adversely affected by both a higher percentage of canal narrowing and a longer duration of canal narrowing after an SCI. Dimar et al. concluded that the tolerance for spinal canal narrowing with a contused cord appears diminished, indicating that an injured spinal cord may benefit from early decompression. They also demonstrated that the longer the spinal cord compression exists after an incomplete cord injury, the worse the prognosis for neurologic recovery.

Carlson et al. also studied the early time-dependent decompression for SCI in 21 beagles and proposed vascular mechanisms of recovery.[5] His results indicated that after precise dynamic spinal cord loading to a point of functional conduction deficit (50% decline in evoked potential amplitude), a critical time period exists during which intervention in the form of early spinal cord decompression can lead to effective recovery of electrophysiologic function in the 1- to 3-hour postdecompression period.

Delamarter et al. also studied spinal cord recovery after immediate and delayed decompression in dogs.[6] They studied 30 dogs with a cable constriction SCI model with periods of compression ranging from 1 hour up to 1 week. Somatosensory evoked potentials, neurologic examination, and histologic and electron microscopy studies were performed. All dogs were paraplegic after the compression of the cord, but the dogs that underwent immediate decompression or decompression within 1 hour of compression recovered the ability to walk as well as bowel and bladder control and had improvement in somatosensory evoked potentials. When compression lasted 6 hours or more, there was no neurologic recovery, and progressive necrosis of the spinal cord was observed. Somatosensory evoked potential recovery by 6 weeks after the decompression was significantly related to the duration of the compression.

Delamarter et al. concluded that longer periods of displacement allowed propagation of the chronic axonal response, resulting in lack of recovery of somatosensory evoked potentials, limited functional recovery, and more extensive tissue damage.[6]

Multiple other animal models of SCI have shown the positive effect of early decompressive surgery to improve neurologic recovery.[7-10]

Human Studies on Timing of Surgery for Spinal Cord Injury

Retrospective human studies have failed to provide convincing data to support the possibility that the neurologic outcome of early spinal surgery is superior to that of delayed spinal surgery. What has been shown is that earlier surgery can be done more safely than was previously thought. A paper in 1987 by Marshall et al. showed deterioration following SCI in 4.9% of 283 SCI patients in this prospective multicenter study.[11] They concluded that early surgery on the cervical spine when cord injury is present appears hazardous. No deteriorations were observed following surgery after the sixth day.

Multiple papers have since been published demonstrating that early spine surgery can be done safely. Mirza et al. studied the changes in neurologic status, length of hospitalization, and acute complications associated with surgery within 3 days of injury versus more than 3 days after the injury.[12] Forty-three patients were followed. Surgery within 72 hours of injury in patients with acute cervical cord injuries was found not to have a higher complication rate. Numbers were too small to conclude that there was definite neurologic improvement in the acute surgery group in comparison to the delayed surgery group, but trends indicated that early surgery may be beneficial. Decreased hospitalizations were observed in the early surgery group. The duration of stay in the ICU and on mechanical ventilation was not statistically different between the two groups. The neurologic status was maintained, and the change in Frankel grade from the preoperative level to the postoperative level was statistically significant in the groups of patients who underwent early surgery (P = .0026) but not in the group of patients who underwent late surgery (P = .30).

Croce et al. also studied early surgery (within 3 days) versus late surgery (after 3 days) in a mix of cervical (163: 83 early, 80 late), thoracic (79: 30 early, 49 late), and lumbar (49: 29 early, 20 late) fractures.[13] Of the 291 patients, there were no differences in injury severity between the early and late groups for each fracture site. What was identified was that the thoracic fracture group showed that early fixation was associated with a lower incidence of pneumonia, a shorter ICU stay, a decreased number of days on a ventilator, and lower charges. Overall, high-risk patients were found to have had lower pneumonia rates and less hospital resource utilization with early fixation. The neurologic status was not an outcome variable in this study; however, the researchers concluded that early fixation resulted in significant resource reductions for patients with neurologic deficits. They concluded that early fixation resulted in a better outcome (not neurologic outcome) and less resource utilization regardless of neurologic deficit.

A retrospective study by Schlegel et al. of 138 patients with acute spine injuries also addressed the issue of timing of surgery.[14] They found no statistically significant difference in the incidence of medical complications in patients with injury severity scores (ISSs) of less than 15 who were operated on within 72 hours or after 72 hours of injury. A separate group of patients with cervical spine injuries with neurologic deficit was analyzed, and it was determined that irrespective of associated injuries, all had fewer complications if they underwent surgery within 72 hours. Morbidity was found to be higher in the neurologic deficit group compared to the neurologically intact group. This study concluded that surgical decompression, reduction, and/or fixation of spine fractures within the first 72 hours are indicated in multiple trauma patients (ISS ≥18) and cervical injuries with neurologic deficits.

A retrospective study by Chipman et al. looked at early surgery for thoracolumbar spine injuries.[15] One-hundred forty-six patients were identified (58 with ISS <15, 88 with ISS ≥15). Early surgery was determined to be within 72 hours or less, and late surgery was more than 72 hours following injury. Chipman was able to conclude that early surgery in severely injured patients with thoracolumbar spine trauma was associated with fewer complications and shorter hospital and ICU lengths of stay, required less ventilator support for noninfectious reasons, and did not increase neurologic deficits.

Schinkel et al. analyzed the German National Trauma Database (N = 8057).[16] Clinical parameters and outcomes of patients with severe thoracic spine injuries (N = 298) were compared to patients undergoing early (<72 hours) versus late (>72 hours) spine stabilization. They were able to show further evidence that early stabilization of thoracic spine injuries in trauma patients reduces overall hospital and ICU stays and improves outcome. The outcome was, overall, not specific for neurologic function.

Kerwin et al. examined the records of the National Trauma Data Bank (NTDB) to determine the efficacy of early surgery (<72 hours) versus late surgery (>72 hours) of 16,812 patients undergoing operative fixation.[17,18] Fifty-nine percent of the surgeries were completed within 3 days of injury. Three hundred seventy-four patients in the late surgery (>72 hours) group were matched to 497 patients in the early surgery group. Kerwin et al. found no significant difference in the presence of SCI between the early and late groups. Complications were significantly higher in the late group (30% vs. 17.5%; P < .0001), yet mortality was similar in the two groups. This study concluded that National Trauma Data Bank records indicate that the majority of patients with spine fractures undergo operative fixation within 3 days and that these patients had fewer complications and required less resources.

A small (N = 27) prospective randomized and controlled study by Cengiz et al. looked at the timing of thoracolumbar spine injuries in early surgery (<8 hours) and late surgery (3 to 15 days) cohorts.[19] They determined that the early group (<8 hours) had significantly shorter overall hospital and ICU stays, fewer systemic complications, and better neurologic improvement than the later group ($P < .05$). They concluded that early surgery may improve neurologic recovery.

Yamazaki et al. analyzed the prognostic factors affecting the outcome of 47 patients with traumatic central cord syndrome.[20] They determined that patient age, admission, Japan Orthopedic Association score, signal change within the cord on MRI, and associated spine diseases were not significant in predicting the patients' recovery. They determined that the anteroposterior diameter of the spinal canal ($P = .0402$) and the interval between injury and surgery ($P < .0001$) were factors that were predictive of excellent recovery. In this series, 13 patients underwent surgery within 2 weeks, and 10 patients underwent surgery after 2 weeks. In the surgical treatment group, timely surgery was found to improve the outcome, while conservative treatment in patients with a low Japan Orthopedic Association score, relatively small anteroposterior diameter of the cord, or signal change within the cord on T2-weighted MRI did not improve.

A small study of 30 patients with spinal cord contusions and complete SCI was done by Zhu et al.[21] Patients underwent internal fixation, laminectomy for epidural decompression, separation of the arachnoid adhesions to restore cerebrospinal fluid flow, and debridement of the spinal cord necrotic tissue with concomitant intramedullary decompression. In this study, all patients recovered some ability to walk. The timing of the operation after injury was determined to be important; the optimal operation time window was identified to be 4 to 14 days after injury.

A study from 1994–1995 performed by Tator et al. reviewed the use and timing of surgery in patients with acute SCI at 36 North American centers.[22] This retrospective multicenter study concluded that there is little agreement on the optimum timing of surgical treatment for SCI. They identified that approximately 66% of patients with acute SCI undergo surgical treatment. They found that only a minority of patients (23.5%) underwent surgery within 24 hours of trauma, and even surgery that is performed within this interval may be too late to reverse some of the secondary injury mechanisms that are identified after SCI. Tator et al. confirmed the need for a randomized controlled trial to assess the optimum timing of decompressive surgery in SCI. This paper also has an excellent discussion of the difficulties in trying to design and conduct a prospective randomized controlled trial of the timing and effectiveness of decompressive surgery after acute SCI. From these difficulties have come multiple evidence-based reviews.

Evidence-Based Reviews

Fehlings and Tator published their evidence-based review of decompressive surgery in acute SCI.[23] The animal model studies that they cited ($N = 16$) were consistent in demonstrating the beneficial effect of early decompressive surgery. The human clinical studies were primarily class III, $N = 17$ (retrospective studies), or class II, $N = 5$ (well-designed comparative clinical studies or prospective series studies). These studies were difficult to compare because of differences in the definitions of early versus late surgeries. The results of the studies of decompressive surgery in patients with acute SCI were mixed, with a trend in the earlier studies (late 1970s to mid-1980s) to favor no difference or late surgery for acute SCI. Since the late 1980s, the results have trended to no difference or early surgery as being possibly beneficial. Multiple class II trials have shown that early decompressive surgery can be performed safely without added morbidity or mortality.

A more recent review by LaRosa et al. using meta-analysis of data obtained through a Medline Search from 1966 to 2000 used a 24-hour window for early surgery compared to those having late surgery or conservative treatment.[24] The analysis included 1687 eligible patients and statistically showed that early decompression resulted in better (neurologic) outcome compared to both conservative ($P < .001$) and late ($P < .001$) management. However, analysis of homogeneity showed that only data on patients with incomplete neurologic deficits who had early surgery were reliable. From this, they concluded that although statistically the percentage of patients with incomplete neurologic deficits improving after early decompression, 89.7% (95% confidence interval), appears to be better than with other modes of treatment when taking into consideration the material available for analysis and the various other factors including clinical limitations, early surgical decompression can be considered only as a practice option for all groups of patients.

A subsequent systematic review by Fehlings and Perrin published in 2006 summarized the results of studies published within the last 10 years (1995–2005).[25] From this review, they had 15 surgical studies and 4 closed reduction studies that provided class II evidence to recommend the following:

- Early surgery (<72 hours) can be performed safely in patients with SCI if they have hemodynamic optimization.
- The data support a recommendation for urgent reduction of bilateral locked facets in a patient with incomplete tetraplegia.
- The data support a recommendation for urgent decompression in a patient with SCI with neurologic deterioration.

Class III evidence was provided to recommend the following:

- Decompression is a reasonable practice option in acute SCI; when possible, except in patients with life-threatening multisystem trauma, it is recommended that urgent decompression be performed within 24 hours of SCI.
- Early (<24 hours) surgery reduces length of stay in patients with acute SCI and may reduce postinjury medical complications. No standard regarding the timing or role of decompression in acute SCI could be determined.

A smaller systematic review by Rutges et al. looked at the neurologic and clinical outcomes with respect to the timing of thoracic and lumbar fracture fixation.[26] They reviewed 10 papers and concluded that early fracture fixation is associated with fewer complications and shorter hospital and ICU stays. They noted that the effect of early treatment on the neurologic outcome remains unclear owing to the contradictory results of the included studies. They also concluded that early thoracic and lumbar fracture fixation results in improvement of clinical outcome, but the effect on neurologic outcome remains controversial.

No Difference in Acute versus Delayed Surgery

Multiple studies have determined no effect of the timing of surgery on improvement of neurologic outcomes. One of the larger retrospective case series (class III evidence) is a study by McKinley et al. involving 779 consecutive patients with acute nonpenetrating traumatic SCI.[27] These patients were obtained from a multicenter National Spinal Cord Injury Database. This study looked at neurologic, medical, and functional outcomes of acute SCI patients undergoing early (<24 hours, 24 to 72 hours) and late (>72 hours) spine surgery versus those treated medically. McKinley et al. concluded that early versus late spine surgery was associated with shorter lengths of stay and reduced pulmonary complications; however, no differences in neurologic or functional improvements were noted between early and late surgical groups.

A retrospective case series by Sapkas and Papadakis of 67 patients with lower cervical spine fractures or fracture-dislocations showed 87% with neurologic deficit.[28] Surgery was early (within 72 hours) in 31 patients and late (>72 hours) in 36 patients. Their results indicated that only patients with incomplete SCI had neurologic improvement after surgery. They found that there were no statistically significant differences in final neurologic outcomes in patients having early surgery compared to delayed surgery; therefore, they concluded that the timing of surgery does not affect neurologic outcomes.

A paper published by Chen et al. in 2009 reviewed 49 patients with surgical treatment for traumatic central cord syndrome.[29] They concluded that surgery could safely be performed in patients with traumatic central cord syndrome; however, factors including type of lesion, timing of surgery within or after 4 days, and surgical approach were not associated with a final American Spinal Injury Association (ASIA) score. The improvement in the ASIA motor score was positively correlated with age at injury.

Vaccaro et al. published their prospective randomized (potentially class II data) study of 62 cervical acute SCI patients undergoing early (N = 34, <72 hours) and late (N = 38, >5 days) surgery.[30] Unfortunately, 20 patients were lost in follow-up. The results showed no significant difference in length of acute postoperative ICU stay, length of inpatient rehabilitation, or improvement in ASIA grade or motor score between early (mean 1.8 days) and late (mean 16.8 days) surgery. They concluded that there was no significant neurologic benefit when cervical spinal cord decompression after trauma is performed in less than 72 hours after injury compared to waiting longer than 5 days.

Bötel et al. analyzed retrospective data on 255 acute SCI patients of whom 178 had surgical decompression and stabilization.[31] Of these, 51.4% had early surgery (<24 hours) and 10.5% had late surgery (>2 weeks). This study did not control for methylprednisolone administration or mechanism of injury (tumor, trauma), and a high reoperation rate of 45.2% was observed, but no neurologic recovery was noted in complete SCI patients. No association of neurologic recovery was associated with the timing of decompressive surgery.

A prospective nonrandomized clinical trial was performed by Vale et al. and published in 1997.[32] This study observed 77 patients, of whom 58 had surgery (11, <24 hours; 13 to 24, 72 hours; 34, >72 hours). All patients were managed with Swan-Ganz and arterial catheters, immobilization, and fracture reduction; systolic blood pressure >85 mm Hg was maintained. Surgical treatment was used in 31 of 35 patients with cervical cord injuries and in 27 of 29 patients with thoracic cord injuries. Early surgery (<24 hours) was performed in 11 patients (7 cervical and 4 thoracic), 9 patients had surgery within 24 to 72 hours (9 cervical and 4 thoracic), and 34 patients had delayed surgery (>72 hours) (15 cervical and 19 thoracic). Researchers found no statistically significant differences between the preoperative routine neurologic examination and the selection for, or timing of, surgery in patients with cervical or thoracic SCI in this series. The 12-month follow-up revealed no statistically significant impact on the timing of surgery with respect to outcome.

Summary

In summary, more recent studies have indicated that acute surgery for SCI can be done safely and without increased complication rates. Lengths of stay, ICU/resource utilization, and economic factors may show potential benefits from early surgery. Animal studies indicate benefit from early decompression of SCI. However, there are still no prospective randomized controlled studies to support the neurologic outcome benefits of early surgery over late surgery for SCI. Intuitively, it makes sense to operate early, but there is an absence of data to support this conclusion.

KEY REFERENCES

Cengiz SL, Kalkan E, Bayir A, et al: Timing of thoracolumbar spine stabilization in trauma patients: impact on neurological outcome and clinical course. A real prospective (RCT) randomized controlled study. *Arch Orthop Trauma Surg* 128:959–966, 2008.

Chen L, Yang H, Yang T, et al: Effectiveness of surgical treatment for traumatic central cord syndrome. *J Neurosurg Spine* 10:3–8, 2009.

Chipman JG, Deuser WE, Beilman GJ: Early surgery for thoracolumbar spine injuries decreases complications. *J Trauma* 56:52–57, 2004.

Fehlings MG, Perrin RG: The timing of surgical intervention in the treatment of spinal cord injury: a systematic review of recent clinical evidence. *Spine (Phila Pa 1976)* 31(Suppl 11):S28–S35, 2006.

Kerwin AJ, Griffen MM, Tepas JJ III, et al: Best practice determination of timing of spinal fracture fixation as defined by analysis of the National Trauma Data Bank. *J Trauma* 65:824–831, 2008.

McKinley W, Meade MA, Kirshblum S, Barnard B: Outcomes of early surgical management versus late or no surgical intervention after acute spinal cord injury. *Arch Phys Med Rehabil* 85:1818–1825, 2004.

Rutges JP, Oner FC, Leenen LPH: Timing of thoracic and lumbar fracture fixation in spinal injuries: a systematic review of neurological and clinical outcome. *Eur Spine J* 16:579–587, 2007.

Schinkel C, Anastasiadis AP: The timing of spinal stabilization in polytrauma and in patients with spinal cord injury. *Curr Opin Crit Care* 14:685–689, 2008.

REFERENCES

The complete reference list is available online at expertconsult.com.

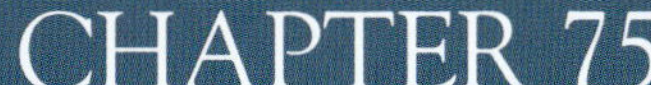

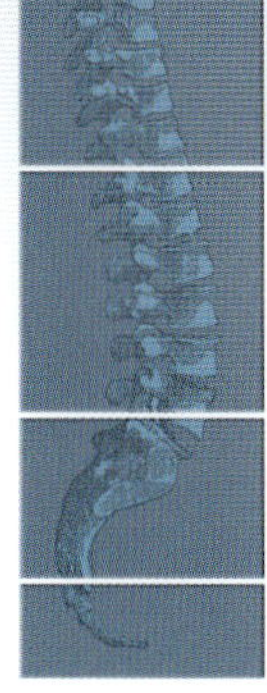

CHAPTER 75

Evaluation of the Cervical Spine after Trauma

Ran Harel | Edward C. Benzel

Unrecognized injury to the cervical spine can produce catastrophic neurologic disability; clinicians are obligated to actively rule out cervical spine injury (CSI). The absence of injury is both difficult and imperative to define. Emergency departments in the United States and Canada are treating more than 13 million trauma victims annually who are at risk for CSI. The guidelines for cervical spine clearance are conflicting, and the management of patients is variable across medical institutions and different countries. Among neurologically intact patients, CSI is detected in 1%, the incidence in blunt trauma patients is 4.3%, and patients suffering a traumatic brain injury have a 5% to 10% chance of having CSI.[1-4]

Recent published studies examined radiation exposure as the cause of cancer. These studies extrapolate from data collected on radiation exposure and secondary malignancies in populations that experienced atomic bombing. Richards et al. compared the use of cervical radiographs combined with head CT to CT of the head and cervical spine. The calculated risk for lifetime cancer was 1:4500 and 1:2400, respectively. They concluded that as a screening procedure for a low-incidence finding, the risks might outweigh the benefits.[5]

Alternative algorithms for cervical spine clearance in several clinical circumstances are presented here. It is emphasized that the schemes that we present are only a few of the many rational approaches to the clearance of the posttraumatic cervical spine.

Clinical Clearance of the Cervical Spine

The proper diagnosis of cervical spine trauma is considered extremely important and therefore results in the liberal use of cervical radiographs. These radiographs are easy to perform, but they expose the patient to ionizing radiation and account for substantial medical health expenses. Several small studies have suggested that patients with blunt trauma have a low probability of injury to the cervical spine if they meet all five of the following criteria: They do not have tenderness at the posterior midline of the cervical spine, they have no focal neurologic deficit, they have a normal level of alertness, they have no evidence of intoxication, and they do not have a clinically apparent, painful injury that might distract them from the pain of a CSI. These studies led to a large trial by the National Emergency X-Radiography Utilization Study Group (NEXUS) regarding criteria for clinical cervical spine clearance. A prospective observational multicenter study in 21 centers in the United States evaluated 34,069 patients with blunt trauma, of whom 4309 patients fulfilled all criteria for clinical clearance. The implementation of the criteria identified all but 8 of the 818 patients who had CSI picked by three-view radiographs. Only 2 of the 8 patients, missed by the clinical evaluation, had significant CSI. Following the outlined clinical algorithm, 12.6% of blunt trauma patients would have avoided the radiography screening.[2]

Stiell et al. proposed a different algorithm (Fig. 75-1) for cervical spine trauma. They studied 8924 patients after blunt head or neck trauma with stable vital signs and a Glasgow Coma Scale score of 15 points, of whom 151 (1.7%) had important C-spine injury. The algorithm consisted of three questions: whether the patient has high-risk factors, whether the patient has low-risk factors, and whether the patient has the ability to rotate the head. The sensitivity of this algorithm was 100% and the specificity was 42.5%, compared to three-view cervical radiograph or 2-week follow-up, reducing the radiography ordering rate to 58.2%.[6]

Stiell et al. compared the use of the NEXUS criteria to those of the Canadian Cervical-Spine Rule (CCR). The sensitivity and specificity for both tests were calculated after evaluation of 8283 Canadian patients suffering from head or neck trauma, 169 of whom (2%) had clinically significant spinal injury. The CCR was more sensitive than the NEXUS (99.4% vs. 90.7%, $P < .001$) and more specific (45.1% vs. 36.8%, $P < .001$) for injury, and its use would have resulted in lower radiography rates (55.9% vs. 66.6%, $P < .001$).[4] The CCR algorithm is statistically superior but is also more complex to remember and implement, thus necessitating screening by well-trained trauma physicians. On the other hand, the NEXUS is less complex and can be utilized by physicians of various specializations.

Rethnam et al. retrospectively analyzed 114 alert trauma patients who had radiographs for cervical spine screening. If the CCR had been utilized, there would have been a 75.8% reduction in the number of patients who received radiographs, and neither of the two CSI patients would have been missed.[7] Grossman et al. surveyed trauma centers in the United States and reported a wide variety of approaches to cervical spine clearance, with significant differences according to the trauma center level.[1] Guidelines from the Eastern Association

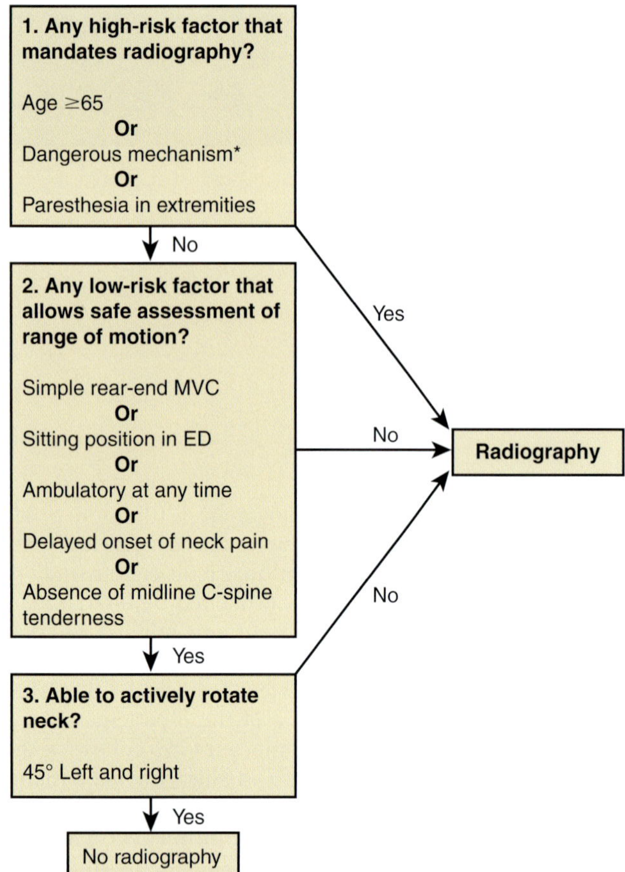

FIGURE 75-1. The Canadian Cervical-Spine Rule algorithm. ED, emergency department; MVC, motor vehicle collision. *Dangerous mechanisms include a fall from ≥1 meter/5 stairs; axial load to head (e.g., diving); high-speed MVC (>100 km/hr), rollover, ejection; motorized recreational vehicles; bicycle collision.

for the Surgery of Trauma (EAST) are based on the NEXUS algorithm.[8,9] Because the best algorithm for cervical clearance is not agreed upon, it seems prudent that trauma centers should have a consensus algorithm implemented by all trauma caregivers.

Radiologic Clearance of the Cervical Spine

Radiographs

The American College of Surgeons Committee on Trauma published recommendations for the initial cervical spine radiographic evaluation in trauma victims. The committee included anteroposterior (Fig. 75-2A), lateral (Fig. 75-2B), and odontoid views of the cervical spine in this evaluation. Optimally, the lateral view images the rostral aspect of the first thoracic vertebra. Lateral films were reported to identify 85% of bony pathology; the addition of anteroposterior and odontoid views increases the sensitivity to 95%.[10,11] However, newer studies utilizing CT and MRI scans in addition to radiographs report a 39% to 94% sensitivity with radiograph alone.[12] Some authors conclude that CT is superior to radiography as a screening tool and should be utilized routinely in severe trauma, with or without radiography.[13,14] Often, conventional lateral radiographs are insufficient, and a swimmer's view may be necessary to image the cervicothoracic junction (Fig. 75-3).

Computed Tomography

Many centers use CT as the first subsequent study following radiography. CT is fast, is readily available, and facilitates patient monitoring (Fig. 75-4). The sensitivity of CT for cervical spine fractures has been reported to be between 90% and 99%, with specificities of 72% to 89%, and studies examining the sensitivity of radiography usually consider CT scan to be the gold standard.[14,15] Nunez et al. compared radiographic screening to CT screening in 88 severe trauma patients. CT depicted 32 fractures that were not identified by radiography, most at the C1-2 and C6-7 regions. One third of these were unstable or clinically important.[13] Link et al. demonstrated that inclusion of the cervicocranial region in the head CT, in addition to a three-view cervical radiograph, revealed additional cervical fractures in 5% of severe head trauma patients.[14] According to EAST recommendations, CT should be utilized, in addition to radiography, for all patients with insufficient imaging of a specific region or evidence of radiographic abnormality, neurologic deficit, or impaired consciousness.[8,9] Patient evaluation with both radiography and CT raised the question of whether the radiographic studies were necessary. In patients with severe trauma, it is difficult to obtain high-quality radiographic studies. Furthermore, imaging the patient delays further studies that may be needed and delivers further radiation to the thyroid. Hashem et al. retrospectively examined the added value of radiography to CT, in patients with CSI admitted to a level 1 trauma center. While CT demonstrated 100% of the pathologies, the sensitivity of radiography was 61%.[16] These data should be considered when the guidelines for cervical spine clearance are being updated.

Magnetic Resonance Imaging

Radiographic and CT images are very sensitive to bony anatomy but are not efficient or sensitive in the detection soft tissue injury. Occurrence of cervical spine ligamentous injury, which is potentially unstable, is estimated to be 0.04% to 0.9%[17]; it is a rare condition but with possible severe consequences. MRI is considered by some to be the gold standard modality for evaluation of soft tissue injury. The images can identify prevertebral hematomas, lesions pressing on the cord such as herniated discs, ossification of the posterior longitudinal ligament, epidural hematoma, and spinal cord contusions or edema (Fig. 75-5). The data that are presented by MRI are a valuable diagnostic tool. Unlike CT, in which axial acquisition is reconstructed to three planes, MRI acquisition is accomplished in three planes, thus reducing the possibility of missing pathology that parallels the acquisition plane. MRI does not deliver radiation and hence reduces potential future risks for cancer. On the other hand, MRI is not always available in some trauma centers; it requires more time and personnel; it requires the use of special ventilator and monitoring techniques; and some immobilization and traction devices will not fit into the MRI or are not MRI compatible. Finally, hemodynamically or respiratory unstable patients should not undergo an MRI.[12,18,19]

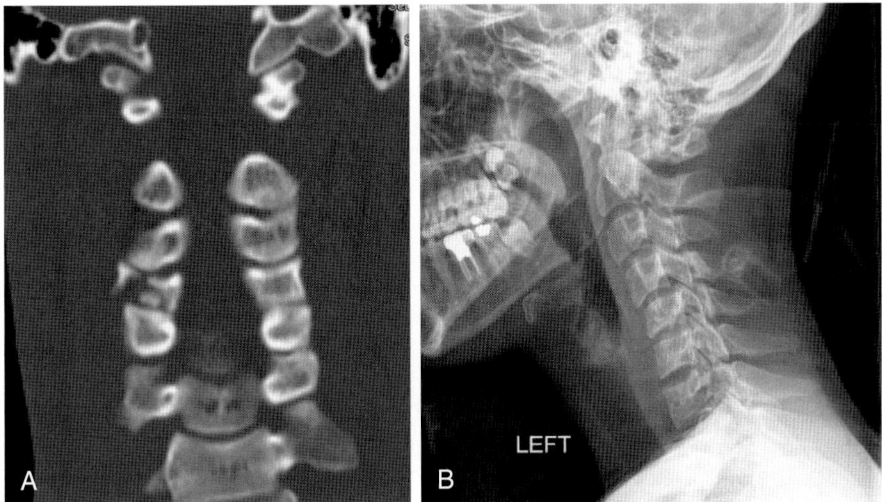

FIGURE 75-2. Anteroposterior CT reconstruction (**A**) and lateral radiograph (**B**) of a patient sustaining right C4 lateral mass fracture-dislocation.

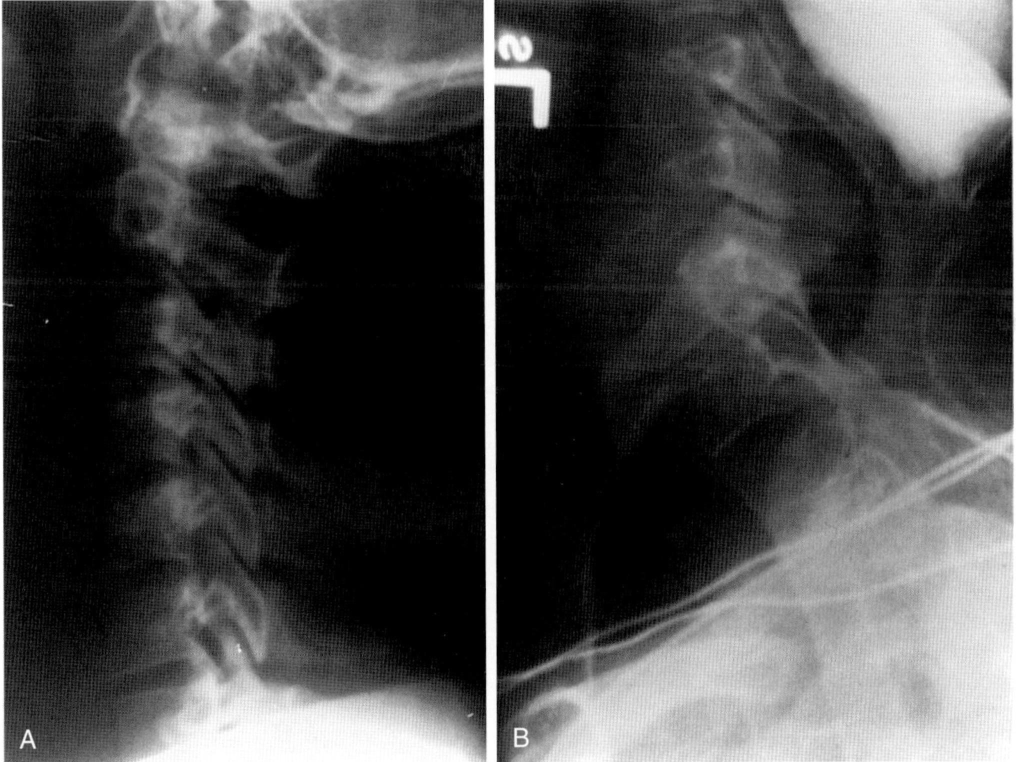

FIGURE 75-3. A, Lateral radiograph that fails to show the cervicothoracic junction. **B,** A swimmer's view showing C7-T1 dislocation.

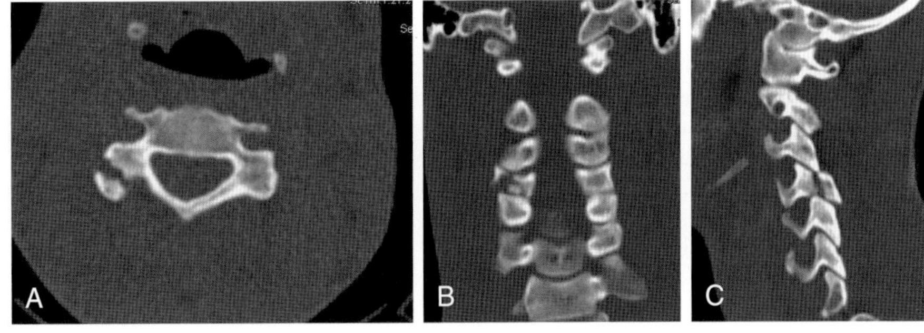

FIGURE 75-4. A, Axial CT of a patient sustaining right C4 lateral mass fracture-dislocation. **B,** Reconstructed coronal CT of a patient sustaining right C4 lateral mass fracture-dislocation. **C,** Reconstructed sagittal CT of a patient sustaining right C4 lateral mass fracture-dislocation.

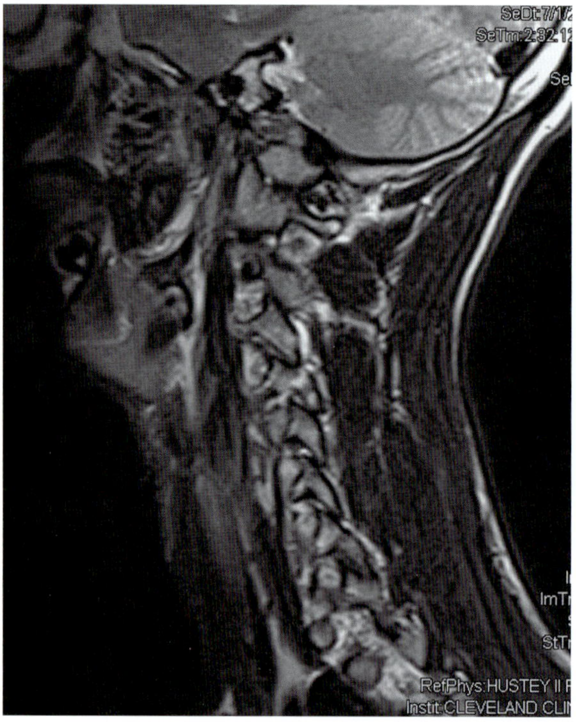

FIGURE 75-5. Sagittal MRI of a patient sustaining right C4 lateral mass fracture-dislocation.

The authors used limited MRI (sagittal T1- and T2-weighted images) as the routine subsequent imaging study in the comatose or obtunded trauma patient. This enabled full visualization of the cervical spine for alignment as well as for identification of soft tissue injury.[20,21] Holmes et al.[22] compared the sensitivity of CT to that of MRI. While MRI was extremely sensitive to spinal cord lesions and ligamentous injury, it missed 45% of vertebral fractures, was 78% sensitive to locked facets, and was 86% sensitive to vertebral dislocation or subluxation. CT was 97% sensitive to vertebral fractures and locked facets, 100% sensitive to vertebral dislocations, and 82% sensitive to subluxation. CT images did not recognize any of the spinal cord injuries but suggested them in a few patients according to the bony damage. Ligamentous injury was reported in 36 patients undergoing CT; 25% of them were inferred by the scan on the basis of bony displacement or angulation. Stassen et al.[23] screened obtunded patients with CT, followed by MRI screening for the patients with negative CTs. They found that 13% of patients with negative CT had positive MRI for ligament injury. These patients were treated by immobilization in a collar and did not undergo surgery. In a review of the literature, MRI detects ligamentous injury in 22.7% of obtunded patients, 80.8% required treatment, and 5.6% required surgical or halo-vest immobilization.[17]

A meta-analysis study assessing the accuracy of MRI in trauma patients demonstrated 97.2% sensitivity and 98.5% specificity.[18] The use of MRI, according to EAST guidelines, is warranted in cases of neurologic deficit only.[8,9] Whether or not MRI should be a part of the routine screening process should be assessed according to level 1 evidence, which is currently unavailable.

Dynamic Studies

Although flexion-extension (FE) lateral radiographs are considered the standard for identifying ligamentous instability, their role should be considered carefully. The EAST recommendation utilizes FE imaging in three situations:[8,9]

1. An alert patient complaining of neck pain with normal radiograph if the patient can move the neck
2. Late examination (i.e., >14 days after the trauma) in an alert patient complaining of neck pain with normal radiograph but with limited motion of the neck (the patient is left in a collar until cleared)
3. An obtunded patient with normal radiograph and CT of the cervical spine (before removal of the collar)

Using FE to clear alert patients following acute trauma requires availability of a technician and a radiologist, delivers ionizing radiation to the patient, and is associated with a high incidence of suboptimal imaging because of body habitus or neck immobility.[24-26] Goodnight et al. retrospectively compared the findings with CT and those with FE views. They found that FE did not provide added value in the face of a negative CT. They concluded that FE views were not efficient.[27] The role of CT in the alert patient for cervical spine clearance is yet to be determined. It should be kept in mind that both CT and FE expose the patient to substantial radiation.

The dispute concerning the use of FE to clear the cervical spine in the obtunded patient is even more intense. Cooper and Ackland[19] compared CT to FE use in obtunded patients. FE studies did not uncover additional injuries that had not already been identified by CT. Griffiths et al. examined the safety and efficacy of FE. They concluded that the examination is safe but did not identify new findings that were not identified by CT.[28] Sliker et al. reviewed the literature concerning FE for clearance of the cervical spine. In 10 studies evaluating the role of FE, 1166 patients were included, 12 of them had CSI, of which 11 were diagnosed by FE, 60% of which required surgical treatment or halo-vest immobilization.[17] The absence of level 1 evidence fosters confusion. The optimal method is yet to be determined.

Cervical Spine Clearance Algorithm

An algorithm for cervical spine clearance was published by EAST,[8,9] but since imaging technology is advancing at a faster pace than the medical guidelines, this algorithm is not uniformly accepted. In addition, the availability of imaging studies and interpreters is not uniform across institutions. Therefore, a universal clearance algorithm is not accepted. The authors will present a proposed algorithm.

Alert Patient

Alert patients could be clinically screened by using either the NEXUS criteria or the CCR algorithm.[2,6] For alert patients who do not qualify for clinical clearance, radiographic clearance should be employed. EAST guidelines are recommended, with the use of anteroposterior, lateral, and open-mouth views. If these are adequate and normal and the patient is neurologically intact and can move the head freely, no further studies are required. Inadequate studies can be supplemented with a swimmer's view or CT scan through the areas of concern. For patients who complain of significant neck pain, FE views should be ordered. If the angle change between flexion and extension is above 30 degrees and no abnormal motion is detected, the cervical spine is cleared. Patients with restricted neck motion should be kept in a hard collar for 10 to 14 days until neck stiffness resolves, and then FE views should be ordered.[8,9] Trauma victims who are expected to require cervical spine CT because of body habitus or mechanism of trauma might not require the use of three-view radiography.[16] Once evidence of injury is found, further studies should be ordered to confirm or reject the findings and to define the characteristics and extent of injury. CT should be ordered to address bony pathology, and either FE studies or MRI should be ordered to define ligamentous injury. After unstable fractures are diagnosed, one should not proceed with FE studies, as they could potentially harm the cord; MRI should be utilized.[8,9,29]

Neurologic Deficit

Perhaps the least controversial clinical scenario is that of the patient with an obvious neurologic deficit. These patients should be evaluated for both bony pathology and soft tissue pathology. Because most will undergo CT and MRI, radiography might not be necessary.[16] The optimal timing for both studies, according to EAST recommendations, is within 2 hours from arrival at the emergency department.[8,9] These recommendations cannot always be followed, depending on personnel and equipment availability, and should be adjusted to provide the best medical treatment according to the resources.

Obtunded and Comatose Patients

Obtunded and comatose patients should be treated as though they have a CSI until sufficient evidence is accrued to confirm or document absence of injury. According to EAST recommendations, trauma victims presenting with altered mental status for whom return of normal mental status is not anticipated for 2 days or more should undergo radiography and CT; if these are normal, an FE study should clear ligamentous injury.[8,9] Multiple authors have challenged this approach. This subset of patients will undergo brain CT, and in many cases sufficient radiographic studies cannot be performed, as the patients are not cooperative and the tubing obscures the cervical spine. Hashem et al. questioned the added information provided by radiography over CT. They concluded that the sensitivity of CT was 100%; hence, radiographic studies are not necessary in these cases,[16] Removing the radiograph from the algorithm reduces both the radiation dose and the time before the patient can be transferred to the CT scanner. Although CT for these patients is generally accepted, opinions regarding the next appropriate steps are highly variable.

Padayachee et al. examined the role of FE studies when added to CT in this subset population of patients. In this study, the FE did not identify any instability that was not recognized by CT.[3] Spiteri et al. reported a series of 87 patients with unstable injuries, two of which were missed by CT. One was detected on FE, and the other was missed. They concluded that although FE studies are safe, they are not warranted because of their low rate of true-positive findings that are not identified by CT.[30] Goodnight et al. reported a series of patients in which all positive FEs after negative CT were negative for ligamentous injury on MRI.[27] These studies do not take into consideration the negative effect of transport to the fluoroscopy unit of these unstable patients, the cost, and the harmful effects of ionizing radiation to the patient and health-care providers.

The most sensitive imaging modality is MRI. MRI is more sensitive to soft tissue than to bony pathology. Holmes et al. studied a cohort of patients who had undergone both CT and MRI. They reported that the sensitivity to osseous fractures was 55%, while the sensitivity to cord injury and ligamentous injury was 100%.[22] MRI in the setting of the polytrauma patient who is ventilated and sedated poses many concerns. These patients are difficult to transport to the MRI suite, special equipment is required to ventilate and monitor them, and they are escorted by professional staff for long periods of time and occupy the MRI scanner and personnel for long durations. In a study examining 173 trauma patients with risk factors for CSI and lack of significant findings in radiography, 36% had soft tissue injury detected by MRI. Of these patients, one was operated upon, and all were placed in either a hard cervical collar or a Minerva jacket.[20] In a study of 121 obtunded or comatose trauma patients who had normal cervical spine radiographs and underwent MRI of the cervical spine as routine screening, 25.6% were found to have sustained significant soft tissue injury, 6.6% were operated upon, and all were treated with a rigid collar.[21] Stassen et al. utilized a protocol containing both CT and MRI for obtunded trauma patients. They reported 25% of patients with negative CT but positive MRI for ligamentous injury. All were treated with a rigid collar.[23]

Sliker et al.[17] reviewed the literature comparing FE studies to MRI for CSI screening. They detected a 0.9% true-positive rate for ligamentous injury using FE studies, of which 0.5% of patients underwent surgery. On the other hand, MRI detected 22.7% of patients with ligamentous injury, but 19.5% when only the obtunded patient population was assessed. Only 1.3% underwent surgery. It is obvious that MRI is very sensitive for the detection of ligamentous injury. The significance of these injuries, however, is uncertain. A meta-analysis examining MRI for cervical spine trauma clearance, encompassing five studies with a total enrollment of 464 patients, reported an incidence of 20.9% MRI abnormalities that were not evident on radiography, with or without CT. Fifteen patients in this cohort underwent surgery. All of these patients were studied with either radiograph or CT prior to the MRI. The authors concluded that while a negative MRI can confirm the absence of ligamentous injury, the false-positive rate has not yet been determined.[18]

It is reasonable to image obtunded patients with CT, with or without cervical radiography. Ligamentous integrity should be demonstrated before final clearance of the cervical spine. That can be done by either dynamic studies or MRI, depending on the institution's resources and availabilities (Fig. 75-6).

Summary

Occult CSI can have devastating sequelae if undetected. Physicians treating traumatized patients must maintain a high level of suspicion when attempting to clear the cervical

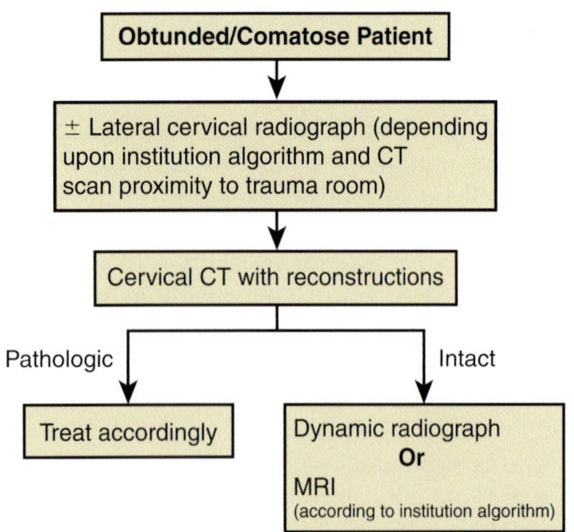

FIGURE 75-6. Proposed algorithm for spinal cord injury in the obtunded or comatose patient.

spine. It cannot be overstated that the completeness of imaging studies is mandatory. The odontoid process and the rostral aspect of T1 must be included in each evaluation. Patients with equivocal neurologic examinations must undergo some form of soft tissue evaluation. The literature comparing one method of screening to another should be evaluated carefully, as new imaging technologies will most likely supercede older technologies; and since no true gold standard exists, one must understand that a sensitivity and specificity that approximate 100% are ideal. We must, however, accept a lesser sensitivity and specificity, since many imaging findings are of minimal, if any, significance. Oversensitive examinations may result in unnecessary workups and treatments.

In summary, the absence of mandating guidelines obligates institutions to establish appropriate algorithms based on current literature and imaging and personnel capabilities.

KEY REFERENCES

Hoffman JR, Mower WR, Wolfson AB, et al: Validity of a set of clinical criteria to rule out injury to the cervical spine in patients with blunt trauma. National Emergency X-Radiography Utilization Study Group. *N Engl J Med* 343(2):94–99, 2000.

Holmes JF, Mirvis SE, Panacek EA, et al: Variability in computed tomography and magnetic resonance imaging in patients with cervical spine injuries. *J Trauma* 53(3):524–529, 2002; discussion 530.

Marion D: *Determination of cervical spine stability in trauma patients (update of the 1997 EAST Cervical Spine Clearance document)*. Chicago, 2000, Eastern Association for the Surgery of Trauma.

Muchow RD, Resnick DK, Abdel MP, et al: Magnetic resonance imaging (MRI) in the clearance of the cervical spine in blunt trauma: a meta-analysis. *J Trauma* 64(1):179–189, 2008.

Stiell IG, Wells GA, Vandemheen KL, et al: The Canadian C-spine rule for radiography in alert and stable trauma patients. *JAMA* 286(15):1841–1848, 2001.

REFERENCES

The complete reference list is available online at expertconsult.com.

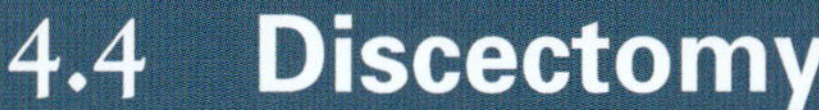

4.4 Discectomy

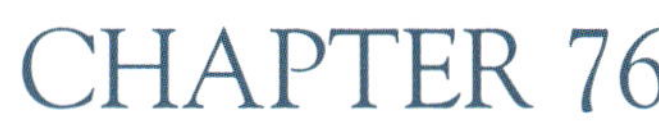

CHAPTER 76

Cervical Discectomy

K. Daniel Riew | Charles H. Crawford III

Indications for Cervical Discectomy

Age-related degeneration as well as trauma can lead to disc pathology requiring surgical excision. Commonly accepted indications for cervical discectomy include myelopathy and persistent radiculopathy that is unresponsive to nonsurgical measures.[1,2] Less commonly accepted indications include axial neck pain and/or headaches[3] that can be attributed to the disc pathology. The pathologic cervical disc can be approached ventrally and dorsally. Both approaches have been in use for over a half century[4-8] and still find utility today.

The dorsal approach is indicated for a soft, foraminal (lateral) disc herniation with radiculopathy.[1] One of the major advantages is that the posterior approach can be performed via a "keyhole" foraminotomy without creating instability at the segment. Disadvantages include the technical challenges (positioning, epidural bleeding, wound complications) and the surgeon's learning curve, as this procedure is less commonly performed than is the more versatile ventral approach in most centers. Additionally, central disc herniations, "hard" disc herniations with uncovertebral bone spurs, and myelopathy are not adequately addressed via this approach. The dorsal approach for a discectomy via a foraminotomy can be accomplished with a small traditional midline incision and a self-retaining retractor[9,10] or with a tubular retractor system.[11]

The ventral approach is very familiar to most spine surgeons. In most patients, the C3-4 level down to the C7-T1 level can be approached via a standard ventrolateral approach. Advantages of the ventral approach include access for central and bilateral foraminal decompression. Although some authors have reported good results for anterior discectomy without interbody fusion, interbody fusion following discectomy has become the standard of care in most centers. Recent trends include the use of allograft along with ventral cervical plates.[12] Cervical disc arthroplasty devices are now available and can be used for postdiscectomy reconstruction; excellent results have been reported in properly selected patients.[13,14]

Anterior Cervical Discectomy

Anterior Cervical Discectomy and Fusion Technique

Preoperative Planning

It may be appropriate in revision settings to get a preoperative otolaryngology consult to evaluate vocal cord paralysis.[15] If a vocal cord paralysis exists, the approach should be made on the ipsilateral side to avoid a potential bilateral paralysis. An approach on the right side may put the recurrent laryngeal nerve at more risk, while a low approach on the left side may put the thoracic duct at risk.

Preoperative Imaging

The preoperative radiographs are examined to identify unique anatomic features. The proper identification of existing instrumentation is especially important to ensure that all needed equipment will be available. Knowledge of the ventral osteophytes can help the surgeon to identify the proper levels during the approach by intraoperative palpation and visualization. The vertebrae are labeled by level, and the anterior-to-posterior distance of the vertebral body (minus the magnification factor) is measured to estimate the graft and screw size. Anatomically "short" necks where the lower cervical levels are at or below the level of the clavicle may alert the surgeon to potential difficulty accessing these lower levels during a standard approach. It may be helpful to list the patient's symptoms (especially left versus right, radiculopathy and/or myelopathy), surgical plan (levels of discectomy), and important comorbidities (smoker, diabetic, etc.). The axial MRI or CT scan should be carefully reviewed for the vertebral artery position, and any anomalies should be carefully noted. The operative site is marked in the holding area.

Intraoperative Procedures

The anesthesiologist administers 10 mg of intravenous decadron to minimize ventral swelling and prophylactic antibiotics (usually cefazolin 1 g) to minimize the risk of infection.

The patient is placed supine on the operating table. Neck flexion should be minimized in moving a patient with a large cervical disc herniation and myelopathy. A folded sheet or an intravenous bag is placed underneath and across the shoulders; sometimes, two sheets will be better. The sheets under the shoulders and the foam doughnut under the head are adjusted to obtain ideal neck extension (it is important to be careful in using two sheets, which may overlordose the cervical spine). It is rare that any support other than the foam doughnut is needed under the head. An unrolled Kerlix is placed around both wrists (NYOH stockinette-style knot) and hung off the bottom of the table to allow pulling down of the arms and shoulders for intraoperative radiographs. Plastic self-adhesive drapes are placed just above the nipple line and along both sides of the neck as low as possible. The side drapes are placed dorsal to the ear and around the circumference above the chin. The upper thorax should be accessible in case of emergency (e.g., vertebral artery injury and necessity for exposure of subclavian artery for proximal control). A half sheet is placed down over the patient's body and legs to prevent accidental contamination via the surgeon's gown touching the bed or patient. Sterile towels are placed over the sterile field and moved away from the center. The inferior towel is usually at the sternal notch; the superior towel is around the chin; the ipsilateral towel is as low as possible; the contralateral towel is several centimeters lateral to midline to accommodate a midline-crossing incision. The carotid tubercle, thyroid cartilage, and cricoid cartilage can be palpated as landmarks. The incision location can also be based on the location of the mandible and clavicle on preoperative radiographs. An incision is marked in a neck crease if possible, crossing midline as needed. Perpendicular lines help during closure. Larger transverse incisions with less retraction (skin stretching) tend to heal better than a smaller incision with stretched skin edges. Vertical incisions leave unappealing scars and can be avoided. The incision should be located in the inferior third of the levels to be decompressed because it is easier to mobilize skin in a cephalad rather than a caudad direction and the disc spaces angle cephalad. The skin is injected with 0.25% Marcaine with epinephrine as early as possible, since the epinephrine takes time to work (ideally 10 minutes). Cut strips of adhesive barrier drape (Ioban) are used to seal the edges after the incision is marked.

A scalpel is used to incise the epidermis and dermis. Leaving an intact corner of dermis at the ends of the wound protects against stretching, thereby allowing for a more cosmetically pleasing closure. Subcutaneous bleeders can be cauterized but will often tamponade with a gently placed Weitlaner retractor that is spread gradually during exposure. Using the cut function on the electrocautery will minimize charred tissue, but small veins will often need the coagulate function. The platysma is cut transversely in line with the incision; sometimes, veins run in the platysma layer and can be dissected bluntly with Metzenbaum scissors or directly coagulated with the cautery. The platysma is undermined cranially and caudally with spreading scissors, blunt finger dissection, and cautery. When multiple segments are being exposed, the platysma should be undermined from the corner of the mandible to the clavicle along the length of the sternocleidomastoid. The interval between the sternocleidomastoid and medial strap muscles is identified. The external jugular vein may be mobilized either laterally or medially. Preserving the sternocleidomastoid fascia by starting the dissection closer to the strap muscles will minimize bleeding. Spreading scissors, blunt finger dissection, and cautery are used to dissect through the interval between the alar fascia (carotid sheath) and the visceral fascia (trachea and esophagus). The carotid pulse can be palpated and kept lateral. In the interval, the ventral cervical spine and longus colli muscles can be palpated. Blunt finger dissection can widen the defect longitudinally, although there may be less bleeding with the spreading scissors technique. Crossing nerves that should be preserved include the glossopharyngeal and hypoglossal nerves at the very top of the approach and the superior laryngeal nerve above the superior thyroid artery. The recurrent laryngeal nerve may be at the bottom of the approach, especially on the right side. It is acceptable to take the inferior, middle, and superior thyroid vessels if necessary. Larger crossing vessels may need to be tied. A wall bleeder can be very difficult to stop if it represents a side-opened vessel; in this case, a bipolar technique will often slow bleeding enough to allow packing with a hemostatic agent and cottonoid patty. A hand-held retractor is placed medially to pull the trachea and esophagus over the midline to see the ventral aspect of the cervical spine. The omohyoid muscle crosses the field around C6 and can be divided with lower-level dissections with no adverse effects. The muscle can be elevated with Metzenbaum scissors underneath and then divided with electrocautery.

The carotid tubercle, usually at C6, and ventral osteophytes can be palpated to estimate levels. The prevertebral fascia is cleared off the discs (hills) and vertebral bodies (valleys) using scissors and forceps with a nick-and-spread technique. The hand-held retractor is then replaced under this layer (Fig. 76-1).

Once the radiology technician is present, a bent 12-mm, 14-mm, or 16-mm spine needle (based on preoperative radiographic measurement) is placed in the disc space of choice. The carotid tubercle and/or ventral osteophytes can be used to predict the level (Fig. 76-2). Dissection can continue while the film is being processed. The sterile draped microscope is then brought into the field. The "valley" of the ventrolateral aspect of the vertebral body above and below the suspected disc is cauterized to get the segmental arteries and perforating branches. The longus colli is elevated off the vertebral body "valley" by using coagulate (cranial and caudal enough to place

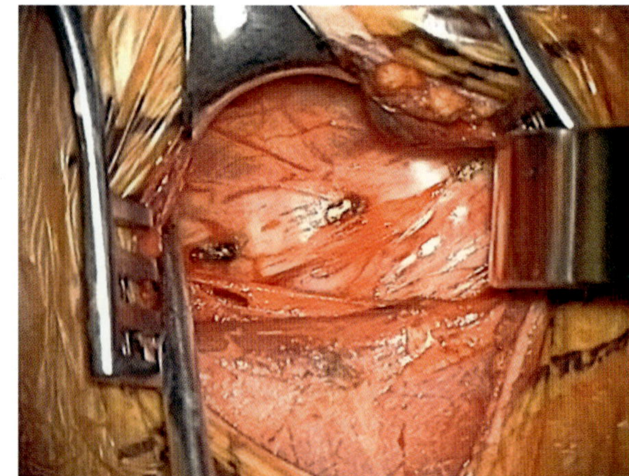

FIGURE 76-1. Prior to elevating the longus colli muscle, one can mark the midline with a Bovie electrocautery. This helps in keeping the decompression centralized and also helps to keep the plate straight.

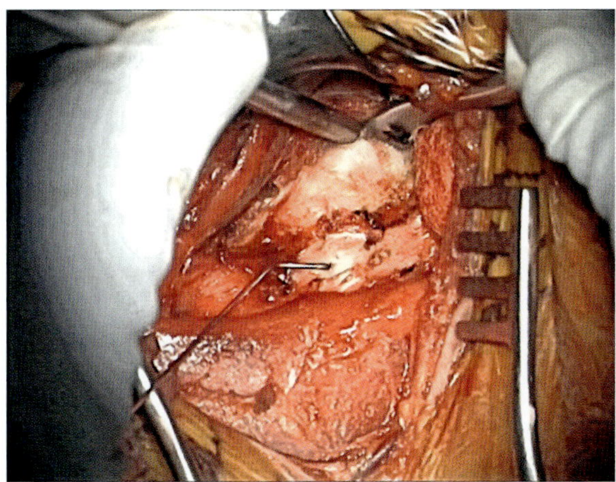

FIGURE 76-2. A safe way to elevate the longus colli muscle is to cauterize it with a bipolar electrocautery and then to elevate it using a Penfield 2 elevator. A spine needle marks the disc space. If one is not sure about the level, it is preferable not to place a needle into a disc space, since that can result in premature disc degeneration if it happens to be at the wrong level. Instead, one can place a pin into the vertebral body or even a staple next to the disc space.

the plate comfortably) and then off the ventral disc "hill." The safe (nonanomalous) position of the vertebral artery should be confirmed on the preoperative axial MRI or CT prior to elevation of the longus. The longus colli in the upper cervical spine (i.e., C3-4 and higher) is less muscular and less well defined. A Penfield 2 can be used to safely elevate the longus at the vertebral body out laterally over the transverse process. Bleeding bone on the front side of the vertebral body under the elevated longus can be coagulated with bone wax used as needed. If bleeding starts from the undersurface of the longus or out laterally, a hemostatic agent and a large cottonoid patty can be used. The self-retaining (Shadowline or similar) retractors are placed underneath the elevated layer of the longus colli. The hand-held retractor is used to move the esophagus so that the self-retaining retractor blade can be safely placed under the longus. An assistant's hand on the medial self-retaining retractor handle can stabilize downward and keep it correctly positioned (Fig. 76-3). The vertebral body just cranial and caudal to the disc space is prepared for insertion of the Caspar retraction posts. Prior to insertion of the Caspar pins, a rongeur or bur is used to remove the ventral osteophytes until they are flat with the ventral surface of the vertebral body. Caspar pins (usually 14 mm or 16 mm based on preoperative and localizing radiographs) are inserted by hand. Careful insertion is important if the patient is very myelopathic or stenotic. The superior post should be farther away from the cranial inferior end plate, but the inferior post is just below the caudal superior end plate. This is due to the angled shape and orientation of the cervical vertebral bodies, and will allow good purchase of the screws. The Caspar pins can be inserted slightly diverging to allow for lordosis. Proper insertion of the Caspar posts is critical. The posts must both be in the center of the vertebral bodies, since going off center with one post may result in vertebral twisting and scoliosis after the Caspar retractor is placed. If the posts are not placed in the center but are both off to one side, the distraction of the interspaces will be asymmetrical and lead to uneven end-plate preparation while the posts are retracting. Excellent visualization of the bodies before placing the posts will help to avoid errors at this step. Centering with reference to the spine is more reliable than centering with reference to the patient's chin and sternal notch. The cranial angulation of the disc space should be parallel to the path of the Caspar pin in the sagittal plane. It can be helpful to identify the disc space with a Bovie or #15 blade if the surgeon is unsure of the location or angle. The posts must diverge or be parallel when inserted to lordose the spine and prevent the cephalad post from entering the end plate, given the upward sloping nature of the end plate. If the Caspar pins are not placed divergently, the threads of the cephalad post may be encountered while burring out the end plate.

A #15 blade is used to cut the width of the ventral anulus (the cutting portion of a #15 blade is 11 mm exactly). Multiple passes are made through the disc, going no deeper than the cutting portion of the blade while turning the blade vertically at the lateral edges of the disc space. The lateral border of the vertebral body is a reasonable guide to determine the location of the vertebral artery. A Penfield 4 can be placed around the edge of the body just for conceptualization. A pituitary rongeur is used to remove initial disc fragments. The Caspar retraction can be increased once the ventral anulus has been excised. A curette (Codman Microsect 4B) can be held like a dagger or a pencil while scraping the disc thoroughly. A side-to-side motion is safe

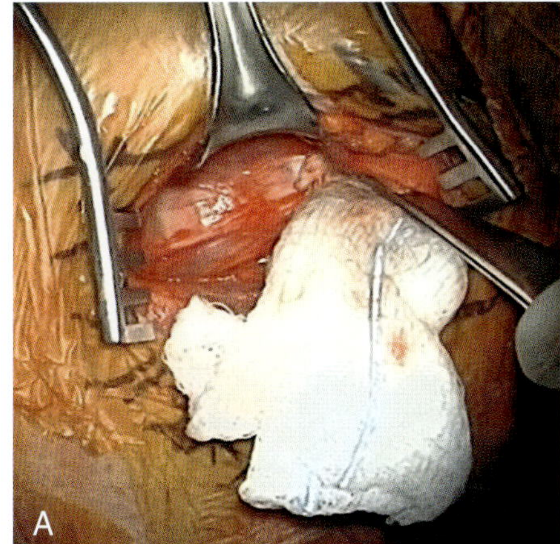

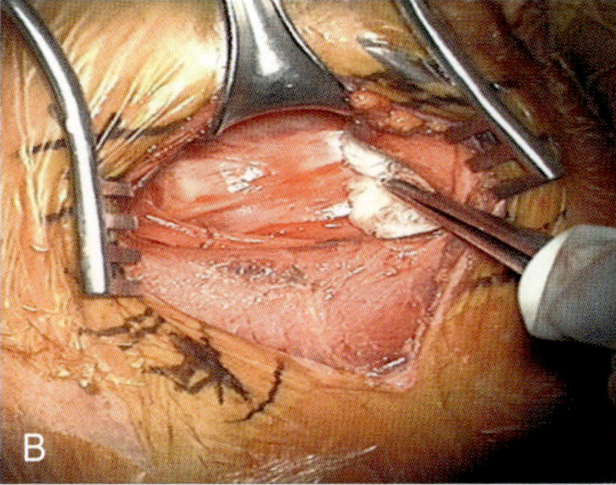

FIGURE 76-3. One way to gently retract the trachea and the esophagus is to place a 4 × 4 sponge cranially and caudally. This helps to slightly retract the trachea and the esophagus away from the operative site. The metal retractor then places less force on the trachea and esophagus at the operative site. The sponge going in (**A**) and the sponge in place (**B**).

as far lateral as the uncovertebral joint allows. The path of the curette should be smile-shaped during the initial passes, not just horizontal. Resting the hand on the patient with all maneuvers will give stabilization and control. A pituitary rongeur is again used to remove numerous pieces of disc and bone and cartilaginous end plate from the field. Keeping the nondominant hand on the patient and using two hands to control the pituitary rongeur will avoid plunging into the canal. A smaller curette (Codman Microsect 2B) can be used to get into foramen by first using a twisting or scooping motion to get the cartilage out of the uncovertebral joint and then using an upward pulling motion to get the uncovertebral process to break and come out of the foramen ventrally. The curette tip should always be kept against the superior vertebral bone medially to prevent accidental injury to an artery. The microscope should be tilted to angle into the intervertebral space optimally. Suction in the nondominant hand should rest on the patient for control and stability while in the disc space. A bur is used to remove the inferior end plate of cephalad vertebrae ventrally. Constant irrigation will keep the field clear. The goal is to make the end plates bleed and flat. The end plates are burred centrally back to the posterior longitudinal ligament (PLL). The last anular fibers can be burred away, leaving longitudinally oriented PLL fibers.

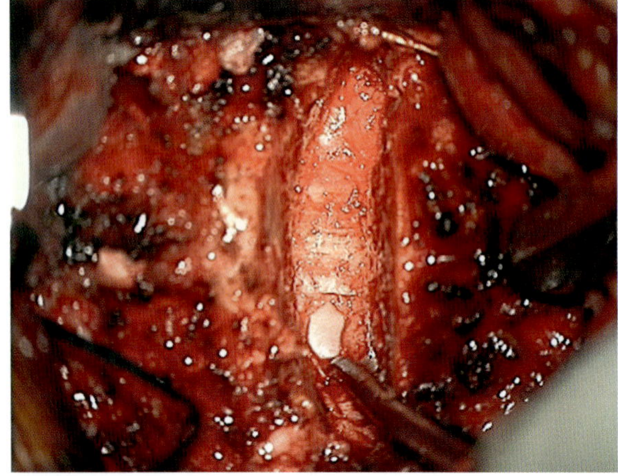

FIGURE 76-4. The central decompression has been completed, and a curette is being used to retract the posterior longitudinal ligament (PLL) in order to visual the dura. While many surgeons prefer to completely resect the PLL, in most discectomy cases, we prefer just to look behind the PLL and to leave it intact. The PLL then acts as a barrier to prevent intrusion of the bone graft and also provide some stability.

The disc space can be squared off by going laterally and taking down some of uncinate bilaterally. The smaller curette can be used to remove any remaining dorsal anular fibers and dorsal osteophyte/PLL if necessary. The PLL may need to be removed only if the surgeon is going after extruded disc. Any remaining dorsal lip of vertebral body can be removed with the bur before the PLL is taken, as the PLL serves as a safety backboard (Fig. 76-4). Inadequate foraminal decompression may lead to residual radicular symptoms. For unciatectomy or wide foraminotomy, the uncinate can be identified by carefully going out of the joint laterally with the 2B curette and turning caudally. A Penfield 4 and then a Penfield 2 can be used to identify the lateral aspect of uncinate (protecting the vertebral artery). With the Penfield held by the assistant, the uncinate can be burred in a ventral-to-dorsal direction. A medial-to-lateral direction is more dangerous, because the bur is then moving toward the vertebral artery, which lies lateral to the uncinate (Fig. 76-5).

After the decompression is complete, a sizer is used to check for the size of interbody graft. A typical graft size is somewhere around 7 to 9 mm and can be estimated from preoperative imaging studies (especially of adjacent healthy levels). If the sizer is not going in smoothly, it is much safer to gently tap it into place with a mallet than to push toward the spinal cord in an uncontrolled manner (Fig. 76-6). In attempting to access C7-T1 when visualization is difficult because of the angle of the disc space and obstruction of the clavicle, it may be necessary to perform a greater end-plate resection of C7 or even a corpectomy if the added end-plate resection results in a weak surface for graft support.

The ventral vertebral bodies are refashioned with a rongeur to smooth out the ventral contour for plate placement. Typically, a structural interbody allograft is placed, followed by a ventral plate. It may be necessary to taper the edges of the graft to facilitate insertion and make it flush with the end plates. After graft placement, no space should be visible between the grafts and the end plates prior to releasing distraction. If necessary, the graft or the end plates can be touched up with the bur.

Once the plate has been inserted, all the landmarks are obscured, and it is very easy for the plate and screws to be misplaced. Some systems allow for drilling of the screw holes while the Caspar pins are still in place marking the midline. The correct plate size should be as short as possible, just spanning the height of the interbody graft, to avoid encroachment on the adjacent discs.

The retractors are then removed, and radiographs are taken. While radiographs are being processed, the wound is

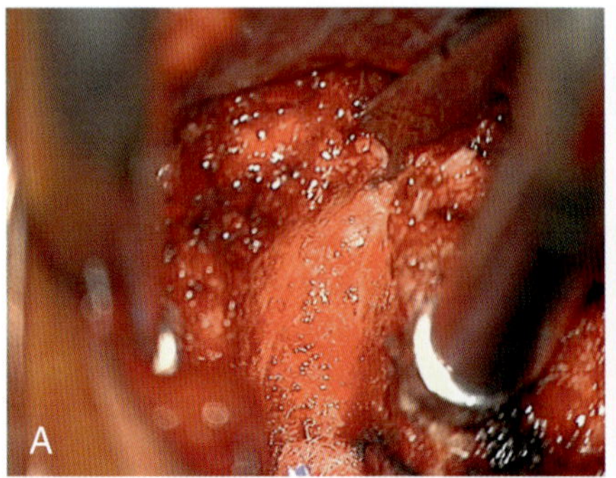

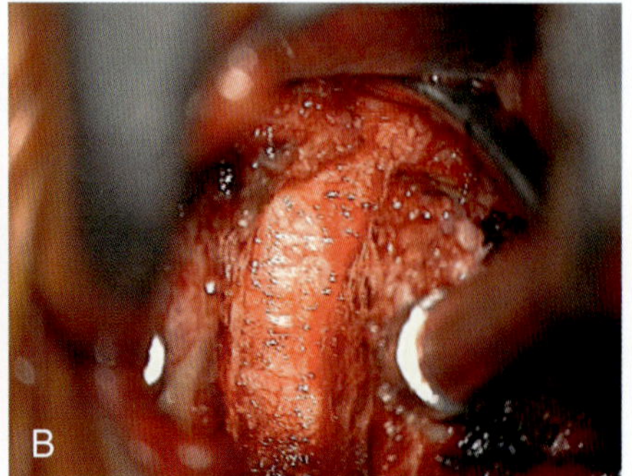

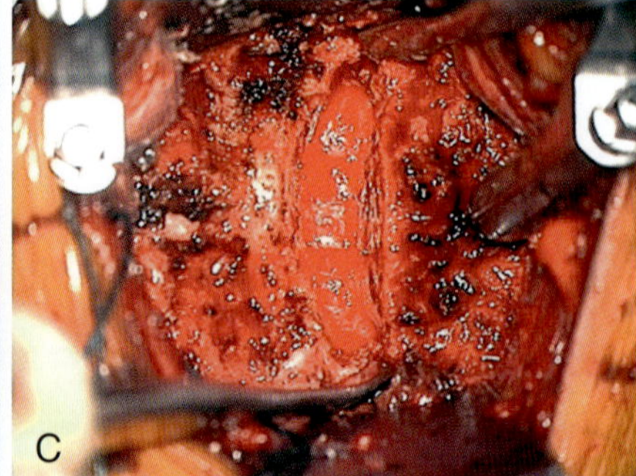

FIGURE 76-5. A, A Penfield 2 is seen at the top of this picture just lateral to the uncovertebral joint. This helps to protect the vertebral artery from injury as one is performing a foraminotomy. **B,** The foraminotomy has been completed, and the Penfield 2 is retracting the vertebral artery. **C,** The width of the decompression from left to right with a Penfield 2 on the right side and a Penfield 4 on the left side.

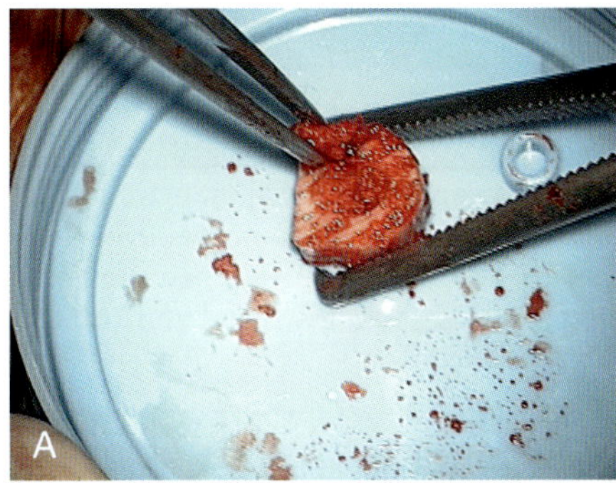

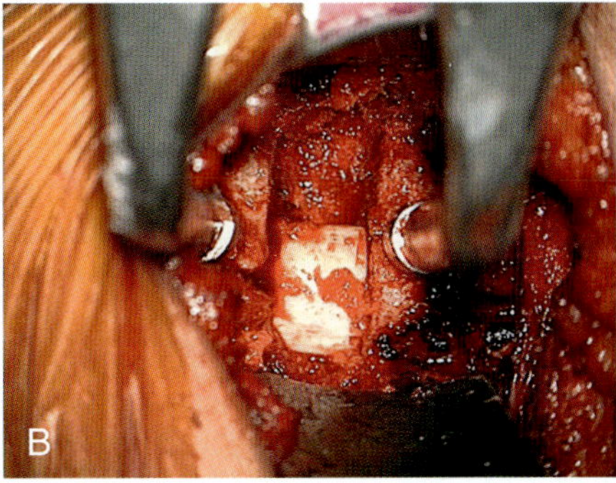

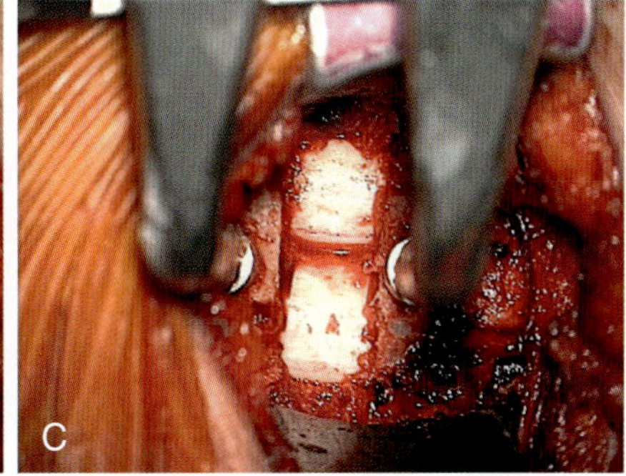

FIGURE 76-6. A, We use a prefabricated allograft that is then packed with local autograft. The local autograft can be obtained from bone shavings as well as any small osteophytes that are removed with a Kerrison punch. With a wide decompression, it is possible to place two bone grafts side by side. By maximally filling the disc space with bone graft, one can achieve high fusion rates. **B,** The first allograft in place. **C,** The second allograft placed next to it.

checked for bleeders, and hemostasis is obtained with hemostatic agents and cottonoids (see Fig. 76-3).

A drain is placed with the internal tip placed in the caudal portion of the wound and the trocar through the skin inferior to the incision. The authors close the platysma with interrupted 3-0 monocryl, and the skin is closed with interrupted 5-0 monocryl.

Postoperative Management

For single-level anterior cervical discectomy and fusion, an appropriately sized soft collar is placed before extubation, and the patient is instructed to wear it as needed for comfort. If the patient is osteoporotic or the construct is more than a single-level anterior cervical discectomy and fusion, a Miami J collar is typically used. Patients are instructed to remove it for eating and cleaning (approximately 1 hour a day) but otherwise to wear it for 6 weeks. Patients are observed overnight in the hospital with a continuous pulse oximeter to watch for airway compromise from postoperative hematoma/seroma. Diet and activity are allowed as tolerated. Drains are typically removed on postoperative day 1 (the goal is <20 mL per 8 hours), prior to discharge.

Complications of Anterior Cervical Discectomy

Complications following anterior cervical discectomy are infrequent but can be life threatening.[16,17] In addition to neurologic deterioration, dural injury, and inadequate decompression with persistent or recurrent symptoms, injuries to vital structures in the neck including the esophagus and the vertebral artery have been reported. These must be promptly recognized and properly treated to minimize patient morbidity. Likewise, postoperative airway compromise must be promptly recognized and emergently treated to avoid patient mortality. Soft tissue swelling associated with prolonged retraction, hematoma, seroma, and implant/graft dislodgement can all contribute to airway compromise. Dysphagia and dysphonia occur following ventral cervical approaches and have traditionally been underreported in the literature. Most of these will resolve with time but in recalcitrant cases should be referred for otolaryngology evaluation.

Vertebral artery injuries require direct repair, stenting, and/or ligation. Immediate bleeding should be controlled with direct pressure. Avoid injecting hemostatic agents directly into the cerebral vascular system. If available, obtain an emergent consultation with a vascular surgeon or interventionalist who can perform an angiogram to assess collateral circulation and potentially stent or occlude the lesion.

Esophageal injuries may not be detected with intraoperative dye.[18] If any suspicion of esophageal injury exists, it is prudent to keep the patient nil per os (NPO) and obtain consultation from a thoracic or head and neck surgeon.

Airway compromise is an emergency with which all personnel caring for postoperative ventral cervical spine surgery patients should be familiar. Voice changes to a high-pitched squeak, difficulty swallowing, and dyspnea are all causes for alarm. Immediate evaluation and treatment are mandatory. Lateral radiographs can help to diagnose implant dislodgement versus hematoma. A tracheostomy and difficult airway cart should be brought to the patient's bedside. Emergent consultation with an anesthesiologist and/or otolaryngologist should be obtained. If time permits, transfer of the patient to the operating suite will allow a controlled environment for evacuation of hematoma and intubation. Sometimes emergent bedside hematoma evacuation and/or cricoidotomy will be necessary.

Dorsal Cervical Discectomy

Dorsal Cervical Foraminotomy and Discectomy Technique

Preoperative Planning

Radiographic assessment is similar to that of ventral discectomy procedures. Imaging studies should be carefully reviewed for pathology and abnormal anatomy. Lateral disc herniations without significant uncovertebral spurring are a common indication for dorsal foraminotomy. Central disc herniations and "disc-osteophyte complexes" are relative contraindications to dorsal foraminotomy. Dorsal cervical wound complications may be reduced by asking the patient to clip the hair from the dorsal neck the night before surgery. Intravenous antibiotics should be administered within 1 hour of making the skin incision. The operative site should be marked in the holding area.

Intraoperative Procedures

Patients are placed prone on the operating table with the neck in flexion. Gardner-Wells tongs are used to apply traction (10 to 20 pounds) via a flexion vector. On the OSI table, three pins should be in place at the superior portion of the bed. The head of the bed should have the pin placed in the superior-most hole, and the foot of the bed should be placed lower in the H-bar to allow for maximum reverse Trendelenburg position (minimizes venous bleeding). Two traction ropes for intraoperative traction (one for flexion and one for extension) can be used if the plan is to instrument and fuse after the discectomy. The flexion vector is usually through the central portal, and the extension vector is over the central groove in the traction H-bar. The flexion position is used for the incision and closure as well as decompression (foraminotomy/discectomy). The extension rope is used in performing a concomitant instrumented fusion to allow lordosis. It can also be used to check the adequacy of the foraminal decompression with the patient's neck extended. The full chest pad is placed in the appropriate position with two iliac crest pads placed at the level of the pelvis and a sling for the legs. A strap or tape across the buttocks will prevent caudal migration of the patient once in reverse Trendelenburg position.

Gardner-Wells tongs are applied symmetrically just above the ears. Pins should affix the bone 1 cm above the superior pole of the external ear. Pins that are placed too ventral will be in thinner bone and may cause a painful hematoma in the temporalis muscle.

After the patient has been flipped prone, a traction cord with 15 pounds of weight is attached to the flexion rope. The arms should be tucked with a sheet at the patient's side with the hands in neutral position. The full chest pad should be at nipple level with female breasts tucked inferior and the chin and neck free from pressure. The iliac pads are placed just below the anterior superior iliac spine. The legs are placed on multiple pillows in the sling with the knees and ankles separated by foam padding. The abdomen hangs free with the patient in reverse Trendelenburg position to decrease venous pressure and minimize bleeding. The hands are checked to make sure they are not pressing directly on anything hard, and foam material is used to pad the hands and bony prominences accordingly. The shoulders are taped down using 3-inch silk tape from around the acromioclavicular joint, down the arms (supporting them from falling downward), then around the foot of the table. Overstretch with excessive force can cause a brachial plexus injury. The dorsal neck is clipped if the patient did not do this the night before, leaving adequate room for the plastic self-adhesive drape to attach without interfering with the exposure. Benzoin or other adhesive is applied prior to placement of the drapes. The surgical area is prepped widely. The warming blanket is taped to the undersurface of the table, ventral to the patient, allowing the heat to rise to the patient. After skin preparation, a half sheet is placed over the legs, and another half sheet is used to cover the end of the bed. Four blue towels are placed around the surgical field. The towels are placed close to the area of the incision. Then a half sheet is placed over the entire area and a small hole is cut out where the incision is to be made. The blue towels are then pulled back to expose the minimum amount of skin necessary to perform the operation. We prefer to prep the skin widely and then drape narrowly. Local anesthetic/epinephrine is injected into the area of the planned incision, and the surgical site is covered with Ioban strips.

A midline skin incision is made with a full-thickness scalpel cut, down into subcutaneous fat. The incision is deepened with electrocautery and while self-retaining retractors are inserted that will aid in hemostasis. Once below subcutaneous fat, it is very important to carefully stay in the midline fascia. The actual median raphe may deviate from the actual physical midline by quite a bit but is visible by carefully using the electrocautery on cut rather than coagulate. Care is used to avoid dissecting into the paraspinal muscles, which would lead to greatly increased bleeding and postoperative pain. Crossing bleeders from the venous plexus can be coagulated. The median raphe usually looks like a white band of fascia approximately 3 to 4 mm wide and can be better visualized with loupe or microscope magnification and lighting. In dissecting deep to the fascia, pink muscles fibers should be avoided. The separation between the paraspinal muscles can sometimes be very fine when they merge centrally in the raphe. At the level of the spinous processes, the muscles span the tips and can be preserved in performing a unilateral foraminotomy/discectomy without fusion. When the plan is to fuse or dissect previously fused levels, the interspinous tissue can be taken with the lateral soft tissue flaps so that only bone remains. This will minimize bleeding by staying out of the vascular muscle. The levels are localized with spine needles on the spinous processes percutaneously prior to incision and/or with a clamp on an exposed spinous process with intraoperative lateral radiograph. Once subperiosteal dissection has been completed with electrocautery down to the level of the lamina, a Cobb elevator is used to strip the soft tissues laterally with a scraping technique.

In performing a foraminotomy, the interlaminar V of the lateral aspect of the desired laminar interspace is the starting point (Fig. 76-7). The interlaminar V points to the affected joint and disc level. A high-speed bur is used with one hand held like a pencil as close to the bottom of the bur as possible for better control. The surgeon's fingers should point down into the wound as a result; the other hand holds a small Frazier suction tip, and the assistant irrigates. The bur is maneuvered in small, circular motions, getting gradually deeper (ventral); in-and-out motions are to be avoided. The inferior articular process of the superior vertebra is burred away, leaving the superior articular process of the inferior vertebra (Fig. 76-8). If the facet joints are arthritic and have large spurs, the foraminotomy hole can become quite deep. Frequent irrigation and suction will maintain visualization. Burring is stopped once soft tissue is seen protruding through the remaining bone at the "floor" or on the "walls" of the foraminotomy or the bone takes on a translucent appearance from becoming so thin (Fig. 76-9).

It is preferable to complete the drilling laterally first, rather than medially, because if the medial cortex if perforated first,

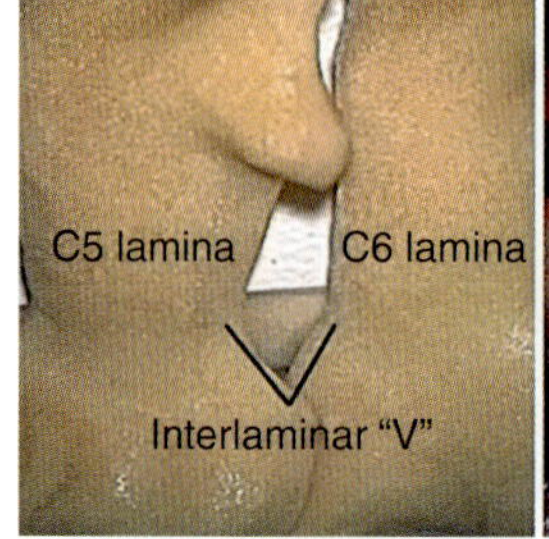

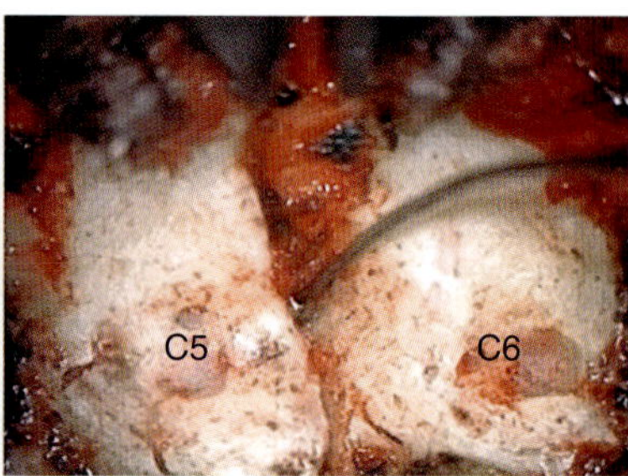

FIGURE 76-7. When performing a dorsal cervical foraminotomy, one must first identify the medial and lateral borders of the foramen. The interspace between the C5-6 lamina is shown as the interlaminar V on the left. On the right, an interoperative picture shows a ball-tipped probe marking the interlaminar V.

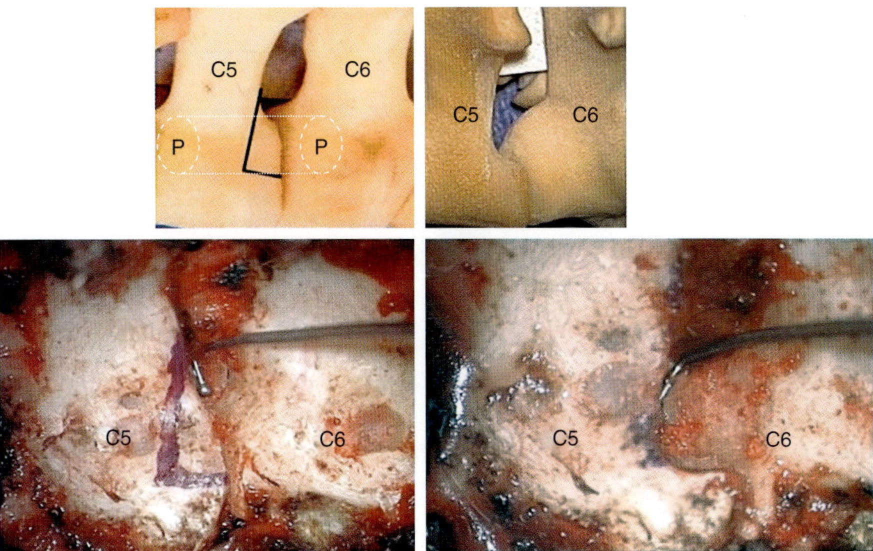

FIGURE 76-8. The first step of the foraminotomy. In the model, an L-shaped resection of the C5 inferior articular facet is to be made. This goes approximately 50% of the distance between the interlaminar V and the lateral margin of the facet. This is because if one resects 50% of the joint, this is approximately where the lateral margin of the pedicle is. The foramen is bounded by the C5-6 pedicles. If one performs a decompression lateral to the pedicle, the foramen will be completely free. On the right-hand side, as the model shows, this L-shaped area has been removed. One then sees the superior margin of the C6 facet.

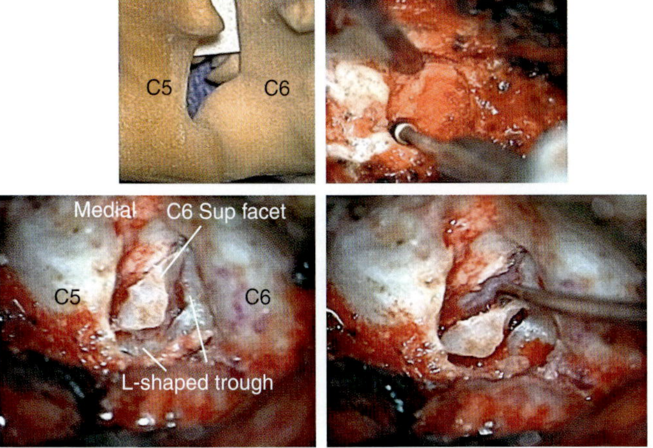

FIGURE 76-9. A high-speed bur is used to resect the triangular piece of bone using an L-shaped trough. Any bone that is overlying the C6 pedicle is then resected.

the engorged vein underneath protrudes while the surgeon is trying to complete the lateral drilling and causes considerable bleeding and difficult visualization.

The suction tip is maintained in the interspace when drilling, to protect the soft tissue overlying the cord in case of a sudden drill "kick" or movement. Alternatively, a curette can be placed into the interspace, hooked into the foramen, to protect the cord. The Codman-Karlin 2B curette is the ideal tool, since it can be held like a pencil, and with a pulling motion, the bone overlying the foramen can be lifted out; the 1-mm Kerrison rongeur is also useful.

The vein that overlies the nerve root tends to bleed profusely, so it is important to understand the maneuvers that can decrease bleeding. Reverse Trendelenburg positioning with the abdomen hanging freely is used to decrease venous pressure. Thrombin-soaked hemostatic gelatin (Gelfoam) and cottonoid patties are packed into the bleeding foraminotomy site, and the decompression is resumed when the bleeding has slowed down.

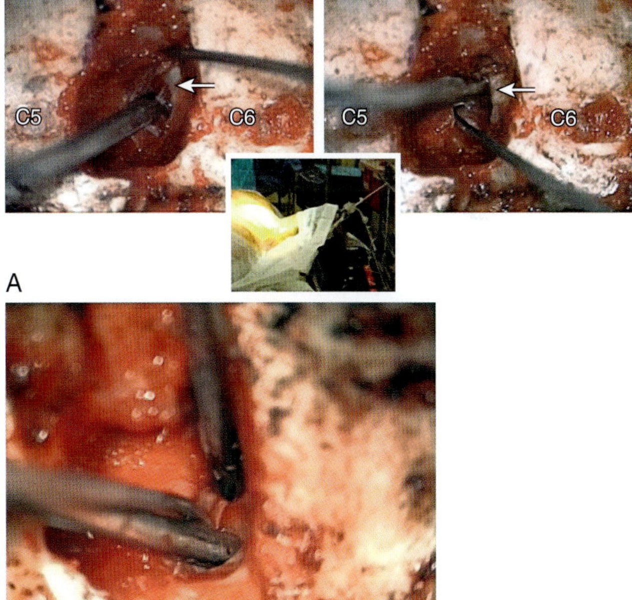

FIGURE 76-10. **A,** The arrows point to the C6 pedicle. The nerve is retracted cranially, and a right-angled ball-tipped probe is utilized to hook the herniated disc fragment. If there is no disc fragment and one is just performing a foraminotomy, after making sure that the foramen is completely open, one should recheck with the neck in full extension. This ensures that even with the patient's neck in full extension, the foramen is still wide open. It should also be noted that the entire foraminotomy and discectomy procedure should be performed with the neck in maximal flexion, which opens up the foramen. **B,** The root is retracted cranially, and the small pituitary rongeurs are used to remove the disc fragment.

The thoroughness of the decompression is assessed by palpating the superior and inferior pedicles with the tip of the Codman curette or a nerve hook. Once the entire interpedicular region has been unroofed, the bony decompression is done (Fig. 76-10).

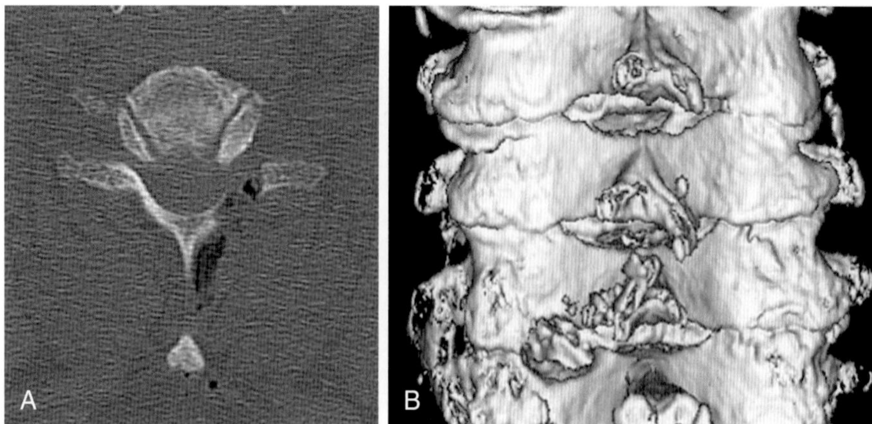

FIGURE 76-11. **A,** Postoperative CT showing a foraminotomy at C6-7. **B,** Three-dimensional reconstructed image of the foraminotomy.

The nerve root can be gently retracted superiorly and the disc material removed with a small nerve hook or pituitary rongeur. Resecting 50% of the cervical facet does not typically require fusion or stabilization (Fig. 76-11).

In closing, a #1 absorbable suture is used for the fascia and muscle. Numerous sutures with small bites are placed in the fascia of the paraspinal muscles deep in an attempt to bring the muscles back together. This combats this incision's tendency to invaginate during healing. It is helpful to tag clamp four to six sutures in the same layer and then tie them before proceeding to a more superficial layer. Meticulous hemostasis and closure of the dead space along with a deep and superficial drain help to prevent postoperative wound complications that are inherent to this approach.

Complications of Dorsal Cervical Discectomy

Similar to anterior cervical discectomy, complications of dorsal cervical discectomy include neurologic deterioration, dural injury, and inadequate decompression with persistent or recurrent symptoms. Air embolism causing stroke was rarely reported in the early literature but has not been reported in recent series in which both the sitting and prone positions were used.

Neurologic deterioration or persistent symptoms should be aggressively investigated and corrected. Evidence of spinal cord injury can prompt consideration of intravenous steroid treatment, although this is controversial. Persistent radiculopathy can arise from a misdiagnosed, unoperated level or from an inadequate decompression. Repeat decompression from either a dorsal or a ventral approach can be successful. Dural injury can result in cerebrospinal fluid leak (pseudomeningocele or fistula). Lumbar drainage can be considered, although local management with fibrin sealant or tissue graft and tight wound closure may be adequate.

Complications associated with cervical discectomy can be minimized with meticulous attention to preoperative planning and the surgical principles described previously.

KEY REFERENCES

Anderson PA, Sasso RC, Riew KD: Update on cervical artificial disk replacement. *Instr Course Lect* 56:237–245, 2007.

Daniels AH, Riew KD, Yoo JU, et al: Adverse events associated with anterior cervical spine surgery. *J Am Acad Orthop Surg* 16(12):729–738, 2008.

Edwards CC II, Karpitskaya Y, Cha C, et al: Accurate identification of adverse outcomes after cervical spine surgery. *J Bone Joint Surg [Am]* 86(2):251–256, 2004.

Lehman RA Jr, Riew KD: Thorough decompression of the posterior cervical foramen. *Instr Course Lect* 56:301–309, 2007.

Rhee JM, Yoon T, Riew KD: Cervical radiculopathy. *J Am Acad Orthop Surg* 15:486–494, 2007.

Riew KD, Buchowski JM, Sasso R, et al: Cervical disc arthroplasty compared with arthrodesis for the treatment of myelopathy. *J Bone Joint Surg [Am]* 90(11):2354–2364, 2008.

REFERENCES

The complete reference list is available online at expertconsult.com.

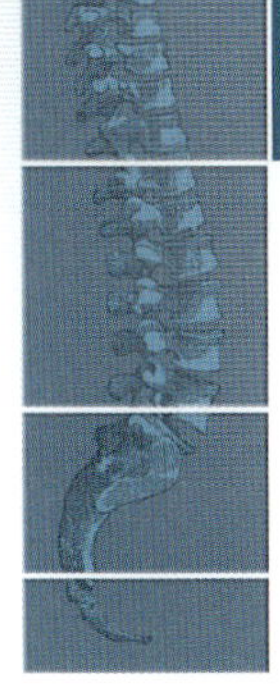

CHAPTER 77

Thoracic Discectomy

Thomas C. Chen | Edward C. Benzel | Paul C. McCormick | Charles B. Stillerman

It has been estimated that up to 20% of the population has a thoracic disc herniation, as evidenced by MRI.[1,2] However, the need for discectomy is relatively rare. Surgery for removal of thoracic disc herniations is thought to constitute less than 4% of all disc operations.[3,4] Historically, these operations have been associated with suboptimal outcomes for various reasons, in part because of diagnostic delays. These delays are a result of the rarity of symptomatic thoracic discs and the lack of a characteristic presentation pattern. It is hoped that a growing awareness of this disorder will lead to better outcomes as a result of earlier treatment. Additionally, there is uncertainty about the natural history of this disease. There is no consensus regarding the indications for disc removal. Most surgeons generally avoid prophylactic surgery for disc herniation; however, this practice has not been based on prospective studies. Generally, surgery is reserved for patients with severe, intractable radicular pain or for those with myelopathy, especially when it is progressive or severe. Finally, there are numerous operations for the removal of these lesions. Regrettably, no universally accepted selection criteria exist to help determine the best operation for each individual situation. Recently, surgical selection guidelines were proposed based on a large series of ventrolateral and lateral operations, the well-documented success of groups using the transpedicular approach, and preliminary experience with newer procedures, including transthoracic thoracoscopy, retropleural thoracotomy, and transfacet pedicle-sparing approaches (Table 77-1).[5-9]

Until the 1950s, laminectomy, with or without disc removal, was the treatment of choice for the surgical management of this disorder. Logue's historical review in 1952 revealed the poor results achieved using laminectomy.[10] Consequently, other methods of performing discectomy were developed. These operations were intended to improve the exposure to the ventral spinal canal throughout the thoracic spine. Although these approaches were successful at improving access to the disc space, they were technically formidable and associated with considerable morbidity. Each of these approaches has a unique set of potential complications; it is important to be aware of them so that they can be avoided. This chapter emphasizes these other methods and focuses on the advantages and disadvantages of each procedure. Fourteen contemporary thoracic disc series are summarized, with special attention given to the reported complications. In closing, a new management paradigm for the treatment of symptomatic thoracic discs is presented.

Surgical Approaches for Thoracic Discectomy

Dorsal Approaches

Laminectomy

The initial approach used for thoracic disc herniation was laminectomy, either with or without disc removal. In 1952, Logue[10] reviewed the thoracic discectomy literature and found that the results were poor. A significant percentage of patients were left paraplegic. Although the precise reasons for these results were not known, it was postulated that laminectomy alone did not significantly reduce the ventral forces created by a thoracic disc herniation acting on the spinal cord.[4] Additionally, when discectomy was performed, spinal cord manipulation was generally poorly tolerated. The limited space available for the spinal cord, as well as the comparatively tenuous blood supply, was thought to increase the

TABLE 77-1

Surgical Approaches for Herniated Thoracic Discs

Surgical Approach	General Indications
Ventral	
Transsternal	Upper thoracic spine Densely calcified centrolateral
Ventrolateral	
Transthoracic/thoracoscopic	Densely calcified centrolateral Selected mildly calcified centrolateral
Retropleural	Selected high-medical-risk static severe myelopathy
Lateral	
A. Extracavitary	
B. Costotransversectomy	A and B, selected densely calcified centrolateral Mildly calcified centrolateral
C. Parascapular	C, upper thoracic spine calcified centrolateral
Dorsolateral	
Transfacet pedicle-sparing/transpedicular	All soft herniated discs Calcified lateral Mildly calcified centrolateral All high-medical-risk except densely calcified centrolateral

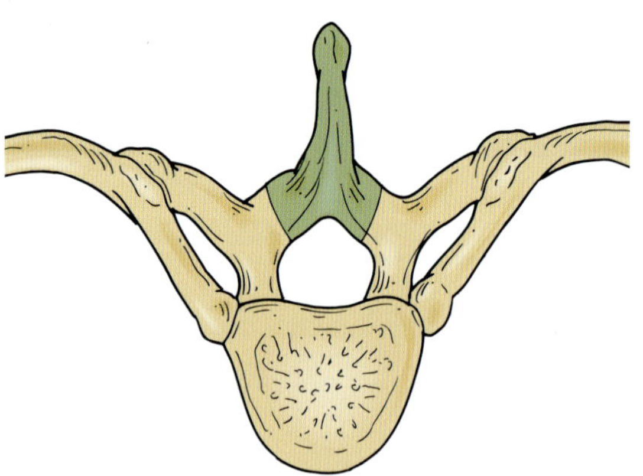

FIGURE 77-1. Laminectomy approach. The lamina and spinous process are removed, often extending above and below the level of disc herniation. This approach has been associated with suboptimal outcomes. It may be used for the management of thoracic spondylosis. (From Stillerman CB, Weiss MH: Principles of surgical approaches to the thoracic spine. In Tarlov EC, editor: *Neurosurgical topics: neurosurgical treatment of disorders of the thoracic spine,* Park Ridge, IL, 1991, AANS, pp 1–19.)

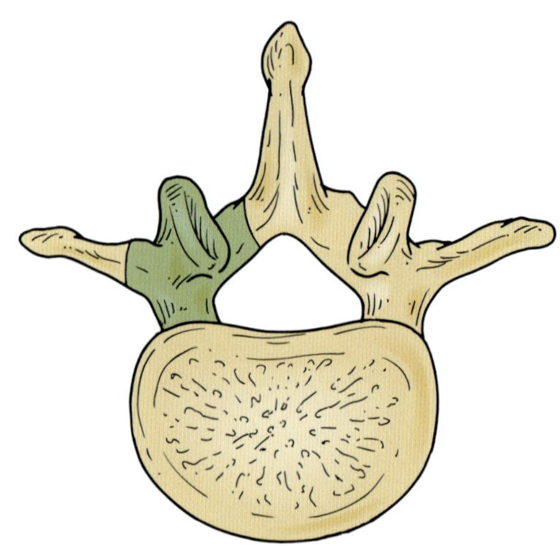

FIGURE 77-2. Transpedicular approach. On the side ipsilateral to the herniation, the facet joint and pedicle flush to the vertebral body are generally removed. A hemilaminectomy may also be performed. (From Stillerman CB, Weiss MH: Management of thoracic disc disease. *Clin Neurosurg* 38:325–352, 1992.)

susceptibility of the thoracic spinal cord to injury during disc removal (Fig. 77-1).

Advantages and Disadvantages

Although laminectomy is technically the simplest decompressive spinal operation, the only indication for its use in thoracic disc disease may be in the treatment of thoracic spondylosis.[11]

Recent Experience

Black described a modified laminotomy/medial facet approach using a unilateral interlaminar laminotomy involving the superior and inferior laminar arches, as well as the medial 2 to 3 mm of the facet joint. The dural edge is exposed to establish boundaries for the cord, and an Epstein stomping curet is used to push the disc downward and away from the cord. This technique was used to remove 11 discs in seven patients. Effective treatment was reported; only one patient reported transient increased weakness compared with preoperative weakness.[12]

Dorsolateral Approaches

Transpedicular Approach

Patterson and Arbit[13] first reported the transpedicular approach in 1978. It was initially performed on three patients with thoracic disc herniations. Two of the patients had complete resolution of their symptoms, and the third markedly improved. Subsequently, several other series have also reported excellent results (Fig. 77-2).

Technique

The patient is placed in the prone position and taped to the table to facilitate rotation away from the surgeon during the disc removal. The spinous process, lamina, and facet joints are exposed using a linear midine incision. Most of the facet joint is removed, as is the pedicle caudal to the disc space. The pedicle is drilled out flush with the vertebral body. A small cavity measuring 1.5 to 2.0 cm in depth is created in the vertebral body to enable depressing the overlying disc away from the ventral dura mater. Additionally, whenever necessary, hemilaminotomies are performed to visualize the dorsolateral dura mater.[11,14-19]

Advantages

This approach is considerably less invasive than most other operations for thoracic disc removal, particularly the transthoracic (TT) and the lateral extracavitary (LECA) approaches. Using this less invasive approach is thought to lessen perioperative pain, shorten hospital stays, and enable earlier return to premorbid activity.[4,8,16,20,21] The surgery avoids problems associated with thoracotomy, rib resection, and extensive muscle dissection. Operating time and blood loss also appear to be less than with other surgeries.

Disadvantages

Critics of this procedure point out the limited ability to visualize across the spinal canal, making decompression of the central and contralateral portions of the disc a relatively blind procedure. Sometimes, difficulty is encountered in managing calcified and intradural disc fragments. We[8,13,16] believe that safety is enhanced by using specially designed thoracic microdiscectomy instrumentation (Fig. 77-3) and endoscopic techniques.[4,8,16] Although some report being able to remove intradural fragments and central, densely calcified discs using the dorsolateral techniques,[5,13,16,19,22] we[4] have not had success with these entities. Dense calcifications involving the dorsal margin of the disc space tend to adhere strongly to the ventral dura mater.[4,17] The possibility of significant dural adherence may lead one to use one of the ventrolateral or lateral procedures in those situations.[4,17]

The final disadvantage of this procedure relates to the removal of the facet-pedicle complex, without the ability to place an interbody graft. It has been reported that patients operated on using the transpedicular approach have somewhat disappointing results from the standpoint of localized

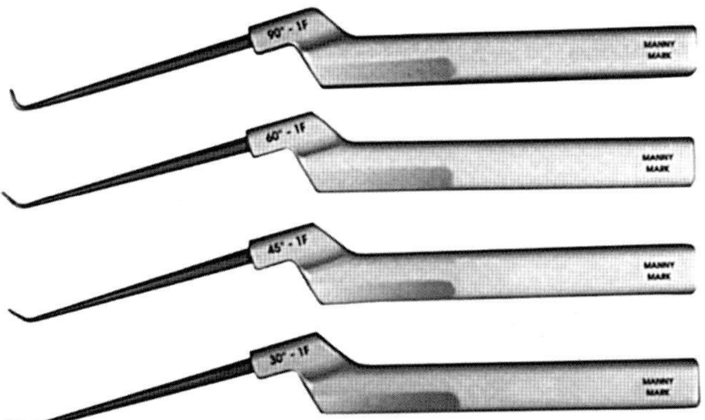

FIGURE 77-3. A selection of the Manny-Mark Stillerman thoracic microdiscectomy instruments. These were developed to facilitate disc removal during a dorsolateral approach without damaging the medially situated spinal cord. (From Stillerman CB, Chen TC, Day JD, et al: The transfacet pedicle-sparing approach for thoracic disc removal: cadaveric morphometric analysis and preliminary clinical experience. *J Neurosurg* 83:971–976, 1995.)

back pain.[8,13,16,19,23] The desire to improve these results led to the development of the transfacet pedicle-sparing approach.[4,8,18] It was postulated that the avoidance of pedicle removal should minimize postoperative back pain. The preliminary experience has suggested that this, in fact, may be the case.

Recent Experience

Bilsky reviewed 20 cases performed between 1982 and 1992 at New York Hospital in which the transpedicular approach was used for thoracic discs (lateral or centrolateral calcified or soft discs). No postoperative instrumentation was used for stabilization; however, no patient suffered from postoperative spinal instability-related pain or delayed kyphosis.[15] Levi et al. have published a contemporary series of 35 patients operated upon via a unilateral transpedicular approach. Good results were obtained in 15 patients, fair results in 11 patients, and no improvement in 8 patients, and 1 patient was paraplegic after surgery. They also did not find evidence of clinical or radiographic instability.[24] Chi et al. describe a mini-open transpedicular thoracic discectomy in which tubular retractors and microscope visualization are used in performing a transpedicular thoracic discectomy. Eleven patients were operated on using the mini-open disectomy approach versus four patients operated on using an open dorsolateral approach. Patients operated on using the mini-open approach had less blood loss and a greater improvement in their modified Prolo score compared with the open procedure. At long-term follow-up, the modified Prolo score was similar for both groups of patients.[25] Jho published a series of endoscopic transpedicular thoracic discectomies in 25 patients. A 1.5-cm trocar is placed at the junction of the lamina and facet via a paramedian incision. The medial portion of the facet, the very lateral portion of the lamina, and the rostral one third of the pedicle are removed using a high-speed drill. A limited amount of spinal cord dura and nerve root are exposed, and then a 70-degree lens endoscope is introduced, allowing for a discectomy to be performed under direct visualization. This surgery was able to be performed on an outpatient or overnight stay basis; no surgery-related complications were reported.[26]

Transfacet Pedicle-Sparing Approach

The transfacet pedicle-sparing approach was developed as a simpler alternative to the formidable ventrolateral and lateral operations for the treatment of thoracic disc disease.[4,8] Initially, morphometric studies were carried out and improved the authors' orientation to the disc space and ventral spinal canal, thereby aiding discectomy. Cadaveric studies demonstrated that a keyhole facetectomy alone, without associated pedicle or lamina removal, did not sacrifice the exposure achieved with the transpedicular approach.[4,8] Although the safety and overall effectiveness of the transpedicular approach have been well documented,[13,16] it was hoped that avoidance of pedicle removal and limiting the amount of facet resected would improve localized back pain results.[8]

Technique

The operation is performed with the patient in the prone position on a radiolucent frame and spinal table. The arms are placed at the sides, and the patient is taped to the table. Anteroposterior (AP) fluoroscopic imaging is used to identify the appropriate disc space. A 4-cm linear skin incision is centered over the disc space. The paraspinal muscles are subperiosteally reflected laterally, exposing the ipsilateral spinous process, lamina, facet joint, and transverse processes above and below the disc space. A small, self-retaining retractor is placed, and the fluoroscope is introduced to verify the correct level and the precise location of the underlying disc relative to the facet joint. Once this relationship is ascertained, a high-speed drill is used to facilitate a partial facetectomy (Fig. 77-4A). Care is taken to preserve the lateral margin of the inferior and superior articular processes of the facet joint and the entire pedicle directly caudal to the disc. When the partial facetectomy is completed, the underlying neuroforaminal fat is coagulated with bipolar cautery. The nerve root, which exits the spinal canal under the more rostral pedicle, is rarely encountered, except in the upper thoracic spine (Fig. 77-4B). The underlying anulus is coagulated and incised. The disc herniation is removed using conventional microdiscectomy techniques (Fig. 77-4C). As with the transpedicular approach, no fusion is required.[8]

Advantages

Advantages of the transfacet pedicle-sparing approach may include diminished operating time, decreased blood loss, and limited bone and soft tissue removal. Like the transpedicular approach, perioperative pain, hospital stay, and return to premorbid activity appear to compare favorably with the more formidable ventrolateral and lateral approaches.[4,17,19] When necessary, multiple disc herniations may be treated.[14] The exposure is identical to that provided by the transpedicular approach. Preservation of the pedicle may improve long-term localized back pain results.[4,17,19]

Disadvantages

The disadvantages are the same as for the transpedicular approach.[13,16] Specially designed thoracic microdiscectomy instrumentation[8] and, on occasion, open endoscopic visualization of the disc and ventral dural mater have been helpful in enhancing safety during the disc removal.[8,16]

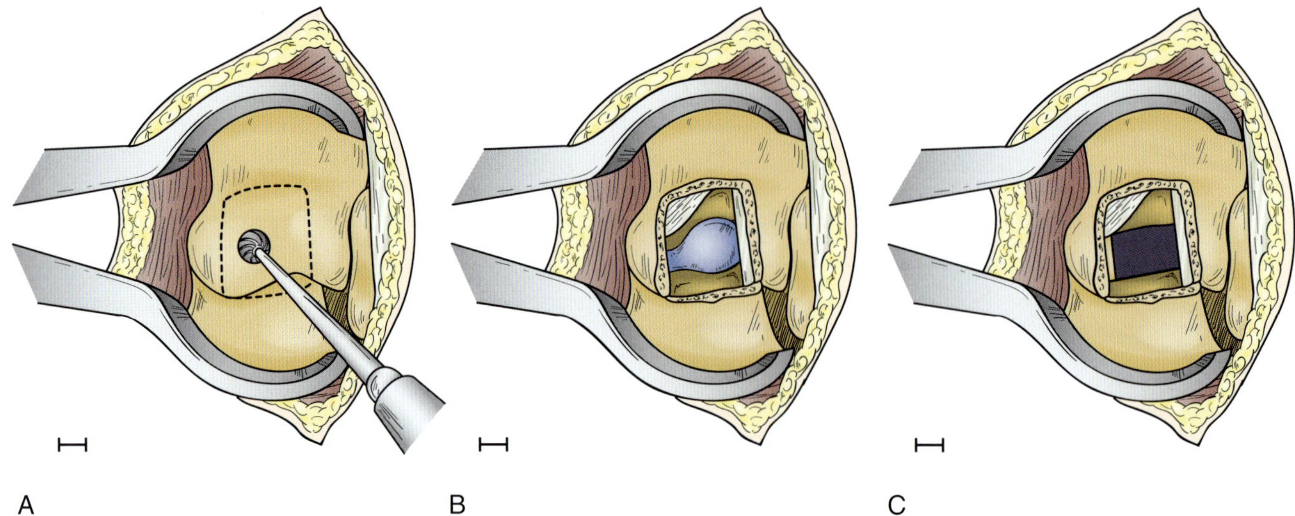

FIGURE 77-4. Transfacet pedicle-sparing approach. Diagrams illustrating surgical sequence. Bar scale represents 0.8 cm = 1 cm. A mesial facetectomy is centered over the disc herniation. **A,** Fluoroscopy is used to limit the amount of bone removed. **B,** On completing the partial facetectomy, the foraminal fat is coagulated and the disc is exposed. **C,** The disc herniation is removed using conventional microdiscectomy techniques. Specially designed thoracic microdiscectomy instruments are helpful to facilitate safety during discectomy. Additionally, open endoscopy can be used to improve visualization of the central and contralateral spinal canal during disc removal. (From Stillerman CB, Chen TC, Day JD, et al: The transfacet pedicle-sparing approach for thoracic disc removal: cadaveric morphometric analysis and preliminary clinical experience. *J Neurosurg* 83:971–976, 1995.)

Recent Experience

Zhang et al. have recently published a series of 18 patients treated with the transfacet pedicle-sparing approach with dorsal instrumentation and fusion. Although the transfacet approach was published with the goal of avoiding dorsal instrumentation, the patients in this series all had additional segmental instrumentation. All patients had good exposure of the disc space and good decompression of the spinal cord. These investigators experienced a complication rate of 33%, with six of the patients requiring additional surgery; five had wound infections or seromas requiring washout and one required revision of a misplaced screw.[27]

Minimally Invasive Approaches

A number of minimally invasive microendoscopic discectomy techniques have been advocated, all using a dorsolateral approach and an endoscope for visualization. Although the series are not large, they have all demonstrated adequate access and visualization with removal of the thoracic discs with decreased morbidity compared with open approaches.[22]

Technique

The basic underlying instrumentation used in all approaches involves a dorsolateral approach, endoscope, and tubular dilators. The patient is usually placed in a prone position; however, Jho has placed the patient in a lateral position for an endoscopic transpedicular thoracic discectomy.[26] The approach used by Fessler et al. involves a prone position on a radiolucent Wilson frame.[28] A localizing radiograph is obtained to determine the level of the thoracic disc. A paramedian skin incision is made at the level of the disc, approximately 3 to 4 cm lateral to the midline. A series of tubular muscle dilators are then placed, and the tubular retractor is placed to form a working port for the endoscope. The endoscope is passed down the center of the tubular retractor. Under endoscopic visualization, the muscle and soft tissue is cleaned off at the level of the transverse process and lateral aspect of the facet. A drill then excises the junction of the transverse process and lateral facet, allowing access to the disc. The pedicle is identified, and drilling of the superior aspect of the caudal pedicle is performed to allow access to the thoracic disc. The disc anulus is identified and cut, and the endoscope is tilted for a 30-degree visualization similar to a transforaminal-type approach. The disc is removed, and a down-going curet or a Woodson elevator is used to push down the disc fragment away from the spinal cord. After the discectomy is performed, the tubular retractor is removed and the wound closed.

Advantages

The main advantages of the minimally invasive approaches are potentially less destruction to the dorsal paraspinal muscles, minimal bone and ligamentous removal, maintenance of disc integrity, avoidance of thoracic fusion, and avoidance of chest entry. The ideal result would be minimal trauma to the adjacent tissue during the approach to the thoracic disc and its removal. As a result, potential recovery time, amount of blood loss, and length of hospital stay would be minimized.

Disadvantages

The main disadvantage of a minimally invasive endoscopic approach is the learning curve and familiarity with the anatomy. This approach should be performed by individuals with facility using the endoscope and previous experience with the open dorsolateral approach. Minimally invasive approaches can turn out to be maximally invasive approaches when the learning curve is steep. Visualization is good at the point of entry and is limited to familiarity with the anatomy seen on the endoscope.

Recent Experience

Two main series using this approach have been published.[22,26] Perez-Cruet et al. have a series of seven patients operated on using a minimally invasive thoracic microendoscopic discectomy (TMED).[22] Results demonstrated no morbidity with this approach, good access, and quick return to work. No case required conversion to an open procedure. Jho reported a series of endoscopic transpedicular approaches also with excellent results. His series is based on a more extensive pedicle takedown, coming in more medially than Perez-Cruet. Results were also excellent for visualization, disc removal, and quick return to work.[26]

Lateral Approaches

Lateral Extracavitary Approach

LECA was developed and refined by Larson.[29] It was first performed for the management of Pott disease. It provides the best exposure to the ventral spinal canal of all lateral operations. Large thoracic discectomy series have documented its safety and efficacy[17,30] (Fig. 77-5).

Technique

The procedure is performed with the patient prone and taped to the table with arms at the side. The skin incision consists of a hockey-stick incision, with the vertical portion centered over the area of pathology[11,18,29,30] (see Fig. 77-5A). Caudally, the incision is gently curved off the midline for 8 to 12 cm, enabling the skin, subcutaneous tissue, and fascial flap to be rotated far laterally. Alternatively, a paramedian lunar-shaped incision may be used. The erector spinae muscles are subperiosteally dissected off the dorsal ribs and transverse processes and flapped medially.[31] The erector spinae muscle complex may be wrapped in a moistened laparotomy pad and gently retracted medially. Intraoperative imaging helps ensure removal of the rib that articulates with the correct disc space (see Fig. 77-5B). Once the proximal 8 to 12 cm of rib is resected, the underlying intercostal nerve is identified and traced into the neural foramen (see Fig. 77-5C). The pedicle caudal to the disc is identified and removed, exposing the lateral aspect of the dura mater (see Fig. 77-5D). At this point, the dorsal third of the disc space is removed. Care is taken to leave intact the dorsal-most margin of disc and the posterior longitudinal ligament (see Fig. 77-5E). The dorsal-caudal quarter of the rostral vertebra is drilled out, as is the dorsal-rostral quarter of the caudal vertebra. This creates a cavity so that the remaining dorsal disc and posterior longitudinal ligament can be gently depressed away from the spinal cord (see Fig. 77-5F). The ventral dura mater can then be inspected either directly, with small dental mirrors, or with an endoscope. The rib, which was resected to facilitate exposure of the disc space, is then fashioned into strut grafts and carefully impacted into the cavity (see Fig. 77-5G). The ventral dura mater and spinal canal are then inspected again to ensure that there is no encroachment by the bone grafts.

Advantages

One major advantage of this procedure is the enhanced safety during the disc removal because of direct visualization of the dura mater before and during the decompression, which is facilitated by the removal of the pedicle.[11,18,29,30] Additionally, because of the extensive amount of rib removed compared with the other lateral procedures, the exposure to the ventral spinal canal is improved. Surgeon orientation is almost truly lateral. By remaining extrapleural, the procedure avoids the complications observed with intrathoracic surgery.[17] These include the need to place a thoracostomy tube and various pulmonary complications (cerebrospinal fluid [CSF]–pleural) fistula, pneumonia, and complications related to the need to take down the diaphragm at the thoracolumbar junction). A ventral strut graft can be placed with relative ease. Finally, in the rare instance of multiple symptomatic discs,[4,32] multiple levels can be exposed.[17,30]

Disadvantages

The major disadvantage of LECA is that it is a formidable operation with a potential for significant perioperative pain.[30] Additionally, there is a potential for a prolonged operating time and considerable blood loss, especially early on in a surgeon's experience. In experienced hands, however, these parameters appear to be comparable to the ventrolateral approaches.[29,30] Densely calcified central discs, intradural fragments, ventral dural tears, or discs that are completely enveloped by the dura mater may be difficult to remove without the need to elevate the dura mater.[4] These conditions may be better treated using a ventrolateral approach. Finally, as is the case with ventrolateral surgeries, we do not generally recommend LECA in the medically high-risk patient.[4]

Lateral Parascapular Extrapleural Approach

Fessler et al.[28] developed a modification of LECA called the lateral parascapular extrapleural approach (LPEA). This operation simplifies removal of a thoracic disc herniation in the upper thoracic spine.

Technique

Patients are placed prone and taped to the table so they can be rotated 15 to 20 degrees away from the surgeon during the decompression. The arms are kept at the sides. A midline incision extends two spinous processes above and below the disc to be removed. Caudally, the incision is gently curved laterally to the scapular line on the side of pathology. To minimize postoperative seroma formation, the incision is carried down to the deep fascia, with only minimal subcutaneous undermining. The rhomboid and trapezius muscles are then dissected off the spinous processes. A myocutaneous flap is rotated toward the medial scapular border. The caudal fibers of the trapezius muscle are transected to reflect the flap. It is important to protect the rostral latissimus dorsi fibers while cutting the inferior portion of the trapezius muscle. The musculocutaneous flap is limited by the skin incision and the medial scapula. The scapula rotates laterally as the trapezius and rhomboid muscles are mobilized. This increases the exposure of the ribs laterally for better orientation to the ventral spinal cord and central disc space.[28,31]

Most of the advantages and disadvantages of LECA are identical to its LPEA modification. The following emphasizes points that are specific to the LPEA surgery.

Advantages

The major advantage of this technique is that it simplifies removal of upper thoracic disc herniations by providing a far lateral orientation to the disc space at this level. This

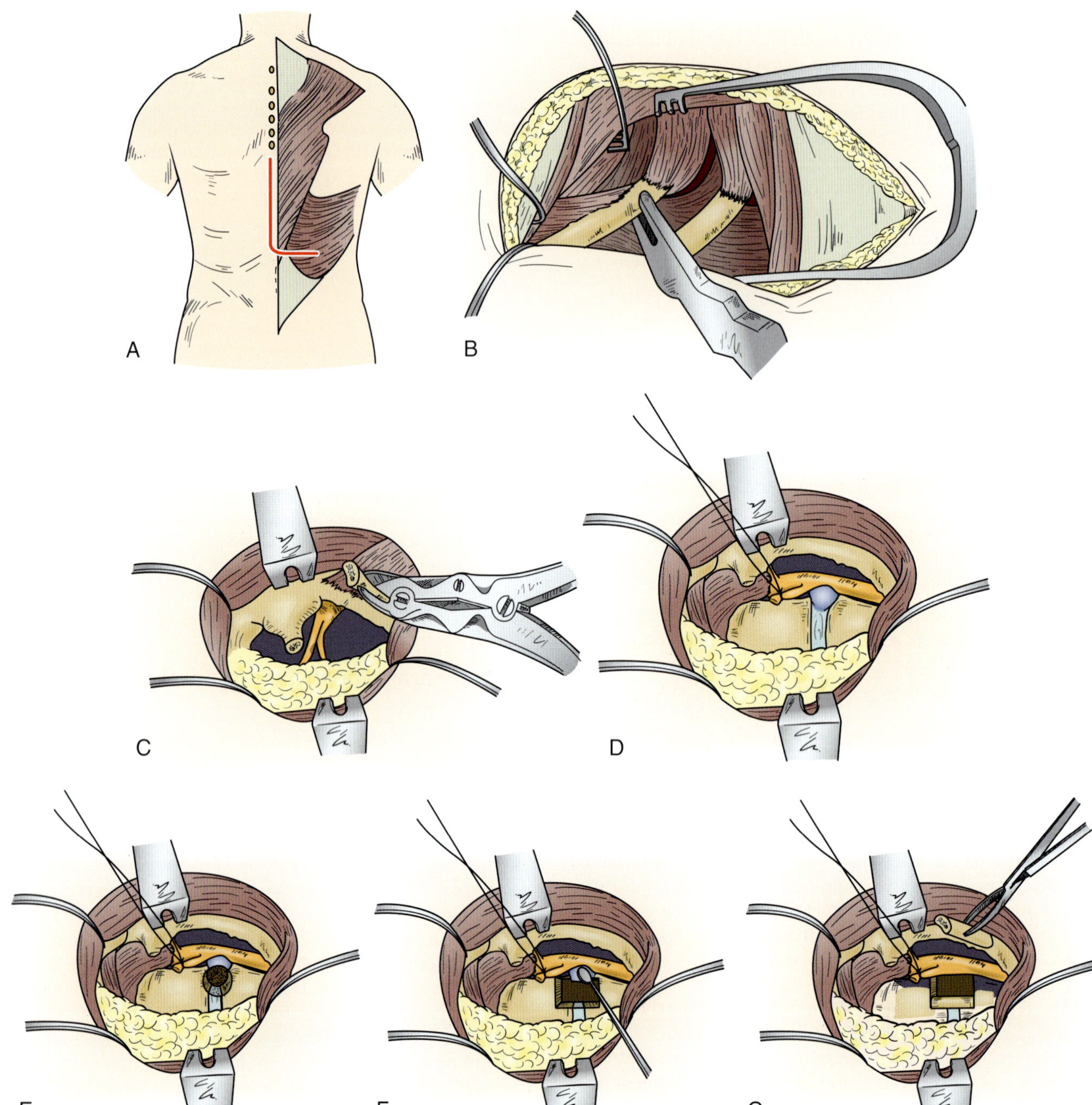

FIGURE 77-5. Lateral extracavitary approach. A hockey-stick–shaped incision centered over the level of disc herniation is generally used. **A**, Caudally, the incision is curved off the midline to maximize the amount of rib that can be exposed and removed. Shorter portions of rib resections create a more dorsolateral orientation to the disc space. Conversely, extensive removal of rib facilitates a more lateral approach to the disc space. The skin, subcutaneous tissue, and fascia are rotated laterally. **B**, The erector spinae muscles are then flapped medially, exposing the underlying rib(s), which are resected flush with the vertebral body. **C**, Removal of the proximal rib head, transverse process, and pedicle directly caudal to the disc space enables exposure of the neural foramen and lateral dura mater. **D,** The intercostal nerve is identified and traced into its respective foramen. This is tagged and cut. Care must be taken to avoid traction on this nerve. **E,** The lateral anulus is incised, and a portion of nucleus is removed, enabling drilling through the disc to the contralateral side. The dorsal portion of the disc, posterior longitudinal ligament, and disc herniation are left intact. A cavity is created by removing a portion of the rostral and caudal vertebral bodies. **F,** The remaining disc and posterior longitudinal ligament are then depressed into this cavity. **G,** Once the ventral dura and spinal canal are directly inspected for retained fragments, the rib that was removed during the exposure is fashioned into struts and gently impacted across the defect. (From Stillerman CB, Weiss MH: Management of thoracic disc disease. *Clin Neurosurg* 38:325–352, 1992.)

far lateral exposure enhances safety during decompression by improving visualization across the ventral spinal canal. Superior mediastinal structures, which may be traumatized with other approaches to the upper thoracic spine, are avoided. Recurrent laryngeal nerve palsies are also avoided.[28]

Disadvantages

Disadvantages include the potential for shoulder morbidity from scapular mobilization, T1 nerve injury, Horner syndrome, sympathectomy, and intercostal neuralgia.

Costotransversectomy

The costotransversectomy approach was initially reported in 1894 by Menard for the treatment of Pott disease.[33] The orientation to the disc space is more dorsal than with either LECA or LPEA. This is the result of a more limited rib resection.

Technique

Different costotransversectomy techniques have been proposed. Patient positioning options vary from prone to modified lateral decubitus.[33] Skin incisions likewise vary and include the paramedian incision along the lateral border of the erector spinae muscles and a semilunar incision. A skin, subcutaneous tissue, and fascial flap may be rotated medially toward the spinous process. The trapezius muscle can be incised in line with the skin incision and retracted medially. The erector spinae muscles are then dissected from their attachments and can be reflected medially. Some surgeons prefer to cut this muscle complex and reapproximate it at the time of closure. From this point, surgical decompression is the same as for LECA.

Advantages

Skin and muscle manipulation and the amount of rib resection are somewhat less than with LECA or LPEA, offering the theoretical advantages of comparatively diminished perioperative pain and a possibly shortened length of hospitalization.

Disadvantages

This is a more dorsal approach than that provided by the other two lateral surgeries. Consequently, the visualization of the central spinal canal is not as good as with those approaches.

Recent Experience

LECA has been augmented by the use of a neuronavigational system for frameless stereotaxy by Kim et al., who used the Stealth surgical navigation system (Stealth Surgical, Gordonsville, VA) to localize the anatomy and provide feedback regarding the dura relative to the disc. Five patients were operated on in this manner with good complete removal of the herniated disc relative to the spinal cord. These investigators cite the advantage of accurate knowledge of the surgical instrumentation relative to the surrounding structures not directly visible in the operating field.[34]

Ventrolateral Approaches

Transthoracic Thoracotomy

The transthoracic thoracotomy approach was first reported independently in 1969 by Perot and Munro[23] and Ransohoff et al.[35] These two groups reported on a combined number of five patients. Despite the limited number of patients initially undergoing this approach, it has developed into one of the surgical cornerstones for the management of symptomatic thoracic disc herniations.[4,19] Two large series of thoracic discectomy patients were compared in 1992.[17] One group primarily used the transthoracic thoracotomy approach, and the other group exclusively used the lateral extracavitary approach. It was determined that these two formidable procedures provided very good results with minimal associated morbidity. Transthoracic thoracotomy provides excellent exposure to the anterior column between T3 and LI (Fig. 77-6).

Technique

The preferred side of approach in the upper thoracic spine is through a right thoracotomy. This avoids the heart as well as the carotid and subclavian arteries. When the disc herniation involves the middle and lower portions of the thoracic spine, most spine surgeons perform a left thoracotomy. Approaching the disc from this side avoids manipulation of the delicate inferior vena cava, which may prove difficult to repair if injured. Additionally, at the thoracolumbar junction the liver is avoided. A double-lumen endotracheal tube may be used to facilitate single-lung ventilation (particularly in the upper thoracic spine). Care is taken to place the patient in a true lateral decubitus position. A bean bag and tape are used to maintain this position so that the patient may be rolled during the decompression. When possible, the area of pathology is centered over the break in the table. All pressure points are padded. A tangential incision is made over the rib to be resected, enabling the removal of additional ribs when necessary. The skin and subcutaneous tissue are incised from the lateral border of the paraspinal muscles to the sternocostal junction (see Fig. 77-6A). The thoracic muscular layers are then incised, and a rib retractor is introduced. It is helpful to verify that the proper rib is being resected by intraoperative AP fluoroscopy. The periosteum of the rib is then incised and exposed using subperiosteal dissection. A Doyen elevator is used to strip the periosteum from the ventral surface of the rib without violating the underlying endothoracic fascia and pleura. Small defects in these layers should be closed primarily; the rib is then resected. Bone edges of the rib are waxed, and the resected portion of rib is saved so that it can be used to form an interbody bone graft on completion of the discectomy. The parietal pleura is then incised along the line of the rib bed, and the wound is held open by introducing a rib spreader (see Fig. 77-6C). The lung is covered with a moistened laparotomy pad and can be gently retracted medially and ventrally. It may be selectively collapsed to facilitate additional exposure of the spinal column. The parietal pleura, which covers the vertebral bodies, is incised. A Cobb elevator can be used to prepare the vertebral bodies. This dissection must avoid injury to the segmental vessels, as well as the sympathetic chain that crosses the middle portion of each vertebral body (see Fig. 77-6D). It may be necessary to ligate or clip these vessels. To expose the dorsolateral disc space, ventral spinal canal, and entire neuroforamen, it is necessary to incise the radiate ligament and to drill off the head of the overlying rib. The overlying transverse process, neurovascular foramen, and rostral and caudal boundaries of the pedicle that is directly caudal to the appropriate disc space are palpated with a small nerve hook. The pedicle can be removed,

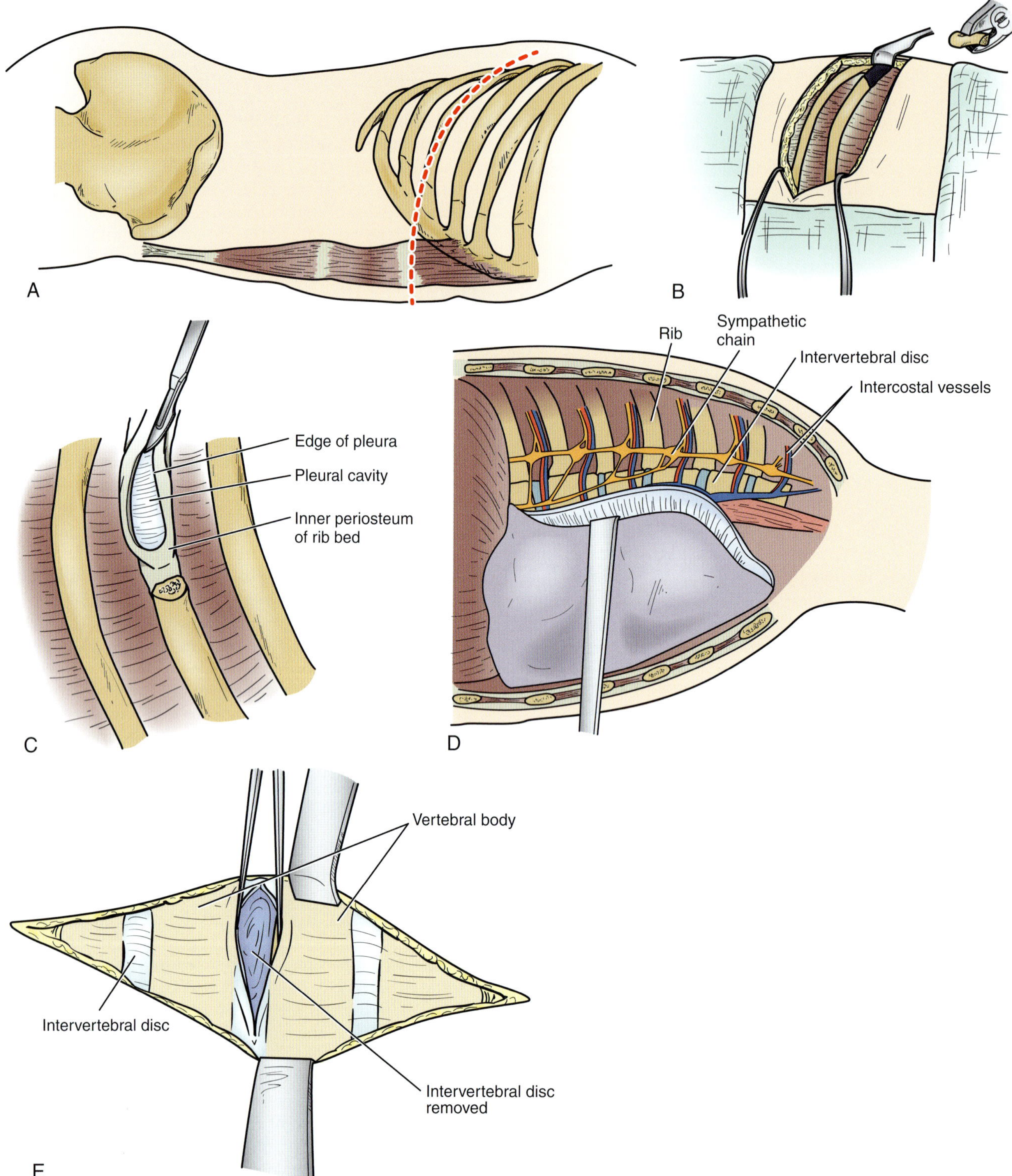

FIGURE 77-6. Transthoracic thoracotomy approach. The patient is placed in the lateral decubitus position. **A**, The incision extends from the border of the paraspinal muscles to the sternocostal junction. The rib is exposed and resected flush with the lateral spinal column. **B**, Removal of the rib head exposes the appropriate disc space and neural foramen. **C,** The pleura are opened in line with the rib bed. The lung is gently retracted, and the parietal pleura overlying the spinal column is incised and carefully reflected. It is often necessary to ligate the intercostal vessels. **D**, The sympathetic chain must be left intact. **E**, The disc space is exposed, and the disc herniation can now be removed. (From Stillerman CB, Weiss MH: Management of thoracic disc disease. *Clin Neurosurg* 38:325–352, 1992.)

exposing the lateral dura mater. When necessary, additional exposure of the neuroforamen can be facilitated by sectioning the intercostal nerve proximal to the dorsal root ganglia. At this point, the surgeon should have precise orientation regarding the location of the ventral floor of the spinal canal. The dorsal portion of the anulus is incised, and the discectomy is carried across the vertebral body approaching the other side. Care is taken to leave intact the most dorsal margin of disc and the posterior longitudinal ligament. A high-speed drill is used to create a small cavity in the dorsal-caudal quadrant of the rostral vertebral body and the dorsal-rostral portion of the caudal vertebral body. Once this cavity has been created, the overlying dorsal disc margin and posterior longitudinal ligament can be incised and gently depressed into the cavity, away from the ventral dura mater. A reverse-angled curet may aid the decompression without manipulating the spinal cord (see Fig. 77-6E). The ventral spinal canal and dura mater should be directly inspected subsequent to placement of bone grafts to ensure that there is no encroachment of the spinal canal. The lung is then expanded under direct visualization. The parietal pleura is closed over a thoracostomy tube.

Advantages

The main advantage of the transthoracic thoracotomy relates to the ventrolateral exposure of the disc space and the ventral spinal canal. This orientation enables improved exposure for the removal of midline densely calcified discs and intradural fragments. Repair of ventral dural tears is also simplified as is interbody bone graft placement. Finally, it is possible to remove more than one disc in the rare situation of multiple symptomatic herniations.[32]

Disadvantages

The main disadvantage is similar to that for the more extensive lateral exposures: this is a formidable operation with significant potential for considerable postoperative pain.[4,17] Because of the visceral exposure, several unique risks are possible. These include CSF–pleural fistulas and pulmonary complications secondary to lung collapse. Additionally, closed chest drainage is required in the postoperative period. Disc herniations that occur at the thoracolumbar junction may require at least partial takedown of the diaphragm. Finally, the operation is technically demanding and may require collaboration with a thoracic surgeon. Patients may have an epidural placed preoperatively prior to surgery for postoperative pain. The chest tube is usually removed 3 to 6 days after surgery, prolonging the time of discharge.

Transthoracic Thoracoscopy

The use of thoracoscopy for the treatment of thoracic disc herniations was reported as early as 1994.[36,37] Subsequently, growing enthusiasm for this procedure has developed, with several surgeons demonstrating proficiency.[38-41] The technique, as described by Rosenthal et al.,[37] uses a right-sided approach. The patient is placed in a lateral decubitus position with the side of access turned upward. Four small incisions are made along the midaxillary line so that four trocars may be inserted in a triangular fashion along this line converging on the disc space. An endoscope with a 30-degree angled lens is introduced through one of the trocars, leaving the other three as working ports. Specially designed long instruments are introduced through the working ports. The rib head and pedicle are removed to expose the dura. At this point, the discectomy proceeds similarly to an open thoracotomy.

Advantages

Proponents of this approach believe that compared with transthoracic thoracotomy, transthoracic thoracoscopy allows for complete disc removal with a reduction in surgical trauma. Thus it is thought to be associated with significantly less pain and morbidity and enables a faster recovery time.[37,38]

Disadvantages

In its present form, this technique has several limitations, including the need for pleural entry with all the attendant risks of intrathoracic surgery (e.g., the need for a postoperative thoracostomy tube). A steep learning curve accompanies this method because of the need to develop techniques requiring new hand-eye coordination skills, limited tactile feedback during the surgery, and difficulties with the three-dimensional visualization during disc removal. Additionally, in an era when growing cost constraints affect surgical methodology, the cost-effectiveness of this procedure must be evaluated from the standpoint of duration of hospitalization, length of surgery, and cost of the instrumentation required. Finally, despite being touted by some as a *minimally invasive* technique for thoracic disc removal, it is important to keep in mind that this operation currently requires multiple stab incisions for the insertion of the camera, two working ports, and, on occasion, a retractor for the diaphragm or an incompletely collapsed lung. In its present form, this procedure is perhaps more invasive than other techniques.[4] The exposure this technique provides is identical to thoracotomy. If this procedure is proven clinically safe and effective over long-term follow-up, it would appear to be best suited as an alternative to open thoracotomy in distinction to being a substitute for the dorsolateral, lateral, and retropleural operations.[4]

Recent Experience

Johnson et al. reported experience with endoscopic thoracic discectomy in 36 patients, which they compared with 8 patients undergoing standard open thoracotomy for thoracic discs. These investigators concluded that patients who underwent thoracoscopic discectomy had shorter operative times, less blood loss, a shorter period of chest tube drainage, less narcotic usage, and shorter lengths of stay. The incidence of complications (minor and major) was felt to be 31% in the thoracoscopic group and greater than 100% (more than one complication per patient) in the thoracotomy/discectomy group. These investigators emphasized that the thoracoscopic discectomy, although safer in experienced hands, had a steep learning curve, which may warrant open surgeries for surgeons not familiar with endoscopic techniques.[42] Rosenthal and Dickman reported on a series of 55 patients who underwent thoracic endoscopic disc removal. There were no neurologic complications from the procedure. They reported a 16% rate of intercostal neuralgia in the endoscopic thoracic discectomy group, versus a 50% rate in the open thoracotomy group. The thorascopic group did not have an increased incidence of a retained disc fragment compared with an open thoracotomy. Surgery time was comparable between the thorascopic group and the open surgery technique. The operative time and hospital discharge were less than for conventional surgery.[6] These investigators also examined the incidence of retained discs and found that the open thoracotomy group had no retained fragments, the thorascopic group had a 4% retention rate, and the open costotransversectomy group had a 13% retention rate.[6] In a series of patients undergoing reoperation for herniated thoracic discs, Dickman et al. found that calcified, large broad-based, centrally located discs were the hardest to remove easily and had higher recurrence rates.[43] Anand and Regan have recently published a report on a series of 100 patients operated on with video-assisted thorascopic surgery with a 2-year follow-up. There were no permanent postoperative neurologic deficits. They found that patients with the most severe presentation (i.e., myelopathy) had the greatest improvement in the Oswestry Disability score. At the end of 2 years, 68 patients responded to the final questionnaire. There was an overall 84% satisfaction rate, with objective long-term clinical success achieved in 70% of the patients after 2 years.[44]

Retropleural Thoracotomy Approach

Retropleural thoracotomy was refined and popularized by McCormick.[5] This surgical option in the management of ventral spinal pathology provides an orientation similar to the other ventrolateral approaches and avoids key complications (Fig. 77-7).

Technique

Like the transthoracic procedures, the side of the approach is determined by the location of the pathology. The patient is placed in the lateral decubitus position on a bean bag with a small roll under the dependent axilla. Lesions that occur at the thoracolumbar junction should be centered over the break in the table. Between T5 and T10, a 12-cm skin incision is made, extending from the dorsal axillary line to a point 4 cm lateral to the dorsal midline over the rib at the level of pathology. For upper thoracic spine lesions, a hockey-stick incision is made that parallels the medial and caudal scapular border (see Fig. 77-7A). The incision is then carried through the scapular muscles (trapezius and rhomboids) to the ribs. The scapula is rotated rostrally to expose the appropriate rib. After the appropriate level is identified, a subperiosteal detachment of intercostal muscles is performed over 8 to 10 cm of rib. The rib is then resected and removed (see Fig. 77-7B). The most proximal 4 cm of rib that has attachments to the vertebral body and transverse process remains intact. Once the rib resection is completed, a well-defined layer of tissue is identified in the rib bed. This layer *is* the endothoracic fascia. It is analogous to the transversalis fascia in the abdomen.

The endothoracic fascia lines the entire chest cavity. The underlying parietal pleura maintains an attachment to the inner chest wall through this layer. There is a potential space between the endothoracic fascia and parietal pleura that may contain loose areolar tissue. The endothoracic fascia is continuous with the inner periosteum of the rib and the thoracic vertebral body. It is important to remember that the thoracic sympathetic chain, the intercostal neurovascular elements, the thoracic duct, and the azygos veins are contained against the thoracic wall and the vertebral bodies within this fascial layer. Once identified, the fascia is incised in line with the rib bed (see Fig. 77-7C). The underlying parietal pleura is bluntly dissected from the undersurface of the endothoracic fascia, in much the same way that the peritoneum is freed from the transversalis fascia. Proximally, the pleura is dissected from the vertebral column. At this point, a table-mounted malleable retractor maintains retraction of a laparotomy pad-covered lung (see Fig. 77-7D). The opening can be further widened by placement of a rib retractor.

The endothoracic fascia should be opened over the remaining 4 cm of proximal rib. The costotransverse ligaments are divided, and the rib head is removed. The fascia and periosteum over the vertebral body are elevated away from the disc space. The intercostal vessels that cross the midvertebral body transversely may be preserved. Once the rib head is resected, the boundaries of the neuroforamen and pedicle are identified and the rostral portion of the pedicle directly caudal to the disc space may be resected. From this point on, the decompression is identical to the other ventrolateral approaches (see Figs. 77-7E and 77-7F). At the thoracolumbar junction, because of the diaphragm and the greater angulation of the ribs, the procedure is modified. A 12- to 14-cm skin incision is usually made over the 10th rib extending from the dorsal axillary line to 4 cm off the midline (see Fig. 77-7A). A 10-cm portion of rib is then exposed and resected and the pleural surface of the diaphragm is identified. It should be noted that the endothoracic fascia is reflected over the diaphragm and tightly applied to its surface.

The initial exposure may be somewhat cramped because of the diaphragm's attachment to the ribs. If the endothoracic fascia is present in the rib bed, it is opened. Caudally, the pleural surface of the diaphragm is depressed and detached from the ventral surface of the T11 and T12 ribs with Cobb elevators. Once this is completed, there is a communication between the retropleural and retroperitoneal space. Medially, the detachment is continued so that the arcuate ligaments are elevated off the quadratus lumborum and psoas muscles. Division of the crus of the diaphragm completes the mobilization of the diaphragm. At this point, table-mounted malleable retractors are inserted as rib spreaders and the proximal 4 cm of rib is then removed. The decompression at this point continues as described earlier.[30]

Advantages

This operation provides exposure to the ventral spinal canal and dura mater that is identical to the intrathoracic operations discussed earlier. However, it avoids pleural entry; thus, many of the significant complications that may arise from these procedures are avoided. Also important is that the retropleural thoracotomy approach provides the shortest direct surgical route to the ventral thoracic and thoracolumbar spine. This may enhance safety during the decompression, as well as enable the surgery to be performed using smaller incisions with less soft-tissue dissection, which should lessen perioperative pain and diminish the length of hospitalization. In contrast to the ventrolateral approaches, the diaphragm can be mobilized quite easily at the thoracolumbar junction without its incision. Additionally, the exposure rendered is obscured by the aorta and vena cava. In contrast to the lateral approaches, exposure to the lateral spinal canal can be achieved without dissection or sacrifice of the intercostal nerve or potential occlusion of the intraforaminal radicular medullary artery. Overall, this procedure appears to offer advantages over the other ventrolateral surgeries (both closed and open) and lateral approaches.[36]

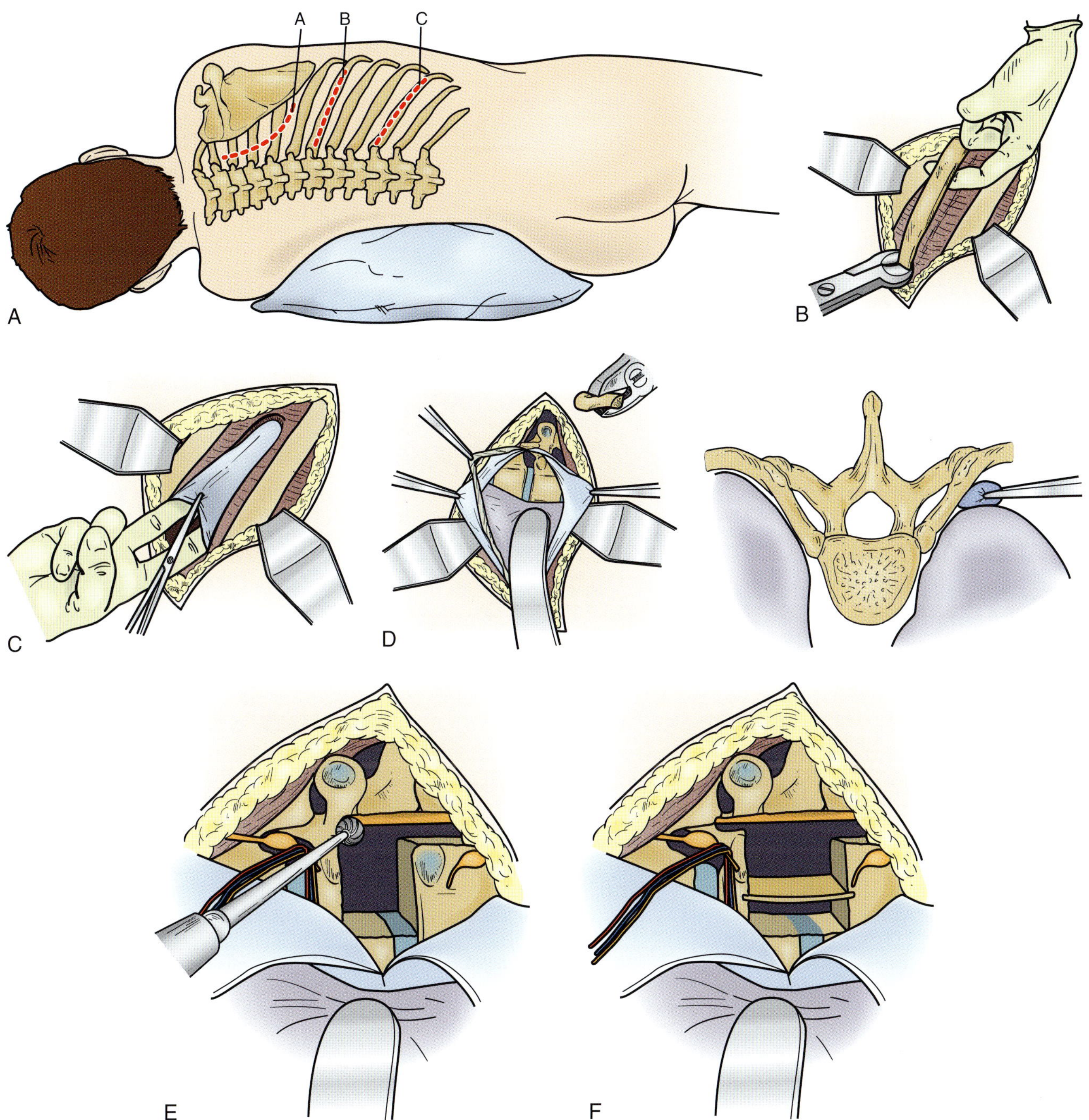

FIGURE 77-7. Retropleural thoracotomy approach. **A,** The patient is placed in the lateral decubitus position. Incision A is used for upper thoracic spine disc herniations. Incision B is used for herniations between T5 and T10. Incision C is used for thoracolumbar herniated discs. The skin incision is extended through the muscle layers and the rib is exposed. **B,** All but the most proximal 4 cm of rib is removed. After rib removal, the well-defined endothoracic fascia is identified within the rib bed. **C,** The endothoracic fascia is then opened in line with the rib bed and the pleura is swept away from the undersurface of the endothoracic fascia. **D,** Proximally, the pleura is dissected off the spinal column. The rib head is removed along with the rostral portion of the pedicle directly caudal to the disc space. **E,** The overlying transverse process can also be removed. This exposes the neural foramen and the lateral dura. **F,** The disc is then removed, the spinal canal and ventral dura are directly examined, and the rib that was removed can be fashioned into strut grafts and impacted across the defect. (From McCormick PC: Retropleural approach to the thoracic and thoracolumbar spine. *Neurosurgery* 37:1–7, 1995.)

Disadvantages

When compared with the dorsolateral operations (transfacet and transpedicular), the orientation to the disc space and ventral spinal canal is more direct. This more direct orientation must be weighed against the more extensive muscle and bone manipulation required by this surgery. If safety and efficacy are demonstrated clinically, the retropleural thoracotomy approach may be ideally suited for disc herniations that cannot be reliably treated using one of the less invasive dorsolateral techniques.

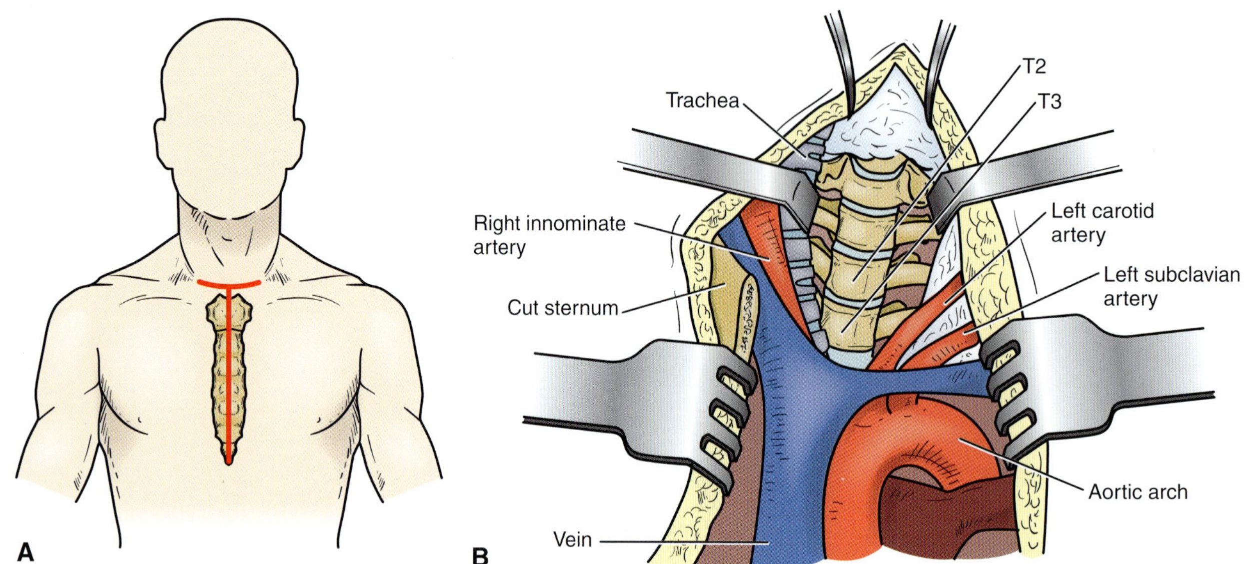

FIGURE 77-8. Transsternal approach. **A,** T-shaped incision with the transverse limb along the lower cervical skin crease and the vertical limb extending along the midline to below the xiphoid process. **B,** The vertebral column is exposed following sternal splitting, dissection, and retraction of the intervening structures. (From Stillerman CB, Weiss MH: Management of thoracic disc disease. *Clin Neurosurg* 38:325–352, 1992.)

Ventral Approaches

Transsternal Approach

The transsternal approach may be an option for the management of midline, densely calcified herniations between T2 and T5 (Fig. 77-8).[11,17] When the surgery requires access to the T4-5 levels, preoperative imaging must define the relationship between the aortic arch and the ventral spinal column.

Technique

This operation is generally performed through a T-shaped skin incision that has its vertical limb extending from the lower cervical skin crease to a few centimeters below the xiphoid process (see Fig. 77-8A). The strap muscles are then divided, and the precervical fascia and pretracheal fascia incised at the level of the sternal notch. The sternum is then split and retracted laterally. After the exposure of the pericardium and thymus, the thymus is retracted to the right, exposing the left innominate vein, which can be sacrificed. The working space is between the left common carotid artery and the innominate artery, trachea, esophagus, and thyroid. Gentle retraction of these structures exposes the ventral region of the spinal column (see Fig. 77-8B). Once the ventral spine is exposed, the disc is removed using standard microdiscectomy techniques that are used during ventral cervical microdiscectomy.[11,17]

Recently, Teng et al. proposed an easy MRI method to measure and categorize individual anatomic variations within the cervicothoracic junction (CTJ). They divided a group of normal patients into three groups based on their lesion relative to the suprasternal notch (STN). In the majority of patients, the T3 vertebra is above the STN, and lesions may be approached via a suprasternal approach. In patients with long necks, this exposure could be carried down one or two vertebral levels lower than those in the short-necked group. In approximately one third of the cases, the lesion is below the STN, and a combined approach involving a manubriotomy and sternotomy is required.[9]

Advantages and Disadvantages

The primary advantage of this approach is the management of thoracic disc herniations that are midline and densely calcified in the upper thoracic spine.[4] The other advantages are similar to those for the ventrolateral approaches. This is clearly a challenging operation with the potential for significant physiologic cost to the patient. Fortunately, disc herniations in the upper thoracic spine are quite rare, constituting just a fraction of symptomatic disc herniations.[4] Most of these herniations can be treated successfully using one of the other, less invasive approaches. In addition to all the disadvantages encountered with the ventrolateral approaches, the transsternal approach has the unique risk of injury to the left recurrent laryngeal nerve and the thoracic duct.[17]

Complications

Thoracic Disc Series

Several independently reported reviews of thoracic disc herniations have appeared in the literature.[1,2,44-47] Many of these reports provide excellent historic perspectives that include surgeries performed before the 1930s. For a better understanding of the overall effectiveness of modern thoracic disc herniation management, a focused review of several large series is presented in Table 77-2.[4] Chen has summarized the results of outcomes of various thoracic disc procedures. Outcomes were measured as improvement in pain control or myelopathy (if present). Duration of surgery, length of hospital stay, and patient satisfaction were reported for the various approaches. Moreover, complications of thoracic discectomy, including paraparesis, instability, dural tear, and pseudomeningocele, were reported.[48] Recently, Stillerman et a1.[4] reported their experience with the operative management of 82 symptomatic herniated thoracic discs.

Thoracic Disc Series 1986 to 1997[5]

Name	Year	Surgical Approach	PTS/Discs	PAIN Back Pre/Post	PAIN Radicular Pre/Post	PAIN Motor Deficit Pre/Post	PAIN Bowel/ Dysfunction Pre/Post	Bladder Complications
Lesoin et al.	1986	Lam 3 MTP 16 TT2	21/22	NR	5/5	16/10	NR	Major 1 (4.5%) Paraparesis permanent Minor 1 (4.5%) Paraparesis transient Total (9%)
Bohlman and Zdeblick	1988	Costo 11 TT8	19/22	13/10	4/1 + NR	14/12	8/2 + NR	Major 2 (9%) 1 paraparesis permanent; 1 wrong level → redo surgery Minor 1 (4.5%) Paraparesis transient Total (13.6%)
Blumenkopf	1988	TT4 TP3	9/#7	7/7	4/4	3/2	1/1	NR
Otani et al.	1988	MCos 23	23/23	NR	NR	23/23	23/18	NR
El-Kalliny et al.	1991	TP8 TT8 Costo 5	21/23	15/11	13/11	10/8	6/NR	Major 3 (13%) 1 paraparesis permanent – TT1 pleural effusion → surgery for CSF leak → TT1 CVA Minor 1 (4.3%) Pleural effusion Total (17.4%)
Singounas et al.	1992	Costo 14 MCos 4	14/14	NR	NR	NR	NR	Major 3 (21.4%) 1 paraparesis; 1 discitis; 1 compound fracture from discitis
Le Roux et al.	1993	TP 20	20/23	17/14	17/16	3/3	1/1	NR
Fessler	1993	LEC 17	17/22	15/10	7/5	8/8		Minor 2 (9%) 1 anesthesia dolorosa; 1 pneumonia
Ridenour et al.	1993 Costo 15	Lam 4 TP12	31/3311/7	12/5	18/9	13/8		Major 3 (9%) 1 increased myelopathy; 1 wrong level additional surgery; 1 incomplete disc removal → redo surgery Minor 3 (9%) 3 superficial wound infection Total (18.2%)
Simpson et al.	1993	MCos 16	21/23	19/19	6/4	4/3	NR	NR
Oppenheim et al.	1993	Costo 8	12/8	7/6	NR	1/1		Major 1 (12.5%) 1 wrong diagnosis progressive weakness; AVM found 3 levels; caudal operated level
Currier et al.	1994	TT19	19/22	15/10	11/7	6/NR		Major 3 (13.6%) 1 nonfatal PE; 1 intraoperative hemodynamic instability vs. tack. + hypotension; 1 spinal instability kyphosis after Lam + TT Minor 10 (41%) 1 incisional hernia; 1 dural tear intraoperative repair + drain; 2 transient urinary retention; 2 UTIs; 4 chronic thoracotomy pain Total (54.5%)
Bilsky and Patterson	1997	TP20	20/20	7/5 MCos 4	6/4	11/11	6/5	Minor 3 (15%) 1 pseudomeningitis; 1 deep wound infection; 1 transient increase in myelopathy

AVM, arteriovenous malformation; *Costo*, costotransversectomy; *CSF*, cerebrospinal fluid; *CVA*, cardiovascular accident; *Lam*, laminectomy; *LEC*, lateral extracavitary; *MCos*, modified costotransversectomy; *MTP*, modified transpedicular; *NR*, not reported; *PE*, pulmonary embolism; *Pre/post*, preoperative signs + symptoms/postoperative patients with resolution or improvement; *TP*, transpedicular; *TT*, transthoracic; *UTI*, urinary tract infection; #7, 7 discs operated (2 treated conservatively), #8, 8 discs operated (4 treated conservatively).

From Stillerman CB, Chen TC, Couldwell WT, et al. Surgical experience in the operative management of 82 symptomatic herniated thoracic discs and review of the literature. *J Neurosurg* 88:623–633, 1998.

TABLE 77-3

Surgical Complications in 82 Thoracic Microdiscectomies

Complication Type	No. of Complications
Death	1 (1.2%)
Loss of spinal integrity	
Stable compression	
Fx: braced	1 (1.2%)
Fx with kyphosis: surgery	1 (1.2%)
Increased weakness	
Transient (resolved 48 hr)	1 (1.2%)
Permanent mild residual deficit	1 (1.2%)
Superficial wound infection	3 (3.7%)
Pneumonia	3 (3.7%)
Seizure	1 (1.2%)
Total	**12 (14.6%)**

Fx, fracture.

From Stillerman CB, Chen TC, Couldwell WT, et al: Surgical experience in the operative management of 82 symptomatic herniated thoracic discs and review of the literature. *J Neurosurg* 88:623–633, 1998.

In this series the overall complication rate was 12/82 (14.6%). Three major complications (3.6%) occurred, consisting of one perioperative death from cardiopulmonary complications in a patient at high medical risk, spinal instability requiring further surgery, and an increase in the severity of a preoperative paraparesis. There were 9/82 (11%) minor complications, which consisted of one transient paraparesis that completely resolved after 48 hours, one compression fracture treated with 3 months of bracing, three superficial wound infections, three pneumonias, and one postoperative seizure. All of the minor complications were treated medically with no sequelae (Table77-3).[4] Results of this series compared with 13 other contemporary series demonstrated a 6.1% major complication rate (16/263) compared with a 3.6% rate (3/82) in the series. This difference was not found to be statistically significant (chi-square test). Although several deaths were reported in earlier studies,[13,14,21,45,49] none occurred in the 13 contemporary review series. The minor complications reported in the review group constituted 8.7% (23/263), compared with 11% (9/82) in the series. The total complication rate reported was 14.8% (39/263) in the review group and 14.6% (12/82) in the series. Like the case with major complications, there was no significant difference in either the total complication rate or minor complication rate.

Based on experience gained with the ventrolateral and lateral surgeries during the course of the series of 82 thoracic discectomies, the well-documented success by others using the dorsolateral transpedicular approach, and the preliminary experience reported with the transthoracic thoracoscopy, retropleural thoracotomy, and transfacet pedicle-sparing approaches, guidelines for selection of a surgical approach have been developed[4] (see Table 77-1).

Special Considerations

Localization

Care must be exercised when attempting to localize a lesion totally on the basis of MRI. For example, the MRI may count the level of the lesion by counting from an end vertebra (i.e., the sacrum or C2). At operation, it is often not possible to count from the end vertebra, so one must count from the rib. In a small but significant percentage of the population, there may be variations in the number of non–rib-bearing lumbar vertebrae or even in the size of the 12th thoracic rib. Therefore, it might be important to reconcile the MRI level with plain films to know the number of nonrib lumbar vertebrae and the size of the 12th rib. Other measures, such as preoperative marking with fluoroscopy, may provide useful information about the level of the herniation.

Failure to Achieve Objective

A thorough review of preoperative studies to determine the size and location of the disc herniation within the spinal canal (i.e., centrolateral vs. lateral, extradural vs. intradural, migration away from the disc space) helps the surgeon determine whether the disc herniation has been completely removed. Examination of the ventral spinal canal with a dental mirror, or through endoscopy, or perhaps the appreciation of the restoration of dural pulsations following the removal of the disc are all means of gaining information on the extent of disc herniation that has been removed. It is important to realize that often a very thin layer of posterior longitudinal ligament remains after the standard removal of the disc. This layer must be fenestrated so that the actual dura is identified to minimize the possibility of a retained disc fragment.

Management of Dural Openings

A CSF leak is not nearly as problematic for the dorsolateral extrapleural approaches as it is for the transthoracic approaches. A CSF–pleural fistula may be difficult to treat. When a dural opening is made during transthoracic surgery, an attempt to achieve a watertight dural closure either primarily or with use of a graft should be made. A small pleural flap may be utilized. Additionally, fibrin glue to reinforce the suture line may be helpful. Using a chest tube with a water seal in instituting spinal drainage avoids creating a CSF–pleural fistula.

New Paradigm for Thoracic Disc Herniations

Based on an evaluation of the aforementioned contemporary series, a management paradigm was developed for treating this disorder[4] (Fig. 77-9). The natural history of the disease, the patient's initial presentation, correlation with MRI findings, and current neurologic examination are crucial to the decision process for surgical versus conservative management. Patients with symptoms from thoracic disc herniations are placed into one of three groups: localized/axial pain, radicular pain, or myelopathy.

Localized/Axial Pain

Patients with back pain alone who do not have myelopathy or severe unrelenting radicular pain constitute a difficult management problem because of the nonspecific nature of

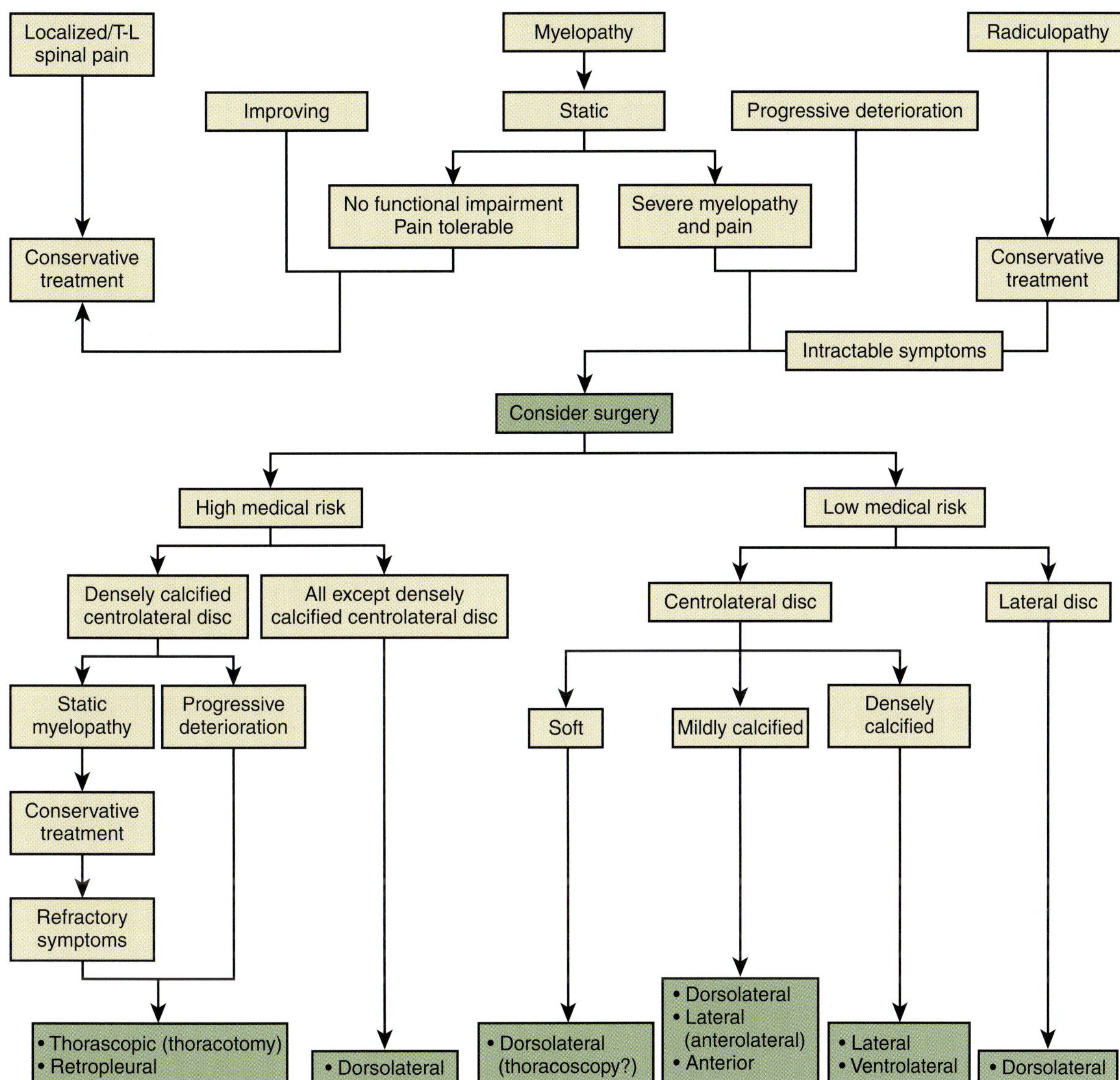

FIGURE 77-9. Management scheme for treating symptomatic thoracic disc herniations. (From Stillerman CB, Chen TC, Couldwell WT, et al: Surgical experience in the operative management of 82 symptomatic herniated thoracic discs and review of the literature. *J Neurosurg* 88:623–633, 1998.)

their pain syndrome. Surgery has a high failure rate in these patients and must be individualized.

Radiculopathy

Patients who are experiencing severe radiculopathy that is refractory to aggressive nonoperative management are evaluated for surgery. This generally consists of a dorsolateral approach for decompression because radiculopathy alone is generally associated with a far lateral disc or an osteophyte.

Myelopathy

Patients with myelopathy who are shown to have a disc herniation are treated based on the status of their neurologic deficit. The following are intended to serve as suggested considerations; the ultimate choice of procedure must be influenced by the surgeon's familiarity and skill with the different approaches. Patients who have a nonsevere static deficit without functional impairment and whose pain is tolerable are treated nonoperatively. Patients who are improving from the standpoint of their myelopathy are likewise treated conservatively. When the myelopathy is either severe and nonprogressive or progressing, the patients are entered into either a high-medical-risk or a low-medical-risk group. In the low-medical-risk group, the parameters influencing the selection of a particular approach include the position of the disc in the spinal canal (centrolateral vs. lateral herniation) and the consistency of the disc (soft vs. mildly calcified vs. densely calcified). Additionally, the location of the calcium in the disc (i.e., ventral vs. dorsal) is important in ascertaining the likelihood of significant dural adherence by the disc material. High-medical-risk patients with severe (static or progressive) myelopathy should undergo dorsolateral decompression unless the disc is midline or central-lateral,[1] large, and densely calcified. Patients with these types of discs are operated on, using either a transthoracic thoracoscopy or retropleural approach, or, on occasion, a transthoracic thoracotomy. The high-medical-risk patients with densely calcified central-lateral discs and static myelopathies are initially treated conservatively. However, if their symptoms prove to be refractory, they are operated on with the same surgical approaches used for patients found to have progressive deterioration in their myelopathy.

Future Trends

Future trends for thoracic discectomy emphasize enhanced imaging, visualization, and smaller incisions. These approaches may be performed dorsolaterally as demonstrated by the minimally invasive endoscopic approaches advocated by Jho[26] and Fessler.[50] Thorascopic endoscopic approaches via a ventrolateral approach are also popular because of the increased visualization provided by the endoscope. Lastly, intraoperative imaging using neuronavigational systems has been advocated to enhance visualization with open procedures.

Summary

The review of contemporary thoracic disc herniation management has illustrated that its treatment still poses a significant problem. Patient outcome has improved considerably from earlier series. Further refinement of management, however, is necessary. The optimal treatment strategy must be designed based on the patient presentation, medical condition, and disc characteristics and the surgeon's familiarity with each approach. Because all of the surgical cornerstones for the treatment of symptoms of thoracic disc herniations have the potential for significant morbidity, there needs to be continued effort in the improvement of *minimally invasive* techniques. It is unlikely that one particular operation will become a panacea for all situations. Therefore, it is important that treating clinicians maintain proficiency in multiple surgical options.

KEY REFERENCES

Brown CW, Deffer PA, Akmakjian J, et al: The natural history of thoracic disc herniation. *Spine (Phila Pa 1976)* 17:S97–S102, 1992.

Maiman DJ, Larson SJ, Luck E, El-Ghatit A: Lateral extracavitary approach to the spine for thoracic disc herniation: report of 23 cases. *Neurosurgery* 14:178–182, 1984.

McCormick PC: Retropleural approach to the thoracic and thoracolumbar spine. *Neurosurgery* 37:1–7, 1995.

Patterson RH Jr, Arbit E: A surgical approach through the pedicle to protruded thoracic discs. *J Neurosurg* 48:768–772, 1978.

Perez-Cruet MJ, Kim BS, Sandhu F, et al: Thoracic microendoscopic discectomy. *J Neurosurg Spine* 1:58–63, 2004.

Perot PL, Munro DD: Transthoracic removal of midline thoracic disc protrusions causing spinal cord compression. *J Neurosurg* 31:452–458, 1969.

Stillerman CB, Chen TC, Couldwell WT, et al: Surgical experience in the operative management of 82 symptomatic herniated thoracic discs and review of the literature. *J Neurosurg* 88:623–633, 1998.

Stillerman CB, Chen TC, Day JD, et al: The transfacet pedicle-sparing approach for thoracic disc removal: cadaveric morphometric analysis and preliminary clinical experience. *J Neurosurg* 83:971–976, 1995.

REFERENCES

The complete reference list is available online at expertconsult.com.

CHAPTER 78

Lumbar Discectomy

Bruce L. Ehni | Krishna Satyan

An estimated 12 million Americans suffer from significant degenerative lumbar disc disease. Approximately one million patients per year undergo surgeries, of which about 200,000 to 300,000 are lumbar discectomies.[1-5] The combination of tremendous volume and a broad spectrum of standard care, including often vague surgical indications, makes lumbar disc pathology an object of legitimate scrutiny. However, proper patient selection and surgical technique can provide excellent and satisfying results for patients and surgeons alike. Neurosurgeons working in this field should remain scrupulously objective in patient selection, abreast of evidence-based outcomes research, and cautious in the selection of new technology.

Lumbar laminectomy for disc hernia or anular prolapse is one of the most common operations performed by North American spine surgeons; it is also one of the most potentially successful. Lumbar laminectomy for herniated lumbar disc has endured considerable analysis and the test of substantial time since its inception 75 years ago and remains a fundamental part of most spine clinical practice. It is a cost-effective procedure for carefully selected patients, being relatively moderate in cost and providing substantial improvement in quality of life.[6]

While lumbar laminectomy may appear unchallenging to a casual observer, the pitfalls and potential complications are numerous. They include distinctions in patient selection, neuroimaging, timing of surgery, and technical nuances in the performance of the surgery and in the subsequent patient follow-up. It is difficult to find a more dissatisfied patient than one who has experienced a poor outcome from lumbar discectomy. Modern outcomes studies show that while short-term outcomes are excellent, long-term outcomes have to be considered as well.

The incidence of lumbar disc hernia peaks between 24 and 45 years of age, with the incidence of surgery most often in patients between 30 to 39 years. Males predominate, at 1.3:1 to 2:1, possibly because of larger mechanical stresses and more tenuous nutritional and waste diffusion through the disc, as will be addressed. Other classically regarded risk factors for disc herniation have included smoking, obesity (BMI >30), sedentary lifestyles, prolonged motor vehicle driving, previous full-term pregnancies, and operating heavily vibrating machinery.[1,4,7,8]

The Twin Spine Study, a research program investigating various environmental factors involved in the etiology and progression of disc degeneration, looked at differing occupational exposures, driving and whole-body vibration exposure, smoking exposure, anthropomorphic factors, heredity, and the identification of genotypes associated with disc degeneration in monozygotic male twins. Although some environmental factors are relevant, as was mentioned, disc degeneration appears to be determined more significantly by genetics. There is a modest correlation with lifting and smoking but little influence from occupational and leisure-time physical loading activities such as sports and resistance training throughout adulthood. The effect of anthropometric factors, such as body weight and muscle strength, appears to be greater than the effect of occupational physical demands. Routine loading and physical demand may actually have some benefits for the disc, physical inactivity being a greater risk factor.[9,10]

The advent of magnification has permitted a small incision, diminished muscle trauma, and reduced manipulation of neural structures. Consequently, outpatient lumbar microdiscectomy has become popular, with success rates equal to those found in initial microdiscectomy studies. Microdiscectomy (by which is understood a small incision, not necessarily use of the microscope) has become standard care, with use of large open incisions now being the exception.

Terminology of disc pathology is of particular importance in the venture of spine surgery and spine clinical research and has important implications for treatment options. The authors endorse the standardization of nomenclature recommended by the combination of the North American Spine Society, the American Society of Spine Radiology, and the American Society of Neuroradiology.[11] Not only do diagnostic radiologists and clinicians need to recognize and utilize the same terms to communicate effectively, but vague or loosely applied terms obscure the results of clinical research. The term *hernia* specifically defines nucleus and/or end-plate cartilaginous tissues escaping the confines of the anulus and residing outside the apophyseal ring. It might not be possible to radiographically determine an anular defect, so the use of the term *hernia* is legitimately broadened to refer to displacement of nucleus, cartilage, fragmented apophyseal bone, or fragmented anulus from its normal location to lie beyond the disc space; disruption of the anulus is implied. Use of the term *anular bulge* or *disc bulge* defines localized or circumferential prominence of an otherwise radiographically intact anulus, not disconnected from the apophyseal ring. It is also useful to add descriptive terms to further define a hernia, such as *protrusion* (broad base), *extrusion* (narrow base or neck), and *sequestrum* (lack of continuity to the disc of origin). The use of the term *rupture* is discouraged as inaccurate unless there is indeed a single violent traumatic event that is clearly the origin of a defect in a previously intact anulus and of resultant disc herniation.[11]

History

A condition that is recognized as sciatica, although not associated with spine abnormality, was described before the time of Alexander the Great.[12] In 1779, Pott[13] was able to associate deformity of the spinal column with sciatic pain. However, it was Lane[14] who described sciatic pain and its origin in a living patient in 1893 and Bailey and Casamajor,[15] in 1911, who described a small series, complete with radiographic studies. Also in 1911, Goldthwait,[16] who thought herniations of the disc were capable of producing sciatic and low back pain, presented a patient with lumbosacral disc hernia and paraplegia. In 1916, Elsberg[17] (who operated on the patients of Bailey and Casamajor and often noted relief after apparently no more than decompressive laminectomy) described it as attributable to a condition of cauda equina radiculitis. Parker and Adson[18] in 1925, Putti[19] in 1927, Dandy[20] in 1929, Mauric[21] in 1933, and others attributed sciatic pain to nerve root involvement within the spinal canal and believed that adjacent vertebral structures were responsible. In 1934, Mixter and Barr[22] published their milestone paper on the pathology and surgical findings associated with a ruptured nucleus pulposus, not only in the lumbar canal but also in the cervical and thoracic canals, complete with their diagnoses of the condition preoperatively.

The surgical procedure of choice for many of these pioneering surgeons was complete laminectomy, which often provided significant relief. Mixter and Barr favored a hemilaminectomy approach, as did Love, for the cases of simple herniated disc that were amenable to preoperative localization.[23] As experience accumulated, it became apparent that dural incision was unnecessary in most cases.

The complicating effect that developmental lumbar stenosis had on the pathology of disc diseases was appreciated in Verbiest's[24,25] reports from 1949 through 1955. Some of the more serious complications of surgery for lumbar disc hernia can be attributed to lack of preoperative appreciation of this anatomic variation and failure to tailor the procedure accordingly.

Working only with myelography and the power of clinical preoperative and subsequent intraoperative observation, the early surgeons were able to learn much and to steadily improve upon the surgical approach to lumbar disc disease. Currently, with the advantages of improved neurodiagnostic modalities in multiple planes, there is no longer much occasion for "surgical exploration," and it should not be common to find an intraoperative surprise. Surgeons should be capable not only of making the preoperative diagnosis but also of adhering to a secure surgical plan, one that should accomplish the goal of radicular or cauda equina decompression with minimal risk of complication or injury. Credit for the use of magnification and small incisions, which has become standard care, is given Williams[26] and Caspar.[27]

Outcomes

Relief of radiculopathic leg pain can be expected in the vast majority of patients who are appropriately selected for lumbar discectomy, with a 75% to 90% success rate.[2,3,28-34] This variability in reported results, which ranged between 75%[2] and nearly 90%[3] for good to excellent results, likely is due to data quality, patient selection, short follow-up, and differing definitions of good outcome.[2] The Asch paper is significant in that outcomes on over 200 patients who were operated on were prospectively determined by six parameters, including the preoperative ODI (Oswestry Disability Index), and the ODI at 1 and 10 days, 6 weeks, and 6 months and at least 12 months postoperatively. One of the most common causes for poor outcome is the poor definition of selection criteria for surgery, which varies remarkably between communities and countries, as much as fourfold or fivefold.[29,35-37] The procedure can be expected, with relative certainty, to relieve radiculopathic leg pain, but relief of back pain cannot be predicted.[38-42] Surgery appears to have the least measurable benefit at L5-S1, intermediate benefit at L4-5, and best results at L2-3 or L3-4, unless the conus is involved or cauda equina syndrome experienced. This may relate to the trend of conservatively treated hernias at upper lumbar levels faring worse than hernias at lower levels.[43]

Recurrent radiculopathy occurs in 5% to 10% of patients,[2,35,40,44] which approaches the lifetime incidence of disc surgery.[29] Less likely causes for failure include perineurial fibrosis and arachnoiditis. The subject of recurrence is important and is covered in depth later in the chapter.

The long-term outcomes of surgery and conservative treatment are similar, but in the short term, surgery provides the prospect of quicker relief than conservative measures do.[35,38,39,44-49] Quicker relief with surgery may translate into reduced economic cost.[6,50,51]

It is difficult to define preoperative findings that are predictive of success or failure, even in the largest series of patients. Part of the problem arises from the instability of results over time, with as many as 40% of patients crossing over from favorable to unfavorable postoperative groups and vice versa.[52] Useful clinical predictors of good outcome from surgery include good underlying health, absence of preoperative comorbidities, absence of previous nonspine surgery or of a workers' compensation claim, young age, the presence of radicular pain to the foot, positive straight-leg raise without back pain, and reflex asymmetry, in approximately descending order of significance.[28,38,39]

Risk factors associated with poor outcome include time off work in excess of 3 months, psychosocial problems including poor educational level, smoking, and possibly obesity. Some authors believe that although obesity complicates anesthesia and convalescence, it might not of itself adversely affect outcome.[28,53] Smoking is a risk factor for chronic low back pain[4,54,55] as well as a risk factor for hernia and poorer outcomes, as has been discussed. Perhaps because of the location of the dorsal root ganglion and because of the difficulty associated with surgically approaching lateral hernias, the probability of good outcome for extraforaminal hernias is not as great as that for paramedian hernia.[31,56]

Radiology, Indications for Discectomy, and Clinical Correlates

Patient selection is critical to good patient outcomes. Technique may not be as important as patient selection in lumbar discectomy. The patient selection pitfalls to be encountered, recognized, and avoided in lumbar discectomy surgery are numerous. Two of the most common errors are the misinterpretation of leg pain of some other origin as being radiculopathy and correlating back pain with an unrelated neuroimaging finding. The most important determinant in favor of proceeding to surgery should be strict correlation between the distribution of the radicular leg pain and the nerve root compression seen on preoperative imaging studies. Performed carefully and correctly, clinical examination can predict findings of neuroimaging and subsequent surgery approximately 70% to 80% of the time.[50,51,57-59]

There has been an increasing realization that information about morphology alone is not enough to make a definitive diagnosis. Radiographic prevalence on MRI of abnormalities in an asymptomatic population is the subject of dozens of papers. MRI-documented disc bulge appears present in up to 81%, protrusion in up to 63%, extrusion in up to 24%, dark disc in up to 83%, disc height loss in up to 56%, anular tears in up to 56%, and Schmorl nodes in up to 19% of asymptomatic volunteer individuals. The numbers are similar in patient populations that are chosen without regard to symptoms.[60,61] It can be said that the potential for finding false-positive indicators is universal, since they are nearly ubiquitous. As MRI scanning power and resolution improve with time, this problem will only grow larger. Also, clinicians and radiologists have different perspectives and perceptions when reading the same study; clinicians are more focused on clear description of the morphology of a particular pathologic finding than radiologists are.[62]

Contrasted MRI may occasionally be necessary. MRI with contrast can demonstrate inflammatory change on the periphery of the hernia, which can be of prognostic value. Contrast is useful to help differentiate nerve sheath tumor from disc material, with which it is often confused in the far lateral location, or other tumors and processes with which a hernia may be confused when it has migrated into unusual locations and into the posterior canal.[63] In the postoperative setting of recurrent radiculopathic pain, contrast will display epidural scar and inflammation around a nonenhancing retained or recurrent nuclear fragment. Occasionally, it is prudent to augment the MRI with CT. CT will show bone anatomy and important bony subtleties that the MRI might not show or might not show well yet that might be important to surgical planning, such as spondylolysis and apophyseal (limbic) fracture. In the case of apophyseal ring fracture, CT is often the best method of examination, while plain radiographs and MRI might not demonstrate the bone of the apophyseal ring.

The synthesis of a decision to operate should be scrupulously clean and based upon a combination of clinical factors and radiographic findings. If MRI and CT do not provide sufficient explanation for a clinical picture, the second-line alternatives of discography and myelography remain. Proponents of discography claim that, through pain provocation, it can provide the specificity that is missing from the purely morphologic information that CT and MR imaging provide. The specificity of discography, however, is far from clear.[64,65] If MR studies fail to provide clear evidence of lumbar disc hernia at the level corresponding with the clinical presentation, myelography may be useful, particularly when no neurologic deficit exists, multiple nerve roots are involved, or a centrally herniated disc affects only a single root.

Regardless of which neuroimaging study is chosen, the findings on the neuroimaging study must be supported by clinical evidence of nerve root compression, given the ubiquitous nature of false-positive findings.

Not only is there great potential for spine MRI scans and other modern neuroimaging to display abnormal findings and poorly interpreted information that have great potential to lead to inappropriate management, but they can also lead to inappropriate, expensive, and disabling behaviors from the patient. Radiologists must take some responsibility for the way in which their reports are used and interpreted. The addition of epidemiologic data and statements may be worthwhile.[66] In an effort to standardize neuroradiologic readings, the North American Spine Society, American Society of Spine Radiology, and American Society of Neuroradiology established a combined task force with recommendations for readings.[11]

Preoperative clinical history may give clues to the anatomic severity of lumbar disc pathology, whether it is an intact anulus (negative exploration or protruding disc at surgery), a ruptured anulus (subligamentous incarceration), or a completely free disc. Vucetic et al. found that shorter duration of leg pain predicted a ruptured anulus; in their series, a 10-week period of symptoms was found in rupture versus a 50-week period found for an intact anulus. Lack of comorbidity predicted a ruptured anulus, with 18% of patients with rupture having prior medical or psychiatric treatment versus 39% of patients with an intact anulus having prior treatment for other diagnoses. Having had previous nonspine surgery was recorded in 32% of patients with a ruptured anulus, while 55% was recorded in patients with an intact anulus. The two groups differed then not only in disc pathology but also in medical, behavioral, and social factors, which undoubtedly plays a role in surgical outcomes.[59]

In practice and as a prerequisite for successful surgery, there should be a strong correlation between the pain, neurologic deficit, and preoperative imaging findings, and this rule should be inflexible. Much of the U.S. population obtains information from the Internet, for which there are no standards regarding quality and content, and at least a third of the available information may be of dubious value and/or distorted by potential commercial gain.[67] Between the power of modern MRI scanning and the influence of the Internet on patients, contemporary spine surgeons must keep their perspectives scientifically valid and treatment goals clear.

Biology of Disc Degeneration

In the well-hydrated discs of youth, the mechanical stresses that are applied to the vertebral column are borne more upon the center of the end plates; but with desiccation, the loads become transmitted more to the periphery of the vertebral body. Ultimately, the anulus bears more load than it is capable of handling, particularly at the posterolateral segment, and hernia occurs. Nutritional support of the living tissue of the disc is dependent on a number of factors, including size of the disc, changes in the vertebral body end plates from which nutritional support diffuses, age-dependent cell density within the disc, and patterns and levels of physical activity that may encourage or discourage diffusion of nutrients to and waste from and through the tissue.[68] The avascular nature of the mature disc also makes it unable to remove and replace degradation products. The mature disc is one of the most sparsely cellular tissues in the body yet with one of the densest extracellular matrices to maintain, dependent on the health of those cells.[69]

The chemical makeup of various tissues of the disc changes with age, potentially increasing in fragility. Collagen is widely distributed in the body, of various compositions; types I, II, III, VI, and IX are found in the nucleus and anulus in both normal and pathologically degenerated discs, but types III and VI are increased in areas of degeneration. Mutations in at least two collagen IX genes, COL9A2 and COL9A3, have been associated with higher likelihood of hernia, and the presence of childhood hernia implies genetic predisposition outside of environmental factors that are commonly held to be responsible.[60,70,71] At a molecular level, collagen cross-links are important to the mechanical stability of the disc, particularly perhaps the anulus. The variety of proteoglycans in the extracellular matrix of the nucleus also change in abundance and structure through life and in their ability to retain hydration of the disc and ability to maintain the electrokinetic environment important to water and nutrient transport. Disc matrix proteins such as fibronectin and elastin throughout the anulus and nucleus also change in age and degeneration.[69]

The most dramatic changes in degenerating discs occur in the loss of hydrostatic pressure as maintained by the negatively charged proteoglycans, in water content, in cell populations, and consequently in cellular biosynthesis and repair. Mechanical stimuli can elicit different cellular responses from similar cells depending on whether the tissue is of the nucleus and inner anulus or outer anulus. The difference potentially amounts to an anabolic response to mechanical stress in nucleus and inner anulus tissues and a catabolic response in outer anulus tissue.[72] Lack of mechanical stimuli or hypomobility of the disc produces changes that may promote degenerative change.[73]

Apart from the molecular changes, the anulus ages as well at a microstructural level. A significant element in the strength of the anulus comes not only from fiber orientation in alternating lamellae, but also interconnectivity between them.[74] With age, decreases in the presence of pyridinoline (by age 65, 50% of that found in younger people) and increases in pentosidine occur within the disc. Decreases in pyridinoline cross-links lead to alterations in the collagen matrix of the disc. Integrity of the anulus deteriorates, perhaps beginning with the translamellar interconnections, leading to delamination of the anulus and ultimately anular tear or fissure. The presence of a tear or fissure does not imply traumatic origin.

Certain proteinases that are not normally present in the healthy disc also begin to appear in aged discs and are at least partially responsible for the degeneration of the extracellular matrix in the anulus, nucleus, and end plate.[75,76] On a macroscopic radiographic level, though, while all the foregoing changes are occurring and fibrous tissue replaces the nuclear mucoid matrix of youth, disc height may yet be preserved, and disc margins remain intact.[64]

The anatomic composition of disc hernia changes with advancing age and perhaps to some extent with gender. In youth, a particular problem of hernia is involvement of the apophyseal ring. The movement of the hernia and anulus avulses the apophyseal ring into the canal, away from its immature attachment to the vertebral body,[77] which often produces more mass effect than will more common nuclear fragments alone. In adolescents and young adults, a hernia is more likely to be composed of nucleus pulposus. As the nucleus becomes more fibrous with age, the percentage of nucleus in the fragments becomes lower, and the likelihood of finding cartilaginous end plate and anulus increases, such that by age 70, a disc hernia is unlikely to contain any nucleus. Women may be found to have higher percentages of cartilaginous end plate than men.[78]

Back Pain

While the topic of discogenic back pain is not the focus of this chapter, lumbar discectomy is often regarded as treatment for lumbar pain, and the association merits brief review here. Low back pain is a poor indicator for discectomy surgery. Diagnosis of the precise disc among many that might be the source of back pain can be difficult, if not impossible, in most cases because neurologic examinations in patients with only back pain and the absence of radiculopathy provide no direction and because radiologic abnormalities do not necessarily correlate with the source of pain. Something like 85% of patients with low back pain cannot be given a legitimate precise diagnosis of its anatomic origin.[44,65] A plain radiographic survey of adults over age 65, examining a cohort of subjects with chronic daily lumbar pain and those without, demonstrates the ubiquity of findings in the discs and facets regardless of pain status. While higher degrees of radiographic severity on plain films may be seen in the pain group as a whole, there is no correlation with the degree of pain experienced.[79]

An anatomic cause is impossible to establish despite modern neuroimaging. In Western medicine, patients expect and press for plain radiographs, despite the widely known lack of correlation with back pain.[66,80] The plain radiographs will often lead to more sensitive imaging studies such as MRI. MRI, in turn, is so sensitive and generally readily accessible that these virtues can in a certain way be looked upon as drawbacks. It is a rare scan that is read as normal or even normal for age, yet it is well known that sizable protrusions and extrusions exist commonly in asymptomatic patients.[9,60,61,64] Therefore, interpretation of the neuroimaging studies must be made in the context of good clinical information. There is "an increasing realization that information about morphology alone is not enough to make a definitive diagnosis."[64] It is difficult for the backache patient (and perhaps even the referring doctor) to conceive that radiographs, MRI, and/or CT-myelogram showing pathology have no relationship to the pain. In fact, just the knowledge of pathology can adversely affect outcome.[80] If present at multiple levels, the presence of a "dark nucleus" on MRI begins to predict a likelihood of back pain, but the pain generator remains unknown, whether it is the anulus, vertebrae, ligaments, fascia, muscles, or facets.[8] The advantage of such sensitivity, of course, is that modern neuroimaging, particularly MRI, has eliminated the need for surgical exploration.

Back surgery on disc hernias as described in this chapter may do little for back pain, and the presence or absence of back pain should have little bearing on the patient's selection for surgery.[42] There are exceptions, however. If a large hernia appears to be responsible for radiographically visible elevation of the posterior longitudinal ligament off the vertebral bodies, particularly in midline,[31] discectomy and the resultant relaxation of tension on the ligament might well result in relief of the resultant back pain. If the hernia is large and midline or if the lumbar spinal canal is shallow and resulting central stenosis of the lumbar canal is caused by disc herniation, the patient may develop a reflexive posture of lumbar flexion (the shopping cart position), which results in lumbar fatigue and pain. The symptoms can often be relieved by surgical decompression of the involved motion segment. In the Maine Lumbar Spine Study, an assessment of the predominant symptom, back pain or leg pain, was made, and improvement in back pain was documentable.[35] However, it should be made clear to the patient without mechanical instability, facing the prospect of simple single-level surgery for degenerative disc disease, that surgery might have no impact on the lumbar pain. Lumbar pain is manageable by other interventions that are outside the scope of this chapter, such as exercises and other conservative measures, injection treatments, and surgical fusion.[81]

Radicular Symptoms

Contemporary outcomes assessment is based on the practical premise that lumbar disc hernia surgery is directed specifically toward radiculopathy. Assessment of the depth of the spinal canal by preoperative imaging is an integral part of the decision to operate. Central spinal canal capacity and the presence or absence of lateral recess stenosis have significant bearing on the presence of nerve root compression and the patient's amenability to surgery. A small bulge or prolapse in one patient with developmental or acquired stenosis can be more damaging to the traversing nerve root or roots than a large extrusion in another patient with a spacious canal.

Radiculopathic leg pain with straight-leg raise and with Valsalva maneuver is more likely to be positive in herniations of L4-5 and L5-S1, where the compression and irritation are more likely to be at the axilla of the nerve root. The femoral stretch test is more likely to be positive at higher lumbar levels.[51] Monoradiculopathic leg pain, or sciatica, is the most useful clinical correlate. It is superior to straight-leg raising, scoliosis, and sensorimotor deficits.[82] Leg pain is often more severe in extraforaminal hernia than in intraforaminal or paramedian hernia, perhaps resulting from direct compression of the dorsal root ganglion by the hernia.[56]

Leg pain is perhaps the most common indicator, and the best indicator, for discectomy. However, conservative measures should be applied for a period of several weeks or longer from onset, if at all possible, prior to consideration for surgery, since long-term outcomes (4 years and more) are similar for conservative and operative care.[38,39,46] In practice, however, the time required for spontaneous resolution of radiculopathy to occur may be more than some patients can bear, so pain becomes an important determinant for surgery. It is commonly accepted that the longer pain and numbness exist prior to decompression, the longer they will last following decompression.[83] Furthermore, there is a legitimate fear that even permanent deafferentation pain can result from untreated compression.[42,84] Inflammation from the disc hernia can adversely affect the nerve root over time and thus affect prognosis.[52] Chronic pathologic changes can occur in the nerve root from prolonged compression, and over time (estimated at 3 to 6 months), there may be irreversible neuropathic changes.[31,42,46] However, literature review and common clinical experience dictate that there is no consensus on what constitutes an appropriate conservative trial, and there is no consensus on what constitutes the factors leading to irreversible nerve root damage. Solid evidence for the hypothesis that delayed surgery impairs results may be debatable.[85] Perhaps this lack of consensus is because there is selection bias to intermediate-level patients without sensorimotor deficit.

The patient's economic imperatives become an important and valid factor in the selection of surgery in the presence of work disability and the requirement for rapid return to work. Surgery provides more rapid relief than conservative measures do.[35] Also, long-term conservative care may ultimately be more expensive than surgery (in properly selected surgical candidates).[50]

Motor and sensory deficits are surgical indicators. It is practical to observe mild motor weakness and to follow for a period of time if stable. Motor deficit that is not improving, however, may be considered a surgical indicator,[42] as should progressively worsening motor deficit[31] and, of course, severe motor deficit.[85]

As will be seen, spontaneous resorption of disc material occurs and should be allowed to progress given the absence of severe motor deficit and the patient's ability to comply. It is, almost paradoxically, a phenomenon that is likely to be more satisfactory and complete in larger hernias, when there is true extrusion, rather than in simple contained anular prolapse. Extrusion past the anulus marshals the processes of inflammation and phagocytosis of the mass.[45,46,86-88]

Disc Resorption

The spontaneous resolution of the initially agonizing symptoms of both back and leg pain as well as the radiographic findings of lumbar disc hernia with time is well established.[7,35,38,39,41,44,47,75,89-95] Several mechanisms may be involved with the phenomenon of regression of disc hernia. Capillaries invade the hernia, and macrophages derived from monocytes migrate out into the hernia and begin a process of phagocytosis. Macrophages are the most commonly found cell type in both acute and chronic disc herniation. Macrophages contain enzymatic lysosomes, which degrade intracellular collagen and other substances present in disc material after phagocytosis. Macrophages also can secrete lysosomes, promoting the breakdown of extracellular substances such as collagen. Both of these mechanisms are closely involved in the regression of herniation. Apoptosis may occur at a higher rate in free disc fragments, another possible mechanism of absorption.

Macrophage activity itself can be a determinant of pain. There is a statistically significant correlation between histologically observed macrophage infiltration of intraoperative disc specimens and postoperative pain grading; patients who harbor inflammatory histology rate postoperative complaints lower than do patients with no evidence of inflammatory reactions.[52,96] The periradicular inflammation that accompanies the hernia characterized by macrophage response also includes an increase in IL-1β and a release of PGE-2.[75]

Discs that are found to have intense perilesional gadolinium enhancement are more likely to regress spontaneously, the thickness of rim enhancement being a strong determinant of spontaneous resorption. Clinical symptom alleviation occurs concordantly with a faster resorption rate. MRI with contrast can be a useful prognostic tool for identifying patients with herniated nucleus pulposus (HNP)–induced sciatica with a benign natural course.[92,93] Ninety-five percent of patients, followed out to 7 years, have decreases in the size of hernia through absorption of the disc. Progression of other disc degenerations occurs in all patients as well.[90]

Role of Surgery

The association between prolonged delay of treatment and poor outcome has been documented.[35,38,39,83,97] In prospective studies of patients having lumbar disc hernia surgery, the duration of leg pain and duration of sick leave are found to be of prognostic value, with leg pain lasting over 8 months predicting a worse outcome, including inability to return to work.[83,98]

Part of the radicular symptomatology of the disc hernia is due not only to the described inflammatory changes, but also to tethering of and ischemic change in the root resulting from periradicular inflammation. As measured by laser Doppler flow, intraneural flow is improved after discectomy.[99,100] Ischemic damage to the root, if present and productive of serious motor deficit, could be expected to have a poor prognosis, better avoided with decompression.

There is good objective evidence that surgery plays a legitimate role in the treatment of acute lumbar radiculopathy from lumbar disc hernia, bringing patients a faster and earlier recovery than would have occurred spontaneously.[35,38,39,44,47-49,101] Nearly universally accepted indications for early surgery include significant motor deficit, unmanageable refractory pain persisting for more than 6 to 12 weeks, and of course cauda equina syndrome.[7] Practicing neurosurgeons have long observed quick resolution of worrisome motor deficit in surgically treated patients.

While patients with worrisome motor deficit may be a small proportion of lumbar disc hernia patients, the cohorts of patients who are willing to accept randomization into prospective randomized controlled trials can be assumed to be underrepresented.

Weber has shown in a prospective randomized study comparing conservative to operative management that surgery produced significantly better outcomes in the short term: 90% versus 60% at 1year, still slightly better with surgery at 4 years, but no difference at 10 years. The study in effect reported a subgroup of patients with moderate indications for surgery. Of the original 280 patients, 67 had what were considered definite indications for surgery and were not randomized, and 87 patients who improved with conservative management were not randomized. One hundred twenty-six patients who could be treated either surgically or conservatively were randomized. The results may be interpreted as showing that if there is clinical uncertainty about the offer of surgery, delaying surgery to observe further clinical progress in these moderately symptomatic patients may delay their recovery but does not produce long-term harm.

Similarly, Peul et al. found that surgery offered short-term benefit. In a randomized prospective trial of early surgery (mean: 2 weeks) versus late surgery (mean: 18 weeks) or conservative treatment, relief of leg pain and recovery was faster in early surgery patients. By 1 year, however, there was a 95% probability of perceived recovery in both the surgically treated cohort and the delayed or conservatively treated cohorts.[47] Osterman found similar results at 2 years.[49] Longer-term results were found by Weber at 4 years,[38,39] the SPORT (Spine Patient Outcomes Research Trial) study at 4 years,[44] and the unrandomized but large and comprehensive Maine Lumbar Spine Study at 10 years.[35] At 1 year and at 4 years, in the prospective randomized multi-institutional SPORT lumbar disc series, patients who were operated on (in both the randomized and nonrandomized cohorts, without regard for intent to treat) maintained greater improvement (in SF-36 Bodily Pain and Physical Function scales and in the ODI) compared to patients patients who were not operated on, although long-term work status was not significantly benefited, as was mentioned. In the short term (3 months), work status was worse in the former group than in the latter, owing to surgical convalescence.[44]

In the Maine lumbar spine study, there did appear to be long-term benefit for patients who received surgery compared to hernia patients who did not. Surgical patients reported resolution or substantial improvement (56% vs. 40%, $P = .006$) and more satisfaction with their current status (71% vs. 56%, $P = .002$). However, work and disability status at 10 years were comparable among those treated surgically or nonsurgically.[35]

With regard to work status, these two large studies agree on lack of long-term surgical benefit.[35,44] On the other hand, a cost-effectiveness analysis performed in concert with the SPORT series resulted in the demonstration of a cost per quality adjusted year of life of approximately $69,000 in 2008 U.S. dollars, supporting the use of surgery as a cost-effective procedure in the short term and for markedly symptomatic patients.

Despite the volume of patients who are seen and treated annually, the breadth of literature on the subject, and these recent high-quality studies, there remains a need for longer-term randomized controlled trials that would address the lifetime consequences of surgery.

In the long term, children may do significantly better than adults following lumbar disc surgery; surgery does not appear to lead to chronic complaints of back pain.[102]

In summary, the ideal patient for discectomy is one with severe, disabling unilateral radiculopathic leg pain without severe sensorimotor loss for whom conservative measures over a period of a few weeks to 2 months have yielded little.[42] A poorer recovery can be expected in the presence of severe persistent sensorimotor loss, once pain has remitted or has acquired the burning deafferentation quality suggestive of nerve root damage. Changes that are induced in the course of back pain through discectomy are unpredictable. The relatively soft and poorly defined nature of these indication guidelines has resulted in widely variable rates of surgery:

as much as a fourfold or fivefold difference between surgeons and between countries.[35-37]

Cauda Equina Syndrome

A somewhat separate issue is the cauda equina syndrome. Bladder and bowel sphincter dysfunction and bilateral neurologic deficits are the strongest indicators for surgery. The outcome for the cauda equina syndrome is better if there is unilateral sciatic pain, worse if there is bilateral sciatica, and very poor if there is saddle hypesthesia. Patients with complete perineal anesthesia are at risk for permanent sphincter dysfunction. The mode of onset of symptoms may also be important, the acute onset of symptoms over hours being thought to be a prognosticator of poorer outcome, particularly bladder function, than is a more insidious onset over days or weeks.[103]

Cauda equina compression often exists in the sensitizing presence of developmental lumbar stenosis and, in the context of this discussion, is the result of acute disc herniation rather than slowly acquired degenerative change such as anular bulge. Unlike with the lesser indications discussed previously, compression of the cauda equina constitutes a medical emergency or urgency and should be relieved as soon as possible after diagnosis.[81,103] If the onset of symptoms is abrupt, the symptoms and prognosis for full recovery are worse than if the symptoms are slower in onset,[103] and by inference, the urgency for decompression is greater. Other poor prognostic signs for the recovery of sphincter control in cases of cauda equina compression include saddle hypesthesia and bilateral radiculopathic leg pain.

In addition to sensitizing patients to the potential for acute cauda equina syndrome, lumbar stenosis can be responsible for unexpected or false localizing findings in the event of disc hernia, for example, producing footdrop from an L12 level.[104] High lumbar hernia also can be symptomatic in the distribution of multiple roots because of their acute angles and the narrow confines of the upper lumbar canal.[104-106] These patients might not fare as well as patients who have disc pathology at more caudal levels if sensorimotor deficit is present. Long-term follow-up (average, 81 months) confirmed worse outcome for patients with hernia at L1-2 and L2-3, only 33% of patients reporting an improvement in their economic or functional status, compared with an 88% rate of improvement at L3-4.[105] Perhaps this is because when lumbar stenosis is present, conventional discectomy via laminotomy increases the risk of damage to the intracanalicular roots because of the narrow confines of the canal. Particularly in the case of large central and calcified hernia at upper lumbar levels, a generous central canal decompression prior to the manipulation and retraction of the lateral thecal sac must be made. An alternative, if the conus terminates above the level in question, is to retrieve a large or calcific hernia through a transdural approach with repair of the ventral and dorsal dura.[106]

Technique

Disc surgery has only a few basic tenets. The object of the surgery is to decompress the nerve root and to leave it freely relaxed and untraumatized, not necessarily to manipulate the disc. The presence of anular prolapse should be differentiated from true hernia; not all abnormal anuli require enucleation, not all bulges are true hernias, and not all nerve root compressions are caused by a true hernia. An injection of irrigant into the disc, as described later, can be done if there is any doubt that the anulus is torn and there is a true hernia in contrast to a bulging but competent anulus. If the disc is merely bulging, it is meddlesome to incise its anulus and to enucleate its contents. The object of the surgery is to remove the compression in a conservative fashion, leaving behind as little encouragement for scar formation as possible. The removal of some bone is necessary in most cases, but overly aggressive or misplaced bone removal can result in subsequent fracture (of the pars) and resultant chronic microinstability or even the risk of overt instability and the necessity of fusion. Patients are rarely symptomatic from multiple levels; therefore, multilevel discectomy should be exceptionally rare and the indications for it very strong (if performed).

The preoperative surgical plan should include an appraisal of the presence or absence of stenosis. In the case of concomitant spinal stenosis, acquired through either spondylosis or congenital stenosis, radiculopathic pain and neurologic deficit may be worse than in a deeper canal, given a similar-sized herniation mass within the canal. Since crowding of the cauda equina already exists and there is an intolerance to further incursion into the canal during the surgery, it is prudent in the course of the operation and in the presence of stenosis to decompress widely prior to manipulating the dural sac to facilitate discectomy.

Open laminectomy and discectomy work as well as microdiscectomy. The advantages to microdiscectomy are the smaller and more comfortable incision and the shortened hospital stay and diminished trauma to the adjacent motion segments and paraspinous musculature. Microdiscectomy requires the use of magnification. The choice of loupes and headlight or microscope is moot. Results from surgery are the same with both techniques.[28,31] Loupes, with the use of a coaxial or near-coaxial headlight, offer the same or nearly the same magnification and the same or nearly the same size incision in the case of microdissection as does the operating microscope. The advantage of the microscope lies in its use by an observer or assistant; the disadvantages are some additional encumbrance and perhaps expense to the patient.

The following discussion assumes that discectomy is the planned end result of the surgery, not to be followed by fusion, in which case restrictions on bone removal would not be as significant. There is insufficient indication for routine spine arthrodesis combined with lumbar disc excision as the primary procedure.[107] While primary lumbar fusion may well be successful in disc hernia,[108] inclusion criteria should be strict and may include both degenerative and isthmic spondylolisthesis, complete facetectomy, and perhaps degenerative scoliosis.[109,110]

Primary disc replacement or dynamic stabilization, like primary fusion for HNP, is not standard care; current thought reflects conservatism. Despite early enthusiasm for disc arthroplasty,[111] it has been found that there may be only a 0.5% incidence of indication in the overall population with the majority in young patients who averaged 38 years of age. Other nonfusion techniques exist with known results. With criteria for arthroplasty tightly confined and given a small number of potentially eligible patients, there is limited use of this technology.[112] Alternatives such as nucleus replacement may ultimately be an option.[113]

Standard paramedian lumbar disc surgery is estimated to take about 75 to 80 minutes, with an average blood loss of about 65 mL, requirement for blood transfusion being a true rarity.[44]

Operative Positioning and Patient Preparation

The disc space is avascular and, as a result, less resistant to infection. There is evidence that the risk of disc space infection may be reduced through the use of perioperative antibiotics.[114]

The preoperative placement of elastic stockings to prevent thromboembolism is recommended.[115] A urinary catheter is usually unnecessary unless the procedure is expected to take more than 2 hours.

Before the skin incision is made, the surgeon should have taken the opportunity to become familiar with the patient's particular anatomy and pathology, and the operation should have been planned. Ideally, the interpretation of the preoperative studies, how they relate to the patient, and the intraoperative plan in brief terms should be committed to the chart. Thus, in the event of the images being unavailable at the time of surgery, the surgeon can proceed unimpaired and prepared for anatomic variation. For example, the surgeon should know whether the patient has L5 or S1 spina bifida occulta.

For most surgeons, the prone position on a frame works well. Often, such devices are inadequate for preventing increased intra-abdominal pressure (and thus increased ventilatory, venous, and cerebrospinal fluid [CSF] pressures) in obese patients. Obese patients are better positioned in such a manner that the abdominal panniculus hangs unimpeded, without bearing any of the patient's weight (e.g., the knee-chest position). The eyes and facial prominences should be well padded and inspected after the patient is turned to the prone position because ocular pressure, or a combination of pressure and hypotension, can lead to blindness.[116] The arms, if held abducted on arm boards, must be well padded over bony prominences and over the ulnar nerves.[117] To prevent costoclavicular compression of the brachial plexus, care should be taken to avoid hyperabduction over 90 degrees at the shoulders and shoulder hyperextension. The radial pulse on each side should be felt. Women should bear the weight of the chest on the ventrolateral rib cage (not on the breasts, which should be moved medially). All skin that is in contact with the frame or with pads on the frame should be protected with a layer of linens; skin should not be allowed to touch the bare occlusive surface of vinyl or silicone rubber cushions. The urinary catheter (if placed) is inspected after the patient has been turned. Male genitalia must not be subject to compression between the approximated thighs. All bony prominences of the legs must be padded; in particular, the toes must bear no weight of the foot. A diminished or absent pedal pulse may indicate femoral artery compression. This can be encountered on a conventional frame as well as in the knee-chest position.[118] The patient, when positioned, should be stable so that vigorous intraoperative manipulation will not cause movement. Hardware in the room, such as IV stands, light sources, carts, tables, and anesthetic equipment, should be arranged to allow easy access for both radiograph equipment and film cassette holders.

Lateral decubitus positioning is occasionally used in obese patients because the intra-abdominal pressure can be kept low, and epidural venous bleeding can be thus kept at a minimum. It may be the favored position if a patient has significant respiratory compromise. The surgeon may have a personal preference for the lateral decubitus position because it can allow greater lumbar flexion than does the prone position, and it allows blood from the wound to drain away from the operative field (rather than be aspirated). Those who favor the lateral decubitus position generally prefer to have the symptomatic side up, because a little table flexion immediately beneath the lumbar segment that is being operated on can help with interlaminar distraction, and the position also helps with visualization. As with the prone position, the patient requires adequate padding and intraoperative support. This may be enhanced in the lateral decubitus position by a beanbag pad.

After the patient has been positioned, a standard scrub is applied, and the patient is draped for surgery in a sterile fashion. A radiograph may be taken at this point, using a radiopaque localizer. If the planned incision is likely to be longer, as in conventional laminectomy, the radiograph can be delayed until an instrument can be applied to one of the exposed spinous processes. In any case, obtaining an intraoperative radiograph is recommended to avoid erroneous interpretation of the level or levels exposed. In obese patients, the spinous processes may be difficult to appreciate on a lateral film, and it may be advantageous to go off the midline to the facet joint in such cases. The point that has been verified by the radiopaque marker should then be visibly marked in the operative exposure before removal of the marker. The authors prefer the use of an interspinous 18-g spine needle just deep to the interspinous ligament as the radiopaque marker, through which indigo carmine dye can be deposited as the needle is withdrawn. Palpation of the iliac crests as a landmark for the L4-5 interspace, percussion of the sacrum to elicit its characteristic sound, and counting interspinous spaces from the desired level to that of the myelogram injection point can all be relied upon to localize the incision. However, these serve only as guides, particularly because skin traction, patient positioning, and body habitus can alter these critical relationships. Microdissection and the use either of the headlight and loupes or of the operating microscope demands accurate placement of the initial skin incision and of all subsequent dissection therefrom.

Developmental spinal stenosis, if present, is a flag of caution, and its presence must be acknowledged with a variation of the standard techniques. The removal of herniated L5-S1 nucleus pulposus that is concurrent with an L5 spondylolysis might not adequately decompress the nerve root if hypertrophic fibrocartilaginous material is responsible for the patient's symptoms.

Standard Technique and Open Laminotomy (Laminectomy)

Although the term *open laminotomy* may imply the absence of visual magnification, some form of low-power magnification is often used. The skin incision for laminotomy for disc herniation is conventionally about three spinous processes in length, 10 to 12 cm for a one-level operation. When performed in this manner, open laminotomy has the advantage of facilitating surgical assistance. Furthermore, illumination is not quite as problematic as with shorter incisions, and the longer incisions have been suggested to be less traumatic to the paraspinous musculature than shorter incisions (that require greater retractor pressure). After the incision has been made, hemostasis is achieved and retractors are placed. As with any incision, tension on the skin retractor should be inspected intermittently throughout the operation because pressure necrosis of the skin edge is a significant source of infectious wound complications. After the skin has been incised, the subcutaneous tissue is divided. This can be accomplished without bleeding or trauma with blunt dissection. The lumbodorsal fascia is then exposed, and for ease of subsequent closure, it is prudent to sweep the subcutaneous fat off a short distance laterally. The fascia is then incised, just lateral to the spinous process, rather than in the midline, which allows the preservation of interspinous ligaments. If the laminotomy is to be performed bilaterally, as in cases of developmental stenosis with superimposed disc hernia, a fascial incision on each side of the spinous processes results in a saved strip, the width of the spinous processes, in the midline, complete with the interspinous ligament.

The paraspinous musculature is then taken down off the spinous processes and the laminae above and below with a sharp periosteal elevator. Performing this step as atraumatically as possible requires division of the tendinous attachments to the caudal lip of the lamina as lateral dissection proceeds. Deep retraction is placed, and again tension should be moderated by consideration for the underlying muscle, its vasculature, and its innervation from the dorsal rami.

With the field prepared for bone work, the overhanging caudal lip of the rostral lamina can be partially removed, allowing for further exposure of the interlaminar ligamentum flavum. The amount of bone removal is at the surgeon's discretion. The hernia and the anulus can be accessed with little or no removal of bone if one is comfortable with the amount of force necessary to retract the nerve root medially.[26,31,119,120] Wider exposure via laminotomy and medial facetectomy, flush with the medial surface of the caudal pedicle, minimizes the need to mobilize the nerve root aggressively. Paramedian discs at higher lumbar levels represent a slightly greater challenge than those at L4-5 and L5-S1 because of the lamina and facet structure. The spinal canal is smaller in caliber, the lamina and facets descend more caudally, the facets are positioned more medially, and the facet clefts are more sagittally oriented than is the case in more caudal segments. Each of these features not only makes it necessary to remove more bone, but also makes progressive removal more risky to the integrity of the pars and the facet. This anatomy becomes particularly important in addressing intraforaminal disc hernia by the midline approach (see later discussion).

It is prudent to initiate the bone removal from a medial to a lateral direction, since there is nearly always less stenosis and more consistent known anatomy medially. With the use of a cutting bur or a Leksell rongeur, a small amount of bone is removed from the medial caudal edge of the rostral hemilamina, just below the spinous process. Here the spinal canal should be at its deepest, and the potential for anatomic confusion and for injury to the spinal canal contents should be the least. The ligamentum flavum attaches to the caudal lip of the rostral lamina and to its inner surface so that the drill or rongeur meets the ligamentum flavum before endangering the dural sac. The ligamentum is then exposed rostrally. It can then be deliberately violated. An incision is made with a sharp knife through its superficial fibers and is completed with a dull instrument, such as a blunt hook or Freer instrument. The blunt dissector is then used to gently palpate within the central canal or lateral recess of the spinal canal, not only feeling for available room, but also potentially identifying and freeing adhesion. This is an important step, for if a simple blunt hook will not fit into a pathologically narrowed lateral recess, it is certain that the foot of a large punch will not fit without damaging the underlying nerve root. With the large instrument, the surgeon loses tactile sensitivity and might not appreciate the compression. The laminar bone is farther removed with a series of punches (of increasingly larger size), removing with it the attached ligamentum flavum.

As will be discussed later under the topic of postoperative perineurial scar formation, a different option to removing the ligamentum is thinning it and incising it so as to leave its undersurface intact as a barrier to scar. In this case, any bone removal would be accomplished superficial to the layer of ligamentum.

As bone removal proceeds rostrally and laterally, the lateral margin of the removal migrates caudally and laterally, in a fashion that makes the defect appear triangular or lung shaped so that the structural integrity of the pars interarticularis is not compromised. Compromise of the pars by an overly aggressive bone removal can result in a pars interarticularis fracture, either during the course of surgery or during convalescence. More than half the bone of the pars, in its lateral dimension, should be left to avoid fracture[121] (Fig. 78-1). As was mentioned earlier, this is particularly important at midlumbar segments, where the pars is narrower and the facet cleft is more sagittally oriented than at lower motion segments. Pars fracture isolates the facet, functionally resulting in complete facetectomy, which increases the failure rate due to back pain and instability.[28]

Alternatively, a minimalist approach can be taken to bone and ligamentum removal as described by Williams.[26] This approach does have the disadvantage of reduced visualization and increased traction upon the nerve root during its medial mobilization. While the amount of bone removal is discretionary, as a rule, decompressive removal should be more generous in the case of concomitant developmental stenosis. At times, it can be minimal when the interlaminar space is large.

Perineurial scar has been blamed for postsurgical failure to relieve sciatica. There are many means of dealing with its development, and more discussion will follow. The ligamentum flavum is one such potential source of fibrosis if it is left in large shreds beneath the lamina. The ligamentum is therefore reasonably dealt with in one of two ways: (1) with minimal fenestration of the ligament, leaving its slick inner surface approximated to the nerve root as a natural barrier[31,119,120]; or (2) with its complete removal from the lateral recess. Because of impaired visualization and mobility of the underlying thecal sac and nerve root sleeve during the surgery and the variable ability to access the lateral recess and its contents with a minimal approach (dependent on the treatment level and concomitant spondylotic enlargement of the facet and lateral recess stenosis), complete flavectomy is usually preferred.

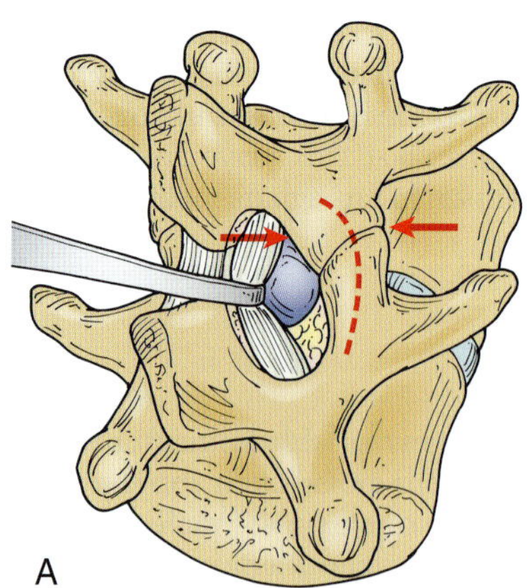

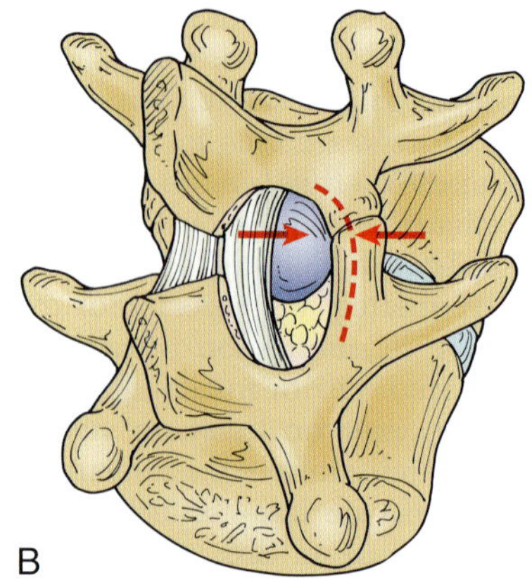

FIGURE 78-1. A, Inadequate bone removal results in necessary excessive nerve root and dural sac retraction. **B,** More generous bone removal reduces the likelihood of nerve root injury. Maintaining pars interarticularis integrity is emphasized. In this regard, bone removal should not extend past the dotted lines.

With angled curettes, removal from the undersurface of the remaining rostral lamina should be thorough. If lateral ligamentum is left in place completely or partially, its raw surface may lead to a significant postoperative fibroblastic response and scar formation, and its continuation with the medial facet capsule contributes to lateral recess and foraminal stenosis, which may be of significance as the disc space narrows postoperatively and with age.

After partial removal of the rostral lamina and ligamentum in this manner, attention is turned to the caudal lamina. The thin rostral lip is removed, again medial to lateral, along with the remaining ligamentum flavum. Care must be taken to avoid compression of the underlying neural elements. Removal of bone in the caudal direction does not need to be as extensive as the rostral removal. It must, however, be extended enough laterally to be flush with the medial side of the pedicle of the caudal vertebra and extended enough caudally to allow ensuing visualization of the disc space, usually a 3- or 4-mm distance from the rostral edge. During the course of bone removal, the underlying epidural fat is protected.

The decompressive approach described here could be described as semihemilaminectomy, medial facetectomy, and hemiflavectomy. Performed as described, it would typically span a distance of 20 to 25 mm longitudinally and 10 to 15 mm laterally. It provides adequate room for nerve root and lateral thecal sac visualization and safe mobilization, yet it does not weaken the motion segment. The amount of bone removed is variable and depends on the motion segment involved, the amount of lumbar flexion afforded during positioning, the amount of spondylotic change present, and the patient's developmental anatomy. Often, little work is required on the bone at the lumbosacral interspace. During the course of bone removal, there is no occasion for blind removal. With strong illumination and adequate exposure and hemostasis, visualization should not present a problem.

The location of the foot of the punch or the edge of the curette and the location of the nerve root sleeve should be well perceived by the operating surgeon. It is worth noting that a risk of dural tear is present in every case. If a scar is present, fixing the dura mater to overlying bone, the risk of a dural tear is increased. The chance of tear is also increased in the elderly (particularly elderly women), in whom the dura mater is thin and in whom a noncompliant scar may be present, even in the absence of prior surgery. An inflammatory response to the hernia itself is often present.[45,86,88] Naturally occurring adhesion may be present, fixing the dorsal dura to overlying laminar bone and ligamentum flavum. For these reasons and as a basic element of prudent use of a bone punch, the space into which the punch foot will sit should be swept with a blunt instrument such as a Woodson or ball-ended dissector. The geometry of the instrumentation involved is crucial because the dura mater can fold over the foot of a punch or the edge of the curette that is not applied closely to the underside of the bone. This is an error that can be worsened if the dura mater is distended under increased intrathecal pressure; as with epidural venous bleeding, its risk can be reduced by careful positioning, with attention paid to intra-abdominal pressure reduction. Piecemeal bone removal is not slowed by cautious inspection. Caution simply requires keeping the eyes on the target, letting the assistant clean the punch, judiciously appreciating the tactile input, and intermittently sweeping the peripheral undersurface of the bone in the direction of the decompression with a dissector.

A dural tear is a significant problem only if it is not cared for properly. In some cases, dural tears are unavoidable, and their occurrence may even be predictable. It is a problem encountered by the best of surgeons. The risk of a tear is high in the elderly with thin and fragile dura as well as ligamentous adhesions to dura, but it is also a risk if the herniated disc fragment has been present long enough to result in dural adhesions. There is also the possibility of natural dural adhesion and of fibrous bands connecting ventral dura (Hofmann ligaments) to the posterior longitudinal ligament, particularly well developed and of potential surgical consequence in the lumbar canal.[122,123]

A mistake is to be cavalier about the occurrence of a CSF leak and not to repair the leak properly. Pinhole dural breaches can and often are successfully treated with fibrin glue, DuraSeal, hemostatic gelatin (Gelfoam), other adhesive substances, and/or indirectly with multilayer tight soft tissue closure. However, larger dural tears of more than 1 mm are best managed with convincing primary suture closure, as they risk spontaneously enlarging and producing CSF fistula and symptomatic pseudomeningocele.

If the tear is dorsal or lateral, it will be problematic for the remainder of the case if not attended to. The defect should be protected from further tearing or from aspiration of nerve roots by the placement of Gelfoam and a cottonoid beneath the suction tip over the tear. It should be exposed, with further bone removal, and repaired primarily with suture in a watertight fashion (preferably immediately after its occurrence). Repair can be tedious and time-consuming at a point in the operation at which much remains to be done. The temptation to delay repair until later is often best resisted. If the repair is one of the last tasks after an unusually lengthy procedure, attention might not be paid to the details of adequately repairing the leak. If the arachnoid is also involved and spinal fluid is being lost, thecal sac collapse occurs, and epidural venous bleeding intensifies because of decreased tamponade. This increased bleeding obscures visualization and blood can enter the thecal sac, possibly resulting in arachnoidal adhesions. Other possible results of unrepaired dural tear include radiculopathies with pain and deficit secondary to herniation of nerve roots through the dural defect, symptomatic pseudomeningocele, the possibility of meningitis, and persistent orthostatic headache complaints.[124-128] In the modern era, with patients conventionally returning home the same or next day, primary repair becomes standard.

Confines of the field often make primary repair difficult, particularly with modern minimal exposures or tubular retractors, but only rarely is it impossible. The needle is more important than the suture size; a tapered needle not much larger than the suture should be used so as not to leave an excessive pinhole of its own. A commonly used suture is 4-0 or smaller, with 6-0 or 7-0 polypropylene suture (Prolene) being the authors' preference (more so for BV-1 or BV-175 needle geometry). A new Ethicon (Johnson and Johnson) suture, Hemo-Seal 5-0 Prolene HS, has a sealing hydrophilic coating. The use of a small pituitary instrument to hold the needle and the use of knot pushers can significantly aid the process, even to the extent that dural repair can be effected through a tubular retractor.[129]

Reinforcement of the durotomy with an onlay of fat, DuraSeal, DuraGen, muscle, fascia, fibrin glue, Gelfoam, Surgicel, polyglactin acid sheet, or mesh,[130] collagen mesh, or the like is prudent but might be ineffective in the long run without the underlying primary repair. Fibrin glue is very effective but short lived, lasting only several days. The authors believe that if a trustworthy repair has been provided, it is advantageous to have the patient ambulatory the day of surgery rather than enforcing bed rest; ambulation will expand the thecal sac, redistribute the caudal nerve elements, and preclude epidural bleeding. With good dural repair, only 1.8% of incidental durotomy patients must return to the operating room.[131] Additional treatment such as lumbar CSF drainage should be considered second line, again being best used to reinforce a good primary suture line repair.

Repaired primarily, CSF leaks incurred intraoperatively have little or no impact on ultimate surgical outcome.[127] Repaired and reinforced carefully, most will heal, but extra consideration should be given host factors that would impair wound healing, such as high CSF pressure anticipated in obesity, connective tissue disorders such as Marfan syndrome and neurofibromatosis, scar tissue, and use of steroids. On occasion, the tear may be located on the ventral aspect of the nerve root sleeve or thecal sac, in which case, while it may be impossible to repair without marked difficulty, it nevertheless does not risk the problems of a dorsal tear and will more than likely tamponade itself.

Preservation of the epidural fat is a worthwhile goal during the development of the interlaminar exposure. Some cases of considerable residual postoperative radiculopathic pain are attributable to epineurial scar formation and the resultant tethering of the nerve root to the adjacent bone and anulus fibrosus. As with hemostasis, attention must be paid to the epidural fat to ensure an optimal outcome. Epidural fat, however, should not be allowed to obscure the field to the detriment of the surgical goal. It is crucial that the nerve root sleeve and the ventral disc space be fully visualized. If necessary, the fat can be pulled off the dorsum of the nerve root sleeve and moved medially, divided gently with the bipolar tips, or rubbed aside and protected with a cotton stamp. When the nerve root and disc pathology is definitively addressed, the fat can be moved back into a protective position.

With the medial aspect of the facet joint and capsule partially removed so that the medial surface of the caudal pedicle can be observed and felt, the need for medial retraction on the nerve root to allow visualization of the disc space should be minimized (see Fig. 78-1B). Before retraction instruments are inserted, room ventral to the nerve root and dural sac must be assessed (Fig. 78-2). With a small-caliber aspiration tip (5 or 7 French), blunt hook, or ball-ended dissector, the nerve root can be mobilized medially, and while doing so, the amount of ventral fibrosis or compression can be determined. This palpation should be gentle, and if resistance to mobilization in this manner is met, the surgeon must determine the cause, as well as a solution to the problem of mobilization. The axilla of the nerve root may straddle a sharp focal prominence of the anulus fibrosus. Forcing the nerve root up and over it may invite neural injury. In such a case, the prominence can be trimmed or impacted down, medial to the nerve root in the axilla, following which the nerve root can be mobilized medially and the disc pathology better addressed. Poor ability to mobilize may reflect a nerve root anomaly such as low origin.

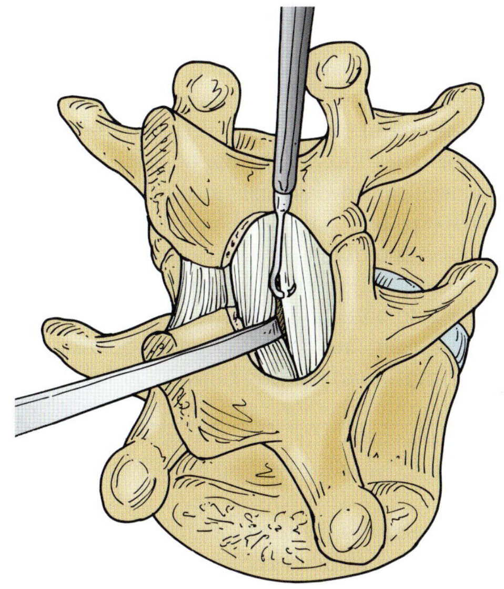

FIGURE 78-2. Adequacy of room is assessed before inserting any retraction device capable of excessive compression of underlying structures.

Overly aggressive retraction of the nerve root out of the lateral recess is potentially traumatizing to the substance of the root directly, as well as disruptive of root blood flow,[99] and can be minimized by partial facet or facet capsule removal. A nerve root retractor with an integral pressure transducer has been described, with the intention of producing retraction which is brief and gentle.[132]

Conjoined nerve roots, low root origins, and interradicular anastomoses often affect the lower lumbar levels and represent something of a surgical challenge for a number of reasons. They can confuse the surgical anatomy, and if the conjoined root is large and pulled or pushed tightly into the lateral recess by the disc pathology, it can be mistaken for the hernia itself.[133] If a low origin from the dura results in a lateral course over the disc space, it can be impossible to safely mobilize to access the disc. Therefore, a thorough decompression of the nerve root may be very difficult to achieve. The presence of a conjoined root should be readily anticipated from modern neuroimaging.

Often, the herniated nucleus pulposus is sequestered beneath the posterior longitudinal ligament rather than being free in the spinal canal or lateral recess. A simple poke with the bipolar tips through the ligament may be all that is necessary to initiate its delivery. Perhaps the most atraumatic method of removing the hernia is to grasp a small slip of the fragment with a pituitary instrument and deliver it slowly up through the ligamentous tear, serially repositioning the instrument to catch more of its bulk while doing so. The residual ligament protects the adjacent nerve root from traction.

Occasionally, the hernia represents a complete nuclear extrusion, and its attempted removal in one piece may force the nerve root medially to such an extent that injury results. It is therefore often optimal to remove it piecemeal. When the prominence has been reduced by removal of some of the herniated disc material, the nerve root is more relaxed, and more room is available for exploration with blunt angled dissecting instruments, such as a ball-ended dissector. The ventral epidural space is thoroughly palpated for any residual fragments by sweeping the dissector over the disc space. The subligamentous space is similarly palpated, as is the neural foramen rostral and lateral to the pedicle. The intervertebral disc space is then thoroughly explored and emptied of nucleus, using a combination of straight and angled pituitary rongeurs. It is often necessary to enlarge the anular tear to permit entrance of the rongeurs into the disc interspace. It is recommended that this be accomplished sharply and generously with a no. 15 or 11 blade on a long handle, fashioning a rectangular window through the anulus fibrosus. After discectomy, the anulus, if otherwise left in the lateral recess, may prolapse or adhere to the nerve root and produce recurrent symptoms.

As was previously mentioned, a special problem of hernia in adolescents and young adults is avulsion of the apophyseal ring with the hernia. The bone and firmly attached anulus, in concert with large mass effect, may make complete effective removal doubtful. Surgical options may be limited to wide decompression. Larger exposure is needed to resect the fractured fragments and disc material.[77,134,135]

To reduce the chances of recurrent disc hernia, all loose nucleus material should be removed. It is neither possible nor desirable to remove all disc material. Overly aggressive curettage with removal of end-plate cartilage and excessive removal of interspace volume can result in a patulous anulus, poor mechanical support of the motion segment, and potential foraminal stenosis or instability. Removal should be limited to loose fragments that are within reach of the anular opening. Approaches range from sequestrectomy alone[26,120] to aggressive curettage of the disc space, which may remain the more common procedure.[136,137] The topics of discectomy volume and of recurrent disc hernia are covered later in the chapter.

Intraoperative ultrasound[138,139] may be useful even when the surgeon believes that removal has been complete. More medially located disc pathology may be difficult to interpret or see.

With the anulus and the cartilaginous end plates being retained, the surgeon must stay focused on an envisioned estimate of the anatomy of the intervertebral space because this is a blind procedure. The majority of vascular and visceral injuries that result from perforation of the ventral anulus occur at L4-5 and L5-S1, although injury can occur at other levels as well.[140-146] The firm ventral and lateral anular margins can usually be palpated with the rongeurs, and the depth of penetration can be controlled. It is possible, however, as a result of ventral anular tears,[143,147-149] that the anulus fibrosus does not adequately restrain the instruments to blind palpation. Tarlov[146] suggests penetrating the anular space to no more than a depth of 1.125 inches and marking the operative instruments at this depth.

Shevlin et al.[150] reported a case in which atraumatic passage of a rongeur to an unusual depth was followed by the observation that irrigating fluid then emptied out the ventral anulus; they suggest this as a sign of potential problems, as occurred with their case. During discectomy and shortly thereafter, any sudden vagal or hypovolemic response should be seriously regarded as indicating possible vascular, ureteral, or intestinal injury. Most often, bleeding from the anular space is not noted in major vascular injuries.

Catastrophic problems occurring as a result of perforation through the ventral anulus are possible, even with skilled surgeons. There is an incidence of 1.6 to 17 per 10,000 cases of ventral perforation with vascular or visceral injury.[5,146,148,151] Body habitus, the operating surgeon's experience, patient positioning, and the type of surgical instrumentation used (including the microscope) do not appear to influence the risk. Good outcome is entirely dependent on early recognition and swift appropriate action. However, the mortality rate may still reach 47% with vascular injury. Vascular injuries during lumbar discectomy may of course result in acute life-threatening hemorrhage but also chronic arteriovenous fistula or pseudoaneurysm formation. The majority of vascular injuries associated with lumbar laminectomy are found at the L4-5 and L5-S1 levels and few higher.[140]

If the anulus fibrosus is simply bulging over a broad area or is partially dislodged from its attachment to the rostral or caudal vertebral lip and does not appear to be torn (permitting expression of the nucleus), it is best left intact. Certainly, if soft disc hernia or prolapse is not seen, the anulus should never be violated. Nerve root decompression can be achieved by removal of overlying bone and ligamentum flavum, allowing the preservation of the motion segment. The decision to violate the posterior longitudinal ligament and anulus can be made with greater assurance by using an intradiscal injection of saline. A small amount of indigo carmine dye, just enough to color the irrigant, and 5 mL of saline are drawn up in a 6- or 10-mL syringe, a 22-gauge spine needle is fitted, and the nuclear space is injected through the anulus. If the irrigant can be observed readily extravasating from the disc space, it can be assumed that the anulus is incompetent and that its contents should, perhaps, be emptied. If the disc accepts only a few milliliters of fluid and no extravasation is observed, the anulus can be assumed to be competent, despite its bulge, and is best left undisturbed.

The unsettling experience of not encountering the expected pathology is not infrequent. The MRI may be dated by several months to the point that involution of hernia may have occurred, or the hernia may be at some distance from its original location, or despite all due care, it may be that the wrong level has been approached. The possibilities can be readily sorted out with thorough inspection and possibly repeated intraoperative x-ray films if necessary. Little harm (other than perhaps medial facetectomy) would come from exposure of the wrong disc unless unnecessary and nontherapeutic discectomy were to follow it.

Intervertebral disc hernia may be encountered at unusual locations within the canal, either distant from the anulus or hidden intradurally. Immediately upon entering the canal, just under the ligamentum, the surgeon might be met with a dorsally migrated epidural fragment of disc material.[152] It is an interesting and occasionally unexpected finding but should not be difficult to remove and trace to its source. More difficult to manage are the rare intradural and intraradicular hernias, which might not be readily apparent either on the MRI or at the tableside. Because of adhesion of the dura to the anulus or posterior longitudinal ligament, a hernia may rarely perforate the dura mater and be located within the thecal sac or within the nerve root itself.[153-156] Another problematic location for hernia may be those that have migrated rostrally to lie well rostral to the disc space. The removal of a large amount of lamina may be necessary. There is further discussion of this problem later.

Adhesion can be a consequence of prior surgery, the result of inflammatory changes incurred by the hernia itself, or a natural occurrence as previously. To find the pathology in these cases requires the surgeon to be vigilant for any discrepancies between what is observed in the field and what was observed on the neuroimaging studies and to simply be aware that such conditions exist. It has been postulated that some cases of surgical failure of benefit may indeed be due to such pathology that has gone unrecognized.[154]

When the ligamentum flavum is aggressively removed, the nerve root decompressed, the fat replaced, and hemostasis obtained, the wound is closed. Irrigating solution is used to flood the wound. A secure, but nonstrangulating, absorbable suture reapproximates the muscle to the midline to eliminate dead space. The fascia is closed in a watertight fashion, and the subcutaneous fat and skin are closed. The surgeon can elect to place a Depo-Medrol–soaked Gelfoam pledget or morphine (Duramorph) over the nerve root before closure or to infiltrate the paraspinous muscle with bupivicaine before closure of the skin.[157]

Microlaminotomy

Microlaminotomy, or microdiscectomy, is the contemporary gold standard treatment of lumbar disc hernia; the use of the larger open incision is waning. Microdiscectomy was introduced in 1977.[27,158] The term *microlaminotomy* denotes the use of a short skin and fascial incision and, by necessity of the short incision, visual magnification of some sort. To accomplish the task accurately and effectively through a microlaminotomy incision, loupes with a magnification power of at least 3.5, with a strong headlight coaxial with the line of sight, or a binocular operating microscope are required. As with the use of loupes, the use of the microscope has certain advantages and disadvantages.

Properly fitted loupes and a coaxial headlight can be worn comfortably for an extended period of time. With loupes, there is no impediment to the surgeon's mobility in the field or in the room. The line of sight can be adjusted to refocus attention on other details in the field without hesitation and without removing hands or instruments from their position or task. Intraoperative radiographs may be obtained with minimum movement of equipment. The disadvantage of loupes is the poor view afforded to surgical assistants.

The most significant advantage of the microscope is the ability of the surgical assistant to obtain a view that is the same as the surgeon's. It is also possible to use a much higher magnification, although for laminotomy this is usually unnecessary. The disadvantage of using a microscope is the encumbrance of the device.

Microlaminotomy has the advantage of decreased postoperative pain. As a result, the complications of postoperative atelectasis and postoperative temperature elevation may be reduced.[27,158,159] The high magnification that is used in its completion encourages gentle tissue handling.

Positioning and preparation are unchanged from those in conventional laminotomy, except that some form of radiographic localization is absolutely required. A spine needle introduced into the interspinous ligament makes an excellent marker, and when the radiograph returns, it can be used to estimate the optimum trajectory to the disc space. The incision can be centered on or placed somewhat above or below the puncture site. In slender adults, a 2- to 3-cm incision is more than adequate, although if necessary, there should be no hesitation to lengthen it. The fascia to the side of the hernia is incised cleanly along the spinous process the same length as the skin incision, and the muscle is stripped subperiosteally, as accomplished with conventional laminotomy. For wound retraction, there is a choice of instruments, including tubular retractors, although most surgeons favor Williams or Caspar retractors.

There is no subsequent difference in technique between open laminotomy and microlaminotomy for the remainder of the surgery, other than the use of magnification. It is possible to perform disc surgery using the operating microscope without removing much, if any, bone, and little ligamentum flavum. In fact, when microlaminotomy was first described by Williams,[26] this approach was recommended. The focus of the operation, however, should be thorough nerve root decompression and the minimization of the chance for recurrent symptoms, rather than an exercise in leaving the least trace. Without a more or less conventional amount of bone removal, the chances of overlooked pathology and a compromised outcome are increased. It is strongly advised, therefore, that microlaminotomy be performed in the same fashion as one would perform a conventional laminotomy. Results from conventional laminotomy and microlaminotomy are similar.[29,101] The theoretical benefit of microdiscectomy is its applicability to outpatient usage.[160-162]

Use of the microscope or high-power loupes is required for optimal treatment of some variants of lumbar disc hernia. One such example is hernia fragment sequestered well rostral to the disc space. There are several approaches to this problem, in which the sequestrum lies directly under laminar bone that the surgeon would prefer to leave undisturbed. It is potentially important to determine as well as possible whether the tissue came from the disc above and migrated down or from the disc below and migrated up, since it would be prudent to arrange an operation that would allow exploration of the responsible anulus. One option is to come up from below, devising an approach from the skin down that is more caudal than conventionally so that the angle of approach will potentially spare laminar bone of the aggressive removal otherwise necessary. Another approach would be to approach it from the motion segment above and remove more of the rostral bone of the caudal lamina than is conventionally required.

A third approach is a translaminar approach to a hernia that has migrated rostrally to lie in the proximal foramen medial to and below the pedicle of the rostral level. This procedure has been described and will be discussed in the section on foraminal hernias.[163-165]

Microendoscopic discectomy, discussed in Chapter 61, is performed through tubular retractors with endoscopic vision. It was introduced in 1997 and has since been demonstrated to be as effective as microsurgical discectomy for treatment of lumbar disc hernia.[166-168]

Complete Laminectomy

Once a popular method of exposure for all disc surgery, complete laminectomy with bilateral removal of the medial facets, laminae, and spinous processes has fallen into disfavor because of its inherently destructive nature. Complete laminectomy deprives the multifidus, rotator, interspinalis, and spinalis muscles of origin and insertion. Some degree of mechanical dysfunction and pain will naturally result. Therefore, complete laminectomy for discectomy should be avoided if possible.

In severe developmental stenosis with superimposed disc hernia or large central adherent disc hernia, however, it may be advisable to perform laminectomy before discectomy to avoid compressive nerve root or cauda equina injury. In some cases of hernia, the nuclear fragment can tear and enter the thecal sac and requires dural incision and repair for its treatment. This is facilitated by complete laminectomy. This is more common with postoperative recurrent hernia than in de novo cases because of epidural fibrosis with tethering of the dura mater. High lumbar disc hernia (at L1-2 or L2-3) may be at the level of the conus medullaris, a structure that is intolerant of retraction and compression. Some consideration may be given to complete laminectomy in the upper lumbar spinal canal if this is thought to be a risk. Finally, in some cases of significant vertebral subluxation complicating disc hernia, a complete laminectomy with discectomy may be required for bilateral decompression before fusion, particularly if reduction cannot be obtained.

As was mentioned in the section on the cauda equina, voluminous high lumbar hernia may be problematic and may require complete laminectomy, since conventional discectomy via laminotomy increases the risk of damage to the intracanalicular roots because of the narrow confines of the canal. This is particularly true in the case of large central and calcified hernias at upper lumbar levels. A generous central canal decompression prior to the manipulation and retraction of the thecal sac must be made, or a transdural approach with repair of the ventral and dorsal dura.[104-106]

Lateral and Far Lateral Hernia

Far lateral disc hernia, with resulting compression of the nerve root in, or lateral to, the intervertebral neuroforamen, occurs in about 10% of all symptomatic anular prolapses or discs.[169-180] Extraforaminal hernia is relatively uncommon, accounting for 0.7% to 11.7% of all lumbar hernias.[169,170,181-184] Most commonly, far lateral disc herniation occurs at L3-4, L4-5, or higher levels. They occur in about equal numbers at L3-4 and L4-5, about half that at L5-S1, and in small numbers at L1-2 and L2-3.[94,169,170,178,182,183,185,186] Lateral hernias occur in older patients more often than the more common dorsolateral hernias do.[51,172,187,188] Lateral hernias are more likely to produce sensorimotor deficit.[109] As a corollary to its frequency at midlumbar and higher lumbar levels, there is some likelihood that patients with ventral thigh pain and sensory deficit, quadriceps weakness, a positive femoral stretch test, and reduced patellar reflex harbor a far lateral hernia. Recognition of this has been facilitated by use of myelography and postmyelographic CT.[189] MRI, particularly the sagittal images, may best demonstrate the pathology.[190,191] Radiculopathic pain may be more severe and back pain less severe than that incurred in paramedian disc hernia because of the location of the sensory root ganglion.[56,109,192]

The exposure of far lateral discs can often be more complicated than that of routine paramedian hernias. Anatomic concerns such as a narrow pars, hypertrophic occluding facets at the rostral level, short vertically oriented pedicles, thickened laminae, enlarged arthrotic facets at the hernia level, and degenerative listhesis can make the exposure difficult and may ultimately affect the judgment about which avenue to take to the pathology.

Preoperative planning is facilitated by classifying the hernia location into one of three areas and judging its accessibility accordingly. First, the lateral hernia may lie within the proximal foramen just at the medial aspect of the pedicle, and in this case can be approached through a modification of the paramedian laminotomy. Second, it may lie in the lateral foramen and must then be approached by means of a lateral facetectomy. Third, it may lie in an extraforaminal location, in which case an extraforaminal or parasagittal approach would be necessary to avoid complete facetectomy. It may be necessary, in a patient with developmental stenosis and therefore unusually large, medially located, and coronal facets to opt for one of the lateral approaches over a more conventional medial facetectomy. Although complete facetectomy has been historically reported to be relatively benign, perhaps more benign at the caudal two levels,[172-174] it may result in delayed instability and failure due to chronic back pain. Consequently, complete facetectomy is avoided when possible.[28,121]

Despite its recognition, it is still difficult to effectively treat a far lateral hernia. The variety of commonly used surgical trajectories is illustrated in Fig. 78-3. The most popular

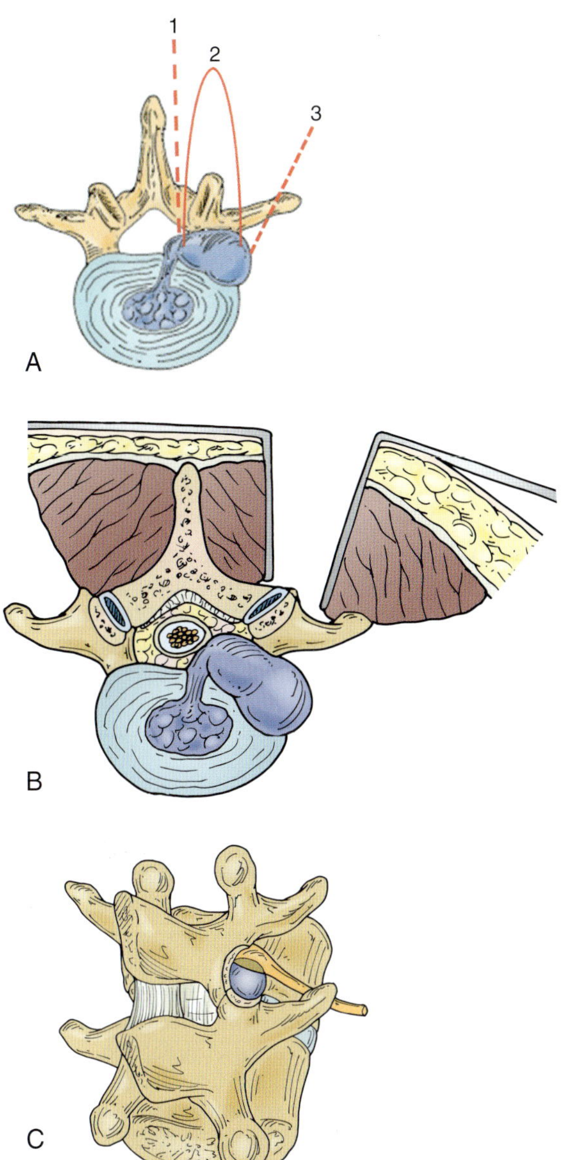

FIGURE 78-3. A, Trajectories achieved by the varieties of exposure for lateral disc hernia. *1,* midline; *2,* interlaminar and extralaminar approach; *3,* paramedian muscle splitting. **B,** Paramedian muscle-splitting approach achieves an optimal angle of exposure to discs situated beyond the pedicle. **C,** For most approaches to a lateral disc hernia, a modest lateral facetectomy is performed, thus providing direct access to the hernia.

approach is a standard midline incision and interlaminar exposure with medial facetectomy.[169,170,172,177,187,188] This approach has the advantages of greater familiarity of the surgeon with surgical anatomy, absence of bleeding, early exposure of the affected nerve root, and the ability to perform discectomy to preclude recurrence. It is most appropriate for a hernia within the proximal foramen. Often, the amount of bone that must be removed to gain exposure to the neuroforamen is greater than that in simple dorsolateral hernias. It helps visualization considerably to tilt the table toward the operator.

On rare occasions, it may be necessary to produce a complete facetectomy in the cases of very large and difficult hernias, such as those including apophyseal ring involvement. While facetectomy may be better tolerated at L5-S1 (where the iliotransverse ligament attaches to L5), partial (medial) facetectomy will nevertheless work best for HNPs at level L5-S1, and complete facetectomy should not be necessary.[173] Higher in the vertebral column, in order to preserve the narrow pars, it may be necessary to augment a medial facetectomy approach with an intertransverse approach.[109,176]

Another option, building on the familiar midline exposure, is the possibility of approaching the hernia in the proximal foramen from an interlaminar approach originating from the contralateral side of the midline and proceeding across the midline and under the facet, minimizing facetectomy.[193] Foraminotomy, with some form of partial facetectomy, is still the most popular surgical option, despite the inherent disadvantage of aggressive bone removal.

Using a modification of the midline approach to address a hernia deeper within the lateral foramen, a slightly different combined interlaminar and extralaminar exposure has also been described by Hood,[175] in which the muscle is not dissected off the spinous processes but rather incised 1 cm lateral to the midline. The facet joint is exposed, and a drill and punch are used to produce a partial lateral facetectomy through which the rostral and caudal pedicles can be palpated. The nerve root, forced dorsally by the pathologic hernia, lies deep to the facet capsule and ligamentum flavum. It can be mobilized and retracted to address the disc hernia. If necessary, the lateral recess and retained disc material within the spinal canal can then be approached through a standard interlaminar route with a minimum of bone removal, thus maintaining the integrity of the facet joint.

In another variation, in which the affected intraforaminal root is exposed in the lateral recess above the foramen, a standard exposure of the affected root through a routine interlaminar midline approach is performed, one level rostral to the neural foramen (e.g., the L4 nerve root compressed in the L4-5 foramen is exposed at L3-4 through a routine interlaminar approach). The nerve root is then followed a short distance with a small amount of bone removal from the rostral edge of the caudal lamina and facet at this level. The extralaminar approach is then used to deal with the nerve root, now identified and protected under a dissector in the neuroforamen.[171]

Di Lorenzo et al. and others[163-165] have reported on a novel approach to proximal intraforaminal disc hernia, producing a small ovoid window through the pars, sparing an isthmus of bone on both its medial and lateral aspects, leaving the inferior facet connected to the pedicle and lamina (Fig. 78-4). The hole that is produced lies directly over the lateral recess or proximal neural foramen where the sequestrum is believed to lie. The benefits are described as not only being directly over the pathology but also producing no disruption of the ligamentum flavum or joint capsule and hence less epidural fibrosis. It does, however, potentially risk pars fracture. At least 3 mm of bone must be left between the hole and the lateral aspect of the pars. It would be hard to enter and clear the disc, and there may be a higher recurrence rate, since the procedure relies on fragment removal alone. The approach is limited to intraforaminal hernia and those fragments that have migrated rostral from the disc space. If it should become necessary to enlarge the hole, the bone removal ends up being more than would be common in a laminotomy from the rostral or caudal motion segment. This approach might not be

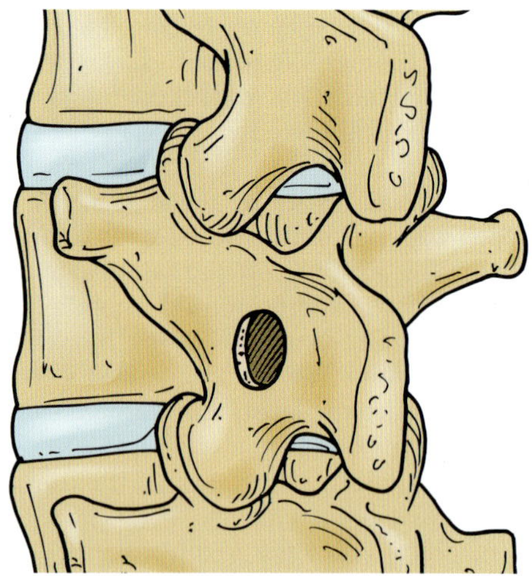

FIGURE 78-4. A translaminar fenestration approach to sequestered fragments migrated rostral to the disc space into the proximal neural foramen has been described.

appropriate for larger hernias and those with apophyseal ring fracture or calcification. The pars must be intrinsically generously wide enough to permit fenestration without compromising its integrity, and the foramen must be large enough, uninvolved by stenosis, to permit manipulation of the root as well as the hernia.

In the foregoing procedures, the paraspinous musculature is removed from the spinous processes or is dissected by using the column approach, 1 cm lateral to midline. Exposure of the neuroforamen is via a trajectory that is almost directly dorsal. Because a dorsal extraforaminal approach provides the same orientation for viewing the intervertebral foramen as the midline approach, it also can require significant bone resection to allow visualization of the pathology.[192]

The midline and paramedian routes are popular and effective, given a conventional approach to the anatomy and surgeons' familiarity. However, they may provide limited access to the intervertebral foramen and the lateral aspect of the vertebral bodies and may require significant bone resection as mentioned. The paramedian, muscle-splitting approach[178-180,194,195] has the advantage of sparing the patient the loss of bone and of providing a somewhat more oblique view of the neuroforamen. It is most useful for hernias that are within the lateral foramen or are extraforaminal. A paramedian skin and fascial incision, about 3 cm from the midline (or further lateral at lower levels), is made just over the natural plane groove between the multifidus and longissimus muscles. Descending through the paraspinous musculature between the transverse processes onto the neuroforamen from a lateral orientation, the surgeon is able to locate the lateral facet and its capsule and perhaps be able to remove only a small amount of lateral facet, if necessary (see Fig. 78-3). The medial transverse processes are exposed, the multifidus muscular attachments to the facet are incised, and the intertransverse muscle and ligament are incised. It is then possible to expose the affected nerve root in the neuroforamen, retract it aside, and address the disc hernia. This is not too dissimilar to the lateral extracavitary approach described by Larson et al.[196] Transforaminal ligaments in the lumbar intervertebral foramen present in over 80% of foramina may be encountered, which could compromise outcome if not recognized and taken down.[197] Although the major advantage is the preservation of the pars interarticularis and the facet joint with little likelihood of instability,[181] it has the disadvantages of surgical unfamiliarity, deeper dissection, possibly poorer visualization, difficulty enucleating the disc space, potential injury to the nerve root within the neuroforamen, and dealing with sequestered fragments beneath the posterior longitudinal ligament.[172,187] The exposure at the lower levels gained by the muscle-splitting approach can be more difficult to achieve than that at higher levels because of the gradually decreasing room available between the confines of the transverse and accessory processes and the sacral ala.[198,199]

O'Brien et al. have described a dorsolateral approach that is farther lateral yet, an incision 10 cm lateral to the midline. A basic tenet of the approach is that of following the lateral branch of the dorsal ramus and the terminal branch of the segmental artery. Both landmarks can be found consistently in the intertransverse space running obliquely across the dorsal surface of the caudal transverse process toward the foramen, with the lateral branch of the dorsal ramus continuing as a guide to the postganglionic root.[192] Minimal soft tissue dissection removal associated with this approach may help to facilitate rapid postoperative mobilization.

Although most intraforaminal disc hernias can be cared for from the midline approach, the surgeon should be familiar with the paramedian and perhaps far lateral approaches. These approaches are indicated when the nerve root is compressed lateral to the neuroforamen[177,192] or when a lateral disc at L4-5 or L5-S1 is encountered. With the availability of these options, there should be little reason to sacrifice the entire facet joint.

Other approaches, such as the ventrolateral retroperitoneal approach and osteoplastic removal and replacement of the pars interarticularis and facet, have been advocated, but they appear to be more complex than warranted, especially with the availability of simpler procedures. Experience has been gained with augmentation of midline and lateral approaches using endoscopy to access the foramen.[57,160,186] No matter which surgical approach is taken, it is wise not to displace the nerve root within the foramen aggressively because the dorsal root ganglion within it is sensitive and its manipulation may worsen the symptoms.[190,191] The historically reported results of treatment for lateral disc hernia are likely similar to those of more classical dorsolateral hernias in patients of the same age-group.[170-173,178,187] However, there may be a lower response rate than that of paramedian disc hernia because of the ganglion issue.[31,56]

Spinal Cysts

Three types of intraspinal cysts at differing sites have been responsible for radiculopathy: synovial cysts of the facet joint, the ligamentum flavum, and the intervertebral disc. Cysts involved with the intervertebral disc (discal cysts) are rare and uncommonly distinguished from other kinds of lesions given their unfamiliarity. Plain films will likely be unrevealing; myelography and CT myelography will show extradural mass effect compressing the spinal nerve as with lumbar disc herniation. MRI demonstrates spherical extradural mass on low-intensity T1-weighted images and high-signal intensity T2-weighted images, with rim enhancement on contrast. If discography is performed, contrast medium may show communication between the intervertebral discs and cyst, but not necessarily. There may be pathologic differences between discal cysts and those arising from the posterior longitudinal ligament (PLL) or anulus.

Such cysts are probably ganglion cysts of either the anulus fibrosus or PLL. They are typically walled in by fibrous connective tissue without a specific cell lining but with frequent myxoid degeneration, and they frequently contain serous fluid that may be bloody by virtue of even mild trauma.[200-202]

Prevention of Perineurial Scar Formation

Throughout the history of lumbar disc surgery, failure has been attributed to scar formation around the nerve root; therefore, the interest in scar formation prevention has been high. At least theoretically, scar formation tethers the root within the otherwise slick interfaces of the lateral recess and sensitizes it to compression, tension, and ischemia, which would otherwise theoretically be asymptomatic.

The evidence for and against the concept of symptomatic scar is conflicting in the modern neuroimaging era.[203] In the circumstance of recurrent hernia following discectomy, fibrosis around the root certainly affects symptoms and reoperation rate. Fibrosis results in unusual anatomic problems, including intraradicular and intradural herniations as mentioned.[153,154] Because of fibrosis and tethering of the dura mater, the presentation of recurrent hernia or prolapse may be polyradicular rather than monoradicular.

Scar tethering the roots could theoretically inhibit the normal sliding movements and could cause pain, numbness, and weakness.[204] Rationally, there would seem to be some impact of both intradural arachnoidal adhesions and extradural scar upon outcome, simply because physiologically, the root sleeves and elements of the cauda equina move with leg and body motion. On the other hand, recent randomized controlled trials showed that neither scar nor the use of the scar-inhibiting barrier Adcon-L had an impact on outcome.[101,205,206]

Determinants of scar formation include soft tissue traumatization and blood left behind in the operative field. Therefore, surgical minimization and cleanliness can be expected to improve outcomes, and these are reasonable and naturally accepted tenets. Gelatin sponge has been reported to increase scar formation. Therefore, the manufacturer recommends its removal from the field after hemostasis is achieved. Urokinase has been used in an animal model to break down the small amount of blood that invariably remains or accumulates after surgery. This has reduced scar formation and lends credence to the theory of blood products being at least partially responsible.[207]

Epidural fat is the principal barrier to scar. It is different from subcutaneous fat, being semifluid without as much connective tissue, allowing roots to move freely in the healthy state.[208] A precept of technically expert surgery is that epidural fat should be treated gingerly and left as intact as possible.[3]

A number of substances have been proposed to reduce scar formation in addition to clean technique. One of the most popular measures is the use of epidural steroids, in use for the last 30 years or so. Epidural methylprednisolone or dexamethasone is commonly used and has been shown in animal models to reduce the epidural scar.[157,209,210] Steroids also have an effect on the disturbed, unmyelinated pain-transmitting C-fibers, which are the most sensitive to the inflammatory milieu of the disc hernia.[98] A combination of systemic and epidural corticosteroids may diminish such damage and improve results with respect to both resolution of pain and preservation of sensation in both the short term and long term.[211]

Free fat grafts taken from the subcutaneous space or paraspinous tissue have also been used for the last 30 years. Fat grafts can be placed in the interlaminar defect dorsally and may prevent the formation of a dorsal scar or "laminectomy membrane" but cannot be placed circumferentially around the nerve root, including its ventral surface. Literature review shows that fat grafts have not been definitively proven to help,[101,204,212,213] but there can be little down side to the application of a small pledget of fat into the interlaminar defect.

In the early postoperative period (within 6 weeks after surgery), the MRI signal intensity of grafted fat decreases, being lower than that of normal subcutaneous fat, but recovers to normal by 1 year after surgery. The total amount of grafted fat used is reduced, but it is alive and remodeled along the shape of the dura mater. There is a remodeling of the grafted fat, which is effective in protecting the spinal nerve. Reoperation with histology on grafted patients shows that grafted fat changes, showing reduction in size of the fat globules, as compared with normal fat tissue.[56,214]

Minimizing disruption of the ligamentum flavum may reduce scar formation,[3,204,215] thereby theoretically relieving the susceptibility to symptomatic tethering and recompression given subsequent anular prolapsed or small recurrent hernia, and facilitating reoperation if necessary.[215] In one method of leaving the deep ligamentum flavum and its smooth inner surface, the bony periphery of the interlaminar space is enlarged cephalad, the ligamentum flavum is thinned to paper thickness starting caudally, and then a lateral slit is produced entering the lateral recess.

Now of only historical significance, carbohydrate polymer in gelatin, Adcon-L, had proven efficacy in the reduction of scar formation around the nerve root, as shown by both animal histologic and human radiographic studies, when placed following discectomy.[216-218] However, there was noted increased incidence of postoperative CSF leakage, and the product was taken off the market.[219,220] Hyaluronic acid has also been used in animal trials[213] and is used in other surgical fields for the purpose of discouraging scar formation, though it has not been used clinically in laminectomy patients. Both agents inhibit the initial influx of inflammatory cells and the ingrowth of fibroblasts, and both agents are biodegradable. Combination carboxymethylcellulose with polyethylene oxide gel preparations are commercially available in Europe and elsewhere, but are not currently available for distribution in the United States. Used in a variety of surgical applications to reduce scar formation, the gel has been used in a randomized controlled trial in microdiscectomy. Blinded outcome assessments at intervals of up to 3-year follow-up demonstrated benefit. The biologically inactive gel does not discourage the formation of scar, but rather encourages its adhesion to dura through a barrier effect.[221]

The interposition of bone wax, silicone rubber, or Dacron sheeting and of fascial graft has also been used; none of these can be recommended, however. Common to the use of these materials is a lack of proven efficacy in the prevention of postoperative residual radiculopathy in large trials.[101]

Recurrence, Loss of Disc Height, and Discectomy Technique

Recurrence of hernia, should it occur, usually occurs within 1 or 2 years of surgery.[2,44,215,222,223] As time passes, the recurrence rate approaches the natural history likelihood that any patient may develop disc hernia. In the Maine lumbar spine study, while at the end of 10 years, 25% of surgical patients had undergone at least one additional lumbar spine operation and 25% of the nonsurgical patients also had at least one lumbar spine operation.[35]

There is broad variability in the reported rate of disc recurrence requiring surgery (as a result of recurrent hernia or secondary degenerative change and stenosis) amongst several series, ranging between 3% and 19.4%.[30,35,40,224,225] This may be the result of several factors, including differences in the definition of a recurrence, confusion with other entities such as foraminal stenosis and segmental instability, differences in technique, differences in postoperative follow-up, and differences in postoperative studies and management.[226,227] When it occurs, recurrent hernia usually occurs within the first 1 or 2 years postoperatively and ultimately approaches the likelihood of hernia in the general patient population.[44,223] The SPORT trial followed 798 surgical patients prospectively for 4 years and found an overall reoperation rate for recurrent hernia of 6% by 1 year, 8% by 2 years, 9% by 3 years, and 10% by 4 years, but half were at the previous level of operation.[44]

Patients in the SPORT study who underwent second operations scored worse outcomes than single-surgery patients and had three times the disability rate, at 8 years. While the outcome for truly recurrent soft disc hernia is as good or nearly as good as initial surgery,[226] the outcome for patients who were reoperated on without the finding of recurrent disc is worse than the outcome of reoperation for recurrent disc at the same level.[222] Operating on scar alone results in the poorest outcomes of potential postoperative radiculopathic entities and is considered futile, and repeat back surgery on an "exploratory" basis is not warranted in any situation and most likely will lead only to further disability[228] and possibly to further scar, instability, and failed back syndrome.

Recurrent disc herniation is mainly found at the first reintervention, the rate of epidural fibrosis and instability increasing with each iteration of repeat surgery along with a consequent decline in long-term improvement.[229] Therefore, a firm clinical diagnosis with strong radiculopathic symptoms and signs in concert with firm concordant radiographic findings should be standard practice.

Height loss after disc hernia and discectomy is pertinent, since it can produce foraminal stenosis, anular bulging, and lateral recess stenosis with delayed onset of recurrent radiculopathy in the same or rostral root distribution. Disc hernia itself may[89] or may not lead to disc space height loss,[230] although it is not known with certainty, since there are no long-term studies of this particular issue in patients who did not undergo surgery. Discectomy resulted in a mean 18% loss of height at 3 months and a 26% loss of height at 2 years in a recent prospective study that measured the clinical outcomes and obtained repetitive CT imaging of the lumbar spine at close intervals for a period of 2 years.[227] The study was designed to find the variables that are responsible for recurrent disc hernia. Loss of disc space height following hernia and hernia surgery is well appreciated; most patients lose about 25% of disc space height. The effect of disc space height loss on long-term outcomes has been examined, and a correlation with low back pain was found, but there is limited evidence that back pain is strongly correlated with disc space collapse.[40] Disc space height loss correlates with enlargement of the end plates and with loss of lumbar flexibility.[75] There may be better evidence that radiculopathy from foraminal stenosis may be a long-delayed result.

It has been stated that bulging anulus should be decompressed rather than violated, in the effort to reduce the chance of recurrence. Most patients with sciatica in fact have contained disc bulge rather than expressed sequestrated disc fragments. As a result, simple sequestrectomy is likely infrequently performed.[137]

Aggressive emptying of the disc space reduces recurrence, according to McGirt et al. in a prospective study specifically addressing the question of recurrence.[227] The percentage of disc material removed does correlate with loss in disc space height, but disc space height loss does not correlate with back pain, leg pain, ODI, or SF-36 at 2 years, although in the longer term, it may.[227] In a prospective outcomes study including five institutions and 2-year follow-up, it was found that those patients with recurrence (10.2%) had less disc volume removed (13% of the disc volume) compared to the patients without recurrence (28% of disc volume removed).[227] Other researchers have also found a relationship between extent of discectomy and potential for recurrent hernia or at least a relationship between preserved disc height and risk of recurrence.[40] In a comprehensive meta-analysis of the literature on the subject, it has been shown that conservative discectomy may result in a shorter operative time, quicker return to work, and decreased incidence of long-term recurrent low back and leg pain but with an increased incidence of recurrent disc herniation compared to aggressive discectomy.[227,231]

Aggressive discectomy has its down side, however, with resulting greater disc space height loss likely producing more postoperative back pain at 3 years than with sequestrectomy alone. This has been shown by Barth et al. in a prospective study of the issue and by others.[3,232-234] Barth did not find recurrence to be higher after conservative discectomy in their series.

According to McGirt et al., 11 of 108 patients suffered recurrent disc hernia (10.2%) at an average of 10.5 months postoperatively. The size of the anular defect and the amount of disc material left at the original surgery were associated with an increased risk of recurrence.[227] The same correlation between the size of the anular defect and the risk of recurrence and between the amount of disc removed and the risk of recurrence has been found by others.[235,236]

As was discussed in the techniques section, a middle ground approach should probably be taken until the matter is better settled; not just sequestrectomy should be performed, but not much aggressive curettage of the disc space either.

As was mentioned, recurrent radiculopathic pain may be due to traction injury of a root fixed in perineurial or arachnoidal scar, or it may be due to recurrent or residual disc hernia or prolapsed anulus. When radiculopathic leg pain reappears or does not remit, repeat neuroimaging is indicated. Optimally, this would be a high-quality MRI without and with gadolinium enhancement. The finding of perineurial scar only is neither a surgical complication nor an indication for revision surgery. However, lateral recess stenosis, anular prolapse, foraminal stenosis, and recurrent or residual disc herniation are all secondary complications that can be responsible for symptoms and are potentially benefitted by revision surgery. The management of repeat or incompletely treated nerve root compression is similar to that of an otherwise untreated hernia, with the exception that there is a variable amount of scar around the nerve root. The fibrosis can make anatomic planes difficult to discern and dissect and can result in unusual anatomic problems, such as intraradicular and intradural herniations, as was mentioned in the section on technique. Also, because of fibrosis and tethering of the dura mater, the presentation may be polyradicular rather than monoradicular. The anatomy is easier to understand if the bony exposure is made wider and fresh dura is identified around the periphery of the exposure.

A time-honored belief was that recurrent hernia required fusion. Fusion is not routinely required in patients undergoing repeat laminectomy and discectomy for recurrent disc herniation. In the absence of objective evidence of spinal instability, recurrent disc herniation may be adequately treated by repeat lumbar laminectomy and discectomy alone.[237]

There is little reason to proceed with fusion unless the motion segment is demonstrably unstable. Of course, the addition of fusion increases the likelihood of its own complications and reoperation rate.[225] Therefore, an initial recurrent disc hernia or secondary stenosis can be treated with conventional laminotomy or microlaminotomy, with good results.[228,237,238] In the case of multiple recurrences, because of the implication of the role of instability, repetitive revision may indicate the need for thorough decompression and fusion.[229] With the need for repetitive revisions, poorer results are encountered.[224]

Management of Complications

In either the prone or the lateral decubitus position, air embolism can occur, though in neither position is it considered to be enough of a risk to warrant invasive line placement. However, if a Doppler monitor is placed, it provides the earliest diagnosis. With paradoxical embolism across a patent foramen ovale, a decrease in arterial carbon dioxide pressure, a decrease in end-tidal carbon dioxide pressure, an increase in arterial carbon dioxide pressure, and subsequent hypotension and tachycardia may all be observed. Proper management consists of ceasing nitrous oxide administration, flooding the field with saline, waxing the bony surfaces, and repositioning the patient quickly to lower the field in relation to the heart.[239]

The incidence of dural tears may be 1.6%[3,240] to 4%,[241] with an incidence of 3% in the SPORT trial.[44] Perhaps the number is more, since ventral tears that are not noted intraoperatively would not be detected. Outcomes studies demonstrate no long-term sequelae when patients are satisfactorily repaired primarily during initial surgery.[127,240-242] The hazard of a dural tear lies not with the nuisance meningeal injury that is sustained, recognized, and repaired adequately at the time of surgery, but rather with injury that is not recognized at surgery, is not adequately repaired, or is acquired postoperatively.

In such cases, hydrostatic pressure and superimposed events such as Valsalva and motion are likely generating or aggravating factors.[243] Long-term postoperative symptoms such as headache reduce daily activity and impair postoperative progress, such that a longer duration of inability to work and long-term functional limitation may be engendered.[242] Delayed or inadequately repaired durotomy risks wound dehiscence and CSF leakage or symptomatic pseudomeningocele. Should they occur, the dura should be repaired as quickly as possible following surgery.[124-126,242]

Pseudomeningocele can cause recurrent back and leg pain, the latter being the result of nerve root herniation into the extradural sac.[125] Good results, with resolution of symptoms by primary closure of the dural defect, can be expected. Ventral dural tear may be a consequence of dural adhesion to the PLL or anulus, in this way perhaps similar to transdural HNP. Generally, ventral dural tear does not require suture closure; however, symptomatic herniation of nerve roots through a ventral defect into the empty disc cavity has been described.[243]

If a spontaneous, unrecognized, or inadequately repaired durotomy complicates the wound postoperatively, an attempt at the use of an autologous blood patch or fibrin glue patch in the treatment of postoperative pseudomeningocele or fistula, if small, is reasonable and potentially successful. The use of closed lumbar drainage for several days placed at a distance from the original incision is also effective.[128] The decision to reoperate and repair the defect is elective and dependent on symptoms in the case of pseudomeningocele but is more urgent in the event of high-volume or persistent fistula, since the soft tissue becomes compromised and has the potential for becoming infected quickly.

A rare complication, cerebellar hemorrhagic venous infarction, has been reported as resulting from durotomy with intraoperative loss of CSF. It is possible that downward cerebellar displacement, or "sag," causes transient stretch occlusion of superior cerebellar veins draining in the rostral direction into the deep venous system. This may cause intracerebellar hemorrhage in patients with insufficient venous collaterals. Remote cerebellar hemorrhage should be considered in a case of neurologic deterioration following lumbar durotomy.[244]

Injury of abdominal organs or viscera occurs in 1.6 to 17 per 10,000 cases.[148] Effective management of visceral or vascular injury requires prompt recognition of its occurrence. Mortality approaches 100% in cases of untreated vascular or visceral injuries.[148] In some reported cases of bowel and ureteral injury, visceral tissue was found in the disc specimen that was submitted for examination. As was mentioned in the section on technique, injury may be suspected intraoperatively because of hypotension, the unexplained egress of irrigation fluid through the anulus and out of the field, or persistent bleeding up through the anulus that is not explained by bone or epidural bleeding. There appear to be no common risk factors predisposing patients to this type of hazard, apart from ventral anular tear. A sound knowledge of retroperitoneal anatomy is useful (Fig. 78-5). Even with treatment, mortality of these injuries is high, at nearly 50%; therefore, if suspected, the injury demands immediate attention.[148] Unfortunately,

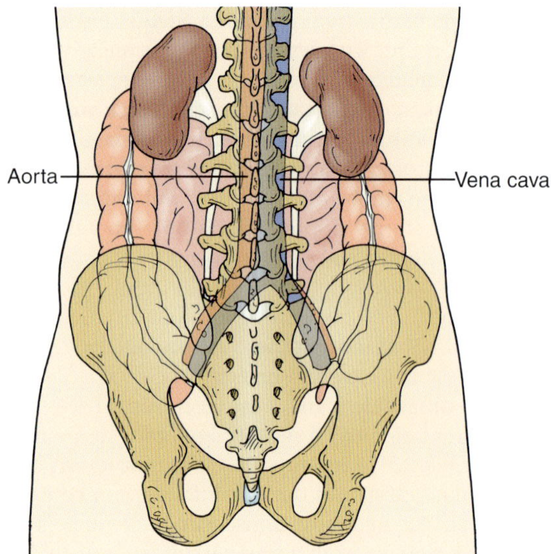

FIGURE 78-5. Abdominal viscera that are at risk through ventral disc penetration.

the initial lack of clinical signs of injury usually accounts for any delay that is encountered, and in a majority of cases, the surgeon fails to recognize perforation of the anulus or ligament and intra-abdominal injury. In convalescence, persistent flank or abdominal pain, ileus, hypotension, and fever may all signal intra-abdominal injury and should be investigated. Plain abdominal radiographs, CT, intravenous pyelogram, angiography, and abdominal ultrasound may all be necessary.

A patient may be sensitized to major vascular injury through one of two or three anatomic variations. Since the anterior longitudinal ligament provides a barrier to the passage of an instrument through the anulus into the retroperitoneum, a high aortic bifurcation results in the iliac vessel lying lateral to the protection of the ligament. A spondylotic ridge may result in attenuation of the ligament.[147] Also, peridiscal inflammation, resulting in fibrosis, can result in adhesion of a large vessel to the anulus. The left iliac artery is the most commonly injured named vessel. Arterial injury is at times large enough, and hypotension is rapid enough, that there might not be time for angiography or scanning. In such cases, immediate laparotomy is indicated purely on clinical suspicion. If the vessel is small and the patient is stable, perhaps having presented with hemorrhage from the disc space, angiography is useful in determining its location prior to laparotomy.[245] There may be an initial lack of clinical signs of vascular injury until significant blood loss has occurred and the patient is in danger of vascular collapse, particularly in healthy young patients with significant cardiovascular reserve (if a small vessel such as a medial sacral vessel has been injured).

Bowel motility is slowed by the use of general anesthesia, but it can also result from the surgery itself, and ileus can affect both the large and small bowel. Usually, it is not a significant problem, but it can last several days and can require nasogastric suction.[246] A more severe form of impaired bowel motility—pseudo-obstruction of the colon (Ogilvie syndrome)—is a life-threatening complication that is characterized by massive cecal distention that can lead to perforation. Bowel sounds are present from areas of active motility, but cecal distention and tenderness are also present. Decompression by colonoscopy is the treatment of choice unless rupture has already occurred.[247]

Infections can be categorized as those involving the bone or the disc interspace and simple wound infections. The risk of wound infection is about 0.5%. A frank wound infection that does not involve the disc space or bone can be managed with drainage and a brief 1- or 2-week course of appropriate antibiotics. Surveillance measures should be taken to rule out a deepening process. Nearly 80% of infections in discectomy patients appear in the first postoperative month. Diabetic, elderly, alcoholic, and immunocompromised patients are at greatest risk. Excessive use of monopolar cautery and excessive tissue trauma and tissue retraction predispose to infectious complication. If extending to the surface, an infected wound may be probed to determine its depth and to drain the purulent material. If probing or scanning demonstrates a wound separation down to the bone, the likelihood of disc interspace involvement is higher.

If disc interspace infection is present, the superficial wound is often well healed, with the nidus of infection contained in the disc space. Marked persistent spastic back pain, marked sedimentation rate elevation, and elevated C-reactive protein levels are clinical and laboratory indicators of disc interspace infection. In these cases, discitis should be assumed until it has been ruled out.[248] The presence of unusually severe pain in the postoperative period, even if the wound is well healed, should prompt a workup for disc interspace infection because superficial evidence of wound infection is unusual. MRI is a very sensitive indicator and can show evidence of infection early in its course. Patients with sedimentation rates of over 45 mm/min and C-reactive protein levels higher than 2.5 mg/L on the fifth or sixth postoperative day are suspected of having disc interspace infections. Although the temperature and peripheral white blood cell count may be elevated, this is not always the case. If disc interspace infection is present, antibiotics should be appropriate for the infectious agent as proven by open or CT-guided biopsy or by peripheral blood culture (which is positive in 25% of cases). Intravenous antibiotics should be administered for a period of 6 weeks. If there is reason to suspect involvement of adjacent vertebral bone, by MRI or CT or by progressive deformity, intravenous antibiotics should be continued for 6 to 8 weeks, followed by oral antibiotics for another 8 weeks. Immobilization is generally recommended.

The radiographic changes of disc interspace infection are often delayed. Optimally, the presence of infection should be recognized before its radiographic appearance. Plain radiographs do not show a change until 6 weeks after the onset of infection, until there is erosion of the subchondral cortical bone. The most sensitive radiographic study early in the course of infection is the MRI scan, which shows (1) a diffuse decrease in the T1 signal from vertebral body bone adjacent to the disc as a result of edema fluid in the marrow; (2) blurring of the margins between vertebral bone, cartilaginous end plates, and disc; and (3) an increased T2 signal in the area of inflammation, particularly in the disc. There may be swelling of paravertebral soft tissues and, with gadolinium infusion, epidural contrast enhancement. Bone scanning and indium-labeled leukocyte scanning are also quite sensitive and positive relatively early in the course of infection.

Staphylococcus aureus can produce, in addition to abscess formation and recurrent neurologic deficit on the basis of space-occupying mass effect, exotoxins with local and distant effects. Toxic shock syndrome is attributable to this, with vascular collapse and encephalopathy. Reportedly, local staphylococcal wound infection after lumbar laminectomy can even result in a cauda equina syndrome, without a compressive mass effect.[249]

Postoperative Course and Postoperative Care

Classically, the first symptom to improve following successful surgery is the pain of radiculopathy, typically followed by improvement in motor function, and finally by resolution of sensory loss.[7,38,39] Sensory loss may be permanent, however, persisting at 10-year follow-up in 35% of Weber's patients.

Impairment of back muscle function due to months of inactivity before surgery may be a factor contributing to prolonged and suboptimal outcome. Surgery itself only superimposes further damage on lumbar paraspinous musculature and does not, by itself, improve function. In a prospective randomized controlled trial of supervised exercise therapy addressing patients who had undergone microdiscectomy, Dolan et al. found that a 4-week exercise program focused on improving strength and endurance of the back and abdominal muscles and mobility of the spine and hips, initiated at 6 weeks postoperatively, provided clear benefit. Outcome measures that improved in the exercise group included paraspinous surface electromyography, pain, disability, back muscle endurance, and lumbar and hip mobility.[250,251]

In another prospective randomized trial of similar design, significant benefit following lumbar disc hernia surgery was demonstrated by a decrease in disability and pain scores at 6 months and 12 months in a group that was randomized to training starting at 4 weeks postoperatively.[252] There is no evidence that activity restriction improves outcomes or avoids complications after lumbar surgery.[235,252]

Dewing et al. reported the outcomes of lumbar discectomy in a population of young, active military personnel, finding not only that 84% were capable of unrestricted return to active service, but that those who did best were special operations personnel and aviators.[253] There is actually little evidence that aggressive physical activity is harmful to disc tissue, whether it is in a degenerative, normal, or postoperative state. In fact, immobilization has been determined to be harmful to the disc, likely through its adverse effect on the diffusion of nutrients and the maintenance of disc tissue homeostasis.[73]

Recurrent symptoms may result from, or be exacerbated by, poor bone and ligamentous healing. Bone healing might not be as important to outcome in discectomy as it would be in attempted fusion, but it is nevertheless significant in bone remodeling postoperatively. Physiologic bone remodeling is important for the reacquisition of normal pars strength and therefore to long-term results and return to preoperative activities. Systemic factors that have been demonstrated to inhibit bone healing and likely to interfere with optimum outcome include smoking, malnutrition, diabetes, rheumatologic conditions, and osteoporosis. Additionally, courses of steroids, nonsteroidal medications, and cytotoxic medications in the perioperative period are to be avoided, particularly the first 2 postoperative weeks.[254] It is suggested that postoperative patients engage in and maintain daily reconditioning, including low-impact aerobic exercises, such as walking and swimming and active range-of-motion exercises.

Conclusions

Surgical discectomy is a cost-effective solution to the problem of short-term pain and disability in carefully selected patients harboring a symptomatic lumbar disc hernia refractory to conservative management.[6,44] In the short term, up to a year postoperatively, the benefits are clear.

Delay in treatment of symptomatic patients may result in a poorer clinical outcome, particularly in those with strong sensorimotor findings. In the longer term, in patients with intermediate-intensity symptoms who accept randomization, benefits become less distinct compared to medical management, such that by 10 years, there may be no discernable difference.

Lumbar disc surgery may appear routine and unchallenging, but pitfalls, potential complications, and the chances for poor outcomes are numerous. Important distinctions in patient selection, neuroimaging, timing of surgery, and technical nuances in the performance of the surgery and in subsequent patient follow-up have been addressed. Keen, objective patient selection is imperative in the offer of lumbar discectomy.

KEY REFERENCES

Atlas SJ, Keller RB, Wu YA, et al: Long-term outcomes of surgical and nonsurgical management of sciatica secondary to a lumbar disc herniation: 10 year results from the Maine lumbar spine study. *Spine (Phila Pa 1976)* 30(8):927–935, 2005.

Battié MC, Videman T, Kaprio J, et al: The Twin Spine Study: contributions to a changing view of disc degeneration. *Spine J* 9(1):47–59, 2009.

Epstein N: Foraminal and far lateral lumbar disc herniations: surgical alternatives and outcome measures. *Spinal Cord* 40(10):491–500, 2002.

Gibson JN, Waddell G: Surgical interventions for lumbar disc prolapse: updated Cochrane Review. *Spine (Phila Pa 1976)* 32(16):1735–1747, 2007.

Weber H: The natural history of disc herniation and the influence of intervention. *Spine (Phila Pa 1976)* 19(19):2234–2238, 1994.

Weinstein JN, Lurie JD, Tosteson TD, et al: Surgical versus nonoperative treatment for lumbar disc herniation: four-year results for the Spine Patient Outcomes Research Trial (SPORT). *Spine (Phila Pa 1976)* 33(25): 2789–2800, 2008.

REFERENCES

The complete reference list is available online at expertconsult.com.

CHAPTER 79

Management of Soft Cervical Disc Herniation: Controversies and Complication Avoidance

Jan Goffin | Jeroen Ceuppens

About 450 years ago, Vesalius described the intervertebral disc.[1] It was not until 1928 that Stookey described a number of clinical syndromes resulting from cervical disc protrusions. These protrusions were thought to be neoplasms of notochordal origin and were incorrectly identified as chondromas.[2] During this same era, other investigators provided a more precise understanding of the pathophysiology of intervertebral disc herniation.[3-5]

Both soft and hard cervical disc herniations can lead to nerve root compression (radiculopathy) and/or compression of the spinal cord (myelopathy). Hard cervical disc herniation is a condition in which osteophytosis is involved. This chapter focuses on pure soft disc herniation, which causes radiculopathy more frequently than myelopathy (Figs. 79-1 to 79-4).

Population-based data from Rochester, Minnesota, indicate that cervical radiculopathy has an annual incidence rate of 107.3 per 100,000 for men and 63.5 per 100,000 for women, with a peak at 50 to 54 years of age. A history of physical exertion or trauma preceded the onset of symptoms in only 15% of cases. A study from Sicily reported a prevalence of 3.5 cases per 1000 population.[6]

The most common cause of cervical radiculopathy (in 70–75% of cases) is foraminal encroachment of the spinal nerve due to a combination of factors, including decreased disc height and degenerative changes of the uncovertebral joints ventrally and the zygoapophyseal joints dorsally (i.e., cervical spondylosis). In contrast to disorders of the lumbar spine, pure herniation of the nucleus pulposus (soft disc herniation) is responsible for only 20% to 25% of cases,[7] although the relative proportion of disc herniation in younger people is significantly higher.[8] Overall, though, in many cases, there is a combination of some spondylosis with a soft disc herniation. Other causes, including tumors of the cervical spine and spinal infections, are infrequent.[6]

A concise strategy for treating soft cervical disc herniations based on former knowledge and new insights is provided in this chapter. Controversies are discussed, including when one operates and, if so, how one does it. Second, an overview of possible complications and how to avoid them is provided.

Controversies

Surgical Indications

Commonly accepted indications for surgery differ, depending on whether a pure soft disc herniation causes radiculopathy without deficit or whether there are neurologic deficits due to nerve root or spinal cord compression.

Data on the natural history of cervical radiculopathy are limited. In the population-based study from Rochester, Minnesota, 26% of 561 patients with cervical radiculopathy underwent surgery within 3 months of diagnosis (typically for the combination of radicular pain, sensory loss, and muscle weakness), whereas the remainder were treated medically.[6] The natural course of spondylotic and discogenic cervical

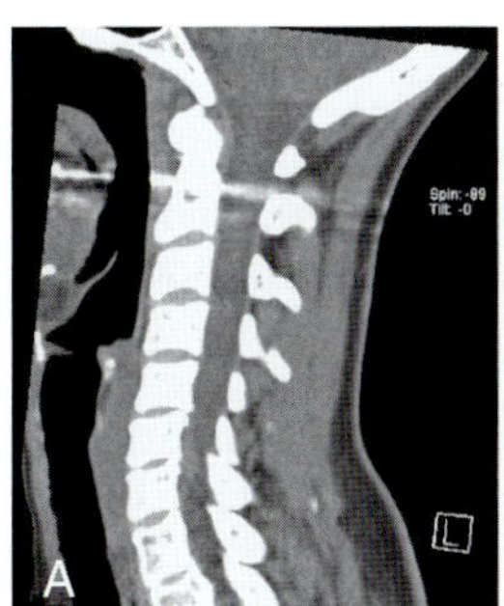

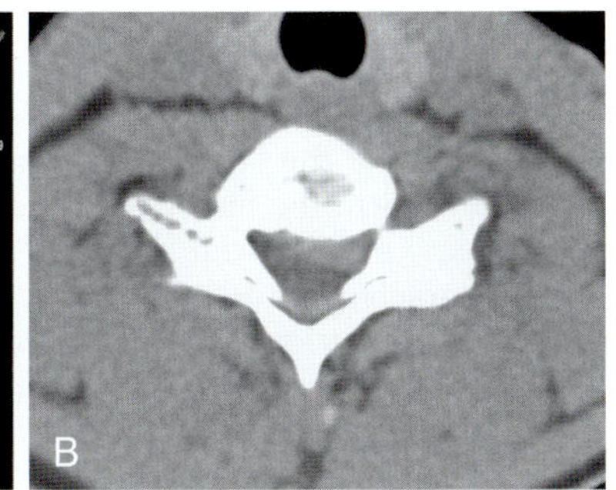

FIGURE 79-1. A and **B,** CT images of C6-7 soft cervical disc herniation.

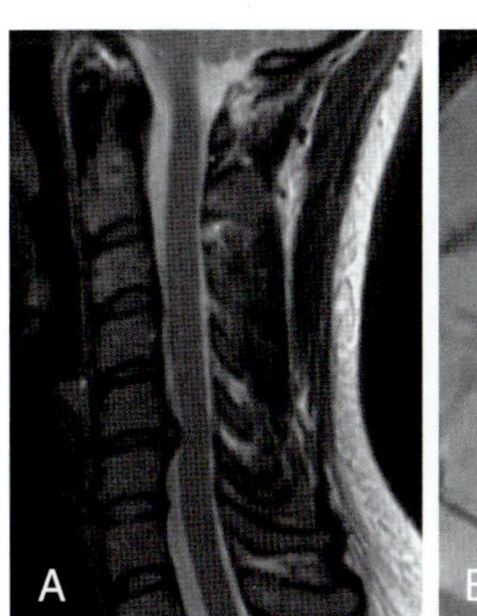

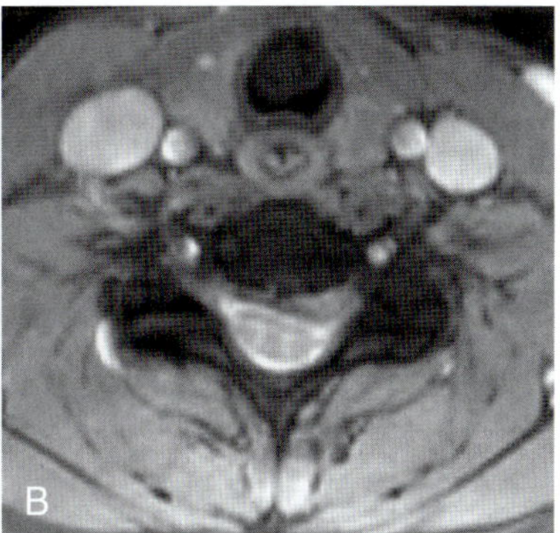

FIGURE 79-2. A and **B,** Magnetic resonance images of C5-6 soft cervical disc herniation.

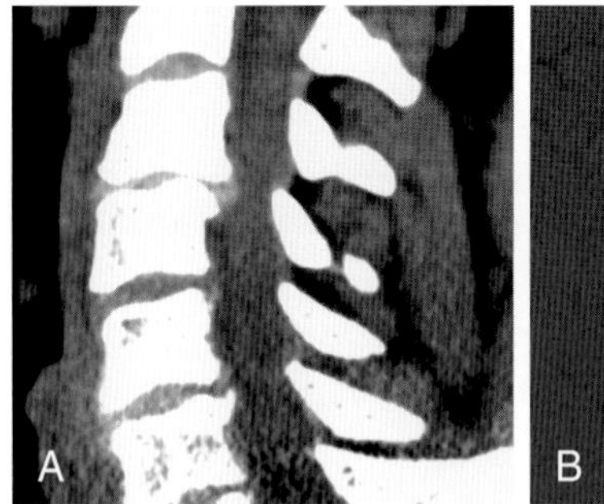
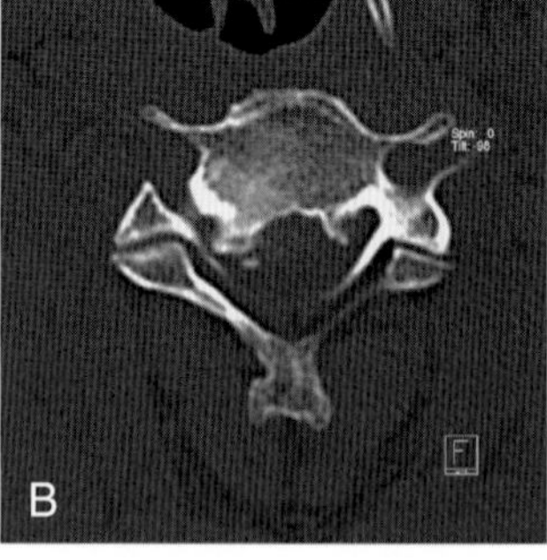

FIGURE 79-3. CT images of C3-4 hard cervical disc herniation.

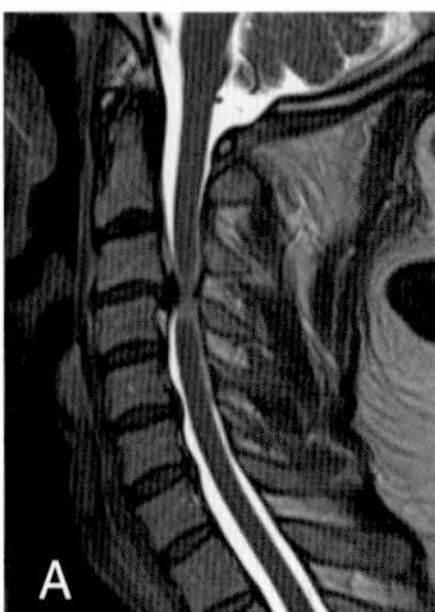
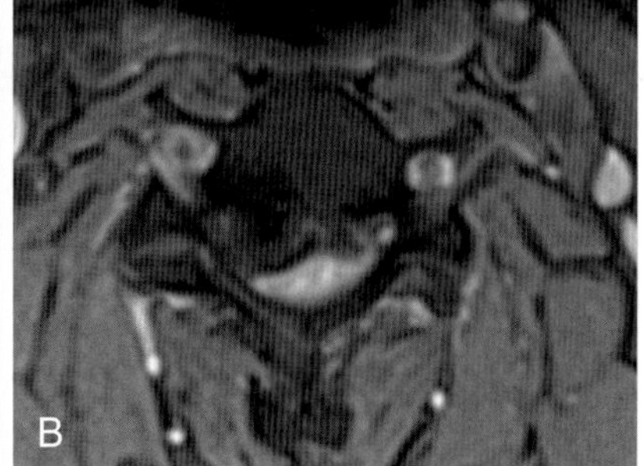

FIGURE 79-4. Magnetic resonance images of C3-4 hard cervical disc herniation.

radiculopathy is generally favorable. In particular, pure soft disc herniations often resolve spontaneously.[8]

The main objectives of treatment are to relieve pain, to improve neurologic function, and to prevent recurrences. None of the commonly recommended nonsurgical therapies for cervical radiculopathy have been tested in randomized, placebo-controlled trials. Therefore, recommendations are derived largely from case series and anecdotal experiences. The patient's preferences should be taken into account in the decision-making process. Analgesic agents, including opioids and nonsteroidal anti-inflammatory drugs, are often used as first-line therapy. Retrospective and prospective cohort studies reported favorable results with interlaminar and transforaminal epidural injections of corticosteroids, with up to 60% of patients experiencing long-term relief of radicular and neck pain and a return to usual activities. However, complications from these injections, although rare, can be serious and include severe neurologic sequelae from spinal cord or brainstem lesions. Given the potential for harm, placebo-controlled trials are needed to assess both the safety and the efficacy of cervical epidural injections. Some investigators advocate the use of short-term immobilization (<2 weeks) with either a hard or a soft collar (either continuously or only at night) to aid in pain control. Cervical traction consists of administering a distracting force to the neck to separate the cervical segments and relieve compression of nerve roots by intervertebral discs. Especially in the absence of night pain, traction therapy may be considered to alleviate pain. Various techniques and durations have been recommended. However, a systematic review stated that no conclusions could be drawn about the efficacy of cervical traction. The same is true for exercise therapy.[6]

Therefore, in appropriate patients, surgery may effectively relieve otherwise intractable symptoms and signs related to cervical radiculopathy, although there are no data to guide the optimal timing of this intervention. For cervical radiculopathy without evidence of myelopathy, surgery is typically recommended when cervical root compression is visualized on MRI or CT myelography with concordant symptoms and signs of cervical root–related dysfunction and when the pain does not disappear despite nonsurgical treatment for at least 6 to 12 weeks. A progressive, functionally important motor deficit represents a more urgent surgical indication. Surgery is definitely recommended in cases in which imaging shows cervical compression of the spinal cord in combination with clinical evidence of moderate to severe myelopathy.[6]

As summarized in a Cochrane review, there are only a limited number of good-quality studies comparing surgical and nonsurgical treatments for cervical radiculopathy. In one randomized trial comparing surgical and nonsurgical therapies among 81 patients with radiculopathy alone, the patients in the surgical group had a significantly greater reduction in pain at 3 months than the patients who were assigned to receive physiotherapy or who underwent immobilization in a hard collar. However, at 1 year, there was no difference among the three treatment groups in any of the outcomes measured, including pain, function, and mood.[9]

Comparing cervical with lumbar (soft) disc herniations, Peul[10] pointed out that in the absence of alarming symptoms related to lumbar disc herniations, surgery is optional, depending on the patient's preference. However, in contrast with lumbar disc herniation, cervical soft disc herniations more frequently justify surgical treatment when refractory radiculopathy is concerned.

Surgical Approach

Multiple surgical approaches to the cervical spinal canal or neural foramina are possible, with associated advantages and disadvantages. Ventral and dorsal options have been described.[11]

The dorsal exposures have three possible advantages in comparison to the ventral approach: (1) Less surgical effort is required in exposing or decompressing multiple levels; (2) additional fusion with or without instrumentation is often not required; and (3) the procedure does not necessarily stiffen the motion segments involved and therefore does not accelerate spondylotic degeneration at adjacent levels, as is thought to occur after (ventral) fusion procedures. Partial hemilaminectomy, with or without foraminotomy, has become a standard dorsal exposure for laterally located cervical disc herniation.[11] Central disc herniations, however, should be approached ventrally.

Technically, the dorsal approach is begun with a small partial hemilaminectomy above and below the level of expected pathology.[11] Removing the caudal margin of the rostral lamina laterally and the attached ligamentum flavum allows for identification of the lateral dural margin and the nerve root origin. Although the major exposure is caudal, it is desirable to also expose the rostral border of the nerve root to allow for its complete identification and achieve some space for the minimal mobilization of the nerve root. Often, there is a small amount of space caudal to the nerve root. This space can be enlarged with a curette or a high-speed drill. Venous bleeding is most common with this approach and should be adequately addressed during exposition of the neural structures. Care must also be taken to ensure that one has enough of the nerve root exposed that the motor root is not confused with extruded disc material. After sufficient exposure of the nerve, the surgeon starts to explore for a disc extrusion, from above or beneath the nerve root. If there is a soft disc extrusion, the posterior longitudinal ligament can be incised with a knife, and a bit of pressure on the above posterior longitudinal ligament occasionally causes the fragment to be milked outward beneath the elevated root. Following this, there is often some additional space so that the foramen can be better explored and enlarged if necessary. If there is only a small, hard bony ridge beneath the nerve root, it might not be necessary to remove this. Often, a simple but thorough decompression of the nerve root dorsally into the foramen provides adequate relief of symptoms. After removal of an extruded cervical disc, it is not necessary or advisable to enter the cervical disc space to remove additional degenerated disc material from behind. Usually, visualizing the interspace would require significant root and spinal cord retraction, which in itself could result in nerve root or spinal cord injury. On the other hand, such additional discectomy is not necessary, since the recurrence rate for a cervical disc herniation without entering the disc space is less than 1% in most series.

Half a century has elapsed since the initial description of ventral cervical discectomy by Bailey and Badgley.[12] Modifications of this technique were described by Robinson and Smith in 1955[13] and by Cloward and the group of Dereymaeker and Mulier, both in 1958.[14,15] Robinson and Smith described an operation for removal of cervical disc material with replacement by a rectangular bone graft, obtained from the iliac crest, to allow for the development of a cervical fusion.[13] With Cloward's method, the discectomy and fusion were performed by a dowel technique. Although numerous modifications have been developed since the 1950s, the great majority of spine surgeons currently use either the Cloward or the Smith-Robinson technique, primarily for herniations that are located on the midline or mediolaterally.[16-25]

Technically, the ventral approach starts with optimal positioning of the patient with the head in slight (hyper-) extension. The side of the incision has been given excessive emphasis because of potential harm to the laryngeal nerve. However, more practical concerns such as previous surgery (and thus potential subclinical vocal cord problems) and the side of the radicular symptoms (as it appears that owing to the surgeon's oblique perspective, contralateral decompression is favored) should dictate the side of incision. After a right- or left-sided approach has been chosen, a transverse skin incision is made. An avascular dissection plane is developed between the esophagus/trachea medially and the sternocleidomastoid/carotid sheath laterally. Hand-held retractors might be utilized to provide initial exposure of the ventral vertebral column and the adjacent longus colli muscles. After removal of the disc and preparation of the end plates according to the technique used (different fusion techniques versus disc replacement; see later discussion), the posterior longitudinal ligament is opened, and the disc extrusion is removed. When myelopathy is present, we advise starting to open the ligament laterally without exerting (additional) pressure on the spinal cord. Finalization of the procedure follows according to technique.

Radiologic evaluation is crucial in decision making. When the abnormality is central, broad based, and dorsal, a ventral procedure is more likely to achieve decompression. On the other hand, with lateral or foraminal nerve root compression, the simpler dorsal keyhole laminoforaminotomy works well. One may consider that the possible additional decompressive effect due to (slight) distraction of the vertebrae (and thus opening of the neuroforamina) in ventral fusion is not obtained via a dorsal approach. Physicians who advocate either procedure exclusively may not always provide the "best" approach.[26]

Ventral Approach: Cervical Discectomy without Bone Fusion versus Cervical Discectomy with Bone Fusion versus Prosthesis

Cervical discectomy with bone fusion (ACDF) as has been described by Cloward [14] and Robinson and Smith[13] has become a routine surgical procedure. Nevertheless, when autografts from the iliac crest are used, the technique has been associated with donor site morbidity such as pain, infection, hematomas, nerve injury, and iliac crest deformity. Graft and fusion problems at the fusion bed may occur, such as nonunion, graft collapse, or dislodgement.[27] In attempts to overcome the graft-related problems, cervical discectomy without bone fusion (ACD) was introduced in 1960 by Hirsch.[28] However, ACD has usually been associated with postoperative neck pain, cervical curve deformity (kyphosis), and lower fusion rates (up to 60%). One can consider that the actual aim of ACD is even to avoid fusion. Hospital stay is an important consideration in the recent era of cost consciousness. In some countries, the debate between advocates of ACDF and of ACD is still ongoing. Abd-Alrahman et al.[27] concluded that the controversial issue in the management of patients undergoing anterior cervical discectomy will continue regarding the choice between ACD and ACDF. Proponents of interbody grafting claim that with ACD, the disc height and the area of the neural foramina at that level will decrease postoperatively, with the potential for persistent symptoms and/or the development of a radiculopathy, and that the kyphosis rate is high. With ACDF, the fusion rate is high, the neck pain is less, the distraction of disc space stretches the ligamentum flavum and reduces its buckling, diminishing the risk for postoperative ongoing or recurrent nerve root compression. Nowadays, ACDF is much more frequently performed than is ACD. ACD should furthermore be limited to patients with a single soft disc without spondylosis.

The option of disc arthroplasty is emerging. Cervical disc arthroplasty or total intervertebral disc replacement (TDR) seems to be a promising nonfusion alternative for the treatment of degenerative disc disease, especially in cases of pure soft disc herniation. TDR is designed to preserve motion, avoid limitations of fusion, and allow patients to quickly return to routine activities. The primary goal of the procedure in the cervical spine is to maintain segmental motion after removing the local pathology and, by doing this, to prevent later adjacent-level degeneration,[29-31] as is sometimes seen after ACDF due to increased motion stress at those adjacent levels. TDR also avoids the morbidity of bone graft harvest, pseudarthrosis, issues caused by ventral cervical plating, and cervical immobilization side effects.[30] The Frenchay (Bristol) prosthesis[32] and the Bryan intervertebral disc prosthesis were the first to be clinically assessed in Europe. The first cervical disc arthoplasty clinical trial in the United States was the Bryan disc study initiated in May 2002 after a European prospective human clinical trial began in 2000.[33] The results of the European clinical trial with the Bryan disc prosthesis, though neither randomized nor controlled, validated the stability, biocompatibility, and functionality predicted by preclinical testing. Although the mechanical rationale seems obvious and TDR thus can be considered an attractive tool for treating cervical soft disc herniation, Peng-Fei and Yu-Hua[34] recently stated that the follow-up time of the studies that have already been published is not (yet) long enough to support the advantage of cervical disc prosthesis technology. On the contrary, Walraevens et al. more recently demonstrated that up to 8 years after surgery with the Bryan disc, maintenance of mobility at the treated level is preserved in the vast majority of cases.[35] Moreover, they argued that the prosthesis seems to protect against acceleration of adjacent-level degeneration. Finally, 90% of all patients were shown to have a clinically good to excellent outcome. Chapter 224D provides further details about this matter (Fig. 79-5).

Recently, Yi et al.[36] reported that ventral cervical foraminotomy, as cervical arthroplasty, can be a valid treatment for unilateral cervical radiculopathy, sharing the same goal of preservation of segmental motion and avoidance of adjacent segment degeneration.

One can finally consider that whereas soft and hard disc herniations are two distinct entities, as was mentioned before, the treatment considerations of the two are similar. In the authors' estimation of optimal ventral surgical treatment, TDR remains optional in pure soft cervical disc herniations, but not so with hard disc herniations.

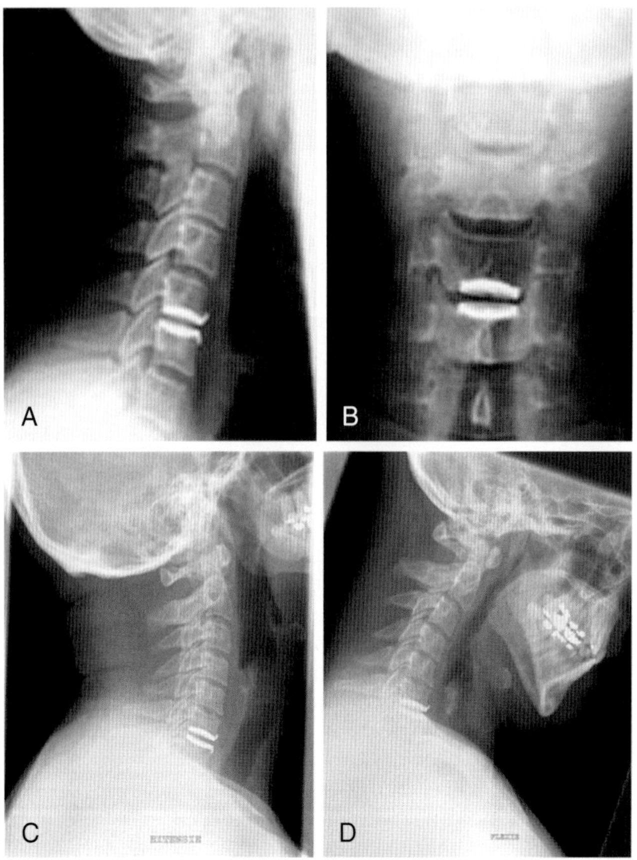

FIGURE 79-5. A–D, Radiographs of Bryan prosthesis with dynamic (flexion-extension) images.

Cervical Discectomy with Bone Fusion Strategies

Several techniques for ACDF are currently performed, mostly depending on the choice of the surgeon. However, there may be differences in perioperative morbidity and short- and long-term outcome. A recently published study by Bhadra et al.[37] analyzed the cost-effectiveness of the three different techniques in comparison to each other and to arthroplasty. Besides a group of arthroplasty patients, they defined three groups of 15 patients each: (1) plate and tricortical autograft; (2) plate, cage, and bone substitute; and (3) cage only. They found that the clinical outcome in terms of a visual analogue scale of neck and arm pain and physical and mental score improvement were comparable with all three techniques. The radiologic fusion rate was comparable to currently available data. Because the hospital stay was longer in the plate and autograft group, the total cost was a maximum with this group. Using a cage alone was the most cost-effective technique in the authors' hands.

The scope of the further discussion is how optimal fusion can be obtained and whether an optimal fusion is clinically relevant.

Autograft?

Autograft is still considered the gold standard in achieving radiographic fusion in one-level anterior cervical discectomy and fusion. Autogenous bone has osteoinductive, osteoconductive, and osteogenic properties.[38] The capacity for rapid regeneration comes mostly from fresh cancellous bone, which contains bone matrix proteins and mineral collagen. An ideal autograft includes strong cortical bone to provide structural support and cancellous bone for augmented incorporation and fusion characteristics. Revascularization of cancellous bone is completed within 2 weeks, whereas it takes 2 months for cortical bone. An additional advantage of autogenous bone graft is that is does not carry transmissible diseases to the host. Cortical and cancellous graft material is generally obtained from the iliac crest.

As was mentioned by Bhadra et al.,[37] autograft as a gold standard is challenged. Seemingly, when rigid instrumentation is used, the inferior fusion rates with allograft can be overcome. Samartzis et al.,[39] found that when autograft (without plate) was compared with allograft with rigid ventral plate fixation in one-level anterior cervical discectomy and fusion, the two methods resulted in statistically equivalently high fusion rates with excellent and good clinical outcomes. The radiographic fusion rate was even higher in the allograft group. They stated also that the use of allograft eliminates complications and pitfalls associated with autologous donor site harvesting. On the other hand, autograft was considered safer in terms of prevention of infection. The specific complication rates related to the plating itself were not addressed. Additionally, the same authors showed in another study [40] that considering autograft in one-level cervical fusion with or without rigid plate fixation, the two methods gave similar results.

Allograft?

Allografts are tissues obtained from cadavers or living donors.[38] They are associated with delayed vascularization and delayed incorporation, perhaps because of antigenic recognition.

Allografts have osteoinductive and osteoconductive properties. However, they have lost their osteogenic property.

To overcome the relatively high collapse rate of allogeneic iliac crest, Martin et al. conducted a study on the efficacy of allogeneic fibula graft[41] on cervical fusion rate. They found that allogeneic fibula is an effective substrate for use in achieving fusion after cervical discectomy. Maximal results were achieved with its use at one level. As a secondary outcome, cigarette smoking appeared to decrease the fusion rates, but not by a statistically significant amount.

As was mentioned earlier, when rigid instrumentation is used, ventral cervical fusions at one level with autograft or with allograft seem to have comparable fusion rates. This therapeutic approach is widely adopted in the United States. Whether similarly increased fusion rates can be obtained when allograft is combined with bone morphogenetic protein (BMP) is hotly debated.

Cage?

Cage fusion technology originated in 1979 from Bagby's work in horses and was first used in humans in around 1990.[42] The principle of distraction-compression, the basic principle of stand-alone intervertebral cage fusion, was introduced. Interbody cages provide initial segmental stability by tensioning the ligament apparatus, which anchors a cage's top and bottom areas to the adjacent end plates. They can be threaded or not.

Titanium cage-assisted ACDF provides long-term stability, increasing lordosis, segmental height, and foraminal height. Polyetheretherketone (PEEK) is a semicrystalline polyaromatic linear polymer that provides a good combination of strength, stiffness, toughness, and environmental resistance. The elastic modulus of the PEEK cage is close to that of bone, which helps to decrease stress shielding and increase bony fusion. The PEEK cage has a deleterious influence on cell attachment and growth and inhibits a stimulatory effect on the protein content of osteoblasts.[43] Trabecular Metal is a porous tantalum biomaterial with structure and mechanical properties similar to those of trabecular bone and with proven osteoconductivity.[44]

Recent studies by Cho et al.[45] and by Chou et al.[43] consistently showed the equivalence of PEEK cages and autografts in ACDF, in terms of fusion rates, clinical improvement, and complication rate. Löfgren et al. recently published a study in which Trabecular Metal showed a lower fusion rate than the Smith-Robinson technique with autograft after single-level ventral cervical fusion without plating. However, no difference was seen in clinical outcomes between the groups. The operative time was shorter with Trabecular Metal implants.[44]

The issue of postoperative image distortion (on CT or MRI) is seldom addressed in the literature, though it should be taken into account in evaluating cage fusions.

To Plate or Not to Plate?

Plating is theoretically designed to improve fusion rates, based on the impending risk of pseudarthrosis in uninstrumented cases. The essential question is twofold: Does instrumentation improve fusion rates, and is pseudarthrosis in uninstrumented cases a significant problem? Furthermore, if pseudarthrosis occurs or is radiographically documented, is it of any clinical relevance? Additionally, focusing on the previously mentioned higher fusion rates in autograft versus allograft, can plating compensate for this difference?

The first question is answered by a number of studies showing higher fusion rates in instrumented autologous and allogeneic grafts, compared with cases without plating, even at one level.[46,47] Second, despite the differences in the reported fusion rates of these procedures, they seem to be similar in their effectiveness of symptomatic relief.[46,48] The proposal that surgical fusion is unnecessary is controversial.

Bhadra et al.[37] tend to answer the final question. Seemingly, plating can compensate for lower fusion rates in allografts in comparison to autografts. The clinical relevance again can be questioned.

As a general appraisal, we state that plating is mostly associated with multilevel pathology, which is rare in pure soft disc herniation cases. In the latter, plating seems to be an issue only when allograft is considered.

Bone Morphogenetic Protein?

Because of the potential risk of pseudarthrosis (0–40%) and late-term destabilization of ventral cervical fusion, means to improve the rate and speed of bone healing seem to be needed. Besides autogenous iliac crest grafts and PEEK cages, BMP containing allograft struts can be considered.[49,50] When consideration is given to BMP, necessity, efficacy, safety, and cost should be taken into account. Tumialan et al.[51] and Buttermann showed the efficacy of BMP.[52] The latter study included 66 patients in whom either autograft (without BMP) or allograft struts augmented with BMP were used to obtain fusion. The autograft (without BMP) nonunion rate was twice as high as that of the allograft with BMP group. Considering safety, the use of BMP may be associated with postoperative swelling and dysphagia. With special techniques—correct packing of the BMP sponges, fibrin glue barriers to limit diffusion of BMP—the risk of postoperative swelling and dysphagia can be decreased to a rate that is comparable to that of ventral cervical fusions in which BMP is not used.[51,53,54] Cahill et al.,[55] on the other hand, found that there remains a higher complication rate with BMP going from wound-related complications to dysphagia and hoarseness. Facing cost, one should consider that a small package of BMP costs about $2500 U.S. Cahill et al. found that the inpatient hospital charges across all categories of fusion were greater if BMP was used. In conclusion, BMP utilization may increase fusion rates and avoid iliac crest harvest complications but seems to increase the overall complication rate. Cost-effectiveness is doubtful. Until there is better evidence on these issues, a cautious approach is certainly in order.

Complication Avoidance

Of utmost importance in avoiding complications with any operation for soft cervical disc herniations is to perform the appropriate operation on the appropriate patient. Correlating the clinical picture with the imaging abnormalities is crucial.[56] It is known that ACDF is one of the most commonly performed spinal procedures. Its outcome is satisfactory in the majority of cases. However, occasional complications can become troublesome and even, in rare circumstances, catastrophic. Although there are several case reports describing such complications, their rate of occurrence is generally underreported, and data regarding their exact incidence in large clinical series are lacking. Meticulous knowledge of potential ACDF-related complications is of paramount importance in order to avoid them whenever possible, as well as to successfully and safely manage them when they happen.[53]

Complications Related to the Dorsal Approach

Since the dorsal approach is worth considering, especially in (lateral) soft cervical disc herniation, some potential problems are worth mentioning. First, one should confirm the correct level to operate. Further, proper visualization of the interlaminar space must be obtained. A high-speed drill can be effective but can damage the spinal cord or exiting nerve, since the amount of ligamentum flavum is occasionally sparse. Venous bleeding commonly occurs and must be dealt with sufficiently for obvious physiologic reasons, as well the minimization of interference with adequate visualization of neural structures. The nerve itself should finally be exposed, in both its sensory and motor component, since the latter can be mistaken for the (soft) herniation and thus may be cut. The authors occasionally choose to insert a drain before closure, although hematomas are rarely reported. Postoperative neck pain is seen more often than after ventral cervical disc surgery.

Complications Related to Cervical Disc Arthroplasty

Besides the intraoperative risks and possible complications that are, for the most part, the same as those seen with ventral discectomy and fusion techniques,[57] one can specifically distinguish disc arthroplasty techniques as specifically being associated with immediate (e.g., malpositioning of the prosthesis), early (e.g., migration), intermediate (e.g., subsidence), and late (e.g., wear debris formation with osteolysis) postoperative complications. The impact of a cervical disc prosthesis and its long-term complications must be elucidated. Such complications can be minimized while providing optimal function by limiting this type of surgery to patients with appropriate indications.

Complications Related to Cervical Discectomy with Bone Fusion

Preoperative Period

In patients with a significant neurologic deficit, the preoperative use of corticosteroids may be considered. However, there are no convincing reports in the literature to support the efficacy of the routine use of corticosteroids in patients undergoing elective decompressive operation.[56] As has been shown for trauma patients,[58] corticosteroids are more likely to induce additional problems, especially in elderly patients, than they are to effectively diminish the risk of spinal cord or nerve injury.

In patients with spinal cord compression, hyperextension of the neck during intubation or preoperative positioning should be avoided. In pure soft disc herniation problems, this situation of risk for spinal cord compression is rarely encountered. However, whenever it is, the patient should be intubated fiberoptically.

Intraoperative Period[56]

Injury to the Laryngeal Nerve(s): Approach Related? On the left side, the recurrent laryngeal nerve loops under the arch of the aorta and is protected in the left tracheoesophagal groove. On the right side, however, it travels around the subclavian artery, passing dorsomedially to the side of the trachea and esophagus. The nerve is vulnerable as it passes from the subclavian artery to the right tracheoesophageal groove. Minor hoarseness after a ventral cervical surgery is common and has been reported in up to one half of patients. In most cases, it resolves spontaneously and is generally due to edema from tracheal intubation or from severe retraction of the larynx. However, permanent laryngeal dysfunction due to injury of the laryngeal nerves may also be the cause of postoperative hoarseness and is estimated to occur in about 1% of cases.

The higher risk of injury to the recurrent laryngeal nerve associated with a right-sided approach, especially in the lower cervical spine—which has never been confirmed in the literature, however—is in the estimation of some surgeons balanced by the convenience of the position for right-handed surgeons. As was stated earlier, more practical concerns should dictate the side of the incision: previous surgery (vocal cord testing should be performed before operating on the opposite side), the side of the radicular symptoms, and the surgeon's routine.

Injury to the Esophagus and Pharynx.[59,60] Likewise, dysphagia due to edema from pressure by retraction blades is common after ventral cervical surgery. In certain cases, however, it may persist as long as several weeks, and in rare cases, it may be permanent. Elderly patients who have had extensive mobilization of the upper esophagus or hypopharynx are more prone to this.

Esophageal or pharyngeal perforation can occur, either as a result of sharp dissection or from the sharp teeth of self-retaining retractors. This complication occurs more frequently in the upper cervical region, in which the wall of the hypopharynx is thinner. If the laceration of the esophagus is recognized intraoperatively, it should be repaired primarily. In the majority of cases, the injury to the esophagus is not recognized during surgery and presents later as a local infection, fistula, sepsis, or mediastinitis.

To avoid injury to the esophagus, dissection below the level of the superficial cervical fascia should be performed with utmost care in a sharp or blunt way. In addition, the longus colli muscles should be freed enough from the ventrolateral side of the superior and inferior vertebral bodies to have the sharp teeth of the self-retaining retractors placed safely under them without risk of dislodgement during the procedure.

The esophagus and other soft tissue structures should be hidden by the retractors to avoid injury by drills during bone removal.

Injury to the Structures in the Carotid Sheath. The carotid artery, the internal jugular vein, and the vagus nerve are at risk of damage in the lateral part of the operative field.

Laceration of these structures is caused by the sharp teeth of retractor blades or during dissection with sharp instruments. For this reason, blunt dissection could be advisable. In most cases, carotid artery lacerations can be repaired primarily. Bleeding from the jugular vein should be controlled by repairing the laceration. In an ultimate case, ligation of the jugular vein should be considered. Injury to the vagus nerve is a very unusual complication, but if transsection is observed intraoperatively, primary anastomosis should be attempted.

Injury to the Vertebral Artery. Far lateral bone removal can damage the vertebral artery and is most likely to occur on the opposite side of the approach. An aggressive dissection of the longus colli muscles can also injure the artery between the transverse processes. Third, an anatomic variation with a midline loop of the vertebral artery into the vertebral body or intervertebral disc can cause problems. Commonly, bleeding can be controlled with gentle compression using a muscle pledget, hemostatic gelatin (Gelfoam), or oxidized cellulose (Surgicel). The risk of neurologic deficit after a unilateral vertebral artery occlusion is low, but this can be encountered if there is a congenital anomaly with absence of anastomosis between the left and the right vertebral arteries.[61] Cases of the Wallenberg syndrome were described in such situations. To avoid this injury, one should identify the midline carefully and proceed with drilling accordingly.

Horner Syndrome. The cervical sympathetic chain is located ventral to the transverse process and ventrolateral to the longus colli muscle. Injury leads to Horner syndrome, which can result from either transsection or retraction of the sympathetic chain. The incidence of permanent injury is less than 1%. To avoid this injury during a ventral approach, the soft tissue dissection should be limited to the medial aspect of the longus colli muscle.[62]

Increased Neurologic Deficit. Increased neurologic deficit is uncommon after ventral cervical surgery but can comprise both the spinal cord and the nerve roots. If neurologic problems are seen immediately after the surgery, the most likely causes are (1) problems related to positioning or manipulation of the neck during intubation, (2) direct surgical trauma to the neural elements, and (3) intraoperative displacement of a graft or cage or severe epidural hematoma. During intraoperative localization, the fluoroscopic localization needle in the disc space can be bent at the tip to avoid inadvertent advancement of the needle into the spinal canal. Nerve root injuries are less common than spinal cord injuries, but for unclear reasons, the C5 nerve root is very sensitive to trauma. Traction caused by decompression in combination with the specific rectangular root entry zone is one of the possible explanations.

If a neurologic deficit is not present immediately after the patient awakens but becomes clear within hours, an epidural hematoma and displacement of the graft are the most frequent possibilities. Using a graft or cage that does not occlude the disc space in its full width allows epidural blood to evacuate ventrally and therefore may limit the risk for epidural hematoma formation. If neurologic worsening occurs within days after the operation, an epidural abscess must be considered in the differential diagnosis.

In an attempt to decrease the potential additional neurologic deficit, one can consider monitoring neurologic function with intraoperative somatosensory evoked potentials. By doing this, spinal cord injury as well as nerve root injury may diminish.[63] Since spinal cord compression is not very common in pure soft cervical disc herniations, the advantage of such a neurophysiologic backup is rather theoretical in this particular indication.

Dural Laceration and Cerebrospinal Fluid Fistula. Dura mater laceration and cerebrospinal fluid leakage may occur during removal of the posterior longitudinal ligament or during drilling. Direct repair is usually not feasible. A piece of Gelfoam with fibrin sealant should be placed over the dural defect, and lumbar subarachnoid drainage should be performed for 4 to 5 days. Attention should be paid when the dorsal cortex or the slope of the uncovertebral joints is encountered. The surgeon must also be aware that the nerve roots are more ventrally located than the spinal cord is.

Postoperative Period[56]

Soft Tissue Hematomas and Respiratory Problems. To prevent prevertebral cervical soft tissue hematomas after a ventral cervical operation, we advocate inserting a drain in the prevertebral space before closure, which should be left in place for 12 to 24 hours. The possibility of a large and compressive hematoma obviously warrants careful monitoring of the patient in the recovery room after the operative procedure. This may be an argument not to discharge a patient too early from the ward.

Postoperative Infection. Both superficial and deep infectious processes can occur after a ventral cervical operation. Superficial infections external to the platysma muscle can be treated by simply opening the incision, followed by dressing changes and administration of appropriate antibiotics and secondary closure. Cellulitis or abscess in the deeper tissues, however, requires a more thorough evaluation.

Bone graft removal in the presence of infection is a complex issue. One option is leaving the graft in place, treating with antibiotics, and following the status of the graft with cervical spine films. Once the graft appears to collapse, removal and replacement with autograft would be indicated. In most cases, bone healing will take place.

Although one can speculate that with cages and/or plates (and TDR) the infection rates may be higher, data in the literature are scarce. Exceptional case reports are described.[64,65]

Finally, rare infectious complications concern epidural abscesses and meningitis. If a patient has delayed progressive postoperative spinal cord dysfunction, with or without evidence of osteomyelitis or systemic signs of sepsis, epidural abscess should always be considered in the differential diagnosis.

Graft or Cage Complications. Bone graft complications include graft collapse, displacement (and subsidence), and nonunion (pseudarthrosis). Elderly patients with osteoporotic bone are most prone to display graft collapse. In case of doubt about the structural integrity of autologous bone, an allograft should be used. However, in younger patients, autologous graft is stronger than allograft in resisting axial compression. Most patients with graft collapse are asymptomatic and do not require reoperation.

Graft Displacement and Subsidence. Graft displacement may require reoperation and has in general been reported to occur in as many as 8% of the patients who undergo surgery for disc herniation. A well-fitting graft and placement with compression may help to reduce this complication.

Subsidence (vertical displacement) is a radiologic finding that most of the time does not cause clinical problems. If subsidence occurs, it mostly does so in the ventral part of the cervical column, not where the width of the neuroforamina can be affected; as such, kyphosis may develop.

Stand-alone cage subsidence appears to occur frequently but, as was stated earlier, does not seem to have significant clinical repercussions.[66] Plating is reported to avoid subsidence, but such has not been shown via clinical studies.[67]

Nonunion. Graft nonunion or pseudarthrosis, which by definition is present when there is radiolucency at the fusion level or more than 2 mm of motion at the fusion site, has been reported in 5% of patients who undergo single-level fusion (and in 15% of multilevel fusions). Despite radiographic nonunion, the majority of these patients are clinically asymptomatic, and reoperation is not indicated. However, persistent neck pain, progressive angulation, and subluxation may mandate graft revision.

Biomechanics: Focus on Kyphosis. Kyphosis after ACD is classic and tends to become greater if the operation is performed on two levels rather than on one level. This could be explained by the fact that after discectomy, the disc space systematically collapses. Collapse occurs ventrally more than dorsally, owing to the dorsal structures of the vertebra (facet joints), which do not collapse, and because of the wedge shape of the cervical disc. This results in a reversal of lordosis or straightening of the cervical curve.[26] Additional fusion (ACDF) is performed to overcome this problem.

Kyphosis is not always uneventful. Neck pain can be associated in a certain number of patients. Furthermore, adjacent-level degeneration seems to be influenced or increased by such deformation.

Long-Term Benefit

Data from prospective observational studies indicate that 2 years after surgery for cervical radiculopathy caused by soft cervical disc herniation (without myelopathy), 75% of patients have substantial pain relief from radicular symptoms (pain, numbness, and weakness).[68,69] Overall improvement of myelopathy symptoms may take longer than recovery from radicular symptoms.[56]

KEY REFERENCES

Bhadra AK, Raman AS, Casey AT, Crawford RJ: Single-level cervical radiculopathy: clinical outcome and cost-effectiveness of four techniques of anterior cervical discectomy and fusion and disc arthroplasty. *Eur Spine J* 18:232–237, 2009.

Carette S, Fehlings MG: Cervical radiculopathy. *N Engl J Med* 353:392–399, 2005.

Chou YC, Chen DC, Hsieh WA, et al: Efficacy of anterior cervical fusion: comparison of titanium cages, polyetheretherketone (PEEK) cages and autogenous bone grafts. *J Clin Neurosci* 15:1240–1245, 2007.

Fountas KN, Kapsalaki EZ, Nikolakakos LG, et al: Anterior cervical discectomy and fusion associated complications. *Spine (Phila Pa 1976)* 32(21):2310–2317, 2007.

Samartzis D, Shen FH, Goldberg EJ, An HS: Is autograft the gold standard in achieving radiographic fusion in one-level anterior cervical discectomy and fusion with rigid anterior plate fixation? *Spine (Phila Pa 1976)* 30:1756–1761, 2005.

Sasso RC, Smucker JD, Hacker RJ, Heller JG: Artificial disc versus fusion. A prospective, randomized study with 2-year follow up on 99 patients. *Spine (Phila Pa 1976)* 32:2933–2940, 2007.

Yue WM, Bronder W, Highland TR: Long term results after anterior cervical discectomy and fusion with allograft and plating: 5-11 year radiologic and clinical follow up study. *Spine (Phila Pa 1976)* 30:2138–2144, 2005.

REFERENCES

The complete reference list is available online at expertconsult.com.

CHAPTER 80

Recurrent Lumbar Disc Herniation

Iain H. Kalfas | Robert Talac

Lumbar discectomy represents the most commonly performed spinal surgical procedure.[1] Approximately 300,000 lumbar discectomy procedures are performed each year in the United States.[2] In general, the clinical outcome for this procedure is favorable, with 80% to 90% of patients undergoing surgery reporting good or excellent results.[3-6]

Despite these favorable results, a relatively small number of patients who have had an initial good outcome following surgery will redevelop symptoms similar to those of their preoperative state owing to a recurrence of herniated disc material at the previous surgical site. The reported incidence of these recurrent lumbar disc herniations ranges from 5% to 15%.[7-11]

The patient with a symptomatic recurrent disc herniation typically undergoes several weeks or months of conservative management. This treatment may be followed by surgical reexploration in those individuals whose symptoms remain unresponsive. Surgery may involve simply removing the reherniated disc material or a fusion and fixation across the affected disc space. Regardless of the management approach, a recurrent disc herniation creates a substantial economic impact.[12] This impact is compounded by time lost from work and the need for many of these patients to be retrained for lighter-duty positions.

Risk Factors for Recurrent Disc Herniations

The risk factors for a primary disc herniation have been noted to include exposure to repetitive lifting, exposure to vibrations, smoking, and a constitutional weakness of the anular tissue.[13-15] Isolated trauma or injury has not been found to be a consistent risk factor, occurring in only 0.2% to 10.7% of adults with a herniation.[14,16] Conversely, Cinotti et al. found that 42% of patients with a recurrent disc herniation related the onset of radicular pain to an isolated injury or precipitating event.[17] Similarly, Suk et al. reported the rate of an isolated injury as a cause of recurrence in 32.1%. This study also noted that 71.4% of the patients with recurrence were males and 57.1% were smokers.[18]

Despite these findings, other studies have found that gender, age, smoking status, level of herniation, and duration of symptoms were generally not associated with higher rates of recurrence.[8,9,17-19] Additionally, the degree of anular incision and the extent of the discectomy (partial or complete) have not been found to affect the potential for recurrence.[9,17-19]

One factor that potentially increases the likelihood of a recurrent disc herniation is diabetes. In general, patients with diabetes have been noted to have lower clinical success rates following the initial lumbar discectomy than do nondiabetic patients. Simpson et al. reported an excellent to good outcome following the initial discectomy of 95% in nondiabetic patients but only 39% in diabetic patients.[20] Mobbs et al. reported success rates of 86% in nondiabetic patients and 60% in diabetic patients.[9] Although these clinical outcome differences were generally felt to be attributable to lower quality-of-life indicators in diabetic patients, Robinson et al. investigated the differences in the proteoglycan profile of the discs in the two groups. This study found that diabetic patients had fewer proteoglycans in the disc material, potentially increasing their susceptibility to recurrent disc prolapse.[21]

Another proposed risk factor is the configuration of the initial disc herniation. Suk et al. and Grane et al. noted that preoperative disc configuration does not affect the rate of recurrence.[18,22] Alternatively, Carragee et al. prospectively evaluated herniated disc configurations along with the rate of reherniation and the rate of reoperation. Disc herniations were divided into four shaped-based groups: (1) fragment-fissure herniations (disc fragment and small anular defect), (2) fragment-defect herniations (large disc fragment with massive dorsal anular tear), (3) fragment-contained discs (incomplete anular tear), and (4) absence of fragment-contained herniations (anular prolapse). Of the four groups, the fragment-fissure type herniations (group 1) were associated with the best outcomes and the lowest rate of reherniation (1%) and required the fewest reoperative procedures (1%). Those with anular prolapse (group 4) were associated with poorer clinical outcomes, with 38% of patients experiencing recurrent or persistent symptoms.[8]

Evaluation of Recurrent Disc Herniation

The patient who presents with a recurrent disc herniation has generally had a period of clinical improvement following the initial discectomy procedure. A retrospective review of 28 patients with recurrent disc herniation found a pain-free interval ranging from 7 to 168 months (mean of 60.8 months).[18] Patients typically report radicular signs and symptoms similar or identical to those of their preoperative clinical state.

Pathologic changes in the ventral epidural space may reflect mass effect due to perineural scarring or recurrent disc herniation.[7,23] Scarring is most pronounced before 9 months and primarily involves the anulus fibrosus.[24] The scar may surround the nerve roots and cause symptoms by means of neural tension, decreased axoplasmic transport, restriction of blood flow, or restriction of venous return.[7]

MRI, with and without gadolinium contrast, is the preferred imaging modality for the assessment of a recurrent disc herniation.[7,10,25,26] The use of contrast material helps to differentiate normal postoperative anatomic changes from a recurrent herniation. Peridural scarring will typically enhance heterogeneously because of its vascular supply. A recurrent disc herniation usually appears as a polypoid mass with a low signal on T1- and T2-weighted sequences. It is usually contiguous with the parent disc unless sequestered. There can be a hypointense rim of the posterior longitudinal ligament and outer anular fibers that outline the herniation. This rim will enhance with contrast administration (Fig. 80-1). The disc itself will not enhance, because it has no blood supply.[7,27]

MRI findings will vary according to the time period during which the study is obtained relative to the primary procedure. In the early (1- to 6-month) postoperative period, MRI demonstrates a high-intensity signal band extending from the nucleus pulposus to the site of anular disruption. This is particularly noticeable in the first 2 months following surgery. The anulus is typically hyperintense, and the nucleus is typically hypointense. There is loss of disc space height. The end plates and marrow will frequently have a low signal on T1-weighted images and a high signal on T2-weighted images, suggesting inflammation and edema. The ventral epidural space initially reveals an increase in soft tissue mass, evidence of tissue disruption, edema, and hemorrhage, with the appearance of mass effect.[10]

Nerve root enhancement with gadolinium in the first few months following surgery is normal. This typically indicates a breakdown of the blood-nerve barrier but usually resolves within 6 months. Postoperative changes at the laminectomy site depend on the extent of surgery, the extent of ligamentum flavum removal, and whether a fat graft was placed in the epidural space. Facet joint enhancement occurs as a local response to dissection and persists long (>6 months) after surgery in more than half of the patients in whom imaging is performed.[7,28,29]

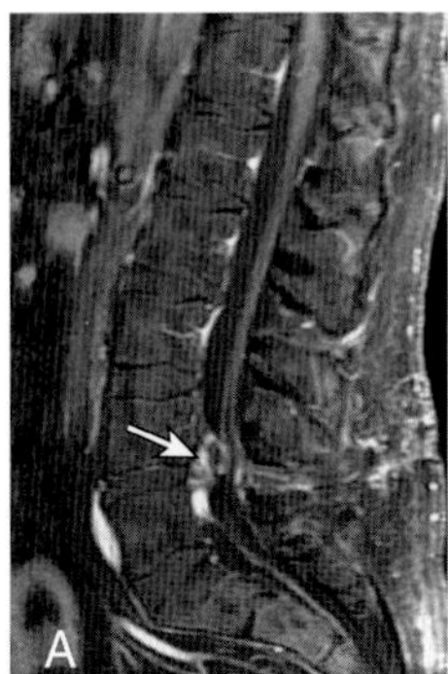

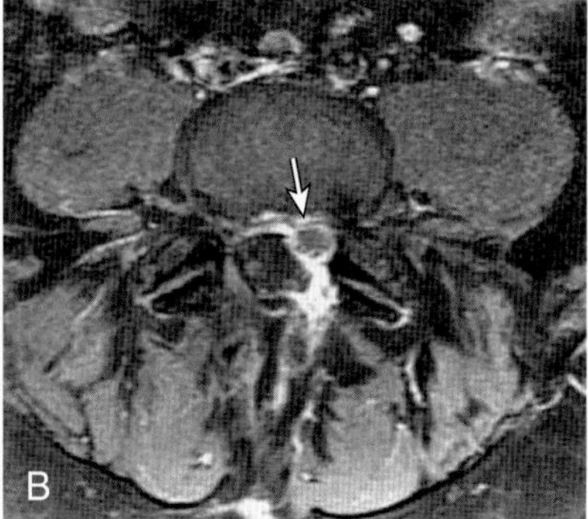

FIGURE 80-1. Sagittal plane (**A**) and axial plane (**B**) MRIs following administration of contrast material demonstrating a recurrent disc herniation on the left side at the L4-5 level. The disc fragment is surrounded by a rim of enhancing scar tissue (*arrows*). The disc fragment itself does not enhance.

Late (>6 months) MRI findings include a low-intensity signal band in the disc space representing a healing anular defect. The mass effect that was seen earlier in the ventral epidural space may have resolved[29] or may persist as a mass-like scar.[23] The laminotomy defect contains mature scar with peripheral enhancement identifying granulation tissue. Facet joint enhancement is visible after contrast administration in approximately half of the patients 6 months postoperatively.[7]

Retraction of the thecal sac toward a soft tissue lesion is suggestive of scar, while displacement away from such a mass is suggestive of a herniated disc.[10] Although a pseudomeningocele may also be seen as a mass, its signal characteristics are different, demonstrating cerebrospinal fluid intensity on T1- and T2-weighted images and often an enhancing fibrous capsule.[7]

Despite the imaging advantages that MRI provides over other techniques, there can be a significant degree of discordance between MRI findings and intraoperative findings. This discordance can occur in 18% to 33% of cases that are proven surgically.[30] As with the initial procedure, the successful outcome of any surgery for recurrent disc herniation depends on close correlation between the clinical and radiographic findings.

Management of Recurrent Disc Herniation

As with patients who present with a primary disc herniation, the initial management of the patient with a recurrence focuses on conservative measures. These treatment options typically include nonsteroidal anti-inflammatory medications, oral steroids, and, in select cases, a trial of epidural or selective nerve-root blocks.

The indications for revision surgery are the persistence of radicular symptoms despite a course of conservative treatment and the presence of a clinically correlative finding on radiographic imaging. It is important to determine that the radiographic finding is actually recurrent disc material rather than perineural scar formation because the clinical outcome of surgery for these two findings is different. Jonsson et al. reported on revision surgery for recurrent disc herniation versus perineural scar formation. Surgery for a recurrent disc herniation was found to yield clinical results that were as good as those of the primary discectomy procedure. However, when only perineural scar was present, the results of revision surgery were not as good.[31]

The most common surgical option used for the management of recurrent disc herniation is a reexploration of the previous surgical site with additional widening of the laminotomy defect and removal of the recurrent disc material. This technique should begin with exposure of normal anatomy immediately above and below the previous laminotomy defect to help orient the surgeon to the pertinent anatomy. Curettes are then used to cautiously dissect the scar from the lateral bony margins. Identification of the medial wall of the pedicles on either side of the disc space allows for further orientation to the neural anatomy. As with the primary procedure, the use of a surgical microscope greatly enhances illumination and visualization of the surgical field.

By using a combination of sharp and blunt dissection, the shoulder of the compressed root is identified and retracted to expose the herniated disc material. The disc fragment is removed, and additional decompression of the root through its foraminal passage is carried out. Spinal fusion and fixation are rarely indicated for a first-time disc recurrence unless segmental instability is present.

Suk et al. reviewed 28 patients who had undergone open conventional discectomy for a recurrent disc herniation. Although the length of the revision surgery was significantly longer than that of the primary procedure, there was no significant difference in length of hospital stay or clinical outcome. Age, gender, smoking, occupation, level of herniation, degree of herniation, and pain-free interval did not affect the clinical outcomes of repeat discectomy.[18]

A limited number of studies have investigated the use of lumbar fusion to manage the patient with a recurrent disc herniation. Chitnavis et al. reported good clinical outcomes in 50 patients with recurrent disc herniation managed by a posterior lumbar interbody fusion.[32] Vishteh et al. reported a good outcome in six patients who were managed with an anterior lumbar interbody fusion.[33] Proponents of discectomy with fusion have proposed that fusion has several theoretical advantages. Specifically, fusion reduces or eliminates segmental motion, immobilizes the spine, and limits mechanical stresses across the degenerated disc space and may lower the potential for any additional herniation at the affected level.

Fu et al. reported on the long-term outcome in patients who had undergone a dorsolateral fusion compared to a comparable group of patients who were managed with only a conventional discectomy. The follow-up period ranged from 6 to 134 months. The clinical outcome was good or excellent in 78.3% of the patients who had undergone conventional discectomy compared to 83.3% of patients who were fused. This difference was not clinically significant. The difference in the postoperative back pain score was also insignificant. However, the fusion group did have significantly higher intraoperative blood loss, length of surgery, and length of postoperative hospitalization compared to the nonfusion group. The study concluded that disc excision alone is the recommended surgical procedure for managing recurrent disc herniation.[34] In the rare case of a recurrent disc herniation that presents with segmental instability (i.e., spondylolisthesis) or in the patient who has had multiple disc herniation recurrences, an interbody or dorsolateral fusion may be a reasonable option to consider.

Conclusion

Recurrent lumbar disc herniations are not uncommon. The clinical presentation of this condition is typically similar to the initial preoperative presentation. The diagnosis is confirmed with contrast-enhanced MRI imaging. Although most patients can be managed successfully with conservative measures, some will eventually require surgical reexploration. Conventional open discectomy as a revision approach for recurrent disc herniation yields a relatively high success rate. The addition of a fusion procedure is best reserved for patients who demonstrate associated segmental instability at the affected level.

KEY REFERENCES

Babar S, Saifuddin A: MRI of the post-discectomy lumbar spine. *Clin Radiol* 57:969–981, 2002.

Carragee EJ, Han MY, Suen PW, et al: Clinical outcomes after lumbar discectomy for sciatica: the effects of fragment type and annular competence. *J Bone Joint Surg [Am]* 85:102–108, 2003.

Erbayraktar S, Acar F, Tekinsoy B, et al: Outcome analysis of reoperations after lumbar discectomies: a report of 22 patients. *Kobe J Med Sci* 48:33–41, 2002.

Jonsson B, Stromqvist B: Clinical characteristics of recurrent sciatica after lumbar discectomy. *Spine (Phila Pa 1976)* 21:500–505, 1996.

Suk KS, Lee HM, Moon SH, et al: Recurrent lumbar disc herniation: results of operative management. *Spine (Phila Pa 1976)* 26:672–676, 2001.

REFERENCES

The complete reference list is available online at expertconsult.com.

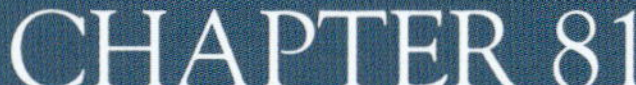

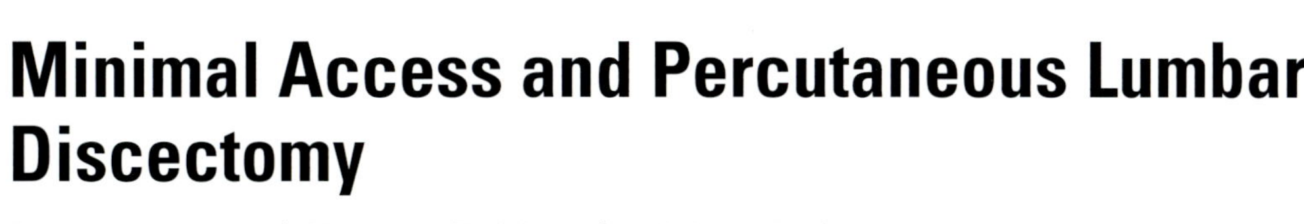

CHAPTER 81

Minimal Access and Percutaneous Lumbar Discectomy

Basem I. Awad | Thomas E. Mroz | Michael P. Steinmetz

Minimal Access Lumbar Discectomy

Lumbar discectomy has become the most common neurosurgical procedure in the United States, with nearly 300,000 procedures performed each year. Herniated lumbar discs and resultant radiculopathy lead to approximately 15 million physician visits per year and have created a financial burden on society exceeding $50 billion annually.[1-3]

Historical Review

The operative treatment of lumbar disc disease has challenged spine surgeons since the first reported case of Dandy in 1929.[4] The operating microscope revolutionized the operation. It improved the ability to visualize the neural elements and disc material, decreased surgical morbidity, and decreased incision size.[5] Yasargil popularized the operating microscope in the mid-1960s, although it was not until the 1970s that the first publications by Yasargil[6] and Caspar began to appear separately.[7] In 1978 Williams reported on 532 patients who had undergone lumbar microdiscectomy through an intralaminar approach.[8] These publications detailed the usefulness of the microscope and the appearance of lumbar microdiscectomy.

Since these early descriptions, surgeons have sought to decrease the incision size and iatrogenic morbidity associated with the operation. Faubert and Caspar in 1991 reported the use of a muscular retractor system[9] rather than subperiosteal dissection to facilitate visualization of smaller operative corridors. The endoscope was also applied for the treatment of spine pathology.[10]

True minimally invasive lumbar microdiscectomy was first described by Foley and Smith[11] in 1997. They reported the use of a microendoscopic discectomy system that entailed the use of tubular dilators to facilitate muscle sparing, a tubular retractor system, and an endoscope coupled with microsurgical techniques and instrumentation. This approach (microendoscopic discectomy) revolutionized minimal access spine surgery and paved the way for minimally invasive surgery (MIS) laminectomy and fusion techniques. The goal of these MIS approaches is to achieve clinical outcomes similar to those of standard approaches yet minimize the iatrogenic injury encountered during the approach to the spine.

This chapter reviews current concepts in minimal access lumbar discectomy. The focus will in large part be on microscopic discectomy, but we will review percutaneous endoscopic discectomy for extraforaminal herniations and other new modalities that may be applied in lumbar disc surgery.

Microsurgical (Microlumbar) Discectomy

General Principles

Microscopic magnification, illumination, and three-dimensional vision have unquestionably increased the accuracy of surgery and reduced tissue trauma.

From a technical standpoint, the microsurgical discectomy technique requires only a small incision with minimum paravertebral muscle dissection. Extradural fat, facets, and laminae can usually be preserved.

The technique requires a blunt paravertebral muscle-splitting approach. Recent evidence has suggested that the approach is characterized by less postoperative pain, shorter hospitalization, and faster return to work.[12] The subperiosteal approach, by contrast, requires a larger incision and the detachment of the tendinous insertions of the paraspinal muscles and their retraction from the spinous process. The paravertebral muscles are rich in proprioceptors and may be injured when retracted. There are reports on the correlation between denervation and retraction-ischemia of the muscles and postoperative pain.[12]

The microsurgical approach to a herniated lumbar disc entails several modifications of the standard approach: surgical planning, positioning of the patient, and intraoperative imaging. Some of these modifications may appear as disadvantages to those surgeons not experienced with microsurgery. The surgical corridor to the target area is very limited, so the localization of the skin incision has to be determined very precisely. Once the skin incision has been placed, there is no way of altering the approach other than by enlarging the incision. The approach uses the same instruments that are used in standard lumbar discectomy but have been modified for use through small tubular retractors. The instruments are usually bayoneted and are of a dark color to reduce glare from the light source. A high-speed drill with a long, tapered, and gradually bent tip is designed to be used through these tubular retractors.

Patient Positioning

The patient is positioned prone on a radiolucent spine table such as the Jackson table. We prefer to place the patient's knees and legs in a sling with the hips flexed rather than on flat boards with the knees and legs extended. This placement increases the interlaminar space and optimizes access (personal experience).

Surgical Technique

Step 1: Localization

The lumbar spine area is prepped and draped in a standard fashion. We prefer to insert a spine needle in the midline at the desired surgical level. This is confirmed on lateral fluoroscopy. The needle tip should point to the disc space. On the basis of the location of the disc space, a vertical paramedian incision is then made through the skin and the fascia one finger breadth from the midline toward the side of pathology. The size of the incision is dependent on the size of tubular retractor to use (typically, 14–19 mm). Generally, the incision should be slightly larger than the working tube.

Step 2: Dilator Insertion

The smallest dilator is then inserted through the incision and is docked on the inferior aspect of the cranial lamina (Fig. 81-1). That is the L4 lamina for an L4-5 disc herniation. This is confirmed with lateral fluoroscopy. Remember that the edge of the lamina is caudal to the disc space. The anatomy should be palpated with the dilator, and a three-dimensional image of the anatomy should be formed in the surgeon's mind. The inferior edge of the lamina is determined as well as the facet/lamina junction. The dilator may then be used to clear soft tissue from the lamina and medial facet. Care should be taken not to allow the dilator to slip into the intralaminar space.

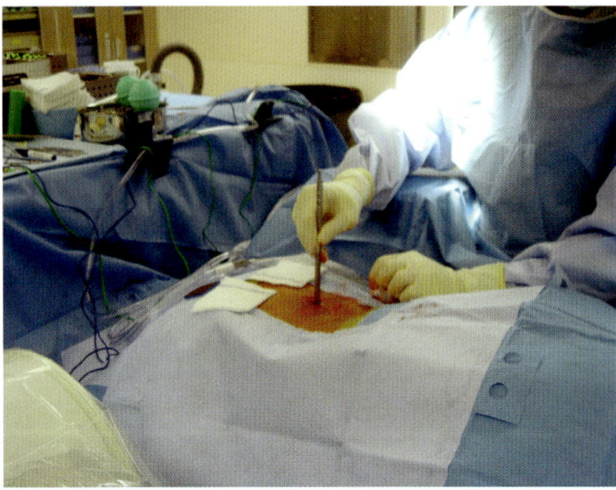

FIGURE 81-1. The smallest dilator has been inserted through a 17-mm skin incision and is docked on the inferior aspect of the cranial lamina (L4 for L4-5 discectomy).

Step 3: Sequential Dilator and Tubular Retraction Insertion

Sequentially place the second, third, and fourth dilators over the initial dilator down to the lamina, and then place the working channel (tubular retractor) over the final dilator (Fig. 81-2). We do not check fluoroscopy after each dilator placed but do so after the last is secured. Continued soft tissue is dissected from the lamina during subsequent dilator placement. The length of the final working tubular retractor is determined from markings on the largest dilator. The length and width of the tube are determined, and the tube is placed over the dilator to dock on the edge of the lamina. Fluoroscopy is used to verify placement of the tube (Fig. 81-3). We then direct the distal end of the tube somewhat medially.

The tube is then fixed to an arm, which is then attached to the operating table (Fig. 81-4). Once it has been attached, the dilators are removed and a corridor is established percutanously to the lamina and interlaminar space. We place a Penfield no. 4 under the edge of the lamina to confirm correct level localization on the lateral image (Fig. 81-5) and also confirm medial-lateral position on the anteroposterior image.

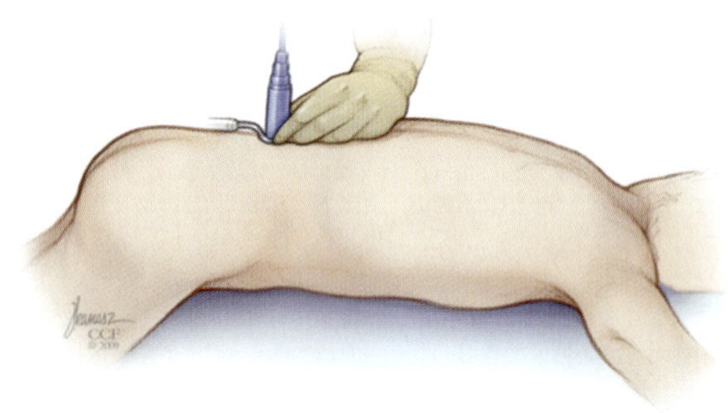

FIGURE 81-2. Following placement of the initial dilator, the other dilators are placed, one over the other, until the final working diameter is reached. Fluoroscopy is used to verify placement, and finally, the working port may be placed over the last dilator. (Copyright Cleveland Clinic Foundation.)

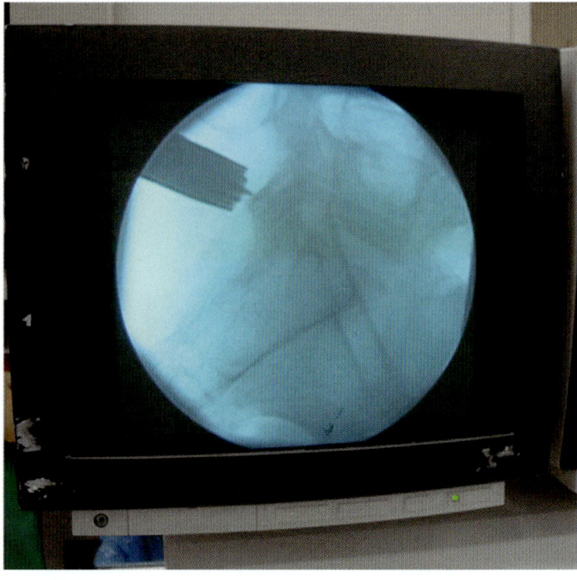

FIGURE 81-3. Fluoroscopy is used to verify tube placement.

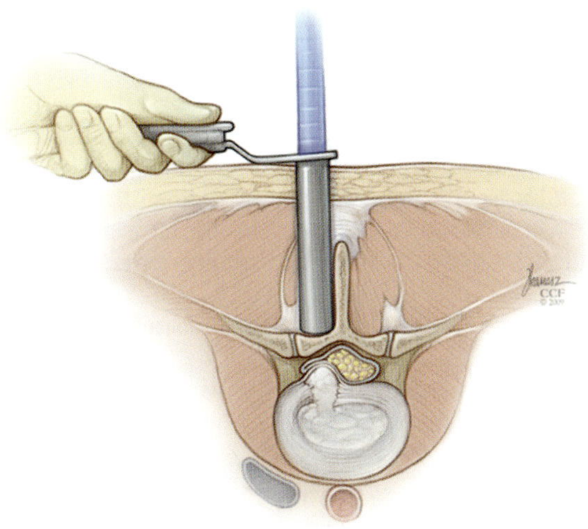

FIGURE 81-4. Demonstration of the port being situated through the muscle-splitting approach and docked on the lamina immediately above the disc herniation. The port is then attached to the table. (Copyright Cleveland Clinic Foundation.)

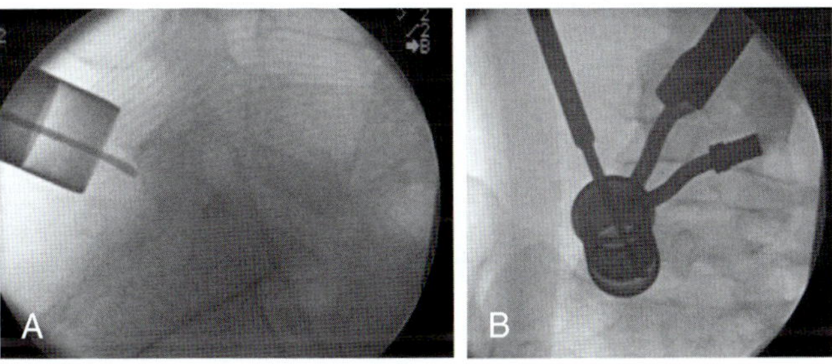

FIGURE 81-5. **A,** Fluoroscopy is then used to verify final positioning prior to beginning the laminotomy. **B,** We place a Penfield no. 4 under the lamina and check both a lateral and an anteroposterior image to verify level localization.

Step 4: Soft Tissue Removal and Laminar Identification

At this point, the operating room microscope or endoscope is brought into the field to provide illumination and magnification. Soft tissue usually will need to be removed from the laminae by using a Bovie with an extended tip and rongeur. The inferior (caudal) edge of the lamina should be identified as well as the medial facet joint (Fig. 81-6). Visualization of the fibers of the facet capsule ensure that one does not inadvertently enter the joint or remove too much of the joint and cause potential instability.

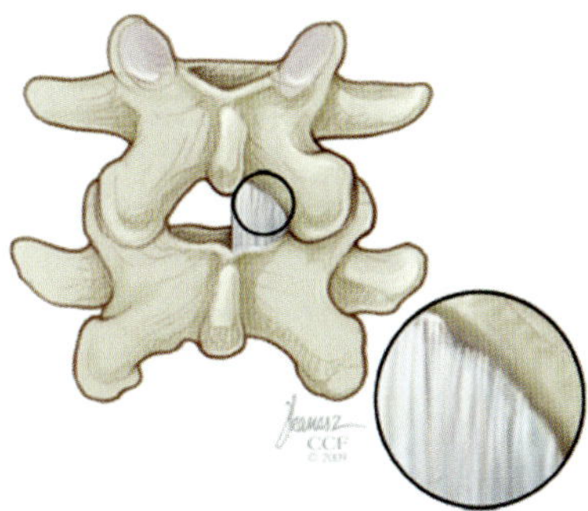

FIGURE 81-6. Once the port is in place and the soft tissue has been cleared, the surgeon should have a clear view of the inferior edge of the lamina and the medial facet joint. (Copyright Cleveland Clinic Foundation.)

If an optimal view is not obtained, the tubular retractor may be angled in any direction. This may be accomplished with the largest dilator. It is critical to keep downward pressure on the tubular retractor before moving, thus preventing soft tissue from creeping under the tubular retractor and obstructing the operative view. It is crucial to remove all soft tissue that is exposed in the operative corridor to maximize the working space within the tubular retractor.

Step 5: Hemilaminotomy and Flavectomy

A small laminotomy and/or facetectomy may be performed with a high-speed drill and match-stick bit. Alternatively, a Kerrison rongeur may be used. The ligamentum flavum is then opened to expose the traversing nerve root and dura mater. This may be performed in multiple ways. We prefer to use an angled curette to access the subligamentous region and remove the remaining ligament with a rongeur.

Step 6: Nerve Root Exploration

The dura and traversing nerve root are then identified. The traversing root is retracted medially by using a Penfield dissector or Love-style retractor. If necessary, the epidural vessels may be bipolar cauterized and divided to identify the disc space.

Step 7: Discectomy and Root Decompression

Once the disc space is visualized, the disc material is removed as for any standard discectomy. We prefer to only remove herniated disc material. If an anulotomy is required, a small one is made in a horizontal fashion (medial/lateral) with a no. 11 blade or a sheathed microknife (Fig. 81-7).

Step 8: Closure

Finally, loosen the flexible arm, and remove the tubular retractor slowly. Any bleeding in the paraspinal musculature may be controlled with bipolar forceps.

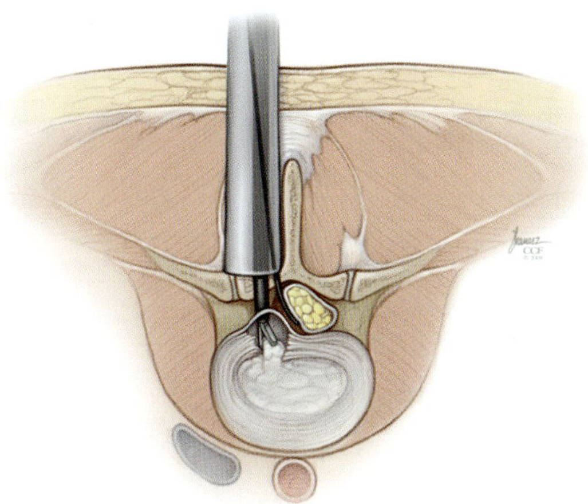

FIGURE 81-7. Once an anulotomy has been made, the offending disc fragment is removed through the port. (Copyright Cleveland Clinic Foundation.)

The fascia is then approximated with one or two interrupted absorbable sutures. The dermal tissue may be closed with interrupted absorbable sutures, and the skin is closed with a running subcuticular absorbable stitch and an adhesive.

Patients are urged to begin ambulating immediately and are discharged within 24 hours, either the same day or the following morning.

Microendoscopic Discectomy for Extraforaminal Lumbar Disc Herniations

Spine endoscopy has been widely used over the last 20 years to treat patients with cervical, thoracic, and lumbar disorders safely and effectively. The most common application has been in the lumbar spine, specifically lumbar discectomy.

General Principles

Extraforaminal lumbar disc herniations (EFDH), otherwise known as far lateral lumbar disc herniations, are relatively rare and make up 1% to 12% of all lumbar disc herniations.[13,14] The surgical treatment of EFDH is more complex than that of the more common dorsolateral or central disc herniation, owing to an increased risk of nerve root injury, postoperative instability from extensive facetectomy, and/or inadequate decompression.

The microendoscopic approach for EFDH can further reduce surgical morbidity by preserving the facet joint stability, providing less chance of nerve root injury while still achieving similar or better outcomes. Despite these advantages, the surgeon faces new challenges. The technique takes surgery from direct line of sight with an open retractor system to one in which surgery is performed through a tubular retractor with visualization of the operative bed on a video monitor placed in front of the surgeon. This requires specialized training and had resulted in a shallow learning curve that must be overcome for proficiency with the procedure.[11,15]

Anesthesia

We prefer to use general anesthesia for microendoscopic discectomy. The operative time for this procedure, especially early in a surgeon's experience, may be prolonged. Use of a general anesthetic will ensure the patient's and surgeon's comfort during the procedure.

Patient Positioning

The patient is positioned prone on a radiolucent operating room table, such as a Jackson table, with the spine flexed. We typically utilize a sling for the legs to optimize interlaminar space and optimize access.

Surgical Technique

Step 1: Disinfection and Localization

The lumbar spine area is prepped and draped in the usual fashion. Fluoroscopy is draped and brought into the operative field, and lateral imaging is performed. A spine needle is inserted into the midline at the level of the affected disc. This needle should aim directly down to the superior end plate of the inferior vertebral body, that is, the superior end plate of the L5 vertebral body for an L4-5 far lateral disc herniation. A set of landmarks may then be used to direct tubular retractor placement. An anteroposterior fluoroscopic image is used next. A horizontal line may be drawn along the caudal edge of the rostral transverse process (L4 in our example), and a second line may be drawn along the superior end plate of the caudal vertebral body (L5). A vertical line may be drawn between these horizontal lines approximately 4.5 cm lateral to the midline on the symptomatic side. This will mark the lateral incision needed for retractor placement as well as the cranial/caudal boundaries.

Step 2: Dilator Insertion

Remove the spine needle, and make a 15- to 22-mm (length determined by the retractor system that is used) vertical skin incision along the vertical mark. The incision length has to match the diameter of the respective tubular retractor, although we typically make the incision a few millimeters longer than the tube diameter. The skin and underlying fascia are incised. The first dilator is directed through the fascial incision to dock on the caudal transverse process, at the junction of the lateral facet, transverse process, and pars interarticularis junction. This requires medial angulation toward the spine. This is confirmed by using lateral fluoroscopy. This first dilator is then used to clear soft tissue from the transverse process, pars, and lateral facet joint.

Step 3: Sequential Dilator and Tubular Retraction Insertion

Insert the sequential dilators over the initial one, followed by the tubular retractor. Secure the flexible arm to the table, attach it firmly to the tubular retractor 180 degrees away from the surgeon, and then remove the sequential dilators to establish a tubular operative corridor. The appropriate positioning is confirmed by fluoroscopy.

Step 4: Endoscope Insertion

Insert the endoscope into the tubular retractor. The endoscope can be placed anywhere within the 360-degree periphery of the tube and can be retracted or extended for variable magnification. This is somewhat limited by the specific endoscope system that is used. The endoscope should initially be placed be in the most retracted position to avoid contact with soft tissue. Blotching the endoscope with soft tissue will dramatically reduce visualization, especially clarity. If this occurs, remove the endoscope from the tubular retractor, and clean the lens using antifog solution and gauze.

Step 5: Focus and Image Orientation

Surgical focusing and orientation are extremely important. To help in this regard, the endoscopic image orientation should be adjusted such that the medial anatomy will be on the top of the video monitor (12 o'clock) and the lateral anatomy on the bottom (6 o'clock). A sucker tip can be place laterally inside the tube to help guide the surgeon regarding lateral and medial orientation.

Step 6: Soft Tissue Removal

Clear the soft tissue from the base of the transverse process and pars interarticularis using an insulated Bovie electrocautery and small pituitary rongeur. This should permit clear visualization of the bony landmarks.

The lower half of the foramen is normally filled with fatty tissue. Small veins coming from the paravertebral plexus cross the foramen to join the epidural veins. The lumbar segmental arteries usually do not cross the foraminal working area. In the case of a disc lesion, this lower part is filled with disc tissue or protruded anulus material.

Coagulate the pars artery, if present, with the bipolar forceps, and divide it with microscissors. Separate soft tissue from the undersurface of the pars, using small, angled microcurettes. This maneuver detaches the medial edge of the intertransverse ligament from the pars and allows for entry into the neuroforamen.

Step 7: Nerve Root Exploration and Decompression

Remove bone from along the inferomedial aspect of the transverse process and the most lateral aspect of the pars with an angled Kerrison rongeur or high-speed drill. This maneuver opens the lateral aspect of the neuroforamen, allowing palpation of the pedicle with a nerve hook or ball-tip probe and straightforward identification of the exiting nerve root as it travels around the pedicle.

When the exiting nerve root has been definitively identified at the level of the pedicle, dissect laterally and caudally along the root, following its caudal course toward the disc by wanding the tubular retractor. If an overhanging articular process is encountered (secondary to coexisting facet hypertrophy), remove the lateral margin of the articular process with the drill or Kerrison rongeur, further exposing the distal course of the nerve root.

Identify the dorsal root ganglion, which makes up the enlargement of the exiting nerve root just lateral and inferior to the neuroforamen. Treat this structure gently, as excessive manipulation of the dorsal root ganglion can produce significant postoperative pain.

Typically, the nerve and ganglion are pushed laterally and cranially by the free disc fragment. Usually, removal of the fragment alone is sufficient for nerve root decompression. But if necessary, enter the interspace for further disc removal. Finally, reexplore the root to confirm that it has been fully decompressed.

Step 8: Closure

Last, irrigate the wound, loosen the flexible arm, and remove the tubular retractor slowly. Any bleeding in the paraspinal musculature may be controlled with the bipolar cautery. Approximate the fascia with one or two interrupted absorbable sutures, close the subcutaneous tissue in an inverted manner, and finally, approximate the skin edges with a subcutaneous suture and adhesive.

Patients are urged to begin ambulating immediately and are discharged within 24 hours, either the same day or the following morning.

Percutaneous Discectomy

The percutaneous dorsolateral approach to a herniated disc allows evacuation of extruded disc material and decompression of the nerve root without entrance into the spinal canal and without destruction of the articular processes and ligamentum flavum.

Historical Review

Percutaneous discectomy promised to change the field of lumbar spine surgery when it was introduced in the late 1970s. Kambin et al.[16,17] and Hijikata[18] separately reported the efficacy of this procedure, that is, percutaneous nucleotomy.

In 1985, Onik et al.[19] reported the technique of automated percutaneous discectomy (APD). This procedure consisted of the insertion of a 2-mm probe into the disc. The device was then able to mechanically facilitate the removal of disc material.

Shortly thereafter, in the late 1980s, Choy et al.[20] introduced percutaneous laser discectomy (PLD). This modification utilized an approach similar to that of APD but used laser energy to remove disc material.

In the 1990s, the intradiscal electrothermal anuloplasty (IDET) procedure was developed by Saal and Saal.[21,22]

The procedure consisted of a percutaneous approach to the site of pathology similar to the approach used by other procedures, such as APD and PLD. The unique feature of the IDET procedure is that it used a navigational catheter with a temperature-controlled thermal resistive coil to heat and absorb the disc material.

Evidence of the superiority of such minimally invasive techniques compared with microdiscectomy remains unclear; this is attributed to the lack of high-quality studies.[23]

Therefore, the percutaneous procedures are highly dependent on patient selection. Patient selection and limited pathology have probably been the single largest factor in preventing the more widespread use of these procedures.

Patient Selection

As was stated previously, appropriate patient selection is the single most important factor with regard to favorable outcome. As in all procedures for disc pathology, candidate patients are those with radiculopathy with little to no back pain. Confirmatory physical examination findings should also be sought, such as a positive straight-leg raise sign. As will all surgical procedures, patients with vague or equivocal symptoms are not candidates for these percutaneous techniques.

In addition, a minimum 6-week course of conservative treatment should be attempted, which may include anti-inflammatory nonsteroidal medications, physical therapy, epidural steroid injections, and other modalities as appropriate.

Radiographic criteria are extremely important in considering percutaneous discectomy. These procedures are appropriate only for patients with a contained disc demonstrated on MRI. This is defined as disc material that is contained by either the anulus fibrosus or the posterior longitudinal ligament. An unfavorable outcome will likely be seen if the procedure is performed on patients with free or extruded discs. In addition, patients with disc herniations compromising more than 50% of the spinal canal with significant thecal sac compression should not be treated by those procedures.

Other radiographic contraindications include spinal stenosis, lateral recess stenosis, and calcified disc herniations.

Needle Placement

The major component of any percutaneous technique or disc decompression is needle placement. The initial needle for essentially all of the aforementioned procedures is passed through the Kambin triangular zone, which is located between the traversing and exiting nerves. We recommend biplanar fluoroscopy for safe passage.

Surgical Technique

The patient is placed prone on a radiolucent spine frame, with the arm away from the side of the body. Care is taken to line up the patient with the C-arm to ensure perfect posteroanterior and lateral views. The spinous process should be centered between the pedicles on the AP view and the end plates parallel in the lateral view.

The sedation is kept light to allow patient feedback. This permits an alteration of trajectory if nerve irritation is encountered. The patient's lumbar region is prepped and draped in the usual fashion. Local anesthetic is infiltrated into the skin and subcutaneous tissue as well.

The fluoroscopy unit is positioned such that an oblique view of the spine is obtained; the gantry angle should be oriented such that the superior articular process (SAP) of the inferior vertebral body crosses the intervertebral disc and divides it into one third medial to the SAP and two thirds lateral to the SAP for the L4-5 and L5-S1 discs. A ratio of half and half is used for the more cephalad lumbar discs.

The fluoroscopic view of the most superior and inferior aspect of each end plate should be superimposed such that the introducer needle can be positioned perpendicular to the disc or parallel with the gantry angle. When this view cannot be obtained, the patient must be repositioned, the cephalocaudal tilt of the C-arm must change, or the entry point of the needle must be altered to correct the malalignment.

Thereafter, a 17-gauge introducer needle is advanced from approximately 8 cm laterally from the midline, using an oblique fluoroscopic projection.

The needle is aimed at the Kambin safe triangle. This triangular working zone is bordered ventrally by the exiting root, inferiorly by the proximal end plate of the lower lumbar segment, and medially by the traversing root and the dural sac. The floor of the triangular working zone is occupied by the intervertebral disc, the vertebral end plate, and the dorsal boundary of the adjacent vertebra[24] (Fig. 81-8).

It is important that the introducer needle be positioned parallel to the vertebral end plate to avoid injury to the end plate. Moreover, the needle should not be placed too lateral (ventral) to the SAP.

A tactile resistance and gritty crunching are encountered when the needle first enters the anulus, and the fluoroscope is then repositioned in a posteroanterior projection. Care should be taken not to advance the needle beyond the disc margins, and if there is any confusion about the position of the needle tip during advancement, the position should be checked fluoroscopically in two orthogonal planes.

The patient may report transient localized back pain as the needle penetrates the anulus. Radicular symptoms are not expected and may indicate a needle position that is too close to the transversing root. The needle position is checked in the posteroanterior projection, confirming the tip position just inside the anulus. Under lateral fluoroscopy, the introducer needle is then advanced minimally to achieve positioning in the nucleus pulposus in the ventral half of the disc. Optimal positioning is with the needle tip between a 12 o'clock and a 3 o'clock position (Fig. 81-9).

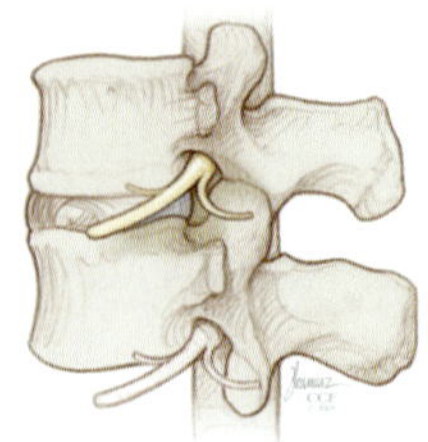

FIGURE 81-8. The Kambin triangle is defined ventrally by the existing nerve root, inferiorly by the proximal end plate of the lower lumbar segment, and medially by the traversing root and dura. The floor is occupied by the intervertebral disc, the end plate, and the dorsal boundary of the adjacent vertebra. (Copyright Cleveland Clinic Foundation.)

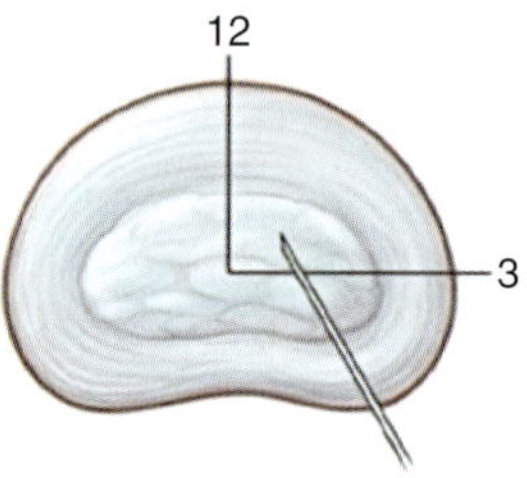

FIGURE 81-9. The needle must be placed in the optimal position in the nucleus pulposus, with the needle tip between a 12 o'clock and a 3 o'clock position as illustrated.

Intradiscal Electrothermal Therapy

The IDET technique involves intradiscal delivery of thermal energy to the internal structure of the disc anulus by way of a catheter placed within the disc for the purpose of shrinking the disc substance and decompressing the nerve root.

The thermal energy is applied into the intradiscal space by means of either a coiled or linear radiofrequency catheter. The catheter with a temperature-controlled thermal resistive coil is inserted through the needle and coiled within the disc space to rest along the inner dorsal anulus under biplanar fluoroscopy (Fig. 81-10). The catheter is then heated to 90 degrees and maintained there for 4 minutes.

Automated Percutaneous Lumbar Discectomy

Automated percutaneous lumbar discectomy (APLD) works by the theory that if the central disc volume is decreased, the pressure transmitted though a rent in the anulus and a bulging disc may be decreased, thereby decreasing pressure on an irritated nerve root.

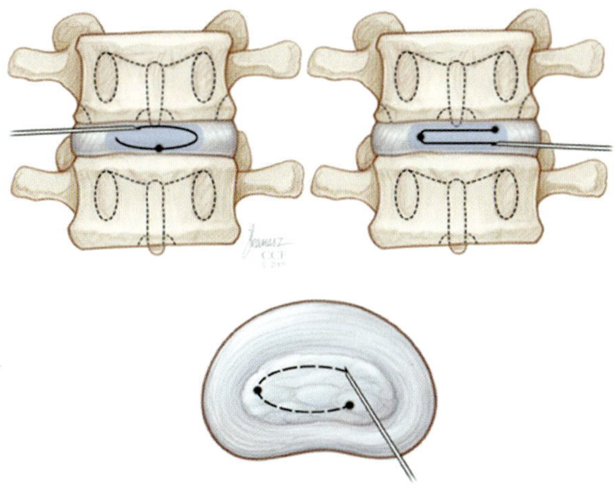

FIGURE 81-10. The course of the catheter along the inner aspect of the anulus and optimal positioning for treatment of the dorsal anulus. (Copyright Cleveland Clinic Foundation.)

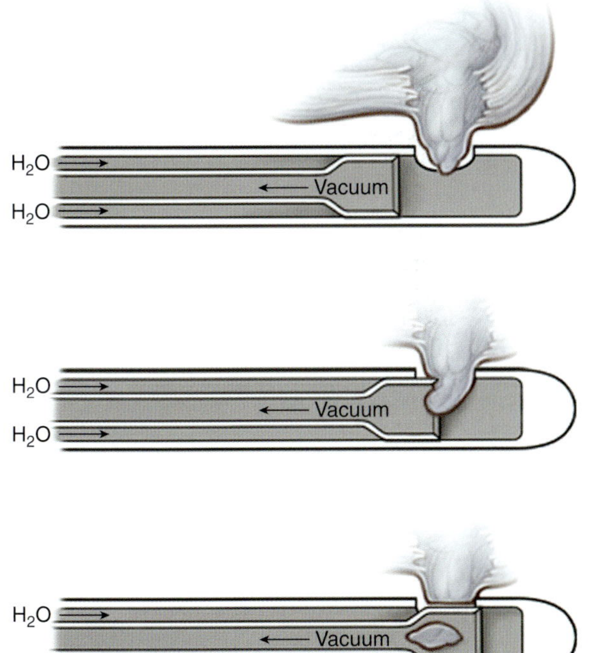

FIGURE 81-11. Illustration of the nucleotome, demonstrating suction through the central bore. The inner cutting sleeve is pneumatically driven across the side port, where the disc material is cut and then aspirated away, suspended in saline.

The APLD probe is inserted by using the percutaneous technique detailed previously. The device is able to decompress the nucleus pulposus by using both a sucking and a cutting action of a side port of the nucleotome. The disc material is then carried away in a saline solution (Fig. 81-11).

Outcomes

These less invasive options do potentially increase the cost of lumbar discectomy; therefore, to be effective, they should at least result in improved clinical outcomes. Unfortunately, the clinical evidence to date has not demonstrated a huge advantage of MIS techniques over standard open ones. However, we do note that the experience gained with these procedures expands one's ability to understand the spinal anatomy through a significantly reduced operative corridor while improving one's skill set for applying these techniques to more complex pathologies such as fusion.

Both retrospective and prospective studies have demonstrated that these MIS procedures are safe and probably at least as effective as their open counterparts. None have demonstrated a significant benefit to the MIS techniques in terms of long-term outcome of leg and back pain. Ryang et al. in 2008 published a prospective randomized study to compare efficiency, safety, and outcome of standard open microsurgical discectomy for lumbar disc herniation utilizing minimal access trocar microsurgical discectomy. They reported that both procedures result in a significant improvement of pain and neurologic deficits, while the differences in operative time, blood loss, and complication rates were statistically not significant in MIS compared to open microdiscectomy.[25] Some studies, however, have shown at least some short-term benefit utilizing MIS techniques. German et al. published a retrospective study that compared the perioperative results following MIS and conventional open lumbar discectomy. No significant difference was seen with regard to leg pain; however, there was a statistically significant difference in length of stay, estimated blood loss, postanesthesia care unit narcotic use, and need for admission to the hospital. These differences were thought to be of only modest significance.[26] Righesso et al. published a prospective randomized study to compare the clinical outcome of open discectomy versus the microendoscopic discectomy. They found a small statistically significant difference between the groups (incision size, length of hospitalization, operative time, and visual analogue scale at 12 hours), but the overall patient outcomes were not affected.[27] Others have demonstrated similar conclusions.[15,28-31]

Recently, a multicenter clinical trial was conducted to compare conventional lumbar to tubular endoscopic discectomy. With 1-year follow-up, we found no benefit for the MIS approach with regard to objective functional outcome scores, while patients rated their back and leg pain worse utilizing subjective pain outcome scores.

Conclusion

Minimal access lumbar microdiscectomy is both safe and effective. Studies have shown that the efficacy of the procedure is high, with reported success rates of 75% to 80%. Studies to date have not demonstrated a significant benefit with regard to pain and neurologic outcomes, although some studies have demonstrated a difference in length of stay, estimated blood loss, postanesthesia care unit narcotic use, and need for admission to the hospital. These differences may be of only marginal significance. The percutaneous procedures are highly dependent on patient selection, which limits the more widespread use of these procedures. Increased experience with minimal access procedures will minimize complications and optimize patient outcomes.

KEY REFERENCES

Foley KT, Smith MM: Microendoscopic discectomy. *Tech Neurosurg* 3: 301–307, 1997.

Kambin P, Brager MD: Percutaneous posterolateral discectomy: anatomy and mechanism. *Clin Orthop Relat Res* 223:145–154, 1987.

Mayer HM, Brock M: Percutaneous endoscopic discectomy: surgical technique and preliminary results compared to microsurgical discectomy. *J Neurosurg* 78:216–225, 1993.

Ryang YM, Oertel MF, Mayfrank L, et al: Standard open microdiscectomy versus minimal access trocar microdiscectomy: results of a prospective randomized study. *Neurosurgery* 62(1):174–181, 2008.

REFERENCES

The complete reference list is available online at expertconsult.com.

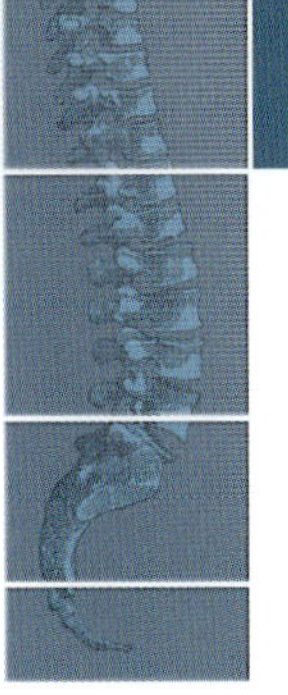

4.5 Arthritides and Related Disorders

CHAPTER 82

Cervical Spondylosis

Varun R. Kshettry

Cervical spondylosis is a ubiquitous degenerative process of aging that can lead to both pain and neurologic impairment. Radiographically, it is observed in about 10% of people by age 25 and in nearly 95% by age 65.[1,2] Multiple authors near the end of the 19th century initially described it as an inflammatory process, possibly infectious in origin, and, therefore, referred to it as *cervical spondylitis*.[3] It was not until 1952 that Brain identified this as a degenerative process of aging and coined the term *cervical spondylosis*. British neurosurgeon Victor Horsley provided the first description of an operation—a C6 laminectomy—for a patient with progressive spastic quadriparesis with presumed cervical spondylotic myelopathy (CSM).[4,5]

Pathology of Cervical Spondylosis and Myelopathy

Degeneration associated with spondylosis begins at the intervertebral disc, unlike degenerative arthritis, which is associated with inflammation of the synovial lining of joints.[1] The nucleus pulposus consists of proteoglycan aggregates that have hydrophilic hyaluronic chains with side chains containing chondroitin sulfate and keratin sulfate. Repeated stress and aging of the nucleus pulposus lead to several changes.[1,6-10] Histologically, there are loss of hydrophilic mucopolysaccharides, increase in keratin sulfate, and loss of water, which lead to disc shrinkage, loss of elasticity, and inequitable distribution of hydrostatic pressure on the anulus with compressive forces. As the disc weakens, surrounding structures are required to bear a greater burden of weight-bearing load and dynamic stresses. As surrounding structures bear greater weight, they undergo reactive changes. End plates, uncovertebral joints, and facet joints form osteophytes as a biomechanical mechanism to increase the weight-bearing surface area.[10-14] The ligamentum flavum and PLL undergo hypertrophy.[15-17] Dorsally, the ligamentum flavum can buckle into the spinal canal as the discs collapse. Ventrally, the anulus bulges into the spinal canal and dissects the PLL of the bone, and the PLL itself hypertrophies. Degenerative changes in the disc occur ventrally first, leading to kyphosis.

Cervical spondylotic changes can lead to spinal canal and intervertebral foramen narrowing that can impinge on the spinal cord centrally or on the exiting nerve roots laterally. Autopsy studies have described histologic changes that are seen in CSM, including white matter demyelination, particularly in lateral corticospinal tracts, gray matter neuronal loss, necrosis, and cavitation.[18,19] Ogino et al. demonstrated that pathologic changes worsened with smaller anteroposterior canal diameter: reduction to 40% to 44% of normal led to mild white matter demyelination; reduction to 22% to 39% correlated with diffuse white matter demyelination and gray matter cavitation; and reduction to 12% to 19% led to white matter gliosis and diffuse gray matter necrosis.[19]

Pathologic changes found in CSM are due to factors that are often divided into static, dynamic, and vascular processes.[1] Static processes are the reactive changes already described stemming from disc desiccation. Dynamic movement in cervical spondylosis may further lead to CSM. During flexion, the spinal cord elongates and may become trapped along ventral osteophytic spurs. With extension, ligamentum buckling may cause dorsal impingement.[1,16,20] An MRI flexion-extension study by Muhle et al. demonstrated increasing spinal stenosis on average during extension compared to flexion.[21] Finally, animal studies demonstrate that the changes that are observed in CSM mimic changes seen in ischemic cord models.[18,22,23] Some authors hypothesize that this occurs because spinal cord compression leads to ischemia at the microcirculation level.[22] Demyelination may also be due to increased susceptibility to ischemia seen in oligodendrocytes.[20,24] While cervical spondylotic changes are seen throughout the subaxial spine, involvement at C5-6 is the most common, followed by C6-7.[25] That this is likely due to the fact that motion is more common at C5-6 and C6-7, where most of flexion and extension in the subaxial spine occur, and motion leads to greater reactive changes.[1,26] Spinal cord compression symptoms may be exacerbated by the fact that C5-7 is a watershed area in the cervical cord, with reduced blood flow and greater potential for spinal cord ischemia.[27,28]

Clinical Syndromes

Axial Pain

Neck pain is a common presenting chief complaint seen by the general practitioner. Contributing anatomic sources of neck pain are multiple and include neck musculature, tendons, ligaments, facet joints, intervertebral discs, craniovertebral junction, and cervical vasculature. Referred pain can be seen with shoulder and temporomandibular joint pathology as well. The intervertebral disc is innervated ventrally by branches from the sympathetic plexus and dorsally by the sinuvertebral nerve, which arises from the ventral nerve root.[29-31] The sinuvertebral nerve also innervates the PLL, the dura, and a substantial portion of the vertebral body periosteum.[1,28] Cervical facet joints are innervated by branches arising from the dorsal ramus.[1]

Axial pain can occur alone or in conjunction with radiculopathy and/or myelopathy. When pain occurs alone, the traditional dictum advocates nonoperative management. However, experience shows that when axial pain accompanies radiculopathy or myelopathy, surgery to ameliorate the latter frequently relieves the former.[29] The most common cause of nondegenerative isolated neck pain is cervical strain resulting from injury to neck muscles, tendons, and ligaments that is frequently seen with whiplash injury.[29] Beliefs about the anatomic source of isolated neck pain in patients with cervical spondylosis vary. The intervertebral disc is commonly cited as the source of axial pain.[32] Tears in the anulus may stimulate the sinuvertebral nerve.[33,34] Additionally, injection of local anesthetic in the disc space can temporarily relieve pain in some patients.[35] The facet joints are another potential source of axial pain.[36,37] Stimulation of subaxial facet joints generates reproducible neck pain patterns in normal volunteers.[38] However, facet steroid injections[39] and percutaneous radiofrequency neurotomy have demonstrated mediocre results.[40,41]

Isolated axial pain that fails to respond to initial conservative therapy can be further evaluated with cervical radiographs. Cervical spondylotic changes on radiograph are ubiquitous in the aging population and include loss of disc height, osteophyte formation, kyphosis, and subluxation.[1,42] Flexion-extension cervical films greatly help in ruling out instability or motion that may be a source of significant pain.

In appropriately selected patients, several studies have demonstrated good results in operative management of axial pain.[31,43-45] These studies utilized provocative discography to localize the level(s) of axial pain and treat symptomatic levels with anterior cervical decompression and fusion (ACDF). Neck pain is common in rheumatoid arthritis and can be secondary to instability or from basilar invagination, and surgery is commonly employed in this population. One must always be alert to the possibility of a C3-4 radiculopathy as a source of axial pain. Unilateral pain should alert the practitioner to look for sensory alterations, ask about paresthesias in this distribution, and look for a positive Spurling sign. C3-4 radiculopathy that causes axial pain generally responds very well to surgical decompression.[46] Pseudarthrosis from previously attempted fusion can also lead to significant axial pain with or without radiculopathy and is a condition that also responds well to reoperation.

Isolated axial pain can be disabling to patients and presents a significant diagnostic and management challenge to the practitioner. The source of neck pain varies from person to person and in many patients is likely multifactorial. Acute neck pain deserves a trial of NSAIDs and short-term muscle relaxants if needed.[47] A temporary soft neck collar can provide comfort as well. Chronic neck pain can be managed with analgesia and physical therapy exercises to strengthen the cervical musculature. Surgery should be reserved for patients with well-accepted indications. Although controversial, surgery may be considered in certain cases of disabling neck pain with positive properly performed discography.

Radiculopathy

Cervical radiculopathy results from compression of an exiting cervical nerve root. This often results from uncovertebral and facet osteophyte formation extending into the neural foramen. Patients often describe a sharp or burning radiating pain in a dermatomal distribution. Nerve compression can also result in paresthesias or impaired sensation in a dermatomal distribution or weakness in the respective myotome. Physical examination is often significant for a positive Spurling sign: Axial compression with lateral bending to the ipsilateral side reproduces the radicular pain. The abduction relief sign—relief of radicular pain by abducting the ipsilateral arm and putting the hand on the head—can help to differentiate radiculopathy from thoracic outlet syndrome or shoulder pathology.[4,48] One must carefully evaluate the radiculopathic complaint and consider alternative etiologies such as peripheral entrapment syndromes, thoracic outlet syndrome, brachial neuritis, shoulder pathology, reflex sympathetic dystrophy, and even angina.[1]

MRI has become the standard for evaluating the neural foramina for radiculopathy. On T2 imaging, individual neural foramina can be evaluated for significant stenosis. With existing hardware, CT myelography is more useful. Dynamic flexion-extension radiographs are invaluable in additionally evaluating for instability to plan operative strategy. In attempting to sort out radiculopathy from peripheral syndromes, electrodiagnostic studies such as electromyography and nerve conduction studies are routinely used.

Radiculopathy without significant weakness deserves an appropriate trial of conservative therapy. This includes analgesia, NSAIDs, and possibly anticonvulsant therapy. Although not FDA approved, anticonvulsant therapy with gabapentin or pregabalin, which has demonstrated benefits in diabetic neuropathy, is now frequently used for radiculopathic pain with good anecdotal results. Epidural steroid injection or localized nerve blocks can provide therapeutic relief, and the latter can help to confirm diagnostic hypotheses.

When conservative therapy fails and the diagnosis of cervical root compression is certain, surgical decompression provides good results. When alignment is well maintained, a minimally destabilizing approach includes dorsal laminoforaminotomy. When fusion is needed, either ACDF or dorsal decompression with fusion provides good results in class III evidence. Persson et al. randomized 81 patients with cervical spondylotic radiculopathy to ACDF, physical therapy, or cervical collar immobilization. Evaluation at 3 to 4 months revealed improved pain scores (using a visual analogue scale) and motor and sensory improvements with surgery compared to nonoperative alternatives. This effect dissipated at 12-month follow-up; however, a disability rating index showed improved return to work and dressing ability at 12 months with surgery.[49,50]

Myelopathy

Patients with myelopathy commonly present with unsteady gait and difficulty with fine motor coordination in the hands.[8,11] Physical examination may demonstrate hyperreflexia below the level of compression, increased muscle tone, clonus, the Babinski sign, the Hoffman sign, and the finger escape sign.[8,51] Some patients may describe the Lhermitte sign (electric shock sensations traveling down the spine with flexion), which is thought to be due to stimulation of the dorsal columns. Hands may demonstrate intrinsic muscle atrophy, which is a classic sign in myelopathy.[51,52] Some patients may complain of urinary retention or spastic detrusor activity leading to frequent urges with or without incontinence. Additional localizing upper motor signs include pectoral muscle reflex, which is suggestive of compression at or above C2-4, and the jaw jerk, which if present suggests a lesion above the foramen magnum.[53,54] Patients with severe cervical spondylosis with canal stenosis can experience central cord syndrome with even minor trauma, particularly in hyperextension injury. Greater motor impairment is seen in the upper extremities and is often accompanied by urinary retention.[55] Burning hands have been described in football injuries and are thought to be a variant of central cord syndrome in patients with congenital canal stenosis.[56] The differential diagnosis for CSM is broad and includes multiple sclerosis, syringomyelia, atrophic lateral sclerosis, subacute combined degeneration, intraspinal tumor, spinal arteriovenous malformation, epidural abscess, Chiari malformation, ossification of the posterior longitudinal ligament, normal pressure hydrocephalus, tabes dorsalis, hereditary spastic paraplegia, and tropical spastic paraparesis.[1,11,57,58] Several grading systems have been developed to classify the severity of CSM in an objective, reliable, and valid assessment that can also be used to measure responsiveness to therapeutic interventions. The Japanese Orthopaedic Association (JOA) scale and the modified version by Benzel et al. are the two most widely used systems and have demonstrated good interobserver and intraobserver reliability.[59-61] Other accepted systems include gait analysis and the short form-36 (SF-36).[62-65]

The gold standard for imaging in CSM has become MRI because it provides the best view of the spinal cord, exiting nerve roots, and CSF signal.[66] CT myelography may be more useful in cases of previous surgery because it is superior to MRI in viewing residual bony anatomy and produces less artifact with existing hardware. The examiner must be aware that the degree of stenosis on imaging frequently does not correlate with clinical impairment. In one study of asymptomatic elderly patients, 26% had some degree of spinal cord impingement on MRI.[11,67] Multiple studies have attempted to correlate spinal cord signal changes on MRI with neurologic recovery after decompression. Several class III studies demonstrate that T2 hyperintensity at a single segment does not predict outcome, but when present at multiple levels or in combination with T1 hypointensity, it does correlate with poor neurologic recovery after surgery.[68-72] Other studies have attempted to correlate the degree of canal stenosis with neurologic recovery after surgery. Most studies demonstrate poorer neurologic recovery in patients with greater radiographic canal stenosis, with most studies using a canal area of 30 to 45 mm^2 as the cutoff to dichotomize groups.[73-76] One study did not corroborate these findings.[77]

Although electrodiagnostic studies are not necessary for diagnosis of CSM, a class I study by Bednarik et al. followed 66 patients (average age 50 years) with radiographic spinal cord compression from cervical spondylosis without clinical myelopathy. These patients were followed for an average of 4 years, during which 19.7% developed CSM. Bednarik et al. found that electromyography and sensory evoked potential abnormalities and, additionally, clinical radiculopathy, when present initially, predicted the development of CSM.[78]

Traditional teaching portrays the natural history of CSM as progressive stepwise neurologic deterioration. However, after initial presentation of neurologic impairment, the natural history is mixed. Some patients remain neurologically stable for long periods of time, with some even improving; others will continue to accrue additional deficits.[79] Many class III studies have tracked the natural history of CSM.[80-83] One of the initial studies by Clarke and Robinson in 1956 retrospectively reviewed 120 patients with CSM: 26 who never underwent surgery plus the preoperative course of 94 patients who eventually underwent surgery. They found that the majority (75%) of patients experienced episodes of neurologic deterioration with intervening periods of stability. Of the smaller cohort that did not undergo surgery, half experienced some degree of neurologic improvement with conservative management.[81] Another study by Nurick in 1972 found that most patients remained neurologically stable after initial deficits, and he advocated surgery for those with progressive symptoms and those older than 60 years of age.[80] One of the only class I studies, by Kadanka et al., demonstrated that 80% of patients younger than 75 years of age with 1 year of mild CSM (defined as modified JOA > 12) remained neurologically stable with conservative management (NSAIDs, rest, cervical immobilization) over 2 to 3 years as measured by the modified JOA scale, a timed 10-meter walk, and video evaluation of ADL performance.[84,85] A 2002 Cochrane review of CSM concluded that there is no clear evidence to support the idea that CSM patients inevitably deteriorate neurologically.[86] However, all of these studies of conservative management excluded patients who underwent early surgery likely because of more severe or progressive forms of CSM. Therefore, these studies have a selection bias toward patients with a more benign natural history and cannot be generalized.[87]

Furthering the decision maker's dilemma, numerous studies demonstrate that increased symptom duration—most studies using between 12 and 24 months as cutoff—portends worse neurologic recovery.[76,88-92] Therefore, it appears that in mild CSM, a conservative management trial is reasonable, but patients with unacceptable neurologic deficits and those with progressive symptoms should be considered for early decompression.

Multiple class III studies demonstrate that the majority of patients either improve or remain neurologically stable, by JOA or Nurick scores, after surgical decompression using both ventral and dorsal approaches.[60,93-99]

Surgical Strategies

Details of surgical technique are covered elsewhere in this book. The following section provides a brief overview of surgical approaches and current evidence regarding their efficacy.

Dorsal Approach

For isolated radiculopathy without myelopathy, dorsal laminoforaminotomy provides an effective alternative to decompress the exiting nerve root.[100] The goal of foraminotomy is to provide additional space to the exiting root without necessarily resecting the offending osteophyte.

Laminectomy is frequently used for multilevel pathology, including multilevel cervical spondylosis, congenital canal stenosis, and dorsal compressive pathology such as ligamentum flavum hypertrophy or ossification. Laminectomy has also been successful for treatment of OPLL.[101] Laminectomy alone is better suited for the straight or lordotic spine but not the kyphotic spine. Long-term studies show that the rate of postoperative kyphosis after isolated laminectomy ranges from 14% to 47%.[102,103] The incidence of postoperative kyphosis increases with loss of lordosis on preoperative radiographs.[103] Particularly concerning is that when multilevel ventral pathology exists, increasing kyphosis may result in further draping of the cord over ventral osteophytes. Laminectomy alone also results in a higher rate of kyphosis than laminoplasty.[104,105] Numerous studies highlight an increased risk of late neurologic deterioration with laminectomy alone compared to ventral or dorsal decompression with fusion.[60,106] However, these same studies are unable to directly correlate kyphosis with development of late neurologic deterioration. One study using dentate ligament sectioning found no additional benefit of such practice.[60]

Laminectomy can be supplemented with arthrodesis when there is concern for the development of kyphosis. Laminoplasty using either a French door or an open-door technique has also been employed with success. Frequently, laminoplasty is supplemented with lateral mass onlay fusion. There currently is no class I or II evidence to suggest superiority between laminoplasty, laminectomy with arthrodesis, anterior cervical corpectomy and fusion (ACCF), or ACDF with plate fixation.

Ventral Approach

When the offending compressive elements are ventral, a ventral approach allows better access for direct decompression. When there are three or fewer diseased levels, ACDF or ACCF may be used. For longer segments, either a dorsal or a combined approach is utilized. Ventral plate fixation and instrumentation have become commonplace but should not be a substitute for good graft technique. Kaiser et al. retrospectively compared 251 patients with ACDF with plate fixation showing a 96% fusion rate for single-level ACDF and a 90% fusion rate for two-level ACDF compared to historical fusion rates for single-level ACDF (91%) and two-level ACDF (72%). Additionally, graft complications with plate fixation were reduced from 6% to 1.3%.[107] A large retrospective review by Caspar et al. found that the reoperation rate for pseudarthrosis was 4.8% for ACDF and 0.7% for ACDF with plate fixation.[108] However, Resnick and Trost performed a systemic review of randomized trials that showed no clear benefit for ventral plate fixation in single-level ACDF.[109] From a biomechanical perspective, plate fixation results in greater preservation of lordosis. Troyanovich et al. calculated that lordosis at the fused segment decreased by 2.5 degrees in ACDF but increased by 5.7 degrees in ACDF with plate fixation.[110]

ACCF is an alternative to ACDF. Traditionally, ACCF demonstrated higher rates of fusion than ACDF without plate fixation.[95] However, ACCF appears to yield results equivalent to those of ACDF with plate fixation.[111] A pooled analysis of 2682 patients by Fraser and Hartl found that two-level ACDF with plate fixation yielded fusion rates (>90%) similar to those of ACCF. For three-level disease, ACDF with plate fixation yielded significantly lower fusion rates (82.5%) than ACCF with plate fixation (96.2%).[112]

Ventral plates vary among manufacturers, and some have more recently produced dynamic plates that allow for motion. Class III studies show no difference in fusion rates between dynamic and rigid fixation plates. However, one study found a higher screw failure rate with rigid fixation but increased dysphagia with dynamic plates.[113]

Cervical disc arthroplasty presents an alternative to fusion with the theoretical benefit of motion sparing at the treated level and the hope of decreasing adjacent segment disease. Mummaneni et al. presented the first randomized controlled trial of 541 patients with single-level cervical disease randomized to arthroplasty versus ACDF without plate fixation. NDI, SF-36, and pain perception scores improved with both groups over a 2-year period. It appears that over the short term, cervical disc arthroplasty is at least as good as traditional fusion without fixation.[114] Similar results have been found with alternative manufacturers.[115,116] However, long-term neurologic outcome and safety are still to be determined.

Summary

Cervical spondylosis is a ubiquitous degenerative process of the aging spine that begins at the intervertebral disc and results in reactive changes that can result in compression of the spinal cord or exiting nerve roots. The symptomatic patient may present with axial pain, radiculopathy, and/or myelopathy. Surgical strategies include both ventral and dorsal approaches for decompression and fusion when indicated. Location of the offending compression, longitudinal extent of compression, and preexisting spinal alignment are all basic factors that determine the best surgical strategy available to the surgeon.

KEY REFERENCES

Al-Mefty O, Harkey HL, Marawi I, et al: Experimental chronic compressive cervical myelopathy. *J Neurosurg* 79(4):550–561, 1993.

Brain WR, Northfield D, Wilkinson M: The neurological manifestations of cervical spondylosis. *Brain* 75(2):187–225, 1952.

Kadanka Z, Bednarik J, Vohanka S, et al: Conservative treatment versus surgery in spondylotic cervical myelopathy: a prospective randomised study. *Eur Spine J* 9(6):538–544, 2000.

Kaptain GJ, Simmons NE, Replogle RE, Pobereskin L: Incidence and outcome of kyphotic deformity following laminectomy for cervical spondylotic myelopathy. *J Neurosurg* 93(Suppl 2):199–204, 2000.

Persson LC, Moritz U, Brandt L, Carlsson CA: Cervical radiculopathy: pain, muscle weakness and sensory loss in patients with cervical radiculopathy treated with surgery, physiotherapy or cervical collar: a prospective, controlled study. *Eur Spine J* 6(4):256–266, 1997.

Shedid D, Benzel EC: Cervical spondylosis anatomy: pathophysiology and biomechanics. *Neurosurgery* 60(1 Suppl 1):S7–S13, 2007.

White AA 3rd, Panjabi MM: Biomechanical considerations in the surgical management of cervical spondylotic myelopathy. *Spine (Phila Pa 1976)* 13(7):856–860, 1988.

Yonenobu K, Abumi K, Nagata K, et al: Interobserver and intraobserver reliability of the Japanese Orthopaedic Association scoring system for evaluation of cervical compression myelopathy, *Spine (Phila Pa 1976)* 26(17):1890–1894, 2001; discussion 1895.

REFERENCES

The complete reference list is available online at expertconsult.com.

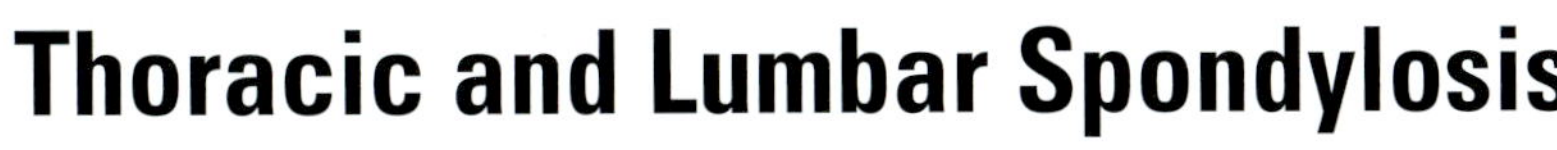

CHAPTER 83

Thoracic and Lumbar Spondylosis

Christopher Wolfla | Michael Martin

Anatomy, Pathophysiology, and Biomechanics

Lumbar and thoracic spondylosis, which can be broadly defined as degenerative destruction or remodeling of the bony elements of the spine, intervertebral discs, facet joints, and/or spinal ligaments, is a progressive age-related disorder. This degeneration secondarily affects the neural structures that are normally protected and supported by the ligamentous and bony elements of the spine as those same elements compress the spinal nerves and thecal sac. The anatomy of the thoracic and lumbar spine as it relates to this process is important not only for understanding the pathophysiology and clinical presentation but also for anatomically sound operative planning and execution. While an exhaustive review of thoracolumbar anatomy is beyond the scope of this chapter, certain anatomic relationships must be emphasized.

The progression of spondylosis in the thoracic and lumbar spine essentially occurs at three points anatomically: the intervertebral disc, the facet joints, and the ligamentum flavum. Each of these structures has its own contribution in a biomechanically intact spine. Therefore, subsequent spondylotic degeneration produces varying clinical pictures depending on the specific structure or combination of structures most involved.

The intervertebral disc is bound ventrally by the anterior longitudinal ligament, dorsally by the posterior longitudinal ligament, and rostrally and caudally by cartilaginous end plates that abut the vertebral bodies. The anulus fibrosus forms the outer ring of the disc and provides most of the structural integrity. A softer, notochord-derived nucleus pulposus forms the center portion of the disc and, although not as strong as the anulus, provides cushioning and some resistance, mainly to axial loads. With aging, the disc progressively desiccates and becomes less elastic, a process that has been termed disc degeneration. In the case of spondylosis, disc degeneration contributes to the overall pathology in several different ways. As the disc desiccates, a process that is demonstrable on MRI by loss of T2 signal (so-called dark disc disease) (Fig. 83-1), it has the potential, by virtue of its innervation by the recurrent sinuvertebral nerve, ventral rami, and rami communicantes, to contribute to back pain.[1] With the loss of hydration, the disc may become incapable of resisting physiologic biomechanical forces, resulting in failure by herniation through a defect in the anulus. This herniation may result in neurologic deficit and/or pain. Even in the absence of true herniation, a broad-based bulge may compress the neural elements, causing symptoms. Apart from symptomatology, the desiccated disc is no longer able to perform a portion of its biomechanical function in the normal movement of the spine. Other elements of the spine must therefore bear the resultant biomechanical stresses, potentially accelerating their degeneration.

Facet joints in the thoracic spine and the lumbar spine are alternatively referred to as zygapophyseal or apophyseal joints. Because they oppose the neural elements, degeneration and hypertrophy may cause compression of spinal roots, the spinal cord, and the thecal sac of the lumbar spine. Each joint is composed of the superior articular process of the caudal vertebra and the inferior articular process of the rostral vertebra. The opposing surfaces are covered with synovium, while the outer surface is covered by fibrous capsule. The joints of the thoracic spine from the C7-T1 joint to the T9-10 joint are typically oriented in the coronal plane and assume a configuration not unlike that of shingles on a roof. The T10-11 joint is often a transition area where the joint orientation becomes slightly tangential to the coronal plane. The portion of the joint that is visible dorsally in the lumbar spine is mostly composed of the inferior articular process of the rostral vertebra; this is readily demonstrated with removal of the joint capsule. The superior articular process of the inferior vertebra forms the ventral and lateral portion of the joint. Because of its location directly adjacent to the exit point of the nerve root laterally and the thecal sac medially, the superior facet process often comprises the point of maximal compression when joint hypertrophy leads to neural compromise. Because innervation of the facets themselves is via medial branches of the dorsal primary rami, degeneration of the facets may produce back pain by this mechanism.[2-4]

Signs and Symptoms

Back Pain

As previously stated, lumbar and thoracic spondylosis may cause back pain. This multifactorial complaint is very common and may occur in the absence of defined spinal pathology. In degenerative spondylosis, however, the generation of pain may be due to facet hypertrophy, disc degeneration,

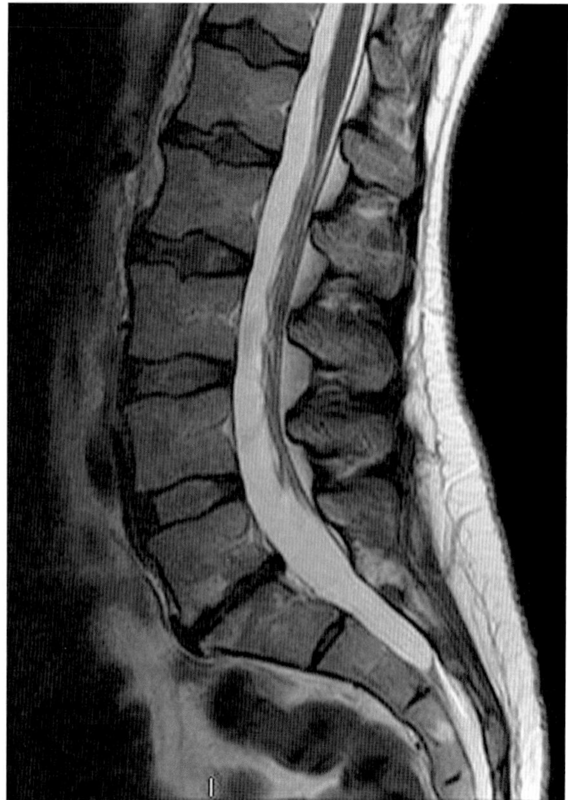

FIGURE 83-1. Sagittal T2-weighted MRI of the lumbar spine illustrating advanced disc degeneration at L5-S1.

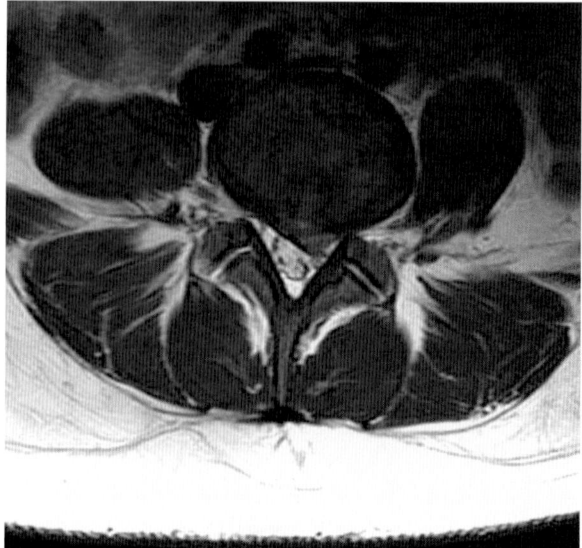

FIGURE 83-2. Axial T2-weighted MRI of the lumbar spine illustrating a left paracentral disc herniation at L4-5, causing compression of the left L5 nerve root.

spinal instability, and/or referred pain from neural compression. These causes are generally difficult to separate from each other; even in the face of overt instability, the so-called pain generator may be protean and difficult to treat.

Nevertheless, the mechanisms by which possible sources of pain in spondylosis affect patients bear discussion. As was mentioned earlier, the intervertebral discs and facet joints are innervated and may cause pain with degeneration.[1-4] Furthermore, as the spine ages, the degenerating facets and increasingly desiccated intervertebral discs lose some of their ability to maintain normal motion and support of the vertebral column. As a result, paraspinal muscles may be recruited to maintain posture, and this may contribute to painful paraspinal muscle spasm.

Radiculopathy

As was mentioned earlier in this chapter, thoracolumbar spondylosis may cause neural compromise by virtue of the location of both the thecal sac and nerve roots adjacent to structures that bear the brunt of the degenerative process. When nerve roots are compromised, radiculopathy may result.

The underlying pathophysiology of radiculopathy is most likely multifactorial. Direct mechanical compression of a nerve root certainly plays some role in the generation of radiculopathy, particularly as removal of the offending lesion frequently results in marked improvement in symptoms. In the lumbar spine, this compression most commonly occurs in the lateral recess and affects the nerve root exiting the next most caudal neural foramen (Fig. 83-2). Thus, a paracentral herniation at L4-5 most commonly affects the L5 nerve root exiting the L5-S1 neural foramen. However, while it is intuitive that a herniated thoracic or lumbar disc causes pain by direct mechanical compression or stretch on the nerve root, many patients have disc pathology that abuts or compresses the neural elements without associated radicular symptoms. Disc material is both immunogenic and inflammatory.[5,6] Animal models have demonstrated that nucleus pulposus material causes an inflammatory reaction and a demonstrable increase in reactive cytokines. Tumor necrosis factor alpha has been proposed as a possible underlying inflammatory factor.[7-10] Both processes have been implicated in symptom generation.

Radiculopathy is not always the result of disc pathology. As the thoracolumbar facet joints hypertrophy as the degenerative process progresses, compression of the ventrally lying nerve roots may occur. This compression generally occurs in the aforementioned region directly adjacent to the exit point of the nerve root laterally and the thecal sac medially, termed the lateral recess (Fig. 83-3). The ligamentum flavum may also hypertrophy, contributing to this compression.

Myelopathy

When spondylotic processes result in compression of the spinal cord, myelopathy may occur. Spondylotic processes in the thoracic spine, including disc pathology, facet hypertrophy, and ligamentum flavum hypertrophy, may cause direct compression of the spinal cord. In the lumbar spine, the situation is somewhat more complex, as the spinal cord in most adults ends in the region of L1-2. Thus, compression from spondylotic pathology at lumbar levels causes symptoms related to compression of the spinal cord, conus medullaris, or nerve roots. Symptoms from pathology at the thoracolumbar junction therefore vary according to the neural structures that are affected, although rarely true thoracic disc herniation can mimic lumbar radiculopathy.[11,12]

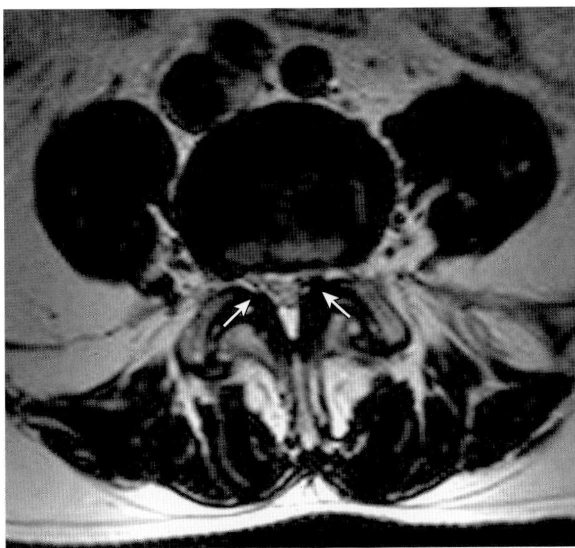

FIGURE 83-3. Axial T2-weighted MRI of the lumbar spine illustrating narrowing of the lateral recesses (*arrows*) due to facet and ligamentum flavum hypertrophy.

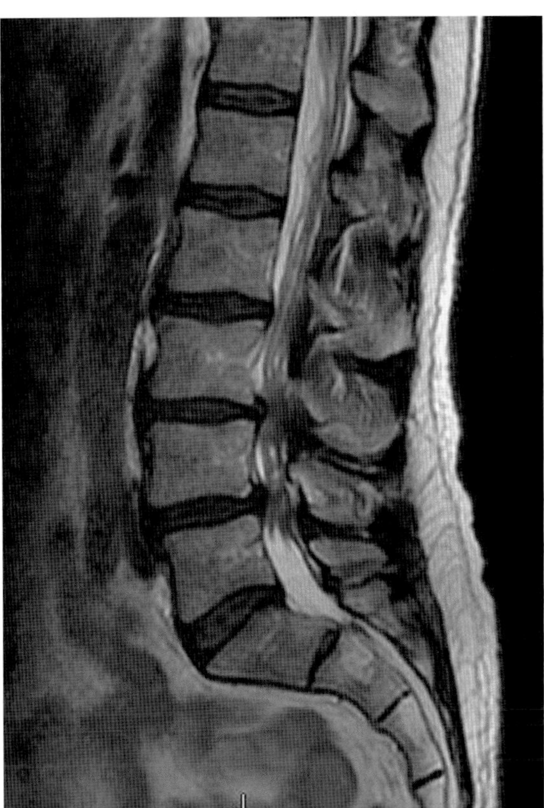

FIGURE 83-4. Sagittal T2-weighted MRI of the lumbar spine illustrating central stenosis at L2-3, L3-4, and L4-5.

Claudication

When spondylotic processes result in compression of the thecal sac below the conus medullaris, neurogenic claudication may result. Most commonly, this occurs as the result of spondylotic spinal stenosis caused by hypertrophy of the ligamentum flavum, by facet arthropathy and subsequent overgrowth, by broad-based intervertebral disc bulges, or by a combination of any of the three. These symptoms are to be distinguished from vascular claudication.[13] Pain often extends down the back of the legs into the calves in neurogenic claudication, while the pain of vascular claudication is often described as being in a "stocking" distribution. With vascular claudication, relief often comes quickly after rest; simply resting does not often help neurogenic claudication. Patients frequently must sit or assume a flexed or stooped posture (the so-called shopping cart sign) to relieve the pain of neurogenic claudication. Vascular problems that cause claudication usually result in diminished or absent peripheral pulses and cool extremities, whereas in neurogenic claudication, the lower-extremity examination may be entirely normal.

Correlative Diagnostics

In general, back pain in the absence of trauma, infection, or possible malignancy, without neurologic symptoms, does not require imaging. The presence of myelopathy, radiculopathy, or claudication symptoms merits diagnostic workup in most instances. Often, in the current era, the first test ordered is MRI without contrast. In the thoracic spine, findings of spinal cord compression are often associated with intervertebral disc herniation. This produces narrowing of the spinal canal and in more advanced disease may demonstrate hyperintensity within the parenchyma of the spinal cord on T2-weighted images. High signal on T2-weighted images is associated with spinal cord injury in the acute care setting; in the outpatient setting, this finding is associated with myelopathy. Ligamentum flavum hypertrophy and facet joint arthropathy that commonly appear on lumbar spine imaging in the setting of spondylosis are often absent in the spondylotic thoracic spine. This may be due to the fact that the thoracic spine is far less mobile than the lumbar spine. Thus, a desiccated thoracic disc does not necessarily cause a reactive hypertrophy of ligaments or joints.

MRI findings in lumbar spondylosis generally differ from those in thoracic spondylosis. Degeneration, as was mentioned earlier in the chapter, may be associated with disc herniation, ligamentum flavum hypertrophy, and facet joint hypertrophy. The summation of these pathologic tissue responses may cause stenosis of the spinal canal in the midline or lateral recesses of the canal (Figs. 83-4 and 83-5). Facet hypertrophy, ligamentum flavum hypertrophy, or broad-based disc bulges (Fig. 83-6) may also contribute to stenosis of the central canal, lateral recesses, or foramina. Extraforaminal disc herniations may cause compression of the exiting nerve root lateral to the neural foramen (Fig. 83-7). As spondylosis progresses and joint arthropathy worsens, increased fluid within the facet capsule itself or the presence of synovial cysts associated with the joints may contribute to compression of the thecal sac and/or nerve roots (Fig. 83-8). In the absence of frank instability, these findings may also portend the development of instability following surgical decompression without stabilization.

Typically, patients with lumbar spondylosis will undergo plain radiographic imaging of the affected area prior to or as a part of their initial evaluation. Most often, anteroposterior (AP), lateral, flexion, extension, and oblique images are obtained. Findings on AP and lateral radiographs include loss

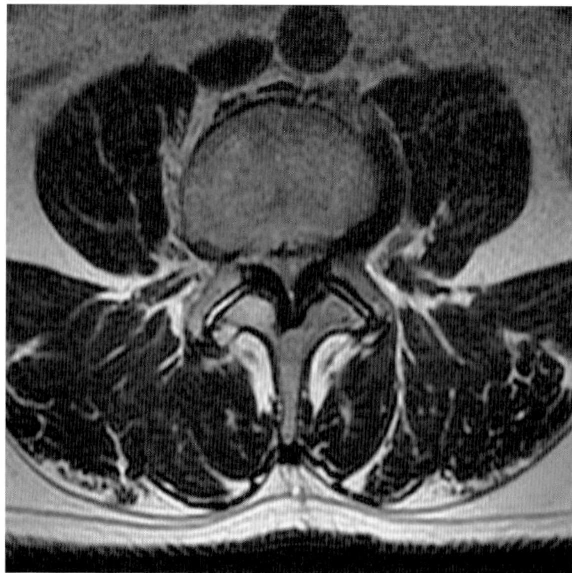

FIGURE 83-5. Axial T2-weighted MRI of the lumbar spine illustrating central and lateral stenosis.

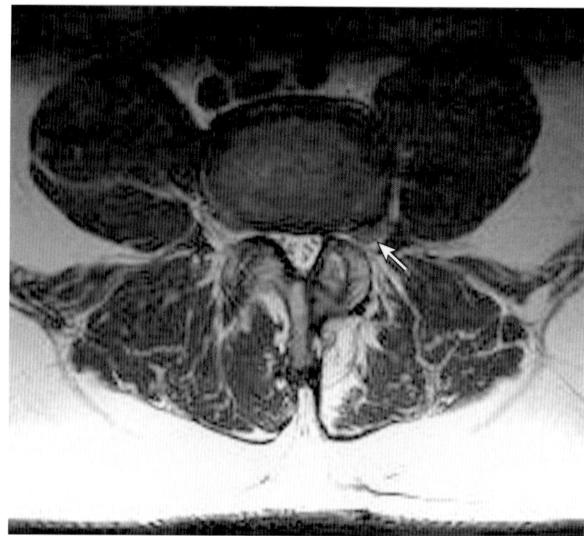

FIGURE 83-7. Axial T2-weighted MRI of the lumbar spine demonstrating an extraforaminal disc herniation at L4-5 on the left (*arrow*).

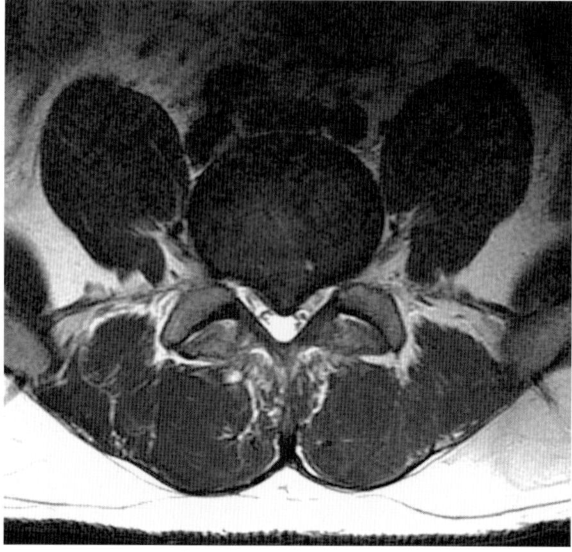

FIGURE 83-6. Axial T2-weighted MRI of the lumbar spine illustrating central stenosis secondary to a large midline disc herniation.

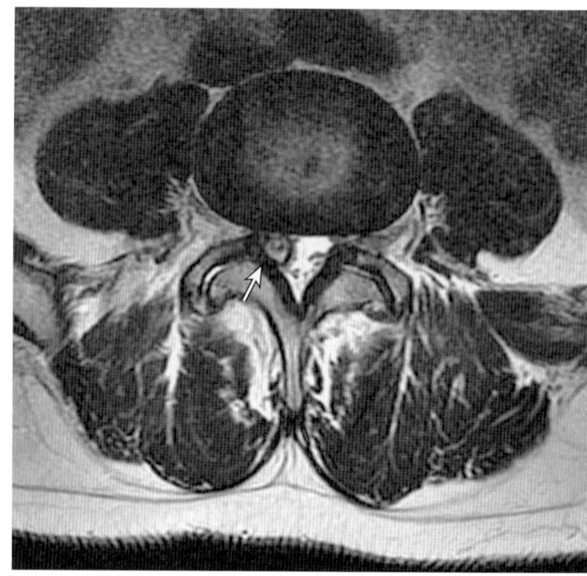

FIGURE 83-8. Axial T2-weighted MRI of the lumbar spine demonstrating a large synovial cyst at L4-5 on the right (*arrow*).

of disc space height, osteophyte formation, and possibly spondylolisthesis (Fig. 83-9). Flexion-extension films are used to assess the movement of the spine in sagittal plane rotation and AP translation, typically to evaluate for excessive translation. In the presence of a defect in the pars interarticularis, oblique radiographs demonstrate discontinuity of the pars (Fig. 83-10). In the presence of lumbar or thoracic spondylosis, attention should also be paid to the alignment of the spinal column as a whole, specifically regarding the presence of scoliosis, kyphosis, or any associated aberration of coronal or sagittal balance.

CT may also be a valuable adjunctive imaging modality in the presence of spondylosis. In patients with questionable bony anatomy, CT may help to define difficult or otherwise obscured anatomic relationships (Fig. 83-11). CT combined with myelography may be particularly helpful when metallic implants from prior surgical procedures obscure the relevant anatomy on MRI or when implanted medical devices prevent the safe acquisition of MRI. CT may also provide invaluable information about pedicle diameters and angles when the placement of spine instrumentation is under consideration. This is particularly important in the thoracic spine, where midthoracic and upper thoracic pedicles may be so small as to prohibit the safe placement of transpedicular instrumentation. It is likewise important in patients with known spondylolysis and spondylolisthesis, in whom CT may demonstrate very small pedicles at the affected level, especially if the listhesis is high grade and long-standing.

Treatment

The management of lumbar spondylosis must be individualized, as many patients have some combination of disc disease, facet hypertrophy, and ligamentum flavum hypertrophy, with

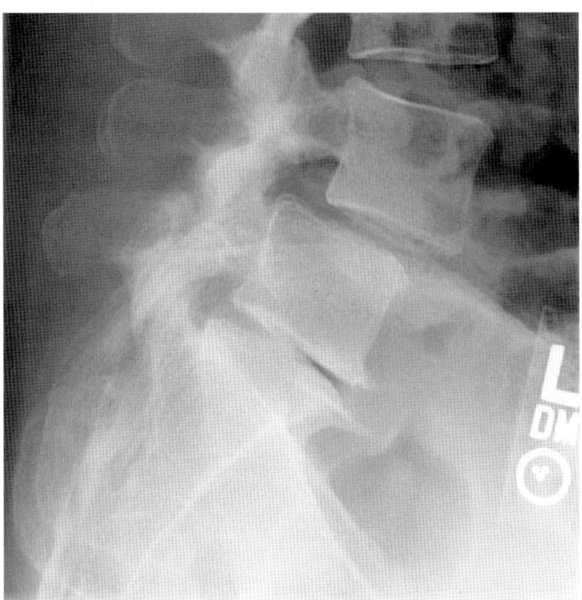

FIGURE 83-9. Lateral radiograph of the lumbar spine demonstrating a degenerative spondylolisthesis at L4-5 with disc degeneration at L5-S1.

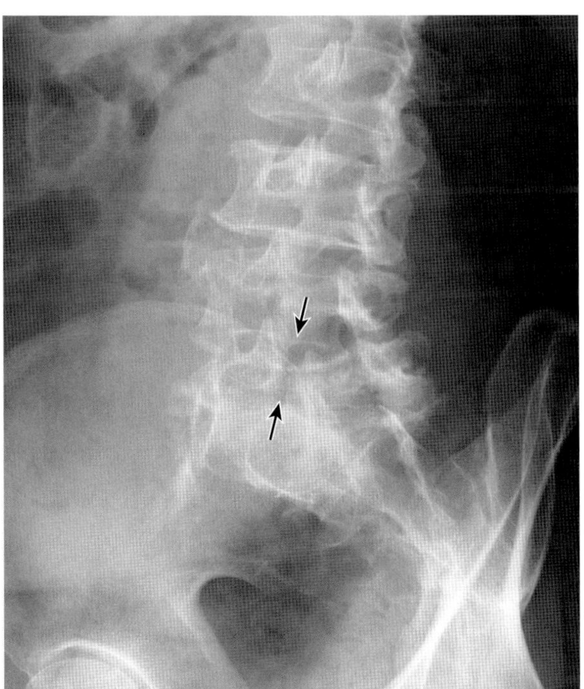

FIGURE 83-10. Oblique radiograph of the lumbar spine demonstrating a fracture of the pars interarticularis of L5 (*arrows*).

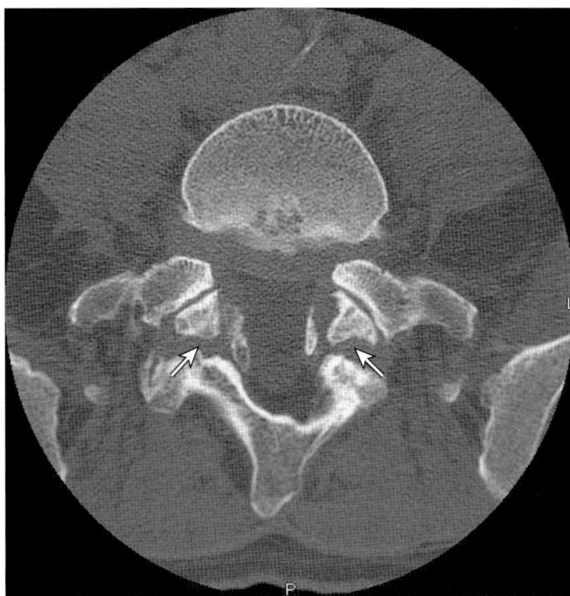

FIGURE 83-11. Axial CT of the lumbar spine demonstrating bilateral fractures of the pars interarticularis of L5 (*arrows*).

or without spondylolisthesis. In many instances, however, treatment may be based on the predominant pathology.

In patients with radiculopathy and minimal weakness from a lumbar disc herniation, a course of medical management including physical therapy, muscle relaxants, nonsteroidal anti-inflammatory medications, and neuropathic pain medication can provide relief. Some patients may obtain relief from epidural steroid injections as well, although data are conflicting and this therapy does not work as well for back pain.[14-16] Patients with acute intractable pain, cauda equina syndrome, or progressive neurologic deficit should be treated with surgery. Surgical treatment of disc herniation with radiculopathy has been the subject of much debate. The well-publicized Spine Patient Outcomes Research Trial was hailed as a definitive study demonstrating similar outcomes for surgical and nonsurgical treatment of lumbar disc herniation causing radiculopathy. However, statistical analysis did not account for crossover and other factors that decreased its validity and the weight of its findings.[17-19] Therefore, while the statistically robust intent to treat analysis showed no advantage of surgical treatment over nonsurgical treatment, the as-treated analysis showed a substantial advantage of surgical treatment over nonsurgical treatment.

In the case of lumbar spinal stenosis, oral agents have not been found to be effective in treating the typically present claudication symptoms, and insufficient evidence exists regarding physical therapy.[20] Epidural steroids may be of benefit for temporary relief.[20] Although the data are limited, patients who are treated nonsurgically with these measures may require surgery 20% to 40% of the time. Of those who do not require surgery, 50% to 70% can expect to have improvement in their pain symptoms with time.[20] Further study that was performed as a part of the aforementioned Spine Patient Outcomes Research Trial demonstrated an improvement in outcome for surgical treatment of symptomatic lumbar stenosis when compared to standard nonsurgical treatment.[21]

Regarding the management of lumbar spondylolisthesis with resultant stenosis, surgical treatment is indicated in patients with instability on flexion and extension radiographs or symptoms of stenosis that are recalcitrant to the previously mentioned nonsurgical treatments. Decompression with fusion with or without instrumentation is currently recommended.[22] The need to reduce the listhesis to normal alignment is not supported in the literature, provided that adequate decompression has been accomplished.[22]

The indications for fusion in patients with lumbar spondylosis in the absence of spondylolisthesis are less well defined. There is some class I evidence to support lumbar fusion in carefully selected patients who have failed conservative therapy, albeit with a moderate amount of benefit over conservative therapy alone.[23,24] There are also data to support the addition of transpedicular instrumentation to aid in fusion.[25] In general, the addition of fusion to simple discectomy should be considered for patients with instability or other structural anomaly or in recurrent herniations with chronic intractable back pain.[26] There are no convincing data to suggest that fusion in addition to decompression for lumbar stenosis conveys any benefit, except in cases of preoperative instability or spondylolisthesis.[27,28]

Consideration must also be given to the possibility of iatrogenic postlaminectomy instability that may be predicted prior to decompression. Postlaminectomy instability is a theoretical risk in all patients, but this risk is increased in patients with marked preoperative instability or deformity.[29,30] If the preoperative imaging suggests that wide (i.e., more than one third of the joint) facetectomy or concomitant laminectomy and discectomy are required for adequate decompression, consideration should be given to adding fusion supplemented with transpedicular instrumentation.[27]

Technique

While a detailed discussion of spine instrumentation techniques as an adjunct to decompression is beyond the scope of this chapter, this section describes the general techniques for spine decompression in the presence of spondylosis. The most important step in decompression of the lumbar spine, however, is the determination of surgical goals, specifically which nerve roots and levels are affected and what the surgical target will be.

Following induction of anesthesia, surgery begins with proper position of the patient in the prone position. Many surgeons prefer the Wilson (Mizuho OSI, Union City, CA) or similar frame when the goal of surgery is decompression, as the frame provides a degree of flexion that can open up the posterior elements of the spine and allow for safer dissection. Once the patient has been positioned, all pressure points must be assessed and appropriately padded. The arms are generally placed on arm boards and abducted no more than 90 degrees. At this point, particularly if the surgery involves only one segment or is a discectomy, many surgeons prefer to obtain radiographs to tailor the location of the incision. Antibiotics and deep venous prophylaxis are instituted prior to the skin incision, and local anesthetic may be injected prior to standard surgical prep.

After standard prepping and draping, an incision is made to the level of the thoracolumbar fascia, which is opened sharply or with electrocautery. A subperiosteal dissection is carried out of the appropriate spinous processes, laminae, and facet joints. For unilateral foraminal decompression or discectomy, unilateral exposure is usually sufficient, while bilateral exposure is usually required for other disease processes. For decompression alone, care is taken to preserve the facet joint capsules. If concurrent transverse process fusion is to be performed, exposure of the corresponding transverse processes is carried out. Attention should be paid to the location and orientation of the pars at each level.

After exposure, radiographic confirmation of the operative level is performed by using plain radiographs or fluoroscopy. It is imperative that an unambiguous and easily identified structure be used as a landmark. The pedicle or transverse process may serve this purpose. Usually, a lateral radiograph is used, though this may be supplemented by AP radiographs in the thoracic region. If an AP radiograph is used to identify a thoracic vertebral level, it is mandatory that the number of ribs be counted on a preoperative radiograph, as variations in the normal number are relatively frequent. Once this has been done, the remaining soft tissue in the area of interest should carefully be removed to expose the intralaminar space. It is here that the techniques for discectomy and laminectomy diverge.

In performing a discectomy, the rostral lamina at the level of interest is undermined by using a curette. This allows safe passage of rongeurs, which are used to accomplish a partial hemilaminotomy. In the case of unusually hard or thick bone, a drill may be used to thin the bone prior to the use of a rongeur. The laminotomy begins on the caudal surface of the more rostral lamina and should be continued to the rostral border of the ligamentum flavum. Care must be taken to avoid excessive thinning or transection of the pars interarticularis. The rongeur or a nerve hook can then be placed under the ligamentum and turned caudally in the epidural space to begin clearing the ligamentum flavum. This is continued until the rostral margin of the inferior lamina is encountered. Variable amounts of this lamina may need to be removed to achieve adequate exposure. More lateral exposure may be obtained by medial facetectomy. Up to one third of the medial portion of the facet may be removed with no increased theoretical risk to the stability of the joint. Removal of bone flush with the superior medial surface of the lower pedicle facilitates positive identification and mobilization of the crossing nerve root. Once the disc space has been identified, epidural veins are coagulated by using bipolar electrocautery. After the disc space has been opened, the herniated fragment can typically be removed with a pituitary rongeur. Calcified or adherent fragments may be delivered into the disc space by using specialized instruments. Care must be taken with the medial portion of the dissection, as a ventral durotomy may prove very difficult to repair. Blind dissection is to be avoided. After all fragments and easily obtainable disc pieces have been removed, the wound is copiously irrigated and closed.

For laminectomy, the exposure must demonstrate the medial facet joints, lamina, and pars interarticularis at each level. Generally, the procedure begins by removal of the spinous processes at each affected level and often the inferior aspect of the next most rostral spinous process, to facilitate exposure. It is typically easiest and safest to approach the target area from the caudal aspect, owing to the angle of the lamina. Ligamentous attachments are dissected free by using curettes to clear the epidural plane. Bony resection is carried out by using rongeurs until the laminae are removed in a caudal-to-rostral fashion. The lateral border of resection is defined by the facet joints and pars interarticularis. As in the discectomy approach described earlier in the chapter, the medial one third of the facet can be removed safely without effect on the biomechanics of the spine. Ligament and bone are removed until the thecal sac is relaxed and the lateral recesses are decompressed. Anatomically, lateral recess decompression includes resection of the medial superior facet process of the caudal vertebra at any given segment until the pedicle and lower exiting nerve root can be visualized. Each foramen should be probed to assess the degree of decompression, and further foraminal decompression should be done as indicated. This must be done with care, as the nerve root is susceptible to injury at this stage. It must also be remembered that complete facetectomy will result in at least the potential for resultant instability.

Expected Outcomes

Following lumbar discectomy, varying degrees of success have been reported. Resolution of both back pain and radicular pain was found in 62% of patients in one large study.[31] Overall satisfaction with the procedure ranges from 69% to 96%, the higher percentage being observed in a 5-year study.[31,32] Up to 3% to 5% of patients may have worsening of motor symptoms, and up to 12% to 15% may have worsening of sensory findings after discectomy.[33] Comparison of technical variations has also yielded conflicting data. While some authors have advocated the so-called sequestrectomy (removal of only the herniated fragment without curettage of the disc space), an analysis of the published literature from 1980 to 2007 showed varying results.[34-37] While patients who had undergone aggressive discectomy demonstrated a lower incidence of recurrent disc herniation than did those with less aggressive removal (3.5% vs. 7%, respectively), they also demonstrated an increase in recurrent back and leg pain (27.8% vs. 11.6%, respectively) when compared with patients who had undergone limited discectomy.[35] Some researchers have suggested that microdiscectomy through minimally invasive tubular systems may be less effective, but results in this study were measured at 1 year postoperatively.[32]

In patients for whom conservative therapy has failed, surgical decompression for lumbar stenosis can improve pain and claudication in up to 80% of cases.[20] Patients who are treated with decompression and fusion for lumbar stenosis with spondylolisthesis may experience relief in back and leg symptoms in up to 86% of cases.[38] Patients with solid fusion have also been shown to do better than those with pseudarthrosis, although this might not achieve true statistical significance.[39]

Outcomes after surgery for spondylosis and related conditions may be influenced by other factors. In general, patients with multilevel disease do worse than those with single-level disease. Patients with underlying mental illness or other psychological impairment might also not do as well, and in the case of psychological impairment, unrealistic expectations must be addressed. Patients with preoperative drug dependency may also have worse outcomes secondary to increased drug tolerance or modified pain responses.

Complications can also arise after surgical treatment for spondylosis. Standard surgical complications such as nonimprovement, bleeding, infection, durotomy, nerve root injury, and, in the case of fusion, nonunion all occur with a finite frequency. Medical complications may also occur. By far the most common complication, however, is incomplete symptom relief. All patients who are being treated with surgery for conditions that arise from spondylotic processes must be counseled that partial relief and failure to improve are possible. Irreversible presurgical damage may preclude complete recovery. In some cases, the purpose of surgery is to stop the progression of disease. Relief of pain or weakness to the premorbid state in patients with long-standing nonprogressive symptoms is in some cases an unrealistic goal.

The importance of identifying coexisting nonspinal conditions that may contribute to the patient's symptoms cannot be overstated. Underlying hip, knee, and vascular pathology may coexist with or even mimic the symptoms of thoracolumbar spondylosis. Peripheral nerve pathology, particularly peroneal nerve pathology, must be distinguished from radiculopathy. Finally, herpes zoster or postherpetic neuralgia may be mistaken for radiculopathy, especially in the thoracic region and especially in the absence of active skin lesions.

Conclusion

Thoracolumbar spondylosis is essentially a disease of repetitive trauma combined with aging effects on the human spine. It is a common condition with a variety of symptoms that may present a nonlinear decision tree with regard to treatment. For much of the treatment, there is a paucity of class I data, underscoring the importance of not only a careful history and physical examination but also a detailed discussion of surgical and nonsurgical options with the patient.

KEY REFERENCES

McCormick PC: The Spine Patient Outcomes Research Trial results for lumbar disc herniation: a critical review. *J Neurosurg Spine* 6(6):513–520, 2007.

McGirt MJ, Ambrossi GL, Datoo G, et al: Recurrent disc herniation and long-term back pain after primary lumbar discectomy: review of outcomes reported for limited versus aggressive disc removal. *Neurosurgery* 64(2):338–344, 2009; discussion 344–345.

Resnick DK, Choudhri TF, Dailey AT, et al: Guidelines for the performance of fusion procedures for degenerative disease of the lumbar spine. Part 9: fusion in patients with stenosis and spondylolisthesis. *J Neurosurg Spine* 2(6):679–685, 2005.

Watters WC 3rd, Baisden J, Gilbert TJ, et al: Degenerative lumbar spinal stenosis: an evidence-based clinical guideline for the diagnosis and treatment of degenerative lumbar spinal stenosis. *Spine J* 8(2):305–310, 2008.

Weinstein JN, Lurie JD, Tosteson TD, et al: Surgical vs nonoperative treatment for lumbar disk herniation: the Spine Patient Outcomes Research Trial (SPORT) observational cohort. *JAMA* 296(20):2451–2459, 2006.

Weinstein JN, Tosteson TD, Lurie JD, et al: Surgical vs nonoperative treatment for lumbar disk herniation: the Spine Patient Outcomes Research Trial (SPORT): a randomized trial. *JAMA* 296(20):2441–2450, 2006.

Weinstein JN, Tosteson TD, Lurie JD, et al: Surgical versus nonsurgical therapy for lumbar spinal stenosis. *N Engl J Med* 358(8):794–810, 2008.

REFERENCES

The complete reference list is available online at expertconsult.com.

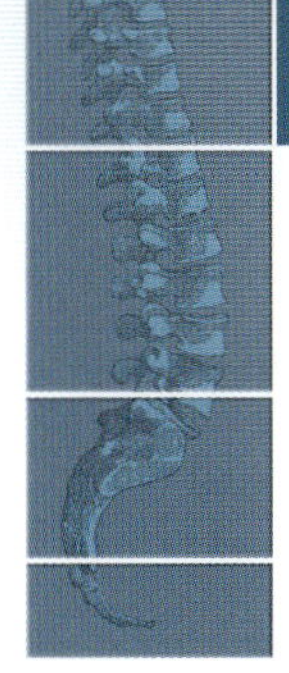

CHAPTER 84

Spondylolisthesis: Sagittal Plane Lumbar Spine Deformity Correction

Ferhan A. Asghar | Charles Kuntz IV

As its name suggests, spondylolisthesis is characterized by a slip in vertebral alignment. However, it is the associated sagittal imbalance that often carries more significance and may result in a symptomatic lumbar kyphosis.[1] This chapter focuses on spondylolisthesis as a condition of lumbar sagittal plane imbalance.

Etiology and Types of Spondylolisthesis

Biomechanically, the motion segment is stabilized by the presence of the intervertebral disc and facet joints. Disruption of this three-joint complex through anatomic variation, either congenital or acquired, results in malalignment. The lordotic lower lumbar spine is continually subjected to gravitational forces that pull the vertebral bodies ventrally.

Spondylolisthesis is also graded in severity from 1 to 5 according to the Meyerding system.[1] Grades 1 and 2 are termed low-grade, while the remainder are considered high-grade (Fig. 84-1).

Several classification systems have been developed, but Wiltse's classification from 1957 remains useful and focuses on the etiology of the slip[2] (Box 84-1). It focuses on the dorsal elements, which counteract the forces discussed previously. The most commonly encountered types are the isthmic and degenerative types, and discussion of these will occupy the bulk of this chapter.

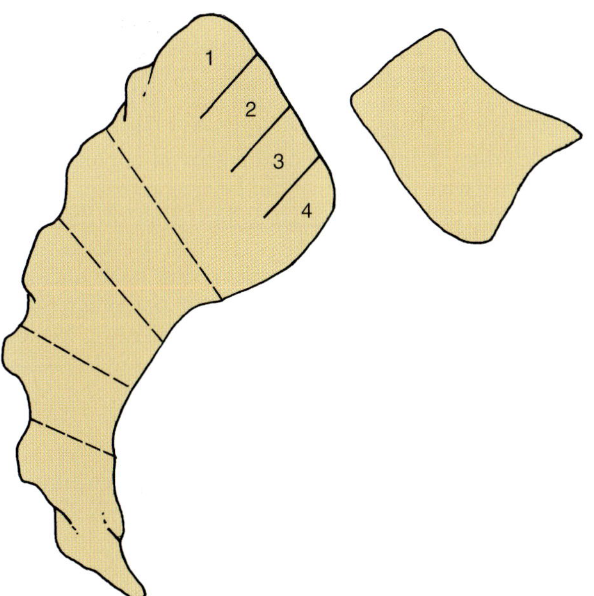

FIGURE 84-1. Meyerding grading system.

Congenital Spondylolisthesis

Congenital spondylolisthesis is more common in females, with a 2:1 ratio. This type is thought to account for 14% to 21% of all cases of spondylolisthesis.

A congenitally dysplastic dorsal arch, which includes the pars interarticularis and facet joints, allows for misalignment across a vertebral segment (Fig. 84-2). These defects are commonly seen at the L5 level (in a case of L5-S1 spondylolisthesis) but may include abnormalities of the sacral ala or superior articular facet.[3]

Three subtypes have been described. In Type A, the facets are horizontally oriented and therefore are unable to act as a buttress to prevent slippage. In Type B, the facets are asymmetrical and sagittally oriented. Type C cases involve other malformations that do not fit into the first two categories.

Neurologic symptoms may occur with relatively little displacement of the vertebral body if the dorsal arch is intact. This is because the arch becomes docked on the ventral vertebral body, compressing the cauda equina as a result. Cauda equina syndrome has been noted.

Isthmic Spondylolisthesis

Isthmic spondylolisthesis (IS) represents the most common form of spondylolisthesis (Fig. 84-3). In contrast to the

BOX 84-1. Wiltse Classification of Spondylolisthesis

- 1: Congenital
- 2: Isthmic
  - 2A: Stress fracture of pars
  - 2B: Elongated pars
  - 2C: Acute fracture of pars
- 3: Degenerative
- 4: Traumatic (involves fracture other than pars)
- 5: Pathologic
- 6: Iatrogenic

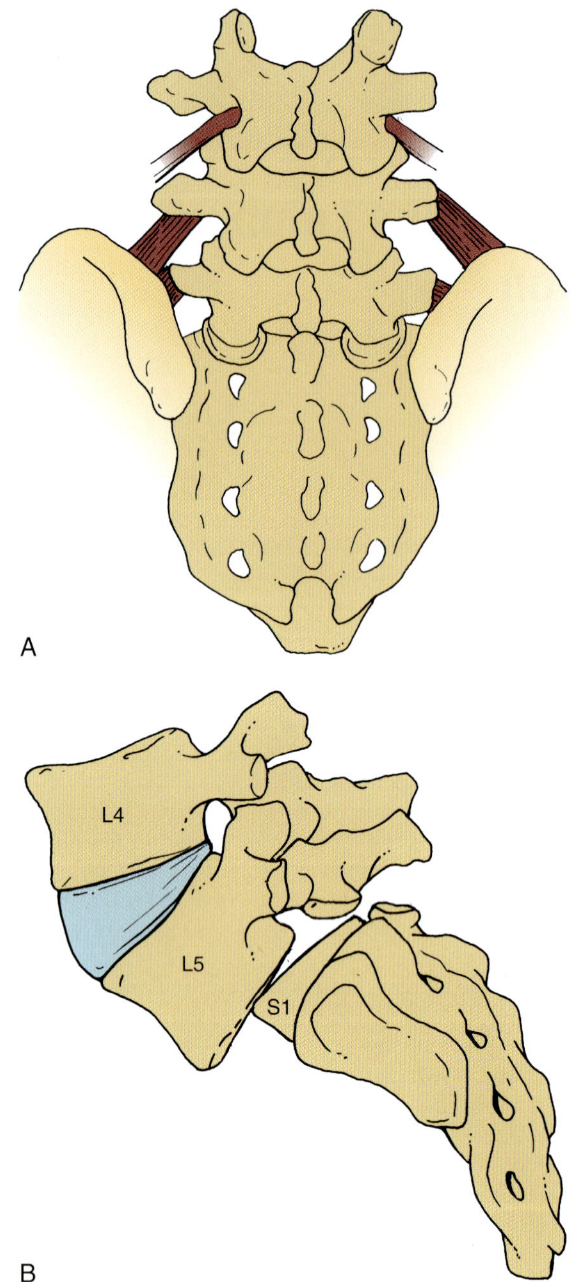

FIGURE 84-2. **A** and **B,** Congenital spondylolisthesis.

congenital form, it is more common in males. Therefore, when found in females, it tends to represent a more significant condition, with more severe symptoms and a higher rate of progression.

IS is most commonly seen at the L5-S1 level. Some consideration has been given to anatomic factors such as pelvic incidence[4-7] and lumbosacral transitional vertebrae.[8]

A modification of the Wiltse classification includes subgrouping of the isthmic category. Type 2A is the commonly seen lytic fatigue fracture of the pars interarticularis. Type 2B spondylolisthesis is seen in the case of an elongated pars, which may result from pars fracture with subsequent union in the distracted position. This should not be confused with a congenitally dysplastic pars. Type 2C is seen in an acute traumatic fracture of the pars.

There is a familial and genetic predisposition to IS. Relatives of IS patients have a 30% or more increased risk of having the disorder.[9-11] Inuit Eskimos have up to a 50% incidence of IS in their population, compared to 6% quoted for the general population and 2.8% in people of African descent.

While genetics plays a role, there is strong evidence for environmental factors in the development of IS. Factors that place increased force across the vertebral column, especially the lower lumbar spine, may result in fatigue fracture of the pars interarticularis, with resultant ventrolisthesis. The bipedal, erect gait of humans places greater stress across the lordotic lower lumbar spine than is seen in animals that have a quadruped gait. Activities that further accentuate the lordosis, such as hyperextension, exacerbate this picture. Therefore, adolescents who are involved in sports such as gymnastics, weight lifting, swimming, and diving have been known to display a higher incidence of symptomatic spondylolysis.[10-12]

Wiltse demonstrated that most cases of spondylolisthesis present before the end of the first decade. Fredrickson demonstrated a 6% incidence of spondylolisthesis in the general population.[10] Saraste noted earlier disc degeneration at the level of the slip, and risk factors for back pain included spondylolysis at the L4 level and greater than 25% slip.[11]

In Frederickson's 45-year follow-up study, only 5% of patients demonstrated progression. However, when the most symptomatic patients are followed, the incidence appears higher, at 20%. When progression occurs in the adult years, it usually results in no worse than a grade 2 slip.[10]

Risk factors associated with progression include skeletal immaturity associated with a high-grade slip. A high slip angle (>50 degrees) may predict progression.[5,13,14] The slip angle is measured between a line drawn along the superior end plate of L5 and the perpendicular to another line drawn along the dorsal vertebral border of S1 (Fig. 84-4). A high angle signifies kyphosis.

Most authors contend that progression of the slip after skeletal maturity occurs as a result of disc degeneration below the level of the slip. Patients may present early or late in life. During adolescence, symptoms relate to the pars fracture and include axial back pain with or without leg pain. In later adult life (after age 50 years), discogenic back pain and radicular leg pain related to worsening foraminal stenosis become a problem. Patients who present early in life are felt to represent a different group than the 6% of the general population with pars defects (who may or may not be symptomatic and have an incidence of back pain that follows that of the general population).[13]

While the pars fracture may or may not heal, once a slip has occurred, it is thought to persist, if not progress, with time. Only a single case report exists documenting spontaneous resolution of a slip in an adolescent patient.[15]

Degenerative Spondylolisthesis

Degeneration of the intervertebral disc and facet joints may lead to degenerative spondylolisthesis (DS). A degenerative disc has been shown to be less capable of resisting shear stress and can place additional stress on the facet joints.[16,17] Degeneration of the facets leads to their inability to guide normal intervertebral motion and maintain alignment. Facet

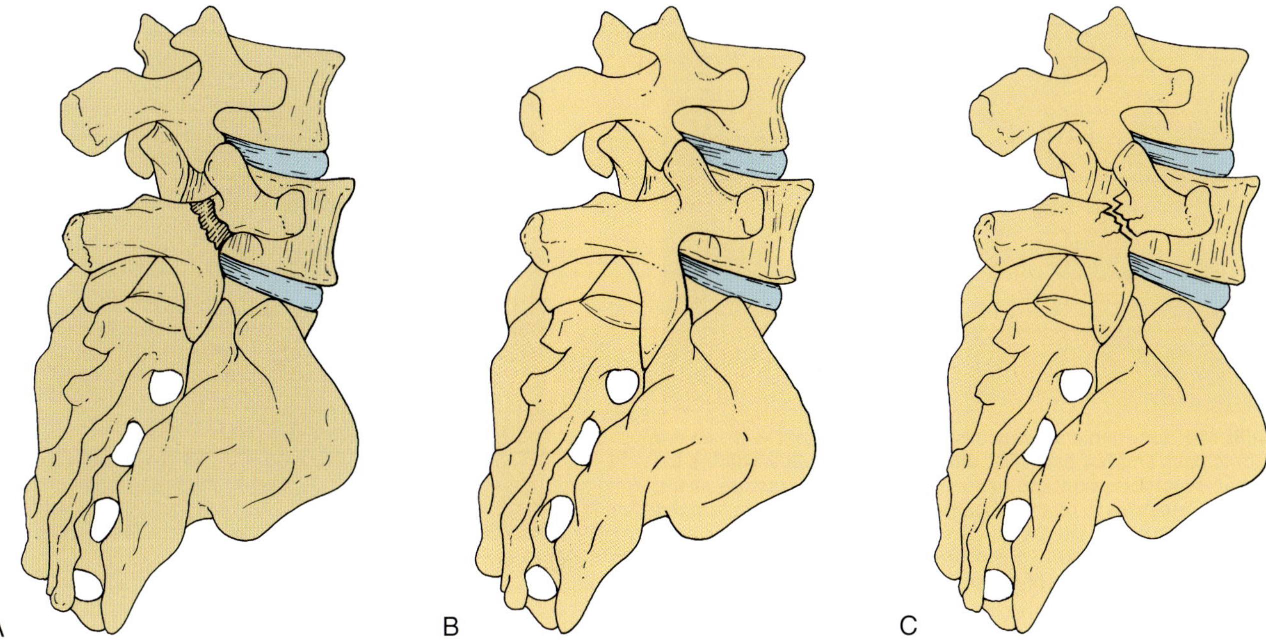

FIGURE 84-3. **A–C,** Isthmic spondylolisthesis.

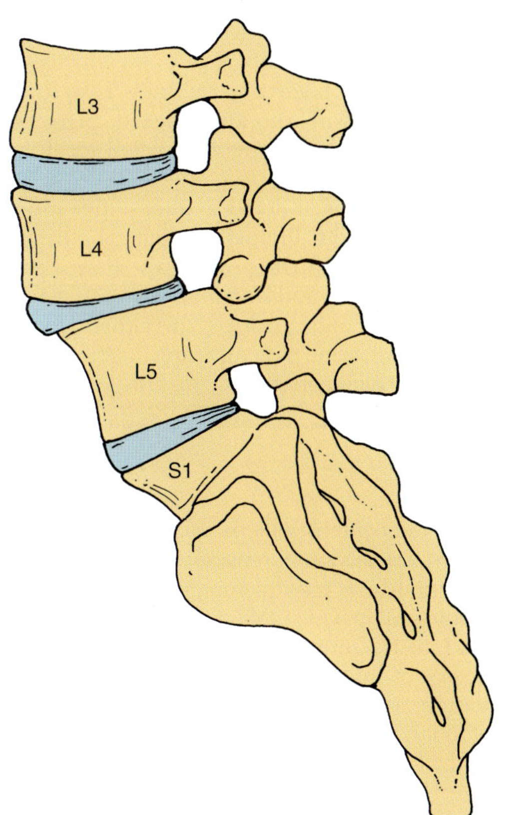

FIGURE 84-4. Horizontal or sagittal facet joint alignment predisposes to degenerative spondylolisthesis.

joint orientation in the sagittal plane predisposes the segment to misalignment (see Fig. 84-4). This is most commonly seen at the L4-5 level, and the presence of strong lumbopelvic ligaments across the L5-S1 interspace is felt to transfer stress to the L4-5 level, resulting in preferential involvement here.[18] Pelvic incidence may also play a role in the development of L4-5 DS.[19]

Traumatic Spondylolisthesis

While an acute fracture of the pars interarticularis would be classified as type 2C, a fracture of any other part of the vertebra (e.g., the pedicles) that results in spondylolisthesis would be classified as type IV.

Pathologic Spondylolisthesis

Tumors, whether primary or metastatic, may result in discontinuity of the vertebral body and dorsal elements via involvement of the pars, facets, or pedicles.

Iatrogenic Spondylolisthesis

An overly aggressive surgical decompression that does not respect the need for preservation of at least half the facet joint and 1 cm of the pars interarticularis places the patient at risk for iatrogenic intraoperative or postoperative fracture and spondylolisthesis (Fig. 84-5). This condition is poorly tolerated and almost uniformly involves revision surgery, which has a higher rate of complications.[20]

Presentation

Patients typically present with a complaint of back and leg pain. The pain is typically mechanical, positional, and activity-related. Leg pain may be radicular and dermatomal in nature or be associated with neurogenic claudication. Such claudication symptoms are seen in DS patients with central stenosis (Fig. 84-6) and include cramping bilateral buttock and thigh pain, "discomfort," or "fatigue." This improves with postural changes, including flexion and rest. Patients tend to

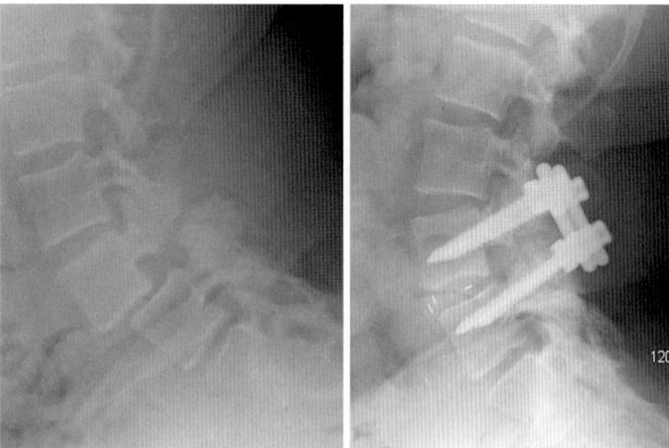

FIGURE 84-5. Iatrogenic spondylolisthesis in a patient with severe chronic back and leg pain who underwent multiple surgeries for lumbar decompression and fusion. Note the pars fracture at the cephalad-most level of the decompression (adjacent to a solid L5-S1 noninstrumented fusion). An interbody construct was chosen for anterior support, given the significant instability noted with complete reduction of the slip simply with prone positioning under anesthesia.

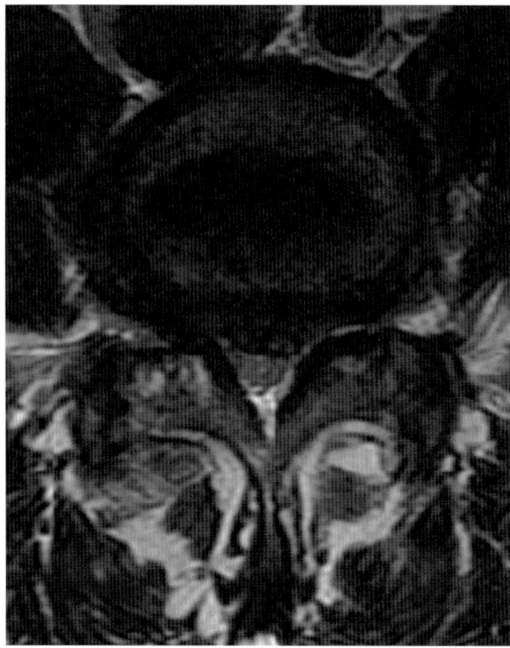

FIGURE 84-6. Stenosis pattern in degenerative spondylolisthesis (DS). Note the central, lateral recess and foraminal stenosis all present in this patient with L4-5 DS with stenosis. The facet joints show severe degenerative changes.

lean on a cart at the supermarket, on a bench at the park, or on furniture and countertops at home. They describe less difficulty going up hills (in a relatively flexed position) than down. They may also be able to ride a bicycle (again placing the lumbar spine in a flexed position) for far longer than they are able to walk. IS patients, on the other hand, commonly suffer from radicular symptoms related to foraminal stenosis (Fig. 84-7). "Pseudoradicular" leg pain has been described in IS patients who demonstrate more of a referred type of leg pain pattern that does not fit a specific dermatome.

On physical examination, IS patients may demonstrate hamstring tightness as the pelvis retroverts to compensate for

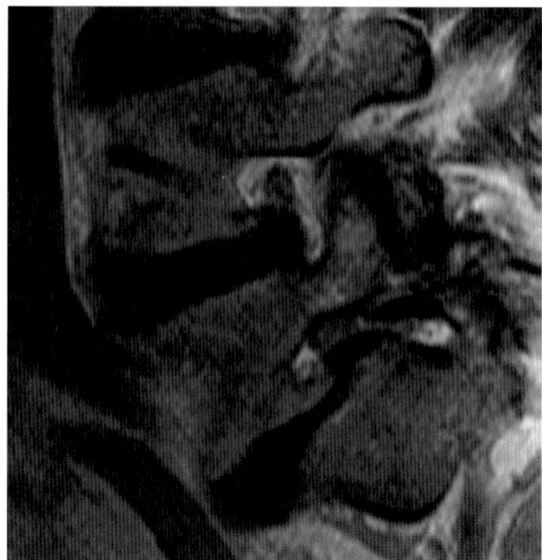

FIGURE 84-7. Foraminal stenosis in isthmic spondylolisthesis.

the lumbosacral kyphosis. As a result of this pelvic malalignment, patients develop flattening of the buttocks. A stepoff may be noted above the LS junction, followed by a proximal compensatory hyperlordosis. Hamstring tightness can result in a waddling gait, as the patient is unable to fully extend the hip to take a long stride. In severe cases, a crouched gait is seen, in which the hamstring tightness is so severe as to necessitate walking with the knees flexed. Signs of neurologic impairment, including numbness and focal weakness, can be seen.

DS patients have been noted to have a higher body mass index.[21] They are often limited in their mobility and may demonstrate difficulty in the physician's office when transitioning between sitting and standing, owing to development of proximal gluteal and quadriceps weakness. Extension is limited and painful, some patients being unable to stand erect during an acute exacerbation.

Imaging

Plain lateral radiographs will show a slip, and this may be more evident on flexion-extension radiographs in cases of dynamic instability. A pars fracture may be visible on anteroposterior or lateral images. Oblique radiographs show the pars en face, and the fracture can be seen as a collar on the "scotty dog." In cases of high-grade slips with compensatory pelvic verticalization, a "heart-shaped" pelvis is seen. Radiographs should be obtained in the upright position, as the slip may reduce in the supine position. Lateral radiographs should be obtained in the true lateral position, as even slight rotation may result in an underappreciation for the degree of slip.[22]

While patients with spondylolysis alone (without listhesis) do not demonstrate radiographic abnormalities in spine morphology, those with IS do have a high lordosis angle, L5 vertebral body wedging, and L4-5 disc wedging. In DS, spine morphology shows wedging of the L5 vertebral body but less wedging of intervertebral discs.[7,23-26]

Adolescents presenting with low back pain commonly have pars fractures that may or may not show on plain radiograph, or even on bone scan or MRI. Single-photon emission computed tomography (SPECT) scans have an increased sensitivity for detection of spondylolysis.[27]

Radiographic predictors of instability include spondylolisthesis, facet widening, end-plate degenerative changes, sagittal facet orientation, and facet sclerosis, widening of the facet being more associated with dynamic instability.[28-30] Lumbosacral transitional anatomy may be a contributor as well.[8]

CT scans can be helpful in showing a pars fracture. To the untrained eye, bilateral pars fractures may appear similar to facet joints. Axial images should be scrutinized carefully in the area of the pars and correlated with sagittally reconstructed images. Three-dimensional reconstructed images are beneficial in demonstrating pathology related to congenital malformations.

MRI scanning is considered for patients with complaints of leg pain or those who are to undergo surgical intervention. Neural compression can be detected in this manner, as can synovial cysts and facet joint effusions, which have a correlation with spondylolisthesis.[28-31] Symptoms can be correlated with degree of intervertebral disc degeneration associated with the spondylolisthesis.[16] In cases of pathologic spondylolisthesis, MRI assists the surgeon in delineation of an associated soft tissue mass and the extent of metastatic spread. The degree of slip cannot be assessed reliably on such scans, and some slips are missed secondary to spontaneous postural reduction in the supine position in the MRI scanner. Newer technology, allowing for functional MRI scans in the upright position, have on occasion detected greater pathology.[14,32]

Nonsurgical Treatment

Nonoperative management of IS patients includes observation with activity restriction and physical therapy for instruction in a flexion exercise program. Bracing with a soft corset, a hard clamshell lumbosacral orthosis, and formal casting have all been employed with success in adolescent patients with a "hot" spondylolysis (i.e., one that is active on bone scan, with physiologic potential for healing, whether fibrous or bony).[33-35]

In the skeletally immature patient, a low-grade slip should be observed with serial radiographs every 6 months until skeletal maturity.[36] Symptomatic patients should have activities restricted, and consideration may be given to bracing. Adolescent patients with high-grade slips or a high slip angle are at risk for progression and are offered surgery.

In DS cases, the first line of treatment includes judicious use of over-the-counter medications with food. The importance of a discussion with patients regarding gastrointestinal side effects of commonly used nonsteroidal anti-inflammatory agents cannot be overstated.

A formal regimen of exercises performed under the dutiful eye of a good physical therapist can be of tremendous benefit, not only in assuaging a patient's acute symptoms but also in training for proper "back hygiene." Patients receive instruction on how to avoid activities or injuries that would contribute to future episodes. Exercises focus on flexion, which limits forces across a painful spondylolysis or a painful facet and can increase neural canal and foraminal dimensions, resulting in improvement of radicular symptoms. Lumbar traction is of variable benefit and may provide a counter to associated muscle spasm.[37] Patients benefit most in acutely painful (<6 weeks) situations. Chiropractic care often employs modalities similar to those of physical therapy but may focus on passive interventions such as mobilization and manipulation, ultrasound, and electrical stimulation.[35,38]

Epidural steroid injections are of significant benefit to the patient with radicular leg pain, with the potential for significant symptomatic relief in an expedited fashion. A series of up to four injections in concert with other treatments can allow patients who would otherwise be considered surgical candidates to avoid surgery.[39]

While nonoperative treatment of DS is often helpful, it has been shown not to be as effective as surgery in the long term.[40] The symptoms associated with chronic conditions such as DS with stenosis do not respond to nonoperative treatment as well as do more acute conditions afflicting the spine, such as disc herniations.

Surgical Treatment

Indications

Indications for surgery include a progressive slip in a skeletally immature adolescent patient, unrelenting back or leg pain for which nonoperative treatment has failed, and progressive neurologic deficit. Patients with primarily leg pain rather than back pain are more likely to benefit from surgery.[41]

A number of surgical options exist, depending on the type of spondylolisthesis, the grade, and the clinical scenario pertaining to the individual patient.

Pars Repair

Adolescents who fail nonoperative treatment and have persistent symptoms from IS may benefit from direct pars repair.[42,43] Surgical candidates should possess a healthy intervertebral disc and have minimal, if any, slip.[16,44] A positive transient response to pars injection suggests that the pars is indeed the pain generator and assists in patient selection. The advantage of such a procedure lies in its ability to spare fusion of a motion segment.

Several technical variations exist for this procedure, ranging from wiring between the spinous and transverse processes to placing a pedicle screw-hook construct and applying compression across the pars fracture, where fibrous tissue is resected and bone graft material is placed over decorticated bone. Care should be taken to avoid injury to the cephalad facet joint during placement of instrumentation and to avoid prominence of implants, which would contribute to the adjacent-segment degeneration.

Decompression Alone

Studies have traditionally not differentiated between patients with dynamic instability as measured on flexion-extension radiographs, as opposed to those with stable slips that show no motion on such radiographs. Thus, comparison of studies is difficult.

Gill described a procedure resecting the mobile dorsal elements of L5 in cases of IS. Further decompression of residual hypertrophic pars and superior facet is required to decompress the L5 nerve root.

Initial studies have demonstrated a 25% to 50% postoperative progression of slips, especially in patients under the age of 30, with resultant poor outcomes[45,46] (Fig. 84-8).

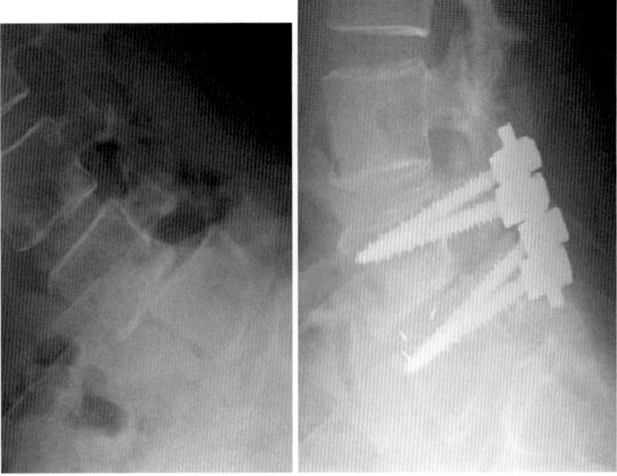

FIGURE 84-8. A 52-year-old female with grade 1 degenerative spondylolisthesis underwent unilateral laminotomy without fusion for unilateral leg pain. One year later, she underwent repeat surgery for leg pain on the contralateral side. Six months later, she had developed a grade 2 spondylolisthesis with unrelenting back and bilateral leg pain, requiring revision decompression, including complete facetectomy for foraminal decompression, and reduction with interbody fusion.

Recent attention to minimally invasive techniques has directed greater focus toward a unilateral approach to laminectomy or toward bilateral laminotomy, with preservation of midline structures as a treatment option for decompression of low-grade slips without dynamic instability.[47]

Fusion Alone

Fusion alone has been more commonly done in IS patients without symptoms of neurologic compression in whom a reduction is not attempted. A single-level L5-S1 instrumented fusion is performed for low-grade slips, and a two-level L4-S1 fusion is done in cases of high-grade slips, owing to difficulty in accessing the L5 transverse process through the slips. Carragee noted that the addition of a decompression to the fusion placed his patients at increased risk for pseudarthrosis and poor outcome.[48]

Decompression and Fusion

Decompression and fusion form the mainstay of surgical treatment for spondylolisthesis. However, the optimal technique for arthrodesis of a low-grade slip is open to individual surgeon preference, ranging from noninstrumented fusion to instrumented dorsolateral fusion to interbody fusion using dorsal-only or ventral-dorsal approaches.

Again, earlier studies showed that patients who underwent a concomitant fusion along with decompression had a lower rate of slip progression and better clinical outcomes. Herkowitz and Kurz published an often-cited early paper that showed improved outcomes in patients who underwent fusion.[46] In a follow-up study, Fischgrund then demonstrated that outcomes correlated with solid fusion and that the addition of instrumentation correlated with achievement of a solid fusion.[49] Multiple studies have similarly confirmed that addition of instrumentation results in improved fusion rates, and this has at times correlated with improved outcomes.[50-52]

Noninstrumented fusion, while beneficial from a short-term cost-analysis perspective, has fallen somewhat out of favor except for elderly or severely osteoporotic patients, who would benefit from shorter operative times and a potentially lower infection rate.[53]

Patients with over 2 mm of dynamic instability on flexion-extension radiographs are likely to have persistent symptoms when a noninstrumented fusion is performed.[54] Instrumented fusion began gaining favor as a technique for maintenance of reduction and achievement of a more robust fusion.[49,55]

A randomized study of patients with DS demonstrated superiority in outcomes for surgically treated patients.[55] While nonsurgical treatment is of benefit in many patients, it tends to be short-lived, and the degree of improvement lags behind that noted after surgery.

The specific approach to fusion, whether dorsolateral or interbody, is the subject of much debate. Various studies point to the superiority of one approach over the other, but the approach that is utilized for low-grade slips remains a matter of surgeon preference.[56-58]

Ventral Surgery

Surgeons have employed ventral stand-alone interbody fusion for cases of spondylolisthesis. However, the majority of data on ventral surgery relate to circumferentially treated patients who undergo dorsal instrumentation with or without formal dorsal supplementary fusion.[59,60] Sacral fractures have been noted that are thought to be secondary to a lack of dorsal tension-band support.[61] Ventral surgery serves primarily as an adjunct to dorsal surgery to enhance fusion and improve alignment.

Bohlman Technique

The Bohlman technique, as well as variations of it, has been employed in high-grade spondylolisthesis. A fibular graft is placed across the L5-S1 interspace from a dorsal approach (Fig. 84-9). Excellent outcomes have been reported with this stabilization technique when accompanied by instrumentation

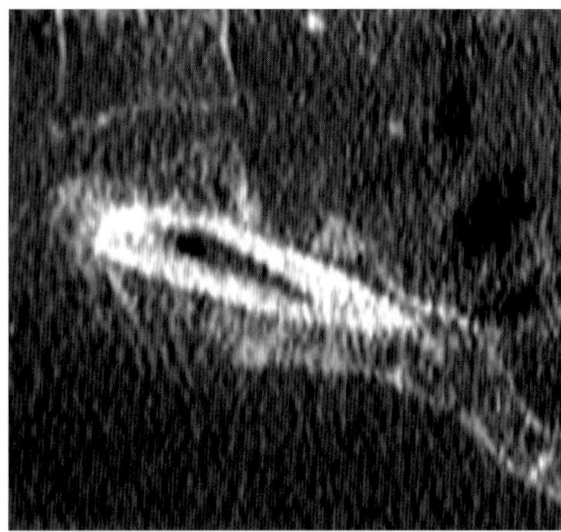

FIGURE 84-9. A fibular interbody graft was placed in this patient with a history of chronic L5-S1 discitis and osteomyelitis, who had developed a progressive grade 2 to 3 slip. Morbid obesity precluded an anterior approach, and extensive epidural phlegmon limited posterior access to the interbody space. Supplementary instrumentation was placed.

from L4 to S1, even without reduction of the slip. Some reduction in slip angle usually occurs with intraoperative prone positioning.[62]

Transsacral screws have also been employed with standard pedicle screw stabilization of L4, followed by screw placement from S1 across the L5-S1 disc space and into the L5 body. Results have been shown to be equivalent to those of a transforaminal lumbar interbody fusion with reduction of the slip.[63] This technique may be employed with or without fibular interbody strut grafting.[64,65]

Gaines Procedure

The Gaines procedure has been utilized in cases of spondyloptosis, or complete dislocation of the vertebrae (grade 5 slip). The L5 vertebra is resected from a ventral approach, thus shortening the spinal column, and the L4 vertebra is then docked onto the sacrum, locking it in place with dorsal instrumentation.[66] A modified Gaines procedure involves excision of the inferior half of the body of L5 ventrally combined with dorsal reduction and fusion.[67] A three-stage shortening procedure for high-grade slips has also been described.[68]

Controversies

Slip Reduction

Historically, high-grade slips have been treated with a reduction prior to stabilization and fusion. Attempts at reduction included the use of preoperative traction, but postreduction casting would not allow sufficient focal control over the subluxed vertebrae to allow for maintenance of correction.[3]

Reduction of a high-grade slip is beneficial in that it allows for a greater surface area of contact between vertebrae available for fusion. An interbody spacer may then be placed, allowing for anterior column support and unloading of stress placed on dorsal instrumentation, with potential for increased fusion rates[56] (Fig. 84-10). Reduction is also associated with greater cosmetic appeal and satisfaction.

Complete reduction has been associated with traction injury to the exiting nerve roots, typically resulting in L5 palsies, which can leave the patient with a devastating bilateral footdrop.

Decompression of the neural elements is essential before any attempt at reduction. Concern arises for traction- or compression-related injury to nerve roots, especially the exiting roots as the vertebral body is reduced dorsally toward the superior articular facet of the vertebra below. Instrumented fusion after decompression allows for visualization of nerve roots during the reduction procedure, and has a lower rate of neural injury, with good results.[49,54,69] Partial reduction of the slip, with a greater emphasis on reduction of the slip angle, may be safely performed (Fig. 84-11).

Recent attention has been drawn toward reduction of lower-grade slips rather than performance of an in situ fusion.

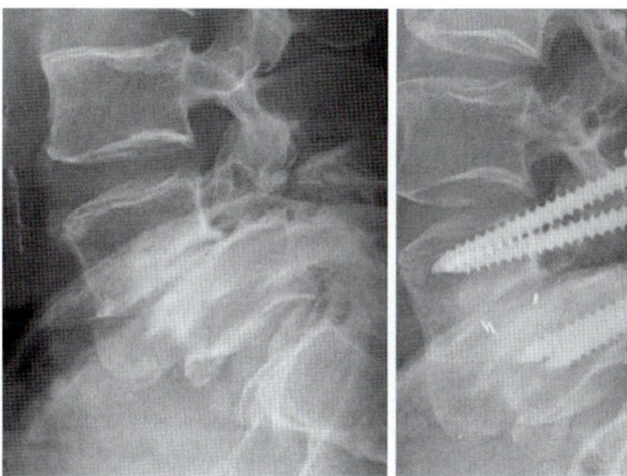

FIGURE 84-11. A 59-year-old with chronic, progressive low back pain and left leg pain presented with a grade 2 to 3 slip. Chosen treatment included decompression and instrumented transforaminal lumbar interbody fusion with partial reduction of the slip.

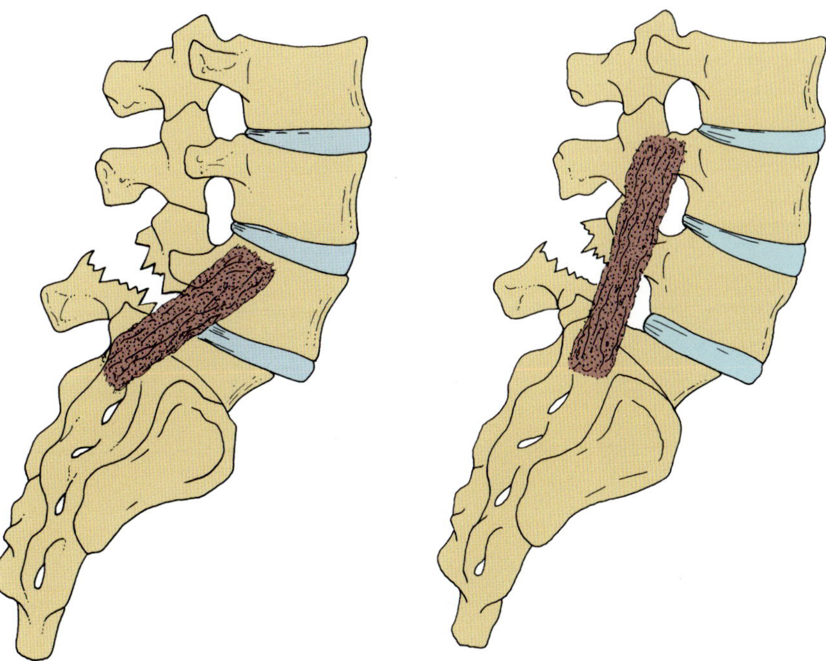

FIGURE 84-10. Reduction of a slip allows for placement of an interbody spacer and decreases stress on posterior instrumentation.

Newer instrumentation includes reduction screws and devices to gradually pull a screw in the slipped vertebral body back into reduction. Other techniques utilize postural reduction in the prone position (with extension of the hips following decompression and instrumentation) and in situ bending of rods.

Instrumentation

The addition of instrumentation to a fusion construct adds significant expense to an operation whose cost is already questioned in many circles. Its legitimacy arises from data that show an improved fusion rate with the use of instrumentation, which is felt to correlate with improved outcomes. Instrumentation is beneficial in achieving and maintaining reduction and in decreasing reliance on external bracing. However, a randomized trial evaluating instrumented fusions in IS patients has not shown improvement in clinical outcome.[48]

Approach: Ventral-Dorsal versus Dorsal Alone

The addition of an interbody fusion may be achieved through a separate ventral-dorsal approach or through a single-incision approach. Ventral approaches afford the opportunity for a more complete discectomy and placement of a larger graft or cage for fusion. Greater restoration of foraminal height and lordosis is possible. Thus, this is appealing in cases of high-grade slips. The lumbosacral junction is often approached with a ventral-dorsal surgery to maximize the fusion rate across this transitional segment. Some authors have found improved outcomes with a combined ventral-dorsal approach, regardless of level treated.[60] There is some evidence that ventral-dorsal fusion may be more cost-effective, as it may contribute to solid arthrodesis and a lower chance for reoperation.[70] For most low-grade slips in patients requiring single-level surgery, however, studies have shown no consistent benefit to the addition of an interbody fusion.[57]

A dorsal-ventral-dorsal approach has been utilized for decompression and sacral dome osteotomy, as well as ventral interbody fusion and reduction, followed by dorsal stabilization.

Short-term studies have evaluated the utility of various "new technologies" in the spine surgeon's armamentarium. These include dynamic stabilization devices such as interspinous distraction devices and pedicle-screw-based devices.[71-76] However, only a small percentage of traditionally treated patients qualify for these procedures, and long-term results are lacking.[71] Novel approaches to interbody fusion, such as the AxiaLIF (TranS1, Wilmington, NC)[77,78] and extreme lateral interbody fusion,[79,80] have been of utility in providing a minimally invasive approach to traditional fusion. Some authors have suggested that the indirect decompression that is achieved through such approaches is sufficient to address stenosis, yet revision surgery for formal decompression has been necessary in a number of cases.[81]

Complications

In an evaluation of over 10,000 surgical cases, the rate of total complications for treatment of DS and IS was 9.2%. The complication rate was higher in patients with high-grade spondylolisthesis, those with a diagnosis of DS, and older patients.[20]

Dural tear is higher in patients undergoing surgery for spondylolisthesis than in those undergoing surgery for other lumbar conditions.[82]

Rates of neural injury are higher in cases of complete reduction of a slip. If a reduction is attempted, the exiting nerve root should be decompressed completely along its length through the foramen. Nerve injury is thought to occur secondary to traction during final stages of a complete anatomic reduction, and recommendations have been made to focus on partial reduction of the slip with a greater focus on reduction of the slip angle and kyphotic deformity. Use of neurologic monitoring with EMG and motor-evoked potentials can help in detecting intraoperative nerve root injury.[69]

Progression of a slip may occur in cases of decompression without fusion. Even in cases of fusion, progression has been noted, especially in noninstrumented cases (in which a pseudarthrosis may be present). Loss of fixation may occur in instrumented cases secondary to osteoporosis in elderly patients (Fig. 84-12).

Pseudarthrosis rates are higher in cases of high-grade slips. A high slip angle (>50 degrees) and the addition of a decompression are risk factors as well.

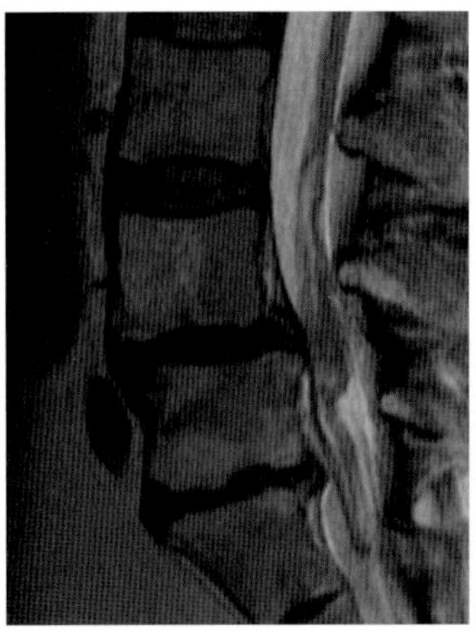

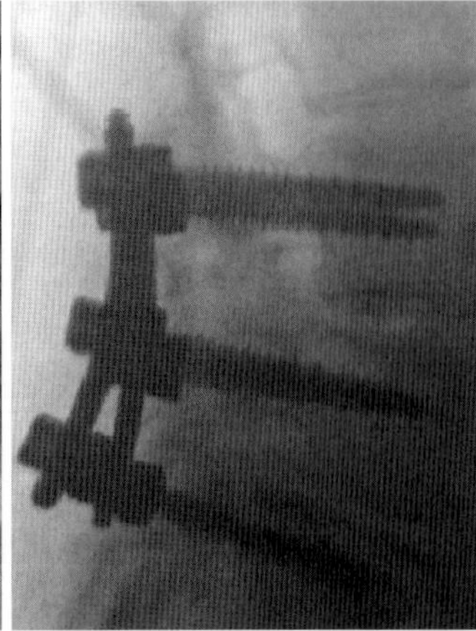

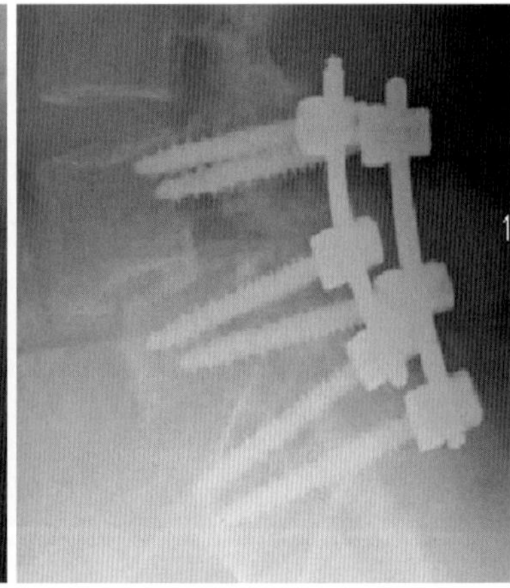

FIGURE 84-12. A 62-year-old female with previously undiagnosed osteoporosis underwent a wide decompression and instrumented posterolateral fusion. Three weeks postoperatively, loss of alignment was noted, with hardware failure, requiring revision anterior-posterior surgery.

Adjacent-segment degeneration may occur at a relatively lower rate in adult low-grade IS compared with other degenerative lumbar spine diseases. Segmental lordosis is significantly correlated with adjacent-segment degeneration, and restoration of normal lordosis may have a role in preventing adjacent-segment degeneration. While interbody fusions (whether performed ventral-dorsal or through a single incision) add to construct stability and in some cases to a higher fusion rate, they have been associated with an increased rate of adjacent-segment degeneration.[83]

DS is often encountered at the L4-5 level, and it is unclear whether an isolated L4-5 fusion ("floating fusion") adjacent to a degenerative L5-S1 segment is adequate or whether inclusion of the L5-S1 segment should be performed.[84]

Hardware failure is a potential complication in multilevel cases and in patients with osteoporosis. Interbody fusion cages are at risk for displacement and subsidence through osteoporotic vertebral end plates. Caution must be utilized in the use of implants in such patients. Care should also be taken to avoid an excessively wide decompression (in the absence of severe foraminal stenosis) that would further destabilize a segment, especially in the case of a spondylolisthesis across a tall and mobile disc space (see Fig. 84-12).

Conclusion

Spondylolisthesis results in focal kyphotic decompensation of the lumbar spine. Recognition and treatment of this sagittal imbalance, in addition to restoration of neural function and spine stability, can result in a high degree of patient satisfaction with surgery when nonoperative treatment fails to provide relief.

KEY REFERENCES

Ben-Galim P, Reitman CA: The distended facet sign: an indicator of position-dependent spinal stenosis and degenerative spondylolisthesis. *Spine J* 7(2):245–248, 2007.

Beutler WJ, Fredrickson BE, Murtland A, et al: The natural history of spondylolysis and spondylolisthesis: 45-year follow-up evaluation. *Spine (Phila Pa 1976)* 28(10):1027–1035, 2003; discussion 1035.

Gaines RW: L5 vertebrectomy for the surgical treatment of spondyloptosis: thirty cases in 25 years. *Spine (Phila Pa 1976)* 30(Suppl 6):S66–S70, 2005.

Fischgrund JS, Mackay M, Herkowitz HN, et al: Volvo Award winner in clinical studies. Degenerative lumbar spondylolisthesis with spinal stenosis: a prospective, randomized study comparing decompressive laminectomy and arthrodesis with and without spinal instrumentation. *Spine (Phila Pa 1976)* 22(24):2807–2812, 1997.

Weinstein JN, Lurie JD, Tosteson TD, et al: Surgical compared with nonoperative treatment for lumbar degenerative spondylolisthesis. Four-year results in the Spine Patient Outcomes Research Trial (SPORT) randomized and observational cohorts. *J Bone Joint Surg [Am]* 91(6):1295–1304, 2009.

REFERENCES

The complete reference list is available online at expert consult.com.

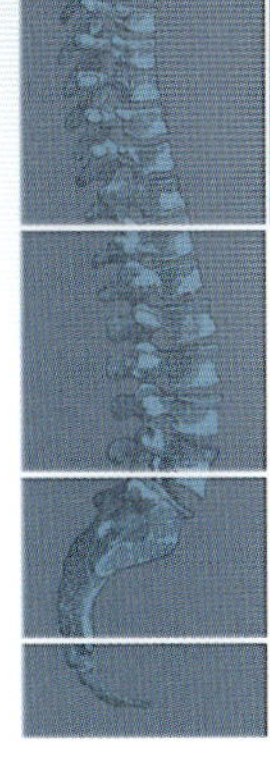

CHAPTER 85

Degenerative Rotatory Scoliosis: Three-Dimensional Thoracic and Lumbar Spine Deformity Correction

Russ P. Nockels | Edward C. Benzel

Degenerative scoliosis is the most common cause of adult scoliosis.[1] It develops de novo during adulthood and is largely due to asymmetrical disc degeneration; the resultant curve has even been referred to as a "discogenic curve."[1] Additionally, it may be related to osteoporosis and associated compression fractures. The apex of this curve is most often present at L2-3 or L3-4 and is usually limited to the lumbar or thoracolumbar regions. Its extent, as illustrated by imaging studies, does not necessarily correlate with symptoms or neurologic deficits, a fact that presents a significant dilemma to the treating physician. Management options are complicated by the wide variety of treatment choices.

When surgery is considered, its rationale must be clearly delineated and based on all possible important factors, including overall spinal balance, bone health, neurologic symptoms, and medical comorbidities. Surgery is indicated in lumbar degenerative rotatory scoliosis for one of three reasons: instability, neural compression, or spinal imbalance.

Instability can take many forms, ranging from mechanical low back pain to overt deformity progression or frank instability. Instability usually manifests through pain of a mechanical nature, pain that is deep and agonizing and is worsened by activity (loading) and improved by rest (unloading). Loss of integrity of the lumbar spinal motion segment to tolerate physiologic loads affects the spine in all planes, which explains the common finding of multiple pathologies presenting in a single patient. These deformities are coupled by the asymmetrical degeneration of the disc and may manifest as spondylolisthesis, oligolisthesis, and fixed sagittal imbalance in addition to the scoliosis.

The treatment for neural compression is often surgical decompression; the treatment for instability is joint immobilization; and the treatment for imbalance is correction. Surgery is a common option for the latter two. Neurogenic claudication (a neurologic syndrome) does not respond to spine fusion. Conversely, mechanical low back pain uncommonly responds to laminectomy. One must separate these clinical manifestations carefully so that surgical management can be specifically tailored to the patient's complaints and to the structural pathology.

As we age, our spines "loosen" somewhat until midlife. Then, at about the age of 55, the degenerative process begins to accelerate, and spinal stiffening occurs (i.e., spine restabilization). This stiffening process, although associated with spinal degeneration and spinal deformation, leads to a progressively more stable spine in most cases. Therefore, this scenario, which is the rule rather than the exception, should mandate a surgically conservative approach in the majority of patients. For example, even with significant spine deformation, a patient with neurogenic claudication may be best managed by a carefully performed decompression procedure, not a radical decompression, deformity correction, fusion, and instrumentation procedure.

Finally, methods of deformity correction and maintenance are described in this chapter. Adjuncts to this aspect of the management of degenerative rotatory scoliosis—such as ventral "release" procedures or orthotic management—are not. In the clinical scenarios presented in this chapter, it is assumed that the patient has a symptomatic and mechanically unstable spine deformity and that adjuncts to the surgical scheme under discussion have been undertaken when appropriate.

Pathophysiology of Disc Degeneration and the Spondylotic Process

Lumbar spondylosis is not a pathologic process; it is but a manifestation of the wear and tear associated with aging, specifically the consequences of loading. It is defined as vertebral osteophytosis secondary to degenerative disc disease[2] and is not an inflammatory process. Noninfectious inflammatory processes are grouped together as arthritides and are excluded from this discussion.

Spondylosis and associated osteophytosis are universally accompanied by degeneration of the intervertebral disc. The intervertebral disc is an amphiarthrodial joint (no synovial membrane) with particular traits that result in a characteristic degeneration pattern. Conversely, arthritides classically involve the synovial membranes of diarthrodial joints (joints lined with synovium and lubricated with synovial fluid, such as facet joints). Facet joints, however, are also affected by the spondylotic process.[3,4]

The degenerative process primarily involves the disc interspace and alters intradiscal dynamics that result in spine deformation. The resultant excessive motion and stresses cause extradiscal soft tissue proliferation. Finally, spine deformation predisposes to further deformation (see the section titled "Osteoporosis"). Osteoporosis contributes to the latter process, with a resultant asymmetrical vertebral body collapse.

Intradiscal Dynamics

Chronically elevated intradiscal pressure causes disc interspace narrowing (collapse), distorting the anulus fibrosus and the facet joint capsule. This in turn accelerates the degenerative process. If disc space degeneration progresses asymmetrically in the coronal plane, a scoliotic deformity may result.

The water content of the disc interspace gradually decreases throughout life, which contributes to alterations in the chemical and anatomic makeup of the disc. Fibroblasts become defective, and the desiccated disc is less effective as a cushion. Fissures then develop in the cartilaginous end plates. Schmorl nodes are manifestations of this pathologic process. Gas may accumulate in the disc (the vacuum phenomenon). An ingrowth of fibrocartilage (mucoid degeneration) with obliteration of the nucleus fibrosus ensues. Relative incompetence of the disc itself and relative instability result, and anulus fibrosus bulging and tension occur as a result of this process.[3]

Disc Deformation

Bulging of the anulus fibrosus results in periosteal elevation and subperiosteal bone formation. Spondylotic ridges (osteophytes) are laid down, and this can result in spinal canal encroachment. These ridges occur most commonly on the concave side of a curvature. Therefore, natural cervical and lumbar lordosis predisposes the spine to osteophyte formation toward the spinal canal, causing spinal canal encroachment. The thoracic region, by virtue of its intrinsic kyphotic posture, is relatively spared this process.

Form follows function, even during the process of degeneration. Therefore, osteophyte formation occurs predominantly on the concave side of a scoliotic curvature (where anulus fibrosus bulging is most significant), while disc herniation occurs commonly on the convex side of a spinal bend. The thin dorsal anulus fibrosus and relatively weak lateral aspect of the posterior longitudinal ligament combine with the migratory tendencies of the nucleus pulposus to encourage dorsolateral disc herniation.[3]

In the laboratory, (1) flexion (causing dorsal nucleus pulposus migration), (2) lateral bending away from the side of disc herniation (causing lateral nucleus pulposus migration), and (3) application of an axial load (causing an increase in intradiscal pressure) are required for the creation of a herniated lumbar disc. A degenerated disc is also necessary as a predisposing factor.[5] This complex loading pattern results in the application of tension on the weakest portion of the anulus fibrosus (the dorsolateral position, the location of the herniation), migration of the nucleus pulposus toward this position, and an asymmetrical increase in intradiscal pressure. The age-related increased frequency of anulus fibrosus tears and a peaking of nucleus fibrosus pressures in people 35 to 55 years of age[4] also predispose to an increased incidence of disc herniation. Asymmetrical collapse of the disc interspace is often a result of the disc degeneration process and places asymmetrical focal stresses on portions of the spine.

Extradiscal Soft Tissue Involvement

Hypertrophy and buckling of the ligamentum flavum, as well as other soft tissue proliferative processes, can result in spinal canal encroachment. Excessive pathologic segmental motion predisposes to this process and is a major factor related to the development of spinal stenosis.

Osteoporosis

Osteoporosis leads to a decrease in bony integrity, and this in turn leads to vertebral body collapse. The presence of thoracic kyphosis predisposes the thoracic spine to ventral vertebral body collapse, whereas asymmetrical disc interspace collapse (which is commonly associated with degenerative disc disease) predisposes to lateral vertebral body collapse. As the overall coronal and sagittal spinal balance worsens, the load shifts to more lateral and ventral supporting elements of the spine, respectively. This dislocation is progressive, subjecting the spine to longer and longer moment arms. Therefore, deformity begets deformity (deformity progression), creating a "vicious cycle" that perpetuates the process. Patients will often seek medical attention when the compensatory spondylotic processes have narrowed the neural canal or the spine has become so immobile that the patient can no longer compensate for the spinal imbalance.

Spinal Configuration

All aspects of spinal configuration should be considered carefully before determination of the surgical approach (which includes application of a spinal implant) for a spine disorder. The thoracic and lumbar regions are affected differently in this regard. Thoracic disc interspace height loss occurs predominantly in the ventral aspect of the disc. This loss results in progression of the natural kyphotic deformity as the degenerative process ensues, thus exaggerating propensities for deformity progression. The rib cage, however, substantially stabilizes the thoracic spine.

The coupling phenomenon (whereby one movement of the spine about or along an axis obligates another movement about or along another axis)[3] plays a significant role in the development of degenerative spine deformations in the lumbar region (whereas it is of minimal significance regarding degenerative deformities in the thoracic region). This is because thoracic degenerative deformities are often oriented in the sagittal plane, whereas degenerative lumbar deformities are usually oriented in the coronal plane (excluding degenerative lumbar spondylolisthesis). The absence of uncovertebral joints (in contrast to the cervical region) and the sagittal orientation of the facet joints (in contrast to the cervical and thoracic regions) create a situation that causes obligatory rotation of the spine in response to lateral bending (coupling) and, commonly, a loss of normal lumbar lordosis. The progression of lateral bending deformities in the lumbar spine (scoliosis) thus predisposes to rotation of the spine (Fig. 85-1), and the influence of an

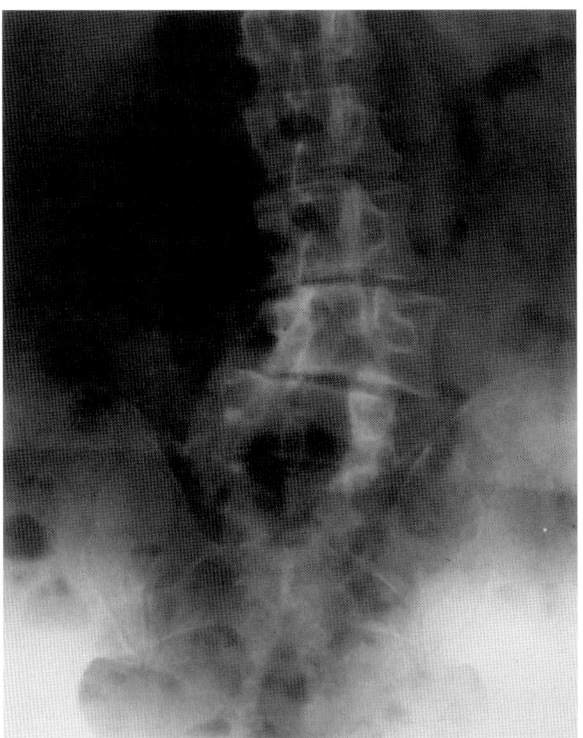

FIGURE 85-1. Radiograph of the lumbar spine of a patient with degenerative rotatory scoliosis. This illustrates that, via the coupling phenomenon, the scoliosis is obligatorily associated with a rotatory deformation of the spine. Note that the spinous processes are rotated toward the concave side of the curvature, in contradistinction to the situation in the cervical spine, in which the coupling phenomenon results in an obligatory rotation of the spinous processes toward the convex side of the curvature.

uncompensated thoracic kyphosis predisposes the lumbar spine to greater "flattening" or loss of the normal lordotic curve.

Not all scoliotic curves are symptomatic, as patients may be able to compensate for these deformities by "rebalancing" the spine through other skeletal structures, such as pelvic tilt. When curve progression can no longer be compensated, the subsequent displacement of the load causes worsening of curve that caused it in the first place. Therefore, lateral bending deformation predisposes to lateral bending deformity progression in the lumbar spine, as the presence of kyphotic deformation predisposes to the progression of kyphotic deformation in the thoracic spine. An asymmetrical loss of height of the lumbar intervertebral disc may progress to an asymmetrical collapse of the vertebral body, as described previously in this chapter. As this scoliotic deformity progresses, it is obligatorily associated with rotation of the spine, with the spinous processes rotating toward the concave side of the curve (coupling).[3] Of note is that because of the aforementioned osteophyte development propensities, osteophytes occur predominantly on the concave side of the curvature.

The obligatory association of rotation and loss of lordosis with lateral bending (coupling) complicates lumbar corrective and spinal instrumentation surgery. Transverse process exposure and dissection can cause injury to underlying nerve roots because of the relative dorsal migration of the root with respect to the transverse processes. Neuroforamina are considerably smaller on the concavity, and the neural structures within the spinal canal will naturally "hug" the lateral wall of the concave curve. This heightens the risk of neurologic injury during placement of instrumentation along the concavity. Therefore, care must be taken both during surgical exposure of the lumbar transverse processes and during placement of spinal instrumentation and subsequent correction.

Operative Treatment

The operative treatment of scoliosis is reserved for patients with refractory pain due to the scoliosis curve, significant curve progression, gait disturbance, and neurologic deficit all leading to a significant limitation of activities of daily living.[6,7] Preoperative preparation should include adequate imaging, as was already mentioned.

Any patient being considered for surgery not should only get detailed radiographic spine imaging but may also need a variety of complementary studies. A dual-energy x-ray absorptiometry scan can provide useful information about bone quality that may affect surgical planning. Patients with suspected pulmonary compromise should be sent for pulmonary function testing, although pulmonary compromise is rare in patients with curves less than 80 degrees.[8] Medical and cardiac risk stratification should be obtained for anyone with a significant medical history. It should be noted that occult cardiac disease can be seen in adult scoliotic patients owing to severe deconditioning and the patient's inability to experience exercise-related stress. Smoking cessation should be pursued, and a general rule of thumb is that elective surgery for deformity correction be offered to patients only after they have quit smoking.

The current approach to the surgical treatment of scoliosis is primarily pedicle screw and rod instrumentation. A recent report comparing hook-rod constructs and pedicle screw-rod constructs found that no pedicle screw patient required revision surgery for instrumentation-related complications and, overall, pedicle screw patients were 89% less likely to require revision surgery.[9] These patients were also found to have better curve correction and maintenance of thoracic kyphosis, and pedicle screw-rod constructs often negated the need for ventral release surgery.[10] However, hooks remain a valuable alternative when pedicle screws are contraindicated.

Goals of surgical correction of scoliosis are correction of coronal and sagittal balance to decrease pain, to decompress the neurologic elements, to correct balance so as to improve function, and to provide cosmesis.[11]

Deformity Correction

A variety of techniques can be used to correct lumbar spine deformities. Deformity correction is accomplished via the application of rotatory or translational forces to the spine along one or a combination of the three axes of the Cartesian coordinate system.[3] It is tempting to use distraction to reduce compression and translational deformations, but this maneuver in the lumbar spine invariably introduces a kyphotic force that can be very injurious to the patient's sagittal balance. Compression is preferable because of its favorable effects on sagittal contour, and is especially useful when combined with interbody devices. Similarly, three- or four-point bending forces can be applied. Finally, bending moments can be applied in either the coronal or sagittal plane to correct spinal curvatures. Complex bending moment forces are often applied.

Methods of deformity reduction and deformity reduction maintenance are discussed in this chapter. When indicated, ventral release procedures can provide the "relaxation" necessary to achieve the desired reduction. There is a growing sense that relatively minor curves in the well-balanced patient may be corrected through ventrolaterally placed interbody devices. Excessive deformity reduction for degenerative lumbar rotatory scoliosis is seldom necessary. Alleviation of symptoms (both for the short and the long term), not necessarily the attainment of a perfectly reduced spine deformity, is the goal of any surgical management scheme. Additionally, except for the presence of the surgical implant and minor residual curve, the spine should appear relatively normal and well balanced in both the coronal and sagittal planes.

Distraction and Compression

Distraction can be applied to the spine to reduce coronal and sagittal plane deformations. Ligamentous or other soft tissue integrity is mandatory for this type of force application to be effective in these circumstances. Distraction via this ligamentotaxis mechanism can be effective as an isolated mechanism of deformity correction.

Distraction force application on the concave side of the curve and compression force application on the convex side of the curve can be used to correct coronal plane deformities. This force couple[3] applies a coronal plane bending moment.

Three- and Four-Point Bending Fixation

Three- and four-point bending of the spine, as defined by White and Panjabi,[12] involves the loading of a long structure (i.e., the spine) with one or two transverse forces on one side and two on the other.[12] In a four-point bending construct, the bending moment is constant between the two intermediate points of force application if all forces are equal. In a three-point bending construct, the bending moment peaks at the intermediate point of force application.

The crossed-rod technique is a complex variant of three- or four-point bending fixation. It is a traditional and common method of thoracic and lumbar kyphotic deformity correction and was first used with Harrington distraction rods. Subsequently, it involved the Luque multisegmental sublaminar wiring technique.[13] Most recently, it has been employed with sequential pedicle screw fixation with universal spinal instrumentation constructs.[14] Regardless of the specific method used, the crossed-rod technique involves sequential and gradual application of kyphosis reduction forces to the spine via moment arms through longitudinal members.

Applied Moment Arm Cantilever Beam Force Application

Applied moment arm cantilever beam constructs are most appropriate in situations in which short-segment constructs are particularly desirable.[3] This type of construct mandates that a significant force be applied by the implant to the spine. Although this type of construct is most often applied for sagittal plane deformities, it can also be used (although uncommonly) for coronal plane deformity correction.

These are constructs that are frequently applied as either flexion or extension bending moments via pedicle screws.[15] They can be used with distraction, compression, or coronal plane bending moment force application and can also be applied with an accompanying ventral dural sac decompression and interbody bone graft placement. Furthermore, they can be applied so that deformity is reduced and compression of the bone graft is achieved. This technique of (1) sequential application of distraction (load bearing), (2) decompression of the dural sac, (3) interbody fusion placement, and (4) compression of the construct to share the load with the ventral spinal elements is termed load-bearing to load-sharing force application. It provides biomechanical advantages (load sharing) as well as clinical advantages.[3]

Short-Segment Parallelogram Deformity Reduction

Short-segment parallelogram deformity reduction is a rigid cantilever beam pedicle fixation technique that applies bending moments for the reduction of lateral translational deformations.[3] This technique is most useful when short-segment fixation is deemed optimal. It involves (1) placement of pedicle screws, (2) appropriate dural sac decompression, (3) attachment of the longitudinal members to the screws (rods), (4) application of a rotatory and distraction force to the rods, (5) maintenance of the achieved spine reduction via rigid cross-fixation, (6) placement of a fusion (interbody and/or lateral), and, finally, (7) compression of the screws so that load sharing is achieved and the interbody bone graft is secured in its acceptance bed.[3] It applies load-bearing to load-sharing forces (Fig. 85-2).

In Vivo Implant Contouring

Segmental relationships can be altered by rod contouring. Employment of in vivo implant contouring for segmental relationship alteration is an effective method of deformity reduction. A multisegmental fixation system can be inserted in such a manner that it conforms to a spine deformity, such as scoliosis. After insertion, rod contouring can be used to "straighten" the spine. Adequate implant-bone juncture security is mandatory. Implant contouring alters the forces applied by the implant to the spine at each segmental level. Typically, this method is used to fine-tune a scoliotic repair to correct for several important hazards. Hooks can overtighten or loosen, infringe on the spinal canal, or migrate laterally or medially.[3] The screw-bone interface is also exposed to significant forces and may loosen. Additionally, the application of significant force through bulky in situ rod benders in close proximity to the spinal canal risks direct trauma to the spinal cord or cauda equina.

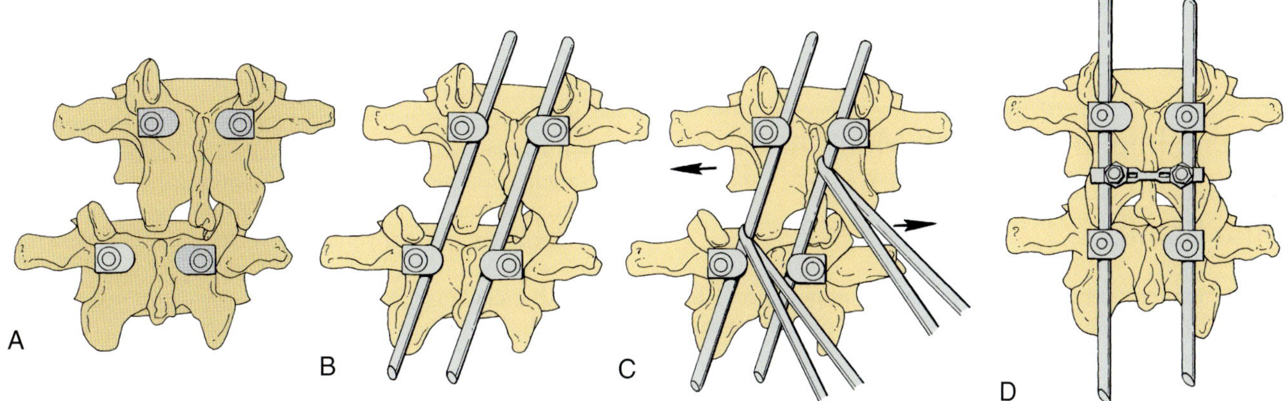

FIGURE 85-2. Short-segment parallelogram deformity reduction. **A,** Lateral translational deformity is reduced by first inserting pedicle screws into each of the pedicles. **B,** Next, rods are attached to each of the screws. **C,** Bending moments are then simultaneously applied to each of the rods by rod grippers. **D,** A rigid cross-member is then used for deformity reduction maintenance and stability augmentation purposes.

Intrinsic Implant Bending Moment Application about the Long Axis of the Spine: The Derotation Maneuver

An obligatory rotatory component coexists with scoliotic deformities (coupling). This phenomenon can be used to an advantage by applying the spine derotation maneuver. Spinal derotation involves conversion of a scoliotic curvature to a kyphotic curvature.[16] The resultant kyphotic curvature can be reduced, if appropriate, via rod contouring. The derotation maneuver is accomplished by first inserting the rods via hooks, screws, or wires, which are relatively loosely attached to the rod (with friction-glide tightness), so that rotation of the rod can occur at its juncture with the hooks, screws, or wires. The attachment should not be so tight as to allow dislodgement (friction-glide tight or "just right tight" is preferable). This allows the hooks, screws, or wires to maintain their relationship with the spinal attachment site. The rods are then simultaneously rotated 90 degrees, which converts a scoliotic deformity to a kyphotic deformity. The rods can be contoured to eliminate an excessive kyphotic curvature. The junctures are then tightened and secured, and cross-fixation is employed to maintain the reduction (Fig. 85-3A).

These maneuvers should be used in a gradual manner so that continuous assessment and reassessment of the implant-spine

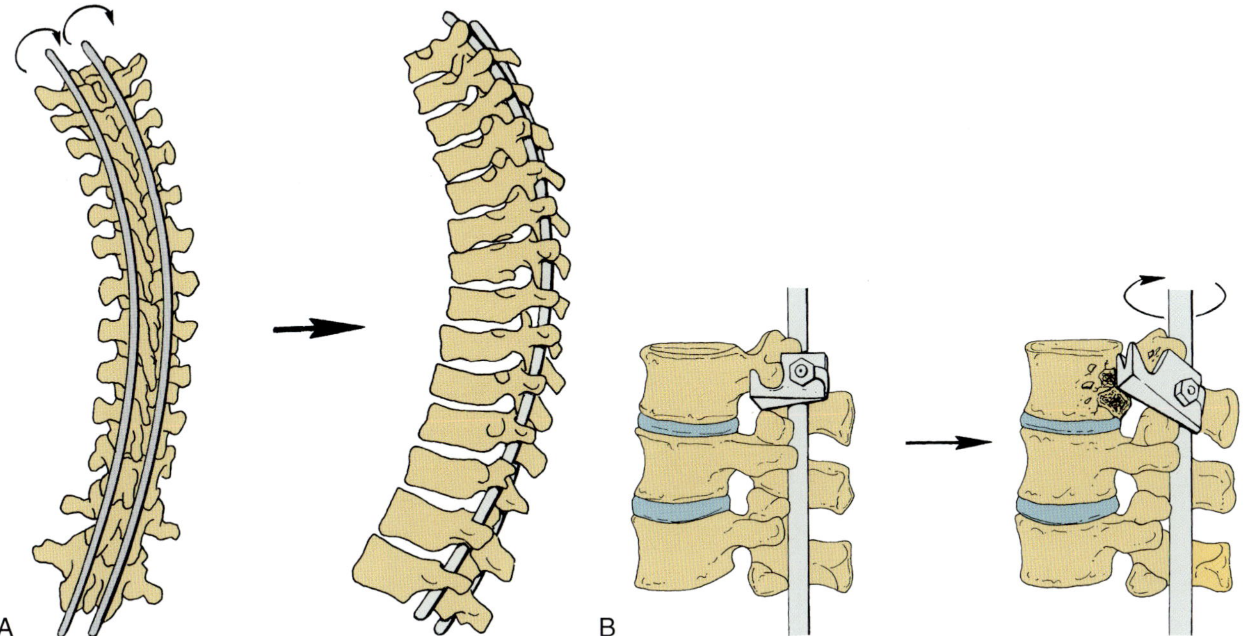

FIGURE 85-3. The derotation maneuver. A scoliotic curvature can be reduced by first attaching contoured rods (contoured to the shape of the deformity) to the affected portion of the spine at multiple attachment sites. Each rod is then rotated gradually and carefully by 90 degrees (*curved arrows*) (**A**). The resultant kyphotic deformity can then be reduced by in situ rod-bending techniques. Care must be taken not to overtighten the hook-rod juncture. If this juncture is overtightened, rotation of the rod may result in hook cutout (**B**).

relationships can be made. For example, a hook might not rotate on the rod during the derotation maneuver, thus placing significant stress on the hook-bone attachment (Fig. 85-3B).

Intrinsic Implant Bending Moment Application about the Axial Axes of the Spine

Intrinsic implant bending moment can be applied in either the sagittal or the coronal plane. One- or two-segment lumbar scoliotic deformations can be partially or completely corrected by this technique. In applying this procedure, pedicle screws are inserted, and the rods are attached to the screws. The screws on the concave side of the curvature are then distracted (usually 1–2 cm), whereas the screws on the convex side of the curvature are compressed. Cross-fixation to maintain the correction is then used (Fig. 85-4). A similar technique can be employed to correct sagittal plane deformities by using rod or plate-screw systems on the lateral aspect of the spine.

One should be cognizant of the type of screw-rod juncture (i.e., variable angle versus fixed angle). The application of distraction forces to a variable-angle screw that is not tightened to a friction-glide extent may result in screw flexion at the screw-rod juncture, which can cause application of an untoward bending moment to the spine. This can be prevented by tightening the screw carefully to friction-glide tightness before applying distraction forces.

Ventral Interbody Correction

A relatively new form of surgical management of lumbar scoliotic deformities involves the placement of ventral-lateral interbody cages.[17] Because these devices result in the distraction of the ventral half of the disc space, they also provide some increase in lumbar lordosis. Although technically easier to place from the spinal convexity, these devices can be placed so as to distract the concavity and therefore reduce the scoliotic curve. When combined with dorsal decompression and instrumentation, these devices theoretically reduce the strain on the dorsal implant in maintaining correction. Anatomic features of the lateral lumbar spine limit application of these devices to the upper lumbar segments—a convenience, since the apex of these deformities is often in this spinal region. Various protocols have been reported, including stand-alone interbody devices used for this purpose, but long-term results are still lacking.

Maintenance of Correction

Implant Selection and Cross-Fixation

It is important to remember that the postoperative spine will undergo forces that are exactly opposite any corrective maneuvers, especially as the patient reloads the spine. Therefore, implant failure, through either breakage or pull-out at the bone interface, can result in loss of deformity correction. A successful surgical plan must therefore oppose these forces through the selection of appropriate implant material and by creating forces within the spine and implant that resist pull-out.

In an effort to allow greater flexibility in construct design and rigidity, several new metallic hybrid rods have recently been used to correct deformities. Cobalt-chrome alloys, for example, are biomechanically superior to titanium rods in maintaining sagittal and coronal correction, produce less imaging artifact than stainless steel rods, and can be used with titanium screws.[18] Recent improvements in pedicle screws include varied thread designs that resist pull-out and hydroxyapatite coating, which improves fixation in osteoporotic bone.

Cross-fixation is the connection of bilaterally placed constructs to each other and can result in a substantial increase in

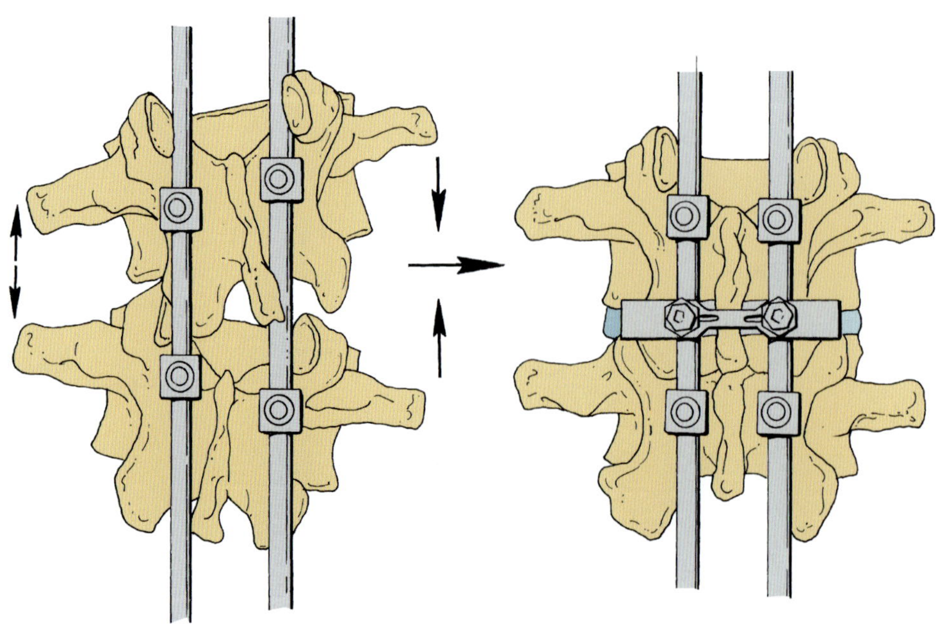

FIGURE 85-4. Intrinsic implant bending moment application. The concave side of a coronal plane curvature is distracted, and the concave side of the curvature is compressed (each ≤2 cm). A rigid cross-member is used to assist in reduction maintenance. A similar technique can be used to correct sagittal plane deformities.

the integrity of the construct. In general, cross-fixation of short constructs is of no significant benefit. However, in selected cases, it can be used to maintain deformity reduction and help prevent implant failure. In such situations, very rigid cross-members should be used because substantial bending moments are applied (resisted) at the cross-member-rod juncture.

With longer constructs, cross-fixation provides a quadrilateral, framelike construct. This is especially valuable when screws are angled in a nonparallel fashion in both the sagittal and coronal planes. By essentially binding the screws both longitudinally and cross-sectionally, rotatory stability and implant-bone juncture integrity are augmented. With long constructs, two cross-members are better than one; however, more than two add very little to construct integrity.[3] Cross-members should be placed approximately at the junction of the thirds of the length of the construct.[3]

Cross-fixation can be used for maintenance of an appropriate interrod width so that hook migration and screw dislodgement from the ilium can be prevented.

Screw Toe-In

By toeing-in pedicle screws, one can increase the length of a pedicle screw and provide much greater resistance to implant failure. Screw toe-in can also play an important role in lateral translational deformity prevention. It can be used with cross-fixation to achieve maintenance of deformity reduction.[3]

Low Lumbar and Lumbosacropelvic Techniques

The distal end of a spinal implant used to reduce an adult deformity has several significant implications. Ending the construct at L5 will certainly result in accelerated degenerative changes at that level. Since many adult deformities have an apex within the lumbar spine, instrumentation and fusion of the lumbosacral junction are common. L5-S1 interbody grafts and ilial-pelvic fixation (iliac screws) have been used as supplemental surgical techniques to combat high L5-S1 pseudarthrosis rates and the poor anatomic configuration of the S1 pedicles for screw fixation. Interbody grafts at the lumbosacral junction whether placed via anterior lumbar interbody fusion or transforaminal lumbar interbody fusion provide circumferential fusion, can help restore disc space and neuroforaminal height, and provide axial loading capacity. If interbody fusion is not used, acquisition of lumbosacral spine stability will indeed be complex and difficult. Surgical alternatives include pedicle fixation with orientation of the S1 screws upward toward the sacral promontory and complex iliac fixation techniques. It should be noted that pedicle fixation in the absence of adequate axial load-supporting capacity places excessive stresses on the implant and the implant-bone juncture. Repetitive loading of such a construct may produce failure at the screw-bone interface or the screw-plate or screw-rod juncture.[3]

Nonrigid lumbosacroiliac techniques, such as the slingshot and Galveston techniques, are cumbersome and involve fixation to predominantly low-density medullary bone. Thus, they may provide inadequate fixation. Prevention of lumbosacral fixation and extension therefore may be inadequate because of poor implant-bone juncture integrity (as was mentioned previously) and because of an inability to apply an adequate moment arm.[19] Furthermore, the ability of these techniques to effectively reduce coronal plane deformities is poor because of their rigid one-piece design.

More rigid iliac screw fixation techniques using bicortical ilial fixation are a more acceptable alternative and are readily available in universal instrumentation systems.[20] They allow the surgeon to use a tripod-like implant geometry for buttressing the sacroiliac segment (Fig. 85-5) and are especially helpful in preventing pull-out of the caudal end of an implant.[3,20] This is particularly important following significant correction of sagittal balance or to counter the long moment arms

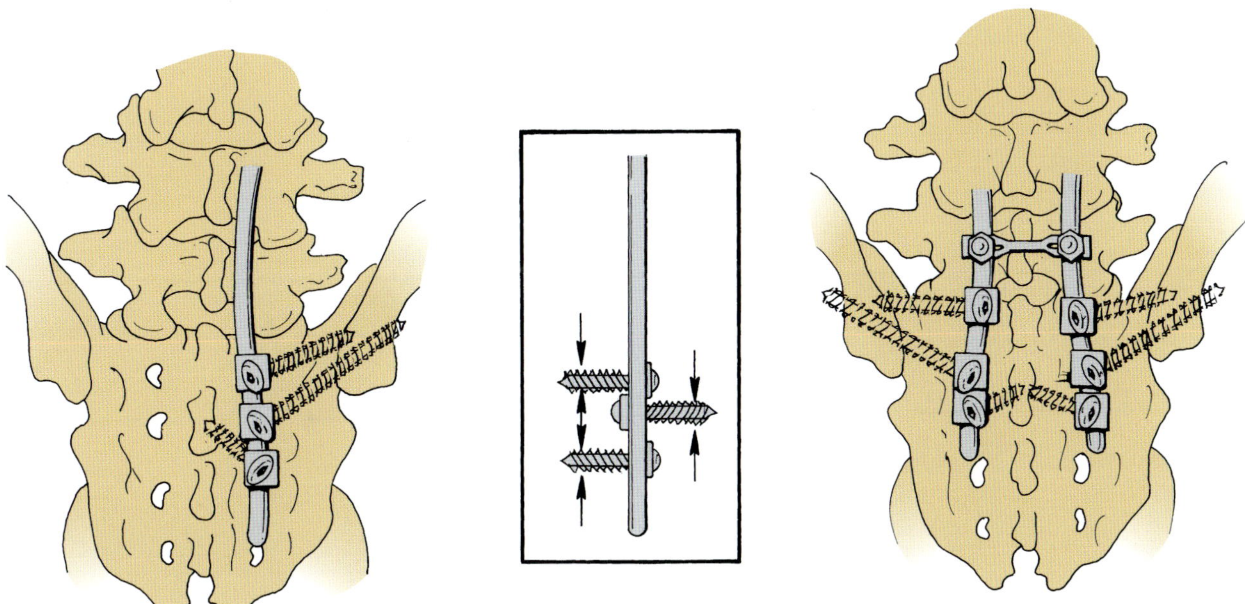

FIGURE 85-5. Bicortical ilial fixation achieves a tripod-like geometry. Rigid cross-fixation can be used to augment the fixation by enhancing the tripod effect.

associated with implants that extend cranially beyond the thoracolumbar junction.

A ventromedial orientation of sacral screws is, in general, superior to a ventrolateral (alar) orientation. Greater bone density and, hence, provision of a stronger implant-bone juncture can be achieved in the region of the midline sacral promontory or the L5-S1 disc interspace.[3,21] Additional implant-sacrum junctures can be used to prevent lumbosacral flexion and extension, including the first sacral lamina (for sublaminar wire fixation), the second dorsal sacral neuroforamina (for hook fixation), and the dorsum of the sacrum itself (via a buttressing effect) (Fig. 85-6).

Lumbosacroiliac fixation techniques should be used with the lumbosacral pivot point in mind. This is defined as the point of intersection of the middle osteoligamentous column (a region of the posterior longitudinal ligament) in the sagittal plane and the L5-S1 intervertebral disc (Fig. 85-7). Constructs that employ lumbosacroiliac fixation via bone screws are most effective in resisting flexion and extension deformation if the ventral extent of the screws extends ventrally to this point (Fig. 85-8).[22]

Clinical Applications

Clinical application of some of the techniques described in this chapter may indeed be difficult and dangerous. Therefore, management options should be carefully considered and individualized. Reduction, fusion, and stabilization procedures are often not indicated despite the presence of a significantly degenerated and deformed spine. In fact, as we age (past approximately 55 years), a spine restabilization process ensues (as a result of osteophyte formation, disc interspace collapse, and calcification). Deformity progression, which has been relentless before this, may slow down or cease. Therefore, attempts at reduction and fusion in this patient population may be ill advised.

Even when reduction and fusion are indicated, the universal application of a single surgical technique to all clinical situations is imprudent. For example, although pedicle fixation is, in general, a useful and efficacious technique, its universal application is inappropriate. For instance, it should not be applied over an unstable segment if ventral axial load-supporting ability is inadequate. Longer techniques or the use of ilial fixation augmentation may be beneficial (Fig. 85-9).

It is also important to remember that the major determinant of clinical success in adult patients undergoing deformity correction is the resultant sagittal contour, as discussed elsewhere.[23,24] Therefore, whatever technique is used to correct a scoliotic deformity, consideration must be given to the effects on global balance. For example, distraction in the lumbar spine along the concavity of the scoliotic curve introduces a potentially deleterious kyphotic force that may result in a painful hypolordosis or a relatively "flat back."

Similarly, several options are available to correct scoliotic deformities. These include distraction, short-segment parallelogram deformity reduction techniques (see Fig. 85-2), the derotation maneuver (see Fig. 85-3), and intrinsic implant bending moment application (see Fig. 85-4). Each procedure is indicated in specific circumstances; however, these indications are currently poorly defined.

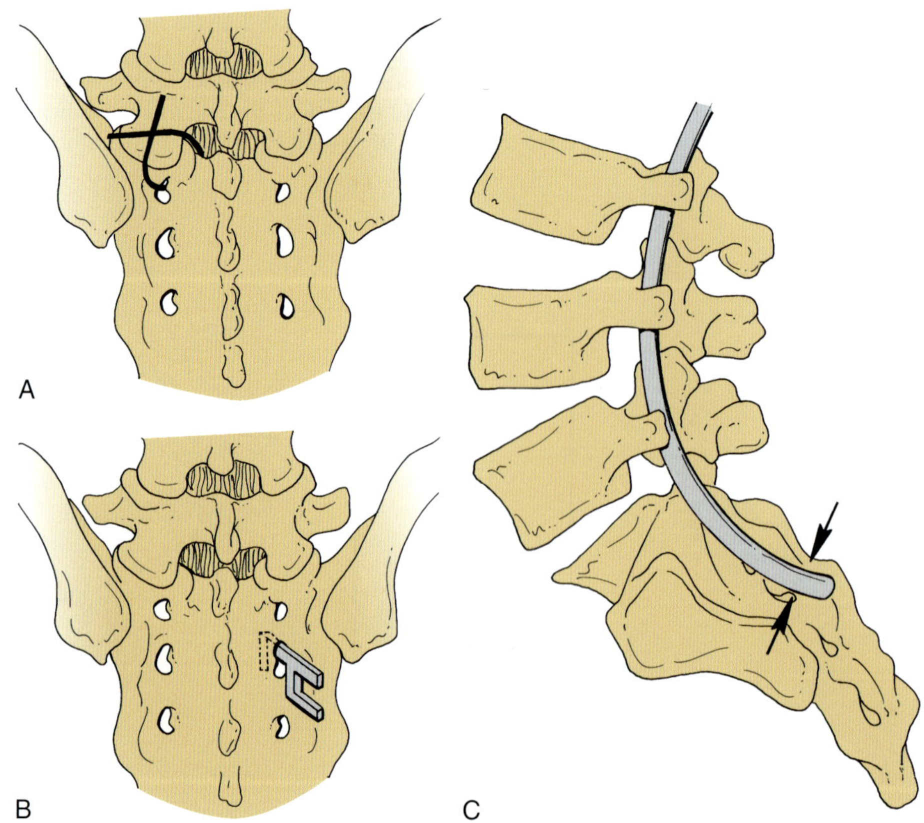

FIGURE 85-6. Additional sacrum fixation techniques. These involve the first sacral lamina for sublaminar wire fixation (**A**), the second dorsal sacral neuroforamina for hook fixation (**B**), and the dorsum of the sacrum itself for buttressing the rod (**C**).

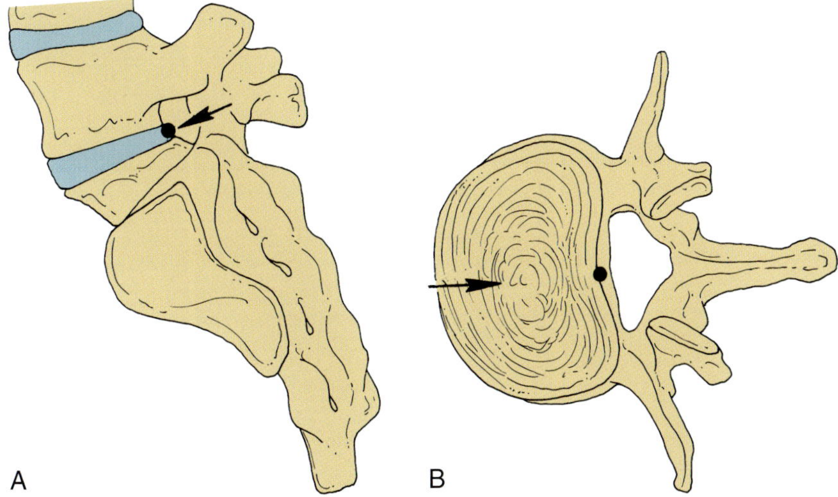

FIGURE 85-7. **A** and **B,** The lumbosacral pivot point is essentially the dorsal aspect of the intervertebral disc. Note that the ilial and sacral screw tips depicted are positioned ventral to the lumbosacral pivot point (*arrows*).

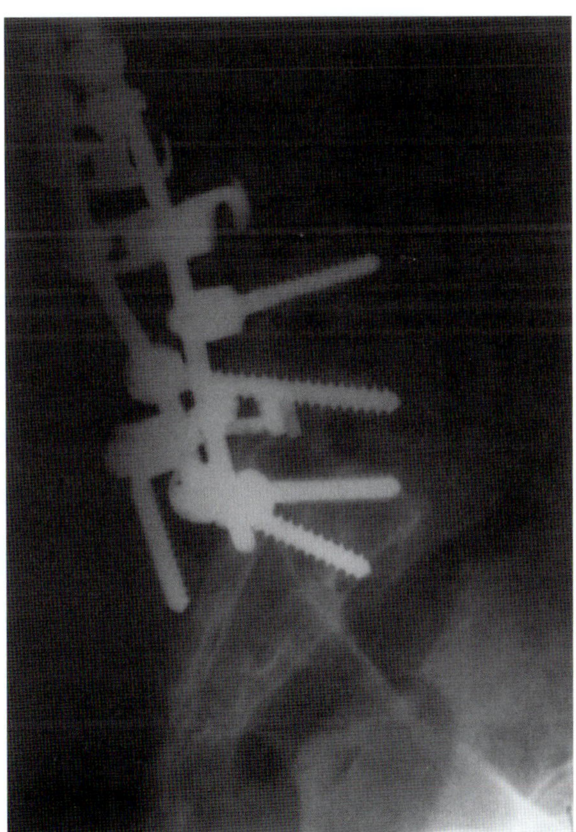

FIGURE 85-8. Use of multiple fixation techniques. Bicortical ilial fixation, laminar fixation, and sacral screw fixation are depicted in a single case.

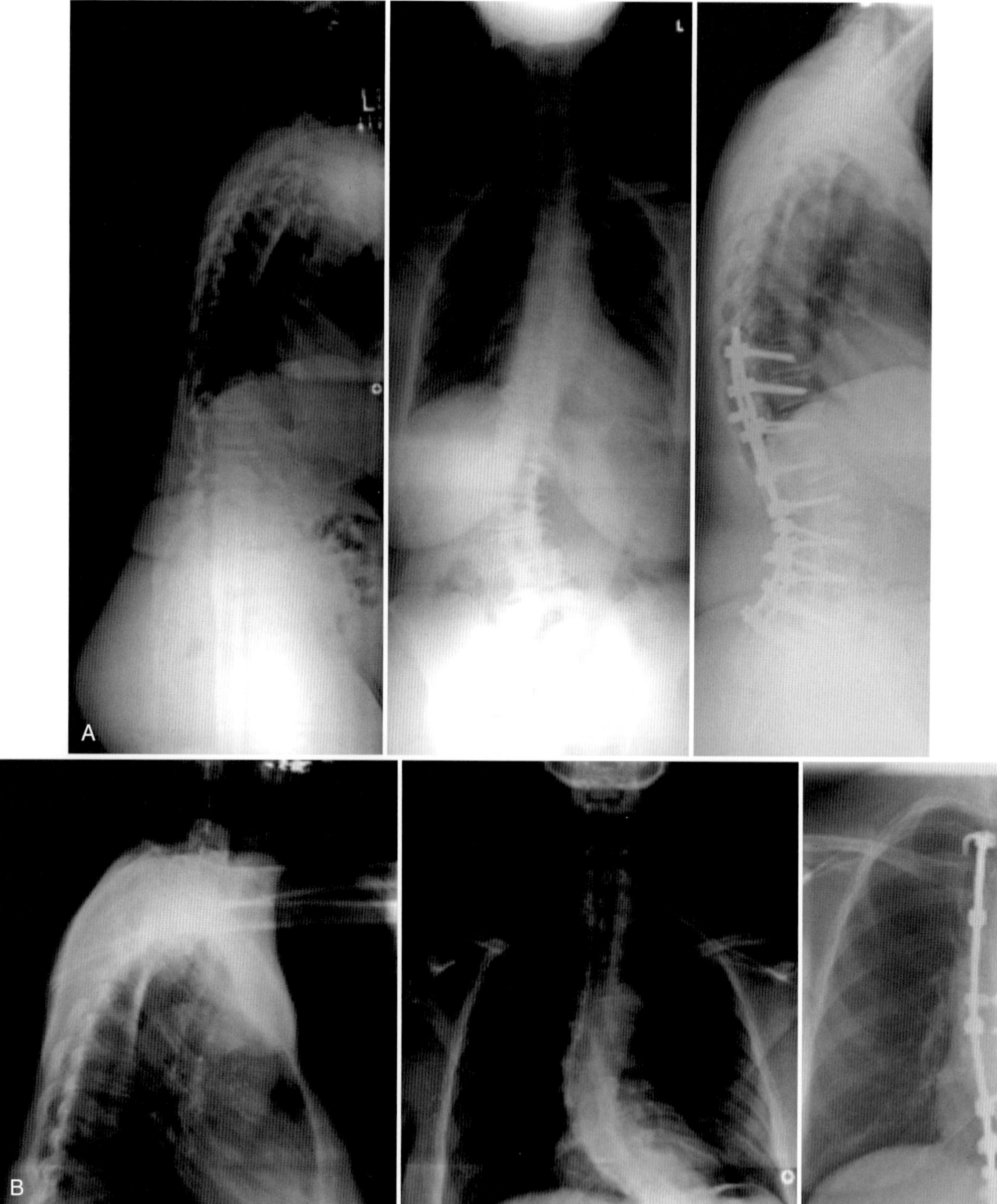

FIGURE 85-9. Preoperative and postoperative standing radiographs of two patients with different biomechanical needs and therefore different surgical goals. **A,** Note that the first patient has only a moderate lumbar scoliotic curve but also requires restoration of lordosis. **B** and **C,** The second patient has a greater-magnitude curve requiring a longer moment arm (pelvis to T4). Also note in the second patient that overall balance is more important than complete correction of the scoliotic curve.

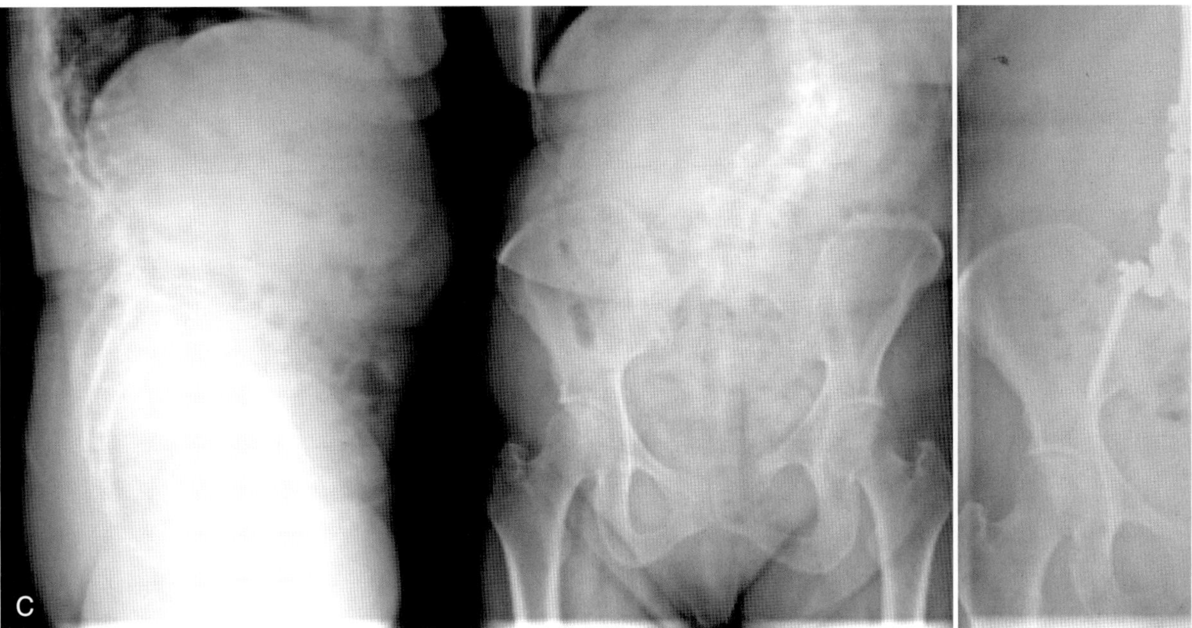

FIGURE 85-9, cont.

KEY REFERENCES

Adams MA, Huton WC: Prolapsed intervertebral disc: a hyperflexion injury. *Spine (Phila Pa 1976)* 7:184–191, 1982.

Cotrel Y, Dubousset J, Guillaumat M: New universal instrumentation in spinal surgery. *Clin Orthop Relat Res* 227:10–23, 1988.

Heary RF, Kumar S, Bono CM: Decision making in adult deformity. *Neurosurgery* 63(3):A69–A77, 2008.

McCord DH, Cunningham BW, Shono Y, et al: Biomechanical analysis of lumbosacral fixation. *Spine (Phila Pa 1976)* 17:5235–8243, 1992.

Rose PS, Lenke LG, Bridwell KH, et al: Pedicle screw instrumentation for adult idiopathic scoliosis. *Spine (Phila Pa 1976)* 34(8):852–857, 2009.

White AA, Panjabi MM: *Clinical biomechanics of the spine*, ed 2, Philadelphia, 1990, JB Lippincott.

REFERENCES

The complete reference list is available online at expertconsult.com.

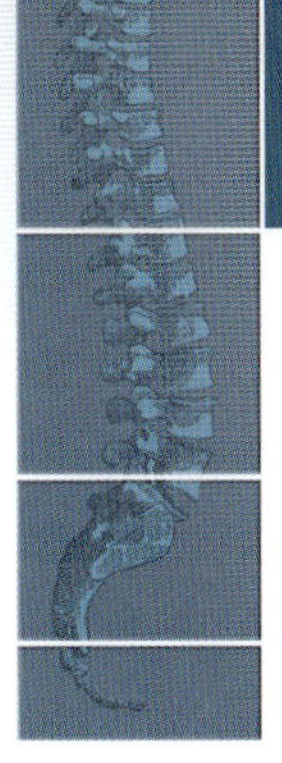

CHAPTER 86

Rheumatoid Arthritis

Robert F. Heary | Daniel S. Yanni | Pinakin R. Jethwa |
Fredrick A. Simeone | H. Alan Crockard

Rheumatoid arthritis is a systemic disease of unknown cause that primarily involves small blood vessels and synovium. A chronic disease, it is generally more common in females. This disorder is characterized by polyarticular symmetrical involvement of the smaller joints of the appendicular skeleton. It destroys the articular joint surfaces and the joint capsules as well as the ancillary ligaments that support the joints.[1] In addition, rheumatoid arthritis can be associated with osteoporosis and erosion and cyst formation in the bone.[2] The extent of myelopathy in patients with rheumatoid arthritis is difficult to evaluate because their disease may be complicated by peripheral joint destruction, peripheral neuropathies, nerve entrapments, and rheumatoid myopathy.[3]

The most common skeletal manifestation of rheumatoid arthritis occurs with the involvement of the metatarsophalangeal joints of the feet. This is followed in frequency by rheumatoid involvement of the cervical spine and the metacarpophalangeal joints of the hands.[4] Cervical spine involvement is very common, and symptoms do not necessarily accompany extensive bony changes of the spine.[5] Rheumatoid involvement of the cervical spine may be present with minimal or no clinical or radiologic expression elsewhere in the body.[4] The major clinical problems result from erosive changes in the cervical spine that lead to pathologic subluxation or dislocation.[6] Involvement of the thoracic and lumbar regions may also occur, although this is much less common.

The three most common lesions that cause neurologic involvement and/or intractable pain are atlantoaxial subluxation, subaxial subluxation, and vertical subluxation of the odontoid process.[7] The onset of cervical spine instability is often insidious. It may be masked by weakness and loss of function associated with peripheral joint disease.[8] Although any synovial joint in the spine may be involved, the earliest changes are usually observed in the upper cervical region.[3] Rheumatoid involvement of the cervical spine appears to begin early and progresses in relationship to peripheral joint involvement. The cervical spine abnormalities are the result of destruction in the joints, ligaments, and bone by synovitis.[2]

Atlantoaxial subluxation represents the most common and significant manifestation of rheumatoid involvement of the cervical spine.[6] The extent of neurologic deficit does not correlate with the degree of subluxation observed on lateral radiographs. This discrepancy may be the result of the formation of a pannus between the dens and the dura mater. This may contribute to spinal cord compression that cannot be visualized on plain radiographs. In 1830, Sir Charles Bell[9] reported the first case of an atlantoaxial subluxation resulting from an inflammatory process. Incompetence of the transverse atlantal ligament was demonstrated pathologically.

The rate of development of neurologic signs and symptoms is usually slow. Numerous large surgical and nonsurgical series of patients with rheumatoid arthritis have demonstrated that the average duration of disease before surgery is 15 to 20 years.[7,8,10-15] Although life expectancy in patients with moderate or severe rheumatoid arthritis is less than that of the general population, the presence of a cervical subluxation does not necessarily influence life expectancy.[14]

The most common clinical finding in rheumatoid involvement of the cervical spine is pain. Typically, this pain is severe and persistent and is usually located in the occipital region[4,10,16,17] or the neck,[18] or it may radiate toward the vertex of the skull.[16] Characteristically, this pain is exacerbated by neck motion.[4,5,19] Tears in the transverse atlantal and alar ligaments and in the atlanto-occipital membrane may give rise to retro-orbital or temporal region pains.[19] Pain in the arms is usually absent. This type of pain helps distinguish these disorders from cervical spondylosis.[20] Neurologic signs and symptoms that are useful for detection of the onset of myelopathy in rheumatoid arthritis patients include neck pain, occipital neuralgia, Lhermitte sign (electric-like shocks produced with neck flexion), and the patient's account of diminished motor ability or a documented worsening in the motor examination from the previous neurologic examination.[21]

Myelopathy may develop as a result of spinal cord compression. This usually occurs in late middle age, following many years of disability.[21] Because of the frequent, severe deforming effects of rheumatoid arthritis in the extremities, the development of long tract signs is useful in detecting myelopathy. These include hyperreflexia and extensor plantar responses.[12,17] Additional signs of myelopathy such as spasticity, presence of a Hoffman sign, and ankle clonus may also be detected. The myelopathy that occurs in rheumatoid arthritis is most likely caused by the effects of compression, stretch, and movement, not by ischemia.[22]

Because of patient selection and referral patterns, there is a marked discrepancy between the incidence of neurologic involvement of rheumatoid disease of the cervical spine in surgical and nonsurgical series. In two large nonsurgical series of more than 2000 patients with rheumatoid arthritis, reported by Smith et al. and Nakano et al., the incidence of cervical myelopathy was less than 3% in each series.[12,14] Interosseous erosive disease of the peripheral joints has been correlated to the severity of involvement of the cervical spine.[18,24]

The executive committee of the American Rheumatism Association established criteria for rheumatoid arthritis that must be applied only to patients with a clear-cut diagnosis. In addition, this committee has adopted a classification of functional capacity that is used in rheumatologic studies.[25]

Ranawat et al. developed a classification based on signs and symptoms.[7] In this surgical series, neurologic deficits were divided into three classes: I, no neurologic deficits; II, subjective weakness, hyperreflexia, and dysesthesias; and III, objective weakness and long tract signs (A, ambulatory, and B, quadriparetic, not ambulatory).

This classification scheme is widely used in many surgical series. The strength of the Ranawat classification system is that it measures a functional, rather than a neurologic, capacity. The ideal classification system has not yet been developed for rheumatoid arthritis patients. In an ideal system, an objective functional score should produce consistent, reliable interobserver and intraobserver results that can be compared among different studies.

Vertebral artery compression leading to vertebrobasilar insufficiency may occur in rheumatoid arthritis. The most common potential sites for mechanical compression of the vertebral artery include the foramen transversarium, the atlantoaxial joint, and the occipitoatlantal joint. Vertebral artery insufficiency may be the result of kinking of the vertebral artery at one of these locations or the involvement of the brainstem by upward migration of the dens.[24] Symptoms that have been attributed to vertebral artery insufficiency secondary to rheumatoid disease of the cervical spine include dizziness, tinnitus, vertigo, diplopia, suboccipital headache, dysphasia, blurring of vision, cortical blindness, nystagmus, transient blackout spells, confusion, and dysarthria.[17,24-26] The frequency with which vertebral artery symptoms may occur is poorly documented. Henderson et al. published nine autopsy cases of severe end-stage rheumatoid arthritis patients with vertical subluxation of the dens that showed the vertebral artery to be patent in all specimens.[22]

The pathologic changes in rheumatoid arthritis of the cervical spine are predominantly secondary to synovitis. Synovitic proliferation destroys the facet joints, erodes and deforms the dens, and weakens the ligamentous attachments.[24] A characteristic pannus may form between the odontoid peg and the ventral dura mater that can compress the spinal cord. This pannus is usually firm, gray-pink tissue that shows end-stage chronic inflammation of synovial tissue.[21] In addition to this proliferation of the synovial tissue, osteoporosis and destruction of cartilage and subchondral bone can occur.[4,26] Localized bone loss around the inflamed joints is the result of prostaglandin and cytokine synthesis during the inflammatory process, which increases bone resorption.[27] Inflammatory destruction of the lateral atlantoaxial joints can lead to vertical translocation of the dens.[24] When the odontoid process herniates through the foramen magnum, it can cause flattening, softening, and atrophy of the medulla.[28]

The specific mechanism by which ischemia causes damage to the spinal cord is unclear. Two separate studies have postulated that intermittent compression of the ventral spinal artery was responsible for the spinal cord injury.[1,12] However, in a necropsy study of nine patients, Henderson et al. demonstrated that the histopathologic changes were localized principally to the dorsal white matter of the spinal cord. In this study, the territory of the ventral spinal artery was spared.[22] O'Brien et al. performed a histologic study of specimens removed during ventral decompressions of the cervicomedullary junction. They determined that repetitive mechanical damage caused by instability at the atlantoaxial joint, rather than an acute compressive effect from an inflammatory pannus, was the cause of spinal cord compression and subsequent axonal injury.[29] In addition, Crockard and Grob have stated that there is no evidence that avascular necrosis or vasculitis is involved in the inflammatory process of rheumatoid arthritis involvement of the spine. They believe that it is the repetitive movement of the unstable atlantoaxial joint against the neuraxis that causes a mechanical "wear-and-tear" phenomenon that leads to the development of a myelopathy.[21]

In rheumatoid arthritis (due to deficient osteogenesis) osteophytes do not form.[1,4,16] This may be contrasted to osteoarthritis that is characterized by the development of osteophytic spurs, which often have a stabilizing effect.[1,16,19]

Imaging Studies

A variety of radiographic imaging modalities are used to image the spine in rheumatoid arthritis. These modalities include plain radiography, CT, myelography, a combination of CT and myelography, CT angiography, MRI, and plain tomography. In addition, dynamic flexion and extension views may be used to augment the information provided by any of these studies. Because the occiput–C1-2 complex is the most frequently involved region of the spine in rheumatoid arthritis, the majority of imaging studies focus attention on this area. When clinically indicated, imaging studies of the subaxial cervical spine and of the thoracic and lumbar spines should also be performed.

In a study by Younes et al., 72.5% of patients who met American College of Rheumatology criteria for rheumatoid arthritis had pathology of the cervical spine identified in at least one imaging modality (plain radiographs, MRI, or CT).[30]

On plain radiographs, small or absent osteophytes, osteoporotic vertebrae, and eroded vertebral end plates characterize rheumatoid arthritis.[4] In the absence of rheumatoid arthritis, degenerative changes are more marked in the lower cervical spine with advancing age. Radiographic changes at the C1-2 level are not present unless a specific process, such as rheumatoid arthritis, is affecting this region. These changes are independent of age.[30] Bland et al. found 86% of patients with classic or definite rheumatoid arthritis to have evidence of cervical spine involvement on plain radiographs. These changes may frequently be asymptomatic and may not be associated with any neurologic deficit.[5] In patients with severe polyarticular rheumatoid arthritis for more than 20 years, Santavirta et al. found radiographic subluxation of the cervical spine in more than 80% of patients.[13]

The most common radiologic abnormality in rheumatoid arthritis is ventral subluxation of the atlas. The atlantodental interval (ADI) measures the distance between the ventral aspect of the dens and the dorsal ring of the atlas. In normal adult patients, this distance is less than 3 mm.[31] An ADI of between 3 and 5 mm in an adult is abnormal and indicates a tear or insufficiency of the transverse atlantal ligament. A separation of greater than 5 mm indicates rupture or attenuation of the alar ligaments in addition to the transverse atlantal ligament.[16] Many studies have shown a poor correlation between abnormalities of the ADI and neurologic deficits. In an innovative study, Boden et al. defined the dorsal atlanto-odontoid interval (AOI) as the distance between the dorsal surface of the dens and the ventral edge of the dorsal ring of the atlas measured along the transverse axis of the ring of the atlas. They demonstrated an excellent correlation between the dorsal AOI and the severity of the neurologic deficit. A dorsal AOI of less than 14 mm correlated significantly with the presence and severity of a neurologic deficit. This dorsal AOI was also found to be a good predictor of neurologic recovery postoperatively. These authors stated that the weak correlation of the ventral ADI with a neurologic deficit may be due to variations in the diameter of the atlas as well as the presence of a pannus behind the odontoid process.[32] Weissman et al. studied 109 patients with rheumatoid arthritis and atlantoaxial subluxations for 5 years. They found that the ADI increased by more than 2 mm in 41%, remained unchanged in 40%, and decreased in 19% by more than 2 mm. Of the patients whose ADI decreased, more than 50% had developed vertical subluxation of the odontoid process.[15] Henderson et al. have stated that vertical subluxation may cause a pseudofixation of the ADI. Interpretation of the ADI must therefore be made in conjunction with measurement of the vertical axial subluxation.[22]

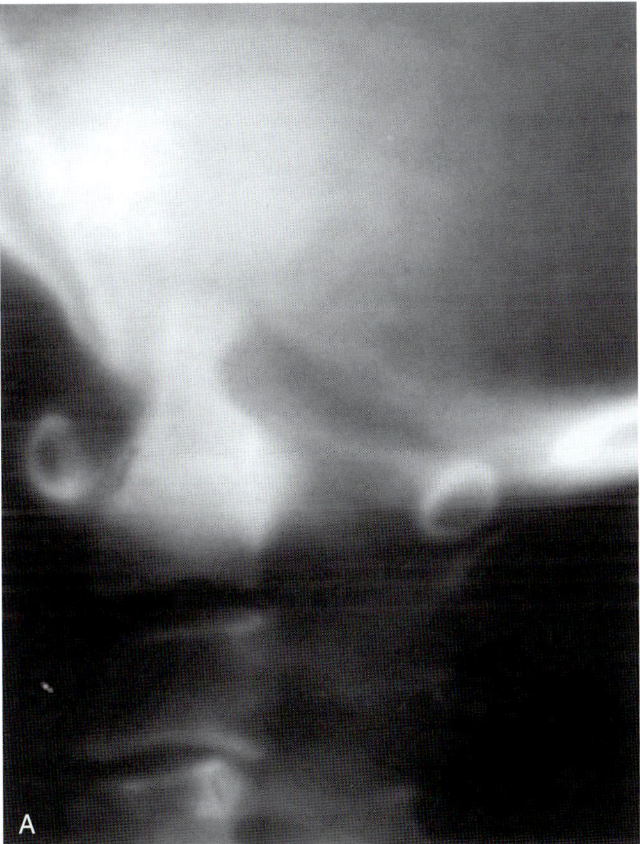

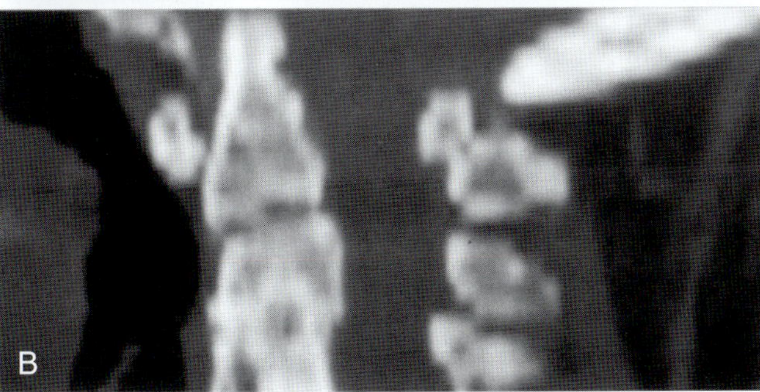

FIGURE 86-1. A, Plain tomogram, lateral view. Vertical subluxation of the odontoid process is clearly demonstrated. The tip of the odontoid is seen dorsal to the clivus in an intracranial position. The arch of the atlas has telescoped down the body of C2. This level of severe bony deterioration can cause the atlantodental interval to actually decrease. **B,** Sagittal reformation of a CT scan (same patient as in **A**). Bony detail and intracranial location of the odontoid are well visualized. The ventral translation of the atlas is more apparent in this view.

Vertical subluxation of the dens is an upward migration of the dens into the foramen magnum (Fig. 86-1). In this location, the dens competes for space with the spinal cord and the brainstem. Vertical subluxation requires the lateral facet joints to be damaged.[12] Vertical subluxation is the second most common upper cervical spine abnormality in rheumatoid arthritis, after atlantoaxial subluxation, and may accompany ventral atlantoaxial subluxation. An increase in the vertical subluxation may actually produce a decrease in the measured ventral atlantoaxial subluxation.[15] In vertical subluxation, the presence of a rheumatoid pannus, together with the invaginated dens, may produce ventral compression of the cervicomedullary junction.[17]

In an attempt to quantify vertical subluxation of the dens, numerous lines and indices have been proposed (Fig. 86-2). These lines are characteristically drawn between bony landmarks that are identifiable on a lateral cervical spine radiograph. The tip of the dens is then measured with respect to the various lines. A McGregor line is drawn from the hard palate to the occiput, and it is probably the most traditional measure.[2] A shortcoming of these lines is that the hard palate, the dorsal edge of the foramen magnum, and the tip of the dens are not always visualized on routine lateral cervical spine radiographs in a patient with vertical subluxation

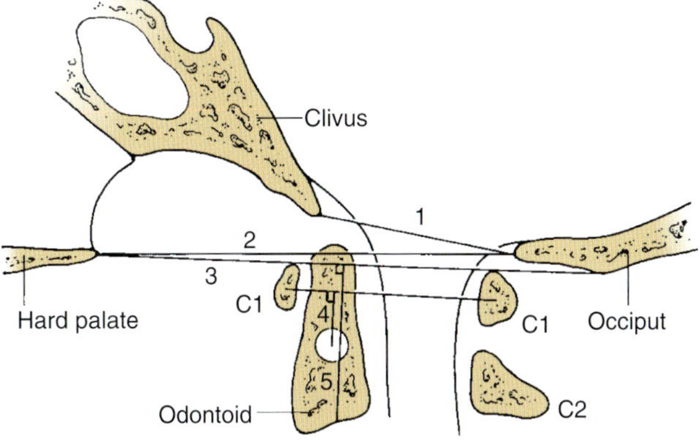

FIGURE 86-2. Common craniometry lines: McRae line (1), Chamberlain line (2), McGregor line (3).

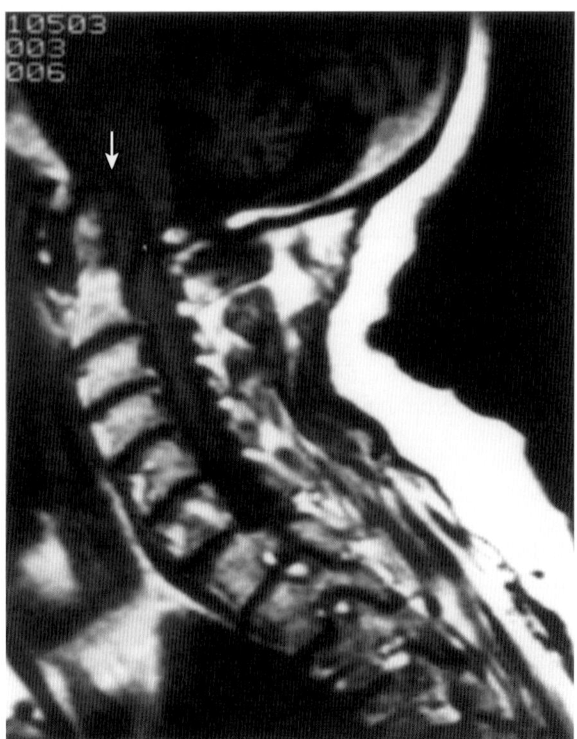

FIGURE 86-3. Sagittal T1-weighted (TR 500/TE 11) MRI image of ventral compression from a large inflammatory pannus (*white arrow*). The cervicomedullary junction is deformed and attenuated by this soft tissue mass.

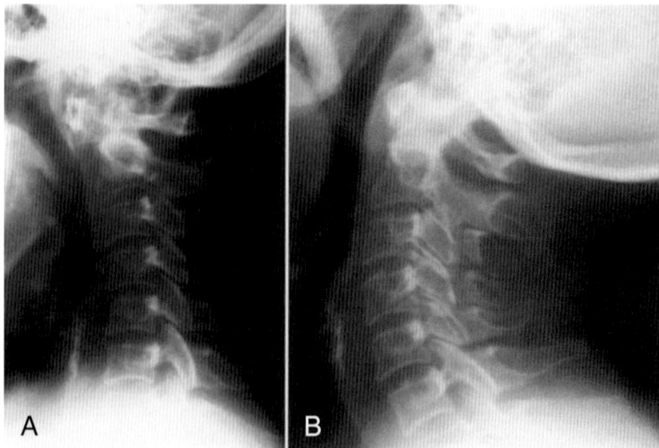

FIGURE 86-4. A, Plain radiograph, lateral flexion view. Significant widening of the atlantodental interval (ADI) with flexion is demonstrated. The occiput-C1 complex translates forward over the C2 vertebra. **B,** Plain radiograph, lateral extension view (same patient as in **A**). The odontoid process is well reduced in extension, with an ADI within normal limits (<3 mm).

of the odontoid. To avoid these difficulties, Ranawat et al. developed an index that measures the distance between the diameter of the ring of the first cervical vertebra to the center of the pedicle of the second cervical vertebra.[7] In men and women with normal cervical spines, this distance measured 17 mm in men and 15 mm in women. No normal patients had an interval of less than 15 mm.

A cervical myelogram provides an indirect visualization of the spinal cord and adjacent structures silhouetted by contrast media in the subarachnoid space.[33] The information obtained by myelography may be augmented by a postmyelogram CT. Computerized myelotomography, with multiplanar reconstruction, can clearly demonstrate the important contribution of proliferative rheumatoid pannus behind the odontoid peg to ventral cervicomedullary compression. In addition, bone windows on the CT scan can demonstrate bony abnormalities.

Currently, MRI is considered the ideal study to demonstrate the level and extent of spinal cord compression.[33,34] The advantages of MRI include direct imaging of the entire length of the spinal cord and the cervicomedullary junction, direct imaging in multiple planes, superior demonstration of soft tissue structures, and the lack of image degradation by bone artifact at the cervicomedullary junction (Fig. 86-3). In addition, MRI is noninvasive (no intrathecal contrast is needed), can be performed on an outpatient basis, does not expose the patient to the dangers of ionizing radiation, and is generally well tolerated.[6,33,35] A limitation of MRI is that it does not image compact bone as accurately as CT.[34]

Furthermore, Dickman et al. have shown that the transverse atlantal ligament can be consistently and clearly visualized with MRI. This determination of a loss of anatomic continuity of the transverse atlantal ligament is useful for operative planning.[36] For patients who are unable to undergo MRI, CT scanning with multiplanar reconstructions provides better information than polytomography. It is important to visualize the neuraxis before surgery; injecting water-soluble contrast into the lumbar subarachnoid space provides additional important anatomic information regarding the flow of cerebrospinal fluid in the upper cervical spine region. Knowledge of the position and course of the spinal vessels, in particular the vertebral arteries, is of extreme importance in many of the surgical approaches to the craniocervical junction. CT angiography provides an excellent means of visualizing the spinal vasculature in relation to the bony anatomy of the upper cervical spine.

Dynamic views of the cervical spine, in flexion and extension, provide useful information about the degree of instability of the occiput–C1-2 complex (Fig. 86-4). These flexion-extension views can be obtained on plain films, tomograms, computerized myelotomography scans, and MRI studies. Dickman et al. recommend routine lateral cervical radiographs in flexion and extension for all patients undergoing transoral surgery.[36] Furthermore, Sharp and Purser recommend lateral flexion and extension radiographs in any patient with severe rheumatoid arthritis undergoing general anesthesia for any surgical procedure.[37] Bell and Stearns have found MRI in flexion and extension to be very useful for demonstrating dynamic changes in spinal cord configuration. They have used this information to determine the proximal extent of fusion required and have stated that it provides an accurate and dynamic study of the relationship between the spinal cord and the surrounding bony and soft tissue structures.[38] Additionally, upright MRI of the cervical spine can help reveal pathology that may be missed at the craniocervical junction in supine position.[39,40]

Operative Indications

As a general rule, the presence of myelopathy or a progressive neurologic deficit continues to be a strong indication for surgical intervention in patients with rheumatoid changes of the cervical spine.*

Likewise, intractable pain is an indication for operative intervention.[2,3,6,11,18,24,29,32] A much more controversial topic is whether a patient with markedly abnormal radiographs, in the absence of pain or progressive neurologic deficit, should undergo surgery. Numerous authors believe that radiologic evidence of an impending neurologic deficit is an indication for surgery.[1,7,41,42] Pellicci et al. believe that radiographic evidence of disease progresses to a greater degree than does neural involvement.[18] As such, they believe that no fusion should be recommended on the basis of a radiographic abnormality or radiographic deterioration alone. Others have supported this more conservative viewpoint.[2,13,19,28] In an intermediate position, Boden et al. stated that only patients with a neurologic deficit underwent surgery in their series. Nevertheless, they recommended surgery for patients with or without a neurologic deficit, if certain radiographic criteria are met.[32]

Crockard reviewed his results with 55 severe end-stage rheumatoid arthritis patients (Ranawat grade IIIB). He found that those patients who are bed-bound for more than 3 months fare extremely poorly, regardless of whether surgical intervention is undertaken. In addition, with these Ranawat grade IIIB patients, mortality rates are unacceptably high in many cases. Therefore, one must question the previously held view that the presence of a myelopathy in a long-term, bed-bound Ranawat grade IIIB patient is an absolute indication for surgery.

Specific Regions of the Spine

Upper Cervical Spine

To fully understand the complex pathologic changes that occur in the occiput–C1-2 region, a thorough understanding of the biomechanics of this region is necessary. The majority of axial rotation occurs in the upper cervical spine. Approximately 60% of the axial rotation of the entire cervical spine and occiput is found in the upper region (occiput–C1-2) and 40% is found in the subaxial region (below C2). There is no axial rotation between the occiput and C1 unless there has been an occipitoatlantal disruption.[44] An extensive amount of axial rotation, 47 degrees, occurs at the C1-2 level.[45] White and Panjabi have identified two distinct reasons why this increased motion can occur at the C1-2 level. First, the articular surfaces of the lateral masses of both C1 and C2 have a convex orientation in the sagittal plane that allows for considerable mobility. Second, a taut yellow ligament is not present between the dorsal elements of C1 and C2. Instead, a loose, readily mobile atlantoaxial membrane connects the dorsal elements of C1 and C2, thereby enhancing the motion capacity of this region.[45] Craniovertebral junction instability in rheumatoid arthritis patients occurs from a combination of bone softening, ligamentous destruction, and inflammatory pannus formation.[46] Unlike the lower cervical spine, the upper cervical spine cannot clearly be divided into ventral and dorsal elements with corresponding mechanical properties.[47] White and Panjabi have defined clinical instability as "loss of the capacity of the spine, under physiologic loads, to maintain relationships between vertebrae so that no spinal cord or nerve root damage occurs and no incapacitating deformity or pain develops."[45] This definition has led to certain anatomic measurements from plain film radiographs that can lead to a suspicion of clinical instability. In adults, a ventral ADI of greater than 3 mm on a lateral radiograph is regarded as potentially unstable. Although less widely used, a dorsal AOI of less than 14 mm is also suspicious for clinical instability.[28] With this basic understanding of the biomechanical relationships of the upper cervical spine, the two most common abnormalities in this region are ventral atlantoaxial subluxation, caused by incompetent ligaments, and vertical subluxation of the odontoid process that occurs because of lateral mass erosion.

Atlantoaxial Subluxation

Ventral atlantoaxial subluxation is the most common abnormality of the spine in rheumatoid arthritis. Classically, atlantoaxial subluxation is considered present if the ADI is greater than 3 mm in an adult or greater than 4 mm in a child.[24] Due to selection biases between surgical and nonsurgical studies of patients with rheumatoid arthritis, there are marked discrepancies in the frequency with which atlantoaxial subluxation occurs. In a large study in the rheumatologic literature on the prevalence of atlantoaxial subluxation in rheumatoid arthritis patients, the authors found that an atlantoaxial subluxation was present in 1 of 30 patients with any evidence of rheumatoid arthritis, in 1 of 15 patients with clinical evidence of the disease, and in 1 of 5 patients with rheumatoid arthritis admitted to the hospital.[37] This last group of patients are those more likely to be seen by a spine surgeon. Indeed, in the study by Weissman et al., ventral atlantoaxial subluxation was found to occur in one fourth to one third of rheumatoid arthritis patients.[15] Disruption of the transverse ligament of the atlas is the most important pathologic abnormality responsible for atlantoaxial instability.[36]

The degree of atlantoaxial subluxation is poorly correlated with clinical evidence of a compressive myelopathy.[33] Similarly, no correlation between the magnitude of an atlantoaxial subluxation and mortality was found in a 10-year follow-up study.[13] In a large radiologic review of 189 rheumatoid arthritis patients with atlantoaxial subluxations, Weissman et al. found the incidence of spinal cord compression to be 11%.[15] These findings underscore the necessity of an accurate history and physical examination to determine which patients with atlantoaxial subluxations demonstrate evidence of neurologic abnormalities related to this radiographic abnormality. A characteristic clinical finding of ventral atlantoaxial subluxation is difficulty in raising the head to the neutral position following downward gaze. This sensation of the head "falling forward" has been referred to as the Sharp-Purser sign.[37] An extremely rare abnormality is dorsal atlantoaxial subluxation. For a dorsal atlantoaxial subluxation to occur, the dens must be destroyed, fractured, or congenitally absent; alternatively, the ventral arch of the atlas must be destroyed or congenitally absent.[15,31,48,49]

Vertical subluxation of the dens can occur simultaneously with a ventral atlantoaxial subluxation. When this occurs, the ADI can appear to actually decrease in size.[50] Isolated

*See references 2, 3, 6, 7, 11, 18, 19, 22, 24, 28, 29, 32, 41, and 42.

ventral subluxation is more common than either vertical subluxation or a combination of ventral subluxation and vertical subluxation. Kraus et al. studied 55 patients with atlantoaxial subluxations who received dorsal fusion and found that none developed subsequent vertical subluxations. They believed that the dorsal fusion operation may have a protective effect in preventing vertical subluxation.[11] This protective effect of dorsal fusion has not been demonstrated in a prospective study. Contrary to the findings of Kraus et al.,[11] we present the case of a patient with rheumatoid arthritis that initially presented with atlantoaxial subluxation that was treated with a Brooks-type fusion. The patient subsequently developed vertical subluxation 6 months after the operation despite fusion at C1-2, which was treated with occipitocervical fusion (see Figs. 86-8 to 86-11).

Vertical Subluxation of the Odontoid

Vertical subluxation of the dens is referred to by a variety of terms, including atlantoaxial impaction, cranial settling, upward migration of the odontoid, pseudobasilar invagination, translocation of the dens, superior migration of the odontoid, basilar invagination, and vertical settling. These terms have been used interchangeably in the medical literature. Vertical subluxation occurs as a consequence of loss of substance of the lateral masses, usually the atlas. However, the lateral masses of the axis and, less commonly, the occipital condyles may also be involved.[22] In vertical subluxation, the ventral arch of C1 gradually articulates with caudal portions of C2, first via the base of the dens and then with the body of C2.[15] If there is more than 18 mm of translocation, the ring of the atlas is usually broken and the base of the axis has migrated within the disrupted ring. Significant vertical subluxation of the dens is generally agreed to be an indication for a fusion operation.[7,13,15-17,28,42]

Neurologic abnormalities are far more common with vertical subluxation of the dens than with atlantoaxial subluxation. The abnormal neurologic symptoms are the result of compression of the brainstem or upper cervical spinal cord. Neurologic abnormalities detected in vertical subluxation of the dens include hyperreflexia, extensor plantar reflexes, limb paresthesias, progressive difficulty with ambulation, a central cordlike syndrome, neurogenic bladder, and lower cranial nerve palsies.[17] Rheumatoid arthritis patients with vertical subluxation are more likely to be symptomatic from spinal cord compression.[13,15,17,28,51]

Lower Cervical Spine

As with abnormalities of the upper cervical spine, the presence of subaxial subluxations of the lower cervical spine varies greatly in reported series. Subaxial subluxation is a gradual process in which there is a forward displacement of one or more vertebral bodies on the vertebral body immediately below (Fig. 86-5). The rheumatoid process attacks the zygapophyseal facet and uncovertebral joints, weakens the supporting ligaments, and erodes the intervertebral discs. These effects loosen the various intervertebral fixations and permit luxation between adjacent vertebral bodies.[1] Subaxial subluxations are usually reducible by traction; however, the reduction is difficult to maintain.[29] Classically, subaxial

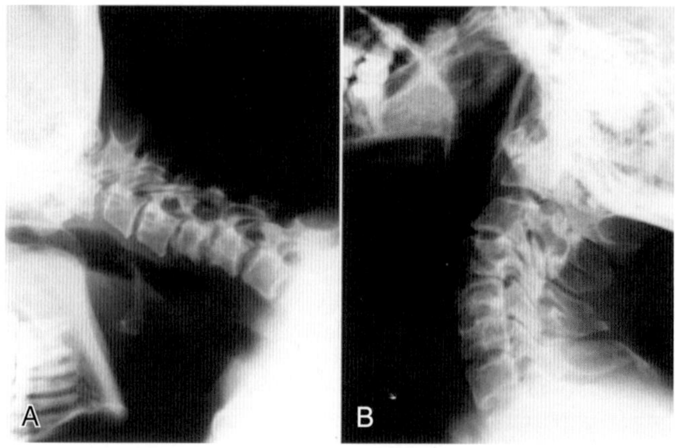

FIGURE 86-5. A, Plain radiograph, lateral flexion view. Multiple subaxial subluxations are seen with neck flexion, producing a "staircase" effect. The vertebral body translates forward with respect to the immediate subjacent vertebral body. Vertical subluxation of the odontoid process is also seen in this view. **B,** Plain radiograph, lateral extension view (same patient as in **A**). Neck extension causes a marked correction in the degree of subaxial subluxations. There is no change in the relationship between the atlas and the axis with neck motion.

subluxation is a translation of one vertebra in relation to an adjacent vertebra of greater than 3.5 mm on a lateral cervical spine radiograph.[31] Boden et al. found that the diameter of the subaxial sagittal spinal canal reflected the presence and degree of a neurologic deficit, more often than did the percentage of vertebral body slip.[32] In addition to the bony luxations, compression from epidural rheumatoid granulations has been reported.[2-4]

Subaxial subluxations are usually late developments in the aggressive forms of rheumatoid arthritis.[4,13] The severity of these subaxial subluxations is also closely related to the duration of rheumatoid disease.[4,14] When compared with patients with atlantoaxial subluxations, the incidence of neurologic deficits is higher in patients with subaxial subluxation, and the final results are poorer.[8]

Typically, subaxial subluxations show a "staircase" appearance with multiple subluxations observed sequentially in the cervical spine.[2,6,12] Subaxial subluxations may result in nerve root impingement from foraminal narrowing.[6] The presence of a subaxial subluxation should be suspected when bizarre weakness of the hands is observed in a patient with rheumatoid arthritis. This may be difficult in patients with long-standing disease who already have crippling deformity of the hands.[52] This subaxial spinal cord involvement may cause myelopathy and may explain why some patients do not respond to surgical decompression at the craniocervical junction.[22] The most common site for subaxial subluxation is at the C3-4 level; however, it often occurs at multiple levels, and these typically lack osteophytes.[2,3,53]

Subaxial subluxations may be present at the time of surgery for an upper cervical instability. The caudal extent of the instrumentation and fusion must therefore be carefully selected to incorporate any segments with a significant subaxial subluxation.[54,55] In an autopsy study of nine patients with severe end-stage rheumatoid arthritis, Henderson et al. found subaxial compression present in eight of the nine patients.[22] More commonly, subaxial subluxations may occur after fusion operations in the upper cervical spine.[3,6,11,53] As a result, it is essential that patients who undergo upper cervical fusions be followed closely with lateral cervical spine radiographs both for evidence of an acceptable bony fusion and for the development of subaxial subluxations. Kraus et al. found a much higher incidence of subaxial subluxations in patients whose upper cervical fusion incorporated the occiput. They postulated that this was because of a longer lever arm that results in higher forces generated at the lower cervical levels and that leads to a subaxial subluxation.[11] Subaxial cervical subluxations in rheumatoid arthritis patients have been associated with quadriplegia, sudden death, and other neurologic complications resulting from damage of the spinal cord or from interference with the flow of the vertebral arteries.[56]

The most accurate radiographic imaging study currently available to detect the site and type of spinal cord compression in subaxial subluxation of the rheumatoid spine is MRI.[13] All patients with subaxial subluxations and atlantoaxial subluxations with neurologic deficits or vertical subluxations of the dens should have an MRI study, if possible.[8] In patients who cannot undergo an MRI, a myelogram followed by a postmyelogram CT scan should be obtained.

Thoracic and Lumbar Spines

Involvement of the thoracic and lumbar spines in rheumatoid arthritis patients is rare. Heywood and Meyers have stated that subcervical rheumatoid spondylitis is more common than is generally believed and have found an incidence of 0.9% in their clinic.[57] Most other series of rheumatoid arthritis patients do not even address the topic of the thoracic and lumbar spines. In a study by Redlund-Johnell and Larsson, of 100 patients with severe rheumatoid arthritis who had previously undergone occipitocervical fusion, four patients with subluxation of the upper thoracic spine were found. These changes in the upper thoracic spine were radiologically similar to the destructive type of subaxial subluxation typically observed in the cervical spine. The authors believed that this upper thoracic subluxation may have been caused by increased motion as compensation for decreased mobility in the cervical spine.[58] The pathogenesis of rheumatoid spondylitis in the thoracic and lumbar spines is believed to be the result of a facet joint synovitis that leads to instability. In addition, involved costovertebral joints can spread their involvement to the disc space, causing a discitis between the disc and the vertebral end plates that can lead to further instability.[57] Rheumatoid granulation tissue causing compression of the thoracic spine has been reported.[59,60] In addition, an extensive inflammatory synovitis of the costovertebral and costotransverse joints can occur in the thorax.[61]

Rheumatoid involvement of the lumbar spine is rarely recognized as a cause of nerve root or cauda equina compression. Intraspinal rheumatoid granulomatous nodules can lead to nerve root compression, causing back and leg pain.[59,62] In addition, rheumatoid granulation tissue can develop in the lumbar facet joints and spread to the periarticular structures to contribute to cauda equina compression.[63,64]

The plain radiographic features of subcervical rheumatoid spondylitis include an ill-defined, blurred, and eroded margin to the vertebral end plates and an ill-defined, eroded facet joint complex.[57] If not specifically sought, these radiographic abnormalities may be easily overlooked. Frequently, rheumatoid arthritis patients have stiff, high-positioned shoulders that may conceal the cervicothoracic junction on conventional radiographs. If clinically indicated, an MRI study allows for better visualization of the cervicothoracic junction and the remainder of the thoracic and lumbar spines.[58]

Surgical Management of the Rheumatoid Spine

Many different operations have been recommended for patients with rheumatoid arthritis of the spine (Fig. 86-6). The various options include a dorsal cervical fusion of C1-2, an occipitocervical fusion, a transoral approach, ventral and dorsal approaches to the subaxial cervical spine, and various combinations of these approaches. With the advent of spinal instrumentation techniques, surgeons have a wealth of different treatment options available to treat rheumatoid arthritis patients. In addition, nonoperative modalities including traction and halo-vest immobilization, as well as adjuvant medical therapies such as steroids, nonsteroidal anti-inflammatory drugs, penicillamine, and methotrexate, enter into the decision-making process.

Most rheumatoid arthritis patients never develop spinal instability and never require spine surgery. As previously described, large studies of patients from rheumatology clinics have demonstrated that the clinical course of rheumatoid arthritis is usually benign. However, the natural history of the disease is that a certain proportion of affected patients eventually require surgery. Pellicci et al. followed 106 patients for more than 5 years and found that diligent use of a supportive collar does not alter the natural history of the disease.[18] Similarly, More and Sen have stated that the realistic treatment goals achieved by conservative measures are pain abatement and reduction of inflammation. The natural history of the disease is not altered.[19] Pellicci's study also documented that rheumatoid involvement of the cervical spine does not appear to shorten life expectancy.[18] These findings are most likely a result of the small number of rheumatoid arthritis patients who develop cervical myelopathy. When cervical myelopathy is established, the natural history without surgical intervention is grave.[2] In addition, the development of a subaxial subluxation or a vertical subluxation in a patient with a preexisting atlantoaxial subluxation has been found to be a poor prognostic sign.[18] The factors that influence the treatment of upper cervical lesions in rheumatoid arthritis are reducibility of the abnormality with traction, the type of compressive lesion (whether of a bony or a soft tissue component), and the direction and mechanics of the spinal cord or brainstem compression.[51]

There is a general agreement among the majority of neurologic and orthopaedic surgeons that intractable pain, progressive neurologic deficit, and the presence of myelopathy are indications for surgical intervention. On the other hand, there is considerable disagreement over surgery for the "risk of instability," which is usually construed by a variety of criteria analyzing radiographic imaging studies of the upper cervical spine.

With appropriate operative indications, the treatment of an isolated atlantoaxial subluxation is a dorsal C1-2 fusion. In these cases, the occiput should not be incorporated into the fusion because the higher complication rate, lower fusion rate, and morbidity associated with the decreased range of neck motion all mitigate against this procedure.

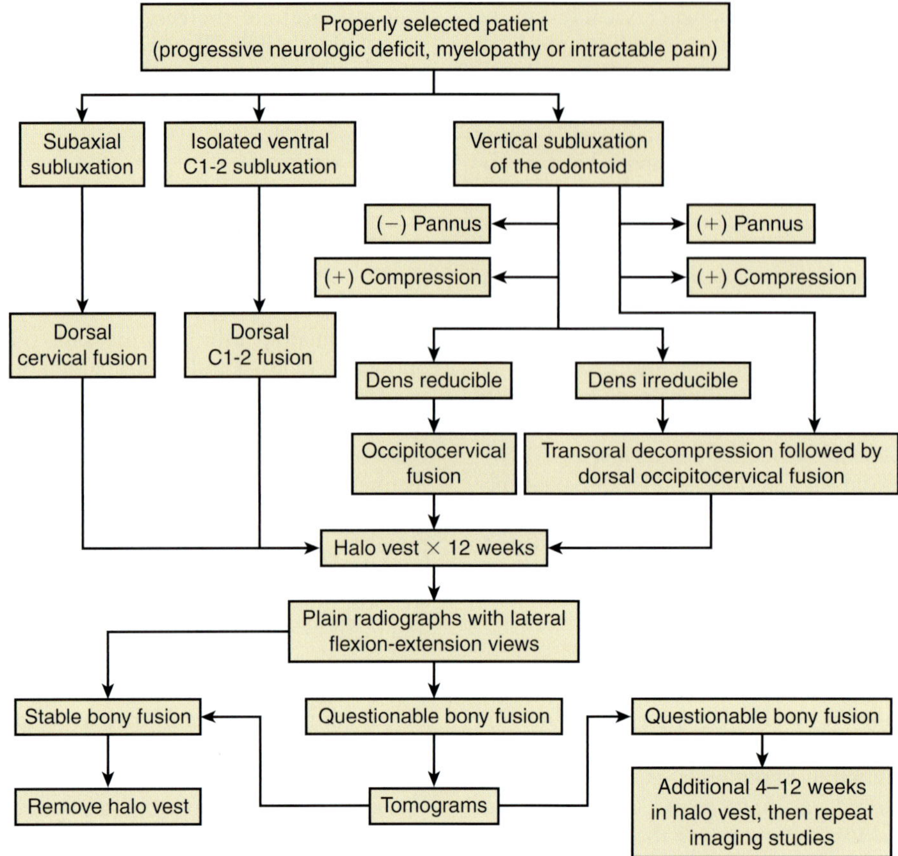

FIGURE 86-6. Algorithm for care of the patient with rheumatoid arthritis.

If vertical subluxation of the dens is present, or a combination of a vertical subluxation with an atlantoaxial subluxation is present, an occipitocervical fusion may be required. To determine whether an occipitocervical fusion alone is adequate, or a ventral decompression is necessary, cervical traction, in addition to the dorsal stabilization, may be used to determine whether the subluxation is reducible.[15,17,46] Transoral decompression may also be deemed necessary if significant soft tissue rheumatoid granulation—that is, a rheumatoid pannus—is responsible for compression of the spinal cord.[65]

Viewpoints in the management of vertical subluxation of the dens are divergent, as has been shown in numerous studies published by Menezes et al.[16,17,51] and Crockard et al.[21,54,65] Menezes et al. maintain that it is the reducibility of a vertical subluxation that is the primary determinant of whether a transoral decompression is necessary. They determined that in 80% of their patients, an adequate reduction of the vertical subluxation could be achieved with traction and, therefore, only a dorsal occipital cervical fusion was necessary. Despite the reducibility, all 45 patients in this series were symptomatic because of compression of the cervicomedullary junction. In addition, these authors have stated that decompression of the cervicomedullary junction, via a transoral approach, is necessary for irreducible lesions. They found that all patients with greater than 20 mm of penetration of the dens through the foramen magnum were unable to have their deformity reduced with cervical traction and required a transoral decompression.[17] Dickman et al. have also recommended a transoral decompressive procedure for irreducible craniovertebral junction compression.[46] Both Menezes et al. and Dickman et al. recommend that the ventral decompressive surgery should be performed first and subsequent dorsal internal fixation later.[17,46] Transoral surgery involves the resection of the dens, the ventral arch of the atlas, the ventral longitudinal ligament, the apical ligament, the alar ligament, the transverse atlantal ligament, and the tectorial membrane.[46] As such, the spine is destabilized after this procedure, necessitating a dorsal fusion. The advantages of the transoral approach to irreducible craniovertebral junction pathology have been described by Menezes and van Gilder. These include performing surgery in an avascular midline plane, accessibility to both bony and soft tissue pathology, and performing surgery with the patient's head in an extended position (which decreases brainstem angulation and compression during the surgery). This approach allows for exposure from the lower half of the clivus to the C2-3 interspace. These authors emphasized the need for a tracheotomy in all transoral surgeries.[51]

Crockard et al. have stressed the contribution of a ventral compressive agent, the rheumatoid pannus, to be as important as any bony deformity in the development of spinal cord compression.[54] Crockard and Grob stated that the overall results of dorsal cervical surgery alone for patients with cervical myelopathy have been unsatisfactory, with excessively high morbidity and mortality rates.[21] For patients with an established myelopathy in whom the pannus has been demonstrated to contribute to the cervicomedullary junction compression, Crockard performs a transoral decompression with a dorsal occipitocervical fusion in a single one-stage operation with the patient in the lateral position. Traditional skull traction is not used at any stage, but the head is held in the Mayfield retractor with a tilt table, which, in effect, functions like skull traction. In Crockard's experience, this one-stage procedure has led to fewer complications and better long-term results than either a two-stage operation or a dorsal fixation procedure alone.[54] Performing both operations at a single sitting avoids the discomfort of prolonged bed rest and the complications associated with prolonged immobilization. In most patients, Crockard has not found it necessary to perform a tracheotomy.[21,54,65]

As with the operative approaches to vertical subluxations, treatment of subaxial subluxations of the cervical spine is varied. Simpson et al. have stated that surgery for subaxial subluxations involves a dorsal fusion and that the role of ventral surgery is unclear in this condition.[6] Santavirta et al. have indicated that reduction of the bony subluxation with a fusion is not adequate in patients with spinal cord compression from subaxial subluxation because rheumatoid granulation tissue in the sublaminar space may continue to compress the neural elements. Therefore, they recommend laminectomy in addition to this fusion procedure.[3] King has stated that a dorsal decompression may relieve the spinal cord compression. It may also, however, worsen spinal instability.[41] At present, the optimal surgical treatment for subaxial subluxation of the rheumatoid cervical spine is unclear. Further experience with the various ventral and dorsal techniques is necessary to clearly delineate which procedure is most advantageous.

Surgical Techniques

Once it has been determined that a patient with rheumatoid arthritis requires a surgical procedure, the ideal operation must be chosen carefully. The most frequent problem in this regard is deciding whether to incorporate the occiput into an upper cervical fusion. Including the occiput into an upper cervical fusion leads to a lower fusion rate and increased morbidity with respect to neck motion. However, it is frequently necessary to arrest the progression of a vertical subluxation of the odontoid. Other operative considerations that are less frequently problematic include the decision of whether to extend the fusion into the subaxial cervical spine when subluxations are present in that region.

It must be remembered that rheumatoid arthritis is a benign disease. As such, a stable arthrodesis is necessary for long-term success in the patient with rheumatoid arthritis. All instrumentation constructs fatigue with time, and only a stable bony fusion provides satisfactory long-term results.

The need for bone grafting in all patients has been challenged. Although it is uniformly agreed that young patients and patients with a reasonable prospect for long-term survival require grafting, Crockard et al.[21,54] and Moskovich et al.[66] contend that the results of arthrodesis in end-stage rheumatoid arthritis patients are very poor. Therefore, they evaluate each case on an individual basis, and in selected situations, perform a fixation procedure without a supplemental bony fusion. This nonfusion approach has not been used by the authors of this chapter.

C1-2 Stabilization

C1-2 stabilization and fusion procedures have been performed since the early 20th century. Techniques have been established, and many modifications of these techniques have been proposed. As new techniques are developed, they must be compared to time-honored, successful procedures that are currently in use. In addition, improved fusion rates and acceptably low complication rates are necessary before a new surgical procedure can be advocated.

Dorsal Techniques

Wire and Cable Fixation

In 1910, Mixter and Osgood described a patient with atlantoaxial instability secondary to a nonunion of an odontoid fracture. They successfully treated this fracture by fixing the dorsal arch of the atlas to the spinous process of the axis using a stout, braided silk thread that had been soaked in tincture of benzoin. This case report represented the first documented C1-2 stabilization procedure.[67] Although not mentioned in the report by Mixter and Osgood, use of bone graft materials to promote a long-term stable bony fusion of the axis and the atlas was soon recognized to be a necessary portion of any upper cervical spine stabilization procedure.

Dorsal wiring methods of C1-2 stabilization require that the dorsal elements be intact. Therefore, any fractures of either the dorsal arch of C1 or the C2 lamina would be contraindications to this method of fixation. Additionally, if there is need for dorsal decompression at these levels, wiring methods cannot be used.

Gallie-Type Fusion

Axial rotation is the major motion that occurs at the C1-2 level. Although this motion is a movement that is clinically important to control, translation is the main pathologic movement at the C1-2 level.[45] Gallie, in 1939, described a method to prevent the recurrence of cervical subluxation at the C1-2 level. He fastened the two vertebrae together with a fine steel wire passed beneath the dorsal arch of the atlas and around the spinous process of the axis. He stated that the risk of a late recurrence could be eliminated if bone grafts were applied to the construct. Gallie used a tricortical bone graft in an onlay fashion.[44] Dickman et al. have described a modification of a Gallie-type C1-2 fusion. In their modification, they interpose a bicortical iliac graft between the dorsal arch of C1 and the lamina of C2.[68] This construct attempts to compress the bone graft between the two bony surfaces of the dorsal elements in an attempt to increase the fusion rate (Fig. 86-7); this type of construct has higher rotational stability as compared with Gallie's original technique.[69]

Brooks-Jenkins Fusion

The next major modification to the Gallie-type C1-2 fusion procedure was proposed by Brooks and Jenkins in 1978. They described a wedge compression arthrodesis of the atlantoaxial joint that was performed by placing sublaminar wires beneath the lamina of C2 and the dorsal arch of C1 bilaterally. Separate bone grafts were placed on each side of the midline and were secured separately. The authors stated that the procedure was rarely indicated in patients with long-standing rheumatoid arthritis or in patients with severe osteopenia. Despite this warning, Brooks-type fusions have been performed frequently for rheumatoid arthritis (Figs. 86-8 to 86-11).[70]

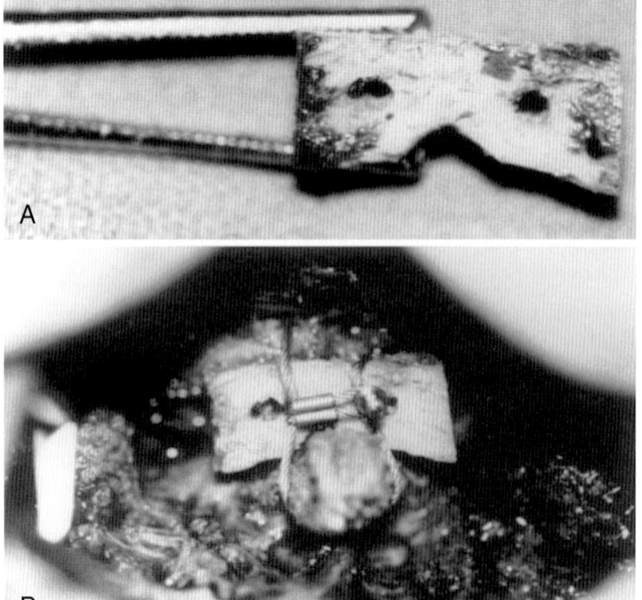

FIGURE 86-7. **A,** Bicortical bone graft harvested from the iliac crest to be interposed between the arch of the atlas and the spinous process of the axis. Holes in the graft allow for the cables to pass through and add further stability to the construct. **B,** A modified Gallie construct using an autogenous bicortical iliac crest graft that is compressed between the dorsal elements of the atlas and the axis with a Songer cable. The free ends of the cable exit the construct through the holes in the graft where they are secured.

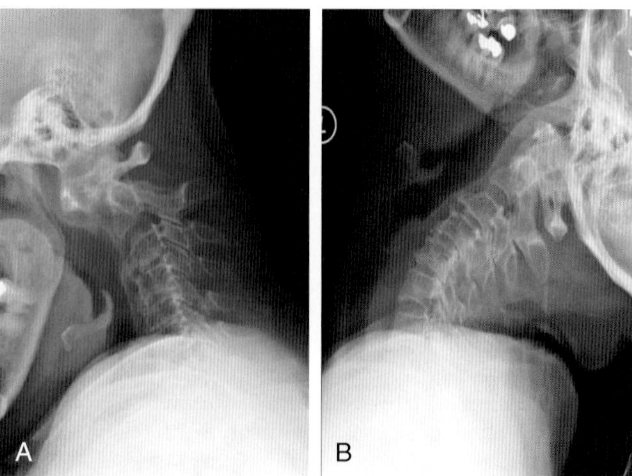

FIGURE 86-8. Preoperative lateral cervical spine radiographs, flexion (**A**) and extension (**B**) views. The atlantodental interval was 19 mm in flexion and 6 mm in extension, signifying significant dynamic instability.

Halifax Interlaminar Clamp

The dangers inherent in both the Brooks-type and the Gallie-type fusions are the necessity to pass the wire beneath the dorsal elements of the upper cervical spine. In doing so, compression from a ventrally located pannus can actually be increased and can lead to neurologic worsening. In an attempt to avoid this complication, techniques were developed that attempted to avoid the need to pass a sublaminar wire. In 1984, Holness et al.[71] reported the use of an interlaminar clamp. This device was originally developed in Halifax, Nova Scotia, Canada, and is commonly referred to as the Halifax clamp. The Halifax clamp involves the bilateral placement of hooks over the dorsal arch of C1 and under the lamina of C2, which are held together by a screw. In their original description, Holness et al. did not advocate routine bone grafting. They did, however, endorse bone grafting in rheumatoid arthritis patients. The Halifax clamp provided numerous advantages, including a decreased risk of dural penetration, a decreased risk of neurologic injury, ease of

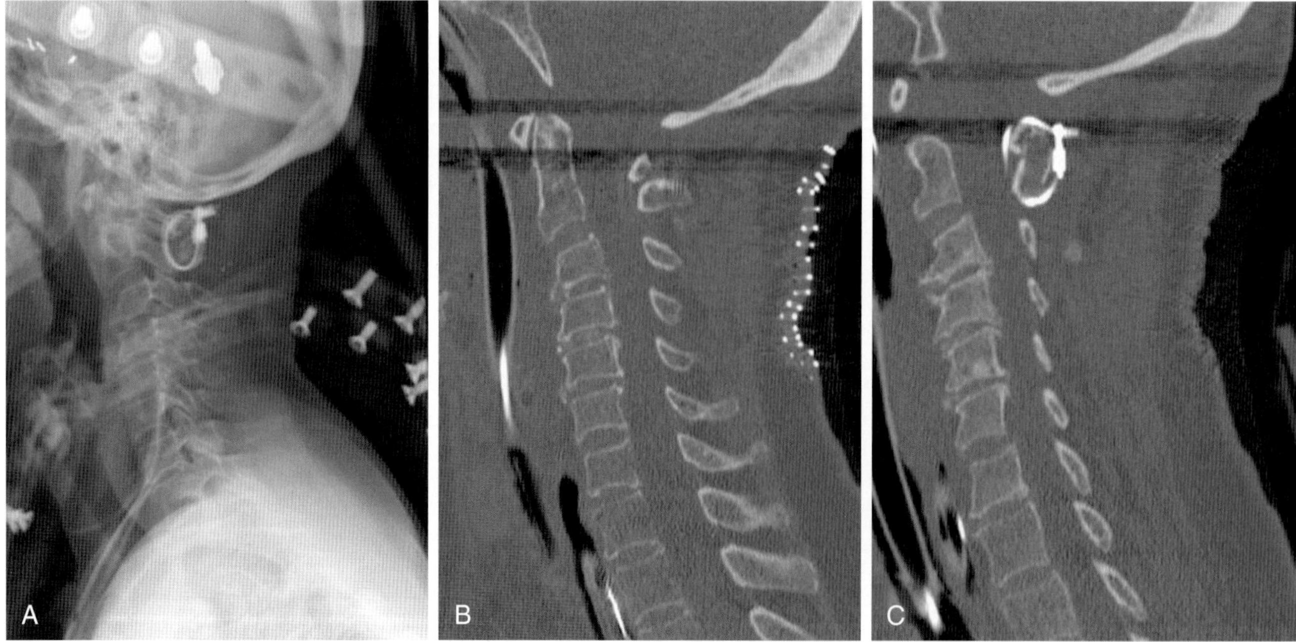

FIGURE 86-9. Postoperative imaging after Brooks-type fusion shows reduction of atlantodental interval to 1.5 mm. **A,** Lateral cervical spine radiograph. **B,** Sagittal reconstruction of CT scan, midsagittal plane. **C,** Sagittal reconstruction of CT scan, parasagittal section through the Brooks-Gallie fusion.

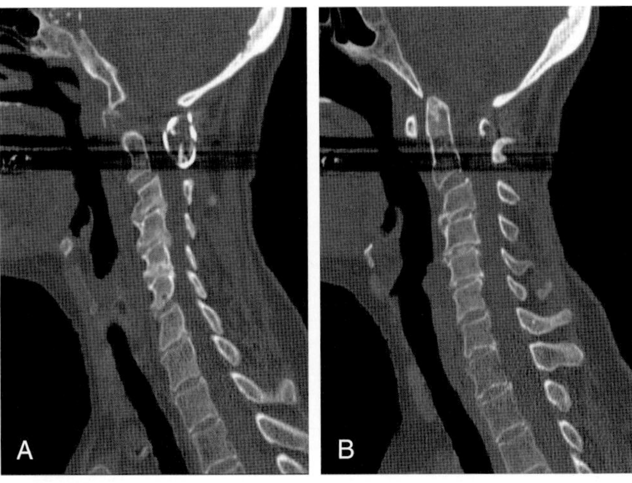

FIGURE 86-10. CT scans of the cervical spine (sagittal reconstructions) taken 6 months after initial C1-2 fusion, showing interval development of vertical subluxation of the odontoid process through the foramen magnum. **A,** Parasagittal section; **B,** midsagittal section.

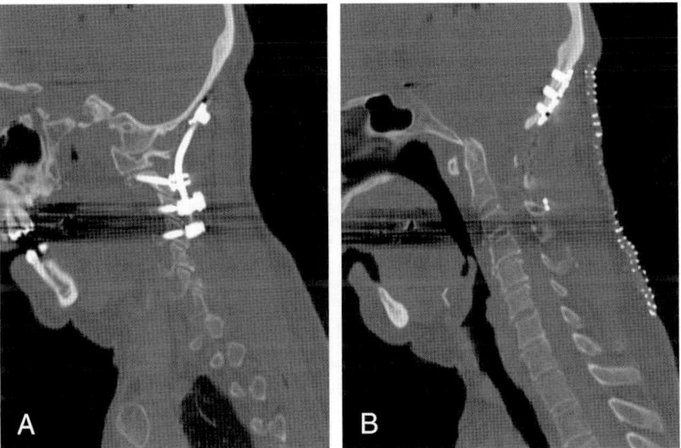

FIGURE 86-11. CT scans of the cervical spine (sagittal reconstructions) in the patient from Figure 86-10 after occipitocervical fusion. **A,** Parasagittal section; **B,** midsagittal section.

use, elimination of wire cutout in osteoporotic bone, and more recently, the development of MRI-compatible clamps to allow for better postoperative imaging.[71] The motion for which the Halifax clamp is particularly suited is the resistance of flexion.[20] In rheumatoid C1-2 ventral subluxation, rotation is the motion that must be controlled, and Halifax clamps do not control rotational movement well. As such, rotational instability can occur, and this can lead to failure.[20,72]

Sonntag described a modification to the Gallie technique providing improved rotational stability without a second sublaminar cable at C2.[68] In the Sonntag technique, a sublaminar cable is passed under the dorsal arch of C1 from caudal to rostral. Next, an iliac crest graft is fashioned in an H configuration and placed between the dorsal arch of C1 and the C2 spinous process. The loop of the cable is then brought over the bone graft and fixed to the C2 spinous process. Sonntag has reported 97% fusion rates using this technique when using a halo vest for 3 months postoperatively and a hard collar for 2 to 3 months thereafter. The use of multistranded cables has reduced the risk of sublaminar passage; however, stand-alone cable fixation is rarely used in modern C1-2 fixation.

Screw Fixation

Transarticular Screw

The optimal mechanical construct to provide internal fixation of the C1-2 segment should consist of a three-point fixation.[21,47] In 1979, Jeanneret and Magerl described the technique of transarticular screw fixation for odontoid fractures with instability.[73] This technique is applicable in reducible subluxations of C1 on C2 and in patients with dorsal element fractures or where a decompressive laminectomy is indicated. This technique limits rotational movement at the atlantoaxial joint (Fig. 86-12).

To avoid vertebral artery injury, it is imperative to have detailed knowledge of its course within the particular patient. Thin-cut CT scans with multiplanar reconstructions are often adequate to identify anomalous vertebral artery location. There is a 19% reported incidence of at least one vertebral artery being in an anomalous location, which would preclude placement of a transarticular screw.[74]

The operation is performed with exposure of the dorsal elements of C1, C2, and the inferior facet of C2 through a midline incision. The dissection is then further carried out to identify the superior border of the C2 lamina and the dorsal and medial surfaces of the pedicle/pars complex. The entry point is selected in the medial half of the inferior facet of C2. A Penfield instrument is placed against the medial surface of the pedicle to provide tactile feedback. Using fluoroscopic guidance, a tract is drilled through the C1-2 facet joint, into the lateral mass of C1 at the dorsal margin of the anterior

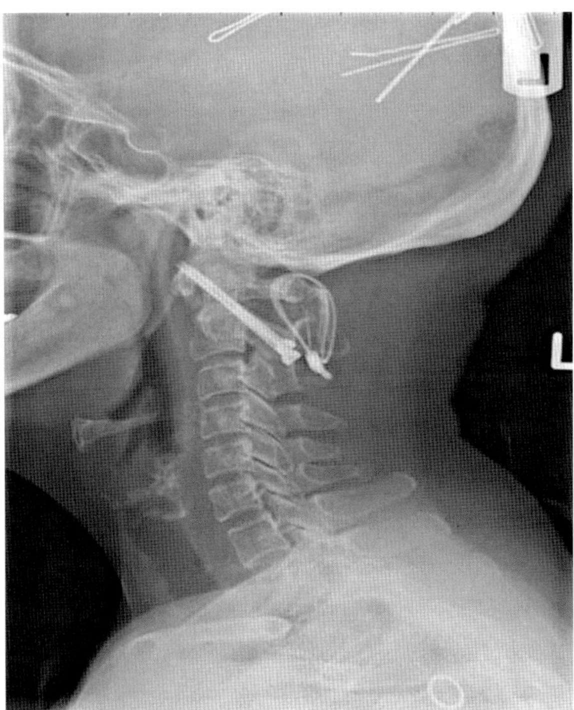

FIGURE 86-12. Lateral radiograph of cervical spine showing posterior C1-2 transarticular screws along with modified Gallie-type construct.

tubercle. After tapping with a 3.5-mm tap, a fully threaded cortical screw is placed through this tract.

Pars and Pedicle Screw

C2 pars screw placement is similar to that of the dorsal transarticular screw placement. The difference in the technique is that the pars screw does not enter into the C1-2 facet joint, making it a significantly shorter screw length (Fig. 86-13). This is typically combined with individual lateral mass screws at C1 connected with dorsal rods. The biomechanical strength of a C1 lateral mass–C2 pars screw has been shown to be comparable to that of the C1-2 transarticular screw.[75-77]

Goel and Laheri described the techniques of C1-2 fixation using C1 lateral mass screws and C2 pedicle screws in 1994.[78] Harms and Melcher modified the techniques using polyaxial screws and rods.[79] The biomechanical strength of this type of construct has been shown to be superior to both C1-2 transarticular screws and C2 pars screws in terms of both insertional torque and pull-out strength.[76] Other advantages of this technique are that (1) anatomic alignment of the C1-2 complex is not necessary prior to instrumentation and that (2) dorsal decompression with laminectomy may be performed, unlike with wiring/clamping techniques. The technique of placing C1 lateral mass screws involves exposing the lateral mass of C1 and the C2 nerve root. The C2 nerve root is protected by retracting it inferiorly. The entry point is the center of the lateral mass and the junction of the lateral mass with the C1 arch. Using fluoroscopic guidance, drilling is started 10 to 15 degrees medially and continues to the posterior border of the anterior tubercle of C1. The trajectory for the C2 pedicle screw is different from that of the C2 pars screw. The entry point for the screw is at a point lateral to the superior margin of the C2 lamina into the superior portion of the C2 pars. The trajectory for drilling the C2 pedicle is 20 degrees superior and 15 to 25 degrees medial from this entry point. The potential risks of the C2 pedicle screw are similar to those of the C1-2 transarticular screw, although the risk of damage to the vertebral artery is somewhat less.[20,80]

C2 Translaminar Screws

Wright described the placement of translaminar screws to stabilize the C1-2 complex in 2003.[81,82] The major advantage of this technique is the decreased risk of damage to the vertebral arteries that exists with the other types of screw fixation described previously. In cases of high-riding vertebral arteries or failed C2 pedicle screw fixation, C2 translaminar screws are a viable option. The screws are placed by first identifying the spinous process, laminae, and lateral masses of C2, as well as the lateral masses of C1. A cortical window is created at the junction of the spinous process and lamina. A hand drill is then used to drill out the contralateral lamina, through which the screw will then be placed. It is advisable to first drill out the smaller lamina because placement of the first screw limits the trajectory of the second.

Biomechanical testing has shown translaminar screws to be stronger in both pull-out strength and insertional torque than C2 pars screws.[77] Complications of this technique include cortical breaching, possibly resulting in cerebrospinal fluid leakage or spinal cord injury. Overall, C2 translaminar screw placement is somewhat safer than placement of other types of screws because the length of the screw is visible within the surgical field.

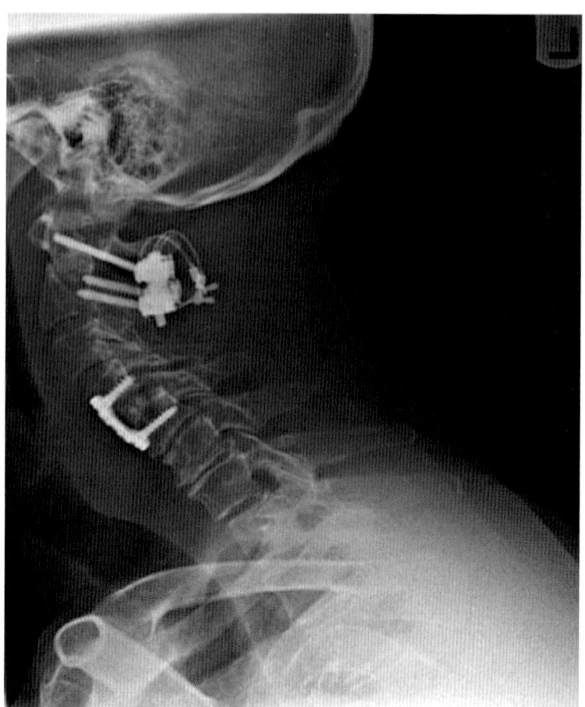

FIGURE 86-13. Lateral radiograph of cervical spine showing fusion construct with C1 lateral mass screws and C2 pars screws. The construct is bolstered with sublaminar wires.

Ventral C1-2 Transarticular Screw

Barbour first described ventral transarticular screw fixation in 1971, but the technique never gained popularity.[83] Koller et al. revisited the feasibility of the procedure in 2006.[84] This is generally used as a salvage procedure in cases of failed dorsal fusion operations. As with dorsal transarticular screws, motion at C1-2 is essentially eliminated.

The use of anteroposterior and lateral fluoroscopic guidance is necessary for placement of ventral transarticular screws. A high ventrolateral retropharyngeal approach is used to expose C2. A K-wire is inserted slightly off the midsagittal line on the inferior aspect of the pinafore of the C2 body. The angle of insertion is toward the lateral rim of C1 but medial to the medial cortical border of the isthmus of C2 in the anteroposterior plane. In the lateral plane, the angle is toward the dorsal border of the vertebral body of C2 via the superior dorsal margin of the Harris ring of C2. A cannulated drill is then used to create the tract with subsequent screw placement using a lag screw.

As with dorsal transarticular screws, it is imperative to have a detailed understanding of the anatomy of the vertebral arteries in this region. Thin-cut multiplanar CT scans are useful in preoperative planning. However, the increasing popularity of CT angiography may help further decrease the risk to the vertebral arteries during this procedure.

The proper screw length and trajectory are necessary to prevent injury to the atlanto-occipital joint. Other potential complications include screw cutout if the entry point is too lateral or not on the inferior border of the vertebral body.

Occipitocervical Fusion

When vertical subluxation of the dens is present, with or without a concurrent atlantoaxial subluxation, an atlantoaxial fusion is not adequate treatment. In these cases, it is necessary to extend the fusion to include the occiput. Inclusion of the occiput in the fusion mass significantly decreases head and neck motion, and as a result, it should not be performed in cases with an isolated ventral atlantoaxial subluxation.

In 1987, Wertheim and Bohlman described a technique for occipitocervical fusion using rigid wiring of the occiput through the external occipital protuberance to the cervical spine by use of large iliac crest bone grafts. This technique avoided the need to penetrate both tables of the skull, allowed for immediate rigid internal fixation, permitted early patient mobilization, and resulted in a successful fusion in all 13 patients in their study. Of note, eight of these patients had rheumatoid arthritis.[85] Modifications of the technique of Wertheim and Bohlman include placement of occipital bur holes to secure the occipital portion of the fusion.[86,87] In addition, Stambough et al. described a technique for occipitocervical fusion in osteopenic rheumatoid arthritis patients using bone in combination with polymethylmethacrylate (PMMA). The authors believed that this technique provided immediate stability and optimized the chances for long-term bony stability.[88] Fusion constructs using PMMA for benign disease are, however, prone to failure because the PMMA inhibits fusion.

In 1986, Ransford et al. described a method of occipitocervical stabilization with an anatomically contoured steel loop secured by occipital and sublaminar wires. This rigid dorsal internal fixation system provides immediate stabilization at the craniocervical junction. The authors stated that the loop system provided the necessary stability to allow the patient to mobilize without major external support. The use of this system was originally described in patients after transoral decompressive surgeries. It has, however, been subsequently widely used for primary occipitocervical surgical stabilizations.[89] A similar modification of this technique incorporates a malleable rod and segmental wiring. This technique, described by Fehlings et al., also provides immediate rigid stabilization, and the authors have stated that it avoids the need for an external orthosis.[55]

Rogers et al. have described a useful clinical tool to help determine which surgical techniques are safest. They have stated that although motor examination may be difficult in patients with severe rheumatoid arthritis, testing of sensation remains relatively straightforward. A loss of proprioception suggests a severe dorsal compressive component, usually at the occipitocervical junction, and passage of sublaminar wires in these cases may be hazardous and may result in neurologic morbidity.[90] Grob et al. described a technique for occipitocervical plating that uses screws into the occiput and the lateral masses in the cervical spine, obviating the need for sublaminar wires. This technique also provides immediate rigid internal fixation and good rotational stability.[91]

Several modifications to the technique of occipital screw placement have been proposed in recent years. Screws can be placed either lateral to the midline or in the midline bony keel.[91,92] Mingsheng et al. reported a method of placing the screws into the diploe paralleling the occipital table.[93] Pait et al. described a technique of placing an "inside-outside" screw by drilling a bur hole and trough in the occipital bone in order to allow for bicortical screw placement while minimizing the risk of dural violation.[87] This technique was reviewed in 21 patients with rheumatoid arthritis; no complications or instrumentation failures were noted in the study.[94]

In a recent review by Winegar et al., several techniques of occipitocervical fusion were compared. Although all methods of fusion were found to have great efficacy, constructs that incorporated rods and screws performed best or near best in all categories studied.[95] It should be noted that there is not adequate inherent stability in any bone-wire or bone-cable constructs, and as a result, external immobilization is advisable whenever these techniques are used. Constructs that incorporate plates and screws or rectangles and cable or wire have greater inherent stability and may diminish the requirements for postoperative external immobilization.

Patients with rheumatoid arthritis and vertical subluxation of the dens, as a general rule, have had long-standing disease and are frequently osteopenic. Thus, it is necessary to evaluate these patients over time to determine the optimal method of fusion and the need for postoperative external support.

Transoral Surgery

In the transoral approach to the odontoid, a midline dorsal pharyngeal incision is made. This allows for exposure of the lower clivus to the level of the C2-3 junction. Depending on the preference of the operating surgeon, splitting the soft palate, performing a tracheotomy, using cervical traction, and using a halo vest postoperatively are all considerations with this surgery. In addition, the transoral decompression can be combined simultaneously with a dorsal cervical stabilization procedure to allow for immediate mobilization of the patient postoperatively.[65] On the other hand, the dorsal stabilization can be performed separately later.[17,46]

Menezes has stated that if the vertical subluxation has caused the dens to penetrate the foramen magnum by greater than 20 mm, an acceptable reduction with prolonged traction cannot be achieved. These patients may require a transoral resection of the dens.[16] In 14 rheumatoid arthritis patients with irreducible vertical subluxation, Menezes and van Gilder found a sequestered odontoid process protruding into the pons intradurally in four cases.[51]

The specific aspects of the surgical procedure are open to debate. However, there appears to be uniform agreement among investigators experienced in this technique that the ventral transoral decompression should precede the dorsal cervical stabilization.[17,46] Postoperative swallowing difficulty is not uncommon after transoral surgery, although the rate is lessened when the procedure is performed without splitting the soft palate.[96]

Subaxial Cervical, Thoracic, and Lumbar Surgery

In cases of subaxial subluxations of the cervical spine, there is not adequate proof that a ventral, dorsal, or combined ventral and dorsal approach is the optimal treatment. Likewise, lesions affecting the thoracic or lumbar spine are so rare that specific treatments must be individualized on a case-by-case basis. Thus, no attempt will be made in this section to analyze the limited information available on these lesions.

Postoperative External Orthoses

There is no consensus in the orthopaedic and neurosurgical literature regarding the optimal type of external orthosis to be used after an upper cervical stabilization procedure. Opinion ranges from the need for postoperative halo vest immobilization for a minimum of 12 weeks, followed by 4 to 8 weeks additional time if flexion-extension views do not show a stable fusion,[41] to no need for any external orthosis postoperatively.[89] The majority of opinions fall into three categories: routine use of the halo vest postoperatively[2,8,41,53,68,88]; routine use of an external orthosis other than the halo vest such as a Minerva jacket, Philadelphia collar, or sternal occipital mandibular immobilizer (SOMI) brace*; and use of a halo vest when fixation is deemed tenuous with a lesser device used when the fixation is considered more secure.[18,28,46,55,85,86]

This lack of agreement regarding the use of external orthoses postoperatively may be the result of varied new surgical procedures currently being developed. In the Magerl transarticular screw fixation of C1-2, if a bone graft is incorporated dorsally, a true three-point fixation can be achieved.[99] Similarly, some occipitocervical fusion techniques also allow for a three-point fixation and thus may eliminate the need for a halo vest.[66,89,100] Long-term follow-up results are needed to determine whether the benefit of improved patient comfort postoperatively in a lesser orthosis outweighs the risk of an inferior fusion rate if the external support is inadequate. The need for the rigid support of a halo vest orthosis may be unnecessary in patients who are able to have a true three-point fixation internally. It should be noted that halo vests have a higher complication rate in elderly patients.[101]

Postoperative Results

Surgery on the rheumatoid cervical spine is indicated for intractable pain, myelopathy, or progressive neurologic deficit. The postoperative results can thus be categorized into neurologic results and bony fusion results. A solid bony arthrodesis is necessary for relief of intractable pain present preoperatively. Likewise, an adequate decompression is necessary for stabilization or improvement of neurologic status postoperatively. Finally, because much of the surgery for rheumatoid arthritis is performed at the occipitocervical junction, postoperative morbidity from systemic problems and postoperative mortality rates must be measured.

Neurologic Outcome

Boden et al. found that the severity of the neurologic deficit present preoperatively was an accurate predictor of the postoperative neurologic status. They also stated that the duration of the neurologic deficit preoperatively did not affect the prognosis for neurologic recovery after the operation.[32] Hultquist et al. found that most of their patients had relief of their pain and amelioration of their neurologic symptoms; however, there was little evidence of improved overall functional capacity. In spite of this, most of their patients expressed great satisfaction in being pain-free postoperatively.[10]

Once again, there is considerable discrepancy in the results of neurologic outcome among reported series. In the review by Menezes et al., all 45 patients with vertical subluxation of the odontoid had an improvement in their functional neurologic grade and amelioration of their neurologic dysfunction.[17] On the other hand, Chan et al. found that no patient with a preoperative myelopathy improved neurologically in the postoperative period.[53]

The lack of improvement in some published series once a myelopathy has been established has led some investigators to recommend that early operative stabilization be considered before the onset of neurologic deficit, when radiographic instability is present. Although all patients in their series had evidence of a neurologic deficit before surgery, Boden et al. have recommended that surgery be performed in neurologically intact patients who have a vertical subluxation of the dens compounding a marked atlantoaxial subluxation.[32] In pain-free neurologically intact patients with severe radiographic abnormalities, the decision to intervene depends on both accurate serial neurologic examinations and accurate serial radiographic imaging studies.

Fusion Outcome

A surgical success with a dorsal cervical fusion operation requires that a stable bony arthrodesis be achieved. A nonunion, also termed *pseudarthrosis*, is more likely to occur in rheumatoid arthritis patients because of the well-documented problems of osteoporosis or osteopenia that occur in these patients. In addition, many of these patients have been on long-term corticosteroid therapy that is also known to inhibit fusion rates.

Moskovich and Crockard have defined the requirements for considering a solid dorsal atlantoaxial fusion a success: lateral flexion and extension radiographs that show no motion and evidence of trabecular bone in continuity between the dorsal elements and the graft.[20] In cases of doubt, plain tomograms or multiplanar CT scan reconstructed images are excellent for determining continuity of the fusion. Chan et al. agreed with this definition, and in addition, they defined a fibrous union as the presence of less than 2 mm of motion on flexion-extension radiographs.[53] Dickman et al. have stressed that patients with fibrous unions must be followed closely for the signs of delayed instability or wire breakage.[68]

In rheumatoid arthritis patients, radiographic determination of an occipitocervical fusion may be difficult. Moskovich et al. have reviewed a series of 152 rheumatoid arthritis patients who underwent occipitocervical stabilization procedures. In 80% of patients, no bone grafting was used to augment the stabilization procedure with a contoured steel loop. To evaluate the occipitocervical complex for postoperative stability, these authors measured the angle between the occiput and the upper cervical vertebrae. The difference in the angle between flexion and extension radiographs provides an indication of stability. This method allows one to determine postoperative stability regardless of whether a bone graft is used to supplement the stabilization procedure.[66]

Variability in the reporting of fusion rates postoperatively in rheumatoid arthritis patients may be a result of discrepancies about whether a given author classifies patients with fibrous union along with the successful bony fusion patients or whether patients with fibrous union are classified along

*See references 17, 20, 21, 66, 70, 72, 73, 89, 97, and 98.

with the nonunion, or pseudarthrosis, patients. When pseudarthrosis occurs after atlantoaxial fusions, it is most common between the dorsal bone graft and the ring of C1.[26,102] The reasons for nonunion at this location include the high cortex-to-medulla ratio of the dorsal ring of C1, which is relatively sclerotic,[20] and frequent erosion of the dorsal arch of C1 in patients with rheumatoid arthritis.[6] In subaxial subluxations, failure of a ventral fusion may be a result of angulation, pseudarthrosis, or collapse of the graft in the bone graft bed.[7] Santavirta et al. believed that ventral procedures for subaxial subluxation often fail because of vertebral body osteoporosis, and they stated that acrylic cement and metal rods are of little use as stabilizers in rheumatoid cervical spines.[13]

Fusion rates vary between 50% to 100% in reported series of atlantoaxial fusions and occipitocervical fusions. Menezes et al. have stated that a stable bony fusion occurred in 100% of their 45 patients with fusion for vertical subluxation of the odontoid.[17] Similarly, all seven rheumatoid arthritis patients of Dickman et al. developed stable osseous unions with a bicortical iliac bone graft in a modified Gallie-type fusion.[68] Tricortical iliac crest bone grafts in dorsal atlantoaxial fusions are associated with a higher rate of fibrous union.[68,103] Fusion rates from 75% to 90% have been reported with Halifax interlaminar clamps,[20,72] a modified Gallie approach,[41,68] and the transarticular screw fixation technique of Magerl.[12,90] Fusion rates between 50% and 75% have been reported with traditional Gallie fusions[13] and after combined transoral and dorsal fusion operations for vertical subluxation of the odontoid.[46]

Many series of upper cervical fusions include rheumatoid patients along with young, healthy trauma patients. As a general rule, victims of trauma have better bone stock and better fusion rates postoperatively when compared with rheumatoid arthritis patients. As previously stated, different external orthoses were used to supplement the internal stabilization procedures in these series, and this can also affect fusion rates.

Mortality

Mortality in rheumatoid arthritis patients varies greatly in reported series. Surgical series must be compared to the natural history of rheumatoid arthritis in patients never subjected to surgical procedures. In a 15-year prospective follow-up study of patients with new-onset rheumatoid arthritis, Corbett et al.[104] found only a small increase in mortality in rheumatoid arthritis patients compared with the general population over the same 15-year period.[105] They found an increased mortality at 15 years in rheumatoid arthritis patients with concurrent heart disease. Males were overrepresented in this study.[104]

Davis and Markley reported the first case of an autopsy-proven death in a rheumatoid arthritis patient secondary to compression of the medulla by herniation of the odontoid process through the foramen magnum.[106] This was followed by two separate case reports by Martel and Abell[102] of autopsy-proven sudden death secondary to atlantoaxial subluxation. As the danger of sudden death was more widely reported, it became apparent that spinal cord damage may not always have been recognized as a cause of death in rheumatoid arthritis patient fatalities in the past. Smith et al. stated that spinal cord involvement may have been responsible for more deaths than had previously been apparent.[14]

Reported mortality rates in the first month postoperatively have varied between 4% and 10%.[11,51,53,66] Many deaths have been attributed to postoperative myocardial infarction; however, it is possible that spinal cord compression may contribute to these deaths. Santavirta et al., while operating on patients with severe rheumatoid arthritis, found that 50% of these patients died over a 10-year follow-up period postoperatively. These authors estimated that the average age of death of these patients was approximately the same as that of other patients with equally severe rheumatoid arthritis.[13] Like the nonsurgical long-term follow-up study of Corbett et al., [104] Santavirta et al. reported a significantly increased rate of death postoperatively when cardiac disease was also present.[13]

The natural history of rheumatoid arthritis has demonstrated that the disease will be present for 15 to 20 years before the need for surgical correction of the abnormalities in the cervical spine. At the time of surgery, these patients are often severely debilitated from the general disease process. Therefore, long-term postoperative mortality must be compared with the mortality of patients with equally severe rheumatoid arthritis who do not require cervical spine operations. The definitive comparative analysis has yet to be completed.

Medical Adjuncts

Patients with long-standing rheumatoid arthritis requiring surgery on the cervical spine have often been treated with glucocorticoid medications for many years. It is well known that these medications exert deleterious effects on bone. Skeletal damage resulting from long-term treatment with supraphysiologic doses of glucocorticoids occur in four ways: inhibition of bone growth, delayed union of fractures, osteoporosis, and osteonecrosis.[107]

Corbett et al. in a 15-year prospective follow-up study of patients with new-onset rheumatoid arthritis, found that long-term use of steroids in rheumatoid arthritis was associated with higher mortality.[104] In addition, Hall et al. have stated that the cumulative dose of steroid is more important with respect to this negative effect than is the daily dose.[100] Santavirta et al. found that patients who had received steroid treatments for greater than 4 years had more fibrous unions and more pseudarthroses in a 10-year follow-up study.[13] Laan et al. found that low-dose prednisone therapy had a deleterious effect on the bone mineral density of postmenopausal women. These postmenopausal patients have an increased risk of developing axial osteopenia and vertebral fractures. A similar bone density loss in men was not demonstrable.[103] In patients with active rheumatoid arthritis, low doses of glucocorticoid can cause marked vertebral trabecular bone loss in the initial month of therapy.[17,103] After cessation of steroid therapy, this bone loss may be partially reversible.[100,108] Papadopoulos et al. found that radiologic progression of atlantoaxial subluxation occurs more rapidly in patients with systemic disease severe enough to require maintenance steroid therapy.[42]

In an attempt to counteract these deleterious effects of glucocorticoids on bone in rheumatoid arthritis patients, prednisone derivatives have been developed. Deflazacort, an oxazolone derivative of prednisone, has been developed and used to reduce the incidence of the catabolic glucocorticoid actions of prednisone and still maintain its beneficial actions. In a randomized double-blind study, deflazacort was found to decrease the amount of corticosteroid-induced osteoporosis.[107]

Another medical adjunct that may be of use is estrogen replacement. In postmenopausal women with rheumatoid arthritis, estrogen replacement is protective with regard to the risk of spinal osteoporosis. Sambrook et al. concluded that estrogen therapy should be considered in postmenopausal women with rheumatoid arthritis who are at risk for osteoporosis.[109]

Additional research is necessary to develop medications that can provide the symptomatic relief of prednisone while eliminating or reducing its harmful side effects on bone in rheumatoid arthritis patients who are predisposed to osteoarthritis by the disease process itself. In a recent review, Klarenbeek et al. concluded that initial treatment for patients diagnosed with rheumatoid arthritis should be with a single disease-modifying antirheumatic drug (DMARD), preferably methotrexate, in combination with a short course of glucocorticoids.[110] Patients that have limited response may then be placed on a tumor necrosis factor-α blocker or placed on a combination of DMARDs (such as sulfasalazine, leflunomide, and hydroxychloroquine).[111,112]

Osteopenia/osteoporosis is a frequently encountered problem in the patient with rheumatoid arthritis. The loss of bone density occurs not only from glucocorticoid use as part of therapy but also from the underlying inflammatory disease.[60,113] Bisphosphonates are currently being studied as useful adjuncts to reduce bony erosion in rheumatoid patients with encouraging preliminary results.[114,115]

Summary

Because the majority of operative interventions on the spine in rheumatoid arthritis patients occur at the C1-2 level, complications must be avoided because there is no effective management for them. Complication avoidance begins with proper patient selection for operative intervention. The authors recommend performing surgery for intractable pain, myelopathy, or progressive neurologic deficit. In the isolated case of an end-stage rheumatoid arthritis patient who has been bed-bound for longer than 3 months, consideration may be given to a nonoperative treatment regimen. However, even with these patients, occasional rewarding results have been achieved surgically. An accurate and thorough history and physical examination, a detailed review of all radiologic imaging studies, and an understanding of the natural history of rheumatoid arthritis of the cervical spine are all necessary. Knowledge of past successes and failures can help optimize results.

Patients with abnormal radiographs in the absence of pain or an abnormal neurologic examination should be followed closely with serial neurologic examinations and radiographic imaging studies. Numerous rheumatologic studies have demonstrated clearly that many of these patients will never require operative intervention and that they may have a life expectancy similar to that of rheumatoid arthritis patients with an equivalent extent of disease with the exception of the spinal involvement.

The radiographic imaging workup can be very extensive. Although this workup is not cost-effective, each of the different imaging modalities provides useful information, both for preoperative planning and for following patients nonoperatively. In a rheumatoid arthritis patient who is suspected of having spinal involvement, the authors routinely obtain plain radiographs, a CT scan, and an MRI study. The plain radiographs allow calculation of the ventral ADI and the dorsal AOI and assessment for any evidence of vertical subluxation of the odontoid. In addition, the subaxial cervical spine can be imaged to look for subluxations. CT scans of the upper cervical spine provide the most accurate bony detail of this region. Identification of the foramen transversaria is best obtained on a CT scan, and this is mandatory if a transarticular C1-2 screw or C2 pars/pedicle screw fixation is contemplated. MRI studies help determine the extent of ventral soft tissue pathology (i.e., rheumatoid pannus) and the extent of spinal cord compression from both the ventral and dorsal directions. MRI is also excellent for screening for abnormalities of the subaxial cervical spine and, if necessary, of the thoracic and lumbar spines also. In cases where MRI cannot be performed, CT myelography should be performed.

A detailed medical evaluation is required for any patient before undergoing surgery. This is best done in conjunction with a rheumatology consultant. When possible, steroids should be tapered or discontinued. This may not be possible in the severely debilitated end-stage rheumatoid arthritis patient with polyarticular disease. In all circumstances, smokers should be strongly advised to quit smoking.

Intraoperative considerations include the routine use of awake fiberoptic intubation. Traction via a halo ring that can later be converted to a halo vest may be preferable to Gardner-Wells traction. Whenever possible, autograft iliac crest is the preferred donor site for fusion operations. In patients with an osteoporotic pelvis who are unable to provide autograft, allograft bone may be used. This may be supplemented with a bone morphogenetic protein preparation; however, this use is not currently approved by the Food and Drug Administration in the United States and its use would be classified as "off-label." Occasionally, one may also consider fixation without a concurrent fusion. It must be remembered that unlike ventral fusion operations in which the bone graft is under compression, dorsal onlay fusions are not under compression. Therefore, the need for long-term rigid immobilization to obtain a stable bony fusion is essential for any dorsal fusion operation. Because these patients are suffering from a benign disease with a potential for long life, PMMA use should be discouraged on rheumatoid arthritis patients.

Following strict operative indications, the operative techniques that the authors recommend are as follows. For an isolated ventral C1-2 subluxation, a modified Gallie operation using bicortical iliac crest graft, advocated by Sonntag and others,[41,68] is used. The numerous other stabilization techniques for isolated C1-2 instability are generally acceptable. An important consideration is that incorporation of the occiput into the fusion construct may increase the risk of a poor result, and this should only be done if clearly indicated. When a vertical subluxation of the dens is present, an occipitocervical fusion with screws into the occipital keel and fixation of the C2 dorsal elements with pars, pedicle, or laminar screws using contoured rods is ideal. These rods can be extended caudally in cases of subaxial subluxation. If the vertical subluxation is irreducible, or if significant ventral pathology causing compression is present, a transoral decompression may be necessary. This transoral decompression should usually be performed before any dorsal surgery. Depending on the patient's physical condition, the ventral surgery may be followed by the dorsal operation in the same sitting, or the dorsal surgery can be performed at a later date. The majority of subaxial subluxations of the cervical spine are best treated with lateral mass fixation. Because thoracic and lumbar spine involvement in rheumatoid arthritis is very rare, the surgical management of these cases must be individualized on a case-by-case basis. As a general rule, ventral pathology should be decompressed and stabilized ventrally and dorsal pathology should be decompressed and stabilized dorsally. The authors routinely use cables over wire or twisted wire constructs. In addition, titanium cables, screws, and rods may be used. It should be recognized, however, that titanium implants are more difficult to work with and fail more easily than traditional steel; also, postoperative neuroimaging studies show significant erosion in the immediate regions of the implant. In addition, bending of the titanium rods at the occipitocervical junction may cause them to weaken.

Postoperatively, the authors recommend using a halo vest for a minimum of 12 weeks. The reasons for halo immobilization include the historically poor fusion results of dorsal cervical fusions in rheumatoid arthritis patients, the osteopenia frequently observed in these patients, and the inability to place the grafts under adequate compressive forces. Therefore, immobilization is the key to obtaining a good bony fusion. After 12 weeks in the halo, plain radiographs are obtained to document a stable osseous arthrodesis. If any question exists, flexion and extension views should be obtained. Multiplanar reconstructed CT scans should be used in cases in which plain radiographs are not able to demonstrate a fusion definitively. If a stable fusion has not been obtained at 12 weeks, the halo should be continued for 4 to 12 additional weeks. Some of the newer techniques such as transarticular C1-2 screw fixation and occipitocervical screw-rod fixation may provide adequate three-point fixation to allow for long-term internal immobilization and thus allow for postoperative external immobilization in a lesser device than a halo.

A nonunion or a pseudarthrosis may require revision surgery. If the initial surgical indication was intractable pain, a postoperative pseudarthrosis may be painful and may require a revision surgery. If surgery was performed for a neurologic deficit, and this has improved, revision surgery may not be necessary. These patients must be followed closely, particularly patients with an asymptomatic fibrous union because some of them develop a delayed bony union. It is preferable to continue using the halo for up to 24 weeks before determining that a nonunion has occurred. In patients with evidence of a successful bony fusion, the external orthosis is removed. It is mandatory to continue to watch these patients closely for development of delayed subaxial subluxations. These subluxations below the level of an upper cervical fusion are not infrequent.

Finally, the majority of surgical procedures on patients with rheumatoid arthritis of the spine are performed in the upper cervical region. Most of the complications arise from difficulties with fusion or instrumentation; these problems are much more common than a worsened neurologic deficit. Several pitfalls can be avoided by operating only when absolutely necessary on patients with intractable pain or a neurologic deficit. In addition, careful preoperative planning allows for use of the appropriate operative procedure that will yield optimal results.

KEY REFERENCES

Cohen MJ, Ezekiel J, Persellin RH: Costovertebral and costotransverse joint involvement in rheumatoid arthritis. *Ann Rheum Dis* 37:473–475, 1978.

Corbett M, Dalton S, Young A, et al: Factors predicting death, survival and functional outcome in a prospective study of early rheumatoid disease over fifteen years. *Br J Rheumatol* 32:717–723, 1993.

Friedman H: Intraspinal rheumatoid nodule causing nerve root compression. *J Neurosurg* 32:689–691, 1970.

Koller H, Kammermeier V, Ulbricht D, et al: Anterior retropharyngeal fixation C1-2 for stabilization of atlantoaxial instabilities: study of feasibility, technical description and preliminary results. *Eur Spine J* 15(9):1326–1338, 2006.

Messina OD, Barreira JC, Zanchetta JR, et al: Effect of low doses of deflazacort vs. prednisone on bone mineral content in premenopausal rheumatoid arthritis. *J Rheumatol* 19:1520–1526, 1992.

REFERENCES

The complete reference list is available online at expert.consult.com.

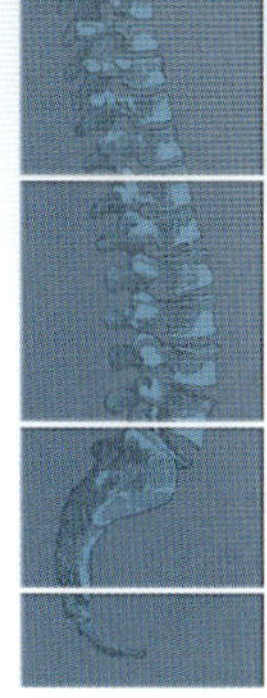

CHAPTER 87

Ankylosing Spondylitis and Related Disorders

C. Philip Toussaint | Russ P. Nockels

Seronegative spondyloarthritis is a group of inflammatory diseases that affect the axial spine, causing progressive pain, deformity, and dysfunction. The common features of seronegative spondyloarthropathies include negative tests for rheumatoid factors, absence of subcutaneous (rheumatoid) nodules, radiologic sacroiliitis with or without spondylitis (often asymmetrical), peripheral inflammatory arthritis, evidence of clinical overlap between group members, and tendency to familial aggregation.[1] Ankylosing spondylitis (AS) is a disabling form of seronegative spondyloarthritis that affects the entheses, where ligaments, tendons, and capsules are attached to the bone. Three processes are observed at the entheses: inflammation, bone erosion, and syndesmophyte (spur) formation. Clinically, this disease is characterized by arthritis of the spine and pelvis, initially manifesting with pain and stiffness and progressing to joint fusion and deformity.[2] Other members of this group of diseases are psoriatic arthritis, reactive arthritis, enteropathic spondylitis, and other undifferentiated forms that do not meet the criteria for a definitive category. Extraskeletal involvement is seen in the iris, myocardium and aorta, lungs, and kidneys.[3-5] Fibrosis of the septum and the atrioventricular bundle may cause conduction defects. Focal necrosis at the root of the aorta often leads to dilation of the aortic ring, causing aortic incompetence. Detailed classification criteria for the entire group of the seronegative spondyloarthropathies have been described by Amor et al.[6] and by the European Spondyloarthropathy Study Group.[7]

Prevalence of seronegative spondyloarthropathies, including AS, are directly correlated with prevalence of HLA-B27 in the population.[8] Over 90% of patients with AS are HLA-B27 positive. The risk of an antigen-positive individual developing AS is under 2%.[9] However, if a patient is antigen-positive and has a family history of AS, the likelihood of developing the clinical syndrome is 20%.[10,11]

The highest prevalence of the disease (4.5%) is found in Canadian Haida Indians, 50% of whose population is HLA-B27 positive. Among Europeans, the prevalence of B27 antigen in the general population ranges between 3% and 13%, and the prevalence of AS is estimated at 0.1% to 0.23%.[1] In the Chinese population, approximately 5% carry the HLA-B27 gene.[2] AS is rare in people of African descent and Australian Aboriginals. Some African populations, such as those in Gambia and Senegal, have a prevalence of HLA-B27 of 3% to 6%, but AS is still rare. Most occurrences of AS in Africans are in HLA-B27-negative individuals.[12] Over 50 subtypes of HLA-B27 have been reported, and each subtype has a different strength of association with AS. Other major histocompatibility complex genes are associated as well with AS and other seronegative spondyloarthritides.[2]

Pathogenesis

The mechanism by which HLA-B27 leads to AS is unknown, but the association of HLA-B27 with AS is one of the strongest genetic associations with any common disease. Other genetic factors are certainly involved, since familial studies have shown that the overall genetic risk of HLA-B27 is less than 50%. Furthermore, first-degree relatives of AS patients are 5 to 16 times more likely to develop AS than are HLA-B27 individuals in the general population.[2]

Population and peptide-specificity analysis of HLA-B27 suggest that it has a pathogenic function related to antigen presentation.[13] Several theories have been proposed to explain these associations, but only one, molecular mimicry, has provided a specific etiologic agent for these diseases. It has been suggested that AS may be triggered by the presentation of certain antigens by enterobacteria. *Klebsiella pneumoniae* shares a sequence of six consecutive amino acids with certain subtypes of the HLA-B27 antigen. Elevated immune responses to *Klebsiella* microbes have been demonstrated in AS patients from 10 different countries. This wide geographic distribution suggests that the same etiologic agent is probably related in producing this condition.[14] Furthermore, HLA-B27 transgenic rats do not appear to develop AS if they are maintained in a germ-free environment.[15] The HLA-B27 antigen may distinguish a group of people whose immune response to such an infectious agent predisposes them to develop spondyloarthropathy through the phenomenon of molecular mimicry.

Pathology

Inflammation occurs initially at the sacroiliac (SI) joint but may also affect entheses, vertebral bodies that are adjacent to intervertebral discs and the peripheral joint synovium.[16]

The lumbar spine is usually involved progressively upward. Skip lesions may occur, especially in women.[17] Hips and shoulders are affected frequently, but peripheral joints are rarely involved.

Although the synovium is the primary site of joint disease in rheumatoid arthritis, the primary site in the spondyloarthritides is less well-defined.[18] It is also thought that enthesitis (inflammation at sites where ligaments, tendons, or joint capsules are attached to bone) is the hallmark of AS and other spondyloarthropathies.[19] Likely, the course of events is more complex than was earlier claimed and may be a combination of enthesitis, synovitis, and subchondral marrow changes, followed by fibrosis, cartilage metaplasia, and ossification; none can thus far be distinguished as a unique hallmark.[20]

In the early stages, chronic inflammatory cells localize to the subchondral bone at the sites of ligament attachment in the SI joints and discovertebral joints, resulting in periarticular osteopenia. Enthesitis at the insertion of the anulus fibrosus on the vertebral bodies in the erosive phase result in square appearance of the vertebrae on lateral radiographs. As the disease progresses, articular cartilage is destroyed by osteoclasts and replaced by granulation tissue, which in radiographs show extensive erosion and destruction of the joint space. In the late stage, granulation tissues are replaced with fibrous tissue that undergoes ossification and completely obliterates the joint, leading to "bamboo" or "poker" spine.[21] Surprisingly, the anterior longitudinal ligament remains free from ossification.

The sequence of events in the synovial joints between the facets, the caudal part of the SI joints, and the peripheral joints resembles rheumatoid arthritis, although the exact target of inflammatory changes and the nature of cellular exudates may differ.[20] Proliferation of synovial tissue and accumulation of plasma cells and lymphocytes at the joint margin lead to the formation of pannus, which infiltrates and destroys the articular cartilage and the subchondral bone. This destruction is followed by fibrosis and, later, by bony ankylosis in the reparative phase.

Clinical Manifestations

The main clinical feature of seronegative spondyloarthritis is inflammatory back pain caused by sacroiliitis and inflammation in the axial skeleton. Peripheral arthritis, enthesitis, and uveitis are often associated as well. Dactylitis, chest wall pain, aortic incompetence together with conduction disturbances, conjunctivitis, and lesions of the lung apices are less common.

AS onset is often in the third decade, with 80% of cases diagnosed prior to age 30. Fewer then 5% are diagnosed after age 45. There is also a gender predominance, with a male-to-female ratio of 2:1.[22]

Juvenile-onset AS, with the onset of symptoms earlier than 16 years, has a higher incidence of hip disease. Patients with hip joint involvement show a faster progression of the spine disease. In the absence of hip disease, there is little difference between juvenile-onset and adult-onset AS in severity of spinal and extraskeletal manifestations.[23]

Inflammatory back pain distinguishes itself from mechanical back pain by insidious onset before age 40, pain persisting for at least 3 months, morning stiffness, and improvement with exercise. Buttock pain typically alternates from side to side. Pain and stiffness in the cervical spine generally start at a later stage.[9] With the progress of the disease, the spine is gradually ankylosed with a generalized kyphotic deformity. To maintain upright posture, the patient hyperextends the hips and flexes the knees. Involvement of the hip joints seriously compromises the compensatory postures. Hyperextension of the cervical spine helps in maintaining the forward gaze. In advanced cases, when the cervical spine becomes ankylosed in flexion, forward gaze and jaw opening are affected. As the disease process immobilizes the spine, the majority of painful symptoms resolve. The inflammatory process tends to become inactive as bony ankylosis sets in, in the late fourth or fifth decade.[24] Spondylodiscitis has a prevalence of 5% to 8% in patients with AS, and most lesions are asymptomatic.[25] In half the cases, there may be multiple lesions. The most common location is in the lower thoracic and upper lumbar region, but the cervicothoracic junction may also be involved. Neither trauma nor infection has been found to be involved in most cases.[25,26] However, owing to a distribution similar to that of thoracolumbar fracture, many researchers believe that these lesions represent pseudarthrosis resulting from the instability of a chronic nonunion, and histologic studies appear to confirm this.[27,28]

The incidence of peripheral joint involvement is 20% to 40%. Peripheral arthritis in AS and related conditions is oligoarticular and asymmetrical and often affects the hips or shoulders. Temporomandibular joint pain and stiffness occur in about 10% of patients. Less frequently involved joints include the knees, ankles, elbows, and wrists. Involvement of the hip joint is more important from the clinical viewpoint, since hip disease is far more disabling than is spinal rigidity.[1] Painful peripheral enthesitis often involves heel insertion of the Achilles tendon and plantar fascia. Other sites of enthesitis include the superior and inferior poles of the patella, tibial tubercle, pubic attachment of the adductor longus, femoral trochanters, humeral epicondyles, and nuchal crests.

The classic diagnostic criteria for the classification of AS are the modified New York criteria. This scheme requires radiographic presence of sacroiliitis and one of the following: back pain and stiffness for more than 3 months that is relieved with exercise and not relieved by rest, limitation of motion of the lumbar spine in the sagittal and coronal planes, or limitation of chest expansion relative to normal values.[29] The limitation of these criteria is that they may exclude patients without clear radiographic abnormality and may delay diagnosis and treatment.[30] Recently, the Assessment of Spondyloarthritis International Society (ASAS) published classification criteria that have been validated and take into account the clinical, laboratory, and radiologic findings[31] (Fig. 87-1). Other classification systems include the European Spondyloarthropathy Study Group and the Amor criteria.[6,7]

Laboratory and Radiologic Features

The HLA-B27 status is important in the early diagnosis of AS and associated conditions, but this test is not helpful in screening chronic low back pain. Erythrocyte sedimentation rate and serum C-reactive protein values may indicate systemic inflammation, but these tests have sensitivities of less than 50%.[32]

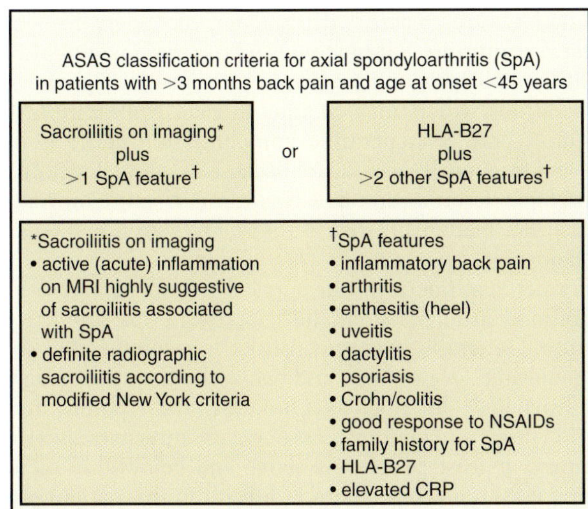

FIGURE 87-1. Assessment of Spondyloarthritis International Society (ASAS) criteria for classification of axial spondyloarthritis (to be applied in patients with chronic back pain and age younger than 45 years at onset of back pain). CRP, C-reactive protein.

On radiographs, a common radiologic feature is squaring of the ventral corners of the thoracic and lumbar vertebrae due to osteopenia at the attachment of the ventral anulus. Vertebral osteopenia also accompanies the loss of normal concavity of the end plates.[33] Symmetrical bilateral patchy areas of osteoporosis along the ill-defined SI joint are often suggestive of early disease. Later, subchondral erosions followed by patchy areas of ossifications develop that eventually lead to obliteration of the SI joint. Ossification extends within the substance of the anulus forming syndesmophytes, which bridges the adjacent vertebral bodies and develops into the bamboo spine in late stages[34] (Fig. 87-2). Dorsal vertebral structures are also ossified. These include the capsule of the facet joints, supraspinous and interspinous ligaments, and ligamentum flavum. In the subaxial cervical spine, extensive ankylosis with varying degrees of kyphosis is seen in the advanced stages. In contrast, the upper cervical spine may demonstrate hypermobility resulting from atlantoaxial instability.[35]

Early diagnosis of AS has been helped, in large part, by the development of MRI, which can detect early signs of inflammation and structural damage to the SI joints and the spine. In particular, increased signal on short-tau inversion recovery and T1 imaging with gadolinium correlate with inflammatory infiltrate.[36] Identification of inflammation at the SI joints is paramount in the early diagnosis of this disease. Various radiographic grading schemes exist for severity of SI and/or spine involvement.[37]

Nonsurgical Management

Treatment of AS should be tailored to the manifestations of the disease. The best combination of treatments includes both pharmacologic and nonpharmacologic treatments. Treatment recommendations have been proposed by a task force made up of the assessment of the ASAS working group and the European League against Rheumatism (EULAR) group.[38]

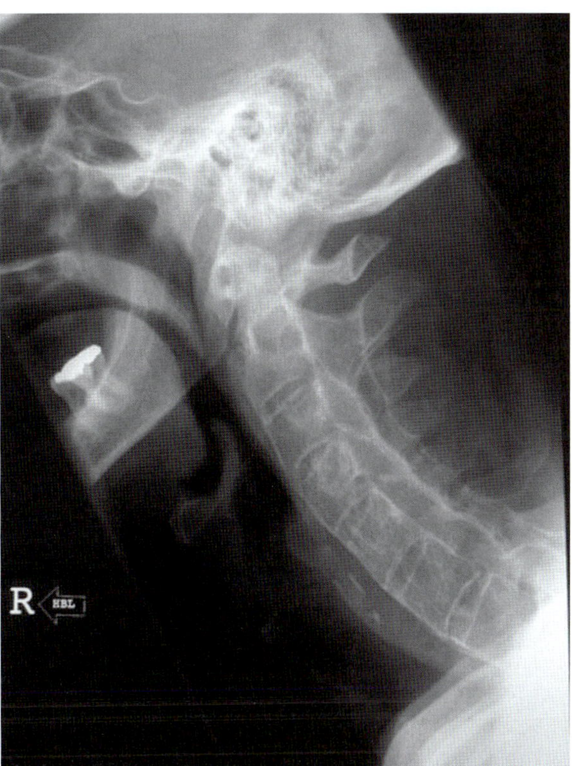

FIGURE 87-2. Typical plain radiograph findings of ankylosis in the cervical spine in a patient with ankylosing spondylitis.

With early diagnosis, nonsurgical treatment, including pharmacologic and physical therapy, can benefit all patients with AS or related conditions. Physical therapy can provide short-term improvement in functionality.[39] Cognitive and behavioral modification may also improve symptoms.[40]

Nonsteroidal anti-inflammatory drugs (NSAIDs) are the first-line agents in the treatment of AS.[41] These medications are symptom-modifying as well as disease modifying.[42] Sulfasalazine has shown clinical benefit in the treatment of peripheral arthritis and spinal stiffness, but there were no statistical improvements in spinal pain, function, or global assessment.[43]

More recently, anti-TNF (tumor necrosis factor) agents have been developed for use in AS patients who failed standard treatments. These include golimumab, infliximab, etanercept, and rituximab. The proinflammatory mediator zTNF is produced by macrophages and activated lymphocytes, and TNF results in increased cytokine expression that results in bone resorption and proteoglycan breakdown. Furthermore, TNF has been shown to be overexpressed in the SI joints in AS patients.[44]

Surgical Management of Ankylosing Spondylitis

Patients with AS often have increased rigidity throughout the spine in addition to poor bone density and osteoporosis, which result in an increased incidence in spine deformity and instability. Therefore, spine surgery in AS patients is often focused on either deformity correction or stabilization of an unstable fracture.

Spine Fractures

As the spine undergoes autofusion through ligamentous ossification and syndesmophytosis, a rigid kyphotic deformity develops that is unable to dissipate energies from a traumatic event.[45-49] Hyperextension is the most often observed mechanism of spine fracture in AS.[50] Spine fractures in AS are pathologic fractures and differ from fractures in the normal spine in many aspects. These fractures (1) often result after trivial trauma, (2) are usually highly unstable and displace more frequently, (3) almost always involve all three columns, (4) are more often associated with neurologic complications, and (5) are associated with epidural bleeding.[51] Because of the syndesmophyte formation, fracture often extends through the disc space.[49,52] Associated conditions, such as peripheral arthritis, may further impair the patient's mobility and increase the incidence of falls.

Neurologic deficit is frequent with these fractures and may be as high as 75%.[46,47] The incidence of spinal cord injury in patients with AS is 11.4 times higher than that in the general population.[50] In a review of 31 consecutive patients with fractures in AS, Olerud et al.[48] reported immediate neurologic impairment in one third of patients, and a further one third subsequently developed neurologic impairment. The secondary neurologic deterioration could be a result of fracture displacement or development of an epidural hematoma. Displacement in hyperextension is considered to be most dangerous for neurologic impairment.[51,53] Because of the kyphotic deformity, the spine tends to displace in hyperextension when the patient lies in a supine position.[48]

The cumulative incidence of spine fractures in patients with AS is approximately 17%, and the incidence of these injuries peaks around the sixth decade of life.[45,54] The midcervical spine is the most frequent site of fracture, followed by the thoracolumbar junction.[48,55] Radiologic demonstration of the fractures may be difficult because of poor bone density and may be missed on plain radiographs.[49] Patients with a history of back or neck pain after trivial trauma or sudden progression of deformity should undergo a thorough radiologic evaluation using CT, and the clinician should have a very high index of suspicion for occult fracture. Multiple fractures are also a strong consideration in patients with AS.

In comparison to the general population, patients with AS and spinal cord injury have poor outcomes. Morbidity is as high as 85%,[52] and mortality rates range from 35% to 50%[13,56,57]; pulmonary complications play a major role relating to decreased chest wall expansion.[49] Vascular injuries such as aortic rupture have been reported in fractures resulting from higher-energy trauma.[58-60]

Because of the frequent incidence of neurologic deterioration, failure of union, or inadequate immobilization at the fracture site with conservative treatment, most surgeons support surgical stabilization as the treatment of choice. A recent study of 122 spine fractures in patients with AS demonstrated that the most common level of fracture was C6-7. Most of these patients (67%) were treated surgically, and the remainder were treated with bracing, secondary to a poor medical condition.[52] If bracing is used, serial imaging should be utilized to recognize persistent movement or progressive subluxation, which may require surgical stabilization. For the most part, nonoperative immobilization alone is difficult and frequently inadequate because of marked instability. Neurologic deterioration may result from fracture movement with simple maneuvers such as transfer to a stretcher[61] or during halo-vest application.[54]

For cervical fractures, the surgical treatment may consist of dorsal, ventral, or combined approaches to stabilize the fracture. Generally, a long construct is recommended spanning multiple levels above and below the fracture.[52] Taggard and Traynelis[62] described a technique of three-point internal fixation combining lateral mass plate and interspinous wiring, spanning at least two levels above and below the fracture. Lateral mass screw placement is difficult in this patient population because the usual landmarks of the facet joints are lost as a result of bony ankylosis. Extrapolation from a recognizable landmark may be necessary to find the point of screw entry. As an additional measure of safety, these authors suggested use of screws that are 14 mm or shorter to avoid nerve root damage.

Combined anterior-posterior stabilization in the cervical spine likely can decrease pseudarthrosis and/or instrumentation failure in patients with poor bone quality. External immobilization using halo or cervicothoracic brace following dorsal surgery is recommended, since immobilization in a cervical collar may result in failed surgical fusion.

Although the subaxial cervical spine is the most common site of fracture in AS, the odontoid process is vulnerable. Bony ankylosis of the atlanto-occipital and/or atlantoaxial joint or the lower cervical spine may make the odontoid susceptible to fracture after minor trauma.[63,64] Spontaneous fracture of the odontoid without history of trauma has also been reported.[65] These injuries may be treated by halo-jacket immobilization alone[66] or in combination with dorsal occipitocervical fusion.

Fractures in the thoracic and lumbar spine involve all three columns and are inherently unstable with a high possibility of secondary neurologic deterioration. Fractures often occur across an ankylosed disc space (Fig. 87-3). Displacements are common, particularly toward hyperextension when the patient is positioned supine.[48,60] Surgical stabilization is therefore mandatory. Stabilization is often attained through long dorsal constructs, three or more segments included above and below the fracture. Anterior column reconstruction is often not needed.[52]

Patients with AS with spine fracture present significant perioperative challenges. First, intubation may be difficult, owing to decreased cervical mobility, instability, or ventral osteophytes.[67] Second, proper positioning can be extremely difficult and requires significant planning. During head positioning, one must take into account the degree of cervical kyphosis and plan accordingly. Cases of spinal cord injury and/or death have been reported with improper head position in patients with AS.[47] With unstable cervical fracture, preoperative halo placement can provide stability for positioning. Neurophysiologic monitoring can provide important information during positioning as well. Increased blood loss should be expected during spine surgery in patients with AS.[68]

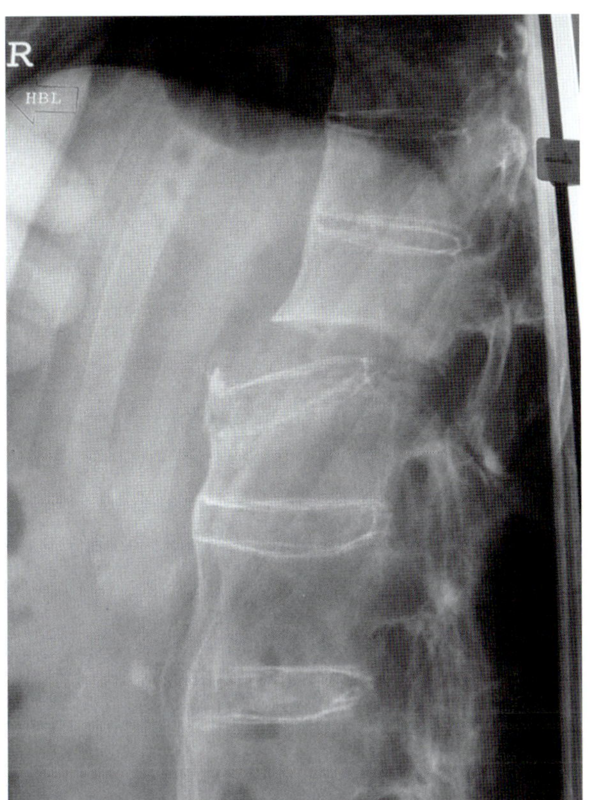

FIGURE 87-3. Plain radiograph of a transdiscal fracture of L1 in a patient with ankylosing spondylitis.

Spine Deformity

A progressive generalized kyphotic deformity, focused at both the cervicothoracic and thoracolumbar junctions, is typical in AS.[69] This kyphotic deformity leads to a shift in the center of gravity both forward and downward, resulting in loss of sagittal balance and difficulty in forward gaze. In the early phase of the disease, patients try to compensate their sagittal balance by hyperextension of the hips and flexion of the knees. Hyperextension of the cervical spine helps to maintain forward gaze. When hips are involved with the disease, fixed flexion deformity develops and further interferes with the sagittal balance. In advanced stages of the disease, the cervical spine is ankylosed, resulting in a global kyphotic deformity, interfering severely with compensation of the gaze angle. Severe kyphotic deformities may produce compression of the abdominal viscera and limitation of the pulmonary function by restriction of the diaphragmatic excursion.

Indications for Deformity Correction

Surgical intervention is indicated when kyphosis is decompensated. This means that the patient cannot maintain a horizontal gaze when the hips and knees are extended and the eyeballs are in the neutral position.[70] In practice, however, the general condition of the patient, the feasibility of correction, and, perhaps above all else, the morale and earnest desire of the patient to accept the risks and rehabilitative measures required for correction become more important decisive factors before surgery is considered. As was mentioned earlier in the chapter, many perioperative challenges exist in these patients.

Preoperative Planning

The correction of complex kyphotic deformities, as seen in advanced AS, requires extensive preoperative planning. The primary goal of surgery is restoration of sagittal balance performed in the safest possible way. Correction may be necessary at the cervicothoracic junction and/or the thoracolumbar spine.

The level of osteotomy to correct a global kyphotic deformity has a disparate effect on gaze angle and sagittal balance. Sagittal balance is restored by redirecting the spine dorsally at the level of osteotomy so that the head lies vertically above the pelvis. The angle by which the spine is redirected at the osteotomy site (the osteotomy angle) for full restoration of the sagittal balance depends on the level of osteotomy. When the osteotomy is performed at a higher level, the osteotomy angle must be greater than that required for osteotomy at a lower level in the spine to achieve the same degree of correction in the sagittal balance.[71,72] In contrast, the visual angle (by which the gaze is redirected forward) will always be the same as the osteotomy angle, irrespective of the level of the osteotomy.

As was mentioned earlier, in the presence of global kyphosis in AS, patients try to extend their hips and flex their knees as much as possible to correct the sagittal balance and to achieve a forward gaze. An estimate of gaze angle and sagittal balance correction from the lateral radiograph taken in this posture will underestimate both these parameters. The simple way to resolve this problem is to take the lateral radiograph while the patient stands with relaxed hips, without making an effort to correct the spine balance or forward gaze. The degree of gaze angle correction needed is determined by the chin-brow to vertical angle (CBVA).[73] The CBVA is an angle between the line drawn from the chin to the brow and a vertical line and is used as a clinical measurement of sagittal balance and its effect on horizontal gaze.[69] The sagittal balance correction is estimated from the degree of dorsal shift of the plumb line required to bring it back to the sacrum. Presence of hip flexion deformity severely affects both the sagittal balance and the gaze angle, and this must be corrected by total hip replacement before spine osteotomy is undertaken.

When both lumbar osteotomy and cervical osteotomy are needed, the lumbar osteotomy is often performed in the first stage, achieving maximum correction of the sagittal balance. Cervical osteotomy is performed subsequently for further modification of the sagittal balance and gaze angle correction.

Thoracolumbar Kyphotic Correction

Three methods are used to correct kyphosis in the thoracolumbar spine in the setting of AS: opening wedge osteotomy, also known as Smith-Peterson osteotomy (SPO); polysegmental wedge osteotomy; and pedicle subtraction osteotomy (PSO). Because these procedures involve resection of stabilizing elements of the spine, they are always supplemented with dorsal instrumentation.

SPO was first introduced by Smith-Petersen et al.[74] and involves two- or three-level osteotomies through the facet joints at the L1-3 levels and closing the gap by osteoclasis of the vertebral body. The wedge is then closed by hyperextension of the spine with manual pressure. This manipulation can cause disruption of the anterior longitudinal ligament and creates a large gap in the ventral aspect of the vertebral column. The main disadvantage of this technique was serious vascular and neurologic complications resulting from sudden elongation of the anterior column during closed osteoclasis maneuver and a large ventral opening of a monosegmental procedure.[5,69,75,76] Mortality rates up to 12% and complication rates up to 50% are not unusual.[70] In general, every 1 mm of facet that is resected results in 1 degree of correction, so each SPO can result in 10 degrees of correction.[77]

The polysegmental wedge osteotomy was developed to reduce disruption at the anterior longitudinal ligament. In this technique, multiple SPOs are performed in the thoracolumbar spine, creating a more gradual correction and small bony defects ventrally. Wilson and Turkell[78] first reported polysegmental osteotomy in one patient in 1949. Mortality rates as low as 4% and complication rates of about 27% have been reported.[70] The total degree of correction that is achieved may be the same as that with open wedge osteotomy, which corresponds to about 10 degrees per level of osteotomy.

PSO, or lumbar closing wedge osteotomy, is a technique in which a transpedicular vertebral wedge resection is performed extending from the dorsal elements through the pedicles into the vertebral body[77] (Fig. 87-4). The wedge is closed by hyperextension of the lumbar spine, hinging on the ventral cortex of the vertebral body. Since there is no elongation of the anterior column, vascular complications are rare. Care must be taken to avoid disrupting the ventral cortical surface, as this may destabilize the segment. The consolidation at the osteotomy site is rapid. This technique was initially described by Scudese and Calabro[79] but was later popularized by Thomasen[80] in 1985. The PSO is typically performed at L2 or L3, as one of these is the typical apex of normal lumbar lordosis (Fig. 87-5). Approximately 30 to 40 degrees of correction may be achieved from a single-level PSO.[81] Kim et al.[82] have reported outcomes on 45 patients with AS and a kyphotic deformity. The average correction was 34 degrees, with improvement of sagittal balance from 94 mm to 8 mm. Complications included ileus in five patients, neurologic deficit in five patients, and visual disturbance in two patients.

Ideally, kyphotic deformity is best corrected when the osteotomy is placed at the site of maximum deformity. It is possible to perform a PSO in both the thoracic and lumbar regions, but thoracic PSOs are technically more difficult and carry a higher risk of neurologic sequelae.[69] In practice, a combination of polysegmental wedge osteotomies and a PSO can provide sufficient sagittal deformity correction.

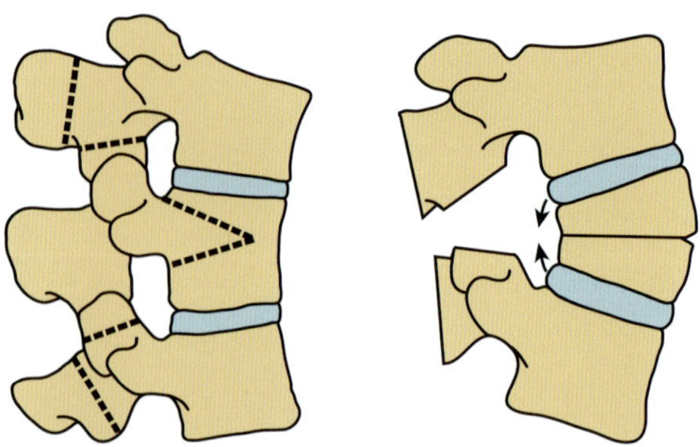

FIGURE 87-4. Schematic showing operative technique of lumbar pedicle subtraction osteotomy in the correction of lumbar kyphosis and sagittal imbalance.

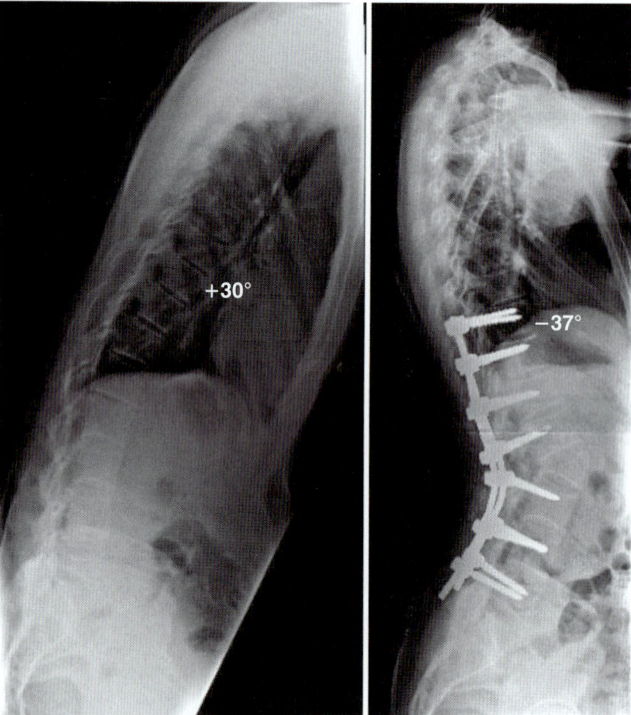

FIGURE 87-5. Preoperative (*left*) and postoperative (*right*) standing radiographs in a patient with ankylosing spondylitis before and after lumbar pedicle subtraction osteotomy.

Cervical Osteotomy

Severe flexion deformity can be seen in the cervicothoracic region in AS, with patients presenting with the characteristic "chin on chest" posture. This results in severe restriction of the forward gaze and interferes with jaw opening. Surgical correction should aim to correct gaze and improvement of jaw opening as well as to improve or maintain sagittal balance. The cervical extension osteotomy is typically performed dorsally at C7-T1. At this level, the vertebral artery is extraspinal, and the spinal canal is relatively wide at this level.

Urist[83] first described a case of cervical osteotomy under local anesthesia with the patient in the sitting position in 1953. Simmons et al.[84] recently published a large retrospective series of patients with AS who underwent cervical extension osteotomy. Over a 36-year period, 131 cases were performed in a sitting position under local anesthesia. CBVA angles were improved on average 37 degrees. The 3-month mortality rate was 3%. Complications included transient C8 radiculopathy (12%), pseudarthrosis (5%), spinal cord injury (2%), and stroke (<1%).

In brief, the spinous processes of C6 and C7 are removed, and a complete laminectomy is performed at C7. The caudal portion of the C6 lamina and the rostral portion of T1 are also removed. The fused C7-T1 facet is removed bilaterally, and the C8 nerve roots are exposed. A portion of the C7 and T1 pedicles is also removed. The head is then extended, breaking the ankylosed anterior column.[69,85] Dorsal instrumentation is placed for stabilization. Preoperative halo application can help to control head position on the table after osteotomy.

Conclusion

AS and associated conditions are chronic diseases that may be effectively treated with disease-modifying medications and physical therapy. Early diagnosis is essential so that treatment can be initiated. In the untreated or treatment-resistant patients, the spine undergoes a transformation in which the spine becomes immobile. At the same time, bone quality is reduced, resulting in a rigid, brittle structure that functions as a long bone. With trivial trauma, this structure is prone to fracture with resulting instability. Neurologic deficits are common following fracture, and spinal cord injury carries significant morbidity and mortality. Chronic stress over the rigid spine results in kyphotic deformity, which can be significantly debilitating. Surgical procedures have been developed to restore balance, but these procedures require much planning and carry significant risk.

KEY REFERENCES

Berens DL: Roentgen features of ankylosing spondylitis. *Clin Orthop Relat Res* 74:20–33, 1971.

Kabasakal Y, Garrett SL, Calin A: The epidemiology of spondylodiscitis in ankylosing spondylitis: a controlled study. *Br J Rheumatol* 35(7):660–663, 1996.

Olerud C, Frost A, Bring J: Spinal fractures in patients with ankylosing spondylitis. *Eur Spine J* 5(1):51–55, 1996.

Smith-Petersen MN, Larson CB, Aufranc OE: Osteotomy of the spine for correction of flexion deformity in rheumatoid arthritis. *Clin Orthop Relat Res* 66:6–9, 1969.

van der Linden S, Valkenburg H, Cats A: The risk of developing ankylosing spondylitis in HLA-B27 positive individuals: a family and population study. *Br J Rheumatol* 22(4 Suppl 2):18–19, 1983.

Wanders A, Heijde D, Landewe R, et al: Nonsteroidal antiinflammatory drugs reduce radiographic progression in patients with ankylosing spondylitis: a randomized clinical trial. *Arthritis Rheum* 52(6):1756–1765, 2005.

Weinstein PR, Karpman RR, Gall EP, Pitt M: Spinal cord injury, spinal fracture, and spinal stenosis in ankylosing spondylitis. *J Neurosurg* 57(5):609–616, 1982.

REFERENCES

The complete list of references is available online at expertconsult.com.

CHAPTER 88

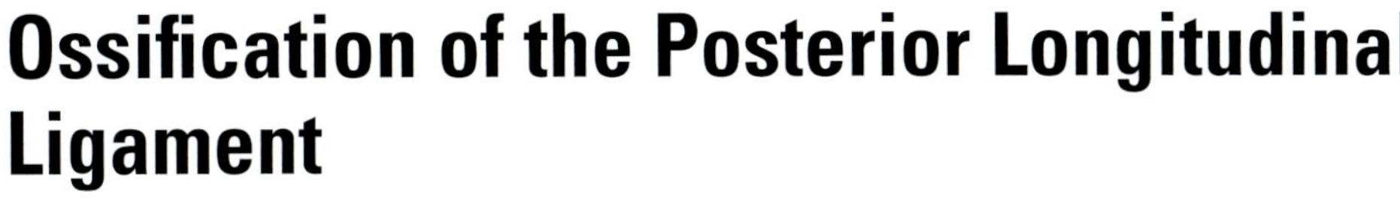

Ossification of the Posterior Longitudinal Ligament

Nancy E. Epstein | Kazuo Yonenobu

Ossification of the posterior longitudinal ligament (OPLL), most typically found in males (2:1) in their mid 50s, contributes to approximately 25% of cervical myelopathy in the North American population and higher percentages in the Asian population.[1,2] Originating as early hypertrophy of the PPL with accompanying punctate ossification centers (early OPLL), these foci coalesce and become loci of frank ossification in the PPL.[1,2] Early OPLL appears in patients in their mid 40s, whereas classic, more ossified OPLL is found in people in their mid 50s and later. OPLL may be managed with either anterior surgery (single/multilevel corpectomies with fusion, with or without combined posterior instrumentation), or posterior surgery (laminectomy with or without fusion or laminoplasty) (Figs. 88-1 to 88-6).

Prevalence of Ossification of the Posterior Longitudinal Ligament

In asymptomatic North Americans, the frequency of OPLL is reportedly 0.12% on plain radiographs, and in the Japanese, it is 2.2%. In Koreans, 0.6% of 11,774 adults demonstrated OPLL involving the C3, C4, and C5 on plain radiographs; 32% had continuous OPLL, 31% segmental OPLL, 31% mixed OPLL, and 5.6% focal OPLL.[3] In the presence of myelopathy, OPLL is evident, using CT and MRI studies in up to 25% of North Americans and in at least 27% of Japanese.[4-6] Seventy percent of cervical OPLLs involve 2.7 to 4 levels, progressing in a caudal-rostral fashion, and the remaining 30% are evenly divided between the proximal thoracic (T1-4) and the proximal lumbar (L1-3) regions.

Genetics of Ossification of the Posterior Longitudinal Ligament

Human Leukocyte Antigen: Probable Site on Genome

Multiple studies increasingly document a genetic correlation among OPLL, diffuse idiopathic skeletal hyperostosis (DISH), and ossification of other ligaments—ossification of the yellow ligament (OYL) and ossification of the anterior longitudinal ligament (OALL).[7,8] In evaluation of 91 sibling pairs of patients with OPLL in 53 Japanese families, the genetic locus for OPLL was found near the human leukocyte antigen (HLA) site on chromosome 6-p. In patients with DISH, 50% have concurrent OPLL and test positive for HLA.[9] In the Chinese population, another susceptibility gene, COL6A1, appears to represent a "common susceptibility gene" for both OYL and OPLL.[10]

Autosomal Dominant Inheritance

An autosomal dominant mode of inheritance is supported by genetic and epidemiologic data from patients with OPLL. OPLL is found in 26.15% of parents and 28.89% of siblings of patients with OPLL, a finding that supports a likely autosomal dominant transmission.[11] A 53% expression rate of OPLL is

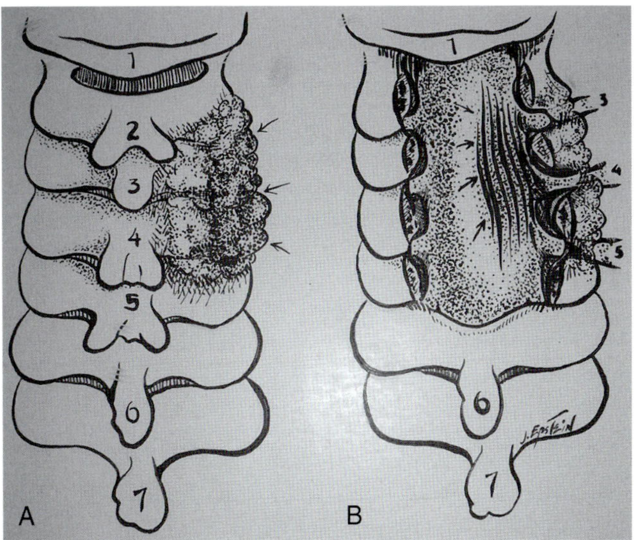

FIGURE 88-1. A, The dorsal illustration of the cervical spine reveals right-sided C2-5 hypertrophied hemilaminae accompanied by arthrotic changes (*arrows*) of the facet joints (C2-3, C3-4, and C4-5). **B,** Following a laminectomy of C2-5, the dorsolateral right-sided cord has been adequately decompressed (*arrows*). Additionally, extended foraminal decompression of the facet joints at the C2-3 through C4-5 levels has skeletonized the exiting C3-5 nerve roots. (Illustrator: Dr. Joseph A. Epstein; copyright: Dr. Nancy Epstein.)

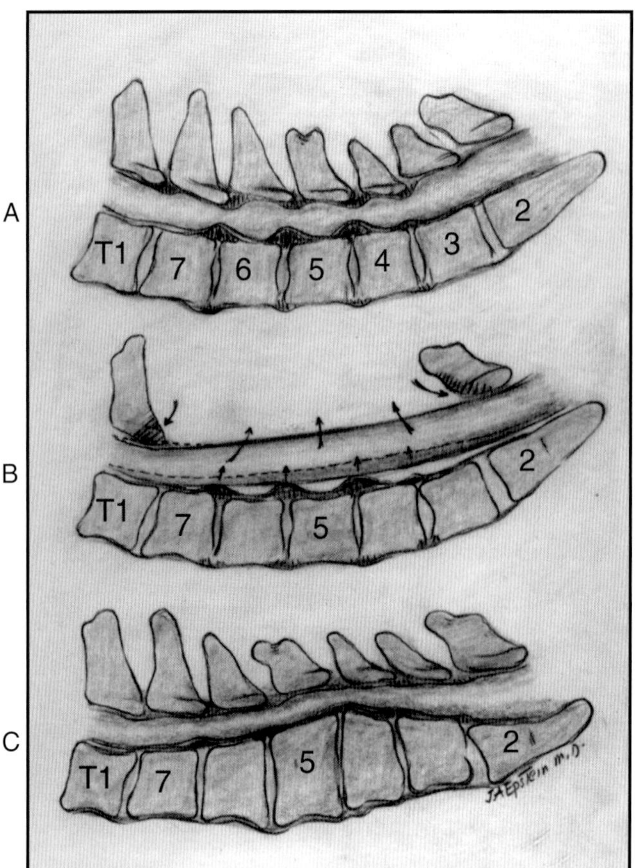

FIGURE 88-2. **A,** Lateral view of the cervical spine from the C2-T1 levels. Note the adequate preservation of the cervical lordotic curvature. Arthrotic degenerative changes, opposite the disc spaces of C4-5, C5-6, and C6-7, result in ventral cord compression. Hypertrophy/ossification of the yellow ligament and shingling of the laminae at the C3-4 through the C6-7 levels simultaneously contribute to dorsolateral cord compression. **B,** In the presence of an adequate cervical lordosis, a C3-7 laminectomy was performed. Note the dorsal migration of the thecal sac/cord away from the multilevel ventrally situated osteophytes following removal of the shingled laminae and hypertrophied/ossified yellow ligament. **C,** Alternatively, when the cervical lordosis is reversed by the presence of marked kyphosis, seen here involving the C4 and C5 vertebrae, laminectomy does not decompress the spinal cord. Rather, the cord remains tethered over the kyphotic deformity. (Illustrator: Dr. Joseph A. Epstein; copyright: Dr. Nancy Epstein.)

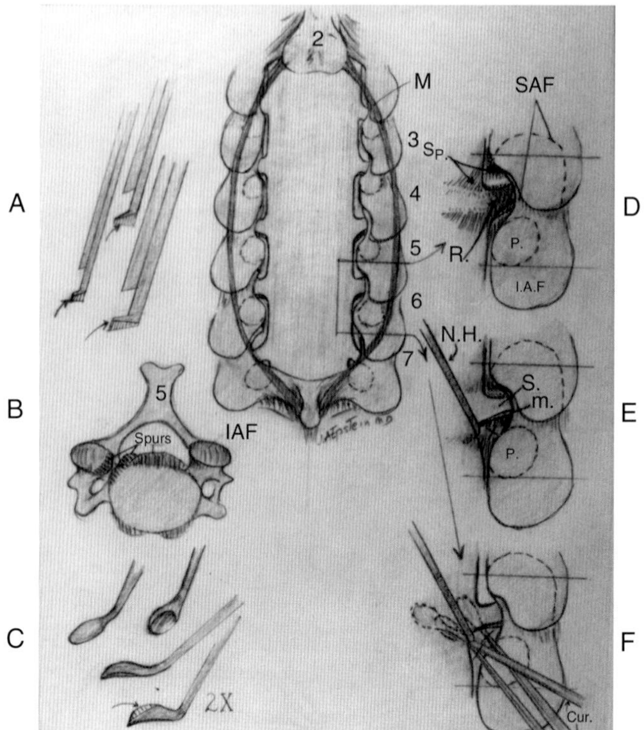

FIGURE 88-3. In the central figure, a cervical laminectomy extends from C3-7 and is accompanied by a medial facetectomy (M) and foraminotomy at every level. **A,** Filed down-biting and 360-degree rotating Kerrison rongeurs (2-mm; 3-mm) are used to remove the 1 to 2 mm of residual lateral bone, which has been thinned down by a 2-mm diamond drill, and perform a medial facetectomy and foraminotomy at each level. **B,** On this axial view of a cervical vertebral level, a ventral osteophyte extends across the base of the spinal canal with right-sided foraminal extension. IAF, inferior articular facet. **C,** Down-biting curets used to resect lateral/foraminal discs and osteophytes. **D,** Following a medial facetectomy and foraminotomy, occasional nerve roots may appear bifid. If bifid, the ventral motor root, invested with a thinner dural sleeve, appears white (Sp). (do not mistake this for disc), whereas the dorsal sensory root (R) appears dark, because it remains within a thicker dural sleeve. Observe how the medial aspects of the superior and inferior articular facets are excised to adequately expose the root that exits above the inferior pedicle (P). SAF, superior articular facet. **E,** A small nerve hook is used to gently retract the axillary portion of the exiting nerve root (S.m.) just parallel to the pedicle. N.H., nerve hook. This occasionally requires filing down the medial aspect of the pedicle with a fine (2-mm) diamond drill or 1-mm Kerrison rongeur. **F,** Once the root has been dissected away from the ventrally situated venous plexus, and the disc and disc space are visualized, small down-biting curets (Cur.) may be introduced into the lateral aspect of the spinal canal. All maneuvers, performed under an operating microscope, should consist of a gentle medial to lateral/inferior sweeping motion, away from the cord. (Illustrator: Dr. Joseph A. Epstein; copyright: Dr. Nancy Epstein.)

observed in patients with two concurrent HLA strands compared with 24% with one strand, which further supports this hypothesis.[8] Autosomal recessive transmission has been suggested when 56% of a patient's siblings with both HLA haplotypes were symptomatic with OPLL, whereas those with only one HLA haplotype were not.[12] Two additional unique genetic factors were identified in 18 patients with OPLL compared with 51 age-matched controls: BamHI 10.0/10.0 kb and HindIII 19.0/19.0 kb genotypes.[7,13]

Other Contributing Factors (Hormones and Proteins)

Genetically modulated hormones and proteins also appear to contribute to the expression of OPLL. Increased concentrations of growth hormone receptors and activins have been shown to enhance OPLL expression/progression.[14,15] Elevated concentrations of bone morphogenetic proteins have resulted in increased osteogenesis in originally nonossified ligaments of OPLL patients (347 families, 1030 relatives).[15] In a more recent study, bone morphogenetic protein 2 (BMP-2) additionally positively correlated with the extent of OPLL progression.[16] Insulin was also correlated with OPLL onset/progression in people with non–type 1 diabetes via direct and indirect stimulation of BMP-2 within the ligament.[17] Fibronectin, a glycoprotein that plays a role in the

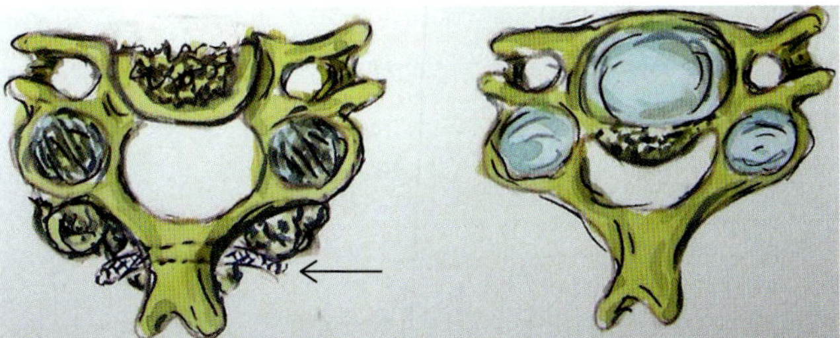

FIGURE 88-4. Cervical ossification of the posterior longitudinal ligament (OPLL) occupying the ventral aspect of the spinal canal (*right*) and circumferential surgery to address that OPLL (*left*). In the right figure there is evidence of the anterior corpectomy graft in place. Posteriorly there is a wire through the base of the spinous process and bone graft applied posterolaterally (*arrow*). (Illustrator: Dr. Joseph A. Epstein; copyright: Dr. Nancy Epstein.)

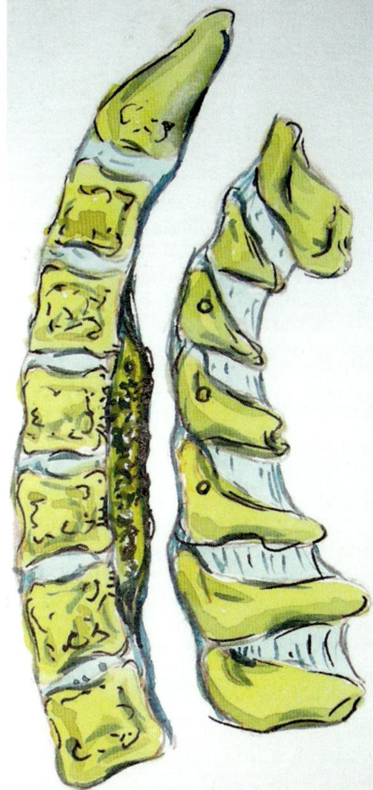

FIGURE 88-5. In the cervical spine, the midline sagittal illustration documents ventral continuous ossification of the posterior longitudinal ligament extending from the inferior aspect of C4 through the midportion of the C7 vertebral body, resulting in marked ventral cord compression. (Illustrator: Dr. Joseph A. Epstein; copyright: Dr. Nancy Epstein.)

development of bony tissues, was also found to be significantly elevated in patients with OPLL or OYL.[18]

Anatomy of Ossification of the Posterior Longitudinal Ligament

Posterior Longitudinal Ligament

The PPL, comprised of collagen fibers with elastin densely concentrated at its center, originates at the base of the clivus

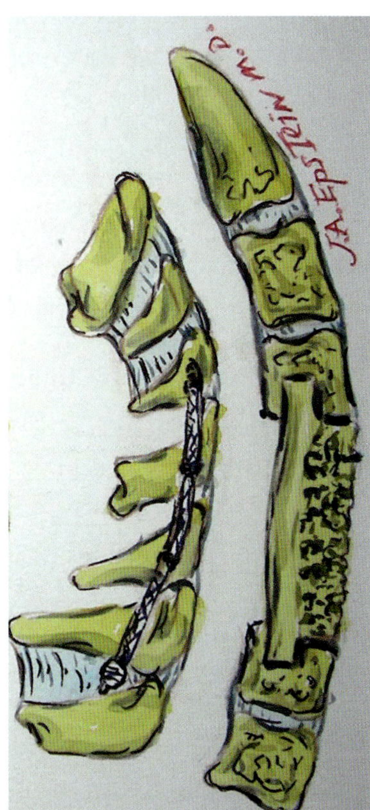

FIGURE 88-6. Multilevel anterior corpectomy and fusion from the C4-7 levels is illustrated here using a reversed iliac crest strut graft and accompanied by posterior C4-7 wiring/fusion. (Illustrator: Dr. Joseph A. Epstein; copyright: Dr. Nancy Epstein.)

and extends to the sacrum. It is attached to each disc anulus, where it is widest, and is narrowest at each midvertebral level; it is 1 to 2 mm thick centrally, thinning out laterally.

Hypertrophied and Ossified Posterior Longitudinal Ligament

Hypertrophy of the PPL is first attributed to fibroblastic hyperplasia followed by increased collagen deposition. The subsequent formation of ossification centers is attributed to progressive mineralization and cartilaginous ingrowth. These centers eventually coalesce, leading to OPLL characterized by mature Haversian canals actively engaged in bone marrow production. OPLL enlarges an average of 0.4 mm per year in its anterior-posterior dimension, and longitudinal expansion occurs at a rate of 0.67 mm per year.

In Vitro Characteristics of Cultured Posterior Longitudinal Ligament in Patients with Ossification of the Posterior Longitudinal Ligament

In patients with OPLL, the PPL is osteogenic.[7,8,13-15] Immunohistochemical evaluation of PPL cells for patients undergoing anterior cervical decompression for cervical disease revealed "up-regulation of proliferating cell nuclear antigen" in patients with OPLL.[19] This finding of increased osteogenicity of the PPL was also confirmed in myelopathic patients with OPLL in North America.[20] Collecting supernatants of PPL obtained intraoperatively from patients with OPLL compared with non-OPLL control patients (with spondylosis) revealed increased osteocalcin synthesis in the OPLL patients. The quantity of osteocalcin induced was determined by incubating these PPL cells with $1.25(OH)_2$ and vitamin D_3 for 72 hours in serum-free medium.[21] Those with OPLL grew to confluence, whereas those with spondylosis alone did not respond to vitamin D_3 priming.

Etiology: Mechanisms of Neural Injury in Ossification of the Posterior Longitudinal Ligament

Two major mechanisms contribute to neural injury in patients with OPLL: direct mechanical compression and indirect ischemic injury. Direct ventral cord compression (acute-surgery related, chronic slow spondylotic/OPLL compression) produces a greater functional loss in the anterior (spinothalamic, motor) and anterolateral (corticospinal) tracts. Indirect injury due to operative distraction, hypotension, or other maneuvers resulting in ischemia produces a disproportionate loss of the posterolateral tracts. Neural injury may begin with edema but is rapidly succeeded by progressive demyelination, myelomalacia, and atrophy. Of interest, many of these changes, particularly with severe OPLL, may occur several levels distal to the focus of major pathology.

Classification of Ossification of the Posterior Longitudinal Ligament

Early Disease

OPLL represents a continuum of maturation that starts with hypertrophy of the PPL and ends with frank ossification.[1,4,6,22] Early OPLL usually originates opposite multiple interspaces in patients in their mid 40s and is often misdiagnosed as multiple disc herniations. However, unlike disc herniations, OPLL begins with retrovertebral extension that can be seen on enhanced MRI studies performed with gadolinium (Gd)-DTPA and as punctate CT-documented ossification. Too often, patients undergo multilevel anterior discectomy and fusion procedures where the PPL is ignored, leading to many retained disc fragments, and in early OPLL, leaving patients with continued symptomatology.

Classic Disease

There are four classic types of mature/classic OPLL[23] (Figs. 88-7 and 88-8). The segmental variant (39%), located behind the vertebral bodies, does not cross the intervening disc spaces. The continuous type (27%) extends from vertebra to vertebra, traversing the disc spaces. The mixed form (29%) simultaneously includes both continuous and segmental elements with "skip" areas. The "other" form (5%) is localized to the disc spaces, with limited degrees of rostral and caudal retrovertebral extension.

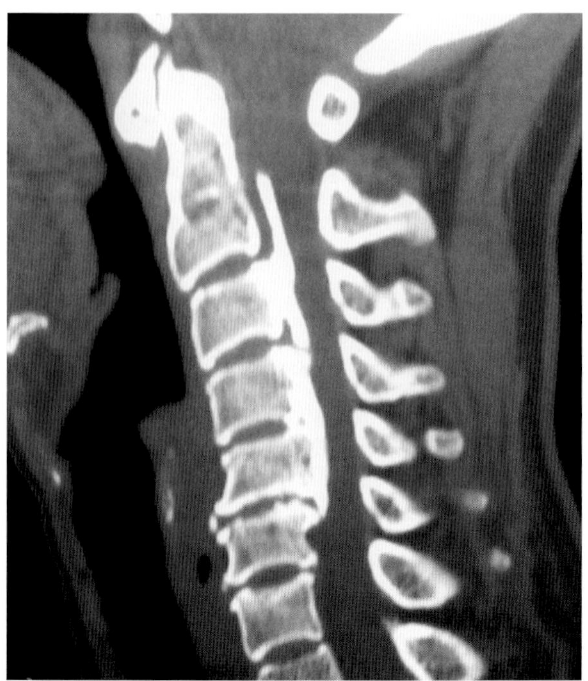

FIGURE 88-7. The midline sagittal two-dimensional CT study (soft tissue image) documents the "mixed" type of ossification of the posterior longitudinal ligament (OPLL). The continuous form of OPLL extends behind the C2-5 vertebral bodies, ending at the C5-6 caudal disc space. Dorsal to the C2 body, the double-layer sign indicative of dural penetrance is most clearly visualized. Observe the hypodense space (representing the dura) separating the C2 vertebral body from the linear ossification that represents intradural OPLL.

Myelopathy Scales

Two major myelopathy scales are used worldwide: the Nurick scale and the Japanese Orthopaedic Association (JOA) scale.

Nurick Scale

The Nurick myelopathy scale offers six grades of neurologic classification.[4,22]

- Grade 0: intact, mild radiculopathy without myelopathy
- Grade I: mild myelopathy
- Grade II: mild to moderate myelopathy
- Grade III: moderate myelopathy
- Grade IV: moderate to severe myelopathy
- Grade V: severe myelopathy, quadriplegic

Japanese Orthopaedic Association Scale

The JOA scale categorizes the severity of myelopathy using a 17-point scale.[24-27] In 2007, the JOA released a new evaluation tool for cervical myelopathy called the Cervical Myelopathy Evaluation Questionnaire (JOA CMEQ).[24-27] The new tool consists of five categories, which include 24 questions devoted to upper extremity motor function, lower extremity motor function, bladder function, cervical spine function, and quality of life. The English version of JOA CMEQ, its calculation software, and users' manual are available at the JOA home page (http://www.joa.or.jp/english/english_frame.html).

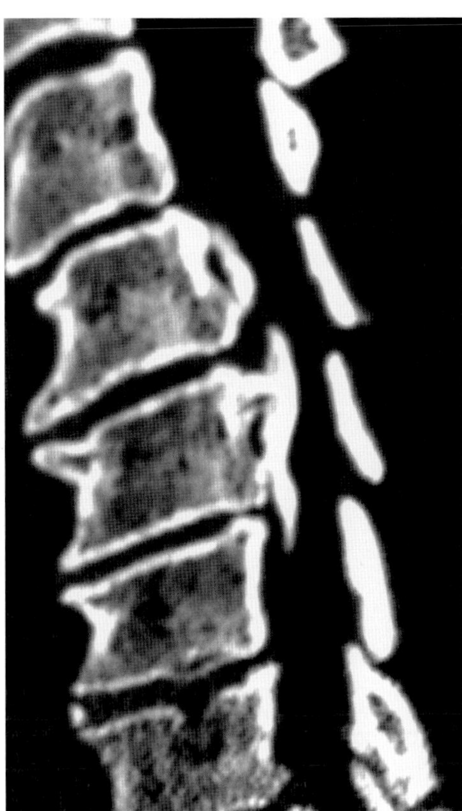

FIGURE 88-8. The parasagittal two-dimensional CT (bone-window) shows classic "segmental" ossification of the posterior longitudinal ligament (OPLL) located along the entire dorsal length of the C4 and C5 vertebral bodies. Also, observe the double-layer sign signified by the hypodense dura visualized between the dorsal aspect of the vertebral bodies and the hyperdense intradural OPLL.

Clinical Presentation of Ossification of the Posterior Longitudinal Ligament

Patients with early OPLL become symptomatic in their mid 40s with mild radiculopathy/myelopathy, whereas those with classic (mature) OPLL are more typically affected in their mid 50s, presenting with more advanced myelopathic syndromes. Males are affected twice as frequently as females. Although most patients become subacutely symptomatic over a progressive 12-month period, 10% present with acute deterioration associated with minor trauma.[28] In a series of 118 OPLL patients, minor trauma resulted in new myelopathy (13 patients), worsening of preexisting myelopathy (7 patients), or no new changes (7 patients). Eighteen of 19 patients with the narrowest cervical canals were most adversely affected.[28] In another series of 91 patients operated on for OPLL, 26 sustaining minor trauma preoperatively experienced major myelopathic deficits postoperatively.[29] Patients with more mobile spines associated with segmental, mixed, and other forms of OPLL exhibited poorer outcomes when compared with those with more rigid spines attributed to continuous OPLL. Typical symptoms included neck/arm pain or dysesthesias (>50% of the patients), and neurologic signs included arm/leg weakness (25%), spasticity, and ataxia.

Patients with OPLL are frequently diabetic or have coexisting hypoparathyroidism, acromegaly, vitamin D–resistant rickets, spondyloepiphyseal dysplasia, DISH, ankylosing spondylitis, OYL, OALL, or myotonic muscular dystrophy.

Neurodiagnostic Studies in Ossification of the Posterior Longitudinal Ligament

Radiography

Based on lateral 6-foot plain radiographs, the normal anteroposterior dimension of the cervical spinal canal should measure 17 mm between the C3-7 levels. In absolute stenosis, the canal is narrowed to 10 mm or less, whereas with relative stenosis, the canal measures between 10 and 13 mm. The extent of OPLL is readily described by the occupancy ratio, which is determined by dividing the thickness of the measured ossified lesion by the anterior/posterior developmental canal diameter. If the ratio is greater than 40%, the risk of myelopathy increases.[2]

Computer-assisted measurements based on plain radiographs may be used to follow the postoperative progression of OPLL.[30] In a multicenter study, lateral radiographs taken immediately as well as 1 and 2 years following posterior decompressions were assessed (131 patients). All radiographs were transformed into digital images and compared. Over 2 years, there was a 56.5% rate of progression, occurring more often in younger patients with the mixed and continuous forms of OPLL.

Magnetic Resonance Imaging

MRI examinations, particularly T1- and T2-weighted MRI studies, performed with and without contrast (Gd-DTPA) demonstrate the spinal column, spinal cord, nerve roots, intrinsic cord disease, and extrinsic cord compression from the occiput through the cervicothoracic junction in the transaxial, coronal, and sagittal planes. On noncontrast MRI studies, hypertrophied PPL often appears opposite multiple disc spaces, demonstrated by accompanying retrovertebral extension appearing slightly hyperintense and enhancing with Gd-DTPA. Classic OPLL is identified on 50% of T1-weighted MRI studies by a hyperintense signal, reflecting the presence of fat within mature Haversian canals actively engaged in bone marrow production. MRI examinations may also help identify disc herniations (hypointense masses) that occur in 81% of cases in conjunction with segmental OPLL.[31]

Ossified OPLL, which appears hypointense on MRI studies, may lead to an underestimation of the true extent of the OPLL and should therefore be combined with plain radiographic and CT-based studies to document the true degree of cord compression more accurately. In a multicenter study, 156 OPLL patients from 16 institutions were followed an average of 10.3 years with plain radiographs, MRI, and CT studies.[32] Of interest, all 39 patients with OPLL occupying greater than 60% of the anteroposterior diameter of the spinal canal were myelopathic, whereas only 49% with OPLL occupying less than 60% of the spinal canal were myelopathic.

Intrinsic cord swelling/edema, myelomalacia, and gliosis produce hyperintense signals on T2-weighted MRI scans and are considered poorer prognostic signs for cervical spondylotic myelopathy (CSM) compared with OPLL.[31,33] Despite the 43% incidence of increased preoperative cord signals on MRI studies that failed to resolve postoperatively, patients with OPLL exhibited better outcomes compared with those with CSM. Dynamic MRI studies may also prove useful in demonstrating "dynamic" compression preoperatively and residual cord compromise postoperatively.

Magnetic Resonance Angiography

Measurement of the interpedicular distance on preoperative CT scans typically dictates the medial/lateral dimension of the surgical trough to be created. It may therefore vary from an average of 14 mm in the Japanese population to 18 to 20 mm in the North American population. Therefore, patients undergoing multilevel anterior corpectomy with fusion (ACF) may benefit from preoperative magnetic resonance angiography studies if the vertebral artery appears to be following an unusually tortuous course. Occasional arterial loops may appear superficially, lateral to the anterior vertebral body margin, extending ventrally as they course between the individual foramen transversarium. Alternatively, loops may be aberrantly medially located lateral to the spinal canal.

The management of vertebral artery injuries is controversial. Direct surgical repair of an injured vessel is often difficult and carries substantial risks, whereas the advent of newer interventional neuroradiologic techniques provides a preferred "endovascular" solution. For injuries that are less than 6 hours old, transient vessel tamponade may be immediately followed by acute stent placement. In those injuries that are more than 6 hours old, endovascular trapping with coils may be performed. Both endovascular alternatives avoid the risk of delayed reopening of the vessel, prevent pseudoaneurysm formation, and limit the potential for cephalad clot propagation and cranial embolization.

Computed Tomography

Noncontrast CT, intravenous-enhanced contrast CT, two-dimensional and three-dimensional reconstructed CT, and myelo-CT studies directly demonstrate punctate ossification characteristic of early OPLL or frank ossification typical of classic OPLL (Fig 88-9; see also Figs. 88-7 and 88-8). CT studies also demonstrate degenerative changes adjacent to levels of prior surgery.[33] (Double-dose intravenous contrast-enhanced CT images may increase resolution of lateral or foraminal root pathology, helping to differentiate postoperative scar [enhancing] from new disc pathology [nonenhancing]). Two-dimensional and three-dimensional noncontrast CT reconstructed images provide a sagittal overview of the extent of cord compression without incurring the risk associated with myelo-CT studies. In particular, younger patients with OPLL and normal-sized spinal cords are at greater risk for acute deterioration following myelography compared with older individuals with OPLL and significant underlying cord atrophy.

Signs of Dural Penetrance on Computed Tomography

Bone-window CT examinations document two major signs of dural penetrance; the double-layer and single-layer CT signs (see Figs. 88-7 to 88-9). The double-layer sign is characterized by a hyperdense line of OPLL directly behind the vertebra, followed

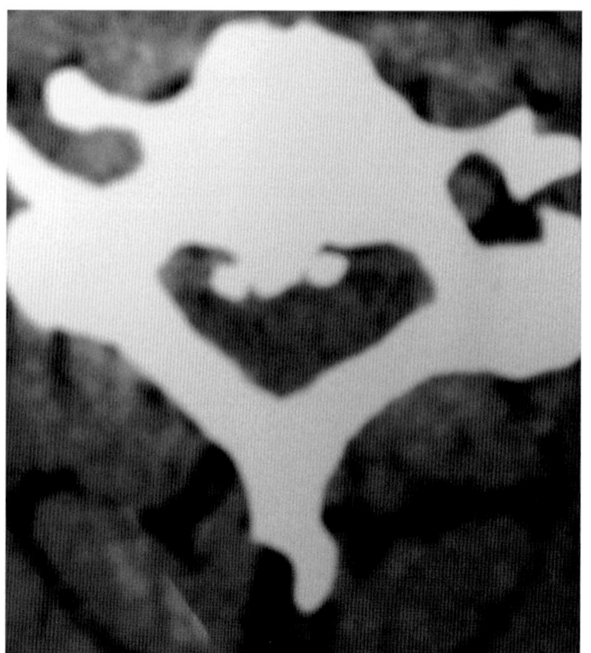

FIGURE 88-9. At the mid-C6 vertebral level, the transaxial CT (soft tissue window) scan documents both the single-layer and C signs produced by ossification of the posterior longitudinal ligament located centrally and toward the right side of the spinal canal.

by a hypodense mass representing penetrated dura, and finally, an intradural hyperdense mass of OPLL.[34,35] The single-layer sign is represented by a large central mass of OPLL. However, when the single mass is lateralized, the resulting positive C sign reflects an imbrication of the lateral dura and a greater likelihood for cerebrospinal fluid (CSF) fistula formation.

The double-layer sign is most highly correlated with absent dura, with CSF fistulas occurring between 52.6% and 84% of the time, whereas the single-layer sign (C sign) produces CSF fistulas 13.6% to 25% of the time. In one series, 10 of 12 OPLL patients with CT-documented double-layer signs developed dural defects at surgery, whereas only 1 of 9 patients showing the single-layer sign developed a CSF leak intraoperatively.[35,36] As anticipated, the greatest focus of OPLL compression in these patients corresponded to the site of dural penetrance. From a series of 197 Korean patients undergoing anterior resection of OPLL, signs of dural penetration were observed in 30.5% of patients: 52.6% with double-layer signs (nonsegmental OPLL) and 13.6% with single-layer signs.[36] For those with double-layer signs, the thicker the central mass of OPLL, the greater the incidence of intraoperative CSF fistula.

The majority of patients with OPLL who exhibit neither the single- nor the double-layer signs should not develop intraoperative CSF fistulas if careful dissection is carried out under an operating microscope. When Epstein performed multilevel simultaneous anterior corpectomies with posterior fusions in 54 OPLL patients, only one demonstrated the double-layer CT sign and one demonstrated the single-layer sign.[34,37] In 85 similar patients, three CSF fistulas resulted, with one double-layer CT sign and two single-layer CT signs.[34] In a more recent series of 110 patients undergoing similar procedures, five CSF fistulas resulted, with three with double-layer CT signs and two with single-layer CT signs.

If CT signs of dural penetrance are observed prior to surgery, then intraoperative fistulas may be anticipated, allowing the surgeon to plan for a complex dural/wound repair. Where dural edges are available, they may be directly sutured using 7-0 Gore-Tex sutures and microdural staplers (rare). More typically, with/without dural margins available, bovine pericardial grafts are applied in an onlay fashion, followed by the application of fibrin sealant, microfibrillar collagen, wound-peritoneal, and lumboperitoneal shunts.

Myelo-Computed Tomography Studies

Myelo-CT studies are now rarely performed, because combined MRI/CT studies are extremely accurate and avoid myelography's inherent risks of precipitating neurologic deterioration. Dorsally and dorsolaterally, myelo-CT studies (dynamic, static) demonstrate shingling of the lamina, OYL, OPLL, spondylosis, and disc pathology contributing to significant cord compression/stenosis. Postoperatively, myelo-CT studies also confirm whether the posterior decompression has been adequate or if further possible anterior surgery is warranted. Following open-door laminoplasty performed in OPLL patients, there was less dorsal shift of the cord but greater cord expansion, the latter factor positively correlating with outcome.[38]

Studies Documenting Fusion Following Multilevel Anterior Cervical Surgery

Fusion criteria, documented on static and two-dimensional CT studies performed immediately postoperatively and repeated at 3, 6, and 12 months postoperatively included (1) the presence of bony trabeculation, (2) lack of bony lucency at the fibula strut allograft/vertebral body interface, and (3) ingrowth of bone centrally into the fibula. Dynamic radiographs additionally revealed (1) less than 3.5 mm of translation, (2) less than 5 degrees of angulation, and (3) less than 1 mm of motion demonstrated between the tips of adjacent spinous processes. An additional criterion for fusion following multilevel ACF performed with fibula strut allograft consists of cephalad or caudad bony ingrowth from the vertebral end plate into the central canal.[39] Eighteen patients with OPLL had, on average, a 2.9-level ACF performed with fresh-frozen fibula strut allografts, accompanied by C2-T1 posterior wiring and fusion (PWF). CT documentation of bony ingrowth and other signs of fusion were observed in 17 (94%) of 18 patients (ingrowth documented utilizing 500–900 Hounsfield units). Bony ingrowth doubled from 3 to 6 months postoperatively, increasing both rostrally (1.5–3.5 mm) and caudally (2.1–4.6 mm). Although early bony ingrowth signaled progression toward fusion, its absence was not pathognomonic for a failure to fuse as observed in the one patient.

Studies Documenting Posterior Fusion

When posterior fusions are performed, whether utilizing wiring techniques (facet wiring, rod-eyelet-cable fusion constructs), lateral mass screws, or pedicle screws, the dynamic radiographic criteria enumerated previously should be met. In such cases, two-dimensional coronal and sagittal CT-based studies should demonstrate continuity between (1) bone graft and underlying laminae and (2) continuity of bone graft and fusion across facet joints.

Diseases Involving Ossification of Ligaments

Diffuse Idiopathic Skeletal Hyperostosis

DISH, an ossifying diathesis involving extensive ossification of the anterolateral aspect of contiguous vertebral bodies, is readily demonstrated on preoperative CT examinations. It typically occurs (15–30% of cases) in adults older than 65 years of age, is often asymptomatic, and is far more prevalent than OALL in North Americans.[9,40] OPLL contributes to the diffuse ligamentous ossification seen in up to 50% of patients with DISH but should only be resected either anteriorly or posteriorly in symptomatic patients.[41,42] DISH often becomes massive before producing dysphagia; therefore, other etiologies of dysphagia must be sought before the surgical resection of DISH, which may result in several months of dysphagia.[42,43]

Ossification of the Anterior Longitudinal Ligament

OALL is defined by initial hypertrophy of the anterior longitudinal ligament, followed by progressive cartilaginous infiltration, and, ultimately, frank ossification. On T1-weighted MRI studies, although the ossified OALL mass appears hypointense, the fat reflecting active bone marrow production occurring within mature Haversian canals is hyperintense.[44] On CT examinations, ventral OALL may become massive but rarely produces dysphagia; therefore, it should be resected only once other etiologies for the symptoms have been eliminated. At surgery, the extent of OALL resection may be assessed on intraoperative lateral radiographs or fluoroscopic images.

Conservative Treatment

Although conservative management of patients with OPLL may include the use of oral nonsteroidal or steroidal agents and very conservative rehabilitation therapy, epidural steroid injections should be avoided due to markedly altered pathology of the spinal canal, which may include obliteration of an epidural space. Bracing is discouraged, because the devices frequently exacerbate rather than relieve symptoms and may inadvertently place the neck in hyperextension or hyperflexion.

Patients with OPLL, whether younger than or older than 65 years of age, with progressive myelopathy, with or without evidence of cord edema, and minimal to no significant medical risk factors are considered good surgical candidates. For those with marked radiographic evidence of cord compromise, operative intervention should be performed prior to the anticipated 10% incidence of even minor cervical trauma, which can precipitate severe and/or permanent myelopathic progression.[28]

In patients with OPLL who are older than 70 years of age with severe myelopathy and significant medical comorbidities, surgery is considered high risk at best. For patients undergoing either multilevel ACF or laminectomies for myelopathy/OPLL, studies have reported that poor prognostic factors include age older than 70; severe myelopathy; cardiovascular or peripheral vascular disease; and a recent trauma history.[45,46] In two of Epstein's initial 44 patients undergoing multilevel circumferential surgery for OPLL, two patients expired from acute or 3-week delayed myocardial infarction.[47,48] Such older patients with significant major comorbidities or fixed deficits should alternatively be managed at comprehensive pain management centers.

Surgical Treatment

Role of Prophylactic Surgery

Asymptomatic patients, younger than 65 years of age, may be considered candidates for prophylactic decompression if severe cervical OPLL is radiographically or physiologically documented. This population, with a longer life expectancy, has a greater risk of inadvertent trauma and resultant irretrievable myelopathy.[28,29] T2-weighted MRI studies demonstrating high cord signals, reflecting cord edema or myelomalacia, may signal the need for surgery. Similarly, abnormal somatosensory-evoked potential (SSEP) responses may indicate subclinical dorsal cord compromise and the need to consider operative intervention. Surgery, performed prior to the onset and/or progression of a neurologic deficit, correlated with better outcomes in 87% of patients in the Saunders series.[45]

Anesthetic Protocol for Patients with Ossification of the Posterior Longitudinal Ligament Undergoing Circumferential Cervical Surgery

Patients undergoing multilevel ACF, posterior stabilization, and halo application for complex OPLL, are managed with a strict anesthetic protocol to avoid emergent hypoxia, reintubation, tracheostomy, and death.[49,50] Awake fiberoptic intubation and positioning are performed first under continuous intraoperative SSEP monitoring.[49] Eliminating cervical motion limits the potential for inadvertent hyperextension or hyperflexion injury to the cord. Following surgery, patients are kept prophylactically intubated the first postoperative night. This eliminates acute respiratory distress, particularly attributable to postoperative tracheal swelling, and the need for emergent reintubation. The following day, patients are evaluated fiberoptically by a skilled anesthesiologist and either electively extubated or kept intubated. Parameters that have to be met prior to extubation include (1) direct fiberoptic evaluation of the trachea and vocal cords for swelling, (2) indirect assessment of swelling performed by letting down the endotracheal cuff checking for an air leak and the ability to verbalize, (3) review of the patient's immediate postoperative CT scan for soft tissue swelling, and (4) assessment of other attendant medical risk factors. If the patient cannot be extubated between postoperative days 1 to 7, elective tracheostomies are scheduled. For 58 patients who underwent, on average, three-level ACF with, on average, 6.5-level PWF, spanning 10 hours, and requiring usually 2.6 units of blood transfusion, fiberoptic extubation was successfully performed the first postoperative day in 40 patients.[49]

For another 15 patients with major risk factors, extubation was delayed until postoperative days 2 to 7, and three required elective tracheostomy (day 7). Seven major risk factors identified in this study were found to positively correlate with delayed extubation or tracheostomy. In descending order, these included (1) surgical time of more 10 hours (12 patients); (2) obesity greater than 220 pounds (12 patients); (3) transfusions of more than four units of blood (10 patients); (4) secondary anterior cervical surgery (9 patients); (5) anterior surgery, including the C2 level (7 patients); (6) four-level ACF (5 patients); and (7) asthma (5 patients). In addition, minor risk factors included advanced age (>65 years), severe preoperative neurologic deficits (Nurick grade IV–V; moderate/severe myelopathy), and an intraoperative CSF fistula. Using this protocol, only one patient required emergent reintubation 20 minutes after being extubated on the third postoperative day. In this case, three major risk factors (prior C4-7 ACF 3 years earlier, asthma, and surgery lasting more than 10 hours [14 hours]) and one minor risk factor (CSF fistula with wound-peritoneal and lumboperitoneal shunts) were identified. Notably, no patients required an emergency tracheostomy. Other factors observed in the literature known to contribute to airway complications included angioedema, recurrent laryngeal nerve palsy, dysphagia with or without esophageal perforation, and new cord injuries.[25,51]

Somatosensory-Evoked Potential and Motor-Evoked Potential Monitoring

Continuous intraoperative SSEP monitoring limits morbidity associated with cervical surgery for OPLL.[42,52,53] SSEP monitoring includes the evaluation of median, ulnar, and posterior tibial responses. Awake fiberoptic nasotracheal intubation and positioning are performed with the patient awake under continuous SSEP monitoring, avoiding any cervical motion (flexion-extension). For patients operated on in the supine position, the chin is taped/distracted slightly superiorly. For patients undergoing surgery in the prone position, the three-pin head holder is applied using local anesthesia (1% lidocaine injection), and the patient is positioned awake. Keeping the patient awake during positioning allows potentials to be more readily compared with prepositioning baseline data. To avoid SSEP changes or loss, inhalation anesthetics (i.e., isoflurane, nitrous oxide) are usually kept at concentrations below 0.4%; an alternative balanced narcotic technique is typically used.

Significant Somatosensory-Evoked Potential Changes

SSEP changes are defined by (1) a 50% decline in the amplitude and (2) a 10% decrease in latency.[52] Such changes are initially observed over 50 seconds for the first recording and are reproduced within 100 seconds. Once reproduced, and not considered false positives, immediate medical and/or surgical resuscitative measures may be initiated. Medical measures include the induction of hypertension, warming of irrigating fluids, decreasing the concentration of inhalation anesthetic, and increasing the oxygen concentration. Surgical resuscitative measures include releasing distraction, removal of an oversized graft, and cessation of manipulation. Epstein demonstrated that no instances of quadriplegia or death were encountered in 100 prospectively SSEP-monitored cervical surgical cases. Eight of 218 previously unmonitored cervical operations resulted in quadriplegia (prior series included eight surgeons).[52] Other series similarly monitored SSEPs and observed 10 new postoperative neurologic deficits in 182 cervical procedures.[54]

Intraoperative Motor-Evoked Potentials and Electromyographic Monitoring

Transcranial motor evoked potentials (MEP) or transcutaneously placed epidural electrodes are typically used to monitor anterior cervical cord function.[55] Complications associated with MEP electrode placement are often minimal (seizures, headache, transient motor deficit), and successful monitoring typically correlates with positive outcomes. In a recent cervical surgical series (1055 patients) combining all three intraoperative monitoring modalities (SSEP [all 1055 patients], MEP [26 patients], and electromyography [EMG; 427 patients]), 34 patients (3.2%) had new postoperative deficits. SSEP sensitivity was 52% (specificity 100%), MEP sensitivity was 96% (specificity 100%), and EMG sensitivity was 46% (specificity 73%).[56]

Risk Factors

Major risk factors that correlated with new neurologic deficits following cervical surgery, including OPLL, are (1) multisegmental surgery, (2) severe preoperative neurologic deficits, (3) age older than 70, and (4) use of instrumentation. In many series, 50% of patients with complete intraoperative loss of potentials may show partial deficits, whereas intraoperative recovery of SSEP potentials is often correlated with eventual neurologic recovery or no deficit. Of the 34 (3.2%) of 1055 patients in Kelleher's series who experienced new postoperative deficits following cervical surgery, 6 had sensory/motor deficits, 7 had new sensory deficits, 9 had motor weakness, and 12 had new root injuries. Of these, 21 fully resolved (average 3.3 months), 9 partially resolved, and 4 were permanent.[56]

Surgical Approaches

Much controversy surrounds whether anterior or posterior surgical approaches are superior for managing cervical OPLL. Anterior surgery offers direct OPLL removal typically through multilevel ACF, whereas posterior procedures allow for indirect dorsal decompression of multilevel pathology employing laminectomy with posterior fusion procedures or laminoplasty. Some authors advocate direct anterior resection of one- to two-level OPLL (111 patients), but in expansive laminoplasty for multilevel OPLL (10 patients), good to excellent outcomes resulting from this approach were being observed in 88% and fair outcomes in 12% of patients.[57]

Posterior Surgical Approach

Older high-risk patients (>65 years) with significant multilevel OPLL but an adequately preserved cervical lordotic curvature or an exaggerated lordosis may be managed with varied posterior surgical decompressive approaches: laminectomy alone, laminectomy with posterior fusion, or laminoplasty.[26,37,58-62] Posterior removal of shingled laminae and a hypertrophied or ossified yellow ligament allows the cord to migrate away from ventrally situated OPLL and spondylotic/osteophytic changes. Nevertheless, posterior surgery is not appropriate in the presence of kyphosis, because removal of the posterior elements will leave the cord tethered over ventral disease.

Laminectomy

Laminectomy may sufficiently decompress the cervical spinal canal in patients with OPLL if the cervical spine is stable and the lordotic curvature is adequately preserved (see Figs. 88-1 to 88-3). Laminectomy and medial facetectomies/foraminotomies should include the resection of 25% or less of the medial aspect of the facet joint to preserve stability; greater than 50% to 75% facet removal correlates with greater pathologic motion/instability.[63] Long-term results of laminectomy for patients with OPLL (44 patients) revealed a neurologic recovery rate of 44.2% 1 year postoperatively, and the rate of 42.9% was nearly unchanged 5 years later.[59] However, outcomes worsened between 5 and 10 years postoperatively. Negative prognostic factors included (1) older age at the time of the original surgery, (2) more severe preoperative neurologic deficits, (3) history of new trauma, and (4) presence of OPLL. Despite OPLL progression in 70% of patients, only one patient experienced significant neurologic deterioration. Additionally, although kyphosis progressed in 47% of patients, it was not significantly correlated with deterioration.

Laminectomy with Posterior Fusion

Cervical laminectomy in conjunction with a posterior fusion is another alternative for the management of OPLL where the lordotic curvature is preserved. In some patients, prophylactic stabilization may be performed to avoid the evolution of instability, whereas in others, instability may already be present. Iatrogenic instability secondary to a failed laminectomy may also contribute to the need for simultaneous fusion.[63] Preoperative documentation of chronic olisthy, partial swan-neck deformity, or hyperlordosis with excessive mobility constitute other reasons for considering posterior fusion.

Limited Laminectomy with Spinous Process-Based Fusions

Utilizing more focal or limited laminectomies (one to three levels), with undercutting and/or removal of the OYL from respective cephalad and caudad laminae, leaves multiple spinous processes intact, which may be used for rod-eyelet-cable–based fusion constructs.[64-67] Advantages of this technique include the avoidance of lateral mass and/or pedicle screws with the accompanying risks of critical breaches (1.4–10.6%) and neurologic/neurovascular injuries.[66,67] In an initial study of 14 patients undergoing one- to two-level focal laminectomy with rod-eyelet-cable–instrumented fusions, maximal 36-Item Short Form Health Survey (SF-36) improvement occurred on five health scales within the initial 6 months postoperatively, and fusions preserved stability and avoided disease progression.[66] In a series of 35 patients undergoing focal laminectomy (one to three levels) with posterior fusion (rod-eyelet-cable construct), patients averaged 65 years of age and exhibited severe myelopathy (Nurick grade IV–V) and cord compression (stenosis, OPLL, OYL, olisthy). Following average two-level laminectomy and seven-level fusions, patients neurologically improved (Nurick grade 0–I; mild radiculopathy, mild myelopathy), exhibiting two transient root injuries, with 100% fusion at 5.2 months postoperatively (dynamic radiographs, CT-documented). Iliac autograft supplemented with beta tricalcium phosphate plus autogenous bone marrow aspirate effectively promoted posterolateral cervical fusion in this series, a finding well documented in posterior iliac crest/posterior cervical and lumbar posterolateral fusion studies.[68-70] When performing these procedures, the use of microfibrillar collagen (Duragen; Integra, Plainsboro, NJ) is also recommended. However, the use of porcine skin hemostatic gelatin (Gelfoam; Pfizer, Morris Plains, NJ), based on the literature and its own insert, is contraindicated, with risks including root compression/neurologic deficits due to severe swelling of the implant, infection, and allergic reactions to the porcine component of the product.[71] In one case, Gelfoam resulted in the delayed (3 weeks) postoperative exacerbation of myelopathy in an elderly female; following the removal of hypertrophied/compressive and adherent Gelfoam, her symptoms resolved. The addition of silver-based dressings (Silverlon; Argentum Medical, Plainsboro, NJ) used with sterile water over a 10-day postoperative period also markedly limited the frequency of wound infections.[72] SF-36 outcomes questionnaires revealed improvement on all 8 health scales, and Odom criteria demonstrated 29 good/excellent outcomes and 6 fair/poor outcomes.[67]

Laminectomy with Facet Fusion, Lateral Mass, and Pedicle Fixation Techniques

Fusion alternatives include facet wiring techniques, insertion of lateral mass screws, and dorsal pedicle screw fixation.[60-62,73,74] Laminectomy with posterior wiring and fusion resulted in high fusion rates without significant complications in Epstein's series of 85 OPLL patients.[37,58] Alternatively, Hamanishi and Tanaka noted no significant difference in outcomes when comparing laminectomy performed in 35 patients without instability to laminectomy with fusion performed in 34 unstable patients.[60] Using the SF-36, Kumar et al. evaluated patient-based outcomes in 25 patients undergoing laminectomy with lateral mass plating for unstable spondylotic myelopathy.[61] No patients exhibited new postoperative instability or increased kyphosis, 80% showed good outcomes, 76% improved on myelopathy scores, and none developed delayed deterioration. Applying lateral mass plates in 43 patients, including 14 with postlaminectomy instability, Wellman et al. encountered no significant complications in 281 screws placed (average, seven screws per patient).[62] However, dorsal decompression with or without fusion did not suffice in a subset of Abumi and Kaneda's patients with significant OPLL.[73] Following the application of pedicle screws for dorsal fixation after 26 laminectomies or laminoplasties, 15 patients required additional anterior procedures. In Abumi et al.'s update 2 years later, postoperative radiographic studies demonstrated that 10 of 190 (5.3%) screws perforated the cortex of the pedicles but did not result in neurovascular complications.[74] Alternatively, of 58 patients with CSM, OPLL, or degenerative disease undergoing dorsal cervical decompressions with posterior pedicle screw–instrumented fusions, 8 developed screw-related complications, including 2 vertebral artery injuries.[75]

Laminoplasty

Some surgeons consider the laminoplasty to be an optimal approach to multilevel OPLL; the more levels of OPLL involved, the more likely a laminoplasty may be performed. Laminoplasty simultaneously offers dorsal decompression while augmenting stability without the need for traditional fusion.[23,26,76] Results of cervical decompression in a goat model using the laminoplasty versus the laminectomy, radiographic and biomechanical results confirmed that laminoplasty was superior in maintaining cervical alignment and avoiding postoperative spinal deformity.[77]

Where OPLL extended up to the C2 level or down to the T1 level, these levels should be included in the original decompression, avoiding further OPLL expansion requiring secondary surgery. In one series, long-term recovery rates of 44.2% were observed after 1 year and 42.9% after 5 years (44 patients undergoing laminectomy); long-term deterioration occurred 5 to 10 years later and correlated with a 32.8% decline in JOA scores.[59] Major negative prognostic factors included advanced age at the time of the original surgery, more severe preoperative myelopathy, and a history of trauma.

For 64 patients who underwent expansive laminoplasty, late recovery rates of 64% were maintained at 10 years with only 14% of patients demonstrating delayed deterioration at 5 to 15 years postoperatively.[78] Of interest, OPLL progressed in only two cases at previously operated sites. When OPLL progression was evaluated over a 5-year period using plain radiographs for 55 postlaminectomy patients, 12 patients (21.8%) demonstrated OPLL progression/thickness; progression was greater in younger patients with continuous or mixed OPLL and was most marked at the C2-4 levels.[79] Long-term follow-up (average, 10.2 years; range, 5–20 years) in 66 patients undergoing laminoplasty for myelopathy/OPLL revealed significantly poorer results for patients with a canal occupancy ratio of greater than 60% and a hill-shaped ossification. Other but lesser negative factors included poorer preoperative clinical status (poorer JOA), postoperative changes in alignment, and older age at the original surgery.[80] In another study with an average 14-year follow-up following open-door laminoplasty for patients with either CSM or OPLL, average JOA scores and recovery rates improved markedly within 3 years postoperatively but showed slight deterioration at 5 years.[81] Notably, although 66% demonstrated OPLL progression, this did not contribute to clinical symptomatic worsening.

Improvement following laminoplasty largely relies on whether there is a sufficient lordotic cervical curvature to allow for dorsal migration of the cord away from ventrally situated OPLL. In one study, comparing preoperative with postoperative myelo-CT studies in 65 patients undergoing laminoplasty for OPLL, a mean dorsal cord shift of greater than 3 mm correlated with good clinical outcomes (range, 0.0–6.6 mm).[76] However, for OPLL lesions located at the rostral or caudal extremes of the canal, decompression had to be extended one level above or below this pathology to maximize dorsal cord migration. In another study involving patients undergoing laminoplasty, a 42% increase in the average postoperative anteroposterior canal diameter (3 years postoperatively), a 96% bone fusion rate, an 83% incidence of preserved range of motion, and significant neurologic improvement (preoperative JOA score, 9; postoperative JOA score, 14.1) were observed.[23] For laminoplasty to be successful in OPLL patients, congenital stenosis had to be largely avoided, because a minimum canal diameter of 17 mm (31 patients) was typically required to achieve adequate cord decompression; in smaller canals, anterior approaches had to be seriously considered.[82]

Limitations of Outcomes with Posterior Decompressions

Lesser-quality clinical outcomes may be observed for patients with severe OPLL undergoing dorsal decompressions (laminectomy with or without fusion, laminoplasty). In one series of OPLL patients, better results were observed following anterior (48 patients) rather than posterior laminoplasty (27 patients) surgical procedures. This included both the mean overall improvement scores (neurosurgical cervical spine scale score of 78% [anterior] versus 46.1% [posterior] decompressions) and long-term follow-up scores (anterior scores rose from 9 and 13, and laminoplasty scores declined from 10.4 to 9.7).[83] Other studies also observed better outcomes following anterior rather than posterior surgery for OPLL.[5,6,47,48]

Increased Ossification of the Posterior Longitudinal Ligament Progression Following Dorsal Decompression

A major concern remains whether dorsal decompression of OPLL increases the rate of OPLL progression. One study radiologically compared OPLL progression rates following 25 laminoplasties, 16 laminectomies, and 56 nonsurgical cases. Although no significant difference was observed in OPLL progression rates following either laminoplasty or laminectomy, both operations increased OPLL's progression compared with those treated conservatively.[84]

Anterior Surgical Approaches

Single-Level Anterior Corpectomy with Fusion

Some surgeons have determined that direct anterior resection of OPLL results in improved postoperative neurologic outcomes when found at one level with retrovertebral extension or two-level discectomy/fusion.[85,86] When patients demonstrated OPLL at one to two interspaces (focal), it was typically accompanied by significant retrovertebral extension and, therefore, one-level corpectomies were the preferred operation. Reoperation rates for 55 OPLL patients undergoing one-level ACF varied according to the type of plates applied: 3 Orion plates, using a fixed-plate/fixed-screw design (Sofamor Danek, Memphis, TN); 12 Atlantis plates, using a fixed-plate variable-screw design (Sofamor Danek); and 40 ABC dynamic plates (Aesculap, Tuttlingen, Germany).[86] The overall failure rates were 7 of 15 (47%) for fixed compared with 4 of 40 (10%) for dynamic plates. The average cephalad migration of the dynamic plates was 6.6 mm (range, 3–10 mm), and the average caudad migration was 5.7 (range, 3–8 mm). The lower failure rate for dynamic plates that allowed several millimeters of rostral and caudal migration indicated that the dynamic design contributed to reduced stress shielding and increased compression, both of which contributed to fusion and stability.

Multilevel Anterior Corpectomy and Fusion

Better outcomes have been reported in some series for OPLL patients undergoing multilevel anterior corpectomy and fusion procedures, rather than posterior operations (see Figs. 88-4 to 88-6).[87-98] In one study, Nurick scores improved in 86% of 93 patients undergoing anterior cervical corpectomy (average score, 1.24), whereas poorer outcomes followed posterior surgery (improvement of only 0.07).[99] In another study comparing the results of ADF in patients with OPLL (27 patients) versus laminoplasty (66 patients), over a mean interval of 6 years postoperatively, ADF resulted in superior neurologic outcomes with patients exhibiting an occupying ratio of 60% or greater. However, this was accompanied by a 15% incidence of graft complications, and additional surgery was required in 26% of patients.[100] Other series include the incidence of major complications that may be associated with multilevel ACF/posterior fusion.[37,47,48,87,88,91,101-103] In 76 patients with OPLL undergoing either nonplated ADF (average, 3.5 levels) or ACF (average, 3 levels), Epstein found a 13% incidence of pseudarthrosis/instability within the first 6 months postoperatively.[88] In another series, 10% of 31 nonplated four-level ACFs also failed acutely.[45] In a third series of 36 patients undergoing two- to four-level ACF (15 performed with plates), the combined perioperative mortality/major morbidity rate was 22%, even though 97% ultimately fused.[104] In a fourth series, involving two-level ACF with fixed anterior plates, a 9% incidence of graft extrusion occurred; the failure rate rose to 50% for three-level plated ACF.[102] In a fifth series, involving one-level ACF (87 patients) and two- to three-level ACF (98 patients), a 98.8% fusion rate, a 3.2% neurologic complication rate, and an 86.5% improvement rate were observed.[105]

Complication Rates

Complication rates were lower when dynamic rather than fixed plates were used to perform multilevel ACF/PWF. When Epstein performed 22 multilevel (two- to four-level) ACFs without anterior plates but added PWF, three graft extrusions resulted.[47] Adding a fixed plate to another 22 of these multilevel constructs resulted in two immediate inferior graft/plate extrusions.[48] When Atlantis plates (Sofamor Danek) were applied in 16 similar patients, three extruded postoperatively (2 patients at 1 month, 1 patient at 4 months). All of these included inferior graft, plate, and screw extrusions.[37] After having performed 25 multilevel ACF/PWFs with dynamic plates, only one patient developed a "partial" pseudarthrosis of the anterior graft demonstrated on sequential CT studies, warranting a second PWF.[86] The average dynamic plate migration for these multilevel ACF/PWF constructs was 6.1 mm (range, 4–10 mm) cephalad and 5.8 mm (range, 4–9 mm) caudad. Dynamic plating similarly appeared to limit stress shielding, promoted graft settling, and fostered fusion in multilevel constructs.[86,92]

Posterior fusions may be completed using posterior wiring and fusion techniques, lateral mass screw/plating systems, or pedicle screw/rod instrumentation. The biomechanical advantage of a posterior construct, or posterior "tension band," has been well documented. In a sagittal plane biomechanical study, Kirkpatrick et al. demonstrated that posterior fusion reduced the range of motion by 62% compared with 24% with strut grafting alone. This percentage was 43% following anterior strut graft and the application of an anterior plate.[101] Posterior spinous process fusions may also readily be performed using a rod-eyelet–braided titanium cable construct, with iliac autograft supplemented with beta tricalcium phosphate applied laterally over the laminae and facet joints.

Cord and Root Injuries

Complications of anterior cervical surgery include a 2% to 10% incidence of quadriplegia and up to a 17% incidence of root injury (typically the C5 root).[12] Root injuries may result from rapid dorsal cord migration, or the so-called untethering effect, more often following a posterior cervical procedure rather than anterior decompression.[45] In one study, 9 of 49 patients undergoing laminectomy and lateral mass screw fixation for OPLL developed postoperative C5 root palsies within 6 hours to 6 days postoperatively. Although there was no increased cord signal observed on T2-weighted MRI studies in these patients, an exaggerated cervical lordosis combined with OPLL indicated that these injuries were due to a tethering effect on the C5 roots themselves.[106] Although less frequent, anterior migration can also occur but may be mitigated by limiting the anterior trough diameter to 14 to 15 mm.[45] Many patients with OPLL in North America are larger individuals and typically require resection of vertebral bodies/discs into the 18- to 20-mm range to achieve adequate decompression. In these cases, therefore, more limited 14- to 15-mm troughs would leave significant amounts of OPLL in place and would likely fail to result in resolution of radicular symptoms.

Outcomes of Circumferential Surgery

Higher rates of successful fusion without plate/graft-related complications were increasingly observed as dynamic plates (ABC; Aesculap, Tuttlingen, Germany) progressively replaced fixed-plated systems. Of 66 patients undergoing simultaneous multilevel ACF (2.6–3.0 levels) with posterior fusions (seven-level; circumferential procedures) for cervical OPLL, 13% of fixed plates (extrusion, fracture, pseudarthrosis) versus only 3.6% of dynamic ABC plates (1 plate; delayed pseudarthrosis) failed.[96] Nurick grades, Odom criteria, and SF-36 outcomes were evaluated in 47 patients undergoing circumferential cervical surgery for OPLL.[97] Patients averaged 54 years of age, exhibited severe myelopathy (average Nurick grade 3.6), and underwent average 2.6-level ACF with seven-level posterior fusions (C2-T1) accompanied by halo placement. Fixed plates (28 plates) and dynamic plates (19 plates) were applied. Determination of fusion was based on both dynamic radiographic and two dimensional–CT studies an average of 5 months postoperatively. At 1 year postoperatively, Nurick grades improved 2.8 to 3.2 points, Odom criteria showed 40 excellent/good and 7 fair/poor outcomes, and SF-36 outcomes revealed moderate improvement on five health scales: social function, bodily pain, role physical, physical function, and role emotional. Minimal additional improvement occurred over the succeeding second year.

Outcomes further improved as increasingly only dynamic plates were used. In a study involving multilevel ACF/posterior fusion using ABC plates in 40 patients, only one patient exhibited a delayed pseudarthrosis, patients fused an average of 6.3 months postoperatively, and there were no longer any plate/graft extrusions.[98] At one postoperative year, Nurick grades improved from a preoperative severe myelopathy (average score, 3.9) to postoperative mild radiculopathy/myelopathy (average score, 0.4), and SF-36 improvement was maximal on role physical, bodily pain, and role emotional health scales.

Anterior Floating Method: An Option for Anterior Resection

The anterior floating method is an alternative technique proposed for ventral OPLL resection where it occupies more than 60% of the spinal canal.[107] This technique includes marked lateral and cephalad/caudad resection and thinning of the vertebral bodies with air drills to avoid CSF fistulas associated with classic ventral OPLL resection. In theory, because this technique frees the ossified dura from its constraints, ventral migration of the remaining dura/OPLL mass allows for adequate spinal cord and nerve root decompression. Although this procedure offers long-term JOA recovery rates of 71%, it does not offer direct resection of the OPLL mass. Therefore, further progression of OPLL accompanied by retethering of the "floating OPLL" mass remains a major concern, as do the technical risks that include vertebral artery and root injury associated with the extreme lateral resection technique.

Summary

Many complex alternatives have been offered concerning the treatment of OPLL. Familiarity with the multiple MRI and CT presentations is critical, but integration of these radiographic data with the patient's clinical and overall medical status is essential if optimal outcomes are to be achieved. As important as knowing when to operate is recognizing those patients who will not benefit from surgery (severe medical comorbidities, previously fixed neurologic deficits). This very complex surgery is multifaceted and requires extensive clinical experience and expertise.

KEY REFERENCES

Abumi K, Kaneda K, Shono Y, et al: One-stage posterior decompression and reconstruction of the cervical spine by using pedicle screw fixation systems. *J Neurosurg* 90(Suppl 1):19–26, 1999.

Epstein NE: An argument for traditional posterior cervical fusion techniques: evidence from 35 cases. *Surg Neurol* 70(1):45–55, 2008.

Epstein NE: Circumferential cervical surgery for ossification of the posterior longitudinal ligament: a multianalytic outcome study. *Spine* 29(12):1340–1345, 2004.

Epstein NE: Evaluation of intraoperative somatosensory evoked potential monitoring during 100 cervical operations. *Spine* 18(6):737–747, 1993.

Fukui M, Chiba K, Kawakami M, et al: Japanese Orthopaedic Association Cervical Myelopathy Evaluation Questionnaire (JOACMEQ). Part 3. Determination of reliability. *J Orthop Sci* 12:21–26, 2007.

Fukui M, Chiba K, Kawakami M, et al: Japanese Orthopaedic Association Cervical Myelopathy Evaluation Questionnaire (JOACMEQ). Part 4. Establishment of equations for severity scores: subcommittee on low back pain and cervical myelopathy evaluation of the clinical outcome committee of the Japanese Orthopaedic Association. *J Orthop Sci* 13:25–31, 2008.

Hida K, Iwasaki Y, Kohanagi I, et al: Bone window computed tomography for detection of dural defect associated with cervical ossified posterior longitudinal ligament. *Neurol Med Chir (Tokyo)* 37(2):173–175, 1997.

Iwasaki M, Okuda S, Miyauchi A, et al: Surgical strategy for cervical myelopathy due to ossification of the posterior longitudinal ligament: part 2: advantages of anterior decompression and fusion over laminoplasty. *Spine* 32(6):654–660, 2007.

REFERENCES

The complete reference list is available online at expertconsult.com.

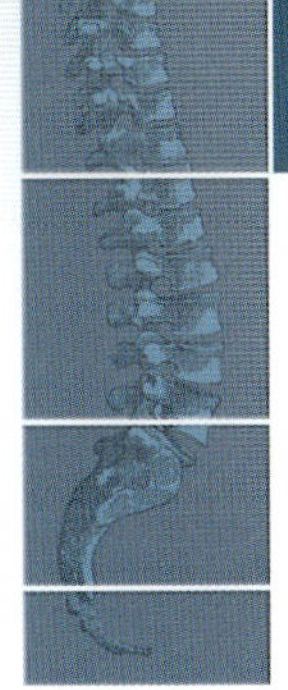

CHAPTER 89

Scheuermann Disease

Daniel Shedid | Isador H. Lieberman

Scheuermann Disease or Kyphosis

In 1920, Holger Werfel Scheuermann, a Danish surgeon, described a rigid kyphosis of the thoracic or thoracolumbar spine occurring in adolescents.[1] The disease, now known as *Scheuermann disease*, manifests itself at puberty and involves ventral wedge formation of one or more vertebral bodies, leading to a rigid kyphotic deformity of the affected segments.[2,3] It is the second most frequent etiologic factor in back pain in children and adolescents following spondylolysis and spondylolisthesis.[4] Scheuermann disease typically involves the midthoracic spine, with the apex at the T7 and T8 vertebrae.[5] Sorenson[6] defined the radiographic diagnosis of Scheuermann kyphosis on the basis of anterior wedging of 5 degrees or more of at least three adjacent vertebral bodies. Scheuermann disease typically involves the thoracic spine but can also occur solely in the thoracolumbar spine in 25% of patients.

Incidence

Scheuermann disease affects between 1% and 8% of the general population.[6,7] In a review of 1384 cadaveric specimens, Scoles et al.[7] reported a prevalence of 7.4%. Scheuermann disease affects the growing, maturing spine and is usually identified in adolescents between 11 and 17 years of age. In Sorenson's review, 58% of those affected were male and 42% were female. There are, however, widely divergent reports regarding the relative gender prevalence. Bradford[8] reported a female-to-male ratio of 2:1. In contrast, Murray et al. reported a 2:1 prevalence in males[9]; 20% to 30% of the patients also have scoliosis. Additionally, there is an increased incidence of spondylolysis in patients with thoracic Scheuermann kyphosis.[10]

A familial occurrence of the disease has been described.[2] Damborg et al.[11] reviewed 35,000 twins and found a prevalence of Scheuermann disease of 2.8% (3.6% in males and 2.1% in females). Both the pairwise and probandwise concordance for monozygotic twins was significantly greater than that for dizygotic twins, and the hereditability was 74%. These findings may indicate a strong genetic contribution to the etiology of the condition.

Pathogenesis

The etiology of Scheuermann kyphosis remains unknown.[8,12,13] Many theories have been proposed to explain the progressive wedge shaping of the involved vertebrae. Scheuermann[1] considered the condition a form of avascular necrosis of the ring apophysis that leads to a growth arrest, resulting in wedging of the ventral portion of the vertebral bodies. However, Bick and Copel[14] later showed that the ring apophysis does not contribute to vertebral growth. Furthermore, avascular necrosis has never been identified in affected vertebral segments of patients with the disease.[8,12,15] Schmorl[16] postulated that herniations of disc material through the vertebral end plates (which now bear his name) lead to a loss of disc height and ventral wedging of the vertebral body. Subsequent studies disproved these early theories but have not yet established a cause.

Osteoporosis may be an etiologic factor in the development of Scheuermann kyphosis. Bradford et al.[17] prospectively studied 12 patients with an extensive osteoporosis workup and iliac crest biopsy. They identified increased levels of serum alkaline phosphatase and urinary hydroxyproline, in conjunction with reduced bone mineral density. However, when compared with age-matched controls, no specific relationship could be identified. The authors postulated that Scheuermann disease may be related to a generalized skeletal disease that presents during the adolescent growth spurt. Gilanz et al.[18] subsequently reported on 20 adolescent patients 12 to 18 years of age with Scheuermann kyphosis and could demonstrate no evidence of osteoporosis (as assessed by quantitative CT).

Mechanical factors have also been postulated in the development of Scheuermann kyphosis.[13,17] Strenuous physical activity has been associated with compression of the vertebrae of patients with this disease.[13] Ogden et al.[19] believe that the term *Scheuermann disease* is a misnomer; these authors state that the changes noted radiographically are altered remodeling responses to abnormal biomechanical stresses and are not secondary to an underlying disease process. They theorized that the kyphosis occurs first and that the ventral vertebral body is then subjected to increased forces that suppress ventral growth and perpetuate the deformity. The reported success of brace treatment lends support to the mechanical theory.[20] Lambrinudi[21] and others have suggested that the upright posture and tightness of the anterior longitudinal ligament of the spine contribute to the deformity. Most investigators believe that the growth plate becomes disorganized first and the emerging kyphosis follows. The kyphosis and growth plate changes may ultimately potentiate each other. The kyphosis likely results in increased pressure on the vertebral end plates ventrally, allowing for uneven growth of the vertebral bodies with wedging (as per Wolff law).

Recently, Fotiadis et al.[22] screened 10,057 students and found 175 children with Scheuermann disease (study group). The length of the sternum was greater in the healthy (control) group. There was a statistically significant difference between the two groups with regard to sternum length. The children with Scheuermann disease were taller in relation to the control group. These authors concluded that the shorter length of sternum than normal has a possible correlation with the appearance of Scheuermann disease. Presumably the shorter length of the sternum increases the compressive forces on the vertebral end plates anteriorly, allowing uneven growth of the vertebral bodies with wedging.

Clinical Features

The onset of Scheuermann disease usually appears around puberty, commonly as kyphosis of the thoracic (type I Scheuermann) or thoracolumbar spine (type II Scheuermann). These two entities differ both in location and by their clinical presentation. The deformity is often attributed to poor posture. This results in a delay in both diagnosis and treatment. Pain is often present; standing, sitting, and heavy physical activity may aggravate the pain (i.e., mechanical pain), which may or may not subside with cessation of growth. Adults who have untreated Scheuermann disease may have severe back pain, especially when the deformity is advanced.

Patients generally present with an angular thoracic or thoracolumbar kyphosis accompanied by a compensatory hyperlordosis of the lumbar spine. Their compensatory lordosis may lead to an increase in pelvic tilt.[3] Frequently, the cervical lordosis is increased with forward projection of the head. The kyphosis is fixed and remains apparent on hyperextension of the spine. In rare instances, advanced thoracic kyphosis can lead to thoracic spinal cord compression and paraparesis.[23] Thoracic disc herniation may also be associated with Scheuermann kyphosis, and the patient may present with signs and symptoms of myelopathy.[2,24,25] Pain, when present, is usually at the site of the thoracic deformity. Sorenson described pain as the major symptom in 50% of patients with advanced disease.[6]

Clinical examination often reveals tight hamstrings as well as a popliteal angle of less than 30 degrees and subtle neurologic findings. Tight hamstrings have recently been implicated as a possible cause of sagittal decompensation.[26]

In addition to the kyphosis of the thoracic spine, affected individuals demonstrate varying degrees of structural scoliosis.[5,15,17] Blumenthal et al.[13] noted lumbar scoliosis in 85% of 50 patients with type I Scheuermann disease. Spondylolysis and spondylolisthesis are also common in the lumbar spine.[2,17] Ogilvie and Sherman[27] observed a 50% incidence of asymptomatic spondylolysis in 18 patients with type I disease. They postulated that the excessive hyperlordosis places stress on the pars of the L4 and L5 vertebrae, resulting in the spondylolysis. Increased cervical lordosis also develops as a compensatory mechanism and causes the head to protrude forward (gooseneck deformity), producing a negative sagittal balance with the C7 plumb line lying posterior to the sacral promontory.[4]

Radiographic Features

Routine radiographic studies obtained for evaluation of the patient with Scheuermann kyphosis should include anteroposterior and lateral radiographs of the entire spine via long films (scoliosis views) and a hyperextension lateral image of the thoracic spine. The lateral radiograph should be obtained with the patient standing, with knees and hips fully extended and arms out and away from the spine. The patient should be looking forward. The lateral radiograph should document the following typical changes of Scheuermann kyphosis:

- Schmorl nodes
- Kyphosis of the involved spinal segment
- Ventral vertebral body wedging
- End-plate irregularity

The abnormal sagittal parameters are determined from the thoracic, thoracolumbar, and lumbar regions of the spine.

Both the vertebral wedging and kyphosis should be measured by the Cobb method. When evaluating serial radiographs to document progression, care should be taken to ensure that the same end-vertebral bodies are measured each time. The normal range of thoracic kyphosis is 20 to 45 degrees on a standing lateral radiograph[28-30] as measured by the Cobb method. Normal kyphosis increases with age and is slightly greater in women than in men.[31,32] Ventral wedge compression of one or more vertebral segments in association with kyphosis is the hallmark radiographic feature in Scheuermann disease.[1] Wedging of at least 5 degrees of three or more vertebrae is diagnostic of Scheuermann disease. The kyphosis in Scheuermann disease is usually incompletely reducible with postural and positional changes. The vertebra with the greatest ventral deformity is located at the apex of the kyphotic curve. The kyphosis may approach 100 degrees in advanced cases with a compensatory hyperlordosis of both the cervical and lumbar spine.[3]

Early in the progression of the disease, the end plates may appear irregular.[3,5,16,33] The changes have been described as moth-eaten and relate to growth retardation rather than to a destructive process.[5] As the disease progresses, the growth plates appear sclerotic, but despite interspace narrowing the change is not associated with interbody fusion. The absence of fusion helps distinguish Scheuermann disease from other kyphotic deformities of the spine.[5,8,13]

An MRI before surgery is recommended to rule out any incidental thoracic disc herniation, epidural cyst, or possible spinal stenosis. The literature has shown such exceptional cases in various reports of neurologic complications in Scheuermann kyphosis.[2,24,25,29] The MRI also assesses the lumbar spine discs, because disc degeneration of the lumbar spine may explain, in some cases, the pain rather than the kyphotic deformity itself.

It is important to differentiate Scheuermann kyphosis from a postural roundback deformity. Adolescents with postural roundback deformity have a slight to moderate increase in the degree of thoracic kyphosis (usually ≤60 degrees), which is less acutely angulated and may be associated with an accentuated lumbar lordosis. This type of kyphosis is flexible and not associated with muscle contractures. There is also a normal appearance of the vertebrae without evidence of wedging, end-plate irregularity, or premature disc degeneration on imaging.[4,33,34]

Natural History

The natural history of Scheuermann disease remains very controversial. The condition tends to be symptomatic during the teenage years. However, in the late teenage years, it often produces less pain. If the residual kyphosis in these patients remains less than 50 to 60 degrees, there is usually little discomfort in adult life.[35] In a long-term follow-up study, Sorenson noted pain in the thoracic region in 50% of patients during adolescence, with the number of symptomatic patients decreasing to 25% by the time of skeletal maturity.[6] Later, other authors offered a contrasting view, stating that adults with Scheuermann kyphosis have a higher incidence of disabling back pain than the normal population.[2,8] Murray et al.[9] performed a study in 67 patients with Scheuermann kyphosis diagnosed by Sorenson's criteria (i.e., physical examination, trunk strength, radiography, a detailed questionnaire, and pulmonary function testing). The patients had an average kyphotic deformity of 71 degrees, and average follow-up was 32 years. An age-matched comparison group was used as a control. Normal or above-normal averages for pulmonary function were found in patients in whom the kyphosis was less than 100 degrees. Patients in whom the kyphosis was greater than 100 degrees and the apex of the curve was in the first to eighth thoracic segments had restrictive lung disease. The authors concluded that patients may have functional limitations but that these did not result in severe limitations due to pain or cause major interference with their lives. Lowe and Kasten state that adults with greater than 75 degrees of kyphosis can have severe thoracic pain secondary to spondylosis that can limit their activity.[36]

In summary, patients experience wide variations in the natural history of Scheuermann kyphosis. Thoracic Scheuermann kyphosis greater than 100 degrees can be associated with reduced pulmonary function. There appears to be a subset of patients with refractory symptoms that justify the risk associated with intensive treatments such as bracing and surgical management.

Treatment

The management of patients with symptomatic Scheuermann kyphosis ranges from observation to combined ventral and dorsal reconstructive surgery. Treatment is based on the severity of the deformity, the presence of pain, and the age of the patient. The recommended treatment should be tailored to the individual on the basis of deformity progression, the severity of the curve, and symptomatology.

Nonsurgical Treatment

Nonoperative treatment is classically indicated during the growth period if thoracic kyphosis exceeds 40 to 45 degrees and if radiologic signs of the disease are present. It includes anti-inflammatory medications, exercise, bracing, and casting.

Anti-inflammatory Medications

Nonsteroidal anti-inflammatory drugs may be useful short-term adjuncts to nonoperative care of adolescents. They may also be considered for longer-term care in adults with spondylosis and back pain.

Exercise

Exercise has never been shown to improve or halt progression of fixed Scheuermann kyphosis.[26] However, a thoracic extension program coupled with an aerobic exercise program does improve conditioning and may alleviate pain. In adults, the exercise program concentrates on stretching the hamstring and pectoral muscles and strengthening the abdominal muscles, which will probably alleviate the back pain but not alter the deformity. Weiss et al.[37] reported pain reduction between 16% and 32% in a group of 351 patients with a painful Scheuermann kyphosis who were treated conservatively with physical therapy, osteopathy, manual therapy, exercises, and psychological therapy.

Bracing

Bracing and casting are of value only in patients with mobile kyphotic deformity and with a sufficient amount of growth remaining.[26] The few available brace treatment studies are retrospective, have different inclusion criteria, and do not have control groups. The initial report of Bradford et al.[38] regarding Milwaukee brace treatment of Scheuermann kyphosis in 75 patients demonstrated a 40% decrease in mean thoracic kyphosis and a 35% decrease in mean lumbar lordosis after an average of 34 months of brace wear. Gutowski and Renshaw[39] reported on the use of Boston lumbar and modified Milwaukee orthoses for Scheuermann kyphosis and abnormal juvenile round back, with an average 26-month follow-up. Of the 75 patients in their group, 31% rejected the brace within 4 months. Compliant patients had an improvement of 27% in the Boston group and 35% in the Milwaukee group. Whether the corrections were maintained over time is not known. Bracing can be expected to provide up to a 50% correction of the deformity, with some gradual loss of correction over time. Sachs et al.[40] followed 120 patients for more than 5 years after discontinuation of the brace and demonstrated that 69% still had improvement of 30 degrees or more.

The Milwaukee brace is the most commonly used brace. It is indicated when the apex of the kyphosis is at or above T8 and for the overweight patient or the female patient with large breasts. The underarm orthosis or thoracolumbosacral orthosis is indicated when the apex of the kyphosis is at or below T9.[34]

The classic prerequisites for brace treatment of Scheuermann kyphosis include a progressive curve beyond 45 degrees. Patients with a kyphosis of up to 65 degrees may be successfully treated. Treatment using a Milwaukee brace was shown to be effective to relieve pain and correct curves less than 74 degrees in skeletally immature patients, but curves greater than 74 degrees have been associated with higher failure rates.[40] Patients must have some flexibility and some remaining growth. Bracing and/or casting is ineffective once the patient's Risser sign is 4 or 5.[26] The brace is typically worn for 23 hours a day for 1 to 2 years.

Surgical Treatment

The indications for surgical intervention remain unclear, because the natural history of Scheuermann kyphosis remains controversial regarding pain, trunk deformity, disability, and self-esteem. The ultimate decision for surgical correction should be individualized. It may relate to the patient's symptoms, self-perception, and sense of self-esteem. The surgeon's training and level of skill in performing a safe, predictable correction also affect the decision-making process.

Surgical indications have evolved over the past 2 decades. The operative indications for Scheuermann kyphosis are similar to those of patients with other deformity types: (1) progression of deformity, (2) neurologic compromise, (3) worsening pain, and (4) cosmesis.[6,40,41] Some authors also list unacceptable trunk appearance as an indication.[36] An adolescent with kyphosis greater than 75 degrees despite a trial of bracing may be a surgical candidate. An adult may become a candidate when severe refractory pain develops secondary to a curve of at least 60 degrees. A formal indication for surgery would be a neurologic complication appearing in the context of Scheuermann disease. The cord compression is more commonly due to thoracic disc lesions. Such complications would require neurologic decompression through an anterior thoracotomy or a posterolateral decompression.[2,24,25]

Biomechanical principles of the correction of the kyphosis include lengthening of the concavity (anterior column) and shortening of the convexity (posterior column). The goal of surgical intervention is a solid arthrodesis throughout the length of the kyphosis; ventral-only, ventral-dorsal, and dorsal-only approaches can accomplish this. Kostuik[42] described a ventral-only approach with interbody fusion and ventral instrumentation with a Harrington distraction system augmented by postoperative bracing. He reported the results in 36 patients, with a mean preoperative reduction from 75.5 to 60 degrees. Subsequently, ventral fusion has not gained significant acceptance for the correction of Scheuermann kyphosis.

Bradford et al. originally reported the correction of deformity by a dorsal instrumentation approach.[43] They noted excellent initial correction of deformity but loss of correction and pseudarthrosis in kyphotic curves exceeding 70 degrees and recommended a combined ventral-dorsal spine arthrodesis. Otsuka et al.,[44] using heavier Harrington compression rods in 10 patients, reported correction from a mean of 71 to 39 degrees at 26-month follow-up. These authors performed dorsal-only surgery if the kyphosis decreased to 50 degrees or less on a hyperextension lateral radiograph. Researchers have attributed the loss of correction after dorsal-only surgery to the fusion being performed on the tension side of the spine, the failure of implants, the lack of ventral support, and inadequate correction of a severe deformity with a short construct.[35]

The correction of deformity by a dorsal instrumentation approach is possible by performing segmental posterior closing-wedge osteotomy across the apex of the kyphosis. Sturm et al.[41] performed surgical instrumentation and fusion on 39 patients with Scheuermann disease. They found that single dorsal internal fixation and fusion was effective in correcting kyphosis (mean correction from 71.5 to 37.7 degrees) and arresting the progression in 30 of 39 patients at 72-month follow-up. The authors argued that a long dorsal fusion is the surgical treatment of choice, obviating the need for ventral approaches.

The role of an additional anterior release is more important in large and rigid curves (75 degrees or greater that do not correct to less than 50 degrees on hyperextension lateral radiographs), which are spanning few levels and are creating an acutely angular deformity, especially in the presence of a bony ankylosis across the anterior aspect of the vertebral bodies and the anterior longitudinal ligament at the apex of the kyphosis.[4] Recently, the combined procedure has been performed at one operative setting; however, some authors still advocate staged procedures. The ventral portion can be performed open or endoscopically.[45-48] The approach is typically performed on the right side to avoid the great vessels. A ventral release and bone graft is performed at all the levels that are wedged or have narrowed disc space. Lim et al.[49] reviewed 23 patients who underwent operative treatment using multisegmental instrumentation for Scheuermann kyphosis. The mean follow-up was 38 months. Preoperative kyphosis averaged 83 degrees. Twenty of the 23 patients (87%) underwent combined anterior release/arthrodesis with posterior arthrodesis/multisegmental instrumentation. The remaining three patients underwent posterior arthrodesis/multisegmental instrumentation. Postoperative total kyphosis averaged 46 degrees and 51 degrees at final follow-up. Lee et al.[50] compared posterior-only treatment (18 patients) results with segmental thoracic pedicle screw constructs versus combined anterior/posterior fusion (21 patients) in patients with Scheuermann kyphosis. The study showed a better degree of kyphosis correction in the posterior-only group and a similar small loss of deformity correction at follow-up between the two groups. They did have a patient who had a permanent paraplegia in the anteroposterior group. They concluded that posterior-only treatment with thoracic pedicle screws achieved and maintained better correction and had significantly fewer complications than with circumferential fusion. Geck et al.[51] reported a series of 17 patients who underwent posterior shortening via segmental osteotomies followed by pedicle screw fixation without loss of kyphosis correction of more than 4 degrees across the instrumented level and no neurologic complications. Lonner et al.[52] reported a large series comparing anteroposterior correction of kyphosis to the posterior-only approach. The authors found comparable initial correction of the deformity between the two groups but a better loss of kyphosis correction at follow-up in the posterior-only group.

Transthoracic endoscopic techniques, compared with thoracotomy, provide a less invasive method of accessing the ventral spinal column, with benefits of an excellent exposure and minimal soft tissue disruption. With the simultaneous technique, staged or subsequent procedures can be eliminated and a circumferential structural release, as well as control of the mobilized spine, can be achieved. This simultaneous technique can be extended for use in correction of a variety of thoracic spinal pathologies.[46]

The precise determination of the vertebrae to include within the instrumented, corrected segment is important. Despite the early recognition that fusing too short results in persistent or recurrent deformity at follow-up,[38] this complication persists in even the most recent series.[36] Selection of fusion levels is integral in decision making, yet no well-established criteria that have been validated with long-term follow-up are available. In the standing patient with kyphosis, the greater the deformity, the greater the compression moment across the thoracic spine.[53] When using operative techniques with claw constructs at the rostral (usually T2-3 and T4-5) and caudal (usually L2-3) ends of the deformity, the remaining levels must be instrumented with the hooks placed in compression toward the apex. Using compression across the apex of the kyphosis lessens the actual bending of the rod and requires less force to be dissipated at either end of the construct. The posterior instrumentation and fusion should extend from the most proximal level of the measured kyphosis to incorporate the first lordotic segment distally as is determined on a standing lateral radiograph. Therefore, the most caudal instrumented vertebra is the one below the first lordotic disc.[4] A recent study by Cho et al.[54] suggested that the distal end of a fusion for thoracic hyperkyphosis should include the sagittal stable vertebra (SSV). The SSV is defined as the most proximal vertebra touched by the posterior sacral vertical line (PSVL). The PSVL is a line drawn vertically from the posterior superior corner of the sacrum on the lateral upright radiograph. Levels that include the first lordotic vertebra but not the SSV frequently lead to postoperative distal junctional kyphosis. It is also important that the fusion should be balanced on either side of the apex of the curve and that the gravity line dropped down from C7 should pass by the middle of the last fused vertebra.[26]

Recently, the trend in the surgical treatment of Scheuermann kyphosis has been toward instrumentation systems involving pedicle screw constructs. Pedicle fixation offers increased biomechanical integrity. However, the insertion of screws safely and reliably can be a technical challenge. Caution must be exercised. The choice of instrumentation system, whether hook or screw, should be left to the surgeon.

The problem of junctional kyphosis at the rostral or caudal end of the fusion mass has received significant attention in the recent literature.[55,56] Factors that may predispose the patient to junctional kyphosis include the following:

- Osteoporosis may be an associated factor for junctional kyphosis at the middle or upper thoracic spine in adults.[55]
- Instrumentation may be too short because of failure to determine the end vertebra accurately.[36] Many authors have reported that the instrumentation and fusion must extend over the entire length of the kyphosis to avoid loss of correction[57] and junctional kyphosis.[58] Instrumentation should not terminate at the middle or low thoracic level.[55]
- Excessive intraoperative dissection of the soft tissues and ligaments of the most rostral and caudal vertebral levels may weaken the construct. Wiring of the spinous processes may diminish the incidence of this complication.[59]
- Some authors have reported that excessive correction of kyphosis may lead to junctional kyphosis.[36]
- Operative techniques using pure cantilever correction of a thoracic kyphosis frequently lead to junctional kyphosis.[32,60]

Junctional kyphosis has been reported with Coutrel-Dubousset instrumentation. It is likely related to sagittal balance and selection of fusion levels.[36,44] Lowe and Kasten[37] found that these patients tend to be in negative sagittal balance. This may be exaggerated by surgery, thus predisposing to junctional kyphosis. The most recent recommendations include fusion levels, the end vertebra of the kyphosis rostrally, and the extent of the fusion to the first lordotic disc beyond the transitional zone distally.[26,36,44] To correct a typical Scheuermann kyphosis adequately, dorsal corrective instrumentation from the T3 to the L2 level is necessary. Recommendations have also been made to limit the correction to 50% or less of the original deformity, in an attempt to prevent proximal junctional kyphosis.[36] Overcorrection should be avoided. The use of contemporary multisegmental rod, hook, and pedicle screw systems has increased the ability of the surgeon to obtain and maintain correction. Long-term follow-up of these newer techniques is needed to assess their efficacy. More in-depth research is needed to analyze the effect of living one's entire life with a 65-degree kyphosis as compared with having it corrected to 35 degrees and possibly subjecting patients to future problems with junctional kyphosis.

The lumbar hyperlordosis tends to improve significantly after correction of the thoracic hyperkyphosis. Jansen et al.[61] measured maximum kyphosis, maximum lordosis, sacral slope, and L5-S1 angle in the preoperative and postoperative standing lateral radiographs of the spine of 30 patients. They showed a significant correlation between kyphosis and lordosis before and after surgery. Surgical correction of thoracic hyperkyphosis gave a predictable spontaneous decrease of lumbar lordosis. Correction of lordosis occurred mainly in the upper segment of lumbar lordosis.

Most surgeons who treat patients with Scheuermann kyphosis favor surgery only in the rare patient with advanced kyphosis refractory to external bracing.[40,58] The dorsal approach is advocated, unless ventral compressive pathology exists. A long dorsal stabilization and internal fixation construct with segmental fixation and the use of autologous fusion provides excellent results.[43,44,48,62] Five cases are provided in the following sections to illustrate the previously mentioned points.

Case One

A male, 16 years and 9 months of age, with a 92-degree Scheuermann kyphosis is shown in Figure 89-1A. On a supine hyperextension lateral, he corrects to 48 degrees (Fig. 89-1B). He is treated with ventral release/discectomy/morselized bone grafting, followed by dorsal instrumentation and fusion. The construct consists of six pedicle hooks/transverse process claws above the apex. Multiple hooks and multiple pedicle screws are placed below the apex. His result at 3½ years following surgery is shown in Figure 89-1C. Clinical appearance before and after surgery is pictured in Figure 89-1D.

Case Two

A female, 12 years and 9 months of age, with a 90-degree Scheuermann kyphosis is presented in Figure 89-2A. On the hyperextension lateral, she corrects to roughly 70 degrees (Fig. 89-2B). She is treated with multilevel ventral release/discectomy/morselized bone grafting with some cages ventrally. Following this treatment, a dorsal fusion and instrumentation with mostly pedicle screws is performed.

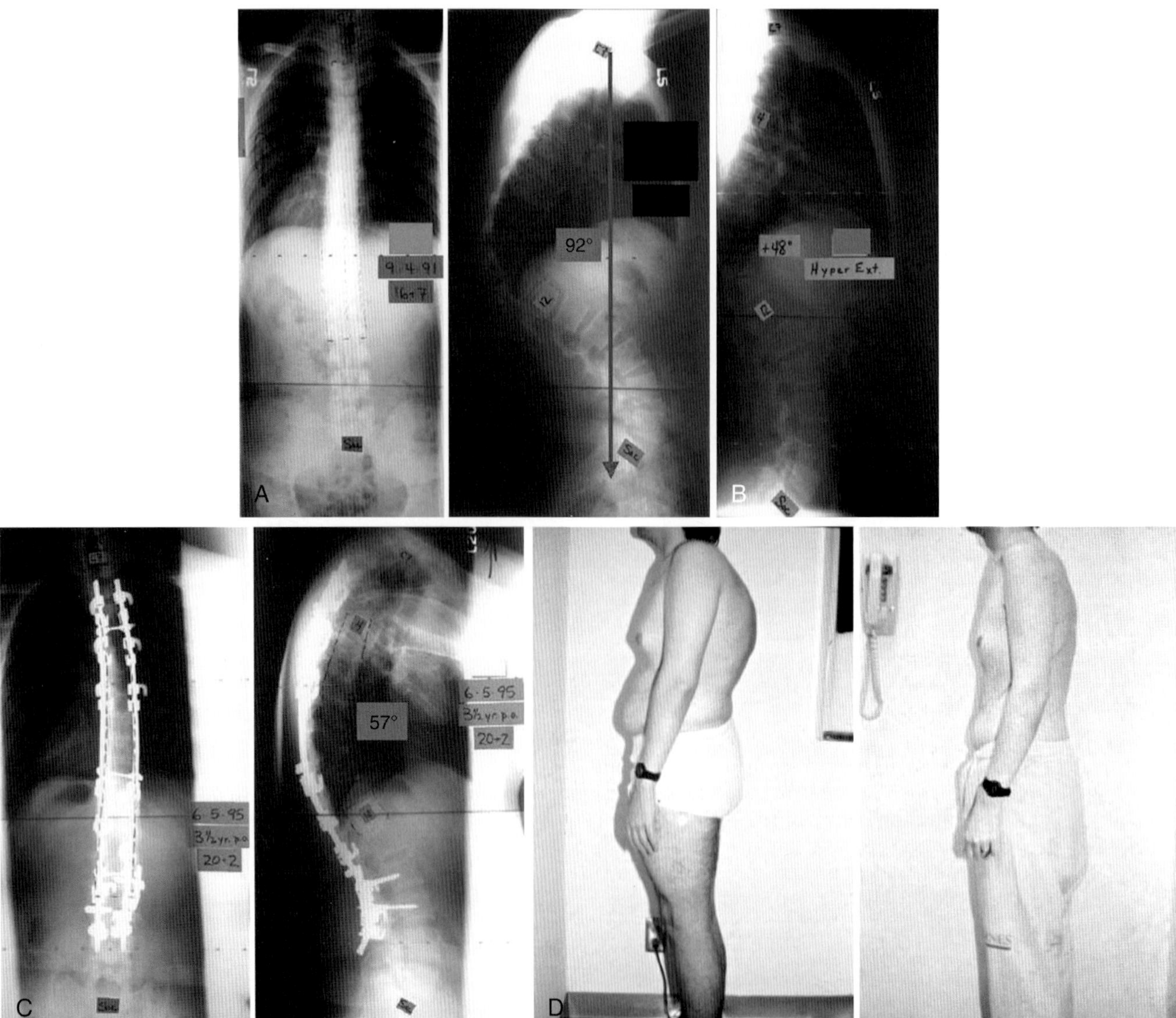

FIGURE 89-1. Case 1: **A,** Upright anteroposterior and lateral preoperative radiographs. **B,** Supine hyperextension radiograph, lateral view. **C,** Upright anteroposterior and lateral radiographs, 3 years following operation. **D,** Preoperative (*left*) and postoperative (*right*) views.

The 2-year postoperative result with correction to 56 degrees of kyphosis is shown in Figure 89-2C. Her preoperative clinical appearance and 2-year postoperative appearance are pictured in Figures 89-2D and E, respectively.

Case Three

A female, 26 years and 6 months of age, initially presented with a 75-degree Scheuermann kyphosis (Fig. 89-3A). Her initial treating surgeons attempted a dorsal-only construct (Fig. 89-3B). This construct failed, and her implants were removed. She subsequently progressed to a 95-degree kyphosis (Fig. 89-3C). With a supine hyperextension maneuver, this deformity only corrected to 85 degrees. She was then treated with a multilevel ventral release, followed by multiple Smith-Peterson osteotomies at essentially all levels and pedicle screw fixation at virtually all levels. Her kyphosis was corrected to 44 degrees (Fig. 89-3D). Her radiographic (see Fig. 89-3D) and clinical results following revision (Fig. 89-3E) and appearance at 1 year, 3 months following operation (Fig. 89-3F) are shown. She is converted from positive to negative sagittal balance.

Case Four

A male, 19 years of age, presented with a 90-degree painful, progressive, and rigid Scheuermann kyphosis (Fig. 89-4A). His main concern was cosmesis. To avoid a front-back-front approach and a thoracotomy scar, a simultaneous anterior endoscopic release with interbody bone grafting and posterior segmental pedicle screw/hook instrumentation with bone grafting was recommended. In the operating room, the patient was positioned prone for the two-team approach (Fig. 89-4B). Correction was obtained by virtue of the multilevel releases with 4 to 5 degrees obtained at each level (Figs. 89-4C–E). Final correction and sagittal balance were achieved and maintained at 45 degrees (Fig. 89-4F). This case illustrates the utility and advantages of the simultaneous approach as an alternative to consider in rigid hyperkyphotic deformities.

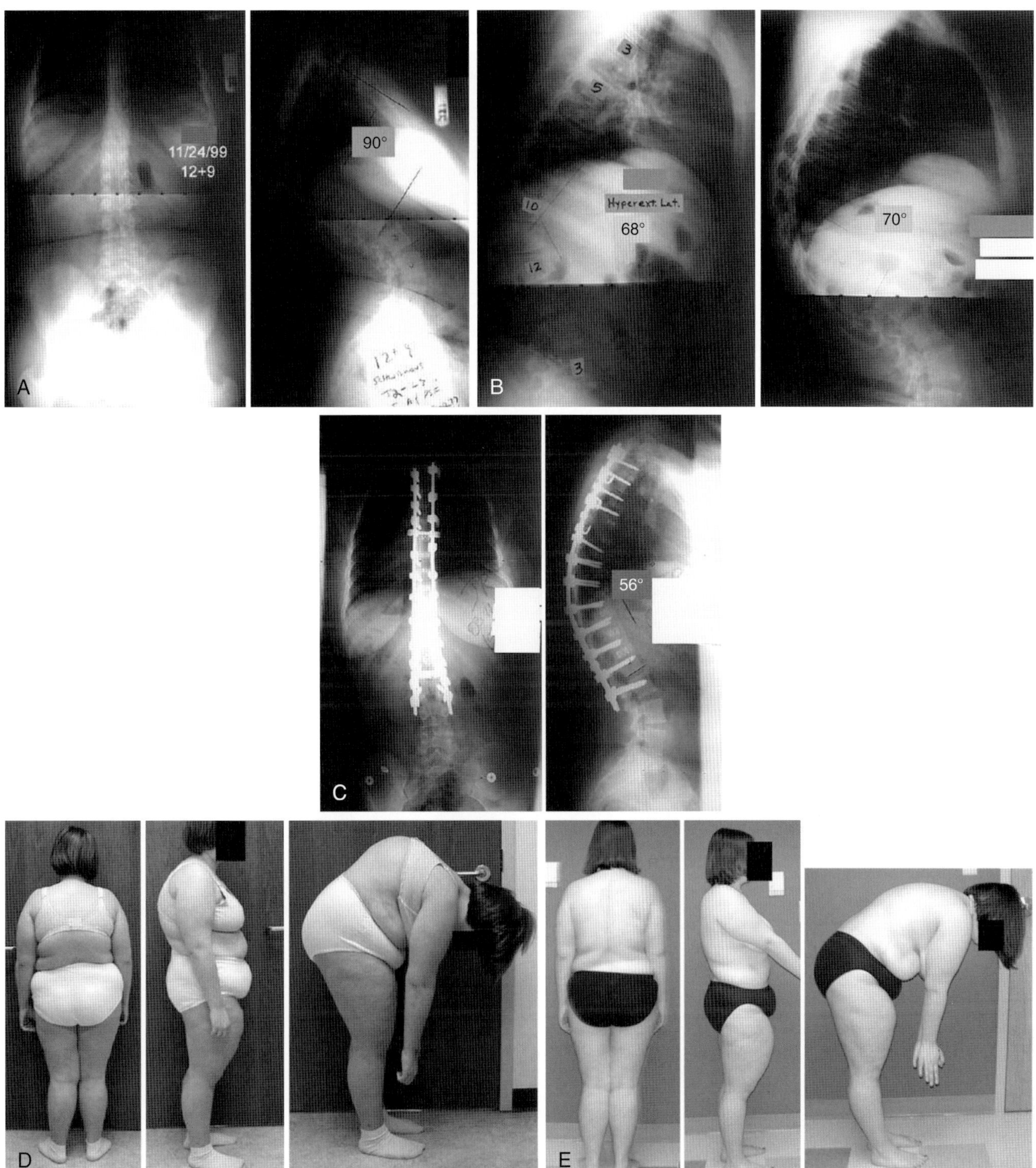

FIGURE 89-2. Case 2: **A,** Upright anteroposterior and lateral preoperative radiographs. **B,** Supine hyperextension radiographs, lateral view. **C,** Upright anteroposterior and lateral radiographs, 2 years following operation. **D,** Preoperative views. **E,** Postoperative views.

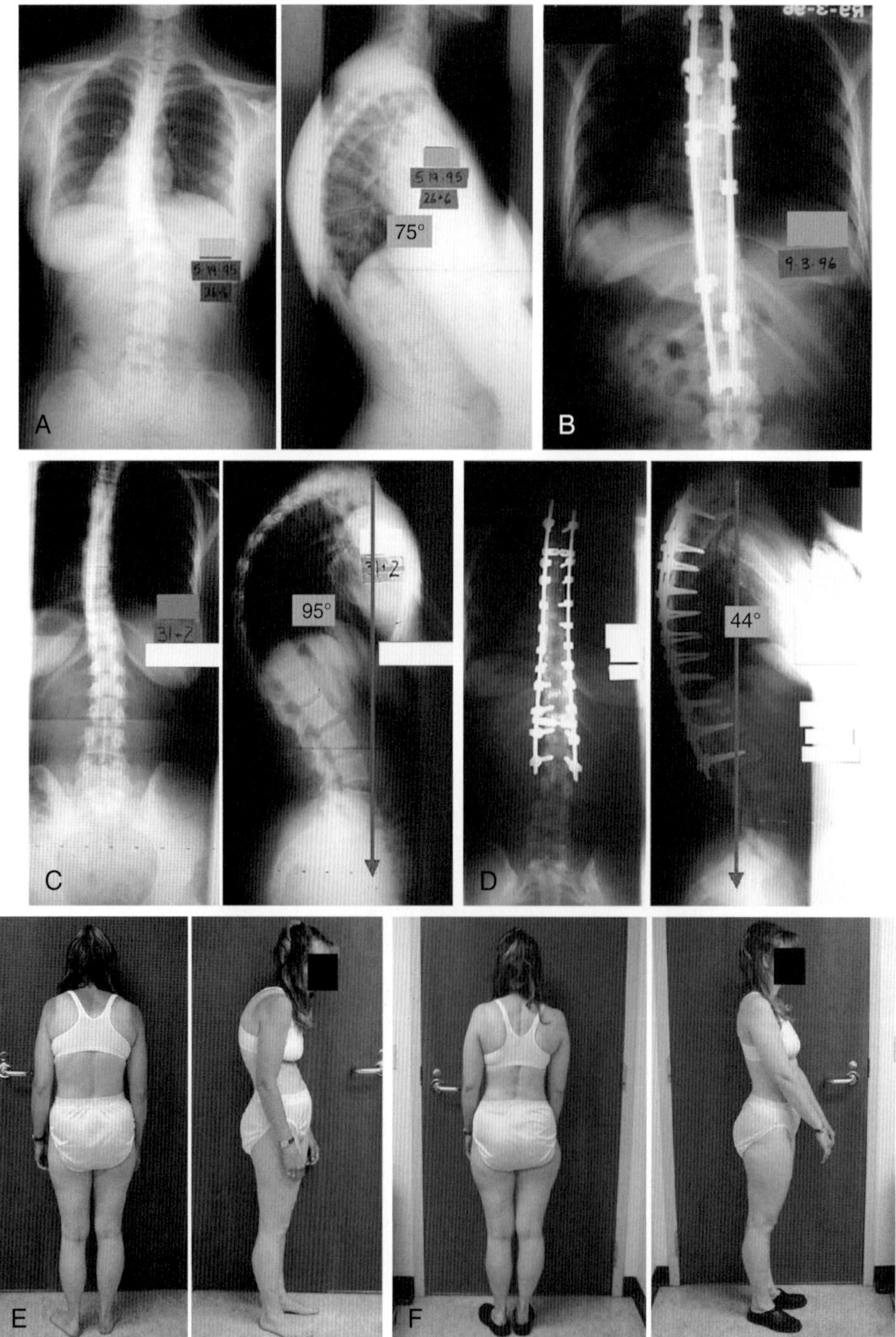

FIGURE 89-3. Case 3: **A,** Initial presentation: upright anteroposterior and lateral radiographs. **B,** Posterior spinal fusion/posterior segmental spinal instrumentation (PSF/PSSI). **C,** Failed PSF/PSSI: upright anteroposterior and lateral radiographs. **D,** Upright anteroposterior and lateral radiographs, after revision reconstruction. **E,** Preoperative views. **F,** Postoperative views.

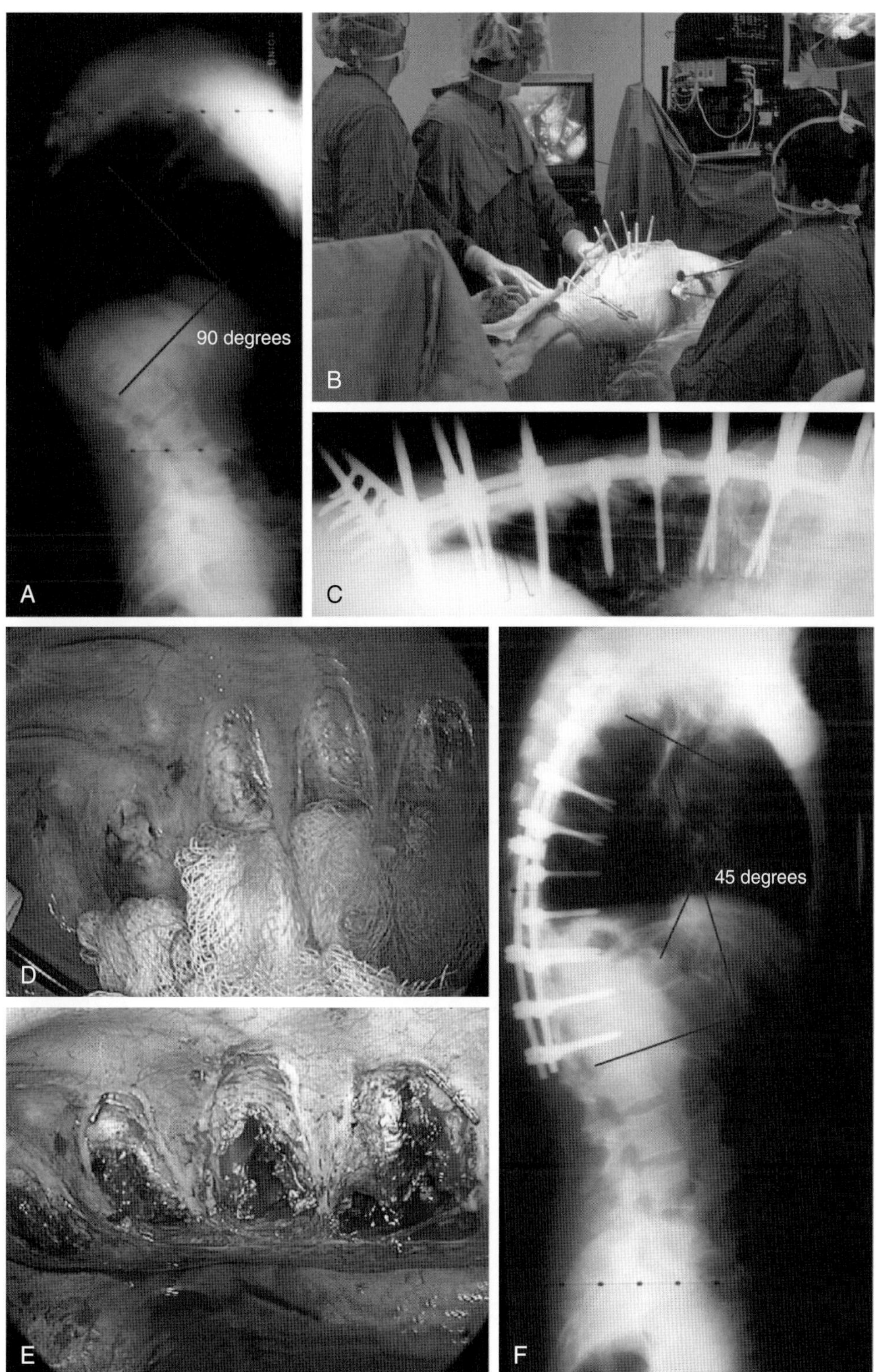

FIGURE 89-4. Case 4: **A,** Preoperative radiograph. **B,** Operating room setup, simultaneous approach. **C,** Intraoperative radiograph. **D,** Precorrection video capture. **E,** Postcorrection video capture. **F,** Postoperative radiograph.

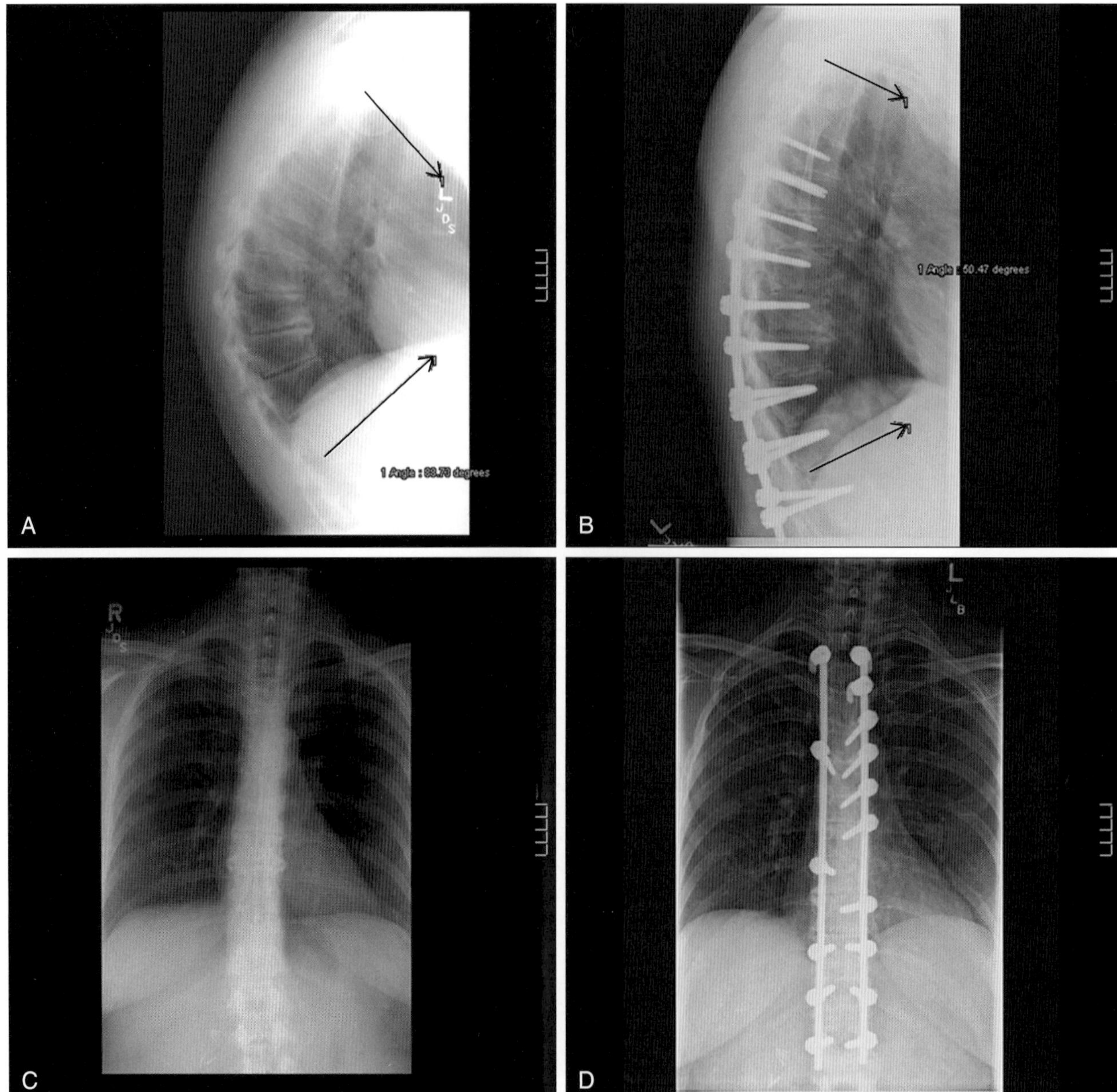

FIGURE 89-5. A–D, Progression is noted in this 59-year-old female with mechanical pain. Multilevel anterior release and fusion followed by posterior T3 to L1 segmental instrumentation correction and fusion (**A,** *arrows*). T3 to T12 curve corrected from 90 degrees to 50 degrees (**B,** *arrows*).

Case Five

A female, 59 years of age, presented with progressive mechanical back pain and rigid Scheuermann kyphosis (Figs. 89-5A and B). A multilevel anterior release and fusion followed by posterior T3 to L1 segmental instrumentation correction and fusion were performed. Postoperatively, her curve (T3 to T12) was corrected from 90 degrees to 50 degrees.

Other Kyphotic Disorders of the Growing Spine

Two other disorders associated with kyphosis occur in the juvenile spine. Roundback deformity is a posture-related kyphosis that is reducible with extension.[39] It is the most common type of thoracic kyphosis identified in patients. Its etiology is unknown but is believed to be related to poor posture during spine maturation.[15] Balderston reported that it is more common in adolescent females and likely represents a compensatory slouch to developing breasts. Postural round back is differentiated from Scheuermann disease by kyphosis that corrects with hyperextension, absence of ventral vertebral deformities, lack of interbody fusion, and absence of compensatory pelvic tilt and hamstring shortening.[8,38] The treatment of postural round back is observation. Occasional exercise and bracing are useful as an adjunct in patients with persistent pain.[15]

Congenital kyphosis of the spine is rare and results from the congenital absence or malformation of one or more vertebral segments.[15] It is characterized by two distinct forms: (1) congenital absence of one or more vertebrae or (2) failure of segmentation of two or more vertebrae.[3] Failure of formation may lead to neurologic compromise. However, failure of segmentation does not, and it is the failure of segmentation that often looks very much like Scheuermann kyphosis clinically and radiographically. Winter described 130 patients with congenital kyphosis of the spine.[53] The female-to-male ratio was 2:1. Eighty-six patients had failure of formation of one or more segments. The treatment of patients with congenital kyphosis revolves around preventing neurologic deterioration and arresting the progressive kyphosis. Bracing is ineffective in young patients. Dorsal instrumentation and fusion is recommended in patients younger than 5 years of age with kyphosis of less than 55 degrees.[15,56] Older patients with advanced kyphosis and neurologic involvement are typically managed with a ventral decompression and release, followed by a dorsal instrumentation and fusion.

Summary

Ultimately, the decision to undergo operative treatment for Scheuermann kyphosis is an individual one between the surgeon and the patient. Potential benefits of the treatment in relieving pain and improving physical appearance and self-esteem, and their related social implications, are weighed against the potential complications of treatment.

KEY REFERENCES

Arlet V, Schlenzka D: Scheuermann's kyphosis: surgical management. *Eur Spine J* 14(9):817–827, 2005.

Betz RR: Kyphosis of the thoracic and thoracolumbar spine in the pediatric patient: normal sagittal parameters and scope of the problem. *Instr Course Lect* 53:479–484, 2004.

Cho KJ, Lenke LG, Bridwell KH, et al: Selection of the optimal distal fusion level in posterior instrumentation and fusion for thoracic hyperkyphosis: the sagittal stable vertebra concept. *Spine (Phila Pa 1976)* 34(8):765–770, 2009.

Damborg F, Engell V, Andersen M, et al: Prevalence, concordance, and heritability of Scheuermann kyphosis based on a study of twins. *J Bone Joint Surg [Am]* 88(10):2133–2136, 2006.

Fotiadis E, Grigoriadou A, Kapetanos G, et al: The role of sternum in the etiopathogenesis of Scheuermann disease of the thoracic spine. *Spine (Phila Pa 1976)* 33(1):E21–E24, 2008.

Geck MJ, Macagno A, Ponte A, et al: The Ponte procedure: posterior only treatment of Scheuermann's kyphosis using segmental posterior shortening and pedicle screw instrumentation. *J Spinal Disord Tech* 20(8):586–593, 2007.

Jansen RC, van Rhijn LW, van Ooij A: Predictable correction of the unfused lumbar lordosis after thoracic correction and fusion in Scheuermann kyphosis. *Spine (Phila Pa 1976)* 31(11):1227–1231, 2006.

Lee SS, Lenke LG, Kuklo TR, et al: Comparison of Scheuermann kyphosis correction by posterior-only thoracic pedicle screw fixation versus combined anterior/posterior fusion. *Spine (Phila Pa 1976)* 31(20):2316–2321, 2006.

Lim M, Green DW, Billinghurst JE, et al: Scheuermann kyphosis: safe and effective surgical treatment using multisegmental instrumentation. *Spine (Phila Pa 1976)* 29(16):1789–1794, 2004.

Lonner BS, Newton P, Betz R, et al: Operative management of Scheuermann's kyphosis in 78 patients: radiographic outcomes, complications, and technique. *Spine (Phila Pa 1976)* 32(24):2644–2652, 2007.

Papagelopoulos PJ, Klassen RA, Peterson HA, et al: Surgical treatment of Scheuermann's disease with segmental compression and instrumentation. *Clin Orthop Relat Res* 386:139–149, 2001.

Papagelopoulos PJ, Mavrogenis AF, Savvidou OD, et al: Current concepts in Scheuermann's kyphosis. *Orthopedics* 31(1):52–58, 2008; quiz 59–60.

Pizzutillo PD: Nonsurgical treatment of kyphosis. *Instr Course Lect* 53:485–491, 2004.

Tsirikos AI: Scheuermann's kyphosis: an update. *J Surg Orthop Adv* 18(3): 122–128, 2009.

Weiss HR, Dieckmann J, Gerner HJ: Effect of intensive rehabilitation on pain in patients with Scheuermnan's disease. *Stud Health Technol Inform* 88:254–257, 2002.

REFERENCES

The complete reference list is available online at expertconsult.com.

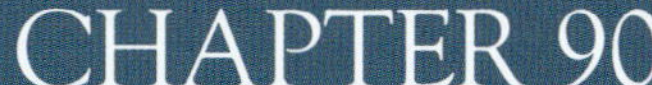

CHAPTER 90

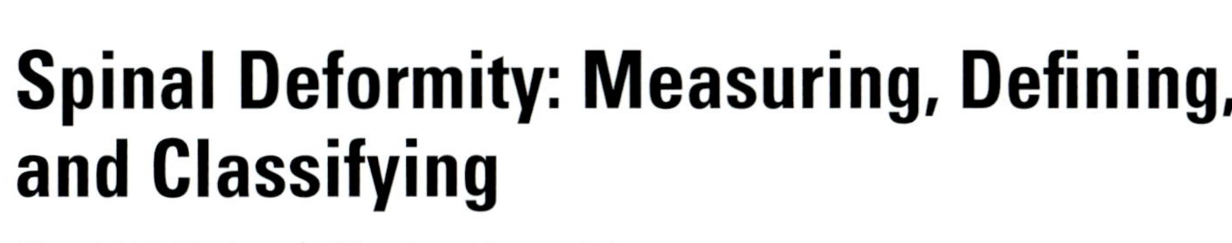

Spinal Deformity: Measuring, Defining, and Classifying

Chad W. Farley | Charles Kuntz IV

The spine is composed of regions with distinct alignment and biomechanical properties that contribute to global alignment. Although regional spinal curves vary widely from the occiput to the pelvis in asymptomatic individuals, global spinal alignment is maintained in a much narrower range for maintenance of horizontal gaze and balance of the spine over the pelvis and femoral heads. Spinal deformity is defined as a deviation from normal spinal alignment.[1,2] Because the human condition is in part defined by the ability to comfortably stand upright and because the treatment of many patients with spinal disorders is directed at restoring this condition, spinal deformity needs to be defined in relation to neutral upright spinal alignment (NUSA) in asymptomatic individuals. NUSA in asymptomatic individuals is defined as standing with the knees and hips comfortably extended, the shoulders neutral or flexed, the neck neutral, and the gaze horizontal. Analysis of spinal alignment involves both clinical and radiographic evaluation. Although there are a myriad of angles and displacements for measuring spinal alignment, our subsequent analysis offers a systematic approach to analyzing regional and global spinal alignment.

Clinical and Radiographic Evaluation of Deformity

To evaluate a spinal deformity, it is necessary to do the following:

1. Perform clinical measurements (facilitated with photographs) in a neutral upright position (standing with the knees and hips comfortably extended, the shoulders and neck neutral) and a forward bend position (standing with feet together, the knees comfortably extended, the hips and spine flexed, and the arms dependent with fingers and palms opposed).
2. Measure occipitocervical and cervical angles and displacements on standard standing anteroposterior and lateral cervical spine radiographs in a neutral upright position (standing with the knees and hips comfortably extended, the shoulders and neck neutral).
3. Measure thoracic, lumbar, sacral, and pelvic angles and displacements, including spinal balance, on standard standing anteroposterior and lateral long cassette radiographs in a neutral upright standing position (standing with the knees and hips comfortably extended, the shoulders neutral or flexed [flexed for lateral radiographs], and the neck neutral).
4. Obtain side-bending (supine) and flexion-extension (standing) radiographs when appropriate for evaluating the flexibility of a deformity curve.

All upright imaging is performed barefoot. In patients with increased or decreased thoracic/lumbar vertebrae, the anomalous vertebrae are included in the appropriate alignment-biomechanical zone. A leg length discrepancy of less than 2 cm is ignored unless the discrepancy significantly contributes to the spinal deformity. When the leg length discrepancy is greater than 2 cm, an appropriately thick lift is placed under the shorter leg.

Coronal Alignment Angles and Displacements

By convention, coronal angles have a positive value. Scoliotic curves are named for the convexity to the right or left. Coronal angulation of the head, shoulders, or pelvis is named for the elevated side: right is right up and left is left up. Schematic illustrations of representative clinical and radiographic measuring techniques for the coronal spinal alignment angles and displacements are detailed in Figures 90-1 and 90-2.

Regional Spinal Alignment

The shoulder tilt angle is defined as the angle subtended by a horizontal reference line and a line drawn through the right and left coracoid processes. Trunk asymmetry (distortions of the torso) is measured using a scoliometer with the patient in a forward bend position (standing with feet together, the knees comfortably extended, the hips and spine flexed, and the arms dependent with fingers and palms opposed). The angle of trunk inclination is the angle between a horizontal reference line and the plane across the back at the greatest elevation of a rib prominence or lumbar prominence. In contrast to radiographic measurements, the shoulder tilt angle and angle of trunk inclination are clinical measurements of the effect of regional spinal deformity on trunk symmetry.

Occipitocervical (O-C2) curves are defined as having an apex from the occiput to C2; a coronal occipital reference

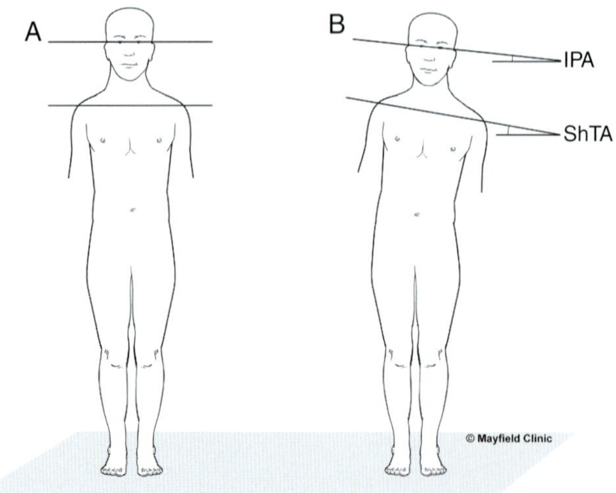

FIGURE 90-1. Schematic illustration showing clinical measurement of the interpupillary angle (IPA) and shoulder tilt angle (ShTA). **A,** Normal IPA and ShTA. **B,** IPA and ShTA with a coronal plane deformity. (Used with permission from the Mayfield Clinic.)

line and the caudal end vertebrae are defined for measuring the Cobb angle.[3]

Cervical coronal curves are defined as having an apex from the C2-3 disc to the C6-7 disc and measured by the Cobb method from the end vertebrae.[3]

The cervicothoracic junction angles are defined from C7 to T1. Cervicothoracic coronal curves are defined as having an apex from C7 to T1 and measured by the Cobb method from the end vertebrae.[3]

Proximal thoracic (T1-2 disc to T5 disc), main thoracic (T5-6 disc to T11-12 disc), thoracolumbar (T12-L1), lumbar (L1-2 disc to L4-5 disc), and lumbosacral (L5-S1) coronal curves are defined as having an apex in the above regions or zones and measured by the Cobb method from the end vertebrae.[3]

The end vertebrae for all coronal curves are defined as the most rostral and caudal vertebrae that maximally tilt into the concavity of the curve. The end vertebrae define the ends of the scoliotic curve. The rostral end vertebra is the first vertebra in the rostral direction from a curve apex whose superior surface is tilted maximally toward the concavity of the curve. The caudal end vertebra is the first vertebra in the caudal direction from a curve apex whose caudal surface is tilted

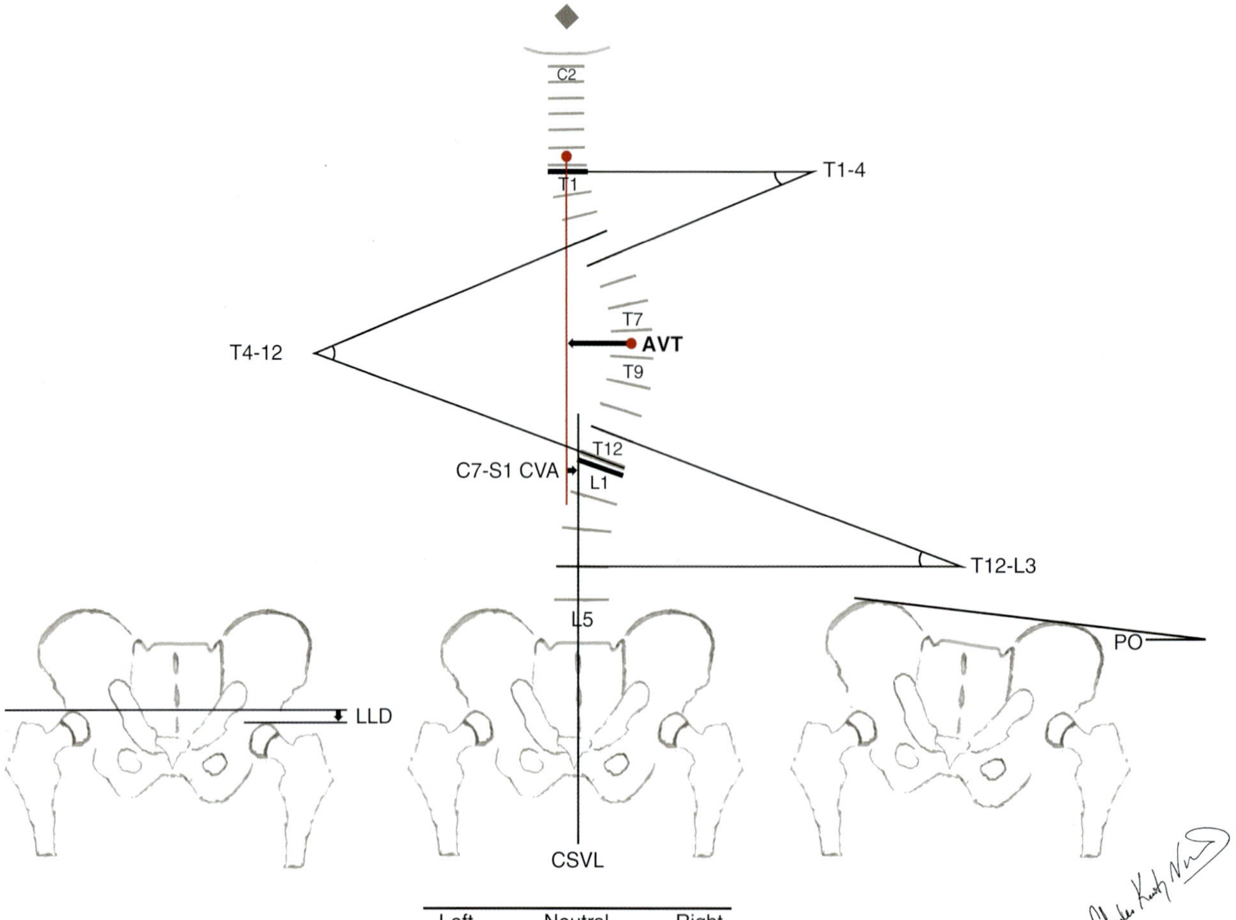

FIGURE 90-2. Schematic illustration of anteroposterior radiographic imaging of the spine from the occiput to the pelvis showing regional and global neutral upright coronal spinal alignment. Radiographic coronal spinal angles and displacements from the occiput to the pelvis are depicted. AVT, apical vertebral translation; CSVL, central sacral vertical line; CVA, coronal vertical axis; LLD, leg length discrepancy; PO, pelvic obliquity. (Used with permission from the Mayfield Clinic.)

maximally toward the concavity of the curve. The apical vertebra or disc of a curve is defined as the most horizontal and laterally deviated vertebra or disc of the curve.[4] Apical vertebral translation is defined as the horizontal distance measured from the C7 plumb line to the center of the apical vertebral body or disc for proximal thoracic and main thoracic curves and from the central sacral vertical line (CSVL) to the center of the apical vertebral body or disc for thoracolumbar and lumbar curves.[4] The CSVL is defined as a vertical reference line drawn through the center of the S1 end plate. Apical vertebral rotation (AVR) is defined by the Nash-Moe classification system.[4,5] (Because AVR is defined on anteroposterior radiographs, AVR is included with the coronal alignment.) Lateral olisthesis is defined by a modified Meyerding classification system.[4,6] For lumbosacral coronal curves, the apical vertebra or disc is defined from L5 to S1; the rostral end vertebra and a horizontal reference line are defined for measuring the Cobb angle (on supine side-bending radiographs, the horizontal reference line may be reconstructed from the standing radiographs).

Pelvic Alignment

Pelvic alignment and morphology are defined by the pelvic obliquity and leg length discrepancy. Pelvic obliquity is defined most frequently as the angle subtended by a horizontal reference line and a line drawn tangential to the top of the crests of the ilium or the base of the sulci of the S1 ala. Pelvic obliquity may result from an intrinsic sacropelvic deformity or leg length discrepancy, or a combination of both. Leg length discrepancy is defined as the vertical distance measured between horizontal lines drawn tangential to the top of the right and left femoral heads.

Global Spinal Alignment

Head tilt is defined by the interpupillary angle (IPA). The IPA is defined as the angle subtended by a horizontal reference line and the interpupillary line. The interpupillary line is defined by a line drawn though the center of the right and left pupils. In contrast to radiographic measurements, the IPA is a clinical measurement of total coronal deformity of the spine and the effect on horizontal gaze.

Coronal spinal balance is defined from the center of C7 and the midpoint of the thoracic trunk to the sacrum. The C7-S1 coronal vertical axis (CVA) is defined as the horizontal distance measured from a vertical plumb line centered in the middle of the C7 vertebral body to the CSVL. The C7-S1 CVA has a positive value when the vertical plumb line is right of the CSVL and a negative value when the vertical plumb line is left of the CSVL. The thoracic trunk–S1 coronal vertical axis (TT-S1 CVA; also known as thoracic trunk shift) is defined as the horizontal distance measured from a vertical plumb line centered at the midpoint of the thorax to the CSVL. The TT-S1 CVA is measured at the midpoint between the rib cage on the left and the rib cage on the right at the level of the main thoracic apical vertebra; if there is no main thoracic apical vertebra, the TT-S1 CVA is measured at the level of T9. The TT-S1 CVA has a positive value when the vertical plumb line is right of the CSVL and a negative value when the vertical plumb line is left of the CSVL.

Sagittal Alignment Angles and Displacements

By convention, kyphosis has a positive value and lordosis a negative value. Schematic illustrations of representative clinical and radiographic measuring techniques for the sagittal and coronal spinal alignment angles and displacements are detailed in Figures 90-3 and 90-4.

Regional Spinal Alignment

Occipitocervical junction angles are defined from the occiput to C2. The occiput-C2 angle is defined as the angle subtended by the McGregor line and a line drawn parallel to the inferior end plate of C2. The McGregor line is drawn from the dorsal rostral aspect of the hard palate to the most caudal point on the midline of the occipital curve.[7] The C1-2 angle is defined as the angle subtended by a line drawn parallel to the inferior aspect of C1 and a line drawn parallel to the inferior end plate of C2.

Cervical lordosis angles are defined from C2 to C7. The C2-7 angle is defined as the angle subtended by a line drawn parallel to the dorsal border of the C2 vertebral body and a line drawn parallel to the dorsal border of the C7 vertebral body.

Cervicothoracic junction angles are defined from C6 to T2, as measured using the Cobb method.[3] The C6-T2 angle is measured from the superior end plate of C6 to the inferior end plate of T2.

Thoracic kyphosis angles are defined from T1 to T12, as measured using the Cobb method.[3] Total thoracic kyphosis is measured from the superior end plate of T1 to the inferior end plate of T12. The proximal thoracic kyphosis is measured from the superior end plate of T1 to the inferior end plate of T5. The main thoracic kyphosis is measured from the superior end plate of T4 to the inferior end plate of T12.

Thoracolumbar junction angles are defined from T10 to L2, as measured using the Cobb method.[3] The T10-L2 angle is measured from the superior end plate of T10 to the inferior end plate of L2.

Lumbosacral lordosis angles are defined from T12-L1 to S1, as measured using the Cobb method.[3] Total lumbosacral lordosis is measured from either the caudal end plate of T12

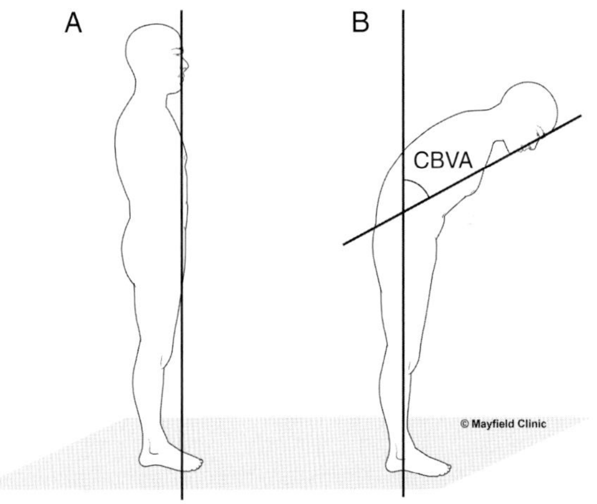

FIGURE 90-3. Schematic illustration showing clinical measurement of the chin-brow to vertical angle (CBVA). **A,** Normal CBVA. **B,** CBVA with a sagittal plane deformity. (Used with permission from the Mayfield Clinic.)

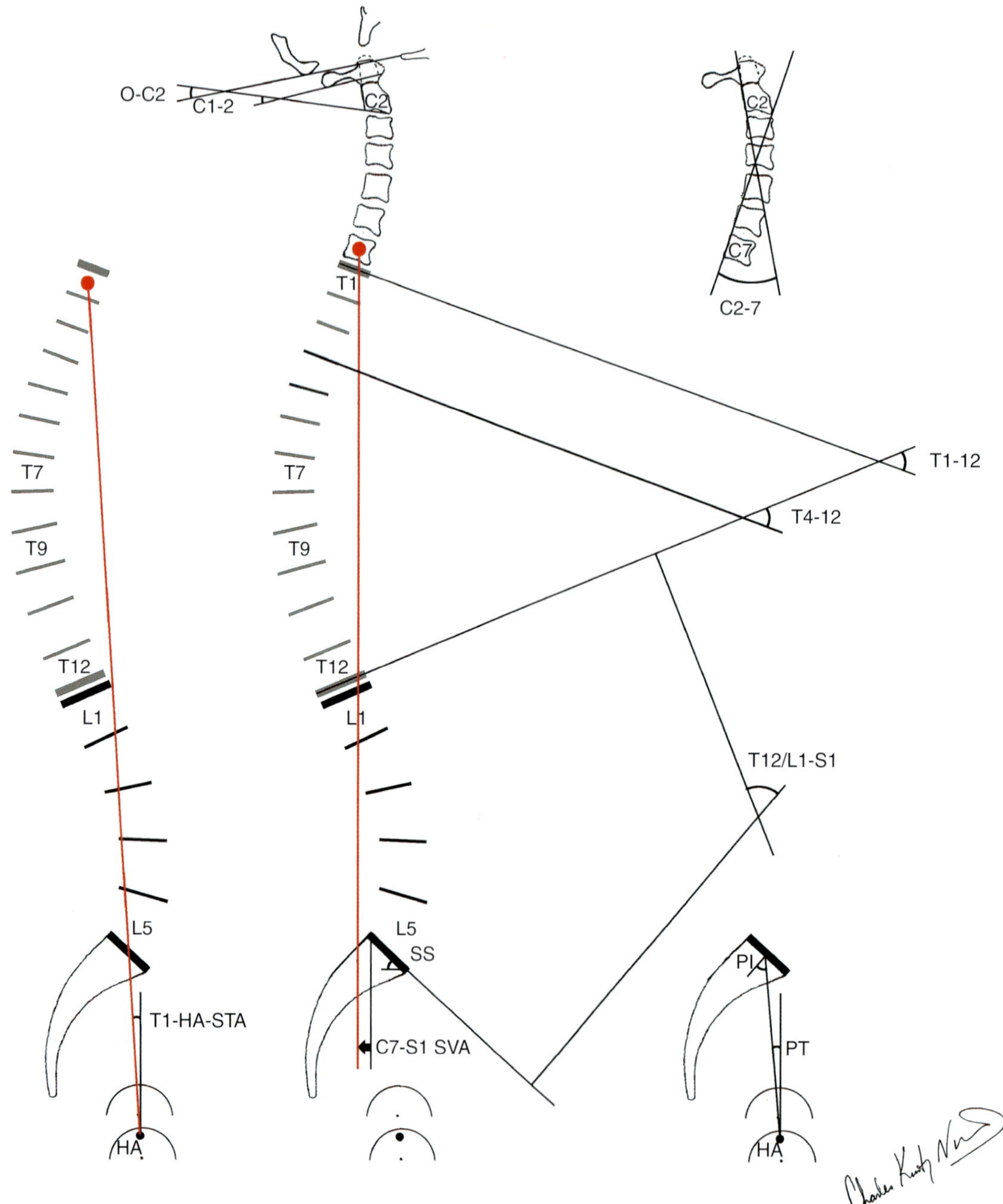

FIGURE 90-4. Schematic illustration of lateral radiographic imaging of the spine from the occiput to the pelvis showing regional and global neutral upright sagittal spinal alignment. Radiographic sagittal spinal angles and displacements from the occiput to pelvis are depicted. HA, hip axis; PI, pelvic incidence; PT, pelvic tilt; SS, sacral slope; STA, sagittal tilt angle; SVA, sagittal vertical axis. (Used with permission from the Mayfield Clinic.)

or the rostral end plate of L1 to the rostral end plate of S1. Lumbar lordosis is measured from the rostral end plate of L1 to the caudal end plate of L5.

Lumbosacral junctional angles are measured from L4 to S1, using the Cobb method.[3] The L4-S1 angle is measured from the rostral end plate of L4 to the superior end plate of S1. The L4-5 angle is measured from the rostral end plate of L4 to the rostral end plate of L5. The L5-S1 angle is measured from the superior end plate of L5 to the rostral end plate of S1.

Ventral and dorsal olisthesis are defined by a modified Meyerding classification system.[4,6]

Pelvic Alignment

Pelvic morphology and rotation are defined by the pelvic incidence, pelvic tilt, and sacral slope. Pelvic incidence (PI) is a constant value unaffected by body posture. The PI is defined as an angle subtended by a line drawn from the hip axis to the midpoint of the sacral end plate and a line perpendicular to the center of the sacral end plate.[8] The hip axis (HA) is defined as the midpoint between the approximate centers of both femoral heads. As PI increases, lumbosacral lordosis must increase to maintain balanced sagittal global spinal alignment. In contrast to the PI, the sacral slope (SS) and pelvic tilt (PT) are posturally dependent values and change with rotation of the pelvis on the hip axis. SS is defined as the angle subtended by a horizontal reference line and the sacral end plate. PT is defined as the angle subtended by a vertical reference line through the HA and a line drawn from the midpoint of the sacral end plate to the HA. PT has a positive value when the midpoint of the sacrum is dorsal to the vertical reference line and a negative value when the midpoint of the sacrum is ventral to the vertical reference line. Geometrically, these pelvic angles produce the following equation: PI = SS + PT.[8] The pelvis rotates on the HA to help maintain balanced sagittal global spinal alignment.

Global Spinal Alignment

Chin-brow to vertical angle is defined as the angle subtended by a vertical reference line and a line drawn parallel to the chin and brow with the neck in neutral or fixed position and the knees and hips extended. In contrast to the radiographic measurements, the chin-brow to vertical angle is a clinical measurement of the total sagittal deformity of the spine and the effect on horizontal gaze.

Sagittal spinal balance is defined from C7, T1, and T9 to the sacrum or HA. The C7-S1 sagittal vertical axis (SVA) is defined as the horizontal distance measured from a vertical plumb line centered in the middle of the C7 vertebral body to the dorsal rostral corner of the S1 end plate. The C7-S1 SVA has a positive value when the vertical plumb line is ventral to the sacral reference point and a negative value when the vertical plumb line is dorsal to the sacral reference point. The T1-HA sagittal tilt angle (STA) is defined as the angle subtended by a vertical reference line through the HA and a line drawn from the midpoint of the T1 vertebral body to the HA. The T9-HA STA is defined as the angle subtended by a vertical reference line through the HA and a line drawn from the midpoint of the T9 vertebral body to the HA. The T1-HA STA and T9-HA STA have a positive value when the T1 or T9 midpoint is ventral to the HA vertical reference line and a negative value when the T1 or T9 midpoint is dorsal to the HA vertical reference line.

Defining Spinal Deformity

Deformity is defined as a deviation from the normal shape or size.[1,2] The eight critically important characteristics of a spinal deformity include patient age; spinal abnormality, including neurologic compromise (e.g., radiculopathy, myelopathy); deformity curve location, pattern, magnitude, and flexibility; pelvic alignment; and global spinal alignment. Spinal deformity may be the primary or a secondary spinal disorder. The deformity may be idiopathic or secondary to known spinal abnormality (e.g., neuromuscular, degenerative, osteoporotic, infectious, traumatic). Spinal deformity may occur in a single plane or in a combination of three planes: coronal, sagittal, and axial. The three basic types of spinal deformity include scoliosis, kyphosis, and lordosis. Each may occur singly or in combination. In combination, coronal and sagittal deformity produces scoliokyphosis and scoliolordosis. Because the human condition is in part defined by the ability to comfortably stand upright and because treatment of many patients with spinal disorders is directed at restoring this condition, spinal deformity needs to be defined in relation to NUSA from the occiput to the pelvis in asymptomatic individuals.

Regional alignment is measured for spinal regions with distinct alignment and biomechanical properties: occipitocervical (OC), cervical (C), cervicothoracic (CT), proximal thoracic (PT), main thoracic (MT), thoracolumbar (TL), lumbar (L), lumbosacral (LS). Spinal deformity is defined by one major structural deformity curve and minor structural deformity curves. Structural curves are defined by their location, magnitude, and flexibility. Deformity major and minor structural deformity curves are classified as scoliotic, kyphotic, lordotic, scoliokyphotic, or scoliolordotic. The major and minor structural curves form a pattern further defining the spinal deformity. The deformity is then finally defined by pelvic alignment and global spinal alignment.

Classification Systems for Thoracic-Lumbar Spinal Deformity

Classification of deformity serves multiple functions. In classifying deformity, a common terminology is established for systematic characterization, allowing clear and concise communication among care providers and more uniform reporting in research. Classification systems can provide a guide for treatment, as in King's initial attempt to guide selection of thoracic fusion levels for thoracic scoliosis. Closely related to this, homogenous cohorts can be compared for outcomes and most beneficial interventions. Natural history studies are also aided by classification systems, enhancing the understanding of spinal pathology. Multiple classification systems are discussed subsequently. For full discussion on the particulars of stratification within each system, the reader is directed to the original publications referenced.

As previously stated, eight critically important characteristics of a spinal deformity should be considered in classification. Simpler classification systems are easier for the physician to use in clinical practice but often incorporate fewer of the critically important spinal deformity characteristics. Although more complicated classification systems incorporate more of the critically important spinal deformity characteristics, these systems are often more complicated for the physician to incorporate into clinical practice.

King et al., in 1983, established the first formal classification system for adolescent idiopathic scoliosis that gained widespread use among spinal surgeons (Table 90-1).[9] Of the eight critically important characteristics of a spinal deformity, the King classification system is limited to adolescent idiopathic scoliosis and only evaluates scoliotic curves in the coronal plane. The classification system focuses on thoracic curves and combined thoracic-lumbar double curves. Scoliotic deformity curve location, pattern, magnitude, and flexibility are included. Pelvic alignment and global spinal alignment are not included. A significant force in the development of this initial spinal deformity classification was the intention to define levels of fusion.[9] This systematic approach served as a baseline from which to begin a more scientific understanding of deformity. The widespread application of the King classification system eventually led specialists to recognize its shortcomings. Classification information was based only on coronal images. The neglect of sagittal and axial

TABLE 90-1

King Classification of Adolescent Idiopathic Scoliosis

Group	Criteria
Type I	S-shaped curve in which both thoracic curve and lumbar curve cross midline Lumbar curve larger than thoracic curve on standing radiograph Flexibility index a negative value (thoracic curve greater than or equal to lumbar curve on standing radiograph, but more flexible on side-bending view)
Type II	S-shaped curve in which thoracic curve and lumbar curve cross midline Thoracic curve greater than or equal to lumbar curve Flexibility index ≥0
Type III	Thoracic curve in which lumbar curve does not cross midline (so-called overhang)
Type IV	Long thoracic curve in which L5 is centered over sacrum but L4 tilts into long thoracic curve
Type V	Double thoracic curve with T1 tilted into convexity of upper curve Upper curve structural on side-bending view

From King HA, Moe JH, Bradford DS, et al: The selection of fusion levels in thoracic idiopathic scoliosis. *J Bone Joint Surg [Am]* 65:1302–1313, 1983.

alignment resulted in correction of spinal deformity in the coronal plane, often ignoring the sagittal and axial plane and producing sagittal deformity, namely the flatback syndrome. At the time of the King classification system development, Harrington rods were the primary instrumentation device and had limited ability to correct or control sagittal curves. Newer three-dimensional segmental instrumentation techniques, including hooks and pedicle screws, came to highlight the three-dimensional aspect of spinal deformity correction that was not fully addressed by the King classification. The King classification has poor applicability to three-dimensional correction of spinal deformity.[10]

Coonrad, in 2000, and Qiu, in 2005, built on the King classification system to develop two new classification systems.[11,12] Of the eight critically important characteristics of a spinal deformity, the Coonrad classification system and Qiu Peking Union Medical College method are limited to idiopathic scoliosis and evaluate scoliotic curves predominantly in the coronal plane. The classification systems include thoracic curves and combined thoracic-lumbar double curves as well as thoracolumbar and lumbar curves. Scoliotic deformity curve location, pattern, magnitude, and flexibility are included. Pelvic alignment and global spinal alignment are not included. The inclusion of thoracolumbar and lumbar scoliotic deformity curve patterns offers an improvement over the King classification system. However, in classification, the continued reliance on coronal alignment with neglect of sagittal alignment remains a significant limitation.

Lenke et al., in 2001, established a new system of classification for adolescent idiopathic scoliosis that included the strengths of the King system and addressed many of its shortcomings (Fig. 90-5).[13] Of the eight critically important characteristics of a spinal deformity, the Lenke classification system is limited to adolescent idiopathic scoliosis. Thoracic and thoracolumbar curves are evaluated in the coronal and sagittal planes, whereas lumbar curves are evaluated in only the coronal plane. Scoliotic deformity curve location, pattern, magnitude, and flexibility are all incorporated. Pelvic alignment and global spinal alignment are not included. The Lenke classification has quickly been adopted for widespread use in treating adolescent idiopathic scoliosis, largely due to the successful accomplishment of its intended goals[13]:

- Comprehensive classification system for adolescent idiopathic scoliosis, including the vast majority of adolescent idiopathic scoliotic deformity curve patterns
- Analysis in both coronal and sagittal planes
- Guide for operative management and selection of appropriate levels for fusion
- Objectivity with good interobserver and intraobserver reliability[14-16]
- System that is relatively practical and easy to understand

Modern classification systems initially were developed for isolated age groups and pathologic conditions (first, adolescent idiopathic scoliosis and, subsequently, adult degenerative deformity). This has been driven in part by the fact that pediatric patients are often minimally symptomatic and treated for anatomic (alignment) reasons, whereas adult and geriatric patients are often significantly symptomatic and treated to relieve symptoms. Adult deformity has features different than adolescent idiopathic scoliosis, including more complex deformity curves with more frequent pelvic and global spinal malalignment. In addition, adult deformity needs to incorporate classification of the degeneration axial skeletal process. Application of adolescent idiopathic classification systems to adult spinal deformity has been particularly problematic and led to the development of adult/geriatric deformity classification systems.

Aebi published an adult scoliosis classification system in 2005 distinguished by classification based on etiology and spinal abnormality (Table 90-2).[17] Of the eight critically important characteristics of a spinal deformity, the Aebi classification system is limited to adult scoliosis. Deformity curve location, pattern, and magnitude are included for descriptive purposes only. Curve flexibility, pelvic alignment, and global spinal alignment are not incorporated. Due to its etiologic foundation, the Aebi classification is uniquely helpful in understanding the natural history of adult deformity of varying etiologies. The Aebi classification provides an alternate insight into adult/geriatric spinal deformity but is lacking in guiding comprehensive classification and treatment.

Schwab et al. presented a classification of adult deformity in 2006 (Table 90-3).[18] Of the eight critically important characteristics of a spinal deformity, the Schwab classification system is limited to adult scoliotic deformity. Thoracic, thoracolumbar, and lumbar curves are evaluated in only the coronal plane, whereas lumbar curves are evaluated in the coronal and sagittal planes. Scoliotic deformity curve location, pattern, and magnitude are included. Spinal abnormality, deformity curve flexibility, pelvic alignment, and global spinal alignment are not incorporated. Classification of the degenerative process is included with a subluxation modifier. Prior established radiographic features with significant patient-reported clinical impact were used as the foundation for this classification.

The Scoliosis Research Society (SRS) classification system for adult spinal deformity, published by Lowe et al. in

Curve Type

Type	Proximal Thoracic	Main Thoracic	Thoracolumbar/ Lumbar	Curve Type
1	Nonstructural	Structural (major*)	Nonstructural	Main thoracic (MT)
2	Structural	Structural (major*)	Nonstructural	Double thoracic (DT)
3	Nonstructural	Structural (major*)	Structural	Double major (DM)
4	Structural	Structural (major*)	Structural	Triple major (TM)
5	Nonstructural	Nonstructural	Structural (major*)	Thoracolumbar/lumbar (TL/L)
6	Nonstructural	Structural	Structural (major*)	Thoracolumbar/lumbar Main thoracic (TL/L-MT)

*Major = largest Cobb measurement, always structural; minor = all other curves with structural criteria applied.

Structural Criteria
(Minor curves)

Proximal thoracic: – Side-bending Cobb ≥ 25°
– T2-T5 Kyphosis ≥ +20°

Main thoracic: – Side-bending Cobb ≥ 25°
– T10-L2 Kyphosis ≥ +20°

Thoracolumbar/lumbar: – Side-bending Cobb ≥ 25°
– T10-L2 Kyphosis ≥ +20°

Location of Apex
(SRS definition)

CURVE	APEX
Thoracic	T2–T11-12 disc
Thoracolumbar	T12-L1
Lumbar	L1-2 disc–L4

Modifiers

Lumbar Spine Modifier	CSVL to Lumbar Apex
A	CSVL between pedicles
B	CSVL touches apical body(ies)
C	CSVL completely medial

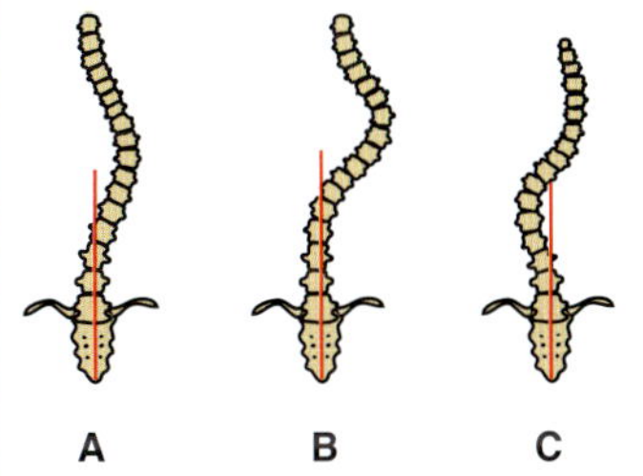

A B C

Thoracic Sagittal Profile T5-12		
–	(Hypo)	<10°
N	(Normal)	10°–40°
+	(Hyper)	>40°

Curve type (1-6) + **Lumbar spine modifier** (**A**, **B**, or **C**) + **Thoracic sagittal modifier** (–, **N**, or +)
Classification (e.g., IB+):______________

FIGURE 90-5. Lenke classification of adolescent idiopathic scoliosis. CSVL, central sacral vertical line; SRS, Scoliosis Research Society. (Used with permission from Lenke LG, Betz RR, Harms J, et al: Adolescent idiopathic scoliosis: a new classification to determine extent of spinal arthrodesis. *J Bone Joint Surg [Am]* 83:1169–1181, 2001.)

2006, is built on the King and Lenke classification systems to include the strengths of the previous classification systems and address the shortcomings (Table 90-4).[19] Of the eight critically important characteristics of a spinal deformity, the classification system is limited to adult spinal deformity. Thoracic, thoracolumbar, and lumbar curves are evaluated in the coronal and sagittal planes. Deformity curve location, pattern, and magnitude as well as global spinal alignment are included. Spinal abnormality, deformity curve flexibility, and pelvic alignment are not incorporated. Classification of the degenerative process in the lumbar spine is included. The SRS classification system has made a significant advance in the classification of adult spinal deformity by including coronal and sagittal plane deformity as well as global spinal alignment. The complexity of the classification system with the exclusion of the evaluation of spinal abnormality, deformity curve flexibility, and pelvic alignment can make this system difficult for the spinal surgeon to use.

A comprehensive classification of spinal deformity, published by Kuntz and colleagues in 2009, was derived from neutral upright spinal measurements in asymptomatic individuals.[20,21] The premise of the CKIV classification system is that because the human condition is in part defined by the ability to comfortably stand upright and because treatment of many patients with spinal disorders is directed at restoring this condition, spinal deformity in this classification is defined in relation to the NUSA from the occiput to the pelvis in asymptomatic individuals (Tables 90-5 and 90-6). Of the eight critically important characteristics of a spinal deformity, the CKIV classification system includes patient age, spinal abnormality, deformity curve location, pattern, magnitude, and flexibility, as well as pelvic alignment and global spinal alignment (Table 90-7). Spinal deformity is evaluated in the coronal, axial, and sagittal planes. Classification of the degenerative axial skeletal process is included by measuring olisthesis. The system places a heavy emphasis on global spinal alignment. Global spinal alignment is evaluated by measuring the effect of a spinal deformity on horizontal gaze and spinal balance. The CKIV classification system in its current form is complicated, but it provides a template for the development of subclassification systems to evaluate and treat spinal deformity of varying abnormalities/etiologies from the infant to geriatric patient.

TABLE 90-2

Abei Classification of Adult Scoliosis

Type	Description	Etiology	PROBLEM LOCATED: In the Spine	PROBLEM LOCATED: Beyond the Spine
Type I	Primary degenerative scoliosis (de novo form), mostly located in the thoracolumbar or lumbar spine, curve apex at L2-3 or L4 most frequently	Asymmetrical disc degeneration and facet joint degeneration	+	
Type II	Progressive idiopathic scoliosis of the thoracolumbar and/or lumbar spine	Idiopathic scoliosis present since adolescence or childhood, progression due to mechanical reasons or bony and/or degenerative changes	+	?
Type III	Secondary deformity scoliosis			
Type III (a)	Secondary adult scoliosis, mostly thoracolumbar and lumbar-umbosacral	Secondary to an adjacent thoracic or thoracolumbar curve of idiopathic, neuromuscular, or congenital origin Obliquity of the pelvis due to leg length discrepancy or hip pathology with secondary lumbar/thoracolumbar curve Lumbosacral transitional anomaly	+	+
Type III (b)	Deformity progressing mostly due to bone weakness with, for example, osteoporotic fracture with secondary deformity	Metabolic bone disease, osteoporosis	+	+

From Aebi M: The adult scoliosis. *Eur Spine J* 14(10):925–948, 2005.

TABLE 90-3

Schwab Classification of Adult Scoliosis

Classification	Radiographic Criteria
Type	
I	Thoracic-only curve (no other curves)
II	Upper thoracic major, apex T4-8
III	Lower thoracic major, apex T9-10
IV	Thoracolumbar major curve, apex T11-L1
V	Lumbar major curve, apex L2-4
Lumbar Lordosis Modifier	
A	Marked lordosis (>40°)
B	Moderate lordosis (0°–40°)
C	No lordosis present (Cobb >0°)
Subluxation Modifier	
0	No intervertebral subluxation, any level
+	Maximal measured subluxation, 1–6 mm
++	Maximal subluxation >7 mm

From Schwab F, Farcy JP, Bridwell K, et al: A clinical impact classification of scoliosis in the adult. *Spine (Phila Pa 1976)* 31(18):2109–2114, 2006.

TABLE 90-4

Scoliosis Research Society Classification of Adult Spinal Deformity

Primary Curve Types

Single thoracic: ST

Double thoracic: DT

Double major: DM

Triple major: TM

Thoracolumbar: TL

Lumbar "de novo"/idiopathic: L

Primary sagittal plane (SP) deformity

Adult Spinal Deformity Modifiers

Regional sagittal modifier (include only if outside normal ranges as listed)

- PT—proximal thoracic (T2-5): ≥ +20°
- MT—main thoracic (T5-12): ≥ +50°
- TL—thoracolumbar (T10-L2): ≥ +20°
- L—lumbar (T12-S1): ≥ −40°

Lumbar Degenerative Modifier (include only if present)

DDD—↓disc height and facet arthropathy based on radiography; include lowest involved level between L1 and S1

LIS—listhesis (rotational, lateral antero, retro) ≥3 mm; include lowest level between L1 and L5

JCT—junctional L5-S1 curve ≥10° (intersection angle superior end plates L5 and S1)

Global Balance Modifier (include only if imbalance present)

SB—sagittal C7 plumb ≥5 cm anterior or posterior to sacral promontory

CB—coronal C7 plumb ≥3 cm right or left of CSVL

Definition of Regions

Thoracic apex: T2–T11-T12 disc

Thoracolumbar apex: T12-L1

Lumbar apex: L1-2 disc to L4

Criteria for Specific Major Curve Types

Thoracic curves

- Curve ≥40°
- Apical vertebral body lateral to C7 plumbline
- T1 rib or clavicle angle ≥10° upper thoracic curves

Thoracolumbar and lumbar curves

- Curve ≥30°
- Apical vertebral body lateral to CSVL

Primary sagittal plane deformity

- No major coronal curve
- One or more regional sagittal measurements (PT, MT, TL, L) outside normal range

CSVL, central sacral vertical line.

From Lowe T, Berven SH, Schwab FJ, et al: The SRS classification for adult spinal deformity: building on the King/Moe and Lenke classification systems. *Spine (Phila Pa 1976)* 31:S119–S125, 2006.

TABLE 90-5

CKIV Neutral Upright Coronal Spinal Alignment Guide: Asymptomatic Individuals

Alignment	Neutral Values (mean, 1 SD) Adult >18 Years*
Regional Spinal Alignment	
Occipitocervical junction angle O-C2 apex	—
Cervical angle C2-3 to C6-7 disc apex	—
Cervicothoracic junction angles C7-T1 apex	—
Proximal thoracic angle T1-2 disc to T5 apex	<20°†
Main thoracic angle T5-6 disc to T11-12 disc apex	<20°†
Thoracolumbar angle T12-L1 apex	<20°†
Lumbar angle L1-2 to L4-5 disc apex	<20°†
Lumbosacral junction angle L5-S1 apex	—
Shoulder tilt angle	1 (2)
Angle of trunk inclination	—
Apical vertebral translation	—
Apical vertebral rotation	<5–10°†
Pelvic Alignment	
Pelvic obliquity	<8°†
Leg length discrepancy	6 (4) mm
Global Spinal Alignment	
Head and shoulder tilt angles Interpupillary angle	0° (1°)
Coronal spinal balance	—
TT-S1 CVA	—
C7-S1 coronal vertical axis	+4 (12) mm

SD, standard deviation.

*Pooled estimates of the mean and variance of the neutral upright coronal spinal angles and displacements from the occiput to the pelvis. Assuming a normal distribution for coronal spinal angles and displacements in the population, the mean ±1SD includes approximately 68% of the population, the mean ±2 SD includes approximately 95% of the population, and the mean ±2.5 SD includes approximately 98.5% of the population.

†Approximately 98.5% of asymptomatic individuals have coronal curves less than the estimated angle. For empty data cells, there was little or no reproducible data.

Used with permission from the Mayfield Clinic.

TABLE 90-6

CKIV Neutral Upright Sagittal Spinal Alignment Guide: Asymptomatic Individuals

Alignment	Neutral Values (mean, 1 SD) Adult >18 Years*
Regional Spinal Alignment	
Occipitocervical junction angle	
O-C2	−14 (7)°
C1-2	−29 (7)°
Cervical lordosis	
C2-7	−17 (14)°
Cervicothoracic junction angle	
C6-T2	—
Total thoracic kyphosis	
T1-12	+45 (10)°
Proximal thoracic kyphosis	
T1-5	+14 (8)°
Main thoracic kyphosis	
T4-12	+41 (11)°
Thoracolumbar junction angle	
T10-L2	+6 (8)°
Total lumbosacral lordosis	
T12–L1-S1	−62 (11)°
Lumbar lordosis	
L1-5	−44 (11)°
Lumbosacral junction angles	
L4-S1	—
L4-5	−17 (5)°
L5-S1	−24 (6)°
Pelvic Alignment	
Pelvic incidence	+54 (10)°
Pelvic tilt	+13 (6)°
Sacral slope	+41 (8)°
Global Spinal Alignment	
Chin-brow to vertical angle	−1 (3)°
Sagittal spinal balance	
C7-S1 sagittal vertical axis (mm)	0 (24) mm
T1-hip axis (HA) sagittal tilt angle (STA)	−1 (3)°
T9-HA STA	−11 (3)°

*Pooled estimates of the mean and variance of the neutral upright sagittal spinal angles and displacements from the occiput to the pelvis. Assuming a normal distribution for sagittal spinal angles and displacements in the population, the mean ±1SD includes approximately 68% population, the mean ±2SD includes approximately 95% population, and the mean ±2.5 SD includes approximately 98.5% of the population. For empty data cells there was little or no reproducible data.

Used with permission from the Mayfield Clinic.

TABLE 90-7

CKIV Classification of Spinal Deformity

Classification of Spinal Deformity*	
Patient age (yr)	
Infantile	0–2
Juvenile	3–9
Adolescent	10–18
Adult	19–60
Geriatric	>60
Spinal Abnormality: scoliotic, kyphotic, lordotic, scoliokyphotic, scoliolordotic, deformity curves	
Major structural deformity curve	Standing deformity curve with greatest deviation from age-appropriate NUSA for 98.5% of asymptomatic population (a spinal deformity has only one major structural deformity curve)
Scoliotic deformity curves	
Scoliotic major structural deformity curve	Greater than age-appropriate NUSA (98.5% of the population)
Minor structural scoliotic curves	remains >25° on side-bending radiographs
Scoliotic curves named for curve apex in spinal zones	
Occipitocervical (OC)	O-C2
Cervical (C)	C2-3 disc–C6-7 disc
Cervicothoracic (CT)	C7-T1
Proximal thoracic (PT)	T1-2 disc–T5 disc
Main thoracic (MT)	T5-6 disc–T11-12 disc
Thoracolumbar (TL)	T12-L1
Lumbar (L)	L1-2 disc–L4-5 disc
Lumbosacral (LS)	L5-S1 (remain >10° on side-bending radiographs)
Kyphotic and lordotic deformity curves	
Kyphotic major structural deformity curve	Greater than age-appropriate NUSA, mean +2.5 SD (98.5% of population)
Lordotic major structural deformity curve	Less than age-appropriate NUSA, mean −2.5 SD (98.5% of population)
Minor structural kyphotic curve	Remain greater than adult NUSA, mean +1 SD on extension radiographs
Minor structural lordotic curve	Remain less adult NUSA, mean −1 SD on flexion radiographs
Kyphotic and lordotic curves named for sagittal angle in spinal zones	
Occipitocervical (OC)	O-C2
Cervical (C)	C2-7
Cervicothoracic (CT)	C6-T2
Proximal thoracic (PT)	T1-5
Main thoracic (MT)	T4-12
Thoracolumbar (TL)	T10-L2
Lumbar (L)	L1-5
Lumbosacral (LS)	L4-S1
Scoliokyphotic and scoliolordotic deformity curves	
Structural scoliotic curve plus structural kyphotic curve in the same spinal zone	
Structual scoliotic curve plus structural lordotic curve in the same spinal zone	
Global Spinal Alignment	
Horizontal gaze	
Balance	
Coronal imbalance (IPA)	Greater than age-appropriate NUSA, mean +2.5 SD
Sagittal imbalance (CBVA)	Greater than or less than age-appropriate NUSA, mean ±2.5 SD
Spinal balance	
Balance	
± Coronal imbalance (C7-S1 CVA)	Greater than or less than age-appropriate NUSA, mean ±2.5 SD
± Sagittal imbalance (C7-S1 SVA)	Greater than or less than age-appropriate NUSA, mean ±2.5 SD
Pelvic Alignment	
Neutral	
Coronal rotation (pelvic obliquity)	Greater than adult, mean +2.5 SD
Sagittal rotation (pelvic tilt)	Greater than or less than adult NUSA, mean ±2.5 SD

Table continues on following page

TABLE 90-7

CKIV Classification of Spinal Deformity—cont.

Recognized Thoracic-Lumbar Deformity Curve Patterns Adapted to the Current Spinal Deformity Classification System

		OC	C	CT PT	MT	TL L	LS
I	MT†,‡	NS	NS	NS	S§	NS	NS
II	Double T†,‡	NS	NS	S§	S§	NS	NS
III	Double major T†,‡	NS	NS	NS	S§	S	NS/S
IV	Double major TL/L†,‡	NS	NS	NS	S	S§	NS/S
V	Triple major†,‡	NS	NS	S§	NS/S§	S§	NS/S
VI	TL/L†,‡	NS	NS	NS	NS	S§	NS/S

C, cervical; CBVA, chin-brow to vertical angle; CT, cervicothoracic; CVA, coronal vertical axis; IPA, interpupillary angle; L, lumbar; LS, lumbosacral; MT, main thoracic; NS, nonstructural curve; NUSA, neutral upright spinal alignment; OC, occipitocervical; PT, proximal thoracic; S, structural curve; SD, standard deviation; SVA, sagittal vertical axis; T, thoracic; TL, thoracolumbar.

*Spinal deformity is classified based on patient age; spinal abnormality; deformity curve location, pattern, magnitude, and flexibility; and global spinal alignment.

†Structural curves are written at the end of the curve pattern, named from cephalad to caudad (s, scoliotic; k, kyphotic; l, lordotic; sk, scoliokyphotic; sl, scoliolordotic). Apical vertebral rotation (AVR) is written as a superscript curve. Greatest olistheses is written as a subscript for structural curves.

‡Global spinal alignment (G) is written at the end of the structural curves (b, balance; ci, coronal inbalance; si, sagittal imbalance). Pelvic alignment (P) is written at the end of the structural curves (n, neutral; cr, coronal rotation; sr, sagittal rotation).

§Major structural curve.

From Kuntz C, Shaffrey CI, Ondra SL, et al: Spinal deformity: a new classification derived from neutral upright spinal alignment measurements in asymptomatic juvenile, adolescent, adult, and geriatric individuals. *Neurosurgery* 63:A25–A38, 2008.

Summary

The spine needs to be evaluated in its entirety prior to formulating a treatment plan. The axial skeleton is composed of spinal regions or zones with distinct alignment and biomechanical properties that contribute to global spinal alignment. Although regional curves vary widely from the occiput to the pelvis in asymptomatic individuals, global spinal alignment is maintained in a much narrower range for maintenance of horizontal gaze and balance of the spine over the pelvis and femoral heads. Spinal deformity is defined as a deviation from normal spinal alignment. Eight critically important characteristics of a spinal deformity include patient age; spinal abnormality to include neurologic compromise (radiculopathy, myelopathy, claudication); deformity curve location, pattern, magnitude, and flexibility; pelvic alignment; and global spinal alignment. Spinal deformity classification systems are evolving to allow surgeons to better evaluate and treat deformity patients. There are multiple classification systems for deformity based on clinical and radiographic evaluation. Deciding which system to apply requires in-depth awareness of the advantages and limitations of each. The objective of this review is to provide the reader with a framework for measuring, defining, and classifying spinal deformity.

KEY REFERENCES

Aebi M: The adult scoliosis. *Eur Spine J* 14(10):925–948, 2005.

Coonrad RW, Murrell GA, Motley G, et al: A logical coronal pattern classification of 2,000 consecutive idiopathic scoliosis cases based on the scoliosis research society-defined apical vertebra. *Spine (Phila Pa 1976)* 23(12):1380–1391, 1998.

King HA, Moe JH, Bradford DS, et al: The selection of fusion levels in thoracic idiopathic scoliosis. *J Bone Joint Surg [Am]* 65:1302–1313, 1983.

Kuntz C, Shaffrey CI, Ondra SL, et al: Spinal deformity: a new classification derived from neutral upright spinal alignment measurements in asymptomatic juvenile, adolescent, adult, and geriatric individuals. *Neurosurgery* 63:A25–A38, 2008.

Lenke LG, Betz RR, Harms J, et al: Adolescent idiopathic scoliosis: a new classification to determine extent of spinal arthrodesis. *J Bone Joint Surg [Am]* 83:1169–1181, 2001.

Lowe T, Berven SH, Schwab FJ, et al: The SRS classification for adult spinal deformity: building on the King/Moe and Lenke classification systems. *Spine (Phila Pa 1976)* 31:S119–S125, 2006.

Qiu G, Zhang J, Wang Y, et al: A new operative classification of idiopathic scoliosis: a Peking Union Medical College method. *Spine (Phila Pa 1976)* 30(12):1419–1426, 2005.

Schwab F, Farcy JP, Bridwell K, et al: A clinical impact classification of scoliosis in the adult. *Spine (Phila Pa 1976)* 31(18):2109–2114, 2006.

REFERENCES

The complete reference list is available online at expertconsult.com.

4.6 Deformity Correction: Principles and Techniques

CHAPTER 91

Spinal Deformity and Correction: The Fundamentals

Michael P. Steinmetz | Edward C. Benzel | Lawrence G. Lenke

Spinal deformity is a three-dimensional alteration of spinal alignment in both the coronal and sagittal planes. Scoliosis, strictly speaking, is a curvature greater than 10 degrees in the coronal (frontal) plane, as determined by measuring the Cobb angle (Fig. 91-1). There are many causes, and the condition may occur throughout life from infancy through adulthood. The type of deformity and patient age at presentation have a significant impact on the ultimate treatment of the condition. These topics will be discussed separately throughout this book and are beyond the scope of this chapter. Surgical treatment of these conditions varies depending on the age of the patient and the degree of the deformity. Adults with spinal deformity often seek surgical consultation for pain associated with the deformity, spinal imbalance, or neurologic signs/symptoms. Children and adolescents are most often sent for surgical evaluation for cosmetic concerns and risk of curve progression. Pain and/or neurologic compromise are rare in this patient cohort. For the purposes of this chapter, the authors will focus on the principles of spinal deformity and not the causes or specific treatments. These principles may be applied to most conditions affecting spinal alignment.

The treatment of spinal deformity is not new. Hippocrates attempted traction scoliosis, and Pare used an iron corset in the 16th century in an attempt to correct a similar deformity.[1] Not until the development of Paul Harrington's rod system in the 1960s did the surgical correction of spinal deformity take off.[2] For the first time, Harrington's distraction rod systems, then compression rod systems, permitted correction and improved arthrodesis of the deformed spine. This development truly revolutionized treatment of these dynamic and complex conditions. Early strategies for fixation focused largely on coronal plane correction. Often excellent results were obtained, but these resulted in flattening of the sagittal plane. Unfortunately, this often led to the development of decompensation in the sagittal plane and subsequent pain. This has been referred to as *flatback* deformity.[3] The next phase in development was the application of hooks, then screws, in the thoracolumbar spine. The use of hooks and screw fixation of the spine permitted a greater control over the spine and corrective maneuvers. Greater degrees of correction could be obtained, fixation was improved, and shorter constructs could be used. Powerful control of individual segments of the spine with three-dimensional correction that was not limited by postoperative bracing became the basis for present-day deformity correction systems.[4]

Treatment Goals

Although the indications and strategies vary, depending on the age of the patient and the deformity encountered, the goals of surgical treatment are essentially the same. The primary goals are to halt curve progression, relieve pain, and improve cosmesis and function. The surgical goals are to obtain a solid arthrodesis with a well-balanced three-dimensional spine.[5] In

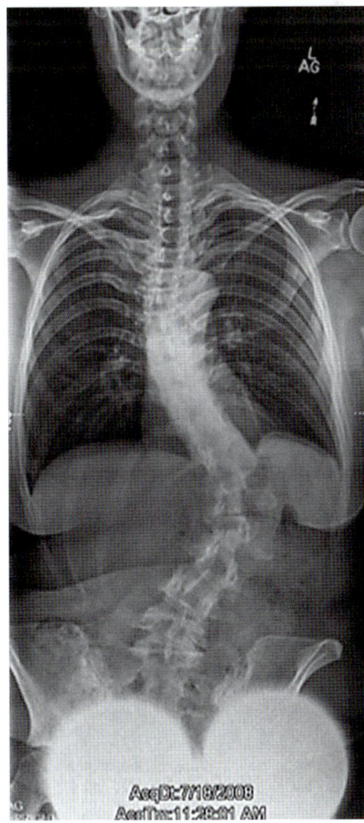

FIGURE 91-1. Scoliosis is defined as a curve greater than 10 degrees in the frontal plane as measured using the Cobb angle.

adolescents, the focus should be on curve correction, improving cosmesis, and halting curve progression. As mentioned earlier, treatment of axial and/or radicular pain is much less of a concern.[6] In adults, the focus is much less on curve correction but rather on balancing the spine and attaining solid arthrodesis and neurologic decompression if required.

General Terms

A unique set of terms may be applied to spinal deformity and should be reviewed briefly. Spinal deformity involves a curvature and obligatory rotation (coronal plane) in either the coronal and/or sagittal planes. Curves in either plane are measured end vertebra to end vertebra. The end vertebra is the most cephalad and most caudal vertebra of a curve (Fig. 91-2). Lines extended along the end plates of the vertebral bodies that are part of the curve in question all converge toward a central point within the concavity of a curve. Lines extended along the end plates of vertebral bodies not involved become divergent. The most rostral or caudal vertebral body visualized is the end vertebra. The neutral vertebra is that vertebra between curves that demonstrates the least rotation. Both pedicles should be relatively symmetrical. The stable vertebra is the vertebra that is bisected by the center sacral vertical line. This line is determined by first drawing a line connecting the most rostral point on each of the iliac crests. A perpendicular drawn from the midpoint of the S1 vertebra superiorly defines this line. Surgeons often use the stable or neutral vertebra when deciding where to end a construct/fusion.

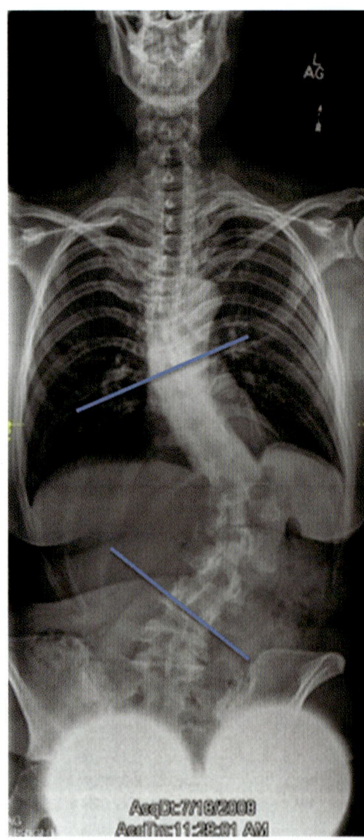

FIGURE 91-2. The end vertebrae are defined (*blue lines*) as the most rostral and caudal vertebrae in the curve.

Spinal balance is critical for optimal biomechanics. This is determined using a plumb line. In the coronal plane, the line is drawn from the center of the C7 vertebral body to the sacrum. This line should fall within 2.5 cm of the center of the sacrum.[7] Deviation greater than this provides evidence of coronal decompensation. This may be determined using 36-inch scoliosis radiographs or directly on the patient, estimating the location of C7 and using the gluteal cleft as the midsacrum. In the sagittal plane, the line should extend from the center of the C7 vertebra and the dorsal aspect of the L5-S1 disc space.[8] On the patient, a plumb line may be drawn from the external meatus of the ear, and the line should fall along the greater trochanter when the spine is balanced.

Spinal curves may be classified as structural or compensatory nonstructural. A structural curve is usually the larger or major curve of the deformity and is closely related to the inciting pathology responsible for the deformity. On bending radiographs, structural curves maintain a significant curve magnitude, generally greater than 25 degrees in the coronal plane. Compensatory curves are countercurves that allow the spine to "compensate" for the structural curve in an attempt to maintain balance. On bending radiographs, compensatory curves are less than 25 degrees, smaller in magnitude than structural curves. Compensatory curves are flexible. Curves are also measured in the sagittal plane. Normal measurements of thoracic kyphosis and lumbar lordosis have been determined. Deviations from these "normal" values may be defined as hyperkyphosis, hypokyphosis, or lordosis. When planning surgical deformity correction, most often the structural curve is instrumented, whereas instrumentation of the compensatory nonstructural curve(s) is avoided or selectively limited. Sagittal curves must be accounted for as well. Hypokyphosis should be addressed in the thoracic spine, even if the Cobb angle of the coronal curve may not be of a significant magnitude.

Causes of Spinal Deformity

Congenital Deformities

Congenital spinal deformities are generally due to defects in either vertebra formation or segmentation. These defects may lead to the formation of hemivertebrae or multiple fused portions of the spine, known as *bars*. The result may be scoliosis or kyphosis, or both. These deformities present early in life, often leading to severe deformities.

Neuromuscular Scoliosis

As the name suggests, neuromuscular scoliosis is due to defects in the neuromuscular system. Examples include muscular dystrophy and cerebral palsy. Children with these disorders are often very limited by the index disease, and many are nonambulatory. The curves are often large and gentle sweeping deformities. Presentation is usually early in life, and correction often involves long fusions, including the pelvis, to improve sitting posture.

Idiopathic Scoliosis

By far the most common type of spinal deformity is idiopathic scoliosis. As the name implies, the cause for the condition is unknown; however, significant evidence suggests genetic influences.[3,9-11] These curves present in adolescence and have a risk of progression during growth of the spine. Surgery is not always required. A discussion of surgical indications is beyond the scope of this chapter and is related to curve magnitude, location, and maturity status of the patient's spine.

Degenerative Deformities

As the spine progresses down the degenerative cascade as defined by Kirkaldy-Willis[12] and does so asymmetrically, deformity may, and often does, occur. Classically, this involves the lumbar spine. Curvature, lateral listhesis, and rotation are usually seen. Patients may present with lumbar axial pain, radiculopathy, and/or neurogenic claudication. Treatment is dependent on the presenting symptomatology. Radicular pain may only require foraminotomy, whereas decompensation and axial mechanical pain may require deformity correction and stabilization.

Iatrogenic Deformities

With the expansion of spinal instrumentation, iatrogenic spinal deformity is frequently encountered. These deformities are often in the sagittal plane and include kyphosis, most often above a previous construct, and lumbar flatback. Others may be seen, but these are the most common. Kyphosis may be due to a fracture above a long lumbar or thoracolumbar construct. These deformities may be complex and difficult to treat due to the prior surgery(ies).

Scheuermann Kyphosis

This type of kyphosis, which may occur solely in the thoracic or thoracolumbar spine, may present at any time between adolescence and adulthood. The cause is thought to involve asymmetrically higher ventral intradiscal pressures, which may lead to focal disc herniation of the end plates, generating Schmorl nodes. There may be injury to the growth plate, disproportional loss of ventral vertebral body height, irregularities of the end plates, and narrowing of the disc interspaces.[11] Patients may present with pain, progression of kyphosis, or cosmetic concerns.

Principles of Deformity Correction

Many techniques are available to the surgeon for the correction of coronal and/or sagittal deformities. In most cases, many techniques are used for the final attainment of a stabilized, balanced spine.

Cantilever Forces

This is probably the most common technique used for the correction of deformity. In general, a rod is bent to the desired contour for optimal alignment and is then connected sequentially to each pedicle screw or hook previously placed. The correction is greater with multiple points of fixation (i.e., multiple pedicle screws or hooks).[13,14] As each screw is sequentially connected to the preformed rod, the spine begins to conform to the rod's contoured design. The spine may be contoured in this manner in both the coronal and sagittal planes.

With rigid curves, the aforementioned technique may not be possible for significant correction. Ventral discectomies/osteotomies may be helpful for more significant correction. Dorsal osteotomies (complete facetectomies), with or without discectomies, also aid in further correction. Moreover, pedicle screws offer greater correction compared with hook constructs.[15] The most difficult task with this correction maneuver is bringing the spine to the rod. Many options exist to aid in reduction and depend on the system used for stabilization. One available option is "reduction screws." These screws have an extra long tulip, in which part of it may be broken off after the rod is secured to the screw. "Persuaders" may also be used, where the rod is pushed to the screw until a "cap" may be inserted. Surgeons must use extreme care in patients with osteoporosis or very rigid curves or when small-diameter pedicle screws have been used. Screws in these circumstances may easily pull out. Lastly, forces may be less on each individual screw if reduction is applied to multiple screws simultaneously as the spine is brought to the contoured implant.

Derotation

Practically speaking, forces applied to the spine (cantilever, compression, distraction) all result in translation of the vertebral bodies. Classically, derotation credited to Cotrel and Dubousset results in translation but not the desired rotation of the apical vertebrae.[16] Newer frame-type constructs are now available in modern deformity instrumentation sets that may actually permit true derotation along with translation.

Classically, this technique is applied to thoracic curves but may be applied throughout the spine. The rod is first bent to the appropriate kyphosis desired in the thoracic spine. This rod is then placed along the concavity of the thoracic curve. Cantilever forces may be used during connection of the rod to the pedicle screws, permitting some correction. (After connection, the rod lies along the concavity, following the curve.) Vice-grip type pliers may then be used to grip the rod in two locations, usually toward the ends of the rod, and then rotation is applied.

Typically, the direction of rotation is toward the concavity, or clockwise. This maneuver translates the apex of the curve toward the midline and into kyphosis. It is best to use monoaxial or uniaxial screws for this maneuver.[17] Some systems have polyaxial screws that make connecting the rod to the screws much easier, but they may then be "locked" as monaxial screws during derotation.

As mentioned previously, new tools that permit true rotation of the apex of a curve are available. A frame is constructed on the sides of the apex of the curve. Connectors are placed on the top of multiple screws along both the concavity and convexity of the curve. These are then connected by longitudinal members and cross connectors, thus creating a frame. This frame may then be rotated (i.e., the convexity is "pushed down" and the concavity is "pulled up") while the spine is translated toward the midline.

Significant forces are applied to the spine during this maneuver. Care must be used in rigid curves or in those with osteoporosis. During derotation, the spine should be continuously assessed. Osteotomies may be necessary for optimal translation. With all corrective maneuvers, the sagittal plane must be assessed following coronal correction. Compression/distraction or in situ bending may be necessary to gain more correction.

Compression

Compression may be applied along any part of a spinal construct. It is a useful technique for both coronal and sagittal corrective maneuvers. Typically, compression is applied along the convexity of a curve. It permits coronal correction to some extent yet also the attainment of lordosis because the force is applied dorsal to the instantaneous axis of rotation. This is important when using compression along with distraction for coronal corrective maneuvers. Compression should be used only where lordosis is desired as well (e.g., in the lumbar curve or with preexisting thoracic hyperkyphosis).

Distraction

Similar to compression, distraction may also be applied along any part of a spinal construct. It is useful for correction in the coronal and sagittal planes. Typically, distraction is applied along the concavity of a curve. It permits coronal correction. One should remember that it also results in kyphosis in the sagittal plane. It is useful along the concavity of thoracic curves where kyphosis is desired (e.g., thoracic hypokyphosis).

Usually, compression and distraction are applied at multiple points along a construct.

In Situ Rod Contouring

Once the rods are connected to all of the bone fixators, hooks, or pedicle screws, the rod may be contoured in situ for "fine-tuning" the correction. Most sets offer in situ benders for both coronal and sagittal bends. Rod contouring should be used for "fine-tuning" and not for major corrective maneuvers. Significant stresses may be applied at the bone-implant interface during bending. Thus, this may result in hook cutout or screw pull-out, especially in the osteoporotic spine.

Ventral Releases

Multilevel discectomies may be performed to increase flexibility and potentially improve the correction attained. Successful arthrodesis may be improved as well. However, these advantages must be weighed against the morbidity associated with the additional procedure(s).

Ventral discectomies may be performed via thoracotomy, or thoracoabdominal or retroperitoneal approaches. The techniques are similar after the spine has been exposed. A complete discectomy is performed back to the dorsal anulus. There is no need to penetrate the dorsal anulus. At times, the anterior longitudinal ligament may need to be resected, especially if it is ossified. This may improve flexibility. Structural or morselized grafts may be used in the interspace. Structural grafts may be useful, especially at L4-5 to level the vertebral end plates and for the attainment of lordosis in the lumbar spine.

With the wide use of pedicle screws, the need for ventral release procedures has been questioned. The additional release procedures expose the patient to increased morbidity, especially pulmonary. It also appears that dorsal-only surgery results in similar outcomes compared with anterior/posterior procedures. Good et al. recently demonstrated that dorsal-only adult scoliosis surgery achieved similar correction to anterior/posterior surgery while decreasing blood loss, operative time, and length of hospital stay, as well as avoiding additional anesthesia. Complications, radiographic outcomes, and clinical outcomes were similar at follow-up of longer than 2 years.[18]

Osteotomies

Osteotomies may be very helpful for correction of coronal and sagittal plane deformities. A wide variety of resections may be performed, but two of the most popular include Smith-Petersen and pedicle subtraction osteotomies. It is beyond the scope of this chapter to discuss these procedures in great detail, but principles will be discussed. Both are mainly used for sagittal correction, but if used asymmetrically, coronal correction may be attained as well.

Smith-Petersen Osteotomy

Smith-Petersen osteotomies (SPOs) were originally described for the treatment of ankylosing spondylitis.[10] Currently, the osteotomy is more widely applied for the treatment of sagittal plane deformities. SPOs are generally indicated for the treatment of gentle "swooping" as opposed to focal "sharp" curves, especially in the thoracic spine (i.e., Scheuermann kyphosis).[19] Approximately 5 degrees of correction may be attained per level. Multiple SPOs may be performed to achieve greater overall correction.

Technically, SPOs involve shortening of the posterior column while lengthening the anterior column. The axis or rotation is based on the middle column. The lower half of the lamina and spinous process of the upper level as well as the upper half of the lamina and spinous process of the lower level are removed. The inferior and superior articulating processes as well as the ligamentum flavum are removed bilaterally. Following placement of screws or hooks, compression may be applied across the osteotomy(ies). As mentioned earlier, this involves shortening the posterior column along the axis of the middle column and lengthens the anterior column. For this to occur and permit correction, the anterior column must not be ankylosed. SPOs are not possible in the face of multiple ventral bridging osteophytes. Careful scrutiny of preoperative imaging is required prior to including SPOs in the plan for deformity correction. Care must be taken to avoid complications during the performance of single or multiple SPOs. Potential major complications directly attributed to the osteotomy include vascular and neurologic complications. Extension or lengthening of the anterior column may include injury to major vascular structures such as the aorta or its vessels. Neurologic complications have been reported in up to 30% of cases.[20] Neurologic complications may be minimized with careful wide osteotomies, including the surrounding lamina, so there is no direct compression of neurologic structures when closing or compressing across the osteotomy. Minor complications include extensive blood loss, especially with multiple SPOs, durotomy, and pseudarthrosis.

Pedicle Subtraction Osteotomy

Thomason introduced pedicle subtraction osteotomy (PSO) in 1985.[21] Similar to SPOs, PSO is largely indicated for the treatment of sagittal plane deformities. It also may be performed asymmetrically for the correction of both coronal and sagittal plane deformities. This type of osteotomy is powerful and able to correct approximately 30 degrees per PSO. It is technically more demanding compared with the SPO and associated with greater morbidity.[19]

PSO is accomplished by first performing a complete laminectomy or equivalent if done through a prior fusion mass (i.e., treatment of flatback syndrome). Next, a complete facetectomy, including the pars interarticularis, is performed. This should result in exposure of the dura, the bilateral existing and traversing nerve roots, and exposure from the pedicles above and below the pedicle to be removed. The pedicle to be removed is thus isolated as an island between the level above and below. The lamina and spinous process should be removed from both the rostral and caudal levels to adequately expose the dura as well as the pedicles above and below. It is necessary to ensure that there is no undue pressure or force on the thecal sac during closure of the osteotomy. Both pedicles may then be removed until flush with the vertebral body. This may be accomplished with rongeurs or a high-speed drill. The exiting nerve root and medial dura must be protected during removal. Often, the cortical wall medial and inferior are left in place for protection of these structures (they are then removed with the dorsal cortical wall of the vertebral body immediately prior to closure of the osteotomy). A wedge may then be performed through the vertebral body for the desired correction.

Various schemes have been developed to not only help determine at which level to perform the osteotomy but also how much of the vertebral body to remove.[22] A rule of thumb is that for every 1 cm of osteotomy, there is 10 degrees of correction in the sagittal plane. Therefore, a dorsal osteotomy of approximately 3 cm permits about 30 degrees of correction.

The vertebral body may be decorticated directly through the pedicles using curets. Rongeurs may be used to remove the decorticated cancellous bone. This must be performed in a wedge shape toward the ventral cortex. Fluoroscopy may be helpful to determine the height of the osteotomy and progression toward the ventral cortex. The lateral vertebral body should be dissected in a subperiosteal fashion toward the ventral cortex. Cottonoids are useful to maintain this dissection. At this point, the osteotomy should be completely decorticated and the height and width should be confirmed both visually and using fluoroscopy. The lateral vertebral body should be removed down to about the level of the ventral cortex. This may be accomplished using rongeurs, down-pushing curets, or osteotomes. Lastly, the dorsal cortex is removed to complete the osteotomy. Pedicle screws should be placed prior to beginning the osteotomy and a temporary rod placed to control the osteotomy until closure is desired. The dorsal cortex is thinned appropriately and may be finally removed with rongeurs, osteotomes, or down-pushing curets. The thecal sac may be carefully retracted (if in the lumbar spine) medially to reach the midline. A tool such as a Woodson elevator may be used to confirm completion of the osteotomy. The osteotomy may then be closed either with the aid of the operating room table or by compression placed across the pedicle screws. This closure should be performed in a controlled fashion with frequent checks of neuromonitoring. If closure is incomplete, confirm lateral vertebral body removal as well as complete dorsal cortex removal.

Morbidity may be high with a PSO. Similar to an SPO, major risks include damage to vascular and neurologic structures. Bleeding may be excessive and continues until the osteotomy is closed.[23]

Vertebral Column Resection

Complete resection of one or multiple vertebral levels and spinal shortening may be required for severe rigid curves, usually more than 80 degrees, fixed trunk translation, or asymmetry between the length of the convex and concave columns to be corrected.[19,24] The goal of vertebral column resection (VCR) is to balance the spine in both planes while shortening the length of the spinal column.

VCR may be performed using a combined anterior/posterior approach or by a dorsal-only strategy.[25,26] The dorsal-only approach may reduce operative time, complications, and effort associated with the combined procedure.

A detailed description of VCR is provided in other chapters but involves complete removal of one or multiple spinal levels. This includes the vertebral body (including intervening discs), pedicles, and all of the dorsal elements. After placement of dorsal instrumentation, the spine may be manipulated into both coronal and sagittal balance. In certain situations, an interbody graft may be used to augment the anterior column and prevent unwanted shortening of the spine and potential spinal cord deficit.

Similar to other osteotomies, the complication rate of a VCR may be high. Bradford and Tribus reported on 24 patients treated with a VCR.[24] They noted 31 complications in 14 of the patients, in which 13% were neurologic but none resulted in paralysis. Significant bleeding may be encountered until final correction is obtained. Recently, Lenke et al.[11] published a report on dorsal VCR patients with a minimum 2-year follow-up. They noted spinal deformity correction rates between 51% and 60% for the various categories of deformity, and more importantly, reported no spinal cord–related complications. However, they did note the complexity of the reconstruction: surgeons should be well versed in spinal deformity surgical treatment before embarking on this technically demanding procedure. A similar report evaluating pediatric and adult VCR patients confirmed these findings.[25]

Summary

Spinal deformity is frequently encountered in everyday practice. These patients require careful consideration of their preoperative signs and symptoms and a search for surgical indications. Preoperative planning, including a clear understanding of curve magnitude, primary and secondary curve structures, flexibility of the curve(s), and potential for spinal balance are paramount. With appropriate indications and spinal balancing and arthrodesis, patient satisfaction is quite high.

KEY REFERENCES

Bess RS, Lenke LG, Bridwell KH, et al: Comparison of thoracic pedicle screw to hook instrumesntation for the treatment of adult spinal deformity. *Spine* 32(5):555–561, 2007.

Cotrel Y, Dubousset J, Guillaumat M: New universal instrumentation in spinal surgery. *Clin Orthop Relat Res* 227:10–23, 1988.

Kim YJ, Bridwell KH, Lenke LG, et al: Results of lumbar pedicle subtraction osteotomies for fixed sagittal imbalance: a minimum 5-year follow-up study. *Spine (Phila Pa 1976)* 32(20):2189–2197, 2007.

Kim YJ, Lenke LG, Cho SK, et al: Comparative analysis of pedicle screw versus hook instrumentation in posterior spinal fusion of adolescent idiopathic scoliosis. *Spine (Phila Pa 1976)* 29(18):2040–2048, 2004.

Lee SM, Suk SI, Chung ER: Direct vertebral rotation: a new technique of three-dimensional deformity correction with segmental pedicle screw fixation in adolescent idiopathic scoliosis. *Spine (Phila Pa 1976)* 29(3):343–349, 2004.

Lenke LG, O'Leary PT, Bridwell KH, et al: Posterior vertebral column resection for severe pediatric deformity. Minimum two-year follow-up of thirty-five consecutive patients. *Spine (Phila Pa 1976)* 34(20):2213–2221, 2009.

Takahashi S, Delécrin J, Passuti N: Surgical treatment of idiopathic scoliosis in adults: an age-related analysis of outcome. *Spine (Phila Pa 1976)* 27(16):1742–1748, 2002.

Thomasen E: Vertebral osteotomy for correction of kyphosis in ankylosing spondylitis. *Clin Orthop Relat Res* 194:142–152, 1985.

Wiggins GC, Ondra SL, Shaffrey CI: Management of iatrogenic flat-back syndrome. *Neurosurg Focus* 15(3):E8, 2003.

Yang BP, Chen LA, Ondra SL: A novel mathematical model of the sagittal spine: application to pedicle subtraction osteotomy for correction of fixed sagittal deformity. *Spine J* 8(2):359–366, 2008.

Yong-Hing K, Kirkaldy-Willis WH: The pathophysiology of degenerative disease of the lumbar spine. *Orthop Clin North Am* 14(3):491–504, 1983.

REFERENCES

The complete reference list is available online at expertconsult.com.

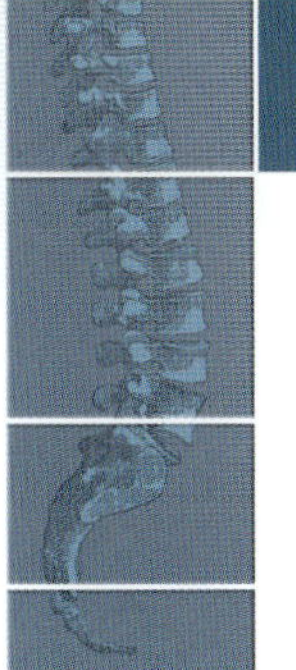

CHAPTER 92

Craniovertebral Junction Deformities

Nathaniel Brooks | Daniel K. Resnick

The craniovertebral junction (CVJ) is subject to deformities caused by trauma, congenital disorders, degenerative disease, infection, and tumors. The goals of management of pathology of the CVJ are to identify instability, decompress neural elements, and provide structural support for the head. Instability can be identified using a number of craniometric and morphometric indices. Many of these criteria were developed in the pre-CT and MRI era, and therefore a description of new indices using "newer" technologies will be presented along with historical ones. The criteria of instability requiring stabilization differ depending on the underlying pathology. For instance, instability caused by acute trauma has very tightly defined criteria for instability as opposed to the chronic instability caused by degenerative disease such as rheumatoid arthritis. The plethora of grading systems causes some confusion regarding management decisions. Attempts have been made to create treatment algorithms for pathology of this complex region; however, high-quality medical evidence relating to many important questions is not available. Therefore, treatment decisions are made with a reliance on a thorough knowledge of the biomechanics, anatomy, and physiology of the CVJ. New technology continues to drive improvement of diagnosis, management, and outcomes of CVJ disease. This chapter will provide a review of the diagnosis and management of this complex region.

Clinical and Radiographic Anatomy of the Craniovertebral Junction

The CVJ consists of the occiput, atlas, axis, and associated ligaments. The CVJ is a compromise between strength and flexibility. The bones and ligaments provide structural support for the head and protect the brainstem and upper cervical spinal cord. Concurrently, these structures allow for significant movement in flexion-extension, lateral bending, and rotational planes. The following discussion is limited to an overview of the anatomic landmarks and indices used to define abnormal relationships because the embryology and anatomy of the CVJ has been presented elsewhere in this text.

The normal relationships among the occiput, atlas, and axis have been studied and are well described. The use of CT with sagittal reconstruction and multiaxial MRI has greatly enhanced the understanding and definition of abnormal anatomic relationships at the CVJ. Various measurements have been described to delineate normal from abnormal pathologies. In other words, there are different indices for trauma, degenerative disease, cranial settling, and basilar impression (Table 92-1).

Trauma

Injury to the CVJ can manifest as ligamentous injury or fracture of the occiput, atlas, or axis. These injuries are as follows: occipital condyle fractures, atlanto-occipital dislocation (AOD), atlas fractures or C1 burst fractures, and C2 fractures of the odontoid or pars interarticularis. Radiographic criteria have been established to help assess clinical stability. Although many of these criteria are used traditionally, they are by no means standardized criteria for each type of injury.[1] Determining instability of these fractures is of primary importance in determining management.

C0 (Occipital Condyle) Fractures

Traditionally, occipital condyle fractures are categorized by the system of Anderson and Montesano.[2] This grades occipital condyle fractures according to occipital fracture (type 1), large condyle fracture (type 2), and avulsion condyle fracture (type 3). The inference from this study is that small condyle fractures represent disruption of the alar ligament. The disruption of the alar ligament has been demonstrated to increase the mobility of the C0-1 joint.[3]

Tuli et al. defined fractures according to evidence of ligamentous instability.[4] Type 1 represents large bony fractures, condensing Anderson and Montesano types 1 and 2 into one group. Type 2 is both small bony fractures of the condyle. The fractures are further subdivided into 2a (stable) and 2b (unstable). Instability is characterized by MRI evidence of alar ligament disruption or CT/radiographic criteria. However, use of MRI to assess disruption of the alar ligament remains controversial.[5]

To simplify the issue, Maserati et al. focused on the C0-1 joint.[6] Determination of instability is made using the elongation of the distance of the C0-1 joint described by Pang.[7] This method is also used to determine AOD and will be more completely described in the next section.

TABLE 92-1

Overview of Craniovertebral Junction Pathology Measurements and Grading Scales*

Trauma

Condyle Fractures	AOD	C1 Burst Fracture	Odontoid Fracture	C2 Pars Fracture
Anderson grade Tuli grade Maserati grade	Condyle-C1 interval Adult >2 mm Child >4 mm Power ratio (BC/AO >1.0) BAI Adult −4–12 mm Child 0–12 mm MRI (showing ligamentous injury)	Distance between C1 lateral mass >8.1 mm (Spence) ADI >3 mm MRI (showing ligamentous injury)	Anderson type	Effendi grade Francis grade

Degenerative Disease

Translational Subluxation	Vertical Translation	Basilar Impression
ADI >3 mm	C1 arch to C2 pedicle distance <13 mm	Clark station McRae line Chamberlain line McGregor line Redlund-Johnell Ranawat Fischgold-Metzger line Wackenheim line MRI/CT

Congenital Disorders†

ADI >3 mm
C1 arch to C2 pedicle distance <13 mm
C1-2 rotary subluxation
Basilar impression measurements (see above)
MRI/CT

ADI, atlantodental interval; AOD, atlanto-occipital dislocation; BAI, basion-axial interval.
*See text for more detail.
†Treatment of abnormal findings is guided by natural history and neurologic findings.

Unstable condyle fractures are a form of AOD and need to be treated as such.[6] However, once instability has been determined, treatment is also not standardized. Fractures without apparent ligamentous disruption can be treated conservatively with a cervical collar or halo vest. Immobilization may be performed if the fracture fragment is large enough and aligned enough to allow bony fusion.[1] If the bony fragment appears small or there is an apparent alar ligament disruption, it may be necessary to perform an occipital cervical fusion because purely ligamentous injury is unlikely to heal by immobilization.[6]

C0-1 Fractures or Atlanto-Occipital Dislocation

In the diagnosis of AOD,vigilant clinical suspicion is most important. The deformity may reduce spontaneously because of recoil of the elastic ligamentous structures. Suspicion should be raised based on the mechanism of injury (e.g., high-velocity crash) or findings on neurologic examination (severe neurologic injury, brainstem or C1-2 level deficits), lateral cervical spine radiograph (obvious separation of the condyle-C1 joint or C1-2 prevertebral swelling), or head CT (subarachnoid hemorrhage around the brainstem or upper cervical spinal cord, or epidural/subdural blood at C1-2).[7-9]

AOD is determined by measurements made from normal plain radiographs. These techniques are the Powers ratio,[10] basion-axial interval (Harris),[11] and the Wholey dens-basion interval (Fig. 92-1). These measurements essentially infer dislocation based on measurement of structures remote from the occipital condyle–atlas joint,[10-12] which can lead to false-negative examinations and lack of interobserver reliability. It has been found that the diagnostic sensitivities for the common tests range from 25% to 50%, with false-negative rates of 50% to 75%. However, the diagnostic sensitivity of the nonstandard indicators (perimedullary blood, tectorial membrane damage, C1-2 extra-axial blood) is 63% to 75%.[7]

An increase in the measurement of the joint distance between the occipital condyle and C1 can be used to determine AOD. This is called the condylar distance. Thin-slice axial CT scanning allowed Pang et al. to calculate that the distance should be less than 4 mm in pediatric patients (Fig. 92-2). This test has been shown in the pediatric population to have a diagnostic sensitivity of 100%.[7] Dziurzynski et al. showed that in adult patients a condylar distance greater than 2 mm was diagnostic of AOD. This has a sensitivity of 92% and specificity of 95%.[13]

If the patient survives the initial injury, he or she should be immediately immobilized. The use of a halo vest to immobilize the patient has been shown to be a safe and effective treatment method to prevent delayed neurologic deterioration while the patient is stabilized and prepared for definitive treatment.[14] Depending on the severity of injury, operative fixation can be performed on an elective basis.[14] The instability of AOD is primarily a ligamentous injury, and therefore internal fixation and fusion is recommended for definitive

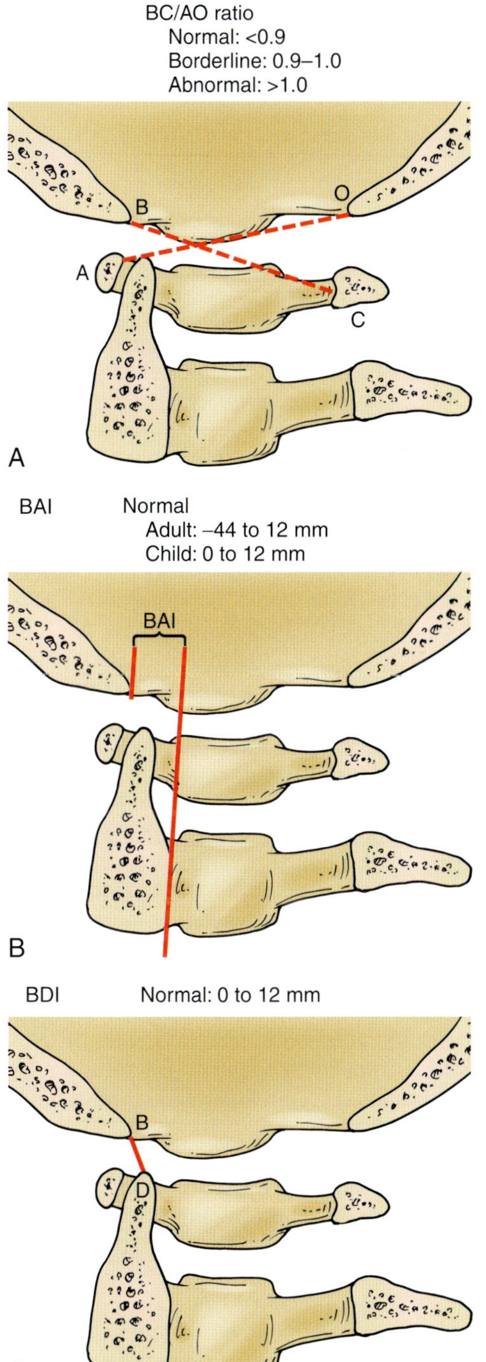

FIGURE 92-1. Classic determination of the atlanto-occipital dislocation. **A,** Power ratio is calculated by measuring distance between the basion (B) and the midpoint of the dorsal arch of C1 (C) as well as the distance between the opisthion (O) and the ventral arch of C1 (A). The normal BC/OA ratio is less than 0.9, borderline is 0.9 to 1.0, and greater than 1.0 is abnormal. Surprisingly, this measure is not sensitive to dislocations in the longitudinal or dorsal direction. **B,** The basion axial interval (BAI) is the distance between the basion and the rostral extension of the dorsal cortical line of the axis. In adults, the basion is between –4 mm and +12 mm. In children, it is between 0 and 12 mm. **C,** The basion dental interval (BDI) is the distance between the basion and the superior cortex of the dens and is less than 12 mm in normal subjects.

treatment. If reduction of the AOD is necessary, it should be done with gentle manual manipulation under fluoroscopic guidance. If the patient has a neurologic examination to follow, the reduction can be performed with the patient under mild sedation. In the anesthetized patient, somatosensory evoked responses may provide some help in determining if reduction is affecting the patient neurologically.

C1 Fractures

Fractures of the atlas (C1) can manifest in multiple ways: isolated ventral or dorsal arch, burst, and lateral mass fractures. Isolated arch fractures are a controversial diagnosis because it is unlikely that a ring can have a fracture in one place without fracturing in another, although they have been described.[15] An axially directed force that translates into C1 through the wedge-shaped occipital condyles causes burst fractures of the atlas. These fractures were first described by Geoffrey Jefferson in 1920.[16] These fractures are detected with an open-mouth odontoid radiograph demonstrating spread of the lateral masses of C1 beyond the lateral borders of the C2 lateral masses. Assessment of the integrity of the transverse ligament is critical in determination of the treatment of C1 burst fractures. Initial assessment of the competence of the ligament was made by a cadaveric study performed by Spence et al.[17] in 1970. Spence showed that the transverse ligament typically failed if the spread between lateral masses was 6.9 mm or more. When corrected for the magnification of the radiographs, this distance should be increased to 8.1 mm.[18] This allows for indirect determination of rupture of the ligament based on plain radiographs. Again, the advent and widespread use of CT and MRI have allowed for direct visualization of ligament integrity. Dickman et al. used MRI to evaluate the transverse ligament and found an abnormal atlantodental interval of 3 mm or more implies the incompetence of the transverse ligament.[19] A ruptured transverse ligament was found in cadaver studies to produce hypermobility at C1-2, increasing flexion-extension (42%), lateral bending (24%), and axial rotation (5%).[20-22]

There is not enough evidence to provide standardized treatment guidelines, but there are recommendations for this treatment of C1 fractures.[23] Isolated ventral or dorsal ring fractures may be treated with cervical immobilization (collar or halo) for 8 to 12 weeks with good results. C1 burst fractures without ligamentous injury can be treated with collar or halo immobilization for 12 weeks. C1 burst fractures with rupture of the transverse ligament may be treated with halo immobilization for 12 weeks or with internal fixation of C1 to C2 with fusion.

C2 Fractures

C2 fractures can be broadly divided into odontoid, C2 body, and pedicle/pars fractures. Odontoid fractures are classified by the system of Anderson and D'Alonzo (Fig. 92-3).[24] Type 1 fractures are rare and are at the distal tip of the odontoid process. Type 2 fractures occur at the base of the odontoid where it meets the body of the axis. Type 3 fractures occur through the body of the axis. The management options for odontoid fractures depend on the type of fracture, the degree of subluxation of the cranial fragment, and the status of the transverse ligament. Type 1 and type 3 fractures

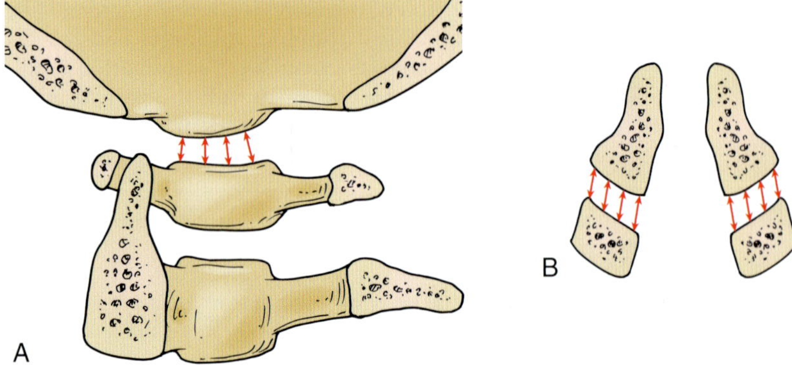

FIGURE 92-2. Condyle–C1 interval. Two images are selected from the midpoint of the joint space in sagittal (**A**) and coronal (**B**) CT reconstructions. Measurements of the joint space are selected at four equidistant points. The average of the measurements in each view should be less than 4 mm in children and 2 mm in adults.

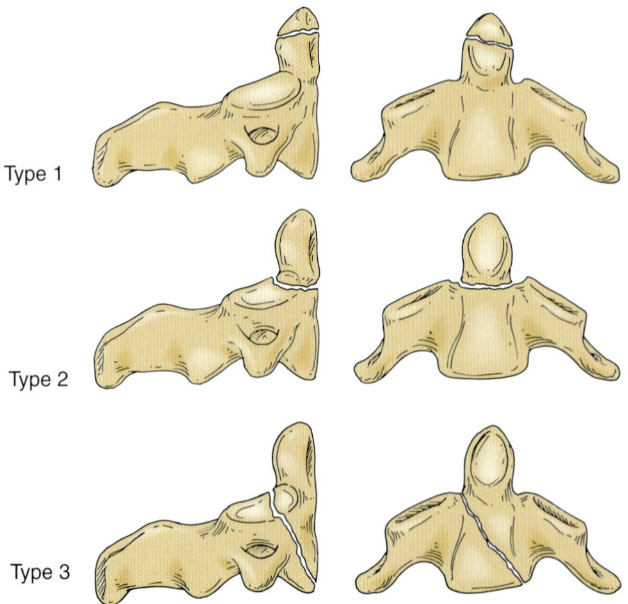

FIGURE 92-3. Odontoid fracture types and management. Type 1 fractures are fractures of the tip of the dens and can be managed in a cervical collar. Type 2 fractures are fractures of the base of the dens, and treatment varies depending on age and distance of displacement. Patients with fractures with greater than 4 to 6 mm of displacement and those older than 55 years of age are less likely to heal with external immobilization and may benefit from surgical stabilization. Type 3 fractures are fractures that extend through the dens and the body of the axis and can be managed in a cervical collar.

are often managed by external immobilization alone, collar or halo. Type 2 fractures can be managed by immobilization or operative intervention depending on patient factors and the degree of subluxation. An increased rate of nonunion has been associated with patient age younger than 60 years and/or subluxation greater than 4 to 6 mm.[25-27] Nonunion rates can be as high as 28%. Type 2a fractures, characterized by comminution of the C2 body, are associated with lower healing rates without surgery.[28,29] C2 pars and pedicle fractures may require surgical intervention, depending on the degree of angulation and distraction between the fragments (see subsequent discussion).[27,29]

Os odontoideum is defined as an ossicle of cortical bone in the position of the odontoid process often attached to the C2 body by a cartilaginous segment (Fig. 92-4). The cause of this remains unclear. There is some evidence to suggest that this is a consequence of old trauma, often at an early age.[30] It is unlikely that this is a failure of fusion during development, because the normal somite pattern of development of the axis does not normally have a site of fusion where the axis meets the body.[31] However, os odontoideum is associated with congenital disorders, such as Down and Morquio syndromes, and spondyloepiphyseal dysplasia. Patients who have neurologic compromise are offered surgical decompression and fusion. Patients with gross instability or narrow canal diameter are also offered surgery. The treatment of incidentally found os odontoideum is controversial. Most authors recommend close follow-up, with surgery reserved for the development of symptoms or radiographic evidence of instability or progressive deformity.[31]

Fractures of the C2 pars interarticularis are called hangman's factures because of the similarity to those seen in judicial hangings.[32] These fractures are also called C2 traumatic spondylolisthesis fractures. These fractures have been classified into three types by Effendi et al. (Fig. 92-5).[33,34] Type 1 fractures are displaced less than 2 mm and minimally angulated, and the C2-3 disc space remains intact. Type 2 fractures have a displaced and angulated body of the axis and a disrupted C2-3 disc space. Type 3 fractures are like type 2 fractures with locked C2 and C3 facets, and the body of the axis is ventrally displaced.

Decisions of treatment of C2 pars fractures are primarily guided by degree of subluxation of C2 on C3. A type 1 fracture without significant ligamentous injury can be treated with immobilization. A halo ring can be used to achieve reduction by extension and capital flexion, reversing the mechanism of fracture. When significant ligamentous injury exists, care must be taken with the use of traction to avoid iatrogenic separation of C2 and C3. In type 2 or 3 fractures, if there is displacement greater than 3 mm, operative intervention may be indicated for reduction and fixation.[25,34,35]

C2 transverse process fractures do not cause instability, but potential injury to the vertebral artery is an area of concern. It is unclear whether aggressive imaging or treatment of these injuries affects patient outcomes, and decisions should be individualized depending on patient symptoms and anatomy.[36]

Degenerative Disease

Abnormalities of bone metabolism, degeneration of synovial joints, or abnormal stresses placed on the CVJ can result in basilar impression. The principles of diagnosis and treatment remain the same, regardless of the cause.

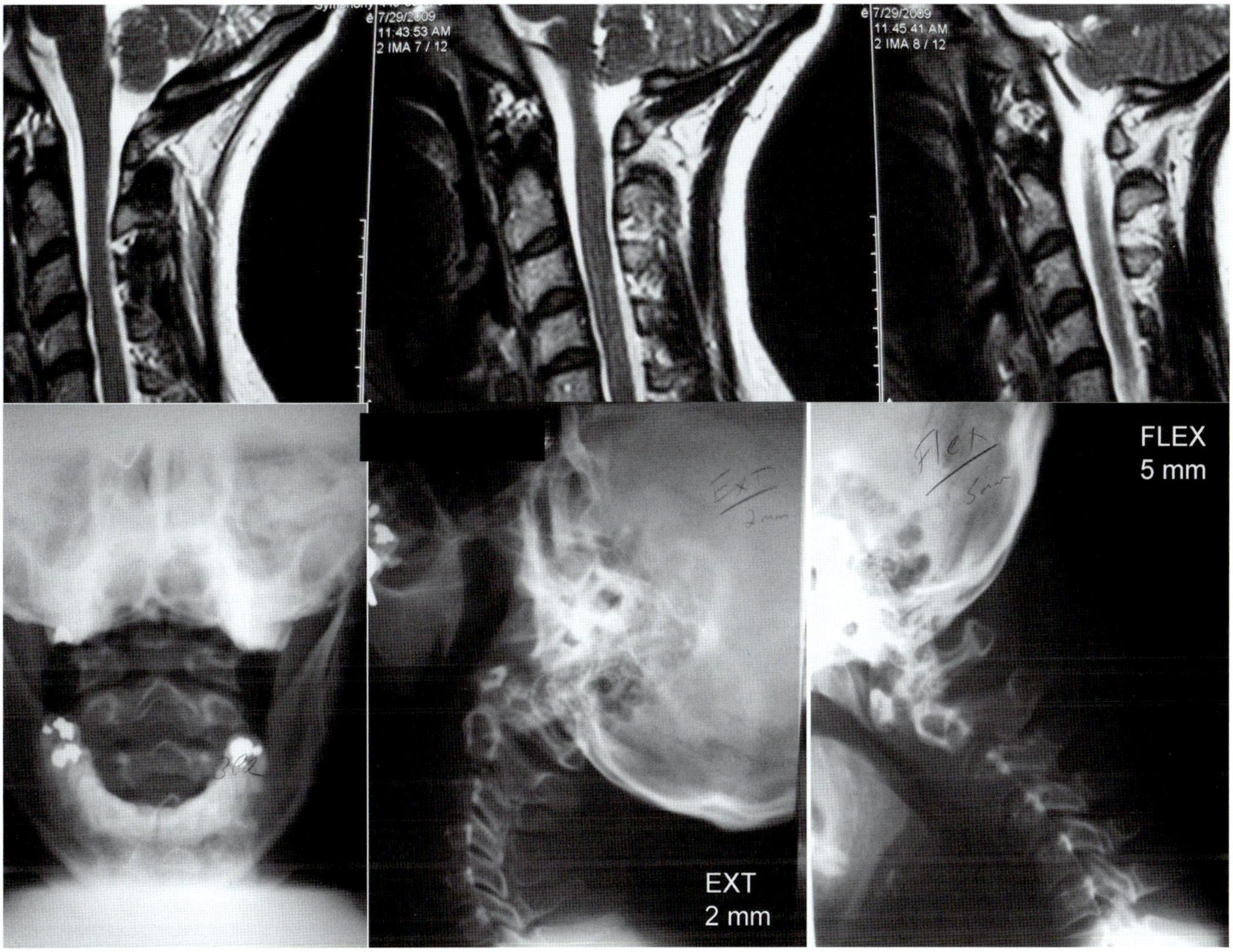

FIGURE 92-4. Os odontoideum is defined as an ossicle of cortical bone in the position of the odontoid process often attached to the C2 body by a cartilaginous segment. The T2-weighted MRI demonstrates hypointensity at the base of the odontoid. The dynamic radiographs demonstrate movement in flexion and extension.

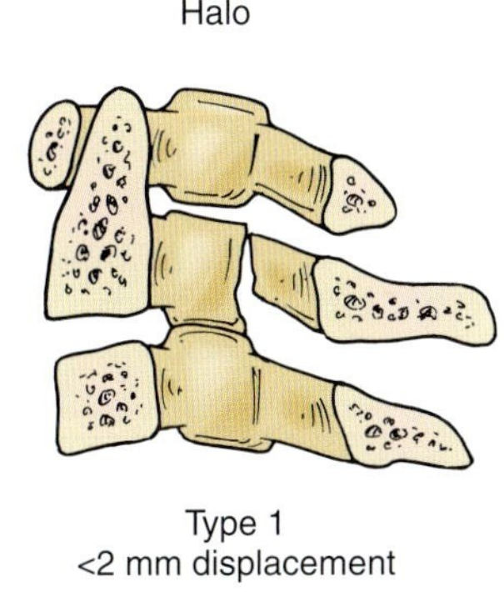

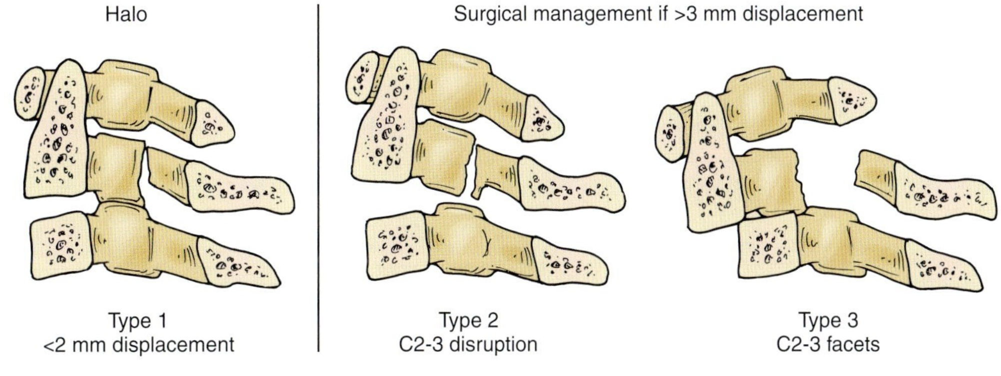

FIGURE 92-5. Effendi classification of C2 traumatic spondylolisthesis. Type 1 fractures are displaced less than 2 mm and minimally angulated. The C2-3 disc space remains intact. Type 2 fractures have a displaced and angulated body of the axis and a disrupted C2-3 disc space. Type 3 fractures are like type 2 fractures with locked C2 and C3 facets.

Rheumatoid arthritis (RA) is the most common degenerative disorder of the CVJ. RA is characterized by destruction of synovial joints. The disease is estimated to affect 0.8% of the Caucasian adult population in the United States, about 2.2 million people. The cervical spine is the second most commonly involved region of the body.[37] The degenerative changes seen in the cervical spine are progressive in nature. Translational subluxation of C1-2 occurs first, followed by vertical subluxation of C1 on C2.[38,39] Compression of the spinal cord and brainstem occurs as the lateral mass joints are eroded by inflammatory synovitis and the odontoid ascends through the atlas and the foramen magnum (Fig. 92-6). Oda et al. found a predictable progression of transverse subluxation to reducible vertical subluxation to irreducible vertical atlantoaxial subluxation.[38] Fujiwara et al. redemonstrated this progression and also noted an association between the severity of RA and the progression of subluxation. Patients with less severe RA develop transverse subluxation, those

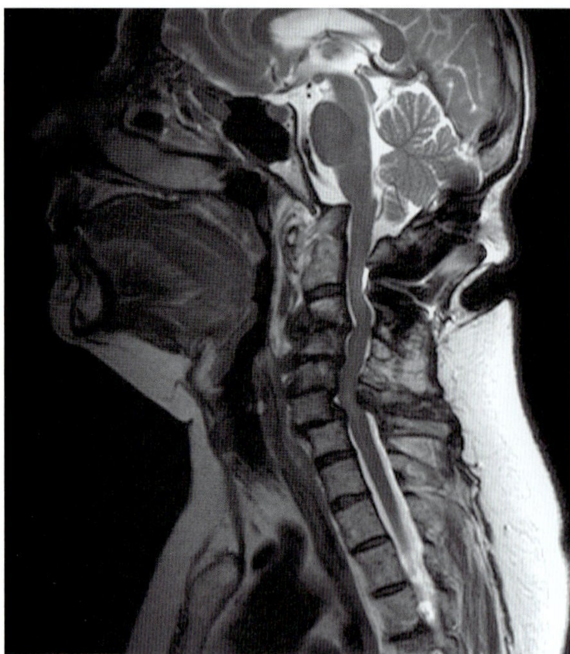

FIGURE 92-6. Basilar impression. This MRI demonstrates the ascension of the odontoid with compression on the medulla and upper cervical spine.

with RA of moderate severity develop a combination of transverse and vertical subluxation, and those with more severe RA develop vertical subluxation.[39] Basilar impression is the ascension of the odontoid process into the posterior cranial fossa and is defined by an abnormal position of the dens with respect to the foramen magnum. As the dens ascends into the posterior fossa, variable symptoms, which include but are not limited to myelopathy and lower cranial nerve deficits, develop. Although motor weakness and sensory changes due to myelopathy are the most common signs, the earliest sign of spinal cord dysfunction is posterior column function.[40]

Determination of transverse C1-2 instability is performed using the anterior dental interval (ADI) (Fig. 92-7A). An ADI greater than 3 mm is considered to be abnormal.[41] Vertical subluxation is measured using the Ranawat method. The vertical distance between the center of the pedicles on the axis to a line connecting the ventral and dorsal arches of the atlas is measured (Fig. 92-7B). If this distance is less than 13 mm in men and 15 mm in women, vertical subluxation is diagnosed.[38]

Many indices are used to screen for basilar impression from plain radiographs. These indices use bony anatomic landmarks and are the Clark station, McRae line,[42] Chamberlain line,[43] McGregor line,[44] Redlund-Johnell criterion,[45] Ranawat criterion,[46] Fischgold-Metzger line,[47] and Wackenheim line.[48] Riew et al. evaluated the sensitivity and specificity of these standard screening measurements.[49] The most sensitive measurement (the test with the fewest false-negative results) is the Wackenheim line, at 88%, and the Clark station, at 83%. The Redlund-Johnell criterion is the most specific measurement (fewest false-positive results) at 76%. The Redlund-Johnell measurement has the highest positive predictive value (PPV) of 68%. The Wackenheim line has a positive predictive value of 48%. The Fischgold-Metzger line has a negative predictive value of 100%. The McRae line has the lowest negative predictive value of 75%. The study also found that identification of bony landmarks is difficult and precludes accurate application of these measurement techniques in many cases. Riew et al. recommend a combination of tests to screen for basilar invagination: the Clark station, the Redlund-Johnell criterion, and the Ranawat criterion (Fig. 92-8).

The goals of treatments of basilar impression are to decompress the brainstem and spinal cord and reestablish support for the head. Decompression of the neural elements can be achieved either directly or indirectly. Indirect decompression is performed via closed reduction through the use of traction and manual manipulation. Long-standing lesions are unlikely to be reducible. However, a trial of craniocervical traction is warranted. Use of a halo ring provides multiple points of skull fixation and allows for fixation to the thoracic vest once the deformity is reduced. Traction is started with a weight of approximately 5 pounds (2.3 kg) and is increased as necessary. Attempted reduction is generally limited for 5 to 7 days because the likelihood of further benefit is limited after this period, and complications related to immobilization

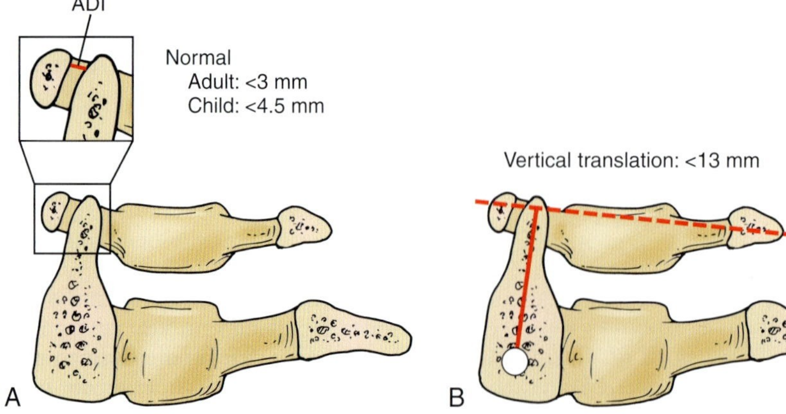

FIGURE 92-7. Assessment of horizontal and vertical translation of C1 on C2. **A,** Horizontal translation is measured using the atlantodental interval (ADI). This is a measurement of the line extending from the dorsal arch of C1 to the ventral cortex of C2. It should be less than 3 mm in adults and 4.5 mm in children. **B,** Vertical translation or subluxation is measured by drawing a line connecting the midpoints of the arch of C1 and then measuring the distance of the perpendicular line between this line and the pedicle. Vertical subluxation exists if this distance is less than 15 mm in males and 13 mm in females. This measurement was described by Ranawat.

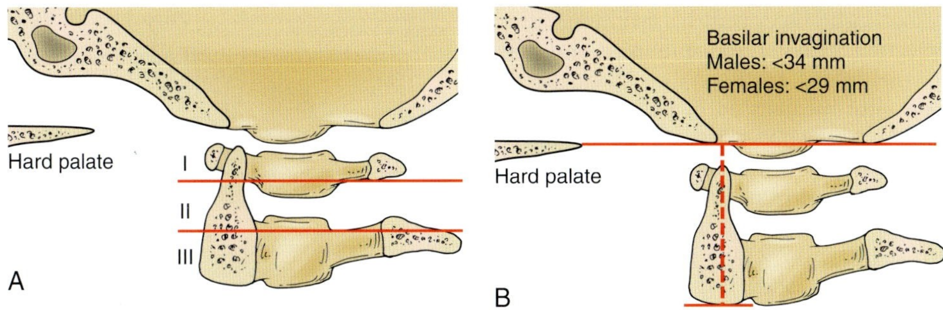

FIGURE 92-8. Measurements of basilar impression. **A,** The Clark station is determined by dividing the C2 body into three equal parts. If the ventral arch of C1 travels into the region of station II or station II itself, basilar invagination is suspected. **B,** The Redlund-Johnell criterion is measured by drawing a line from the tip of the hard palate to the rim of the occiput. A second line is drawn from the midpoint of the caudal margin of the body of C2. Basilar invagination is diagnosed if the measurement is less than 34 mm in men and 29 mm in women. The Ranawat classification is described in Figure 92-7B. The combination of these measurements should be used to screen for basilar invagination, and if suspected, an MRI should be performed to evaluate for evidence of neurologic compression.

increase.[37] Special beds have been designed to help prevent complications of immobilization.

The ventral rheumatoid pannus often resolves once the C1-2 junction is fused, which can indirectly decompress the brainstem and spinal cord.[50,51] However, occasionally a ventral transoral approach needs to be used to obtain adequate decompression.[52-56] Intraoperative image guidance may be used to help with the decompression in a region where anatomic landmarks have been distorted.[57-59]

Congenital Disorders

CVJ abnormalities are common in a number of congenital disorders. These disorders can be broadly grouped as connective tissue disorders (Down syndrome); Klippel-Feil syndrome; osteochondrodysplasias (e.g., achondroplasia); mucopolysaccharidoses (e.g., Morquio and Lesch-Nyhan syndromes); and skeletal dysplasias (i.e., osteogenesis imperfecta); as well as other disorders of development: Goldenhar syndrome, Conradi syndrome, and Klippel-Feil triad.[60-64] The incidence of atlantoaxial subluxation is about 20% in Down syndrome[65] and 50% in Morquio syndrome.[66] The anatomic abnormalities produced by these disorders and the natural history of these can help guide treatment decisions. The following will review the more common disorders of Down syndrome, Morquio syndrome, and achondroplasia to help delineate some concepts. Description and management of other mentioned syndromes can be found in the listed references.[37,67-70]

CVJ abnormalities in these patients have variable causes. C1-2 subluxation is likely related to ligamentous laxity that is a common consequence of connective tissue disorders, such as Morquio syndrome and Lesch-Nyhan syndrome, and it is also a component of Down syndrome. Aberrant ossification of the dens occurs; this could be due to ligamentous laxity and disturbances in blood supply during development because of inordinate mobility.[71,72] Patients with skeletal dysplasias, such as osteogenesis imperfecta, have abnormal collagen deposition, resulting in brittle bones that easily develop multiple microfractures. Accumulation of these microfractures leads to ascension of the dens and medial skull base, causing basilar invagination.[72]

Treatment of these lesions is guided by symptoms and the syndrome involved. For example, many children with Down syndrome have asymptomatic increased ADIs and atlanto-occipital hypermobility.[73,74] The usual measurements of CVJ instability may not apply to patients with Down syndrome. Large cohort studies have not demonstrated increased rates of neurologic injury in children with Down syndrome and abnormal ADIs as compared with their peers without abnormal ADIs. These studies also do not demonstrate a protective effect of restricted activity.[74,75] Reduction and stabilization of the CVJ is probably not indicated unless the patient has clear signs of brainstem or upper cervical spinal cord compression.[73,76]

Morquio syndrome and other skeletal dysplasias are often found to have an os odontoideum and ligamentous laxity.[77] The cartilaginous os odontoideum deforms with flexion and extension. Radiographically, C1-2 instability manifests as changes in the ADI and is a late finding in affected children. By the time this is seen, myelopathy is nearly always present. These patients benefit from prophylactic fusion prior to the onset of myelopathy. The ideal age for this operation has not been determined. Ransford et al.[77] suggest that the surgery be performed at 4 years of age unless myelopathic signs develop earlier. Dorsal occipitocervical fusion can result in complete ossification of the dens, which supports the role of ligamentous laxity in the formation of os odontoideum.[72]

The treatment of patients with congenital disorders of the CVJ varies depending on the syndrome, symptomatology, and relevant anatomy. The natural history of the disorder takes precedence in treatment and also the particular anatomy of the lesion. Traction should be used if there is a suspicion that the lesion is reducible. Use of a halo ring allows for application of corrective forces and subsequent fixation when reduction is completed. If a lesion proves to be irreducible, either after a trial of reduction or radiography, surgery is indicated to decompress the brainstem and spinal cord and to stabilize the CVJ.

Infection: Atlantoaxial Rotatory Subluxation and Fixation

Infection may lead to a rare syndrome termed *atlantoaxial subluxation* or *atlantoaxial rotary fixation.* It was originally described by Bell[78] in 1830 but was named after Grisel,[79] a French otolaryngologist who described this syndrome after upper respiratory infection. It is more common in children who present with torticollis and the head in a "cock-robin" position. There is no clear mechanism of pathogenesis for this entity, although it is associated with infection, trauma, head and neck surgery, RA, Down syndrome, Morquio disease, and other congenital cervical anomalies.[80] Battiata et al.[81] hypothesize a baseline ligamentous laxity along with an inflammatory response to an infectious process. Pang et al. hypothesize that rather than ligamentous laxity, there is increased friction of the C1-2 joints.[80]

The diagnosis is made by the clinical presentation along with findings of rotation of C1 on C2 seen on axial CT imaging. It is important to differentiate the presentation from muscular torticollis that has other etiologies. Pang et al. have used a dynamic CT scanning protocol to diagnose and grade the degree of pathologic "stickiness" of C1 on C2.[80,82] Type I shows movement of less than 20% with movement of the head away from the affected side. Type II is less sticky, and C1 moves on C2 greater than 20%. Type III allows movement of C1 on C2 past midline but still remains abnormal compared with normal controls. MRI can be performed to evaluate for infectious etiology.

Primary treatment of atlantoaxial rotary fixation involves traction and muscle relaxants. Traction can be performed using a head halter. Once a reasonable amount of clinical reduction has been achieved, the patient can be placed in a cervical collar and treated with muscle relaxants for 2 weeks. Any infection needs to be treated completely to help prevent recurrence.[54] Patients whose condition does not reduce or continues to recur may need more aggressive treatment. Closed reduction under general anesthesia can be used in selected cases. Operative C1-2 fixation and fusion can be used to permanently prevent recurrence. Surgical intervention is controversial. None of the patients in Menezes' series of 52 patients required fusion.[54]

The outcomes of treatment have recently been shown by Pang et al.[83] to be associated with the degree of rotary fixation seen with dynamic CT imaging. Patients with type I disease were more likely to have difficult reductions and recurrences than those with type III disease. Patients with type I disease were also more likely to require surgical correction. Delay in treatment also was associated with difficulty in reduction.

Tumors

Tumors of the CVJ produce signs and symptoms of neural element compression and mechanical instability (pain and progressive deformity). The treatment of these tumors depends on prognosis, symptoms, and anatomic configuration. The most common presentations of adults are myelopathy, radiculopathy, and occipitocervical pain.[84] The presentations of children in descending frequency are occipitocervical pain, paresthesias or dysesthesias of the hands, cranial nerve palsies (most commonly diplopia), and myelopathy.[85] The most commonly encountered tumors in this region are chordomas and meningiomas, but other primary tumors—osteoblastoma, eosinophilic granuloma, plasmacytoma, chondrosarcoma, and Ewing sarcoma—also occur. Metastatic tumors, including breast tumors and paragangliomas, have also been encountered.[84-86]

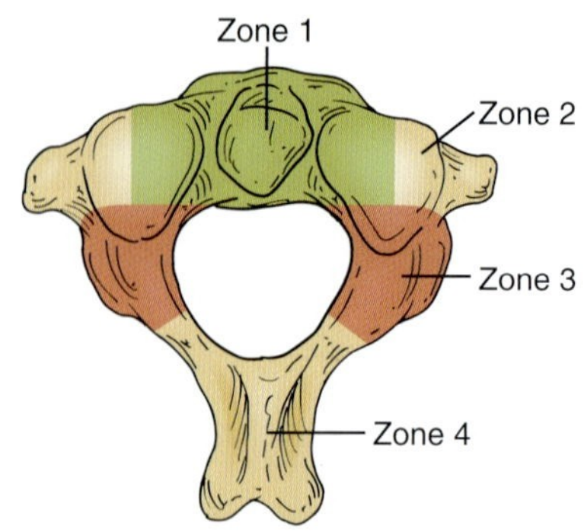

FIGURE 92-9. Surgical approaches and anatomic zones for tumor resection at the craniocervical junction as described by Menezes and Piper. Zone 1 tumors are in the ventral midline involving the axis, atlas, and lower clivus and are best accessed by the transoral approach, with or without division of the palate or the mandible. Zone 2 tumors are more ventrolateral and often involve the lateral mass of C1 and C2. They are best accessed using a retropharyngeal approach. Zone 3 tumors are located dorsal to the lateral mass and may extend into the occipital condyle or dorsal fossa. These tumors are best accessed using a far lateral approach. However, this approach may not be good for later instrumention of the spine. Zone 4 tumors are in the dorsal midline and are resected through a standard midline approach.

Treatment of patients with CVJ tumors involves decompression of neural structures and then determining if surgery has destabilized the CVJ to the point that fusion is necessary. The first step is to determine the direction of the surgical approach. Piper and Menezes divide the axis into four zones that help guide the surgical approach for tumor resection (Fig. 92-9).[84] Zone 1 tumors are in the ventral midline involving the axis, atlas, and lower clivus and are best accessed by the transoral approach, with or without division of the palate or the mandible. Zone 2 tumors are more ventrolateral and often involve the lateral mass of C1 and C2. They are best accessed using a retropharyngeal approach. Zone 3 tumors are located dorsal to the lateral mass and may extend into the occipital condyle or dorsal fossa. These tumors are best accessed using a far lateral approach. However, this approach may not be good for later instrumention of the spine. Zone 4 tumors are in the dorsal midline and are resected through a standard midline approach.[84]

Determining the need for stabilization of the spine and timing of that stabilization is not entirely straightforward. It can be helpful to think about the area of resection to give some criteria for stabilization.

Ventral Odontoid Resection

Dickman et al. performed a biomechanical study of transoral odontoidectomy and concluded that resection of the ventral C1 ring, odontoid, and transverse ligament causes increased motion of C1 on C2 and acute/chronic instability.[53] The conclusion from this study was that ventral odontoid resection requires subsequent dorsal fixation. Menezes[87] reported that a minority of patients undergoing odontoidectomy could go without dorsal stabilization. Disagreement also exists regarding the timing of dorsal stabilization. Menezes delayed fixation for 1 week postsurgery and maintained patients in a halo to allow for wound healing and assessment of instability. Crockard and Stevens[71] recommended performing the dorsal stabilization at the time of ventral resection. An increased incidence of infection has not been seen due to immediate dorsal surgery after a transoral resection.[88]

Lateral Condyle Resection and Lateral Mass Resection

Biomechanical studies have shown a significant increase in hypermobility with resection of greater than 50% of the condyle. Resection of the condyle affected the stability of the C1-2 junction as well.[89] Based on their retrospective case series, Shin et al. recommended an occipital cervical fusion if greater than 50% of a condyle is resected or if the C1 or C2 lateral masses are resected.[86]

Deformity Reduction

Reduction of deformity can be performed by either closed or open methods depending on the anatomic configuration. Successful closed reduction with axial traction can sometimes obviate the need for open ventral decompression, or in some cases of trauma, such as traumatic spondylolisthesis, closed reduction can potentially obviate the need for surgical intervention. Closed reduction is achieved with the use of axial traction with a halo fixator. In some cases, manual manipulation under fluoroscopic guidance is used for reduction. The halo is applied carefully, and the force of pin application is tailored to patient age and underlying pathology. Children younger than 2 years of age or with underlying pathology affecting the skull may not be candidates for a halo ring, and the use of a custom-built Minerva device may be preferable. Children 2 to 4 years of age should have an eight-point halo fixation with an MRI-compatible device. The pins should be tightened to between 1 to 1⅓ pounds of torque.[90] The maximum pin torque is 4 pounds for children who are 5 years of age. Traction should be initiated with low weight (4 pounds) in 5-year-old children, and it should not exceed 7 pounds.[54] Halo application and traction are performed under general anesthesia or moderate sedation in some cases. Fluoroscopy, plain radiographs, or even CT or MRI may be used to determine if reduction has been achieved.[91]

Patients who have long-standing degenerative disorders or tumors are generally not candidates for preoperative reduction. These patients require direct surgical decompression via the appropriate surgical route. This can be aided with the use of computerized stereotactic navigation.[58,92] After the decompression, reduction of the deformity can be achieved by direct manipulation and appropriate shaping of implants and postoperative immobilization.

Summary

Surgical pathology of the CVJ is quite complex. Treatment of traumatic causes of deformity in primarily guided by clinical suspicion and identification of instability followed by stabilization. Management of degenerative disease is guided by the natural history and symptomatology. Congenital abnormalities also are guided by the natural history of the disease and symptoms. Tumor management is guided by tumor location and management of subsequent instability related to tumor debulking. Although technically challenging, appropriate preoperative consideration of the biologic, biomechanical, and pathophysiologic factors associated with CVJ surgery increases the likelihood of a favorable clinical outcome.

KEY REFERENCES

Bono CM, Vaccaro AR, Fehlings M, et al: Measurement techniques for upper cervical spine injuries. *Spine (Phila Pa 1976)* 32(5):593–600, 2007.

Menezes AH: Craniovertebral junction database analysis: incidence, classification, presentation, and treatment algorithms. *Childs Nerv Syst* 24(10):1101–1108, 2008.

Menezes AH: Craniovertebral junction neoplasms in the pediatric population. *Childs Nerv Syst* 24(10):1173–1186, 2008.

Pang D, Nemzek WR, Zovickian J: Atlanto-occipital dislocation–part 2: the clinical use of (occipital) condyle-C1 interval, comparison with other diagnostic methods, and the manifestation, management, and outcome of atlanto-occipital dislocation in children. *Neurosurgery* 61(5):995–1015, 2007; discussion 1015.

Riew KD, Hilibrand A, Palumbo MA, et al: Diagnosing basilar invagination in the rheumatoid patient. The reliability of radiographic criteria. *J Bone Joint Surg [Am]* 83:194–200, 2001.

REFERENCES

The complete reference list is available online at expertconsult.com.

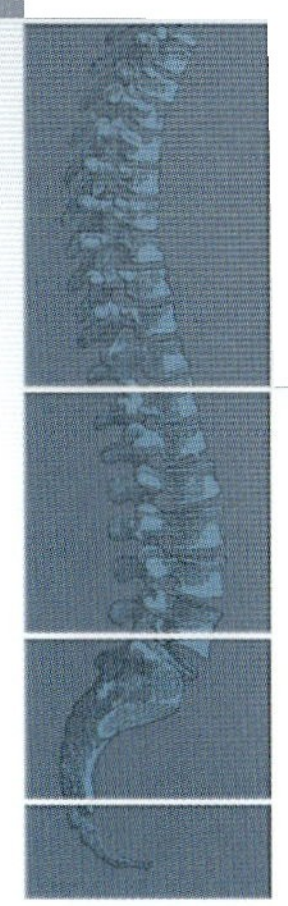

Subaxial Cervical Deformities

Paul M. Arnold | Harel Arzi | Dennis J. Maiman

A deformity of the cervical spine may result from a variety of etiologies, including trauma, degenerative disease, congenital anomaly, infection, tumor, muscle denervation and neuromuscular disease,[1] as well as iatrogenic causes such as surgery and irradiation. Cervical deformities may also occur in patients with systemic arthritides such as ankylosing spondylitis and rheumatoid arthritis.[2] Likewise, patients with primary neurologic disorders such as athetoid cerebral palsy, spasmodic torticollis, and other movement disorders, as well as patients with neuromuscular disorders, are predisposed to develop cervical deformity due to degeneration. Patients with bone disorders such as osteogenesis imperfecta and spondyloepiphyseal dysplasia may also develop deformity involving the cervical region. Patients often present with complaints of neck pain, myelopathy, radiculopathy, or neck deformity with loss of mobility.

Subaxial cervical deformities most commonly occur in the sagittal plane, primarily as kyphosis, although hyperlordosis or a mixed swan-neck deformity can also be observed. Deformity in the coronal plane, manifesting as a scoliosis or angulation, is uncommon in the cervical region when compared with the thoracic and lumbar regions.[3] Most cervical coronal deformities are the result of congenital vertebral anomalies.

Congenital vertebral lesions can be categorized as defects of segmentation and defects of formation. By far, the most common congenital defects of the subaxial cervical vertebrae are the defects of segmentation associated with Klippel-Feil syndrome. Anomalies of vertebral formation are uncommon in the subaxial region of the spine. In the rare cases of hemivertebra of the cervical region, an angular coronal plane deformity may occur, with a risk of neurologic involvement, especially in a skeletally immature person. Trauma or postsurgical changes theoretically could produce a deformity with a coronal component. In practice, however, this is rare. Compensatory curves, which are occasionally observed in response to upper thoracic deformities, must be distinguished from a primary deformity affecting the cervical spine. Deformities in the coronal plane in adults are usually not severe and are infrequently associated with significant pain or neurologic symptoms. As a result, surgical treatment is rarely contemplated.

Significance of Cervical Kyphosis

A considerable variation in the degree of cervical lordosis can be observed in the average patient population. Degenerative changes associated with aging typically produce a straightening of the spine, but the limits of normality are not established.[4] After examining a group of asymptomatic patients, Gore et al. concluded that the normal cervical spine has a lordotic curve measuring approximately 15 to 20 degrees from C1 to T1.[5] Generally, cervical kyphosis is defined as a ventral or kyphotic angulation of 5 degrees or more. The incidence of straightening or kyphosis increases with age for two reasons: (1) the cervical discs contribute to the normal lordotic curve, and (2) the loss of disc height and formation of osteophytes associated with degenerative changes produce a straightening of the spine. In some patients, increases in thoracic kyphosis associated with aging may produce a compensatory increase in cervical lordosis. Load transmission in the cervical spine is thought to be mostly in the posterior column; loss of sagittal alignment may occur if this axis is shifted ventrally.

After performing cadaver studies, Breig first called attention to the motion and degree of elongation of the spinal cord that occur during flexion and extension movements of the cervical spine.[6] According to his measurements, there may be as much as a 45- to a 75-mm change in length of the spinal cord as a result of flexion and extension. Furthermore, there is relative motion of the cord in relation to the underlying vertebrae. Flexion movements produce tensile forces within the cord and elongation, whereas extension causes shortening or compression of the cord. Flexion also produces a decrease in the anteroposterior dimension of the spinal cord, but because of straightening of the dura and ligamenta flava, the available canal diameter is actually increased. Extension has the opposite effect. Changes in the normal configuration of the spinal canal caused by osteophyte formation, disc changes, or facet hypertrophy have the potential to compress or stretch the cord. Instability that results from ligamentous laxity, particularly when associated with a short, angular kyphotic segment, has an increased likelihood of inducing trauma to the spinal cord or adjacent nerve roots. The vascular supply could be decreased, leading to ischemia, which could in turn lead to neuronal loss and myelomalacia. Frequently, examination of the spinal cord in the axial projection demonstrates flattening that is most marked at the kyphotic segment. The potential for neurologic deficit arising from kyphosis without actual compression is small but certainly not nonexistent.

The degree to which these dynamic changes are clinically manifest is difficult to determine. Current imaging studies are performed with the patient recumbent and with the cervical spine in a neutral or slightly extended position, and the images produced are static. Although flexion-extension MRI has

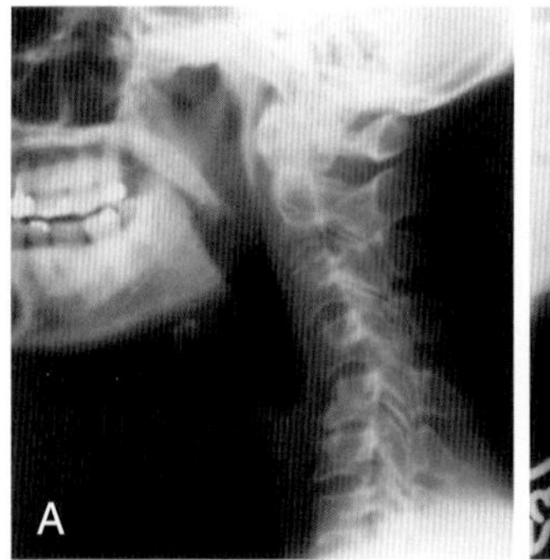

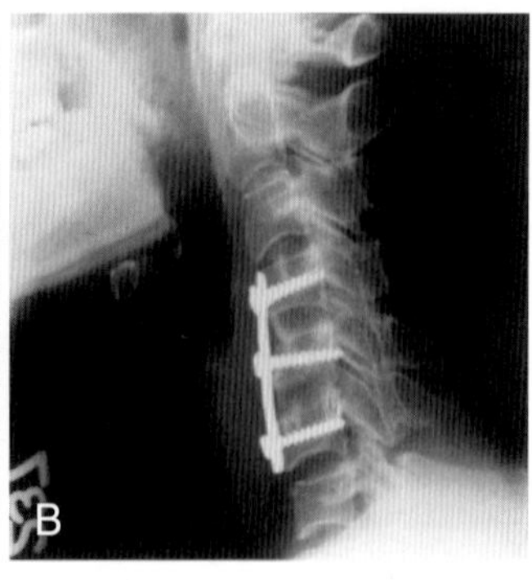

FIGURE 93-1. **A,** Lateral cervical radiograph of a 53-year-old woman presenting with refractory posterior neck pain 6 months after a fall in which she had hyperflexion of her neck. Note the angulation and persistent fanning of the spinous processes at C4-5. **B,** Postoperative radiograph demonstrating anterior interbody fusion augmented with plate fixation. The disc at C5-6 was markedly degenerative with osteophytes narrowing the canal and was, therefore, included in the fusion. The patient had immediate relief of her pain, and this has been maintained over 2 years of follow-up.

been advocated, especially to evaluate craniocervical junction instability, it has yet to receive widespread clinical use.

The significance of cervical kyphosis in the production of chronic muscle fatigue and dorsal neck pain is unclear. Although many patients demonstrate reversal of normal cervical lordosis on plain radiographs, a very small number actually have refractory neck pain as a result of the deformity per se. Nonetheless, an occasional patient appears to have pain on this basis and requires careful evaluation and consideration for deformity correction and fusion (Fig. 93-1).

Postlaminectomy Kyphosis

Kyphosis is a well-recognized complication of laminectomy of the cervical spine.[7-15] The detachment of the dorsal paraspinous muscles, removal of the dorsal osseoligamentous complex, and occasional disruption of the facet complexes have all been recognized as potential causes of the development of a kyphotic deformity after laminectomy.[16]

The reported incidence of kyphosis after cervical laminectomy has been quite variable, although it is considerably more common in the pediatric group. The incidence of postlaminectomy kyphosis in series of pediatric patients ranges from 33% to 100%. Many of these patients, however, have other factors that predispose them to spinal deformity, such as bony tumors, neurofibromatosis, or irradiation. A recent series, which excluded these confounding factors, noted an incidence of kyphotic deformity of 53% in children.[7] Although the data are mixed, it appears that a younger age and a greater number of segments treated with laminectomy are associated with higher rates of deformity. Injury or resection of the facet joints also increases the probability of kyphosis. Laminectomy of C1 has a relatively low tendency to result in spinal deformity. Although it has not been conclusively demonstrated that the performance of laminoplasty, as recommended by Raimondi et al.,[17] reduces the likelihood of postlaminectomy kyphosis in children, many neurosurgeons who routinely perform cervical procedures on children perform laminoplasty, and some report evidence suggestive of benefit.[18] Prophylactic fusion should also be considered for patients undergoing laminectomy who are at high risk for developing kyphosis.[15] Dorsal fusions are much more effective at preventing kyphosis than at correcting it (Fig. 93-2).

The incidence of postlaminectomy kyphosis in adults is relatively uncommon in the absence of an additional predisposing factor such as facet joint damage, prior ligamentous instability, ventral column compromise, neurologic deficit, or irradiation.[19,20] Adult cases are, nonetheless, seen in any busy practice specializing in spinal problems (Fig. 93-3). A recognition of the significance of this finding in terms of the probability of progression, the potential for symptoms, and the

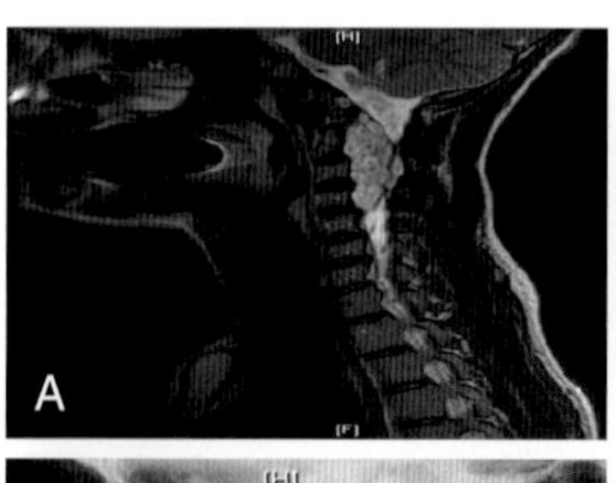

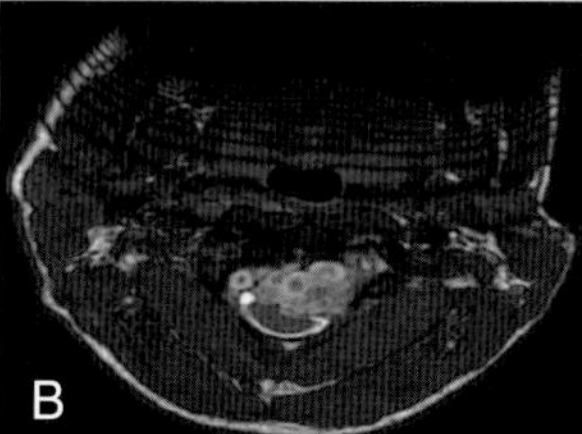

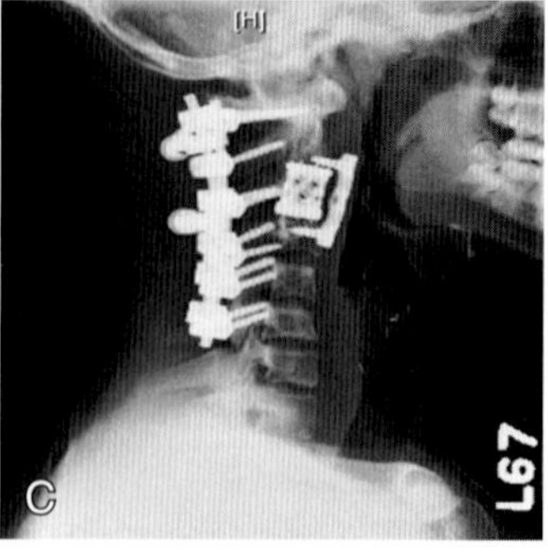

FIGURE 93-2. MRIs, sagittal (**A**) and axial (**B**), show a large neurofibroma from C2 to C4. The patient underwent cervical laminectomy and C3 vertebrectomy to resect the tumor. A posterior fusion (**C**) was performed to prevent kyphosis.

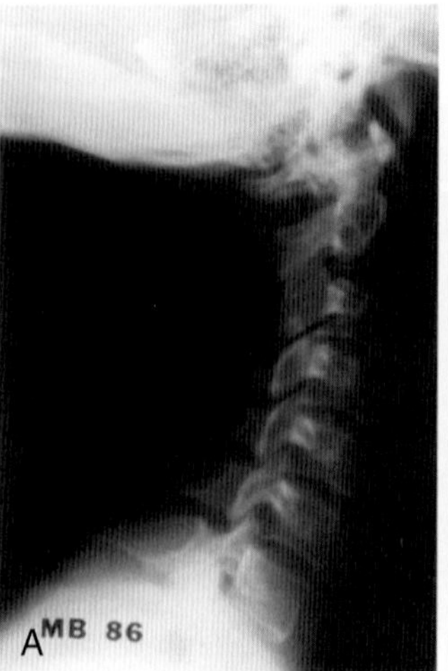

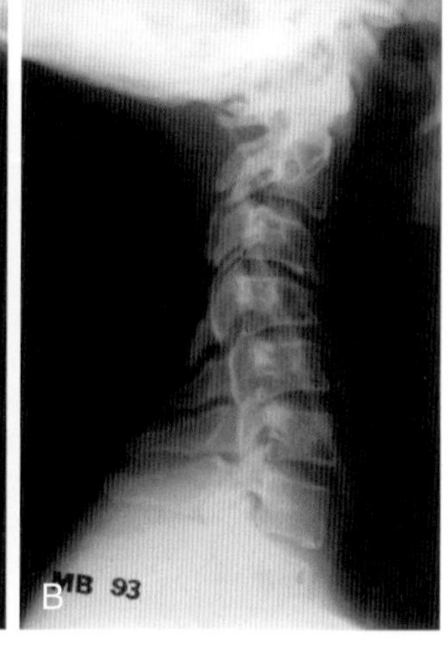

FIGURE 93-3. **A,** Postoperative lateral cervical radiograph obtained after a C1-4 cervical laminectomy in a 20-year-old woman with long-standing shunted hydrocephalus. Surgery was performed to address progressing myelopathy that appeared to be related to dural fibrosis and stenosis causing spinal cord compression in the upper cervical spine. The patient improved after surgery. **B,** Lateral cervical radiograph 7 years later demonstrating the interval development of postlaminectomy kyphosis in this skeletally mature patient. At the time of this follow-up, the patient was exhibiting recurrent symptoms of myelopathy and dorsal neck pain.

appropriate therapeutic options is essential for optimal management. Patients with the greatest risk of postlaminectomy kyphosis are those that have preoperative instability as well as those with straightening of the cervical spine. Additional risk factors include multilevel laminectomy, extensive facetectomy, and resection of the musculature at C2. Iizuka noted that removal of the semispinalis cervicis muscle attachment at C2 could lead to loss of alignment and kyphosis.[21]

In adults, when postlaminectomy kyphosis is mild, it is usually well tolerated, especially when there is associated stiffening of the spine from degenerative changes leading to loss of disc height and development of buttressing osteophytes. Progressive deformity, especially in a previously straight or lordotic spine, warrants close observation or consideration of treatment. Some surgeons routinely manage all cervical laminectomy patients in a hard cervical collar for several weeks postoperatively in an attempt to minimize the development of a postoperative deformity.

Surgical Correction of Cervical Kyphosis

Preoperative Assessment

Patients who present with kyphotic deformity of the cervical region generally have complaints of pain, neurologic symptoms, or both. Less frequently, they cite problems relating to the deformity itself, such as difficulty raising their head, looking forward, or opening their mouth. This latter group of patients encompasses those patients with the more severe deformities.

The preoperative evaluation of all such patients should include a careful neurologic assessment to look for subtle signs of myelopathy or radicular involvement. Plain cervical spine radiographs with flexion-extension views provide information about the deformity, including the levels involved, the severity, and whether it appears fixed or rigid. Neuroradiologic imaging with MRI or myelography and postmyelographic CT is important for evaluating spinal cord compression and the dimensions of the spinal canal. Assessment of the bony and ligamentous anatomy is also possible with these studies. Three-dimensional reconstructive CT has also been useful in assessing kyphosis, because bony detail, amount of deformity, and spinal canal encroachment can be visualized on one image (Fig. 93-4). The degree of spinal instability can also be assessed. Standing long-cassette films are helpful for evaluating overall sagittal spinal balance in patients with severe deformity. Concomitant thoracic kyphosis or fixed flexion contracture of the hip must be evaluated before consideration is given to "lordosing" a cervical kyphosis.

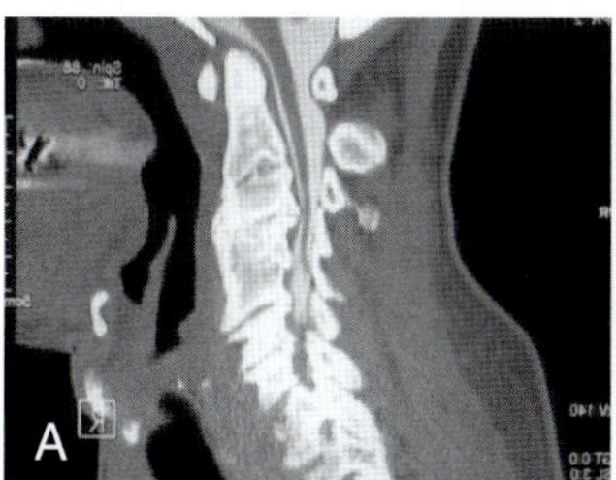

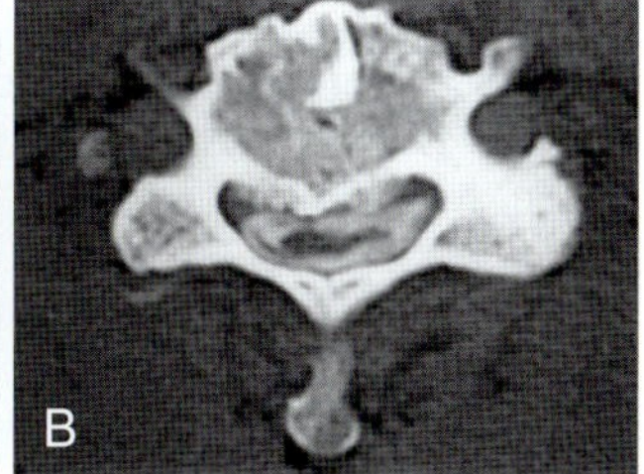

FIGURE 93-4. **A** and **B,** Three-dimensional reconstruction CT shows degenerative kyphosis with multilevel stenosis. This 62-year-old man had cervical myelopathy and required a combined anterior/posterior procedure. His neck pain and paresthesias resolved, and his weakness and myelopathy improved.

Most patients whose deformities do not reduce with neck extension should be given a trial of traction before surgery to determine the reducibility of the kyphosis. An exception to this is patients with minor deformity (which can often be reduced intraoperatively) or those with an obviously fixed kyphosis (e.g., ankylosing spondylitis). Traction is applied either with tongs or with a halo ring. Cervical halters are generally unsatisfactory because for most deformities, traction needs to be sustained to be effective. The amount of weight to apply is a matter of clinical judgment. We generally begin with 5 to 10 pounds and increase the weight in a stepwise fashion, with regular assessment of neurologic function and patient tolerance and radiographic visualization of the degree of reduction. Weights of more than 5 pounds per level are usually not required. Close neurologic observation is imperative during traction because patients may demonstrate neurologic worsening, which necessitates immediate discontinuation of traction. The optimal duration of traction is unclear; we usually apply traction for 48 hours or less before scheduled surgery.

If surgery is contemplated primarily for the treatment of pain believed to be the result of the deformity, other confounding conditions should be ruled out. In selected patients, psychological screening may also be worthwhile for obtaining objective data regarding the likelihood of surgical success.

Surgical Techniques

The choice of operative technique for cervical deformity must be predicated on the type and severity of the deformity to be treated, etiology of the deformity, bone quality, neurologic symptomatology, posterior column integrity, rigidity of the spine, and experience of the surgeon. The indications for a ventral approach, a dorsal approach, or a combined ventral and dorsal approach are not absolute. Goals of surgery may include progression of further kyphosis, long-term spinal stability, restoration of sagittal balance, neural decompression, establishment of a posterior tension band, and reconstruction of the anterior column.

Ventral Surgery

A ventral approach is preferred for cases in which there is insufficient anterior column height or insufficient ability to bear an axial load, such as with collapse of a ventral bone graft or compression fracture, with ventral pathology such as tumor or associated spondylotic bars producing myelopathy, or with a deformity that is rigid or incompletely reducible. Anterior surgery may also be indicated for focal areas of deformity. In addition, ventral surgery may be safer for the treatment of postlaminectomy kyphosis because surgery can be performed through an unoperated field (Fig. 93-5). The ventral approach has other advantages, including the ability to decompress the spinal cord ventrally and to use ventral interbody strut grafts that are loaded in compression, thereby enhancing fusion.[22]

In these cases, a ventral release, with or without ventral decompression of the spinal canal, is performed. If appropriate, the kyphotic deformity is then reversed, with reestablishment of some lordotic curve. Reversal of kyphosis

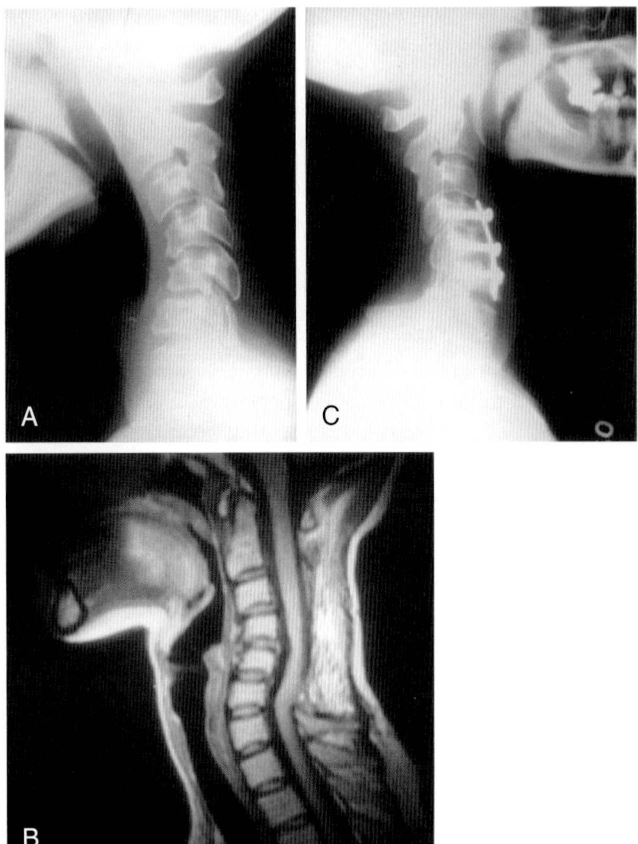

FIGURE 93-5. Standing lateral cervical radiograph (**A**) and sagittal T1-weighted MRI scan (**B**) of a 38-year-old woman with severe dorsal neck pain and subtle signs of myelopathy. The patient had undergone cervical laminectomy several years previously. Note the development of a postlaminectomy swan-neck deformity in an adult. Anterior interbody fusion and plating (**C**) was performed to restore lordosis with resolution of the patient's pain and neurologic symptoms. On this film, performed 6 months postoperatively, there is slight kyphosis at C3-4 that may progress and will bear watching.

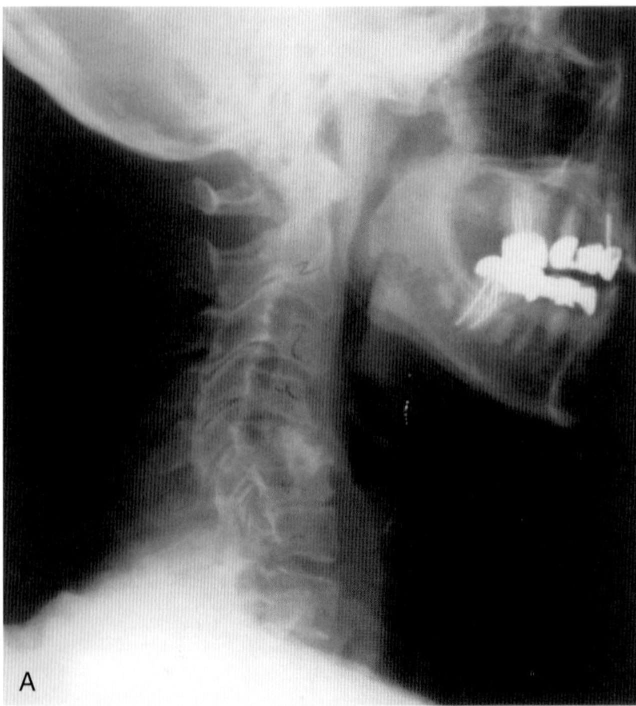

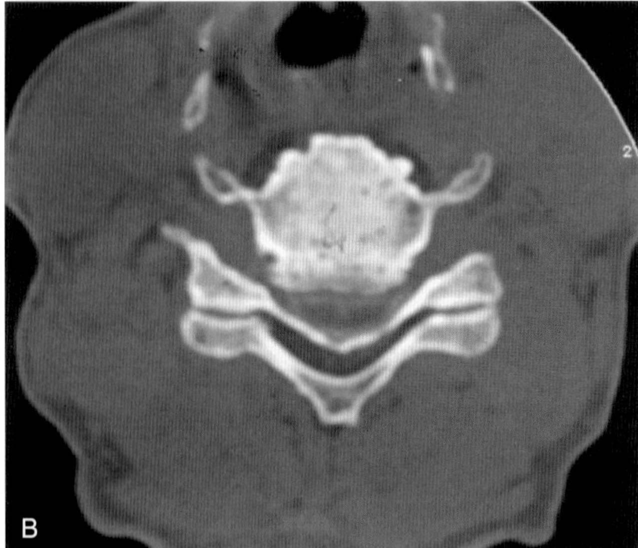

FIGURE 93-6. A, Lateral cervical radiograph of a 71-year-old woman presenting with myelopathy. A kyphosis is observed from C4 to C6. **B,** CT myelogram at C5-6 demonstrating tight "circumferential" stenosis with shingling of the laminae. Because of the combination of dorsal and ventral cord compression, a posterior laminectomy was performed from C4 to C6 before repositioning the patient supine and carrying out C5 and C6 corpectomy, strut grafting, and anterior Caspar plate fixation from C4 to C7. The involved area progressed to solid fusion after immobilization in a rigid collar. Partial improvement of the myelopathy was observed.

should not be attempted in the face of significant radiologic evidence of spinal cord impingement unless surgical decompression is first performed (Fig. 93-6). As noted previously, extension of the cervical spine decreases the anteroposterior dimension of the spinal canal while increasing the thickness of the spinal cord. With a severe, rigid angular kyphotic deformity, dorsal decompression by means of laminectomy and foraminotomy should be considered before ventral osteotomy.

The surgical techniques for ventral decompression and fusion of deformity are quite similar to those used in the treatment of trauma or degenerative disease. Fiberoptic nasotracheal intubation is preferred to allow dental occlusion and maximal proximal exposure that is unimpeded by the mandible. The patient is positioned supine in traction with as much extension as is possible, as determined preoperatively. This may be facilitated by a roll placed dorsally in the cervical region. In cases in which spinal cord compression is observed, methylprednisolone as a 30-mg/kg IV bolus over 15 minutes followed by 5.4 mg/kg per hour continuous IV infusion can be given, although this is a controversial issue. If the patient awakens neurologically intact, the infusion is stopped. Otherwise, the infusion is continued for 23 hours. Prophylactic antibiotics are administered. When bicortical ventral fixation plates are used, C-arm fluoroscopy is routine. Plain radiography or fluoroscopy is also invaluable for assessing the degree of reduction and for graft placement. An intraoperative radiograph is performed at this time to assess spinal alignment. Significant deformity reduction is often evident following the placement of tong traction and general anesthesia. If autologous bone graft is to be used, the donor site and cervical region are prepared simultaneously. The incision is centered at the middle of the deformity to be treated. A transverse incision placed in a skin crease is preferred for short (one to three) segment fusions or in people with short, thick necks. An incision along the ventral margin of the sternocleidomastoid muscle is used for longer fusions. Exposure of the ventral aspect of the spine is accomplished as described by Cloward[23] and Smith and Robinson.[24]

Dissection of the medial attachments of the longus colli muscles and placement of self-retaining retractors is followed by incision of the anulus fibrosus at the affected disc levels. The Caspar vertebral body distractor (Aesculap, San Francisco, CA) that uses screw posts placed into the vertebral bodies is a useful aid for reducing the kyphosis and placing ventral strut grafts (Fig. 93-7). Excess intervertebral traction, however, may be injurious to the compromised spinal cord and thus should be used judiciously. The distraction posts are placed parallel to the vertebral end plates. After osteotomy or ventral release of anular attachments, the posts are used to effect reduction by positioning them in a parallel configuration. This maneuver realigns the spine and allows application of the retractor.[25] The retractor then maintains the reduction and allows further distraction force to be applied. After a bone graft is inserted, the retractor is removed and a plate is applied. This technique should not be used if there is evidence of dorsal compression by laminae, ligaments, or other pathology.

The decompression is tailored according to the results of preoperative imaging. In some cases, multilevel discectomy with multiple interbody bone grafts is preferred. This is useful for kyphotic deformities extending over several motion segments. Plate fixation can then be segmental to provide greater rigidity. Alternatively, when there is a bony encroachment on the canal, trough corpectomy with strut grafting is performed. A strut graft spanning two disc spaces with an additional ventral interbody graft at the level above or below can also be used when required (Fig. 93-8). Alternatively, the cancellous bone obtained from the decompression can be morselized and placed in a cage, allowing anterior column reconstruction with the associated morbidity of iliac crest grafting or the small risks associated with allograft (Fig. 93-9). This type of mixed construct provides the maximum number of sites for screw placement and allows for greater fixation and optimal reestablishment of lordosis. If two or more vertebral bodies are replaced, consideration should be given to adding dorsal fixation.[26]

Locking and nonlocking plates and slotted plates are used. For multisegment constructs, the latter system often provides more flexibility and is easier to apply. The variability in screw angulation allowed by the Caspar plate is helpful when plates are extended to C2 or C3. Fluoroscopy can be an aid to kyphosis reduction and plate application regardless of which system is used. Fluoroscopic control is highly desirable when screws

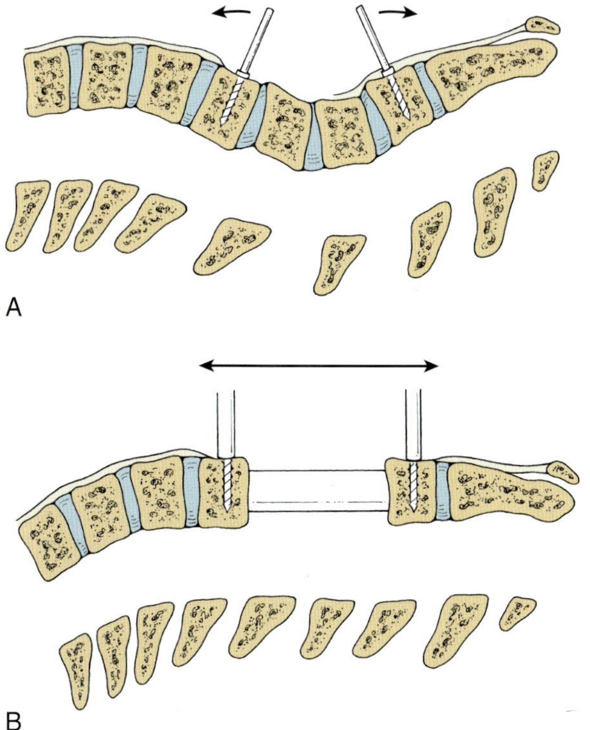

FIGURE 93-7. Use of the Caspar vertebral body distraction retractor to help maintain correction of kyphosis. **A,** Initially, the distraction posts are inserted parallel to the end plates of the vertebral bodies. **B,** When the deformity is corrected and the retractor is applied on the posts, it maintains a more normal alignment as the site is prepared for strut grafting. Although the posts may be used as "handles" to aid in performing a reduction, this must be done with caution, or fracture of the vertebral body can result.

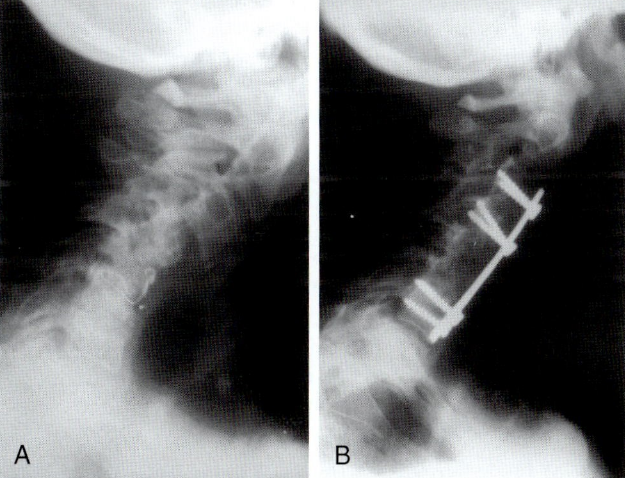

FIGURE 93-8. A, Lateral cervical radiograph of a 70-year-old man with a painful, rigid cervical kyphosis resulting from multiple failed previous attempts at anterior interbody fusion. Complaints included occipitocervical pain and an inability to maintain the head in an upright position. **B,** Lateral radiograph obtained 18 months postoperatively demonstrating solid fusion with partial correction of the kyphotic deformity by means of corpectomy and osteotomy with strut grafting from C4 to C7, interbody grafting at C3 to C4, and ventral plating. Postoperatively, the patient was immobilized in a halo orthosis for 12 weeks.

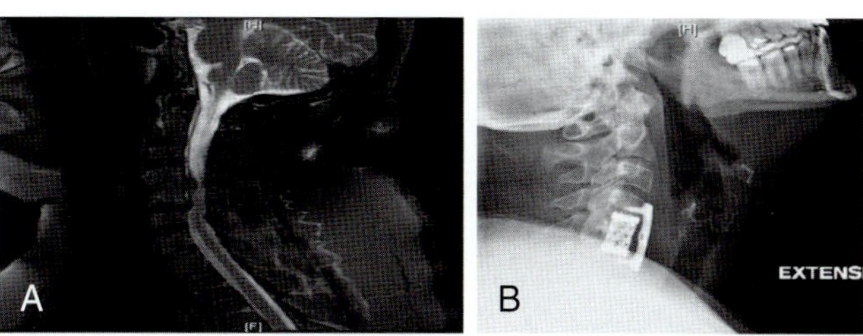

FIGURE 93-9. A, A 45-year-old woman with straightening of the cervical spine and cervical myelopathy. **B,** She underwent C5 vertebrectomy and C4-6 anterior fusion with autograft and mesh cage.

are placed into the dorsal vertebral body cortex. Steinmetz et al. recently reported a series of 14 patients treated ventrally for postsurgical kyphosis. They used intraoperative neck extension, as well as a dynamic, ventrally placed implant with multiple fixation points, to restore lordosis. They corrected 11 of 12 patients with this method (average 20-degree correction) with minimal complications.[27]

In most cases, postoperative immobilization is achieved with a rigid cervical collar that is worn for 6 weeks to 3 months. A halo vest or Minerva jacket may be used in cases in which fixation is suboptimal or when fusion is expected to be delayed. Patients with severe osteoporosis, high-grade instability noted preoperatively, or failed prior attempts at fusion perhaps should be included in this group. Herman and Sonntag also noted the occasional need for halo immobilization in some high-risk patients after this type of procedure.[28]

Complications

The potential complications associated with the ventral approaches are well known and include vocal cord palsy, hoarseness or dysphagia, injury to visceral structures (such as the esophagus or trachea), graft displacement, screw loosening or fracture, wound complications (such as infection), hematoma (which may be sufficient to cause respiratory embarrassment), and dehiscence.[29] The incidence of a number of complications can be reduced by periodically releasing or removing the retraction during the operation. Also, for procedures involving the lower cervical spine, a left-sided approach may reduce the likelihood of vocal cord paralysis in the event that there is a nonrecurrent right inferior laryngeal nerve.

Overdistraction of the cervical spine and placement of a strut graft that is too long for the corpectomy defect is a common technical error. This situation preloads the construct, making telescoping, graft collapse, or displacement more likely. When a ventral plate is used, there must be no encroachment of the plate on the adjacent disc spaces, and screws must be placed appropriately. Meticulous sizing of the bone graft and any ventral plate is critical for avoiding complications and for long-term success.

Dorsal Fixation and Fusion Techniques

Dorsal fusion for cervical kyphotic deformity is primarily indicated as a prophylactic measure after laminectomy or when the deformity is the result of dorsal ligamentous insufficiency associated with the preservation of axial integrity of the anterior column, such as is seen acutely after ligamentous trauma (Fig. 93-10). Posterior surgery is also indicated in patients requiring a posterior osteotomy, as in cases of ankylosing spondylitis. In these cases, usually performed at the cervicothoracic junction, the C7 lamina and pedicles are removed.[30] In these cases, the kyphosis usually significantly or completely reduces with neck extension. Dorsal fusion is accomplished via standard techniques, including interspinous wiring or lateral mass wire or plate fixation. Abumi et al.[31] recently reported a series of patients with cervical kyphosis who underwent placement of cervical pedicle screws to maintain correction. Dorsal surgical approaches for rigid or incompletely reducible kyphotic deformities have limited application and are biomechanically less sound. Nevertheless, certain circumstances may warrant their use as the sole operative treatment, especially if fusion in situ is being performed. More often, dorsal fusions are

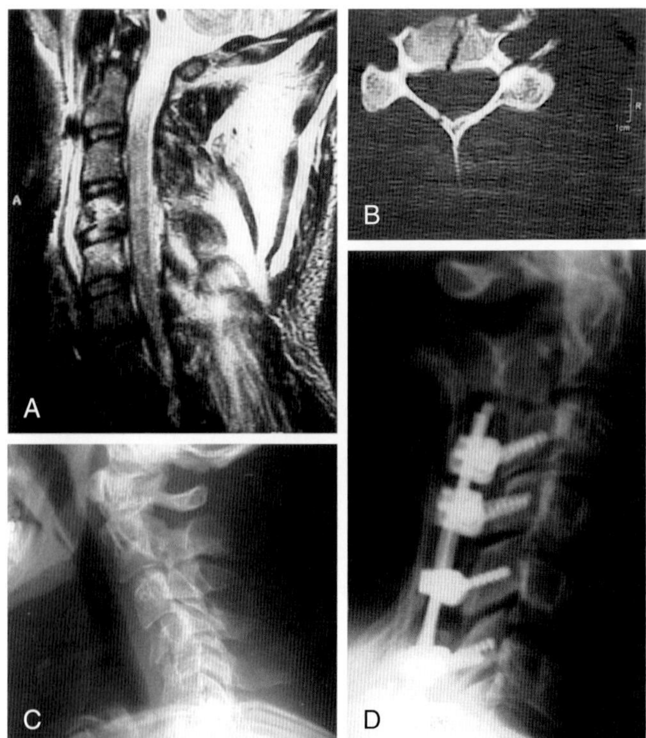

FIGURE 93-10. A 22-year-old male involved in a motor vehicle accident was neurologically normal, but had C4 and C5 fractures with normal alignment (**A** and **B**). The patient required anticoagulation and was placed in a halo. Three weeks later, he began experiencing neck pain, and a plain radiograph revealed kyphosis (**C**). His anticoagulation was reversed, and a posterior cervical fusion was performed (**D**).

performed in conjunction with a dorsal decompression and ventral procedures when treating severe deformity associated with spinal cord compression.[11,32]

Postlaminectomy kyphosis is corrected less well by dorsal fixation and fusion than by ventral techniques. If this approach is to be used, lateral mass plates or interfacet wiring, combined with iliac strips or rib grafts, are used. In the early 1990s, lateral mass fixation became the preferred fixation method because it provided greater rigidity than wire fixation.[33] Complications associated with screw placement are uncommon if meticulous care is used to select screw entry points and the screws are angled appropriately rostrally and laterally to avoid the nerve root and vertebral artery. However, it must be cautioned that a deformity or prior surgery may obscure the anatomic landmarks so that great care is required for satisfactory screw placement. Frameless stereotaxy may be used in patients with previous surgery where standard landmarks may be lost. Bicortical purchase does not appear to be necessary for successful fixation in most cases. Fehlings et al. obtained successful fusion results using lateral mass plates without additional bone graft.[33] This study, however, was heavily weighted with posttraumatic cases, so careful consideration should be given to the use of autologous bone graft in deformity cases. Patients with cervical spine trauma and injury to the posterior ligamentous complex may also benefit from a posterior cervical procedure. Injury reduction can occur with the use of traction or in the operating room. The facets may need to be drilled off to achieve reduction. Lateral mass or pedicle screw fixation may be used to achieve fixation and fusion, and these constructs have been found to be biomechanically superior to ventral procedures.[34]

Combined Ventral and Dorsal Decompression and Fusion

Combined procedures involving both an anterior and a posterior approach are occasionally indicated, especially for the correction of rigid deformities (Fig. 93-11). Other indications include cases of both anterior and posterior compression with radiculopathy secondary to foraminal stenosis as a prominent feature, cases in which severe slippage is associated with incompetent posterior ligamentous structures, and cases of trauma when there is compromise of the anterior and posterior columns (Fig. 93-12). Mummaneni et al. had good results in a series of 30 patients who underwent circumferential fusion for a variety of etiologies causing multilevel cervical kyphosis, including fractures, tumors, and degenerative disease.[35]

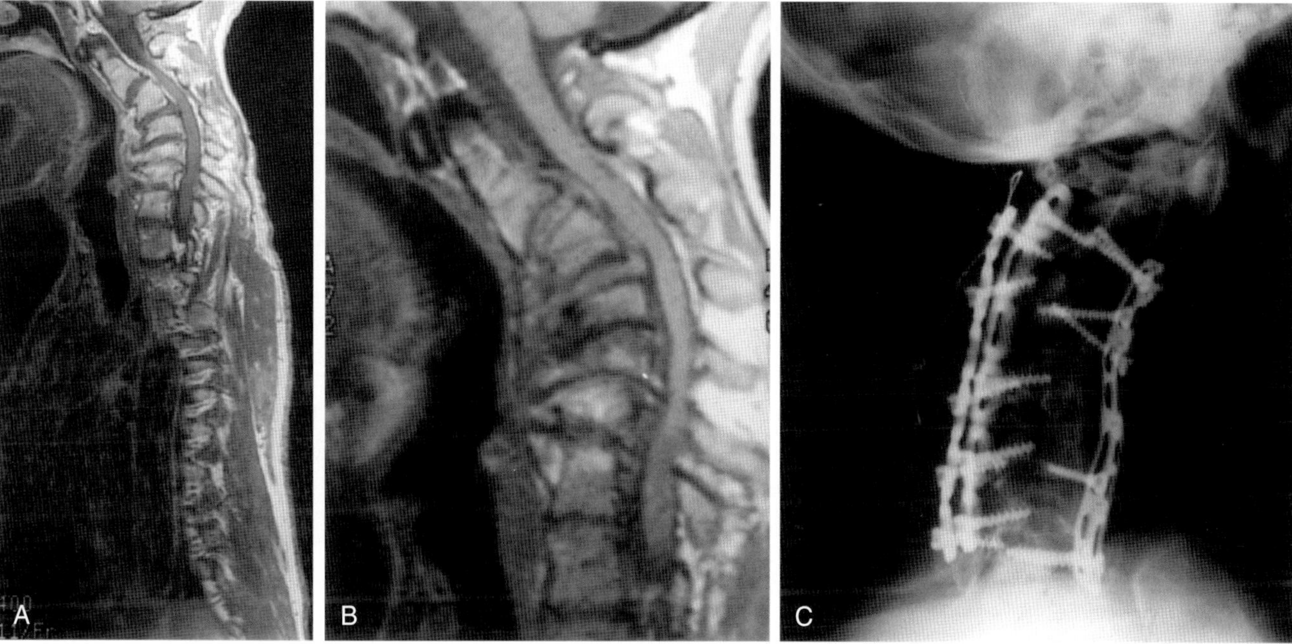

FIGURE 93-11. This 38-year-old right-handed man presented with progressive cervical myelopathy. He had a history of a cerebral palsy–like condition associated with mild spasticity, joint contractures, and thoracolumbar scoliosis. **A,** A sagittal T1-weighted MRI image demonstrated a kyphotic deformity of the cervical spine with associated thoracic lordoscoliosis. **B,** A detailed sagittal MRI image of the cervical region demonstrated spinal cord impingement at multiple sites. Minimal preoperative reduction of this relatively rigid kyphosis was noted with cervical traction. **C,** An anteroposterior decompression and fusion with internal fixation was performed from C2 to C7 using titanium instrumentation. The kyphosis correction was a secondary goal of surgery and was partial. The patient, who required aids for ambulation preoperatively, now walks independently.

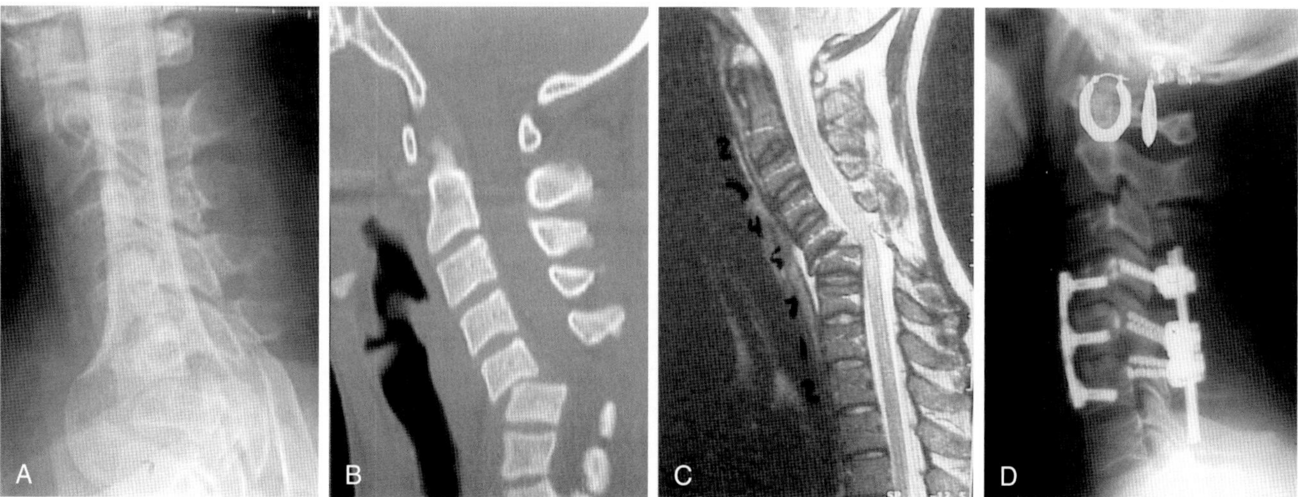

FIGURE 93-12. A 41-year-old woman who was involved in a motor vehicle accident complained of lower extremity painful dysesthesia. She was densely paraparetic with weakness in her distal upper extremities. Radiographic workup included plain radiography (**A**), CT (**B**), and MRI (**C**). Postoperative radiograph shows reduction of deformity and solid fusion (**D**).These studies revealed severe kyphosis at C5-6, with injury to the anterior and posterior columns. She underwent a combined anterior/posterior procedure. She is able to ambulate independently, and her dysesthetic pain has resolved.

Patients with ankylosing spondylitis may present with a severe, rigid cervical kyphosis that limits the ability to look forward, and in some severe cases, this kyphosis may limit jaw opening secondary to contact with the chest. Correction of this type of deformity requires osteotomy with resection of a portion of the posterior elements. Different methods have been described for this procedure,[36-38] the most notable being the one advocated by Simmons,[30,38] in which a posterior decompression is performed under local anesthesia at the C7-T1 level, with the patient in the seated position. The spine is fractured by forcibly extending the neck, which is held in traction by a halo ring. Usually, the fracture in these patients occurs at the junction between the vertebral end plate and the disc. Simmons advocates that the procedure be performed with the patient awake to provide for patient feedback during kyphosis reduction. Other surgeons have performed the procedure using a general anesthetic and have monitored evoked potentials.

Summary

Deformity of the cervical spine is generally observed in the context of degenerative disease with its concurrent ligamentous laxity, loss of disc height, and bony remodeling. Another relatively common circumstance is postlaminectomy kyphosis that tends to affect younger patients. Deformity resulting from congenital anomalies is uncommon in the lower cervical region. Surgical procedures may be indicated to treat neurologic symptoms (myelopathy) rather than the deformity itself. Ventral procedures are preferred in most cases of spinal cord compression or when the deformity is rigid. In irreducible kyphosis in which movement occurs across the angulated segment, decompression, combined with strut grafting and fusion in situ, may allow stabilization or improvement of neurologic symptoms. Severe kyphotic deformity may occasionally require correction for postural reasons. There is a small group of patients with neck pain and cervical deformity who benefit from reduction and fusion, although the methods to clearly identify patients suitable for surgery are not standardized. Management of these patients requires a thorough assessment of the anatomic, neurologic, and biomechanical factors contributing to the deformity. Careful patient selection is required for this difficult group.

KEY REFERENCES

Arnold PM, Bryniarski M, McMahon J: Posterior stabilization of subaxial cervical spine trauma: indications and techniques. *Injury* 36:S36–S43, 2005.

Deutsch H, Haid RW, Rodts GE, et al: Postlaminectomy cervical deformity. *Neurosurg Focus* 15:1–5, 2003.

Fassett DR, Clark R, Brockmeyer DL, et al: Cervical spine deformity associated with resection of spinal cord tumors. *Neurosurg Focus* 20:1–7, 2006.

Hoh DJ, Khoueir P, Wang MY: Management of cervical deformity in ankylosing spondylitis. *Neurosurg Focus* 24:1–10, 2008.

Kaptain GJ, Simmons N, Replogle RE, et al: Incidence and outcome of kyphotic deformity following laminectomy for cervical spondylotic myelopathy. *J Neurosurg Spine* 93:199–204, 2000.

Mummaneni PV, Dhall SS, Rodts GE, et al: Circumferential fusion for cervical kyphotic deformity. *J Neurosurg Spine* 9:515–521, 2008.

Simmons ED, DiStefano RJ, Zheng Y, et al: Thirty-six years experience of cervical extension osteotomy in ankylosing spondylitis: techniques and outcomes. *Spine (Phila Pa 1976)* 31:3006–3012, 2006.

Steinmetz MP, Kager CD, Benzel EC: Ventral correction of postsurgical cervical kyphosis. *J Neurosurg Spine* 98:1–7, 2003.

Stewart TJ, Steinmetz MP, Benzel EC: Techniques for the ventral correction of postsurgical cervical kyphotic deformity. *Neurosurgery* 56(1):191–195, 2005.

REFERENCES

The complete reference list is available online at expertconsult.com.

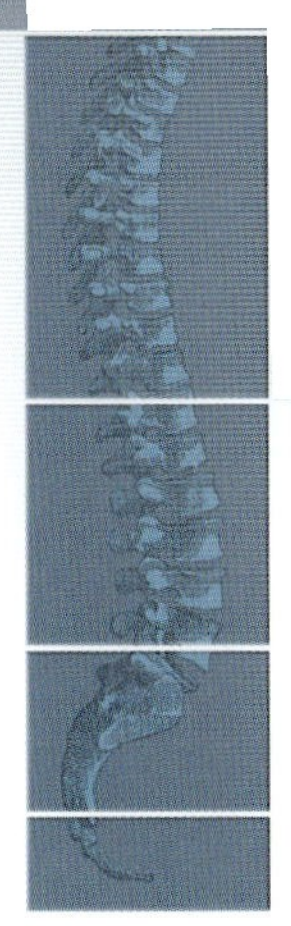

Cervical Facet Dislocations: A Ventral Surgical Strategy for Decompression, Reduction, and Stabilization

Ron Riesenburger | Simcha J. Weller | Sait Naderi | Edward C. Benzel

Much controversy surrounds the management of subaxial cervical subluxations resulting from facet fracture-dislocation.[1-11] An initial attempt at closed reduction using skeletal traction is not without risk.[12-18] The most serious complication of cervical traction and closed reduction is the retropulsion of disc fragments into the spinal canal and resultant spinal cord compression (Fig. 94-1). Several reports of neurologic deterioration after closed reduction in the setting of concurrent disc herniation have been described.[19-23] In addition, late instability is relatively common in patients treated with closed reduction alone, because of the concomitant presence of significant ligamentous disruption associated with these injuries.

The surgical technique for the open reduction of unstable cervical dislocations varies from surgeon to surgeon. Most reports have described dorsal reduction techniques.[20,21,24-29] However, the ventral surgical approach for reduction has its advocates.[30] Several small series have been published that describe the technique of ventral reduction of locked facets.[19,31-35] Because of the popularization of dorsal fixation techniques (e.g., lateral mass plating and spinous process wiring), ventral reduction has not been widely used in clinical practice. However, an increasing concern has been raised regarding the danger associated with the dorsal reduction of a cervical spine dislocation in the presence of a ventral disc herniation.[19,21-24] Furthermore, because of the common coexistence of significant dorsal bony and soft tissue disruption, a three-vertebral segment (two-motion segment) dorsal fixation is commonly required to stabilize a two-vertebral segment (one-motion segment) instability. In addition, in dorsal reduction of locked facets, it is commonly necessary to remove a significant portion of the involved facet(s), thus often mandating a three-vertebral segment dorsal fixation procedure. Conversely, ventral reduction may be followed by arthrodesis of only a single-motion segment, thus sparing additional motion segments from arthrodesis.

Kwon et al.[36] concluded that both ventral stabilization and dorsal stabilization for unilateral cervical facet injuries were valid treatment options. In this randomized study of 42 patients with unilateral cervical facet injuries, patients on whom a ventral approach was used had a lower rate of wound infection, had a higher rate of radiographically demonstrated union, and healed in a more lordotic sagittal alignment. However, they also more frequently had signs of dysphagia and voice changes in the early postoperative period in comparison to the group treated with dorsal stabilization. Patients undergoing a ventral approach should be informed of these (and all other) risks.

Surgical Technique

Discectomy

The standard ventromedial approach is used through a transverse skin incision. After radiographic confirmation of the operative level, a discectomy is performed. A special consideration in the case of facet dislocation is the ventral translation (ventrolisthesis) of the rostral vertebral body on its caudal counterpart. This is often associated with some degree of kyphotic angulation and a resultant obscuration of the disc space, necessitating removal of the ventral aspect of the caudal end plate of the rostral vertebral body with a high-speed air drill (Fig. 94-2). Care must be taken not to remove so much of the vertebral body as to preclude ventral screw-plate fixation. After exposure of the disc space, a standard discectomy is performed. The posterior longitudinal ligament is always removed, thus exposing the dura mater and ensuring adequate decompression.

Reduction

After completion of the discectomy, deformity reduction is attempted. Often, simple distraction is successful, because a potentially significant obstruction to reduction (the disc and anulus fibrosus) has been removed. However, if this maneuver fails, one of two intraoperative maneuvers may be used to facilitate reduction through the ventral approach: the interbody spreader technique or the vertebral body post technique. Failure to use either technique appropriately may result in failure of reduction.

Interbody Spreader Technique

A Cloward interbody spreader, or an equivalent device, is inserted into the disc interspace at a 30- to 40-degree angle (Fig. 94-3A). Failure to place this device at an angle results in achieving only distraction force application (as simple distraction with tongs achieves). This does not result in the

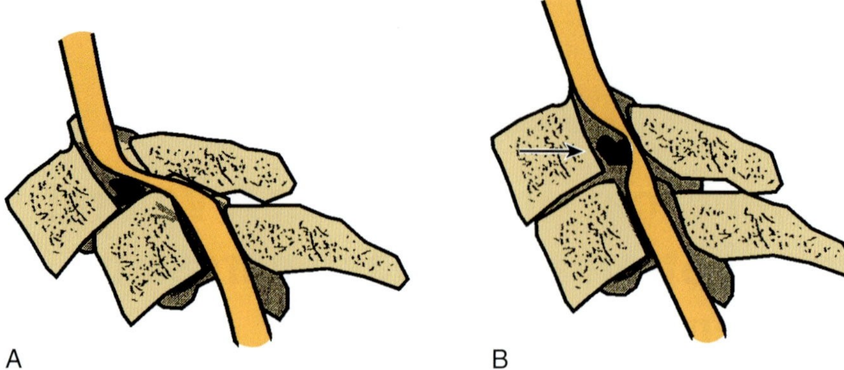

FIGURE 94-1. A typical bilateral facet dislocation with disc extrusion. **A,** Note that the spinal cord is compressed predominantly by the dislocated caudal vertebral body and rostral lamina before reduction. **B,** After reduction, the large fragment of extruded disc has been retropulsed into the spinal canal (*arrow*), resulting in spinal cord compression. (From University of New Mexico, Division of Neurosurgery, with permission.)

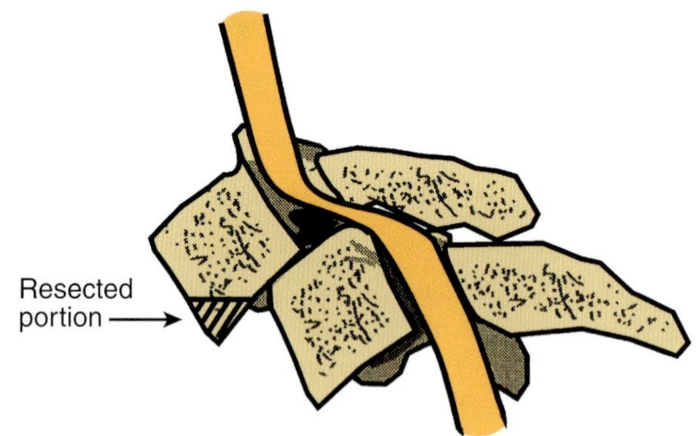

FIGURE 94-2. The ventrocaudal aspect of the rostral vertebral body obscures visualization of the disc interspace, necessitating partial resection. (From University of New Mexico, Division of Neurosurgery, with permission.)

application of a bending moment, which is required for reduction with this technique.

While distraction is gradually applied with the disc interspace spreader (applied in the midvertebral body region) (Fig. 94-3B), the spreader is rotated rostrally. This applies a bending moment to the dislocated vertebral body while the facet dislocation is reduced by distraction. If the locked facets are disengaged, the vertebrae should realign. Distraction is then relaxed in the aligned position, and the spreader is removed (Fig. 94-3C).

For bilateral facet dislocations, the intervertebral spreader should be placed in the midvertebral body region. For unilateral dislocations, the spreader should be placed on the side of the dislocation to facilitate the application of a torque about the long axis of the spine via the spreader. Placement of the intervertebral spreader too far ventrally may result in fracture of the end plate.

Vertebral Body Post Technique

If the aforementioned technique fails, the vertebral body post technique may be attempted. This technique uses a vertebral body distractor post. It is important to remember that parallel distraction via the vertebral body posts is equivalent to simple traction, in that these techniques do not apply a bending moment.

The vertebral body post technique usually involves placing the posts at an angle with respect to each other (Fig. 94-4A). This facilitates the application of a bending moment that unlocks the facets before the application of distraction forces (Fig. 94-4B). Distraction should then allow for complete disengagement of the locked facets. Manual reduction via the placement of the dorsally directed pressure on the rostral vertebral body encourages reduction if the facets have been adequately disengaged (Fig. 94-4C). Relaxation of the distraction forces then allows reengagement of the facets in a normal position. The placement of dorsally directed pressure on the rostral vertebral body, as described previously, may also be applied with the interbody spreader technique.

As an aside, unilateral facet dislocation reduction through a ventral approach may be achieved in a similar manner with the application of torque about the long axis of the spine, thus facilitating the reduction of the rotatory component of the deformity (Fig. 94-5). This tends to reduce the rotational component of the dislocation.

Special Considerations

In contemplating a ventral approach to the dislocated and unstable cervical spine, at least four factors must be considered: (1) the advantage of first performing a ventral discectomy before an attempt at reduction, (2) the feasibility of achieving a reduction by using a ventral approach, (3) the potential need for an accompanying dorsal procedure (failure of ventral reduction), and (4) the ability to obtain a stable construct through an isolated ventral approach. We emphasize that each of these factors must be thoroughly addressed preoperatively.

Ventral Decompression before Reduction

The incidence of extruded cervical disc herniation associated with cervical spine injury has been reported to be 0.7% to 42%.[19-21,23,37] Reduction of the dislocation with the potential for retropulsion of disc material into the reduced and realigned spinal canal may result in significant spinal cord encroachment.

Several authors have recommended a ventral decompression before reduction when they suspect the potential for

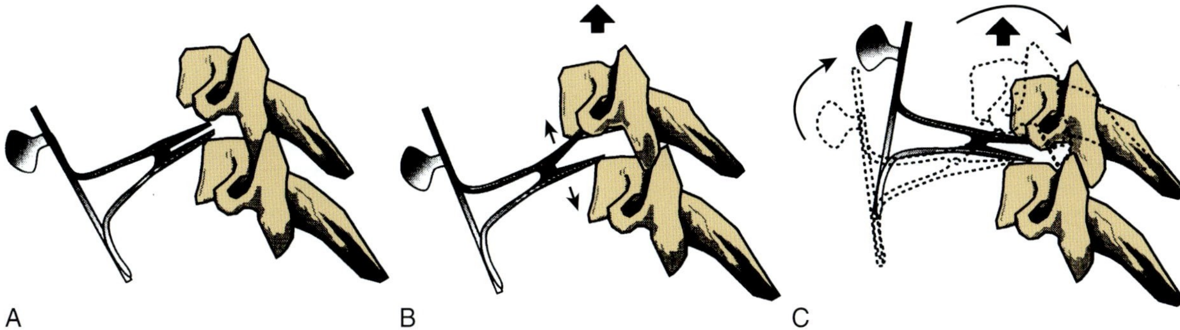

FIGURE 94-3. The interbody spreader technique for reduction of locked facets. After completion of discectomy, the spreader is placed into the disc interspace at a 30- to 40-degree angle. **A,** Note that the blades of the spreader should be placed deep enough to provide an adequate bending moment. **B,** The application of traction (*thick arrow*) and the simultaneous opening of the appropriately placed spreader (*thin arrows*) create a bending moment and distraction of the disc interspace. **C,** The application of a dorsally directed force by the spreader on the ventrocaudal aspect of the rostral vertebral body results in the realignment of the disengaged vertebrae. (From University of New Mexico, Division of Neurosurgery, with permission.)

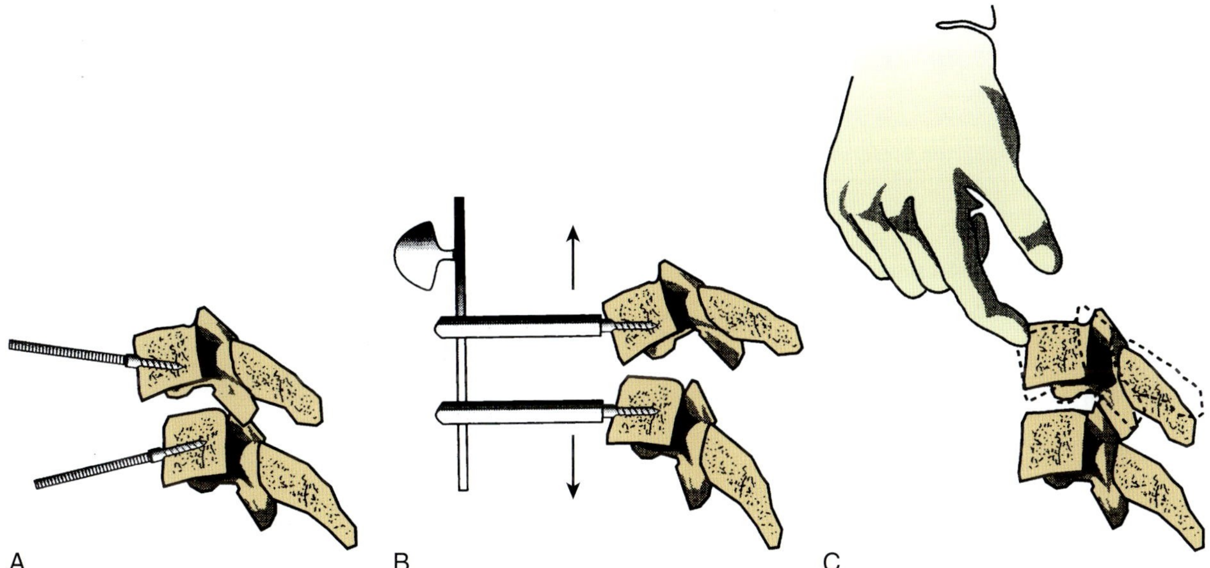

FIGURE 94-4. The vertebral body distractor post technique. **A,** Placement of the posts at an angle with respect to each other allows for the application of a bending moment that helps disengage the dislocated facet joints. **B,** The application of distraction forces (*arrows*) results in realignment. Relaxation of the distraction can lead to reengagement of the facets in their normal position. **C,** Relaxation can be aided by the application of a dorsally directed force on the rostral vertebra. (From University of New Mexico, Division of Neurosurgery, with permission.)

reduction-induced spinal cord encroachment.[19-21,23,38] This relatively uncommon event may occur with either open or closed reduction strategies and is avoided by the removal of the potentially offending disc before reduction (see Fig. 94-1). Although magnetic resonance imaging (MRI) is useful in predicting this event, it probably is not universally accurate. In fact, MRI may demonstrate the absence of intracanalicular disc fragments. Nevertheless, disc material could be retropulsed through a disrupted anulus into the spinal canal during reduction.[20]

Reduction Feasibility

Previous reports have addressed the ventral reduction of cervical spine dislocations.[18,19,31-34] The only relatively large series of ventral reductions of locked facets was by de Oliviera,[32] who reported ventral reduction in 15 cases. He reported no failure with this interbody spreader technique. An understanding of the case-specific anatomy and fundamental biomechanical principles allows ventral reduction to be much more successful than was generally thought. The key is facet joint disengagement before an attempt at reduction. This requires the application of a bending moment to the unstable motion segment, followed by distraction, reduction, and finally relaxation of the distraction.

Failure of Ventral Reduction

The failure of attempts at ventral deformity reduction is a reality. Therefore, it behooves the spine surgeon to appropriately counsel the patient and family preoperatively regarding the possible need for a combined ventral and dorsal (and possibly an additional ventral) approach. Although the latter might seem to be an excessive amount of surgical intervention, it

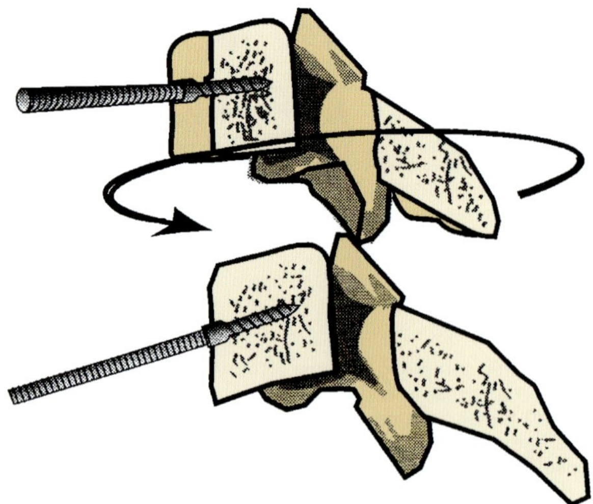

FIGURE 94-5. Appropriately placed posts and the application of torque about the long axis of the spine (*arrow*) can reduce the rotational component of a deformity. (From University of New Mexico, Division of Neurosurgery, with permission.)

provides the greatest chance for preservation and improvement of neurologic function. Significant comminution of the facets appears to be a risk factor for failure of ventral reduction. Therefore, in patients with this risk factor, consideration should be given to a dorsal reduction and arthrodesis if a disc herniation is not present.

Stability Acquisition Using a Ventral Approach

Some authors have addressed the concern for stability acquisition in the circumferentially unstable spine (severe three-column injury)[39] via an isolated ventral approach.[40] Most of these concerns have been directed at dislocations involving two or more motion segments (one or more vertebral body fractures) or after the use of dynamic fixation systems (nonfixed moment arms). However, with one-motion segment circumferential instability, the short bending moment applied by the implant (short implant) by way of the spine allows for greater stability acquisition potential.

Summary

A ventral approach to cervical dislocation and instability may be appropriate in more cases than was previously thought. The ventral approach facilitates (1) ventral decompression before reduction (thus minimizing the chance for iatrogenic neurologic injury), (2) single-motion segment fixation (in contrast to two-motion segment fixation using a dorsal approach), and (3) stability acquisition through the application of effective ventral fixation techniques (Fig. 94-6).

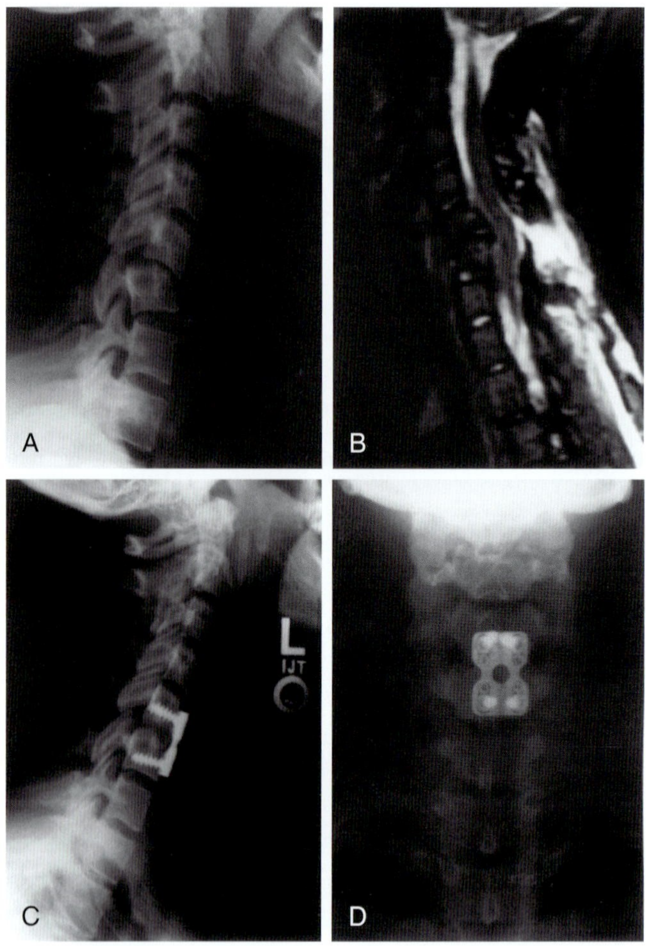

FIGURE 94-6. Lateral cervical radiograph of a neurologically intact 18-year-old woman who was involved in a diving accident, demonstrating a bilateral C5-6 facet dislocation (unilateral jumped facet, contralateral perched facet). Note the significant focal kyphosis with resultant obstruction of ventral access to the disc space (**A**). Preoperative T2-weighted sagittal magnetic resonance image demonstrating a traumatic disc herniation at the level of the dislocation (**B**). Postoperative lateral (**C**) and anteroposterior (**D**) radiographs after ventral decompression, reduction, and stabilization.

KEY REFERENCES

Benzel E, Kesterson L: Posterior cervical interspinous compression wiring and fusion for mid to low cervical spinal injuries. *J Neurosurg* 70:893–899, 1989.

Eismont FJ, Arena MJ, Green BA: Extrusion of an intervertebral disc associated with traumatic subluxation or dislocation of cervical facets. *J Bone Joint Surg [Am]* 73:1555–1560, 1991.

Hadley MN, Fitzpatrick BC, Sonntag VKH, Browner CM: Facet fracture dislocation injuries of the cervical spine. *Neurosurgery* 30:661–666, 1992.

Kwon BK, Fisher CG, Boyd MC, et al: A prospective randomized controlled trial of anterior compared with posterior stabilization for unilateral facet injuries of the cervical spine. *J Neurosurg Spine* 7:1–12, 2007.

Ordonez BJ, Benzel EC, Naderi S, Weller SJ: Cervical facet dislocation: techniques for ventral reduction and stabilization. *J Neurosurg* 92(Suppl 1):18–23, 2000.

REFERENCES

The complete reference list is available online at expertconsult.com.

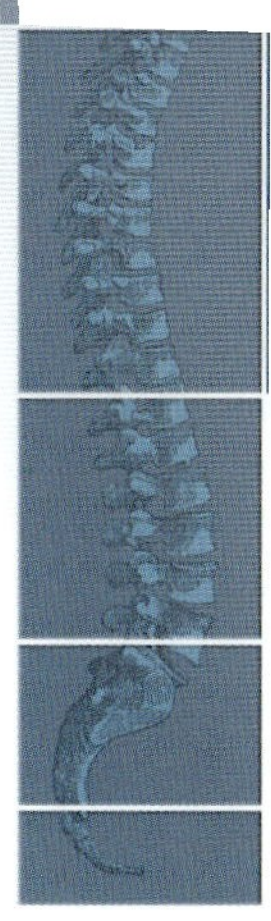

Kyphotic Cervical Deformity

Nathaniel Brooks | Michael P. Steinmetz | Christopher D. Kager | Alexander R. Vaccaro | Edward C. Benzel

Kyphotic cervical spine deformity can be caused by advanced degenerative disease, systemic arthritides, trauma, neoplastic disease, and postsurgical (iatrogenic) causes.[1] The most common cause is postsurgical.[2]

Subaxial cervical deformities most commonly occur in the sagittal plane and primarily develop a kyphotic deformity. Scoliotic coronal plane deformities are uncommon in the cervical spine. However, when they do occur, it is most often a result of congenital vertebral anomalies.

The postsurgical development of cervical kyphosis can follow both ventral and dorsal approaches. Following ventral approaches, kyphosis may develop secondary to pseudarthrosis or failure to restore anatomic cervical lordosis during surgery. Ventral discectomy without graft placement is associated with a 33% rate of kyphosis.[3] Following dorsal surgery, kyphosis may develop and progress secondary to disruption of the dorsal elements (interspinous ligaments, laminae, and facet joints). The incidence of kyphosis after laminectomy ranges from 14% to 47%.[4,5]

Cervical kyphosis is biomechanically unfavorable for the cervical musculature. The kyphosis will tend to progress as axial loads of the head produce a bending moment through the moment arm of the cervical spine.[6] This will often produce mechanical pain that improves when the patient is supine.[7] Often, excessive degeneration of the cervical discs occurs that contributes to cervical pain. As the kyphosis progresses, the patient's field of view, swallow, and respiration may be affected. The patient may develop low back pain and accelerated degeneration by hyperlordosing the lumbar spine to accommodate for the cervical deformity.

Clinical Presentation

Patients often present with mechanical neck pain. This pain is typically worse in the upright position and with exertion and improved with rest and recumbancy. Patients can also present with radiculopathy or myelopathy from compression on neural elements. As the kyphosis worsens, there is increased stress on the ventral spinal cord from tethering of the cord by the dentate ligaments. This may adversely affect the spinal cord vasculature and lead to worsened myelopathic symptoms.[8,9] Patients with severe deformity may present with swallowing dysfunction and in some cases nutritional deficiency, compromise of horizontal gaze, and compromised breathing.[10,11]

Clinical Evaluation

The clinical examination should elicit the degree of deformity, the overall sagittal and coronal balance, and whether there is some flexibility of the deformity. It is important to evaluate the patient's overall posture and gait, which can provide important clues as to the degree of deformity.

The deformity should be evaluated radiographically as well. Evaluate the cervical deformity using static upright and dynamic (flexion-extension) radiographs. The thoracic spine should be evaluated if deformity is suspected at the cervicothoracic junction. By using radiographs, the sagittal angle of the deformity may be measured (Fig. 95-1), and other abnormalities may be identified, such as subluxation and pseudarthrosis. Pseudarthrosis and existing fusion can be better clarified by using thin-cut CT scan. The ability of the alignment of the cervical spine to be reduced can also be assessed with extension or supine radiographs. Standing long-cassette radiographs can be useful to assess overall sagittal balance. In designing the treatment strategy, thoracic hyperkyphosis, lumbar hyperlordosis, and ankylosed joints must be taken into account.

All patients should be evaluated with preoperative MRI or CT myelography to evaluate for any compressive pathology. Compressive pathology can be addressed with a variety of modalities depending on the direction of compression. If ventral compressive pathology is present, this must be decompressed prior to correction of the deformity.

Deformity Correction Strategies

The cervical spine may be exposed to coronal plane, rotational, axial (subsidence), or, most commonly, sagittal plane deformation stresses. It is important to establish goals of treatment prior to surgery. Decompression of the neural elements should be the first priority. Most commonly, the surgical approach will address the compression directly, but occasionally, this is dealt with indirectly by deformity correction. Ferch et al.[12] demonstrated an association of improved myelopathy with restored lordosis in cervical kyphotic deformity patients. Fusion at abnormal levels may also prevent damage to the cord from micromotion.

Sagittal plane deformity may be addressed ventrally,[13-18] dorsally,[19-21] or both.[18,19,22-27] If there is imaging evidence

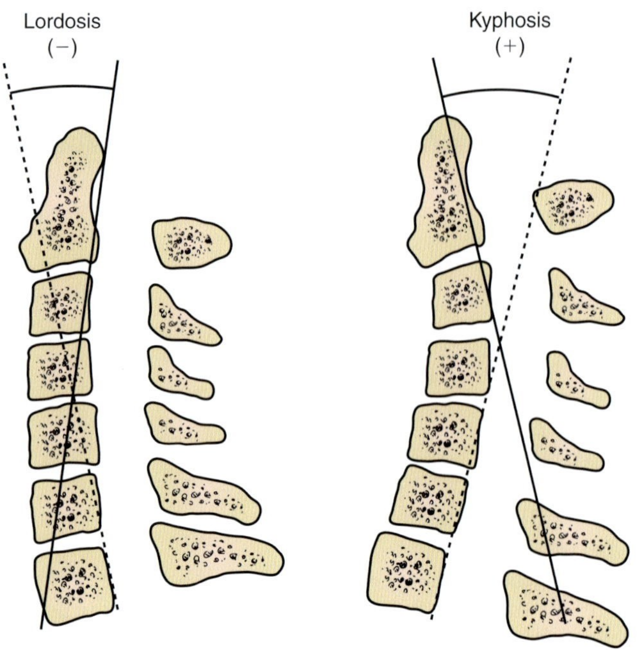

FIGURE 95-1. Measuring the angle of lordosis and kyphosis. Although these angles can be measured segmentally, they can also be calculated by using the bodies of C2 and C7 for an overall measurement of sagittal angle. A negative angle is lordotic; a positive angle is kyphotic.

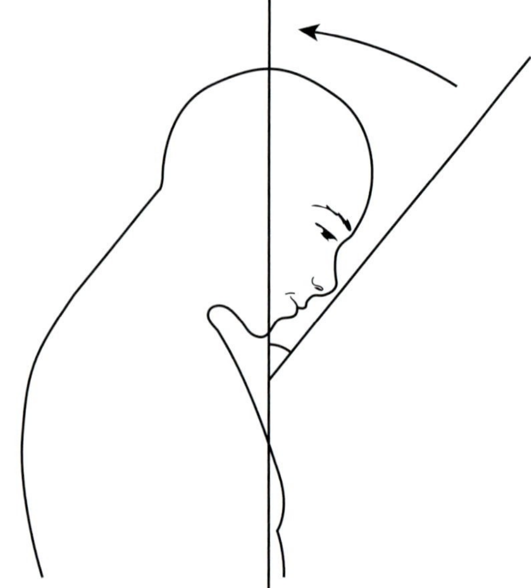

FIGURE 95-2. Chin-brow vertical angle. Although there is not an optimal degree of correction, this angle should be reestablished nearer to 0 degrees so that the patient can see the horizon but not so high that the patient is unable to see where his or her feet are going.

of ventral compression, then a ventral procedure should be considered. If the deformity is fixed ventrally without dorsally fused joints, then a ventral decompression with fusion can be used to correct the kyphosis. If the dynamic radiographs demonstrate normal movement and a normal lordosis can be achieved in extension, then a dorsal surgical reconstruction can adequately address the pathology. If the deformity is fixed owing to dorsally fused joints (ankylosing), then a dorsal osteotomy can be used to correct the kyphosis.[10,11,28] Finally, a flexible deformity can be corrected posturally or with traction and then be fused dorsally.

The goal for restoration of sagittal alignment is unclear. A definition of normal lordosis does not exist. However, Gore et al. measured lordotic angles in the cervical spine of patients with osteoarthritis using the perpendicular of the C2 and C7 vertebral bodies. Lordosis of 16 to 22 degrees was observed in men and 25 degrees in women.[29] However, it is likely that if a patient is not restored to neutral or a lordotic posture, the deformity will continue to progress over time. Another useful measure, especially in rigid cervical kyphosis (e.g., ankylosing spondylosis), is the chin-brow vertical angle, which will help to determine whether the patient will be able to see the horizon (Fig. 95-2). Finally, overall sagittal and coronal balance is important. Ideally, the head should be balanced over the sacrum.

Traction

Traction can be used as the initial tool in the evaluation of the surgical approach to kyphosis. If the deformity can be corrected with traction, then dorsal fixation can be used to hold the correction for fusion. Traction can be applied for a trial of 3 to 5 days. Muscle relaxants may be utilized to aid in the reduction process. Typically, the patient is taken to the operating room with the traction applied. If traction has not reduced the deformity after 5 days, it is unlikely to be of benefit.

Ventral Strategies

The ventral approach to the cervical spine is common and has low morbidity. It allows ventral decompression, deformity correction, and reconstruction with corpectomy grafts, multilevel ventral cervical grafts, or a combination of both. This approach also allows for a greater ability to manipulate the spine compared to the dorsal approach.

The ventral strategy uses both posture and biomechanical principles to correct the cervical deformity. Initially positioning the head on a towel or foam doughnut with the neck in a neutral or only slightly extended position allows adequate exposure for the approach but without compromising the spinal cord. After the decompression is complete, the towel or doughnut can be removed, allowing further extension of the cervical spine (Fig. 95-3).

Distraction posts should be placed into the vertebral bodies in a convergent manner (Fig. 95-4A). This will allow distraction on the posts to provide further lordosis (Fig. 95-4B).

Long-segment corpectomies, greater than two vertebral bodies, have been used to correct ventral deformity. However, the authors believe that long-segment corpectomies should be avoided. Biomechanical studies show that three-segment corpectomies allow more movement than two-level corpectomies do.[30] Long-segment corpectomies are more likely to fail at the terminal end because of the amount of force at the terminal screw-bone interface. Vaccarro et al. found that the early failure rate of two-segment corpectomies was 9% compared with 50% for three-segment corpectomies.[31] In straight or kyphotic spines, corpectomies do not maintain as much sagittal angle correction as they do in lordotic spines.[32]

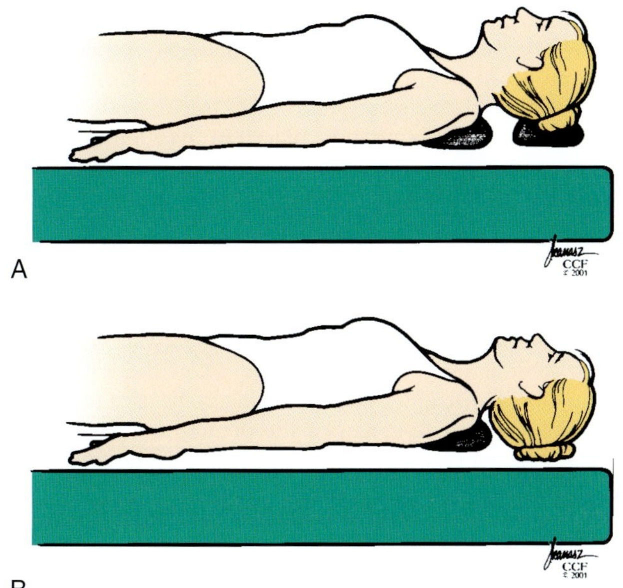

FIGURE 95-3. Use of padding to aid in deformity correction. **A,** Place padding beneath the patient's head prior to decompression to keep the spine neutral or slightly extended. **B,** Once decompression is complete, remove the padding to allow the neck to be further extended. (Copyright Cleveland Clinic Foundation.)

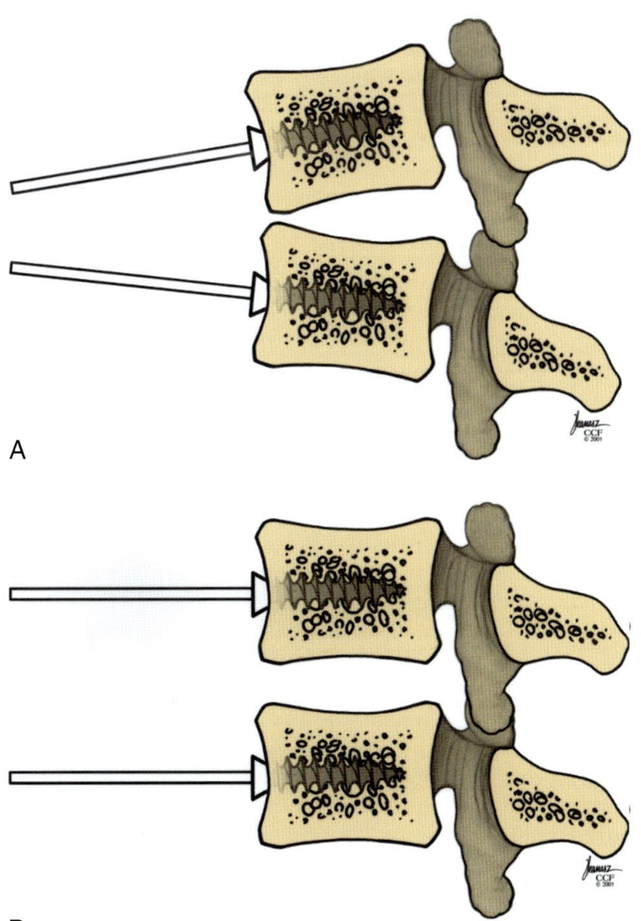

FIGURE 95-4. Distraction after placement technique to improve lordosis. **A,** Posts should be placed so that they converge. **B,** Distraction on the posts then allows for reestablishing kyphosis. (Copyright Cleveland Clinic Foundation.)

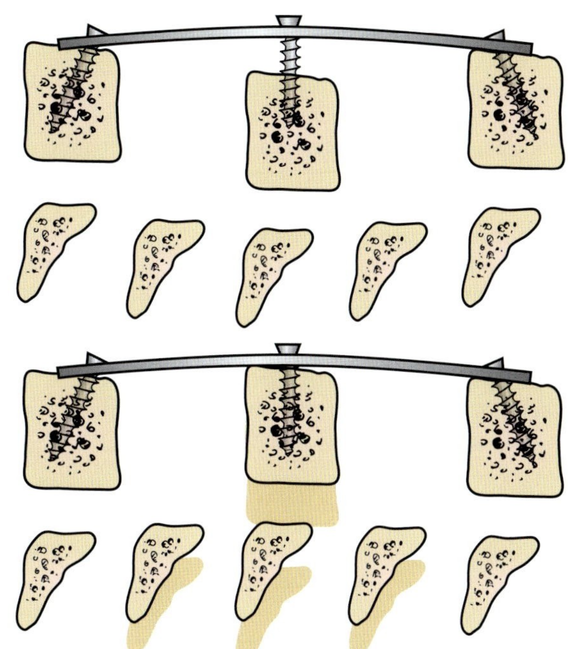

FIGURE 95-5. Leaving a vertebral body as an intermediate point of fixation is beneficial in providing an additional point of fixation to improve the lordosis of the construct and rigidity. (Copyright Cleveland Clinic Foundation.)

An alternative method for ventral correction is multilevel discectomy and fusion and/or a combined short-segment corpectomy. Leaving an intermediate vertebral body allows adequate decompression and provides additional intermediate fixation points for security of fixation and deformity correction (Fig. 95-5). Wei-bing et al.[33] showed that two-level corpectomies had a higher rate of plate and graft migration requiring reoperation than did a combined construct of one-level anterior cervical discectomy and fusion (ACDF) plus one-level corpectomy. Oh et al.[34] did not show a difference in clinical outcome between single-level corpectomy versus two-level ACDF.

The degree of correction required must be considered preoperatively to help plan the number of levels to be involved for deformity correction. Although this is often simply estimated, some recent studies may be helpful. Cabraja et al.[35] found that a ventral or two-level corpectomy achieved a segmental correction of 6.2 degrees and an overall cervical lordosis correction of 8.8 degrees. However, using ventral correction only, they found that there was an approximately 2-degree loss of correction over an average 33-month follow-up period. Ferch et al.[12] demonstrated that a ventral only approach can improve overall lordosis an average of 11 degrees. Eighty-five percent of the patients in their series were restored to neutral or lordotic alignments.

Dorsal Strategies

It is uncommon to use a dorsal strategy alone to correct cervical deformity because it is difficult to reduce a kyphotic deformity and achieve adequate lordosis from a dorsal approach alone. But if the deformity is flexible and no ventral decompression is required, then it should be possible to correct the deformity from a dorsal approach alone. If there is evidence of ventral compression, then a combined approach should be considered.

The deformity should be reduced, with traction begun prior to the operation and continued into the operating room if deemed appropriate. This maintains alignment and control during the course of instrumentation and rod contouring. The patient's head should be held in a three-point head holder to maintain reduction. Alignment should be confirmed clinically by examining the patient's head position prior to draping and radiographically with a lateral radiograph or fluoroscopy.

There are many instrumentation choices. The most common method is lateral mass fixation at the levels of C3-6. The C7 lateral masses are often not large enough to hold a screw, and screw placement often makes it difficult to align rods across the cervicothoracic junction. Lateral mass fixation might not be an optimal stabilizing anchor in some patients.[20,23,36]

If no decompression is performed, interspinous wiring can be performed. However, this is performed less commonly, owing to the advent of lateral mass instrumentation.

It is also possible to use cervical pedicle screws for the dorsal correction of cervical deformity. Abumi et al.[19] have demonstrated their usefulness in deformity correction, achieving a correction from 28.4 to 5.1 degrees of kyphosis with all patients achieving solid fusion. It should be emphasized that lordosis was not achieved with the dorsal procedure alone. Kotani et al.[37] have demonstrated that these screw systems are biomechanically equivalent to combined ventral plate and dorsal wiring.

If dorsal decompression is not necessary, the spinous processes and lamina can remain intact as a surface area for fusion.

Combined Strategies

In general, combined ventral and dorsal approaches allow improved deformity correction because they allow ventral lengthening with dorsal shortening. In fixed (or inflexible) deformity with ankylosed dorsal elements, a combined ventral and dorsal approach may be required. Also, if the deformity involves the cervicothoracic junction, a combined approach should be considered. The addition of a dorsal construct aids in preventing deformity progression at the cervicothoracic junction by using a long moment arm strategy.[38]

Identifying the goals of the operation is key to planning a combined approach. Decompression of neural elements is the first priority. The subsequent goal should be deformity correction. These two goals are often managed concurrently. The use of lordotic grafts or well-shaped corpectomy struts aids in deformity correction. Consideration must then be given to where the spine is fused. If the spine is fused primarily ventrally, then the deformity can be corrected ventrally. The length of the construct and degree of deformity may necessitate additional dorsal instrumentation. Rarely, a dorsal only approach can be performed, but the degree of correction is limited. To achieve correction of a spine that is fused ventrally and dorsally, both sides must be released. This necessitates "540-degree" surgery, starting with a dorsal release, followed by ventral release, deformity correction, instrumentation and arthrodesis, and then a subsequent dorsal instrumentation and arthrodesis.

Ankylosing spondylosis often requires a 540-degree procedure. A dorsal osteotomy is performed first. Some authors have proposed performing a C7-T1 osteotomy under local anesthesia in the seated position.[39] After the osteotomy is performed, the patient can be placed in the supine position, and a ventral corpectomy or multilevel ACDF can be performed to allow decompression and ventral release for the correction of the deformity. Ventral instrumentation can then be applied. Careful attention should be paid to the patient's chin-brow vertical angle, which can help to determine whether the patient will be able to look to the horizon and in front of himself or herself when walking. Owing to the large moment arm above and below the level of the fusion, dorsal instrumentation should also be used to prevent later deformity. The stages of the operation often need to be tailored depending on the basis of the anatomy of the deformity.

If the deformity is to be corrected by using a 540-degree approach, a ventral decompression and release should be performed without graft or instrumentation. The patient may then be positioned prone to expose the dorsal cervical spine. At this point, an assistant may adjust the head holder to achieve the appropriate alignment that should be determined with the aid of fluoroscopy and direct visualization. The dorsal instrumentation may then be placed and contoured to secure deformity correction. Rib or iliac crest bone graft can then be harvested to provide autogenous bone graft. The patient will then again be placed supine, and the ventral strut graft can be placed and secured with ventral instrumentation. Utilizing this combined approach, Abumi et al.[19] were able to improve preoperative kyphosis of 30.8 degrees to 0.5 degrees at final follow-up.

Extension Osteotomy

Some cervical kyphotic deformities, for example, ankylosing spondylosis, may produce an extreme fixed flexion deformity at the cervicothoracic junction. This deformity can be treated with an extension osteotomy at the cervicothoracic junction.[28,39,40] The procedure as initially described was performed under local anesthesia with the patient awake and sitting.[11,28,39] However, this was primarily due to early limitations in intubating patients with severe kyphotic deformity. Subsequently, the procedure has been described under general anesthesia in the prone position with intraoperative nerve monitoring.[11] Positioning the patient remains a significant challenge, owing to the degree of deformity. Positioning often requires additional padding and table adjustment to gain access for a dorsal approach. The head must be placed in a halo frame and attached to an adjustable head holder.

After positioning the cervicothoracic junction is exposed. A wide laminectomy is performed at C7 with partial laminectomy at C6 and T1. The spinous process of C6 is removed. The ankylosed C7 and T1 facet joints are then removed to expose the C8 nerve roots beyond the foramina. Then the C6 and T1 pedicles are removed to avoid impingement (Fig. 95-6). One surgeon then adjusts the head while the other surgeon watches for evidence of impingement or subluxation. Electrophysiologic monitoring continues as the deformity is corrected. If a change is

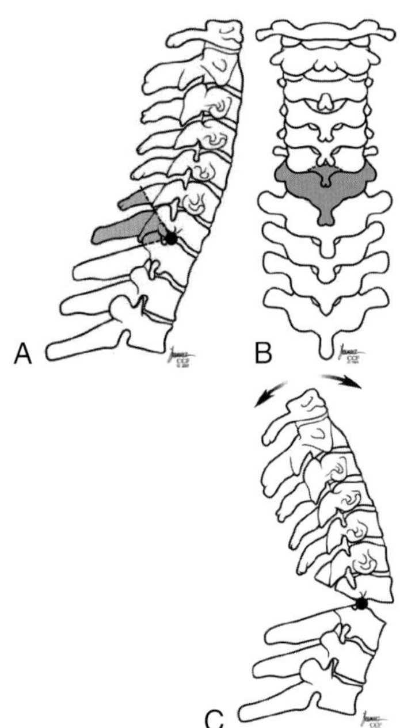

FIGURE 95-6. An extended wedge osteotomy can be used to correct severe deformity. **A** and **B**, A laminectomy of C7 is performed along with partial laminectomies of C6 and T1 (*shaded area*), including spinous processes. The ankylosed C7-T1 facet joints, as well as a portion of the C6 and T1 pedicles, are removed bilaterally. **C**, The spine is then extended about the fulcrum of the posterior aspect of C7 and T1 (*dot*). During this maneuver, the spine will fracture ventrally at C7-T1, so care must be taken to maintain meticulous control. (Copyright Cleveland Clinic Foundation.)

noted, leads should be checked, and blood pressure should be optimized. If the signals do not correct, the dura should be evaluated for compression. If none of these correct the signals, the deformity can be returned to its original alignment. A wake-up test can also be considered.

As the kyphosis is corrected, a fracture will eventually develop ventrally. This is the most difficult portion of the operation to control. Various instrumentation and techniques have been used to try to control this portion of the reduction, including articulated halo jackets,[28] prebent loops and wires,[41] temporary malleable rods,[42] and hinged rods.[43] Tokala et al.[44] described a more ventrally based wedge osteotomy to try to allow a more controlled closure.

Other surgeons have described using a ventral release prior to the dorsal osteotomy to help control the correction.[45-47] However, this can be a difficult approach in patients with severe chin-on-chest deformities.

Instrumentation Techniques

Ventral cervical plates, either constrained or nonconstrained, can be used for multilevel fusions and will allow stabilization for fusion and also achieve lordosis.[48] Dynamic ventral fixation devices allow sagittal correction along with controlled deformation in the axial plane.[6] The controlled subsidence encourages bone healing via Wolff's law and also off-loads stresses at the screw-bone interface. Nunley et al.[49] found that there was improved clinical outcome with dynamic plates rather than fixed plates.

There are many options for dorsal instrumentation. Interspinous wiring may be used, but lateral mass fixation has been shown to provide greater rigidity than wire fixation alone.[36] Lateral mass and cervical pedicle screws have similar biomechanical stability and have been shown to be superior in resisting axial rotation compared to cervical laminar hooks.[50] There have not been studies looking specifically at fusion rates using lateral mass screws. Cervical pedicle screws are more difficult and dangerous to place but may increase load sharing across the disc space compared to lateral mass screws.[51]

Interbody and corpectomy grafts are often used for deformity correction. The choice of grafts includes autologous iliac crest, which has a fusion rate of 98% to 100%,[52] but there is a risk of persistent donor site morbidity.[53] The allograft fusion rate using fibula is 86.6% when combined with instrumentation.[54] The use of titanium cage with autologous graft has been reported to have a fusion rate of 97.8%.[55] Other options include cages made of polyetheretherketone or carbon fiber filled with morselized autologous or allograft bone. Corpectomy grafts are more prone to technical failures, particularly at the distal end of long constructs. Sasso et al.[56] demonstrated increased failure rates with long (more than two-body) corpectomy constructs.

Bone morphogenic protein-2 can be used to promote fusion. However, its use in the ventral neck is associated with significant soft tissue swelling in 23% to 37% of patients.[53] It is used primarily to promote dorsal arthrodesis.

Intraoperative Neurologic Monitoring

There are multiple methods to monitor intraoperative neurologic function. The Stagnara wake-up test has been described as the gold standard.[11,41] The wake-up test definitively determines the patient's neurologic function; however, it does take expert anesthesia to administer, and because it takes time to perform, the critical time window for reversal of deficit may be missed.

Electrophysiologic recording allows for intraoperative monitoring of neurologic function. The most common modalities used are somatosensory-evoked potentials (SSEPs) and motor-evoked potentials (MEPs). SSEPs record continuously; they evaluate primarily information from the dorsal columns. MEPs record intermittently from the corticospinal tracts. These modalities are sensitive to the types of anesthetics used. A common anesthetic protocol is induction with propofol combined with remifentanil and maintenance of general anesthesia with isoflurane. Paralytic and nitrous agents should be avoided.

Care must be taken in interpreting neurologic monitoring. The use of SSEPs alone should be avoided, as there can be significant postoperative neurologic deficits despite normal intraoperative recordings.[57,58] MEPs can be used also and have a high sensitivity and specificity, but there are inconsistent data regarding correlation of MEP changes to neurologic outcome.[40,59] A 20% decrease in amplitude of the MEPs is considered a significant neurologic change. In the event that this occurs, technical problems should be assessed, and hemodynamic parameters should be optimized. If the amplitude remains decreased, the surgical maneuver preceding the change should be reversed.[60]

Outcomes

Clinical

There have been no randomized clinical trials evaluating the clinical outcome of cervical deformity correction. In studies in which horizontal gaze was restored, patients were satisfied with their outcomes.[44,61] Cabraja et al.[35] found a statistically significant improvement in visual analogue scale and modified Japanese Orthopaedic Association Scale for patients receiving ventral or dorsal surgery for deformity correction. The study did not find a difference between the ventral and dorsal groups. Using a combined surgical approach, Nottmeier et al. described preoperative symptom improvement of 97.5%.[62]

Radiographic

By using a ventral only approach, overall cervical lordosis was improved in the ventral group by 9 to 32 degrees, and segmental lordosis by 6.2 degrees.[62] However, the 2 degrees of ventral correction was lost over an average of 33-month follow-up.[35]

By using a dorsal only approach, approximately 6.5 to 54 degrees of improvement in overall lordosis can be achieved.[35,63] The chin-brow vertical angle can be corrected an average of 35 to 52 degrees.[63]

Nottmeier et al.[62] reviewed their combined approaches and found that they had an average correction of 22 degrees. They showed a fusion rate of 97.5%.

Complications

Complications of the correction of cervical kyphosis are greater in the deformity correction patient. This is because these cases often involve larger exposures, and in many cases, the patients have had prior surgery.

Complications of the ventral approach include vocal cord palsy, dysphagia, tracheal or esophageal injury, vertebral artery injury, graft failure or displacement, hardware failure, and fracture and wound complications. Overall operative and perioperative complications of 22% to 33% have been reported.[52,54]

Complications from the dorsal approach include hardware failure or fracture, nonunion, vertebral artery injury, and wound complications (infection, hematoma). The morbidity from the dorsal approach is greater than that of a ventral approach, and patients have considerably greater pain in the postoperative period

The dorsal wedge osteotomy for the correction of flexion deformity has a potential high incidence of morbidity.[11] Complications include infection and respiratory and cardiovascular problems. There is a potential for vertebral artery injury during the osteotomy or neurologic injury during deformity correction. The resultant neurologic injury may range from minor nerve root irritation to spinal cord compression and quadriplegia. After deformity correction, there is risk of subluxation of C7 on T1, with resultant bony nonunion.

Circumferential fusion has a complication rate of about 32% to 33%.[22,26] These complications can include neurologic deficits, wound infection, plate dislodgement, pseudarthrosis, dysphonia, requirement of tracheostomy and PEG tube, and death. Many of these are early transient complications, with about 5% persisting long term.[26]

Conclusion

Deformity of the cervical spine has multiple causes, the most common being prior surgery. Patients may present with symptoms related to the deformity itself (e.g., swallowing dysfunction) or with neurologic deficit. If deformity is causing symptoms, it should be corrected. Surgical goals should be decompression of neural elements, restoration of lordotic alignment, and prevention of further deformity. Controversy remains regarding the optimal approach to achieve these goals, and some situations may require combined approaches (Fig. 95-7). The ventral approach has been found to be most beneficial in restoring sagittal alignment. However, the dorsal approach has been shown to be beneficial in maintaining alignment. There is more likelihood of having perioperative complications in this type of surgery, but many of these complications are transient. The majority of patients have both relief of their mechanical symptoms and improvement of their neurologic function.

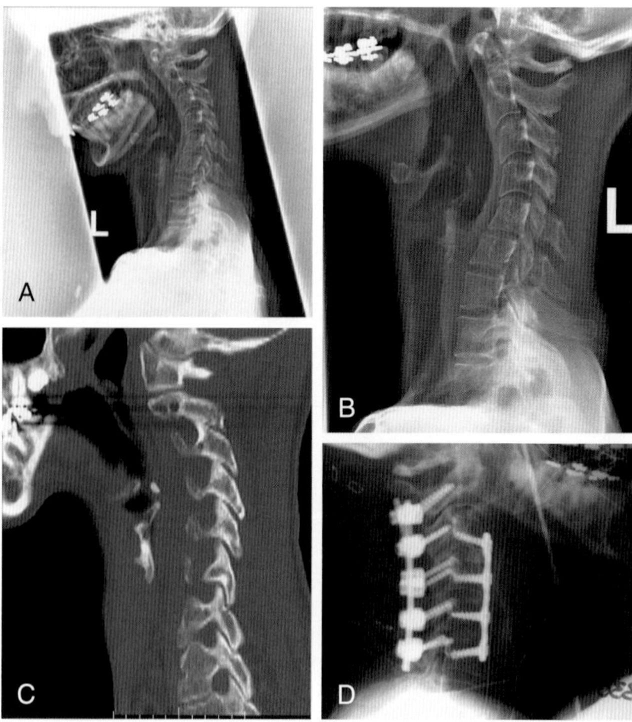

FIGURE 95-7. **A,** A 60-year-old woman with mechanical neck pain and cervical kyphosis 8 years after cervical laminectomy. **B,** Dynamic extension radiograph, showing that the kyphosis is inflexible. **C,** The CT scan demonstrates ankylosed joints. On MRI imaging (not shown), there was no evidence of compression. The case was managed with a "540-degree" procedure starting dorsally to release the ankylosed joints and to place dorsal C2 pars and lateral mass screws. The patient was then placed into a supine position, and multilevel ventral interbody grafts were placed. Adjustment of intraoperative positioning was used to induce lordosis, and a lordotic ventral plate was placed. Intermediate points of fixation were also used to improve lordosis. The patient was then replaced in the prone position, and posterior rods were placed. **D,** The postoperative radiograph demonstrates that the patient had improved alignment, and clinically, her mechanical neck pain and kyphosis improved.

KEY REFERENCES

Cabraja M, Abbushi A, Koeppen D, et al: Comparison between anterior and posterior decompression with instrumentation for cervical spondylotic myelopathy: sagittal alignment and clinical outcome. *Neurosurg Focus* 28(3):E15–E19, 2010.

Etame AB, Wang AC, Than KD, et al: Outcomes after surgery for cervical spine deformity: review of the literature. *Neurosurg Focus* 28(3):E14–E21, 2010.

Hoh DJ, Khoueir P, Wang MY: Management of cervical deformity in ankylosing spondylitis. *Neurosurg Focus* 24(1):E9, 2008.

Kaptain GJ, Simmons N, Replogic RE, et al: Incidence and outcome of kyphotic deformity following laminectomy for cervical spondylotic myelopathy. *J Neurosurg Spine* 93:199–204, 2000.

Koller H, Hempfing A, Ferraris L, et al: 4- and 5-level anterior fusions of the cervical spine: review of literature and clinical results. *Eur Spine J* 16(12):2055–2071, 2007.

Mummaneni PV, Dhall SS, Rodts GE, Haid RW: Circumferential fusion for cervical kyphotic deformity. *J Neurosurg Spine* 9(6):515–521, 2008.

REFERENCES

The complete reference list is available online at expertconsult.com.

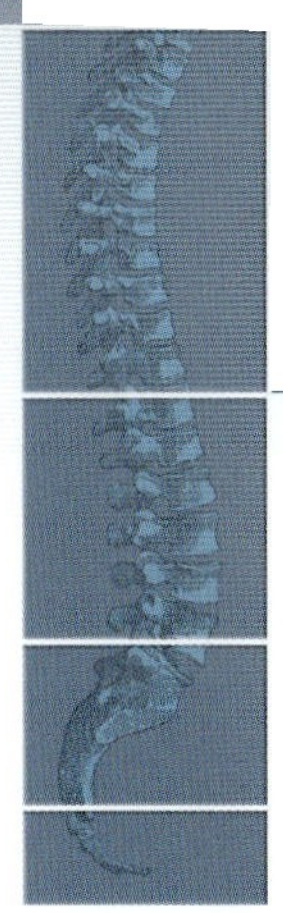

Scoliotic Cervical Deformity

Harminder Singh | George M. Ghobrial | James S. Harrop

The vertebral or spinal column provides humans with the ability to maintain an upright posture, protects the neural and visceral organs (i.e., heart, lungs, abdominal contents), and aids with mobility. The cervical spine provides a transition from the rigid thoracic spine to the cranium and provides the ability to alter position to improve swallowing function and optimize hearing and sight. Numerous forces, both internal and external, may affect the structure and position of the cervical spine such that it becomes deformed or is altered from its normal anatomic alignment.

Spinal deformities are more often encountered in the thoracic and lumbar spine. However, the cervical spine may also develop structural deformities secondary to congenital disorders,[1] neuromuscular diseases,[2,3] trauma,[4] neoplastic disease,[5] or previous spine surgery.[6] These deformities may also occur in patients with systemic arthritides such as ankylosing spondylitis and rheumatoid arthritis. This chapter reviews the normal subaxial cervical anatomy, alignment, biomechanical properties, etiologies of scoliotic deformity, and treatment strategies.

Anatomy of the Cervical Spine

The cervical spine consists of seven vertebrae (C1-7) (Fig. 96-1).[7] C1 and C2 are anatomic and functionally unique, which allows for the transition and attachment of the cervical spine to the cranium. These vertebrae (C1-2) are not considered when discussing the subaxial cervical spine (C3-7).

Vertebral Body and Disc

The size of the subaxial cervical vertebral bodies (C3-7) generally increases from rostral to caudal (see Fig. 96-1). The exception is the C6 body, which is slightly decreased in size compared with C5.[8-10] This increase in the vertebral body's width, depth, and total end-plate cross-sectional area allows greater loads to be supported and forces to be dispersed.[11] The majority of these physiologic loads are carried through the ventral cervical vertebral body in a flexion posture, whereas the loads are carried through the dorsal elements (articular columns) in extension.[10]

The intervertebral disc connects the vertebral end plates and is composed of the cartilaginous end plate, anulus fibrosus, and nucleus pulposus. The disc heights are not symmetrical, with the ventral height being greater than the dorsal height (see Fig. 96-1). This contributes to the lordotic curvature of the cervical spine.[9,12]

The pedicles are horizontal columns of bone that connect the vertebral body to the dorsal elements (Fig. 96-2). The cervical pedicles have an elliptical shape, with the height being greater than the width.[11,13] The cortical bone surface of the cervical pedicles is similar on the rostral and caudal portion, but the lateral wall thickness is significantly less than the medial wall thickness.[14] These pedicles insert into the vertebral body with transverse angle ranges from −8 to +11 degrees from the horizontal and sagittal angles ranging from 40 to 29 degrees.[11]

Articulations

There are four articular surfaces between adjacent vertebral segments in the subaxial cervical spine, one set located on the vertebral body and another set involving the dorsal elements. The articulations located on the rostral, lateral dorsal aspect of the vertebral body are termed the *uncovertebral* or *Luschka* joints. These "joints" articulate with the caudal, dorsal, lateral aspect of the rostral vertebral body (Fig. 96-3).[8] The heights of the uncinate process gradually increase as one descends the spine at each segment from C3-7, whereas the length and width remained relatively constant.[13] These joints are actually believed to be degenerative clefts and not true joints because they are not present at birth and develop during adolescence.[15,16]

The dorsal elements of the cervical spine allow a large degree of mobility due to a pair of segmental articulations in the form of facet joints (see Fig. 96-3). These are apophyseal joints and are composed of a loose but strong capsule and synovial lining. The cervical facet joints are oriented at approximately 45 degrees in the coronal plane and 80 to 90 degrees in the sagittal plane.[8,17] This facet orientation permits a large degree of sagittal plane motion, flexion, and extension but limits or restricts translation and lateral movements or bending.[8,18]

Ligaments

The anterior longitudinal ligament (ALL) and the posterior longitudinal ligament (PLL) are the two major ligaments in the cervical spine and are attached directly to the vertebral

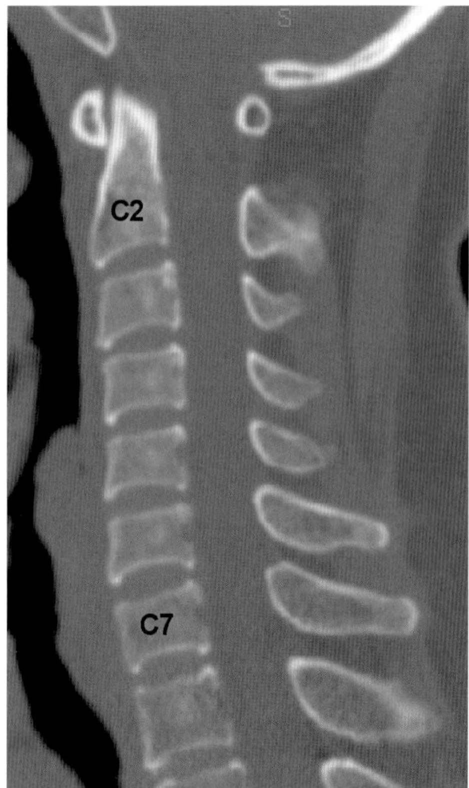

FIGURE 96-1. A sagittal CT reformatted image of the cervical spine. The rest of the cervical spine vertebral bodies, C3-7, increase in size ventrally to caudally with the exception of C6, which is slightly decreased. Also, note that the disc spaces are increased ventrally compared with dorsally, particularly at C5-6, increasing the overall lordosis of the cervical spine.

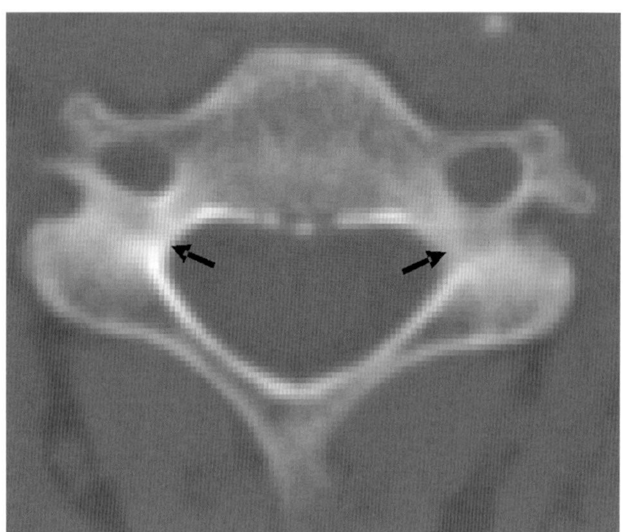

FIGURE 96-2. Axial CT scan of the cervical spine. The cervical pedicles (*arrows*) are horizontal columns of bones that connect the vertebral bodies to the dorsal elements.

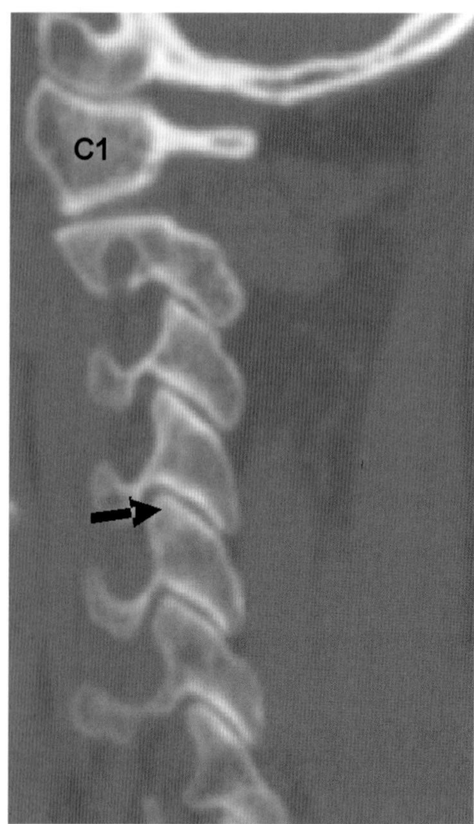

FIGURE 96-3. Lateral portion of sagittal CT reformat images of cervical spine from occiput to thoracic junction. Note the facet joints (*arrow*) articulate with approximately a 45-degree angulation. This provides for a great degree of mobility in flexion and extension.

body. The ALL is a fibrous band that attaches to the edges of the vertebral bodies (C2 to sacrum) and that is diminished in width at the disc spaces. It provides significant support and resists cervical extension.[19] The PLL also is continuous from C2 to the sacrum but differs from the ALL in that it narrows over the vertebral bodies and then widens at the disc interspace where it is interwoven with the anulus fibrosus. This ligament resists flexion and has half the strength of the ALL.[19]

Numerous other ligaments also support the dorsal cervical spine. These include the ligamentum flavum and the capsular and interspinous ligaments. The ligamentum flavum extends from the undersurface of the lamina to the adjacent rostral lamina. This ligament has the highest amount of elastin in the human body. It also has a baseline amount of strain in the neutral position such that with extension, the ligament does not relax and buckle into the spinal canal. The capsular ligaments attach circumferentially around the facet joints and are the strongest ligaments in the cervical spine. The interspinous ligament is a relatively weak ligament that spans between adjacent spinous processes.

Normal Cervical Alignment

The cervical spine permits head rotation, flexion, and extension to maintain the line of sight while also placing the cranium over the pelvis and supporting a balanced upright posture. Hardacker et al. demonstrated that a plumb line dropped from the tip of the odontoid process would fall ventral to the seventh cervical vertebra, hence sagittal balance[20] (Fig. 96-4).

It is difficult to define spine deformity based on clinical observation alone. Gross deformities may be determined through observation of the relationship of the tragus to the spinous process of C7 in the sagittal plane. However, these physical

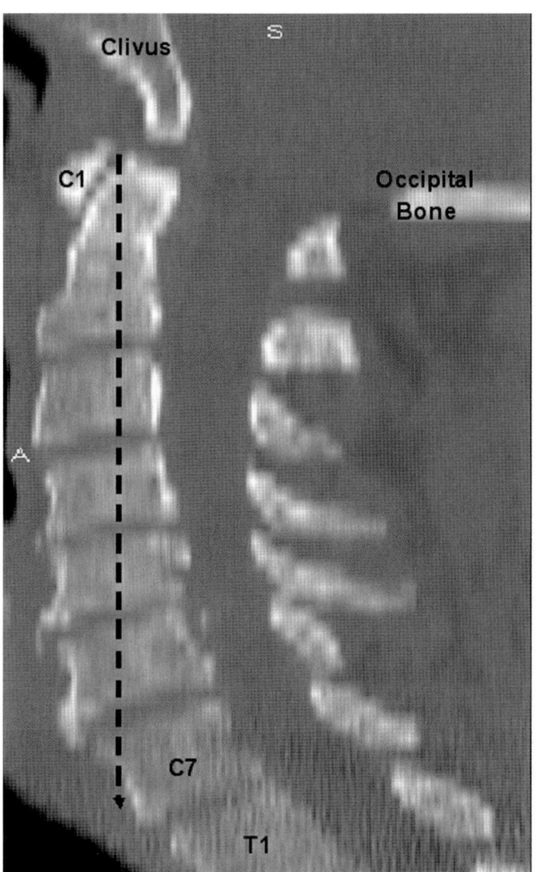

FIGURE 96-4. A plumb line drop from the tip of the odontoid process, which falls ventral to the seventh cervical vertebra typically between 0 and 2 cm.

examination findings have been found to be inaccurate in most circumstances. In general, surface contour has not been shown to correlate with vertebral body location and position.[21,22] Therefore, radiographs are essential to attempt to understand and document spinal alignment objectively.

At present, there is no accepted standard measurement algorithm for sagittal or coronal cervical spinal curvature. The most commonly used method is the Cobb angle technique that places parallel lines from the caudal and rostral aspects of the vertebral bodies and then measures the intersection angle of these perpendicular lines[23] (Fig. 96-5A). Inaccuracy of the Cobb method has been reported because it is based on the noncuboidal shape of the vertebral bodies, where the vertebral body end plate–to–dorsal cortical angle is greater than 90 degrees.[24] Harrison used tangential lines to the dorsal vertebral bodies (Fig. 96-5B) and calculated the "normal" cervical (C2-7) lordosis to be 26 degrees (C2 and C7).[24] Based on these results and engineering principles, he concluded that the tangential technique is more accurate at assessing the cervical angle than the Cobb method, which from C1-7, overestimated, and from C2-7, underestimated the lordosis.[24]

Cervical Alignment—Neutral

The length of the cervical spinal canal measured in the sagittal plane during flexion (kyphotic posture) is greater than during extension (lordotic posture).[25] Therefore, the normal cervical lordosis allows the neural elements to traverse the spinal canal through a shorter course without ventral compression. The lordotic curvature may also protect against neural injury because axial loads are dispersed dorsally onto the facet joints and large articular pillars, rather than the vertebral body (as seen in kyphosis).

A number of disease processes affect the spine, in particular the thoracic and lumbar spine's sagittal balance, which in turn affects the entire spine's sagittal balance. The flexibility of the cervical spine allows it the ability to compensate for misalignment of the thoracic and lumbar spine. Therefore, an increased lordotic cervical posture has been observed when there was a concurrent exaggerated thoracic kyphosis.[14,20,26-28] This compensation permits the maintenance of the overall sagittal balance (i.e., head over the pelvis).

Hardacker et al. measured the cervical curvature of 100 volunteers and recorded the mean total cervical lordosis alignment (foramen magnum to C7 inferior end plate) as 40 degrees (standard deviation of 9.7 degrees) where the majority of the lordotic curve was at the C1-2 junction and only 6 degrees was present from C4 to C7.[20] Despite no patient having an overall cervical kyphotic posture, 39% had a segmental kyphotic angle greater than 5 degrees, typically at C4-5 and C5-6, based on individual segmental angles analysis.[20] Gore et al.[29] also measured mean lordotic angles in the cervical spine of osteoarthritis patients from perpendicular lines of the C2 and C7 bodies and observed a 16- to 22-degree lordosis for men and a 15- to 25-degree lordosis in women. Others have measured the C2-7 lordotic curvature to be approximately 14 degrees.[30,31] Although numerous studies have shown a wide range for cervical lordosis, slight head extension (0–13.9 degrees) has been shown not to affect the cervical spine alignment.[32]

Overall, there is not an accepted range defined as "normal" for cervical posture. Although definitive angles have not been calculated, studies have shown that due to aging and degenerative changes, the cervical spine has an increase in the lordotic angle.[20,29,33] This lordotic angle increases with aging,[20] from approximately 15 degrees in the third decade to 22 to 25 degrees in the seventh decade.[29]

Cervical Alignment—Dynamic Movement

The cervical spine, also, allows a great degree of flexibility, and dynamic images (flexion and extension radiographs) permit an assessment of the intersegmental motion related to this flexibility. Flexion and extension radiographs of normal individuals have shown that the greatest motion occurs at C4-5 and C5-6 and the least at C2-3.[25,33-35] Lin et al.[35] further demonstrated that the spine moved from a lordotic position in extension to a nearly parallel position with flexion, such that all intervertebral differences in angular displacement were less than 7 degrees and translation was less than 0.6 mm. The total range of motion (ROM) from C2 to C7 was reported from 50 degrees to greater than 90 degrees with a normal gaussian distribution and a mean of 67 degrees.[35] This ROM is affected by the stiffening of the spine, which occurs throughout the normal aging process.[36]

Degenerative Changes

Cervical spondylotic myelopathy is a pathologic process that affects the aging spine. Gore et al. showed that 90% of asymptomatic males, age 60 to 65 years, had degenerative changes

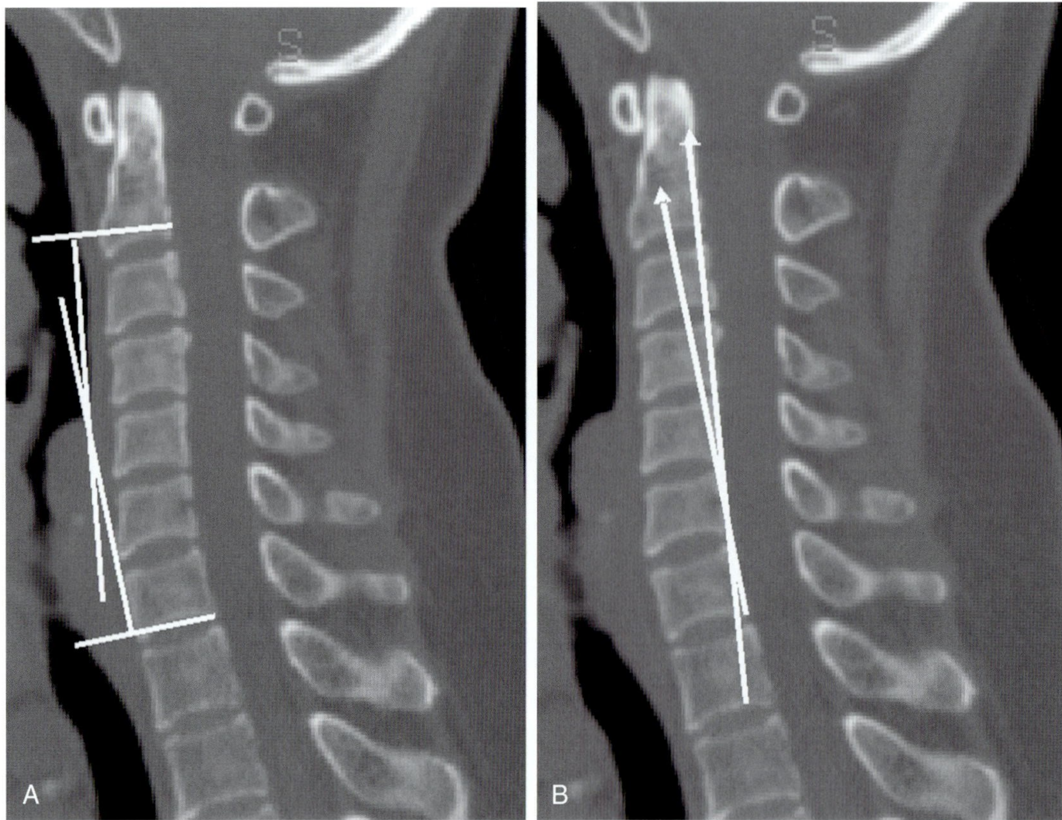

FIGURE 96-5. A, Cobb lines are drawn from the caudal end plate of the rostral body and from the caudal end plate of the caudal vertebral body. Perpendicular lines are drawn and the angle of intersecting lines is measured. **B,** Harrison tangential lines to the dorsal vertebral bodies typically performed at C2 and C7.

on cervical roentgenographic studies.[29] As a result of aging, the vertebral discs dehydrate, and the vertebral column loses height (Fig. 96-6). This loss of height results in a decreased tension of the ligamentum flavum. The loss of tension on the ligament causes it to shorten and results in buckling of the ligament into the spinal canal, with possible spinal cord compression. Also, degenerative and osteophytic changes take place in the facet joints, along with the vertebral disc space junction. The result is a stiffening or rigidity of the cervical spine and a decreased ROM. Holmes illustrated this by showing that the spine segments with the greatest motion migrate from C5-6 to C4-5 with aging.[33]

The overall alignment of the cervical spine should not assume a kyphotic posture due to the normal aging process (see Fig. 96-6). Gore et al. showed that, despite the decrease in the intervertebral distance, the overall lordotic curve (C2-7) increased with aging in 200 asymptomatic adults.[29]

Biomechanical Principles of the Cervical Spine

The position, posture, and motion of the cervical spine are complex processes that direct and manipulate forces on and around the spine. These forces allow the cervical spine to maintain an upright and lordotic posture. Due to the significant mobility of the cervical spine, the displacement of loads can be variable through different anatomic structures depending on the position of the spine during loading. For example, applied axial loads, with the spine in extension, are dispersed through the facet and dorsal articular column, whereas in flexion the vertebral body supports the majority of the load.

The point or position in the vertebral body that all other points rotate about when a movement occurs is termed the *instantaneous axis of rotation* (IAR). This is not a static point but rather is dynamic and changes with position, posture, and direction of movements. Also, each segment has a unique IAR for every movement; it is influenced by spine alignment, anatomy, muscle, and loads exerted. White and Panjabi[10] theorized that in the sagittal plane for flexion and extension, the IAR is located in the ventral portion of the vertebral body. Therefore, each vertebral body has its own IAR for each directional movement. The summation of all the IAR movements dictates spinal column orientation and motion (Fig. 96-7).

These forces that act on the spinal column have both a direction and a magnitude and are therefore referred to as force vectors. The perpendicular distance between a force vector and the IAR is defined as the lever or moment arm. The combination of the force vector and the lever arm results in a bending moment about the IAR. Therefore, the IAR can be thought of as a fulcrum, such that with flexion all points ventral to it come together and all points dorsal spread apart[8] (see Fig. 96-7).

The muscle and ligament complexes of the cervical spine have a significant effect on the support, motion, and stability of the cervical spine. The effectiveness of each ligament

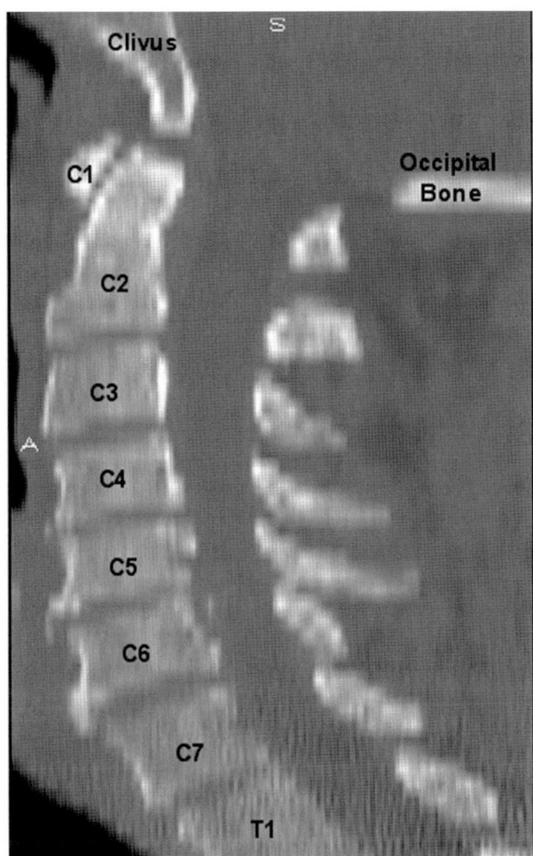

FIGURE 96-6. CT reformatted sagittal images of degenerative cervical spine. Note the osteophyte formations and loss of disc height.

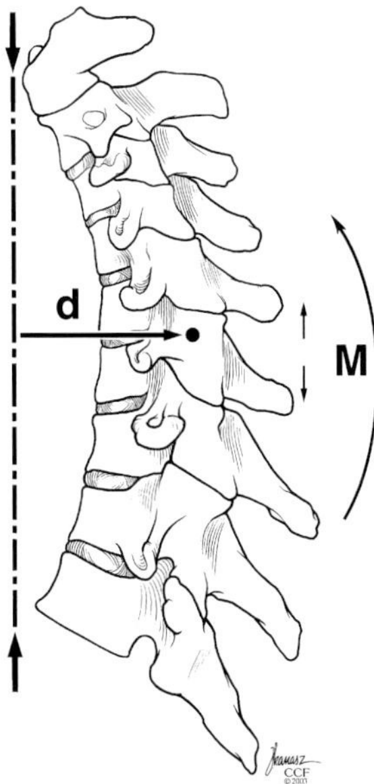

FIGURE 96-7. The instantaneous axis of rotation (IAR), dot in figure, is defined as the position of the vertebral body that all other points rotate about when movement occurs. The perpendicular distance (*d*) between the force vector and the IAR is defined as a lever or moment arm (*M*). The combination of both the force vector and lever arm results in a bending moment about the IAR. (Copyright Cleveland Clinic Foundation.)

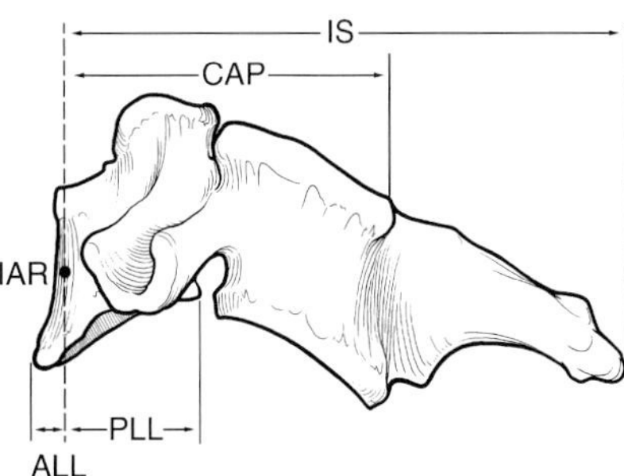

FIGURE 96-8. The lever arm of the ligaments to the instantaneous axis of rotation (IAR) greatly influences the stability of the spine. The weaker interspinous ligaments work at the greatest distance from the IAR and therefore provide significant resistance to gravitational influences. Although the dorsal elements have weaker ligaments in general, they have much longer lever arms on which they act, therefore providing a substantial dorsal tension band. ALL, anterior longitudinal ligament; CAP, capsular ligaments; IS, interspinous ligaments; PLL, posterior longitudinal ligament.

is not only related to the strength of that ligament but also to the moment arm through which the ligament acts[8,37] (Fig. 96-8). A weaker ligament with a longer level arm might provide more support and strength to the spine than a very strong ligament located on the spinal column, with a short lever arm.

Multiple studies have illustrated the importance of intact and functioning cervical musculature to support and maintain the cervical lordosis. Nolan and Sherk performed a biomechanical analysis of the extensor musculature of the cervical spine and demonstrated that the semispinalis muscle acted as a dynamic stabilizer and the removal of its attachments resulted in the loss of cervical lordosis.[38] Iizuka et al.[39] reattached the semispinalis cervicis muscle after laminoplasty and found that attachment of the extensor musculature on serial MRIs correlated with a maintained cervical lordosis in the postoperative period.

The majority of the cervical spine's ligamentous and muscle complexes support and attach to the dorsal aspect of the spine. These structures, along with the laminae, provide a lever arm, which allows the cervical spine to maintain a lordotic curve. Panjabi showed that without muscular support, the osteoligamentous cervical spine would buckle and fail at only one fifth the weight of the human head.[40,41] These cervical spine specimens (C0-T1) failed with increasing loads of only 11 N,[40] whereas in vivo load testing has shown load ranges from 53 to 1175 N.[42,43] These data have to be taken in the context that in vitro models comparing segmental vertebral body motions do not correlate well with in vivo data.[41]

The human body's center of gravity is located approximately 4 cm ventral to the sacrum. Therefore, in the sagittal plane, this center of gravity is ventral to the vertebral body. In the standing individual, a plumb line dropped from the tip of the odontoid process falls slightly ventral (0–2 cm) to the ventral surface of the C7 vertebral body (see Fig. 96-4). The cervical IAR is also located ventral to the vertebral bodies. Therefore, there is a constant attraction or force drawing or pulling the spine toward the center of gravity. Newton's first law states that an object at rest tends to stay at rest while an object in motion tends to stay in motion with the same speed and in the same direction unless acted on by an unbalanced force. Therefore, as long as the spine has the ability to resist against these gravitational forces through a strong tension band in the form of the dorsal musculoligamentous complex, the spine will maintain a lordotic curvature. Otherwise, the cervical spine will gravitate to its lowest energy state or a kyphotic posture, which implies that the cervical spine, without resisting forces, would prefer to be located at the center of gravity or zero energy state.

The strong muscles and ligaments of the cervical spine are able to maintain this lordotic posture against the gravitational forces due to their increased distance or greater lever arm relative to the IAR (see Fig. 96-8). This increased distance creates a mechanical advantage that the muscles and ligaments use to maintain a lordotic curvature. If the muscles and ligaments are weakened either due to congenital diseases or iatrogenic causes (postsurgical), such a dorsal "anchor" has a less substantial effect. Then, despite the mechanical advantage provided by the increased lever arm, the cervical spine will migrate further ventrally and the result will be a loss of the lordotic curvature. The ventral migration toward the IAR causes the lever arm that the compromised dorsal muscles and ligaments are acting through to be shorter (Fig. 96-9). The shorter lever arm and the weakened dorsal tension band, ligaments, and muscles fail to provide ample support. This in turn results in further progression of the kyphotic deformity.

This cycle of impaired muscles and shorter lever arm continues until a significant deformity with possible neurologic findings results. This sequence may be illustrated in individuals with Marfan syndrome. In this disorder, the affected patients have an increased laxity of their ligamentous structures and therefore are at an increased risk for abnormal cervical alignment. Hobbs et al.[27] confirmed this by showing that 36% of patients with this disorder had absence of the normal cervical lordosis.

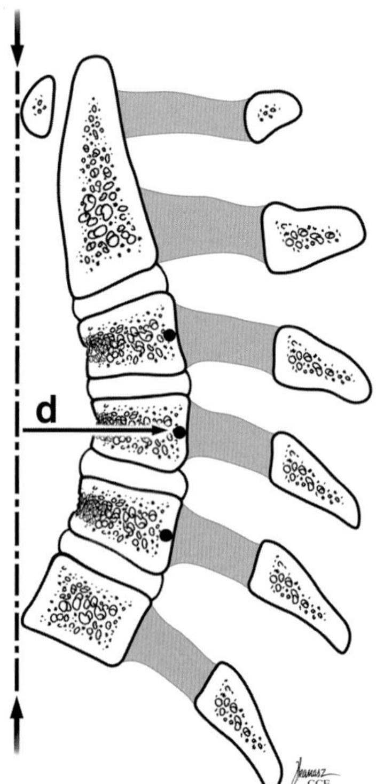

FIGURE 96-9. The dorsal migration of the instantaneous axis of rotation (*d*) causes the lever arms of the dorsal muscle and ligaments to be shorter, therefore weakening the dorsal tension band. (Copyright Cleveland Clinic Foundation.)

Etiologies of Cervical Deformity

Subaxial cervical deformities can develop in any plane or direction but most commonly occur in the sagittal plane, primarily as a kyphotic deformity, and rarely as coronal plane abnormalities (i.e., scoliosis). Cervical and cervicothoracic scoliosis are extremely rare disorders and only sparse reports of their occurrences are available in the literature. However, there are multiple causes for kyphotic deformities, resulting either through congenital or acquired disorders. Congenital disorders (Klippel-Feil syndrome, hemivertebrae),[44-46] systemic disorders (dystrophic dystonia, Larsen syndrome),[47-51] and neuromuscular disorders (Marfan syndrome, Prader-Willi syndrome)[27,52] can all result in cervical deformities. Acquired kyphotic cervical spine disorders may be secondary to spinal tumors (neurofibromatosis),[53] occupational exposures,[54] iatrogenic causes (postlaminectomy, pseudarthrosis),[55,56] and traumatic injuries.

This discussion focuses on cervical scoliotic deformities, their etiologies, and their treatment.

Cervical and Cervicothoracic Scoliosis

Smith defined cervical and cervicothoracic scoliosis as a structural curvature of the cervical or cervicothoracic region resulting from an osseous abnormality such as a block vertebra or unilateral bar that is visible on either anteroposterior or lateral radiographs (Fig. 96-10).[44,45] Other etiologies include a failure of segmentation, block vertebrae, a failure of formation, hemivertebrae, or a combination of these anomalies.[44,45] Cervical scoliosis is occasionally associated with unilateral congenital nerve defects in the upper extremity.[46] This disorder typically occurs in children, and they present early due to cosmetic concerns of malpositioning of the head. Cervical spine alignment abnormalities do not have the ability to form a rostral compensatory curve because the head is the rostral terminus of the spine.

Congenital Scoliosis

The origin of congenital scoliosis may be environmental or genetic, or the condition may result from a combination of factors. Environmental factors, genetics, vitamin deficiency, chemicals, and drugs, singly or in combination, have all been implicated in the development of vertebral abnormalities. Whatever the cause, the physiologic injury occurs early in the embryologic period, well before the development of cartilage and bone. The resulting defects can lead to full or partial fusion or lack of development of the vertebrae, which, in turn, can cause a curvature that may be progressive during the growth of the child.[57]

The body of literature describing congenital cervical scoliosis is found in the form of case reports. Winter and House[46] describe two cases of congenital cervical scoliosis associated with a unilateral progressive nerve deficit in the upper extremity. A unilateral spina bifida was present in both cases. The patients were treated with a fusion at 2 and 5 years. Poole and Briggs[58] describe a "cranio-facio-cervical scoliosis complex" in

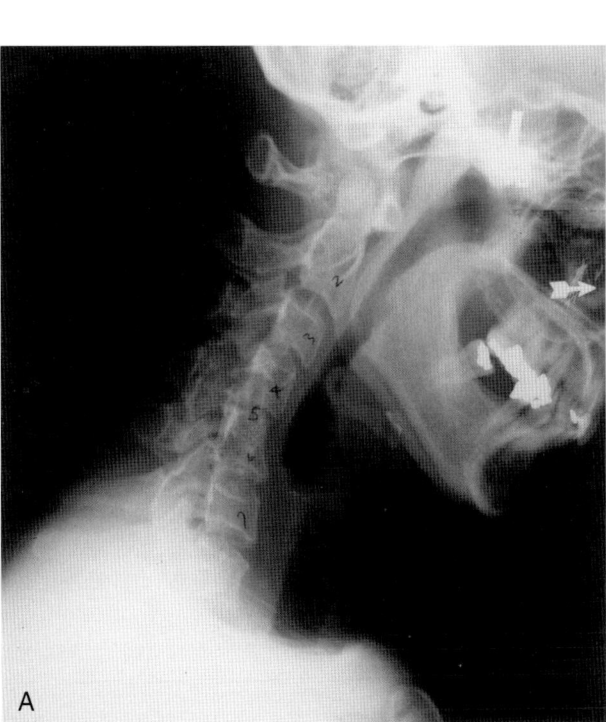

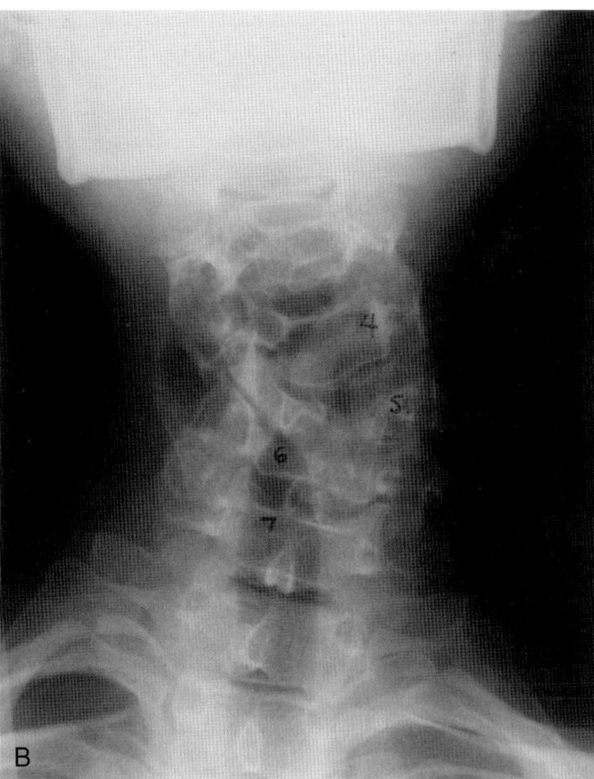

FIGURE 96-10. Adult patient presenting with radiculopathy who is noted to have a congenital hemivertebra and kyphotic deformity (**A**) and resultant scoliosis, as seen on the anteroposterior radiograph (**B**).

six cases, all presenting with facial asymmetry, vertical orbital dystopia, and torticollis. Five of the six patients had hemifacial microsomia. Four of the six had symptomatic cervical scoliosis.

Ruf et al.[59] evaluated three patients treated with hemivertebra resection for congenital cervical scoliosis presenting with torticollis. Surgery was performed by the dorsal-ventral-dorsal approach at a mean age of 9 years. The mean Cobb angle was 29 degrees prior to operating, 5 degrees postoperatively, and 6 degrees on follow-up. Torticollis improved by 16 degrees to an average of 1 degree postoperatively and 3 degrees on follow-up examination.

Svantesson et al.[60] analyzed 320 patients in Sweden with juvenile rheumatoid arthritis and found that 17 (5.3%) had scoliosis predominating in the thoracic and lumbar spine, with minimal cervical involvement. Twelve of the 17 had a curvature greater than 20 degrees. Torticollis was seen in 3 of the 17 patients and was associated with increased cervical curvature.

Marfan Syndrome

Scoliosis is a common presentation in Marfan syndrome and may require surgical intervention. Children with the disorder and a spinal deformity may also have a concurrent serious cardiac abnormality. Spontaneous dissection of the aortic root is a potential danger and patients should be monitored by a cardiologist prior to any surgical intervention. Cardiac surgery may be necessary prior to any spinal surgery.

The incidence of scoliosis in patients with Marfan syndrome ranges from 55% to 64% among reported case series.[61] There is a predilection for thoracic and lumbar spine involvement, and cervical scoliosis is a rare entity in Marfan syndrome. It is proposed that connective tissue laxity in conjunction with early puberty in this population causes earlier peak growth velocity that results in pelvic malpositioning or rotation. The resulting malpositioned pelvis may predispose to scoliosis.[61]

The coronal spinal deformity or scoliosis associated with Marfan syndrome has a clinical presentation similar to idiopathic scoliosis, with the exception of a higher prevalence of triple major curvature and double thoracic curvature. Sponsellar et al. noted that an adolescent curvature exceeding 40 to 50 degrees had a higher likelihood to progress into maturity, suggesting that treatment goals should be to prevent curvature of adolescence from exceeding 40 degrees.[62]

Sponsellar et al. further monitored 14 patients with coronal curves less than 45 degrees, treated for an average of 21 hours daily with a brace for at least 2 years or until skeletal maturity. He reported a 17% "success rate" where success was defined as prevention of curvature from exceeding 45 degrees or progression of curvature below 5 degrees. This "success rate" drastically contrasts to the 45% to 63% success rate for bracing patients with idiopathic scoliosis.[63] Progression of curvature averaged 6 to 8 degrees per year with a final average curvature of 49 degrees.[62] These data suggest that for adolescent patients with curvature greater than 40 degrees, bracing would be ineffective at preventing disease progression. However, bracing may still be an option for those with curvature ranging from 15 to 25 degrees.

In an additional retrospective review, 39 patients with Marfan syndrome who underwent deformity correction surgery at two institutions demonstrated the technical difficulties with instrumentation and inherent comorbidity due to cardiopulmonary insufficiency.[63] Pseudarthrosis was noted in 10%, and there was an additional instrumentation fixation failure rate of 21%. Infection was as high as 8%. Experience with operating on this rare population demonstrates the need for preoperative CT evaluation of the bony anatomy for assessment of its adequacy for fixation.[63]

Halo traction is a well-recognized adjunct in addition to ventral and dorsal release and fusion for correcting severe, complex, rigid scoliotic curves. However, caution should be applied when using halo traction in patients with Marfan or other connective tissue disorders. Halo traction creates more tension in the cervical spine than the thoracolumbar spine. This, in addition to the laxity of the connective tissue in Marfan, can cause worsening of existing cervical kyphosis after the traction.[64]

Jeune Syndrome

Jeune syndrome, also known as asphyxiating thoracic dystrophy, is characterized by a small, narrow chest with varying degrees of limb shortness. The prognosis is grim due to neonatal respiratory distress.[65] In a case series involving 13 patients, thoracic malformations tended to become less severe with age, although the majority of patients' height was found to be below the third percentile by adulthood.[65] A variety of pelvic abnormalities, a high rate of dwarfism, and predominantly thoracic skeletal dysplasia all are thought to contribute to scoliosis.

Patients with Jeune syndrome have a high rate of proximal cervical stenosis and should undergo screening with cervical spine films at birth.[66] Significant stenosis or instability may require decompression and cervico-occipital fusion.

Larsen Syndrome

Larsen syndrome is a rare congenital disease typically presenting with multiple congenital hip dislocations, "dish" facies (a term for a saddle nose and hypertelorism), and less commonly cervical scoliosis and kyphosis.[67] Larsen syndrome may have early-onset scoliosis that is very rigid and requires early intervention. Cervical kyphosis and subluxation may be lethal in affected patients, and screening radiographs are important. Upper airway abnormalities are an anesthesia concern.

Literature pertaining to coronal spinal deformity correction is entirely retrospective by way of case reports. One case report by Hosoe et al.[67] describes a 12-year-old girl who presented with bilaterally dislocated hips and right thoracic curvature with a Cobb angle of 77 degrees. Abnormal thoracic lordosis and lumbar hyperlordosis were present. Minimal cervical scoliosis also was evident radiographically. A dorsal spinal fusion from T4 to L2 resulted in improved thoracic scoliosis from 77 to 28 degrees and improvement of deformity in the sagittal plane as well. On 15-year follow-up, the patient was asymptomatic in her spine and hips. The significance of hip dislocations is that the associated flexion contracture of the hips is thought to have an influence on spinal sagittal alignment. In this case, spinal surgery preceded hip surgery. The position of the pelvis after spinal fusion is unpredictable. Secondly, the effect of abnormal muscle forces to the hips due to spinal deformity makes hip surgery technically difficult.[68]

Jarcho-Levin Syndrome

Jarcho-Levin syndrome is a congenital disorder occasionally marked by scoliosis. It is characterized most commonly by the presence of rib and vertebral defects at birth. This syndrome most commonly presents in infancy and is characterized by identification of a short neck, trunk, and stature. Skeletal survey characterizes multiple vertebral anomalies at different levels of the spine, including "butterfly vertebrae," hemivertebrae, and fused hypoplastic vertebrae. Unfortunately, the associated small size of the thorax in newborns frequently leads to respiratory compromise and death in infancy.[69]

Jarcho-Levin syndrome results in a thoracic volume depletion deformity due to shortness of the thoracic cavity, due to either a spondylocostal dysostosis variant or spondylothoracic dysplasia. The former has chaotic congenital scoliosis with varied combination of missing and fused ribs. Although spondylocostal dysostosis has a benign reputation in the literature for respiratory complications, respiratory insufficiency is nevertheless common and one death is known from respiratory failure. Spondylothoracic dysplasia seldom has significant scoliosis but has a mortality rate approaching 50% from respiratory complications due to thoracic insufficiency syndrome. In spite of severe restrictive respiratory disease, adult survivors of spondylothoracic dysplasia appear to do well clinically for unknown reasons. Cerebrocostomandibular syndrome is characterized by scoliosis, micrognathia, and thoracic insufficiency syndrome, due to an "implosion" deformity of the thorax from congenital pseudarthrosis of the dorsal ribs.[66]

Klippel-Feil Syndrome

Klippel-Feil syndrome is a congenital disorder of spinal segmentation distinguished by the bony fusion of ventral cervical vertebrae. Feil subclassified patients presenting with Klippel-Feil syndrome into three groups. Group I included patients with fusion of cervical and upper thoracic vertebrae with synostosis. Group II included patients with congenital fusion of the vertebrae in the cervical spine only. Group III included patients with cervical vertebral fusions as well as associated lower thoracic or upper lumbar fusion.[70] Scoliosis, mirror movements, and otolaryngologic, kidney, ocular, cranial, limb, and/or digit anomalies are often associated. Mutations in *GDF6* are associated with vertebral segmentation defects in Klippel-Feil syndrome.[71]

Wildervanck syndrome, or cervico-oculo-acoustic syndrome, refers to Klippel-Feil syndrome with the additional findings of congenital sensorineural deafness and Duane retraction syndrome (characterized by deficits with abduction and adduction of the eye).[72] Wildervanck syndrome is the most common abnormality to overlap with Duane retraction syndrome. The fact that Klippel-Feil syndrome has been shown to overlap with Noonan, Turner, and Wildervanck syndromes should warrant a comprehensive examination by the clinician to rule out alternative diagnoses.[72]

Thomsen et al. reviewed data from 57 patients with Klippel-Feil syndrome treated over 25 years. He found that scoliosis in patients with group I had a Cobb angle of 31 degrees at the level of deformity. Patients in groups II and III had Cobb angles of 9 and 23 degrees, respectively. With isolated cervical spine involvement, there was the least risk of scoliosis. Still, 70% of the patient population demonstrated scoliosis.[70]

Cervical Spine Dysmorphisms

Cervical spine dysmorphisms (CSDs) occur in a heterogeneous group of patients unified by the presence of congenital defects that result from malalignment, formation, or segmentation of the cervical spine, thus generating disability. This problem requires comprehensive evaluation of patients with a diagnosis of scoliosis, correlating clinical and radiologic findings and the presence of numerous abnormalities of other systems to give an appropriate syndrome diagnosis and multidisciplinary management of these patients with the aim to give them an integral rehabilitation treatment increasing their quality of life. Santillan Chapa et al. described clinical and radiologic findings in children with diagnosed CSD. They studied 47 consecutive outpatients of the Pediatric Rehabilitation Division in Instituto Nacional de Rehabilitacion with diagnosed scoliosis. Sixteen patients (34%) had diagnosed CSD. The most frequently seen syndromes were Klippel-Feil (19%), Wildervanck (4.3%), neurofibromatosis (4.3%), Morquio (2.1%), Stickler (2.1%), and Williams (2.1%). The researchers found CSD in 34% of the group studied, greater than in the medical literature.[73]

Morquio syndrome, or mucopolysaccharidosis IVA, is a genetic deficiency of N-acetylgalactosamine-6-sulfate sulfatase that results in accumulation of lysosomal mucopolysaccharides. This accumulation occasionally manifests as cervical scoliosis among a varied presentation of skeletal dysplasias.[74] Stickler syndrome is an autosomal dominant connective tissue disorder marked by ocular involvement. Obvious skeletal and facial deformities are present. Cervical dysmorphism is highly likely by adulthood.[75]

Neuromuscular Scoliosis

Scoliosis is seen in a variety of neurologic disorders at different levels of the nervous system, from peripheral nerves to the CNS.[76] As seen in poliomyelitis, spina bifida, cerebral palsy, spinal muscular atrophy as well as rarer conditions, disorders of the segmental efferent nervous system result in the development of scoliosis secondarily.[76] The goal of deformity correction is to stabilize the spine without the loss of motor or sensory function, with the torso balanced over a level spine.[77]

Surgical stabilization is the standard treatment of neuromuscular spinal deformities. The debate persists today regarding the necessity for extending the construct and arthrodesis to the sacrum. Studies suggest a similarity initially between patients with fusions distally to either the lumbar spine or sacrum. One view is that with higher grade curvature and pelvic obliquity, suprapelvic fusion results in an increased loss of correction on long-term follow-up.[78] On the other hand, McCall and Hayes demonstrate in long-term follow-up of 55 patients who underwent instrumentation and fusion to L5 only that a comparable degree of deformity correction is maintained.[77]

Congenital muscular torticollis is due to fibrosis of one or both of the heads of the sternocleidomastoid muscle. Asymmetrical forces acting on the cervical spine during the developmental phase in all likelihood contribute to the incidence of cervical scoliosis in torticollis patients.

Idiopathic Scoliosis

Adolescent idiopathic scoliosis (AIS) is the most common form of scoliosis because of its exclusionary diagnosis. AIS is diagnosed as a coronal curvature of the spine greater than 10 degrees with a rotational component and no other etiologic explanation in a child 9 years of age or older. If the child is younger than 9 years of age, the diagnosis is referred to as early-onset scoliosis.[69] Despite years of research, the etiology of AIS is poorly understood.[76] Indeed, the pathogenesis is multifactorial. Wynne-Davies[79] screened 114 first-, second-, and third-degree relatives of patients with AIS to indicate a dominant or multiple gene inheritance pattern. Work by Robin and Cohen[80] suggested autosomal inheritance.

Historically, treatment options for AIS included exercise, in-patient rehabilitation, braces, and surgery. Evidence suggests that the use of scoliosis intensive rehabilitation and braces can alter the natural history of the condition. However, no prospective controlled studies compare the natural history with surgical treatment.[81] Genome-wide association studies have successfully identified single nucleotide polymorphisms related to the severity of curve progression.[69]

Traumatic Scoliosis

Scoliosis can occur in the acute setting of trauma. Shen and Samartzis[82] describe a 7-year-old boy with the development of scoliosis following a motor vehicle crash. The patient was without motor or sensory deficits on examination and had intact rectal tone and normal volition. An upright radiograph demonstrated a traumatic scoliosis with widening of the dorsal elements, a so-called "Chance fracture" or "flexion-distraction" injury. The patient underwent a dorsal spinal fusion and stabilization with realignment. Follow-up examination and radiographs demonstrated a solid fusion, full ROM, and absence of pain.

Purely ligamentous flexion-distraction injuries, as seen in the previously described case, can be difficult to heal with bracing alone and can result in a dramatic acute traumatic scoliosis.[82] Surgical fixation is needed to achieve stabilization through arthrodesis. Unilateral cervical jumped fractures can also present with scoliosis. Treatment is closed (via traction) or open (via surgery) reduction of the fracture, depending on the neurologic status of the patient and a review of appropriate imaging, followed by halo or instrumented fixation.

Treatment Strategies for Cervical Scoliosis

Treatment options vary depending on the degree of curvature, the anatomic abnormalities, and the age and medical condition of the patient. Bracing is the least invasive technique but unfortunately is not an optimal treatment strategy, because most deformities are due to segmental, formation, and developmental disorders, and, therefore, are usually associated with a large curve. In the few patients with a scoliotic angle less than 30 degrees that passively correct past the neutral plane, bracing is the best treatment option.[44,45] These patients must be able to wear their brace for extended periods and be followed clinically with serial imaging and clinical examinations for signs of curve progression.

Unfortunately, most patients present with severe curves (i.e., >40 degrees), rigidity, severe torticollis, and lateral tilting that does not respond to bracing.[44,45] Smith et al.[44,45] advocated operative treatment strategy for these patients via a dorsal fusion of the structural portion of the curve. Surgical dissection must be meticulous because the incidence of bone abnormalities and absent lamina has been reported to be as high as 30%.[45] Fortunately, these curves are usually flexible due to the young age of the patient population and can be manipulated intraoperatively. Smith,[45] using this dorsal arthrodesis technique, had a solid fusion in 20 of 21 patients, with an average follow-up of 17 years. If the curves are stiff and rigid, the use of traction preoperatively increases the mobility of the spine. Winter[83] had two cases of cervical scoliosis with associated arm paralysis and advocated early surgical intervention for progressive spinal deformity. Deburge[84] reported one patient with a cervical scoliosis secondary to a hemivertebra and Klippel-Feil syndrome that was treated with a staged ventral and dorsal procedure.

With the advent of segmental pedicle screw fixation that enables more powerful corrective forces, Suk et al. reported that an additional ventral procedure may be unnecessary even in severe cervical scoliotic deformities. Thirty-five scoliosis patients treated by pedicle screw fixation and rod derotation were retrospectively analyzed after a minimum follow-up of 2 years. Residual coronal decompensation was observed in only three patients postoperatively. The authors concluded that dorsal segmental pedicle screw fixation without ventral release in severe scoliosis had satisfactory deformity correction without significant loss of curve correction.[85]

Summary

Cervical spine deformities result from a variety of causes. They may result in and present with mechanical neck pain and/or progressive neurologic deficit. If the patient is symptomatic or quality of life is threatened as a result of the deformity, surgical correction should be considered. Emphasis should also be placed on the prevention of further deformity, such as restoring lordosis after a ventral decompression procedure or using dorsal fusion and/or instrumentation after an extensive dorsal decompression. Overall, the correction of cervical deformities is rewarding because the majority of patients obtain relief of their mechanical symptoms and enjoy an improvement of neurologic function.

KEY REFERENCES

Hilibrand AS, Tannenbaum DA, Graziano GP, et al: The sagittal alignment of the cervical spine in adolescent idiopathic scoliosis. *J Pediatr Orthop* 15:627–632, 1995.

Hobbs WR, Sponseller PD, Weiss AP, Pyeritz RE: The cervical spine in Marfan syndrome. *Spine (Phila Pa 1976)* 22:983–989, 1997.

Smith MD: Congenital scoliosis of the cervical or cervicothoracic spine. *Orthop Clin North Am* 25:301–310, 1994.

Smith MD, Lonstein JE, Winter RB: Congenital cervicothoracic scoliosis. A long term follow-up study. *Orthop Trans* 16:165–170, 1992.

Weiss HR: Is there a body of evidence for the treatment of patients with adolescent idiopathic scoliosis (AIS)? *Scoliosis* 2:19, 2007.

White AA III, Johnson RM, Panjabi MM, et al: Biomechanical analysis of clinical stability in the cervical spine. *Clin Orthop Relat Res* 109:85–96, 1975.

Wynne-Davies R: Genetic aspects of idiopathic scoliosis. *Dev Med Child Neurol* 15:809–811, 1973.

REFERENCES

The complete reference list is available online at expertconsult.com.

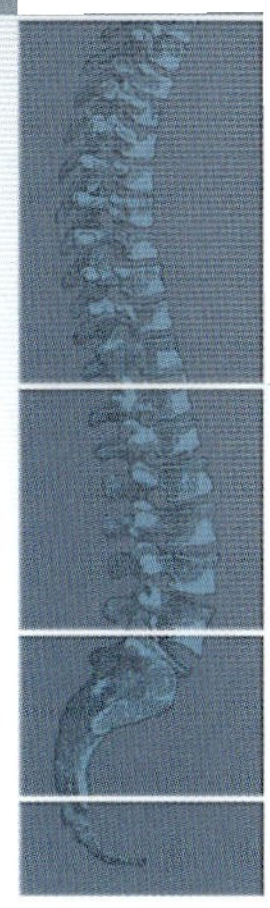

Adult Thoracic and Lumbar Deformity

Joshua E. Heller | Kai-Ming G. Fu | Justin S. Smith | Christopher I. Shaffrey

Deformity of the spine implies abnormality of proper spinal alignment that can lead to pain, instability, and neurologic and/or physiologic dysfunction. The deformity can occur in any plane (axial, coronal, or sagittal) and often involves a combination of abnormalities in multiple planes, as demonstrated by the patient in Figure 97-1. An accurate and accepted nomenclature is useful for describing deformities. Table 97-1 defines some common terms used in deformity and is in part adapted from the work of the Scoliosis Research Society (SRS) Terminology Committee and Working Group on Spinal Classification.[1,2] Spinal deformity is a broad term that encompasses a variety of pathologies. Scoliosis is defined classically as "lateral curvature of the spine." However, the pathophysiology of scoliosis can create a three-dimensional deformity involving abnormal spinal curvature (coronal deformity), rotation (axial deformity), and often kyphosis (sagittal deformity). Abnormal spinal profile in the sagittal plane (kyphosis or lordosis) can result in sagittal imbalance. In uncompensated hyperkyphosis, the normal upright posture of head over pelvis and feet (sagittal balance) is shifted forward. Spondylolisthesis is a regional abnormality in the sagittal plane in which one vertebra is displaced ventrally or dorsally in relation to an adjacent level.

Spinal deformity has multiple causes, including, but not limited to, (1) unknown factors likely related to genetic presusceptibility (as in adolescent idiopathic scoliosis), (2) congenital abnormalities, (3) neuromuscular conditions (i.e., cerebral palsy, spinal cord injury), or (4) conditions associated with spinal cord dysfunction such as myelomeningocele. Deformity can also result as a consequence of trauma (i.e., posttraumatic kyphosis), infection, malignancy, degeneration, or iatrogenic causes. Table 97-2 lists some of these causes. The goal of deformity surgery, despite the etiology, is the relief of the patient's symptoms while achieving a balanced spine.

Conditions often detected and treated in the pediatric population, such as adolescent idiopathic scoliosis, Scheuermann kyphosis, congenital scoliosis, neuromuscular scoliosis, and scoliosis associated with other congenital syndromes (syndromic), are discussed in greater detail elsewhere in this text. This chapter will focus on the clinical and radiographic diagnosis, classification, and nonoperative management of adult thoracic and lumbar spinal deformity, with attention paid to scoliosis and kyphosis. Symptomatic deformity in adults is most frequently a consequence of advanced degenerative disease and is termed *degenerative* or *de novo* scoliosis. Curves are thought to result as a consequence of asymmetrical degeneration of lumbar discs and facet joints.[3] The operative techniques used in treatment of adult thoracic and lumbar deformity are discussed in a later chapter.

Clinical Evaluation of the Adult Patient with Spinal Deformity

A thorough history is critical in the evaluation of adult patients with thoracic and lumbar deformity. It is important to understand what symptoms are most pressing for the patient. For example, if the predominant symptom is pain, determining if the pain is axial versus radicular is essential. Aggravating and ameliorating factors should be elucidated. Care should be taken to document symptoms of neurogenic claudication or radiculopathy. Symptoms of bowel and bladder dysfunction should be evaluated. Discrete physical weakness should be identified. In patients with significant thoracic components, pulmonary status may need to be addressed. A patient's comorbidities should be evaluated and the presence of osteoporosis or osteopenia should be ascertained.

Key components of the physical examination include an assessment of the patient's gait, a musculoskeletal evaluation, and a thorough neurologic examination. Signs of myelopathy such as hyperreflexia, clonus, and an impaired gait may be present in patients with severe thoracic or concomitant cervical disease. Other conditions that may contribute to the deformity such as a leg length discrepancy should be sought. The cosmetic appearance of the deformity is also a considerable factor in the psychosocial well-being of the patient. The importance of appearance is accepted in children but has yet to be thoroughly evaluated in adults.[4,5]

Diagnostic Imaging

Diagnostic imaging is crucial in the evaluation and management of patients with thoracic or lumbar deformity. A multimodal approach, including MRI and CT, is often used. However, much information can be elucidated from standard radiographs.

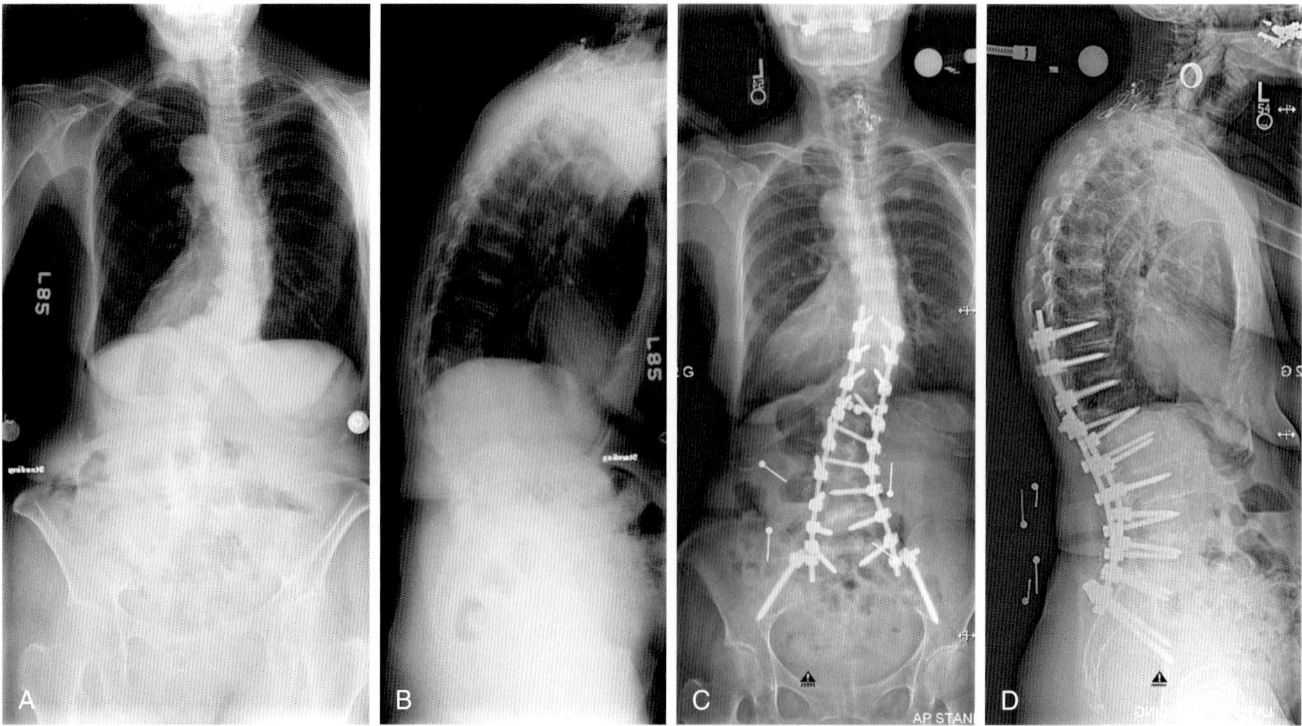

FIGURE 97-1. Preoperative and postoperative radiographs of a 78-year-old woman presenting with back pain and neurogenic claudication. **A,** Preoperative standing posteroanterior (PA) film demonstrating thoracic and thoracolumbar scoliosis. **B,** Preoperative lateral film demonstrating concomitant positive sagittal alignment resulting from a loss of lumbar lordosis. PA (**C**) and lateral (**D**) postoperative standing films demonstrating improvement in coronal and sagittal planes after the patient was treated with a T10-sacrum instrumented fusion with multiple Smith-Petersen osteotomies.

Conventional Radiographs

Standing frontal (anteroposterior or posteroanterior) and sagittal (lateral) whole spine (i.e., 14 × 36-inch long cassette or digitally stitched) radiographs are required in the proper evaluation of patients with spinal deformity. Radiographs should show the occiput and shoulders superiorly and the pelvis, including femoral heads, inferiorly.[6] Standing views should be taken in a standardized position with the patient's hips and knees in extension to remove potential compensation of sagittal imbalance. Frontal radiographs are oriented with the patient's right side on the right side of the screen or view box. This orientation allows the observer to view the film as if he or she is standing behind the patient examining the spine, or as he or she would see it while performing surgery using a dorsal approach. Sagittal radiographs are oriented with the patient facing right. Proper orientation of full-length scoliosis radiographs is demonstrated in Figure 97-2.

A comparison between the degree of deformity between weight-bearing and non–weight-bearing films (i.e., supine) gives some information regarding the rigidity of the deformity. Additional views to help determine stiffness of the deformity can be useful. These views include supine lateral bending films, bending films over a bolster, fulcrum bending films, and push and traction views. In the evaluation of spondylolisthesis, dynamic lateral views, shown in Figure 97-3, of the lumbar spine are used to help determine the degree of instability. Additional plain radiographic views that are useful in deformity include oblique views to visualize the pars interarticularis, the Ferguson view to better visualize the sacral region, and the Stagnara or Leeds view (an oblique view through the apical region of a scoliotic curve that accounts for rotation) to better visualize the pedicles.

Advanced Imaging

Advanced imaging has become nearly standard in the evaluation of patients with deformity. Common modalities include CT, CT myelography, CT angiography, and MRI. MRI gives excellent soft tissue detail and is useful in demonstrating disc disease, spondylotic changes, and intraspinal anomalies. MRI should be obtained in all cases associated with neurologic compromise unless contraindicated. CT gives excellent bony detail and is extremely useful in preoperative planning. CT myelography has the added benefit of providing intraspinal information in addition to high-resolution bony detail. CT angiography and MR angiography are useful in the evaluation of vascular anatomy, which may have surgical approach implications.

Advances in imaging software such as multiplanar rendering (MPR) allow the surgeon to view multislice CT and MRI data in multiple and adjustable planes. This allows for more accurate preoperative measurement of pedicle diameter and a greater appreciation of the disease process, as shown in Figure 97-4. Three-dimensional reconstructions can easily be created to aid in operative planning. It is also possible to have models of an individual patient's spine fabricated and surgery simulated prior to the patient reaching the operating room.[7,8] In our opinion, thin-cut CT myelography plus MPR provides extremely useful information in operative planning for deformity.

TABLE 97-1

Glossary of Terms Frequently Used in Deformity

Term	Meaning
Scoliosis	Lateral curvature of the spine (now recognized to be a three-dimensional deformity)
Kyphosis	Dorsal convex angulation of the spine
Hyperkyphosis	Kyphosis greater than the normal range
Hypokyphosis	Kyphosis of the thoracic spine less than the normal range
Lordosis	Ventral convex angulation of the spine
Hyperlordosis	Lordosis greater than the normal range
Hypolordosis	Lordosis of the cervical or lumbar spine less than the normal range
Kyphoscoliosis	Nonidiopathic scoliosis associated with an area of true hyperkyphosis
Lordoscoliosis	Scoliosis associated with an area of lordosis
Major curve	Curve with the largest Cobb measurement on upright long cassette radiograph of the spine
Minor curve	Any curve that does not have the largest Cobb measurement on upright long cassette radiograph of the spine
Structural curve	Measured spinal curve in the coronal plane in which the Cobb measurement fails to correct past zero on supine maximal voluntary lateral side-bending radiograph
Compensatory curve	Minor curve above or below a major curve that may or may not be structural
End vertebrae	Vertebrae that define the ends of a curve in a frontal or sagittal projection
Cephalad end vertebra	First vertebra in the cephalad direction from a curve apex whose superior surface is tilted maximally toward the concavity of the curve
Caudad end vertebra	First vertebra in the caudad direction from a curve apex whose inferior surface is tilted maximally toward the concavity of the curve
Neutral vertebra	Vertebra without axial rotation (in reference to the most cephalad and caudal vertebrae that are not rotated in a curve)
Apical vertebra	In a curve, the vertebra most deviated laterally from the vertical axis that passes through the patient's sacrum (central sacral line)
Apical disc	In a curve, the disc most deviated laterally from the vertical axis of the patient that passes through the sacrum (central sacral line)
Stable vertebra	Thoracic or lumbar vertebra cephalad to a lumbar scoliosis that is most closely bisected by a vertically directed central sacral line assuming the pelvis is level. Alternatively, both pedicles of this vertebra should lie between vertical reference lines drawn from the sacroiliac joints.
Central sacral line (central sacral vertical line)	Vertical line in a frontal radiograph that passes through the center of the sacrum (identified by suitable landmarks, preferably on the first sacral segment)
C7 plumb line	Vertical line in a frontal radiograph drawn from the center of C7 (i.e., spinous process) down, which is used to measure compensation (coronal balance) relative to the central sacral line
	Vertical line in a lateral radiograph drawn from the C7 centroid

TABLE 97-2

Etiology of Deformity

Deformity	Etiology
Idiopathic scoliosis Infantile (2 months to 3 years of age) Juvenile (3 to 10 years of age) Adolescent (>10 years of age) Adult (after skeletal maturity)	Unknown factors likely related to genetic presusceptibility subtype classified by age of onset
Congenital scoliosis	In utero derangement of vertebral formation or segmentation
Neuromuscular scoliosis	Result of neurologic injury such as spinal cord injury, cerebral palsy, or conditions associated with spinal cord dysfunction (myelomeningocele, tethered cord, spinal dysraphisim)
Posttraumatic deformity	Following fracture with progressive vertebral collapse and angulation
Postinfectious deformity	Following vertebral osteomyelitis/discitis with vertebral destruction following tuberculosis infection (Pott disease)
Degenerative scoliosis and kyphosis	Consequence of advanced degenerative changes
Iatrogenic deformity	Consequence of previous interventions (i.e., laminectomy)

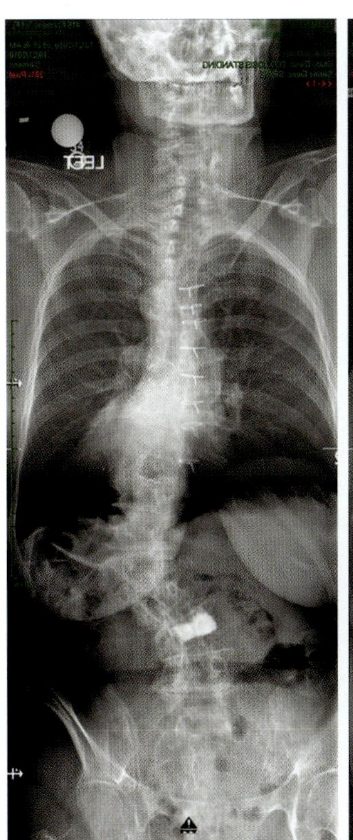

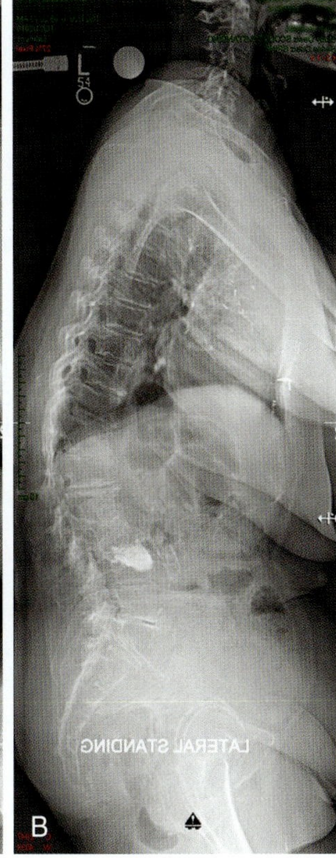

FIGURE 97-2. Proper orientation for standing posteroanterior (**A**) and lateral (**B**) radiographs of an adult patient with scoliosis. Both the occiput and femoral heads are clearly visible.

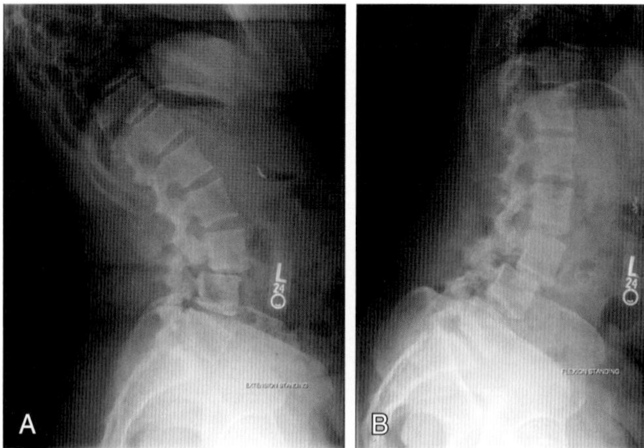

FIGURE 97-3. Examples of dynamic extension (**A**) and flexion lateral (**B**) radiographic views demonstrating spondylolisthesis of L3 over L4.

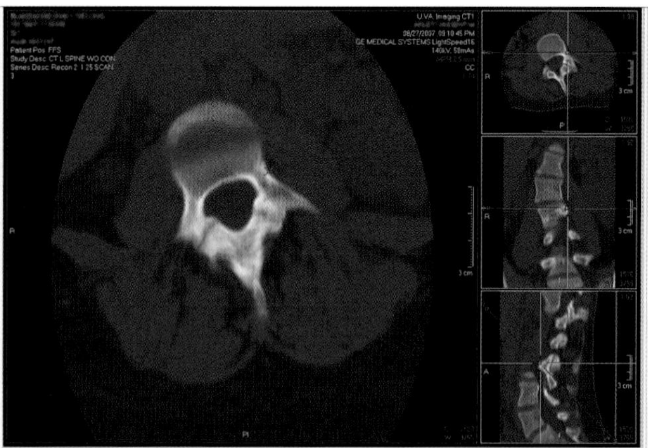

FIGURE 97-4. CT lumbar spine in a patient with scoliosis and a pars defect. Multiplanar rendering is used to better visualize the pathology.

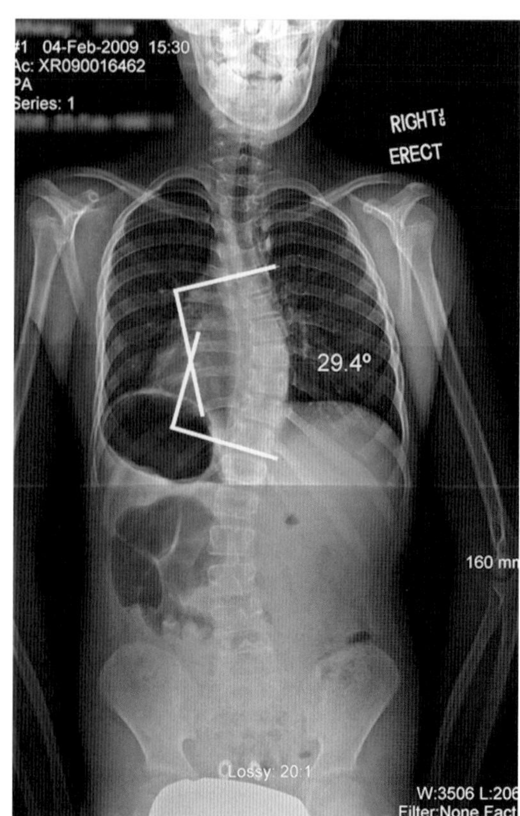

FIGURE 97-5. Cobb method used to determine degree of scoliosis.

Diagnostic Imaging Conventions and Measurements

The location of a sagittal or coronal deformity is defined by the location of the apex of the curve. The apex is the disc or vertebra that is maximally displaced and minimally angulated. A deformity is considered thoracic if it has an apex between the T2 and the T11-12 disc, thoracolumbar if the apex lies between the T12 and L1 vertebrae, and lumbar if the apex is at or distal to the L1-2 disc.[6] In scoliosis, the curve is described based on the side of its convexity. Convex to the right is known as dextroscoliosis, and convex to the left is known as levoscoliosis. Rarely is there just a single curve in scoliosis. The largest curve is called the "main" curve, which is typically structural (e.g., the curve does not correct completely on bending radiographs). Compensatory curves develop in response to the main structural curve and serve the purpose of maintaining spinal balance. Compensatory curves may or may not be structural.

Curve degree is measured via the Cobb method as illustrated in Figure 97-5. Originally described by John Cobb in 1948, the technique involves selecting vertebrae maximally tilted into the curve (end vertebrae). Lines are drawn parallel to the superior end plate of the cephalad end vertebra and the inferior end plate of the caudal end vertebra. If the end plates are not clearly visualized, an alternative technique is to use the pedicle margins as the basis for these lines.[9] Bisecting perpendicular lines from the end-plate lines are drawn and the angle determined. The Cobb technique is classically thought to have an inherent error of 3 to 5 degrees; therefore, a change in angle between consecutive films has to be greater than 5 degrees to be considered a true change. Intraobserver error ranges between 1% and 5%, and interobserver error can be as high as 10 degrees.[10] Modern Picture Archive and Communication Systems (PACS) workstations and image viewers have tools to measure Cobb angles digitally. To date, studies comparing Cobb angle measurements of primary and secondary curves on digital radiographs and traditional radiographs have shown no statistical difference in the intraobserver or interobserver variance between the two techniques.[11-13] New systems that automatically measure the Cobb angle and determine rotation are currently under development and may be able to reduce intraobserver and interobserver variability.[14] Proximal and distal neutral vertebrae (not rotated in the axial plane) as well as stable vertebrae (vertebrae above and below the end vertebra that is bisected by the central sacral vertical line [CSVL]) should also be determined because these are used to help select fusion levels in operative planning.

The Cobb method, although initially described for measurement of coronal deformity, is also used to measure degree of lordosis and kyphosis in the sagittal plane. In patients with a normal spinal profile, thoracic kyphosis typically measures between 30 and 35 degrees and lumbar lordosis ranges

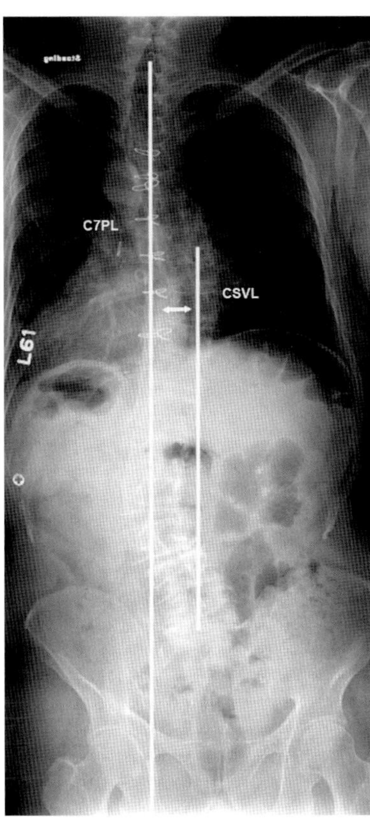

FIGURE 97-6. Coronal balance as determined on a frontal radiograph by measuring the distance between the central sacral vertical line (CSVL), a line drawn up through the center of the sacrum parallel to the edge of the film, and the C7 plumb line (C7PL), a vertical line drawn down from the midportion of the C7 vertebral body. By convention, a difference with the C7PL to the left is considered negative and a difference toward the right is positive.

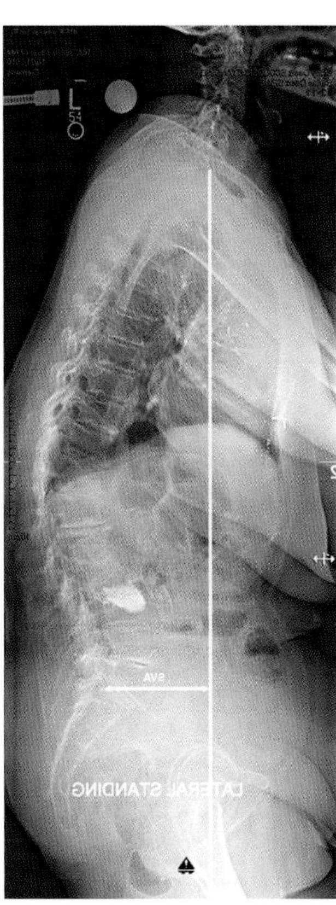

FIGURE 97-7. Sagittal balance is determined on a lateral radiograph by measuring the distance between the C7 plumb line (C7PL), drawn from the centroid (geometric center of the vertebrae) of C7 down and the dorsal/rostral corner of the sacrum. This difference is known as the sagittal vertical axis (SVA) offset. The balance is considered positive if the C7PL falls ventral to this reference point and negative if it falls dorsal to it.

between 35 and 50 degrees. Approximately two thirds of the total lordosis of the lumbar spine occurs at L4-S1.[15]

Spinal balance in the coronal and sagittal planes is determined through the use of vertical reference lines. The CSVL is a line drawn up through the center of the sacrum parallel to the edge of the film (e.g., perpendicular to the floor). The C7 plumb line (C7PL) on a frontal radiograph is a vertical line drawn down from the midportion of the C7 vertebral body (approximated by the spinous process, or more accurately through determination of the centroid). Coronal balance, demonstrated in Figure 97-6, is determined by measuring the distance between these reference lines. By convention, a difference with the C7PL to the left is considered negative and a difference toward the right is positive.

Sagittal balance, shown in Figure 97-7, is determined on a lateral radiograph by measuring the distance between the C7PL, drawn from the centroid (geometric center of the vertebrae) of C7 down and the dorsal/rostral corner of the sacrum. This difference is known as the sagittal vertical axis (SVA). The balance is considered positive if the C7PL falls ventral to this reference point and negative if it falls dorsal to it. Normal mean SVA offset is +0.5 cm and lies within a tight range between −1.0 and +1.0 cm.

Axial rotation on plain radiographs can be determined using the Nash-Moe method. The Nash-Moe method categorizes vertebral rotation into five grades based on the location of the pedicle in relation to the lateral aspect of the vertebral body.[16] CT measurement of rotation may be more reliable than standard radiographic techniques.[17]

Overall sagittal balance of the patient is greatly affected by relationship of the spine to the pelvis.[18] An adult patient with thoracic hyperkyphosis or loss of lumbar lordosis attempts to compensate for spinal sagittal imbalance through pelvic retroversion and hip extension, thereby attempting to bring his or her head back over the center of the pelvis. In the operative planning for deformity, including fusion to the sacrum or pelvis, spinopelvic relationships, including these compensatory mechanisms, should be taken into account. Figure 97-8 demonstrates the spinopelvic measurements, including pelvic tilt, sacral slope, and pelvic incidence. Pelvic tilt (a measure of the degree of pelvic retroversion [e.g., compensation for sagittal imbalance]) is the angle determined between a vertical reference line drawn up from the center of the femoral heads (femoral head axis) and a line drawn from the femoral head axis to the midpoint of the sacral end plate. If femoral heads are not perfectly aligned on a lateral radiograph, the location of the femoral head axis is approximated by the midpoint of a line connecting the geometric center of each femoral head. Sacral slope simply is the angle of a line drawn along the sacral end plate and the horizontal. Pelvic incidence is measured by determining the angle between a line drawn perpendicular to the sacral end plate at its midpoint and a line from the femoral head axis

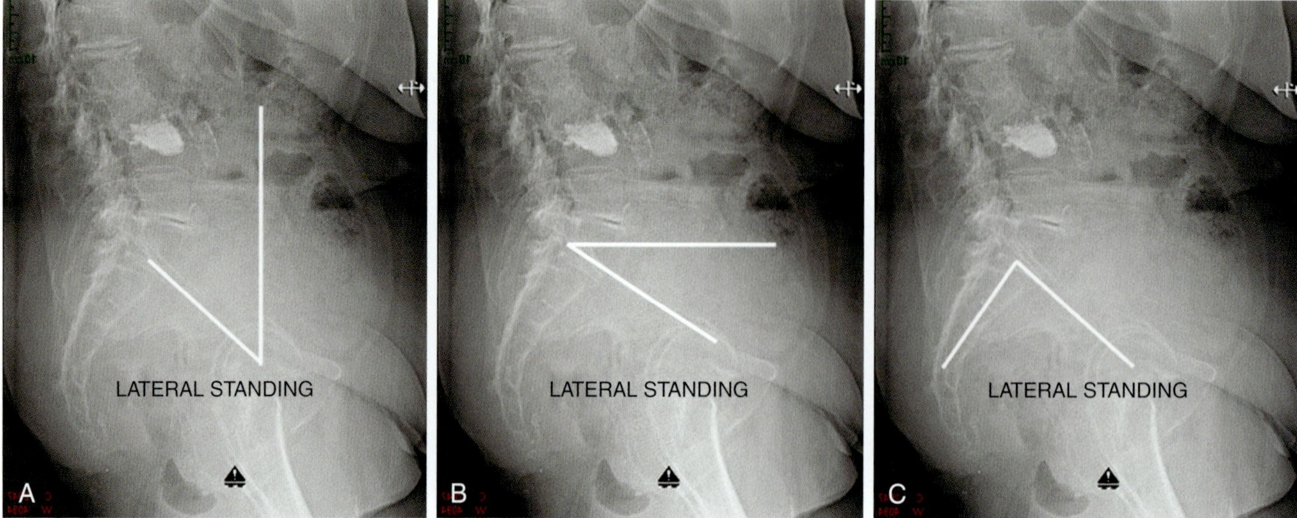

FIGURE 97-8. Demonstration of spinopelvic parameters used in surgical decision making. **A,** Pelvic tilt is the angle determined between a vertical reference line drawn up from the center of the femoral heads (femoral head axis) and a line drawn from the femoral head axis to the midpoint of the sacral end plate. **B,** Sacral slope is the angle subtended by a line drawn along the sacral end plate and a horizontal reference line. **C,** Pelvic incidence is measured by determining the angle between a line drawn perpendicular to the sacral end plate at its midpoint and a line from the femoral head axis to this point.

to this point. The pelvic incidence is equal to the pelvic tilt plus the sacral slope.[19]

$$\text{Pelvic incidence (PI)} = \text{Pelvic tilt (PT)} + \text{Sacral slope (SS)}$$

This relationship is important in operative decision making. For example, a patient may have a sagittal balance that appears closer to normal but is in fact maximally compensating by increasing the pelvic tilt. This would be evident by a high pelvic tilt (generally >25 degrees) and a decreased sacral slope. Not taking this compensation into account could lead to continued symptoms due to undercorrection in the sagittal plane.

The relationship between pelvic incidence and lumbar lordosis has been determined in normal subjects. It can be approximated by the pelvic incidence + 9 degrees (±9).[19]

$$\text{Lumbar lordosis (LL)} = \text{Pelvic incidence (PI)} + 9°(\pm 9)$$

This information can be used in patients with flat back deformity of the lumbar spine to calculate the degree of lumbar lordosis that needs to be recreated to regain proper lordosis.

Scoliosis Classification

Classification systems in spinal deformity are useful in that they can facilitate communication, allow comparison of similar cases, and provide a framework for an evidence-based approach to understanding prognosis and guiding management.[20,21] The need for a reliable adult classification system distinct from established pediatric scoliosis classification systems (i.e., King-Moe, Lenke) has recently been recognized.[22,23] Pediatric classification systems, when introduced, predominantly aimed to help select fusion levels for the correction of deformity in adolescent idiopathic scoliosis. In contrast, adult classification systems need to address a "wide variability in segmental, regional, and global alignment" plus incorporate the clinical symptoms affecting the patient in order to be clinically useful.[24]

Aebi Classification

In 2005, Max Aebi proposed classifying adult scoliosis into four groups based on the apparent etiology of the disease (Table 97-3).

Type I: primary degenerative ("de novo") scoliosis due to asymmetrical disc and facet joint degeneration occurring most commonly in the lumbar or thoracolumbar region (apex at L2-3 or L3-4 most frequently)

Type II: progressive idiopathic scoliosis due to continued progression of a curve that has existed since childhood or adolescence

TABLE 97-3

Aebi Classification of Adult Scoliosis

Type	Description	Etiology
I	Primary degenerative scoliosis, apex at L2, L3, or L4	Asymmetrical disc degeneration and facet joint degeneration
II	Progressive idiopathic scoliosis	Progression due to mechanical or degenerative changes of an already present adolescent scoliosis
III (a)	Secondary adult scoliosis	Secondary to an adjacent thoracic or thoracolumbar curve; obliquity of the pelvis with secondary lumbar/thoracolumbar curve
III (b)	Deformity progressing mostly due to bone weakness	Metabolic bone disease, osteoporosis

Modified from Aebi M: The adult scoliosis. *Eur Spine J* 14:925–948, 2005.

Type IIIa: secondary adult scoliosis with deformity due to a preexisting condition either intrinsic to the spine (i.e., an adjacent curve present since childhood or adolescence) or due to a condition extrinsic to the spine (i.e., pelvic obliquity caused by a leg length discrepancy)

Type IIIb: secondary adult deformity progressing due to bone weakness (i.e., caused by osteoporotic compression fracture)[25]

Schwab Classification

In 2006, Frank Schwab introduced a classification system for adult scoliosis based on "high impact clinically significant radiographic parameters" through a prospective study of 947 adult patients with deformity.[26] He justified this approach to classification through previous studies that demonstrated the "impact" of radiographic parameters on self-assessed function.[27-29] Interestingly, sagittal imbalance through a loss of lumbar lordosis and lumbar vertebra obliquity, not the Cobb angle on frontal radiographs, most closely correlated with pain scores on self-assessment. Other "impact" radiographic factors included global imbalance, apical level of scoliotic deformity, and intervertebral subluxation.

The original Schwab system categorizes patients into five groups based on location of the apex of the main (major) curve on standing frontal full-length radiographs (Box 97-1). The scheme then further classifies patients through the use of two modifiers accounting for degree of lumbar lordosis and subluxation on either frontal or sagittal radiographs, because these factors were found to have the highest clinical significance. In 2007, the classification system was modified to account for patients with deformity in the sagittal plane alone through the addition of a sixth group. In addition, a global balance modifier was added; this factor has been increasingly recognized as being "high impact"[30] (see Box 97-1).

Apical Level

The six groups of the Schwab classification are as follows:

Type I: patients with thoracic-only scoliosis, with no thoracolumbar or lumbar curvature

Type II: patients with an upper thoracic major curve, apex T4-8, with a thoracolumbar or lumbar minor curve

Type III: patients with a lower thoracic major curve, apex T9-10, with a thoracolumbar or lumbar minor curve

Type IV: patients with a thoracolumbar major curve, apex T11-L1, with any other minor curve

Type V: patients with a lumbar major curve, apex L2-4, with any other minor curve

Type K: patients with sagittal deformity alone

In instances of double major curvature, the lower curve is considered the major curve, for purpose of classification.

Lordosis Modifier

Lumbar lordosis of T12-S1 is determined using the Cobb method, and patients are assigned to three groups.

Group A: marked lumbar lordosis (>40 degrees)

Group B: only moderate lordosis (0–40 degrees)

Group C: no lordosis (Cobb >0 degrees; i.e., flat back)

BOX 97-1. Schwab Adult Classification of Adult Deformity

Type

Location of the deformity (apical level of the major curve *or* sagittal plane only)

- Type I: thoracic-only scoliosis (no thoracolumbar or lumbar component)
- Type II: upper thoracic major, apex T4-8 (with thoracolumbar or lumbar curve)
- Type III: lower thoracic major, apex T9-10 (with thoracolumbar/lumbar curve)
- Type IV: thoracolumbar major curve, apex T11-L1 (with any other minor curve)
- Type V: lumbar major curve, apex L2-4 (with any other minor curve)
- Type K: deformity in the sagittal plane only

Lordosis Modifier

Sagittal Cobb angle from T12 to S1

- A: marked lordosis, 40 degrees
- B: moderate lordosis, 0–40 degrees
- C: no lordosis (0 degrees)

Subluxation Modifier

Frontal or sagittal plane (ventral or dorsal), maximum value

- 0: no subluxation
- +: subluxation, 1–6 mm
- ++: subluxation, 7 mm

Global Balance Modifier

Sagittal plane C7 offset from dorsal/rostral corner S1

- N: normal (0–4 cm)
- P: positive, 4–9.5 cm
- VP: very positive, 9.5 cm

From Schwab F, Lafage V, Farcy JP, et al: Surgical rates and operative outcome analysis in thoracolumbar and lumbar major adult scoliosis: application of the new adult deformity classification. *Spine (Phila Pa 1976)* 32:2723–2730, 2007.

Subluxation Modifier

Schwab found olisthesis in either the frontal or sagittal plane to have similar clinical impacts. As a modifier for his classification system, maximal olisthesis on either frontal or sagittal view radiographs (at any level), determined in millimeters, is used to separate patients into three groups:

Group 0: no subluxation

Group +: 1 to 6 mm of subluxation

Group ++: more than 7 mm of subluxation

Global Balance Modifier

Sagittal balance is determined through measurement of the SVA offset (C7PL to dorsal/rostral corner of the sacrum, as described earlier). Patients are divided into three groups:

N: normal (0–4 cm)

P: positive (4–9.5 cm)

VP: very positive (>9.5 cm)

Since its introduction, the authors of the Schwab classification system have been examining the scheme with regard to how the type of deformity and modifiers relate to rates of surgery, surgical approach, use of osteotomies, and fusion extension to the sacrum, as well as to predictors of outcome and complications.[24,31] They found that modifiers of the classification had significant variation in surgical rates as the grade of modifier increased.[24] As lordosis is lost, surgical rates increase significantly (group A, 37%, group C, 51%; $P = .05$). With increasing subluxation (0–++), the operative rate increases from 35% to 52% ($P < .05$). Similarly, as sagittal balance increases from N to P to VP, surgical rate significantly increases 39%, 46%, and 58%, respectively (N vs. VP; $P = .02$). Loss of lumbar lordosis, lordosis modifiers B and C, and marked subluxation (modifier ++) were associated with more circumferential surgery. Sagittal imbalance was associated with higher rates of dorsal-only surgery. Osteotomies were also used more frequently in cases of sagittal imbalance and increasing loss of lumbar lordosis. Higher rates of fixation to the sacrum were found to be associated with loss of lumbar lordosis (groups B and C) and with increasing positive sagittal balance ($P = .0006$).[24]

In evaluating the system in terms of surgical outcome, the authors found that patients with no lordosis (modifier C) had the greatest disability prior to surgery, showed the greatest improvement with dorsal-only procedures, and had the least disability at 1-year follow-up.[24] Patients most likely to obtain significant benefit through surgery had higher grades of deformity through the classification modifiers and a higher degree of disability before surgery (high Oswestry Disability Index [ODI] score; low SRS and SF-12 scores). They propose that patients with less morbidity prior to surgical intervention have less of an opportunity to improve and may be more affected by the significant morbidity associated with surgery.[31]

Scoliosis Research Society Classification

In 2006, the SRS introduced and validated a classification system for adult deformity with the intention of providing an organizational structure for spinal deformity to permit comparison of similar cases and provide a framework for an evidence-based approach to operative and nonoperative management (Box 97-2).[20] The classification categorizes patients into seven types based on the major curve type on standing radiographs. Modifiers are added for deformity in the sagittal plane, degenerative changes in the lumbar spine, and global balance in the sagittal and coronal planes.

Major Curve Types

The system identifies six major coronal curve types, plus a seventh additional type:

Single thoracic (ST)
Double thoracic (DT)
Double major (DM)
Triple major (TM)
Thoracolumbar (TL)
Lumbar "de novo"/idiopathic (L)
Sagittal deformity without concurrent coronal deformity, or primary sagittal plane deformity (SP)

Sagittal Modifiers

A regional sagittal modifier is included in the SRS system to account for excessive kyphosis in each of the four regions of the spine. These are listed only if the regional degree of kyphosis exceeds the normal range.

BOX 97-2. Scoliosis Research Society Classification System for Adult Deformity

Primary Curve Types
- Single thoracic (ST)
- Double thoracic (DT)
- Double major (DM)
- Triple major (TM)
- Thoracolumbar (TL)
- Lumbar "de novo"/idiopathic (L)
- Primary sagittal plane deformity (SP)

Adult Spinal Deformity Modifiers

Regional sagittal modifier (include only if outside normal range, as listed)
- Proximal thoracic (PT; T2-5): 20 degrees
- Main thoracic (MT; T5-12): 50 degrees
- Thoracolumbar (TL; T10-L2): 20 degrees
- Lumbar (L; T12-S1): 40 degrees

Lumbar degenerative modifier (include only if present)
- Two-disc height and facet arthropathy based on radiograph; include lowest involved level between L1 and S1
- Listhesis (rotational, coronal, or sagittal) 3 mm; include lowest level between L1 and L5
- Junctional L5-S1 curve 10 degrees (intersection angle superior end plates L5 and S1)

Global balance modifier (include only if imbalance present)
- Sagittal C7 plumb 5 cm ventral or dorsal to sacral promontory
- Coronal C7 plumb 3 cm right or left of CSVL

Scoliosis Research Society definition of regions
- Thoracic: apex T2–11-12 disc
- Thoracolumbar: apex T12-L1
- Lumbar: apex L1-2 disc–L4

Criteria for specific major curve types

1. Thoracic curves
- Curve 40 degrees
- Apical vertebral body lateral to C7 plumb line
- T1 rib or clavicle angle 10 degrees upper thoracic curves

2. Thoracolumbar and lumbar curves
- Curve 30 degrees
- Apical vertebral body lateral to CSVL

3. Primary sagittal plane deformity
- No major coronal curve
- One or more regional sagittal measurements (PT, MT, TL, L) outside normal range

CSVL, central sacral vertical line.
From Lowe T, Berven SH, Schwab FJ, et al: The SRS classification for adult spinal deformity: building on the King/Moe and Lenke classification systems. *Spine (Phila Pa 1976)* 31:S119–S125, 2006.

Proximal thoracic (PT) T2-5 for kyphosis: greater than or equal to 20 degrees
Main thoracic (MT) T5-12 for kyphosis: greater than or equal to 50 degrees
Thoracolumbar (TL) T10-L2 for kyphosis: greater than or equal to 20 degrees
Lumbar (L) T12-S1 for kyphosis (loss of lordosis): greater than or equal to −40 degrees

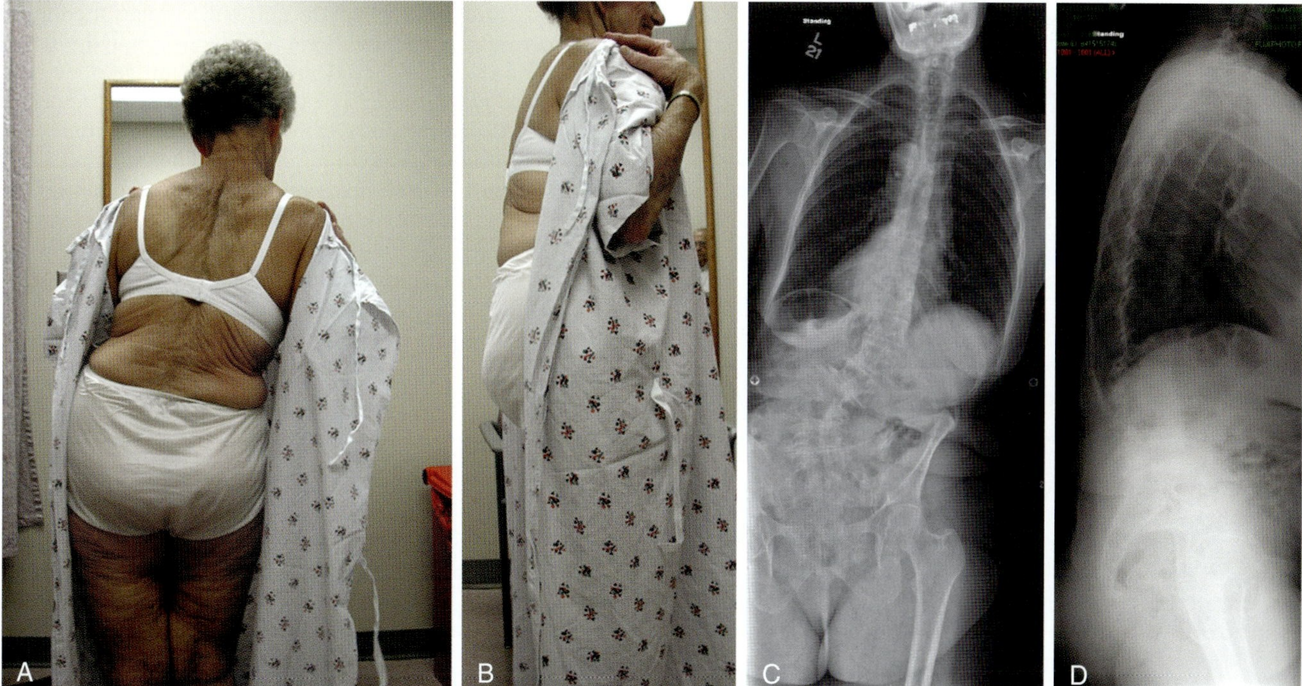

FIGURE 97-9. Clinical frontal (**A**) and lateral (**B**) photographs, as well as posteroanterior (**C**) and lateral (**D**) upright radiographs of a 70-year-old woman with back and leg pain. The patient has degenerative scoliosis. Using the Schwab classification system, the patient has a type V lumbar major curve, type B moderate lordosis modifier, + subluxation modifier, and N (normal) global balance modifier. Thus, it is type VB + N. Using the Scoliosis Research Society classification system, the patient has an L lumbar "de novo" curve, with degenerative disc disease (DDD), listhesis (LIS), and coronal balance (CB) modifiers. Thus, it is type L DDD LIS CB.

Lumbar Degenerative Modifiers

Lumbar degenerative change modifiers were included in the system because it has been recognized that degenerative changes within the lumbar spine are often responsible for the presenting clinical symptoms in adult patients with deformity.[20] Modifiers included in the system account for the following conditions:

- Degenerative disc disease: evidence of decreased disc height and facet arthropathy on radiograph (L1-S1)
- Listhesis: greater than 3 mm in any plane (rotational, coronal, sagittal) (L1-5)
- Junctional L5-S1 curve: greater than 10 degrees

Global Balance Modifier

The global balance modifier was included to describe imbalance in either the coronal or sagittal planes. A sagittal balance modifier is included if the sagittal C7PL lies greater than or equal to 5 cm either ventral or dorsal to the sacral promontory. A coronal balance modifier is included if the coronal C7PL lies greater than or equal to 3 cm to either side of the CSVL.

The SRS system was evaluated for interobserver variability through the analysis of 14 expert surgeons' choice of classification of 25 radiographic cases. There was good interobserver reliability for primary curve type ($\kappa = 0.64$), regional sagittal modifier ($\kappa = 0.73$), degenerative lumbar modifier ($\kappa = 0.65$), and global balance modifier ($\kappa = 0.92$). These same surgeons were queried regarding selection of fusion levels for operative intervention. Although there was good agreement on selection of the caudal level ($\kappa = 0.77$), there was significantly higher variability in choice of cephalad level ($\kappa = 0.56$).[20]

Figure 97-9 shows a case example of a patient with adult degenerative scoliosis. This patient demonstrates how to use both the Schwab and SRS classification systems properly.

Initial Management of Adult Thoracic and Lumbar Deformity

Indications for operative intervention in adult deformity include worsening pain, worsening neurologic function, progression of the deformity clinically and radiographically, and failure of nonoperative management. Predictive models are being developed to determine which patients will receive the most benefit through operative versus nonoperative approaches to deformity.[31] In most instances, conservative management is attempted before proceeding with surgery (often prior to referral to a spine surgeon), although evidence to support many of the modalities used is lacking. Nonoperative strategies include pain management with oral analgesics and nonsteroidal anti-inflammatory drugs, fluoroscopic-guided steroid injections (epidural steroid injection, facet joint blocks, selective nerve root block), physical therapy to increase core strength (including strategies to help unload the spine such as aquatic therapy), and nonconventional therapies such as massage and acupuncture.[32] Bracing has not been shown to be of considerable benefit in adult deformity and may lead to deconditioning.[32,33]

In 2010, Glassman et al. evaluated the costs and benefits of nonoperative management for adult scoliosis in a cohort of 123 patients. The researchers used data collected prospectively over a 2-year period. They divided patients into three groups based on degree of disability: low-symptom (ODI ≤ 20), mid-symptom (ODI 21 to 39), and high-symptom (ODI ≥ 40). Fewer total resources were used by the low-symptom group; however, all groups used substantial resources. Modalities included medications, exercise therapy, injections, physical therapy, chiropractic care, bed rest, and bracing. None of these treatments demonstrated benefit as measured by health-related quality of life (HR-QOL) scores. Patients who received no treatment actually showed slightly better outcomes over the 2-year period than patients who had some form of nonoperative therapy. The mean cost of treatment was $4418 in the first year and $6397 in the second year. There was no significant difference in treatment cost between the groups.[34]

Several recent papers have demonstrated significant, long-term benefit for the surgical management of patients, including the elderly, with adult deformity.[35-37] Smith et al., in a recent retrospective review of prospectively collected multicenter data for adult deformity, evaluated 206 patients treated surgically for deformity. Patients were divided into groups based on age: 25 to 44 years, 45 to 64 years, and 65 to 85 years. Risks and benefits were assessed through evaluation of complications suffered (minor and major) and through accepted measures of health status, disability, and pain (HR-QOL, ODI, SF-12, SRS-22 questionnaire, Numeric Rating Scale [NRS]). In each of the age groups evaluated, outcome measures improved significantly on 2-year follow-up. The oldest group of patients at baseline had the greatest degree of disability and pain as well as the worst health status of the groups. The eldest group also experienced the highest rate of surgical complications, having close to four times the number of minor complications and five times the number of major complications when compared to the youngest age group.[37] Despite this, the group with the oldest patients at 2 years had measures of disability, pain, and health status indistinguishable from the other groups.[37] These results suggested that elderly high-risk patients may stand to gain disproportionately greater improvement in disability and pain."[37] However, the degree of disability has to be weighed against an individual's comorbidities and risk of surgical complications. Conservative management should be attempted initially in most cases.

Factors that can affect outcome should be addressed prior to intervention. Smoking is a relative contraindication to spinal fusion procedures, because it leads to higher rates of pseudarthrosis. In his recent evaluation of reoperation after primary fusion for adult spinal deformity, Mok found that smoking was a significant risk factor for revision.[38] Patients who smoke should make every attempt not only to quit but to wean themselves from nicotine dependence. Bone health, especially in elderly patients, needs to be considered and maximized.[39] A bone mineral density scan should be obtained in patients suspected of being osteopenic or osteoporotic, and medical therapy to increase bone density started if indicated. The vitamin D level should be checked, and supplementation with vitamin D and calcium should be started in many patients. Patients with significant medical comorbidities should have appropriate clearance for operative intervention. Finally, patients suspected of having some respiratory compromise should have pulmonary function tests and an evaluation by a pulmonologist.

Summary

Clinical and radiographic evaluation of adult thoracic and lumbar deformity is complex, and it is important for the clinician treating these patients to have an appreciation of the current approaches, including an understanding of the classification systems. Selection of fusion level, choice of approach (ventral or dorsal, or both), need for osteotomies for deformity correction, need for pelvic fixation, and need for screw augmentation should all be considered prior to proceeding to the operating room. Patient factors will dictate many of these decisions, and there is often more than one correct way to proceed. Techniques for the surgical management of adult deformity will be discussed in a later chapter.

KEY REFERENCES

Aebi M: The adult scoliosis. *Eur Spine J* 14:925–948, 2005.

Bridwell KH, Baldus C, Berven S, et al: Changes in radiographic and clinical outcomes with primary treatment adult spinal deformity surgeries from two years to three- to five-years follow-up. *Spine (Phila Pa 1976)* 35:1849–1854, 2010.

Lenke LG, Betz RR, Harms Jr, et al: Adolescent idiopathic scoliosis. *J Bone Joint Surg [Am]* 83:1169, 2001.

Smith JS, Shaffrey CI, Glassman SD, et al: Risk-benefit assessment of surgery for adult scoliosis: an analysis based on patient age. *Spine (Phila Pa 1976)* 36(15):1218–1228, 2011.

Smith JS, Shaffrey CI, Kuntz CIV, et al: Classification systems for adolescent and adult scoliosis. *Neurosurgery* 63:A16–A24, 2008.

Stokes IA: Three-dimensional terminology of spinal deformity. A report presented to the Scoliosis Research Society by the Scoliosis Research Society Working Group on 3-D terminology of spinal deformity. *Spine (Phila Pa 1976)* 19:236–248, 1994.

REFERENCES

The complete reference list is available online at expertconsult.com.

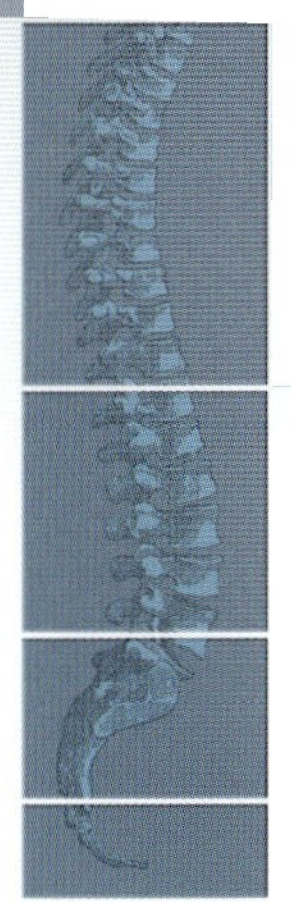

An Approach for Treatment of Complex Adult Spinal Deformity

R. Douglas Orr

Complex spinal deformities arise from numerous pathologies. In some cases, they manifest as large-magnitude curves associated with idiopathic scoliosis or kyphosis. Such deformities may be the result of secondary deformity from neuromuscular disease, congenital anomalies, infection, or trauma. The two major groups in terms of volume are decompensated deformities that are due to degenerative change in the preexisting curve and iatrogenic deformities.

The range of normal for cervical lordosis, thoracic kyphosis, and lumbar lordosis is quite variable.[1-3] Varying degrees of scoliosis can be tolerated depending on many other factors. As a result, spinal balance apparently is more important in terms of symptoms and progression than the magnitude of scoliosis or kyphosis. A review by Kuntz et al.[1] showed that there is only a narrow range of spinal balance and that this is highly conserved.

Clinically, spinal balance can be assessed by examining the head position of a standing patient in relation to the pelvis. In the lateral view, a plumb line from the ear canal should pass through or behind the greater trochanter. In the anteroposterior view, a plumb line from the inion should pass between the posterior superior iliac spines. Radiographically on a long cassette film, one can use either the C7 vertebral body or the odontoid as the starting point for a plumb line. Use of the odontoid as a marker allows assessment of cervical deformity in overall spinal balance. A plumb line from the odontoid should pass dorsal to the center of rotation of the hip in the lateral plane and should fall between the medial borders of the S1 pedicle in the anteroposterior plane. A plumb line from the C7 vertebral body should pass through the L5-S1 disc space. Figure 98-1 shows preoperative anteroposterior (see Fig. 98-1A) and lateral (see Fig. 98-1B) views of a patient with decompensated kyphoscoliosis with loss of both sagittal and coronal balance. Postoperative views of the same patient show restoration of balance (see Figs. 98-1C and D).

In many patients with spinal deformity, in particular, in adults, the clinical picture can be complex, and the decision-making process can seem daunting. When a patient with a complex deformity presents for evaluation, it is often difficult to know where to start. Having a systematic approach to assessment and planning of treatment makes treatment easier. A complex problem can be made easier to understand if it is broken down into its component parts. The author uses a four-part process to do this, and this chapter uses this framework to discuss the treatment of complex spinal deformity. The four components are *problems*, *goals*, *options*, and *plans*.

Define the Problem

Although it may seem simplistic, it is important to begin the process by defining the problem. In contrast to idiopathic adolescent scoliosis, in which the predominant focus is on the magnitude and progression of the deformity, there are more factors to consider in adult deformity. One key clinical difference in adult deformity is that adults generally seek treatment for the symptoms of the deformity rather than the deformity itself.[4] As a result, the deformity is viewed within the context of the symptoms it produces. In addition, comorbidities need to be considered. In many cases, the patient will already have had other spine procedures.

The first step is a detailed history. What is the main presenting problem? How does it affect the quality of life? How has it changed over time? If the effect on quality of life is relatively minimal, what is the likelihood of the problem progressing? In many patients, nonoperative treatment may be a viable option even in the presence of significant deformities. It is also important to understand the patient's perception of the problem. In the author's experience, some patients present with few symptoms but desire aggressive treatment because of fear that progression of the problem will lead to paralysis or death. Other patients present seeking information or to establish a relationship with a practitioner in case symptoms worsen.

Comorbidities are an important part of the history if one is considering surgery. In addition to cardiovascular and pulmonary conditions, nutritional status and risk factors for osteoporosis should be considered. If the patient has had prior surgery, it is important to know what was done. It is also important to know why the surgery was performed and what the short-term and longer-term outcome of the surgery was. Prior investigations and operative reports are very valuable in the assessment if they can be obtained. In some cases, the deformity may be iatrogenic.

The physical examination should include a detailed neurologic examination. Examination of spinal alignment and balance is important. Loss of sagittal and coronal balance is associated with increased symptoms and seems to have a higher risk of progression.[5-7]

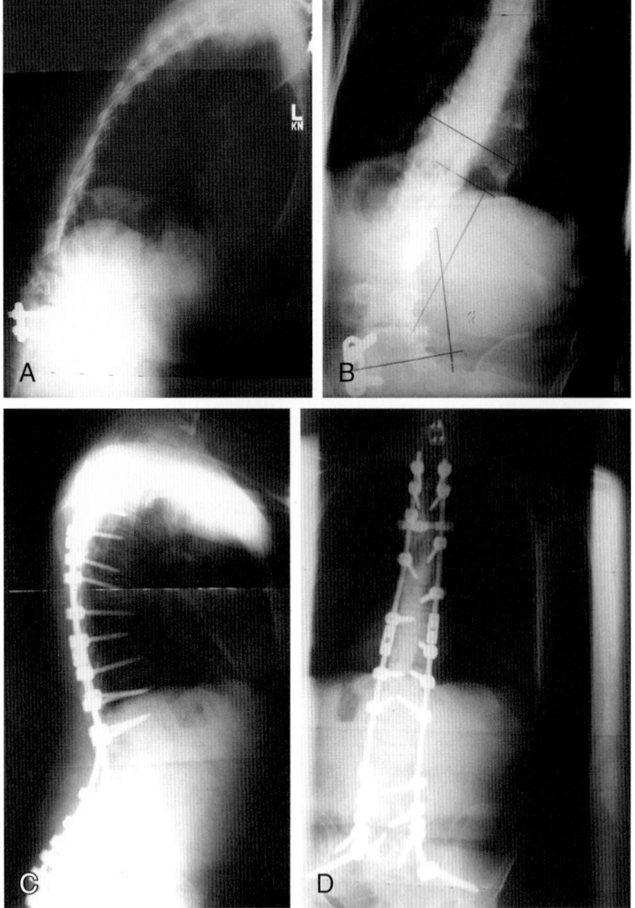

FIGURE 98-1. **A,** Preoperative anteroposterior view of a 58-year-old woman with decompensated kyphoscoliosis. There is a lateral trunk shift. **B,** Preoperative lateral view. The C7 vertebra is significantly in front of the L5-S1 disc space. **C** and **D,** Postoperative anteroposterior (**C**) and lateral (**D**) films. A plumb line from C7 would not pass through the L5-S1 disc space in both planes.

Imaging studies are an integral part of defining the problem. Conventional radiographs in the standing position including the entire spine and pelvis are the standard method of assessing deformity. Lateral bending films can assess the flexibility of the coronal deformity. Supine films (often done with a bolster under the apex of the deformity) can help assess the flexibility of sagittal plane deformities. MRI is the investigation of choice for assessing the status of the discs and the neural axis. CT provides excellent assessment of the bony anatomy, and the use of sagittal and coronal reformatting allows a more detailed assessment of the bony architecture. If a patient has had prior surgeries, CT is a sensitive and specific method of assessing fusion status. Myelography with or without CT may make assessment of the neural axis easier in large deformities. Bone scan has historically been used for assessment of pseudarthrosis but has been largely supplanted by CT in the author's practice.

In patients in whom surgery is being considered and comorbidities are present, general and specialty medical consultation for preoperative optimization should be used.[8] Nutritional and bone health status are often overlooked in the workup and can have significant effects on outcome.[9-12] Bone mineral density testing can help to assess bone health, although the presence of degenerative changes in the spine may artificially increase bone mineral density of the spine.[13,14] Vitamin D testing and supplementation in the preoperative period should be considered, especially in regions or cultures where there is little direct sun exposure.[15,16] In large-magnitude thoracic deformities, pulmonary function testing should be done for risk assessment.[17]

Goals

After the problem has been defined, the next step is to decide on the goals of treatment. It is important to assess the patient's goals for treatment as well as the practitioner's goals. Are these goals achievable and at what risk? Patients with minimal symptoms in daily life who have limits with high-level activities may desire a level of function that is not achievable. Alternatively, for a patient with low demands and expectations, simpler nonoperative treatments may provide an appropriate quality of life without the risks associated with addressing the deformity.

Prevention of progression is a common goal in treatment of deformity. In adult deformity, progression is unpredictable for many conditions, and progression of symptoms may or may not correlate with progression of deformity.[18-20] As a result, prevention of progression is an uncommon indication for treatment after skeletal maturity.[21-23]

Generally, the goals of surgical treatment are to relieve compression of neural elements, stabilize instabilities, and correct and maintain the correction of the deformity. These goals need to be accomplished while minimizing risk in the short term and the long term. A primary end result of deformity treatment should be the restoration of sagittal and coronal balance. Outcome studies have shown weak, if any, correlation between correction of the Cobb angle and outcome but have shown clear correlation with spinal balance and outcome.[6,7,24-27]

Osteoporosis

Osteoporosis is common in patients with spinal deformity. It may be associated with vertebral fractures leading to increased deformity.[21,28] It also may have an effect on outcome of surgery.[11,29] Although osteoporosis does not affect bone healing, it does affect the holding power of spine instrumentation.[30-32] For this reason, assessment of osteoporosis is an important step when considering surgery. Although there is no quoted level of bone density beyond which surgery is not an option, the risks of failure increase with higher degrees of bone loss. Preoperative optimization of bone health with vitamin D testing and supplementation as required and pretreatment with teriparatide have been advocated,[16] but no studies have looked at outcomes of these interventions. Animal studies have suggested that teriparatide may improve healing of fusions.[33,34]

Options

Decompression Alone

In patients with a stable balanced spine with isolated radiculopathy, one option may be to consider an isolated decompression. Generally, compressive pathology occurs on the concavity of the deformity.[35] If a single level can be identified either on the basis of clinical symptoms or with nerve root blocks, an isolated decompression may be a reasonable option. There is a risk that decompression may exacerbate deformity in these patients. Previous studies showed that the results of decompression alone in the presence of scoliosis may not be as good as decompression in a normally aligned spine.[36-38] Many of these studies were done with more extensive decompression than would be done at the present time. Decompression alone is not an option in the presence of a rotatory subluxation or spondylolisthesis at the apex of the deformity. Anecdotally, decompressions of a keyhole or laminotomy type are associated with a lower risk of progression of deformity.[39,40] This option may be particularly good in elderly patients with an isolated radiculopathy and relatively minimal axial back pain.

Fusion without Instrumentation

In patients with severe osteoporosis, use of pedicle screw instrumentation may be contraindicated. In these patients, an option may be fusion without instrumentation. This procedure is reserved for patients with stable balanced deformities. Generally, fusion without instrumentation is used in patients who are much older, more frail, and less able to tolerate extensive procedures. There is little or no literature on this procedure, and consequently it is difficult to compare it with other techniques.

Limited Fusion

In many patients, symptoms can be isolated to a single level of pathology. An example would be a degenerative spondylolisthesis and a degenerative scoliosis. In these patients, it may be reasonable to treat only the symptomatic level. This is a controversial treatment. In a more recent study, reasonably good results were obtained with single-level fusion for degenerative spondylolisthesis in degenerative scoliosis. A few patients needed further surgery, and few if any had progression of deformity.[41] Some authors have criticized this technique as having an unacceptably high rate of failure.[42] However, there are no controlled trials comparing it with more extensive fusion; the literature contains few articles.[43,44]

One more recent trial[45] looked at surgeons whose practice contained more than 50% deformity cases and showed that these surgeons were more likely to perform fusion of more levels than surgeons whose practice contained less than 50% deformity cases. The authors implied that the surgeons with more deformity cases were more likely to select a correct course; however, there was no clinical correlation in this study. It is perhaps equally valid to suggest that the surgeons with more deformity cases were more likely to perform fusion of excess levels.

Instrumented Correction and Fusion

In most patients with complex deformity, some form of instrumented correction and fusion is performed. Multiple options are available, and each option has advantages and disadvantages. The end result should be a stable balanced spine with a solid biologic fusion. Any technique that achieves this goal is a reasonable option.

In most cases, pedicle screw instrumentation is the mainstay of instrumented fusion. Pedicle screws allow better correction of most deformities.[46-50] Pedicle screws are extremely versatile and have excellent holding power. They can exert or resist forces in multiple planes. Pedicle screws tend to be weakest in pull-out.[51] As a result of their versatility, pedicle screws have become the main type of instrumentation used. Hooks and wires are less commonly used because they are more technically demanding and less versatile. Hooks and wires are relatively strong in pull-out but need intact posterior elements.

Obtaining solid biologic fusion is of utmost importance in the long-term. Fusion can be achieved through interbody, dorsal, or dorsolateral fusion. Interbody techniques generally have a higher fusion rate.[52-54] In the lumbar spine, dorsolateral fusion is biomechanically superior and more effective than laminar onlay fusion.[55] In the thoracic spine, dorsal fusion is more typically performed. The biology of fusion, choice of bone graft or bone graft substitute, and use of extenders are discussed elsewhere. In complex surgery with the high risk of fusion failure, the choice of bone graft and bone graft substitutes is of great importance. The use of bone morphogenetic protein in deformity seems to lead to significantly higher fusion rates. Limited evidence suggests that it is cost-effective in this indication.[56-58]

Selection of rostral and caudal levels is the first step in determining an operative plan. Generally, the construct should begin and end at a neutral vertebra in both the sagittal and the coronal planes. In complex or degenerative deformities, it is often more difficult to determine these levels than in an idiopathic scoliosis. The presence significant disc degeneration or instability below a neutral vertebra would generally necessitate extension of the fusion beyond this.[59,60] Perhaps the most controversial question is whether or not to end a fusion at the L5 vertebra. Numerous studies have been performed and reached conflicting results.[61-65]

A series of studies by Lenke et al.[61,62] looked at this question and concluded that if the L5-S1 disc is relatively normal on MRI and the L5 vertebral body does not have an oblique takeoff, preserving the L5-S1 motion segment is a reasonable option. In these patients, the incidence of repeat surgery to fuse the 5/1 level was lower than the incidence of repeat surgery for pseudarthrosis. In the presence of significant L5-S1 disc degeneration or oblique takeoff or instability at L5-S1, the incidence of repeat surgery to fuse the 5/1 level was higher than the incidence of surgery for pseudarthrosis.

Numerous factors must be looked at in considering the upper stop point of the construct. The thoracolumbar junction represents a transition from the mobile lumbar spine to the stiffer thoracic spine. Constructs extending up from the sacrum to the lumbosacral junction can create a stress riser if stopped at the junction. Typically, it has been considered acceptable to stop such a construct at L2, but constructs longer than this should extend to T10[59,60,66,67]; however, a more recent study has called this into question. In this study, there seemed to be no clearly defined level at which the risk of subsequent surgery was lessened.[66] In deciding to stop in the lower thoracic spine, one must also consider whether this stop point is at the apex of the thoracic kyphosis. In patients in whom a fusion stops at the apex of the thoracic kyphosis, there is significant risk of proximal junctional kyphosis. It may be preferable in these patients to extend the construct up into the upper thoracic spine, typically T4 or T5.[59,60]

Long fusion constructs to the sacrum have a high incidence of failure because of pseudarthrosis at L5-S1. This pseudarthrosis is due to numerous biomechanical and anatomic factors. The S1 pedicle is more cancellous and has a short anteroposterior diameter, and the holding power of S1 pedicle screws is less than at other levels. In addition, forces at this level are magnified because of the relatively large lever arm exerted by the pelvis.[65,69] Many strategies have been suggested to increase the fusion right at L5-S1. Primary among these strategies is the use of interbody fusion through either a ventral or a dorsal approach.[65] This strategy has been shown to decrease pseudarthrosis.

More recent studies have assessed anterior lumbar interbody fusion and compared it with posterior lumbar interbody fusion or transforaminal lumbar interbody fusion. None of these techniques showed clear superiority in these studies.[68-71] McCord et al.[72] analyzed alternative fixation techniques at the lumbosacral junction; this study led to the concept of the *pivot point*, which is the region of the dorsal aspect of the anulus fibrosus at L5-S1. Fixation at the lumbosacral junction should extend ventral to this pivot point to provide increased stability. Sacral alar screws, S2 screws, iliac bars and screws, and iliosacral screws have been suggested for this procedure. Biomechanical studies showed increased rigidity with the use of iliac or sacroiliac screws, and clinical studies suggested that these two fixation types are superior to sacral alar or S2 screws.[70-77] In a longitudinal series by Kostuik and Musha,[65] pseudarthrosis rates were decreased from 83% to 3% by the use of interbody fusion and iliac fixation.

Many authors have advocated increasing deformity correction through the use of anterior releases and fusions.[78,79] It is believed that this approach increases correction and increases the fusion rate. However, more recent studies have called this into question.[80-82] With the use of segmental pedicle screw fixation and alternative release techniques, equivalent deformity correction can be obtained through purely dorsal procedures without the morbidity[83] of an anterior release. These studies compared more traditional open anterior release techniques. With the advent of new or less invasive procedures and the use of interbody fusions through a direct lateral approach, the morbidity of anterior releases may be significantly less. Such minimal access lateral approaches and fusion techniques have been shown to give good correction, high fusion rates, and reasonably good clinical results.[84-86] In the author's practice, these techniques have replaced traditional open releases and fusions. The use of these techniques at the L4-5 level should be considered cautiously. The anatomic corridor is small,[87,88] and there is a relatively high rate of L3 neurapraxia.[86] The author no longer uses minimal access lateral techniques for the L4-5 level.

Instrumentation in Osteoporosis

The presence of osteoporosis increases the failure rate of instrumented constructs in deformity surgery. Osteoporosis compromises the holding power of the implants leading to this increased failure rate. Numerous strategies have been mediated to lessen this failure risk, and Hu[29] summarized them well in a review article. Essentially, these strategies all are methods of dispersing or decreasing forces across the construct. Increasing the number of fixation points decreases the stress on each element of the construct. Cement augmentation of pedicle screws has been shown to increase their pull-out resistance. Generally, it is unnecessary to perform cement augmentation of all fixation points; only the points at the ends of the construct need to be reinforced with cement. There is relatively more loss of cancellous than cortical bone in osteoporosis, and fixation that uses cortical bone is relatively stronger. As a result, laminar hooks may be a good option in a kyphosis construct, which is likely to fail in pull-out. If correction can be obtained through osteotomies or releases, loads on the hardware are more likely to be neutral, and the construct is less susceptible to hardware failure.[12,29,89,90]

Osteoporosis has been considered a relative contraindication to the use of interbody fusions. Biomechanical studies by Cunningham and Polly[91] showed that use of interbody fusion increases the strength and rigidity of constructs. Interbody grafts or cages placed asymmetrically can be used to obtain correction, allowing the hardware to be in neutral and decreasing the risk of hardware failure.[92]

Interspinous Spacers

Interspinous spacers such as the X-Stop (Medtronic, Memphis, TN) are indicated for treatment of spinal stenosis in the absence of deformity. In the U.S. Food and Drug Administration (FDA) studies, scoliosis was an exclusion criterion. It has been suggested that these spacers may be used in an off-label manner for the treatment of stenotic symptoms in the presence of deformity.[93] The author has used interspinous spacers in rare cases of patients with severe medical comorbidities and significant deformity who would not tolerate traditional surgery. The results have been mixed, but there have been few complications. Further studies are warranted.

Osteotomies

Osteotomies are powerful tools in the treatment of complex deformity. Many of these deformities are very rigid, and in patients who have undergone previous surgery, the deformity may be fixed owing to fusions. Osteotomies are generally used to correct sagittal plane deformities but may also be used to correct coronal and biplanar deformities. They can be very technically demanding but can give excellent clinical results.

The simplest osteotomies to perform are facet resection osteotomies as described by Ponte or Smith-Petersen. There is confusion as to nomenclature of these osteotomies. Smith-Petersen et al.[94] described a procedure where the facet was resected and the disc released leading to a pivot at the dorsal corner of the vertebral body, causing closure of the osteotomy dorsally and extension through the disc space ventrally. This procedure was originally described in ankylosing spondylitis. The more common facet resection and closure through a mobile disc was first described by Wilson and Turkell[95] but has been widely attributed to Ponte.[96] For clarity, the author uses facet resection osteotomy.

These osteotomies can be used anywhere there is a mobile disc. Correction of 5 to 10 degrees of kyphosis can readily be obtained, and multiple levels can be used.[97,98] Some coronal correction can be obtained as well. Facet resections can also be used to increase the correction of the coronal deformity. A facet resection osteotomy augmented by an interbody fusion can increase the amount of correction obtained through this technique. An example is shown in Figure 98-2.

If larger degrees of correction are required, a pedicle subtraction osteotomy can be considered. This is a closing wedge osteotomy performed by removing the posterior elements of the pedicle and a portion of the vertebral body. First described by Scudese and Colabro,[99] this is a very powerful technique that allows routine correction of 30 degrees or more.[97,98] It has typically been performed at lumbar levels[100-102] but can be performed safely in the thoracic spine as well.[103,104] These procedures are technically demanding and associated with significant complications.[105-107] Clinical results are very good. Biplanar correction can also be achieved allowing correction of deformity in more than one plane.[100-102]

Two basic types of pedicle subtraction osteotomy have been described. In the first type, osteotomes are used to create a wedge, which is then removed. The alternative procedure is a decancellation osteotomy. In this procedure, the vertebra is decancellized, the dorsal wall is reduced into the cavity, the lateral wall is osteotomized, and the osteotomy is closed.[108] No comparison studies of these two techniques exist. Figure 98-3 shows the preoperative and postoperative radiographs of a patient with a posttraumatic kyphosis treated with a pedicle subtraction osteotomy to restore lumbar lordosis.

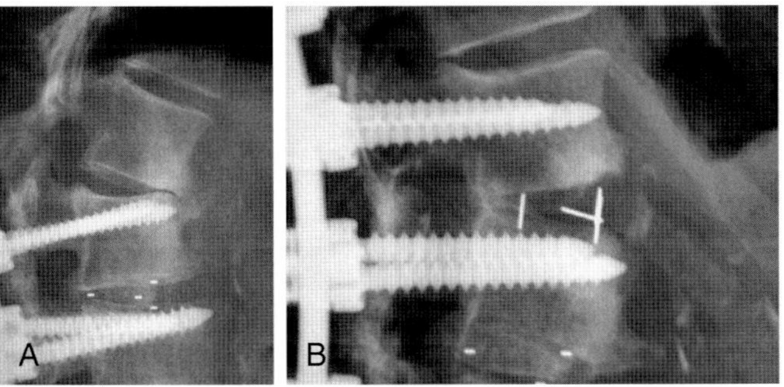

FIGURE 98-2. A, Preoperative lateral view of focal kyphosis above a previous fusion. **B,** Postoperative lateral view shows approximately 20 degrees of correction with facet resection osteotomy and interbody implant.

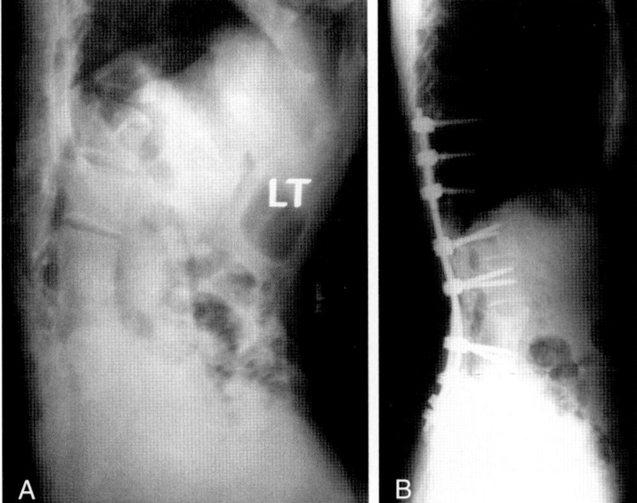

FIGURE 98-3. A, Preoperative lateral view of a 38-year-old woman 20 years after operative treatment of L5 burst fracture shows significant lumbar kyphosis in a fused spine. **B,** Postoperative film shows correction through L3 pedicle subtraction osteotomy.

Vertebral Column Resection

In some very complex high-magnitude deformities, complete resection of one or more vertebral segments may be required to correct deformity. This procedure is called a *vertebal column resection*. It can be done through a combined anteroposterior or a dorsal-only approach.[97,102,109,110] This technique may be used in an apical kyphectomy for spina bifida.[111] This procedure can be used for both kyphosis and scoliosis and may be used to obtain biplanar correction. In some cases, the anterior column is reconstructed with a graft or cage implant; in other cases, the spinal column is shortened. These procedures are also associated with significant risks. Reasonably good clinical results have been reported.[97,101,109,112-115]

Plans

After the specific problem has been defined and the goals of surgery established, the operation should be planned. Careful preoperative planning and communication of the plan to the operative team make the procedure more efficient and safer.

In the preoperative period, steps should be taken to ensure the patient is optimally prepared for surgery. The author considers smoking cessation to be mandatory for all such procedures. Preoperative consultation with a hematologist for blood management may help optimize hemoglobin before surgery.[116] Studies have suggested an increased risk of thrombotic complications with the use of erythropoietin analogues, so the risks and benefits must be balanced.[117,118] Preoperative medical cardiology and pulmonology consultations should be obtained as indicated.[8,17]

If a combined anteroposterior approach is being considered, one must decide whether to use a single-day or staged multiday approach. Single-day procedures have the advantage of only a single anesthetic and recovery period but can result in very long procedures with excessive blood loss. Single-day procedures may also be more demanding on the surgeon. Staged procedures may be less physically demanding for the patient and the surgeon. Studies that have compared single-day and multiday approaches showed no clear benefit of one over the other.[119-124] It is the author's practice to do most of these procedures as a single-day surgery but to stage them if the procedure is particularly complex or complications arise.

Complex surgeries often require large inventories of implants. It is important to coordinate with equipment suppliers to ensure an adequate supply of appropriate implants is available. The plan should include determining whether any special implants or instruments are required for the procedure. These sets should be present before beginning the procedure. If an access surgeon is being used for the approach, the appropriate sets for this surgeon should be obtained as well.

Neurologic monitoring should be considered for all of these procedures. At the author's institution, somatosensory-evoked and motor-evoked potentials are used for all spinal deformity cases. Stimulated electromyographic monitoring is used for minimal access lateral lumbar approaches. Neurologic monitoring has been shown to decrease the risk of neurologic injury.[125,126] If motor-evoked potentials are to be used, this should be communicated to the anesthesiologist to ensure that neuromuscular blockade is not used during the procedure.

Intraoperative red blood cell salvage is routinely used in complex surgery to reduce the use of autologous blood donation.[127-129]

Intraoperative imaging is facilitated by the use of a radiolucent table. Radiographs obtained intraoperatively in both sagittal and coronal planes allow an estimate of correction obtained and implant placement. Intraoperative fluoroscopy may be used to guide implant placement. CT-based navigation systems have been shown to increase accuracy of screw placement, particularly in significant deformities.[130,131] Clinically, however, freehand placement of pedicle screws has been shown to be safe and effective.[132-134] The author prefers to use freehand techniques for placement of pedicle screws in most primary cases and to use fluoroscopy or navigation in complex or revision instrumentation.

Numerous techniques have been described for determining the magnitude of angle needed to be corrected in the sagittal plane to restore balance. Perhaps the simplest way to do this is to cut a 3-foot film at the level of the planned osteotomy, balance the head over the pelvis, and measure the subtended angle. With the advent of digital radiography, printed 3-foot films are becoming rare, and this is no longer as good an option. A second option is to measure the angle subtended between a vertical line at the pivot point of the planned osteotomy and either the C7 or the C1 vertebral body. An osteotomy higher in the lumbar spine requires a greater angle of correction for a given amount of linear translation of the head.[135] Ondra et al.[135-137] described two mathematical models for determining osteotomy correction. Although these models are effective, the author finds them cumbersome to use in clinical practice.

It is generally recommended to overcorrect sagittal deformity by 5 to 10 degrees to compensate for loss of hip extension that occurs with aging. This recommendation applies to constructs extending to the sacrum. Aging patients with a normal lumbar spine are able to compensate for the loss of hip extension by rotating the pelvis through the lumbar spine. Patients who have fusions extending to the sacrum have lost this compensation. The loss of hip extension prevents normal stride through with gait; when this occurs, a patient who is able to stand in neutral sagittal balance is forced to walk in positive sagittal balance to have a normal gait. Preoperative examination of these patients should include careful assessment of the range of motion of the hip. Treating hip flexion contractures through either physical therapy or surgical releases may need to be considered before osteotomies.

Even with an extensive preoperative workup, it is sometimes difficult to predict how much correction of the deformity will be obtained at the time of surgery and with successive stages of the surgery. Consequently, operative plans are often flexible. Anterior interbody fusions with lordotic graft or cages may provide significant correction in patients with collapsed discs. Positioning on a four-post frame in the prone position often provides significant correction of a deformity that did not seem flexible. If one is planning a pedicle subtraction osteotomy through a level with mobile discs, it may be advisable to obtain an intraoperative lateral radiograph after the facet resection to determine if sufficient correction has been obtained through these methods to eliminate the need for pedicle subtraction osteotomy.

Outcomes of Complex Surgery for Adult Deformity

It is difficult to use the literature to assess the outcomes of complex deformity surgery and make generalizations. The wide range of presenting symptoms, deformity magnitude and flexibility, previous surgery, and comorbidities make it impossible to identify a homogeneous patient population. In addition, a wide variety of surgical techniques may be used to address similar problems. Randomized controlled surgical trials are essentially nonexistent. Most studies are retrospective case reviews.

Yadla et al.[138] performed a systematic review of outcomes of surgery for lumbar scoliosis. They showed that at a minimum 2-year follow-up there was consistent improvement in radiographic and clinical outcomes. The Oswestry Disability Index (ODI) showed an average 15.7 decrease. The Scoliosis Research Society (SRS)-30 showed a mean postoperative decrease of 23.1. These authors showed a relatively high (40%) complication rate.

Using a prospectively collected database, Daubs et al.[139] analyzed 46 patients older than 60 years who underwent a procedure in the thoracic or lumbar spine with more than five levels. Average ODI scores improved from 49 to 25 for a 49% improvement. The overall complication rate was 37%, with 20% of complications being defined as major.

In a prospective cohort study, Alpert et al.[140] used the 36-item Short Form Health Survey (SF-36) to assess 68 adults undergoing surgery for spinal deformity. These authors showed significant increases in physical function, social function, bodily pain, and perceived health change. They did not show a difference comparing patients older than 40 years with younger patients, and there was no difference in outcome observed in patients with complications.

In a matched cohort analysis, Glassman et al.[141] compared patients with major complications, minor complications, and no complications. They noted no difference in scores on the SRS, SF-36, ODI, or visual analogue scale. There was a decrease in general health (12-item Short Form Health Survey [SF-12]) at 1 year for the group with major complications.

Li et al.[142] performed a retrospective case-control study of 83 patients older than 65 years with scoliosis. Of these patients, 34 underwent surgery, and 49 were managed nonoperatively. The patients managed operatively were noted to have significantly less pain, better health-related quality of life, and better self-image and were more satisfied with treatment compared with conservatively treated patients. There was no difference in ODI or the physical and mental components of SF-12. The magnitude of preoperative deformity was not predictive of whether operative or nonoperative treatment was performed.

Two further studies have looked at operative versus nonoperative care. In a retrospective analysis of 55 patients, Kluba and Dikmenli[143] showed that 24 patients who underwent operation had more significant pathology and symptoms preoperatively. At an average of 4 years postoperatively, surgical patients had better activity levels and less analgesic use but no difference in axial back pain. Two articles from the Spinal Deformity Study Group used prospectively collected data on nonmatched cohorts to look at leg pain and disability[144] and quality of life[145] and showed that at 2 years the operative patients were better off than the nonoperative patients despite having more disability, leg pain, and lower quality of life preoperatively.

Smith et al.[146] performed a risk benefit analysis based on patient age for surgical treatment of adult scoliosis. They showed that although the risks were higher for older patients, these patients had a disproportionately greater improvement in pain and function.

Conclusions

The presenting clinical symptoms and radiographic abnormalities of complex spinal deformity span a wide range, and decision making is often quite complex. Many patients are treated adequately with nonoperative approaches. Surgical options are varied and range from minimal decompressive procedures to extensive anteroposterior reconstructions. Focusing on the patient's presenting symptoms and goals for treatment helps determine the treatment course. The surgeries involved can be technically demanding with high complication rates but have reasonably good clinical outcomes. Detailed preoperative planning and a multidisciplinary approach to preoperative and postoperative care are important to minimize morbidity.

KEY REFERENCES

Bess S, Boachie-Adjei O, Burton D, et al: Pain and disability determine treatment modality for older patients with adult scoliosis, while deformity guides treatment for younger patients. *Spine (Phila Pa 1976)* 34:2186–2190, 2009.

Bridwell KH: Decision making regarding Smith-Petersen vs. pedicle subtraction osteotomy vs. vertebral column resection for spinal deformity. *Spine (Phila Pa 1976)* 31(Suppl 19):S171–S178, 2006.

Bridwell KH, Glassman S, Horton W, et al: Does treatment (nonoperative and operative) improve the two-year quality of life in patients with adult symptomatic lumbar scoliosis: a prospective multicenter evidence-based medicine study. *Spine (Phila Pa 1976)* 34:2171–2178, 2009.

Glassman SD, Bridwell K, Dimar JR, et al: The impact of positive sagittal balance in adult spinal deformity. *Spine (Phila Pa 1976)* 30:2024–2029, 2005.

Hu SS: Internal fixation in the osteoporotic spine. *Spine (Phila Pa 1976)* 22(Suppl 24):43S–48S, 1997.

Mok JM, Hu SS: Surgical strategies and choosing levels for spinal deformity: how high, how low, front and back. *Neurosurg Clin N Am* 18:329–337, 2007.

Pekmezci M, Berven SH, Hu SS, et al: The factors that play a role in the decision-making process of adult deformity patients. *Spine (Phila Pa 1976)* 34:813–817, 2009.

Yadla S, Maltenford MG, Ratliff JK, et al: Adult scoliosis surgery: a systematic review. *Neurosurg Focus* 28:E3, 2010.

REFERENCES

The complete reference list is available online at expertconsult.com.

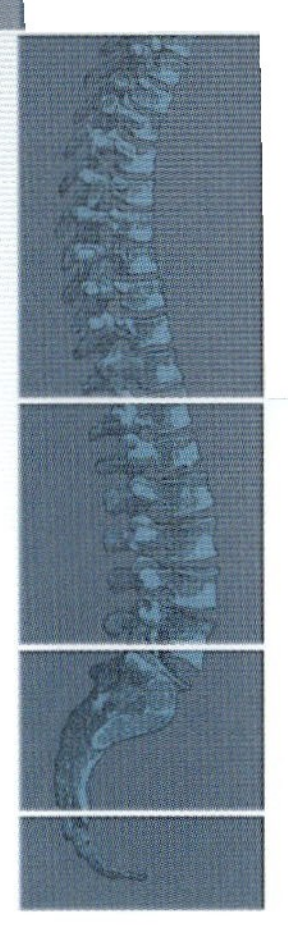

Deformity Surgery for Ankylosing Spondylitis

J. Patrick Johnson | Darren L. Bergey | Michael Weisman | Robert S. Pashman

Ankylosing spondylitis (AS) is an inflammatory disease that can lead to painful disability and deformity.[1] AS is characterized by a strong heretability factor, with most of the risk for susceptibility being connected to the presence of certain genes.[2] The pathogenesis is thought to be immune-mediated joint erosion and bone proliferation that primarily affects the axial skeleton, including ligaments and articulations of the pelvis and spinal column. Inflammation of the vertebral joints and intervertebral disc spaces leads to ossification and fusion of the spine characterized by syndesmophyte formation, ankylosis, and the classic hallmark appearance of "bamboo spine." Concomitant osteoporosis causes the spine to become brittle and susceptible to fracture and progressive spinal deformity. The etiopathogenesis of AS is under intense scrutiny at present, with current efforts under way to determine the exact roles of the mixture of genetic susceptibility, chronic inflammation, and bone-forming pathways.[3]

Surgery to correct related deformity is necessary when conservative management is insufficient and traumatic instability, persistent degenerative radiculopathy, persistent axial pain, or significant deformity is present. This chapter details the presentation and sequelae of AS and focuses on considerations and options in the surgical management of AS deformity.

Clinical Presentation

AS is a chronic lifelong disease that affects men two to three times more frequently than women, and manifests clinically between the ages of 20 and 30.[4] The prevalence of AS is between 0.5% and 1.3% and varies due to definition of the cases (pure AS vs. spondyloarthritis), screening criteria, ethnicity, and presence of the major histocompatability complex class I molecule HLA-B27.[5] Although there is a strong correlation between the prevalence of HLA-B27 and AS, it is suspected but not proven that several non HLA-B27 genes are related to the disease progression.

The primary clinical axial spine symptom of AS from chronic inflammatory sacroiliitis is low back pain.[6] The pain may be unilateral or bilateral and may include radicular symptoms extending into the buttocks or thigh that rarely extend below the knee. Symptoms are usually worse in the morning and improve with activity, distinguishing AS from mechanical low back pain. It is not uncommon for this back pain to awaken the patient at night, further distinguishing AS from other causes of chronic back pain. In children, of course, AS may present with peripheral arthritis.

Ankylosing spondylitic spinal deformity results from progressive flexion and kyphosis of the lumbar, thoracic, and cervical spine as patients attempt to unload stress from painful spondylitic facet joints.[7] Autofusion in kyphosis results in a fixed flexion deformity and global sagittal imbalance with ventral displacement of the patient's center of gravity. Compensatory flexion contractures of the hips and knees may develop as the patient attempts to maintain an erect posture and adequate field of vision. These strains lead to osseous remodeling, further kyphosis, and progressive deformity.

Inflammation and new bone formation drive vertebral column remodeling in AS.[8] Indeed, the first two spinal lesions in AS described by Andersson[9] and Romanus and Yden[10] are inflammatory in nature. Andersson lesions appear as a spondylodiscitis that destroys the central portion of the intervertebral disc and adjacent vertebral body. Romanus lesions are erosive changes at the ventral and dorsal vertebral end plates that appear on radiographs as "shiny corners." In late disease, these Romanus lesions lead to destruction and rebuilding of the cortex, resulting in squaring of the vertebral bodies.

Other inflammatory lesions are also characteristic of AS.[6] Enthesopathy, or inflammation of the ligamentous insertion points, characterizes AS throughout the axial spine. Indeed, enthesitis is the cause of both Andersson and Romanus lesions. Synovitis occurs at zygapophyseal, costovertebral, and costotransverse joints. Inflammation then promotes ectopic bone formation within affected ligaments, resulting in ossification of spinal ligaments and within intervertebral discs, end plates, and apophyseal structures. Formation of new ectopic bone leads to formation of syndesmophytes (bridging the ossified nucleus pulposus at each disc level) or enthesophytes (osseous outgrowths that do not bridge structures). Therefore, advanced AS is characterized by universal syndesmophytosis and squared vertebral bodies with kyphotic deformity that is aptly termed "bamboo spine." It is this propensity of AS patients to make new bone that may not be affected by newer biologic agents that provide remarkable symptom relief. This is the challenge to our understanding of the fundamental nature of this disease.[3]

Osteoporosis in AS is particularly challenging. Early papers hinted of osteoporosis as a late finding, but more recent studies have demonstrated that spinal osteoporosis is found even in early AS without peripheral osteoporosis.[11] This axial osteoporosis is linked to early inflammatory remodeling of the spine. Syndesmophyte formation may also correlate with lower bone mineral density of the spine.[12] Paradoxically, dual-energy x-ray absorptiometry (DEXA) scans in advanced AS may overestimate bone mineral density due to the increased mineral concentration in syndesmophytes, which provide no real functional support. CT can help correlate osteoporosis and disease duration. The clinical consequences of this osteoporosis are profound. Patients with early AS and mild osteoporosis have a fracture prevalence five times greater than in the normal population.[13]

The combination of inflammation and osteoporosis promotes AS fractures and is paradoxically related to ossification. Ossification of the disc space occurs centripetally through the anulus fibrosus, and only rarely is the center of the disc involved. This incomplete ossification leads to formation of polysegments in the spine, with resulting long lever arms of force. The combined stress concentration from loss of polysegmental spinal motion and secondary osteopenia predisposes patients to spinal fracture and nonunion. Aseptic spondylodiscitis, presenting as focal pain with coexisting erosive sclerotic changes in adjacent vertebral bodies, is noted at these sites.[14] It is uncertain whether aseptic spondylodiscitis is a primary inflammatory process or the result of trauma. Radiographically, the appearances of spondylodiscitis, pseudarthrosis, and discitis are similar.

Acute traumatic fractures, particularly in the cervical spine, are also widely reported.[6] Again, osteoporosis and stress forces due to long, stiff lever arms enhance the susceptibility of the AS patients to acute spinal fracture. The lifetime incidence of acute traumatic fractures is believed to be approximately 14%.[15,16] It is reported that 75% of fractures occur in the cervical or cervicothoracic junction, 14% in the thoracic spine, and 5% in the lumbar spine.[17,18] Cervical fractures commonly involve both anterior and posterior columns, leading to higher rates of mortality and neurologic complications in AS than in non-AS patients.[19,20] Even minor trauma such as a simple slip and fall can cause a major spinal fracture and neurologic injury, with the rate of neurologic deficit ranging from 53% to 83%.[21] There should be a high index of suspicion in any AS patient with acute onset of new focal pain or deformity, including any newly observed loss of height. Occult fractures must be suspected any time an abrupt change occurs in the patient's condition, and CT is often required to fully evaluate the symptomatic areas. Undiagnosed or poorly managed spinal fractures can contribute to worsening kyphosis and deformity, particularly if the fractures heal in flexion.

Spinal deformity leads to disability and subsequent mortality.[6] Chin-on-chest deformity seen with fixed cervical flexion significantly hinders forward vision, swallowing, hygiene, and self-esteem. The combination of debilitating disease, deformity, and limited treatment options makes managing these deformities difficult. Although the surgical management of AS deformity is technically challenging and not without risks, the psychological and functional impairment of progressive deformity warrants surgical correction and stabilization when conservative options have been exhausted.

Surgical Management

General Principles

Because AS can lead to severe flexion deformities of the spine, the goal in treatment of these patients is early recognition and adequate medical therapy in an attempt to control the disease progress and prevent associated deformities. However, patients may still become grossly deformed and functionally disabled. Spinal osteotomy may be indicated to correct the deformity and achieve upright posture.

The initial evaluation of the AS patient with deformity involves identifying the primary area in need of correction. Physical examination involves assessing the patient while seated, supine, and upright with hips fully extended. A primary cervical deformity demonstrates cervical flexion while the patient is supine. In contrast, a hip or thoracic/lumbar deformity corrects while the patient is sitting or supine.

Accurate measurement of the deformity is required for surgical planning. Simmons advocates the chin-brow to vertical (CBV) angle as the most effective and reproducible measurement of deformity.[22] The CBV can be evaluated on photographs and is the angle created by (1) the vertical axis of the patient standing with hips and knees extended and (2) the line drawn from the chin to the brow. A greater CBV angle correlates with greater compromise of horizontal gaze and is a critical marker for the degree of deformity (Figs. 99-1A and B).

Normal CBV is 0 degrees but can exceed 90 degrees in severe chin-on-chest deformity. A final corrected angle of approximately 10 degrees of flexion is generally recommended.[23] Radiographic evaluation with 36-inch plain radiography is highly recommended.[24] Osseous anatomy for instrumentation, existing stenosis requiring decompression, and evaluation of soft tissue or vascular structures like the vertebral arteries can be better delineated on the CT and MRI studies necessary for preoperative planning.[25-27] Flexion and extension radiographs can evaluate for instability (particularly atlantoaxial instability) sometimes present in AS.

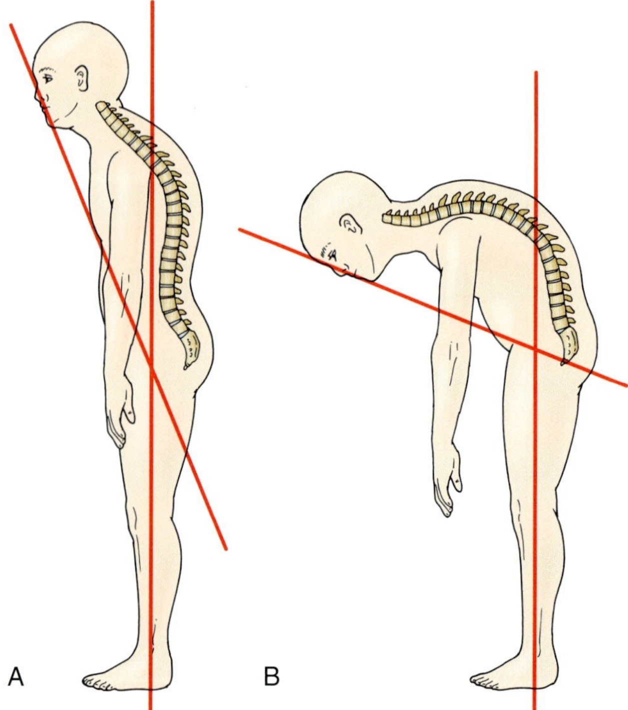

FIGURE 99-1. Measurement of sagittal plane deformity with chin-to-brow to vertical angle: **A**, Lesser deformity; **B**, greater deformity.

The technique and location of the osteotomy depends on the region of the spinal deformity that maximally influences sagittal alignment. Overall spinal balance as well as the hips must be evaluated to delineate the primary site of deformity. In some patients, more than one site may contribute to the deformity. The common sites of deformity include the cevicothoracic junction, midthoracic spine, thoracolumbar spine, and hip joints.[6] Assuming equal deformity at these levels, lumbar correction surgery should be considered prior to cervical correction surgery because of the lower rate of complications.[28]

The site of correction depends on the site of deformity. Deformities isolated to the lumbar spine are corrected by a lumbar osteotomy procedure. The osteotomy is preferred below the level of the conus medullaris and is usually performed at L3 to avoid acute angular correction at the cord level.[22] Most thoracolumbar kyphotic deformities can be addressed through a single lumbar osteotomy. The correction should be planned so that the plumb line from C7 falls within the body of S1. Even in cases in which the thoracic kyphosis is greater than normal, a compensatory lumbar osteotomy may correct sagittal plane malalignment and allow the patient to have forward gaze with the hips and knees fully extended. In cases of severe thoracic kyphosis, where the lumbar and cervical lordosis have been at least partially maintained, thoracic osteotomy by a combined ventral and dorsal approach may be indicated. It is important to note that due to fixed cervical deformity, overcorrection of the gaze angle can cause significant gait difficulty. When the primary deformity is at the cervicothoracic junction with a chin-on-chest deformity, an osteotomy of the cervical spine is indicated. The C7-T1 junction is the preferred location because it places the osteotomy below the entrance of the vertebral arteries into the transverse processes at C6 and uses the relatively large spinal canal–to–cord area ratio to safely obtain correction.

The influence of severe hip flexion contractures, with or without associated hip joint disease, is critical in the preoperative assessment. Soft tissue release about the hips, or more commonly, total hip joint arthroplasty, may be sufficient in itself to allow the patient to stand reasonably upright and see straight ahead, irrespective of the spinal deformity.[29] These procedures should be performed prior to any larger surgical correction of spinal deformity.

Diligent presurgical screening is paramount since AS patients frequently have multiple comorbidities.[24] Preoperatively, patients with a fixed thoracic deformity should be screened for cardiac and pulmonary abnormalities that can be associated with extra-articular manifestations of AS. Although pulmonary function abnormalities secondary to decreased thoracic expansion have not carried anesthetic risk for most patients, 10% will have cardiac pathology, generally either aortic stenosis or conduction abnormalities.[30] Nonsteroidal anti-inflammatory agents may need to be halted prior to surgery to reduce the risk of pseudarthrosis and nonunion. Nutrition should be optimized, sometimes with tube feeding or parenteral nutrition in extreme cases, especially with postoperative risks of swallowing difficulty.

Surgical Correction

The major categories of osteotomies for AS deformity include the Smith-Petersen osteotomy (SPO), polysegmental wedge osteotomy (PWO), and pedicle subtraction osteotomy (PSO). A note is provided regarding ventral release and osteotomy.

Smith-Petersen Osteotomy

Smith-Petersen and Larson first proposed their osteotomy for the correction of flexion deformity for rheumatoid arthritis in the lumbar spine on six patients in 1945.[31] Since that time, the Smith-Petersen osteotomy (SPO), also known as the opening wedge osteotomy and extension osteotomy, has been used extensively and optimized for AS. It has been reported primarily in the lumbar and cervical spine.

Smith-Petersen originally performed a V-shaped wedge resection osteotomy at the L1, L2, and L3 levels (Fig. 99-2).[31] In the original operation, the L2 spinous process was removed completely along with the articular processes of L1, L2, and L3. This dorsal osteotomy wedge was then closed and the deformity corrected via forceful manual manipulation through hyperextension. This maneuver used the middle column (e.g., the posterior longitudinal ligament) as a fulcrum and caused disruption of the anterior longitudinal ligament with a monosegmental opening wedge and extension of the anterior column. Local bone grafts were placed across the osteotomy sites, and the patient was immobilized in a postoperative cast for 2 months followed by a back brace for 1 year. Detailed results were not described.

In 1973, McMaster and Coventry reported on 17 patients with an SPO of the lumbar spine using a plaster case with a turnbuckle and hip spica immobilization for postoperative correction (no instrumentation was used).[28] They reported an impressive 39-degree correction average, which has been replicated by other authors.[32] Twelve of the 17 patients had complications, including 2 deaths and 5 neurologic deficits.

The SPO has also been commonly employed in the cervical spine. In 1953, Mason et al. reported successful correction of flexion deformity of the cervicothoracic spine in a patient with AS.[33] They performed the osteotomy distal to C7 to avoid damage to the vertebral arteries. In 1958, Urist reported a successful osteotomy at the cervicothoracic junction in a patient awake under local anesthesia.[34] However, it was Simmons that elaborated on the SPO in the first large case series of 42 patients in 1977.[22]

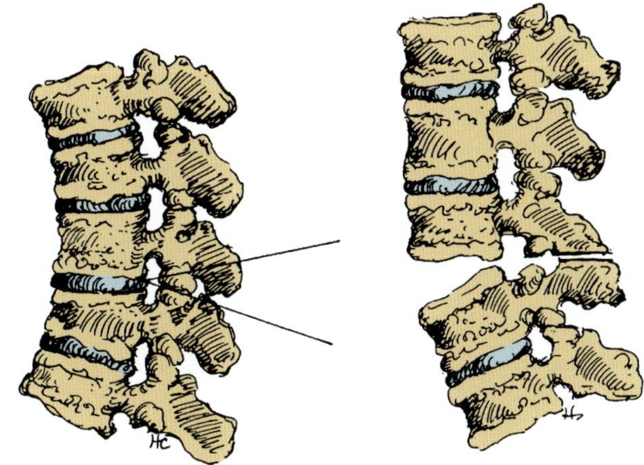

FIGURE 99-2. Illustration of Smith-Petersen lumbar osteotomy technique.

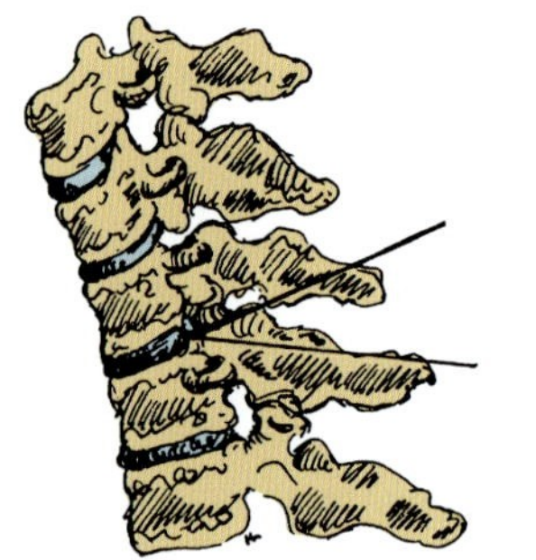
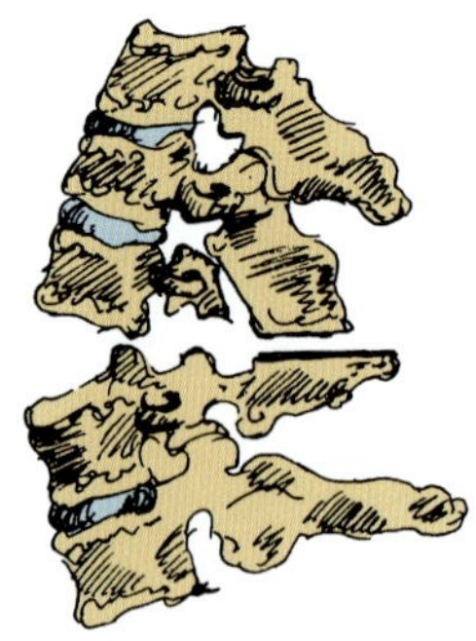

FIGURE 99-3. Illustration of Smith-Petersen cervical osteotomy technique.

The Simmons SPO modification involved a wide laminectomy from C6 to T1, with osteotomy at the C7-T1 space (Fig. 99-3).[22] Simmons resected the entire dorsal arch of C7, the inferior half of C6, and the upper half of T1. The laminae were undercut and foraminotomies performed to prevent impingement of the C8 nerve root. Following bony decompression, Simmons extended the neck and "cracked" the anterior column. Simmons performed the procedure under local anesthesia with halo control and then fixed the halo to a body cast that was worn for 4 months. There were no mortalities, and C8 weakness was the primary morbidity, occurring in 18 patients, with five permanent deficits.

Some authors have performed an initial ventral release prior to a cervical SPO.[35,36] Mummaneni et al. have described a staged ventral-dorsal-ventral procedure for cervical osteotomy.[37] This consists of a ventral release (C5-6 discectomy and partial wedge resection of C5 and C6 vertebral bodies), followed by a dorsal SPO with controlled correction supplemented by a screw-rod construct, and finally a ventral placement of iliac autograft in the opening wedge defect with a cervical plate and screws.

Several adjustments of the original SPO technique have since become standard. General anesthetic is now frequently used with controlled halo correction, followed by either an intraoperative wake-up test or spinal cord monitoring. Lateral mass screws are used in the cervical spine, with pedicle screws the method of choice elsewhere for internal fixation. Indeed, modern instrumentation is now ubiquitous in deformity surgery. Halo and vest supplementation may or may not be used. Neurologic compression is now minimized by adequate decompression and undercutting of the lamina prior to closure of the osteotomy site and rigid stabilization. Despite these modifications, subluxation caused by rupture of the posterior longitudinal ligament has been associated with nonunion, high neurologic complications, and mortality.[38] Although the SPO remains in common use, some surgeons prefer other alternatives.

Polysegmental Wedge Osteotomy

In 1949, Wilson and Turkell reported the first polysegmental wedge osteotomy (PWO) on a patient with thoracolumbar kyphotic deformity attributed to AS.[39] Correction was achieved by multiple closing wedges of dorsal lumbar osteotomies including the interlaminar space and by trimming the facet processes. In contrast to the SPO, a PWO leaves the anterior longitudinal ligament (ALL) intact and generates a more gradual multisegment curvature. In the 1980s, Zielke et al. advocated polysegmental lumbar dorsal wedge osteotomies with internal fixation.[40,41] He first used Harrington rods and laminar hooks and, more recently, transpedicular screws.

Several authors have demonstrated good results with the PWO. Van Royen et al. reported a mean correction of 36.3 degrees overall (9.5 degrees per level) in 21 patients treated with PWOs in the thoracic and lumbar spine.[42] At last follow-up, however, there was a mean loss of 10.7 degrees, with a significant rate of pedicle fractures, deep wound infections, and pseudarthrosis. Hehne and Zielke described 177 patients with AS and 44-degree overall correction (9.5 degrees per segment) without resulting pseudarthrosis and no loss of correction over the long term.[41] Chen reported an average correction of 25.8 degrees overall (5 degrees per level) with a 25% pseudarthrosis rate.[43] These results suggest that PWOs are reasonable when gradual correction is necessary over multiple levels. There may be concern for insufficient correction, however, especially if the intervertebral discs are calcified.[44]

PWOs are relevant in thoracic osteotomies. Note that thoracic osteotomies are rarely required in patients with AS. As stated previously, if the thoracic kyphosis is mild or moderate and associated with a flat or kyphotic lumbar spine, the deformity can be addressed with a lumbar spine osteotomy. The rare patient has severe thoracic kyphosis with minimal loss of lumbar or cervical lordosis. This is the patient in whom a thoracic osteotomy may be indicated.

Smith-Petersen pointed out in 1945 that single-stage dorsal thoracic osteotomy correction is compromised by stiffness of the costovertebral joints.[31] An alternative involves a two-stage procedure that consists of a first-stage transthoracic approach creating osteotomies through the ossified thoracic disc spaces. Ventral interbody fusion is performed with an autogenous cancellous bone graft. This is followed at the same sitting or 1 week later by PWOs with segmental instrumentation. Dural adhesions to the lamina that formed during the inflammatory phase of the disease can be encountered during dorsal osteotomy and likewise may make passage of sublaminar wires used in the Luque technique more difficult. Hook-rod or screw-rod compression instrumentations are alternatives commonly used today. The approach is similar to that used for severe juvenile kyphosis.[45,46]

Pedicle Subtraction Osteotomy

The pedicle subtraction osteotomy (PSO), also known as the decancellization procedure, eggshell osteotomy, or closing wedge osteotomy, has been well described in the literature.[47-49] Today, the PSO is primarily performed at the upper lumbar and more recently in the cervicothoracic junction. The PSO is a mainstay in correcting deformity due to iatrogenic kyphosis, traumatic kyphosis, rheumatoid arthritis, and AS.

A PSO involves first removing a wedge of the dorsal elements and bilateral pedicles, followed by resection of the dorsal vertebral cortex as well as the cancellous bone of the vertebral body (Fig. 99-4). The ALL and ventral cortex of the vertebral body are left intact. In contrast to the SPO, the ALL is the fulcrum for closure and results in three-column bone-on-bone closure. Closure effectively shortens

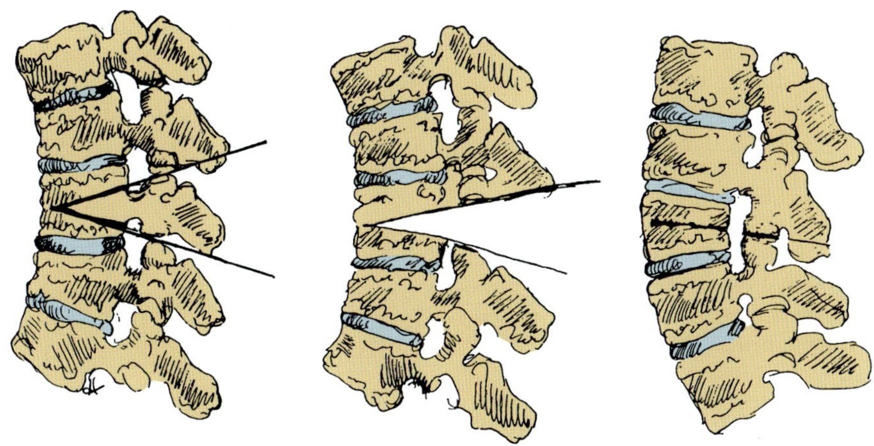

FIGURE 99-4. Illustration of pedicle subtraction osteotomy technique.

the spinal canal and achieves angular correction at a single level. Moreover, removal of the pedicle creates a "superforamen," which transmits the nerve roots from the adjacent segments and decreases the chance for root compression. Generous undercutting and decompression of the supra- and subadjacent laminar edges are performed to ensure adequate space for the redundant dura that may be produced during closure of the osteotomy. Segmental spinal fixation using screw-rod or hook-rod constructs is used to allow for immediate patient mobilization. The surgical table is carefully extended, closing the osteotomy. If necessary, closure can be augmented by pressure on the patient's shoulders or legs and by compression between the pedicle screws once the rods are placed. A wake-up test or neuromonitoring is routinely performed to assess neurologic function. Finally, a local bone graft is applied and augmented with iliac crest autograft or banked bone, as needed.

The PSO has several advantages. The removal of the dorsal aspect of a single ventral body closes the vertebral body with the hinge at the anterior column rather than the middle column. The resulting bone-on-bone contact in all three columns (lateral masses included) theoretically improves the likelihood of fusion. Furthermore, as the spine is effectively shortened, the PSO avoids stretching the major vessels and soft tissue ventral to the spine, which can occur using an SPO.

The PSO is generally well tolerated in the lumbar spine. Thomasen reported 12 to 50 degrees of correction in 11 patients, with 5 of the 11 having a correction of less than 35 degrees.[48] Other reports show corrections of 30 to 40 degrees in the lumbar spine.[50] The ability to correct all three columns through a single dorsal approach, correction of more than 30 degrees at a single level, and correction through a prior fusion mass make the PSO a favored procedure in the lumbar spine.

PSOs of the cervicothoracic junction deserve special focus. Recently, Samudrala et al. reported on eight patients who underwent PSO for correction of CT junction kyphosis, achieving a mean correction of 35 degrees, restoration of forward gaze, and significant reduction of pain.[51] As with Simmons' cervical SPO for AS, the site for a cervical PSO is recommended at C7-T1 since the spinal canal is relatively wide, the C8 roots are mobile, and the vertebral artery is rostral to the C7 foramen transversarium. The modern cervical PSO offers a dorsal fusion system in the cervicothoracic junction that avoids stretch injury to critical ventral structures such as the trachea and esophagus while promoting fusion through all three columns.

Ventral Release and Osteotomy

Some authors advocate using an initial ventral release prior to SPOs.[24] Ventral release and osteotomy have the advantages of allowing a controlled correction with neck extension without the abrupt fracture from an SPO. The osteotomy is controlled to a specific site, whereas correction of SPO can lead to a fracture at a random, undesired level. Finally, ventral exposure allows for placement of a structural graft.

Ventral exposure in AS may be inappropriate in some cases. Ventral exposure may be unnecessary since an ankylosed, osteoporotic spine often will fracture without excessive force. Chin-on-chest deformity also limits the exposure and operative corridor with a ventral approach. Finally, syndesmophyte formation limits a surgeon's ability to distinguish normal from abnormal anatomic landmarks of the disc spaces. The added risk of patient repositioning and extended anesthesia must also be considered. Finally, the use of standard dorsal screw-rod instrumentation provides greater mechanical stability than ventral constructs.[52,53]

Anesthesia, Neuromonitoring, and Intraoperative Care

Although local anesthesia has been reported in the treatment of these spinal deformities, general anesthesia is preferred.[54,55] With endotracheal intubation, the airway access is secured, allowing for the procedure to be performed in a prone rather than sitting position, which facilitates placement of instrumentation, reduces the risk of air embolism, and ensures patient comfort. Intubation is facilitated by the use of fiberoptic guidance where cervicothoracic kyphosis complicates easy passage of the endotracheal tube. Awake intubation allows for constant neurologic monitoring and limits the risk of neurologic injury.

The ability to monitor neurologic function is critical in deformity correction since neurologic injury can occur due to translation of the spine or by compression on closing of the osteotomy. McMaster has described using the Stagnara wake-up test as the gold standard for intraoperative neurologic evaluation.[23] However, anesthetic limitations often hinder timely and safe wake-up during a prolonged procedure, especially during a period when critical neural compression may go unrecognized.

Neuromonitoring is a useful adjunct for any deformity correction. Somatosensory-evoked potentials (SSEPs) and motor-evoked potentials (MEPs) are routine in complex spine procedures. SSEPs provide monitoring of the dorsal column but do not provide information regarding motor pathways, and several reports have demonstrated postoperative neurologic deficits despite normal intraoperative SSEPs.[56] MEP monitoring, in contrast, evaluates the corticospinal tracts. Langeloo et al. evaluated MEP monitoring in 16 patients undergoing SPO using a 20% decrease in MEP measurements as a threshold.[57] Langeloo addressed any MEP decreases by first evaluating for technical problems and optimizing hemodynamics. Persistent decreases were addressed by reversing the surgical maneuver that preceded the MEP change. In his 16 patients, he found 9 events in 7 patients. One patient had spontaneous recovery of MEP amplitude without sequelae. In six patients, the cervical extension maneuver preceded the MEP change. Upon change, the extension was reversed, leading to recovery in five of the six patients. One patient did not recover MEPs and had persistent C6 cord injury despite reversing the maneuver and performing a secondary ventral decompression the same day. There were no cases of stable intraoperative MEPs with postoperative neurologic sequelae.

Intraoperative care of the patient varies depending on the deformity, the patient's comorbidities, and surgeon comfort. After the patient has been anesthetized and intubated, the operating table must be modified accordingly. In cases of thoracic or lumbar deformity, the table is flexed into a position where the apex of the table is under the primary spinal deformity. Bolsters are used to free the abdomen and protect bony prominences and peripheral nerves in the extremities. For cervical deformity, the patient may be placed in either a halo or Mayfield pin fixation. Cell saver autotransfusion is a useful adjunct in settings where blood loss may hinder patient safety. Finally, intraoperative image guidance provides live feedback and facilitates the osteotomy as well as placement of instrumentation safely away from vital structures to reduce iatrogenic injury while minimizing radiation to the surgeon.

Internal Fixation

Early reports of correction often used external immobilization with either a halo cast or halo vest without internal fixation. However, the lack of supplemental internal fixation poses the risk of delayed subluxation with potential neurologic injury or pseudarthrosis, particularly in the situation of an SPO. McMaster compared 12 SPO patients with halo immobilization alone with 3 patients with a halo body cast with internal Luque rod and wiring fixation.[23] He found four cases of postoperative C7-T1 subluxation and two cases of nonunion in the patients treated with halo immobilization alone, compared with no cases of subluxation or pseudarthrosis in patients treated with internal fixation. Similarly, Belanger et al. reported on 26 SPO patients, 7 with halo vest alone and 19 with internal fixation.[58] There were five cases of subluxation reported, all of which occurred in the patients treated with halo vest alone.

Modern screw-rod constructs are the mainstay of deformity correction. The use of dorsal wiring has been well described, although the use of sublaminar wires in the thoracic spine represents a high risk of cord injury with limited immobilization. Multilevel fixation is crucial given the long lever arms and osteoporosis prominent in AS.[59]

Complications

It has been stated in review of several series that mortality has varied from 8% to 10%, and neurologic complications have occurred in up to 30% of patients. However, these quotes may be misleading. We performed an analysis of the 14 largest series consisting of five or more cases reported. A total of 427 cases were found with a 4% incidence of neurologic complications and a 5% mortality rate.[30,31,33,48,55,60-68] In the single largest study, 177 patients reported by Hehne and Zielke, there was a 2.3% mortality rate and a 2.3% rate of irreversible root lesions.[41] Based on the authors' review of the published data and their own experience, it appears that neurologic complications and mortality can be greatly lessened if not prevented altogether by careful attention to four critical factors: (1) avoiding compression of neurologic tissue, (2) monitoring neurologic function during the osteotomy, (3) using internal fixation, and (4) avoiding translational displacement at the osteotomy site.

Complications related to surgical correction are related to patient, site, and procedure attempted. Van Royen and De Gast identified 856 patients surgically treated for thoracolumbar kyphotic deformity in 41 articles from 1945 to 1998 using SPO, PWO, and PSOs in the lumbar spine for AS.[44] They classified three main categories of complications (1) loss of correction and implant failure, (2) vascular complications, and (3) neurologic complications. Loss of correction and implant failure are related to osteoporosis and present as implant loosening and pullout. This failure places additional stress on the fusion construct and remaining instrumentation, increasing the likelihood of nonunion and loss of correction. Vascular complications, primarily rupture of the aorta and its branches, were found in 0.9% (4 of 450 patients) of lumbar SPO at L1-2 and L2-3, but not below L3.[66,69,70] Finally, neurologic deficit due to displacement of the vertebral body was reported in six patients with SPO (2.7%) and in one patient treated by PSO (2.0%).[48,71,72]

Correction of cervical deformity in AS has its own set of complications. In 2008, Hoh et al. reviewed the literature for case series of at least 10 patients with AS who underwent cervical SPO.[24] The review found 5 of 183 patients had significant spinal cord injury (1 paraparesis, 1 hemiparesis, and 3 tetraparesis), several cases of transient postoperative weakness with spontaneous recovery, and 35 cases of C8 sensory disturbances with most resolving over several months.[23,26,57,58] Six deaths were noted within 3 months of the operation. Other complications included postoperative dysphagia and pseudarthroses as reported by Simmons et al. and McMaster only in cases treated without internal fixation.[23,26]

Summary

Deformity in AS is progressive and ultimately debilitating. Inflammation is a major factor leading to structural remodeling of the spine, although only a few of the pathways involved in the new bone formation that is widespread in this disease are known. In order to halt the spiral to deformity, neurologic decline, and loss of function, surgical treatment must be considered when conservative measures have failed. A grasp of the surgical indications, options, and techniques is essential to optimize AS therapy.

Acknowledgment. The authors acknowledge Helen Cambron, RN, FNP-C, for her illustrative contribution to this chapter.

KEY REFERENCES

Hehne HJ, Zielke K: Polysegmental lumbar osteotomies and transpedicled fixation for correction of long-curved kyphotic deformities in ankylosing spondylitis: report on 177 cases. *Clin Orthop Relat Res* 258:49–55, 1990.

Samudrala S, Vaynman S, Thiayananthan T, et al: Cervicothoracic junction kyphosis: surgical reconstruction with pedicle subtraction osteotomy and Smith-Petersen osteotomy. Presented at the 2009 Joint Spine Section Meeting. Clinical article. *J Neurosurg Spine* 13:695–706, 2010.

Simmons ED, DiStefano RJ, Zheng Y, et al: Thirty-six years experience of cervical extension osteotomy in ankylosing spondylitis: techniques and outcomes. *Spine (Phila Pa 1976)* 31:3006–3012, 2006.

Tokala DP, Lam KS, Freeman BJ, et al: C7 decancellisation closing wedge osteotomy for the correction of fixed cervico-thoracic kyphosis. *Eur Spine J* 16:1471–1478, 2007.

van Royen BJ, de Kleuver M, Slot GH: Polysegmental lumbar posterior wedge osteotomies for correction of kyphosis in ankylosing spondylitis. *Eur Spine J* 7:104–110, 1998.

REFERENCES

The complete reference list is available online at expertconsult.com.

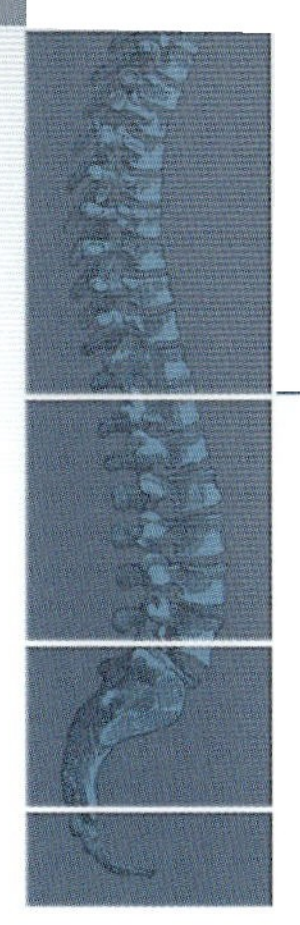

Pediatric Spinal Deformities and Deformity Correction

Brian J. Williams | Justin S. Smith | Christopher I. Shaffrey

Pediatric spinal deformity can result from congenital anomalies, neuromuscular disorders, genetic conditions, connective tissue disorders, skeletal dysplasia, and developmental (idiopathic) causes.[1,2] Each category of spinal deformity has a typical behavior dictated by the pathophysiology of the underlying condition.

Scoliosis, kyphosis, and lordosis refer to deviations from normal spinal alignment. In the coronal plane, the spine is normally straight. In the sagittal plane, the thoracic region is kyphotic (range, 20–40 degrees), the lumbar region is lordotic, and the transition over the thoracolumbar region is relatively straight (Fig. 100-1).[3] Scoliosis, curvature in the coronal plane, is also associated with transverse rotation, as well as with pathologic lordosis or kyphosis (Figs. 100-2 and 100-3).[3-5] Therefore, the terms *lordoscoliosis* and *kyphoscoliosis* are frequently used to characterize the three-dimensional nature of a deformity. When more than one pathologic curvature exists along the length of the spine, the primary (or major) curve is designated on the basis of its size and rigidity. The secondary (or minor) curve(s), even if compensatory, may be rigid or have a "structural" component. Surgical planning should address the magnitude and flexibility of all the curves in all three planes.

Growth of the Spine

Pediatric spinal deformities are usually not clinically evident at birth. However, they progress in proportion to spinal growth. Therefore, anticipating and modifying the growth potential of the vertebral elements composing the deformity is essential. Two periods of rapid growth occur in children: the first between birth and 3 years and the second during the adolescent years. The timing and duration of the adolescent growth spurt can be determined by monitoring the growth velocity (Fig. 100-4). The spine grows heterogeneously; that is, during the adolescent growth spurt, the thoracic spine grows 1.2 cm per year and, in contrast, the lumbar spine grows 0.6 cm per year. Thus, the effect of spinal fusion on future growth can be estimated, although it should be remembered that a spine with scoliosis grows with progressive deformity. Apical vertebral growth exacerbates the deformity with further rotation, displacement, and tilting of the vertebrae.

Predicting growth around the time of puberty is based on physical and radiographic examinations. In girls, Tanner stage 2, the development of pubic hair and breast buds, marks the onset of the growth spurt and typically precedes menarche. Skeletal age at this stage is approximately 11.5 years. The growth spurt ends at a skeletal age of 14 years, or approximately 1.5 years after menarche. For boys, Tanner stage 3, when the pubic hair becomes curly, corresponds to the onset of the growth spurts. The skeletal age is approximately 13

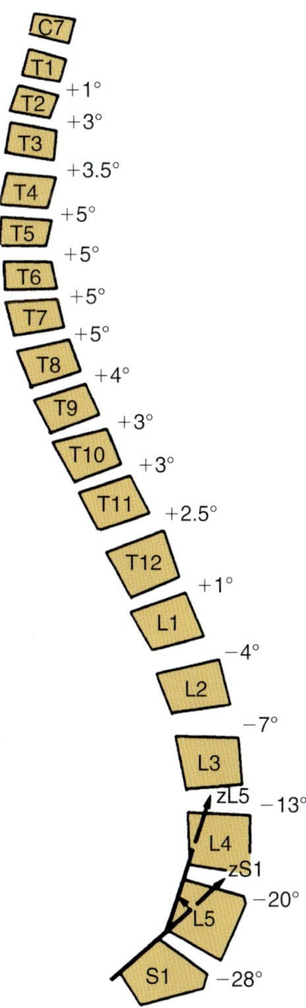

FIGURE 100-1. Spinal sagittal alignment is shown with the segmental angulation between vertebrae. (From Bernhardt M, Bridwell KH: Segmental analysis of the sagittal plane alignment of the normal thoracic and lumbar spines and thoracolumbar junction. *Spine* [Phila Pa 1976] 14:717–721, 1989, with permission.)

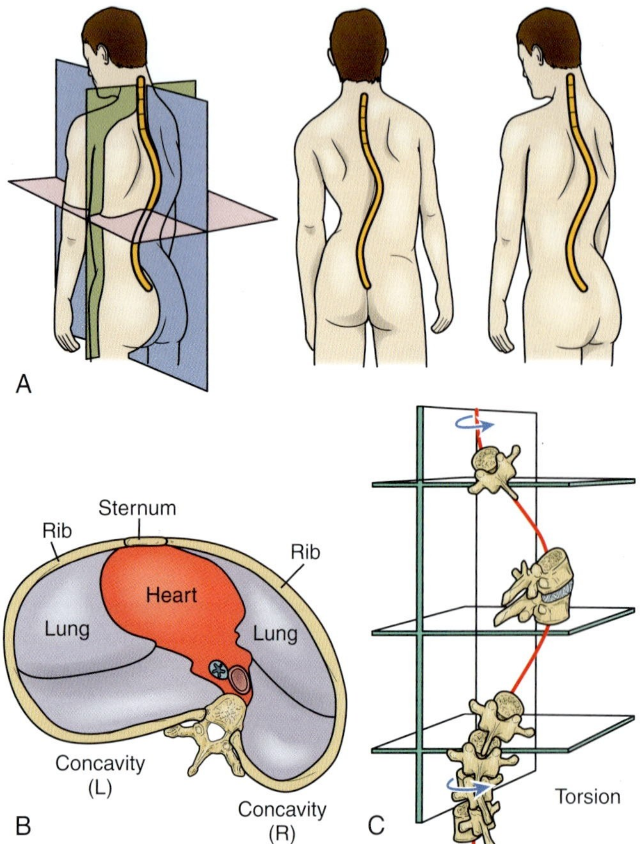

FIGURE 100-2. **A,** Idiopathic scoliosis is a three-dimensional deformity, typically associated with thoracic hypokyphosis or lordosis. **B,** The rib cage deforms so that the right dorsal rib angle becomes more prominent, and the left breast projects forward. The star-shaped body is the inferior vena, which is positioned next to the aorta in the posterior mediastinum. **C,** The end vertebrae of the scoliosis are most tilted, whereas the apical vertebrae are most rotated and laterally translated.

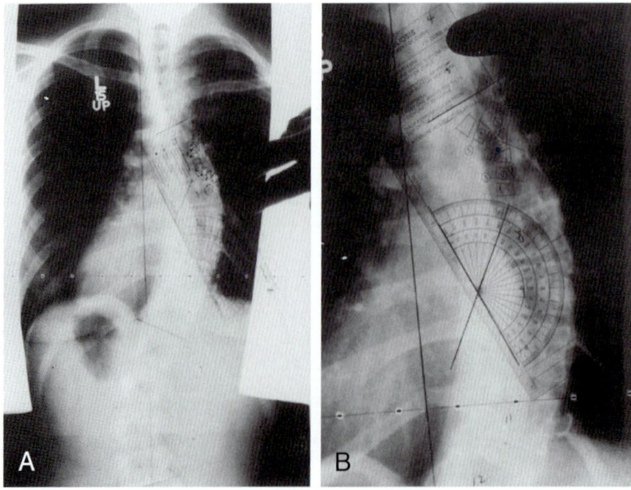

FIGURE 100-3. **A,** The Cobb angle for scoliosis measurement is formed by the intersection of perpendicular lines drawn to the end plates of the most tilted vertebrae. **B,** In this case, the Cobb angle measures 52 degrees.

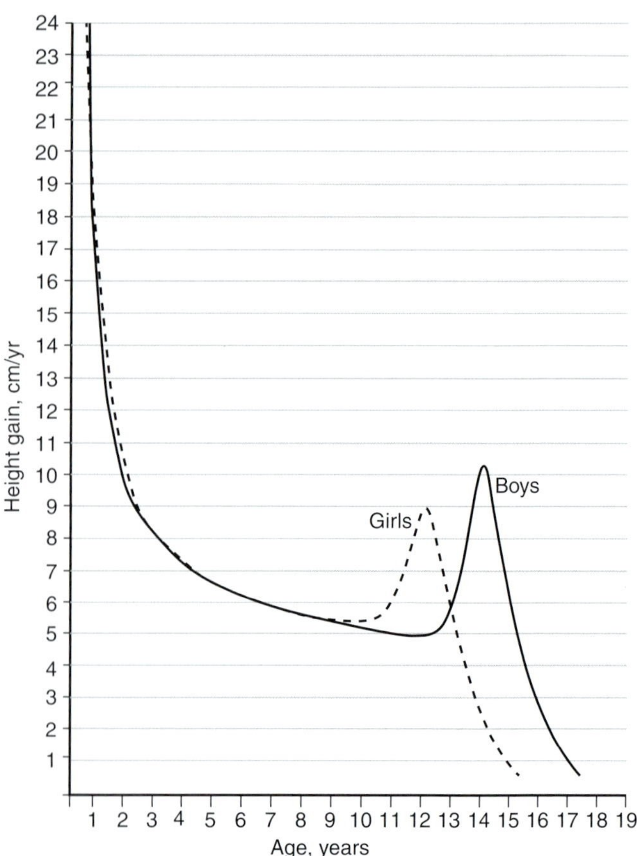

FIGURE 100-4. Growth velocity can be plotted by measuring height gain per year. The greatest velocity and propensity for scoliosis progression occur during the adolescent growth spurt.

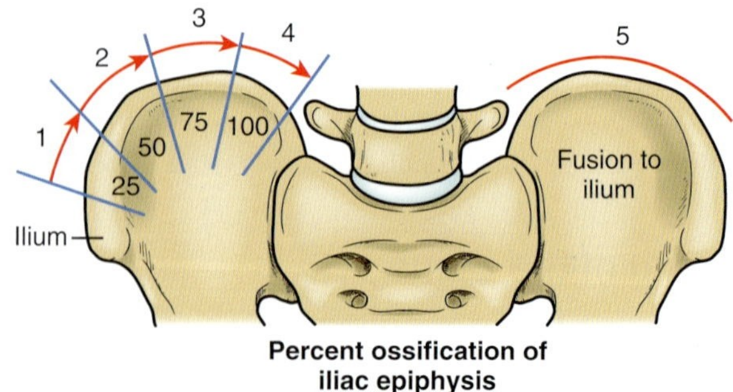

FIGURE 100-5. The Risser stage of iliac ossification can be used to estimate remaining maturity and growth.

years and continues until 18 years. A growth rate chart is the ideal means of monitoring growth, but realistically this is not always feasible to obtain. Otherwise, the surgeon should consider physical findings such as the Tanner stage, in conjunction with historical information regarding the onset of menarche or the appearance of axillary hair in boys.

Several methods for this assessment of skeletal maturity have been reported, including Risser stage, presence of triradiate cartilage, and hand films.[6-10] The Risser stage is a method based on the degree of iliac ossification, with stages 1 through 4 corresponding to sequential ossification of each quarter of the iliac crest from ventral to dorsal[11] (Fig. 100-5). Stage 4 reflects completion of spinal growth, and stage 5 is defined as fusion to the ilium. Alternatively, hand films can be obtained for the assessment of skeletal maturity, without the need to expose the pelvis to radiation, as is required for both the Risser stage and assessment of the triradiate cartilage.[8,9]

The rib–vertebral angle difference (RVAD) is another measure that can guide decision making in pediatric spinal deformity. This measure is an important prognostic indicator for infantile scoliosis.[12] The RVAD is the difference between the angles formed by a line along the rib head and perpendicular to the base of the apical vertebra on the right and left sides of the spine. Spontaneous resolution of the scoliosis is expected in 85% to 90% of the cases if the RVAD is less than 20 degrees, but progression is expected with an RVAD greater than 20 degrees.[12]

Evaluation

Clinical Evaluation

Initial evaluation should begin with a detailed history, including the prenatal, birth, and cognitive and motor developmental history.[9] Details of the suspected spinal disorder should be documented, including symptoms, deficits, onset, and progression, as well as disability and the quality of life. Past medical history can be a significant contributor, especially with congenital spinal disorders, which can be associated with other anomalies.[13]

Physical examination should include assessment of the head, entire spine, and extremities, including the skin; it should also encompass a detailed neurologic examination, including strength, tone, gait, coordination, sensation, and physiologic and pathologic reflexes. For example, neurofibromatosis may be suggested by the presence of café au lait spots or freckling, and underlying anomalies such as diplomyelia or lipomeningocele can be evidenced by patches of hair or skin dimpling. Nonambulatory patients should be examined for evidence of decubitus ulceration, which may affect surgical planning. Posture should be assessed and may include sitting, standing, and walking.

The scoliometer or inclinometer is used to quantify the rib prominence and paralumbar prominence. A scoliometer reading greater than 5 degrees is associated with a scoliosis of at least 10 degrees (Fig. 100-6).

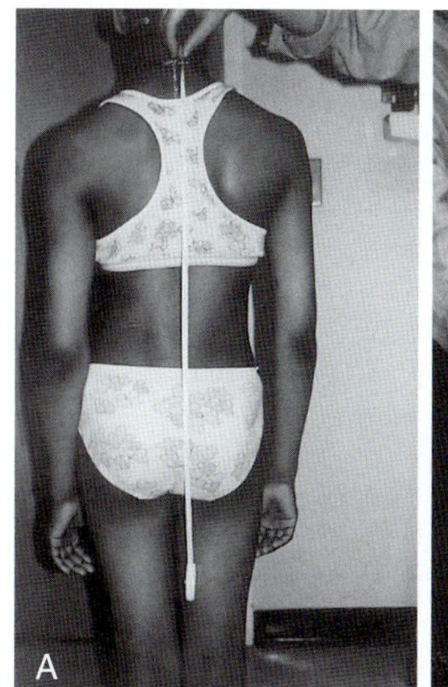

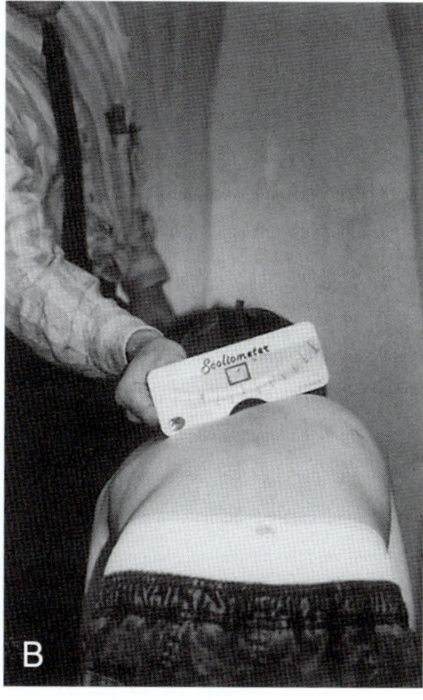

FIGURE 100-6. Body asymmetry produced by scoliosis is assessed by noting (**A**) the balance of the head and trunk over the pelvis by plumb line measurements, the level of the shoulders and iliac crests, and the definition of the waist and (**B**) the rib rotation by scoliometer (inclinometer) measurement.

Imaging Evaluation

Initial evaluation of suspected spinal deformity often includes full-length (36-inch) posteroanterior (PA) and lateral spinal radiographs to assess global and regional spinal alignment. PA images evaluate for scoliosis, with measures including Cobb angle and coronal balance. Coronal balance is typically measured as the distance between a vertical line from the center of the C7 vertebral body (C7 plumb line) and the central sacral vertical line (CSVL) (Fig. 100-7). Lateral full-length spinal radiographs can be used to assess for regional kyphosis and lordosis and for global sagittal balance. Sagittal balance is typically measured as the distance between a vertical line from the center of the C7 plumb line and the dorsal rostral corner of the S1 vertebral body. If the C7 plumb line is ventral to the dorsal rostral corner of the S1 vertebral body, the sagittal balance measure is reflected as a positive value, and if dorsal, it is reflected as a negative value.

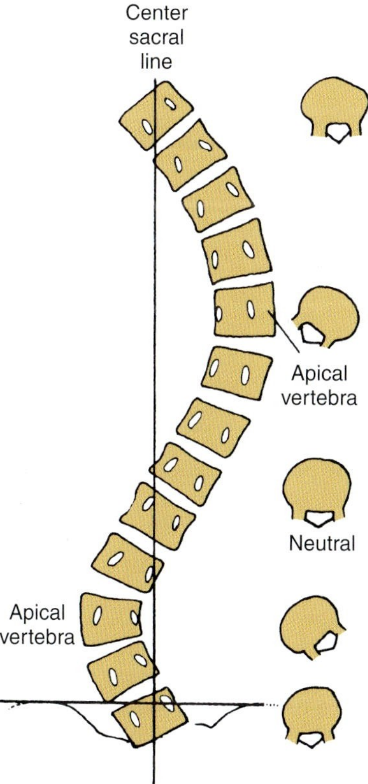

FIGURE 100-7. The center sacral line is the perpendicular to a horizontal line across the iliac crest, passing vertically through the sacral spinous processes. Vertebrae bisected by the center sacral line are designated as stable vertebrae.

The flexibility of scoliotic curves can be assessed with side-bending PA films to the left and to the right. Alternatively, the same information may be obtained with the patient placed over a bolster or with the use of traction. The flexibility of kyphotic deformities can be assessed with a bolster placed under the apex of the kyphosis, and the flexibility of

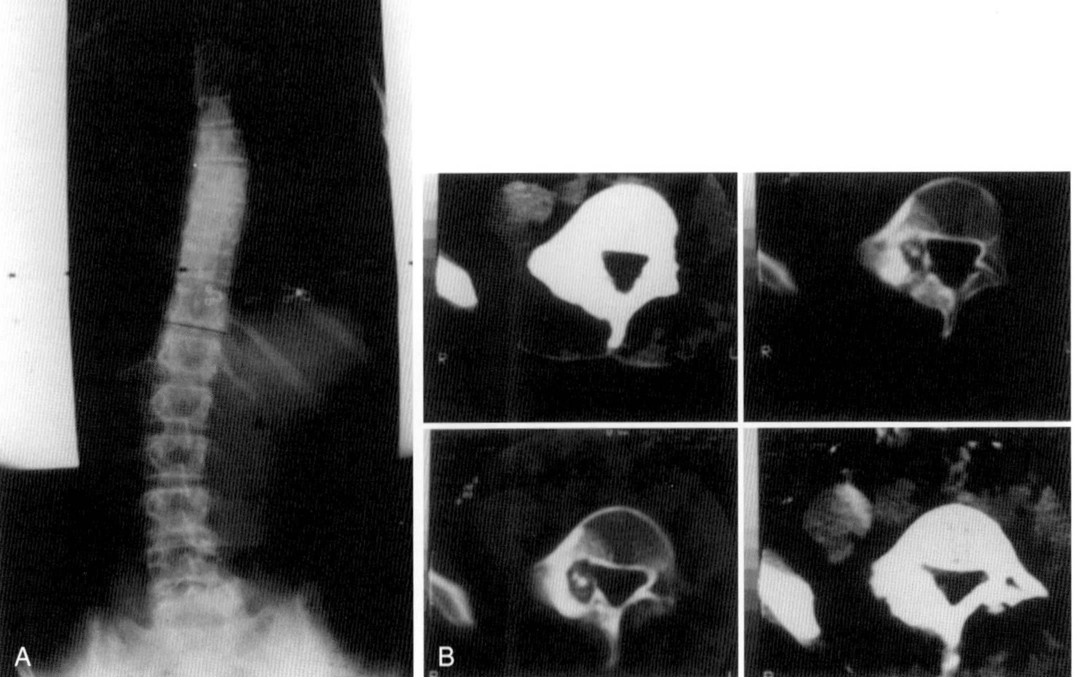

FIGURE 100-8. **A,** A 13-year-old girl presented with upper back pain and a right thoracic scoliosis. **B,** Due to a history of pain, a bone scan and CT scan were obtained, revealing an osteoid osteoma in the T8 pedicle.

lordotic deformities may be assessed with the spine and pelvis placed in flexion.

CT imaging provides greater detail of the bony anatomy and a three-dimensional view of complex deformities; such information may facilitate planning of surgical treatment.[14,15] CT clearly defines congenital deformities with underlying anomalies, such as hemivertebra or unsegmented bars that may be occult on plain-film radiographs (Fig. 100-8).

In the setting of spinal deformity, MRI can be used to evaluate for central canal and foraminal stenosis, as well as for underlying abnormalities, which may warrant treatment or alter surgical planning. Associated abnormalities, such as tethered cord, syringomyelia, and tumors, occur in up to 15% to 38% of congenital spinal deformity patients[16-21] (Fig. 100-9). Although MRI is often used as an adjunct in the imaging evaluation of pediatric spinal deformity, several specific indications necessitate this evaluation, including severe pain; neurologic findings, including motor weakness, muscle atrophy, and upper motor neuron signs; early-onset scoliosis with a Cobb angle greater than 20 degrees; atypical scoliosis curve patterns (e.g., left thoracic curves, sharp angular curves, congenital deformities, and curves that are >70 degrees); scoliosis curves with a rapid progression (>1 degree per month); neurofibromatosis; deformity associated with myelomeningocele; and lack of apical lordosis in idiopathic scoliosis[9,22] (Fig. 100-10).

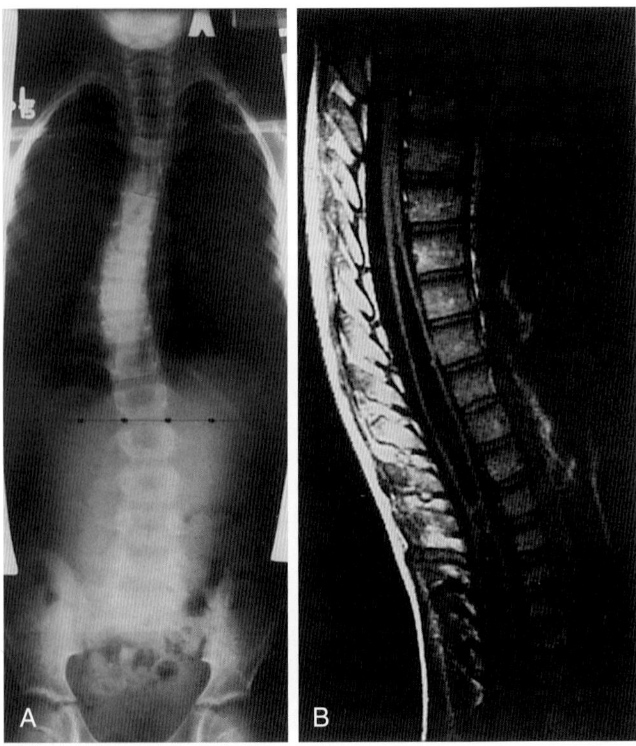

FIGURE 100-9. **A,** A 10-year-old boy with a left thoracic curve has a normal neurologic examination. **B,** Because of the atypical features (male gender and left thoracic curve) an MRI scan was obtained, demonstrating syrinx.

Idiopathic Scoliosis: Early Onset and Adolescent Onset

Idiopathic scoliosis has a familial tendency and a bimodal frequency distribution. With the early-onset type the majority of

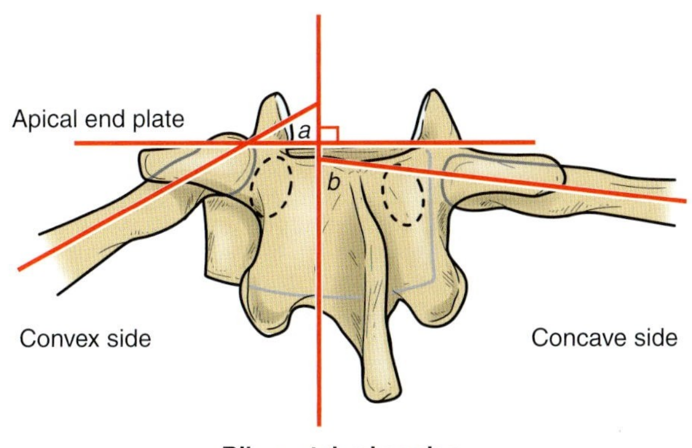

FIGURE 100-10. Dorsal view of apical vertebrae from a left thoracic, infantile curve. The rib–vertebra angles are formed between a perpendicular to the vertebral end plates and a line along the corresponding rib head. The rib–vertebral angle difference (RVAD) is calculated by subtracting the convex angle (*a*) from the concave angle (*b*): RVAD = *b*–*a*.

cases occur in infancy and a second major peak arises during adolescence. Idiopathic scoliosis is divided into two groups: early onset (<5 years) and late onset (5 years to skeletal maturity).[23,24] The most common type is adolescent idiopathic scoliosis (AIS).

The diagnosis of AIS is one of exclusion. In idiopathic scoliosis, deformity is the most common reason for referral. Occasionally, low-grade, activity-related back pain can result from lumbar curves or curves greater than 40 degrees. Atypical cases demand further evaluation to establish a diagnosis.[9,22]

The prevalence of AIS with a curve of at least 10 degrees is 2% to 3% of the adolescent population. Curves in excess of 20 degrees have a prevalence of 0.3% to 0.5%, whereas the prevalence of curves in excess of 40 degrees is 0.1%.

Curves originating before the age of 5 years can exceed 100 degrees and affect both the cardiac and pulmonary systems. Thus, treatments are predicated by patient age and degree of deformity.

Adolescent Idiopathic Scoliosis

Clinical Features

AIS occurs more frequently in girls than in boys. The typical curve pattern is a right thoracic curve with a compensatory left lumbar curve. Patients typically present with physical deformity from body asymmetry, such as a trunk shift, unlevel shoulders, rib prominence, and breast or waist asymmetry. Screening has traditionally been a means of identifying these curves; however, there is no evidence that this has changed clinical outcomes.

The natural history of AIS was studied thoroughly by Weinstein, who followed a cohort of patients for over 40 years, and by Collis and Ponseti.[25–28] Factors that correlate with progression of idiopathic curves include physiologic younger age, female gender, curve magnitude, and double curves. During the adolescent years, curves typically progress an average of 1 degree per month and curves in excess of 50 degrees have a high risk of progression even after skeletal maturity. Finally, there is a significant inverse relationship between the pulmonary vital capacity and magnitude of thoracic scoliosis. Thoracic curves greater than 70 degrees are associated with a vital capacity less than predicted for size.

Classification

Lenke et al. developed the currently most commonly applied classification for AIS.[29,30] Based on both coronal and sagittal radiographs, it was developed to aid in determination of the appropriate vertebral levels to be included in an arthrodesis. The classification system includes six curve types (numbered 1 through 6), a lumbar spine modifier (A, B, or C) that is based on deviation of the apical lumbar vertebra, and a sagittal plane modifier (−, N, or +).

The structural curve types are main thoracic (type 1), double thoracic (type 2), double major (type 3), triple major (type 4), thoracolumbar/lumbar (type 5), and thoracolumbar/lumbar main thoracic (type 6). The left and right side-bending radiographs determine which curves are structural and nonstructural. The lumbar spine modifier is determined on the basis of the relationship of the center CSVL to the lumbar curve on the coronal radiograph. The lumbar modifiers quantify the amount of lumbar curve as A (minimal), B (moderate), and C (large). The CSVL either (A) runs through the lumbar vertebra to the stable vertebrae, (B) runs between the medial border of the lumbar concave pedicle and the concave lateral margin of the apical vertebrae, or (C) falls completely medial to the entire concave lateral aspect of the apical vertebrae. The sagittal thoracic modifier describes overall thoracic kyphosis: hypokyphosis (−), a curve less than +10 degrees; normal (N), a curve +10 to +40 degrees; or hyperkyphosis (+), a curve more than +40 degrees.

Treatment

Bracing is the traditional nonsurgical treatment for idiopathic scoliosis; however, the evidence supporting its benefit is primarily from uncontrolled observational studies, and patient compliance varies significantly. There is no standardization of indications for bracing, how it should be used, or the optimal type of brace. For a scoliotic curve with an apex at or below T7, a thoracolumbosacral orthosis may be used. For curves with an apex above T7, a cervicothoracolumbosacral orthosis may be used. In general, one should anticipate that bracing will stabilize the deformity rather than correct it.

Bracing may be indicated in patients with AIS for curves greater than 20 degrees that have progressed more than 5 degrees. Adolescents with significant remaining growth potential who have curves between 25 degrees and 40 degrees may also warrant bracing, despite no documented progression.[31] Bracing is typically stopped in adolescents if the curve progresses to surgical dimensions (45–50 degrees) or when skeletal maturity is reached.

Surgery for AIS is often recommended in growing children once curves reach 45 degrees. Surgery is also recommended for skeletally mature teenagers for curves greater than 50 degrees, because curves of this severity have a high risk of progression in adult life.[25,26,32] The goals of surgery include stopping curve progression, restoring alignment, balancing the spine in all anatomic planes, and minimizing the number

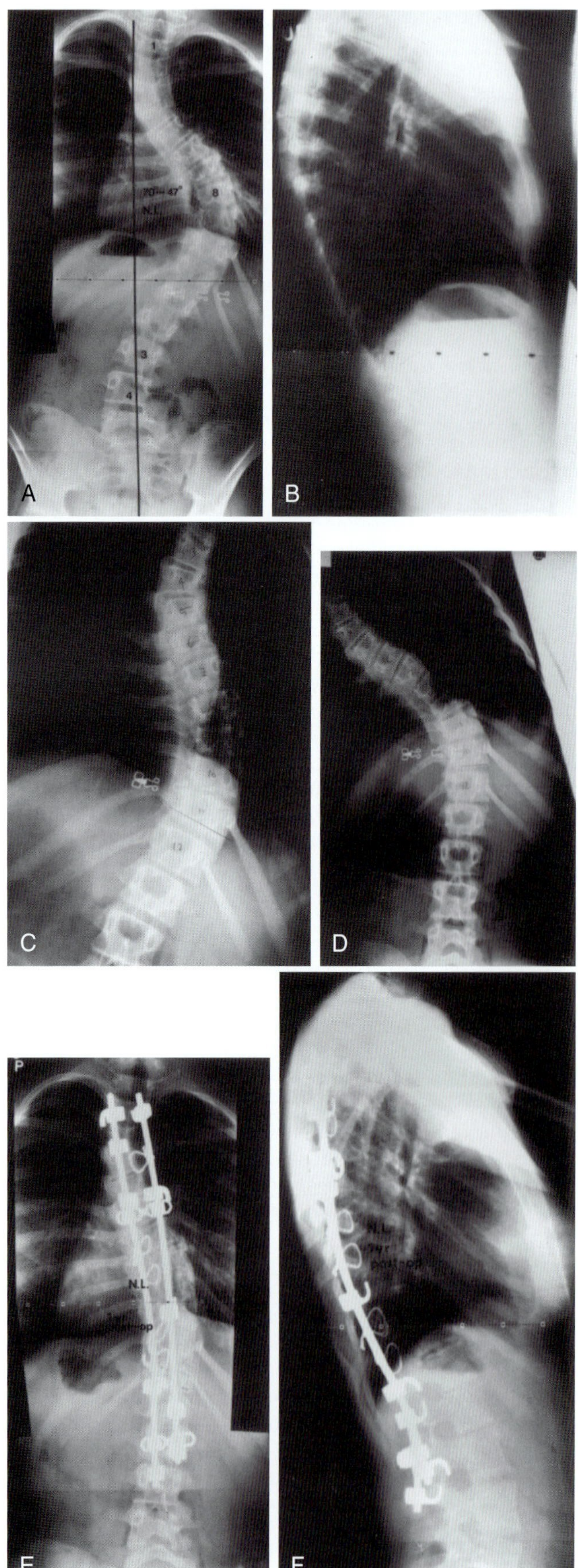

FIGURE 100-11. **A,** Twelve-year-old female, Tanner stage 2, and Risser stage 0. The upper thoracic curve measures 45 degrees with the right shoulder down and the lower thoracic curve, 70 degrees. The stable vertebra is L3 and the neutral vertebra is T12. **B,** Sagittal contours are relatively normal. **C,** Right side-bending film shows correction of the lower thoracic curve to 47 degrees. **D,** Left side-bending film shows complete correction of the fractional lumbar curve, whereas the upper thoracic curve reduces to 35 degrees. The L1-2 space opens to the right on this film. **E,** Surgical correction involved ventral discectomies from T7 to T11 followed by dorsal instrumentation and fusion from T2 to L2. Distraction was used across the concavities, apical translation with sublaminar wires, and compression over the convexities. **F,** Final correction shows balanced residual curves of 30 degrees and normal sagittal contours.

of vertebral levels that are fused (Figs. 100-11 to 100-13). Current dorsal instrumentation systems include hooks, wires, and/or pedicle screws that are typically connected with dual rods (Figs. 100-14 to 100-16). Pedicle screw instrumentation of pediatric patients in experienced hands has been shown to be safe.[33–37] Regardless of the instrumented system selected, the ultimate success of the procedure depends on achieving solid bony fusion.

Early-Onset Scoliosis

Clinical Features

Idiopathic scoliosis typically develops during late childhood (juvenile type) and can create serious cosmetic and functional problems. Pulmonary compromise is an additional concern in the rare cases of scoliosis developing before 5 years of age. According to the study of Nilsonne and Lundgren, severe curves (>100 degrees) resulted in death from cardiac or pulmonary causes in 60% of cases.[38] This significant morbidity and mortality underscores the importance of identifying these patients early. Because idiopathic infantile scoliosis is so rare, meticulous examination of these patients and radiography are mandatory to exclude congenital or neurologic causes of the scoliosis. Routine brainstem and spinal cord MRI is reasonable for excluding CNS abnormalities in patients younger than 8 years presenting with a spinal deformity of greater than 20 degrees.

In comparison with adolescent and juvenile idiopathic scoliosis, the curves in infantile scoliosis are commonly (in 50–75% of patients) left thoracic curves, with boys more commonly affected than are girls. Increased risk of curve progression is associated with double curves, large curves, and significant rotational deformity. Mehta found that risk of progression was related to the RVAD.[12] This angle is formed by a line along the rib head perpendicular with the base of the apical vertebra (see Fig. 100-12). If the difference between the angles on the concave and convex sides exceed 20 degrees, then progression is probable.

Treatment

In general, bracing or casting is the preferred treatment modality. If these approaches are contraindicated or fail, then

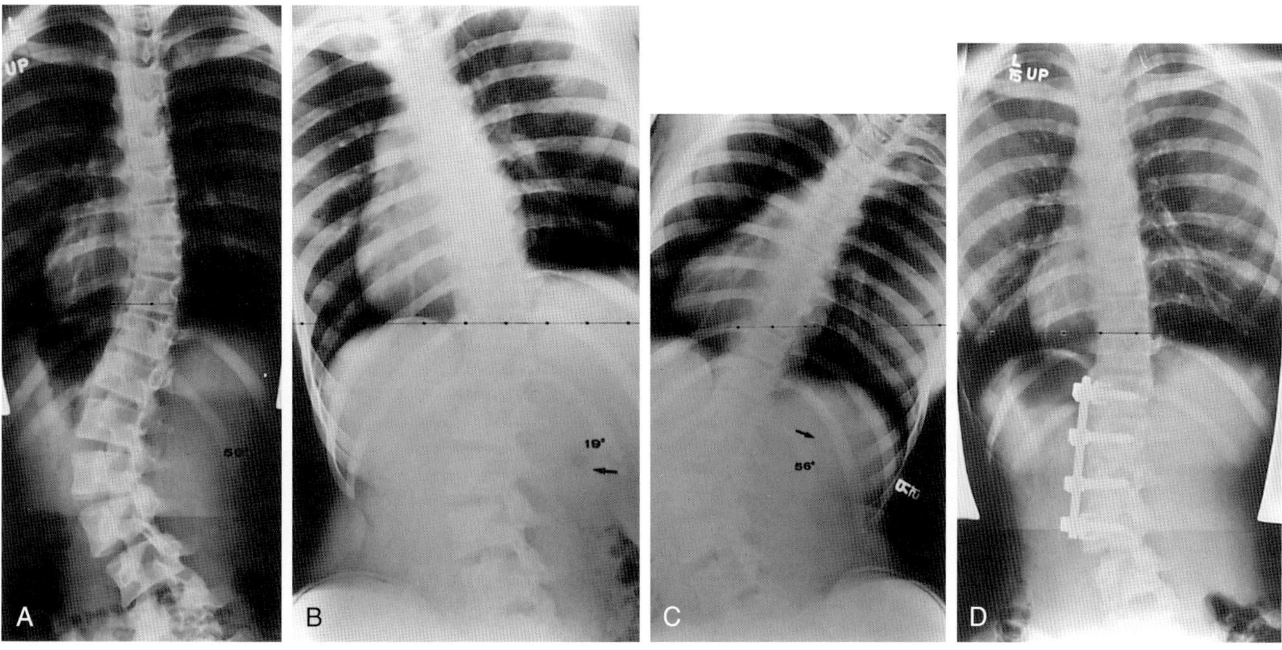

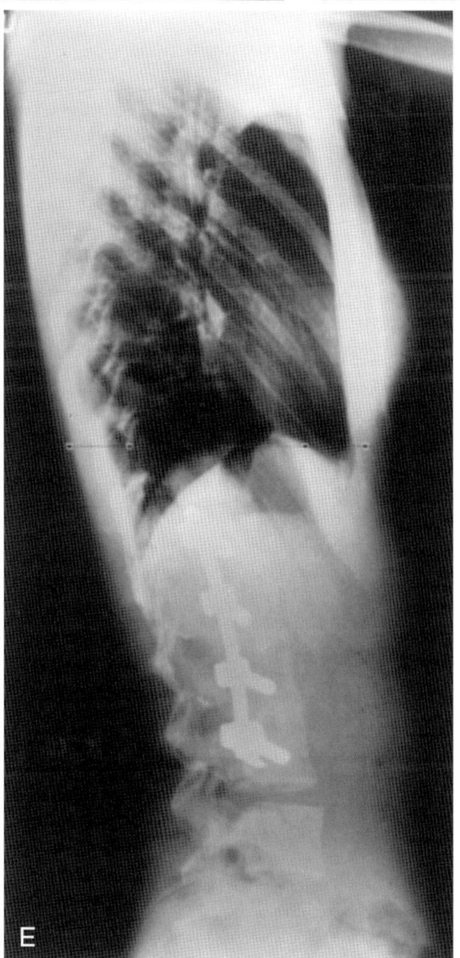

FIGURE 100-12. A, Thirteen-year-old female with 50-degree left lumbar idiopathic scoliosis. Vertebral ring apophyses are visible, signifying further spinal growth potential. **B,** Left side-bending film shows the curve is flexible, correcting to 19 degrees. **C,** L3-4 opens to the left on the right side-bending film. (*Arrows* indicate direction of bending.) **D,** Treatment consisted of ventral instrumentation from T12 to L3 using vertebral body screws and rods. Residual scoliosis measures 25 degrees with preservation of three lumbar discs. **E,** Sagittal contours were normalized postoperatively.

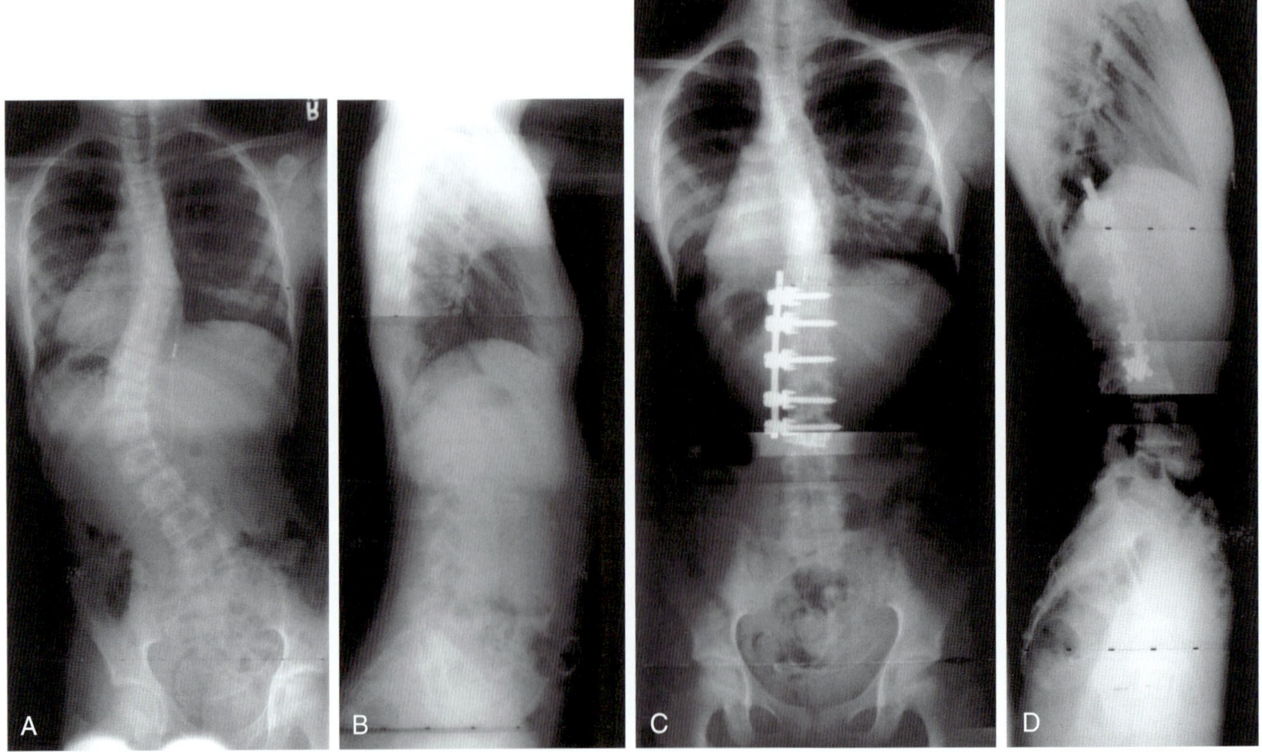

FIGURE 100-13. Sixteen-year-old female. Posteroanterior (**A**) and lateral (**B**) radiographs reveal a 61-degree lumbar curve and compensatory flexible thoracic curve. **C,** Treatment consisted of ventral release and instrumentation from T11 to L3 with near-complete correction of the lumbar curve. Three lumbar discs were preserved. **D,** She maintained normal lumbar lordosis postoperatively.

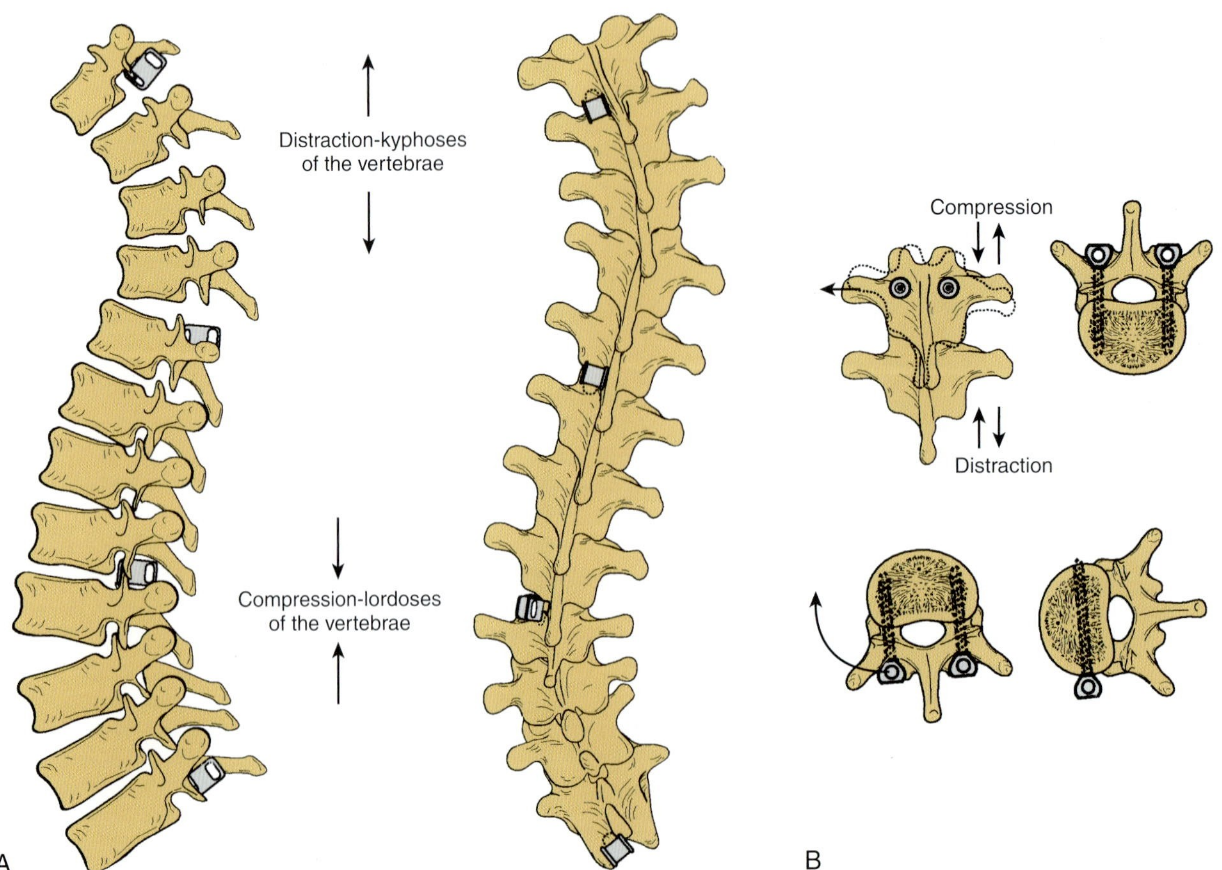

FIGURE 100-14. Implant-derived forces. **A,** Distraction across the concavity corrects scoliosis and produces kyphosis. Similarly, compression across the convexity reduces scoliosis and produces lordosis. **B,** Hooks and pedicle screws can be employed for sagittal or coronal tilting of the vertebrae as the axial force (distraction or compression) is applied. In addition, rotational forces can be exerted with pedicle and vertebral body screws.

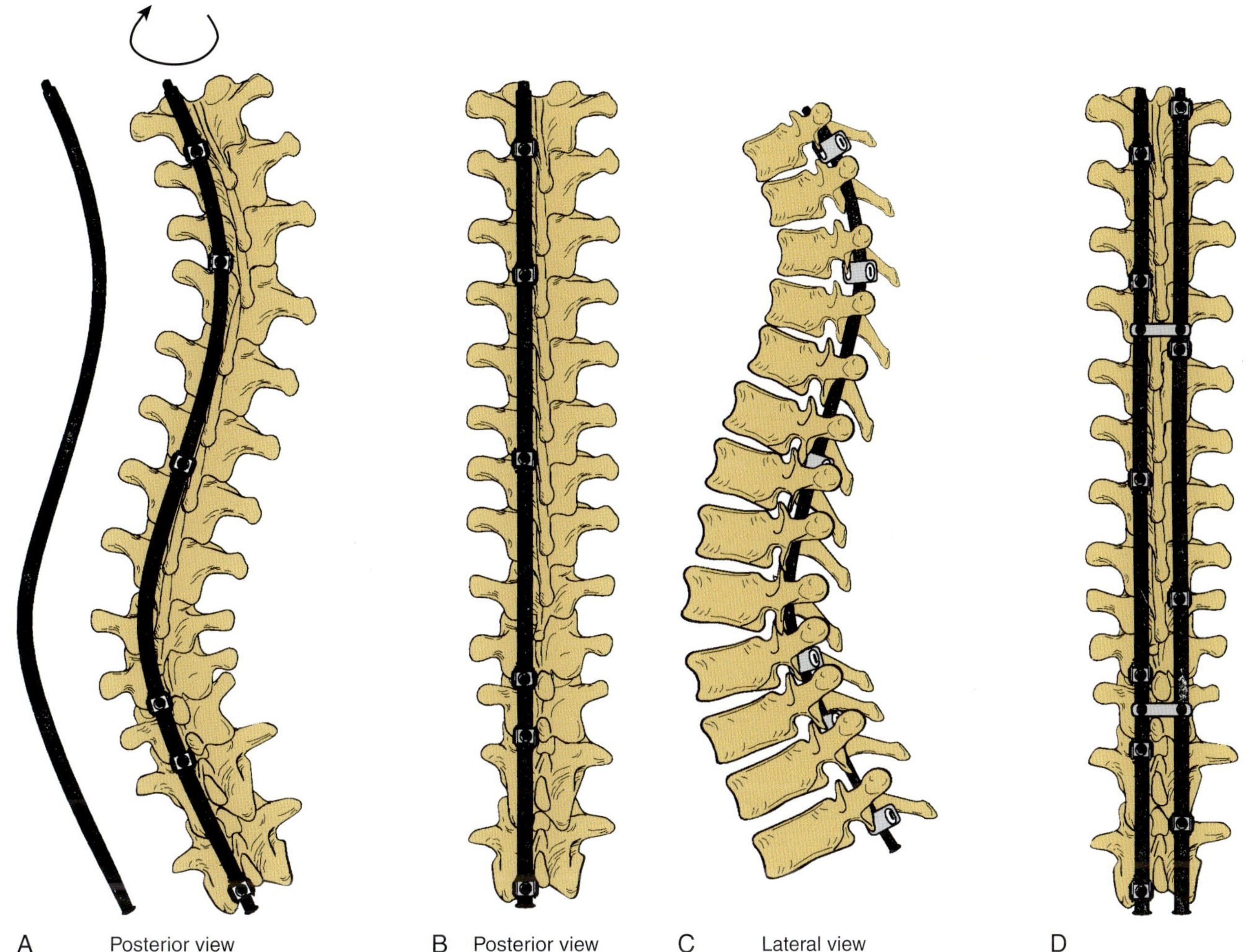

FIGURE 100-15. Scoliosis correction by rod rotation. **A,** Hooks are placed on the end, intermediate, and apical vertebrae to produce segmental forces. The rod is contoured to fit the scoliosis, placed within the hooks, and rotated to the left. **B,** This rotation converts the right lordoscoliosis into thoracic kyphosis and the left lumbar scoliosis into lumbar lordosis. **C,** The right hooks are inserted to apply compression across the thoracic convexity and lumbar distraction across the concavity. **D,** The two rods are linked with two cross-connectors to produce a rigid construct with 10 points of fixation to the spine.

surgical treatment may be required. Observation is a reasonable course of action until the curve reaches 30 degrees, due to the difficulty of bracing and casting small children. Curves less than 35 degrees with an RVAD of less than 20 degrees have a good response to bracing, whereas curves greater than 45 degrees with RVAD greater than 20 degrees have a poor prognosis for avoiding further progression and surgery. If the early-onset curve fails to be halted by several attempts at casting or bracing, surgery should be considered once the curves exceed 55 to 60 degrees.

Spinal instrumentation without fusion is the preferred technique for patients younger than 9 years of age.[39-49] Serial distraction is carried out every 6 to 9 months with the ratcheted distraction rod. The patient is protected in a brace at all times, and once adolescence is reached, a formal instrumentation and fusion is carried out. Complications with this technique are common and include hook dislodgement, rod breakage, skin breakdown, and early fusion without bone graft. Despite the frequent complications, subfascial instrumentation for early-onset or juvenile scoliosis is a reasonable alternative to the inevitable cardiopulmonary problems associated with curve progression. Some surgeons perform ventral discectomy over the apical segments as the initial procedure, followed by dorsal subcutaneous rod insertions. This makes sense in the more severe curves and in the presence of thoracic lordosis.

Congenital Disorders

A broad range of congenital spinal disorders occur.[50] Although many of these may not be evident at birth, each is thought to result from errors during development.[51] Congenital spine anomalies most commonly occur sporadically and have an incidence of approximately 1 per 1000 to 2000.[52-54] However, not all congenital spinal disorders are sporadic.

Congenital spinal malformations are not infrequently accompanied by associated anomalies, most frequently the organ systems affected develop at a similar phase of embryogenesis. Genitourinary anomalies are the most common, occurring in up to 25%.[55] The cardiovascular system also develops anomalies, including ventricular septal defects, atrial septal defects, dextrocardia, and tetralogy of Fallot, in approximately 10% of cases.[16]

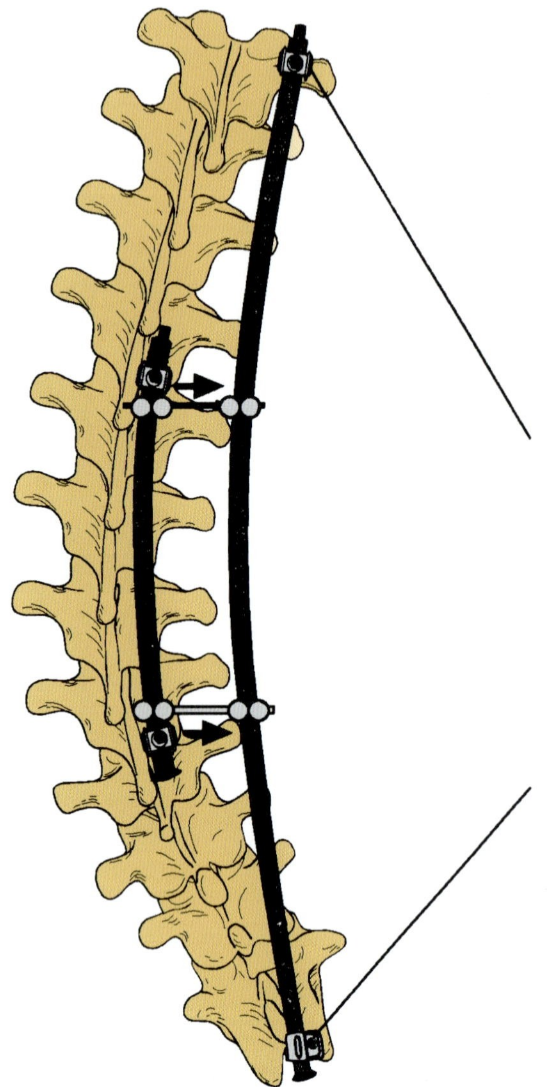

FIGURE 100-16. Two-rod translation. If the curve is rigid, a short rod across the apex can be translated to a longer rod attached to the end vertebrae. Threaded cross-fixation devices are designed to produce transverse traction and apical translation to the midline.

Congenital Scoliosis

Scoliosis is an abnormal curvature of the spine in the coronal plane. Congenital scoliosis is distinguished by the presence of anomalous vertebrae at birth. Although the vertebral abnormality is present at birth, typically no evidence of deformity presents until the growth phases of childhood or adolescence. Balanced spine anomalies may go undiagnosed until adulthood or are discovered incidentally. Infantile idiopathic scoliosis and juvenile idiopathic scoliosis also present with scoliosis in childhood, but these are distinguished from congenital scoliosis by their lack of vertebral anomalies.[56]

The presentation of congenital scoliosis varies and depends on the type and level of the spine anomaly, their number, and the degree of deformity. At the extremes, anomalies can result in rapidly progressive scoliosis with significant morbidity in early childhood or can result in minimal or no deformity throughout life. Approximately one quarter of patients with congenital scoliosis can be expected to experience no progression; one half progress slowly; and one quarter progress rapidly.[50] With advancements in CT and MRI have come concomitant advances with classification and improvements in the surgical management.

The normal vertebral body has growth plates on the superior and inferior surfaces, and normal spine growth occurs as a balanced process between these plates. Congenital spine anomalies can result in absent or deficient growth at one or more end plates and may affect the vertebral level asymmetrically, resulting in unbalanced growth. Lateral asymmetry of growth can produce scoliosis, AP asymmetry of growth can result in kyphotic or lordotic deformity, and combinations of asymmetrical growth can produce kyphoscoliosis or lordoscoliosis.

Congenital abnormalities of the spine are classified based on embryologic development of the spine, with categories including failures of formation, failures of segmentation, and mixed anomalies[9,57] (Fig. 100-17). Failures of formation can range from mild wedging to complete absence of a vertebral body. The most common cause of congenital scoliosis is a hemivertebra, which typically consists of a wedged vertebral body with a single pedicle and hemilamina (Figs. 100-18 to 100-20). Failures of segmentation result in unilateral or bilateral bony fusion between vertebrae.[58,59] The most common is the unilateral unsegmented bar, consisting of a bony block including the disc space and facet joints (Fig. 100-21). Among the various complex combinations of vertebral anomalies that can coexist is the unsegmented bar with contralateral hemivertebra, which can result in significant progressive scoliosis.[60]

The degree to which hemivertebrae result in spinal deformity is based on several factors: the vertebral level and the degree of segmentation. For example, a hemivertebra located at the thoracolumbar or lumbosacral junction can produce substantial deformity. Segmentation refers to the extent of normal disc formation above and below the vertebral body. A fully segmented hemivertebra has a normal disc space at the superior and inferior end plates, allowing for near-normal longitudinal growth. This near-normal capacity for unilateral growth, coupled with the lack of growth capacity on the contralateral side, can result in significant deformity. A semisegmented vertebra lacks a disc space at either the superior or inferior end plate. This would be expected to produce relatively balanced growth, although lateral differences in growth may still exist and can result in some degree of scoliosis. A nonsegmented vertebra lacks adjacent disc spaces and is fused to the adjacent vertebrae. Although the wedge shape of a nonsegmented vertebra can produce some degree of deformity, it typically is not progressive.

Unilateral unsegmented bars, resulting from failure of segmentation of two or more vertebrae, are another common cause of congenital scoliosis. Since unilateral unsegmented bars contain no growth plate, asymmetrical, unbalanced growth takes place from the contralateral growth plate, resulting in the potential for deformity.

An understanding of the natural history of congenital spine anomalies is important in order to define optimal treatment strategies. Of 202 patients with congenital scoliosis, 11% were nonprogressive, 14% had limited progression, and 75% progressed significantly.[56] The type of anomaly is an important factor in the likelihood of progression. The most severe congenital scolioses may result from a unilateral unsegmented bar with a contralateral hemivertebra at the same level. The

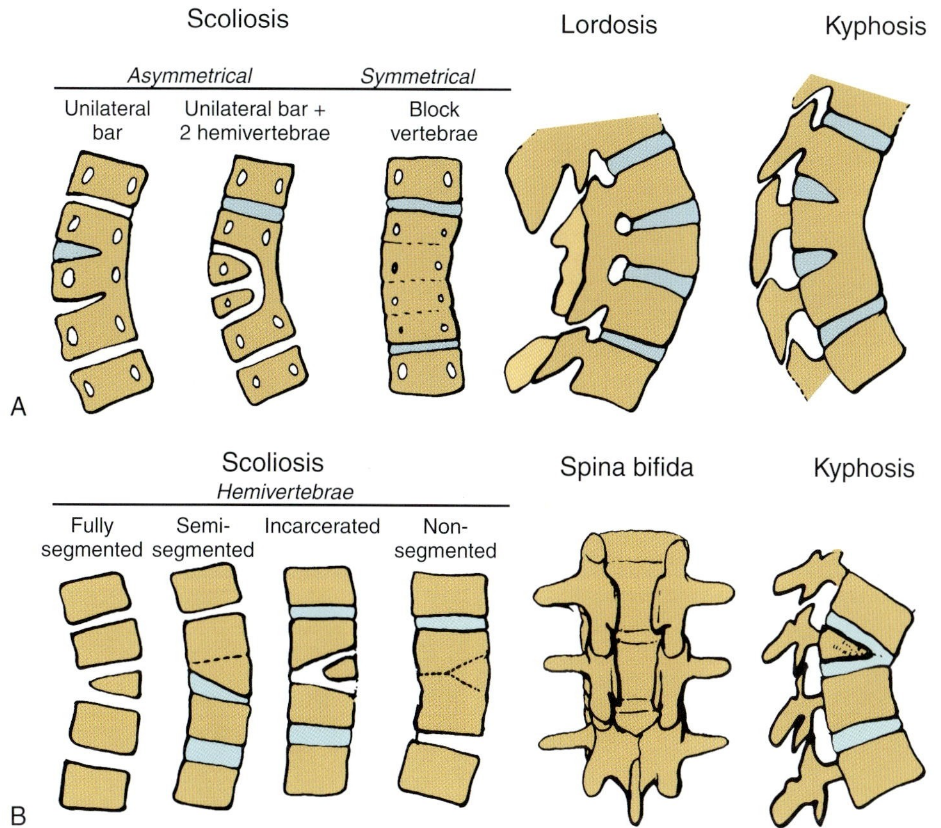

FIGURE 100-17. A, Defects of segmentation; **B,** defects of formation.

significant potential for this combination of anomalies to produce deformity argues for treating the patient immediately, without allowing for a period of observation.[56,61] Patient age is also an important factor in determining capacity for deformity progression, with the greatest risk typically arising during the preadolescent growth spurt. Cases in which deformity presents in the first years of life are often associated with significant growth imbalance and are at high risk of significant deformity.

In cases of severe or progressive congenital scoliosis, surgery is often the most effective treatment. Surgical options include hemivertebra excision, convex hemiepiphysiodesis, fusion in situ, spinal instrumentation, and thoracoplasty with vertical expansion prosthetic titanium rib (VEPTR).[50] Hemivertebra excision offers the ability to directly address the biomechanical decompensation and can provide immediate and often significant deformity correction.[62-64] Convex hemiepiphysiodesis involves excision of the disc and fusion on the convex side of the curve and relies on remaining growth potential on the side of the concavity.[65] Although in situ fusion with casting or bracing has been the traditional treatment, the use of dorsal instrumented arthrodesis has become more popular in cases requiring fusion. Patients with progressive curves and congenital rib fusions may benefit from thoracoplasty and VEPTR.[44,46] It is important to recognize the surgical morbidity that can accompany complex reconstructions for congenital scoliosis. Reames et al. reported a modern series of more than 2000 patients from the Scoliosis Research Society treated for congenital scoliosis, in which the morbidity rate was more than 10% and the mortality rate was 0.3%.[66]

Dysplastic Spondylolisthesis

Spondylolisthesis is the malalignment of one vertebral body relative to an adjacent level. The most widely accepted classification of spondylolisthesis describes five types, including dysplastic (type I), isthmic (type II), degenerative (type III), traumatic (type IV), and pathologic (type V).[67] Dysplastic spondylolisthesis is a congenital disorder that results from a defect in the facet complex, typically L5-S1, that permits pathologic movement. The development of spondylolisthesis is extremely rare in infancy and usually requires ambulation.

Clinical presentations for dysplastic spondylolisthesis may include back or leg pain, paresthesias, weakness, and, rarely, bowel or bladder incontinence. In general, more severe malalignment is more likely to be associated with neurologic deficit. Younger patients with skeletally immature spines are at higher risk of slip progression.

Initial treatment of dysplastic spondylolisthesis should be nonoperative, unless there has been documented progression in a young patient or a slippage more severe than 50% of the initial presentation. Surgical treatment includes decompression with fusion in situ or decompression, fixation with pedicle screws, and fusion. Instrumentation facilitates partial or complete reduction but is associated with an increased rate of new neurologic deficit.[68]

Congenital Lordosis

Congenital lordosis results from dorsal defects in segmentation and is much rarer than other congenital spinal deformities.[69] Congenital lordosis is usually accompanied by a

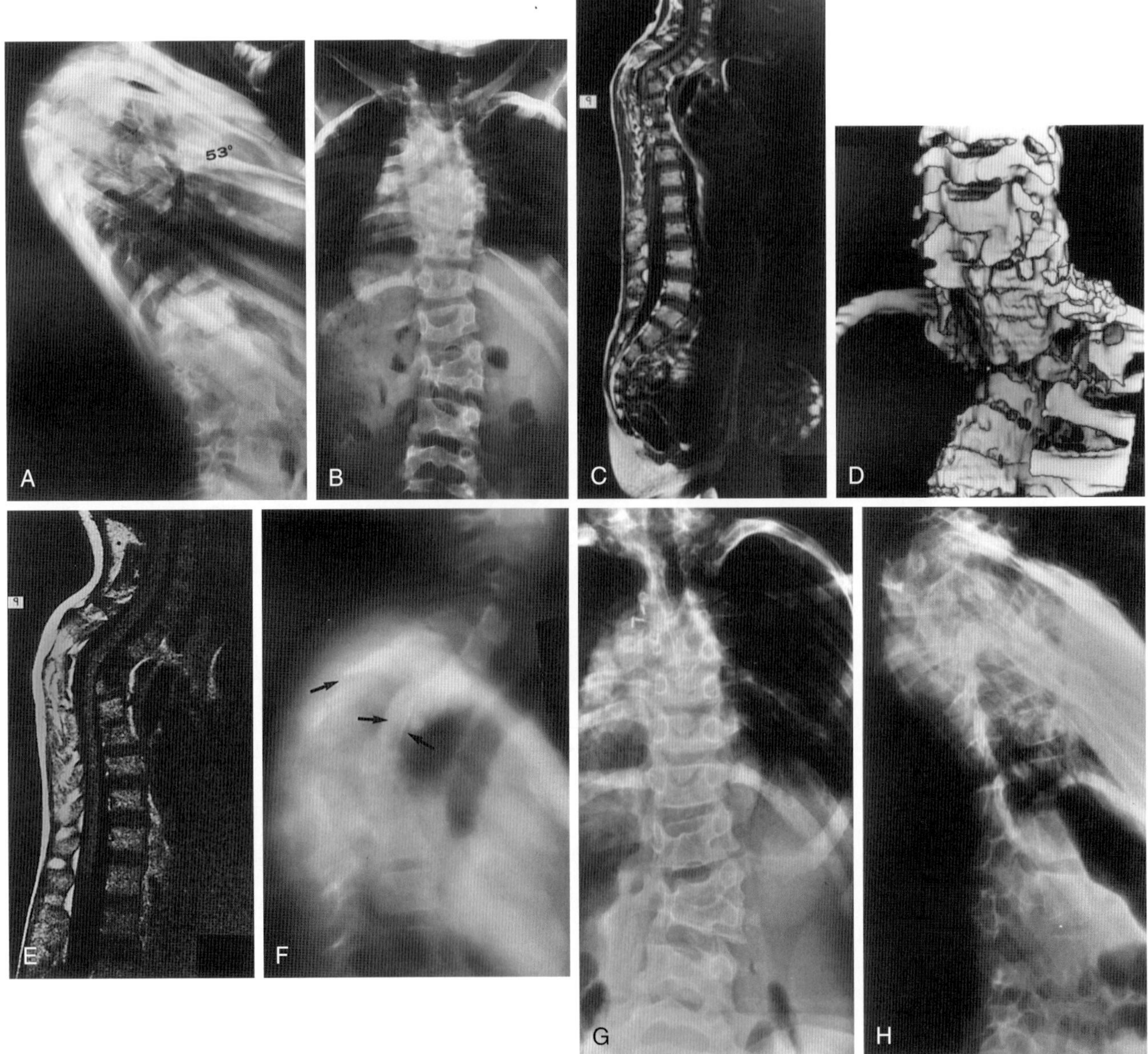

FIGURE 100-18. **A,** Eight-year-old male presented with severe cervicothoracic kyphosis measuring 53 degrees secondary to a congenital left hemivertebra at T2. Clonus and hyperreflexia were noted. **B,** Posteroanterior radiograph shows multiple vertebral anomalies; however, head and trunk alignment are satisfactory. **C,** MRI reveals spinal cord impingement and narrowing of the canal. **D,** Three-dimensional CT demonstrates the left dorsal location of the hemivertebra, behind. Decompression and hemivertebrectomy was performed via a high left thoracotomy and T3 rib resection. The scapula was elevated for this approach, and the T3 rib was used as a strut graft. **E,** Postoperative MRI shows the canal has been widened and the cord decompressed. **F,** Tomogram demonstrates the ventral strut graft (*double arrows*) and a dorsal laminar defect (*single arrow*) that was addressed by dorsal autogenous grafting 2 weeks later. The patient was confined in a halo cast for 3 months followed by a cervicothoracic orthosis for 3 months. Neurologic symptoms resolved after the decompression. Frontal (**G**) and lateral (**H**) alignment 1 year postoperatively.

concomitant coronal plane deformity (lordoscoliosis) due to a dorsolateral unsegmented bar. The incidence of neurologic deficits with congenital lordosis is much lower than with congenital kyphosis.

Congenital Kyphosis

Congenital kyphosis is a sagittal plane deformity resulting from vertebral anomalies, including failures of formation and segmentation.[9] Congenital kyphosis often results in neurologic deficit without treatment. There are three distinct types: failure of formation of the vertebral body (type I), failure of segmentation of the vertebral body with ventral unsegmented bar (type II), and mixed failure of formation and segmentation (type III).[70] Type I is the most common and the one that most frequently results in severe deformity and neurologic deficits. Type II produces less deformity and is considerably less likely to result in neurologic deficit. The severity of kyphosis produced with type II depends on the differential growth between ventral vertebral and dorsal structures. Type III is very rare and is thought to behave in a fashion similar to type I.

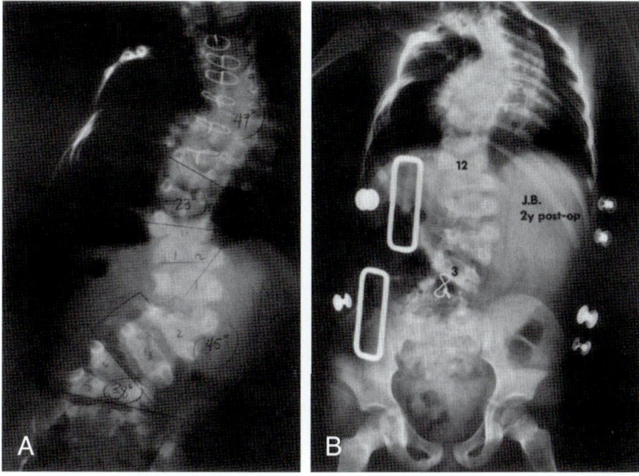

FIGURE 100-19. **A,** Two-year-old male with Goldenhar syndrome (oculoauriculovertebral dysplasia) has multiple organ system anomalies, including vertebral, cardiac, and renal anomalies and Sprengel deformity. The L5 hemivertebra was addressed to reduce the right trunk shift. **B,** Frontal radiograph 2 years after hemivertebrectomy shows some improvement. A brace is currently employed to maintain the trunk alignment.

In general, nonoperative treatment is not recommended for congenital kyphosis because of the significant risk of neurologic deficits with progression. Dorsal fusion alone is adequate in patients younger than 5 years with kyphosis less than 55 degrees. Combined ventral and dorsal procedures are often required in older patients or those with kyphosis greater than 55 degrees. Surgical correction of congenital kyphosis can be associated with significant risk of morbidity and mortality. Adverse events are associated with kyphosis greater than 60 degrees and spinal cord compression evident on preoperative imaging.[71]

Neuromuscular Disorders

Cerebral Palsy

Among nonambulatory cerebral palsy patients, approximately 70% develop scoliosis by the age of 15 years.[72] Although these curves can progress into adulthood, the greatest progression occurs intuitively during the times of peak growth (~2–4 degrees per month).[73,74] These deformities are typically long sweeping curves that include pelvic obliquity and may also include significant kyphosis or hyperlordosis. Although braces may be used to temporarily treat these deformities, many patients ultimately require surgical intervention.[75] Surgical correction often includes long segmental instrumentation including pelvic fixation. Significant pelvic and hip contractures should be treated prior to spinal fusion, since pelvic fixation could exacerbate these conditions.

Neuromuscular Dystrophies and Myopathies

Both scoliosis and sagittal plane deformities are common among patients with primary disorders of the nervous system or muscular system, or both. The Scoliosis Research Society has classified neuromuscular scoliosis including categories of upper motor neuron pathology (e.g., cerebral palsy, Rett syndrome), lower motor neuron and mixed pathology (e.g., Charcot-Marie-Tooth atrophy, spinal muscular atrophy, spinal cord injury, myelomeningocele), and primary myopathies (e.g., Duchenne muscular dystrophy, myopathies).[76]

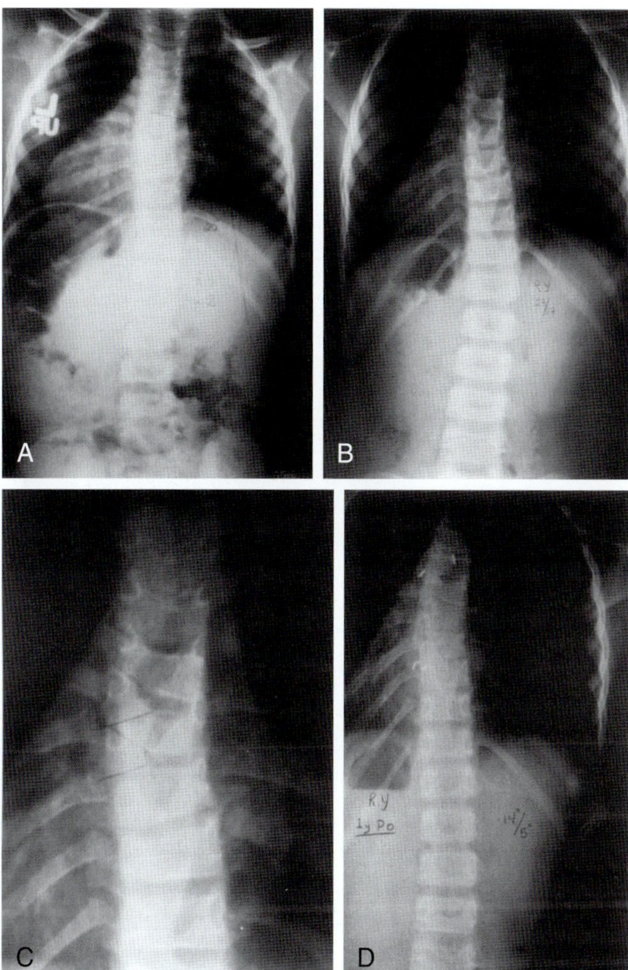

FIGURE 100-20. **A,** Two-year-old female with left thoracic 20-degree scoliosis resulting from hemivertebrae. **B,** Eighteen months later, the curve measured 28 degrees and a compensatory 17-degree right thoracolumbar curve had developed. **C,** Focused thoracic films show fully segmented contiguous hemivertebrae. Treatment consisted of convex hemiepiphyseodesis from T6 to T10 via a ventral and dorsal approach. **D,** One year postoperatively, reduction of deformity resulted from concave growth. The right thoracic curve measured 14 degrees and the left thoracolumbar curve, 5 degrees.

The risk of deformity depends on the severity of the underlying disorder. For example, almost all patients with Duchenne muscular dystrophy develop collapsing deformity and many require surgical treatment after becoming nonambulatory. Up to 70% of patients with severe cerebral palsy develop scoliosis by the age of 7.[72,77] Among patients with myelomeningocele at L3 or above, at least 70% develop significant deformity. By the time these deformities develop, many of these patients are nonambulatory and may suffer from significant comorbidities, including osteopenia, pulmonary compromise, and malnutrition.

Nonoperative treatments for neuromuscular deformities include bracing and wheelchair seating systems that provide support for the head, trunk, pelvis, and extremities. Although

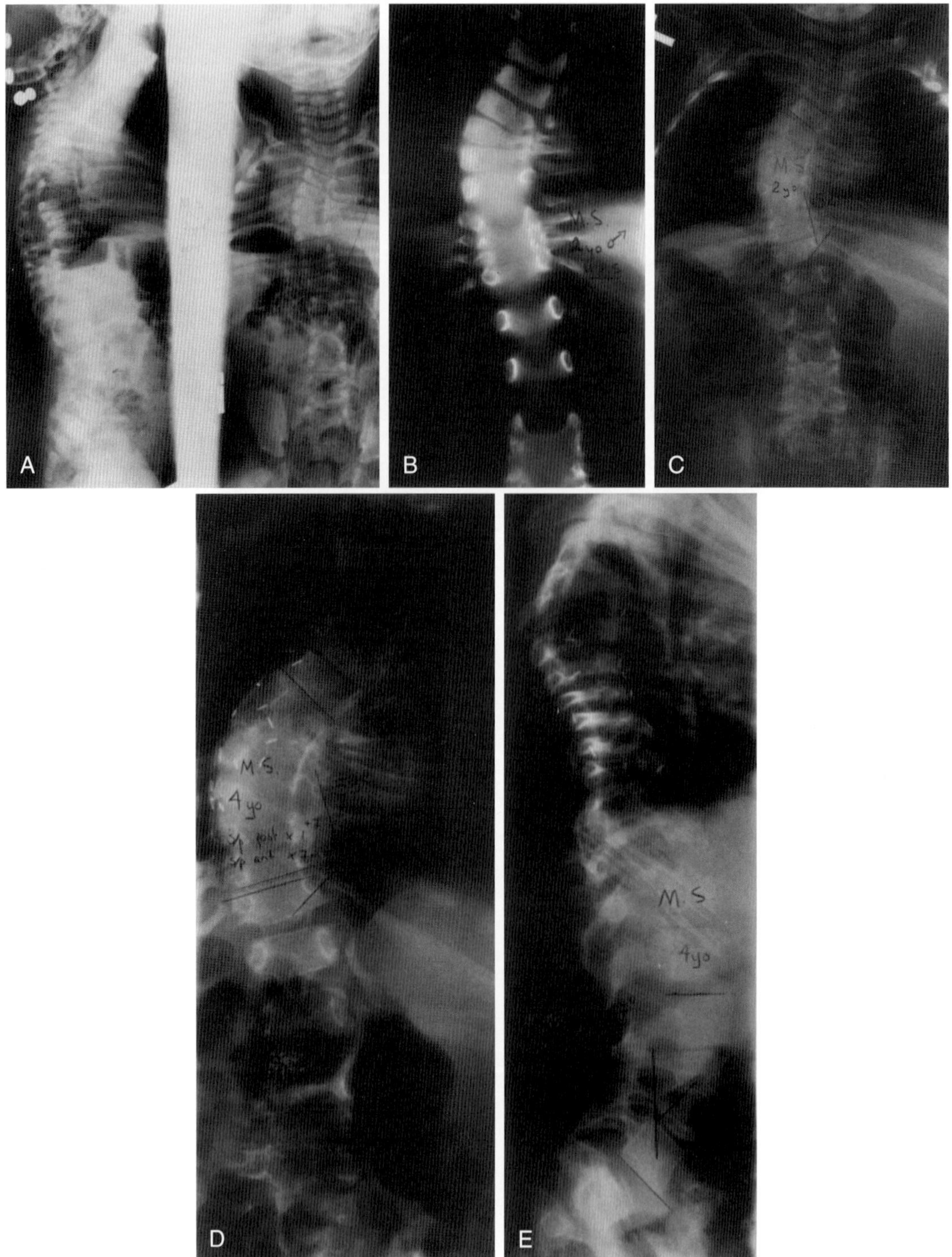

FIGURE 100-21. A, Progressive lordoscoliosis developed in a 2-year-old male with multiple pterygium syndrome. **B,** Focused thoracic films show the segmentation defect with open disc spaces on the convex side of the deformity. **C,** When the thoracic curve reached 52 degrees, a dorsal fusion was carried out from T4 to T8. Progression continued because of further ventral growth, and thus left thoracotomy and discectomy were carried out from T5 to T8. **D,** Nineteen months after the initial procedures and 7 months after the ventral discectomy, the scoliosis measures 58 degrees. **E,** Lateral radiograph shows the thoracic lordosis and lumbar dorsal synostoses. In the presence of thoracic lordosis, a combined ventral and dorsal arthrodesis should have been done initially.

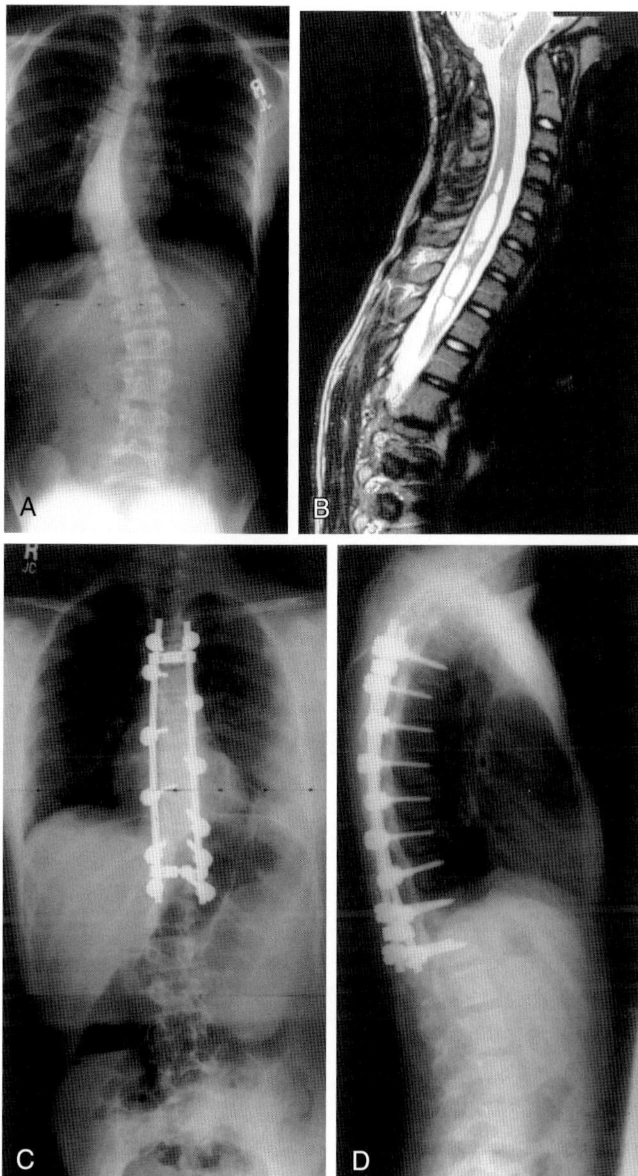

FIGURE 100-22. **A,** Twelve-year-old female. **B,** Because she had a neurologic deficit, an MRI was performed, revealing a complex cervicothoracic syrinx. After the syrinx was treated, she underwent T4-12 instrumented fusion with pedicle screws. Postoperative anteroposterior (**C**) and lateral (**D**) images show near-complete correction of structural curve with normal sagittal plane balance.

several studies suggest that bracing does not correct the deformity,[75,78-82] it can support young children and flexible deformities (e.g., hypotonic myopathies, some types of cerebral palsy, spina bifida, and spinal muscular atrophy) (Fig. 100-22).

Goals of surgery include improving quality of life through alleviation of pain, improving seated spinal balance, preventing further pulmonary compromise, improving GI function, stabilizing spinal deformity, and facilitating patient care.

Neuromuscular curves are often sweeping and involve significant portions of the spine. Indications for surgical intervention are not precisely defined, but typically curves greater than 50 degrees are considered for surgical treatment. Bracing can be used in an attempt to delay surgical treatment if the curve is flexible. Occasionally fusion may be required for curves less than 50 degrees. Ambulatory status and often significant comorbidities of this patient population result in significant morbidity and mortality associated with surgical correction. A recent series by the membership of the Scoliosis Research Society of 4657 patients with neuromuscular scoliosis who underwent surgical correction demonstrated overall morbidity and mortality rates of 18% and 0.3%, respectively.[66]

Several muscular dystrophies and myopathies are associated with developmental anomalies of spinal alignment. Surgical treatment typically includes fusion with segmental instrumentation and incorporating the pelvis for pelvic obliquity greater than15 degrees. Patients with these disorders have a higher incidence of malignant hyperthermia when exposed to anesthetic agents. Depolarizing agents should not be used if neuromuscular blockade is necessary for surgery, and nondepolarizing agents should be used. It is essential to perform a thorough cardiac and pulmonary evaluation for these patients due to the incidence of associated anomalies. Pulmonary compromise can result from spinal deformity and decreased muscle function. Despite an increase in complication rates when vital capacity falls to less than 40% of predicted, it is possible to perform successful surgery, with the caveat that the patient may require a tracheostomy for long-term ventilation.[83-86] Deformity correction is unlikely to improve pulmonary function but may slow its progression.[87] Preoperative assessment of cardiac function is important in patients with neuromuscular deformity, particularly Duchenne muscular dystrophy and myotonic dystrophy. For Duchenne muscular dystrophy, steroid treatment offers the potential to prolong ambulation and delay the onset of scoliosis.[88]

KEY REFERENCES

Archer IA: Surgical treatment of late-onset idiopathic thoracic scoliosis. The Leeds procedure. *J Bone Joint Surg [Br]* 69(5):709–714, 1987.

Dickson RA: Conservative treatment for idiopathic scoliosis. *J Bone Joint Surg [Br]* 67(2):176–181, 1985.

Dickson RA, Ferguson RL: Medical and congenital comorbidities associated with spinal deformities in the immature spine. *J Bone Joint Surg [Am]* 89(Suppl 1):34–41, 2007.

Hedequist DJ, Hall JE, Emans JB: The safety and efficacy of spinal instrumentation in children with congenital spine deformities. *Spine (Phila Pa 1976)* 29(18):2081–2086, 2004; discussion 2087.

Lenke LG, Betz RR, Harms J, et al: Adolescent idiopathic scoliosis: a new classification to determine extent of spinal arthrodesis. *J Bone Joint Surg [Am]* 83(8):1169–1181, 2001.

Sanders JO, Browne RH, McConnell SJ, et al: Maturity assessment and curve progression in girls with idiopathic scoliosis. *J Bone Joint Surg [Am]* 89(1):64–73, 2007.

Smith JS, Abel MF, Shaffrey CI, et al: Decision making in pediatric spinal deformity. *Neurosurgery* 63(Suppl 3):54–68, 2008.

Weinstein SL, Zavala DC, Ponseti IV: Idiopathic scoliosis: long-term follow-up and prognosis in untreated patients. *J Bone Joint Surg [Am]* 63(5):702–712, 1981.

REFERENCES

The complete reference list is available online at expertconsult.com.

INDEX

Page numbers followed by b, f, or t indicate boxes, figures, or tables, respectively. "E" pages appear online only on Expert Consult.

B

C

D

E

F

G

H

J

K

M

O

Q

R

S

T

U

W